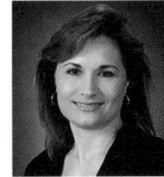

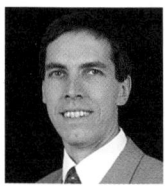

Kurt S. Schulz, DVM, MS, Diplomate ACVS, Associate Professor of Small Animal Surgery, University of California, Davis; Staff Surgeon, Animal Medical Center of New England, Nashua, New Hampshire. Dr. Schulz has an extensive research program and speaks internationally on arthroscopy, canine elbow dysplasia, joint replacement, and management of osteoarthritis. He served as Chief of Small Animal Surgery at the University of California Davis from 1999 to 2003 and currently serves on the board of examiners for the American College of Veterinary Surgeons. His other publications include: Small Animal Arthroscopy and the Pet Lovers Guide to Canine Joint Disease and Osteoarthritis. He is an active member of the Veterinary Orthopedic Society, AO-Vet, and the ACVS.

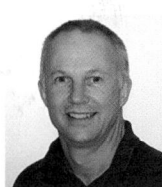

Howard B. Seim, III, DVM, Diplomate ACVS, Associate Professor and Chief of Small Animal Surgery, Department of Clinical Sciences, Colorado State University. Dr. Seim has garnered accolades for his teaching ability. He was co-recipient of the 1993 Merck AGVET Award for Creative Teaching and was awarded Colorado State University's N. Preston Davis Award for Instructional Innovation in 1995. Dr. Seim has been teaching for 25 years and has been an active student, intern, and resident advisor. Dr. Seim is well recognized for his knowledge of and experience in the field of neurosurgery. He has presented innumerable scientific papers in this field and has authored or co-authored many book chapters. Dr. Seim has obtained funding for a variety of research projects, particularly developing implants for spinal fusion and disk replacement. He has been a member of the Editorial Review Board of the *Journal of the AVMA, Veterinary Surgery,* and the *Journal of Feline Medicine and Surgery.* Dr. Seim served on the ACVS's Examination committee from 1991 to 1995 and as a member of their Board of Regents from 1998 to 2000.

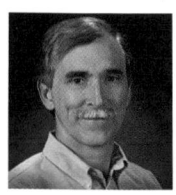

Michael D. Willard, DVM, MS, Diplomate ACVIM, Professor, Department of Small Animal Medicine and Surgery, College of Veterinary Medicine, Texas A&M University. Dr. Willard is an internist with a special emphasis on gastroenterology, endoscopy, pancreatology, and hepatology. Dr. Willard has received several awards for teaching excellence since 1987, among them the 1994 National Norden Award. In addition, he has numerous clinical presentations and has conducted some research in gastroenteric problems. Dr. Willard is a past Secretary of the specialty of Internal Medicine and a past President of the Comparative Gastroenterology Society. He serves as a reviewer for several veterinary journals. He has contributed numerous journal articles and several monographs and book chapters.

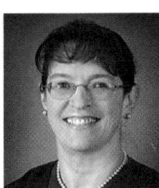

RADIOLOGY CONSULTANT
Anne Bahr, DVM, MS, Diplomate ACVR. Assistant Professor and Chief of Radiology, Department of Large Animal and Clinical Sciences, Texas A&M University. Dr. Bahr is the Assistant Chair of the 2006 Radiology Examination Committee. She reviewed all of the imaging chapters and offered her expertise on the radiologic techniques featured throughout *Small Animal Surgery.*

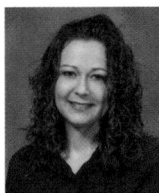

ANESTHESIA CONSULTANT
Gwendolyn L. Carroll, MS, DVM, Diplomate ACVA. Professor, Anesthesiology, Department of Small Animal Medicine and Surgery, College of Veterinary Medicine, Texas A&M University. Dr. Carroll's primary interest is perioperative analgesia. She is also certified in acupuncture by the International Veterinary Acupuncture Society. Dr. Carroll is a member of the ACVA and the International Veterinary Academy of Pain Management. She has authored several refereed publications and book chapters, as well as a text on small animal pain management. She was responsible for reviewing and verifying most anesthetic regimens and dosages included throughout *Small Animal Surgery.*

Kim Knap, BS, CVT, CCRP, Technician, Orthopedic Services, University of Illinois. Kim contributed to Chapter 12, Fundamentals of Physical Rehabilitation, and to physical rehabilitation strategies throughout the Orthopedics and Neurology sections of this text.

Special thanks to **Ralph Hamor** for reviewing the ophthalmologic surgery section and to **Curtis Dewey** for reviewing the neurosurgery section.

Special thanks to **Dr. Chris Orton,** who contributed to the original cardiovascular chapter in Edition 1.

THIRD EDITION

SMALL
ANIMAL
SURGERY

THIRD EDITION

SMALL ANIMAL SURGERY

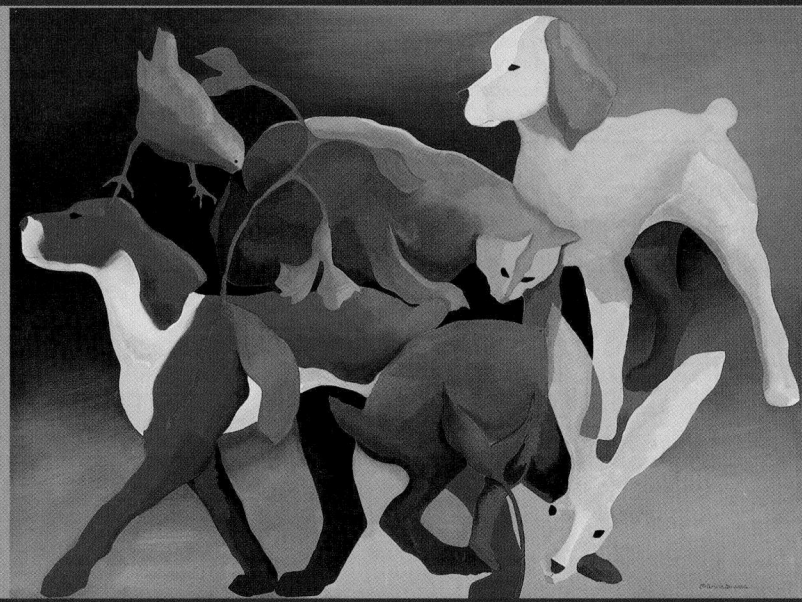

THERESA WELCH FOSSUM, DVM, MS, PhD

Diplomate ACVS
Tom and Joan Read Chair in Veterinary Surgery;
Director of Cardiothoracic Surgery and Biomedical Devices,
Michael E. DeBakey Institute;
Professor of Surgery
Texas A&M University
College of Veterinary Medicine
College Station, Texas

LAURA PARDI DUPREY
DONALD O'CONNOR
Medical Illustrators

With more than 2100 illustrations

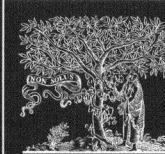

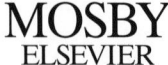

11830 Westline Industrial Drive
St. Louis, Missouri 63146
Small Animal Surgery

ISBN-13: 978-0-323-04439-4
ISBN-10: 0-323-04439-5

Notice

Knowledge and best practice in this field are constantly changing. As new research and experience broaden our knowledge, changes in practice, treatment and drug therapy may become necessary or appropriate. Readers are advised to check the most current information provided (i) on procedures featured or (ii) by the manufacturer of each product to be administered, to verify the recommended dose or formula, the method and duration of administration, and contraindications. It is the responsibility of the practitioner, relying on their own experience and knowledge of the patient, to make diagnoses, to determine dosages and the best treatment for each individual patient, and to take all appropriate safety precautions. To the fullest extent of the law, neither the Publisher nor the Editors assumes any liability for any injury and/or damage to persons or property arising out or related to any use of the material contained in this book.

The Publisher

Previous editions copyrighted 2002, 1997

ISBN-13: 978-0-323-04439-4
ISBN-10:   0-323-04439-5

Publishing Director: Linda Duncan
Veterinary Publisher: Penny Rudolph
Developmental Editor: Shelly Stringer
Publishing Services Manager: Pat Joiner
Senior Project Manager: Rachel E. Dowell
Design Direction: Amy Buxton

Printed in China

Last digit is the print number: 9   8   7   6   5   4   3   2   1

This book is dedicated to my husband (Matt Miller)
and sons, Chase and Kobe,
who made a personal sacrifice while it was being written;
to fellow practitioners throughout the world;
and to all veterinary students.

This third edition of *Small Animal Surgery* has undergone significant changes to reflect cutting-edge information in a more user-friendly format than ever before. Now including an e-dition, this text offers a new and dynamic way of learning in addition to the traditional text. We are extremely proud of this third edition and hope you will find that we have accomplished our goals.

In keeping with the previous editions, we have maintained our initial goals of providing (1) a limited number of contributors, (2) an excellent and consistent art program, and (3) a precise and consistent format that varies minimally between chapters.

Throughout the text, you will find that we have updated procedures with new information published since the previous editions were printed, and in many cases we have added descriptions of entirely new procedures that were either rarely used or not used when the previous editions were published. It was our goal to make sure that we produced the most state-of-the-art book possible. Although it has always been our desire to provide clinically useful information rather than a monologue of research on a given topic, we have addressed the need for a review of recent research by providing up-to-date references and a suggested reading list at the end of each chapter. The suggested reading list contains a short description of the article and why the author thought it relevant. In the e-dition, the references and selected reading list are directly linked to the original article for easy access by the reader.

We were lucky to enlist the aid of many of the same surgeons from the previous editions in this revised edition. As with previous editions, the bulk of this book was written by five surgeons and an internist. Dr. Howard Seim and I were responsible for Part I, *General Surgical Principles,* while Dr. Mike Willard contributed to the endoscopy and minimally invasive material throughout the text. Dr. Cheryl Hedlund and I were responsible for Part II, *Soft Tissue Surgery,* and Drs. Ann Johnson and Kurt Schulz provided the material encompassed in Part III, *Orthopedics.* Dr. Howard Seim contributed Part IV, *Neurosurgery.* Dr. Gwen Carroll provided the chapter on pain management (Chapter 13). New to this edition, Dr. Anne Bahr reviewed all of the imaging sections and provided her expertise along with many new figures. Lastly, Dr. Mike Willard reviewed and provided his perspective on many of the chapters so that we might provide the most up-to-date information on the medical management of surgical disease.

FORMAT

While we have added significant new information to the text, we have also revised the formatting. Additionally, we condensed the minimally invasive surgery into one basic chapter and have located the description of minimally invasive procedures in the specific chapter where they are applicable (for example, thoracoscopic pericardiectomy follows surgical pericardiectomy). We believe that readers will find this new format practical and easy to follow.

To maintain a reasonable size textbook, some of the less commonly performed procedures detailed in the second edition are now presented in a fully searchable format in the e-dition for easy reference.

As with previous editions, we believe that to be successful, surgeons must have detailed knowledge of the important issues regarding diagnosis, an awareness of potential diagnoses, and a thorough appreciation of preoperative concerns relative to the animal's disease or condition. These sections are each outlined in the text. Additionally, anesthetic concerns, surgical anatomy, wound healing, postoperative concerns, and potential complications are detailed. The surgical technique itself is described in detail, which provides the reader with a comprehensive and thorough description of each procedure. The surgical procedure is discussed in an *italicized typeface and is printed as blue text* to make it easy to distinguish from the rest of the text.

The previous editions garnered much praise for using a consistent and user-friendly format. We have maintained that format here, expanding upon it where appropriate. Because we know that veterinary practitioners are busy, we have used tables throughout the text to provide easy reference and to reduce the amount of time spent searching for drug doses and other important information. Again, to prevent excessive duplication of material throughout the text, we have in some instances referred readers to other pages; however, when we have done so we have attempted to provide a specific page number for reference to help you find the information as quickly and easily as possible.

GENERAL FORMAT

This book comprises 41 chapters and is organized into four parts. The first 14 chapters of Part I, *General Surgical Principles,* were written with veterinary medical students and practitioners in mind. The information contained within these chapters is the information we teach our students in their introductory surgery courses. Found within these chapters is detailed information on the basics of sterile technique, surgical instrumentation, suturing, preoperative care, and rational antibiotic use. We have updated the sterile technique section to include new advances in scrubless and/or waterless prep solutions that veterinary surgeons will find useful. Chapter 11 contains information on postoperative care, including nutrition for surgical patients. Because nutrition affects many body systems and is an important adjunct to case management, we have included detailed information on techniques for hyperalimentation in this chapter. Chapter 12 is a new chapter that details the basics of physical rehabilitation in veterinary patients. We believe that physical rehabilitation is underutilized in many veterinary practices. In addition to this basic chapter, specific recommendations for physical rehabilitation can be found throughout the orthopedic and neurologic chapters. We have also expanded Chapter 13, Perioperative Mutlimodal Analgesic Therapy, with important information for practitioners. Chapter 14 is a new chapter that describes the basic principles of minimally invasive surgery, including instrument selection and care and basic techniques. As previously noted, we have moved specific minimally invasive procedures to the appropriate chapter of this book because we felt this would make the material more relevant and useful to busy practitioners. We have also expanded descriptions of minimally invasive techniques throughout the text. With the addition of Kurt Schulz as an author of this edition, we have greatly expanded arthroscopy in Part III and have added details regarding many new orthopedic procedures.

Parts II, III, and IV contain information on soft tissue surgery, orthopedic surgery, and neurosurgery, respectively. These chapters are divided into a section detailing general principles and a section on specific diseases. The *General Principles and Techniques* portion begins with definitions of procedures and terms relevant to the organ system detailed. Next are sections detailing information on preoperative concerns and anesthetic considerations. This is followed by a discussion on antibiotic use (including recommendations for antibiotic prophylaxis) and a brief description of pertinent surgical anatomy. Anatomy is too often neglected in surgical textbooks, or because of formatting is not well correlated with the techniques in a given chapter. As with the previous editions, we have circumvented this problem by including it as a separate and consistent heading under *General Principles and Techniques*. Surgical techniques that are broadly applicable to a number of diseases are also detailed in this section. However, if a surgical procedure is specific to a particular disease, the description of the technique will be found instead with the specific disease description. Brief discussions on healing of the specific organ or tissue as well as suture material and special instruments follow the surgical techniques descriptions. The final headings in the *General Principles and Techniques* section are *Postoperative Care and Assessment, Complications,* and *Special Age Considerations.*

The *Specific Diseases* portion of each chapter begins with definitions and, when relevant, synonyms for the disease or techniques are given. Next, general considerations and clinically relevant pathophysiology are detailed. This information is meant to provide practical material for case management, rather than serving as a supplemental text for pathophysiology. The discussions of diagnoses are detailed and include information on signalment and history, physical examination findings, diagnostic imaging, and pertinent laboratory abnormalities. Sections on differential diagnoses

and medical management of affected animals are consistently provided. These are followed by a detailed description of the relevant surgical techniques. We have attempted to detail most commonly used techniques, although we may have noted our preference for a particular method. Information on positioning patients for a given procedure is often neglected in surgical textbooks; to avoid this we have provided this information as a separate and consistent heading. The remainder of the *Specific Diseases* section deals with postoperative care of the surgical patient, potential complications, and prognosis.

GENERAL CHAPTER FORMAT

I.   General principles and techniques
   A. Definitions
   B. Preoperative management
   C. Anesthesia
   D. Antibiotics
   E. Surgical anatomy
   F. Surgical technique
   G. Wound healing
   H. Suture materials and special instruments
   I. Postoperative care and assessment
   J. Complications
   K. Special age considerations
II. Specific diseases
   A. Definitions
   B. General considerations and clinically relevant pathophysiology
   C. Diagnosis
      1. Clinical presentation
         a. Signalment
         b. History
      2. Physical examination findings
      3. Diagnostic imaging
      4. Laboratory findings
   D. Differential diagnosis
   E. Medical management
   F. Surgical treatment
      1. Preoperative management
      2. Anesthesia
      3. Surgical anatomy
      4. Positioning
   G. Surgical technique
   H. Suture materials and special instruments
   I. Postoperative care and assessment
   J. Complications
   K. Prognosis

ANESTHESIA PROTOCOLS

In most surgery textbooks, anesthesia is either totally neglected or is included in separate chapters near the end of the book. Busy practitioners often find it difficult to access this information and correlate it with the cases on which they are working. Therefore, recommendations for anesthetizing animals with a particular disease or disorder are found in the *Specific Diseases* section of each chapter. As with the first edition, Dr. Gwen Carroll served as our anesthesia consultant for this revision. Gwen was responsible for reviewing the general anesthesia information for each organ system included in the *General Principles and Techniques* sections. Also included in this book are numerous suggested anesthetic protocols, including drug dosages. Although we recognize that many veterinarians have established protocols that they prefer and with which they are comfortable, the protocols provided in this book have proved to be a handy resource for both students and doctors.

REFERENCES

As with the previous editions, rather than provide a long list of available references, we have chosen to provide a limited number of references. It was our feeling that with the ready availability of computerized bibliographic information, laundry lists of references are no longer necessary. In order to make room for newer references, we have removed many references more than 6 years old from this edition, unless the reference was thought to be a "classic." Additionally, we have listed selected references under the heading *Suggested Reading*. These references are followed by a short description of why the authors found this article to be useful or valuable.

NEW TO THIS EDITION

We have added many new procedures, particularly in surgery of the joints, including detailed descriptions of TPLO and total hip replacement, as well as more advanced procedures. Although we debated the practicality of including advanced procedures in this textbook, we decided that practitioners would benefit greatly from a better understanding of the procedures, even though they likely would choose to refer these cases to a specialist.

With this in mind, we have marked some procedures as "advanced" to forewarn readers of the difficulty of the procedure. While the difficulty of any procedure lies primarily with the experience of the surgeon, the procedures marked "advanced" and denoted with the icon are ones that the authors find particularly challenging and thus would recommend that they be performed by someone with advanced training or special expertise in that area.

E-DITION

An exciting new feature to the third edition of *Small Animal Surgery* is the optional e-dition website. The e-dition offers online access to the complete book, plus content that is updated weekly. The frequently updated e-dition keeps information current and provides additional learning tools to the user. The e-dition contains the complete text with full search capabilities and updates throughout the life of the third edition. It also provides case studies, aftercare instructions, and abstracts of relevant articles. The e-dition (textbook plus online access) is sold as a stand-alone product.

In addition to a fully searchable text, the e-dition offers several user-friendly tools that will enhance the learning experience. A few key e-dition capabilities include note-taking, saving searches, and viewing the extensive image collection with a lightbox function that allows the user to save images to PowerPoint presentations. Users will also be able to watch video clips and study animations of surgical procedures.

SPECIAL FEATURES

It has always been our intent to make this book as user-friendly as possible. For this reason, we have expanded the NOTE boxes, which highlight important concerns, key concepts, and precautions. We have also expanded the use of tables and boxes that provided antibiotic, anesthetic, and analgesic protocols. The tables and boxes are color-coded and are identified by distinct icons for easy access.

As in the first edition, we have included hundreds of summary tables and boxes for key clinical information. To facilitate ease of access and to promote comprehension, we have created unique logos and color schemes for tables and boxes with similar types of information:

 Analgesics/Pain Management

 Anesthetics/Sedation

 Antibiotics

 Calculations

 Classifications of Disease

 Clinical Signs

 Complications

 Diagnosis and Differential Diagnosis

 Etiology

 General

 General Treatment

 Key Points

ART PROGRAM

We were extremely privileged to work with our original illustrator, Laura Pardi DuPrey, on this third edition. In addition to being an incredibly skilled artist, she has an extremely broad-based and detailed knowledge of anatomy. We also welcomed a new artist, Don O'Connor, to this edition. Don created many new illustrations that greatly enhanced the orthopedic chapters. You will find that the illustrations in this text are exceptionally clear and accurate. We have added many new illustrations, and revised many more, in our attempt to make this book among the best illustrated textbooks in veterinary medicine.

We have added new artwork to existing procedures, and you will find that there are more color illustrations in this edition than in the last. In fact, 75% of the illustrations in this edition are in full color. The artwork in the orthopedic section, in particular, has been vastly redone.

INDEX

We felt that an extensive index was mandatory. The index of *Small Animal Surgery* is thorough and exhaustive. Additionally, we have avoided cross-referencing readers to separate entries in the index. Rather, we have opted to duplicate page sources each time a topic is listed because we believe that this is the most useful format for practitioners.

ACKNOWLEDGMENTS

A textbook of this nature takes the input and hard work of a great number of people to ensure that it is a quality reference. Special thanks to Shelly Stringer, Developmental Editor; Stacy Beane, Editorial Assistant; Penny Rudolph, Veterinary Publisher; and all the others at Elsevier who worked on this proj-

ect. We thank them for their enthusiasm, words of encouragement, and vision, and most of all for their belief in this book. Without them, this edition would not have been possible.

We would also like to thank our mentors and colleagues, who have instilled in us a love of surgery and a dedication to our profession. Without you, this book would not have become a reality. I would particularly like to thank Dr. Phil Hobson, whose vision, support, and words of encouragement I continue to hold dear.

To all of you who purchased previous editions, we appreciate your input and recommendations. We particularly welcome your suggestions on how to improve future editions. We hope you find this edition a worthy effort.

I would like to once again thank my fellow contributors on this book. I am blessed to have been able to work with some of the best and most dedicated surgeons in veterinary medicine. This edition was no less of an undertaking than the previous editions, and your dedication and hard work made it a timely and worthwhile addition to the veterinary literature. Many thanks!

Finally, I would like to acknowledge the support and encouragement of my wonderful family: my husband, Matt Miller; my sons, Chase and Kobe Miller; my mother, Marian Smith; and my mother-in-law, Diane Miller.

Advances are continuously being made in the field of small animal surgery. The third edition of *Small Animal Surgery* is designed to grow with each of these new developments through the *Small Animal Surgery e-dition* website, a constantly evolving counterpart to this revised textbook. This resource is readily available to purchasers of the *Small Animal Surgery e-dition* or those who upgrade to web access. Resources of the *Small Animal Surgery e-dition* include the complete revised *Small Animal Surgery* text as well as a host of enhanced features not possible in a printed textbook.

Below is an introduction to each of the supplemental features found on the *Small Animal Surgery e-dition* website. These features form the core of the *Small Animal Surgery e-dition* but, just as small animal surgery continues to evolve, so does this interactive resource.

COMPLETE ONLINE, SEARCHABLE TEXT

The *Small Animal Surgery* online component allows the entire textbook to be searchable.

The accompanying search engine enables users to **instantly locate all content** related to a given topic.

CONTINUOUS CONTENT UPDATES

Ongoing updates provide users with cutting-edge information on new developments in small animal surgery throughout the life of the third edition. These updates are accessible directly from corresponding sections in the text.

INTERACTIVE REFERENCES

All of the bibliographic material for *Small Animal Surgery* is presented in a searchable format that is directly linked, through PubMed, to the original full-text articles and abstracts referenced in the creation of the third edition.

CASE PRESENTATIONS

Online users can access documented case studies that provide current information drawn from material in the text and other online resources. The cases include histories, presenting symptoms, test results, diagnoses, and treatment options, as well as pertinent clinical photographs and radiographs.

VIDEO CLIPS

Important techniques, procedures, and concepts from *Small Animal Surgery* are supported by high-quality video clips accessible directly from the corresponding sections.

ELECTRONIC IMAGE COLLECTION

Every image from the third edition of *Small Animal Surgery* is viewable in the electronic image collection. Users can review key points from the text and customize PowerPoint presentations with supporting material taken directly from the third edition.

CLIENT INFORMATION SHEETS

Aftercare instructions for many of the procedures found throughout *Small Animal Surgery* are provided in PDF format. This feature gives practitioners easy access to handouts that are designed to give clients important information pertaining to their pets.

RARELY PERFORMED PROCEDURES

Many rarely performed procedures that appeared in the second edition of *Small Animal Surgery* are now presented in a fully searchable format in the e-dition. The online text directly links users to detailed guidelines for performing uncommon surgical techniques, accompanied by illustrations and other supplemental materials wherever possible.

FRACTURE PLANNER

Users interested in improving their mastery of orthopedic surgery can use this dynamic interactive program to create an accurate diagnostic assessment and viable surgical plan. Surgeons can show their surgical plan to clients before surgery so clients know better what to expect, or after surgery to explain to clients what was done. Students can use this interactive study tool to determine what surgical approach can be taken to successfully effect an orthopedic repair.

CONTENTS

DETAILED CONTENTS

CHAPTER 1

Principles of Surgical Asepsis

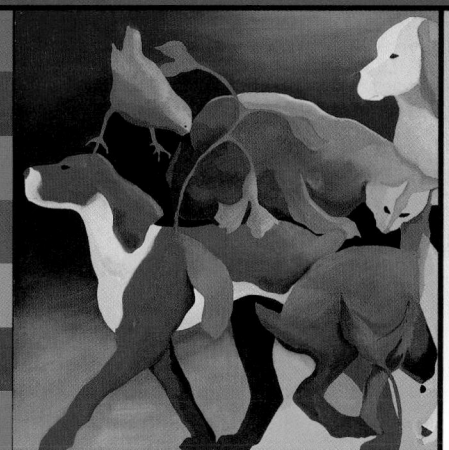

Whenever dermal integrity is disrupted, such as during surgery, microorganisms have access to inner tissue. The bacteria that contaminate surgical wounds generally originate from the patient's endogenous flora, from operating room personnel, and from the environment. Rules of aseptic technique must be followed to prevent wound contamination. These rules are not simply guidelines; they are laws of the operating room, and breaking them subjects patients to the risk of infection or disease.

Aseptic technique is defined as the methods and practices that prevent cross contamination in surgery. It involves proper preparation of the facilities and environment (see Chapters 3 and 4), surgical site (see Chapter 6), surgical team (see Chapter 7), and surgical equipment (see Chapters 2 and 8).

Infection first requires microorganisms being introduced into the surgical wound. The source of the microorganisms may be **exogenous** (i.e., the air, surgical instruments, surgical team, or patient) or **endogenous** (i.e., organisms that originate in the patient's body). It is impossible to eliminate all microorganisms from the surgical wound and sterile field; however, aseptic technique limits the patient's exposure to a number of microorganisms that is not detrimental. Rules of aseptic technique and reasons for them are listed in Table 1-1. "No pathogen has yet developed resistance to aseptic technique."

PREPARATION OF SURGICAL PACKS

Regardless of the sterilization technique used, instruments and linens (e.g., towels, gowns, and drapes) must be cleaned of gross contamination. Instruments should be cleaned manually or with ultrasonic cleaning equipment and appropriate disinfectants as soon as possible after surgery (see Chapter 8), and linens should be laundered. The procedure for wrapping items is based on enhancing the ease of sterilization and preserving the sterility of the item, not on convenience or personal preference.

Packaging materials (e.g., wrapped or container systems) allow penetration of the sterilization agent and maintenance of sterility after sterilization. Materials for maintaining sterility of instruments during transport and storage include wrapped perforated instrument cassettes, peel pouches of plastic or paper, sterile container systems, and sterilization wraps (which can be either woven or unwoven). Packaging materials should be designed for the type of sterilization process being used (Table 1-2). Items sterilized by pressurized steam or other methods (e.g., ethylene oxide, plasma) must be wrapped in a specific manner (see p. 9). Packaging materials also should be appropriate for the items being sterilized (Table 1-3). For example, nonpaper materials should be used to package sharp instruments, which can easily puncture paper packaging. Metal closures (e.g., staples, paper clips) that might puncture packaging materials should not be used.

Sterile container systems are typically rigid, boxlike devices made from heat-resistant and steam-sterilizable high-performance plastic or other materials in which instruments can be placed and sterilized. Rigid containers were first developed in Germany in the mid-1890s. The main function of these early containers was to transport sterile instruments and dressings. In that era it was not unusual for sterile supplies to be kept in a few containers for an entire day's operating schedule. At the Association of Operating Room Nurses Congress in 1980, the concept of "rigid packaging for sterilization" was introduced in the United States. With time, sterilization containers have gained the confidence of hospital professionals. They are both durable and cost-effective, aid in pack organization, and tend to protect instruments better than wraps. Closed container systems require filters (in the lid only or both the lid and bottom of the container) and latches, seals, and/or tamper-resistant seals. Rigid containers may be a good choice if the sterilization chamber is large enough to accommodate them and if current storage space is sufficient to accommodate the new configuration. There are dozens of different container sizes and shapes to accommodate most commonly used instruments including scopes, drills, and cameras.

The original sterilization wraps were 140-thread-count muslin cloth. Advantages of these cloths included that they were soft, reusable, inexpensive, and absorbent, and could

TABLE 1-1

Rules of Aseptic Technique

RULE	REASON
Surgical team members remain within the sterile area.	Movement out of the sterile area may encourage cross contamination.
Talking is kept to a minimum.	Talking releases moisture droplets laden with bacteria.
Movement in the operating room (OR) by all personnel is kept to a minimum; only necessary personnel should enter the operating room.	Movement in the OR may encourage turbulent airflow and result in cross contamination.
Nonscrubbed personnel do not reach over sterile fields.	Dust, lint, or other vehicles of bacterial contamination may fall on the sterile field.
Scrubbed team members face each other and the sterile field at all times.	A team member's back is not considered sterile even if wearing a wraparound gown.
Equipment used during surgery must be sterilized.	Unsterile instruments may be a source of cross contamination.
Scrubbed personnel handle only sterile items; nonscrubbed personnel handle only nonsterile items.	Nonscrubbed personnel and nonsterile items may be a source of cross contamination.
If the sterility of an item is questioned, it is considered contaminated.	Nonsterile, contaminated equipment may be a source of cross contamination.
Sterile tables are only sterile at table height.	Items hanging over the table edge are considered nonsterile because they are out of the surgeon's vision.
Gowns are sterile from midchest to waist and from gloved hand to 2 inches above the elbow.	The back of the gown is not considered sterile even if it is a wraparound gown.
Drapes covering instrument tables or the patient should be moisture proof.	Moisture carries bacteria from a nonsterile surface to a sterile surface (strike-through contamination).
If a sterile object touches the sealing edge of the pouch that holds it during opening, it is considered contaminated.	Once opened, sealed edges of pouches are not sterile.
Sterile items within a damaged or wet wrapper are considered contaminated.	Contamination can occur from perforated wrappers or from strike-through from moisture transport.
Hands may not be folded into the axillary region; rather, they are clasped in front of the body above the waist.	The axillary region of the gown is not considered sterile.
If the surgical team begins the surgery seated, they should remain seated until the surgery has been completed.	The surgical field is sterile only from table height to the chest; movement from sitting to standing during surgery may increase cross contamination.

easily be draped over trays. However, because they were woven, bacteria could penetrate the pack. Most hospitals double-wrap packs when using cloth to reduce contamination of surgical instruments. In the 1960s, nonwoven materials were introduced that provided a more effective microbial barrier that was also water resistant. However, the material used for these wraps was derived from cellulose and was not particularly strong. Hence, sequential (double) wrapping was still necessary. The introduction of polypropylene allowed the development of wraps possessing strength, barrier, and repellent properties. Currently the most preferred nonwoven technologies used in the medical market are spunlaced and SMS. Spunlaced nonwovens are made by entangling polyester fibers with a layer of wood pulp, whereas SMS materials feature a composite of three layers—spunlace, meltblown, and spunbonded—normally using a polypropylene resin and then being stacked together. These products provide excellent protection from microbial contamination. However, despite the fact that the barrier efficacy of a single sheet of wrap has improved over the years, using multiple wrap layers is still common practice because of the rigors of handling packs and the consequences of bacterial contamination.

Before packing, instruments are separated and placed in order of their intended use. If steam or gas sterilization is used, the selected wrap should be penetrable by steam or gas, impermeable to microbes, durable, and flexible. Commonly used wrapping materials, the advantages and disadvantages of each, and the sterilization techniques with which each is compatible are listed in Table 1-4.

To ensure maximum penetration, specific guidelines should be followed when preparing packs for steam and gas

TABLE 1-2

Types and Use of Sterilization Packaging Materials Based on Sterilization Method

STERILIZATION METHOD	PACKAGING MATERIAL REQUIREMENTS	ACCEPTABLE MATERIALS
Steam autoclave	Should allow steam to penetrate	Paper Plastic Cloth Paper peel packages Wrapped perforated cassettes
Dry heat	Should not insulate items from heat Should not be destroyed by temperature used	Paper bags Aluminum foil Polyfilm plastic tubing Wrapped perforated cassettes
Unsaturated chemical vapor	Vapors should be allowed to precipitate on contents Vapors should not react with packaging material Plastics should not contact sides of sterilizer	Wrapped perforated cassettes Paper Paper peel pouches

Modified from Miller CH, Palenik CJ: *Infection control and management of hazardous materials for the dental team,* ed 2, St Louis, 1998, Mosby.

 TABLE 1-3

Packing Materials Based on Device Type

MEDICAL DEVICE	STERILIZATION METHOD	SUGGESTED PACKAGING MATERIAL
Stainless steel instrument(s) Instrument set(s)	Steam	140-count muslin SMS Woven cotton/polyester-blend fabrics Pouches
Endoscopic instrument(s) Instrument set(s)	Plasma Ethylene oxide (EtO)	Plasma: SMS, polyester-blend fabrics, low-temp SMS pouches EtO: 140-count muslin, SMS, polyester-blend fabrics, some crepe-type papers, thermoplastic polymers (Tyvek)
Glass syringes or other medical devices made of glass	Steam EtO Plasma	Steam: SMS pouches EtO/plasma Low-temp SMS pouches Thermoplastic polymers

sterilization. Presterilization wraps for steam sterilization comprise two thicknesses of two-layer muslin or nonwoven (i.e., paper) barrier materials. The poststerilization wrap (i.e., the wrap used after sterilization and the proper cool down period) is a waterproof, heat-sealable plastic dust cover; this wrap is not necessary if the item is to be used within 24 hours of sterilization. Small items may be wrapped, sterilized, and stored in heat-sealable paper or plastic peel pouches. Items to be gas sterilized are wrapped in heat-sealable plastic peel pouches or tubing or muslin wrap. When plasma sterilization is used, items should be wrapped in heat-sealable Tyvek-Mylar pouches or polypropylene wraps.

Time, temperature, and humidity recommendations for steam, ethylene oxide, and plasma sterilization are given in Chapter 2.

For steam and gas sterilization, instruments should be organized on a lint-free (huck) towel placed on the bottom of a perforated metal instrument tray. Instruments with boxlocks should be open when autoclaved. A 3- to 5-mm space between instruments is recommended for proper steam or gas circulation. Complex instruments should be disassembled when possible, and power equipment should be lubricated (see Chapter 8) before sterilization. If the item has a lumen, a small amount of water should be flushed

TABLE 1-4

Advantages and Disadvantages of Wrapping Materials for Pack Preparation

MATERIAL	ADVANTAGES	DISADVANTAGES	STERILIZATION METHOD
Cotton muslin; 140 or 270 thread counts	Durable, flexible, reusable, easily handled	Requires double layer and double wrap, generates lint, not moisture resistant	Steam, ethylene oxide (EtO)
Nonwoven barrier material (i.e., paper)	Inexpensive	Single use, memory, not as durable, not moisture resistant, requires double wrap	Steam, EtO
Nonwoven polypropylene fabric*	Flexible, durable, excellent bacterial barrier, puncture resistant, lint free	Single use, requires double wrap	Steam, EtO
Paper/plastic pouches† (heat sealed)	Convenient, long shelf life, water resistant	Instruments may puncture pouch	Steam, EtO
Plastic pouches‡ (heat sealed)	Convenient, long shelf life, waterproof, more puncture resistant	Instruments may puncture pouch	Plasma, EtO

*Spunguard.
†Made of paper and Mylar.
‡Made of Tyvek and Mylar.

through it immediately before steam sterilization because water vaporizes and forces air out of the lumen; conversely, moisture left in tubing placed in a gas sterilizer may reduce the action of the gas below the lethal point. Containers (e.g., saline bowl) should be placed with the open end facing up or horizontal; containers with lids should have the lid slightly ajar. Multiple basins should be stacked with a towel between them. A standard count of radiopaque surgical sponges should be included in each pack. A sterilization indicator (see p. 13) should be placed in the center of each pack before it is wrapped. Solutions should be steam sterilized separately from instruments using the slow exhaust phase (see Table 2-2, p. 11).

> NOTE: Immersing instruments for long periods of time in any solution can prove damaging. Never leave instruments in any solution for longer than 20 minutes. Do not immerse instruments with tungsten carbide inserts (gold handles) in solutions containing benzyl ammonium chloride (BAC) because this chemical is known to loosen the tungsten carbide.

Linens may be steam sterilized. The maximum size and weight of linen packs that can be steam sterilized effectively are 12 × 12 × 20 inches and 6 kg, respectively. Closely woven table drapes should be packed separately. Layers of linen are alternated in their orientation to permit steam penetration. As with instruments, a sterilization indicator (see p. 13) should be placed in the center of each pack.

Wrapping Instrument Packs

Instrument packs should be wrapped so that they can be easily unwrapped without breaking sterile technique (Fig. 1-1).

Folding and Wrapping Gowns

Gowns must be folded so that they can be easily donned without breaking sterile technique (Fig. 1-2).

Folding and Wrapping Drapes

Drapes should be folded so that the fenestration can be properly positioned over the surgical site without contaminating the drape (Fig. 1-3).

HANDLING AND STORAGE OF STERILIZED INSTRUMENTS AND EQUIPMENT

After removal from the autoclave, packs are allowed to cool and dry individually on racks. Placing the packs on top of each other during cooling may promote condensation of moisture, resulting in strike-through contamination. Strike-through contamination occurs when moisture carries bacteria from a nonsterile surface to a sterile surface. When the sterile packs are completely dry, they should be stored in waterproof dust covers in closed cabinets (rather than uncovered on open shelves) to protect them from moisture or exposure to particulate matter (i.e., dust-borne bacteria). Excessive handling of sterile supplies should be avoided, especially if the items are pointed or have sharp edges. Sterile items should be handled gently and should be protected from bending, crushing, or compression forces that could break a seal or puncture the package. Sterile packs should be

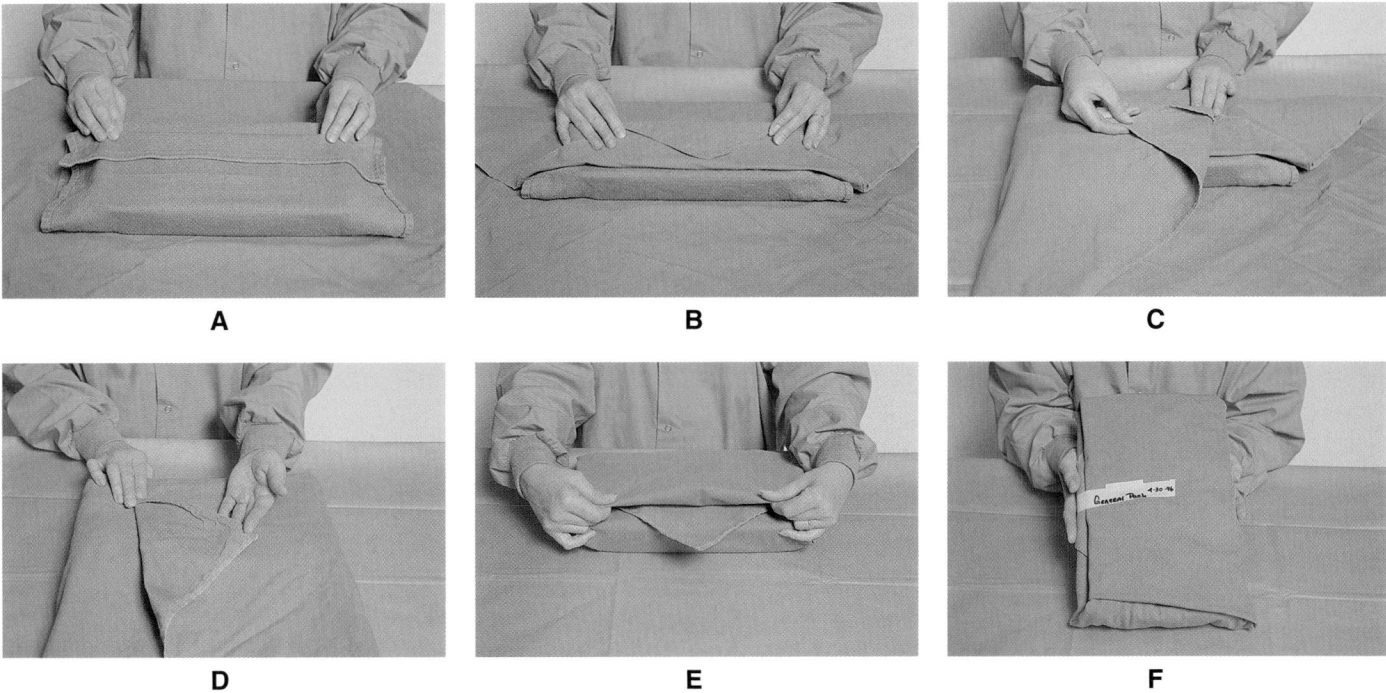

FIG. 1-1
Wrapping an instrument pack. **A,** Wrap the instrument pack in a clean huck towel. Place a large, unfolded wrap in front of you and position the instrument tray in the center of the wrap so that an imaginary line drawn from one corner of the wrap to the opposite corner is perpendicular to the long axis of the instrument tray. **B,** Fold the corner of the wrap that is closest to you over the instrument tray and to its far edge. Fold the tip of the wrap over so that it is exposed for easy unwrapping. **C,** Fold the right corner over the pack. **D,** Fold the left corner similarly. **E,** Turn the pack around and fold the final corner of the wrap over the tray, tucking it tightly under the previous two folds. **F,** Wrap the pack in a second layer of cloth or paper in a similar manner. Secure the last corner of the outer wrap with masking tape and a piece of heat-sensitive indicator tape.

stored away from ventilation ducts, sprinklers, and heat-producing light. The ideal environmental conditions are low humidity, low air turbulence, and a constant, controllable room temperature.

Sterile Shelf Life

The use of published expiration dates for sterilized items in various types of wrappers (Table 1-5) is controversial. Events, not time, contaminate products. It recently was shown that if items are packaged, sterilized, and handled properly, they remain sterile unless the package is opened, gets wet, is torn, has a broken seal, or is damaged in some other way (i.e., event-related expiration). The length of time an item is considered sterile depends on a number of factors: (1) the type and configuration of the packaging materials; (2) the number of times a package is handled before use; (3) the number of personnel who may have handled the package; (4) whether the package was stored on open or closed shelves; (5) the condition of the storage area (e.g., cleanliness, temperature, and humidity); and (6) the method of sealing and whether dust covers were used (Association of Operating Room Nurses, 2000). To effectively use an event-related expiration

system, appropriate protocols must be adopted for sterilizing and handling items.

Handling Sterilized Items

In the future, sterile packs will not have an expiration date; they will have the date on which the item was sterilized and a control lot number for tracing a nonsterile item. Heat-sealed, waterproof dust covers will be placed on items not routinely used. All packages will state: "Sterility guaranteed until the package is damaged or opened." These items will have to be stored in a manner that does not compromise packaging and sterility, and they will need to be rotated in such a way that the item processed first is used first.

If a sterile pack is damaged, it should not be used. Damage is defined as wraps that have moisture present; packs that have been placed in a dusty environment or stored near the source of an air current; items that have been dropped, bent, crushed, compressed, torn, or punctured; or packs that have a broken seal. Education of surgery personnel must include training in ways to protect sterile items from events that cause loss of sterility. The integrity of sterilized items must be carefully assessed to identify damaged goods, and

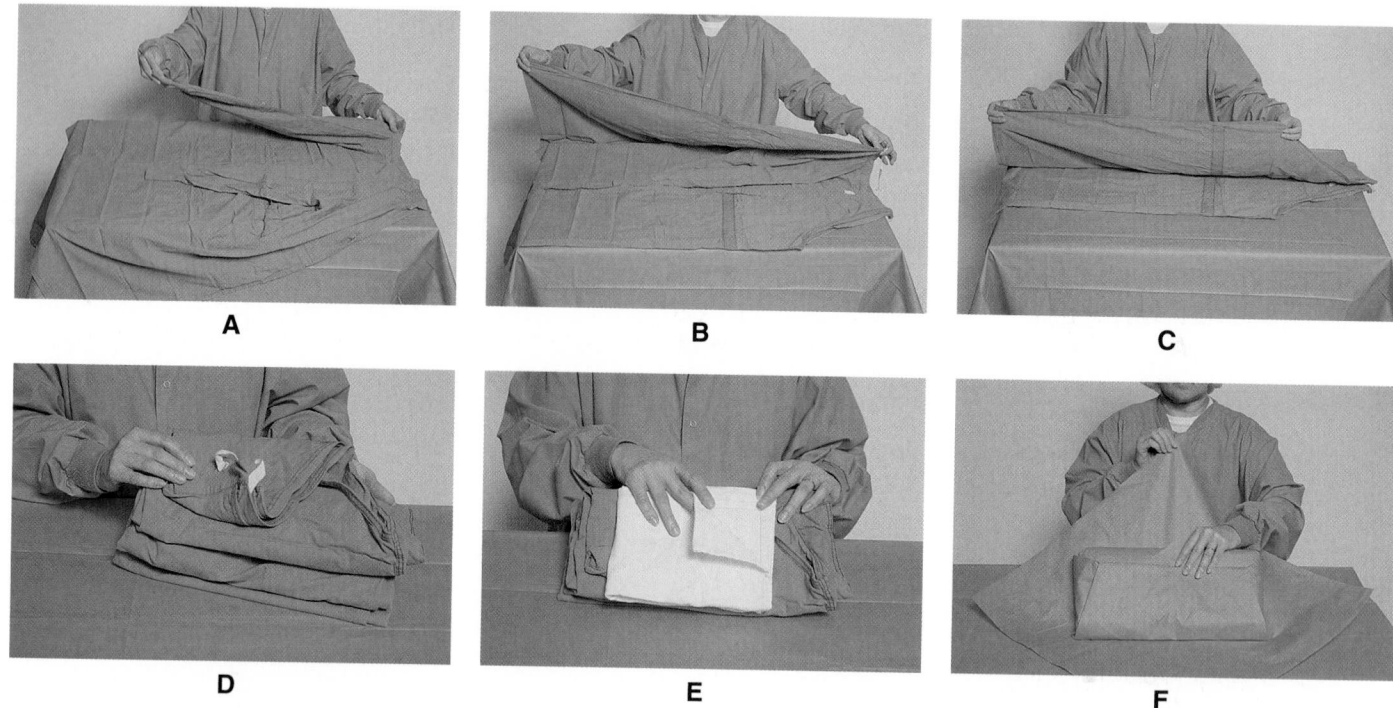

FIG. 1-2
Folding and wrapping surgical gowns. **A,** Place the gown on a clean, flat surface with the front of the gown facing up. Fold the sleeves neatly toward the center of the gown with the cuffs of the sleeves facing the bottom hem. **B,** Fold the sides to the center so that the side seams are aligned with the sleeve seams. **C,** Fold the gown in half longitudinally (the sleeves will be inside the gown). **D,** Starting with the bottom hem, fanfold the gown toward the neck. **E,** Fold a hand towel in half horizontally, and fanfold it into about four folds. Place it on top of the folded gown, leaving one corner turned back so that it can be easily grasped. **F,** Wrap the gown and towel in two layers of paper or cloth wrap as described in Fig. 1-1.

plastic dust covers must be removed or wiped clean before reaching the surgical area.

Unwrapping and Opening Sterile Items

Sterile items are wrapped in a manner that allows operating room personnel to unwrap the item without contaminating it. There are three popular methods of distributing sterile items.

Unwrapping large sterile linen/paper/polypropylene packs that cannot be held during distribution. If the pack is too large, cumbersome, or heavy to be held during distribution, it may be opened onto a Mayo stand or back table. Place the pack on the center of the Mayo stand or back table and open each folded layer by pulling it toward you (this prevents your hand and arm from extending over the sterile area). Handle only the edge and underside of the wrap. Follow the same procedure for each fold. When the pack is open, have a sterile team member place it on the sterile table.

There is disagreement over the correct way to open double-wrapped sterile packs—outer layer only or both layers—and there is evidence to support both techniques. The rationale for opening the outer layer only is that this technique elimi-

nates the risk of microbial shedding from the circulating nurse's hands and arms onto the contents of the sterile package. The rationale for opening both wrappers is that when the outer surface of the inner wrapper is opened, it may become contaminated by dust particles and debris from the outer wrapper; if this inner wrapper is opened by the circulating nurse, the possibility of contamination is reduced. The decision on which technique to use must be based on the technical expertise of personnel and on barrier quality.

Unwrapping sterile linen/paper packages that can be held during distribution. These packs may be opened and placed on a sterile table as described in Fig. 1-4, or after opening, they may be grasped by a sterile team member.

Unwrapping sterile items in paper/plastic or plastic peel-back pouches. Identify the edges of the peel-back wrapper and carefully separate them. Peel the edges of the wrapper back slowly and symmetrically to ensure that the sterile item does not come in contact with the torn edge of the wrapper (the torn edge of a peel-back wrapper is unsterile). If the item is small, place it on the sterile area as described above, being careful not to lean across the sterile table. If the item is long or cumbersome, have a sterile

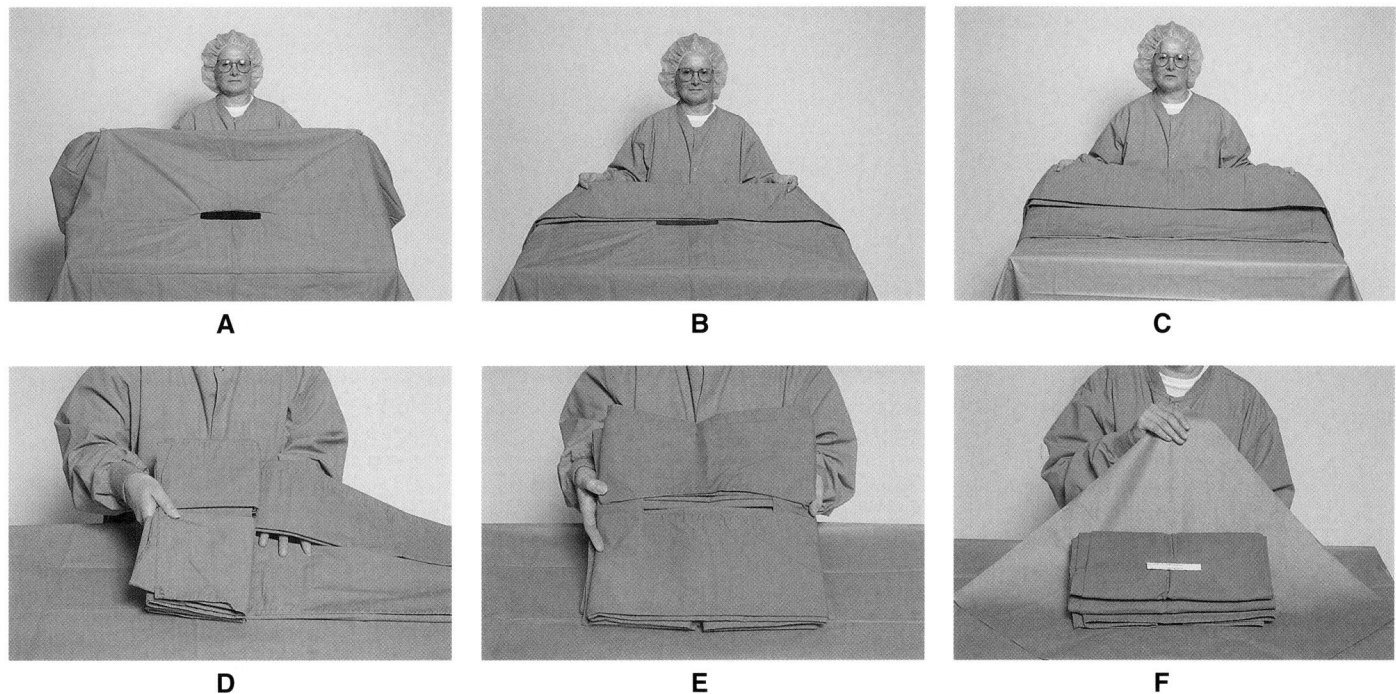

FIG. 1-3
Folding and wrapping drapes. **A,** Lay the drape flat with the ends of the fenestration perpendicular to you and the sides of the fenestration parallel to you. **B,** Grasp the edges of the drape nearest you and fanfold the drape to the center. The edge of the drape should be exposed (dorsal) so that it can be easily grasped during unfolding. **C,** Turn the drape around and fanfold the other half the same way. **D,** Fanfold one end of the drape to the center (the fingers are through the fenestration); repeat with the other end. **E,** If the drape has been folded properly, the fenestration is on the ventral outermost aspect. **F,** Fold the drape in half, and wrap it in two layers of paper or cloth wrap as described in Fig. 1-1.

TABLE 1-5

Recommended Storage Times for Sterilized Packs

WRAPPER	SHELF LIFE
Double-wrapped, two-layer muslin	4 weeks
Double-wrapped, two-layer muslin, heat sealed in dust covers after sterilization	6 months
Double-wrapped, two-layer muslin, tape sealed in dust covers after sterilization	2 months
Double-wrapped nonwoven barrier materials (i.e., paper)	6 months
Paper/plastic peel pouches, heat sealed	1 year
Plastic peel pouches, heat sealed	1 year

Sterilized items from hospitals that have adopted event-related sterility assurance have an indefinite shelf life (see p. 5 Sterile Shelf Life).

team member grasp it and gently pull it from the peel-back wrapper, taking care not to brush the item against the peeled edge of the wrapper. Scalpel blades and suture material are opened in a similar manner.

POURING SOLUTIONS INTO BASINS

Solutions (i.e., sterile saline and antiseptics) are poured into basins. The basin should be held away from the surgical table by a sterile team member to prevent the nonsterile assistant's hand and arm from extending over the sterile area. The solution is poured without splashing, taking care to prevent it from dripping down the container onto the sterile person's hand. The solution container should not touch the sterile basin.

Reference

Association of Operating Room Nurses: Standards, recommended practices and guidelines: recommended practices for selection and use of packaging systems, Denver, 2000, The Association.

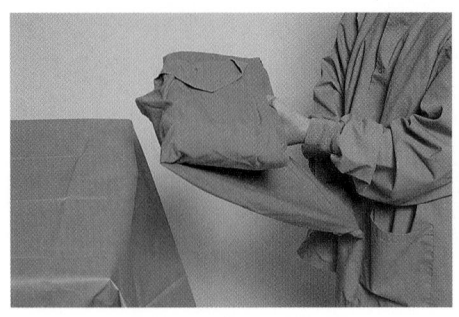 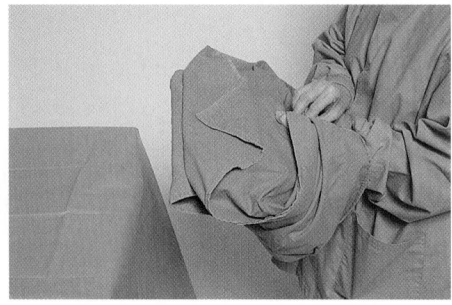 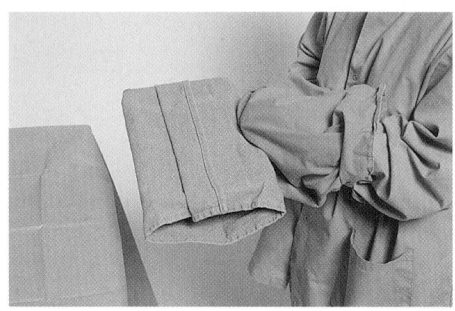

A   B   C

FIG. 1-4
A, To unwrap a sterile linen pack that can be held during distribution, hold the pack in your left hand if you are right-handed (and vice versa). **B,** Using your right hand, unfold one corner of the wrap at a time, being careful to secure each corner in the palm of your left hand to prevent them from recoiling and contaminating the contents. **C,** Hold the final corner with your right hand; your hand should be completely covered by the wrap. When the pack is fully exposed and all corners of the wrap have been secured, gently set the pack on the sterile field, being careful not to allow your hand and arm to reach across or over the sterile field.

Suggested Reading

Broder BD: *Wrap it up, I'll take it (to Surgery)!* Infection control today at www.infectioncontroltoday.com; 2006, Virgo Publishing.

Harter B: *Getting wrapped up in packaging choices,* Infection control today at www.infectioncontroltoday.com; 2006, Virgo Publishing.

CHAPTER 2
Sterilization and Disinfection

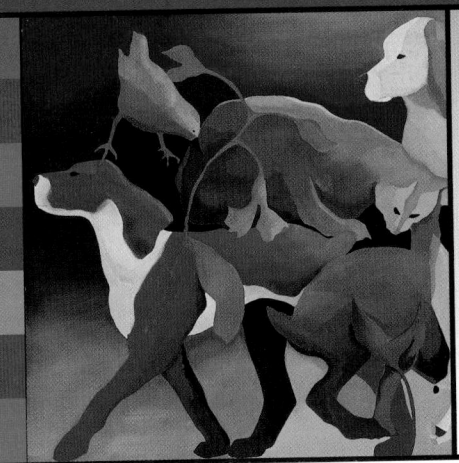

Sterilization is the destruction of all microorganisms (bacteria, viruses, and spores) on an item. It usually refers to objects (e.g., instruments, drapes, catheters, and needles) that come in contact with tissue or enter the vascular system. **Disinfection** is the destruction of most pathogenic microorganisms on inanimate (nonliving) objects, whereas **antisepsis** is the destruction of most pathogenic microorganisms on animate (living) objects. Neither procedure claims to kill or inactivate all microorganisms, even when used properly. **Antiseptics** are used to kill microorganisms during patient skin preparation and surgical scrubbing (see Chapters 6 and 7); however, the skin is not sterilized. **Cleaning** is usually restricted in meaning to the physical removal of surface contaminants, usually with detergents or soap and water, ultrasound, or other methods. Although cleaning does remove soils and bacteria, it does not kill or inactivate viruses or bacteria.

DISINFECTION

Disinfection usually involves the use of liquid compounds, such as phenol or its derivatives, alcohols, halides, aldehydes, quaternary ammonium compounds, chloroform, ethylene oxide (EtO), heavy metal ions, or dyes. Selection of the appropriate disinfectant depends on the desired result; some disinfectants are effective at destroying a limited number of microorganisms; others are effective at killing all organisms, including spores. Common disinfectants, their uses, and necessary precautions are listed in Table 2-1.

STERILIZATION

Any equipment or supplies that come in contact with body tissues or blood must be sterile. Methods of sterilizing surgical instruments or other equipment include steam, chemicals, plasma, and ionizing radiation. The reliability of any sterilization method depends on the number, type, and inherent resistance of microorganisms on the items to be sterilized and whether other materials (e.g., soil, oil) are present on the items that may shield against or inactivate the sterilizing agent. Commonly used sterilization processes have a variety of advantages and disadvantages. For example, the steam autoclave, a 200-year-old sterilization technology,

is an effective sterilization process, but its high temperature and moisture make it unusable for many of today's devices. Likewise, dry-heat sterilization has process temperatures that cannot be tolerated by most devices.

Low-temperature, low-moisture processes, such as sterilization by EtO gas or hydrogen peroxide gas plasma, must be used for many medical devices (see pp. 11 and 12). Increasingly, operating room (OR) personnel are being asked to sterilize equipment more quickly and efficiently and with lower cost. Advanced sterilization systems that enable more rapid availability of wrapped, sterile devices and instruments may result in more rapid turnover of the OR suite and less "downtime" between procedures. Swift and efficient sterilization of expensive heat-and moisture-sensitive medical and surgical devices (i.e., cameras, fiberoptic cables, and rigid endoscopes) is particularly advantageous when costs of such equipment may limit their duplication in most veterinary practices. A low-temperature hydrogen peroxide gas plasma sterilization system that provides terminal sterilization of sophisticated instruments in 55 minutes is useful for such devices.

Steam Sterilization

Saturated steam under pressure is a practical and dependable agent for sterilization of heat-tolerant medical supplies and packaging. Steam rapidly destroys all known microorganisms by means of coagulation and cellular protein denaturation. To ensure the destruction of all living microorganisms, the correct relationship between temperature, pressure, and exposure time is critical. If steam is contained in a closed compartment and the pressure is increased, the temperature also increases, provided the volume of the compartment remains the same. If items are exposed long enough to steam at a specified temperature and pressure, they become sterile. The unit used to create this high-temperature, pressurized steam is called an autoclave. Certain types of microorganisms have more inherent heat resistance than do other organisms. Spores of thermophilic aerobes and anaerobes are the most resistant forms of life to moist heat known. Virus particles are much less tolerant to steam sterilization than are spores.

TABLE 2-1

Common Disinfectants Used in Veterinary Practice

AGENT	PRACTICAL USE	DISINFECTANT PROPERTIES	ANTISEPTIC PROPERTIES	MECHANISMS OF ACTION	PRECAUTIONS
Alcohol: isopropyl alcohol (50%–70%); ethyl alcohol (70%)	Spot cleaning; injection site preparation	Good	Very good	Protein denaturation, metabolic interruption, and cell lysis	Corrosive to stainless steel; volatile
Chlorine compounds: hypochlorite	Cleaning floors and countertops	Good	Fair	Release of free chlorine and oxygen	Inactivated by organic debris; corrosive to metal
Iodine compounds: iodophors (7.5%) scrub solution	Cleaning dark-colored floors and countertops	Good	Good	Iodination and oxidation of essential molecules	Stains fabric and tissue
Glutaraldehyde: 2% alkaline solution	Disinfection of lenses and delicate instruments	Good; sterilizes	None	Protein and nucleic acid alkylation	Tissue reaction odor (rinse instruments well before using)

Sterilization failure may occur if packs are wrapped too tightly or are improperly loaded in the autoclave or gas sterilizer container. Instrument packs should be positioned vertically (i.e., on edge) and longitudinally in an autoclave. Heavy packs should be placed at the periphery, where steam enters the chamber. A small amount of air space is allowed between the packs to facilitate the flow of steam (1 to 2 inches between the packs and away from the surrounding walls). Linen packs are loaded so that the fabric layers are oriented vertically (i.e., on edge). These packs are not stacked because the increased thickness reduces penetration of the steam. Close supervision and exact standards for preparing, packaging, and loading of supplies are necessary for effective steam and gas sterilization. Sterilization indicators should be used (see p. 13).

Types of Steam Sterilizers

Gravity displacement sterilizer. The most commonly used steam sterilizer in veterinary practice is the gravity (or "downward") displacement sterilizer (Fig. 2-1). This sterilizer works on the principle that air is heavier than steam. Supplies to be sterilized are loaded into the inner chamber. A narrow, outer jacket-type chamber surrounds the inner chamber. Pressurized steam from the narrow, outer chamber enters the inner chamber and surrounds the supplies. Air in the inner chamber is pulled downward by gravity to the floor and exits through a temperature-sensitive valve. As steam accumulates and the temperature increases, the steam-release valve closes. Because the function of this sterilizer is based on the ability of air to move to the bottom of the autoclave, careful wrapping (see p. 4) and loading of supplies are critical (see previous discussion). The minimum time and temperature standards for a gravity displacement sterilizer are 10 to 25 minutes at 270° to 275° F (132° to 135° C) or 15 to 30 minutes at 250° F (121° C). Table 2-2 shows the recommended sterilization times for commonly sterilized items.

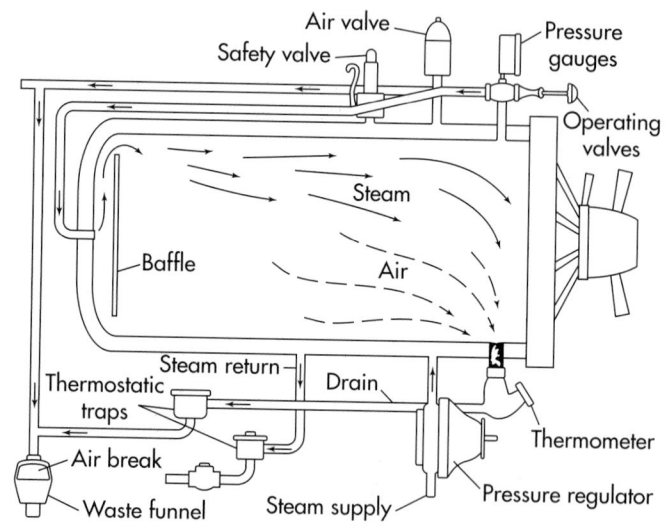

FIG. 2-1
Gravity displacement autoclave.

Prevacuum sterilizer. The prevacuum sterilizer relies on air being actively pulled out of the inner chamber, thereby creating a vacuum. Steam is injected into the chamber to replace the air. This method of sterilization provides greater steam penetration in a shorter time than the gravity displacement sterilizer. The minimum time and temperature standard for a prevacuum sterilizer is 3 to 4 minutes at 270° to 275° F (132° to 135° C).

Flash sterilizer. Emergency or "flash" sterilization is performed when an unwrapped, nonsterile item must be sterilized quickly. A gravity displacement sterilizer is used for this purpose. The item is placed unwrapped in a perforated metal tray and sterilized according to the manufacturer's time and temperature recommendations. With detachable handles, sterilized items are transported to the OR in the

TABLE 2-2

Exposure Periods for Sterilization in Gravity Displacement Sterilizers

ITEM	MINIMUM TIME REQUIRED (MIN) 250°-254° F (121°-123° C)
Scrub brushes (in dispensers, cans, individually wrapped)	30
Dressings (wrapped in muslin or paper)	30
Glassware (empty, inverted)	15
Instruments (wrapped in double thickness muslin)	30
Instruments combined with suture, tubing, porous materials (wrapped in muslin or paper)	30
Metal instruments only (unwrapped)	15
Linen—maximum size 12 × 12 × 20 inches (6 kg wrapped)	30
Needles (individually packaged in glass vials or paper, lumens moist)	30
Needles (unwrapped, lumens moist)	15
Rubber catheters, drains, tubing (wrapped in muslin or paper; lumens moist)	30
Rubber catheters, drains, tubing (unwrapped; lumens moist)	20
Utensils (wrapped in muslin or paper, on edge)	20
Utensils (unwrapped, on edge)	15
Syringes (unassembled, individually packaged in muslin or paper)	30
Syringes (unassembled, unwrapped)	15
Suture—silk, cotton, nylon (wrapped in paper or muslin)	30
Solutions: 75–250 ml	20 (slow exhaust)
500–1000 ml	30 (slow exhaust)
1500–2000 ml	40 (slow exhaust)

metal tray. It is difficult to deliver flash-sterilized devices aseptically; the tray is hot, wet, and unwrapped, which means it collects dust, debris, and microorganisms more readily than dry, cool trays with biobarrier protection. This type of sterilization should be used only in emergencies when no alternative is available. The minimum time and temperature standard for a gravity flash sterilizer is 3 minutes at 270° to 275° F (132° to 135° C) for metal or nonporous items (i.e., items without a lumen) and 10 minutes at the same temperature for metal items with lumens, porous items (e.g., rubber, plastic), and autoclavable power tools sterilized together.

Chemical (Gas) Sterilization

Ethylene oxide. EtO is a flammable, explosive, gas that kills microorganisms by altering their deoxyribonucleic acid (DNA) through alkylation. Equipment that cannot withstand the extreme temperature and pressures of steam sterilization (i.e., endoscopes, cameras, plastics, and power cables) can safely be sterilized with EtO. Flexible endoscopes typically require special preparation with EtO caps that prevent rupture of the outer plastic layer. The process is enhanced by heat and moisture, with the optimum temperature ranging from 120° to 140° F (49° to 60° C) and the optimum humidity level from 20% to 40%. The time required for sterilization depends on the concentration of EtO, humidity level, temperature, and density and type of materials to be sterilized. Most items are sterilized at 54.4° C (130° F) for approximately 2.5 hours; heat-sensitive items are sterilized at 37.8° C (100° F) for approximately 5 hours. The manufacturer's recommendations for EtO exposure time must be followed. Compact, tabletop units are available that have combinations of ventilation and purge systems (e.g., Anprolene, Anderson Products, Haw River, N.C.).

It is critical for the safety of the patient and hospital personnel that all materials sterilized with EtO be aerated appropriately. The specific aeration time necessary for surgical items depends on many variables, including the composition and size of the item, its preparation and packaging, the type of EtO sterilizer used, the type of aerator used, and the temperature penetration pattern of the aerator's chamber. The manufacturer's guidelines should be followed, but generally aeration in a well-ventilated area for a minimum of 7 days, or 12 to 18 hours in an aerator, is sufficient.

Items should be clean and dry before EtO sterilization; moisture and organic material bond with EtO and leave a toxic residue. If an item cannot be disassembled and all surfaces cleaned, it cannot be sterilized. Items are packed

TABLE 2-3

Alternatives to the Use of Ethylene Oxide*

PRODUCT (VENDOR)	APPLICATION	COMMENTS
Sterrad (Advanced Sterilization Products)	Enclosed sterilization processor with 45-minute cycle time	Generates hydrogen peroxide gas plasma from 58% hydrogen peroxide solution
Steris 20 (Steris Corp.)	Sterilization in 12 min at 50–55° C; instruments ready for use in patients in <30 min	0.2% peracetic acid (diluted from 35%)

*Modified from EPA Region 9: Replacing ethylene oxide and glutaraldehyde, *Environmental Best Practices for HealthCare Facilities,* Nov. 2002, ICAHD Environment of Care Standards.

 BOX 2-1

Routes of Exposure to Ethylene Oxide

- Inhalation of ethylene oxide gas in air
- Skin, eye, or mucous membrane contact with the liquid or with ethylene oxide absorbed in solid materials
- Oral—residual ethylene oxide in ingested material
- Intravenous—leaching of ethylene oxide from inadequately aerated medical devices inserted intravenously

and loaded loosely in the sterilizer to allow gas circulation. Complex items (e.g., power equipment) are disassembled before processing (see p. 52). Items that cannot be sterilized with EtO include acrylics, some pharmaceutical items, and solutions.

The environmental and safety hazards associated with EtO are numerous and severe. The manufacturer's guidelines for equipment use should be followed carefully to prevent injury to the patient or hospital personnel (Box 2-1 and Table 2-3). The acute (short-term) effects of EtO in humans consist mainly of central nervous system (CNS) depression and irritation of the eyes and mucous membranes. Chronic (long-term) exposure to EtO in humans can cause irritation of the eyes, skin, and mucous membranes, and problems in the functioning of the brain and nerves. Some human cancer data show an increase in the incidence of leukemia, stomach cancer, cancer of the pancreas, and Hodgkin's disease in workers exposed to EtO. However, these data are considered to be limited and inconclusive because of uncertainties in the studies. The Environmental Protection Agency (EPA) has classified EtO as a Group B1, probable human carcinogen.

Plasma Sterilization

Plasma sterilization is a low-temperature sterilization technique that has become the method of choice for sterilizing heat-sensitive items (see Table 2-3). Conventional sterilization techniques (e.g., autoclaves, ovens, chemicals like EtO) rely on irreversible metabolic inactivation or on breakdown of vital structural components of the microorganism. Plasma sterilization operates differently because it uses ultraviolet (UV) photons and radicals. An advantage of the plasma method is the possibility of sterilizing at relatively low temperatures (50° C), preserving the integrity of polymer-based instruments, which cannot be subjected to autoclaves and ovens. Furthermore, plasma sterilization is safe, both for the operator and the patient, in contrast to EtO.

Vapor phase hydrogen peroxide sterilization is a form of plasma sterilization that uses hydrogen peroxide to process instruments quickly and efficiently. Instruments can be sterilized at low temperatures (i.e., below 122° F [50° C]) and short time intervals (i.e., 45 minutes), and they are immediately available because aeration is not required. Items for sterilization must be wrapped in nonwoven polypropylene fabric or plastic (Tyvek-Mylar) pouches (see Table 1-2 on p. 3). Items that can be sterilized with this process are stainless steel, aluminum, brass, silicone, Teflon, latex, ethyl vinyl acetate, Kraton, polycarbonate, polyethylene (high density and low density), polyolefin, polyurethane, polypropylene, polyvinyl chloride (PVC), and polymethylmethacrylate. An important shortcoming of plasma sterilization is its dependence on the actual "thickness" of the microorganisms to be inactivated because UV photons need to reach the DNA. Any material covering the microorganisms (e.g., packaging) will slow down the process. Items that cannot be sterilized safely include linen, gauze sponges, wood products (including paper), endoscopes, some plastics, liquids, items that cannot be disassembled, items that cannot be completely dried, items with copper or silver solder or that use bisphenole epoxy, tubes and catheters longer than 12 inches, and tubes and catheters less than 1 to 3 mm in diameter. Special adapters (H_2O_2 boosters) are required for use with devices with lumens to ensure that the sterilant gains access to these areas.

Ionizing Radiation

Most equipment available prepackaged from the manufacturer has been sterilized by ionizing radiation (i.e., cobalt 60). This process is restricted to commercial use because of its expense. Items commonly used in the OR that are sterilized with ionizing radiation include suture material, sponges, disposable items (i.e., gowns, drapes, and table covers), powders, and petroleum goods. Resterilization by other means may not be possible for prepackaged sterilized items that have been opened but not used because an alternate technique could damage the item and create a health hazard.

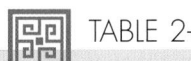 TABLE 2-4

Alternatives to the Use of Glutaraldehyde*

PRODUCT (VENDOR)	APPLICATION	COMMENTS
Cidex OPA (Advanced Sterilization Products)	High level disinfection in 12 min at 20° C	0.55% OPA solution: exposure limits not yet determined
Sporox II (Sultan Chemists)	High level disinfection in 30 min at 20° C	7.5% hydrogen peroxide
Sterilox (Sterilox Tech, Inc)	Cycle time is 10 min for high level disinfection	System generates hypochlorous acid Currently used in Europe as a chemical sterilant

*Modified from EPA Region 9: Replacing ethylene oxide and glutaraldehyde, *Environmental Best Practices for HealthCare Facilities,* Nov. 2002, ICAHD Environment of Care Standards.

Cold Chemical Sterilization

Chemicals used for sterilization must be noncorrosive to the items being sterilized. Glutaraldehyde is a saturated dialdehyde that has gained wide acceptance as a high level disinfectant and chemical sterilant. It is noncorrosive to metals, rubbers, and plastics and provides a means of sterilizing delicate lensed instruments (i.e., endoscopes, cystoscopes, and bronchoscopes). The biocidal activity of glutaraldehyde is a consequence of its alkylation of sulfhydryl, hydroxyl, carboxyl, and amino groups, which alters RNA, DNA, and protein synthesis within microorganisms. Most equipment that is safe for immersion in water is safe for immersion in 2% glutaraldehyde. Glutaraldehyde products are marketed under a variety of brand names and are available in a variety of concentrations, with and without surfactants (Table 2-4). For the high level disinfection of endoscopes, a 2% glutaraldehyde solution without surfactant is recommended.

Items for sterilization should be clean and dry; organic matter (e.g., blood, saliva) may prevent penetration of crevices or joints. Residual water causes chemical dilution. Complex instruments should be disassembled before immersion. Immersion times suggested by the manufacturer should be adhered to closely (e.g., 2% glutaraldehyde: 10 hours at 68° to 77° F [20° to 25° C] for sterilization; 10 minutes at the same temperature for disinfection). After the appropriate immersion period, instruments should be rinsed thoroughly with sterile water and dried with sterile towels to prevent damaging the patients' tissues. The major problem associated with glutaraldehyde is that it is a known respiratory and dermal irritant and sensitizer, and adverse health effects may occur in exposed workers. Failure to rinse disinfected equipment thoroughly, leaving residual glutaraldehyde on the endoscope, has led to serious conditions, including chemical colitis, pancreatitis, and mucosal damage in human patients. Ortho-phthalaldehyde (OPA) is a new alkylating agent that contains 0.55% 1,2-benzenedicarboxaldehyde. It has shown superior mycobactericidal activity compared with glutaraldehyde with less contact time required. There are limited "in use" data available regarding this product.

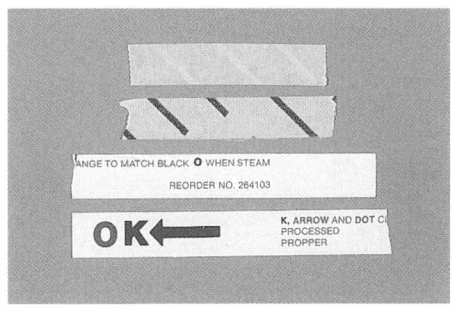

FIG. 2-2
Tape and indicator strips for steam sterilization. The diagonal stripes on the tape *(top)* turn from tan to black. The "K" arrow and dot on the indicator strips *(bottom)* turn from white to black to match "O."

STERILIZATION INDICATORS

Simply placing an item in a sterilizer and initiating the process does not ensure sterility. Failure to achieve sterility may be the result of improper cleaning (if an item cannot be disassembled and all surfaces cleaned, it cannot be sterilized), mechanical failure of the system used, improper use of equipment, improper wrapping, poor loading technique, or failure to understand the concepts of sterilization processes.

Sterilization indicators allow monitoring of the effectiveness of sterilization. Indicators undergo either a chemical or biologic change in response to some combination of time and temperature. Chemical indicators, which are available for steam, gas, and plasma sterilization, generally are paper strips or tape impregnated with a material that changes color when a certain temperature is reached (Figs. 2-2 to 2-4). The chemical responds to conditions such as extreme heat, pressure, or humidity, but does not reflect the duration of exposure, which is critical to the sterilization process. Therefore it is important to remember that chemical indicators do not indicate sterility—only that certain conditions for sterility have been met. The indicators are placed in the center of each pack and on the outside of the item to be sterilized.

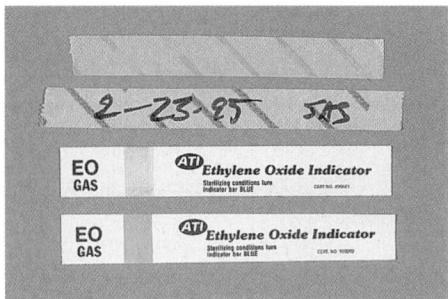

FIG. 2-3
Tape and indicator strips for EtO sterilization (before→after).
Tape: yellow→red. Strips: yellow→blue.

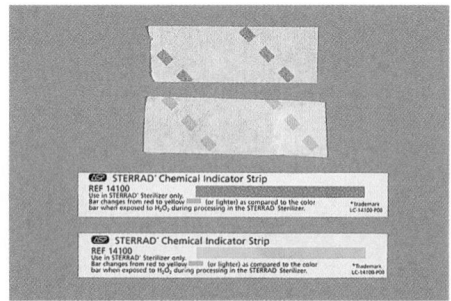

FIG. 2-4
Tape and indicator strips for plasma sterilization (before→
after). Tape: red→yellow. Strips: red→yellow.

Some autoclaves have a temperature-time graph on the control panel. This indicator method is reliable for measuring the temperature reached and the length of time that each load is exposed to that temperature. A written record can be kept of each processed load.

Use of a biologic indicator is the surest way to determine sterility. A strain of highly resistant, nonpathogenic, spore-forming bacteria (*Bacillus stearothermophilus* for steam, *Bacillus subtilis* for gas), which is contained in a glass vial or a strip of paper, is placed in the load of goods to be sterilized. After the sterilization cycle is complete, the vial or strip is recovered and cultured; growth of the organism documents inadequate sterilization. Biologic indicators should be used at least weekly to test the effectiveness of the sterilization process.

Sterilization indicators should not be relied on heavily because of the problems mentioned above. There is no substitute for close supervision of personnel, a general understanding of sterilization processes, and maintaining high standards for preparing, packing, and loading supplies.

Suggested Reading

McDonnell G, Russell AD: Antiseptics and disinfectants: activity, action, and resistance, *Clin Microbiol Rev* 12:147, 1999.
This is a comprehensive review of the common antiseptics and disinfectants used in hospital settings. Known mechanisms of microbial resistance are reviewed, with emphasis on the clinical implications of these reports.

Moisan M, Barbeau J, Crevier MC et al: Plasma sterilization: methods and mechanisms, *Pure Appl Chem* 74:349, 2002.
This article reviews the mechanisms of plasma sterilization as an alternative to conventional sterilization techniques.

Ulualp K, Hamzaoglu I, Ulgen SK et al: Is it possible to resterilize disposable laparoscopy trocars in a hospital setting, *Surg Lap Endo Percutaneous Tech* 10:2, 2000.
This article investigated the safety of hospital disinfection of disposable laparoscopic instruments of complex structure with 2% glutaraldehyde and EtO. The authors determined that disinfection was not effective and might result in nosocomial disease transmission by bacteria, fungi, and viruses.

CHAPTER 3

Surgical Facilities, Equipment, and Personnel

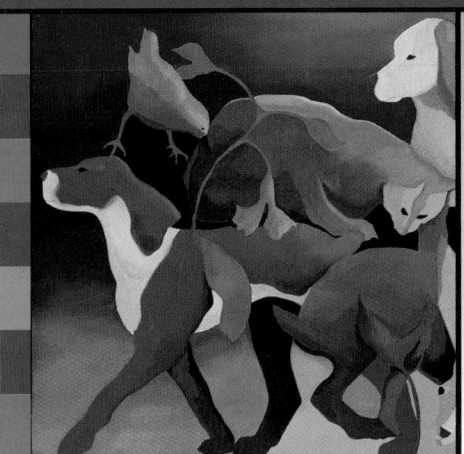

A variety of physical layouts are suitable for modern operating rooms (ORs) and surgical areas, but the goals of all designs are patient safety and work efficiency. The surgical area should be close to the anesthesia and surgical preparation area, critical care, radiology, and central supply. However, it should be isolated from general traffic flow (i.e., examination rooms, offices, reception area, and wards). In large facilities, such as universities and surgical referral centers, the anesthesia and surgical preparation area should be a separate working unit that is isolated from general hospital traffic.

STRUCTURE AND DESIGN OF THE SURGICAL AREA

Because of the constant danger of contamination to surgical patients, the surgical area is clearly delineated into "clean," "mixed," and "contaminated" areas. Clean areas include the ORs, scrub sink areas, and sterile supply rooms. Mixed areas include the hallways between the ORs and nurses' stations, instrument and supply processing areas, storage areas, and utility rooms. Contaminated areas include anesthesia and surgical preparation rooms, dressing rooms, lounges, and offices.

A commonly used floor plan is one in which the surgical suites are arranged around a central work station for OR nurses. Easy access to each OR from the work station ensures efficient traffic flow, which reduces cross contamination between areas. Clean areas should be restricted to clean traffic, and contaminated areas to contaminated traffic. Individuals entering a clean area from a contaminated area must don proper surgical attire (see Chapter 7); the ideal location for moving from a contaminated area to a clean one (or vice versa) is through a locker room. Surgical personnel who leave a clean area and enter a contaminated area must cover their clothing before they leave and discard these items when they return to the clean area. Doors between clean and contaminated areas should be kept closed at all times. Food and drink are permitted only in contaminated areas. Movement of clean and sterile supplies and equipment should be separated as much as possible from movement of contaminated supplies and equipment by space, time, and traffic patterns.

Soiled linen and trash should be kept in a contaminated area, and patients should be clipped and vacuumed in a contaminated area before transport to a clean area (e.g., the operating room).

> NOTE: To prevent contaminating the surgical suite, clip the patient and perform the initial surgical preparation in a separate area.

DESCRIPTION AND FUNCTION OF ROOMS IN THE SURGICAL AREA

Dressing Room

The dressing room is used by surgical personnel for changing into proper surgical attire. It should have closed cabinets for storing scrub suits, shoe covers, masks, and caps and a separate area for hanging street clothes. A hamper for dirty laundry should be available to minimize the carrying of contaminated linen through the hospital.

Anesthesia and Surgical Preparation Room

The anesthesia induction and surgical preparation room should be adjacent to the surgical area yet out of major hospital traffic patterns. This room should be supplied with equipment and medications that may be necessary in an emergency (i.e., defibrillator, endotracheal tubes, suction, oxygen, and crash cart). It also should have anesthetic equipment (machines and drugs), laryngoscopes, clippers (mounted on the wall or hanging from the ceiling), vacuums (large canister or central), skin preparation materials (antiseptic soaps, alcohol, sterile gauze sponges), sharps containers, needles and syringes, and monitoring equipment, all of which should be readily available to ensure efficient anesthesia and preoperative patient preparation.

> NOTE: Drugs and equipment necessary for an emergency can be stored in a mobile crash cart; this facilitates movement from the anesthesia preparation room to the OR and to recovery.

Preparation counters and surfaces should be impervious and easily cleaned and disinfected. Stainless steel preparation tables with built-in sinks are ideal. Gas scavenger systems should be present at each anesthesia preparation table. General lighting is supplied by main overhead fluorescent lights, which are supplemented by a spotlight directed at each preparation table. A sink designated for cleaning anesthetic hoses, endotracheal tubes, and rebreathing bags, plus a plastic rack for draining and drying rebreathing bags and hoses, should be available. An erasable anesthesia-surgery scheduling board, easily visible to anesthesia and surgical personnel, should list the day's procedures.

Temperature in the preparation room should be kept between 62° and 68° F (17° and 20° C) and humidity at 50% or less to reduce microbial growth. Gurney surfaces should be padded, and circulating water and/or warm air blankets should be used to prevent hypothermia. Well-constructed gurneys should be available for patient transportation. They should be made of stainless steel or other easily cleaned materials, have relatively large wheels with bearings that can be easily lubricated, and have rubber bumpers mounted on the corners to prevent damage to doors and walls. An adhesive microfilm dust pad should be placed at the doorway between the anesthesia preparation room and the surgical area to collect dust, hair, and other particulates on gurney rollers, shoes, and anesthetic equipment.

Anesthesia Supply Room

The anesthesia supply room should be adjacent to the anesthesia and surgical preparation room. Equipment necessary to keep anesthesia machines working properly, extra endotracheal tubes, anesthetic monitoring equipment, oxygen "E" tanks, hoses, catheters, and airway connectors are stored here. This room may also have a cabinet for storing nongaseous anesthetic agents, and it may be a convenient location for storing large oxygen tanks that supply oxygen to each anesthesia preparation table and to the OR.

Nurses' Work Station

The nurses' work station should be centrally located in the surgical area (i.e., the clean area). An autoclave (for flash sterilization), an incubator and/or blanket warmer (for irrigation fluids and for towels to wrap patients after surgery), a refrigerator (for medications and solutions), and formalin containers are kept in this area. A daily surgery log, operating room protocols, and a telephone also are kept at the work station. Soiled instruments may be sent to a central supply area, or may be decontaminated, washed, lubricated, and wrapped or packaged for resterilization here. This area should be divided into two separate areas to prevent cross contamination of clean supplies if it is used for decontaminating and wrapping instruments.

Sterile Instrument Room

The sterile instrument room is a clean area that houses all sterilized and packaged instruments and supplies. It commonly is near the nurses' work station. Surgery personnel

assemble items necessary for a particular case from supplies in this room. Items should be logically arranged on shelves (e.g., alphabetical order) and routinely checked for "outdates" (i.e., time-related expiration; see p. 5) and package integrity (i.e., event-related expiration; see p. 5).

Equipment Room

Large pieces of equipment, such as anesthesia machines, lasers, monitoring equipment, operating microscopes, and portable surgery lights, can be stored in an equipment room. Equipment should be kept free of dust and cleaned routinely using the protocol described for OR disinfection (see p. 19). The equipment room is a valuable area because it eliminates storage of large, expensive pieces of equipment in hallways, where they could be damaged or create a hazard.

Housekeeping Supply Room

Supplies used to decontaminate and clean surgical suites may be stored in the supply room or closet. Cleaning equipment and supplies stored here must be restricted to use in the OR to prevent cross contamination from other hospital areas.

Scrub Sink Area

Scrub sink areas should be centrally located for the OR suites. Antiseptic soap in an appropriate dispenser (i.e., foot activated), scrub brushes (i.e., sterilized reusable brushes or a disposable polyurethane brush-sponge combination, unless brushless scrub solutions are used [see Chapter 7]), and fingernail cleaners should be kept within easy reach at each scrubbing station. Deep stainless steel sinks equipped with knee-, elbow-, or foot-operated water activators are ideal. With reusable brushes, the dispensing container and clean brushes must be detached and autoclaved regularly. The scrub sink area must be located away from wrapped sterile supplies because of possible contamination by water droplets and spray from the sinks. Scrub sinks should never be used to clean equipment or instruments or to dispose of body fluids.

Gowning and Gloving Area

Gowning and gloving can be done outside or inside the operating room. Controversy exists over which location results in the least cross contamination, but no evidence supports one location over another.

> NOTE: If the operating room is small or if several people are scrubbing in, gowning and gloving in a separate area may help prevent contamination of personnel, sterile supplies, or the prepped surgical site.

Operating Room

ORs are individual rooms where surgeries are performed. The room should be large enough to allow personnel to move around sterile equipment without contaminating it and to accommodate the large pieces of equipment necessary for some procedures. Some suppliers that offer both lights and tables (e.g., Skytron, Grand Rapids, Mich.; Berchtold Corp., Charleston, S.C.) are now supplying voice and touch screen activation, video monitors, cameras, power booms, and more for an integrated OR that is efficient and multifunctional. Integrated OR suites can be custom-configured to be minimal or extravagant and may be built from scratch or retrofitted.

The OR should be uncluttered and simple so that no areas trap dust or are difficult to clean. Floors, ceiling, walls, and other surfaces should be smooth, nonporous, and constructed of fireproof materials. Smooth surfaces can be thoroughly cleaned and disinfected, and prevent trapping of biologic material that could cross contaminate. Surface materials should be able to withstand frequent washing and cleaning with strong disinfectants.

Ventilation systems for surgical suites should be designed to provide positive air pressures in the OR and lower air pressures in adjoining corridors. Ideal ventilation systems deliver a minimum of 15 to 20 air exchanges per hour. Positive pressures inside the OR reduce likelihood of contaminated air from adjacent corridors mixing with OR air. Scavenging systems that pull anesthetic gases out of the OR air should be installed in each OR. The OR environment should be kept at a constant humidity and temperature. Humidity is controlled to minimize static electricity and microbial growth; the ideal level is 50% or lower. Air temperature is maintained at 62° to 68° F (17° to 20° C).

General lighting in the OR is supplied by main overhead fluorescent lights, which are supplemented by one, or preferably two, halogen spotlights. Surgery lights are designed to emit a soft white light that is high intensity, low heat, and true color, and that has shadow reduction without glare. Options include single, double, and triple light-head configurations in wall, ceiling, and stand mounts. Surgical lights are generally ceiling mounted. Track lighting should be avoided because dust and bacteria may become trapped in the tracks. Rotation capabilities are important; most lights rotate 360 degrees at the light-head axis, but some are even more flexible. Many lights can incorporate cameras in them. Fiberoptic headlamps worn by many surgeons are now available in comfortable, lightweight models that virtually eliminate shadowing of the surgical site (Fig. 3-1).

Stainless steel operating tables should be fully adjustable for height (hydraulic mechanism) and degree of tilt. Tabletops should be either a flat, one-piece surface or have V-trough capabilities. Table options vary not only in the types of procedures that can be performed on them, but also in imaging capabilities, mobility, and availability of accessory options. Tables that provide full-function tilt, Trendelenburg's, reverse Trendelenburg's, and other positioning capabilities are particularly useful. Tables with removable leg sections are convenient for orthopedic procedures. Specialized tables are available for intraoperative imaging where 100% of the tabletop is radiolucent.

Portable V-troughs and insulating table pads should be available. Patient body temperature must be maintained

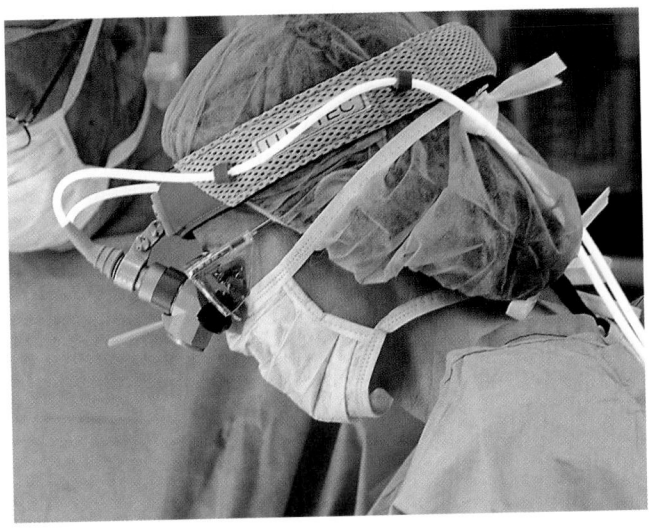

FIG. 3-1
Fiberoptic headlamp.

during surgery, especially if the animal weighs less than 10 kg or if the surgical procedure will last longer than 2 hours. Body temperature usually is maintained by using a warm-air circulating device (e.g., Bair Hugger, Arizant Healthcare, Inc., Prairie, Minn.). Special tabletop attachments that allow the anesthesiologist to see the patient's head should be provided so that the patient can be monitored without contaminating the surgical field.

An instrument table (i.e., Mayo stand) or back table should be available. The table should be large enough to accommodate all instrumentation required for the surgical procedure. Instrument tables should be made of stainless steel and should be adjustable in height. A kick bucket is used by surgical team members to discard soiled sponges during surgery. The bucket frame should have wheels so that it can be moved easily (i.e., kicked) about the operating room. Plastic bag liners for kick bucket containers facilitate clean-up.

Suction (portable or piped in) should be available in each OR. Suction units with disposable containers are reliable, easily cleaned, and cost-efficient. Suction hoses should not be reused unless they are sterilized because they are a common source of surgical wound contamination. Other accessory equipment, such as physiologic monitors, the anesthesia supply cart, intravenous stands, and sitting stools, should be available. Each OR should be provided with a radiographic view box, preferably flush mounted to facilitate cleaning. Portable imaging devices are optimal for evaluating placement of orthopedic implants. The OR should have a wall clock for determining elapsed time, particularly when vascular occlusion is necessary.

Supply cabinets with tight-fitting doors (to minimize dust accumulation) should be located in each OR for storing suture material, dressings, sponges, scalpel blades, and frequently used instruments. Doors to the OR should be kept closed to reduce the mixing of OR air with corridor air.

Postoperative Recovery Area

The postoperative recovery area should be adjacent to the surgical area, yet separate from other hospitalized patients. Patients should be placed in individual, heated cages and carefully monitored until recovery is complete. Patients that require intensive care should be taken directly to the critical care facility. Temperature in the recovery room should be warmer than in the OR (i.e., 70° to 77° F [21° to 25° C]). Warming cabinets with a supply of warm fluids and blankets should be available. Analgesic medications and any equipment or medications that may be necessary in an emergency (i.e., defibrillator, laryngoscopes, endotracheal tubes, suction, oxygen, and the crash cart) should be available.

Minor Procedures Surgery Room

A separate room adjacent to the anesthesia preparation area should be designated for minor contaminated surgical procedures (i.e., lacerations, biopsies, wound management, dental procedures, and endoscopy). The room should be equipped with an operating table, spotlight, gas and suction lines for anesthesia equipment, suture material, antiseptic preparation materials, and instrument packs for minor surgery. Because of the nature of surgical procedures performed in this room, it should be properly cleaned and disinfected after each surgical procedure and at the end of each surgery day (see Chapter 4).

PERSONNEL

Responsibilities and functions of every member of the surgical team should be clearly defined in writing. This is done to clarify the job description and establish the accountability of each employee. These policies must be carefully followed and strictly enforced to ensure safe and efficient operation of the surgical area. All staff members should be evaluated periodically. Provision should be made for training programs, educational self-improvement, and information dissemination, and current books, periodicals, and audiovisual tapes of new procedures and techniques should be available.

The surgeon's role is to guide the flow and scope of what happens in the OR during surgery. Surgical assistance often is provided by a veterinary technician. Surgical assistants carry out functions that assist the surgeon in performing a safe operation, including developing a working knowledge of the procedure being performed, providing retraction and hemostasis, and manipulating instrumentation and tissues into proper position to complete the surgical task. A knowledgeable surgical assistant is invaluable.

An anesthesiologist is responsible for meticulous monitoring and adjustment of the patient's physiologic status during surgery. Anesthesiologists are trained to render immediate care in a physiologic crisis. Occasionally the surgeon and anesthesiologist must work together to carefully time surgical maneuvers, as in cardiothoracic surgery. A properly trained anesthesiologist allows the surgeon to concentrate on the surgical procedure.

Operating Room Supervisor and Surgical Technician

In large facilities, the OR supervisor oversees technicians working in the surgical area. It is this individual's responsibility to organize work schedules, train new staff, set policies for the surgical area, implement and enforce policies, and develop educational programs and seminars. The OR supervisor also participates in the day-to-day technical aspects of running a surgical area (i.e., circulates, opens surgical packs, and retrieves special instruments).

In a small facility (i.e., one that has only one OR), the OR supervisor assumes all the tasks of the surgical technician mentioned above. The supervisor may also have other technical tasks to perform as a veterinary technician, such as administering anesthetic, providing restraint, and serving as receptionist. The qualifications of a well-educated technician include graduation from an approved veterinary technician program and 1 to 2 years of basic training in a veterinary practice or veterinary teaching hospital.

Suggested Reading

Loonam JE, Millis DL: Choosing surgical lighting, *Compend Cont Educ Pract Vet* 25:537, 2003.

CHAPTER 4

Care and Maintenance of the Surgical Environment

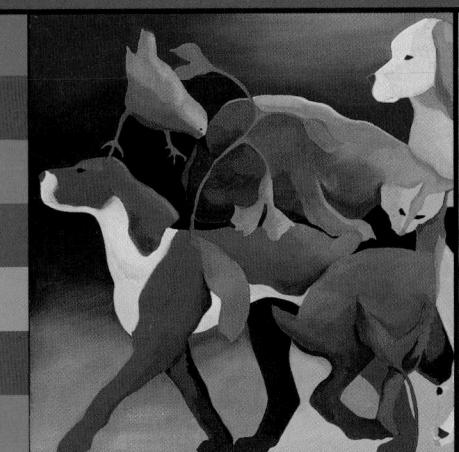

Surgery puts patients at risk for nosocomial (hospital acquired) infections unless strict environmental, equipment care, and maintenance standards are established and followed. Because most surgical infections develop from bacteria entering the incision site during surgery, proper preparation of the surgical environment is crucial to reducing the likelihood of infection.

The operating room (OR) is considered a clean area (see Chapter 3), and appropriate attire must be worn by all personnel entering or leaving it (see Chapter 7). To keep the surgical environment as free of microorganisms as possible, routine cleaning and disinfection should be performed. The term **cleaning** refers to removal of soil (i.e., blood, serum, urine, or pus); the term **disinfection** refers to treatment of surfaces, materials, and equipment with chemicals to reduce bacterial numbers. Cleaning and disinfection usually are performed simultaneously, except when a large amount of organic material or other body fluids are present.

DAILY CLEANING ROUTINES
Operating Room

At the beginning of each surgery day, all horizontal surfaces, lights, OR equipment, and furniture should be damp dusted with a lint-free cloth and hospital-grade disinfectant (Box 4-1). After each surgical procedure, areas contaminated by organic debris (e.g., floors, doors, counters, equipment, and operating table) should be cleaned and disinfected. If biohazards (i.e., infectious diseases or chemotherapeutic agents) were encountered during surgery, special precautions should be taken during cleaning and disinfection (i.e., specific disinfectant, cleaning time, and disinfectant contact time).

At the close of each day, operating tables, counters, lights, equipment, floors, windows, cabinets, and doors should be cleaned and disinfected in preparation for the next day's activities. Linen and waste bags should be collected, the linen laundered, and waste disposed of properly. Kick buckets should be disinfected and lined with new plastic bags. Surgical lights and monitoring and anesthetic equipment are cleaned and disinfected according to manufacturers' specifications. Wheels and coasters of all movable equipment and

 BOX 4-1

Daily Care and Maintenance of the Operating Room

At the Beginning of Each Day
- Wipe flat surfaces of furnishings and lights with a cloth dampened with a disinfectant solution.

After Each Surgical Procedure
- Collect used instruments and place them in a cool water and detergent or enzymatic solution.
- Collect waste materials and soiled linens and place them in the proper containers.
- Wipe instrument and surgical tables, stands, kick buckets, and heating pads with a disinfectant.
- If necessary, clean the floor (move the surgical table and clean under it if body fluids have collected there).

After the Last Surgical Procedure of the Day
- Clean and disinfect kick buckets.
- Check ceilings, walls, cabinet doors, counter surfaces, and all furniture and clean as necessary.
- Clean and care for individual items (i.e., monitoring devices, anesthesia equipment, surgical lights) according to the manufacturer's instructions.
- Wipe counter surfaces and cabinet doors with a disinfectant solution.
- Wipe instrument and surgical tables, stands, heating pads, and light fixtures with a disinfectant solution. Disassemble the surgical table if necessary to clean it thoroughly.
- Check supplies and restock as necessary.
- Roll wheeled equipment (e.g., surgical table, monitoring devices) through a small amount of disinfectant solution placed on the floor.
- Wet vacuum or damp mop the floor.

gurneys are cleaned and disinfected. The OR should be restocked with commonly used instruments, suture material, gauze sponges, needles, and syringes, and the floor wet vacuumed or damp mopped. Wet vacuuming is preferred because mops are a major source of infection. If mops are used, mop heads should be laundered and dried daily. They should be rinsed between uses and soaked in disinfectant.

BOX 4-2

Daily Care and Maintenance of the Scrub Room and Sinks

Between Scrubbing Sessions
- Dispose of wrappings from packs.
- Dispose of debris in sinks.

After the Last Surgical Procedure of the Day
- Remove waste and clean waste receptacles with a disinfectant. Line waste receptacles with a plastic bag.
- Check supplies and restock.
- Clean and refill soap dispensers.
- Wipe counter surfaces, cabinet doors, walls adjacent to sink, and switch plates.
- Scrub and disinfect sinks.
- Wet vacuum or damp mop the floor.

 BOX 4-3

Daily Care and Maintenance of the Patient Preparation Area

Between Patient Preparations
- Discard waste material (e.g., feces).
- Properly dispose of urine and clean the sink.
- Remove hair from clipper blades and lubricate according to manufacturer's instructions.
- Check walls, counters, and cabinet doors and clean with a disinfectant if necessary.
- Vacuum and clean the floor as necessary to remove hair clippings.

At the End of the Day
- Remove waste and clean waste receptacles with a disinfectant. Line waste receptacles with a plastic bag.
- Wipe light fixtures and supply lines with a disinfectant.
- Clean clippers according to manufacturers' instructions.
- Vacuum the floor to remove hair clippings. Change the filter in the vacuum. Wipe the outside of the vacuum, the hose, and the nozzle with a disinfectant.
- Check the walls and ceiling and clean as necessary.
- Check supplies and restock.
- Wipe counter surfaces, cabinet doors, walls adjacent to sink, and switch plates with a disinfectant.
- Scrub and disinfect sinks.
- Wet vacuum or damp mop the floor.

Scrub Sinks

Scrub sink areas need special attention during the day because water (a vehicle for bacterial contamination) frequently is splashed on floors and walls, and blood and other organic debris can be tracked from the scrub sink area to the surgical suite (Box 4-2). This area should be cleaned as needed throughout the day (i.e., floors mopped, used scrub brushes and fingernail cleaners removed, soap dispensers cleaned, and sinks and walls washed), and it should be disinfected at the end of the day.

Anesthesia and Surgical Preparation Room

Sinks, vacuum canisters, trash buckets, gurneys, and anesthesia preparation tables should be kept clean of organic debris and disinfected as necessary throughout the day (Box 4-3). Hair removed during patient preparation should be vacuumed from surgical tables and floors. Blood, urine, feces, tissue, serum, and purulent material should be contained and discarded. Needles and other sharp instruments should be disposed of in appropriate containers. Discarded biohazard materials should be disposed of in color-coded bags or should be clearly marked as a biohazard.

Plumbing fixtures, floors, cabinets, anesthetic equipment, utility rooms, furniture, and other equipment should be cleaned and disinfected daily. At the end of the day, the sink in the preparation area should be disinfected and a cup of disinfectant solution poured down the drain. The inner surface of garbage containers should be disinfected. Bags and filters of portable vacuums should be removed and replaced as necessary; the outside surfaces of the vacuum (including the hose and nozzle) should be wiped clean and disinfected. Clippers should be cleaned according to manufacturers' instructions. Floors should be wet vacuumed or damp mopped and supplies restocked. If a mop is used, the mop bucket should be emptied and cleaned, and all cleaning equipment and supplies should be returned to a designated storage closet.

Recovery Room

Cages, sinks, trash buckets, and gurneys should be cleaned of organic debris and disinfected as needed throughout the day. Plumbing fixtures, floors, cabinets, anesthetic equipment, utility rooms, furniture, and other equipment should be cleaned and disinfected daily as described in the previous section.

After a surgical patient has vacated a recovery room cage, it must be carefully disinfected before being used by the next patient. Before the cage is disinfected, padding, paper, and organic matter should be removed. Disinfectant should be sprayed on all surfaces of the cage, including the door. Dry organic matter should be scrubbed with a brush until it is released. Lastly, the area in front of the cage should be cleaned and disinfected. Linen (i.e., pads, blankets, and heating blanket covers) should be laundered before reuse. Plastic circulating water heating blankets should be cleaned and disinfected. This protocol helps maintain a consistently low level of microbes in the surgical recovery area, which reduces the incidence of nosocomial infections. However, some infectious diseases (e.g., parvovirus) require special precautions.

WEEKLY AND MONTHLY CLEANING ROUTINES

Surgical suites should be emptied of movable equipment and thoroughly cleaned once a week. Shelves of supply cabinets, walls, windows, windowsills, ceilings, light fixtures, surgical tables, utility and supply carts (and castors), utility rooms, equipment storage areas, and infrequently used equipment also should be cleaned and disinfected. OR floors should be wet vacuumed at least weekly, and the grills of ventilation ducts vacuumed. Walls, floors, and ceilings should be mopped once a month, and wheels and other movable parts of equipment and gurneys should be lubricated.

Suggested Reading

Neil JA, Nye PF, Toven LA: Environmental surveillance in the operating room, *AORN J* 82:43, 2005.

Recommended practices for high-level disinfection, *AORN J* 81:402, 2005.

CHAPTER 5

Preoperative and Intraoperative Care of the Surgical Patient

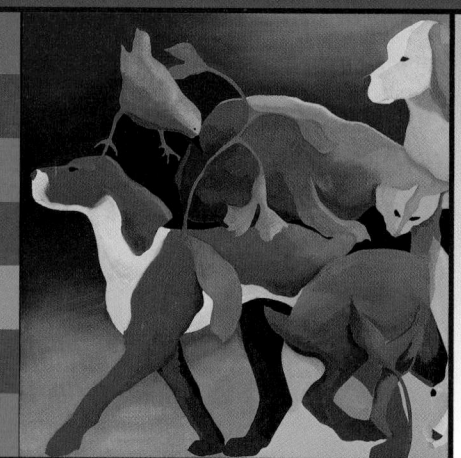

The selection and preparation of surgical patients require attention to a number of details. The patient should always receive a complete physical examination, followed by the appropriate laboratory work-up. A thorough history helps determine the extent of the physical and laboratory examinations. Obtaining preoperative information also allows comparison of the animal's status before and after surgery (e.g., ability to micturate before and after spinal surgery). General assessment and stabilization of the surgical patient are discussed here; preoperative considerations for specific diseases are provided throughout the text.

HISTORY TAKING

A thorough history from the owner or caregiver aids in evaluation of the underlying disease process and identification of other abnormalities that might affect the outcome of surgery. Although in emergencies an abbreviated history often is necessary, a thorough history eventually should be obtained. The history should include the signalment, diet, exercise, environment, past medical problems, recent treatment (especially antiinflammatory, antimicrobial, and potentially nephrotoxic or hepatotoxic therapy), and evidence of infection. Before embarking upon a detailed chronology of endless detail, the presenting complaint should initially be described from the standpoint of (1) When did the current problem start? (2) What did the problem look like when it first began? and (3) Has the problem gotten better, worse, or stayed the same (and a brief explanation of how)? After this information has been obtained, then one has a framework in which the details will hopefully make sense.

Questions should be framed so as to avoid vague responses and to obtain specific information. For example, "When was your dog last vaccinated?" is a better question than "Is your dog current on his vaccinations?" Vomiting, diarrhea, altered appetite, exposure to toxins or foreign bodies, coughing, exercise intolerance, and other abnormalities should be noted. Animals with a history of seizures must be identified so that drugs that precipitate seizures (e.g., acepromazine) can be avoided.

PHYSICAL EXAMINATION

The animal should be systematically evaluated during the physical examination, and all body systems should be included. The animal's general condition (body condition, attitude, and mental status) should be noted. Traumatized animals should have a neurologic examination (see Chapter 36) and an orthopedic examination (see Chapter 31) in addition to evaluation of the respiratory, gastrointestinal, cardiovascular, and urinary systems. Emergencies may allow only a cursory examination until the animal has been stabilized. Evaluation of the preanesthetic physical status (Table 5-1) is one of the best determinants of the likelihood of cardiopulmonary emergencies during or after surgery; the more deteriorated the physical status, the higher the risk of anesthetic and surgical complications.

LABORATORY DATA

The animal's physical status and the procedure to be performed dictate the extensiveness of the laboratory work-up. Determination of the hematocrit, total protein (TP), blood urea nitrogen (BUN) or preferably a serum creatinine, and urine specific gravity may suffice for young, healthy animals undergoing elective procedures (e.g., ovariohysterectomy and declawing) and in healthy animals with localized disease (e.g., patellar luxation). If the animal is older than 5 to 7 years, even with a physical status of I or II (see Table 5-1), or has systemic signs (e.g., dyspnea, heart murmur, anemia, ruptured bladder, gastric dilation-volvulus, shock, and hemorrhage), and if the anticipated surgery time is longer than 1 to 2 hours, a complete blood count (CBC), serum biochemistry profile, and urinalysis should be done.

The necessity for additional laboratory data is dictated by the animal's presenting signs and underlying disease (Table 5-2). Identification of associated or underlying disease influences preoperative management, the surgical procedure performed, the prognosis, and postoperative care. Animals with neoplasia should be evaluated for metastasis (e.g., with thoracic radiographs, abdominal ultrasound, and/or lymph node aspiration). Those with cardiac disease should have thoracic radio-

TABLE 5-1

Rating of Physical Status in Surgical Patients

PHYSICAL STATUS	ANIMAL'S CONDITION	EXAMPLES
I	Healthy with no discernible disease	Patient came for elective procedure (e.g., ovariohysterectomy, declaw, and castration)
II	Healthy with localized disease or mild systemic disease	Patellar luxation, skin tumor, cleft palate without aspiration pneumonia
III	Severe systemic disease	Pneumonia, fever, dehydration, heart murmur, anemia
IV	Severe systemic disease that is life threatening	Heart failure, renal failure, hepatic failure, severe hypovolemia, severe hemorrhage
V	Moribund; patient not expected to live longer than 24 hours with or without surgery	Endotoxic shock, multiorgan failure, severe trauma

 TABLE 5-2

Brief Considerations for Selected Clinical Pathologic Findings

LABORATORY ABNORMALITY	COMMENTS	MAJOR DIFFERENTIAL DIAGNOSES
High blood urea nitrogen (BUN)	Obtain urine specific gravity before initiating fluid therapy; measure serum creatinine concentration	Prerenal azotemia, primary renal disease, postrenal azotemia
Low BUN		Hepatic insufficiency (e.g., portosystemic shunt, cirrhosis), severe polyuria-polydipsia, low-protein diet
High alanine aminotransferase (ALT)	ALT may be normal in some animals with severe hepatic disease	Hepatic disease: the magnitude of the increase in ALT is neither diagnostic for any particular disease nor prognostic; severe muscle disease can cause minor increases in ALT
Low albumin	Substantial inconsistencies between laboratories, methodology used to measure albumin in people can severely underestimate canine albumin concentration	Hepatic disease, loss from kidneys or gastrointestinal tract, severe exudative cutaneous lesion (e.g., burn); lack of nutrition is not the sole cause for a serum albumin <2.0 g/dl
High serum alkaline phosphatase (SAP)	Commonly elevated in young growing animals or caused by steroids or anticonvulsants; falsely elevated with severe lipemia or severe bilirubinemia (>8 g/dl).	Hepatic disease, steroid therapy, extrahepatic biliary obstruction, some neoplasms; many dogs with increased SAP as the only biochemical abnormality do not have clinically significant disease
High bilirubin	Exposure to fluorescent light may degrade bilirubin	Hepatocellular disease, extrahepatic biliary obstruction, intrahepatic cholestasis, hemolytic anemia, severe sepsis
High calcium	It is probably best to measure ionized serum calcium because serum albumin concentrations can have a substantial effect on total serum calcium concentrations, masking hypercalcemia	Paraneoplastic syndrome (lymphosarcoma, anal sac adenocarcinoma), primary hyperparathyroidism, calciferol-containing rodenticides, hypervitaminosis D, hypoadrenocorticism, granulomatous disease, chronic renal failure
Low calcium	Artificially low in animals with low albumin	Renal disease (especially acute), pregnancy (eclampsia), hypovitaminosis D, hypoparathyroidism
High phosphorus	Normal in young, growing dogs	Renal failure (acute and more severe chronic)
Low phosphorus		Refeeding syndrome, excessive insulin—especially in ketoacidotic cats (can cause hemolysis)
High creatinine	Emaciated animals have a falsely reduced serum creatinine	Renal disease, uroabdomen, muscle trauma (very minor elevations)

Continued

TABLE 5-2

Brief Considerations for Selected Clinical Pathologic Findings—cont'd

LABORATORY ABNORMALITY	COMMENTS	MAJOR DIFFERENTIAL DIAGNOSES
High glucose	Stress may increase glucose to 200–400 mg/dl in cats	Diabetes mellitus
Low glucose	Delayed separation of red blood cells (RBCs) falsely lowers glucose	Hepatic disease, insulinoma, hypoadrenocorticism, extrahepatic neoplasms, septicemia or toxemia, starvation of neonates
High sodium	Primarily caused by loss of free water	Vomiting, diarrhea, renal failure, diabetes insipidus, inappropriate fluid therapy, adipsia for any reason
High potassium	Thrombocytosis may falsely elevate potassium; hemolysis increases potassium in selected breeds	Hypoadrenocorticism, severe renal failure, uroabdomen, selected drugs
Low potassium		Vomiting, diarrhea, diuretic therapy, chronic renal failure (especially in cats), inappropriate fluid therapy, refeeding syndrome
High total CO_2		Usually means metabolic alkalosis due to vomiting gastric contents, excessive diuretic administration, sodium bicarbonate administration, inappropriate fluid therapy. Can also mean a compensated respiratory acidosis (exceedingly rare)
Low total CO_2		Usually means metabolic acidosis from any of a number of causes, rarely means compensated respiratory alkalosis
High eosinophils		Parasitism (heartworm, gastrointestinal), eosinophilic diseases, mast cell tumor, hypersensitivities
High basophils		Parasitism (heartworm), mast cell tumors
High lymphocytes	Can be found in young animals	±Lymphosarcoma, ±feline leukemia virus, chronic lymphocytic leukemia, some dogs with ehrlichiosis
Low lymphocytes		Severe stress, lymphangiectasia, chylothorax, acute viral diseases
High RBCs	Some breeds (e.g., greyhounds) normally have higher packed cell volume (PCV) (e.g., 55%) than other breeds	Dehydration, polycythemia, hypoxia (right to left shunts)

graphs, cardiac ultrasound scans, and/or electrocardiograms (see Chapter 27). In endemic areas, the patient's heartworm status should be checked before surgery. Traumatized animals should have thoracic radiographs so that the diaphragm, pleural space, and lungs can be evaluated for conditions such as pulmonary contusion, pneumothorax, or diaphragmatic hernia. Although economic considerations are important, a thorough preoperative examination is cost-effective because it often prevents or predicts costly complications.

NOTE: Remember that there are age-related differences in hematologic and serum biochemical values in dogs. Growth and maturation of puppies influences some of these values such that they diverge greatly from those for adults (e.g., WBC count, RBC count, hematocrit, alkaline phosphatase activity, hemoglobin, calcium, phosphorus, protein, and globulin concentrations).

DETERMINATION OF SURGICAL RISK

Once the history, physical examination, and laboratory tests have been completed, the surgical risk can be estimated and a prognosis given (Table 5-3). An excellent prognosis should be given if the potential for complications is minimal and there is a high probability that the patient will return to normal after surgery. If there is a high probability of a good outcome but some potential for complications, a good prognosis is warranted. If serious complications are possible but uncommon, if recovery may be prolonged, or if the animal may not return to its presurgical function, a fair prognosis is warranted. If the underlying disease or the surgical procedure is associated with many or severe complications (or both), if recovery is expected to be prolonged, if the likelihood of death during or after the procedure is high, or if the animal is unlikely to return to its presurgical function, a poor prognosis should be given. A guarded prognosis is often given when the outcome is highly variable or unknown.

TABLE 5-3

Guidelines for Determining Surgical Prognosis

PROGNOSIS	CRITERIA
Excellent	• Potential for complications is minimal • High probability that patient will return to normal after surgery
Good	• Some potential for complications • High probability of a good outcome
Fair	• Serious complications are possible, but uncommon • Recovery may be prolonged • Animal may not return to its presurgical function
Poor	• Underlying disease or surgical procedure is associated with many or severe complications • Recovery is expected to be prolonged • Likelihood of death during or after the procedure is high • The animal is unlikely to return to its presurgical function
Guarded	• Outcome is unknown or uncertain

 BOX 5-1

Calculation of Volumes Needed for Blood Transfusion or Bicarbonate Therapy

Blood Transfusion

Blood needed (ml) = Recipient's weight (kg) ×
$$\frac{\text{Desired PCV} - \text{Recipient PCV}}{\text{Donor's PCV}} \times 70 \text{ (cat) or } 90 \text{ (dog)}*$$

Note: A rough estimate is 2.2 ml of blood/kg of body weight increases the recipient's PCV by 1%.

Bicarbonate Therapy

Bicarbonate needed (mEq) = 0.3 ×
Base deficit† (mEq) × Body weight (kg)

Give one half intravenously (IV) over 10 to 15 minutes and reevaluate; give remainder over 4 to 6 hours if necessary or give 1–2 mEq/kg IV; repeat only if indicated based on assessment of acid-base balance and potassium concentration.

Note: Because carbon dioxide is an end product of bicarbonate administration, ensure adequate ventilation.

*Total blood volume is estimated at 90 ml/kg for dogs and 70 ml/kg for cats.
†Some calculate the base deficit as the difference between the desired bicarbonate and the actual bicarbonate (rather than the normal bicarbonate and the actual bicarbonate). Animals that are acidotic enough to require bicarbonate therapy need continual monitoring.
PCV, Packed cell volume.

Occasionally the risk of the surgical procedure may outweigh its potential benefits. For example, removal of an apparently benign skin mass may not be warranted in an animal with hepatic or renal dysfunction. Likewise, patients with thoracic metastases may not benefit from removal of the primary tumor (e.g., limb amputation for osteosarcoma). Quality of life must be considered for veterinary patients; those with severe, debilitating, untreatable disease may not benefit from surgery. However, for some patients surgery may improve the quality of life even if length of life is limited.

CLIENT COMMUNICATION

Communication with the client is extremely important to ensure the owner's satisfaction after surgery. Owners should be informed before surgery of the diagnosis, surgical or nonsurgical options, potential complications, postoperative care, and cost. Although cost cannot always be predicted because of unanticipated complications, owners should be kept apprised of the animal's status and of procedures that may affect the initial cost estimate. If the disease is hereditary, neutering should be recommended. A waiver signed by the owner, authorizing surgery and accepting anesthetic and surgical risks, is mandatory and should be placed in the medical record.

PATIENT STABILIZATION

Patients should be stabilized as thoroughly as possible before surgery. Occasionally, stabilization is impossible, and surgical intervention must be done rapidly; however, replacing fluid deficits and correcting acid-base and electrolyte abnormalities before induction of anesthesia usually are justified.

Intravenous fluids are indicated for all animals undergoing general anesthesia and surgery, including healthy animals having elective procedures. The need for perioperative antibiotics is dictated by the animal's disease and the procedure being performed. Recommendations for antibiotic prophylaxis and therapy are given with discussions of specific diseases throughout this text. Perioperative antibiotic use is discussed in Chapter 10.

The patient history, clinical signs, physical examination findings, and total carbon dioxide (CO_2) are helpful in identifying significant acid-base abnormalities. The blood pH, arterial oxygen partial pressure (PaO_2), arterial carbon dioxide partial pressure ($PaCO_2$), and bicarbonate concentration may be measured to determine the extent of such abnormalities. If the animal is notably acidemic (arterial pH <7.2), efforts to optimize ventilation and capillary perfusion should be instituted. As a result of production and retention of CO_2 in the tissue, correcting base deficits with sodium bicarbonate without concurrent ventilatory and hemodynamic support may be detrimental; most acidotic patients do not require bicarbonate administration. The amount of bicarbonate necessary to give for a given base deficit can be calculated using the formula in Box 5-1.

The patient's nutritional state often is critical in chronically diseased animals. Preoperative parenteral or enteral hyperalimentation (see Chapter 11) is sometimes recommended to improve nutritional status before surgery. For example, in patients with cleft palate, cleaning particulate

TABLE 5-4

Methods for Supplementing Oxygen

MODE OF OXYGEN DELIVERY	INDICATION	OXYGEN FLOW RATE	FRACTION OF INSPIRED OXYGEN
Face mask	Short-term emergency stabilization	6–10 L/min (be sure face mask fits well)	35%–55%
Flow-by	Short-term emergency stabilization; face mask not tolerated	6–8 L/min	25%–45%
Tent or Elizabethan collar canopy	Nasal catheter not tolerated; oxygen cage not available	0.75–1 L/min	30%–40%
Nasal catheter	Postoperative oxygen delivery; prolonged delivery	1–6 L/min; 50-100 ml/kg/min	30%–50%
Intratracheal catheter	Upper airway obstruction; nasal catheter not tolerated	50 ml/kg/min	40%–60%
Oxygen cage	Prolonged delivery of oxygen; limited access to patient		40%–50%

matter from the nasal cavity, administering the appropriate antibiotics, and providing enteral hyperalimentation for several weeks before surgery may reduce infection and improve wound healing.

Traumatized patients must be evaluated swiftly to detect life-threatening abnormalities. The cardiovascular and respiratory systems should be assessed by evaluating the pulse quality and rate, respiratory rate and effort, mucous membrane color, and capillary refill time. The heart should be auscultated for evidence of murmurs or an arrhythmia, and the lungs should be evaluated for crackles or wheezes. Diminished heart or lung sounds suggesting the presence of pleural fluid or air or a diaphragmatic hernia should be noted. Oxygen therapy should be given to animals that appear to be in respiratory distress or have other signs of oxygen deprivation (see Oxygen Therapy). Initial assessment of the urogenital system should include palpation of the bladder to rule out obstruction and determination of the animal's ability to urinate. During the initial examination, the animal's level of consciousness and ability to ambulate should be noted (see Chapter 36).

Needle thoracentesis should be performed in severely dyspneic animals suspected of having a pleural cavity disease (i.e., pneumothorax or pleural effusion). Tube thoracostomy (see p. 899) and/or oxygen supplementation by means of an oxygen cage, nasal insufflation (see Oxygen Therapy), or mask may be necessary. Thoracic radiographs should be taken after the condition of severely dyspneic patients has been stabilized. Abdominal abnormalities (i.e., hemorrhage, uroabdomen, bile peritonitis, and mesenteric avulsion) are common in traumatized animals. The animal's ability to void and the urine's characteristics should be noted. Uroabdomen should be identified (i.e., abdominal pain, peritoneal effusion, or postrenal azotemia, or all three) and treated appropriately (see p. 678). Early recognition of peritonitis is important for reducing patient morbidity and improving

survival. Diagnostic peritoneal lavage may be useful in patients suspected of having peritonitis (see p. 335).

OXYGEN THERAPY

Clinical signs of hypoxia include dyspnea, cyanosis, tachycardia, tachypnea, postural changes, anxiety, and/or central nervous system depression. If clinical signs, arterial blood gases, pulse oximetry, or the patient's disease suggest hypoxia, supplemental oxygen may be administered via mask, tent, flow-by, or nasal catheter, or the animal may be placed in an oxygen cage or tent.

NOTE: Remember that patients can be hypoxic without showing signs of cyanosis because greater than 5 g/dl of deoxygenated hemoglobin must be present in the circulation before cyanosis can be detected. The patient must have a PCV of approximately 15% to have 5 g hemoglobin/dl.

Flow-by oxygen may be the easiest way to provide supplemental oxygen in an emergency situation (Table 5-4). The oxygen line is placed within 1 to 3 cm of the patient's nose and mouth, which creates a small area where the fraction of inspired oxygen (F_IO_2) is increased. However, because it requires a care provider to be present to hold the oxygen line and to ensure that the patient does not move away from it, and because a high oxygen flow rate is required, it is not always practical or the best choice. Furthermore, it is not nearly as effective as the other methods described below.

Face mask delivery of oxygen is a useful short-term method to provide supplemental oxygen. With an oxygen flow rate of 6 to 10 L/min and a well-fitted mask, an F_IO_2 of 0.35 to 0.55 may be achieved (see Table 5-4). Be aware that face masks may not be tolerated (especially in severely dyspneic animals) and are often difficult to fit well to the faces of

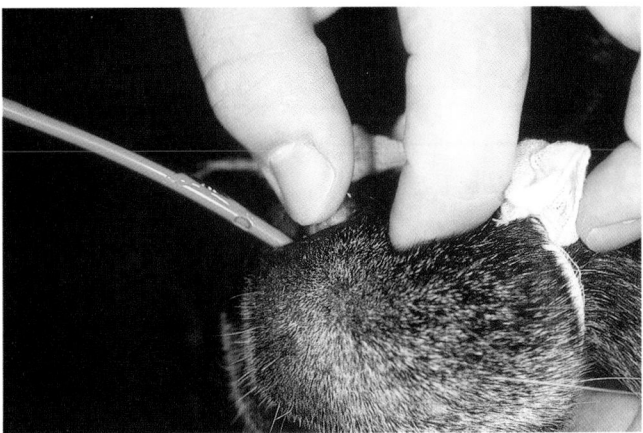

FIG. 5-1
To facilitate placement of the oxygen catheter in the nostril, push the dorsal aspect of the nose up slightly.

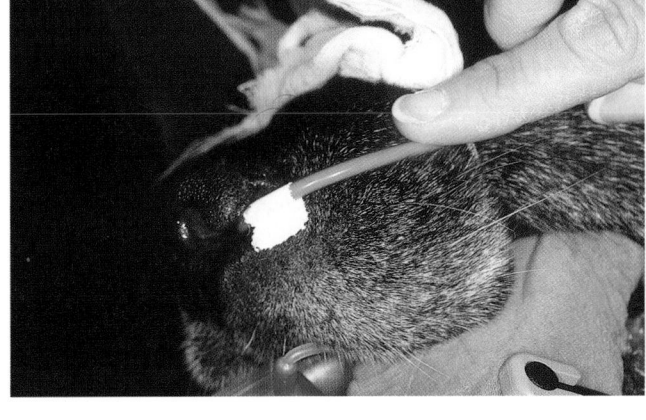

FIG. 5-2
Suture or glue the oxygen catheter to the external nares.

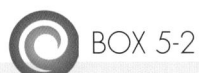 BOX 5-2

Nasal Oxygen Insufflation

1. Select a small, red rubber feeding tube (3.5–5 Fr for cats; 5–8 Fr for dogs) to serve as a catheter and lubricate the tip with lidocaine gel.
2. Place one or two drops of local anesthetic (e.g., 2% lidocaine or proparacaine) in the nostril.
3. Premeasure the catheter to the medial canthus of the eye or the caudal ramus of the mandible.
4. Elevate the dorsal aspect of the nose and feed the lubricated catheter into the nostril the predetermined distance.
5. Suture or glue (e.g., VetBond) the catheter to the external naris and muzzle, and over the frontal sinus or along the jaw. With cats, do not allow the tube to touch the whiskers.
6. Place an Elizabethan collar on the animal.
7. Attach the tube to an oxygen source and administer humidified oxygen to maintain oxygen saturation at greater than 90%; typically start at 50 ml/kg/minute and adjust as necessary.*

*Gastric distention may occur if the flow rate is too high.

cats and brachycephalic dogs. An alternative is to use an Elizabethan collar covered with plastic wrap to create an oxygen-enriched environment. The end of the oxygen tube should be fed up through the collar and secured. To allow elimination of CO_2, make a small hole in the plastic wrap.

Nasal catheters may be used when more prolonged oxygen delivery is desired than can be achieved with flow-by or face mask techniques (Figs. 5-1 and 5-2; Box 5-2). Other advantages of nasal catheter delivery of oxygen are that it permits access to the patient without loss of the oxygen-rich environment (versus an oxygen cage), and it is well tolerated in most patients. When necessary, bilateral catheters can be placed. The appropriate oxygen flow rate is based upon assessment of the degree of respiratory distress, the patient's respiratory rate and pattern, and the patient's size. The recommended initial therapeutic dose for unilateral nasal oxygen supplementation is approximately 50 to 100 ml/kg/min. These flow rates can achieve a tracheal F_1O_2 of approximately 50%. Although high gas flow rates can be administered through a single nasal catheter, these high flow rates may be associated with patient discomfort. In such cases, administering oxygen through bilateral nasal catheters may be justified. A recent study showed that although F_1O_2 and PaO_2 could be increased with higher total oxygen flow rates, the increase is the same whether the higher flow is delivered through one nasal catheter or two. Thus the use of bilateral nasal catheters appears to be beneficial primarily in improving patient comfort (Dunphy et al, 2002). When oxygen is administered via nasal catheter for prolonged periods (i.e., greater than 6 to 12 hours), it should be humidified. Intratracheal catheters may be used in animals that will not tolerate an intranasal catheter (see Table 5-4).

An oxygen cage provides a sealed environment in which the F_1O_2, ambient temperature, and humidity can be controlled. An ambient temperature of 70° F and a relative humidity of 40% to 50% is desired. The major disadvantage of an oxygen cage is that it isolates the patient from the clinician because each time the oxygen cage door is opened there is a loss of the oxygen-rich environment.

FLUID THERAPY

Fluid therapy should be initiated if hemorrhage or shock is suspected. The normal blood volume of dogs is approximately 90 ml/kg and that of cats is about 70 ml/kg. Treatment of acute hypovolemia is intended to establish a circulating blood volume that allows adequate tissue perfusion. Generally, hypovolemic patients can be given polyionic isotonic fluid intravenously in the first hour (60 to 90 ml/kg in dogs, 45 to 60 ml/kg in cats) without adverse effects; however, patients with pulmonary, cardiovascular, or severe renal disease may be less tolerant of rapid fluid administration. Commonly, half the calculated shock dose is administered

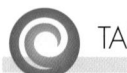 TABLE 5-5

Blood and Fluid Products: Indications for Use and Doses

PRODUCT	INDICATIONS	INFUSION RATE
Isotonic crystalloid solutions*	Shock Dehydration Maintenance	Dogs: Up to 90 ml/kg (to effect) Cats: Up to 60 ml/kg (to effect) Maintenance rate is approximately 66 ml/kg/day for a 10 kg dog; larger dogs need less (e.g., 44 ml/kg/day for a 40 kg dog), whereas smaller dogs need more (e.g., 81 ml/kg/day for a 5 kg dog)
Hetastarch	Shock Hypoalbuminemia	Dogs: 10–20 ml/kg/hr (shock) Cats: 10–15 ml/kg/hr over 10-15 min (shock) 5–10 ml/kg (can repeat) or constant-rate infusion (1–2 ml/kg/hr) up to 20 ml/kg/day (hypoalbuminemia)
Dextran 70	Shock Hypoalbuminemia	Dogs: 10–20 ml/kg/hr (shock) Cats: 10–15 ml/kg/hr (shock) 5–10 ml/kg (can repeat) or constant-rate infusion (1–2 ml/kg/hr) up to 20 ml/kg/day (hypoalbuminemia)
25% Human serum albumin	Shock Hypoalbuminemia	5–25 ml/kg; maximal volume 2–4 ml/kg (bolus or slow push) 0.1–1.7 ml/kg/hr as a constant rate infusion‡
7% Hypertonic saline†	Shock Hypoalbuminemia	4 ml/kg over 5 min, then isotonic crystalloids (10–20 ml/kg/hr) to effect
Fresh whole blood	Anemia Hemorrhage Coagulopathy Shock	10–22 ml/kg (see also Box 5-1); in general, 2 ml/kg will raise the PCV by 1% For shock: 22 ml/kg/hr maximum
Stored whole blood	Anemia Hemorrhage	10–22 ml/kg (see also Box 5-1); in general, 2 ml/kg will raise the PCV by 1%
Packed red blood cells	Anemia Hemorrhage	6–10 ml/kg and then reassess the patient's PCV to determine if more is necessary; in general, 1 ml/kg will raise the PCV by 1%
Platelet-rich plasma	Thrombocytopenia Coagulopathy	1 unit/3–10 kg
Fresh-frozen plasma	Coagulopathy Hypoproteinemia DIC	10–20 ml/kg; then reassess serum albumin or AT III concentration to determine if more is necessary
Cryoprecipitate	Von Willebrand's disease Hemophilia	1 unit/5–15 kg
Oxyglobin	Anemia Shock	Dogs: 15–30 ml/kg at a maximum rate of 10 ml/kg/hr Cats: 5–10 ml/kg at a maximum rate of 5 ml/kg/hr

bid, Twice daily; *CVP*, central venous pressure. *PCV*, packed cell volume; *DIC*, disseminated intravascular coagulation. *AT III*, antithrombin III.
*Monitor CVP to prevent fluid overload.
†To prolong the effect of hypertonic saline, hetastarch or other colloid may be administered simultaneously. Do not exceed the maximum rate for either fluid.
‡From Mathews KA, Barry M: The use of 25% human serum albumin: outcome and efficacy in raising serum albumin and systemic blood pressure in critically ill dogs and cats, *J Vet Emerg Crit Care* 15:110, 2005.

over 15 to 30 minutes, and the patient is carefully reassessed for changes in vital signs. If hemodilution is not a concern, balanced electrolyte solutions (i.e., lactated Ringer's solution, Normosol-R) may be given. The duration of action of infused crystalloids is short, with only approximately 10% of the solution remaining in the intravascular space at 1 hour.

Hypertonic saline solutions are beneficial for reducing total fluid requirements, limiting edema, and increasing cardiac output (Table 5-5). Adding a colloid (i.e., hetastarch; see Table 5-5) to the hypertonic saline prolongs the effect of the

volume expansion. However, animals with protein-losing nephropathy or enteropathy quickly lose the albumin they receive from plasma, making this an expensive and poorly effective therapy in these patients; hetastarch is better in such patients. Colloids should also be considered for animals that are hypoproteinemic (i.e., total solids less than 4.5 g/dl). Fresh-frozen plasma (see Table 5-5) is beneficial for patients in need of coagulation factors because of consumption or dilution (e.g., when large doses of synthetic colloids have been given). Transfusions (i.e., whole blood or packed red

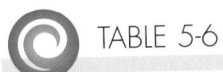 TABLE 5-6

Sliding Scale for Potassium Supplementation

SERUM POTASSIUM (mEq/L)	mEq KCl TO ADD TO 250 mL FLUID	MAXIMAL FLUID INFUSION RATE* (ml/kg/h)
<2.0	20	6
2.1–2.5	15	8
2.6–3.0	10	12
3.1–3.5	7	16

*Do not exceed 0.5 mEq/kg/h

cells) may be necessary in anemic patients. Animals with a preoperative packed cell volume (PCV) less than or equal to 20% usually benefit from blood transfusions. The major preoperative concern in anemic patients is maintaining oxygen-carrying capacity, and this requires blood transfusion. The amount of donor blood necessary can be estimated by the formula presented in Box 5-1. In selected cases, when red blood cells are not available or are contraindicated, administration of a synthetic hemoglobin solution (e.g., oxyglobin) may be considered.

Crystalloid Solutions

Crystalloids are solutions containing electrolyte and nonelectrolyte solutes capable of entering all body fluid compartments. Examples include **Normosol-R, lactated Ringer's solution, 5% dextrose, Plasma-lyte A**, and **normal saline (0.9%)**. Supplementation of these fluids with KCl may be necessary if the patient is hypokalemic or is likely to become so (e.g., from vomiting). A sliding scale for potassium addition to parenterally administered fluids is provided in Table 5-6.

The choice of fluid to administer depends on the nature of the disease process and the composition of the body fluid losses. Patients that are vomiting gastric contents may become hypokalemic or hypochloremic, and have a metabolic acidosis (see p. 409); making 0.9% NaCl with 20 to 30 mEq KCl per liter added a reasonable choice. If the vomitus is not primarily stomach contents, lactated Ringer's may be used initially while awaiting laboratory results.

Hypertonic saline (7%) can be used for restoration of intravascular volume in patients with severe hypovolemic shock or head trauma. Its use requires preexisting normal hydration and thus hypertonic saline is primarily useful in dogs or cats with sudden development of hypovolemia rather than hypovolemia from untreated dehydration. If it is given too rapidly, hypotension may occur and can be fatal (see Table 5-5). Lower doses should be used in patients with cardiac disease, and central venous pressure should be monitored during administration. Hypertonic saline should be avoided in patients with severe dehydration and hyperosmolar conditions. It is given as a rapid IV bolus (1 ml/kg/minute) at a dose of 4 to 6 ml/kg.

Colloid Solutions

Colloids are large-molecular-weight substances (e.g., plasma, dextrans, and hetastarch) that are restricted to the plasma compartment because of their size. These solutions are often used in animals in shock or that are severely hypoalbuminemic (i.e., serum albumin <1.5 g/dl). Factors that influence the duration and volume of intravascular expansion associated with artificial colloids are the species of animal, dose, specific colloid formulation, preinfusion intravascular volume status, and microvascular permeability (DiBartola, 2000). After administration, plasma rapidly disappears from the intravascular space. Artificial colloids, however, contain molecules that vary in molecular weight; the smaller molecules are rapidly excreted, whereas the larger molecules remain in the circulation and are gradually hydrolyzed or removed by the reticuloendothelial system. The benefits of colloid therapy include rapid volume expansion with low volume administration as compared with crystalloids.

> NOTE: Use colloids judiciously as studies have suggested that their use may be deleterious in patients with sepsis, capillary leak syndrome, and adult respiratory distress syndrome after trauma (DiBartola, 2000).

Albumin has a molecular weight of approximately 69,000 and is typically given to small animal patients as stored or fresh frozen plasma (FFP), stored whole blood, or fresh whole blood. Because it equilibrates with the interstitial space rapidly, relatively large volumes must be given to achieve a sustained rise in plasma colloid osmotic pressure (COP). Plasma can be administered at a rate of 4 to 6 ml/min. **Human serum albumin (HSA)** can be used for volume expansion. In a recent study of 37 dogs receiving HSA, administration of this colloid effectively increased serum albumin, total solids, and COP in critically ill dogs and was associated with relatively few complications (Chan et al, 2004). In another study of 66 critically ill animals (64 dogs and 2 cats) receiving 25% HSA (Plasbumin), a significant increase in serum albumin, total solids, and blood pressure was noted after administration without serious adverse reactions (Mathews and Barry, 2005). Despite the aforementioned studies, use of HSA in dogs and cats is controversial because safety and efficacy have not been definitively determined in large multicenter trials.

The artificial colloids used most frequently in the United States are **hetastarch** and **dextran 70**. Recommended dosages for both is 20 ml/kg/day (see Table 5-5). All of the commonly used artificial colloids can cause abnormal coagulation when large doses are given, when they are given repeatedly, or when there is reduced intravascular degradation. These coagulopathies may be associated with a reduction in factor VIII and von Willebrand's factor. The low-molecular-weight dextrans (e.g., dextran 40) may be associated with acute renal failure and should not be used.

Blood Products

Whole blood is the blood product most commonly transfused into dogs and cats. It contains donor blood plus anticoagulant. Although no standards have been established for the volume of blood that constitutes 1 unit, a human collection system generally contains approximately 450 ml of blood and 63 ml of anticoagulant and is designated as 1 unit. Whole blood contains red blood cells, clotting factors, proteins, and platelets. The initial dose is 10 to 22 ml/kg (see Table 5-5).

Packed red cells are the red cells and a small amount of plasma that remains after most of the plasma has been removed. Approximately 200 ml of packed red cells is obtained from 450 ml of whole blood. Because packed red cells do not contain clotting factors or platelets, they are typically used to treat anemia. The initial dose is 6 to 10 ml/kg (see Table 5-5). **Fresh-frozen plasma (FFP)** is the plasma obtained from a unit of whole blood plus the anticoagulant. If frozen at $-30°$ C, clotting factors contained in FFP remain viable for approximately 1 year, whereas albumin is preserved for 5 years. The dose of plasma that is required to increase the albumin concentration of blood by 1 g/dl is approximately 45 ml/kg, which makes its use in many hypoproteinemic animals cost prohibitive. It is typically used to treat coagulopathies that arise from a congenital deficiency of clotting factors (e.g., von Willebrand's disease or hemophilia). The dose is 10 to 20 ml/kg. **Platelet-rich plasma** and platelet concentrates are prepared from fresh whole blood by slow centrifugation. The platelets are then suspended in plasma for transfusion. Transfused platelets may be rapidly destroyed in patients with immune-mediated thrombocytopenia. **Cryoprecipitate** is a concentrated source of von Willebrand's factor, factors XIII and VIII, and fibrinogen. It is primarily used to treat the corresponding clotting disorders (i.e., von Willebrand's disease and hemophilia).

Whole blood transfusions are readily available in many practices. Whole blood should be serotyped to avoid allergic reactions in dogs and cats. Typing sera are available for six blood types in dogs (dog erythrocyte antigen [DEA] 1.1, 1.2, 3, 4, 5, 7) and three in cats (A, B, AB). The most antigenic canine blood type appears to be DEA 1.1. A DEA 1.1-negative dog that has been previously sensitized with DEA 1.1-positive blood will develop an acute hemolytic transfusion reaction after repeated transfusions of type DEA 1.1-positive blood, thus blood typing of blood donor and patient before the first transfusion is generally recommended or at least before a second transfusion if only DEA 1.1-negative blood donors are used (Giger et al, 2005).

More than 99% of domestic cats in the United States are type A; however, cats develop naturally occurring antibodies against foreign blood types that result in premature destruction of transfused red cells, clinically severe transfusion reactions, and neonatal isoerythrolysis. Type B cats that are given type A blood typically develop a rapid, potentially fatal transfusion reaction following even a single transfusion of a small volume of blood (Knottenbelt, 2002). Type A cats given type B blood may develop a mild transfusion reaction that is often not clinically apparent; however, the PCV typically falls to pretransfusion levels within a few days of the transfusion (Stieger et al, 2005). Type A and type AB kittens born to a type B queen receiving anti-A alloantibodies through the colostrum are at risk for developing isoerythrolysis during the first few days of life. Type AB is extremely rare in domestic cats, and blood from a type A donor is adequate. Cross-matching should be performed to detect antibodies in the plasma of the recipient or donor.

In a massive hemorrhage, blood may be given as rapidly as possible. In stable patients, starting with a low dose (i.e., 0.25 ml/kg) to ascertain whether a transfusion reaction is likely is wise (see Table 5-5). If no adverse reaction is noted, the rate can be increased. A dosage of 4 ml/kg/hr has been recommended as the upper limit in patients with heart disease. The volume of whole blood or packed red blood cells necessary to elevate the patient's PCV to the desired level (generally 25% to 30% in dogs and 20% in cats) can be calculated using the formula in Box 5-1. Transfusion reactions may be acute or chronic. Acute reactions may be immunologic (acute hemolytic reaction, febrile nonhemolytic reaction, urticaria) or nonimmunologic (hypocalcemia, hyperkalemia, air embolism, endotoxic shock). Minor transfusion reactions (febrile, nonhemolytic, urticaria) may be treated with short-acting glucocorticoids (methylprednisolone succinate, 30 mg/kg IV once; or dexamethasone, 4 to 6 mg/kg IV once) and antihistamines (diphenhydramine at 2 mg/kg IV, as required). The transfusion can often be continued at a slower rate while the patient is being carefully observed. Antihistamines are often given before administration of blood or plasma products to help prevent mild reactions. If a hemolytic reaction occurs, the transfusion should be stopped immediately and treatment as indicated above (glucocorticoids, antihistamines) initiated. In a recent retrospective study of 81 cats receiving 112 units of blood products, transfusion reactions occurred in 3 cats (Castellanos et al, 2004). Two of these reactions were mild febrile events, but a fatal reaction occurred in one type B cat that received type A blood. In another study, 11 acute transfusion reactions were seen in 126 cats that received blood transfusions (Klaser et al, 2005).

Hemoglobin-based, oxygen-carrying fluid or blood substitutes have been approved for use in dogs. **Oxyglobin** (Biopure Corp., Cambridge, Mass.) is an ultrapurified, polymerized hemoglobin of bovine origin that can be stored at room temperature for up to 2 years. Typing and cross-matching are not necessary with Oxyglobin use. After treatment, a transient discoloration of the mucous membranes, sclera, urine, and sometimes skin occurs and vomiting may occur in some patients. The oxygen-carrying effects of Oxyglobin last up to 3 days in circulation. The recommended dose in dogs is 15 to 30 ml/kg IV up to a maximum rate of 10 ml/kg/hr (see Table 5-5). Generally an initial dose of 10 ml/kg is advised. Although not currently labeled for cats, an initial dose of 5 to 10 ml/kg at a rate of 5 ml/kg/hr has been recommended (Haldane et al, 2004). Patients should be monitored closely for signs of volume overload during administration, and these solutions should be used cautiously in patients with poor ventricular function.

Intraoperative Fluid Therapy

Intraoperative fluid therapy must take into consideration the effects of anesthesia and surgery on fluid hemodynamics. A dosage rate of 10 to 15 ml/kg/hr of crystalloid fluids during surgery is generally recommended to offset hypotension and maintain perfusion during anesthesia. Lower rates (5 ml/kg/hr) may be adequate for healthy patients undergoing elective procedures. Prewarming fluids, especially for young or small patients, is recommended.

If blood losses exceed 10% of the blood volume in an animal with a normal PCV and total protein, blood replacement during surgery is indicated. Although an awake animal may tolerate acute blood loss of up to 25% of their total blood volume, anesthetized animals are less tolerant of rapid blood loss. Blood loss during surgery should be calculated by counting blood-saturated sponges and cotton-tipped applicators and monitoring blood suctioned from the field. As a general rule of thumb, a blood-soaked sponge (4 × 4) will contain 5 to 10 ml of blood, whereas a premoistened (with sterile saline) blood-soaked laparotomy sponge will contain up to 50 ml of blood (Kudnig and Mama, 2003). To estimate the amount of blood lost in aspirated fluids, the PCV of the aspirated fluid can be multiplied by the volume of fluid aspirated and this figure divided by the PCV of the patient.

References

Castellanos I, Couto C, Gray TL: Clinical use of blood products in cats: a retrospective study (1997-2000), *J Vet Intern Med* 18:529, 2004.

Chan DL, Rozanski EA, Freeman LM et al: Retrospective evaluation of human albumin in critically ill dogs, *Inter Vet Emerg Crit Care Symposium* (abstract), 2004.

DiBartola SP: Fluid therapy in small animal practice, ed 3, Philadelphia, 2006, WB Saunders.

Dunphy ED, Mann FA, Dodam JR et al: Comparison of unilateral versus bilateral nasal catheters for oxygen administration in dogs, *J Vet Emerg Crit Care* 12:245, 2002.

Giger U, Stieger K, Palos H: Comparison of various canine blood-typing methods, *Am J Vet Res* 66:1386, 2005.

Haldane S, Roberts J, Marks SL et al: Transfusion medicine, *Compendium* July 502, 2004.

Klaser DA, Reine NJ, Hohenhaus AE: Red blood cell transfusion in cats: 126 cases (1999), *J Am Vet Med Assoc* 226:920, 2005.

Knottenbelt CM: The feline AB blood group system and its importance in transfusion medicine, *J Feline Med Surg* 4:69, 2002.

Kudnig ST, Mama K: Guidelines for perioperative fluid therapy, *Compendium* 25:102, 2003.

Mathews KA, Barry M: The use of 25% human serum albumin: outcome and efficacy in raising serum albumin and systemic blood pressure in critically ill dogs and cats, *J Vet Emerg Crit Care* 15:110, 2005.

Stieger K, Palos H, Giger U: Comparison of the various blood-typing methods of the feline AB blood group system, *Am J Vet Res* 66:1393, 2005.

Suggested Reading

Engelhardt MH, Crowe DT: Comparison of six non-invasive supplemental oxygen techniques in dogs and cats, *Inter Vet Emerg Crit Care Symposium* (abstract), 2004.

The authors determined the amount of time required to reach the highest concentration of oxygen at the patient's face using various techniques. Their findings may provide some guidelines for oxygen supplementation in emergency situations.

Harper EJ, Hacket RM, Wilkinson J et al: Age-related variations in hematologic and plasma biochemical test results in beagles and Labrador retrievers, *J Am Vet Med Assoc* 223:1436, 2003.

Age-related variations in hematologic and serum biochemical values of two breeds over their entire lifespan are reported.

Logan CK, Callan MB, Drew K et al: Clinical indications for the use of fresh frozen plasma in dogs: 74 dogs (October through December 1999), *J Am Vet Med Assoc* 218:1449, 2001.

Guidelines for administration of fresh frozen plasma were developed based upon use of FFP in critically ill dogs.

Preparation of the Operative Site

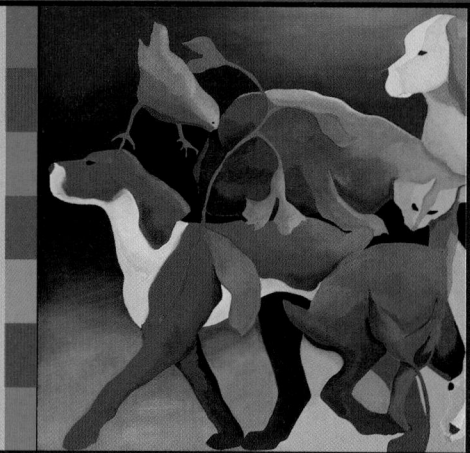

Endogenous microbial flora (particularly *Staphylococcus aureus* and *Streptococcus* spp.) are the most common source of surgical wound contaminants. Normal or resident organisms live in the skin's superficial cornified layers and outer hair follicles. Resident canine flora include *Staphylococcus epidermidis, Corynebacterium* spp., and *Pityrosporum* spp.; *S. aureus, Staphylococcus intermedius, Escherichia coli, Streptococcus* spp., *Enterobacter* spp., and *Clostridium* spp. are transient pathogens. Eliminating exposure to this flora is extremely important during surgery. Although it is impossible to sterilize skin without impairing its natural protective function and interfering with wound healing, preoperative preparation reduces the number of bacteria and the likelihood of infection. **Antisepsis** is the prevention of sepsis by preventing or inhibiting the growth of resident and transient microbes. An **antiseptic** is a product with antimicrobial activity that formerly may have been referred to as an "antimicrobial agent." An **antiseptic agent** is an agent capable of producing antisepsis.

Although perioperative infections have typically been thought to be caused by free-moving, individual microorganisms or small isolated groups of microorganisms, it is now known that if bacteria establish a presence in the body of any duration, they generally form a highly complex, self-regulating, bacterial community known as a biofilm matrix (Paulson, 2005). Bacterial biofilm complexes cause challenging infections, which generally are both difficult and expensive to treat. To form a clinically significant biofilm, bacteria must attach to tissue or an inanimate surface, such as a metal implant, a catheter, or suture in a patient's body and then attract and attach to other bacterial cells. Because normal skin residents typically do not elicit an immune response from the patient, such infections may initially go unrecognized and untreated. Bacteria in a biofilm matrix are 500 to 1500 times more resistant to antibiotic therapy than are free-moving (planktonic) bacteria because bacteria in a biofilm are more metabolically efficient, which limits their uptake of antibiotics (Paulson, 2005). Thus it is imperative that veterinarians and their staff be proactive in preventing infections during surgery by using proper techniques and solutions to prepare the skin for surgery.

DIETARY RESTRICTIONS

In adult animals, food intake generally is restricted 6 to 12 hours before induction of anesthesia to prevent intraoperative or postoperative emesis and aspiration pneumonia. Access to water generally is not curtailed. Operations of the large intestine (see Chapter 19) often require specialized preparations (i.e., dietary restriction for 48 hours) or enteric antibiotics (i.e., oral kanamycin, neomycin, or penicillin G), or both. Food should not be withheld for more than 4 to 6 hours in young animals because hypoglycemia could occur.

EXCRETIONS

The animal should be allowed to defecate and urinate shortly before induction of anesthesia. Colonic surgery may require enemas. An empty urinary bladder often facilitates abdominal procedures. If urine is not evacuated naturally, the bladder may be manually expressed with the animal under general anesthetic, or a sterile urethral catheter may be passed into the bladder.

TREATMENT OF HAIR

Before a patient is prepared for surgery, the patient's identity, surgical procedure to be performed, and surgical site should be verified. In some cases, bathing the animal the day before surgery to remove loose hair, debris, and external parasites may be warranted. Whenever possible, infections remote to the surgical site should be identified and treated before elective operations, and elective operations should be postponed on patients with remote site infections until the infection has resolved.

Hair should be removed as close to the time of surgery as possible, and hair removal should always occur outside the room where the surgical procedure will be performed (e.g., in the prep room). Removal of hair the night before surgery is associated with a significantly higher superficial skin infection rate than removing the hair immediately before surgery (Mangram, 1999). The surgical site should be noted, and hair should be liberally clipped around the proposed incision site so that the incision can be extended within a sterile field (Fig. 6-1). The prepared area should be large enough to accommodate extension of the incision, additional incisions

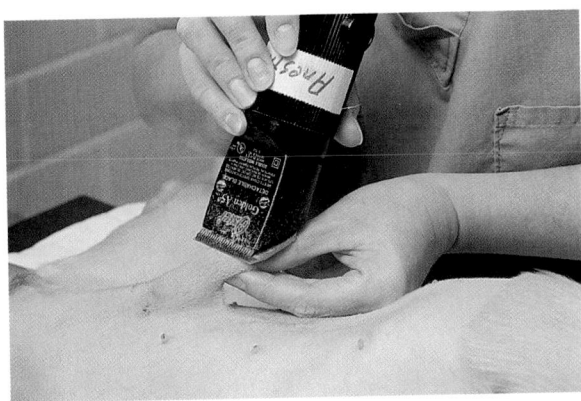

FIG. 6-1
Liberally clip hair around the proposed incision site so that the incision can be extended within a sterile field. In male dogs be sure to clip the prepuce.

(if necessary), and all possible drain sites. It also must be large enough that inadvertent wound contamination is avoided if the drapes move during the procedure. A general guideline is to clip at least 20 cm on each side of the incision. The hair can be removed most effectively with an electric clipper and a No. 40 clipper blade. Patients with dense hair coats may be clipped first with a coarser blade (No. 10); the higher the blade number, the shorter the remaining hair. Clippers should be held in a "pencil grip," and initial clipping should be done with the hair growth pattern. Subsequent clipping should be against the pattern of hair growth to obtain a closer clip. Depilatory creams are less traumatic than other hair removal methods, but they induce a mild dermal lymphocytic reaction. They are most useful in irregular areas where adequate hair removal is difficult. Razors occasionally are used for hair removal (e.g., around the eye), but can cause microlacerations in skin that may increase irritation and promote infection.

After hair removal is complete, loose hair is removed with a vacuum. For limb procedures, in which exposure of the paw is unnecessary, the paw can be excluded from the surgical area by placing a latex glove over the distal extremity and securing it to the limb with tape (Fig. 6-2). The glove should be covered with tape or Vetrap. The foot is then "draped out" of the sterile field (see p. 36). To enhance manipulation of limbs during surgery, a hanging-leg preparation may be done. The limb is circumferentially clipped and then hung from an intravenous (IV) pole during prepping to allow all sides to be scrubbed.

Before the animal is transported to the surgical suite, the incision site is given a general cleansing scrub, and ophthalmic antibiotic ointments or lubricants are placed on the cornea and conjunctiva. Recent studies suggest that using *clean*, rather than sterile, supplies for this initial cleansing prep does not influence infection rates if the skin is intact (Cheng et al, 2001). Thus there should be no lesions, eruptions, abrasions, irritations, rashes, dermatitis, burns, denuded or traumatized areas, or other similar medical condi-

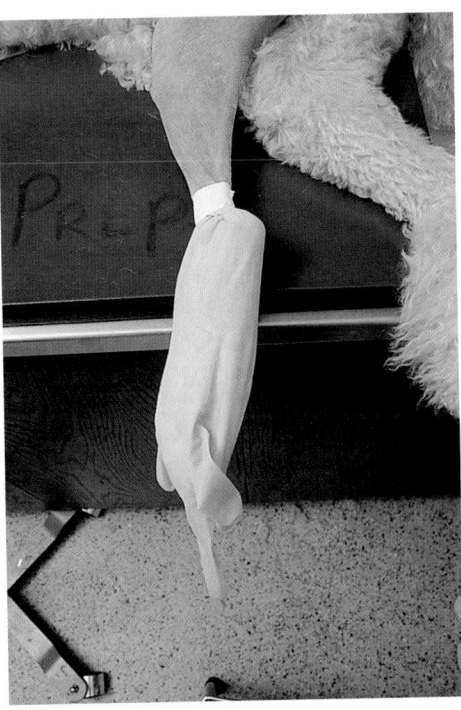

FIG. 6-2
For limb procedures that do not require exposure of the paw, exclude the paw from the surgical area by placing a latex glove over the distal extremity and securing it to the limb with tape. Wrap the glove with tape or Vetrap.

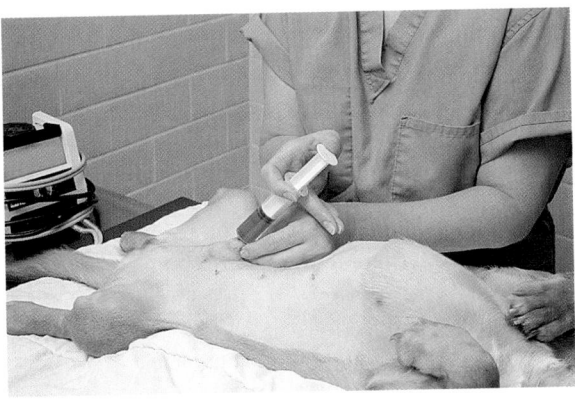

FIG. 6-3
Flush the prepuce of male dogs with antiseptic solution before performing the sterile preparation.

tions that could provide a portal of entry for a pathogen. In male dogs undergoing abdominal procedures, the prepuce should be flushed with an antiseptic solution (Fig. 6-3). The skin is scrubbed with germicidal soaps to remove debris and reduce bacterial populations. The area is lathered well until all dirt and oils have been removed. This is a generous scrub that often encompasses the hair surrounding the operation site to remove unattached hairs and dander that may be disturbed during draping.

Commonly used scrubbing solutions are iodophors, chlorhexidine (CHG), alcohols, hexachlorophene, and qua-

TABLE 6-1

Properties of Antiseptics Used for Preoperative Skin Preparation

ANTISEPTIC	MODE OF ACTION	ACTIVITY	EXAMPLES
Iodine/iodophors (povidone-iodine [PVI])	Penetration of the cell wall and oxidation and replacement of intracellular molecules with free iodine; *iodophors* are solutions of iodine with a surfactant or stabilizing agent that liberates free iodine	Wide range of bacteria, tubercle bacilli, and some spores (e.g., clostridia); activity is greatly reduced by the presence of organic material (pus and exudates)	10% PVI = Betadine
Alcohol (isopropyl alcohol [IPA])	Rapidly denatures bacterial cell wall proteins and biomolecules (DNA, RNA, lipids)	Wide range of bacteria, tubercle bacillus, and many fungi and viruses	70% IPA
Chlorhexidine (CHG)	Disrupts cell membrane and precipitates cellular contents	Wide range of bacteria; more effective against gram-positive bacteria than gram-negative bacteria; minimal activity against tubercle bacteria, *Mycobacterium* spp. and fungi	4% CHG = Hibiclens, Betasept
Alcohol-based solutions	Combination of above listed mode of actions	Broad spectrum activity due to the combination of several antiseptics with different modes of action	2% CHG + 70% IPA = ChloraPrep; 83% ethanol + zinc pyrithione = ACTIPREP; PVI (0.7% available iodine) + 74% IPA = DuraPrep

ternary ammonium salts. Alcohol is not effective against spores, but produces a fast kill of bacteria and acts as a defatting agent. Using alcohol by itself is not recommended, but it is commonly used in conjunction with CHG or povidone-iodine (PVI; see later discussion). Hexachlorophene and quaternary ammonium salts are less effective than other available agents and are no longer recommended for preoperative skin preparation. It is important to avoid abrading the skin by excessive scrubbing with gauze sponges.

POSITIONING

Before the sterile application of the epidermal germicide, the animal is moved to the operating room, positioned so that the operative site is accessible to the surgeon, and secured with ropes, sandbags, troughs, tape, or vacuum-activated positioning devices. When these restraints are applied, interference with respiratory function and peripheral circulation and with the musculature and its innervation must be prevented. Monitoring devices should be connected or the connections rechecked after positioning of the patient. The animal generally is placed on a water circulating heating pad and/or a warm-air circulating blanket or tubes are placed adjacent to or over the patient. Warm-air circulating blankets (e.g., Bair Huggers) may be more effective in maintaining body temperature during surgery than water circulating heating pads. If electrocautery is to be used, the ground plate should be positioned under the patient. If a hanging-leg preparation is to be done, the limb should be carefully suspended with tape from an IV pole.

STERILE SKIN PREPARATION

The purpose of the preoperative skin preparation is to (1) remove soil and transient microorganisms from skin, (2) reduce the resident microbial count to subpathogenic levels in a short period of time and with the least amount of tissue irritation, and (3) inhibit rapid rebound growth of microorganisms. "Sterile" preparation begins after positioning of the animal has been completed. Gauze sponges are sterilized in a pack, along with bowls into which the germicides can be poured. Handle sponges with sterile sponge forceps or a gloved hand using aseptic technique. Use your dominant hand to perform the sterile preparation, and your less dominant hand to retrieve sponges from the preparation bowl. Transferring sterile sponges to the dominant hand before scrubbing the animal helps ensure that the hand picking up the sponges is not contaminated during the procedure.

Begin scrubbing at the incision site, usually near the center of the clipped area. Use a circular scrubbing motion, moving from the center to the periphery. Do not return sponges from the periphery to the center because bacteria could be transferred onto the incision site; discard sponges after reaching the periphery. Frequently, when PVI (Table 6-1) and alcohol are used, the site is scrubbed alternately with each solution three times to allow 5 minutes of contact time. However, using alcohol (isopropyl alcohol; IPA) between the PVI scrubs reduces the contact time of PVI with skin and may diminish its efficacy. Excess solution on the table or in body "pockets" should be blotted with a sterile towel or sponges. When the final PVI scrub is fin-

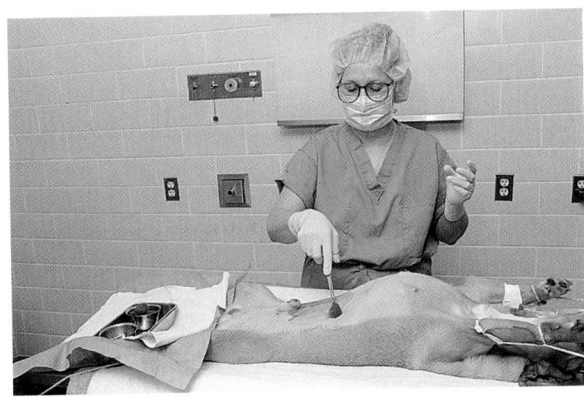

FIG. 6-4
If using povidone-iodine, spray or paint a 10% solution on the operative site after preparation has been completed.

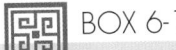

BOX 6-1

Characteristics of an Ideal Preoperative Antiseptic

The ideal agent would:
- Kill all bacteria, fungi, viruses, protozoa, tubercle bacilli, and spores
- Be hypoallergenic
- Be nontoxic
- Have residual activity
- Not be absorbed
- Be nontoxic and be able to be used repeatedly and safely
- Be safe to use on all parts of the body and in all body systems

ished, a 10% PVI solution should be sprayed or painted on the operative site (Fig. 6-4). In one study of human obstetric patients, PVI applied as a spray and left to dry for 3 minutes was as effective as the traditional scrub-paint technique in reducing abdominal wall bacteria before abdominal surgery (Moen, 2002). If CHG (see Table 6-1) is the preparation solution, it remains in contact with the skin at the end of the preparation procedure or may be rinsed with saline. Because CHG binds to keratin, contact time is less critical than with PVI. Two 30-second applications have been advocated as being adequate for antimicrobial activity. With the new one-step alcohol-based solutions (e.g., ACTIPREP; Healthpoint, Ltd, Ft. Worth, Tex.; ChloraPrep, Medi-Flex, El Paso, Tex.; DuraPrep, 3M, St. Paul, Minn.), the solution is applied with a sterile applicator, working from the center outwards and once a uniform application has been applied, the site is allowed to dry approximately 2 to 3 minutes before draping or use of an electrosurgical unit.

NOTE: Prevent pooling of alcohol or alcohol-based solutions, particularly if electrocautery is being used, as these solutions are flammable. Do not drape until the solution is thoroughly dried.

Characteristics of an ideal preoperative antiseptic are given in Box 6-1. Alcohol-based solutions that require shorter prep times than previously used solutions (i.e., PVI or CHG) are now being marketed. Alcohol is an effective antimicrobial, but its lack of persistence when used alone has reduced its effectiveness as a skin prep solution. Alcohol-based solutions are ones in which an agent such as PVI, CHG, or zinc pyrithione is added to provide a persistent effect in reducing the baseline number of bacteria. These solutions appear to have better antimicrobial activity than PVI, CHG, or alcohol alone. In human clinical studies, 2% CHG plus IPA (ChloraPrep; Medi-Flex; see Table 6-1) showed significantly better residual antimicrobial activity than 70% IPA alone or 2%

CHG alone (Hibbard, 2005). In other studies, ChloraPrep (83% ethanol + zinc pyrithione) had significantly better immediate antimicrobial activity than 4% CHG (Hibiclens) or PVI (e.g., Betadine). DuraPrep solution (PVI plus IPA) was found to provide a greater decrease in the number of positive skin cultures immediately after disinfection and in bacterial regrowth and colonization of epidural catheters when compared with PVI alone (Bimbach et al, 2003). It appears that an antiseptic containing a combination of two antiseptics with different mechanisms of action consistently and significantly demonstrates better antimicrobial activity than a single antiseptic alone. The efficacy of combining two antiseptics with two different antimicrobial activities is additive. Alcohol-based solutions that have an additive (e.g., zinc pyrithione) to prolong their residual activity (e.g., ACTIPREP) have also been shown to be more effective than PVI or CHG in clinical studies. Comparison of three skin preparations (PVI or 4% CHG with either saline or 70% IPA rinse) showed no significant difference in the percentage of bacterial reduction for surgical times up to 8 hours in dogs (Osuna, DeYoung, Walker, 1990); however, significantly more skin reactions occurred with PVI than with CHG. Approximately 50% of dogs prepared with iodophors in this study developed erythema, edema, papules, wheals, and/or weeping of serum from the skin. As skin disinfectants in dogs undergoing ovariohysterectomy, 0.3% stabilized glutaraldehyde (SG) plus alcohol or SG plus water were compared with 4% CHG (Lambrechts et al, 2003). All three solutions were found to be safe and effective.

DRAPING

Once the patient has been positioned and the skin prepared, the animal is ready to be draped. If electrocautery is to be used, sufficient time should elapse between skin preparation and the application of drapes to permit complete evaporation of flammable substances from the skin (e.g., alcohol, defatting agents). If an abdominal incision extends to the pubis in male dogs, the prepuce should be clamped to one side with a sterile towel clamp (Fig. 6-5). The purpose of

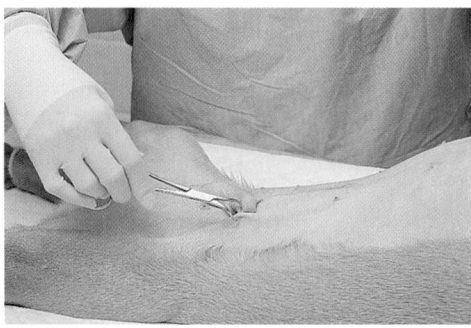

FIG. 6-5
If an abdominal incision extends to the pubis in male dogs, clamp the prepuce to one side with a sterile towel clamp.

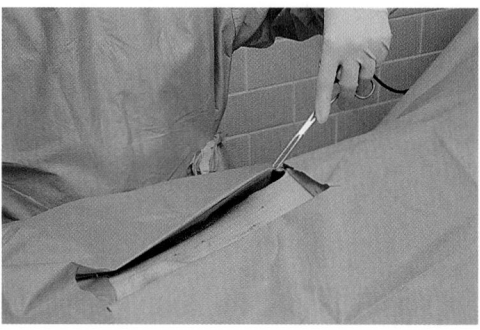

FIG. 6-7
If the drape does not have a fenestration, cut one to the appropriate size. The edges of the drape can be secured to the field drapes with Allis tissue forceps (not towel clamps). Do not put holes through the outer drape.

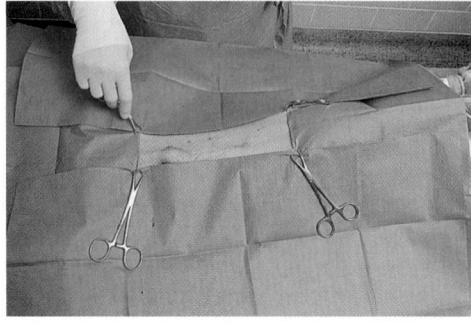

FIG. 6-6
Secure field drapes at the corners with sterile Backhaus towel clamps. The tips of the towel clamps are considered nonsterile once they have been placed through the skin and should be handled appropriately.

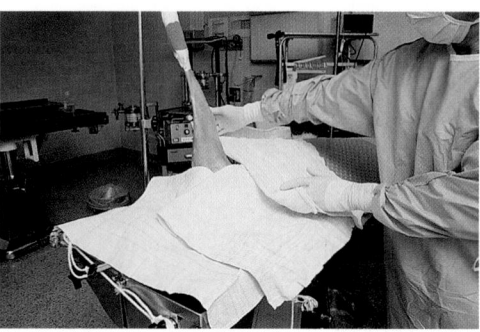

FIG. 6-8
When performing a hanging-leg preparation, place field drapes around the limb and secure them with towel clamps.

drapes is to create and maintain a sterile field around the operative site. Draping is performed by a gowned and gloved surgical team member and begins with placement of field drapes (quarter drapes) to isolate the unprepared portion of the animal. These towels should be placed one at a time at the periphery of the prepared area. Field drapes may be huck towels or disposable, nonabsorbent towels. Drapes should not be flipped, fanned, or shaken because rapid movement of drapes creates air currents on which dust, lint, and droplet nuclei can migrate. Drapes, supplies, and equipment that extend over or drop below table level should be considered nonsterile because they are not within the surgeon's visual field, and their sterility cannot be verified.

Once the towels have been placed, they should not be readjusted toward the incision site because this carries bacteria onto the prepared skin. Towels are secured at the corners with sterile Backhaus towel clamps (Fig. 6-6). The tips of the towel clamps, once placed through the skin, are considered nonsterile and should be handled appropriately. Generally, field towels do not cover the edges of the table,

and care should be taken not to brush a sterile gown against this nonsterile field. Once the animal and incision site are protected by field drapes, final draping can be performed (Fig. 6-7). A large drape is placed over the animal and the entire surgical table to provide a continuous sterile field. Cloth drapes should have an opening of the appropriate size and position that can be placed over the incision site while the drape covers the remaining surfaces.

To drape a limb, field drapes should be placed and secured as described above to isolate the surgical site or the proximal aspect of the limb if the leg is hung (Fig. 6-8). The unprepared area of the limb is held by a nonsterile member of the surgical team, and the tape holding the elevated limb is cut. The limb is presented to the sterile surgical member so that it may be taken with a hand in a sterile stockinette or towel. The limb should not be turned loose until it is securely held by the sterile surgical team member. If a stockinette is used, it should be carefully unrolled down the limb and secured with towel clamps. If a sterile towel is used, the limb should be carefully wrapped with the towel before it is

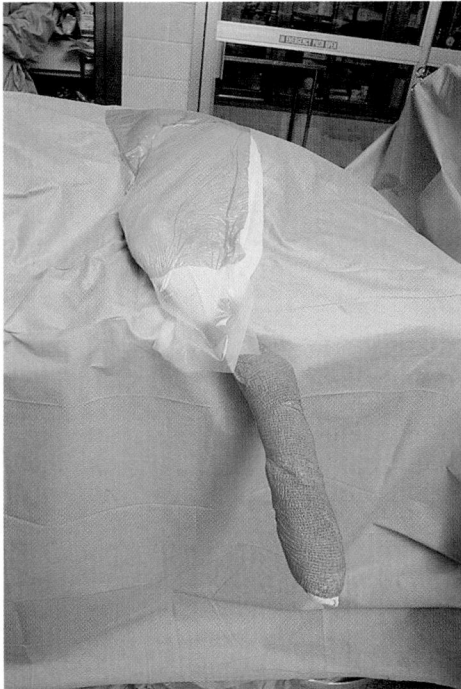

FIG. 6-9
The limb is placed through a fenestration of a lap or fanfold drape, and the drape is secured. A plastic adhesive drape has been applied to the skin and surrounding drapes.

secured to the skin with a towel clamp. Water-impermeable (disposable) towels (plus the towel clamp) should then be covered with sterile Kling. If a cloth towel is used, it (and the towel clamp) should be covered with sterile Vetrap. The limb is now ready to be placed through a fenestration of a lap or fanfold drape and the drape secured (Fig. 6-9). The end of the stockinette is wrapped with sterile Vetrap.

To reduce skin exposure and subsequent contamination during surgery, additional skin draping, or "toweling-in," can be performed after the skin incision has been made. Plastic adhesive drapes can be applied to the skin and surrounding drapes for the same purpose. After the animal and nearby nonsterile surfaces have been covered with sterile drapes, the instrument tray can be arranged, and surgery can begin.

References

Bimbach DJ, Meadows W, Stein DJ et al: Comparison of povidone iodine and DuraPrep, an iodophor-in isopropyl alcohol solution, for skin disinfection prior to epidural catheter insertion in parturients, *Anesthesiology* 98:164, 2003.

Cheng SM, Espin S, Garcia M et al: Literature review and prevalence survey on the use of surgical clean preparation kits, *SSM (AORN)* 7:40, 2001.

Hibbard JS: Analysis comparing the antimicrobial activity and safety of current antiseptic agents: a review, *J Infusion Nursing* 28:194, 2005.

Lambrechts NE, Huter K, Picard JA et al: A prospective comparison between stabilized glutaraldehyde and chlorhexidine for preoperative skin antiseptics in dogs, *Vet Surg* 33:636, 2003.

Mangram AJ, Horan TC, Pearson ML et al: Guidelines for prevention of surgical site infection, 1999, *Infect Control Hosp Epide* 20:250, 1999.

Moen M, Noone MB, Kirson I: Povidone-iodine spray technique versus traditional scrub-paint technique for preoperative abdominal wall preparation, *Am J Obstet Gynecol* 187:1434, 2002.

Osuna DJ, DeYoung DJ, Walker RL: Comparison of three skin preparation techniques in the dog. I. Experimental trial, *Vet Surg* 19:14, 1990.

Osuna DJ, DeYoung DJ, Walker RL: Comparison of three skin preparation techniques. II. Clinical trial in 100 dogs, *Vet Surg* 19:20, 1990.

Paulson DS: Efficacy of preoperative antimicrobial skin preparation solutions on biofilm bacteria, *AORN Journal* 81:491, 2005.

CHAPTER 7

Preparation of the Surgical Team

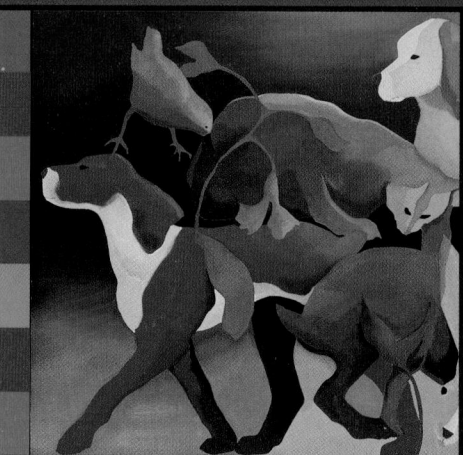

Surgical personnel are a major cause of microbial contamination during surgery. Careful preparation of the surgical team and nonsterile personnel reduces the number of bacteria in the surgical suite, but does not eliminate them. A correlation has been noted between the number of people, their movements, and the number of airborne bacteria in a surgical suite. To minimize contamination during surgery, strict guidelines should be followed regarding surgical attire for all surgical room personnel, including observers. If possible, surgical room personnel should be reduced to only those essential for anesthesia or surgical support.

SURGICAL ATTIRE

All those entering the operating room (OR) suite should be appropriately clothed, regardless of whether surgery is in progress. To minimize microbial contamination from OR personnel, scrub clothes rather than street clothes should be worn in the operating suite. With two-piece pant suits, loose-fitting tops should be tucked into the trousers. Tunic tops that fit close to the body may be worn outside the trousers. The sleeves of the top should be short enough to allow the hands and arms to be scrubbed. Pants should have an elastic waist or drawstring closure. Nonscrubbed personnel should wear long-sleeved jackets over their scrub clothes. Jackets should be buttoned or snapped closed during use to minimize the risk of the edges inadvertently contaminating sterile surfaces. Scrub clothes should be laundered between wearings and changed if they become visibly soiled or wet to prevent transfer of microorganisms to the surgical environment. Wearing scrub clothes outside the surgical environment increases microbial contamination. If a scrub suit must be worn outside the surgery room, a laboratory coat or single-use gown should be used to cover it. If a scrub suit becomes visibly soiled, contaminated, and/or penetrated by blood or other potentially infectious material, it should be changed.

Other surgical attire includes hair coverings, masks, shoe covers, gowns, and gloves. Hair is a significant carrier of bacteria; when left uncovered, it acts as a filter and collects bacteria. Because shedding from hair has been shown to affect the surgical wound infection rate, complete coverage is necessary. Even when surgery is not in progress, caps and masks should be worn in the surgical suite. Caps should completely cover all

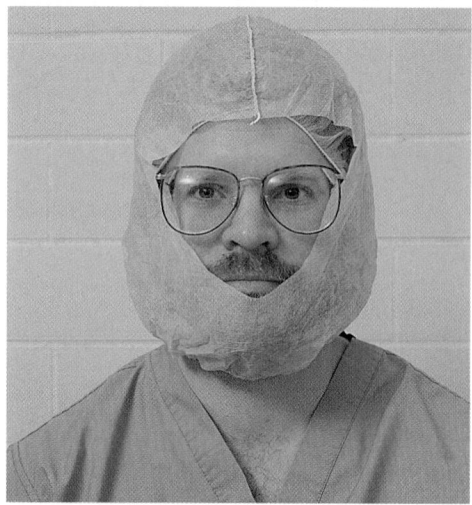

FIG. 7-1
Facial hair and sideburns should be covered with a hood.

hair, and masks should cover the mouth and nostrils. Sideburns and beards require hoods (Fig. 7-1) for complete coverage. Skullcaps that fail to cover the side hair above the ears and the hair at the nape of the neck should not be worn.

Any footwear that is comfortable can be worn in the surgery area. Shoe covers should be donned when first entering the surgical area and should be worn when leaving it to keep shoes clean. New shoe covers are donned upon returning to the surgical area. Shoe covers generally are made of reusable or disposable materials that are water repellant and that are tear resistant. The use of shoe covers has not been shown to decrease the risk of surgical infections or to decrease bacteria counts on the OR floor in human hospitals (Mangram, 1999). However, because of the abundance of animal hair in veterinary hospitals, changing shoe covers immediately before entering the surgical theater may decrease the amount of hair tracked into the OR by surgical room personnel.

Masks constructed from lint-free material containing a hydrophilic filter web sandwiched between two outer layers should be worn whenever entering a sterile area. Their major function is to filter and contain droplets of microorganisms expelled from the mouth and nasopharynx during talking, sneezing, and coughing. Masks must be fitted over the mouth and nose and be secured in a manner that prevents venting. The dorsal aspect of the mask is secured by shaping the reinforcing top edge tightly around the nose. All individuals entering restricted areas of the OR suite should wear a mask when open sterile items and equipment are present.

Surgical gowns may be reusable and made of woven materials (usually cotton), or they may be disposable. Disposable (single-use) gowns are nonwoven and are made directly from fibers rather than yarn. Loosely woven, all-cotton fabric, type 140 muslin commonly is used to make reusable gowns. This fabric is instantly permeable to bacteria when it becomes wet. A more expensive alternative, 270 pima cloth that has been treated to produce a durable, water-repellant finish, provides a better bacterial barrier. Fifty/fifty polyester/cotton blend cloth is available as a tightly woven fabric that resists bacterial penetration. Laundering woven gowns widens the fabric pores, diminishing their effectiveness as microbial barriers. Nonwoven gown materials include olefins and polyesters. The number of microorganisms isolated from the surgical environment is lower when disposable, nonwoven materials are used.

SURGICAL SCRUB

The surgical scrub is a procedure for cleaning the hands and forearms to reduce the number of bacteria that come in contact with the wound through scrubbed personnel during surgery. All sterile surgical team members perform a hand and arm scrub before entering the surgical suite. The objectives of a surgical scrub are mechanical removal of dirt and oil, reduction of the transient bacterial population (i.e., bacteria deposited from the environment), and residual depression of the skin's resident bacterial population (i.e., bacteria persistently isolated from the skin) during the procedure. Relying on gloves alone (without a surgical scrub) to prevent microbial contamination is not recommended because many surgical gloves have holes at the completion of surgery, and the percentage may increase for long or difficult surgeries. A recent study at two veterinary institutions found that the overall incidence of glove defects was 23.3% (Character et al, 2003). Significantly more defects occurred in non–soft tissue procedures and in gloves worn on the nondominant hand. Eighty-four percent of all defects occurred in procedures lasting greater than 60 minutes. Importantly the individual performing the surgery was not able to accurately predict the presence of a defect in their gloves.

> NOTE: Given the high rate of glove defects in longer surgical procedures (especially orthopedic procedures), you may wish to consider changing gloves every 60 minutes or double gloving.

Antimicrobial soaps or detergents used for scrubbing should be rapid acting, broad spectrum, and nonirritating, and should inhibit rapid rebound microbial growth. Some hand scrubs can bind with the stratum corneum, resulting in residual activity. Because bacteria proliferate under gloves, particularly if the gloves are damaged during surgery, persistent chemical activity is desirable. The most commonly used surgical scrub solutions are chlorhexidine gluconate, povidone-iodine, and hexachlorophene (Table 7-1). However, new alcohol-based, waterless

 TABLE 7-1

Common Antimicrobial Soaps Available for Surgical Scrubs

ANTIMICROBIAL SOAP	MECHANISM OF ACTION	PROPERTIES
Chlorhexidine gluconate	Disruption of cell wall and precipitation of cell proteins	• Broad spectrum (more effective against gram-positive than gram-negative bacteria or fungi) • Good virucide • Residual activity because it binds to keratin • Not inactivated by organic material • May be less irritating to skin than iodophors
Hexachlorophene	Disruption of cell wall and precipitation of cell proteins	• Bacteriostatic for gram-positive cocci • Minimal activity against gram-negative bacteria, fungi, or viruses • Not inactivated by organic material • Cumulative (nullified by alcohol) • May be neurotoxic
Iodophors (e.g., povidone-iodine)	Cell wall penetration, oxidation, replaces microbial contents with free iodine	• Broad spectrum (gram-negative and gram-positive bacteria, fungi, and viruses) • Some activity against spores • Inactivated by organic material • Requires minimum of 2 minutes of skin contact
Parachlorometaxylenol (PCMX)	Disruption of cell wall and enzyme inactivation	• Broad spectrum (more effective against gram-positive than gram-negative bacteria, fungi, or viruses) • Slow onset of action
Triclosan	Disruption of cell wall	• Broad spectrum (ineffective against many *Pseudomonas* spp.) • Minimally affected by organic material
Alcohol-based solutions	Combination of above	• Broad spectrum (gram-negative and gram-positive bacteria, fungi, and viruses)

and/or brushless solutions are now on the market and preferred by many practitioners. Most experts agree that although using the bristle end of a scrub brush under the nails may still be a good idea, the time-honored convention of vigorously scrubbing off the uppermost layers of skin with a brush is not only unnecessary, but also unwise. These brushless solutions generally have a very rapid kill and require a shortened contact time compared with traditional povidone-iodine or chlorhexidine solutions. There are several such solutions on the market including Triseptin (Healthpoint, Ltd, Ft. Worth, Tex.), Avagard (3M Medical, St. Paul Minn.), and Endure 450 (Ecolab Inc., St. Paul, Minn.); these solutions have routinely shown greater efficacy than chlorhexidine or povidone-iodine in clinical trials (Parienti et al, 2002; Seal and Paul-Cheadle, 2004). One study found that a waterless hand preparation was associated with less skin damage and lower microbial counts, was less costly, and was preferred by more surgical personnel than a traditional surgical scrub (Larson et al, 2001). Endure 450 incorporates APT, a patented system of adjuvants and potentiators that works synergistically with ethyl alcohol to extend persistent residual antimicrobial protection for up to 6 hours Avagard is a waterless, brushless hand antiseptic composed of 1% chlorhexidine and 61% w/w ethyl alcohol. Triseptin is a brush-free, alcohol-based formula that quickly removes surface dirt and inactivates microorganisms. It contains emollients that help reduce drying and maintain skin integrity. Preservatives help prolong persistence. Although traditional hand scrubs generally take 5 to 10 minutes (see later discussion), alcohol-based solutions generally use two 90-second scrubs (Box 7-1; Fig. 7-2).

The surgical scrub physically separates microbes from skin and inactivates them through contact with the antimicrobial solution. The traditional accepted methods of performing a surgical scrub are the anatomic timed scrub (i.e., 5-minute scrub) and the counted brush stroke scrub (strokes per surface area of skin). These methods are described in Box 7-2 (Fig. 7-3). Recommendations vary regarding the number of times to lather and rinse during the scrub, the number of strokes per surface area, and the time spent on each surface area; however, both methods ensure sufficient exposure of all skin surfaces to friction and antimicrobial solutions. If the hands and arms are grossly soiled, the scrub time should be extended or the brush counts increased; however, skin irritation or abrasion should be avoided because this causes bacteria residing in deeper tissues (e.g., around the base of hair follicles) to become more superficial, increasing the number of potentially infective organisms on the skin surface. The contact time between the antimicrobial soap or detergent and the skin should be based on documentation of a product's efficacy in the scientific literature. A 5- to 7-minute scrub for the first case of the day, followed by a 2- to 3-minute scrub between subsequent operations, generally is adequate. Products such as Alcare (STERIS Corp.) or the brushless solutions mentioned above are available for use as a supplement to the initial scrub or as a reentry scrub. A reentry scrub is any scrub following the first scrub of the

 BOX 7-1

Traditional Surgical Scrub Procedure

- Locate scrub brushes, antibacterial soap, nail cleaners.
- Remove watches and rings.
- Wet hands and forearms thoroughly.
- Apply 2–3 pumps of antimicrobial soap to hands and wash hands and forearms.
- Clean nails and subungual areas with a nail cleaner under running water.
- Rinse arms and forearms.
- Apply 2–3 pumps of antimicrobial soap to hand and forearm.
- Apply 2–3 pumps of antimicrobial soap to the sterile scrub brush.

Anatomic Timed Method	Counted Brush Stroke Method
Note starting time; scrub each side of each finger, between fingers, and back and front of the hand for 2 minutes.	Apply 30 strokes (one stroke consists of up and down or back and forth motion) to the very tips of your fingers and thumb.
Proceed to scrub the arms, keeping the hand higher than the arm.	Divide each finger and thumb into four parts and apply 20 strokes to each of the four surfaces, including the finger webs (see Fig. 7-3, *A*).
Scrub each side of the arm to 3 inches above the elbow for 1 minute.	Scrub from the tip of the finger to the wrist when scrubbing the thumb, index, and small fingers.
Total scrub time is 2 to 3 minutes per hand and arm.	Divide your forearms into four planes and apply 20 strokes to each surface (see Fig. 7-3, *B*).

- Rinse the scrub brush well under running water, and transfer the brush to your scrubbed hand. Do not rinse the scrubbed hand and arm at this time.
- Repeat the process on your other hand and arm.
- When both hands and arms have been scrubbed, drop the scrub brush in the sink.
- Starting with the fingertips of one hand, rinse under water by moving your fingertips up and out of the water stream and allowing the rest of your arm to be rinsed off on the way out of the stream.
- Always allow the water to run from your fingertips to your elbows (see Fig. 7-3, *C*).
- Never allow your fingertips to come below the level of your elbows.
- Never shake your hands to get rid of excess water; allow the water to drip from your elbows.
- Rinse off your other hand similarly.
- Hold your hands upright and in front of you so that they can be seen, and proceed to the gowning and gloving area.

day. For immediate reentry with clean hands, the hands are dried with a sterile towel. A palm full (5 g) of solution is dispensed in one hand, and the solution is spread on both hands and forearms and rubbed into the skin until it is dry (approximately 1 to 1½ minutes). A smaller amount of solu-

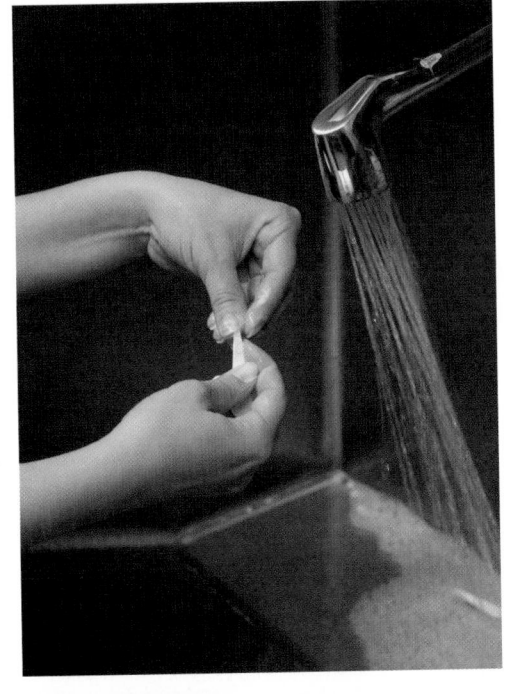

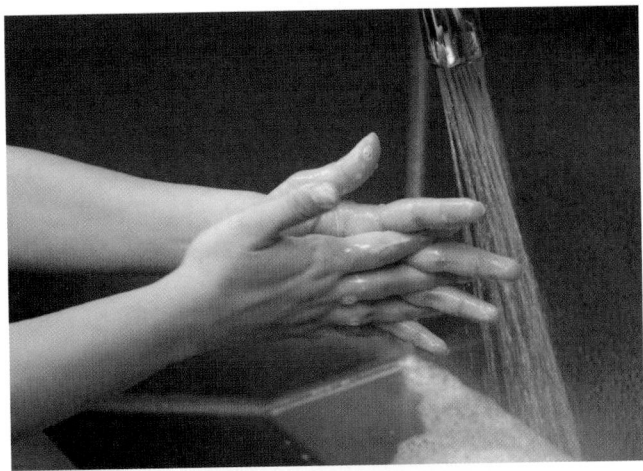

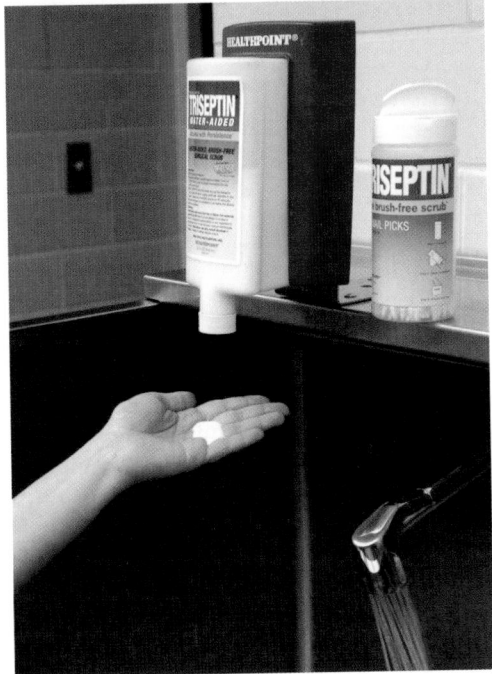

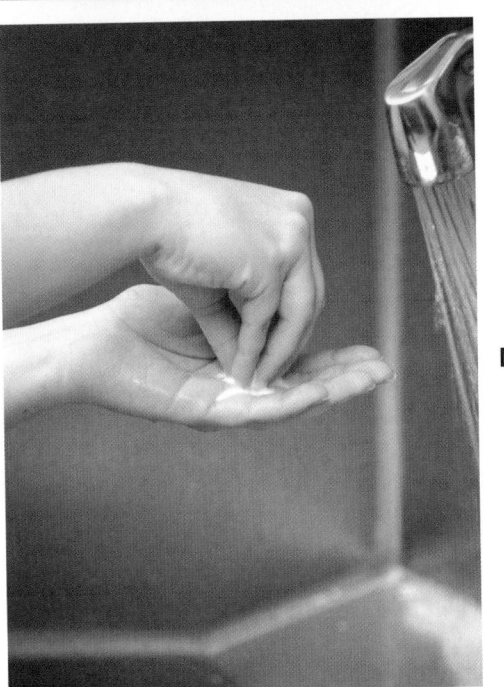

FIG. 7-2
When using a brushless surgical scrub solution: **A,** Clean under your fingernails with a nail pick. **B,** Wet your hands and arms. **C,** Dispense the appropriate amount of solution (e.g., Triseptin, ¼ oz) into the palm of your hand by depressing the foot pump. **D,** Insert and twist the fingertips of your opposite hand into the solution for several seconds. Transfer the solution to your opposite hand and repeat this step with fingers of your other hand.

Continued

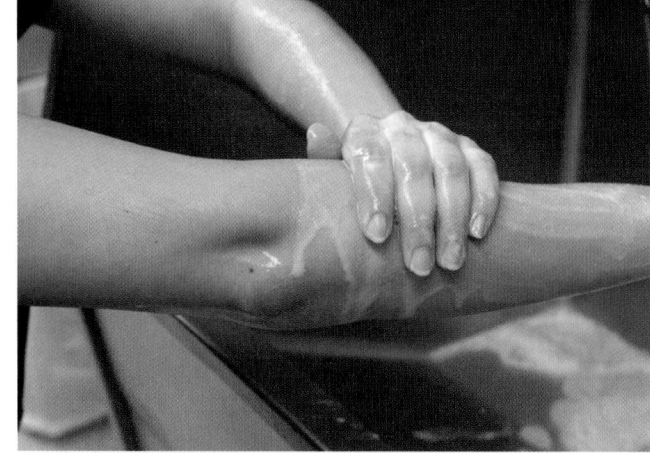

E

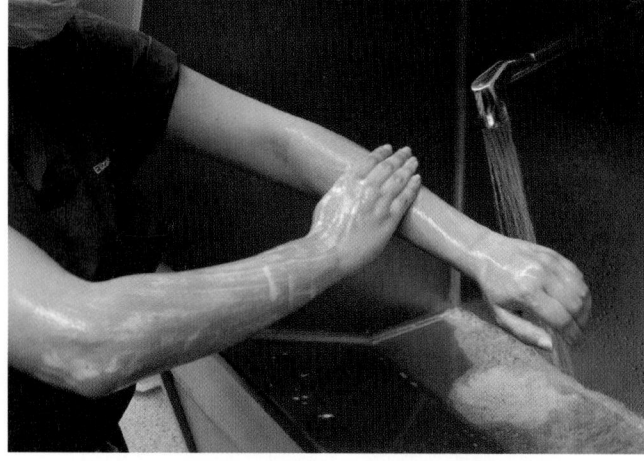

F

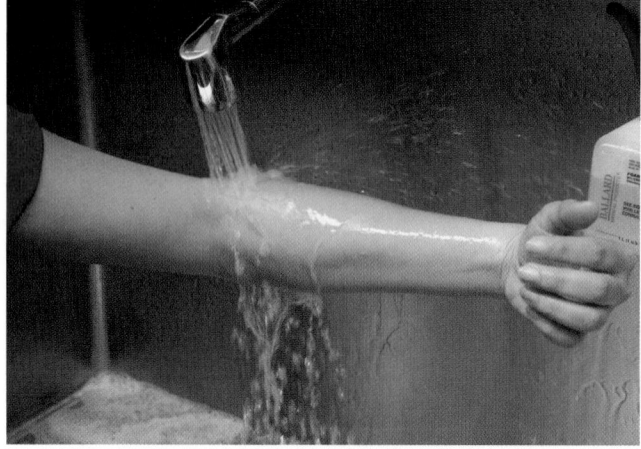

G

FIG. 7-2, cont'd
When using a brushless surgical scrub solution: **E,** Rub your hands together, moving up the forearms to slightly past the elbows. **F,** Add water throughout the wash to create additional lather. **G,** Rinse thoroughly and repeat steps B-F. Stop below the elbows on the second application. Total scrub time: 3 minutes.

tion is then dispensed into one hand, spread over both hands to wrists, and rubbed into the skin until it is dry (approximately 30 seconds).

Before scrubbing, all jewelry (including watches) should be removed from the hands and forearms because it is a reservoir for bacteria. Fingernails should be kept short, clean, natural, and healthy. Recent studies found no increase in microbial growth related to wearing freshly applied nail polish; however, nail polish that is obviously chipped or worn longer than 4 days is associated with the presence of greater numbers of bacteria and has been associated with infections (Arrowsmith et al, 2001; Edel et al, 1998). Artificial nails (e.g., bondings, tips, wrappings, tapes) should never be worn. A higher number of gram-negative microorganisms have been cultured from the fingertips of personnel wearing artificial nails than from personnel with natural nails, both before and after hand washing. Fungal growth between artificial nails and the natural nail has also been reported and can contaminate the surgical wound. Hands and forearms should be free of open lesions and breaks in skin integrity because skin infections may contaminate surgical wounds.

Once the scrub has been started, nonsterile items cannot be handled. If the hands or arms are inadvertently touched by a nonsterile object (including surgical personnel), the scrub should be repeated. During and after scrubbing procedures, the hands should be kept higher than the elbows. This allows water and soap to flow from the cleanest area (hands) to a less clean area (elbows). In most cases a single scrub brush can be used for the entire procedure. No difference in effectiveness has been documented between sterilized reusable brushes and disposable polyurethane brush-sponge combinations.

When the scrub has been completed, the hands and arms should be dried with a sterile towel. Pick up the sterile towel from the table, taking care not to drip water on the gown beneath it, and step back from the sterile table. Hold the towel lengthwise and, using a blotting motion, dry one hand and arm, working from hand to elbow with one end of the towel (Fig. 7-4). Bend over at the waist when drying the arms so that the end of the towel does not brush against your scrub suit. Once the hand and arm are dry, bring the dry hand to the opposite end of the towel. Dry the other hand and arm in a similar manner. Drop the towel into the proper receptacle or on the floor if a receptacle has not been provided. Do not lower your hands below waist level.

GOWNING

Gowns serve as a barrier between the skin of the surgical team member and the patient. They should be constructed of a material that eliminates the passage of microorganisms between sterile and nonsterile areas (see p. 39). They should

**Surgical Hand Antisepsis/Hand Rub
With an Alcohol-based Surgical Hand-Rub***

A standardized protocol for alcohol-based surgical hand rubs should follow the manufacturer's written instructions and include, but may not be limited to, the following:
1. Wash hands and forearms with soap and water if they are visibly soiled or contaminated with blood or saliva. Dry thoroughly.
2. Using running water, clean under the fingernails of both hands using a nail cleaner or pick.
3. Dispense the manufacturer-recommended amount of the surgical hand-rub product. Apply the product to the hands and forearms, following the manufacturer's written instructions. Some manufacturers may require the use of water as part of the process.
4. Rub thoroughly until dry.
5. Repeat the product application process if indicated in the manufacturer's written instructions.

*Modified from: Recommended practices for surgical hand antisepsis/hand scrubs. In *Standards, recommended practices, and guidelines,* Denver, 2004, AORN Inc.

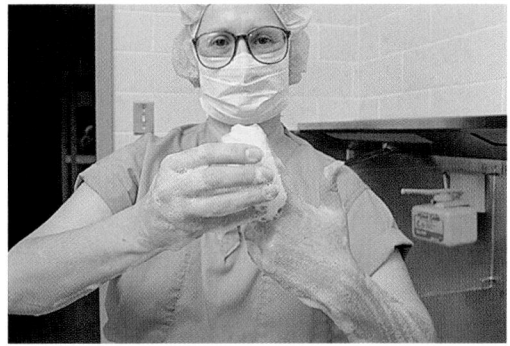

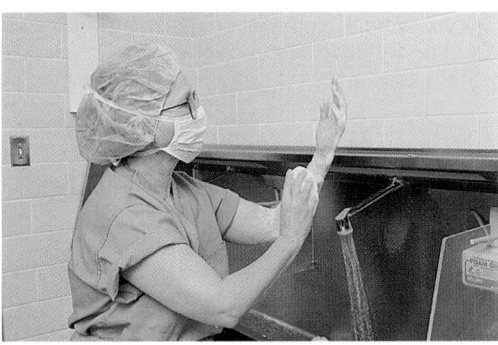

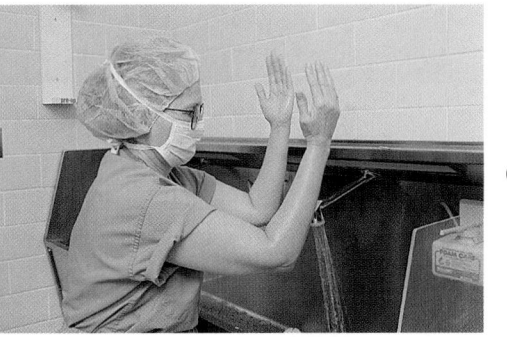

FIG. 7-3
When using a traditional scrub technique: **A,** Divide each finger and thumb into four parts and scrub each of the four surfaces, including the finger webs. **B,** Divide your forearm into four planes and scrub each surface. **C,** When rinsing, always allow the water to run from your fingertips to your elbows.

be resistant to fluid, lint, stretching, pressure, and friction (especially in the forearm, elbow, and abdominal areas) and should be comfortable, economical, and fire resistant. Gowns are available as disposable (single use) or reusable.

The technique of gowning is described below and illustrated in Fig. 7-5. Gowning and gloving should be done from a surface separate from other sterile supplies (the surgical table) or the surgical patient to prevent dripping water onto the sterile field and contaminating it. Gowns are folded so that the inside of the gown faces outward. Grasp the gown firmly and gently lift it away from the table. Step back from the sterile table to allow room for gowning. Hold the gown at the shoulders and allow it to gently unfold. Do not shake the gown because this increases the risk of contamination. Once the gown is open, identify the armholes and guide each arm through the sleeves. Keep your hands within the cuffs of the gown. Have an assistant pull the gown up over your shoulders and secure it by closing the neck fasteners and tying the inside waist tie (see Fig. 7-5, *A*). If a sterile back gown is used, do not secure the front tie until you have donned sterile gloves (see Fig. 7-5, *B*).

GLOVING

Latex rubber gloves are barriers between the surgical team member and the patient; however, they are not a substitute for proper scrubbing methods. If the glove of a properly scrubbed hand is perforated during a surgical procedure, bacteria are rarely cultured from the punctured glove. Lubricating agents for latex gloves, such as magnesium silicate (talcum) or low cross-linked cornstarch, allow gloves to slide more easily onto the hand. However, these agents cause considerable irritation to various tissues, even if gloves are vigorously rinsed in sterile saline before surgery.

Therefore the surgeon should use gloves in which the inner surfaces have been lubricated with an adherent coating of hydrogel. In one study, potentially pathogenic gram-positive bacteria were cultured from the water droplets collected from surgeons after scrubbing (Heal et al, 2003). It was thought that these organisms were from the scrub room tap water. It has also been demonstrated that gram-positive bacteria strike through the glove wrappings within 2 minutes of wetting the paper. Optimally, gloves should not be dropped onto the opened gown pack before scrubbing and should not be placed onto a sterile field until the surgeon's arms have been dried.

Gloving can be performed by three separate methods: (1) gloving yourself using a closed method; (2) gloving yourself using an open method; and (3) assisted gloving.

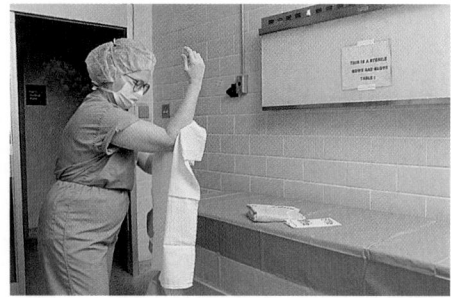

FIG. 7-4
When drying your hands and arms, use one end of the towel to dry one hand and arm (work from hand to elbow). Then bring the dry hand to the opposite end of the towel and dry the other hand and arm in a similar manner.

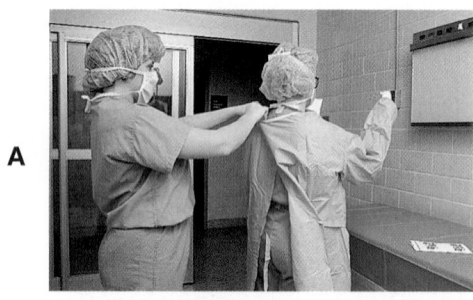

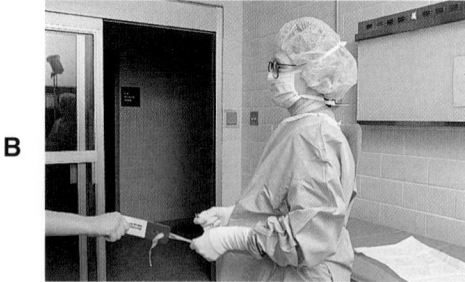

FIG. 7-5
A, Have an assistant pull the gown up and over your shoulders, and secure it by closing the neck fasteners and tying the inside waist tie. **B,** If a sterile back gown is used, do not secure the front tie until you have donned sterile gloves.

CLOSED GLOVING

The closed method of gloving ensures that the hand never comes in contact with the outside of the gown or glove (Fig. 7-6).

OPEN GLOVING

The open method of gloving is used when only the hands need to be covered (as for urinary catheterization, bone marrow biopsy, or sterile patient preparation) or during surgery when one glove becomes contaminated and must be changed. This method should not be used routinely for gowning and gloving (Fig. 7-7). The procedure used when both gloves are donned is shown in Fig. 7-8.

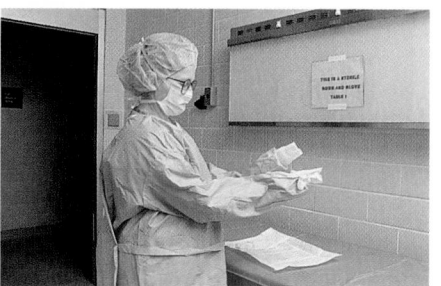

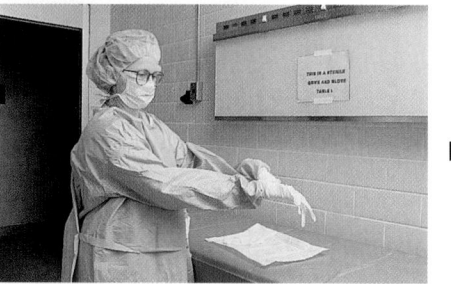

FIG. 7-6
Closed gloving. **A,** Working through the gown sleeve, pick up one glove from the wrapper. Lay the glove palm down over the cuff of the gown with the thumb and fingers of the glove facing toward your elbow. **B,** Grasp the cuff of the glove with your index finger and thumb. With the index finger and thumb of the other hand (within the cuff), take hold of the opposite side of the edge of the glove. Lift the cuff on the glove up and over the gown cuff and hand. Turn loose and come to the palm side of the glove and take hold of the gown and glove, pulling them toward the elbow while pushing the hand through the cuff and into the glove. Proceed with the opposite hand using the same technique.

ASSISTED GLOVING

The steps involved in assisted gloving are shown in Fig. 7-9.

REMOVING GLOVES ASEPTICALLY

The procedure for removing gloves in an aseptic manner is described in Fig. 7-10.

MAINTAINING STERILITY DURING SURGERY

The techniques described in this chapter for gowning and gloving minimize the risk of the operative team contaminating the surgical field. However, vigilance is necessary to prevent contamination of gowns or gloves. Once gowned, the surgical team members should always face the sterile field, and they should not touch or lean over a nonsterile area. The arms and hands should remain above waist level and below shoulder level. The arms should not be folded; they should be clasped in front of the body, above the waist. Scrubbed personnel should avoid changing position levels; they should be seated only if the entire surgical procedure will be performed at this level.

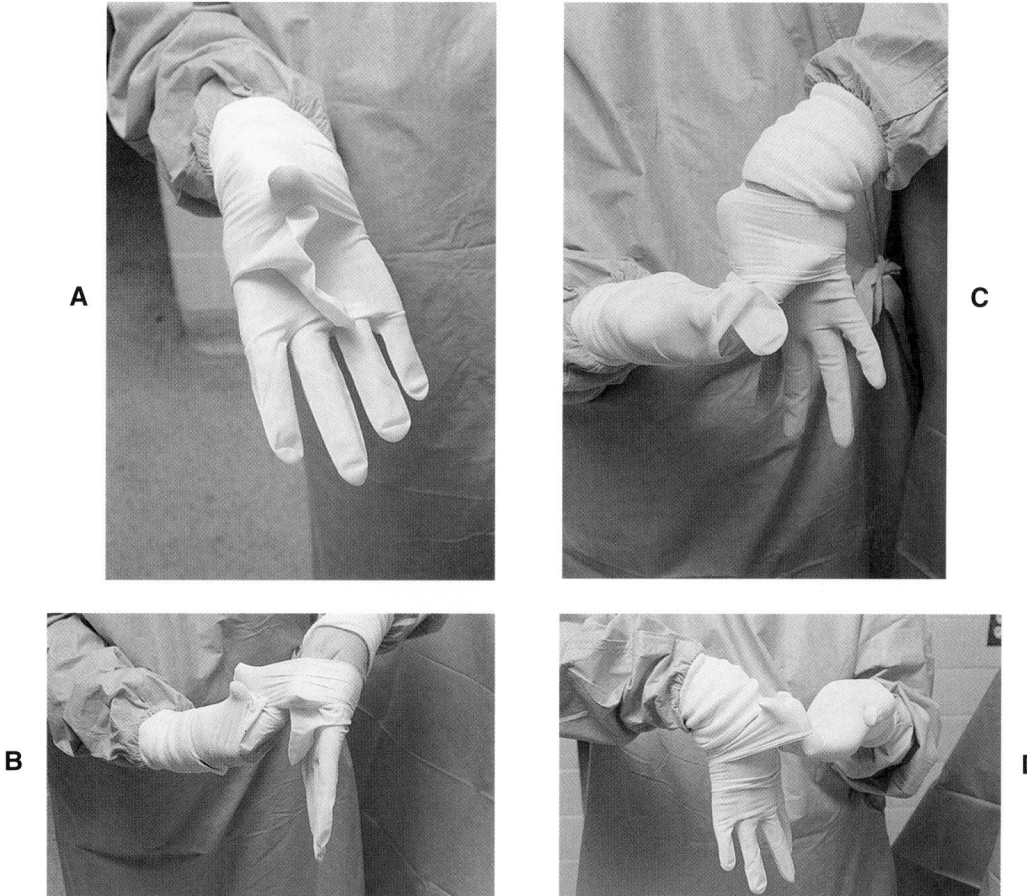

FIG. 7-7

Open gloving when one hand is sterile. **A,** Open the glove wrapper and pick up the correct glove at the folded edge with your sterile hand. Gently put your hand into the glove until your fingers are in the fingers of the glove. Place your thumb inside or near the thumb of the glove and hook the cuff of the glove over your thumb. Let go of the glove. **B,** Place the finger of your sterile hand under the cuff at the palm of the glove. **C,** Bend the wrist of the hand being gloved 90 degrees. **D,** Gently walk your fingers around the cuff until they are at the front of the cuff and at the same time pull the cuff up and over your gown.

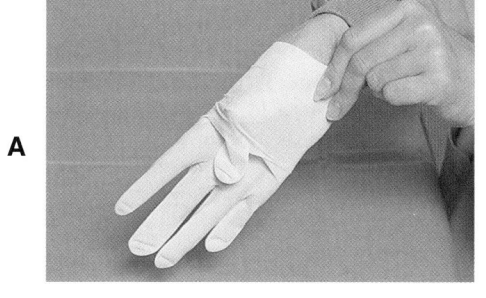
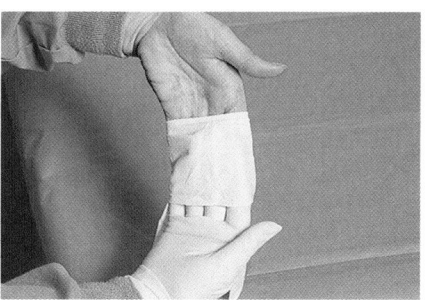

FIG. 7-8

Open gloving when neither hand is sterile. **A,** Pick up one glove by its inner cuff with the opposite hand. Slide the glove onto the opposite hand; leave the cuff down. **B,** Using the partly gloved hand, slide your fingers into the outer side of the opposite glove cuff. Slide your hand into the glove and unfold the cuff; do not touch your bare arm as the cuff is unfolded. With the gloved hand, slide your fingers under the outside edge of the opposite cuff and unfold it.

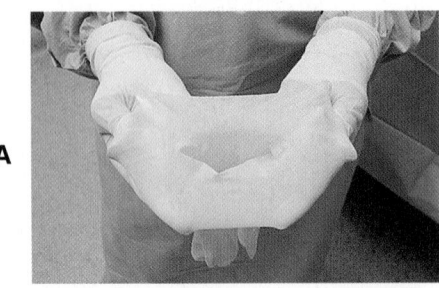

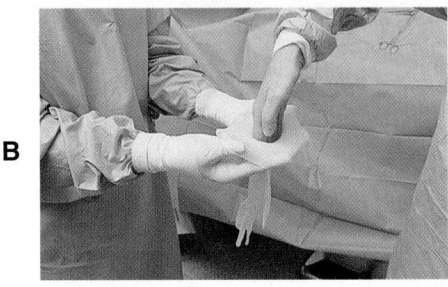

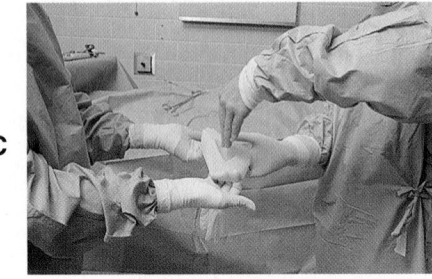

FIG. 7-9
Assisted gloving. **A,** Have the assistant pick up one glove and place his or her fingers and thumb under the cuff of the glove. **B,** With the thumb of the glove facing you, slip your hand into the glove; then have the assistant bring the cuff of the glove up and over the cuff of your gown and gently let it go. **C,** Have the assistant pick up the other glove. Assist by holding the cuff of the glove open with the fingers of your sterile hand while putting your ungloved hand into the open glove. The assistant's thumbs are kept under the cuff while you thrust your hand into it.

The front of the gown should be considered sterile from the chest to the level of the sterile field; the back of the gown is not considered sterile (even if a sterile back or wraparound gown is used) because it cannot be seen by the scrubbed individual. The sleeves should be considered sterile from 2 inches above the elbow to the stockinette cuff. Because the stockinette cuff collects moisture (making it an ineffective microbial barrier), it is considered nonsterile and should be covered by sterile gloves at all times. The neckline, the shoulders, and the area under the arms should also be considered

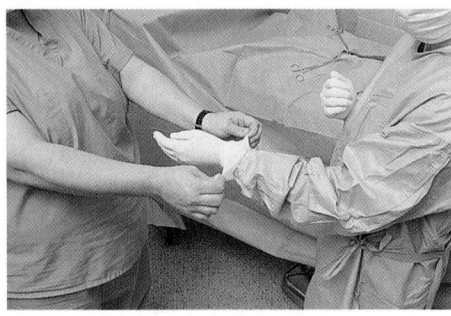

FIG. 7-10
To remove gloves aseptically, the nonsterile assistant grasps the glove near the cuff (being careful not to touch the gown) and pulls it gently from the fingertips. Regloving should be performed using the assisted gloving technique described in Fig. 7-9.

nonsterile because they may be contaminated by perspiration or by collar and shoulder surfaces rubbing together during head and neck movements.

References

Arrowsmith VA, Mauder JA, Sargent RJ et al: Removal of nail polish and finger rings to prevent surgical infection, *Cochrane Database of Systematic Reviews* 1:1, 2001.

Character BJ, McLaughlin RM, Hedlund CS et al: Postoperative integrity of veterinary surgical gloves, *J Am Anim Hosp Assoc* 39:311, 2003.

Edel E, Houston S, Kennedy V et al: Impact of a 5-minute scrub on the microbial flora found on artificial, polished, or natural fingernails of operating room personnel, *Nursing Research* 47:54, 1998.

Heal JS, Blom AW, Titcomb D et al: Bacterial contamination of surgical gloves by water droplets spilt after scrubbing, *J Hosp Inf* 3:136, 2003.

Larson EL, Aieloo AE, Heilman JM et al: Comparison of different regimens for surgical hand preparation, *AORN J* 73:412, 2001.

Mangram AJ, Horan TC, Pearson ML et al: Guidelines for prevention of surgical site infection, 1999, *Infect Control Hosp Epide* 20:250, 1999.

Parienti JJ, Thibon P, Heller R et al: Hand rubbing with an aqueous alcoholic solution vs. traditional surgical hand-scrubbing and 30-day surgical site infection rates, *JAMA* 288:722, 2002.

Seal LA, Paul-Cheadle D: A systems approach to preopoerative surgical patient skin preparation, *Am J Inf Cont* 32:57, 2004.

Suggested Reading

Association of Operating Room Nurses: Standards, recommended practices, and guidelines: recommended practices for surgical hand scrubs, Denver, 2000, The Association.

CHAPTER 8
Surgical Instrumentation

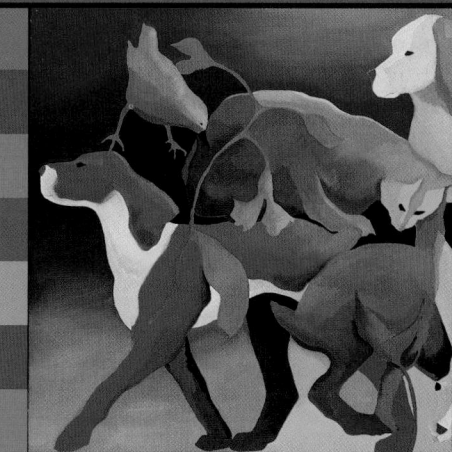

INSTRUMENT CATEGORIES

Each type of surgical instrument is designed for a particular use and should be used only for that purpose. Using instruments for procedures for which they are not designed (e.g., using Metzenbaum scissors to cut suture or tissue forceps to hold bone) may dull or break them.

Scalpels

Scalpels are the primary cutting instrument used to incise tissue (Fig. 8-1). Reusable scalpel handles (No. 3 and 4) with detachable blades are most commonly used in veterinary medicine; however, disposable handles and blades are available. Disposable scalpels with a locking retractable shield are designed to minimize the risk of surgical blade injuries while passing blades between procedural steps and during disposal (BD Bard-Parker, Franklin Lakes, N.J.). Blades are available in various sizes and shapes, depending on the intended task. A No. 10 blade is most commonly used in small animal surgery.

Scalpels usually are used in a "slide cutting" fashion, which means that the direction of pressure applied to the knife blade is at a right angle to the direction of scalpel pressure. When incising skin, the scalpel blade should be kept perpendicular to the skin surface. Scalpels can be held with a pencil grip, fingertip grip, or palmed grip. The pencil grip allows shorter, finer, and more precise incisions than with the other grips because the scalpel is at a 30- to 40-degree greater angle to the tissue (Fig. 8-2). However, this angle reduces cutting edge contact, making this grip less useful for long incisions. The fingertip grip offers the best accuracy and stability for long incisions.

Scissors

Scissors come in a variety of shapes, sizes, and weights and generally are classified according to the type of point (e.g., blunt-blunt, sharp-sharp, or sharp-blunt), the blade shape (e.g., straight or curved), or the cutting edge (plain or serrated) (Fig. 8-3). Curved scissors offer greater maneuverability and visibility, whereas straight scissors provide the greatest mechanical advantage when cutting tough or thick tissue. Metzenbaum (also called Metz, Nelson, delicate, or tissue

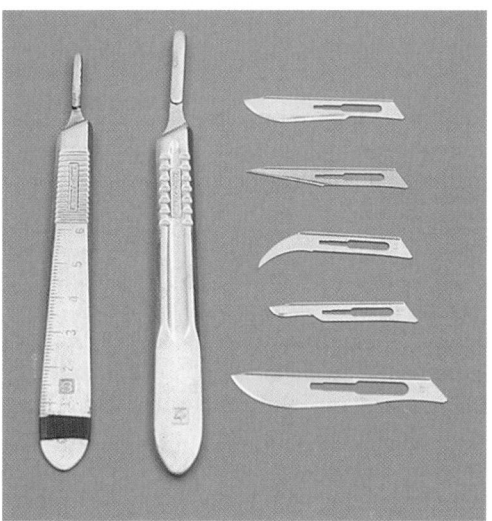

FIG. 8-1
Scalpel handles (*left,* No. 3; *right,* No. 4) and blades *(top to bottom)*: No. 10, 11, 12, 15, and 20.

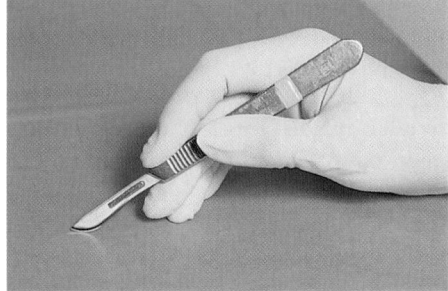

FIG. 8-2
Scalpels generally are held with a pencil grip because it allows short, fine, precise incisions.

scissors) or Mayo scissors are most commonly used in surgery; the former are more delicate and should be reserved for cutting delicate tissue and for blunt dissection. Mayo scissors are used for cutting heavy tissue, such as fascia. Suture scissors, not tissue scissors, should be used to cut sutures. The

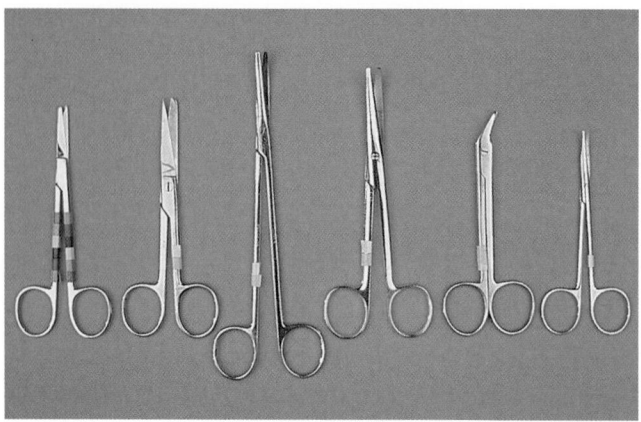
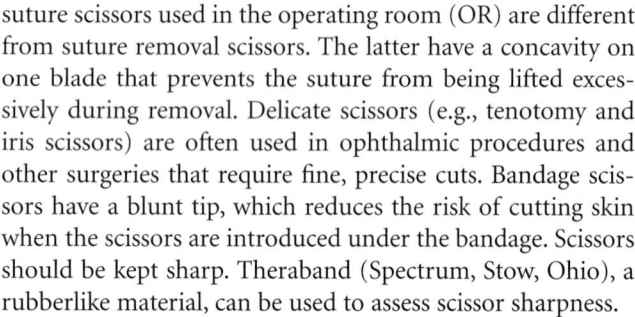

FIG. 8-3
Scissors. *Left to right:* Stitch (suture removal), sharp-blunt, Metzenbaum, Mayo, wire, tenotomy.

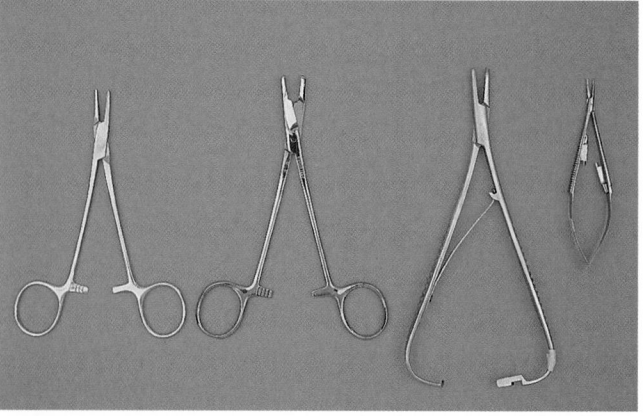

FIG. 8-4
Needle holders. *Left to right:* Mayo-Hegar, Olsen-Hegar, Mathieu, Castroviejo.

suture scissors used in the operating room (OR) are different from suture removal scissors. The latter have a concavity on one blade that prevents the suture from being lifted excessively during removal. Delicate scissors (e.g., tenotomy and iris scissors) are often used in ophthalmic procedures and other surgeries that require fine, precise cuts. Bandage scissors have a blunt tip, which reduces the risk of cutting skin when the scissors are introduced under the bandage. Scissors should be kept sharp. Theraband (Spectrum, Stow, Ohio), a rubberlike material, can be used to assess scissor sharpness.

Scissors may be used for sharp cutting or blunt dissection. They are held with the tips of the thumb and ring finger through the finger rings and with the index finger resting on the shanks near the fulcrum. The ring finger or thumb should not be allowed to "fall through" the handle; the rings should be kept near the distal finger joint. Most scissors are designed for use with a right-handed grip so that the natural pushing of the thumb and pulling of the fingers in a gripping motion applies maximal shear and torque to the blades. When used in the left hand, the thumb blade is positioned such that a grasping motion that pushes with the thumb causes loss of shear and torque forces. It takes considerable practice for a left-handed surgeon to use right-handed scissors. However, most instrument companies manufacture left-handed instruments.

Direction, control, and accuracy in cutting depend on the stability of the tissue between the blades of the scissors and of the scissors in the operator's grip. The more obtuse the angle between the blades when cutting, the less the scissors stabilize the tissue and the less accurate the cut. Using the end of the blade stabilizes tissue more securely and allows a more precise cut. Scissors should not be completely closed if the incision is to be continued because the result is a ragged incision; the scissors should be nearly closed, advanced, and nearly closed again. Blunt dissection (i.e., separation of tissue by inserting the points and opening the handles) may be used to separate muscles and fat. Blunt dissection should not be used in tougher tissue or where precise cuts are possible.

Needle Holders

Needle holders grasp and manipulate curved needles (Fig. 8-4). Size and type of needle holder are determined by characteristics of the needle to be held and location of tissue to be sutured. Heavier, larger needles require wider, heavier jawed needle holders. If needle holders are used to hold suture, the jaws should be finely serrated or smooth to prevent damaging the suture by fraying or cutting it. Long needle holders facilitate working in deep wounds. High-quality needle holders are made of noncorrosive, high-strength alloy and have a glare-free finish. The tips are hardened by coating them with a diamond surface or by fusing tungsten carbide to the face. Tungsten carbide inserts may be replaced when they become damaged or fail to hold suture adequately.

Most needle holders have a ratchet lock just distal to the thumb (e.g., Mayo-Hegar, Olsen-Hegar types), but some (e.g., Castroviejo type) have a spring and latch mechanism for locking. Mayo-Hegar needle holders are commonly used in veterinary medicine for manipulating medium to coarse needles. Olsen-Hegar needle holders are used similarly, but have scissor blades that allow suture to be tied and cut with the same instrument. The disadvantage of Olsen-Hegar needle holders is that expertise is required to prevent cutting the suture during tying. Mathieu needle holders have a ratchet lock at the proximal end of the handles of the needle holder, which permits locking and unlocking simply by progressively squeezing the handles together.

Needles generally should be placed perpendicular to the needle holder because this allows greatest maneuverability. When needles are placed at an angle, the handles must move through a wide arc during suturing. A needle generally is grasped near its center to allow it to be advanced through tissue with greater force and less risk of breakage. When the needle is grasped near the eye or swage, maximum needle length is available for suturing, and there is less risk of needle slippage; however, the needle is more likely to bend or break unless delicate tissue is being sutured. Conversely, holding the needle near the pointed end allows the greatest driving

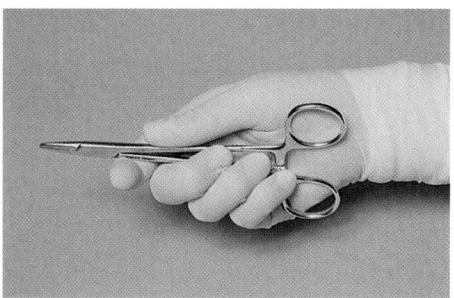

FIG. 8-5
A palmed grip provides a strong driving force but less precision.

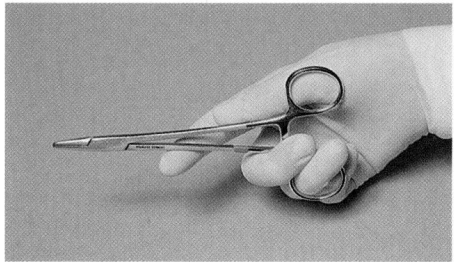

FIG. 8-6
A thenar grip provides good mobility, but releasing the needle holder by applying pressure with the ball of the thumb to the upper ring causes the handles to "pop" apart. This causes some movement of the needle in the tissue being sutured.

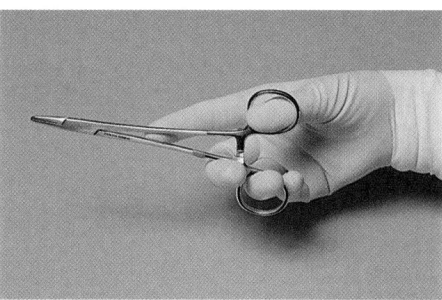

FIG. 8-7
The thumb-ring finger grip allows for the most precision of all grips and is preferable when suturing delicate tissue.

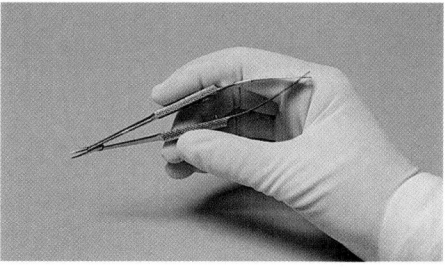

FIG. 8-8
A pencil grip is used with Castroviejo needle holders.

force when suturing tough tissue, but extracting the needle is difficult.

Needle holders may be held using a palmed grip (no fingers are placed in the rings, and the upper ring rests against the ball of the thumb [Fig. 8-5]), a thenar grip (the upper ring rests on the ball of the thumb, and the ring finger is inserted through the lower ring [Fig. 8-6]), a thumb-ring finger grip (thumb is placed through the upper ring and ring finger through the lower ring [Fig. 8-7]), or a pencil grip (the index finger and thumb rest on the shafts of the needle holders [Fig. 8-8]), which is used with Castroviejo needle holders. The palmed grip is most advantageous for suturing tough tissue that requires a strong needle-driving force; however, the needle cannot be released and regrasped after a stitch without changing to another grip, making suturing less precise.

> NOTE: Left-handed surgeons cannot palm right-handed instruments because the boxlock closes rather than opens with pressure.

The thenar grip allows the needle to be released and regrasped for extraction without changing grips. Although it allows mobility, releasing the needle holder by exerting pressure on the upper ring with the ball of the thumb causes the needle holder handles to "pop" apart, and some needle movement occurs during this process. The greatest advantage of a thumb-ring finger grip is that it allows precision when releasing a needle. Although slower than the palmed or thenar grip, it is preferred when tissue is delicate or when precise suturing is required.

Tissue Forceps

Tissue (thumb) forceps are tweezerlike, nonlocking instruments used to grasp tissue (Fig. 8-9). The proximal ends are bonded together to allow the grasping ends to spring open or be squeezed shut. They are available in various shapes and sizes; tips (grasping ends) may be pointed, flat, round, smooth, or serrated or may have small or large teeth. Tissue forceps with large teeth should not be used to handle tissue easily traumatized. Smooth tips are recommended with delicate tissue, such as blood vessels. The most commonly used tissue forceps (e.g., Brown-Adson forceps) have small serrations on the tips that minimize trauma, but facilitate holding tissue securely.

Tissue forceps generally are used in the nondominant hand. They should be held so that one blade functions as an extension of the thumb and the other blade functions as an extension of the opposing fingers (i.e., pencil position [Fig. 8-10]). Holding the shanks in the palm greatly limits maneuverability. When forceps are not in use, they can be palmed and held with the ring and little fingers, leaving the index and middle fingers free.

Tissue forceps are used to *stabilize* tissue and/or *expose* tissue layers during suturing. During suturing, tissue forceps

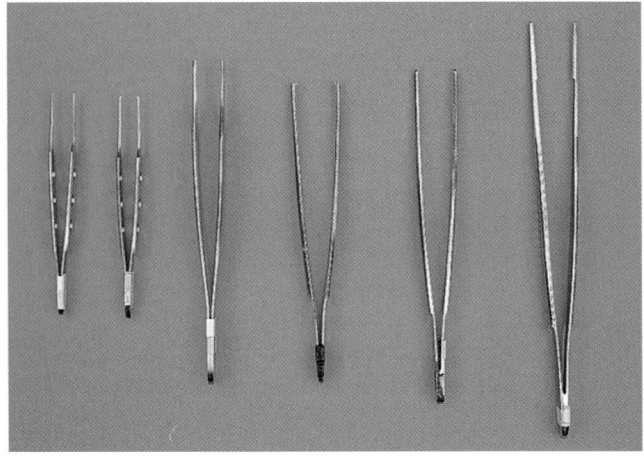

FIG. 8-9
Tissue forceps. *Left to right:* Bishop-Harmon (smooth tip), Bishop-Harmon (toothed), Brown-Adson, 132 tissue, serrated, DeBakey.

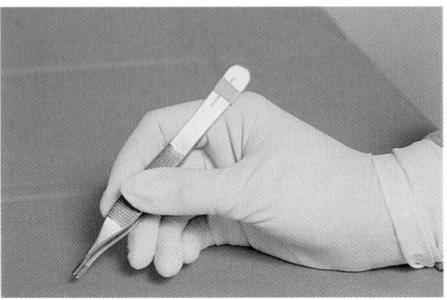

FIG. 8-10
Holding tissue forceps with a pencil grip provides greater maneuverability than with other grips.

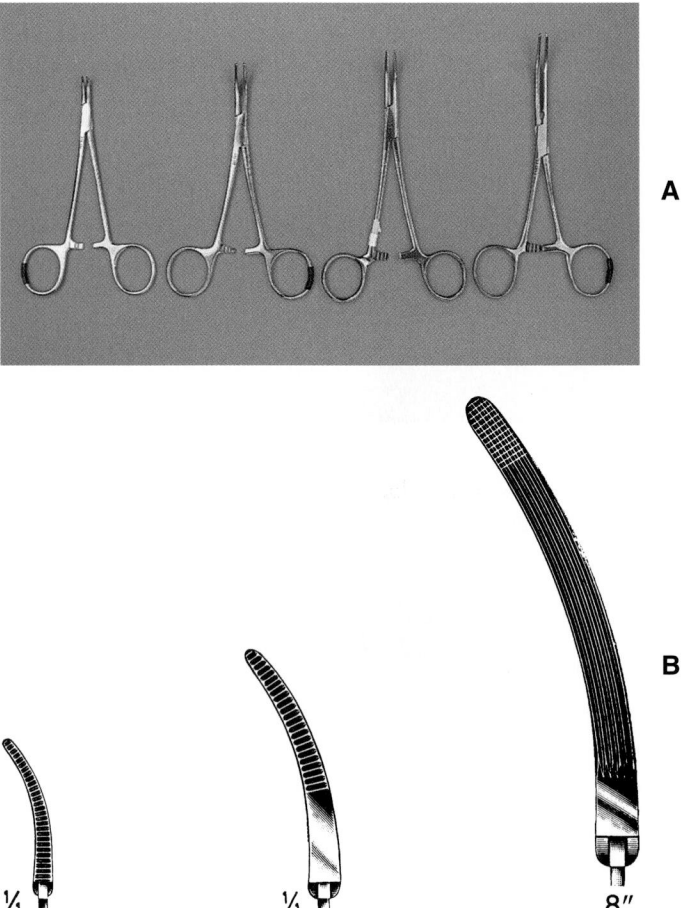

FIG. 8-11
A, Hemostat forceps *(left to right)*: Mosquito, Kelly, Crile, Rochester-Carmalt. **B,** Jaw detail of hemostatic forceps *(left to right)*: Mosquito, Kelly, Rochester-Carmalt.

are used on the far side of the wound to grasp the layer above the one being sutured. This layer is retracted upward and outward with the forceps, exposing the layer to be sutured. The needle point can then be placed at the desired level. Before the needle is driven completely through the tissue, the forceps should be moved from the superficial layer to grasp the layer being sutured. This layer can then be lifted to expose the needle's exit as it is passed through the tissue. The tissue layer on the near side being sutured is grasped and lifted to expose the desired needle entrance site. After the needle point has been placed at the desired site, the tissue forceps are moved and used to retract the more superficial layer, thereby exposing the exit site. When needles are grasped during suturing, they should be grasped perpendicular to the shaft.

Hemostat Forceps

Hemostat forceps are crushing instruments used to clamp blood vessels (Fig. 8-11). They are available with straight or curved tips and vary in size from smaller (3-inch) mosquito hemostats with transverse jaw serrations to larger (9-inch) angiotribes. The serrations on the jaws of larger hemostat forceps may be transverse, longitudinal, diagonal, or a com-

bination of these. Longitudinal serrations are generally gentler to tissue than cross serrations. Serrations usually extend from the tips of the jaws to the boxlocks, but in Kelly forceps, transverse (i.e., horizontal) serrations extend only over the distal portion of the jaws. Similarly sized Crile forceps have transverse serrations that extend the entire length of the jaw. Kelly and Crile forceps are used on larger vessels. Rochester-Carmalt forceps are larger crushing forceps often used to control large tissue bundles, such as during an ovariohysterectomy. They have longitudinal grooves with cross grooves at the tip ends to prevent tissue slippage. Specialized cardiovascular forceps (e.g., Satinsky forceps) allow occlusion of only a portion of the vessel. Serrations of cardiovascular clamps provide tissue compression without cutting delicate vessel walls. Large teeth at the tip ends of some forceps (i.e., Oschner) help prevent tissue slippage within forceps.

Curved hemostats should be placed on tissue with the curve facing up. As little tissue as possible should be grasped to minimize trauma, and the smallest hemostat forceps that accomplish the job should be used. To prevent having fingers momentarily trapped in the rings of hemostats, fingertips should be placed on the finger rings or fingers should be inserted into rings only as far as the first joint.

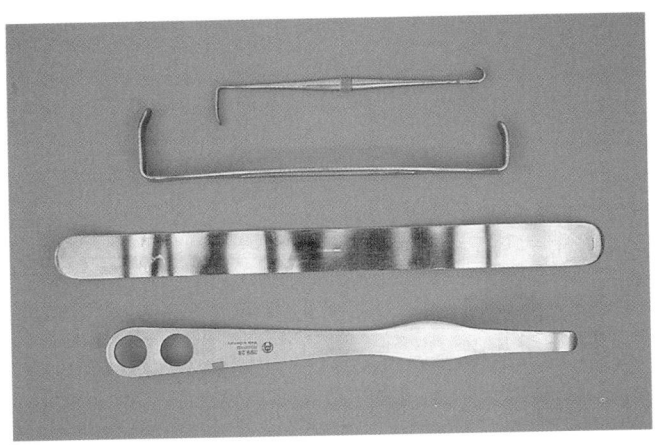

FIG. 8-12
Hand-held retractors. *Top to bottom:* Senn, Army-Navy, malleable, Hohmann.

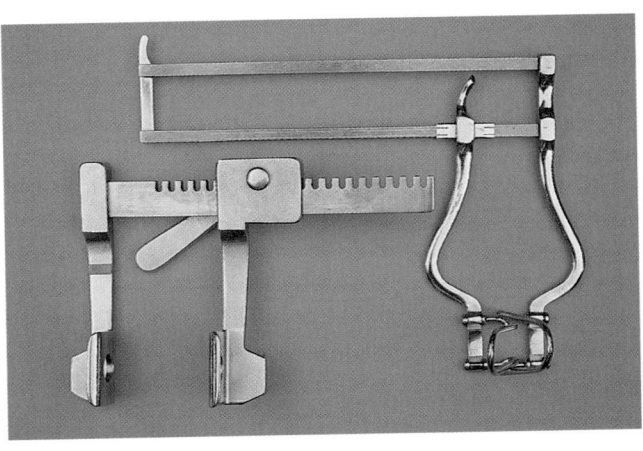

FIG. 8-14
Self-retaining retractors: *Left,* Finochietto; *right,* Balfour.

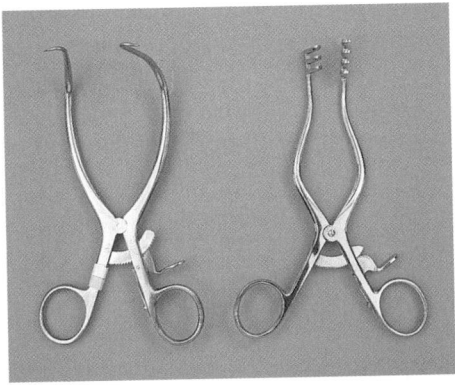

FIG. 8-13
Self-retaining retractors: *Left,* Gelpi; *right,* Weitlaner.

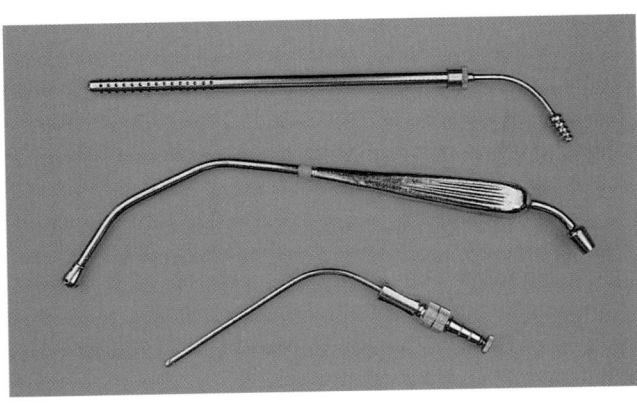

FIG. 8-15
Suction tips. *Top to bottom:* Poole, Yankauer, Frazier.

Retractors

Hand-held retractors (Fig. 8-12) and self-retaining retractors (Fig. 8-13) are used to retract tissue and improve exposure. The ends of hand-held retractors may be hooked, curved, spatula-shaped, or toothed. Some hand-held retractors may be bent (i.e., malleable) to conform to the structure or area of the body being retracted. Senn (rake) retractors are double-ended retractors. One end has three fingerlike, curved prongs; the other end is a flat, curved blade. Self-retaining retractors maintain tension on tissue and are held open with a boxlock (e.g., Gelpi, Weitlaner retractors) or other device (e.g., a set-screw, such as in Balfour and Finochietto retractors [Fig. 8-14]). Balfour retractors generally are used to retract the abdominal wall, and Finochietto retractors are commonly used during thoracotomies.

Miscellaneous Instruments

Instruments are available to suction fluid (Fig. 8-15), clamp drapes or tissues (Fig. 8-16), cut and remove pieces of bones (rongeurs [Figs. 8-17 and 8-18]), hold bones during fracture repair (Fig. 8-19), scrape surfaces of dense tissue (curettes), remove periosteum (periosteal elevators [Fig. 8-20]), cut or shape bone and cartilage (osteotomes and chisels [Fig. 8-21]),

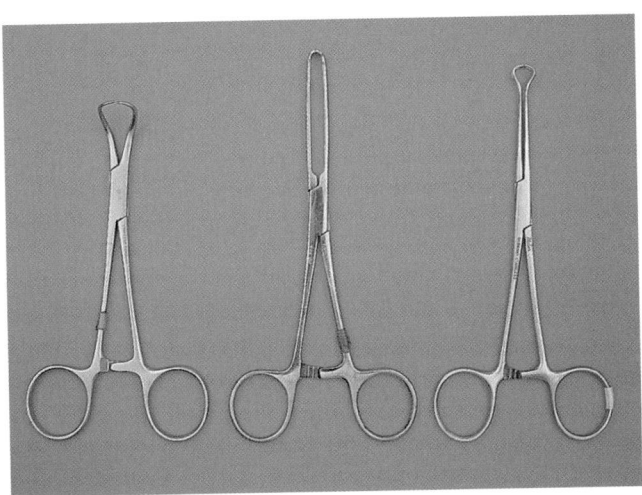

FIG. 8-16
Clamps and forceps. *Left to right:* Backhaus towel clamp, Allis tissue forceps, Babcock forceps.

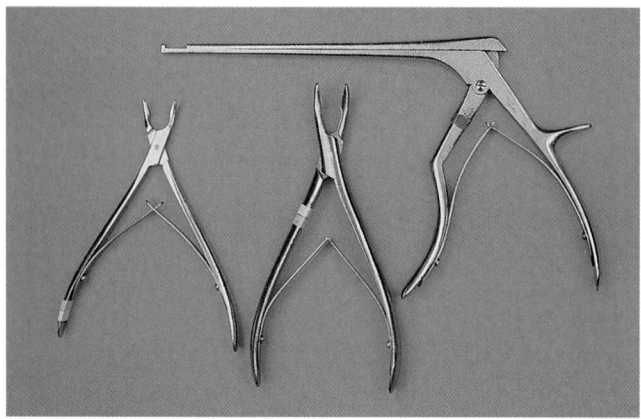

FIG. 8-17
Rongeurs. *Left to right:* Lempert, Ruskin, Kerrison.

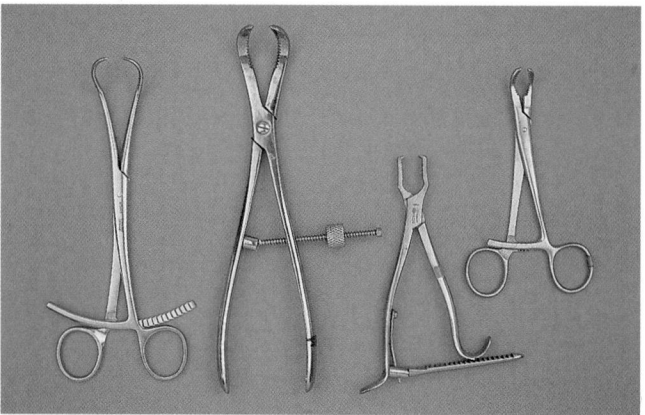

FIG. 8-19
Bone-holding forceps. *Left to right:* AO reduction forceps, large speed-lock reduction forceps, Lane bone-holding forceps, small clamshell reduction forceps.

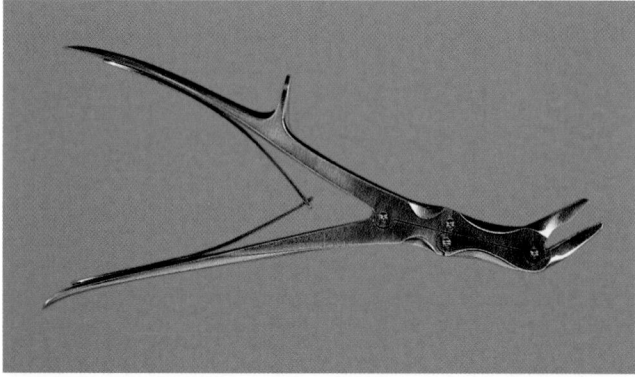

FIG. 8-18
Duck-bill double-action rongeurs.

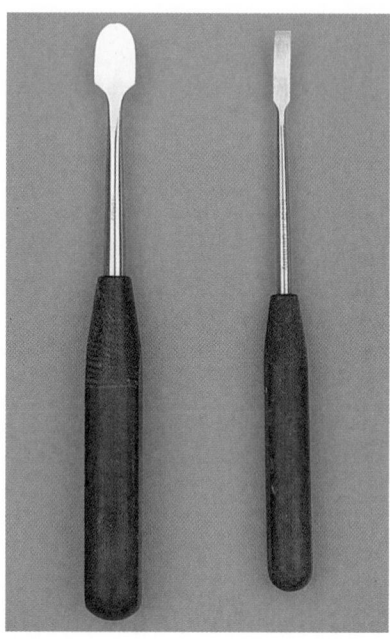

FIG. 8-20
Periosteal elevators. *Left,* AO-round edge; *right,* AO-curved blade, straight edge.

and bore holes in bone (trephines). Magnifying loupes are useful when precise cutting or suturing of tissue is necessary (e.g., cardiovascular or neurologic surgery) and when relatively small tissues are handled (e.g., ureteral anastomoses). Numerous other specialized instruments have been developed to facilitate specific surgical procedures. Some instruments used in orthopedic and neurologic procedures are shown in Figs. 8-22, 8-23, and 8-24. Other orthopedic instruments are described in Chapter 31.

INSTRUMENT CARE AND MAINTENANCE

Good surgical instruments are valuable investments. They must be used properly and receive routine care and maintenance to prevent corrosion, pitting, and discoloration (Table 8-1). Instruments should be rinsed in warm water immediately after the surgical procedure to prevent blood, tissue, saline, or other foreign matter from drying on them. If instruments cannot be immediately cleaned, they should be kept moist under a wet towel.

Many manufacturers recommend that instruments be rinsed, cleaned, and sterilized in distilled or deionized water because tap water contains minerals that may discolor and stain the instruments. If tap water is used for rinsing, instruments should be dried thoroughly to prevent staining. Water

with high mineral counts left to sit on an instrument can cause stains; therefore it is important to dry instruments thoroughly after cleaning. Instruments with several components should be disassembled before cleaning. Delicate instruments should be cleaned and sterilized separately.

Cleaning

Ultrasonic and enzymatic cleaning methods (e.g., a hemolytic enzyme solution such as HaemoSol) effectively and efficiently clean instruments. Enzymatic solutions are typically used to remove proteinaceous materials from general surgical instruments and endoscopic equipment. Soiled instruments should be washed in cleaning solution to remove all

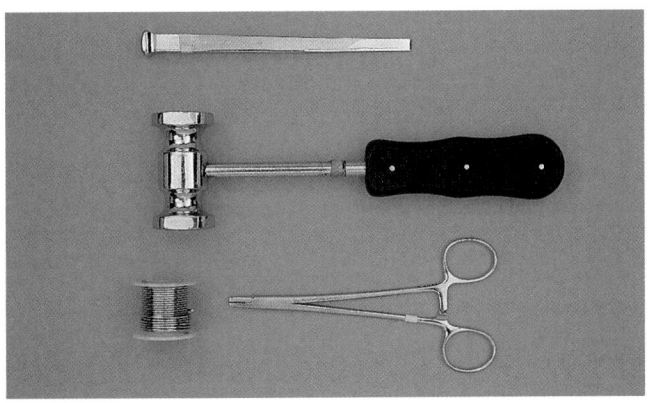

FIG. 8-21
Orthopedic equipment. *Top to bottom:* Chisel, mallet, orthopedic wire, and wire twisters.

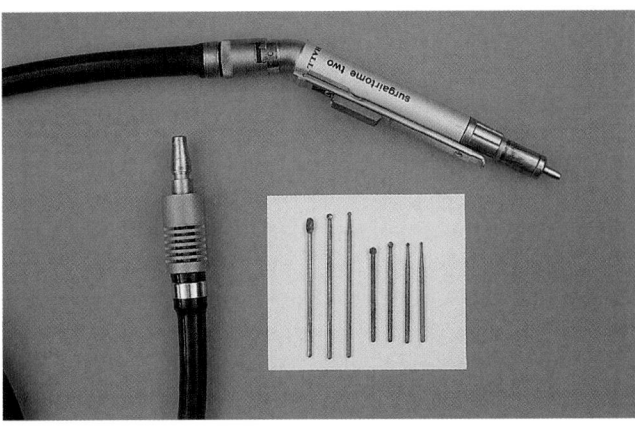

FIG. 8-23
Hall air drill and assorted bits.

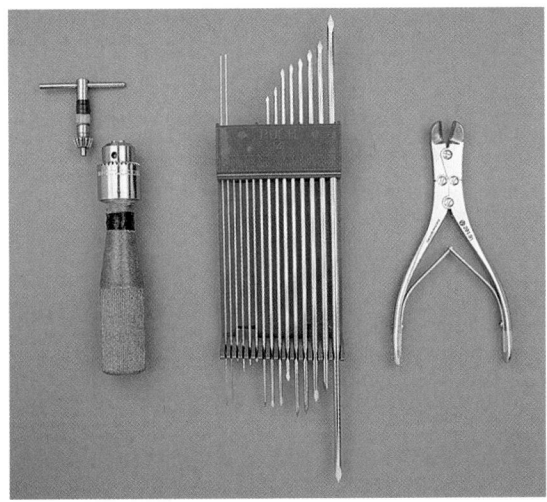

FIG. 8-22
Orthopedic equipment. *Left to right:* Jacobs chuck and key, Steinmann pins and Kirschner wires (pin caddy), bone cutter.

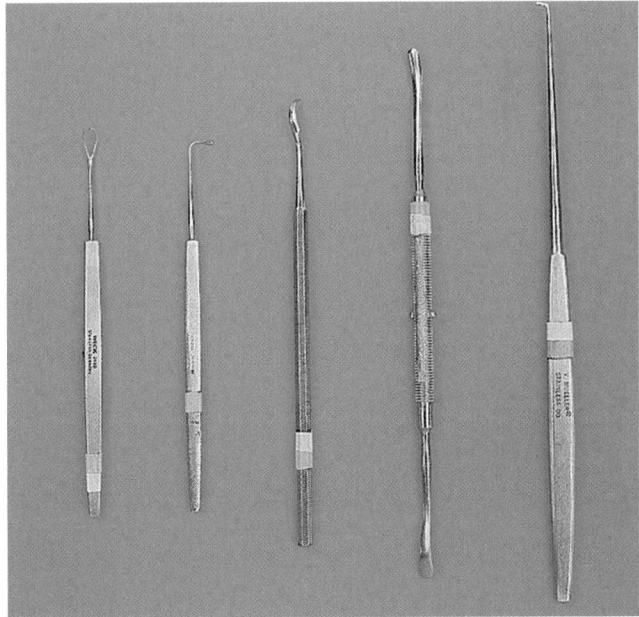

FIG. 8-24
Neurosurgery equipment. *Left to right:* Lens loop; small nerve root retractor; tartar scraper; Freer dissector; large right angle nerve root retractor.

visible debris before being put in an ultrasonic cleaner. Use a soap with a neutral pH (between pH 7 and 8); low pH detergents corrode the protective surface of stainless steel if not fully rinsed off, whereas high pH detergents corrode or cause "browning" of instruments and may impair function.

> NOTE: Do not use Betadine solution, dish soap, laundry soap, or hand scrubbing solutions to clean instruments because these will cause spotting and corrosion.

Dissimilar metals (e.g., chrome and stainless steel) should not be mixed in the same ultrasonic cycle. All instruments should be placed in the ultrasonic cleaner with ratchets and boxlocks open. Instruments should not be piled on top of each other because delicate instruments could be damaged.

They should be removed from the cleaner and rinsed and dried at completion of the cycle. If an ultrasonic cleaner is unavailable, instruments should be cleaned as thoroughly as possible. Use an instrument cleaning brush to remove debris from the jaw serrations, teeth, and hinged areas. Various specialized instrument brushes are available (e.g., Frazier suction tube brushes, laparoscopic brushes, bone reamer brushes, and endoscopic brushes) along with general instrument cleaning brushes. A soft nylon brush or toothbrush may also be used; rasps and serrated areas may require a wire brush. Dry surgical instruments on a clean paper towel. Place the fine tips of surgical hemostats face up on towels to prevent damaging them.

TABLE 8-1

Causes of Instrument Corrosion, Pitting, or Discoloration

TYPE AND CAUSE OF DAMAGE	SOLUTION
Corrosion	
• Excessive moisture left on the surface of the instrument or in the instrument pack	• Preheat the autoclave; allow instruments to cool slowly; check autoclave valves for leaks
• Rinsing with tap water; deposition of alkali earth on walls of autoclave, which deposits on instruments	• Use distilled or deionized water during sterilization; clean autoclave with acetic acid periodically
• Prolonged exposure to enzymatic cleaning solutions	• Do not expose carbon steel instruments to enzymatic cleaners for longer than 5 minutes
Pitting	
• Exposing instruments to saline or foreign materials	• Rinse instruments with distilled water immediately after the procedure
• Detergent residue on instruments during autoclaving	• Avoid detergents with chloride base, which form hydrochloric acid when combined with steam
• Use of alkaline detergents that remove the chromium oxide coat	• Use detergents that have a pH near 7
• Simultaneously cleaning metals of dissimilar composition in an ultrasound cleaner	• Separate instruments made from dissimilar metals during cleaning
Rust Deposition	
• Deposition of iron on instrument from tap water	• Use distilled or deionized water during cleaning, rinsing, and sterilization
• Deposition and oxidation of carbon particles on stainless steel instruments when they are sterilized with chrome-plated instruments that have exposed metal	• Separate the two types of steel during sterilization; replace plated instruments that are peeling or imperfect
Spotting	
• Condensation and slow evaporation of water droplets containing sodium, calcium, and/or magnesium on instruments	• Follow instructions for autoclave use; open door after steam has been exhausted; check valves or gaskets; use distilled or deionized water

Lubricating and Autoclaving

Autoclaving is not a substitute for proper instrument cleaning. Instruments with boxlocks, hinges, and power equipment should be lubricated before autoclaving. Only surgical lubricants should be used because they are steam-penetrable; industrial oils interfere with steam sterilization and should not be used. *It is no longer recommended to use a lubricant bath because the solution may contain bacteria from instruments previously dipped into it. A lubricant spray is advised.* Instruments generally are grouped into packs or kits according to their use (Tables 8-2 and 8-3). Before autoclaving, instruments should be wrapped in cloth or placed on a cloth inside a fenestrated pan to absorb moisture. Instruments should be sterilized with boxlocks or hinges open.

NOTE: NEVER lock an instrument during autoclaving; this prevents steam from reaching and sterilizing overlapping metal surfaces. Hinge areas of forceps and hemostats can expand and crack when exposed to heat during autoclaving if they are locked.

The chamber should not be overloaded, and stacking of instruments should be avoided to prevent damage to delicate instruments. Kits should be double wrapped (see p. 5) and sealed with tape (e.g., autoclave tape), and a monitor (e.g., OK sterilization indicators, Sterrad chemical indicator strip) should be added before autoclaving (see p. 13). Rapid cooling of instruments should be avoided to prevent condensation. Additional information on autoclaving and other methods of sterilization can be found in Chapter 2. Stains should be distinguished from rust (Table 8-4). Stains can be removed, whereas rust causes permanent damage.

NOTE: To determine if a brown or orange discoloration is a stain or rust, use the eraser test. Rub a pencil eraser over the discoloration. If the eraser removes discoloration and the metal underneath is smooth and clean, this is a stain. If a pit mark appears under the discoloration, this is corrosion or rust (Spectrum surgical instruments).

TABLE 8-2

Suggestions for a Basic Soft Tissue Pack*

INSTRUMENT	QUANTITY
Halsted-mosquito hemostats, curved, 5-inch	2
Halsted-mosquito hemostats, straight, 5-inch	2
Kelly hemostats, curved, 5½-inch	2
Crile forceps, straight, 5½-inch	2
Rochester-Carmalt hemostats, curved, 7¼-inch	4
Mayo-Hegar or Olsen-Hegar needle holders, 7-inch	1
Brown-Adson tissue forceps	1
Allis tissue forceps, 5 × 6 teeth, 6-inch	4
Backhaus towel clamps, 5¼-inch	4
Metzenbaum scissors, curved, 8-inch	1
Mayo scissors, curved, 8-inch	1
Suture scissors, sharp-blunt, straight, 5-inch	1
Instrument tray	1
Senn retractors	2
Blade handle, No. 3	1
Ovariohysterectomy "spay" hook	1
Saline bowl	1
Radiopaque sponges (4 × 4 inches)	20

*For spaying, laparotomy, or wound repair.

 TABLE 8-3

Suggestions for a Basic Orthopedic Pack*

INSTRUMENT	QUANTITY
Jacobs chuck and key	1
Hohmann retractor	2
Army-Navy retractor	2
Periosteal elevator	1
Wire twister	1
Medium pin cutter	1
Kern or Lane bone-holding forceps	2
Reduction forceps	1
Orthopedic wire (18, 20, and 22 gauge)	1 each size
Kirschner wires	2 each size
Intramedullary pins	2 each size

*Augmented with a general pack (see Table 8-2).

 TABLE 8-4

Trouble-Shooting Stain Guide for Surgical Instruments*

STAIN COLOR	CAUSE
Brown/orange	High-pH detergents, chlorhexidine, or improper soaking of instruments. May also be caused by soaking in tap water.
Dark brown	Low-pH instrument solutions. The brownish-colored film may also be caused by a malfunctioning sterilizer. Similar localized stain spots may be a result of baked-on blood.
Bluish black	Reverse plating, when instruments of different metal (e.g., chrome and stainless steel) are ultrasonically processed together. Additionally, exposure to saline, blood, or potassium chloride will cause this.
Multicolor	Excessive heat by a localized hot spot in the sterilizer. The rainbow-colored stain can be removed.
Light- and dark-colored spots	Water droplets drying on the instruments. Slow evaporation leaves sodium, calcium, and magnesium deposits.
Bluish gray	Liquid (cold) sterilization solutions being used beyond manufacturer's recommendations.
Black	Contact with ammonia or a solution containing ammonia.
Gray	A liquid rust remover being used in excess of manufacturer's recommendations.
Rust†	Dried blood that has become baked on the serrated or hinged areas of surgical instruments. This organic material, once baked on, may appear dark in color. Also can be caused by soaking in tap water.

*Modified from Spectrum, surgical instruments, repairs, instrument accessories; www.spectrumsurgical.com.
†See box for how to distinguish rust from stains.

Cold Sterilization

Cold sterilization is used for some instruments, but does not guarantee sterility. Instruments that cannot be autoclaved are best sterilized using alternate means (e.g., ethylene oxide or plasma sterilization; see p. 11). Solutions that contain benzyl ammonium chloride (BAC) should not be used with instruments that have tungsten carbide inserts because BAC dissolves tungsten.

DRAPING AND ORGANIZING THE INSTRUMENT TABLE

Instrument tables should be height adjustable to allow them to be positioned within reach of surgical personnel. The instrument table should not be opened until the animal has been positioned on the surgical table and draped. Large, water-impermeable table drapes should cover the entire instrument table. To open these drapes, the drape and outer wrap are positioned on the instrument table. The exposed underneath surface of the drape is gently grasped, and the ends and then the sides are unfolded. Once the drape has been opened, nonsterile personnel should not reach over it. Mayo stands often are used in procedures that require additional instruments, such as bone plating; specially designed stand covers are available for these tables. After the instrument pack has been opened (see p. 6), instruments should be positioned so that they can be readily retrieved. The layout generally is determined by the surgeon's preference, but grouping similar instruments (i.e., scissors and retractors) facilitates their use. Whenever a body cavity is opened, sponges should be counted at the beginning of the procedure (before the incision is made) and again before closure to ensure that none have been inadvertently left in the cavity. Contaminated instruments or soiled sponges should not be placed back on the instrument table.

CHAPTER 9

Biomaterials, Suturing, and Hemostasis

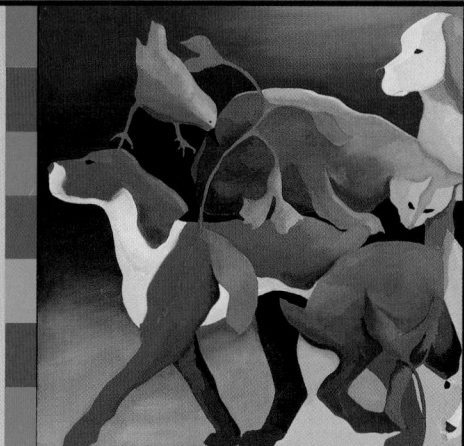

SUTURES AND SUTURE SELECTION

Suture plays an important role in wound repair by providing hemostasis and support for healing tissue. Different tissues have differing requirements for suture support, and they heal at different rates; some tissues need support for only a few days (e.g., muscle, subcutaneous tissue, skin), whereas others require weeks (fascia) or even months (tendon) to heal. Individual patient variation further affects suture choice: healing of wounds may be delayed by infection, obesity, malnutrition, neoplasia, drugs (steroids), and collagen disorders. In rapidly healing tissue, choosing a suture that will lose its tensile strength at about the same rate as the tissue gains strength and that will be absorbed by the tissue so that no foreign material remains in the wound is ideal. Minimally invasive surgical techniques (see Chapter 14) put additional demands on the performance of surgical sutures. Not only must good knot security be maintained, but the surface lubricant must ensure ease of manipulation, minimal tissue drag, and good biocompatibility with minimal inflammatory responses. Subjective preferences, such as familiarity with the material and availability, need also to be taken into consideration.

Suture Characteristics

The ideal suture is easy to handle; reacts minimally in tissue; inhibits bacterial growth; holds securely when knotted; resists shrinking in tissue; is noncapillary, nonallergenic, noncarcinogenic, and nonferromagnetic; and absorbs with minimal reaction after the tissue has healed. Unfortunately, such an ideal suture does not exist. Therefore surgeons must choose a suture that most closely approximates the ideal for a given procedure and tissue to be sutured. A wide variety of suture and needle combinations are available.

Suture size. The smallest diameter suture that will adequately hold the mending wounded tissue should be used to minimize trauma as the suture is passed through the tissue and to reduce the amount of foreign material left in the wound. A suture need be no stronger than the sutured tissue. The most commonly used standard for suture size is the USP (United States Pharmacopeia), which denotes dimensions from fine to coarse (with diameters in inches) according to a numeric scale, with 12-0 being the smallest and 7 the largest. Sutures were originally sized 0 to 3, but as materials advanced and sutures thinner than 0 were developed, extra 0s had to be added. The USP uses different standards for surgical gut and for other materials (Table 9-1). The smaller the suture size, the less tensile strength it has. Stainless steel wire usually is sized according to the metric or USP scale or by the Brown and Sharpe (B and S) wire gauge (see Table 9-1).

Flexibility. The flexibility of a suture is determined by its torsional stiffness and diameter, which influence its handling and use. Flexible sutures are indicated for ligating vessels or performing continuous suture patterns. Less flexible sutures (e.g., wire) cannot be used to ligate small bleeders. Nylon and surgical gut are relatively stiff compared with silk suture; braided polyester sutures have intermediate stiffness.

Surface characteristics and coating. The surface characteristics of a suture influence the ease with which it is pulled through tissue (i.e., the amount of friction or "drag") and the amount of trauma caused. Rough sutures cause more injury than smooth sutures. Smooth surfaces are particularly important in delicate tissues, such as the eye. However, sutures with smooth surfaces also have disadvantages: they require greater tension to ensure good apposition of tissues, and they have less knot security (see p. 60). Braided materials have more drag than monofilament sutures. Braided materials often are coated to reduce capillarity (see later discussion) and provide a smooth surface. Teflon, silicone, wax, paraffin-wax, and calcium stearate are used for coating sutures.

Capillarity. Capillarity is the process by which fluid and bacteria are carried into the interstices of multifilament fibers. Because neutrophils and macrophages are too large to enter the interstices of the fiber, infection may persist, particularly in nonabsorbable sutures. All braided materials (e.g., silk) are capillary; monofilament sutures are less capillary. Coating reduces the capillarity of some sutures. Capillary suture materials should not be used in contaminated or infected sites.

Knot tensile strength. Knot tensile strength is measured by the force (in pounds) that the suture strand can withstand before it breaks when knotted (Box 9-1). Sutures should be as strong as the normal tissue through which they

TABLE 9-1

Suture Sizes

SYNTHETIC SUTURE MATERIALS (USP)	SURGICAL GUT (USP)	BROWN AND SHARPE WIRE GAUGE	METRIC GAUGE	ACTUAL SIZE (MM)
10-0			0.2	0.02
9-0			0.3	0.03
8-0			0.4	0.04
7-0	8-0	41	0.5	0.05
6-0	7-0	38-40	0.7	0.07
5-0	6-0	35	1	0.1
4-0	5-0	32-34	1.5	0.15
3-0	4-0	30	2	0.2
2-0	3-0	28	3	0.3
0	2-0	26	3.5	0.35
1	0	25	4	0.4
2	1	24	5	0.5
3,4	2	22	6	0.6
5	3	20	7	0.7
6	4	19	8	0.8
7		18	9	0.9

USP, United States Pharmacopeia.

 BOX 9-1

Terminology Used to Describe Suture Characteristics*

- Absorbable—Progressive loss of mass and/or volume of suture material; does not correlate with initial tensile strength
- Breaking strength—Limit of tensile strength at which suture failure occurs
- Capillarity—Extent to which absorbed fluid is transferred along the suture
- Elasticity—Measure of the ability of the material to regain its original form and length after deformation
- Fluid absorption—Ability to take up fluid after immersion
- Knot-pull tensile strength—Breaking strength of knotted suture material (10%–40% weaker after deformation by knot placement)
- Knot strength—Amount of force necessary to cause a knot to slip (related to the coefficient of static friction and plasticity of a given material)
- Memory—Inherent capability of suture to return to or maintain its original gross shape (related to elasticity, plasticity, and diameter)
- Plasticity—Measure of the ability to deform without breaking and to maintain a new form after relief of the deforming force
- Pliability—Ease of handling of suture material; ability to adjust knot tension and to secure knots (related to suture material, filament type, and diameter)
- Straight-pull tensile strength—Linear breaking strength of suture material
- Suture pullout value—The application of force to a loop of suture located where tissue failure occurs, which measures the strength of a particular tissue; variable depending on anatomic site and histologic composition (fat, 0.2 kg; muscle, 1.27 kg; skin, 1.82 kg; fascia, 3.77 kg)
- Tensile strength—Measure of a material or tissue's ability to resist deformation and breakage
- Wound breaking strength—Limit of tensile strength of a healing wound at which separation of the wound edges occurs

*From Lai SY, Becker DG: Sutures and needles, e-medicine, Topic 38, 2004.

are being placed; however, the tensile strength of the suture should not greatly exceed the tensile strength of the tissue.

Relative knot security. Relative knot security is the holding capacity of a suture expressed as a percentage of its tensile strength. The knot-holding capacity of a suture mate-

rial is the strength required to untie or break a defined knot by loading the part of the suture that forms the loop, whereas the suture material's tensile strength is the strength required to break an untied fiber with a force applied in the direction of its length (see Box 9-1).

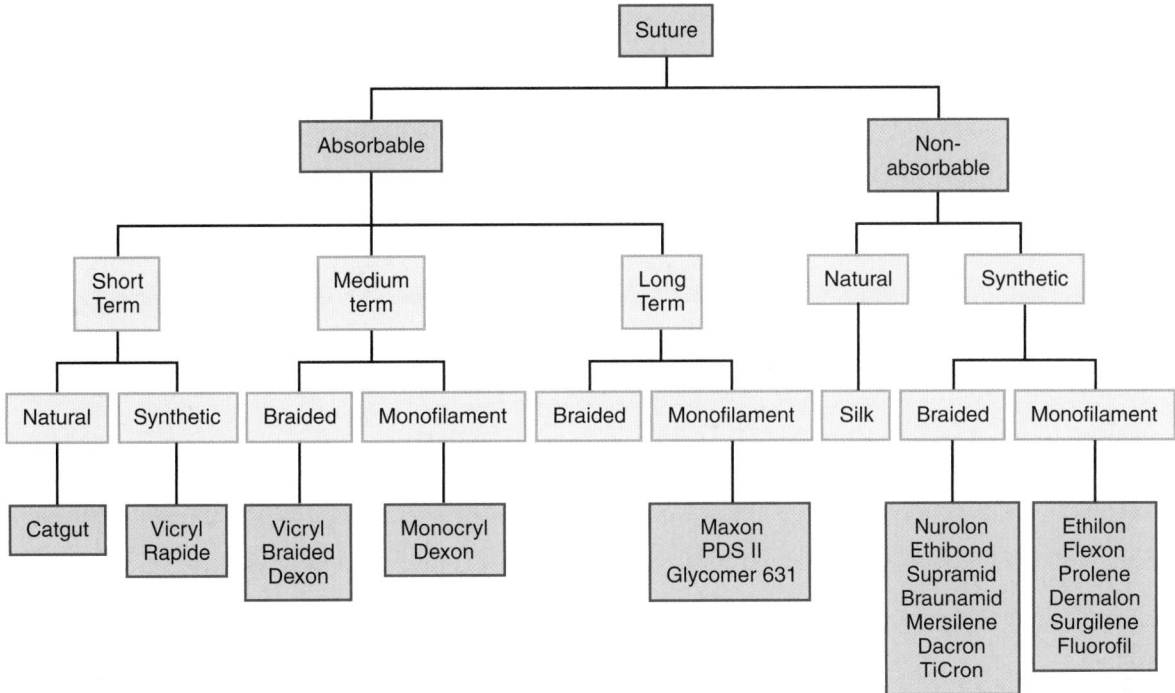

FIG. 9-1
Characteristics of sutures used in veterinary medicine.

Specific Suturing Materials

Suture materials may be classified according to their behavior in tissue (absorbable or nonabsorbable), their structure (monofilament or multifilament), or their origin (synthetic, organic, or metallic) (Fig. 9-1 and Table 9-2). Two major mechanisms of absorption result in the degradation of absorbable sutures. Sutures of biologic origin, such as surgical gut, are gradually digested by tissue enzymes and phagocytized, whereas sutures manufactured from synthetic polymers are principally broken down by hydrolysis. Nonabsorbable sutures are ultimately encapsulated or walled off by fibroblasts.

Monofilament sutures are made of a single strand of material. They have less tissue drag than multifilament sutures and do not have interstices that may harbor bacteria. Care should be used in handling monofilament sutures because nicking or damaging them with forceps or needle holders weakens them and predisposes them to breakage. Multifilament sutures consist of several strands of suture that are twisted or braided together. Multifilament sutures generally are more pliable and flexible than monofilament sutures. They may be coated to reduce tissue drag and enhance handling characteristics (see previous discussion).

Absorbable Suture Materials

Absorbable suture materials (e.g., surgical gut, polyglycolic acid [Dexon], polyglactin 910 [Vicryl], polydioxanone [PDS II], polyglyconate [Maxon], and poliglecaprone 25 [Monocryl]) lose most of their tensile strength within 60 days and eventually disappear from the tissue implantation site because they have been phagocytized or hydrolyzed (see Fig. 9-1 and Table 9-2). The time to loss of strength and for complete absorption varies among suture materials.

Catgut (surgical gut). The word *catgut* is derived from the term *kitgut* or *kitstring* (the string used on a kit, or fiddle). Misinterpretation of the word *kit* as referring to a young cat led to the use of the term catgut. Surgical gut actually is made from the submucosa of sheep intestine or the serosa of bovine intestine and is approximately 90% collagen. It is broken down by phagocytosis and, compared with other suture materials, elicits a notable inflammatory reaction. Plain surgical gut loses strength rapidly after tissue implantation. "Tanning" (cross-linking of collagen fibers), which occurs by exposure to chrome or aldehyde, slows absorption. Surgical gut is available as plain, medium chromic, or chromic; increased tanning generally implies prolonged strength and reduced tissue reaction. Surgical gut is rapidly removed from infected sites or areas where it is exposed to digestive enzymes and is quickly degraded in catabolic patients. The knots may loosen when wet.

Synthetic absorbable materials. Synthetic absorbable materials (e.g., polyglycolic acid, polyglactin 910, polydioxanone, polyglyconate, poliglecaprone 25, and glycomer 631 [BIOSYN]) generally are broken down by hydrolysis. Polyglycolic acid is braided from filaments extracted from glycolic acid. It loses 35% of its tensile strength by 14 days and 65% by 21 days. Polyglycolic acid is available in both coated and uncoated forms. Polyglactin 910 is a multifilament suture made of a copolymer of lactide and glycolide with polyglactin 370. It is coated with calcium stearate. Its rate of loss of tensile strength is similar to that of polyglycolic acid. Polydioxanone and polyglyconate are monofila-

TABLE 9-2

Characteristics of Suture Materials Commonly Used in Veterinary Medicine

GENERIC NAME	TRADE NAME	MANUFACTURER	SUTURE CHARACTERISTICS	REDUCTION IN TENSILE STRENGTH*	COMPLETE ABSORPTION (DAYS)	RELATIVE KNOT SECURITY†	TISSUE REACTION‡
Chromic surgical gut (catgut)	–	–	Absorbable Multifilament	33% at 7 days	60	– Wet	+++
Polyglactin 910	Vicryl	Ethicon	Absorbable Multifilament	35% at 21 days; 60% at 14 days	56-70	++	+
	Vicryl Rapide			50% at 5-6 days; 100% at 2 weeks	42	++	+
	Vicryl Plus	Ethicon		25% at 2 weeks; 50% at 3 weeks	56-70	++	+
Polyglycolic acid	Dexon "S" (uncoated)	Davis & Geck	Absorbable Multifilament	35% at 14 days	60-90	++	+
	Dexon II (coated)			65% at 21 days			
Polydioxanone	PDS II	Ethicon	Absorbable Monofilament	14% at 14 days	180	++	+
				31% at 42 days			
Polyglyconate	Maxon	Davis & Geck	Absorbable Monofilament	30% at 14 days	180	++	+
				45% at 21 days			
Poliglecaprone 25	Monocryl	Ethicon	Absorbable Monofilament	40%-50% at 7 days	90-120	++	+
				70%-80% at 14 days			
Glycomer 631	Biosyn	Davis & Geck	Absorbable Monofilament	25% at 2 weeks	90-110	++	+
				60% at 3 weeks			
Silk	Perma-Hand	Ethicon Davis & Geck	Nonabsorbable Multifilament	30% at 14 days 50% at 1 year	>2 years	–	+++
Polyester	Mersilene (uncoated) Ethibond (coated) Dacron (uncoated) Ti●cron (coated)	Ethicon Ethicon Davis & Geck Davis & Geck	Nonabsorbable Multifilament			–	++
Polyamide (Nylon)	Ethilon (monofilament) Nurolon (multifilament) Dermalon (monofilament) Surgilon (multifilament)	Ethicon Ethicon Davis & Geck Davis & Geck	Nonabsorbable Monofilament or multifilament	30% at 2 years (monofilament) 75% at 180 days (multifilament)		+	–
Polypropylene	Prolene Surgilene Fluorofil	Ethicon Davis & Geck Mallinckrodt Veterinary	Nonabsorbable Monofilament			+++	–
Polybutester	Novafil	Davis & Geck	Nonabsorbable Monofilament			++	–
Polymerized caprolactam	Supramid Braunamid Vetcassette II	S. Jackson B. Braun Melsungen Ag Mallinckrodt Veterinary	Nonabsorbable Multifilament			++	++ (if coating breaks)
Stainless steel wire	Flexon (multifilament)	Davis & Geck Ethicon	Nonabsorbable Monofilament or Multifilament			+++	–

*Values given are approximate. Actual loss of tensile strength may vary depending on suture and tissue.
† (–), Poor (<60%); (+), fair (60% to 70%); (++), good (70% to 85%); (+++), excellent (>85%).
‡ (–), Minimal to none; (+), mild; (++), moderate; (+++), severe.

ment sutures that retain their tensile strength longer than polyglycolic acid or polyglactin 910. Polydioxanone suture has a 14% loss of tensile strength in 14 days, 31% in 42 days, and complete absorption in 6 months. Calcinosis circumscripta has been associated with polydioxanone suture in dogs. Glycomer 631 is synthetic absorbable suture prepared from a polyester that is composed of glycolide (60%), dioxanone (14%), and trimethylene carbonate (26%). It is a monofilament suture that maintains approximately 75% of its USP tensile strength at 2 weeks and 40% at 3 weeks postimplant. Absorption is complete between 90 and 110 days.

Polyglactin 910 and polyglycolic acid are more rapidly hydrolyzed in alkaline environments, but are relatively stable in contaminated wounds. Polyglycolic acid, polyglactin 910, and poliglecaprone 25 may be rapidly degraded in infected urine; polydioxanone, polyglyconate, and glycomer 631 are acceptable for use in sterile bladders and those infected with *E. coli*. However, use of any suture that is degraded via hydrolysis may be risky when the bladder is infected with *Proteus* spp. (see also p. 677). A recent study found that all monofilament absorbable sutures degraded within 7 days in *P. mirabilis*–inoculated urine (Greenberg et al, 2004).

Absorbable suture materials cause minimal tissue reaction, and the time to loss of strength and to absorption is fairly constant in different tissue. Infection or exposure to digestive enzymes does not significantly influence the rate of absorption of most synthetic absorbable sutures. Poliglecaprone 25 is a pliable, synthetic absorbable, monofilament suture made from a co-polymer of glycolide and epsilon caprolactone. Because it lacks stiffness, it has little "memory" and good handling characteristics. Vicryl Rapide (polyglactin 910) is a new rapidly absorbed, synthetic braided suture that has an initial strength that is comparable to nylon and gut. However, the tensile strength declines to 50% in 5 to 6 days, and it is completely absorbed in 42 days. This suture is indicated for superficial closure of mucosa, gingival closure, and periocular skin closure. Vicryl Plus is a new suture that was designed to reduce bacterial colonization on the suture. It has been coated with an antibacterial agent, triclosan.

Nonabsorbable Suture Materials

Organic nonabsorbable materials. Silk is the most common organic nonabsorbable suture material used. It is a braided multifilament suture made by a special type of silkworm and is marketed as uncoated or coated. Silk has excellent handling characteristics and often is used in cardiovascular procedures; however, it does not maintain significant tensile strength after 6 months and therefore is contraindicated for use in vascular grafts. It should also be avoided in contaminated sites; one silk suture may reduce the number of bacteria required to induce infection in a wound from 10^6 to 10^3.

Synthetic nonabsorbable materials. Synthetic nonabsorbable suture materials (see Table 9-2) are marketed as braided multifilament threads (e.g., polyester or coated caprolactam) or monofilament threads (e.g., polypropylene, polyamide, polyolefins, or polybutester). They typically are strong and induce minimal tissue reaction. Nonabsorbable suture materials, which consist of an inner core and an outer sheath (e.g., Supramid), should not be buried in tissue because they may predispose to infection and fistulation. The outer sheath frequently is broken, which allows bacteria to reside under it.

> NOTE: Cable ties should NEVER be implanted in the body (e.g., used to ligate ovarian pedicles) because toxic substances are released during their degradation, and their use may result in abscess or tumor formation.

Metallic sutures. Stainless steel is the metallic suture most commonly used. It is available as a monofilament or multifilament twisted wire. Tissue reaction to stainless steel generally is minimal, but the knot ends evoke an inflammatory reaction. Stainless steel has a tendency to cut tissue and may fragment and migrate. It is stable in contaminated wounds and is the standard for judging knot security and tissue reaction to suture materials.

Surgical Needles

A variety of needle shapes and sizes are available; selection of a needle depends on the type of tissue to be sutured (e.g., penetrability, density, elasticity, and thickness), the topography of the wound (e.g., deep or narrow), and the characteristics of the needle (i.e., type of eye, length, and diameter). Needle strength, ductility, and sharpness are important factors in determining the handling characteristics and use of a needle. The amount of angular deformation a needle can withstand before becoming permanently deformed is called surgical yield. Ductility is the needle's resistance to breaking under a specified amount of bending. The sharpness of a needle is related to the angle of the point (see p. 62) and the taper ratio of the needle. The sharpest needles have a long, thin, tapered point with smooth cutting edges. Most surgical needles are made from stainless steel wire because it is strong and corrosion free, and does not harbor bacteria.

The three basic components of a needle are the attachment end (i.e., swaged or eyed end), the body, and the point (Fig. 9-2, *A*). Eyed needles must be threaded, and because a double strand of suture is pulled through the tissue, a larger hole is created than when swaged suture material is used. Eyed needles may be closed (i.e., round, oblong, or square) or French (i.e., with a slit from the inside of the eye to the end of the needle for ease of threading) (Fig. 9-2, *B*). Eyed needles are threaded from the inside curvature. With swaged sutures, the needle and suture are a continuous unit, which minimizes tissue trauma and increases ease of use.

The needle body comes in a variety of shapes (Fig. 9-2, *C*); the tissue type and depth and the size of the wound determine the appropriate needle shape. Straight (Keith) needles generally are used in accessible places where the needle can be manipulated directly with the fingers (e.g.,

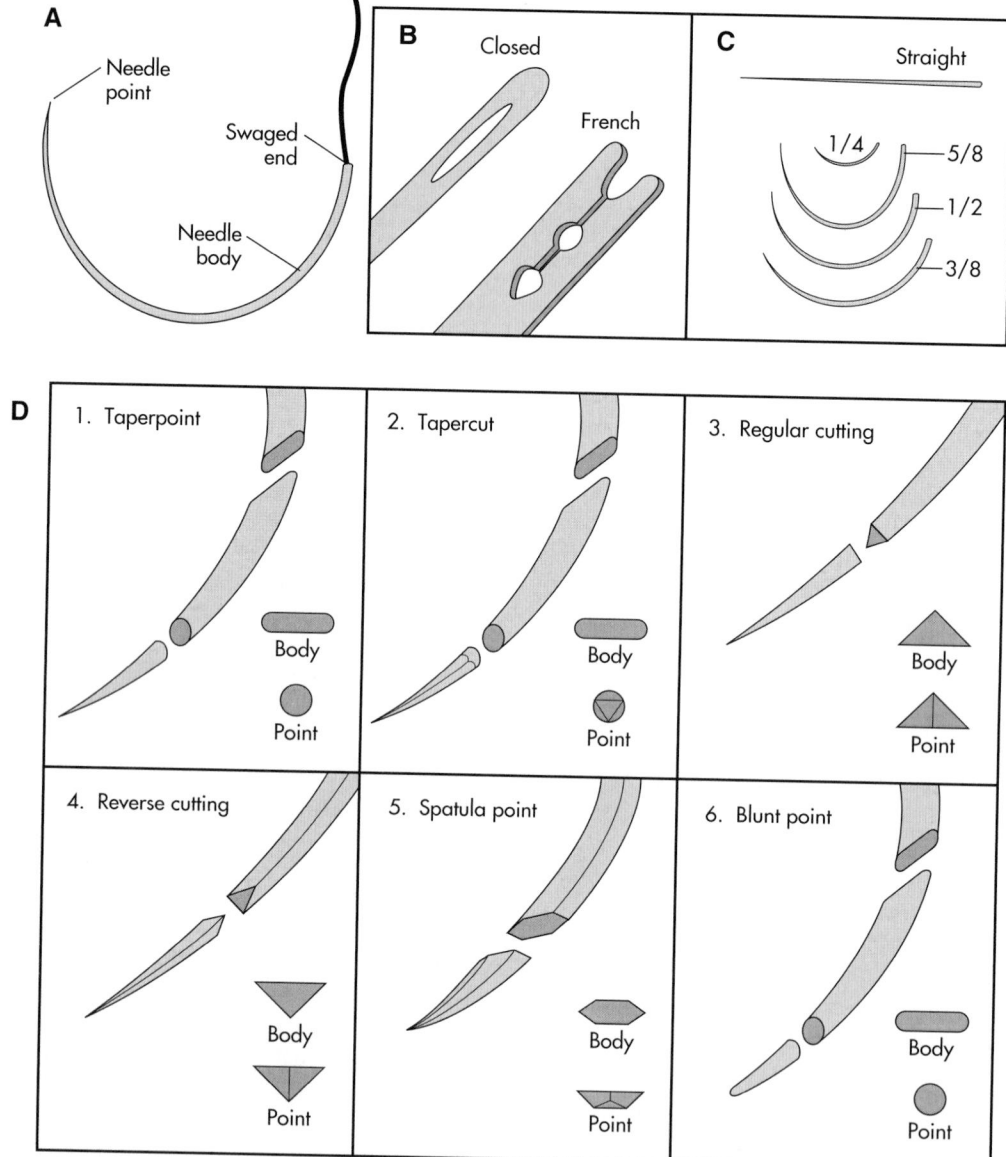

FIG. 9-2
A, Basic components of a needle. **B,** Types of eyed needles. **C** and **D,** Needle body shapes and sizes.

placement of purse-string sutures in the anus). Curved needles are manipulated with needle holders. The depth and diameter of a wound are important when selecting the most appropriate curved needle. One-fourth (¼) circle needles are primarily used in ophthalmic procedures. Three-eighths (⅜) and one-half (½) circle needles are the most commonly used surgical needles in veterinary medicine (e.g., for abdominal closure). Three-eighths circle needles are more easily manipulated than one-half circle needles because they require less pronation and supination of the wrist. However, because of the larger arc of manipulation required, they are awkward to use in deep or inaccessible locations. A one-half circle or five-eighths (⅝) circle needle, despite requiring more pronation and supination of the wrist, is easier to use in confined locations.

The needle point (i.e., cutting, taper, reverse cutting, or side cutting) (Fig. 9-2, *D*) affects the sharpness of a needle and the type of tissue in which the needle is used. Cutting needles generally have two or three opposing cutting edges. They are designed to be used in tissues that are difficult to penetrate, such as skin. With conventional *cutting needles,* the third cutting edge is on the inside (i.e., concave) curvature of the needle. The location of the inside cutting edge may promote "cut out" of tissue because it cuts toward the edges of the wound or incision. *Reverse cutting* needles have a third cutting edge on the outer (i.e., convex) curvature of the needle; this makes them stronger than similarly sized conventional cutting needles and reduces the risk of tissue cut out. *Side cutting needles* (i.e., spatula needles) are flat on the top and bottom. They generally are used in ophthalmic procedures. *Taper needles* (i.e., round needles) have a sharp tip that pierces and spreads tissues without cutting them. They generally are used in easily penetrated tissues, such as the intestine, subcutaneous tissue, or fascia. *Tapercut needles*, which are a combination of a reverse cutting edge tip and a taperpoint body, generally are used for suturing dense, tough fibrous tissue, such as a tendon, and for some cardiovascular procedures, such as vascular grafts. *Bluntpoint needles* have a rounded, blunt point that can dissect through friable tissue without cutting. They occasionally are used for suturing soft, parenchymal organs, such as the liver or kidney.

Suture Selection for Different Tissue Types

Considerations for suture selection include the length of time the suture will be required to help strengthen the wound or tissue, the risk of infection, the effect of the suture material on wound healing, and the dimension and strength of the suture required.

Abdominal closure. Monofilament sutures should be used in skin to prevent wicking or capillary transport of bacteria to deeper tissue. Synthetic monofilament nonabsorbable sutures (e.g., Prolene, Novafil, and Fluorofil) generally have good relative knot security and are relatively noncapillary. Polymerized caprolactam (Supramid, Vetafil) has good handling characteristics, but because it is braided it should not be buried in deeper tissue. Absorbable sutures (e.g., PDS or Maxon) may be used in skin, but they should be removed because absorption requires contact with body fluids. Subcutaneous sutures are used to obliterate dead space and reduce tension on skin edges; absorbable suture material (e.g., PDS II, Maxon, Monocryl) is preferred.

The rectus fascia may be closed with either an interrupted or a continuous suture pattern; however, most surgeons routinely close the rectus fascia with a simple continuous suture pattern. When using an interrupted pattern, numerous suture materials are adequate; however, suture that is rapidly removed (e.g., surgical gut) should be avoided in catabolic (i.e., hypoalbuminemic and malnourished) patients. When a continuous suture pattern is used, a strong monofilament suture with good knot security should be used (e.g., PDS II, Maxon, Prolene, or Novafil). One size larger suture than would normally be used is preferred for a continuous suture pattern. The knots should be tied carefully, and three or four square knots (six or eight throws) should be placed. Absorbable suture (e.g., PDS II or Maxon) may be preferable to prevent large amounts of foreign material from remaining permanently in the incision.

Muscle and tendon. Muscle has poor holding power and is difficult to suture. Absorbable or nonabsorbable suture material may be used. Sutures placed parallel to the muscle fibers are likely to pull out. Suture material used for tendon repair should be strong, nonabsorbable, and minimally reactive. Suturing with a taper or taper-cut needle generally is less traumatic. The largest suture that will pass without trauma through the tendon should be used.

Parenchymal organs. Parenchymal organs, such as the liver, spleen, and kidneys, generally are sutured with ab-sorbable monofilament sutures. Multifilament sutures should be avoided in areas of contamination, and sutures with increased drag (e.g., Dexon or Vicryl) may tend to cut through tissue.

Hollow viscus organs. Absorbable sutures generally are recommended in hollow viscus organs, such as the trachea, gastrointestinal tract, or bladder, to prevent tissue retention of foreign material once the wound is healed. Also, nonabsorbable suture may be calculogenic when placed in the urinary bladder or gallbladder. Dexon suture rapidly dissolves when incubated in sterile urine (6 days) or infected urine (3 days). See also under Synthetic Absorbable Materials section.

Infected or contaminated wounds. If possible, sutures should be avoided in highly contaminated or infected wounds because even the least-reactive nonabsorbable sutures elicit some degree of infection in tissue contaminated with either *Escherichia coli* or *Staphylococcus aureus*. Multifilament nonabsorbable sutures (e.g., silk or polyester) should not used in infected tissue because they potentiate infection and may fistulate. Absorbable suture material is preferred; however, surgical gut should be avoided because its absorption in infected tissue is unpredictable. Synthetic monofilament nylon and polypropylene sutures may elicit less infection in contaminated tissue than metallic sutures.

Vessels and vascular anastomoses. Vessels should be ligated with absorbable suture material. Vascular anastomosis are typically performed with monofilament nonabsorbable suture material such as Prolene. Nonabsorbable suture should also be used for vascular grafts. Arterial anastomoses may be performed in an end-end (Fig. 9-3, *A*) or end-side fashion (Fig. 9-3, *B*). Arteriotomies may be closed using a vertical (Fig. 9-4, *A*) or transverse (Fig. 9-4, *B*) method.

Reduction of blood loss from a vascular anastomosis (e.g., when a polytetrafluoroethylene [PTFE] graft is used) can be affected by suture choice, even when a technically perfect anastomosis has been performed. This is because bleeding may occur from the needle holes. Sutures having a needle-to-suture ratio of 2:1 or 3:1 are associated with more bleeding than when the needle-to-suture diameter ratio is 1:1. Theoretically, this allows the suture to completely fill the graft needle hole and control bleeding.

OTHER BIOMATERIALS
Tissue Adhesives

Cyanoacrylates (e.g., N-butyl and isobutyl-2-cyanoacrylate) are commonly used for tissue adhesion during some procedures, such as declawing, tail docking, and ear cropping. Products advocated for use in veterinary patients include Tissueglue, Vetbond, and Nexabond. These adhesives rapidly polymerize in the presence of moisture and produce a strong, flexible bond. Adhesion of the contact tissue generally takes less than a minute, but may be prolonged with excessive hemorrhage. Persistence of the glue in the dermis may result in granuloma formation or dehiscence, and placement in an infected site may be associated with fistula-

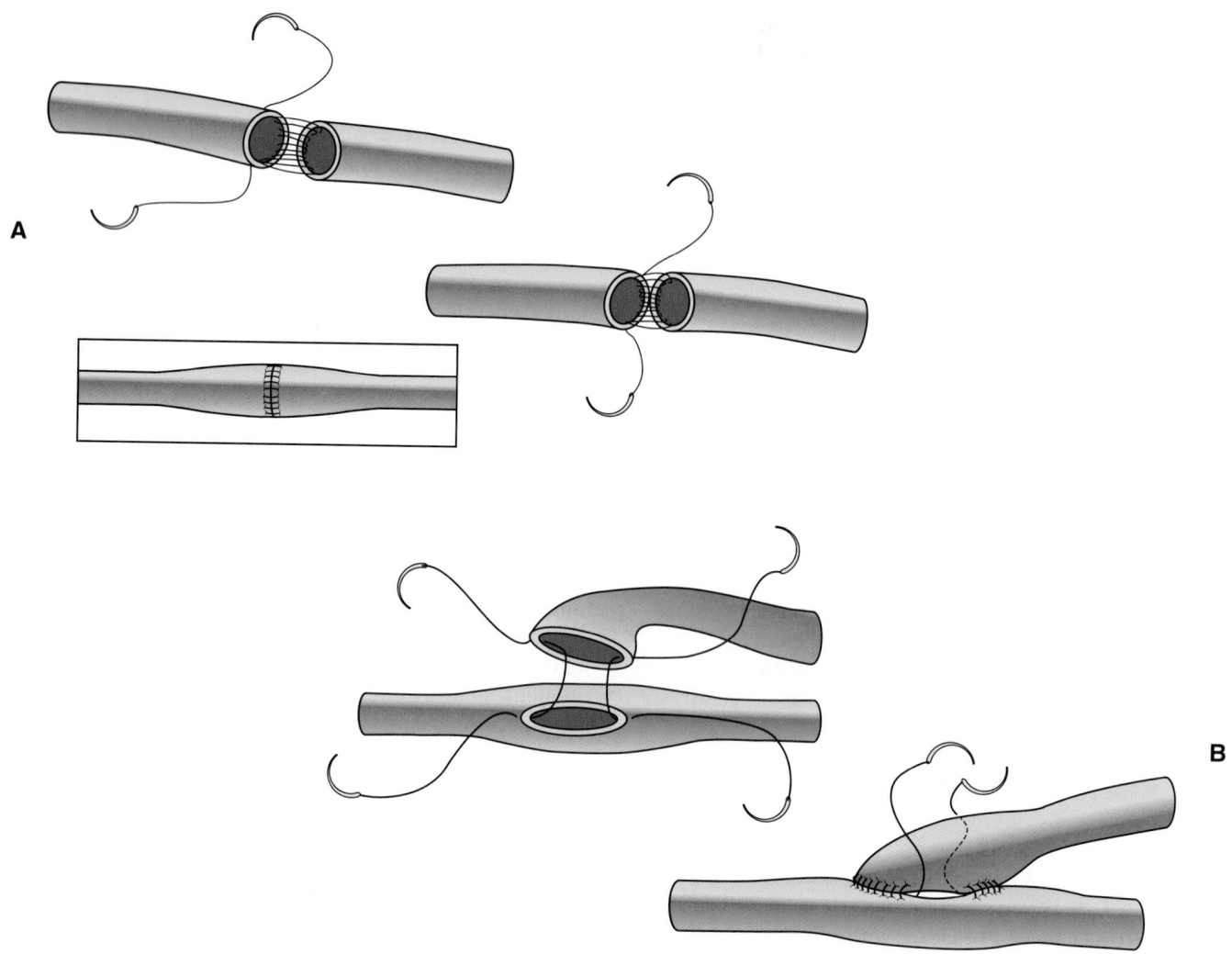

FIG. 9-3
To perform an end-end arterial anastomosis, **A,** approximate the vessel ends and place two stay sutures at equidistant points (usually at the corners) between the ends. Use these sutures to hold the vessel steady and rotate the vessel if required while the anastomosis is being performed. Place over and over sutures at 2 mm intervals, 2 mm from the edge of the vessel beginning at the posterior wall (away from the surgeon) and continuing to the anterior wall. If stenosis is a concern, spatulate the ends. **B,** For an end-side anastomosis, place sutures initially at the cranial (head) and caudal aspect (toe) of the two ends. Perform the anastomosis circumferentially, beginning with the posterior wall first and progressing to the anterior wall.

tion. Heat generated during the procedure may cause tissue burns. Cyanoacrylate adhesives cause an intense inflammatory reaction within subcutaneous tissue and should never be applied within deep wounds.

Dermabond (2-octylcyanoacrylate) is an adhesive to which special plasticizers have been added to provide flexibility. It reaches maximum bonding strength within 2½ minutes and is equivalent in strength to healed tissue at 7 days after repair. It is marketed for humans as a replacement for sutures that are 4-0 to 5-0 or smaller in diameter for incisional or laceration repair. Adhesives should not be used on bite wounds, severely contaminated wounds, ulcers, puncture wounds, mucous membranes, near the eye, or in areas of high

moisture content. They are most useful when they are used on wounds that close spontaneously, have clean or sharp edges, and are located on clean, nonmobile areas. Wounds in which the edges are separated more than 5 mm by the underlying skin tension are unlikely to stay closed with tissue adhesives alone and should be supported with subcutaneous sutures. Reliable closure of lacerations longer than 5 cm is also uncertain when tissue adhesives alone are used.

To apply tissue adhesives, clean the wound and control bleeding. Absolute dryness is not required. Hold the wound together with the edges slightly everted with tissue forceps. Apply the adhesive by lightly wiping the applicator tip over the area (at least 5 mm beyond the skin edges) in the direc-

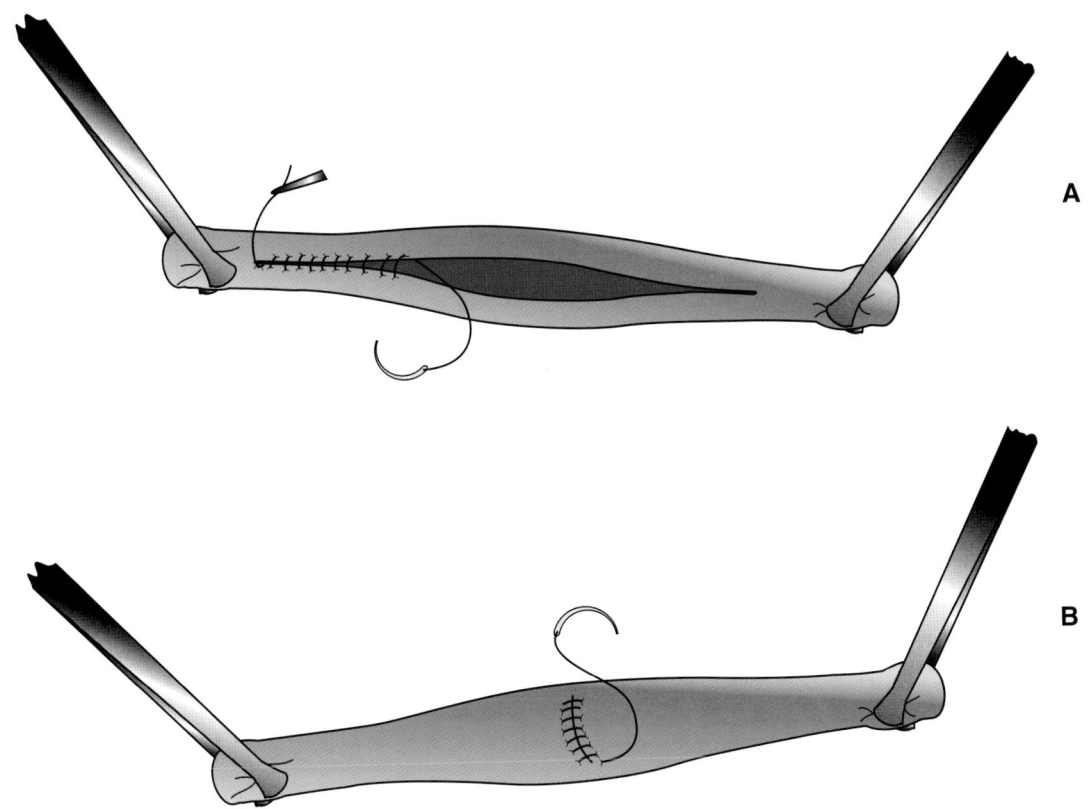

FIG. 9-4
An arteriotomy may be closed **(A)** vertically or **(B)** transversely.

tion of the long axis of the wound. Apply three to four thin layers successively; avoid a droplet or a single thick layer. Hold the wound edges together for about 60 seconds after the last adhesive application to ensure that the adhesive has time to set fully. Remove adhesive applied to unwanted areas by using petroleum jelly or acetone. Do not cover with ointment, bandage, or a dressing. After 24 hours, gently wash the area with plain water, but do not scrub, soak, or expose it to moisture for any length of time. The adhesive will spontaneously slough off in 5 to 10 days.

Adhesive Surgical Membranes

Adhesive surgical membranes or tapes designed for wound closure are available; however, there have been few reports of their use in veterinary patients. One study of the use of an adhesive polyurethane membrane for skin closure in cats found that it was quicker and easier to apply than sutures (Court and Bellenger, 1989). It adhered strongly to skin and provided adequate support. Histologically, wounds closed with the polyurethane membrane were characterized by milder inflammatory reactions and greater vascular infiltration than sutured wounds.

Staples and Ligating Clips

Clips (e.g., hemoclips or ligaclips) may be used for vessel ligation. They are particularly useful when the vessel is difficult to reach or when several vessels must be ligated. How-

ever, ligating clips are not recommended for use on vessels larger than 11 mm in diameter. The vessel should be dissected free of surrounding tissue before the clip is applied, and 2 to 3 mm of vessel should extend beyond the clip to prevent slippage. The vessel should be one-third to two-thirds the size of the clip.

Staples (e.g., Michel clips, Proximate Plus skin staples) are used to appose wound edges or attach drapes to the skin. When staples are used for skin closure, the staple must be appropriately bent so that it cannot be easily removed by the animal. A special staple remover facilitates clip removal after healing. Skin closure by metal staples is quick and economical. An additional advantage of staples is their low level of tissue reactivity; wounds with staple closure exhibit resistance to infection similar to minimally reactive suture. *When placing staples, hold the wound edges together with tissue forceps. Place the stapling device gently (not firmly or with pressure) against the skin surface and slowly squeeze the trigger.* Stainless steel staples are commonly used in thoracic anastomoses (e.g., pulmonary resection or right atrial tumor resection) and gastrointestinal anastomoses (see p. 453).

Autologous Fibrin Glue

Autologous fibrin glue is a biologic adhesive made of fibrinogen, factor XIII, fibronectin, thrombin, apoprotinin, and calcium chloride. It is made from the patient's blood before surgery. In humans, uses of the glue include fixation of skin grafts (i.e., without sutures) and stabilization of gastrointestinal and nerve anastomoses. It also has been used as a preclot material on vascular grafts and as a seal for sutured vascular anastomoses. There is limited experience with the use of fibrin glue in small animals.

Surgical Mesh

Surgical mesh may be used to repair hernias (e.g., perineal hernias) or reinforce traumatized or devitalized tissue (abdominal hernias). Occasionally, it is used to replace excised, traumatized, or neoplastic tissue (see p. 895). Surgical mesh is available in nonabsorbable forms (e.g., Mersilene [polyester] fiber mesh and Prolene [polypropylene] mesh) or absorbable forms (e.g., Vicryl [polyglactin 910] and Dexon [polyglycolic acid]) and in woven and knitted forms. Although surgical mesh generally is elastic, it does not stretch significantly as the patient grows and thus should be used cautiously in immature patients. Fibrous tissue grows through the mesh interstices. New surgical mesh has been developed that has a thin, bioresorbable fabric layer that effectively separates the strong, supportive mesh from underlying tissue (Proceed Mesh, Ethicon). It is being advocated for use in the abdominal cavity. Nonabsorbable mesh placed in contaminated wounds may extrude or fistulate and should be removed when the tissue has healed and the mesh is no longer required for support. A recent study determined that implantation of polypropylene mesh facilitated the reconstruction of large tissue defects and was not associated with any serious complications (Bowman et al, 1998).

COMMON SUTURE TECHNIQUES
Suture Patterns

Suture patterns can be classified as interrupted or continuous by the way they appose tissue (e.g., appositional, everting, or inverting) or by which tissues they primarily appose (e.g., subcutaneous or subcuticular). Appositional sutures (e.g., simple interrupted sutures) bring the tissue in close approximation; everting sutures (e.g., continuous mattress sutures) turn the tissue edges outward, away from the patient and toward the surgeon. Inverting sutures (e.g., Lembert, Connell, and Cushing sutures) turn tissue away from the surgeon, or toward the lumen of a hollow viscus organ.

Subcutaneous and subcuticular patterns. Subcutaneous sutures are placed to eliminate dead space and provide some apposition of skin so that less tension is placed on skin sutures (Fig. 9-5, *A*). Subcutaneous sutures generally are placed in a simple continuous manner; however, in some instances, such as when drainage might be necessary, simple interrupted sutures are preferable. Subcuticular closure may be used in place of skin sutures to reduce scarring or eliminate the need for suture removal in such cases as castration or a fractious patient. The suture is begun by burying the knot in the dermis (see p. 70). The suture is advanced in the subcuticular tissue, but in contrast to a continuous subcutaneous line, the bites are parallel to the long axis of the incision (Fig. 9-5, *B*). The suture line is completed with a buried

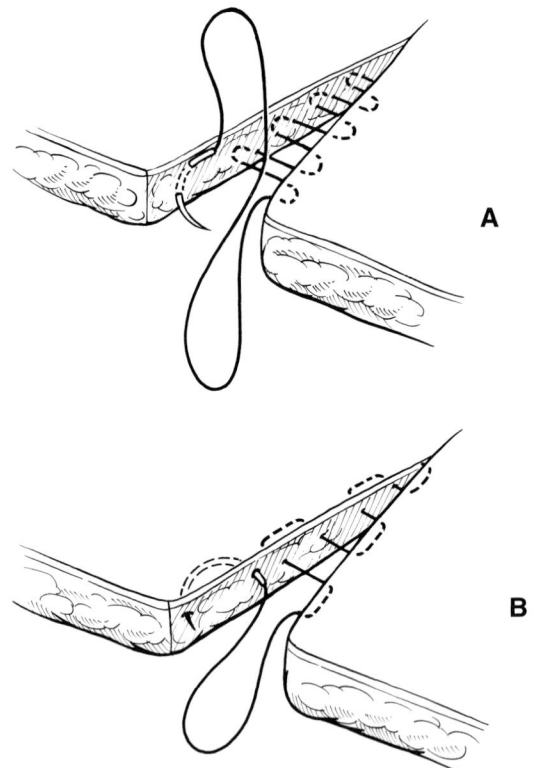

FIG. 9-5
Suture patterns. **A,** Subcutaneous. **B,** Subcuticular.

knot. Absorbable suture material is preferred for subcuticular suture patterns.

Interrupted Suture Patterns

Simple interrupted pattern. A simple interrupted suture is made by inserting the needle through tissue on one side of an incision or wound, passing it to the opposite side, and tying (Fig. 9-6, *A*). The knot is offset so that it does not rest on the incision, and the ends of the suture are cut (for skin sutures, the ends are left long enough to allow them to be grasped during removal). The sutures should be placed approximately 2 to 3 mm away from the skin edge. Right-handed surgeons place sutures from right to left in a horizontal fashion; left-handed surgeons do the opposite.

Simple interrupted sutures are easy and quick to place. They are appositional unless excessive tension is applied; then inversion may occur. Inversion of skin results in poor healing, therefore care should be taken to ensure that skin sutures are loose and the edges are apposed. The primary advantage of simple interrupted sutures is that disruption of a single suture does not cause the entire suture line to fail. However, simple interrupted sutures take more time than continuous patterns and result in more foreign material (knots) in the wound.

Horizontal mattress pattern. Horizontal mattress sutures are placed by inserting the needle on the far side of

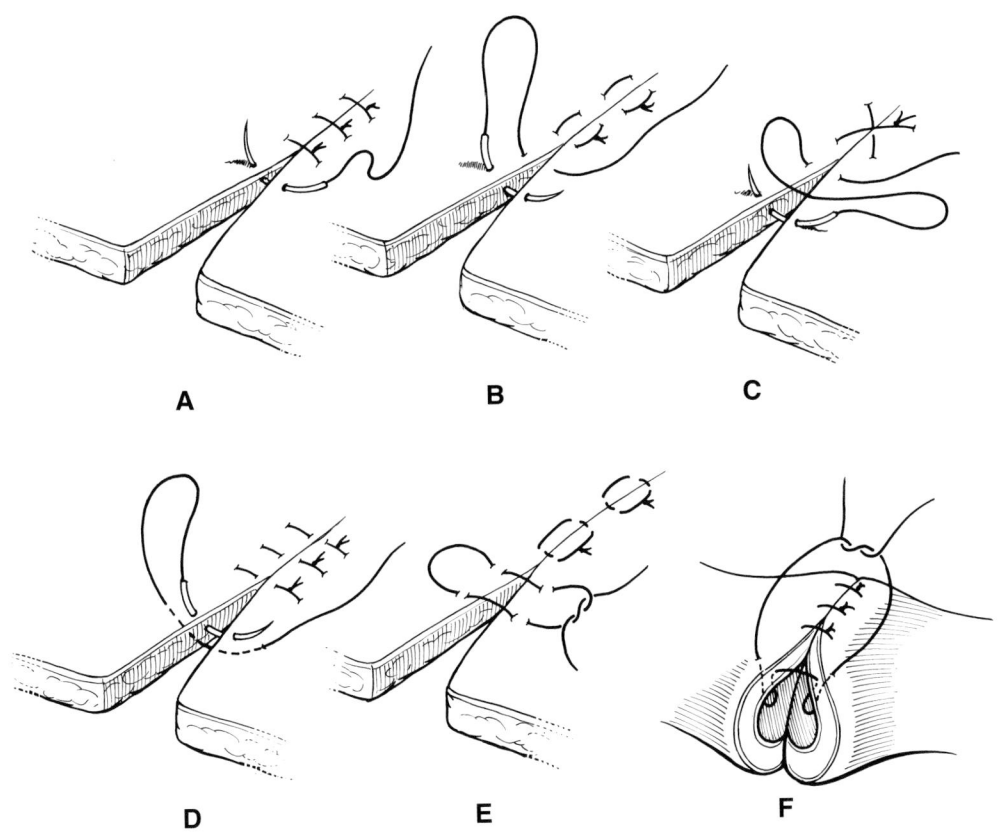

FIG. 9-6
Interrupted suture patterns. **A,** Simple interrupted. **B,** Horizontal mattress. **C,** Cruciate.
D, Vertical mattress. **E,** Halsted. **F,** Gambee.

the incision, passing it across the incision, and exiting it on the near side, as described for a simple interrupted suture (Fig. 9-6, *B*). The needle is then advanced 6 to 8 mm along the incision and reintroduced through the skin on the near side. It then crosses the incision, exiting from the skin on the far side, and the knot is tied. Horizontal mattress sutures generally are separated by 4 to 5 mm. They are used primarily in areas of tension and can be placed rapidly; however, they often cause tissue eversion. Care should be exercised to appose, rather than evert, tissue margins, and the suture should be angled through the tissue so that it passes just below the dermis. Mattress sutures can be modified to form a cross over or under the incision (cruciate sutures) (Fig. 9-6, *C*).

Vertical mattress pattern. To place a vertical mattress suture, the needle is introduced approximately 8 to 10 mm from the incision edge on one side, passed across the incision line, and exited at an equal distance on the opposite side (Fig. 9-6, *D*). The needle is reversed and inserted through skin on the same side, approximately 4 mm from the skin edge, and the knot is tied. Vertical mattress sutures are stronger than horizontal mattress sutures when used in areas of tension. Placement of vertical mattress sutures is relatively time-consuming, but eversion of the skin margins is less of a problem than with horizontal mattress sutures. When two vertical mattress sutures are placed in a parallel fashion be-

fore they are tied, the pattern is known as a Halsted suture (Fig. 9-6, *E*).

Gambee pattern. Gambee sutures are used in intestinal surgery to reduce mucosal eversion. The suture is introduced the same as a simple interrupted suture from the serosa through the muscularis and mucosa to the lumen (Fig. 9-6, *F*). It is then returned from the lumen through the mucosa to the muscularis before it crosses the incision. After crossing the incision, it is introduced in the muscularis and is continued through the mucosa to the lumen. The needle is then reintroduced through the mucosa and muscularis to exit from the serosal surface, and the suture is tied. Gambee sutures reduce mucosal inversion and may reduce wicking of material from the intestinal lumen to the exterior.

Continuous Suture Patterns

Simple continuous pattern. A simple continuous suture consists of a series of simple interrupted sutures with a knot on either end; the suture is continuous between the knots (Fig. 9-7, *A*). To begin a simple continuous suture line, a simple interrupted suture is placed and knotted, but only the end that is not attached to the needle is cut. The needle is directed through skin perpendicular to the incision. The resulting suture line has a suture perpendicular to the incision line below the tissue and advances forward above it. If both

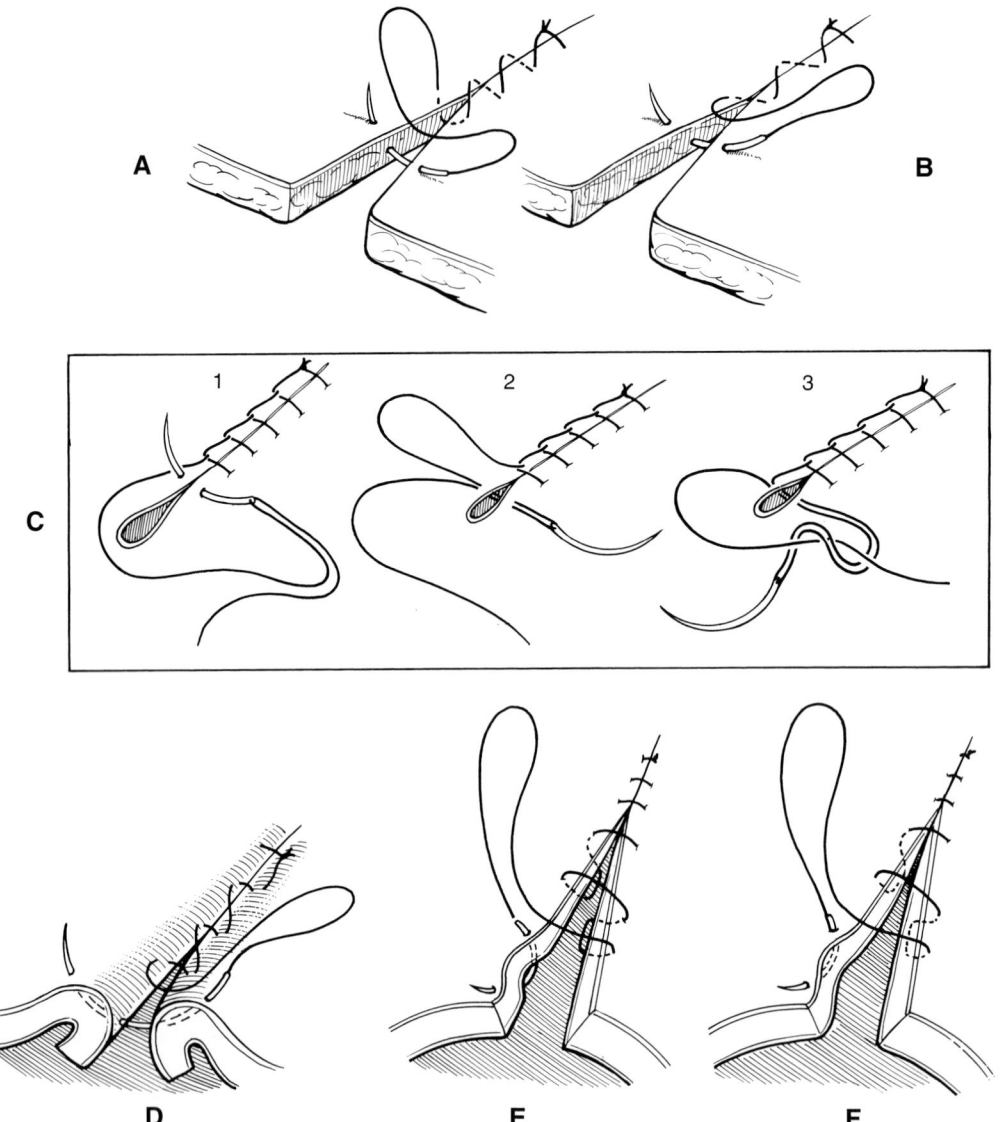

FIG. 9-7
Continuous suture patterns. **A,** Simple continuous. **B,** Running. **C,** Ford interlocking (C2 and C3 illustrate how to end the suture line). **D,** Lembert. **E,** Connell. **F,** Cushing.

the deep and superficial portions of the suture line advance, the suture is called a running suture (Fig. 9-7, *B*). To end a continuous suture, the needle end of the suture is tied to the last loop of suture that is exterior to the tissue. If an eyed needle is used, the needle is advanced through the tissue, and the short end of the suture is grasped. A loop of suture is pulled through with the needle, and this loop is tied to the single end on the contralateral side.

Simple continuous suture lines provide maximum tissue apposition and are relatively air tight and fluid tight compared with a series of simple interrupted sutures. Simple continuous suture lines frequently are used to close the linea alba and subcutaneous tissue. Care should be taken when placing continuous suture lines in areas where tightening of the suture may result in a purse-string–like effect, such as with an intestinal anastomosis.

Ford interlocking pattern. Ford interlocking sutures are modifications of a simple continuous pattern in which each passage through the tissue is partly locked, as shown in Fig. 9-7, *C.* To terminate this suture pattern, the needle is introduced in the opposite direction from that used previously (near to far), and the end is held on that side. The loop of the suture formed on the opposite side is tied to the single end. Locked suture patterns may be placed quickly and may appose tissue better than a simple interrupted pattern. However, they use a large amount of suture and may be difficult to remove.

Lembert pattern. A Lembert pattern is a variation of a vertical mattress pattern applied in a continuous fashion. It is an inverting pattern that often is used to close hollow viscera. The needle penetrates the serosa and muscularis approximately 8 to 10 mm from the incision edge and exits

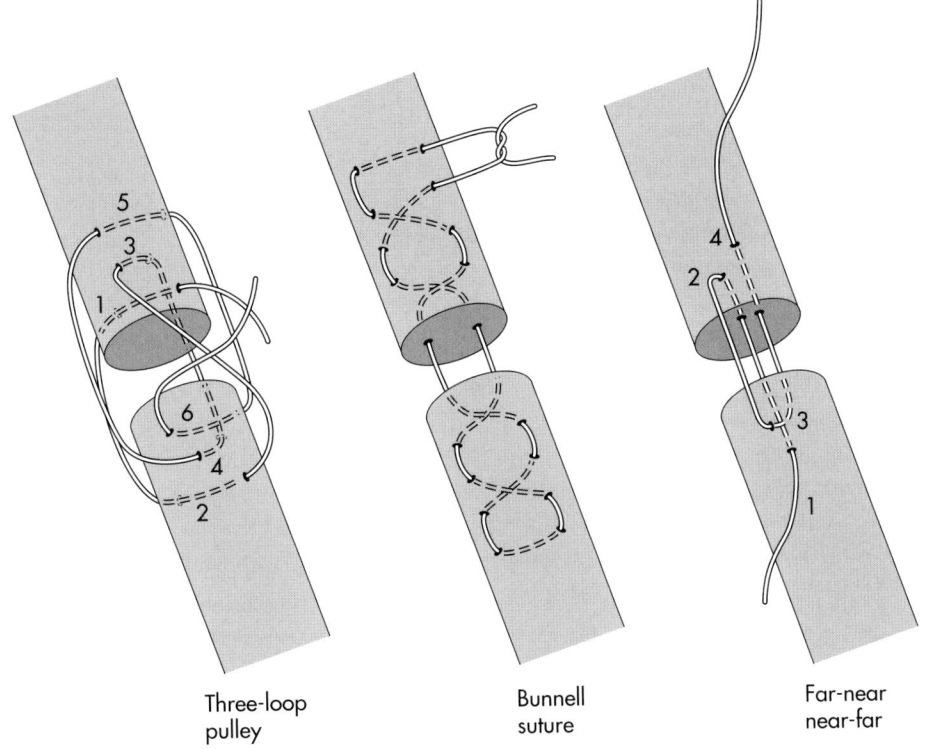

Three-loop   Bunnell   Far-near
pulley   suture   near-far

FIG. 9-8
Tendon sutures.

near the wound margin on the same side. After passing over the incision, the needle penetrates approximately 3 to 4 mm from the wound margin and exits 8 to 10 mm away from the incision. This pattern is repeated along the length of the incision (Fig. 9-7, *D*).

Connell and Cushing patterns. These patterns are infrequently used to close hollow organs because they cause tissue excessive inversion. They were historically used because they provided a watertight seal. The Connell and Cushing patterns are similar, except that a Connell pattern enters the lumen, whereas a Cushing pattern extends only to the submucosal area (Fig. 9-7, *E* and *F*). It was previously thought to be important that sutures not penetrate into the lumen of the bladder because these sutures might be calculolytic; however, with the rapidly absorbed monofilament sutures available today, this is no longer a real concern. The suture line is begun with a simple interrupted or vertical mattress suture. The needle is advanced parallel to the incision and introduced into the serosa, passing through the muscular and mucosal surfaces. From the deep surface (the lumen with a Connell suture), the needle is advanced parallel along the incision and returned through the tissue to the serosal surface. Once outside the viscera, the needle and suture are passed across the incision and introduced at a point that corresponds to the exit point on the contralateral side. The suture is then repeated. The suture should cross the incision perpendicularly. When the suture is tightened, the incision inverts. A Parker-Kerr suture is a modification of the Cushing and Lembert patterns that has been advocated for

closing the stump of hollow viscera. It is seldom used because it also causes excessive tissue inversion.

Tendon Sutures

Sutures may be used to approximate severed ends of a tendon or to secure one end of a tendon to bone or muscle.

Three-loop pulley suture. The three-loop pulley pattern is made with three loops oriented approximately 120 degrees to each other. The initial loop is placed perpendicular to the long axis of the tendon ends in a near-far fashion (Fig. 9-8). The second loop is placed in a plane 120 degrees from the first, at a point midway between the near and far positions. The final loop is placed in a far-near pattern 120 degrees from the first two sutures. In a recent study, the three-loop pulley pattern was found to be more resistant to gap formation during tensile loading and was quicker to place than two locking loop sutures (Moores et al, 2004).

Bunnell suture. A modified Bunnell suture pattern may be used to appose severed tendons. The needle is passed from one side of the proximal end of the severed tendon and crossed diagonally across the tendon to the opposite side, where it exits (see Fig. 9-8). The suture is reintroduced approximately 1 mm distal to the exit site and crossed diagonally to the other side of the tendon, where it exits from the severed end. It is introduced into the distal portion of the severed tendon from the cut end, and two cruciate sutures are placed. The suture exits at the severed end of the distal portion of the tendon and is reintroduced into the proximal tendon. The pattern is repeated in this portion of the tendon, with the suture exiting near the original entrance site. The tendon ends are apposed and the suture tightened.

This pattern is used less often than in the past because it is difficult to place and may damage the tendon's microcirculation. Ischemia resulting from the suture may cause the suture to pull out or may result in death of the tendon ends. The resultant gap must then be filled with fibrous tissue.

Far-near–near-far suture. A far-near–near-far suture may be used in flat tendons. The needle is passed through the tendon perpendicular to and 5 mm from the severed tendon end (see Fig. 9-8). The needle then enters the distal section of the severed tendon in the same vertical plane 2 mm from the tendon edge. It is looped back to the proximal section of tendon, where it enters 2 mm from the severed edge. The suture is again looped back to the distal section of the tendon to enter 5 mm from the severed tendon edge. The suture ends are pulled taut and tied with a surgeon's knot. This pattern minimally disrupts blood flow and provides good resistance to tension because all suture passes are in the same vertical plane.

Knot Tying

The knot is the weakest point of a suture. A knot consists of at least two throws laid on top of each other and tightened. The throws can be joined parallel, as in a square knot (Fig. 9-9), or crosswise, as in a granny knot (see Fig. 9-9). Correct knot-tying technique is important, because incorrectly tied knots (e.g., tumbled knots, half-hitches [see Fig. 9-9], or granny knots) may lead to dehiscence. Factors that influence knot security are the material coefficient, the length of the cut ends, and the structural configuration of the knot. The most reliable configuration for a knot is superimposition of squared knots. A surgeon's knot (see Fig. 9-9) cannot be tightened and can withstand only a slight strain on the suture loop. Although it often is used in areas of tension, it generally is not recommended for use with coated or monofilament materials and should be avoided unless tissue tension is such that use of the standard square knot would result in poor tissue apposition. It should never be used to ligate vessels.

A recent study of the effect of the knot-tying method on the structural properties of nonabsorbable suture materials used for extraarticular stabilization of joints recommended that a surgeon's knot be avoided when using No. 2 polypropylene, 27-kg fishing line, or 27-kg leader material because the knot reduced the stiffness of the suture (Huber et al, 1999). Conversely, clamping the first throw of a square knot had no adverse effect on the acute properties of the sutures tested and actually increased the stiffness of leader material. Multifilament sutures generally have better knot-holding properties than monofilament materials; however, coating the suture to reduce drag reduces knot security. To prevent strangulating tissue, excessive tension should be avoided when tying knots (except when ligatures are applied for hemostasis). Excessively tight skin sutures cause the patient discomfort and increase the likelihood that the animal will remove the sutures prematurely.

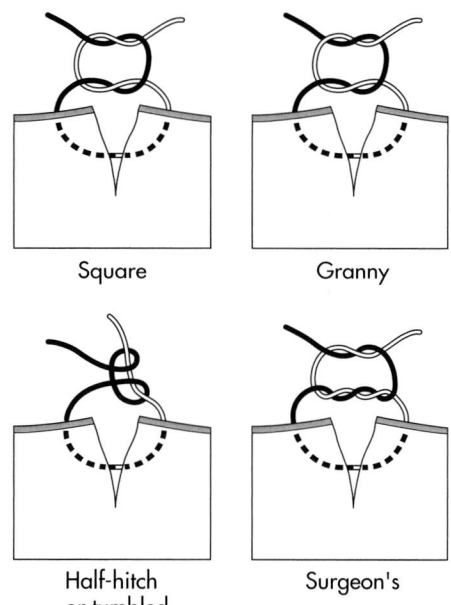

FIG. 9-9
Types of knots.

Instrument ties. In veterinary medicine, instrument ties (Fig. 9-10) are more commonly used than hand ties because there is less waste of the suture. The first loop is made as shown in Fig. 9-10, after which the suture should not be lifted or have uneven pressure applied to either end, or the throw will loosen. If one end is pulled with greater tension than the other, a half-hitch will form (see Fig. 9-9). Opposing suture ends should be pulled perpendicular to the long axis of the incision. Lifting one hand causes the suture to tumble, forming a sliding two half-hitch knot. Failure to correctly cross the hands results in a granny knot.

Hand ties. Hand ties are particularly useful in confined or hard to reach areas or when sutures have been preplaced, as in a thoracotomy closure. Hand ties generally require that suture ends be left longer than for an instrument tie. A one-handed or two-handed technique may be used. The two-handed technique generally allows better control and accuracy; however, the one-handed technique is more useful in confined areas. Techniques for tying one-handed and two-handed knots are shown in Figs. 9-11 and 9-12.

Burying the knot. The knots of subcutaneous and subcuticular suture patterns often are buried to reduce irritation caused by the knots rubbing against more superficial tissue. Fig. 9-13 presents a detailed description of this procedure.

Suture Removal

Skin sutures generally should be removed once healing is sufficient to prevent dehiscence, usually within 10 to 14 days after surgery. However, prolonged healing, such as in extremely debilitated animals, may require that the sutures be left in place longer. Also, if fibrosis is desired (e.g., as with an aural hematoma), delaying suture removal may be considered.

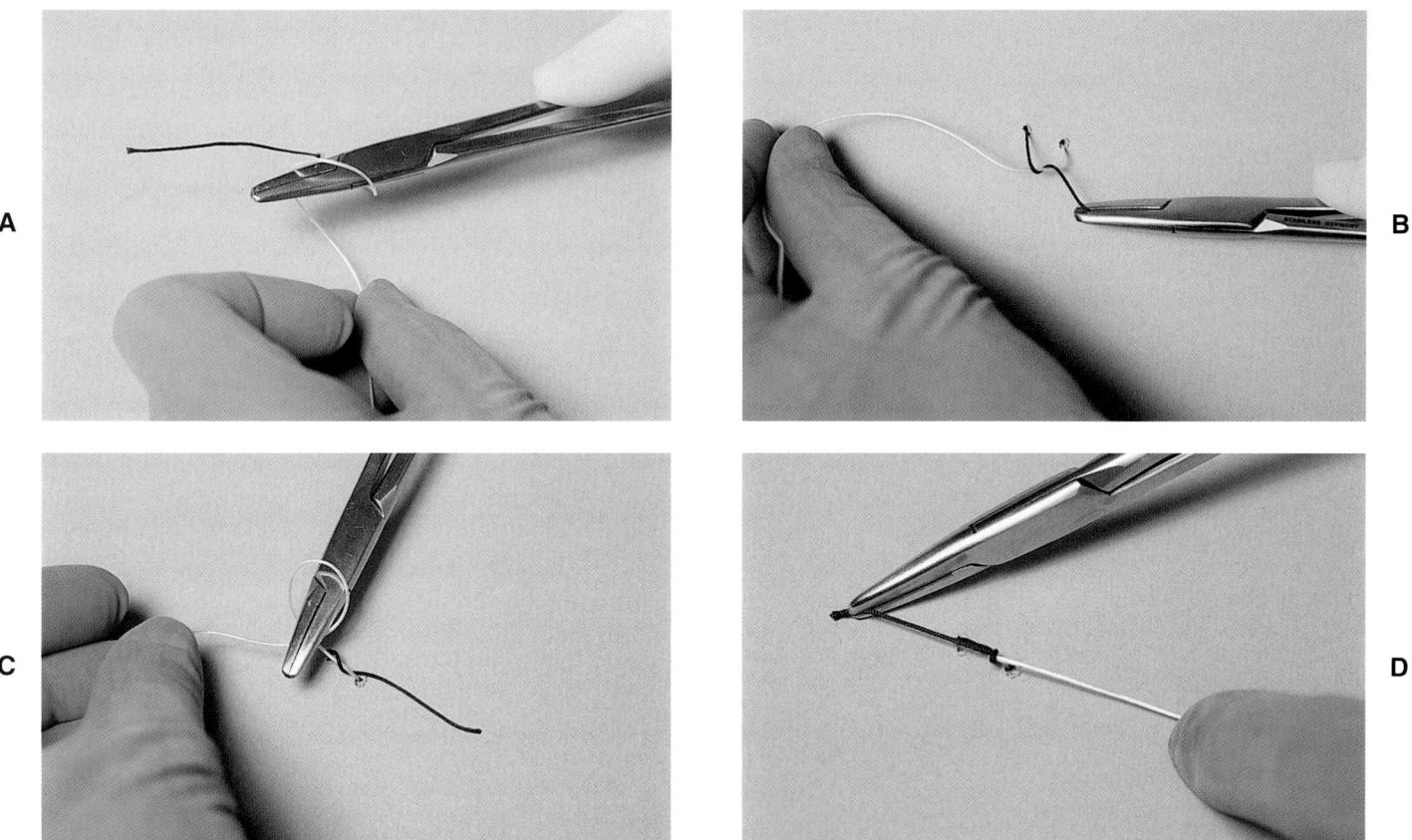

FIG. 9-10
Instrument tie. **A,** Place the tips of the needle holders between the two strands of suture. Wrap the strand nearest you (*white,* or long end) around the needle holders to form a loop and grasp the end of the far piece of suture (*black,* or short end) in your needle holders. **B,** Bring the short end toward you (through the loop) by reversing your hands and tighten the suture gently. **C,** For the second throw, wrap the strand farthest from you (*white,* or long end) over the needle holders to form a loop, grasp the end of the suture nearest you (*black,* or short end), and **(D)** pull it through the loop, snugging it down gently to prevent tightening the suture excessively. Keep your hands low and parallel when tightening the suture to prevent causing the knot to tumble.

HEMOSTATIC TECHNIQUES AND MATERIALS

Hemostasis is a complex process that involves platelet activation and circulating clotting factors. Numerous diseases or conditions may interfere with clotting in surgical patients. The reader is referred to a veterinary medicine text for an in-depth discussion of normal clotting and alterations of clotting caused by disease. Obtaining hemostasis allows appropriate visualization of tissue during the procedure and prevents a life-threatening hemorrhage. A low pressure hemorrhage from small vessels can be controlled by applying pressure to the bleeding points with gauze sponges. Once a thrombus has formed, the sponge should be gently removed to prevent disrupting clots. Soaking the sponge with saline before removal may also help prevent clot disruption.

Large vessels must be ligated. Double ligatures are recommended for larger vessels, particularly arteries. Transfixation ligatures (Fig. 9-14) may be indicated for larger vessels to prevent the ligature from slipping off the vessel end. Using the smallest suture possible for vessel ligation improves knot security. A surgeon's throw should not be used for vessel ligation (see p. 70).

Electrosurgery

Electrocoagulation, or vascular coagulation, is widely used for hemostasis. It generally is used in vessels less than 1.5 to 2 mm in diameter; larger vessels should be ligated (see previous discussion). The term *electrocautery* often is used erroneously to mean electrocoagulation. *Electrocautery* refers to direct current (electrons flowing in one direction) whereas *electrosurgery* uses alternating current. During electrocautery, current does not enter the patient's body. Only the heated wire comes in contact with tissue. In electrosurgery, the patient is included in the circuit and current enters the patient's body.

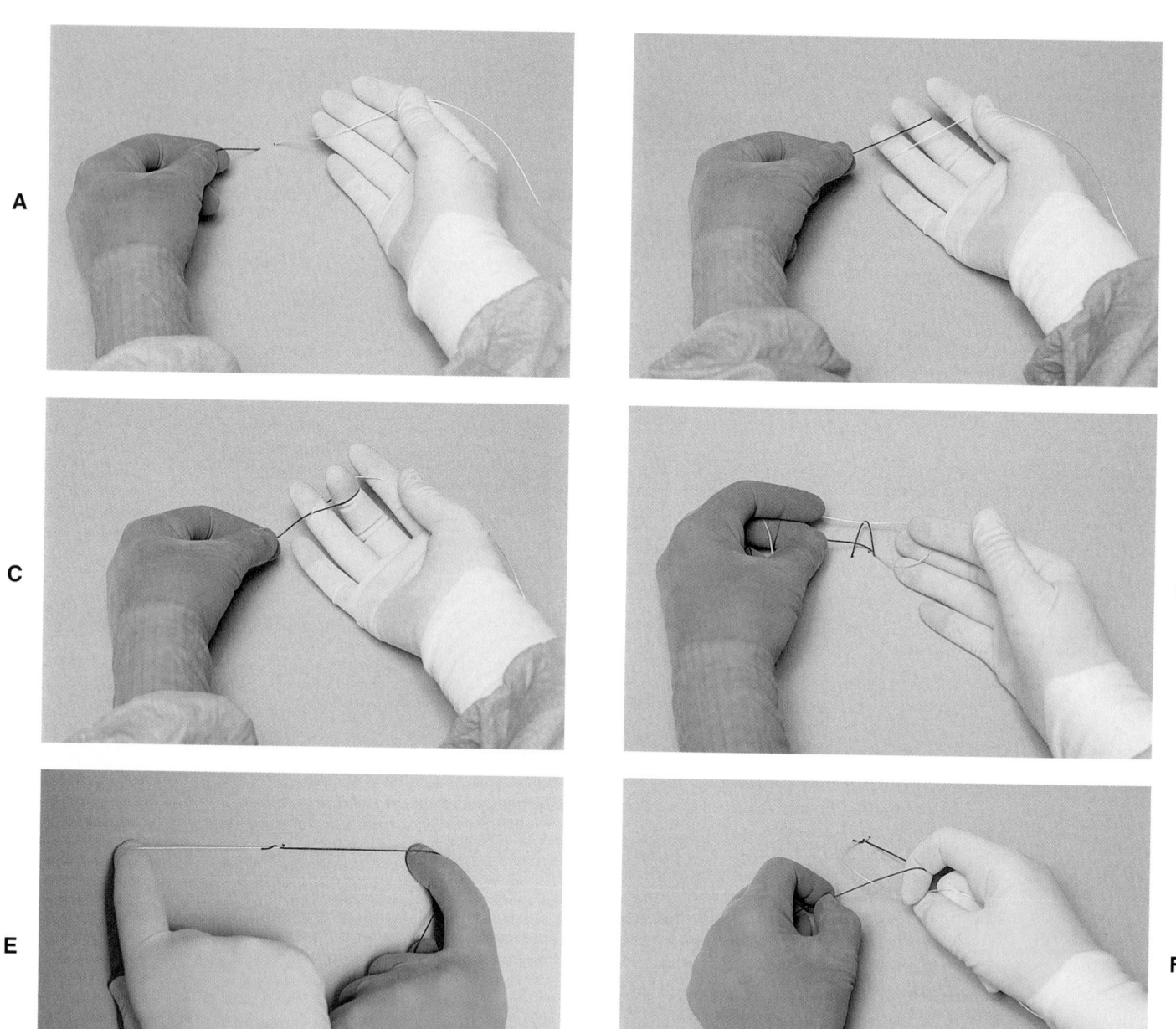

FIG. 9-11
One-handed square knot (right-handed). **A,** Reflect the right suture *(white)* between the three fingers of your right hand *(white glove)* and hold it between your index finger and thumb. **B,** Hold the left suture *(black)* in your left hand *(dark glove)* and pass it between the index finger and second finger of your right hand. **C,** Flex the distal phalanx of the second finger of your right hand and draw the left strand to the right of the right strand. Extend the tip of the second finger so that the white strand is drawn with it through the loop. **D,** Pull the right strand through the loop by the tips of the second and third fingers of your right hand. **E,** Cross your hands and apply even tension to the two strands. **F,** Place the index finger of your right hand between the right *(black)* and left *(white)* strands so that the left-hand strand forms a loop with the right. Flex the distal phalanx of your right index finger. (Modified from Knecht CD et al: *Fundamental techniques in veterinary surgery,* ed 2, Philadelphia, 1981, WB Saunders.)

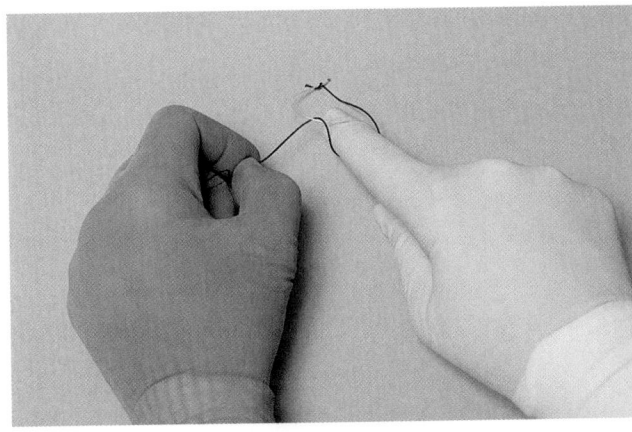

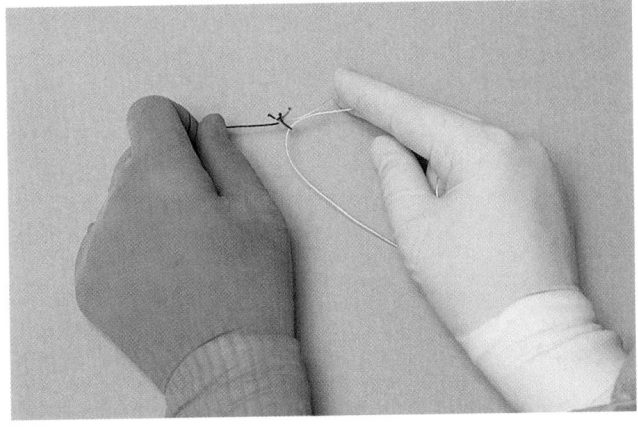

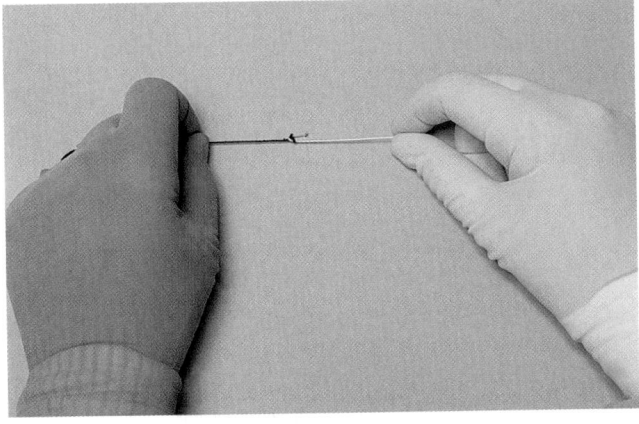

FIG. 9-11, cont'd
One-handed square knot (right-handed), continued. **G,** Extend the distal phalanx of your right index finger to draw the right-hand strand through the loop. **H,** Pull the right strand through the loop and **(I)** apply even tension to complete the square knot. (Modified from Knecht CD et al: *Fundamental techniques in veterinary surgery,* ed 2, Philadelphia, 1981, WB Saunders.)

Standard electrical current alternates at a frequency of 60 cycles per second (Hz). Because nerve and muscle stimulation cease at 100,000 cycles/second (100 kHz), an electrosurgical generator takes 60 cycle current and increases the frequency to more than 200,000 cycles per second. This affords minimal neuromuscular stimulation without a risk of electrocution. On the "cut" setting, a constant waveform is produced that vaporizes or cuts tissue. When an intermittent waveform (coagulation) is used instead of tissue vaporization, a coagulum is produced. High heat produced rapidly causes vaporization; low heat produced more slowly creates a coagulum.

High quality, modern electrosurgery units have a blend setting. A cut cycle on blend produces an intermittent waveform that has a much higher duty cycle than the coagulation duty cycle, and produces more heat than pure cut. Consequently, some coagulation occurs with the cut cycle (and vice versa). Direct contact of the electrode with the tissue produces lower heat sufficient to coagulate. The use of the arc between the electrode and tissue produces higher heat and consequently a cutting or vaporization action.

If an adequate low-impedance ground pad is not present, alternate paths to ground can be inadvertently used by the circuit, resulting in burns. Most modern electrosurgery units have circuitry to eliminate this danger, but safe practices are important. The amount of current multiplied by the time of current and divided by the area of the return path is proportional to the probability of a burn. Hence a small ground pad or an alternate path to ground (i.e., through an ECG pad) can easily produce a severe burn. It is worth remembering that in an AC current circuit the only difference in the grounding pad and the active electrode is their impedance, size, and conductivity. *To reduce the risk of a burn, use a large pad placed on well vascularized tissue that is close to the operative site.* Keeping the electrodes clean and free of eschar will enhance performance by maintaining lower resistance within the surgical circuit.

> NOTE: Research studies have confirmed that the smoke plume given off during electrocautery can contain toxic gases and vapors, such as benzene, hydrogen cyanide, formaldehyde, bioaerosols, dead and live cellular material (including blood fragments), and viruses. Thus the Occupational Safety and Health Administration recommends that smoke evacuation systems be used to reduce potential acute and chronic health risks to patients and personnel.

Electrosurgery may be done with monopolar or bipolar devices.

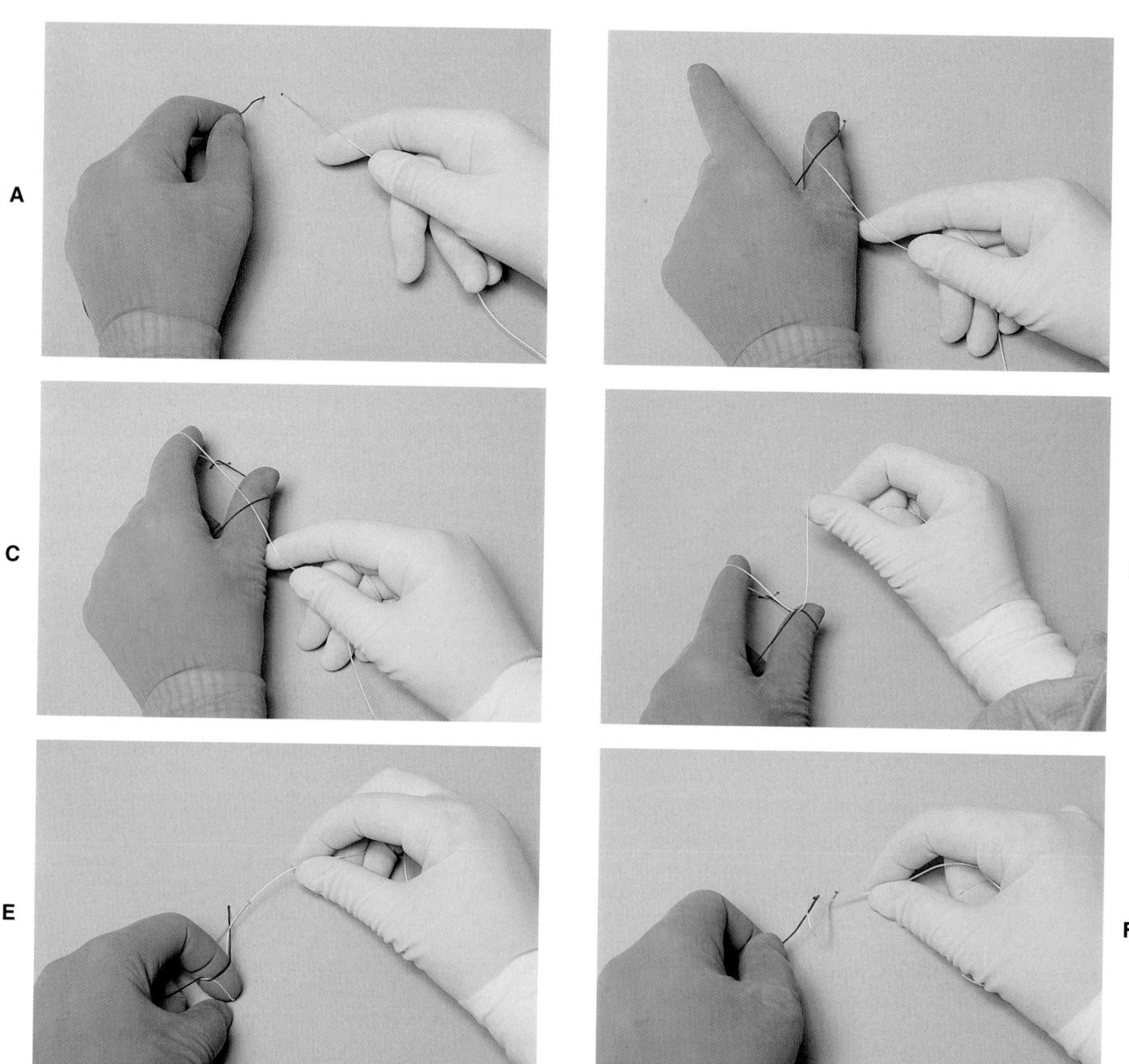

FIG. 9-12
Two-handed square knot (right-handed). **A,** Extend the index finger of your right hand *(white glove)* as a bridge and place the right *(white)* strand over it. Hold the left *(black)* strand in the palm of your left hand *(dark glove)*. **B,** Pass your left thumb below and around the right strand and then to the left of the left strand. **C,** Introduce your left index finger between the crossed strands (with your left thumb). **D,** Carry the right strand to your left index finger and thumb and **(E)** using your left index finger and thumb, carry it through the loop. **F,** Return the suture to your right hand. (Modified from: Knecht CD et al: *Fundamental techniques in veterinary surgery,* ed 2, Philadelphia, 1981, WB Saunders.)

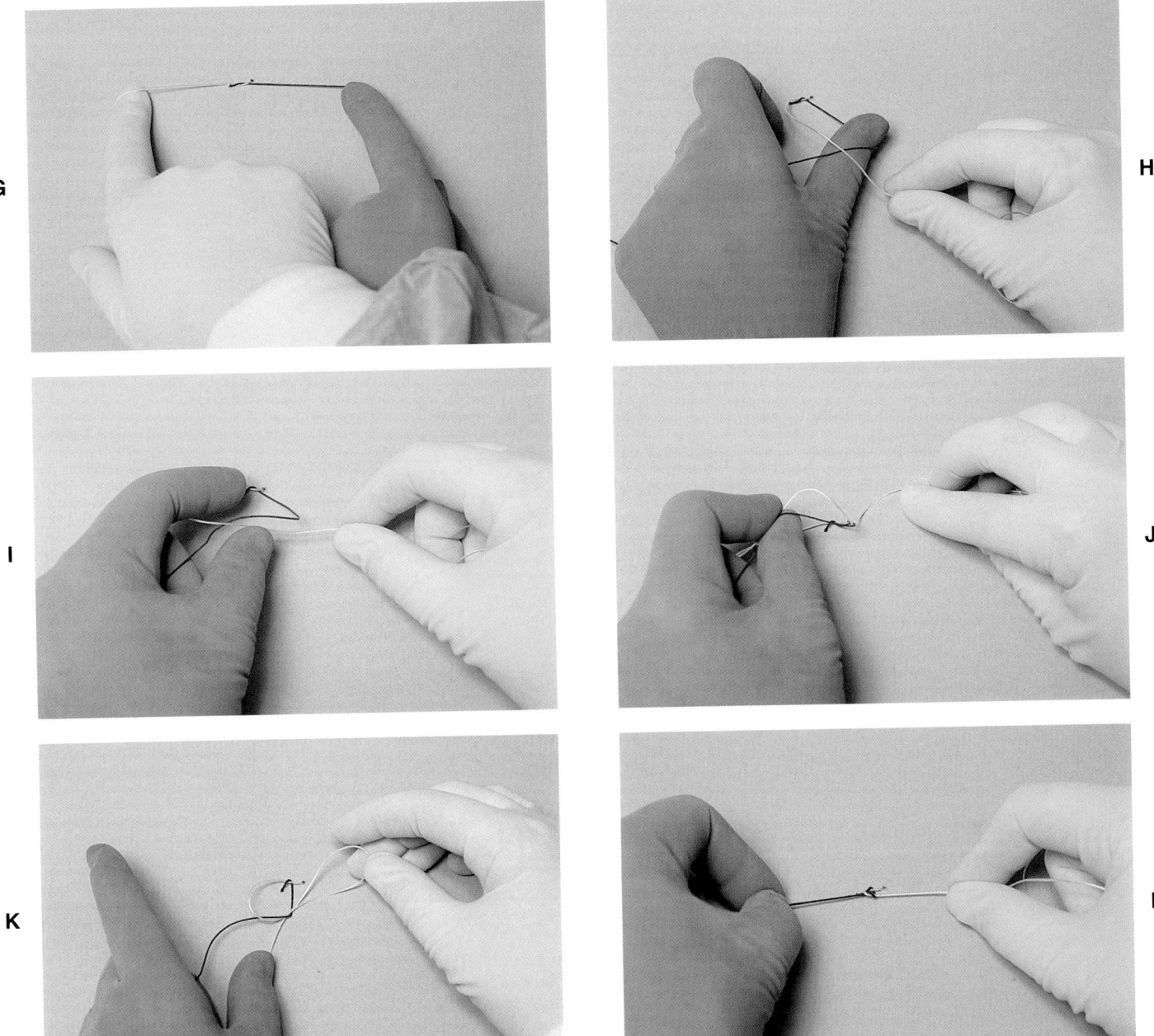

G   H   I   J   K   L

FIG. 9-12, cont'd
Two-handed square knot (right-handed), continued. **G,** Cross your hands and apply even tension to the suture ends. **H,** Place your left thumb between the two strands and make a loop with your right hand. **I,** Place your left index finger through the loop and use it and your left thumb to grasp the left *(white)* strand and **(J)** pull or push it through the loop. **K,** Pass the left strand from your left hand to your right thumb and index finger after passing it through the loop and **(L)** apply even tension to the suture strands to tighten the square knot. (Modified from: Knecht CD et al: *Fundamental techniques in veterinary surgery,* ed 2, Philadelphia, 1981, WB Saunders.)

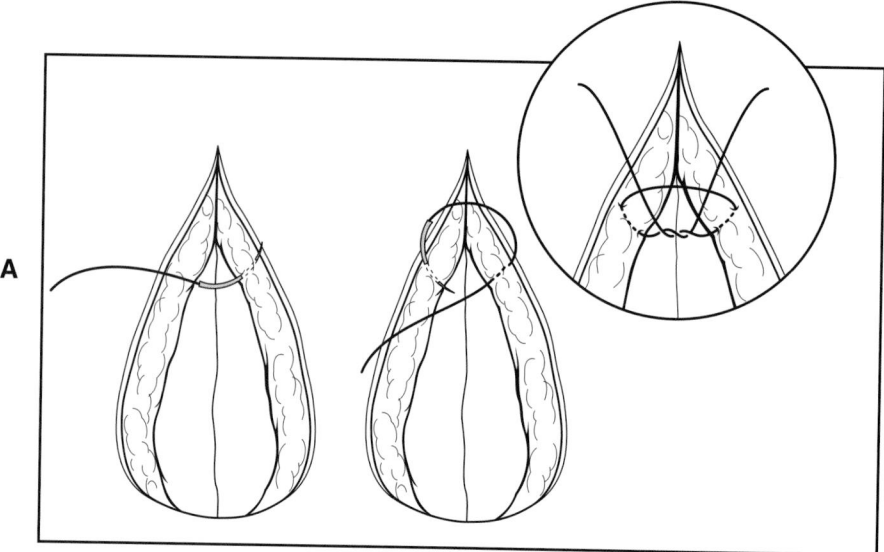

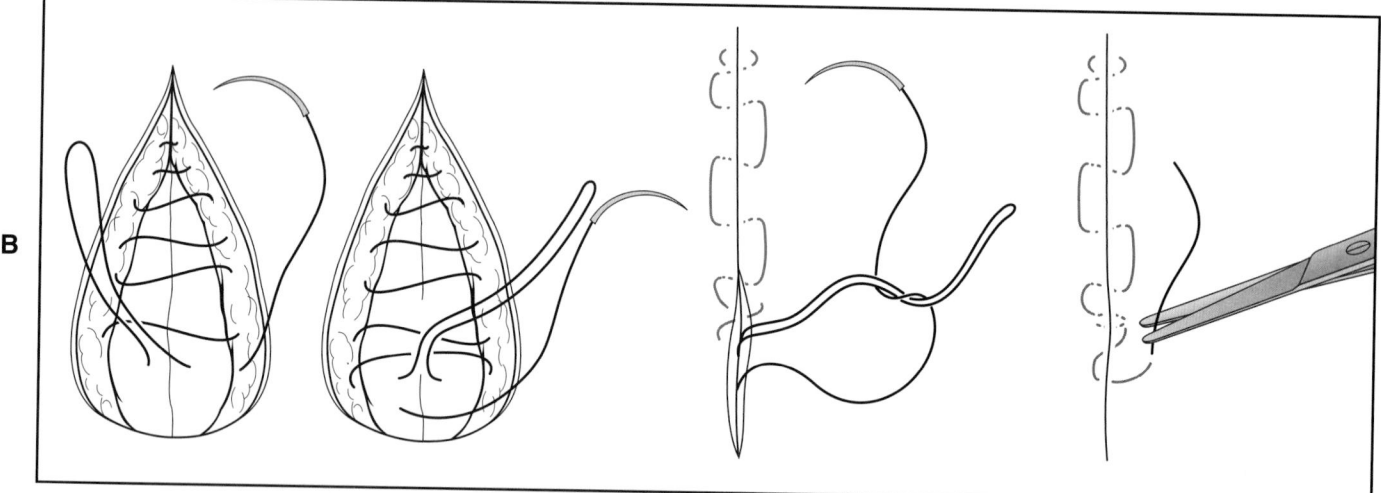

FIG. 9-13

A, To bury a simple interrupted suture, introduce the needle deep in the far subcutaneous tissue and pass it toward the dermis. Then pass it across the incision line and reintroduce it in the near subcutaneous tissue at the dermis, exiting deep in the incision line. **B,** To bury a knot at the end of a continuous suture line, lift a loop of suture from the incision line, introduce the needle from deep to superficial on one side, pass it across the incision, and insert it from superficial to deep in the tissue near the loop. Alternately, after the continuous pattern is completed, advance the needle 2 to 3 mm to the opposite side. Place a vertical bite from the mid-dermis down to subcutaneous tissue. Then insert the needle on the opposite side, vertically aiming up from the subcutaneous tissue, exiting at the mid-dermis within 2 to 3 mm of the commissure. Create a 2 cm loop of suture between the two vertical bites. Take a third vertical bite parallel to the first, initiating in the mid-dermis, but exiting deeper in the subcutaneous layer. Bring the needle up between the exposed loop and final suture crossing the incision. Apply tension to the exposed loop to tighten the horizontal sutures and appose the wound margins, then tie the free suture end to the exposed loop with four to five throws to complete the knot and close the wound. Trim the loop 2 to 3 mm above the knot. Insert the needle close to the knot, aiming to exit the dermis at least 1 cm lateral to the incision. As tension is applied to the suture, the knot is pulled deeper into the tissue, below the dermis. Finally, under tension, trim the free end of suture flush with the skin.

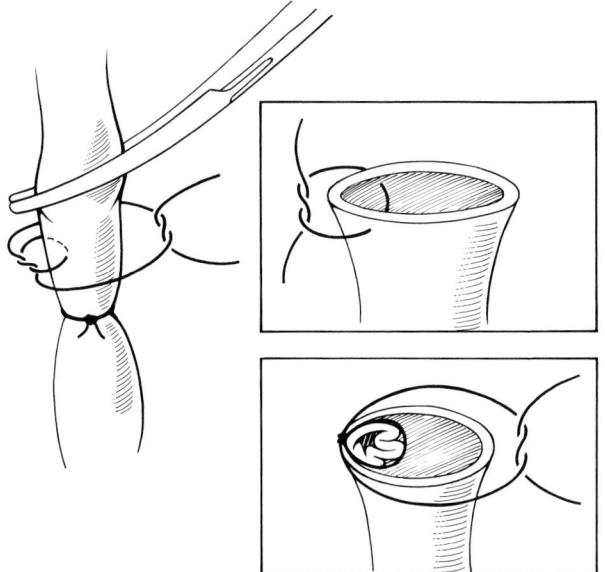

FIG. 9-14
To place a transfixation ligature on a vessel, introduce the needle through the previously ligated tissue. Place a single throw in the suture on the near side, then tie the suture (two square knots) on the opposite side of the vessel.

Monopolar electrosurgery. Monopolar electrosurgery is the most commonly used method of electrosurgery. It involves the flow of current from an active electrode (handpiece) through the patient to a ground plate. The small surface area of the handpiece concentrates the current density, increasing the temperature of the contact tissue and causing coagulation. The larger surface area of the ground plate reduces the current density so that minimal tissue heating occurs. Good contact of the ground plate to the patient (see p. 73) is essential to prevent thermoelectric burns; conduction gel usually is placed on the ground plate to enhance contact. The tip of the handpiece generally is frequently touched to a hemostat that has been applied to the bleeding vessel; however, with modern electrosurgical equipment this practice is not necessary. The standard flat-tipped electrode is designed to create an eschar or coagulum directly on tissue. When there is direct contact of the tip with the tissue, the cutting cycle will use far less voltage to accomplish the same coagulation as the coagulation cycle produces.

With monopolar coagulation, the field must be relatively dry and the electrode kept clean and free of debris.

NOTE: Do not activate the generator while the active electrode is touching or in close proximity to another metal object. The instrument (particularly in body cavities) when energized can seek its own pathway to the return electrode, resulting in patient injury. Gloves can sometimes act in a capacitance function and allow burns to the surgeon.

Bipolar electrosurgery. Bipolar electrosurgery involves the use of a forcepslike handpiece. Current passes from one tip through the tissue being held between the forceps to the opposite tip. The tips must be held approximately 1 mm apart for a current to be generated. Bipolar coagulation is used when precise coagulation is necessary to prevent damage to adjacent structures, such as in thyroidectomy or ophthalmic procedures.

Hemostatic Agents

Substances available to control hemorrhage during surgery include bone wax and hemostatic materials made of gelatin or cellulose. Bone wax is a sterile mixture of semisynthetic beeswax and a softening agent (i.e., isopropyl palmitate). It may be pressed into cavities in bone (e.g., the mandibular foramen) or applied to the bone surface to inhibit bleeding. It is poorly resorbed and should be used sparingly because it may act as a physical barrier to healing and promote infection.

Surgicel (Johnson and Johnson) is made of oxidized regenerated cellulose. When saturated with blood, it becomes a gelatinous mass that provides a substrate for clot formation. It can be cut to the desired size and placed on an area of hemorrhage. Surgicel is absorbed by the body, but removal is recommended because it may inhibit callus formation and promote infection. It is not activated by tissue fluids other than blood and therefore should be used only at sites of hemorrhage. Gelfoam (Pharmacia and Upjohn) is an absorbable gelatin sponge that can be used in a similar fashion to Surgicel. When applied to an area of hemorrhage, Gelfoam swells and exerts pressure on the wound; absorption occurs over 4 to 6 weeks. Gelfoam may cause granuloma formation and should not be left in infected sites, the brain, or areas with a high risk of infection. SurgiFlow Hemostatic Matrix and Vetspon (Novartis Animal Health) are also hemostatic products made from absorbable gelatin sponge. They are indicated for surgical procedures (except urologic and ophthalmic) when control of capillary, venous, and arteriolar bleeding by pressure, ligature, and other conventional procedures is ineffective or impractical. These products should not be used in closure of skin incisions as they may interfere with healing.

QuickClot is a zeolite hemostatic agent that has been shown to significantly reduce bleeding in a lethal model of complex groin injury in swine. It speeds coagulation of blood, even in large wounds, by physically adsorbing the liquid from blood, thereby concentrating the clotting factors and encouraging rapid clotting (Alam et al, 2004). Thrombin may also be mixed with Gelfoam in a wound that is bleeding excessively because of a coagulopathy.

References

Alam HB, Chen Z, Jaskille A et al: Application of zeolite hemostatic agent achieves 100% survival in a lethal model of complex groin injury in swine, *J Trauma-Injury Inf Crit Care* 56:974, 2004.

Greenberg CB, Davidson EB, Bellmer DD et al: Evaluation of the tensile strengths of four monofilament absorbable sutures after immersion in canine urine with or without bacteria, *Am J Vet Res* 65:847, 2004.

Moores AP, Owen MR, Tarlton JF: The three-loop pulley suture versus two locking-loop sutures for the repair of canine Achilles tendon, *Vet Surg* 33:131, 2004.

Suggested Reading

Tan RHH, Bell RJW, Dowling BA et al: Suture materials, composition and applications in veterinary wound repair, *Aust Vet J* 81:140, 2003.

A comprehensive review of suture materials and their properties is given for large and small animals.

Surgical Infections and Antibiotic Selection

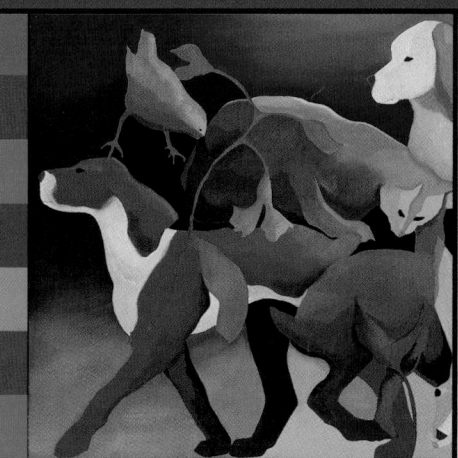

The golden age of modern antibiotic therapy began with the discovery and mass production of penicillin in 1941. Since then, many potentially fatal infections have been prevented through the use of antibiotics; however, these drugs are commonly misused. The widespread use of prophylactic antibiotics in surgical patients has resulted in de-emphasis of surgical asepsis and the development of antibiotic-resistant bacteria. The accumulation of resistant bacteria in hospitals and the associated increase in bacterial infections have been accentuated by prolonged, extensive surgical procedures, increased invasiveness of supportive measures, lengthy hospital stays, inappropriate use of antibiotics, increased survival of geriatric and debilitated patients, and use of immunosuppressive drugs.

Antibiotic selection often is based on preconceived bias and tradition rather than on actual or expected bacterial flora. Antibiotic therapy may be prophylactic or therapeutic in nature. Prophylactic antibiotic therapy should be used only when indicated by a likelihood of infection or when infection would be catastrophic; selection of prophylactic antibiotics should be based on expected bacterial flora in the targeted tissue. Selection of therapeutic antibiotics ideally is based on culture and susceptibility results. However, this often is not possible, and initial selection is based on expected flora, with a subsequent change in antibiotics, if necessary, based on the clinical response or on culture and sensitivity results. Inappropriate use may render antibiotics ineffective or cause serious morbidity and mortality from toxicity or the development of resistant microbes.

Bacterial survival in a host depends on the bacterial virulence and numbers, host immunocompetence, and wound factors that deactivate host defenses (e.g., presence of blood clots, ischemic tissue, pockets of fluid, or foreign material). Successful antibiotic therapy requires reduction of bacterial numbers to the point where the host defenses are effective. With competent host defenses, bacteriostatic agents that slow protein synthesis or prevent bacterial replication are adequate (see later discussion). However, when the host defenses have been compromised, either directly or because of deleterious wound factors, bactericidal concentrations of antibiotics are typically required. In addition to use of the

appropriate antibiotics, wound factors may need to be corrected through wound débridement, drainage, or removal of foreign material to achieve a successful outcome.

> NOTE: Some antibiotics are bacteriostatic at low concentrations and bactericidal at higher concentrations. If susceptibility testing has been done, use an antibiotic to which the bacteria are susceptible regardless of whether it is bacteriostatic or bactericidal.

MECHANISMS OF ANTIBIOTIC ACTION

When antibiotics inhibit bacterial growth, they are noted as being *bacteriostatic*; when they kill bacteria, they are noted as being *bactericidal*. The distinction between bactericidal and bacteriostatic classifications of antibiotics is relative and depends on the ratio between the MBC (minimum bactericidal concentration) and the MIC (minimum inhibitory concentration). The MIC, generally expressed in micrograms per milliliter (μg/ml), is the lowest concentration of a drug that inhibits visible bacterial growth; it is the concentration necessary to inhibit bacterial growth in the patient's plasma or tissue. The MBC is the lowest concentration that kills 99.9% of bacteria in plasma or tissue. Antibiotics with a small MBC to MIC ratio (i.e., less than 4) are classified as bactericidal because plasma and tissue levels that kill 99.9% of the bacteria typically are achieved. Conversely, it may be difficult to achieve plasma or tissue levels that kill bacteria if drugs have a large MBC to MIC ratio; such drugs are considered bacteriostatic.

The antibiotic must kill bacteria without harming the host. When the dose required to kill bacteria is greater than can be tolerated by the host or achieved in the plasma and tissue, the bacteria are considered "resistant" to that drug. Because the distribution of antibiotics in body tissue varies, culture and susceptibility results may be misleading. For example, a urinary tract infection that is "marginally sensitive" to a particular antibiotic based on susceptibility testing may be successfully treated if the antibiotic is concentrated in urine. Conversely, if the infection involves the central nervous system (CNS) and if the particular antibiotic does not penetrate the blood-brain barrier, treatment is unlikely to succeed. An effective antibiotic is one that reaches the target tissue and then inhibits or kills the microorganism.

Antibiotics typically are classified according to their mechanism of action. They may destroy or alter the bacterial cell wall or inhibit its synthesis, or inhibit protein or deoxyribonucleic acid (DNA) synthesis.

Destruction of Bacterial Cell Walls

Antibiotics that inhibit synthesis or promote destruction of bacterial cell walls include the β-lactam ring antibiotics (e.g., penicillins, cephalosporins, carbapenems, and monobactams), vancomycin, bacitracin, polymyxin, and the antifungal drugs nystatin, amphotericin B, and the imidazoles. β-Lactams function by binding to penicillin-binding proteins (PBPs) in the cell wall, thereby impairing cell wall synthesis, which in turn reduces its strength and rigidity,

ultimately causing increased permeability and cell lysis. β-Lactam antibiotics tend to be bactericidal.

Penicillins are generally effective against gram-positive aerobes and gram-positive and gram-negative anaerobes. Resistance to penicillins is mediated by bacterial penicillinases (a type of β-lactamase), decreased permeability of the cell wall to penicillins as a result of altered porin size, and altered PBP structure such that the penicillin does not bind to the altered PBP (e.g., methicillin-resistant staphylococci). Penicillinase inhibitors (e.g., clavulanic acid) may be combined with penicillins (e.g., amoxicillin or ticarcillin plus clavulanic acid) to enhance their activity.

The cephalosporins (Table 10-1) are more effective than penicillins against gram-negative rods (e.g., Enterobacteriaceae), but may be inactivated by cephalosporinases (a type of β-lactamase). Most are poorly effective against anaerobes (cefoxitin is an exception). First-generation cephalosporins are effective against most gram-positive and

 TABLE 10-1

Cephalosporin Drugs Commonly Used in Veterinary Medicine

DRUG NAME	BRAND NAME	INDICATIONS	DOSAGE
First-Generation Cephalosporins			
Cephalexin	Keflex	Wide spectrum of activity against gram-positive organisms; variable against gram-negative organisms, poor activity against anaerobic infections	22–44 mg/kg; PO; bid-tid
Cephalothin	Keflin	As above	22–44 mg/kg; IV, IM, SC; bid-tid
Cefazolin	Kefzol	As above	22 mg/kg; IV, IM, SC; bid-tid
Cefadroxil	Cefa-tabs	As above	22–35 mg/kg; PO; bid-tid
Second- and Third-Generation Cephalosporins			
Cefotetan	Cefotan	Anaerobes and gram-negative bacilli (e.g., septic peritonitis, *Escherichia coli*)	30 mg/kg; IV; tid 30 mg/kg; SC; bid
Cefoxitin	Mefoxin	Anaerobes and gram-negative bacilli (e.g., septic peritonitis)	*Dogs:* 30–40 mg/kg; IV; tid *Cats:* 22–33 mg/kg; IV, IM; tid-qid
Cefotaxime	Claforan	Wide spectrum of activity against both gram-negative and gram-positive organisms; most active in this group against staphylococci; reaches good concentrations in spinal fluid	*Dogs:* 20–80 mg/kg; IV, IM, or SC; tid *Cats:* 20–80 mg/kg; IV, IM, or SC; tid
Ceftazidime	Fortaz	Effective against *Pseudomonas aeruginosa*	30–40 mg/kg; IV, SC; tid-qid
Cefixime	Suprax	Limited activity against most gram-positive organisms; can be given orally; use lower dose for urinary tract infections and higher dose for other infections	5–12 mg/kg; PO; qd-bid
Cefoperazone	Cefobid	Effective against Enterobacteriaceae	22–50 mg/kg; IV or IM; bid-tid
Ceftriaxone	Rocephin	Often used in CNS infections and borreliosis	50 mg/kg IV, SC, IM, bid
Ceftiofur	Naxcel	Activity against gram-positive organisms; can be given once a day for urinary tract infections, twice a day for systemic infections; not effective against enterococci	2.2–4.4 mg/kg; SC; qd-bid (use 4.4 mg/kg for soft tissue infections)

PO, Oral; *IV,* intravenous; *IM,* intramuscular; *SC,* subcutaneous; *qd,* once a day; *bid,* twice a day; *tid,* three times a day; *qid,* four times a day.

some gram-negative organisms. Second-generation cephalosporins have greater activity against gram-negative bacteria and anaerobes, but have no additional efficacy against gram-positive organisms. Third-generation cephalosporins are highly effective against more than 90% of gram-negative bacteria, but they often are less active against gram-positive organisms than first-generation cephalosporins. Some third-generation cephalosporins have specific gram-negative spectra, and it is important to note that just because one third-generation cephalosporin is effective in a particular patient does not mean that another third-generation cephalosporin will be effective, or vice versa. **Ceftiofur** is a third-generation cephalosporin with prolonged antibacterial activity because its major metabolite is active; however, it does not have a broad spectrum of activity against serious gram-negative infections. **Cefepime** (Maxipime) is a fourth-generation cephalosporin that is unique among the cephalosporins because of its broad spectrum of activity, which includes gram-positive cocci, enteric gram-negative bacilli, and *Pseudomonas aeruginosa*. Resistance to cephalosporins is mediated by the same mechanisms that cause resistance to penicillins.

Imipenem (Table 10-2) and aztreonam are newer β-lactam antibiotics that are highly resistant to β-lactamases. They are as effective against gram-negative organisms as aminoglycosides, but are not nephrotoxic. **Imipenem** (a carbapenem) has the broadest antibacterial spectrum of any systemic antimicrobial and is effective against most clinically relevant bacterial species, including gram-negative and gram-positive anaerobes and aerobes. It is not active against methicillin-resistant staphylococci or resistant strains of *Enterococcus faecium*. Imipenem should be used only for severely ill patients who fail to respond to other antibiotics. Its broad spectrum of activity is likely to encourage abuse, resulting in the emergence of resistant bacteria. **Aztreonam**, a synthetic monobactam, is unaffected by bacterial β-lactamase. It is highly effective against many gram-negative aerobes, but has little activity against anaerobes. It has no activity against gram-positive bacteria and must be used in combination with other drugs to achieve broad-spectrum activity.

Inhibition of Protein Synthesis

Chloramphenicol, tetracycline, erythromycin, and clindamycin bind to bacterial ribosomes, causing reversible inhibition of protein synthesis. **Chloramphenicol** has broad spectrum activity against streptococci, staphylococci, *Brucella* spp., *Pasteurella* spp., and anaerobes, but poor activity against *Pseudomonas* spp. It is highly lipophilic and readily enters cells, the CNS, and the eye. The drug may cause idiosyncratic fatal anemia in humans, but dogs and cats usually experience only a mild, transient anemia, if that. Oral chloramphenicol

TABLE 10-2

Dosages of New or Commonly Used Antibiotics in Veterinary Medicine

GENERIC AND TRADE NAMES	DOSAGE
Azithromycin (Zithromax)	*Dogs:* 5–10 mg/kg; PO; qd or bid for 5–20 days *Cats:* 5–15 mg/kg; PO; qod to qd to bid for 3–5 days
Clindamycin (Antirobe)	*Dogs:* 11 mg/kg; PO, SC, or IV; bid to tid *Cats:* 5–22 mg/kg; PO or SC; bid to qd
Gentamicin (Gentocin)	*Dogs:* 4.4–6.6 mg/kg; IV, SC, or IM; qd (preferably in the morning) *Cats:* 2.2–4.4 mg/kg IV, SC, or IM; qd
Amikacin (Amiglyde-V)	20–25 mg/kg; IV, SC, or IM; qd (preferably in the morning)
Ticarcillin plus clavulanate (Timentin)	50 mg/kg; IV; tid to qid
Imipenem-cilastatin (Primaxin)	3–7.5 mg/kg; IV* or IM†; tid or qid (or up to every 4 hr for multidrug resistant bacteria)
Enrofloxacin (Baytril)‡	*Urinary tract infection:* 2.5 mg/kg; IV, IM, SC, PO; bid *Deep tissue infection:* 7–20 mg/kg; IV, IM, SC, PO; qd *Septicemia:* 30 mg/kg; IV; qd
Difloxacin (Dicural)	5–10 mg/kg; PO; qd (use higher dose for organisms with higher MIC)
Orbifloxacin (Orbax)	2.5–7.5 mg/kg; PO; qd (use higher dose for organisms with higher MIC)
Vancomycin (Vancocin, Vancoled)	*Dogs:* 10–20 mg/kg; IV; qid (infuse over 30–60 minutes) *Cats:* 15 mg/kg; IV; bid or tid (infuse over 30–60 minutes)
Metronidazole (Flagyl)	7.5–10 mg/kg; PO or IV; bid to tid (dilute and give slowly over 20 minutes)

PO, Oral; *qd,* once a day; *qod,* every other day; *IV,* intravenous; *SC,* subcutaneous; *IM,* intramuscular; *bid,* twice a day; *tid,* three times a day; *MIC,* minimum inhibitory concentration; *qid,* four times a day.
*For infusion (imipenem-cilastatin injection), administer over 20–30 minutes.
† For IM injection (suspension), reconstitute with 1% lidocaine.
‡When given IV, enrofloxacin is typically diluted and given over 10 to 20 minutes. Recent reports suggest that enrofloxacin may be associated with blindness in cats when doses greater than 5 mg/kg are used. It can be given as a single IV injection daily.

was taken off the market for a time, but currently both the injectable and the oral forms are available.

The **tetracyclines** are effective against many gram-positive and gram-negative bacteria, including *Chlamydia* spp., rickettsiae, spirochetes, *Mycoplasma* spp., bacterial L-forms, and some protozoa. They usually are ineffective against staphylococci, enterococci, *Pseudomonas* spp., and Enterobacteriaceae. Tetracyclines are distributed well to most tissues, although not to the CNS, and they achieve good intracellular concentrations. Products containing calcium chelate tetracyclines interfere with oral absorption. Binding of the drugs to calcium can be a problem in young or pregnant animals, and tooth discoloration and inhibited bone growth can occur.

> NOTE: Tetracyclines are caustic, and it is critical that the patient drink water immediately after swallowing a tablet or capsule (in the case of doxycycline, the patient may eat nondairy food). Otherwise the tablet may lodge in the esophagus and cause esophagitis and even a benign stricture (especially in cats).

Erythromycin is readily absorbed from the upper gastrointestinal system and diffuses well throughout most tissue; however, it has a narrow spectrum of activity and may be associated with nausea and vomiting because of its prokinetic activity. New derivatives include clarithromycin (Biaxin), azithromycin (Zithromax), and dirithromycin (Dynabac). Azithromycin (see Table 10-2) is active against aerobic bacteria, such as staphylococci and streptococci, and anaerobes. It also has good activity against *Mycoplasma* spp. and intracellular organisms, such as *Bartonella* spp., *Toxoplasma* spp., and atypical mycobacteria. Oral absorption of azithromycin is high, and it is well tolerated. The drug achieves extremely high tissue concentrations and needs to be given only once daily.

Clindamycin, a semisynthetic derivative of lincomycin, has a limited spectrum of activity compared with erythromycin. It is active against gram-positive pathogens, including staphylococci, streptococci, clostridia, several *Actinomyces* spp., and some *Nocardia* spp. It is extremely effective against many anaerobic bacteria. Clindamycin often is used to treat infections resistant to penicillins and erythromycin or in patients that cannot tolerate those drugs. It is effective against staphylococcal osteomyelitis but ineffective against gram-negative bacteria.

The **aminoglycosides** (e.g., amikacin, gentamicin, kanamycin, neomycin, netilmicin, and tobramycin) also disrupt protein synthesis, but bind irreversibly to bacterial ribosomes and are bactericidal. They are effective against gram-negative and gram-positive bacteria, including Enterobacteriaceae and pseudomonads, and have a synergistic effect with β-lactam antibiotics. Their activity is reduced in necrotic tissue because of free nucleic acid material. Anaerobes are resistant to aminoglycosides because they lack the receptor necessary for transport ParnTO the bacterial cell. Aminoglycosides are polar and therefore lipid insoluble, meaning they have limited dis-

tribution in the extracellular and cerebrospinal fluids. However, distribution into the pleural fluid, bone, joints, and peritoneal cavity is good. None of the aminoglycosides are well absorbed orally. They are "concentration-dependent" rather than "time-dependent," meaning that they can be given at higher doses at longer intervals (e.g., once daily), a dosing schedule that maintains effectiveness but reduces renal toxicity. Dehydration, electrolyte loss, preexisting renal disease, and concurrent use of other nephrotoxic drugs (e.g., nonsteroidal antiinflammatory drugs [NSAIDs]) increase the nephrotoxicity of aminoglycosides. Ototoxicosis and neuromuscular blockade are other possible adverse effects. Using a combination of a β-lactam and an aminoglycoside is often synergistic, plus it helps prevent bacteria from becoming resistant to these drugs.

> NOTE: A β-lactam drug should never be mixed in the same syringe, vial, or intravenous (IV) line with an aminoglycoside because mixing the two can result in a chemical reaction that inactivates one or both of the drugs.

Inhibition of DNA Synthesis

Fluoroquinolones (e.g., enrofloxacin, difloxacin, ciprofloxacin, ofloxacin, marbofloxacin) (see Table 10-2) and potentiated sulfas (e.g., trimethoprim-sulfa) inhibit DNA synthesis. Fluoroquinolones inactivate DNA gyrase, preventing uncoiling of the DNA molecule during DNA replication and transcription to messenger ribonucleic acid (mRNA). They are rapidly bactericidal and are effective for soft tissue infections, pneumonia, osteomyelitis, and urinary tract infections caused by gram-negative organisms and staphylococci. They also are effective against *Rickettsia rickettsii* and possibly L-form bacteria, but are variably effective against gram-positive cocci, especially enterococci (except staphylococci) and anaerobic bacteria. An additional reported advantage is activity against *Pseudomonas aeruginosa,* but recent reports suggest that higher than normal doses are required to achieve this effect. The dose of enrofloxacin varies depending on the target tissue (see Table 10-2). Although the development of resistance to fluoroquinolones initially was considered unlikely, some pseudomonads, *Escherichia coli, Enterococcus,* and *Staphylococcus* spp. have become resistant. In one human hospital, 80% of methicillin-resistant *staphylococcus aureus* (MRSA) developed resistance to ciprofloxacin within 1 year of its introduction in patients. Outbreaks of MRSA are occurring worldwide. In the United States and Europe, the prevalence of MRSA was less than 3% in the early 1980s, but rose as high as 40% in the 1990s. Infections caused by MRSA have become a significant global health issue with serious consequences for all areas of human hospitals, especially operative rooms and intensive care units. Indiscriminate use of antibiotics probably will continue the development of resistant strains in both human and veterinary hospitals.

Possible side effects of antibiotic use include vomiting, CNS effects in animals of all ages, and cartilage lesions in developing animals.

> NOTE: When given IV, enrofloxacin must be given slowly in a diluted solution or the patient may experience morbidity or even death.

Oral ciprofloxacin is much less expensive than enrofloxacin, but it is also much less bioavailable in dogs (approximately 30% to 40%) than in people (approximately 70% to 80%). Therefore it is commonly underdosed when administered to dogs. Marbofloxacin has a broad spectrum of activity against the major pathogens encountered in surgical infections. It is safe in dogs, and a single IV injection of 2 to 4 mg/kg maintains plasma concentrations above the MIC for Enterobacteriaceae and staphylococci for 12 to 24 hours.

Trimethoprim-sulfonamide combinations are effective for the treatment of osteomyelitis, prostatitis, pneumonia, tracheobronchitis, pyoderma, and urinary tract infections. These combination drugs are bactericidal and function by inhibiting sequential steps in folate synthesis. Also, combination therapy is less likely to result in the development of resistant strains. Trimethoprim-sulfonamide combinations have a broad spectrum of activity, including most streptococci, many staphylococci, and *Nocardia* spp. They have usually not been effective against pseudomonads. Possible side effects include keratoconjunctivitis sicca, thrombocytopenia, anemia, bone marrow suppression, vomiting, hypersensitivity (i.e., vasculitis or arthritis), and hepatic disease. Some breeds, such as Doberman pinschers and rottweilers, and some families of dogs seem more likely to suffer side effects.

CAUSES OF ANTIBIOTIC FAILURE AND MECHANISMS OF ANTIBIOTIC RESISTANCE

Successful antibiotic drug therapy is based on administering the appropriate dose to the site of infection so that the bacteria there are killed or suppressed sufficiently to allow the patient's immune system to control the infection. Factors that contribute to antibiotic failure include inappropriate dose (i.e., excessive or suboptimal), frequency, or route of administration; inadequate length of treatment; inappropriate antibiotic selection (i.e., not based on culture and sensitivity results); inability of the antibiotic to alleviate the cause of infection (i.e., foreign body or implant); inability of the antibiotic to reach the target tissue in sufficient doses (e.g., cross the blood-brain barrier); antibiotic resistance by bacteria (see later discussion); depressed host immunity (i.e., concurrent severe or debilitating illness); pharmacokinetics of the drug; drug reactions; antibiotic antagonism; and incorrect diagnoses (i.e., viral diseases or foreign bodies).

Antibiotic resistance may be the result of enzymatic destruction of the antibiotic (e.g., some bacteria produce β-lactamases, which inhibit β-lactam drugs), alteration of bacterial permeability to the antibiotic (e.g., streptococci have a natural permeability barrier to aminoglycosides, which may be overcome if a cell wall–active drug, such as a β-lactam, is used simultaneously), alteration of the structural target for the antibiotic (e.g., resistance to aminoglycosides can develop through alteration of the protein composition of the bacterial ribosome that serves as the receptor in susceptible organisms), or development of alternative metabolic pathways that bypass the reaction antagonized by the particular antibiotic.

SURGICAL INFECTIONS
Classification of Surgical Wounds

Surgical wounds are classified by degree of contamination to help predict the likelihood that infection will develop. Bacterial infection is defined as having more than 10^5 bacteria per gram of tissue. The classification scheme was developed by the National Research Council (Table 10-3) to provide a basis for comparison between types of wounds and between institutions. Although this scheme is helpful, there is some overlap and inconsistency between and within groups. The infection rate for all types of surgical wounds is approximately 5%. Further classification of surgical wounds by degree of contamination results in significant differences in infection rates. There is typically a clear correlation in humans between the four categories of wound contamination (clean, clean-contaminated, contaminated, and dirty) and the surgical site infection rate. Risk index scores have been developed to better predict a person's risk of acquiring a surgical site infection. Procedure-related factors that have definitively been associated with a higher risk of infection in humans include hair removal the day before surgery, duration of surgery, and antibiotic prophylaxis. The "infection/inflammation" rate in a recent study of dogs and cats that had undergone surgery (1000 interventions) was 5.8%, whereas the "infection" rate was 3% (Eugster et al, 2004). *Infection* was defined as the presence of purulent drainage, an abscess, or a fistula, whereas *infection/inflammation* was used when the wound was "infected" or when greater than three of the following signs were present simultaneously: redness, swelling, pain, heat, serous discharge, and wound dehiscence. In this study, "infection" was associated with three major risk factors (duration of surgery, increasing number of persons in the operating room, and a dirty surgical site) and one protective factor (antimicrobial prophylaxis). The outcome "infection/inflammation" was associated with six significant factors (duration of anesthesia, duration of postoperative intensive care unit stay, wound drainage, increasing patient weight, dirty surgical site, and antimicrobial prophylaxis).

Clean wounds (see Table 10-3) have a published infection rate that varies from zero to 4.4%. In this category, wounds most likely to result in postoperative infection are those associated with severe trauma with multiple fractures, traumatic procedures (i.e., carpal arthrodesis), or fractures of the distal radius or tibia that require plating. It has been commonly believed that antibiotic prophylaxis does not reduce the infection rate except when surgery is performed by students or when the procedure lasts longer than 90 minutes.

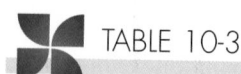

TABLE 10-3

Wound Classification System*

CLASSIFICATION	DESCRIPTION	PROCEDURE TYPE (EXAMPLES)
Clean	Nontraumatic, noninflamed operative wounds in which the respiratory, gastrointestinal, genitourinary, and oropharyngeal tracts are not entered	Exploratory laparotomy Elective neuter Total hip replacement PDA
Clean-contaminated	Operative wounds in which the respiratory, gastrointestinal, or genitourinary tract is entered under controlled conditions without unusual contamination; an otherwise clean wound in which a drain is placed	Bronchoscopy Cholecystectomy Small intestinal resection Enterotomy
Contaminated	Open, fresh, accidental wounds; procedures in which gastrointestinal contents or infected urine is spilled or a major break in aseptic technique occurs	Bile spillage during cholecystectomy or biliary diversion procedures Open cardiac massage Cystotomy with spillage of infected urine Lacerations
Dirty	Old traumatic wounds with purulent discharge, devitalized tissue, or foreign bodies; procedures in which a viscus is perforated or fecal contamination occurs	Excision or drainage of an abscess Peritonitis Perforated intestinal tract Ruptured gallbladder caused by necrotizing cholecystitis Bullae osteotomy for otitis media

PDA, Patent ductus arteriosus.
*National Research Council, Division of Medical Sciences.

However, one study determined that perioperative administration of antimicrobials effectively reduced the postoperative infection rate in dogs undergoing elective orthopedic surgery (Whittem et al, 1999). In this study, the antibiotics (penicillin G or cefazolin) were given within a 30-minute period before the first surgical incision and repeated every 90 minutes until surgery was complete. Antibiotics were not continued after the procedure was finished.

Another study showed no significant difference in the infection rate between animals with clean wounds that received appropriate perioperative antibiotic prophylaxis and those that received no antibiotic prophylaxis (Brown et al, 1997). Is this study, perioperative prophylaxis consisted of initiation of the drug less than 2 hours before surgery and discontinuation less than 24 hours after the procedure. However, the same study noted that animals that received antibiotics that were not given according to the aforementioned prophylaxis protocol and those that received only postoperative antibiotics had a higher rate of infection than the group that did not receive any antibiotics. This underscores the importance of using prophylactic antibiotics correctly. In a recent study, animals that were given antibiotic prophylaxis were 6 to 7 times less likely to develop surgical site infection than patients without prophylaxis (Eugster et al, 2004). Therefore it seems that prophylactic antibiotics are indicated in some clean procedures; however, it is imperative that they be given at induction and discontinued within 24 hours of the procedure (preferably at the end of surgery).

Clean-contaminated wounds (see Table 10-3) are identified when nonsterile luminal organs are entered without significant spillage of contents. Included in this category are procedures in which a minor break in aseptic technique occurs, such as perforation of a surgical glove. The published infection rate for this type of surgical wound is 4.5% to 9.3%; clean-contaminated fractures of the pelvis and long bones become infected most frequently. Antimicrobial prophylaxis is indicated in clean-contaminated wounds, and the choice of antibiotic is based on anticipated flora. In one study of 239 dogs and cats that had clean-contaminated surgical procedures, intact males and animals with concurrent endocrinopathies were found be at higher risk of developing postoperative wound infection (Nicholson et al, 2002). Total surgery and total anesthesia time were longer in animals that developed postoperative wound infection. No other factors were statistically significant.

Contaminated wounds (see Table 10-3) have a published infection rate that varies from 5.8% to 28.6%; contaminated fractures of long bones and the pelvis, and contaminated urogenital procedures most frequently become infected. Antibiotic prophylaxis is indicated for contaminated wounds, and drug selection is based initially on anticipated bacterial flora and modified according to culture and sensitivity results. These wounds are not infected initially, but have the potential to become so. The fate of contaminated wounds can be notably altered by early management. Delicate débridement, copious lavage, and antibiotic therapy can convert these wounds to clean ones, whereas inadequate therapy often results in a dirty, infected wound.

Dirty wounds (see Table 10-3) are those in which gross infection is present at the time of surgical intervention (e.g., traumatic wounds with retained devitalized tissue, foreign bodies, or fecal contamination). Management of this type of wound requires antibiotic therapy (initial selection is based on anticipated flora and later modified by bacterial culture and sensitivity results), copious lavage, débridement, drainage, and possibly use of wet-to-dry bandages to further débride the wound during the early postoperative period.

Classifications of Surgical Infections

Infections can plague surgical patients in four major settings: (1) with primary surgical disease (e.g., osteomyelitis that occurs secondary to an open fracture; pyometra; peritonitis that occurs secondary to gastrointestinal perforation; or prostatic abscessation), (2) as a complication of a surgical procedure not commonly associated with infection, (3) as a complication of support procedures, and (4) with prosthetic implants. The bacteria that cause infections associated with primary surgical diseases are characteristic of the nonsterile source (e.g., skin, urinary tract, or gastrointestinal tract). These infections are subject only to surgical treatment and not surgical prevention. Initial antibiotic selection is based on expected bacterial flora and later modified by culture and sensitivity results.

Sites of surgical procedures not normally associated with infection become infected when bacteria are introduced from nonsterile surfaces, such as the skin, gastrointestinal tract, or urinary tract, to sterile tissue. All surgical procedures result in some bacterial contamination. Development of infection depends on the number and virulence of the bacteria, the competence of host defenses, and the amount of tissue damage and dead space resulting from the procedure. Infections can be minimized through meticulous surgical technique, copious wound lavage, closure of dead space, and appropriate antibiotic prophylaxis.

Infection may be a complication of support procedures, particularly when extensive support procedures are performed in debilitated, traumatized, or immunocompromised patients. Intravenous catheters may be associated with sepsis, which persists until the catheters are removed. Patients with prolonged intravenous catheterization should be monitored carefully for infection. Cephalic catheters typically should be changed every 48 to 72 hours (although with proper care, they may be used for longer periods if necessary); jugular catheters often last for 7 to 10 days if managed properly. Urinary catheters are a common source of infection in perioperative patients when the duration of catheterization is greater than 2 to 3 days; proper care and maintenance of the catheter can reduce this risk. Bacterial culture of urinary catheter tips to diagnose catheter-associated urinary tract infections was not reliable in a recent study, and it was recommended that it only be used as an initial screening tool (Smarick et al, 2004). Patients with indwelling urinary catheters are not protected from infection by systemic antibiotics. Indwelling urinary catheters should be connected to closed drainage systems to help prevent ascending infection. Prolonged endotracheal intubation promotes the development of infection through the presence of a foreign body,

disruption of the mucociliary apparatus, and disruption of an effective cough reflex.

Prosthetic implants are foreign substances used to support, rebuild, or in some fashion mimic the function of an anatomic structure (i.e., total hip replacement, polypropylene mesh, nonabsorbable suture, vascular prostheses, metallic implants, or polymethylmethacrylate bone cement). The presence of foreign material in contaminated or infected wounds significantly increases the chance for chronic infection and implant rejection. Antibiotic treatment is seldom successful until the implant is removed because implants inhibit medications and defense mechanisms from reaching bacteria, partly because of the formation of biofilms. Biofilm forms when bacteria adhere to surfaces in aqueous environments and begin to excrete a slimy, gluelike substance that can anchor them to the surface of medical implants and tissue. A biofilm can be formed by a single bacterial species, but more often biofilms consist of many species of bacteria, along with fungi, algae, protozoa, debris, and corrosion products. Once anchored to a surface, biofilm microorganisms are extremely resistant to antibiotics.

If sterile, biocompatible implants are placed using appropriate aseptic surgical technique and antibiotic prophylaxis, infection and subsequent implant rejection are rare. Transient bacteremia (e.g., such as occurs with ultrasonic dental prophylaxis) may seed porous implants (i.e., methylmethacrylate) with bacteria and cause an infection. Therefore patients with surgical implants that require such procedures should be treated beforehand with prophylactic antibiotics.

Prevention of Surgical Infections

Preventing infection of the surgical wound is the primary objective of aseptic surgery. Factors that may determine if microbial contamination of a surgical wound occurs include host factors (i.e., age, physical condition, nutritional status, diagnostic procedures, concurrent metabolic disorders, and nature of the wound), operating room practice, and the characteristics of bacterial contaminants. Patients older than 10 years of age may be predisposed to infection because of an inability to mount an appropriate immune response or the presence of concurrent debilitating disorders, such as hyperadrenocorticism, diabetes mellitus, or protein-losing enteropathy. Patients younger than 1 year of age may be predisposed because of an underdeveloped immune system. Patients with protein-calorie malnutrition (see Chapter 11) are at increased risk, especially if hypoproteinemic. Diagnostic procedures (i.e., urethral catheterization, thoracocentesis and abdominocentesis, and intravenous catheterization), immunosuppressive therapy (i.e., with corticosteroids or cancer chemotherapy), long periods of hospitalization, previous antibiotic therapy, remote infections, and wound or body cavity drains may also predispose an animal to infection. Surgical duration is a risk factor for infection; in a recent study it was determined that the risk for infection doubled every 70 minutes during the surgical procedure (Eugster et al, 2004).

NOTE: Duration of surgery (and anesthesia) should be minimized in small animal surgery, and particular care should be taken in teaching hospitals where anesthesia and surgery times are often prolonged beyond that required by the surgical procedure itself.

Local conditions at the surgical site (i.e., presence of necrotic tissue, hematoma, serum pockets, local infection, foreign bodies, or dead space) may influence the patient's susceptibility to infection because they allow bacterial proliferation and inhibit the normal host response. A recent study identified the duration of anesthesia as a risk factor for postoperative wound infection, independent of the duration of surgery (Beal et al, 2000). Therefore long patient preparation times should be minimized to reduce postoperative infections. In addition, diagnostic imaging procedures such as myelography, ultrasonography, or radiography should be minimized in the immediate perioperative period.

Perioperative hypothermia should be minimized because it may reduce the patient's innate resistance to bacterial infections. However, in the study by Beal et al, no statistically significant difference in temperature was found between patients that developed wound infections and those that did not. In one study, animals that received propofol were 3.8 times more likely to develop postoperative wound infections than animals that did not receive the drug (Heldman et al, 1999). This was thought to be because of contamination of the propofol by hospital personnel, therefore propofol should be prepared and handled using strict aseptic technique, and any unused drug should be discarded promptly.

Operating room practices (i.e., principles of aseptic technique, sterilization and disinfection, preparation of the surgical environment, gowning and gloving, and preparation of the surgical patient, operative site, and surgical team) are important in preventing surgical wound infection and are discussed in Chapters 1 through 7. Considerable evidence supports the assumption that endogenous bacteria (i.e., bacteria from the patient) account for most wound infections. In a recent study it was found that the risk of surgical site infection increased 1.3 times for each additional person in the surgical suite (Eugster et al, 2004).

Proper atraumatic tissue handling and instrument use are also important in preventing infection. Traumatized tissue supports bacterial growth and has impaired host defenses. Traumatized or necrotic tissue also has reduced oxygen content, which permits the growth of anaerobic bacteria. Phagocytosis and humoral immunity are significantly diminished when tissue integrity is interrupted during surgery. Inexperienced surgeons cause more tissue trauma than experienced surgeons, resulting in greater susceptibility to infection.

The characteristics of bacterial contaminants may influence surgically acquired infection. The agents most likely to cause surgical wound infection are environmentally resistant bacteria. Such infections generally are acquired during hospitalization and are referred to as *nosocomial* infections. Surgical wounds are a common site for nosocomial infections. Overuse of antibiotics, indwelling catheters (i.e., intravenous or urinary), diagnostic procedures (i.e., transtracheal wash, thoracocentesis, abdominocentesis), advanced age (i.e., older than 10 years), and chronic debilitating disease are risk factors for nosocomial infections. Prevention of nosocomial infection requires control of endogenous flora (i.e., patient preparation [see Chapter 6]), diminished bacterial transmission (i.e., hand washing, gloves, disinfection, and sterilization [see Chapters 2, 7, and 8]), control of the hospital environment (i.e., maintaining proper cleaning, disinfection, and hospital sterilization protocols [see Chapter 4]), and rational antibiotic use, which is based on patient need plus culture and sensitivity results.

PROPHYLACTIC AND THERAPEUTIC USE OF ANTIBIOTICS
Prophylactic Use

Prophylactic antibiotics must be present at the surgical site during the time of potential contamination to prevent growth of contaminating pathogens. Surgical procedures that warrant use of prophylactic antibiotics are listed in Box 10-1. Antibiotics are not a substitute for proper aseptic tech-

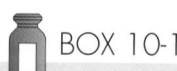 BOX 10-1

Examples of Surgical Procedures That Warrant Prophylactic Antibiotics

General Indications
- Surgery time longer than 90 minutes
- Prosthesis implantation (e.g., mesh, pacemaker, vascular prosthesis, bone cement)
- Patients with a preexisting prosthesis (e.g., total hip, pacemaker, bone cement) undergoing surgical procedures (e.g., dental prophylaxis, traumatic wounds, colorectal surgery)
- Severely infected or traumatized wounds

Orthopedic Procedures
- Total hip replacement
- Open fracture repair
- Extensive fracture repair
- Other elective procedures

Respiratory Procedures
- Resection of infected lung lobe or lobes
- Closure of esophagobronchial fistula

Gastrointestinal Procedures
- Colonic anastomosis or colectomy
- Strangulation or obstruction
- Pancreatic abscess
- Gastric resection for gastric dilation-volvulus
- Anal and rectal surgery
- Esophageal surgery
- Perineal herniorrhaphy
- Hepatobiliary surgery with infection

Urogenital Procedures
- Renal, ureteral, bladder, or urethral surgery with infected urine

nique, meticulous and atraumatic tissue handling, careful hemostasis, judicious use of sutures, preservation of the blood supply, elimination of dead space, and anatomic apposition of tissues.

Rational selection of antibiotics for antimicrobial prophylaxis requires that the most likely contaminating microorganism(s) be identified and that they be susceptible to the drug used. Empiric selection of drugs is necessary for antimicrobial prophylaxis. Antibiotic selection should be based on clinical experience plus published studies of the microbiology of small animal infection. Empiric selection of an antibiotic to prevent or treat infection requires a drug that is effective against at least 80% of the probable pathogens. The pathogens usually responsible for postoperative wound infection in small animal surgical patients are *Staphylococcus* spp. (especially *S. aureus*), *E. coli*, and *Pasteurella* spp. (especially in cats). The organisms most likely associated with surgical procedures are listed in Table 10-4 according to body system. Special considerations in the selection and administration of prophylactic antibiotics are presented in Box 10-2. Cefazolin has no adverse effects on platelet aggregation, bleeding time, platelet count, platelet size, prothrombin time, or activated partial thromboplastin time and therefore is a good choice for use as a perioperative antibiotic in dogs with conditions predisposing to hemostatic complications. Intravenous prophylactic antibiotics should be given no earlier than 30 minutes to an hour before the first surgical incision, and they should optimally be discontinued at the end of the surgical procedure or at least within 24 hours (see Box 10-2).

Therapeutic Use

Therapeutic use of antibiotics is based on clinical judgment, knowledge of the antibiotic's mechanism of action (see previous discussion), and microbiologic factors. When an anti-

biotic is indicated, the goal is to choose a drug that is selectively active for the most likely infecting microorganism or microorganisms, has the least toxicity, kills bacteria at the site of infection, and does not negatively influence the host's immune system. Therapeutic antibiotics are indicated in surgical patients with overwhelming systemic infection (i.e., septicemia or bacteremia); when infection is present at the surgical site or in a body cavity (i.e., wound infection, pyothorax, or abdominal abscess); or with any contaminated or dirty surgical procedure listed in Box 10-1. Generally, antibiotic therapy is instituted before surgery and continued for at

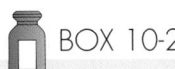 BOX 10-2

Considerations for Selection and Administration of Prophylactic Antibiotics

Antibiotic Selection
- Determine system involved and most likely organism (see Table 10-4)
- Cefazolin attains appropriate concentrations to prevent bacterial growth of the most common contaminants

Timing of Antibiotic Administration

Thirty minutes to 1 hour before first surgical incision

Cefazolin Dose

22 mg/kg

Routes of Antibiotic Administration

Intravenous; may repeat every 1.5 to 2 hours, depending on length of surgery

Duration of Antibiotic Administration

Discontinue immediately after closure of surgical wound or within 24 hours

 TABLE 10-4

Organisms Most Commonly Isolated From Various Body Systems

PROCEDURE, SYSTEM, OR CONDITION	LIKELY PATHOGENS
Thoracic surgeries (pulmonary and cardiovascular procedures)	*Staphylococcus* spp., gram-negative bacilli
Orthopedic surgeries (e.g., total hip replacement, prolonged internal fixation)	*Staphylococcus* spp.
Gastric and upper intestinal surgeries (high-risk patients)	Gram-positive cocci, enteric gram-negative bacilli, anaerobes
Biliary tract surgeries (high-risk patients)	Enteric gram-negative bacilli, anaerobes (especially *Streptococcus* spp., *Clostridium* spp.)
Colorectal surgeries	Enteric gram-negative bacilli, anaerobes (especially *Bacteroides* spp., *Streptococcus* spp.)
Urogenital system (e.g., with pyometra, endometritis)	*Escherichia coli*, *Streptococcus* spp., anaerobes
Deep, penetrating wounds (e.g., wounds less than 6 hr old, bite wounds)	Anaerobes, facultative bacteria
Dentistry (patients with valvular heart disease)	*Staphylococcus* spp., *Streptococcus* spp., facultative bacteria, anaerobes

least 2 to 3 days after apparent resolution of the infection; the maximum duration of therapy depends on the drug's toxicity and the disease treated.

Special considerations in the selection and administration of therapeutic antibiotics are listed in Box 10-3. The success of antibiotic therapy initially is determined by observing the patient's response for a minimum of 2 to 3 days. If the animal's condition has not improved by then, one must question if the antimicrobial therapy is correct. It will be necessary to reinvestigate whether the original diagnosis is correct; the culture and sensitivity results are accurate; the pathogen is susceptible to the antibiotic; the proper dosage, route, and frequency are being used; a foreign body or undrained focus of infection is present; a new infection is superimposed on the original infection; and/or the host's defense mechanism is severely compromised. With most surgical infections, antibiotic therapy needs adjunctive therapy to be effective. This may mean drainage of accumulations of serum, pus, or blood from surgical wounds or body cavities, concurrent débridement of necrotic tissue, continued lavage of infected wounds, removal of foreign bodies or infected implants, removal of urinary calculi, removal of pus from an abdominal abscess, débridement of chronic osteomyelitis, or drainage of suppurative arthritis.

References

Beal MW, Brown DC, Shofer FS: The effects of perioperative hypothermia and the duration of anesthesia on postoperative wound infection rate in clean wounds: a retrospective study, *Vet Surg* 29:123, 2000.

Brown DC, Conzemius MG, Shofer F et al: Epidemiologic evaluation of postoperative wound infections in dogs and cats, *J Am Vet Med Assoc* 210:1302, 1997.

Eugster S, Schawalder P, Gaschen F et al: A prospective study of postoperative surgical site infections in dogs and cats, *Vet Surg* 33:542, 2004.

Heldman E, Brown DC, Shofer F: The association of propofol usage with postoperative wound infection rate in clean wounds: a retrospective study, *Vet Surg* 28:256, 1999.

Nicholson M, Beal M, Shofer F et al: Epidemiologic evaluation of postoperative wound infection in clean-contaminated wounds: A retrospective study of 239 dogs and cats, *Vet Surg* 31:577, 2002.

Papich MG: Antibacterial drug therapy: focus on new drugs, *Vet Clin North Am Small Anim Pract* 28:215, 1998.

Smarick SD, Haskins SC, Alrdich J et al: Incidence of catheter-associated urinary tract infection among dogs in a small animal intensive care unit, *J Am Vet Med Assoc* 224:1936, 2004.

Whittem TL et al: Effect of perioperative prophylactic antimicrobial treatment in dogs undergoing elective orthopedic surgery, *J Am Vet Med Assoc* 215:212, 1999.

Suggested Reading

Albarellos G, Montoya L, Ambros L et al: Multiple once-daily dose pharmacokinetics and renal safety of gentamicin in dogs, *J Vet Pharmacol Therap* 27:21, 2004.

The authors tested six healthy adult dogs and found that once daily administration of 6 mg gentocin/kg body weight safely resulted in therapeutic levels of the antibiotic.

Barker CW, Zhang W, Sanchez S et al: Pharmacokinetics of imipenem in dogs, *Am J Vet Res* 64:694, 2003.

In a study on six healthy dogs, imipenem was rapidly and completely absorbed after SC and IM administration.

Bidgood TL, Papich MG: Comparison of plasma and interstitial fluid concentration of doxycycline and meropenem following constant rate intravenous infusion in dogs, *Am J Vet Res* 64:1040, 2003.

In a study of six beagles, interstitial fluid concentrations of doxycycline were lower than blood levels because of protein binding.

Boothe DM, Boeckh A, Boothe HW et al: Tissue concentrations of enrofloxacin and ciprofloxacin in anesthetized dogs following a single intravenous administration, *Vet Therap* 2:120, 2001.

In a study of four anesthetized dogs, enrofloxacin was present in all tissues examined after IV administration, but was lowest in trachea, articular cartilage, fat, tendon, and aqueous humor.

Frazier DL, Thompson L, Trettien A et al: Comparison of fluoroquinolone pharmacokinetic parameters after treatment with marbofloxacin, enrofloxacin, and difloxacin in dogs, *J Vet Pharmacol Therap* 23:293, 2000.

 BOX 10-3

Considerations for Selection and Administration of Therapeutic Antibiotics

Antibiotic Selection

- Determine system involved and most likely pathogen, to establish primary therapy (see Table 10-4).
- Obtain representative samples for Gram's stain, cytologic studies, and culture and susceptibility testing (e.g., fluid, tissue, implants, necrotic debris). It is best to obtain samples for culture before administering antibiotics, if this wait does not put the patient at inappropriate risk.
- Ensure that antibiotic reaches target tissue.
- If several antibiotics are effective, select the one that is least expensive, least toxic, and most convenient to administer. If the patient will be discharged while still receiving antibiotics, it is often best to choose an orally administered drug.

Timing of Antibiotic Administration

As soon as samples have been obtained, begin empiric antibiotic therapy.

Dose

Follow recommended doses carefully.

Routes of Antibiotic Administration

Treat for 2–3 days and then reassess animal's condition; if improving, continue therapy; if not improving, reevaluate and consider changing antibiotics.

Duration of Antibiotic Administration

Duration depends on effect of antibiotic, toxicity, and disorder being treated; give for at least 2–3 days after apparent resolution of the infection.

Marbofloxacin had the longest plasma half-life, and difloxacin had the lowest urine concentrations.

Gelatt KN, van der Woerdt A, Ketring KL et al: Enrofloxacin-associated retinal degeneration in cats, *Vet Ophthal* 4:99, 2001.

Seventeen animals with apparent retinal degeneration from enrofloxacin were studied; a few animals regained their vision.

Mealey KL: Penicillins and beta-lactamase inhibitor combinations, *J Am Vet Med Assoc* 218:1893, 2001.

This is a good review of the β-lactamases and the inhibitors that are used in combination with penicillins: clavulanate, sulbactam, and tazobactam.

Melendez LD, Twedt DC, Wright M: Suspected doxycycline-induced esophagitis with esophageal stricture formation in three cats, *Fel Pract* 28:10, 2000.

Doxycycline appeared to be responsible for esophagitis and subsequent esophageal stricture in three cats, probably because the medication stayed in the esophagus as opposed to rapidly passing into the stomach.

Moore KW, Trepanier LA, Lautzenhiser SA et al: Pharmacokinetics of ceftazidime in dogs following subcutaneous administration and continuous infusion and the association with in vitro susceptibility of *Pseudomonas aeruginosa*, *Am J Vet Res* 61:1204, 2000.

In a study of 10 healthy dogs, administering ceftazidime at 30 mg/kg SC or at a CRI at 4.1 mg/kg/hr resulted in serum levels sufficient to treat *Pseudomonas aeruginosa*.

Morgan MR, Gaynor JS, Monnet E: The effects of sodium ampicillin, sodium cefazolin, and sodium cefoxitin on blood pressures and heart rates in healthy, anesthetized dogs, *J Am Anim Hosp Assoc* 36:111, 2000.

These antibiotics were found to be safe in a study of 40 healthy, anesthetized dogs.

Rebuelto M, Albarellos G, Ambros I et al: Pharmacokinetics of ceftriaxone administered by the intravenous, intramuscular or subcutaneous routes to dogs, *J Vet Pharmacol Therap* 25:73, 2002.

In a study of six dogs receiving 50 mg ceftriaxone/kg body weight, giving the drug SC or IM, once to twice daily should be effective in treating most susceptible infections.

Rodriques J, Poeta P, Martins A et al: The importance of pets as reservoirs of resistant *Enterococcus* strains, with special reference to vancomycin, *J Vet Med* 49:278, 2002.

In a study from Portugal, vancomycin-resistant enterococci were not isolated from dogs.

Shamir MH, Leisner S, Klement E et al: Dog bite wounds in dogs and cats: a retrospective study of 196 cases, *J Vet Med* 49:107, 2002.

In a study of 185 dogs and 11 cats that were bitten by other dogs, mortality only occurred with thoracic or abdominal injuries.

Trepanier LA, Danhof JT, Watrous D: Clinical findings in 40 dogs with hypersensitivity associated with administration of potentiated sulfonamides, *J Vet Int Med* 17:647, 2003.

Samoyeds and miniature schnauzers were overrepresented, and clinical signs became evident 5 to 36 days after starting the drug. Fever and thrombocytopenia were the most common signs, but there were many other problems associated with sulfa drug administration.

van den Hoven R, Wagenaar J, Walker R: In vitro activity of difloxacin against canine bacterial isolates, *J Vet Diagn Invest* 12:218, 2000.

Difloxacin had activity similar to enrofloxacin, but was more bactericidal against *Staphylococcus intermedius* than was enrofloxacin.

CHAPTER 11

Postoperative Care of the Surgical Patient

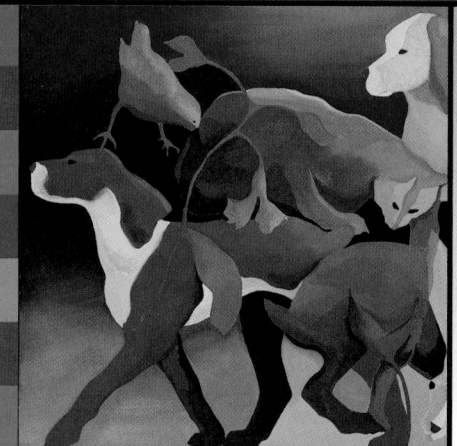

Care of the surgical patient does not end when the procedure is finished. The postoperative care of surgical patients often determines the ultimate outcome; with critical patients, it may determine whether they survive. Postoperative care involves normalizing homeostasis, controlling pain (see Chapter 13), and recognizing complications early. Early recognition of potentially catastrophic conditions facilitates treatment and ultimately recovery. Recommendations for postoperative care are included throughout this textbook with information on the treatment of specific diseases; general recommendations for animals undergoing surgery are presented in this chapter.

After surgery, patients should be moved to a quiet recovery room where they can be observed. Geriatric patients, ill or debilitated patients (e.g., those with renal dysfunction, hepatic disease, vomiting, or diarrhea), and patients that underwent a long surgical procedure should be maintained on intravenous (IV) fluids until they are able to eat and drink. Close attention must be paid to fluid administration rate and urinary losses to prevent volume depletion, severe electrolyte imbalances, and/or acid-base disorders. Temperature, pulse, and respiration should be monitored at least hourly (more frequently in critical patients) until the temperature is normal and the animal is alert. Hypothermic animals may need to be actively rewarmed with heated cages, hot water bottles or gloves, warmed blankets, or warm-air circulating blankets. Recumbent animals should be alternated between left and right lateral recumbency or placed in sternal recumbency until they are able to sit or stand without assistance. Evaluation of hematocrit, blood gases, blood pressure, and/or oxygen saturation may be necessary. Oxygen supplementation by means of an oxygen cage, nasal insufflation (see p. 27), or mask should be considered for hypoxemic patients (i.e., those with an arterial oxygen partial pressure [PaO_2] under 80 mm while breathing room air). Patients unable to urinate without assistance (e.g., patients with intervertebral disk disease) require special care; treatment of animals with neurologic disease is discussed in Chapters 36 to 41.

Anesthesia, toxic or metabolic disorders, primary brainstem disease, or increased intracranial pressure may cause central nervous system (CNS) depression. Patients with delayed recovery from anesthetic episodes should be evaluated for increased intracranial pressure, particularly those with preexisting CNS disease or trauma. Seizures, which are paroxysms of abnormal brain function, may occur after surgery as a result of the anesthetic drugs (i.e., ketamine), diagnostic procedures (i.e., myelography), primary intracranial disease that occurs secondary to intracranial surgery, or secondary effects of other disease processes on brain function (e.g., portosystemic shunts, hypocalcemia after thyroid or parathyroid surgeries, or hypoglycemia associated with insulinomas). Most seizures are short-lived and resolve before treatment can be instituted; however, patients in status epilepticus or with cluster seizures should be treated immediately, even if the primary cause has not been ascertained.

Mechanical ventilation may be necessary after surgery in some animals, such as those with severe hypoxemia (PaO_2 less than 50 to 60 mm Hg), severe hypercarbia (arterial carbon dioxide partial pressure [$PaCO_2$] more than 50 to 60 mm Hg], or increased intracranial pressure. Volume-cycled or pressure-cycled ventilators may be used. The respiratory rate and tidal volume should be adjusted to maintain the $PaCO_2$ between 30 and 40 mm Hg and the PaO_2 more than 60 mm Hg. Excessive airway pressures should be prevented. The PaO_2 generally is five times the fractional concentration of inspired oxygen (F_IO_2) (e.g., if a patient is breathing 40% oxygen, the expected PaO_2 would be 200 mm Hg); values less than this may suggest gas exchange impairment. Depending on the degree of impairment, additional treatment, such as positive end-expiratory pressure (PEEP), may be necessary. PEEP increases the functional residual capacity and volume for gas exchange, lessening alveolar collapse. PEEP can be provided with sophisticated equipment or by placing the expiratory limb of the breathing circuit under water. The pressure against which the patient breathes (usually 2 to 5 cm H_2O) depends on the depth the expiratory limb extends under water.

Hemorrhage may be due to surgery or underlying disease. Severe hemorrhage reduces the circulating blood volume and oxygen-carrying capacity, eventually resulting in cardiovascular collapse. Clinical signs of severe hemorrhage may be obvious, but occult hemorrhage into a body cavity may be hard to recognize. Pale mucous membranes, a slow capillary refill time, weak pulses, and a high heart rate are nonspecific signs of hemorrhage, but these parameters should be monitored closely after surgery. The hematocrit should be evaluated frequently if bleeding is a concern; however, acute blood loss often occurs without a change in the hematocrit. Although normal animals can lose approximately 10% of their blood volume without severe consequences, many postoperative patients are unable to tolerate this much hemorrhage. Ongoing hemorrhage should be eliminated or minimized and blood volume replaced. The choice of replacement product is dictated by onset of the deficit, clinical signs, and potential for complications. If hemodilution is not a concern, a balanced electrolyte solution may be given (e.g., Normosol-R). Two to three times the volume of blood lost may be given rapidly (not to exceed 60 to 90 ml/kg). Central venous pressure may be monitored to assess volume replacement, especially in patients with substantial cardiac disease. Packed cell volume (PCV) and total solids should be evaluated at frequent intervals after resuscitation. The optimum PCV in critical patients is 25% to 35%. A slightly lower than normal PCV reduces blood viscosity, effectively reducing afterload and improving cardiac output. If the PCV is 20% or lower or if hemodilution or ongoing hemorrhage is likely to cause the PCV to fall below 20%, blood products should be administered (see Box 5-1, p. 25). Fresh, whole blood replaces red cell mass, plasma proteins, platelets, and clotting factors. If the animal is not hypoproteinemic, packed red blood cells may be given. All blood products should be administered through a filtered administration set. Patients that are hypoproteinemic but not anemic may be given plasma or other colloidal solutions, such as hetastarch, to increase the plasma oncotic pressure (see p. 28).

> **NOTE:** Fluids containing calcium should not be used to dilute or flush lines containing blood products because clotting may occur in the tubing.

NUTRITIONAL MANAGEMENT OF THE SURGICAL PATIENT

An important component of postoperative care is nutritional support of debilitated or anorexic patients. Malnutrition is defined as the progressive loss of lean body mass and adipose tissue because of an inadequate intake of or increased demand for protein and calories. Possible consequences of protein-calorie malnutrition (PCM) are organ and muscle atrophy, impaired immunocompetence, ineffective wound healing, anemia, hypoproteinemia, diminished resistance to infection, and death. For these reasons, patients with PCM require nutrient supplementation during treatment of the underlying disorder.

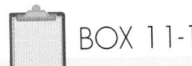

BOX 11-1

Diagnosis of Protein-Calorie Malnutrition*

- Weight loss of more than 10% normal body weight
- Anorexia or hyporexia (i.e., suboptimal intake of nutrients) for more than 5 days or an expected decrease in nutrient intake of more than 5 days
- Increased nutrient loss (i.e., through vomiting, diarrhea, severe wounds, or burns)
- Increased nutrient needs (i.e., due to trauma, surgery, infection, burns, or fever)
- History of chronic illness
- Serum albumin concentration less than or equal to 2.5 g/dl

*These are findings that suggest PCM. The more of these findings that are present, the more likely it is that PCM is present. However, not all of these will be found in a patient with PCM, and not every patient with one of these findings will have PCM.

A variety of conditions can cause PCM, including starvation, anorexia, malabsorption syndromes, severe trauma, surgical stress, sepsis, large surface area burns, and various types of malignancies. Surgery, postoperative complications, and surgically induced anorexia also increase metabolic demand for protein and calories. PCM shows no age, sex, or breed predisposition; it is common in all severely ill animals, with an incidence ranging from 25% to 65%.

Diagnosis of PCM is possible if three or more of the criteria listed in Box 11-1 are present. A physical examination may reveal a poor hair coat, pressure sores or wounds that will not heal, tissue wasting, skeletal muscle atrophy, emaciation, or all of these. Additional physical findings vary depending on the cause of malnutrition. Thoracic and abdominal radiographs of malnourished patients generally are nonspecific. Imaging techniques occasionally reveal an underlying cause for the patient's hyporexia, anorexia, or emaciation, such as an intestinal obstruction or an abdominal or thoracic mass. Biochemical changes with PCM may include hypoproteinemia, anemia, hypoglycemia, hyperglycemia, hyperlipidemia, or a combination of these. Other changes may be related to the specific underlying disease.

Prevention and Treatment of Malnutrition

Nutritional supplementation and identification and appropriate treatment of the underlying disease are the goals of treatment for malnourished patients. Hyperalimentation is the administration of adequate nutrients to malnourished patients or those at risk of malnutrition. Enteral hyperalimentation provides nutrients to a functional gastrointestinal tract by means of a nasoesophageal, pharyngostomy, esophagostomy, gastrostomy, or enterostomy tube; parenteral hyperalimentation provides nutrients intravenously.

Predicting malnutrition (e.g., on the basis of prolonged postoperative anorexia or the early stages of a possibly chronic disorder) and supplementing nutrients before they are depleted help prevent malnutrition in hospitalized patients. The specific treatment depends on the patient's calculated energy needs, the dietary formula chosen, and the route of administration (i.e., enteral, parenteral, or partial parenteral). Basal energy requirement (BER) is based on body weight; maintenance energy requirement (MER) is determined from the BER and the number and severity of clinical problems (i.e., cage rest, postsurgical stress, trauma, cancer, sepsis, or major burn). These calculations are based on specific patient data and are applied to the formulas shown in Fig. 11-1.

Diets for enteral use. The ideal enteral diet formula should be well tolerated and readily digested and absorbed, contain essential nutrients, be readily available and inexpensive, have a long shelf life, and be easy to use. Generally, diets should be isotonic (i.e., approximately 300 mOsm/L), should have a caloric density of approximately 1 kcal/ml, should include fiber at 1 to 1.5 g/100 kcal, and should provide approximately 16% of total calories as protein (i.e., protein content of at least 4 g/100 kcal) and approximately 30% as fat. Diets for enteral use are generally categorized as monomeric (sometimes called "elemental") or polymeric. Monomeric diets usually use crystalline amino acids as the protein source, glucose and oligosaccharides as the carbohydrate source, and safflower oil as the essential fatty acid source. They generally have twice the normal osmolality, can be used in patients with malabsorptive or inflammatory gastrointestinal disorders (e.g., short bowel syndrome, severe inflammatory bowel disease), and are expensive. A commonly used commercially available monomeric elemental diet is Vivonex HN; its composition is shown in Table 11-1.

Polymeric enteral diets contain large-molecular-weight proteins, carbohydrates, and fats; approach isotonic osmolality; require normal gastrointestinal digestive processes; supply about 1 kcal/ml; and are more economical than monomeric diets. These diets include blenderized diets, commercially available partially hydrolyzed diets, and commercially available liquid diets (Tables 11-1 and 11-2). Commercial polymeric diets are available in a variety of osmolalities, caloric densities, and compositions. Examples of commonly used commercial polymeric diets and their compositions are listed in Table 11-1. These diet formulas are indicated for malnourished patients with intact digestive and absorptive function or those suspected of having a food allergy; they also should be used for patients that must be fed through small-diameter tubes, such as nasoesophageal, esophagostomy, gastroduodenostomy, or enterostomy tubes. A prospective multicenter study evaluated the use of polymeric liquid enteral diets for nutritional support in seriously ill or injured dogs and cats and found them to be effective at maintaining good nutritional status (Crowe et al, 1997). Patients fed 7 days or longer maintained body weight, plasma protein concentrations, and serum albumin concentrations, and their attitude and strength improved.

The most cost-effective, well-balanced diets for enteral administration are those blenderized from prescription pet food or homemade diets. Caloric density and protein content vary with the diet chosen. Examples of blenderized diets and their compositions are given in Table 11-2. Blenderized diets can be administered through tubes with a diameter of size 8 French (Fr) or larger; a commercially available liquid diet is recommended when feeding through smaller diameter tubes (i.e., 5 Fr).

Diets for total parenteral nutrition. Diets available for total parenteral nutrition (TPN) should be customized to meet an animal's protein, carbohydrate, and fat requirements; caloric needs are calculated as described in Fig. 11-1. A common composition is 8.5% amino acids with electrolytes (protein source), 10% to 20% lipids (fat source), and 50% dextrose (carbohydrate source). B-complex vitamins are added at 1 to 2 ml/L. A recent study suggested that parenteral nutrition does not directly contribute to an increase in oncotic pressure; however, the indirect effects (associated with attenuating protein turnover and providing a supply of amino acids and energy) are not known (Chan et al, 2001). TPN can affect nitrogen balance, accelerate wound healing, and improve the patient's recovery from severe PCM. Possible problems include catheter management (i.e., sterile placement, maintaining sterility of the catheter entrance, and routine changing of infusion sets), expensive equipment (i.e., infusion pump), expensive feeding formulas, technical problems (i.e., routine patient monitoring during administration, proper diet preparation, and storage), and sepsis. In addition, if the gastrointestinal tract is not adequately stimulated by luminal nutrients and hormonal or neurovascular mechanisms, the intestines and pancreas may atrophy. Intestinal mucosal compromise predisposes intestinal mucosa to bacterial translocation into the portal circulation and possibly sepsis. These problems make parenteral hyperalimentation less desirable than enteral hyperalimentation.

Diets for partial parenteral nutrition. These diets are made with the same ingredients used for TPN except that 5% dextrose in water is used instead of 50% dextrose because it is only necessary to provide 50% of the patient's caloric need. The use of D5W instead of D50W means fluid composition will be determined by patient size. Smaller patients generally have 25% of their calories come from D5W, whereas 50% of their calories come from 20% lipid emulsion to allow for smaller volumes of fluid to be administered each day; larger patients may be the reverse. Partial parenteral nutrition (PPN) tends to be much less expensive and much less work than TPN.

Oral feeding is preferable to parenteral nutrition if adequate nutrients can be consumed to meet protein and caloric requirements. Several techniques have been used successfully to coax an animal to eat. If the owners can manage the patient at home, it may eat better there. Petting and vocal reassurance are also helpful, albeit time-consuming. Highly palatable foods or food coverings, such as gravy, may stimulate the appetite. Warming foods (e.g., in a microwave oven)

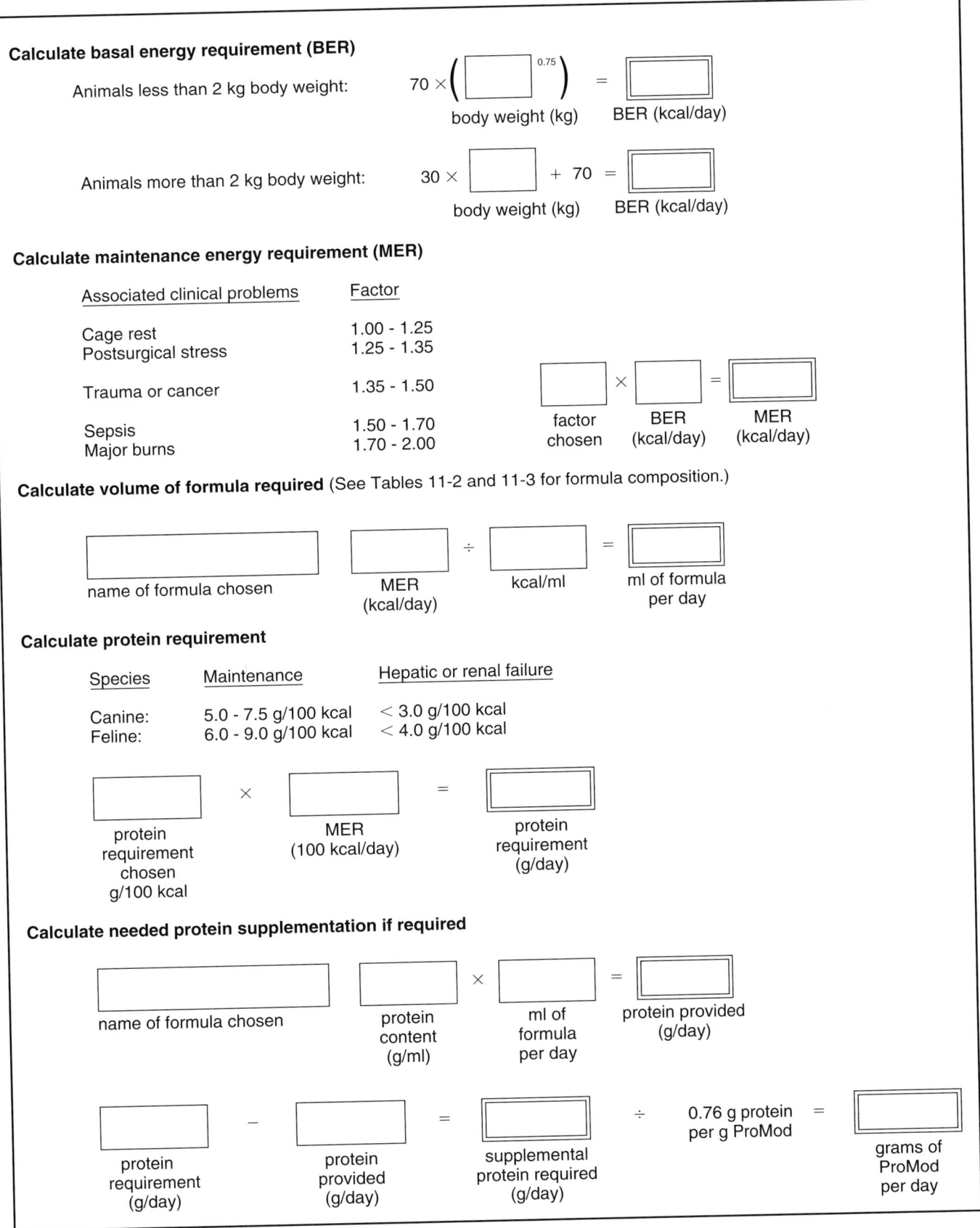

FIG. 11-1

Formulas used to calculate basal and maintenance energy requirements for dogs and cats.

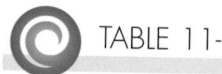

TABLE 11-1

Commercially Available Diets and Their Composition*

PRODUCT	CALORIC CONTENT (kcal/ml)	PROTEIN CONTENT (g/100 kcal)	(g/ml)	FAT CONTENT (g/100 kcal)	OSMOLALITY (mOsm/kg)
Polymeric Diets					
Jevity	1.06	4.2	0.045	3.48	300
Osmolite HN	1.06	4.2	0.037	3.68	300
Impact	1.00	5.6	0.056	2.80	375
Vital HN	1.00	4.7	0.042	1.08	500
Clinicare canine/feline	1.00	8.6	0.086	4.6	310
ProMod	1.48	0.76	N/A	N/A	N/A
Monomeric Diets					
Vivonex HN	1.00	4.60	N/A	0.90	810

N/A, Not applicable.

*These figures should be used for the energy requirement calculations in Fig. 11-1.

increases aroma and palatability. Supplementing potassium (i.e., 0.5 to 1 mEq/kg per os), vitamin B complex (in maintenance fluids), and/or zinc may increase appetite. Drugs that may stimulate appetite and their recommended dosages are listed in Box 11-2. These drugs are rarely adequate for stimulating a severely anorexic animal to eat sufficiently, but they may stimulate partly anorexic patients to resume eating.

METHODS OF PROVIDING HYPERALIMENTATION
Total Parenteral Nutrition

TPN is indicated when the intestine cannot adequately absorb nutrients, such as occurs with massive small bowel resection, greatly impaired small intestine motility, or severe malabsorption. Severe, prolonged pancreatitis and severe malnutrition are also possible indications. For placement of TPN catheters, patients should be tranquilized or anesthetized.

> NOTE: Designate the catheter as a dedicated-use or sole-use catheter and do not use it for obtaining blood samples or administering other medications unless there are severe extenuating circumstances.

Insert a 16-gauge, 18-cm, single- or double-lumen silicone elastomer catheter into the right or left external jugular vein. Position the catheter tip in the cranial vena cava and create a subcutaneous tunnel such that the catheter hub emerges on the dorsum of the neck. Anchor the catheter to the vein, to subcutaneous tissue along the tunnel, and to skin at the exit point with 4-0 to 5-0 nonabsorbable monofilament suture. Attach an extension set to the catheter hub, and bandage the catheter in place with sterile gauze, cast padding, and self-adherent wrap. After each use flush the catheter with heparinized saline (0.9% sterile saline with 1 IU/ml heparin).

The predetermined nutrient formulation (based on calculations described above and in Fig. 11-1 and Table 11-1) should be administered using an infusion pump. Generally, 50% of the calculated nutrient requirement should be administered the first day and 100% the second day. Initially, serum electrolyte, phosphorus, glucose, albumin, serum lipid, PCV, and blood urea nitrogen (BUN) levels should be evaluated daily, and body weight and temperature should be checked twice daily. In patients receiving TPN for several weeks, biochemical monitoring is often decreased to once every 2 to 3 days, depending upon the patient's condition. Every 2 days the neck bandage should be removed, the catheter entrance site cleaned with a povidone-iodine or chlorhexidine solution, the extension and administration sets changed, and a new bandage applied. Complications associated with TPN include catheter kinking and displacement, phlebitis, thrombosis, sepsis, hyperglycemia, hypophosphatemia, hyperlipidemia, azotemia, and electrolyte imbalances. If sepsis is suspected, it may be necessary to replace the IV catheter, although antibiotic therapy occasionally is sufficient. If a new catheter is placed, the tip of the old catheter should be submitted for culture and susceptibility testing.

Partial Parenteral Nutrition

PPN can be administered through a peripheral catheter because the partial parenteral solution is not as hypertonic as TPN solution. Although a dedicated catheter is ideal, it is not as important with PPN as it is with TPN. PPN is generally administered for less than a week, as opposed to TPN, which may occur for weeks in some patients. Patients receiving PPN initially are monitored once a day in the same way as patients receiving TPN. Complications (e.g., sepsis, phlebitis, hyperglycemia, or other metabolic derangements) are much less common with PPN than with TPN (Zsombor-Murray and Freeman, 1999) (Box 11-3).

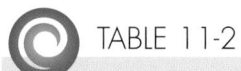

TABLE 11-2

Blenderized Diets for Dogs and Cats

Homemade Diets

Liquid Diet for Dogs

INGREDIENTS	NUTRIENT AVAILABILITY
1 jar (2.5 oz) baby food	1 kcal/ml
1 cooked egg	
15 ml corn oil	
15 ml corn syrup	
100 ml water	

Liquid Diets for Cats

INGREDIENTS	NUTRIENT AVAILABILITY
Equal parts egg yolk, strained baby food, and water	1.1 kcal/ml
3 oz egg yolk	1.5 kcal/ml
3 oz strained baby food	
3 oz water	
1 tsp cooking oil	
1 T corn syrup	

Prescription Diets

NAME OF PRODUCT	AMOUNT OF DIET	AMOUNT OF WATER ADDED	PROTEIN CONTENT		FAT CONTENT	
			(kcal/ml)	(g/100 kcal)	(g/ml)	(g/100 kcal)
Feline a/d	1 can*	none	1.2	8.75	0.105	5.5
	1 can*	1 can‡	0.6	4.38	0.053	2.75
Feline p/d	½ can†	¾ cup§	0.8	9.29	0.074	6.22
Feline k/d	½ can†	1¼ cup‖	0.9	4.36	0.039	7.54
Feline c/d	½ can†	1¼ cup‖	0.62	8.87	0.055	5.96
Canine a/d	1 can	none	1.2	8.75	0.105	5.5
	1 can	1 can	0.6	4.38	0.053	2.75
Canine k/d	½ can	1¼ cup‖	0.62	3.06	0.019	5.29
Canine u/d	½ can	1¼ cup‖	0.66	1.94	0.013	5.13
Canine i/d	½ can	1¼ cup‖	0.57	5.86	0.033	3.41

Preparation of Prescription and Homemade Diets

Ingredients

Mix the appropriate quantity of each ingredient (see chart above).

Preparation

Blend at high speed for 60 seconds.
Strain twice through kitchen strainer (1-mm mesh).

Advantages

Provides all required nutrients, low cost, appropriate protein and branched-chain amino acid content, normal stool consistency, manageable viscosity for 8 Fr catheter or larger.

Disadvantages

Cannot be used if the lumen diameter of the feeding tube is smaller than 8 Fr.

*1 can is equal to 156 g.
‡1 can is equal to 156 ml.
†½ can is equal to 224 g.
§¾ cup is equal to 170 ml.
‖1¼ cup is equal to 284 ml.

BOX 11-2

Drugs Used as Appetite Stimulants

Cyproheptadine (Periactin)

Cats: 2 mg/cat given orally (PO)

Diazepam (Valium)

Cats*: 2–5 mg/cat PO or 0.2 mg/kg intravenously (IV)
Dogs: 0.2 mg/kg IV

Oxazepam (Serax)

Cats: 2.5 mg/cat PO

Vitamin B$_{12}$ (Cobalamin)

Dogs: 100 to 200 mg, SC or IM or IV
Cats:
for inappetence: 50–100 μg/day PO, SC, IV, or IM
for cobalamin deficiency: <5 kg give 250 μg/cat IV, IM,
or SC, once weekly
>5 kg give 500 μg/cat IV, IM,
or SC, once weekly

*Rarely causes hepatic necrosis in cats.

 BOX 11-3

Partial Parenteral Nutrition for 10 to 25 kg Dogs

Calculation of Calories to Be Delivered by PPN

Resting energy requirement: (Body weight [(kg] × 30) +
70 = ___ kcal/day*
Calories to be administered: Resting energy requirement
÷ 2 = ____ kcal given daily by PPN

Formulation of PPN Solution†:

[Calories to be administered ÷ 3] ÷ 0.17 kcal/ml =
___ ml of 5% dextrose in water needed
[Calories to be administered ÷ 3] ÷ 0.34 kcal/ml =
___ ml of 8.5% amino acids needed
[Calories to be administered ÷ 3] ÷ 2 kcal/ml =
___ ml of 20% lipid emulsion needed
Parenteral B-complex vitamins = 2 ml/L of solution
___ ml of PPN solution to be given daily

Modified from Compendium of Continuing Education, 21(6):520,
1999.
*For animals with serious illnesses or extreme hypermetabolism, this
number may be increased by a factor of 1.2–1.5.
†For dogs and cats <10 kg give 25% of calories from 5% dextrose,
25% of calories from amino acids, and 50% from lipids.

Enteral Hyperalimentation

Enteral hyperalimentation is practical, safe, easy, economical, physiologic, and well tolerated, and has minimal morbidity in patients with a functional gastrointestinal tract. Enteral hyperalimentation is indicated in any animal with overt or impending PCM. Such patients include those that are hypermetabolic (e.g., patients with severe burns, sepsis, postsurgical stress, trauma, or cancer) and those with chronic anorexia or malnutrition, as evidenced by a greater than 10% loss of normal body weight. Enteral hyperalimentation can also be used whenever 5 to 7 days of anorexia are anticipated, such as after oral, pharyngeal, esophagogastric, duo-

 BOX 11-4

Tube Diameter Used Based on Route of Administration of Enteral Diets

5 Fr Tube Diameter
• Nasoesophageal
• Enterostomy (jejunostomy)

8 Fr or Larger Tube Diameter
• Esophagostomy
• Gastrostomy (typically 16 Fr or larger)

denal, pancreatic, or biliary tract surgery; during postoperative management of cancer patients, particularly if chemotherapy is instituted; and when the patient's mental status prevents self-feeding, such as with head trauma or after brain surgery.

Although enteral hyperalimentation is desirable for most patients with actual or pending PCM, infusion of nutrients into the intestines may be contraindicated in patients with severe adynamic ileus, small bowel obstruction, or lymphosarcoma in which enteral administration of nutrients results in a marked worsening of vomiting or diarrhea, such that it is difficult to maintain fluid-electrolyte balance or the patient becomes substantially more uncomfortable. In these patients, nutrients should be delivered parenterally.

Generally, oral administration of food is more efficient, easier, and safer and allows greater flexibility in formula composition. However, the further aboral materials are delivered, the less efficient the assimilation and digestion of nutrients, and the greater the care necessary in choosing formula composition. Route of administration dictates the diameter of the feeding tube (Box 11-4), which in turn dictates the usable feeding formulas. Various formulas have different viscosities and particulate matter size (see previous discussion). The most common routes of administration for enteral hyperalimentation are oral, nasoesophageal, pharyngostomy, esophagostomy, gastrostomy, gastroduodenostomy, and enterostomy routes. Each route has its indications, contraindications, advantages, disadvantages, and complications.

Nasoesophageal Intubation

Nasoesophageal intubation is easy, effective, and efficient. The availability of small-bore, soft rubber (polyvinyl chloride), and Silastic feeding tubes (i.e., 5 Fr) and of low-viscosity, nutritionally complete liquid diet formulations (see Table 11-1), in addition to patient tolerance of tube placement, have made nasoesophageal feeding popular. Advantages of nasoesophageal tubes include ease of placement, acceptance by patients, ease of tube care and feeding, patients' ability to eat and drink around the tube, and flexibility that allows tube removal anytime after placement. The major disadvantages of nasoesophageal tubes are the small size of the tube, inadvertent tracheal placement, and premature removal by the patient. Rarely, a patient may vomit out a nasoesophageal tube and bite off the tip. Placement of a nasoesophageal tube is indi-

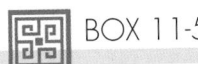

BOX 11-5

Recommended Tube Sizes for Nasoesophageal Placement

Cats, dogs smaller than 15 kg: 5 Fr × 91 cm
Dogs larger than 15 kg: 8 Fr × 91 cm

cated in patients with PCM that will not undergo pharyngeal, esophageal, or gastric surgery. Nasoesophageal tubes can be left in place for several weeks, are well tolerated, and are easy to remove. The patient can drink and swallow around the tube, eliminating the need for repeated orogastric intubation. Light general anesthesia may be necessary to place a nasoesophageal tube, but a topical anesthetic or light sedation usually suffices.

Instill proparacaine hydrochloride (0.5 to 1 ml; 0.5%) into the nasal cavity and elevate the head to encourage the local anesthetic to coat the nasal mucosa. Repeat the application of the local anesthetic to ensure adequate anesthesia of the nasal mucous membrane. If the patient will not tolerate nasal intubation, heavily sedate it and administer topical lidocaine (e.g., 1 to 2 ml of 2% lidocaine) or use light general anesthesia. Select an appropriate-size feeding tube (Box 11-5). Estimate the length of tube to be placed in the esophagus by measuring the tube from the nasal planum, along the patient's side, to the seventh or eighth intercostal space. Place a tape marker on the tube once the appropriate measurement has been taken. Do not allow the feeding tube to pass through the lower esophageal sphincter because this may result in sphincteric incompetence, esophageal reflux of hydrochloric acid, and esophagitis. Before passing the tip of the tube, lubricate it with 5% viscous lidocaine and hold the patient's head in a normal functional position (i.e., prevent hyperflexion or hyperextension). Identify the prominent alar fold and direct the tube from a ventrolateral location in the external nares to a caudoventral and medial direction as it enters the nasal cavity (Fig. 11-2). When the tube has been introduced 2 to 3 cm into the nostril, contact with the median septum at the floor of the nasal cavity can be felt. Push the external nares dorsally to facilitate opening of the ventral meatus. Elevate the proximal end of the tube and advance it into the oropharynx and esophagus. It generally will "drop" into the oropharynx and stimulate a swallowing reflex. Several methods can be used to confirm esophageal placement: (1) check for negative pressure, (2) inject 3 to 5 ml of sterile saline through the tube and see if a cough is elicited, (3) inject 6 to 12 ml of air and auscultate for borborygmus at the xiphoid, or (4) visualize tube placement using a chest radiograph. If the patient requires general anesthesia, visually confirm correct tube placement. Once satisfied that the tube has been properly placed, suture it to the nose and head to prevent removal by the patient. In cats, it is important that the tube not contact the whiskers; position it directly over the dorsal aspect of the nose and forehead (Fig. 11-3),

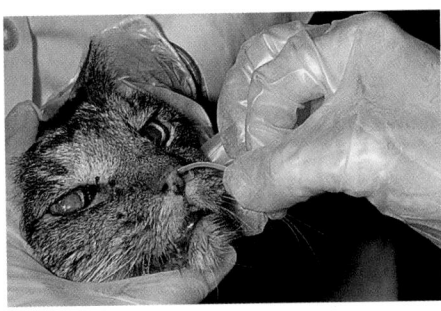

FIG. 11-2
Direct the nasoesophageal tube from ventrolateral in the external nares to caudoventral and medial as the tube enters the nasal cavity.

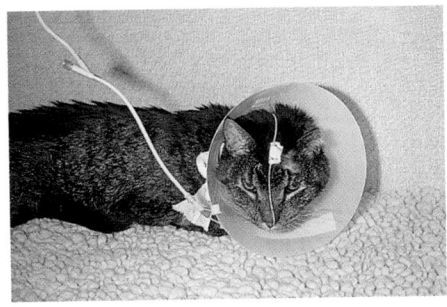

FIG. 11-3
In cats, secure nasoesophageal feeding tubes to the dorsal nasal midline and forehead.

and secure it with a Chinese finger-trap friction suture (see Fig. 30-8 on p. 901). In dogs, secure the tube to the lateral aspect of the nose and dorsal nasal midline with a Chinese finger-trap friction suture or cyanoacrylate glue. Place a column of water in the tube before capping it to prevent air intake, reflux of esophageal contents, or occlusion of the tube by diet.

NOTE: Use an Elizabethan collar immediately after surgery until it is determined if the patient will tolerate the nasoesophageal feeding tube.

Esophagostomy Tube

Esophagostomy tube feeding is indicated in anorexic patients with disorders of the oral cavity or pharynx and in anorexic patients with a functional gastrointestinal tract distal to the esophagus. It is contraindicated in patients with primary or secondary esophageal dysfunction, such as with esophageal stricture, after esophageal surgery or removal of an esophageal foreign body, or with esophagitis or megaesophagus. Advantages of esophagostomy tubes include ease of placement, acceptance by patients, large-bore tubes that allow blenderized diets, ease of tube care and feeding, patients' ability to eat and drink around the tube, and flexibility that allows tube removal anytime after placement. Esophageal tube placement eliminates the coughing, laryngospasm,

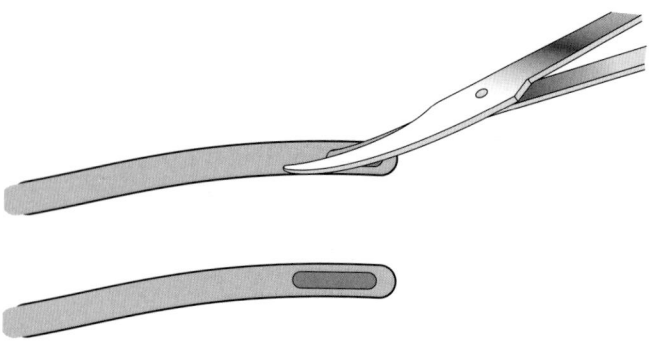

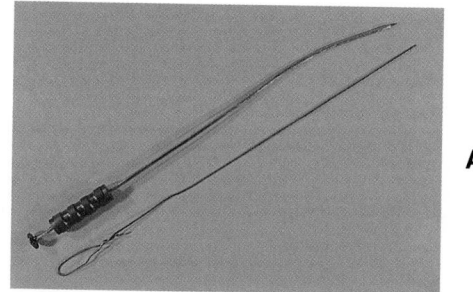

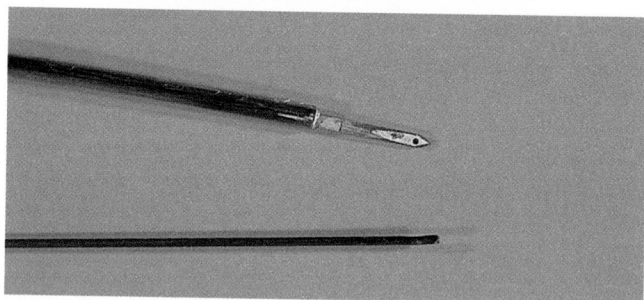

FIG. 11-4
For esophagostomy tube, enlarge the lateral openings of the tubes 3 to 4 mm to encourage a smooth flow of blended diets.

FIG. 11-5
A, Eld feeding tube placement device and stylet. **B,** Activated spring-loaded blade *(top)* and stylet *(bottom)*. (From Devitt CM, Seim HB III: Clinical evaluation of tube esophagostomy in small animals, *J Am Anim Hosp Assoc* 33:55, 1997.)

partial airway obstruction, and aspiration occasionally associated with pharyngostomy tubes. The major disadvantages of esophagostomy tubes are the need for general anesthetic for tube placement and the fact that some animals manage to scratch the tubes out.

Anesthetize the animal and place it in right lateral recumbency (left side uppermost). The tube may be placed on either the right or left side of the midcervical region; however, the esophagus lies left of the midline, making left-sided placement more desirable. Prepare the midcervical area from the angle of the mandible to the thoracic inlet for aseptic surgery. Place a speculum to hold the mouth open, and premeasure a 20 to 24 Fr polyvinyl chloride feeding tube from its insertion point to the level of the seventh or eighth intercostal space (ensuring midesophageal to caudal-esophageal placement), and mark it. Enlarge the two lateral openings of the feeding tube to encourage smoother flow of a blended diet (Fig. 11-4). Generally an Eld feeding tube placement device (Fig. 11-5) is used; however, in cats and small dogs, a curved Rochester-Carmalt hemostat can be used to place the tube. Place the oblique tip of the Eld instrument shaft into the oral cavity to the level of the midcervical region (i.e., equidistant from the angle of the mandible and the point of the shoulder). Palpate the tip as it bulges through the cervical skin. Make a small skin incision over the tip of the device and activate the spring-loaded instrument blade until it is visible through the skin incision (Fig. 11-6, A and B). Using the tip of the scalpel blade, carefully enlarge the incision in the subcutaneous tissue, cervical musculature, and esophageal wall to allow penetration of the instrument shaft (see Fig. 11-6, B). Place a 2-0 nonabsorbable suture through the side holes of the feeding tube and the hole in the instrument blade. Tighten the suture until the tip of the instrument blade and the tip of the feeding tube are in close apposition (Fig. 11-6, C). Retract the blade into the instrument shaft so that the tip of the feeding tube enters the instrument shaft (i.e., deactivating the instrument blade), and lubricate the tube and the instrument shaft. Retract the instrument and pull the feeding tube

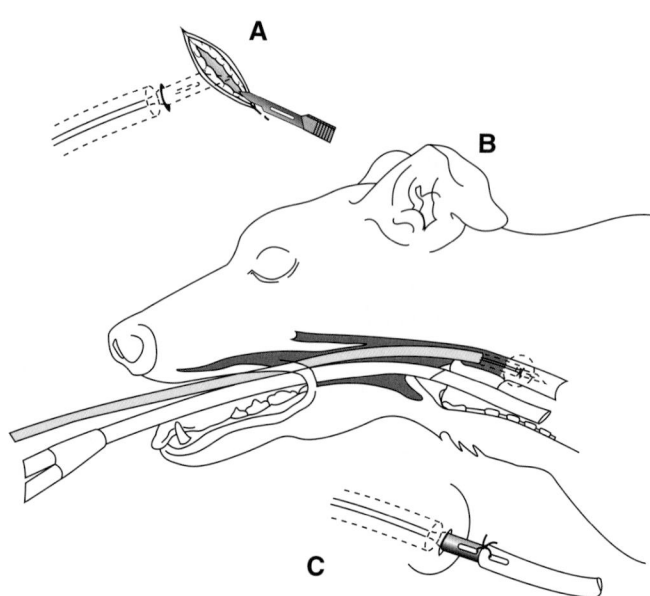

FIG. 11-6
Esophageal tube placement. **A,** Place the instrument shaft in the oral cavity and palpate the tip as it bulges the cervical skin; make an incision over the tip. **B,** Activate the instrument blade until it is visible through the skin incision; enlarge the incision to allow penetration of the instrument shaft. **C,** Use 2-0 nonabsorbable suture (e.g., nylon) to secure the tip of the feeding tube to the tip of the blade; retract the blade so that the tip of the feeding tube contacts the instrument shaft.

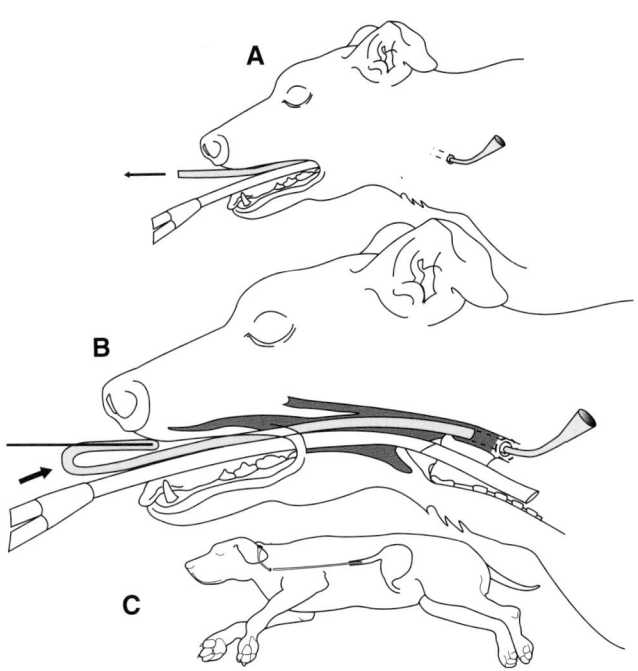

FIG. 11-7
Esophageal tube placement (continued from Fig. 11-6).
A, Retract the instrument and pull the feeding tube into the oral cavity. **B,** In dogs, place a stylet into one of the lateral holes of the feeding tube and against its tip; advance the tube into the esophagus. **C,** The esophageal tube should lie in the midesophageal region.

into the oral cavity to its predetermined measurement (Fig. 11-7, A). Remove the suture to free the feeding tube from the instrument blade and, in dogs, place a stylet through one of the side holes of the feeding tube and against its tip (Fig. 11-7, B). Lubricate the tube and advance it into the esophagus until the entire oral portion of the feeding tube disappears (Fig. 11-7, C) and the tube passes down the esophagus without twisting or bending. Carefully retract the stylet from the oral cavity to ensure its release from the tube. In cats, do not use a stylet. Instead, lubricate the tube and advance it into the esophagus with the thumb and forefinger until the tube is out of reach. Use a mosquito hemostat to advance the tube as far into the esophagus as possible. Manipulate the part of the tube that exits the cervical region to ensure proper passage into the esophagus. Secure the tube to the cervical skin with a Chinese finger-trap friction suture of No. 1 nonabsorbable suture (see Fig. 30-8 on p. 901). Leave the exit point of the tube exposed, or bandage it loosely. Place a column of water in the tube, and cap the exposed end with a 3-ml syringe.

NOTE: In dogs and cats, a small diameter, rigid endoscope can, if necessary, be used to direct the tube into the esophagus and ensure that there are no kinks or other problems.

Most patients tolerate esophagostomy tubes, and Elizabethan collars are seldom necessary. Esophagostomy tubes can be safely removed immediately after placement or can be left in place for several weeks or months. The tube exit site may require light bandaging and periodic cleaning with an antiseptic solution. The tube is removed by cutting the finger-trap suture and gently pulling the tube. No further exit wound care is necessary; the hole seals in 1 or 2 days and is healed by 4 to 5 days. In rare cases, esophageal contents leak from the stoma site.

Complications associated with esophagostomy tube placement include early removal by the patient or vomiting the tube up and chewing off the end. Esophageal perforation has occurred in cats, but is unlikely if a stylet is not used. Esophageal perforation has not been reported in dogs. Significant complications (e.g., esophagitis, esophageal stricture, esophageal diverticulum, subcutaneous cervical cellulitis) appear to be very rare. Reflux esophagitis can occur from improper tube placement (i.e., through the lower esophageal sphincter), or the tube itself can irritate esophageal tissue. Midesophageal placement of soft rubber or Silastic tubes notably reduces the incidence of esophageal injury and reflux esophagitis.

Pharyngostomy Tubes

A pharyngostomy tube may be considered whenever nutritional supplementation must be provided to anorexic patients (i.e., those with PCM) or to patients that are unable or reluctant to ingest food orally (i.e., patients with cleft palate, mandibular or maxillary fractures, or oral neoplasia). Pharyngostomy tubes should not be used for nutritional management of patients with esophageal disorders, such as esophagitis, esophageal stricture, recent esophageal surgery, removal of an esophageal foreign body, or esophageal neoplasia. The major advantage of a pharyngostomy tube over a nasoesophageal tube is tube diameter; pharyngostomy tubes generally are 20 to 24 Fr and therefore accommodate a wider variety of diets. The major disadvantage of pharyngostomy tubes is the ease with which the inexperienced person can malposition the tube (especially in smaller patients such as cats) such that the tube touches the larynx and elicits gagging and retching. For this reason, esophagostomy tubes (see previous discussion) are typically easier to properly place and maintain than pharyngostomy tubes.

NOTE: Pharyngostomy tubes are passed into the midesophagus; do not place them through the lower esophageal sphincter.

For tube placement, anesthetize the patient and position it in lateral recumbency with the incision site uppermost. Aseptically prepare an area 4 cm square just caudal to the angle of the mandible. Hold the mouth open with a mouth speculum. Premeasure a 24 Fr polyvinyl chloride feeding tube from the insertion point to the level of the seventh or

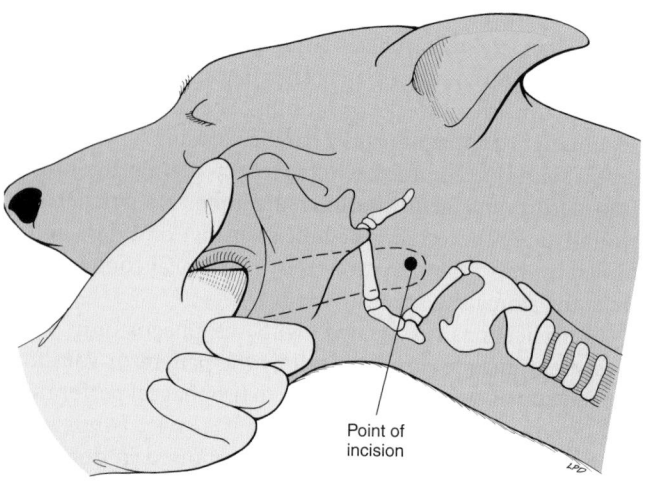

FIG. 11-8
Proper location of pharyngostomy tube exit relative to the hyoid apparatus.

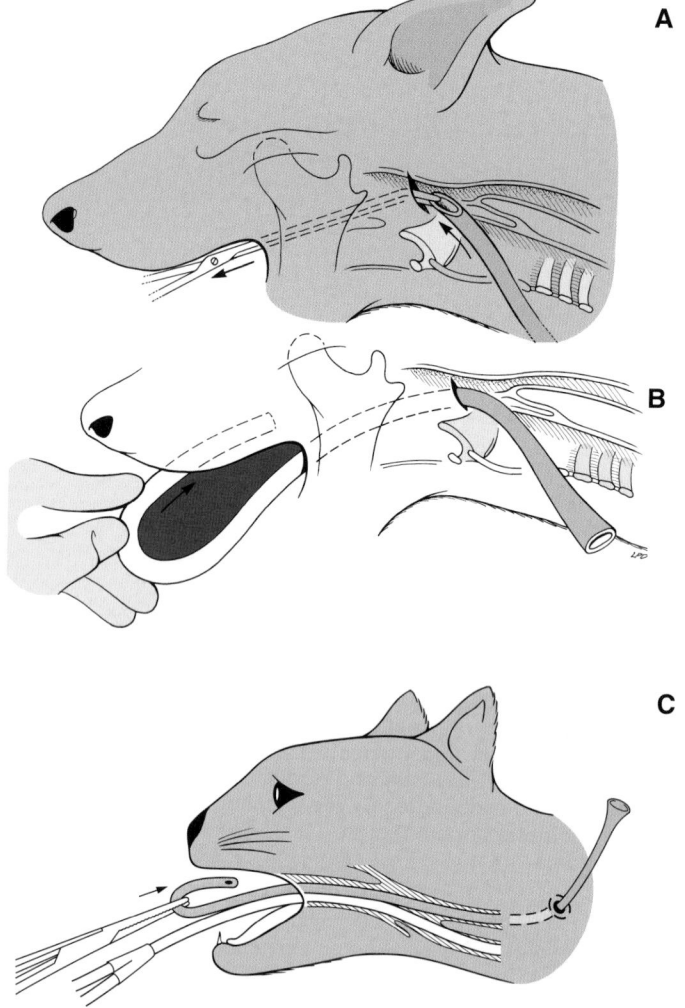

FIG. 11-9
Placement of a pharyngostomy tube. **A,** Pass a long forceps into the mouth to the point of tube entrance; incise over the instrument tip, grasp the tip of the tube, and pull the tube out through the mouth. **B** and **C,** Reinsert the tip of the tube into the mouth and pass the tube to its premarked midesophageal location (white tube is an endotracheal tube).

eighth intercostal space and mark it, ensuring midesophageal placement. Position an index finger in the pharynx, near the base of the tongue (Fig. 11-8), and palpate the epiglottis, arytenoid cartilages, and hyoid apparatus. Flex the orally located index finger toward the lateral aspect of the neck to identify the junction of the intrapharyngeal ostium and laryngopharynx (this is the proper location for the pharyngostomy tube exit). In general, the tube should be inserted as far back and as far up as possible. Apply enough pressure to the lateral pharyngeal wall to create an externally visible bulge. Substitute large, curved forceps (e.g., curved Rochester-Carmalt forceps) for the index finger to maintain the bulge. Make a 1- to 2-cm skin incision over the bulge and use curved forceps to bluntly dissect subcutaneous tissue, pharyngeal muscle, and pharyngeal mucosa until the index finger or forceps becomes visible. If the index finger rather than forceps is being used to maintain the bulge, replace it with curved forceps, grasp the tip of the pharyngostomy tube, and pull it through the incision into the oral cavity and out of the mouth (Fig. 11-9, A). Reinsert the tip of the tube into the mouth and pass it into the midesophagus (i.e., the premarked location on the feeding tube) (Fig. 11-9, B) as described for esophagostomy tube placement. Secure the tube at its exit point with a Chinese finger-trap friction suture (see Fig. 30-8 on p. 901) and to the patient's neck to encourage the tube to remain dorsal. Place a column of water in the tube, and cap it with a 3-ml syringe. When the tube is no longer required, cut the Chinese finger-trap friction suture, pull the tube, and allow the pharyngeal wound to heal by contraction and epithelialization.

If the pharyngostomy tube is placed ventral and medial to the intrapharyngeal ostium and laryngopharynx, partial airway obstruction, coughing, and gagging may result. If the end of the tube is placed through the lower esophageal sphincter, reflux esophagitis may occur. Vomiting up the tube has also been reported.

Gastrostomy Tubes

Gastrostomy tubes are indicated in patients with a functional stomach and gastrointestinal tract that are anorexic or are undergoing operations of the oral cavity, larynx, pharynx, or esophagus. These tubes are contraindicated in patients with primary gastric disease, such as gastritis, gastric ulceration, or gastric neoplasia. The advantages of gastrostomy tubes include ease of placement, patient tolerance, availability of large-bore feeding tubes, ease of feeding and tube care, and the fact that oral feeding can begin while the tube is in place. Disadvantages include the need for specialized equipment (e.g., an endoscope) and general anesthesia, invasion of the peritoneal cavity, and the fact that, depending on the placement technique, the tube cannot be removed for at least 10 to 12 days (i.e., to encourage adhesion formation between the stomach and the abdominal wall). Very large dogs may be problematic in that it can sometimes be difficult to achieve a good adhesion between the stomach and the abdominal wall when placing a gastrostomy tube with a device or an endoscope (i.e., it is hard to have the stomach in apposition to the body wall without any movement in these patients). In such circumstances, it may be best to place the gastrostomy tube surgically, or endoscopically but then percutaneously place sutures through the abdominal wall that incorporate the gastric wall, thus preventing such movement. Also, tubes placed blindly using a spring-loaded device can be malpositioned such that they are placed at the lower esophageal sphincter (resulting in vomiting and gastroesophageal reflux) or so far caudally in the stomach that the stomach may pull off the tube when it is filled with food. Very rarely the tube may be associated with gastric bleeding. Recently, low-profile gastrostomy ports have been recommended for use in animals for which long-term nutritional management or medication administration is anticipated (Elliott et al, 2000; McCrackin et al, 2000).

Gastrostomy tubes can be placed percutaneously without the aid of an endoscope, percutaneously with the aid of an endoscope or other device, or by laparotomy. Percutaneous placement can be done with or without gastropexy.

Percutaneous gastrostomy tube placement with gastropexy. The advantages of this technique include ease of tube placement; ease of finding the stomach in an anorexic patient; quick placement; no need for special equipment, such as an endoscope or feeding tube placement device; an immediate seal between the stomach wall and the body wall (with surgical gastropexy); and confirmation of proper placement during the procedure. The tube can be removed safely at any time after placement.

Anesthetize the animal and perform standard skin preparation of the left paralumbar fossa. Prepare the left flank area for aseptic surgery and drape the area. Have a nonsterile assistant pass a large-bore, stiff plastic tube into the stomach. The surgeon, who is sterile, palpates the left flank area until the end of the stomach tube can be palpated and grasped (Fig. 11-10, A). Manipulate the tube to a location 2 to 3 cm caudal to the thirteenth rib and 2 to 3 cm distal to the transverse processes of the lumbar vertebrae. Hold the tube stable and make a skin incision over the end of the stomach tube. Bluntly dissect the subcutaneous tissues and abdominal muscles to expose the wall of the stomach over the tube; take care not to enter the lumen of the stomach (Fig. 11-10, B). Place a purse-string suture in the stomach wall around the tube (Fig. 11-10, C). Use a No. 11 scalpel blade to puncture the stomach wall by punching the blade into the lumen of the tube; make the incision large enough to accommodate the selected tube easily. Place a 20 to 24 Fr Foley catheter into the lumen of the stomach and inflate the bulb (Fig. 11-11, A). Place traction on the purse-string suture and slowly withdraw the stiff stomach tube from the oral cavity.

Place gentle traction on the Foley catheter to bring the inflated bulb against the stomach wall (Fig. 11-11, B). Snugly tie the purse-string suture around the Foley catheter. Place three to four simple interrupted 2-0 absorbable sutures (i.e., PDS or Maxon) from the stomach wall to the body wall to firmly pexy the stomach in place. Close the subcutaneous tissue and skin around the existing Foley catheter, push the Foley catheter 1 to 2 cm into the stomach lumen, and secure the Foley catheter to the skin with a Chinese finger-trap friction suture of No. 1 nonabsorbable suture (Fig. 11-11, C).

Percutaneous gastrostomy tube placement without gastropexy. Advantages of this technique are that no special instrumentation is required for placement, and it is easy to perform. Disadvantages are that the stomach is not pexied to the body wall (early removal by the patient could result in peritonitis), the novice can easily place the tube incorrectly so that it is either too far orad or too far caudad in the stomach, it is possible to penetrate and trap omentum or mesentery, and tube placement can be confirmed only endoscopically or radiographically.

Position the patient and prepare it as described above. Prepare a 20 Fr Pezzer (mushroom-tip) urinary catheter in the following manner. Cut off and discard the dilated proximal end of the tube. Cut off 1.5 cm of the remaining tube and set this piece aside for use as an external flange. Cut the remaining proximal end of the tube at a sharp angle. Cut a strand of No. 1 Braunamid to the length of the prepared feeding tube. Pass a stiff, large-bore stomach tube or feeding tube placement device (Fig. 11-12, A) into the stomach until it can be palpated bulging against the left body wall 1 to 2 cm caudal to the last rib and 2 to 3 cm distal to the transverse processes of lumbar vertebrae two or three. If a stomach tube is used, pass an 18-gauge hypodermic needle through the skin into the lumen of the stomach tube. Place a strand of No. 1 suture through the needle, into the stomach tube, and out through the mouth. Remove the stomach tube. If a feeding tube placement (Eld) device is used (see esophagostomy tube placement above), activate the device and thread the No. 1 suture through the hole in the instrument blade (Fig. 11-12, B). Retract the blade into the instrument shaft and withdraw the instrument out through the mouth (Fig. 11-12, C). In each case the No. 1 suture enters the stomach through the left flank and exits through the oral cavity. Thread the end of the suture exiting the oral cavity through the narrow end of an 18-gauge sovereign catheter and tie it to the proximal end of the prepared Pezzer urinary catheter (i.e., the feeding tube) (Fig. 11-12, D). Pull the Pezzer catheter tightly into the flange of the catheter and lubricate it. Pull the No. 1 suture exiting the left flank until the catheter tip exits the skin (Fig. 11-12, E). Enlarge the skin incision to 3 to 4 mm, allowing easy delivery of the catheter. Pull the catheter until the mushroom tip is snugly against the body wall, ensuring a seal between the stomach wall and the body wall. Secure the catheter to the skin with a Chinese finger-trap suture using No. 1 nonabsorbable suture (e.g., Novafil).

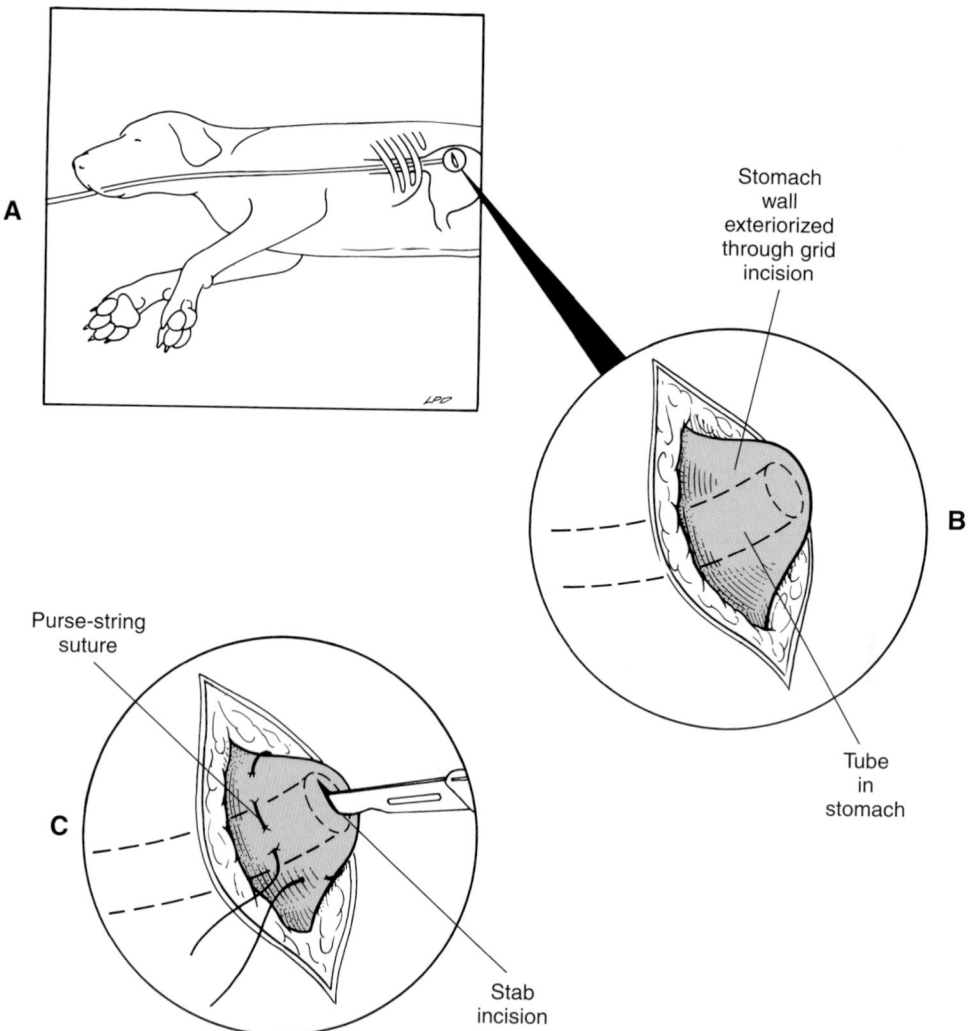

FIG. 11-10

Percutaneous gastrostomy tube placement with gastropexy. **A,** Pass a large-bore, stiff plastic stomach tube into the stomach. Palpate the end of the tube at the flank. **B,** Grasp the tube and move it to a point 2 to 3 cm caudal to the thirteenth rib and 2 to 3 cm distal to the transverse processes of the lumbar vertebrae. Secure the tube with thumb and finger, make an incision through the skin and subcutaneous tissue, and bluntly dissect the abdominal muscles to expose the gastric wall over the tube. **C,** Place a purse-string suture in the gastric wall around the tube and puncture the wall with a scalpel blade.

Percutaneous endoscopic gastrostomy tube placement. The advantage of endoscopic placement is that the tube is under direct visualization throughout placement and the stomach is submaximally insufflated, which tends to displace omentum and intestines so that when the gastrostomy tube is placed it does not penetrate omentum or mesentery. If a pexy is not done, no early, permanent seal is formed between the stomach wall and the body wall, and a 10- to 12-day wait is required before the tube can be removed.

Perform percutaneous endoscopic tube placement without gastropexy as described for percutaneous placement without gastropexy, except place the No. 1 suture from the left flank and out through the oral cavity with the aid of an endo-

scope. Pass the endoscope into the stomach, and insufflate the stomach with air. Make a 1-mm skin incision in the left flank 1 to 2 cm caudal to the last rib and 2 to 3 cm distal to the transverse spinous processes of lumbar vertebrae two or three. Thrust an 18-gauge needle through the skin incision and into the stomach lumen. Pass the strand of No. 1 suture through the needle and into the stomach, retrieve it endoscopically, and bring it out through the mouth. Once the strand of suture is entering the left flank and exiting the oral cavity, place the feeding tube as described for percutaneous surgical placement without gastropexy.

Gastrostomy tube placement by laparotomy.
This procedure generally is performed when tube placement

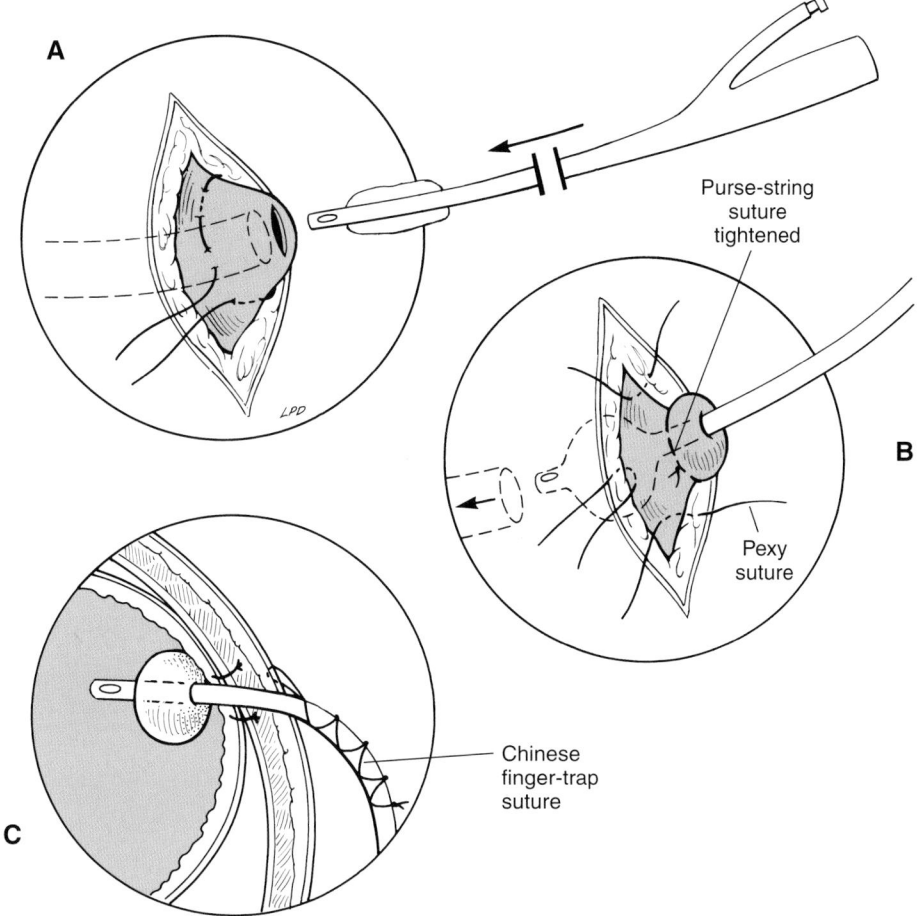

FIG. 11-11
Percutaneous gastrostomy tube placement with gastropexy (continued from Fig. 11-10).
A, Place the Foley or Pezzer catheter into the lumen of the stomach and into the tube.
B, Tighten the purse-string suture, remove the stomach tube, inflate the bulb of the Foley catheter, and suture the gastric wall to the abdominal wall. **C,** Note the proper tube placement of the inflated Foley catheter, the gastropexy, and the Chinese finger-trap friction suture to secure the tube in place

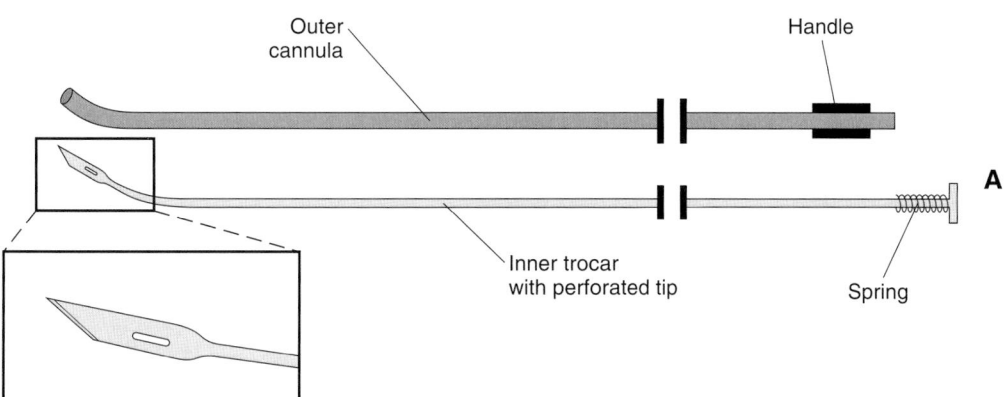

FIG. 11-12
A, Schematic view of a device designed to place gastrostomy tubes without endoscopy. The trocar *(lower)* is placed through the cannula *(upper)*. The cutting tip *(detailed insert)* is not extended until the device has been properly placed.

Continued

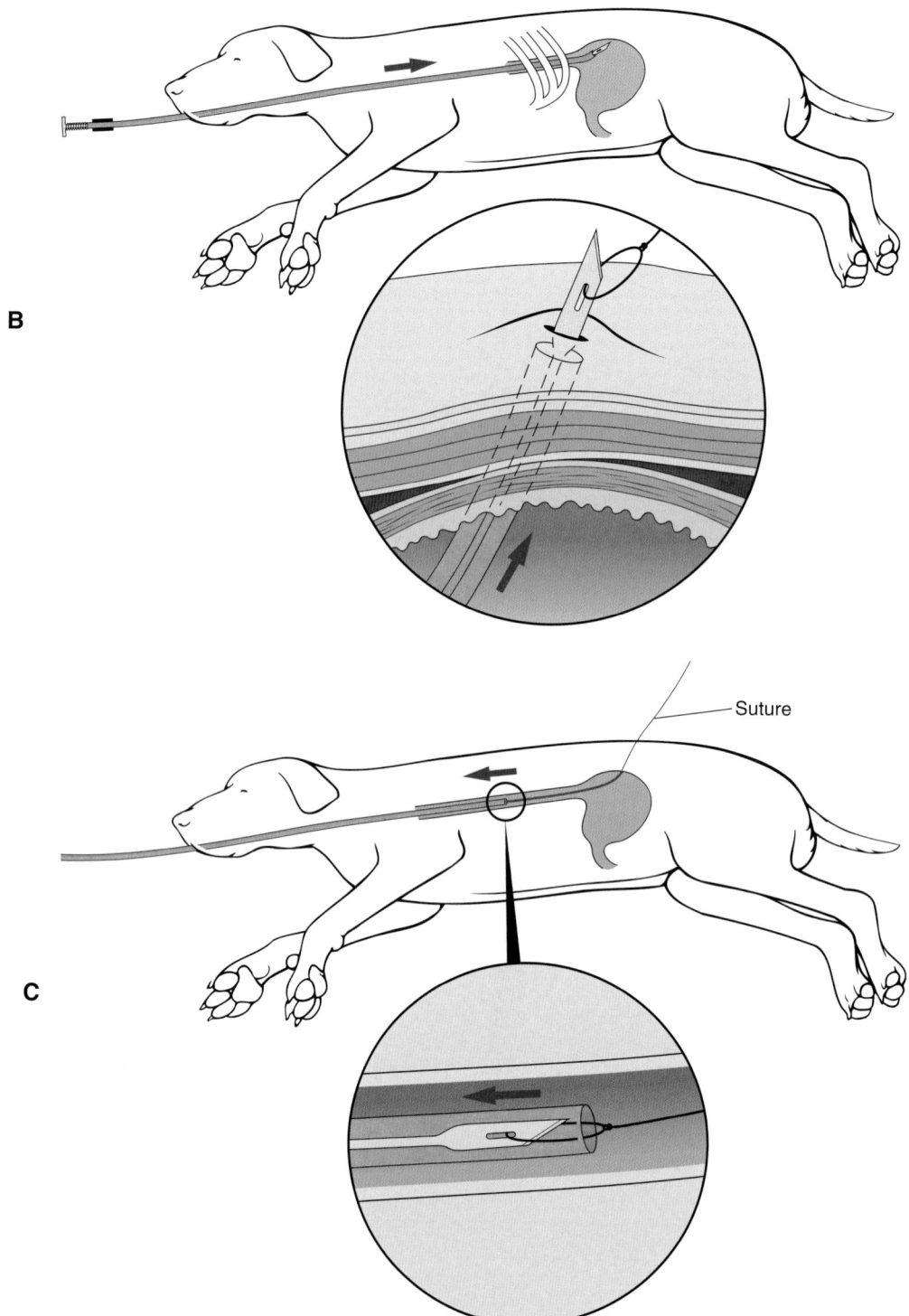

FIG. 11-12, cont'd
B, Schematic view showing how the device is placed in an animal receiving a gastrostomy tube. Note that the tip of the device ultimately arrives at a point 2 to 3 cm caudal to the last rib and 2 to 3 cm distal to the transverse processes of lumbar vertebrae two or three. Push the trocar tip through the cannula so that the blade tip extends through the skin *(insert),* and tie a suture to the tip. **C,** Retract the entire device (cannula and trocar) through the mouth, bringing the suture with it.

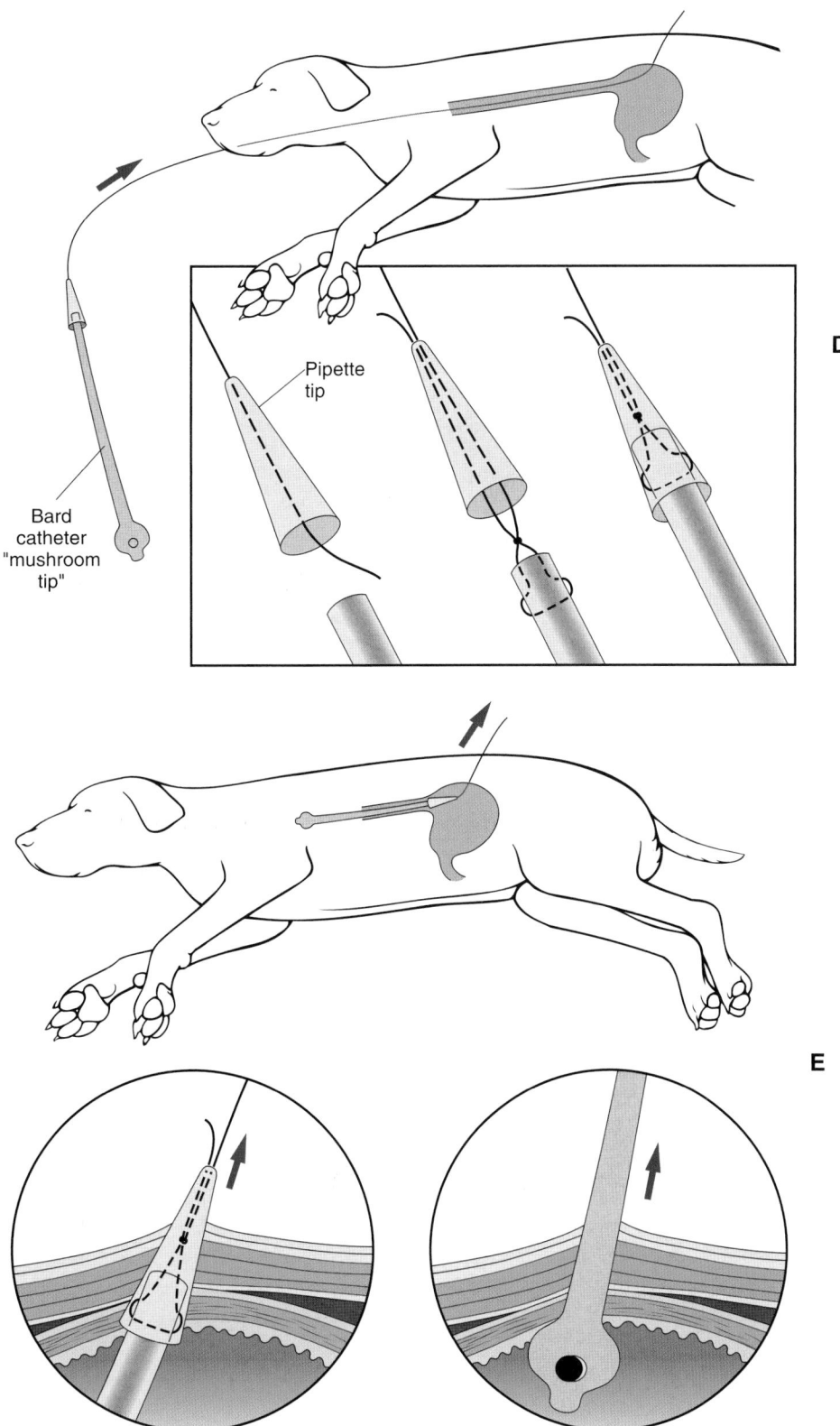

FIG. 11-12, cont'd
D, Fasten the end of the suture that is brought out of the mouth to the tip of a mushroom-tip catheter. Note how a pipette tip is placed where the suture attaches to the tip of the catheter. **E,** Pull the suture through the skin, pulling the mushroom-tip catheter into the stomach. The pipette tip facilitates passage of the catheter through the abdominal wall. Withdraw the catheter until the mushroom tip is against the gastric mucosa; the stomach is pulled snugly against the abdominal wall.

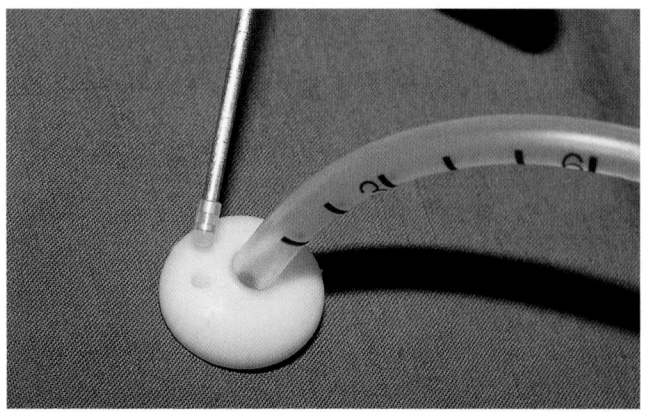

FIG. 11-13
Detail of the tip of the Gauderer Genie low-profile percutaneous endoscopic gastrostomy tube showing a small depression in the umbrella tip with the rod that fits into this depression.

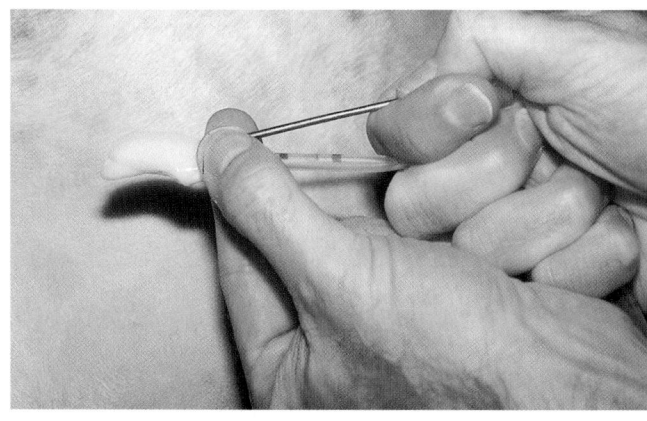

FIG. 11-15
Retract the low-profile percutaneous endoscopic gastrostomy tube, causing the umbrella tip to deform; this makes it easier to push this assembly through the previously established stoma.

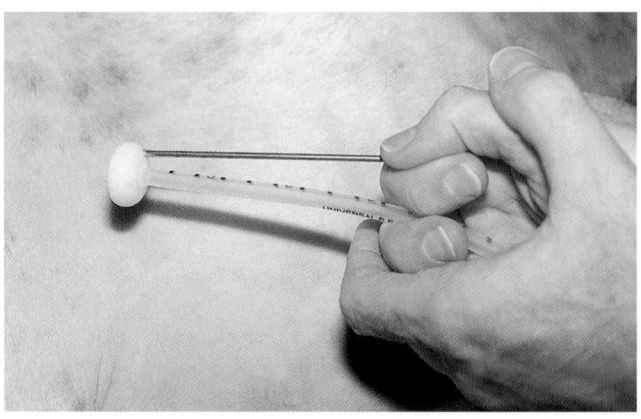

FIG. 11-14
Detail of the assembled low-profile percutaneous endoscopic gastrostomy tube and rod shown in Figure 11-13.

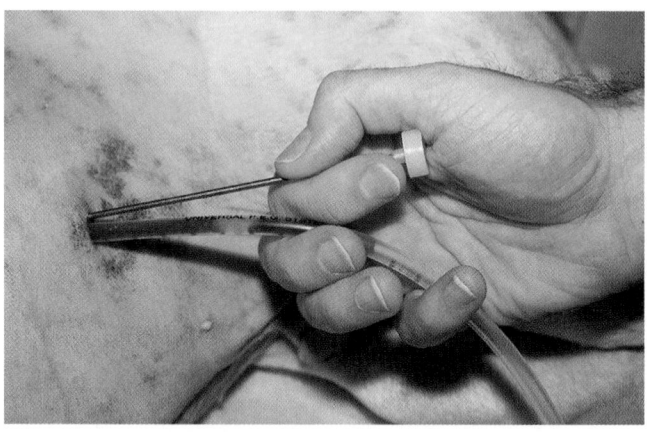

FIG. 11-16
Insert the tip of the low-profile percutaneous endoscopic gastrostomy tube completely into the stomach via the stoma. Remove the rod while holding the tube stationary; the umbrella tip reassumes its normal configuration.

is ancillary to another abdominal procedure, such as biopsy or removal of an abdominal mass.

Pass the distal end of a 20 Fr Foley or Pezzer catheter (i.e., bulb or mushroom tip) into the abdominal cavity through a stab incision in the left body wall. Exteriorize the stomach and place a purse-string suture in the ventrolateral wall of the body of the stomach. Make a stab incision in the center of the purse-string suture with a No. 11 scalpel blade and place the distal end of the feeding catheter in the lumen of the stomach. Tighten the purse-string suture around the catheter and inflate the catheter bulb (i.e., Foley catheter) with saline. Place gentle traction on the catheter to bring the body of the stomach in close apposition to the left body wall. Pexy the stomach wall to the abdominal wall with four 2-0 or 3-0 synthetic absorbable sutures. Secure the feeding tube to the skin with a Chinese finger-trap suture of No. 1 nonabsorbable suture (e.g., Novafil). Close the abdomen routinely.

Low-profile gastrostomy tube devices. Low-profile gastrostomy tube devices are available in different configurations and generally serve two main functions. First, some owners prefer to use them when a percutaneous endoscopic gastrostomy tube will be required for some time because the low-profile devices do not have a long tube exiting the body, which makes them esthetically more appealing. Tubes that do not "dangle" from the body may also be easier to care for (i.e., they are less likely to be pulled out or chewed out by the patient). Second, and perhaps the major value of low-profile devices, is that they allow quick and easy replacement of gastrostomy tubes that have inadvertently been pulled out or have so deteriorated that they must be replaced. The low-profile device is inserted into the stoma made by the first gastrostomy tube (Figs. 11-13 through 11-16). However, such stomas close rapidly (i.e., <24 hours) after removal of the gastrostomy tube; therefore, speed is of the essence. If the patient cannot be seen within several hours after removal of the first gastrostomy tube, a relatively large-diameter sterile red latex male urinary catheter or the like should be placed in the stoma to prevent it from closing down until the low-profile device can be placed. Some systems, such as the Gauderer Genie percutaneous endoscopic gastrostomy system with a Ponsky nonballoon replacement gastrostomy tube, allow the clinician to decide whether to make the device a low-profile one or to leave the tube long, mimicking the original percutaneous endoscopic gastrostomy tube.

> NOTE: If you need to replace a gastrostomy tube but do not have a low-profile device, simply insert the string through the existing gastrostomy tube before removal and use it to place a second, regular gastrostomy tube.

The most catastrophic complication associated with gastrostomy tubes is leakage of stomach contents into the abdomen with subsequent generalized peritonitis. This may occur if there is premature tube removal, when overfeeding large breed dogs (i.e., a very heavy stomach can pull the stomach off the tube), or secondary to improper placement of a low-profile tube when trying to replace an old gastrostomy tube. This complication can generally be prevented by using a technique that results in a sutured pexy of the stomach to the body wall (i.e., percutaneous surgical placement with gastropexy or by laparotomy). Other complications of gastrostomy tubes include vomiting, peristomal infection (relatively common, although often minor and easily managed), and migration of the tip of the catheter into the pylorus. Pezzer catheters last longer (weeks to months) in the stomach than Foley catheters because the balloons of Foley catheters disintegrate. As noted previously, low-profile gastrostomy devices (e.g., Flexiflo gastrostomy tubes, Ross Laboratories, Columbus, Ohio) may be better tolerated by owners when tubes are meant to remain in place for some time, such as in dogs with chronic renal failure. The low-profile tubes, although more expensive initially, last longer than either Pezzer or Foley catheters, and the less-frequent replacement may offset the initial high cost (Elliott et al, 2000).

Enterostomy Tube

Enterostomy feeding tubes are indicated in patients with gastric, intestinal, or pancreatic disease and in patients having biliary tract surgery in which the intestinal tract distal to the disease or surgical site is functional. Immediate feeding of a highly digestible, low-bulk diet in patients undergoing colonic surgery or that will undergo colonic surgery can be accomplished using an enterostomy feeding tube. Patients with preexisting PCM that must have major abdominal surgery are candidates for early enteral hyperalimentation by means of an enterostomy tube.

Celiotomy or laparoscopy is required for placement of an enterostomy feeding tube. A 5 Fr, 90-cm infant feeding tube is recommended for cats and for small and medium size dogs. An 8 Fr feeding tube may be used in large and giant breed dogs.

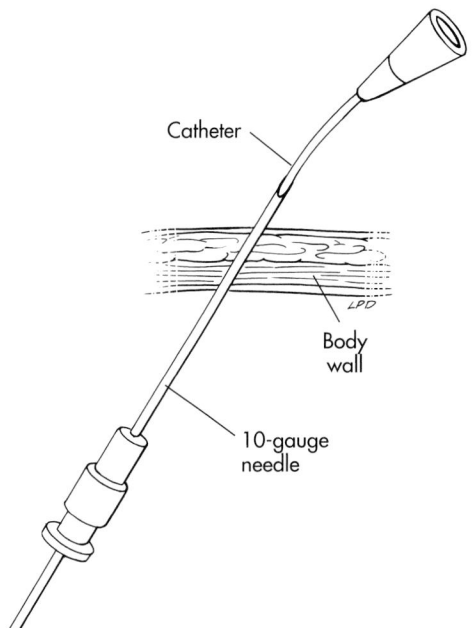

FIG. 11-17
For placement of an enterostomy tube, a 10-gauge hypodermic needle facilitates transabdominal placement of a 5 Fr feeding tube.

Bring the distal tip of the feeding tube into the abdominal cavity through a 2- to 3-mm stab incision made on the right or left body wall with a No. 11 scalpel blade or a 10-gauge hypodermic needle (Fig. 11-17). Select a segment of proximal jejunum and identify the normal direction of flow of ingesta (i.e., aboral and oral end). Ensure that the selected intestine is easily mobilized to the feeding tube entrance on the body wall. Make a 1- to 1.5-cm linear incision in the seromuscular layers of the antimesenteric border of the selected jejunal segment (Fig. 11-18, A). Use a No. 11 scalpel blade to enter the lumen of the jejunum at the most aboral end of the incision. Insert the distal end of the feeding tube through the incision and pass 10 to 12 inches (25 to 30 cm) of the tube in an aboral direction into the jejunal lumen. Position the exiting portion of the tube in the 1- to 1.5-cm seromuscular incision, and suture it in this "tunnel" by inverting the seromuscular layer over the tube with three or four Cushing sutures of 4-0 or 5-0 synthetic absorbable suture material (i.e., Maxon, PDS) (Fig. 11-18, B and C). Pexy the jejunal tube exit site to the exit site at the body wall with four to five simple interrupted sutures of 4-0 absorbable suture; secure the feeding tube to the skin using a Chinese finger-trap friction suture of 2-0 nonabsorbable material (e.g., Novafil).

Patients with enterostomy feeding tubes can be fed immediately after surgery. The exit point of the feeding tube should be incorporated into a body bandage to prevent premature removal by the patient, technical staff, or client. A column of water should be kept in the tube between uses.

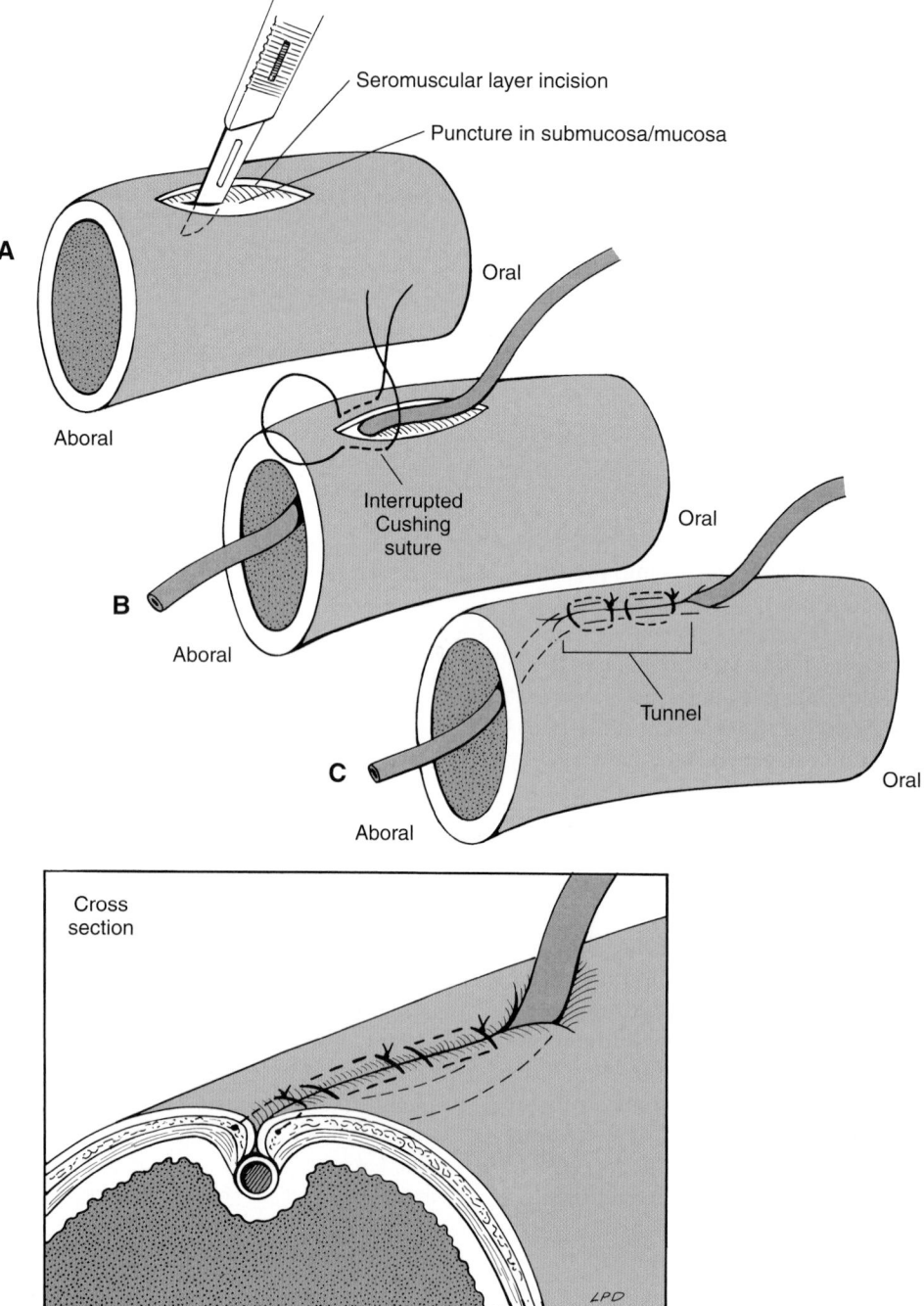

FIG. 11-18
Placement of an enterostomy tube. **A,** Make a 1- to 1.5-cm linear incision in the seromuscular layers of the antimesenteric border of the selected jejunal segment; use the tip of a scalpel blade to puncture a hole in the aboral aspect of the seromuscular incision. **B** and **C,** Place the distal end of the feeding tube through the incision; lay the exiting portion of the tube in the 1- to 1.5-cm seromuscular incision and construct a "tunnel" by inverting the seromuscular layer over the tube with three or four Cushing sutures of 4-0 absorbable material.

Possible complications include premature removal, tube-induced jejunal perforation, peritoneal leakage, and subcutaneous leakage. Subcutaneous leakage can be prevented by securely fixing the tube to the skin, and peritoneal leakage is prevented by taking care to include a 360-degree jejunal-abdominal wall pexy.

CALCULATION OF RATE AND VOLUME OF FEEDING

Once the number of calories necessary to meet the patient's total caloric requirement has been calculated, the rate and volume of feeding are determined based on the route of administration (e.g., oral, nasoesophageal, esophagostomy, pharyngostomy, gastrostomy, or enterostomy). When feeding into the stomach (i.e., oral, nasoesophageal, esophagostomy, pharyngostomy, and gastrostomy tubes), the amount fed is determined by the patient's stomach capacity. The normal canine and feline gastric capacity is approximately 80 ml of fluid per kilogram of body weight. However, anorexic patients can typically accommodate only 30 to 40 ml/kg of body weight when feeding begins. A gradual increase over 2 to 3 days allows the stomach to accommodate progressively larger volumes. The patient should have a minimum of three feedings daily; however, if vomiting and abdominal distention occur, the volume should be reduced and the number of daily feedings increased. In animals that routinely vomit after administration of the diet through a nasoesophageal, esophagostomy, or gastrostomy tube, it is often advantageous to drip commercially prepared liquid diets into the tube as a constant rate infusion (CRI). Simultaneous administration of antiemetics and/or gastric prokinetic agents may also be beneficial.

When feeding into the small intestine (enterostomy tubes), the rate and volume must be carefully regulated to prevent overdistention. Each patient is unique in the amount of fluid the small intestine will accommodate; guidelines for feeding by enterostomy tube are presented in Box 11-6. These are only guidelines; however, some patients require a longer adjustment time (5 to 7 days), whereas others allow total volume feeding in 2 to 3 days. Signs of overfeeding include vomiting, diarrhea, abdominal distention, or cramping, or all of these. Diluting the diet concentration and reducing the rate and volume of administration generally resolve these complications.

COMPLICATIONS

Three types of complications can occur with enteral hyperalimentation: mechanical complications, gastrointestinal complications, and metabolic complications. In most cases, complications can be prevented by proper tube placement technique; by using an appropriate-diameter, soft rubber feeding tube and the proper diet; by carefully calculating feeding schedules; and by proper tube management during and between feedings. A recent study evaluating complications and prognostic factors associated with TPN in cats suggested that mechanical and septic complications were infrequent and not associated with an increased mortality rate; however, the

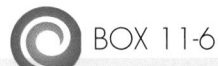 **BOX 11-6**

Guidelines for Feeding Via an Enterostomy Tube

- Calculate total caloric requirement.
- Give ¼ of the calculated volume during the first 24 hours; a minimum of four to five feedings per day is recommended.*
- Give ½ of the calculated volume during the second 24 hours in four to five feedings.*
- Give ¾ of the calculated volume during the third 24 hours in four to five feedings.*
- Give the entire calculated volume during the fourth 24 hours in four to five feedings.*

*Continuous feeding by means of an infusion pump is preferred.

mortality rate in this study was more than 50%, with most cats being euthanized or dying of their primary illness or complications associated with their illness (Pyle et al, 2004).

Mechanical Complications

Mechanical complications include inadvertent placement of the tube in the trachea (nasoesophageal, esophagostomy, and pharyngostomy tubes) or peritoneal cavity (gastrostomy or enterostomy tubes), gut perforation by the feeding tube (gastrostomy and enterostomy tubes), regurgitation or vomiting of the tube (nasoesophageal, esophagostomy, and pharyngostomy tubes), esophageal irritation (nasoesophageal, esophagostomy, and pharyngostomy tubes), gastric outflow obstruction (gastrostomy tubes), infection at the tube exit site, occlusion of the tube, or removal of the tube by the patient. Inadvertent placement of feeding tubes in the trachea or peritoneal cavity can be prevented by paying careful attention during tube placement. If there is any question about the tube's location, a small amount of sterile aqueous contrast material should be injected through the feeding tube and a radiograph taken. Gut perforation has been virtually eliminated by use of small-bore, Silastic or soft rubber enterostomy feeding tubes. In cats, esophageal perforation (esophagostomy tube) has been eliminated by discontinuation of the use of a stylet during tube placement. Premature tube removal by the patient can usually be prevented by adequate mechanical restraint (e.g., bandaging and an Elizabethan collar) and secure attachment of the tube to its exit site (i.e., Chinese finger-trap friction sutures). The use of small-bore, soft rubber feeding tubes has improved patient tolerance. Esophagitis that occurs secondary to placement of a nasoesophageal, esophagostomy, or pharyngostomy tube has been reported; however, use of Silastic or soft rubber feeding tubes has reduced esophageal irritation. Also, midesophageal placement effectively eliminates reflux esophagitis.

Infection at the tube site can be minimized by proper tube management. The area should be kept clean and covered with a loose bandage. Care should be taken when feeding the patient to prevent diet formula from contaminating the exit site. Rhinitis secondary to placement of a nasoesophageal tube has been reported, but use of small-bore, soft-rubber tubes has minimized this.

Small-bore feeding tubes (3 to 5 Fr) can become occluded with the diet formula. This is best prevented by using a commercial liquid diet rather than a blenderized diet preparation. Taking care to flush material out of the tube when feeding is finished and capping the tube to maintain a column of water also help prevent occlusion by gastrointestinal reflux. Large-bore feeding tubes accept blenderized diets, but similar precautions should be taken to prevent occlusion. If a tube becomes occluded, flexible endoscopy forceps can be passed into the tube to remove the clogged material. If endoscopy forceps are unsuccessful, a carbonated liquid, such as cola, can be infused into the tube; the effervescence of the liquid and its acid pH may encourage removal of clogged material. If this is unsuccessful, tube replacement may be necessary.

Gastrointestinal Complications

Common gastrointestinal complications of enteral nutritional therapy include vomiting, cramping, abdominal distention, diarrhea, or all of these. The most common causes are feeding too rapidly, feeding too large a volume, and feeding diets with a high osmolality. Treatment is aimed at reducing the rate and volume fed or diluting the diet formula.

Metabolic Complications

The most common metabolic complication of enteral nutritional therapy is hyperglycemia that occurs secondary to rapid absorption of glucose. Insulin may be used to control the hyperglycemia; however, it is rarely necessary. In the rare case in which insulin is required, the clinician should start with a very low dose and closely monitor the patient, anticipating that the need for insulin will disappear as the patient adapts. There is not a dose of insulin that has been well established by experience to use in such cases. One might try 0.25 to 0.5 unit of regular insulin/4.5 kg body weight in dogs. Cats tend to be more sensitive to the effects of insulin than dogs, but a similar dose might be tried. Patients, especially emaciated animals, must be carefully monitored for hypophosphatemia, hypokalemia, and hyperkalemia.

Complications associated with PPN have been infrequently reported. One study found that the most common metabolic complication was hyperglycemia, followed by lipemia and hyperbilirubinemia (Chan et al, 2002). Most complications were mild and did not require discontinuation of PPN.

> NOTE: Use insulin with care in cats; they are very sensitive to it.

References

Chan DL, Freeman LM, Lobato MA et al: Retrospective evaluation of partial parenteral nutrition in dogs and cats, *J Vet Intern Med* 16:440, 2002.

Chan DL, Freeman LM, Rozanski EA et al: Colloid osmotic pressure of parenteral nutrition components and intravenous fluids, *J Vet Emerg Crit Care* 11:269, 2001.

Crowe DT et al: The use of polymeric liquid enteral diets for nutritional support in seriously ill or injured small animals: clinical results in 200 patients, *J Am Anim Hosp Assoc* 33:500, 1997.

Elliott DA, Riel DL, Rogers QR: Complications and outcomes associated with use of gastrostomy tubes for nutritional management of dogs with renal failure: 56 cases (1994-1999), *J Am Vet Med Assoc* 217:1337, 2000.

McCrackin MA, Stiffler KS, Schmiedt CW: One-step placement of a percutaneous, nonendoscopic, low-profile gastrostomy port in cats, *J Am Vet Med Assoc* 217:1636, 2000.

Pyle SC, Marks SL, Kass PH: Evaluation of complications and prognostic factors associated with administration of total parenteral nutrition in cats: 75 cases (1994-2001), *J Am Vet Med Assoc* 225:242, 2004.

Zsombor-Murray E, Freeman LM: Peripheral parenteral nutrition, *Comp Cont Educ* 21:512, 1999.

Suggested Reading

Chandler ML, Guilford WG, Payne-James J: Use of peripheral nutritional support in dogs and cats, *J Am Vet Med Assoc* 216:669, 2000.

A comparison of total parenteral and partial parenteral nutrition. Peripheral venous thrombosis is discussed along with how to prevent this complication.

Hewitt SA, Brisson BA, Sinclair MD et al: Evaluation of laparoscopic-assisted placement of jejunostomy feeding tubes in dogs, *J Am Vet Med Assoc* 225:65, 2004.

This paper describes how to place a jejunostomy tube laparoscopically. The authors recommended this technique in dogs that did not require a laparotomy for other reasons.

Ireland LM, Hohenhaus AE, Broussand JD et al: A comparison of owner management and complications in 67 cats with esophagostomy and percutaneous endoscopic gastrostomy feeding tubes, *J Am Anim Hosp Assoc* 39:241, 2003.

This study found that owners were comfortable with use of esophagostomy and gastrostomy tubes. They concluded that esophagostomy tubes were excellent alternatives to gastrostomy tubes.

Pyle S, Marks S, Kass P: Evaluation of complications and prognostic factors associated with administration of total parenteral nutrition in cats, 75 cases (1994-2001), *J Am Vet Med Assoc* 225:242, 2004.

A study of 75 cats given TPN, which shows that a history of weight loss, hypoalbuminemia, chronic renal failure, and protracted hyperglycemia were all associated with a poor prognosis, as was multiple concurrent diseases.

Salinardi BJ, Harkin KR, Bulmer BJ et al: Comparison of complications of percutaneous endoscopic versus surgically placed gastrostomy tubes in 42 dogs and 52 cats, *J Am Anim Hosp* 42:51, 2006.

When analyzed on a species basis (just dogs or just cats), there was no difference in the rate of complications between the two techniques; however, when dogs and cats were combined into one large group, endoscopically placed tubes had a higher complication rate and greater severity of complication score.

von Werthern CJ, Wess G: A new technique for insertion of esophagostomy tubes in cats, *J Am Anim Hosp Assoc* 37:140, 2001.

This paper describes the use of a specially devised applicator that allows rapid esophagostomy tube placement.

CHAPTER 12
Fundamentals of Physical Rehabilitation

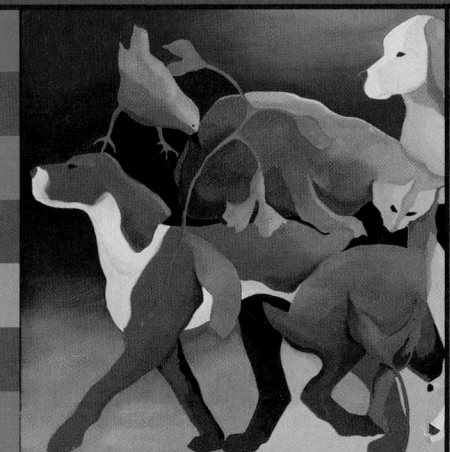

DEFINITIONS

Physical rehabilitation is a veterinary derivative of the human-oriented profession of physical therapy. The term rehabilitation stems from the Latin word *rehabilitare* meaning "to restore ability." Physical rehabilitation is primarily used to treat orthopedic and neurologic disease and encompasses the use of physical or mechanical agents, such as light, thermotherapy (heat and cold), water, electricity, massage, and exercise. Other terms used to describe physical rehabilitation are canine rehabilitation, physical therapy, and physiotherapy.

GENERAL CONSIDERATIONS

Physical therapy is the conventional standard of care in human medicine and has proved to maximize the overall physical recovery of patients. Used in conjunction with standard medical and surgical treatment plus proper pain management (see Chapter 13), rehabilitation can facilitate early and more complete recovery from surgery and trauma. Advances in veterinary medicine have led to a longer life expectancy for most domestic pets, which in turn has increased the number of animals with chronic discomfort, disease, and geriatric maladies; physical rehabilitation modalities provide options for treatment and symptomatic relief of these patients, resulting in an improved quality of life. Applications of physical rehabilitation in veterinary medicine include treating patients with chronic osteoarthritis; promoting postoperative recovery or conservative management of orthopedic or neurologic patients; treating severely debilitated patients; allowing interaction with oncology patients having extended hospitalization times (i.e., for radiation therapy), which enhances their mental health and happiness; enhancing condition, strength, and performance in canine athletes or working dogs; aiding weight loss in obese patients; and promoting bonding and/or obedience in family pets.

Objectives of physical rehabilitation are to maximize recovery from disease processes and surgical procedures while improving function and overall well-being of the patient. These objectives may be realized by improving joint range of motion (ROM), decreasing pain, providing more complete recovery of injured and inflamed neurologic and musculoskeletal tissues, preventing disuse atrophy of affected musculature, improving function of weak and paralyzed limbs, preventing soft tissue contracture and fibrosis, and providing positive physiologic outcomes for patients and owners. Physical rehabilitation protocols include the use of multiple treatment modalities and must be individualized to both patient and client.

TREATMENT MODALITIES
Cryotherapy and Hypothermia

Cryotherapy and **hypothermia** are terms for the therapeutic application of cold. Cold is the thermal agent of choice for managing the acute phase of tissue injury because it minimizes inflammatory processes and provides analgesia. Lowering the temperature of skin and underlying tissue causes vasoconstriction, reduces blood flow, and decreases sensory and motor nerve conduction velocity. Cryotherapy is commonly used to treat postoperative inflammation, musculoskeletal trauma, and muscle spasm, and to minimize secondary inflammation following therapeutic exercise. It induces a temperature change in the affected tissue of between 1° and 4° C intramuscularly and 12° and 13° C at the skin surface as heat is removed from the body. Typically, the return to baseline temperature occurs in 15 to 30 minutes, allowing a significant period of analgesia and inflammation and/or edema reduction. Ice packs, ice massage with homemade ice popsicles, running cold water over the affected tissue, cold water immersion, or a cold compression unit may all be used for hypothermia application.

First, apply a towel over the site to protect the skin. Apply an ice pack (a freezer bag filled with crushed ice), cold compress, or iced towel to the affected site. If possible, secure the ice pack with a compression wrap to hold the pack in place, compress tissues, and protect the rest of the body from the pack.

Application time for a medium to large dog is 15 to 20 minutes, repeated as often as every 4 hours.

Continue the applications for at least the first 72 hours after a surgical procedure or injury to allow the acute inflammatory phase to resolve.

Hypothermia is relatively safe, but should not be used in patients with cold sensitivities. The patient's reaction should be closely observed and therapy terminated if they appear uncomfortable. The skin should be observed for signs of frostbite; pale or white skin after application indicates possible tissue damage.

> NOTE: Take particular care when applying cryotherapy in animals with decreased or absent sensation and those with metal implants.

Heat therapy and Hyperthermia

Hyperthermia or heat application is the thermal agent of choice in the management of chronic injuries, but should not be used on tissues that are actively inflamed. Physiologically, superficial heat causes cutaneous vasodilation, increased nerve conduction velocity, muscle relaxation, elevated pain threshold, increased enzymatic and metabolic activity, and increased connective tissue extensibility. Superficial heat is commonly used to reduce extremity joint stiffness and increase connective tissue elasticity before stretching or exercise; however, to adequately heat deeper tissue, ultrasound or diathermy may be more appropriate.

First, apply an insulating layer to the affected area. Secure the hot packs (either commercially prepared packs or hot towels) to the limb with straps. Alternatively, use a warm bath, whirlpool, underwater treadmill, or swimming pool. To treat deeper tissue, use therapeutic ultrasound (see later discussion). Apply heat to a medium-sized to large dog for 15 to 20 minutes and as frequently as every 4 hours before exercise or stretching to promote plastic changes to the tissue and increase joint mobility. Observe the skin condition during and after application for adverse effects.

Hyperthermia should not be used over any area of acute inflammation as it may exacerbate hemorrhage and edema. Other contraindications to using hyperthermia are animals with decreased or absent sensation, poor thermoregulation, or bleeding disorders. Heat should not be applied over a pregnant uterus, malignancies, or areas of active infection. Tissue burn may occur if the animal is unable to dissipate the heat or if excessive heat is used for prolonged periods.

Therapeutic Ultrasound

Therapeutic ultrasound units are designed to emit sound waves into tissue, providing the thermal effect of local deep tissue heating. The thermal form of therapeutic ultrasound is effective for treating chronic tendonitis, limited ROM secondary to tissue contracture, myositis, bicipital tendonitis, and muscle spasm. Ultrasound enhances blood flow to aid healing, increases tissue temperature to reduce pain, and promotes tissue stretching. Ultrasound units may also be set for low intensity, continuous or pulsed modes to promote healing in acute (used within 2 weeks after injury) or chronic wounds. **Phonophoresis** is the use of therapeutic ultrasound to enhance the delivery of topically applied drugs.

Treatment protocols and technical support are generally provided when therapeutic ultrasound units are purchased. Variables to consider include frequency, intensity, and duty cycle. Ultrasound beams are collimated and *frequencies* in the megahertz (MHz) range are used. *Intensity* is the rate of energy delivery per unit area, indicated as watts per centimeter squared (W/cm^2). Higher intensities induce greater and faster temperature increases. *Duty cycle* is the percent of time that the sound is emitted during one pulse period. Other factors to consider include the treatment area, duration of treatment, and treatment schedule. The optimal treatment area is one that is twice the size of the transducer head. Typical treatment time is 5 minutes for an area approximately twice the size of the selected transducer head; however, some units will preset the time necessary based on the intensity of other settings. Treatment schedules initially may include daily treatment (up to 10 days), followed by less frequent application as the condition improves.

Clip the hair to allow ultrasound penetration into the underlying tissue. Apply a commercially prepared water-soluble coupling gel to the treatment area. For deep lesions, set the frequency for 1 MHz, which heats at depths between 2 and 5 cm. Treat superficial lesions with a frequency of 3 MHz. Set the intensity from 0.5 to 2 W/cm^2 based on the amount of soft tissue present; the more soft tissue, the higher the required setting. Consider also patient tolerance when setting the intensity. Typically set the duty cycle range from 5% to 50% based on the desired tissue effect.

Duration of treatment varies based on the area and sound head size selected as outlined above.

Move the sound head over the skin no faster than about 4 cm/s (Fig. 12-1). Be careful to move the transducer head continually over the entire area in varying patterns to prevent hot spots and potential tissue damage.

Precautions must be taken to prevent tissue burns with therapeutic ultrasound. Patients with decreased circulation, sensation, or awareness are at higher risk for tissue burns. Contraindications to therapeutic ultrasound include tumors, acutely inflamed tissue, infected tissue, and painful areas.

> NOTE: Take care to avoid direct ultrasound exposure to bony prominences and over metal implants, physes, the heart, a gravid uterus, or the testes.

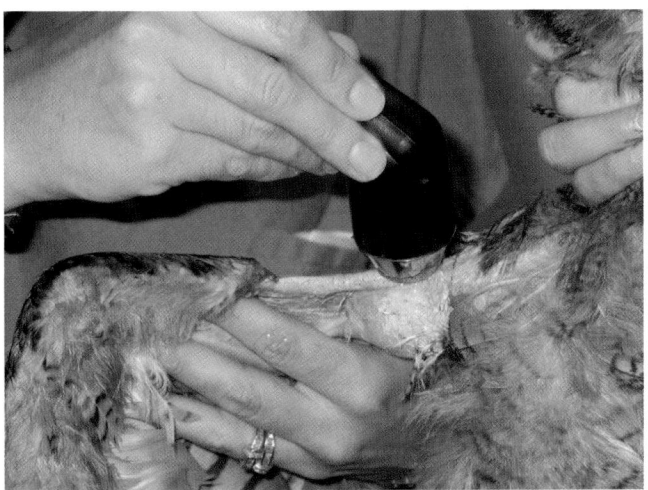

FIG. 12-1
Photograph showing therapeutic ultrasound being applied to the pterygium ligament of an owl.

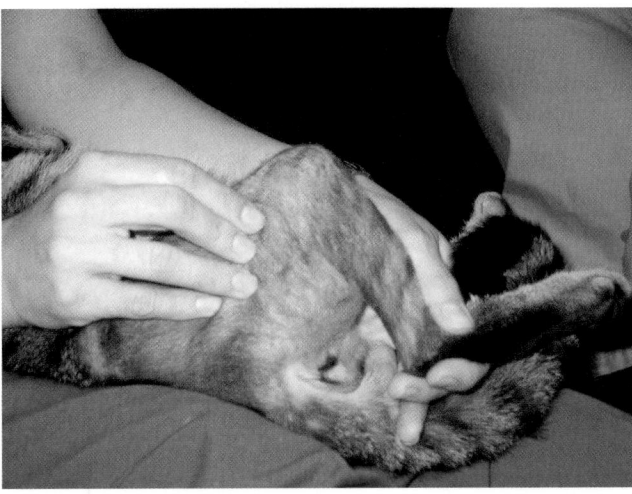

FIG. 12-2
Proper technique for stifle flexion. Note the decreased angle of flexion caused by muscle trauma after surgery to stabilize a distal femoral fracture.

Massage

Massage is the gentle manipulation of muscles and soft tissues. It is effective in both moving fluid into the lymphatic system and moving fluid from the extremities to the central body core in patients with distal extremity edema. Massage is also hypothesized to have a circulatory-based effect that promotes movement of fluid from damaged tissue and replacement with new blood-borne nutrients. Because massage results in movement within and between multiple tissue layers, it can help mobilize and soften adhesions, limit and relieve muscle and tendon contracture, and decrease fibrosis. Massage is most effective in relaxing muscles and soft tissue before exercise. Muscle spasms and associated pain may be relieved by massage. It may be used to help postoperative patients maintain mobility; to promote pain-free exercise in animals with chronic conditions, such as osteoarthritis; and as therapy for enhancing performance in competitive dogs. Massage is typically applied following hyperthermia and before stretching or exercising and may be limited to one area or applied to the entire body. Owners may be taught to successfully perform massage.

Start massage by gently petting or stroking the affected limb using moderate pressure.

This relaxes the dog and allows the therapist to assess the tissue by noting muscle tone, presence of swelling or masses, and temperature differentials.

Beginning at the distal portion of the affected area and moving proximally, gently manipulate and apply pressure to the soft tissue and muscles. Next, apply gentle pressure, then knead and squeeze the tissue. Increase the intensity and duration of massage as the animal's tolerance and comfort level improve.

Most massage sessions start at 5 minutes duration and can be as long as 15 to 30 minutes depending on the severity of the condition.

Passive Range of Motion and Stretching

Range of motion (ROM) refers to the full motion that a joint may be moved through. **Passive range of motion** (PROM) is the artificial manipulation of a joint through a pain-free ROM. Stretching is often performed in combination with PROM to increase joint flexibility and soft tissue extension. Immobilization is detrimental to the health of articular cartilage, ligaments, bone, and muscle. PROM is vital to maintaining joint integrity by helping to minimize soft tissue and muscle contracture, articular cartilage damage, and tissue atrophy. PROM also enhances synovial movement for cartilage nutrition and improves blood flow and sensory awareness of joints and limbs.

Typically PROM is indicated for animals that are unable or not allowed to actively move an extremity. PROM can be applied to severely debilitated/recumbent patients to minimize complications associated with decreased circulation. This technique is often used to treat muscle soreness from weekend overactivity and as a warm-up for other exercises. PROM is not a substitute for active ROM because it will not prevent muscle atrophy, increase strength, or assist in circulation.

Place your hands above and below the joint and gently flex and extend the joint while supporting the limb. Manipulate the joint(s) through a pain-free ROM (Figs. 12-2 and 12-3). Slowly extend and flex the joint beyond the pain-free ROM to stretch the tissue. Do not force the motion beyond a comfortable level. Hold the stretch for 15 to 30 seconds. Return the joint to normal. Repeat the stretch up to 20 times per

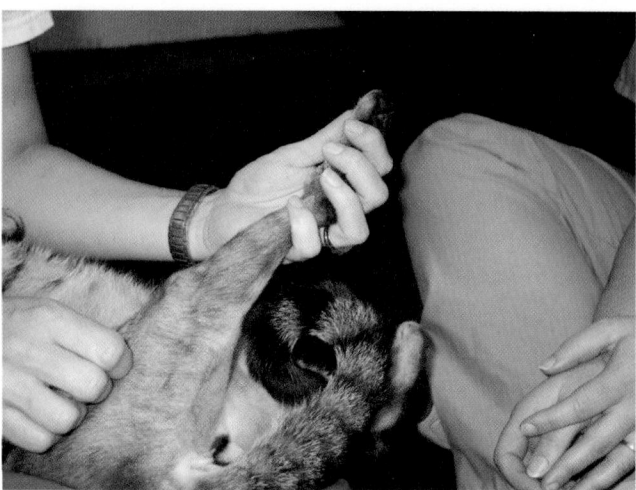

FIG. 12-3
Proper technique for stifle extension.

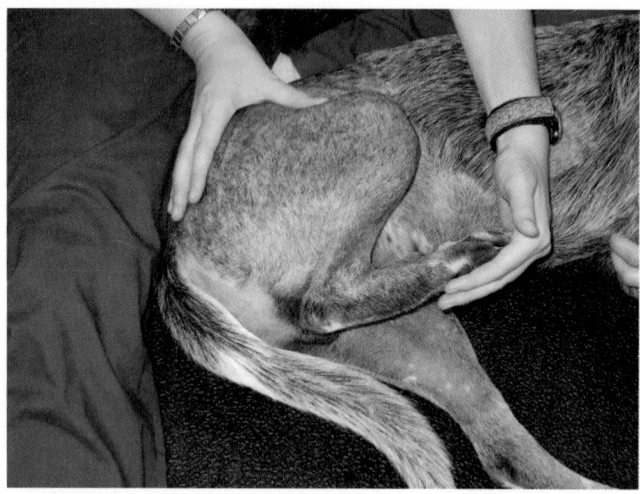

FIG. 12-4
A simple method of flexing all joints of the pelvic limb in one movement.

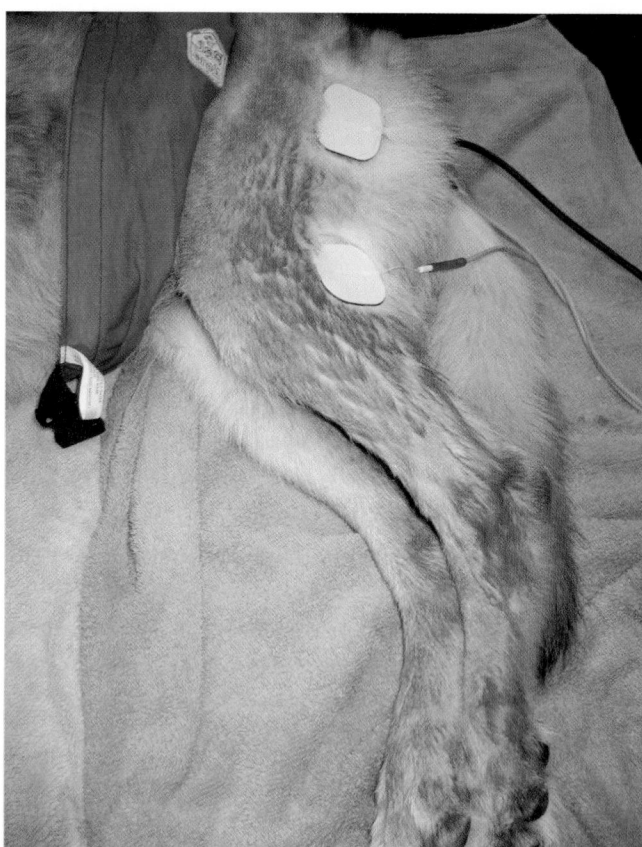

FIG. 12-5
Electrical stimulation being performed on the semimembranosus and semitendinosus muscle of a German shepherd dog with degenerative myelopathy.

session. Manipulate all joints of the affected limb for maximal benefit (Fig. 12-4). Monitor the patient before, during, and after treatment for changes in pain, active ROM, or quality of movement.

> NOTE: Do not use PROM when motion may result in injury or instability or if stretching is uncomfortable for the patient. Take care to prevent disruption of soft tissue repairs.

Neuromuscular Electrical Stimulation

Neuromuscular electrical stimulation (NMES) is the application of an electrical current to tissue to promote healing. The NMES devices are generally pulsed current stimulators, which may use either alternating or direct current waves. These devices may be set for wave form, amplitude (magnitude of one electrical wave), pulse duration (time during which the charge flows in both directions), phase duration (time current flows from baseline in one direction and back), pulse rate (number of pulses delivered per second), duty cycle (ratio of on time to total cycle time), ramp (allows gradual increase or decrease in amplitude), and polarity.

NMES is most frequently used to rehabilitate patients with orthopedic and neurologic disease. Effects of NMES include increasing ROM, increasing muscle strength, and improving muscle tone; decreasing edema and enhancing circulation; and decreasing muscle spasms and pain. It improves muscle strength by increasing muscle contractile proteins and improves muscle endurance by increasing vascularity, aerobic capacity, and mitochondrial size. Electrical muscle stimulation may be used to reeducate denervated muscle. **Iontophoresis** is the use of electrical stimulation to enhance transdermal medication administration.

Clip and prepare the skin over the motor point with alcohol. Apply gel to the skin, and place the electrode (Fig. 12-5). Locate the approximate motor point (area where the motor

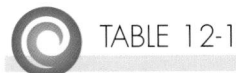 TABLE 12-1

Common Neuromuscular Stimulation Protocols

PROBLEM	WAVELENGTH	AMPLITUDE/ MUSCLE RECRUITMENT	PULSE DURATION	FREQUENCY	DUTY CYCLE	TREATMENT TIME
Muscle strengthening	Biphasic	Motor	150–250 μsec	30–50 pps	Interrupted, 1:3 or 1:5	10–20 min once or twice daily, 3–5 days/wk
Muscle reeducation	Biphasic	Motor	100–400 μsec	30–50 pps	Interrupted, 1:1 or 1:2	10–20 min once or twice daily, 3–5 days/wk
Acute pain LFC		Motor	2–50 μsec	50–100 pps	Continuous	20–30 min, no residual effect
Chronic pain LFC		Sensory	>150 μsec	2–4 pps	Continuous	30–45 min
Edema		Motor	100–400 μsec	30–50 pps	Continuous	

LFC, Low frequency current.

nerve enters the muscle) for the targeted muscle. With the current on, move the electrode to identify the precise motor point. Mark the point for future reference. Select the parameters for the electrical stimulation. First select a wavelength.

The wavelength helps determine overall patient comfort. Commonly, symmetrical biphasic and symmetric triphasic wavelengths are chosen because smooth and regular wavelengths are most comfortable.

Select either motor recruitment or sensory recruitment.

Recruitment determines the intensity of the contraction. For motor recruitment, NMES elicits an actual visible contraction. Sensory recruitment uses a lower intensity current that the patient can feel without causing the muscle to actually move.

Set the pulse duration, which is directly proportional to the duration of the contraction. Set the frequency (which defines the number of pulses of electricity per second) to determine the rate at which the muscle fibers are stimulated. Set the duty cycle to 1:1 to enhance endurance or 1:3 or 1:5 for muscle strengthening. Set the ramp to control patient comfort.

The ramp is the gradual rise and decay of the current that elicits the contraction. A gradual ramp means that the current gradually works up to the peak instead of abruptly generating current to the tissue. This allows the patient to gradually acclimate to each contraction.

One muscle may be selected for treatment to promote joint motion, or opposing muscle groups may be treated if joint motion is not desired. Generally NMES is applied for 15 to 20 minutes, one to five times per week (but can be performed as often as twice daily for 5 days per week; Table 12-1). Muscle soreness may occur with aggressive application of NMES. NMES is most effective when used to enhance contraction and strength during or immediately before active exercise.

> NOTE: Take care when using NMES over areas with impaired sensation or skin irritation or over a gravid uterus. NMES is contraindicated over the heart or carotid sinus, in animals with pacemakers or seizures, and over tumors or infected areas.

Therapeutic Exercise

Therapeutic exercise (TE) is the art of encouraging an animal to exercise appropriate muscle groups and to perform voluntary active motion of the affected joint or limb. This is achieved by using creative exercises that incorporate the environment and other tools. TEs may be assisted by the rehabilitator or owner. The goals of TE can be numerous, including to improve the animal's pain-free ROM; limb usage, muscle mass, and strength: and to enhance its overall ability to function. It may also minimize the potential for additional injury, improve physical fitness for events or competitions, maximize the potential to return to working duties, improve cardiovascular fitness, and provide a sense of well-being and involvement for both owner and pet. The basic concepts underlying successful application of TE include varying the animal's routine, individualizing exercises to fit the patient, allowing patient progress to guide increases in activity, and most importantly, using one's imagination to make exercise fun for the owner and pet.

TE choices vary depending on the stage of tissue repair and the animal's endurance. Setting a realistic goal for each patient is important. The exercise plan should be matched to the animal's progress. Exercise intensity may be increased by increasing the number of sessions, the number of repetitions per session, the overall intensity, and/or the speed of the activity. Although many therapeutic exercises require minimal equipment, there are also many assisting devices, such as thera-balls, balance boards, weights, thera-bands (elastic bands used to provide resistance to specific muscle groups), tunnels, cavaletti rails, treadmills (land and underwater), and swimming pools, available.

The key to successful TE is controlling the situation. The animal should be secured with a very short leash, in heel position, and be attentive to the handler. Sling support should be used for any animal with a healing bone or unstable fixation. The risks of causing damage to a surgical repair and other medical concerns need to be evaluated when deciding on the level of TE. Care must be taken to avoid potentially problematic situations, such as visible wildlife, slippery flooring, and the presence of children or other dogs. If the owner does not have control of the pet and cannot perform the exercises in a controlled and safe manner, cage rest or inpatient rehabilitation may be the only viable options.

Standing exercises. Therapeutic standing exercises are recommended for debilitated and recumbent animals.

Support the animal by holding it physically under the abdomen or pelvis or use a sling, cart, or wheelchair. Assist the animal to stand for brief intervals (seconds to minutes as tolerated) (Fig. 12-6). Repeatedly help the animal move from a seated or down position to a standing position. Encourage the animal to support as much weight as possible before providing assistance. Be sure to allow sufficient rest intervals between exercises. As the animal's strength and endurance increase, reduce the amount of assistance provided and increase the duration of activity.

Balancing exercises. Balancing exercises are used to encourage early limb usage, build muscle, and improve proprioception and body awareness. Balancing exercises allow the animal to build confidence and understand that using the leg is no longer painful. Balancing sessions may be started as early as 24 hours postoperatively. Sessions typically start at 1 to 2 minutes twice a day, and increase to a maximum of 5 to 8 minutes twice a day.

Begin the exercise by placing the animal in a standing position on a stable, nonslippery surface and very gently shift its weight from side to side (Fig. 12-7). To increase the challenge, place the animal on an unstable surface, such as a couch cushion, water bed, exercise roll, or ball (Fig. 12-8). Eventually work up to using a balance board or raft on water as stamina and endurance increase.

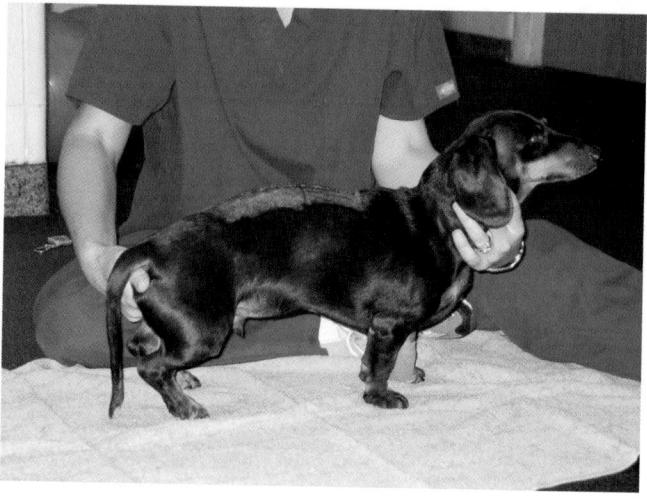

FIG. 12-6
When performing standing exercises on a dog after surgery, take care to ensure the surface is not slippery and the patient is supported.

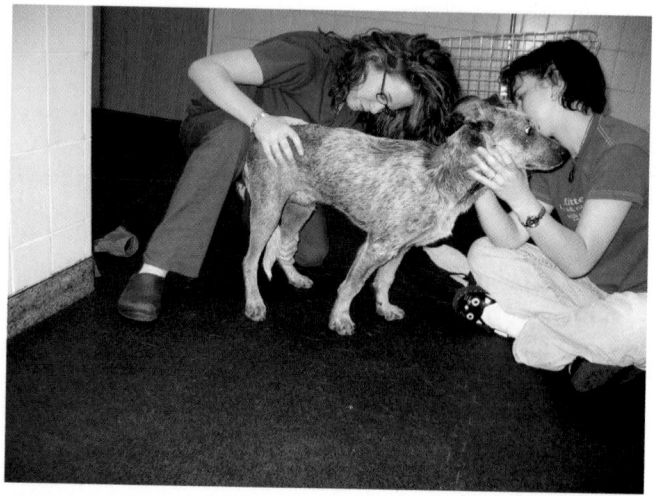

FIG. 12-7
Balance exercises may begin on a flat, stable surface.

Sit-to-stand/stand-to-down exercises. Repetitive sit-to-stand exercises are useful for strengthening the semimembranosus, semitendinosus, and quadriceps muscles. Repetitive down-to-stand exercises are useful for strengthening the biceps and triceps muscles. Both exercises are effective in improving active ROM and function of periarticular structures. Severely debilitated patients can also benefit from assisted sit-to-stand or down-to-stand exercises by using a sling or other device to help them through the motions of standing. These exercises can typically be started immediately after most surgical procedures.

With the animal on a short leash, encourage it to stand and then sit or lie down as squarely (symmetrically with no lean-

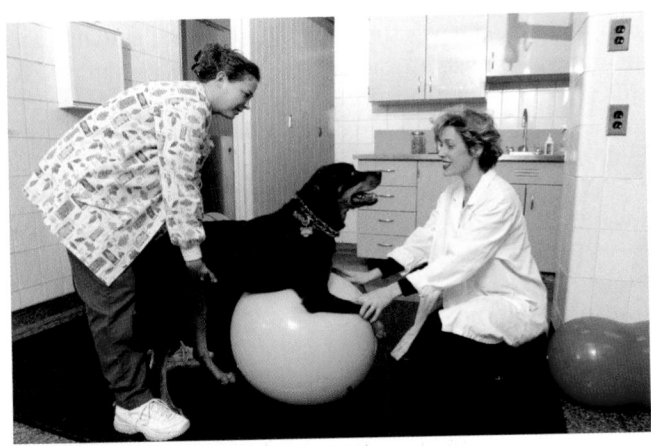

FIG. 12-8
To increase the challenge of balancing exercises, you may place only the unaffected limbs on an exercise ball.

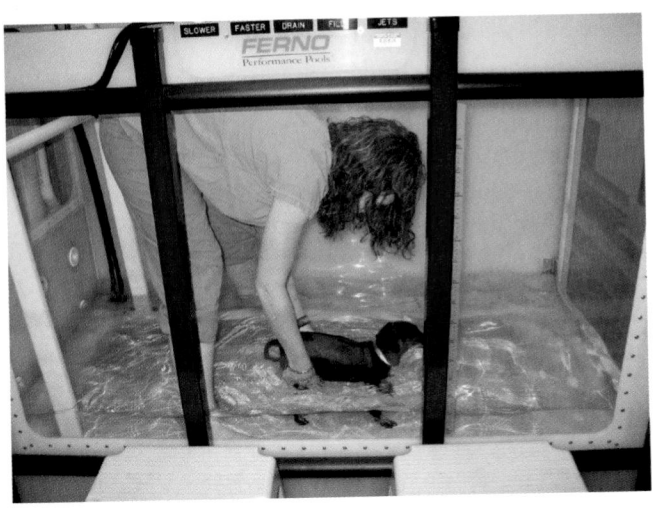

FIG. 12-9
Gait patterning.

ing to the side) as possible. Allow the animal to then rise by pushing off of both limbs equally.

Training and encouragement with treats may be necessary initially. Placing the animal in a corner or against a wall may help square up the sit position.

Start with 1 to 5 repetitions twice a day. Do not add repetitions until the pet sits or lies down squarely and symmetrically. Then add 5 repetitions per session until the animal is performing 20 to 30 exercises each session.

Gait training or patterning. Gait training or patterning exercises are used to encourage an animal to move its limbs in a walking motion. Also called "assisted walking," this type of exercise can help reeducate the afferent nervous pathway or change a gait abnormality. The exercise is generally applied to nonambulatory animals needing assistance to stand. Gait training can be performed immediately after most surgical interventions.

Assist the animal to stand using a sling, harness, or cart. Move the affected limbs slowly in a walking pattern, ensuring each foot contacts the ground appropriately with each step.

This exercise may be performed with the animal on the land treadmill (LTM).

Alternatively, place the animal in the underwater treadmill (see p. 120), where the water supports the patient's weight and move the legs through a normal walking pattern. Perform the exercises as long as the animal will tolerate them, twice or three times daily (Fig. 12-9).

Ground/land treadmill. LTMs are manufactured specifically for dogs, but with proper training, cats may be acclimated. Safety features include side rails and in some cases an overhead hook for a harness. The therapist should be familiar with the manufacturer's instructions before using the equipment. The speed and incline control offered with the treadmill are helpful for rehabilitating orthopedic patients. Decreased breaking and propulsive forces afforded by the treadmill greatly decrease the concussive forces felt by the joints. In some cases, the distraction of an unfamiliar environment encourages early weight bearing on the affected limb. Because the animal is able to walk in a constrained area, gait patterning can be performed with less effort on the part of the therapist. Assistive devices, such as thera-bands, weights, and off-loading can be used while the animal is on the treadmill. Animals on the treadmill may be more easily evaluated for lameness and stride length alterations. Athletic patients can be worked on the treadmill until the occult lameness becomes more evident.

Slowly introduce the animal to the treadmill. Depending on the patient, start treadmill exercise for 5 to 10 minutes as early as 12 hours after surgery. Consider the injury, surgical repair, and previous levels of activity when instituting treadmill therapy.

Generally, the frequency of treadmill sessions is one to two times a day for 3 to 5 days per week, depending on the patient and owner.

Increase session length as tolerated by the animal.

By 4 to 6 weeks after surgery, most animals can typically sustain a 20- to 30-minute session.

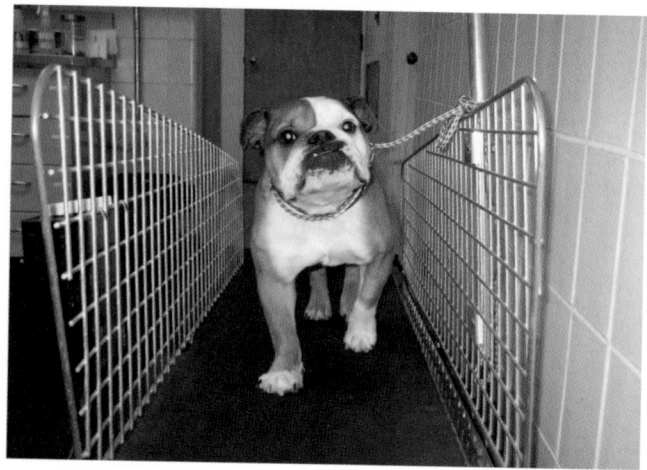

FIG. 12-10
Patient on the LTM after surgery for a ruptured cranial cruciate ligament.

Observe the patient carefully for progressive lameness after each session and decrease session length if lameness is noted (Fig. 12-10).

Controlled walks. The importance of slow, controlled, sling-supported leash walking cannot be overemphasized. Controlled leash walks allow the pet to move its limbs through a good active ROM while strengthening periarticular structures and helping to build muscle. Controlling the speed is a great way to encourage a patient that is reluctant to use the limb to place it on the ground. The slower an animal walks, the more difficult it is to "cheat." At slower paces, quadrupeds do not possess the momentum necessary to hold the leg up and maintain balance for long periods. Walks can take place anywhere, but challenge can be added by using an LTM or an underwater treadmill (UWTM) or by varying the terrain or surface.

Start slow leash walking for most patients after surgery at 10 minutes per session. Generally plan for 3 sessions daily, 5 to 7 days per week.

Leash walking may be increased to 60 minutes depending on the level of athleticism of the animal and the patience of the owner.

Cavaletti rails and obstacle work. Cavaletti rails are rails that are placed in a row for an animal to walk or trot over. The rails can be elevated and secured in a frame to increase the effort necessary to traverse the obstacle. Other obstacles, such as broomsticks, landscape timbers, or terrain (e.g., stepping onto and off of curbs, walking in deep sand or tall grass), may be used. Obstacle work is limited only by the therapist's imagination and encourages the animal to actively flex and extend joints, thereby improving active ROM and simultaneously stretching and strengthening periarticular structures. These exercises are easy for owners to perform at home and are generally fun for the patient. Typically, obstacle work is gradually incorporated into an exercise program, and its frequency is increased as dictated by patient tolerance.

Weaving and circles. Moving an animal through weaving patterns and circles encourages more thoughtful active ROM and navigation on the part of the patient. When an animal with orthopedic disease turns, it is encouraged to shift weight onto the affected limb and use periarticular musculature that is not used in a normal forward motion. Similarly in patients with neurologic disease, circling helps reeducate the afferent nervous pathway to adjust to shifts of weight and changes of directions. Weaving and circles are very simple and effective exercises that produce noticeable results. Postoperative orthopedic patients can begin controlled weaving and circles once the fixation is deemed stable; neurologic patients can begin weaving and circles once they are ambulatory.

Hills. Ascending and descending hills is another effective home exercise. Walking the animal up an incline strengthens the quadriceps, semitendinosus, semimembranosus, and gluteal muscles. Descending a hill requires the dog to flex the hock, hip, and stifle.

Start with gentle slopes and control the speed of the animal's activity at all times. Progress to steeper and longer inclines as the animal improves.

Stair climbing. Stair climbing is useful to improve strength and power in the rear limb's extensor muscles, active ROM, balance, and coordination. Descending stairs is also effective for improving forelimb muscle strength and ROM. Stair climbing is instituted after the animal is comfortable with leash walks and inclines and declines. For fracture patients, the fracture should be stable or healed and the lameness improving before stairs are included in the exercise program. The animal's activity should be controlled with a short leash and possibly a sling at all times during climbing.

Start stair climbing by having the animal ascend and descend 5 to 7 steps; gradually increase to 2 to 4 flights of stairs daily. Maintain a slow pace to encourage the animal to place each leg appropriately. Observe the patient carefully for signs of fatigue because stair climbing may be a challenging exercise for some.

Wheelbarrowing and dancing. Wheelbarrowing increases strength, proprioception, coordination, and balance in the forelimbs; dancing has a similar effect on the rear limbs. These exercises are optional for therapists and owners alike, but are typically reserved for patients later in the recovery process or those that are healed but not yet fully functional.

Muzzle the dog before exercising until the animal is comfortable with the procedure. To perform the wheelbarrowing technique, place your hands under the rear limbs, close to the abdomen, and lift the limbs off the ground, forcing the animal's weight onto its forelimbs. Move the dog forward, encouraging steps with the forelimbs. To perform the dancing technique, lift the forelimbs off the ground and encourage the animal to walk on its hindlimbs.

Jogging. Jogging is not typically started unless the fixation is considered sufficiently stable or the fracture has healed. This exercise is often reserved for athletic patients.

Begin by adding intermittent jogging spurts during the controlled leash walk or TE sessions; then increase the duration of jogging according to the animal's tolerance level. Observe carefully that the lameness does not worsen with jogging.

Pulling or carrying weights. Pulling or carrying weights is also typically reserved for late in the recovery process. Exercising with weights is very effective for recovering neurologic patients and for working dogs. Weights add resistance and result in muscle building for all areas of the body. Dogs may be harnessed to sleds or carts to pull weights. Care must be taken to ensure that the harness is well padded to prevent injury. Soft, pliable, neoprene wrist weights ranging from ½ to 2 lb may be placed on selected limbs. Leg weights should be introduced carefully and increased as tolerance permits to prevent injury. Special canine back packs made for hiking can be used to load weight onto the animal during exercise; the weights may be placed symmetrically or asymmetrically depending on the exercise. Weights may also be used during other exercise to increase exercise tolerance, strength, and stamina.

Controlled ball and Frisbee playing. Fetching is a goal-based exercise that can be used to bring working dogs back to full function. This exercise is not used until the fracture is healed or affected joint is stable. The unique combination of a burst of energy in a controlled environment enhances the animal's agility, power, speed, and muscle strength.

Start with a few repetitions in a small fenced area or with the dog on a leash, and gradually work up to longer distances and more repetitions as tolerated by the patient.

Toy batting and tug-of-war. Occasionally, animals with neurologic deficits of the forelimbs can be difficult to rehabilitate. Some techniques that are effective in encouraging forelimb use include toy batting, toy holding, tug-of-war, and controlled play. Toy batting and holding encourage the animal to use the limb differently than walking. The animal must focus on limb movement to grasp or hold the toy. Using a bone or "kong" filled with a treat intensifies the patient's desire to secure the toy. These exercises are particularly effective for feline patients. Projecting a laser light or using a fishing pole to move an attached furry, catnip-filled mouse encourages batting activities. Controlled tug-of-war can also be used to enhance forelimb balance.

For all of these activities, start with short sessions and work up gradually as tolerance and stamina improve.

Aversion techniques. Occasionally the therapist will find it necessary to use aversion techniques to force weight bearing. Aversion techniques should not be used until it is determined that there is no medical reason for the patient to

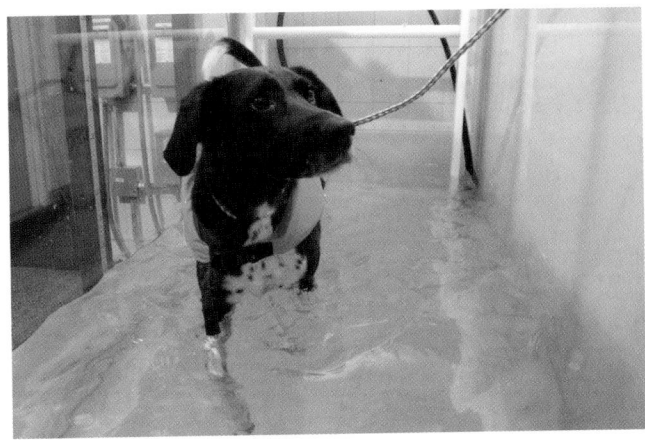

FIG. 12-11
A large, rambunctious, nonambulatory paraparetic patient being exercised independently on the underwater treadmill. The buoyancy supports his weight while he strengthens his rear limb muscles.

avoid using the limb. Syringe caps have been taped to the unaffected foot to encourage the animal to bear weight on the affected limb. Another tactic is to use a thera-band to restrain the contralateral limb. As the patient moves the normal limb forward, pressure may be applied to the band. This resistance causes the animal to increase the stride length of the normal limb and unbalances it enough to cause the animal to place the affected limb on the ground. Usually aversion techniques only need be repeated once or twice because once the animal realizes that the limb is useable, it will bear weight on it.

Aquatic Therapy

Aquatic therapy involves exercising in water to improve muscle strength and endurance, ROM, and agility while offering a safe nonconcussive exercise environment for earlier postoperative or postinjury intervention. General indications for aquatic therapy include rehabilitation of osteoarthritic patients, postoperative orthopedic cases, and animals with neurologic disease. Working dogs and athletes may benefit from aquatic therapy used for conditioning and training. Aquatic therapy is also helpful for cardiovascular and obese patients because it provides a controlled exercise environment.

Inherent properties of water (i.e., buoyancy, hydrostatic pressure, viscosity, and surface tension) make it an excellent therapeutic tool. *Buoyancy* or upward thrust of water acting on the animal causes an apparent decrease in weight and creates an environment of reduced gravity. This environment decreases concussive forces on joints, allowing earlier intervention and faster recovery, enables ataxic or weak patients to stand and ambulate with confidence, allows debilitated and painful patients to exercise more comfortably (Fig. 12-11), and protects fractures stabilized with implants from concussion. *Hydrostatic* or fluid pressure is directly proportional to the depth of immersion and provides a constant pressure, which relieves pain and edema. *Viscosity,* a measure

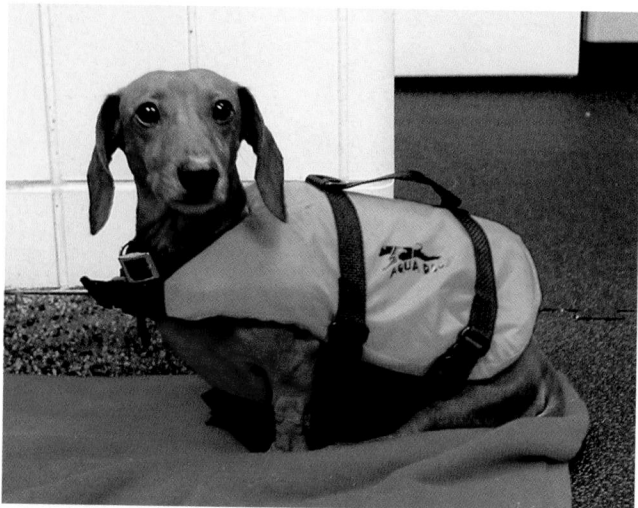

FIG. 12-12
Life vests are essential for patient safety with any type of aquatic therapy. Several companies now make vests designed specifically for dogs.

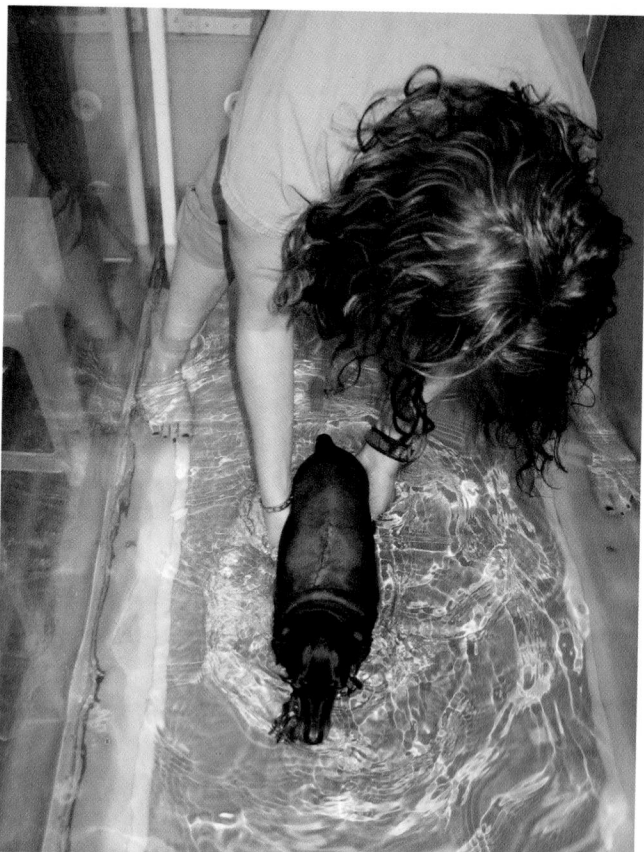

FIG. 12-13
Gait patterning in a postoperative hemilaminectomy patient. This technique is much easier with the water buoyancy supporting the patient's weight.

of the resistance caused by the cohesion of water molecules, provides resistance that strengthens musculature and improves active ROM. Viscosity also helps stabilize the patient's position, reducing patient anxiety. Resistance to movement is slightly greater at the water surface due to surface tension, making movement more difficult for the animal when the limb comes out of the water. Raising the water height to submerge the moving part will minimize drag, whereas lowering water height will maximize resistance to motion. Water is 25 times more effective than air as a heat conductor, thus appropriate selection of water temperature enhances the effects of thermotherapy.

Aquatic therapy can be as simple as using a nearby waterway or a wading pool or as elaborate as a UWTM or swimming pool. Assistive devices, such as life vests (Fig. 12-12), are available to help make aquatic therapy safe and effective. UWTMs may be equipped with jets, which can provide additional resistance for athletes or aquatic massage for a debilitated patient that appears uncomfortable. Weights, therabands, splints, and children's water wings can be used in the water if additional resistance is desired.

Disadvantages of aquatic therapy include the initial cost and upkeep for a pool or UWTM. Daily tasks include chemical checks and adjustments, filter cleaning, pump checks, and pool cleaning and disinfecting. Complete water change, chemical balancing, and filtration system cleaning must be performed weekly. Cultures should be performed every 2 to 4 weeks. Although routine maintenance measures may be burdensome in a busy practice, the rewards of a safe and useful aquatic exercise system are numerous.

Caution must be taken to prevent wound infection when using a UWTM; proper maintenance and an understanding of the healing process decrease this risk. Minimally, postoperative patients must have a fibrin seal over the incision before beginning aquatic exercise. Aquatic therapy should not

be initiated in patients with the potential for deleterious consequences of infection, such as those with implants, until the incision has healed. Some animals are afraid of water and a panicked patient who thrashes uncontrollably during swimming (even if only for a second) can destroy a surgical fixation. However, slow introduction of the activity coupled with understanding animal behavior and animal training will allow therapists to accommodate most patients. Because it is always possible for an animal to aspirate water or drown, they should never be left unattended.

Underwater treadmill. Typically UWTM units are designed with a walk-through exercise chamber, a filtration and heating system, and a holding tank. The water is heated, chlorinated, and recirculated. Most units can be filled to allow the animal to swim in a small area. Some units have incline treadmills, jets for resistance and turbulence, or are portable. A UWTM is a tremendous asset to any rehabilitation facility because it can be an integral part of all stages of therapy for a wide range of patients. The buoyancy of water supports the weight of severely debilitated patients, making it much easier to perform functional gait patterning (Fig. 12-13) or positioning of the body during exercise. In many cases, a patient that feels safe and confident in the water will demonstrate much better function than when on land. For example, motor function is regularly observed earlier in neurologic patients in the UWTM than is apparent on land. Mildly debilitated or postoperative patients can safely ambulate in a UWTM, maximizing function, achieving more extensive active ROM, and strengthening muscle. Abnormalities in gait can be corrected. Therapeutic jets can be used in all types of patients to relax and warm up the muscles before exercise.

Once normal limb usage returns, most dogs no longer need rehabilitation. However, canine athletes and working dogs can be assisted in returning to a higher functional level using the unique properties of the UWTM. Resistance can be applied with weights, water wings, jets, and changing water levels to provide an environment for increasing muscle strength and endurance. Walking, jogging, and running are controlled in this environment and can be monitored to record miles per hour and total miles.

Fit the patient with a flotation device. Begin the session by introducing the patient to the unit and the unfilled exercise chamber. Fill the water to the desired level (selected based on the desired effects of buoyancy, ROM, and resistance for each individual patient).

Filling the UWTM such that the water level reaches the animal's sternum or higher provides maximum buoyancy, hydrostatic pressure, and resistance and is used for patients with severely debilitating disease, edema, and unstable fixations, and for those patients that are athletic. Shallow water provokes an exaggerated active ROM of the limbs and should be used when fixations are stable.

Start with very short sessions of 1 to 2 minutes daily and increase the sessions by 5-minute increments every couple of days as tolerated.

The patient's athletic ability sets the maximum amount of time, but it is not unusual to have sessions last 60 minutes in those that are fit.

Use the perceived exertional rating system (Box 12-1) as a guide for patient tolerance.

Swimming. Swimming is great exercise for most minimally debilitated and healthy patients. The primary benefit of swimming is the elimination of concussive forces to the body and joints (Fig. 12-14). Swimming provokes an exaggerated active ROM, especially in the forelimbs; however, only a few pets will actually paddle or move their hindlimbs while swimming. Swimming is an excellent cardiovascular exercise, particularly for athletic animals receiving therapy for conditioning. Swimming is often used when the patient is completely healed, and therapy is concentrated on restoring normal function, stamina, and muscle mass.

Fit the patient with a flotation device. Gradually enter the water with the patient to minimize fear and encourage

BOX 12-1

Perceived Exertion for Walking or Running

0–Not tired at all—no signs of exertion, panting, agitation, or abnormal gait.
1–Slightly tired—may be beginning to show early signs of exertion, no signs of panting or agitation, no change in gait
2–A little tired—may be showing early signs of exertion, very early panting, no to minimal agitation, no change in gait
3–Slightly tired—just beyond 2
4–Getting more tired—moderate signs of exertion, panting consistently but not labored breathing, mild agitation, no change in gait
5–Increasingly tired—just beyond 4
6–Tired—obvious signs of exertion, panting hard, mild labored breathing, moderate agitation, moving slowly or reluctantly
7–Really tired—obvious signs of exertion, panting very hard, moderate labored breathing, moderate agitation, occasional stumbling <35%
8–Really tired—obvious signs of exertion, panting very hard, moderate labored breathing, moderate agitation, more frequent stumbling 35%–75%
9–Very, very tired—obvious signs of exertion, severe labored panting and labored breathing, severe agitation, can barely carry normal gait, mistakes made >75%–100%
10–Exhausted—obvious signs of exertion, open-mouth breathing where animal cannot catch their breath, extreme agitation, collapse

Based on modified OMNI Scale of perceived exertion for walking/running.

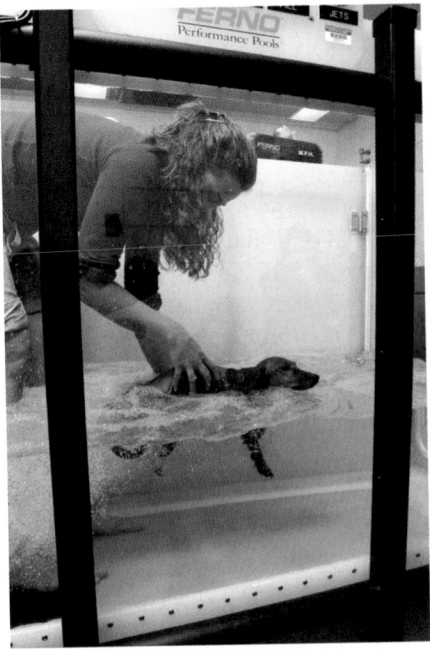

FIG. 12-14
A postoperative hemilaminectomy patient swimming in an underwater treadmill unit. In the water the dog can exercise independently without the fear of falling.

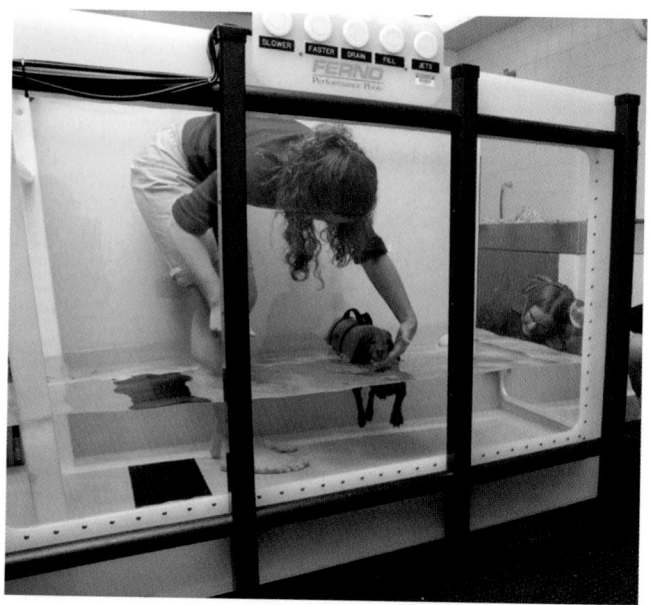

FIG. 12-15
The combination of life vests, compassion, and an understanding of animal behavior can often make the initial fear of the swimming experience short lived.

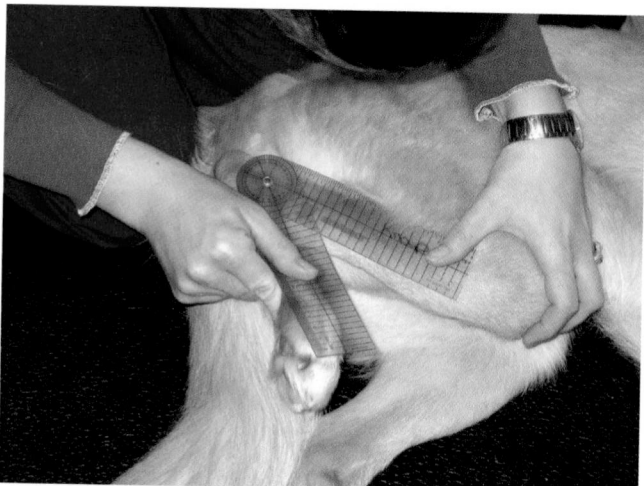

FIG. 12-16
Goniometric measurement of the tarsus in flexion.

acclimation to the pool and surroundings (Fig. 12-15). If possible, gradually lower the patient into the water until swimming movements begin. Begin sessions with brief intervals (e.g., 20 to 30 seconds, two to three times daily) and gradually increase by 30-second intervals every 2 to 3 days, as tolerated.

Maximum session time is determined by the patient's level of fitness and perceived exertion.

Measuring Outcomes in Rehabilitation

Historically, orthopedic patient postoperative care consisted of 6 to 12 weeks of cage rest. Although most surgeons felt the outcomes of fracture healing or other procedures were acceptable, with recent interest in rehabilitation it has become apparent that more can be done to enhance functional outcome. Frequently, patients are athletes, working dogs, and irreplaceable family members. Because physical therapy is the standard of care in human medicine, owners often demand a similar level of care with more rapid and complete return to function for their pets than might be achieved with cage rest alone. It has become the veterinary team's duty to use all modalities at their disposal to return pets to their former level of activity. Coincident with increased owner expectations, veterinarians and therapists must also become more familiar with objective outcome measures of physical function, including force plate analysis, lameness scores, pain assessment, perceived exertional scoring, disability indexes, goniometric measurements, muscle girth measurements, electromyography (EMG), and dual energy x-ray absorptiometry (DEXA) analysis. These measurements allow therapists to monitor progress and adjust rehabilitation treatment plans accordingly. Achieving a measurable outcome is a great motivator for owners. Most importantly, attention to outcome data lends credibility to the field of rehabilitation and provides a foundation for future improvement.

An ideal rehabilitation evaluation includes a thorough history and general examination, followed by a systematic approach to an orthopedic or neurologic exam (see p. 931 and 1358), and incorporates joint goniometry, muscle girth measurements, gait analysis, body condition scoring, and radiographs or DEXA. Obtaining complete historical data may be simplified by developing a questionnaire seeking information about the pet's normal activity and lifestyle, limb involvement, onset of the problem and its association with trauma, and activities that exacerbate it. It is also important to discuss specific treatments, duration of treatment, and expected outcomes before embarking on a rehabilitation protocol. Finding out what motivates and/or scares the pet may be essential to the success of rehabilitation.

Rehabilitation evaluations should include a complete set of goniometric measurements.

Use a commercially available goniometer to measure the angles of greatest comfortable flexion and extension. Begin with the unaffected limb and record the measurements for all joints (Fig. 12-16). Place one limb of the goniometer along the long axis of the long bone proximal to the joint and the other limb of the goniometer along the long axis of the long bone distal to the joint. Be sure the center of the goniometer is located over the isometric point of the joint. Relax the patient before measuring the joint angles. If necessary, have an assistant restrain the animal. Limit measurement variation by having the same person take the measurements consistently. Use measurement from the contralateral unaffected limb as a comparison. While moving the joint through the ROM, note the "end feel."

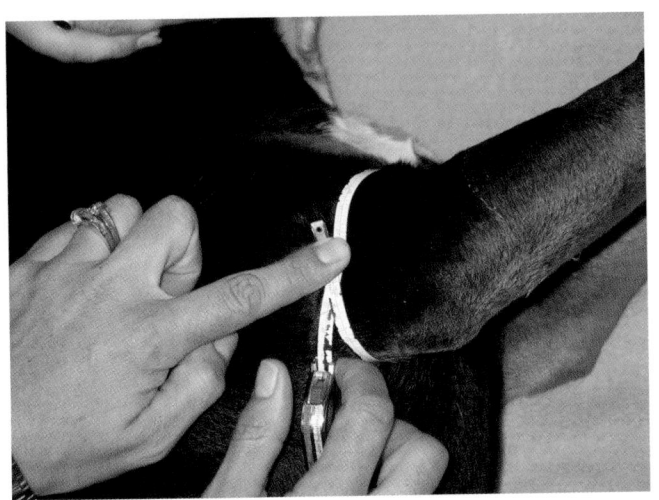

FIG. 12-17
Circumferential measurement of the proximal forelimb.
Collecting actual measurements is an easy and inexpensive
way to document progress.

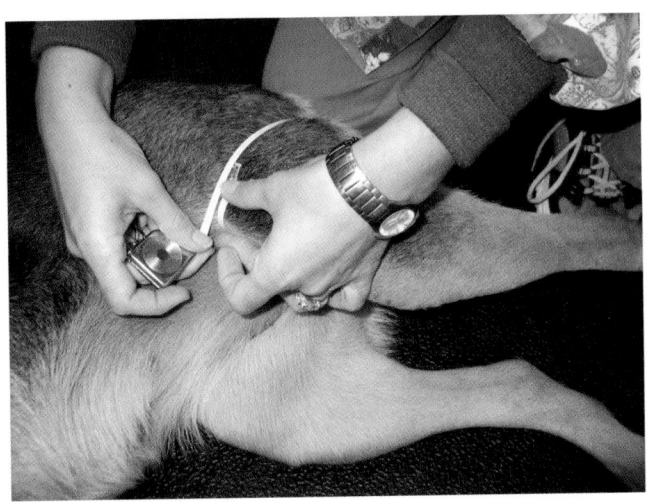

FIG. 12-18
Circumferential measurement of the proximal hind limb.

"End feel" is the description of resistance palpated by either extreme flexion or extension.

Girth measurement involves measuring and recording the circumference of a body part, area of musculature, or joint, but is most frequently used to estimate muscle mass. Muscle mass may also be estimated with ultrasound, computed tomography, magnetic resonance imaging, and DEXA. Girth measurement is inexpensive, is easily performed, and provides an objective number for sequential evaluation of the affected limb and comparison of the affected limb to the normal limb. It is an accurate tool for determining lean body mass and body condition scores. There is a margin of error, which is minimized by consistency in measurement location and evaluator. Other variables include hair coat, limb position, body condition, sedation, point of measurement, and the patient's body stance at time of measurement.

To measure the circumference of the proximal forelimb, position the limb in a standing angle. Locate the distal third of the humerus using the greater tubercle and olecranon as landmarks (Fig. 12-17). Encircle the area with a measuring tape, taking care to maintain a consistent tension on the tape. To measure the circumference of the antebrachium, locate the proximal fourth of the radius using the lateral epicondyle of the humerus and styloid process of the ulna as landmarks. To measure the circumference of the proximal rear limb, locate the proximal fourth of the femur using the patella and greater trochanter as landmarks (Fig. 12-18). To measure the circumference of the distal portion of the rear limb, measure at the proximal fourth of the tibia using the tibial plateau and malleoli as landmarks.

Body condition scoring systems are effective for monitoring patient weight loss or gain (Table 12-2). Many patients are obese and should benefit from rehabilitation by losing weight. Habitual use of a body condition scoring system by trained personnel provides another method of documenting progress during rehabilitation.

Subjective gait analysis should be performed on a non-slippery surface, such as grass, rubber flooring, or cement.

Examine the patient at all gaits as they walk toward and away from you; also view them from the sides and at a stand and a sit. Walk the patient in varying sized circles. Exercise athletes or patients with intermittent lameness on the LTM to appreciate subtle lameness. Use a consistent lameness scoring system with a numeric score for overall function (Box 12-2).

After subjective gait analysis, it is advantageous to collect an objective gait analysis. Systems such as a force plate or a Gait analysis systems are costly, but allow the observer to document a patient's lameness with an objective numeric value. Some advanced systems can measure stride length and center of gravity, and can even determine weight bearing on a single digit of the paw.

Because pain can significantly limit rehabilitation success, it is important to observe and document pain with a scoring system (Box 12-3; see also Chapter 13). Pain should be recorded daily and appropriate adjustments should be made to modalities and medications to assure the patient is as comfortable as possible.

Disability indices (DI) may also be used to document function (Box 12-4). The staff should be trained to understand the meaning of each level and should document the index daily. Perceived exertional scales (PES) may be used to measure exertion (see Box 12-1). These scoring systems are effective in determining the appropriate intensity of exercises for the individual animal. The PES score should be documented at several intervals before, during, and after the exercise session. Overexertion may be detrimental to recovery.

TABLE 12-2

Body Condition Chart

Use the scores on this chart to record body condition on questionnaires.

1 Thin dog		• Ribs, lumbar vertebrae, and pelvic bones easily visible • No palpable fat • Obvious waist and abdominal tuck • Prominent pelvic bones
2 Underweight dog		• Ribs easily palpable • Minimal fat covering • Waist easily noted when viewed from above • Abdominal tuck evident
3 Ideal dog		• Ribs palpable, but not visible • Waist observed behind ribs when viewed from above • Abdomen tucks up when viewed from side
4 Overweight dog		• Ribs palpable with slight excess fat covering • Waist discernible when viewed from above, but not prominent • Abdominal tuck apparent
5 Obese dog		• Ribs not easily palpable under a heavy fat covering • Fat deposits over lumbar area and tail base • Waist barely visible to absent • No abdominal tuck—may exhibit obvious abdominal distention

From Millis DL, Levine D, Taylor RA: *Canine rehabilitation and physical therapy,* St. Louis, 2004, Saunders.

 BOX 12-2

Lameness Scoring

Evaluation at a Walk

0 Walks normally
1 Slight lameness
2 Obvious weight-bearing lameness
3 Severe weight-bearing lameness
4 Intermittent non–weight-bearing lameness
5 Continuous non–weight-bearing lameness

Lameness Evaluation at a Trot

0 Trots normally
1 Slight lameness
2 Obvious weight-bearing lameness
3 Severe weight-bearing lameness
4 Intermittent non–weight-bearing lameness
5 Continuous non–weight-bearing lameness

Developing a Treatment Plan

Although rehabilitation plans can be generally grouped based on effectiveness for specific problems, it is important to fine tune the plan to suit the individual animal. Variables such as fixation stability, severity of disease, stoicism, breed characteristics, training level, lifestyle, and behavior can significantly affect the success of rehabilitation.

 BOX 12-3

Pain Scoring System

0 No signs of pain during palpation of affected joint
1 Signs of mild pain during palpation of joint
2 Signs of moderate pain during palpation
3 Signs of severe pain during palpation
4 Dog will not allow examiner to palpate joint

To develop a rehabilitation plan, first complete a thorough evaluation of the patient and make a problem list. Based on the problem list, select and try the most potentially effective modalities initially to determine the patient's ability to accept the modality. After selecting appropriate exercises, write a detailed inpatient and home exercise plan (Table 12-3 and Box 12-5). Determine the proportion of home exercises versus intensive inpatient rehabilitation based on the patient's function; generally the more debilitated the patient, the more inpatient rehabilitation is required.

On days when the patient receives inpatient therapy, home exercises need not be performed.

Demonstrate each exercise to the owner and observe them performing the exercise with their pet. Explain why each

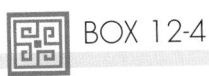

BOX 12-4

Disability Indexes

Disability Index

Paraparesis/Paraplegia; Tetraparesis/Tetraplegia; Hemiparesis/Hemiplegia; Monoparesis/Monoplegia

Stage 1: Paralysis With No Voluntary Limb Movements

0–No limb movement and absent deep pain
1–No limb movement and present deep pain
2–No limb movement but voluntary tail movement

Stage 2: Non–Weight-Bearing Voluntary Limb Movements

3–Minimal non–weight-bearing activity of one limb (one joint)
4–Non–weight-bearing activity in more than one joint <50% of the time
5–Non–weight-bearing activity in more than one joint >50% of the time

Stage 3: Voluntary Limb Movement With Occasional Weight Bearing

6–Weight-bearing activity of the limb <10% of the time
7–Weight-bearing activity of the limb 10%–50% of the time
8–Weight-bearing activity of the limb >50% of the time

Stage 4: Weight-Bearing Movements With Decreased Motor Strength

9–Weight-bearing activity 100% of the time, but with reduced strength and mistakes made >90% of the time, including crossing of the limbs, knuckling of the paws, standing on the dorsum of the paws, and falling
10–Weight-bearing activity 100% of the time, but with reduced strength and above mistakes made 50%–90% of the time
11–Weight-bearing activity 100% of the time, but with reduced strength and mistakes made <50% of the time

Stage 5: Normal Motor Strength With Ataxia

12–Ataxic gate with normal strength, but mistakes made >50% of the time, including lack of coordination, crossing of hind limbs, skipping steps, bunny-hopping, and knuckling of the paws
13–Ataxic gait with normal strength, but mistakes made <50% of the time
14–Normal gait

From Olby NJ, DeRisio L, Munana KR et al: Development of a functional scoring system in dogs with acute spinal cord injuries, *AJVR* 62:1624, 2001.

Table 12-3

Sample Inpatient Exercise Protocol for Routine Postoperative TPLO

ALL TREATMENTS BID	DAY 1 TO DAY 14	DAY 15 TO DAY 24	DAY 25 UNTIL HEALED	HEALED TO RETURN TO FUNCTION
Heat therapy		10 min	10 min	
Massage	5 min	5 min	5 min	
Passive ROM/stretching (repetitions)	20* repetitions	20* repetitions	10–15* repetitions	Stop when ROM normal
Electrical stimulation†	10 min	10 min	10 min	10 min
Therapeutic exercise: total time	10 min	15 min	15 min	25–45 min
Walk/land treadmill	10 min	5 min	5 min	10+ min
Balancing	+	+	+	+
Obstacles	+	+	+	+
Weaving				+
Circles				+
Hills				+
Stairs				+
Jog/run				+
Underwater treadmill		10 min	10 min	15+ min
Swimming				5–10 min
Hypotherapy	15 min	15 min	15 min	PRN

TPLO, Tibial plateau leveling osteotomy.
*Passive ROM to all joints of the affected limb.
†Electrical stimulation: to be performed on semimembranosus/semitendinosus muscle groups for femur fractures in patients with muscle atrophy. See p. 114 for specifications.

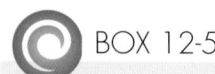

BOX 12-5

Outpatient Home Exercise Protocol for Animals After a TPLO Procedure

Day 0 to Day 14; Perform Twice Daily

1. Gently massage the affected limb for 5 minutes
2. Perform PROM to all joints of the affected limb for 20 repetitions
3. Perform balancing exercises for 3 minutes as tolerated
4. Perform controlled leash walk with sling support for 8 minutes. Walk in a straight line on nonslippery, nonconcussive surfaces such as grass
5. Follow the exercise session with 15 minutes of cryotherapy

Return 3 days a week for twice daily inpatient therapy as outlined above.

Day 15 to 24

1. Apply a warm compress to the affected limb for 10 minutes
2. Gently massage the affected limb for 5 minutes
3. Perform PROM exercises on all joints of the limb for 20 repetitions
4. Perform balancing exercises for 3 minutes as tolerated
5. Perform controlled leash walks with sling support for 15 minutes; during these walks, encourage walking over obstacles and add a limited amount of gradual weaving, vary surfaces of the walk, but try to remain on less concussive surfaces such as grass
6. Have the pet perform five repetitive sit-to-stand exercises; encourage them to sit as square as possible or try to have them sit in a corner
7. Apply a cold compress for 15 minutes after the exercise session

Return 3 days a week for twice daily inpatient therapy as outlined above.

Day 25 Until Healed

1. Apply a warm compress to the affected limb for 10 minutes
2. If the pet is still not consistently using the limb, you should continue massage and ROM exercises as previously described; if they are using the limb, you may discontinue these modalities
3. Place the hind limbs on a mildly unstable surface, such as a couch cushion, and perform balancing exercises for 3 minutes
4. Perform controlled leash walks with sling support for 15 minutes; during these walks, encourage walking over many obstacles and add several weaves and turns; vary surfaces of the walk, but try to remain on less concussive surfaces such as grass

5. Have the pet perform 10 repetitive sit-to-stand exercises; encourage them to sit as square as possible or try to have them sit in a corner
6. If the pet is showing signs of lameness, apply a cold compress for 15 minutes after the exercise session

Return 2–3 days a week for twice daily inpatient therapy as outlined above.

Healed to Return to Function (for an average, fit, nonworking pet)

1. In most cases discontinue heat therapy, massage, and PROM
2. Elevate the front limbs with an exercise ball and perform balancing exercises for 3–5 minutes; add 1 minute each week
3. Continue leash walks for 20–25 minutes; add 5 minutes each week until a maximum of previous activity
   a. Continue obstacle work, increasing the height and number of obstacles.
      Continue weaves and sharpen turns.
      Vary surfaces of the walk, trying to maximize active ROM.
      Add hills and stairs to the walk. Start with a few and increase as stamina increases.
   b. Add 30-second spurts of jogging or running to the walk. Increase jogging time by 30 seconds each week.
4. Have the pet perform 15 repetitive sit-to-stand exercises, encourage them to sit as square as possible or try to have them sit in a corner; add 5 a week until muscle mass is adequate and the patient can sit nicely square again
5. If the pet is showing signs of lameness, apply a cold compress for 15 minutes after the exercise session

Return 2–3 days a week for twice daily inpatient therapy as outlined above.

TPLO, Tibial plateau leveling osteotomy.

---

exercise is important and how it relates to the functional outcome. Plan an evaluation schedule; depending on the problem, evaluations may be daily, weekly, or monthly.

As a general rule, the more changes you expect to occur, the more frequently evaluations should be performed.

Modify the treatment plan as necessary as the patient progresses.

Specific Concerns for Rehabilitating Fracture Patients

Concerns specifically related to fracture patients include the type of fracture fixation used (internal vs. external fixation), stability of the fixation, fracture location, and potential for infection. The therapist has a responsibility to safely exercise the patient without compromising the surgical outcome. In early fracture patient rehabilitation, overactivity can cause implant failure. Conversely, failure to use the leg may cause delayed healing, soft tissue contracture, excessive scar tissue, limited ROM, and muscle atrophy.

Most fractures treated with bone plates, interlocking nails, or external fixators are sufficiently stable for patients to bear weight on them immediately after surgery. Controlled walking, use of the LTM, and most TEs are generally safe and effective and encourage weight bearing and prevent loss of ROM and muscle atrophy. Because of infection concerns, UWTM exercise and other hydrotherapies are best delayed until the incision is healed. However, occasionally the benefits of aquatic therapy started 48 hours after surgery to encourage early weight bearing outweigh the risks of infection. Compromise of the fracture fixation is a concern and all exercise must be controlled. Slings should be used at all times during therapy, and owners should be advised regarding potential catastrophic effects of falls. If the owner or caregiver cannot perform the exercises in a controlled manner or is unable to control the dog, cage rest or inpatient therapy is a better option.

Typically the exercise plan for the average size dog should consist of 10 to 15 minutes of exercise twice daily for the first 4 weeks, and then the exercise may gradually be increased to two 30-minute sessions daily until the fracture is healed (see Chapter 32 for suggested treatment plans for each bone). At that time, exercise should be increased according to patient tolerance until the functional outcome is acceptable for the surgeon, therapist, and owner.

Specific Concerns for Rehabilitating Neurologic Patients

Optimally, rehabilitation of neurologic patients begins immediately after injury or surgery and starts slowly, progressing as the patient improves (see Chapters 38 to 40 for suggested therapy tables). A paralyzed patient without deep pain may be treated with warm compresses applied to extremities, followed by PROM and massage of the affected limbs. Electrical stimulation should follow the warm-up and precede active exercise. Assisted standing and balancing exercises should begin on a nonslippery, stable surface, such as a rubber floor or mat, followed by UWTM with gait patterning. If a UWTM is not available, a wading pool or bathtub filled with warm water may be substituted, or alternatively sling-supported LTM walks may be used. A wheelchair (Fig. 12-19) or one person is necessary to support the animal's weight with a sling, and an assistant gait patterns the affected limbs. Assistive devices, such as thera-bands, can be used to advance the limbs if the patient is not cooperative or is aggressive. All sessions should be kept relatively short (i.e., <30 minutes total) and should be performed consistently 2 to 3 times a day. Extreme care must be taken to protect the stability of the spine and surgical site.

For a paralyzed patient with deep pain sensation, it is vital to stimulate sensation and encourage functional movement. Warm compresses, PROM, and massage should be used as a warm-up. Electrical stimulation is helpful for muscle reeducation and to combat muscle atrophy. Assisted standing and balancing exercises should challenge the patient by being

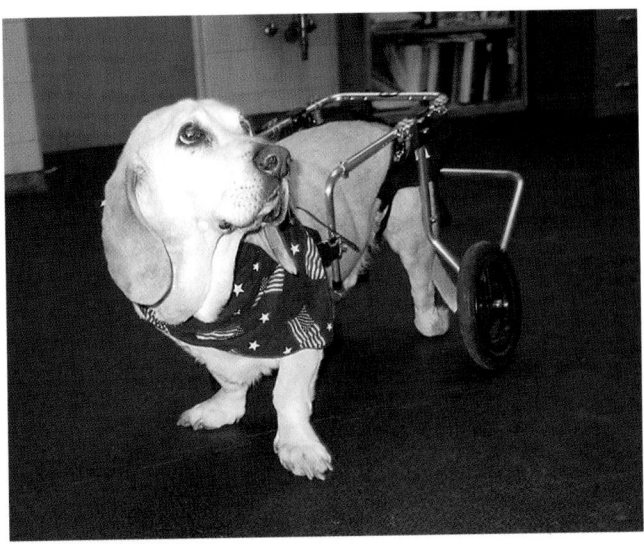

FIG. 12-19
A paretic patient acclimated to a wheelchair or cart. The cart can be used as a therapy tool in the absence of aquatic therapy or as an ambulation aid at home if improvement is not expected.

performed on a slightly unstable surface to provide additional afferent feedback. Appropriate surfaces include pillows, cushions, air mattresses, or a waterbed. The ability to push off when falling off center returns before motor function and can be detected with these exercises. As the patient improves, increasingly unstable surfaces, such as thera-balls or balance boards, may be used. Gait patterning is an important part of therapy. Sessions should be performed 2 to 3 times daily, gradually increasing session time to a maximum of 40 to 45 minutes as tolerated.

Therapy for weakly ambulatory patients should focus on building strength, stamina, and balance. Warm-ups and TEs are described above. The UWTM is particularly useful for increasing strength and allowing the therapist to encourage proper foot placement. Splints can be used for a portion of the session to encourage proper paw placement. Although swimming is an option, often patients will only move their front limbs in a swimming environment, which is not therapeutic for regaining rear limb function. Sessions are generally performed twice a day, with the length of session increasing as tolerated. As the patient progresses, weaving, circles, and small hill climbing can be added to improve their ability to balance and walk at the same time. Owners can be taught to perform some exercises at home, and intensive therapy can be provided on an outpatient basis.

Specific Concerns for Rehabilitating Osteoarthritic Patients

Osteoarthritic patients are often treated medically with individualized combinations of weight loss, nonsteroidal antiinflammatory drugs (NSAIDs), chondroprotective agents, and controlled minimally concussive exercise (see Chapter 33).

Rehabilitation provides excellent therapy for osteoarthritic patients, and exercise coupled with calorie restriction encourages weight loss. Many therapeutic modalities offer the opportunity for minimally concussive, controlled exercises that strengthen periarticular tissue, improve muscle mass and flexibility, and promote comfortable function.

After a thorough evaluation of the patient, dietary recommendations and a personalized exercise program, including inpatient therapy and home exercise, should be developed (see Table 12-3 and Box 12-5). Exercise tolerance and ability of each patient must be considered when developing the program. The goal is to comfortably exercise each patient to the individual level of tolerance. Commonly, patients are treated with heat therapy, massage, PROM, and therapeutic exercises. Treadmill exercise is effective in these patients because it limits the braking and propulsive forces used in walking. The UWTM can provide complete therapy when warm water, therapeutic jet massage, and walking in the buoyant environment are combined. Swimming is therapeutic for fit patients. Inpatient exercise sessions should include weekly weight assessment. Comfort and function are often maintained with one to two sessions weekly.

Home-based therapies include heat therapy, massage, and PROM, followed with a controlled leash walk in the yard or on another low-impact surface. TEs, such as sit-to-stands, weaving, and balancing are incorporated to improve function of the affected joints and muscles.

Specific Concerns for Rehabilitating Patients After Joint Surgery

Patients with joint diseases requiring surgery make up a substantial portion of the caseload for most surgical facilities. Rehabilitation programs are beneficial before and after surgical intervention, especially in osteoarthritic patients. It is possible that increasing fitness before surgery results in a more complete postoperative recovery. Intensive rehabilitation after surgery encourages weight-bearing activity and strengthens existing muscle and periarticular tissue, which helps patients compensate for the affected limb or joint. Therapists developing rehabilitation programs for postoperative patients should work closely with the surgeon and must consider the disease, surgical procedure, and postoperative stability of the joint and surrounding tissue.

Animals with extracapsular stabilizations for cruciate-deficient stifles and femoral head and neck ostectomies (see pp. 1244 and 1275) can typically begin aggressive rehabilitation immediately. The primary goal immediately after surgery is to get the patient to bear weight on the affected limb. Massage, PROM, stretching, balancing exercises, and mild TEs, followed with cryotherapy to curb inflammation and ease discomfort, are useful. Once weight bearing is achieved, the focus shifts to improving active ROM and increasing muscle mass in the semimembranosus, semitendinosus, and gluteal muscles. It is generally safe to be aggressive with muscle gain relatively soon after surgery. Sit-to-stands, treadmill exercise at an incline, obstacles, weights applied just proximal to the tarsus, thera-bands for additional resistance,

and dancing are all useful modalities. Once the incision is healed, controlled UWTM exercise may be added to the program. Initially the water level should be high to support most of the patient's weight, minimizing concussion and the potential for falling. An animal with a femoral head ostectomy that has no risk for implant infection but intensive need to develop adequate hip ROM may begin UWTM or swimming once the fibrin seal is formed over the incision. After lameness resolves, the water level can be decreased to hock level to maximize active ROM. Sessions are initially brief, but can typically be increased to 15 to 20 minutes per session within the first few weeks. As function improves, exercise times are gradually increased. Animals with extracapsular repairs for cruciate-deficient stifles may start swimming if they have tolerated the UWTM for 5 days with no progressive signs of lameness.

Similarly, animals with joint disease treated with bone or cartilage fragment removal, such as osteochondrosis, fragmented coronoid process, and ununited anconeal process (see pp. 1176, 1197, and 1209), can be rehabilitated aggressively because the joints are relatively stable. These patients are treated initially with massage and aggressive PROM and/or stretching. Walking and TEs to encourage weight bearing and active ROM are incorporated in the treatment plan. Wheelbarrowing, obstacle work, balancing exercises, stand-to-downs, and weaving are also useful TEs. UWTM sessions can begin when the incision is sealed or healed, depending on immediacy of the need for therapy. Initially the water level should be high to support weight, but it is gradually lowered to maximize active ROM. Once lameness is resolved, the water level may be increased to maximize resistance and promote muscle strengthening. Swimming can be very beneficial as it encourages exaggerated active ROM in the forelimbs.

Animals treated for joint disease with corrective osteotomies (see pp. 1011, 1029, and 1220) should be treated as described for fracture patients (see previous discussion), whereas animals treated with reconstructive joint procedures for patella luxation or luxated joints (see pp. 1289, 1297, and 1301) should be subjected to a more conservative rehabilitation program to allow time for tissue healing. Therapy should begin immediately after surgery, but progression of time and intensity of exercises are initially limited. A sling should be used, not to support the animal's weight, but to provide a safety net to prevent or cushion a fall. Initial therapy includes massage, PROM, and mild TEs, followed with cryotherapy to curb inflammation and alleviate discomfort. As healing and lameness improve, exercise time may be gradually increased. After the incision is healed, controlled UWTM exercise may be instituted. Water level should support most of the patient's weight to minimize concussion and incidence of falls. Sessions should be initially brief, but slowly increased to 15 minutes. Swimming is not typically considered to be sufficiently controlled exercise for these patients. Until the osteotomy and soft tissue are healed, the primary goal for the therapist is to maintain flexibility and muscle mass, and enhance patient comfort. After healing is deemed sufficient to prevent implant failure, more aggressive rehabilitation may be instituted.

Patients with stabilized intraarticular fractures are often a challenge for the therapist. Depending on the complexity of the fracture, reduction and stability may be compromised. Although rehabilitation is essential to restoring ROM and function, in some cases it is not feasible until fracture healing is safely progressing. Again, communication with the surgeon is necessary to prevent complications. If conservative rehabilitation is allowed, massage, PROM, and stretching are indicated to restore ROM and limit muscle atrophy. Balancing exercises work well because they are nonconcussive and encourage a mild, controlled contraction of periarticular muscles. Therapeutic ultrasound may be warranted if joint contracture occurs. Therapeutic exercises should be chosen to concentrate on affected muscle groups. The UWTM may offer a safer modality for walking and promoting active ROM.

Animals with total joint replacements (see pp. 1157 and 1257) require conservative rehabilitation to prevent costly and/or catastrophic complications. The therapist must work closely with the surgeon to develop appropriate rehabilitation programs. A sling should be used at all times to prevent falls or inappropriate limb positioning. Rehabilitation is generally started 48 hours after surgery and is limited to massage, PROM, electrical stimulation, balancing exercises, and 5-minute controlled walks. After the incision is healed, controlled UWTM exercise may be initiated. The water level should support most of the patient's weight to minimize concussion and incidence of falling. Sessions should be brief for the entire recovery period. Swimming is not typically considered to be a sufficiently controlled exercise for these patients.

Suggested Reading

Millis DL, Levine D, Taylor RA: *Canine rehabilitation and physical therapy,* St Louis, 2004, WB Saunders.
This is a comprehensive textbook that provides a basic understanding of canine rehabilitation for both veterinarians and therapists. The text includes in-depth discussions of therapeutic modalities and the application of those modalities in patient rehabilitation.

CHAPTER 13

Perioperative Multimodal Analgesic Therapy

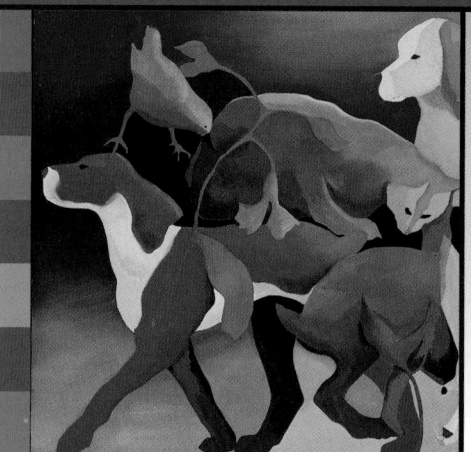

Pain is now considered the fourth (or fifth if you measure blood pressure) vital sign. The American Animal Hospital Association (AAHA) has determined that a comprehensive analgesic program is necessary for hospitals that are seeking AAHA accreditation (see p. 150 under Selected References and Videos). A thorough physical examination requires evaluation of the patient's pain. There are several different types of pain scoring systems, each with its own advantages and disadvantages. A combination of (1) physiologic responses; (2) anticipated pain caused by the procedure, trauma, or disease; (3) the animal's behavior; and (4) its response to therapy is used to determine if a patient is painful.

In cats, the most reliable physiologic variables for evaluating pain are blood pressure and cortisol. However, physiologic signs of pain are not very specific; they can increase because of stress, disease, and numerous drugs. Be aware that when one uses preconceived ideas regarding how painful a procedure should be (or how an animal should respond to that disease, trauma, or procedure) to guide therapy, personal bias may result in the patient being denied appropriate analgesic therapy. Individual variation greatly impacts patient response and should always be considered. Behavioral response, a subjective determination, is relied on more than any other single variable when determining the presence of pain. Pain behaviors are not very adaptive, so these signs may come late in the progression of disease once all the coping mechanisms have been exhausted. Regardless of the scoring system chosen, it is helpful to do in-house training with staff so that interobserver variation can be minimized. If on examination the patient is determined to have pain, treatment and reevaluation should be undertaken.

NOTE: Do not spend much time convincing yourself that a patient is painful. Treat them for pain and if there is no improvement or if there are unwanted side effects (very rare), discontinue or change the therapy.

In most instances it is better to start analgesic therapy before a potentially painful event rather than attempt to regain control of a painful situation once it occurs. This is known as preemptive therapy. The efficacy of preemptive analgesia is related to stopping or obtunding "windup" (the volley of afferent impulses in the spinal cord that result from stimulation of a nociceptor). Preemptive therapy should be followed by scheduled maintenance therapy. It is important to realize that one regimen will not work for all situations or all patients. There are different types of pain, and pain is regulated in several ways. **Customized multimodal therapy** is the best technique for providing optimal analgesia.

Most current analgesic therapies are designed to provide optimum analgesia and the most rapid return to normal function. Analgesic therapy may inhibit afferent nociceptive impulses at the brain and spinal cord (e.g., opioids and ketamine), interrupt neural impulse conduction (e.g., local anesthetics), or prevent nociceptor sensitization that accompanies inflammation (e.g., nonsteroidal antiinflammatory drugs [NSAIDs]). Additional therapies tried in patients with chronic pain may include antiviral medications (e.g., amantadine), antiepileptic drugs (e.g., gabapentin) and antidepressants (e.g., amitriptyline). Physical medicine techniques are also used to improve comfort and ensure return to function. These techniques are briefly described later. Current American Veterinary Medical Association (AVMA) guidelines for the use of alternative or complementary therapies should always be consulted (see p. 145 under Selected References and Videos).

Analgesic requirements should be anticipated and incorporated into each patient's anesthetic management. Comprehensive reviews of pain assessment for dogs and cats are available in the veterinary literature. If you are just beginning to incorporate analgesic therapy into your anesthetic regimen, you may benefit from a more exhaustive examination of pain recognition than is offered here. There are several resources available, including a website for the International Academy of Pain Management (http://www.cvmbs.colostate.edu/ivapm).

Generally the extent of postoperative pain is determined by integrating the surgeon's expectations of a procedure's painfulness with the patient's behavioral and physiologic responses to surgery and by observing the individual patient's response to the analgesic therapies. Table 13-1 provides an estimate of the pain judged to be associated with

TABLE 13-1

Estimates of Pain Associated With Various Types of Surgery*

MOST PAINFUL	MODERATELY TO SEVERELY PAINFUL	MILDLY TO MODERATELY PAINFUL
Thoracotomies (particularly median sternotomies), amputations, ear resections, pelvic fracture repair, nephrectomy, cervical disk surgery	Mastectomy, mandibulectomy, thoracic or lumbar disk surgery, stabilization of a fractured femur or humerus, cranial abdominal procedures	Tracheotomy; aural hematoma; stabilization of a fractured radius, ulna, tibia, or fibula; castration; caudal abdominal procedures; dental cleaning; extraction

Modified from Carroll GL: *Small animal pain management*, Lakewood, Colo, 1998, American Animal Hospital Association Press.
*The practitioner's expectations of the level of pain should not be grounds for denying a patient analgesic relief.

 TABLE 13-2

Behavioral and Physiologic Responses to Pain

RESPONSE	SIGNS OF PAIN
Behavioral responses	*Vocalization:* Groaning, whining, growling, purring *Facial expression:* Fixed stare, glazed or squinted eyes, dilated pupils, furrowed brow *Body posture:* Hunched, rigid, prayer position or other abnormal position *Activity:* Restless or restricted movement, trembling *Attitude:* Aggression, fearfulness, timidity, comfort seeking *Appetite:* Decreased *Urinary and bowel habits:* Increased urination, failure in house training or failure to use litter box *Grooming:* Loss of hair coat sheen, unkempt appearance *Guarding and self-mutilation:* Protects wound or limb; fails to bear weight; may lick, chew, or rub surgical area
Physiologic responses	*Cardiovascular system:* Increased heart rate and blood pressure, vasoconstriction *Pulmonary system:* Increased respiratory rate, shallow breathing, splinting *Digestive system:* Inappetence, salivation; possibly vomiting, diarrhea or constipation, evacuation of anal glands *Musculoskeletal system:* Tense muscles, muscle tremors *Immune system:* Diminished resistance, stress leukogram; increased metastasis *Neuroendocrine system:* Increased catabolism, decreased anabolism

Modified from Carroll GL: *Small animal pain management*, Lakewood, Colo, 1998, American Animal Hospital Association Press.

different types of surgery. However, an individual patient's response to a particular procedure may not be consistent with one's preconceived idea of how painful a procedure should be; therefore patients that appear painful should be given analgesic therapy. Table 13-2 provides a summary of animals' behavioral and physiologic responses to pain. If there is any question of whether a patient is in pain, treat it. Perioperative analgesia has a strong beneficial effect on surgical outcome (e.g., less self-mutilation or faster return of appetite). Be sure to monitor the animal's response to therapy and change or discontinue your treatment if the drug or technique you have chosen produces undesirable side effects or does not promote clinical improvement.

PAIN MANAGEMENT

Good perioperative nursing care is imperative. To promote well-being, keep your patients dry and warm, avoid clipper burns, remove dried blood, check bandages for tightness, position patients so that pressure is not placed on surgical sites, and turn patients that are unable to turn themselves. A dry, warm, quiet environment should be provided both for induction of an anesthetic and for recovery from surgery. During induction of anesthesia, be sure to use adequate intraoperative and postoperative padding and position patients in such a way as to lessen postoperative pain from areas that were not operated on but that may be injured during the anesthetic period (e.g., ischemia of the skin and underlying tissue, neural deficits). Lubricate the eyes. Prevent corneal, oral, lingual, tracheal, or dental injuries during induction and recovery. Before recovery, empty the bladder to prevent postoperative discomfort.

Preventing sleeplessness and anxiety in the perioperative period enhances postoperative pain management because anxiety and pain are closely related. Pain is intensified in an anxious patient, and tranquilizers or sedatives may reduce perioperative anxiety and make the experience less distressing. Tranquilization may also be necessary to curtail activity in rambunctious patients; tranquilization, not pain, should be used to restrict movement. However, to prevent masking signs of pain, do not use tranquilizers such as acepromazine or diazepam alone in patients with pain; administer an analgesic before or at the same time as the tranquilizer.

Tranquilizers and Sedatives

Few tranquilizers in veterinary medicine provide anxiolysis. Acepromazine (Table 13-3) is an excellent tranquilizer for an acutely distressed or dysphoric dog or cat. Use cau-

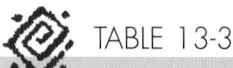 TABLE 13-3

Tranquilizers and Sedatives

DRUG	DOSAGE (mg/kg)	ROUTE
Acetylpromazine	0.25–0.5 (not to exceed 1 mg total dose per dog)	IV, SC, IM
Diazepam (Valium)	0.2	IV
Midazolam (Versed)	0.2	IM, IV
Xylazine (Rompun)*	0.1–0.5	IV, IM, SC
Medetomidine (Domitor)*	0.001–0.005	IV, IM, SC

IV, Intravenous; *SC*, subcutaneous; *IM*, intramuscular.
*Use with caution; postoperative doses and duration are not well established, and profound cardiac depression may occur.

tion in administering acepromazine to dogs or cats that are hypovolemic or hypotensive, have clotting disorders, or have a history of seizures. Benzodiazepines (i.e., diazepam, midazolam; see Table 13-3) do not provide reliable tranquilization in young healthy dogs and cats. These drugs disinhibit learned behavior and may cause excitement. However, benzodiazepines do achieve sedation in very young, very old, or critically ill dogs and cats. They often are used in these patients because few significant cardiopulmonary effects are associated with their administration. Diazepam and midazolam provide more predictable sedation when administered with an opioid or sedative. Flumazenil is a specific benzodiazepine antagonist; it generally is titrated to effect (e.g., if a cat with hepatic lipidosis who received a benzodiazepine is having a delayed recovery, flumazenil may be used to speed recovery).

α_2-Agonists (e.g., xylazine, medetomidine; see Table 13-3) provide reliable sedation and profound analgesia; the sedation outlasts the analgesia. Cardiopulmonary depression is dose dependent. Xylazine is the classic α_2-agonist, and medetomidine is a newer α_2-agonist. Because these drugs may have profound cardiopulmonary effects (i.e., bradycardia, hypoventilation, and hypertension followed by hypotension), perioperative use of α_2-agonists generally is reserved for young adult healthy dogs and cats, and low doses of xylazine or medetomidine have been used as sedatives for postoperative anxiety. α-Antagonists (e.g., yohimbine, atipamezole, and tolazoline) antagonize the effects of α_2-agonist drugs, but antagonism of α_2-agonists is not without risk in patients with pain. Therefore it may be prudent to titrate the antagonists to effect, as necessary.

Anesthetics

Current anesthetic practices rely on induction agents, such as propofol and etomidate, and inhalation agents, such as isoflurane and sevoflurane, which offer speedy induction and recovery but provide no analgesia. It is imperative to supplement these anesthetic techniques with appropriate analgesia.

Analgesics

Good postoperative pain management should begin before surgery. Preemptive administration of an opioid obtunds windup (the hyperexcitable state caused by sensitization by prior noxious stimuli) (see p. 135), whereas administration of a local anesthetic prevents windup. If a patient is in pain, administering an analgesic before induction of anesthesia facilitates patient handling and manipulation and improves the patient's comfort. Preoperative administration of an analgesic also reduces the inhalant requirement during surgery. If an analgesic is administered preoperatively, it may need to be repeated postoperatively depending on the drug's duration of action. The ideal duration of postoperative analgesic administration has not been determined for most surgeries in dogs and cats, but it is reasonable to provide at least 2 or 3 days of therapy after most major procedures. Several options are available for perioperative administration of an analgesic. Systemic drugs may be administered on a schedule (Table 13-4, e.g., every 4 hours), by continuous infusion (e.g., fentanyl and lidocaine), or by continuous absorption (e.g., transdermal fentanyl; Table 13-5). Local and regional techniques with local anesthetics and opioids may also be used. An analgesic should be administered according to its duration of activity rather than "as needed." Pharmacokinetic and pharmacodynamic information provides a rational defense against "as needed" medication. If a patient must demonstrate pain before an analgesic is given, it is much more difficult to gain control of the pain. In that instance, the clinician will generally need to administer higher doses than would have been necessary if given on schedule (preventing peaks and troughs).

Opioids

If an opioid analgesic is used, it should be chosen before surgery. Optimally a single opioid analgesic agent is used throughout the perioperative period. Unless it is contraindicated, the same analgesic agent should be used after surgery that was used before and during surgery. The two primary considerations for choosing an opioid analgesic are efficacy and duration. Some opioids are indicated for mild to moderate pain (e.g., buprenorphine), whereas others are more beneficial for moderate to severe pain (e.g., morphine, hydromorphone, and methadone). For opioids of short duration (e.g., butorphanol and fentanyl), the ease and expense of redosing and method of redosing should be considered. In most cases intravenous injection is preferred when an intravenous port is available to avoid painful intramuscular injections.

Opioid agonists and agonist-antagonists commonly used perioperatively include morphine, hydromorphone, methadone, oxymorphone, fentanyl, butorphanol, and buprenorphine. Most opioids currently used in veterinary medicine are "scheduled." *Schedule* relates to the potential for abuse and the liability of a drug to cause dependence. Schedule I drugs have a high potential for abuse and no currently ac-

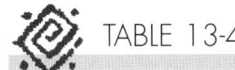 TABLE 13-4

Commonly Used Systemic Opioid Analgesics*

DRUG	USES	DOSAGE (mg/kg)†	ROUTE	DURATION
Butorphanol	Elective reproductive surgery, caudal abdominal procedures, gallbladder surgery, bile peritonitis, distal limb fractures	0.2–0.4	IV, SC, IM	2–3 hr
Buprenorphine	Elective reproductive surgery, caudal abdominal procedures, distal limb fractures	0.005–0.015	IV, IM	4–8 hr
Fentanyl	A premedicant; too short acting for analgesia; see text for information on continuous rate infusion (CRI) and transdermal application	0.002–0.010	IV, SC, IM	Less than 1 hr
Morphine	Thoracotomies, amputations, pelvic fractures, ear ablations	0.2–1.0	IV,‡ SC, IM	3–4 hr
Hydromorphone	Thoracotomies, amputations, pelvic fractures, ear ablations	0.1–0.2	IV, SC, IM	3–4 hr
Methadone	Thoracotomies, amputations, pelvic fractures, ear ablations	0.1–0.5	IV (dog), IM, SC	3–4 hr
Oxymorphone	Thoracotomies, amputations, pelvic fractures, ear ablations	0.05–0.1	IV, SC,§ IM	3–4 hr

Modified from Carroll GL: How to measure perioperative pain, *Vet Med* 91:353, 1996.
IV, Intravenous; *SC*, subcutaneous; *IM*, intramuscular.
*Dosage and duration are based on clinical experience and may need to be individualized to a particular situation and patient. Higher doses may be necessary for recalcitrant pain.
†Lower dosages are used for intravenous routes and in cats.
‡Hypotension may occur with intravenous administration of morphine; the drug also may be associated with excitement in cats.
§Subcutaneous administration may be less efficient.

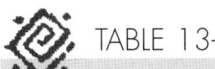 TABLE 13-5

Guidelines for Fentanyl Patch Dosing*

BODY WEIGHT (kg)	PATCH SIZE (μg/hr) †
Under 3.2	12: Use of patch not recommended‡
3.2–6.8	25
6.8–18.2	50
18.2–27.3	75
Over 27.3	100

*Guidelines are not well established generally; transdermal fentanyl patches should deliver 1 to 4 μg/kg/hr.
†Generic fentanyl patches are now available.
‡The pharmacokinetics and safety of the 12-μg/hr patch (pediatric) have not been determined in veterinary patients and this patch is currently not recommended for juvenile patients; covering or cutting a portion of the 25-μg/hr patch affects delivery.

cepted medical use, whereas Schedule V drugs have the least potential for abuse and in some circumstances may be available without a prescription order.

Morphine. Morphine (Schedule II; see Table 13-4) is the prototype opioid agonist and is indicated for moderate to severe pain. The onset of action is approximately 15 to 30 minutes, and the duration of action is 3 to 4 hours. Cardiovascular effects include vagally induced bradycardia, direct depression of the sinoatrial node, and slowed atrioventricular (AV) conduction. Morphine does not sensitize the myocardium to catecholamines. Ventilation is directly depressed (a dose-dependent effect) through inhibition of central respiratory centers. Morphine also alters the rhythm of breathing. Hypoventilation may cause increased intracranial pressure as a result of elevated arterial carbon dioxide partial pressure ($PaCO_2$). Nausea and vomiting result from stimulation of the chemoreceptor trigger zone. Morphine may cause hypothermia and miosis in dogs, and mydriasis and hyperthermia in cats. Histamine may be released when the drug is administered intravenously (IV); slow IV administration minimizes this risk. Morphine is administered as continuous IV infusions in human pain management and is being used clinically in veterinary medicine. It frequently is used for epidural administration (see p. 139 and Table 13-6). Recently, morphine has been used intraarticularly to provide analgesia for stifle surgery. For intraarticular injection, morphine (0.1 mg/kg; diluted as needed with saline to fill the joint space) provides good analgesia; the analgesia obtained is comparable with that provided by epidural morphine, but not quite as good as

TABLE 13-6

Dosages and Duration of Epidural Drugs*

DRUG	USES	DOSAGE†		ONSET	DURATION
		Canine	**Feline**		
Lidocaine (2%)‡	Motor and sensory block: abdominal and hindlimb procedures	1 ml/3.4 kg (T5)§ 1 ml/4.5 kg (T13–L1)§	1 ml/4.5 kg (T5)	10 minutes	1–1½ hr
Bupivacaine (0.25% or 0.5%)‡	Motor and sensory block: abdominal and hindlimb procedures	1 ml/4.5 kg§	1 ml/7 kg	20–30 min	4–6 hr
Fentanyl	Sensory block: abdominal and hindlimb procedures	0.001 mg/kg diluted in saline	–	4–10 min	6 hr
Morphine	Sensory block: thoracotomies, forelimb and hindlimb amputations, cranial and caudal abdominal procedures, hindlimb and pelvic fractures	0.1 mg/kg (preservative free)	0.1 mg/kg (preservative free)	25 minutes	About 20 hours
Buprenorphine	Sensory block: abdominal and hindlimb procedures	0.003–0.005 mg/kg diluted with saline	–	30 min	12–18 hr
Oxymorphone	Sensory block: abdominal, pelvic, and hindlimb procedures	0.1 mg/kg diluted in saline	0.05–0.1 mg/kg diluted in saline	15 min	About 10 hr

Modified from Carroll GL: How to manage perioperative pain, *Vet Med* 91:353, 1996.
*Dosage, onset, and duration are based on clinical experience; each patient should be evaluated individually. Reduce the dose by half for spinal administration of local anesthetics; reduce the epidural dose in geriatric, obese, and pregnant animals and in those with space-occupying lesions of the spinal cord or conditions in which venous engorgement is expected.
†Volume for dilution should be less than 0.3 ml/kg; do not exceed 6 ml/dog or 1.5 ml in cats.
‡Avoid the head down position after an epidural with a local anesthetic.
§A block to T1 leads to intercostal nerve paralysis; a block to C5–C7 leads to phrenic nerve paralysis.

that achieved with intraarticular bupivacaine. Preservative-free morphine has also been used successfully for pain in patients with corneal laceration or ulceration. Oral morphine has low bioavailability, but oral preparations, including sustained-release products, are available. When determining oral dosing, begin with a low dose and adjust it to fit individual needs.

Hydromorphone. Hydromorphone (Schedule II; see Table 13-4) is indistinguishable from morphine in effects and duration, although histamine release is not reported. Hydromorphone is used for moderate to severe pain and has replaced oxymorphone in many practices because of limited availability of oxymorphone in the United States.

Oxymorphone. Oxymorphone (Schedule II; see Table 13-4) is similar to morphine, but does not cause histamine release. It is appropriate for moderate to severe pain and is particularly useful in managing critically ill patients that require intraoperative analgesic supplementation to reduce the amount of inhalant required. Although oxymorphone causes sedation, panting, and sometimes hypothermia, it seems to cause less vomiting than morphine or hydromor-

phone in dogs and cats. Oxymorphone has been variably available in the United States for the last several years.

Methadone. Methadone (Schedule II; see Table 13-4) is similar in action (but lacks histamine release) and duration to morphine. The duration of action in humans is longer than morphine, but in dogs and cats the duration is about 4 hours. There is potentially less vomiting and sedation than with morphine. Dose rates have been reported for the dog (0.1-0.5 mg/kg, IM, IV) and cat (0.1-0.3 mg/kg, IM).

Fentanyl. Fentanyl, a synthetic opioid (Schedule II; see Table 13-4), is an effective analgesic. It has a quicker onset of action than morphine but a short duration of action. In veterinary medicine, fentanyl is used for intraoperative management of critically ill patients in balanced anesthetic techniques (e.g., fentanyl and midazolam are used as a constant-rate infusion [CRI] for pericardiectomy, see p. 777). Fentanyl can be administered intravenously, intramuscularly, epidurally (see Table 13-6), transmucosally, and transdermally (generic available; see Table 13-5). When used for pain management, fentanyl must be administered as a CRI epidurally or transdermally because of its short duration of action. For

CRI, a loading dose is administered (dogs, 2 μg/kg given IV; cats, 1 to 2 μg/kg given IV), followed by an infusion (dogs, 1 to 6 μg/kg/hour given IV; cats, 1 to 4 μg/kg/hour given IV); the duration of analgesia is the duration of the infusion plus 30 minutes. When used for its minimal alveolar concentration (MAC) sparing effect in unstable dogs, a much higher dose is used (i.e., fentanyl 0.8 μg/kg/min, IV plus midazolam 8 μg/kg/min, IV). Transcutaneous fentanyl administration is commonly used in dogs and cats (see Table 13-5).

For transdermal administration of fentanyl, clip the hair over the lateral thorax or dorsal cervical region (in cats, the axillary area is also a good location) without damaging the skin. Locate the patch carefully so that during surgery the patch and the skin below it will not be exposed to increased heat (avoid direct contact with a warm water circulating blanket). Do not clean the site with alcohol or surgical scrub. Handle the patch by the edge or wear gloves to prevent contact with the membrane. Hold the patch in place for 2 minutes; in dogs, bandage the site (in cats, covering the patch may not be necessary). Do not use tissue adhesive to increase the adhesiveness of the patch to the skin because the glue will interfere with the membrane and alter absorption. After placing the patch, allow sufficient time for plasma concentrations to reach therapeutic levels (about 24 hours in dogs and 12 hours in cats).

Drug delivery from the patch may vary, and patients should be observed regularly for signs of breakthrough pain or side effects, such as ventilatory depression. Altered drug delivery has been documented in patients in whom the patch was covered. Transdermal fentanyl may provide up to 72 hours (dog) or 96 hours (cat) of analgesia, and fever may increase absorption of fentanyl from a patch. To remove the patch, wear gloves, fold the patch on itself, and flush it down a toilet in the presence of a witness. Fentanyl may cause bradycardia, ventilatory depression, and skeletal muscle rigidity.

Codeine. Codeine (variable schedule depending on the formulation) may be used orally in dogs for mild to moderate pain. In healthy dogs, Tylenol 4 (60 mg of codeine and 300 mg of acetaminophen), dosed at 1 to 2 mg codeine/kg of body weight and given orally three times a day has been recommended for pain, but it should not be used in dogs with hepatic disease or in those prone to Heinz body anemia. Codeine without acetaminophen (1-4 mg/kg PO every 1 to 6 hours) may be administered to dogs with hepatic disease or to those prone to Heinz body anemia. The codeine-acetaminophen combination is strictly contraindicated in cats.

Buprenorphine. Buprenorphine (Schedule III; see Table 13-4) is a partial μ-opioid agonist. Its onset of action is about 30 minutes and its duration is 4 to 8 hours. Buprenorphine's affinity for μ-receptors causes prolonged duration of action and difficulty associated with antagonism. It is used for mild to moderate pain in veterinary patients because buprenorphine has little intrinsic activity. Buprenorphine causes little sedation or dysphoria in dogs and cats. Its prolonged duration of action makes it useful if redosing is problematic. Because of the pH of saliva, buprenorphine is 100% bioavailable in cats if delivered transmucosally, but not orally; bioavailability in dogs after transmucosal administration is unknown, but may be more consistent with that seen in people.

Butorphanol. Butorphanol (Schedule IV; see Table 13-4) is a mixed agonist-antagonist. It has a low affinity for μ-receptors (i.e., it is not a complete antagonist), a moderate affinity for κ-receptors (produces analgesia), and minimal affinity for σ-receptors (decreased incidence of dysphoria). Because butorphanol is a mixed agonist-antagonist, it can attenuate the efficacy of subsequently administered agonists. One advantage of butorphanol is that analgesia is achieved with minimal ventilatory depression; additional doses do not produce additional depression. The ceiling effect on ventilation is accompanied by a modest ability to reduce anesthetic requirements. Generally, butorphanol is administered for mild to moderate pain in dogs and cats. However, because butorphanol has minimal effects on the biliary and gastrointestinal tracts, it is particularly effective for visceral pain, such as bile peritonitis and pancreatitis. Another advantage of butorphanol is that it is available in an oral preparation. Oral butorphanol (0.4 mg/kg up to 1 mg/kg given three times daily for 2 to 3 days) has been particularly useful in cats after onychectomy. Oral butorphanol is used in small dogs, but the cost may be prohibitive in larger dogs.

Opioid antagonists. Ventilatory depression and sedation caused by opioids may be reversed with opioid antagonists. Opioids should be antagonized carefully in patients with pain because the antagonist also reverses analgesia. Patients in pain may breathe shallowly; they usually ventilate better when comfortable. Patients that have had a thoracotomy or high abdominal procedure may have small tidal volumes because they guard themselves from the pain incurred during breathing. Although an opioid may depress ventilation, its analgesic effect is more likely to reduce splinting, allowing larger tidal volumes and improved ventilation. In human beings, antagonism of opioids with naloxone, an opioid antagonist, has been associated with catecholamine release, hypertension, dysrhythmias, and even a fatal outcome. Dilution of naloxone with saline and slow IV titration reduce the likelihood of untoward side effects. Agonist-antagonists, such as nalbuphine and butorphanol, are preferable to naloxone for opioid antagonism because they are associated with fewer reversal side effects than naloxone. Some analgesia may also be preserved. Titration of a 1:10 diluted solution of nalbuphine (20 mg/ml diluted to 2 mg/ml) appears to antagonize sedation and respiratory depression, maintain some analgesia, and prevent the dangerous side effects associated with high-dose naloxone reversal. Butorphanol may also be used for antagonism of μ-opioids, such as oxymorphone.

Dissociative Anesthetics

Although ketamine does not provide visceral analgesia, it may provide profound somatic analgesia. Ketamine (Schedule III) may be used in low doses (1 to 2 mg/kg given IV) for changing bandages on burns or wounds. Since ketamine is an N-methyl-D-aspartic acid (NMDA) receptor antagonist, it may be used successfully in the treatment of chronic pain. NMDA receptor antagonists also prevent or reverse central sensitization and decrease wound hyperalgesia. In dogs and cats, ketamine at a dosage of 1 to 2 mg/kg, IV or IM or 0.5 mg/kg, IV may be administered, followed by 2 to 10 μg/kg/min IV as a CRI. The side effects of ketamine, which are dose related, include emergence delirium, increased salivation and lacrimation, cardiovascular stimulation, increased regurgitant fraction in patients with mitral insufficiency, increased intracranial pressure, increased intraocular pressure, seizures, and bronchodilation.

Constant Rate Infusions

Several drugs previously discussed may be administered as a single agent CRI (e.g., fentanyl, morphine, ketamine, and lidocaine [dogs only; see later discussion]). For patients with unremitting pain, drugs from different classes may be combined to provide the best analgesia with the fewest side effects. In general, analgesic therapy relies heavily on opioids to which other drugs may be added if necessary.

Fentanyl, lidocaine, and ketamine (FLK) may be used in combination for animals in severe pain. An electronic spreadsheet that may be added to a personal handheld device or computer is provided in the e-dition of this book. This spreadsheet can be used to help determine the quantity of each drug to add to a given volume and the rate at which the mixture should be administered by CRI. Dosages for FLK are given in Box 13-1. A morphine, lidocaine, and ketamine (MLK) CRI (see Box 13-1) has been used to significantly decrease the MAC of isoflurane-anesthetized dogs (Muir et al, 2003).

α_2-Agonists

α_2-Agonists (e.g., xylazine and medetomidine) cause dose-dependent sedation, cardiopulmonary depression, and analgesia; their use as anxiolytics was discussed previously under Tranquilizers and Sedatives. Sedation appears to outlast analgesia, which is provided through a nonopioid system. α_2-Agonists are not scheduled drugs. They are appropriate for sedation and chemical restraint in healthy dogs and cats, but care should be used if administering them for perioperative analgesia. Very low doses of α_2-agonists may increase analgesia and sedation when administered concurrently with an opioid. As a result, microdoses of α_2-agonists have been used during anesthetic recovery if oxygen is available.

Caution has been advocated when using α_2-agonists postoperatively because postsurgical doses and duration have not been well established, and profound cardiac depression may occur. Xylazine and medetomidine have been reported to provide analgesia for acute pain in dogs and cats. However, because profound cardiopulmonary depression may occur (particularly if the drug is used concurrently with an opioid), oxygen must be available. α_2-Antagonists (e.g., yohimbine, tolazoline, and atipamezole) antagonize the effects of α_2-agonists, but their use may be associated with side ef-

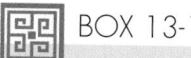 BOX 13-1

Dosages for FLK and MLK CRIs

Fentanyl, Lidocaine, Ketamine (FLK) CRI	
Fentanyl	1–5 μg/kg/hr, IV
Lidocaine	25–50 μg/kg/min, IV
Ketamine	2–5 μg/kg/min, IV

Morphine, Lidocaine, Ketamine (MLK) CRI	
Morphine	3.3 μg/kg/min, IV
Lidocaine	50 μg/kg/min, IV
Ketamine	10 μg/kg/min, IV

fects (e.g., arrhythmias and central nervous system stimulation), particularly in animals in pain.

Local Anesthesia and Analgesia

Adjuncts to opioid administration generally involve local anesthetics. Lidocaine is commonly administered as a continuous IV infusion in human beings to supplement opioid therapy for recalcitrant pain. Subantiarrhythmic doses of lidocaine (5 to 30 μg/kg/minute given IV) can supplement opioid analgesia in dogs when the latter is insufficient. Lidocaine CRI is not recommended in cats. Generally, local anesthetics are used in regional techniques and are more effective when given before surgical stimulation. Local anesthetic prevents windup, which is probably responsible for the reduction of postoperative pain past that expected based on pharmacokinetics. Several local anesthetic techniques are effective in obtunding pain, including ring blocks, splash blocks, local infiltration, brachial plexus blocks, regional anesthetics, intercostal blocks, interpleural blocks, and epidurals. These techniques also reduce inhalant requirements, which facilitate intraoperative patient management. The two most commonly used local anesthetics in small animal practice are lidocaine and bupivacaine. Bupivacaine lasts longer than lidocaine, but also has a longer onset of action. In dogs, the total dose of bupivacaine should not exceed 2 mg/kg. Lower doses (not more than 1 mg/kg) can be used in cats. If mixing lidocaine and bupivacaine to provide immediate and sustained analgesia, the doses of each should be adjusted. Typically, lidocaine (1 mg/kg in the dog; 0.5 mg/kg in the cat) and bupivacaine (1 mg/kg in the dog; 0.5 mg/kg in the cat) will provide sufficient coverage perineurally for the immediate and postoperative period.

Regional techniques. Regional local anesthetics often aid recovery and allow the patient to adjust to the onset of discomfort. Sufficient time must be allowed for tissue to absorb local anesthetics. Wound perfusion and infiltration is the simplest technique for providing wound analgesia, but the efficacy in infected wounds is poor. Effective local infiltration is used for incisional pain, nerve pain (amputation), onychectomy, and ear ablation. Intralesional and intraarticular infusion pumps (e.g., PainBuster; I-Flow Corp., Lake Forest, CA; Fig. 13-1) are systems providing continuous infusion of a local anesthetic directly into the surgical wound. The main advantage to this system is that it can be used in outpa-

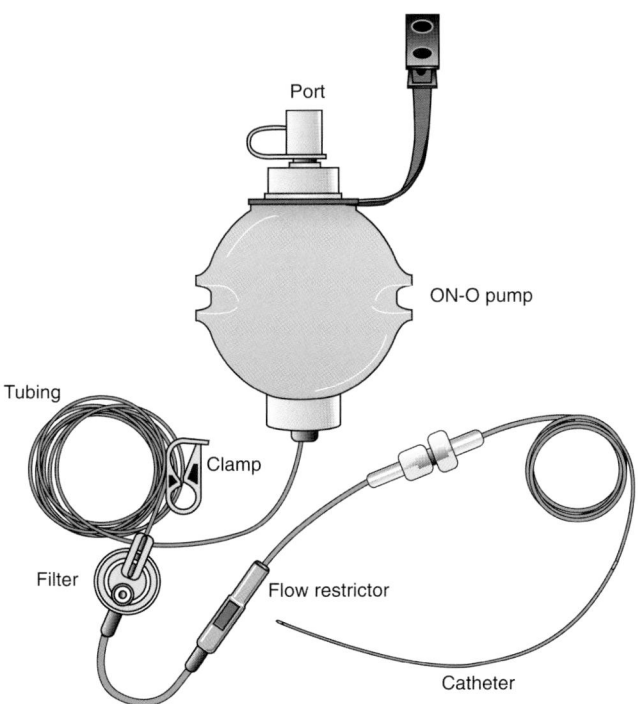

FIG. 13-1
PainBuster for intralesional instillation of local anesthetic in orthopedic or soft tissue surgery.

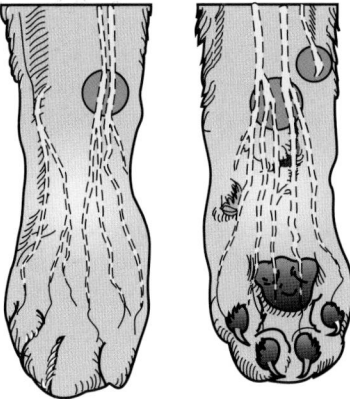

FIG. 13-2
Nerve block for onychectomy. The median and palmar branches of the ulnar nerve are blocked medial to the accessory carpal pad; the dorsal branch of the ulnar nerve is blocked lateral and proximal to the accessory carpal pad. The superficial radial nerve branches are blocked at the dorsomedial aspect of the proximal carpus.

tient surgery. Their effectiveness in veterinary patients is still being determined. When performing local anesthetic blocks, the maximum dose for each species should not be exceeded.

Blocks for incisional pain. The skin area to be incised is instilled with local anesthetic before you make the surgical incision (e.g., line block for a cesarean section).

Ring blocks. Ring blocks instill a line of local anesthetic around the distal limb, digit, or tail (e.g., before an onychectomy).

To block the distal radial, median, and dorsal and palmar branches of the ulnar nerve, use a slightly more difficult technique. Block the median and palmar branches of the ulnar nerve medial to the accessory carpal pad. Block the dorsal branch of the ulnar nerve lateral and proximal to the accessory carpal pad. Block the superficial radial nerve branches at the dorsomedial aspect of the proximal carpus (Fig. 13-2).

Splash block. Splash blocks splash the surgical area with the local anesthetic and allow it to remain in contact with the tissue for 15 to 20 minutes (e.g., after an ear ablation).

Brachial plexus anesthesia. Brachial plexus anesthesia blocks the distal foot up to the elbow region (radial, median, ulnar, musculocutaneous, and axillary nerves) (e.g., before carpal arthrodesis) (Fig. 13-3). Brachial nerve plexus block may be accomplished before surgery.

After clipping and sterile preparation, insert the needle (22-gauge, 3-inch needle in the dog) into the axillary area medial to the shoulder joint (at the point of the shoulder)

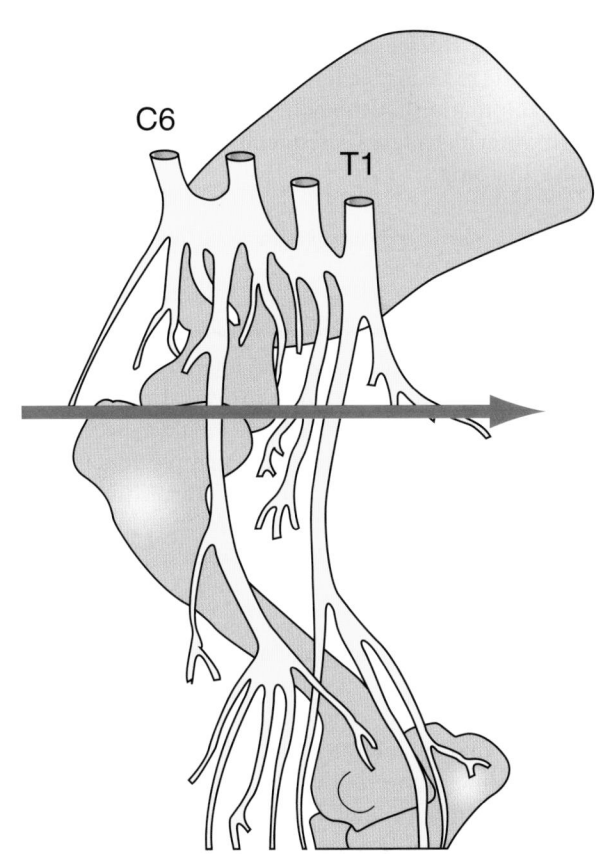

FIG. 13-3
Brachial plexus nerve block.

and lateral to the ribs. Direct the needle toward the costochondral junction and parallel to the vertebral column. Aspirate and inject the local anesthetic as the needle is withdrawn. Use 10 to 15 ml of 2% lidocaine (do not exceed maximum dose) to provide up to 2 hours of anesthesia with a 10-minute onset.

NOTE: For perioperative analgesia, bupivacaine provides longer analgesia. A similar technique (1.5-inch needle) is used for cats. The maximum dose of bupivacaine may be calculated and enough used to cover the area.

Median, ulnar, musculocutaneous, radial nerve (MUMR) block. MUMR is a modification of the brachial plexus block. It may be used to desensitize the area below the elbow (e.g., before distal radial fracture) (Fig. 13-4).

Palpate these nerves, if possible. Block the median, ulnar, and musculocutaneous nerves by injecting local anesthetic proximal to the medial epicondyle of the humerus between the biceps and triceps; palpate the brachial artery and the nerves in its proximity. Aspirate before injecting to avoid the brachial artery. Block the radial nerve, which is proximal to the lateral epicondyle between the brachialis and triceps, and inject below the triceps at approximately the same level of the brachial artery on the other side.

Blocks for nerve pain. Direct visualization allows local anesthetic to be instilled into the nerve (e.g., during limb or digit amputation). Although technically more difficult to perform, brachial plexus anesthesia may be used for pre-emptive analgesia.

With amputation, infiltrate the femoral nerve or brachial plexus before nerve incision.

Intraarticular bupivacaine block. Intraarticular bupivacaine block provides analgesia after stifle surgery (see p. 1262) and has been employed in several different joints that are easily aspirated (e.g., elbow, shoulder; see p. 1145). Distention of the joint is noxious and may result in increased respiratory and heart rate (e.g., after stifle arthroscopy [0.5%, diluted if necessary to fill the joint]).

Intercostal and interpleural blocks. Intercostal and interpleural blocks are used singly or together to manage thoracotomy pain (e.g., for thoracotomy). Intercostal and interpleural administrations of bupivacaine hydrochloride have proven efficacious after thoracotomy, especially when combined with systemic opioid administration. If intercostal (preoperatively) and interpleural (intraoperatively and postoperatively) blocks are both used, adjust the bupivacaine dosage to stay below a total dose of 2 mg/kg in 6 to 8 hours.

Intercostal nerve blocks may also be used to place a chest tube in a conscious animal. Intercostal nerve blocks have been used for many years and are considered safe, although possible complications include pneumothorax, motor blockade and ensuing respiratory failure, and drug toxicity.

For intercostal analgesia, selectively block the intercostal nerves supplying the thoracotomy incision site by blocking two nerves cranial to the incision site, and two nerves caudal to the incision. Make the injection just caudal to each of five ribs near the intervertebral foramen (Fig. 13-5).

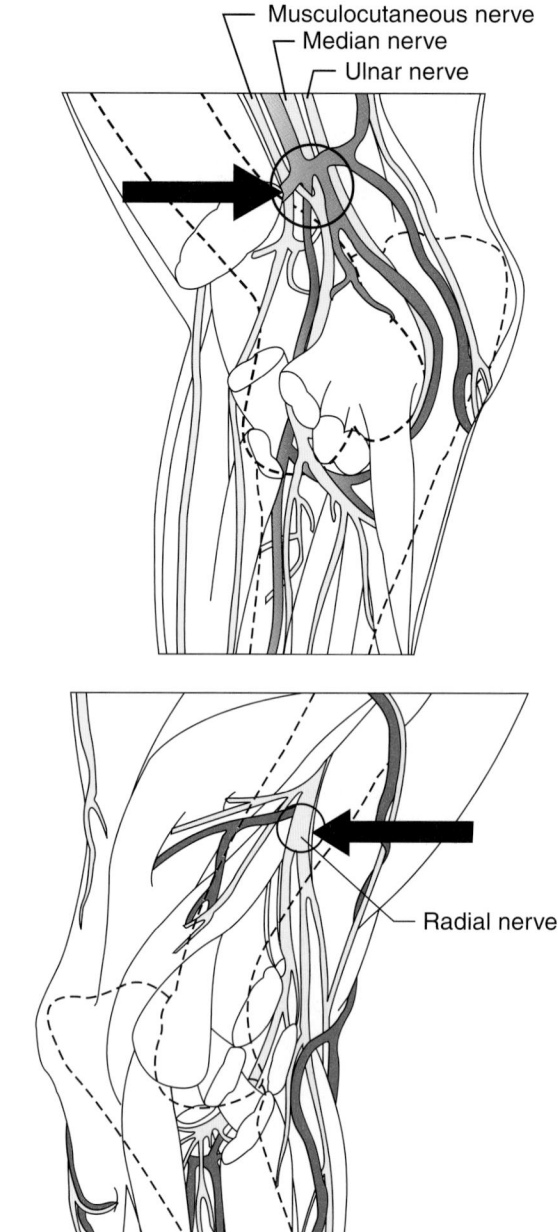

FIG. 13-4
A median, ulnar, musculocutaneous, and radial (MUMR) nerve block.

Interpleural analgesia is an alternative to intercostal neural blockade and offers prolonged analgesia without multiple needle sticks. If a chest tube is present, additional bupivacaine may be administered postoperatively (e.g., every 6 hours). After administering the bupivacaine, place the affected side down for 15 minutes. Bupivacaine stings and should be administered slowly to an awake patient. The possible complications of interpleural analgesia are similar to those for intercostal analgesia. Interpleural analgesia should not be used if the pericardium is open, and it is unlikely to be effective in pyothorax.

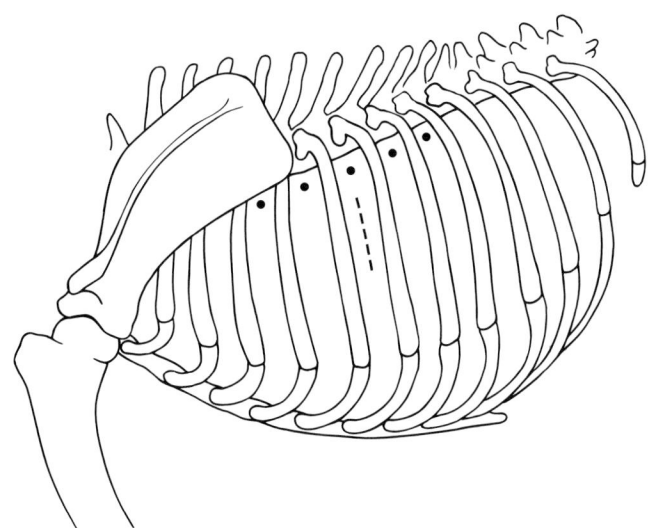

FIG. 13-5
Intercostal nerve blocks.

Infraorbital block. Infraorbital block provides anesthetic to the ipsilateral canine teeth and incisors (e.g., before maxillectomy). This procedure may be accomplished by lifting the lip on the affected side and palpating the infraorbital foramen through the buccal mucosa above the upper third premolar. In dogs, the caudal maxillary alveolar nerve branch (caudal maxillary teeth), middle maxillary alveolar nerve (middle maxillary teeth), and rostral maxillary alveolar nerve (upper canine teeth and incisors) are desensitized.

Being careful to avoid the infraorbital artery and vein, insert the needle just inside the infraorbital foramen (Fig. 13-6, A); aspirate and inject (0.25 to 0.5 ml of local anesthetic—always calculate maximum dose). To block the caudal and middle maxillary alveolar nerves, estimate the length of the infraorbital canal by palpating the distance from the infraorbital foramen to the caudal ventral margin of the bony orbit. Insert a 22- or 25-gauge needle into the infraorbital canal in a caudal-dorsal direction, keeping the syringe parallel to the long axis of the jaw to the predetermined depth; there should be no resistance. Aspirate and inject (0.25 to 0.5 ml local anesthetic—always calculate maximum dose).

NOTE: In cats, the infraorbital foramen is ventral to the eye at the junction of the zygomatic arch and maxilla; it is difficult to palpate (Fig 13-6, *B*).

Mandibular nerve block. The alveolar branch of the mandibular nerve (Fig. 13-7) may be desensitized by two methods: transcutaneous and transoral (e.g., before mandibulectomy).

For the transcutaneous approach, clip the hair and prepare the skin ventromedial to the angle of the mandible. Palpate the medial mandibular foramen with one hand, introducing the needle through the skin with the other. When the needle is palpated near the foramen, aspirate and inject 0.25 to 0.5 ml local anesthetic, being careful not to exceed the maximum dose. For the transoral approach, palpate the mandibular foramen on the medial side of the mandible with one hand and introduce the needle from the medial surface of the mandible with the second hand.

NOTE: In the case of mandibular blocks, self-trauma may occur when the tongue, lips, and inner surface of the cheek are bitten because of a lack of sensation.

Epidurals. Epidural administration of analgesics and anesthetics is useful for intraoperative management of high-risk patients, perioperative analgesia, cesarean section, caudal anesthesia and analgesia, and in some cases for thoracotomies and forelimb amputations. Epidural anesthesia is easily accomplished and provides hours of relative comfort (e.g., before cesarean section, thoracotomy, or amputation) (see Table 13-6). Specific contraindications to epidurals include hemorrhagic diathesis and sepsis. Epidural administration of local anesthetics, but not opioids, is contraindicated with hypovolemia; pretreatment with fluids may improve the hemodynamic response, making performance of an epidural with a local anesthetic in a hypovolemic patient less risky. The dose of local anesthetic should be reduced in geriatric, pregnant, and obese patients and those with space-occupying lesions or conditions in which venous engorgement is expected. The dose of local anesthetic should also be reduced by 50% if cerebrospinal fluid (CSF) is encountered when performing an epidural.

Epidurals may be safely administered to dogs with locally desensitized skin (i.e., lidocaine) and neuroleptanalgesia (e.g., opioid plus tranquilizer), but general anesthesia usually is required for safe epidural administration in cats. Supplies needed include a spinal needle, sterile gloves, an appropriate dose and volume of the selected drug, a syringe to administer the drug, a test syringe for air or for air and saline, and a fenestrated drape (eye drape). In conscious patients, a syringe and needle with lidocaine are also necessary to desensitize the skin and subcutaneous tissue immediately dorsal to the lumbosacral space. When performing an epidural in dogs, the spinal cord variably ends at L6-L7; the dural sac ends at L7-S1. In cats, the cord and dural sac usually extend one vertebra more caudal (cord termination may be as caudal as S3), therefore dural punctures are more likely in cats than in dogs.

To perform an epidural, clip the area over L7-S1 and perform a sterile skin prep. Note that the dorsal process of L6, not L7, is most prominent. Place the animal in sternal recumbency with the rear limbs flexed and pulled cranially; patients

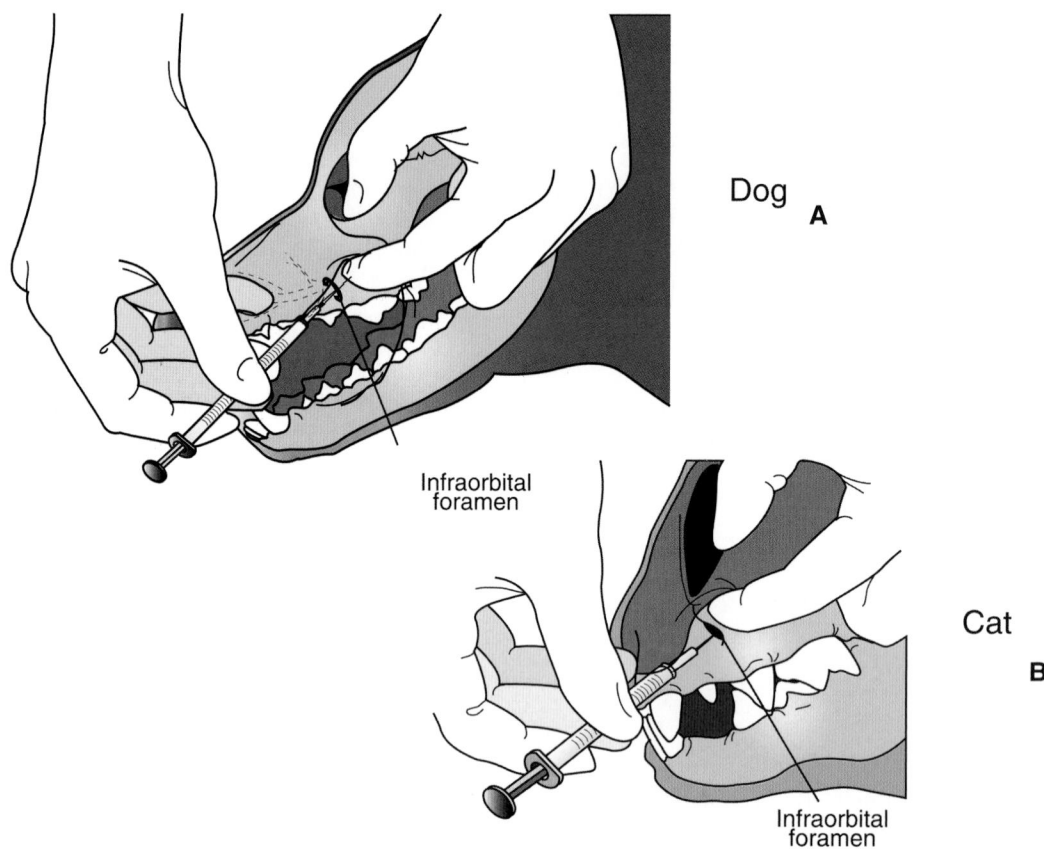

Dog **A**

Infraorbital
foramen

Cat
B

Infraorbital
foramen

FIG. 13-6
A and **B,** An infraorbital block.

may alternately be placed in lateral recumbency. Palpate the landmarks (the right and left cranial dorsal iliac spines, the spinous process of L7, and the median sacral crest; Figs. 13-8 and 13-9); insert the spinal needle through the skin with the bevel craniad. Penetrate the skin on the dorsal midline perpendicular to the skin in the center of the space between L7 and S1. As an alternative, penetrate the skin on the dorsal midline immediately behind and parallel to the spinous process of L7. If one method is unsuccessful, try the other method. Advance the needle through the subcutaneous tissue, the supraspinous ligament, the interspinous ligament, and the ligamentum flavum into the epidural space. In dogs (but not in cats), a pop or change in resistance to the advancement of the needle usually is apparent as the ligamentum flavum is penetrated. If the spinal needle strikes bone during advancement, the caudal aspect of the spinous process of L7 or the cranial aspect of S1 may have been encountered. In that case, withdraw the needle slightly, alter the angle of the needle's penetration craniad or caudad (based on the position of the needle in reference to L7 or S1), and gently advance it off the edge of the bone. If this is unsuccessful, remove the needle, palpate the landmarks, and try again. To confirm needle placement, remove the stylet and check for CSF or blood; no CSF should be encountered when per-

forming an epidural. Gentle aspiration may be performed. If CSF is encountered, reduce the dose of local anesthetic by 50%; if blood is encountered, replace the stylet and reposition the needle. In dogs, there should be no resistance to an injection of 0.5 ml of air (0.5 ml of air and 0.5 ml of saline may be used while watching the fluid line for resistance); use less in cats (0.1 to 0.2 ml of air). After the appropriate epidural drug has been slowly injected, replace the stylet, remove the needle, and position the patient with the affected side (operative site) down. A similar procedure is followed when placing an epidural catheter; the bevel of a Tuohy needle directs the catheter craniad and facilitates catheter placement. Before injecting the epidural drug into the catheter, confirm correct placement by aspiration to guard against catheter migration and inadvertent intravenous or intrathecal injections. Clearly label the catheter and injection port to prevent injection of drugs intended for systemic administration.

NOTE: A similar procedure is followed when placing an epidural catheter; the bevel of a Tuohy needle directs the catheter craniad and facilitates catheter placement.

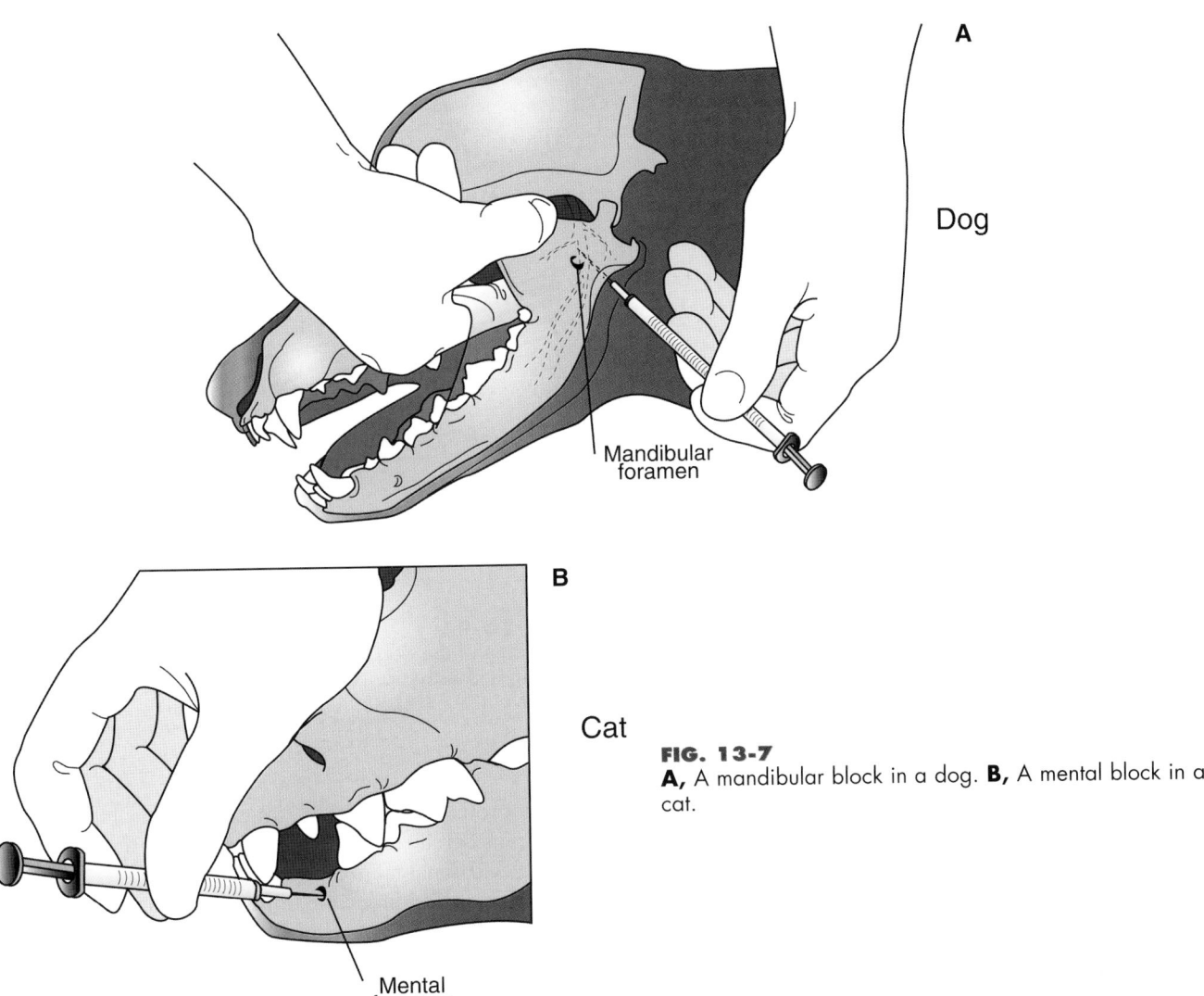

A

Dog

Mandibular
foramen

B

Cat

FIG. 13-7
A, A mandibular block in a dog. **B,** A mental block in a
cat.

Mental
foramen

The "hanging drop" technique is an alternate method of performing an epidural in small animals. The hanging drop involves similar sternal positioning and skin preparation. *Once the spinal needle and stylet have penetrated the skin, remove the stylet and apply saline to the hub. Slowly advance the needle.* When the epidural space is penetrated, the saline will be sucked into the needle and epidural space. If the dural sac is penetrated, CSF will push the drop out of the needle. Alternatively, if blood is encountered, blood will be visualized in the hub.

Once the spinal needle and stylet have penetrated the skin, remove the stylet and apply saline to the hub. Slowly advance the needle.

Complications associated with epidurals or epidural catheterization are rare and usually not serious, but can include infection, hemorrhage, and failure to produce analgesia or anesthesia. Local anesthetic administration results in sensory and motor blockade, whereas opioid administration affects only sensory function. Local anesthetic administration results in no or mild sedation, minimal nausea and

vomiting, and occasionally urinary retention. Opioid administration may cause notable sedation, nausea, vomiting, urinary retention, and/or pruritus. If urinary retention occurs, the bladder should be catheterized rather than expressed. With respect to cardiopulmonary function, epidural administration of a local anesthetic may result in a decrease in heart rate, cardiac output, and blood pressure. Postural hypotension can be expected. Local administration at appropriate doses usually does not impair the respiratory system, but excessive doses can cause respiratory failure or convulsions or both. Keep the head elevated after local anesthetic administration. Opioid administration at appropriate doses produces minimal changes in heart rate, cardiac output, or blood pressure, but may cause early and late respiratory depression. The respiratory depression can be antagonized. Preservative-free morphine has an extended duration and may be used for caudal abdominal and hindlimb procedures. Since morphine is not lipid soluble, it migrates craniad and provides analgesia for cranial abdominal or thoracic procedures, or forelimb amputations. In the case of epidural morphine, the patient should be watched for respi-

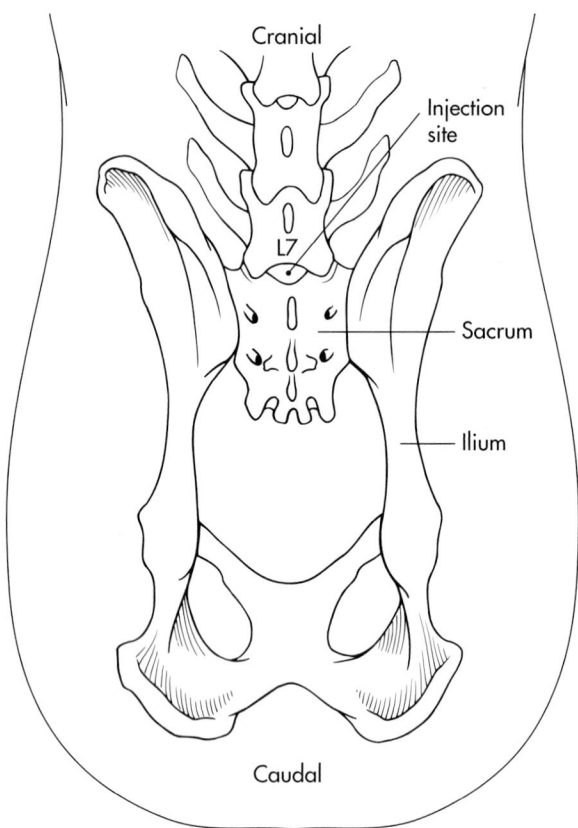

FIG. 13-8
Dorsal view of a dog showing palpable landmarks for injection of an epidural anesthetic or analgesic.

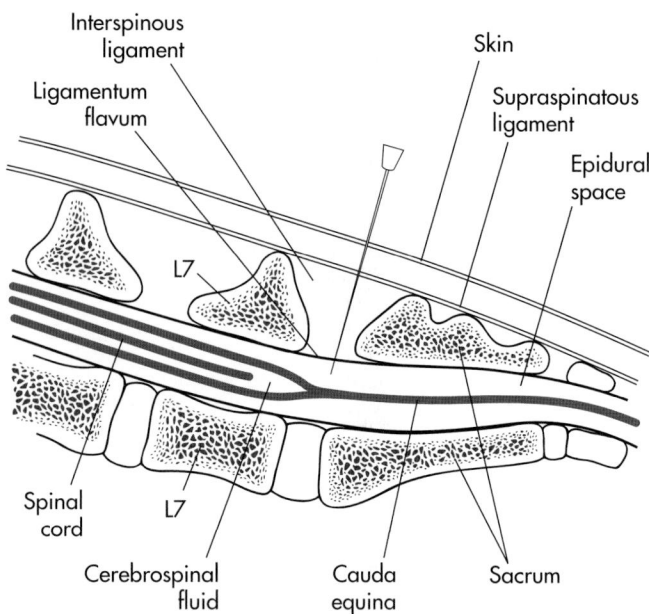

FIG. 13-9
Anatomy of the dog pertinent to placement of a needle for epidural anesthesia. Note the placement of the needle.

ratory depression following the epidural administration because of systemic uptake; similarly, after several hours the patient should be observed for respiratory depression as a result of the spread of the opioid to the brain. Opioids may be combined with local anesthetics for epidural administration in selected cases. If opioids are combined with local anesthetics, the overall volume should be considered to prevent cranial migration of the local anesthetic, which may result in paralysis of the intercostals and phrenic nerve.

Nonsteroidal Antiinflammatory Drugs

The use of NSAIDs should be restricted to those that are approved for use in the target species in this (Table 13-7) or other (Table 13-8) countries. Even though a diligent effort has been made to provide current information regarding mechanisms of action, safety, and efficacy of NSAIDs, the rapid advances in knowledge dictate that there will be new developments that are omitted from this chapter. For example, the previous belief that NSAIDs act peripherally through either constitutive cyclooxygenase (COX)-1 or inflammatory COX-2 is an oversimplification. Historically, COX-1 has been considered constitutive and mainly responsible for housekeeping functions (e.g., renoprotection,

gastroprotection, blood clotting), whereas its inhibition was considered responsible for most side effects (e.g., gastric ulcers, renal failure, and blood dyscrasias). COX-2 has been considered inducible in inflammation and its inhibition considered responsible for most therapeutic effects (e.g., analgesia and antiinflammatory). Therefore drugs were developed with greater COX-2 specificity, believing them to be safer. Although COX-1 is mostly constitutive and COX-2 is mostly inflammatory, there is still much to learn regarding their mechanisms of action. COX-2 inhibitors are more gastroprotective, but may also have side effects since COX-2 is constitutive in the kidney, brain, and reproductive tract. In chronic inflammation, the role of COX-1 may also be important. Recent discovery in dogs and humans of COX-3, a COX isoform derived from the same gene as COX-1, may explain the action of acetaminophen and dipyrone.

In addition to COX inhibition, there is also a 5-lipooxygenase (LOX) inhibitor available for dogs. When considering the arachidonic acid cascade, some believe that if the COX pathway (e.g., responsible for thromboxane and prostaglandin formation) is inhibited, the arachidonic acid will be shunted to the lipoxygenase pathway, which is responsible for production of leukotrienes and other inflammatory mediators.

Until an NSAID has been widely used, its idiosyncratic and toxic reactions may not be fully known despite prerelease testing by drug companies. Improved reporting of adverse drug reactions to the Food and Drug Administration (FDA) Center for Veterinary Medicine (CVM) and continued pharmacovigilance conducted by the industry will assist

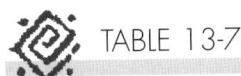 TABLE 13-7

Commonly Used NSAIDs Approved for Use in the United States

NSAID	INDICATION*	DOSE	FORMULATION	SPECIES
Carprofen	Preoperative†	1–2 mg/kg, PO bid or 4 mg/kg, SC	Chewable tablet, caplet, injectable	Dog
Carprofen	Osteoarthritis	1–2 mg/kg, PO bid or 4 mg/kg, SC	Chewable tablet, caplet, injectable	Dog
Deracoxib‡	Preoperative†	3–4 mg/kg/d PO for up to 7 days	Chewable tablet	Dog
Deracoxib‡	Osteoarthritis	1–2 mg/kg/d PO	Chewable tablet	Dog
Etodolac	Osteoarthritis	10–15 mg/kg qd PO	Tablet	Dog
Firocoxib	Osteoarthritis	5 mg/kg PO qd	Chewable tablets	Dog
Meloxicam	Osteoarthritis	0.2 mg/kg, PO, IV, SC followed by 0.1 mg/kg/day PO	Suspension, injectable	Dog
Meloxicam	Preoperative†	0.3 mg/kg, SC once (too high); ↓ to 0.2 mg/kg, SC	Injectable	Cat
Tepoxalin	Osteoarthritis	10–20 mg/kg PO followed by 10 mg/kg/day	Rapidly disintegrating tablet	Dog

Dispense with client information sheet.
*NSAIDs should only be used in young, adult, healthy, normovolemic, normotensive patients without history of renal or liver disease, or bleeding diathesis; see text for other conditions that limit the use of NSAIDs (e.g., pregnancy). See United States prescribing information for side effects.
†Recommend intraoperative fluid administration and postoperative rather than preoperative administration.
‡Only approved for use in dogs weighing greater than 2 kg.

 TABLE 13-8

Available NSAIDs Approved for Use in Other Countries

NSAID	INDICATION*	DOSE	SPECIES	CAUTIONS
Carprofen	Preoperative†	1–2 mg/kg SC ONCE	Cat	Once only; give fluids; off label
Ketoprofen	Postoperative	1–2 mg/kg SC, IM, IV; followed by 0.5–1 mg/kg, PO, SC up to 4 days	Dog	Hemorrhage; give fluids; off label
Ketoprofen	Postoperative	1–2 mg/kg SC, IM; followed by 0.5–1 mg/kg, PO, SC up to 4 days	Cat	Hemorrhage; give fluids; off label
Meloxicam	Perioperative†	0.1–0.2 mg/kg, SC, PO followed by 0.05–0.1 mg/kg, PO for 1–3 days	Cat	Give fluids; off label
Meloxicam	Osteoarthritis	0.1–0.2 mg/kg, SC, PO then 0.05–0.1 mg/kg, PO for 1–3 days, then 0.025 mg/kg, PO or 0.1 mg/cat, 2–3 times/wk	Cat	Off label
Meloxicam	Perioperative†	0.2 mg/kg, PO followed by 0.1 mg/kg/d PO for 2–3 days	Dog	Off label

Dispense with client information sheet.
*NSAIDs should only be used in young, adult, healthy, normovolemic, normotensive patients without history of renal or liver disease, or bleeding diathesis; see text for other conditions that limit the use of NSAIDs (e.g., pregnancy).
†Advise postoperative use rather than preoperative.

practitioners in making appropriate decisions about NSAID administration. However, the onus of determining the risk to benefit ratio for each patient will rest with the individual practitioner.

NSAIDs produce analgesia and reduce inflammation and fever. NSAIDs have been historically used for treating chronic pain and are only now being investigated for acute pain. NSAIDs have not been used extensively in cats because of toxicity. Most NSAIDs are marketed as oral preparations and have not been approved for perioperative pain management. NSAIDs may be associated with clotting problems (inhibition of platelets), gastrointestinal ulceration and perforation, and possibly renal or liver damage, which has limited their utility for perioperative administration. Since hypotension and hemorrhage during anesthesia cannot be accurately predicted, the perioperative use of NSAIDs should be saved for postoperative administration. It is important to maintain visceral perfusion when using NSAIDs, even if it means administering IV fluids. There are two NSAIDs approved in the United States for perioperative use in dogs (i.e., carprofen and deracoxib) and one in cats (i.e., meloxicam). NSAIDs should be used only in healthy, young adult, normotensive, normovolemic animals with no evidence of gastric ulceration, bleeding diathesis, or compromised liver or renal function, and with proven efficacy and safety in the target species.

In breeding and pregnant females, the use of NSAIDs during estrus should be avoided. COX-2 is probably necessary for normal reproduction. COX-2 may be necessary for ovulation, implantation, and placental development. Prostaglandins induce luteolysis and cause myometrial contractions. In very young and very old patients, the ability to metabolize and excrete NSAIDs may be compromised, so extra care should be taken when prescribing NSAIDs for those populations.

NSAID treatment should not be initiated if steroid or other NSAID therapy is ongoing. Appropriate "washout" periods have not been established, so other classes of analgesics (e.g., opioids) should be administered during a respectful interval. The elimination half-life is known for most NSAIDs and may be used to guide washout.

NSAIDs may interact with other drugs in several ways. NSAIDs are highly protein bound. Drugs with a narrow therapeutic index (e.g., digoxin, cisplatin, methotrexate, and oral anticoagulants) offer the greatest risk by increasing risk of toxicity from the NSAID or the other drugs. NSAIDS may decrease the effectiveness of other drugs, such as diuretics, ACE inhibitors, or β-blockers. When co-administered with some drugs (e.g., corticosteroids, heparin, and aminoglycosides), the risk of side effects from the NSAID is increased.

Gastrointestinal disorders are the most commonly recognized side effect of NSAIDs. NSAID agents that are more COX-2–specific may offer protection from inflammation with less gastrointestinal damage. It may be prudent for veterinarians to add drugs to the NSAID regimen for treatment and prophylaxis of ulcers; if they are used in cats, care should be taken to prevent constipation.

The most important safety precaution when using NSAIDs is client education. A careful history should be taken to ensure that other NSAIDs or corticosteroids are not being co-administered. The smallest effective dose of NSAID should be used. Intermittent administration will be appropriate for some patients, similar to the way that humans take NSAIDs (e.g., after a hard play day). Owners should be cautioned to administer only veterinarian prescribed NSAIDs and to administer the NSAIDs no more frequently than prescribed. Most importantly, owners should be advised to discontinue administration of the NSAID and contact the veterinarian in the case of inappetence, vomiting, diarrhea, or lethargy.

Miscellaneous Drugs

There are adjunctive drugs (Table 13-9) to the typical analgesics that we employ, particularly for chronic or neurogenic pain. Nonopiate μ-agonists (e.g., tramadol), antiepileptics (e.g., gabapentin), antidepressants (e.g., amitriptyline and fluoxetine), and antivirals (e.g., amantadine) offer additional options for patients with refractory pain. Tramadol is a nonopioid μ-agonist serving as an analgesic. Tramadol functions as a selective serotonin and norepinephrine uptake inhibitor, which explains why it is not completely antagonized with naloxone. Concomitant use of tramadol with other drugs that affect serotonin concentration should be avoided. Tramadol may cause serotonin syndrome if used with monoamine oxidase inhibitors (selegiline, *l*-deprenyl, isoniazid), selective serotonin reuptake inhibitors (fluoxetine), or antidepressants (amitriptyline). Effects from S-adenosyl-methionine may be additive. It is not scheduled in the United States, but has potential for human abuse. The adverse effects are similar to those of other opioids. Tramadol may lower the seizure threshold.

Other Treatment Options

Few controlled studies have examined the outcome of complementary and alternative therapies for pain management. Physical rehabilitation (e.g., massage, exercise, and hydrotherapy) may provide for earlier return of function and maintenance of range of motion, and may reduce fibrosis and muscle atrophy (see Chapter 12). Alternative therapies (e.g., acupuncture, magnetic therapy, chiropractic therapy, holistic herbal therapy, and nutraceuticals) may be considered by some veterinarians and owners for patients that have not responded to conventional therapy. The American Veterinary Medical Association has published guidelines for alternative and complementary veterinary care.

POSTOPERATIVE PATIENT EVALUATION

Generally, patients should be treated for pain for 1 to 3 days after surgery. The same variables that are monitored to determine if a patient needs analgesia are monitored to assess the efficacy of treatment. Heart rate, respiration, blood pressure, body temperature, mucous membrane color, and pain score should be monitored in postoperative patients. Successful analgesic therapy often causes these variables to nor-

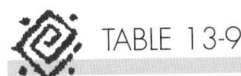 TABLE 13-9

Adjunctive Drugs and Herbs Used As Analgesics

DRUG/HERB (CLASS)	DOSE*	INDICATIONS	SIDE EFFECTS
Amantadine (antiviral)	Dog and cat: 3 mg/kg, PO qd	In conjunction with an opioid or NSAID for chronic pain	
Gabapentin (antiepileptic)	Dog and cat: 1.25–10 mg/kg PO BID (begin with low dose)	In conjunction with an opioid or NSAID for chronic pain or neuropathic pain	Lethargy
Amitriptyline (tricyclic antidepressant)	Dog and cat: 0.5–1 mg/kg, PO qd	In conjunction with an opioid or NSAID for chronic pain or neurogenic pain; muscle relaxant	Weight gain; drowsiness; do not administer with monoamine oxidase inhibitors or serotonin uptake inhibitors
Tramadol (nonopiate μ-agonist)	Dog: 2–5 mg/kg, PO bid, tid Cat: 1–2 mg/kg, PO bid	Chronic pain (mild to moderate); may be used in conjunction with NSAID or opioid	Similar to opioid, but less intense; seizures; may cause serotonin syndrome if used with serotonin uptake inhibitor or with MAO inhibitor
Drynaria 12 (herb)	1 tablet/12 kg, PO, bid	Osteoarthritis, pain (mild to moderate)	Use as an adjunct; not in pregnancy
Corydalis 5 (herb)	1 tablet/12 kg, PO, bid	Pain (mild to moderate), spasm	Monitor liver; use as an adjunct; not in pregnancy

*Doses are not well established.

malize. Additional physiologic measurements should be taken as dictated by the patient's status. Analgesia may cause the patient to be sedate, but it should be arousable; it is appropriate for the animal to sleep. It may be difficult to assess the amount of pain in a heavily sedated animal accurately. As the effects of sedatives and anesthetics diminish or if analgesics are used that do not cause sedation, it usually becomes easier to evaluate the patient's status. The patient should be monitored for normal behavior, such as eating, drinking, urinating, and defecating (and, with cats, appropriate use of the litter box), grooming, and attention to the environment, all of which indicate that the patient is not in severe pain.

References

Carroll GL, Simonson SM: Recent developments in nonsteroidal antiinflammatory drugs in cats, *J Am Anim Hosp Assoc* 41:347-354, 2005.

Curry SL, Cogar SM, Cook JL: Nonsteroidal antiinflammatory drugs: a review, *J Am Anim Hosp Assoc* 41:298-308, 2005.

Muir WW, Wiese AJ, Philip A et al: Effects of morphine, lidocaine, ketamine, and morphine-lidocaine-ketamine drug combination on minimum alveolar concentration in dogs anesthetized with isoflurane, *Am J Vet Res* 64:1155-1160, 2003.

Selected References and Videos (see e-dition for links)

Information regarding accreditation standards may be found at AAHA's website: http://www.aahanet.org/Stand/Index.html

JAVMA, Vol 209, No 6, September 15, 1996 or http://www.vet-task-force.com/Guidelines.htm

Mathews KA: Relieving pain, Guelph, Ontario, Canada, 1998, Jonkar Computer Services, The Center for the Study of Animal Welfare, University of Guelph.

This is an interactive software program that demonstrates how to assess and treat postoperative pain in dogs and cats.

Mathews KA: Pain H.U.R.T.S. Guelph, Ontario, Canada, 2003, Jonkar Computer Services.

This software program addresses pain management, including physiology, pathophysiology, and origin of pain. Pain recognition, assessment, and treatment in several species, including the dog and cat, are reviewed.

Pain management. MES Companion CD-ROM. Teton New Media, 2000.

This illustrated guide shows how pain management techniques are performed and reviews pain management therapies.

CHAPTER 14

Principles of Minimally Invasive Surgery

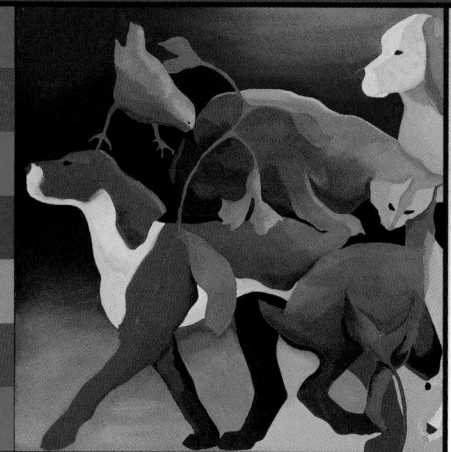

Minimally invasive surgery is increasingly becoming an accepted diagnostic and therapeutic tool in veterinary practices. Although some minimally invasive procedures are more commonly being done by veterinary internists, many procedures are now being performed by surgeons. This chapter provides a brief overview of endoscopic techniques, including underlying principles and a description of equipment used in these procedures. Specific techniques (e.g., thorascopic pericardiectomy and removal of osteochondritis dissecons [OCD] lesions) will be found in the relevant chapter for that system, disease, or condition.

DEFINITIONS AND TERMINOLOGY

Endoscopy is the use of an instrument (i.e., an endoscope) to visualize the interior of an organ or other area that otherwise cannot be examined without surgery. **Flexible endoscopy** uses an endoscope, which is flexible (usually plastic) and designed to bend to look and/or move around corners. The degree of flexibility depends upon the instrument, but being able to make 180°-plus bend (i.e., retrace its course while being advanced) is typical for most flexible scopes. Most endoscopes have a *handle* (i.e., where the scope is held by the operator), an *insertion tube* (i.e., the part that is inserted into the patient), and an *umbilical cord* (i.e., the part that attaches the scope to the light source and video processor. The *biopsy channel* is the passage that serves to allow one to place instruments through the scope (i.e., biopsy forceps, foreign body retrieval forceps, aspiration tubes, cytology brushes, etc.). *Immersible scopes* are those that can have their handles placed in water without risk of damage.

Rigid endoscopy uses a plastic or metal scope that cannot bend. A lens at the tip of the scope may allow one to look back on oneself, but when advancing the scope, the tip of the scope cannot change directions from the rest of the scope. An *obturator* is a device placed through a hollow endoscope to facilitate insertion of the scope into the organ desired (e.g., colon).

Instrumentation refers to the insertion of an endoscope, arthroscope, or other tool into the joint. *Triangulation* refers to successful visualization of the hand instruments through the scope in a manner that is conducive to performing biop-

sies or therapeutic procedures within the body cavity or joint. All equipment inserted into the body or joint is done so through *portals* or holes established through the skin and soft tissue. Portals are defined by their use. The scope is inserted through a *scope* or *camera portal*, whereas power and hand tools are inserted through an *instrument portal*. *Cannulas* are metal tubes that maintain the portals and protect the instruments.

Gastroduodenoscopy is endoscopy of the esophagus, stomach, and duodenum (and occasionally the upper jejunum). **Colonoscopy** is endoscopy of the colon. **Ileoscopy** is endoscopy of the ileum and is performed in conjunction with colonoscopy. **Proctoscopy** refers to examination of the anus and rectum. **Bronchoscopy** is endoscopy of the trachea and bronchi, whereas **laryngoscopy** is examination of the pharynx and larynx. **Rhinoscopy** generally refers to placing an endoscope through the anterior nares and examining the nasal passages. It may or may not include using an endoscope to examine the choanae. **Cystoscopy** is endoscopy of the urinary bladder and may include retrograde cystoscopy (i.e., advancing the scope through the urethra and into the bladder) or transabdominal placement (i.e., placing the scope through a cannula that has been inserted through the abdominal wall and the bladder wall). **Vaginoscopy** is endoscopy of the vagina. **Laparoscopy** is endoscopy of the peritoneal cavity and may be diagnostic (i.e., concerned with biopsy of organs) or interventional (i.e., used to perform minimally invasive surgery, such as gastropexy or placing a jejunostomy tube). **Thoracoscopy** is endoscopy of the pleural cavity and likewise may be diagnostic or interventional.

Arthroscopy is the technique of endoscopy of a joint. Arthroscopes are always used through specifically designed *cannulas*. Other instruments and fluid outflow devices may be used with or without cannulas. Fluid flowing into the joint is referred to as *inflow* or *ingress*; fluid flowing out of the joint is referred to as *outflow* or *egress*. Repeat arthroscopic examination of a joint that has been previously scoped is referred to as *second-look arthroscopy*. In all endoscopies, a *"red out"* or a *"white out"* refers to having the viewing tip of the endoscope so close to the surface of what is being examined that one cannot focus on the surface (a blur occurs) or to having debris on the viewing end of the scope.

ENDOSCOPY: GENERAL PRINCIPLES, EQUIPMENT, AND TECHNIQUES

Endoscopy is used to take biopsies of organs, remove foreign objects, examine the interior surface of hollow structures, and perform procedures typically done by more invasive surgery. This technique is valuable only when it eliminates the need for more invasive surgery. However, if for any of a number of reasons tissue samples obtained endoscopically are inadequate for diagnosis, unacceptable trauma occurs during endoscopic removal of foreign objects, or mucosal surfaces cannot be adequately examined endoscopically, then endoscopy ceases to be useful. Unfortunately for some practitioners, endoscopy has been more of a "hobby" than an important procedure to be learned and practiced diligently, and patients have suffered as a result. Flexible endoscopy of the upper gastrointestinal tract in particular can be much more difficult to properly perform than is widely appreciated, especially in regard to taking a biopsy of the mucosa. Much as is the case for a hemilaminectomy, if the veterinarian is not seriously trained in the first place or is not going to perform the procedure often enough to maintain expertise, then it might be best if patients were referred for this procedure.

INDICATIONS
Flexible Endoscopy

Although flexible endoscopy of the alimentary and the respiratory tracts occasionally is performed to dilate a stricture, control hemorrhage, remove part or all of an organ, insert a tube, or remove a foreign object, its primary use in veterinary medicine is to visualize and obtain tissue or cytologic samples of the mucosa (Box 14-1). Biopsy should always be performed regardless of the gross mucosal appearance unless a specific contraindication exists, such as coagulopathy or increased risk of perforation. Tissue samples obtained by flexible endoscopy usually are limited to the mucosa and adjacent submucosa as opposed to the full-thickness samples obtained surgically. However, samples obtained endoscopically appear adequate for diagnosis in at least 80% to 90% of patients with gastric or intestinal infiltrative disease (e.g., inflammatory bowel disease, histoplasmosis, and neoplasia). Endoscopy cannot diagnose disorders that are beyond its reach (e.g., focal carcinoma of midjejunum), nor can endoscopy reliably diagnose infiltrates that are too deep in the mucosa for the endoscopic biopsy forceps to reach (a problem more likely with scopes that have smaller biopsy channels, such as 2 mm or smaller) or those that are hard, densely fibrotic lesions (e.g., pythiosis or scirrhous carcinoma).

Cytologic studies from endoscopic brushings or washes are occasionally diagnostic for disorders such as cancer, histoplasmosis, prototheosis, and eosinophilic enteritis. In fact, histoplasmosis occasionally has been diagnosed cytologically when it was missed histologically. However, most inflammatory bowel diseases, especially lymphocytic-plasmacytic disorders, cannot be definitively diagnosed through cytologic methods. Washings are especially useful in the respiratory tract to diagnose inflammatory or infiltrative problems, but they may also be useful when looking for gastric *Ollulanus tricuspis* infestation or duodenal giardiasis.

Rectal and gastric polyps can be removed endoscopically, although endoscopic snares fitted for electrocautery are required. However, because rectal polyps usually are found close to the rectum, surgical removal is typically easier and more certain to remove the entire polyp. Endoscopic polypectomies should be attempted only if the practitioner has been trained in endoscopic electrocautery; inappropriate use of electrocautery can damage or destroy the endoscope and/or video processor.

Percutaneous placement of gastrostomy feeding tubes can be done with or without endoscopy (see p. 100). Endoscopic placement of such tubes is indicated when the nonendoscopic apparatus for placement cannot be safely passed through the esophagus, such as when esophageal stricture or dilation is present, or when the endoscope is already in the stomach for some other purpose. Endoscopic placement includes insufflation of the stomach, which is advantageous because insufflation helps prevent other abdominal organs from becoming trapped between the stomach and the abdominal wall.

Endoscopic dilation of benign esophageal strictures, such as those caused by postesophagitis scarring, is preferred to surgical resection. Strictures can recur after either method, but surgery may be associated with greater postprocedural morbidity and mortality and has a higher recurrence rate.

Severe upper gastrointestinal hemorrhage and persistent vaginal hemorrhage are indications for endoscopy. Preoperative endoscopy may help determine if surgery is indicated and ensure that all bleeding sites are located. Intraoperative endoscopy is indicated to find bleeding gastric mucosal lesions that are difficult to detect from the serosal surface; large ulcers may be missed when the stomach is examined only through a gastrostomy incision. Severely hemorrhaging lesions may require endoscopic electrocautery or injection with alcohol. Endoscopy may also detect small mucosal tumors indiscernible from the serosal surface.

Rigid Endoscopy

Rigid endoscopy can be used for the gastrointestinal and respiratory tracts, urinary bladder, peritoneal cavity, pleural cavity, and joints. The indications for rigid endoscopy include many of the same as for flexible endoscopy (see Box 14-1), but rigid endoscopy (especially laparoscopy, thoracoscopy, and arthroscopy) is more often used for interventional procedures than is flexible endoscopy.

BOX 14-1

Primary Indications for Endoscopic Procedures in Dogs and Cats

Gastroduodenoscopy

- Gastric and intestinal biopsy/cytology for diagnosis of infiltrative disorders
- Identification of a mass or of ulceration, erosion, or *Physaloptera* infestation
- Identification and removal of foreign objects
- Placement of a gastrostomy tube
- Location of lesions (e.g., ulcer, site of bleeding) before or during surgery

Esophagoscopy

- Identification and removal of foreign objects
- Diagnosis and dilation of strictures
- Diagnosis of esophagitis
- Biopsy of tumors

Proctoscopy and Colonoileoscopy

- Biopsy of the colon, ileum, or cecum for infiltrative disorders, especially infiltrative rectal lesions
- Identification of occult whipworm infestation
- Removal of polyps
- Diagnosis of ceco-colic intussusception

Laryngoscopy

- Identification of laryngeal paralysis
- Identification of elongated soft palate
- Location and removal of foreign objects
- Biopsy of a mass

Cystoscopy

- Diagnose ectopic ureters
- Biopsy proliferative lesions in urethra and bladder, especially carcinomas

Thoracoscopy

- Identify/biopsy masses and other infiltrative lesions, including lung biopsy
- Identify bullae and determine location
- Assist in placing chest tubes in animals with severe pyothorax
- Determine if thoracotomy is appropriate, and if so, the best approach
- Perform minimally invasive surgery, such as pericardiectomy, ligation/resection of PRAA

Bronchoscopy

- Identification of lesions (e.g., collapsed trachea, *Oslerus osleri* infestation)
- Bronchoalveolar lavage or brushing of trachea/bronchus for cytology/culture
- Identification and removal of foreign objects
- Identification of lung lobe torsion
- Biopsy of mucosa (e.g., with chronic bronchitis)

Rhinoscopy

- Identification and removal of foreign objects
- Biopsy/cytology of mass lesions and mucosa for infiltrative disorders
- Identification and biopsy of aspergillomas
- Identification of source of epistaxis or chronic nasal discharge

Posterior Nares Examination

- Identification and removal of foreign objects
- Cytology/culture of the caudal nares
- Identification of and biopsy of proliferative disorders
- Identification of nasal mites

Laparoscopy

- Examination and biopsy of abdominal viscera
- Determine if celiotomy is warranted (e.g., is there evidence of metastasis that means surgery cannot be curative?)
- Perform minimally invasive interventional surgery, such as gastropexy, placement of jejunostomy tube, ovariohysterectomy, and removal of retained testicle

Arthroscopy

- Identification/biopsy of lesions
- Removal of loose bodies (cartilage fragments, bone fragments, torn meniscus)
- Topical management of osteoarthritis—abrasion arthroplasty, microfracture
- Joint lavage for sepsis
- Arthroscopic assisted fracture repair
- Arthroscopic assisted joint stabilization

PRAA, Persistent right aortic arch.

When used for diagnosis, the tissue samples obtained by rigid colonoscopy can be almost as deep and large as full-thickness samples obtained surgically. Rigid biopsy instruments can typically procure large, deep colonic or rectal samples that include relatively large amounts of submucosa. Therefore rigid endoscopy is often appropriate even when dense, fibrotic, submucosal lesions are suspected.

Foreign Bodies

Both rigid and flexible endoscopy are commonly used to remove foreign objects, and rigid endoscopy is typically the preferred way to remove most esophageal foreign objects. Most esophageal, nasal, tracheal, and laryngeal foreign objects—and many gastric and duodenal foreign objects—can be removed endoscopically without undue risk to the patient. Objects that are out of reach of the endoscope, that cannot be firmly grasped or trapped by endoscopic devices, or that may cause severe damage if endoscopic removal is attempted (e.g., linear foreign objects that have been present for several days and objects with sharp edges or points that cannot be covered during removal) should usually be removed surgically.

BOX 14-2

Comparison of Flexible and Rigid Endoscopes

Flexible

- Greater access to more sites in viscus organs
- More expensive than rigid scopes
- Easier to damage
- Requires substantial training to use properly

Rigid

- Less expensive than flexible scopes
- Usually more durable
- Easier to learn to use
- Capable of larger biopsies than with flexible scopes
- Excellent for removing foreign objects and protecting mucosa
- Of the viscus organs, can access only the esophagus, descending colon, larynx, nose, and trachea
- Can be used in the peritoneal, pleural, and joint spaces

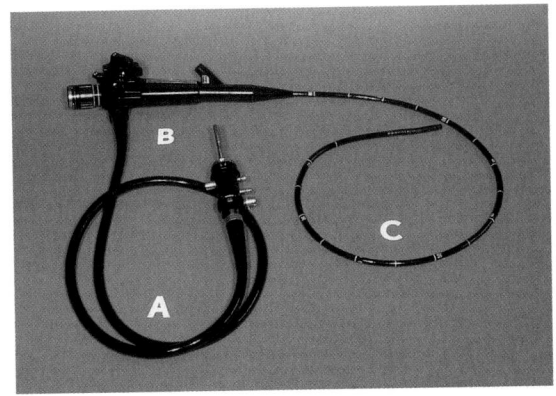

FIG. 14-1
Flexible gastroduodenoscope showing the umbilical cord **(A)**, which attaches the scope to the light source; the handle **(B)**; and the insertion tube **(C)**, which is introduced into the animal.

EQUIPMENT
Flexible Endoscopes

Endoscopes. The equipment needed depends on the type of endoscopy and the body system to be investigated. Basically, there are rigid and flexible endoscopes available in a large assortment of sizes and lengths; both types have advantages and disadvantages (Box 14-2). The flexible endoscopes most often used in veterinary medicine are gastroduodenoscopes, bronchoscopes, and colonoscopes. Flexible scopes have a handle, an insertion tube, and an umbilical cord (Fig. 14-1). Bronchoscopes usually have a 2- to 6-mm outer diameter, gastroduodenoscopes a 7.9- to 10-mm outer diameter, and colonoscopes a 10- to 16-mm outer diameter. All scopes should have a biopsy-suction channel (usually 2 mm in diameter for bronchoscopes and 2 to 3.2 mm for gastroduodenoscopes and colonoscopes). Gastroduodenoscopes and colonoscopes have four-way deflection of the tip of the scope and an air-water channel that is used to insufflate air and wash off the viewing lens; bronchoscopes typically have only two-way deflection of the tip and do not have an air-water channel. The insertion tube typically has a working length of 40 to 60 cm in bronchoscopes, 100 to 135 cm in gastroduodenoscopes, and 130 to 220 cm in colonoscopes.

The ideal assortment of flexible scopes should include one bronchoscope (4- to 5-mm diameter), one pediatric gastroduodenoscope (<7.9-mm diameter with a 2-mm channel), and one regular gastroduodenoscope (8.5- to 9.8-mm diameter with a 2.8-mm channel). This assortment allows optimum instrumentation for almost every case. If you wish to purchase a fourth scope, you may want to consider a 1.6-m pediatric colonoscope or an ultrathin bronchoscope or ureteroscope. If you can purchase only two scopes, which will be used for both alimentary and respiratory tract work, consider a bronchoscope (4- to 5-mm diameter) and a gastroduodenoscope (8.5- to 9-mm outer diameter with a 2.8-

mm channel). If you want only one scope and your clinic wishes to perform both respiratory and alimentary tract endoscopy, a 7.9-mm outer diameter pediatric gastroduodenoscope is the best compromise. If you wish to obtain only one scope and it will be used only for alimentary tract endoscopy, a 8.5- to 9-mm outer diameter scope with a 2.8-mm channel is preferable.

Biopsy/cytology equipment. Biopsy and foreign body retrieval forceps for flexible scopes come in various shapes. The size of the forceps depends on the size of the biopsy-aspiration channel; the larger the channel, the bigger and stronger the biopsy or retrieval device that can be used. If possible, a scope with a 2.8-mm channel should be used for most alimentary tract endoscopy in dogs and for cats weighing more than 3.2 kg. The tissue sample obtained through a 2.8-mm channel can be more than twice the size of a sample obtained through a 2-mm channel. These larger pieces of alimentary tissue often contain the full thickness of the mucosa and some submucosa. I prefer fenestrated biopsy forceps in an ellipsoid, alligator jaw configuration without a needle (Fig. 14-2). Disposable biopsy forceps are widely used in human medicine, but seem to have few advantages in veterinary medicine because the sharpness of the forceps is rarely important in obtaining good mucosal samples.

Brushes used to obtain samples for cytology and culture typically consist of a brush in a plastic tube. This brush can be manually extended out the tip of the plastic tube once the tip of the brush assembly has been advanced through the endoscopic biopsy channel and is near the tissue to be sampled. However, it is possible for such a brush assembly to be contaminated because it is passed through the endoscopic channel. There are brush assemblies made for when it is absolutely critical that a noncontaminated sample be obtained (typically for culture). These brushes consist of an extendable brush that is within an extendable tube that is in

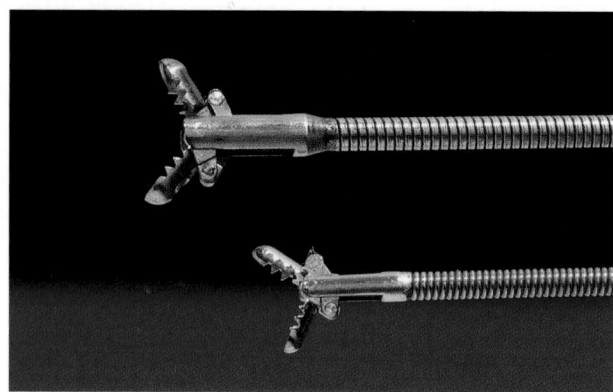

FIG. 14-2
Detail of flexible biopsy forceps with an ellipsoid, alligator jaw configuration. The upper forceps is used for a 2.8-mm channel, the lower one for a 2.2-mm channel. (From Willard MD: Colonoscopy, proctoscopy, and ileoscopy, *Vet Clin North Am* 31:657, 2001.)

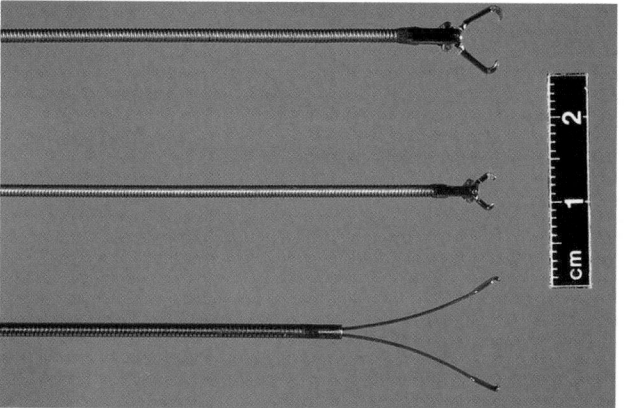

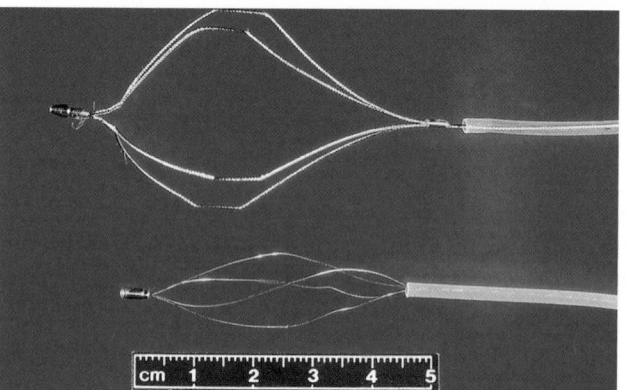

FIG. 14-3
A, Tips of three commonly used foreign body retrieval forceps. *Top to bottom:* Shark's tooth forceps, rat's tooth forceps, and coin retrieval forceps. The coin retrieval and rat's tooth forceps can pass through a 2-mm channel; the shark's tooth forceps requires a 2.8-mm channel. **B,** At top is a 4-wire basket that works well because of the extreme flexibility of the wires. The 4-wire basket below does not open as widely and has wires so firm it is difficult to ensnare the foreign body.

yet another tube. The tip of the outermost tube is typically plugged so that there is no chance of contamination when the scope is passed through the biopsy channel of the endoscope. Once the tip of the brush assembly is near the site to be cultured, the innermost tube is extended out the end of the outermost tube, and then the brush is extended out the tip of the innermost tube. Brushes for diagnostic purposes should never be cleaned and reused, as opposed to biopsy forceps, which can be used repeatedly.

Interventional tools for flexible endoscopes. A variety of special retrieval instruments are necessary to reliably remove most commonly encountered foreign objects. The most useful devices are a coin retrieval (W-type) forceps, a shark's tooth forceps (especially useful for firmly grabbing cloth), and a 4-wire basket (Fig. 14-3). An alligator jaws forceps is similar to a shark's tooth and is also useful. The basket should be made of very flexible wire to facilitate passage over and around an object; however, this quality also makes it easier to bend the wire and ruin the basket. Other retrieval devices include wire snares, 3-wire grabbers, magnetic-tip probes, and forceps with nonskid rubber; these instruments are seldom required.

There are balloons and bougies specifically designed to dilate esophageal strictures. Despite earlier pronouncements that ballooning is superior to bougienage, success is more dependent upon the skill of the operator. Therefore the operator should use the equipment that he/she is trained to use. Esophageal dilation balloons come in two major configurations, "over the wire" or "through the endoscope channel." It is important to use these as opposed to a more round balloon, such as is found on endotracheal tubes.

A variety of flexible endoscopic biopsy instruments, snares, knives, and probes have electrocautery capability. The electrocautery snares are most commonly used because they allow removal of esophageal, gastric, and colonic polyps; they can also be used to make three or four quadrant

"cuts" into esophageal strictures to aid in ballooning difficult lesions.

NOTE: Use of these instruments by untrained individuals can damage or destroy the video processor and cause substantial patient morbidity; therefore they should only be used if the operator is trained in their use.

Rigid Endoscopes

Colonoscopes. Rigid colonoscopes (typically human sigmoidoscopes) and proctoscopes are plastic or metal tubes of variable size and length that have an obturator and light source. Air can be insufflated into the colonic lumen with a colonoscope, but not with most proctoscopes. A better examination of the colonic lumen is possible with longer scopes of larger diameter. The minimum recommended

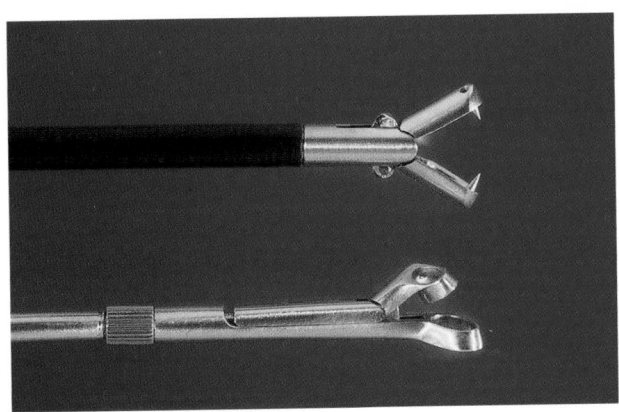

FIG. 14-4
Tips of two types of rigid biopsy forceps. The upper forceps is a human uterine biopsy forceps, also known as a "clamshell" or "double-spoon" forceps. The lower forceps has a smaller upper punch that fits into a larger lower cup with a shearing action, much like the blades of a scissors. (From Tams TR: *Small animal endoscopy,* ed 2, St Louis, 1999, Mosby.)

working length for colonoscopes is 25 cm, and 35 cm is preferred. Most dogs, except the toy breeds, tolerate a 15-mm inner diameter scope, but a 19- to 25-mm-diameter scope should be used whenever possible. Rigid scopes must allow simultaneous viewing of the mucosa and insufflation of air. Unlike flexible scopes, rigid colonoscopes do not allow simultaneous insufflation and biopsy. A suction tube that can be inserted through the lumen is important for removing residual feces and debris. A variety of anoscopes and proctoscopes in different lengths (usually 90 to 120 mm) and diameters (usually 14 to 22 mm) should be available. Biopsy forceps used with rigid colonoscopes and proctoscopes should have a shearing or "scissorlike" tip that cuts the mucosa (i.e., a small punch that fits into a larger diameter cup) rather than the "clamshell" or "double-spoon" tip that grasps and tears tissue (Fig. 14-4). Grasping forceps (such as would be used for esophageal foreign bodies) must be strong and preferably have large ridges to aid in obtaining a strong purchase on foreign objects.

Laryngoscopes. Laryngoscopy requires having an assortment of various sized rigid laryngoscopic blades in straight and curved configurations. Flexible scopes can be used, but are seldom necessary.

Rigid endoscopy with special additional equipment needs. Rigid cystoscopy, laparoscopy, thoracoscopy, and arthroscopy require an outer cannula (usually with a trocar), which is inserted into the cavity to be examined, plus a viewing telescope (also responsible for directing light), which is inserted through the cannula into the cavity. The same equipment can be used for rhinoscopy, if the patient is large enough. However, not all rhinoscopy is done with this equipment.

Laparoscopes/thoracoscopes. Most telescopes used for laparoscopy and thoracoscopy are 5 mm in diameter. There are a variety of angles of view at the tip, ranging progressively from 0° (i.e., looking straight ahead) to 30°

(a commonly used telescope that effectively allows one to look behind lesions) to scopes that can look back on themselves (i.e., angles of view of 270° or greater). These 5-mm and smaller diameter scopes are used for double puncture procedures (i.e., the telescope is placed through one cannula while other instruments [e.g., biopsy forceps, Babcock forceps, etc.] are placed through additional cannulas), meaning that at least two punctures are made into the cavity. Smaller diameter instruments are available, but are not commonly used for canine or feline laparoscopy or thoracoscopy. Larger diameter (10-mm) telescopes exist, and some have a channel that allows insertion of an instrument (e.g., biopsy forceps, grasping forceps, scissors, etc.) while viewing through the scope. Such scopes are called operating endoscopes and can be used in single-puncture or double-puncture laparoscopy and thoracoscopy.

Laparoscopy requires a means of insufflating the abdomen (i.e., Veress needle) and both laparoscopy and thoracoscopy require a trocar/cannula assembly to insert the telescope into the appropriate cavity. There are various types of cannulas, but it is generally desirable to have at least one cannula with an air port on it so that the Veress needle can be removed from the animal and the insufflation line hooked up to the cannula (i.e., one less piece of equipment remaining into the abdomen). It also is desirable to have at least one threaded cannula, which is "screwed" into the thoracic or abdominal wall, to eliminate the risk of the cannula inadvertently being withdrawn. The type of biopsy forceps depends upon the nature of the biopsy. A liver biopsy is best taken with "clamshell" or "double-spoon" forceps (see Fig. 14-4); a biopsy from the pancreas is best accomplished with a punch type of forceps. In general, TruCut needles are only used for the kidney and some masses; they are not recommended for hepatic biopsies unless there is a focal mass (such lesions should generally have been aspirated via ultrasound before endoscopy). Various other forceps (e.g., Babcock), hemostats, aspiration tubes, needle holders, scissors, etc., should also be available, and electrocautery is particularly important when performing thoracoscopy. Because thoracoscopy is almost always a two person operation, requiring coordination between endoscopists, video capability is typically an absolute requirement (as opposed to most other endoscopies in which it is helpful but not critical), the exception being arthroscopy, in which it is also absolutely required.

Cystoscopes. Most cystoscopy is retrograde as opposed to transabdominal, except in cats, in which only transabdominal cystoscopy is possible. Small diameter flexible scopes (e.g., bronchoscopes) can be used, but rigid telescopes are usually preferred. The rigid telescopes used for retrograde cystoscopy of dogs are usually 10 to 22 Fr in diameter. Cannulas are very important in cystoscopy because they allow concurrent infusion of a fluid (e.g., physiologic saline) around the telescope during examination, which dilates the urethra and bladder and washes away blood, mucus, and other debris.

Rhinoscopes. Rigid rhinoscopy typically uses the same telescopes as cystoscopy and arthroscopy because of the need for small diameter equipment. The cannulas used for cystoscopy are especially useful because patients presented for rhinoscopy often have mucoid or bloody nasal discharge that obscures visualization. Infusion of cold saline during the procedure often washes away the mucus, allowing better visualization. However, the small size of the nasal cavity in cats and some small dogs limits the use of cannulas because they enlarge the diameter of the instrument being inserted into the nose. Therefore a variety of instruments have been used for rhinoscopy, including flexible and rigid scopes.

Arthroscopes. See later discussion on p. 155.

EQUIPMENT CARE

Endoscopes (especially flexible) are easily damaged. Therefore access to endoscopic equipment should be limited to a few essential individuals, including those who set it up and clean it (Box 14-3). When not in use, flexible scopes should be hung vertically on a rack. If it is absolutely necessary to store a flexible endoscope in its carrying case, extreme care must be taken to ensure that the insertion tube is not caught between the edges of the case (a common way that fiber bundles are broken). Newer flexible scopes are immersible, including the handle; however, older fiberoptic scopes can be severely damaged if water penetrates the handle through a seam during the endoscopic procedure or cleaning. Water must not be splashed on the light source or other electronic equipment, and surge protectors should be used. Only water-soluble jelly should be used as a lubricant on a flexible instrument; petroleum-based substances can shorten the life span of the rubber or plastic coverings.

The insertion tube must not be bent into an acute angle, especially at the junction of the insertion tube and the handle, or the fiber bundles can be broken. Care must be taken to prevent taking a biopsy of the insertion tube when taking a biopsy with the tip of the scope maximally retroflexed. An instrument should *never* be forced through the biopsy channel, especially when the tip of the scope is notably deflected. If fine, rough material (e.g., sand) is aspirated into the biopsy channel, it can tear the channel and cause a leak when a biopsy instrument is inserted. The insertion tube, especially the tip, should not be allowed to strike a hard surface.

> NOTE: Always use a mouth gag; *never* introduce the insertion tube into the mouth of an unanesthetized animal.

The scope should be cleaned after each procedure, and the manufacturer's recommendations should be followed explicitly. Generally, a leakage test should be performed first because it is much less expensive to repair a leaking scope before water leaks into the insertion tube and damages fiberoptics or electronics. Next, all water should be expelled from the air-water channel, and the suction and biopsy channels should be cleaned with an approved detergent or cleaner. Anytime a disinfectant is used on a flexible scope, only chemicals recommended by the manufacturer should be used. A brush is used

 BOX 14-3

Basic Cleaning of Flexible Endoscopes*

- Perform leakage test *first*.
- Aspirate approved detergent through biopsy channels.
- Brush biopsy channels and reaspirate.
- If appropriate, aspirate disinfectant solution through biopsy channels.
- Aspirate distilled water and then alcohol through biopsy channels.
- Aspirate air until biopsy channels are dry.
- Clean air-water and suction valves.
- Lubricate air-water and suction valves.
- Flush all water out of air-water channel.
- Clean exterior of scope with approved detergent and water.
- Clean and dry biopsy and foreign body retrieval forceps.

*Always see manufacturer's recommendations.

to remove adherent material from the biopsy channel. After these channels have been cleaned, alcohol and then air is aspirated through the channels until they are dry. Cleansing and disinfection of flexible scopes usually is adequate; sterilization is rarely necessary. If sterilization is necessary, use only approved cold-sterilization solutions or ethylene oxide.

> NOTE: Review the manufacturer's recommendations and be sure to use ethylene oxide caps, if necessary. Never subject flexible scopes to heat and especially not to autoclaving.

Rigid scopes usually are more resistant to damage than flexible equipment and require relatively simple care, such as washing in an approved detergent solution. Care must be taken to avoid hitting or scratching the lenses in the tips of some rigid scopes, such as cystoscopes. Small diameter rigid scopes (e.g., cystoscopes and rhinoscopes) are easily bent, so care must be taken when handling and storing them. Sterilization of rigid equipment may involve autoclaving (*if* the scope is designated by the manufacturer as one that can withstand autoclaving), but hydrogen peroxide plasma sterilization is preferred.

Care of the arthroscope is given on p. 156.

ANTIBIOTICS

Preprocedural administration of antibiotics is not required for routine endoscopies, including cystoscopy and laparoscopy, unless the patient has valvular cardiac defects or prosthetic implants, or is severely immunosuppressed. Esophageal ballooning is associated with bacteremia, and prophylactic use of antibiotics in such cases is reasonable, although not of proven use. Use of antibiotics after foreign body removal may be reasonable if significant ulceration or perforation has occurred.

For antibiotic usage during arthroscopy, see p. 157.

PROCEDURES

Four basic principles apply to most endoscopic procedures:

1. Advance the scope only if you can see where you are going.
2. If you cannot see what is happening (i.e., a condition known as a "red out"), back the scope out a little rather than advancing it, or insufflate a little air into the lumen (or do both).
3. Unless you need to look at a specific lesion, aim the scope toward the center of the lumen.
4. Do not insert the endoscope into your patient any harder than you would want a physician to insert it into you.

There are very few exceptions to these rules. Beware of excessive insufflation of the alimentary tract or abdomen, as both can impair respiration and/or venous return. Using too large of a scope can obstruct the respiratory tract. In general, the largest scope that can *safely* be used allows better visualization, larger biopsy samples, and use of better foreign body retrieval devices. The following sections describe selected techniques that might be performed in a variety of locations.

Biopsies

With flexible instruments, the largest biopsy instrument possible should be used. Better pieces of alimentary mucosa usually can be obtained if the organ is not excessively distended with air. Biopsies of both grossly normal and apparently diseased mucosa should be taken. Always note the difficulty involved in taking a biopsy of a particular lesion; some infiltrative lesions (i.e., scirrhous carcinomas and pythiosis) characteristically produce so much dense connective tissue that the flexible biopsy forceps cannot "bite" into the tissue and tear off an adequate piece. Such a finding may be an indication for full-thickness biopsy. Proliferative lesions can exist below the mucosa so that only normal-appearing mucosa is seen overlying a mass effect; in such cases repeated biopsies in the same spot (i.e., "drilling for oil") sometimes allow you to reach the underlying lesion. A biopsy is often best performed when the opened biopsy instrument can be pushed against the mucosa at a near 90° angle. In the intestines, the turn and suction technique often is used to achieve such an angle.

Biopsy of gastrointestinal mucosa

Advance the biopsy forceps through the channel, then open the jaws of the forceps and withdraw it until the opened jaws are flush with the tip of the endoscope. Flex the tip of the scope so that it is turned into the mucosa at as close to a 90° angle as possible; suction air out of the intestine, thereby drawing mucosa into the jaws of the forceps. Advance the forceps into the mucosa until moderate resistance is felt (do not advance the forceps so much that the cable on the instrument begins to bow excessively) and close the jaws. Be sure to straighten the tip of the endoscope before withdrawing the forceps.

At this time, it appears best to routinely obtain at least eight biopsies of each part of the alimentary tract to try to ensure that (1) sporadic and scattered lesions are sampled and (2) some tissue samples will be oriented optimally to maximize histologic interpretation. Intestinal, nasal, and gastric fundus and body mucosa are relatively "soft" and easy to biopsy. Pyloric and antral mucosa are tougher, and the mucosa may need to be grasped more firmly to pull off an adequate piece. Normal canine esophageal mucosa is so tough it is almost impossible to obtain an adequate tissue sample with routine flexible forceps. Normal tracheal mucosa is so thin it is difficult to obtain an adequate sample for histopathologic studies.

Using a needle, carefully retrieve mucosal samples from the biopsy forceps and place them mucosal side up on a plastic sponge, cucumber slice, or piece of formalin-soaked paper without distorting them.

Gastric, colonic, and nasal mucosa are relatively sturdy, but small intestinal mucosa is delicate and must be handled carefully to avoid artifacts.

Place the sponge, cucumber slice, or piece of paper with the biopsies on it in a vial of neutral buffered formalin, and do not allow the samples to dry out excessively before they are fixed.

Cytologic Preparations

Make cytologic preparations (i.e., squash preps) by putting a small piece of mucosa between two glass slides.

Press the slides together and then pull them apart either vertically or horizontally. As an alternative, use an endoscopic brush; lightly rub the extended brush against the lesion (do not cause hemorrhage) and then rub it against a glass slide. For cytologic studies of very fibrotic lesions that can be obtained only with rigid forceps, scrape the cut surface of the sample with a scalpel blade and make a squash preparation of the material obtained.

Washes

Insert a sterile polyethylene or similar tube through the biopsy channel, position the tip of the tube as desired, instill the solution (usually physiologic saline solution or Hank's buffered salt solution), and apply suction. Do not place the tip of the tube too close to the mucosa and use only modest negative pressure, or you may end up occluding the end of the tube with tissue. As an alternative, aspirate the sample directly through the endoscopic biopsy channel.

Foreign Body Removal

Each foreign object must be considered individually, because an ill-planned endoscopic removal may be more damaging to the patient (e.g., perforate the tract) than the foreign object (Box 14-4). It is also possible to "grab" a foreign object and find that it can be neither removed nor released, neces-

BOX 14-4

Advantages and Disadvantages of Endoscopic Removal of Foreign Objects

Advantages
- Often much quicker than surgery
- Often less stressful to the patient
- Reduced tissue trauma, morbidity, and recovery time

Disadvantages
- Cannot remove all objects
- Can hurt animal with careless technique
- Requires an assortment of expensive foreign body retrieval forceps

sitating surgery to retrieve the endoscope. There are numerous techniques for foreign body removal, but some basic principles always apply:

1. *Always radiograph the animal shortly before inducing anesthesia.* Some foreign objects that have been present for weeks pass out of reach of the scope just before the procedure is performed. In the same manner, some foreign objects will perforate the organ just a few hours after admission to the clinic. Finding air or water in the thorax or abdomen means that perforation may have occurred, and that one should analyze the fluid (i.e., looking for evidence of sepsis) or perform a contrast radiographic procedure (e.g., contrast esophagram) using an iodide-based contrast agent.

2. *Do not just grab the object and pull.* The object may need to be repositioned or turned to allow the forceps to obtain the best grasp on it. It may also be necessary to orient the object to make it easier to pull through the sphincters.

3. *Select the retrieval forceps that allows the firmest grasp on the object.* Rigid retrieval forceps typically allow the tightest grasp on an object.

4. *When an object has been snared, do not pull it out against undue resistance.* Resistance is expected at the lower esophageal sphincter (gastric cardia), the base of the heart, the thoracic inlet, and the cricopharyngeal area. If inappropriate resistance is noted, it may be better to release the object and perform surgery.

5. *Consider an overtube if there are sharp edges or if you need to dilate the lower esophageal sphincter.*

Postendoscopy care. Special care is not necessary after routine biopsy of the alimentary or respiratory tracts. Slight hemorrhage is expected after most procedures, especially those that biopsy mucosa. Most hemorrhage is minor or stops spontaneously shortly after the procedure if the coagulation system is normal. Preprocedural coagulation testing is generally done only when (1) there is a reason to suspect the integrity of the coagulation system (e.g., petechiae, spontaneous bleeding, and hepatic disease) or (2) one will perform biopsies during laparoscopy or thoracoscopy. However, nasal biopsies can be associated with severe hem-

orrhage, at times requiring ligation of the ipsilateral carotid artery. When laparoscopy has been used to perform a biopsy on a parenchymatous organ, such as the liver or kidneys, observe the patient closely for 2 to 4 hours to ensure that excessive hemorrhage does not occur. Also observe the patient for any evidence of infection. If excessive hemorrhage persists, which is quite rare, repeat endoscopy may be necessary to find the bleeding lesion and cauterize it. If excessive hemorrhage continues for an inappropriately long time after routine biopsy, a coagulopathy should be considered.

After a foreign object has been removed, the mucosa should be reevaluated for erosion or ulceration and other foreign objects or lesions. If there is any possibility of perforation, radiograph the appropriate body cavity to look for pneumothorax or pneumoperitoneum. Antibiotic regimens effective against aerobic and anaerobic bacteria often are useful in such cases. Such a regimen might be enrofloxacin, 15 mg/kg given IV once daily, plus either amoxicillin (22 mg/kg SC) or clindamycin (11 mg/kg IV) given two or three times a day, respectively. If severe ulceration is a factor, it may be useful to bypass the affected portion with a feeding tube and use antacids (e.g., ranitidine [2.2 mg/kg IV] or famotidine [0.5 mg/kg IV] given twice a day) or protectants (e.g., Carafate, 0.5 to 1 g given two to four times a day PO), or both.

It is important to watch for postprocedure dyspnea and/or hypoxia after performing bronchoalveolar lavage in patients with substantial pulmonary disease. In patients that are already marginally oxygenated, it is sometimes best to perform brushings for cytology and culture as opposed to washes.

ARTHROSCOPY: GENERAL PRINCIPLES, EQUIPMENT, AND TECHNIQUES

Procedures that may be performed arthroscopically are developing rapidly as surgeons adapt and develop techniques used in other species, particularly humans and horses. The most common arthroscopically performed procedure is fragment removal for diseases such as OCD (see p. 1178) or fragmented coronoid process (FCP, see p. 1201). Other common procedures include treatment of meniscal injuries (see p. 1286), synovial biopsies, tenotomy (see p. 1196), and arthroscopic assisted fracture repair. Techniques are being developed for joint stabilization.

INDICATIONS

Arthroscopy may be indicated for either the diagnosis or treatment of joint disease (Fig. 14-5 and Boxes 14-5 and 14-6). Arthroscopy is vastly superior to radiography in the diagnosis of joint diseases because it allows direct visualization of the cartilage and soft tissue structures, provides magnification, and enables biopsy of virtually all structures within the joint (Fig. 14-6). The most significant diagnostic advantage of arthroscopy is the operator's ability to assess the condition of the

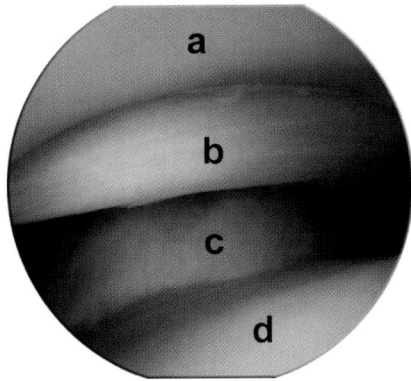

FIG. 14-5
Arthroscopic view of a normal shoulder joint. *a,* Glenoid cavity. *b,* Medial collateral ligament. *c,* Subscapularis ligament. *d,* Humeral head. (From Beale et al: *Small animal arthroscopy,* Philadelphia, 2003, Saunders.)

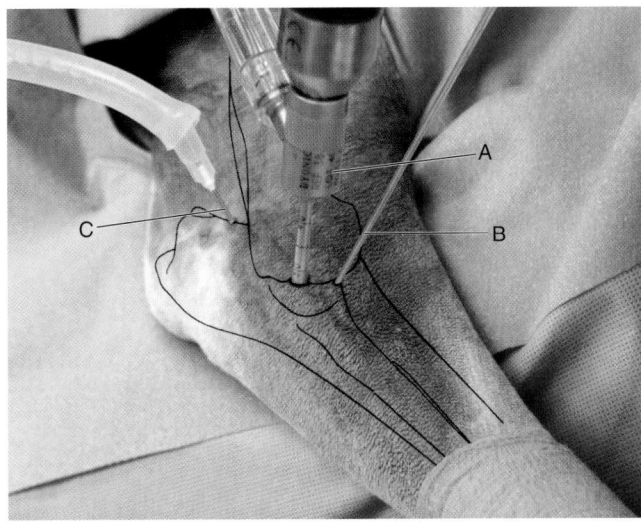

FIG. 14-6
Arthroscopy of the elbow joint. *A,* Arthroscope and scope portal. *B,* Hand instrument and instrument portal. *C,* Outflow needle. (From Beale et al: *Small animal arthroscopy,* Philadelphia, 2003, Saunders).

 BOX 14-5

Common Diagnoses With Arthroscopy

Shoulder	**Hip**
OCD	Osteoarthritis
Osteoarthritis	Labral tearing and avulsion
Biceps disease	Tearing of the ligament of
Medial collateral tearing	the femoral head
Lateral collateral tearing	
	Knee
Elbow	OCD
FCP	Cruciate disease
OCD	Osteoarthritis
UAP	Meniscal disease
Osteoarthritis of the me-	
dial compartment	**Tarsus**
	OCD
Carpus	Chip Fractures
Osteoarthritis	
Chip fractures	

OCD, Osteochondritis dessicans; *FCP,* fragmented coronoid process; *UAP,* ununited anconeal process.

 BOX 14-6

Common Arthroscopic Procedures

Shoulder

Fragment removal—OCD
Osteoarthritis treatment—microfracture, abrasion
Biceps tenotomy
Soft tissue shrinkage for instability

Elbow

Fragment removal—OCD, FCP
Osteoarthritis treatment—microfracture, abrasion

Carpus

Fragment removal—chip fractures
Osteoarthritis treatment—microfracture, abrasion

Hip

Osteoarthritis assessment

Knee

Fragment removal—OCD
Osteoarthritis treatment—microfracture, abrasion
Meniscal treatment
Cruciate

Tarsus

Fragment removal OCD
Osteoarthritis treatment—microfracture, abrasion

cartilage surface. Recent studies have demonstrated that radiology poorly reflects the condition of cartilage in canine osteoarthritis, whereas arthroscopy enables specific grading and determination of the extent of cartilage injury.

EQUIPMENT

Arthroscopes are differentiated by diameter (1.9, 2.3, 2.7 mm, and larger), length (short, long) and angle. Arthroscopes in common use in small animal arthroscopy include any of the diameters and lengths listed above with the vast majority having a 30° angle (Fig. 14-7). The diameter applies to the telescope portion alone and does not include the diameter of the arthroscope cannula, which is necessary for use. The selection of diameter is based on the size of the joint and surgeon preference, with larger scopes providing more

rigidity and greater field of view and smaller scopes causing less iatrogenic damage and having greater mobility. Cameras are available as 1 or 3 chip and must be used with a specific camera box that processes the image for the television screen. For general use, 1-chip cameras provide excellent

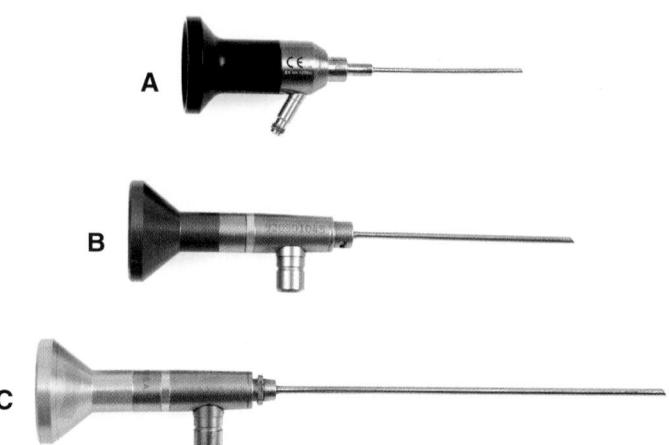

FIG. 14-7
Arthroscopes for small animal procedures. **A,** 1.9-mm short arthroscope. **B,** 2.3-mm short arthroscope. **C,** 2.7-mm long arthroscope. (From Beale et al: *Small animal arthroscopy,* Philadelphia, 2003, Saunders.

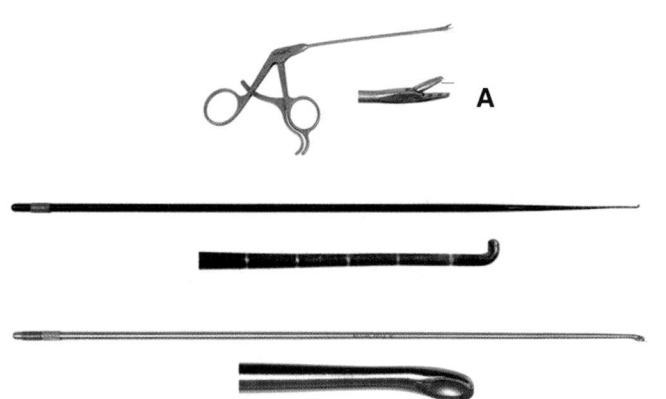

FIG. 14-8
Hand instruments for small animal arthroscopy. **A,** Grasping forceps. **B,** Right angle probe. **C,** Microcurette.

resolution and recording capabilities and 3-chip cameras are generally only necessary for higher-end video or still image work. Medical grade monitors are recommended to provide a bright, clear, and accurate image. Most new light sources use xenon lamps, which provide increased light intensity and higher color temperature than halogen and therefore provide higher visual clarity and color rendition. Xenon light sources are more expensive than halogen, but are generally recommended for superior image quality.

Video images may be obtained using either analog or digital equipment. With increasing availability of video editing on personal computers, use of digital recording devices has become more practical.

Fluid flow helps maintain joint distention, aids in clearing blood and other debris from the joint, and decreases the risk of contamination. Fluid may be delivered to the joint either by means of gravity or from an arthroscopic pump. Fluid outflow is provided by either a disposable needle or a specific outflow cannula.

The majority of arthroscopic therapy is performed with hand instrumentation (Fig. 14-8). These tools and power tools are inserted into the joint through an instrument portal that may be used with or without a cannula. Hand instruments include probes, knives, curettes, and forceps. The most commonly used probes are right angled and may have calibration marks for measurement of lesions. Numerous styles of knives and curettes are available for manipulations of soft tissue. The most common forceps used in small animal arthroscopy are graspers for removal of hard or soft tissue and biters for débridement of soft tissue.

Power instruments are not necessary for basic small animal arthroscopy, but will increase efficiency and enhance the capabilities of the operator. The most common power instrument used is a shaver. These motorized hand tools have numerous tip designs, including burrs, sharp cutters, and aggressive cutters. Additional power instruments include electrocautery and radiofrequency. Electrocautery tips specific for use in arthroscopy are available for some electrocautery generators. Alternatively, cautery may be performed by use of a radiofrequency unit. These units, which are available in both bipolar and monopolar designs, have also been advocated for soft tissue ablation and collagen shrinkage.

EQUIPMENT CARE

The telescope is the most fragile and expensive portion of the arthroscopy equipment. It may be damaged during the surgery or at any other time by cracking or scratching the lens or by bending. Specific protocols should be established for handling of the arthroscope to prevent any damage. It is advisable to have small cases for each arthroscope that can secure the arthroscope, cannula, and trocars for sterilization and storage. The cases should be sturdy and have a means of securing the instruments within the case. The arthroscope should be placed back in the case immediately after use to prevent damage while the remainder of the surgical table is cleared. Any junctions on the arthroscope, including those between the light post and scope or between the eye piece and telescope, should be checked regularly for tightness. If these junctions become loose, they may permit fluid to leak in, which may impede light or image transmission. Bending of an arthroscope may be evident by the appearance of a black crescent at the periphery of the field of view. Severe bending will result in complete obliteration of the view. If bending occurs, the instrument should be sent to a qualified repair facility versus attempting to straighten the instrument, which may result in permanent damage.

Arthroscopes should be cleaned by hand with an enzymatic cleaner and distilled water as soon as possible after the procedure to remove blood or other body fluids or tissue. The lens and eye piece may be gently cleaned with a cotton ball and distilled water. The cannulas and trocars are similarly cleaned. Sterilization may be performed by several methods. Cold ster-

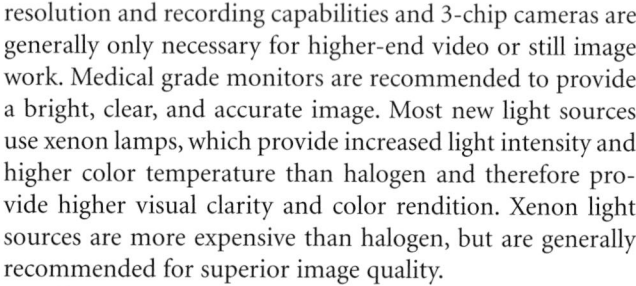

ilization is performed by placing the arthroscope, cannula, and trocars in a 14-day glutaraldehyde solution (e.g., Cidex, by Johnson & Johnson) for no more than 30 minutes. The arthroscope may also be sterilized by ethylene oxide gas, Steris, or Sterad, depending upon the recommendations of the manufacturer. Most arthroscopes are not autoclavable; even those that are will not last as long if they are repeatedly autoclaved as a result of gradual destruction of the glue.

The camera head, with its associated lens and prism, and the cable may be damaged by dropping or mishandling. The camera cord contains relatively delicate wires and the connection may have fine pins. The camera cord should never be bent or wound too tightly, and the cap should always be placed back on the connector when not in use. Camera heads may be sterilized by autoclave, ethylene oxide gas, or cold sterilization according to manufacturer's recommendations.

The light cable may be sterilized by ethylene oxide gas, soaking, or autoclaving, depending on the manufacturer's recommendations. The light cable is composed of numerous glass fibers that may be broken if the cable is bent or wound too tightly. The fiberoptic cable will also heat up significantly and should never be placed directly against the patient because it may cause burning.

Hand instruments should be cared for using routine cleaning and sterilization techniques. These instruments should be inspected during each use for damage or dull edges. The care of power instruments varies based on the tool and manufacturer, although as a rule it is recommended to gas sterilize electrical power instruments.

ANTIBIOTICS

The minimally invasive nature and high volume of fluid flow used with arthroscopy result in a very low risk of infection. Antibiotics are typically administered only on a perioperative basis during these procedures. A first generation cephalosporin (cephalexin, 22 mg/kg, IV) should be given at induction and discontinued after the procedure.

GENERAL PROCEDURES

The most commonly performed arthroscopic procedures are diagnostic visualization and fragment removal (see Box 14-6). When performing diagnostic arthroscopy, it is critical that a complete and repeatable method to document the procedure be routinely performed using either still or video imaging, or preferably both. For best results, make a short video of the entire joint (approximately 15 to 20 seconds in length, depending on the joint) and then take still images of any abnormal findings. This results in a record of all joints examined while producing a minimum of electronic data. The images are valuable for showing lesions to pet owners and for use as a reference for follow-up evaluation of the case.

NOTE: Anticipate that as a beginning arthroscopist you may not be able to successfully remove all fragments, and thus be prepared to perform an arthrotomy.

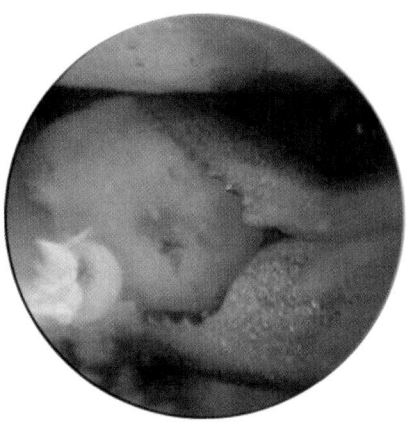

FIG. 14-9
Fragment removal in canine elbow arthroscopy. (From Beale et al: *Small animal arthroscopy*, Philadelphia, 2003, Saunders).

Fragment removal varies depending on the joint being treated and the specific disease (Fig. 14-9). The most critical points for successful fragment removal include establishment of suitable joint portals, use of appropriate hand instruments, and development of excellent arthroscopic hand-eye skills. The establishment of suitable portals allows good visualization of the fragment, easy removal and insertion of the instrument, and enhanced ability to manipulate the fragment.

SPECIFIC PROCEDURES

Arthroscopy of specific joints can be found in the chapter detailing procedures for conditions affecting that joint. For arthroscopy of the shoulder, see p. 1178; for the elbow, see p. 1201; for the hip, see p. 1235; for the stifle, see p. 1258.

POSTARTHROSCOPY CARE

Because of the minimally invasive nature of arthroscopy, small animal patients undergoing this procedure require little specific postoperative care. Specific instructions depend upon the disease being treated and condition of the joint. Arthroscopy portals are generally closed only with skin sutures, although some small portals may not require closure. Regardless of closure method, moderate postoperative drainage from these incisions due to the large volumes of fluid used in the procedure may be seen. Although many animals are administered nonsteroidal antiinflammatory medications for treatment of the primary disease, most patients will not require postoperative analgesics for pain associated with the arthroscopic procedure itself. Exercise restriction is indicated for several days to a week to permit the portals to heal and may be prescribed for longer periods, depending on the underlying disease.

Suggested Reading

Austin B, Lanz OI, Hamilton SM et al: Laparoscopic ovariohysterectomy in nine dogs, *J Am Anim Hosp Assoc* 39:391, 2003.

Laparoscopic ovariohysterectomy took a median of 60 minutes and had few complications.

Beale BS, Hulse DA, Schulz KS et al: Small animal arthroscopy, Philadelphia, 2003, WB Saunders.

This comprehensive textbook on arthroscopy has detailed information regarding instrumentation and techniques involving small animal arthroscopy. It also contains a thorough discussion of the indications and disease processes treated.

Cannizzo KL, McLoughlin MA, MaHon JS et al: Evaluation of transurethral cystoscopy and excretory urography for diagnosis of ectopic ureters in female dogs: 25 cases (1992-2000), *J Am Vet Med Assoc* 223:475, 2003.

This paper showed that cystoscopy was more accurate than excretory urography for diagnosis of ectopic ureters in dogs.

Devitt CM, Cox RE, Hailey JJ: Duration, complications, stress, and pain of open ovariohysterectomy versus a simple method of laparoscopic-assisted ovariohysterectomy in dogs, *J Am Vet Med Assoc* 227:921, 2005.

The laparoscopic technique was associated with less pain.

Dupre GP, Corlouer JP, Bouvy B: Thoracoscopic pericardiectomy performed without pulmonary exclusion in 9 dogs, *Vet Surg* 30:21, 2001.

Pericardiectomy is one of the more commonly performed interventional thoracoscopic procedures and has advantages over open pericardiectomy. The procedure does not need pulmonary exclusion.

Gualtieri M: Esophagoscopy, *Vet Clin North Am* 31:605, 2001.

This is an excellent overview of endoscopic diagnosis and treatment of esophageal disease, which also includes some advanced information about esophageal strictures.

Hewitt S, Brisson BA, Sinclair MD et al: Evaluation of laparoscopic-assisted placement of jejunostomy feeding tubes in dogs, *J Am Vet Med Assoc* 225:65, 2004.

Placing a jejunostomy feeding tube is one of the more useful interventional laparoscopic techniques. The authors recommend this technique in dogs that did not require a laparotomy for other reasons.

Jergens AE, Andreasen CB, Hagemoser WA et al: Cytological examination of exfoliative specimens obtained during endoscopy for diagnosis of gastrointestinal tract disease in dogs and cats, *J Am Vet Med Assoc* 213:1755, 1998.

This paper explains how to use cytology for quick diagnosis of some infiltrative disorders of the gastrointestinal tract.

Kovak JR, Ludwig LL, Bergman PJ et al: Use of thoracoscopy to determine the etiology of pleural effusion in dogs and cats: 18 cases (1998-2001), *J Am Vet Med Assoc* 221:990, 2002.

This paper showed that thoracoscopy was beneficial in diagnosis of malignant and inflammatory causes of pleural effusion in 18 patients.

Leib MS, Baechtel MS, Monroe WE: Complications associated with 355 flexible colonoscopic procedures in dogs, *J Vet Intl Med* 18:642, 2004.

This paper documents the safety of colonoscopy and discusses the more common, minor problems that may be encountered.

Leib MS, Dinnel H, Ward DL et al: Endoscopic balloon dilation of benign esophageal strictures in dogs and cats, *J Vet Med* 15:547, 2001.

This retrospective study of 18 dogs and 10 cats showed that a median of two procedures was required for resolution, and only one animal had a perforation.

Mansell J, Willard MD: Biopsy of the gastrointestinal tract, *Vet Clin North Am* 33:1099, 2003.

This paper discusses endoscopic biopsy in detail, including equipment, technique, and common mistakes.

Miura T, Maruyama H, Sakai M et al: Endoscopic findings on alimentary lymphoma in 7 dogs, *J Vet Med Science* 66:577, 2004.

A cobblestone appearance was often seen, and it was easy to confuse the lesion with the condition caused by inflammatory bowel disease.

Monnet E, Twedt DC: Laparoscopy, *Vet Clin North Am* 33:1147, 2003.

An excellent overview of the technique and possible uses of laparoscopy for diagnostic and therapeutic purposes.

Rawlings CA, Mahaffey MB, Bement S et al: Prospective evaluation of laparoscopic-assisted gastropexy in dogs susceptible to gastric dilatation, *J Am Vet Med Assoc* 221:1576, 2002.

Laparoscopic gastropexy is a widely used procedure that is easy to perform.

Schulz KS et al: Self-retaining braces for canine arthroscopy, *Vet Surg* 31:77, 2004.

This article describes braces that are useful for positioning patients for arthroscopy.

Smith A, Posner LP, Goldstein RE et al: Evaluation of the effects of premedication on gastroduodenoscopy in cats, *J Am Vet Med Assoc* 225:540, 2004.

This study showed that hydromorphone, butorphanol, and medetomidine were acceptable premedicants in cats that were later induced with ketamine and maintained with isoflurane.

Tams TRL: Gastrointestinal endoscopy: instrumentation, handling technique, and maintenance. In Tams TR, editor: *Small animal endoscopy*, ed 2, Philadelphia, 1999, Mosby.

A good discussion of basic endoscopic equipment and care.

Willard MD: Colonoscopy, proctoscopy, and ileoscopy, *Vet Clin North Am* 31:657, 2001.

This paper gives an overview of the technique, equipment, and application of endoscopy of the lower gastrointestinal tract.

Willard MD, Lovering SL, Cohen ND et al: Quality of tissue specimens obtained endoscopically from the duodenum of dogs and cats, *J Am Vet Med Assoc* 219:474, 2001.

This paper documents the importance of training to obtain high quality endoscopic biopsies of the duodenum.

CHAPTER 15
Surgery of the Integumentary System

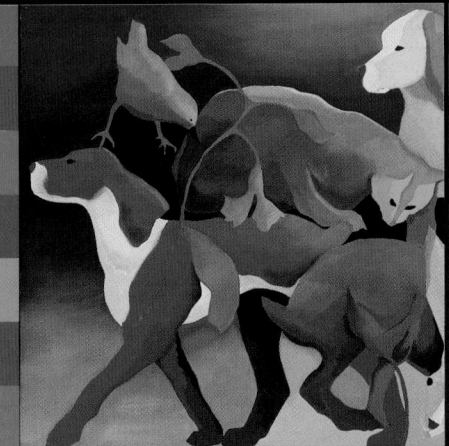

GENERAL PRINCIPLES AND TECHNIQUES

WOUND MANAGEMENT

SURGICAL ANATOMY

The skin is composed of epidermis, dermis, and associated adnexa. The outermost layer (i.e., epidermis) is thin but protective; it is especially thin in areas with abundant hair and slightly thicker in areas without much hair. The thickest epidermis is on the nose and footpads, where it is keratinized. The epidermis is avascular, receiving nourishment from fluid penetrating the deeper layers and from dermal capillaries. The thicker, vascular dermis lies deep to the epidermis, which it nourishes and supports. The dermis is composed of collagenous, reticular, and elastic fibers surrounded by a mucopolysaccharide ground substance. Fibroblasts, macrophages, plasma cells, and mast cells are found throughout this layer. The dermis contains blood and lymph vessels, nerves, hair follicles, glands, ducts, and smooth muscle fibers. The hypodermis, or subcutis, lies below the dermis.

Musculocutaneous vessels are the primary vessels supplying skin in human beings, apes, and swine; however, dogs and other loose-skinned animals lack musculocutaneous vessels. Musculocutaneous vessels run perpendicular to the skin's surface, whereas vessels supplying canine and feline skin approach and travel parallel to the skin and are direct cutaneous vessels. For this reason, some human pedicle grafting techniques have limited application in dogs and cats. Terminal arteries and veins branch from direct cutaneous vessels and form subdermal (deep) plexus, cutaneous (middle) plexus, and subpapillary (superficial) plexus. The subdermal plexus supplies hair bulbs and follicles, tubular glands, the deeper portion of the gland ducts, and arrectores pilorum muscles. The cutaneous plexus supplies sebaceous glands and reinforces capillary networks around hair follicles, tubular gland ducts, and arrectores pili muscles. The subpapillary plexus lies on the outer layer of dermis, and capillary loops from this plexus project into and supply the epidermis. The capillary loop system is poorly developed in dogs and cats compared with human beings and swine, which is why canine skin does not usually blister with superficial burns.

The subdermal plexus is of major importance to skin viability. In areas where there is a panniculus muscle (cutaneous trunci, platysma, sphincter colli superficialis, sphincter colli profundus, preputialis, supramammarius muscles), the subdermal plexus lies both superficial and deep to it. Therefore surgeons must undermine the fascial plane beneath the cutaneous musculature to preserve the integrity of the subdermal plexus. Where the panniculus is absent, such as in the extremities, the subdermal plexus runs in the deep surface of the dermis, requiring that one undermine well below the dermal surface.

WOUND HEALING

Wound healing is a preferred biologic process that restores tissue continuity after injury. It is a combination of physical, chemical, and cellular events that restore wounded tissue or replace it with collagen. Wound healing begins immediately after injury or incision. The four phases of wound healing are inflammation, débridement, repair, and maturation. Wound healing is dynamic; several phases occur simultaneously. The first 3 to 5 days are the lag phase of wound healing because inflammation and débridement predominate, and wounds have not gained appreciable strength. Healing is influenced by host factors, wound characteristics, and other external factors.

Stages of Wound Healing

Inflammatory phase. Inflammation is a protective tissue response initiated by damage. This phase is characterized by increased vascular permeability, chemotaxis of circulatory cells, release of cytokines and growth factors, and cell activation (macrophages, neutrophils, lymphocytes, and fibroblasts). Hemorrhage cleans and fills wounds immediately after injury. Blood vessels constrict for 5 to 10 minutes to limit hemorrhage, but then dilate and leak fibrinogen and

159

BOX 15-1

Growth Factors Important in Wound Healing

BFGF	Basic fibroblast growth factor
EGF	Epidermal growth factor
KGF	Keratinocyte growth factor; also known as growth factor 7
PDGF	Platelet-derived growth factor
TGF-α and TGF-β	Transforming growth factor
VEGF	Vascular endothelial cell growth factor

clotting elements into wounds. Vasoconstriction is mediated by catecholamines, serotonin, bradykinin, and histamine. The extrinsic coagulation mechanism is activated by thromboplastin released from injured cells. Platelet aggregation and blood coagulation form a clot that ensures hemostasis and provides a scaffold for cell migration. Platelets also release potent chemoattractants and growth factors (epidermal, platelet-derived, transforming growth factors: α and β) that are necessary in later stages of wound healing (Box 15-1). Fibrin and plasma transudates fill wounds and plug lymphatics, localizing inflammation and "gluing" wound edges together. Fibronectin dimers within the clot become covalently cross-linked to fibrin and to themselves in the presence of activated factor XIII, forming a provisional extracellular matrix. This blood clot formation stabilizes the wound's edges and provides limited wound strength. It also provides an immediate barrier to infection and fluid loss, and a substrate for early organization of the wound. Scabs form when the blood clot dries; they protect wounds, prevent further hemorrhage, and allow healing to progress beneath their surface. Inflammatory phase cells such as platelets, mast cells, and macrophages secrete growth factors or cytokines, which initiate and maintain the proliferative phase of healing. Inflammatory mediators (i.e., histamine, serotonin, proteolytic enzymes, kinins, prostaglandins, complement, lysosomal enzymes, thromboxane, and growth factors) cause inflammation that begins immediately after injury and lasts approximately 5 days. White blood cells leaking from blood vessels into wounds initiate the débridement phase.

Débridement phase. An exudate composed of white blood cells, dead tissue, and wound fluid forms on wounds during the débridement phase. Chemoattractants encourage neutrophils and monocytes to appear in wounds (approximately 6 hours and 12 hours after injury, respectively) and initiate débridement. Neutrophils increase in number for 2 to 3 days. They prevent infection and débride organisms and debris by phagocytosis. Degenerating neutrophils release enzymes and toxic oxygen products that facilitate the breakdown of bacteria, extracellular debris, and necrotic material, and they stimulate monocytes. Monocytes are essential for wound healing; neutrophils are not. Monocytes are major secretory cells synthesizing growth factors that participate in tissue formation and remodeling. Monocytes become macrophages in wounds at 24 to 48 hours. Macrophages secrete

collagenases, removing necrotic tissue, bacteria, and foreign material. They may coalesce and form multinucleated giant cells with phagocytic functions. Macrophages also secrete chemotactic and growth factors. Growth factors (i.e., platelet-derived growth factor, transforming growth factor-α, transforming growth factor-β, fibroblast growth factor, and interleukin-1) can initiate, maintain, and coordinate formation of granulation tissue. Chemotactic factors (i.e., complement, collagen fragments, bacterial endotoxins, and inflammatory cell products) direct macrophages to injured tissue. Macrophages also recruit mesenchymal cells, stimulate angiogenesis, and modulate matrix production in wounds. Platelets release growth factors important for fibroblastic activity. Lymphocytes appear later in the débridement phase than neutrophils and macrophages. They secrete soluble factors that may stimulate or inhibit migration and protein synthesis by other cells. However, they usually improve the rate and quality of tissue repair. Although healing is severely impaired when macrophage function is suppressed, neutropenia and lymphopenia do not inhibit healing or the development of wound tensile strength in sterile wounds.

Repair phase. The repair phase usually begins 3 to 5 days after injury. Macrophages stimulate deoxyribonucleic acid (DNA) and fibroblast proliferation. Cytokines, in concert with extracellular matrix molecules, stimulate fibroblasts in the surrounding tissue to proliferate, express appropriate integrin receptors, and migrate into wounds. Fibroblasts are stimulated by transforming growth factor-β to produce fibronectin, which facilitates cell binding and fibroblast movement. Platelet-derived growth factor and basic fibroblast growth factor are also involved. A tissue oxygen content of approximately 20 mm Hg and slight acidity also stimulate fibroblast proliferation and collagen synthesis. Fibroblasts originate from undifferentiated mesenchymal cells in surrounding connective tissue and migrate to wounds along fibrin strands in the fibrin clot. Fibroblasts migrate into wounds just ahead of new capillary buds as the inflammatory phase subsides (2 to 3 days). They invade wounds to synthesize and deposit collagen, elastin, and proteoglycans that mature into fibrous tissue. Orientation initially is haphazard, but after 5 days tension on wounds causes fibroblasts, fibers, and capillaries to orient parallel to the incision or wound margin. Wound fibrin disappears as collagen is deposited. Collagen synthesis is associated with an early increase in wound tensile strength. As the wound matures, there is a notable increase in the ratio of type I (mature) to type III (immature) collagen. The amount of collagen reaches a maximum within 2 to 3 weeks after injury. As the collagen content of a wound increases, the number of fibroblasts and the rate of collagen synthesis decrease, marking the end of the repair stage. The fibroblastic interval of healing lasts 2 to 4 weeks, depending on the nature of the wound. Fibroblast migration and proliferation, collagen production, and capillary ingrowth are delayed if macrophages are absent.

Capillaries invade wounds behind migrating fibroblasts by the process of angiogenesis. Angiogenesis is complex, relying on interaction of extracellular matrix with cytokines that stimulate migration and proliferation of endothelial cells. Stimulus for angiogenesis probably includes macrophage production of mitogenic and chemotactic factors for endothelial cells, and low oxygen tension and increased lactic acid, which affect cytokine production. Basic fibroblast growth factor and vascular endothelial growth factor are specific angiogenic factors. Capillary buds originate from existing blood vessels with columns of capillary endothelial cells migrating toward the site of injury and uniting with other capillary buds or disrupted vessels. New capillaries increase oxygen tension in wounds, augmenting fibroplasia. Mitotic activity in adjacent mesenchymal cells increases as blood begins to flow in new capillaries. Lymphatic channels develop similar to capillary buds but more slowly. Lymphatic drainage of wounds is poor during early healing. The combination of new capillaries, fibroblasts, and fibrous tissue forms bright red, fleshy granulation tissue 3 to 5 days after injury.

Granulation tissue is formed at each wound edge at a rate of 0.4 to 1 mm/day. Unhealthy granulation tissue is white and has a high fibrous tissue content with few capillaries. Granulation tissue fills defects and protects wounds. It provides a barrier to infection, a surface for epithelial migration, and a source of special fibroblasts (i.e., myofibroblasts), which are important in wound contraction. Myofibroblasts are believed to contain proteins (actin and myosin) that contribute to wound contraction. Myofibroblasts are not found in normal tissue, incised and coapted wounds, or tissue surrounding a contracting wound.

Epithelium is an important barrier to external infection and internal fluid loss. Epithelial repair involves mobilization, migration, proliferation, and differentiation of epithelial cells. *Epithelialization* begins almost immediately (24 to 48 hours) in sutured wounds with good edge to edge apposition because there is no defect for granulation tissue to fill. Epithelialization begins in open wounds when an adequate granulation bed has formed (usually 4 to 5 days). In partial-thickness skin wounds, epidermal migration over the wound surface begins almost immediately from both the wound margins and epidermal appendages, such as hair follicles and sweat glands. Epidermal cells at the margin of the wound undergo phenotypic alteration that includes retraction on intracellular monofilaments, formation of peripheral cytoplasmic actin filaments, and temporary dissolution of the desmosomes and hemidesmosomes, which release keratinocytes to migrate beneath the eschar at the junction between any remaining necrotic tissue and extracellular matrix of the viable connective tissue. The epidermal cell path of migration is determined by integrins expressed on the membranes of migrating epidermal cells. Chalone, water-soluble glycoproteins found in the epidermis, inhibits epithelial mitosis in normal tissue but is diminished in wounds, which allows epithelial cells along wound margins to divide and migrate across the granulation tissue. Other growth factors secreted by platelets, macrophages, and fibroblasts may also be involved. Increased basal cell mitotic activity occurs as early as 24 to 48 hours after wounding.

Epithelial migration is random, but guided by collagen fibers. Migrating epithelial cells enlarge, flatten, and mobilize, losing their attachments to the basement membrane and other epithelial cells. Basal cells at wound edges develop microvilli and extend broad, thin pseudopodia over the exposed surface of collagen bundles. They develop intracytoplasmic microfilaments and selectively fix antiactin and antimyosin antibodies. Epithelial cells in the layers behind these altered cells migrate over them until they contact the wound surface. Cells continue to slide forward until the wound surface is covered. The migrating cells move under scabs and produce collagenase, which dissolves the base of the scab so it can be shed. Contact on all sides with other epithelial cells inhibits further cell migration (contact inhibition). Initially, new epithelium is only one cell layer thick and fragile, but it gradually thickens as additional cell layers form. After a basement membrane has been established, epithelial cells become plump, develop mitoses, and proliferate, restoring the normal, stratified, squamous epithelium architecture. Some hair follicles and sweat glands may regenerate, depending on the depth of skin damage. Epithelial migration also occurs along suture tracts, which may lead to a foreign body reaction, sterile abscess, or scarring or all of these. Epithelialization of suture tracts can be minimized by early removal of sutures. New epithelium usually is visible 4 to 5 days after injury. Epithelialization occurs faster in a moist environment than in a dry one. It will not occur over nonviable tissue. Epithelial migration is energy dependent and related to oxygen tension. Anoxia prevents epithelial migration and mitosis, whereas hyperbaric oxygen therapy may enhance migration. Wet-dry bandages (see p. 186) débride newly formed epithelium, delaying reepithelialization.

Wound contraction reduces the size of wounds subsequent to fibroblasts, reorganizing collagen in granulation tissue and myofibroblast contraction at the wound edge. Contraction occurs simultaneously with granulation and epithelialization, but is independent of epithelialization. Wound contraction involves a complex interaction of cells, extracellular matrix, and cytokines. Significant fibroblastic invasion into the wound is necessary for contraction to begin. Centripetal, full-thickness skin edges are pulled inward by contraction, and wounds may be noticeably smaller by 5 to 9 days after injury. During wound contraction, the surrounding skin stretches (intussusceptive growth) and the wound takes on a stellate appearance. Contraction progresses at a rate of approximately 0.6 to 0.8 mm/day. Wound contraction stops when wound edges meet, when tension is excessive, or when myofibroblasts are inadequate. Wound contraction is limited if skin around wounds is fixed, inelastic, or under tension, and it is inhibited if myofibroblast development or function is impaired. Contraction can also be impaired by antiinflammatory steroids, antimicrotubular drugs, and local application of smooth muscle relaxants. If wound contraction stops before granulation tissue is covered, epithelialization may continue and cover the wound.

Maturation phase. Wound strength increases to its maximum level because of changes in the scar during the maturation phase of wound healing. Wound maturation begins once collagen has been adequately deposited in wounds (17 to 20 days after injury) and may continue for years. The cellularity of granulation tissue is reduced as cells die. There is also a reduction in collagen content of the extracellular matrix. Collagen fibers remodel with alteration of their orientation and increased cross-linking, which improves wound strength. Fibers orient along lines of stress. Functionally oriented fibers become thicker. Type III collagen gradually decreases, and type I collagen increases. Nonfunctionally oriented collagen fibers are degraded by proteolytic enzymes (matrix metalloproteinases) secreted by macrophages, epithelial cells, endothelial cells, and fibroblasts within the extracellular matrix. The most rapid gain in wound strength occurs between 7 and 14 days after injury as collagen rapidly accumulates in the wound. Wounds gain only about 20% of their final strength in the first 3 weeks after injury. Slower increase in wound strength then occurs, but normal tissue strength is never regained in wounds; only 80% of original strength may be regained. As the number of capillaries in fibrous tissue declines, the scar becomes paler. Scars also become less cellular, flatten, and soften during maturation. Collagen synthesis and lysis occur at the same rate in maturing scars.

Moist Wound Healing

A moist wound environment allows optimal healing. Wound fluid is allowed to remain on the wound, keeping it moist. In a moist environment, débridement is hastened and selective, granulation tissue formation is promoted, and epithelialization is faster. Allowing wound fluid to remain in contact with wounds fosters autolytic débridement by endogenous enzymes that break down necrotic, but not healthy, tissue. Autolytic débridement occurs within 72 to 96 hours under an occlusive bandage. White blood cell phagocytosis decreases bacterial load and removes necrotic debris. White blood cells migrate more readily in a moist environment. Wound fluid also contains cytokines and growth factors that stimulate granulation tissue, angiogenesis, and reepithelialization. Chemotactic factors in wound fluid attract neutrophils and macrophages that secrete additional enzymes, cytokines, and growth factors. Moist wounds limit infections because more white blood cells are found in the wound, and there is improved phagocytosis and a lower pH. Scabs do not form with moist wound healing; therefore white blood cells are not trapped in the scab, and topical medications better penetrate the wound. If the animal is receiving systemic antibiotics, wound fluids may contain antibiotics, which help prevent or control infection. Low oxygen tension under an occlusive bandage stimulates macrophage activity, fibroblast proliferation, and capillary ingrowth. The rate of epithelialization is twice as fast for wounds kept moist with occlusive dressings than for air-exposed wounds. Epithelial cells travel faster and a shorter distance for epithelialization to occur in moist environments; in air-exposed wounds, migrating epidermal cells must travel beneath a crusted scab and devitalized dermis to reach their destination. Hydrophilic, occlu-

sive, or semiocclusive bandages help keep a wound warm and moist. Increased warmth enhances enzymatic activity. A moist wound is less painful and pruritic, tissues do not desiccate, and scar formation is less. Potential disadvantages of moist wound healing include bacterial colonization (not infection) of the wound surface, folliculitis, and maceration of the wound border.

Host Factors Affecting Wound Healing

Old animals tend to heal slowly, probably because of concurrent disease or debilitation. Malnourished animals and those with serum protein concentrations below 1.5 to 2 g/dl may have delayed wound healing and diminished wound strength. Hepatic disease may cause clotting factor deficiencies. Hyperadrenocorticism delays wound healing because of excess circulating glucocorticoids. Animals with diabetes mellitus have delayed wound healing and a predisposition to wound infections. Uremia occurring within 5 days of injury impairs healing by altering enzyme systems, biochemical pathways, and cellular metabolism. Obesity is associated with a higher incidence of postoperative wound infections in human beings. The risk of postoperative wound infection in dogs and cats increases as the duration of anesthesia increases (Beal et al, 2000). Cats heal differently than dogs. Sutured wounds in cats are only half as strong as similar wounds in dogs after 7 days of healing (Bohling et al, 2004). Cat wounds healing by secondary intention heal slower; produce less granulation tissue, which is more peripherally located; and heal more by contraction of wound edges than dogs (Bohling et al, 2004).

Wound Characteristics Affecting Wound Healing

Intact surfaces, such as periosteum, fascia, tendon, and nerve sheath, do not support granulation tissue, so when exposed these surfaces slow wound healing. Fenestration or drilling holes in exposed cortical bone may improve granulation by releasing osteogenic or other factors. Foreign material in wounds (e.g., dirt, debris, sutures, and surgical implants) can cause intense inflammatory reactions interfering with normal wound healing. Release of enzymes designed to degrade foreign bodies destroys wound matrix, prolongs inflammation, and delays the fibroblastic phase of tissue repair. Soil may contain infection, potentiating factors that inhibit antibiotics, leukocytes, and antibodies. Exposure of the wound to antiseptics delays healing and may predispose to infection. Warmth (30° C [86° F]) allows wounds to heal more quickly and with greater tensile strength than if they are at room temperature. A moist wound promotes recruitment of vital host defenses and cells, encouraging wound healing. Bandages help keep wounds warm and moist. Wounds (incisions) created with sharp surgical instruments heal faster and with less necrosis at the wound margin than those made with scissors, electroscalpels, or lasers. Wound infection interferes with the repair phase of healing. Contaminated tissues become infected if invasive bacteria multiply to 10^5 organisms per gram of tissue. Development of wound infection depends on the degree of tissue trauma, amount of foreign material present, delay between injury and treatment, and effectiveness of host defenses. Bacterial toxins and associated inflammatory infiltrates cause cell necrosis and vascular thrombosis. Wound exudates can separate tissue layers and further delay healing. Inflammation caused by infection further compromises vasculature, causing additional necrosis.

Healing depends on blood supply, which delivers oxygen and metabolic substrates to cells. Impairment of blood supply by trauma, tight bandages, or wound movement slows healing. Macrophages resist hypoxia, but epithelialization and fibroblastic protein synthesis are oxygen dependent. Collagen synthesis requires 20 mm Hg partial pressure of oxygen (Po_2). Hyperbaric oxygen therapy increases tissue oxygen and produces more rapid gains in wound strength. Accumulation of fluid in dead space delays healing because the hypoxic fluid environment of a seroma inhibits migration of reparative cells into wounds. Fluid mechanically prevents adhesion of flaps or grafts to the wound bed.

Recruitment, proliferation, and cellular function in wound healing are controlled by growth factors; proteins synthesized and released by cells involved in wound healing. Numerous growth factors have been identified, including platelet-derived growth factor, epidermal growth factor, fibroblast growth factor, and type-transforming growth factor. Platelet-derived growth factors are found in granules, whereas macrophages must be stimulated to synthesize and release growth factors.

Fibronectins are glycoproteins critical to wound healing. They stimulate cell attachment and migration and are found in soluble form in plasma and in insoluble form in connective tissue matrix. Macrophages, endothelium, fibroblasts, and epithelium synthesize and release fibronectin. Fibronectin in the coagulum probably assists initial migration of cellular elements (macrophages and epithelium) into wounds. It binds bacterial cell wall components, collagen, actin, thrombospondin, heparan sulfate, hyaluronic acid, fibrin, cell surface receptors, and other fibronectin molecules. Fibronectin may also be important in providing an early wound healing matrix and in interlinking cellular and matrix components during healing. Fibronectin in wounds declines as healing nears completion. Proteoglycans are also important in all phases of wound healing. The matrix during cell migration contains elevated concentrations of nonsulfated glycosaminoglycans (i.e., hyaluronate). As wound maturation progresses, more sulfated glycosaminoglycans (i.e., chondroitin sulfate and heparan sulfate) appear.

External Factors Affecting Wound Healing

Radiation therapy and some drugs delay wound healing. Corticosteroids depress all phases of wound healing and increase chances of infection. Vitamin A and anabolic steroids may reverse the effects of corticosteroids on wound healing. Antiinflammatory drugs suppress inflammation, but have little effect on wound strength. Aspirin may delay blood clotting. Some chemotherapeutic drugs (e.g., cyclophosphamide, methotrexate, and doxorubicin) inhibit wound healing. Radiation therapy can profoundly inhibit wound healing, de-

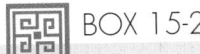

BOX 15-2

Fundamentals of Wound Management

Temporarily cover the wound to prevent further trauma and contamination.
Assess the traumatized animal and stabilize its condition.
Clip and aseptically prepare the area around the wound.
Culture the wound.
Débride dead tissue and remove foreign debris from the wound.
Lavage the wound thoroughly.
Provide wound drainage.
Promote healing by stabilizing and protecting the cleaned wound.
Perform appropriate wound closure.

pending on dose and time of exposure relative to the time of injury. It reduces the quantity of blood vessels, affects collagen maturation, and causes increased dermal fibrosis. Therefore chemotherapeutic drugs and radiation therapy should be avoided for 2 weeks after surgery. Vitamin A, vitamin E, and aloe vera may promote healing in irradiated wounds. Exposure to pico-tesla electromagnetic field treatment improves strength of sutured wounds and speeds contraction of open wounds in rats (Trostel et al, 2003). Hyperbaric oxygen therapy increases dissolved oxygen in plasma, which stimulates growth of new capillaries; therefore it may be useful for treatment of ischemic wounds. Ultrasonography and phototherapy (low-powered laser) shorten the inflammatory phase of healing and enhance release of factors that stimulate the proliferative stage of repair. Use of controlled subatmospheric pressure dressings helps remove interstitial fluid, which allows tissue decompression, helps remove tissue debris, and promotes wound healing (see p. 173).

MANAGEMENT OF OPEN OR SUPERFICIAL WOUNDS

Wounds should be covered with a clean, dry bandage immediately after injury or when the animal is brought for treatment to prevent further contamination and hemorrhage (Box 15-2). Life-threatening injuries should be treated and the animal's condition stabilized before further wound management is undertaken. When appropriate during stabilization, bandages should be removed and the wound assessed and classified as either contaminated or infected and as an abrasion, laceration, avulsion, puncture, crush, or burn wound. The "golden period" is the first 6 to 8 hours between wound contamination at injury and bacterial multiplication greater than 10^5 organisms per gram of tissue. A wound is classified as infected rather than contaminated when bacterial numbers exceed 10^5 organisms per gram of tissue. Infected wounds often are dirty and covered with a thick, viscous exudate.

Abrasions are superficial and involve destruction of varying depths of skin by friction from blunt trauma or shearing forces. Abrasions are sensitive to pressure or touch and bleed minimally. A laceration is created by tearing, which damages skin and underlying tissue. Lacerations may be superficial or deep and have irregular edges. Avulsion wounds are characterized by tearing of tissues from their attachments and creation of skin flaps. Avulsion injuries on limbs with extensive skin loss are called degloving injuries. A penetrating or puncture wound is created by a missile or sharp object, such as a knife, pellet, or tooth that damages tissue. Wound depth and width vary depending on the velocity and mass of the object creating the wound. The extent of tissue damage is directly proportional to missile velocity. Pieces of hair, skin, and debris can be embedded in wounds. Crush injuries can be a combination of other types of wounds with extensive damage and contusions to skin and deeper tissue. Burns may be partial- or full-thickness skin injuries caused by heat or chemicals (see p. 228).

Wounds less than 6 to 8 hours old with minimal trauma and contamination are treated by lavage, débridement, and primary closure. Generally, the sooner treatment begins, the better the prognosis. Penetrating wounds should not be primarily apposed without surgical exploration. Severely traumatized and contaminated wounds, wounds older than 6 to 8 hours, or infected wounds should be treated as open wounds to allow débridement and reduction of bacterial numbers. Most wounds are surgically apposed after infection has been controlled; however, some wounds heal by contraction and epithelialization (healing by secondary intention).

Often anesthesia is required for initial wound inspection and care. The objective of open wound care is to convert the open, contaminated wound into a surgically clean wound that can be closed. Aseptic technique, gentle tissue handling, and hemostasis are essential. Severely contaminated or infected wounds should be cultured after initial inspection. The area surrounding the wound should be widely clipped and prepped. The wound may be protected from clipped hair and detergents by applying a sterile, water-soluble lubricant (K-Y Jelly) or by placing saline-soaked sponges in the wound and covering with a sterile pad or towel. As an alternative, the wound may be temporarily closed with sutures, towel clamps, staples, or Michel clips. Hair may be clipped from the wound margin with scissors dipped in mineral oil to prevent hair from falling into the wound. Povidone-iodine or chlorhexidine gluconate skin scrubs are used to prepare clipped skin. The detergents in antiseptic scrubs cause irritation, toxicity, and pain in exposed tissue and may potentiate wound infection. Alcohol kills and fixes exposed tissue on contact and should be used only on intact skin.

Initial wound management begins with removal of gross contaminants and copious lavage using a warm, balanced electrolyte solution, sterile saline, or tap water (500 to 1000 ml) (Table 15-1). Sterile isotonic saline or a balanced electrolyte solution (lactated Ringer's solution) is the preferred lavage solution. Tap water is effective and less detrimental than distilled or sterile water, although it causes some hypotonic tissue damage (cellular and mitochondrial swelling). Wound lavage reduces bacterial numbers mechanically by loosening and flushing away bacteria and associated necrotic debris. Lavage may be facilitated by the use of noncytotoxic wound cleansers (e.g., Constant Clens; Kendall). Generally, these cleansers are applied to loosen debris and soften necrotic tissue during bandage changes; they act as a surfactant, disrupting the ionic bonding of particles and organisms to the wound and allowing them to be easily rinsed off with saline or balanced electrolyte solutions. Lavage following application, however, is not necessary. Antibiotics or antiseptics (e.g., chlorhexidine or povidone-iodine; see p. 169) in the lavage solution reduce bacterial numbers; however, these agents may damage tissue. Antiseptics have little effect on bacteria in established infections. Lavaging is preferred to scrubbing the wound with sponges. Sponges inflict tissue damage that impairs the wound's ability to resist infection and allows residual bacteria to elicit an inflammatory response.

Bacteria are effectively removed from the wound surface by high-pressure lavage using a 35- or 60-ml syringe and an 18-gauge needle, which generates approximately 7 to 8 psi of pressure. The syringe may be connected to a bag of fluid with a three-way stopcock and intravenous tubing to facilitate refilling. Higher pressure (70 psi), generated by pulsatile lavage instruments (i.e., Water Pik [Teledyne], Surgilav, or Pulsavac débridement system), is more effective in reducing bacterial numbers and removing foreign debris and necrotic tissue, but may drive bacteria and debris into loose tissue planes, damage underlying tissue, and reduce resistance to infection. Bulb syringes do not generate enough pressure to remove bacteria and debris adequately.

Débridement

Healing is delayed if necrotic tissue is left in the wound. Devitalized tissue is removed from the wound by débridement. Débridement involves removal of dead or damaged tissue, foreign bodies, and microorganisms that compromise local defense mechanisms and delay healing. The goal of débridement is to obtain fresh clean wound margins and wound bed for primary or delayed closure. Devitalized tissue is removed by surgical excision, autolytic mechanisms, enzymes, wet-dry bandages (see p. 186), or biosurgical methods. The extent of devitalized tissue usually is obvious within 48 hours of injury.

Surgical débridement. Devitalized tissue should be surgically excised in layers beginning at the surface and progressing to the depths of the wound. This can be done by sharp dissection, electrosurgery, or laser. Bones, tendons, nerves, and vessels must be preserved, but bone sequestra should be removed because they may prevent complete granulation of the wound (especially with metacarpal and metatarsal degloving injuries) and predispose the wound to infection. Muscle should be débrided until it bleeds and contracts with appropriate stimuli. Contaminated fat should be liberally excised because it is easily devascularized and harbors bacteria, but cutaneous vessels must be spared to maintain the viability of overlying skin. As an alternative, the entire wound can be excised *en bloc* if sufficient healthy tissue surrounds the wound and vital structures can be preserved. The danger of surgical débridement is removal of an excessive amount of possibly viable tissue. With penetrating wounds or punctures, it

TABLE 15-1

Suggested Wound Cleansers

CLEANSER	ADVANTAGE	DISADVANTAGE
Commercial cleansers: Constant Clens (best)	Surfactant breaks the bonds between foreign bodies and the wound surface Convenient	Most ionic surfactants and many non-ionic surfactants have been shown to be toxic to cells, delay wound healing, and inhibit the wound's defense mechanisms Expense
Tap water	Availability Inexpensive Ease of application	Hypotonic Cytotoxic trace elements Not antimicrobial
Balanced electrolyte solution: Lactated Ringer's solution (LRS) Normosol	Isotonic Least cytotoxic	Not antimicrobial
Normal (0.9%) solution	Isotonic	Slightly more acidic than LRS Not antimicrobial
0.05% Chlorhexidine (1 part stock solution to 40 parts sterile water or LRS) or (~25 ml stock solution per liter)	Wide antimicrobial spectrum Good residual activity Not inactivated by organic matter	Precipitates in electrolyte solutions More concentrated solutions are cytotoxic and may slow granulation tissue formation *Proteus, Pseudomonas,* and *Candida* are resistant Corneal toxicity
0.05% Chlorhexidine with Tris EDTA	Makes bacteria more susceptible to destruction by lysozymes, antiseptics, and antibiotics. Rapidly lyses *P. aeruginosa, E. coli,* and *Proteus vulgaris* Increases antimicrobial effectiveness approximately 1000 fold.	Precipitates in electrolyte solutions More concentrated solutions are cytotoxic and may slow granulation tissue formation Corneal toxicity
0.1% povidone-iodine (1 part stock to 100 parts LRS) or (~10 ml stock to 100 ml LRS)	Wide antimicrobial spectrum	Inactivated by organic matter Limited residual activity Cytotoxic at concentrations greater than 1% Contact hypersensitivity Thyroid disorders if absorbed

may be necessary to enlarge the wound to assess the extent of injury and allow débridement. Electrosurgery or a high-powered carbon dioxide laser can be as effective as sharp surgical débridement of devitalized tissue. They have the advantage of providing simultaneous hemostasis, which helps prevent débridement of normal tissue. Low-level laser therapy has been advocated to stimulate wound healing in chronic wounds by shortening the inflammatory phase and enhancing the release of factors that stimulate the proliferative stage of repair. Increased collagen deposition and endothelial cell, fibroblast, and myofibroblast proliferation are the most significant effects.

Surgical débridement of obviously devitalized tissue is often combined with autolytic débridement to remove surface contaminants and tissue of questionable viability. After surgical débridement, wounds often are treated as open wounds with hydrophilic dressings and bandages. Provision of adequate wound drainage and a viable vascular bed is important to wound healing. The wound should be closed when it appears healthy or when a bed of healthy granulation tissue has formed, unless wound closure by contraction and epithelialization is anticipated.

Autolytic débridement. Autolytic débridement is often preferred over surgical débridement in wounds with questionable tissue viability. Autolytic débridement is accomplished by maintaining a moist wound environment with hydrophilic, occlusive, or semiocclusive bandages (see pp. 176-188), which allow exudates or wound fluid with its endogenous enzymes and growth factors to remain in contact with the wound. Maintaining the enzymes in the wound allows significant débridement.

Enzymatic débridement. Enzymatic débriding agents are used as an adjunct to wound lavage and surgical débridement. They are beneficial in patients that are poor anesthetic risks or when surgical débridement may damage healthy tissue necessary for reconstruction. Enzymatic agents break down necrotic tissue and liquefy coagulum and bacterial biofilm, allowing better antibiotic contact with wounds and enhanced exposure for development of cellular and humoral immunity; they do not damage living tissue if used properly.

Burned skin, necrotic bone, and connective tissue are not digested by available enzymes. Enzymes must remain in contact with the wound for an adequate time to produce the desired effect. Local tissue irritation may occur with enzyme use. Granulex V (Bertek Pharmaceuticals, Research Triangle Park, N.C.) is an enzymatic débriding agent containing pancreatic trypsin, balsam of Peru, and castor oil. Trypsin débrides and liquefies protein, but can cause local inflammation and pyrogenic reactions; balsam of Peru stimulates capillary beds to increase wound circulation; castor oil improves epithelialization by reducing epithelial desiccation and cornification. Travase ointment (Flint Laboratories, Division of Travenol Laboratories, Deerfield, Ill.) contains *Bacillus subtilis* protease as a débriding enzyme. Preparation H (Whitehall Laboratories, New York, N.Y.) is a hemorrhoid medication that has traditionally been composed of a water-soluble live extract of yeast (brewer's yeast, *Saccharomyces cerevisiae*) sometimes used on granulating wounds. It stimulates oxygen consumption, angiogenesis, epithelialization, and collagen synthesis in wounds and has been called the wound respiratory factor. This live yeast cell derivative is recommended in wounds with healthy granulation tissue and in the proliferative phase of repair. Some formulations of Preparation H no longer have live yeast extracts. Collagenase (Santyl, Smith & Nephew, Largo, Fla.); papain-urea (Accuzyme, Healthpoint, Fort Worth, Tex.; Kovia, Stratus Pharmaceuticals, Inc, Kendall, Fla.); and papain, urea, and chlorophyllin (Ziox, Stratus Pharmaceuticals, Inc, Kendall, Fla.) are other effective enzymes often used to débride burn wounds.

Bandage débridement. Dressings that are allowed to dry on the wound, such as wet-to-dry bandages or dry-to-dry bandages, adhere to the wound surface and pull the debris and strip the superficial layers off the wound bed when removed. Débridement is nonselective with the removal of healthy tissue in addition to necrotic tissue and debris. This technique is inferior to enzymatic débridement with collagenase and fibrinolysin. Advances in veterinary wound management have made this technique outmoded and contraindicated, especially during the proliferative stage of wound healing.

Biosurgical débridement. Maggot therapy using greenbottle fly larvae (*Lucilia sericata*) débrides wounds as the maggots secrete proteolytic digestive enzymes into the wound. Sterile medicinal maggots (Monarch Laboratories, LLP, Irvine, Calif.) are bred specifically for biosurgery. A single maggot may consume up to 75 mg of necrotic tissue each day. They require an optimal temperature, an oxygen supply, and a moist wound. Maggot therapy is best suited to necrotic, infected, or chronic nonhealing wounds. The maggots remove necrotic tissue, disinfect the wound, and promote granulation tissue formation. Medicinal maggots are applied to the wound at a density of five to eight per square centimeter. A hole is cut into a self-adhesive hydrocolloid dressing that matches the wound dimensions. This dressing is applied to the wound to prevent the maggots from crawling onto intact skin and absorbs wound secretions. The dressing is covered to trap the maggots in the wound, changing absorbent layers as necessary. Maggots are usually applied for two 48-hour cycles each week.

ANTIBIOTICS

Selective use of antibiotics may help prevent or control integument infections after injury or surgery. Minimally or moderately contaminated wounds less than 6 to 8 hours old may be cleaned and closed or treated without antibiotics. Severely contaminated, crushed, and/or infected wounds or wounds older than 6 to 8 hours typically benefit from antibiotic therapy. Contaminated wounds and those with established infection should be cultured before antibiotics are given, and antibiotic selection should ultimately be based on culture and susceptibility testing. Ideally, quantitative bacterial counts should be performed before grafts or flaps are placed over granulating wounds. Reconstruction should be delayed if bacterial counts are greater than 10^5 organisms per gram of tissue.

Systemic antibiotics should be given if there is a high risk of bacteremia or disseminated infection. A broad-spectrum antibiotic should be administered while awaiting culture results. Antibiotic blood levels should be present at the time of surgery when antibiotics are used prophylactically for clean or clean contaminated procedures. Prophylactic antibiotics optimally are given intravenously when anesthesia is induced (see Chapter 10). Contamination occurring during surgery usually is limited to the patient's skin flora; therefore drugs effective against gram-positive skin flora, especially staphylococci (see p. 87), should be selected (e.g., 22 mg/kg cefazolin given intravenously).

TOPICAL WOUND MEDICATIONS
Topical Antimicrobials and Antibiotics

Antimicrobial agents and antibiotics eliminate or reduce the number of microorganisms in a wound that destroy tissue. Topical rather than systemic antibiotics are preferred for open wounds. Mildly or moderately contaminated wounds do not benefit from combined topical and systemic antibiotic therapy; however, combined therapy is advantageous in heavily contaminated wounds. Antibiotics applied within 1 to 3 hours of contamination often prevent infection. Benefits of topical drugs should outweigh their cytotoxic effects. Antibiotics used effectively as topical ointments or added to lavage solutions are penicillin, ampicillin, carbenicillin, tetracycline, kanamycin, neomycin, bacitracin, polymyxin, and cephalosporins. Once infection is established, topical and systemic antibiotics have no beneficial effect in preventing suppuration of wounds undergoing closure. Wound coagulum prevents topical antibiotics from reaching effective levels in tissues deep in the wound and also prevents systemic antibiotics from reaching superficial bacteria. These wounds must be débrided to allow antimicrobial access to bacteria.

Advantages of topical antibiotics over antiseptics in wound management include selective bacterial toxicity, efficacy in the presence of organic material, and combined efficacy with systemic antibiotics. Disadvantages include expense, narrower antimicrobial spectrum, potential for bacterial resistance, creation of "super infections," systemic or local toxicity, hypersensitivity, and increased nosocomial infections. Antibiotic solutions are preferable to ointments and powders. Ointments liberate antibiotics slowly and may be occlusive, promoting growth of anaerobic bacteria. Powders act as foreign bodies and should not be used.

Triple antibiotic ointment. Triple antibiotic ointment (bacitracin, neomycin, polymyxin) is effective against a broad spectrum of pathogenic bacteria commonly infecting superficial skin wounds. However, its efficacy against pseudomonads is poor. Zinc bacitracin is responsible for enhancing reepithelialization of wounds, but can retard wound contraction. Because these drugs are poorly absorbed, systemic toxicosis (nephrotoxicity, ototoxicity, neurotoxicity) is rare. The ointment is more effective for preventing infections than for treating them.

Silver sulfadiazine. Silver sulfadiazine in a 1% water-miscible cream (Silvadene, Hoechst Marion Roussel, Kansas City, Mo.) is effective against most gram-positive and gram-negative bacteria and most fungi. It also serves as an antimicrobial barrier, can penetrate necrotic tissue, and enhances wound epithelialization. It is the drug of choice to treat burn wounds. In vitro toxicity to human keratinocytes and fibroblasts and inhibition of polymorphonuclear cells and lymphocytes have been shown. These wound-retardant effects of silver sulfadiazine are reversed when it is combined with aloe vera. A slow-release hydrogel ointment or dressing is available (SilvaSorb, Medline Industries, Inc, Mundelein, Ill.; Silvadex SR, Royer Biomedical Inc, Frederick, Md.). Ointments remain effective for up to 3 days, whereas dressings may be left in place for 7 days. Only a small amount of silver is released slowly from its molecular lattice over a sustained period, reducing cytotoxic effects of ionic silver and making it nonstaining, nonirritating, and nonsensitizing while maintaining its antimicrobial effects. These products are also hydrophilic, helping to maintain a moist wound environment and absorbing exudates.

Nitrofurazone. Nitrofurazone (Furacin) has broad-spectrum antibacterial and hydrophilic properties. It has little effect against *Pseudomonas* spp. Its polyethylene base gives it hydrophilic properties, enabling it to draw body fluid from wound tissue, which helps dilute tenacious exudates so they can be absorbed into bandages. Nitrofurazone delays wound epithelialization. It loses some of its antibacterial effects in the presence of organic matter.

Gentamicin sulfate. Gentamicin sulfate is available as a 1% ointment or powder (Garamycin), but solutions are preferred. Products with an oil-in-water cream base slow wound contraction and epithelialization. It is especially effective in controlling gram-negative bacterial growth (*Pseudomonas* spp., *Escherichia coli*, Proteus organisms). It is often used before and after grafting and for wounds that have not responded to triple antibiotic ointment. Gentamicin in an oil-in-water cream base may initially inhibit wound contraction and epithelialization. However, gentamicin in an isotonic solution does not inhibit contraction; it promotes epithelialization.

Cefazolin. Cefazolin is an effective antimicrobial against gram-positive and some gram-negative organisms. Topical cefazolin (the combined systemic and topical dose should not exceed 22 mg/kg) provides high levels of antibiotic in wound fluid. The drug's minimum inhibitory concentration is prolonged in wounds when it is applied topically compared with systemic administration. Topically administered cefazolin is 95% bioavailable and rapidly absorbed; therefore systemic levels equal wound fluid levels within 1 hour.

Mafenide. Mafenide (hydrochloride or acetate) is a topical sulfa compound available as an aqueous spray. It has a spectrum against gram-negative bacteria, including *Pseudomonas* and *Clostridium*, and is particularly useful on severely contaminated wounds.

Other Topical Agents

Antiinflammatory agents are used to prevent progressive inflammatory damage. Topical steroids may inhibit epithelialization, wound contraction, and angiogenesis. Production of exuberant granulation tissue may be reduced by one or two applications of corticosteroids. Topical anesthetics may be used to reduce the animal's pain. Lidocaine or bupivacaine applied topically reduces traumatic and postoperative pain and may decrease the need for systemic analgesics. Hydrophilic agents cause diffusion of fluids through wound tissues to the surface or into the bandage. This dilutes the tenacious coagulum and debris on the wound surface and allows easier absorption. Copolymer flakes (Avalon Copolymer Flakes), dextranomer (Debrisan), and maltodextrin NF (Intracell) are hydrophilic agents that absorb tissue fluid with minimal tissue reaction. An organic acid combination of malic, benzoic, and salicylic acids (Derma Clens) enhances fluid absorption by devitalized tissue to promote its separation from wounds. Underlying healthy tissue is not damaged by acids, and the 2.8 pH discourages microbial growth. Hexamethyldisiloxane acrylate copolymer (No Sting Barrier Film) produces a uniform, transparent, colorless, fast-drying, noncytotoxic film that serves as a skin protectant type of dressing. Applied in a thin layer to clean, dry skin every third day, it allows inflammation to resolve quickly and prevents tape from causing epidermal striping and skin irritation. Hydroxyethylated amylopectin (Facilitator; Ridge Pharmaceuticals, Idexx Laboratories, Greensboro, N.C.) is a similar product used in place of a bandage on superficial lesions. This water-soluble product is placed in a thin layer (1 drop spread over 2 square inches) over the wound and allowed to dry. It reduces wound drying and itching and accelerates healing. Neither of these products should be used with other topicals as they may inhibit adherence of the film to the skin.

Aloe vera. Aloe vera gel is extracted from the aloe vera leaf and contains 75 potentially active constituents. Aloe vera has been used on burns because of its antibacterial activity against *Pseudomonas aeruginosa*. It also inhibits fungal growth. The antiprostaglandin and antithromboxane properties of aloe vera medications are beneficial in maintaining vascular patency and thus helping avert dermal ischemia.

Aloe vera medications may also stimulate fibroblastic replication. Aloe vera has the ability to penetrate and anesthetize tissue. Acemannan, a component of aloe vera extract gel, promotes wound healing (see later discussion). It is also found in other preparations. Allantoin, another component of aloe vera extract gel, stimulates tissue repair in suppurating wounds and resistant ulcers by promoting epithelial growth. Use on full-thickness wounds is discouraged because of its antiinflammatory effects. Aloe vera counteracts the inhibitory effects of silver sulfadiazine when the two are combined.

Acemannan. Acemannan (Carravet, Veterinary Products Laboratories, Phoenix, Ariz.; or Carrasorb, Carrington Laboratories, Irving, Tex.) is available as a topical wound hydrogel or a freeze-dried gel form. It is indicated for managing superficial and deep partial-thickness burns, lacerations, dermal ulcers, abrasions, and nonhealing wounds. Acemannan is a β-(1,4) acetylated mannan derived from the aloe vera plant that enhances early stages of healing. Acemannan stimulates macrophages to secrete interleukin-1 and tumor necrosis factor alpha, which enhance fibroblast proliferation, neovascularization, epidermal growth and motility, and collagen deposition to form granulation tissue. Acemannan may also bind growth factors, prolonging their stimulating effect on formation of granulation tissue. The freeze-dried form enhances healing over exposed bone and has hydrophilic properties, which help cleanse the wound and reduce wound edema. The most effective time to begin topical application is in the early inflammatory stage of healing, with daily application under a bandage continuing into the repair stage of healing. The greatest effects are seen in the first 7 days of application. Excess granulation tissue can occur, especially with the freeze-dried form, which inhibits wound contraction.

Tripeptide-copper complex. (glycyl-L-histidyl-lysine (L-phenylalanine) tripeptide- and tetrapeptide-copper complexes). This tripeptide-copper complex (Iamin-Vet Skin Care Gel, Covington, GA) stimulates wound healing and is a chemoattractant for mast cells, monocytes, and macrophages, which stimulate débridement, angiogenesis, collagen synthesis, and epithelialization. Copper is needed by enzymes involved in collagen cross-linking. The best time to begin tripeptide-copper complex application is the late inflammatory and early repair phases, with treatment continuing into later repair phase. It has been effective in accelerating wound healing in chronic, ischemic open wounds (Canapp et al, 2003). Its greatest effect is in the first 7 days of its use. Exuberant granulation tissue may be a problem with this agent.

D-glucose polysaccharide (Maltodextrin NF). Maltodextrin (Intracell, Macleod Pharmaceutical, Fort Collins, Colo.) is available in a hydrophilic powder or gel form containing 1% ascorbic acid for use on contaminated and infected wounds as a wound healing stimulant. It is reported to stimulate healing by supplying glucose for cell metabolism via hydrolysis of its polysaccharide component. Its hydrophilic property draws fluid through the tissue, keeping it moist. Maltodextrin is chemotactic and pulls neutrophils,

lymphocytes, and macrophages into the wound. Maltodextrin also has antibacterial and bacteriostatic properties. It reduces odor, exudates, swelling, and infection, and it may enhance early granulation tissue formation and epithelialization. After débridement and lavage, a 5- to 10-mm layer of maltodextrin is applied to the wound and covered with a bandage from the early inflammatory stage into the repair stage of healing. Daily bandage changes, lavage, and reapplication are recommended.

Honey and sugar. Honey is an old agent that has seen renewed interest. Proposed benefits include enhancing wound débridement, reducing edema and inflammation, promoting granulation tissue formation and epithelialization, and improving wound nutrition. It has an antibacterial effect through its enzymatic production of hydrogen peroxide from glucose, its hypertonicity, low pH, inhibin content, and other unidentified components. Honey increases collagen content, accelerates collagen maturation resulting from cross-linking, and maintains optimal pH conditions for fibroblast activity. Honey contains a wide range of amino acids, vitamins, and trace elements in addition to readily assimilable sugars that stimulate tissue growth. It also has a deodorizing effect. Not all honey is created equal and only medicinal honey is recommended for use (Medihoney, Medihoney Pty Ltd, Richlands, Australia, or raw sterilized Manuka honey, Summerglow Apiaries Ltd, Hamilton, N.Z.). Sugar has similar hypertonic effects, but does not have the inherent antiinflammatory and wound stimulation effects. Sugar is applied in a 1-cm-thick layer, and the wound is bandaged after débridement and lavage. Honey is applied by impregnating sterile gauze, which is then positioned on the wound and covered with a thick, absorbent bandage. Frequency of dressing changes depends on how rapidly the honey or sugar is diluted by exudates, varying from one to three times daily. They are indicated in the inflammatory and early repair phases of healing. These dressings are discontinued when débridement is complete, a healthy granulation bed is present, and epithelialization has begun. Honey has been used primarily on burn wounds. In one pig study, histopathologic findings showed that honey balm–treated burns entered the repair phase of healing 10 days sooner than those treated with silver sulfadiazine; wounds were moister and more elastic, and had less edema and reddening than those treated with saline or silver sulfadiazine (Kabala-Dzik et al, 2004). The scientific merit of related studies has been questioned.

Phenytoin. Phenytoin is an anticonvulsant prescribed for human epileptics. Used topically it seems to enhance healing without side effects (minimal systemic absorption) by enhancing gene expression of platelet-derived growth factor in macrophages and monocytes, and stimulating fibroblast proliferation and angiogenesis. It may also facilitate collagen deposition and maturation, decrease collagenase activity, and antagonize glucocorticoid activity. It acidifies the environment and increases blood supply, reducing bacterial numbers and promoting granulation tissue. The powder is applied to a clean, débrided wound and the area is bandaged.

Growth factors. Application of growth factors to stimulate more rapid healing has been investigated. Application of growth factors assumes the wound is deficient in specific growth factors. Knowing which factor is deficient in what amount at what time is nearly impossible in the complex healing process. Evidence indicates that applying single growth factors to wounds is not as effective as the combination of growth factors that the body produces. Allowing these factors to remain on the wound in the wound fluid under an occlusive or semiocclusive bandage is preferred to adding exogenous growth factors. A few growth factors are available commercially including recombinant human-derived platelet-derived growth factor (Regranex, Ortho-McNeil Pharmaceutical, South Raritan, N.J.) and equine recombinant growth hormone (Equigen, Pfizer Animal Health, Sydney, Australia).

Hydrolyzed bovine collagen. Hydrolyzed bovine collagen powder has hydrophilic properties. The moist environment created by the product is beneficial in stimulating early wound epithelialization. There is little histologic evidence of an inflammatory reaction in dogs. The collagen matrix provided serves as a lattice for ingrowth of fibroblasts, thus facilitating the repair phase of wound healing. It is probably most effective when used in the late inflammatory and early repair phases of healing.

Solcoseryl. Solcoseryl (Solco Basle Ltd, Birsfelden, Switzerland) is a protein-free dialysate and ultrafiltrate derived from calf blood with claims of improved healing. It stimulates fibroblast proliferation and migration and promotes differentiation of monocytes to macrophages. The inflammatory reaction is enhanced with subsequent migration and proliferation of fibroblasts. Use should occur in early stages of wound healing to stimulate the inflammatory response. After wound contraction slows and epithelialization predominates, application of this product should stop as it will inhibit epithelialization.

Ketanserin. Ketanserin (Vulketan gel, Janssen Animal Health, Beerse, Belgium) is a selective serotonin inhibitor that competitively antagonizes serotonin-induced vasoconstriction and platelet aggregation. It also antagonizes the serotonin-induced suppression of wound macrophages and thus allows a strong and effective inflammatory response within wounds. Efficacy is best in wounds with impaired circulation or at peripheral sites.

Bioactive glass. Bioactive glass is a novel treatment that stimulates an inflammatory reaction that is detected microscopically, without overt gross signs of inflammation. Intraincisional application or placement before wound closure increases early wound breaking strength.

WOUND CLEANSING SOLUTIONS

Wound cleansing solutions should have ideal antiseptic properties with minimal cytotoxicity. They are used primarily in the initial phases of wound management to decrease bacterial load and rid wounds of necrotic tissue and debris. Once the wound is clean, balanced electrolyte or physiologic saline solutions are ideal for cleansing it (see Table 15-1). Tap water is not an ideal wound cleanser, but is acceptable to initially remove dirt and debris when there is severe contamination. Tap water's hypotonicity causes cell swelling, which can cause significant cell destruction and delay wound healing with prolonged use. Antiseptic solutions are used early in wound management to reduce bacterial numbers and reduce chances of infection. They are contraindicated in clean wounds because all antiseptics have some cytotoxic effects and may do more harm than good.

Commercial Wound Cleansers

Read the label carefully when selecting a commercial wound cleanser; many are a combination of agents that are contraindicated for use in wounds because of cytotoxic effects. Some ingredients to avoid include hydrogen peroxide, sodium hypochlorite, and hydrochlorous acid. The cleansing activity of many of the available cleansers depends on a surfactant that breaks the bonds between foreign bodies and the wound surface. Most ionic surfactants and many nonionic surfactants are toxic to cells, delay wound healing, and inhibit the wound's defense mechanisms. An in vitro study done to compare the performance of some of the available commercial wound cleansers (e.g., Constant Clens, Shur-Clens, Saf-Clens, Cara-Klenz, and Ultra-Klenz) on human fibroblasts, red blood cells, and white blood cells concluded that Constant Clens (Kendall Co) was the most biocompatible (Rodeheaver, 2001).

Chlorhexidine Diacetate

The preferred wound lavage and wetting solution is 0.05% chlorhexidine diacetate because of its wide spectrum of antimicrobial activity and sustained residual activity. It has antibacterial activity in the presence of blood and other organic debris, has minimal systemic absorption and toxicity, and promotes rapid healing. A 0.05% solution is created by diluting one part of stock solution with 40 parts of sterile water. Chlorhexidine forms heavy precipitates in electrolyte solutions, but this neither delays wound healing nor interferes with antibacterial activity. More potent solutions may slow formation of granulation tissue with prolonged wound contact. Residual activity may last as long as 2 days, and effectiveness increases with repeat application. Potential drawbacks of chlorhexidine include resistance to *Proteus, Pseudomonas,* and *Candida,* and corneal toxicity.

Povidone-Iodine

A 1% or 0.1% povidone-iodine solution (10% stock solution diluted 1:10 or 1:100, respectively) is used frequently for wound lavage because of its wide spectrum of antimicrobial activity. Iodine compounds are active against vegetative and sporulated bacteria, fungi, viruses, protozoa, and yeasts. A 0.1% solution is recommended. This concentration kills bacteria within 15 seconds, and there is no known bacterial resistance. Povidone-iodine is a water-soluble, strongly acidic (pH 3.2) iodophor produced by combining molecular iodine with polyvinylpyrrolidone. Frequent reapplication (every 4 to 6 hours) is required when it is used as a wetting solution because residual activity lasts only 4 to 8 hours, and organic matter (i.e., blood and serous exudate) inactivates the free iodine in povidone-iodine. Iodine absorption through the skin and mucous membranes may cause excess systemic iodine concentrations and transient thyroid dysfunction. The low pH of povidone-iodine can cause or intensify metabolic acidosis when the solution is absorbed. Scrubbing wounds with povidone-iodine detergents damages tissue and potentiates infection. Contact hypersensitivities may occur in as many as 50% of dogs scrubbed with povidone-iodine compounds. Povidone-iodine at 0.5% is cytotoxic to fibroblasts.

Tris EDTA

Tris EDTA (disodium calcium salt of ethylenediamine tetraacetic acid buffered with tris [hydroxymethyl] aminomethane) added to lavage solutions increases permeability of gram-negative bacteria to extracellular solutes and leakage of intracellular solutes. Tris-EDTA solution is prepared by adding 1.2 g of EDTA and 6.05 g of tris to 1 L of sterile water. Sodium hydroxide is used to adjust the pH of the solution to 8, and the solution is mixed and autoclaved for 15 minutes. Treated bacteria are more susceptible to destruction by lysozymes, antiseptics, and antibiotics. Tris EDTA in sterile water rapidly lyses *P. aeruginosa*, *E. coli*, and *Proteus vulgaris*. The addition of tris EDTA to a 0.01% chlorhexidine gluconate solution increases antimicrobial effectiveness approximately 1000 fold. Antimicrobial synergism against *E. coli* occurs between tris EDTA and penicillin, oxytetracycline, and chloramphenicol. Similarly, tris EDTA and gentamicin, oxytetracycline, polymyxin B, nalidixic acid, or triple sulfonamide have synergistic activity against *P. vulgaris*.

Other Solutions

Acetic acid at 0.25% or 0.5% occasionally is used as a lavage solution. Its antibacterial effect is achieved by lowering wound pH. Wound acidification is beneficial in wounds that contain urea splitting organisms, such as *Pseudomonas* spp.; however, resistance to acetic acid may develop. Acetic acid is more cytotoxic to fibroblasts than bacteria. Hydrogen peroxide and Dakin's solution should not be used as wound lavage solutions. Hydrogen peroxide, even in low concentrations, damages tissue and is a poor antiseptic. It is an effective sporicide; therefore it may be beneficial if clostridial spores are suspected. Hydrogen peroxide dislodges bacteria and debris from wounds by effervescent action. Dakin's solution is a 0.5% solution of sodium hypochlorite (1:10 dilution of laundry bleach). It releases free chlorine and oxygen into tissue, killing bacteria and liquefying necrotic tissue. However, even at half or quarter strength, Dakin's solution is detrimental to neutrophils, fibroblasts, and endothelial cells and therefore should not be used as a wound lavage solution.

OTHER WOUND TREATMENT METHODS

Experimentally, pulsed electromagnetic field treatment of open wounds enhances wound epithelialization and may promote early wound contraction without adverse effects on perfusion or tensiometric, histologic, clinicopathologic, or electroencephalographic parameters. A pulsed electromagnetic field generates complex multiform pulses of oscillating electromagnetic fields in the ultra low–frequency range (0.5 to 18 Hz). Treatment for 60 minutes (magnetic field unit activated 20 minutes, deactivated 20 minutes, activated 20 minutes) was given twice daily for 21 days. A frequency of 0.5 Hz was used for the first 4 days, 3 Hz for 5 days, and 8 Hz for the last 13 days. Both ultrasonography and phototherapy delivered by low-intensity lasers shorten the inflammatory phase of healing and enhance release of factors stimulating the proliferative stage of repair. Exposure to pico-tesla electromagnetic field treatment improves the strength of sutured wounds and speeds contraction of open wounds in rats (Trostel et al, 2003).

ASSESSMENT OF SKIN VIABILITY

Skin circulation may deteriorate for 5 days after surgery because of edema and other factors. Skin viability is clinically assessed by color, warmth, pain sensation, and bleeding. Viability may also be assessed by dyes, transcutaneous oxygen or carbon dioxide, laser Doppler velocimetry, ultrasonic Doppler flow detection, and scintigraphy. Nonviable skin is black, bluish black, or white, and the area may be nonpliable, cool, and devoid of sensation. Normal skin is warm, pliable, and pink with normal capillary refill (difficult to assess) and pain sensation. Areas of questionable viability often are blue or purple, and capillary refill and sensation are poor.

Intravenous injection of vital stains fluorescein (10 mg/kg) or xylenol orange (90 mg/kg) has been used to assess vascular integrity of skin, but has not been better than visual observation. Transcutaneous oxygen (Po_2) or carbon dioxide (Po_2) monitoring allows immediate evaluation for ischemia, but requires prolonged, quiet recumbency, and transcutaneous oxygen or carbon dioxide sensors left in place longer than 3 hours may cause superficial burns. Skin generally survives if a transcutaneous Po_2 value of approximately 60 mm Hg is maintained. Transcutaneous Po_2 values of 30 to 60 mm Hg may be associated with partial or complete survival. Transcutaneous Pco_2 values are lower at the base of skin flaps (approximately 53 mm Hg) than at the apex (approximately 106 mm Hg), where ischemia is most apt to occur. Laser Doppler velocimetry is an indicator of capillary blood flux that may give an accurate assessment of local circulation. Probes must be placed away from major vessels to monitor relative blood flow, volume, and velocity, factors that vary with species, site, and instrumentation. Ultrasonic Doppler flow detection is a noninvasive, inexpensive means of determining blood flow and predicting viability in an area. Two sounds usually are heard with each arterial pulse, but only one sound is heard with proximal occlusion or stenosis. Areas of nonviable tissue may also be identified by evaluating the area with scintigraphy after injection of technetium 99m methylene diphosphate.

INTEGUMENTARY SURGERY

The fundamental surgical principles for reconstructive surgery are listed in Box 15-3. Incisions made with scalpel blades cause less tissue trauma than those made with scissors, electrosurgery, or lasers. The CO_2 laser is the best suited

BOX 15-3

Fundamental Surgical Principles for Reconstructive Surgery

- Use strict asepsis in preparation of surgical team, room, and instruments and during surgery.
- Handle tissue gently.
- Preserve vascularity.
- Remove necrotic tissue.
- Maintain hemostasis.
- Approximate tissue anatomically without tension.
- Obliterate dead space.
- Use appropriate suture materials and implants.

BOX 15-4

Predictive Major Risk Factors for Postoperative Surgical Site Infection

Increasing American Society of Anesthesiologists' preoperative assessment score ≥3
Increasing duration of anesthesia (~30% increase for each hour)
Increasing duration of surgery (doubles every 70–90 minutes)
Increasing number of persons in operating room (1.3 times higher/person)
Dirty classification of wound site
No preoperative or intraoperative antimicrobial prophylaxis (6–7 times more likely)
Increasing duration of postoperative intensive care stay (1.16 times for each additional day)
Wound drain (foreign materials reduce number of microorganisms required for infection by 10^4)
Increasing patient weight

Modified from Eugster S, Schawalder P, Gaschen F et al: A prospective study of postoperative surgical site infections in dogs and cats, *Vet Surg* 33:542-550, 2004.

laser for skin incisions; it creates wounds that hemorrhage minimally because vessels are sealed. Skin edges should be manipulated atraumatically using skin hooks or fine-tooth forceps. The deep or subdermal plexus must be preserved during dissection and excision to ensure skin survival. It is important to undermine at the level of the subcutaneous fat to prevent transection of the subdermal plexus. To prevent transecting the direct cutaneous arteries that supply the subdermal plexus, dissection should be performed under the cutaneous muscles (i.e., panniculus, preputialis, supramammarius, platysma, and sphincter colli muscles) or in the distal extremities in the deep dermal layer. Risk of infection after surgery is diminished by antimicrobial prophylaxis, but increased by several factors (Box 15-4) (Eugster et al, 2004).

Sutures

A suture acts as a foreign body in wounds. A buried suture greatly reduces the critical number of bacteria required to cause infection because the suture causes direct irritation,

harbors bacteria, and generates ischemic islands of tissue. The smallest and fewest sutures possible should be used to close a wound. Approximating sutures should be used to bring tissue edges into anatomic apposition. A 3-0 or 4-0 absorbable suture (e.g., polyglyconate, polydioxanone, poliglecaprone 25, glycomer 631, or polyglactin 910) with a swaged taper point needle should be used to close subcutaneous and subcuticular tissue. A 3-0 or 4-0 monofilament, nonabsorbable suture (e.g., nylon, polypropylene, or polybutester) with a reverse cutting needle is preferred for most skin sutures. Skin sutures should be placed at least 0.5 cm from the wound margins. Interrupted sutures are preferable to continuous skin sutures because continuous patterns lead to reduced microcirculation. Suture tension should just appose edges as loosely approximated wounds are stronger during the first 21 days.

Staplers

Skin stapler used to appose skin edges are less time consuming to place than sutures; however, it is more difficult to correctly align skin edges, and staples are less secure than sutures. Apply skin staples perpendicular to the incision after aligning and apposing the edges with thumb forceps; then apply moderate pressure before the trigger is compressed. Space staples approximately 6 mm apart. Recently, absorbable staples composed of polyglycolic-polylactic acid copolymers have been introduced for subcuticular closure and are meant to replace cutaneous closure by other methods (Fick et al, 2005). These staples are degraded by hydrolysis, losing 60% of their holding strength in 14 days and having a tissue half-life of 10 weeks. Subcuticular staples are applied after aligning the skin edges with forceps and then firing the stapler in the subcuticular tissue. Staples are spaced approximately 1 cm apart. Subcuticular staples incite less inflammation than subcuticular polyglactin 910 sutures or skin staples; therefore they have a less detrimental effect on wound healing (Fick et al, 2005).

Tissue Adhesives

Cyanoacrylate tissue adhesives may be used in selected procedures to facilitate skin closure or secure drains. They are often used to hold skin in apposition following onychectomy, tail docking, and ovariohysterectomy in population control programs. Adhesives allow a quick cosmetic closure with less risk of infection or scarring when used properly. Initial wound strength is less than sutured wounds (5-0 nylon), but strength at 5 to 7 days is equivalent or greater with adhesives. Sometimes skin sutures and adhesives are used together to reduce the number of sutures used. Of the nonabsorbable tissue adhesives, N-butyl or isobutyl-2 cyanoacrylates are preferred to propyl or methyl cyanoacrylates because they are less toxic. These adhesives should not be placed within the wound or incision but rather over the apposed surface to prevent foreign body reactions. An absorbable sterile methoxypropyl cyanoacrylate tissue adhesive is now available (Tissumend II Sterile, Innovative Products in Veterinary Medicine, Phoenix, Ariz.). It may be used externally and internally, with trials having been performed on lung, liver, spleen, kidney, and cornea. It has hemostatic properties, enhances healing, is nonreactive, and absorbs via hydrolysis in 60 to 90 days.

Fibrin tissue glues reduce hemorrhage when vessels are anastomosed, provide a barrier to microleakage, reduce suture line tension following intestinal anastomosis, and have an adhesive effect, improving tensile strength after skin edges are apposed with sutures. Two-component fibrin glues are mainly composed of bovine or human thrombin and concentrated fibrinogen, duplicating the final stages of the coagulation cascade.

Drains

Dead space allows seepage and accumulation of blood and serum in a warm moist environment that is ideal for bacterial proliferation. Dead space may be eliminated by layered wound closure when adequate tissue is available, by suture obliteration, by compression bandages, or by drainage. Leaving a wound open provides optimal drainage for an animal's injury. Implanting drains allows evacuation of potentially harmful fluids (e.g., blood, pus, and serum) from wounds and helps eliminate dead space. Drains often are necessary for treatment of bite wounds, lacerations, skin avulsions or separations, mastectomies, seromas, abscesses, and hygromas. Drains may help maintain contact between a flap or graft and its bed. Drains may be either passive or active. Passive drains (e.g., Penrose drains) depend on gravity for fluid evacuation, whereas active drains require a vacuum. Penrose drains are used most commonly to drain subcutaneous spaces. Active drains increase drain efficiency and reduce drain-related infection. They are especially useful in draining deep wounds and after grafting. Negative pressure can be applied to active drains intermittently or continuously; continuous suction reduces chances of drain occlusion with fibrin or blood clots and encourages tissue apposition. Active drains may be open, with an air vent into the wound, or closed. With vented drains (e.g., sump) there is a danger of retrograde contamination of particulate matter and bacteria passing through the air vent into the wound. Filtered vents reduce the risk of contamination. Closed active drains are preferable to Penrose drains (Fig. 15-1).

Penrose drains or passive tube drains should be used in clean wounds only if the exposed end and wound can be covered with a sterile compressive dressing or bandage. Superficial, passive drains should be secured to the skin at the dorsal aspect of the wound by direct visualization or blind suture placement. They should be exited through a stab incision at least 1 cm from the primary incision and positioned such that they allow maximum flow by gravity.

Many portable, closed suction systems are commercially available (e.g., Snyder Hemovac). An effective closed suction drain can easily be made using a butterfly catheter and an evacuated tube or syringe. The syringe adapter is removed from the plastic tubing, and the tube is fenestrated before the drain is placed in the wound. After wound closure, the needle is inserted into the evacuated tube (5 to 10 ml) to apply

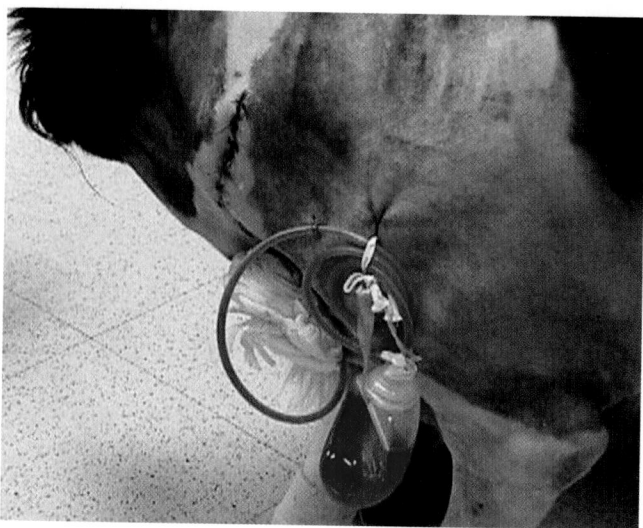

FIG. 15-1
A closed suction drain is being used to evacuate an abscess between the thoracic wall and scapula.

suction. As an alternative, the needle can be removed, the tube fenestrated, and the adapter attached to a syringe with suction applied. Active collection systems should be emptied frequently to maintain constant negative pressure. The collection reservoir is replaced or emptied when it loses negative pressure or fills with fluid. Most collection systems lose pressure as they become more than half full. Initial collection may simply remove air from the wound as the vacuum is established, and fluid drainage may not occur until several reservoir changes. The volume of fluid collected should be measured and recorded. For prolonged drainage, collection tubing (if possible) and reservoir should be changed every 48 to 72 hours.

The smallest diameter and fewest number of drains with the fewest number of exit holes should be used to prevent complications. Drains should not exit or lie directly under the primary incision. No part of the drain should be in contact with haired skin. Secure drains to the skin so they cannot be removed prematurely or allowed to retract into the wound. Drains should be protected with a bandage that is changed before "strike through" occurs. Strike through is the saturation of a bandage with fluid that wets both inner and outer surfaces. An Elizabethan collar or bucket can prevent self-inflicted drain or bandage damage. The animal should be kept in a clean, dry environment and have limited exercise. Tissue fragments, fibrin, or viscous exudates may cause drain malfunction. Drains are foreign bodies and cause drainage until removed. They should be removed when the discharge is serosanguineous and the volume has diminished to one fourth or more of the original drainage. Most wound drains can be removed after 2 to 5 days. Closed suction drains placed under grafts usually are removed after 48 to 72 hours, when drainage has diminished. Be careful when removing drains to prevent disrupting the skin–wound bed interface. Culturing the buried tip of the drain as it is removed allows monitoring for residual infection or development of nosocomial contamination or infection. Apply a bandage after drain removal to absorb any residual drainage and stabilize the wound site.

> NOTE: All drains should be protected by a bandage.

The major disadvantage of drains is that they serve as retrograde conduits for skin contaminants to enter the wound. Drains also impair tissue resistance to infection and may disrupt graft adherence. Drains made from latex incite more inflammatory reaction than those of Silastic or silicone. Drains reduce the number of microorganisms required to cause infection by 10,000 fold. To prevent incisional dehiscence and herniation, drains should not exit from primary incisions.

A new method of wound drainage using an open-cell foam and subatmospheric pressure has been described (V.A.C., Kinetic Concepts, Inc, San Antonio, Tex.). Medical-grade, open-cell, polyurethane ether foam dressing with pore sizes between 400 and 600 μm fitted with an evacuation tube is cut to the specific wound configuration and placed into the wound defect. Exposed viscera are covered with mesh and/or omentum, and major vessels with adjacent soft tissue, before the foam is positioned. The wound site is bandaged, and the tubing is connected to a collection reservoir. The reservoir is connected to a vacuum pump and subatmospheric pressure (125 mm Hg) is applied continuously or intermittently for cycles of approximately 5 minutes on and 2 minutes off. Continuous suction may be less painful and is often applied during the initial 48 hours of use. The foam is changed every 48 hours (except initially after grafting) to prevent tissue ingrowth, and the bandage is changed as necessary. Fluid is pulled from the wound, creating a moist environment and reducing local tissue swelling. Animal studies showed increased blood flow, increased rate of granulation tissue formation, more rapid reduction in numbers of microorganisms, and greater flap survival following application of this vacuum system (Morykwas et al, 1997). In addition, this system facilitates readhesion of degloved tissue, flaps, and grafts. Application of this technique has facilitated healing of chronic wounds, acute wounds, flaps, and grafts (Argenta and Morykwas, 1997). Complications may include pain, excessive ingrowth of granulation tissue, and visceral erosion.

Tourniquets

Tourniquets help control hemorrhage of distal extremities, improving visualization and reducing operating time. However, tourniquets should not be used on traumatized limbs or those with vascular injury or circulatory compromise. Pneumatic tourniquets with pressures below 300 mm Hg for less than 3 hours should be used. The limb should be elevated for about 5 minutes or exsanguinated with a rubber bandage before the tourniquet is applied. Exsanguination is contraindicated with local suppuration, deep venous thrombosis, or neoplasia. Pressure is more evenly applied if two or

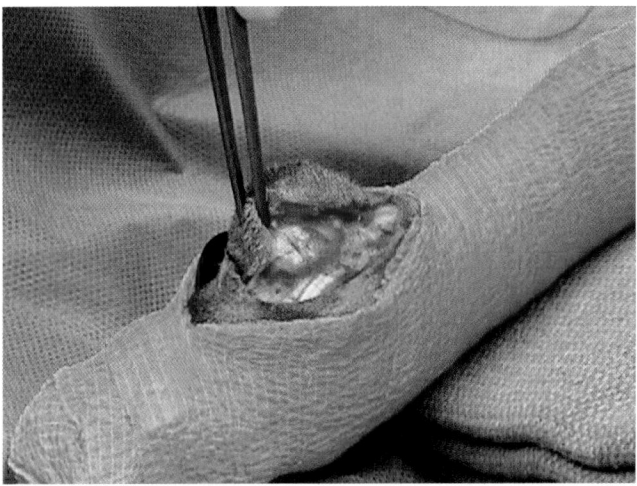

FIG. 15-2
Sterile elastic wrap may be used as a short-term tourniquet. An incision made in the elastic wrap allows access to the lesion for excision.

three layers of orthopedic padding are placed under the tourniquet. The tourniquet cuff should be applied at a point of maximum circumference, where nerves and blood vessels are protected against direct compression. Although of dubious value, releasing the tourniquet 10 minutes for every hour of inflation has been recommended. For a short-term tourniquet (as an alternative to or in combination with a pneumatic tourniquet), apply sterile elastic wrap (Vetrap). Apply it from the digits proximally without excess tension, and then incise it beginning at the toes to expose the surgical area (Fig. 15-2). Complications of tourniquet use are ischemia, hypoxia, or acidosis of local tissue; neurapraxia; and muscle damage.

WOUND CLOSURE

Wounds may be closed immediately (primary wound closure); within 1 to 3 days after injury, when they are free of infection but before granulation tissue has appeared (delayed primary wound closure); or after the formation of granulation tissue (secondary closure); or they may be allowed to contract and epithelialize (healing by secondary intention). Wounds closed in the presence of contamination, necrotic tissue, excessive tension, or dead space are apt to dehisce, often with the loss of additional tissue because of bacterial toxins and pressure necrosis. If there is any doubt whether a wound should be closed, it is best to leave it open. Factors that affect the decision to close wounds include the following:

1. *Amount of time that has elapsed since injury.* Wounds older than 6 to 8 hours are initially treated with bandages.
2. *Degree of contamination.* Obviously contaminated wounds should be thoroughly cleansed and initially treated with bandages.
3. *Amount of tissue damage.* Wounds with substantial tissue damage have reduced host defenses and are more likely to become infected; therefore they initially should be treated with bandages.

4. *Completeness of débridement.* Wounds should remain open if the initial débridement was conservative and if further débridement is necessary.
5. *Status of the wound's blood supply.* A wound with questionable blood supply should be observed until the extent of nonviable tissue is determined.
6. *The animal's health.* Animals unable to tolerate prolonged anesthesia are best treated with bandages until their health improves.
7. *Extent of tension or dead space.* If excessive tension or dead space is present, wounds should be bandaged to prevent dehiscence, fluid accumulation, infection, and delayed wound healing.
8. *Location of the wound.* Large wounds in some areas (e.g., limbs) are not amenable to closure.

Primary healing occurs with clean, incised wounds that are held together. Healing is initiated by movement of epithelial cells from the two edges of the wound toward the center that usually meet within 4 to 7 days of the incision. Primary wound closure is infrequently indicated following trauma. It should *only* be performed if less than 6 to 8 hours (within the golden period) have elapsed since injury; there is minimal tissue contamination, loss, or trauma; the wound is suitably cleaned by lavage and débridement; there is good hemostasis; and there is no tension or dead space. Traumatic wounds contaminated by feces, saliva, purulent exudate, or soil should not be closed primarily. *Delayed primary closure* is indicated for mildly contaminated, minimally traumatized wounds that require some cleansing and débridement or when the wound is older than 6 to 8 hours. Wounds are first lavaged and débrided to control local contamination or infection. These wounds should be treated with bandages after injury and before closure. Delayed primary closure allows staged débridement and maximum wound drainage. The wound should be surgically closed after bandaging and débridement for 3 to 5 days when it appears clean.

Lavage the wound with a balanced electrolyte solution or sterile saline to remove debris and reduce bacterial numbers (see p. 169). Next, thoroughly explore the wound. Anastomose transected tendons in clean wounds (see p. 69). Primarily appose large motor nerves that are transected sharply and cleanly; otherwise, delay nerve repair for 2 to 3 weeks until the wound has healed. If excessive dead space surrounds a wound, use Penrose or suction drains. Appose subcutaneous tissues with 3-0 or 4-0 buried interrupted or continuous approximating sutures (e.g., polydioxanone, polyglyconate, glycomer 631, or poliglecaprone 25). Bring the skin edges into apposition with buried walking sutures (see p. 197) or subcuticular sutures (e.g., 3-0 or 4-0 polydioxanone, polyglyconate, or poliglecaprone 25). Use approximating sutures in skin (e.g., 3-0 or 4-0 polypropylene, polybutester, or nylon).

Wounds with considerable tissue loss, contamination, or infection, or those older than 6 to 8 hours should be treated as open wounds. Initially, they should be lavaged, explored, and débrided. Tendons, ligaments, and vessels may be damaged beyond repair. Identifiable tendon ends should be tagged. Apply a hydrophilic bandage (see p. 176) that immobilizes the area and promotes formation of a healthy granulation bed. The wounds will initially begin healing by contraction and epithelialization and may heal completely (*healing by secondary intention*). Healing by secondary intention often is less expensive and results in normal-appearing skin if contraction is complete. Body wounds are more apt than leg wounds to completely close by secondary intention. Disadvantages of healing by secondary intention include contracture with disfigurement, incomplete healing, and fragile epithelial scars with large wounds. Alternatively, healthy wounds may be repaired by *secondary closure* or by use of a flap or graft. Secondary closure occurs at least 3 to 5 days after injury, after a healthy granulation bed has formed. Granulation tissue helps control infection in the wound and fills tissue defects. Secondary closure is appropriate when the wound is severely contaminated or traumatized; when epithelialization and contraction will not completely close the wound; or when healing by secondary intention is undesirable. Secondary closure involves resecting the granulation bed and skin margins, lavaging the wound, and apposing skin edges. Secondary closure also can be accomplished by resecting skin margins, débriding the surface of the healthy granulation bed, and apposing skin edges over the granulation tissue. Wound closure in the presence of granulation tissue is somewhat difficult because the tissue is thickened and not pliable. Excising the entire granulation bed gives a more cosmetic closure. If secondary closure is not possible, a flap or graft can be applied over the defect. After wound closure, an absorbent, nonadherent bandage should be applied to support the wound and absorb exudate. Bandages should be changed once or twice daily if a passive drain is used; if little drainage is expected and if drains are not used, once every 3 to 4 days may be adequate.

POSTOPERATIVE CARE AND ASSESSMENT

Postoperative wound care should optimize healing and be tailored to the type of wound. Wounds should be evaluated frequently for infection, tension, fluid accumulation, dehiscence, and necrosis. They may be evaluated visually and with ultrasonography, which helps detect and localize fluid accumulation. An ultrasound scan allows monitoring of wound depth and width and identifies blood clots, edematous regions, granulation tissue, scar tissue, epidermis, and eschar. Wounds should be protected with clean, dry bandages. Bandages act as a barrier against exogenous bacteria and support the wound during the first few days after surgery. Healing, sutured wounds become increasingly resistant to bacterial penetration. The patient and its environment should be kept clean, and adequate nutrition should be provided. Analgesics (see Chapter 13) and antibiotics (see Chapter 10) should be used postoperatively as necessary.

Infection may be suspected if the patient has fever, leukocytosis, anorexia, or depression or all of these. Although these abnormalities can be a normal response to stress and surgery and do not indicate infection, they generally are more exaggerated with infection than with nonseptic inflammation. If infection is suspected, samples should be collected for culture and cytology. If a surgical wound becomes infected, the sutures should be removed and the incision treated as an open wound with appropriate bandages (see p. 177). Topical or systemic antibiotics (see previous discussion) are used to control infection based on the results of susceptibility testing. The wound may be closed after the infection has resolved.

Sutures should be removed from wounds in 7 to 14 days, even though the wound has regained only 20% to 30% of its original strength. Scarring and infection associated with sutures are greater when sutures are left for longer periods. Most complications are prevented by using good surgical and wound management techniques. Potential complications include inflammation, edema, seroma and hematoma formation, drainage, infection, dehiscence, necrosis, granulomas, contracture, and failure to heal. *Seromas* are caused by excessive dead space or motion. They are prevented by closing dead space, using drains, and applying bandages to immobilize and support the wound. Seromas are treated by immobilizing the area and applying a pressure bandage. Large seromas may be drained, although this increases the risk of infection. Dehiscence may occur if tissue necrosis occurs; if sutures are placed too close to the margin; if tension exceeds suture strength; if sutures absorb too quickly; or if sutures strangulate and cut through tissue. Dehiscence may also occur secondary to self-trauma, infection, severe cough, hypoproteinemia, hypovolemia, or administration of drugs that interfere with healing. Wounds that dehisce may be allowed to heal by secondary intention or may be débrided and resutured. A *granuloma* is a chronic inflammatory process that may be caused by foreign material. Contracture or excess scar formation occurs most commonly at sites of motion (e.g., elbow or stifle) or body orifices. Contracture limits motion and may be disfiguring. Scar revision or excision is necessary when contracture interferes with activities. Wounds may fail to heal when the area is infected or has been irradiated or when the animal has received chemotherapy or is severely debilitated or malnourished.

References

Argenta LC, Morykwas MJ: Vacuum-assisted closure: A new method for wound control and treatment: Clinical experience, *Ann Plast Surg* 38:563, 1997.

Beal MW, Brown DC, Shofer FS: The effects of perioperative hypothermia and the duration of anesthesia on postoperative wound infection rate in clean wounds: a retrospective study, *Vet Surg* 29:123, 2000.

Bohling MW, Henderson RA, Swaim SF et al: Cutaneous wound healing in the cat: a macroscopic description and comparison with cutaneous wound healing in the dog, *Vet Surg* 33:579, 2004.

Canapp SO, Farese JP, Schultz GS et al: The effect of topical tripeptide-copper complex on healing of ischemic open wounds, *Vet Surg* 32:515, 2003.

Eugster S, Schawalder P, Gaschen F et al: A prospective study of postoperative surgical site infections in dogs and cats, *Vet Surg* 33:542-550, 2004.

Fick JL, Novo RE, Kirchhof N: Comparison of gross and histological tissue responses of skin incisions closed by use of absorbable subcuticular staples, cutaneous metal staples, and polyglactin 910 suture in pigs, *Am J Vet Res* 66:1975, 2005.

Kabala-Dzik A, Stojko R, Szaflarska-Stojko E et al: Influence of honey-balm on the rate of scar formation during experimental burn wound healing in pigs, *Bull Vet Inst Pulawy* 48:311, 2004.

Morykwas MJ, Argenta LC, Shelton-Brown EI et al: Vacuum-assisted closure: a new method for wound control and treatment. Animal studies and basic foundation, *Ann Plast Surg* 38:553, 1997.

Rodeheaver GT: Wound cleansing, wound irrigation, wound disinfection. In Krasner DL, Rodeheaver GT, Sibbald GR, editors: Chronic wound care: a clinical source book for healthcare professionals. Wayne, Pa, 2001, HMP Communications.

Trostel CT, McLaughlin RM, Lamberth JG et al: Effects of pico-tesla electromagnetic field treatment on wound healing in rats, *Am J Vet Res* 64:845, 2003.

Suggested Reading

Dart AJ, Dowling BA, Smith CL: Topical treatments in equine wound management, *Vet Clin Equine* 21:77, 2005.

Products described are useful in both equine and small animal wounds.

Diana A, Preziosi R, Guglielmini C et al: High-frequency ultrasonography of the skin of clinically normal dogs, *J Am Vet Med Assoc* 65:1625, 2004.

Evaluation of 26 normal dogs comparing ultrasonography and histopathology found that epidermis, dermis, and subcutaneous layers are distinguishable with ultrasonography.

Faria MCF, de Almeida FM, Serrao ML et al: Use of cyanoacrylate in skin closure for ovariohysterectomy in a population control programme, *J Feline Med Surg* 7:71, 2005.

Use of N-butyl cyanoacrylate tissue adhesive in 27 cats allowed quicker closure and similar healing when compared with 25 cats closed with simple interrupted nylon sutures.

Ferguson MWJ, O'Kane S: Scar-free healing: from embryonic mechanisms to adult therapeutic intervention, *Phil Trans R Soc Lond B* 359:839, 2004.

Experimentally subtle alterations in the ratio of growth factors present during adult wound healing can result in scar-free healing at an accelerated rate and without adverse effects.

Gillette RL, Swaim SF, Sartin EA et al: Effects of a bioactive glass on healing of closed wounds in dogs, *Am J Vet Res* 62:1149, 2001.

This study involving nine beagles with three matched bilateral skin incisions showed that bioactive glass caused increased histologic signs of inflammation and has the potential for increasing tissue strength.

Maiti SK, Hoque M, Kumar N et al: Sutureless closure of skin wounds, *Indian J Anim Sci* 74:470, 2004.

This study used goats to compare skin closure with silk, nylon, and n-butyl-2 cyanoacrylate.

Mathews KA, Binnington AG: Wound management using honey, *Compend Cont Educ Vet Pract* 24:53, 2002.

This article reviews the effects of honey on a wound and two cases in which it was used.

Mison MB, Steficek B, Lavagnino M et al: Comparison of the effects of CO_2 surgical laser and conventional surgical techniques on healing and wound tensile strength of skin flaps in the dog, *Vet Surg* 32:153, 2003.

Three pairs of identical skin flaps were made and evaluated for hemostasis, wound healing, and strength. Findings included better hemostasis, partial necrosis of wound edges, and more extensive inflammatory response with laser incisions making them more susceptible to complications, such as dehiscence.

Park W, Kim WH, Lee CH et al: Comparison of two fibrin glues in anastomoses and skin closure, *J Vet Med Assoc* 49:385, 2002.

These glues are found useful for hemostasis following vascular anastomosis or partial splenectomy and have an adhesive effect in the early stage of skin incision closure.

Rozaini MZ, Zuki ABZ, Noordin M et al: The effects of different types of honey on tensile strength evaluation of burn wound tissue handling, *Intern J Appl Res Vet Med* 2:290, 2004.

This experimental study on rats showed that skin treated with Manuka honey had the highest skin tensile strength when compared with similar control wounds and those treated with silver sulfadiazine cream and other honeys.

Sangwan V, Singh AP, Nagpal SK et al: Comparative evaluation of skin closure with tissue adhesive and subcuticular sutures in female dogs: a microscopic study, *Indian J Vet Surg* 25:86, 2004.

This study used catgut for subcuticular sutures and cyanoacrylate tissue adhesive; results showed similar healing with histologic and histochemical evaluation.

Seguin B, McDonald DE, Kent MS et al: Tolerance of cutaneous or mucosal flaps placed into a radiation therapy field in dogs, *Vet Surg* 34:214, 2005.

Twenty-six client owner dogs were evaluated to find that flaps that were part of a planned therapy had a better clinical outcome than those created to correct a complication or failure of radiation therapy.

Swaim SF, Hinkle SH, Bradley DM: Wound contraction: basic and clinical factors, *Compend Cont Educ Pract Vet* 23:20, 2001.

Principles of wound contraction are reviewed, and things that impede or improve contraction are discussed in this well-illustrated article.

Tan THH, Bell RJW, Dowling BA et al: Suture materials: composition and applications in veterinary wound repair, *Aust Vet J* 81:140, 2003.

This review includes useful charts listing properties and indications of commonly used suture materials.

Theoret CL: Growth factors in cutaneous wound repair, *Compend Cont Educ Pract Vet* 23:383, 2001.

This is an up-to-date review of the stages of wound healing and the interaction of cytokines and growth factors.

Zachos TA, Bertone AL: Growth factors and their potential therapeutic applications for healing of musculoskeletal and other connective tissues, *Am J Vet Res* 66:727, 2005.

This review concentrates primarily on bone, cartilage, and connective tissue healing and available products that influence healing.

BANDAGES

No single type of bandage provides the optimum environment for all wounds or for total healing of a particular wound. Bandages provide wound cleanliness, control the wound environment, reduce edema and hemorrhage, eliminate dead space, immobilize injured tissue, and minimize scar tissue. They also provide comfort, absorb and allow characterization of wound secretions, and give an aesthetic appearance. Bandages keep wounds warm, which improves

 BOX 15-5

Desirable Characteristics of Wound Dressings

Removes exudates and toxic components
Maintains high humidity at the wound-dressing interface
Allows gaseous exchange
Provides thermal insulation
Relieves pain
Protects from secondary infection
Protects from particulate or toxic contaminants
Allows dressing removal without wound trauma

 BOX 15-6

Hydrophilic Contact Layers

Hypertonic saline	Hydrogel
Calcium alginate	Hydrocolloid
Polyurethane foam	Some topical medications

wound healing and facilitates oxygen dissociation (Box 15-5). Covering wounds with a bandage promotes an acid environment at the wound surface by preventing carbon dioxide loss and absorbing ammonia produced by bacteria. An acid environment increases oxygen dissociation from hemoglobin and subsequently increases oxygen availability in wounds.

Bandages should be comfortable and clean. Uncomfortable bandages annoy patients, who may then mutilate the bandage or wound or both. Pressure should be applied over and distal to wounds, rather than proximal to them, to minimize venous or lymphatic compromise. When outer layers of a bandage become wet, bacteria readily pass from the outer surface and colonize wounds. Wounds bandaged with adherent or nonhydrophilic contact layers are generally unbandaged, inspected, and treated daily; however, wounds with excessive tissue damage, exudate, or established infection may require bandage changes twice or three times daily. Adherent bandages should be changed more frequently if the gauze is saturated with exudate and slides on the wound during bandage changes. Bandages applied over wounds with healthy granulation tissue and support bandages used to immobilize fractures may need changing only once every 2 to 4 days. Hydrophilic bandages (Box 15-6) are designed to be left on the wound for 3 to 7 days depending on the characteristics of the contact layer and the amount of exudate being produced. Analgesia or anesthesia may be required for initial bandage changes.

WOUND BANDAGING MATERIALS

Bandages have three basic layers: the contact dressing (i.e., primary layer), the intermediate (i.e., secondary layer), and the outer (i.e., tertiary) layer.

Contact (Primary) Layer

The contact layer touches the wound surface and should remain in contact with it during movement. It is used to débride tissue, deliver medication, transmit wound exudate, or

BOX 15-7

Factors in Contact Layer Selection

Phase of wound healing
Amount of exudates
Wound location and depth
Presence or absence of eschar
Amount of necrosis
Presence of infection

 BOX 15-8

Factors That May Affect Wound Contraction

Stimulate or Enhance	Inhibitors
Acemannan	Corticosteroids
Tripeptide copper complex	Silver sulfadiazine
Occlusive hydrogel dressings	Mafenide acetate
Equine amnion	Hydrocolloid dressings
Pulsed electromagnetic field radiation	Porcine small intestine submucosa
Adjustable horizontal mattress sutures	Thick skin grafts or flaps
Skin stretchers	

Modified from Swaim SF, Hinkle SH, Bradley DM: Wound contraction: basic and clinical factors, *Compend Cont Educ Pract Vet* 23: 20-34, 2001.

form an occlusive seal over the wound. The contact layer should minimize pain and prevent excess loss of body fluids (Boxes 15-5 through 15-8, Tables 15-2 and 15-3). It may be adherent or nonadherent, and occlusive or semiocclusive (Table 15-4). Adherent contact layers that stick to the wound surface are no longer recommended because wound débridement is nonselective, with normal healing tissue being damaged when the bandage is removed. Bleeding and pain also occur when they are removed. Nonadherent contact layers traditionally have been selected when granulation tissue has formed, but current wound care standards recommend use of hydrophilic nonadherent contact layers for all wounds. These products are very absorptive; they create a moist environment to facilitate healing and reduce the frequency of bandage changes (usually once every 3 to 7 days). Semiocclusive bandages allow air to penetrate and exudate to escape from the wound surface. They are the most commonly used bandages in veterinary medicine. Occlusive bandages are impermeable to air and fluid. They are used on less exudative wounds to keep tissue moist. Semiocclusive bandages are less likely to macerate adjacent normal tissue.

Dry adherent. This type of contact layer is no longer recommended. The disadvantages of a dry adherent contact layer are that it is painful to remove; viable cells may be removed with necrotic debris; and the wound may desiccate. In the past, a dry adherent contact layer was selected when the wound surface had loose necrotic tissue and foreign material or a large amount of low-viscosity exudate that did not aggregate. An absorbent, wide-mesh gauze was used without a cotton filler. Dry gauze absorbs exudate and adheres to necrotic tissue and debris. The bandage was removed after the primary layer had absorbed fluid and debris, and dried.

Wet adherent. This type of contact layer is no longer recommended, as débridement is nonselective, normal cells are damaged, and the wound is allowed to dry. In the past, a wet adherent contact layer was used when the wound surface had necrotic tissue, foreign matter, or a viscous exudate. Sterile, wide-mesh gauze soaked with saline was applied to the wound. A 0.05% solution of chlorhexidine diacetate (Nolvasan solution) was sometimes used as a wetting solution. The fluid diluted the exudate so that it could be absorbed by the intermediate layer of the bandage. Necrotic tissue and foreign material adhered to the gauze as it dried and was removed with the bandage. Wet bandages absorb faster than dry bandages and are more comfortable. Potential disadvantages of a

wet adherent contact layer are pain and tissue damage during bandage changes, bacterial proliferation, tissue maceration, and strike through (exudate absorption through outer bandage layer). Rewetting the dried dressing with warm saline facilitates removal and reduces pain during bandage changes.

Adherent film or skin sealant. Transparent liquids that are spread in a thin layer over the wound dry, creating a film or bandage that acts as a barrier between the skin or granulating wound and the external environment (see p. 167; Facilitator or No Sting Barrier Film). They are made from natural ingredients, primarily hetastarches and water. These films are generally permeable to water vapor and occlusive to bacteria and water. They are nonirritating and do not stain. They prevent skin irritation from exudates, urine, or feces contamination. They may be used alone over wounds or with a bandage. Reapplication is necessary every 3 to 4 days.

Nonadherent. Nonadherent contact layers do not stick to the wound surface, and most are semiocclusive. They are used to promote moist wound healing. Nonadherent contact layers retain moisture to promote epithelialization and prevent wound dehydration. They allow excess fluid to drain, preventing tissue maceration. Traditionally, wide-mesh gauze impregnated with petrolatum (Adaptic or Xeroform), polyethylene glycol (Furacin Dressing or Aquaphor), or petrolatum-based antibiotic ointment is used as the nonadherent contact layer when wounds have newly formed granulation tissue and some exudate, but are not epithelialized. Petrolatum gauze slows epithelialization. Polyethylene glycol is a hydrophilic, water-soluble substance that serves as the base of some ointments and prevents adherence and increases capillarity. Xeroform is a semiocclusive dressing composed of fine-mesh gauze impregnated with 3% bismuth tribromophenate and petrolatum. It allows egress of fluid and bacteria from wounds through the mesh. Fibrin from the wound bed causes temporary bonding of the dressing to wounds as the dressing dries. It is inexpensive and associated with low infection rates, but painful to remove.

TABLE 15-2

Guide to Dressings Based on Purpose

PURPOSE OF PRODUCT	SUGGESTED PRODUCTS
Cleanse wound	Noncytotoxic commercial cleanser; balanced electrolyte or saline solution
Absorb exudate	Absorption beads, pastes, powders, and pads: Alginates Foams Hydrocolloids Hydrogels Composite dressings
Autolytic débridement: Cover wound to allow endogenous enzymes in wound fluid to self-digest eschar and fibrinous slough	Same as above, plus transparent films
Chemically débride devitalized tissue	Enzymatic débridement agents: Granulex, live yeast Preparation-H
Add moisture to wound	Hydrogel Hypertonic saline dressing Medicinal honey
Maintain moist wound environment	Hydrophilic ointments Foam Hydrocolloids Hydrogels Transparent films
Fill dead space	Absorption beads, pastes, powders, and tapes: Alginates Hydrocolloid Hydrogel Foam
Reduce swelling to improve perfusion	Hypertonic saline
Prevent contamination	Biguanide-impregnated antimicrobial gauze Occlusive Semiocclusive
Reduce bacterial numbers	Biguanide-impregnated antimicrobial gauze Antibiotics
Cover and protect wound	Non-adherent, hydrophilic dressing with appropriate intermediate and outer bandage layers
Protect surrounding skin from moisture and trauma	Moisture barrier ointments Skin sealants Transparent film dressings Bandage
Reduce odor	Vapor-permeable film or polyurethane foam with activate charcoal

Epithelialization is rapid. Nonadherent dressing without petrolatum (a cotton nonadherent film dressing such as Telfa pads or a rayon-polyethylene dressing such as Release) should be used once epithelialization begins. These dressings do not adhere to the wound surface and cause minimal pain.

Another type of nonadherent contact layer is an *occlusive dressing.* Occlusive dressings are impermeable to air. They are used on healthy wounds with minimal exudation during the repair phase of healing. Occlusive dressings accelerate wound epithelialization and collagen synthesis by maintaining a moist wound environment. They require less frequent changes than other types of bandages. Some types of occlu-

sive dressings have a hydrocolloid, adhesive layer (Dermaheal or DuoDerm). Other occlusive, nonadherent contact layers include polyurethane films, hydrogels, and hydrophilic beads, flakes, powders, and pastes. Polyurethane films and hydrogels are transparent, expensive, and contraindicated in infected wounds. Polyurethane films are used on flat, granulating surfaces. Hydrophilic polymers rapidly absorb large amounts of wound fluid and are indicated for deep, granulating, and/or infected wounds.

New nonadherent contact layers are now available to facilitate moist wound healing through all phases of healing. These dressings control the wound environment and are sometimes referred to as *interactive dressings.* They are indi-

TABLE 15-3

Guide to Dressings Based on Wound

WOUND	OBJECTIVE	WOUND CHARACTERISTICS	DRESSING TO CONSIDER
Acute mild contamination and tissue damage	Hemostasis, débride, reduce contamination, provide moist environment	Hemorrhaging Less than 6–8 hr old	Calcium alginate Hydrogel, hydrocolloid
Acute moderate to severe contamination and tissue injury	Reduce contamination, débride Provide moist environment	Gross dirt and debris in wound; contusions, avulsions, ischemia and less than 6–8 hr	Hydrogel, hydrocolloid
Exposed muscle, fascia, subcutaneous tissue	Provide moist environment Encourage granulation	Clean wound	Calcium alginate, hydrogel
Necrotic	Promote débridement Provide moist environment Absorb exudates	Dry eschar or slough Excessive exudate and surface devitalized	Hypertonic saline or hydrogel Hydrogel or calcium alginate
Granular	Provide moist environment Encourage granulation	Irregular or incomplete granulation, minimal to moderate exudate	Calcium alginate, hydrogel
Need epithelialization	Provide moist environment to promote and protect resurfacing	Healthy granulation tissue: pink, smooth dry moist	Hydrogel sheet, hydrocolloid Foam

vidually designed to meet the different environmental stages found in the different phases of wound healing. No single dressing will produce the optimum microenvironment for all wounds or for all stages of wound healing on a single wound. The appropriate contact layer is selected based on the phase of wound healing, amount of exudate, wound location and depth, presence or absence of an eschar, and amount of necrosis or infection. Moist wound healing is promoted by incorporating hydrophilic materials that are placed on the wound bed or in the wound cavity. Hydrophilic dressings include hypertonic saline, calcium alginate, polyurethane foam, hydrogel, hydrocolloid, and some topical medications. Hydrophilic materials should not extend onto normal skin to prevent maceration of tissue adjacent to the wound. Barrier ointments or skin sealant adhesive films may be applied adjacent to the wound to prevent maceration if necessary. Some products with adhesive borders designed for people do not adhere around animal wounds well because of higher skin lipid concentrations and rapid hair regrowth. Most nonadherent, hydrophilic contact layers are highly absorbent, requiring bandage changing only every 3 to 7 days; this is sometimes difficult for veterinarians who are accustomed to changing bandages once or twice daily. Product costs are higher, but with fewer bandage changes, the overall cost is comparable to more frequently changed wet-dry bandages.

> NOTE: No single dressing will produce the optimum microenvironment for all wounds or for all stages of wound healing on a single wound.

Transparent vapor-permeable films. Transparent film dressings (e.g., OpSite, Tegaderm, Polyskin II, and Bioclusive) are thin, transparent moisture-retentive dressings made of polyurethane. They are comfortable, water resistant, and allow wound inspection without dressing removal. They are adhesive to dry skin but nonadhesive to wounds. They are semipermeable, transmitting oxygen, water vapor, and carbon dioxide but occlusive to water and bacteria (e.g., *Pseudomonas, Staphylococcus,* and *E. coli*). Drainage collects under the membrane. The moist environment accelerates healing. Uses include superficial or partial-thickness wounds with few or no exudates and dry necrotic eschars to provide a moist autolytic débridement. They are not used on infected or exudative wounds or thin, fragile skin. They may be used during the entire healing period. They are applied so they extend at least 2 cm beyond the wound margins. Applying a skin sealant on intact surrounding skin before dressing application helps prevent maceration and skin stripping. They do not adhere well to areas with skin folds or unshaved hair; they are better suited to people than animals. Adherence can be improved around the perimeter with vapor-permeable film spray.

Hypertonic saline. Curasalt (Tyco Health Care Kendall, Mansfield, Mass.) is a hypertonic saline dressing with 20% sodium chloride. Hypertonic saline dressings are indicated for infected, necrotic, and heavily exudative wounds and eschars. Eschars should be cross-hatched before application. Loosely woven gauze or umbilical tape is impregnated with hypertonic saline to make these dressings. They should be used in the inflammatory stages of healing during the first few days of wound care. Osmotic action desiccates bacteria

TABLE 15-4

Contact Layer Wound Dressings

TYPE	TRADE NAME	INDICATION	ACTION
Adherent Dressings			
Wet-dry	—	Inflammatory phase, high-viscosity exudate	Absorbs, débrides, hydrates, disrupts granulation tissue Change qd to tid
Dry-dry	—	Inflammatory phase, low-viscosity exudate	Absorbs, débrides, disrupts granulation tissue Change qd to tid
Antimicrobial sponge or roll gauze	Kerlix A.M. D. (Kendall)	All phases	Kills surface bacteria, prevents bacterial penetration of bandage
Hypertonic saline	Curasalt (Kendall)	Inflammatory and débridement phases Necrotic, infected, heavy exudates	Osmotic action desiccates bacteria and necrotic tissue Nonselective débridement Decreases edema, resulting in increased perfusion Change every 1–3 days, apply only once or twice
Adhesive Dressings			
Semipermeable films	OpSite (Smith & Nephew) Tegaderm (3M) Polyskin II (Kendall) Bioclusive (J & J)	Low- and high-exudate wounds with granulation tissue. Covering for sutured wounds	Adhesive sticks to skin around wound; may have a thin nonadherent contact layer. Creates a moist environment. Accelerates epithelialization; permeable to water vapor, but occlusive to bacteria and water Change every 1–3 days
Skin protectant films	No Sting Barrier Film (3M) Facilitator (Blue Ridge Pharmaceuticals)	Skin irritation, chronic wounds, burns, hot spots	Forms a film over surface. Protects skin from urine, feces, and tape; allows rapid healing Reapply every 3–4 days
Semiocclusive to Occlusive Nonadherent Dressings			
Calcium/calcium-sodium alginate (pad, ribbon, fiber)	Kaltostat (BritCair) Sorbsan (Steriseal) Tegagel (3M) Curasorb (Kendall) Curasorb ZN (with zinc) (Kendall)	Transition from inflammatory to repair phase, heavy exudate; burns; lacerations; incisions; biopsy	Pad forms a gel when absorbing exudate, which cleans the wound; it also is hemostatic and encourages epithelialization and granulation Do not use overexposed tendon, bone, or necrotic tissue Cover with semiocclusive pad Change every 5–7 days
Petroleum impregnated:	Jelonet (Smith & Nephew) Adaptic (J & J)	Early repair phase, viscous to sanguineous exudate	Increases wound contraction, absorbs bacteria and exudate, delays epithelialization Change every 1–3 days
With 0.5% chlorhexidine acetate	Bactigras (Smith & Nephew)		
With 3% bismuth tribromophenate	Xeroform (Sherwood Medical) Xerofoam (Kendall) Adaptic + Zerofoam (J & J)		

TABLE 15-4

Contact Layer Wound Dressings—cont'd

TYPE	TRADE NAME	INDICATION	ACTION
With 5% scarlet red	Scarlet Red (Sherwood)		Protects against contamination; stimulates epithelialization
Rayon/polyethylene glycol (sheets, gel) or cotton (pad) Perforated polyester film with cotton	Release Pads (J & J) Telfa Pads (Kendall)	Early to midrepair phase when epithelialization begins, sanguineous exudate to dry; sutured wounds; minor lacerations	Increases wound contraction, absorbs bacteria and exudate; may promote exuberant granulation Change every 1–3 days
Polyurethane film	Allevyn (Smith & Nephew) Tegaderm (3M) Polyskin II (Kendall) OpSite (Smith & Nephew)	All healing phases. Partial thickness injuries; wounds with granulation tissue and minimal exudate; may use as covering for hydrogel or hydrophilic pastes or powders	Increases epithelialization; may cause tissue maceration and bacterial proliferation Change every 1–3 days
Hydrocolloid (sheet, paste, powder; some are semiocclusive)	Granuflex (Convatec) Duoderm (Convatec) Tegasorb (3M) Comfeel (Coloplast) Dermaheal (Solvay) Nu-Derm (J & J)	Early repair phase; healthy granulation tissue bed with advanced wound contraction and little to moderate exudate; pressure sores; burns; cavity wounds; degloving	Increases epithelialization and comfort; adhesiveness may reduce contraction; use until granulation tissue fills wound; promotes granulation and may cause hypergranulation; gas permeable, but has water impermeable coating or is totally impermeable; if infection develops under dressing discontinue Change every 2–3 days
Hydrogel (mesh, paste, gel, sachets)	Curafil & Curagel (Kendall) Intrasite Gel (Smith & Nephew) BioDres (DVM Pharmaceuticals Geliperm (Geistlich) Carravet (Carrington Labs) Tegagel (3M) Nu-gel (J & J) Solugel (J & J)	Inflammatory, débridement, and repair phases; dry, sloughing, or necrotic wounds; abrasions; blisters; superficial wounds Use with minimal exudates	Absorbs fluid; keeps wound moist; permits autolytic débridement; increases collagenase activity in burns Discontinue when granulation tissue fills the wound; may promote exuberant granulation Promotes contraction Can use to deliver topicals: acemannan (Carravet), hyaluronic acid, chondroitin sulfate (Tegaderm), silver, and metronidazole Change bandage every 4–7 days
Particulate dextranomers; hydrophilic material (beads, flakes, powders, paste)	Alavon Copolymer Flakes (Summit Hill) Intracell (Technivet) Intrasite Cavity Filler (Smith & Nephew)	Deep granulating wounds or high exudate or transudate; donor sites; chronic ulcers	Absorbs fluid; keeps wound moist; may be chemotactic; accelerates epithelialization; inhibits anaerobic bacteria and removes organisms by capillary action; antimicrobials can be added Discontinue when healthy granulation develops or wound is dry Some biodegradable; rinse others from wound Replace every 1–3 days

Continued

TABLE 15-4

Contact Layer Wound Dressings —cont'd

TYPE	TRADE NAME	INDICATION	ACTION
Foam			
Polyurethane (liquid, sachet, pad)	Lyofoam (Seton) Allevyn Cavity (Smith & Nephew) Hydrasorb Foam Sponge (Kendall) Sof-Foam (J & J) Tielle (J & J)	Inflammatory or repair phase; deep wounds with little exudate; inguinal or axillary wounds	Absorbent; acts as a filler or stent; comfortable; may cause maceration Reduces granulation Promotes epithelialization and contraction Change every 3–7 days
Silicone Foam Also gel dressing	Cavi-Care (Smith & Nephew) CicaCare (Smith & Nephew) Silastic gel (Dow Corning)	Same as for polyurethane foam	Same as for polyurethane foam May prevent or reduce formation of exuberant granulation tissue
Biologic Dressings			
Amnion, peritoneum, grafts, cultured epithelium collagen dressings	Fibracol (J & J) Collasate (PRN) Collamend (VPL) Skin Temp (BioCore) FasCURE (Loveland)	Inflammatory to repair phase	Reduces pain, heat, water loss, and contamination; stimulates epithelialization, collagen synthesis, and granulation; increases contraction (amnion); reduces bacterial numbers; controls exudates Provides scaffold Experimental results are mixed
Porcine small intestinal submucosa (SIS)	Vet BioSIS (Cook Veterinary Products)		
Porcine bladder extracellular matrix	Acell (Acell Vet, Inc.)		
Silicone membrane and porcine collagen	Biobrane (UDL Laboratories, Inc.)	Early to midrepair phase when epithelialization begins, sanguineous exudate to dry; sutured wounds; minor lacerations	Increases wound contraction, absorbs bacteria and exudate; transparent and conforms, but may adhere
Miscellaneous Dressings			
Activated charcoal	Activate (3M) Actisorb (J & J)	Débridement to repair phase with severe infection	Adsorbs bacteria and reduces odor Provides moist wound healing Prevents formation of exuberant granulation
Iodine-containing slow release	Iodoflex (Smith & Nephew) Iodosord (Smith & Nephew) PRN Wound Dressing (PRN)	Early in inflammatory phase of repair; contaminated wounds	Decreases bacterial numbers; 1% available iodine; potential cytotoxicity
Silver impregnated	Silverlon (Argentum) Acticoat (Westaim Biomed) Actisorb (J & J) Aquacel AG (Convatec)	Inflammatory to repair phase with high bacterial load; burns	Reduces bacteria; strips facilitate drainage Change every 3–4 days
Maltodextrin: powder or gel	Intracell (Macleod Pharm)	Débridement; slow-healing wounds	Cleanses and promotes healing in contaminated and infected wounds; hydrophilic; chemotactic to WBCs; yields glucose to promote healing; antibacterial and bacteriostatic

and necrotic tissue, and reduces edema, resulting in improved perfusion. Débridement is nonselective, so use is limited to one or two applications. Bandages should be changed at least every 3 days to prevent saline dilution and dependent on the amount and character of the exudates. These dressings quickly convert a nasty, sloughing, and necrotic wound to a moderately exudating and granulating wound. They are used before placement of calcium alginate, hydrogel, or foam dressings.

Hydrogel. Hydrogels, or water polymer gels, are modified cross-linked polysaccharide formulations (gelatin or polysaccharide) available as gels, dry or hydrated sheets, or impregnated gauze. They are hydrophilic and swell when interacting with aqueous solutions; they will contain about 90% to 95% water when hydrated. Gels are moisture retentive, nonadherent, nonocclusive, and highly comfortable, giving a cool, soothing effect and some pain relief. They are highly absorptive, creating a moist wound environment that promotes débridement, granulation, and epithelialization. They are used to treat dry, sloughing, or necrotic wounds and abrasions, lacerations, burns, and minor skin irritations. They are very effective in hydrating a wound and they increase collagenase activity to facilitate autolytic débridement and promote granulation. Excessive granulation may occur. These products do not inhibit wound contraction. They may be used as a vehicle for antibiotics or other antimicrobials, including metronidazole, silver sulfadiazine, acemannan (Carravet, VPL, Phoenix, Ariz.; Carrasorb, Carrington Lab, Irving, Tex.), and hyaluronic and chondroitin sulfate (Tegaderm, 3M). Dressings should be cut to the size of the wound to prevent maceration of adjacent tissue and bandaged. Bandages are changed every 4 to 7 days.

Hydrocolloids. Hydrocolloids are biocompatible hydrophilic polymers, such as sodium carboxymethylcellulose or hydroxyethylcellulose with pectins and gelatin or embedded in an elastic mesh. They may be occlusive or semiocclusive adhesive pads (not to wound bed), pastes, or powders. Pads consist of an inner (often adhesive) layer of thick absorbing hydrocolloid, and an outer, thin, water-resistant, bacterial impervious, polyurethane film. They are flexible and highly absorbent, and adhere to both wet and dry tissue. Wound exudates are absorbed, and the hydrocolloid swells, forming a gel on the wound surface. The gel expands, filling the wound cavity, keeping it moist. Hydrocolloids maintain a moist wound environment, promote autolytic débridement, and insulate the wound bed. They increase epithelialization and comfort, but adhesiveness to surrounding tissue may reduce contraction and cause hypergranulation. Dressings are useful on partial- or full-thickness wounds with clean or necrotic bases, including pressure sores, minor burns, or granulating wounds with necrotic tissue. They are also used to hold other dressings in place. They are not intended for heavily exudative or infected wounds. Hydrocolloid pads should extend 2 cm beyond the wound onto normal skin that is protected with a skin sealant to prevent maceration if necessary. Cavitary wounds should be loosely packed with a filler agent to fill dead space before applying a hydrocolloid pad.

The hydrocolloid dissolves as it absorbs fluid, forming a yellow-colored fluid. Bandage changes are typically needed every 3 to 5 days; bandages are changed when exudates begin to leak or the dressing loosens. Wound inspection is difficult through the opaque pads. Use of these dressings should be discontinued if infection develops under them.

Some hydrocolloid dressings have an adhesive layer and are occlusive (Dermaheal or DuoDerm). The hydrocolloid adheres to skin around the wound, and the dressing over the wound interacts with the wound fluid to create a nonadherent, occlusive hydrocolloid gel. These dressings are used on wounds with an established granulation tissue bed, advanced contraction, minimal fluid production, and initial epithelialization. The wound should first be lavaged and dried. The hydrocolloid dressing then is warmed between the palms to make it soft and pliable. The dressing is cut to an appropriate size and shape to cover the wound, and the protective film is removed. The dressing is applied with light pressure until it adheres to the skin. Adherence is a problem in dogs and cats, but may be improved by clipping the hair adjacent to the wound. It may be necessary to apply a light intermediate and outer bandage layer to hold the hydrocolloid dressing in place over mobile areas. The dressing is removed after 2 to 3 days when the outer surface of the hydrocolloid feels like a fluid-filled blister or if leakage occurs. The gel is lavaged or wiped from the wound, and a new dressing is applied. Wounds dressed with hydrocolloid contact layers are less painful and epithelialize more rapidly than wounds covered by semiocclusive, nonadherent dressings; however, wound contraction is reduced. The dressings are not transparent, which makes wound monitoring difficult.

DuoDerm is an oxygen-impermeable dressing used to treat dermal ulcers, burns, abrasions, and graft donor sites. Its outer layer is polyurethane foam that is impermeable to oxygen and water; its inner layer is a hydrocolloid polymer complex that is occlusive and hydrophilic. Oxygen impermeability promotes the rate of epithelialization and collagen synthesis and lowers the pH of wound exudate, thereby potentially reducing bacterial counts. The dressing does not adhere to the wound bed and is comfortable. Fluid accumulates under the dressing. The dressing should be discontinued when epithelialization is complete.

Calcium alginate. Calcium alginates are nonocclusive, nonadhesive, hydrophilic, moisture-retaining dressings. They are classified as fibrous dextranomers. Calcium alginate products are derived from salts of alginic acid obtained from algae Phaeophyceae found in seaweed, forming pads, ropes, ribbons or packing whose fibers are either calcium sodium alginate or pure calcium alginate. Calcium alginate is used as a hemostatic agent for lacerations, postoperative wounds, donor sites, nasal sinuses, or dental alveoli; a formulation in combination with zinc improves this ability. It is used as a wound filler or dressing, which stimulates granulation in wounds after they have been débrided and absorbs exudate. Calcium alginate may also increase epithelialization. They are appropriate during the inflammatory or repair phases of healing for wounds with moderate-to-large amounts of exudates; application to dry or low exudative wounds allows them to adhere and is contraindicated. Ion exchange with the exudates causes a biodegradable viscous hydrogel to form on the surface of the wound; it absorbs up to 20 to 30 times its weight in wound fluid. The released calcium ions and a phospholipid surface promote the activation of prothrombin in the clotting cascade. Placement of calcium alginate dressings over exposed muscle, tendon, bone, or dry necrotic tissue is not recommended.

Apply to the wound and change the dressing from every day to once every 5 to 7 days. The pad can be premoistened if the wound is somewhat dry; lavage to loosen and replace with a hydrogel dressing if it adheres to the wound.

The gel forming on the surface is easily lavaged away.

Foams. Polyurethane foam dressings (e.g., Hydrosorb, Kendall, Massfield, MA) are highly absorbent, hydrophilic dressings with a nonadherent contact surface. Some have adhesive borders to adhere to normal adjacent skin. They are highly conforming, vapor permeable, and an effective barrier to bacterial penetration. They are designed to protect and cushion a variety of wounds, especially those in difficult areas. Products vary in conformability, permeability, and absorbency. They maintain a moist wound environment and support autolytic débridement. Their use is versatile, being appropriate for partial- or full-thickness wounds with small-to-moderate amounts of exudates, moist necrotic wounds, or clean granulating wounds. They promote epithelialization, are easy to apply, and the foam pads can be cut to fit the wound dimensions. The foam should be wetted with saline or medications if the wound is mildly exudative, or it can be used with another contact layer to prevent adherence. Dressing changes are recommended every 1 to 5 days depending on wound exudation. Also available are silicone foams (e.g., Cavi-Care, Smith & Nephew, Lhargo, FL), which are formed in situ and used for large cavity wounds. Components are mixed immediately before use. This produces a slightly exothermic reaction and over a period of 2 to 3 minutes the material expands to approximately four times its original volume. It becomes a soft, spongy foam conforming to the contours of the wound cavity. It is removed, rinsed, and repositioned in the wound twice daily and replaced weekly.

Antimicrobial gauze dressing: polyhexamethyl biguanide–impregnated dressing. Sterile gauze sponges impregnated with polyhexamethyl biguanide (Kerlix AMD sponge, Kendall) may be used alone or on top of another contact layer. Impregnated roll gauze is also available (Kerlix AMD roll, Kendall). Polyhexamethyl biguanide is a polymeric biguanide with antimicrobial action against gram-positive and gram-negative bacteria. Susceptibility to biguanides varies among bacterial species, with greater efficacy noted against gram-positive bacteria. Polyhexamethyl biguanide is rapidly bactericidal at high concentrations, causing disruption of bacterial cytoplasmic membranes with leakage and precipitation of cell contents. It is tissue compatible and does not have any apparent negative effects on wound healing. It is similar to chlorhexidine and is used in contact lens solutions, disinfectants, antiseptics, and other products to control bacterial growth. Dressings impregnated with polyhexamethyl biguanide resist bacterial colonization on wounds and have prolonged local activity. Environmental bacteria are inhibited from penetrating the bandage to gain access to the wound, and bacteria on the wound are inhibited from contaminating the environment. Both gauze sponges and rolls are available. Premoisten the gauze if it is used as a packing material.

Other antimicrobial dressings. Dressings impregnated with iodine, silver, activated charcoal, and antibiotics are also available to aid in the prevention and control of infection. Iodine is found in cross-linked polymerized dextran dressings. As the dressing hydrates in the moist wound environment, elemental iodine is released to exert an antibacterial effect and to interact with macrophages to produce TNF-α and IL-6. The slow release is designed to maintain adequate levels of active iodine for about 48 hours.

Silver chloride–coated nylon dressings (Silverlon, Argentum, Chicago, IL; Acticoat antimicrobial barrier, Westaim Biomedical, Exetor, NH; Actisorb Silver 220, Johnson & Johnson) release silver from the dressing over time to kill bacteria. Bacterial susceptibility includes *E. coli*, *Klebsiella pneumoniae*, *P. aeruginosa*, *Streptococcus* spp., and *Staphylococcus* spp. The rate of silver release varies with the product used. Wound packing strips are also available that will facilitate drainage while enhancing healing. Use these during the inflammatory to repair phases of wound healing. Moisten the dressing before application and change every 3 to 4 days.

Activated charcoal dressings (Activate, 3M, St. Paul, MN; Actisorb, Johnson & Johnson, New Brunswick, NJ) provide a moist wound healing environment, absorb bacteria, prevent exuberant granulation tissue formation, and may reduce wound odor. They are intended for heavily infected wounds during the débridement phase to the repair phase of wound healing.

Antibiotic-impregnated collagen sponges have been used in human surgery for some time. One product, Collatamp G (Schering Plough, Union, NJ), is made from denatured type 1 bovine collagen impregnated with gentamicin. In addition to its antibacterial effects, it exerts a hemostatic effect by causing the adhesion and aggregation of platelets and bridge proteins. High levels of antibiotic are released at the implant site, whereas serum levels remain below toxic levels.

Bioactive dressings. Bioactive dressings are composed of materials that originate from living tissue. Bioactive dressings include those derived from fibroblasts by tissue cell cultures, artificial skin derived from keratinocytes, and extracellular matrix dressing derived from the submucosal layers of the porcine small intestine or urinary bladder. Biologic dressings include skin grafts, amniotic membrane, and peritoneum. Collagen dressings are derived from bovine or swine material and rendered nonantigenic as a result of enzymatic purification. They are available in sheets, particles, pastes, or gels. They are believed to accelerate wound repair by the provision of a matrix for cellular migration. They are used most often on large avulsion wounds as a scaffold for tissue ingrowth. Extracellular matrix scaffolds have an angiogenic effect and recruit stem cells to migrate into the acellular scaffold to reconstruct and remodel severely damaged or missing tissue. Chitin, a polymeric N-acetyl-D-glucosamine, is a component of skeletal material of crustaceans and insects and found in fungi and bacterial cell walls. It has been prepared as an artificial type of skin. Other preparations include sponge, cotton, flake, and nonwoven fabric.

Biobrane is an expensive, temporary wound dressing composed of an ultrathin, semipermeable silicone membrane bonded to a flexible, knitted nylon fabric with pores. The two layers are covalently bonded to porcine collagen peptides to increase wound adherence. Biobrane is flexible and stretches to conform to the area. It is incorporated into the wound and therefore is comfortable. The wound can be seen through the dressing, and minimal fluid collects. The dressing is removed when epithelialization is complete or infection is detected. Biologic dressings may serve as contact layers on wounds with minimal exudate.

Intermediate (Secondary) Layer

The intermediate layer of a bandage is an absorbent layer that removes and stores deleterious agents (e.g., blood, serum, exudate, debris, bacteria, and enzymes) away from the wound surface. Bacterial growth is retarded if the bandage allows fluid evaporation and exudate becomes concentrated. The intermediate layer should have capillarity for absorption and should be thick enough to collect fluid. The intermediate layer also pads the wound from trauma, splints the wound to prevent movement, and holds the contact layer against the wound. Absorbent cotton, combine roll (Gamgee, 3M, St. Paul, MN), or cast padding (Specialist cast padding or Kerlix rolls) may be used. Enough pressure must be applied during application of this layer to eliminate spaces between the wound and contact layer, and between the contact layer and intermediate layer. Such spaces allow fluid to accumulate, which promotes tissue maceration; however, excessive compression impairs absorption and interferes with blood supply and wound contraction. The outer layers of the intermediate layer can be made nonabsorptive by applying petrolatum, which inhibits environmental fluid from reaching the wound.

Outer (Tertiary) Layer

The tertiary layer holds the other bandage layers in place and protects them from external contamination. Roll gauze (Conform Stretch Bandages, Kling, or Kerlix AMD), stockinette (Specialist tubular stockinette), surgical adhesive tape, or a reusable polypropylene dressing holder or spandex garment is used for the outer bandage layer. Surgical adhesive tape is most commonly used. Porous tape allows fluid evaporation and promotes dryness, but allows surface bacteria to contaminate the wound when it becomes wet. Conversely, wound bacteria can migrate through taped bandages and contaminate the environment. Using antimicrobial roll gauze (Kerlix AMD) to compress the intermediate bandage layer helps control bacteria on the wound surface and helps prevent environmental organisms from migrating through the bandage to the wound. Waterproof tape protects the wound from environmental fluids, but creates an occlusive bandage that may lead to tissue maceration. It should be used only in areas predisposed to getting wet (e.g., the feet), and it often is used in combination with porous tape. Elastic adhesive tapes (Elastikon porous adhesive tape or Vetrap) apply pressure, conform to the area, and immobilize it. Support rods or splints may be incorporated into the outer layer of the bandage if additional immobilization is required. Premade dressing holders (Tapeless Wound Care Products; Veterinary Sales and Marketing, Phoenix, Ariz.; www.vsmllc. com) may also be used to stabilize and protect intermediate and contact layers of the bandage. They are made of breathable, nonwoven polypropylene fabric and fixed in position with Velcro fasteners. They are nonadhesive, require no tape, and are reusable, washable, and nonconstrictive. Anatomically designed, they are available in different sizes for the hip, elbow or shoulder, head, abdomen, thorax, and legs. Spandex garments may also be used to protect bandages or serve as the outer bandage layer. Custom-made or modified garments, such as children's T-shirts, can be used to protect or replace the tertiary layer of bandages applied to the body or head. Elizabethan collars, side or body bars, and tape hobbles are used frequently to protect bandages from the patient.

TYPES OF BANDAGES

When applying bandages, appropriate materials of adequate width should be used to prevent a tourniquet effect. Porous materials allow air to circulate and moisture to escape. All bandages should be applied as smoothly as possible to prevent ridges and lumps, which may cause irritation and skin necrosis. Each turn of the bandage should overlap the previous turn by 50%. It is sometimes advantageous to unroll elastic tapes and allow them to relax before encircling a body part to prevent application of excessive pressure. Owners must be instructed on proper bandage care. Bandages should be evaluated frequently for signs of slippage or strike through. The surface of all bandages should be kept clean and dry. Patients should be observed for discomfort, swelling, hypothermia, skin discoloration, dryness, or odor, which may indicate that the area has been bandaged improperly. Bandages applied too tightly impair circulation and damage soft tissue. Digits should be exposed when extremity bandages are applied to allow sensation and circulation to be monitored. Loose bandages cause pressure sores or slippage. Patients should be restrained from chewing at the bandage, and exercise should be limited to short leash walks. When the patient is outside, bandages should be covered with a plastic bag or other waterproof material to protect them from dirt and moisture. The waterproof material should be removed within 30 minutes to prevent excess accumulation of moisture under the bandage.

Signs of pain, excessive licking or chewing at the bandage, and swelling may indicate a malfunctioning or malfitted bandage, which should be replaced to prevent serious complications. Bandages that apply too much or uneven pressure, especially over bony prominences, may lead to ischemia and pressure necrosis. If deep tissues are affected, amputation of a limb may be necessary. Skin grafting or flaps may be necessary to reconstruct more superficial injuries.

Absorbent Bandages

Absorbent bandages are indicated for open contaminated and infected wounds. Absorbed debris is removed from the wound surface to allow better healing. The contact layer is an absorbent hydrophilic material (see Boxes 15-6 through 15-8 and Tables 15-2 and 15-3) followed by an absorbent intermediate layer (Kerlix rolls) to hold the pad in place. The thickness of the intermediate absorbent wrap varies with the amount of expected drainage. An elastic contouring wrap (i.e., Conform Stretch Bandages or Kling) is placed over the absorbent wrap to conform the bandage and apply slight pressure. Adhesive or elastic tape is the final covering. Depending on the absorbency of the contact layer, bandage changes range from daily—or more often if strike through occurs—to once every 3 to 7 days.

Adherent Bandages

The types of adherent bandages are wet-dry, wet-wet, and dry-dry. These bandages have been replaced in favor of newer hydrophilic products that promote moist wound healing and selective débridement, and provide enormous absorbency.

Wet-dry. Wet-dry bandages are the most common type of adherent bandage used in veterinary medicine. Wet bandages assist débridement by liquefying coagulum and absorbing necrotic debris while leaving viable tissue intact. The principle of a wet saline bandage is that, as the sponges dry, wick action pulls debris and exudate into the sponge and away from the wound. Features of wet-dry bandages are that (1) antimicrobials can be used in the wetting solution; (2) a physiologic environment can be maintained; (3) comfort is maintained; and (4) exudate is removed. However, bacteria may flourish in a moist environment, and tissue maceration may occur. Most importantly, débridement is nonselective, normal healing tissue is damaged, and dressing removal is often painful. Topical antibiotics used in conjunction with a wet bandage should be in a water-soluble form and placed in the solution used to wet the sponges.

Place several layers of sterile gauze sponges over the wound and soak them with saline or a 0.05% to 0.1% chlorhexidine solution. Cover the wet sponges with an absorbent bandage. Change the bandage daily or more often if strike through occurs. To remove the primary layers of the bandage (dry gauze sponges), moisten the sponges with saline and lift them from the wound.

Removal of the primary bandage layer may cause bleeding or oozing. A nonadherent bandage generally is indicated after 3 to 5 days of wet-dry bandaging.

Wet-wet. A wet-wet bandage is similar to a wet-dry bandage except that the contact layer is expected to remain wet and is not allowed to dry before bandage removal. The bandage can be kept moist between bandage changes by inserting a fenestrated drain between layers of gauze and injecting fluid into the bandage every 4 to 6 hours. A wet-wet bandage is used to transport heat and enhance capillary movement of exudate from the wound. It creates a moist environment to help clean the wound, but has little débrid-

ing capacity. This type of bandage is used on wounds with large amounts of viscous exudate and little debris or necrotic tissue. The disadvantages of wet-wet bandages include increased management time, tissue maceration that promotes infection, and environmental contamination of the wound by bacteria if fluid reaches the bandage surface. After 3 to 5 days, a healthy granulation bed should have formed, and the wet-wet bandage is replaced with a nonadherent bandage.

Dry-dry. Dry-dry bandages are used on wounds with loose necrotic tissue and debris or a large amount of low-viscosity exudate.

Apply a dry, wide-mesh gauze to the wound, then an absorbent intermediate layer and tape. Leave the bandage in place until absorbed fluid and debris have dried in the intermediate layer.

Dry-dry bandages are painful to remove, viable cells may be dislodged with necrotic debris, and tissue may desiccate.

Nonadherent Bandages

Wet-dry, wet-wet, and dry-dry bandages should be replaced with nonadherent bandages. However, if used initially in wound management, they are exchanged for nonadherent bandages when drainage becomes serosanguineous and granulation tissue forms on the wound. The contact layer is a nonadherent pad (i.e., Release or Telfa) followed by an intermediate absorbent wrap (Kerlix rolls) to hold the pad in place. The thickness of the intermediate absorbent wrap varies with the amount of drainage expected.

Place an elastic contouring wrap (Conform Stretch Bandages or Kling) over the absorbent wrap to conform the bandage and apply slight pressure. Place adhesive tape as the final covering. Change the bandage every 1 to 3 days or as necessary.

Occlusive Bandages

Occlusive bandages allow wound fluid and normal body moisture to accumulate and prevent external fluid contamination of the wound. Bandages become occlusive when the outer layer is waterproof adhesive tape, rubber, or plastic. Another type of occlusive bandage is a hydrocolloid material that serves as a nonadherent contact layer (Dermaheal or DuoDerm) (see discussion of wound dressing materials, p. 176). Occlusive dressings are beneficial in speeding the rate and quality of healing in comparison with dressings that allow wound desiccation. However, wound contraction is reduced when hydrocolloid dressings that adhere to wound edges are used. Occlusive bandages are used to retain moisture over partial-thickness wounds without necrosis or infection. Maceration of normal skin surrounding the wound may be a problem.

Tie-Over Bandages

The contact and absorbent layers of a bandage can be held in place with a tie-over bandage when the wound is in an area inaccessible to standard bandaging techniques (e.g., the hip, shoulder, axilla, or perineum).

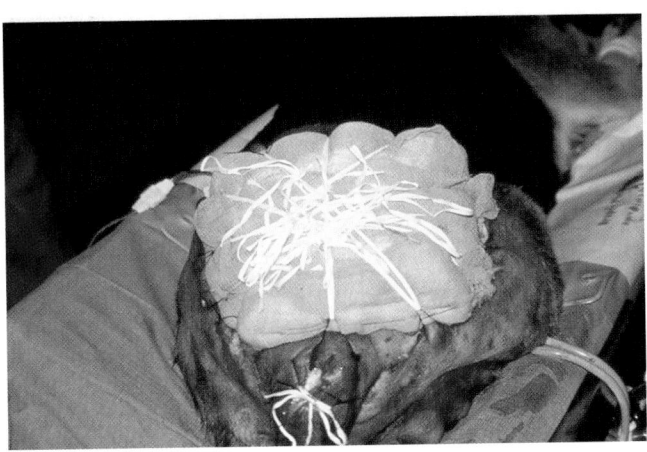

FIG. 15-3
Apply several sutures or skin staples with loose loops around the periphery of wounds to create a tie-over bandage in areas inaccessible to standard bandaging techniques. Apply the primary and secondary bandage layers, then hold the tertiary layer in position by lacing umbilical tape or heavy suture through the loose skin sutures or staples.

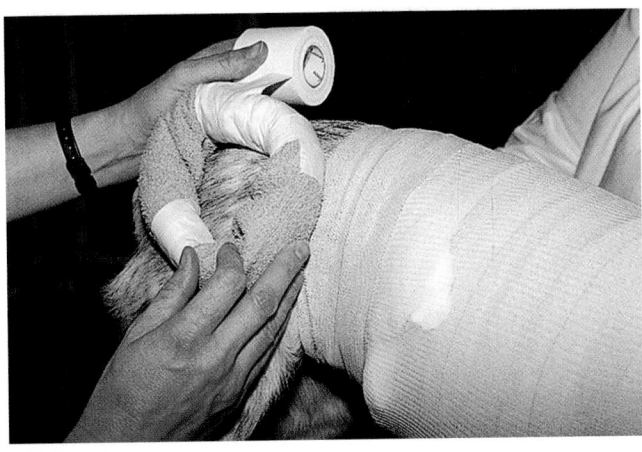

FIG. 15-4
Pressure relief bandage applied over the greater trochanter in a dog. The bandage is made from a firmly rolled towel that is cut, taped, and applied over the bony prominence.

Place several sutures (e.g., 2-0 nylon, 0 nylon, or polypropylene) in the skin surrounding the wound, tying them with a loose loop. Apply an adherent or nonadherent contact layer and an intermediate bandage layer on the wound. Hold these layers in place by lacing sterile gauze or umbilical tape through the loose skin sutures. As an alternative, staple long strands of suture 2 to 3 cm from the wound edges around the periphery of the wound, then tie or clamp these sutures over the bandage to hold it in place. Cover the area with an outer bandage layer if possible (Fig. 15-3).

Stabilizing Bandages

Stabilizing bandages help immobilize fractures to minimize further tissue damage during transport for definitive fracture fixation. These bandages are heavily padded and often are referred to as Robert Jones bandages (see p. 946 for application technique). After fracture fixation with splints, external fixators, or internal fixation, stabilizing bandages may be used to support injured tissue, reduce swelling, and treat open wounds. The type of wound and condition of the tissue determine the type of bandage applied to the wound.

Postoperative or Closed Wound Bandages

Bandages may be applied to areas without an open wound to absorb fluid from a drain or incision line, to support the incision, to compress dead space, to apply pressure, or to prevent trauma or contamination. These bandages improve the patient's comfort by supporting wounds.

Place a nonadherent, absorbent dressing over the incision line and several layers of wide-mesh, absorbent gauze over drains. Determine the thickness of the intermediate layer based on the amount of drainage expected. Be sure to use adequate padding over the end of the drain to prevent strike

through. Assess the character and amount of drainage with each bandage change.

Incisions expected to have minimal drainage may be protected from environmental contaminants with a nonadherent absorptive pad, which is incorporated into an adhesive polyurethane film dressing (e.g., Polyskin II or OpSite).

Pressure Bandages

Pressure bandages facilitate control of minor hemorrhage, edema, and excess granulation tissue. Direct application of a corticosteroid ointment to the wound may help control excess granulation tissue. The more convex the surface, the greater the pressure exerted by the dressing on the tissue.

Apply an absorbent, nonadherent contact layer over the area of hemorrhage or excess granulation tissue. Use a thick, absorbent intermediate layer and elastic adhesive tape for the outer bandage layer. Wrap the elastic tape carefully to prevent excess pressure, which can impair arterial, venous, and lymphatic circulation and cause tissue necrosis or nerve damage. Check for discomfort, swelling, hypothermia, dryness, or odor, which may indicate that the area has been bandaged too tightly. Remove the bandage within 24 to 48 hours if it was applied to control hemorrhage.

Pressure Relief Bandages

Bandages designed to prevent pressure over an area (usually a bony prominence) are used to treat or prevent pressure sores (see p. 238). Preventing pressure encourages healing over bony prominences. Most pressure relief bandages use a doughnut-shaped bandage, foam, or pipe insulation (Fig. 15-4) to distribute pressure around rather than over the wound. The bandage should be large and thick enough to prevent pressure over the bony prominence. A circular opening may be created in the bandage and used to treat the wound without removing the entire bandage.

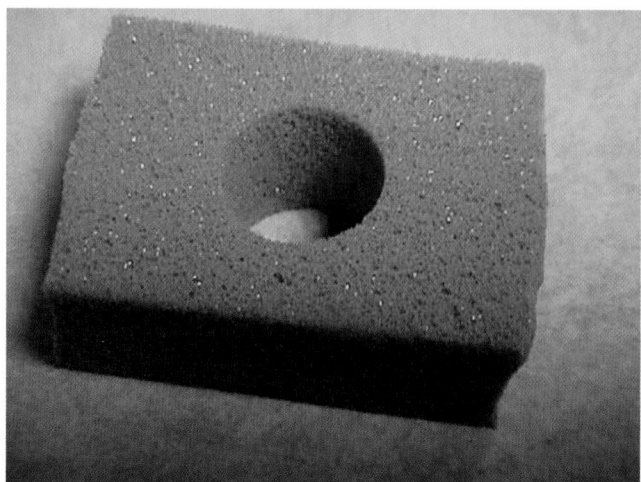

FIG. 15-5
A hole has been cut through this foam sponge (Temperfoam; HiTech Foam, Lincoln, Neb.) to distribute pressure around a pressure sore or wound.

A doughnut-shaped bandage may be created from cast padding, medium-density foam sponge (Temperfoam, HiTech Foam, Lincoln, Neb.) or a towel (Figs. 15-4 and 15-5). Create a doughnut- shaped bandage by rolling a towel or cloth into a tight cylinder, securely taping it to maintain the roll, and forming it into an appropriately sized circle. Create a doughnut-shaped bandage from cast padding by folding several layers together and cutting a hole in the center to accommodate the bony prominence or to surround the wound. Create a doughnut opening in thick foam by cutting a hole in the center to accommodate the bony prominence or to surround the wound. Center the doughnut-shaped bandage over the lesion or bony prominence and secure it to the skin with tape so that it does not slip.

These bandages may be difficult to maintain in position, and taping directly to the skin may cause skin irritation. Pipe insulation bandages usually are used to protect the olecranon.

Create bandages from foam rubber pipe insulation tubes by splitting the tube and cutting a hole where the bony prominence will lie. If necessary, use two or three thicknesses of pipe. Stack and tape the pieces of pipe together. When using the bandage over the olecranon, first pad the cranial surface of the radiohumeral joint with cast padding to prevent joint flexion and to keep the dog from lying in sternal recumbency. Then tape the cast padding and pipe insulation in place. Use a spica type of bandage (see discussion on bandaging extremities, p. 189) if necessary to hold the bandage in position. When using the doughnut to redistribute pressure from a wound, first apply the contact and intermediate layers of the bandage, then incorporate the doughnut in the outer bandage layer.

BANDAGING TECHNIQUES
Bandaging the Thorax and Abdomen

The thorax and abdomen often are bandaged to cover wounds, surgical incisions, or drainage devices. These bandages should be applied firmly, but without constricting the chest or abdomen. Abdominal pressure bandages occasionally are used when abdominal hemorrhage is suspected. Their effectiveness lasts only 1 to 2 hours, and they should be removed within 4 hours. When placing an abdominal pressure bandage, bandage layers should be applied firmly. A rolled towel can be placed along the midline to reinforce the bandage before tape is applied.

Apply a nonadherent contact layer over the incision or wound. Place several layers of sterile gauze sponges (Kerlix AMD) over the end of Penrose drains. Hold the contact layer in position with combine rolls, cast padding, or cotton. Use padding, gauze, and tape rolls 3 to 6 inches wide. Wrap the padding circumferentially around the torso with slight pressure. Overlap each wrap by approximately one half to one third the width of the roll. Increase the thickness of the intermediate layer with increasing amounts of expected drainage. Reduce rostral or caudal slipping of the bandage by wrapping the intermediate and outer bandage layers between the legs and over the shoulders or hips in a crisscross fashion. Encircle the torso with one wrap of bandage material, then direct the bandage from the right inguinal area (axillary area) to the left perineal area (shoulder area). Encircle the torso again and continue across the right perineal area (shoulder area), through the left inguinal area (axillary area), to the left flank (thorax). Repeat the crisscross pattern several times. Also reduce slippage by adhering ½ to 1 inch of tape to the hair. Do not wrap the bandage so tightly that thoracic expansion is inhibited. Hold the intermediate layer in place with elastic gauze (Kling) or stockinette. Cut a length of stockinette (3 inches for cats and small dogs; 4 to 6 inches for medium and large dogs) slightly longer than the length of the body from head to rump. Cut small holes in the stockinette to accommodate the legs. Place the stockinette over the head, and pull the front legs through the leg holes before rolling the stockinette caudally. Pull the hind legs through the leg holes. Secure the bandage with tape. Alternately the bandage can be secured with a premade reusable bandage holder (Tapeless Wound Care Products, Veterinary Sales and Marketing, Phoenix, Ariz.; www. vsmllc.com). In male dogs, cut a hole in the bandage to accommodate the prepuce or divert urine with a catheter to keep the bandage dry. During bandaging, manipulate the ends of the tube drains so that they can be easily accessed for aspiration or infusion.

Bandaging the Head

Most head bandages are placed to protect an ear that has been traumatized or has surgical incisions. Similar bandages can be used to cover the eye. Head bandages may interfere with breathing if they are applied too snugly or with neck flexion. A properly applied bandage should allow insertion of the fingers between the bandage and chin to allow room for neck flexion without airway obstruction. If the bandage is too tight, an incision can be made partway across the bandage under the chin. Leaving one ear out of the bandage helps to keep the bandage from sliding. Extreme caution should be used when removing the bandage to prevent laceration or amputation of the pinna.

Apply 1-inch porous tape directly to the edge of the pinna to form a stirrup (see Figure 17-22 on p. 311). Fold the ear over an absorbent pad or gauze sponges onto the dorsum of the head, and wrap the tape around the head to secure the ear in position. Using a similar technique, pad and place the opposite pinna over the first pinna if indicated. Place a nonadherent contact layer over an incision or place gauze sponges over the end of a passive drain. Hold the pinna and contact layers in position with 2- to 3-inch cast padding or cotton roll. Encircle the head, passing the rolls of bandage material cranial and caudal to the opposite ear unless both ears are immobilized. Starting under the chin, wrap loosely and overlap each wrap by approximately one third the width of the roll. Cover this intermediate bandage layer with overlapping wraps of elastic gauze or stockinette. To prevent slippage, secure the bandage in position with elastic tape attached to the skin and hair at the cranial and caudal edges of the bandage. Alternately the bandage can be secured with a premade reusable bandage holder (Tapeless Wound Care Products, Veterinary Sales and Marketing, Phoenix, Ariz.; www.vsmllc.com). During bandaging, manipulate the ends of the tube drains so that they can be easily accessed for aspiration or infusion. If it will be necessary to medicate the ear, cut holes in the bandaging over the external acoustic meatus.

Bandaging the Extremities

A soft padded extremity bandage is used to cover abrasions, lacerations, or incisions and can be modified to accommodate splints for joint or bone immobilization. Modifications of the basic padded bandage may be necessary to allow immobilization, prevent slippage, or protect digits. Immobilization is accomplished by placing a spoon splint, molded thermoplastic splint, fiberglass splint, or aluminum rods between the intermediate and outer bandage layers. These materials may sometimes replace the outer layer. It is important to ensure adequate padding at the ends of the splint material to prevent skin irritation. Placing additional padding over possible pressure points under a splint or bandage increases the pressure on these points when compressed; therefore it is better to use a doughnut pad to redistribute the pressure to a larger area surrounding the pressure point (see Figs. 15-4 and 15-5).

Begin by applying a 1-inch porous tape stirrup to the dorsal and ventral or medial and lateral surfaces of the paw (Fig. 15-6, A). Extend stirrups 3 to 8 inches beyond the digits to help prevent the bandage from slipping distally. If necessary,

use a loose layer of elastic gauze to help secure the stirrups. Insert small pledgets of cotton or other absorbent material between the digits and the metatarsal-metacarpal pads and digital pads. Apply an appropriate contact layer over the wound (see p. 176). Snugly apply cast padding around the paw beginning at the level of the second and fifth digital pads. Wrap obliquely so that the third and fourth digits protrude slightly beyond the bandage (Fig. 15-6, B). Overlap the cast padding (2 to 3 inch width) one half to two thirds of its width as it is advanced up the leg. Continue the bandage to the proximal radius and ulna (tibia and fibula) or above the elbow (stifle), depending on the site of the injury. Use enough padding to create the bulkiness necessary for protection. Snugly wrap elastic gauze (2 to 3 inch width) over the cast padding to conform the padding to the limb, overlapping each turn by one half the width of the material. Separate the tape stirrups and attach them to their respective sides of the bandage (Fig. 15-6, C). Apply an outer layer of elastic tape (2 to 3 inch width), overlapping one half the width with each turn (Fig. 15-6, D). Alternately the bandage can be secured with a premade reusable bandage holder (Tapeless Wound Care Products, Veterinary Sales and Marketing, Phoenix, Ariz.; www.vsmllc.com). Avoid overstretching the tape to prevent compromising limb circulation. Check exposed digits three and four frequently for swelling, coolness, and discomfort; remove the bandage and evaluate the limb if these signs are observed.

Eliminate pressure from digital pad injuries by using a triangular piece of medium-density foam (Temperfoam, HiTech Foam, Lincoln, Neb.) cut to the size of the carpal or tarsal pad or a medium-density foam doughnut to protect carpal or tarsal pad injuries (see Fig. 15-5).

Placing a solid foam pad outside the intermediate bandage layer before the outer tape layer is placed helps to relieve pressure from the digits.

Similarly, place the doughnut before applying the outer bandage layer.

Pressure can be further minimized by incorporating a metal splint into the outer bandage layer or by creating a localized crutch or "clamshell" splint. Two metal paw splints, one on the bottom and one on the top of the paw, are placed so they extend beyond the digits and bandage approximately 1 inch. The splints are then secured with tape to create the "clamshell" splint.

Slippage can be prevented by extending the bandage to encircle the shoulder and thorax (hip and caudal abdomen), creating a spica type of bandage (Fig. 15-7). This bandage immobilizes the shoulder or hip in addition to the more distal joints and often incorporates splint material. The intermediate and outer bandage layers crisscross cranial and caudal to the affected limb and caudal and cranial to the contralateral limb, as described on p. 188, for abdominal and thoracic bandages. The bandage is reinforced with splint rod, fiberglass casting tape, or thermoplastic splint material

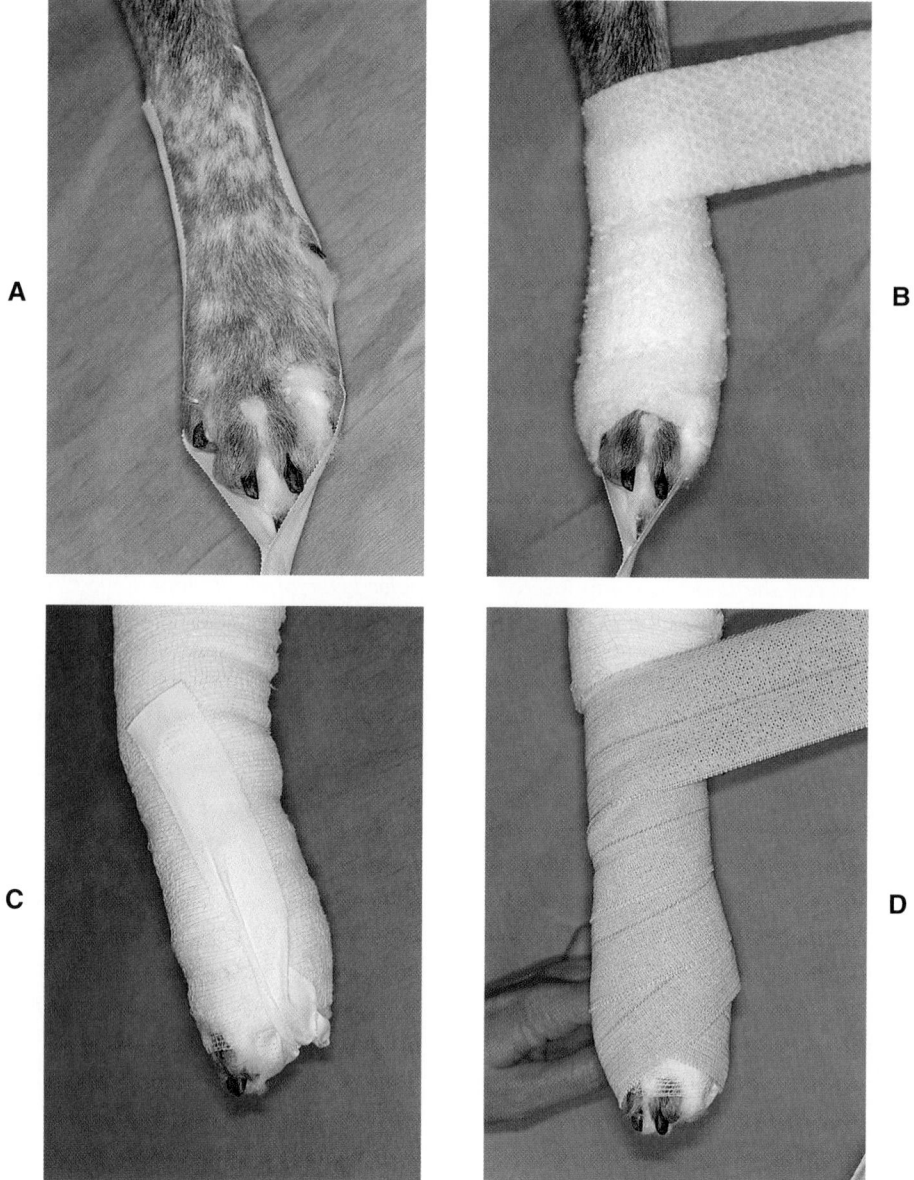

FIG. 15-6
A, For a leg bandage, apply a 1-inch porous tape stirrup to the dorsal and ventral or medial and lateral surfaces of the paw. Insert an absorbent material between the digits and the metacarpal or metatarsal and digital pads. **B,** Apply cast padding or cotton over an appropriate contact layer, overlapping wraps by one half to two thirds the width of the roll. Keep the third and fourth digits exposed. Conform the padding to the limb by applying elastic gauze. Apply a splint for greater immobilization between the padding and elastic gauze (optional). **C,** Fold the tape stirrups over the gauze. **D,** Apply an outer layer of 2- to 3-inch-wide elastic tape, overlapping one half of the width of the tape with each turn.

if fractures are to be temporarily stabilized or if additional wound immobilization is desired.

Temporary immobilization of injuries below the elbow or stifle can also be accomplished by applying a Robert Jones bandage or a modified Robert Jones bandage. A Robert Jones bandage is a large, bulky bandage that provides stabilization by applying compression to a thick cotton layer

(see p. 946). A modified or light Robert Jones bandage has much less cotton padding, making it less bulky. Modified Robert Jones bandages are used to reduce limb edema after surgery.

Onychectomy, digit amputation, or pad reconstruction may benefit from a bandage to protect the digits and reduce hemorrhage. In these cases, stirrups should be applied later-

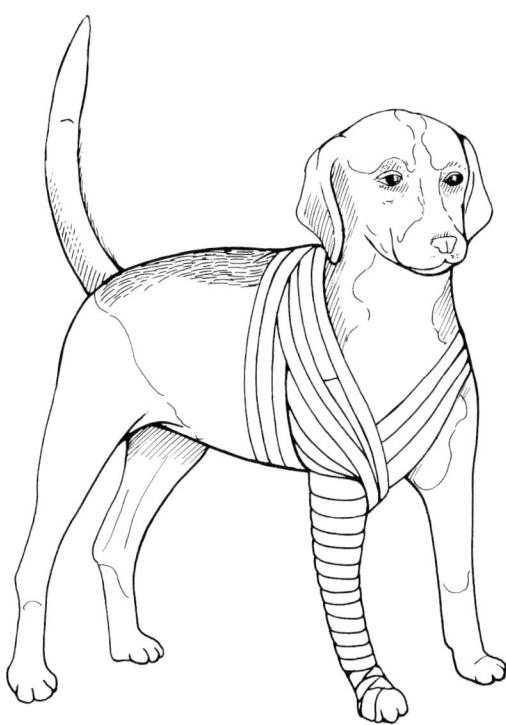

FIG. 15-7
For proximal extremity lesions, continue the bandage up the leg, around the chest or abdomen, and between the legs to create a spica type bandage.

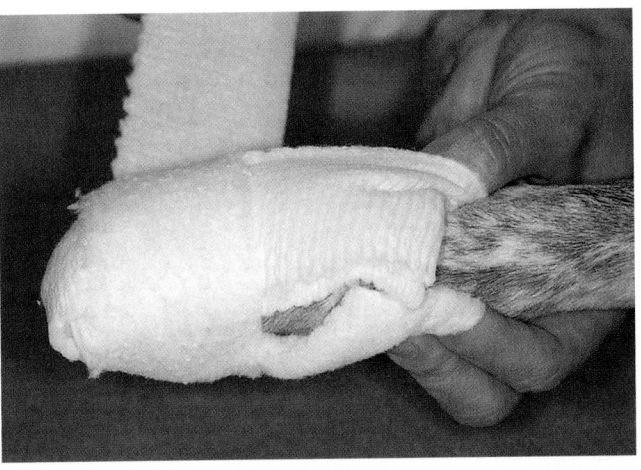

A

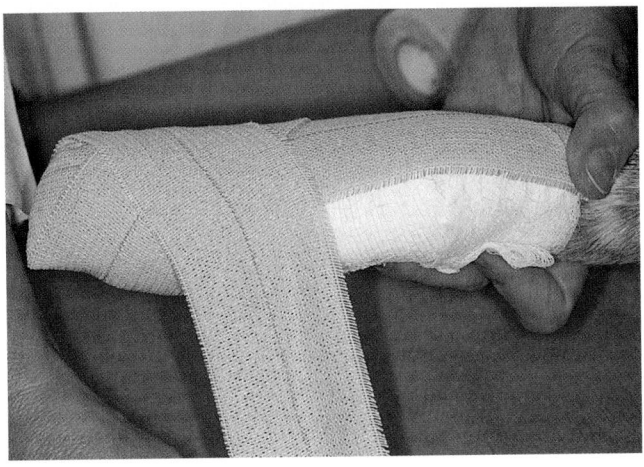

B

FIG. 15-8
A paw bandage is placed in a manner similar to a leg bandage, except that the digits are covered. **A,** After placing stirrups and the contact layer, reflect cast padding over the digits from dorsal to ventral and then ventral to dorsal. Then wrap the padding around the distal limb. **B,** Conform the bandage to the limb with elastic gauze and secure the bandage with elastic tape in a similar fashion.

ally and the digits covered with gauze sponges or a nonadherent contact layer.

Reflect layers of 2-inch cast padding from dorsal to ventral and then ventral to dorsal over the end of the paw (Fig. 15-8, A). Extend the cast padding in a spiral pattern to the midradius and midulna (tibia and fibula). Leave the proximal ends of the tape stirrup exposed to aid bandage removal. Cover the cast padding with elastic gauze. Fold the tape stirrups to their respective sides. Cover the bandage with tape from the distal extremity to the proximal hair (Fig. 15-8, B). As an alternative, Tubegauz or Finger BOB (B. Braun Veterinary Care, Bethlehem, Pa.), a thin, elastic stockinette, may be used to cover the contact layer and cast padding. It is applied with or without a "bale," or metal cage cylinder. Insert the foot in the bale covered with Tubegauz, grasp the stockinette proximally, pull the bale to the end of the foot using a slight rotating motion, and twist 180° to 360°. Push the bale up, and pull it down the limb to add additional layers of stockinette. Cover the stockinette with tape. Increase tension by increasing the rotation of the bale along the long axis of the leg. Avoid applying the stockinette too tightly. Remove the bandage by incising the proximal aspect to expose the proximal ends of the tape stirrups. Pull the tabs of the stirrup down the leg to loosen and remove the bandage.

Suggested Reading

Anderson DM, White RAS: Ischemic bandage injuries: a case series and review of the literature, *Vet Surg* 29:488, 2000.

Eleven cases are retrospectively reviewed with complications occurring with a variety of bandages and often requiring grafting or amputation.

Dart AJ, Cries L, Jeffcott LB et al: Effects of 25% propylene glycol hydrogel (Solugel) on second intention wound healing in horses, *Vet Surg* 31:309, 2002.

The experimental study using eight horses found no beneficial effects.

Ducharme-Desjarlais M, Celeste CJ, Lepault E et al: Effect of a silicone-containing dressing on exuberant granulation tissue formation and wound repair in horses, *Am J Vet Res* 66:1133, 2005.

Silicone dressing was used on five horses and compared with a nonadherent permeable control dressing. It was found to prevent exuberant granulation tissue more effectively.

Lee WR, Tobias KM, Bemis DA et al: In vitro efficacy of a polyhexamethylene biguanide-impregnated gauze dressing against bacteria found in veterinary patients, *Vet Surg* 33:404, 2004.

Impregnated gauze dressings reduced bacterial growth, especially gram-positive species. They are used to reduce wound contamination by bacterial pathogens.

Reimer SB, Schulz KS, Mason DR et al: Effects of a whole-body spandex garment on rectal temperature and oxygen consumption in healthy dogs, *J Am Vet Med Assoc* 224:71, 2004.

This snug spandex garment did not cause overheating and may be useful to cover wounds or incisions.

Senel S, McClure SJ: Potential applications of chitosan in veterinary medicine, *Adv Drug Deliv Rev* 56:1467, 2004.

Veterinary applications for chitosan, including wound healing, bone regeneration, analgesic, and antimicrobial effects are reviewed.

Simpson AM, Beale BS, Radlinsky MA: Bandaging in dogs and cats: basic principles, *Compend Cont Educ Pract Vet* 23:12, 2001.

This article reviews traditional bandaging techniques, but does not include a discussion of interactive dressings.

Stashak TS, Farstvedt E, Othic A: Update on wound dressings: indications and best use, *Clin Tech Equine Pract* 3:148, 2004.

Current dressing and wound care options are presented with inclusion of a useful chart.

Swaim SF, Hinkle SH, Bradley DM: Wound contraction: basic and clinical factors, *Compend Cont Educ Pract Vet* 23:20, 2001.

The numerous factors affecting wound contraction and methods to manage them are reviewed in this well-illustrated paper.

Swaim SF, Gillette RL, Sartin EA et al: Effects of hydrolyzed collagen dressing on the healing of open wounds in dogs, *Am J Vet Res* 61:1574, 2000.

Powdered collagen appeared hydrophilic and resulted in greater epithelialization than wounds treated with semiocclusive nonadherent pads alone in this experimental study involving nine dogs.

Swaim SF, Marghitu DB, Rumph PF et al: Effects of bandage configuration on paw pad pressure in dogs: a preliminary study, *J Am Anim Hosp Assoc* 39:209, 2003.

Seven bandage configurations were evaluated with pressure data. The most pressure was relieved from the pads with a "clamshell" configuration bandage and additionally, by placing a compressible foam sponge on the carpal pad, pressure was relieved from the digital pads.

Winkler JT, Swaim SF, Sartin EA et al: The effect of a porcine-derived small intestinal submucosa product on wounds with exposed bone in dogs, *Vet Surg* 31:541, 2002.

This prospective experimental study found no contraindication to use and no evidence that this product affects epithelialization, contraction, or time to complete healing in wounds with exposed bone compared with controls.

YoungSam K, JungWoo R, KwangHo J: A comparison of hydrocolloid (Duoderm®) and hydrogel (Nu-Gel®) occlusive dressing materials in the treatment of full-thickness skin wounds in dogs, *J Vet Clinics* 20:294, 2003.

When comparing hydrocolloid, hydrogel, and saline dressings in canine wounds, those dressed with hydrogel healed faster with more epithelialization and contraction.

PRINCIPLES OF PLASTIC AND RECONSTRUCTIVE SURGERY

SKIN TENSION AND ELASTICITY

Reconstructive surgery is commonly performed to close defects that occur secondary to trauma, to correct or improve congenital abnormalities, or after removal of neoplasms. A variety of reconstructive procedures are available; it is important to select the appropriate technique or techniques to prevent complications and avoid unnecessary cost. Although large lesions, particularly those on the trunk, often heal by contraction and epithelialization (see p. 161), wound closure may be preferable. Large or irregular defects sometimes can be closed using relaxing incisions or "plasty" techniques (e.g., V-to-Y plasty, Z-plasty). Large defects or those on the extremities may require that tissue be mobilized from other sites. Pedicle flaps are tissues that are partly detached from the donor site and mobilized to cover a defect (see p. 205); grafts involve the transfer of a segment of skin to a distant (recipient) site (see p. 224). Careful planning and meticulous, atraumatic surgical techniques are necessary to prevent excessive tension, kinking, and circulatory compromise. The amount of skin available for transfer varies between sites on the same animal and between breeds. Little skin can be mobilized in the extremities, whereas advancing adjacent tissue often can close large defects over the trunk. The character of the recipient bed influences the choice of reconstructive technique. Properly developed and transferred local flaps can survive on avascular beds, whereas grafts and distant flap transfers require vascular beds (i.e., healthy granulation tissue, muscle, periosteum, and paratenon).

Hirudiniasis, or the attachment of leeches to skin, can help in reconstructive and microvascular surgery. Leeches are recommended only for tissues with impaired venous circulation. The medicinal leech is *Hirudo medicinalis*. After a blood meal, a leech can go for months without eating. Leeches produce a small bleeding wound that mimics venous outflow. The leech eats an average of 5 ml of blood, but blood oozes from the wound for 24 to 48 hours after the leech detaches because of anticoagulants and vasodilator substances introduced into the wound. There is a significant risk of infection with *Aeromonas hydrophila* when leeches are used.

TENSION LINES AND TENSION RELIEF

The location of the wound, elasticity of surrounding tissue, regional blood supply, and character of the wound bed should be considered when planning reconstructive surgery. Grasping and lifting the skin in the proposed flap or graft area and allowing it to retract spontaneously assesses skin tension and elasticity. Evaluating the amount of tension that can be tolerated by tissue is subjective. Apposing incision edges under too much tension causes incisional discomfort and pressure necrosis, resulting in sutures "cutting out" (see p. 197) and partial or complete incisional dehiscence. Methods of reducing tension include undermining wound edges, selecting appropriate suture patterns, and using relief incisions, skin stretching, and tissue expansion. In addition, the animal is always positioned for surgery, such that mobile skin is not pinned against the table; using pads and flexing the appropriate joints accomplish this. If these methods do not allow primary ap-

position, wounds may be allowed to heal by secondary intention or may be reconstructed with flaps or grafts.

Tension Lines

Tension lines are formed by the predominant pull of fibrous tissue within the skin. General lines of tension have been mapped in animals, but breed, conformation, gender, and age variations occur (Fig. 15-9). Tension causes incised skin edges to separate and widens linear scars (Fig. 15-10). Incisions should be made parallel to tension lines. Incisions and wounds along tension lines heal better, faster, and with more aesthetic results, whereas those made across tension lines tend to gape. Incisions made at an angle to tension lines take a curvilinear shape. Incisions made across tension lines require more sutures for closure and are more likely to dehisce than those made parallel to tension lines. Traumatic wounds should be closed in the direction that prevents or minimizes tension. Wound edges should be manipulated before closure to determine which direction the suture line should run to minimize tension (Fig. 15-11). If tension is minimal, a wound should be closed in the direction of its long axis. The direction of closure should prevent or minimize the creation of "dog ears," or puckers, at the ends of suture lines.

Tension Relief

Skin is undermined by using scissors to separate the skin or panniculus muscle (or both) from underlying tissue. Undermining skin adjacent to a wound is the simplest tension-relieving procedure. It releases skin from underlying attachments so that its full elastic potential can be used as it is stretched over the wound. Skin should be undermined deep to the panniculus muscle layer to preserve subdermal plexus and direct cutaneous vessels that run parallel to the skin surface (Fig. 15-12). Where there is no panniculus muscle layer (middle and distal portion of the extremities), the skin should be undermined in the loose areolar fascia deep to the dermis to preserve the subdermal plexus. Elevated skin should include a portion of the superficial fascia with the dermis to preserve the direct cutaneous arteries. In areas where skin is closely associated with an underlying muscle,

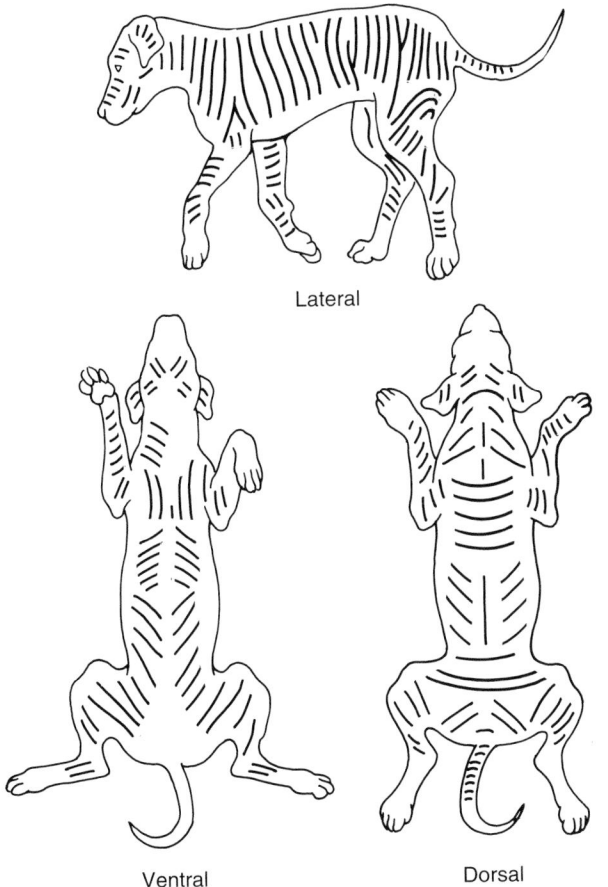

FIG. 15-9
Approximate skin tension lines in dogs. (Modified from Irwin DHG: Tension lines in the skin of the dog, *J Small Anim Pract* 7:595, 1966.)

Lateral

Ventral

Dorsal

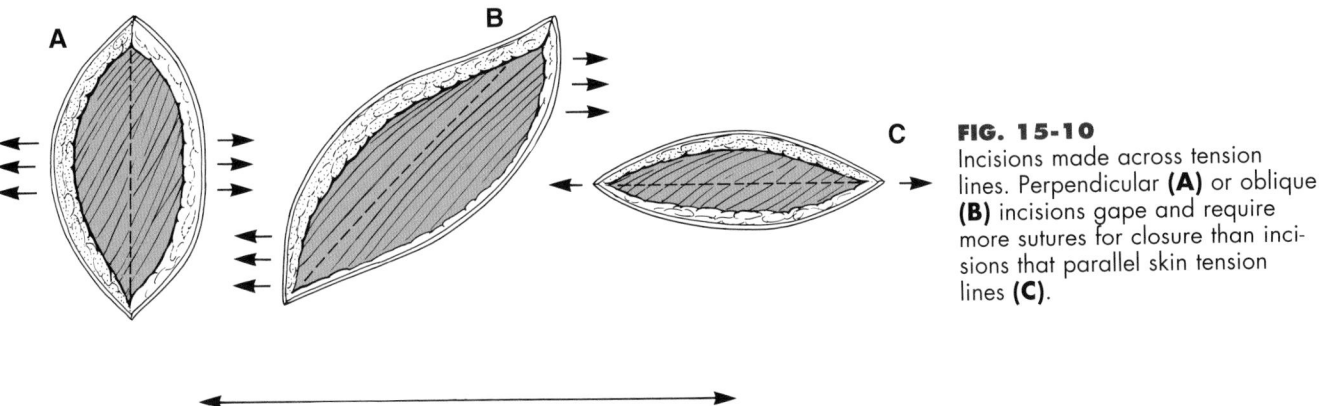

FIG. 15-10
Incisions made across tension lines. Perpendicular (**A**) or oblique (**B**) incisions gape and require more sutures for closure than incisions that parallel skin tension lines (**C**).

Skin tension line

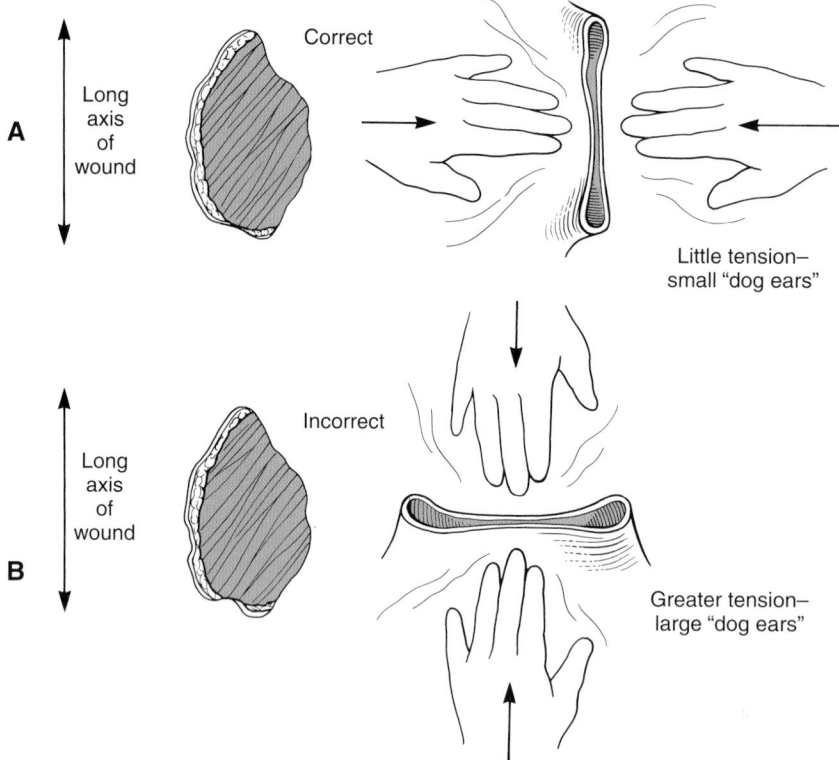

FIG. 15-11
Wound edges should be manipulated to determine the direction of least tension and minimal "dog ear" formation. **A,** Wound edges showing little tension and small "dog ears." **B,** Wound edges showing greater tension and large "dog ears."

FIG. 15-12
Before wound closure, use scissors to undermine skin and subcutaneous tissue or skin and panniculus muscle and to separate them from the underlying tissue.

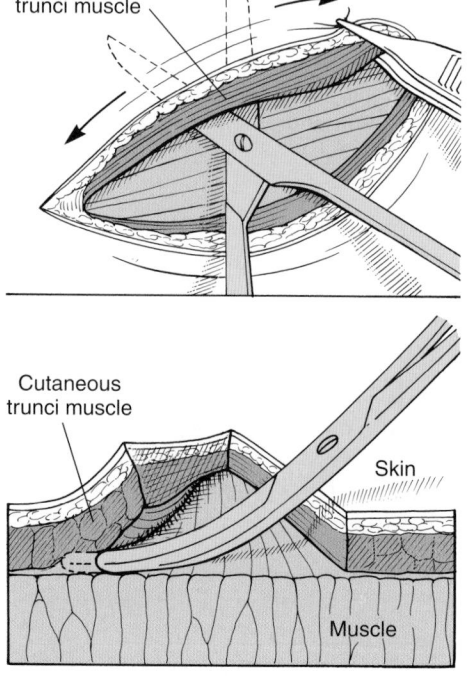

a portion of the outer muscle fascia should be elevated with the dermis rather than dissecting these structures. Prevent subdermal plexus injury by using an atraumatic surgical technique, including cutting skin with a sharp scalpel blade instead of scissors and avoiding crushing instruments (e.g., Allis tissue forceps). Brown-Adson thumb forceps, skin hooks, or stay sutures should be used to manipulate skin. Tissue layers are separated by repeatedly inserting Metzenbaum scissors with the blades closed, opening the blades, and then withdrawing the scissors in an open position. Tissue is snipped with the scissors as necessary. As an alternative, the partly opened scissors can be advanced along the cleavage plane without snipping. While undermining, determine if tension relief is adequate by periodically attempting to approximate the skin edges.

Bleeding usually is insignificant during undermining. Excessive bleeding may be controlled with electrocoagulation or ligation; however, skin tension and bandaging usually control hemorrhage and prevent seromas. Undermining areas near wound margins associated with delayed wound closure requires that the epithelialized skin edge be separated from the granulation tissue. The skin should be excised with a scalpel blade at the junction of normal skin and new epithelium. The incision should be continued through the granulation tissue at the normal cleavage line of subcutaneous fascia, deep to the subdermal plexus. Wound closure under excessive tension, rough surgical technique, and division of direct cutaneous arteries interfere with cutaneous circulation and may cause skin necrosis, wound dehiscence, or infection. Surgical manipulation of recently traumatized skin should be minimized until circulation improves. Resolution of contusions, edema, and infection indicates improved skin circulation.

Skin Stretching and Expansion

Skin stretching and expansion is a technique used in reconstructive surgery that takes advantage of the skin's ability to stretch beyond its natural or inherent elasticity, by the processes of mechanical creep and stress relaxation, when continuous tension is applied. During this process, dermal collagen fibers are stretched, and tissue fluid is slowly displaced from around collagen fibers, which are straightening and compacting longitudinally in the direction of the stretching force. Skin can be prestretched hours to days before surgery to allow closure with less tension at the time of the procedure. Presuturing, adjustable sutures, skin stretchers, and skin expanders are used in this technique (Fig. 15-13). Presuturing is performed 24 hours before surgery to prestretch the skin. Lidocaine, sedation, or general anesthesia is administered before suture placement to relieve discomfort. Tension sutures (interrupted Lembert or vertical mattress sutures of 2-0 or 0 monofilament, nonabsorbable suture material) are placed to imbricate skin on apposing sides of the lesion (see Fig. 15-13). Sutures are placed 3 to 5 cm from the proposed incision site. The sutures exert their effect primarily on healthy skin immediately adjacent to the proposed surgical site, and they are not adjustable. Presuturing is effective only in areas where elastic skin is limited (i.e., extremities). An adjustable horizontal suture can be used to stretch skin over a wound gradually. This is a continuous intradermal suture (2-0 nylon, polypropylene, or polybutester) anchored at one or both ends with a button secured on the skin surface with a split shot fishing weight. On succeeding days, traction on the suture advances the wound edges over the wound, and new weights are applied to maintain tension. These sutures are used primarily on limb wounds in which the wound edges cannot initially be apposed.

The skin stretcher (X-Banders) is a noninvasive device capable of stretching skin both adjacent to and distant from the surgical site. More skin can be stretched or recruited using this technique than by presuturing or tissue expanders. Skin stretchers are most effective on the neck and trunk. Self-adherent skin pads with a thin coat of additional cyanoacrylate adhesive are applied to clipped, clean, dry skin adjacent to and distant from the surgical site, depending on the amount of stretching needed. Pads are placed 1 to 2 cm from the wound margin with their long axis perpendicular to the direction of skin tension. Elastic connecting cables are attached to pads on one side of the wound and stretched before they are attached to the pads on the opposite side of the wound. An additional row or tier of pads and cables can be placed more distant from the wound if further skin recruitment is required. The cables are adjusted every 6 to 8 hours to generate the optimal high-tension load to accelerate skin stretching or deformation. Sufficient skin may be recruited within 24 to 48 hours, although 96 hours may be required. Pads are peeled from the skin or removed with glue solvent before surgery. Little or no undermining generally is required after skin stretching. Skin stretchers are also used before removal of a mass or after surgery when incisions are closed under excessive tension. Application of a skin stretcher helps alleviate tension and prevent dehiscence (see Fig. 15-13). Pads generally are removed 3 to 5 days after surgery.

Tissue expanders are inflated in subcutaneous tissue to stretch overlying skin, allowing creation of larger flaps for closing defects. They are beneficial in overcoming tissue shortage and obtaining skin with desirable qualities. Tissue expanders reduce dermal thickness and temporarily increase epidermal mitosis. Subcutaneous fat and muscle adjacent to the tissue expander atrophy, and neurapraxia may occur. Tissue expanders have an inflatable bag and reservoir made of silicone elastomer. Although expensive, they are available in various sizes and shapes (e.g., Intravent Intraoperative Tissue Expanders and Radovan Tissue Expander). Careful planning is required for optimal expansion and reconstruction. The base of the expander should approximate the size of the donor site. The incision for insertion of the expander should be made parallel to tension lines at the leading edge of the future flap, or skin adjacent to the site will be inappropriately stretched. The device is placed subcutaneously and inflated with saline.

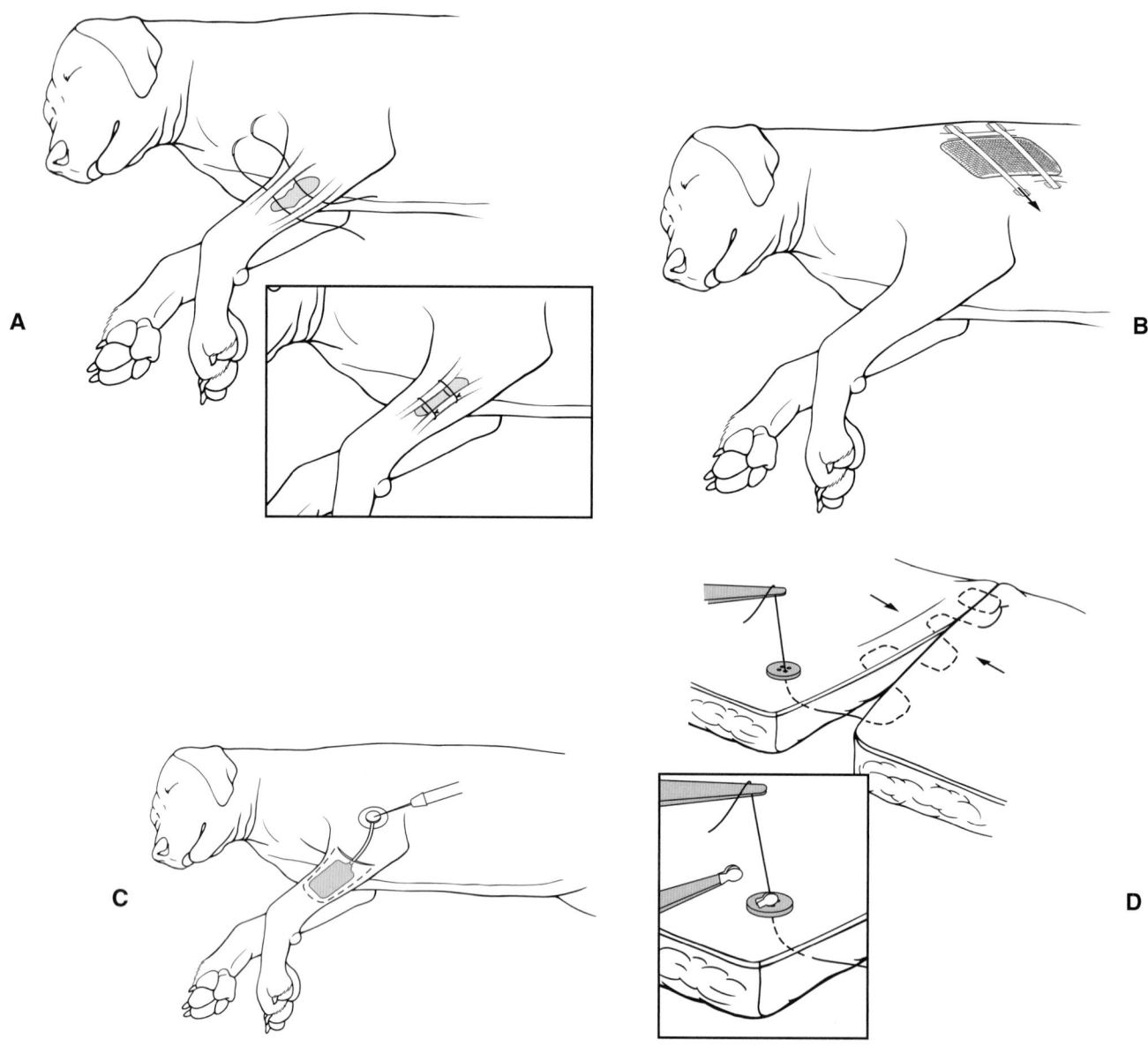

FIG. 15-13
Methods for recruiting skin to close wounds under tension include using presuturing **(A)**, skin stretchers **(B)**, inflatable tissue expanders **(C)**, and adjustable sutures **(D)**.

Rapid expansion requires intermittent intraoperative short-term inflation of the expander. It involves inflating the expander for 2 to 3 minutes, deflating and letting the tissue rest for 3 to 4 minutes, and then repeating the cycle two or three times before creating a flap. Gradual expansion involves injecting to a given pressure or volume at intervals spanning days to weeks (usually every 2 to 7 days). Inflation at injection is continued until the skin feels tense or looks blanched or until discomfort is perceived. When the tissue is sufficiently stretched to allow reconstruction, the device is removed and a skin flap is created to close the defect. Complications of tissue expanders include pain, seroma formation, scar widening, infection, dehiscence,

skin necrosis, and implant failure, and they should not be used in previously irradiated tissue. Axial pattern flaps (see p. 211) are preferable to tissue expanders.

SUTURE PATTERNS
Subdermal Sutures
Subdermal fascia is strong and tolerates tension better than subcutaneous tissue or skin. Sutures placed in subdermal or subcuticular tissue reduce tension on skin sutures and bring skin edges into apposition. These sutures also reduce scarring. For subdermal and subcuticular sutures, 3-0 or 4-0 polydioxanone, poliglecaprone 25, or polyglyconate suture with a buried knot is used.

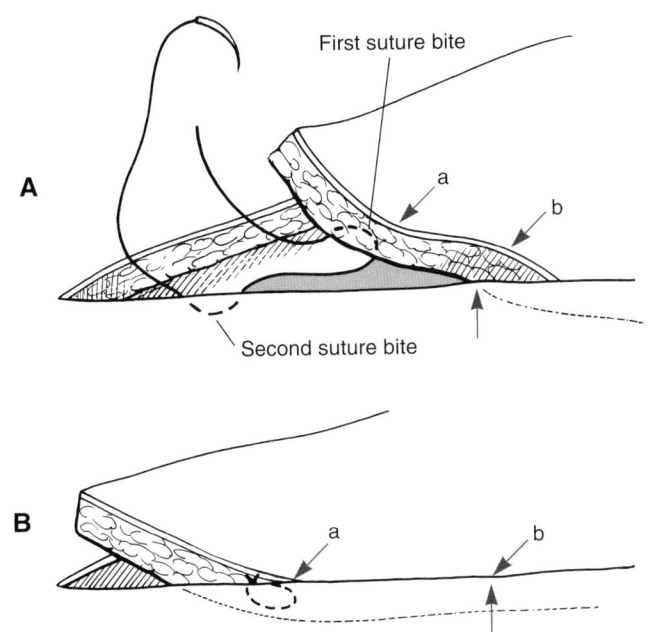

FIG. 15-14
Use walking sutures to advance skin toward the center of the wound. **A,** Place the suture through the fascia of the body wall at a distance closer to the center of the wound than the bite through the subdermal fascia or deep dermis. **B,** Note that the distance from *a* to *b* increases because of skin stretching when the suture is tied.

Walking Sutures

Walking sutures move skin across a defect, obliterate dead space, and distribute tension over the wound surface. Skin is advanced toward the center of the wound by placing rows of interrupted, subdermal sutures beginning at the depths of the wound. The suture (e.g., 2-0 or 3-0 polydioxanone, poliglecaprone 25, or polyglyconate) should be placed through fascia of the body wall at a distance closer to the center of the wound than the bite through the subdermal fascia or deep dermis (Fig. 15-14). Walking sutures do not penetrate the skin surface. Tying the suture advances skin toward the wound center. Walking sutures are placed no closer than 2 to 3 cm apart. Successive rows of walking sutures further advance the skin toward the center of the wound. Sutures are placed on both sides of the defect to advance undermined skin toward the center. The number of walking sutures should be minimized to prevent creating subcutaneous loculi or compromising circulation. Subdermal and skin sutures are used to complete wound closure.

External Tension-Relieving Sutures

External tension-relieving sutures help prevent sutures from cutting out, which occurs when pressure on skin within the suture loop exceeds the pressure that allows blood flow. Pressure is reduced by spreading it over a larger area of skin. Placing sutures farther from the skin edge or using mattress or cruciate sutures helps disperse pressure. Other suture patterns that help relieve tension include alternating wide and narrow bites using simple interrupted sutures or placing "far-near-near-far" or "far-far-near-near" sutures. The standard tension-relieving suture is the vertical mattress suture. A tension-relieving row of vertical mattress sutures should be placed 1 to 2 cm away from the primary row of sutures apposing the skin edges. The vertical mattress sutures (2-0 to 0 polypropylene, polybutester, or nylon) are placed while the skin is approximated with towel clamps or skin hooks before apposition of the skin edges with approximating sutures (e.g., 3-0 or 2-0 polypropylene, polybutester, or nylon). Tension-relieving vertical mattress sutures usually can be removed by the third day after surgery, when fibrin has stabilized the wound edges. Horizontal mattress sutures with or without rubber tubing stents may be used; however, they have a greater potential for impairing local cutaneous blood flow.

PREVENTION OF "DOG EARS"

"Dog ears," or puckers, may be prevented or corrected at the end of a suture line by unequal suture spacing or by resecting a small ellipse or triangle of skin. Placing sutures close together on the convex side of the defect and farther apart on the concave side of the wound may prevent dog ears (Fig. 15-15, *A*). Dog ears may be corrected by outlining with an elliptic incision, removing redundant skin, and apposing the skin edges in a linear or curvilinear fashion (Fig. 15-15, *B*). As an alternative, the dog ear may be incised in the center to form two triangles; one triangle should be excised and the other used to fill the resultant defect (Fig. 15-15, *C* and *D*), or both triangles may be excised and the edges apposed, creating a linear suture line (Fig. 15-15, *E*). Thin elastic skin is less prone to the formation of dog ears than thick skin. Many dog ears flatten without excision.

RELAXING INCISIONS

Relaxing incisions, or incisions made near a defect to allow apposition of skin edges, are beneficial in allowing skin closure around fibrotic wounds or over important structures or before radiation therapy after extensive tumor excision. They are rarely indicated except on legs, around the eyes and anus, or to cover tendons, ligaments, nerves, vessels, or implants.

Simple Relaxing Incisions

Relief incisions heal by contraction and epithelialization in 25 to 30 days. Some relaxing incisions surrounded by loose elastic tissue can be closed primarily after the wound is approximated.

Begin undermining at the edge of the defect at the point of maximum skin tension and continue until the edges can be apposed under tension. Close the wound and make a relaxing incision at the point where undermining stopped or where tension lines are observed (Fig. 15-16, A). Begin the incision at the point of maximum skin tension and extend it as necessary to relieve excess tension. If neces-

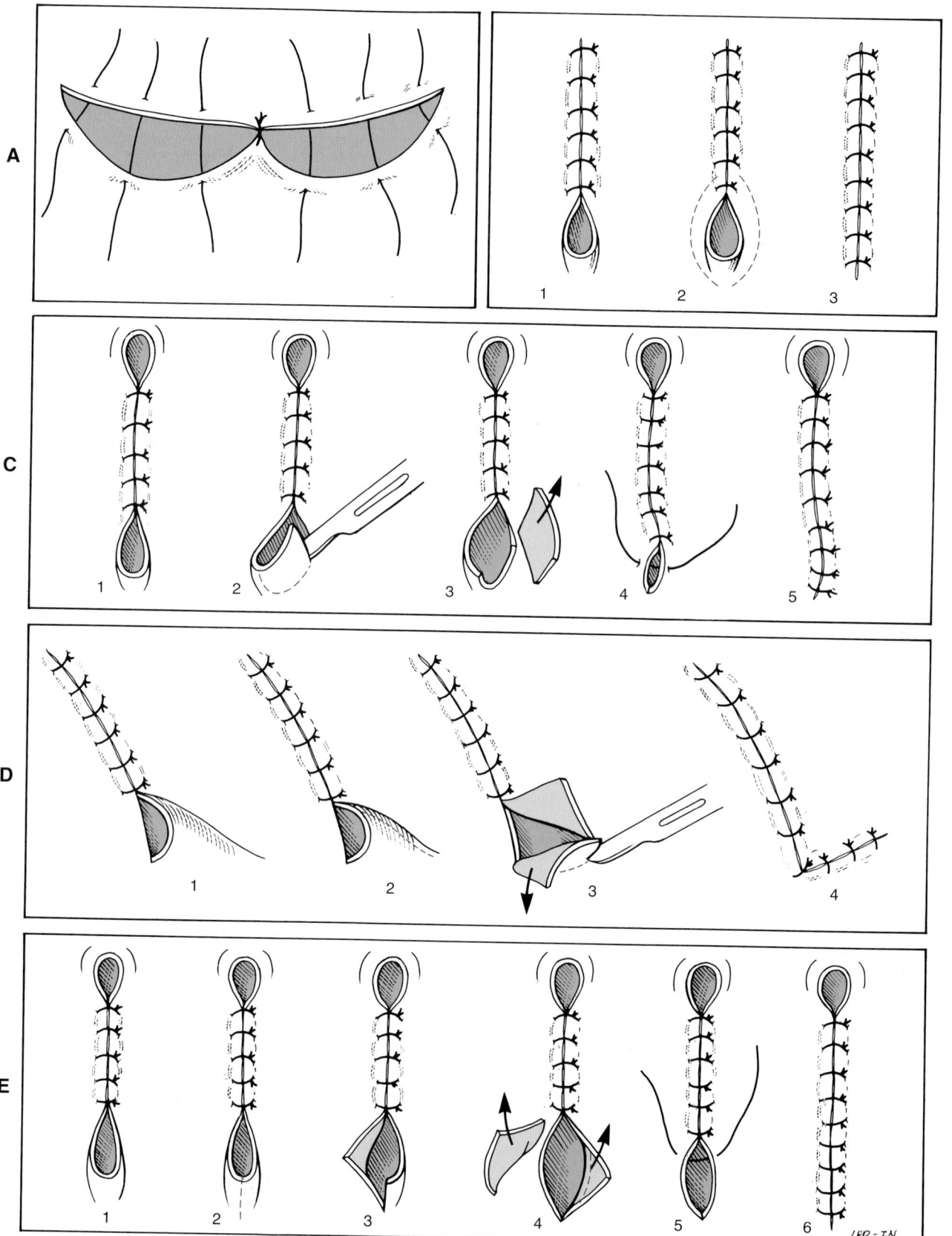

FIG. 15-15
Prevent or correct "dog ears" or puckers at the end of suture lines by using unequal suture spacing **(A)**, or by resecting an elliptic segment of skin **(B)**, or one large triangle **(C** and **D)**, or two smaller triangles **(E)** of skin.

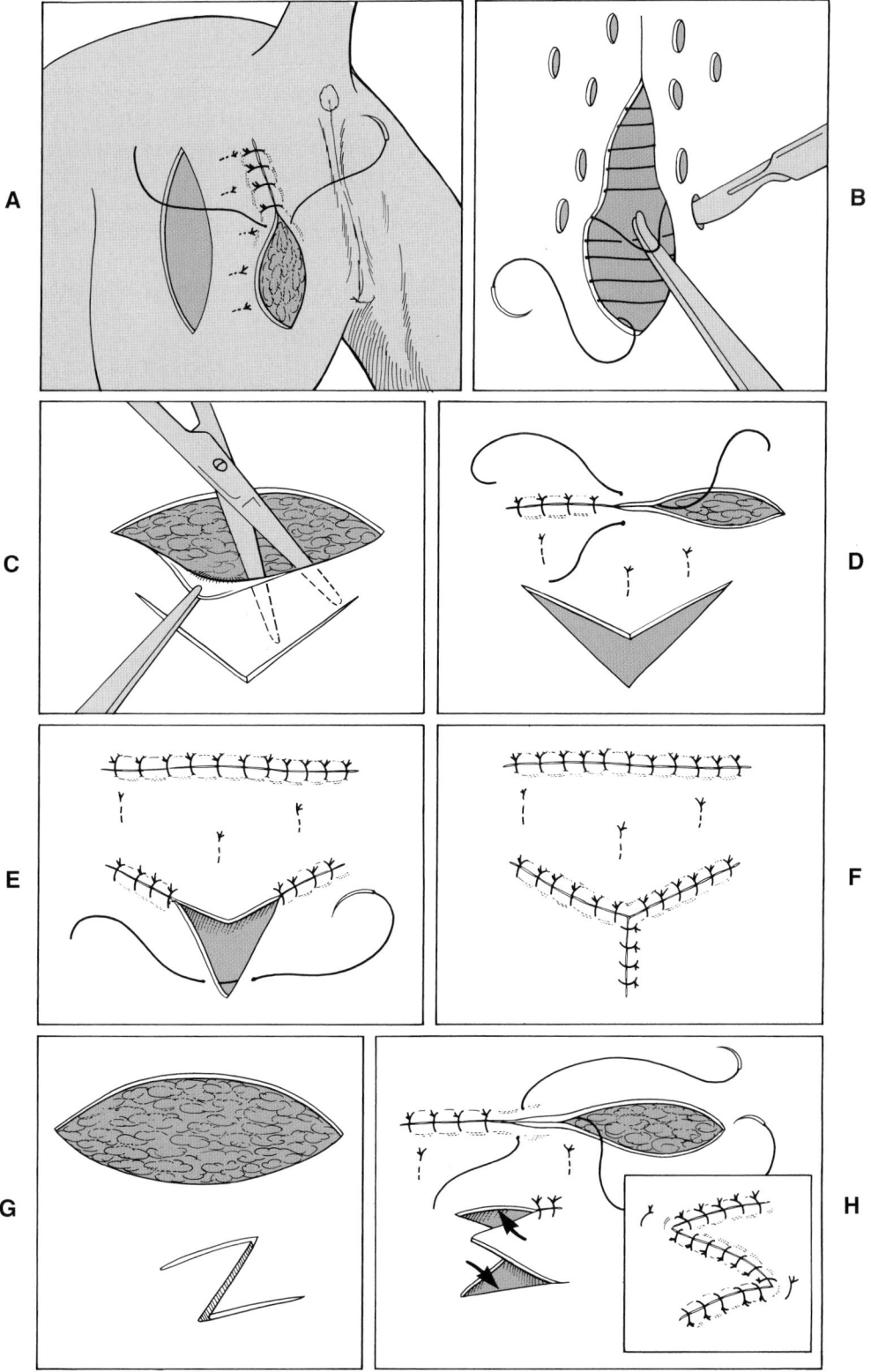

FIG. 15-16
Make relaxing incisions near the defect to allow skin apposition. **A,** After undermining the skin, unilateral or bilateral simple relaxing incisions are made adjacent to the wound. **B,** After preplacing a continuous subcuticular suture pattern, multiple punctate incisions are made parallel to the wound. **C** through **F,** V-to-Y plasty provides an advancement flap to cover the wound. **G** and **H,** A Z-plasty can be made adjacent to or involving the wound to allow wound closure.

sary, make the relief incision before skin closure. Place a nonadherent pad over the relief incisions and suture line, followed by a padded bandage. Initially, change the bandage every 1 or 2 days.

Multiple Punctate Relaxing Incisions

Multiple punctate relaxing incisions are small, parallel, staggered incisions made in skin adjacent to a wound to allow closure with reduced tension (Fig. 15-16, *B*).

Undermine skin around the wound and place a continuous subdermal suture pattern. Tighten the suture, starting at one end of the incision and working toward the other end. If the skin edges do not appose in an area, make a small incision approximately 1 cm long in adjacent skin on either side of the wound, approximately 1 cm from the wound. If excessive tension persists, make a second row of incisions 0.5 to 2 cm lateral to the first row. Tighten the suture to appose the wound edges; continue the procedure along the length of the wound. Place skin sutures to appose the original wound, then place a nonadherent bandage. Change the bandage daily during the early stages of healing and less often as healing progresses.

Tension-relieving incisions heal by secondary intention. Multiple punctate relaxing incisions are more cosmetic than single relaxing incisions but provide less relaxation and have a higher risk of causing significant circulatory compromise.

V-to-Y Plasty

V-to-Y plasty is a type of relaxing incision that provides an advancement flap to cover a wound. It is used to close chronic, inelastic wounds or wounds that would distort adjacent structures if closed under tension. It is commonly used in eyelid surgery. A V-shaped incision is made approximately 3 cm from the wound (Fig. 15-16, *C*). The original wound is closed after undermining skin (Fig. 15-16, *D*). The V relief incision is closed in the shape of a Y. Closure is begun at the ends of the V until tension develops (Fig. 15-16, *E*). The remainder of the relief incision is closed as the stem of the Y (Fig. 15-16, *F*).

Z-Plasty

Z-plasty is a technique that lengthens or relaxes an incision. The Z may be incorporated into the wound, or a separate Z may be made adjacent to the wound to facilitate closure with less tension. The central limb of the Z is the wound or primary incision. The two arms of the Z are made the same length as the central limb (Fig. 15-16, *G*). The angles of the Z can vary between 30° and 90°, but 60° is advised. Larger angles give more length gain (45° gives approximately a 50% increase; 60° approximately a 75% increase). Length is gained along the original central limb of the Z when the flaps of the Z are transposed (Fig. 15-16, *H*). A Z-shaped incision is made with the central arm of the Z parallel to the direction length is needed. The flaps are undermined before transposition and suturing (Fig. 15-16, *I*).

SKIN BIOPSY

Skin biopsies are required to diagnosis some dermatologic problems, skin infections, and tumors. With chronic dermatitis, biopsy is sometimes useful only to rule out other disorders such as neoplasia. Secondary skin infections should be eliminated before biopsy, if possible. Biopsies of chronic skin abnormalities should include multiple samples of representative lesions. Usually biopsy of abnormal skin is sufficient, but samples of normal skin are helpful for comparison when evaluating scaling disorders (primary seborrhea, depigmenting or hyperpigmenting lesions, and alopecia).

Administer a short-acting anesthetic or inject lidocaine around the lesion (0.5 to 1 ml/site but less than 1 ml of 2% lidocaine/10 lb of body weight). Clip the hair, carefully leaving approximately ¼ inch and avoid inflicting skin trauma. When the primary problem is dermatologic, and not infectious or neoplastic, do not scrub or disinfect biopsy sites because this may adversely affect the pathologist's interpretation. Scrubbing may interfere with identification of the type of keratin and presence of surface crust, scales, microorganisms, or parasites. Mark the lesions by circling or drawing a 2- to 3-cm line in the direction of the hair growth with an indelible marker. Perform the biopsy with a sharp 6- or 8-mm biopsy punch and a small, sharp-sharp scissors or scalpel blade for cutting the specimen from the subcutaneous tissue. Hold the skin taut around the biopsy site with the thumb and forefinger. Place the punch perpendicular to the skin surface with the lesion in the center. Rotate the punch in one direction while applying moderate pressure until a pop is felt or to the hub of the punch. Apply gentle pressure for hemostasis. Grasp and gently retract the specimen with small tissue forceps; then transect the attached subcutaneous tissue. Blot blood from the specimen, and place it on a tongue depressor or cardboard marked with the direction of hair growth to prevent curling. Appose skin edges (3-0 or 4-0 monofilament nonabsorbable suture) with a single suture.

Alternatively for bullae, nodules, or deep lesions, make a wedge or elliptic-shaped incision around the lesion or at the junction of normal and abnormal tissue with a scalpel blade. Laser biopsies are not advised as laser-induced artifacts may make small specimens nondiagnostic.

Specimens of tumors can be obtained by incisional, excisional, or needle core biopsies.

Unlike specimens collected for dermatologic disorders, clip the hair and prepare it for aseptic surgery. Perform incisional biopsies such as skin biopsies using a punch or elliptic incision through both normal and abnormal tissue. Perform needle core biopsies using a TruCut biopsy instrument with samples taken from peripheral and central areas of the mass.

Excisional biopsies are described below and should include all previous biopsy incisions, punctures, and needle tracts.

Immediately after collection, place samples in fixative (10% neutral buffered formalin) to preserve their integrity. Make sure the pathologist can orient the specimen correctly and if necessary mark with ink or sutures. Provide a gross description of the lesion because evidence of erythema is lost in the fixative.

It is usually wise to also submit tissue for bacterial and/or fungal culture.

REMOVAL OF SKIN TUMORS

Before a tumor is removed, skin tension and elasticity should be assessed, but excessive tumor manipulation should be avoided. The direction of skin tension lines, shape of the excision, and method of closure should be planned before surgery. A large area should be clipped and aseptically prepared for surgery, especially if there is a chance that skin flaps may be needed for closure. Excision of skin tumors should include the tumor, previous biopsy sites, and wide margins of normal tissue in three dimensions (i.e., length, width, and depth). For benign tumors, remove the tumor and 1 cm of normal tissue; for malignant tumors, a margin of more than 2 to 3 cm may be necessary for complete local excision. These margins are taken in all dimensions, including the deep margin if feasible. Induration of the periphery of the lesion resulting from a fibroplastic host response may help identify the gross limits of the tumor. The margin distance should be greater for aggressive, infiltrative tumors (i.e., mast cell tumors, melanomas, squamous cell carcinomas, soft tissue sarcomas, feline mammary adenocarcinomas, hemangiopericytomas, and infiltrating lipomas). Tumor invasion is affected by the type of surrounding tissue. Tissue easily infiltrated by tumor cells (i.e., fat, subcutaneous tissue, muscle, and parenchyma) should be resected with the tumor. Cartilage, tendon, ligaments, fascia, and other collagen-dense, vascular-poor tissues are resistant to neoplastic invasion and therefore often are spared during resection. Excision of infiltrative or aggressive tumors should extend at least one fascial layer below the detectable tumor margins. Radical tumor excision (i.e., removal of an entire compartment or structure, amputation, or lobectomy) is indicated for poorly localized tumors or those with high-grade malignancy.

> NOTE: Excision of infiltrative or aggressive tumors should include greater than 2 to 3 cm of "normal" tissue around the lesion. Extend the dissection at least one fascial layer below the detectable tumor margins.

Perform resections as atraumatically as possible to protect adjacent tissue and to prevent tumor seeding. Use a length to width ratio of 4:1 when making elliptic incisions around a tumor to minimize "dog ear" formation. As the ellipse is started through all layers (skin, subcutaneous tissue, and fascia or muscle) place a suture through them to maintain alignment and prevent retraction of one layer from the others. When removing multiple masses from the same animal, first remove lesions believed benign and change instruments

and gloves (drapes if necessary) after removal of each mass to prevent spreading tumor cells from one site to another. Ligate the blood supply as early as possible to prevent systemic spread of tumor cells or substances (i.e., histamine and heparin). Irrigate the wound bed after tumor incision. Biopsy regional lymph nodes to stage the disease. Replace tumor-contaminated (or possibly contaminated) instruments, drapes, and gloves before wound closure. If radiation therapy is anticipated, mark resection margins within the wound using metallic staples to facilitate planning radiation therapy. Mark tumor margins with sutures or dyes and submit all resected specimens for histologic evaluation. Place the sample in approximately 10 parts formalin to 1 part tissue.

Adequate fixation with 10% neutral, buffered formalin requires that specimens be less than 5 to 10 mm wide. Identification of the tumor type is imperative in determining the appropriate postoperative therapy and the prognosis.

> NOTE: Local tumors most often recur because the surgical margins for the original tumor were inadequate; be sure to mark tumor borders.

REMOVAL OF IRREGULAR SKIN DEFECTS

Although it is advisable to remove skin lesions with an elliptic skin incision to facilitate closure, some lesions cause irregularly shaped defects because of their size or location. Skin elasticity and tension lines should be assessed before excision and closure.

Circular Defects

Circular excision of lesions saves the most normal skin compared with other excision patterns. Skin tension lines may convert defects of other shapes into circular defects. Circular defects are difficult to close because "dog ears" tend to develop. They may be closed using a variety of techniques. The linear, combined V, and bow tie techniques are preferred. Conversion of a circular defect by a fusiform or elliptic excision with a 4:1 length to width ratio resects more skin than necessary (156%). The linear technique may be used for small defects when skin edges can be apposed without the formation of large "dog ears Sutures are placed parallel to the direction of skin tension lines, beginning at the center of the defect. The "dog ears" at each end of the suture line are excised and the remaining defects apposed (Fig. 15-17, *A*).

The combined V technique is used when skin apposition causes "dog ears," and limited skin is available for reconstruction. This technique does not remove additional normal skin. Two equilateral triangles are designed on opposite sides of the circular defect with the central axis 45° from the long axis (tension lines) of the defect. The sides of each triangle are incised such that the vertex of the V points to the longitudinal axis of the defect. The skin flaps are rotated and sutured to convert the circular defect into a smaller, irregular fusiform defect. Edges of the converted defect are apposed with approximating sutures (Fig. 15-17, *B*). The

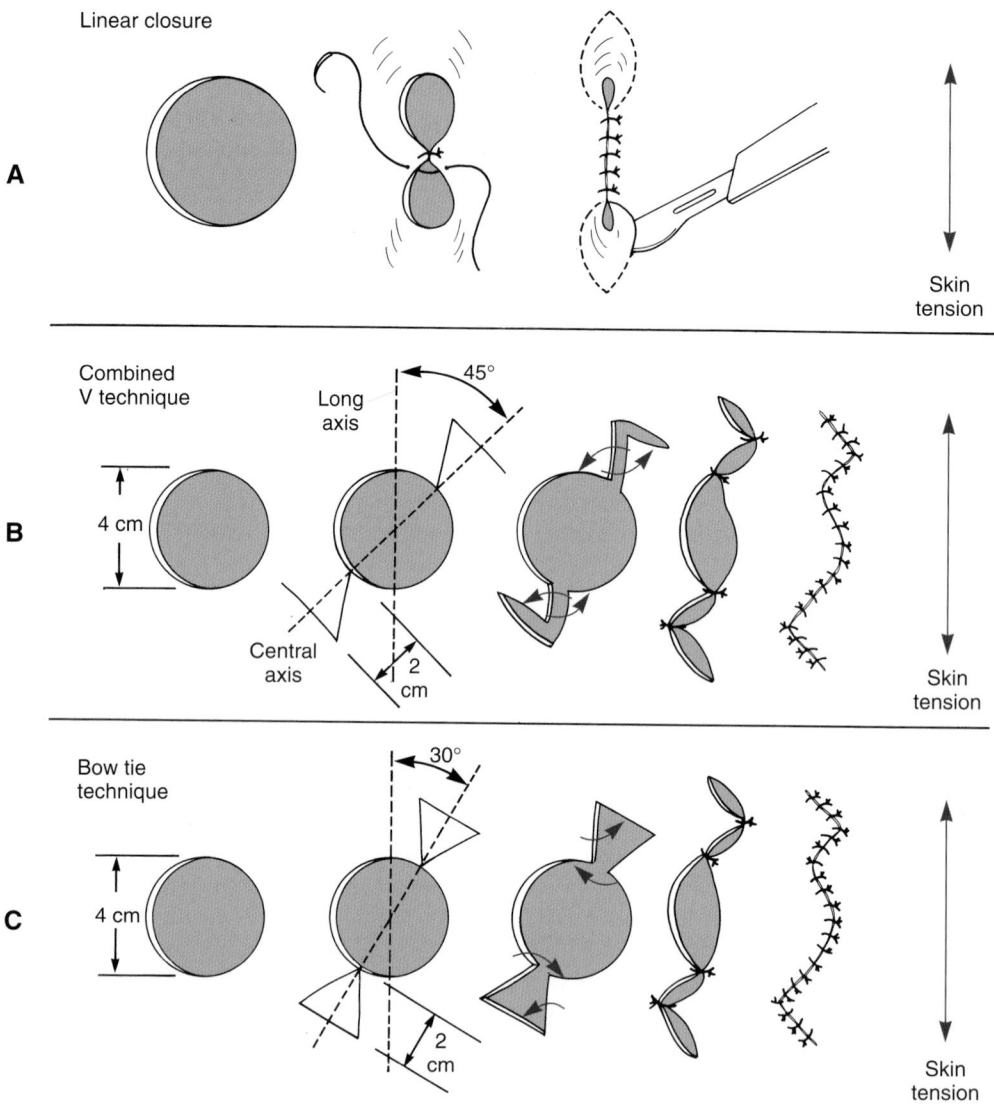

FIG. 15-17
Closure of small circular defects. **A,** Use a linear closure if the skin edges can be apposed without creating large "dog ears." **B,** Use a combined V technique when limited skin is available for reconstruction. **C,** Use a bow tie technique when abundant skin is available.

bow tie technique is used when skin apposition results in large "dog ears" and abundant skin surrounds the defect. This technique removes 36% additional skin. Two equilateral triangles are removed from opposite sides of the circular defect, with the central axis of each triangle 30° from the long axis of the skin tension lines. The flaps are transposed and sutured into their new positions to shorten the sides of the original circle and transform the shape of the defect (Fig. 15-17, *C*).

Triangular Defects

Triangular lesions may be closed by shifting local tissue or rotating flaps. A simple closure technique is to begin at each point of the triangle and suture toward the center of the defect to create a Y-shaped suture line (Fig. 15-18, *A*). A ro-

tational flap is a semicircular or three quarter circular flap of skin that is rotated about a pivot point into the defect (Fig. 15-18, *B*). Rotational flaps are used when skin is available on only one side of the defect or when moving skin from one side of the defect results in distortion of adjacent structures (i.e., near the eye or anus). Bilateral rotational flaps are used when little movable skin is available, but it is movable on two sides of the defect. Flaps should be sufficiently large (about 4:1 length to width ratio) to prevent tension on surrounding tissue. If tension is noted, a backcut into the base of the flap may ease tension and allow the flap to move by a combination of rotation and transposition (Fig. 15-18, *C*). Tension may also be relieved by removing a small triangle of skin (Bürow's triangle) at the end of the semicircle opposite the defect.

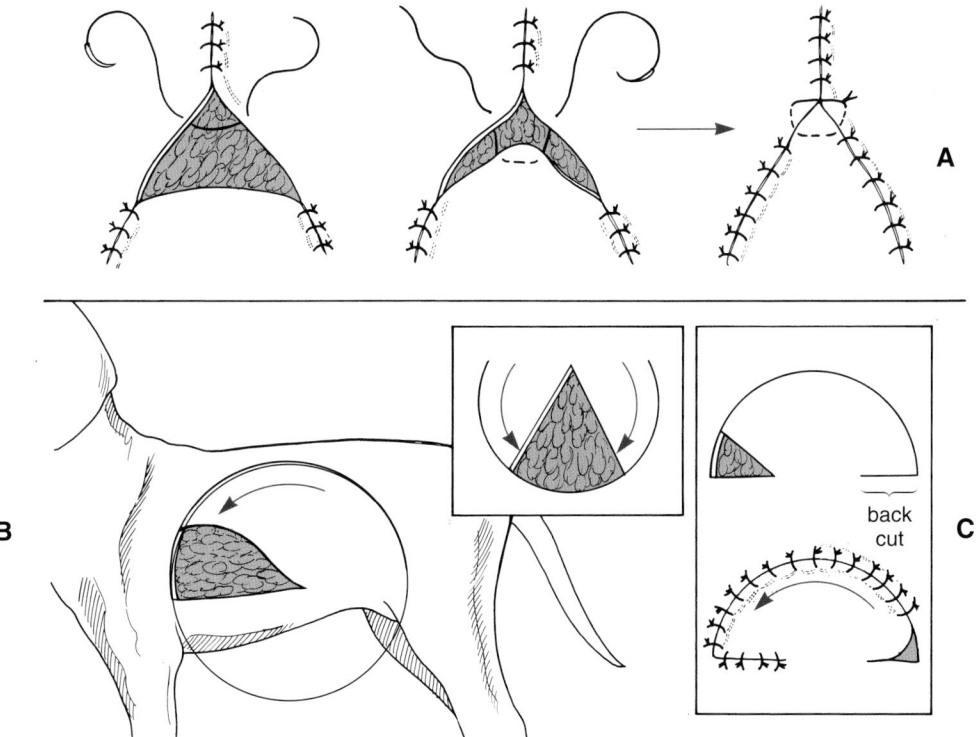

FIG. 15-18
Repair of triangular defects. **A,** Close the defect as a Y by beginning at each point and suturing toward the center. **B,** Create one or two rotational flaps at the defect edge. **C,** A backcut or excision of Bürow's triangle may be necessary to relieve tension at the base of the flap.

Square and Rectangular Defects

Square or rectangular defects may be closed using centripetal, unilateral, or bilateral advancement flaps or rotational flaps. Centripetal closure begins with suture closure at each corner of the defect and advances toward the center to form an X suture line (Fig. 15-19, *A*). This technique should be used when skin is available on all four sides of the defect. A unilateral or single-pedicle advancement flap should be used to close defects with mobile skin on only one side and in the same plane as the defect. Parallel incisions are made from two corners of the defect at least as long as the width of the defect, and skin is undermined and advanced over the defect (Fig. 15-19, *B*). If necessary, relaxing incisions are made at the base of the flap. An H-plasty or a double-pedicle advancement flap is used to close large defects that have mobile skin available on two sides of the defect (Fig. 15-19, *C*). A rotational or transposition flap is used to cover defects that have mobile skin on only one side of the defect and available skin in a plane different from that of the defect (Fig. 15-19, *D*). These flaps become effectively shorter with increasing rotation. They should be longer than the defect to achieve adequate coverage without tension. The width of the flap base should at least equal the width of the defect. The diagonal from the pivot point of the flap to the farthest corner of the defect should be equal to the diagonal from the flap's

pivot point across the flap. A "dog ear" forms at the base of the flap opposite the pivot point.

Fusiform Defects

Fusiform, or elliptic, defects are closed by first placing a suture across the widest part of the defect. Continue to divide each remaining segment in half with subsequent sutures to achieve a linear closure without "dog ears" (Fig. 15-20).

Crescentic Defects

In crescentic defects, one side is longer than the other. These defects are closed beginning at the midpoint. Each remaining segment is divided in half with subsequent sutures, and sutures on the convex side are spaced closer together than sutures on the concave side. "Dog ears" are removed as necessary (Fig. 15-21).

Suggested Reading

Aitken ML, Patnaik AK: Comparison of needle-core (Trucut) biopsy and surgical biopsy for the diagnosis of cutaneous and subcutaneous masses: a prospective study of 51 cases (November 1997-August 1998), *J Am Anim Hosp Assoc* 36:153, 2000.
Needle-core biopsy specimens accurately predicted surgical biopsy results.

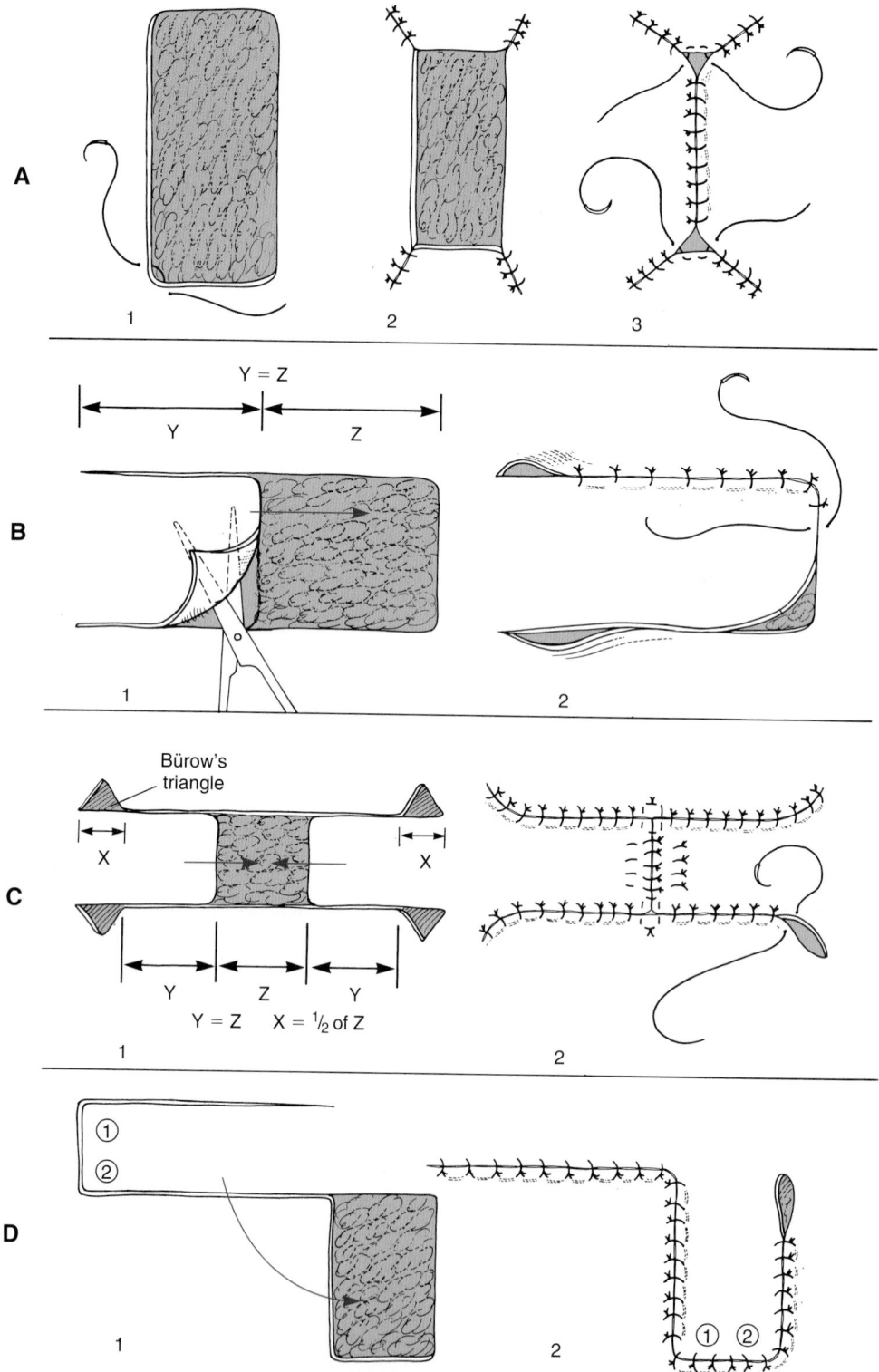

FIG. 15-19

Repair of square or rectangular defects. **A,** Close from the corners and advance to the center to form an X suture line. Use a unilateral **(B)** or bilateral **(C)** advancement flap to close defects with mobile skin on only one or two sides of the defect. **D,** Use a rotational or transposition flap to cover defects with mobile skin in a plane different from the defect.

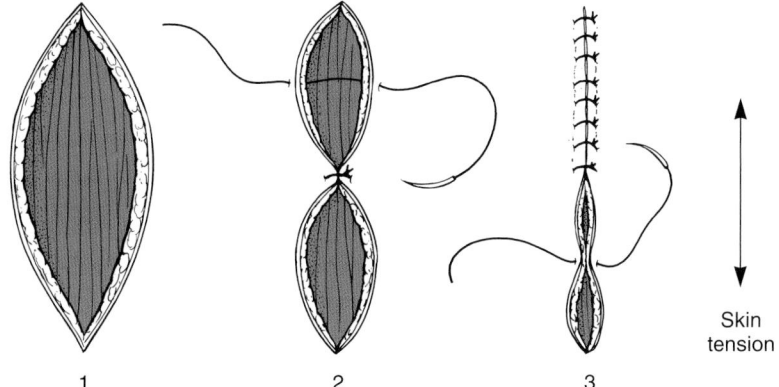

FIG. 15-20
Close fusiform defects *(1)* by placing the first suture across the widest part of the wound.
Continue to divide each segment of the defect in half with subsequent sutures *(2 and 3)*.

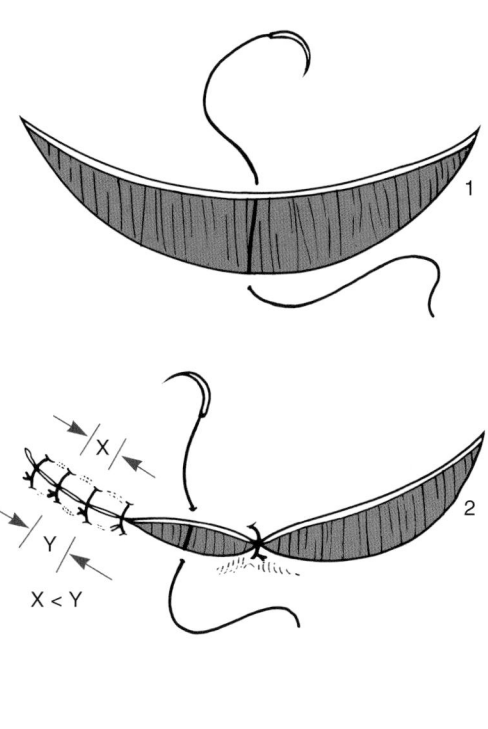

FIG. 15-21
Close crescent defects by *(1)* beginning at the midpoint and dividing each segment of the defect in half with subsequent sutures *(2 and 3)*. Space sutures closer on the convex than the concave aspect of the defect.

McEntee MC, Samii VF, Walsh P et al: Postoperative assessment of surgical clip position in 16 dogs with cancer: a pilot study, *J Am Vet Med Assoc* 40:300, 2004.
Results suggest that clips are potentially useful in identifying the tumor bed and determining the radiation treatment fields.

Pavletic MM: Use of an external skin-stretching device for wound closure in dogs and cats, *J Am Vet Med Assoc* 217:350, 2000.
The mechanism of skin stretching and the results from 24 animals where an external stretching device was used are presented.
Pavletic MM: *Atlas of small animal reconstructive surgery,* ed 2, Philadelphia, 1999, WB Saunders.
Helpful descriptions and illustrations of fundamental techniques are presented.
Rizzo LB, Ritchey JW, Higbee RG et al: Histological comparison of skin biopsy specimens collected by use of carbon dioxide or 810-nm diode lasers from dogs, *J Am Vet Med Assoc* 225:1562, 2004.
Multiple skin samples were collected from four dogs; evaluation determined that carbon dioxide lasers caused less thermal injury than 810-nm diode lasers.
Simpson AM, Ludwig LL, Newman SJ et al: Evaluation of surgical margins required for complete excision of cutaneous mast cell tumors in dogs, *J Am Vet Med Assoc* 224:236, 2004.
Results from a prospective trial involving 21 dogs suggest that a 2-cm lateral margin and a deep margin of 1 fascial plane appear to be adequate for complete excision of grade I and II mast cell tumors.
Swaim SF, Henderson RA: *Small animal wound management,* ed 2, Philadelphia, 1997, Williams & Wilkins.
A textbook with in-depth descriptions of fundamental and advanced reconstructive techniques.

PEDICLE FLAPS

Pedicle flaps are "tongues" of epidermis and dermis that are partly detached from donor sites and used to cover defects. The base or pedicle of the flap contains the blood supply essential for flap survival. Pedicle flaps often allow immediate coverage of a wound bed and prevent the prolonged healing, excessive scarring, and contracture associated with healing by secondary intention. They can be classified in various ways based on the location, blood supply, and tissue formation. A specific flap may be classified in more than one way. Most flaps are called *subdermal plexus flaps;* however, those with direct cutaneous vessels are called *axial pattern flaps.*

Flaps that remain attached to the donor bed by only the direct cutaneous vessels and subcutaneous tissue are *island flaps.* Flaps created adjacent to the defect in loose elastic skin are *local flaps. Interpolation flaps* are rectangular flaps that are rotated into a nearby rather than adjacent defect. Those created at a distance from the defect are *distant flaps,* which usually require multiple-stage reconstruction. Flaps that include tissue other than skin and subcutaneous tissue are called compound or composite flaps and may include muscle (myocutaneous), cartilage, or bone.

Increasing the width of a pedicle flap does not increase the surviving length of the flap. However, narrowing the base of the pedicle by backcut techniques increases the possibility of necrosis. The base of flaps should be slightly wider than the width of the flap body. Multiple small flaps may be preferable to a large flap if circulation is questionable. Delaying flap transfer 18 to 21 days after initial creation may improve circulation and survival in ischemic flaps (delay phenomenon). Flaps must be fixed to the edges of the recipient bed with no tension to allow revascularization and healing. Donor sites should have enough skin to permit primary closure and skin transfer to the recipient site. Donor sites with excessive motion and stress should be avoided. Reconstruction should be planned so that the color and direction of hair growth after transfer of flaps or grafts to the recipient site are similar to those of the donor site.

Hyperbaric oxygen treatment may improve survival of the flap or graft. Hyperbaric oxygen treatment consists of breathing 100% oxygen in a chamber where pressure is maintained at greater than 1 atm absolute or greater than sea level pressure. Hyperbaric oxygen therapy hyperoxygenates hypoxic tissue, stimulates fibroblasts, and enhances tissue revascularization.

Venous congestion in a flap may be suspected if the flap becomes dusky or bluish in color; if capillary return is quicker than normal; and if rapid or dark bleeding occurs in response to a needle prick. Venous congestion may lead to failure of the flap or graft.

ADVANCEMENT FLAPS

Advancement flaps are local subdermal plexus flaps. They include single-pedicle, bipedicle, H-plasty, and V-Y advancement flaps (see Figs. 15-16, 15-18, and 15-19). Flaps are formed in adjacent, loose, elastic skin that can be slid over the defect. An advancement flap is developed parallel to lines of least tension to facilitate its forward stretch over a wound. It does not bring additional loose skin to the wound. Advancement flap stretching is opposed by retractive forces that may lead to dehiscence.

ROTATIONAL FLAPS

Rotational flaps are local flaps that are pivoted over a defect with which they share a common border. They are semicircular and may be paired or single. They may be used to close triangular defects without creating a secondary defect. A curved incision is created, and the skin is undermined in a stepwise fashion until it covers the defect without tension (see Fig. 15-18).

TRANSPOSITION FLAPS

Transposition flaps are rectangular, local flaps that bring additional skin when rotated into defects. A Z-plasty is a modified transposition flap (see Fig. 15-16, *G* and *H*). Ninety degree transposition flaps are aligned parallel to the lines of greatest tension to obtain the bulk of the flap required to cover the defect. The donor site is easily closed because minimal tension lines are perpendicular to the suture line. The width of the flap equals the width of the defect (see Fig. 15-19, *D*). The length of the flap is determined by measuring from the pivot point of the flap to the most distant point of the defect; the length decreases as the arc of rotation increases past 90° because of kinking and skin folding. "Dog ears" occur but flatten with time. Other useful transposition flaps include the forelimb fold and flank fold flaps (Figs. 15-22 through 15-25). The size and length of skin fold flaps vary with body conformation and which three of the four flap attachments are severed. The four attachments are medial and lateral attachments to the upper limb and dorsal and ventral attachments to the trunk. Often a margin of the defect to be closed serves as one of the incisions. Skin fold flaps can be harvested bilaterally to close large axillary and sternal or inguinal wounds. Creation of these flaps begins by grasping the loose skin extending from the elbow to the body wall or flank to determine the amount of skin that can be harvested as a flap. Symmetric lateral and medial incisions are first outlined and then made. These incisions are connected with a crescentic incision made proximal to the elbow (stifle). The flap is elevated from the triceps or quadriceps, transposed, and sutured to the prepared wound bed. The donor site is apposed after flap transposition. Other elbow or flank fold flap configurations can be created for coverage of defects involving the lateral thorax, abdomen, hip, stifle, shoulder, or elbow by severing either the dorsal or ventral body wall attachments. (Figs. 15-23 and 15-25). The flank fold flap supplied by the lower branches of the ventral branch of the deep circumflex iliac artery can be considered an axial pattern flap. Similarly, if the elbow fold flap includes the lateral thoracic artery, it should be considered an axial pattern flap as well. A novel transposition flap can be created from scrotal skin after prescrotal castration and positioned in the perineum and thigh.

INTERPOLATION FLAPS

A variation of the transposition flap, the interpolation flap differs in that it lacks a common border with the wound; this leaves an area of interposed skin between the donor bed and the recipient wound. The flap is created in the same way as a transposition flap except that the length of the interpolation flap must include the length of the intervening skin segment (see Fig. 15-19). The subcutaneous tissue on the segment of flap overlying the intervening skin is left exposed. After approximately 14 days, this redundant segment of the flap is resected and the incised edges are sutured. As an alternative, a bridge incision can be made connecting the donor and recipient beds to facilitate flap transfer, which eliminates the need for a second surgical procedure.

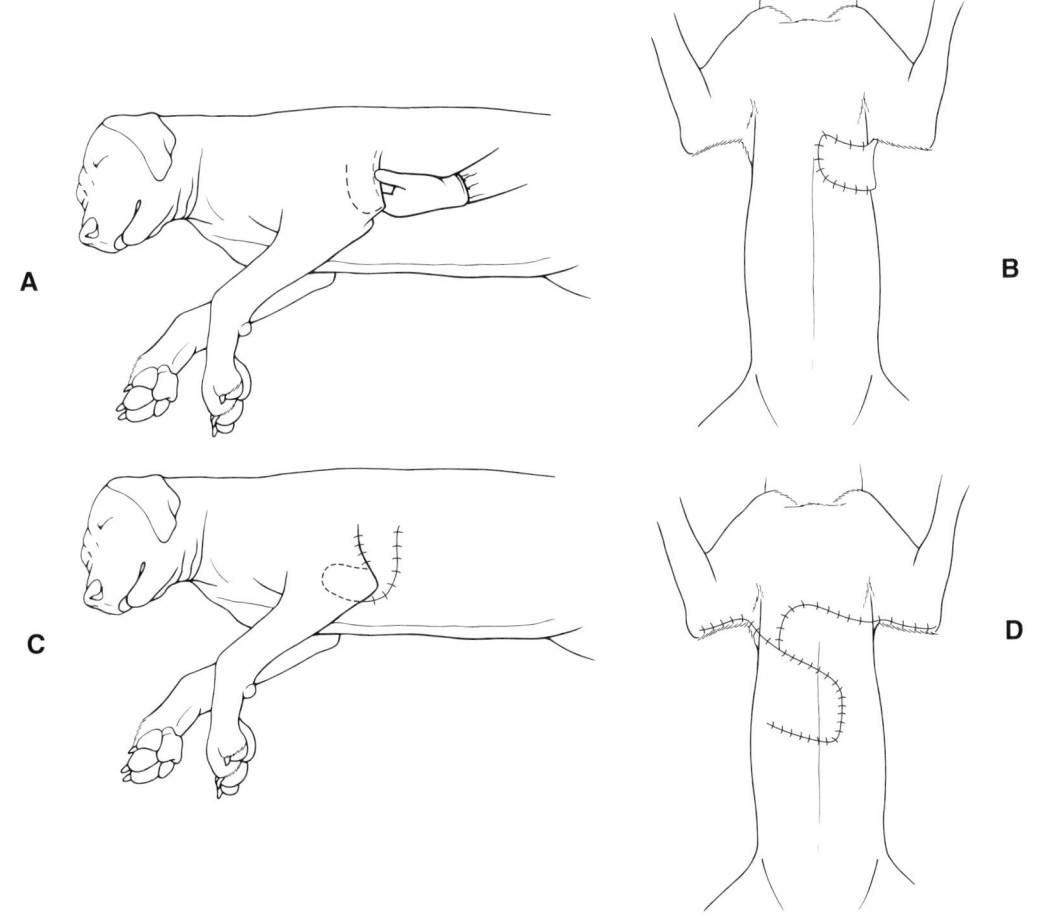

FIG. 15-22
The forelimb skin fold is harvested to close axillary or sternal wounds. **A,** Grasp loose skin from the elbow to the body wall to determine the amount of skin that can be harvested. Dashed lines indicate incision to create lateral and medial skin incisions to define the width of the flap, then connect the incisions with a crescent-shaped incision proximal to the elbow. **B** and **C,** Elevate, transpose, and suture the flap into the wound, then close the donor site. **D,** Create bilateral flaps to close larger wounds.

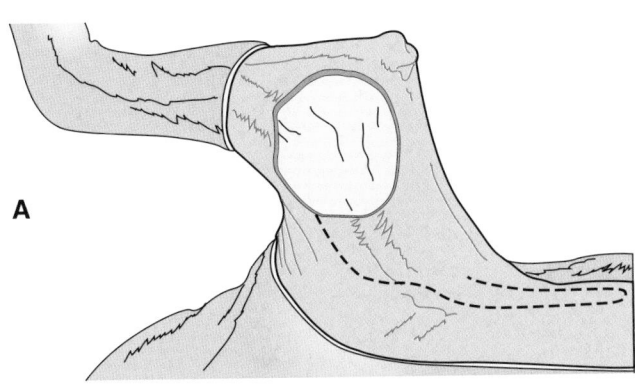

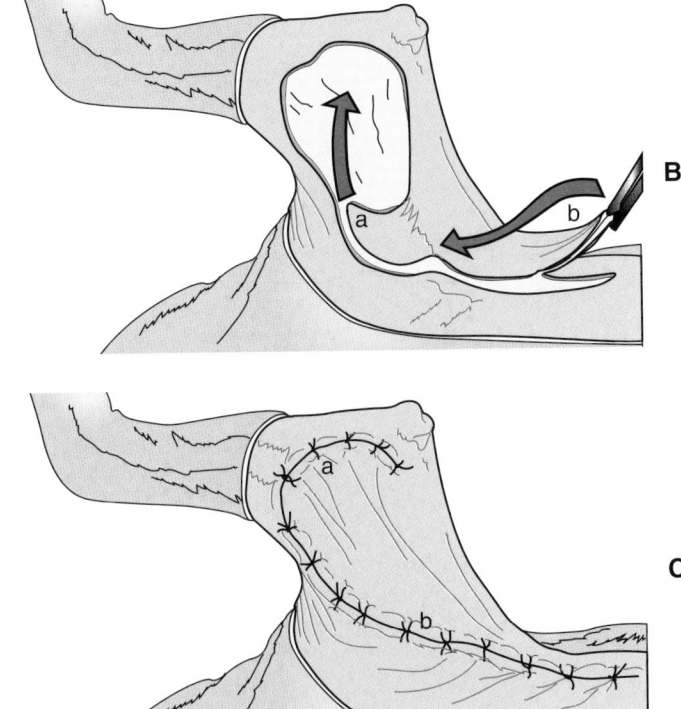

FIG. 15-23
This elbow fold flap is being created to close a defect on the medial aspect of the proximal forelimb. **A,** The dashed line indicates the incision of the ventral body wall attachment of the fold. **B,** The flap is elevated and prepared for transposition. **C,** The flap is sutured into position and the donor site is closed.

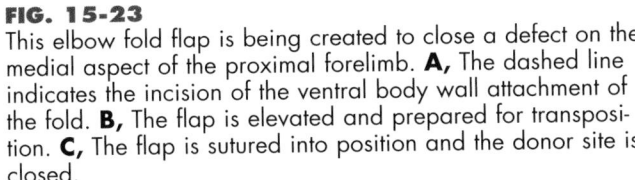

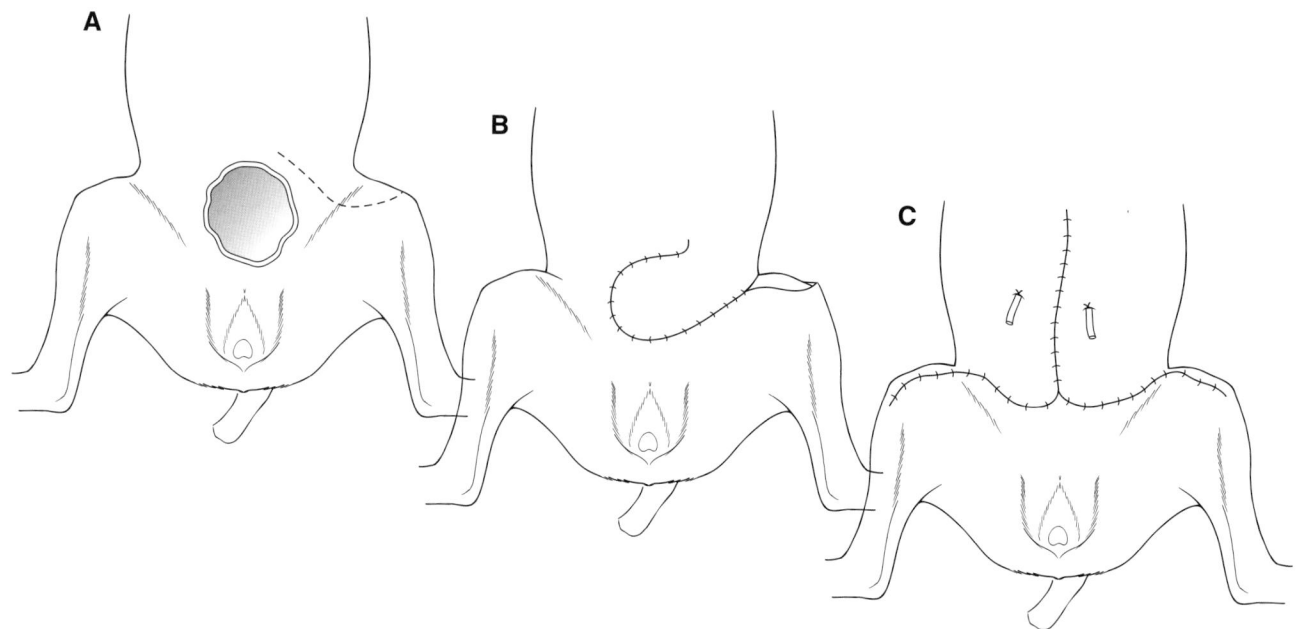

FIG. 15-24
The flank skin fold is harvested to close inguinal wounds. **A,** Loose skin from the flank is incised to create a flap (dashed line). **B,** Create lateral and medial skin incisions to define the width of the flap; then connect these incisions with a crescent-shaped incision proximal to the stifle; transpose and suture to defect. **C,** Create bilateral flaps to close larger wounds.

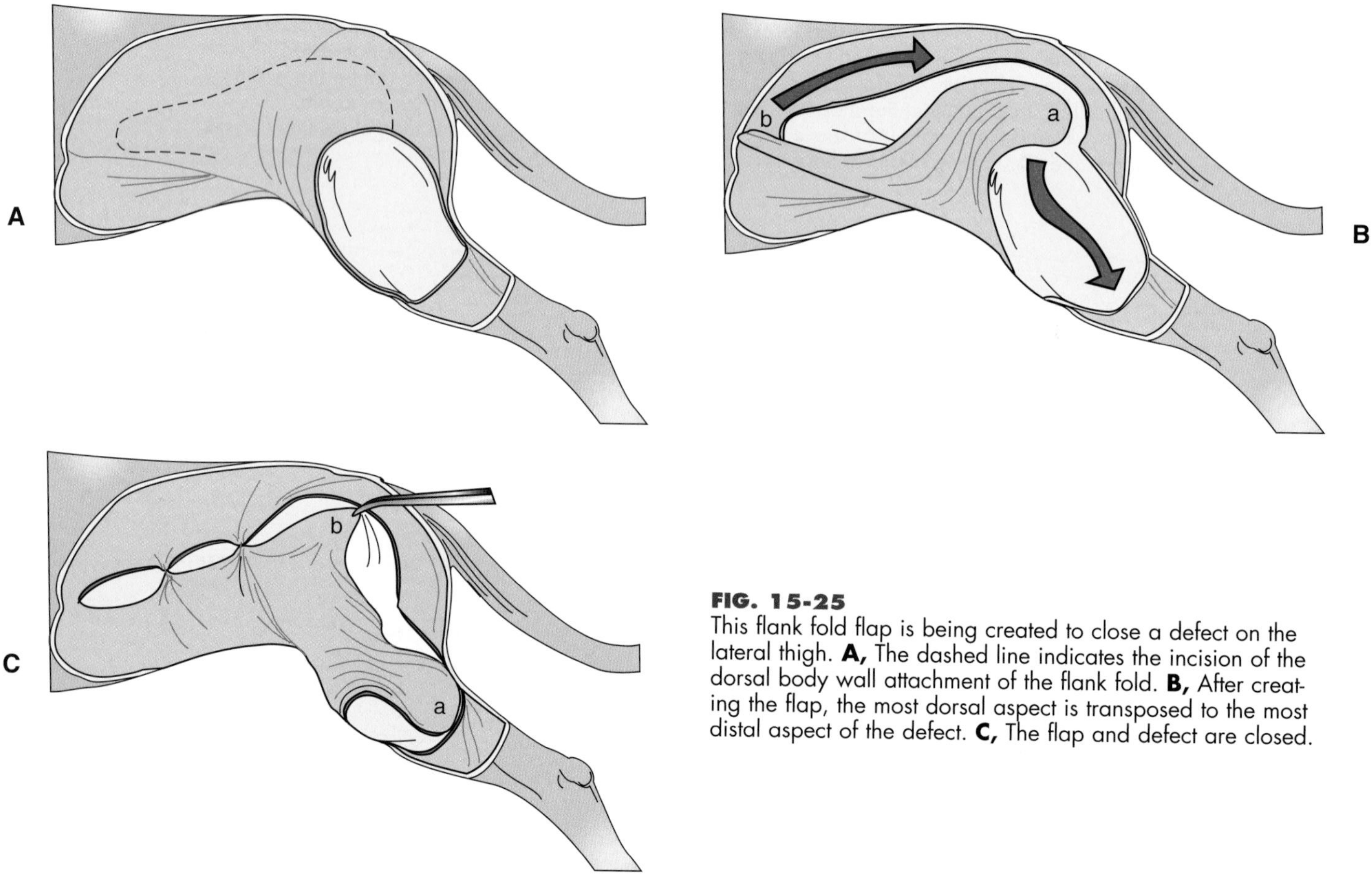

FIG. 15-25
This flank fold flap is being created to close a defect on the lateral thigh. **A,** The dashed line indicates the incision of the dorsal body wall attachment of the flank fold. **B,** After creating the flap, the most dorsal aspect is transposed to the most distal aspect of the defect. **C,** The flap and defect are closed.

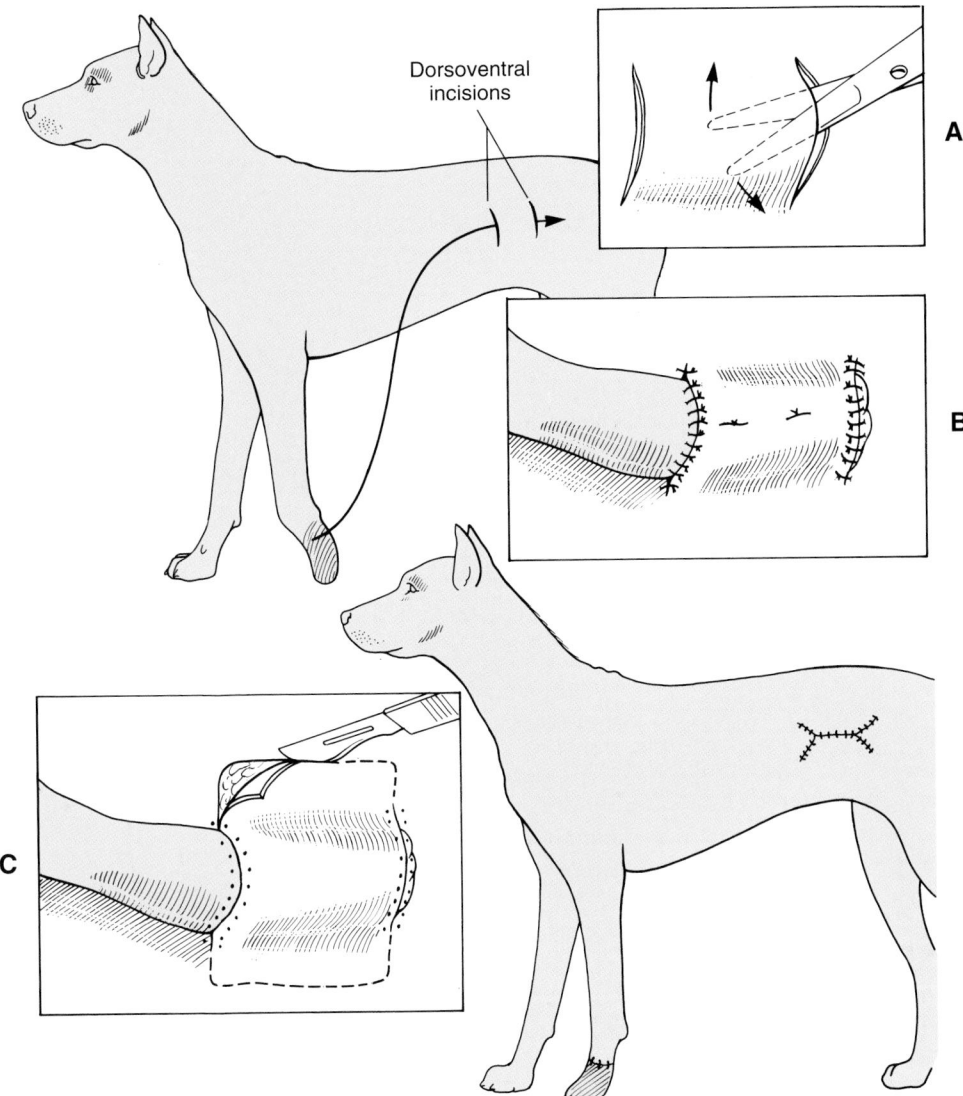

FIG. 15-26
Pouch flap. **A,** Make two parallel dorsoventral incisions and undermine skin to create a pouch. **B,** Position the limb inside the pouch and suture the edges of the defect to the flap. **C,** After 2 to 3 weeks, release the limb and cover the remainder of the defect. Make two horizontal incisions to free the flap, then suture it to the remaining edges of the defect. Close the donor site.

POUCH AND HINGE FLAPS

Pouch flaps (bipedicle flaps) and hinge flaps (single-pedicle flaps) are direct, distant flaps useful for reconstructing lower extremity skin defects, although axial pattern or mesh grafts are more commonly used. Reconstruction using the pouch or hinge flap requires three stages: (1) débridement and granulation, (2) flap creation and healing, and (3) flap release. After a healthy bed of granulation tissue has formed, the skin on the limb and ipsilateral thoracoabdominal area is prepared for aseptic surgery. The limb is positioned along the animal's side, and two parallel dorsoventral incisions are made at locations that allow complete coverage of the defect (Fig. 15-26, *A*).

Create a flap 1 to 2 cm wider than the defect to accommodate elastic contraction and stretching of the flap.

If pad tissue is absent, only a single cranial incision is necessary.

Undermine the flap beneath the cutaneous trunci muscle, and place the foot within the pouch. Appose skin at the wound edges with the edges of the flap using interrupted approximating sutures (e.g., 3-0 or 4-0 polypropylene, polybutester, or nylon). Place three to four interrupted sutures through the skin of the flap into the granulation tissue to immobilize the flap over the defect. Place two or three retain-

ing or tension-relieving sutures through the skin adjacent to the flap on the limb and body wall to help prevent the limb from shifting ventrally and placing tension on the flap. Bandage the limb against the body for 14 days, and change the bandage every 3 to 4 days. As an alternative, cut an access window over the flap, allowing evaluation and wound care without removal of the entire bandage. Place a patch bandage over the access window between treatments. Release the limb from the pouch by making two horizontal incisions (dorsal and ventral) an appropriate distance from the paw to allow coverage of the palmar aspect of the defect (Fig. 15-26, B).

Delayed release of the flap by dividing the pedicles in stages encourages flap survival.

Incise half of the lower pedicle, followed by release of the remaining half in 2 to 3 days. Two days later, begin delayed division of the upper pedicle in a similar fashion. Lavage the medial aspect of the paw to remove exudate and débride if necessary. Trim freed flap edges and suture to the opposing wound border with each division. Lavage the donor site and close with interrupted approximating sutures (e.g., 3-0 to 4-0 polypropylene or nylon) (Fig. 15-26, C).

Although this technique is successful in covering distal extremity skin defects, some animals may not tolerate the limb being positioned against the body wall, and temporary joint stiffness and muscle atrophy may occur.

AP TUBED PEDICLE FLAPS

A tubed pedicle flap uses a multistaged procedure to "walk" an indirect, distant flap to a recipient site. The tube is made wider and longer (2 to 3 cm) than the recipient bed because these tubes contract as a result of decreased elasticity and fibrosis before transfer.

To create the tube, make two parallel incisions through the skin in an area where remaining skin can be reapposed without excess tension (Fig. 15-27, A). Undermine skin between the two incisions. Suture incised edges of the flap together with approximating sutures (e.g., 3-0 or 4-0 polypropylene or nylon), creating a tube attached at both ends. Appose the edges of the donor site with approximating sutures (e.g., 3-0 or 4-0 nylon or polypropylene). After 18 to 21 days, transect one end of the tube and transpose it to the recipient bed.

Transection can also be done in stages; half of the tube is incised and resutured in place, then 2 days later the remainder of the tube is transected and then transposed.

As an alternative, transpose the end of the tube nearer the donor site, and transect the other end of the tube and transpose it over the defect (Fig. 15-27, B) after an additional 18 to 21 days. Incise the tube and unroll it as needed to cover the defect, and suture the edges of the tube to the edges of the defect (Fig. 15-27, C). Appose skin edges at the tube's

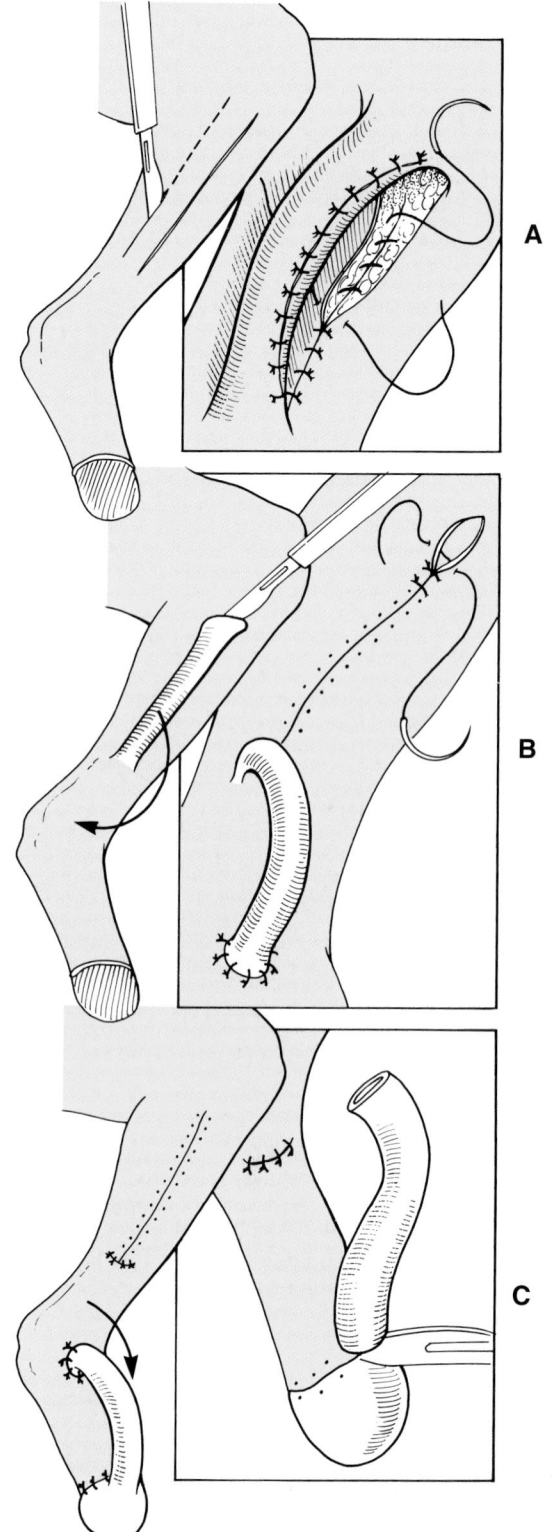

FIG. 15-27

Tubed pedicle flap. **A,** Make two parallel incisions in mobile skin. Create a tube by suturing the edges together and appose the donor site. Note: The tube may need to be created more proximally on the limb than illustrated to have sufficiently mobile skin to close the donor site defect. **B,** Approximately 3 weeks later, advance the tube toward the defect by severing one end of the tube and suturing it nearer the defect. **C,** After another 3 weeks, sever the other end of the tube and use it to cover the defect or advance it closer to the defect.

origin. Transect the remaining end of the tube after 18 to 21 days to complete coverage of the defect if necessary.

The disadvantage of this technique is the number of stages and time required to accomplish wound closure.

AXIAL PATTERN FLAPS

Axial pattern flaps are pedicle flaps that include a direct cutaneous artery and vein at the base of the flap. The terminal branches of these vessels supply the subdermal plexus. They have better perfusion than pedicle flaps with a circulation from the subdermal plexus alone. Axial pattern flaps are elevated and transferred to cutaneous defects within their radius. They usually are rectangular or L-shaped flaps. Axial pattern flaps have been described using the caudal auricular artery branches, the superficial temporal artery, the omocervical artery (superficial cervical), the thoracodorsal artery, the lateral thoracic artery, the superficial brachial artery, the cranial superficial epigastric and caudal superficial epigastric arteries, the deep circumflex iliac artery, the genicular artery, and the lateral caudal arteries as direct cutaneous arteries in dogs (Fig. 15-28). Although similar flaps can be created in cats, only the thoracodorsal, caudal superficial epigastric, caudal auricular, superficial cervical, superficial temporal artery axial pattern, and reverse saphenous conduit flaps have been evaluated. Axial pattern flaps require careful planning, measuring, and mapping on the skin surface to minimize errors. Positioning is important to ensure that skin and underlying landmarks are in normal anatomic position. Limbs are placed in relaxed

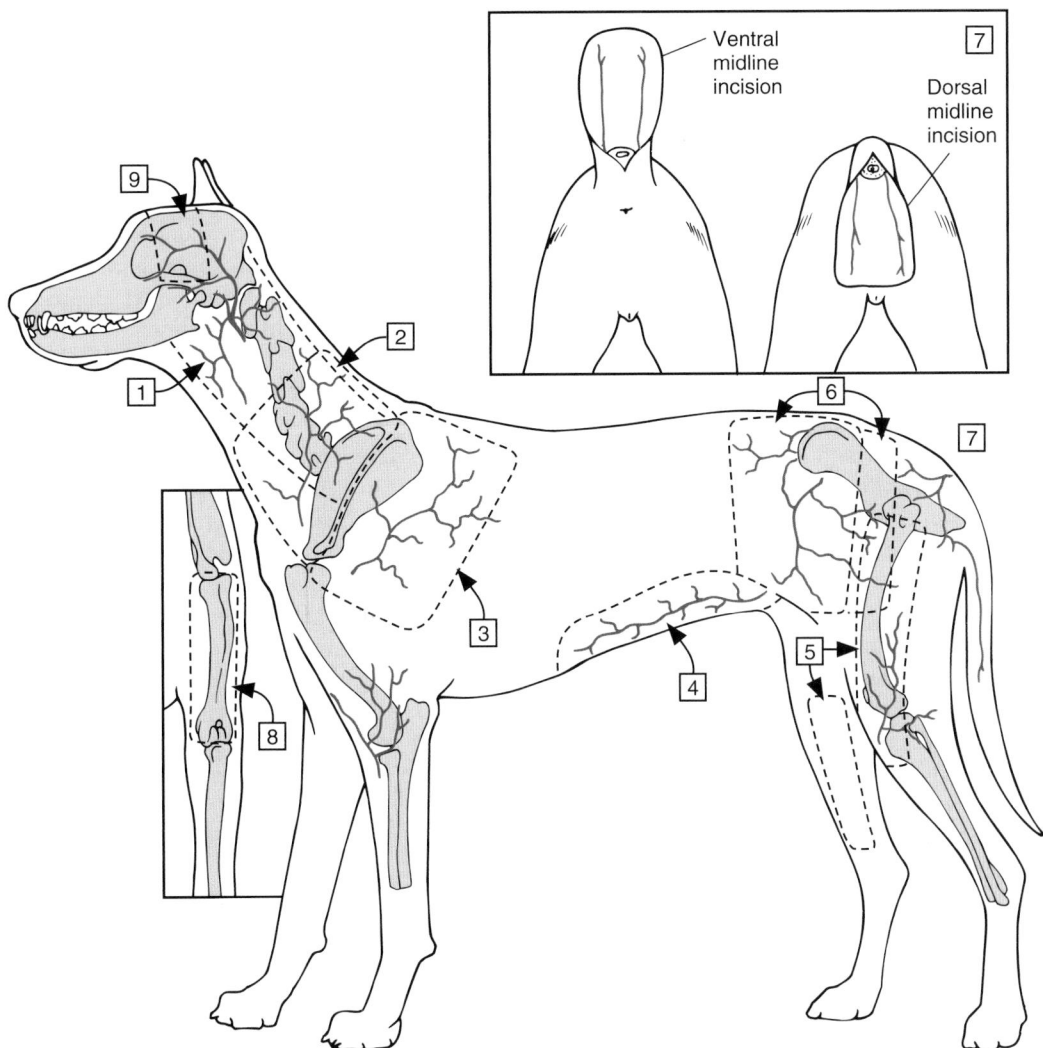

FIG. 15-28
Direct cutaneous vessels used in axial pattern flaps. *1,* Caudal auricular; *2,* omocervical; *3,* thoracodorsal; *4,* caudal superficial epigastric; *5,* medial genicular; *6,* deep circumflex iliac; *7,* superficial lateral caudal *(inset); 8,* superficial brachial *(inset); 9,* superficial temporal. Dashed lines outline anticipated flaps corresponding with each direct cutaneous vessel (neither a cranial superficial epigastric flap nor a reverse saphenous conduit flap is shown).

extension, and thoracoabdominal skin is grasped, lifted, and allowed to retract spontaneously to normal position before the flaps are outlined. Axial pattern flaps can be modified to create island arterial flaps by severing the cutaneous pedicle but preserving the direct cutaneous artery and vein. Island flaps have the potential for use as a free flap for transfer and microvascular anastomosis.

Axial pattern flaps are used most commonly to facilitate wound closure after tumor resection or trauma. The survival rate for axial pattern flaps is approximately twice that for subdermal plexus flaps of comparable size. Axial pattern flaps also provide durable, full-thickness skin that can be transposed primarily without the need for a vascular bed or postoperative immobilization. Complications include wound drainage, partial dehiscence, distal flap necrosis, infections, and seroma formation. The cosmetic results are good.

Caudal Auricular Axial Pattern Flap

The sternocleidomastoideus branches of the caudal auricular artery and vein may be used to reconstruct ipsilateral or contralateral defects involving the head and neck. The sternocleidomastoideus branches are located between the lateral aspect of the wing of the atlas and the vertical ear canal and are directed caudodorsally. The caudal auricular artery is located approximately 1 cm caudal to the base of the scutiform cartilage of the pinna (a palpable depression at the midpoint between the base of the ear and the wing of the atlas).

Position the forelimb in relaxed extension so that the scapula is perpendicular to the trunk. Outline the flap with the base centered over the lateral aspect of the wing of the atlas (see Fig. 15-28). Draw a caudal incision line parallel to the base at a point rostral to the scapular spine, which will provide a flap long enough to cover the defect. Then draw dorsal and ventral lines that connect the base and the caudal incision line at a width that allows closure of the donor site.

In cats, the dorsal border is nearer the dorsal midline. The width of the flap approximates that of the central third of the lateral aspect of the cervical area.

Incise the dorsal, ventral, and caudal lines and elevate the flap deep to the platysma (sphincter colli superficialis) muscle until the sternocleidomastoideus branches of the caudal auricular artery are identified. Rotate the flap into the defect, place drains, and appose skin edges. If there is interposing skin between the donor and recipient sites, make a bridge incision to connect the sites or partly tube the flap to span the interposing skin.

Superficial Temporal Artery Axial Pattern Flap

A cutaneous branch of the superficial temporal artery allows formation of an axial pattern flap that can be used to cover defects involving the face and head, especially the maxillofacial area. This flap is also used in oral reconstruction after partial maxillectomy. The superficial temporal artery lies in a subcutaneous position at the base of the zygomatic arch and extends rostrally along the zygomatic arch.

Position the animal in ventral recumbency. Mark the base of the flap caudally at the caudal aspect of the zygomatic arch and rostrally at the lateral orbital rim. Outline the flap by making two parallel lines; extend one line from each of these points dorsally and laterally to the middle of the dorsal orbital rim of the contralateral eye. Limit the width of the flap to the orbits and ears. Connect the parallel lines (see Fig. 15-28). Incise the outlined flap and elevate it with the frontalis muscle, which is a thin muscle overlying the temporalis muscle. Transpose the flap. Eliminate dead space with Penrose or closed suction drains and close the defects.

Omocervical Axial Pattern Flap (Superficial Cervical Axial Pattern Flap)

Omocervical axial pattern flaps are used for defects involving the face, head, ear, shoulder, neck, and axilla. By making a bridging incision between the angle of the jaw and the cranioventral edge of the donor site and creating a parapharyngeal tunnel, a staged, extended flap can be passed into the mouth to reconstruct oronasal defects caudal to the third premolar. They incorporate the superficial cervical branch of the omocervical artery and associated vein. Vessels originate adjacent to the prescapular lymph node at a site corresponding to the cranial shoulder depression and course dorsally just cranial to the scapula.

Position the patient in lateral recumbency with the forelimb in relaxed extension perpendicular to the trunk. Draw a line over the scapular spine to identify the caudal incision. Draw the cranial incision line parallel to the scapular spine at a site equal to the distance between the scapular spine and the cranial shoulder depression at the cranial edge of the scapula. Extend the lines to and continue along the dorsal midline. Extend the flap to the contralateral scapulohumeral joint if necessary. As an alternative, create a right-angle design incorporating the skin over the dorsal aspect of the opposite scapula. Large omocervical flaps may require ligation of the opposite omocervical direct cutaneous artery and vein. Incise the outlined flap and undermine deep to the sphincter colli superficialis muscle. Transpose the flap. Eliminate dead space with Penrose or closed suction drains and close the defects.

Thoracodorsal Axial Pattern Flap

Thoracodorsal axial pattern flaps are preferable to omocervical flaps because they are more robust. They are used to cover defects involving the shoulder, forelimb, elbow, axilla, and thorax (Fig. 15-29). In cats, the thoracodorsal flap extends to the carpus. In dogs, distal limb coverage depends on the body conformation and limb length. The flap is based on a cutaneous branch of the thoracodorsal artery and associated vein located at the caudal shoulder depression at a level parallel to the dorsal border of the acromion.

from the caudal aspect of the shoulder joint running horizontally and slightly ventrally on the lateral thoracic wall ventral to the thoracodorsal artery. It arises from the axillary artery close to the caudal border of the first rib. Deep branches supply the axillary lymph node, the ventral portion of the latissimus dorsi muscle, and part of the deep pectoral muscles. More superficial cranial branches to the elbow skin fold supply this axial pattern flap. The distribution of this vessel varies slightly between breeds.

Position the patient in lateral recumbency with the forelimb in relaxed extension perpendicular to the trunk. Palpate the caudal aspect of the shoulder joint and identify the origin of the thoracodorsal artery (see previous discussion) to estimate the location of the lateral thoracic artery in a more ventral location. Draw the flap with the ventral border along the dorsal border of the deep pectoral muscle and the dorsal border parallel to this line with the artery in the center. Incise along these lines extending toward but not including the second mamma. Connect the parallel lines caudally, undermine the flap deep to the cutaneous trunci, and transpose up to 90° to cover the defect. Place a closed suction drain, secure the flap to the defect, and appose the donor site.

Superficial Brachial Axial Pattern Flap

Superficial brachial axial pattern flaps are used to cover defects involving the antebrachium and elbow. These flaps depend on a small branch of the brachial artery located 3 cm proximal to the elbow (superficial brachial artery).

Position the patient in dorsal recumbency with the leg suspended in an elevated position. Outline the flap by drawing parallel to the humeral shaft two lines that extend dorsally and gradually converge at or below the greater tubercle. Center the base of the flap over the anterior third of the flexor surface of the elbow. Elevate the flap to the base, being especially careful to preserve the subdermal plexus, superficial brachial vessels, and cephalic vein. Rotate the flap into the defect, place drains, and appose skin edges. Flap length and survival preclude use of this flap to cover wounds in the carpal area.

Caudal Superficial Epigastric Axial Pattern Flap

The caudal superficial epigastric axial pattern flap is a versatile flap that is used to cover defects involving the caudal abdomen, flank, prepuce, perineum, thigh, and hind leg. In cats, the flap extends over the metatarsal area. In dogs with long bodies and short limbs, it may extend to or below the level of the tibiotarsal joint. The flap includes the three to four caudal mammary glands and is supplied by the caudal superficial epigastric artery and associated vein that pass through the inguinal ring.

Position the patient in dorsal recumbency. Outline the flap with the ventral midline as the location of the medial incision.

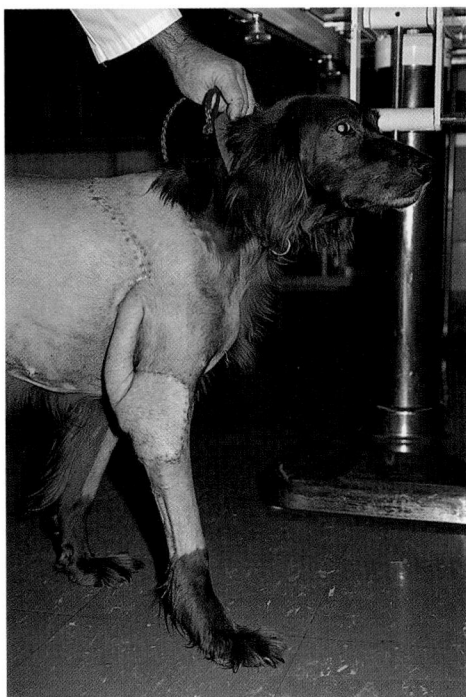

FIG. 15-29
A thoracodorsal axial pattern flap has been tubed and applied over an elbow wound.

Position the patient in lateral recumbency with the forelimb in relaxed extension perpendicular to the trunk. Outline the flap by drawing a line over the scapular spine to mark the cranial incision (see Fig. 15-28). Draw the caudal incision line parallel to the scapular spine at a site approximately twice the distance from the acromion to the caudal shoulder depression. Extend the lines to and continue along the dorsal midline. Create an L flap for extended coverage by extending the dorsal incision line by about 50% and creating a parallel incision line beginning at the approximate midpoint of the caudal incision line. Incise the outlined flap and undermine deep to the cutaneous trunci muscle. Transpose the flap. Create a tube or make a bridge incision as needed for distant transposition. Eliminate dead space with Penrose or closed suction drains and close the defects.

> NOTE: Flaps extended ventral to the contralateral scapulohumeral joint usually survive. Development of long thoracodorsal axial pattern flaps may require division of the opposite cutaneous branches of the thoracodorsal artery and vein.

Lateral Thoracic Axial Pattern Flap

The lateral thoracic axial pattern flap is similar to the thoracodorsal flap, but smaller with a less extensive approach. It is used to cover the elbow. The lateral thoracic artery extends

In male dogs, incorporate the base of the prepuce. Mark a parallel lateral incision at a distance equal to the distance from the mammary teats to the midline. Determine the number of mammary glands to include in the flap based on the size of the defect. Create the flap by connecting the two parallel lines between the first and second or second and third glands with a crescent-shaped incision. Undermine the flap at the level of the external abdominal oblique aponeurosis, deep to the supramammarius muscle. Make the flap wider as needed to cover the defect if abundant loose, elastic skin is available for closure. Transpose the flap, place drains, and appose skin edges.

> NOTE: Concurrent ovariohysterectomy is recommended because transposed glands remain functional. Later, mammae may be resected if their appearance is objectionable.

Cranial Superficial Epigastric Axial Pattern Flap

The cranial superficial epigastric flap is smaller and less versatile than the caudal superficial epigastric axial pattern flap; however, it can be quite useful for closure of large skin defects overlying the sternum. The flap is kept small because these vessels are short, and some flap necrosis is expected. The flap may include mammary glands three, four, and possibly five. In males, the flap ends cranial to the prepuce. Although there is some variability, the cranial superficial artery penetrates the medial aspect of the rectus abdominis muscle at the junction between the second and third mammary glands. Cranial and caudal superficial epigastric artery anastomoses occur between or near the third and fourth mammary glands. The positioning and creation of the flap are similar to those for the caudal superficial epigastric flap. The base of the flap is located in the hypogastric region, where the cranial epigastric vessel enters the skin lateral to the abdominal midline, and a few centimeters caudal to the cartilaginous border of the ventral thorax (xiphoid process).

Outline the flap with the ventral midline as the location of the medial incision. Mark a parallel lateral incision at a distance equal to the distance from the mammary teats to the midline. Determine the number of mammary glands to include in the flap based on the size of the defect. Create the flap by connecting the two parallel lines between the fourth and fifth glands or caudal to the fifth gland with a crescent-shaped incision. Undermine the flap at the level of the external abdominal oblique aponeurosis, deep to the supramammarius muscle. Ligate branches of the caudal superficial epigastric artery as necessary. Transpose the flap, place drains, and appose skin edges. Create an island flap by making a crescent-shaped incision between the second and third mammary glands. Use caution during dissection and manipulation to prevent trauma, kinking, or stretching of the cranial superficial epigastric vessels.

Deep Circumflex Iliac Axial Pattern Flap

The dorsal branch of the deep circumflex iliac vessel is used in flaps to cover defects involving the caudal thorax, lateral abdominal wall, ipsilateral flank, lateral lumbar area, medial or lateral thigh, greater trochanter, and pelvic area. The dorsal and ventral branches of the deep circumflex iliac artery originate at a point cranioventral to the wing of the ilium.

Position the patient in lateral recumbency with the hindlimb in relaxed extension perpendicular to the body. Outline the flap by first drawing a line midway between the cranial border of the wing of the ilium and the greater trochanter. For the cranial incision, draw a second line parallel to the first line and equal to the distance from the iliac border to the caudal line. Extend the lines to the dorsal midline and create an L extension, if needed, to cover the defect (see Fig. 15-28). Incise the outlined flap. Elevate the flap below the level of the cutaneous trunci muscle. Transpose the flap, place drains, and appose skin edges.

The ventral branch of the deep circumflex iliac artery is used in flaps to cover defects of the lateral abdominal wall and as an island flap for pelvic and sacral defects.

Make the reference lines as for the previous flap. Draw the caudal incision line extending distally cranial to the border of the femoral shaft. Extend the cranial incision line down the flank and thigh region parallel to the caudal flap border. Connect the two lines above the patella. Elevate the flap below the level of the cutaneous trunci muscle. Incise the outlined flap. Transpose the flap, place drains, and appose skin edges.

The flank fold flap is a variation of the ventral deep circumflex iliac axial pattern flap (see p. 206) developed for transposition into inguinal defects.

Genicular Axial Pattern Flap

Genicular axial pattern flaps are used to cover defects involving the lateral and medial tibia and potentially the tibiotarsal joint. These flaps are dependent on the short genicular branch of the saphenous artery and medial saphenous vein.

Position the patient in lateral recumbency. Mark a point 1 cm proximal to the patella and 1.5 cm distal to the tibial tuberosity (see Fig. 15-28). Extend these two points dorsally parallel to the femoral shaft, ending at the base of the greater trochanter. Connect the parallel lines dorsally. Incise the outlined flap. Elevate the flap and rotate it to cover the defect. Place drains and appose skin edges.

Although circulation usually is sufficient, this is not a robust flap.

Reverse Saphenous Conduit Flap

Reverse saphenous conduit flaps are used for defects at or below the tarsus. They are created by ligating and dividing the vascular connection between the femoral artery and vein and the saphenous artery and medial saphenous vein. Reverse blood flow occurs because of anastomoses between the cranial branch of the saphenous artery and the perforating metatarsal artery (via medial and lateral plantar arteries), the cranial branch of the lateral saphenous vein, and other venous connections with the cranial and caudal branches of the medial saphenous veins distal to the tibiotarsal joint. Preoperative angiography ensures the presence and function of the saphenous artery, medial saphenous vein, and femoral artery and vein.

Position the patient in lateral recumbency with the affected limb down. Roughly outline the flap by marking a line across the central third of the inner thigh at or slightly above the level of the patella. Make parallel lines 0.5 to 1 cm cranial and caudal to the branches of the saphenous artery and medial saphenous vein. Make the transverse incision as marked to expose the saphenous vessels and nerve. Ligate and transect the saphenous artery and medial saphenous vein at their junction with the femoral artery and vein. Extend the incisions distally as marked in a slightly converging fashion. Undermine deep to the saphenous vessels by elevating a portion of the medial gastrocnemius muscle fascia with the flap. Ligate and divide the peroneal (fibular) artery and vein. Do not elevate the flap beyond the anastomosis between the cranial branch of the medial saphenous vein and the cranial branch of the lateral saphenous vein. Rotate or partly tube the pedicle transfer to the defect. As an alternative, make a bridge incision between the donor site and the wound. Place drains and appose the defects.

Lateral Caudal Axial Pattern Flap

The lateral caudal arteries of the tail may be used to reconstruct areas involving perineum and caudodorsal trunk defects. The largest source of skin is from the proximal third of the tail. The tail skin may also be used as a tube flap to cover defects on the hind leg. The lateral caudal vessels are bilateral and are located in the subcutaneous tissue of the tail. The lateral caudal arteries arise from the caudal gluteal arteries and have several anastomotic branches with the median caudal artery. Use of this flap requires tail amputation.

Make a dorsal midline incision along the length of the tail to cover dorsocaudal defects (see Fig. 15-28). Make a ventral midline skin incision to cover defects on the hind leg. Dissect the subcutaneous tissue from the deep caudal fascia, preserving the right and left lateral caudal arteries and veins. Amputate the tail at the third or fourth caudal intervertebral space (see p. 248). Transpose the skin flap over the defect, place drains, and appose skin edges.

Suggested Reading

Anderson DM, Charlesworth TC, White RAS: A novel axial pattern skin flap based on the lateral thoracic artery in the dog, *Vet Comp Orthop Traumatol* 17:73, 2004.
The creation of this flap is described for use in the region of the caudal elbow.

Aper R, Smeak D: Complications and outcome after thoracodorsal axial pattern flap reconstruction of forelimb skin defects in 10 dogs, 1989-2001, *Vet Surg* 32:378, 2003.
This retrospective study involving 10 dogs reports distal flap necrosis in 70%. Other complications included infection, seroma, edema, bruising, and partial dehiscence.

Dundas JM, Fowler JD, Shmon CL et al: Modification of the superficial cervical axial pattern skin flap for oral reconstruction, *Vet Surg* 34:206, 2005.
This experimental study investigated the flap anatomy and creation of an extended flap to repair oronasal defects.

Hunt GB, Tisdall PLC, Liptak JM et al: Skin-fold advancement flaps for closing large proximal limb and trunk defects in dogs and cats, *Vet Surg* 30:440, 2001.
Various incisions are described to allow more versatile use of flank and elbow fold flaps.

Lascelles BDX, White RAS: Combined omental pedicle grafts and thoracodorsal axial pattern flaps for the reconstruction of chronic, nonhealing axillary wounds in cats, *Vet Surg* 30:380, 2001.
Ten cats with chronic nonhealing axillary wounds were débrided and then successfully reconstructed, with complete healing occurring with only minimal complications.

Leonatti S, Tobias KM: Skin reconstruction techniques: axial pattern flaps, *Vet Med* 99:862, 2004.
Frequently used axial pattern flaps are reviewed and well illustrated.

Lidbetter DA, Williams FA, Krahwinkel DJ et al: Radical lateral body-wall resection for fibrosarcoma with reconstruction using polypropylene mesh and a caudal superficial epigastric axial pattern flap: a prospective clinical study of the technique and results in 6 cats, *Vet Surg* 31:57, 2002.
This technique was successful in achieving local tumor control with acceptable patient morbidity.

Matera JM, Tatarunas AC, Fantoni DT et al: Use of the scrotum as a transposition flap for closure of surgical wounds in three dogs, *Vet Surg* 33:99, 2004.
The scrotum was useful for closing defects in the perineal and thigh regions after tumor excision.

Pavletic MM: *Atlas of small animal reconstructive surgery*, ed 2, Philadelphia, 1999, WB Saunders.
Illustrations and brief technique descriptions are presented.

Seguin B, McDonald DE, Kent MS et al: Tolerance of cutaneous or mucosal flaps placed into a radiation therapy field in dogs, *Vet Surg* 34:214, 2005.
Results from a clinical study involving 26 dogs are presented. Flaps that were part of the planned therapy fared better than those that were created to correct a complication or failure of radiation therapy.

Teunissen BD, Walshaw R, Hauptman JG et al: Evaluation of primary critical ischemia time for deep circumflex iliac cutaneous flap in cats, *Vet Surg* 33:440, 2004.
Flaps were studied in 13 cats with variable ischemia time and then replaced; all flaps survived.

Vasconcellos CHDC, Matera JM, Dali MLZ: Clinical evaluation of random skin flaps based on the subdermal plexus secured with sutures or sutures and cyanoacrylate adhesive for reconstructive surgery in dogs, *Vet Surg* 34:59, 2005.
Closure techniques were compared in 15 dogs after tumor removal; the use of a combination of adhesives and sutures allowed accurate margin apposition with good cosmetic outcome, and fewer sutures were needed.

COMPOSITE FLAPS

Flaps composed of skin with muscle, bone, or cartilage are termed composite flaps. The pinna has been used as a composite flap to cover maxillofacial defects. Numerous myocutaneous flaps, with or without attached bone segments, have been used to facilitate reconstructive surgery.

MYOCUTANEOUS AND MUSCLE FLAPS

Muscle flaps with overlying skin (myocutaneous flaps) or without skin (muscle flaps) may be created to facilitate herniorrhaphy, to cover soft tissue defects, to contribute circulation to fractures, and to combat infection. They should be used only when reconstruction with local flaps (see p. 205), axial pattern flaps (see p. 211), or free grafts (see p. 224) is not feasible. These flaps must be sufficiently large to cover the defect and have an easily accessible and constant dominant vascular supply. Donor sites should be easily closed. Muscles in dogs and cats that may be sacrificed without loss of function include the cutaneous trunci, gracilis, trapezius, sternohyoid, sternothyroid, deep pectoral, anconeus, ulnaris lateralis, humeral head of the flexor carpi ulnaris, sartorius, semitendinosus, rectus femoris, cranial tibial, long digital extensor, and portions of the latissimus dorsi.

MYOCUTANEOUS FLAPS

Myocutaneous flaps described in the veterinary literature include latissimus dorsi, cutaneous trunci, gracilis, semitendinosus, and trapezius muscles. These muscles are superficial, allowing easy access and elevation, and have direct cutaneous arteries exiting the muscle surface to supply overlying skin. A vascular pedicle sufficient to maintain circulation is required to facilitate flap rotation into defects. Increased rotation may impair circulation and require that the flap length be reduced. Distant transfer of gracilis, latissimus dorsi, transverse abdominis, and some trapezius flaps is possible with microvascular anastomosis.

> NOTE: Development of myocutaneous flaps requires the presence of direct cutaneous arteries exiting the muscle surface to supply the overlying skin.

Platysma Myocutaneous Flap

The platysma muscle is a well-developed muscle originating from the middorsal tendinous raphe of the neck and skin. It courses longitudinally toward the mouth over the parotid and masseter to the lips and ventrally to the midline. The platysma myocutaneous flap used to cover defects involving the head and neck is identical to the caudal auricular axial pattern flap (see p. 212).

Latissimus Dorsi Myocutaneous Flap

The latissimus dorsi muscle is a flat, triangular muscle overlying the dorsal half of the lateral thoracic wall. It originates from thoracolumbar fascia of the thoracic and lumbar spi-nous processes and from muscular attachments to the last two or three ribs. The aponeurosis of the latissimus dorsi inserts on the major teres tuberosity of the humerus. The muscle flexes the shoulder, drawing the limb caudally. The ventral portion of the muscle is supplied by branches of the thoracodorsal artery (dorsal and lateral thoracic arteries), which penetrate the muscle and supply the cutaneous trunci muscle and skin. Intercostal arteries supply segmental branches to the dorsal portion of the latissimus dorsi muscle and the overlying cutaneous trunci muscle. Latissimus dorsi myocutaneous flaps are bulky because they contain the cutaneous trunci muscle and skin, subcutaneous fat, and latissimus dorsi muscle. They are best suited for thoracic defects, although they may be used for forelimb defects. Anatomic landmarks are the ventral border of the acromion, adjacent caudal border of the triceps muscle, head of the last rib, and distal third of the humerus that corresponds to the axillary skin fold (Fig. 15-30).

With the patient in lateral recumbency and the forelimb in relaxed extension perpendicular to the trunk, plan and outline the flap with a marking pen.

Draw a line from the caudal border of the triceps muscle to the vertebral attachment of the last rib. Draw a parallel line caudodorsally from the axillary skin fold and connect them to outline the flap (see Fig. 15-30). Incise skin and extend the incision through the underlying latissimus dorsi muscle. The muscle flap equals the size of the skin flap. Elevate the latissimus dorsi and skin as a unit. Isolate, ligate, and divide the lateral intercostal vessels deep to the latissimus muscle. Identify and preserve the thoracodorsal artery and vein. Transpose the flap to the desired location without occluding the thoracodorsal vessels. If necessary, make a bridge incision or partial tubing of the flap for transposition. Place Penrose or closed suction drains at the donor site and beneath the flap at the recipient site. Secure the flap in position and close the donor site.

The latissimus dorsi may be used alone as a muscle flap; it is harvested in a similar manner without the skin for this purpose.

Cutaneous Trunci Myocutaneous Flap

The cutaneous trunci muscle arises from the pectoralis profundus and forms a thin leaf covering most of the dorsal, lateral, and ventral walls of the abdomen (see Fig. 15-30). It is more closely associated with skin than underlying structures. Blood supply is from small muscular branches and direct cutaneous arteries supplying the overlying skin. The cutaneous trunci overlying the latissimus dorsi muscle receives two to four short, direct cutaneous branches of the thoracodorsal artery caudal to the border of the triceps muscle. Elevating the cutaneous trunci muscle with skin helps preserve the subdermal plexus. Cutaneous trunci myocutaneous flaps are more pliable and elastic than latissimus dorsi myocutaneous flaps and are preferred for forelimb flaps.

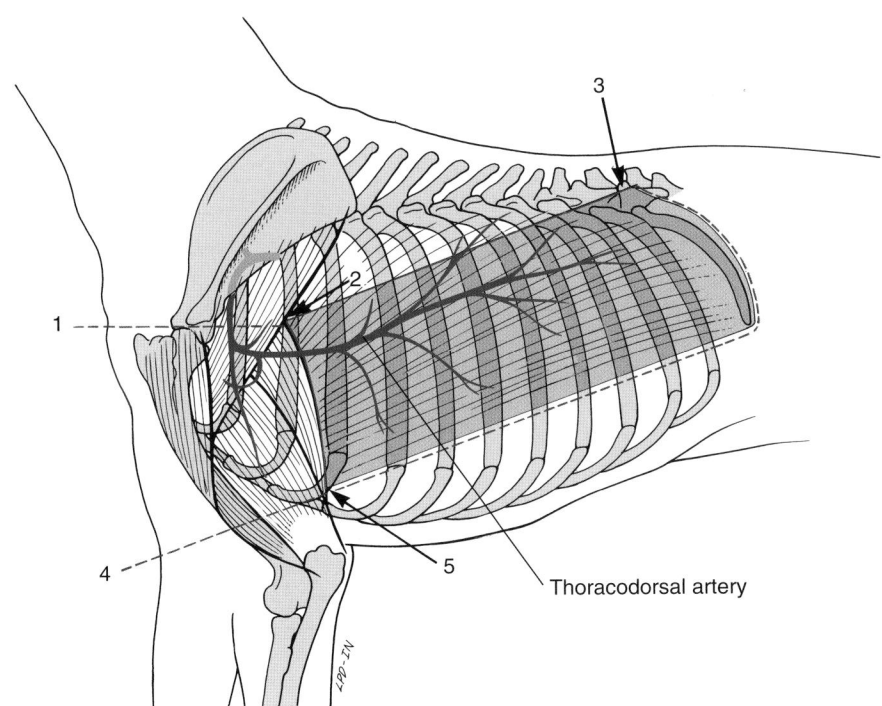

FIG. 15-30
Landmarks for the latissimus dorsi and cutaneous trunci myocutaneous flaps. *1*, Ventral border of the acromion; *2*, adjacent caudal border of the triceps muscle; *3*, vertebral attachment of the last rib; *4*, distal third of the humerus; and *5*, axillary skin fold. To construct the flaps, draw a line from *2* to *3* and a second parallel line from *5*. Incise and connect the two parallel lines dorsally.

Thoracodorsal artery

Plan and outline the flap in the same way as for a latissimus dorsi myocutaneous flap. Incise the skin as outlined, but do not extend the incision beyond subcutaneous tissue between the cutaneous trunci and latissimus dorsi. Elevate the cutaneous trunci by dissecting the loose subcutaneous tissue. Ligate and divide branches of the proximal lateral intercostal direct cutaneous vessels. Transpose the flap to its desired location without occluding the thoracodorsal vessels. If necessary, make a bridge incision or partial tubing of the flap for transposition. Place Penrose or closed suction drains beneath the flap at recipient and donor sites. Secure the flap in position and close the donor site.

Trapezius Osteomyocutaneous Flap

Trapezius osteomyocutaneous flaps generally are used for defects in the neck, cranial thorax, or proximal thoracic limb; however, they may be transferred to distant sites with microvascular anastomosis. The trapezius is a thin, triangular muscle divided into cervical and thoracic parts. The cervical part of the trapezius is overlapped by the cleidocervicalis muscle and the thoracic part by the latissimus dorsi muscle. The muscle originates from the median raphe of the neck and supraspinous ligament from the level of the third cervical vertebra to the ninth thoracic vertebra and inserts on the scapular spine. It acts to elevate and abduct the forelimb. Lameness and scapular fractures may occur when this flap is used. Only the scapular spine and not the scapular body remains viable. The bone in this flap is weak and should be used as a source of osteogenesis rather than support. Dorsal, caudal, and cranioventral borders of the flap are 2 cm ventral to the dorsal midline, 2 cm caudal to the scapular spine, and a line between the acromion and transverse process of the third cervical vertebra, respectively.

Make a triangular skin incision over the cervical part of the trapezius muscle (Fig. 15-31). Incise the origin of the cervical part of the trapezius on the dorsal midline. Dissect the incised trapezius from the cleidocervicalis and omotransversarius muscles, preserving the attachment to the scapular spine and the prescapular branch of the superficial cervical vascular pedicle. Dissect the caudal half of the supraspinatus muscle from its attachment on the scapular spine and body. Incise the deltoideus and thoracic part of the trapezius attachments to the scapular spine. Dissect the cranial half of the infraspinatus from the scapular spine and body. Create a bone flap using an air-powered burr or saw. Dissect the medial attachments of the subscapularis and serratus ventralis muscles from the bone flap. Elevate the osteomusculocutaneous flap and transfer it to the recipient site, preserving the prescapular branch of the superficial cervical vascular pedicle. Place a Penrose drain at the donor site and close the defect with approximating sutures (for muscle, use 2-0 or 3-0 polydioxanone or polyglyconate suture; for subcutaneous tissue, use 3-0 or 4-0 polydioxanone or polyglyconate suture; for skin, use 3-0 or 4-0 nylon or polypropylene suture). Apply a bandage over the donor and recipient sites for support and fluid absorption.

MUSCLE FLAPS

Muscle flaps may be transposed beneath skin to fill defects, repair hernias, and treat paralysis. Many muscles have been used to facilitate adjacent visceral repair and to fill defects. Using muscle in reconstruction is limited by the tissue avail-

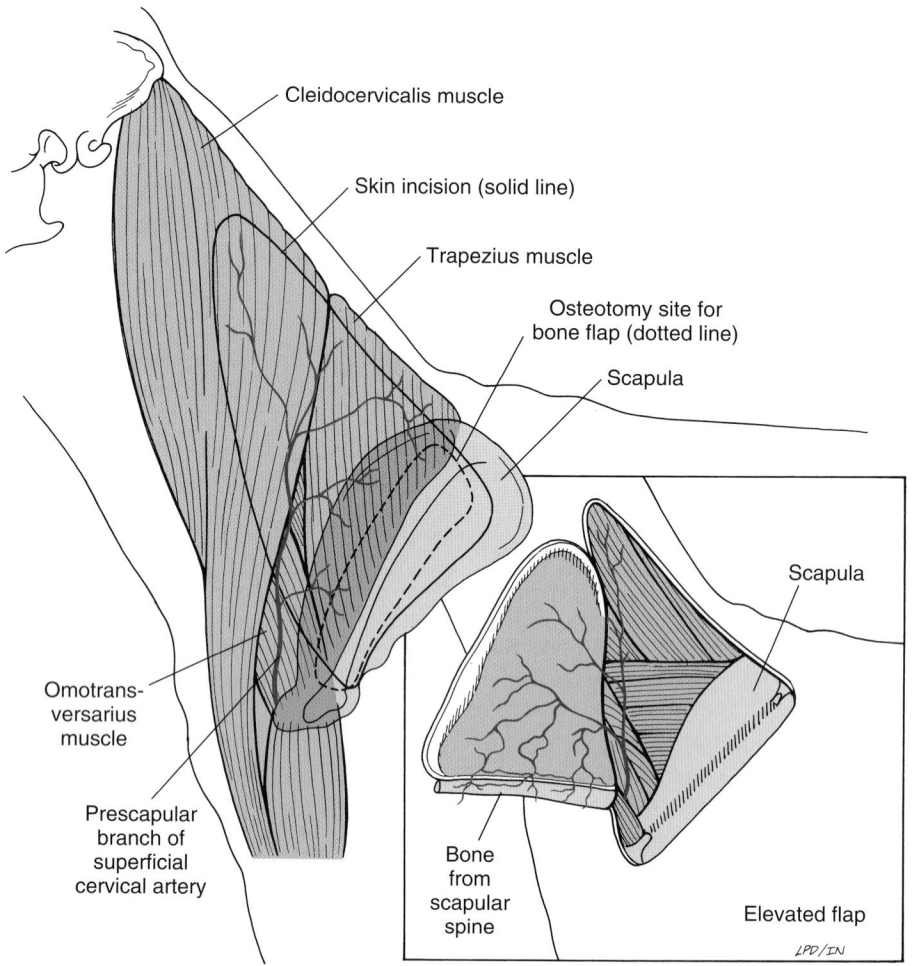

FIG. 15-31
Outlined trapezius osteomyocutaneous flap for regional reconstruction. The inset shows the flap ready for relocation.

able and the surgeon's imagination. Muscles are capable of contributing circulation to areas of ischemia caused by trauma or radiation therapy. They may also provide support, facilitate return of function, improve cosmesis, and reduce wound contamination and sepsis. The latissimus dorsi may be used with or without a cutaneous flap to cover thoracic wall defects (see previous discussion). The muscle flap may be used with mesh or other implants to give support and is sutured to adjacent muscle or fascial planes. Diaphragmatic hernia repair has been facilitated by using the transversus abdominis muscle. The internal obturator, superficial gluteal, and semitendinosus muscles have been used in perineal hernia repair (see p. 517). Caudal abdominal hernias or defects can be reinforced with pectineus or sartorius muscle flaps. Esophageal repair may be facilitated by use of intercostal, diaphragm, sternocephalicus, or sternothyroideus muscles (see p. 381). The sternohyoideus and sternothyroideus muscles may be used to cover laryngotracheal defects. Biceps femoris or deep gluteal muscle flaps are sometimes used to cushion the femoral head and neck ostectomy site (see p. 1242). Reconstruction of distal antebrachial, carpal, and metacarpal injuries can be assisted by transposition of the humeral head of the flexor carpi ulnaris. The semitendinosus has been used to reconstruct tibial defects.

External Abdominal Oblique Muscle Flap

The external abdominal oblique muscle is elastic and mobile and may be used to facilitate repair of defects in the abdominal wall or caudal thoracic wall. This flap may be used to fill defects larger than 10 × 10 cm in medium-size dogs. The external abdominal oblique muscle is a long, flat muscle covering the ventral half of the lateral thoracic wall and lateral abdominal wall. Its fibers are directed caudoventrally. It is divided into a costal part arising from the fifth to thirteenth ribs and a lumbar part arising from the last rib and the thoracolumbar fascia. It has a wide aponeurosis that inserts on the linea alba and cranial pubic ligament and contributes to the external rectus fascia, external inguinal ring, and prepubic tendon. The cranial branch of the cranial abdominal artery supplies the middle zone of the lateral abdominal wall and is accompanied by the cranial hypogastric nerve and satellite vein. The deep branch of the deep cir-

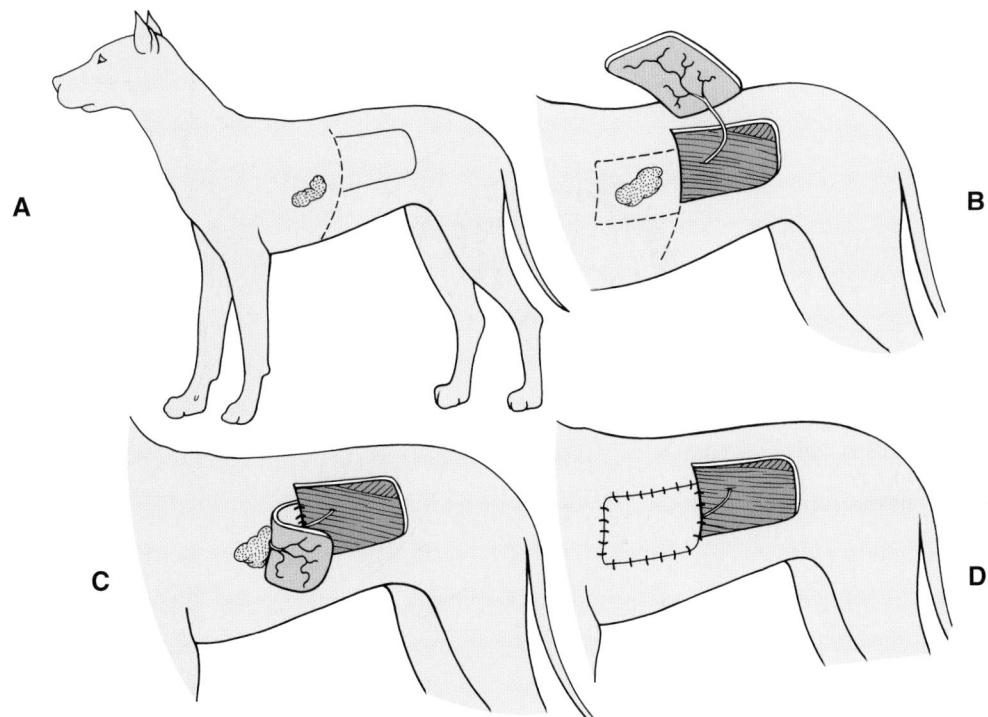

FIG. 15-32
An external abdominal oblique flap is created to reconstruct defects involving the caudal thorax or abdominal wall. **A,** Make a paracostal incision from the epaxial muscles toward the ventral midline, beginning 5 cm caudal to the thirteenth rib. **B,** Incise the lumbar fascial edge of the external abdominal oblique muscle and undermine it, preserving the neurovascular pedicle. **C** and **D,** Transpose and suture the muscle over an adjacent defect.

cumflex artery anastomoses with the cranial and caudal abdominal arteries and is the main supply to the caudodorsal fourth of the abdominal wall. It is accomplished by a satellite vein and joined by the lateral cutaneous femoral nerve.

Make a paracostal skin incision from the level of the epaxial muscles to the ventral midline, beginning 5 cm caudal to the thirteenth rib. Identify and divide the lumbar fascial edge of the external abdominal oblique muscle, leaving a 0.5- to 1-cm margin of fascia along the muscular edge (Fig. 15-32). Undermine the lumbar external abdominal oblique muscle. Identify and preserve the neurovascular pedicle (branches of the cranial abdominal artery and cranial hypogastric nerve and satellite vein) in a craniodorsal location caudal to the thirteenth rib. Divide the dorsal fascial attachment and sever the lumbar external abdominal oblique muscle at the level of the thirteenth rib. Transpose the flap to an adjacent defect. Overlap the defect with the flap, and suture the inner fascial surface with 2-0 polydioxanone or polyglyconate using a simple interrupted pattern. Place Penrose or closed suction drains, and appose the defect edges.

Cranial Sartorius Muscle Flap

Cranial sartorius muscle flaps are used to repair prepubic tendon ruptures or femoral hernias when tissue trauma, retraction, and fibrosis preclude adequate anatomic reapposi-

tion. This type of flap may also be used to cover femoral trochanteric ulcers. In the dog, the sartorius muscle consists of two long, flat, straplike muscles on the craniomedial surface of the thigh. In the cat, the sartorius muscle has only one belly and an origin and insertion similar to that of the dog. The feline sartorius muscle has one or more large vascular pedicles entering either the origin or insertion of the muscle and other smaller pedicles. In dogs, the origin of the cranial part of the sartorius is the crest of the ilium and the thoracolumbar fascia. The cranial sartorius inserts on the patella with the rectus femoris of the quadriceps. A single major vascular pedicle, branches of the femoral artery and vein, enters the proximal one third of the muscle caudally. The muscle acts to extend the stifle and flex the hip.

Incise the skin of the medial thigh over the cranial sartorius extending to the inguinal region, and dissect subcutaneous tissue to expose the muscle (Fig. 15-33, A). Isolate the muscle by blunt and sharp dissection from the caudal sartorius and quadriceps femoris muscles and other tissue. Transect the muscle distally at its insertion on the tibia and elevate it to its vascular pedicle, which enters the proximal one third of the muscle caudally. Rotate the flap up to 180° into adjacent defects. As an alternative, create an island muscle flap by subperiosteal elevation of the muscle's ilial origin. Suture muscle borders to adjacent fascial planes to cover the defect

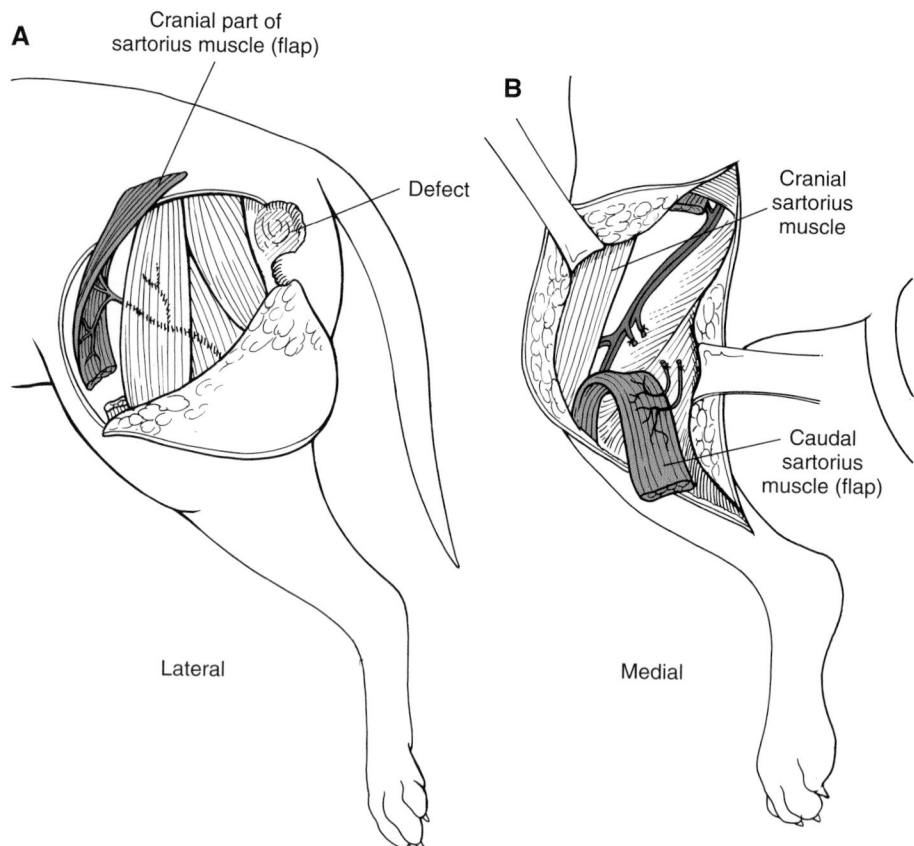

FIG. 15-33
A, Use a cranial sartorius muscle flap to reconstruct prepubic tendon ruptures, femoral hernias, or femoral trochanteric ulcers. **B,** Elevate a caudal sartorius muscle flap to cover defects over the tibia or metatarsus.

with absorbable suture material (e.g., 2-0 or 3-0 polydioxanone, poliglecaprone 25, or polyglyconate). Place Penrose or closed suction drains in the donor and recipient sites, and close the defect or defects.

Caudal Sartorius Muscle Flap

Caudal sartorius muscle flaps can be rotated distally to cover defects over the tibial or metatarsal area. These flaps may facilitate fracture repair when healing is impaired by osteomyelitis or poor circulation. Preoperative angiography ensures that the saphenous artery is not the primary source of circulation to the traumatized area and distal extremity. The caudal sartorius muscle originates from the cranial ventral iliac spine and adjacent ventral border of the ilium. It inserts on the cranial border of the tibia in common with the gracilis muscle. The caudal sartorius muscle has a segmental blood supply with a dominant vascular pedicle off the saphenous artery and medial saphenous vein at the distal third of the muscle belly. It acts to flex the hip and stifle.

Make a skin incision on the medial aspect of the thigh along the length of the caudal sartorius, and dissect subcutaneous tissue to expose the muscle (Fig. 15-33, B). Transect the caudal sartorius muscle approximately 4 cm distal to its origin on the ilium. Double ligate and transect the saphenous artery and medial saphenous vein where they join the femoral

artery and vein. Prevent traumatizing the saphenous vessels in the medial tibial region and along the caudal border of the muscle. Transect the caudal sartorius near the tibial crest for complete mobilization. This creates an island muscle flap dependent on the saphenous artery and medial saphenous vein. Extend the skin incision and further mobilize the vascular pedicle as needed. Transfer the flap to the desired location and secure. Place a Penrose or closed suction drain, and close the defects at the donor recipient sites.

Flexor Carpi Ulnaris Muscle Flap

The humeral head of the flexor carpi ulnaris muscle is useful for reconstructing injuries involving the tissues of the antebrachial, carpal, or metacarpal areas. The humeral head of the flexor carpi ulnaris lies cranial to the ulnar head of the flexor carpi ulnaris except distally, where the tendon lies caudally. The origin of the humeral head is the medial epicondyle of the humerus; its insertion is the accessory carpal bone. The blood supply to the proximal portion of the muscle is from varying pedicles of the recurrent ulnar, ulnar, and deep antebrachial arteries. A vascular pedicle from the caudal interosseous artery enters the distal end of the humeral head on its deep face near the accessory carpal bone. There are intramuscular anastomoses between the proximally coursing branches of the caudal interosseous artery and the descending branches of the ulnar and deep ante-

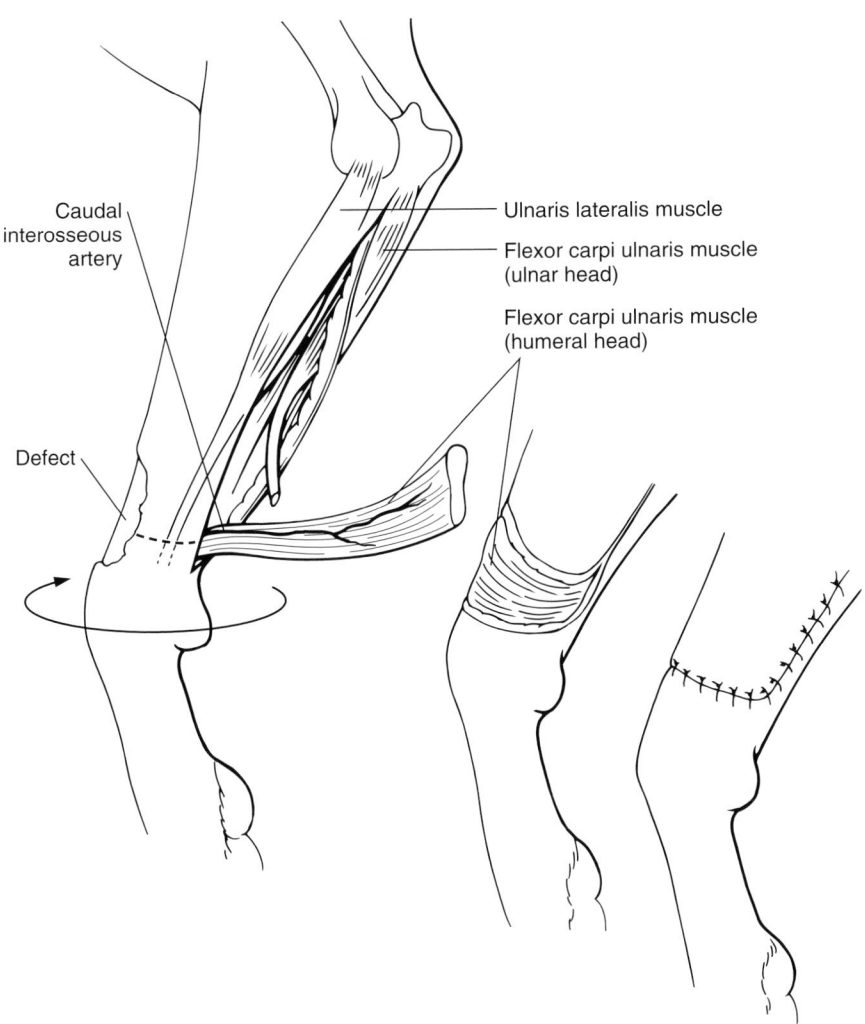

Caudal
interosseous
artery

Defect

Ulnaris lateralis muscle

Flexor carpi ulnaris muscle
(ulnar head)

Flexor carpi ulnaris muscle
(humeral head)

FIG. 15-34
Use a flexor carpi ulnaris flap with the
caudal interosseous vascular pedicle
entering the muscle on the deep surface
near the tendon of insertion to cover
wounds in the antebrachial, carpal, or
metacarpal areas.

brachial arteries. The action of the flexor carpi ulnaris is to flex the carpus.

Incise along the caudolateral aspect of the antebrachium from just below the elbow extending 1 to 2 cm distal to the accessory carpal bone to expose the muscle. Incise the antebrachial and carpal fascia to identify the humeral head lying between the ulnar head of the flexor carpi ulnaris caudally and the ulnaris lateralis laterally. Transect the distal tendon of the ulnar head to completely expose the humeral head. Dissect the fascial attachments of the humeral head and transect at the junction of the proximal and middle third of the muscle (Fig. 15-34). Make a bridge incision to the wound and rotate the muscle medially or laterally into the wound. Appose the muscle to the surrounding viable tissue, and place drains as needed. Apply a moist, nonadherent bandage over the exposed muscle if the wound is not immediately covered with skin.

Temporalis Muscle Flap

Temporalis muscle flaps are used to close orbitonasal defects or to improve cosmesis after orbital exenteration. The temporalis muscle is fan shaped and arises from the tem-

poral fossa, inserting on the mandibular coronoid process. The temporal and masseter muscles fuse between the zygomatic arch and the coronoid process. The temporal branches of the superficial temporal artery, cranial deep temporal artery, and caudal deep temporal artery supply the temporalis muscle. The blood supply enters the muscle near its narrow insertion on the mandible and runs in a ventrodorsal direction, paralleling the muscle fibers. The muscle closes the mandible in conjunction with the masseter and medial pterygoid muscles.

Make a cranial to caudal incision centered over the orbit to expose the temporalis muscle (Fig. 15-35). Preserve the superficial temporal artery. Dissect and transect the temporalis fascia from the zygomatic arch. Incise and subperiosteally elevate the desired portion of temporalis muscle. Rotate the flap around its insertion to the recipient site, resecting the zygomatic arch and lateral orbital ligament as needed. Secure the flap over the defect with approximating sutures (e.g., 2-0 or 3-0 polydioxanone, poliglecaprone 25, or polyglyconate). Obliterate dead space with Penrose or closed suction drains and close cutaneous defects routinely.

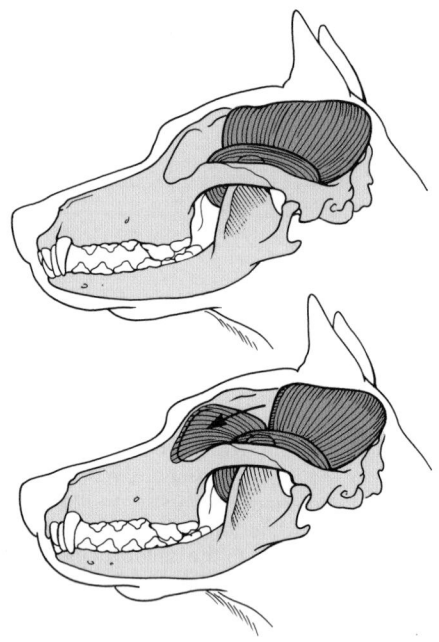

FIG. 15-35
Use a temporalis muscle flap to close orbitonasal defects.

Suggested Reading

Baines SJ, Gardner J, Allnutt R et al: The deep pectoral muscle flap in the cat: its vascular supply and potential use, *Vet Comp Orthop Traumatol* 13:141, 2000.

This cadaver study defines the vascular anatomy of the deep pectoral muscle with a dominant pedicle based on the lateral thoracic artery and finds a wide arc of rotation feasible for advancement to the chest wall, sternum, axilla, and medial forelimb. No live animal trials have been done.

Canapp SO, Mann FA, Henry CJ et al: The use of a latissimus dorsi muscle flap for scapular reconstruction in a cat following fibrosarcoma excision, *J Am Anim Hosp Assoc* 37:283, 2001.

This flap was successful in reconstructing a site that had eight previous surgeries for tumor recurrence.

Chambers JN, Purinton PT, Allen SW et al: Flexor carpi ulnaris (humeral head) muscle flap for reconstruction of distal forelimb injuries in two dogs, *Vet Surg* 27:342, 1998.

The distal end of the humeral head of the flexor carpi ulnaris was successfully used to cover wounds in the carpal and metacarpal areas.

Monnet E, Rooney MB, Chachques JC: In vitro evaluation of the distribution of blood flow within a canine bipedicled latissimus dorsi muscle flap, *Am J Vet Res* 64:1255, 2003.

Blood flow in the predominant perforating artery found at the level of the fifth intercostal space improves perfusion to the middle part of the latissimus dorsi.

Pavletic MM: Plastic and reconstructive surgery, *Vet Clin North Am Small Anim Pract* 20:127, 1990.

This is a good review article with illustrations.

Puerto DA, Aronson LR: Use of a semitendinosus myocutaneous flap for soft-tissue reconstruction of a grade III B open tibial fracture in a dog, *Vet Surg* 33:629, 2004.

A mycocutaneous flap was created by elevating the origin of the semitendinosus and rotating it distally to allow one-stage reconstruction of a tibial fracture and associated soft tissue defect.

Vnuk D, Babic T, Stejskal M et al: Application of a semitendinosus muscle flap in the treatment of perineal hernia in a cat, *Vet Record* 156:182, 2005.

This case report describes transection of the muscle at midbelly and rotation ventral to the anus to aid in herniorrhaphy.

OMENTAL FLAPS

Omental flaps may be used to cover soft tissue defects, contribute to circulation and drainage, enhance healing, control adhesion, and combat infection, similar to muscle flaps. Although less durable than muscle flaps, they stimulate formation of granulation tissue to allow earlier wound closure with skin flaps or grafts. They are especially useful for chronic nonhealing wounds involving the thorax, abdomen, and inguinal and axillary areas and can be used for facial and distal extremity wounds if extended omental lengthening or microvascular transfer is used. In dogs and cats, the omentum is a thin, double sheet of mesothelium that folds on itself in the caudal abdomen. It attaches ventrally to the greater curvature of the stomach and dorsally to the pancreas and spleen. The omental blood supply is from peripheral vessels of the right and left gastroepiploic arteries.

Two methods may be used to mobilize the omentum. One involves creating a vascular pedicle involving either the right or left gastroepiploic artery; the other involves releasing the omentum from the pancreas and then lengthening it with an inverted L-shaped incision. Both methods require a ventral midline celiotomy. The multiple vessel ligations required for the former technique increase the risk of hematoma formation, which may affect omental flap viability.

Create a vascular pedicle based on either the right or left gastroepiploic artery by ligating the segmental gastric arteries as they leave the gastroepiploic artery and enter the greater curvature of the stomach. Ligate either the right or left gastroepiploic artery, depending on which side of the body the omentum is needed. Incise additional attachments to the pancreas and spleen, and ligate vessels as necessary to harvest an appropriate length of omentum for transposition.

To perform the other lengthening technique, retract the dorsal omental leaf cranially and exteriorize the spleen. Release the dorsal leaf from the pancreas using sharp dissection, and ligate or cauterize vessels as encountered. Ligate and transect the one or two vessels originating from the splenic artery close to the spleen. Extend the dorsal leaf caudally, unfolding the omentum. Begin the inverted L-shaped incision on the left side just caudal to the gastrosplenic ligament (Fig. 15-36). Double ligate and transect omental vessels when encountered as you extend the incision across one half to two thirds of the omentum's width. Continue the incision caudally, parallel to the remaining omental vessels, along two thirds the length of the omentum. Ligate or cauterize vascular branches as encountered. Rotate the omentum caudally to fully extend the pedicle.

After the omentum has been mobilized, make a small incision (2 to 3 cm) through the lateral abdominal wall near

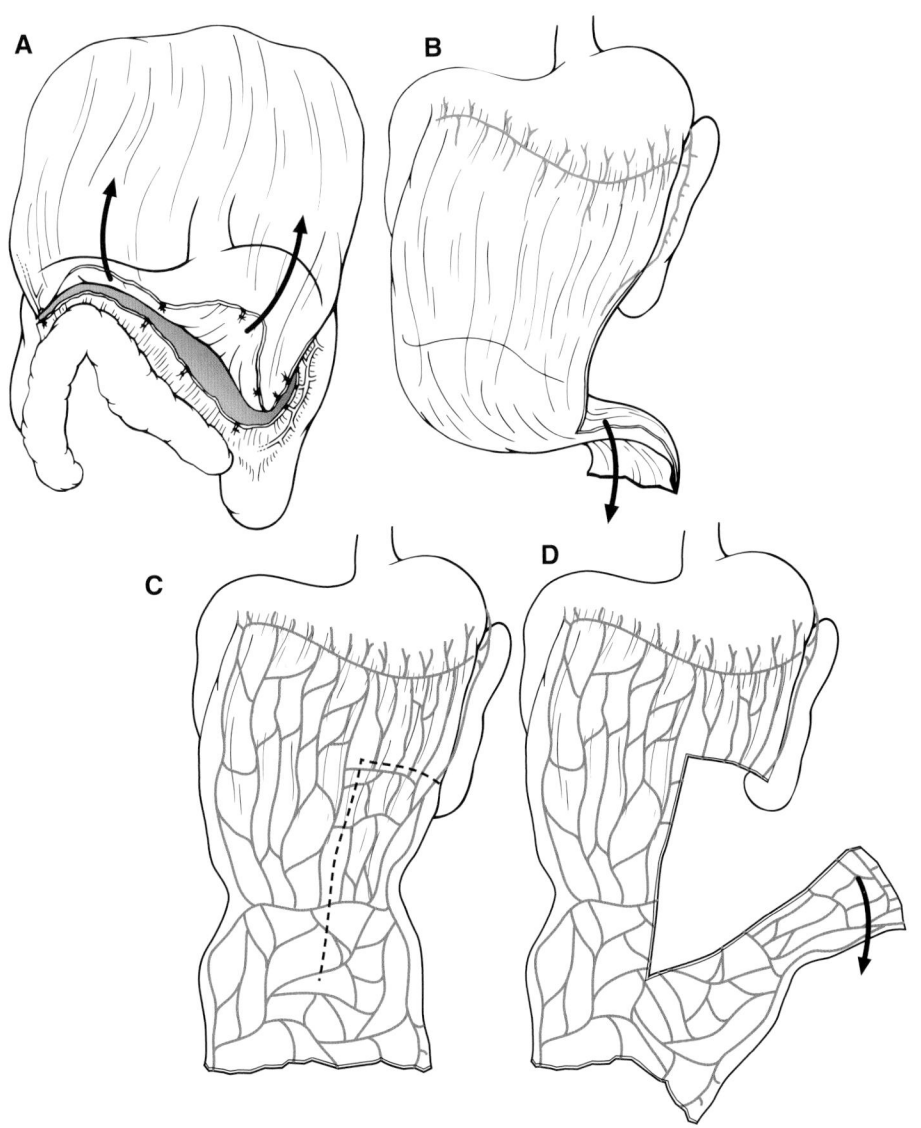

FIG. 15-36
Omental extension. **A,** Exteriorize the omentum and spleen, then retract the dorsal leaf cranially and free it from its pancreatic attachments. **B,** Extend the dorsal leaf of the omentum caudally. **C,** Make an inverted L-shaped incision just caudal to the gastrosplenic ligament. **D,** Rotate the left side caudally to achieve full extension.

the wound or several centimeters from the celiotomy for distant wounds. Create a subcutaneous tunnel to the wound, transpose the omentum through this tunnel, and secure it to the wound with interrupted absorbable sutures. Take care when handling and transposing the omentum to keep it warm and moist and to prevent occlusion of remaining omental vessels to maintain its viability.

Possible complications after omental transposition include seroma formation, herniation through the omental exit hole, and flap necrosis.

MICROVASCULAR FLAP TRANSFER

Specialized training and equipment are necessary to successfully perform microvascular transfers. The required equipment includes an operating microscope with good optics, 9-0 to 11-0 suture material, approximating and atraumatic vascular clamps, microscissors, jeweler's for-

ceps, ophthalmic needle holders, vessel dilators, and coupling devices. Most axial pattern skin flaps and muscle flaps can be used for microvascular transfer if vessels in the flap are large enough and if vessels of similar size are available near the wound bed. Peripheral angiography of the recipient site is advised to ensure that recipient vessels are present and functioning. Recipient vessels that have been used clinically for free flap transfer include the ulnar artery and cephalic vein in the forelimb; the cranial tibial artery and the dorsal branch of the medial saphenous vein or the plantar branch of the medial saphenous artery and its vena comitans in the hind leg; and the left infraorbital and superior labial arteries for palatal reconstruction. Anastomosis of recipient vessels should occur outside the area of trauma.

Once the location of the vascular pedicle has been identified during creation of the flap, magnifying loupes and the operating microscope are used to identify and isolate the vessels. Vessel clamps are applied, and the vessels are ligated and transected proximal to the clamps. At the recipient bed, the wound undergoes final débridement, and the vessels are identified and isolated in a similar manner. End-to-end anastomosis is preferred to end-to-side anastomosis because it is technically easier. Vessel ends are irrigated with heparinized saline, and excessive periadventitial tissue is removed. Arteries and then vein are anastomosed. Failure of flap transfer occurs if vessels are kinked or if they thrombose.

Suggested Reading

Calfee EF, Lanz OI, Degner DA et al: Microvascular free tissue transfer of the rectus abdominis muscle in dogs, *Vet Surg* 31:32, 2002.

This experimental study determined that the rectus abdominis muscle could be successfully transferred to serve as a bed for skin grafting.

Degner DA, Walshaw R, Fowler JD et al: Surgical approaches to recipient vessels of the fore- and hindlimbs for microvascular free tissue transfer in dogs, *Vet Surg* 34:297, 2005.

Six forelimb and 12 hindlimb approaches were developed and described for isolation before transfer.

Jackson AH, Degner DA, Jackson IT et al: Deep circumflex iliac cutaneous free flap in cats, *Vet Surg* 32:341, 2003.

This three phase experimental and clinical study found the flap promising, but there was concern about tolerable ischemia time as 4/6 flaps failed in one phase.

Lanz OI, Broadstone RV, Martin RA et al: Effects of anesthesia on microcirculatory blood flow in free medial saphenous fasciocutaneous flaps in dogs, *Vet Surg* 30:374, 2001.

Ten dogs were used to determine that epidural anesthesia combined with general anesthesia did not improve microcirculatory flow in pelvic limb free flaps.

Sereda CW, Lanz OI, Cross AR et al: Concurrent use of a medial saphenous fasciocutaneous free tissue flap and external skeletal fixation for treatment of a distal antebrachial injury in a dog, *Vet Surg* 32:238, 2003.

This is a case report of carpal arthrodesis performed with an extra skeletal fixator and concurrent free tissue transfer to cover the wound.

Teunissen BD, Walshaw R, Hauptman JG et al: Evaluation of primary critical ischemia time for deep circumflex iliac cutaneous flap in cats, *Vet Surg* 33:440, 2004.

Flaps were studied in 13 cats with variable ischemia time and then replace; all flaps survived.

⬛AP SKIN GRAFTS

Skin grafts are the transfer of a segment of free dermis and epidermis to a distant recipient site. They may be full thickness (epidermis and entire dermis) or partial thickness (epidermis and a variable portion of the dermis). They are used for defects that cannot be reconstructed by direct apposition or skin flaps (usually limb and large trunk defects). Skin graft survival depends on absorption of tissue fluid and revascularization. *Autografts* (grafts from the same animal) are most useful; however, *allografts* (grafts from the same species, also called homografts) and *xenografts* (grafts from different species, or heterografts) that eventually are rejected may be used to temporarily cover and protect large burned or denuded areas. Making templates of the defect and graft and drawing reference lines on the skin are helpful in planning reconstruction.

Successful graft healing, or graft "take," is dependent on the establishment of arterial connections and adequate drainage. This must occur by the seventh or eighth postoperative day, or the graft will die. The graft bed must supply adequate vasculature for the graft. Healthy granulation tissue or a fresh, clean wound free of infection and debris may serve as the graft bed. Healthy muscle, periosteum, and peritenon can support a skin graft. Bone, cartilage, tendon, and nerve that are denuded of their overlying connective tissue do not support grafts. Poor graft take occurs over avascular fat, crushing injuries, infected tissue, irradiated tissue, old or hypertrophic granulation tissue, and chronic ulcers. Chronic granulation tissue should be excised to allow new granulation tissue to form before grafting (approximately 4 to 5 days). The surface of healthy granulation tissue may be débrided by excising a thin layer (0.5 to 2 mm) with a blade or by rubbing with a gauze sponge before grafting. If bleeding persists, hemorrhage may be controlled with pressure or pinpoint electrocoagulation. The graft bed should be covered with moistened sponges while preparing the graft. A graft adheres to its bed by fibrin contraction soon after being placed. Fibrous tissue forms after fibroblasts, leukocytes, and phagocytes invade the area. The strength of graft adherence increases as fibrous tissue forms; by the tenth postoperative day, a firm union has occurred. Good graft contact with the graft bed is essential to adherence and graft take. To achieve good contact, the graft bed must be free of debris and irregularities. Immobilizing the graft with sutures and bandages minimizes graft movement over the wound and facilitates adhesion. Use of subatmospheric pressure drainage (see p. 173), which improves graft contact with the recipient bed and drainage, is being advocated to facilitate graft survival. Improperly applied or wrinkled bandages or those that apply excess pressure or abrade the graft can result in graft necrosis. Bandages should be well padded and bulky to restrict limb motion.

Plasmatic imbibition initially nourishes the graft and keeps the graft vessels dilated until the graft revascularizes. Capillary action pulls the fibrinogen-free, serumlike fluid and cells from the graft bed into the dilated vessels of the graft. Absorption of hemoglobin products gives the graft a bluish black color. The absorbed fluid diffuses into the interstitial tissue of the graft, causing edema; edema reaches its maximum at 48 to 72 hours after grafting. As venous and lymphatic drainage improves, fluid is taken away from the graft, and the edema regresses. Anastomosis of graft vessels with graft bed vessels of similar sizes *(inosculation)* may begin within 1 day of grafting. Vascular buds from the graft bed follow the fibrin scaffold to meet preexisting severed graft vessels. Vascular anastomoses form, and blood flow to the graft begins. Initially blood flow is sluggish and disorganized, but it improves and approaches normal by the fifth or sixth day. Fluid accumulations (i.e., seroma or hematoma) inhibit inosculation. Grafts may also be revascularized by the ingrowth of new vessels from the bed into the graft. New vessels form by endothelial sprouting and anastomosis with another sprout or formed vessel. Vascular sprouts may be found within the lower layers of the graft in 48 to 72 hours. New vascular connections remodel, differentiate, and mature until a system of arterioles, venules, and capillaries forms. New lymphatic vessels develop in the graft and establish lymphatic drainage by the fourth or fifth postoperative day.

Fluid accumulation within or under the graft and movement of the graft prevent good vascular connections from developing between the graft and the bed. A nonadherent, hydrophilic bandage should be placed immediately after grafting and left undisturbed for 24 to 72 hours to facilitate graft immobilization, fluid absorption, and graft adhesion and to protect the graft from trauma. The frequency of bandage changes depends on the wound and varies from daily to every 3 to 4 days for at least 3 weeks. Grafts are pale when initially placed in a wound. They appear black and blue during the next 48 hours. The dark colors fade and a light reddish tinge appears by 72 to 96 hours. The entire graft should be red 7 to 8 days after surgery if graft survival is complete. Normal color gradually returns by the fourteenth day. Persistently pale areas are avascular and will undergo necrosis and slough. Black coloration indicates dry ischemic necrosis. Do not resect areas of questionable viability.

The most common causes of graft failure are separation from the graft bed, infection, and movement. They cause graft failure by disrupting the delicate fibrin bonds that bind the graft to the bed. Without adherence, revascularization and organization are impossible. Hematoma or seroma formation under the graft is a common cause of graft failure. Fluid mechanically separates the graft from its bed, impairing nutrition and revascularization. Meticulous hemostasis during graft bed preparation helps prevent hematomas and seromas. Nonexpanded mesh grafts, closed suction drainage, and vacuum-assisted drainage (see p. 172) are the best methods of facilitating drainage. Mesh grafts have an advantage of not requiring placement of a tube that may disrupt graft adhesion and healing. Vacuum-assisted drainage has an advantage of promoting good contact between the graft and the recipient bed, and continuous drainage. The initial bandage change is recommended 24 to 72 hours after grafting to detect and drain fluid accumulation under the graft. The danger of fluid accumulation is greater than the risk of moving the graft during bandage manipulations. Infection is detrimental to graft survival because bacteria may cause dissolution of fibrin attachments or produce sufficient exudate to lift a graft from the recipient bed. Plasminogen activators and proteolytic enzymes released by bacteria disrupt the fibrin seal. β-Hemolytic streptococci and pseudomonads produce large amounts of plasmin and proteolytic enzymes. *Pseudomonas* spp. also produce elastase, which breaks down elastin; elastin adheres to fibrin, facilitating graft adhesion.

Donor site skin should have hair the same color, texture, length, and thickness as the hair surrounding the recipient site. The donor site should have enough skin to allow closure without tension after graft removal. Hair follicles may be damaged during graft harvesting and preparation or by poor graft revascularization. Removal of subcutaneous tissue may damage the base of hair follicles and reduce hair regrowth. Hair regrowth usually is noticed within 2 to 3 weeks after grafting; however, hair color may be altered after grafting. Split-thickness grafts result in sparse hair regrowth. Hair regrowth with strip, punch, and expanded mesh grafts is patchy. Full-thickness sheet grafts and nonexpanded mesh grafts result in the best hair regrowth and cosmetic appearance.

Reinnervation of grafts depends on the type and thickness of the graft, the amount of scar tissue formation, and the innervation of surrounding tissue. Return of sensation is greatest in flaps, less in full-thickness grafts, and least in split-thickness grafts. Reinnervation occurs from the margins of the graft. Pain is the first sensation to return, followed by touch, and last, temperature discrimination.

FULL-THICKNESS SKIN GRAFTS

Full-thickness skin grafts include the epidermis and entire dermis. They are indicated to cover large defects on flexor surfaces, thus preventing contracture and distal extremity defects (Fig. 15-37). After healing, full-thickness grafts resemble normal skin in hair growth, color, texture, and elasticity. They become pliable, movable, and durable. Full-thickness grafts take and split-thickness grafts. The disadvantages of full-thickness grafts include planning, tedious removal of subcutaneous tissue, and areas of nonviability. Full-thickness grafting techniques include meshes, plugs, strips, and sheets of skin.

Sheet Grafts

Sheet grafts are indicated to prevent contracture of defects on the distal aspect of the limbs and over flexor surfaces. They should be used only over uninfected granulation beds and when minimal fluid production is expected because fluid accumulation or drains prevent graft adhesion. Sheet grafts are less flexible, less expansive, and less conforming than mesh grafts. The donor site is the skin of the lateral thoracic wall, back, shoulder, or other areas with abundant skin. The lateral thoracic wall is the preferred donor site because the skin is relatively thin and well haired.

Aseptically prepare the surgical sites. Débride, lavage, and control hemorrhage in the graft bed before placing the graft. Make a pattern of the defect using a sterile towel or paper template. Using the pattern of the defect as a guide, harvest a segment of skin about 1 cm larger than the pattern from the donor site with the hair oriented in the proper direction. Excise all subcutaneous tissue from the graft with a scalpel blade during harvest or it will interfere with revascularization (Fig. 15-38). As an alternative, excise the graft, stretch it, and fix it to a piece of stiff card-

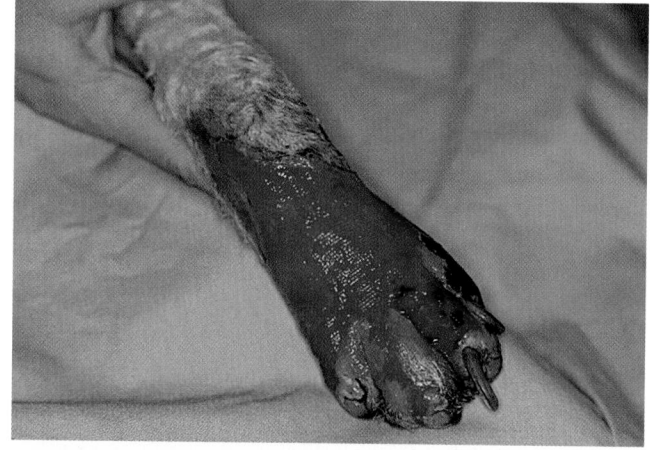

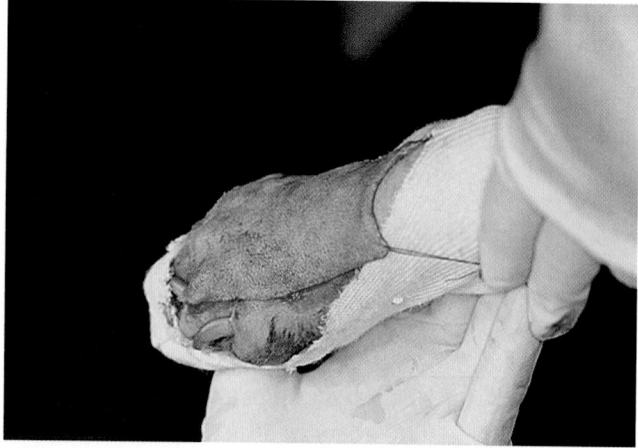

FIG. 15-37
A, Injuries involving the distal extremities commonly require grafting. Grafts should be applied over healthy granulation tissue. **B,** A full-thickness sheet graft has been applied over the wound.

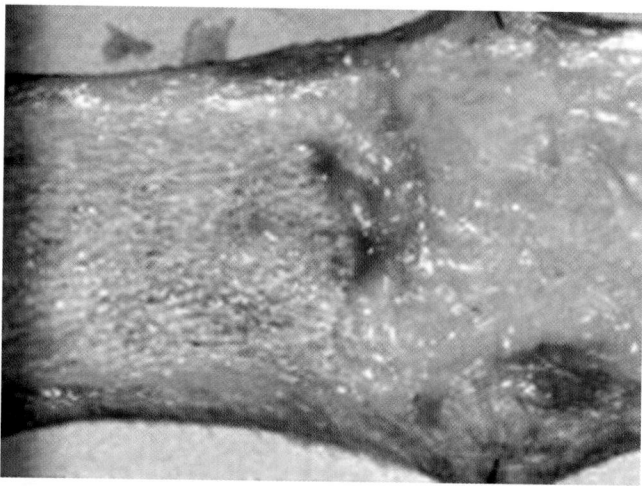

FIG. 15-38
Subcutaneous tissue has been removed from half of the graft to expose hair follicles.

bandage that restricts the patient's motion. Change the evacuation tube as needed. Change the bandage, evaluate the graft 24 to 48 hours after surgery, and continue rebandaging as needed for 21 days.

Where the graft overlaps skin edges, it will necrose and peel off when sutures are removed at 7 to 10 days.

Plug, Punch, or Seed Grafts and Strip Grafts

Plug, punch, or seed grafts and strip grafts are placed in a prepared granulation tissue bed. They are indicated for limb wounds and wounds with low grade infection or irregular surfaces. They are best used on smaller wounds in areas not subjected to excessive wear or external trauma. These grafts are difficult to immobilize after implantation. The initial bandage change after surgery is delayed for 3 to 5 days to prevent displacing the grafts. Wounds that are parallel to the long axis of the limb lend themselves to strip grafting. Plugs and strip grafting are easy to perform and require no special equipment. However, excessive bleeding from the graft bed may float plugs out of the recipient site or delay revascularization. The cosmetic appearance is poor because of epithelial scarring and sparse hair growth, which result because the wounds heal by epithelialization from each graft and wound edge.

Prepare the graft bed by débriding and treating it as an open wound for several days. Harvest plugs of skin from the donor site with a 5- or 6-mm biopsy punch or tent the skin with a bent hypodermic needle or curved suture needle and resect a small piece of tissue. Harvest 5-mm-wide strips of skin freehand for strip grafting. Remove subcutaneous tissue from the dermis (see Fig. 15-38). For plugs, make small, slitlike pockets in the granulation tissue (2 to 4 mm deep,

board or drape it over the index finger, and then remove subcutaneous tissue with a Metzenbaum scissors. Keep grafts moist by periodically submerging them in a bowl of saline or lactated Ringer's solution; this also rinses off fat fragments and helps identify remaining subcutaneous tissue. Keep the donor site moist with saline-soaked sponges while placing the graft. Place the graft in the defect with the hair properly oriented and with uniform contact with the recipient bed. Overlap the skin edges with the graft to ensure complete wound coverage and to prevent the skin edges from curling underneath. Tack the graft in position with interrupted sutures. Place a closed suction drain beneath the graft or make one or more stab incisions to promote drainage. Appose the edges of the graft and wound with staples or simple interrupted or continuous sutures (e.g., 3-0 or 4-0 nylon or polypropylene) placed 3 to 4 mm apart. Close the donor site by undermining and apposing wound edges or using a pedicle flap. Bandage the graft site with a nonadherent, hydrophilic, absorbent

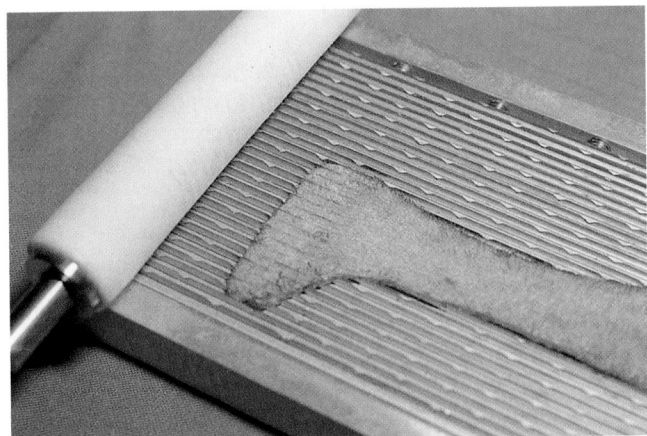

FIG. 15-39
After a skin graft has been harvested, it can be meshed (dermal side down) using a mesh graft expansion unit.

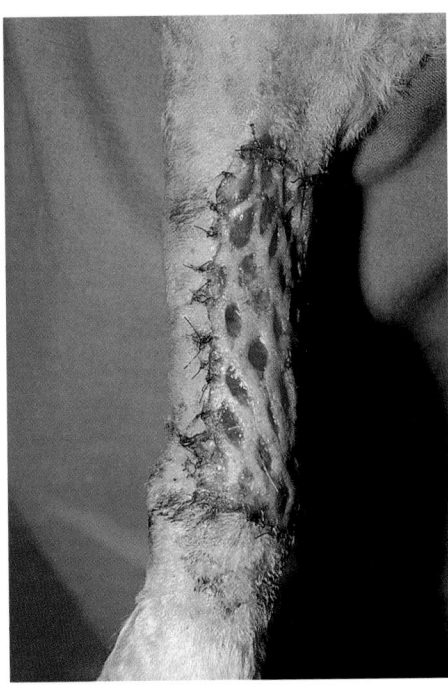

FIG. 15-40
Skin grafts may be meshed by making small, full-thickness incisions through the graft. The incisions are aligned in parallel rows.

5 to 7 mm apart), almost parallel to the wound surface. Insert a plug in each pocket after controlling hemorrhage, holding it in position with gentle pressure for 1 to 2 minutes. As an alternative, cut holes in the granulation tissue with a 4-mm skin biopsy punch (about 2 mm smaller than the punch used for harvesting the graft) approximately 1 to 2 cm apart, and insert the skin plugs into these holes. Make grooves 2 mm wide and 3 to 5 mm apart for strip grafting. After hemorrhage has been controlled, lay a skin strip in each groove and anchor it with an interrupted suture at each end. Bandage and splint the graft site with nonadherent, hydrophilic, absorbent materials. Excise and reappose the donor site or treat it as an open wound with bandages. Change the graft bandage 3 to 4 days after surgery, taking care not to dislodge any of the grafts. Rebandage the area as needed until healing is complete. Bandages should be bulky and restrict motion.

Mesh Grafts

Mesh grafts may be either full-thickness or split-thickness grafts in which parallel rows of staggered slits have been cut. Meshing a sheet graft allows drainage, flexibility, conformity, and expansion. The degree of expansion is directly related to the length of the slits; longer slits equal greater expansion. As the graft is expanded, it shortens in the perpendicular plane. A sheet graft is meshed with a special mesh graft expansion unit (Fig. 15-39) or freehand (Fig. 15-40). Freehand slits are made in a sheet graft when it is fixed to cardboard after subcutaneous tissue has been removed. Slits are made with a No. 11 or No. 15 scalpel blade and should be approximately 5 to 15 mm long and 2 to 6 mm apart and oriented in staggered rows. Mechanically meshed grafts are more expansible because they expand in more than one direction; those meshed with freehand slits expand in only one direction. Cosmesis is improved if the slits are placed parallel to the skin tension lines.

A nonexpanded, full-thickness mesh graft is recommended for most grafting needs because it may be used under a wide range of circumstances, has a high success rate, and has a good cosmetic appearance. Meshing allows a graft to conform and adhere to irregular surfaces and allows placement on graft beds with exudation or blood. Meshing allows drainage, which facilitates graft adherence. The cosmetic appearance is as good as that with sheet grafts (Fig. 15-41). Survival is 90% to 100% when grafts are applied on healthy granulation beds and managed properly. Expanded mesh grafts are indicated when donor sites are limited and defects are large. They should be cut longer than the defect to account for shortening with expansion. A diamond-shaped pattern with tufts of hair between epithelial scars results when a mesh graft is expanded. This may not be cosmetically acceptable.

SPLIT-THICKNESS SKIN GRAFTS

Split-thickness skin grafts are composed of epidermis and a variable thickness of dermis. Feline skin is too thin for split-thickness grafting. Graft take with split-thickness grafts is similar to that with full-thickness grafts. Split-thickness grafts are less durable and more subject to trauma than full-thickness grafts, and hair growth may be absent or sparse. Also the graft may appear scaly. Hair regrowth at the donor site of thick split-thickness grafts may also be sparse if the site is allowed to heal as an open wound rather than being resected. Skin of the lateral thoracic wall, back, shoulder, or another area with abundant skin may be used as the donor

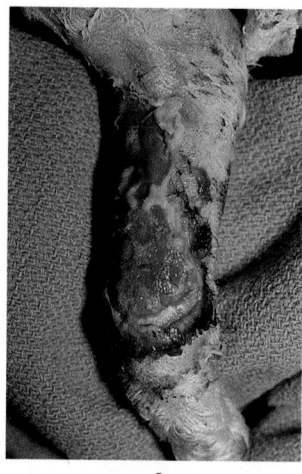 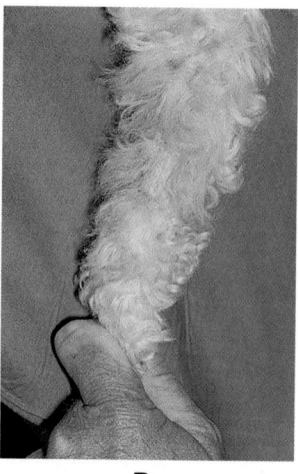

FIG. 15-41
A, Skin graft in Fig. 15-40 at 6 days; note partial graft loss.
B, Cosmetic appearance after 100 days is good.

site. However, the flexibility of the abdominal wall and the irregularity of the thoracic wall make graft harvesting difficult. The relatively firm, flat surface over the epaxial muscles lateral to the dorsal spinous processes, lateral thigh, and arm muscles are better sites for harvesting skin.

Aseptically prepare the surgical sites. Débride, lavage, and control hemorrhage in the graft bed before placing the graft. Harvest the split-thickness graft with a dermatome or free-hand. Inject sterile saline subcutaneously under the donor site to elevate the skin, and reduce contour irregularities. If using a dermatome, lubricate the skin surface with sterile mineral oil or water-soluble gel. Pull the skin in opposite directions over the donor site to make it taut. Harvest the graft. Using a scalpel, make a partial-thickness incision perpendicular to the skin surface. Then holding a modified safety razor almost parallel to the skin surface, begin cutting. Place stay sutures in the cut edge of the graft to apply traction while cutting. Change blades as they become dull. Place the graft on the bed with hair growth oriented in the proper direction. Overlap the wound edges with the graft by 2 to 4 mm. Anchor the graft in place with interrupted sutures or skin staples. Irrigate under the graft with saline or thrombin. Apply a nonadherent, absorbent bandage with a splint to immobilize the area. Use a tie-over bandage if necessary. Holes inadvertently perforating the graft will allow drainage and eventually heal. After harvest and grafting, excise the donor site and close it or manage it as an open wound with bandages. Perform the first bandage change 24 to 48 hours after surgery. Drain the area if a seroma or hematoma has formed by making a small incision in the graft and aspirating. Expect the graft overlapping the skin to necrose. Rebandage the area and change the bandage only as needed because movement of the graft bed interferes with revascularization.

NOTE: Increased pain is expected when the graft site is managed as an open wound; however, the wound will reepithelialize in approximately 3 weeks and additional split-thickness grafts can be harvested from the same site if necessary.

STAMP GRAFTS

Stamp grafts are square patches of split-thickness skin applied to a granulating wound. The graft bed and graft are prepared and managed in the same manner as for other split-thickness grafts. The graft is cut into patches ranging from 5 mm² to 25 mm². Patches are spaced 1 to 10 mm apart in graft bed depressions. These grafts are particularly susceptible to movement and easily displaced by bandages.

Suggested Reading

Aragon CL, Harvey SE, Allen SW et al: Partial-thickness skin grafting for large thermal skin wounds in dogs, *Compend Contin Educ Pract Vet* 26:200, 2004.
This article describes the indications, advantages, disadvantages, and technical aspects of partial-thickness skin grafting and provides case-based examples of its application.

Pavletic MM: *Atlas of small animal reconstructive surgery*, ed 2, Philadelphia, 1999, WB Saunders.
This is a good pictorial guide to reconstructive surgery.

SURGICAL MANAGEMENT OF SPECIFIC SKIN DISORDERS

BURNS AND OTHER THERMAL INJURIES

Burns occur when heat energy is applied at a faster rate than tissue can absorb and dissipate it. Fires, electric heating pads, hair dryers, scalding water, steam, hot cooking oil, exhaust systems, and hot pipes are common sources of thermal burns in domestic animals. The extent of injury is influenced by the temperature of the heat source, duration of contact, and tissue conductance. In man, temperatures above 113° F (45° C) can cause coagulation necrosis and irreversible skin damage; a temperature of 158° F (49° C) for only 1 second causes a full-thickness burn. A transition zone separates completely devitalized tissue from uninjured tissue. The area in direct contact with the heat coagulates; cellular proteins denature and blood vessels coagulate. The transition zone is characterized by reduced blood flow, intravascular sludging, and potentially reversible tissue damage. Progressive dermal ischemia may occur in this area because of release of vasoactive substances (e.g., thromboxane A_2, histamine, leukotrienes, prostaglandins, oxygen free radicals), tissue edema, desiccation, and bacterial invasion. The transition zone is surrounded by an area of hyperemia where minimal damage occurs and healing is complete. It can be difficult to determine the burn depth and area of involvement because the depth of injury is not uniform, and the skin surface often is leathery and covered by dry coagulum. Eschar is the residue of skin elements that have been coagulated by the heat. It is composed almost entirely of tough, denatured collagen fibers. Scabs contain dead cells and flimsy fibrin and, unlike eschar, are not a strong protective covering.

Superficial *(first-degree)* burns affect only epidermis. The area is painful, thickened, erythematous, and desquamated. Healing occurs rapidly (within 3 to 6 days) by epithelialization from stratum germinativum or adnexal dermal structures. Unlike human skin, canine skin does not act as an organ for heat dissemination; dogs therefore do not have the rich superficial vascular plexus that human beings do. For this reason, dogs show less erythema with superficial burns than people do. Superficial partial-thickness burns are moist, blanch with pressure, and are sensitive to pain. They usually heal within 3 weeks because of epithelialization from deeper portions of the skin appendages. Healing usually is complete and occurs without grafting.

Deep partial-thickness *(second-degree)* burns cause major destruction of the dermis. The only remaining adnexal epithelium is in the upper layers of the subcutaneous fat. Subcutaneous edema and notable inflammation occur, and the hair does not epilate easily. Progressive damage during the first 24 hours results from the heat of injury and the release of proteolytic enzymes, prostaglandins, and vasoactive substances. Although these burns frequently heal without grafting, healing takes months, and scarring may be extensive. Healing occurs by reepithelialization from deep adnexa and wound margins. The burn must be protected against trauma and contamination while healing. Ineffective therapy may allow a second-degree burn to progress to a third-degree burn, especially if bacterial infection occurs.

Full-thickness *(third-degree)* burns form a dark brown, insensitive, leathery eschar. All skin structures are destroyed, and hair epilates easily. Third-degree burns are less painful than first- or second-degree burns because nerves have been destroyed. Superficial vascular thrombosis and deep vascular permeability cause subcutaneous edema and necrosis. Healing occurs by contraction and reepithelialization unless the wound is reconstructed. Some indication of injury depth may be obtained by elevating the eschar. First- and second-degree burn eschars split when elevated and bent to reveal underlying epidermis or dermis; third-degree burns may not split, or the split may extend to subcutaneous tissue. Early eschar removal is important as a necrotic eschar quickly becomes colonized on its deep surface and serves as a nidus of infection.

Burns that extend beyond the dermis are sometimes classified as *fourth-degree burns.* They have the same characteristics as third-degree burns but with additional tissue damage extending into the muscle and bone. Healing by secondary intention or reconstruction is usually required.

Burn wounds are sterile or colonized only by superficial bacteria during the first 24 hours. The large volume of dead tissue provides an excellent medium for bacterial growth, and occlusion of local blood supply impairs delivery of humeral and cellular defense mechanisms and systemic drugs to the wound. Superficial bacteria proliferate and invade the deeper tissue under the eschar within 4 to 5 days of injury. Initially, most organisms are gram-positive cocci, but by 3 to 5 days, the wound is colonized with gram-negative bacteria, typically *Pseudomonas* spp. Early removal of eschar and application of topical antibiotics are necessary to minimize progression of damage.

Burns frequently cause shock and multiple organ failure because of fluid loss, fluid shifts, electrolyte imbalances, protein losses, myocardial depression, increased peripheral vascular resistance, and increased blood viscosity. Cardiac abnormalities, immunosuppression, anemia, renal failure, liver failure, and disseminated intravascular coagulation sometimes occur. More severe systemic signs are associated with large burn surface areas. Respiratory distress may occur from smoke inhalation (corrosive gases and chemical irritants), thermal burns of the upper airway, and carbon monoxide and cyanide poisoning. Smoke inhalation causes pulmonary edema with vascular congestion, interstitial edema, and atelectasis. Pneumonia often occurs several days after smoke inhalation.

Burns from contact rather than fire may not be immediately recognized. Moisture and flattening of the hair coat may be noted a few days after injury. This is rapidly followed by hair and skin loss, which makes demarcation of the burn area obvious. Burns may be prevented during surgery by using circulating warm water pads or bags inflated with circulating warm air (42° C [107.6° F] or lower) rather than electrical wire element pads. Thermal burns may also be caused by gloves or bottles filled with hot water. Anesthetized or hypothermic animals are particularly susceptible to burns from hot water bottles because of reduced circulation associated with vascular constriction. The longer the exposure, the greater the risk of burns. Burns may also be prevented by properly grounding patients when using electrosurgical units.

TREATMENT

The first priority in treating burns is to minimize tissue loss by administering first aid and preventing shock. Prevention of septic complications by good wound management is the next priority. Meticulous care immediately after injury to ensure adequate perfusion, hydration, and wound protection from trauma and infection may prevent progression of tissue damage and allow salvage of injured tissue. Early wound débridement and reconstruction are important to minimize morbidity. Cooling affected areas immediately after thermal injury (within 2 hours) may limit extension of tissue destruction. The area should be lavaged with cold water, or cold packs should be applied to the wound; however, it is important to prevent systemic hypothermia. Analgesics should be given as necessary to alleviate pain (e.g., see Chapter 13). Vital signs, mental status, hematocrit, total protein, urine output, central venous pressure, electrolytes, blood gases, and daily body weight should be monitored.

The size of the burn area can be estimated by measuring the area of burned skin with a metric ruler, dividing that area by the animal's total surface area (see Table 15-5), and multiplying by 100. As an alternative, a rough estimate can be gained using the rule of nine: each forelimb of the animal represents approximately 9% of the total body surface area (TBSA); each rear limb is 18% (two nines); and the dorsal and ventral thorax and abdomen are each 18%. Animals with partial-thickness burns involving less than 15% TBSA require minimal supportive therapy, whereas those with burns involving more than 15% TBSA require emergency supportive care. Euthanasia should be considered for those with burns involving more than 50% TBSA. Shock doses of lactated Ringer's solution or hypertonic saline solution should be administered to minimize and reverse signs of shock. The amount of isotonic fluid required during the first 24 hours may be estimated using the formula 3 to 4 ml/kg/percentage TBSA burned. Hypertonic saline solutions are beneficial in reducing total fluid requirements, limiting edema, and increasing cardiac output. Hypertonic saline (4 ml/kg bolus) plus lactated Ringer's solution (1 ml/kg/percentage TBSA burned) may be administered. When giving hypertonic saline, the serum sodium concentration should not exceed 160 mEq/L. Nonprotein colloid solutions (i.e., dextran 70, hetastarch) given in the early postburn period (16 to 24 hours after injury) may improve survival and reduce edema formation (see p. 29). Administration of protein colloids (i.e., fresh frozen plasma or albumin) to hypoproteinemic patients should be delayed for 8 to 12 hours to allow the stabilization of membrane permeability and increased lymph return that reduces protein loss. Protein colloids given within the first 8 to 12 hours are lost into the burn wound and worsen edema formation. Dogs with partial-thickness burns involving 20% TBSA may lose 28% of their plasma volume during the first 6 hours. Trans-fusions (i.e., whole blood and packed red blood cells) may be necessary in anemic patients.

Respiratory distress should be treated by giving oxygen (mask, nasal insufflation, tracheostomy tube) and bronchodilators. The half-life of carbon monoxide is reduced with oxygen therapy. Continuous positive pressure ventilation may be necessary in some animals. Tracheostomy (see p. 825) and mechanical ventilation are indicated in patients with upper airway swelling or severe tracheobronchial secretions. The trachea and bronchi should be suctioned if necessary. Systemic antibiotics should be administered if bronchopneumonia occurs (see p. 30).

Aggressive nutritional support counters the increased metabolic demand and protein losses that occur in burn patients (see Chapter 11). Animals with moderate to severe wounds should be fed a high-protein, high-calorie diet. Early enteral feeding is important in preventing gastroduodenal ulceration. Histamine H_2 receptor antagonists should be given if gastroduodenal ulceration is suspected (see p. 435).

BURN WOUND MANAGEMENT

Removal of dead tissue is essential to the control of sepsis and promotion of a viable vascular bed suitable for surgical closure. Necrotic tissue may be débrided from burn wounds with dissection, autolytic, bandage, enzyme, or biosurgical techniques (see p. 164). Autolytic, enzymatic, and biosurgical débridement spare viable tissue that may be removed by

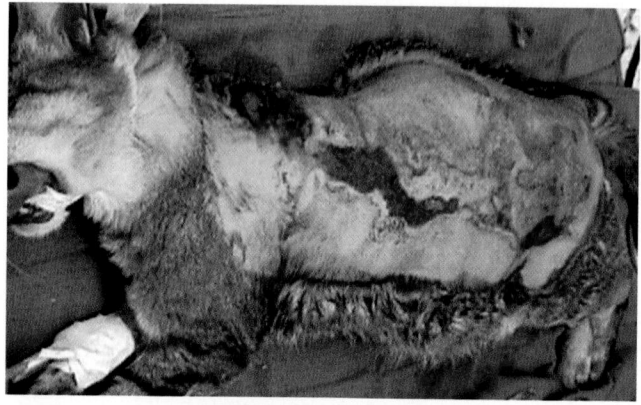
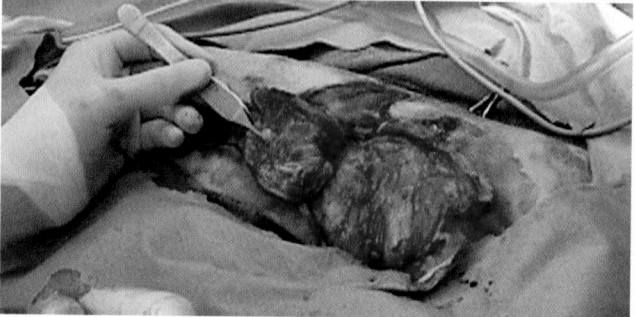
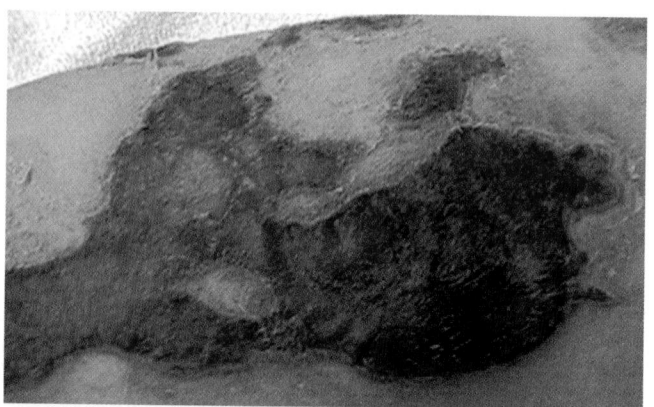
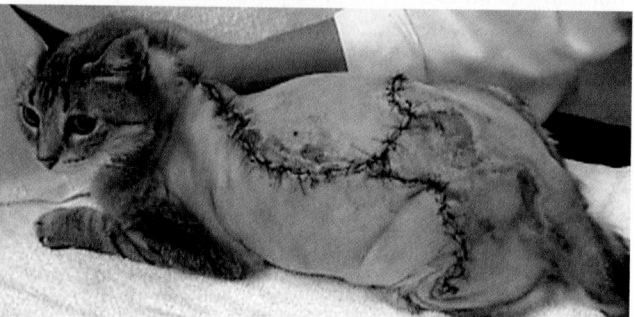

FIG. 15-42
A, This cat received a thermal burn several days before presentation. **B,** Close-up appearance of an area of the burn showing varying degrees of discoloration and a distinct line of demarcation. **C,** The eschar is being surgically removed, exposing the subcutaneous tissue. **D,** Postoperative appearance after excision and flap advancement to close the defect.

surgical excision or bandages, but results vary; the best results are obtained with endogenous or exogenous enzymes on a moist, pliable eschar. Loose and obviously devitalized tissue in partial-thickness burns may be removed with scissors, hydrotherapy, or gauze sponge abrasion. With full-thickness burns, sharp excision to muscle fascia is necessary. Early burn excision is recommended to minimize secondary infections and systemic effects (e.g., endotoxins and blood loss). Application of negative pressure wound therapy (Vacuum Assisted Closure [VAC], Kinetic Concepts, Inc, San Antonio, Tex.) may prevent progression of partial-thickness burns by reducing edema and improving circulation.

TABLE 15-5

Burns: Calculation of Total Body Surface Area

CONVERSION CHART BODY WEIGHT (kg) TO TOTAL BODY SURFACE AREA (m²)			
kg	**m²**	**kg**	**m²**
1.0	0.10	26.0	0.88
2.0	0.15	27.0	0.90
3.0	0.20	28.0	0.92
4.0	0.25	29.0	0.94
5.0	0.29	30.0	0.96
6.0	0.33	31.0	0.99
7.0	0.36	32.0	1.01
8.0	0.40	33.0	1.03
9.0	0.43	34.0	1.05
10.0	0.46	35.0	1.07
11.0	0.49	36.0	1.09
12.0	0.52	37.0	1.11
13.0	0.55	38.0	1.13
14.0	0.58	39.0	1.15
15.0	0.60	40.0	1.17
16.0	0.63	41.0	1.19
17.0	0.66	42.0	1.21
18.0	0.69	43.0	1.23
19.0	0.71	44.0	1.25
20.0	0.74	45.0	1.26
21.0	0.76	46.0	1.28
22.0	0.78	47.0	1.30
23.0	0.81	48.0	1.32
24.0	0.83	49.0	1.34
25.0	0.85	50.0	1.36

From Swaim SF: *Surgery of traumatized skin: management and reconstruction in the dog and cat*, Philadelphia, 1980, WB Saunders. Total body surface area = $Weight^{0.425} \times Height^{0.725} \times 0.007184$ ($m^2 = kg^{0.425} \times cm^{0.725} \times 0.007184$) or Total body surface area = $0.1 \times Weight (kg)^{2/3}$

Small burn wounds can be excised and closed primarily (Fig. 15-42). Closure is achieved by skin advancement or skin flaps. Larger wounds may be allowed to heal by contraction and epithelialization, or they may be grafted. Healing by secondary intention may take months or may be incomplete, and the resulting scar may be cosmetically unacceptable. For these reasons, many large burns are débrided, allowed to form a healthy granulation bed, and then reconstructed using rotating skin flaps, axial pattern flaps, tissue expansion, or grafts. Early wound closure reduces wound management and secondary infection, and shortens hospitalization. Scars are fragile and may erode and bleed easily. Squamous cell carcinomas occasionally occur in burn scars.

Estimate the burn depth and calculate the size of the burn in relationship to the TBSA obtained from a weight conversion chart (see previous discussion and Table 15-5). Clip the wound and surrounding hair before gently lavaging with an antiseptic solution (e.g., 0.05% chlorhexidine diacetate). Cover the wound with a topical aloe vera compound or silver sulfadiazine (see p. 167). If treatment is begun soon after the burn, use aloe vera or dipyridamole (thromboxane synthetase blocker) to help preserve patency of the dermal vasculature, then apply a hydrophilic bandage. After the first 24 hours, apply water-soluble, 1% silver sulfadiazine cream (Silvadene cream) to the wound once or twice daily or a slow-release silver sulfadiazine dressing (SilvaSorb) once every 3 to 7 days (see p. 167). Silver sulfadiazine is bactericidal with activity against gram-positive and gram-negative bacteria and Candida organisms. Alternatively, apply medicinal honey to the wound (see p. 168). Bandage the wound, and aseptically manage it during subsequent bandage changes performed at intervals appropriate for the contact layer and amount of exudation (see Boxes 15-5 through 15-9 and Tables 15-2 and 15-3). Medicinal honey bandages may require bandage changes several times daily. Remove the proteinaceous gel from the surface of the wound during bandage changes and before reapplication of topicals. Use gentle hydrotherapy to remove debris and clean the wound.

 BOX 15-9

Suggested Burn Wound Bandage Contact Layer

Eschar present—needs softening and débridement	Hypertonic saline or hydrogel dressing with silver sulfadiazine *and* biguanide-impregnated gauze
Eschar gone—needs further débridement	Hydrogel or hydrocolloid dressing *and* biguanide-impregnated gauze
Eschar gone—needs granulation	Hydrogel or calcium alginate *and* biguanide-impregnated gauze
Needs epithelialization	Polyurethane foam pad *and* biguanide-impregnated gauze

Suggested Reading

Aragon CL, Harvey SE, Allen SW et al: Partial-thickness skin grafting for large thermal skin wounds in dogs, *Compend Contin Educ Pract Vet* 26:200, 2004.

This article describes the indications, advantages, disadvantages, and technical aspects of partial-thickness skin grafting and provides case-based examples of its application.

Johnson RMJ, Richard R: Partial-thickness burns: identification and management, *Adv Skin Wound Manage* 16:178, 2003.

An overview of evaluation and management of partial-thickness burns in people is presented.

Kabala-Dzik A, Stojko R, Szaflarska-Stojko E et al: Influence of honey-balm on the rate of scar formation during experimental burn wound healing in pigs, *Bull Vet Inst Pulawy* 48:311, 2004.

In this pig study, histopathologic findings showed that honey-balm treated burns entered the repair phase of healing 10 days sooner than those treated with silver sulfadiazine; wounds were moister, more elastic, and had less edema and reddening than those treated with saline or silver sulfadiazine.

Murphy KD, Lee JO, Herndon DN: Current pharmacotherapy for the treatment of severe burns, *Expert Opin Pharmacother* 4:369, 2003.

The review concentrates on the pathophysiology and medical management of the systemic problems associated with burns in people.

Smith ML: Pediatric burns: management of thermal, electrical and chemical burns and burn-like dermatologic conditions, *Pediatr Ann* 29:367, 2000.

Causes, initial care, and wound management are discussed.

ELECTRICAL INJURIES

Electrical burns occur when current touches one point on the body, with or without an exit point. Chewing on electrical cords is the most common cause of electrical injury in small animals. Resistance to electrical current flow is greatest in bone and least in nerves (from greatest to least resistance, the order is bones, fat, tendon, skin, muscle, blood, and nerve). Low-voltage electrical current (<1000 V) follows the path of least resistance, which usually is along blood vessels. Low-voltage burns char tissue at the initial site, which decreases conductivity and limits further current flow, minimizing further injury. The initial contact point with high-voltage currents (>1000 V) negligibly decreases conductivity; therefore, injury is extensive. Tissue necrosis occurs from vascular thrombosis and release of vasoactive substances. Tissue damage may be massive because of deep extension of the generated heat. Immediate death can result from respiratory paralysis or ventricular fibrillation, and tetany can result in spinal fractures.

Animals often are found collapsed in a tonic state with an electrical cord in the mouth. The body stiffens from contraction of striated muscles while receiving the electric current. Generalized tonoclonic activity with vomiting and defecation also can occur. If the animal survives, the tonic state resolves when the cord is removed from the mouth, although the animal may be weak and ataxic for a short period. Burns primarily occur on the lips, gums, palate, or tongue. These areas initially may appear charred, pale gray, or tan. Edema develops after 1 to 2 days. The extent of injury may not be apparent for 2 to 3 weeks. Pulmonary edema frequently occurs, causing dyspnea and moist rales.

TREATMENT

Affected patients should be examined frequently for pulmonary edema. Pulmonary edema may be treated with diuretics (i.e., furosemide, 2.5 to 5 mg/kg given intramuscularly or intravenously once or twice a day) and aminophylline (10 mg/kg given intravenously or intramuscularly three times a day). Morphine (1 mg/kg given intramuscularly or subcutaneously) may be given to dogs to reduce anxiety. Ventilatory support is needed if there is no response to medication.

Repair of damaged tissue should be delayed until the full extent of the injury is known. Technetium scans of muscle are helpful in determining viability. Minor burns may be allowed to heal by secondary intention. Oronasal fistulae must be repaired (see p. 356). Large lip wounds should be repaired to prevent oral drying and improve cosmesis.

Suggested Reading

Smith ML: Pediatric burns: management of thermal, electrical and chemical burns and burn-like dermatologic conditions, *Pediatr Ann* 29:367, 2000.

Causes, initial care, and wound management are discussed.

FROSTBITE

Severe or prolonged cold may cause necrosis of exposed tissue. The extremities (i.e., ear, tail, scrotum, mammary glands, digits, and flank folds) are most commonly affected because of the sparse hair coat and poor peripheral circulation in these areas. Frozen tissue is pale, hypoesthetic, and cool. Thawed viable tissue is hyperemic, painful, and scaly. Nonviable tissue undergoes dry gangrene or mummification and sloughs. Superficial injuries involve skin and subcutaneous tissue, whereas deep injuries extend beyond the subcutaneous tissues. Ice crystals form in intracellular and extracellular spaces, causing cell damage and death.

TREATMENT

The affected body parts should be rapidly rewarmed in warm water (39° to 42° C [102° to 107.6° F]) for about 20 minutes to improve circulation. Affected areas become erythematous and edematous, form large vesicles, and often are painful, necessitating analgesics (see Chapter 13). Topical aloe vera or silver sulfadiazine should be applied to the affected areas. Bandages are used to prevent self-trauma. Conservative therapy should be continued until viable tissue can be distinguished from nonviable tissue (i.e., 3 to 6 weeks). Necrotic tissue should then be débrided and the area reconstructed if necessary. Healing may be complete beneath the mummified tissue.

CHEMICAL INJURIES

Chemical burns from strong acids or alkalis or special chemicals destroy tissue by denaturing proteins or interfering with cell metabolism. The mechanism of injury is usually a direct chemical reaction rather than actual thermal injury, although thermal damage can result from an exothermic reaction. Mechanisms of injury include oxidation, reduction, corrosion, dehydration, denaturation, and vesication. The severity of injury depends on the type of chemical and its strength; the volume involved, the contact time, and the depth of penetration; the chemical's mechanism of action; and the total area of contact. Corrosives (i.e., sodium-containing drain and oven cleaners, and phenol disinfectants) denature proteins, resulting in erosion and ulceration. Dehydrating chemicals (i.e., sulfuric and hydrochloric acids) desiccate tissue, and oxidizing agents (i.e., chromic acid, hypochlorite, and potassium permanganate) coagulate protein. Denaturizing agents (i.e., picric acid, tannic acid, acetic acid, formic acid, and hydrofluoric acid) fix or stabilize tissue by the formation of salts. Vesicants (i.e., dimethyl sulfoxide, cantharides, halogenated hydrocarbons, and gasoline) liberate tissue amines (histamine, serotonin), causing blisters.

TREATMENT

Resultant burns should be flushed with large volumes of water immediately after chemical exposure to remove the chemical and prevent further injury. Dry chemicals should be dusted off before irrigation. Flushing dilutes the chemical and dissipates the heat of chemical reactions. Do not immerse the area in water as this may spread chemical damage. After flushing with water, neutralizing agents, if used, are applied with gauze sponges, which are loosely wrapped over the area for 20 minutes. Attempting to neutralize alkaline injuries with acidic solutions (and vice versa) is dangerous and may lead to thermal injury from the resulting exothermic reaction. The animal should be prevented from licking the wound to prevent chemical burns of the tongue, oropharynx, and esophagus. Antimicrobials and bandages should be applied as described for thermal burns (see p. 231). Early débridement may prevent further chemical penetration and tissue destruction, but excessive tissue removal should be avoided.

Alkali

Lye (sodium hydroxide), cement (calcium, sodium, and potassium hydroxide) and many detergents produce saponification of fat and liquefaction necrosis of tissues, leaving them with a soapy feel. Irrigation should continue until the "soapy" texture is gone. Some alkalis, such as a common fertilizer—anhydrous ammonia, penetrate the skin quickly and may require extensive irrigation for many hours.

Acid

Acids cause destruction by cell dehydration and production of acid albumins. Irrigate exposed skin with large volumes of water. Muriatic acid and sulfuric acid should be neutralized with soap before flushing. Hydrofluoric acid (risk in petroleum factories, glass etching, air condition cleaning, and chemical manufacturing) must be neutralized to stop penetration; irrigate with aqueous benzalkonium chloride or apply calcium gluconate gel, which precipitates residual fluoride ion. If pain persists, 10% calcium gluconate should then be injected into and around the lesion (0.5 ml/cm^2). Early local excision and grafting is indicated if pain continues or to prevent continued tissue damage. Calcium ions trapped as calcium fluoride may lead to hypocalcemia if hydrofluoric acid burns are extensive.

Special chemicals include phenol, phosphorus, and petroleum products such as gasoline and tar. Phenol has an anesthetic effect on the skin and is not water soluble. It is rapidly absorbed through the skin and may cause central nervous system depression, hypothermia, hypotension, intravascular hemolysis, and death. A lipophilic solvent, such as polyethylene glycol, propylene glycol, glycerol, or vegetable oil, is used to cleanse the area. White phosphorus is used in insecticides, fertilizers, and incendiaries. It is lipophilic and is converted to phosphoric acid on contact with tissue. Its high penetrability may lead to systemic toxicity, causing damage to the liver and kidneys and depressed calcium levels. Phosphorus particles can also ignite when in contact with the air. Therefore, copious lavage followed by wet soaks to prevent ignition is recommended. Rinsing the area with dilute 0.5% to 1% solution of copper sulfate results in the formation of a blue-gray cupric phosphide coating over the residual phosphorus particles to help prevent ignition and identify particles. An ultraviolet light can also be used to identify particles for removal. Gasoline's hydrocarbons act as a fat solvent and can damage skin, leading to absorption and systemic toxicity, causing multiorgan injury. Tar products cause thermal injuries. Cold water is used to cool the material, which is then dissolved and removed with a petrolatum-based ointment. If a petrolatum solvent is used, the burn may absorb it, leading to toxicity.

Suggested Reading

Smith ML: Pediatric burns: management of thermal, electrical and chemical burns and burn-like dermatologic conditions, *Pediatr Ann* 29:367, 2000.
Causes, initial care, and wound management are discussed.

RADIATION INJURY

Radiant energy from roentgen ray tubes, radioactive elements, luminous bodies, fluorescent substances, or the sun may cause injury. In animals, radiation injury usually is a consequence of radiation therapy to cure or control tumors. Effects of radiation therapy on normal tissue are related to the energy of the ionizing radiation, number of fractions given, total dose, and time elapsed following radiation. There are four degrees of radiation injury: (1) cutaneous erythema, (2) superficial epidermal (dry) desquamation, (3) moist desquamation from loss of basal layers of epidermis, and (4) necrosis with dermal destruction and irreversible ulceration. Cutaneous erythema occurs during the first week of therapy as a result of dilation of capillaries and increased vascular permeability. Superficial epidermal or dry desquamation occurs with doses less than 30 Gy and is characterized by pruritus, scaling, and increased melanin pigmentation. Moist desquamation occurs with doses greater than 40 Gy, being characterized by discomfort, bullous formation, epidermal sheds, edema, and fibrin exudates. Reepithelialization will occur within 10 days with moist desquamation if the wound does not become infected. Ulcers associated with moist desquamation often heal after therapy but recur. Higher doses of radiation lead to dermal destruction and irreversible ulceration.

Radiation injury may also be classified as early (acute) or late (chronic) changes. Early, or acute, injury is characterized by the development of edema, erythema, tenderness, and desquamation in the irradiated area within 1 to 4 weeks of radiation therapy. The skin may be either moist or dry. Acute injuries are due to depletion of rapidly dividing cells, occurring in renewing tissues, such as mucosa, epidermis, hair follicles, and sebaceous glands. Late, or chronic, injury occurs in nonrenewing tissue, such as bone, nerves, and sometimes skin. Late injury is marked by dryness, pigmentation, induration, loss of pliability, atrophy or thinning, telangiectasia, keratosis, a decrease in adnexal structures, ulceration, progressive fibrosis, and a progressive decrease in circulation. Capillaries dilate and decrease in number and arteries sclerose as fibrous tissue increases and skin elasticity is lost. These changes are slow and progressive. Late injury may become evident weeks to years after radiation therapy. Radiation impairs soft tissue healing by (1) microvascular obliteration, (2) excessive fibrosis, and (3) disruption of cellular proliferation. Proliferating microvasculature, epithelial cells, fibroblasts, and myofibroblasts are damaged. After 1 year, the epidermis is thin, dry, and semitranslucent; hair follicles and sebaceous glands are usually absent. Much of the collagen and subcutaneous adipose tissue are later replaced by atypical fibroblasts and dense fibrous tissue that may cause induration of skin and limit movement. Eccentric myointimal proliferation of small arteries and arterioles may progress to thrombosis or complete obstruction. Ischemic ulcers are often a consequence of these vascular changes. Chronic changes to skin make it thin, hypovascular, extremely painful, and easily injured by slight trauma or infection. Irradiated tissue cannot tolerate the same degree of bacterial contamination as normal tissue, and antibiotics are not delivered in effective concentrations because of compromised microcirculation. The goal of treatment is to transform the chronic wound into an acute wound state.

> NOTE: When excising tissue that has been irradiated, be sure to submit all excised tissue for histologic examination.

Incision into previously radiated tissue should be avoided because healing is inhibited. Avoid or minimize surgical manipulations that may further compromise tissue. If surgery is to follow radiation therapy, it should be performed 2 to 8 weeks after therapy, when radiation inflammation is subsiding and tissue circulation is still sufficient for healing.

TREATMENT

For acute radiation injury, treatment involves keeping the area clean, applying topical medications (a hydrogel containing acemannan, silver sulfadiazine, or aloe vera cream), and preventing self-mutilation. Cleanse the area with normal saline or a mild soap solution and rinse thoroughly to prevent irritation. Apply hydrophilic topicals that absorb water and act as mild lubricants. Sometimes protective ointments or gels (A & D ointment) are applied to protect dry lesions. Reduce itching with colloidal oatmeal bath (Aveeno Bath), cornstarch, or 1% hydrocortisone cream. Moist desquamation injuries may also benefit from astringent soaks, antibiotics, and moisturizers. Avoid any products with alcohol or menthol because they remove natural lipid and worsen the skin's reaction. Experimentally, growth factors, orgotein, topical vitamin C, NSAIDs, and helium-neon lasers have been used to treat acute radiation injuries. Apply hydrophilic bandages to provide a moist wound healing environment (see Box 15-6). Most acute injuries heal within 10 to 14 days after conclusion of radiation therapy.

For chronic radiation injury, débridement of ulcers should be conservative, removing only necrotic tissue. Evaluating bleeding edges is not a reliable method of determining viability. Continual assessment and débridement are necessary to avoid removing tissue that will heal. Use topical antibiotics on irradiated wound beds after débridement because this tissue may have decreased resistance to infection and poor regional vascularity, leading to unreliable delivery of systemic antibiotics to the wound. Complete excision of all irradiated tissue may be necessary with chronic radiation wounds. Submit all excised tissue to determine if neoplasia is present. Wound closure is most successful when vascularized myocutaneous, cutaneous, muscle, or omental flaps are used. Flaps are created outside the irradiated area and transposed over the wound. Healing by secondary intention and free grafts are apt to fail because of impaired vascularity. Hyperbaric oxygen therapy may improve healing by increasing the oxygen gradient in the wound or damaged tissue. Consider using subatmospheric drainage devices (see p. 172), and apply hydrophilic bandages to encourage optimal healing (see Box 15-6).

Suggested Reading

Mendelsohn FA, Divino CM, Reis ED et al: Wound care after radiation therapy, *Adv Skin Wound Care* 15:216, 2002.
Effects of radiation and topical products available for wound care are reviewed.

Teknos TN, Myers LL: Surgical reconstruction after chemotherapy or radiation: problems and solutions, *Hematol Oncol Clin North Am* 13:679, 1999.
The effects of therapy on tissue are discussed, and surgical recommendations are made.

ANIMAL BITE WOUNDS AND ABSCESSES

Bites inflicted on one animal by another may be provoked or unprovoked. Bites often cause crushing, tearing, and avulsion injury that is more severe to the underlying tissue than is apparent from the often minor-appearing skin laceration or puncture. This is because canine and feline skin is freely movable, and the bite pressure is high (150 to 450 psi). The most commonly affected sites are the neck, limbs, head, chest, shoulder, abdomen, and perineal regions. Multiple wounds are common. Mortality associated with bite wounds is less than 10% and is more common with thoracic bite wounds. Mortality is generally due to either infection or concurrent trauma; the wound is contaminated with the attacker's oral flora and bacteria, hair, and other debris from the skin and environment. Devitalized tissue, dead space, compromised blood supply, and serum accumulate, creating a prime environment for bacterial growth. This type of environment is synergistic to anaerobic bacterial growth. Wound infection is common if treatment is delayed. Cat bites are more likely to become infected than dog bites. Common aerobic isolates from bite wounds include *Pasteurella multocida*, *Staphylococcus* spp., *Enterococcus* spp., and *E. coli*; common anaerobic isolates include *Bacillus* spp., *Clostridium* spp., and *Corynebacterium* spp. (Box 15-10). Severe infections may occur after inoculation with *Mycobacterium*, *Pythium*, or *Sporotrichosis* organisms.

Culture all wounds and identify organisms present and their antimicrobial susceptibility. Initial antibiotic therapy before susceptibility data are available is based on whether organisms identified are gram-positive or gram-negative. Cephalosporins and penicillins are appropriate for many wounds as they have a good spectrum of activity and enter wound sites quickly when given intravenously. If gram-negative organisms are identified, consider aminoglycosides or fluoroquinolones. Metronidazole can be given if an anaerobic infection is suspected.

Manage bite wounds by clipping and scrubbing a wide area around the wound followed by copious lavage and cleaning of the wound (see p. 169). Explore full-thickness punctures and lacerations to remove debris and devitalized tissue and to determine the extent of the injury.

Penetration of the abdominal or thoracic cavity necessitates exploration of the cavity to identify and treat concurrent visceral injury. Ultrasonography and radiographs may help evaluate the wounds.

Close wounds presented in the "golden period" (within 6 to 8 hours of injury) with minimal contamination and tissue trauma primarily after thorough cleaning.

Most wounds should be managed with bandages (see p. 176) to optimize drainage and allow autolytic débridement. After 3 to 5 days, most acute wounds will be healthy enough for delayed primary closure with or without placement of closed suction drains. More chronic bite wounds may require bandaging for a longer period. These wounds are closed secondarily (after the appearance of granulation tissue) or allowed to heal by secondary intention.

Closure of severely contaminated, infected, or traumatized wounds and sealing or healing of punctures often cause abscessation.

Treat abscesses by first clipping and aseptically preparing a wide area around the swelling or draining tract. Then using aseptic technique, open the abscess by lancing or enlarging the tract's opening. Obtain cultures. Thoroughly lavage the abscess cavity and débride necrotic tissue. Place a drain or leave the wound open to facilitate drainage and apply a bandage.

> NOTE: Treat bite wounds with hydrophilic bandages for 3 to 5 days to prevent wound complications.

 BOX 15-10

Normal Oral Flora of Dogs and Cats

Gram-positive	Gram-negative
Bacillus spp.	*Pasteurella multocida*
Corynebacterium spp.	*Enterobacter aerogenes*
Staphylococcus aureus	*Escherichia coli*
Staphylococcus epidermidis	*Pseudomonas fluorescens*
Staphylococcus saprophyticus	*Acinetobacter calcoaceticus*
Streptococcus spp.	*Caryophanon* spp.
Actinomyces spp. (anaerobic)	*Neisseria* spp.
	Moraxella spp.
	Mycoplasma spp.

Suggested Reading

Armbrust LJ, Biller DS, Radlinsky MG et al: Ultrasonographic diagnosis of foreign bodies associated with chronic draining tracts and abscesses in dogs, *Vet Radiol Ultrasound* 44:66, 2003.
This retrospective study of six dogs found that no foreign bodies were identified with radiographs, 2/4 with fistulograms, and 1/6 with ultrasound. A hyperechoic structure believed to be a foreign body was identified in 5/6; these were confirmed surgically.
Griffin GM, Holt DE: Dog-bite wounds: bacteriology and treatment outcome in 37 cases, *J Am Anim Hosp Assoc* 37:453, 2001.
This prospective study found that 86% had multiple wounds and 57% of wounds were full thickness with avulsion of underlying tissue and dead space. Aerobic bacteria were isolated from 65%, and 15% had positive anaerobic cultures.

SNAKEBITE

Snakebites can cause severe local tissue damage and systemic effects. Snake venom is an extremely complex mixture of enzymes, proteins, and peptides; venom composition varies between species, individual snakes, and the bite itself. Venomous snakes in the United States include the Crotalidae (pit vipers) and Elapidae (coral snakes) subfamilies. The Crotalidae subfamily includes the copperhead, cottonmouth water moccasin, and rattlesnake. Pit vipers have a triangular head with facial pits between the nostrils and eyes, and vertically elliptic pupils (Box 15-11). Their fangs are hollow, retractable teeth (hinged) near the rostral maxilla. Coral snakes, along with many nonpoisonous snakes, have round heads, no pits, and round pupils. Coral snakes have small fangs that are fixed in the cranial maxilla. Their short fangs allow them to hang from animals they bite. Nonvenomous snakes have teeth, but no fangs.

Coral snake venom is primarily neurotoxic and hemolytic, causing moderate tissue reaction and pain at the puncture sites. There is a delay of several hours before the onset of systemic signs, which worsen gradually over 18 hours. The effects may last 7 to 10 days. Neurotoxicity caused by coral snake venom is characterized by central nervous system depression, vasomotor instability, and muscle paralysis. Coral snake envenomation may cause lethargy, tremors, ptosis, dysphonia, incoordination, and hematuria. Larger doses may cause vomiting, salivation, defecation, and generalized parasympathetic stimulation, followed by paralysis and death. The primary cause of death is respiratory paralysis.

Crotalid (pit viper) venoms are primarily enzymatic in activity (i.e., phospholipase A, phosphatases, exopeptidase, hyaluronidase, L-amino acid oxidase, proteases, and endopeptidase). These venoms are hematotoxic, vasculotoxic, and necrogenic. They alter the resistance and integrity of blood vessels, cause hypotension and bleeding, affect cardiac dynamics and nervous system function, and produce respiratory depression and myonecrosis. Bites most commonly occur on the face and legs. Bites correlate with the snakes' nonhibernating periods and times of day when owners are most likely to be walking with the pet. Signs of envenomation vary and depend on the species of snake, the volume of venom, and the size of the victim. The bite of a pit viper usually produces two puncture marks surrounded by edema. The fang marks may bleed. Erythema, edema, and pain are immediate local effects. Envenomation has not occurred if these signs are not seen within 20 minutes of the bite; envenomation does not occur in approximately 20% to 25% of bites. Progressive swelling and sometimes local hemorrhage occur with moderate to severe envenomation. Tissue discoloration caused by petechiae and ecchymosis occurs, followed by local tissue necrosis. Tissue damage varies with the depth of the bite and the amount of venom injected. Systemic signs of crotalid envenomation usually are lethargy, vomiting, diarrhea, hypotension, and shock. Other signs may include anorexia, salivation, thirst, lymph node pain, weakness, bradycardia or tachycardia, generalized tremors, coma, tachypnea, pulmonary edema, urinary and fecal incontinence, paralysis, convulsions, and hemorrhage. Venom-induced coagulation defects may be severe (activated clotting time greater than 120 seconds). Other common laboratory abnormalities include echinocytosis (burr cells), leukocytosis, and thrombocytopenia. Serious effects of envenomation, such as respiratory paralysis and acute renal failure, may not develop for several hours; therefore, animals should be monitored for a minimum of 24 hours after being bitten.

TREATMENT

Treatment goals include neutralizing the venom, treating systemic effects and wounds, and reconstructing tissue defects (see Box 15-11). The animal should be supported with intravenous fluids. Corticosteroids may help treat shock and reduce edema and pain. However, corticosteroid use is controversial because it may enhance venom toxicity. Antihistamines are often given. Broad-spectrum antibiotics are used to inhibit wound infection. Additional supportive care may include analgesics, sedatives, transfusions, and oxygen.

The bite wound should be immobilized and excitement or exertion avoided. The wound should be lavaged and cleaned with antiseptics or germicidal soaps. The use of tourniquets or incision, suction, or manipulation of the bitten area is rarely helpful and must be done immediately after the bite to have any beneficial effect. These techniques also can easily cause additional tissue damage. A tourniquet, if applied, should be placed 10 cm proximal to the fang marks, should be lightly constrictive, and should be released for 60 to 90 seconds every 30 minutes. However, tourniquets can prevent dilution of the venom and reduce tissue perfusion, thereby promoting ischemia and tissue necrosis.

The site should be clipped to facilitate examination for fang marks. Hospitalization and observation for systemic signs are indicated. Hemograms, coagulation profiles, urinalysis, and serum biochemical analyses should be moni-

---

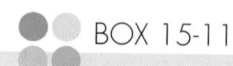 BOX 15-11

Snakebites: Key Points

Pit Vipers: Copperhead, Cottonmouth Water Moccasin, Rattlesnake

- Characteristics: Triangular heads with facial pits between eyes and nostrils, elliptic pupils, hollow fangs
- Usually bitten during spring and summer months
- Most commonly bitten on head; sometimes neck and legs
  - Verify bite by identifying two fang marks
  - May be bitten more than once
- Signs: swelling, depression, tachypnea, bleeding punctures, petechial/ecchymotic hemorrhages, cardiac arrhythmias.
- Expect: leukocytosis, hemolytic anemia, thrombopenia, echinocytosis, abnormal coagulation, elevated fibrin split products
- Treatment:
  - Supportive care: fluids and analgesics; ± antiinflammatories, antihistamines, antibiotics ± oxygen, blood products, hetastarch, antiarrhythmic drugs, etc.
  - Antivenin: expensive and of questionable value
  - Wound: Mobilize; clip, aseptically prepare, and lavage wound; débride necrotic tissue

DO NOT USE TOURNIQUETS, SUCTION, OR AN INCISION TO REMOVE VENOM!

tored every 6 to 12 hours, depending upon the severity of the envenomation. Persistent decreased platelet counts and prolonged clotting times suggest progressive venom activity. Myoglobinuria indicates rhabdomyolysis, and hemoglobinuria indicates hemolysis. The electrocardiogram should be monitored. The circumference of the edematous area around the bite should be measured and recorded to monitor progression.

Antivenin (Antivenin Crotalidae Polyvalent or North American Coral Snake Antivenin) should be administered only if a snakebite is known to have occurred. It should be administered as soon as possible to limit tissue necrosis and prevent systemic reactions. Pretreating with antihistamines and skin testing the animal with antivenin before intravenous administration may prevent anaphylactic reactions. However, the correlation between intradermal skin testing and the predictability of early antivenin reactions is poor. Recommended antivenin doses range from 1 to 5 vials. The number of vials used is directly related to the clinical signs, the animal's body fluid volume, and the location of the bite. Snakebites on digits or in small animals may require 50% more antivenin than those found elsewhere on the body or in larger animals. Although it is not known how long antivenin can be given after envenomation and still be effective, administration after 8 hours is considered of questionable value. Some evidence in mice and rabbits indicates that antivenin may have some benefit for at least 60 hours after envenomation. In human beings, antivenin is given until pain associated with the bite is relieved. This end point is difficult to determine in animals; therefore antivenin should be given until serial examinations and coagulation profiles suggest that the animal's condition is stable. Necrotic tissue should be treated as an open, infected wound (see p. 163). Bandages that support moist wound healing and débridement (see p. 176) should be applied until healthy granulation tissue has formed. Then nonadherent absorbent bandages (see p. 177) should be used and the wound allowed to heal by secondary intention or reconstructed with flaps or grafts.

Suggested Reading

Hackett TB, Wingfield WE, Mazzaferro EM et al: Clinical findings associated with prairie rattlesnake bites in dogs: 100 cases (1989-1998), *J Am Vet Med Assoc* 220:1675, 2002.

Data from these cases concluded that most bites occur on the head in the late afternoon, swelling is the primary sign, and raised questions about the benefit of antivenin.

Willey JR, Schaer M: Eastern diamondback rattlesnake (*Crotalus adamanteus*) envenomation of dogs: 31 cases (1982-2002), *J Am Anim Hosp Assoc* 41:22, 2005.

This study reports signs, laboratory findings, and treatment finding that 88% of surviving and 50% of nonsurviving dogs received antivenin.

PRESSURE SORES

Animals incapable of or unwilling to change positions are prone to pressure sores because pressure is exerted on bony prominences when animals lie down (Table 15-6). Pressure sores form when animals (especially large dogs) are recumbent for long periods because of paralysis, fractures, injuries, or illness. Pressure sores may also develop under improperly fitted or padded casts and bandages. Pressure on the wound pushes wound edges apart, complicating healing. They can be prevented by providing well-padded bedding (i.e., water mattress, air mattress, egg-crate-type foam-rubber mat, artifical sheepskin mat, and fleece), by repositioning the animal frequently, and by keeping the animal clean and dry. Bony prominences should be checked daily for signs of an impending ulcer (i.e., hyperemia, moisture, and easily epilated hair) (Box 15-12). The lateral humeral epicondyle, tuber calcaneus, greater femoral trochanter, tuber coxa, and ischiatic tuberosity are most susceptible to pressure sores (Box 15-13). Less common sites are the acromion of the scapula, lateral tibial condyle, lateral malleolus, olecranon, and sternum. Soft tissues, including skin, loose connective tissue, fat, deep fascia, and periosteum, cover these prominences. All intervening tissues are compressed when pressure is exerted on a bony promi-

 TABLE 15-6

Pressure Sore Classification and Treatment

CLASSIFICATION	DESCRIPTION	TREATMENT
Grade I	Dark red erythema with superficial to partial-thickness skin loss	Wound cleansing, débridement, bandaging, healing by secondary intention
Grade II	Full-thickness skin loss (ulcer) extending into the subcutis	Wound cleansing, surgical or bandage débridement, bandaging, and healing by secondary intention or wound excision and primary closure, delayed primary closure, or secondary closure
Grade III	Ulcer extends through subcutis to deep fascia overlying bony prominences; edges may be undermined	Treatment as for grade II, but drains may be necessary with undermined edges; muscle flaps or myocutaneous flaps and partial excision of the bony prominence may be necessary
Grade IV	Ulcer extends to bone; osteomyelitis or septic joint (or both) may be present	Treatment as for grade III, but sinus tracts and pockets may need to be excised or opened

BOX 15-12

Prevention and Treatment of Pressure Sores

Prevention

- Keep pressure off vulnerable sites.
- Bedding: vinyl covered, thick egg-crate type of foam rubber with artificial sheepskin mat; water mattress or air mattress with fleece
- Keep clean and dry to prevent urine scalds
- Change animal's position every 1 to 5 hr
  - Rotate from right lateral, to sternal, to left lateral
  - Place in a sling for 2 to 4 hours daily
  - Support pelvic area in wheeled carts
- Apply properly padded and fitted bandages, splints, and casts
  - Do not apply extra padding over pressure points (actually increases pressure)
  - Use doughnut type of pad (see p. 187)
  - Reduce weight bearing: foam pad, clamshell splint, or extension splints
- Apply skin toughening agents (Pad Toughening Compound, Island Pharmacy Services, Woodruff, Wisc.)
- Provide good hygiene
  - Inspect skin daily
  - Reduce local skin moisture
  - Whirlpool baths
  - Clip perineal area if incontinent
- Physical therapy: passive range of motion, massage, hydrotherapy, local hyperthermia and hypothermia, ultrasonography, neuromuscular stimulation (see Chapter 12)

- Provide good nutrition: high-protein, high-carbohydrate diet with vitamin supplements
- Surgery: amputation, wedge osteotomy, arthrodesis or phalangeal fillet techniques for nerve or musculoskeletal abnormalities

Treatment

- Follow the prevention guidelines above
- Keep pressure off the wound
- Cleanse wound
- Débride and drain wound as necessary
- Apply appropriate topical medications (see p. 166)
  - Antibiotics
  - Acemannan products: stimulate macrophages to produce cytokines and growth factors
  - D-glucose polysaccharide: antibacterial, bacteriostatic, and provides glucose for cell metabolism
  - Tripeptide-copper complex: attracts mast cells and macrophages to stimulate healing
- Apply bandages that promote moist wound healing (see p. 176)
- Allow healing by secondary intention or transpose flaps to cover wound

 BOX 15-13

Common Pressure Sore Sites

Most Common	Less Common
Lateral humeral epicondyle	Acromion of scapula
Tuber calcaneus	Lateral tibial condyle
Greater femoral trochanter	Lateral malleolus
Tuber coxae	Olecranon
Ischiatic tuberosity	Sternum

nence. Typically, repeated trauma and inflammation are mild, and protective callus develops. Prolonged or severe compression leads to soft tissue ischemia and cell death. Biochemical changes (oxygen free radicals, thromboxane) occur in ischemic tissue and contribute to necrosis. Elevated tissue thromboxane levels cause vasoconstriction, platelet aggregation, and ischemia to exacerbate already compromised tissue circulation. Persistent neutrophilia causes an ongoing inflammation, leading to a chronic wound.

As pressure sores begin developing, blood vessels dilate and inflammatory edema of skin and subcutaneous tissue occurs. If trauma persists, tissues break down, causing a hematoma or an open sore. Untreated hematomas are not absorbed because the surrounding tissues have been damaged. The fluid is mucinous and yellow to red. Tissues

thicken around the hematoma, forming a false bursa (hygroma). The wall of the hygroma is thick and tough, composed of granulation tissue and collagen. The lining of this sac is pale and smooth or rough with irregular, villuslike projections extending into the lumen. Open sores may involve the epidermis and dermis or may extend through subcutaneous tissue and fascia to bone. Osteomyelitis or septic arthritis may develop. Diagnostic imaging may be helpful in determining the extent of soft tissue injury (ultrasound or computed tomogrpahy (CT) and presence of osteomyelitis or skeletal abnormalities (radiographs, CT, magnetic resonance imaging [MRI]).

TREATMENT

Treatment and prevention are similar (see Box 15-12). Early pressure sores are treated by padded bedding (water mattress, air mattress, egg-crate type of foam-rubber mat, artifical sheepskin mat, and fleece), bandaging the limb or using slings or side bars to eliminate pressure over the bony prominence, and changing the recumbent animal's position every 1 to 5 hours. A well-padded, doughnut type of bandage or pipe insulation bandage should be applied to prevent trauma (see p. 187). In addition, the skin must be kept clean and dry. Treatment for open or chronic pressure sores is similar, but the response is poorer (see Table 15-6). Open wounds should be treated with topical agents (see p. 163) and with bandages that promote moist wound healing (see p. 176), which encourages débridement and granulation. When deep ulcers are present, dead space should be drained and infected tissue and bone surgically should be débrided.

Small superficial wounds may heal by secondary intention. However, healing by secondary intention may not provide a surface durable enough to prevent reinjury. Secondary closure is performed after healthy granulation tissue has formed in large, deep wounds. Skin edges should be undermined and apposed if possible. Skin flaps (i.e., local advancement, transposition, axial pattern, or musculocutaneous [see pp. 205 to 222]) and grafts (see pp. 224 to 228) may be necessary for a tension-free closure. Suture lines should not be positioned over bony prominences. A well-padded bandage and a soft padded bed should be used to protect the site during healing. Ulcers may recur if the cause goes uncorrected.

Suggested Reading

Swaim SF: Pressure-related wounds: prevention and treatment, *NAVC Clinician's Brief* December 8, 2003.
A concise, well-illustrated, updated review.

ELBOW HYGROMA

A hygroma is any chronic tissue swelling that contains serous fluid. An elbow hygroma (elbow seroma, olecranon bursitis) is a fluid-filled cavity surrounded by dense fibrous connective tissue that occurs over the lateral aspect of the olecranon (Fig. 15-43). Caused by chronic trauma, elbow hygromas often occur bilaterally as painless swellings. Most occur in young dogs (6 to 18 months old) of large breeds before a protective callus forms over the bony prominence; however, they may occur in older animals with neuromuscular disease. Some dogs with thin skin and sparse subcutaneous fat are predisposed to hygromas. Others with hip dysplasia or pain from other orthopedic disease may exert excess pressure on the elbows while positioning themselves in sternal recumbency. Elbow hygromas vary in size, becoming larger and thicker with repeated trauma. They usually are sterile initially, but bacteria may be introduced during aspiration. Infected hygromas are painful. Small, painless hygromas are cosmetic problems that persist if not treated. Hygromas also occur over other bony prominences (i.e., tuber calcaneus, greater trochanter, tuber coxa, tuber ischium, external occipital protuberance, and thoracic vertebral dorsal spinous processes).

TREATMENT

The primary treatment for elbow hygromas is elimination of repeated elbow trauma. Affected animals should be housed on yielding surfaces with soft, thick padding and bandaged (see Box 15-12). A spica type of bandage or elbow splint may be necessary to prevent slippage (see p. 949). Most acute lesions regress slowly if repeated trauma is eliminated. The hygroma retains its ability to produce a fluid transudate until all granulation tissue and connective tissue undergo fibrosis. Aspiration of the hygroma is of little benefit and may

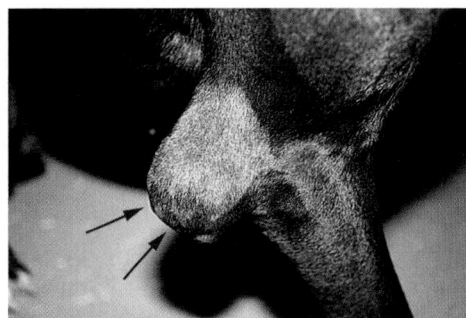

FIG. 15-43
Elbow hygroma in a dog. Note the fluid-filled swelling over the olecranon *(arrows)*.

introduce bacteria. Although surgery should be avoided if possible, development of a fibrous capsule or infection may necessitate it. Infection requires drainage and administration of appropriate antibiotics. Prolonged drainage may be obtained by placing closed suction or Penrose drains in the hygroma. Nonhealing wounds and infection are complications of drains. The advantage of this technique is that the protective callus is preserved. Drains should not be used on ulcerated hygromas.

For nonulcerated (infected or sterile) hygromas, prepare the limb for aseptic surgery and make several dorsal and ventral stab wounds into the hygroma cavity. Probe the cavity, breaking down fibrous septa, and lavage it. Place several Penrose drains or one or more fenestrated closed suction drains in the hygroma cavity and secure them. Apply a non-adherent, absorbent bandage with a "doughnut" (see p. 187) to relieve pressure, absorb drainage, and prevent trauma. Change the bandage daily. Remove the drains when drainage becomes minimal and scar tissue adherence occurs (i.e., 2 to 3 weeks). Continue to bandage the elbow for at least 1 week after removing the drains or until healing is complete.

When all conservative treatment attempts have failed, hygromas are occasionally surgically excised if fibrous tissue, fistulae, or infection develop without a large, fluid-filled cavity. The naturally protective callus is removed during excision, and postoperative management often is complicated. Incisions may dehisce and ulcerate, bandages are difficult to maintain, and recurrence is common. Wounds that dehisce may not heal. Small hygromas can be excised and the defect closed by undermining and advancing local tissue until skin edges can be approximated with interrupted sutures. Complete excision of fibrous tissue is ideal; however, when this is not possible because of the size of the lesion, the cavity lining should be débrided and lavaged, and Penrose drains should be placed before closure. Incision and suture lines are positioned medial or lateral to the olecranon and other bony prominences if possible. It is difficult to excise large hygromas and close the wound without using skin flaps (i.e., axial pattern [see p. 211], pedicle [see p. 205], or myocutaneous [see p. 216]). The limb should be bandaged for a minimum of 4 weeks. An external coaptation splint (i.e., spica bandage; see p. 949) protects and pads the elbow.

LICK GRANULOMA

Lick granulomas (acral lick dermatitis, acral pruritic nodule, acropruritic granuloma, psychogenic dermatoses, and neurodermatitis) are self-induced by continuous licking or chewing. They usually are single and unilateral and may occur anywhere, although the cranial and medial aspects of the carpus-metacarpus and the cranial and lateral aspects of the tarsus-metatarsus are most commonly affected. Less frequent sites include the stifle, tibia, flank, and tail base. They usually occur in older, male, large breed dogs, especially Labrador retrievers, golden retrievers, German shepherds, German shorthair pointers, Great Danes, Saint Bernards, and pit bulls. Although wounds, foreign bodies, infections, and musculoskeletal pain may be initiating factors, most lick granulomas are believed to be psychogenic (obsessive-compulsive disorder) and associated with boredom, inactivity, or environmental change. A cycle of obsessive licking and secondary pruritus and infection develops that is difficult to interrupt. The lesion is sparsely haired, thickened, firm, ulcerated, erythematous, and surrounded by a hyperpigmented halo (Figs. 15-44 and 15-45). Secondary furunculosis and apocrine hidradenitis contribute to enlargement and inflammation of the lesion. Superficial tissue may erode and expose bone. Lameness sometimes results from the mechanical presence of the mass or from underlying periostitis. Dermatologic examination, skin scraping, fungal culture, biopsy, radiographs, electrodiagnostics, allergy testing, thyroid function testing, and/or hypoallergenic diet trials may be necessary. Diagnostic imaging may reveal periosteal proliferation secondary to soft tissue inflammation or associated arthritis, osteomyelitis, osteosarcoma, or foreign bodies. Biopsy to rule out neoplasia and deep cultures to determine bacterial involvement and antimicrobial sensitivity are recommended. Expected histopathology results include cellulitis, dermal fibroplasias, epidermal hyperplasia with compact hyperkeratosis, furunculosis, and vertical collagen streaking.

TREATMENT

Previously recommended treatments have included activity or environmental modification, bandaging, collars, muzzles, topical antichew agents, glucocorticoids, orgotein, radiation therapy, cryosurgery, surgical excision, behavior modifying drugs (phenobarbital, diazepam, hydroxyzine, naltrexone, hydrocodone), cobra venom, acupuncture, and other medications (i.e., fluocinolone acetonide, flunixin meglumine, dimethyl sulfoxide, proteolytic enzymes, and progestogens). The results have been inconsistent, and recurrence is common.

Treatment should be individualized and initiated before the lesion becomes chronic and unresponsive. Initially, administer long-term antibiotic therapy (45 to 90 days) based

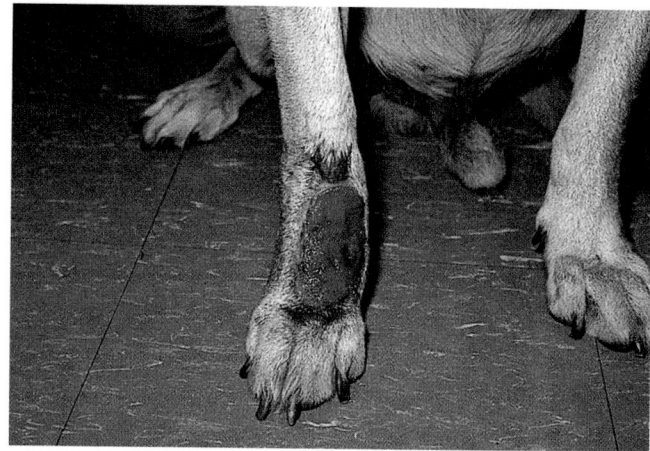

FIG. 15-44
Lick granulomas often occur in the carpal-metacarpal or tarsal-metatarsal area. They are sparsely haired, thickened, firm, ulcerated, erythematous, and surrounded by a hyperpigmented halo.

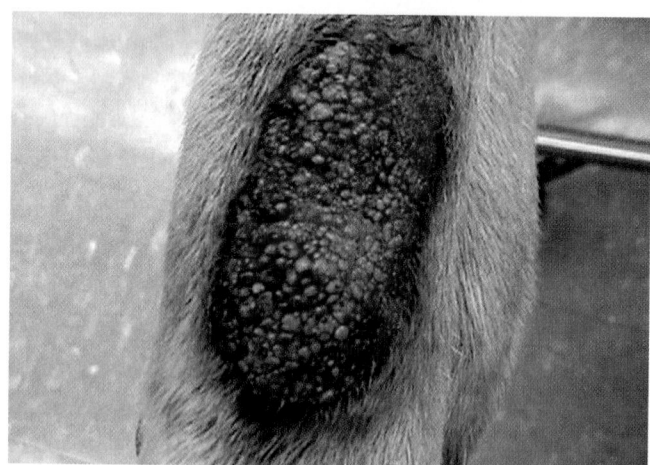

FIG. 15-45
Close-up view of a chronic lick granuloma.

on culture and susceptibility results and use bandages and restraint devices. Periodic CO_2 laser cross-hatching of the granuloma surface may help to eliminate hair embedded in the granulation tissue and facilitate control of infection. If an underlying cause is identified, it should be treated or eliminated, especially such things as allergies, and behavior should be modified.

Treatment investigations involving behavior modification have shown beneficial results using serotonin reuptake-blocking drugs (clomipramine, 0.25 to 1 mg/kg/day; fluoxetine hydrochloride, 0.1 to 1 mg/kg/day; sertraline hydrochloride, 1 mg or less/kg/ day; amitriptyline, 1 to 3 mg/kg twice a day; or imipramine, 2 to 4 mg/kg/day PO) and electronic stimulation. Although not commonly performed, surgical excision of a lick granuloma followed by reconstruction using direct apposition, flaps, or grafts is possible. The surgical site should be protected with a bandage until suture removal.

However, the lesion usually recurs at the same or a different site unless the causative factor or factors are eliminated.

Suggested Reading

Lynch AK: Successful treatment of lick granuloma with chiropractic therapy, *Aust Vet Pract* 33:176, 2003.
This case report describes a thoracic wall lesion that resolved after one adjustment.

DERMOID SINUS (PILONIDAL SINUS)

A dermoid sinus or cyst is a tubular skin indentation that extends ventrally as a blind sac from the dorsal midline. It is a neural tube defect caused by incomplete separation of skin and the neural tube during embryonic development. Sinus depth varies; some are superficial whereas others extend to the supraspinous ligament or dura mater. Multiple or single draining tracts may be identified, especially in the cervical region. Cervical sinuses generally are attached to the dorsal spinous process of the second cervical vertebra. They are most common in Rhodesian ridgebacks, occurring along the dorsal midline cranial and caudal to the midline ridge. They also have been reported in a Shih Tzu, Yorkshire terrier, English bulldog, Siberian husky, Great Pyrenees, chow chow, boerboel, springer spaniel, golden retriever, Kerry blue terrier, and boxer. Because the lesion is believed to be hereditary (complex dihybrid mode of inheritance) in Rhodesian ridgebacks, affected animals should be neutered.

Lesions can be recognized at a young age as openings on the dorsal midline with protruding hair or a whorl of hair. A tube or cord is palpated in the subcutaneous tissue when a skin fold is elevated in the area of the sinus. The cord is 1 to 5 mm in diameter and courses toward the spine. Cystlike subcutaneous swellings may also be palpated. The lumen of the sinus is filled with inspissated sebum, exfoliated keratin debris, and hair. Periodic plugging of the sinus opening leads to cellulitis, infection, and abscessation. Myelitis, meningomyelitis, or encephalitis can occur if the infected sinus extends to the spine. Sinuses should be classified as one of five types (Table 15-7).

Congenital dermoid sinuses have also been reported on the dorsal nasal midline of golden retrievers, spaniels, and English bull terriers. Presenting signs are usually a fluctuant, nasal swelling and intermittent discharge. An opening or "nasal pit" is usually found immediately behind the nasal planum. It courses caudally and extends through an incomplete suture into the nasal septum. Embryogenesis of these sinuses is not completely understood, but is believed to be a failure of the foramen cecum to close during maturation of the skull. The foramen cecum is a canal in the frontal bone at the base of the skull, which allows an outpouching of the meninges into the prenasal space and into contact with the somatic ectoderm. Dogs are usually presented in early adulthood for treatment of sebaceous discharge or secondary infection from the sinus. The sinus may be difficult to identify, and diagnostic imaging may be helpful in determining its caudal extent.

Differential diagnoses include foreign bodies, sebaceous cysts, abscesses, epidermal inclusion cysts, follicular reten-

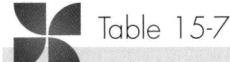

Table 15-7

Classification of Dermoid Sinus Involving the Neck and Back

Type I	Tract extends as far as the supraspinatus ligament or nuchal ligament and attaches there.
Type II	Tract does not extend to the ligament, but is attached by a fibrous band.
Type III	Tract does not extend to or attach by fibrous band to the ligament.
Type IV	Tract attaches to the dura mater.
Type V	Sinus has no connection to the skin surface.

tion cysts, and intracutaneous cornifying epitheliomas. Samples should be collected for cytologic studies and microbial culture and sensitivity testing. Metrizamide fistulography and myelography may reveal spinal communications, especially in conjunction with CT or MRI. Excised tissue should be submitted for histologic examination to rule out other causes of draining tracts. The histology of the dermoid sinuses is consistent with normal skin plus adnexa.

TREATMENT

Dermoid sinuses may be resected if they are associated with drainage or neurologic signs. Treat with antibiotics before surgery if the sinus is infected. Strict asepsis is essential to prevent postoperative meningitis if the sinus extends to the dura. Incomplete excision may occur if the sinus attaches to the dura and causes a chronic draining lesion. Successful treatment of nasal dermoid sinuses requires complete surgical excision with careful dissection between the nasal bones into the nasal septum. They usually terminate in the septum, but may communicate with the dura. Complications include recurrence if incompletely excised, abscesses, and meningitis. The prognosis is good with complete surgical excision. The prognosis is guarded if neurologic signs occur before surgery.

Clip and aseptically prepare a large area around the sinus. Position the dog in ventral recumbency with the spine or nose deviated dorsally; then make an elliptic incision around the sinus opening. Carefully dissect the sinus to its origin and free its attachment. Divide or split the nuchal ligament if necessary. Perform a laminectomy or hemilaminectomy (see pp. 1409-1415) if the sinus tract extends to the dura. Lavage thoroughly before closure. If the nuchal ligament has been transected, reappose it with a locking loop or modified Bunnell suture pattern (see p. 69). Appose muscles and deep tissue with interrupted absorbable sutures to eliminate dead space (e.g., 3-0 or 4-0 polydioxanone or polyglyconate). If a large amount of dead space is still present, place a closed suction drain at the site. Appose subcutaneous tissue and skin routinely. Submit tissue samples for culture and sensitivity testing and histologic evaluation. Give analgesics and antibiotics, and bandage the site after surgery. Neuter affected animals.

Suggested Reading

Anderson DM, White RAS: Nasal dermoid sinus cysts in the dog, *Vet Surg* 31:303, 2002.

Six cases are reported with draining tracts on the bridge of the nose near the planum that resolved after complete surgical excision. The article also reviews and makes comparison to the human condition.

Bailey TR, Holmberg DL, Yager JA: Nasal dermoid sinus in an American cocker spaniel, *Can Vet J* 42:213, 2001.

This is an unusual case; the sinus was more caudal than is typical and communicated with the left frontal sinus and rostral cerebral dura.

Burrow RD: A nasal dermoid sinus in an English bull terrier, *J Small Anim Pract* 45:572, 2004.

This dog was older than others, and signs were recognized after trauma.

Cornegliani L, Jommi E, Vercelli A: Dermoid sinus in a golden retriever, *J Small Anim Pract* 42:514, 2001.

This is the first report of a dermoid sinus in this breed.

Salmon Hillbertz NHC: Inheritance of dermoid sinus in the Rhodesian ridgeback, *J Small Anim Pract* 46:71, 2005.

Data from 57 litters and 492 offspring found 82 dermoid sinuses (frequency of 8% to 10%) and suggests a dihybrid mode of inheritance.

Tshamala M, Moens Y: True dermoid cyst in a Rhodesian ridgeback, *J Small Anim Pract* 41:352, 2000.

This case would be classified as a Type V dermoid sinus.

INTERDIGITAL PYODERMA

Interdigital pyoderma (granuloma, acne, furunculosis, folliculitis) is a bacterial pododermatitis that may coexist with other conditions. Sometimes erroneously called an interdigital cyst, pododermatitis may be caused by parasites, allergies, mycoses, irritants, neoplasms, and metabolic, neurologic, or autoimmune disease. Bacterial infections usually occur secondary to demodicosis, allergy, hypothyroidism, or hyperglucocorticoidism. Immunosuppression is suspected in some animals. The primary bacterial pathogen is *Staphylococcus intermedius;* secondary opportunistic bacteria include *Proteus* spp., *P. aeruginosa,* and *E. coli.* The condition is seen frequently in West Highland White and Scottish terriers, Pekingese, and English bulldogs.

Varying degrees of pruritus, pain, paronychia, swelling, erythema, and hyperpigmentation are common. Papules, pustules or nodules, draining tracts, and ulcers may be present. Chronic infections may produce interdigital fibrosis and pyogranulomas. Antibiotic and steroid therapy may cause remission, but recurrence is common. The underlying cause should be identified and treated. Diagnostics include hematologic and serum biochemistry profiles, urinalysis, skin scraping, culture and sensitivity testing, cytologic studies, and biopsy. Consider referring animals that do not respond to conservative treatment to a dermatologist.

TREATMENT

Conservative surgical treatment involves incision, exploration, and débridement of all fistulous tracts. Lesions should be medicated with antibacterial agents (e.g., chlorhexidine, povidone-iodine, and nitrofurazone) and bandaged for 24 to 48 hours. Subsequently, they should be soaked with an antibacterial solution for 15 to 20 minutes twice daily. Oral antibiotics based on sensitivity testing are administered for 6 to 8 weeks. Lesions that fail to respond to this treatment may require fusion podoplasty (see p. 258).

REDUNDANT SKIN FOLDS

Redundant skin is characteristic of some breeds and is exacerbated by obesity. Chronic skin overlap or apposition creates skin folds of varying depths. Commonly involved areas include the labia, face, vulva, tail head, and leg folds, with severity and frequency varying with breed and conformation. Pyoderma occurs in the skin fold recesses (intertriginous dermatitis) because they provide a poorly ventilated, dark, warm, moist environment that permits the accumulation of surface debris, such as sebum, saliva, tears, urine, or feces. Sebum contains fatty acids that are both bacteriostatic and fungistatic; however, excessive accumulation of sebaceous material allows surface bacteria within the skin fold to proliferate. Coagulase-positive *Staphylococcus* spp. are most commonly involved, but other organisms include streptococci, coliforms (*E. coli,* pseudomonads, *Proteus* spp., etc.), and yeasts, such as *Malassezia* and *Candida* spp. Friction at contact points, retention of secretions, and bacterial proliferation cause skin maceration and superficial ulceration. In addition to impairing the cutaneous barrier, immune function may be impaired. Affected areas become painful and foul smelling, causing the animal to further traumatize the area by scooting, rubbing, licking, or scratching. The severity of clinical signs is affected by coexisting skin disease.

Skin fold resection is the most effective treatment for skin fold pyoderma (see later discussion). First, medical therapy should reduce infection, inflammation, and secretions or exudates. Medical therapy consists of clipping hair from the folds and surrounding area, applying topical antibacterial solutions and medicated soaps, using antiseborrheic shampoos and astringents, and giving appropriate systemic antimicrobials. Culture and sensitivity testing is necessary to select appropriate antimicrobials. Corticosteroids sometimes are necessary to reduce pruritus-induced self-trauma. Weight reduction is beneficial for obese animals. Continuous medical therapy is palliative, not curative. The surgical site must be kept clean, dry, and protected from trauma. Continued antimicrobial therapy may be necessary. General complications of skin fold resection and reconstruction are self-trauma, infection, dehiscence, and pyoderma recurrence.

LIP FOLDS

Breeds with excessive mandibular labial tissue (large pendulous lips) (e.g., spaniels, Saint Bernards, Newfoundlands, Labrador retrievers, golden retrievers, and Irish setters) most commonly have lip fold dermatitis. It may also occur after partial maxillectomy or mandibulectomy. The fold usually

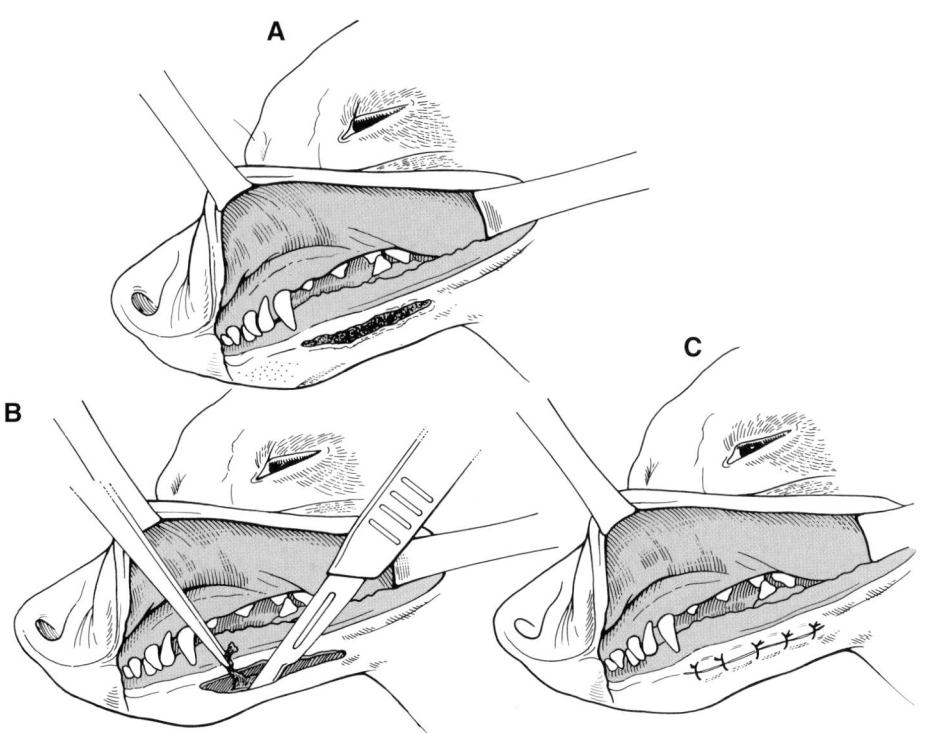

FIG. 15-46
A, Cheiloplasty for lip fold dermatitis. **B,** Make an elliptic incision and excise the infected skin. **C,** Appose healthy skin edges with approximating sutures.

occurs behind the mandibular canine tooth, where food and saliva accumulate. Affected dogs rub and paw the face, and the skin becomes inflamed and thickened. Halitosis and pruritus are the most common presenting complaints.

Lip Fold Resection (Cheiloplasty)

Position the anesthetized animal in dorsal recumbency to allow access to both lips. Clip and aseptically prepare the mandibular area (Fig. 15-46, A). Make an elliptical incision around the affected area, paralleling the horizontal ramus of the mandible (Fig. 15-46, B). The incision may involve the mucocutaneous junction. Elevate and remove the outlined skin segment, preserving underlying muscles. Control hemorrhage with ligation, electrocoagulation, and pressure. Assess the adequacy of resection and excise additional skin if necessary. Lavage the site and appose subcutaneous and subcuticular tissue with continuous or interrupted approximating monofilament absorbable sutures (e.g., 3-0 or 4-0 polydioxanone, poliglecaprone 25, glycomer 631, or polyglyconate). Place interrupted appositional sutures in the skin (e.g., 3-0 or 4-0 polypropylene or nylon) (Fig. 15-46, C). Use an Elizabethan collar or bucket to prevent self-inflicted trauma to the surgical site. Keep the area clean and dry, removing food and saliva as necessary.

Antidrool Cheiloplasty

Dogs whose face and neck are constantly wetted by saliva are candidates for this procedure. Antidrool cheiloplasty (cheilopexy) reduces the loss of food and saliva from the lateral vestibules of the oral cavity when there is excessive eversion or denervation of the lower lip. This is accomplished by suspending the lower lip from the inside of the upper cheek. Oral function usually is normal after surgery, but inflammation and infection occasionally occur at the surgical site. Permanent flap adhesion and cheek scars are expected.

Position the anesthetized patient in lateral recumbency. Clip the lateral face, lavage the oral cavity, and aseptically prepare the skin for surgery. Grasp the lower lip 2 to 3 cm rostral to the commissure, and elevate it dorsally until the lip is taut when the dog's mouth is completely opened (Fig. 15-47, A). The site of maximum tautness usually is near the level of the caudal root of the upper fourth premolar. Beginning near an imaginary line between the medial canthus of the eye and the commissure, make a 2.5 to 3 cm, horizontal, full-thickness incision through the maxillary skin at the site of tautness (Fig. 15-47, B). Adjust the length of the incision to match the breed size. Control hemorrhage with ligation or electrocoagulation. The dorsal labial vein lies just dorsal to the proposed incision site. Use scissors to remove a 2-mm strip of mucosa adjacent to the mucocutaneous junction of the lower lip, beginning 2 cm rostral to the commissure and extending 2.5 cm (Fig. 15-47, C). Create 0.5- to 0.75-cm mucosal and skin flaps by undermining on each side of the incision (Fig. 15-47, D). Place stay sutures at the rostral and caudal aspects of the flaps. Evert the flaps through the cheek incision with the stay sutures (Fig. 15-47, E). Secure and bury the flap edges in the cheek skin incision with three to four preplaced vertical mattress sutures (e.g., 2-0 or 3-0 polypropylene or nylon) (Fig. 15-47, F and G). Place additional approximating skin sutures if necessary to achieve good skin apposition. Reposition the patient and

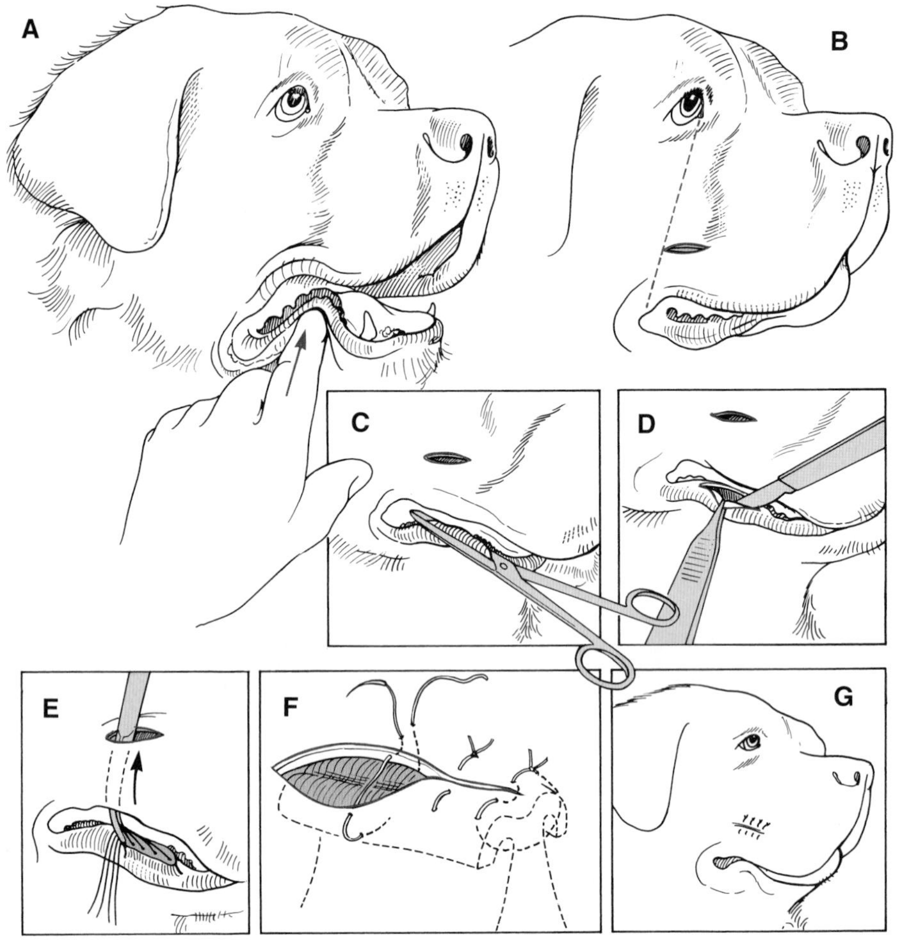

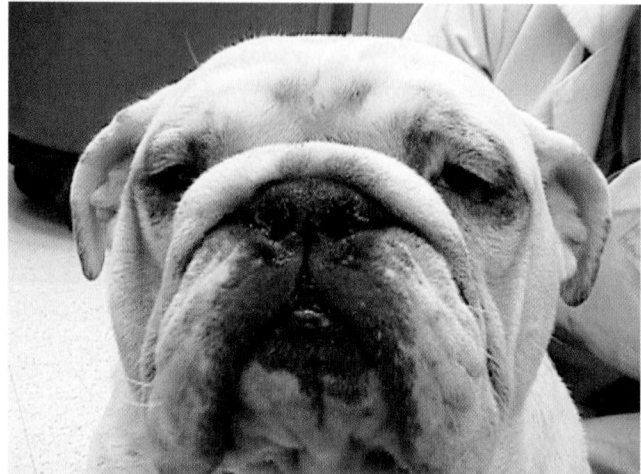

FIG. 15-47
A, For cheiloplasty in dogs that drool excessively, elevate the everted lip dorsally until it is taut when the dog's mouth is opened maximally. **B,** Make a 2.5- to 3-cm horizontal, full-thickness incision through the maxillary skin at the site of tautness near the upper fourth premolar. **C,** Remove a 2-mm-wide strip of mucosa 2.5 cm long from the mucocutaneous junction of the lower lip beginning 2 cm rostral to the commissure. **D,** Create 0.5- to 0.75-cm flaps. **E,** Evert the flaps through the skin incision. **F** and **G,** Secure with vertical mattress sutures.

FIG. 15-48
This English bulldog has a severe facial fold with pyoderma; the nares have been resected.

repeat the procedure on the other side. Lavage the oral cavity with water after meals. Fit the dog with an Elizabethan collar or bucket to prevent self-inflicted trauma if necessary. Remove sutures at 21 days. Delay suture removal because constant lip movement may interfere with healing. Do not permit retrieving or chew toys for 2 months after surgery.

NASAL FOLDS

Brachycephalic breeds (i.e., English bulldogs, French bulldogs, Pekingese, Boston terriers, pugs, and Persian cats) characteristically have facial or nasal skin folds across the bridge of the nose. Prominent folds cause pyoderma and a foul odor (Fig. 15-48). Hair rubbing on the cornea is associated with keratitis, ulceration, epiphora, pain, and blepharospasm. Facial folds remain moist and become stained secondary to epiphora. Fold resection and ophthalmic medications are necessary. Excision of too much skin may cause ectropion or promote dehiscence.

Nasal Skin Fold Resection

Position the patient in ventral recumbency. Protect the eyes with a petrolatum-based ophthalmic ointment. Clip and aseptically prepare the dorsum of the nose and lips. Estimate the amount of skin that must be resected to eliminate the skin folds without causing excess tension or ectropion. Make an elliptical incision around or through the skin folds in unmacerated tissue. Keep the caudal incision approximately 1 cm away from the medial canthus. Undermine and remove the outlined skin segment. Avoid traumatizing the nasolabialis muscle and facial vessels during dissection. Control hemorrhage with ligatures, electrocoagulation, and pressure. Lavage the area with sterile saline. Bury three or four interrupted sutures in the subcutaneous and subcuticular tissues to align and appose the

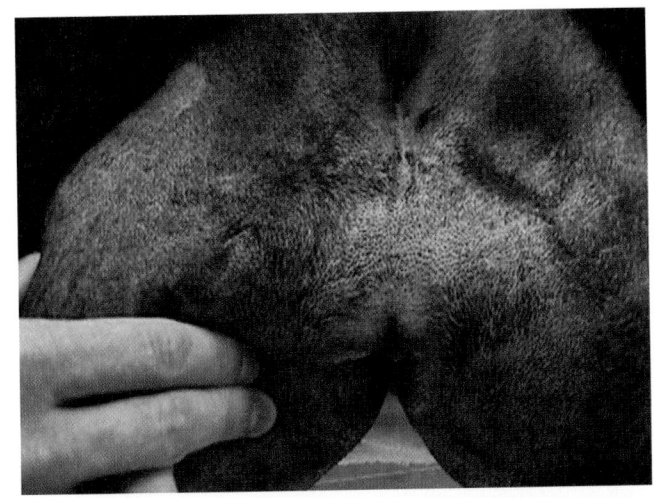

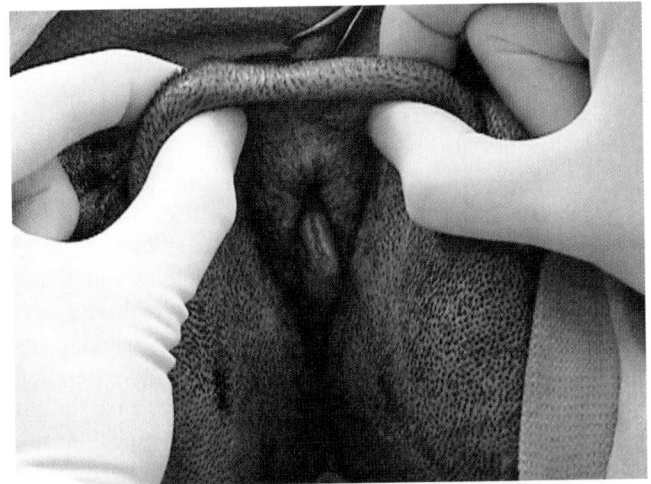

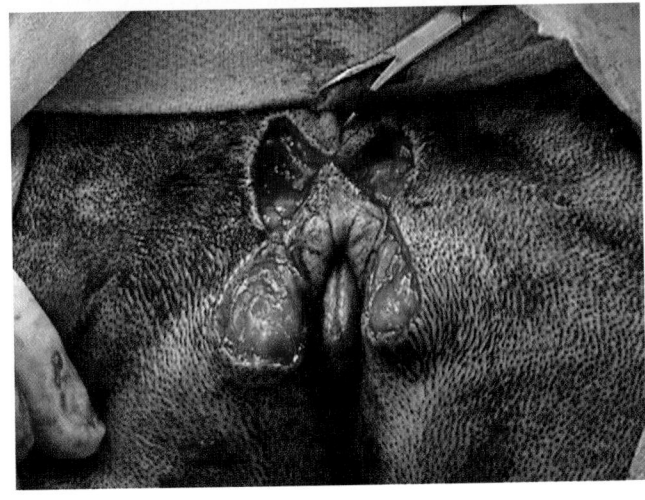

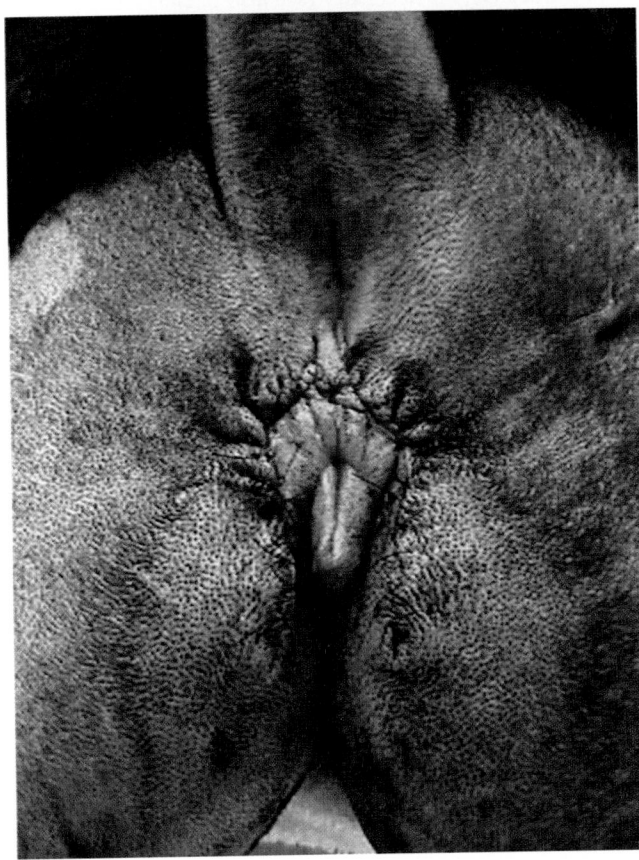

FIG. 15-49
A, The vulva is completely obscured by the adjacent skin fold. **B,** The skin is evaluated to determine the amount to be resected. **C,** Skin has been resected and tacked into place to determine if resection was adequate. **D,** Appearance of vulva following reconstruction.

skin edges and assess the adequacy of resection. Resect more skin if skin recesses remain. If necessary, undermine the skin edges to allow apposition without tension. Place additional interrupted, subcuticular sutures (e.g., 4-0 polydioxanone, poliglecaprone 25, glycomer 631, or polyglyconate) with buried knots. Use approximating skin sutures (e.g., 4-0 nylon or polypropylene), and cut the ends short to prevent further corneal irritation. Place an Elizabethan collar or bucket to prevent self-trauma. Keep the site free of exudates and ocular discharge. Continue to medicate the eyes.

VULVAR FOLDS

Vulvar skin folds occur in obese females and those with infantile, recessed vulvas (Fig. 15-49). Urine and vaginal secretions are trapped by the skin fold, resulting in superficial perivulvar dermatitis. Clinical signs include perineal pain, odor, vaginitis, urinary tract infection, urinary incontinence, and pollakiuria. Skin fold pyoderma should be resolved medically before surgery. Episioplasty is a vulvar reconstructive procedure that removes the skin fold (see p. 721 for a description of the technique). Excessive suture line tension may cause dehiscence. Other complications include inflammation, swelling, infection, and recurrent perivulvar dermatitis. Perivulvar dermatitis recurs if the amount of skin excised is inadequate. Urinary incontinence may persist if associated with other abnormalities. Prognosis is good following surgery because most clinical signs are expected to improve.

TAIL FOLDS

Redundant skin often overlaps deformed terminal caudal vertebrae ("screwtails," "corkscrew" tails, ingrown tails). Tail fold pyoderma occurs most commonly in brachycephalic breeds, but has also been reported in Schipperke dogs and Manx cats. The skin fold may be several inches deep with severe pyoderma. The depth of the folds varies with the animal's size, amount of fat, abundance of skin, and degree of vertebral deviation. Fecal contamination, licking, and scooting exacerbate the condition. Signs include perineal pruritus, pain, odor, ulcers, and fistulous tracts. Differential diagnoses should include perianal fistula, anal sacculitis, perianal tumors, trauma, and foreign bodies. Draining tracts should be probed or a fistulogram performed to determine their site of origin. To remove all skin recesses at the tail head, complete caudectomy is necessary (see also p. 248).

Tail Fold Resection

Give perioperative antibiotics based on skin fold culture and sensitivity results. Scrub the skin folds separately from the remainder of the surgical field. Resect the tail and skin folds en bloc, taking care during dissection to avoid penetrating the skin folds or traumatizing the rectum. Manipulate the tail with bone holding forceps or towel clamps. Ankylosis or severe ventral deviation may make the vertebrae immobile. Transect the tail cranial to the deviated vertebrae with Gigli wire or a bone cutter if the intervertebral space cannot be located. Smooth sharp bone edges with rongeurs or a bone rasp. Lavage thoroughly and insert Penrose or closed suction drains before apposing the subcutaneous tissues with absorbable sutures (e.g., 3-0 or 4-0 polydioxanone, poliglecaprone 25, glycomer 631, or polyglyconate). Drains should exit ventral to the incision and lateral to the anus. Close the skin with nonabsorbable sutures (e.g., 3-0 or 4-0 nylon, polybutester, or polypropylene). Keep the area clean and free of exudate and fecal contamination by applying warm, moist compresses two or three times daily for 15 to 20 minutes. Remove drains in 3 to 5 days.

Alternatively, in animals whose breed standards relish the tail fold, the deviating terminal caudal vertebrae can be removed and the skin fold salvaged. The severity of the pyoderma is decreased following vertebrectomy.

Suggested Reading

Crawford JT, Adams WM: Influence of vestibulovaginal stenosis, pelvic bladder, and recessed vulva on response to treatment for clinical signs of lower urinary tract disease in dogs: 38 cases (1990-1999), *J Am Vet Med Assoc* 221:995, 2002.
This study uses ratios to evaluate and categorize vestibulovaginal stenosis. Those with severe stenosis and recessed vulva did not respond well to vulvoplasty.
Hammel SP, Bjorling DE: Results of vulvoplasty for treatment of recessed vulva in dogs, *J Am Anim Hosp Assoc* 38:79, 2002.
Data from 34 affected dogs are reported; improvement was seen in 82% with greatly reduced incidences of urinary tract infections, vaginitis, and external irritations.
Lightner BA, McLoughlin MA, Chew DJ et al: Episioplasty for the treatment of perivulvar dermatitis or recurrent urinary tract infections in dogs with excessive perivulvar skin folds: 31 cases (1983-2000), *J Am Vet Med Assoc* 219:1577, 2001.
Complete resolution of vulvar dermatitis and urinary tract infections was seen following surgery in all but one case. Relapse occurred in one following weight gain.

SURGERY OF THE TAIL

CAUDECTOMY

Caudectomy, or amputation of a portion of the tail, which is performed to comply with breed standards or tradition, is ethically and morally controversial. *Therapeutic caudectomy* is indicated for traumatic lesions, infection, neoplasia, and possibly perianal fistula. The tail should be amputated with 2 to 3 cm of normal tissue margins when resecting tumors or traumatic lesions. Amputation should be performed near the anus if the end of the tail chronically bleeds because of repeated abrasion or chewing. Amputation near the base is recommended for avulsed tails and if necessary for tail fold pyoderma and perianal fistula.

CAUDECTOMY IN PUPPIES

Cosmetic caudectomy (i.e., tail docking) in puppies is performed between 3 and 5 days of age. Traditionally, anesthesia has not been used; however, better understanding of pain and its management dictates the use of local anesthesia, with or without sedation. A ring block with lidocaine (less than the toxic dose of 10 mg/kg) at the tail base is commonly performed. Another protocol for sedation and analgesia begins with intranasal diazepam (0.1 mg/100 g) followed 3 minutes later by intranasal ketamine hydrochloride (1 mg/100 g) and then 5 minutes later by a local anesthetic ring block proximal to the proposed incision. If a caudectomy is not performed during the first week of life, it should be delayed until the puppy is 8 to 12 weeks old and performed using general anesthesia. The desired tail length should be determined by referring to breed standards and consulting with the owner (Table 15-8). Healing after a caudectomy in puppies usually is uncomplicated. Puppies rarely irritate the surgical site, but bitches may lick sutures out within a few days.

Have an assistant restrain the puppy. Clip and aseptically prepare the proposed site of resection. Retract the tail's skin toward the tail head, immobilize the tail between the thumb and index finger, and apply pressure to help control hemorrhage (Fig. 15-50, A). Palpate the desired transection site. Transect the tail between adjacent caudal vertebrae with Mayo scissors, nail trimmers, scalpel blade, or a tail docker/ cutter (Tail Docker/Cutter, electrosurgery, or laser). You may use scissors to assist with skin retraction. Place the ventral blade at the desired transection site. Position the dorsal blade more distally at an oblique angle. Rotate the blades into a perpendicular position while maintaining firm contact

TABLE 15-8

Tail Docking Guidelines

BREED	LENGTH*
Sporting Breeds	
Brittany spaniel	Leave 1 inch
Clumber spaniel	Leave ¼ to ⅓ of length
Cocker spaniel	Leave ⅓ of length (approximately ¾ inch)
English cocker spaniel	Leave ⅓ of length
English springer spaniel	Leave ⅓ of length
Field spaniel	Leave ⅓ of length
German shorthaired pointer	Leave ⅖ of length
German wirehaired pointer	Leave ⅖ of length
Sussex spaniel	Leave ⅓ of length
Vizsla	Leave ⅔ of length
Weimaraner	Leave ⅗ of length (approximately 1½ inches)
Welsh springer spaniel	Leave ⅓ to ½ of length
Wirehaired pointing griffon	Leave ⅓ of length
Working Breeds	
Bouvier des Flanders	Leave ½ to ¾ inch
Boxer	Leave ½ to ¾ inch (two vertebrae)
Doberman pinscher	Leave ¾ inch (two vertebrae)
Giant schnauzer	Leave 1¼ inch (three vertebrae)
Old English sheepdog	Leave one vertebra (close to body)
Rottweiler	Leave one vertebra (close to body)
Standard schnauzer	Leave 1 inch (two vertebrae)
Welsh corgi (Pembroke)	Leave one vertebra (close to body)
Terrier Breeds	
Airedale terrier	Leave ⅔ to ¾ of length†
Australian terrier	Leave ⅖ of length
Fox terrier	Leave ⅔ to ¾ of length†
Irish terrier	Leave ¾ of length
Kerry blue terrier	Leave ½ to ⅔ of length
Lakeland terrier	Leave ⅔ to ¾ of length
Miniature schnauzer	Leave ¾ inch
Norwich terrier	Leave ¼ to ⅓ of length
Sealyham terrier	Leave ⅔ to ½ of length
Soft-coated Wheaten terrier	Leave ½ to ¾ of length
Welsh terrier	Leave ⅔ to ¾ of length†
Toy Breeds	
Affenpinscher	Leave ⅓ inch (close to body)
Brussels griffon	Leave ¼ to ⅓ of length (approximately ⅓ inch)
English toy spaniel	Leave ⅓ of length (approximately 1½ inches)
Miniature pinscher	Leave ½ inch (two vertebrae)
Silky terrier	Leave ⅔ of length (approximately ½ inch)
Toy poodle	Leave ½ to ⅔ of length (approximately 1 inch)
Yorkshire terrier	Leave ⅓ of length (approximately ½ inch)
Nonsporting Breeds	
Miniature poodle	Leave ½ to ⅔ of length (approximately 1⅛ inches)
Schipperke	Close to body
Miscellaneous Breeds	
Standard poodle	Leave ½ to ⅔ of length (approximately 1½ inches)
Cavalier King Charles spaniel (optional)	Leave ⅔ of length with white tip
Spinoni Italiani	Leave ⅗ of length

*When docking is performed at less than 1 week of age.
†The tip of the docked tail should be approximately level with the top of the skull when the puppy is in show position.

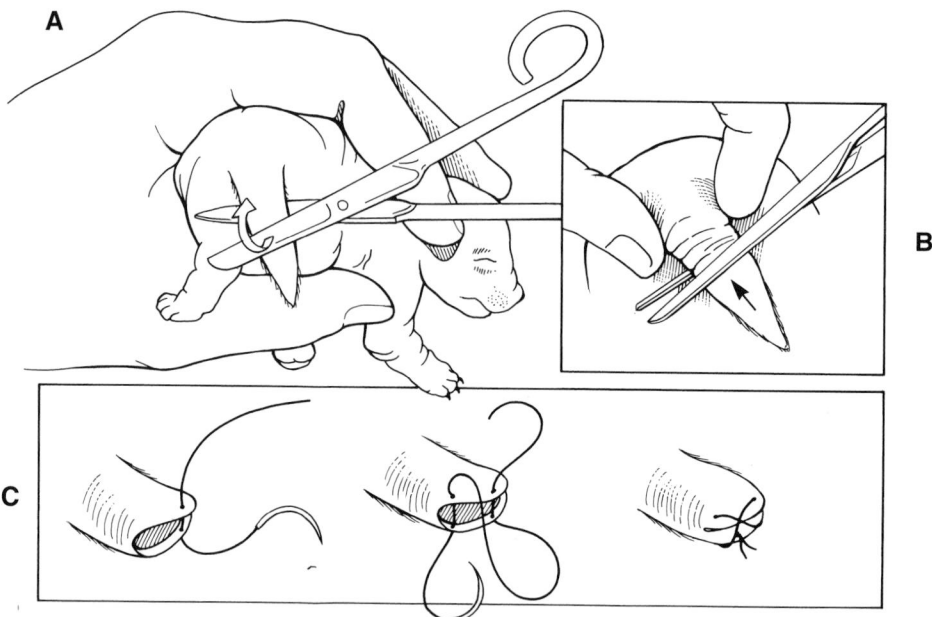

FIG. 15-50
Caudectomy in a puppy. **A,** Retract the tail's skin toward the tail head and immobilize the tail between the thumb and index finger. **B,** Rotate the scissors toward the tail head to push the skin toward the body. Transect the tail through the desired intervertebral space. **C,** Appose the skin edges with approximating sutures.

with the skin to push the skin cranially; maintaining the scissors in this position, transect through an intervertebral space (Fig. 15-50, B). Control hemorrhage with pressure or electrosurgery. Extend the retracted skin over the remaining tail, assess the tail length, and resect more if necessary. Appose skin edges with two or three approximating sutures (e.g., 4-0 nylon or polypropylene) or absorbable tissue adhesive (Fig. 15-50, C).

CAUDECTOMY IN ADULTS

A caudectomy in dogs older than 1 week requires general or epidural anesthesia. The surgical site should be observed for swelling, draining, inflammation, and pain. Healing after caudectomy is uncomplicated if excess skin tension and self-trauma are prevented. The site should be protected with a bandage or restraining device if necessary. Complications include infection, dehiscence, scarring, fistula recurrence, and anal sphincter or rectal trauma. Incisions that dehisce after partial amputation may heal by secondary intention, which usually leaves a hairless scar. Reamputation may be necessary to relieve irritation and improve cosmesis.

Partial Caudectomy

Wrap the distal tail with gauze or insert it into an examination glove and secure the covering with tape. Clip a generous area near the amputation site and aseptically prepare it for surgery. Place the patient in a perineal position or lateral recumbency. Position a tourniquet proximal to the transection site. Retract the skin toward the tail head. Make a double V incision in the skin distal to the desired intervertebral tran-

section site. Orient the V to create dorsal and ventral skin flaps that are longer than the desired tail length (Fig. 15-51, A). Identify and ligate the medial and lateral caudal arteries and veins slightly cranial to the transection site (Fig. 15-51, B). Incise soft tissue slightly distal to the desired intervertebral space and disarticulate the distal tail with a scalpel blade. If bleeding occurs, place a circumferential ligature around the distal end of the remaining tail or re-ligate the caudal vessels (Fig. 15-51, C). Appose subcutaneous tissue and muscle over the exposed vertebrae with interrupted approximating sutures (e.g., 3-0 polydioxanone, poliglecaprone 25, glycomer 631, or polyglyconate). Position the dorsal skin flap over the caudal vertebrae (Fig. 15-51, D). Trim the ventral skin flap as needed to allow skin apposition without tension. Appose skin edges with approximating sutures (e.g., 3-0 or 4-0 nylon or polypropylene with a reverse cutting needle) (Fig. 15-51, D). Protect the surgical site with a bandage or by placing an Elizabethan collar or bucket over the animal's head.

Complete Caudectomy

Anesthetize the patient; clip and aseptically prepare the entire perineum and tail head area. Position the animal in ventral recumbency. Make an elliptic incision around the tail base (Fig. 15-52, A). Incise subcutaneous tissues to expose the muscles. Separate the attachments of the levator ani, rectococcygeus, and coccygeus muscles to the caudal vertebrae (Fig. 15-52, B). Ligate the medial and lateral caudal arteries and veins before or after transection. Transect the tail by disarticulation with a scalpel blade at the second or

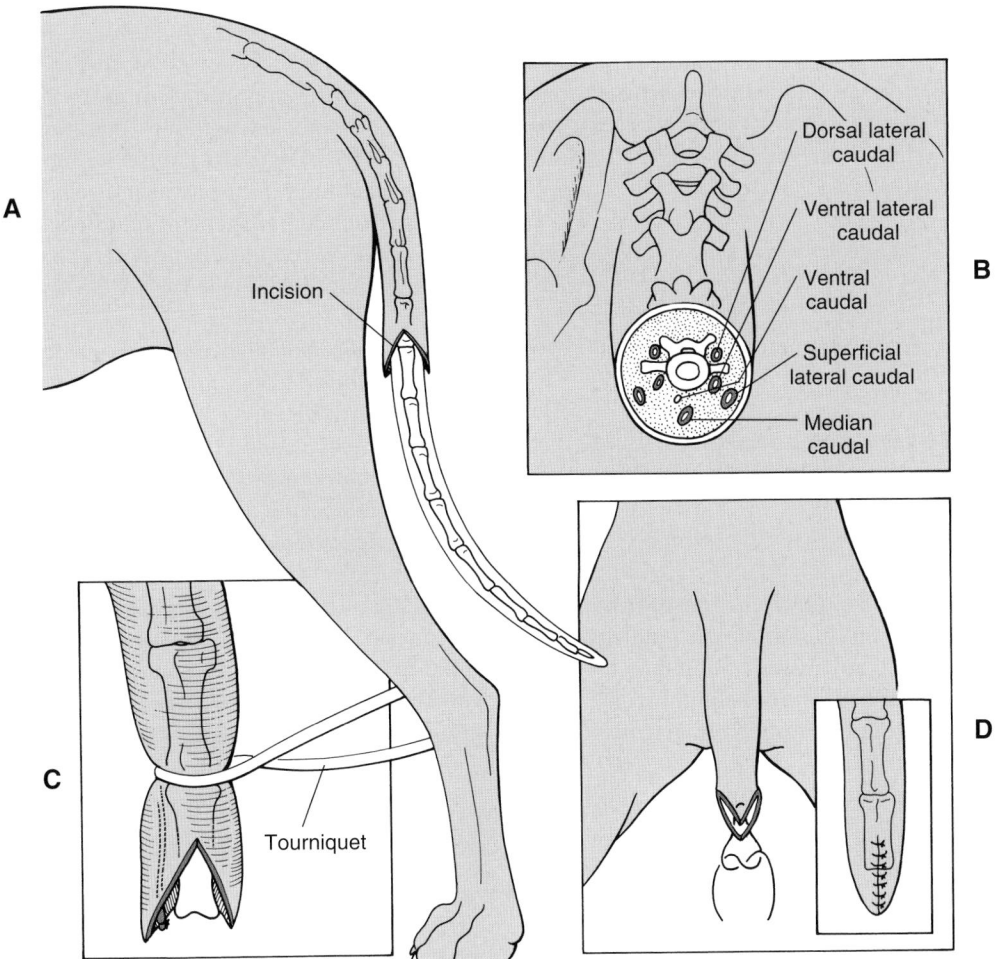

FIG. 15-51
Partial caudectomy in an adult. **A,** Retract the tail's skin toward the tail head and make a double V incision in the skin distal to the desired transection site. **B,** Ligate the medial and lateral caudal arteries and veins. **C,** Transect the soft tissue distal to the desired intervertebral space. Transect the tail through the desired intervertebral space. A proximally placed tourniquet assists hemostasis. **D,** Appose soft tissue and skin with approximating sutures.

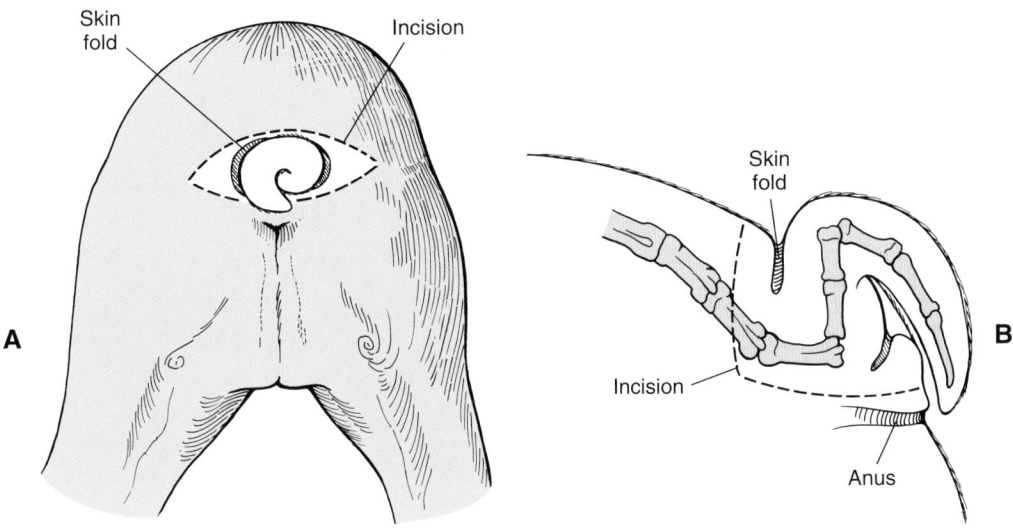

FIG. 15-52
Complete caudectomy with tail fold pyoderma requires **(A)** an elliptic incision around diseased skin and **(B)** deep dissection to locate the caudal vertebrae rostral to the vertebral deviation.

third caudal vertebra. Lavage the site after hemostasis is achieved. Appose the levator ani muscles and subcutaneous tissue with simple interrupted or continuous suture patterns (e.g., 3-0 or 4-0 polydioxanone, poliglecaprone 25, glycomer 631, or polyglyconate). Excise redundant skin if necessary and appose skin edges with approximating, non-absorbable sutures (e.g., 3-0 or 4-0 nylon, polybutester, or polypropylene). As an alternative, the tail fold may be preserved; however, skin fold pyoderma may persist.

SURGERY OF THE DIGITS AND FOOTPADS

BIOPSY

Diagnosis of dermatologic conditions of the claw may require biopsy if history, physical examination, cytology, and cultures have not yielded an answer. Submission of an avulsed or sloughed claw is usually not helpful because claw matrix is absent. Punch biopsies are often not diagnostic and owners are often reluctant to allow distal phalanx (P3) amputation to achieve a definitive diagnosis. The described

technique yields appropriate samples of the claw epithelium to allow diagnosis without onychectomy (Mueller and Olivry, 1999). Dewclaws should be biopsied when affected and present to prevent postoperative lameness.

After induction of general anesthetic, the paws designated for biopsies are clipped, but not scrubbed to prevent removing important pathologic surface clues.

Apply a tourniquet to decrease hemorrhage. Position an 8-mm diameter biopsy punch parallel to the long axis of the claw 1-2 mm distal to the claw fold. Rotate the punch slowly in one direction deep into the tissue (Fig. 15-53). Initially, cut through the horn of the claw, then through the bone of the distal phalanx and laterally through normal skin on the lateral aspect of the claw fold. Transect the base of the biopsy with a scalpel blade or iris scissors. Control hemorrhage with pressure. Mark the haired surface for identification and place the specimen in formalin. Place interrupted sutures (3-0 to 4-0 monofilament nonabsorbable) to appose the skin and cover the exposed bone. Give analgesics postoperatively as the animal will experience pain.

Claws may not grow back normally after the biopsy.

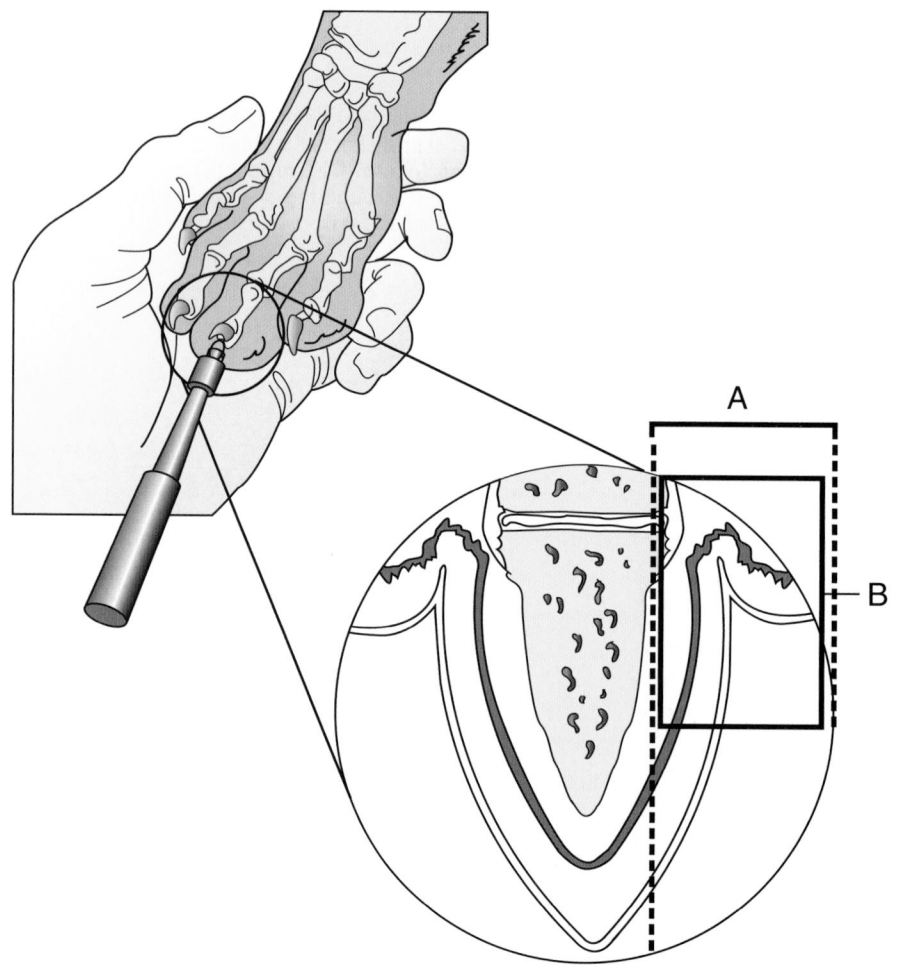

FIG. 15-53
A, Position an 8-mm-diameter biopsy punch parallel to the long axis of the claw 1 to 2 mm distal to the claw fold. Rotate the punch slowly in one direction deep into the tissue initially through the horn of the claw, then through the bone of the distal phalanx and laterally through normal skin on the lateral aspect of the claw fold. **B,** *Inset,* claw segment biopsied.

ONYCHECTOMY

Onychectomy (i.e., declawing) is removal of the third digital phalanx (P3) (Fig. 15-54, *A*). *Elective onychectomy* usually is performed between 3 and 12 months of age to prevent cats from scratching furniture or people. Usually only the forelimb claws are removed. Although it is recommended that declawed cats be kept indoors because the procedure interferes with a cat's ability to protect itself, those with hindlimb claws can climb to escape some dangers. Alternatives to elective onychectomy are to glue a vinyl cap to each claw every 6 to 8 weeks (SoftPaws) or perform deep digital flexor tenectomy (see p. 254). Vinyl caps blunt the claws to render them less damaging. Onychectomy or more extensive digit amputation may be required to remove infected nail beds and neoplasms. The most common nail bed tumors are squamous cell carcinomas, melanomas, soft tissue sarcomas, osteosarcomas, and mast cell tumors. Complete excision may require that adjacent phalanges be removed with the affected claw. Onychomycosis, usually caused by *Trichophyton mentagrophytes,* produces dry, cracked, brittle, and deformed nails with inflamed alopecic nail beds. Follicular infections with *Demodex* spp. and staphylococci produce similar lesions.

Onychectomy is performed with the patient under general anesthetic with multimodal analgesia (Box 15-14). Perioperative analgesia (butorphanol, oxymorphone, meloxicam) is recommended for a minimum of 24 to 48 hours after surgery. Additional perioperative analgesia may be provided by blocking regional nerves with 0.5% bupivacaine (Ringwood and Smith, 2000). Sensory innervation to the feline forepaw is provided by the dorsal and palmar branches of the radial, median, and ulnar nerves. These branches are blocked at four sites using 0.1 to 0.2 ml of 0.5% bupivacaine at each site (not to exceed a total dose of 5 mg/kg), which provides 4 to 6 hours of analgesia.

Perform the nerve blocks after induction of anesthesia and preparation of the paw for onychectomy. Fully extend the

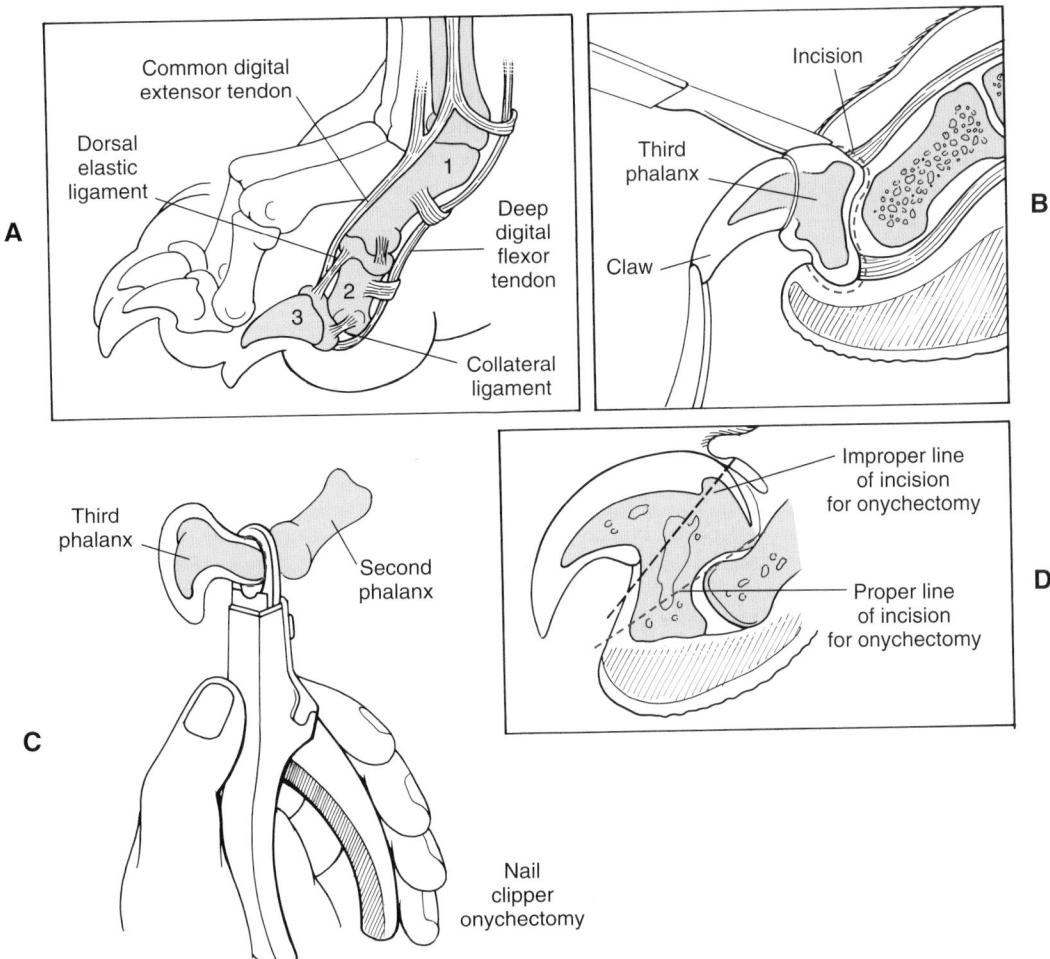

FIG. 15-54
A, Distal phalangeal anatomy for onychectomy. **B,** Dissection onychectomy disarticulates the third phalanx by transecting tendons, ligaments, and other soft tissue attachments.
C, Nail clipper onychectomy should remove the entire ungual crest, but often leaves a portion of the ventral flexor process of P3. **D,** Proper and improper lines of transection.

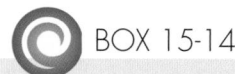

BOX 15-14

Multimodal Therapy for Onychectomy

Premed: Opioid*

Butorphanol; 0.2–0.4 mg/kg, SC, IM, repeat q 4–6 hr; if switch to oral tablets, use 1 mg/kg PO, or
Buprenorphine; 7–14 mcg/kg, SC, IM, TM, repeat q 6 hr, or
Hydromorphone; 0.05 to 0.1 mg/kg, SC, IM, repeat q 4 hr, or
Fentanyl patch; 4 mcg/kg/hr; place patch 6–12 hr before surgery; analgesia lasts 72–96 hr.

Plus an Anticholinergic

Glycopyrrolate; 0.011 mg/kg SC, IM, or
Atropine; 0.04 mg/kg SC, IM

+/-Tranquilizer

Acepromazine 0.05 mg/kg SC, IM

Induction: Give to effect
Propofol; 4–6 mg/kg, IV, or
Thiopental; 8–10 mg/kg, IV, or
Diazepam/ketamine (diazepam 0.27 mg/kg IV plus ketamine 5.5 mg/kg IV)
Maintenance: Isoflurane or sevoflurane in oxygen

Adjuncts: Local anesthetic block (see also Chapter 13, p. 137)
NSAID (e.g., meloxicam: see Chapter 13, p. 142)

*With all opiates, watch for breakthrough pain or side effects and adjust dose accordingly. Do not mix agonists.

carpus and palpate the superficial digital flexor tendon along the palmar aspect of the paw. Block the median nerve with 0.15 ml of bupivacaine injected just medial to the superficial digital flexor tendon at a point approximately one third the distance between the carpal pad and the first digital pad (Fig. 15-55, A). Block the palmar branches of the ulnar nerve at about the same level along the lateral aspect of the superficial digital flexor tendon using 0.15 ml bupivacaine (see Fig. 15-55, A). Block dorsal digital nerves II through V by inserting the needle from lateral to medial just distal to the carpus. Inject 0.2 ml of bupivacaine as the needle is withdrawn, being careful to block dorsal digital nerve V, which lies lateral to metacarpal V (Fig. 15-55, B). Inject 0.1 ml of bupivacaine to block dorsal digital nerve I. Locate this nerve by inserting the needle from distal to proximal to the point of articulation between metacarpals I and II.

Dissection Onychectomy

In cats, either a scalpel or a guillotine type nail clipper, electrosurgery, or CO_2 laser may be used to remove the third phalanx. There is little scientific documentation of the advantages or disadvantages of laser techniques. The dissection technique is used for canine onychectomy. Clipping hair from the paw and around the toes is advised in dogs and long-haired cats. Although most germinal cells are located in the ungual crest, the entire process must be removed to prevent claw regrowth.

FIG. 15-55
Sites for nerve blocks of sensory innervation to the feline forepaw. **A,** Extend the carpus and palpate the superficial digital flexor tendon along the palmar aspect of the paw. Block the median nerve with 0.15 ml of bupivacaine just medial to the superficial digital flexor tendon. Similarly block the palmar branches of the ulnar nerve along the lateral superficial digital flexor tendon. **B,** Block dorsal digital nerves II–V by inserting the needle from lateral to medial just distal to the carpus. Inject 0.2 ml of bupivacaine as the needle is withdrawn. Block dorsal digital nerve I at the articulation between metacarpal I and II with 0.1 ml of bupivacaine.

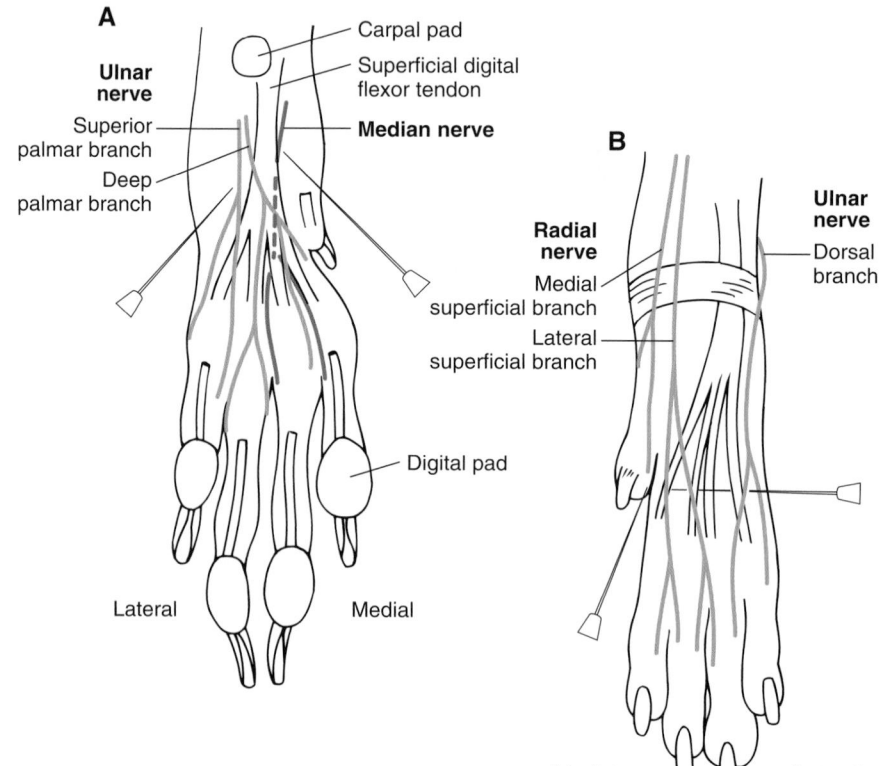

Aseptically scrub the paw, digits, and nails for surgery. Block the regional nerves to each front paw. Position the animal in lateral recumbency and apply a tourniquet below the elbow to minimize blood loss and improve visualization. In cats, tourniquet application above the elbow may damage the radial, median, or ulnar nerves because feline arm muscles lack protective bulk. As an alternative, have an assistant compress the brachial artery with a thumb or index finger against the humeral shaft by applying pressure just cranial to the triceps muscle on the medial aspect of the brachium. Drape the feet. Extend the claw by grasping the tip with a towel clamp or grasping forceps or by pushing up on the digital pad. Circumferentially incise the hairless, cuticle-like skin away from the claw near the articulation between the second and third phalanges (see Fig. 15-54, B). Transect the common digital extensor tendon and dorsal ligaments with a No. 11 or No. 12 scalpel blade. Follow the contour of the proximal end of P3 to transect the deep digital flexor tendon and dissect the phalanx from the digital pad and other soft tissue attachments (i.e., joint capsule, collateral ligaments, and other tendons). Avoid cutting the digital pad. Remove all 10 claws from the front paws for elective onychectomy. Appose skin edges with a bandage, single interrupted cruciate sutures, or cyanoacrylate absorbable tissue adhesive (e.g., Tissuemend II Adhesive). Do not place sutures through the digital pads. Apply tissue adhesives over the apposed surface of the skin and not between the cut edges.

Alternatively, some do not appose the tissue following onychectomy, especially in kittens.

Apply a bandage from the paw to the distal antebrachium (see p. 189) and remove the tourniquet.

Nail Clipper Onychectomy

Prepare the paws for surgery as described in the section on Dissection Onychectomy. Trim the claws to facilitate positioning the nail trimmer in the interphalangeal space. Position a sharp, guillotine type of nail clipper (Resco nail shears) around the claw (see Fig. 15-54, C). Extend the claw by grasping the tip with a towel clamp or grasping forceps. Position the blade dorsally at the joint space and transect the extensor tendon or tendons. Rotate the blade ventrally with continuous contact with the skin. Lift the claw dorsally to close the joint space and deviate the flexor process ventrally. After ensuring that the digital pad is proximal to the line of transection and the instrument is in the joint space, close the instrument to amputate the phalanx. Inspect the articular surfaces for complete excision of P3 (see Fig. 15-54, D). If a small portion of the palmar aspect of P3 remains, grasp it with a thumb forceps and carefully dissect it from the digital pad with a scalpel blade or sharp-sharp scissors. Some prefer to retain this portion of P3, especially in large cats, to maintain deep digital flexor function. Remove all 10 claws from the front paws for elective onychectomy. Appose skin edges with a single interrupted suture or absorbable tissue adhesive. Apply a bandage from the paw to the distal antebrachium (see p. 189) and remove the tourniquet.

Postoperative Care and Complications

Mild bleeding should be expected when the bandage is removed after 12 to 24 hours; if bleeding persists, the bandage should be reapplied for 2 to 3 days. Shredded paper, instead of litter, should be used for 2 weeks while the nail beds heal. Sutures usually are removed by the cat within a week. Convalescence is more rapid in young, growing cats than in older or obese cats. Owner satisfaction with this procedure is high. Complications (i.e., pain, hemorrhage, pad damage, lameness, swelling, infection, claw regrowth, second phalanx protrusion, and palmigrade stance) occur in 50% of patients. Cutting the digital pads prolongs postoperative pain and lameness. Early postoperative pain is more common after blade onychectomy than after the nail clipper procedure. Hemorrhage is most common in older animals and when wounds are not apposed. Late postoperative complications are more common when nail clippers are used. Nonabsorbable tissue adhesives may cause postoperative lameness (frequently nonweight bearing) and infections and may be extruded from the wounds as a foreign body. Improper tourniquet use may cause neurapraxia, tissue necrosis, and lameness. The radial nerve is most often affected, but signs usually resolve in 6 to 8 weeks. Tight bandages can result in ischemic necrosis of the paw (Fig. 15-56). Incomplete removal of the germinal cells in the dorsal aspect of the ungual crest allows claw regrowth. If only a small remnant of the flexor process remains, claw regrowth is not anticipated. Claw regrowth should be suspected if draining tracts develop. The regrown claw usually is deformed. Flexor tendon contracture pulling the paw and digits in fixed flexion has been reported (Cooper et al, 2005). Chronic pain evidenced by behavioral changes—such as decreased activity, decreased appetite, or increased aggression—is sometimes seen and may be caused by the wind-up pain phenomenon associated with unsatisfactory perioperative analgesia (see p. 132).

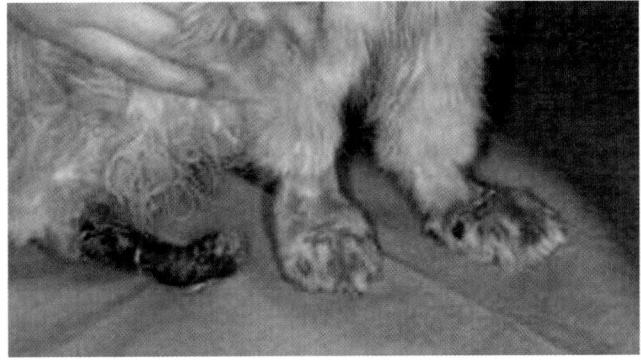

FIG. 15-56
This cat was not confined after onychectomy and its bandages got wet and were left on longer than desired. All four paws were injured, with the right rear leg requiring amputation.

DEEP DIGITAL FLEXOR TENECTOMY

The deep digital flexor tendon inserts on the flexor process of the third phalanx and is needed to flex the phalanx. Claws remain retracted after the deep digital flexor tendons have been severed, which limits the cat's ability to scratch; however, the nails become thick and blunt and must be trimmed regularly. Hemorrhage, infection, and lameness may occur postoperatively. Tenectomy of the superficial digital flexor (which inserts on the proximal aspect of P2) instead of the deep digital flexor results in an abnormal flat-footed stance. Problems may include persistent lameness and ability to scratch, interphalangeal joint immobility, fibrosis, pain, and claw ingrowth into the digital pads. Owners are frequently dissatisfied because of the cat's continued ability to scratch, the unaesthetic appearance of the thickened claws, the long-term lameness, and the necessity for nail clipping, which is difficult to accomplish. Cats may require an onychectomy to relieve clinical signs. For these reasons, this technique is not routinely recommended.

Anesthetize the cat and position it in dorsal or lateral recumbency. Clip and aseptically prepare the paws. Apply a tourniquet below the elbow to minimize hemorrhage. Make a 3- to 5-mm skin incision over the palmar surface of the second phalanx (P2), near the P2-P3 interphalangeal joint and digital pad (Fig. 15-57, A). The glistening white tendon of the deep digital flexor lies directly beneath the skin. Dissect under the tendon with mosquito hemostats or small scissors (Fig.

15-57, B). Excise a 5-mm segment of tendon with a scalpel blade, electrosurgery blade, or laser (Fig. 15-57, C). Appose the skin edges with an interrupted suture or absorbable tissue adhesive as for onychectomy. Repeat the procedure on each digit, and trim each claw.

Use torn paper rather than litter for 2 weeks. Limit activity and discourage jumping for 1 week.

DEWCLAW REMOVAL

The dewclaw is the first digit of the canine rear paws. The first and second phalanges of the digit are inconsistent. Dewclaws are absent in some dogs and double in others. Great Pyrenees and Briards must have double rear dewclaws to meet breed standards. In other breeds, loosely attached dewclaws are removed to prevent trauma during hunting or grooming (Box 15-15). Often only the rear dewclaws are removed. Dewclaws should be removed at 3 to 5 days of age, at the same time as the caudectomy. Hemorrhage is more excessive after 5 days of age, and anesthetics are necessary. Complications include hemorrhage, pain, infection, and dehiscence. Premature suture removal may cause scarring. Bandages applied too tightly may cause swelling or ischemic necrosis.

Dewclaw Removal in Puppies

Aseptically prepare the medial aspect of the paw. Have an assistant cup the puppy in his or her hands and immobilize the paw. Facilitate restraint and analgesia by giving a sedative

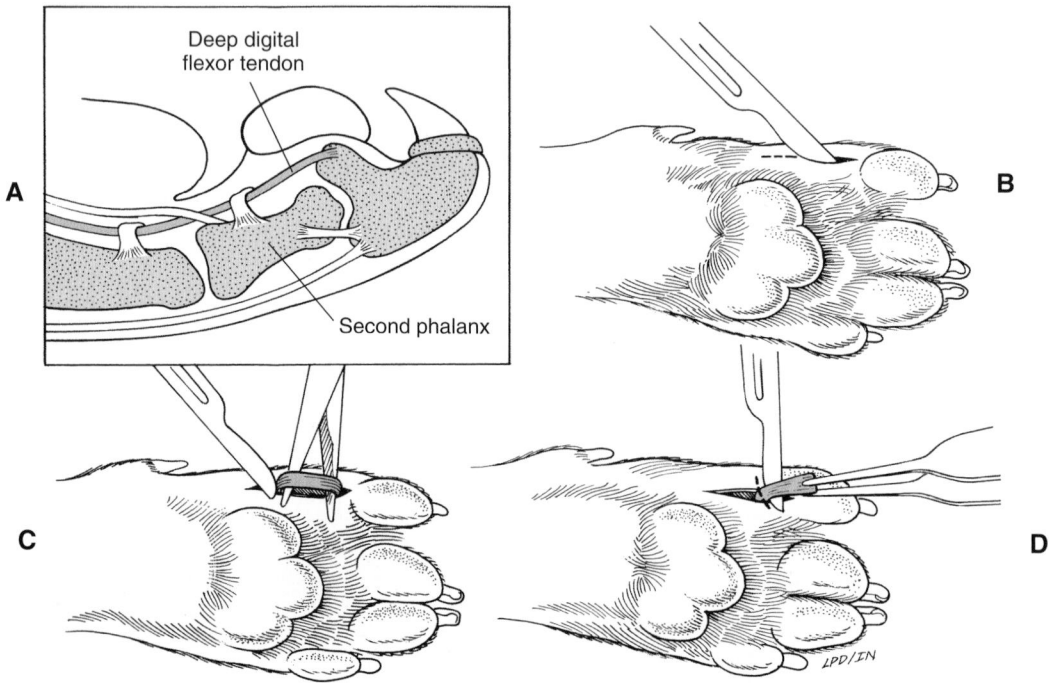

FIG. 15-57
Deep digital tenectomy. **A,** Make a 3- to 5-mm incision over the palmar surface of the second phalanx. **B** and **C,** Elevate and excise a 5-mm segment of deep digital flexor tendon. The inset shows the relationship of the deep digital flexor tendon to P1, P2, and P3.

or local anesthetic or both (see p. 137). Abduct the digit and transect the web of skin attaching the dewclaw to the paw with Mayo scissors, electrosurgery, or laser (Fig. 15-58, A). Disarticulate the metatarsal (carpal)-phalangeal joint or transect the bone near the metatarsal or metacarpal bone with a scalpel blade or Mayo scissors, electrosurgery, or laser. Control hemorrhage with pressure or electrocautery. Appose skin margins with a single approximating suture or absorbable tissue adhesive or allow healing by secondary intention.

Dewclaw Removal in Adults

If dewclaw removal is not performed within the first week of life, it should be delayed until after 3 months of age and performed using a general anesthetic. It is convenient to remove dewclaws at the time of neutering.

 BOX 15-15

Breeds Recommended for Dewclaw Removal

- Alaskan malamute
- Basset hound*
- Belgian malinois
- Belgian sheepdog
- Belgian tervuren
- Bernese mountain dog
- Boxer
- Cardigan Welsh corgi
- Chesapeake Bay retriever
- Dalmatian
- Dandie Dinmont terrier
- Kerry blue terrier
- Komondor
- Lakeland terrier
- Norwegian elkhound
- Papillon
- Puli*
- Rottweiler
- Shetland sheepdog
- Siberian husky
- Silky terrier
- Saint Bernard
- Vizsla
- Weimaraner

*Removal optional.

Position the patient in lateral recumbency. Clip and aseptically prepare the paws for surgery. Make an elliptic incision around the base of the digit where it articulates with the metatarsal or metacarpal bone (Fig. 15-58, B). Abduct the digit and dissect subcutaneous tissue to the metacarpophalangeal or metatarsophalangeal joint. If the first and second phalanges are firmly attached, free them with a No. 11 blade. Ligate the dorsal common and axial palmar digital arteries. Disarticulate the metacarpophalangeal or metatarsophalangeal joint with a scalpel blade. The results are less cosmetic when bone cutters are used to transect the first phalanx near the metacarpophalangeal or metatarsophalangeal joint. Appose subcutaneous tissue with 3-0 or 4-0 simple continuous or interrupted approximating sutures using absorbable suture material (i.e., polydioxanone, polyglyconate, poliglecaprone 25, glycomer 631, polyglactin 910, or chromic catgut). Appose the skin with interrupted approximating sutures (i.e., 3-0 or 4-0 nylon or polypropylene) (Fig. 15-58, C). Apply a soft, padded bandage to protect the surgical site for 3 to 5 days. Remove sutures at 7 to 10 days.

DIGIT AMPUTATION

Digit amputation is performed because of neoplasia, chronic bacterial or fungal infections, osteomyelitis, or severe trauma (Fig. 15-59). Affected digits are swollen and painful with thickened, dystrophic, or absent claws. Occasionally a digit is amputated to facilitate salvage of a weight-bearing pad or portion of the paw. The primary weight-bearing digits are the third and fourth digits. The level of amputation is determined by the site of the lesion and the disease process. General anesthesia is required. Complications include hemor-

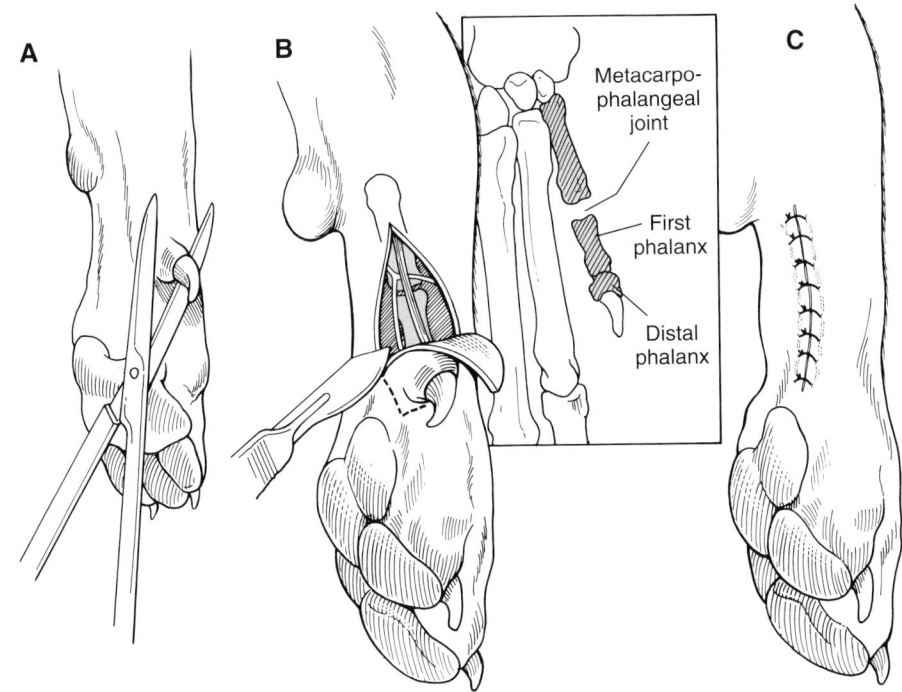

FIG. 15-58
Dewclaw removal. **A,** In puppies, abduct and transect the dewclaw with scissors, disarticulating at the metatarsal (carpal)-phalangeal joint. **B,** In adults, make an elliptic incision around the base of the dewclaw, dissect subcutaneous tissue, and ligate the dorsal common and axial palmar arteries. Then disarticulate the joint or transect P1 with bone cutters *(inset)*. **C,** Appose subcutaneous tissue and skin with approximating sutures.

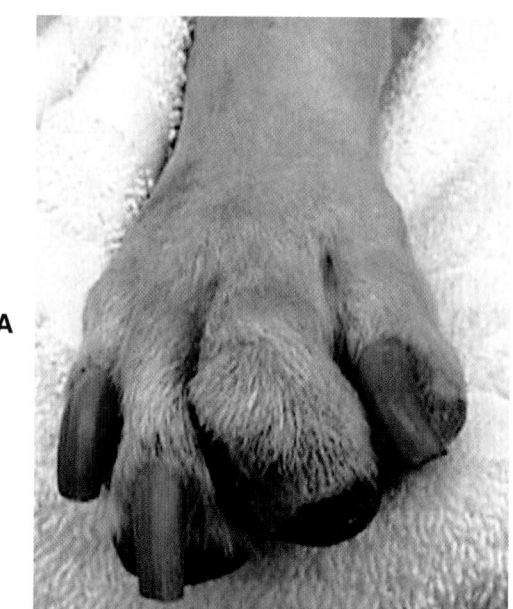
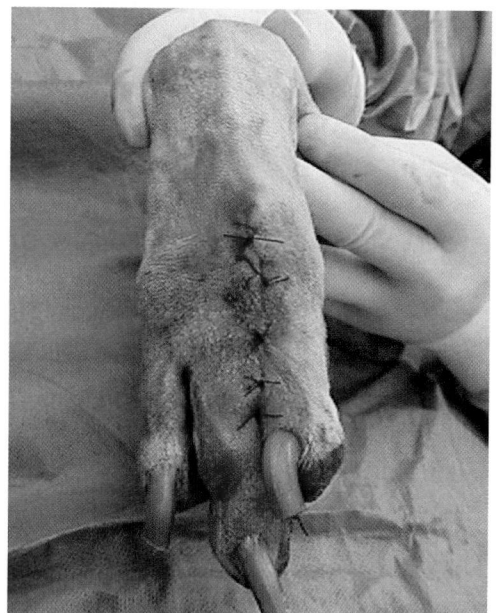

FIG. 15-59
A, A melanoma caused this digit to enlarge and the nail was lost. **B,** The digit was amputated and the adjacent toes were fused.

rhage, infection, dehiscence, and recurrence. Tight bandages may cause swelling or ischemic necrosis. Lameness results if more than two digits or the third or fourth digit is removed. Low-grade, persistent lameness after amputation of the third or fourth digit may occur with resection through the middle to distal region of P1 or P2.

Digital tumors occur in older dogs (mean age of 10 years) and more rarely in cats (mean age 12.7 years) and often are initially misdiagnosed as infections. They occur most often in male large- to medium-breed dogs (10 to more than 30 kg). Bone invasion is common. Clinical signs include lameness, digit swelling and ulceration, and a fixed protruding, deviated, or lost nail. Tumors must be differentiated from paronychia. Squamous cell carcinomas, malignant melanomas, soft tissue sarcomas, osteosarcomas, and mast cell tumors are common digital tumors. Squamous cell carcinomas, mast cell tumors, and melanomas arising in the subungual epithelium are aggressive and sometimes metastatic. Black dogs are predisposed to subungual squamous cell carcinomas. The 1-year survival rate after digital amputation varies from 45% to 100%, depending on the tumor type. Digital tumors in cats are often metastatic from pulmonary neoplasia, commonly involve weight-bearing digits, and can involve more than one toe (Gottfried et al, 2000). Cats with digital tumors should be carefully evaluated for primary disease. In one study involving digital carcinomas in cats, digital amputation was rarely palliative because of the development of additional lesions and a median survival of only 67 days (Gottfried et al, 2000).

Clip and aseptically prepare the paw for surgery. Position the dog in ventral or lateral recumbency with the leg suspended. Place a tourniquet and drape the area. Release the aseptically prepared paw into the sterile field. Begin a dorsal skin incision at the distal end of the appropriate metacarpal (metatarsal) or the proximal end of the first phalanx. Make a transverse encircling incision at the appropriate interphalangeal joint (inverse Y incision) (Fig. 15-60, A and B). Preserve the digital pad if only the third phalanx is removed. Transect the flexor and extensor tendons, ligaments, and joint capsule. Ligate the digital arteries and veins with 3-0 or 4-0 absorbable suture. Disarticulate with a scalpel blade or transect the phalanx with bone cutters. Include the sesamoid bones with the excision. Suture the extensor tendon to the dorsal surface of the pad when it is preserved. Appose subcutaneous tissues over the end of the bone with interrupted absorbable sutures (e.g., 3-0 or 4-0 polydioxanone, poliglecaprone 25, glycomer 631, or polyglyconate). Appose skin with approximating sutures (e.g., 3-0 or 4-0 nylon or polypropylene) (Fig. 15-60, C). Apply a padded bandage and, if necessary, an Elizabethan collar or bucket. Keep the bandage clean and dry. Change the bandage in 2 to 3 days or as needed to evaluate the wound. Remove the bandage and sutures after 7 to 10 days.

FOOTPAD INJURIES

The footpad is the toughest area of the canine skin and is designed to absorb shock, standing, and abrasive forces. The stratum corneum usually is pigmented, thick, and keratinized, with a rough surface of conical papillae. Footpad inju-

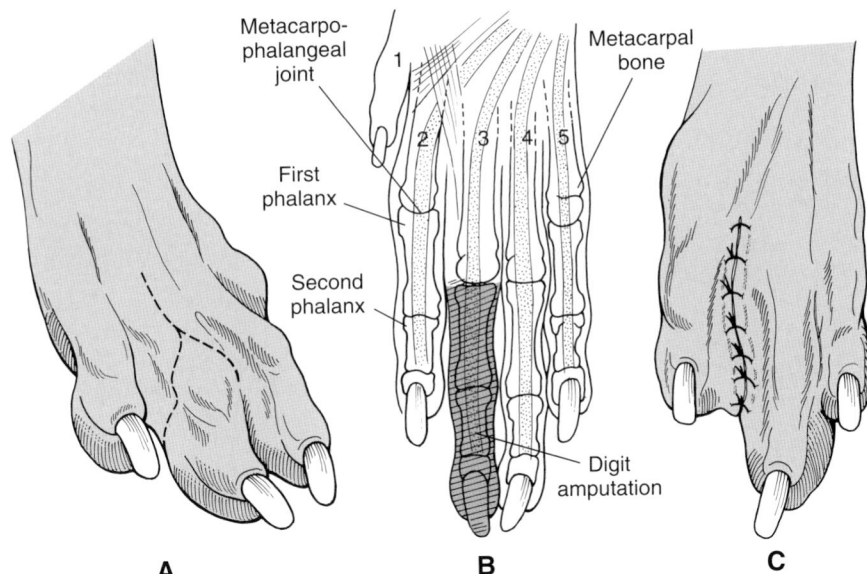

FIG. 15-60
Digit amputation. **A,** Begin the skin incision dorsally and extend it laterally on each side of the involved digit. **B,** Ligate the digital vessels and transect the tendons, ligaments, and joint capsule to disarticulate the digit between P3–P2, P2–P1, or P1–metacarpal (tarsal). **C,** Appose subcutaneous tissue over the end of the bone and approximate skin edges.

ries include laceration, degloving, abrasion, avulsion, burns, and tumors. Injuries may not heal well as a result of the weight-bearing forces and pad loss. Weight-bearing areas without pads may ulcerate.

Superficial Pad Loss

Wounds with superficial pad loss are allowed to heal by secondary intention and treated with nonadherent, absorbent, or semiabsorbent bandages and a spoon splint. A functional pad is maintained if epithelial tissue remains at the periphery and the wound is able to heal by contraction and epithelialization. Splinting the paw promotes healing because wound contractile forces are antagonized by weight bearing, which pushes the wound edges apart. Aloe vera extract gel has a positive effect on early stages of paw pad healing. Acemannan-containing hydrogel wound dressing also stimulates wound healing. Bandaging and splinting the paw should be continued until reepithelialization and some keratinization occur. Exercise should be restricted while the limb is bandaged. After the bandage has been removed, exercise may be gradually allowed on nonabrasive surfaces.

Lacerations

Improperly managed simple lacerations can become chronic nonhealing wounds because forces applied on the pads during standing or walking flatten and spread the pad, separating the lacerated edges. Proper management of lacerated pads includes lavage, suturing, and bandaging. If the wound extends through the entire thickness of the pad, exposing the digital flexor tendons, place a closed suction or Penrose drain under the pad that emerges through skin adjacent to the pad. Acute lacerations should be thoroughly lavaged and minimally débrided. Old, severely contaminated, or infected lacerations need hydrophilic bandages for several days.

Débride the edges of chronic lacerations to remove necrotic tissue and provide a bleeding edge for apposition. Appose deep layers of the pad with buried simple interrupted absorbable sutures (e.g., 3-0 and 4-0 polydioxanone, poliglecaprone 25, glycomer 631, or polyglyconate). Appose epithelial edges with interrupted approximating sutures (simple, vertical mattress, far-near-near-far) (e.g., 2-0 or 3-0 polypropylene or nylon), taking bites several millimeters from the cut edge. After closure, protect the pad with a nonadherent, thick, absorbent bandage with a foam sponge, and a spoon splint or clamshell splint (see p. 189). Change the bandage every 1 to 3 days, depending on the amount of drainage. Remove the sutures after 10 to 14 days and reapply the splint and bandage for 3 to 4 days. Remove the splint but rebandage the paw for an additional 3 to 6 days to allow the wound to strengthen. As an alternative, protect the pad with a commercial boot after suture removal (Dog Bootie). Restrict exercise while the limb is bandaged. Gradually institute exercise on a nonabrasive surface after bandage removal.

Paw Salvage

Degloving or crushing injuries to the paw may result in a nonfunctional paw. Amputation or multiple surgical procedures are required to maintain paw function when injury is severe. Free grafts, axial pattern flaps, or thoracic wall pouch flaps may be used to replace skin. Indoor cats and small dogs that walk primarily on carpets may function well on grafted skin that does not have pads; however, most dogs require salvage or replacement of the metacarpal-metatarsal pad. Replacement of metatarsal, metacarpal, or weight-bearing digital pads may be achieved by transposing adjacent pads, segmental digital pad grafts, or microneurovascular free digital or carpal pad transfer (Fig. 15-61). Tissue should not be transposed over a pad injury caused by tendon malfunction, bone malalignment, or nerve

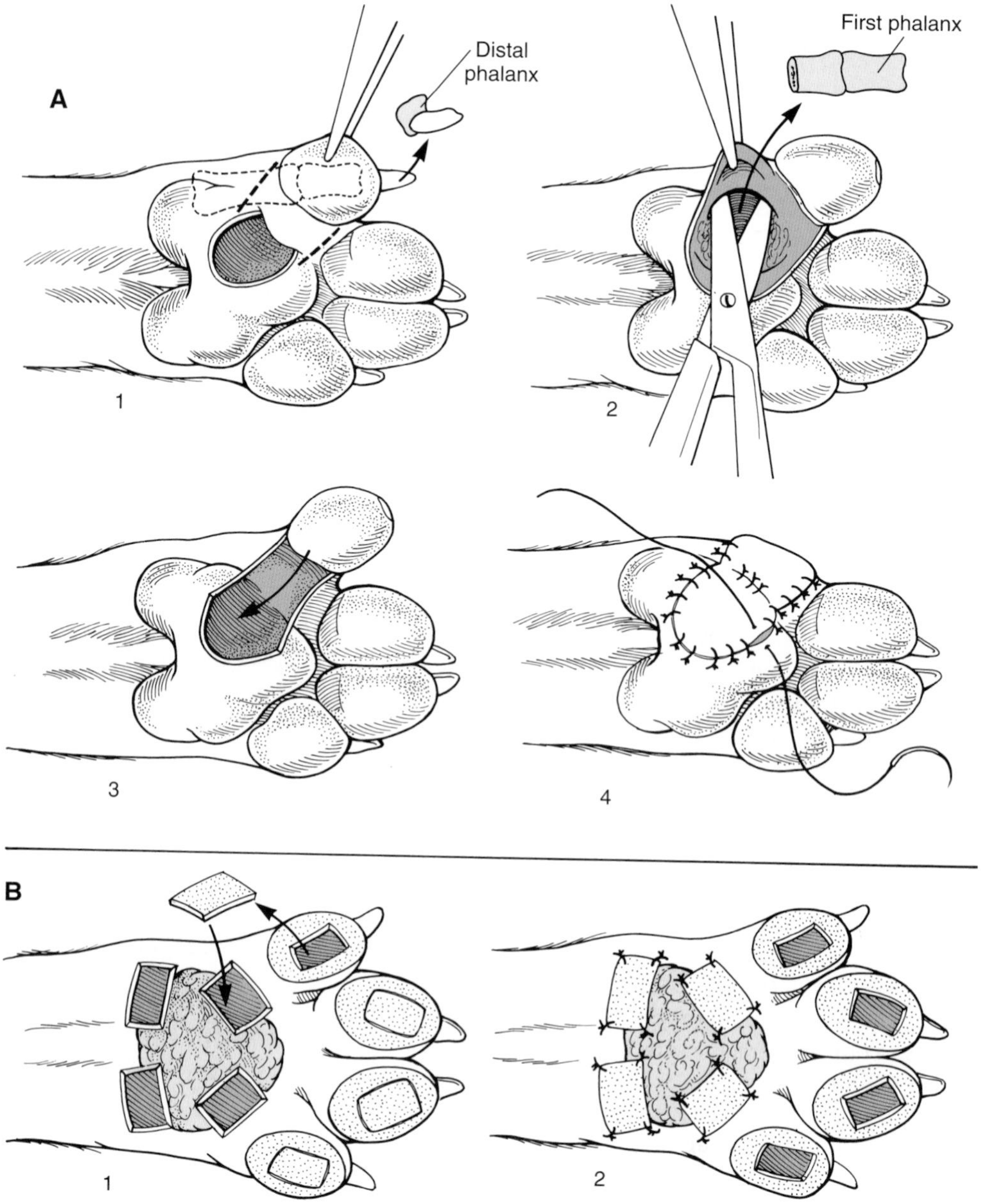

FIG. 15-61
Replacement or salvage of weight-bearing pads. **A,** Partly or completely replace a pad by removing P3 and P2 from digit two or five and transposing the pad and skin to the injured area (phalangeal fillet technique). **B,** The metacarpal or metatarsal pad may be salvaged by grafting from digital pads. Place the free segmental graft on a healthy granulation bed and across the skin pad junction. Donor sites are apposed with approximating sutures if tissue is pliable or allowed to heal by secondary intention under a protective bandage.

damage until the cause is corrected. A digital pad is transposed to replace a portion of the metatarsal or metacarpal pad. The phalanges of digit two or five are removed through a palmar incision. The digital pad is maintained on a pedicle of skin and is transposed to the metatarsal-metacarpal pad. As an alternative, severe trauma to all digits may necessitate digital amputation and transposition of the metatarsal or metacarpal pad over the bone ends to provide a weight-bearing surface. Free segmental digital pad grafts (6 × 8 mm) sutured into recessed recipient beds in granulation tissue allow pad reepithelialization with a tough, keratinized, and effective weight-bearing surface. Microneurovascular pad transfer requires specialized instrumentation and training. The paw should be bandaged after surgery as described above for lacerations.

AP FUSION PODOPLASTY

Fusion podoplasty is a salvage procedure used to treat severed flexor tendons or chronic interdigital pyoderma and to reconstruct the paw after digit amputations. Fusion podoplasty is not recommended on all four paws during a single surgery because of the prolonged operative time and postoperative discomfort.

Clip and aseptically prepare the paw. Position the anesthetized patient in dorsal or lateral recumbency. Secure a tourniquet around the distal limb. Excise the interdigital web and skin between the digital and metacarpal-metatarsal pads. Preserve 2 to 3 mm of skin adjacent to the nail. Prevent damage to the digital vessels and nerves during dissection. Control hemorrhage with electrocoagulation, pressure, and ligation. Thoroughly lavage the wound. Suture the digital pads in apposition with simple interrupted sutures (e.g., 3-0 polypropylene or nylon). Approximate the digital and metacarpal-metatarsal pads with simple interrupted sutures; direct apposition of epithelial edges may not be possible. Before the last few pad sutures are inserted, place a small closed suction or Penrose drain across the paw deep to the sutures. Approximate adjacent skin edges dorsally with simple interrupted sutures (e.g., 3-0 polypropylene or nylon). Leave a gap between skin edges at the end of the digits to allow drainage. Repeat the procedure on the opposite paw if indicated. Remove the tourniquet.

Following amputation of the third or fourth digit or both (see p. 255), the weight-bearing portion of the foot is reconstructed with the second and fourth or fifth digits. The digits and tumor are removed *en bloc* with the digital pads while the metacarpal or metatarsal pads are preserved.

Close the defect in three layers. First appose the interosseous muscles of the adjacent digits with 3-0 or 4-0 monofilament absorbable interrupted sutures, next appose the subcutaneous tissue on both the palmar (plantar) and dorsal surfaces with absorbable sutures. Finally, appose the dorsal skin remaining on the second digit with the dorsal skin of the fourth or fifth digit and then the plantar or palmar skin between the digits with 3-0 or 4-0 monofilament nonabsorbable appositional sutures.

Apply an antibiotic ointment and then a nonadherent, absorbent bandage and spoon splint or clamshell type of splint extending from the paw to the elbow or hock. For patients with interdigital pyoderma, change the bandage and splint daily until drainage diminishes, usually within 10 to 14 days. Remove the drain and extend the interval between bandage and splint changes to every 2 to 3 days. Soak the paw in an antiseptic solution before rebandaging if a pseudomonad infection is suspected. Remove sutures between 10 and 21 days after surgery, but continue bandaging until granulation is complete.

Additional débridement may be indicated if nonhealing wounds or draining tracts persist after surgery.

After digit amputation, change the bandage and splint every 3 to 5 days and remove sutures between 10 and 14 days after surgery.

When healing nears completion, a lighter bandage or a paw bootie (Dog Bootie) allows transition between a heavy-splinted bandage and full weight bearing. Lameness is expected after digit amputation with fusion podoplasty for 4 or more weeks. Infection may persist in animals with interdigital pyoderma.

References

Cooper MA, Laverty PH, Soiderer EE: Bilateral flexor tendon contracture following onychectomy in 2 cats, *Can Vet J* 46:244, 2005.

Gottfried SD, Popovitch CA, Goldschmidt MH et al: Metastatic digital carcinoma in the cat: a retrospective study of 36 cats (1992-1998), *J Am Anim Hosp Assoc* 36:501, 2000.

Mueller RS, Olivry T: Onychobiopsy without onychectomy: description of a new biopsy technique for canine claws, *Vet Dermatol* 10:55, 1999.

Ringwood B, Smith JA: Anesthesia case of the month, *J Am Vet Med Assoc* 217:1633, 2000.

Suggested Reading

Carroll GL, Howe LB, Peterson KD: Analgesic efficacy of preoperative administration of meloxicam or butorphanol in onychectomized cats, *J Am Vet Med Assoc* 226:913, 2005.

Data from 138 cats find that improved analgesia was provided by meloxicam compared with butorphanol.

Gaynor JS: Chronic pain syndrome of feline onychectomy, *NAVC Clinician's Brief* April: 11, 2005.

Treatment and prevention of chronic pain are presented.

Gordon WJ, Conzemius MG: Analgesia after onychectomy in cats, *Vet Med* 100:46, 2005.

This is a good review with a nice drug chart.

Liptak JM, Dernell WS, Rizzo SA et al: Partial foot amputation in 11 dogs, *J Am Anim Hosp Assoc* 41:47, 2005.

Amputation of one or more weight-bearing digits with fusion podoplasty to adjacent digits in some dogs allowed limb salvage.

Mison MB, Bohart GH, Walshaw R et al: Use of carbon dioxide laser for onychectomy in cats, *J Am Vet Med Assoc* 221:651, 2002.

This study compares the use of the laser to the scalpel for performing declaws in 20 cases.

Romans CW, Gordon WJ, Robinson DA et al: Effect of postoperative analgesic protocol on limb function following onychectomy in cats, *J Am Vet Med Assoc* 227:89, 2005.

Twenty-seven cats were divided into three groups to compare the effects of topical bupivacaine, IM butorphanol, or a fentanyl patch on postoperative pain with the aid of pressure platform gait analysis.

Swaim SF, Marghitu DB, Rumph PF et al: Effects of bandage configuration on paw pad pressure in dogs: a preliminary study, *J Am Anim Hosp Assoc* 39:209, 2003.

Results from the evaluation of seven bandage configurations indicated that clamshell bandages resulted in the least pad pressure, and placement of a thick foam pad to protect the major weight-bearing pad helped to alleviate pad pressure.

Swiderski J: Onychectomy and its alternatives in the feline patient, *Clinical Techniques in Small Animal Practice* 17:158, 2002.

This is a good review of options, pros, and cons, but is not illustrated.

CHAPTER 16
Surgery of the Eye

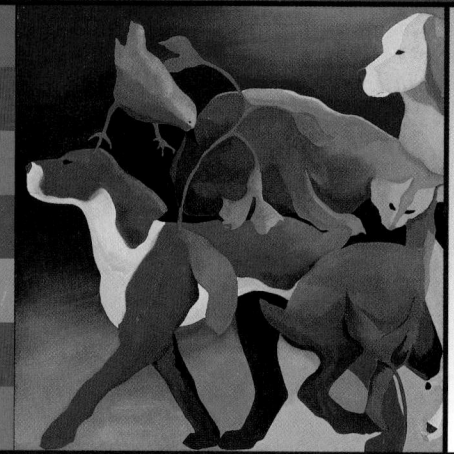

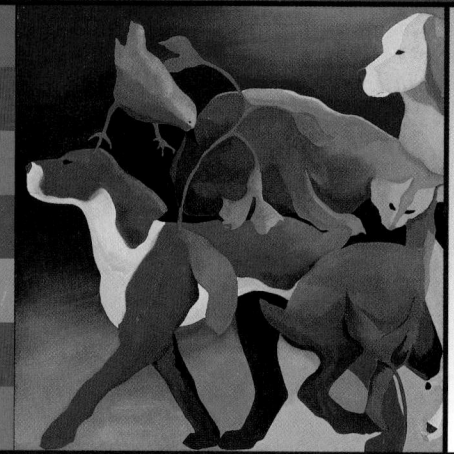

GENERAL PRINCIPLES AND TECHNIQUES

DEFINITIONS

Proptosis is the outward displacement of the eye from its normal position in the orbit. **Enucleation** is the removal of the globe and nictitating membrane. **Exenteration** is removal of the globe, nictitating membrane, orbital contents, and lid margins. **Entropion** is inversion or inward turning of the eyelid's edge. **Ectropion** is eversion or outward turning of the edge of the eyelid.

PREOPERATIVE CONCERNS

Some periocular and ocular procedures are performed by general practitioners; however, many are typically referred to veterinary ophthalmologists. Surgical conditions commonly managed by general practitioners include emergency procedures (i.e., traumatic proptosis; minor lid, conjunctival, and corneal lacerations; and penetrating wounds or ulcers) and entropion or ectropion repair, tumor removal, and enucleation. Complicated or severe periocular or corneal problems and intraocular procedures should be performed by persons with specialized training in veterinary ophthalmology.

Successful ophthalmic surgery requires a correct diagnosis, appropriate choice of surgical procedure, attention to detail, and proper instrumentation and equipment. Each animal should be thoroughly evaluated for concurrent and contributing abnormalities. This should include a complete physical examination and appropriate diagnostics. A complete blood count (CBC) and serum chemistry panel are typical preanesthetic tests in older patients (see Chapter 5). If there is a heart murmur in an older patient, then thoracic radiographs, echocardiography, and/or electrocardiography (ECG) may be appropriate, depending upon the patient. Ultrasonography, computed tomography (CT), and magnetic resonance imaging (MRI) are helpful in defining orbital and retrobulbar disease (Mason et al, 2001). The normal flora of the conjunctival sac, lacrimal ducts, and tarsal glands includes potential pathogens so perioperative antibiotics are reasonable. Periocular tissues rapidly become inflamed and swollen when manipulated. This swelling can be

minimized by preoperative topical or systemic corticosteroids or topical nonsteroidal antiinflammatories (NSAIDs). It is advantageous to dilate the pupil before some intraocular procedures. Preoperative pupil dilation (mydriasis) is achieved with topical tropicamide or 1% atropine. Sodium flurbiprofen 0.03%, a topical NSAID, assists in maintenance of pupillary dilation.

PREPARATION OF THE SURGICAL SITE

Liberally apply artificial tears or antibiotic ophthalmic ointment in both eyes to protect the corneas before clipping and preparing the skin and periocular tissue. Clip an area around the surgical site using a No. 40 clipper blade and electric clipper. Do not use a vacuum to remove the clipped hair; rather, gently brush it away or use adhesive tape to collect it to prevent damaging the delicate eyelid tissue. Irrigate the conjunctival sac with eyewash or physiologic saline with an added 10% povidone-iodine (1 part povidone-iodine to 50 parts eyewash) solution. Using cotton-tipped applicators or soft surgical sponges soaked in a diluted antiseptic solution, prepare the skin for aseptic surgery. Do not use soap, detergents, or alcohol, which may damage the cornea. After surgery, protect the surgical site from rubbing, pawing, or scratching by administering analgesics, applying a protective collar, and sometimes bandaging the paws or head.

> NOTE: Identification of tissue layers and accurate placement of sutures are facilitated by using a magnifying loupe or an operating microscope.

Improving access to the anterior aspect of the eye in small dogs can be accomplished by retrobulbar injection of 0.9% saline after the dog is anesthetized. Exposure is improved by the saline forcing the globe further rostrad in the orbit or to rotate it. Injections immediately behind the globe push the globe forward; injections external to the retrobulbar muscles rotate the globe laterally.

Insert the needle caudal to the junction of the lateral orbital ligament and dorsal aspect of the zygomatic arch, and direct it toward the retrobulbar space in a ventromedial direction toward the opposite mandibular joint. Alternatively, insert the needle beneath the zygomatic arch at the level of the lateral canthus and direct it rostral to the vertical portion of the ramus of the mandible toward the orbital fissure. Once the desired effect is achieved, stop the injection; the saline is generally absorbed in 30 to 60 minutes. Take care to avoid causing retrobulbar hemorrhage or penetrating the globe.

ANESTHETIC CONSIDERATIONS

Anesthetic selection should be appropriate for the animal's age and condition. General anesthesia is most appropriate. Analgesic administration preoperatively leads to a smoother and less painful recovery. Regional anesthetic blocks may be beneficial for some procedures to facilitate perioperative analgesia and reduce the need for intraoperative systemic drugs. Preoperative administration of atropine (0.02 to 0.04 mg/kg) or glycopyrrolate (0.005 to 0.011 mg/kg) or both minimizes the oculorespiratory cardiac reflex as does adequate oxygenation. The oculorespiratory cardiac reflex, which results in bradycardia and respiratory depression, can be precipitated by ocular pressure massage, intraorbital injections, and manipulation of the extraocular or eyelid muscles. Use thiopental sodium (8 to 12 mg/kg IV to effect) or propofol (6 mg/kg IV to effect) for induction, and isoflurane or sevoflurane and oxygen for maintenance of anesthesia in healthy animals. Neuromuscular blocking agents (i.e., pancuronium 0.06 mg/kg IV, duration approximately 20 to 40 minutes; or atracurium 0.3 mg/kg IV) are used for intraocular procedures to reduce extraocular muscle tone and improve eye position. Ventilation must be supported if the patient is paralyzed. A train-of-four should be available to monitor neuromuscular blockade. Nondepolarizing neuromuscular agents may be antagonized (e.g., edrophonium) once after at least one twitch has returned. Monitoring equipment is especially advantageous because the head is covered in the sterile field and not accessible for detecting palpebral reflexes or lingual pulse. Application of topical analgesics, such as lidocaine or morphine sulfate, following surgery reduces pain and blepharospasm (Stiles et al, 2003). A smooth, quiet recovery is necessary to prevent trauma to the operated eye.

Most general anesthetics lower intraocular pressure through actions on the central nervous, respiratory, and circulatory systems. The decrease in pressure is directly related to the depth of anesthesia. Drugs that produce an increase in the arterial blood pressure, central venous pressure, episcleral venous pressure, or extraocular muscle tone will result in a moderate increase in intraocular pressure. These effects are transient because the aqueous humor dynamics rapidly return pressures to normal.

General anesthesia is also associated with reduced tear production. Applying a corneal lubricant every 90 minutes or frequent application of an eyewash or balanced salt solution during general anesthesia is important, especially when anticholinergics are administered. Using eyewash or balanced salt solutions is preferable for corneal or intraocular procedures to prevent ointments from gaining intraocular

access. Using ointments before eyelid surgery may make them slippery. Always use ointments in the unoperated eye. Reduced tear production may persist for 24 hours postoperatively, so continued application of lubricant ointment is recommended for 1 to 2 days postoperatively (Herring et al, 2000).

ANTIBIOTICS

Potential pathogens in the normal flora of the conjunctiva, lacrimal glands, and tarsal glands is one reason perioperative antibiotics are often administered to animals having periocular or ocular surgery. Most often the bacteria recovered from corneal ulcers are *Staphylococcus* and *Streptococcus* spp., which are sensitive to most antibiotics. Administration of corticosteroids for their local and systemic antiinflammatory and immunosuppressive properties is another reason for antibiotic administration. Ophthalmic preparations containing bacitracin, polymyxin, and neomycin are often chosen for perioperative prophylaxis. Other frequently used topical antibiotics include chloramphenicol, gentamicin, and tobramycin. Generally, systemic antibiotics are given for eyelid, intraocular, and orbital surgeries, whereas topical antibiotics are used for conjunctival and corneal surgeries. Systemic antibiotics should be given such that there are therapeutic blood levels at the time of surgery (see Chapter 10).

SURGICAL ANATOMY

The eyelids and orbit house and protect the eye (Fig. 16-1). Eyelids are mobile folds of skin that block light and protect the cornea. The upper lid is slightly larger and more mobile than the lower lid. The upper and lower lids join at the medial and lateral commissures, which are stabilized by the medial and lateral palpebral ligaments. The width of the opening between the lids is controlled by opposing groups of muscles; the orbicularis oculi muscle closes the palpebral fissure while the fissure is widened by the levator palpebrae superioris, pars palpebralis of the sphincter colli profundus muscle, and smooth muscles of the periorbita. The upper and lower *lacrimal puncta*, which drain tears, open onto the bulbar surfaces of the lid margins 2 to 5 mm from the medial commissure. The *lacrimal caruncle* is located near the medial commissure. It projects fine, small hairs; has sebaceous glands; and may be pigmented. Long hairs known as *cilia* project from the upper lid margin, while the lower lid is devoid of cilia. There is a tuft of long tactile hairs at the dorsal medial margin of the orbit, which corresponds to man's eyebrows.

Glands in the lid margins are similar to glands found elsewhere in skin. Sebaceous glands open into follicles of the cilia on the upper lid. Both upper and lower lids have specially modified sebaceous glands—the *tarsal glands* (meibomian glands). Duct openings of these glands are found in a shallow furrow immediately caudal to the mucocutaneous junction. The tarsal glands produce an oily tear film and are usually visible through the conjunctiva. Sometimes very fine hair originates from these glands. This condition is called *distichiasis*. *Ciliary glands* (apocrine sweat glands) secrete

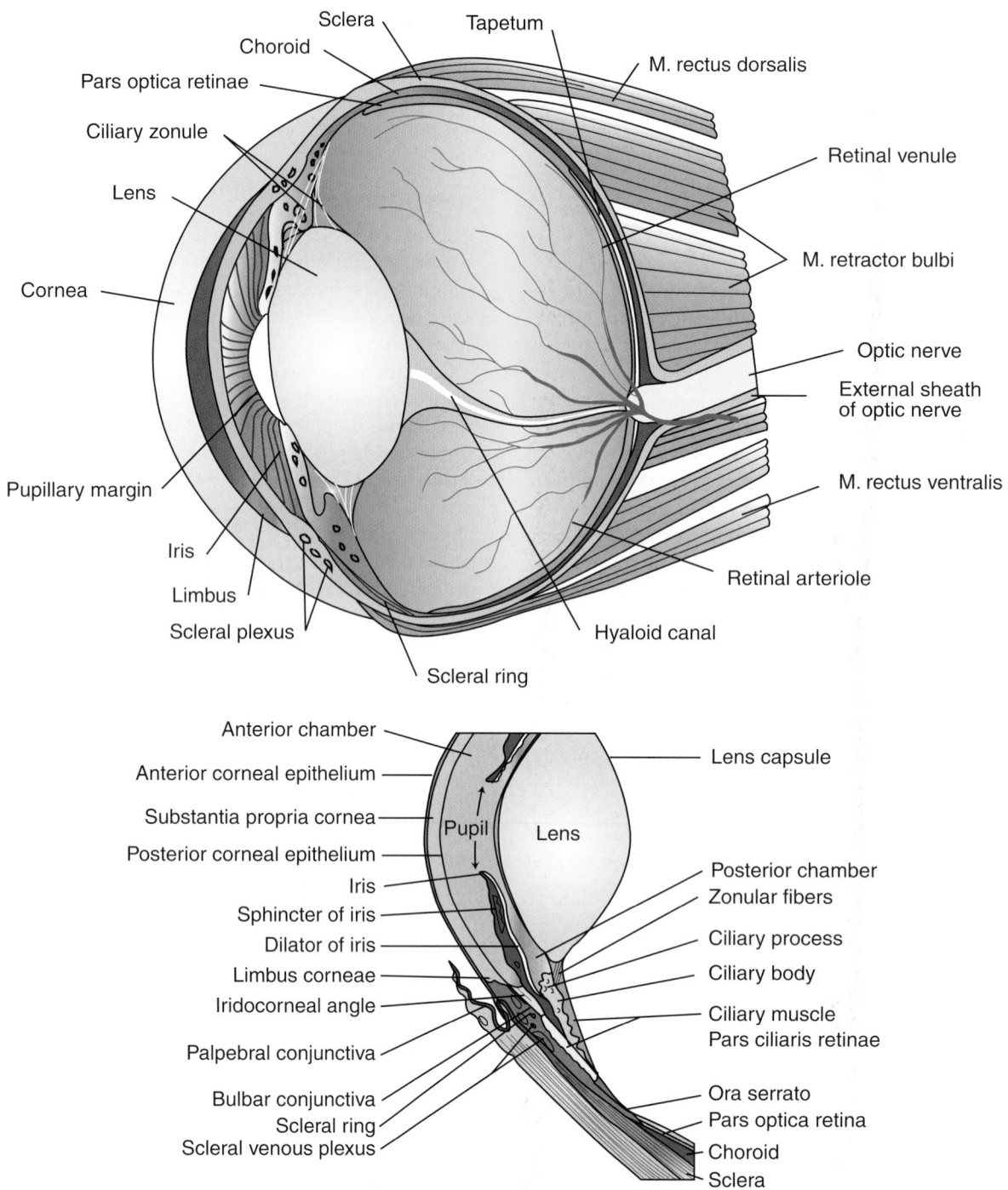

FIG. 16-1
Ocular and periocular anatomy.

into hair follicles, sebaceous glands, or directly onto the lid margin.

The special mucous membrane on the inner aspect of the lids is called *palpebral conjunctiva*. At the level of the orbital rim, the palpebral conjunctiva reflects onto the eye to become the *bulbar conjunctiva*. The palpebral conjunctiva has goblet cells, whereas the bulbar conjunctiva is thinner and without goblet cells. Lymphatic nodules are found throughout the conjunctiva, but are especially prominent on the

bulbar surface of the third eyelid. Lymphatic drainage from the conjunctiva empties into the parotid lymph nodes. The third eyelid arises as a fold from the ventromedial aspect of the conjunctiva. It is very mobile, being able to cover the entire anterior face of the cornea. A T-shaped piece of hyaline cartilage stiffens the third eyelid. The superficial gland of the third eyelid, a mixed seromucous gland that contributes significantly to the tear film, surrounds the base of the cartilage.

The orbit is the cavity containing the eye and ocular adnexa. The bony orbital margin (frontal, lacrimal, and zygomatic bones) encompasses approximately four fifths of the orbit's circumference, with the remainder being completed by the orbital ligament. The orbital ligament is a thick fibrous band connecting the zygomatic process of the frontal bone with the frontal process of the zygomatic bone. Both the orbicularis oculi muscle and lateral palpebral ligament attach to the orbital ligament. The medial wall and part of the roof of the orbit are bony (frontal, lacrimal, presphenoid, and palatine bones). There are five foramina in the medial wall: the optic canal, orbital fissure, lacrimal canal, and two small ethmoidal foramina. The optic canal is rostral in the orbit and traversed by the optical nerve and internal ophthalmic artery. The orbital fissure between the basisphenoid and presphenoid bones gives passage to the oculomotor, trochlear, abducent, and ophthalmic nerves; the anastomotic branch of the external ophthalmic artery; and the orbital venous plexus. The retractor bulbi muscle originates in the orbital fissure. The rostromedial continuation of the orbit is the lacrimal canal through which the nasolacrimal duct travels. The *nasolacrimal duct* connects to the two canaliculi, whose two puncta are found at the medial canthus. There is a fossa for the lacrimal gland in the ventral surface of the zygomatic process of the frontal bone where the orbital ligament originates. The lateral wall and floor are formed by soft tissue, the medial pterygoid muscle, the temporal muscle, and the zygomatic gland. The maxillary artery and nerve cross the floor of the orbit near its apex. The orbital fat body is present at the caudal pole of the eye, surrounding the optic nerve and spaces between extraocular muscles. This fat serves as a cushion and permits rotation and retraction of the eye. The extraocular muscles insert on the sclera and function to rotate and retract the eye. These muscles include the rectus muscles (dorsal, ventral, medial, and lateral), the oblique muscles (dorsal and ventral), and the retractor bulbi muscle. The orbit, extraocular muscles, and other orbital structures are covered with fascia (periorbital, muscular, and bulbar).

The contents of the eye are surrounded by an external fibrous coat; the transparent, multilayered cornea; and the white, opaque sclera (Fig. 16-2). The two meet at the corneoscleral junction or limbus. The *cornea* is usually less than 1 mm thick, is covered by a precorneal tear film, and has four layers: epithelium with its basement membrane, stroma, Descemet's membrane (basement membrane of endothelium), and endothelium. The *sclera* has three layers: episclera (vascular layer), sclera proper (collagen fibers and fibroblasts), and lamina fusca (collagen bundles that intermingle with the choroids and ciliary body). The sclera is covered anteriorly by the conjunctiva; posteriorly, muscles insert around vessels and nerves, which penetrate its surface. The middle or vascular coat is the *uvea*, which consists of three continuous parts: the choroid, ciliary body, and iris. The *iris* is seen through the cornea and regulates the size of the centrally located pupil. The *ciliary body* is a thick circular mound at the level of the limbus, which regulates the shape of the lens. The folds of the internal surface of the ciliary body are the ciliary processes. The *choroid* lines, and is firmly attached to, the sclera. The *retina* lines the internal surface of the choroid to the level of the ciliary process. The retina is the nervous coat of the eye. Zonular fibers attach the equator of the lens to the ciliary process. The *lens* is transparent and elastic.

The interior of the eye is divided into chambers. The *vitreous chamber* located posterior to the lens is filled with the transparent jellylike vitreous body. The space between the cornea and lens is filled with aqueous humor and divided into two chambers. The *anterior chamber* is the space between the cornea and the iris, and the *posterior chamber* is a narrow space between the iris and lens.

SURGICAL TECHNIQUES
Eyelid Laceration Repair

Lacerated eyelids are commonly associated with bite wounds and automobile injuries. They should be repaired as soon as possible to protect the cornea and maintain an effective blink reflex. Healing of lid lacerations by secondary intention may result in considerable fibrosis and distortion of the eyelids and lid margin. Direct reapposition is possible if one third or less of the lid margin is missing. More extensive injuries require advancement flaps or grafts for repair. Preservation of the eyelid margin and its associated structures is essential for normal eyelid function. No matter how thin a flap of tissue has been created by a laceration running parallel to the eyelid margin, it should not be excised (Fig. 16-3). If these flaps do not survive, the eyelid margin can be reconstructed.

Apply topical ophthalmic ointment to keep the tissue moist before surgical repair. Thoroughly irrigate and gently cleanse the wound with a dilute Betadine or chlorhexidine solution. Identify the mucocutaneous junction, meibomian glands, tarsal plate, orbicularis muscle, and palpebral conjunctiva. Convert simple lacerations to a V-shaped defect with judicious wound débridement (scarify necrotic margins and smooth jagged edges) (Fig. 16-4, A). Place a mattress suture (5-0 to 6-0 absorbable) in the tarsal plate at the mucocutaneous junction to ensure proper anatomic alignment of the eyelid margin and conjunctiva (Fig. 16-4, B). Continue this suture in the subconjunctival tissue as a simple continuous suture pattern (4-0 to 6-0 absorbable) to appose the conjunctiva (Fig. 16-4, C). Take care that knots and suture ends do not abrade the cornea by positioning them subcutaneously. Place a marginal skin suture, ensuring that the lid margin has perfect alignment (see Fig. 16-4, D). Use a simple interrupted or cruciate suture (4-0 to 6-0 nonabsorbable) with the knot ends directed away from the cornea to close the skin (Fig. 16-4, E). Space remaining skin sutures approximately 2 mm apart. If the nasolacrimal duct has been damaged by the trauma near the medial canthus, stent it by first cannulating the canniculus and duct with 0 to 2-0 monofilament suture and then passing polyethylene or Silastic tubing over the suture and securing it to the skin near the medial canthus and lateral of the nostril (see insert Fig. 16-4).

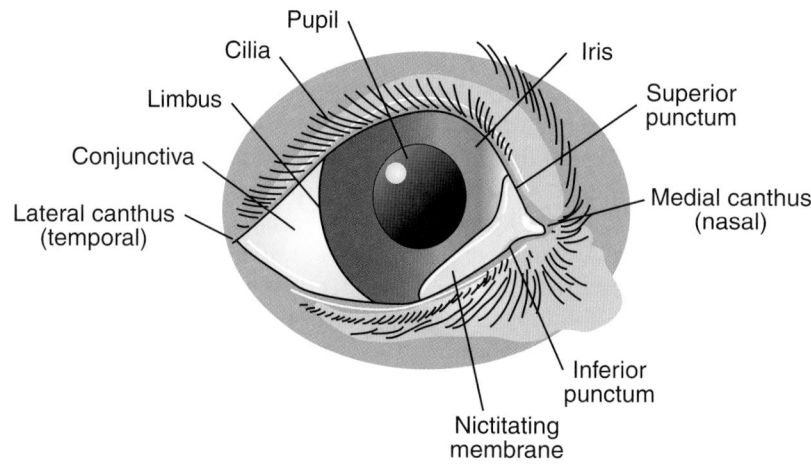

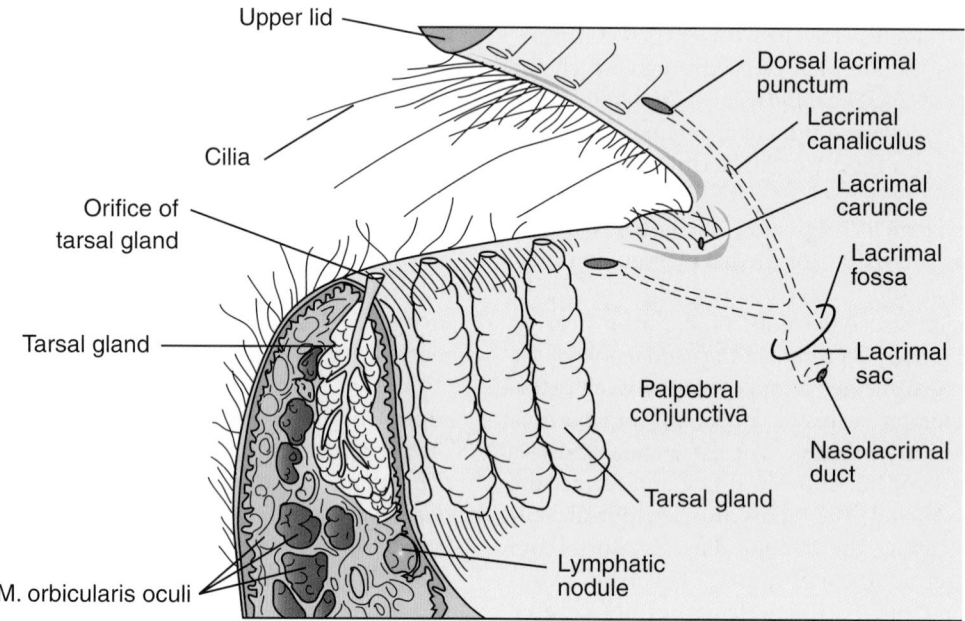

FIG. 16-2
Intraocular anatomy.

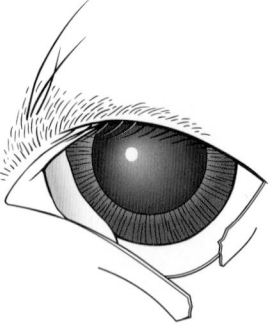

FIG. 16-3
Eyelid laceration involving the lid margin. Preserve even thin strips of tissue to avoid lid margin reconstruction.

A complete temporary tarsorrhaphy may be indicated to protect the cornea after repair of extensive eyelid injuries because of impaired eyelid functions and blink reflex.

Medicate the wound with an ophthalmic antibiotic ointment for 5 to 7 days and monitor for blepharospasm, tearing, or mucopurulent discharge, which may indicate that a corneal ulcer has formed. Remove sutures at 10 to 14 days. Leave the cannula in place for 4 to 6 weeks.

Conjunctival and Corneal Lacerations

Conjunctival lacerations without eyelid lacerations rarely require surgical repair because they heal rapidly. They are allowed to heal by secondary intention after debris has been

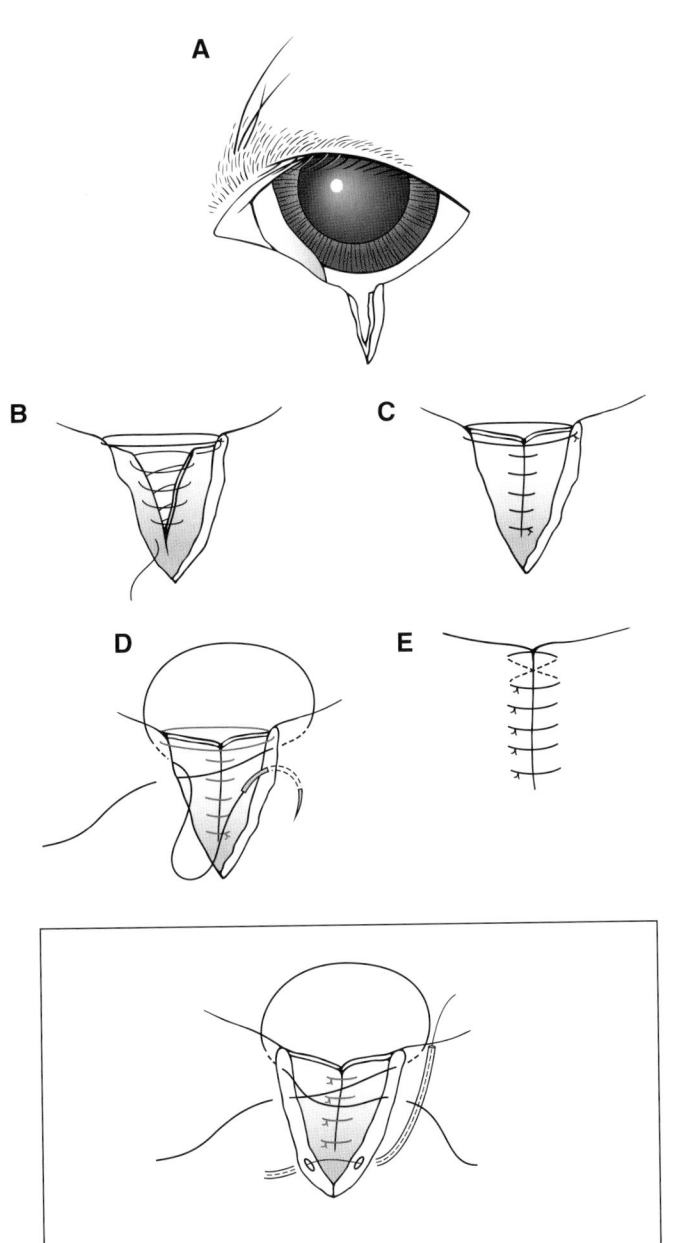

FIG. 16-4
Eyelid laceration. **A**, Repair eyelid lacerations perpendicular to the lid margin by first placing a mattress suture in the tarsal plate (**B** and **C**) at the mucocutaneous junction to accurately align the eyelid margin and conjunctiva, and then appose the conjunctiva with a simple continuous suture pattern. **D** and **E**, Appose the skin beginning at the eyelid margin with a cruciate suture, keeping suture ends away from the cornea. *Inset*, If the nasolacrimal duct is damaged near the medial canthus, first stent it with monofilament suture to guide polypropylene or Silastic tubing through the duct, and then appose the conjunctiva and skin.

removed and topical antibiotics applied. Conjunctival wounds 7 to 8 mm in diameter or larger should be sutured (6-0 to 7-0 absorbable) using a continuous suture pattern. Undermining and sliding adjacent conjunctiva facilitates closure of large wounds. Apply topical ophthalmic antibiotics to prevent infection.

Corneal lacerations or perforations are surgical emergencies and should be corrected as soon as they are discovered.

Use eyewashes rather than topical ointments during preparation because petrolatum-based ointments may cause severe uveitis if they are absorbed into the anterior chamber. Evaluate the intraocular structures for evidence of additional trauma. Remove foreign material embedded in the cornea with irrigation, forceps, and minimal dissection.

Seal perforations less than 1 to 2 mm with a tissue adhesive (n-butyl cyanoacrylate or absorbable methoxypropyl cyanoacrylate monomer) permanently or temporarily. Remove all necrotic or friable corneal tissue. Dry the surface of the cornea with cellulose sponges or warm air. Using a 30-gauge needle or similar applicator, apply a small volume of adhesive directly to the wound in a smooth, thin layer.

Adhesive polymerization occurs within a few seconds, and it becomes very hard. Tissue adhesive may also be useful on deep ulcers and descemetoceles. The adhesive has low tissue toxicity, is bacteriostatic, and inhibits corneal stroma melting. The adhesive is extruded (2 to 4 weeks) as the cornea heals or it may be excised at definitive repair. Application of a soft bandage contact lens reduces discomfort. When the laceration is small (1 to 2 mm), with a formed anterior chamber and no iris prolapse, and when the eye does not seem to be painful, the condition can be managed medically.

Perform a Seidel test to determine if small lacerations can be sealed by placing sodium fluorescein on the cornea; then, without irrigation, observe to see if a clear river of aqueous is running through the fluorescein (which indicates that the anterior chamber is not sealed). Use suture repair to treat lacerations that leak aqueous and those that are long and deep or have a prolapsed iris. Lavage and reposition a viable iris if possible and excise any necrotic iris with iris scissors or an electroscalpel. If the iris prolapse is more than 12 hours old, protract it to fresh iris and amputate close to the corneal surface. Wait several minutes for clotting and vessel sealing before replacing the iris within the anterior chamber. Lavage the anterior chamber with balanced saline solution. Re-form the anterior chamber with a viscoelastic agent (1% sodium hyaluronate or 2% hydroxypropylmethylcellulose). Place the viscoelastic agent between the cornea and iris and between the iris and anterior lens capsule. Perform lens extraction if the anterior lens capsule has ruptured or if the lens is luxated or subluxated. Irrigate the cornea with a balanced electrolyte solution during the procedure to prevent drying. Appose the cornea with 6-0 to 9-0 polyglactin 910 or nylon simple interrupted or continuous suture. Place sutures 1 mm apart, penetrating 75% to 90% of the thickness of the cornea, with sutures entering and emerging perpendicular to the surface 1 to 2 mm from the wound edge (Fig. 16-5). Remove the viscoelastic material from the anterior chamber. Re-form the anterior chamber by injecting balanced saline solution as the last suture is placed. Observe for leaks at the repair site as the anterior chamber is rein-

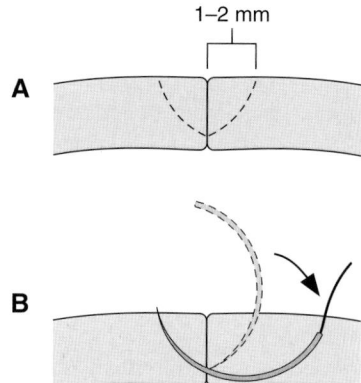

FIG. 16-5
Corneal sutures should penetrate 75% to 90% of the cornea, with sutures entering and emerging perpendicular to the surface and at a distance of 1 to 2 mm from the wound edge. **A,** Desired width and depth of corneal sutures. **B,** Insert the needle so it penetrates the cornea perpendicular to the surface; then it is tipped upward before entering the opposite corneal edge so it emerges from the cornea perpendicular and 1 to 2 mm from the wound edge.

flated and place additional sutures as necessary to achieve a watertight seal. Perform a temporary tarsorrhaphy if additional support is desired (see below). Administer systemic, subconjunctival, and topical antibiotics; topical atropine; systemic corticosteroids; and antiprostaglandin drugs as needed. Apply a restraint collar and restrict exercise for 10 to 14 days. Remove the tarsorrhaphy sutures at 14 days and the corneal sutures at 21 days.

> NOTE: Corneal apposition must be precise to reestablish an airtight and fluid-tight seal in the anterior chamber. Asymmetric or shallow sutures will result in wound gapping and leakage.

> NOTE: *Never* touch or vigorously flush the corneal endothelium.

Temporary Tarsorrhaphy

Temporary tarsorrhaphy may be performed after correction of entropion, ectropion, lacerations, or mass removal to help prevent wound contracture during healing.

Place horizontal mattress sutures at the lid margins to appose them, using partial-thickness bites oriented parallel or perpendicular to the lid margin (Fig. 16-6).

Conjunctival Flap

Conjunctival flaps are used to treat deep corneal ulcers, descemetoceles, and ruptures. Sometimes conjunctival flaps are placed over small intestinal submucosal grafts that serve as a

scaffold and provide tectonic support (Bussieres et al, 2004). Conjunctival flaps are typically harvested from the bulbar conjunctiva and adhere quickly to the cornea to provide a protective covering that brings blood vessels and fibroblasts to facilitate healing. The flap permanently adheres to the injured site, where a heavy, opaque scar may develop. Plan the flap so that it is a few millimeters larger than the defect it must cover.

Prepare a thin sliding conjunctival flap by grasping the conjunctiva with ophthalmic forceps approximately 2 mm from the limbus. Apply traction to tent the conjunctiva and incise near the cornea with a pair of tenotomy scissors (Fig. 16-7, A). Elevate the cut edge, dissecting toward the fornix with tenotomy scissors to create a thin flap (Fig. 16-7, B). Position the flap over the defect after it has been débrided to remove any melting or necrotic cornea, and any corneal epithelium. Place two sutures (6-0 to 9-0 absorbable) through the flap and half the depth of the limbus. Then place two additional sutures from the flap to the edges of the cornea, penetrating approximately 75% to 90% of the depth of the cornea (Fig. 16-7, C).

It is important to get epithelial-to-epithelial apposition without flap overlap.

Close the conjunctival donor site with a continuous suture pattern. Medicate the eye with ophthalmic antibiotics and atropine if indicated. Trim the flap 4 to 6 weeks after surgery once the corneal lesion has healed, allowing the corneal attachment to atrophy and undergo fibrosis, thus minimizing scar formation. Alternatively, create a conjunctival bridge graft as shown in Fig. 16-7, D and E. Loose and excess conjunctiva can also be trimmed from the cornea to reduce the vascular reaction and subsequent scar, but do not remove the conjunctiva from the former corneal ulcer or defect.

Scar remodeling occurs over several months, and final results vary from an insignificant opacity to a dense leukoma.

Third Eyelid Flap

Third eyelid flaps serve as physiologic bandages to support and protect the cornea after trauma. They are easier to create than conjunctival flaps, but should not be used as the sole means of support for treating deep corneal ulcers or descemetoceles.

Exteriorize and extend the third eyelid by grasping it with forceps and elevating it. Pass a cutting needle with swaged-on 3-0 or 4-0 suture monofilament absorbable through the upper eyelid in the dorsolateral conjunctival fornix (Fig. 16-8, A). Direct the needle through the external surface of the third eyelid under the crossbar of the T-shaped cartilage and exit through the external surface of the third eyelid on the opposite side of the cartilage. Alternatively, to absolutely prevent any chance of the suture rubbing on the cornea, direct the suture around the cartilage, but do not

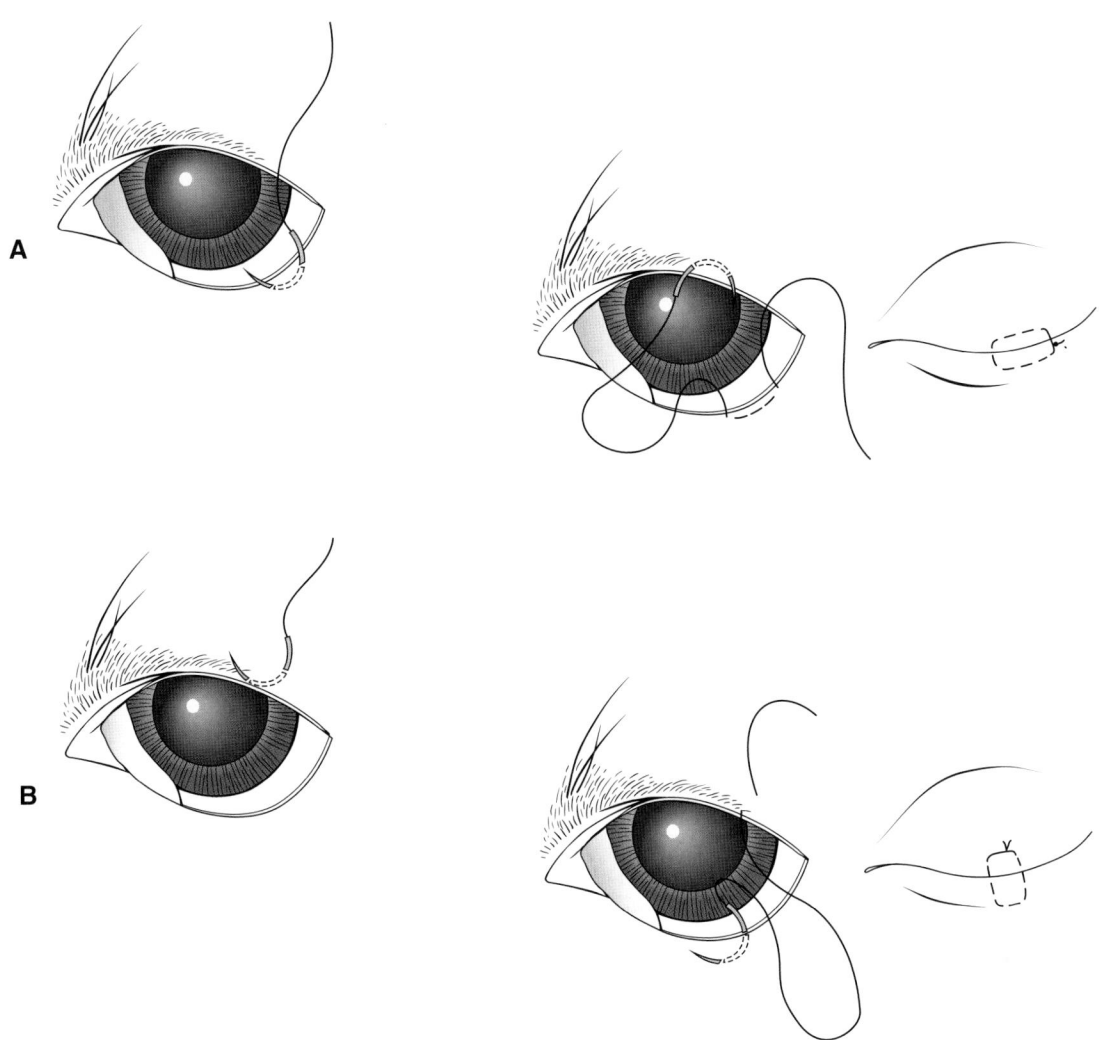

FIG. 16-6
Temporary tarsorrhaphy. **A,** Temporary closure of the eyelid achieved by orienting horizontal mattress suture parallel or perpendicular to the eyelid margin **(B)**. Sutures do not penetrate the full thickness of the eyelid.

penetrate the conjunctiva on the bulbar surface of the third eyelid (Fig. 16-8, B). Direct the suture back through the dorsolateral conjunctival fornix and out the upper eyelid. Apply tension on the suture, pulling the third eyelid over the cornea. Tie the suture over a stent, with the ends long enough to tie a bow so that the cornea may be inspected periodically (Fig. 16-8, C). As an alternative, use double-armed 3-0 to 0 nonabsorbable suture and begin by placing the suture midway along the length of the third eyelid and then through the fornix.

Enucleation or Exenteration

Enucleation is the removal of the globe, the nictitating membrane, and the lid margins. **Exenteration** is removal of the globe, nictitating membrane, orbital contents, and lid margins. Enucleation is indicated after severe ocular trauma,

intractable glaucoma, endophthalmitis, panophthalmitis, intraocular neoplasia, congenital defects, or intractable infections. Exenteration is indicated for intraorbital neoplasia or ocular neoplasia that has extended beyond the globe. Owners often are resistant to either procedure despite the predicted improvement for the animal.

Begin enucleation with a lateral canthotomy by incising 1 to 2 cm laterally from the junction of the upper and lower eyelid margins with scissors or a scalpel blade. Grasp the conjunctiva near the limbus with thumb forceps and make a 360° perilimbal incision (Fig. 16-9, A). Separate the conjunctiva, Tenon's capsule, and extraocular muscle from the sclera with curved Metzenbaum or enucleation scissors or an electrosurgical unit (Fig. 16-9, B). Remove the lacrimal gland located beneath the orbital ligament if it was not removed

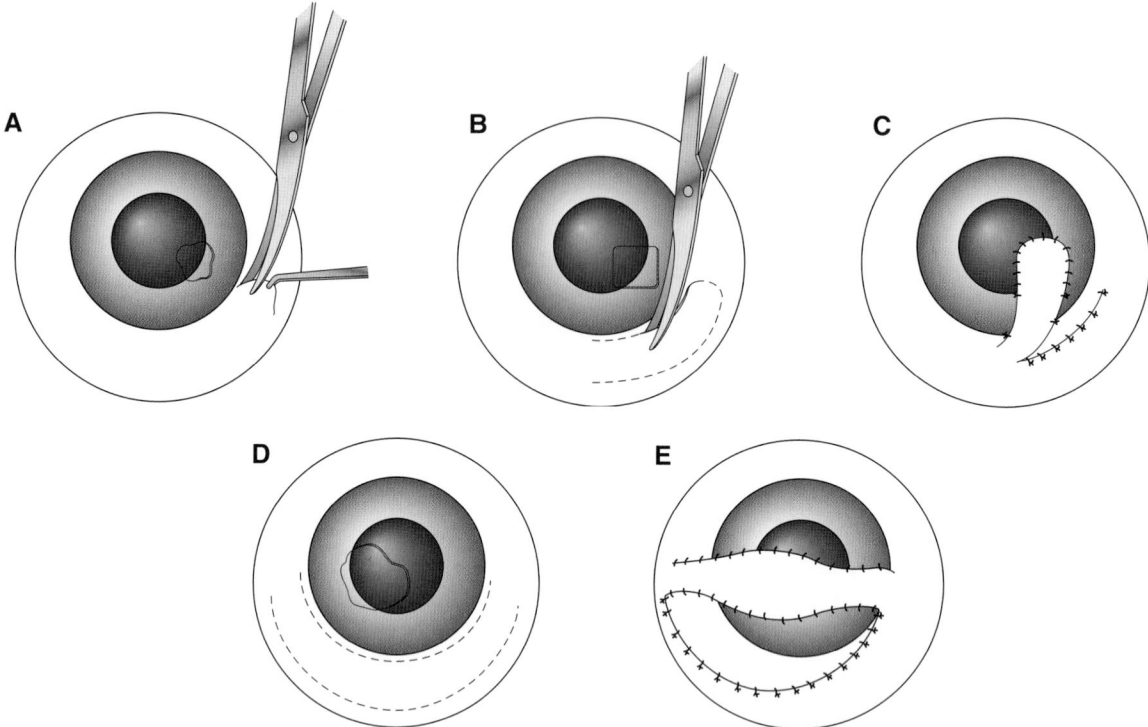

FIG. 16-7
Conjunctival flap. **A,** Prepare a thin sliding conjunctival flap by grasping the conjunctiva with ophthalmic forceps approximately 2 mm from the limbus; apply traction and incise with tenotomy scissors **(B)**. **C,** Elevate the flap, and rotate to cover the corneal defect. Place two sutures from the flap through half the depth of the limbus, then place additional continuous sutures. **D** and **E,** A bipedicle flap can be created and transposed for large corneal defects in a similar manner.

FIG. 16-8
Third eyelid flap. **A,** Pass a cutting needle through the upper eyelid in the dorsolateral conjunctival fornix. Exteriorize and extend the third eyelid with forceps and direct the needle through the external surface of the third eyelid, around the cartilage crossbar but not through the third eyelid on the bulbar surface. **B,** Direct the suture through the dorsolateral conjunctival fornix and out the upper eyelid. **C,** Tie the suture over a stent with a bow to allow release and periodic corneal inspection.

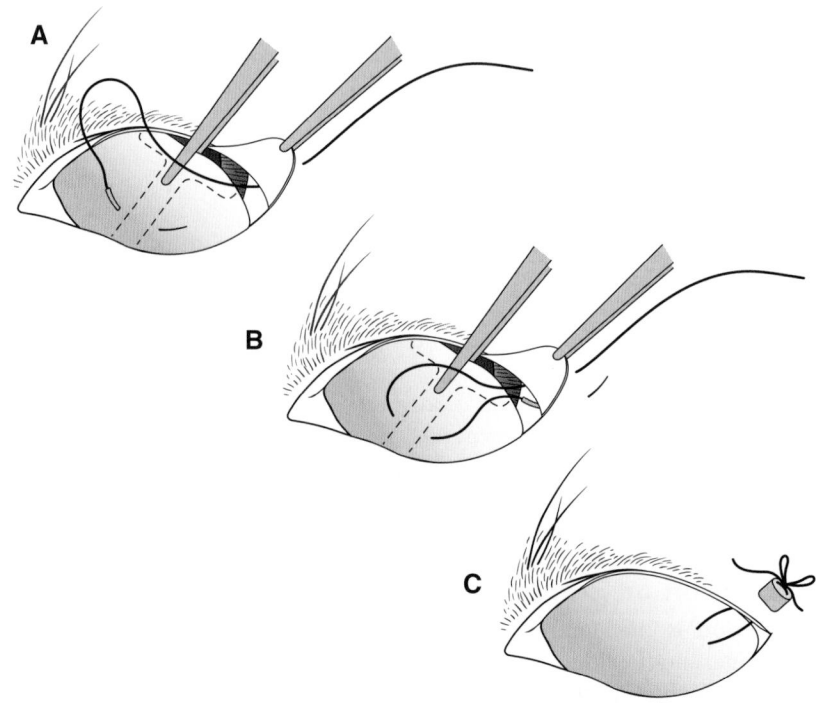

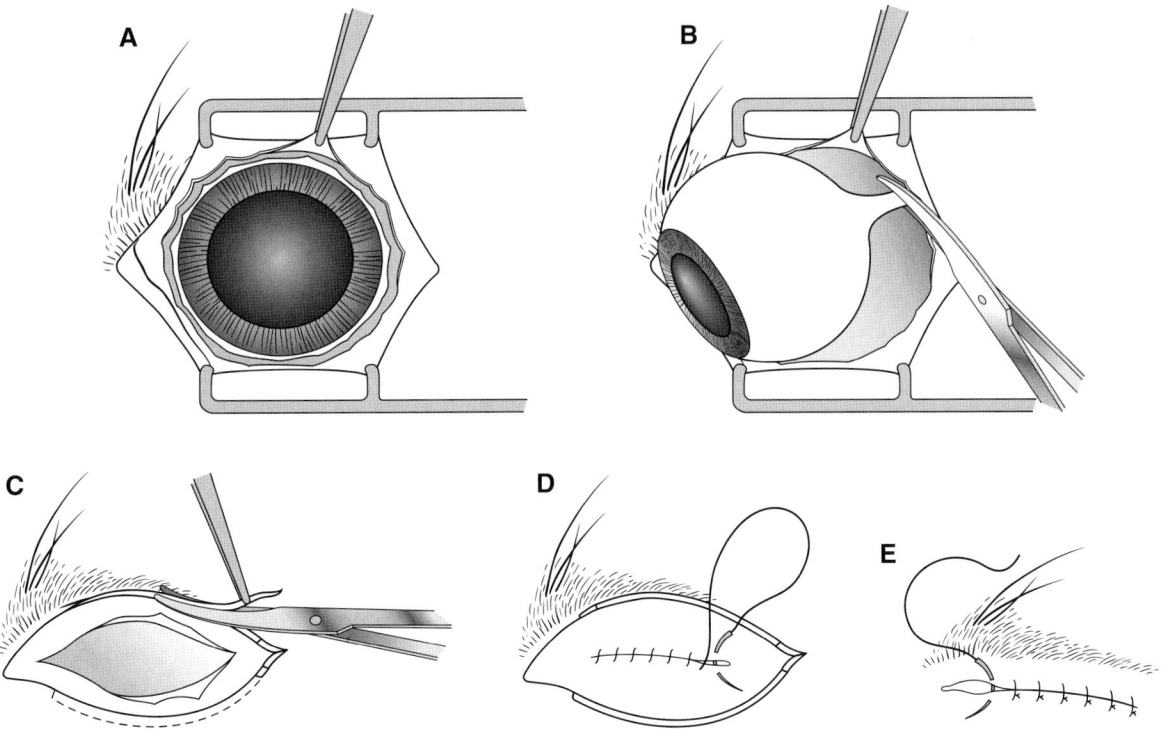

FIG. 16-9
Enucleation. **A,** Perform a lateral canthotomy, then grasp the conjunctiva at the limbus and make a 360° perilimbal incision. **B,** Separate the conjunctiva, Tenon's capsule, and extra-ocular muscles from the sclera, then sever the optic nerve. Attempts to ligate or visualize the optic nerve before severing results in excessive tension on the optic chiasm and may lead to blindness in the other eye. **C,** Excise 3 to 4 mm of the eyelid margins. **D,** Close the conjunctiva, Tenon's capsule, and orbital septum. **E,** Appose the subcutaneous tissue and skin of the eyelid margins.

with the globe. After freeing these attachments to the globe, sever the optic nerve with curved Metzenbaum or enucleation scissors (see Fig. 16-9, B). Avoid excess traction on the optic nerve because injury to the optic chiasm may damage vision in the remaining eye.

Attempts to ligate or visualize the optic nerve before severing it lead to excessive traction and may damage the optic chiasm.

Control hemorrhage with gentle pressure or calcium alginate. Excise the third eyelid and its gland. Excise 3 to 4 mm of the eyelid margins, stopping at the medial canthus (Fig. 16-9, C). Avoid the angularis oculi vein located superficial and medial to the medial canthal tendon. Insert an orbital prosthesis if appropriate after scarifying its surface to facilitate orbital retention. Close the conjunctiva, orbital septum, and Tenon's capsule with a simple continuous pattern using 3-0 absorbable suture (Fig. 16-9, D). Appose subcutaneous tissue with 3-0 or 4-0 absorbable appositional sutures and close the lid margins with 3-0 or 4-0 nonabsorbable appositional sutures (Fig. 16-9, E). Alternatively, begin the enucleation by suturing the eyelids together then incising circumfer-

entially 4 to 6 mm from the eyelid margin. Then with blunt dissection continue the incision under the conjunctival fornices and onto the globe under the bulbar conjunctiva. Excise the eyelid margins and entire palpebral, fornix, and bulbar conjunctivae and nictitating membrane en bloc. This variation reduces the chance of orbital contamination and infection from the conjunctiva and cornea.

Exenteration is performed much like enucleation, except that it begins by suturing the eyelids together and then excising their margins and conjunctiva, together with the globe, extraocular muscles, lacrimal gland, and zygomatic salivary gland. Surgical dissection is along the orbital walls, external to the extraocular muscles. In animals in which wide excision is necessary to remove all diseased tissue (i.e., neoplasia), creation of skin flaps may be necessary to allow primary wound closure.

NOTE: Cosmesis can be improved by using mesh or spherical orbital implants or by transposing the temporalis muscle to the orbit to prevent concavity after either enucleation or exenteration.

HEALING OF THE EYE

Healing of the eyelid skin and mucosa occurs as in other parts of the body. Superficial injuries to the cornea are quickly covered by epithelium. Epithelial cells lose cilia, flatten, and begin migration over a corneal wound defect within 1 hour. Fibronectin found in the defect temporarily helps maintain adhesion between the epithelial cells and extracellular matrix. After the defect has been covered, contact inhibition assists in halting epithelial migration. The entire cornea can be reepithelialized in 7 to 10 days. Once the cells have covered the defect, mitosis occurs and the multilayered epithelial surface is reconstituted. Attachment of the epithelium to the underlying basement membrane may be fragile for 6 to 8 weeks.

Uncomplicated stromal wounds undergo avascular healing, but in infected or destructive lesions vascular healing occurs as in other parts of the body. If the wound extends to the corneal stroma, the hydrophilic barrier of the corneal epithelium is lost, fluid is imbibed by the collagen fibril of the stroma, and corneal edema results. Within 24 hours, chemotaxis of leukocytes from the tear film and limbus coat the bottom of the lesion. Stromal keratocytes become reactive, transform into fibroblasts, and migrate into the lesion. Fibroblasts then produce collagen fibrils that are randomly deposited into the corneal wound. Macrophages move into the area to remove cellular debris after about 48 hours; they later transform into keratocytes. Collagen fibers in the regenerating stroma are irregular and decrease corneal transparency. Scar density decreases but the scar does not disappear over succeeding weeks. Release of various enzymes (collagenases, proteases) from degenerating corneal cells, leukocytes, and certain bacteria causes dissolution of the corneal stroma and can potentiate progression of the ulcer. Healing of the stroma takes several weeks to months. Vascularization is necessary to fill the defect with deep corneal ulcers. Cellular infiltration is more extensive, and blood vessels from the limbal plexus invade. This results in granulation tissue, loss of lamellar architecture, loss of corneal transparency, and scarring. Damaged corneal nerves gradually regenerate and sensation returns slowly to the affected area.

Corneal endothelium is very delicate tissue, and if it is damaged, permanent opacity may result. The elastic Descemet's membrane retracts and curls toward the anterior chamber, exposing stroma when damaged. Neighboring endothelial cells slide in to cover the area, and a new Descemet's membrane is formed. Endothelium may not cover extensive lesions and an area of swollen and edematous stroma persists.

SUTURE MATERIALS AND SPECIAL INSTRUMENTS

Ophthalmic surgery requires specialized equipment and ophthalmic or microsurgical instruments that are delicate, fragile, and often expensive. Magnification using head loupes (1.5× to 4×) or an operating microscope is recommended for most ophthalmic procedures. A focal light source is recommended to reduce reflections. Hand-held, battery-operated cautery units are ideal for controlling minor hemorrhage. Use cellulose sponge wedges for penetrating ocular wounds to avoid lint. Cryotherapy and laser equipment is useful for treatment of extraocular tumors and distichiasis. Absorbable and nonabsorbable small-gauge, soft-suture material (4-0 to 10-0) with swaged-on needles is used for most procedures. Use 4-0 to 6-0 soft pliable sutures for lids, 5-0 to 7-0 for conjunctiva, and 6-0 to 10-0 for cornea. Spatula or cutting micropoint needles are recommended for corneal suturing. Ophthalmic scalpel blades, forceps, scissors, needle holders, and retractors (specula) are also recommended because they are specially designed to be delicate, with fine tips and unique curves for specific purposes.

POSTOPERATIVE CARE AND ASSESSMENT

Recovery should be slow, calm, and smooth to prevent vocalizing, head thrashing, rubbing, or scratching the surgical site. Prevention of self-trauma by the patient is critical to prevent or minimize swelling of the eyelids, subconjunctival hemorrhage, hyphema, and anterior uveitis. Analgesics are essential to prevent pain and pruritus that might encourage the patient to rub and scratch the eye. Perioperative tranquilizers (acepromazine 0.03 to 0.1 mg/kg IM or SC) are also beneficial to prevent self-trauma. The eye is protected with an Elizabethan collar, which extends 4 to 8 cm beyond the animal's nose. Sometimes an eye bandage, paw bandages, or hobbles are also appropriate, but less effective than a collar. Frequent topical ocular medications may be necessary.

Assess surgical sites for anatomic alignment, inflammation, and edema. Sutures at the eyelid margin should have their knots external to the "gray line" to prevent corneal contact. Inflamed and swollen eyelids may develop temporary entropion. Chemosis (conjunctival edema) is expected when conjunctiva is incised or manipulated, but responds to corticosteroids and antiinflammatory medications. Medicate eyelid repairs with an ophthalmic antibiotic ointment for 5 to 7 days, and monitor for blepharospasm, tearing, or mucopurulent discharge, which may indicate that a corneal ulcer has formed. Epiphora may also indicate injury or fusion of the lacrimal canaliculi. Remove sutures at 10 to 14 days. Leave a stenting cannula in the lacrimal canaliculi for 4 to 6 weeks.

Evaluate the eye daily following corneal injuries. Laceration or ulceration of the cornea stimulates corneal nerve endings, causing pain and secondary iridocyclitis (reflex miosis, conjunctival and anterior uveal hyperemia, and altered blood-aqueous barrier). Following corneal incision or laceration repair, one should administer systemic, subconjunctival, and topical antibiotics; topical atropine; 10% phenylephrine; systemic corticosteroids; and antiprostaglandin drugs as needed. Use nonsteroidal antiinflammatory agents (i.e., carprofen) to reduce postoperative iridocyclitis, pain, and conjunctival and eyelid swelling. Use mydriatics

(1% atropine) daily to treat secondary uveitis and reduce the frequency as uveitis resolves. Begin topical corticosteroids after 10 to 14 days to reduce scarring if the cornea is fluorescein stain negative. Administer topical 20% acetylcysteine or autogenous serum to progressive corneal ulcers. Continue topical medications for 4 to 6 weeks, but discontinue systemic medications after 7 to 10 days if the anterior uveitis has resolved. Apply a restraint collar, and restrict exercise for 10 to 14 days. Remove the tarsorrhaphy sutures at 14 days and the corneal sutures at 21 days. When absorbable sutures are used, they do not need to be removed. Two to six weeks after application of tissue adhesives to small punctures or corneal ulcers, the adhesive is absorbed or extruded *en masse* or in fragments. Failure to seal the defect usually results from excessive adhesive application.

Partial temporary tarsorrhaphy is sometimes performed in conjunction with conjunctival flaps to reduce eyelid trauma to the surgical site, reduce exposure, provide pressure on the flap site, permit topical medication, allow patient vision, and facilitate daily ophthalmic examinations. Topical medications are administered to treat the corneal ulcer and secondary anterior uveitis. Complete advancement and pedicle conjunctival grafts are usually trimmed and the limbal base severed with the aid of topical anesthetic about 4 to 6 weeks postoperatively. Trimming the conjunctiva adhered to the cornea is not necessary unless excessive and protruding mucosa is present. These flaps will gradually conform to the corneal curvature and usually become pigmented. Check nictitating membrane flaps daily or every few days for proper positioning and adjust the position as necessary.

Following enucleation or exenteration, swelling and hemorrhage are minimized by applying cold compresses and counter pressure with an eye bandage. Antibiotics are appropriate if preexisting infections are present or if an ocular or orbital prosthesis is implanted.

COMPLICATIONS

The eyelid margin may not be perfect and may appear irregular or notched after repair of lacerations, entropion or ectropion, and tumor removal. Scar tissue at the eyelid margin can cause chronic irritation of the conjunctiva and cornea. Cicatricial scarring after trauma near the lid margin or overcorrection of entropion may cause ectropion. Failure to adequately correct entropion or ectropion results in persistent clinical signs. Corneal ulcers may occur following trauma to the cornea associated with lacerations or abrasions and periocular surgery. Blepharospasm, tearing, or mucopurulent discharge may indicate ulceration. Epiphora may also be a sign of unrecognized injury to the lacrimal canaliculi. Severe pruritus often occurs if inflammation persists because of infection, tissue trauma, or large or tight sutures. Pruritus may result in rubbing and self-trauma by the patient.

Complications following full-thickness corneal lacerations with iris prolapse include corneal edema, dense corneal scar formation, hyphema, hypopyon, anterior and posterior synechiae, iris deposits on the anterior lens capsule, cataract formation, and phthisis bulbi. Vision may be adversely affected with corneal scarring, the degree depending on the location and density of the scar. Phthisis bulbi is commonly secondary to severe anterior uveitis. These complications are minimized by adequate postoperative control of iridocyclitis. Corneal tissue adhesives may fail to seal an injury if too much is applied. The eyelids may adhere to the cornea if not retracted until the adhesive dries. Application of adhesives on small descemetoceles is contraindicated and may cause perforation.

Although success exceeds 90%, conjunctival flaps may fail if there is inadequate corneal wound débridement and if necrotic and infected tissue remains. Other causes of flap failure may be poor technique and local bacterial infections. Aqueous leakage under the flaps prevents adherence of the flap to the wound bed. Sutures occluding blood vessels in the flap may cause flap necrosis.

Nictitating membrane flaps may inhibit delivery of topical medications to the corneal surface; therefore, systemic medications are often used. Complications of nictitating membrane flaps include eyelid necrosis, corneal irritation from suture contact, cartilage deformation, and persistent protrusion following release. Eyelid swelling is expected. If suture contacts the cornea, the animal will be painful and have blepharospasm.

Complications following globe removal may include swelling due to hemorrhage, infection, and extrusion of the intraorbital prosthesis. Contracture of the orbital space and concavity of the permanent tarsorrhaphy may be noticeable without the use of a prosthesis, especially in short-haired dogs and cats. Glandular secretions or orbital swelling may be noted if the lacrimal gland or nictitating membrane glandular tissue persists. Occasionally, small fistulae develop from retained conjunctiva, resulting in small amounts of brown fluid that stain the eyelids. Rarely, orbital emphysema occurs because of communication with the nose through the nasolacrimal duct.

References

Bussieres M, Krohne SG, Stiles J et al: The use of porcine small intestinal submucosa for the repair of full-thickness corneal defects in dogs, cats and horses, *Vet Ophthalmol* 7:352, 2004.

Herring IP, Pickett JP, Champagne ES et al: Evaluation of aqueous tear production in dogs following general anesthesia, *J Am Anim Hosp Assoc* 36:427, 2000.

Mason DR, Lamb CR, McLellan GJ: Ultrasonographic findings in 50 dogs with retrobulbar disease, *J Am Anim Hosp Assoc* 37:557, 2001.

Stiles J, Hondra CN, Krohne SG et al: Effect of topical administration of 1% morphine sulfate solution on signs of pain and corneal wound healing in dogs, *Am J Vet Res* 64:813, 2003.

Suggested Reading

Gelatt KN, Gelatt JP: *Small animal ophthalmic surgery,* Oxford, 2001, Butterworth-Heinemann.
This is an easy to understand surgical reference book.

Slatter D: *Fundamentals of veterinary ophthalmology,* ed 3, Philadelphia, 2001, WB Saunders.
This is a general textbook on ophthalmology, which includes medical and surgical conditions.

Stiles J, Townsend W, Willis M et al: Use of a caudal auricular axial pattern flap in three cats and one dog following orbital exenteration, *Vet Ophthalmol* 6:121, 2003.
This report describes the flap technique and complications associated with its use.

Vygantas KR, Whitley RD: Management of deep corneal ulcers, *Compend Contin Educ Pract Vet* 25:196, 2003.
This review article discusses both medical and surgical management.

SPECIFIC DISEASES

ENTROPION

DEFINITIONS

Entropion is inward rolling of the eyelid margin, which may be developmental, spastic, or cicatricial.

GENERAL CONSIDERATIONS AND CLINICALLY RELEVANT PATHOPHYSIOLOGY

Entropion may affect the entire length of the lid margin, but is usually restricted to one area. It can be developmental or conformational, spastic, or cicatricial. Developmental entropion may not show up until later in life. Developmentally affected breeds often have specific areas of the eyelid that are involved. Spastic entropion infrequently occurs secondary to pain and blepharospasm associated with corneal foreign bodies, ulceration, chronic conjunctivitis, blepharitis, and keratitis. Cicatricial entropion is associated with eyelid scarring. Hair rubs on the cornea, causing irritation, epiphora, blepharospasm, photophobia, conjunctivitis, corneal ulceration, and vascularization.

DIAGNOSIS
Clinical Presentation

Signalment. Developmental or conformational entropion is a common condition in purebred dogs and is also seen in cats. Chinese Shar-Peis, Labrador retrievers, English bulldogs, chow chows, rottweilers, Saint Bernards, golden retrievers, Irish setters, Great Danes, English springer spaniels, American cocker spaniels, toy and miniature poodles, bull mastiffs, Chesapeake Bay retrievers, Norwegian elkhounds, and several sporting breeds are predisposed.

History. Animals have a history of epiphora and mucopurulent ocular discharge, rubbing the eyes, and photophobia. Signs may be intermittent early in the course of the condition. Developmental entropion usually affects both eyes, usually at the lateral aspect of the lower lid. Some animals will have both entropion and ectropion. Corneal foreign bodies, ulceration, chronic conjunctivitis, blepharitis, and keratitis may cause spastic entropion. Cicatricial entropion occurs after eyelid injury. Vision may be impaired in severe cases.

Physical Examination Findings

Diagnosis is made when inversion of the eyelid(s) is identified. The affected area is usually restricted to one portion of the eyelid margin, but the entire lid margin is involved in severe cases. In addition to epiphora and mucopurulent ocular discharge, there may be blepharospasm, eyelid discoloration, and excoriation. Breeds with abundant forehead skin (e.g., Chinese Shar-Pei, chow chow, bloodhound mastiff, and basset hound) commonly have both ptosis and entropion of the upper eyelid. Chronic cases may have corneal ulceration and vascularization. The conjunctiva may be reddened and inflamed.

Diagnostic Imaging

Imaging is unnecessary unless concurrent problems exist.

Laboratory Findings

No specific changes are expected in the CBC, chemistry panel, or urinalysis. Corneal ulceration may be identified on staining.

DIFFERENTIAL DIAGNOSIS

Entropion must be differentiated from enophthalmus and phthisis bulbi, which may mimic entropion but are not associated with pain and epiphora. Distichiasis, trichiasis, ectopic cilia, imperforate lacrimal puncta, dacryocystitis, and corneal injuries are other causes of epiphora. Corneal ulceration, distichiasis, ectopic cilia, and severe uveitis are other causes of blepharospasm.

MEDICAL MANAGEMENT

A nonsurgical method of treating entropion includes subcutaneous injection of an antibiotic such as procaine penicillin, which provides temporary eyelid margin eversion and relief from trichiasis and blepharospasm. The larger the volume injected, the greater the eyelid margin eversion. Surgical correction is generally required. Corneal ulcers and conjunctivitis are treated medically. Treatment of the underlying cause of spastic entropion sometimes relieves the spasm, although surgery is often necessary for correction.

SURGICAL TREATMENT

Various methods of treating entropion have been described. Selection of technique is based on the species, severity, and position of the abnormality.

Preoperative Management

Initiate treatment for corneal ulcers and conjunctivitis before surgery. Before anesthetizing the animal, evert the lid to estimate the amount of skin to be removed.

Anesthesia

See p. 261.

Surgical Anatomy

See p. 261.

Positioning

Position animals with bilateral entropion in ventral recumbency; those with unilateral lateral entropion may be positioned in lateral recumbency.

SURGICAL TECHNIQUES

Success is greater and complications fewer if there is minimal tissue trauma, accurate tissue resection, and good hemostasis.

Eyelid Tacking

Entropion in the neonate or young animal (up to 20 weeks of age), especially Shar-Pei puppies, may be temporarily everted to a more normal position using a drop of tissue adhesive to glue adjacent skin surfaces together, thereby rolling the eyelid margin outward, or by placement of inverting Lembert sutures. Treatment of Shar-Pei puppies at 2 to 4 weeks of age and maintenance of a normal position for 10 to 20 days may effectively resolve the inversion.

Using 3-0 or 4-0 absorbable or nonabsorbable suture (e.g., polypropylene), insert the needle into the skin and through the tarsal plate and orbicularis muscle 3 mm from the eyelid margin. Exit the needle 5 mm from its insertion to complete the first bite (Fig. 16-10). Position the second bite over the rim of the orbit with the needle directed away from the eye. Pass the needle through the skin, subcutaneous tissue, and orbital fascia and exit, creating a second 5-mm bite (see Fig. 16-10). Do not penetrate the eyelid margin or conjunctiva. Tie the suture, inverting a furrow of skin. Place additional sutures (3 to 14) as necessary to correct both upper and lower lid entropion. Alternatively, place skin staples after inverting the skin. Place a few drops of surgical glue within the created furrow to reduce tension on the suture line. This keeps the sutures in place longer and helps keep them from being rubbed out.

The tacking procedure is repeated in young dogs until maturity, if necessary, to prevent corneal damage. Permanent correction by excision of tissue is delayed until the animal reaches adult or near-adult conformation. Tacking may be used for spastic entropion to provide relief from corneal irritation until the primary cause is corrected.

Excisional Procedures

In severe cases or in mature animals, skin resection is necessary to correct entropion. In extreme cases, stellate rhytidectomy to remove skin from the dorsal region of the head or brow suspension with sutures has been used successfully. Various adaptations of the Hotz-Celsus or "pinch" procedure is the most commonly used procedure to provide definitive surgical correction for chronic or recurring entropion. The amount of eversion is determined by the amount of skin removed and proximity of the incision to the lid margin. The closer the incision is to the lid margin, the more pronounced the eversion. Concurrent distichiasis should be treated at the time of entropion repair using the tarsoconjunctival resection technique or cryoablation.

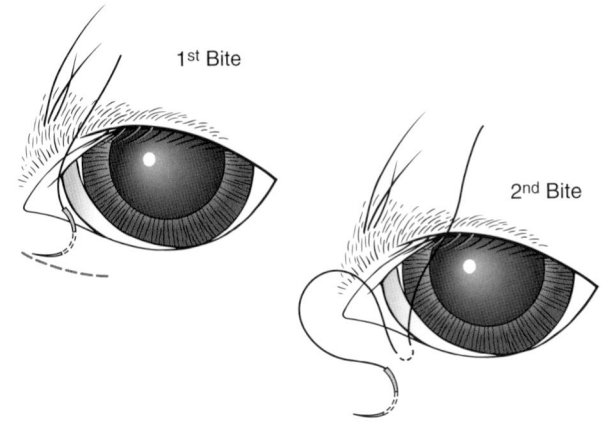

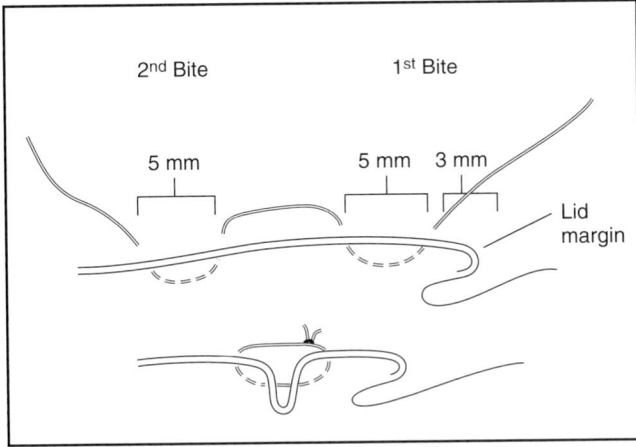

FIG. 16-10
Entropion-eyelid tacking. Use Lembert sutures in the neonate to temporarily evert the eyelid margin. The first bite is 5 mm wide and begins 3 mm from the eyelid margin *(inset)*. Position the second 5-mm-wide bite over the rim of the orbit, biting into the orbital fascia. Tie the suture, inverting a furrow of skin. A few drops of surgical glue placed within the created furrow minimize tension on the sutures and helps maintain their position if the patient rubs at the eyes.

Estimate the size of the ellipse to be removed by tenting the skin in the area of entropion with thumb forceps (Fig. 16-11, A). Stabilize the eyelid by placing a Jaeger eyelid plate into the conjunctival fornix under the affected eyelid and gently pull and stretch the lid (Fig. 16-11, B).

Some surgeons place a curved Halsted or Crile forceps across the skin to be excised.

Using a No. 15 blade, incise along the length of the entropion, beginning 1 to 3 mm from the lid margin (see Fig. 16-11, B). Make a second, crescent-shaped skin incision a distance from the first incision sufficient to correct the entropion.

The amount of surgical correction should allow for 0.5 to 1 mm of additional eversion of the eyelid margin that occurs with healing.

Remove the strip of skin. Do not remove orbicularis muscle or conjunctiva. Close the defect (Fig. 16-11, C and D) beginning

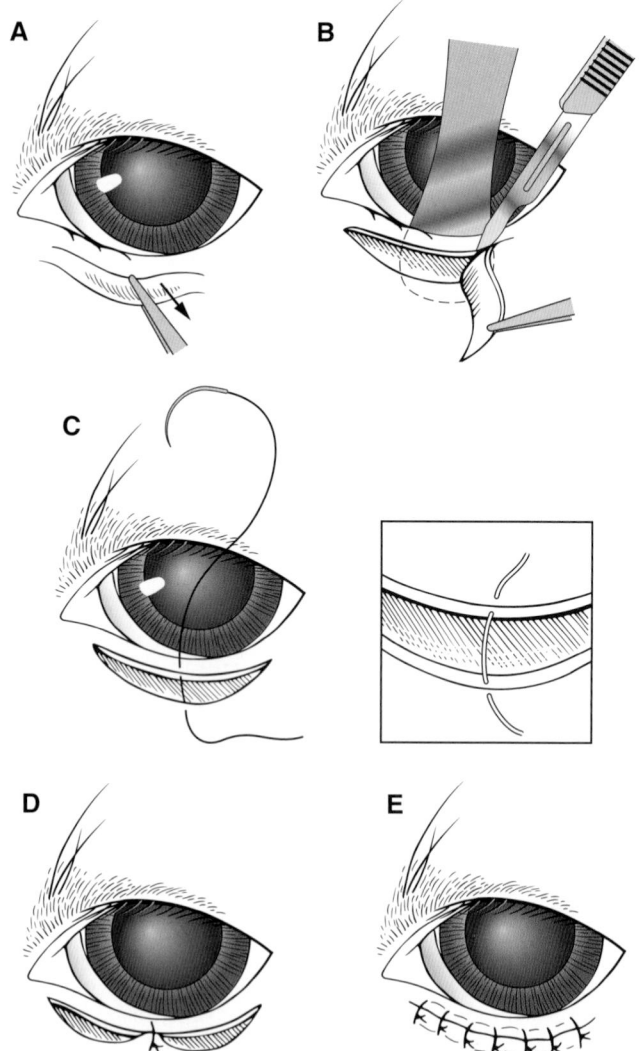

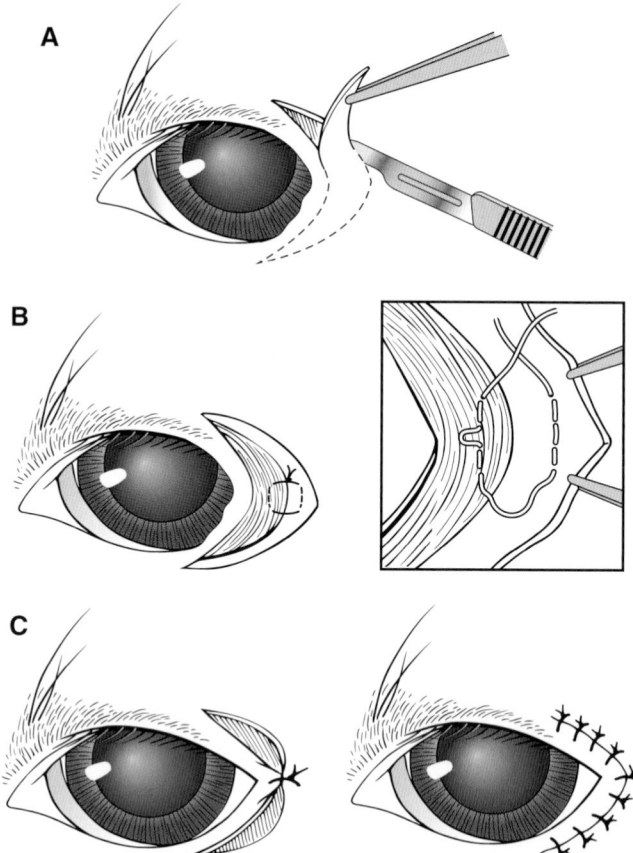

FIG. 16-11
Hotz-Celsus procedure for entropion repair. **A,** Using thumb forceps, tent the skin in the area of the entropion to estimate the size of the ellipse to be removed. **B,** Stabilize the lid by placing a Jaeger eyelid plate into the conjunctival fornix. Incise along the length of the entropion beginning 3 mm from the lid margin and remove a crescent-shaped piece of skin. **C,** Begin closing the defect at the center of the wound with a simple interrupted split-thickness skin suture *(inset).* **D** and **E,** Place additional sutures 2 to 3 mm apart.

at the center with simple interrupted split-thickness 4-0 to 6-0 nonabsorbable skin sutures to allow more precise skin apposition (see inset, Fig. 16-11, C). Split the distance of the remaining defect when placing additional sutures so that ultimately sutures are spaced 1.5 to 3 mm apart (Fig. 16-11, E). Cut suture ends that are directed toward the eye short (2 mm) to prevent corneal irritation.

An arrowhead modification of the Hotz-Celsus procedure is performed when lateral canthus inversion is the predominant component of the entropion. This procedure is performed using a V-shaped or arrowhead resection at the lateral canthus rather than an elliptic incision (Fig. 16-12).

FIG. 16-12
Arrowhead modification of the Hotz-Celsus procedure is performed when the lateral canthus is inverted. **A,** Make a V-shaped or arrowhead resection at the lateral canthus. **B,** Place a horizontal suture from the deep fascia overlying the orbital ligament to fascia beneath the skin. **C,** Begin skin closure at the center of the wound, then place additional sutures 2 to 3 mm apart.

In addition, a subcutaneous lateral canthal tension suture is placed to anchor and stabilize the lateral canthus in a more lateral position (see Fig. 16-12). A horizontal mattress suture is placed into the lateral canthal fascia and orbicularis muscle deep to the skin incision and fascia overlying the orbital ligament. In other cases, a lateral canthal tenectomy will relieve tension at the lateral canthus.

An alternative to the technique of elliptic skin excision is to use a Y-to-V correction (Fig. 16-13). This technique is recommended for cicatricial entropion.

Place an eyelid plate or sterile tongue depressor into the lower conjunctival fornix for support. Make a Y-shaped incision with the arms of the Y extending just beyond the affected segment of the eyelid. Determine the length of the stem of the Y incision by applying traction to the skin flap until the eyelid margin is in a normal position (see Fig. 16-13). Undermine the skin flap, resecting any scar tissue present, then suture the point of the flap to the most distal aspect of the incision. Appose the remainder of the skin with approximating sutures (4-0 to 6-0 nonabsorbable).

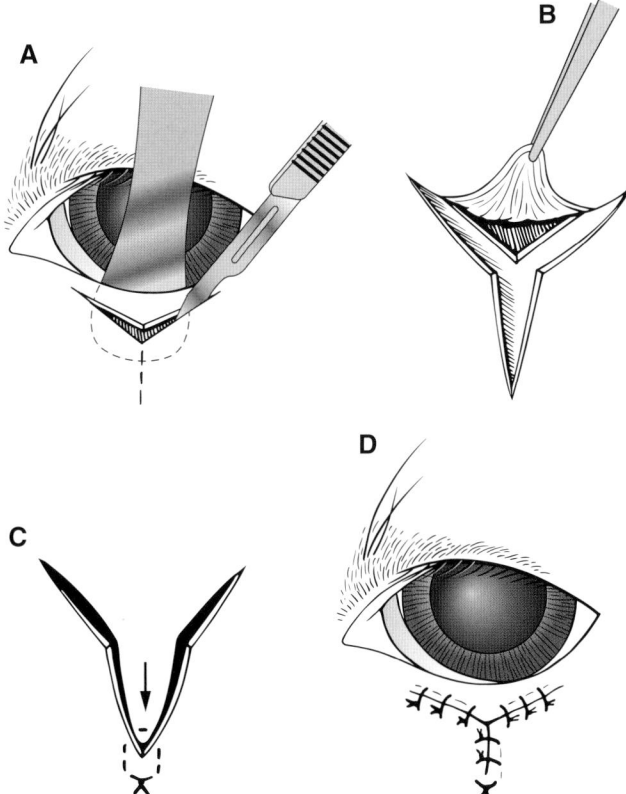

FIG. 16-13
Y-to-V correction for cicatricial entropion. **A,** Make a Y-shaped incision with the arms of the Y extending just beyond the affected segment of eyelid. Apply traction to the skin flap until the margin of the eyelid is in normal position to determine the length of the Y-stem incision. **B,** Undermine the flap and remove scar tissue. **C,** Suture the point of the flap to the most distal aspect of the incision. **D,** Appose the remainder of the incision.

Small focal areas of entropion may also be treated with removal of a circular rather than an elliptical piece of skin. This "trephine" technique is accomplished using a 6-to 7-mm skin biopsy punch. The circular defect is closed as described with the "pinch" technique.

The tarsal pedicle procedure is used in animals that need additional lid eversion because of the severity of the condition or its recurrence.

Make a curvilinear incision 3 to 4 mm distal and parallel to the lid margin in the area of entropion. Deepen the incision to the orbicularis oculi muscle. Make two parallel incisions at right angles to the lid margin through the orbicularis oculi muscle and the tarsus. Dissect the pedicle from the skin and palpebral conjunctiva to its base at the lid margin. Using tenotomy scissors, create a tunnel through the subcutaneous tissues distal to the pedicle.

The tunnel's length depends on the severity of the entropion and the degree of eversion required.

Place a cruciate or Bunnell suture pattern in the pedicle using double-armed, nonabsorbable suture material (e.g., nylon

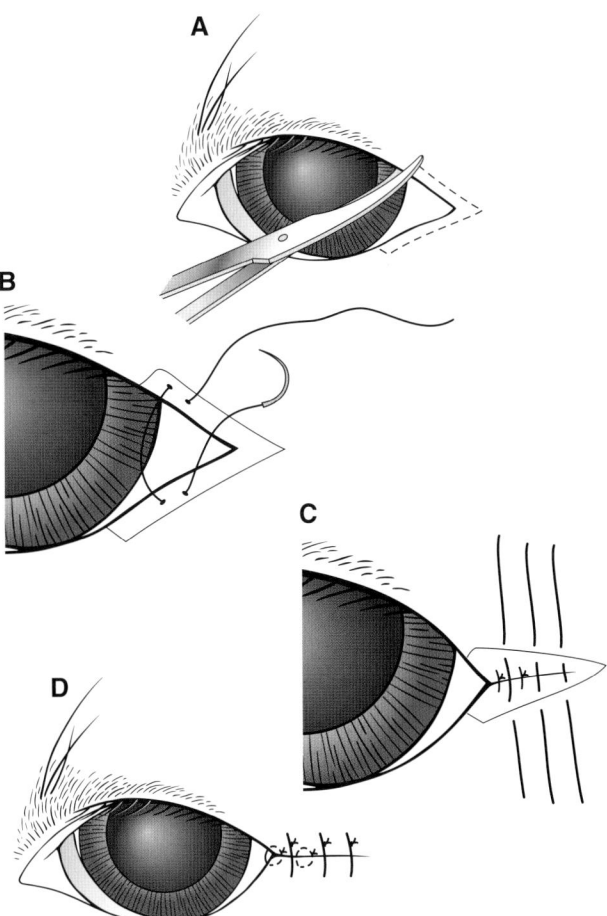

FIG. 16-14
Permanent lateral tarsorrhaphy. **A,** Excise upper and lower lid margins at the lateral canthus, removing a V-shaped segment of skin. **B,** Place intradermal or subcuticular sutures to realign the skin edges. **C** and **D,** Place skin sutures to precisely align the eyelid margins and appose the skin.

or polypropylene). Pass the suture ends through the subcutaneous tunnel, skin, and a piece of elastic band. Tie the suture with enough tension to evert the lid margin the desired amount. Create more than one pedicle if the entropion is long and not corrected by one pedicle. Excise overlapping skin edges, and then appose the skin.

Permanent lateral tarsorrhaphy can be combined with other procedures to correct entropion associated with enlarged palpebral fissures (Fig. 16-14). Facial skin fold excision, lateral canthoplasty, and medial canthoplasty procedures have also been described to aid entropion correction. A medial canthoplasty is generally preferred in brachycephalic breeds to correct the nasal entropion, protect the cornea from facial folds, and correct lagophthalmos.

SUTURE MATERIALS AND SPECIAL INSTRUMENTS

Use fine (4-0 to 6-0) nonabsorbable suture material swaged onto a fine cutting needle. Ophthalmic instruments are useful, including a needle holder, thumb forceps, entropion clamp or

Jaeger eyelid plate, and tenotomy scissors. A skin biopsy punch can be used when entropion affects only a small area.

POSTOPERATIVE CARE AND ASSESSMENT

Recover the animal quietly to prevent trauma to the surgical sites. Protect the area after surgery by applying a restraint collar (Elizabethan collar). Give analgesics as needed for the first 2 to 3 days. Apply antibiotics and corticosteroids topically after surgery. Use antibiotics (without steroids) and mydriatics if corneal ulceration is present.

Following eyelid tacking procedures, apply topical antibiotic ointment for 10 to 14 days and leave sutures for 2 to 3 weeks or until suture abscesses or granulomas are recognized. Most Shar-Pei puppies respond to the tacking procedure.

Following excision techniques, expect minimal eyelid swelling postoperatively, which should resolve within 48 hours. As a result of inflammation and edema, ectropion may be present postoperatively; therefore delay assessment of the adequacy of correction until swelling subsides (5 to 7 days). If undercorrection has occurred, repeat the procedure. Repeat surgery is more commonly necessary when the initial procedure is performed in young and growing animals. Remove the sutures at approximately 10 days. Maintain the Elizabethan collar for 2 to 3 days after suture removal if the animal wants to scratch the site. Corneal lesions usually resolve rapidly after surgical correction. Treat purulent secondary bacterial conjunctivitis with topical antibiotics.

COMPLICATIONS

Complications include undercorrection or overcorrection. Correction of severely affected animals, especially Shar-Peis, should be performed by an experienced ophthalmologist or surgeon. If the incisions are placed too far from the eyelid margin, there is a tendency for undercorrection. There is a greater chance of suture damaging the cornea if incisions are made too close to the eyelid margin or if suture ends are long. A completely normal eyelid contour may not always be possible. Incisions for medial entropion may damage the lower lacrimal punctum and canaliculus if made deeper than the orbicularis oculi muscle. Removal of the orbicularis oculi muscle increases hemorrhage, postoperative edema, and infection. Breeds with excessive forehead skin folds complicate entropion surgery by requiring concurrent resection, which may alter appearance. Self-trauma may result in dehiscence.

PROGNOSIS

Although achieving a completely normal eyelid contour is not always possible, signs associated with entropion resolve following appropriately selected and performed entropion procedures.

Suggested Reading

Gelatt, KN, Gelatt JP: *Small animal ophthalmic surgery,* Oxford, 2001, Butterworth-Heinemann.

This is a general textbook on ophthalmology, which includes medical and surgical conditions.

Hamilton HL, McLaughlin SA, Whitley RD et al: Diagnosis and blepharoplastic repair of conformational eyelid defects, *Compend Cont Educ Pract Vet* 22:588, 2000.

This is a well illustrated review of several techniques for entropion and ectropion correction.

McCallum P, Welser J: Coronal rhytidectomy in conjunction with deep plane walking sutures, modified Hotz-Celsus and lateral canthoplasty procedure in a dog with excessive brow droop, *Vet Ophthalmol* 7(5):376, 2004.

This case report describes radical skin resection to facilitate entropion repair in a bloodhound.

Slatter D: *Fundamentals of veterinary ophthalmology,* ed 3, Philadelphia, 2001, WB Saunders.

This is a general textbook on ophthalmology, which includes medical and surgical conditions.

Van der Woerdt, Alexandra: Adnexal surgery in dogs and cats, *Vet Ophthalmol* 7:284, 2004.

This review article summarizes procedures appropriate for adnexal surgery. No illustrations are included.

ECTROPION

DEFINITIONS

Ectropion is eversion of the lower eyelid.

GENERAL CONSIDERATIONS AND CLINICALLY RELEVANT PATHOPHYSIOLOGY

Ectropion may be a developmental condition or one acquired secondary to scar tissue formation or fatigue of the orbicularis oculi muscle. In some breeds, the eyelids and palpebral fissure are excessive in size. In some large and giant breeds of dogs, the laxity of the lower eyelid may vary with fitness and age. The drooping eyelid allows tears to escape (epiphora) and exposes the conjunctiva to drying and trauma. This leads to tear staining and development of chronic keratitis, conjunctivitis, and keratoconjunctivitis. Some of the pathology is associated with an impaired blink reflex, preocular film defects, and impaired tear movement to the medial conjunctival sac.

DIAGNOSIS
Clinical Presentation

Signalment. The predisposition to having droopy eyelids is seen in breeds such as Saint Bernards, bloodhounds, cocker spaniels, and basset hounds. Other frequently affected breeds include Great Danes, Newfoundlands, and mastiffs.

History. Developmental ectropion is usually breed-associated (St. Bernard, bloodhound, cocker spaniel) and may be seen in dogs with loose facial skin. Intermittent or physiologic entropion is seen in large hunting breeds (golden retriever, Irish setter, Labrador retriever). These dogs appear normal in the morning, but have droopy eyelids late in the day. Signs of ectropion include exposed conjunctiva, epiphora, conjunctivitis, or keratitis.

Physical Examination Findings

Diagnosis is made when "out turning" of the lid is recognized. Some animals have abnormally large eyelids and palpebral fissures. Central ectropion may also be associated with lateral canthal entropion. Signs of ectropion include exposed conjunctiva, epiphora, conjunctivitis (congestion and inflammation), or keratitis. Corneal neovascularization and pigmentation are seen in severe cases. Exfoliative blepharitis may be caused by epiphora.

Diagnostic Imaging

Diagnostic imaging is unnecessary unless concurrent problems exist.

Laboratory Findings

No specific changes are expected in the CBC, chemistry panel, or urinalysis. Corneal ulceration may be identified on staining.

DIFFERENTIAL DIAGNOSIS

Ectropion must be differentiated from eyelid trauma. Other causes of epiphora include distichiasis, trichiasis, ectopic cilia, imperforate lacrimal puncta, dacryocystitis, and corneal injuries. Conjunctivitis may also be caused by microorganisms, parasites, allergens, foreign bodies, toxins, or precorneal film deficiency.

MEDICAL MANAGEMENT

Treat corneal ulcers and conjunctivitis as described on p. 270.

SURGICAL TREATMENT

Developmental ectropion and ectropion caused by scar tissue that causes conjunctival or corneal lesions may be corrected by a variety or combination of surgical techniques. Surgical correction of intermittent ectropion is contraindicated. The goal of surgery is to provide a relatively normal length to the lower eyelid; most procedures shorten and strengthen the lid. Selection of technique is based on the species, severity, and position of the abnormality. Most procedures involve the lateral one half of the lower eyelid and lateral canthus to avoid the nasolacrimal apparatus and nictitating membrane. Correction is required less frequently than with entropion, and only when it causes conjunctivitis, corneal vascularization or pigmentation, or exfoliative blepharitis from epiphora.

Preoperative Management

Initiate treatment for corneal ulcers and conjunctivitis before surgery. Before anesthetizing the animal, estimate the amount of skin to be removed.

Anesthesia

See p. 261.

Surgical Anatomy

See p. 261.

Positioning

Position animals with bilateral ectropion in ventral recumbency; those with unilateral lateral ectropion may be positioned in lateral recumbency.

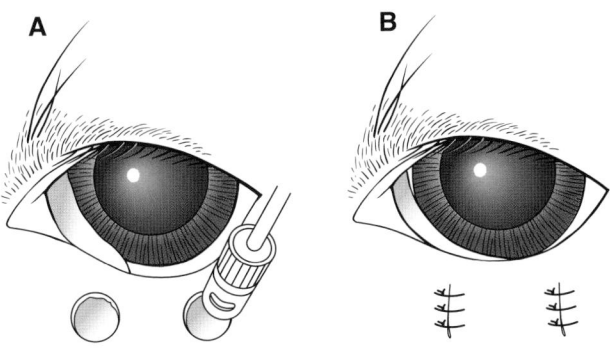

FIG. 16-15
Trephination for mild ectropion correction. **A,** Use a skin biopsy punch to remove several small circles of skin 3 to 4 mm from the eyelid margin. **B,** Place sutures to close the defect and realign the skin edges in a vertical direction.

SURGICAL TECHNIQUES

Success is greater and complications fewer if there is minimal tissue trauma, accurate tissue resection, and good hemostasis.

> NOTE: Always estimate the amount of excess skin to be resected before administering preoperative sedation or anesthetic.

Trephination

Trephination is used when ectropion is mild.

Using a skin biopsy punch (5 to 7 mm), remove one or more circles of skin distal (3 to 4 mm) to the affected portion of the eyelid margin. Appose the skin edges with two to four sutures (4-0 to 6-0 nonabsorbable suture) such that the closure is perpendicular to the lid margin (Fig. 16-15).

Wedge Resection

Wedge resection is used for mild to severe cases of ectropion. The size of the wedge should be slightly smaller than the extent of eyelid shortening and correction anticipated as an additional 0.5 to 1 mm correction occurs with fibrosis.

Resect a triangular full-thickness wedge of skin from the lateral aspect of the lower eyelid near the lateral canthus. Mark the site of incision laterally by nicking or crushing, then manipulate the redundant lid laterally with thumb forceps to determine the amount of lid margin to resect (Fig. 16-16, A). Make the sides of the excised triangle twice the length of the base of the triangle to facilitate apposition. Excise this segment of skin as a triangle with its base at the lid margin (Fig. 16-16, B). Appose the conjunctiva using a simple continuous pattern of absorbable suture with knots buried between conjunctiva and skin (Fig. 16-16, C). Align and accurately appose the eyelid margin with a simple interrupted or cruciate suture, then place additional skin sutures (4-0 to 6-0 absorbable), positioning and cutting suture ends so that they do not rub on the cornea (Fig. 16-16, D).

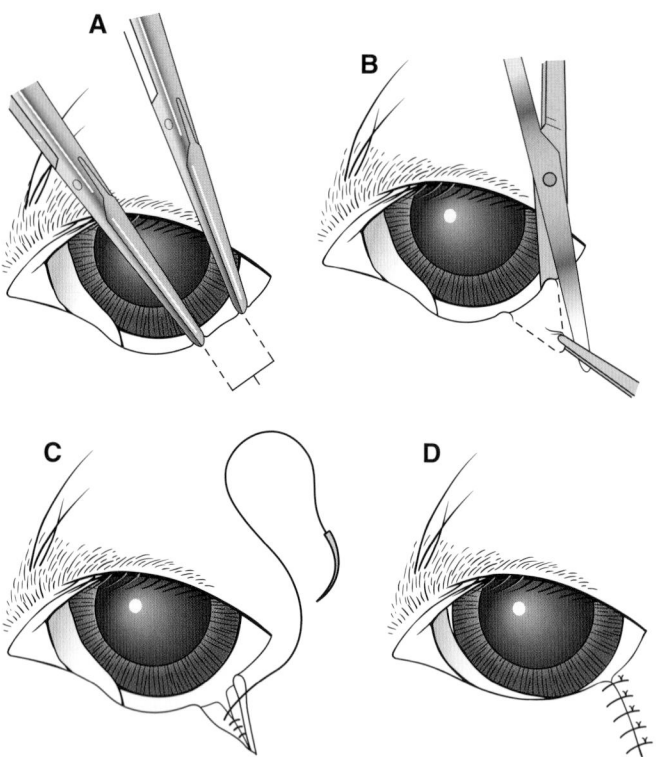

FIG. 16-16
Wedge resection for ectropion correction. **A,** Mark the width of resection by nicking or crushing the eyelid margin. **B,** Excise a triangle of skin with the base at the lid margin. For good apposition, the sides of the triangle should be twice the length of the base. **C,** Appose the conjunctiva using a simple continuous pattern. **D,** Align and accurately appose the lid margin with a simple interrupted skin suture, then place additional skin sutures.

Conjunctival Resection

Conjunctival resection may be performed alone or in combination with other ectropion procedures to improve cosmetic results.

Grasp the palpebral conjunctiva in the ventral fornix with forceps; elevate and then clamp parallel to the lid margin with hemostats for 30 seconds. Remove the hemostats and excise the defined area of the conjunctiva. Appose the incised edges with a simple continuous pattern of absorbable suture (4-0 to 6-0).

V-Y Correction

A V-Y correction is commonly used for cicatricial ectropion from wounds, tumor excision, or overcorrection of entropion when resection of a small wedge of tissue is insufficient. It is especially useful for lesions with a broad contracting scar. This procedure tightens but does not substantially shorten the eyelid margin.

Make a V-shaped incision distal to and slightly wider than the area of the ectropion (Fig. 16-17, A). Begin the incision about 1 mm from the eyelid margin. Undermine the flap to near its

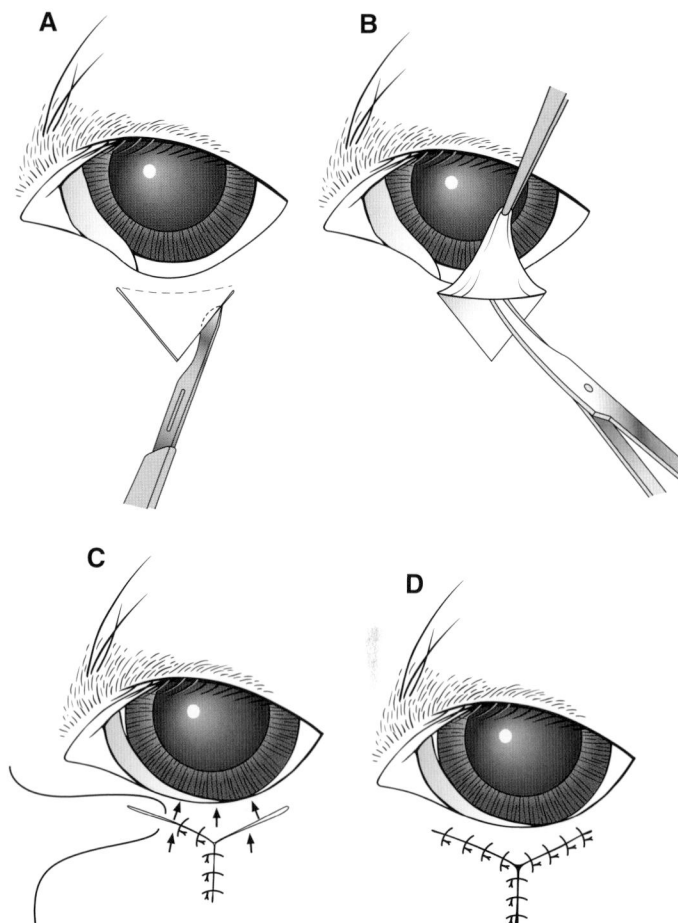

FIG. 16-17
V-to-Y ectropion correction. **A,** Make a V-shaped incision distal and slightly wider than the ectropion area. **B,** Undermine the flap to near the eyelid margin and remove scar tissue if present. **C,** Beginning at the most distal aspect of the V, begin placing sutures from medial to lateral, creating the stem of the Y. **D,** Close the arms of the Y when the desired position of the lid is obtained.

base on the eyelid and remove any scar tissue (Fig. 16-17, B). Beginning at the most distal aspect of the V incision, begin placing sutures (4-0 to 6-0 nonabsorbable) from medial to lateral, creating the stem of the Y (Fig. 16-17, C). The length of the stem of the Y depends on how much elevation the lid margin requires to return it to a normal position (estimated as defect + 2 to 3 mm). When the desired position of the lid has been obtained, appose the arms of the Y (Fig. 16-17, D).

A temporary tarsorrhaphy (see Fig. 16-17) may be needed to help prevent contracture along the suture lines during healing. Severe cases of cicatricial ectropion may attain more release using a Z-plasty with the central limb of the Z coinciding with the line of traction of the scar (p. 200).

Modified Kuhnt-Szymanowski Procedure

The modified Kuhnt-Szymanowski procedure reduces the risk of scarring the lid margin and damaging cilia or meibomian glands in animals with atonic ectropion.

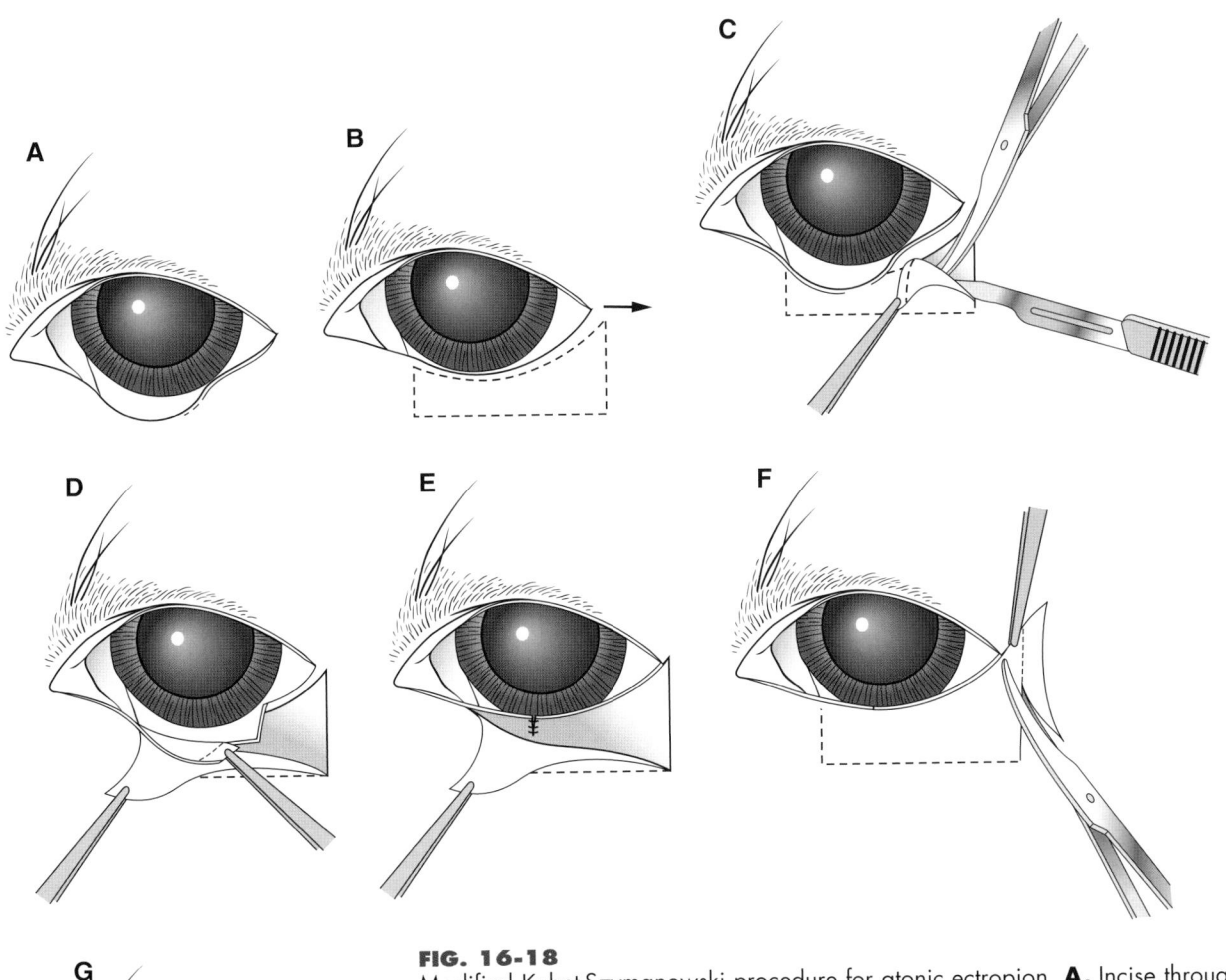

FIG. 16-18
Modified Kuhnt-Szymanowski procedure for atonic ectropion. **A,** Incise through skin and orbicularis oculi muscle 3 mm distal and parallel to the lid margin along the lateral half to three fourths of the lower lid. **B,** Continue the incision dorsolaterally 1 cm beyond the lateral canthus. Make a second incision from the termination of this incision 1.5 cm distally. **C,** Undermine this flap of tissue. **D,** Remove redundant lid by excising a wedge of lid margin and tarsoconjunctiva near the medial aspect of the first incision. **E,** Close the tarsoconjunctiva with a simple continuous suture pattern beginning at the lid margin. **F,** Pull the skin and muscle flap dorsolaterally, and excise a triangle of the excess skin laterally. **G,** Appose the skin with interrupted appositional sutures.

Incise through the skin and orbicularis oculi muscle 3 mm distal and parallel to the lid margin along the lateral one half to three fourths of the lower lid (Fig. 16-18, A). Continue the incision dorsolaterally 1 cm beyond the lateral canthus (Fig. 16-18, B). Make a second incision from the termination of this incision near the lateral canthus 1.5 cm distally (Fig. 16-18, C). Undermine this flap of tissue. Remove redundant lid tissue by excising a wedge of lid margin and tarsoconjunctiva near the medial aspect of the first incision (Fig. 16-18, D). Close the tarsoconjunctiva with a simple continuous suture pattern (4-0 to 6-0 absorbable) beginning at the lid margin (Fig. 16-18, E). Then pull the skin and muscle flap dorsolaterally and excise a triangle of the excess skin laterally (Fig. 16-18, F). Close the skin with interrupted appositional sutures (4-0 to 6-0 nonabsorbable) (Fig. 16-18, G).

Lateral Blepharoplasty

Lateral blepharoplasty can be performed for animals with combined entropion-ectropion. This procedure combines the Hotz-Celsus technique for entropion with creation of a lateral ligament from the orbicularis oculi muscle.

Excise a pinch of redundant skin from both the upper and lower eyelids, which meet at the lateral canthus (Fig. 16-19, A). Extend the incision laterally from the lateral canthus to the temporal bone. Dissect a corresponding strip of orbicularis oculi muscle from both the upper and lower excision sites, which remain attached at the lateral canthus. Using 4-0 absorbable suture material (e.g., polydioxanone), suture the ends of the muscle pedicles together and retract them laterally. Then tack the muscle pedicles to

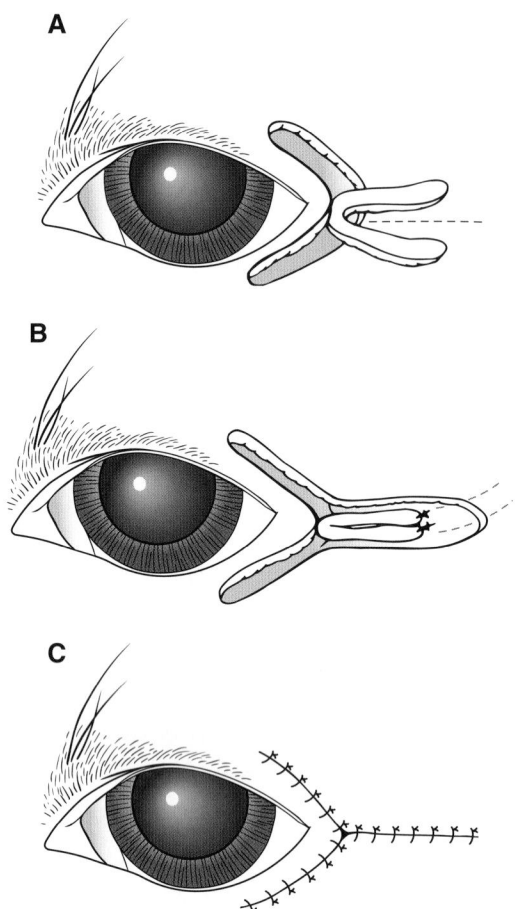

FIG. 16-19
Lateral blepharoplasty for animals with combined entropion-ectropion. **A,** Excise an ellipse of skin from the upper and lower lids, which meets at the lateral canthus. Extend the incision laterally to the temporal bone. Dissect a corresponding strip of orbicularis oculi from both the upper and lower excision sites, which remains attached at the lateral canthus. **B,** Suture the muscle pedicles together, retract them laterally, and suture them to the periosteum over the temporal bone. **C,** Place appositional sutures to appose the skin.

*the periosteum over the temporal bone (Fig. 16-19, B).
Place appositional sutures (4-0 to 6-0 nonabsorbable) to
close the skin (see Fig. 16-19, C).*

SUTURE MATERIALS AND SPECIAL INSTRUMENTS

Use fine (4-0 to 6-0) nonabsorbable suture material swaged onto a fine cutting needle. Ophthalmic instruments including a needle holder, thumb forceps, entropion clamp or Jaeger eyelid plate, and tenotomy scissors are useful. A skin biopsy punch can be used when ectropion affects only a small area.

POSTOPERATIVE CARE AND ASSESSMENT

Recover the animal quietly to prevent trauma to the surgical sites. Protect the area after surgery by applying a restraint collar (Elizabethan collar). Give analgesics as needed for the first 2 to 3 days. Apply topical antibiotics and corticosteroids after surgery. Use antibiotics and mydriatics if corneal ulceration is present. Treat purulent bacterial conjunctivitis with topical antibiotics. Expect minimal eyelid swelling postoperatively, which should resolve within 48 hours. Reserve assessment of the correction for 5 to 7 days, at which time swelling secondary to inflammation and edema subsides. If undercorrection has occurred, repeat the procedure. Repeat surgery is more commonly necessary when the initial procedure is performed in young and growing animals. Remove the sutures at approximately 10 days. Maintain the Elizabethan collar for 2 to 3 days after suture removal if the animal wants to scratch the site. Corneal lesions usually resolve rapidly after surgical correction.

COMPLICATIONS

Complications include undercorrection or overcorrection. Slight undercorrection is desired. Overcorrection causes entropion, which may increase corneal and conjunctival damage. There is a greater chance of suture damaging the cornea if incisions are made too close to the eyelid margin or if suture ends are long. A completely normal eyelid contour may not always be possible. Removal of the orbicularis oculi muscle increases hemorrhage, postoperative edema, and infection. Self-trauma may result in dehiscence.

PROGNOSIS

Although achieving a completely normal eyelid contour is not always possible, most signs associated with ectropion resolve following appropriately selected and performed ectropion procedures.

Suggested Reading

Gelatt KN, Gelatt JP: *Small animal ophthalmic surgery,* Oxford, 2001, Butterworth-Heinemann.
This is a general textbook on ophthalmology, which includes medical and surgical conditions.
Hamilton HL, McLaughlin SA, Whitley RD et al: Diagnosis and blepharoplastic repair of conformational eyelid defects, *Compend Cont Educ Pract Vet* 22:588, 2000.
This is a well illustrated review of several techniques for entropion and ectropion correction.
Slatter D: *Fundamentals of veterinary ophthalmology,* ed 3, Philadelphia, 2001, WB Saunders.
This is a general textbook on ophthalmology, which includes medical and surgical conditions.
Van der Woerdt A: Adnexal surgery in dogs and cats, *Vet Ophthalmol* 7(5):84, 2004.
This review article summarizes procedures appropriate for adnexal surgery. No illustrations are included.

PROTRUSION OF THE THIRD EYELID GLAND

DEFINITIONS

Protrusion, prolapse, or eversion of the gland of the nictitating membrane (cherry eye, hyperplasia, adenitis, adenoma, haws) is caused by enlargement of the gland.

GENERAL CONSIDERATIONS AND CLINICALLY RELEVANT PATHOPHYSIOLOGY

The pathogenesis has not been determined, but may be associated with primary or secondary adenitis, fascial attachment abnormalities, or specific pathogens affecting the glands. The condition is not caused by primary inflammation, neoplasia, or hyperplasia. Keratoconjunctivitis sicca occurring after protrusion (sometimes years later) suggests involvement of both the lacrimal and nictitans glands. The hypertrophied, protruding gland, which extends beyond the leading edge of the nictitans, becomes abraded and dry—resulting in secondary inflammation and swelling. Protrusion may be unilateral or bilateral. Adenitis is found on histologic examination.

DIAGNOSIS
Clinical Presentation

Signalment. The breeds most often affected are American and English cocker spaniels, English bulldogs, beagles, Pekingese, Boston terriers, Basset hounds, Shih Tzus, and Lhasa apsos. Most are first affected at a young age (usually younger than 1 year). The condition is more common in dogs than in cats. Burmese is the most commonly affected cat breed.

History. Owners notice a mass, tearing, and/or ocular irritation. The condition usually begins unilaterally, but may eventually become bilateral.

Physical Examination Findings

Presenting signs include an obvious reddish mass protruding from behind the third eyelid near the medial canthus, conjunctivitis, epiphora, and local irritation.

Diagnostic Imaging

Imaging is not necessary to diagnose this condition, but may be indicated as part of the preoperative work-up if the animal is older or if concurrent disease conditions are present, such as cardiovascular or renal disease.

Laboratory Findings

Minimum data base findings are nonspecific and usually normal. Cytology of the protruding gland may reveal inflammation.

DIFFERENTIAL DIAGNOSIS

Differentials include neoplasia, hyperplastic lymphoid follicles, and malformation of the nictitating membrane.

MEDICAL MANAGEMENT

Topical antibiotics with or without corticosteroids can be used to treat early, mild cases. Reducing inflammation and edema of the conjunctiva allows the gland to return to its normal position and size. However, topical treatment is often unsuccessful.

SURGICAL TREATMENT
Preoperative Management

Clipping the periocular area is not required unless there are other abnormalities. The periocular area is scrubbed and then rinsed with saline. Exudates are removed from the corneal and conjunctival surfaces with a sterile cotton-tipped applicator and the area is irrigated with a dilute antiseptic solution (0.5% povidone-iodine). See page 260.

Anesthesia

See p. 261.

Surgical Anatomy

The nictitating membrane is a roughly triangular fold of mucosa located in the medial canthus. The base of the triangle is its free or leading margin. Bulbar (posterior) and palpebral (anterior) surfaces are confluent with the conjunctival mucosa. A T-shaped piece of cartilage lies within the membrane, with the "arms" of the T along the leading margin. This cartilage supports the membrane and helps support the corneal contour and protect it. The superficial gland of the nictitating membrane (nictitans gland, gland of the third eyelid) surrounds the base of the cartilage and produces seromucoid tears. Excretory ducts leave the gland and emerge in the middle section of the bulbar mucosa surface. It produces 25% to 40% of the total tears. Lymphoid follicles found primarily on the bulbar surface of the nictitans appear as raised translucent spots. Blood supply to the nictitating membrane is from branches of the internal maxillary artery. The nictitating membrane is important in protecting the cornea, spreading the tear film, and contributing essential mucin to the preocular film. See p. 262.

Positioning

Position the animal in lateral or dorsal recumbency.

SURGICAL TECHNIQUES

Although both removal and replacement techniques have been used, replacement is recommended to reduce the incidence of keratoconjunctivitis sicca later in life. Goals of surgical treatment include replacing the protruding gland behind the leading margin of the nictitans, maintaining nictitans mobility, and preserving glandular tissue and excretory ducts. Not all goals are met by each technique. Described techniques include anchoring the nictitans to oblique muscles, equatorial sclera, periorbital fascia, or periorbital rim—or creating an envelope or pocket in adjacent mucosa and covering it with or without scarification of the surface. Anchoring procedures interfere with mobility, whereas pocket procedures may damage excretory ducts. Anchoring procedures may be more successful for more extensive and chronic protrusions. Pocket procedures may be more effective in young animals and those with mild protrusions. The described technique is a pocket procedure.

Place eyelid retractors to maximize exposure. To replace the prolapsed gland, grasp and extend the third eyelid with thumb forceps, then make 1-cm-long parallel incisions through the bulbar conjunctiva ventral and dorsal to the free margin of the gland (Fig. 16-20, A). Separate the mucosa from underlying submucosa at the incision edge nearest the

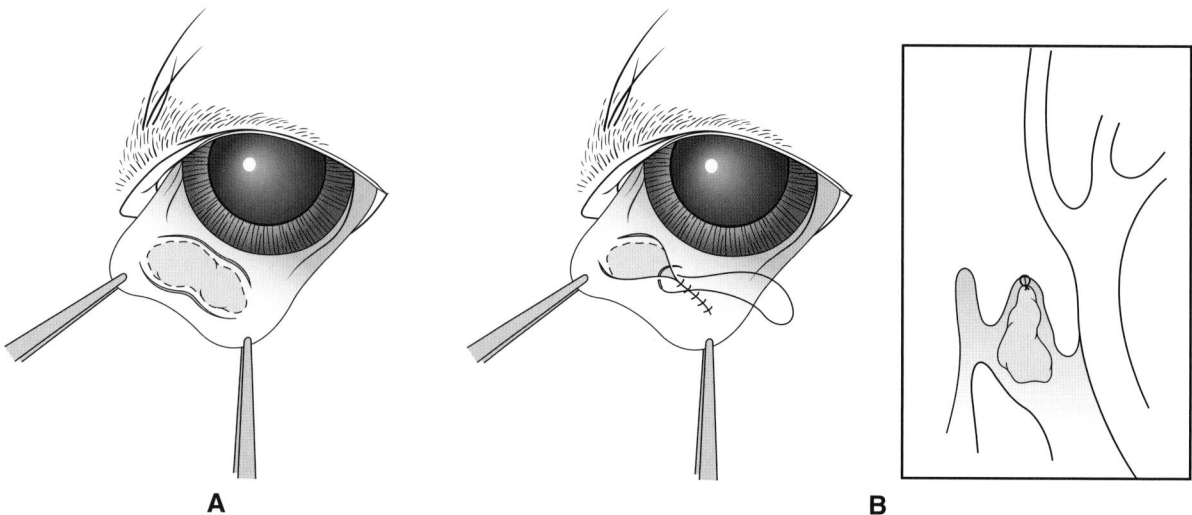

FIG. 16-20
Prolapse of the gland of the third eyelid is corrected by making 1-cm-long parallel incisions through the bulbar conjunctiva ventral and dorsal to the free margin of the gland **(A)**.
B, Return the gland to a normal position by apposing these incisions over the gland using a simple continuous suture pattern with buried knots.

leading margin and at the incision edge nearest the base of the nictitans. Return the gland to its normal position by suturing the two incisions together over the gland (Fig. 16-20, B). Use a simple continuous (5-0 to 7-0) or interrupted (4-0 to 5-0) suture pattern of absorbable suture with buried knots. As an alternative, scarify the conjunctiva over the gland and place a purse-string suture around the conjunctiva of the fornix and around the gland. Apply downward pressure to the gland as the suture is tied, burying it in mucosa. Begin and end suture placement in the fornix so that the knot is away from the cornea. An anchor suture may be necessary with either technique to keep the third eyelid from protruding or riding away from the globe until inflammation and swelling resolve. Place a single anchor suture through the third eyelid and anchor it to the anterior ventral fornix and periosteum of the orbital rim (Fig. 16-21).

NOTE: Removal of the gland of the nictitating membrane frequently results in keratoconjunctivitis sicca and therefore is not recommended.

SUTURE MATERIALS AND SPECIAL INSTRUMENTS

An eyelid retractor, ophthalmic forceps, and tenotomy or Stevens scissors are helpful.

POSTOPERATIVE CARE AND ASSESSMENT

Apply antibiotic or combined antibiotic and corticosteroid ointment topically several times daily for 5 to 7 days. Large, chronic gland protrusions may take several weeks to return to normal. Observe for mobility or distortion of the nictitans and recurrence. There is limited distortion and displacement of the nictitans base, limited to no restriction of movement, and less risk of suture failure with the pocket technique. Anchoring techniques may result in entropion, restricted nictitans movement, and reprotrusion if the suture fails or is inadequately anchored.

PROGNOSIS

Prognosis is good if the protrusion is acute and mild. Chronic protrusions are more difficult to replace and are more likely to recur. Keratoconjunctivitis sicca occurs in approximately 14% of eyes treated by replacement compared with 48% if the gland is partially removed. Recurrence does not preclude additional surgery several weeks later to replace the gland.

Suggested Reading

Gelatt KN, Gelatt JP: *Small animal ophthalmic surgery,* Oxford, 2001, Butterworth-Heinemann.
This is an easy to understand surgical reference book.
Slatter D: *Fundamentals of veterinary ophthalmology,* ed 3, Philadelphia, 2001, WB Saunders.
This is a general textbook on ophthalmology, which includes medical and surgical conditions.

TRAUMATIC PROPTOSIS

DEFINITIONS

Traumatic ocular proptosis is defined as the forward displacement of the eye by a traumatic episode with entrapment of the palpebral margins behind the eye.

GENERAL CONSIDERATIONS AND CLINICALLY RELEVANT PATHOPHYSIOLOGY

Blunt head trauma, bite wounds, retrobulbar hemorrhage, orbital fractures, or restraint of exophthalmic animals can cause acute forward displacement of the globe beyond the bony orbit and eyelids. Once displaced, contraction and in-

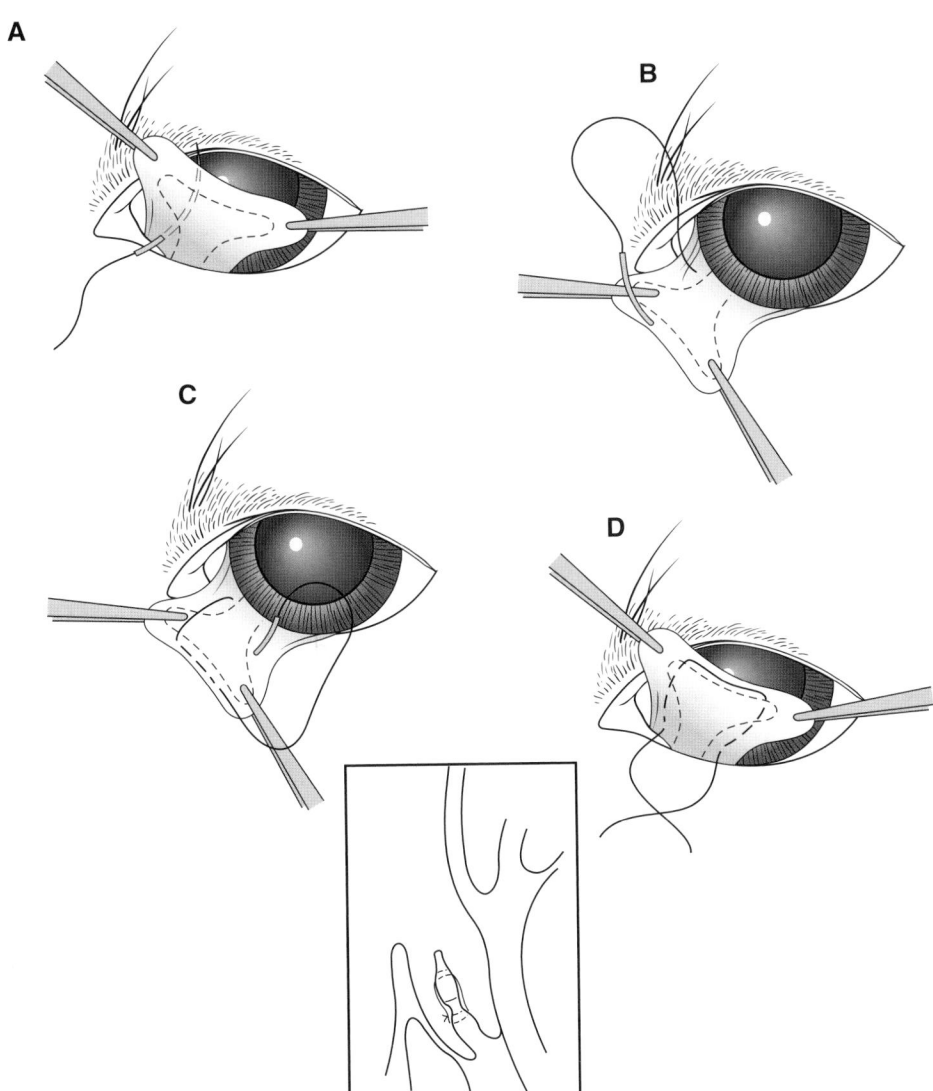

A

B

C

D

FIG. 16-21
An anchor suture helps keep the third eyelid from protruding until inflammation and swelling resolve. **A,** Exteriorize the third eyelid with forceps, and insert the needle from the external surface of the third eyelid around the internal surface of one arm of the cartilage "T." **B,** Pass the needle beneath the conjunctiva to the other arm of the cartilage "T." **C,** Direct the needle around the cartilage arm, exiting the third eyelid on the external surface, anchoring it to the conjunctiva in the ventral fornix and periosteum of the orbital rim. **D,** Tie to secure the anchoring suture.

ward rolling of the eyelids and spasms of the orbicularis oculi muscle prevent return of the prolapsed globe to its normal position. Ocular muscle damage, venostasis, chemosis, subconjunctival hemorrhage, and corneal drying occur. Proptosis occurs more commonly in brachycephalic breeds because they have shallow orbits and large palpebral fissures. The trauma to produce proptosis in these breeds is less than in mesocephalic and dolichocephalic breeds. Proptosis in other dog breeds and cats requires considerable trauma and is often associated with skull and mandibular fractures. The longer the cornea is exposed, the more extensive the damage to the epithelium and stroma, and the more severe the retrobulbar hemorrhage and edema. Pressure and stretching may damage the optic nerve and papillary pathways. In addition, the ocular rectus and oblique muscles are frequently avulsed, resulting in strabismus.

DIAGNOSIS

Visual inspection of the face is diagnostic. Diagnosis of concurrent injuries requires a thorough physical examination and imaging. Assessment of blood loss and physiologic pa-

rameters requires a CBC, serum chemistries, electrolytes, and blood gas analysis.

Clinical Presentation

Signalment. Any animal may suffer proptosis with severe trauma; however, it is seen most commonly in brachycephalic breeds (Pekingese, Lhasa Apso, Shih Tzu, Boston terrier, pug). Sexually intact males are more often affected.

History. The condition is associated with blunt trauma, bite wounds, or forceful restraint.

Physical Examination Findings

Perform a thorough physical examination assessing the animal for shock and life-threatening injuries. Auscultate the chest for evidence of pneumothorax, hemothorax, and contusions. Palpate the skull carefully for evidence of fracture crepitance and subcutaneous emphysema. Perform an ophthalmic examination as thoroughly as possible. The size of the resting pupil and the light-induced pupillary reflexes can help to assess whether there is damage to the optic nerve and pupillary pathways. A widely dilated pupil with limited or no light pupillary reflexes signals neural damage. A nonvisual eye with mydriasis or no visual pupil, hyphema, and optic nerve damage are unfavorable prognostic signs.

Diagnostic Imaging

Imaging the thorax may reveal concurrent pneumothorax, pleural fluid, and pulmonary contusions. Imaging of the skull may reveal fractures of the orbit and mandible.

Laboratory Findings

Hematologic and serum biochemical profile results are non-specific. The animal may be anemic if significant hemorrhage has occurred.

DIFFERENTIAL DIAGNOSIS

Other possible causes of extreme exophthalmos include glaucoma, inflammatory disease, and an intraocular or retrobulbar mass.

MEDICAL MANAGEMENT

Stabilize the animal and treat other injuries. Immediately and frequently apply topical solutions to the exposed cornea to keep it moist and minimize damage.

SURGICAL TREATMENT

This is a surgical emergency, and replacement of the globe should not be delayed unnecessarily.

Preoperative Management

Keep the eye moist with an irrigating solution until the animal is anesthetized. Lubricate the eye with a sterile viscous lubricant or antibiotic ointment. Administer intravenous corticosteroids to treat or prevent optic neuropathy and orbital edema (methylprednisolone sodium succinate, 30 mg/kg; then give 15 mg/kg at 2 and 6 hours). Quickly prepare the area surrounding the eye for aseptic surgery after induction.

Anesthesia

Short-acting, easily reversible anesthesia is recommended because of the possibility of thoracic and abdominal injuries.

Surgical Anatomy

See p. 261.

Positioning

Position the animal in lateral or ventral recumbency.

SURGICAL TECHNIQUES

Replace the globe into the orbit and suture the eyelids together. Enucleate the eye if the globe is ruptured or the optic nerve is severed (see p. 267). In questionable cases, replace the globe and enucleate later if necessary.

Evert and retract the eyelids (Fig. 16-22, A), and then apply gentle retrograde pressure on the globe with a lid plate; scalpel handle; or similar smooth, flat instrument or a moist-

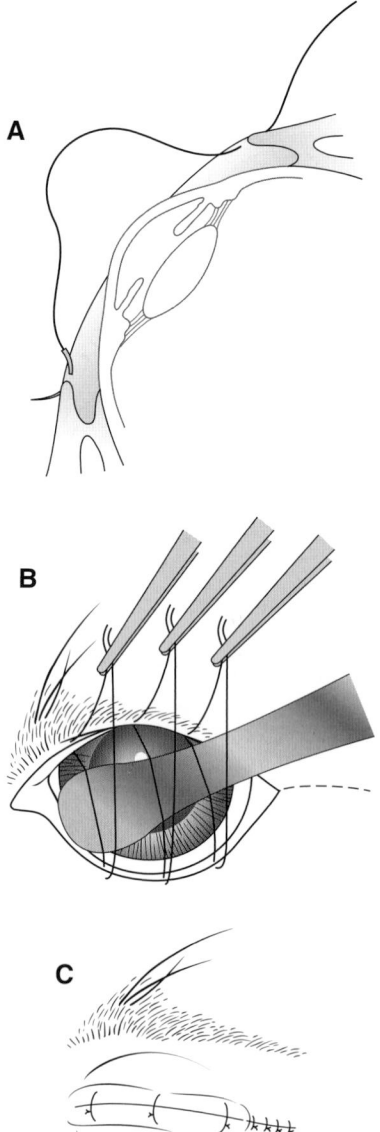

FIG. 16-22
Proptosis. **A,** Evert and retract the eyelids with preplaced temporary tarsorrhaphy sutures. **B,** Apply gentle retrograde pressure on the globe with a lid plate or scalpel handle to replace it within the orbit. A lateral canthotomy is usually necessary to evert the eyelid margins and allow for accurate suture placement. **C,** Maintain reduction by tying temporary tarsorrhaphy sutures.

ened cotton ball (Fig. 16-22, B). Accomplish lid eversion with either preplaced temporary tarsorrhaphy sutures or a strabismus hook (see Fig. 16-22, A). If necessary, perform a lateral canthotomy to allow replacement of the globe. Flush the conjunctival fornices with a balanced electrolyte solution. Maintain reduction with a temporary tarsorrhaphy using three or four sutures and stents to prevent pressure necrosis (see Fig. 16-22, C). To prevent corneal abrasion, place split-thickness sutures through the eyelids with the suture exiting near the meibomian gland openings and tie on the dorsal surface. Leave the medial canthus open to facilitate adminis-tration of topical medications. Close the lateral canthotomy incision in two layers. Perform a permanent partial tarsor-rhaphy in brachycephalic dogs with macropalpebral fissures to prevent recurrence of proptosis and exposure keratitis.

SUTURE MATERIALS AND SPECIAL INSTRUMENTS

A lid plate, Stevens tenotomy or strabismus scissors, and strabismus hook facilitate the procedure. Use 2-0 to 4-0 non-absorbable suture.

POSTOPERATIVE CARE AND ASSESSMENT

Monitor for pain, mucopurulent exudate, malaise, and/or pyrexia. Medicate with ophthalmic atropine, antibiotics, and corticosteroids if the cornea is intact. Administer intrave-nous corticosteroids to treat or prevent optic neuropathy and orbital edema (methylprednisolone sodium succinate, 30 mg/kg; then give 15 mg/kg at 2 and 6 hours). Alternatively or in addition, a retrobulbar injection of corticosteroids can be given at the time of surgery (10 mg of triamcinolone). Diuretics may help reduce excessive orbital fluids. Give anal-gesics as needed (see Chapter 13). Apply cold compresses for 48 to 72 hours, then apply warm compresses to help relieve local discomfort and lid swelling after surgery. Apply an Elizabethan collar to prevent self-trauma. Canthotomy su-tures should be removed 10 to 14 days after surgery. Tarsor-rhaphy sutures are generally removed 10 to 28 days after surgery, but can be removed sooner if persistent pain, muco-purulent exudate, malaise, or pyrexia develops. Replace and maintain tarsorrhaphy sutures for 2 to 3 weeks if the lids do not meet after initial suture removal; this will allow further regression of orbital swelling.

PROGNOSIS

The prognosis for sight and a cosmetically acceptable eye depends on the duration and severity of the prolapse. The prognosis is better if the prolapse is mild, the duration short, the pupil miotic, hyphema absent, extraocular muscle damage minimal, the fundic examination normal, and the patient visual. If positive direct or consensual reflexes have not returned within a week, it is likely that there is perma-nent ocular damage. Blindness occurs in approximately 60% to 70% of dogs and 100% of cats. Postproptosis stra-bismus occurs in 36% of dogs, most frequently as a result of avulsion of the medial rectus muscle. If only a few muscles are avulsed, deviation of the globe may correct itself over 6 to 9 months. Blindness, lagophthalmos, deviation of the globe, corneal ulcers or perforations, keratitis, hyphema, phthisis bulbi, and glaucoma are ocular sequelae to trau-matic proptosis.

Suggested Reading

Gelatt KN, Gelatt JP: *Small animal ophthalmic surgery,* Oxford, 2001, Butterworth-Heinemann.
This is an easy to understand surgical reference book.

Slatter D: *Fundamentals of veterinary ophthalmology,* ed 3, Philadelphia, 2001, WB Saunders.
This is a general textbook on ophthalmology, which includes medical and surgical conditions.

LID MASSES

DEFINITIONS

Eyelid masses may be inflammatory or neoplastic.

GENERAL CONSIDERATIONS AND CLINICALLY RELEVANT PATHOPHYSIOLOGY

Neoplastic masses are common in dogs; most are benign (sebaceous adenomas, benign melanomas, histiocytomas, papillomas) and are associated with the meibomian glands. Sebaceous (tarsal) adenoma is the most common eyelid tu-mor in dogs. Sebaceous adenomas grow rapidly and appear histologically malignant, but are clinically benign. Although less common (10%), malignant eyelid tumors include squa-mous cell carcinomas, adenocarcinomas, basal cell carcino-mas, hemangiosarcomas, or fibrosarcomas. Eyelid tumors are rare in cats but when identified are most commonly (60%) squamous cell carcinomas. Other eyelid tumors in cats include fibrosarcoma, adenocarcinoma, basal cell carci-noma, melanoma, and hemangiosarcoma. Eyelid masses cause discomfort, interfere with eyelid function, and may cause keratitis.

DIAGNOSIS
Clinical Presentation

Signalment. The average age of dogs presenting with eye-lid neoplasia is 8 years, whereas cats are usually 10 years old. Beagles, Siberian huskies, and English setters appear to have a higher risk of eyelid neoplasia.

History. A mass on the eyelid or secondary ocular irrita-tion is noted. Most are slow growing, but some malignant tumors will grow rapidly. An ocular discharge, periocular excoriation, conjunctivitis, and encrusted or hemorrhagic regions on the eyelid may be noticed.

Physical Examination Findings

A mass is visualized or palpated on the skin of the eyelid, eyelid margin, or conjunctiva. Evert the lid and inspect the palpebral surface to identify tarsal gland or meibomian gland tumors. Approximately 10% of canine malignant lid tumors are locally invasive. Conjunctivitis, blepharitis, ocu-lar discharge, periocular excoriation, encrusted hemorrhagic lid margins, and corneal irritation may be present.

Diagnostic Imaging

Thoracic and/or abdominal radiographs or abdominal ultra-sonography may be performed to evaluate for metastasis.

Laboratory Findings

Findings are nonspecific and reflect the age and other disease conditions of the animal. Cytology may help differentiate inflammatory from neoplastic lesions. Inflammatory lesions should be cultured. Histopathologic evaluation of all excised masses should be performed for definitive diagnosis.

DIFFERENTIAL DIAGNOSIS

Inflammatory conditions must be differentiated from neoplastic conditions. Histopathology is necessary to make a definitive diagnosis.

MEDICAL MANAGEMENT

Chemotherapy, radiation therapy, or immunotherapy may be appropriate therapy for some tumors alone, in combination, or as an adjunct to surgery. Treatment of squamous cell carcinomas in cats often combines surgery with radiation therapy.

SURGICAL TREATMENT

Eyelid tumors that are growing or that cause clinical signs should be excised. Wide margins are required when removing melanomas or squamous cell carcinomas. Laser surgery, cryosurgery, hyperthermia, immunotherapy, photodynamic therapy, chemotherapy, and radiation therapy are additional therapeutic possibilities for eyelid tumors and have been used with varying success. Eyelid lesions can be excised and margins directly apposed when less than one third of the eyelid margin is involved. More eyelid can be resected in some breeds like cocker spaniels that have considerable eyelid length. Less than expected amounts of lid are resectable in other breeds, such as the Doberman, collie, miniature poodle, and cats because of tight-fitting eyelid fissures. The lateral canthal ligament may be divided to relieve tension if necessary.

Preoperative Management

Initiate treatment for corneal ulcers and conjunctivitis before surgery. Estimate the amount of skin to be removed before anesthetizing the animal. Place a bland petroleum-based ointment on the cornea and conjunctival surfaces to collect debris and hair during preparation. Remove eyelid hair with small clippers or by shaving. The periocular area is scrubbed with a 1:50 povidone-iodine solution and then rinsed with saline. Do not use normal scrubs or alcohol because they can irritate the cornea and conjunctiva. Remove ointment and exudates from the corneal and conjunctival surfaces with a sterile cotton-tipped applicator, and irrigate the area with a dilute antiseptic solution (0.5% povidone-iodine) (see p. 260).

Anesthesia

See p. 261.

Surgical Anatomy

See p. 261.

Positioning

Ventral or lateral recumbence allows access to the eyelids.

SURGICAL TECHNIQUES

Masses on the eyelid skin are excised as tumors elsewhere on the body with an elliptical or circular incision. Closure is at 90° to the eyelid margin on the lower lid and parallel to the upper lid margin to reduce the scar tissue effect on lid movement. Partial-thickness skin defects can also be closed using Z-plasty, transpositional, pedicle, advancement, and rhombic type of flaps.

Expose masses arising from the conjunctiva by everting the lid with chalazion clamps. Incise the conjunctiva surrounding the mass with tenotomy scissors, then allow the palpebral conjunctival defect to heal by secondary intention.

Full-thickness excisions are performed when the mass involves the lid margin.

Stabilize the lid, and provide hemostasis with a chalazion clamp (Fig. 16-23, A). If a chalazion clamp is not available, a sterile tongue depressor can be used to support and stabilize the lid. Using a No. 15 Bard-Parker blade or a No. 64 Beaver blade, make a wedge or house-shaped incision around tumors involving less than one third of the eyelid margin (Fig. 16-23, B). Remove the tumor and 1 to 2 mm of normal skin on each side. Control hemorrhage with pressure or point electrocautery. Close the lid in two layers as described for laceration repair. Make a lateral canthoplasty incision or a semicircular incision approximately the length of the eyelid margin to create a sliding flap to allow closure without tension if necessary (see Fig. 16-23, C). Make an elliptical incision around masses that do not involve the lid margin or conjunctiva, are less than 25% of the eyelid length, and are no wider than 4 to 5 mm. Close the skin with interrupted sutures (4-0 to 6-0 nonabsorbable) (Fig. 16-23, D). Secondary ectropion may result if too large a lesion is removed by elliptic excision. If ectropion is noted during closure, use an advancement or rotational flap in lieu of direct appositional closure.

> NOTE: The suture at the eyelid margin is the most critical for lid alignment and to reduce the likelihood of a notch developing.

Masses involving more than one third the length of the eyelid margin require advancement flaps for reconstruction. A single-pedicle advancement flap and a lip-to-lid flap are options for reconstruction.

After resecting the mass, create a single-pedicle advancement flap by extending distally the medial and lateral incisions perpendicular to the eyelid margin (Fig. 16-24, A). Undermine and mobilize as much conjunctiva adjacent to the defect as possible to line the flap. Advance the flap to the lid margin, aligning it carefully with the remaining lid and suturing it in place (4-0 to 6-0 nonabsorbable) (Fig. 16-24, B and C). Suture conjunctiva and skin at the new lid margin with a simple continuous pattern (6-0 absorbable) (Fig. 16-24, D).

As an alternative, a semicircular incision at the lateral canthus may be used to advance the lateral lid margin of the upper or lower lid centrally (see Fig. 16-24, *B*). Other flaps,

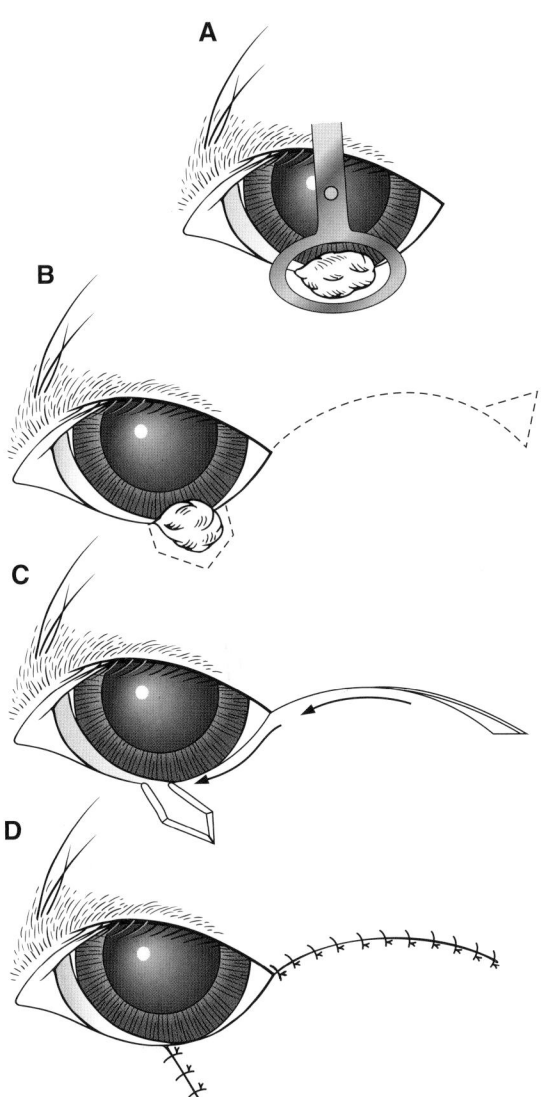

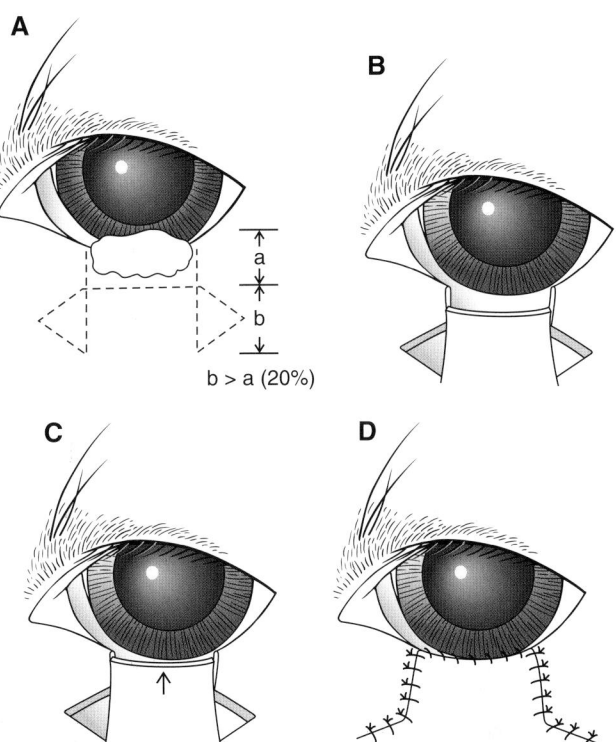

FIG. 16-24
Reconstruction of the eyelid margin using an advancement flap for a mass involving more than one third the eyelid margin length. **A,** Resect the mass with a rectangular incision, including 2-mm margins of normal skin. Create an advancement flap by extending distally the medial and lateral incisions. Remove triangles of tissue on each side of the flap to prevent dog ears. Undermine and mobilize conjunctiva.
B and **C,** Advance the flap to the lid margin, aligning it carefully. **D,** Suture conjunctiva and skin at the new lid margin with a simple continuous pattern. Place interrupted sutures to appose the remaining incision.

FIG. 16-23
Eyelid mass resection. **A,** Stabilize the lid and provide hemostasis with a chalazion clamp. **B,** Make a wedge or house-shaped incision around tumors involving less than one third of the eyelid margin. Make a semicircular lateral canthoplasty incision approximately the length of the eyelid margin if necessary to relieve tension. **C,** Advance the skin flap to appose the edges of the defect. **D,** Appose the conjunctiva and skin in separate layers and appose the lateral canthus incision.

including rotational, Z-plasty, bucket handle, and cross-lid flaps, can also be created to close defects.

Use a lip-to-lid flap to repair large defects created by mass removal or trauma with a mucocutaneous subdermal plexus flap. The flap can be used to replace part or all of the lower lid and can be modified to reconstruct the upper lid.

AP *Mark two parallel incisions on the upper lip at a 45° to 50° angle to a line bisecting the medial and lateral canthi of the palpebral fissure. Make the distance between the incisions slightly wider than the defect*

(Fig. 16-25, A). Make a full-thickness lip incision along the marked lines (Fig. 16-25, B). Split the oral mucosa at a level sufficient to replace the excised conjunctiva. Carefully dissect the skin from the remaining oral mucosa to allow sufficient pedicle length to reach the lid defect without tension. Appose the oral mucosa with simple interrupted or continuous sutures (3-0 to 5-0 absorbable) (Fig. 16-25, C). Create a bridge incision by incising from the midpoint of the lid defect to the cranial aspect of the donor site. Rotate the flap into position, then appose the oral mucosa of the flap to the remaining conjunctiva with buried interrupted or continuous sutures (4-0 to 6-0 absorbable). Complete the transfer by suturing the skin of the flap to the remaining lid and then reapposing the skin at the lip margins using 4-0 to 5-0 nonabsorbable suture (Fig. 16-25, D). To prevent vascular compromise, do not attempt to correct skin folds and puckers at the initial reconstruction. If desired, remove the cutaneous transfer pedicle after 4 to 6 weeks. If necessary, revise the new eyelid margin for a more cosmetic appearance.

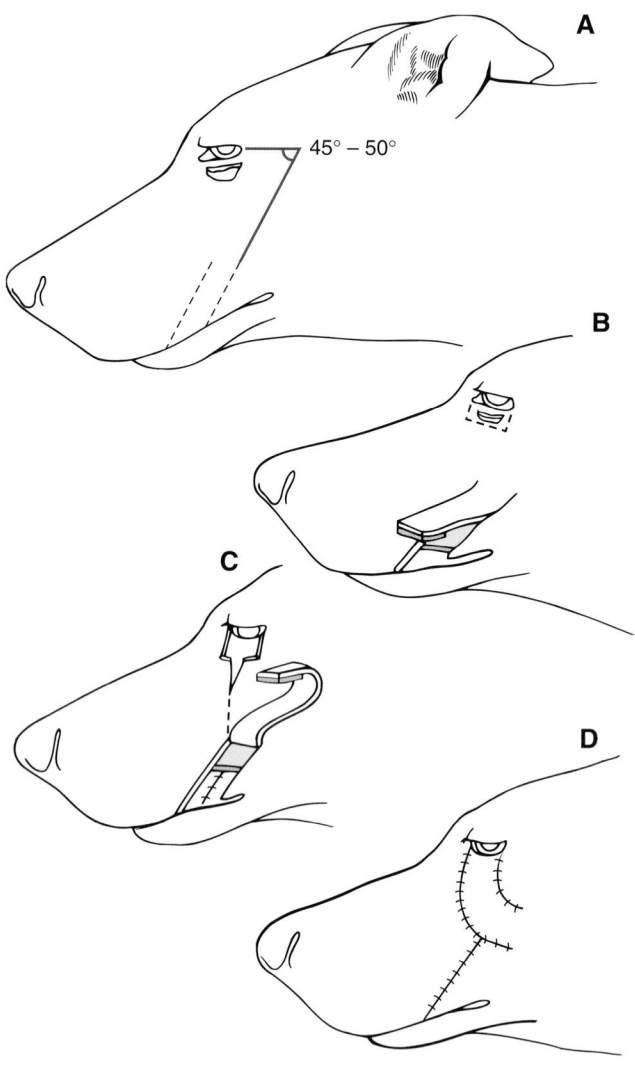

FIG. 16-25

Lip-to-lid reconstruction of large eyelid defects provides a mucocutaneous junction for the new lid margin. **A,** Mark two parallel incisions on the upper lip at a 45° to 50° angle to a line bisecting the medial and lateral canthi. **B,** Make two full-thickness lip incisions along the marked lines slightly wider than the defect. Split the oral mucosa at a level sufficient to replace the excised conjunctiva. **C,** Dissect the skin from the remaining mucosa a sufficient length to allow transposition of the pedicle. Create a bridge incision from the midpoint of the lid defect to the cranial aspect of the donor site. **D,** Rotate the flap into position and suture the oral mucosa to the remaining conjunctiva. Complete the transfer by suturing the skin flap into position and repairing the lip defect.

SUTURE MATERIALS AND SPECIAL INSTRUMENTS

Use fine (4-0 to 6-0) nonabsorbable suture material swaged onto a fine cutting needle. Ophthalmic instruments, including a needle holder, thumb forceps, chalazion or entropion clamp, Jaeger eyelid plate, and tenotomy scissors, are useful.

POSTOPERATIVE CARE AND ASSESSMENT

Recover the animal quietly to prevent trauma to the surgical site. Protect the area after surgery by applying a restraint collar (Elizabethan collar). For larger blepharoplastic procedures, a temporary tarsorrhaphy provides protection and minimizes tension on the suture lines as they are healing. Give analgesics as needed for the first 2 to 3 days (see Chapter 13). Apply antibiotics and corticosteroids topically after surgery. Use antibiotics and mydriatics if corneal ulceration is present. Treat purulent secondary bacterial conjunctivitis with topical antibiotics (without steroids). Expect minimal eyelid swelling postoperatively, which should resolve within 48 hours. Apply cold and warm compresses to reduce eyelid swelling and promote circulation if major reconstruction or grafts were used. Reserve assessment of the repair for 5 to 7 days when swelling as a result of inflammation and edema subsides. Remove the sutures at approximately 10 days. Maintain the Elizabethan collar for 2 to 3 days after suture removal if the animal wants to scratch the site. Hair growing on skin flaps that have been advanced into large defects needs periodic clipping to prevent corneal irritation and ulcers.

Dehiscence following repair occurs with rubbing, scratching, or excess tension. A "v" notch in the eyelid margin may occur if alignment is not maintained. Tumor recurrence is also a complication.

PROGNOSIS

Prognosis depends on the type of tumor identified and its biologic behavior. Histologically, 20% to 30% of eyelid neoplasms in dogs are malignant. Comparison of recurrence rates of all eyelid tumors in dogs was 30 months after surgical excision and 8 months after cryotherapy. In cats, the rate of recurrent eyelid malignancy is very high and the prognosis is poor.

Suggested Reading

Bussieres M, Krohne SG, Stiles J et al: The use of carbon dioxide laser for the ablation of meibomian gland adenomas in dogs, *J Am Anim Hosp Assoc* 41:227, 2005.

CO_2 laser ablation of meibomian glands is described in 12 dogs. Healing by secondary intention resulted in a good cosmetic result, although with magnification all dogs had an eyelid scar with margin irregularity.

Gelatt KN, Gelatt JP: *Small animal ophthalmic surgery,* Oxford, 2001, Butterworth-Heinemann.

This is an easy to understand surgical reference book.

Schmidt K, Bertani C, Martano M et al: Reconstruction of the lower eyelid by third eyelid lateral advancement and local transposition flap after an "en bloc" resection of squamous cell carcinoma in 5 cats, *Vet Surg* 34:78, 2005.

This case series describes a technique for removal of more than 50% of the lower eyelid.

Slatter D: *Fundamentals of veterinary ophthalmology,* ed 3, Philadelphia, 2001, WB Saunders.

This is a general textbook on ophthalmology, which includes medical and surgical conditions.

CHAPTER 17
Surgery of the Ear

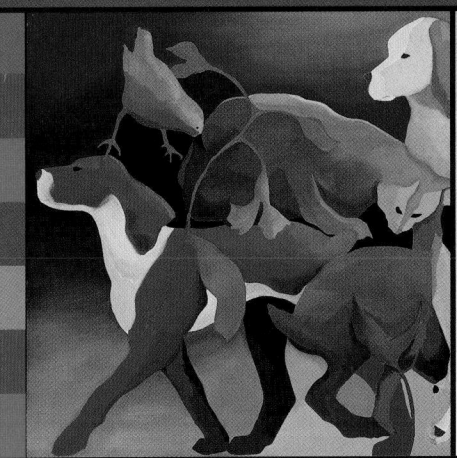

GENERAL PRINCIPLES AND TECHNIQUES

DEFINITIONS

Otitis externa is inflammation of the vertical or horizontal ear canal or both; **otitis media** is inflammation of the tympanic cavity and membrane. **Otitis interna** is inflammation of the inner ear that typically causes vestibular disease in dogs. It is nearly always caused by extension of infection into the petrosal bone from otitis media.

PREOPERATIVE CONCERNS

To anticipate surgical complications in animals undergoing ear surgery, it is imperative to determine the extent and severity of disease. Thickening and calcification of the ear canal indicate irreversible inflammatory disease. A sharp pain response on deep palpation of the ear may indicate middle ear infection, whereas a head tilt may indicate severe pain in the ear on the lower side or otitis media or interna (see p. 304). The latter conditions should be suspected if the head tilt is associated with circling, nystagmus, and/or vestibular dysfunction (loss of balance). Facial nerve deficits in patients with chronic otitis externa (i.e., poor palpebral reflex, lip droop, and facial spasms), suggest that the facial nerve is embedded in the horizontal canal or that serious concurrent middle ear disease also is present. Such abnormalities should be noted before surgery to avoid confusion with problems caused by intraoperative trauma during total ear canal ablation.

Otoscopic examination should determine if the tympanic membrane is intact and should define the severity of change in the horizontal and vertical canals. Always inspect both ear canals, even if the animal has unilateral clinical signs. Skull radiographs should be taken to determine if concurrent middle ear disease or neoplasia exists (see p. 301). Proliferation of cartilage or bone around the horizontal ear canal should be noted. After radiographs have been taken, the ear should be cleaned; however, if the tympanic membrane has ruptured, do not use chlorhexidine in a solution stronger than 0.2%, nondilute iodine or iodophors, ethanol, benzalkonium chloride, or some aminoglycosides. Drugs and solu-

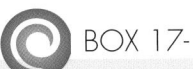 **BOX 17-1**

Partial List of Drugs and Solutions That May Be Used to Flush the Ear in Animals With a Ruptured Tympanic Membrane

- Aqueous penicillin
- Carbenicillin
- Cefmenoxime
- Ceftazidime
- Ciprofloxacin
- Clotrimazole
- Enrofloxacin
- Fluocinolone (aqueous form)
- Miconazole
- Nystatin
- Ofloxacin
- Silver sulfadiazine solution (0.1%)
- Squalene (Cerumene)
- Ticarcillin
- Tolnaftate
- Tris-EDTA

tions that may be used in animals with a ruptured tympanic membrane are listed in Box 17-1.

The owner's expectations must be considered before planning surgery in animals with ear disease. Always question owners as to their perception of the dog's hearing before surgery because total ear canal ablation (TECA) may diminish hearing and be unacceptable. Most owners of dogs with severe, chronic otitis externa or media do not report substantial changes in their pets' hearing after this procedure, probably because notable hearing loss already had occurred before surgery. Similarly, brainstem-auditory evoked responses reveal that auditory function declines minimally after total ear canal ablation in dogs with chronic otitis externa.

> NOTE: Be sure that the owner is aware of the dog's hearing deficits before surgery. This reduces owner dissatisfaction associated with any perceived hearing loss after surgery.

ANESTHETIC CONSIDERATIONS

Most animals undergoing ear surgery are healthy, and a variety of anesthetic protocols can be used. Ear surgery is painful, particularly TECA, vertical canal resection, and lateral canal resection. Although butorphanol (0.2 to 0.4 mg/kg

A BOX 17-2

Selected Anesthetic Protocols for Ear Surgery

Dogs

Premedication

Give atropine (0.02–0.04 mg/kg SC or IM) or glycopyrrolate (0.005–0.011 mg/kg SC or IM) plus hydromorphone (0.1–0.2 mg/kg SC or IM; see text)

Induction

Thiopental sodium (10–12 mg/kg IV) or propofol (4–6 mg/kg IV)

Maintenance

Isoflurane or sevoflurane

Cats

Premedication

Give atropine (0.02–0.04 mg/kg SC or IM) or glycopyrrolate (0.005–0.011 mg/kg SC or IM) plus butorphanol (0.2–0.4 mg/kg SC or IM) or buprenorphine (5–15 μg/kg IM); if a tranquilizer (e.g., acepromazine) is used, a μ-agonist (e.g., hydromorphone) may be used with it

Induction

Use chamber induction with isoflurane or sevoflurane; or thiopental sodium or propofol at dose given above for dogs; or diazepam plus ketamine (0.27 mg/kg and 5.5 mg/kg, respectively; see text) combined and administered IV to effect

Maintenance

Isoflurane or sevoflurane

SC, Subcutaneous; *IM,* intramuscular; *IV,* intravenous.

given subcutaneously or intramuscularly) and buprenorphine (5 to 15 μg/kg given intramuscularly) are common premedicants in dogs, hydromorphone (Box 17-2) appears to be a better analgesic for dogs undergoing ear surgery. Saturating the surgical site with bupivacaine hydrochloride (splash block; use a volume sufficient to cover the area, but do not exceed 2 mg/kg in the dog) before closing the incision after resections or ablations may increase the patient's comfort in the early postoperative period; however, this technique should always be used in conjunction with other analgesics. The area should not be flushed after a splash block for at least 20 minutes. In cats, a variety of anesthetic protocols (i.e., chamber induction with isoflurane or sevoflurane; thiopental or propofol; or a combination of ketamine and diazepam (0.27 mg/kg and 5.5 mg/kg, respectively, combined and administered IV to effect) can be used after premedication with butorphanol or buprenorphine to achieve anesthesia for ear surgery (see Box 17-2). Ketamine should not be given to cats with neurologic or renal dysfunction. In the absence of contraindications, a small ketamine bolus (0.5 mg/kg, IV) followed by a ketamine constant rate infusion (CRI) (2 to 10 μg/kg/min, IV) may facilitate intraoperative management and decrease postoperative pain in dogs or cats that have chronically painful ears. In dogs, a fentanyl, lidocaine, ketamine (FLK) or morphine, lidocaine, ketamine (MLK) CRI may be used intraoperatively for management or postoperatively for analgesia (see p. 136). Other useful CRI in dogs include fentanyl and lidocaine; a fentanyl, but not lidocaine, CRI may be used in cats. Use of a continuous, local infusion of bupivacaine for postoperative analgesia in dogs undergoing TECA was not found to increase the degree of postoperative analgesia (Radlinksy et al, 2005).

Postoperative analgesics should be given after ear surgery. If hydromorphone was used as a premedicant, it should be readministered 3 to 4 hours later (0.05 to 0.1 mg/kg given intravenously, subcutaneously, or intramuscularly). If the animal appears dysphoric or anxious, tranquilization may be necessary; however, tranquilizers should be used only in animals that have been given sufficient analgesics. If acepromazine is not contraindicated by hypotension or seizures, low doses may be given (0.025 to 0.05 mg/kg given subcutaneously, intramuscularly, or intravenously; do not exceed 1 mg).

ANTIBIOTICS

Preoperative antibiotics are recommended in animals undergoing aural surgery. Severe infection should be treated for several weeks before surgery with systemic and/or topical antibiotics, depending on the site of the infection. Otitis externa is best treated with topical therapy because systemic antimicrobials are unlikely to achieve therapeutic concentrations within the fluid and exudates of the external ear canal. Commercially produced topical products typically contain one or more active ingredients (antibacterial, antifungal, and antiinflammatory) in various combinations plus a vehicle and various solubilizers, stabilizers, and surfactants. In contrast, systemic antibiotics are indicated in otitis media because the highly vascularized mucous membrane lining the tympanic cavity of the inflamed middle ear promotes diffusion of drugs from the blood to the bulla. Packing the bulla with an antibiotic ointment may be used in conjunction with systemic antibiotics if systemic antibiotics alone do not resolve the infection. The choice of systemic antibiotics for treating the middle ear compartment is preferably based on culture and susceptibility testing (Table 17-1). Cultures of deep tissues taken during surgery often are more useful than preoperative cultures.

Findings in a recent study support the concept that initial treatment of otitis externa can be empirically based on historical information of the most common isolates and their susceptibility patterns in conjunction with examination of stained otic swab samples (Graham-Mize and Rosser, 2004). When treatment failures occur, repeat examination and modification of the treatment may be aided by repeat cytology of otic exudate and by submitting cultures. *Malassezia* spp. and *Staphylococcus intermedius* are typically the most common microbial isolates identified in dogs with otitis externa. Most *S. intermedius* are susceptible to cephalothin and oxacillin (Peterson et al, 2002). Most other bacterial isolates are susceptible to a number of antimicrobials; however, *Pseudomonas aeruginosa* and *Enterococcus* spp. are often fairly resistant bacte-

⌗ TABLE 17-1

Percentage of Common Microbial Isolates Susceptible to a Tested Antimicrobial in Dogs With Chronic Otitis Externa*

BACTERIAL ISOLATE	ANTIBIOTIC† (PERCENT OF SUSCEPTIBILITY)
Pseudomonas aeruginosa	Ceftazidime (71%)
Enterococcus spp.	Ampicillin (100%) Augmentin (87.5%) Tetracycline (83%) Penicillin (62.5%)
Staphyloccocus intermedius	Cefoxitin (100%) Cephalothin (100%) Oxacillin (100%) Ceftiofur (98%) Clavamox (98%) Gentamicin (98%) Clindamycin (96%) Enrofloxacin (90%) Tribrissen (88%) Tetracycline (72%)
Corynebacterium spp.	Cefoxitin (95%) Cephalothin (95%) Gentamicin (95%) Clindamycin (95%) Tetracycline (95%) Azithromycin (95%) Ampicillin (95%) Enrofloxacin (90%) Augmentin (86%) Ceftiofur (86%) Tribrissen (86%)
Streptococcus group G	Ampicillin (100%) Cefoxitin (100%) Penicillin (100%) Ceftiofur (96%) Gentamicin (93%) Oxacillin (67%) Tetracycline (60%) Enrofloxacin (60%) Clindamycin (60%)
Proteus mirabilis	Ampicillin (100%) Clavamox (100%) Gentamicin (100%) Cefazolin (100%) Ticarcillin (100%) Cefoxitin (100%) Cephalothin (100%) Amikacin (93%) Ceftiofur (93%) Enrofloxacin (60%)

*From Graham-Mize CA, Rosser EJ: Comparison of microbial isolates and susceptibility patterns from the external ear canal of dogs with otitis externa, *J Am Anim Hosp Assoc* 40:102, 2004.
†Only antibiotics with susceptibilities greater than 50% are listed.

ria (see Table 17-1). If possible, ototoxic antibiotics should be avoided (i.e., gentamicin, kanamycin, neomycin, streptomycin, tobramycin, amikacin, and polymyxin B). Tris-EDTA solution (see p. 302) may be beneficial in some animals with resistant infections.

SURGICAL ANATOMY

The ear is composed of three parts: (1) the inner ear, which consists of a membranous and a bony labyrinth and functions for hearing and balance; (2) the middle ear, which is formed by the tympanic cavity and connects to the pharynx via the auditory tube (eustachian tube); and (3) the external ear, which is formed by the auditory meatus and a short canal (Fig. 17-1). The inner ear is located within the osseous labyrinth of the petrous part of the temporal bone. The middle and external ears are separated by the tympanic membrane, and the opening of the horizontal canal into the middle ear is known as the external acoustic meatus. The three auditory ossicles (stapes, malleus, and incus) connect the tympanic membrane to the inner ear. The tympanic cavity is air-filled and in dogs is composed of a small dorsal epitympanic recess and a large ventral tympanic bulla. In medium-size dogs, the long axis of the tympanic cavity is about 15 mm. The auditory ossicles are found in the middle portion of the tympanic cavity. Vibrations of the tympanic membrane are transmitted through the chain of these auditory ossicles to the perilymph fluid within the vestibule. The middle ear also connects to the nasopharynx via the auditory tube (commonly referred to as the eustachian tube). Nasopharyngeal polyps (see p. 314) may extend from nasopharynx into the tympanic cavity and can extrude into the external ear canal.

The feline tympanic cavity is divided into two compartments by a thin, bony septum that arises along the cranial aspect of the bulla and curves to attach to the midpoint of the lateral wall (Fig. 17-2). The larger ventromedial compartment is an air-filled tympanic bulla. For complete drainage of the middle ear of cats, this bony septum often needs to be perforated. Most of the lateral wall of the smaller craniolateral compartment is formed by the tympanic membrane. These compartments communicate through a narrow fissure located dorsally near the cochlear window. Near this fissure, the postganglionic sympathetic nerves form a plexus on a structure known as the promontory. Because of their vulnerable location, these nerves are often traumatized during surgical curettage of the feline middle ear, causing Horner's syndrome (see p. 300). The tympanic membrane normally is thin and semitransparent, but may thicken or rupture when diseased. The facial nerve exits the stylomastoid foramen caudal to the ear and courses ventral to the horizontal canal close to the middle ear.

The external ear varies in size and shape among dog breeds. The auricular cartilage determines the appearance of the canine pinna. The base of the ear is composed of a number of ridges that are important landmarks for ear surgery (Fig. 17-3). These include the tragus, lateral crus of the helix, pretragic incisure, and intertragic incisure. The external opening of the vertical canal is known as the external auditory meatus. Numerous muscles attach to the cartilage of the ear, allowing it to move to localize sound. The external ear canal consists of an initial vertical part and a shorter horizontal canal that runs medially. The vertical part and most of the horizontal part of the canal are cartilaginous; however, the deepest part (near the tympanic membrane) is os-

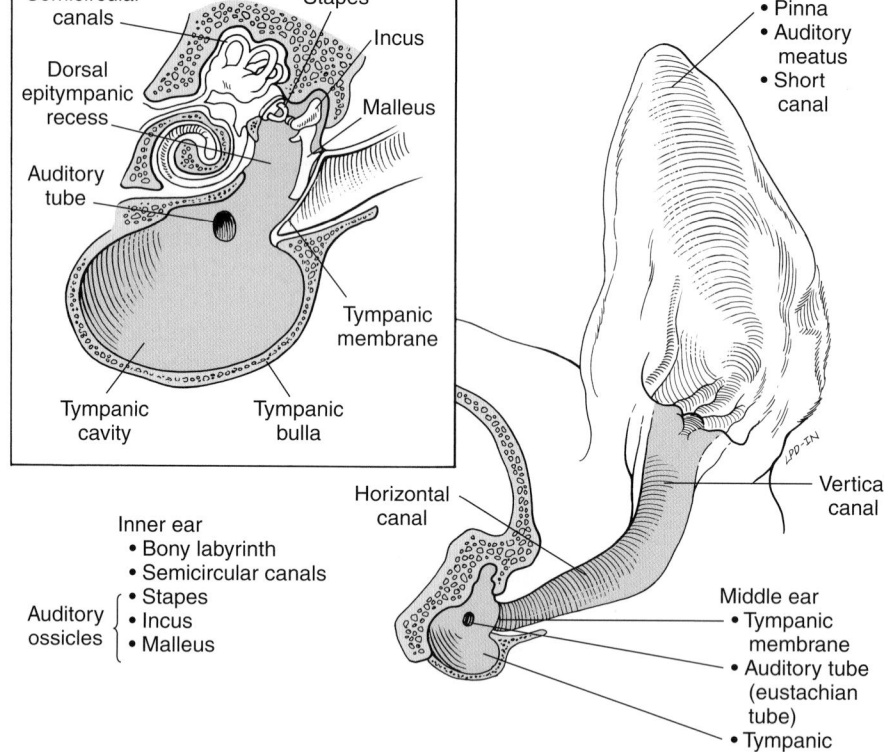

FIG. 17-1
Anatomy of the ear.

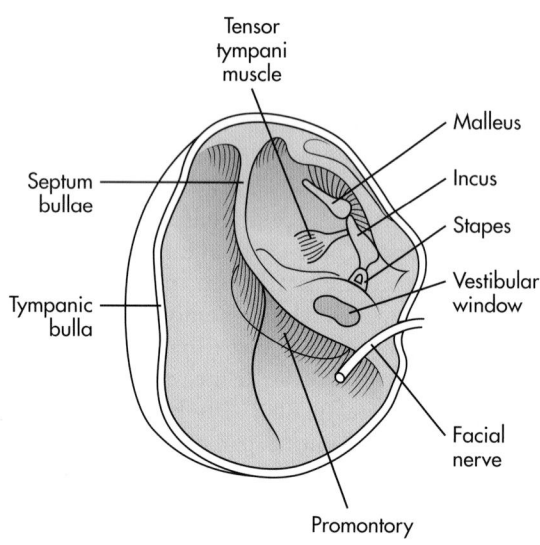

FIG. 17-2
Feline tympanic cavity.

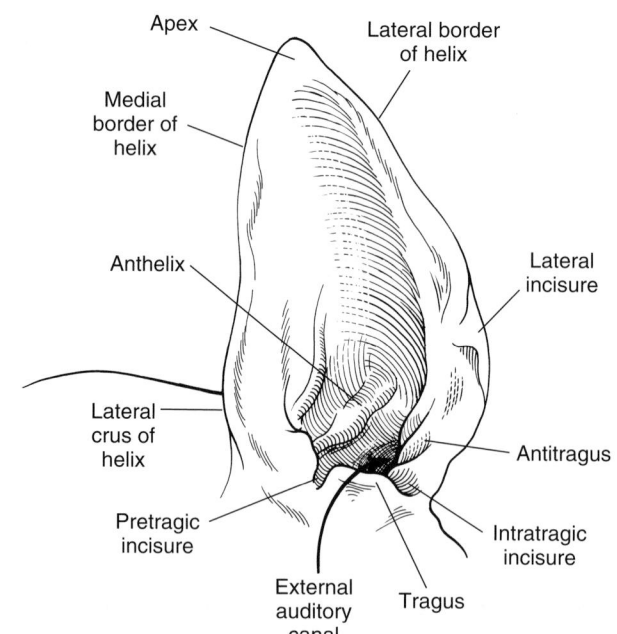

FIG. 17-3
Landmarks of the external ear in dogs.

seous. The parotid salivary gland overlies the auricular cartilage, forming the vertical canal.

SURGICAL TECHNIQUES

Numerous surgical techniques have been described for the treatment of ear disease in dogs and cats. Only the more commonly performed procedures are described here. When performing a lateral canal resection or vertical canal ablation, be sure you are prepared to perform a total ear canal ablation if the opening of the horizontal canal is stenotic or too narrow to allow adequate drainage.

Lateral Ear Canal Resection

Lateral ear canal resection increases drainage and improves ventilation of the ear canal. It also facilitates placement of topical agents into the horizontal canal. Lateral ear canal resection is indicated in patients with minimal hyperplasia of the ear canal epithelium or small neoplastic lesions of the lateral aspect of the vertical canal. It should not be performed in animals with obstruction or stenosis of the horizontal ear canal or concurrent otitis media (unless performed in conjunction with ventral bulla osteotomy; see p. 298), or in patients with severe epithelial hyperplasia. Dogs with underlying disease (e.g., hypothyroidism and primary idiopathic seborrhea) often respond poorly to this surgery. Owner counseling is extremely important before performing a lateral ear canal resection. Most studies have shown that owner satisfaction is low when lateral ear canal resection is performed for chronic otitis externa in dogs. In one study the outcome of surgery was unacceptable in 86.5% of cocker spaniels (Sylvestre, 1998). A modification of the original technique for lateral ear resection, described by Lacroix, established a "drainboard" and is known as a Zepp procedure (Fig. 17-4). The drainboard restricts hair growth at the horizontal canal opening.

> NOTE: Make sure the owner understands that lateral ear canal resection is not a cure and that medical management of the ear probably will be necessary for the remainder of the animal's life.

Clip the entire side of the face and both sides of the pinna. Gently flush the ear and remove as much debris as possible. Position the animal in lateral recumbency with the head elevated on a towel and prepare the pinna and surrounding skin for aseptic surgery. Place quarter drapes around the ear with the entire pinna draped into the surgical site. Stand at the ventral aspect of the dog's head and position a forceps into the vertical ear canal to determine its ventral extent. Mark a site below the horizontal ear canal that is half the length of the vertical ear canal (Fig. 17-5, A). Make two parallel incisions in the skin lateral to the vertical ear canal that extend from the tragus ventrally to the marked site (Fig. 17-5, B). These incisions should be 1½ times the length of the vertical ear canal. Connect the skin incisions ventrally

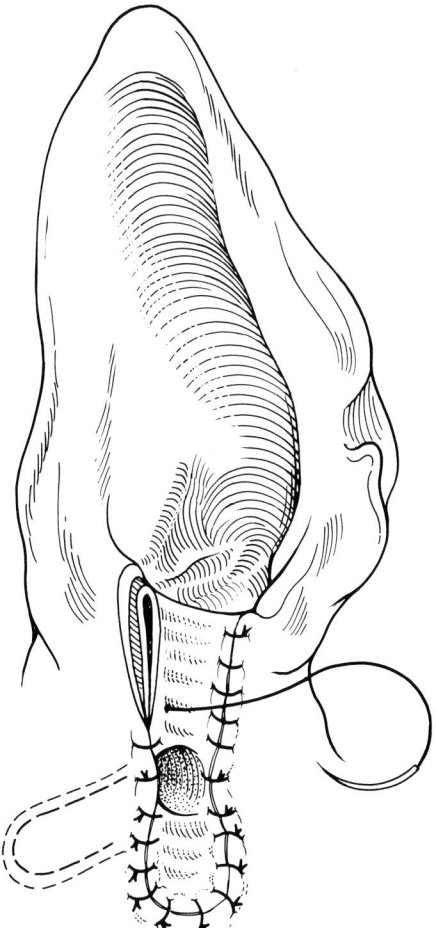

FIG. 17-4
Lateral ear resection (Zepp procedure).

and, using a combination of sharp and blunt dissection, reflect the skin flap dorsally—exposing the lateral cartilaginous wall of the vertical ear canal. During dissection, stay as close as possible to the cartilage of the ear canal to prevent inadvertently damaging the facial nerve. Note the parotid gland at the ventral extent of the incision and avoid damaging it. Standing at the dorsal aspect of the animal's head, use Mayo scissors to cut the vertical canal (Fig. 17-5, C). Place one blade of the scissors in the canal at the pretragic or tragohelicine incisure at the cranial (or medial) aspect of the external auditory meatus and, with the scissors at a 30° angle, incise the canal ventrally to the level of the horizontal canal. Repeat the process beginning at the intertragic incisure (caudal or lateral aspect of the external auditory meatus). Do not allow the incisions to converge toward the lateral aspect of the canal, or the drainboard will be too narrow. Be sure to extend the incisions as far distally as the beginning of the horizontal canal, or the drainboard will not lie flat against the skin. Reflect the cartilage flap distally, and inspect the opening of the horizontal canal; if indicated, obtain cultures (Fig. 17-5, D). Occasionally the opening can be widened by making two small cuts at the cranial and caudal aspects. Resect the distal half of the cartilage flap to

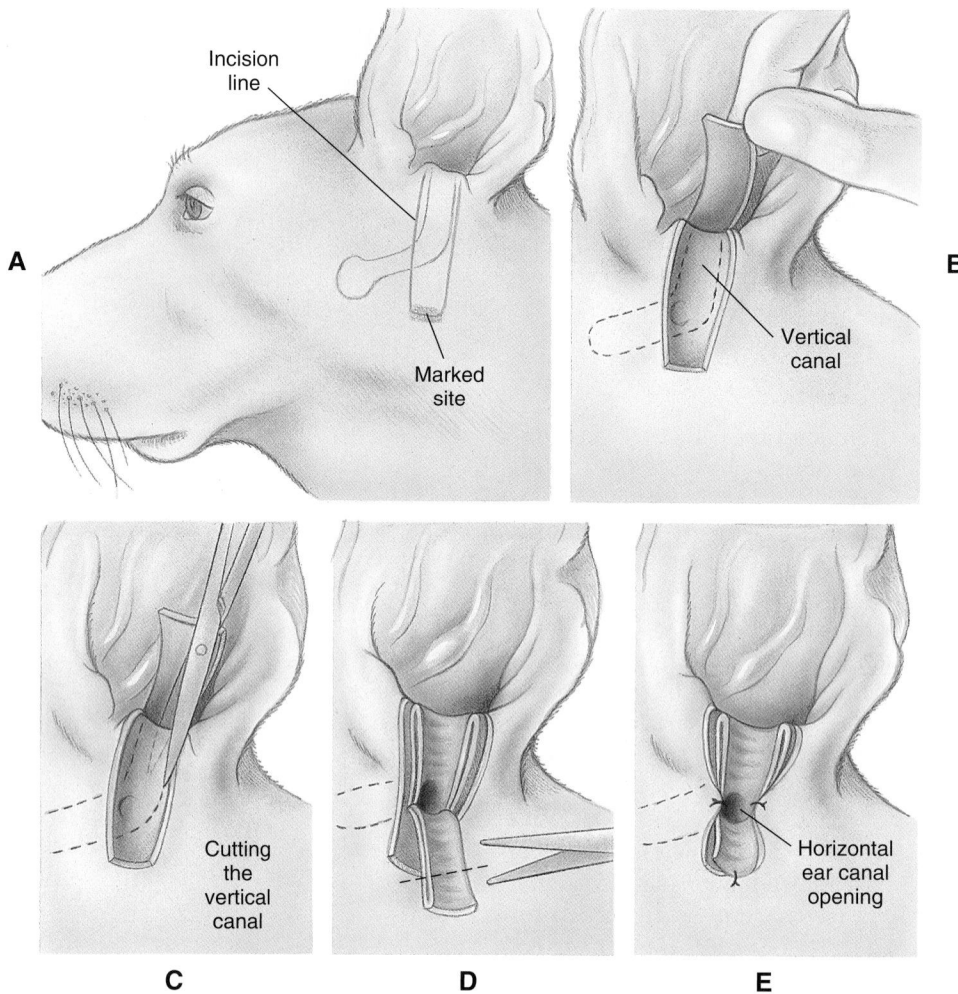

FIG. 17-5

Lateral ear canal resection. **A,** Mark a site one half the length of the vertical ear canal below the horizontal ear canal. **B,** Lateral to the vertical ear canal, make two parallel incisions that extend from the tragus ventrally to the marked site. **C,** Connect the skin incisions ventrally, and reflect the skin flap dorsally, exposing the lateral cartilaginous wall of the vertical ear canal. Use Mayo scissors to cut the vertical canal. **D,** Reflect the cartilage flap distally, and inspect the opening of the horizontal canal. Resect the distal half of the cartilage flap to make the drainboard, and remove the skin flap. **E,** Place sutures from the epithelial tissue to the skin. Begin suturing at the opening of the horizontal canal, then suture the drainboard.

make the drainboard and remove the skin flap. The ligament between the horizontal and vertical flaps usually acts as a hinge to allow the drainboard to lie flat, but in some cases scoring the cartilage on the ventral aspect of the drainboard facilitates this. Place absorbable or nonabsorbable monofilament sutures (3-0 or 4-0) from the epithelial tissue to the skin (Fig. 17-5, E). Begin suturing at the opening of the horizontal canal first, then suture the drainboard. Last, suture the cranial and caudal aspects of the medial wall of the vertical ear canal to the skin (see Fig. 17-5, E).

Vertical Ear Canal Ablation

Vertical canal ablation can be performed when the entire vertical canal is diseased but the horizontal canal is normal. It may be the technique of choice when neoplasia is con-fined to the vertical canal or in some animals with chronic otitis externa. Total removal of the vertical canal may result in less postoperative exudation and pain. This technique may also provide a better cosmetic appearance of the ear than lateral ear canal resection when an abundance of hyperplastic tissue is present in and around the vertical canal (Fig. 17-6).

Position and prepare the animal as for a lateral ear canal resection. Make a T-shaped incision with the horizontal component parallel and just below the upper edge of the tragus (Fig. 17-7, A). From the midpoint of the horizontal incision, make a vertical incision that extends to the level of the horizontal canal. Retract the skin flaps, reflect loose connective tissue, and expose the lateral aspect of the vertical ear canal

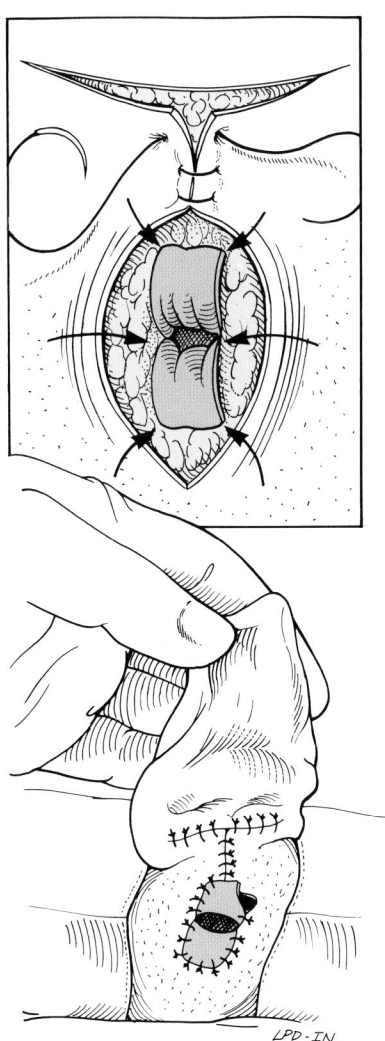

FIG. 17-6
Vertical ear canal resection may be performed when the entire vertical canal is diseased but the horizontal canal is normal.

(Fig. 17-7, B). Continue the horizontal incision through the cartilage around the external auditory meatus with a scalpel blade. Remove as much of the diseased tissue on the medial surface of the pinna as possible, but avoid damaging the major branches of the great auricular artery. Use curved Mayo scissors to dissect around the proximal and medial aspects of the vertical canal. During dissection, stay as close as possible to the cartilage of the ear canal to prevent inadvertently damaging the facial nerve. Free the entire vertical canal from all muscular and fascial attachments (Fig. 17-7, C). Transect the vertical canal ventrally 1 to 2 cm dorsal to the horizontal canal and submit it for histologic examination (Fig. 17-7, D). Incise the remnant of the vertical canal cranially and caudally to create dorsal and ventral flaps (Fig. 17-7, E). Reflect the ventral flap downward, and suture it to the skin for a drainboard using absorbable or nonabsorbable monofilament sutures (2-0 to 4-0). Suture the dorsal flap to the skin and close the subcutaneous tissue with an

absorbable suture material (2-0 or 3-0). Then close the skin in a T shape (Fig. 17-7, F).

Total Ear Canal Ablation

TECA is indicated in animals with chronic otitis externa that has failed to respond to appropriate medical management in cases of severe calcification and ossification of the ear cartilage, or when severe epithelial hyperplasia extends beyond the pinna or vertical ear canal (Fig. 17-8). The procedure commonly is performed on animals in which lateral ear resections have failed, and it may also be beneficial to those with severely stenotic ear canals. Occasionally, neoplasia of the horizontal canal can be treated by TECA. In a recent study in cats, TECA was performed in 41% of cases because of neoplasia (typically ceruminous gland adenocarcinoma; see p. 312), whereas half of the cats had it performed because of chronic inflammatory or polypoid (see p. 314) disease (Bacon et al, 2003). Because of the potential for serious complications, this surgery should not be performed on animals with mild disease or by surgeons unfamiliar with the anatomy of the ear. A high percentage of dogs that undergo TECA have associated skin disease, such as seborrhea, atopy, or food or contact allergy dermatitis. The skin disease should be treated before resorting to surgery because effective dermatologic therapy usually benefits the ears also. If the skin condition is unresponsive, TECA is preferred over lateral ear resection (see p. 293) and should be performed in conjunction with a lateral bulla osteotomy (see p. 298).

> NOTE: Most animals with severe, chronic otitis externa have concurrent otitis media. Removing the avenue for drainage of exudative material by performing a TECA without treating the otitis media is disastrous. Therefore always perform a bulla osteotomy in conjunction with a TECA for otitis externa and media.

Pinna deformity after TECA in cats may be a source of dissatisfaction for some owners. A recently reported technique using a single-pedicle advancement flap at the base of the pinna during a modified TECA may facilitate upright ear carriage and improve the cosmetic result, and thus enhance owner satisfaction (McNabb and Flanders, 2004; Fig. 17-9).

Position the animal in lateral recumbency with the head elevated with a towel. Prepare the pinna and surrounding skin for aseptic surgery. Make a T-shaped incision with the horizontal component parallel and just below the upper edge of the tragus (Fig. 17-10, A). From the midpoint of the horizontal incision, make a vertical incision that extends to just past the level of the horizontal canal (see Fig. 17-10, A). Retract the skin flaps, reflect loose connective tissue, and expose the lateral aspect of the vertical canal. Continue the horizontal incision around the opening of the vertical ear canal with a scalpel blade (Fig. 17-10, B). Use curved Mayo

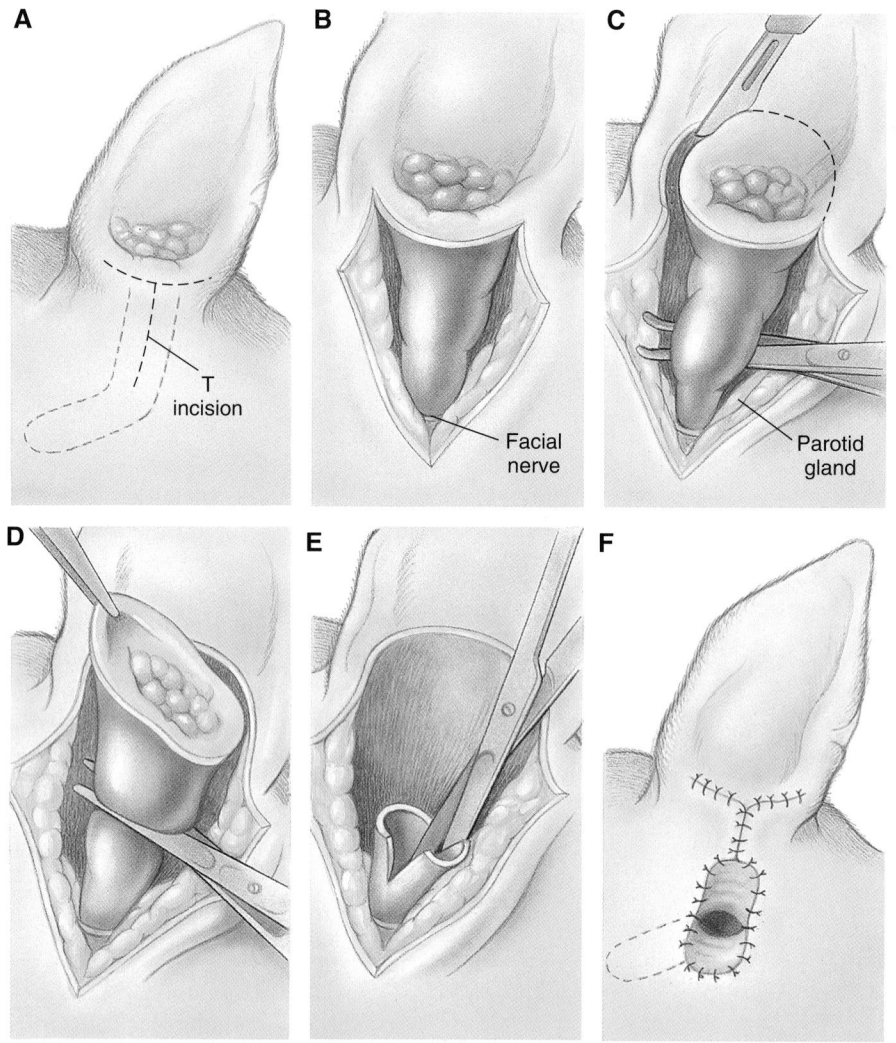

FIG. 17-7

Vertical ear canal ablation. **A,** Make a T-shaped incision with the horizontal component parallel and just below the upper edge of the tragus. From the midpoint of the horizontal incision, make a vertical incision that extends to the level of the horizontal canal. **B,** Retract the skin flaps, reflect loose connective tissue, and expose the lateral aspect of the vertical canal. **C,** Continue the horizontal incision through the cartilage around the external auditory meatus with a scalpel blade. Use curved Mayo scissors to dissect around the proximal and medial aspects of the vertical canal. Free the entire vertical canal from all muscular and fascial attachments. **D,** Transect the canal ventrally 1 to 2 cm dorsal to the horizontal canal and submit the canal for histologic examination. **E,** Incise the remnant of the vertical canal cranially and caudally to create dorsal and ventral flaps. **F,** Reflect the ventral flap downward and suture it to the skin for a drainboard. Suture the dorsal flap to the skin and close the subcutaneous tissue. Then close the skin in a T shape.

scissors to dissect around the proximal and medial aspects of the vertical canal (Fig. 17-10, *C*). During dissection, stay as close as possible to the cartilage of the ear canal to prevent inadvertently damaging the facial nerve. Avoid damaging the major branches of the great auricular artery at the medial aspect of the vertical canal. Identify the facial nerve as it courses caudoventrally to the horizontal canal (gently retract it if necessary). If the facial nerve is trapped within thickened, calcified horizontal canal tissue, carefully dissect the nerve from the horizontal canal. Continue the dissection to the level of the external acoustic meatus (Fig. 17-10, *D*). Excise the horizontal canal attachment to the external acoustic meatus with a scalpel blade, rongeur, or Mayo scissors, but be careful to avoid damaging the facial nerve. Remove the entire ear canal, and obtain deep cultures around or just inside the external acoustic meatus. Submit the ear for histologic examination. Use a curette to carefully remove secretory tissue that is adherent to the rim of the external acoustic

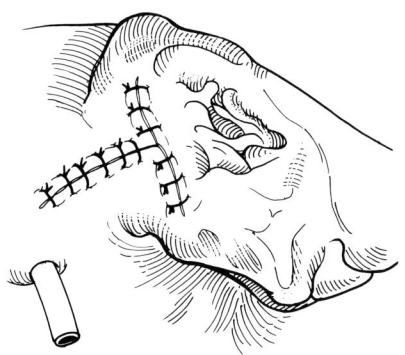

FIG. 17-8
Total ear canal ablation.

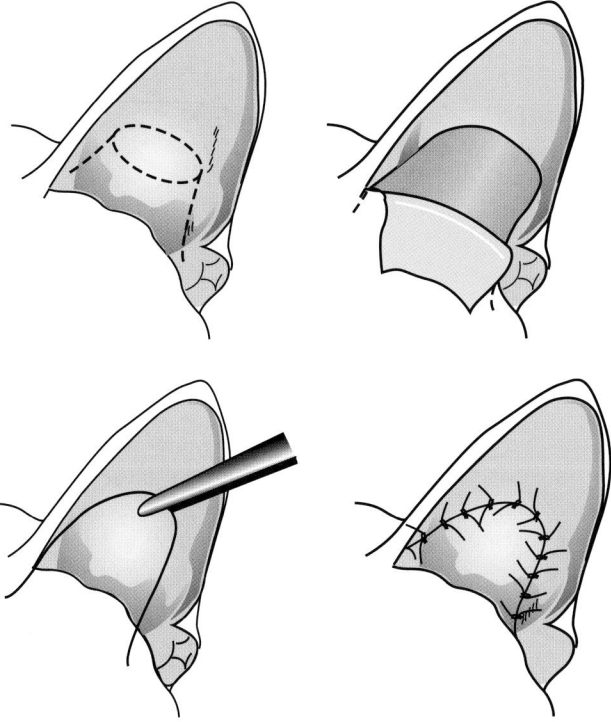

FIG. 17-9
To perform a modified TECA in a cat, make a vertical incision at the cranial and caudal ends of an elliptic incision centered around the external auditory meatus. Dissect the single-pedicle advancement flap ventrally, allowing exposure of the subcutaneous tissue over the vertical ear canal. After lateral bulla osteotomy and excision of the ear canal, pull the top of the advancement flap to the base of the pinna to determine if further release of the flap is necessary to reduce tension on the pinna. Suture the flap to the base of the pinna.

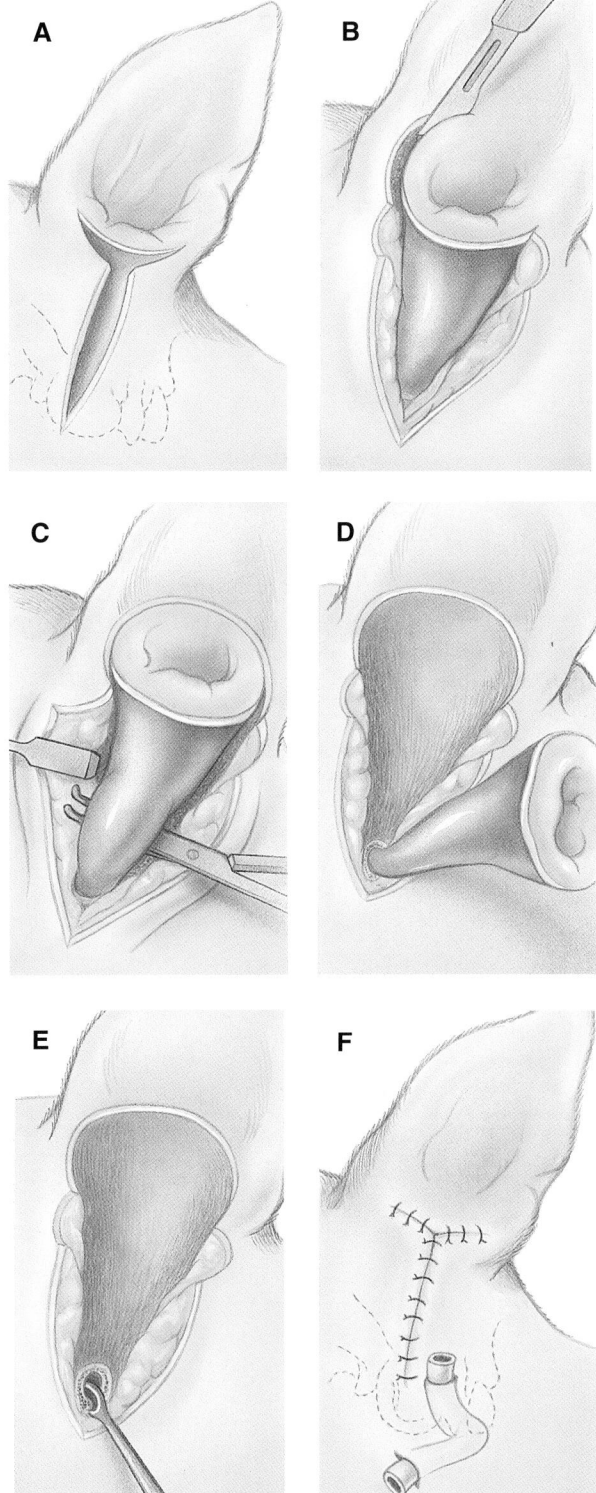

FIG. 17-10
Total ear canal resection. **A,** Make a T-shaped incision with the horizontal component parallel and just below the upper edge of the tragus. From the midpoint of the horizontal incision, make a vertical incision that extends to just past the level of the horizontal canal. **B,** Retract the skin flaps, reflect loose connective tissue, and expose the lateral aspect of the vertical canal. Continue the horizontal incision around the opening of the vertical ear canal with a scalpel blade. **C,** Dissect around the proximal and medial aspects of the vertical canal. **D,** Continue the dissection to the level of the external acoustic meatus. **E,** Excise the horizontal canal attachment to the external acoustic meatus with a scalpel blade, rongeur, or Mayo scissors, and use a curette to carefully remove secretory tissue that is adherent to the rim of the external acoustic meatus. **F,** If desired, place a Penrose drain. Close the subcutaneous tissue and skin.

meatus (Fig. 17-10, E). Be sure to remove all epithelial tissue in this region, or chronic fistulation will occur. Perform a lateral bulla osteotomy (see later discussion). Flush the area with sterile saline solution before closure. Close the subcutaneous tissue with absorbable suture (2-0 or 3-0), and close the skin in a T shape (Fig. 17-10, F). If drainage is desired, use blunt dissection to exit a Penrose drain (¼ to ½ inch wide) or soft rubber tubing ventral to the incision in a dependent area (through a separate stab incision) or use closed suction drainage (e.g., butterfly catheter and Vacutainer tube). The end of the drain near the tympanic cavity may be secured with a single suture of chromic catgut (4-0 or 5-0). Secure the drain to the skin at the exit site.

Lateral Bulla Osteotomy

Lateral bulla osteotomy exposes the tympanic cavity so that exudate and secretory epithelium can be removed, which improves drainage. It should be performed in conjunction with TECA in animals with chronic otitis externa and middle ear disease. Although a lateral bulla osteotomy affords less exposure to the tympanic cavity than a ventral osteotomy, it does not require that the animal be repositioned and is preferred when performed in conjunction with TECA.

Bluntly dissect the tissue from the lateral aspect of the bulla using a small periosteal elevator. Avoid damaging the external carotid artery and maxillary vein that travel just ventral to the bulla. Rongeur the lateral and ventral aspects of the bulla until the caudal aspect of the middle ear canal is exposed (Fig. 17-11). Extend the bony excision as needed to fully visualize the contents of the tympanic cavity, but avoid sharp dissection and curettage of the rostral aspect of the osseous ear canal to reduce the risk of retroauricular vein damage. Use a curette to remove infected material, but avoid curetting in the rostral (dorsal) or rostromedial area of the tympanic cavity so as not to damage the auditory ossicles or inner ear structures. Gently irrigate the cavity with saline to remove all remaining debris.

Ventral Bulla Osteotomy

Ventral bulla osteotomy allows increased exposure of the tympanic cavity and can be performed alone or in conjunction with lateral ear resection. It is the technique of choice when middle ear neoplasia is suspected in cats that have nasopharyngeal polyps (see p. 314). This technique provides better drainage of the bulla than does lateral bulla osteotomy and allows both bullae to be opened without repositioning the animal.

Place the patient in dorsal recumbency, and prepare a generous area surrounding the angle of the mandible for aseptic surgery. Palpate the bulla immediately caudal and medial to the vertical ramus of the mandible. Draw an imaginary line connecting the mandibular rami and a second imaginary line along the long axis of the ventral aspect of the head (Fig. 17-12, A). In dogs, make a 7- to 10-cm incision (3 to 5 cm

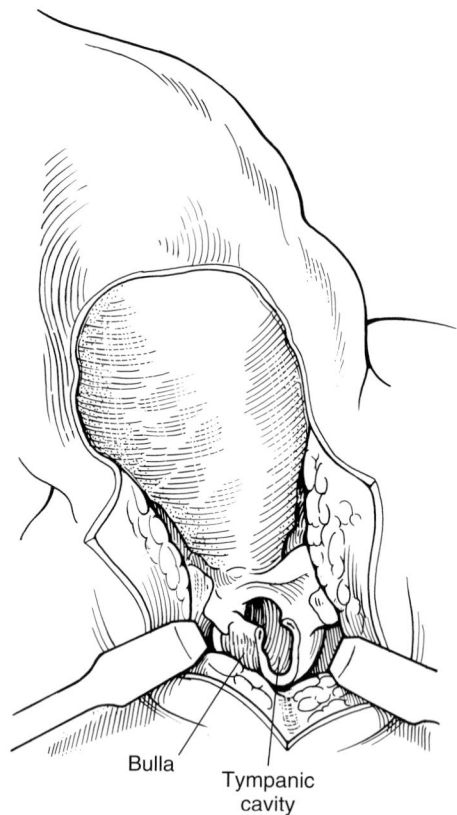

FIG. 17-11
Lateral bulla osteotomy.

Bulla   Tympanic cavity

in cats) parallel to the midline of the animal and centered 2 cm toward the affected side from where these imaginary lines intersect (see Fig. 17-12, A). Incise the platysma muscle, retract the linguofacial vein if necessary, and deepen the incision by bluntly dissecting the digastricus muscle (lateral) from the hyoglossus and styloglossus muscles (medial). Avoid damaging the hypoglossal nerve, located on the lateral aspect of the hyoglossus muscle. Confirm the location of the bulla and use self-retaining retractors (i.e., Gelpi or Weitlaner) to spread the digastric and glossal muscles and retract them from the bulla (Fig. 17-12, B). Palpate the bulla craniomedial to the cornu process of the hyoid bone and caudomedial to the angle of the mandible. Bluntly dissect tissues from the ventral surface of the bulla and use a Steinmann pin to make a hole in its ventral aspect. Enlarge the opening with a small rongeur (i.e., Lempert). Examine the interior of the bulla for inflammatory debris, neoplastic tissue, or foreign bodies, and obtain samples for culture, sensitivity, and histopathologic examination. In cats, be sure to examine both compartments of the bulla (see the discussion on surgical anatomy, pp. 291 and 292, and Fig. 17-2). Flush the cavity with warm saline, and if evidence of infection is noted or if continued drainage is anticipated, place a small, fenestrated drain tube in the cavity and exit it through a separate stab incision. Suture the fenestrated portion of the drain tube to the bulla with small chromic gut suture (4-0 to

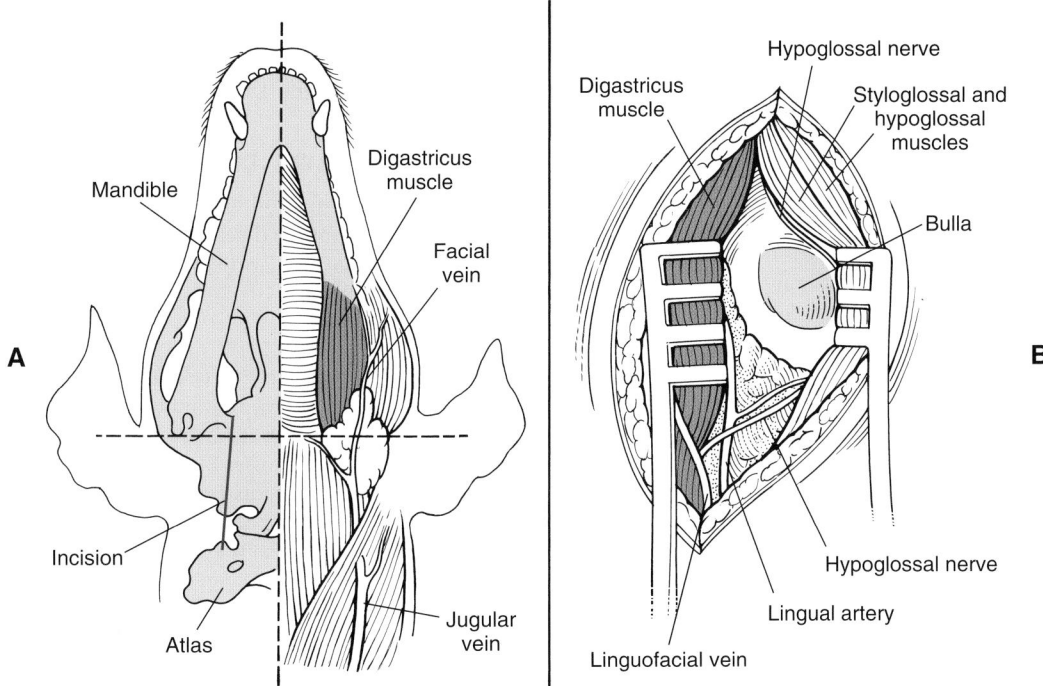

FIG. 17-12
Ventral bulla osteotomy. **A,** For ventral bulla osteotomy, draw an imaginary line connecting the mandibular rami and a second imaginary line along the long axis of the ventral aspect of the head. Make a 7- to 10-cm incision parallel with the midline of the neck and centered 2 cm toward the affected side from where these imaginary lines intersect. **B,** Incise the platysma muscle, retract the linguofacial vein if necessary, and deepen the incision by bluntly dissecting the digastricus muscle (lateral) from the hypoglossal and styloglossal muscles (medial). Confirm the location of the bulla, and use self-retaining retractors to spread the digastricus and glossal muscles and retract them from the bulla.

6-0). Depending on the amount of exudation, remove the drain in 3 to 7 days.

HEALING OF THE EAR

Hyperkeratinization of the epidermis and hyperplasia of the dermis and epidermis of the ear canals occur secondary to chronic infection or inflammation. Sebaceous glands become less numerous and active, and apocrine tubular glands distend and increase secretion. Healing of the surgical techniques previously described is routine unless incisional infections develop that cause dehiscence. Such wounds are best left open to granulate unless they are very large.

SUTURE MATERIALS AND SPECIAL INSTRUMENTS

Electrosurgery is useful for ear surgery because numerous vessels are encountered. Small curettes simplify removal of the epithelial tissue on the bony rim at the external acoustic meatus. An assortment of various sized rongeurs (e.g., Cleveland, Lempert, Kerrison, and Ruskin) or an air-driven burr is needed to remove the lateral and caudal aspects of the bulla when performing a TECA. A Freer elevator is useful for reflecting soft tissue attached around the ventrolateral wall of the bulla. Retractors, such as Senn or Army-Navy, are

helpful to aid in visualization of deep structures. A Steinmann pin, hand chuck, and rongeurs are necessary for ventral bulla osteotomy (unless the bone has been eroded by infection or neoplasia). Self-retaining retractors are useful when performing a ventral bulla osteotomy to allow retraction of the muscles superficial to the bulla. Culture swabs (both aerobic and anaerobic) should be available whenever ear surgery is performed. Monofilament suture (i.e., polydioxanone, polyglyconate, poliglecaprone 25, polypropylene, or nylon) should be used to suture the epithelial tissue of the canal to the skin. Absorbable suture should be used for subcutaneous sutures.

POSTOPERATIVE CARE AND ASSESSMENT

Postoperative analgesics should be given after ear canal resection or ablation (see the discussion on anesthetics on p. 290), and tranquilizers may be administered if the animal appears dysphoric or anxious (see p. 290). A bandage should be placed over the ear or ears, and an Elizabethan collar or sidebar should be used to prevent bandage removal or ear mutilation. If swelling is excessive, a hot pack can be applied to the side of the face several times a day for the first few days after surgery. Antibiotics should be based on culture results and continued for 3 to 4 weeks. Penrose drains generally can be removed in 3 to 7 days, and sutures can be removed in 10 to 14 days.

> NOTE: Monitor these patients closely after surgery. Bandages or excessive swelling, particularly after bilateral TECA and lateral bulla osteotomy, may impair respiration.

COMPLICATIONS

Complications other than inadequate drainage and continued otitis externa are uncommon after lateral ear resection or vertical ear canal ablation. Clinical signs associated with otitis externa may not be relieved in dogs with underlying dermatologic disease that cannot be effectively managed. If the opening of the horizontal canal is insufficient for drainage or if these techniques are performed in animals with concurrent middle ear disease without treating the middle ear infection, the result is persistent or recurrent signs of otitis externa. Facial nerve palsy is a rare complication of vertical ear canal ablation. Complications of TECA (i.e., superficial wound infections, facial nerve paralysis, vestibular dysfunction, deafness, chronic fistulation or abscessation, and avascular necrosis of the skin of the pinna) are potentially more serious than with the other techniques discussed in this chapter. Facial nerve paralysis, which usually resolves within a few weeks of surgery, is caused by stretching or retraction of the nerve; however, permanent damage occurs if the nerve is transected or severely stretched. Facial nerve paralysis was reported to occur in 56% of cats after TECA (Bacon et al, 2003). This complication was permanent in approximately one fourth of them. Facial nerve damage may result in loss of the blink response and parasympathetic nerve innervation to the lacrimal glands. The eye should be kept moistened with artificial tears or an ophthalmic lubricant to prevent corneal ulceration. If normal lid function does not return within 4 to 6 weeks or if ulceration of the eye occurs because of chronic drying, enucleation may be indicated; however, this is seldom necessary.

> NOTE: Facial nerve paralysis, vestibular dysfunction, and Horner's syndrome all may be caused by otitis media and interna or by surgery. The presence of these abnormalities before surgery must be noted to avoid having them considered as surgical complications.

Signs of middle and inner ear disease may persist after surgery, but if they worsen acutely, an abscess of the tympanic cavity should be suspected. Superficial wound infections are common and are attributed to surgical manipulation of infected tissue, inadequate closure of dead space, inadequate drainage, and resistance to antibiotics. In cats, surgical curettage of the tympanic cavity may cause a transient Horner's syndrome, which usually resolves in 2 to 3 weeks (see discussion on surgical anatomy, p. 291).

> NOTE: Warn owners that Horner's syndrome and facial nerve paralysis are common in cats after ventral bulla osteotomy but that both are typically transitory.

SPECIAL AGE CONSIDERATIONS

Young cats with middle or inner ear signs or a previous history of respiratory disease should be examined for nasopharyngeal polyps (see pp. 314-316).

References

Bacon NJ, Gilbert RL, Bostock DE et al: Total ear canal ablation in the cat: indications, morbidity, and long-term survival *J Small Anim Pract* 44:430, 2003.

Graham-Mize CA, Rosser EJ: Comparison of microbial isolates and susceptibility patterns from the external ear canal of dogs with otitis externa, *J Am Anim Hosp Assoc* 40:102, 2004.

McNabb AH, Flanders JA: Closure of total ear canal ablations in 6 cats: 2002-2003, *Vet Surg* 33:435, 2004.

Peterson AD, Walker RD, Bowman MM et al: Frequency of isolation and antimicrobial susceptibility patterns of *Staphylococcus intermedius* and *Pseudomonas aeruginosa* isolates from canine skin and ear samples over a 6-year period (1992-1997), *J Am Anim Hosp Assoc* 38:407, 2002.

Radlinsky MG, Mason DE, Roush JK et al: Use of a continuous, local infusion of bupivacaine for postoperative analgesia in dogs undergoing total ear canal ablation, *J Am Vet Med Assoc* 227:414, 2005.

Sylvestre AM: Potential factors affecting the outcome of dogs with a resection of the lateral wall of the vertical ear canal, *Can Vet J* 39:157, 1998.

Suggested Reading

Smeak DD, Inpanbutr N: Lateral approach to subtotal bulla osteotomy in dogs: pertinent anatomy and procedural reviews, *Compend* 27:377, 2005.

This article provides an excellent review of ear anatomy and a detailed procedural description of exposure of the tympanic cavity during lateral bulla osteotomy.

SPECIFIC DISEASES

OTITIS EXTERNA

DEFINITIONS

Otitis externa is an inflammation of the epithelium of the horizontal and vertical ear canals and surrounding structures (i.e., external auditory meatus and pinna). **Swimmer's ear** is a term used to describe otitis externa that occurs after swimming or bathing.

GENERAL CONSIDERATIONS AND CLINICALLY RELEVANT PATHOPHYSIOLOGY

Otitis externa is common in both dogs (3.9% to 20% of hospital admissions) and cats (2% to 6.6% of hospital admissions). It may be associated with other dermatologic diseases, particularly allergic or immune-mediated skin disease (i.e., food allergy dermatitis, atopy, and contact dermatitis) or systemic diseases (i.e., endocrinopathies, such as hypothyroidism or Sertoli cell tumors). Bacterial infections, foreign bodies (e.g., foxtails), parasites (e.g., *Otodectes cynotis*, *Demodex canis*, *Sarcoptes scabiei*, *Notoedres cati*, and ticks), fungi, yeasts (e.g., *Malassezia pachydermis*), or neoplasia also may be the cause. *O. cynotis* is responsible for more than 50% of cases of otitis externa in cats.

Predisposing conditions for otitis externa include excessive moisture or increased humidity in the ear canal, a narrow canal conformation, or obstruction of the canal. The normal ear canal is inhabited by bacteria (i.e., *Staphylococcus* and β-*Streptococcus* spp.). High humidity and temperature promote moisture retention in the ear, which allows maceration of the epithelial lining and fosters secondary bacterial colonization. It has been proposed that in chronic otitis externa the apocrine glands increase in size, number, and secretory activity, whereas the sebaceous glands decrease in number and become less active. However, the dog may not have a common physiologic pathway for progressive changes as previously thought. Cocker spaniels with otitis externa have been shown to have distinct differences in pathologic characteristics of the horizontal ear canal compared with other breeds. They more commonly have ceruminous tissue responses, whereas other breeds have predominantly fibrosis (Angus et al, 2002).

The bacteria most often isolated from the ears of dogs with chronic otitis externa are *Corynebacterium* spp., *Escherichia coli*, *Proteus mirabilis*, *P. aeruginosa*, and *S. intermedius*. *Pasteurella multocida* and *S. intermedius* are commonly isolated from the ears of cats. In some animals chronic otitis externa may cause secondary changes in the ear canal (i.e., epithelial hyperplasia and ossification of chronically inflamed tissue) that perpetuate the infection and make medical management difficult because of constriction of the external ear canal lumen. In addition, ulceration and secondary infection with pyogenic bacteria, yeast, and/or fungi commonly occur.

DIAGNOSIS
Clinical Presentation
Signalment. Dogs and cats of any breed or age may develop otitis externa, but some groups are at higher risk. Dogs with long, pendulous ears (e.g., spaniels and basset hounds) and those with abundant hair in the ear canal (e.g., poodles) are commonly affected. Of the erect-eared dogs, German shepherds are most frequently affected. Spaniel breeds, particularly cocker spaniels, may have abnormal keratinization and increased sebaceous gland secretion of the pinna or ear canal or both. Chronic bacterial infection and hyperplastic changes in the sebaceous glands and epithelial lining of the ear often lead to scarring and ear canal obstruction.

History. Animals with otitis externa may be presented for evaluation of acute or chronic signs. If a foreign body is lodged in the ear, head shaking and scratching at or near the ear are typical. Head shaking and ear scratching are also common among animals with parasitic infections and acute bacterial infections. A purulent, odoriferous discharge may be noted with chronic infections. The animal may constantly rub its head on objects and may seem to be in pain when the head or ear is touched.

Physical Examination Findings
Palpation of the ear may suggest thickening or calcification of the ear canal. A thorough otoscopic examination should be performed even if it requires tranquilization. Examination of the ear canal often is difficult if hyperplasia or exudation is present; general anesthesia may be necessary to allow meticulous inspection. The extent of involvement of the vertical and horizontal ear canals and the status of the tympanic membrane should be determined. Purulent yellow or cream-colored exudates may be associated with gram-negative infections, particularly *Pseudomonas* and *Proteus* spp. Dark brown or black exudates are more commonly associated with yeast infections or those caused by *Staphylococcus* or *Streptococcus* spp. A bloody exudate may be suggestive of neoplasia. A definitive diagnosis requires examination of exudate collected during the procedure by placing sterile swabs into the canal through the otoscope cone. The exudate should be examined for parasites, bacteria, fungi, and yeast; bacterial and fungal cultures should be performed if indicated. The ear should be flushed with a bulb syringe or soft catheter, and alligator forceps should be available to remove foreign bodies and debris. Biopsy of the external ear canal may allow diagnosis of neoplasia and some allergic conditions.

> NOTE: Perform a complete dermatologic examination in all animals with otitis externa unless an obvious cause is found, such as a foreign body.

Diagnostic Imaging
Skull radiography or cross-sectional imaging should be performed to determine if concurrent otitis media is present; cross-sectional imaging is preferred because of the lack of superimposition and the increased sensitivity in detecting abnormalities (see p. 305). Because improper obliquity or angulation of the skull for radiographs or malpositioning of the tongue can result in an inadequate study, false negatives or underestimation of the extent of middle ear disease is common with radiographs. Calcification of the external auditory canal is commonly noted with chronic otitis externa (Fig. 17-13); this finding may influence the choice of surgical techniques. Occasionally imaging signs suggestive of neoplasia are found, such as bony lysis of the petrous temporal bone. Computed tomography (CT) findings with otitis externa include mineralization of the ear canal, narrowing of the lumen of the external ear canal, and soft tissue attenuating material within the lumen of the ear canal. CT may also be useful for evaluation of abscess formation following a TECA. Uptake of contrast may be noted in areas of infection (abscessation, fistulous tracts). Canalographic evaluation of the external ear canal has been proposed as a mechanism to

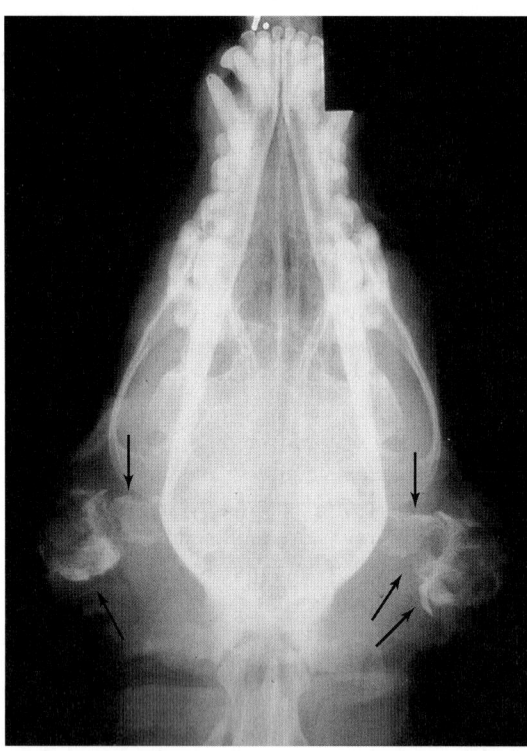

FIG. 17-13
Calcification of the external ear canals *(arrows)* in a dog with chronic otitis externa. (Courtesy L. Homco, Ithaca, N.Y.)

help delineate the status of the tympanic membrane before medical or surgical therapy in dogs (Eom, 2000).

Laboratory Findings

Specific laboratory abnormalities are not found. Thyroid function tests should be performed if hypothyroidism is suspected.

DIFFERENTIAL DIAGNOSIS

The diagnosis of otitis externa usually is simple; however, differentiation of the various causes may be difficult. It is important to identify treatable underlying causes of otitis externa before considering surgical intervention; optimal results require appropriate treatment of underlying diseases. In some cases, surgery is unnecessary if the underlying cause is treated. Concurrent otitis media should be identified in animals that are to undergo surgery for otitis externa.

> NOTE: Lateral ear canal resection and vertical canal ablation often fail if concurrent dermatologic or middle ear disease is not resolved.

MEDICAL MANAGEMENT

Treatment of otitis externa involves identifying the underlying or perpetuating causes, cleaning and drying the ear, and using appropriate topical medications (see p. 290). Because ceruminous material impairs the ability of topical medica-

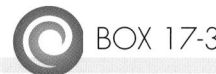 **BOX 17-3**

Otic Preparations

Tris-EDTA Solution (0.05 mol/L Tris, 0.003 mol/L EDTA)

24.2 g Tris (base)
4.8 g ethylenediamine tetraacetic acid (EDTA) (disodium salt)
3900 ml distilled water
100 ml white vinegar (5% acetic acid)
Adjust pH to 8 with additional vinegar (30–50 ml)
Autoclave and store sterile

Silver Sulfadiazine Solution (0.1%)

0.1 g silver sulfadiazine powder
100 ml distilled water
Mix to dissolve

tions to reach the infection and may inactivate some drugs, the ears must be thoroughly cleaned before treatment. The status of the tympanic membrane (intact versus ruptured) should be ascertained. Many topical agents are available for treatment of otitis externa, and most contain various combinations of antibiotics and parasiticidal, antiinflammatory, and/or antifungal agents. The reader is referred to a dermatology or medicine text for an in-depth discussion of the use of these various agents. Medications that can be used in animals with a ruptured tympanic membrane are listed in Box 17-1. The combination of Tris-EDTA and an antimicrobial has a synergistic effect against some bacteria implicated in otitis externa (Box 17-3). Ototoxicity of the various agents should be taken into account before they are used, particularly if the tympanic membrane has been ruptured. Silver sulfadiazine solution (0.1%; see Box 17-3) can be used without an intact tympanic membrane. Persistence of clinical signs after treatment of otitis externa may suggest concurrent otitis media. Targeted systemic antibiotics, administered for 6 to 8 weeks, are indicated for treatment of otitis media (see p. 290).

SURGICAL TREATMENT

Surgical therapy of otitis externa should be considered when medical management fails or in cases involving proliferative growths or stenotic canals. The surgical alternatives in animals with otitis externa that do not have middle ear involvement include a lateral ear canal resection (see p. 293), vertical ear canal ablation (see p. 294), or TECA (see p. 295). If concurrent otitis media exists, a lateral ear canal resection in conjunction with a ventral bulla osteotomy (see p. 298) or a TECA with lateral bulla osteotomy (see p. 298) can be performed.

Preoperative Management

Preoperative antibiotic therapy is recommended. Bacterial cultures should be performed if purulent discharge is present, and the appropriate antibiotics should be initiated before surgery. If no discharge is present, perioperative antibiotics (see p. 290) may be given intravenously immediately before the surgical procedure or may be administered during surgery but after intraoperative cultures have been obtained. Based on culture and susceptibility testing, cefazolin may be a poor choice for perioperative prophylaxis in dogs undergoing TECA and bulla osteotomy (Hettlich et al, 2005). In the aforementioned study, antibiotics with overall susceptibility rates greater than 75% included imipenem, gentamicin, and amoxicillin-clavulanic acid. Cefazolin, tetracycline, and trimethoprim-sulfonamide all had an overall susceptibility of less than 50%. Amoxicillin-clavulanic acid or cephalothin may be a reasonable choice for prophylaxis because most *S. intermedius* are susceptible to them and *S. intermedius* is a common isolate of ear samples. Culture and susceptibility testing is advised if *P. aeruginosa* infections are suspected because *P. aeruginosa is* typically resistant to many antibiotics. See also Table 17-1 on p. 291 for a list of antimicrobial susceptibilities to bacteria found in dogs with chronic otitis externa.

Anesthesia

See p. 289 for anesthetic recommendations for animals with ear disease.

Surgical Anatomy

See p. 291 for a description of the surgical anatomy of the ear canal.

Positioning

See pp. 293 to 295 for positioning for the various surgical procedures.

SURGICAL TECHNIQUE

The choice of surgical techniques depends on the severity and extent of the disease. See pp. 293 to 299 for a description of the surgical techniques used in animals with ear disease. A discussion of the indications and contraindications for each procedure is provided.

SUTURE MATERIALS AND SPECIAL INSTRUMENTS

See p. 299 for a discussion of appropriate suture materials and instruments for surgery of the ear.

POSTOPERATIVE CARE AND ASSESSMENT

Postoperative pain is common in animals that have undergone ear surgery. See p. 290 for a discussion of analgesic therapy in these patients. After administration of adequate analgesics, tranquilizers may be given if the animal appears dysphoric or anxious (see p. 290). The ear should be bandaged after surgery to minimize contamination of and trauma to the surgical site. Animals often shake their heads excessively after ear surgery and may try to paw or scratch at the bandage. Close supervision in the early postoperative period and use of an Elizabethan collar or sidebar are recommended.

PROGNOSIS

Chronic otitis externa is a difficult disease to treat with medical therapy or surgery. A poor surgical outcome may be the result of technical failures (e.g., not making the horizontal canal opening large enough with lateral ear canal resection or vertical ear canal ablation), lack of owner compliance in continuing to treat the ear (with lateral ear canal resection or vertical ear canal ablation), unrealistic expectations on the part of the owner, unrecognized middle ear disease, faulty diagnoses (e.g., not recognizing neoplasia as the underlying cause), or failure to treat the underlying disease or perpetuating cause. Surgical procedures designed to increase drainage (i.e., lateral ear canal resection and vertical ear canal ablation) often fail in animals with untreated dermatologic disease or unrecognized middle ear disease. A Zepp procedure results in a satisfactory outcome in less than half of patients; however, this may be related to the fact that the procedure is often done in dogs with chronic otitis externa in which TECA would have been the preferred technique. A properly performed TECA combined with a lateral bulla osteotomy resolves clinical signs in most animals.

COMPLICATIONS

Partial or complete facial nerve paralysis occurs in some animals after TECA; however, this complication is less likely when the surgeon is experienced in performing the procedure. Other complications include persistent infection (dissecting cellulitis, prolonged wound drainage, incisional dehiscence, periauricular abscess formation), nystagmus, head tilt, postural abnormalities, and loss of hearing (see p. 300).

References

Angus JC, Lichtensteiger C, Campbell KL et al: Breed variations in histopathologic features of chronic severe otitis externa in dogs: 80 cases (1945-2001), *J Am Vet Med Assoc* 222:1000, 2002.

Eom KD, Lee HC, Yoon JH: Canalographic evaluation of the external ear canal in dogs, *Vet Radiol Ultrasound* 41:231, 2000.

Hettlich BF, Boothe HW, Simpson RB et al: Effect of tympanic cavity evacuation and flushing on microbial isolates during total ear canal ablation with lateral bulla osteotomy in dogs, *J Am Vet Med Assoc* 227:748, 2005.

Suggested Reading

Sylvestre AM: Potential factors affecting the outcome of dogs with resection of the lateral wall of the vertical ear canal, *Can Vet J* 39:157, 1998.

Records of 60 dogs that had a resection of the lateral wall of the vertical ear canal (Zepp procedure) were examined. The outcome of surgery was unacceptable in 55% of the cases. Breed was the only factor that could be correlated with outcome.

Vogel PL, Komtebedde J, Hirsch DC et al: Wound contamination and antimicrobial susceptibility of bacteria cultured during total ear canal ablation and lateral bulla osteotomy in dogs, *J Am Vet Med Assoc* 214:1641, 1999.

Thirteen dogs undergoing TECA and lateral ear canal resections were evaluated prospectively to detect contamination of wound sites from surgical handling of excised tissue during the procedure. Cefazolin was effective against only 70% of the bacterial isolates.

OTITIS MEDIA AND INTERNA

DEFINITIONS

Otitis media is inflammation of the middle ear; **otitis interna** is inflammation of the inner ear. **Myringotomy** is a surgical puncture of the tympanic membrane to relieve pressure or obtain samples for analysis. **Otoliths** are mineral opacities within the tympanic bullae. The auditory tube is also known as the **eustachian tube**.

GENERAL CONSIDERATIONS AND CLINICALLY RELEVANT PATHOPHYSIOLOGY

Otitis media may occur secondary to bacterial, yeast, or fungal infection; neoplasia; trauma; or the presence of a foreign body. Otoliths have also been reported within the tympanic cavity of dogs and may or may not be associated with clinical signs (Ziemer et al, 2003). In cats, inflammatory or nasopharyngeal polyps (see p. 314) are additional causes of otitis media. Congenital palatine defects may also be associated with middle ear disease in dogs and cats (Gregory, 2000). The most common cause in both dogs and cats is bacterial infection; more than half of animals with chronic end-stage otitis externa have documented evidence of otitis media at surgery. Consequently, pathogens cultured from the middle ear are similar to those cultured from the ears of animals with otitis externa (i.e., *Staphylococcus* spp., *Streptococcus* spp., *Pseudomonas* spp., *E. coli*, and *P. mirabilis*). In addition to spreading across the tympanic membrane to the middle ear, infections may ascend from the pharynx via the auditory tube or may reach the inner ear via the bloodstream. Bilateral otitis media usually is indicative of bacterial infection. Otitis media may lead to otitis interna (Box 17-4).

Inflammatory or nasopharyngeal polyps are benign masses that may be located in the nasopharynx, auditory tube, or tympanic cavity, or all three. In rare cases, they may rupture the tympanic membrane and protrude into the external ear canal. When located in the tympanic cavity, they often cause signs of unilateral otitis media. These polyps may occur as a result of ascending infection from the pharynx or may arise as a result of chronic otitis media. Polyps thought to be congenital in origin have also been reported in kittens.

Neoplasia originating in the middle ear is uncommon in both dogs and cats. In dogs, tumors that originate in the external ear canal and then extend into the tympanic cavity are more common than primary middle ear tumors. Benign tumors of the middle ear cavity of dogs (i.e., papillary adenomas and fibromas) have been more commonly reported than malignant tumors. Epidermoid cysts (cholesteatomas)

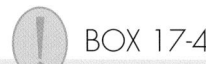

BOX 17-4

Clinical Signs Associated with Otitis Interna (Vestibular Dysfunction)

- Head tilt to affected side
- Circling to affected side
- Falling to affected side
- Rolling to affected side
- Nystagmus (horizontal or rotary) with fast component away from affected side
- Asymmetric ataxia with strength preserved
- Positional or vestibular strabismus with the eyeball ipsilateral to the lesion deviated ventrally
- Postural reactions (except for the righting reflex)

occur in the canine middle ear. These cysts often are associated with chronic otitis media and must be differentiated from neoplastic lesions. In cats, squamous cell carcinoma is the most common tumor of the middle and inner ear. Other tumors found in the feline middle ear have included fibrosarcoma, anaplastic carcinoma, lymphoblastic lymphosarcoma, and ceruminous gland adenocarcinoma.

DIAGNOSIS
Clinical Presentation

Signalment. Most animals that develop otitis media secondary to otitis externa are middle-aged. Older animals more commonly develop neoplasia of the middle ear, and young cats are more apt to have nasopharyngeal polyps. There is no known breed or gender predisposition in cats to nasopharyngeal polyps or in either dogs or cats to neoplastic middle ear disease. Canine breeds predisposed to otitis externa (see p. 301) also have a higher incidence of otitis media. Primary secretory otitis media was recently reported in Cavalier King Charles Spaniel dogs that presented with pain localized to the head or cervical area and/or neurologic signs, suggesting that this is an important differential in this breed when the aforementioned clinical signs are present (Stern-Bertholtz et al, 2003).

History. The history and clinical signs of animals with otitis media do not differ substantially from those of animals with otitis externa alone (see p. 301). Affected animals commonly scratch or paw at their ears, and they may shake their heads excessively. The ear may have an odor, and animals often appear to be in pain on manipulation or palpation of the ears or adjacent skull. A history of chronic, poorly responsive otitis externa is common. Some animals come for evaluation of vestibular signs caused by otitis interna (see Box 17-4). Pain during eating or when the mouth is opened may be noted, especially in cats with neoplastic middle ear disease. Ipsilateral facial nerve paralysis also is common in animals with middle ear neoplasia. In rare cases, neoplastic lesions of the middle ear may extend into the nasopharynx, causing gagging, retching, or dyspnea, or all three. Cats with nasopharyngeal polyps often have nasal discharge, sneezing,

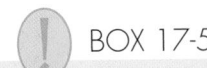

BOX 17-5

Clinical Signs Associated With Facial Nerve Paralysis

- Diminished palpebral reflex
- Widened palpebral fissure
- Drooping of the ear and lip
- Excessive drooling
- Blepharospasm
- Elevation and wrinkling of the lip
- Caudal displacement of the labial commissure
- Elevation of the ear on the affected side

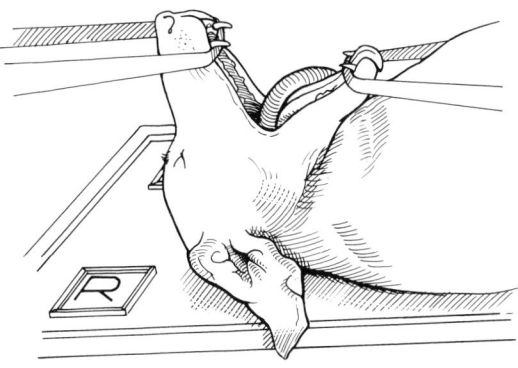

FIG. 17-14
Positioning for a frontal open-mouth projection.

or stridor (see p. 314). If a pharyngeal polyp is present concurrently, dysphagia and/or dyspnea may be noted. Some nasopharyngeal polyps become so large that they protrude to the edge of the soft palate and cause gagging. Cats that have sinonasal disease with nasal exudate often have concurrent otitis media (which may be clinically silent). Evaluation of the external and middle ears in such cats is warranted. Deafness may be reported with bilateral disease, but loss of hearing is seldom evident with unilateral lesions.

Physical Examination Findings

Discharge from the external auditory canal, hyperplasia, and ulceration of the aural epithelial tissue often are obvious on physical examination in animals with otitis media and externa. Neurologic abnormalities referable to the inner ear or facial nerve paralysis (Box 17-5) are not found in most animals with otitis media. Horner's syndrome may occur as a result of damage to the sympathetic trunk as it courses through the middle ear. Clinical signs associated with the syndrome are ptosis, miosis, enophthalmos, and protrusion of the third eyelid.

Otoscopic examination of these patients often requires general anesthesia. The tympanic membrane may be ruptured, or it may bulge outward because of purulent material, blood, or serum. However, an intact tympanic membrane does not rule out middle ear disease. Abundant mucus in the middle ear cavity has been associated with adenomatous lesions. The normal tympanic membrane appears shiny and is gray or white; it becomes opaque with infection. If the tympanic membrane has ruptured, samples for cytologic studies and culture can be taken directly from the middle ear. Otherwise, samples can be obtained using a 20-gauge, 3½-inch spinal needle inserted through the ventral half of the tympanum (myringotomy). If the opening is too small, it may be enlarged with a small cannula.

Inflammatory polyps (see p. 314) usually appear as pedunculated, smooth, shiny, light pink masses. The oral cavity of animals with inflammatory polyps or neoplastic masses should be carefully examined because extension into the pharynx may occur. Neoplastic lesions may be friable, but they often are difficult to differentiate grossly from chronically infected tissue.

Diagnostic Imaging

The most valuable radiographic view for evaluating animals suspected of having otitis media is the frontal open-mouth projection (also known as the rostrocaudal open-mouth view) in which the animal is placed in ventrodorsal recumbency with the head flexed 80° to 90° to the cassette and table (Fig. 17-14). The mouth is held open with gauze strips hooked on the upper and lower canine teeth, and the x-ray beam is centered on the temporomandibular joints. The tongue and endotracheal tube must be retracted from the field of view with gauze secured to the lower mandible. The tympanic bullae and their contents are demonstrated with this view. The most common findings with middle ear disease are opacification of the air-filled tympanic cavities and thickening and sclerosis of the walls of the bullae (Fig. 17-15). Lateral oblique views (Fig. 17-16) with the head tilted 10° to 15° show individual bullae, whereas ventrodorsal or dorsoventral views show the external ear canals and the architecture of the petrous temporal bones. Lysis or periosteal reaction of the bullae and petrous temporal bone should increase suspicion of neoplasia. A soft tissue mass in the pharyngeal region on the lateral view may be noted in cats with inflammatory polyps.

NOTE: Radiography is not a sensitive indicator of middle ear disease; CT is more sensitive. Nearly one fourth of animals with middle ear disease will have normal appearing bullae on radiographs.

CT is particularly useful for diagnosis of otitis media, evaluation of nasopharyngeal polyps, and determination of the extent of otitis externa or neoplasia (Fig. 17-17). Due to collapse of the pharynx when the animal is under anesthesia, it may be difficult to identify a nasopharyngeal polyp using cross-sectional imaging techniques; reformatted sagittal images may be better. Direct visualization is always recommended after cross-sectional imaging examinations to better evaluate for the possibility of a nasopharyngeal

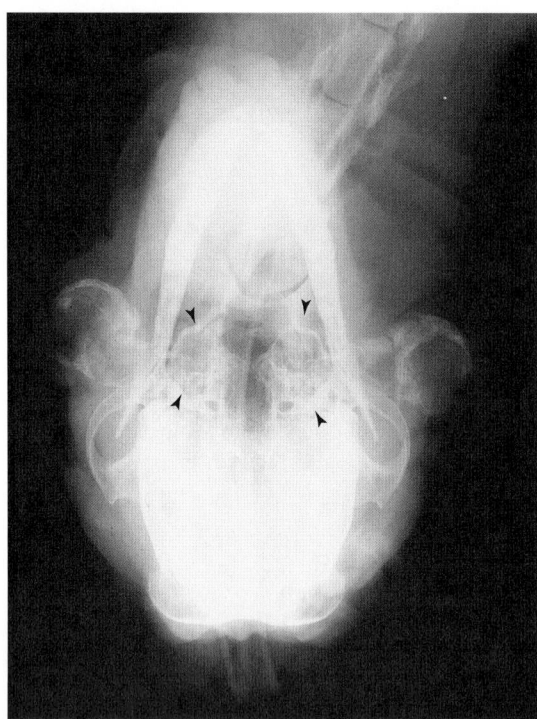

FIG. 17-15
Frontal open-mouth projection showing opacification, thickening, and sclerosis of the bullae *(arrows)*. (Courtesy L. Homco, Ithaca, N.Y.)

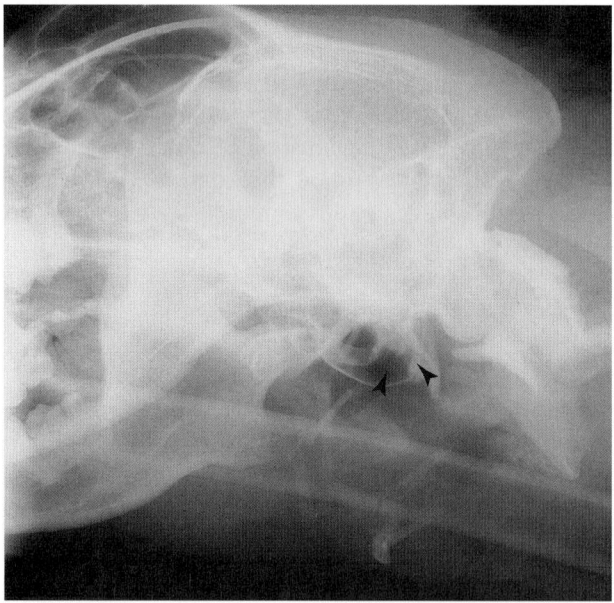

FIG. 17-16
Lateral oblique radiograph of a dog with unilateral otitis media. Note the thickened wall of the left bulla *(arrows)* compared with the normal, thin-walled right bulla. (Courtesy L. Homco, Texas A&M University.)

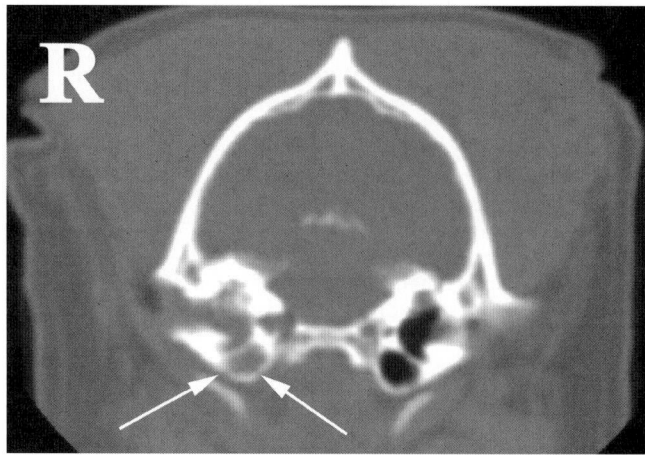

FIG 17-17
CT axial image of a dog. There is increased soft tissue attenuating material within the right tympanic bulla *(arrows)* without derangement of the bony aspect of the bulla in a dog with otitis media.

polyp. On a well-positioned study, both bullae should appear symmetric. The tympanic bullae and external ear canal lumens should be filled with air, and the wall of the tympanic bulla should be thin and well defined. In animals with otitis media, thickening and irregularity of the tympanic bullae is often seen. Other findings may include lysis of the tympanic bulla, a soft tissue attenuating material within its lumen, and signs of otitis externa. Evaluation of the bone of the bullae is more difficult using magnetic resonance imaging (MRI), but it can be used to identify soft tissue changes that occur with otitis media and has the additional advantage of providing evaluation of the brain in animals with signs of otitis interna.

Laboratory Findings
Specific laboratory abnormalities are uncommon.

DIFFERENTIAL DIAGNOSIS

Differential diagnoses for disease of the middle and inner ear cavity include bacterial, fungal, or yeast infection; inflammatory polyps; neoplasms; foreign bodies; trauma; sebaceous gland and ceruminous gland hyperplasia; paraoral abscesses; and idiopathic vestibular disease. Otitis media is common in animals with otitis externa, but because the clinical signs are similar, the former often goes unrecognized.

MEDICAL MANAGEMENT

The most important aspect of the treatment of otitis media is removing infected tissues or exudate, neoplasms, polyps, or foreign bodies from the tympanic cavity. The external ear canal should be cleaned, and concurrent otitis externa must be treated (see p. 302). Medical management of animals with acute otitis media consists of myringotomy, cultures of middle ear contents, irrigation of the tympanic cavity, and topical and systemic antibiotics. The mean volume of the middle ear cavity in mesaticephalic dogs (e.g., Labradors, retrievers, and Cocker spaniels) is approximately 1.5 ml (DeFalque et al, 2005). Many veterinary dermatologists recommend starting an oral fluoroquinolone pending culture and susceptibility results. If no improvement is seen in 3 to 4 weeks, ventral bulla osteotomy should be considered.

SURGICAL TREATMENT

Surgery often is necessary to distinguish between the various possible causes of middle ear disease. Surgical treatment of otitis media caused by infection includes bulla osteotomy, culture of affected tissue or exudate, drainage, and long-term antibiotics. Benign neoplastic or inflammatory lesions usually can be removed by a bulla osteotomy; however, Horner's syndrome is a common, short-term complication of this procedure in cats (see p. 300). Neoplasia of the bulla warrants a poor prognosis.

NOTE: If neurologic signs are present before surgery, be sure to warn the owner that they may persist after surgery.

Preoperative Management

Preoperative antibiotics may be given; however, intraoperative cultures often are performed in animals with middle ear disease. In such patients intravenous antibiotics should be given immediately after culture results have been obtained.

Anesthesia

See p. 289 for anesthetic recommendations for animals with ear disease. Chamber or mask induction should not be used in dyspneic animals (i.e., some cats with nasopharyngeal polyps). Because nitrous oxide increases middle ear pressure, it should be avoided in animals with middle ear disease.

Surgical Anatomy

The middle ear is composed of the tympanic cavity and its contents and the auditory tube. See p. 291 for a description of the surgical anatomy of the ear.

Positioning

The animal is positioned in lateral recumbency for a lateral bulla osteotomy and in dorsal recumbency for a ventral bulla osteotomy.

SURGICAL TECHNIQUE

Approach the middle ear by means of a lateral bulla osteotomy (see p. 298) in conjunction with TECA (see p. 295) or through a ventral bulla osteotomy (see p. 298).

SUTURE MATERIALS AND SPECIAL INSTRUMENTS

See p. 299 for a description of surgical supplies necessary for a bulla osteotomy.

POSTOPERATIVE CARE AND ASSESSMENT

Cats with concurrent upper airway disease (i.e., nasopharyngeal polyps) may have respiratory distress after extubation and may require supplementary oxygen. Oxygen may be given by mask or nasal insufflation in these animals.

PROGNOSIS

Animals with bacterial otitis media may have persistent neurologic signs despite surgical treatment. Many cats with otitis interna before surgery will have permanent head tilts after surgery; however, these cats often have a normal level of activity despite their neurologic dysfunction. The prognosis for benign tumors is good, but surgical cures are rare with malignant tumors because of their extensive nature at the time of diagnosis. Inflammatory polyps may recur if they are simply removed from the external ear using traction (see p. 315). Recurrence is less likely if traction and bulla osteotomy are performed.

References

DeFalque VE, Rosenstein DS, Rosser EJ: Measurement of normal middle ear cavity volume in mesaticephalic dogs, *Vet Radiol Ultrasound* 46:490, 2005.

Gregory SP: Middle ear disease associated with congenital palatine defects in seven dogs and one cat, *J Small Animal Pract* 41:398, 2000.

Stern-Bertholtz W, Sjostrom L, Hakanson NW: Primary secretory otitis media in the Cavalier King Charles spaniel: a review of 61 cases, *J Small Anim Pract* 33:253, 2003.

Ziemer LS, Schwarx T, Sullivan M: Otolithiasis in three dogs, *Vet Radiol Ultrasound* 44:28, 2003.

Suggested Reading

Bischoff MG, Kneller SK: Diagnostic imaging of the canine and feline ear, *Vet Clin Small Anim* 34:437, 2004.

This review details the techniques, including appropriate positioning, for animals undergoing radiographs, CT, or MRI for diseases of the ear. Findings in normal and diseased ears are reviewed.

Gotthelf RN: Diagnosis and treatment of otitis media in dogs and cats, *Vet Clin Small Anim* 34:469, 2004.

This is a general review of the treatment of otitis media. Detailed techniques for flushing the bulla are given.

AURAL HEMATOMAS AND TRAUMATIC LESIONS OF THE PINNA

DEFINITION

An **aural (auricular) hematoma** is a collection of blood within the cartilage plate of the ear.

GENERAL CONSIDERATIONS AND CLINICALLY RELEVANT PATHOPHYSIOLOGY

Aural hematomas may occur in dogs or cats and usually are characterized as fluctuant, fluid-filled swellings on the concave surface of the pinna. The entire concave surface of the pinna may be involved or only part of it. The cause of aural hematomas is not well understood; however, in many cases they appear to be the result of head shaking or scratching at the ear caused by pain or irritation associated with otitis externa. The latter is usually bacterial in dogs and due to *O. cynotis* infestation in cats. Head shaking may cause sinusoidal wave motions in the ear, resulting in fracture of the cartilage. The hematoma appears to originate from branches of the great auricular artery within the fractured auricular cartilage rather than between the skin and cartilage as was initially postulated. Some animals that develop aural hematomas do not have evidence of concurrent ear disease; hematoma formation in some patients may be associated with increased capillary fragility (e.g., Cushing's disease).

The ear may be lacerated as a result of fighting or other trauma. These wounds may be superficial, involving the skin on one surface of the ear only, or may perforate the cartilage and involve both skin surfaces. Depending on the severity of the wounds, some may be left to heal by secondary intention, whereas others will have a more cosmetic appearance if sutures are placed. In rare cases, a portion of the ear may be avulsed, resulting in an unacceptable cosmetic deformity.

DIAGNOSIS
Clinical Presentation

Signalment. Dogs and cats with otitis externa have a greater risk of developing aural hematomas.

History. A history of violent head shaking and/or acute or chronic otitis externa (see p. 301) may be noted; some animals may have no history of previous ear disease.

Physical Examination Findings

Hematomas initially appear fluid filled, soft, and fluctuant, but eventually may become firm and thickened as a result of fibrosis. The ear may then develop a "cauliflower" appearance.

Diagnostic Imaging

Skull radiographs may be indicated if underlying otitis externa or media (or both) has predisposed the animal to aural hematoma.

Laboratory Findings

Specific laboratory abnormalities are uncommon.

DIFFERENTIAL DIAGNOSIS

Aural hematoma is diagnosed during the physical examination; however, the underlying ear disease must be diagnosed and treated to reduce the likelihood of recurrence.

MEDICAL MANAGEMENT

Underlying ear disease should be appropriately treated (see pp. 290, 302, and 306). Needle aspiration of aural hematomas has been attempted (with and without concurrent injection of a corticosteroid); however, recurrence is common with this technique.

SURGICAL TREATMENT

Numerous techniques have been described for surgical treatment of aural hematomas. The goals of surgery are to remove the hematoma, prevent recurrence, and retain the natural appearance of the ear (i.e., minimize thickening and scarring). The most commonly used procedure involves incising the tissue overlying the hematoma, evacuating blood clots and fibrin, and holding the cartilage in apposition with sutures until scar tissue can form. As an alternative, drains or cannulas have been used to provide drainage for several weeks during the healing process. To prevent enlargement or fibrosis, hematomas should be treated soon after they occur, preferably within several days. Use of the carbon dioxide laser has been reported for treatment of aural hematomas (Dye et al, 2002). The laser is used to make an incision into the hematoma to allow for evacuation of blood; then multiple, small incisions are made over the surface of the hematoma to stimulate adhesion formation. No sutures are placed.

Linear lacerations that involve only one skin surface may be left to heal by secondary intention or may be sutured. The laceration should be cleaned and the edges débrided if necrotic tissue is present. The skin margins can be apposed with simple interrupted sutures. If a flap of tissue has been elevated away from the cartilage, it should be sutured. Sutures are placed through the skin at the margins of the wound; sutures also should be placed through the skin and cartilage at the center of the flap to obliterate any dead space where fluid might collect. Full-thickness injuries through the ear margin should be sutured. The skin on both sides of the defect may be sutured with simple interrupted sutures, or as an alternative, a vertical mattress suture may be used to appose the skin and cartilage on one side of the ear and simple interrupted sutures used to appose the skin on the opposite side of the ear (Fig. 17-18).

Preoperative Management

Concurrent otitis externa (see p. 302) should be treated simultaneously. Appropriate cultures should be submitted and the ear canal cleaned and flushed.

Anesthesia

Animals with aural hematomas usually are healthy, and a variety of anesthetic protocols can be used. Tranquilization may be necessary upon recovery from anesthesia once sufficient analgesics have been provided (see p. 290). See p. 290 for the anesthetic management of animals with ear disease.

Surgical Anatomy

Structural support of the pinna is provided by cartilage interposed between the two skin surfaces. Branches of the great auricular arteries and veins supply the pinna. These main vessels are located along the convex surface of the ear, and small branches penetrate the scapha to supply the concave surface. The sensory innervation to the ear is supplied by the second cervical nerve (convex surface) and by the auriculotemporal branches of the trigeminal nerve (concave surface).

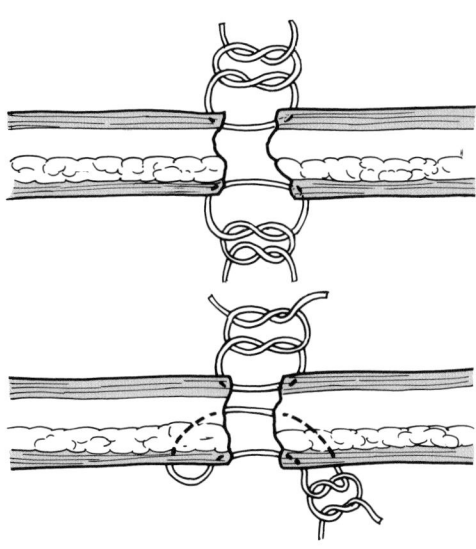

FIG. 17-18
Suture placement for repair of pinna lacerations.

Positioning

Patients generally are placed in lateral recumbency for aural hematoma and laceration repair.

SURGICAL TECHNIQUES
Aural Hematomas

Make an S-shaped incision on the concave surface of the ear and expose the hematoma and its contents from end to end (Fig. 17-19). Remove the fibrin clot and irrigate the cavity. Place ¾- to 1-cm long sutures through the skin on the concave surface of the ear and underlying cartilage. Place the sutures parallel to the major vessels (vertical rather than horizontal). They may be placed through the cartilage without incorporating the skin on the convex surface of the ear, or they may be full thickness. Place an ample number of sutures so that no pockets are left in which fluid can accumulate. Do not ligate the branches of the great auricular artery visible on the convex surface of the ear. Do not suture the incision closed; it should gap slightly to allow for continued drainage. Place a light protective bandage over the ear, and support the ear over the animal's head (see p. 311 under Postoperative Care and Assessment). Remove the bandage and sutures in 10 to 14 days.

If minimal fibrin is present, a teat cannula or drain can be placed in lieu of the above procedure (Fig. 17-20, *A*).

Trim half of the collar of the cannula to allow the tube to rest comfortably against the ear (Fig.17-20, B). Aspirate the contents of the hematoma using a large needle (14 or 16 gauge) inserted into the hematoma at its most distal margin. Insert the cannula through the needle hole, and suture it to the ear. (The cannula is placed in the most distal aspect of the hematoma, even in erect-eared animals, to prevent

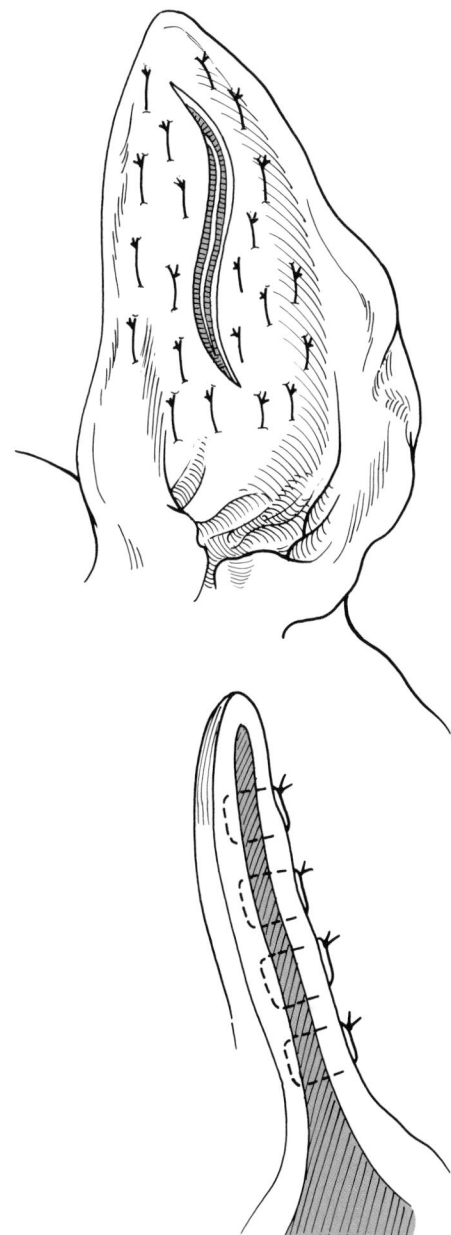

LPD - IN

FIG. 17-19
Sutures should be placed vertically rather than horizontally for aural hematoma repair. They may be placed through the cartilage without incorporating the skin on the convex surface of the ear, or they may be full thickness.

drainage from entering the concha.) Do not bandage or support the ear over the top of the head.

A one-fourth-inch fenestrated latex drain can be used instead of a teat cannula (Fig. 17-20, *C*).

Make a stab incision in the proximal and distal limits of the hematoma. Empty the hematoma of fluid and fibrin, and use a mosquito or alligator forceps to bring the drain into the hematoma cavity. Suture the ends of the drain to the skin

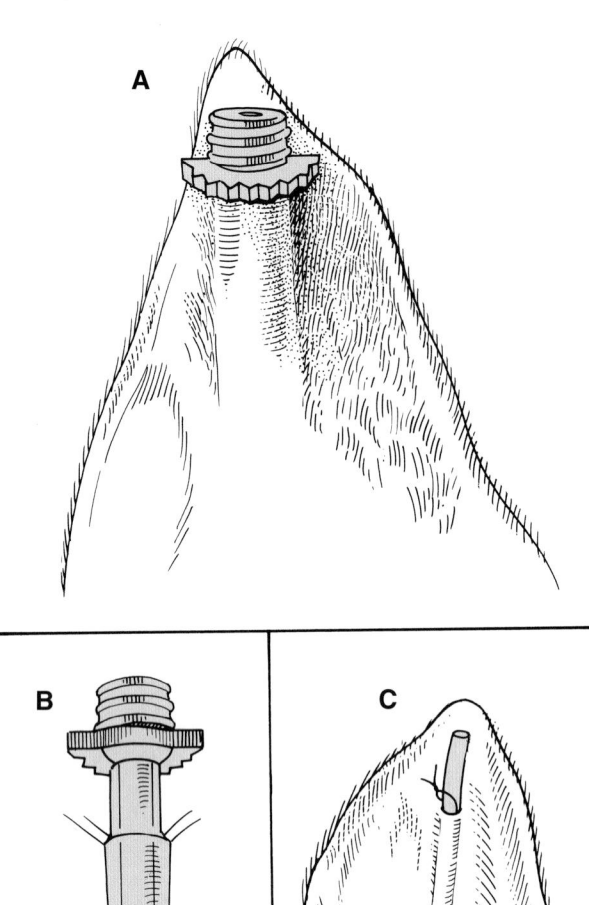

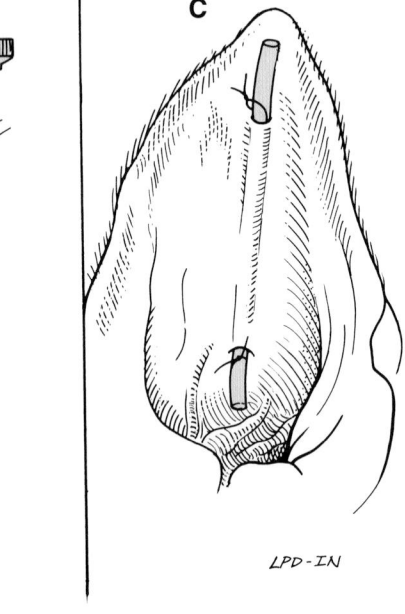

LPD-IN

FIG. 17-20
A, If minimal fibrin is present, a teat cannula can be used for aural hematoma repair. **B,** Trim half of the collar of the cannula to allow the tube to rest comfortably against the ear. **C,** As an alternative, a one-fourth-inch fenestrated latex drain can be used.

where they protrude from the cavity. Place a light bandage over the ear (see p. 311 under Postoperative Care and Assessment).

Avulsions of the Ear Margin

Small avulsions of the ear margin may be treated by resecting surrounding tissue to restore a normal ear contour. The skin edges are sutured over the cartilage using a continuous suture pattern. Larger defects of the ear may be repaired using a pedicle flap obtained from the side of the neck in dogs with pendulous ears or from the dorsum of the head in dogs with erect ears.

> NOTE: Defects of the ear margins can be repaired for cosmetic reasons, but repair should be delayed after excision of neoplasms until it has been determined that recurrence is unlikely.

Prepare the ear and donor site for aseptic surgery. Débride the margins of the ear defect. Place the ear on the donor site and incise the skin, extending the limbs of the incision 0.5 to 1 cm longer than the defect (Fig. 17-21, A). Suture the flap to the skin on the convex surface of the ear (Fig. 17-21, B). Place a nonadherent dressing over the wound and leave the ear bandaged for 10 to 14 days. Then sever the flap from the donor site in the shape of the defect on the concave side of the ear (Fig. 17-21, C). Gently fold the flap over the ear margin and suture it to the skin (Fig. 17-21, D). Remove skin sutures in 10 to 14 days.

SUTURE MATERIALS AND SPECIAL INSTRUMENTS

Monofilament, nonabsorbable (polypropylene or nylon) or absorbable (polydioxanone, poliglecaprone 25, or polyglyconate) suture material (3-0 or 4-0) should be used to suture the ear. Other materials that may be used in animals with aural hematomas are Dr. Larson's plastic teat tubes or Silastic medical-grade tubing.

POSTOPERATIVE CARE AND ASSESSMENT

A bandage can be used to protect the ear from contamination and self-inflicted trauma after hematoma repair. Maintaining bandages on the head can be difficult. One method is to place short strips of tape on the rostral and caudal margin of the convex surface of the pinna (Fig. 17-22, A). The tape should extend beyond the ear border. Longer pieces of tape are placed on the concave surface of the pinna so that these tape pieces contact the tape on the convex surface (Fig. 17-22, B). The ear is placed over the top of the head (cotton can be placed between the ear and the top of the head to support the ear), and a nonadherent pad is placed over the incision (Fig. 17-22, C). The long pieces of tape are applied to the skin. Cast padding and Kling are applied over the ear (the unaffected ear on the other side is not incorporated into the bandage), and Vetrap or stockinette (cut a hole for the unaffected ear) can be placed as the external layer (Fig. 17-22, D). The bandage can then be secured to the head cranially or caudally with Elastikon or 1-inch tape that is applied to both the hair and bandage.

> NOTE: Be sure to check head bandages periodically to ensure that they are not too tight and are not restricting breathing.

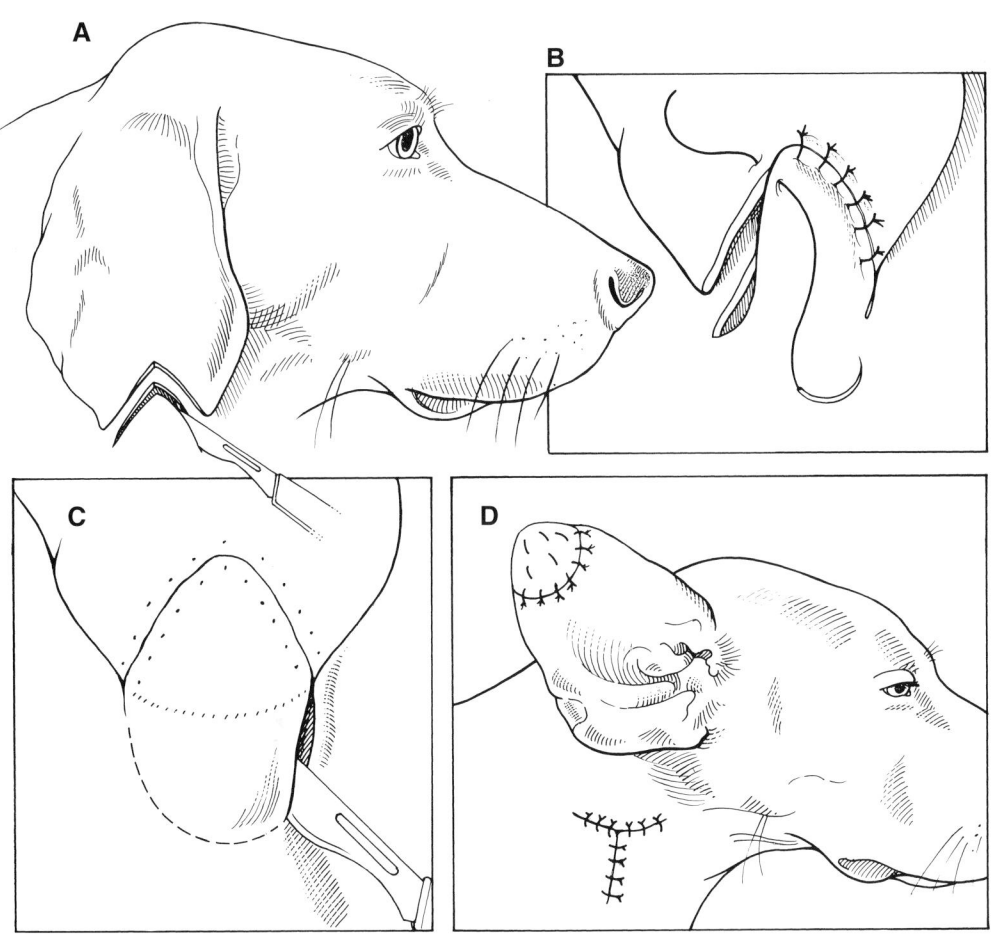

FIG. 17-21
Repair of pinnal defects.
A, Place the ear on the donor site and incise the skin, extending the limbs of the incision 0.5 to 1 cm longer than the defect. **B,** Suture the flap to the skin on the convex surface of the ear. **C,** After 10 to 14 days, sever the flap from the donor site in the shape of the defect on the concave side of the ear. **D,** Gently fold the flap over the ear margin, and suture it to the skin.

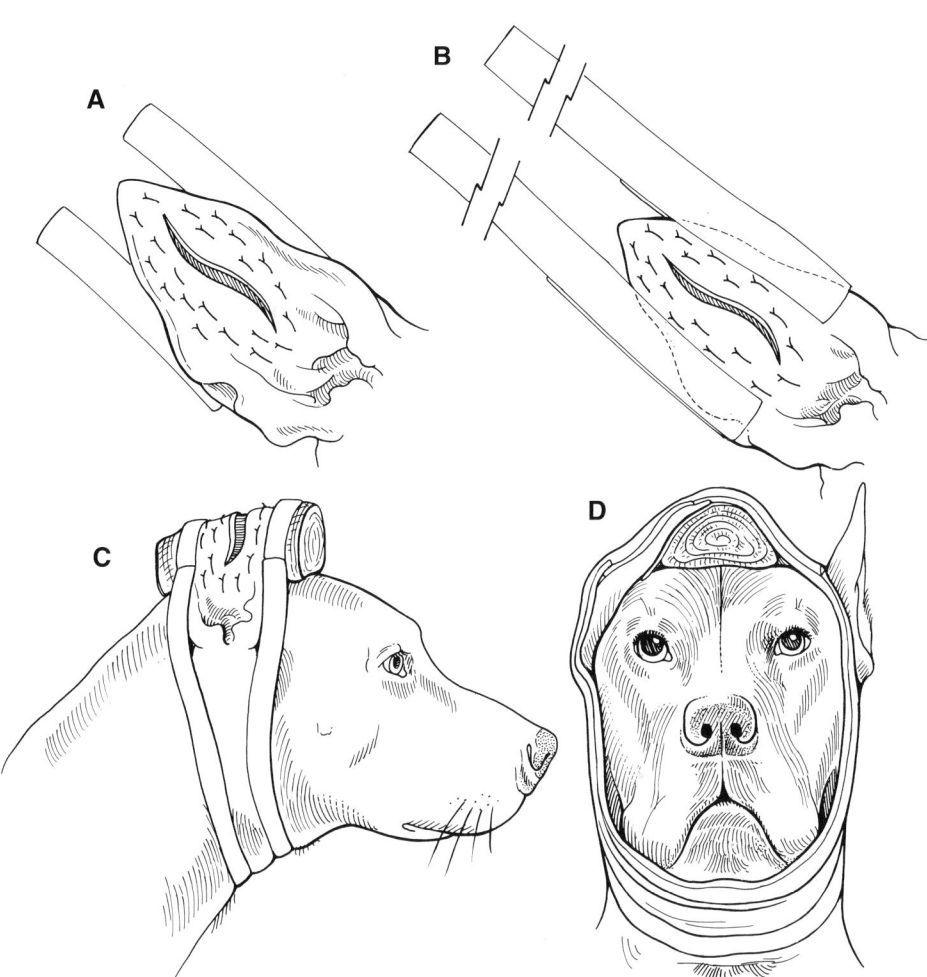

FIG. 17-22
Bandaging the ear after a surgical procedure. **A,** Place short strips of tape on the rostral and caudal margins of the convex surface of the pinna. **B,** Use longer pieces of tape on the concave surface of the pinna so that these tape pieces contact the tape on the convex surface. **C,** Place the ear over the top of the head and place a non-adherent pad over the incision. **D,** Apply cast padding and Kling over the ear, then use Vetrap or stockinette as an external layer.

PROGNOSIS

Aural hematomas seldom recur if they are properly treated and if any underlying ear disease is appropriately treated.

Reference

Dye TL, Teaque HD, Ostwald DA et al: Evaluation of a technique using the carbon dioxide laser for the treatment of aural hematomas, *J Am Anim Hosp Assoc* 38:385, 2002.

NEOPLASIA OF THE PINNA AND EXTERNAL EAR CANAL

DEFINITION

The **pinna** is the portion of the ear that projects outward from the skull.

GENERAL CONSIDERATIONS AND CLINICALLY RELEVANT PATHOPHYSIOLOGY

Neoplasms of the external ear canal are relatively uncommon in dogs and cats; however, they may arise from any structure that lines or supports the ear canal. Aural tumors in the dog and cat can be histologically benign or malignant. The most common tumors of the external ear canal arise from the ceruminous glands (ceruminous gland adenomas or adenocarcinomas). Squamous cell carcinoma, basal cell tumors, and mast cell tumors may also be found. Benign aural conditions include inflammatory polyps (see p. 314), basal cell tumors, papillomas, histiocytomas, and ceruminous gland adenomas. Aural tumors tend to be more aggressive in cats than in dogs. Most canine ceruminous gland tumors are benign, but such tumors in cats are usually malignant.

Although tumors of the external ear canal are more common than those arising in the internal or middle ear cavities, clinical signs of middle or inner ear disease may predominate if these tumors extend through the tympanic membrane (see p. 305). Neoplasms of the external ear frequently are associated with concurrent bacterial and yeast infections. It has been hypothesized that chronic otitis causes hyperplasia, which eventually may induce dysplastic and neoplastic changes. The mere presence of a tumor in the ear canal often obstructs drainage, resulting in otitis externa.

Any tumor that affects the skin may arise on the pinna, but the most common tumor of the pinna in cats is squamous cell carcinoma. These tumors most often are diagnosed in older cats, particularly white ones. The association between a lack of protective pigmentation and the occurrence of these tumors suggests that solar radiation may be a causative factor. Although these tumors are highly invasive, metastasis is uncommon. If metastasis does occur, it usually is to the regional lymph nodes and lungs. Tumors may also be noted on the nares and eyelids. Other tumors of the pinna of dogs and cats are melanoma, fibrosarcoma, basal cell tumor, fibroma, lymphoma, histiocytoma, papilloma, and mast cell tumor.

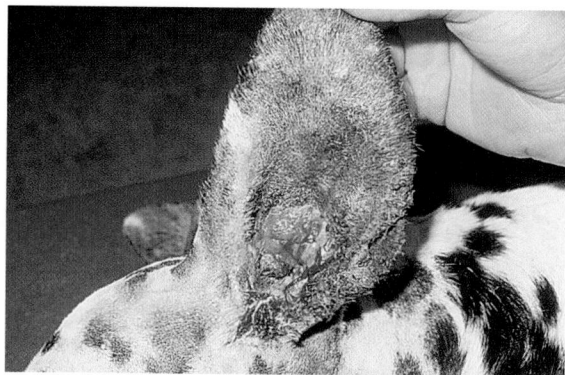

FIG. 17-23
Ceruminous gland adenocarcinoma on the pinna of a 6-year-old dog presented for treatment of chronic otitis externa.

DIAGNOSIS
Clinical Presentation

Signalment. Most neoplastic lesions of the external ear are found in middle-aged or older animals. Older male cats may be at increased risk of developing ceruminous gland tumors of the ear canal. Squamous cell carcinoma of the pinna occurs almost exclusively in older white-eared cats or multicolored cats with little pigmentation of the pinna.

History. The history of a patient with a tumor arising from the external ear canal usually differs minimally from that of a patient with primary bacterial otitis externa (see p. 301). The history of cats with squamous cell carcinoma often is insidious and begins with the owner intermittently noticing crusty, eczematous lesions at the edge of the ear.

Physical Examination Findings

Small, pedunculated masses of the external ear canal suggest ceruminous gland hyperplasia or adenomas, papillomas, or inflammatory polyps. Infiltrative masses suggest ceruminous gland adenocarcinoma (Fig. 17-23). Squamous cell carcinoma usually originates on the tips of the ears, where little hair is present, and initially may appear as hyperemic skin. As the lesions progress, erosion, ulceration, crusting, and thickening become noticeable (Fig. 17-24). The ear may bleed with mild trauma.

Diagnostic Imaging

Radiographic signs of neoplasia (i.e., bony lysis of the petrous temporal bone) may be noted on skull radiographs of animals with neoplasia of the external ear canal. Cross-sectional imaging is more sensitive for detection and evaluation of the extensiveness of lesions (Fig. 17-25). Although metastasis usually occurs late in the course of the disease, pulmonary metastasis may be noted with some ear tumors, therefore thoracic radiographs are recommended.

Laboratory Findings

The diagnosis of ear neoplasia requires that a biopsy be taken of the lesion.

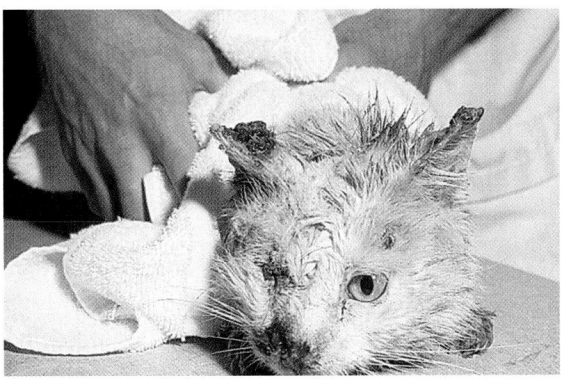

FIG. 17-24
Squamous cell carcinomas on the ear tips of a cat. Note the crusting and the thickened appearance of the pinna.

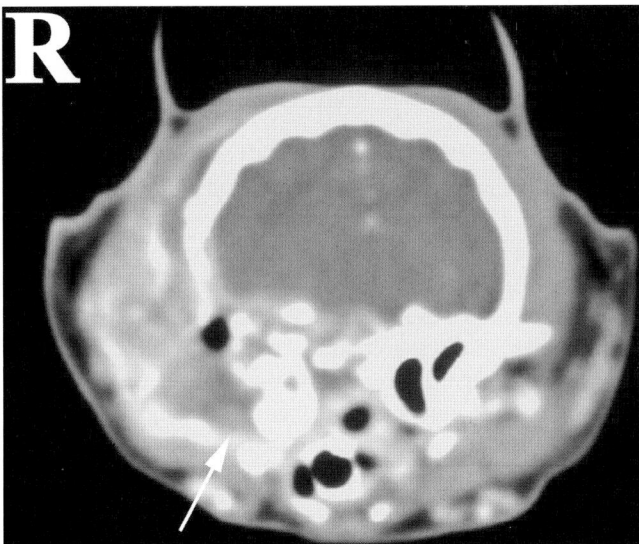

FIG. 17-25
Contrast enhanced CT axial image of a cat. Notice the destruction of the right tympanic bulla *(arrow)* and the ventral aspect of the calvarial vault. There is irregular contrast enhancement of the surrounding tissue. Necropsy revealed a squamous cell carcinoma with invasion into the calvarial vault.

DIFFERENTIAL DIAGNOSIS

Neoplastic lesions of the ear pinna must be differentiated from nonneoplastic lesions, such as dermatitis caused by insect bites or immune-mediated lesions. A biopsy should be taken for suspicious lesions to improve the chances of an early, complete resection.

MEDICAL MANAGEMENT

Squamous cell carcinoma may be prevented or reduced by applying sunscreens to nonpigmented areas of the ear and preventing physical exposure to ultraviolet radiation. Cryotherapy and radiation are alternatives to surgical removal of the pinna. Cryotherapy may be curative in small, superficial tumors, but local recurrence is common. Radiation therapy is less disfiguring than surgical removal of the lesions and is a viable alternative for small, superficial tumors and preneoplastic lesions.

SURGICAL TREATMENT

For neoplasms of the external ear canal, vertical ear canal ablation or TECA usually is required (see pp. 293 to 299). Local treatment options for pinnal squamous cell carcinoma include surgical resection, cryosurgery, and photodynamic therapy. For cats with more aggressive or advanced disease, systemic chemotherapy may provide limited improvement in survival times. The aim of surgical treatment of squamous cell carcinoma is to remove the neoplasm with a wide margin of normal surrounding skin. This may require pinnectomy alone or a vertical ear canal ablation and removal of the pinna. The owner should be prepared for the resulting cosmetic deformity.

Preoperative Management

If concurrent otitis externa is present, perioperative antibiotics based on culture results should be given. Preoperative cytologic studies can help determine if radical resection is necessary when neoplasia is suspected.

Anesthesia

See p. 289 for anesthetic recommendations for animals with ear disease.

Surgical Anatomy

See p. 291 for a description of the surgical anatomy of the ear canal and pinna.

Positioning

Positioning for ear surgery is described with the discussion of surgical techniques on pp. 293 to 298.

SURGICAL TECHNIQUE

The most important aspect of surgery of ear neoplasms is to achieve wide margins to prevent local recurrence; this may require removal of the entire pinna and ear canal. If aggressive surgical therapy cannot provide clean margins, adjunctive therapy (i.e., radiation) should be considered. See pp. 293 to 299 for a description of surgical techniques commonly used for diseased or neoplastic ears.

> NOTE: Malignant ear tumors must be excised with wide margins of normal tissue. The owner should be advised of the resulting cosmetic defect before surgery.

For pinnectomy, remove the affected portion of the ear and suture the remaining skin over the exposed cartilage. For small tumors on the central portion of the convex surface of the pinna, resect the neoplasm and mobilize the skin around the defect by undermining between the cartilage and skin.

Suture the skin margins or, if necessary, leave the defect open to heal by secondary intention under a light bandage. For small tumors on the concave surface of the ear, repair the skin defect by elevating a flap from surrounding skin and rotating it into the defect. Suture the flap to the wound margins. After 10 to 14 days, transect the flap and suture the edge to the defect. Close the donor site primarily.

SUTURE MATERIALS AND SPECIAL INSTRUMENTS

See p. 299 for a discussion of suture materials and surgical instruments for ear surgery.

POSTOPERATIVE CARE AND ASSESSMENT

An Elizabethan collar or sidebar should be used to prevent the animal from mutilating the ear after surgery. Ear surgery is painful, and postoperative analgesics such as hydromorphone should be provided (see p. 290). If the animal appears dysphoric or anxious, tranquilizers may be given once the patient has received adequate postoperative analgesics (see p. 290).

PROGNOSIS

For malignant ceruminous gland tumors of the external ear, ablation is seldom curative, and adjunctive therapy (radiation therapy) should be considered. Local recurrence of squamous cell carcinomas is common if wide margins are not obtained at surgery. The prognosis is poor with squamous cell carcinoma of the middle and inner ear; however, amputation of the pinna for squamous cell carcinoma of the ear margin may be curative.

Suggested Reading

Fan TM, de Lorimer LP: Inflammatory polyps and aural neoplasia, *Vet Clin Small Anim* 34:489, 2004.
Contains a comprehensive review of aural tumors and their treatment.

INFLAMMATORY POLYPS

DEFINITION

Inflammatory polyps are benign, fibrous, pedunculated masses that may be found in the oropharynx, middle ear, or external ear canal. They are also known as nasopharyngeal, middle ear, or otopharyngeal polyps.

GENERAL CONSIDERATIONS AND CLINICALLY RELEVANT PATHOPHYSIOLOGY

Inflammatory polyps are the second most common cause of nasopharyngeal disease in cats, after lymphoma. Although less commonly diagnosed, inflammatory polyps of the ear canal may also occur in dogs. The cause is not known; however, both infections (i.e., upper respiratory infection and chronic otitis media) and congenital causes have been theorized to be associated with their formation. The latter theory suggests that they are aberrant growths associated with remnants of the branchial arches. Others believe that they are more likely related to inflammation. The origin of polyps is unclear, but they may arise from the mucosa of the nasopharynx, eustachian tube, or middle ear. It is most likely that they arise from the middle ear or auditory tube at its junction with the tympanic cavity and then migrate to the nasopharynx (via the eustachian tube) or external ear (via the tympanic membrane).

DIAGNOSIS
Clinical Presentation

Signalment. Inflammatory polyps tend to occur in young cats (<2 years of age); however, they have been reported in cats as old as 15 years of age. No breed or sex predisposition has been identified in cats. Dogs are typically male and middle-aged to older (although clinical signs may be present for months or even years before evaluation).

History. Most cats present for evaluation of dysphagia or upper respiratory signs, such as stertorous respiration, nasal discharge, sneezing, voice change, and/or dyspnea. Occasionally the animal may be presented for an acute onset of head tilt, nystagmus, and/or vestibular imbalance. Clinical signs may be present for months before evaluation.

Physical Examination Findings

Most inflammatory polyps are unilateral, although they may be bilateral. These masses tend to be pink and pedunculated, but may be ulcerated to varying degrees. Polyp extension into the external canal may appear as a dark ceruminous mass on otoscopic examination or they may be red, pink, or white. These masses are often covered by mucus and/or blood. The tympanic membrane may appear distorted and discolored if the mass has not extended through it. Evidence of upper respiratory obstruction is present in most affected cats, and in some cats secondary infections, such as nasal discharge, rhinitis, and/or sinusitis, may be noted.

Evaluation of the area dorsal to the soft palate may be done with a dental mirror and a Snook hook. However, much better visualization of the nasopharynx is possible with endoscopes. The easiest method is to retroflex a small-diameter flexible endoscope over the soft palate. This technique has the advantage of allowing excellent visualization and also provides an opportunity to obtain biopsies and brush samples for cytology and culture if a mass is not present. Another option is to insert a rigid endoscope, which has a near 180° view into the mouth, until one can see back over the soft palate. This is rarely done because there is little other use for rigid endoscopes with such a field of vision. Lastly, one can make a stab incision through the skin and into the pharynx (in about the same position as one would place a pharyngostomy tube) and insert a small-diameter rigid endoscope with a 0°-degree field of view. Rigid endoscopic procedures have the disadvantage of not allowing the operator to obtain biopsies or brushings of the affected area.

Diagnostic Imaging

Well positioned, lateral radiographic images of the pharyngeal region are the most useful for diagnosing nasopharyngeal polyps. CT may also be useful and may help determine

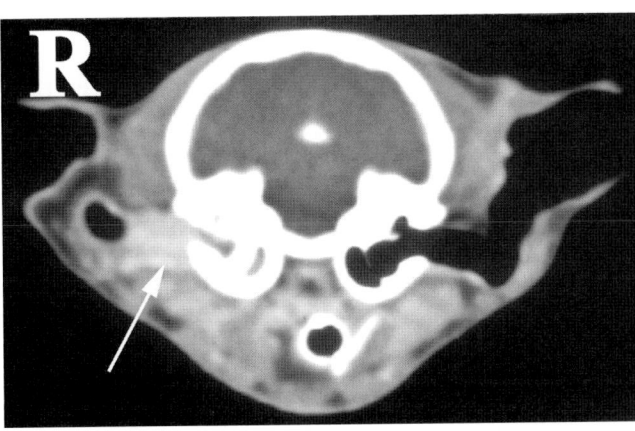

FIG. 17-26
Contrast enhanced CT axial image of a cat. There is a contrast enhancing mass within the right external ear canal *(arrows)* and increased soft tissue within the right tympanic bulla. A polyp was removed at surgery.

the extent of involvement and whether the condition is unilateral or bilateral before surgery (Fig. 17-26). On CT, a soft tissue attenuating mass may be seen extending from the middle ear into the lumen of the external ear canal. Alternately a soft tissue mass may be seen in the nasopharyngeal region (although collapse of the pharyngeal region during anesthesia can hinder this evaluation). Nasopharyngeal polyps, rather than neoplasia, should be suspected in young animals with a soft tissue mass in the nasopharyngeal region.

Laboratory Findings
Specific laboratory abnormalities are uncommon.

DIFFERENTIAL DIAGNOSIS
Polyps should be differentiated from neoplastic masses, particularly in older cats. Other differentials include upper respiratory tract infections, nasal foreign bodies, otitis externa/media, and fungal diseases.

MEDICAL MANAGEMENT
Treatment of concurrent infections should be instituted following appropriate microbial cultures. Surgical removal of the masses is indicated, as medical management has been uniformly unsuccessful in eliminating these polyps. If traction alone is used, concurrent treatment with an antiinflammatory (e.g., prednisolone, 1 to 2 mg/kg/day for 2 weeks followed by a tapered dose for an additional 2 weeks) may reduce the recurrence rate.

SURGICAL TREATMENT
Surgical procedures advocated for removal of polyps include traction-avulsion of the mass, ventral bulla osteotomy, lateral ear canal resection, TECA combined with lateral bulla osteotomy, and myringotomy. The best results

are seen when a ventral bulla osteotomy is performed (see p. 298); with this procedure the recurrence rate is less than 2% (Donnelly and Tillson, 2004). Although traction has been used to remove masses when there is no evidence of otitis media (see above under Medical Management), performing a ventral bulla osteotomy in conjunction with this procedure is recommended to decrease the recurrence rate. Ventral bulla osteotomy should *always* be performed if there is evidence of middle ear disease on radiographs or cross-sectional imaging.

Preoperative Management
If severe respiratory obstruction is present, a temporary tracheostomy may be necessary; however, this is rarely required. Antimicrobial therapy should await results of microbial cultures.

Anesthesia
Anesthetic management of animals undergoing ear surgery is provided on p. 289. Care must be used when intubating animals that have oropharyngeal masses; occasionally a smaller endotracheal tube than is typically used for intubation may be necessary. The cuff on the tube should be carefully checked to ensure its function and to prevent blood and other debris from entering the trachea during surgery.

Surgical Anatomy
Anatomy of the ear is detailed on p. 291.

Positioning
The animal is positioned in dorsal recumbency for ventral bullae osteotomy (see p. 298).

SURGICAL TECHNIQUES
Ventral bulla osteotomy is described on p. 298. In cats, the bullae should be entered through the larger ventromedial compartment. Most polyps are found in the dorsolateral compartment. Removal of the septum at its most lateral aspect may help prevent damage to the sympathetic trunk. Cultures should be taken of the bullae and the polyp. The polyp, epithelial lining, and associated exudate should be carefully removed with thumb forceps. The polyp should be submitted for histopathology.

SUTURE MATERIALS AND SPECIAL INSTRUMENTS
Ventral bullae osteotomy can be performed using a small Steinmann pin and a hand chuck or an air drill. The opening is typically enlarged with a rongeur (e.g., Kerrison or Lempert).

POSTOPERATIVE CARE AND ASSESSMENT
The animal should be evaluated for seroma formation after surgery. These seromas rarely require drainage. Surgical curettage of the tympanic cavity frequently causes a transient Horner's syndrome in cats, which usually resolves in 2 to 3 weeks (see discussion on surgical anatomy, p. 291). Horner's

syndrome is rare in dogs after this procedure, probably reflecting the difference in the anatomy of the tympanic cavity between the two species.

PROGNOSIS

The prognosis is excellent with complete removal of the polyp. Nasopharyngeal polyps may be less likely to recur than aural ones. Horner's syndrome typically resolves within a few weeks. Rarely, temporary or permanent vestibular signs (i.e., nystagmus and head tilt) may occur. Transient facial nerve paralysis is uncommon, but may occur after bulla osteotomy (see p. 300).

Reference

Donnelly KE, Tillson DM: Feline inflammatory polyps and ventral bulla osteotomy *Compend* 26:446, 2004.

Suggested Reading

Morris DO: Medical therapy of otitis externa and otitis media, *Vet Clin Small Anim* 34:541, 2004.

This article provides an extensive review of medications used to treat ear disease. Indications and contraindication of the various agents are discussed.

Pratschke KM: Inflammatory polyps of the middle ear in dogs, *Vet Surg* 32:292, 2003.

The presenting history, clinical signs, and outcome of five dogs having middle ear polyps are reported. Surgical removal of aural polyps had a good prognosis.

CHAPTER 18
Surgery of the Abdominal Cavity

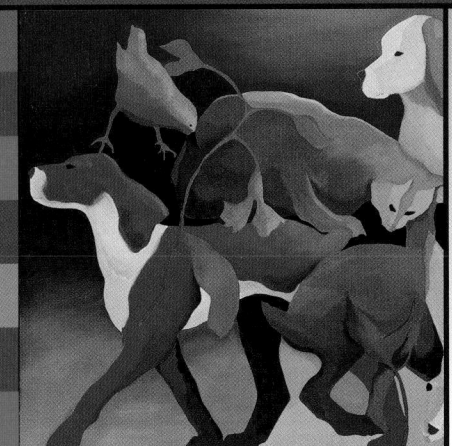

DEFINITIONS

Celiotomy is a surgical incision into the abdominal cavity; the term **laparotomy** often is used synonymously, although it technically refers to a flank incision. A sudden onset of clinical signs referable to the abdominal cavity (e.g., abdominal distention, pain, and vomiting) is called an **acute abdomen**.

PREOPERATIVE CONCERNS

Celiotomy is performed for various reasons; it may be indicated for diagnostic (e.g., biopsy of an organ) and/or for therapeutic reasons. Many animals undergoing abdominal exploratory surgery have chronic disease, but some patients require emergency abdominal surgery because of acute clinical signs. Some conditions are life threatening (e.g., gastric dilation-volvulus, colonic perforation, and severe hemorrhage), and appropriate therapy must be started promptly. Conditions that require surgery must be differentiated from those that can be managed medically. Although surgery that is obviously unnecessary must be avoided, surgery cannot always be delayed until one is certain the patient will benefit from it.

The decision to operate is based on the history and physical examination findings, radiographic and ultrasonographic studies, and laboratory analyses. Physical examination can be unreliable in predicting severity of abdominal trauma. The inaccuracy associated with examining patients with acute abdominal disease, particularly that associated with trauma, can be attributed partly to the patient's condition at the time of examination and to delayed development of clinical signs associated with some injuries. Depressed or lethargic animals may not show pain during abdominal palpation. Clinical signs of hemorrhage often are inapparent immediately after trauma; delays of 3 to 4 hours between injury and development of shock and collapse are common in patients with hepatic or splenic lacerations. Therefore animals that have suffered traumatic injuries should be closely observed for at least 8 to 12 hours. Life-threatening hemorrhage becomes apparent before this time in most cases. However, animals with traumatic bilious peritonitis may not have overt clinical signs for weeks. Likewise, traumatic mesenteric avulsion is seldom associated with clinical signs until peritonitis develops, usually several days after injury. Sensitive diagnostic tests, such as diagnostic peritoneal lavage (see p. 335), may help identify patients with significant abdominal trauma before overt clinical signs develop.

NOTE: Be aware that overt clinical signs associated with mesenteric avulsions or rupture of the biliary tract may not become evident for 1 to 2 weeks after injury.

Preoperative management of most animals undergoing exploratory laparotomy is dictated by the underlying abdominal disease. General observations include noting the animal's attitude and posture, temperature, respiratory rate and effort, and heart rate and rhythm. Abdominal auscultation, percussion, and palpation plus rectal examination are indicated. Serial examinations are important to detect trends or deterioration in the patient's status. An intravenous catheter should be placed for fluid and drug administration, and blood samples should be drawn. Useful initial blood work in an animal with acute abdomen includes complete blood count (CBC), platelet count, serum total protein and glucose concentrations, and blood urea nitrogen (BUN). Other laboratory tests (e.g., serum biochemistry profile and clotting parameters) can be performed, depending on the animal's condition and the suspected underlying disease. Urine may be collected by means of cystocentesis or catheterization for urinalysis. An indwelling urinary catheter may be used to quantitate urinary output if necessary. Abdominal radiographs may detect peritoneal fluid (i.e., uroabdomen and peritonitis) or abnormal accumulations of air. Animals with acute abdominal signs of uncertain cause should have diagnostic peritoneal lavage (see p. 335) if radiographs are nondiagnostic. Electrolyte and hydration abnormalities should be corrected before surgery.

BOX 18-1

Selected Anesthetic Protocols for Relatively Healthy Animals With Peritonitis

Premedication

Atropine (0.02–0.04 mg/kg SC or IM) or glycopyrrolate (0.005–0.011 mg/kg SC or IM) plus hydromorphone (0.1–0.2 mg/kg SC or IM) or butorphanol (0.2–0.4 mg/kg SC or IM) or buprenorphine (5–15 μg/kg IM)

Induction

Thiopental sodium (10–12 mg/kg IV) or propofol (4–6 mg/kg IV) or diazepam plus ketamine (0.27 mg/kg and 5.5 mg/kg, respectively) combined and administered IV to effect

Maintenance

Isoflurane or sevoflurane

SC, Subcutaneous; *IM,* intramuscular; *IV,* intravenous.

NOTE: If you note free air in the abdominal cavity of an animal that has suffered a recent traumatic injury, consider exploratory surgery; this finding may indicate rupture or perforation of the gastrointestinal tract.

ANESTHETIC CONSIDERATIONS

The anesthetic management of animals with abdominal disease depends on the underlying disease. Animals with peritonitis that are not in shock can be premedicated with an anticholinergic and opioid (i.e., hydromorphone, butorphanol, or buprenorphine), and induced with thiopental, propofol, or a combination of diazepam and ketamine given intravenously to effect (Box 18-1). Box 18-2 provides suggested anesthetic protocols for animals that are in shock or that are debilitated.

ANTIBIOTICS

The appropriate use of antibiotics in patients undergoing abdominal surgery depends on the underlying disease, the animal's overall general health, and the length and type of surgical procedure (see Chapter 10).

SURGICAL ANATOMY

The rectus sheath is composed of an external and internal leaf (Fig. 18-1). The external leaf is formed by the aponeurosis of the external abdominal oblique muscle and a portion of the aponeurosis of the internal abdominal oblique muscle. The aponeurosis of the transversus abdominis muscle joins the external leaf near the pubis (see Fig. 18-1). The internal leaf consists of a portion of the aponeurosis of the internal abdominal oblique muscle, the aponeurosis of the transversus abdominis muscle, and the transversalis fascia. The internal leaf disappears in the caudal third of the

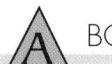 BOX 18-2

Selected Anesthetic Protocols for Animals With Peritonitis That Are Debilitated or in Shock

Dogs
Premedication and Induction

Hydromorphone (0.1 mg/kg IV) plus diazepam (0.2 mg/kg IV). Give in incremental doses and intubate if possible. If necessary, give etomidate (0.5–1.5 mg/kg IV). As an alternative, if the patient has not been vomiting or is not debilitated, use mask induction or give thiopental or propofol at reduced doses.

Maintenance

Isoflurane or sevoflurane.

Cats
Premedication

Butorphanol (0.2–0.4 mg/kg SC or IM) or buprenorphine (5–15 μg/kg IM) or hydromorphone (0.05–0.1 mg/kg SC or IM).

Induction

Diazepam (0.2 mg/kg IV) followed by etomidate (0.5–1.5 mg/kg IV). As an alternative, if the patient has not been vomiting, use mask or chamber induction or give thiopental or propofol at reduced doses. If ketamine is not contraindicated, reduced doses of diazepam and ketamine may also be used.

Maintenance

Isoflurane or sevoflurane.

IV, Intravenous; *SC,* subcutaneous; *IM,* intramuscular.
Note: Use etomidate with caution in animals with renal insufficiency (see text).

---

abdomen where the aponeurosis of the internal abdominal oblique muscle joins the external leaf, leaving the caudal rectus abdominis muscle covered only by a thin sheet of transversalis fascia and peritoneum (see Fig. 18-1).

NOTE: The linea alba is easier to locate near the umbilicus because it becomes thinner near the pubis.

SURGICAL TECHNIQUES

The abdomen generally is explored by means of a ventral midline incision. In most animals the entire abdomen, including the inguinal areas and caudal thorax, should be prepared for aseptic surgery to allow extension of the incision into thoracic or pelvic cavities if necessary. Prepping too small an area is a common mistake, particularly for abdominal exploration in trauma patients. To visualize all abdominal structures adequately, the incision must extend from the xiphoid process to the pubis. If only a specific abdominal structure will be examined, a shorter incision can be made. A caudal abdominal incision extending from umbilicus to pubis is adequate for bladder exploration;

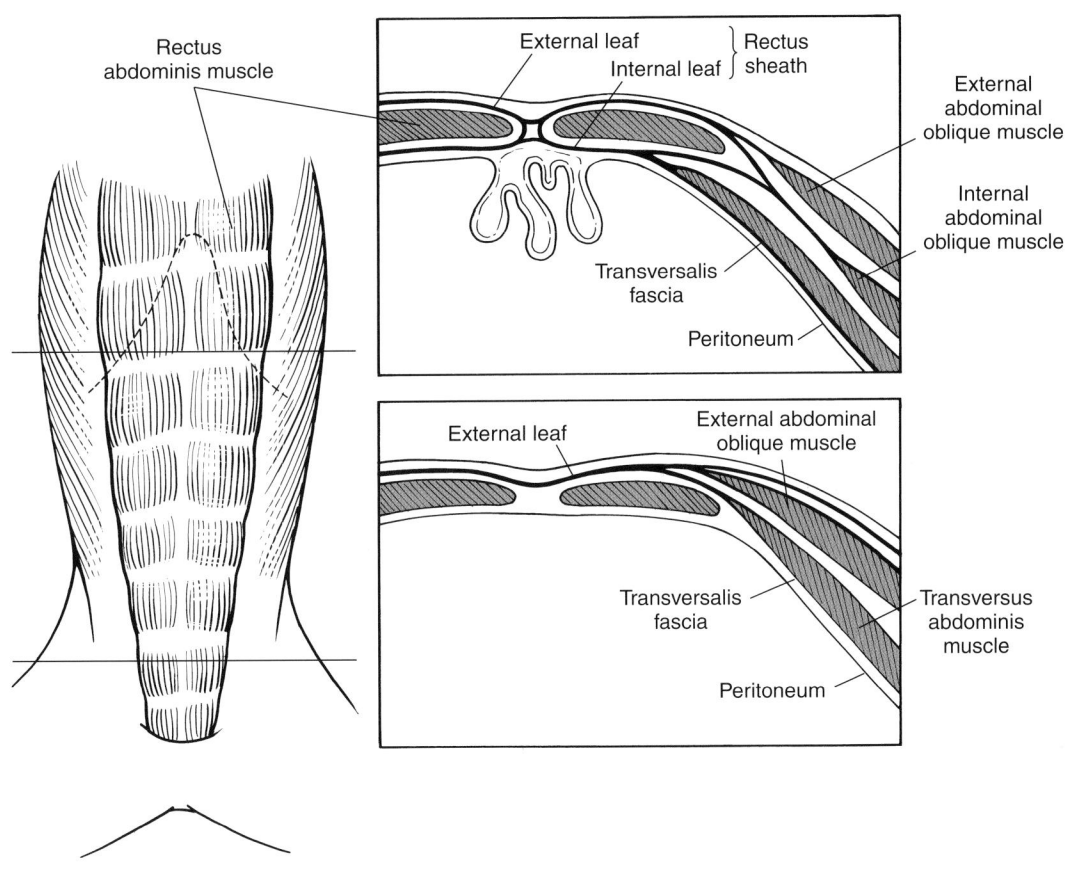

FIG. 18-1
Anatomy of the rectus sheath.

similarly, a cranial abdominal incision (i.e., umbilicus to xiphoid process) allows evaluation of the liver and stomach. Occasionally the midline incision is extended laterally at the xiphoid process (1 cm caudal to the last rib) to facilitate exposure of the liver, biliary system, and diaphragm. A paracostal (paralumbar) celiotomy can be used to expose the kidneys and adrenal glands; it is most commonly used for unilateral adrenalectomy.

> NOTE: Always count surgical sponges before making the incision and before abdominal closure to help ensure that none are inadvertently left in the abdominal cavity.

Ventral Midline Celiotomy in Cats and Female Dogs

With the patient in dorsal recumbency, make a ventral midline skin incision beginning near the xiphoid process and extending caudally to the pubis (Fig. 18-2, A). Sharply incise the subcutaneous tissue until the external fascia of the rectus abdominis muscle is exposed. Ligate or cauterize small subcutaneous bleeders and identify the linea alba. Tent the abdominal wall, and make a sharp incision into the linea alba with a scalpel blade. Palpate the interior surface of the

linea for adhesions. Use scissors to extend the incision cranially or caudally (or both) to near the extent of the skin incision. Digitally break down the attachments of one side of the falciform ligament to the body wall or excise it and remove it entirely if it interferes with visualization of cranial abdominal structures. Clamp the cranial end of the falciform ligament and ligate or cauterize bleeders before removing it.

Ventral Midline Celiotomy in Male Dogs

With the patient in dorsal recumbency, place a towel clamp on the prepuce and clamp it to the skin on one side of the body (Fig. 18-2, B). Drape the tip of the prepuce and clamp outside the surgical field. Make a ventral midline skin incision beginning at the xiphoid process and continuing caudally to the prepuce. Curve the incision to the left or right of the penis and prepuce (i.e., the side opposite the clamped prepuce), and extend it to the level of the pubis (see Fig. 18-2, B). Incise the subcutaneous tissue and fibers of the preputialis muscle to the level of the rectus fascia in the same plane as the skin incision. Ligate or cauterize large branches of the caudal superficial epigastric vein at the cranial aspect of the prepuce. Retract incised skin and subcutaneous tissues laterally, and locate the linea alba and external fascia of the rectus abdominis muscle. Do not attempt to locate the caudal linea alba until subcutaneous tissues have been incised and the

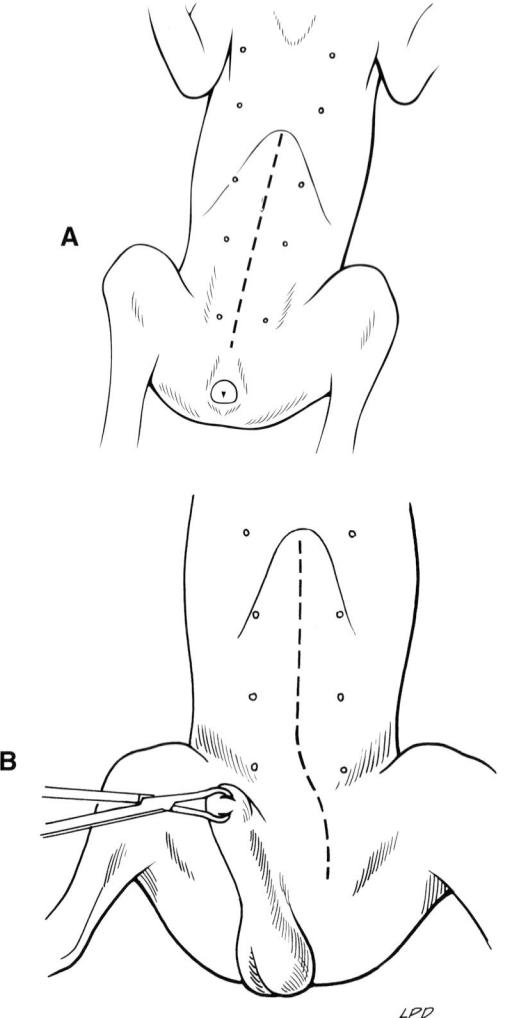

FIG. 18-2
Ventral midline celiotomy. **A,** In cats and female dogs. **B,** In male dogs.

abdominal musculature fascia has been identified. Tent the abdominal wall and make a sharp incision into the linea alba with a scalpel blade. Palpate the interior surface of the linea for adhesions. Use scissors to extend the incision cranially or caudally (or both) to near the extent of the skin incision.

Paracostal Celiotomy

Position the animal in lateral recumbency, and place a rolled towel or sandbag between the animal and the operating table. Make a skin incision from the ventral vertebral column to near the ventral midline. Center the incision halfway between the wing of the ilium and the last rib. Extend the incision through the external abdominal oblique muscle with scissors. Separate internal abdominal oblique and transversus abdominis muscle fibers and expose the peritoneal and transversalis fascia. Tent the peritoneum and sharply incise it with scissors.

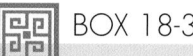 **BOX 18-3**

Systematic Exploration of the Abdominal Cavity

1. Explore the cranial quadrant.
   * Examine the diaphragm (including the esophageal hiatus) and the entire liver (palpate the liver).
   * Inspect the gallbladder and biliary tree; express the gallbladder to determine its patency.
   * Examine the stomach, pylorus, proximal duodenum, and spleen.
   * Examine both pancreatic limbs (palpate gently), the portal vein, hepatic arteries, and caudal vena cava.
2. Explore the caudal quadrant.
   * Inspect the descending colon, urinary bladder, urethra, and prostate or uterine horns.
   * Inspect the inguinal rings.
3. Explore the intestinal tract.
   * Palpate the intestinal tract from the duodenum to the descending colon and observe the mesenteric vasculature and nodes.
4. Explore the gutters.
   * Use the mesoduodenum to retract the intestine to the left, and examine the right "gutter." Palpate the kidney and examine the adrenal gland, ureter, and ovary.
   * Use the descending colon to retract the abdominal contents to the right. Examine the left kidney, adrenal gland, ureter, and ovary.

Abdominal Exploration

Systematically explore the entire abdomen.

Various techniques may be used; however, every surgeon should develop a consistent pattern to ensure that the entire abdominal cavity and all structures are visualized and/or palpated in each animal (Box 18-3).

Use moistened laparotomy sponges to protect tissue from drying during the procedure. If generalized infection is present or if diffuse intraoperative contamination has occurred, flush the abdomen with copious amounts of warmed, sterile saline solution.

Historically, many different antiseptics (i.e., povidone-iodine and chlorhexidine) and antibiotics have been added to lavage fluids. Povidone-iodine is the most widely used antiseptic; however, this practice has not shown a beneficial effect in repeated experimental and clinical trials and may be detrimental in animals with established peritonitis because the carrier—polyvinylpyrrolidone—inhibits macrophage chemotaxis. Similarly, there is no substantial evidence that adding antibiotics to lavage fluid benefits patients treated with appropriate systemic antibiotics. Room temperature lavage fluids should not be used in anesthetized patients. Heated lavage fluids have been proven to be effective in increasing the temperature in dogs (Nawrocki et al, 2005).

Remove the lavage fluid and blood and inspect the abdominal cavity before closure to ensure that all foreign material and surgical equipment have been removed. Perform a sponge count and compare it with the preoperative count to ensure that surgical sponges have not been left in the abdominal cavity.

Abdominal Wall Closure

The linea alba may be closed with simple interrupted sutures or a simple continuous suture pattern. The simple continuous technique does not increase the risk of dehiscence when properly performed (i.e., secure knots and appropriate suture material), and it allows for rapid closure. Preferably strong, absorbable suture material (i.e., polydioxanone, polyglyconate, and poliglecaprone 25) should be used for continuous suture patterns, and six to eight knots should be placed at each end of the incision line. Monofilament, nonabsorbable suture material (i.e., nylon and polypropylene) has been associated with suture sinus formation and should be avoided. Surgical gut and stainless steel wire should not be used for continuous suture patterns.

On each side of the incision, incorporate 4 to 10 mm of fascia in each suture. Place interrupted sutures 5 to 10 mm apart, depending on the animal's size. Tighten sutures sufficiently to appose but not enough to strangulate tissue because overly tight sutures adversely affect wound healing. Incorporate full-thickness bites of the abdominal wall in the sutures if the incision is midline (i.e., through the linea alba; Fig. 18-3). Do not incorporate the falciform ligament between the fascial edges. If the incision is lateral to the linea alba and if muscular tissue is exposed (i.e., paramedian incision), close the external rectus sheath without including muscle in the sutures. Do not attempt to include peritoneum in the sutures. Close subcutaneous tissue with a simple continuous pattern of absorbable suture material, and reappose the preputialis muscle fibers. Use nonabsorbable sutures (simple interrupted or continuous appositional pattern; see Chapter 9) or stainless steel staples to close the skin. Place skin sutures without tension.

For paracostal celiotomy, close the individual muscle layers with synthetic absorbable suture material in a continuous or interrupted pattern. Attempt to eliminate dead space between muscle layers. Appose subcutaneous tissue with absorbable suture in a continuous or interrupted pattern and close the skin with nonabsorbable suture in a simple interrupted or continuous pattern.

HEALING OF THE ABDOMINAL WALL

The ability of tissue to hold sutures without tearing depends on the tissue's strength and the orientation of collagen fibrils. Skin and fascia are strong, whereas muscle and fat are weak. Peritoneum heals rapidly across the incision and does not contribute to wound strength; therefore closure of this layer is not beneficial. Experimental and clinical studies in dogs suggest that suturing peritoneum may increase the incidence of postoperative intraabdominal adhesions.

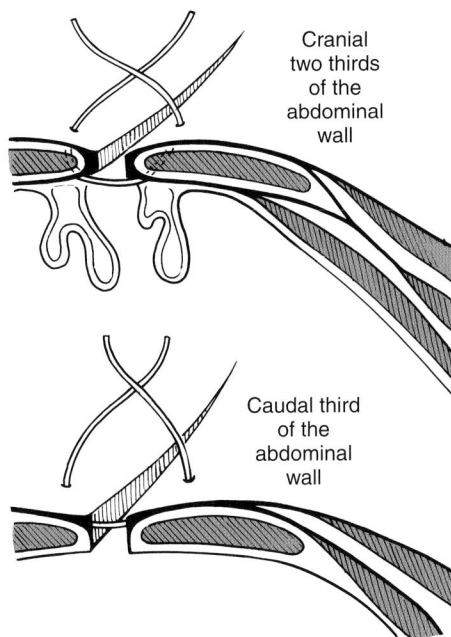

FIG. 18-3
To close a midline incision, incorporate full-thickness bites of the linea alba (or the external sheath only) in the sutures.

> NOTE: Make sure to incorporate fascia in the linea closure. Because the holding layer of abdominal incisions is fascia rather than muscle, dehiscence is common if the rectus fascia is not incorporated in sutures.

SUTURE MATERIALS AND SPECIAL INSTRUMENTS

Useful instruments for celiotomy include Balfour abdominal retractors, Poole or Yankauer suction tips, malleable retractors, and Mixter (right-angle) forceps. Laparotomy pads and 4 × 4 sponges should have radiopaque markers. See the previous discussion on abdominal wall closure for choice of suture material.

POSTOPERATIVE CARE AND ASSESSMENT

The abdominal incision should be checked twice daily for redness, swelling, or discharge. If the animal licks or chews at the incision, an Elizabethan collar or sidebar should be used to prevent iatrogenic suture removal. Early signs of altered wound healing are inflammation and edema. Swelling and serosanguineous drainage from the incision are consistent signs of acute incisional dehiscence. Dehiscence usually occurs 3 to 5 days after surgery, when minimal healing has occurred and the sutures have weakened; however, it may occur earlier if knots were tied improperly or if fascia was not incorporated into the sutures. Evisceration usually causes sepsis and severe blood loss secondary to mutilation of exposed intestine; it must be treated promptly. The abdomen should be bandaged, fluid therapy initiated, and broad-spectrum antibiotics given while the animal is prepared for surgery. If technical failure is suspected, such as poor knot tying or improper suturing, the entire suture line should be removed and replaced. Débridement of the wound edges is unnecessary and delays wound healing. The intestine should be closely inspected for viability, and damaged sections resected if appropriate (see p. 450). The abdominal cavity should be lavaged copiously with warmed, sterile saline. Open abdominal drainage (see p. 336) should be considered in animals with generalized peritonitis. Wound disruption after 10 to 21 days usually causes hernia formation rather than evisceration. Hernial repair in these animals may require excision of fibrotic tissue. Subsequent closure requires that tissue layers be accurately apposed.

COMPLICATIONS

Dehiscence (incisional hernias) may occur if improper surgical technique is used (see the above discussion). The most common causes of wound dehiscence in the early postoperative period are suture breakage, knot slippage or untying, or sutures cutting through tissue. A higher rate of dehiscence may be seen in animals with wound infections, fluid or electrolyte imbalances, anemia, hypoproteinemia, metabolic disease (e.g., hyperadrenocorticism and diabetes mellitus), immunosuppression (e.g., feline immunodeficiency virus [FIV] and feline leukemia virus), or abdominal distention or in those that have been treated with corticosteroids, chemotherapeutic agents, or radiation. Suture sinus formation has been reported with nonabsorbable suture material. Such cases require surgical resection of affected tissue and removal of offending sutures.

SPECIAL AGE CONSIDERATIONS

Healing may be delayed in debilitated, very young or very old, or hypoproteinemic animals; chromic gut suture should not be used for abdominal wall closure in these patients.

Reference

Nawrocki MA, McLaughlin RM, Hendrix PK: The effects of heated and room-temperature abdominal lavage solutions on core body temperature in dogs undergoing celiotomy, *J Am Anim Hosp Assoc* 41:61, 2005.

SPECIFIC DISEASES

UMBILICAL AND ABDOMINAL HERNIAS

DEFINITIONS

External abdominal hernias are defects in the external wall of the abdomen that allow protrusion of abdominal contents; **internal abdominal hernias** are those that occur through a ring of tissue confined within the abdomen or thorax (i.e., diaphragmatic hernia and hiatal hernia). External abdominal hernias may involve the abdominal wall anywhere other than the umbilicus, inguinal ring, femoral canal,

or scrotum. **Umbilical hernias** occur through the umbilical ring. The contents of **true hernias** generally are enclosed in a peritoneal sac; **false hernias** allow protrusion of organs outside a normal abdominal opening, therefore the contents seldom are contained in a peritoneal sac. **Omphaloceles** are large midline umbilical and skin defects.

Abdominal hernias may be defined according to their location (i.e., ventral, prepubic, subcostal, hypochondral, paracostal, or lateral). The cranial pubic ligament formerly was called the *prepubic tendon*.

GENERAL CONSIDERATIONS AND CLINICALLY RELEVANT PATHOPHYSIOLOGY

Abdominal hernias generally occur secondary to trauma, such as vehicular accidents or bite wounds; however, they occasionally occur as congenital lesions. Congenital cranial abdominal hernias (i.e., cranial to the umbilicus) have been reported in association with peritoneopericardial diaphragmatic hernias in dogs and cats. Abdominal hernias are false hernias because they do not contain a hernial sac. When associated with blunt trauma, they arise as a result of rupture of the wall from within caused by an increase in intraabdominal pressure while the abdominal muscles are contracted. The most common sites for traumatic abdominal hernias are the prepubic region and the flank. Cranial pubic ligament hernias often occur in association with pubic fractures (Fig. 18-4). Paracostal hernias may allow migration of abdominal contents along the thoracic wall (see Fig. 18-4). In rare cases the abdominal contents enter the chest through defects in the intercostal muscles.

Umbilical hernias usually are congenital, caused by flawed embryogenesis (see Fig. 18-4). Umbilical vessels, the vitelline duct, and the stalk of the allantois pass through the umbilical ring in the fetus, but this aperture closes at birth, leaving an umbilical cicatrix. If the aperture fails to contract or is too large or improperly formed, a hernia results. These hernias are lined by a peritoneal sac and are considered true hernias. The cause of umbilical hernias is seldom known, but most are thought to be inherited. Many male dogs with umbilical hernias are also cryptorchid. Omphaloceles allow abdominal organs to protrude externally (eviscerate). The abdominal contents initially are covered by amniotic tissue, but this membrane covering is easily ruptured. Most affected neonates either die or are euthanized at birth.

DIAGNOSIS
Clinical Presentation

Signalment. Most animals with umbilical or abdominal hernias are young. Umbilical hernias are believed to be heritable in some breeds (i.e., Airedale, basenji, and Pekingese). Cranial ventral abdominal hernias associated with peritoneopericardial diaphragmatic hernias may be inherited in weimaraners.

History. A history of trauma is common with abdominal hernias. The hernia initially may be overlooked, whereas more obvious or life-threatening injuries are treated. Small umbilical hernias often are not noticed until the animal is examined for neutering. If strangulation or intestinal ob-

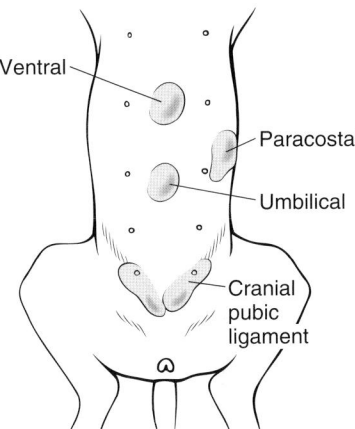

Ventral

Paracostal

Umbilical

Cranial
pubic
ligament

FIG. 18-4
Location of abdominal and umbilical hernias.

struction occurs, the animal may be presented for treatment of vomiting, abdominal pain, anorexia, and/or depression.

Physical Examination Findings

Abdominal structures (i.e., organs or omentum) in the subcutaneous space or between muscle layers usually cause asymmetry of the abdominal contour. The size of the swelling may not correspond to the size of the hernia, particularly if the intestine has migrated into the hernia. The swelling should be palpated carefully to discern the contents of the hernia (i.e., intestine, bladder, or spleen) and to locate the abdominal defect. These patients should be thoroughly examined to determine whether a concurrent abdominal, thoracic injury, or abnormality exists. Rupture of the cranial pubic ligament often is difficult to palpate because of subcutaneous swelling and pain.

Umbilical hernias usually manifest as a soft ventral abdominal mass at the umbilical scar. Deep palpation of the swelling reveals the size of the umbilical ring and helps characterize hernial contents. The hernial ring is not palpable in some animals because the ring closes subsequent to herniation of falciform fat or omentum. Occasionally intestine or other abdominal structures can be palpated; they generally can be reduced into the abdominal cavity. If the umbilical sac is warm or painful and the contents are irreducible, intestinal strangulation or obstruction should be suspected.

> NOTE: Be sure to evaluate dogs with congenital hernias for other defects (e.g., cryptorchidism with umbilical hernias; ventricular septal defects and pericardial diaphragmatic hernias with cranial abdominal hernias).

Diagnostic Imaging

Radiographs should be taken in animals with abdominal hernias. Routine ventral dorsal and lateral views may show an associated abdominal or thoracic injury (e.g., abdominal fluid or diaphragmatic hernia). Abdominal radiographs may help confirm a hernia (i.e., subcutaneous intestinal loops and loss of the ventral abdominal stripe) when the abdominal wall defect cannot be palpated because of swelling or pain. Radiographs generally are not indicated in small umbilical hernias. Ultrasound examination may also help define contents of hernias.

Laboratory Findings

Laboratory abnormalities are uncommon with umbilical hernias unless strangulation or intestinal obstruction is present. Abnormalities associated with abdominal hernias vary depending on the severity of concurrent internal injuries.

DIFFERENTIAL DIAGNOSIS

Most hernias are diagnosed on physical examination. Differential diagnoses for abdominal swellings include abscesses, cellulitis, hematomas or seromas, and neoplasia.

MEDICAL MANAGEMENT

Initial treatment of animals with abdominal hernias is directed toward diagnosing and treating shock, and concurrent life-threatening internal injuries.

SURGICAL TREATMENT

Most abdominal hernias can be repaired by suturing torn muscle edges or by apposing the disrupted abdominal wall edge to the pubis, ribs, or adjacent fascia. Synthetic mesh must be used to repair the defect in rare cases. Some hernias (i.e., intestinal strangulation, urinary obstruction, and concurrent organ trauma) require emergency surgical correction. However, the extent of devitalized muscle may not be apparent initially; in stable patients surgical correction may be delayed until muscle damage can be accurately assessed. The most common complications are hernia recurrence and wound infection. Abdominal hernias secondary to bite wounds usually are contaminated; wound infection and dehiscence of the skin or hernial repair (or both) are common. Mesh should not be placed in these hernias, and the wounds should be drained. Treatment of infected wounds includes cultures, drainage, antibiotics, and/or flushing. Abdominal exploration should be performed at herniorrhaphy to diagnose concurrent abdominal organ injury (i.e., mesenteric avulsion, gastric or intestinal perforation, diaphragmatic herniation, and bladder rupture).

Many umbilical hernias resolve spontaneously in young animals or are small and are not corrected until the animal is neutered. Spontaneous closure may occur as late as 6 months of age. Intestinal strangulation is most likely when the hernial defect is about the size of intestine and the hernial sac is large. Strangulation is unlikely in very small or large defects. If abdominal viscera in the hernia cannot be reduced, surgery should be performed as soon as possible.

Preoperative Management

Preoperative care depends on the animal's status and concurrent injuries. Hydration and electrolyte abnormalities should be corrected before surgery.

Anesthesia

If there are no concurrent abdominal injuries or disease, a variety of anesthetic protocols can be used to anesthetize the animal. See Box 18-2 for anesthetic management of animals that are in shock or are debilitated. See also subsequent chapters for detailed information about anesthetic management of patients with specific diseases (i.e., renal, pancreatic, and hepatic).

Surgical Anatomy

The abdominal wall is composed of four muscle layers (the external and internal abdominal oblique muscles, the rectus abdominis muscle, and the transversus abdominis muscle). Abdominal hernias may occur at insertions or attachments of these muscles or through muscle bellies themselves. The cranial pubic ligament (prepubic tendon) is a band of transverse fibers that connects the iliopectineal eminence and pectineal muscle origin of one side with those on the other side. This ligament attaches the rectus abdominis muscle to the pelvis.

Positioning

For ventral hernias, the animal is placed in dorsal recumbency and the area around the hernia is prepared for aseptic surgery. Repair of ruptures of the cranial pubic ligament may be facilitated by placing the animal in dorsal recumbency with the rear limbs flexed and pulled cranially.

SURGICAL TECHNIQUES
Abdominal Hernias

For most abdominal hernias, perform a ventral midline abdominal incision to allow the entire abdomen to be explored. Assess the extent of visceral herniation. Reduce the herniated contents, and amputate or excise necrotic or devitalized tissue around the hernia. Close the muscle layers of the hernia with simple interrupted or simple continuous sutures. If a large area of devitalized tissue is removed, use synthetic mesh, such as Marlex or Prolene, to close the defect (do not place mesh in infected sites). Fold the edges of the mesh over, and suture the folded edges to viable tissue using simple interrupted sutures. Injuries to the cranial pubic ligament can be difficult to repair. If necessary, drill holes in the pubic bone to anchor the sutures.

Paracostal hernias. *Make a midline incision or make one directly over the hernia. Explore the hernia, and suture the torn edges of the transverse, internal, and external abdominal oblique muscles. Incorporate a rib in the suture if muscle has been avulsed from the costal arch.*

Cranial pubic ligament hernias. *Make a ventral midline skin incision, and identify the ruptured tendon and its pubic insertion. Evaluate the inguinal rings and vascular lacuna; these hernias may extend into the femoral region as a result of rupture of the inguinal ligament. Reattach the free edge of the abdominal wall to the cranial pubic ligament with simple interrupted sutures. As an alternative, suture the*

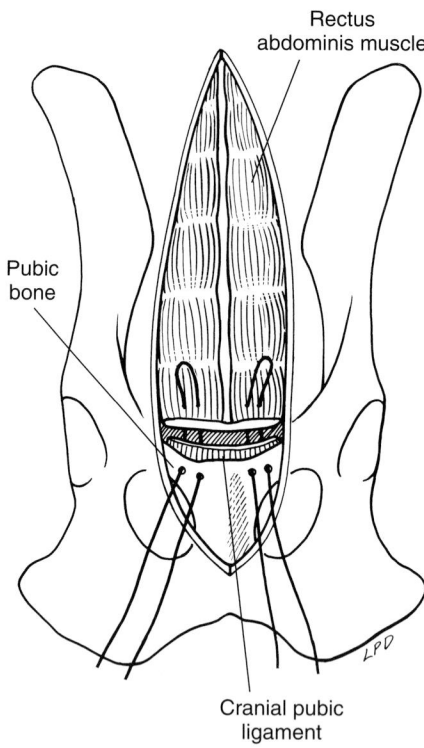

FIG. 18-5
To repair injuries to the cranial pubic ligament, it may be necessary to anchor the ligament to the pubis by drilling holes in the pubic bone through which sutures can be placed.

tendon remnant to the muscle fascia and periosteum covering the pubis or anchor it to the pubis by drilling holes in the pubic bone through which sutures can be placed (Fig. 18-5). If the hernia extends into the femoral region, it may be necessary to suture the body wall to the medial fascia of the adductor muscles. When doing so, take care to avoid damaging the femoral vessels or nerves.

Umbilical Hernias

For umbilical hernias, palpate the hernial ring, reduce the abdominal contents if possible, and incise the skin over the umbilicus. If the hernia contains only fat or omentum, ligate the hernial neck and excise the sac and its contents. As an alternative, if adhesions are not present, invert the sac and its contents into the abdominal cavity. Do not débride the wound margins. Suture the edges of the defect with monofilament, synthetic, absorbable suture (i.e., polydioxanone, polyglyconate, or poliglecaprone 25) in a simple interrupted pattern. If the hernial contents cannot be reduced, make an elliptic incision around the swelling to prevent damaging the contents. Incise the hernial sac, and replace the contents in the abdominal cavity. If the contents are irreducible or if strangulation or intestinal obstruction is present, extend the abdominal defect on the midline. Explore the abdomen, and inspect the intestines for viability before closing the defect. Umbilical hernia repair seldom requires mesh implantation.

SUTURE MATERIALS AND SPECIAL INSTRUMENTS

Strong, absorbable suture (polydioxanone, polyglyconate, and poliglecaprone 25) or nonabsorbable suture (polypropylene and nylon) should be used to repair abdominal or ventral hernias. Marlex and Prolene synthetic mesh may be used to repair some large defects.

POSTOPERATIVE CARE AND ASSESSMENT

The postoperative care of these patients is dictated by the presence of concurrent injuries or disease. The patient should be kept quiet, and the wound should be checked frequently for infection or dehiscence. Vomiting, fever, and/or leukocytosis may indicate peritonitis (see p. 331).

PROGNOSIS

The prognosis generally is good, and recurrence is uncommon. When recurrence occurs, it generally is noted within a few days of surgery. Most animals have excellent long-term results when appropriate techniques are used.

Suggested Reading

Shaw SP, Rozanski EA, Rush JE: Traumatic body wall herniation in 36 dogs and cats, *J Am Anim Hosp Assoc* 39:35, 2003.
Traumatic body wall hernias were commonly associated with bite wounds in dogs (54%) and cats (40%). Seventy-three percent of dogs and 80% of cats survived to hospital discharge.

INGUINAL, SCROTAL, AND FEMORAL HERNIAS

DEFINITIONS

Inguinal hernias are protrusions of organs or tissue through the inguinal canal adjacent to the vaginal process. **Scrotal hernias** occur when inguinal ring defects allow abdominal contents to protrude into the vaginal process adjacent to the spermatic cord. **Femoral hernias** occur through a defect in the femoral canal.

GENERAL CONSIDERATIONS AND CLINICALLY RELEVANT PATHOPHYSIOLOGY

Inguinal hernias may arise from a congenital abnormality of the inguinal ring or may be caused by trauma (Fig. 18-6). An inguinal ring defect allows abdominal contents (e.g., intestine, bladder, and uterus) to enter subcutaneous spaces. Congenital hernias may be associated with other abnormalities, such as umbilical hernias, perineal hernias, and cryptorchidism. Whether inguinal hernias are heritable in most breeds is unknown; neutering is recommended in dogs with nontraumatic hernias until the genetics of this condition become known.

The causes of inguinal herniation in small animals are poorly understood. Both neutered and intact male and female dogs may develop nontraumatic inguinal hernias. They may be unilateral or bilateral; unilateral inguinal hernias occur more commonly on the left side. Sex hormones have been incriminated in the formation of inguinal hernias in

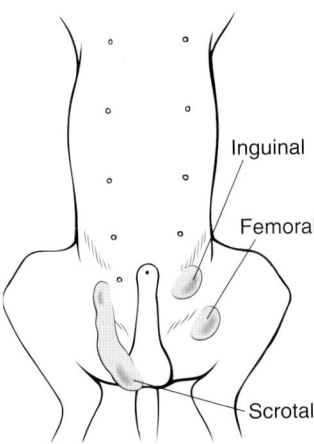

FIG. 18-6
Location of inguinal, femoral, and scrotal hernias.

mice, but their role in dogs is unclear. Pregnancy and obesity may be associated with the formation of an inguinal hernia. Traumatic inguinal hernias may occur as a result of a congenital weakness of the musculature or an abnormality of the inguinal ring.

Scrotal hernias are rare, indirect hernias (see Fig. 18-6). They usually are unilateral, and strangulation of abdominal contents is common. Little is known about the cause and heritability. A congenital defect or trauma may predispose some dogs to hernia formation. An increased incidence of testicular tumors has been reported in conjunction with scrotal hernias.

Femoral hernias are rare in dogs and cats. They occur when abdominal contents or fat protrude through the femoral canal, caudomedial to the femoral vessels (see Fig. 18-6). They may be mistaken for inguinal hernias. Femoral hernias may occur after trauma and avulsion of the cranial pubic ligament, or they may result if the origin of the pectineus muscle is transected from the pubis during subtotal pectineal myectomy.

DIAGNOSIS
Clinical Presentation

Signalment. Nontraumatic inguinal hernias are most often reported in intact, middle-aged female dogs or young male dogs (under 2 years of age). Inguinal hernias presumably arise in young male dogs because late testicular descent delays closure of the inguinal ring. Breeds that are predisposed to this condition include Pekingese, cairn terrier, basset hound, basenji, and West Highland white terrier. Older bitches may be predisposed to develop inguinal hernias because they have a relatively large-diameter ring with a short canal. Inguinal hernias are rare in cats. Scrotal hernias have been reported most commonly in chondrodystrophic dogs, particularly Shar-Peis. No breed or sex predisposition has been reported for femoral hernias.

History. Animals with inguinal hernias may be brought in because of a painless swelling in the inguinal region or for vomiting, lethargy, pain, and/or depression if the hernial contents are incarcerated. Small hernias often go unnoticed unless organ entrapment or incarceration occurs. Omentum is the most common organ present in canine inguinal hernias. The uterus often is in hernias of affected intact females. These hernias often are chronic and do not cause clinical signs until pregnancy or pyometra develops.

Animals with scrotal and femoral hernias usually are presented for evaluation of scrotal or medial thigh swelling, respectively, or for vomiting and pain if intestinal incarceration occurs.

Physical Examination Findings

Physical characteristics of the swelling vary according to hernial contents and degree of associated vascular obstruction. Often a soft, painless, unilateral or bilateral swelling is noted in the inguinal region. If intestinal strangulation has occurred or if a gravid uterus or urinary bladder is in the hernia, the swelling may be large, fluctuant, and painful. Finding nonviable small intestine is more common in young male dogs (under 2 years of age) with nontraumatic hernias than in older animals. Associated vascular or lymphatic obstruction (or both) may cause testicular and spermatic cord edema. Concurrent abnormalities may be noted, such as perineal hernia or cryptorchidism. Unilateral inguinal hernias are more common than bilateral hernias. Bilateral hernias occur more commonly in young dogs, and careful palpation of the contralateral inguinal region for occult hernias is recommended in all dogs.

A scrotal hernia usually appears as a firm, cordlike mass that extends into the caudal aspect of the scrotum. Pain and bluish-black tissue discoloration may be noted if intestinal strangulation has occurred. Femoral hernias cause swelling on the medial aspect of the thigh that may extend into the inguinal region. The swelling is located caudal to the inguinal ligament and ventrolateral to the pelvic brim.

Diagnostic Imaging

Abdominal radiographs may help identify herniation of a gravid uterus, intestine, or bladder in an inguinal hernia. Loss of the caudal abdominal stripe may be noted in affected animals. Ultrasonography is useful with scrotal hernias to assess the viability of testicular blood flow and to help determine if spermatic cord torsion or a hydrocele is present.

Laboratory Findings

Laboratory abnormalities are uncommon unless intestinal incarceration has occurred.

DIFFERENTIAL DIAGNOSIS

Differentiation of mammary tumors, lipomas, lymphadenopathy, hematomas, abscesses, and/or mammary cysts from inguinal hernias is facilitated by placing the animal on its back and attempting to reduce the contents of the swelling. Incarceration of intestine may prevent reduction and makes differentiation of these abnormalities difficult. Differential diagnoses for scrotal hernias include trauma, testicular or scrotal neoplasia, orchitis, and severe scrotal inflammation or swelling. Differential diagnoses for femoral hernias include neoplasia, abscesses, and lymphadenopathy. Femoral and inguinal hernias may be difficult to distinguish from each other before surgery.

> **NOTE:** Do not mistake the caudal abdominal fat pad in obese cats for an inguinal hernia.

MEDICAL MANAGEMENT

The animal's condition should be stabilized before surgery.

SURGICAL TREATMENT

Prompt surgical correction is recommended to prevent complications associated with intestinal strangulation or pregnancy. Undescended testicles should be removed during repair of an inguinal hernia. Necrosis of ipsilateral descended testicles may occur secondary to vascular obstruction and requires orchiectomy. If a gravid uterus is contained in the inguinal hernia, the animal can be spayed, or if the fetus is viable and termination of the pregnancy is not desired, an attempt can be made to reduce the uterus and close the inguinal ring. However, parturition or uterine enlargement may be associated with recurrence.

> **NOTE:** Neuter animals with inguinal hernias. Warn owners of intact female dogs that the hernia may recur if the dog is bred or develops pyometra.

Preoperative Management

If intestinal incarceration or strangulation is suspected, antibiotics should be given before surgery.

Anesthesia

If the animal is healthy, a variety of anesthetic protocols can be used safely. For patients in which nonviable intestine is present see Box 18-2. See p. 445 for additional anesthetic recommendations for animals undergoing intestinal surgery. Anesthetic protocols for pregnant animals can be found on p. 706.

Surgical Anatomy

The inguinal canal is a sagittal slit in the caudoventral abdominal wall through which pass the genital branch of the genitofemoral nerve, artery, and vein; the external pudendal vessel; and the spermatic cord (males) or round ligament (females) (Fig. 18-7). The vascular structures are located in the caudomedial aspect of the canal. The inguinal canal is bounded by the internal and external inguinal rings. The internal inguinal ring is formed by the caudal edge of the internal abdominal oblique muscle (cranial), the rectus abdominis muscle (medial), and the inguinal ligament (lateral and caudal); the external inguinal ring is a longitudinal slit in the aponeurosis of the external abdominal oblique muscle. Direct hernias happen when peritoneal evagination oc-

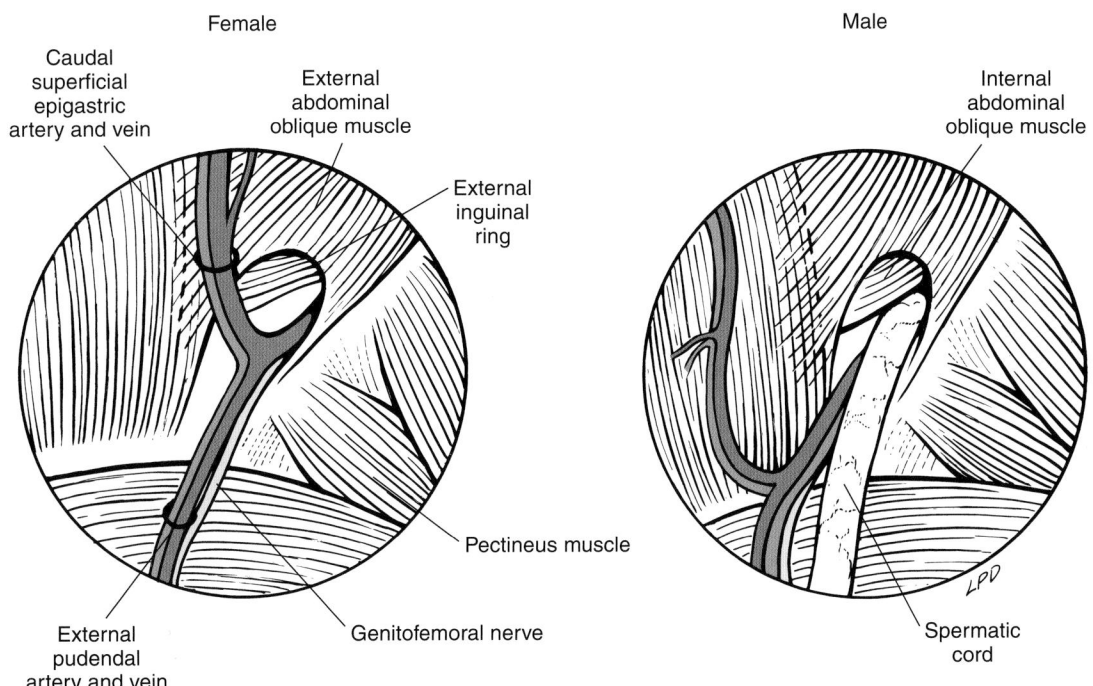

FIG. 18-7
Components of the inguinal canal.

curs as a separate, distinct outpocketing from the vaginal process; indirect hernias are protrusions through the normal evagination of the vaginal process.

Positioning

The animal is positioned in dorsal recumbency, and the caudal abdominal and inguinal areas are prepared for aseptic surgery.

SURGICAL TECHNIQUES

The goal of surgery is to reduce the abdominal contents and close the external inguinal ring so that herniation of abdominal contents cannot recur. The approach for inguinal hernias depends on whether the hernia is unilateral or bilateral; if the contents can be reduced; and if intestinal strangulation or concurrent abdominal trauma is a factor. Although an incision can be made parallel to the flank fold directly over the lateral aspect of the swelling, a midline incision usually is preferred in female dogs because it allows palpation and closure of both inguinal rings through a single skin incision. Inguinal hernias usually can be closed without using prosthetic materials. Occasionally, repair of recurrent or large traumatic defects requires placement of synthetic mesh (see p. 324) or a cranial sartorius muscle flap (see p. 219). Bilateral orchiectomy is recommended with scrotal hernias to lessen recurrence.

Inguinal Hernias

Make a caudal abdominal midline skin incision in female dogs cranially from the brim of the pelvis (Fig. 18-8). Deepen the incision through subcutaneous tissue to the ven-

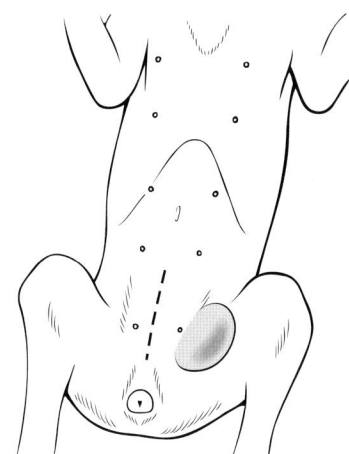

FIG. 18-8
Incision for repair of an inguinal hernia.

tral rectus sheath. Expose the hernial sac by bluntly dissecting beneath mammary tissue, and identify the hernial sac and ring (Fig. 18-9, A). Reduce the abdominal contents by twisting the sac and milking the contents through the ring; or if necessary, incise the hernial sac and make an incision in the craniomedial aspect of the ring to enlarge it (Fig. 18-9, B). After reducing the abdominal contents, amputate the base of the hernial sac, and close it with horizontal mattress sutures in a simple continuous suture pattern or an inverting suture pattern (i.e., Cushing plus Lembert) (Fig. 18-9, C and D). Close the inguinal ring with simple interrupted sutures of

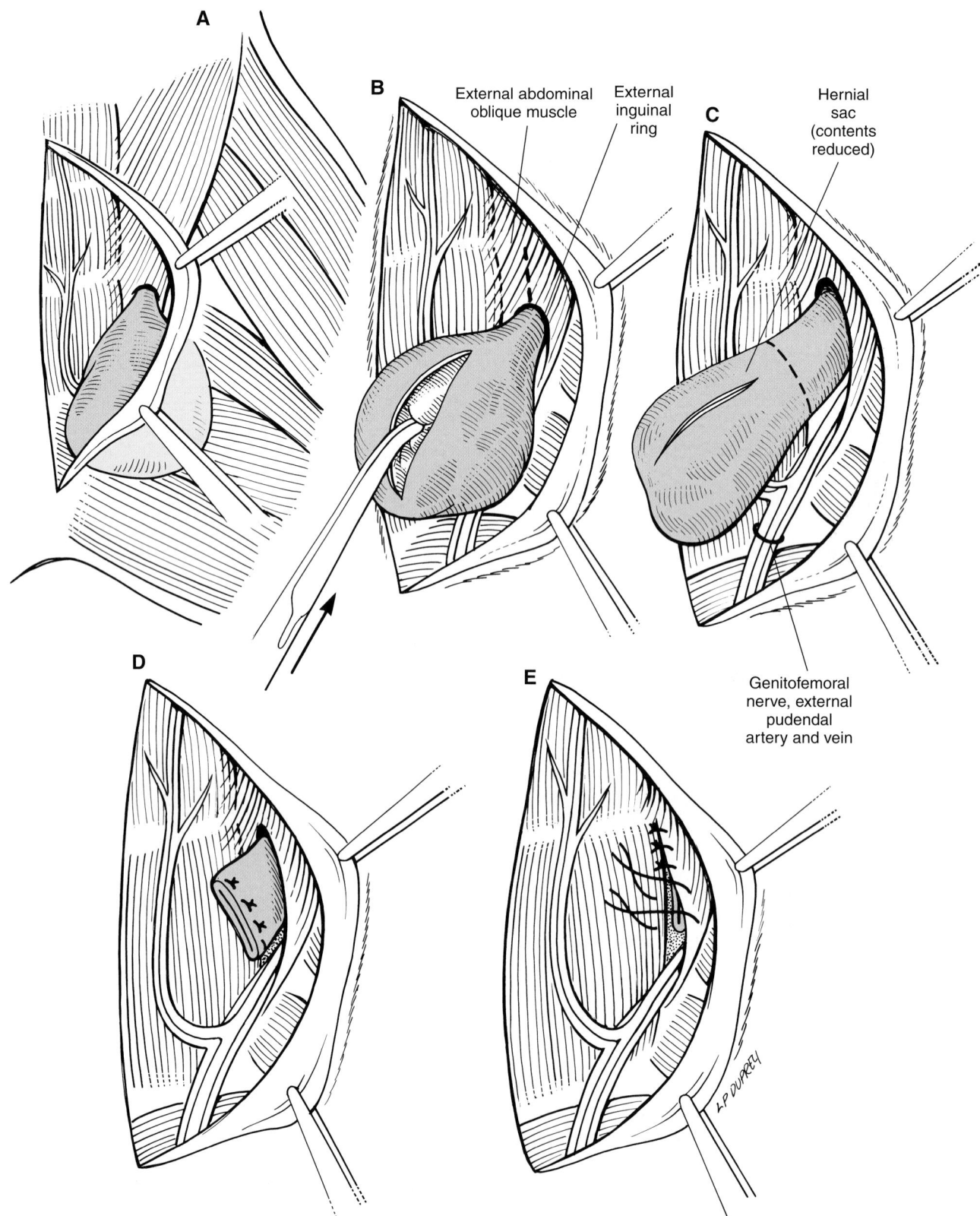

A

B

External abdominal oblique muscle

External inguinal ring

C

Hernial sac (contents reduced)

D

E

Genitofemoral nerve, external pudendal artery and vein

L.P. DURREY

FIG. 18-9
Inguinal hernia repair. **A,** Bluntly dissect beneath mammary tissue and identify the hernial sac and ring. **B,** If necessary, incise the hernial sac. **C,** Reduce the hernial contents and amputate the base of the sac. Close the sac **(D)** and the inguinal ring **(E).**

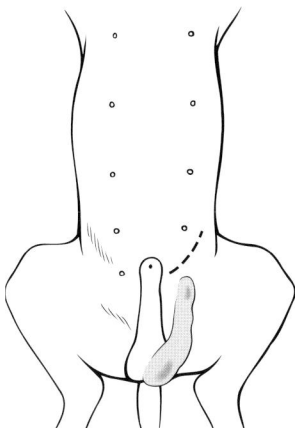

FIG. 18-10
Incision for scrotal hernia repair.

absorbable or nonabsorbable synthetic suture material (Fig. 18-9, E). Avoid compromising the external pudendal vessels and genitofemoral nerve, which exit from the caudomedial aspect of the ring (or the spermatic cord in intact male dogs). Palpate the contralateral ring, and close it if necessary before skin closure.

If the hernial contents cannot be reduced, perform a celiotomy and explore the abdominal contents. Expose the inguinal ring as described above, and reduce the hernial contents (enlarge the inguinal ring if necessary). Resect nonviable intestine, or perform an ovariohysterectomy and close the inguinal ring (or rings).

Scrotal Hernias

Incise the skin over or lateral to the inguinal ring and parallel to the flank fold (Fig. 18-10). Expose the hernial sac, and reduce the abdominal contents (incise the hernial sac if necessary). If hernial repair is performed in conjunction with orchiectomy (preferred), open the hernial sac and ligate the contents of the spermatic cord (Fig. 18-11, A). Remove the testicle after disrupting the ligament of the tail of the epididymis, and ligate the hernial sac at the level of the internal inguinal ring (Fig. 18-11, B). If castration is not performed, make an incision into the hernial sac (parietal vaginal tunic) and evaluate the hernial contents (Fig. 18-11, C). Reduce the herniated contents and place a transfixing ligature or several horizontal mattress sutures in the hernial sac to reduce the size of the vaginal orifice (Fig. 18-11, D). Partly close the external inguinal ring with interrupted sutures (Fig. 18-11, E). Do not compromise the spermatic cord or vascular structures at the caudomedial aspect of the ring.

If the hernial contents cannot be reduced or if viscera are strangulated and necrotic, perform a midline celiotomy as described previously. After resecting the intestine, expose the inguinal ring and repair the hernia. Perform a scrotal ablation if the vaginal process and scrotum have been severely contaminated.

Femoral Hernias

Incise the skin parallel to the inguinal ligament, and expose the hernial sac. Reduce the contents and ligate the hernial sac as high in the femoral canal as possible. If the inguinal ligament is intact, close the femoral canal by placing sutures between the inguinal ligament and the pectineal fascia. Do not damage or compromise the neurovascular structures of the femoral canal (Fig. 18-12). Close the subcutaneous tissue and skin. If abdominal organs have strangulated, perform a midline celiotomy. Reduce the abdominal contents, then invert and ligate the sac. Dissect laterally from the skin incision to the femoral canal and close the femoral canal defect as described above.

SUTURE MATERIALS AND SPECIAL INSTRUMENTS

Monofilament absorbable (polydioxanone, polyglyconate, poliglecaprone 25) or nonabsorbable (polypropylene or nylon) suture material should be used to close the hernial ring. Multifilament nonabsorbable suture may be associated with a higher incidence of wound infection. Mesh can be used as an overlay to reinforce the primary hernia repair (see p. 324).

POSTOPERATIVE CARE AND ASSESSMENT

Routine use of drains is not recommended; however, hernial sites should be assessed postoperatively for evidence of infection or the formation of a hematoma or seroma. If abscessation occurs, prompt removal of skin sutures, drainage, and topical therapy are indicated to prevent dehiscence of the hernia repair. Exercise should be restricted to leash walks for several weeks. An Elizabethan collar may be necessary to prevent the animal from licking at the surgical site. Postoperative testicular swelling may indicate compromise of testicular lymphatic or vascular drainage (or both). With femoral hernias, hobbles may be necessary during healing to prevent limb abduction, and femoral nerve function should be assessed postoperatively. Nerve deficits or severe pain may indicate compromise of the femoral nerve during the repair; reoperation is warranted in such cases.

PROGNOSIS

The prognosis is excellent unless intestinal leakage and perforation occur. The overall complication rate in one study of 35 dogs with inguinal hernias was 17% with a mortality rate of 3% (Waters et al, 1993).

PERITONITIS

DEFINITIONS

Primary generalized peritonitis refers to spontaneous inflammation of the peritoneum without any preexisting intraabdominal pathologic condition. **Secondary generalized peritonitis** occurs in conjunction with an intraabdominal pathologic condition and may be further classified as infectious or noninfectious.

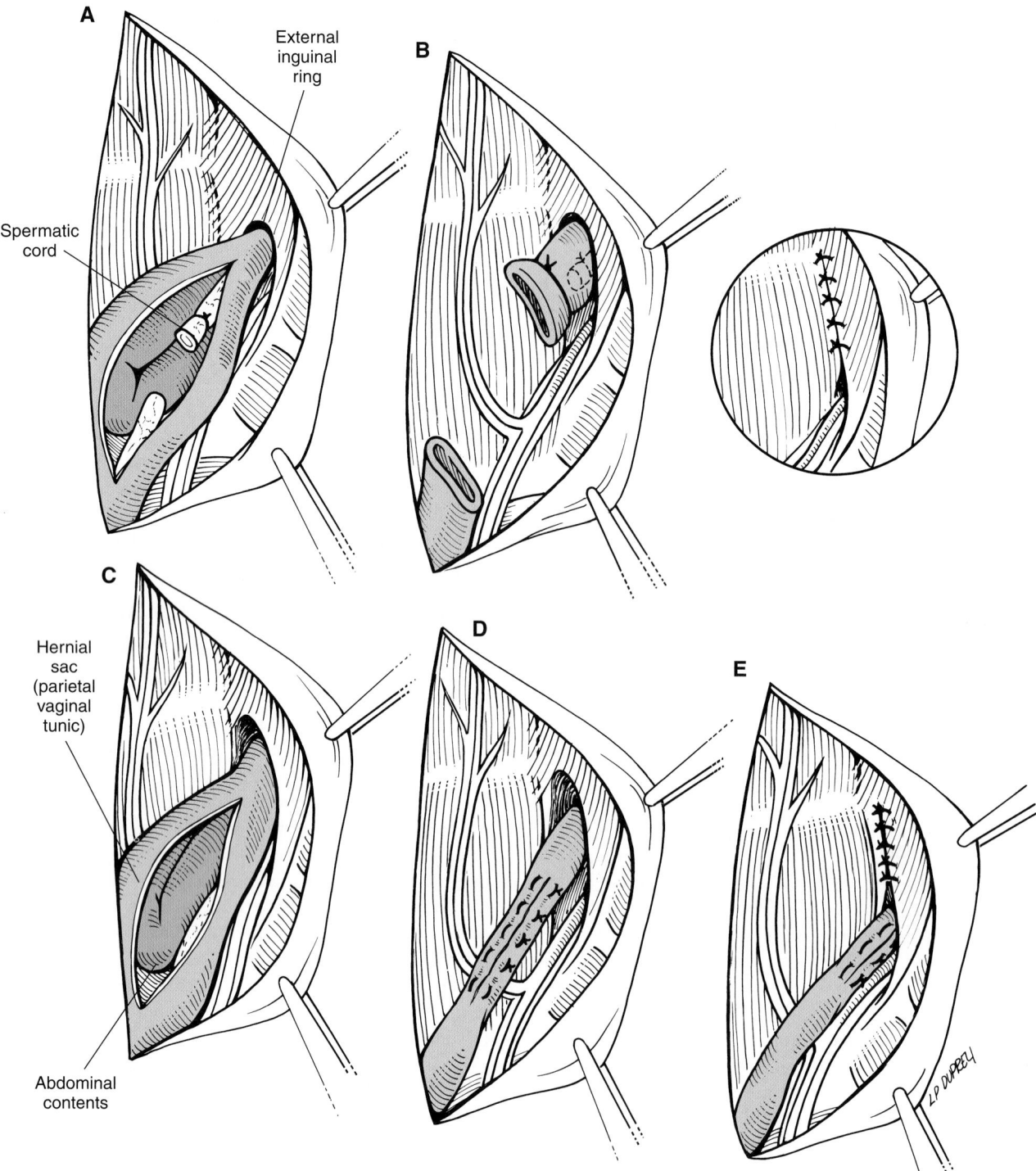

A
External inguinal ring

Spermatic cord

B

C
Hernial sac (parietal vaginal tunic)

Abdominal contents

D

E

FIG. 18-11
Scrotal hernia repair in conjunction with orchiectomy. **A,** Open the hernial sac and ligate the contents of the spermatic cord. **B,** Remove the testicle, and ligate the hernial sac at the level of the internal inguinal ring. If castration is not performed, make an incision into the hernial sac **(C),** reduce the contents, and reduce the size of the vaginal orifice **(D). E,** Partly close the external inguinal ring.

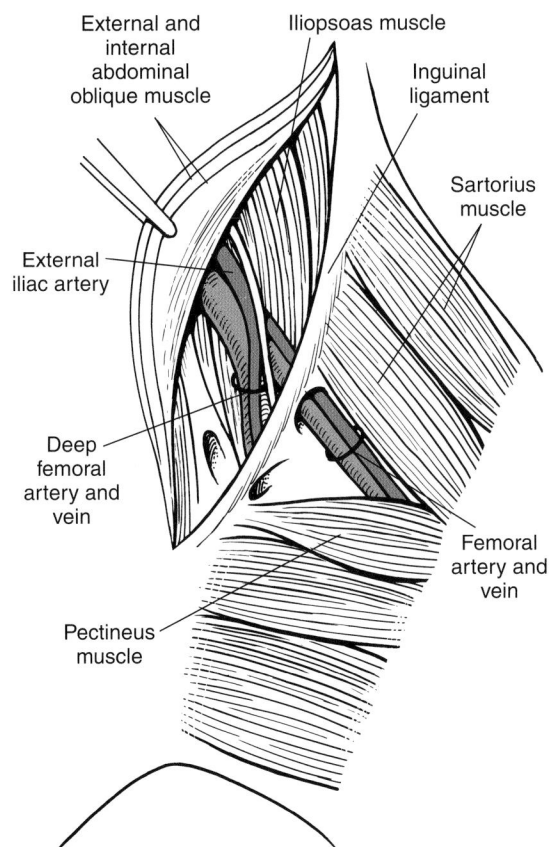

FIG. 18-12
Neurovascular structures of the femoral canal.

External and internal abdominal oblique muscle
Iliopsoas muscle
Inguinal ligament
Sartorius muscle
External iliac artery
Deep femoral artery and vein
Pectineus muscle
Femoral artery and vein

GENERAL CONSIDERATIONS AND CLINICALLY RELEVANT PATHOPHYSIOLOGY

Secondary generalized peritonitis is the predominant form of peritonitis in dogs and usually is caused by bacteria. Most cases arise through contamination from the gastrointestinal tract, often secondary to surgical wound dehiscence. Other causes include gallbladder perforation, rupture, or necrosis; gastric or intestinal foreign bodies; intussusception; mesenteric avulsion; gastric dilation-volvulus; necrotizing cholecystitis; pancreatic abscessation; prostatic abscesses; or foreign body penetration of the body wall. Acute staphylococcal peritonitis following cystocentesis has been reported in a dog (Specht et al, 2002). Primary generalized peritonitis occurs in cats and is associated with feline infectious peritonitis.

DIAGNOSIS
Clinical Presentation

Signalment. Any age, gender, or breed of dog or cat may develop peritonitis. It is particularly common in young animals that have perforating foreign bodies and in those that suffer abdominal injury, such as vehicular trauma or bite wounds.

History. The history often is nonspecific. The animal may not show signs of illness for several days after the traumatic episode. Mesenteric avulsions often do not cause clinical signs of peritonitis for 5 to 7 days after the injury. Animals with traumatic bile peritonitis may be asymptomatic for several weeks after the injury. Most animals are presented for treatment of lethargy, anorexia, vomiting, diarrhea, and/or abdominal pain.

> NOTE: Be sure to evaluate any sick intact female dog for pyometra.

Physical Examination Findings

Abdominal palpation often causes pain in affected dogs. The pain may be localized, but generalized pain is more common, and the animal often tenses or "splints" the abdomen during palpation. Cats with septic peritonitis may be less likely to show evidence of pain on abdominal palpation than similarly affected dogs (Costello et al, 2004). Vomiting and diarrhea may be noted. Abdominal distention may be noted if sufficient fluid has accumulated. Pale mucous membranes, prolonged capillary refill times, and tachycardia may indicate that the animal is in shock. Dehydration and arrhythmias may also occur.

Diagnostic Imaging

The classic radiographic finding in animals with peritonitis is loss of visceral detail with a focal or generalized "ground glass" appearance (Fig. 18-13). The intestinal tract may be dilated with air or fluid or both. Free abdominal air may occur as a result of rupture of a hollow organ and sometimes from infection with gas-producing anaerobes. A more localized peritonitis may occur secondary to pancreatitis and can cause the duodenum to appear fixed and elevated ("sentinel loop"). Ultrasonography is useful for localizing fluid accumulation and assisting in obtaining a sample for analysis. Abdominal radiography and ultrasonography should be performed before diagnostic peritoneal lavage (see p. 335). Ultrasonography is also a valuable tool to evaluate the abdomen and surgical site in dogs. A recent study suggested that most abdominal organs can be assessed ultrasonographically 24 hours postoperatively; the limiting factor to evaluation of the abdomen was pain, not air (Weinstein et al, 2005).

Laboratory Findings

The most common laboratory finding in animals with peritonitis is notable leukocytosis; however, the neutrophil count may be normal or low in some cases. The predominant cell type is the neutrophil, and a left shift is often but not always apparent. Other abnormalities may include anemia, thrombocytopenia, dehydration, hypoglycemia, hyperbilirubinemia, and/or electrolyte and acid-base abnormalities. The activity of circulating anticoagulant proteins (protein C and antithrombin) was found to be significantly lower in dogs with naturally occurring sepsis compared with controls in a recent study (de Laforcade et al, 2003). Bile peritonitis usually causes elevations of alkaline phosphatase, alanine transaminase, and total bilirubin concen-

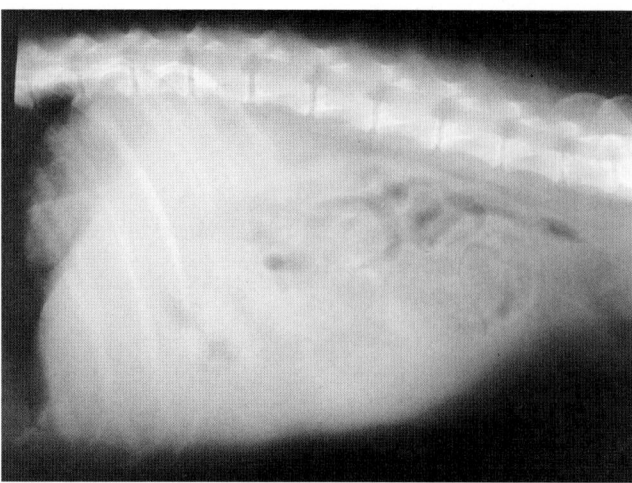

FIG. 18-13
Lateral radiograph of an animal with peritoneal effusion. Notice the lack of visceral detail.

 BOX 18-4

Estimating the TNCC and Amount of Blood in Abdominal Fluid

The total nucleated cell count (TNCC) of abdominal fluid can be estimated using the following formula:

$$X = NC \times OP^2$$

where:
X = TNCC
NC = number of nucleated cells per microscopic field
OP = objective power of the lens; the objective power chosen should allow visualization of 1–10 cells per microscopic field

The amount of blood in the abdominal cavity can be estimated using the following formula:

$$X = \frac{L \times V}{P-L}$$

where:
X = Amount of blood in the abdominal cavity
L = Packed cell volume (PCV) of the returned lavage fluid
V = Volume of lavage fluid infused into the abdominal cavity
P = PCV of the peripheral blood before intravenous infusion of fluids

trations (see p. 571). See p. 678 for a description of laboratory abnormalities associated with uroabdomen.

Little or no abdominal effusion may be seen in early cases of peritonitis. When effusion is present, abdominocentesis should be performed (see p. 335) and fluid retrieved for analysis. See pp. 678 and 571 for fluid analysis of animals with uroabdomen and bile peritonitis, respectively. Toxic degenerative neutrophils with intracellular or extracellular bacteria are indicative of bacterial peritonitis. Leukocyte morphology and the presence of bacteria are more important than leukocyte numbers. If total nucleated cell counts (TNCC) are performed, they should be done on fluid that has been placed in an ethylene diamine tetraacetic acid (EDTA) (lavender top) tube (Box 18-4). Bacteria are sometimes not seen in patients with bacterial peritonitis, especially if they have been receiving antibiotics. Differentiating between these effusions and those caused by pancreatitis may be difficult because large numbers of degenerative white blood cells can be seen with both. A concentration difference greater than 20 mg/dl between blood and peritoneal fluid glucose concentration has been reported to reliably differentiate between septic peritoneal effusions and nonseptic peritoneal effusions in dogs and cats (Bonczynski et al, 2004). Lactate concentrations greater than 2.5 mmol/L were indicative of septic peritoneal effusions in dogs in another study; however, lactate concentrations were not accurate tests for detecting septic peritoneal effusions in cats (Levin et al, 2004).

After abdominocentesis the amount of blood in the abdominal cavity can be estimated by observing the lavage sample. A red color reflects the presence of red blood cells, and a deep red color usually indicates severe hemorrhage. If newsprint cannot be read through the plastic tubing, hemorrhage is significant; if print can be seen through the tubing, only moderate or minimal hemorrhage is present. The amount of blood in the abdominal cavity can be estimated using the equation shown in Box 18-4. Surgical intervention is indicated when the packed cell volume (PCV) of lavage samples taken within 5 to 20 minutes of each other increases substantially or if an animal in shock does not respond to aggressive fluid therapy.

DIFFERENTIAL DIAGNOSIS

Advanced peritonitis with significant accumulation of abdominal fluid is not difficult to diagnose. The difficulty usually arises in determining the cause of the effusion or infection. Early peritonitis, before the onset of overt clinical signs, is difficult to diagnose and may require diagnostic peritoneal lavage (see p 335).

MEDICAL MANAGEMENT

The goals of management of animals with peritonitis are to eliminate the cause of the contamination, resolve infection, and restore normal fluid and electrolyte balances. Food should be withheld if the animal is vomiting. Intravenous fluid replacement therapy should be initiated as soon as possible, particularly if the animal is dehydrated or appears to be in shock (in dogs, 60 to 90 ml/kg/hr; in cats, 40 to 60 ml/kg/hr). Synthetic colloids, such as hetastarch and dextran 70 (see pp. 28 and 334), may be beneficial, particularly if vasculitis is present. Hypokalemia (Table 18-1) and hyponatremia may be present and require intravenous supplementation. Hypoglycemia is common in animals with septic shock (systemic inflammatory response syndrome), and glucose may need to be added to the fluids (i.e., 2.5% to 5%

Table 18-1

Intravenous Potassium Supplementation Guidelines

SERUM POTASSIUM* (mEq/L)	mEq KCl/L OF FLUID	MAXIMAL INFUSION RATE† (ml/kg/hour)
<2.0	80	6
2.1–2.5	60	8
2.6–3.0	40	12
3.1–3.5	28	16

*If serum potassium is not available, add potassium to a total concentration of 20 mEq/L.
†Do not exceed 0.5 mEq/kg/hr.

 BOX 18-5

Sodium Bicarbonate Therapy

1–2 mEq/kg given intravenously; repeat only if indicated based on assessment of acid-base balance and potassium concentration.
The following formula can also be used:
0.3 × Base deficit (mEq) × Body weight (kg)
Give half of this dose intravenously over 10 to 15 minutes and reevaluate. If the remainder is needed, administer over 4 to 6 hours.

dextrose). Standard shock therapy should be initiated (i.e., fluid replacement and antibiotics, with or without soluble corticosteroids). If severe metabolic acidosis is present, bicarbonate therapy may be indicated (Box 18-5).

Broad-spectrum antibiotic therapy should be initiated as soon as the diagnosis is made. *Escherichia coli, Clostridium* spp., and *Enterococcus* spp. are commonly isolated from animals with peritonitis, and ampicillin plus enrofloxacin (Box 18-6) typically is an effective antimicrobial combination. However, amikacin plus either clindamycin or metronidazole (see Box 18-6) may be necessary. A second-generation cephalosporin (e.g., cefoxitin [see Box 18-6]), may also have a reasonable gram-negative and anaerobic spectrum. If renal compromise is present in an animal with a resistant bacterial infection, imipenem may be considered (see Box 18-6). The initial antibiotic therapy should be altered according to the aerobic and anaerobic culture results of lavage fluid or cultures obtained at surgery. Septic peritonitis typically causes disseminated intravascular coagulation (DIC). Plasma administration to replace clotting factors is probably one of the most beneficial therapies in such patients.

Low-dose heparin (Box 18-7) increases survival and significantly reduces abscess formation in experimental peritonitis. The inflammatory process in peritonitis is associated with an outpouring of fibrous exudate that causes intraabdominal loculation of bacteria. The loculated bac-

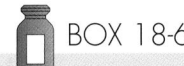 BOX 18-6

Antibiotic Therapy in Animals With Peritonitis

Ampicillin
22 mg/kg IV, tid or qid

Metronidazole (Flagyl)*
10 mg/kg IV, tid

Enrofloxacin (Baytril)*†
10–15 mg/kg IV, qd

Cefoxitin (Mefoxin)†
30 mg/kg IV, tid

Amikacin (Amiglyde-V)
20–25 mg/kg IV, qd

Imipenem (Primaxin)
3–7.5 mg/kg IM, slow IV, tid or qid

Clindamycin (Antirobe)
11 mg/kg IV, tid

IV, Intravenous; *tid*, three times a day; *qid*, four times a day; *bid*, twice a day; *qd*, once a day.
*Dilute and give slowly over 20 minutes.
†Recent studies suggest that enrofloxacin may be associated with blindness in cats when dosages greater than 5 mg/kg are used.

 BOX 18-7

Adjunctive Therapy in Dogs With Peritonitis

Heparin
50–100 U/kg, SC, bid or tid

Plasma (fresh frozen)
10–20 ml/kg, then re-assess the plasma ATIII activity. Repeat as needed to increase the ATIII to near-normal concentrations.

Heparin (low molecular weight [LMW]) (Dalteparin)
100–150 U/kg SC, qd to bid*

Heparin-Activated Plasma
Put the first heparin dose (50–100 U/kg) in the plasma and incubate for 30 minutes before administration. Once antithrombin III (AT III) levels are more than 60%, continue heparin subcutaneously. If additional plasma is needed, incubation with heparin is not necessary.

SC, Subcutaneous; *bid*, twice a day.
*Research into LMW heparin use in dogs and cats is ongoing, and this recommendation might change.

teria are protected from host defense mechanisms and antibiotics that may not be able to penetrate the fibrin clots. Although the exact mechanism of its beneficial effect is still unknown, it appears indicated in patients with severe peritonitis. Heparin may also be incubated with plasma and given to animals with DIC (see Box 18-7). Low molecular weight heparin (enoxaparin, dalteparin) differs from unfractionated heparin in its mechanism of action and may be more effective; however, large clinical studies are lacking.

SURGICAL TREATMENT

Abdominocentesis (see later discussion) is the percutaneous removal of fluid from the abdominal cavity, usually for diagnostic purposes although it may also be therapeutic. Indications include shock without apparent cause, undiagnosed disease with signs involving the abdominal cavity, suspicion of postoperative gastrointestinal dehiscence, blunt or penetrating abdominal injuries (i.e., gunshot wounds, dog bites, or vehicular injury), and undiagnosed abdominal pain. A multifenestrated catheter will enhance fluid collection. Physical and radiographic examinations should precede abdominocentesis to detect instances in which it may be unsafe and to guide needle placement. Four-quadrant paracentesis may be performed if simple abdominocentesis is unsuccessful in retrieving fluid. It is similar to simple abdominocentesis except that multiple abdominal sites are assessed by dividing the abdomen into four quadrants through the umbilicus and tapping each of these four areas. Alternatively, ultrasound may be used to identify small amounts of fluid and allow collection of a sample for evaluation. Diagnostic peritoneal lavage should be performed in animals suspected of having peritonitis if the above methods are unsuccessful in obtaining fluid for analysis (see p. 335).

Exploratory surgery is indicated when the cause of peritonitis cannot be determined or when bowel rupture, intestinal obstruction (e.g., bowel incarceration and neoplasia), or mesenteric avulsion is suspected. Serosal patching and plication reduce the incidence of intestinal leakage, dehiscence, or repeated intussusception (see p. 457). Animals that require surgery and have peritonitis secondary to intestinal trauma (disruption of mesenteric blood supply, bowel perforation, chronic intussusception, foreign body) often are hypoproteinemic. The role that protein levels play in healing intestinal incisions is not understood. However, most surgeons are concerned that hypoproteinemic patients may not heal as quickly as patients with normal protein levels, despite the fact that similar complication rates are typically seen among euproteinemic and hypoproteinemic animals. Most experimental evidence has shown that retardation of wound healing is only seen with severe protein deficiencies (less than 1.5 to 2 g/dl).

Although the practice of lavaging the abdominal cavity of animals with peritonitis is controversial, lavage generally is indicated with diffuse peritonitis. Lavage should be done with care in animals with localized peritonitis to prevent dissemination of infection. When lavage is performed, as much of the fluid as possible should be removed because fluid inhibits the body's ability to fight off infection, probably by inhibiting neutrophil function. Historically, many different agents have been added to lavage fluids, especially antiseptics and antibiotics. Povidone-iodine is the most widely added antiseptic; however, its use may be contraindicated with established peritonitis. Furthermore, no beneficial effect of this agent has been shown in repeated experimental and clinical trials in animals. Although a great many antibiotics have been added to lavage fluids over the years, there is no substantial evidence that their addition benefits patients being treated with appropriate systemic antibiotics. Warmed sterile physiologic saline is the most appropriate lavage fluid.

Open abdominal drainage (OAD) (see p. 336) is useful for managing animals with peritonitis. Reported advantages include improvement in the patient's metabolic condition secondary to improved drainage, fewer abdominal adhesions and abscesses, and access for repeated inspection and exploration of the abdomen. With this technique the abdomen is left open, and sterile wraps are placed around the wound. The frequency of wrap changes depends on the amount of fluid drained and external soiling. Complications of open abdominal drainage include persistent fluid loss, hypoalbuminemia, weight loss, adhesion of abdominal viscera to the bandage, and contamination of the peritoneal cavity with cutaneous organisms. Closed-suction drainage may also be effective in dogs and cats with generalized peritonitis.

Preoperative Management

Animals with peritonitis that are in shock should be stabilized before surgery. Preoperative management of peritonitis is similar to that described in the previous discussion on medical management. The nutritional management of animals with peritonitis is extremely important; if the patient is debilitated, vomiting, or unlikely to resume eating for several days after surgery, enteral or parenteral hyperalimentation should be considered (see Chapter 11).

Anesthesia

Animals with peritonitis often are endotoxic and/or hypotensive. Small amounts of endotoxins are normally absorbed from the intestine and transported via the portal system to the liver, where they are removed and destroyed by hepatocytes. Hypotension in dogs is associated with intense portal vasoconstriction. This vasoconstriction causes breakdown of the intestinal mucosal barrier, allowing more intestinal endotoxin to be absorbed. If hepatic function is impaired, a common condition in septic animals, small doses of endotoxin that normally would be harmless may be lethal. For these reasons, hypotension should be corrected before and prevented during and after surgery in animals with peritonitis. Animals with a total protein level under 4 g/dl or an albumin level under 1.5 g/dl may benefit from perioperative colloid administration. Colloids may be given preoperatively, intraoperatively, or postoperatively (or all three) for a total dose of 20 ml/kg/day (dog) or 10 to 15 ml/kg/day (cat). If colloids are given during surgery (7 to 10 ml/kg), acute intraoperative hypotension should be treated with crystalloids.

Dobutamine or dopamine (Box 18-8) may be given during surgery for inotropic support. Dobutamine is less arrhythmogenic and chronotropic than dopamine and is preferred if the patient is hypotensive and anuric. If the patient is anuric and normotensive, low-dose dopamine (0.5 to 1.5 µg/kg/min given intravenously) plus furosemide (0.2 mg/kg given intravenously) may be preferable. These patients should be monitored for arrhythmias or tachycardia.

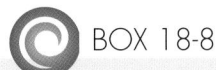 BOX 18-8

Inotropic Support of Hypotensive Animals

Dobutamine
2–10 μg/kg/minute IV

Dopamine
2–10 μg/kg/minute IV

IV, Intravenous.

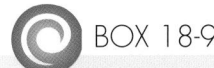 BOX 18-9

Anticholinergics for Bradycardia

Atropine
0.02–0.04 mg/kg IV, SC, or IM

Glycopyrrolate
0.005–0.011 mg/kg IV, SC, or IM

IV, Intravenous; *SC*, subcutaneous; *IM*, intramuscular.

Hepatic necrosis occurs during sepsis, reducing hepatic function. The pathogenesis of hepatic necrosis is uncertain, but may be caused by hypotension and hypoxia. Patients with hepatic necrosis may have diminished ability to metabolize drugs, and prolonged duration of action or altered function of drugs may result. Acepromazine should not be used in animals with peritonitis if severe hepatic dysfunction (or hypotension) is suspected (see p. 531). A benzodiazepine (e.g., diazepam or midazolam) plus an opioid (e.g., hydromorphone) are useful IV premedicants in patients with hepatic dysfunction (see p. 531). Diazepam used alone may disinhibit some behaviors, and it should be used with caution in hypoalbuminemic patients. Most opioids have little or no adverse effect on the liver; however, morphine should not be given intravenously to dogs with hepatic dysfunction because it may cause hepatic congestion secondary to histamine release and hepatic vein spasm. Although some opioid analgesics may have prolonged action when hepatic function is reduced, their effects can be antagonized. Barbiturates (e.g., thiopental) should be used cautiously or avoided in patients with significant hepatic dysfunction.

Preoxygenation before induction is recommended to reduce hypoxia secondary to respiratory depression. Anesthetic protocols for relatively healthy patients with peritonitis are provided in Box 18-1. Balanced anesthesia (e.g., an opioid and a benzodiazepine for induction) should be used in patients that are in shock or debilitated (see Box 18-2). Propofol may cause hypotension secondary to vasodilation, decreased cardiac output, and respiratory depression in some patients. Medetomidine is contraindicated because it causes vasoconstriction and secondarily decreases perfusion to vital organs, even at very low doses. Ketamine may have direct cardiodepressant effects associated with poor contractility, decreased cardiac output, and hypotension in debilitated patients. An anticholinergic may be given if the animal is bradycardic (Box 18-9). Etomidate should be used cautiously in animals with adrenal insufficiency because a single induction dose of this agent has caused adrenal insufficiency in dogs and cats. Etomidate has also caused hemolysis as a result of the propylene glycol. Clinically, hemolysis seems to be a greater problem in cats than in dogs. When contemplating etomidate use in cats, the benefit of cardiovascular stability should be weighed against this risk.

Surgical Anatomy

The surgical anatomy of the abdominal cavity is described on p. 318.

Positioning

For abdominocentesis and diagnostic lavage, the abdomen should be clipped and prepared aseptically. These procedures may be performed with the animal in lateral recumbency or standing.

SURGICAL TECHNIQUES
Abdominocentesis

Insert an 18- or 20-gauge, 1½-inch plastic over-the-needle catheter (with added side holes) into the abdominal cavity at the most dependent part of the abdomen. Do not attach a syringe; instead allow the fluid to drip from the needle and collect in a sterile tube. If sufficient fluid is obtained, place it in a clot tube and an EDTA tube, submit samples for aerobic and anaerobic culture, and make four to six smears for analysis. If fluid is not obtained, apply gentle suction using a 3-ml syringe.

It is difficult to puncture the bowel by this method because mobile loops of bowel move away from the tip of the needle as it strikes them. Perforations created by a needle this size usually heal without complications. The major disadvantage of needle paracentesis is that it is insensitive in finding small volumes of intraperitoneal fluid, and thus a negative result can be meaningless. At least 5 to 6 ml of fluid per kilogram of body weight must be present in the abdominal cavity of dogs to obtain positive results in most cases using this technique.

Diagnostic Peritoneal Lavage

Make a 2-cm skin incision just caudal to the umbilicus and clamp or ligate any bleeders to prevent false positive results. Spread loose subcutaneous tissue, and make a small incision in the linea alba. Hold the edges of the incision with forceps while the peritoneal lavage catheter (Stylocath) without the trocar is inserted into the abdominal cavity (Fig. 18-14). Direct the catheter caudally into the pelvis. With the catheter in place, apply gentle suction. If blood or fluid cannot be aspirated, connect the catheter to a bottle of warm sterile saline and infuse 20 ml/kg of fluid into the abdominal cavity. When the calculated volume of fluid has been delivered, roll the patient gently from side to side, place the bottle on

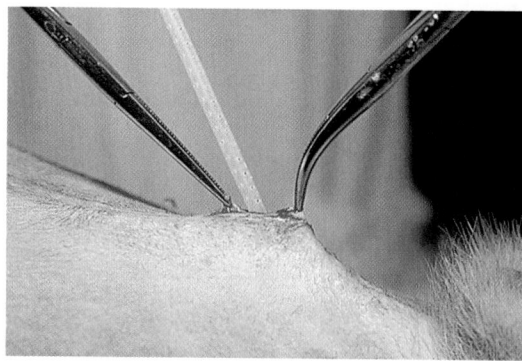

FIG. 18-14
Diagnostic peritoneal lavage.

the floor, vent it, and collect the fluid by gravity drainage. Do not be surprised if you do not retrieve all of the fluid, particularly in dehydrated animals.

Alternatively, place an over-the-needle catheter into the abdomen as above and infuse a crystalloid solution. Remove the catheter and gently palpate the abdomen. Thirty minutes later, perform single or four-quadrant abdominocentesis.

Exploratory Laparotomy

Perform a ventral midline incision from the xiphoid process to the pubis (see pp. 318 to 321). Obtain a sample of fluid for culture and analysis. Explore and inspect the entire abdomen. Find the source of infection and correct it. Break down adhesions that may hinder drainage. Lavage the abdomen with copious amounts of warm, sterile saline if the infection is generalized. Remove as much necrotic debris and fluid as possible. Close the abdomen routinely or perform open abdominal drainage.

Open Abdominal Drainage

After completing the abdominal procedure, leave a portion of the abdominal incision (usually the most dependent portion) open to drain. Generally, make the opening just large enough to allow a gloved hand to be inserted. Close the cranial and caudal aspects of the incision with monofilament suture using a continuous suture pattern. Place a sterile laparotomy pad over the opening, then place a sterile wrap over the laparotomy pad. Change the wrap at least twice daily initially with the animal standing; sedation is seldom necessary (use sterile bandage materials and wear sterile gloves). The volume of drainage dictates the number of wrap changes needed. Break down adhesions to the incision that may interfere with drainage. Abdominal lavage may be attempted, but is seldom necessary. Place a diaper over the wrap to reduce contamination from urine. Assess the fluid daily for bacterial numbers and cell morphology. When the bacterial numbers have declined and the neutrophil morphology is normal (nondegenerative), close the incision (generally in 3 to 5 days). If the opening is small, it may be left to heal by secondary intention.

SUTURE MATERIALS AND SPECIAL INSTRUMENTS

Monofilament synthetic nonabsorbable suture (polypropylene or nylon) or slowly absorbable suture (polydioxanone or polyglyconate) should be used to close the abdomen in animals with peritonitis. Braided suture (Dacron, silk, braided nylon) or suture that may be rapidly degraded (chromic gut) should not be used.

POSTOPERATIVE CARE AND ASSESSMENT

Fluid therapy should be continued postoperatively in most animals with peritonitis and is mandatory in those being managed with an open abdomen. Electrolytes, acid-base, and serum protein should be assessed in the postoperative period and corrected as necessary. Nasal oxygen may benefit septic animals. Ensuring that patients with peritonitis have an adequate caloric intake postoperatively often is difficult. An animal's energy requirement is much greater after injury or illness than at rest. Generally the formula (30 × weight [kg]) + 70 is used to calculate a resting animal's energy requirement. Postoperatively the metabolic rate of dogs and cats increases 25% to 35% over resting levels. With mild trauma the increase in the energy requirement is 35% to 50%; with sepsis 50% to 70% more calories can be required. The factor 1.5 has been used to estimate the energy requirement of ill or injured dogs and cats. Meeting these caloric requirements in dogs with intestinal disease is particularly difficult and may require enteral or parenteral nutritional support (see Chapter 11). If hypoproteinemia becomes severe, plasma transfusions should be considered. Postoperative analgesia is recommended (see Chapter 13).

PROGNOSIS

The prognosis for animals with generalized peritonitis is guarded; however, with proper and aggressive therapy, many survive. The overall mortality in two recent studies of dogs with peritonitis was 21% and 29% (Winkler and Greenfield, 2000; Staatz et al, 2002). The mortality rates reported in animals with generalized peritonitis treated with open abdominal drainage have varied from 20% to 48%. Animals with a lower preoperative alanine transaminase (ALT) and gammaglutamyl transferase (GGT) may have a better prognosis (Winkler and Greenfield, 2000).

References

Bonczynski JJ, Ludwig LL, Barton LJ et al: Comparison of peritoneal fluid and peripheral blood pH, bicarbonate, glucose, and lactate concentration as a diagnostic tool for septic peritonitis in dogs and cats, *Vet Surg* 32:161, 2003.

Costello ME, Drobatz KJ, Aronson LR et al: Underlying cause, pathophysiologic abnormalities and response to treatment in cats with septic peritonitis: 51 cases (1990-2001), *J Am Vet Med Assoc* 225:897, 2004.

De Laforcade AM, Freeman LM, Shaw SP et al: Hemostatic changes in dogs with naturally occurring sepsis, *J Vet Int Med* 17:674, 2003.

Levin GM, Bonczynski JJ, Ludwig LL et al: Lactate as a diagnostic test for septic peritoneal effusions in dogs and cats, *J Am Anim Hosp Assoc* 40:364, 2004.

Specht A, O'Toole T, Kent M et al: Acute staphylococcal peritonitis following cystocentesis in a dog, *J Vet Emerg Crit Care* 12:183, 2002.

Staatz AJ, Monnet E, Seim HB: Open peritoneal drainage versus primary closure for the treatment of septic peritonitis in dogs and cats: 42 cases (1993-1999), *Vet Surg* 31:174, 2002.

Weinstein J, Beck K, Quinn M et al: Evaluation of the abdomen using ultrasound following a ventral midline celiotomy, *Vet Radiol and Ultrasound* 46:337, 2005.

Winkler KP, Greenfield CL: Potential prognostic indicators in diffuse peritonitis treated with open peritoneal drainage in the canine patient, *Vet Emerg Crit Care* 10:259, 2000.

Suggested Reading

Mueller MG, Ludwig LL, Barton LJ: Use of closed-suction drains to treat generalized peritonitis in dogs and cats: (1997-1999), *J Am Vet Med Assoc* 219:789, 2001.

Closed-suction drains were effective in the treatment of generalized peritonitis in dogs and cats. No important complications were associated with their use.

HEMOPERITONEUM

DEFINITIONS

Hemoperitoneum or hemoabdomen is the abnormal accumulation of blood in the peritoneal cavity.

GENERAL CONSIDERATIONS AND CLINICALLY RELEVANT PATHOPHYSIOLOGY

Hemoperitoneum is associated with many diseases. Determination of the cause of the effusion requires a careful examination of the animal, coupled with consideration of potential diagnoses. Trauma (vehicular accidents, falls, kicks) is a common cause in both dogs and cats. Neoplasia is the most common cause of nontraumatic hemoabdomen in dogs and cats. Splenic neoplasia (see p. 631) is particularly common in dogs, although rupture of other tumors (e.g., hepatic) may also cause hemoabdomen. Nontraumatic rupture of adrenal gland tumors has been reported in dogs and was associated with life-threatening hemorrhage (Whitemore et al, 2001). Nonmalignant disease associated with nontraumatic hemoperitoneum includes benign neoplasms, primary hepatobiliary disease, gastric dilation-volvulus (see p. 427), splenic torsion (see p. 629), liver lobe torsion, and intoxication with vitamin K antagonists.

DIAGNOSIS
Clinical Presentation

Signalment. Young male mixed breed dogs are more likely to be evaluated because of trauma; older dogs are more likely to have underlying neoplasia. Similar findings are true in cats.

History. A history of trauma may be present. With neoplasia, the history often is nonspecific. It should be ascertained whether there is a previous history of hemorrhage. Other important historical findings include previous surgery or diagnostic procedures, presence of previously diagnosed abdominal masses, access to toxins or rodenticides, and administration of medications.

Physical Examination Findings

The animal should be carefully observed for external signs of trauma. Other findings may include abdominal distention (possibly with the presence of a fluid wave), abdominal tenderness, discoloration or bruising of the abdominal wall, and/or bulging of the umbilicus. Intraabdominal hemorrhage may cause severe hemorrhagic shock, or the animal may appear clinically normal.

Diagnostic Imaging

The classic radiographic finding in animals with hemoabdomen is loss of abdominal detail with a focal or generalized "ground glass" appearance. Both lateral views and a ventrodorsal view are recommended to help detect abdominal masses; however, ultrasonography is generally more sensitive when large quantities of fluid are present. A rapid sonographic technique to detect the presence of free abdominal fluid after motor vehicle accidents was recently reported (Boysen et al, 2004). Transverse and longitudinal views were obtained at each of four sites (just caudal to the xiphoid process, on the midline over the urinary bladder, and at the left and right flank regions). The technique was simple and rapid and could be performed by veterinary clinicians with minimal previous ultrasonographic experience. Ultrasonography is useful for localizing fluid accumulation, and it may assist fluid retrieval and evaluation of abdominal organs for enlargement (i.e., neoplasia) or evidence of trauma. The presence of metastatic disease may also be noted ultrasonographically.

Thoracic radiographs should be taken in animals with suspected or confirmed neoplasia. In animals with trauma, thoracic radiographs should be taken to look for diaphragmatic hernia (see p. 904) or other thoracic trauma. CT is useful for detecting neoplasia and is considered the gold standard for diagnosis of carcinomatosis in humans; however, ultrasonography may actually detect masses that are smaller than can be visualized with CT.

Laboratory Findings

Hemoperitoneum is diagnosed by finding nonclotting bloody fluid in the abdomen that has been retrieved by abdominocentesis (see p. 335). The PCV and total solids of the fluid should be determined and the fluid carefully examined for bacteria or neoplastic cells. If bacteria or degenerative neutrophils are noted, microbial culture is warranted. Other parameters that may be useful include creatinine, bilirubin, lactate, glucose, and lipase. Nonneoplastic effusions typically have lower lactate concentrations and higher glucose concentrations than neoplastic effusions (Nestor, 2004).

Peripheral blood should be evaluated for anemia, but the CBC may not reflect the degree of bleeding for several hours after trauma. In a recent study, 97% of dogs presenting with acute nontraumatic hemoabdomen were anemic and 76% were hypoalbuminemic (Pintar et al, 2003). A clotting profile should be performed in animals with nontraumatic hemorrhage. Abnormal hemostatic profiles are common in dogs with splenic hemangiosarcoma (see p. 633) and may be seen in animals with other types of malignancies and coagulopathies.

NOTE: Clinicopathologic abnormalities in dogs with hemoabdomen are typically similar regardless of the cause of the abdominal bleeding.

DIFFERENTIAL DIAGNOSIS

Hemoabdomen must be differentiated from other causes of peritoneal effusion (e.g., peritonitis; see p. 329) based on results of fluid analysis (see pp. 332 and 571). Once hemoabdomen has been diagnosed, the underlying cause must be determined.

MEDICAL MANAGEMENT

Rapid action must often be taken to save the life of an animal that has a hemoabdomen. Intravenous fluid replacement therapy (see p. 27) should be initiated as soon as possible, particularly if the animal is in shock (in dogs, 60 to 90 ml/kg/hr; in cats, 40 to 60 ml/kg/hr). Blood transfusions may be required if the PCV falls below 20%. Application of a tight abdominal bandage or compress may help attenuate or arrest the bleeding; however, arterial or hepatic hemorrhage is unlikely to be stopped by this method. Abdominal compresses should only be used short term while the animal is being stabilized and other definitive measures are being taken. Oxygen therapy via a nasal catheter or oxygen cage should be considered to optimize tissue oxygenation (see p. 27). Typed and cross-matched blood should be available for transfusion, if needed (see p. 30). In an emergency situation in which blood typing is not possible, dogs may be given dog erythrocyte antigen 1.1 negative blood. All cats should be blood typed before transfusion because of the risk of fatal reactions when nonspecific blood is given (see p. 30) Trauma patients with hemoabdomen that stabilize after medical management often do not require surgery.

SURGICAL TREATMENT

Surgery is indicated when the source of bleeding cannot be determined or effectively controlled or when evaluation and removal of intraabdominal neoplasia are required. A routine ventral abdominal incision should be performed. Suction is useful to remove the blood and help identify any sites of active bleeding. Although transfusion of suctioned blood back into the patient is not generally recommended, use of a cell saver system—which removes clots and activated blood components from red cells—will allow blood to be salvaged and safely autotransfused. The kidneys, liver, and spleen should be carefully examined for trauma. Severe bleeding from the spleen or evidence of splenic neoplasia is an indication for splenectomy (see p. 626). Nephrectomy (see p. 639) may be required if severe bleeding from the kidney is noted. Clotting agents, such as platelet gel or commercial products (see p. 65), may help control bleeding from the liver. If these are not successful, partial hepatectomy (see p. 536) may be required.

Preoperative Management

Animals with hemoabdomen that are in shock should be stabilized before surgery (see p. 332). Every effort should be made to correct fluid, acid-base, electrolyte, and cardiovascular abnormalities before inducing anesthesia. Blood transfusions should be given if the PCV is less than 20, the animal is hypoxic as a result of anemia, or ongoing bleeding is expected.

Anesthesia

Preoxygenation of these patients is recommended to reduce hypoxia secondary to respiratory depression or anemia. Anesthetic principles are similar to those given under peritonitis (see p. 334).

Surgical Anatomy

The surgical anatomy of the abdominal cavity is described on p. 318.

Positioning

The animal is placed in dorsal recumbency for a midline exploratory celiotomy. The entire abdomen and caudal chest should be prepped for aseptic surgery.

SURGICAL TECHNIQUES

The procedure for an exploratory laparotomy is given on p. 320. If neoplasia is suspected, biopsies or the entire mass should be submitted for histopathology.

SUTURE MATERIALS AND SPECIAL INSTRUMENTS

Monofilament synthetic, absorbable suture should be used to close the abdomen in these animals.

POSTOPERATIVE CARE AND ASSESSMENT

Fluid therapy should be continued postoperatively in most animals. Electrolytes, acid-base, and serum protein should be assessed in the postoperative period and corrected as necessary. Postoperative analgesia is recommended (see Chapter 13).

PROGNOSIS

The prognosis for animals with hemoabdomen depends on the underlying disease. Dogs with malignant splenic hemangiosarcoma seldom survive longer than 4 months after surgery without adjuvant chemotherapy.

References

Boysen SR, Rozanski EA, Tidwell AS et al: Evaluation of a focused assessment with sonography for trauma protocol to detect free abdominal fluid in dogs involved in motor vehicle accidents, *J Am Vet Med Assoc* 225:1198, 2004.

Nestor DD, McCullough SM, Schaeffer DJ: Biochemical analysis of neoplastic versus nonneoplastic abdominal effusions in dogs, *J Am Anim Hosp Assoc* 40:372, 2004.

Pintar J, Breitschwerdt EB, Hardie EM et al: Acute nontraumatic hemoabdomen in the dog: a retrospective analysis of 39 cases (1987-2001), *J Am Anim Hosp Assoc* 39:518, 2003.

Whitemore JC, Preston CA, Kyles AE et al: Nontraumatic rupture of an adrenal gland tumor caused intra-abdominal or retroperitoneal hemorrhage in four dogs, *J Am Vet Med Assoc* 219:329, 2001.

CHAPTER 19
Surgery of the Digestive System

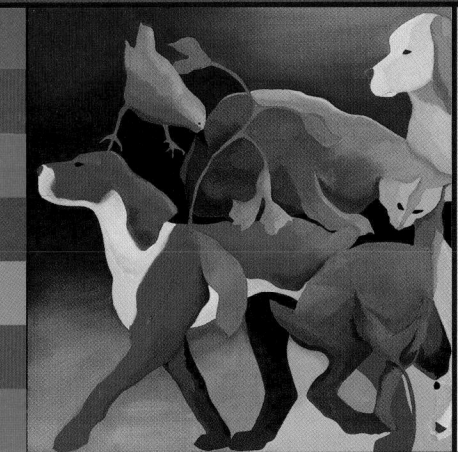

Surgery of the Oral Cavity and Oropharynx

DEFINITIONS

Maxillectomy is removal of a portion of the maxilla, and **mandibulectomy** is removal of a portion of the mandible. **Tonsillectomy** is excision of one or both tonsils. **Glossectomy** is excision of a portion of the tongue. **Cheiloplasty** is performed to alter the shape of the lip, generally to reduce drooling. **Mucoceles** are subcutaneous collections of saliva or mucus (or both). **Ranulas** are collections of fluid from the mandibular or sublingual salivary glands that occur beneath the tongue on either side of the frenulum.

PREOPERATIVE MANAGEMENT

Surgical diseases of the oral cavity and oropharynx are common in dogs and cats. They include congenital and traumatic abnormalities, foreign bodies, neoplasia, salivary gland disease, and dental disease. Patients with oral cavity or oropharyngeal disease may have drooling, dysphagia, anorexia, bleeding from the mouth, and/or fetid breath. Some animals are asymptomatic until the lesions become large or are discovered on routine physical examination. Others are presented for treatment of a mass, oral hemorrhage, oral pain, difficulty eating, nasal regurgitation, chronic rhinitis, dyspnea, or all of these. They may have a history of dental disease, weight loss, or trauma. The diagnosis is based on the history, clinical signs, physical examination, cytologic studies, radiographs, ultrasonography, computed tomography (CT), magnetic resonance imaging (MRI), and/or biopsy.

Before major surgery is performed, a thorough physical examination, complete blood cell count (CBC), and serum biochemical profile should be performed; urinalysis and electrocardiography (ECG) may be appropriate, too. Animals undergoing maxillectomy or mandibulectomy and those predisposed to coagulopathies should have the coagulation system checked (i.e., platelet count and mucosal bleeding time) and blood cross matching done before surgery. Skull radiography, MRI, or CT images usually can determine the extent of the lesion. Thoracic radiographs are indicated to evaluate for metastasis, cardiac size, and pulmonary disease. The teeth of animals with periodontal disease should be cleaned several days before major reconstructive surgery to improve tissue health and reduce oral bacterial numbers. Nutrition should be maintained by tube feeding if necessary (see Chapter 11). Animals with oronasal fistulae can be fed via feeding tubes to reduce the chances of rhinitis and inhalation pneumonia before surgery. Metabolic abnormalities should be corrected. Mature animals should fast for 12 to 18 hours before induction of anesthesia (pediatric patients fast 4 to 8 hours). After induction and orotracheal intubation, the mouth should be flushed with dilute Betadine or chlorhexidine solution to reduce bacterial numbers.

ANESTHESIA

Preemptive analgesics and local nerve blocks (infraorbital, maxillary, mandibular, mental, or palatine nerves; bupivacaine 0.5%, 0.1 to 0.5 ml per site; see also Chapter 13) should be used to minimize pain associated with major oral reconstructive surgery. An orally placed endotracheal tube can sometimes hinder oral cavity and oropharyngeal surgery; in these cases, endotracheal intubation can be performed through a pharyngotomy (see p. 99) or tracheotomy incision (see p. 825). It is important that the endotracheal tube and its cuff prevent blood and fluid from entering the lower airways. One or two gauze sponges can be placed in the oropharynx around the endotracheal tube to help absorb fluids. Postoperative swelling of the oral mucous membranes may obstruct the glottis; this can be minimized by pretreatment with corticosteroids (e.g., dexamethasone, 1 to 2 mg/kg given subcutaneously or intramuscularly before induction of anesthesia or intravenously at induction). Most animals with oral disease are healthy, and numerous anesthetic protocols can be used (Box 19-1). Blood, hypertonic saline, and/or colloids should be available in the event of severe

BOX 19-1

Selected Anesthetic Protocols for Use in Animals With Oral Disease

Premedication

Give atropine (0.02–0.04 mg/kg SC or IM) or glycopyrrolate (0.005–0.011 mg/kg SC or IM) plus hydromorphone* (0.1–0.2 mg/kg SC or IM) or butorphanol (0.2–0.4 mg/kg SC or IM), or buprenorphine (5–15 µg/kg IM)

Induction

Thiopental (10–12 mg/kg IV) or propofol (4–6 mg/kg IV) to effect or a combination of diazepam and ketamine (diazepam 0.27 mg/kg plus 5.5 mg/kg ketamine IV) titrated to effect

Maintenance

Isoflurane or sevoflurane

SC, Subcutaneous; *IM*, intramuscular; *IV*, intravenous.
*May use 0.05 mg/kg in cats.

 BOX 19-2

Prophylactic and Therapeutic Antibiotics for Oral Surgery

Cefazolin (Ancef, Kefzol)

22 mg/kg IV, bid to tid

Ampicillin

22 mg/kg PO, IV, IM, or SC, tid to qid

Clindamycin (Antirobe)

11 mg/kg PO, bid

Metronidazole (Flagyl)

10–15 mg/kg PO, bid

IV, Intravenous; *PO*, oral; *IM*, intramuscular; *SC*, subcutaneous; *bid*, twice a day; *tid*, three times a day; *qid*, four times a day.

hemorrhage. Placement of two cephalic catheters allows simultaneous administration of blood and inotropes if necessary. Evaluation of the arterial blood pressure during surgery is warranted, and acetylpromazine should be avoided. Specific recommendations for anesthetizing animals with concurrent organ dysfunction (i.e., hepatic failure or renal failure) appear in the chapters discussing general techniques for the organ system of concern.

ANTIBIOTICS

The oral cavity and oropharynx are contaminated (aerobic, facultative, and anaerobic bacteria); saliva is antimicrobial, and blood supply to this region is excellent. For these reasons, infections after oral surgery are rare. One dose of a prophylactic antibiotic effective against gram-positive aerobes and anaerobes (e.g., ampicillin and clindamycin) may be given at anesthetic induction (Box 19-2). Therapeutic antibiotics (e.g., cefazolin plus metronidazole; amoxicillin plus clavulanic acid; and clindamycin; see Box 19-2) are indicated in debilitated or immunosuppressed patients and those with severe periodontal disease.

SURGICAL ANATOMY

The oral cavity is divided into the vestibule and the oral cavity proper. The vestibule is the cavity lying outside the teeth and gums, but inside the lips and cheeks. The ducts of the parotid and zygomatic salivary glands open in the dorsocaudal part of the vestibule. The oral cavity proper is the area bounded by the hard palate and a small part of the soft palate dorsally, by the dental arches laterally and rostrally, and by the tongue and adjacent mucosa ventrally. The tongue is attached to the floor of the oral cavity by the lingual frenulum. The oropharynx extends from the level of the palatoglossal arches to the caudal border of the soft palate and the base of the epiglottis. Dorsally the oropharynx is bounded by the soft palate and ventrally by the root of the tongue. The palatine tonsils are found in the lateral wall of the oropharynx.

The blood supply to this region originates from branches of the common carotid arteries. The paired major and minor palatine arteries are important (Fig. 19-1). Two or three vessels emerge from the major palatine foramen at the caudal edge of the fourth upper premolar and course rostrally, midway between the midline and the dental arcade. The right and left major palatine arteries anastomose caudal to the incisors. The minor palatine arteries enter the palate caudal to the last molar and lateral to the major palatine artery, then course caudomedially to ramify in the caudal hard palate and soft palate. The major blood supply to the mandible is via the mandibular alveolar artery, which enters the mandibular canal on the medial surface of the mandible (see Fig. 19-1). The entry point is where an oblique line connecting the last molar tooth and the angular (muscular) process (which is hidden beneath the pterygoid muscle) meet. The mandibular alveolar artery ends at the middle mental foramen, where it branches to form the caudal, middle, and rostral mental arteries and exits via the mental foramina. The mandibular canal also transmits the mandibular vein and the mandibular alveolar nerve.

> NOTE: Infection is rare and healing is rapid after surgery of the oral cavity because of its excellent blood supply.

SURGICAL TECHNIQUE

Atraumatic surgical technique is important for reducing tissue damage and swelling and encouraging rapid healing (Box 19-3). Hemorrhage is expected and should be controlled with pressure and vessel ligation. Electrosurgery

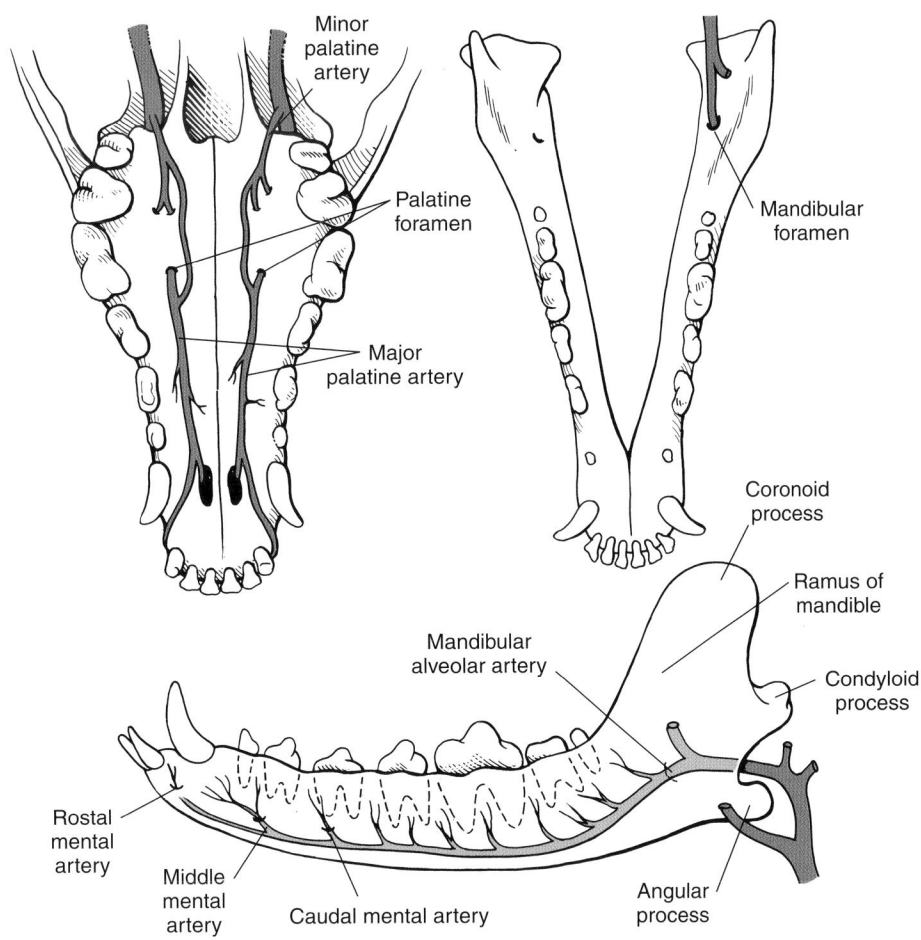

FIG. 19-1
The major blood supply to the maxilla is via the major and minor palatine arteries and to the mandible via the mandibular alveolar artery.

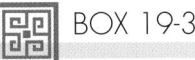 BOX 19-3

Principles of Oral Surgery

- Use atraumatic technique.
- Control hemorrhage using pressure and ligation.
- Prevent tension; make flaps 2 to 4 mm larger than the defect.
- Support flaps; do not suture over defects.
- Use appositional sutures (e.g., simple interrupted, simple continuous, cruciate, vertical mattress patterns).

should be used sparingly because excessive use delays healing and may cause dehiscence. Electrocoagulation should be applied only to discrete, isolated areas. The possibility exists that flammable gases (i.e., oxygen) leaking around the endotracheal tube could be ignited when electrosurgery or laser surgery is used.

Tension-free closure is imperative to prevent wound dehiscence and a subsequent oronasal fistula. Flaps created dur-

ing reconstructive procedures should be approximately 2 to 4 mm larger than the defect, and major vessels entering these flaps must be preserved. Tension on these flaps should be minimized by adequate mobilization. Flaps should be manipulated with skin hooks or stay sutures to minimize trauma. Suture lines should be placed over connective tissue or bone, rather than the defect, to help support mucosal flaps. Cleanly incised edges of tissue should be apposed with a two-layer closure in an appositional suture pattern (simple interrupted, simple continuous, cruciate, or vertical mattress patterns). Monofilament suture material (i.e., 4-0 or 3-0 poliglecaprone 25, polyglyconate, polydioxanone, or polypropylene) minimizes wicking and tissue reaction. A temporary acrylic obturator can be cemented or wired to the teeth to protect healing tissues in the occasional case in which tongue or pharyngeal muscle activity is apt to break down the suture line.

Biopsy Techniques

Impression smears or aspirates should be obtained from oral lesions before incisional or excisional biopsy. Cytologic studies may allow a tentative diagnosis that is helpful in planning further diagnostics; however, it must be realized that many oral lesions have inflamed surfaces secondary to the oral bacterial flora. Therefore one should not hesitate to obtain a deeper and larger biopsy if only inflamed, necrotic tissue is found. An incisional biopsy using a core needle or wedge biopsy technique should be performed if the definitive diagnosis will change the course of therapy. A TruCut or Vim-Silverman needle can be used to obtain small cores from several areas of the mass, whereas wedge biopsies should be performed from nonnecrotic areas of the mass when larger pieces of tissue are needed. A loop or needle electrode of an electrosurgical unit is useful in obtaining oral biopsies. However, the specimen will be nondiagnostic if too much current is applied, especially to a small sample. Tissue coagulation can be prevented by keeping the power setting on the electrosurgical unit as low as possible. Diseased tissue often is friable and difficult to appose with sutures after a biopsy; however, pressure over the cut area usually is sufficient to control hemorrhage. Silver nitrate cautery can be used if necessary. An excisional biopsy (e.g., partial maxillectomy, mandibulectomy, tonsillectomy, glossectomy, or lip resection) should be performed and the area reconstructed if the definitive histologic diagnosis will not alter the course of therapy. All specimens should be submitted for histologic evaluation.

> NOTE: Avoid areas of superficial necrosis when obtaining biopsies; sample deeper, viable tissue instead.

Temporary Carotid Artery Ligation

Some surgeons perform temporary carotid artery occlusion before maxillectomy to minimize blood loss.

To do so, place the animal in dorsal recumbency and prepare the ventral cervical area for surgery. Expose the trachea through a 5- to 8-cm ventral cervical midline incision. Palpate the carotid pulse and exteriorize the carotid sheath. Separate the common carotid artery from the vagosympathetic trunk and internal jugular vein. Temporarily occlude the carotid artery with a vascular clamp or tie. Repeat the procedure on the opposite carotid artery. Temporarily appose skin with a continuous suture pattern or staples during the maxillectomy procedure. After maxillectomy, reopen the cervical wound and remove the vascular clamps or ties. Lavage the area thoroughly and appose the sternohyoid muscles, subcutaneous tissue, and skin in separate layers.

> NOTE: Temporary carotid artery ligation may not be safe in cats or in severely anemic dogs. Perform with caution.

Partial Maxillectomy

Maxillectomy is most often performed to resect an oral neoplasm (Fig. 19-2). Varying amounts of the maxilla and hard palate may be excised, depending on the gross and radio-

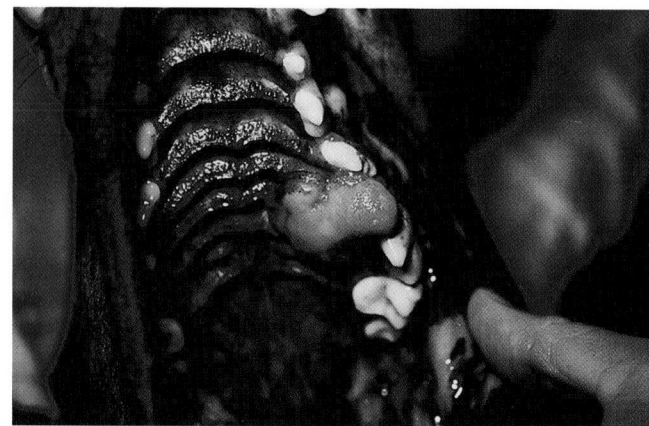

FIG. 19-2
An odontogenic tumor involving the maxillary dental arcade, palate, and maxilla.

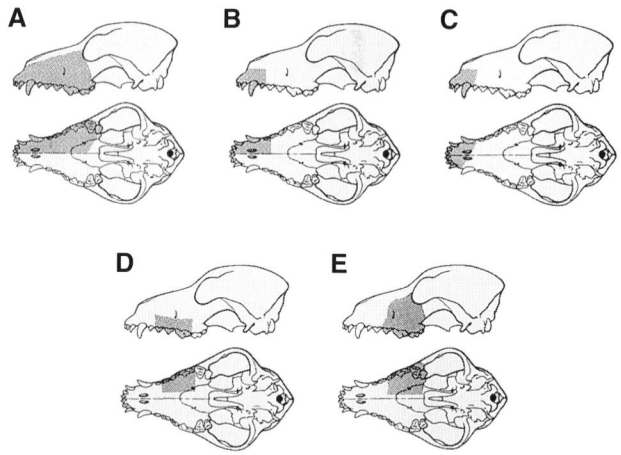

FIG. 19-3
Areas resected with partial maxillectomy techniques.
A, Hemimaxillectomy. **B,** Rostral hemimaxillectomy.
C, Premaxillectomy (bilateral rostral hemimaxillectomy).
D, Central hemimaxillectomy. **E,** Caudal hemimaxillectomy.

graphic, CT, or MRI extent of the lesion. Depending on the area being resected, partial maxillectomies may be classified as hemimaxillectomies (rostral, central, or caudal) or premaxillectomies (bilateral rostral) (Figs. 19-3 and 19-4). Hemimaxillectomy, without a definition of site, usually refers to removal of one entire maxilla. Partial maxillectomies can be combined with nasal planectomy and dorsolateral approaches through the skin (Lascelles et al, 2004). Partial maxillectomy is limited by the surgeon's ability to reconstruct the oronasal defect; lesions that cross the midline of the palate are difficult to reconstruct.

Clip and aseptically prepare the maxillary and nasal skin. Flush the mouth with antiseptic solution. Place the patient in dorsal recumbency for lesions of the premaxilla and open the

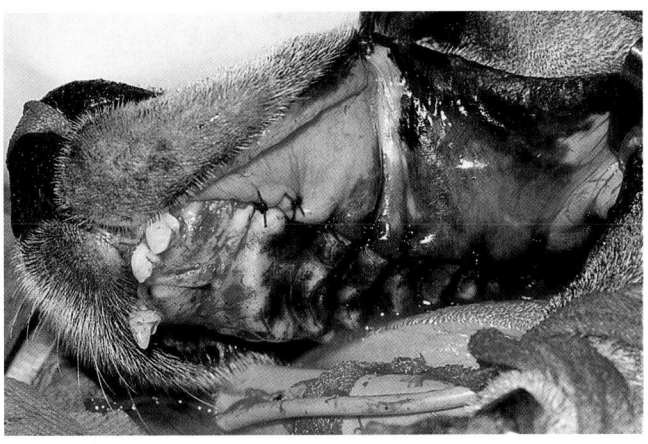

FIG. 19-4
Appearance of the oral cavity of a dog after a rostral hemi-maxillectomy. A buccal flap has been advanced across the defect and secured with apposition sutures.

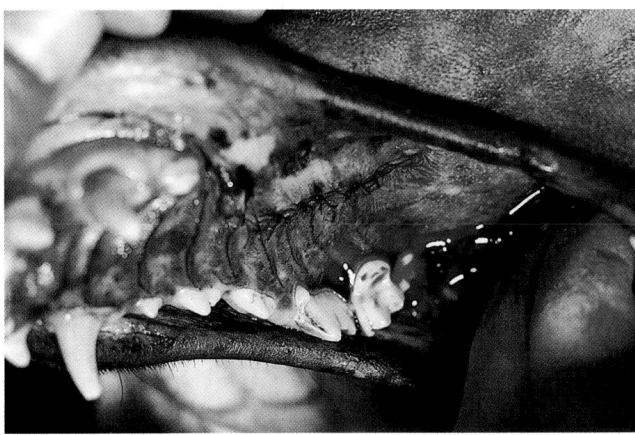

FIG. 19-6
A buccal mucosal flap was advanced over the defect evident in Fig. 19-5 and secured with approximating sutures.

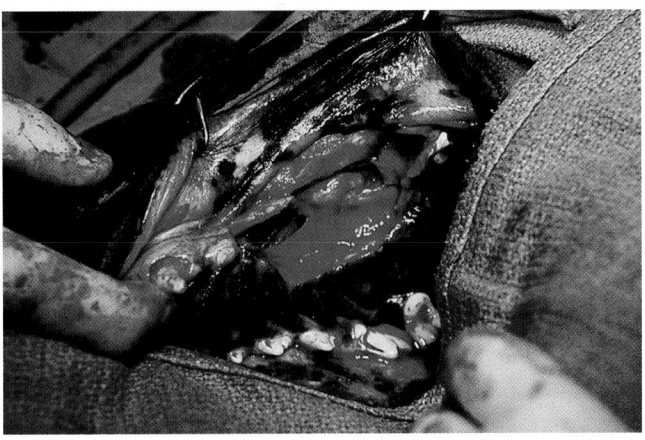

FIG. 19-5
A central hemimaxillectomy was performed to remove the lesion shown in Fig. 19-2 and an additional 1 to 2 cm of normal tissue. Note that the nasal cavity is exposed.

mouth to its maximum extent by placing a mouth speculum or by taping the mouth open. Place the patient in lateral or dorsal recumbency for lesions caudal to the premaxilla. Determine the extent of resection based on the size of the soft tissue lesion and the radiographic, CT, or MRI degree of bony involvement. Generally, excise the mass and a minimum of 1 to 2 cm of normal soft tissue and bone on all borders. Remove the mass en bloc by first making mucosal incisions (buccal, gingival, and hard palate) around the tissue to be resected. Avoid rectangular excision because the corners are susceptible to dehiscence. Using a periosteal elevator, undermine and reflect the gingival and palatal mucosa.

Use an oscillating saw or an osteotome and mallet to cut the maxilla, incisive bone, and/or palate. Resect all premolar and molar teeth for lesions extending to the third premolar because of the outward turn of the dental arch. When performing a caudal maxillectomy, remove a portion of the

zygomatic arch and orbit if necessary to obtain clean borders. Elevate the tissue block and sever any remaining soft tissue attachments to complete the resection and expose the nasal cavity (Fig. 19-5). Remove involved nasal turbinates with rongeurs and hemostats if disease extends into the nasal cavity. Control hemorrhage by ligating identifiable vessels and applying pressure to other areas. Isolate and ligate the major palatine and infraorbital artery and vein if they are included in the resection site. Use bone wax or electrofulguration to help control bone hemorrhage. Lavage and inspect the defect to ensure that all grossly diseased tissue has been excised. Close the defect by elevating a buccal mucosal flap from the adjacent cheek or lip (Fig. 19-6). Elevate enough buccal mucosa and submucosa to allow a tension-free approximation with the gingival and palatal mucosa. Place the first layer of simple interrupted sutures in the submucosa with the knot directed toward the nasal cavity. Place a second layer of interrupted approximating sutures (i.e., simple, cruciate, or vertical mattress) to accurately appose buccal mucosa to the palatal and gingival mucosa.

A double-flap technique may be used to close premaxillectomy defects to provide mucosa on both the nasal and oral surfaces. However, an epithelial surface on the nasal aspect of the flap is not necessary because the connective tissue surface of the flap is covered with respiratory epithelium within 1 to 2 weeks.

If carotid artery occlusion was performed, release the occlusion after the defect has been closed.

Partial Mandibulectomy

Mandibulectomy is most often performed to resect an oral neoplasm. Occasionally, mandibular fractures are also treated by partial mandibulectomy. Varying amounts of mandible may be excised, depending on the extent of the

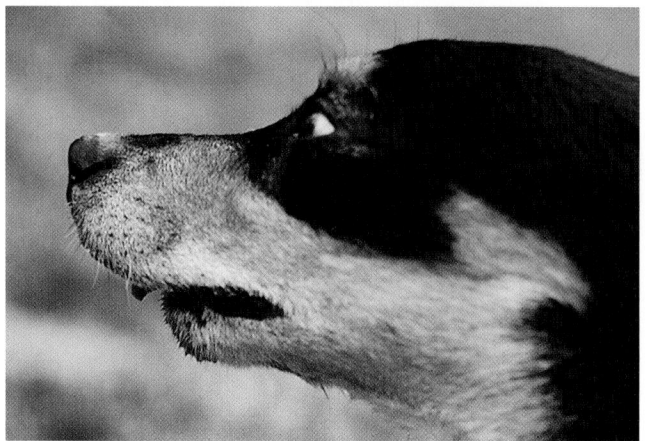

FIG. 19-7
Postoperative appearance after rostral mandibulectomy. Note that the tongue is barely apparent despite the short mandible.

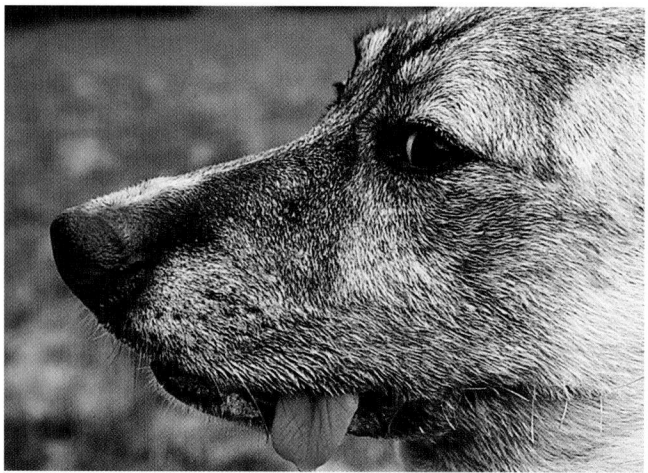

FIG. 19-9
Postoperative appearance after hemimandibulectomy in which cheiloplasty was not performed. Although the tongue is movable, it protrudes from the oral cavity.

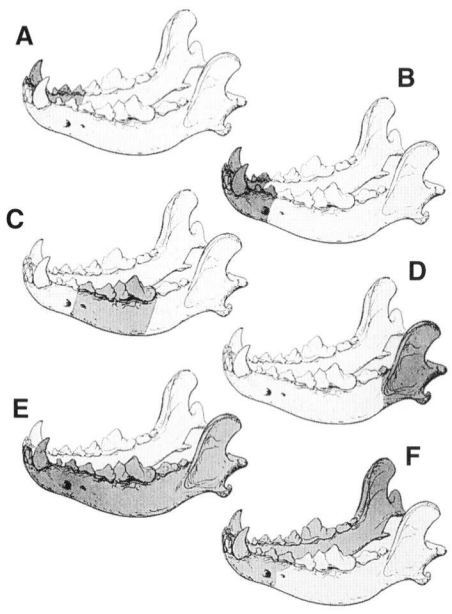

FIG. 19-8
Areas resected with partial mandibulectomy techniques. **A,** Rostral hemimandibulectomy (unilateral rostral hemimandibulectomy). **B,** Rostral mandibulectomy (bilateral rostral hemimandibulectomy). **C,** Central hemimandibulectomy. **D,** Caudal hemimandibulectomy. **E,** Total hemimandibulectomy. **F,** Three-quarter mandibulectomy.

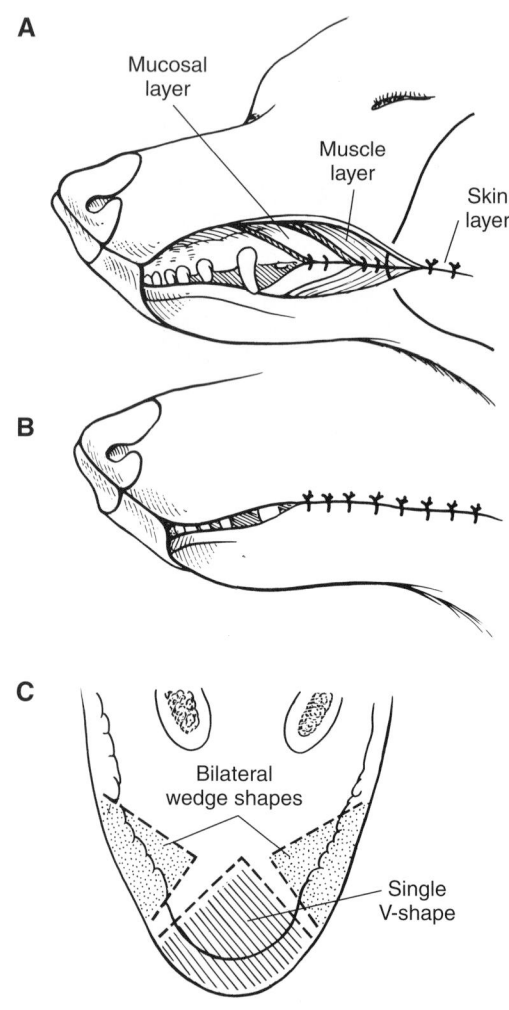

FIG. 19-10
Cheiloplasty. **A,** Excise the lip margins to the level of the second premolar. **A** and **B,** Appose the incised lip margins in three layers (oral mucosa, muscle and connective tissue, and skin). **C,** To improve cosmesis after rostral mandibulectomy, excise redundant skin from one or more of the indicated sites.

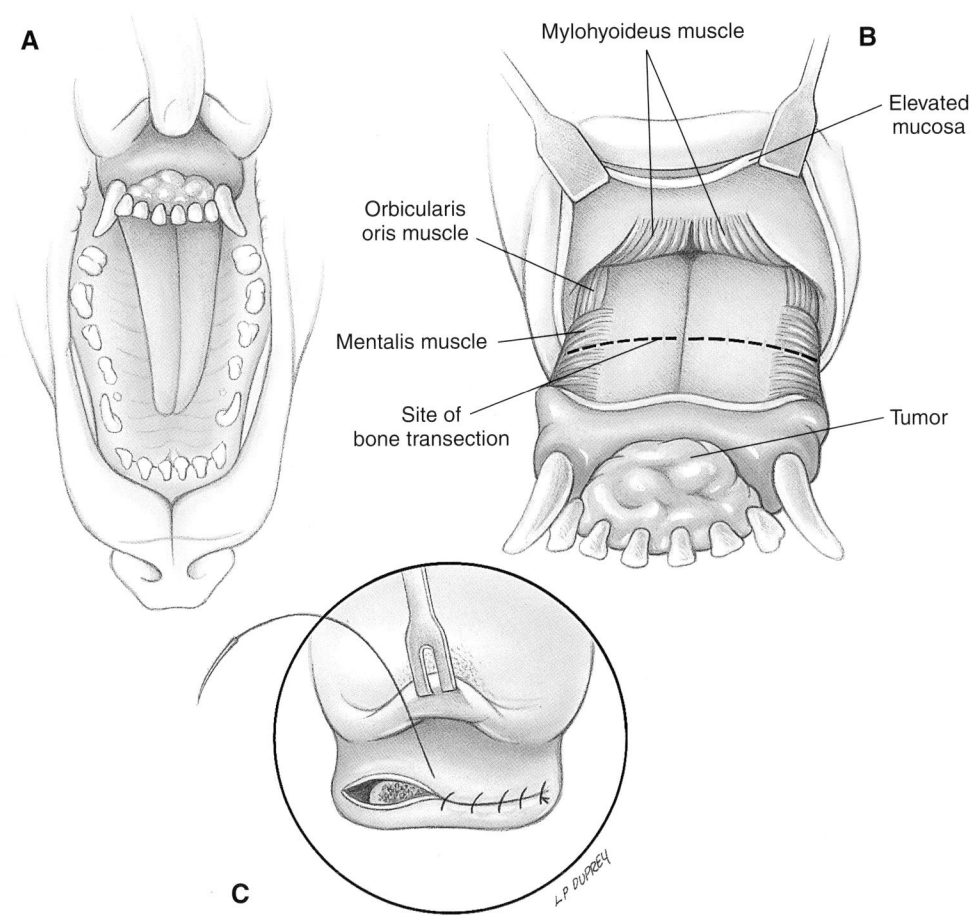

A

Mylohyoideus muscle

B

Elevated mucosa

Orbicularis oris muscle

Mentalis muscle

Site of bone transection

Tumor

C

L-P DUPREY

FIG. 19-11
Rostral mandibulectomy.
A, Position the patient in dorsal recumbency. **B,** Incise the mucosa 1 to 2 cm from the lesion, exposing the underlying muscles. Elevate the muscles and transect the bone (broken line). **C,** Appose the labial and sublingual mucosa after en bloc excision.

tumor or lesion (Fig. 19-7). Depending on the extent of resection, hemimandibulectomies may be classified as rostral, rostral-bilateral, central, caudal, or total (Fig. 19-8). These techniques may be combined when more extensive resection is necessary. After mandibulectomy, cheiloplasty (commissuroplasty) may be performed to minimize excessive drooling and lateral protrusion of the tongue (Fig. 19-9). It is accomplished by removing the mucocutaneous junction of the upper and lower lip to the level of the second premolar or canine tooth. The commissure is advanced rostrally during closure. The upper and lower lip margins are apposed in three layers (oral mucosa, muscle and connective tissue, and skin) (Fig. 19-10). Opening the mouth fully during the first 2 weeks may cause dehiscence. Tension-relieving button sutures or a loose tape muzzle may be used to help prevent this. During rostral mandibulectomies, redundant skin and mucosa may be eliminated by excising and apposing V-shaped wedges. The base of the V is along the mucocutaneous junction (see Fig. 19-10).

Position the patient in lateral, sternal, or dorsal recumbency with the neck extended (Figs. 19-11, A and 19-12, A). Clip and aseptically prepare the skin of the lateral face and ventral mandible. Flush the mouth with antiseptic solution. Determine the amount to be resected based on the size of the soft tissue lesion and the radiographic, CT, or MRI evidence

of bony involvement. Generally, excise the mass and a minimum of 1 to 2 cm of normal soft tissue and bone on all borders. Retract the commissure and lip to give maximum exposure. If necessary, improve visualization by incising the commissure to the level of the mandibular angle (Fig. 19-12, B). Begin en bloc resection by first incising mucosa (buccal, gingival, and sublingual) around the diseased area (Figs. 19-11, B and 19-12, B). Using a periosteal elevator, undermine and reflect the gingival mucosa to expose the lateral and ventral aspects of the ramus. Transect or elevate and retract muscles (mentalis, orbicularis oris, buccinator, mylohyoideus, geniohyoideus, genioglossus, masseter, digastricus, temporalis, and pterygoideus) attached to the portion of the mandible being resected (Figs. 19-11, B and 19-12, C and D). Use an oscillating saw or an osteotome and mallet to transect the ramus and separate the symphysis. As an alternative, use a Gigli wire to transect the ramus. Complete a total hemimandibulectomy by incising the joint capsule and disarticulating the temporomandibular joint (Fig. 19-12, C). Locate the temporomandibular joint by rotating the mandible and palpating the articulation. Ligate or cauterize the mandibular artery (see Fig. 19-12, D). Sever any remaining soft tissue attachments to complete the resection. Avoid traumatizing the lingual frenulum or sublingual and mandibular salivary ducts. Contour the ostectomy sites with bone rongeurs, removing sharp bone and tapering the edges to facilitate

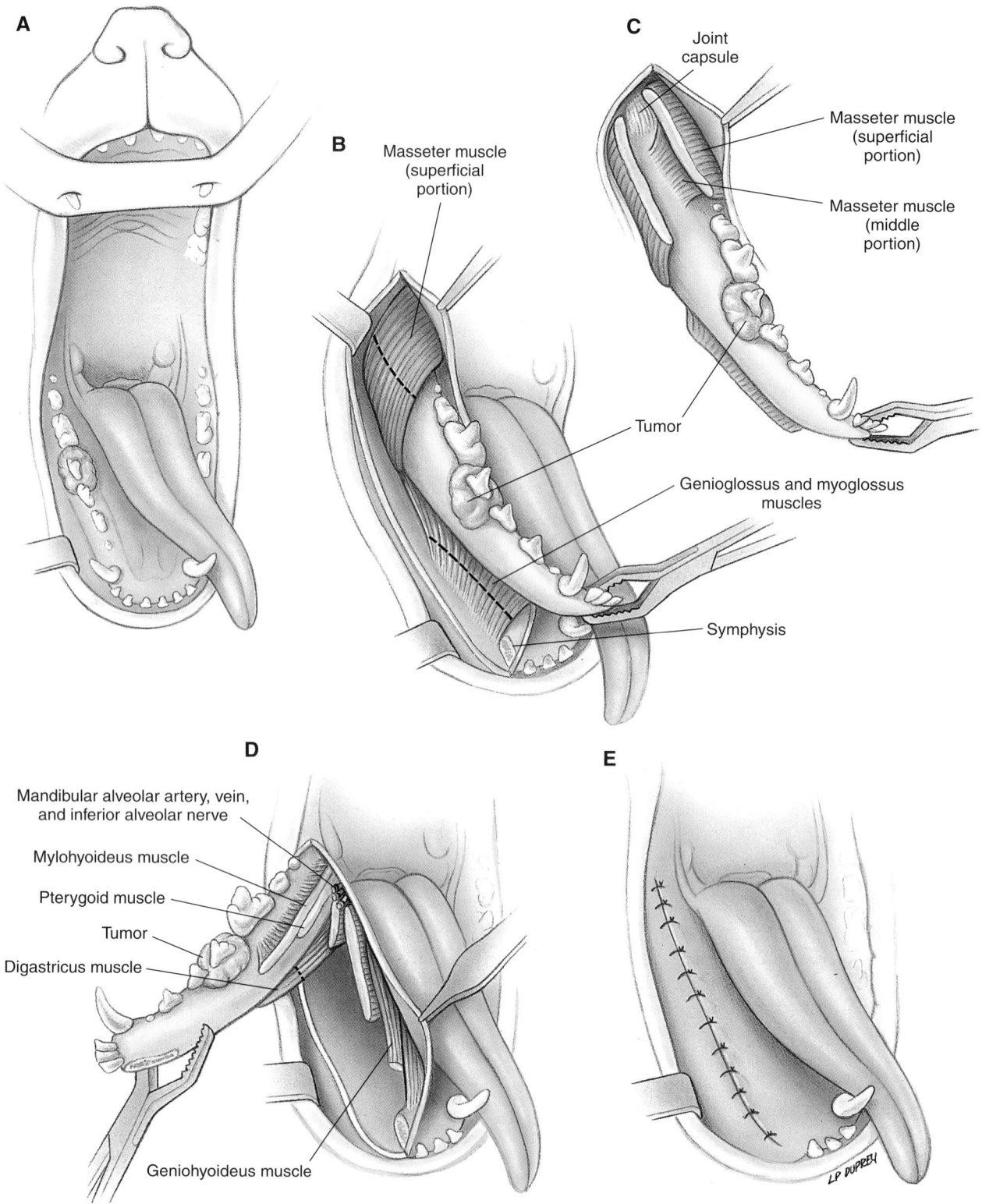

FIG. 19-12

Total hemimandibulectomy. **A,** Position the patient in ventral recumbency. **B,** Incise the mucosa 1 to 2 cm from the lesion. Incise the commissure to allow better exposure of the caudal mandible. Separate the mandibular symphysis and identify and transect (broken line) the muscles. **C,** Dissect and transect the lateral mandibular muscles and expose the temporomandibular joint. **D,** Dissect and transect the medial muscles of the mandible and identify the mandibular artery entering the mandibular foramen. Ligate the mandibular vessels, disarticulate, and remove the mandible. **E,** Appose the buccal and sublingual mucosa with approximating sutures.

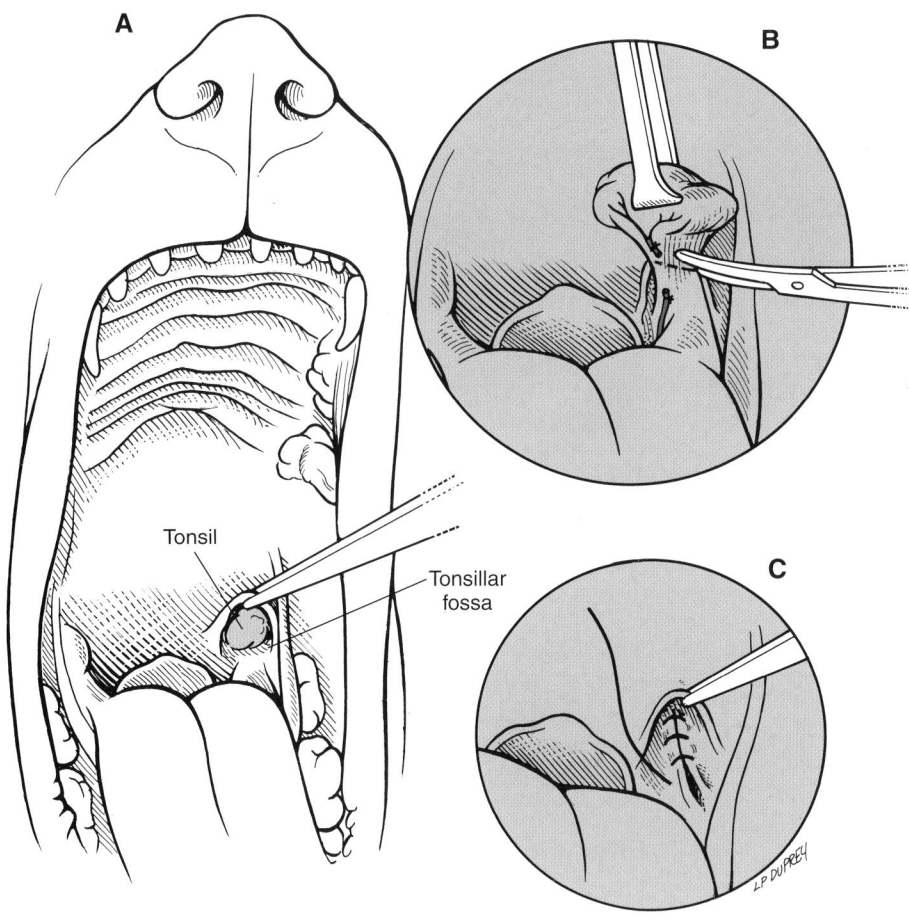

Tonsil

Tonsillar fossa

FIG. 19-13
Tonsillectomy. **A,** The palatine tonsils are located in the dorsolateral pharynx. **B,** During tonsillectomy evert the tonsil from the crypt, ligate the tonsillar vessels, and begin transection along the base. **C,** Close the crypt with a simple continuous pattern to help control hemorrhage.

closure. Close the defect by elevating a mucosal flap from the adjacent lip or cheek (Figs. 19-11, C and 19-12, E). Elevate enough mucosa and submucosa to allow a tension-free approximation with the gingival and sublingual mucosa. Place the first layer of simple interrupted sutures in the submucosa with the knots buried. Place a second layer of interrupted approximating sutures (simple, cruciate, or vertical mattress) to accurately appose the labial, sublingual, and gingival mucosa. As an alternative, use a single-layer, simple continuous or interrupted suture pattern.

> NOTE: It is not necessary to stabilize the remaining mandible after mandibulectomy. However, cortical bone grafts have been used to improve the animal's appearance.

Tonsillectomy

When neoplasia of the palatine tonsils is suspected, a biopsy should be taken or the neoplasm removed. Squamous cell carcinoma and lymphosarcoma are the most common tumors of the tonsils, and it is very doubtful that either will be cured with surgery alone. Enlarged tonsils occasionally are removed if they contribute to airway obstruction or dysphagia and in cases of unresponsive chronic tonsillitis. However, ton-

sillitis is usually secondary to other diseases (e.g., esophageal dysfunction), and removing the tonsils rarely effects a cure.

Administer dexamethasone (1 to 2 mg/kg IV) at the time of induction to minimize postoperative swelling and edema. Position the animal in ventral recumbency with the maxilla suspended from an IV stand or similar device. Open the mouth maximally, and secure it open with tape or gauze. Locate the tonsil in the tonsillar fossa or crypt on the dorsolateral wall of the oropharynx just caudal to the palatoglossal arch (Fig. 19-13). Retract the edge of the tonsillar crypt caudodorsally to expose the tonsil. Grasp the tonsil at its base with an Allis tissue forceps or hemostat, and retract it from the crypt. Transect the hilar mucosa at the base of the tonsil with Metzenbaum scissors or a tonsillectomy snare. Ligate the tonsillar artery as it enters the caudal aspect of the tonsil. (Some surgeons excise the tonsil using electrosurgery or laser surgery.) Appose the edges of the tonsillar crypt with a simple continuous suture pattern of 3-0 or 4-0 monofilament absorbable suture to minimize hemorrhage.

Glossectomy

The primary reason for partial tongue amputation is neoplasia, which usually occurs on the margin or base of the tongue. The most common tongue tumor is squamous cell

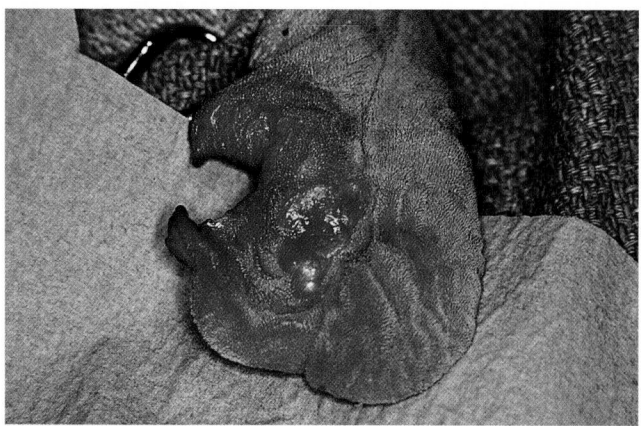

FIG. 19-14
Appearance of a squamous cell carcinoma of the tongue in a dog.

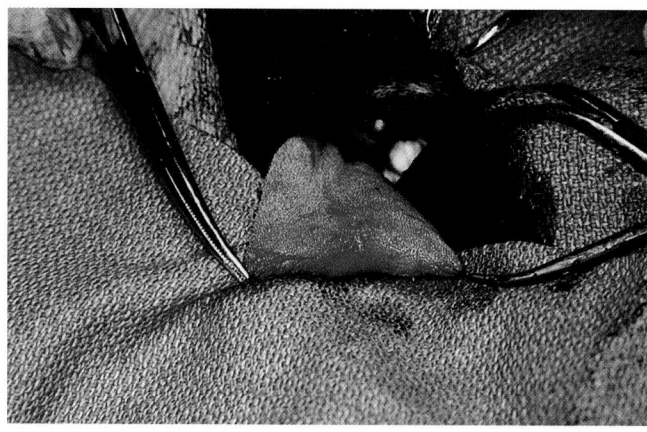

FIG. 19-15
Postoperative appearance of the tongue in Fig. 19-14 after partial glossectomy. The glossectomy was completed by apposing epithelial edges with a simple continuous suture pattern.

carcinoma (Fig. 19-14); others include malignant melanoma, granular cell myeloblastoma, and mast cell tumor. Most lacerations of the tongue are amenable to repair with a one-layer or two-layer closure rather than amputation. Other reasons for tongue surgery include abscess drainage, glossitis, severe trauma, and congenital ankyloglossia (limited tongue movement) (Temizsoylu and Avki, 2003). Tongue lesions are associated with signs of drooling, malodor, dysphagia, and sometimes dyspnea.

Glossectomies are classified as partial (involving only the free tongue), subtotal (entire free tongue and part of the genioglossus and geniohyoid muscles), near total (greater than 75% of tongue), and total (100% of tongue) glossectomies (Dvorak et al, 2004). Glossectomy is considered major if more than the free portion of the tongue is removed. Amputation of 40% to 60% of the rostral tongue usually is well tolerated. Amputation at the base of the tongue or total glossectomy makes eating and drinking difficult; however, the animal can learn to suck in food and water, or chunks of food can be tossed to the base of the tongue. Hyperptyalism following major glossectomy occasionally occurs; improvement may be seen with bilateral sialoadenectomy.

When performing glossectomy, resect the diseased portion of the tongue and a minimum of 2 cm of normal tissue after placing a noncrushing clamp across the base of the tongue. When a total glossectomy is performed, a clamp is not used. Wedge the incision so that slightly more tongue muscle than dorsal or ventral mucosa is excised. Control hemorrhage by ligation, pressure, or electrosurgery. Use through-and-through horizontal mattress sutures as needed to control hemorrhage. Appose the epithelial edges with a simple continuous suture pattern using 3-0 or 4-0 monofilament absorbable suture (Fig. 19-15). Place a feeding tube when major glossectomies are performed (see pp. 96-107).

> **NOTE:** Dogs seem to adapt better than do cats to tongue amputation. A feeding tube may be required until the animal learns to eat after the procedure.

Pharyngotomy

Pharyngotomy is performed to allow endotracheal intubation or tube feeding. For a description of the technique, please see p. 99 and Figs. 11-8 and 11-9.

Salivary Gland Excision

The salivary glands most often are removed to treat salivary mucoceles or neoplasia, and the mandibular and sublingual salivary glands are most often removed to treat cervical, sublingual, and pharyngeal salivary mucoceles. Neoplasms (usually adenocarcinomas or carcinomas) occur most frequently in the parotid (50% dogs, 19% cats) and mandibular (30% dogs, 59% cats) salivary glands. (Hammer et al, 2001). Salivary gland excision is described on pp. 370 to 372.

HEALING OF THE ORAL CAVITY AND OROPHARYNX

The oral cavity and oropharyngeal mucosa heal more rapidly than skin because phagocytic activity (primarily monocytes rather than polymorphonuclear leukocytes) and epithelialization are more extensive and occur earlier in mucosa. An excellent mucosal blood supply, warmer temperatures, higher metabolic activity, and a higher mitotic rate contribute to rapid healing of mucosa. Apposed wounds reepithelialize within a few days, and defects heal by secondary intention.

SUTURE MATERIALS AND SPECIAL INSTRUMENTS

Special instruments that may facilitate surgical procedures of the oral cavity include periosteal elevators, an oscillating saw or osteotome and mallet, Gigli wire, rongeurs or bone cutters, vascular bulldog clamps, vascular ties, tissue hooks, Metzenbaum scissors, noncrushing clamps (Doyen intestinal forceps), and Penrose drains. Although many suture materials may be used in the oral cavity and oropharynx, 3-0 or 4-0 polydioxanone, polyglyconate, or poliglecaprone 25 (monofilament absorbable) and 3-0 or 4-0 polypropylene or nylon (monofilament nonabsorbable) are preferred.

POSTOPERATIVE CARE AND ASSESSMENT

After oral surgery, gauze sponges should be removed from the caudal pharynx, and the nasopharynx should be suctioned. Extubation should be delayed until a well-developed swallowing reflex is present. Patients should be recovered in a slightly head down position, and the tube should be removed with the cuff slightly inflated to help ensure that blood clots are expelled through the mouth rather being aspirated or swallowed. These patients should be monitored for airway obstruction or pain, and analgesics provided as necessary (for opioid analgesics see Table 13-4 on p. 133; for nonsteroidal antiinflammatory drugs [NSAIDs], see Tables 13-7 and 13-8 on p. 143; and for adjunctive drug therapy see Table 13-9 on p. 145). Elizabethan collars or similar restraining devices should be used on some animals to prevent disruption of the surgical site. Occasionally an acrylic oral splint is used to protect the surgical site.

> NOTE: Be sure to suction the oral cavity and oropharynx before extubation. Extubate with the cuff partially inflated, and monitor for airway obstruction during recovery.

Oral intake should not be allowed for the first 8 to 12 hours after surgery (except in pediatric patients at risk for hypoglycemia); hydration should be maintained with intravenous fluids. Water should be offered after 12 hours and the animal observed for signs of dysphagia, pain, or regurgitation. If no serious problems are identified, soft food may be offered between 12 and 24 hours after surgery. Gruel is unnecessary and may seep between sutures, inhibiting healing. Hand feeding (tossing meatballs) and watering may be necessary for 1 to 2 weeks following major glossectomy, until the animal is trained to suck water and prehend food without a tongue. Feeding through a gastrostomy, pharyngostomy, or esophagostomy tube occasionally is necessary for animals with severe wounds or those unwilling to eat within 3 days after surgery (see Chapter 11). Soft food should be fed until the wound has healed, and the animal should be prevented from chewing on sticks, toys, or other hard surfaces. Healing should be evaluated at 3 to 5 days, 2 weeks, and 4 weeks after surgery. Additional reconstruction may be necessary if areas of partial dehiscence do not heal by secondary intention or if an oronasal fistula remains after 4 to 6 weeks. Animals with neoplasia should be evaluated every 3 to 6 months for tumor recurrence.

Epistaxis, serous to mucoid nasal discharge, and pain are expected after a maxillectomy. Crusting of the nares and epiphora may occur when the nasolacrimal duct is transected. Subcutaneous emphysema occasionally occurs when a large portion of the nasal cavity is exposed. Emphysema, crusting, and nasal discharge are short-term sequelae that usually resolve in days to weeks. Cosmesis usually is good, with a slight facial concavity and lip elevation after lateral maxillectomy. Removal of a canine tooth causes more noticeable concavity. Premaxillectomies involving all incisors and one or both canine teeth produce ventral drooping of the nose and displacement of the maxillary lip caudal to the mandibular canine teeth unless further reconstruction (e.g., cantilever technique) is performed (Pavletic, 1999). Extensive premaxillectomies (caudal to the first premolar) shorten the nose and may cause an obvious prognathic appearance (protrusion of the lower jaw).

> NOTE: Dogs do better after hemimandibulectomies than do cats. Warn owners that some cats refuse to eat after this procedure and may require a feeding tube.

Cosmesis and function after partial mandibulectomy are good (see Fig. 19-7). Mandibular "drift" and instability occur more often when the osteotomy is caudal to the second premolar. The remaining hemimandible may deviate medially, producing malocclusion, clicking of the teeth, and/or trauma to the palatal or gingival mucosa. Most animals adapt, and serious problems seldom occur. The involved canine tooth may be pulled or shortened if erosion or ulceration develops. Rostral mandibulectomy (bilateral) caudal to the third or fourth premolar may cause difficulty with prehension and is less cosmetic. Tongue protrusion may occur, but most patients are able to keep the tongue retracted. Cheiloplasty may decrease drooling and lateral tongue protrusion in animals after partial mandibulectomies or maxillectomies.

COMPLICATIONS

Minor swelling of the skin and mucous membranes should be expected after partial maxillectomy or mandibulectomy, but should resolve within 2 to 3 days. Infection is possible because the oral cavity is contaminated. However, infection is rare if the blood supply is maintained and good surgical technique used. Partial dehiscence may occur 3 to 5 days after surgery if tissue is severely traumatized, blood supply is inadequate, or excessive motion or tension affects any area of the repair. Sometimes appearances that are unacceptable to owners may be modified with further cosmetic reconstruction following maxillectomy or mandibulectomy. The most common postoperative complication after tonsillectomy is hemorrhage. Regrowth of tonsillar tissue may occur if excision is incomplete. After pharyngotomy, complications of airway obstruction and aspiration pneumonia may be seen if the pharyngostomy tube is located cranial or ventral to the epihyoid bone. Apparent hyperptyalism following major glossectomy occasionally occurs; improvement may be seen with bilateral sialoadenectomy. Tumor recurrence or metastasis is always possible after any oncologic surgery.

SPECIAL AGE CONSIDERATIONS

Pediatric patients with congenital cleft palate should be fed with a tube until they are 8 to 12 weeks old and may be more safely anesthetized. Pediatric patients are at higher risk of hypothermia and hypoglycemia, therefore they should not fast for more than 4 to 8 hours. Neoplasia is more common in geriatric patients; they should be thoroughly evaluated before surgery for concurrent disease and metastasis.

References

Dvorak LD, Beaver DP, Ellison GW et al: Major glossectomy in dogs: a case series and proposed classification system, *J Am Anim Hosp Assoc* 40:331, 2004.

Hammer A, Getzy D, Ogilvie G et al: Salivary gland neoplasia in the dog and cat: survival times and prognostic factors, *J Am Anim Hosp Assoc* 37:478, 2001.

Lascelles BDX, Henderson RA, Seguin B et al: Bilateral rostral maxillectomy and nasal planectomy for large rostral maxillofacial neoplasms in six dogs and one cat, *J Am Anim Hosp Assoc* 40:137, 2004.

Pavletic MM: Nasal reconstruction techniques. In *Atlas of small animal reconstructive surgery*, ed 2, Philadelphia, 1999, WB Saunders Co.

Temizsoylu MD, Avki S: Complete ventral ankyloglossia in three related dogs, *J Am Vet Med Assoc* 223:1443, 2003.

Suggested Reading

Lascelles BDX, Thomson MJ, Dernell WS et al: Combined dorsolateral and intraoral approach for the resection of tumors of the maxilla of the dog, *J Am Anim Hosp Assoc* 39:294, 2003.

This paper describes a combined dorsal skin incision and intraoral maxillectomy approach for removing tumors involving the caudal maxilla. A bipedicle flap of skin, buccal mucosa, and associated soft tissue of the lateral aspect of the nasal cavity is created. Better exposure, more aggressive margins, and improved outcome are possible using this technique variation.

SPECIFIC DISEASES

CONGENITAL ORONASAL FISTULA (CLEFT PALATE)

DEFINITIONS

A **congenital oronasal fistula** is an abnormal communication between the oral and nasal cavities involving the soft palate, hard palate, premaxilla, and/or lip. The **primary palate** consists of the lip and premaxilla. Incomplete closure of the primary palate is a **primary cleft** or **cleft lip** (harelip). The **secondary palate** consists of the hard and soft palates. Incomplete closure of either of these structures is a **secondary cleft** or **cleft palate**. Animals may also have unilateral or

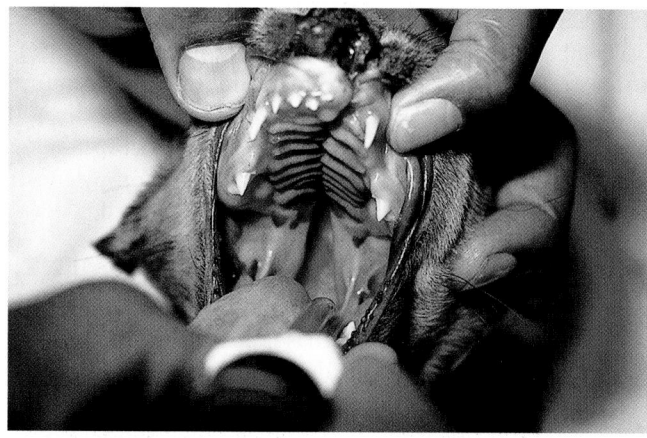

FIG. 19-16
A puppy with a cleft extending through the primary and secondary palate.

bilateral failure of the soft palate to fuse with the nasopharyngeal wall. This is termed a **lateral cleft of the soft palate** or **lateral cleft or hypoplastic soft palate**.

GENERAL CONSIDERATIONS AND CLINICALLY RELEVANT PATHOPHYSIOLOGY

Congenital palatal defects result when the two palatine shelves fail to fuse during fetal development (Fig. 19-16). The most critical time for development and closure of the fetal palate appears to be 25 to 28 days of gestation in dogs. Incomplete closure of either the primary or secondary palate is attributed to inherited (recessive or irregular dominant, polygenic traits), nutritional (inadequate folic acid), hormonal (steroids), mechanical (*in utero* trauma), and toxic (including viral) factors. Primary cleft palate alone is rare; however, secondary cleft palate may occur alone or in combination with primary clefts. Some affected neonates are unable to nurse effectively and die soon after birth. Others contaminate their nasal cavity with saliva and food. Signs of rhinitis and other respiratory infections are common. Middle ear disease that is often clinically unrecognized is sometimes associated with congenital clefts (Gregory, 2000).

DIAGNOSIS
Clinical Presentation

Signalment. Dogs, particularly brachycephalic breeds, are more commonly affected with cleft palate than cats. Purebred dogs have a higher incidence than mixed breeds. Breeds at high risk for cleft palate include Boston terriers, Pekingese, bulldogs, miniature schnauzers, beagles, cocker spaniels, and dachshunds. Siamese cats have a higher incidence than other cat breeds. Females are more commonly affected than males. The cleft is present at birth, although it is not always recognized immediately.

History. A history of difficulty nursing, nasal regurgitation, nasal discharge, and failure to thrive are common problems. Signs related to incomplete separation of the oral and nasal cavity include drainage of milk from the nares during or after nursing; gagging, coughing, or sneezing (or all three) while eating; poor growth; and respiratory infection (i.e., rhinitis and aspiration pneumonia).

Physical Examination Findings

All puppies and kittens should be checked on initial presentation for evidence of a cleft palate. Diagnosis of congenital oronasal fistula is made by visual examination. Incomplete closure of the lip is easily recognized when the patient is first examined; however, a thorough oral examination is required to identify incomplete closure of the premaxilla, hard palate, or soft palate. Anesthesia may be necessary to thoroughly assess the soft palate. A secondary cleft may occur without a primary cleft. Patients may be thin and stunted. Abnormal respiratory sounds are auscultated if aspiration pneumonia is present.

> NOTE: Be sure to thoroughly evaluate affected neonates for concurrent congenital anomalies.

Diagnostic Imaging

Radiographic examination of the skull is not necessary; however, thoracic radiographs are useful in evaluating for aspiration pneumonia typically characterized by interstitial to alveolar infiltrates within the ventral aspect of the lungs. It should be noted that middle ear disease can be seen in association with defects in the palate; thus imaging of the tympanic bullae may be indicated (Gregory, 2000).

Laboratory Findings

Laboratory abnormalities are not present unless the animal has aspiration pneumonia or is cachectic.

DIFFERENTIAL DIAGNOSIS

Traumatic or acquired clefts, rhinitis, nasal foreign body, and aspiration pneumonia are potential differential or concurrent diagnoses.

MEDICAL MANAGEMENT

Affected patients should be tube fed to maintain an adequate nutritional status and reduce the incidence of aspiration pneumonia until they are old enough for surgery. Aspiration pneumonia may be treated with antibiotics, fluids, oxygen, bronchodilators, and/or expectorants. Use of corticosteroids is controversial for acute aspiration and of no benefit for chronic aspiration. A tracheal wash or brushing for culture and sensitivity testing should be performed if aspiration pneumonia is severe. Broad-spectrum antibiotics with efficacy against anaerobes (Box 19-4) are indicated for severe aspiration or purulent rhinitis. Animals with severe rhinitis may benefit from having the nasal infection treated before surgical closure of the defect. Cultures should be obtained from the nasal cavity after anesthetizing the patient, and the nose and oral cavity

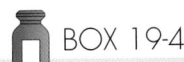
BOX 19-4

Antibiotic Treatment of Aspiration Pneumonia

Chloramphenicol (Chloromycetin)
Dogs: 50 mg/kg PO or IV, tid to qid
Cats: 20–50 mg/kg PO, IV, or SC bid to qid

Cefazolin
22 mg/kg IV, tid

Enrofloxacin
7–20 mg/kg PO or IV (must be given diluted and slowly over 30 minutes), qd*

Ampicillin
22 mg/kg IV, IM, or SC, tid to qid

Ticarcillin plus clavulanic acid (Timentin)
50 mg/kg IV, tid to qid

Amikacin (Amiglyde-V)
20–25 mg/kg IV, qd

Clindamycin (Antirobe, Cleocin)
11 mg/kg PO or IV, bid to tid

PO, Oral; *IV,* intravenous; *tid,* three times a day; *qid,* four times a day; *IM,* intramuscular; *SC,* subcutaneous; *bid,* twice a day; *qd,* once a day.
*Can cause blindness in cats receiving high doses.

flushed of debris and exudate. To prevent recontamination of the nasal cavity with food, the animal should be given nothing by mouth for 10 to 14 days. Nutrition can be provided via tube feeding (e.g., esophagostomy or gastrostomy tube; see pp. 97 and 100, respectively) during this time.

SURGICAL TREATMENT

Most animals with defects of the primary and secondary palate are euthanized or die. Surgical treatment generally is delayed until the patient is at least 8 to 12 weeks of age to allow growth and easier access to the palate. Older patients seem to have less friable tissue that holds sutures better. Palatoplasty performed before 16 weeks of age may hinder maxillofacial growth and development. Although rare, a narrower maxilla and occlusal problems may result. The primary goal of repairing a cleft palate is to reconstruct the nasal floor. Several procedures may be necessary before the entire cleft is permanently reconstructed. This is a hereditary defect; affected patients should be neutered.

Preoperative Management

Pediatric patients should not fast longer than 4 to 8 hours. After induction of anesthesia and placement of a cuffed endotracheal tube, the nasal and oral cavities should be flushed with saline and a dilute antiseptic solution. Perioperative antibiotics may be given intravenously at induction of anesthesia if the animal is not already receiving them. Poorly nourished animals should be fed through a gastrostomy or esophagostomy tube for several days before surgery.

Anesthesia

Puppies and kittens are better able to metabolize drugs after 8 weeks of age, making them better anesthetic risks. Special precautions should be taken to prevent hypothermia and hypoglycemia in young patients. Intubation through a pharyngotomy (see p. 99) or tracheotomy incision (see p. 825) may facilitate repair of secondary clefts. Pharyngotomy generally is preferred if it allows adequate visualization of the defect. General anesthetic recommendations for animals undergoing oral surgery are provided on p. 339. Guarded tracheostomy tubes should be used to prevent kinking during the procedure. Care should be taken to prevent and recognize dislodgment of the anesthetic tubing from the endotracheal tube during oral manipulations.

Surgical Anatomy

The major palatine arteries emerge from the major palatine foramen midway between the midline and caudal edge of the upper fourth premolar (see Fig. 19-1). The main artery courses rostrally equidistant between the lingual border of the teeth and the palatal midline to anastomose with the major palatine artery of the contralateral side caudal to the incisors. The minor palatine arteries enter the palate at the level of the last molar, caudal and slightly lateral to the major palatine foramen. The minor palatine arteries course caudomedially and ramify in the caudal hard palate and soft palate. The soft palate is also supplied by branches of the ascending pharyngeal artery.

Positioning

To facilitate repair of a secondary palate defect, the animal should be positioned in dorsal recumbency with the mouth maximally opened. Ventral or dorsal recumbency may be used for a primary palate repair.

SURGICAL TECHNIQUE

The first step in the repair of combined primary and secondary clefts is to separate the oral and nasal cavities by reconstructing the nasal floor. After separation the lip defect is reconstructed. Areas where flaps were harvested for closure of primary or secondary clefts are allowed to heal by secondary intention. Granulation and epithelialization usually are complete within 2 to 3 weeks.

Closure of Hard Palate Defects

The two procedures most often used to repair secondary clefts are sliding bipedicle flaps and overlapping flap techniques. Sliding bipedicle flaps (von Langenbeck technique) are created to close hard palate defects. The disadvantage of this technique is that the repair is unsupported and directly over the defect.

Incise the margins of the defect, and make bilateral releasing incisions along the margins of the dental arcade (Fig.

19-17, A). Elevate the mucoperiosteal layer on both sides of the defect with a periosteal elevator (Fig. 19-17, B). Avoid damaging the major palatine arteries. Control hemorrhage with pressure and suction. Appose the nasal mucosal edges or periosteum at the margin of the defect with buried interrupted sutures (knots within the nasal cavity) if possible. Slide the elevated mucoperiosteal flaps across the defect and appose with simple interrupted sutures (Figs. 19-17, C and D). Allow the denuded hard palate near the dental arcades to heal by secondary intention.

A variation of this technique in which a partial-thickness rather than a full-thickness incision of the mucoperiosteum is made without exposure of the palatal bone may reduce maxillofacial deformity.

An alternate technique for repair of hard palate defects is the overlapping "sandwich" technique (Figs. 19-18 and 19-19). This technique is advantageous because it does not place the repair over the palate defect.

Incise one margin of the defect separating the oral and nasal mucosa (see Fig. 19-19, A). Elevate the mucoperiosteum at this edge approximately 5 mm. At the opposite side of the defect, create a mucoperiosteal rotational flap large enough to cover the defect with its base hinged at the margin of the palatal defect (see Fig. 19-20, B). Begin the incision near and parallel to the dental arcade, creating a flap 2 to 4 mm larger than the defect. Make perpendicular incisions at the rostral and caudal end of the incision extending to the cleft. Elevate this mucoperiosteal flap, taking care not to disrupt the margin of the defect (see Fig. 19-19, B). Dissect carefully around the palatine artery to release it from fibrous tissue. Rotate the flap across the defect (see Fig. 19-19, C). Place the edge of the flap under the mucoperiosteal flap on the opposite side. Preplace and then tie a series of horizontal mattress sutures to secure the flaps in position (see Fig. 19-19, D).

> NOTE: Warn owners that several operations may be necessary to completely close large hard palate defects.

Closure of Soft Palate Defects

Incise the margins of the cleft to separate the oral and nasal mucosae. Continue incisions made in the margins of hard palate clefts caudally into the soft palate (see Fig. 19-19, D). Isolate the nasal mucosa, palatal muscles, and oral mucosa. Appose the palatal edges in three layers beginning caudally and working rostrally to a point adjacent to the caudal or midpoint of the tonsil. First appose the nasal mucosa using a series of simple interrupted sutures with nasally oriented knots or use a simple continuous pattern. Then appose the palatal muscle and connective tissue with a simple continuous suture pattern. Last, appose the oral mucosa with a simple continuous or interrupted suture pattern. Make tension-relieving incisions in the oral mucosa

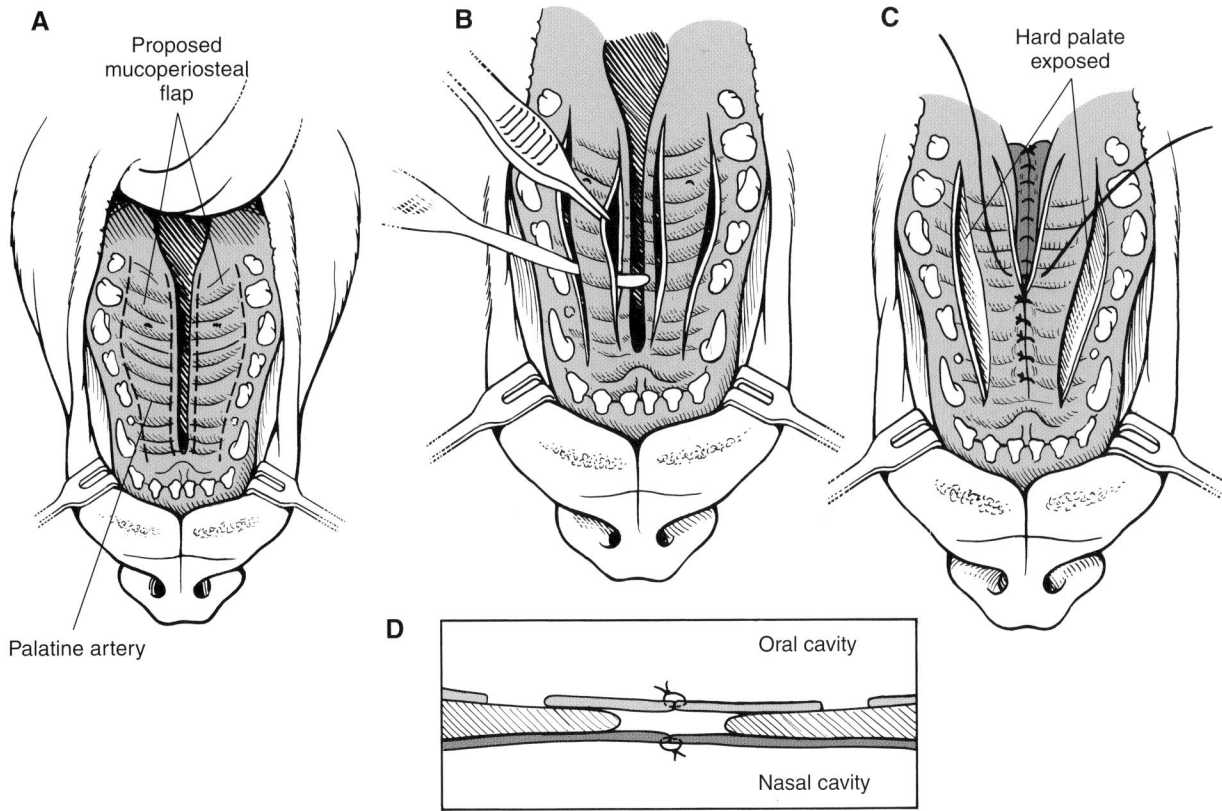

FIG. 19-17
A sliding bipedicle flap repair may be used to repair a congenital oronasal fistula. **A,** The dotted lines represent the mucoperiosteal incisions necessary to create two sliding flaps. **B,** The mucoperiosteum is elevated from the hard palate with the major palatine artery. **C,** The nasal mucosa and mucoperiosteum are apposed in two layers over the defect in the hard palate. **D,** Cross-sectional view of the repair.

from the lingual aspect of the last molar to near the tip of the soft palate.

An overlapping flap technique, rotational flaps from the hard or soft palate, and nasal or nasopharyngeal mucosal flaps can also be used to repair soft palate defects. Correction of lateral soft palate clefts generally includes an oropharyngeal/nasopharyngeal mucosal flap. Some surgeons fracture the pterygoid hamulus (where the palatal muscles attach) with an osteotome to reduce tension on the soft palate.

AP   Closure of Primary Clefts

Cosmetic repair of primary clefts can be very complicated, requiring elaborate planning to achieve a successful outcome (Fig. 19-20, *A*).

Create a mucosal flap to separate the nasal cavity from the oral cavity (Fig. 19-20, B). If the cleft extends into the premaxilla, evaluate the gingival mucosa of the deciduous incisors and pull them if necessary. Suture the buccal or gingival mucosal flap to the nasal mucosa. Use a freehand modified Z-plasty for reconstruction of the lip defect (Fig. 19-20, C).

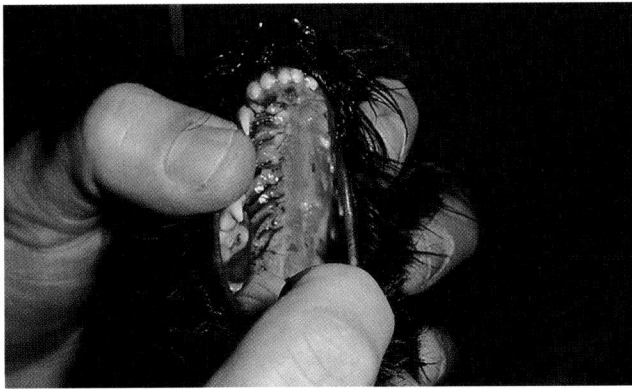

FIG. 19-18
The secondary palate of the puppy in Fig. 19-16 was repaired with an overlapping flap technique. The defect over the hard palate was allowed to heal by secondary intention.

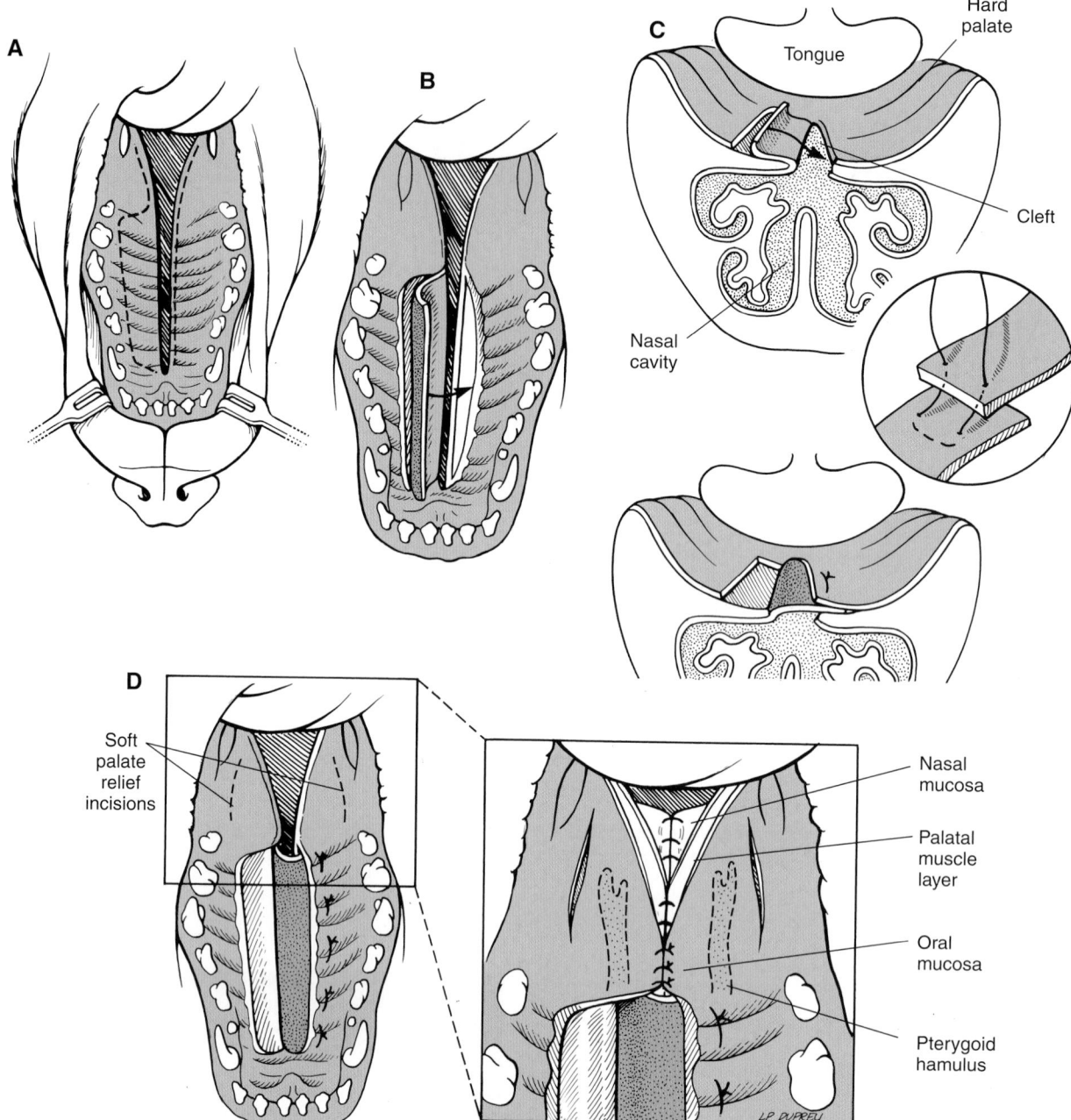

FIG. 19-19

A congenital oronasal fistula may be repaired with an overlapping flap technique. **A,** The dotted lines represent the incisions necessary to allow soft tissue closure. **B** and **C,** Elevate the mucoperiosteal flap and rotate it medially to cover the hard palate defect. Insert the edge of this flap between the hard palate and the mucoperiosteum on the opposite side of the defect. Secure the flaps in position with horizontal mattress sutures *(inset).* **D,** Complete the repair by apposing the incised edges of the cleft soft palate in three layers. Make lateral relief incisions (broken lines) to reduce tension on the repair.

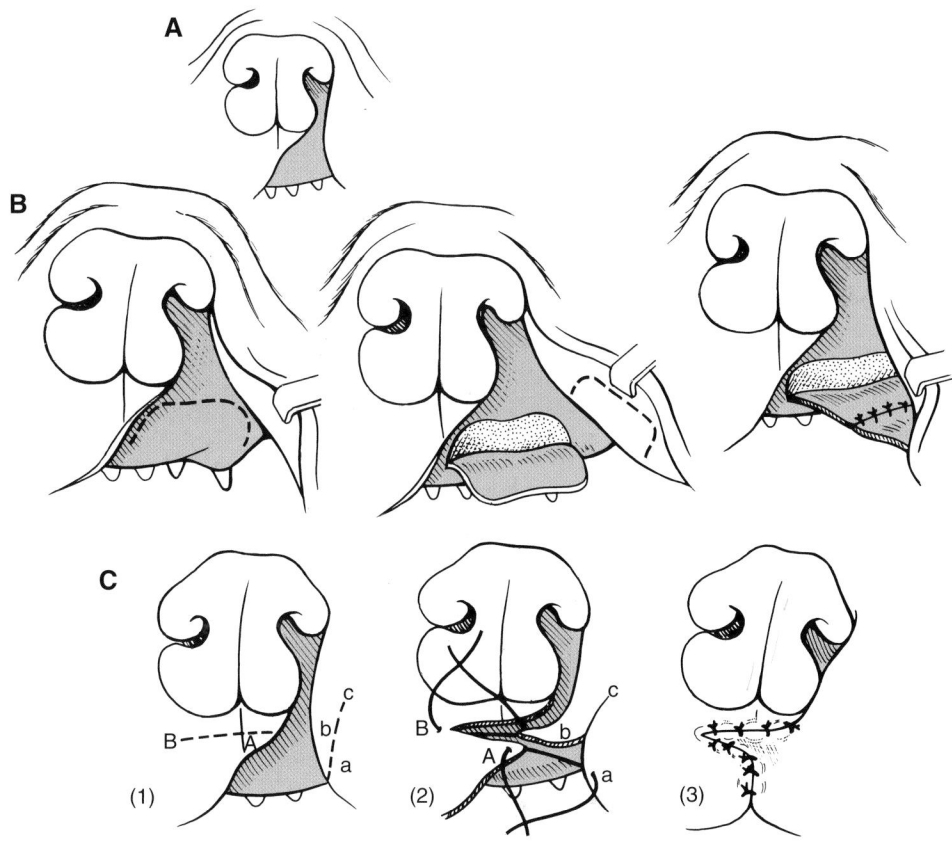

FIG. 19-20
A, Schematic drawing of a repair of a primary cleft palate involving the lip, premaxilla, and nostril. **B,** Create a flap from the nasal wall and suture it to a labial mucosal flap to separate the nasal cavity from the oral cavity. **C,** Repair the cleft lip with one or a series of Z-plasties: *(1)* Make incisions from A to B and a to c; *(2)* place a suture between A and a, and B and b, to transpose the flaps; *(3)* place additional sutures as needed.

Close the lip defect so that the distance from the ventral nostril to the free ventral edge of the lip is the same on both sides. Make multiple small flaps if necessary for a cosmetic closure. Place a layer of sutures in the fibromuscular layer (orbicularis oris muscle and connective tissue) before skin closure.

POSTOPERATIVE CARE AND ASSESSMENT

Soft food should be fed for a minimum of 2 weeks after surgery, and chewing on hard objects (e.g., bones, sticks, and chew toys) should be prevented. Gastrostomy or esophagostomy feeding for 7 to 14 days may facilitate healing. Reevaluation at 2 weeks may require anesthesia to identify small defects.

COMPLICATIONS

Dehiscence and subsequent incomplete healing of oronasal fistulae are the most common complications. Dehiscence usually occurs within 3 to 5 days of surgery, but may occur later. Early dehiscence may occur if tension is excessive, blood supply is poor, or the tissue is traumatized. Motion of the tongue against the repair and particulate matter in the surgical site can also lead to dehiscence. Early dehiscence of the lip occurs if the orbicularis oris muscle has not been apposed. Contraction of the unapposed muscle during lip movement causes excess tension on the suture line. Tissues are friable after dehiscence, therefore repair of early dehiscence should be delayed for 4 to 6 weeks to allow tissues to revascularize and regain strength. Late dehiscence is a result of growth-induced stress on the repair and is best treated after the patient matures.

PROGNOSIS

The prognosis is good for animals with successful cleft palate repair; however, several operations may be required. Chronic rhinitis and aspiration pneumonia persist if large defects are not repaired. Untreated patients with small clefts may have few clinical signs.

References

Gregory SP: Middle ear disease associated with congenital palatine defects in seven dogs and one cat, *J Small Anim Pract* 41:398, 2000.

Leenstra TS et al: Palatal surgery without denudation of bone favours dentoalveolar development in dogs, *Int J Oral Maxillofac Surg* 24:440, 1995.

Suggested Reading

Headrick JF, McAnulty JF: Reconstruction of a bilateral hypoplastic soft palate in a cat, *J Am Anim Hosp Assoc* 40:86, 2004.
This report describes soft palate reconstruction using a hard palate mucoperiosteal flap and two pharyngeal mucosal flaps.

ACQUIRED ORONASAL FISTULAE

DEFINITION/SYNONYMS

Acquired oronasal fistulae (traumatic cleft palate, palatal defect) are abnormal communications between the nasal and oral cavities caused by trauma or disease.

GENERAL CONSIDERATIONS AND CLINICALLY RELEVANT PATHOPHYSIOLOGY

Acquired palatal defects are most often caused by dental disease (Fig. 19-21). An oronasal fistula results when a deep maxillary periodontal pocket progresses to the apex of the tooth, lysing bone between the apex of the alveolus and the nasal cavity or maxillary sinus. A fistula may also result from trauma (i.e., bite wounds, gunshot wounds, blunt trauma to the head, or electrical burns) or may be a complication of surgery (e.g., mass excision or ventral rhinotomy), radiation, or hyperthermic treatment of oral lesions. Foreign bodies lodged between the dental arcades may cause pressure necrosis of the hard palate and subsequent development of an oronasal fistula (Fig. 19-22). Ingested food that passes through the fistula into the nasal cavity may be expelled from the nostril by sneezing. Chronic rhinitis is common.

DIAGNOSIS

Clinical Presentation

Signalment. Any breed or gender may acquire an oronasal fistula. Oronasal fistulae that occur secondary to dental disease or tumors are seen more often in middle-aged and older animals. Oronasal fistulae that develop secondary to trauma may occur at any age.

History. An oronasal fistula should be suspected in patients with chronic rhinitis and a history of dental disease, trauma, or previously treated oral tumors. Common clinical signs are sneezing and chronic unilateral serous or mucopurulent nasal discharge.

Physical Examination Findings

The diagnosis of an oronasal fistula can be made by identifying an abnormal communication between the oral and nasal cavities (see Figs. 19-21 and 19-22). Small fistulae associated with periodontal disease are not easily identified unless the area around the involved tooth is explored with a narrow dental probe. If passing the probe into the gingival pocket causes epistaxis, a fistula is present. The palatal aspect of the maxillary canine tooth is a common site for an oronasal fistula. Anesthesia generally is required to probe periodontal pockets.

Diagnostic Imaging

Skull radiography or cross sectional imaging may identify underlying causes of fistulae, such as periapical abscesses, advanced periodontal disease, maxillary neoplasia (see p. 361), or broken or retained tooth roots. Lysis, especially of the laminae dura around tooth roots, is indicative of periapical abscesses.

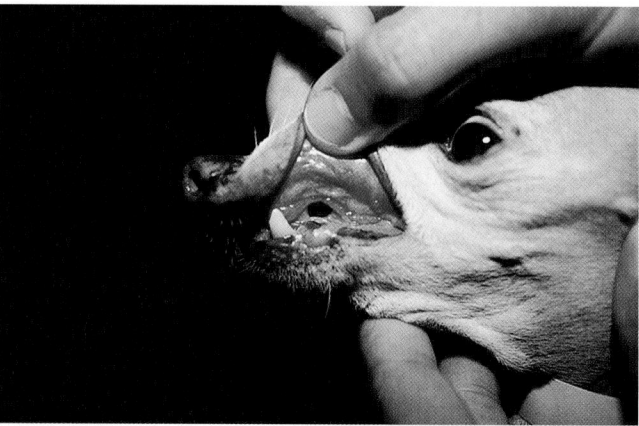

FIG. 19-21
An oronasal fistula that occurred from loss of the canine tooth.

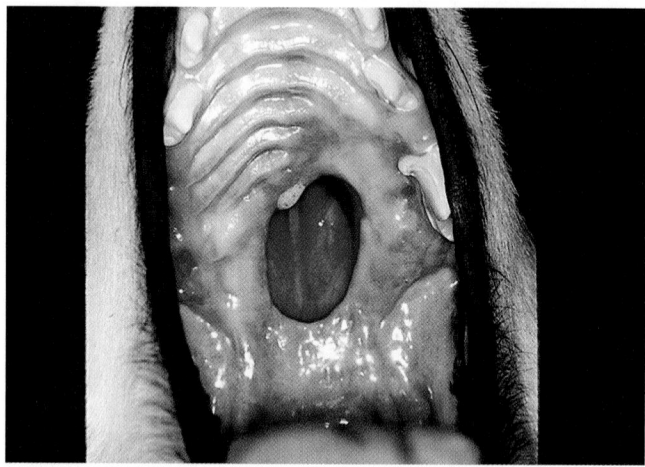

FIG. 19-22
An acquired oronasal fistula caused by a foreign body that lodged between the dental arcades.

Laboratory Findings

Inflammatory changes on a CBC may be seen secondary to rhinitis or aspiration pneumonia.

DIFFERENTIAL DIAGNOSIS

Differential diagnoses include any disease that causes chronic rhinitis (e.g., fungal disease, nasal foreign body, congenital oronasal fistula, and invasive oral neoplasia) and congenital clefts. These conditions generally can be differentiated based on physical examination, imaging, and/or histopathologic examination. Histopathologic evaluation should be performed to distinguish fistulae that occur secondary to neoplasia from those associated with infection or trauma.

MEDICAL MANAGEMENT

Broad-spectrum antibiotics effective against anaerobes (e.g., chloramphenicol, amoxicillin plus clavulanic acid, and clindamycin) should be given if severe purulent rhinitis is present (see Box 19-4). Such animals may benefit from having the nasal infection treated before closure of the defect. With the patient under general anesthetic, cultures should be obtained from the nasal cavity, and the nose and oral cavity flushed of debris and exudate. To prevent recontamination of the nasal cavity with food, the animal should be given nothing by mouth for 10 to 14 days. Nutrition can be provided via tube feeding (e.g., tube gastrostomy, p. 100, or esophagostomy, p. 97) during this time.

SURGICAL TREATMENT

Most oronasal fistulae require surgical reconstruction, although small or traumatic fistulae occasionally heal spontaneously. A variety of surgical techniques have been described for repair, including simple suturing of the fistula edges, mucosal flaps, mucoperiosteal flaps, double reposition flaps, orbicularis oris axial pattern flaps (Bryant et al, 2003), palatal island flaps (Smith, 2001), and two-staged tongue flaps. Successful repair of oronasal fistulae requires a well-supported, airtight, tension-free closure. Flap techniques are more successful than direct apposition of the fistula edges because of less tension and increased support for the repair. Teeth involved in the fistula should be extracted several weeks before reconstruction of the defect. Central lesions may require that normal teeth be extracted to allow creation of adequate mucosal flaps. If the fistula is of dental origin, it may be necessary to perform a limited maxillectomy (at least 5 mm from each margin) to remove necrotic or diseased bone. Traumatic oronasal fistulae may require stabilization of the maxilla and hard palate with small pins or wire. Interdental wiring (see p. 1016) using the carnassial teeth or the canine teeth (or both) can help bring bone edges into apposition. Areas where flaps were harvested heal by secondary intention in 2 to 3 weeks. Acrylic, Silastic, or metal obturators may also be fitted over the defect.

Preoperative Management

Pediatric patients should not fast for longer than 4 to 8 hours. After anesthetic induction the nasal and oral cavities should be flushed with saline-diluted antiseptic solution. Aggressive management of rhinitis (see previous Medical Management section) may reduce infection and improve the tissues' ability to hold a suture.

Anesthesia

General anesthetic recommendations for animals undergoing oral surgery are provided on p. 339. Intubation through a pharyngotomy (see p. 99) or tracheotomy incision (see p. 825) may facilitate repair of large or centrally located oronasal fistulae. Pharyngotomy generally is preferred if it allows adequate visualization of the defect. Care should be taken to prevent and recognize dislodgment of the anesthetic tubing from the endotracheal tube during oral manipulations.

> NOTE: Use guarded tracheostomy tubes to prevent kinking during oral procedures.

Surgical Anatomy

The surgical anatomy of the hard palate is discussed on p. 352.

Positioning

The patient should be positioned in lateral recumbency for repair of oronasal fistulae associated with the dental arcade. Dorsal recumbency with the mouth opened maximally facilitates repair of more centrally located fistulae involving the secondary palate.

SURGICAL TECHNIQUE
Direct Apposition

Direct apposition of the fistula should be performed only if the fistula is very small.

Débride the fistula to healthy, bleeding mucosal edges (Figs. 19-23, A and B). Incise or débride the margin of the fistula and elevate the edges enough to allow approximation without excess tension. Appose the mucosa with interrupted appositional sutures (i.e., simple, cruciate, or vertical mattress pattern) (Fig. 19-23, C).

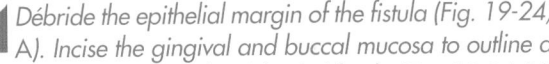

Single-Layer Flap Repair

Débride the epithelial margin of the fistula (Fig. 19-24, A). Incise the gingival and buccal mucosa to outline a flap 2 to 4 mm larger than the débrided fistula (Fig. 19-24, B). Make these incisions perpendicular to the dental arcade. Elevate the gingival mucosa with a periosteal elevator. Then undermine the buccal mucosa until the flap can be advanced across the defect without tension (Fig. 19-24, C). Using a rongeur, remove infected alveolar and maxillary bone. Expose approximately 1 to 2 mm of the hard palate at the medial aspect of the fistula by excising 1 to 2 mm of mucoperiosteum. Lavage the surgical site with saline. Suture the gingival-buccal flap to the mucoperiosteum of the hard palate in an interrupted approximating pattern (i.e., simple, cruciate, or vertical mattress) using monofilament, absorbable (3-0 to 4-0) sutures.

Inclusion of the angularis oris artery, which arises from the facial artery caudal to the commissure of the lips, during flap creation yields a mobile, strong flap with a good blood supply that may extend to the ipsilateral canine or across the palate to the opposite dental arcade (Bryant et al, 2003).

Rotational Flap Repair

A rotational or advancement flap may be created from the hard or soft palate (Figs. 19-24, D to G), or an overlapping technique similar to that described for repair of congenital oronasal fistulae may be used (see p. 352).

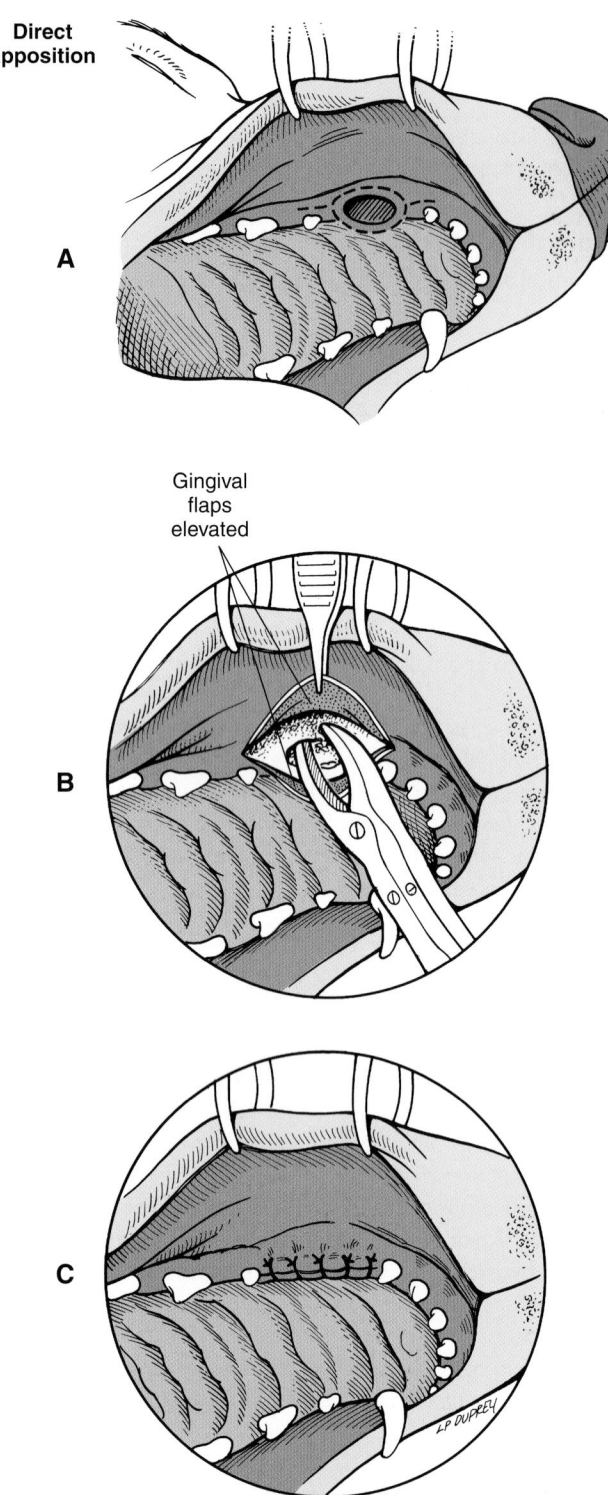

Direct apposition

Gingival flaps elevated

FIG. 19-23
Small fistulae may be repaired with a direct appositional technique. **A,** Incise the mucosa around the fistula. **B,** Elevate the gingival flaps and débride the edges of the fistula. **C,** Appose the mucosa over the defect.

Create a flap 2 to 4 mm larger than the débrided fistula. To ensure a good blood supply, incorporate the major or minor palatine artery in palatal flaps. Transpose and suture the flap over the defect (see Figs. 19-24, D to G).

> Granulation tissue fills the defect over the hard palate, and the area reepithelializes within a few weeks.

Double-Flap Repair

Double-flap techniques may be used with large dental fistulae and with fistulae located in more central areas of the palate. Double-flap techniques provide a mucosal surface on both the oral and nasal sides of the fistula. If buccal flaps are planned to close large central defects, extraction of teeth may be necessary. The extraction sites should be allowed to heal before reconstruction. Do not débride the palatal epithelial margin during débridement of the fistula because this edge serves as the base of the mucoperiosteal flap and must remain continuous with the nasal mucosa to be effective.

Create a flap in the mucoperiosteum 2 to 4 mm larger than the débrided fistula (Figs. 19-25 to 19-27). Elevate the flap without disrupting the palatal margin of the fistula. Fold the flap over the defect, and suture it to the gingival mucosa with interrupted, approximating, monofilament, absorbable sutures for the first layer of closure (see Fig. 19-25). This flap provides "nasal" mucosa. Create a rotational mucoperiosteal flap 2 to 4 mm larger than the defect for the second layer of closure (see Fig. 19-25). Appose this flap to the gingival mucosa with approximating 3-0 to 4-0 sutures. To ensure a good blood supply, incorporate the major palatine artery in palatal flaps. As an alternative, create one or two mucoperiosteal flaps 2 to 4 mm larger than the defect (see Fig. 19-27, A). Transpose and suture the flap in place for the first layer of the closure (see Fig. 19-27, B). This flap provides "nasal" mucosa. Cover this layer with a mucosal flap (gingival and buccal) to provide the "oral" mucosal layer of the closure (see Fig. 19-27, C and D). Allow the denuded hard palate to heal by secondary intention.

POSTOPERATIVE CARE AND ASSESSMENT

Intravenous fluids should be provided until the animal begins eating and drinking (usually within 24 hours of surgery). Soft food should be fed for 2 to 3 weeks, and chewing on hard objects (i.e., toys or sticks) must be prevented to avoid dehiscence or perforation of the flap separating the oral and nasal cavities. If the animal paws at the mouth, an Elizabethan collar should be used. Severe rhinitis should be treated with antibiotics (see Box 19-4). Healing should be evaluated 2 and 4 weeks after surgery.

COMPLICATIONS

Most oronasal fistulae are successfully repaired if flaps can be apposed without tension and with a good blood supply. Dehiscence and recurrence of the oronasal fistula

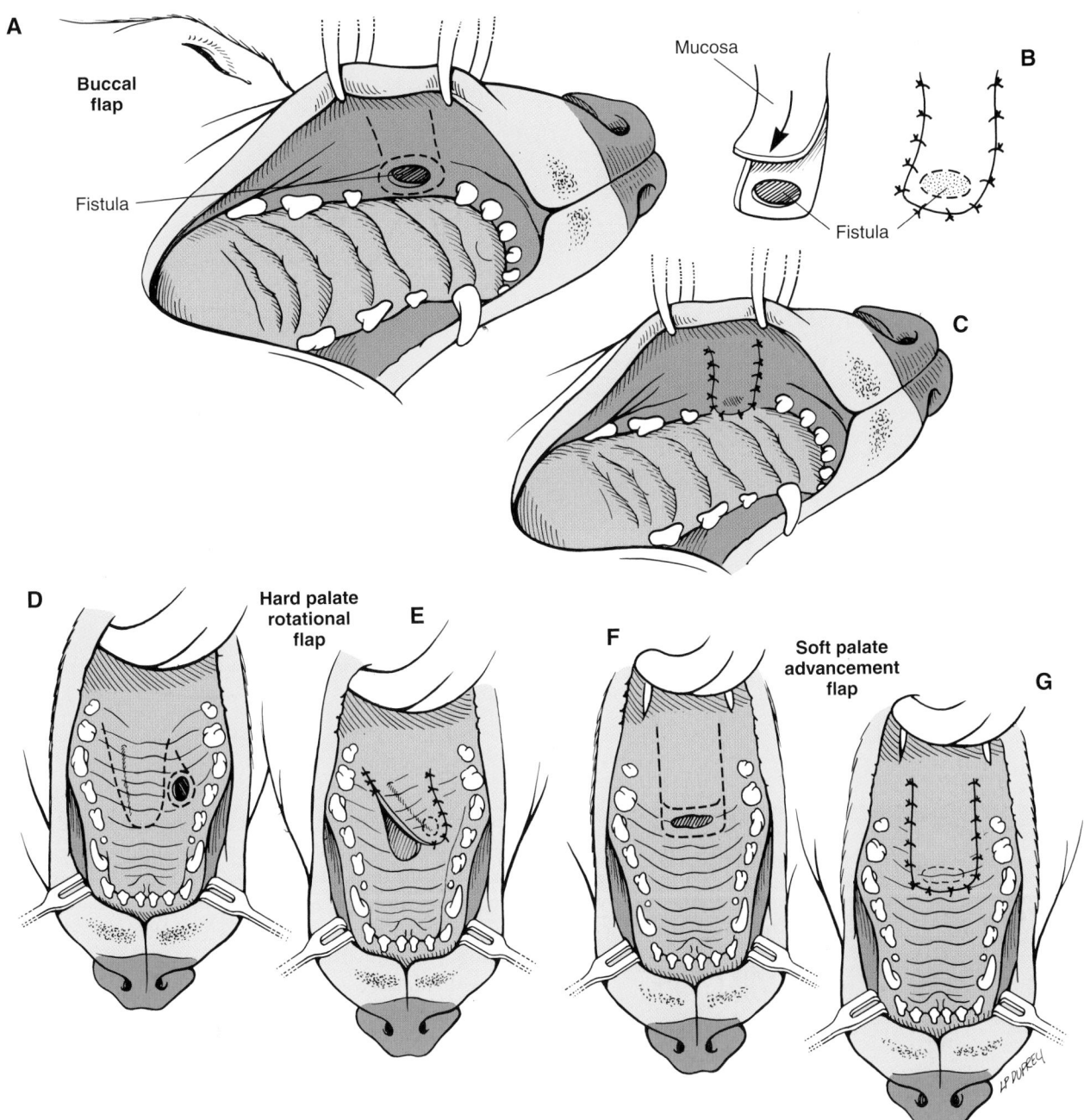

FIG. 19-24

Single-flap technique for fistula repair. **A,** Incise mucosa around the fistula to create the buccal flap *(dashed line),* then débride the fistula. **B** and **C,** Advance a buccal flap over the defect and suture into place. **D** and **E,** After débriding the fistula, create a hard palate rotational flap *(dashed line)* and rotate the mucoperiosteal hard palate flap over the defect. Suture the flap to surround the mucoperiosteum. **F** and **G,** To repair lesions at the junction of the hard and soft palates, débride the defect, then create and close the defect with a soft palate advancement flap *(caudal dashed line).*

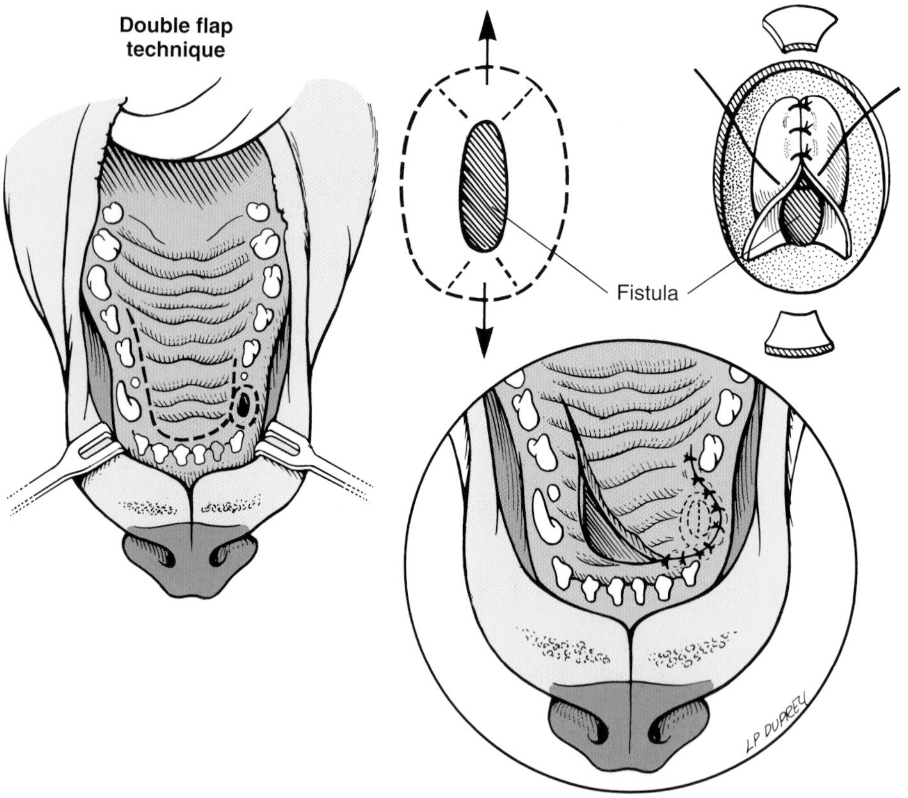

**Double flap
technique**

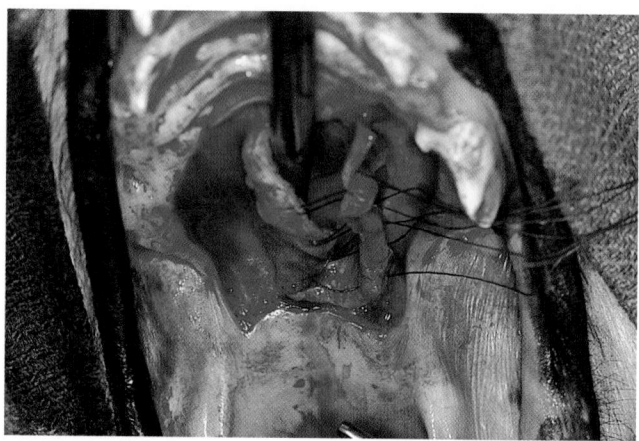

FIG. 19-25
A double-layer flap technique may be performed using tissue surrounding the fistula and a flap from the mucoperiosteum of the hard palate. Create the first flap *(gingival dashed line)* by rotating the gingival margins of the fistula medially and apposing with sutures *(top insert)*. Cover this flap *(bottom insert)* with a rotational mucoperiosteal hard palate flap *(palatal dashed)*.

Fistula

FIG. 19-26
Intraoperative photograph showing repair of an oronasal fistula using a double-layer flap technique. The margins of the fistula have been elevated and rotated medially to cover the defect. This flap was later covered with a flap created from the buccal mucosa.

are expected if conditions for healing are not ideal. Motion of the tongue against the repair and particulate matter in the surgical site can also lead to dehiscence. Tension, poor blood supply, infection, poor débridement, lack of flap support, and traumatic technique may inhibit healing. Additional attempts to repair recurring fistulae should be delayed 4 to 6 weeks to allow sites of previous flap harvesting to heal, revascularize, and mature before additional flaps are created. Rhinitis should resolve after the fistula has healed if irreversible mucosal changes have not occurred.

PROGNOSIS

Traumatic clefts may heal spontaneously in 2 to 4 weeks. Signs of rhinitis caused by regurgitation of food into the nasal cavity may be controlled with chronic antibiotic therapy. The long-term prognosis for most patients with nontraumatic fistulae is poor when surgical correction is not possible because fistulae do not heal without surgical reconstruction.

References

Bryant KJ, Moore K, McAnulty JF: Angularis oris axial pattern buccal flap for reconstruction of recurrent fistulae of the palate, *Vet Surg* 32:113, 2003.

Smith MM: Island palatal mucoperiosteal flap for repair of oronasal fistula in a dog, *J Vet Dent* 18(3):127, 2001.

Double-flap technique

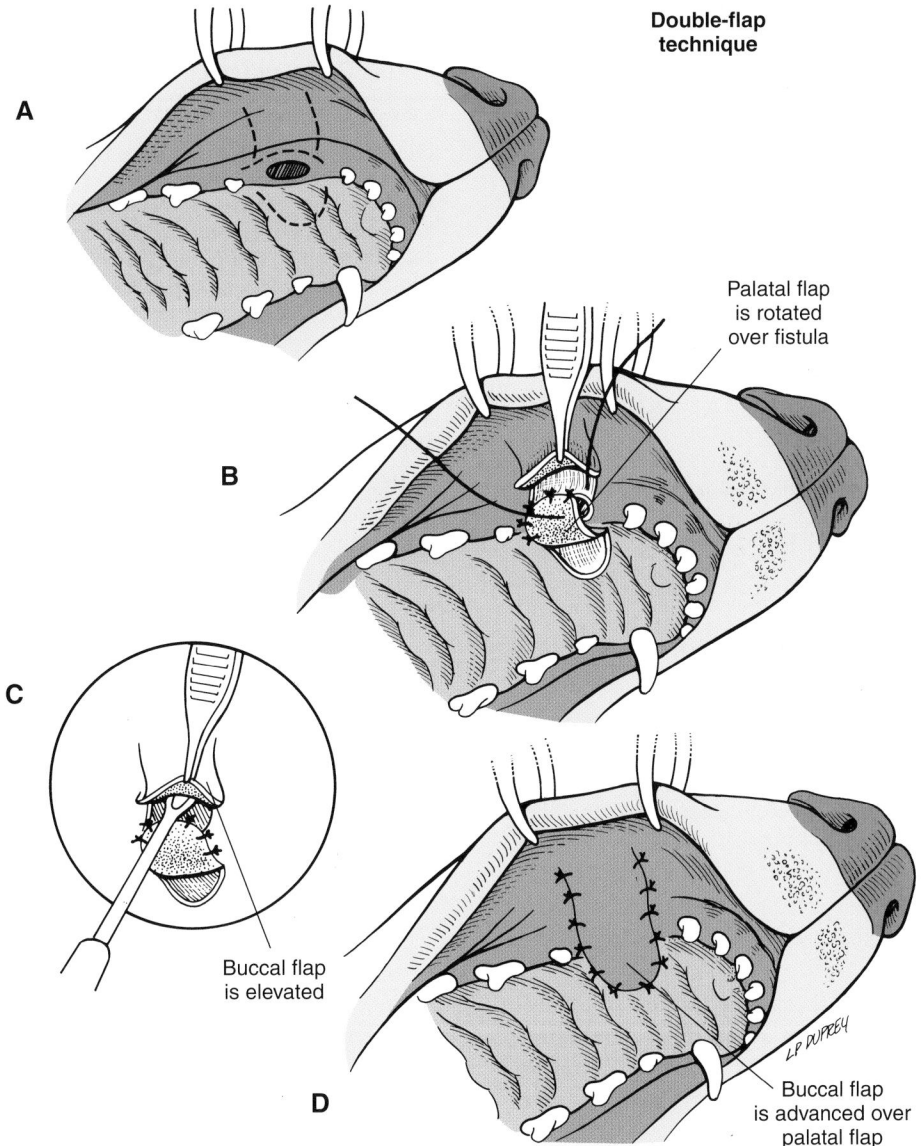

A

B Palatal flap is rotated over fistula

C Buccal flap is elevated

D Buccal flap is advanced over palatal flap

LP DUPREY

FIG. 19-27
A double-layer flap technique for fistula repair may be performed using a mucoperiosteal hard palate flap *(palatal dashed line)* and a buccal flap *(buccal dashed lines)*. **A** and **B,** Create a flap from the mucoperiosteum of the hard palate *(palatal and gingival dashed lines)*; rotate and suture to gingival margin. **C** and **D,** Cover it with a second flap created from the buccal mucosa *(inset)*, then advance and suture over the first flap.

ORAL TUMORS

DEFINITIONS

Oral tumors encompass those neoplasms that arise from the gingiva, buccal mucosa, labial mucosa, tongue, tonsils, or dental elements. Malignant melanoma is also known as *melanosarcoma;* ameloblastoma is also referred to as *adamantinoma.*

GENERAL CONSIDERATIONS AND CLINICALLY RELEVANT PATHOPHYSIOLOGY

The oral cavity is the fourth most common site of neoplasia in dogs and cats; oral tumors account for 5% (dogs) to 7% (cats) of all malignant tumors in these species. Oral tumors occur 2.6 times more often in dogs than in cats. Malignant oral tumors have a higher relative risk of occurring in male than in female dogs. Oral tumors originate from the mucosa, tongue, periodontium, odontogenic tissue, mandible, maxilla, tonsils, and lips, spreading by direct extension or invasion of adjacent bone and cartilaginous tissue. Metastasis occurs by lymphatics or blood to the regional lymph nodes and lungs. All tumors should be clinically staged according to the TNM classification system (primary tumor, regional lymph nodes, and metastasis) described by the World Health Organization (Box 19-5).

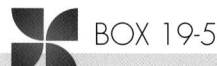

BOX 19-5

Clinical Stage Classification System for Canine and Feline Tumors of the Oral Cavity*

The following are the minimum requirements for assessing the T, N, and M categories (if these cannot be met, the symbols TX, NX, and MX should be used).

   T categories: Clinical and surgical examination
   N categories: Clinical and surgical examination
   M categories: Clinical and surgical examination, radiography of the thorax

T: Primary Tumor

   Tis—Preinvasive carcinoma (carcinoma in situ)
   T0—No evidence of tumor
   T1—Tumor less than 2 cm maximum diameter
   T1a—Without bone invasion
   T1b—With bone invasion
   T2—Tumor 2 to 4 cm maximum diameter
   T2a—Without bone invasion
   T2b—With bone invasion
   T3—Tumor greater than 4 cm maximum diameter
   T3a—Without bone invasion
   T3b—With bone invasion
   The symbol m added to the appropriate T category indicates multiple tumors.

N: Regional Lymph Nodes (RLN)†

   N0—No evidence of regional lymph node involvement
   N1—Movable ipsilateral nodes
   N1a—Nodes not considered to contain growth‡
   N1b—Nodes considered to contain growth‡
   N2—Movable contralateral or bilateral nodes
   N2a—Nodes not considered to contain growth‡
   N2b—Nodes considered to contain growth‡
   N3—Fixed nodes

M: Distant Metastasis

   M0—No evidence of metastasis
   M1—Distant metastasis (including distant nodes) detected; specify site or sites

Stage Grouping

	T	N	M
I	T1	N0, N1a, or N2a	M0
II	T2	N0, N1a, or N2a	M0
III§	T3	N0, N1a, or N2a	M0
	Any T	N1b	
IV	Any T	Any N2b or N3	M0
	Any T	Any N	M1

*Modified from document VPH/CMO/80.20, World Health Organization, 1980; reproduced with permission.
†The regional lymph nodes are the cervical, submandibular, and parotid nodes.
‡ (−), Histologically negative; (+), histologically positive.
§Any bone involvement.

The most common malignant canine tumors are malignant melanoma, squamous cell carcinoma (SCC), and fibrosarcoma; squamous cell carcinoma is the most common malignant oral tumor in cats. Other malignancies are listed in Box 19-6. Benign oral tumors are rare in cats. The most common benign oral neoplasms in dogs are epulides; other benign oral lesions are listed in Box 19-6.

Malignant melanomas are the most common malignant oral tumor in dogs; they rarely occur in cats (Box 19-7). Melanomas are rapidly growing, white-gray or brown-black tumors that are firm and vascular. They usually occur on the gingiva and are characterized by early local invasion. Some types are easily mistaken at histology for fibrosarcoma. Metastasis to the regional lymph nodes and lungs occurs in 80% of cases. Wide surgical excision using partial maxillectomy, mandibulectomy, tonsillectomy, or glossectomy is recommended. Radiation therapy may be used, but there is a high rate of recurrence. The response to radiotherapy may be better if concurrent hyperthermia is used, but the high rate of metastasis makes long-time survival unlikely (Proulx et al, 2003). Administering cisplatin or carboplatin before radiation therapy provides better local control than radiation therapy alone (Freeman et al, 2003). Chemotherapy and immunotherapy are of minimal benefit in treating malignant melanomas; however, research continues into the use of immunotherapy and biologic response modifiers.

SCC is the most common malignant oral tumor in cats and the second most common malignant oral tumor in dogs (Box 19-8). Increased risk of SCC in cats has been associated with flea control products, diet, and environmental tobacco smoke (Bertone et al, 2003). These tumors occur on the gingiva, lip, tongue, or tonsil. The masses are red, friable, vascular, and sometimes ulcerated. Most tumors in the rostral oropharynx are locally invasive, often invading bone, and have a low metastatic potential, whereas those in the caudal oropharynx tend to be more infiltrative and metastasize more rapidly. Canine gingival SCC tends to be highly invasive and osteolytic, but has a low rate of metastasis. Feline gingival SCC has a poorer prognosis than canine SCC. Wide resection is recommended for gingival tumors. They are radiosensitive, and combining radiotherapy with hyperthermia has been effective. Investigations into the use of chemotherapy alone or as an adjunct to surgery continue (De Vos et al, 2005). Tonsillar SCC grows rapidly and is associated with early local invasion and a high rate of lymph node and lung metastasis. These tumors occur most often in male urban dogs; tonsillar SCC has rarely been reported in cats. The prognosis for these tumors is guarded. SCCs may also occur on the tongue.

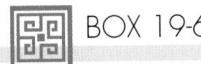 BOX 19-6

Types of Oral Tumors

Malignant
- Malignant melanoma
- Squamous cell carcinoma
- Fibrosarcoma
- Osteosarcoma
- Lymphosarcoma
- Mast cell tumor
- Gingival hemangiosarcoma
- Neurofibrosarcoma
- Anaplastic sarcoma
- Chondrosarcoma
- Myxosarcoma
- Invasive nasal tumors
- Transmissible venereal tumor
- Histiocytic neoplasia

Benign
- Epulides
- Viral papillomatosis
- Odontogenic tumors: adamantinoma* (ameloblastoma)
- Fibroma
- Peripheral giant cell granuloma
- Chondroma
- Lipoma
- Hemangioma
- Plasma cell tumor

*Biologic behavior is unpredictable.

 BOX 19-7

Characteristics of Oral Malignant Melanomas

- Most common malignant oral tumor in dogs (approximately 20%)
- Rare in cats
- Most common on gingiva
- More common in male dogs
- Mean age of affected animals is 9 to 11 years (10.3)
- Breeds with pigmented oral mucosa, cocker spaniels, and German shepherds may be predisposed
- Metastasis is common
- Prognosis is poor; median survival is 8 to 9 months

 BOX 19-8

Characteristics of Oral Squamous Cell Carcinomas

- Most common tumor in cats (approximately 70%)
- Second most common tumor in dogs (with fibrosarcoma) (approximately 15%)
- Occur on the gingiva, lip, tongue, or tonsil
- Biologic behavior varies with location and species; regional lymph node involvement is common with tongue and tonsillar squamous cell carcinomas

 BOX 19-9

Characteristics of Oral Fibrosarcomas

- Second most common malignant oral tumor in dogs (with squamous cell carcinoma)
- Occur most commonly on the gingiva and hard palate
- More common in large breeds (i.e., more than 20 kg) and male dogs
- Younger dogs may be affected (mean age under 7 years)
- Locally invasive; high metastatic potential in dogs under 2 years of age

median tumor control time with radiation alone may be as long as 12 months. Aggressive postoperative radiation therapy has improved survival times, but cryotherapy is believed to stimulate recurrence.

Osteosarcomas account for approximately 10% of canine mandibular and maxillary tumors. They are locally aggressive and have a high metastatic potential. The response to conventional therapies (i.e., surgery, radiation, and chemotherapy) is poor, although survival is longer than with appendicular osteosarcoma.

The epulides are the most common benign oral neoplasms, accounting for 30% of all canine oral neoplasms (Box 19-10). They are rare in cats. These tumors are firm gingival masses that arise from the periodontal ligament. There are three types of epulides: fibromatous, ossifying, and acanthomatous. Fibromatous epulides are noninvasive, firm, smooth, pink masses that originate at the gingival sulcus and may be single or multiple, and pedunculated or sessile (Fig. 19-28). The primary cell type is periodontal ligament stroma. Ossifying epulides are similar to fibromatous epulides except that they have large amounts of osteoid matrix in the stroma of the periodontal ligament. They are firm and difficult to cut. Malignant transformation to osteosarcoma has been reported. Acanthomatous epulides are classified as benign masses, but they are often locally aggressive and sometimes difficult to differentiate histologically from SCC. They are the most common type of epulis and frequently infiltrate

Fibrosarcomas are found primarily in dogs (Box 19-9). They most commonly occur on the maxillary gingiva and hard palate, and appear as pink-red, firm, smooth, multilobulated masses that often are attached to underlying tissue. Local infiltration with bony involvement is common, but distant metastasis is uncommon. Local recurrence is high with any treatment; wide surgical resection is recommended. Most fibrosarcomas are poorly responsive to chemotherapy. Fibrosarcomas generally are radioresistant, although the

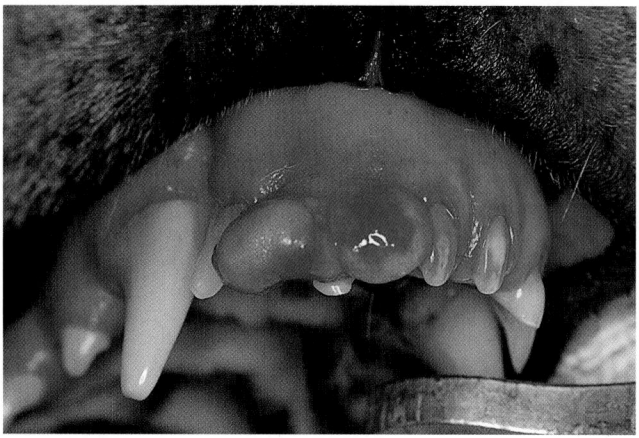

FIG. 19-28
Appearance of a fibromatous epulis surrounding the maxillary incisors in a dog.

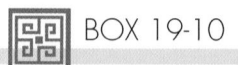 BOX 19-10

Characteristics of Epulides

- Most common oral tumor in dogs (approximately 30%)
- Mean age about 8.2 years
- More common in large-breed dogs (i.e., more than 20 kg)
- Do not metastasize
- Acanthomatous epulis is most common form

bone, causing lysis. Acanthomatous epulides most often occur rostral to the mandibular canine teeth. They are primarily composed of epithelial cells arranged in sheets and cords intimately associated with the underlying stroma and invading bone. Wide surgical excision is recommended even though they are radiosensitive. They recur locally if not treated adequately.

Ameloblastomas (adamantinomas) are benign tumors that arise from the dental lamina. They usually occur in younger dogs and involve the rostral mandible. Ameloblastomas develop as intraosseous tumors and are locally invasive and nonmetastasizing. Odontomas are rare, benign odontogenic tumors that arise from the dental follicle and cause induction of both enamel and dentin in the lesion. Dentigerous cysts appear as closed cavities or sacs with one or more teeth embedded in the cyst wall. They arise within islands of odontogenic epithelium and are described as benign, nonneoplastic lesions; however, they may represent an early stage of malignant epithelial tumor development.

Oral papillomas are benign tumors caused by a papillomavirus or papovavirus in young dogs. They occur primarily on the buccal and gingival mucosa, appearing as multiple gray-white pedunculated lesions. Papillomas spontaneously regress within 2 months in most dogs as immunity to the viral agent develops. Surgical resection is necessary only to confirm the diagnosis or in dogs that are dysphagic as a result of many large papillomas. Some animals have been treated with autogenous vaccines, but this is not recommended because malignant skin tumors may develop at the site of inoculation.

DIAGNOSIS
Clinical Presentation

Signalment. Breeds that appear to be predisposed to oral tumors include boxers, German shepherds, golden retrievers, cocker spaniels, poodles, German shorthaired pointers, collies, Old English sheepdogs, and Weimaraners. Oral tumors are generally observed in middle-aged or older animals (older than 7 to 10 years). Exceptions to this include oral papillomatosis (typically occurs in dogs 1 year old or younger) and fibrosarcoma (mean age of occurrence of approximately 5 years).

Melanomas are more common in males (the reported male to female ratio has been as high as 4:1) with an average age of onset of 9 to 11 years. Breeds with pigmented oral mucosa, cocker spaniels, and German shepherds appear to have an increased incidence. SCCs usually occur in cats of either gender older than 10 years of age. Nontonsillar SCCs are most common in small-breed dogs of either gender between 8 and 10 years of age. Fibrosarcomas occur more commonly in large-breed dogs, particularly Doberman pinschers and golden retrievers. Males are affected more often than females (2:1). For fibrosarcomas, the age of onset is younger (4 to 5 years) in large-breed dogs (more than 25 kg) than in smaller dogs (8 years or older). Oral osteosarcomas most often affect the mandible and occur in females more often than in males (1.8:1). Fibromatous epulides are common in boxers.

NOTE: Remember, not all melanomas are pigmented; amelanotic melanomas may be easily confused with other oral tumors.

History. Oral tumors often are large when recognized by an owner; however, some are found during yearly examinations or routine dentistry. Neoplasia should be suspected during dentistry if teeth are excessively mobile. Affected animals frequently are presented for evaluation of a visible mass, oral bleeding, difficulty eating, or halitosis. Anorexia, weight loss, loose or displaced teeth, salivation, facial deformity, and/or nasal discharge may also be noted. A history of recent tooth extraction may precede rapid growth of a mass at the extraction site. Clinical signs in dogs with tonsillar SCC may be related to oropharyngeal obstruction (i.e., dyspnea, anorexia, cough, or drooling), and a large ventral cervical swelling may be associated with lymph node metastasis.

Physical Examination Findings

Oral tumors arising from the rostral portion of the oral cavity generally are easily viewed; however, examination for tonsillar or caudal oropharyngeal tumors may require sedation or anesthesia. General anesthetic often is necessary to define the extent of disease. The surface of growing neoplasms may appear ulcerated, infected, and necrotic. Regional lymph nodes should be evaluated for evidence of enlargement, nodularity, and adherence to surrounding tissue.

> NOTE: When you first observe the tumor, measure it and record its location, particularly if treatment is to be delayed.

Diagnostic Imaging

Three-view thoracic radiographs should be obtained to look for pulmonary metastasis and concurrent pulmonary or cardiovascular disease. Ventrodorsal and both lateral radiographic views should be taken because tumors may be missed on a single lateral view as a result of recumbent atelectasis. Further therapy may not be indicated if metastasis is noted. Skull radiographs, CT, or MRI studies are performed with the patient under general anesthetic and are used to assess the extent of the lesion and bony involvement. Malignant tumors show a tendency for irregular, destructive, or aggressive bone loss, whereas bone production predominates in benign tumors.

Laboratory Findings

Laboratory examination of animals with oral tumors should include a CBC, chemistry profile, and bleeding time. In older dogs and those with evidence of renal or cardiac disease, urinalysis and ECG are appropriate. Other than anemia of chronic blood loss, abnormalities related to the tumor are uncommon.

DIFFERENTIAL DIAGNOSIS

Granulation tissue secondary to foreign body, trauma, or infection; eosinophilic granuloma complex; and gingival hyperplasia are the primary differential diagnoses. Other differentials include leishmaniasis and dental disease. Fluctuant swellings in the sublingual and pharyngeal area may be salivary mucoceles (see p. 367) or congenital cysts. Other differential diagnoses include nasopharyngeal polyp, osteomyelitis, and feline plasma cell gingivitis-pharyngitis. Cytologic or histologic analysis of masses may be necessary to differentiate neoplastic from some nonneoplastic oral lesions.

MEDICAL MANAGEMENT

Cytologic analysis of the tumor and draining lymph nodes is indicated before surgery. Excisional or incisional biopsy (see p. 341) usually is necessary to determine the prognosis and treatment. Treatment modalities other than surgery that have been used alone or in combination for oral tumors include radiotherapy, hyperthermia, chemotherapy, cryosurgery, immunotherapy, and photodynamic therapy. SCCs are radiosensitive and are successfully treated by this radiotherapy. Fibrosarcomas are radioresistant. Melanomas may be sensitive to radiotherapy, but distant metastasis frequently renders it ineffective. Radiation-induced tumors occur in up to 20% of the irradiated sites. The prognosis after treatment with chemotherapy, immunotherapy, hyperthermia, and photodynamic therapy needs further investigation. Refer to an oncology text for additional information about these techniques.

SURGICAL TREATMENT

Treatment protocols must be based on the tumor type, site, extent, and stage; the patient's age and health; and treatment limitations. Early, aggressive therapy offers the best chance of success in treating oral malignancies. Aggressive surgical excision (e.g., mandibulectomy and maxillectomy) may be curative for gingival tumors if resection is completed before metastasis occurs. Because most gingival tumors invade bone, mandibulectomy or maxillectomy usually is necessary. Shaving the tumor down to bone generally results in recurrence. Caudal tumors and those crossing the midline may be unresectable, or the area may be difficult to reconstruct successfully with flaps. Excision of the middle and caudal maxilla is limited by the size of mucosal flap that can be created. Mandibulectomy is limited by the medial and caudal extent of the tumor (see p. 343). Tumors invading the sublingual musculature and caudal pharynx may not be resectable. Tumor extension into the lip necessitates full-thickness lip resection with partial maxillectomy (see p. 342) or mandibulectomy.

> NOTE: Owners often think that their pets will be unacceptably disfigured after major oral resections. It may help to show them pictures of animals that have had procedures similar to the one you are recommending for their pet.

Preoperative Management

Perioperative antibiotics are indicated for oral tumors, which often have focal areas of necrosis and infection (see p. 340). Debilitated animals may require IV fluids and enteral or parenteral hyperalimentation before surgery.

Anesthesia

General anesthetic protocols for animals undergoing oral surgery are given on p. 339. Sedation or general anesthetic may be required for fine-needle aspiration, depending on the location of the tumor and the animal's disposition. General anesthetic generally is recommended for biopsy because of subsequent bleeding. Surgical excision of tumors requires general anesthetic with inhalant anesthetics. Because most affected animals are old, isoflurane is the inhalant anesthetic of choice. Cuffed endotracheal tubes, preferably guarded to prevent kinking, should be used. Intubation may be accomplished through a pharyngotomy (see p. 99) or tracheotomy (see p. 825) if necessary to facilitate surgery. Nerve blocks provide analgesia and reduce the amount of other anesthetic drugs needed during surgery (see Chapter 13). Sterile sponges should be placed in the caudal oropharynx to prevent aspiration of blood.

Surgical Anatomy

The surgical anatomy of the oropharynx is discussed on p. 340.

Positioning

Mandibular lesions usually are resected with the patient in lateral recumbency. Maxillary lesions may be resected with the patient in lateral or ventral recumbency.

AP SURGICAL TECHNIQUE

Identify the soft tissue and/or bone to be resected and remove them according to the techniques for maxillectomy, mandibulectomy, glossectomy, and tonsillectomy described on pp. 342 to 348. Radiographing the excised segment before wound closure may help determine whether adequate bone was removed; however, tumor growth up the mandibular foramen may necessitate wider margins than radiographic evaluation of bone destruction might predict. Intraoperative cytologic evaluation often is more beneficial in determining the adequacy of resection. Submit excised tissue for histologic analysis. If additional bone is excised, mark the caudal border to allow determination of whether additional resection is necessary (i.e., if this margin contains a tumor). Concurrent or prior excision of regional lymph nodes (mandibular, parotid, and medial retropharyngeal) is important in staging the disease.

POSTOPERATIVE CARE AND ASSESSMENT

Sponges should be removed from the caudal oropharynx, and the oral cavity and nasopharynx suctioned before anesthetic recovery. Analgesics (i.e., hydromorphone, butorphanol, or buprenorphine; see Table 13-4 on p. 133) should be provided postoperatively. Soft food and water may be offered the day after surgery. Intravenous fluids may be discontinued when the animal maintains hydration by drinking. Dogs are seldom reluctant to eat after surgery; however, cats may require 2 to 3 days to adapt. The patient should be reevaluated 1 and 2 weeks after surgery to assess healing. Sutures usually are extruded or sloughed 2 to 4 weeks postoperatively. Facial swelling usually resolves within 3 to 7 days after surgery. Thoracic radiographs may be taken at 3, 6, and 12 months postoperatively to evaluate for metastases, and oral examinations should be performed regularly to look for tumor recurrence. After partial maxillectomy or mandibulectomy, excessive dental tartar may accumulate on the teeth of the opposite dental arch. Owner satisfaction after partial mandibulectomy or maxillectomy usually is good.

COMPLICATIONS

Tumor recurrence and dehiscence are the most common complications after major oral reconstruction. Overall, tumor recurrence after resection with tumor-free margins is less than 40%. Recurrence in these cases is due to the presence of a multifocal tumor, development of a new tumor, or inadequate pathologic assessment. Dehiscence occurs in less than one third of cases with major reconstruction. Suture line tension, excessive use of electrocautery, ischemic necrosis of a mucosal flap, excessive flap movement, infection, and tumor recurrence are major causes of dehiscence. Dehiscence occurs more often if surgery is combined with radiotherapy or chemotherapy because these adjuvant therapies may inhibit wound healing.

PROGNOSIS

The prognosis for oral tumors depends on the type of tumor, its biologic behavior, and the stage of disease. The prognosis is good for benign oral tumors, whereas the prognosis for malignant oral tumors is poor. The best chance for cure or control of malignant or benign oral tumors is surgical resection and reconstruction. Elimination of local disease is essential. Overall the 1-year survival rate is approximately 50%, with a median survival time of 8 months for dogs with malignant maxillary tumors. For malignant mandibular tumors the overall 1-year survival rate is 45%, with a median survival time of 11 months. Dogs with tumors rostral to the maxillary canine or the first mandibular premolar teeth have a better prognosis. This may be because of earlier recognition, altered tumor behavior based on location, or prevalence of tumor type.

SCCs respond best to surgery because they are localized and usually have not metastasized. In dogs, more than 50% of SCCs are controlled locally for a year or more, and the mean survival time is approximately 13 to 19 months. Reports of 1-year survival rates vary from 50% to 91%. Fibrosarcomas are localized, but are aggressive and difficult to resect completely. Recurrence of up to 80% in the first year after resection has been reported. The mean postexcision survival time varies from 10 to 14 months, and 1-year survival rates vary from 21% to 50%. Melanomas have the poorest prognosis because they metastasize early. Fewer than 20% of affected animals are disease free 1 year after surgery, and the mean survival time is 9 months. Reported median survival times vary from 8 to 10 months. Tumors arising from the tongue have a poor prognosis. They are controlled locally in only 25% of animals 1 year after resection or radiation therapy.

References

Bertone ER, Snyder LA, Moore AS: Environmental and lifestyle risk factors for oral squamous cell carcinoma in domestic cats, *J Vet Intern Med* 17:557, 2003.

De Vos JP, Burm AGD, Focker AP et al: Piroxicam and carboplatin as a combination treatment of canine oral nontonsillar squamous cell carcinoma: a pilot study and a literature review of a canine model of human head and neck squamous cell carcinoma, *Vet Comparative Oncol* 3:16, 2005.

Freeman KP, Hahn KA, Harris D et al: Treatment of dogs with oral melanoma by hypofractionated radiation therapy and platinum-based chemotherapy (1987-1997), *J Vet Intern Med* 17:96, 2003.

Proulx DR, Ruslander DM, Dodge RK et al: A retrospective analysis of 140 dogs with oral melanoma treated with external beam radiation, *Vet Radiol Ultrasound* 44:352, 2004.

Suggested Reading

Boria PA, Murry DJ, Bennett PF et al: Evaluation of cisplatin combined with piroxicam for the treatment of oral malignant melanoma and oral squamous cell carcinoma in dogs, *J Am Vet Med Assoc* 224:388, 2004.

This is a report of a prospective nonrandomized clinical trial involving 25 dogs. Combined treatment was found to have antitumor activity but renal toxicity must be monitored.

Dhaliwal RS, Tang KN: Parathyroid hormone-related peptide and hypercalcaemia in a dog with a functional keratinizing ameloblastoma, *Vet Comparative Oncol* 3:98, 2005.

This case report describes resolution of hypercalcemia after hemimandibulectomy.

Kuntsi-Vaattovaara H, Verstraete FJM, Newsome JT et al: Resolution of persistent oral papillomatosis in a dog after treatment with recombinant canine oral papillomavirus vaccine, *Vet Comparative Oncol* 1:57, 2003.

This is a case report of a dog whose papillomas did not spontaneously regress or respond to surgery.

Schmidt BR, Glickman NW, DeNicola DB et al: Evaluation of piroxicam for the treatment of oral squamous cell carcinoma in dogs, *J Am Vet Med Assoc* 218:1783, 2001.

This is a prospective case series involving 17 dogs. Treatment results included complete remission (1), partial remission (2), and stable disease (5).

SALIVARY MUCOCELES

DEFINITIONS

A **salivary mucocele** *(sialocele, salivary cyst, honey cyst)* is a collection of saliva that has leaked from a damaged salivary gland or duct and is surrounded by granulation tissue. A **cervical mucocele** is a collection of saliva in the deeper structures of the intermandibular space, the angle of the jaw, or the upper cervical region. A **sublingual mucocele (ranula)** is a collection of saliva in the sublingual tissue caudal to the openings of the sublingual and mandibular ducts, and a **pharyngeal mucocele** is a collection of saliva in the tissue adjacent to the pharynx. A **zygomatic mucocele** is a collection of saliva ventral to the globe. **Complex mucoceles**, consisting of two or more types, occur in some animals. **Marsupialization** is the process of incising a mucocele and suturing the edges to the mucosa. The interior of the mucocele suppurates and gradually closes by granulation.

GENERAL CONSIDERATIONS AND CLINICALLY RELEVANT PATHOPHYSIOLOGY

Tearing of a salivary gland or duct results in leakage of saliva into the surrounding tissue. Salivary mucoceles are not cysts. Cysts are cavities lined by epithelium, whereas the granulation tissue lining of a mucocele is produced secondary to inflammation caused by free saliva in the tissues. The cause

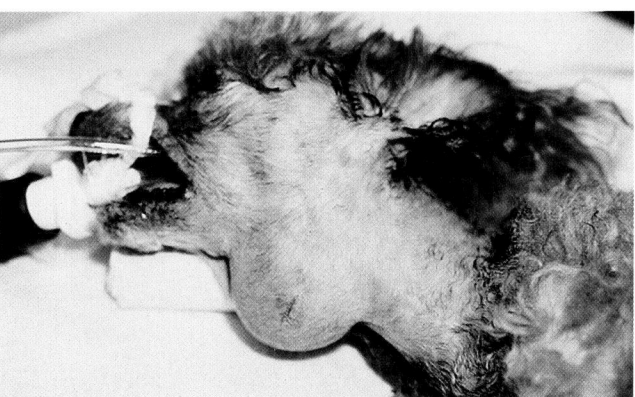

FIG. 19-29
Cervical mucocele in a dog.

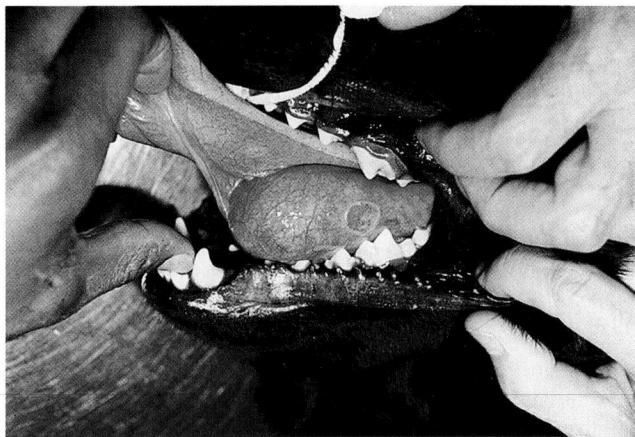

FIG. 19-30
Intraoperative appearance of a sublingual mucocele (ranula) located lateral to the tongue in the sublingual tissue. Note the ulcer from mucosal entrapment between teeth.

of salivary mucoceles is rarely identified, although blunt trauma (choke chains), foreign bodies, and sialoliths have been suggested. The sublingual salivary gland is most commonly involved. Saliva takes the path of least resistance, most commonly accumulating in the cranial cervical or intermandibular (Fig. 19-29), sublingual (Fig. 19-30), or pharyngeal tissues (Fig. 19-31). Saliva irritates the tissue and causes inflammation. The swelling may be firm and painful initially, but the animal usually is asymptomatic. Granulation tissue forms in response to the inflammation and prevents saliva from migrating further. The diagnosis of salivary mucocele is based primarily on the history, clinical signs, and cytologic findings. Radiographs may determine which gland is involved, and histopathologic examination is diagnostic.

DIAGNOSIS
Clinical Presentation

Signalment. Dogs are more frequently affected than cats. All breeds are susceptible, but some reports indicate that poodles, German shepherds, dachshunds, and Australian

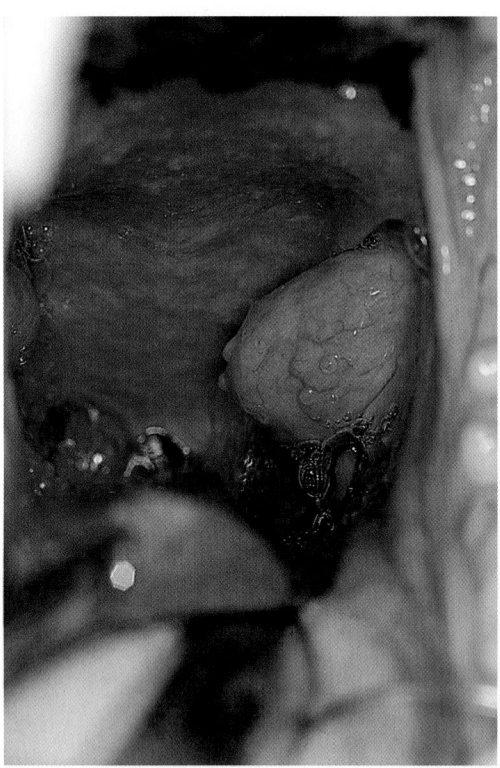

FIG. 19-31
Pharyngeal mucocele in a dog.

silky terriers are more commonly affected. There is a slight predisposition for males to be affected. Any age animal may develop a mucocele.

History. Clinical signs depend on the location of the mucocele. Most dogs have cervical or intermandibular mucoceles and are asymptomatic. These animals usually are presented for treatment with a history of a gradually developing, fluctuant, painless mass. Patients with a sublingual mucocele (i.e., ranula) may have abnormal prehension and oral bleeding, which is caused by trauma during chewing. Respiratory distress and dysphagia are common in patients with pharyngeal mucoceles. Swelling in the oropharyngeal area may cause abnormal tongue movements and may interfere with eating or breathing, and swelling in the orbital area with zygomatic mucoceles may cause enophthalmos and divergent strabismus.

> NOTE: Ask the owners where they first noticed the swelling because this may help you determine the affected side.

Physical Examination Findings

The parotid and mandibular glands are easily palpated. The sublingual gland occasionally is palpable in a cooperative or sedated patient. Palpation of the glands is expected to be normal and without discomfort. Most mucoceles are soft and fluctuant, whereas tumors and abscesses generally

are firm. Mucoceles are painless except during the acute phase of swelling. It sometimes is difficult to identify the affected side when mucoceles are located on the ventral midline or intermandibular space. Examining these animals in dorsal recumbency often allows the mucocele to gravitate to the affected side. Palpation of some cervical mucoceles causes the sublingual tissues to bulge on the affected side. Concurrent sublingual and cervical mucoceles originate from the side where the sublingual mucocele is found. Blood-tinged saliva may occur in patients with sublingual mucoceles because teeth often traumatize the mucocele. Periorbital facial swelling, enophthalmos, and periocular pain are signs of a zygomatic mucocele. Optic neuropathy may occur secondary to pressure from zygomatic mucoceles.

> NOTE: Animals with pharyngeal mucoceles often are presented for treatment in acute respiratory distress. Institute appropriate therapy rapidly or they may die.

Diagnostic Imaging

Survey radiographs rarely help except in cases involving sialoliths, foreign bodies, or neoplasia. Thoracic radiographs are indicated to evaluate for metastasis if neoplasia is suspected. Sialography (i.e., injecting iodinated, water-soluble contrast agent into a salivary duct) is difficult and usually unnecessary to confirm the diagnosis or determine the site of origin. In some cases, particularly pharyngeal mucoceles, cross-sectional imaging can be used to better evaluate the location and extensiveness of the lesion.

Laboratory Findings

Laboratory abnormalities are rare. Salivary gland function and duct patency can be evaluated by placing a drop of topical ophthalmic atropine solution on the tongue to stimulate saliva flow; however, it may be difficult to distinguish flow from individual ducts. Paracentesis should be performed under aseptic conditions to prevent infection of the mucocele. Aspiration of a clear, yellowish, or blood-tinged, ropy, mucoid fluid with a low cell count is consistent with saliva. Staining a smear with a mucus-specific stain, such as periodic acid-Schiff (PAS), confirms the presence of saliva. An elevated white blood cell count may indicate concurrent sialoadenitis.

DIFFERENTIAL DIAGNOSIS

Sialoadenitis, sialadenosis, salivary neoplasia, sialolith (calcium phosphate or carbonate), cervical abscess, foreign body, hematoma, cystic or neoplastic lymph nodes, tonsil cyst, thyroglossal cyst, cystic Rathke's pouch, and branchial cysts may cause swellings in the same region as mucoceles. Occasionally, mucoceles may be difficult to distinguish from cysts or tumors. Histopathologic examination is necessary to diagnose salivary gland tumors and to differentiate a congenital cyst from a mucocele. Congenital cysts have an epithelial lining, whereas mucoceles are lined by granulation tissue.

Salivary neoplasia presents as a mass in older animals and is associated with halitosis, weight loss, dysphagia, exophthalmos, Horner's syndrome, sneezing, and dysphonia. The mandibular gland is most commonly affected in cats and the parotid in dogs, and simple adenocarcinoma is the most common histologic type (Hammer et al, 2001).

Animals presenting with chronic oropharyngeal abscesses typically have draining tracts, cervical swelling, dysphagia, and oral pain (Griffiths et al, 2000). A history of fighting, penetrating trauma, or chewing on sticks is common with abscesses.

MEDICAL MANAGEMENT

Emergency aspiration of the mucocele may be necessary for animals in respiratory distress. Repeated drainage or injection of cauterizing or antiinflammatory agents does not eliminate mucoceles; however, it complicates subsequent surgery by leading to abscessation or fibrosis. Mucoceles rarely resolve without surgery.

SURGICAL TREATMENT

Complete excision of the involved gland-duct complex and drainage of the mucocele are curative. The side of origin of the mucocele may be determined by oral examination, palpation, sialography, or exploration of the mucocele.

> NOTE: If you are having trouble identifying the affected side in an animal with a cervical mucocele, place the animal on its back. The contents of the mucocele often gravitate to the side of the affected gland.

Preoperative Management

Animals with pharyngeal mucoceles may be presented for treatment in acute respiratory distress, and rapid intubation may be necessary. Intubation may not be possible through the mouth, and a temporary tracheostomy may be required. Once these animals have been intubated they generally are stable, and surgical excision of the salivary glands and drainage of the mucocele can be delayed while further diagnostics are performed, if necessary. Intravenous antibiotics may be given at induction of anesthetic, but are not essential.

Anesthesia

Most animals undergoing salivary gland excision for mucoceles are healthy, and a variety of anesthetic protocols can be used. General anesthetic recommendations for animals undergoing oral surgery (i.e., for ranulas or pharyngeal mucoceles) are listed on p. 339. Oral intubation may be difficult in patients with large pharyngeal mucoceles (see previous discussion), and placement of the endotracheal tube by means of tracheostomy often is necessary to allow adequate visualization of the lesion.

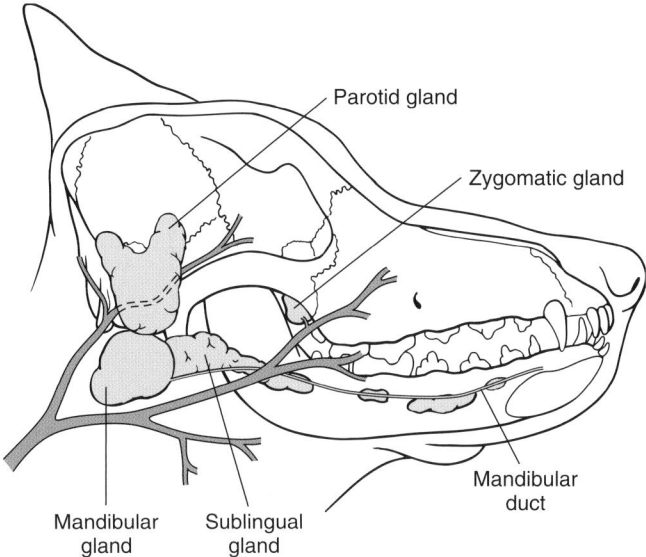

FIG. 19-32
Surgical anatomy of the salivary glands. The parotid gland lies ventral to the ear canal. The mandibular gland is ventral to the parotid gland, lying between the maxillary and linguofacial veins. The sublingual gland follows the rostral course of the mandibular duct toward the oral cavity. The zygomatic gland is protected by the zygomatic arch.

Surgical Anatomy

Dogs and cats have four major pairs of salivary glands of surgical significance (Fig. 19-32). They are the parotid, mandibular, sublingual, and zygomatic glands. The parotid gland is a triangle-shaped serous gland located ventral to the horizontal ear canal. Numerous arteries, veins, and nerves are closely associated with the medial aspect of the gland. The parotid duct papilla is located on the mucosal surface of the cheek at the level of the upper carnassial tooth (fourth premolar). The mandibular gland is large and ovoid, and lies within a fibrous capsule caudal and ventral to the parotid gland. It is located between the linguofacial and maxillary veins as they merge to join the external jugular vein. The mandibular duct runs with the sublingual gland toward the floor of the mouth and opens on a small papilla lateral to the rostral border of the frenulum (Box 19-11). The sublingual gland is divided into a monostomatic and a polystomatic portion. The monostomatic portion originates on the rostroventral border of the mandibular gland. The ducts from this portion of the sublingual gland course with the mandibular duct, but often open on separate papillae. The polystomatic portion is divided into several loosely connected lobules that surround the mandibular duct and lie immediately beneath the oral mucosa, secreting directly into the oral cavity. The zygomatic gland, an irregularly ovoid gland, is located on the floor of the orbit ventrocaudal to the eye and medial to the zygomatic arch. The zygomatic gland has several ducts that run ventrally and open on a fold of mucosa lateral to the last upper molar tooth. The major zygomatic duct usually

BOX 19-11

Oral Openings of the Salivary Gland Ducts

Parotid Duct
- Labial mucosa at level of upper carnassial tooth

Mandibular Duct
- Papilla lateral to the rostral border of the frenulum

Sublingual Duct
- Opens with the mandibular duct near the lingual frenulum

Zygomatic Gland
- Lateral to the last upper molar tooth

---

can be identified at this location about 1 cm caudal to the parotid papilla.

Positioning

Salivary gland excision is performed with the animal in lateral recumbency. Ventral recumbency and maximum opening of the mouth facilitate marsupialization of pharyngeal mucoceles and ranulas.

SURGICAL TECHNIQUE
Mandibular and Sublingual Salivary Gland Excision

The mandibular and sublingual salivary glands are excised together because the sublingual gland is intimately associated with the mandibular salivary gland duct; removal of one would traumatize the other. Removal of glands on the involved side is all that is necessary for mucocele resolution; however, both pairs of mandibular and sublingual glands may be resected without risk of xerostomia. If it is not clear from which side the mucocele originated, make a stab incision in the mucocele and digitally palpate the lumen. The unaffected side is rounded and smooth. The affected side has a tract or tunnel toward the site of leakage.

Position the patient in lateral recumbency. Place a pad under the neck to rotate the ventral aspect dorsally and fix the neck in an extended position. Locate the mandibular salivary gland between the linguofacial and maxillary veins as they join the external jugular vein (Fig. 19-33, A). Incise the skin, subcutaneous tissue, and platysma muscle from the angle of the mandible caudally to the external jugular vein to expose the fibrous capsule of the mandibular gland (Fig. 19-33, B). Avoiding the branch of the second cervical nerve that crosses the capsule, incise the capsule and dissect it away from the mandibular and monostomatic sublingual salivary glands. Ligate the artery (branch of the great auricular artery) and vein as they are encountered on the dorsomedial aspect of the gland. Continue dissecting cranially, following the mandibular duct, sublingual duct, and polystomatic sublingual glands toward the mouth (see Fig. 19-33, B). Incise

the fascia between the masseter and digastricus muscles. Expose the entire mandibular and sublingual salivary gland complex by retracting the digastricus muscle and applying caudal traction on the mandibular gland. If necessary, perform digastricus muscle myotomy or tunnel the caudal sublingual gland duct complex under the digastricus muscle to improve visualization. Dissect (digital and sharp) rostrally until the lingual branch of the trigeminal nerve is identified and only ducts remain in the complex. Avoid traumatizing the lingual or hypoglossal nerves. Try to identify the gland-duct defect causing the mucocele because failure to identify this defect may indicate that the mucocele originated from the contralateral gland-duct complex. Ligate and transect the mandibular sublingual gland-duct complex just caudal to the lingual nerve.

Traction on the gland-duct complex may cause the ducts to tear. If this occurs near the point of proposed transection or on the oral aspect of the gland-duct defect, no further dissection is needed. However, if the tear occurs before the gland-duct defect or when the defect has not yet been identified and if glandular tissue is identified orad to the tear, further resection of glandular tissue is recommended to prevent recurrence.

Lavage the surgical site before closure. Appose the digastricus muscle if it has been incised with horizontal mattress or cruciate sutures. Close the dead space with a few sutures in the capsule and deep tissue. Routinely appose superficial muscles, subcutaneous tissue, and skin. Following excision, submit the glands and ducts to rule out neoplasia and submit a portion of the mucocele wall to rule out congenital cysts.

Drain cervical mucoceles by making a stab incision at the most dependent point; place a closed suction or Penrose drain if desired. Protect the drain with an absorbent bandage. Change the bandage and cleanse discharge from the neck as needed to prevent excoriation of the skin. Maintain the drain for 1 to 5 days, removing it when there is minimal discharge. Allow the stab incision to heal by secondary intention. Redundant skin resumes its normal appearance within several weeks. Drain sublingual mucoceles (ranulas) by excising an elliptical, full-thickness section of the mucocele wall. Suture the granulation tissue lining to the sublingual mucosa (marsupialization) to encourage drainage for several days (Fig. 19-34). Drain pharyngeal mucoceles by aspiration or marsupialization. Excise redundant pharyngeal tissue to prevent airway obstruction after evacuation of the mucocele.

Marsupialized ranulas contract and heal quickly by secondary intention. After bilateral mandibular and sublingual salivary gland excision, dogs still have sufficient saliva to adequately moisten their food.

Zygomatic Gland Excision

Zygomatic gland excision is required for zygomatic mucoceles, unresponsive infections, inflammatory conditions, and neoplasia.

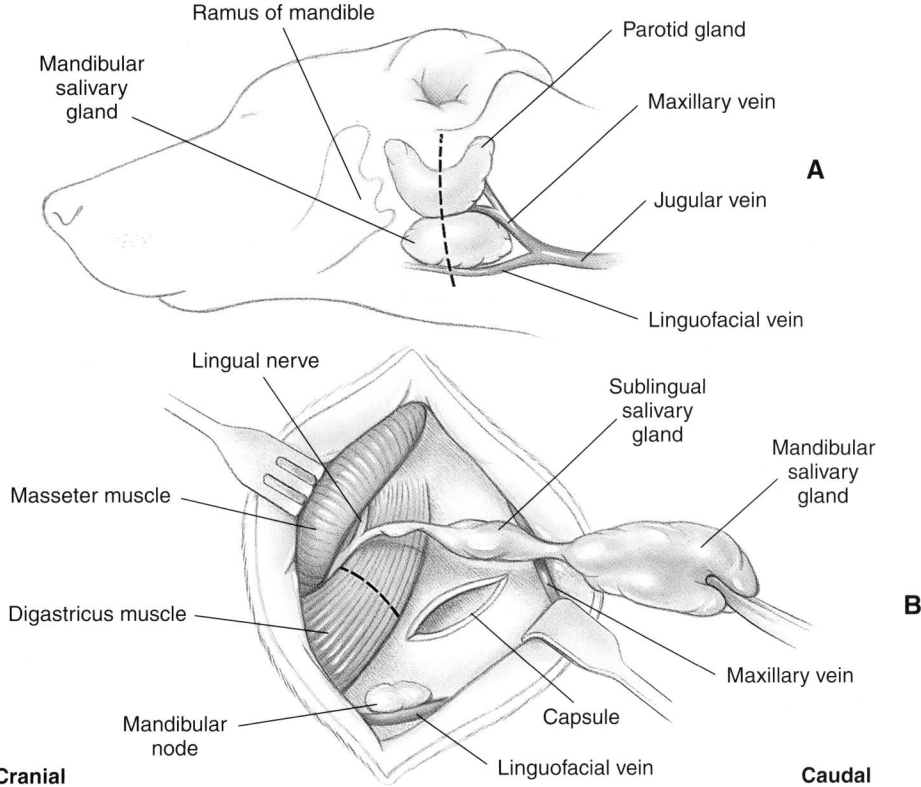

FIG. 19-33
Excision of the mandibular and sublingual salivary glands. **A,** Make an incision ventral to the external ear canal and over the mandibular salivary gland at the junction of the linguo-facial and maxillary veins. **B,** Dissect the mandibular salivary gland after incising the cap-sule. Apply caudal traction on the mandibular gland and dissect the duct and sublingual gland until the lingual nerve has been identified. Transect the digastricus muscle *(dashed line)* to aid dissection if necessary.

Position the patient in lateral or ventral recumbency. Protect the animal's eye from irritants with ophthalmic ointment. Incise the skin and subcutaneous tissues over the dorsal rim of the zygomatic arch. Incise the palpebral fascia, retractor anguli oculi muscle, and orbital ligament, and elevate them dorsally with the skin and globe. Further expose the gland by partly removing the zygomatic arch with rongeurs or by osteotomy. Retract the globe dorsally to expose the perior-bital fat and underlying zygomatic gland. Remove the gland by blunt dissection (the gland is friable). Avoid the ventrally located anastomotic branch between the deep facial and external ophthalmic veins. Drain the mucocele if present. If possible, replace the zygomatic arch by securing the bone with sutures placed through predrilled holes. Lavage the area and appose the palpebral fascia to the zygomatic peri-osteum with sutures. Close subcutaneous tissues and skin.

Parotid Gland Excision

Parotid gland excision occasionally is performed for neoplasia, fistula, chronic infection, or mucocele. The triangle-shaped gland is located at the base of the auricular cartilage.

Position the patient in lateral recumbency. Incise the skin from 1 to 2 cm ventral to the external acoustic meatus to a

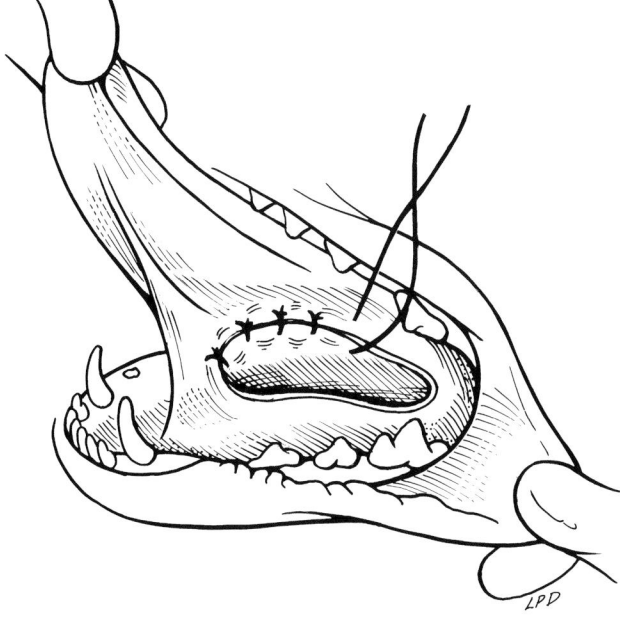

FIG. 19-34
Marsupialization of a ranula. After excising an elliptical piece of mucosa and granulation tissue from the mucocele wall, suture the mucosa to the lining of the mucocele.

point midway between the ramus of the mandible and the bifurcation of the jugular vein. Incise the platysma muscle to expose the parotidoauricularis muscle, vertical ear canal, and parotid salivary gland. Sever and retract the parotidoauricularis muscle from its vertical ear canal attachment. Ligate and divide the caudal auricular vein. Begin dissection of the parotid gland at its dorsocaudal angle. Separate the parotid from the mandibular gland ventrally. Continue dissection between the gland and the vertical ear canal. Avoid traumatizing the facial nerve at the base of the horizontal ear canal. Ligate and divide the superficial temporal vein (a branch of the maxillary vein) coursing through the gland. Cauterize or ligate small vessels on the gland's medial surface. Ligate and transect the parotid duct as it leaves the gland. Lavage the area. Reappose the parotidoauricularis muscle. Complete closure by apposing subcutaneous tissues and skin. Ligation of the parotid duct may be an alternative treatment for parotid mucoceles or fistulae.

Ligating the duct proximal to the disruption, near the body of the gland, causes glandular atrophy.

POSTOPERATIVE CARE AND ASSESSMENT

Histologic assessment of the excised gland rules out neoplasia as a cause of the mucocele. Change bandages daily if a Penrose drain has been placed. Depending on the amount of drainage, remove the drain 24 to 72 hours after surgery or when drainage is minimal. Allow the drain site to heal by secondary intention. Soft food should be fed for 3 to 5 days after ranula marsupialization or drainage of pharyngeal mucoceles.

COMPLICATIONS

Postoperative complications after salivary gland resection are uncommon, but may include seroma formation, infection, and mucocele recurrence. Seromas can form in the dead space created by removal of the glands; they typically resorb and do not need aspiration or drainage. Infection is rare if aseptic technique is used. Mucoceles recur if the side of mucocele origin was misdiagnosed or if an inadequate gland was excised. Regional lymph nodes are sometimes mistaken for salivary glands. Dissection may be difficult if the mucocele was previously infected or injected. Attention to anatomic detail during surgery should minimize recurrence and complications associated with salivary gland excision.

PROGNOSIS

In rare cases, a mucocele resolves without surgery. The prognosis is excellent if the disease is accurately diagnosed and if excision is complete.

References

Griffiths LG, Tiruneh R, Sullivan M et al: Oropharyngeal penetrating injuries in 50 dogs: a retrospective study, *Vet Surg* 29:383, 2000.

Hammer A, Getzy D, Ogilvie G et al: Salivary gland neoplasia in the dog and cat: survival times and prognostic factors, *J Am Anim Hosp Assoc* 37:478, 2001.

Suggested Reading

Boydell P et al: Sialadenosis in dogs, *J Am Vet Med Assoc* 216:872, 2000.

This prospective study includes 13 dogs with enlarged salivary glands, retching, and gulping who responded to treatment with phenobarbital.

Canapp SO, Cohn LA, Maggs DJ et al: Xerostomia, xerophthalmia and plasmacytic infiltrates of the salivary glands (Sjögren's-like syndrome) in a cat, *J Am Vet Med Assoc* 218:59, 2001.

This case report describes a syndrome that may be a primary autoimmune disease or a connective tissue disorder.

Gibbon KJ, Trepanier LA, Delaney FA: Phenobarbital-responsive ptyalism, dysphagia, and apparent esophageal spasm in a German shepherd puppy, *J Am Anim Hosp Assoc* 40:230, 2004.

This case report includes a review of 44 reported cases of salivary gland enlargement. This syndrome of phenobarbital-responsive hypersialosis (sialadenosis) has been suggested to be a form of epilepsy.

Sozmen M, Brown PJ, Whitbread TJ: Idiopathic salivary gland enlargement (sialadenosis) in dogs: a microscopic study, *J Small Anim Pract* 41:243, 2000.

Primarily a histologic review, this report gives some clinical information on 13 cases. Sialadenosis presents with a variety of signs including dysphagia, inappetence, and a submandibular mass or swelling that may be unilateral or bilateral.

Surgery of the Esophagus

GENERAL PRINCIPLES AND TECHNIQUES

DEFINITIONS

Esophagotomy is an incision into the esophageal lumen; **esophagectomy** is partial resection of the esophagus. **Esophagostomy** is the creation of an opening in the esophagus for placement of a feeding tube. **Regurgitation** is the passive expulsion of undigested food or fluid from the esophagus. **Vomiting** is a centrally mediated reflex that causes expulsion of food or fluid from the stomach or duodenum or both.

PREOPERATIVE MANAGEMENT

The esophagus carries food, water, and saliva from the pharynx to the stomach. Although less common than intestinal obstruction, esophageal obstruction may occur in dogs and cats associated with foreign bodies, strictures, or masses. Esophageal surgery may be indicated if function is interrupted by obstruction or perforation (Box 19-12).

Diagnosis of esophageal disorders is based on history, clinical signs, radiography, and/or endoscopy. The predominant clinical signs of esophageal pathology are typically regurgitation or dysphagia (Box 19-13). The history can be used to try to distinguish vomiting from regurgitation, but this is not always easy to do. *Regurgitation* is classically a passive process whereas *vomiting* usually is preceded by salivation, vigorous retching, and abdominal contractions. Regurgitated material generally consists of undigested food and saliva, whereas vomited material may contain bile or di-

BOX 19-12

Possible Surgical Diseases of the Esophagus

- Foreign bodies
- Tumors
- Perforation
- Hiatal hernia
- Fistulae*
- Gastroesophageal intussusception*
- Diverticula*
- Cricopharyngeal achalasia
- Strictures

*Rare

BOX 19-13

Clinical Signs of Esophageal Disease

- Regurgitation
- Coughing
- Dysphagia
- Dyspnea
- Ptyalism
- Fever
- Altered appetite
- Weight loss

gested blood. However, some animals vomit material that looks just like regurgitated material, and not all vomiting animals have the previously listed signs. If a patient has the classic signs of vomiting, then it is usually vomiting. However, if it does not have the classic signs of vomiting, it can be hard to know whether it is vomiting or regurgitating.

Some patients with esophageal disease have respiratory signs (especially coughing, but also pulmonary crackles, mucopurulent nasal discharge, and/or fever suggestive of aspiration pneumonia) without any history of regurgitation or spitting up. Anytime a dog presents with pneumonia, aspiration must be a differential, even if there is no history of throwing up. A patient with esophageal disease may have a normal, ravenous, or depressed appetite, and some patients lose weight.

Distention of the cervical esophagus may occur in patients with severe esophageal weakness. Compressing the thorax while the nostrils are occluded occasionally demonstrates cervical esophageal distention in animals with megaesophagus. Abnormalities of prehension and swallowing may sometimes be noted by observing the animal while it is eating. Masses and foreign bodies may sometimes be palpated in the cervical esophagus. Rarely esophageal perforations may cause septic mediastinitis producing fever, mediastinal or pleural effusion, respiratory distress, and eventual death.

Definitively diagnosing esophageal disease and then defining the type may require a variety of techniques. Survey radiographs of the esophagus extending from the caudal portion of the oral cavity to the stomach should be assessed for foreign bodies, esophageal dilation with gas or liquid, periesophageal fluid or gas opacities, and aspiration pneumonia. The esophagus is not radiographically visible in most normal dogs and cats; however, small amounts of swallowed air may sometimes be seen in the cranial cervical and cranial thoracic esophagus. Mediastinitis, pneumome-

diastinum, and/or pleural effusion suggest esophageal perforation. Contrast fluoroscopic examination of the esophagus is indicated if survey radiographs are nondiagnostic; a reasonable number of dogs with esophageal weakness do not have obvious abnormalities on plain radiographic studies. Fluoroscopic examination allows evaluation of swallowing, motility, and gastroesophageal sphincter function. Barium sulfate paste may be used if fluoroscopy is not available, but information on motility will not be ascertained. Also, barium sulfate paste may cause complications if aspirated. Liquid barium sulfate is the first choice for use in performing an esophagogram and is relatively safe if aspirated (except in large quantities). Food mixed with barium may reveal some partial obstructions that would be missed with liquid barium sulfate.

> NOTE: Use aqueous iodinated contrast if esophageal perforation is suspected. Do not use barium sulfate in such cases. Nonionic iodinated contrast agents (such as iohexol or iopamidol) are the safest. Ionic iodinated contrast will cause fulminate pulmonary edema if aspirated.

Esophagoscopy is indicated if plain radiographs reveal what may be a mass or foreign body, or if esophageal obstruction, tumor, hiatal hernia, or inflammation is suspected. During esophagoscopy, mucosal lesions may be identified and a biopsy taken; foreign bodies can be removed or advanced into the stomach. Esophagotomy or partial esophagectomy may be performed as a diagnostic and therapeutic procedure if a definitive diagnosis cannot be made by other means (p. 376).

Treatment for aspiration pneumonia, esophagitis, and nutritional debilitation should be initiated before surgery (Box 19-14). For mild esophagitis, antacids (e.g., famotidine; Box 19-15) with or without gastric prokinetics (e.g., metoclopramide; see Box 19-15) are administered, and food and water are withheld for 24 to 48 hours to reduce esophageal irritation. Water should be offered first. If there is no regurgitation, a low-fat, high-protein gruel that will enhance lower esophageal sphincter tone, speed gastric emptying, and reduce reflux should be fed for 3 to 4 days. Soft food should be fed for an additional 5 to 7 days, and then the animal should be gradually returned to its normal diet. For severe esophagitis, aggressive antacid therapy (e.g., omeprazole; see Box 19-15) and more potent gastric prokinetic therapy (e.g., cisapride; see Box 19-15) are often necessary. Oral intake of food and water may need to be withheld for 7 days or longer. Hydration should be maintained with intravenous fluids; nutritional support may require a gastrostomy tube (see p. 100). Oral feeding with a low-fat gruel should be initiated as described for mild esophagitis and continued for 10 to 14 days. Sucralfate slurries may be beneficial for patients with reflux esophagitis. Sucralfate selectively binds and protects denuded mucosa and reduces esophageal inflammation (see Box 19-15). Antibiotics effective against

BOX 19-14

Preoperative Management of Patients With Esophageal Disorders

- Withhold food: Mature animals—12 to 18 hours; pediatric animals—4 to 8 hours
- Correct fluid, electrolyte, and acid-base imbalances
- Give prophylactic antibiotics (i.e., ampicillin, cephalosporins), if appropriate
- Support nutrition
- Treat esophagitis and aspiration pneumonia

 BOX 19-15

Treatment of Esophagitis

Cimetidine (Tagamet)

5–10 mg/kg PO, IV, SC, tid to qid

Ranitidine (Zantac)

2.2 mg/kg PO, IV, IM, bid

Famotidine (Pepcid)

0.5 mg/kg PO, qd to bid

Omeprazole (Prilosec)

0.7–1.5 mg/kg PO, qd

Metoclopramide

0.2–0.4 mg/kg PO, IV, tid

Cisapride (pharmacy compounded)

0.1–0.5 mg/kg PO, bid

Sucralfate* (Carafate)

0.5–1 g PO, tid to qid

PO, Oral; IV, intravenous; SC, subcutaneous; tid, three times a day; bid, twice a day; qid, four times a day; qd, once a day.
*Carafate impairs absorption and/or reduces bioavailability of cimetidine; give at different intervals.

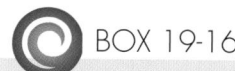 BOX 19-16

Treatment of Aspiration Pneumonia

Bronchodilators

Aminophylline

Dogs: 5–11 mg/kg PO, IM, IV (if given IV, give slowly over 5 minutes), tid
Cats: 5 mg/kg PO, bid to tid

Theophylline (extended release)

Dogs: 5–30 mg/kg PO, qd to bid, depending upon the product
Cats: 10–25 mg/kg PO, qd, depending upon the product

Terbutaline (Brethine, Bricanyl)

Dogs: 1.25–5 mg/dog SC, PO, bid to tid
Cats: 0.625 mg/cat SC, PO, bid

Antimicrobials

Ampicillin

22 mg/kg IV, IM, SC, tid to qid

Clindamycin (Antirobe, Cleocin)

11 mg/kg PO, IV, bid to tid

Enrofloxacin (Baytril)

7–20 mg/kg PO, IV (diluted and given slowly over 30 minutes) qd

Amikacin (Amiglyde-V)

20–25 mg/kg IV, qd

PO, Oral; IM, intramuscular; IV, intravenous; SC, subcutaneous; tid, three times a day; bid, twice a day; qid, four times a day.

oral contaminants (e.g., ampicillin, amoxicillin, and clindamycin; Box 19-16) are often administered, but are of unknown effectiveness. Concurrent corticosteroid therapy (e.g., prednisone, 1.1 mg/kg given orally once daily) may reduce the risk of stenosis caused by severe esophagitis; however, the benefit of this therapy is unknown.

Treatment of aspiration pneumonia should be started before esophageal surgery, unless there is an esophageal foreign object, in which case it should be removed as soon as possible. If aspiration is observed while the animal is anesthetized, the airway should be suctioned to remove irritants. Fluid therapy is indicated for animals that are severely dyspneic or in shock. Nasal oxygen supplementation should be provided to dyspneic animals, and positive pressure ventilation may be necessary for unresponsive patients. Bronchodilators (i.e., aminophylline, oxtriphylline, and terbutaline sulfate) may reduce bronchospasms and ventilatory muscle fatigue in these patients (see Box 19-16). Corticosteroids, such as prednisone (0.25 mg/kg given intravenously twice a day), may be beneficial if the animal is in shock or severely dyspneic; however, these drugs should be used with caution because they may interfere with host defense mechanisms. Expectorants (e.g., guaifenesin) occasionally are used in animals with productive coughs. Systemic antibiotic therapy is indicated in animals with pulmonary infection or sepsis. Broad-spectrum antibiotics (or combinations of antibiotics) effective against gram-negative and anaerobic bacteria should be used (e.g., clindamycin, ampicillin, or cefazolin plus either enrofloxacin or amikacin; see Box 19-16). Culture and sensitivity should be done, if possible. Aerosol therapy and coupage facilitate both delivery of antibiotics to the respiratory tree and elimination of excessive respiratory secretions.

ANESTHESIA

Fluid, electrolyte, and acid-base imbalances should be corrected before induction of anesthetic. If feasible, mature animals should fast for 12 to 18 hours before esophageal surgery; however, young puppies and kittens may fast for shorter periods (4 to 8 hours) to prevent hypoglycemia. Selected anesthetic protocols for patients in stable condition undergoing

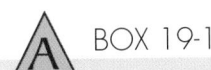 BOX 19-17

Selected Anesthetic Protocols for Use in Animals With Cervical Esophageal Disorders

Premedication

Give atropine (0.02–0.04 mg/kg SC or IM) or glycopyrrolate (0.005–0.011 mg/kg SC or IM) plus hydromorphone* (0.1–0.2 mg/kg SC or IM) or butorphanol (0.2–0.4 mg/kg SC or IM), or buprenorphine (5–15 µg/kg IM).

Induction

Thiopental (10–12 mg/kg IV) or propofol (4–6 mg/kg IV). As an alternative, use a combination of diazepam and ketamine (diazepam 0.27 mg/kg plus 5.5 mg/kg ketamine IV) titrated to effect.

Maintenance

Give isoflurane or sevoflurane.

SC, Subcutaneous; *IM*, intramuscular; *IV*, intravenous.
*May use 0.05 mg/kg in cats.

cervical esophageal surgery are listed in Box 19-17. Procedures on the thoracic esophagus require modification of general anesthetic protocols to accommodate compromised function of the respiratory and cardiovascular systems. General recommendations for anesthesia in patients undergoing thoracic surgery are provided on p. 867. A mechanical ventilator is recommended. Nitrous oxide should not be used after the thorax is open because large pulmonary shunts may develop during lateral thoracotomy because the "up lung" receives most of the ventilation and the "down lung" receives more perfusion. Compressing the up lung and increasing inflation pressures to 20 to 30 cm H_2O can minimize shunts. The tidal volume (15 ml/kg) must be adequate to expand the lungs during thoracotomy. The inspiratory time should be kept between 1 and 1½ seconds because a prolonged inspiratory time may collapse alveolar capillaries and impede venous return. The respiratory rate should be 6 to 10 breaths per minute. See p. 868 for recommendations for analgesics for patients undergoing thoracotomy. After induction of anesthesia, suctioning secretions and ingesta from the obstructed esophagus may help prevent aspiration and minimize contamination of the surgical site.

ANTIBIOTICS

Perioperative antibiotics may be given to prevent infection of periesophageal tissues. Prophylactic intravenous antibiotics should be given when anesthesia is induced and repeated 2 to 3 hours later. A third dose may be given 8 hours after the second dose. Broad-spectrum antibiotics effective against anaerobes are recommended (i.e., clindamycin, ticarcillin plus clavulanic acid, and cefoxitin). Animals with preoperative perforation or severe esophageal trauma should be treated with therapeutic antibiotics (see Box 19-16). Specimens collected from the surgical site or perforation should be submitted for bacterial culture and susceptibility testing. The duration of antibiotic therapy varies according to the source of infection and the contaminating organisms, but they generally should be continued for a minimum of 2 weeks.

SURGICAL ANATOMY

The cervical and proximal thoracic portions of the esophagus lie to the left of the midline; however, the esophagus lies slightly to the right of the midline from the tracheal bifurcation to the stomach. The layers of the esophageal wall include the mucosa, submucosa, muscularis, and adventitia. The submucosa is the holding layer of the esophagus and must be incorporated with all sutures. The normal canine esophagus has linear mucosal striations throughout its length. The distal portion of the feline esophagus usually has circular mucosal folds that form a herringbone pattern with positive contrast.

NOTE: Because the esophagus lacks a serosal layer, early fibrin sealing of esophagotomy sites may occur more slowly than in other areas of the gastrointestinal tract.

The vascular supply of the cervical esophagus is from branches of the thyroid and subclavian arteries. Bronchoesophageal arteries and segmental branches from the aorta supply the thoracic esophagus. The abdominal esophagus is supplied by branches from the left gastric and left phrenic arteries. Intramural branches ramify and anastomose in the submucosal layer. Collateral blood flow from the cervical and abdominal portions of the esophagus can provide the thoracic esophagus with adequate blood flow if the intramural esophageal vascular system is intact.

SURGICAL TECHNIQUE

Abnormalities of the cervical esophagus are approached using a ventral midline cervical incision. Thoracic esophageal abnormalities at the base of the heart are approached using a right lateral thoracotomy and those cranial or caudal to the heart with a left cranial or caudal thoracotomy. The abdominal esophagus is approached through a ventral midline celiotomy. Hair should be clipped from the entire ventral cervical area for surgery of the cervical esophagus and from the entire hemithorax for approaches to the thoracic esophagus. The skin should be aseptically prepared for surgery. Atraumatic meticulous technique must be employed to ensure rapid healing without dehiscence or stricture (Box 19-18).

Approach to the Cervical Esophagus

Position the patient in dorsal recumbency (Fig. 19-35, A). Incise the skin on the midline, beginning at the larynx and extending caudally to the manubrium. Incise and retract the platysma muscle and subcutaneous tissue. Separate the paired sternohyoid muscles along the midline to expose the underlying trachea (Fig. 19-35, B). Retract the thyroidea ima vein with the sternohyoid muscle or ligate it. If access to the

BOX 19-18

Principles of Esophageal Surgery

Use atraumatic meticulous technique because healing is challenged by there being no serosa, no omentum, segmental blood supply, constant motion and bolus distention, intolerance of longitudinal stretching
Choose the most advantageous approach
Preserve vasculature; dissect sparingly
Suction the lumen before incising
Make incision through healthy tissue
Make longitudinal esophagotomy incisions
Inspect for contralateral perforations or necrosis
Resect only 3 to 5 cm during esophagectomy

Incorporate submucosa with all sutures
One-layer closure: keep knots extraluminal
Two layer closure—inner layer: intraluminal knots; outer layer: extraluminal knots
Tension-relieving techniques: circumferential myotomy, gastric advancement, phrenic nerve interruption, "pexy" sutures
Seal and support with a harvested omental flap or muscle flap
Treat esophagitis with H_2 receptor antagonists and/or proton pump inhibitors and/or gastric prokinetics

caudal cervical esophagus is necessary, separate and retract the sternocephalicus muscles. Retract the trachea to the right to expose the adjacent anatomic structures, including the esophagus, the thyroid gland, the cranial and caudal thyroid vessels, the recurrent laryngeal nerve, and the carotid sheath (vagosympathetic trunk, carotid artery, and internal jugular vein) (Fig. 19-35, C). Pass a stomach tube or esophageal stethoscope to facilitate identification of the esophagus and lesion. After completing the definitive procedure, lavage the surgical site with warm sterile saline and return the trachea to its normal position. Close the incision by apposing the sternohyoid muscles using absorbable suture (3-0 or 4-0) in a simple continuous pattern. Appose subcutaneous tissue in a simple continuous pattern with 3-0 or 4-0 absorbable suture. Use nonabsorbable suture (3-0 or 4-0 monofilament) and an appositional suture pattern to appose the skin.

Approach to the Cranial Thoracic Esophagus via a Lateral Intercostal Thoracotomy

Position the patient in right lateral recumbency over a rolled towel placed perpendicular to the long axis of the body (Fig. 19-36, A). Choose the appropriate intercostal space incision based on the radiographic location of the abnormality (Figs. 19-36, B, C, and D).

Most abnormalities cranial to the base of the heart can be accessed through an incision in the left third or fourth intercostal space (the technique for thoracotomy is described on p. 871).

Identify the esophagus in the mediastinum dorsal to the brachiocephalic trunk (Fig. 19-36, E). Identification may be aided by passage of a stomach tube or by palpating the abnormality. Dissect the mediastinal pleura overlapping the esophagus to just above and below the proposed surgical site. Preserve the branch of the internal thoracic vein and the costocervical vein, which cross the cranial esophagus.

Approach to the Esophagus at the Heart Base via a Right Lateral Thoracotomy

The approach is the same as that for the cranial esophagus except that the incision is made through the right fourth or fifth intercostal space (Fig. 19-37, A and B).

Identify the esophagus, located just dorsal to the trachea in the mediastinum (Fig. 19-37, C). Dissect and retract the azygous vein from the esophagus to allow adequate exposure. Ligate the azygous vein if necessary to adequately expose the esophagus. Close the same as described for intercostal thoracotomy (see p. 873).

Approach to the Caudal Esophagus via a Caudal Lateral Thoracotomy

Position the patient in lateral recumbency as described above for cranial lateral thoracotomy. Perform a caudal lateral thoracotomy (Fig. 19-38, A).

Although the caudal esophagus can be approached through an incision in either the left or right eighth or ninth intercostal space, the left ninth space is preferred.

Expose the caudal esophagus by transecting the pulmonary ligament and packing the caudal lung lobes cranially. Identify the esophagus, which is just ventral to the aorta (Fig. 19-38, B). Identify the dorsal and ventral vagal nerve branches on the lateral aspect of the esophagus and protect them.

Esophagotomy

Pack off the esophagus from the remainder of the field with moistened laparotomy pads. Suction material from the cranial esophagus before making the esophagotomy incision to minimize contamination of the surgical site. If ingesta and secretions have not been completely suctioned, occlude the lumen cranial and caudal to the proposed esophagotomy site with fingers or noncrushing forceps. Place stay sutures adjacent to the proposed incision site to stabilize, aid manipulation, and prevent trauma to the esophageal edges. Make a stab incision into the lumen of the esophagus and extend the incision longitudinally as necessary to remove the foreign body or observe the lumen. Make the incision over the foreign body if the esophageal wall appears normal. If the wall appears compromised, make the incision caudal to the lesion or foreign body. Remove foreign bodies with forceps, taking care to prevent further esophageal trauma (tearing or perforation). Examine the esophageal lumen. Obtain culture specimens from necrotic and perforated

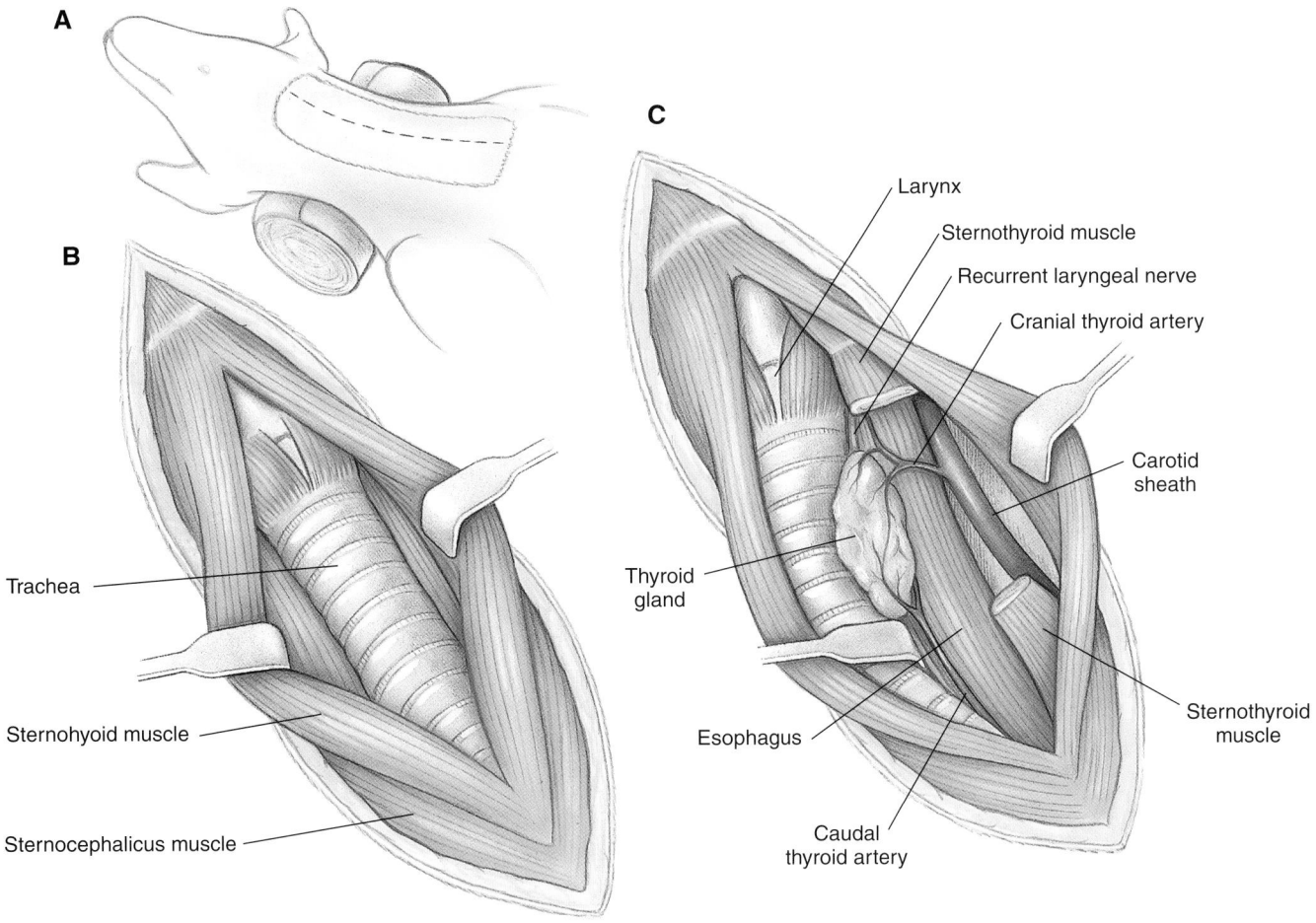

FIG. 19-35
Approach to the cervical esophagus. **A,** Position the patient in dorsal recumbency with the neck resting on a rolled towel. **B,** Incise the skin from the larynx to the manubrium, and separate the sternohyoid muscles to expose the trachea. **C,** Retract the trachea to the right to expose the esophagus, thyroid, carotid sheath, and recurrent laryngeal nerve.

areas. Débride and close perforations surrounded by healthy tissue that involve less than one fourth the circumference of the esophagus. Identify large necrotic areas or extensive perforations and perform a resection and anastomosis (see later discussion).

Esophagotomy incisions may be closed with a one- or two-layer closure. A two-layer simple interrupted closure results in greater immediate wound strength, better tissue apposition, and improved healing after esophagotomy, but takes longer to perform than single-layer techniques.

Place each suture approximately 2 mm from the edge and 2 mm apart. Incorporate the mucosa and submucosa in the first layer of a two-layer simple interrupted closure. Place sutures so that the knots are within the esophageal lumen (Fig. 19-39, A and B). Incorporate the adventitia, muscularis, and submucosa in the second layer of sutures with the knots tied extraluminally (Fig. 19-39, C). When a one-layer closure is used, pass each suture through all layers of the *esophageal wall and tie the knots on the extraluminal surface. Check closure integrity by occluding the lumen, injecting saline, applying pressure, and observing for leakage between sutures.*

Partial Esophagectomy

Esophagectomy is performed to remove devitalized or diseased esophageal segments. Benign strictures should be dilated endoscopically if possible, with surgery reserved as a salvage procedure. Periesophageal tissue must be dissected from around the abnormal area to allow resection of diseased tissue and mobilization of normal esophagus; however, extensive dissection should be avoided to preserve vasculature. Excessive tension along the anastomosis may cause dehiscence. Although 20% to 50% of the esophagus has been resected and primarily anastomosed without tension-relieving techniques, resection of more than 3 to 5 cm risks anastomotic dehiscence. Partial myotomy is recommended to relieve anastomotic tension when resecting large segments of the esophagus (Fig. 19-40). Circumferential myotomy is a

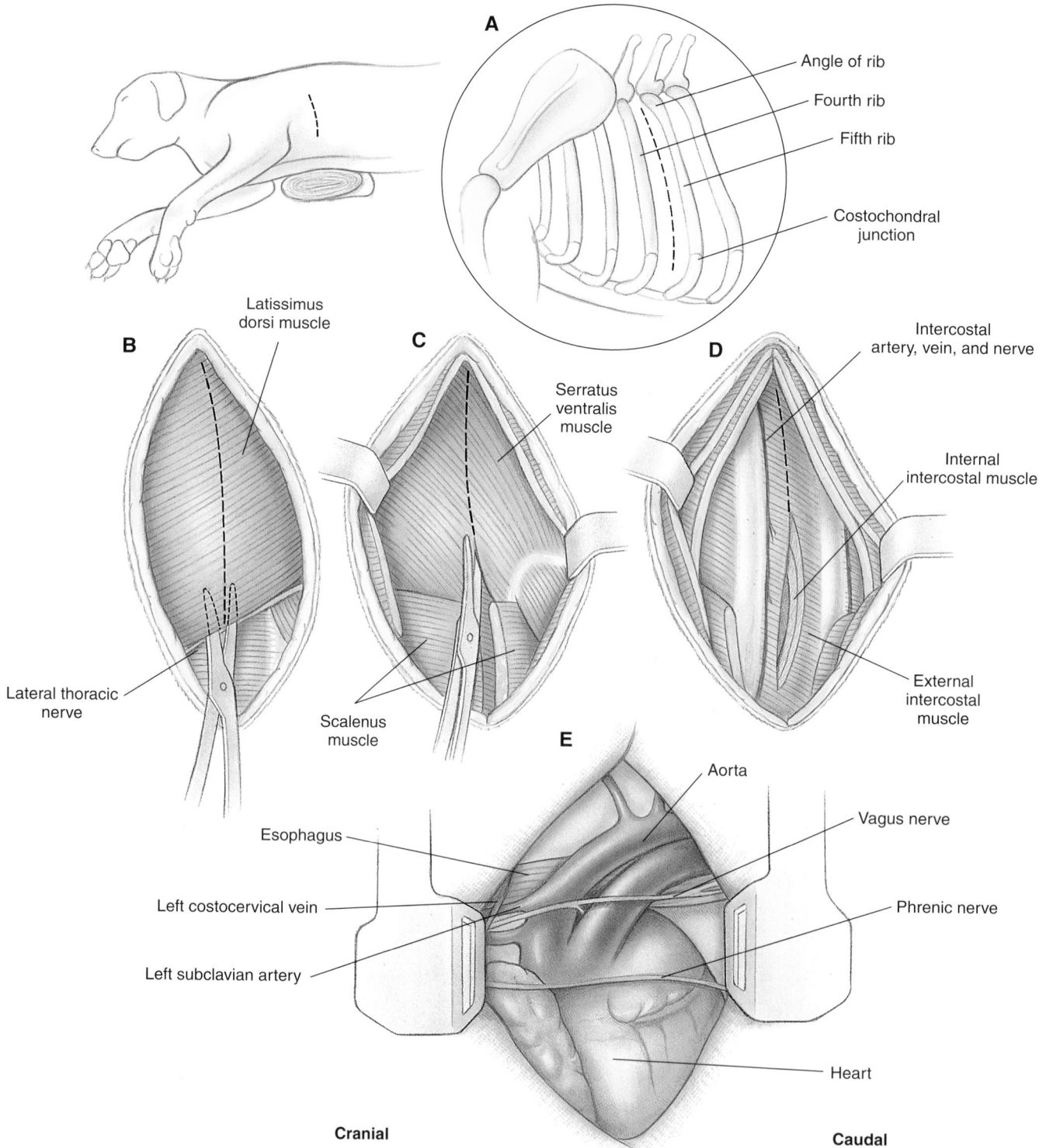

A, Angle of rib

Fourth rib

Fifth rib

Costochondral junction

B, Latissimus dorsi muscle

Lateral thoracic nerve

C, Serratus ventralis muscle

Scalenus muscle

D, Intercostal artery, vein, and nerve

Internal intercostal muscle

External intercostal muscle

E, Aorta

Esophagus

Left costocervical vein

Left subclavian artery

Vagus nerve

Phrenic nerve

Heart

Cranial

Caudal

FIG. 19-36

Approach to the cranial thoracic esophagus. **A,** Position the patient in right lateral recumbency over a rolled towel placed perpendicular to the long axis of the body. Select the appropriate incision site based on the radiographic location of the lesion *(inset)*. **B,** Identify and transect the latissimus dorsi muscle *(dashed line)*. **C,** Identify and transect or retract the serratus ventralis *(dashed line)* and scalenus muscles. **D,** Expose and incise the intercostal muscles *(dashed line)*. **E,** Position rib retractors and identify the thoracic viscera.

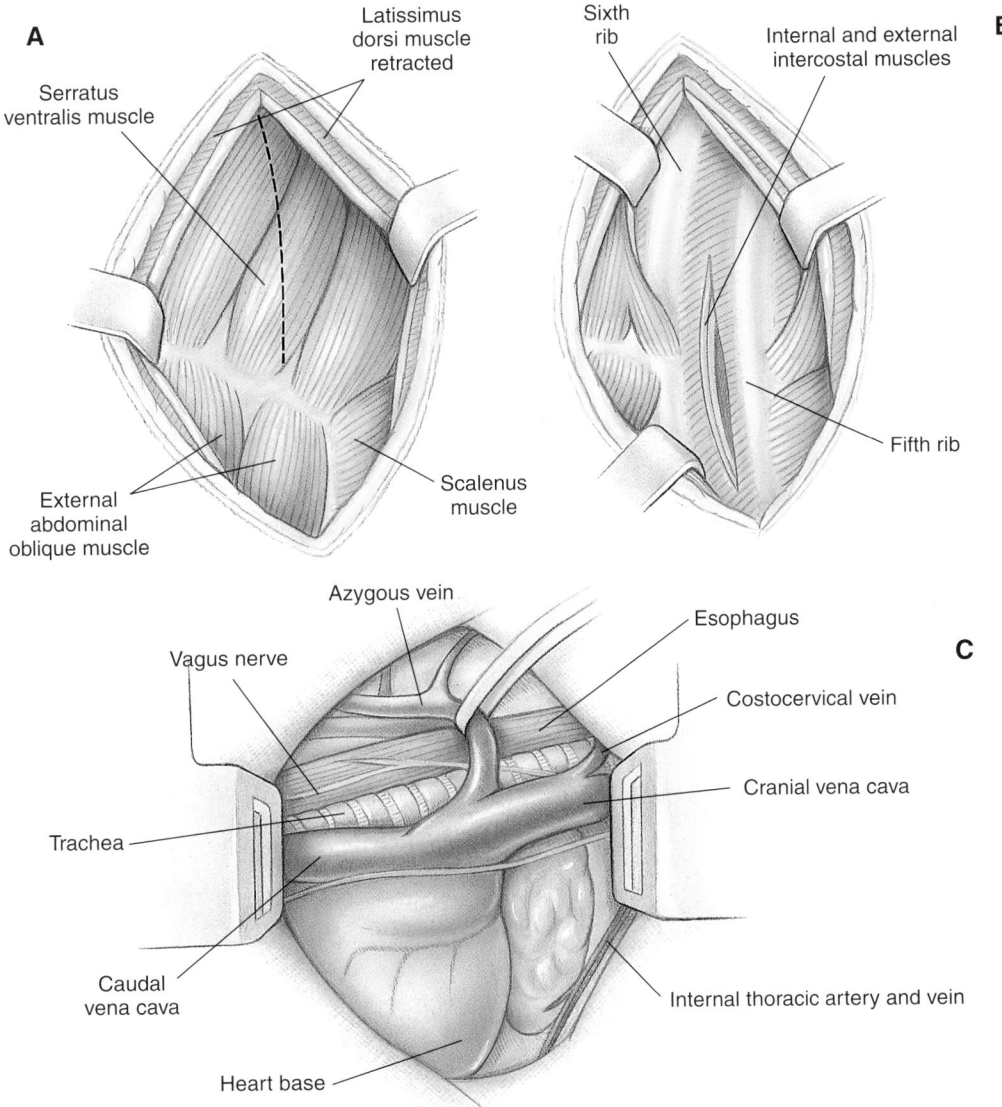

FIG. 19-37
Approach to the esophagus at the heart base. **A,** Make an incision through the right fourth or fifth intercostal space. Identify and transect or retract the latissimus dorsi, serratus ventralis *(dashed line)*, scalenus, and external abdominal oblique muscles. **B,** Incise the intercostal muscles. **C,** Expose the thoracic viscera.

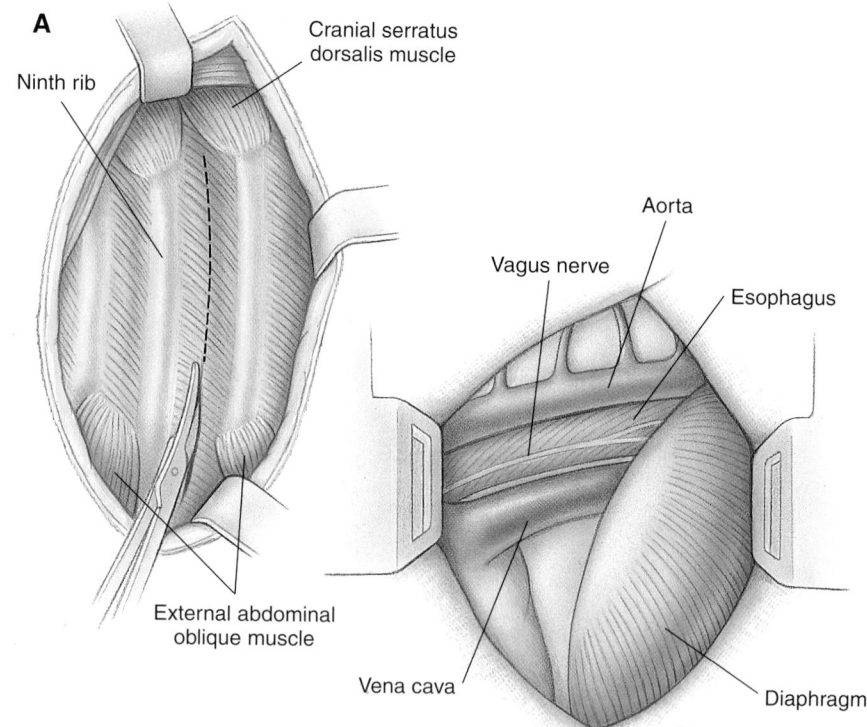

FIG. 19-38
To approach the caudal thoracic esophagus, position the animal in right lateral recumbency and make an eighth or ninth intercostal space incision. **A,** Identify and transect or retract the latissimus dorsi, cranial serratus dorsalis, external abdominal oblique, and intercostal muscles *(dashed line)*. **B,** Identify the diaphragm and other thoracic viscera.

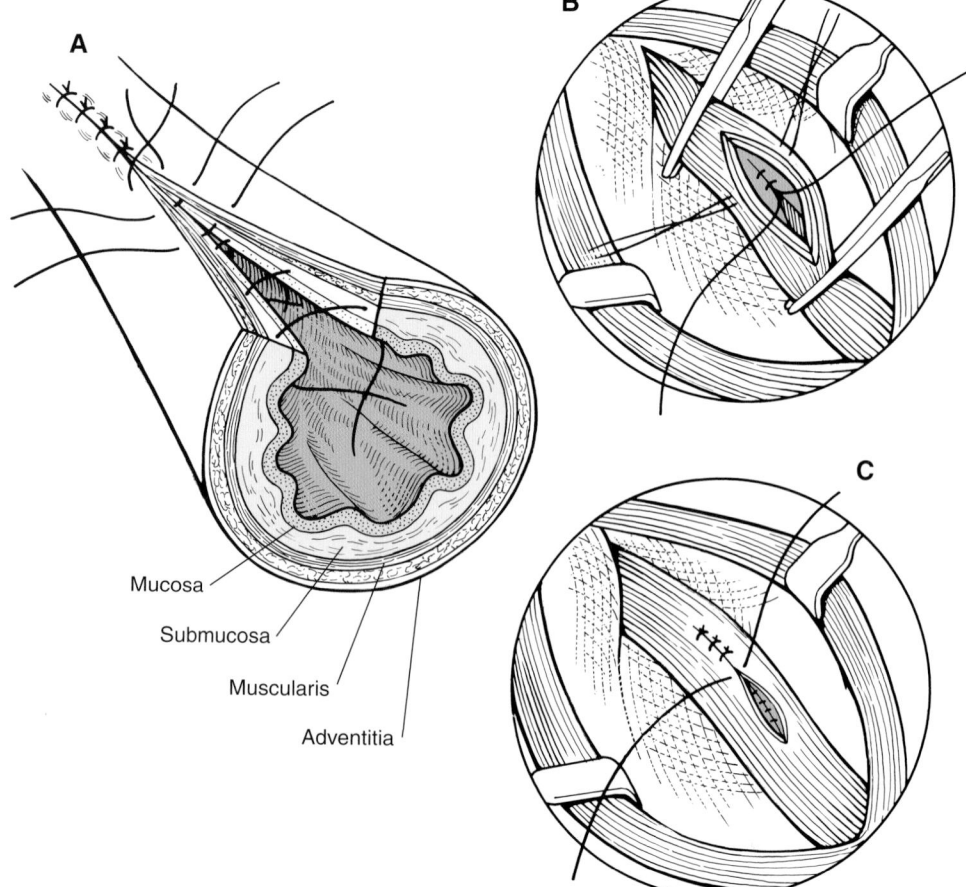

FIG. 19-39
Esophagotomy closure. **A** and **B,** Close the mucosa and submucosa with simple interrupted sutures so that the knots are intraluminal. **A** and **C,** Appose the adventitia and muscularis with a second layer of simple interrupted sutures oriented with extraluminal knots.

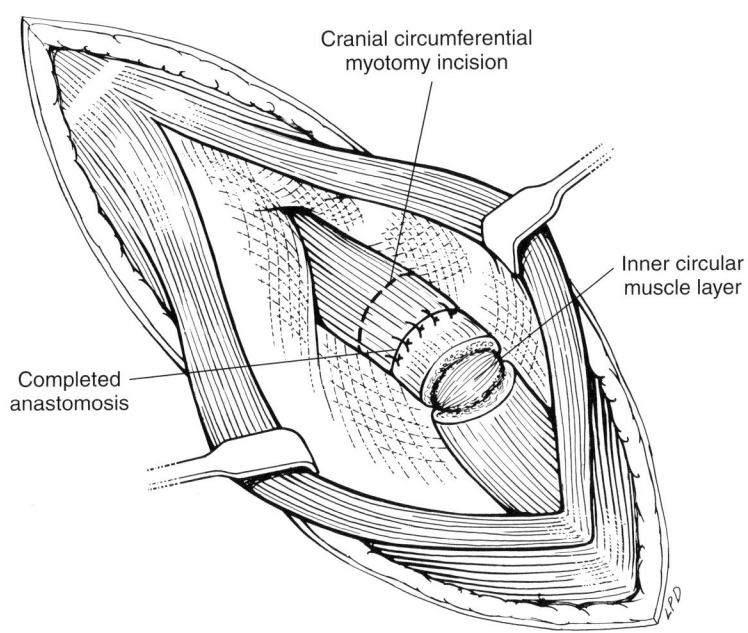

Cranial circumferential
myotomy incision

Inner circular
muscle layer

Completed
anastomosis

FIG. 19-40
Tension-relieving esophageal myotomy is performed
2 to 3 cm cranial and caudal to the anastomosis.

partial-thickness myotomy through the longitudinal muscle layers 2 to 3 cm cranial and caudal to the anastomosis. The inner circular muscle layers are not incised to prevent damaging the submucosal blood supply. Injection of saline into the muscularis may aid identification of the different muscle layers. The myotomy gap heals by secondary intention without stricture or dilatation. Mobilizing the stomach cranially through an enlarged esophageal hiatus can also help reduce tension across the anastomosis. Other tension-relieving techniques include interruption of the phrenic nerve and placement of "pexy" sutures between the esophagus and the prevertebral fascia. Esophageal replacement may be necessary if segments of more than 3 to 5 cm are resected. Many replacement techniques have been described, including microvascular anastomosis of the colon or small intestine to the esophagus, gastric tubes, skin tubes, and various prostheses. Replacement of the esophagus requires specialized training, techniques, and equipment.

For esophagectomy, occlude and stabilize the esophagus with fingers (scissor action of middle and index fingers) or noncrushing forceps. Resect the diseased portion of the esophagus (Fig. 19-41). Suction debris from the lumen of the remaining esophagus. Place three equally spaced stay sutures at each end of the remaining esophagus to facilitate gentle handling of the esophagus and help maintain apposition and alignment of the transected ends (see Fig. 19-41). Bring the esophageal ends into apposition with the stay sutures, and suture the ends together using a one- or two-layer closure as described for esophagotomy. Place sutures in the contralateral (far) wall first and then in the more accessible ipsilateral (near) wall. When using a two-layer closure, appose the esophagus in the following four steps: (1) appose the adventitia and muscularis of the contralateral wall

around approximately one half of the esophageal circumference (Fig. 19-42, A); (2) appose the mucosa and submucosa of the contralateral wall (Fig. 19-42, B); (3) appose the mucosa and submucosa of the ipsilateral wall (Fig. 19-42, C); and (4) appose the adventitia and muscularis of the ipsilateral wall (Fig. 19-42, D). Check the integrity of the closure by occluding the lumen, injecting saline, applying pressure, and observing for leakage between sutures.

An end-to-end circular stapling device may reduce operating time and contamination of the surgical field, but this technique may have a greater potential for stricture formation.

Place a purse-string suture in the cranial esophageal remnant. Insert the anvil and tie the purse string around the instrument shaft. Place a second purse-string suture around the distal resection site and secure it. Appose the esophageal ends by tightening the stapler's wing nut. Activate the instrument and then remove it with a rotating motion. Close the access incision for placement of the stapling device with a linear stapler (see p. 454).

Support or Patching Techniques

Augmentation of esophagotomy or esophagectomy sites with omentum or muscle can aid healing by supporting, sealing, and revascularizing the surgical site. Muscle pedicles from the sternohyoid, sternothyroid, intercostal, diaphragm, or epaxial muscles can be mobilized and sutured over the primary repair or esophageal defect (Fig. 19-43, *A*). As an alternative, omentum can be mobilized from the abdomen, brought through a rent in the diaphragm, and sutured over the esophageal site (Fig. 19-43, *B*). Pedicles from the gastric wall and pericardium have also been used.

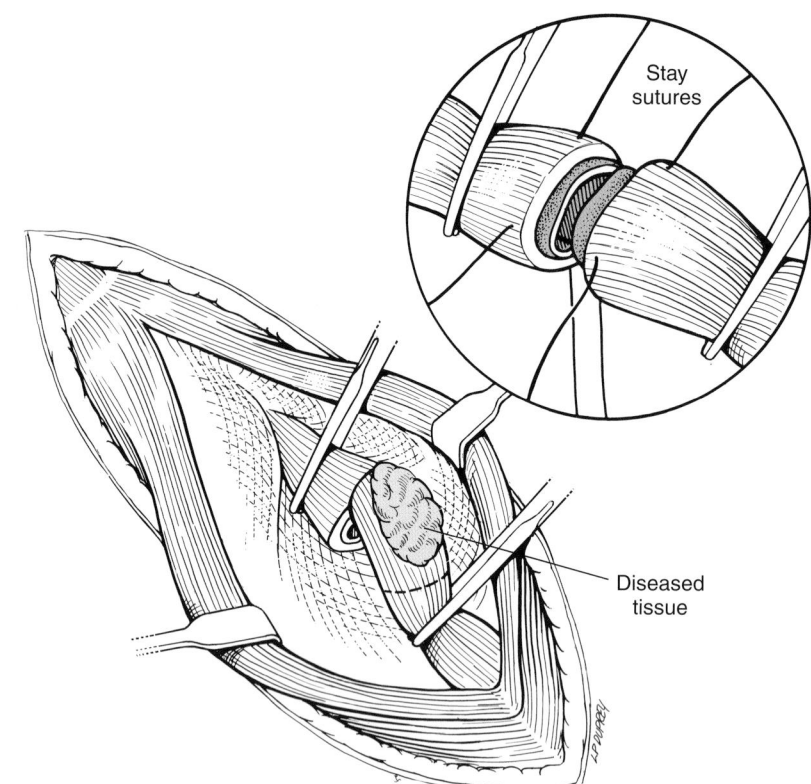

FIG. 19-41
For partial esophagectomy, occlude the esophageal lumen with noncrushing forceps and mobilize and resect the diseased esophagus *(dashed line)*. Place stay sutures to manipulate the esophageal ends *(inset)*. Anastomose the ends as shown in Fig. 19-42.

FIG. 19-42
During partial esophagectomy, appose the ends with two layers of sutures in a four-step procedure. **A,** First, appose the adventitia and muscularis on the far side with simple interrupted sutures and extraluminal knots. **B,** Second, appose the submucosa and mucosa on the far side with simple interrupted sutures using intraluminal knots. **C,** Third, appose the near-side submucosa and mucosa. **D,** Last, appose the near-side muscularis and adventitia.

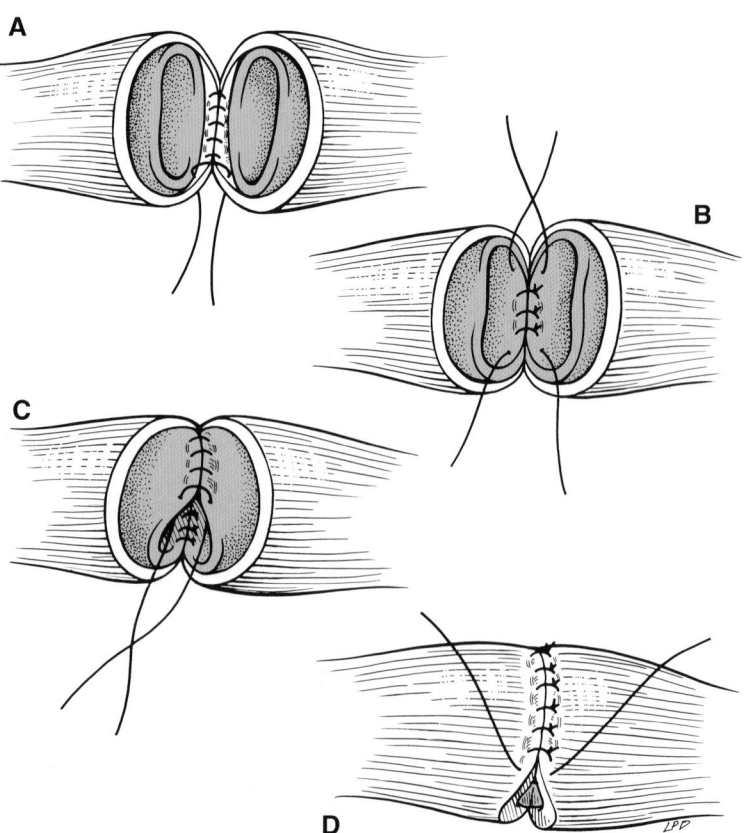

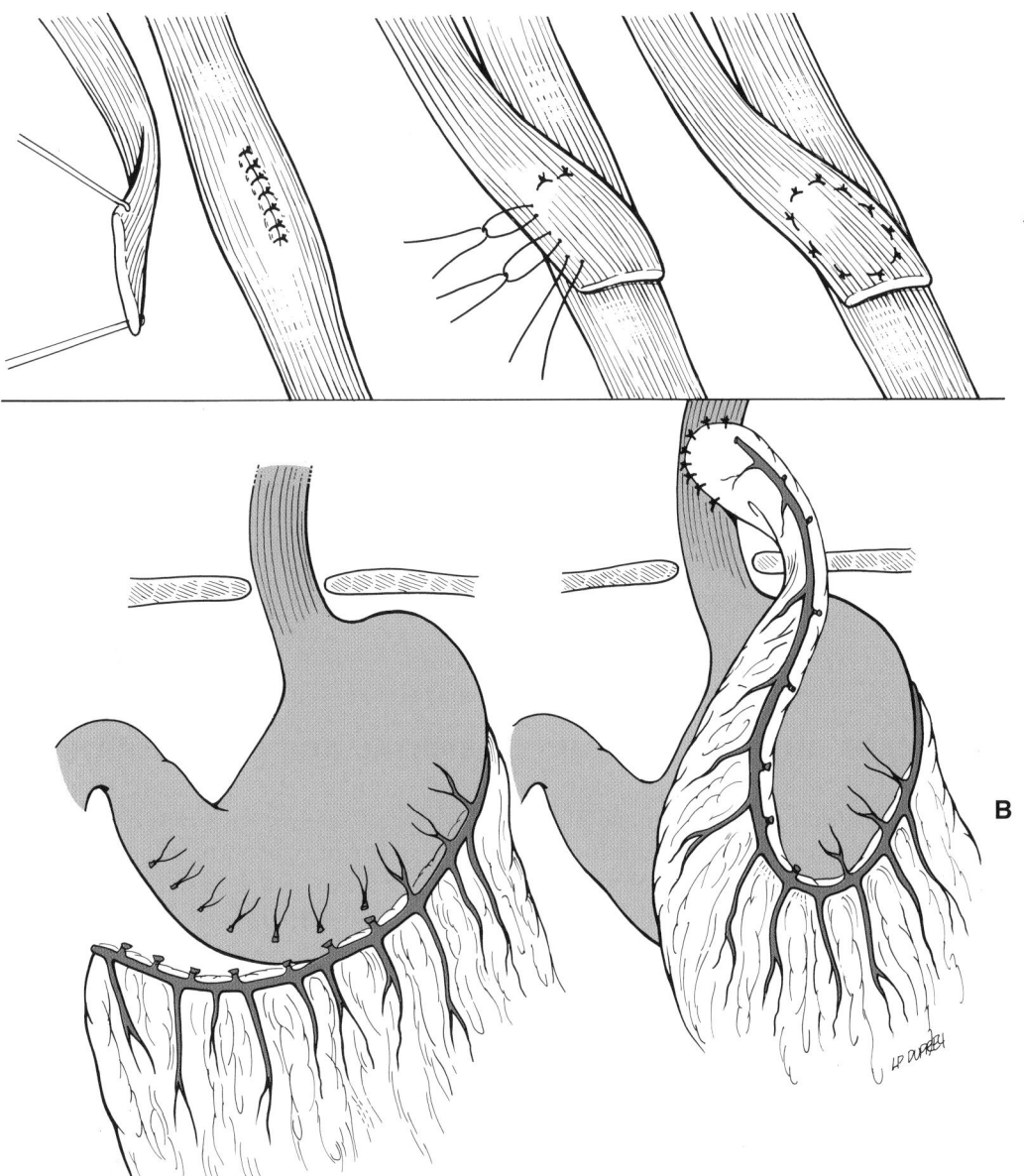

FIG. 19-43
Patching the esophagus. **A,** Mobilize muscle adjacent to the esophagus and suture it over an esophageal incision to create an esophageal patch. **B,** As an alternative, mobilize omentum from the greater curvature of the stomach, pass it through an incision in the diaphragm, and suture it over the esophageal closure to create an omental patch.

Esophagostomy

Feeding tubes placed in the midcervical esophagus are associated with fewer complications than pharyngostomy or nasogastric feeding tubes. The techniques for esophagostomy tube placement are described on p. 97. Tubes are positioned rostral to the gastroesophageal junction to reduce gastroesophageal reflux. Ostomy wounds heal by secondary intention after removal of the tube without evidence of stricture or esophagocutaneous fistula.

HEALING OF THE ESOPHAGUS

The esophagus is subject to constant movement from swallowing and respiration. This continuous motion may interfere with healing and must be overcome with good surgical technique. Although large segments of the esophagus have been resected successfully, the esophagus does not tolerate longitudinal stretching well and may dehisce if tension is excessive. Complications (especially dehiscence, stricture, fistulation) are common after esophageal surgery. The high complication rate has been blamed on the lack of serosal covering, lack of omentum, segmental blood supply, constant motion, and distention with passage of food boluses. Careful surgical technique and patient management can minimize most of the possible complicating factors.

SUTURE MATERIALS AND SPECIAL INSTRUMENTS

In addition to a general pack, other requirements may include special forceps (i.e., noncrushing Doyen forceps), delicate hemostats (i.e., Adson), Metzenbaum scissors, retractors (for the cervical approach, Gelpi retractors; for the thoracic approach, Finochietto retractors; malleable retractors), and tubes (chest tube, gastrostomy tube, stomach tube). A suction unit and laparotomy pads should also be available. Surgical stapling equipment (e.g., linear stapler, circular end-to-end stapler, ligate-and-divide vascular stapler, and skin stapler) is beneficial but optional. Monofilament absorbable suture (polydioxanone, polyglyconate, or poliglecaprone 25 with a swaged-on taper point needle) and nonabsorbable suture (polypropylene, nylon with a reverse cutting needle) (3-0 or 4-0) are recommended in the esophagus.

POSTOPERATIVE CARE AND ASSESSMENT

After esophageal surgery, analgesics should be provided as described for thoracotomy patients on p. 868. Air and fluid must be evacuated via a thoracostomy tube or needle thoracentesis after thoracic procedures. Unless periesophageal or thoracic infection is anticipated, thoracostomy tubes generally can be removed within 8 to 12 hours after esophageal surgery. Nasal oxygen may benefit animals after thoracotomy (see Table 5-4 on p. 26).

Oral intake should be withheld for 24 to 48 hours. Intravenous fluids should be continued until oral intake resumes. Water may be offered 24 hours postoperatively if the esophagus is in good condition and if regurgitation or vomiting does not occur. Blenderized food (gruel) may be offered during the next 24 hours if no vomiting or regurgitation occurs after water consumption. Blenderized food should be continued for 5 to 7 days, and then the animal should be gradually returned to its normal diet over the next week. If oral intake is not anticipated or possible within 48 to 72 hours after surgery, feeding should be performed via a gastrostomy tube (see p. 100).

Esophagitis and aspiration pneumonia should be treated as described in the discussion on preoperative considerations (p. 373). Patients undergoing esophageal surgery should be closely monitored for fever and neutrophilia, which may indicate infection secondary to leakage. Dysphagia and regurgitation that occur 3 to 6 weeks after surgery may indicate esophageal stricture formation. It is extremely important that clients be informed of possible complications before and after surgery (Box 19-19).

COMPLICATIONS

Infection, regurgitation, pneumonia, esophagitis, dehiscence, fistula, stricture, and recurrence of disease are possible complications of esophageal surgery. Common errors in treating

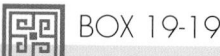

BOX 19-19

Client Education and Communication

- Regurgitating or vomiting can cause aspiration pneumonia, which can be fatal if not controlled.
- Surgery may not resolve all clinical signs of esophageal disease.
- Preventing oral intake, tube feeding, or feeding from an elevated platform such that the patient must be almost vertical to the floor may be necessary.
- Esophageal healing is poor compared with other parts of the gastrointestinal tract; therefore, leakage, infection, dehiscence, and stricture are more common.
- Foreign bodies may perforate the esophagus or great vessels during extraction, with fatal results.
- Dogs should not be fed bones.

esophageal disorders include delayed identification of esophageal foreign bodies, perforation, or aspiration pneumonia; failure to control esophagitis; inappropriate surgical approach; and failure to patch or support the esophagus appropriately.

SPECIAL AGE CONSIDERATIONS

Care must be used in anesthetizing young animals for esophageal surgery. Surgery is often performed in animals with persistent right aortic arches (see p. 405) or hiatal hernias (see p. 396) at 8 to 16 weeks of age. Perioperative hypothermia and hypoglycemia are common problems in these pediatric patients and may be life threatening.

Suggested Reading

Ranen E, Shamir MH, Shahar R et al: Partial esophagectomy with single layer closure for treatment of esophageal sarcomas in 6 dogs, *Vet Surg* 33:428, 2004.

This retrospective study describes resection pedunculated esophageal masses without anastomosis using a one-layer esophageal closure. Various sarcomas were diagnosed, with survival ranging from 2 to 16 months with one dog still living.

SPECIFIC DISEASES

ESOPHAGEAL FOREIGN BODIES

DEFINITION

Foreign bodies are inanimate objects that may cause obstruction of the esophageal lumen to varying degrees.

GENERAL CONSIDERATIONS AND CLINICALLY RELEVANT PATHOPHYSIOLOGY

The most common foreign bodies found in the esophagi of dogs and cats are bones, although sharp metal objects (e.g., needles and fish hooks), rawhide chew toys, balls, string, and an assortment of other objects have lodged there. Foreign bodies lodge in the esophagus because they are too large to pass or they have sharp edges that become embedded in the

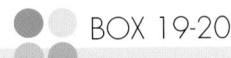

BOX 19-20

Esophageal Foreign Bodies: Key Points

History of roaming or garbage eating is a diagnostic clue
Common location: thoracic inlet, heart base, or diaphragm
Suspect perforation, pressure necrosis, aspiration pneumonia, fistula
Most are identified or suspected from survey radiographs
Most patients with esophageal perforations will have pleural effusion or pneumothorax; contrast radiographs are rarely necessary
If you use radiographs to find perforations, use iodinated contrast media
Most can be removed during esophagoscopy; do not use force
Fatal hemorrhage can occur if a sharp object penetrates the wall
If the mass cannot be retrieved per mouth, then advance object into stomach if possible
Radiograph the patient after endoscopic removal to look for signs of perforation (pneumothorax)
Feeding tubes may be required
Postoperative strictures may occur with or without surgery

esophageal mucosa. Foreign bodies are most commonly found at the thoracic inlet, at the base of the heart, or in the epiphrenic (diaphragm) area because extraesophageal structures limit esophageal dilatation at these sites. The persistence of a foreign body (acting as a bolus) in the esophagus stimulates peristaltic activity. If the foreign body puts excessive pressure on the esophagus or if it remains at one location for several days, pressure necrosis may occur and can cause perforation. If esophagitis occurs, it may interfere with esophageal motility and lower esophageal sphincter function. Food that does not pass the obstruction accumulates and may be regurgitated or may cause proximal esophageal distention. Distention disrupts normal neuromuscular function and reduces peristalsis. Esophageal perforation and aspiration pneumonia (see p. 374) are the major complications possible.

Sharp objects may abrade or lacerate the esophageal mucosa, causing irritation and inflammation of the underlying tissue (esophagitis). Sharp objects may also perforate the esophageal wall and allow bacteria, ingesta, and secretions to contaminate the periesophageal tissue. Occasionally, sharp objects perforate the esophageal wall and one of the great vessels at the base of the heart, causing severe hemorrhage. Foreign bodies may penetrate the esophageal wall and establish a fistula with the trachea, bronchi, pulmonary parenchyma, or skin (Box 19-20).

DIAGNOSIS
Clinical Presentation

Signalment. Indiscriminate eaters (dogs) are more commonly affected than more particular eaters (cats). Although any breed of dog or cat may have an esophageal foreign body, small-breed dogs are more frequently affected because their esophagus is smaller. Cats, having a tendency to play and hunt, more commonly have string or needle foreign bodies than bones. Foreign bodies may occur in an animal of any age, but are most common during the first 3 years of life.

History. Animals may be presented for treatment within minutes of foreign body ingestion (especially when it is seen, as commonly occurs with fish hooks) or weeks later. An acute onset of dysphagia or regurgitation (or both) is the most common initial sign. Other signs may include gagging, excessive salivation, retching, inappetence, restlessness, depression, dehydration, and respiratory distress. Clinical signs vary somewhat depending on the duration, location, and type of obstruction. Patients with acute obstructions generally show excess salivation and gag or regurgitate soon after eating. Weight loss and emaciation sometimes are seen in patients with long-term esophageal obstruction. Patients with complete obstruction regurgitate both solids and liquids, whereas those with partial obstruction may retain liquids. Esophageal pain may cause anorexia. Foreign bodies that impinge on the upper airways may cause acute respiratory distress. Sharp foreign bodies or those that have caused necrosis of the esophageal wall allow leakage of saliva and ingesta into the surrounding tissue, causing inflammation and infection. These patients are likely to be anorexic, febrile, and/or dyspneic as a result of pleural effusion. Hypovolemic shock can occur if a foreign body penetrates a major vessel adjacent to the esophagus. A history of being fed bones, getting into garbage, or roaming is consistent with foreign body ingestion. Fish hook ingestion is typically obvious from the history.

> **NOTE:** Strive to differentiate between vomiting and regurgitation; acute-onset regurgitation is strongly suggestive of an esophageal foreign body.

Physical Examination Findings

Most patients are normal to slightly depressed and dehydrated on physical examination. If the foreign body is lodged in the cervical esophagus, it may sometimes be palpated. Poor body condition may be a factor if the patient has been anorexic or regurgitating for several weeks. Abnormal lung sounds may be auscultated in patients with aspiration pneumonia. Animals that are in severe pain may drool because they refuse to swallow.

Diagnostic Imaging

Most foreign bodies (probably 99%) can be seen as a density on good quality survey radiographs (Fig. 19-44) provided that they are radiopaque, but it is not always obvious that they are in the esophagus. Esophageal masses and foreign bodies may be poorly demarcated densities that closely resemble pulmonary masses. Foreign bodies usually are found at or cranial to the thoracic inlet, the base of the heart (approximately 10%), and the diaphragm (approximately 85%). In addition to the foreign body, there may be an adjacent soft tissue opacity, and a dilated, air-filled cranial esophagus may be seen. Pneumonia and tracheal distortion may also be present. Patients should be closely examined for signs of

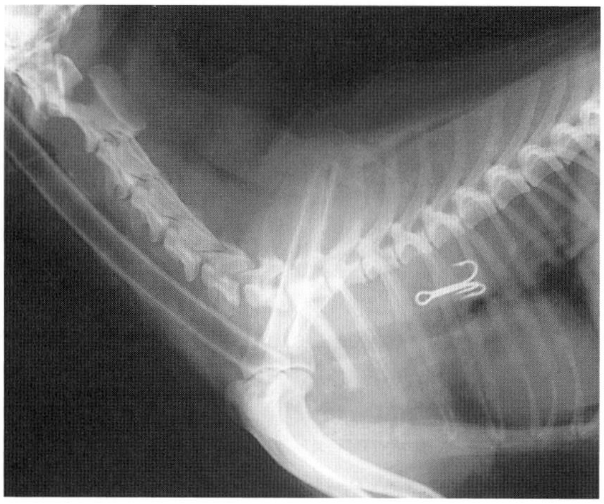

FIG. 19-44
Lateral thoracic radiograph showing a treble fish hook esophageal foreign body at the base of the heart in a dog.

subcutaneous emphysema, pneumomediastinum, pleural effusion, or pneumothorax, each of which suggests esophageal perforation. If pleural effusion is seen, it must be analyzed cytologically to see if it is consistent with infection secondary to perforation.

Esophagograms are rarely necessary to identify foreign bodies and perforations. Water-soluble, organic, iodine contrast materials or iohexol are recommended if contrast radiographs will be done in a patient that is suspected of having an esophageal perforation. Nonionic iodinated contrast agents are the safest because they will not cause pulmonary edema if aspirated or if there is a bronchoesophageal fistula. Ionic, iodinated contrast agents should be avoided in these situations. However, one does not generally do a contrast radiograph to look for perforation (see later discussion on endoscopy), and the presence of a foreign body may mask identification of a perforation during an esophagogram. If a bronchoesophageal fistula is suspected, an iodinated contrast agent should not be used because its hypertonicity may cause pulmonary edema. Foreign bodies can also be diagnosed endoscopically, which is usually the next step after finding a suggestive density on radiographs.

NOTE: If available, endoscopy generally is of greater value than radiographic contrast studies in diagnosing esophageal foreign bodies because the foreign body can potentially be removed during the endoscopic procedure.

Laboratory Findings

Laboratory findings are normal with acute obstructions. Perforations usually cause neutrophilic leukocytosis. Hypoglycemia may be seen in young patients that are unable to eat or in septic shock (or both).

DIFFERENTIAL DIAGNOSIS

Vascular ring anomalies, extraluminal masses, esophageal neoplasia, strictures, esophagitis, gastroesophageal intussusception, esophageal diverticula, hiatal hernias, megaesophagus, and cricopharyngeal dysfunction are other possible causes of regurgitation that must be differentiated from esophageal foreign bodies. Radiographs of pulmonary tumors and esophageal masses can perfectly mimic radiographs of esophageal foreign bodies.

SURGICAL TREATMENT

It is very important to take a radiograph just before induction of anesthesia to ensure that the foreign body has not moved and that there is no sudden evidence of perforation; this is true before endoscopy and surgery.

Most esophageal foreign bodies (probably 90%) can be successfully removed endoscopically. Rigid endoscopes (i.e., colonoscopes) are preferred, assuming that they are long enough. Rigid endoscopes allow one to use rigid grasping forceps, which in turn allow better manipulation and grasping than is available with forceps inserted through flexible endoscopes. The rigid scopes also offer some degree of protection to the esophagus; the foreign body is partially drawn up into the scope during removal so that it does not traumatize the esophageal mucosa. The major advantage to flexible endoscopes is that some esophageal foreign bodies are out of reach of rigid scopes; but the retrieval devices used in flexible endoscopes do not offer the operator as much control or power as do the rigid endoscopic forceps. Surgical removal of esophageal foreign bodies should be elected if (1) there is obvious perforation (i.e., preoperative pneumothorax or pleural exudate, (2) endoscopy cannot retrieve the foreign body, or (3) a fish hook is deeply embedded such that the point and barb are obviously completely through the wall of the esophagus and free to lacerate thoracic vessels. After removal of the foreign body, the esophagus must be carefully reevaluated endoscopically and the chest reradiographed to look for evidence of perforation. Perforations generally should be managed with débridement and surgical closure (see p. 377); however, small perforations occasionally may be allowed to close on their own.

Preoperative Management

Therapy to correct significant dehydration and electrolyte and acid-base imbalances should be initiated before surgery. Prophylactic antibiotics should be given (see p. 375).

Anesthesia

Anesthetic management of patients undergoing esophageal surgery is described on p. 374. Deep general anesthetic or muscle relaxants that reduce esophageal tone facilitate endoscopic manipulations. Nitrous oxide should not be used in these patients. Animals with pneumonia should be given oxygen before induction of anesthesia, and frequent ventilation and high inspired oxygen concentrations should be used during surgery.

Surgical Anatomy

The surgical anatomy of the esophagus is described on p. 375.

SURGICAL TECHNIQUE

Foreign bodies may be removed by extracting them endoscopically with grasping instruments, pulling them out using a balloon catheter, and advancing them into the stomach where they can be allowed to dissolve or be removed by gastrotomy (see p. 411), or by performing an esophagotomy (see p. 376) or a partial esophagectomy (see p. 377).

Endoscopic Removal of Esophageal Foreign Bodies

After examining the radiograph taken just before anesthetic induction, carefully advance the rigid endoscope down the esophagus to the level of the foreign body.

The larger the diameter of the endoscope, the better the visualization and the more the esophageal lumen will be dilated (which can aid in removing the foreign object).

Position the patient such that the neck is extended so that the endoscope will not put undue pressure on the trachea or the nearby vessels (if a flexible scope is used, positioning of the neck is not as important). Only advance the scope while observing through it so as not to push the scope into the foreign object and cause further trauma. Insufflate with minimal amounts of air and only if necessary; insufflating too much air might rupture weakened areas in the esophagus, cause a gastric dilatation that cannot be relieved by stomach tube due to obstruction of the esophagus, or it may cause a tension pneumothorax. Once the foreign object is found, aspirate any fluid or debris surrounding it so as to enhance visualization. After examining the object, grasp it firmly and then gently manipulate it to free it from the esophagus (there are typically points of the foreign object protruding into esophageal defects). Once it is freed, draw it as far as possible up into the rigid scope, and then remove the scope and foreign object as one unit. If there is severe trauma to the esophageal mucosa, put in a gastrostomy tube (see p. 100).

If the foreign object cannot be grasped, it can sometimes be pushed into the stomach *if* the endoscopist *knows* that there are no sharp objects or structures that could cause perforation. If necessary, a water-soluble lubricant can be applied around the foreign object to facilitate this maneuver. Forcing an object that is firmly embedded in the esophageal wall is contraindicated because doing so may cause perforation or enlargement of a preexisting perforation. Once in the stomach, the foreign object may be removed by gastrotomy (see p. 411) or, in the case of bones, allowed to dissolve. However, do not administer antacids, or the stomach will not be able to dissolve the bone.

Fish hooks can usually be removed with rigid scopes, depending upon the size of the barb (hooks with very large barbs often cannot be torn out of the mucosa) and whether the barb has been pushed all the way through the wall of the esophagus such that it could lacerate thoracic vessels when it is pulled back into the esophagus. The technique varies a little, depending upon whether the point of the hook is pointed craniad or caudad.

If the point of the hook is pointed caudad, then firmly grasp the hook at the bend such that when it is pulled, the point of the hook is pulled straight out, parallel with the esophageal lumen.

The barb will tear through the esophageal wall, leaving a small defect.

If the point of the hook is pointed craniad, firmly grasp the eye of the hook with the rigid forceps. Next, advance the rigid endoscope until the rim of the scope rests on the bend of the hook. Then holding the eye of the hook so that the shaft remains parallel with the lumen of the esophagus and the rigid scope, advance the scope and the rigid grasping forceps as one unit, tearing the hook out of the mucosa.

Balloon Catheter–Assisted Removal of Foreign Objects

An alternative to grasping the foreign body is to pass a balloon catheter distal to the object (Figs. 19-45 and 19-46). The esophageal lumen is then dilated beyond its normal size by inflating the balloon, and the object is disengaged from the esophageal wall by endoscopic manipulation if necessary and removed as the catheter is pulled out through the mouth. This procedure is advisable only for foreign bodies with a relatively smooth contour. After nonsurgical foreign body removal, radiographs may be taken to look for evidence of perforation (e.g., pneumomediastinum and pneumothorax).

Surgical Removal of Esophageal Foreign Objects

Foreign bodies can be surgically removed by performing an esophagotomy (see p. 376) or a partial esophagectomy (see p. 377). Distal esophageal foreign bodies occasionally are removed by a gastrotomy.

Make an incision midway between the greater and lesser curvature. Direct a forceps into the distal esophagus, grasp the object, pull it into the stomach, and remove it.

An esophagotomy or a partial esophagectomy is performed when foreign bodies cannot be removed by other means, when the risk of esophageal perforation or laceration is high, or when there is evidence of mediastinitis, pleuritis, or esophageal necrosis.

Débride all esophageal disruptions as necessary and close in one or two layers as for esophagotomy (see p. 376).

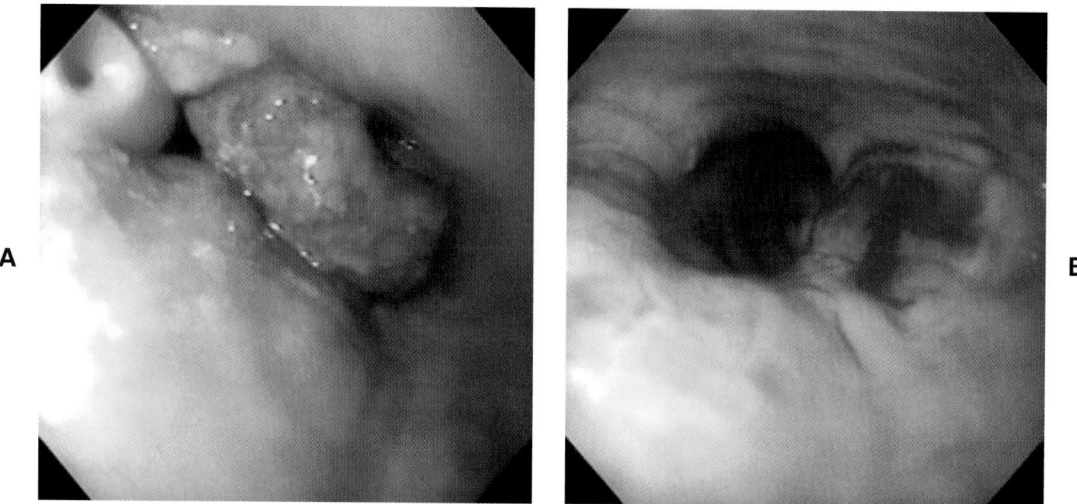

FIG. 19-45
A, Endoscopic appearance of a piece of liver lodged in the esophagus. Note the tip of a Foley catheter, which is being passed to retrieve it. **B,** After retrieval of the foreign body, ulceration of the mucosa was visible (3 o'clock).

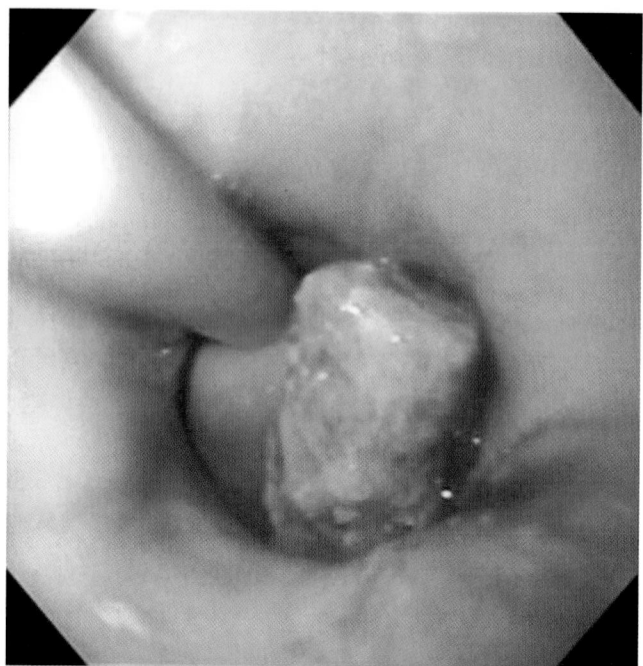

FIG. 19-46
Smooth esophageal foreign bodies can be removed by balloon retraction during endoscopy. Dilate the esophagus, pass the catheter distal to the foreign body, then inflate the balloon and withdraw the catheter and foreign body.

Abnormal communications between the alimentary and respiratory tracts (i.e., bronchoesophageal or tracheoesophageal fistula) must be closed. Partial or complete pulmonary lobectomy (see p. 875) is required with some bronchoesophageal fistulae.

SUTURE MATERIALS AND SPECIAL INSTRUMENTS

Endoscopes (both flexible and rigid, but preferably rigid), endoscopic grasping forceps, or ballooned-tipped catheters (i.e., Foley catheter) are necessary for nonsurgical foreign body removal. Thoracic retractors are necessary for surgical removal of intrathoracic foreign bodies. Noncrushing intestinal forceps to occlude the esophageal lumen may be necessary for esophagotomy or esophagectomy procedures.

POSTOPERATIVE CARE AND ASSESSMENT

All patients should be observed carefully for 2 to 3 days for signs of esophageal leakage and infection. Esophagitis and aspiration pneumonia should be treated as described on p. 373. Antibiotics should be continued for several days if the esophageal mucosa is severely eroded or lacerated, and especially if a fish hook was removed. Intravenous fluids should be continued until feeding resumes. To prevent delays in healing, all oral intake (food, water, medications) should be withheld for a minimum of 24 hours after removal of the foreign bodies that cause substantial erosion or ulceration. If no regurgitation is seen, water and then a bland gruel should be introduced gradually. Animals with minimal esophageal trauma may be offered water within 24 to 48 hours, followed by small meals of gruel. After 3 to 7 days of gruel feeding, soft, moist food should then be offered for 5 to 7 days, followed by a gradual return to a normal diet. Animals with moderate to severe esophageal trauma should avoid oral intake for 3 to 7 days. In debilitated patients or those requiring no oral intake for longer than 3 days, gastrostomy feeding tubes should be placed (see p. 100). Severe esophagitis should be treated with H_2-antagonists or proton pump inhibitors to reduce gastric acidity. Sucralfate may be considered. Antibiotics effective against oral anaerobes (ampicillin, amoxicillin, clindamycin; see Box 19-16) are used, and corticosteroids may help prevent cicatrix formation. Analgesics may be necessary to control pain (see Table 13-4 on p. 133).

COMPLICATIONS

Complications of foreign body removal include esophagitis, ischemic necrosis, dehiscence, leakage, infection, fistulae, esophageal diverticula, and stricture formation. Esophageal perforation may lead to mediastinitis, pleuritis, and pyothorax. Prolonged duration of clinical signs and increased numbers of immature neutrophils may suggest esophageal perforation; however, perforation is best diagnosed radiographically.

PROGNOSIS

Removal of a foreign body is essential. The prognosis is good if perforation has not occurred; however, it is guarded if perforation has resulted in mediastinitis or pyothorax (or both). Ischemic necrosis or perforation of the esophagus may occur after foreign body removal. Leakage of saliva and ingesta into the mediastinum or pleural cavity usually causes severe inflammation, infection, and death.

Suggested Reading

Cohn LA, Stoll MR, Branson KR et al: Fatal hemothorax following management of an esophageal foreign body, *J Am Anim Hosp Assoc* 39:251, 2003.

This dog died when the bulb of a gastrostomy tube was retrieved endoscopically from the stomach. The hemorrhage was due to avulsion of small arterial branches, which in turn may have been due to medial necrosis caused by prior disruption of blood flow as a result of the esophageal foreign body.

Nawrocki MA, Mackin AJ, McLaughlin R et al: Fluoroscopic and endoscopic localization of an esophagobronchial fistula in a dog, *J Am Anim Hosp Assoc* 39:257, 2003.

This case report describes endoscopic localization of a fistula in a diverticulum after foreign body removal and placement of a guidewire, which assisted surgical isolation.

Moore AH: Removal of oesophageal foreign bodies in dogs: use of the fluoroscopic method and outcome, *J Small Anim Pract* 42:227, 2001.

The authors report 65 admissions for esophageal foreign body, of which 51 of 61 were successfully removed by manipulating forceps under fluoroscopic guidance.

ESOPHAGEAL STRICTURES

DEFINITION

Benign esophageal strictures *(stenosis, cicatrix)* are bands of intraluminal or intramural fibrous tissue that may completely or partly obstruct the esophagus.

GENERAL CONSIDERATIONS AND CLINICALLY RELEVANT PATHOPHYSIOLOGY

Benign esophageal strictures may be caused by esophagitis secondary to esophageal foreign bodies, gastroesophageal reflux during anesthesia, surgery, trauma, or caustic agents (e.g.,

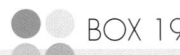

BOX 19-21

Esophageal Strictures: Key Points

Strictures form when the mucosa is traumatized
Suspect if there has been an anesthetic episode during the previous month or if the patient has been receiving tetracycline or doxycycline
Signs may begin immediately after injury
Often missed by survey radiography and sometimes by contrast radiography
Esophagoscopy is diagnostic, but inexperienced endoscopists can miss lesions in larger animals
Strictures may be multiple and extensive but are usually single
Most occur near the lower esophageal sphincter
Treat for esophagitis and pneumonia if indicated
Balloon dilation results in a satisfactory outcome in most patients, but some patients need multiple balloonings
Most can eat canned or dry food after treatment
Strictures may recur

tetracycline, doxycycline, and acid or alkaline agents). The risk of developing a stricture after an anesthetic episode is reported as 0.7% (Wilson and Walshaw, 2004), and 65% of animals with strictures have been associated with an anesthetic episode (Melendez et al, 1998). Most strictures are single, but occasionally they are multiple and most occur near the lower esophageal sphincter (Box 19-21). Strictures occur more commonly after circumferential esophageal trauma. To produce a stricture, esophageal damage must involve the muscular layers and affect most of the circumference in a focal area. The mucosal defect is then replaced by epithelial migration. The gap in the muscle is filled by fibrous connective tissue, and the width of the scar is reduced by wound contraction and collagen remodeling. This leads to narrowing of the esophageal lumen, which may cause obstruction. The degree of obstruction varies, depending on the severity of the original lesion. Peristaltic waves carrying food boluses are disrupted by the obstruction. In cases of partial obstruction, part of each bolus passes the obstruction and moves down the esophagus. The other portion of the bolus accumulates proximal to the obstruction, and the proximal esophagus may eventually distend. If distention occurs and is severe, it may disrupt normal neuromuscular function and reduce peristalsis. The accumulated food and secretions frequently are regurgitated.

Factors related to the development and severity of esophagitis following reflux include the duration of esophageal contact; acidity; presence of enzymes, such as pepsin; effectiveness of esophageal clearance; and mucosal resistance to injury. Once esophagitis develops, a vicious cycle can occur in that the esophageal inflammation decreases lower esophageal sphincter tone, predisposing to additional reflux, which exacerbates the inflammation, and so on. Gastroesophageal reflux may occur during anesthesia when protective mechanisms are diminished and the gastroesophageal sphincter loses tone. Anticholinergics, thiopental, propofol, opioids, and inhaled anesthetics decrease the lower esophageal sphincter pressure in dogs. Prolonged fasting is associated with a more acidic reflux and a higher incidence of gastroesophageal reflux (Wilson and Walshaw, 2004). Gastric acid can damage the esophagus severely if not neutralized by saliva or removed by peristalsis within a few minutes. Signs of regurgitation may become evident within a few days or weeks after surgery because of stricture formation.

DIAGNOSIS

Clinical Presentation

Signalment. Any age, breed, or gender of dog or cat may be affected.

History. Regurgitation is the most common presenting sign, and stricture should be suspected in animals experiencing frequent regurgitation with a history of previous esophageal trauma, surgery, anesthetic episode, or treatment with a tetracycline derivative. Some animals retain fluids but regurgitate solids. Pain may be experienced when solid food becomes lodged in the stricture by forceful esophageal peristaltic waves. Regurgitation or vomiting often begins within 2 weeks of an anesthetic episode. Vomiting and regurgitation are often associated with eating, ptyalism, gagging, and dysphagia. Weight loss, coughing, and aerophagia may also be recognized.

Physical Examination Findings

Although animals with esophageal strictures may be thin and depressed, the physical examination usually is normal. Occasionally the cervical esophagus is dilated. There may be putrid breath secondary to decay of material retained in the esophagus. Patients with aspiration pneumonia may be febrile and have increased respiratory rate and effort, crackles, wheezes, and increased lung sounds.

Diagnostic Imaging

Esophageal strictures can be difficult to identify. Positive contrast esophagograms facilitate diagnosis (Fig. 19-47). Partial strictures are more readily identified if barium is mixed with food and observed fluoroscopically. There may or may not be dilatation of the esophagus proximal to an abrupt narrowing. It may be difficult to determine the extent of a stricture radiographically.

Esophagoscopy. Esophagoscopy allows visualization of the lesion. The mucosa sometimes is inflamed and has erosions and ulcers; sometimes it appears normal but with a compromised diameter (Fig. 19-48). In other cases, the stricture is a ring of white fibrous tissue that narrows the esophageal lumen and fails to distend with insufflation. In severe cases, it may be impossible to advance the scope beyond the stricture, and gastric overdistention can be a significant complication of esophagoscopy if the scope cannot be passed into the stomach to suction excess air. Biopsy and histologic examination rule out stricture that has occurred secondary to neoplasia.

Laboratory Findings

Animals with esophageal strictures show no specific laboratory abnormalities unless aspiration pneumonia is present.

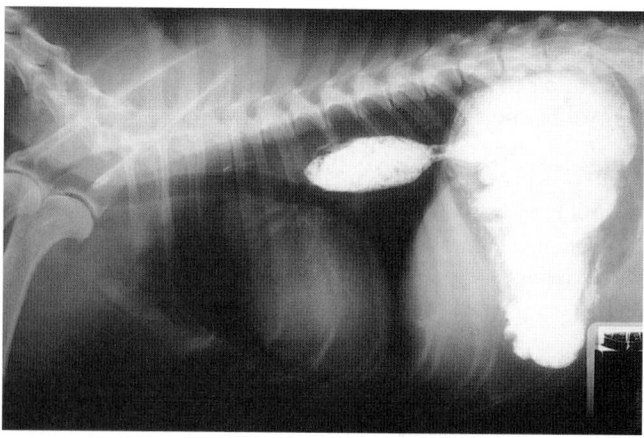

FIG. 19-47
Radiographic appearance of an esophageal stricture after administration of barium. Notice the accumulation of contrast in the distal thoracic esophagus just cranial to the diaphragm.

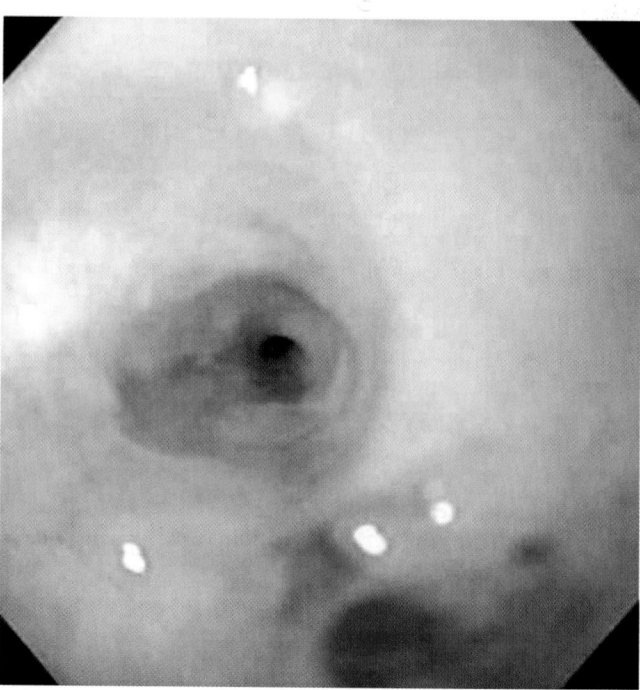

FIG. 19-48
Endoscopic appearance of a distal esophageal stricture subsequent to anesthesia and surgery to remove mammary tumors.

DIFFERENTIAL DIAGNOSIS

Vascular ring anomalies, extraluminal masses, esophageal neoplasia, foreign bodies, esophagitis, gastroesophageal intussusception, esophageal diverticulum, hiatal hernias, megaesophagus, and cricopharyngeal dysfunction are other possible causes of regurgitation that must be differentiated from esophageal stricture.

MEDICAL MANAGEMENT

The goals of treatment are to resolve regurgitation and maintain nutrition and hydration by oral feeding. Treat esophagitis (see p. 373) and aspiration pneumonia (see p. 374) as previously described (see Boxes 19-15 and 19-16). Soften food by adding water until it is liquid enough to pass through the obstruction. A gastrostomy tube will allow feeding if the stricture is severe. Alter the environment so foreign bodies, which may become lodged at the stricture, are avoided.

SURGICAL TREATMENT

Strictures are treated by correcting the cause and then reducing the narrowing with balloon catheter dilation or bougienage. Balloon catheter dilation is the preferred method for dilation of esophageal strictures because there is less chance of perforation and fewer dilations are required. Laser incision of the scar tissue at several sites around the circumference can be used to augment dilation in severe cases. Partial esophagectomy usually is not necessary and may not be possible, depending on the length of the stricture. Resistant cervical strictures may be corrected by the creation of a traction diverticulum.

Preoperative Management

Animals should fast before esophageal dilation. Treatment for esophagitis and aspiration pneumonia should be initiated as necessary before stricture treatment (see p. 373). Dilation of esophageal strictures is associated with bacteremia in people, and preprocedure antibiotics are recommended although there are no data on their effect on outcome in dogs and cats.

Anesthesia

General anesthetic is required for esophageal dilation or bougienage. Recommendations for an anesthetic in patients with esophageal disorders are given on p. 374.

Surgical Anatomy

The surgical anatomy of the esophagus is discussed on p. 375.

Positioning

Balloon dilatation and bougienage generally are performed with the patient in lateral recumbency.

SURGICAL TECHNIQUE
Bougienage

Bougienage involves the dilation of a stricture using blunt dilators that are graduated in size. A thoroughly lubricated, small, tapered probe (dilator) is pushed through the stricture. The initial dilator is followed by a graduated series of successively larger probes until the desired lumen size is achieved or excess resistance is encountered. Some types of dilators are passed over guide wires. This technique is best done under direct endoscopic visualization, but can be done with fluoroscopic guidance. Bougienage also exerts a longitudinal shearing force at the stricture site that can be more traumatic than is usual with balloon dilation. However, data from human medicine suggest that success is more related to the training of the endoscopist than the type of equipment (i.e., bougienage versus balloon dilation) used.

> NOTE: It is advised that you be trained in this technique before attempting it as it is possible to perforate the esophagus if you do it improperly.

Balloon Dilation

There are two main techniques: placing a balloon catheter through the biopsy channel of the endoscope and through the stricture (Leib et al, 2001), or running the balloon catheter down and over a previously placed guide wire.

The guide wire technique involves more work, but may be somewhat safer.

First, endoscopically place a guide wire through the stricture site. Use a wire that is stiff at one end and floppy at the other. Insert the floppy end of the wire through the scope's biopsy channel and through the stricture. Then withdraw the endoscope from the patient while continually feeding the wire into the patient, thus removing the endoscope from around the wire while the latter is kept in the stricture. Next, place the balloon in the stricture by running the balloon catheter over the wire while observing it endoscopically. Once the balloon is positioned so that the middle of it is near the center of the stricture, inflate the balloon with fluid or air (depending on the type of balloon) and deflate it after a minute. If (1) the stricture is very mature and thick, and the balloon cannot rupture the stricture, or (2) ballooning is typically associated with excessive trauma and reformation of the stricture, it may be advantageous to incise mature fibrotic strictures at three or four sites around the circumference of the esophagus using an electrosurgical or laser unit before dilation.

This should cause the stricture to rupture more evenly at three or four sites as opposed to causing a major, deep rupture at just one site.

The balloon must stay in the stricture during this process. If the balloon is not correctly positioned, it will migrate out of the stricture as it is inflated and the stricture will not be dilated. Progressively larger balloons may be used until the desired degree of dilation has been achieved. The amount of dilation necessary is subjective and should not be overly ambitious. Most small animals will be functional if the esophageal lumen is opened up to 10 mm; larger animals may need to be opened up to 15 or even 20 mm. Repeat the dilation as often as necessary to attain a satisfactory outcome. Many animals only require 1 dilation, but some require more (15 or more). If multiple dilations are required, they are usually done 2 to 3 times weekly until the stricture no longer re-forms.

> NOTE: Cause as little trauma as possible during dilation to lessen the likelihood of stricture reformation. In particular, try not to tear off or aspirate any more esophageal mucosa than is absolutely necessary.

The goal is to open the stricture just enough so that the patient is functional and can eat soft food, not just gruel. It is often not possible to completely eliminate the stricture. These patients are often at risk for esophageal foreign bodies at the site of the stricture because there is usually some degree of lumen compromise remaining.

Failure of dilatory therapy may necessitate esophageal resection or replacement. Stents are sometimes inserted in people, but have not been particularly successful in dogs.

SUTURE MATERIALS AND SPECIAL INSTRUMENTS

When dilating an esophageal stricture, balloons specifically designed for use in the esophagus should be used (e.g., Max-Force TTS High Performance Balloon Dilation Catheter, Boston Scientific Microvasive, Natick, Mass.). An electrosurgical unit adaptable to laparoscopic sites or a laser unit is advantageous with mature fibrotic strictures.

POSTOPERATIVE CARE AND ASSESSMENT

Continue to monitor for regurgitation and aspiration pneumonia. Superficial mucosal tears are expected following dilation. However, patients should be monitored closely for signs of perforation, which include dysphagia, subcutaneous emphysema, pneumothorax, pneumomediastinum, and mediastinitis. Nasal oxygen may benefit these animals postoperatively, and analgesics (see Chapter 13) should be provided if necessary (esophageal lesions are surprisingly painful). If perforation is suspected, one should verify with thoracic radiographs, put in a gastrostomy tube, and administer antibiotics. Monitor for hemorrhage; although rare it can be excessive, requiring transfusion. Diverticulum formation is another complication that may develop (see later discussion on this page).

If the procedure has caused a substantial mucosal tear, therapy for esophagitis (antacids, prokinetics, sucralfate, and antibiotics) may be administered (see Boxes 19-15 and 19-16). Antibiotic therapy intuitively makes sense, but there are no data showing that it has an effect on outcome. Corticosteroids (e.g., prednisolone, 1.1 mg/kg given orally once a day) may be administered to help prevent stricture reformation, but the efficacy of this treatment on outcome is unknown. Steroids have also been endoscopically injected intralesionally. Preexisting esophagitis and aspiration pneumonia should be treated as described on p. 373. Placement of a gastrostomy tube (see p. 100) may be beneficial in these patients so that oral feeding can be avoided for 7 to 10 days, but the patient can be kept in a positive nitrogen balance during healing. When oral feeding resumes, feed small, frequent meals of a soft (not gruel) consistency.

PROGNOSIS

Most patients (approximately 85%) with esophageal strictures can be helped by dilation, but strictures may reform. Most animals are able to tolerate canned or dry food without regurgitation, but some require gruel. Thin stricture bands may require only a single dilation; however, patients with severe or long strictures often require multiple dilations. There is a more guarded prognosis if strictures are several centimeters long; if there is dense, thick, mature fibrous tissue; or if severe esophagitis is persistent. Prognosis is worse if perforation occurs. Resection of long strictures may result in dehiscence caused by excessive anastomotic tension.

References

Leib MS, Dinnel H, Ward DL et al: Endoscopic balloon dilation of benign esophageal strictures in dogs and cats, *J Vet Int Med* 15:547, 2001.

Melendez LD, Twedt DC, Weyrauch EA et al: Conservative therapy using balloon dilation for intramural, inflammatory esophageal strictures in dogs and cats: a retrospective study of 23 cases (1987-1997), *Eur J Comparative Gastroenterol* 3(1): 31, 1998.

Wilson DV, Walshaw R: Post anesthetic esophageal dysfunction in 13 dogs, *J Am Anim Hosp Assoc* 40:455, 2004.

Suggested Reading

Han E, Broussard J, Baer KE: Feline esophagitis secondary to gastroesophageal reflux disease: clinical signs and radiographic, endoscopic, and histopathologic findings, *J Am Anim Hosp Assoc* 39:161, 2003.

Three cats had chronic esophagitis due to reflux. Radiographs revealed poor motility and esophageal dilation, whereas endoscopy revealed ulcers, hyperemia, and an abnormal lower esophageal sphincter.

Sellon RK, Willard MD: Esophagitis and esophageal strictures, *Vet Clin North Am Small Anim Pract* 33:945, 2003.

This is a recent review of the diagnosis and therapy of these two disorders.

Wilson D, Evans A, Miller R: Effects of preanesthetic administration of morphine on gastroesophageal reflux and regurgitation during anesthesia in dogs, *Am J Vet Res* 66:386, 2005.

Administering morphine as a preanesthetic increased the incidence of gastroesophageal reflux during the following anesthesia.

ESOPHAGEAL DIVERTICULA

DEFINITIONS

Esophageal diverticula are saclike dilatations that produce pouches in the wall of the esophagus. A **pulsion diverticulum** is a herniation of the mucosa through the muscular layers of the esophagus. These diverticula are produced by exaggerated intraluminal pressure in association with abnormal regional peristalsis or when obstruction interferes with normal peristalsis. **Traction diverticula** are distortions, angulations, or funnel-shaped bulges of the full-thickness wall of the esophagus caused by adhesions resulting from an external lesion.

GENERAL CONSIDERATIONS AND CLINICALLY RELEVANT PATHOPHYSIOLOGY

Esophageal diverticula are rare. They may be acquired or congenital and are found most commonly in the distal cervical esophagus cranial to the thoracic inlet or in the distal thoracic esophagus just cranial to the diaphragm (epiphrenic). Congenital diverticula are believed to develop as a result of a congenital weakness of the esophageal wall, abnormal separation of tracheal and esophageal embryonic buds, or eccentric vacuole formation in the esophagus. Acquired forms are classified as pulsion or traction diverticula based on their cause. *Pulsion diverticula* are most common in the epiphrenic area, but can form cranial to any diseased esophageal segment. Many conditions may initiate the formation of diverticula, including esophagitis, esophageal stenosis, foreign bodies, vascular ring anomalies, neuromuscular dysfunction, and hiatal hernias. The esophageal mucosa herniates secondary to increased intraluminal pressure, accumulation of food, and esophageal inflammation. The wall of a pulsion diverticulum consists of only esophageal epithelium and connective tissue.

Traction diverticula occur after an inflammatory process involving the trachea, bronchi, lymph nodes, or other extraesophageal structures. Inflammation causes fibrous tissue to form between the esophagus and the diseased structure. As the fibrous tissue matures, it contracts and pulls an area of the esophagus outward to form a pouch. Most traction diverticula occur in the cranial and midthoracic esophagus. The wall of a traction diverticulum consists of adventitia, muscle, submucosa, and mucosa.

DIAGNOSIS
Clinical Presentation

Signalment. Any age, breed, or gender of dog or cat may be affected.

History. Small diverticula can be asymptomatic. Large, multilobulated diverticula usually are associated with clinical signs. Diverticula may result in esophageal impaction, chronic esophagitis, and rupture of the diverticulum wall, with resultant mediastinitis or the formation of an esophagotracheal-bronchial fistula. Clinical signs may include distress or gasping after eating, postprandial regurgitation, intermittent anorexia, fever, weight loss, thoracic or abdominal pain, and respiratory distress.

Physical Examination Findings

The physical examination is normal if the diverticulum is asymptomatic. Abnormal lung sounds may be auscultated if aspiration pneumonia has developed.

Diagnostic Imaging

Radiographs should be performed with the neck in an extended position to diminish "normal" esophageal redundancy in young and brachycephalic breeds. Diverticula appear as air-filled or food-filled masses in the area of the esophagus. An esophagogram usually demonstrates a deviation or outpouching of the esophageal lumen that fills partly or completely with contrast material. Esophagoscopy is helpful in confirming the radiographic diagnosis and identifying associated esophagitis, strictures, or other abnormalities. The esophageal wall may be very thin, and esophagoscopy must be performed with care.

NOTE: Dogs and cats with generalized megaesophagus tend to have greater outpouching of the esophageal wall cranial to the base of the heart. Do not misdiagnose these animals as having diverticula.

Laboratory Findings

Esophageal diverticula do not produce any specific laboratory abnormalities. Laboratory findings consistent with pyothorax (see p. 923) may result if the diverticulum has ruptured. Neutrophilia may be present if aspiration pneumonia has developed.

DIFFERENTIAL DIAGNOSIS

Esophageal hiatal hernia, gastroesophageal intussusception, stricture, neoplasia, extraluminal masses, vascular ring anomalies, esophageal foreign body, esophagitis, and megaesophagus are other possible causes of regurgitation.

SURGICAL TREATMENT

Persistent underlying causes of the diverticula must be identified and treated. Asymptomatic, small diverticula may be treated by feeding a soft, bland diet with the animal in an upright position to prevent food accumulation in the pouch. Large diverticula should be surgically excised.

Preoperative Management

Esophagitis and aspiration pneumonia should be treated preoperatively as described on p. 373. Prophylactic antibiotics are indicated if esophageal resection is considered likely.

Anesthesia

Anesthetic recommendations for animals undergoing cervical esophageal surgery are discussed on p. 375. Anesthetic recommendations for thoracotomy are given on p. 867.

Surgical Anatomy

The surgical anatomy of the esophagus is described on p. 375.

Positioning

Patients are positioned in dorsal or lateral recumbency, depending on the site of the diverticulum. Radiographs are important to help determine the best surgical approach. Diverticula in the cervical esophagus are approached via a ventral cervical midline incision with the animal in dorsal recumbency. Thoracic diverticula usually are approached via a lateral thoracotomy. Occasionally a median sternotomy or thoracic wall flap may be necessary to approach diverticula at the thoracic inlet or cranial mediastinum.

SURGICAL TECHNIQUE

After identifying the diverticulum, isolate it from surrounding structures with blunt and sharp dissection, and then pack it off with laparotomy pads. Partial lung lobectomy may be necessary if adhesions cannot be easily separated. Position a TA (thoracoabdominal; linear) or GIA (gastrointestinal anastomosis) stapling device along the base of the diverticulum and fire. Transect and remove the diverticulum without contaminating the surgical site. If stapling equipment is not available, suction the esophageal lumen and place noncrushing forceps across the proposed transection site. Transect the diverticulum, and appose the edges as for esophagotomy with a one- or two-layer simple appositional pattern (see p. 377). Lavage the surgical site and, if possible, mobilize and place omentum over the incision. Thoracostomy tubes may be placed in animals having thoracotomies to evacuate residual air and fluid.

POSTOPERATIVE CARE AND ASSESSMENT

After surgery, these patients should be monitored for esophagitis and aspiration pneumonia and treated appropriately (see p. 373). Postoperative esophagoscopy and esophagograms may be indicated if problems are detected. Regurgitation that occurs secondary to persistent esophagitis is a possible problem. Infection as a result of contamination of the surrounding tissue during surgery, dehiscence, or leakage at the surgical site are other possible problems. Postoperative analgesics should be provided to control pain (see p. 868 for recommendations after thoracotomy).

PROGNOSIS

Asymptomatic patients often continue to do well without surgery; feeding them in an upright position to prevent food accumulation in the diverticula may be helpful. Clinical signs may be difficult to control in symptomatic patients with medical therapy alone. If surgery is not possible, such patients should be treated for esophagitis and fed soft food in an upright position. The prognosis with surgical correction is good if thoracic contamination is prevented and good esophageal apposition is achieved.

ESOPHAGEAL NEOPLASIA

DEFINITION

Esophageal neoplasia is any abnormal, noninflammatory proliferation of cells in the esophagus.

GENERAL CONSIDERATIONS AND CLINICALLY RELEVANT PATHOPHYSIOLOGY

Esophageal neoplasia is rare and usually malignant. Tumors are often locally invasive and metastasize through lymphatic and hematogenous routes. The most common types of tumors are sarcomas, SCCs, and leiomyomas. Leiomyomas have been reported at the lower esophageal sphincter in aged beagles. These tumors usually are advanced by the time clinical signs are recognized. Primary esophageal carcinomas are of unknown etiology. Primary esophageal sarcomas (os-teosarcoma, fibrosarcoma) often are located in the vicinity of parasitic granulomas caused by *Spirocerca lupi*. The life cycle of *S. lupi* involves a coprophagous beetle that is eaten by the dog or a transport host that is subsequently eaten by the dog. Regional tumors from the thyroid, thymus, heart base, or lung may invade the esophagus secondarily.

Esophageal tumors initially cause partial obstruction of the esophagus, which may interfere with motility and lead to dilatation of the proximal esophagus. As the tumor enlarges, signs of complete esophageal obstruction become apparent. Most esophageal tumors are locally invasive and metastasize to the draining lymph nodes.

DIAGNOSIS
Clinical Presentation

Signalment. In cats, SCCs usually are seen in females in the middle third of the esophagus just caudal to the thoracic inlet. Most esophageal tumors occur in dogs and cats over 6 to 8 years of age.

History. Chronic progressive signs of obstructive esophageal disease in middle-aged and older animals suggest esophageal neoplasia. Animals with primary tumors may be asymptomatic until the mass becomes large enough to cause almost complete obstruction. These animals may be brought in with regurgitation, lethargy, depression, drooling, dysphagia, anorexia, weight loss, and/or fetid breath. In animals with secondary tumors, clinical signs may include regurgitation, dyspnea, palpable masses, and/or systemic and local tumor effects.

Physical Examination Findings

The physical examination usually is normal. Some animals are thin, and a dilated cervical esophagus may be identified. Hypertrophic osteopathy and spondylosis deformans may be noted, especially with *S. lupi*–induced sarcomas. Some will have pyrexia, submandibular swelling, pale mucous membranes, melena, salivation, cough, neurologic signs, and weight loss. Crackles from aspiration pneumonia may be detected.

Diagnostic Imaging

Aerophagia (swallowing of air), displacement of the esophagus, and megaesophagus may be signs of esophageal neoplasia. Survey thoracic radiographs may be normal or may reveal a soft tissue opacity in the plane of the esophagus or mediastinum (Fig. 19-49). This density may be impossible to distinguish from an esophageal foreign body in some cases. The esophagus may retain air cranial to the tumor. The lungs should be evaluated for metastatic lesions. Contrast esophagograms may demonstrate an intraluminal mass (mucosal irregularities, filling defects, or stricture) with primary tumors, or an impinging mural or extraluminal mass with smooth mucosal margins and no filling defect with secondary tumors. Fluoroscopic studies may reveal abnormal motility. Signs of spondylosis and spondylitis may be detected at the ventral aspect of the cervical and thoracic vertebrae. Dogs with *S. lupi* infestation commonly have spondylosis

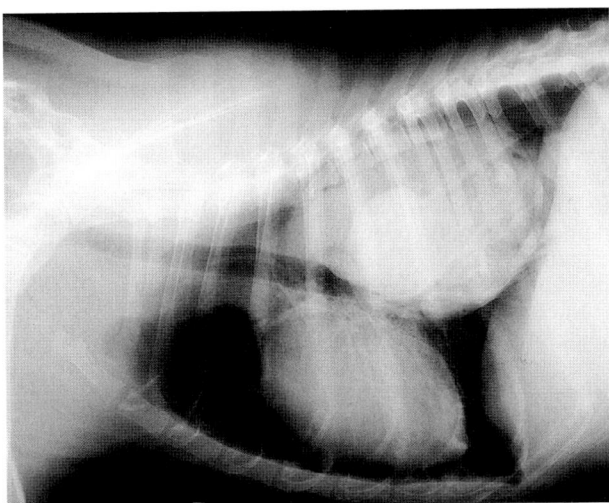

FIG. 19-49
Lateral thoracic radiograph of an 8-year-old dog with a large esophageal carcinoma. Notice the soft tissue opacity mass in the plane of the distal thoracic esophagus.

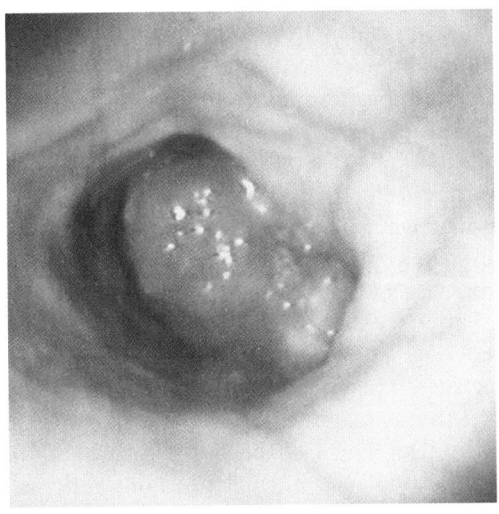

FIG. 19-50
Appearance of an intraluminal mass on esophagoscopy. Esophagoscopy allows biopsy of such masses.

deformans or spondylitis of the cervical or thoracic vertebrae with or without hypertrophic osteopathy. CT scans may help determine the degree of esophageal wall involvement. Esophagoscopy allows direct visualization of intraluminal masses and a biopsy for definitive diagnosis (Fig. 19-50). An adult *S. lupi* worm occasionally is seen protruding into the lumen from the mass. Identification of a granuloma with a nipplelike orifice is characteristic of spirocercosis. Extraluminal masses cannot be visualized unless they have eroded into the lumen. It is difficult to inflate the lumen if it is impinged on or has been invaded by extraluminal masses.

Laboratory Findings

Laboratory values may indicate chronic disease or paraneoplastic syndromes. Animals with spirocercosis-associated sarcomas may have neutrophilic leukocytosis (82%) and microcytic anemia (30%) (Ranen et al, 2004). *S. lupi* eggs may be detected on a fecal sedimentation test, but usually are difficult to find. A histologic diagnosis of esophageal sarcoma in addition to detecting *S. lupi* eggs in feces, esophageal nodular granulomas, or spondylitis of the caudal thoracic vertebrae is considered diagnostic of spirocercosis-associated sarcomas (Ranen et al, 2004).

DIFFERENTIAL DIAGNOSIS

Esophageal stricture, extraluminal masses, vascular ring anomalies, esophageal foreign body, esophagitis, gastroesophageal intussusception, esophageal diverticulum, hiatal hernia, and megaesophagus are other possible causes of regurgitation. The clinical signs of ptyalism, odynophagia, and sialadenopathy associated with *Spirocerca* lesions appear similar to the clinical signs in dogs with salivary gland necrosis and necrotizing sialometaplasia syndrome (Berry, 2000).

SURGICAL TREATMENT

Early diagnosis is important before metastasis or extensive esophageal involvement has occurred. Partial esophagectomy with end-to-end anastomosis is indicated when approximation can be accomplished without excess tension.

Preoperative Management

S. lupi–associated esophageal granulomas often resolve after treatment with doramectin (200 mg/kg given subcutaneously at 14-day intervals for three treatments) (Berry, 2000). Complete resolution of the esophageal nodules was confirmed by endoscopy in all dogs. None of the dogs experienced adverse effects to the drug. Chemotherapy, radiation therapy, or photodynamic therapy may be beneficial in some animals.

Anesthesia

Anesthetic recommendations for animals undergoing cervical esophageal surgery are provided on p. 374. Selected anesthetic protocols for animals undergoing thoracic surgery are provided on p. 867.

Surgical Anatomy

The surgical anatomy of the esophagus is described on p. 375.

SURGICAL TECHNIQUE

Esophagectomy is described on p. 377. Refer to p. 384 for a description of suture material and special instruments for esophageal surgery.

POSTOPERATIVE CARE AND ASSESSMENT

The patient should be monitored for esophagitis and aspiration pneumonia and treated as needed postoperatively (see p. 373). Nasal oxygen may benefit these animals, and analgesics should be provided to control pain. See p. 384 for recommendations for postoperative care of animals undergoing esophageal surgery. Dehiscence caused by excessive tension at the anastomosis and tumor recurrence are possible complications of esophageal surgery. Continue doramectin treatment in animals with spirocercosis.

PROGNOSIS

Most esophageal tumors are advanced at the time of diagnosis and do not respond well to radiation therapy or chemotherapy. Radiation therapy may be palliative, but radiation-induced esophagitis and damage to the heart, lungs, and great vessels are possible sequelae that are poorly tolerated. Photodynamic therapy may palliate some nonresectable tumors. Resection may be curative for leiomyomas, but for other malignancies the prognosis is guarded for cure or palliation because resection is difficult as a result of the advanced nature of most tumors at the time of detection.

References

Berry WL: *Spirocerca lupi* esophageal granulomas in 7 dogs: resolution after treatment with doramectin, *J Vet Intern Med* 14:609, 2000.

Ranen E, Lavy E, Aizenberg PS et al: Spirocercosis-associated esophageal sarcomas in dogs. A retrospective study of 17 cases (1997-2003), *Vet Parasitol* 119:209, 2004.

Suggested Reading

Jacobs TM, Rosen GM: Photodynamic therapy as a treatment for esophageal squamous cell carcinoma in a dog, *J Am Anim Hosp Assoc* 36:257, 2000.

Reduction of tumor size was seen after each of three treatments. Nutrition via gastrostomy tube and oral alimentation were successful in maintaining the dogs until euthanasia 9 months after initial treatment.

Ranen E, Shamir MH, Shahar R et al: Partial esophagectomy with single layer closure for treatment of esophageal sarcomas in 6 dogs, *Vet Surg* 33:428, 2004.

Marginal resection allowed palliation of signs for 1 to 13 months and survival was 2 to 16 months.

HIATAL HERNIA

DEFINITION

Hiatal hernias are protrusions of the abdominal esophagus, gastroesophageal junction, and sometimes a portion of the gastric fundus through the esophageal hiatus into the caudal mediastinum cranial to the diaphragm.

GENERAL CONSIDERATIONS AND CLINICALLY RELEVANT PATHOPHYSIOLOGY

Hiatal hernias usually are caused by congenital abnormalities of the hiatus that allow cranial movement of the abdominal esophagus and stomach (Box 19-22). The phrenicoesophageal ligament is lax or stretched and allows the gastroesophageal junction to be displaced through the hiatus into the caudal mediastinum. Malpositioning or lack of sup-

BOX 19-22

Hiatal Hernia: Key Points

Most are congenital rather than acquired
Shar-Peis and English bulldogs are most commonly affected
Some are asymptomatic
Symptomatic animals have regurgitation and esophagitis
Herniation may be intermittent, making radiographic diagnosis challenging
Herniorrhaphy includes hiatal reduction, esophagopexy, and left-sided gastropexy
Surgery is usually most appropriate for younger symptomatic animals; older symptomatic animals are usually best treated medically
Treat for esophagitis initially after surgery
Prognosis is usually good after repair

port of the gastroesophageal sphincter reduces gastroesophageal sphincter pressure and leads to gastroesophageal reflux. Gastroesophageal reflux and subsequent esophagitis and megaesophagus are responsible for most of the clinical signs. Hiatal hernia occasionally occurs secondary to trauma and has occurred concurrently with severe respiratory distress. Trauma may damage diaphragmatic nerves and muscles, resulting in hiatal laxity and subsequent herniation. In patients with upper respiratory obstruction, reduced intrathoracic pressure during inspiration has been theorized to contribute to esophageal reflux and visceral herniation. Hiatal hernia has been reported with tetanus.

With hiatal hernias, the stomach commonly slides in and out of the thorax. If the hernia is large enough, other abdominal viscera may also be cranially displaced into the thorax. Various types of hiatal abnormalities have been described (Fig. 19-51). In patients with sliding or axial hiatal hernias, the gastroesophageal junction is located within the thoracic cavity. In patients with paraesophageal or rolling hiatal hernias, the gastroesophageal junction usually is located in a normal position, and the gastric fundus or other abdominal viscera are displaced through the hiatus and located in the thorax. Some hiatal hernias are a combination of sliding and paraesophageal hernias, with the gastroesophageal junction and gastric fundus both displaced.

DIAGNOSIS
Clinical Presentation

Signalment. Hiatal hernias may occur in a variety of dog and cat breeds; however, male Shar-Peis and English bulldogs appear to be predisposed to this condition. Most symptomatic animals have signs relating to congenital hiatal hernia before reaching 1 year of age, although diagnosis may occur later. Patients with acquired hernias may develop signs at any age.

History. Regurgitation is the primary clinical sign in symptomatic individuals, but many patients are asymptomatic. Other signs may include vomiting, hypersalivation,

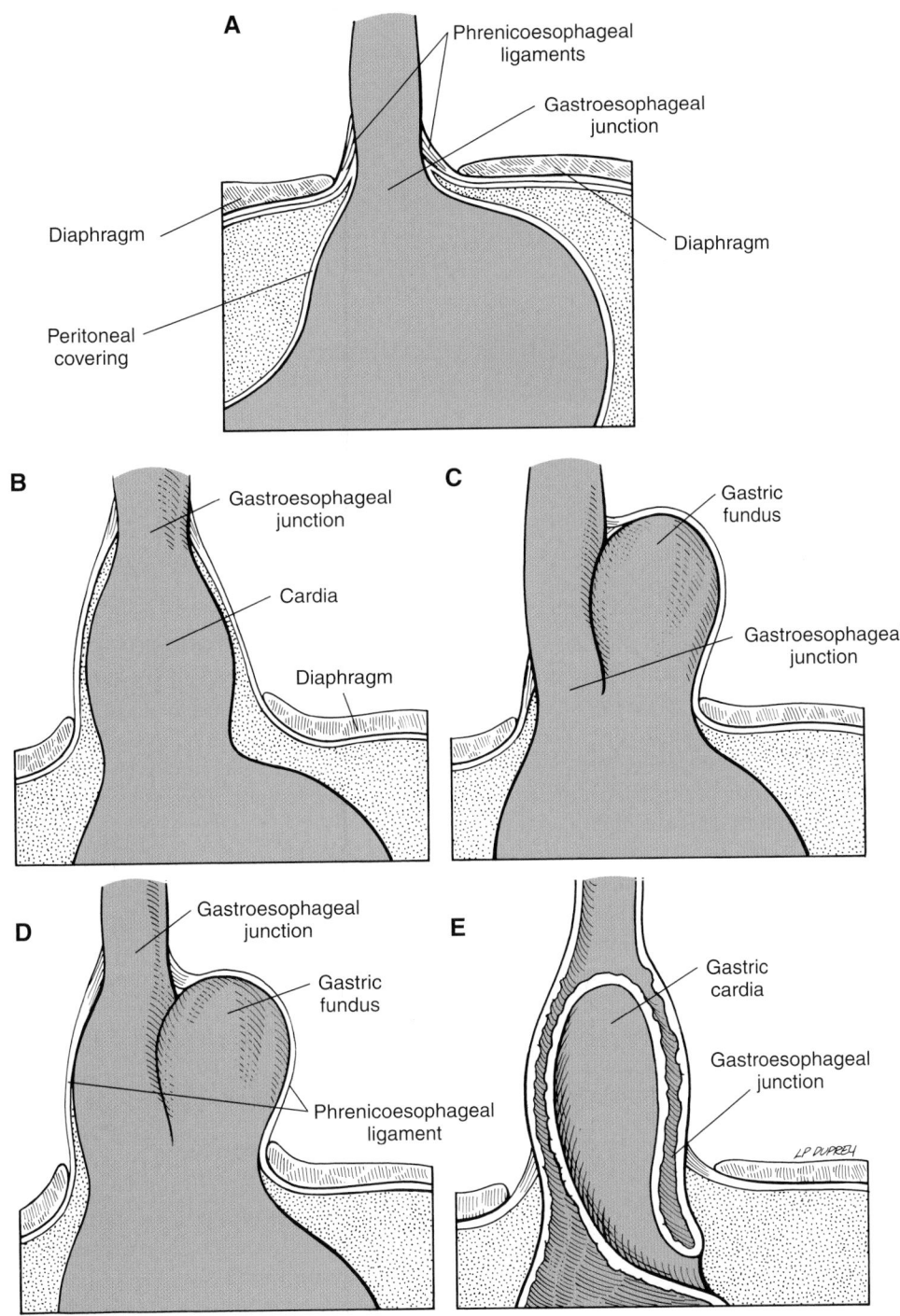

FIG. 19-51
Diagrams of a normal gastroesophageal junction (**A**) and hiatal abnormalities (**B** through **E**). **B,** Sliding or axial hiatal hernia. **C,** Paraesophageal or rolling hiatal hernia. **D,** Combination sliding and paraesophageal hernia. **E,** Gastroesophageal intussusception.

dysphagia, respiratory distress, hematemesis, anorexia, and weight loss. Severe dyspnea or trauma may have occurred.

Physical Examination Findings

Affected patients may be thin on physical examination. Abnormal lung sounds are auscultated with aspiration pneumonia.

Diagnostic Imaging

Hiatal hernias usually appear as a soft tissue or soft tissue/gas-filled mass near the esophageal hiatus in the caudodorsal thoracic region on survey radiographs (Fig. 19-52). However, with sliding hernias, several radiographs may be necessary to identify the herniation, which may be intermittent.

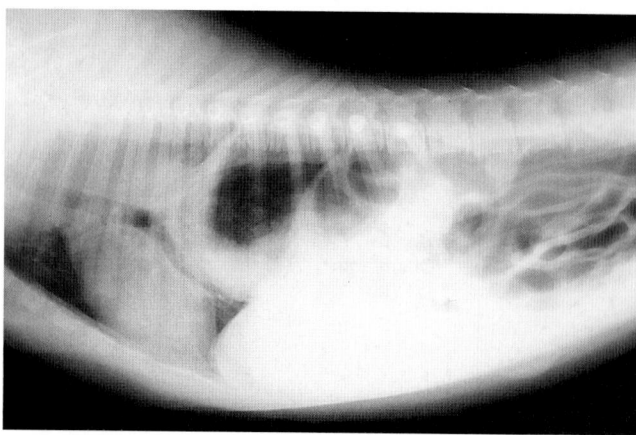

FIG. 19-52
Lateral radiograph of a 12-week-old Shar-Pei with a hiatal hernia. Note the air-filled mass (stomach) in the caudal thorax.

Intermittent hernias are particularly common in cats. The presence of gas in the herniated portion aids in identification of the mass as herniated stomach. Varying degrees of megaesophagus and pneumonia may be noted. A positive contrast esophagogram should show the gastroesophageal junction, rugal folds, or both cranial to the hiatus. Occasionally, strictures may be identified. Fluoroscopy may demonstrate hypomotility, delayed clearing of the distal esophagus, or gastroesophageal reflux. Compressing the abdomen during fluoroscopy may help identify hernias. Esophagoscopy can detect the hernia and esophagitis (inflammation, mucosal erosion), gastric reflux, and strictures. Gastric mucosa that has entered the thoracic cavity can sometimes be identified. Some hiatal hernias are intermittent (sliding) and require multiple radiographs or fluoroscopy (or both) to diagnose. Do not confuse hiatal hernias with peritoneopericardial (see p. 907) or traumatic (see p. 903) diaphragmatic hernias, despite their sometimes having a similar radiographic appearance. Hiatal hernias typically are located in the plane of the caudal mediastinum.

Laboratory Findings

Hematologic and serum chemistry results are nonspecific in affected animals.

DIFFERENTIAL DIAGNOSIS

Esophageal stricture, neoplasia, extraluminal masses, vascular ring anomalies, esophageal foreign body or perforation, esophagitis, esophageal intussusception, esophageal diverticulum, and megaesophagus are other possible causes of regurgitation.

SURGICAL TREATMENT

Affected patients may benefit from medical treatment for gastroesophageal reflux or esophagitis (see p. 373); however, surgery generally is recommended in symptomatic, young animals with congenital disease that does not respond to 30

days of appropriate medical treatment. A number of surgical techniques have been described for correcting hiatal hernias. Diaphragmatic hiatal reduction and plication, esophagopexy, and left-sided fundic gastropexy are described here. Gastropexy is probably the most important step in the repair. Displacing the terminal esophagus slightly caudally with a left-sided gastropexy increases barrier pressure at the gastroesophageal junction, and reflux disease often resolves after the procedure (Pratschke et al, 2001). If esophagitis is severe and if oral intake is to be withheld for several days, a gastrostomy tube (see p. 100) allows early alimentation without further esophageal irritation. Some surgeons perform sphincter-enhancing procedures, such as a Nissen fundoplication (antireflux procedure), instead of the aforementioned techniques. However, fundoplication or other antireflux procedures are only indicated in patients with evidence of gastroesophageal reflux. In dogs and cats, primary incompetence of the caudal esophageal sphincter has not been documented in association with hiatal hernia; therefore antireflux procedures are not routinely recommended.

Preoperative Management

Reflux esophagitis and aspiration pneumonia should be treated before induction of anesthesia (see p. 373). Feeding frequent, small meals of high-protein/low-fat foods may be beneficial. If megaesophagus is present, feeding affected animals in a standing, upright position may reduce regurgitation.

Anesthesia

Positive pressure ventilation may be necessary if pneumothorax is created during hiatal manipulations. Nitrous oxide should not be used in these patients. Negative intrathoracic pressure is reestablished by thoracentesis or tube thoracostomy after hiatal manipulations are complete. See p. 374 for anesthetic recommendations for patients undergoing esophageal surgery and p. 867 for recommendations for patients undergoing thoracic surgery.

Surgical Anatomy

The esophageal hiatus is one of three openings in the diaphragm. The esophageal hiatus is more centrally located than the caval foramen (located ventrally) or aortic hiatus (located dorsally). The esophagus passes through the esophageal hiatus, along with the vagal nerve trunks and esophageal vessels. The esophageal hiatus is surrounded by the phrenicoesophageal ligament, the thickened collagen fibers of which are weakened, stretched, or in some way defective in hiatal hernias. The terminal 1 to 2 cm of the esophagus is expected to lie within the abdominal cavity caudal to the diaphragm. The esophagogastric junction and gastroesophageal sphincter, which are in the abdomen, regulate movement of ingesta between the esophagus and the stomach.

Positioning

Patients are positioned in dorsal recumbency, and the caudal thorax and ventral abdomen are prepared for aseptic surgery.

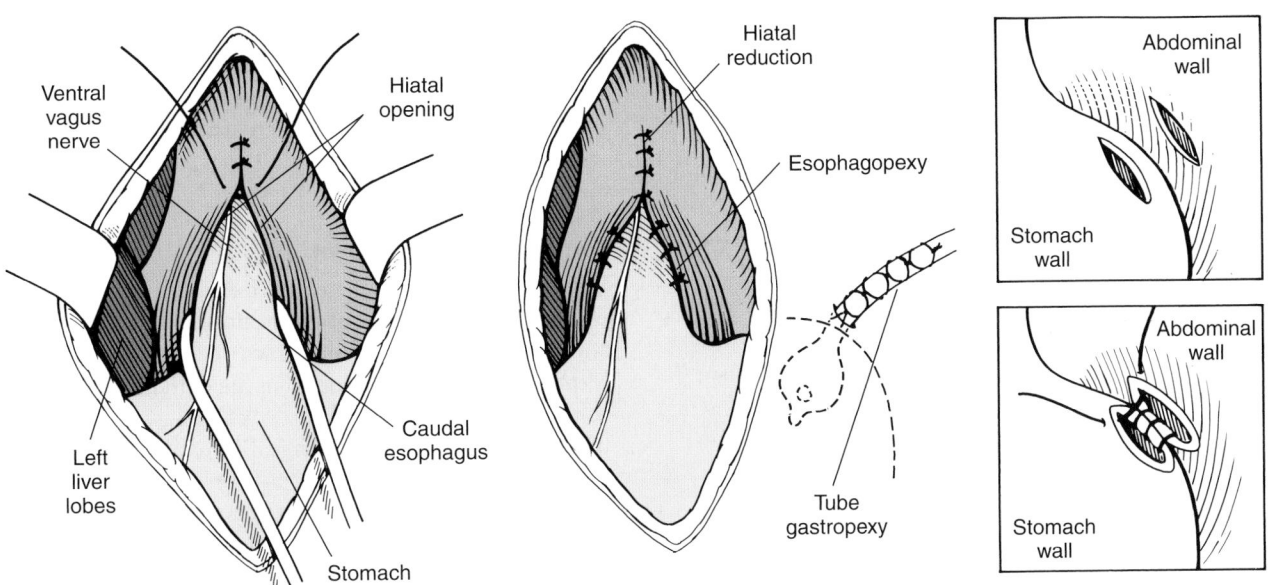

FIG. 19-53
Reduce hiatal hernias and reduce the size of the esophageal hiatus with plicating sutures. Suture the esophagus to the diaphragm (esophagopexy) and perform a tube or incisional *(inset)* gastropexy at the fundus.

SURGICAL TECHNIQUE

Make a cranial ventral midline incision extending caudal to the umbilicus to expose the diaphragm and stomach. Retract the left lobes of the liver medially to expose the esophageal hiatus. Pass a stomach tube (28 to 32 French) to help identify and manipulate the esophagus. Grasp the stomach and reduce the hernia with gentle traction. Examine the hiatus. Dissect the phrenicoesophageal membrane, freeing the esophagus from the diaphragm ventrally. Preserve the vagal trunks and esophageal vessels during dissection. Place an umbilical tape sling around the abdominal esophagus to displace it caudally and facilitate manipulations. Perform a diaphragmatic hiatal plication-reduction, esophagopexy, and left-sided fundic gastropexy. Accomplish diaphragmatic hiatal plication-reduction by excoriating or débriding the margins of the hiatus and then place three to five sutures (2-0 polydioxanone or polypropylene) to appose the edges and narrow the hiatus (Fig. 19-53). Perform plication around a large stomach tube (28 to 32 French) (Fig. 19-53). Reduce the hiatus to 1 or 2 cm, a size that allows passage of one finger. Accomplish esophagopexy by placing sutures (3-0 or 2-0 polydioxanone or polypropylene) from the remaining margin of the hiatus through the adventitia and muscular layers of the abdominal esophagus. Complete the repair with either a left-sided tube gastropexy or incisional gastropexy (see pp. 417 to 420). Fix the fundus with slight to moderate caudal traction to prevent cranial movement of the gastroesophageal junction into the thorax. Evacuate air from the chest by thoracentesis or tube thoracostomy, and lavage and close the abdomen.

POSTOPERATIVE CARE AND ASSESSMENT

Patients should be monitored after surgery for dyspnea caused by pneumothorax, and air should be evacuated from the thorax as necessary. Nasal oxygen may benefit dyspneic animals. Analgesics should be provided as necessary to control pain (see Table 13-4 on p. 133). Affected animals may continue to regurgitate after surgery because of persistent esophagitis. Treatment of esophagitis and aspiration pneumonia should be continued postoperatively (see p. 373). Feed small portions of low-fat, high-protein softened or liquefied food three to five times day. Feeding from an elevated platform may be beneficial in animals with concurrent megaesophagus. Postoperative esophagoscopy may benefit patients with persistent clinical signs by identifying persistent herniation, obstruction, or ulceration.

COMPLICATIONS

Dysphagia is common for several days; however, if it continues beyond that time, the hiatus may have been overreduced, requiring reoperation. Infection may occur if the esophageal or gastric lumen is penetrated with sutures or tubes. Possible problems after antireflux procedures include gastric dilatation, necrotic gastritis, and acute death.

PROGNOSIS

The prognosis without surgery is good in asymptomatic patients and those that respond to medical therapy; however, symptomatic patients that do not respond to medical therapy and are not surgically repaired may develop severe esophagitis and stricture. The prognosis with surgery is good; however, aspiration pneumonia must be controlled for a favorable outcome. Patients with gastroesophageal sphincter incompetence may benefit from additional antireflux procedures.

Reference

Pratschke KM, Bellenger CR, McAllister H et al: Barrier pressure at the gastroesophageal junction in anesthetized dogs, *Am J Vet Res* 62:1068, 2001.

Suggested Reading

Hardie EM, Ramirez O, Clary EM et al: Abnormalities of the thoracic bellows: stress fractures of the ribs and hiatal hernia, *J Vet Intern Med* 12:279, 1998.
Twenty one dogs were identified with these problems secondary to cardiopulmonary, neuromuscular, or metabolic disease.
Pratschke KM, Fitzpatrick E, Campion D et al: Topography of the gastro-oesophageal junction in the dog revisited: possible clinical implications, *Res Vet Science* 76:171, 2004.
This study using greyhounds and beagles found a lack of consistency in topographical anatomy and found no abdominal esophagus in most dogs.

GASTROESOPHAGEAL INTUSSUSCEPTION

DEFINITION

Gastroesophageal intussusception (*esophageal intussusception, gastroesophageal invagination, esophageal invagination*) is the invagination of the gastric cardia into the distal esophagus with or without the spleen, duodenum, pancreas, and omentum.

GENERAL CONSIDERATIONS AND CLINICALLY RELEVANT PATHOPHYSIOLOGY

Gastroesophageal intussusception can be confused with esophageal hiatal hernia (see Fig. 19-51, *E*). However, the gastroesophageal junction does not move cranially into the thorax as with a sliding hiatal hernia, and the cardia is within the esophageal lumen rather than external to the esophagus as with a paraesophageal hiatal hernia. Gastroesophageal intussusception usually occurs in immature animals with megaesophagus. The etiology of gastroesophageal intussusception is unknown. Idiopathic megaesophagus or incompetency of the gastroesophageal sphincter mechanism or abnormal esophageal motility and subsequent regurgitation may predispose an animal to this disorder. Vomiting and retching cause the esophagus to dilate. Experimental work in puppies has shown that vomiting can cause invagination of the gastric cardia into the esophagus. A large or lax esophageal hiatus may be necessary to allow the gastric cardia to move cranially into the esophagus. Entrapment or strangulation of the invaginated stomach occurs, causing esophageal obstruction, continued regurgitation, and rapid fluid loss. Discomfort is caused by stretching of gastric mesenteric attachments and esophagitis. Severe respiratory distress is caused by the greatly enlarged esophagus compressing the pulmonary parenchyma or by aspiration pneumonia (or both). Cardiovascular collapse occurs secondary to obstruction of venous return and eventually of the arterial blood supply. The resulting congestion, inflammation, and necrosis contribute to the animal's deterioration.

DIAGNOSIS
Clinical Presentation

Signalment. Although several breeds have been reported with gastroesophageal intussusception, German shepherds and other large-breed dogs seem to be at increased risk. More cases have been reported in males than in females. The condition is most common in young dogs, usually under 3 months of age. Gastroesophageal intussusception has been reported in cats.

History. In most cases there is acute onset of clinical signs (i.e., regurgitation, vomiting, dyspnea, hematemesis, abdominal discomfort, rapid deterioration, or death) with rapid deterioration and death within 1 to 3 days if the condition is not treated immediately. Signs may mimic those of aspiration pneumonia, making diagnosis difficult. Affected animals often have a history of esophageal disease (50%). At least three cases (2 cats and 1 dog) have been reported with chronic, intermittent clinical signs, including recurrent vomiting and regurgitation, and lethargy. These chronic cases may be secondary to a sliding intussusception.

Physical Examination Findings

Animals may be thin and may show pain on abdominal palpation. Signs of shock may be noted (i.e., poor capillary refill, pale mucous membranes, labored breathing, tachycardia, and thready pulse).

Diagnostic Imaging

Radiographs show a dilated distal esophagus with a luminal soft tissue mass (Fig. 19-54). Rugal folds may be associated with the soft tissue mass. The trachea may be deviated ventrally, and signs of aspiration pneumonia may be apparent. The normal gastric gas bubble usually seen in the cranial abdomen may be absent or diminished in size. The intussusception can be outlined by either positive or negative contrast studies; however, this may be difficult to perform as these patients are often severely dyspneic. Esophagoscopy reveals a dilated esophagus with a large soft tissue mass having gastric rugal folds in the distal esophageal lumen. Esophagitis may be apparent. It may not be possible to advance the endoscope into the distal esophagus or stomach.

Laboratory Findings

Laboratory findings are nonspecific and related to dehydration and shock.

DIFFERENTIAL DIAGNOSIS

Esophageal hiatal hernia, neoplasia, extraluminal masses, esophageal foreign body, and esophageal diverticulum are differential diagnoses.

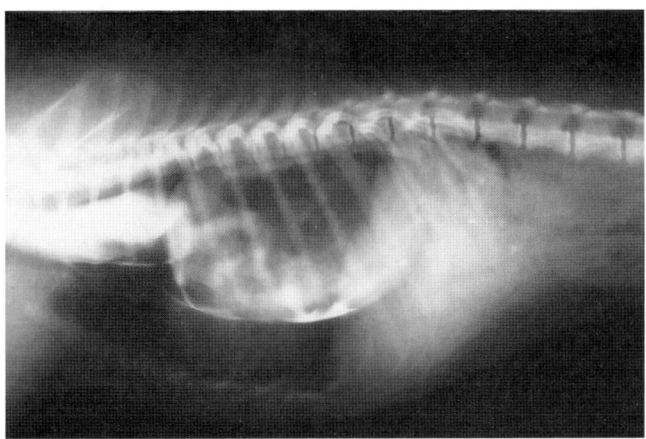

FIG. 19-54
Radiograph of a dog with a gastroesophageal intussusception. Note the luminal soft tissue mass in the dilated distal esophagus.

SURGICAL TREATMENT

Surgical intervention should be performed as soon as possible after diagnosis. Stabilization of the patient's condition and treatment for shock should be performed before induction of anesthesia; however, surgical treatment should not be delayed in acute cases.

Preoperative Management

Before induction of anesthesia, shock treatment should be initiated (i.e., administration of fluid therapy and broad-spectrum antibiotics, with or without steroids), and electrolyte and acid-base abnormalities should be identified and corrected if possible. An ECG also should be performed before induction of anesthesia.

Anesthesia

Anesthetic recommendations for animals undergoing esophageal surgery are provided on p. 374.

Surgical Anatomy

The surgical anatomy of the esophageal hiatus is discussed on p. 398.

Positioning

The animal is positioned in dorsal recumbency, and the caudal thorax and ventral abdomen are prepared for aseptic surgery.

SURGICAL TECHNIQUE

Make a ventral midline abdominal incision from the xiphoid process to several centimeters caudal to the umbilicus. Explore the abdomen, and locate the duodenum and stomach. Apply gentle traction on the duodenum and stomach to reduce the intussusception. If necessary, digitally dilate or enlarge the esophageal hiatus to allow
complete reduction of the intussusception. Examine the distal esophagus, the stomach, and any other involved viscera for evidence of vascular thrombosis, avulsion, ischemia, or necrosis. Resect devitalized tissue. Reduce the size of the esophageal hiatus to 1 to 2 cm if it is too large or lax (see p. 399). Perform an incisional gastropexy (see p. 417) at the gastric fundus to prevent recurrence. In addition to the fundic gastropexy, an incisional right or pyloric antrum gastropexy is sometimes performed. Lavage and close the abdomen. Place a feeding tube if esophageal disease is severe.

POSTOPERATIVE CARE AND ASSESSMENT

Fluids should be continued after surgery, and acid-base and electrolyte imbalances corrected. Nasal oxygen may benefit dyspneic animals. Postoperative analgesics should be provided (see Table 13-4 on p. 133) and oral intake withheld initially to encourage resolution of esophagitis and gastritis (see p. 373). After 24 to 48 hours, water can be offered. If vomiting or regurgitation does not occur, small amounts of low-fat, high-protein gruel can be offered several times a day. If megaesophagus is present, the animal should be fed in an upright position or through a gastrostomy tube. However, esophageal weakness may not resolve, especially in young animals. Treat esophagitis as necessary (see Box 19-15). Gastrostomy tube feeding may be helpful. Deterioration and death may occur if the condition is not recognized and treated promptly. Devitalization of a portion of the esophagus or stomach may occur as a result of preoperative vascular compromise. Dysphagia is common for several days after surgery; however, persistent dysphagia may occur if the hiatus is overly narrowed by surgery. Such patients require reoperation.

PROGNOSIS

Antemortem diagnosis is rare in acute cases (mortality approaches 95%), therefore few cases of gastroesophageal intussusception have been diagnosed and treated successfully. Recurrence is not expected if incisional gastropexy is performed and esophagitis is controlled. Prognosis in chronic intermittent cases is fair if reduction is maintained and if esophageal disease is manageable.

Suggested Reading

Martinez NI, Cook W, Troy GC et al: Intermittent gastroesophageal intussusception in a cat with idiopathic megaesophagus, *J Am Anim Hosp Assoc* 37:234, 2001.
This is the case report of a cat that was cured by reducing the intussusception with a stomach tube during endoscopy, and then performing an incisional gastropexy.
Pietra M, Pinna S, Fracassi F et al: Intermittent gastroesophageal intussusception in a dog: clinical features, radiographic and endoscopic findings and surgical management, *Vet Res Communications* 27 (Supplement 1):783, 2003.
This is a case report of a pug that was cured with gastropexy. Endoscopic pictures are included.

CRICOPHARYNGEAL ACHALASIA

DEFINITION

Cricopharyngeal achalasia *(congenital cricopharyngeal achalasia, cricopharyngeal dysphagia, cricopharyngeal dysfunction, cricopharyngeal asynchrony)* is one type of pharyngeal dysphagia. The condition is characterized by interruption of passage of a bolus from the oropharynx through the cranial esophageal sphincter into the cervical esophagus because of failure of the sphincter to open correctly.

GENERAL CONSIDERATIONS AND CLINICALLY RELEVANT PATHOPHYSIOLOGY

Cricopharyngeal achalasia is a rare cause of dysphagia; however, it is important to differentiate it from other forms of oropharyngeal dysphagia because the former is treatable. There are a number of swallowing disorders, and their treatment varies. The cause of cricopharyngeal achalasia is unknown, but appears to be a congenital derangement in the coordination of the swallowing reflex. The cause probably is neurologic because transecting the pharyngeal branch of the tenth cranial nerve can reproduce the disorder. Cricopharyngeal achalasia is characterized by inadequate relaxation of the cricopharyngeal muscle and/or lack of coordination with pharyngeal muscle contractions during swallowing. This disrupts the cricopharyngeal phase of swallowing, causing food to remain in the pharynx, and produces gagging, regurgitation, aspiration, and coughing. Repeated attempts to swallow are made until retained pharyngeal contents are swallowed, regurgitated, or aspirated. Food remaining in the pharynx may be aspirated into the trachea during inspiration, eliciting a cough and causing pneumonia. The small amount of food that succeeds in passing from the oropharynx into the proximal esophagus passes normally into the stomach.

In normal swallowing, food is grasped by the teeth and formed into a bolus by rapid tongue movements. The bolus is pushed up and back by the base of the tongue into the oropharynx. The pharyngeal muscles (hyopharyngeal, pterygopharyngeal, palatopharyngeal muscles) contract and force the bolus through the relaxed upper esophageal sphincter (cricopharyngeal, thyropharyngeal muscles) into the cervical portion of the esophagus. The cricopharyngeal muscle contracts after the bolus passes. Cricopharyngeal muscle tone is linked to deglutition and the respiratory cycle. During swallowing the airways are protected by the soft palate (which closes the nasopharynx) and the epiglottis (which flips back to close the glottis).

DIAGNOSIS
Clinical Presentation

Signalment. The condition is rare. It seems to be more common in springer and cocker spaniels and miniature poodles, but has been seen in a variety of breeds. Signs of dysphagia begin at weaning, although in rare cases animals may not be diagnosed until they are older.

History. Most dogs appear normal until they begin eating solid food. At that time, repeated unsuccessful attempts to swallow are noted, with gagging, retching, and expulsion of saliva-covered food. Regurgitation occurs immediately after swallowing. Other signs may include aspiration, coughing, excess salivation, and nasal reflux during eating. Most patients have a voracious appetite, but some fail to thrive, become anorexic, and lose weight.

Physical Examination Findings

Affected animals may appear normal or stunted at the time of examination. Some patients are emaciated. The animal should be observed eating and drinking to confirm dysphagia and to characterize it as oral or pharyngeal. Patients with oral dysphagia have difficulty with prehension and bolus formation. Those with pharyngeal dysphagia have difficulty transporting the bolus into the esophagus. Patients with cricopharyngeal dysphagia usually have more difficulty with solid food, whereas those with other types of pharyngeal dysphagias may have more difficulty (i.e., may aspirate more readily) when swallowing liquids. Swallowing attempts may trigger the animal to cough, gag, and choke. A neurologic examination is performed to rule out cranial nerve deficits and concurrent neuromuscular abnormalities. Signs of concurrent aspiration pneumonia, rhinitis, laryngeal paralysis, or megaesophagus may be present.

Diagnostic Imaging

Survey thoracic radiographs should be evaluated for aspiration pneumonia and esophageal size. Definitive diagnosis requires fluoroscopic or cinefluoroscopic evaluation of swallowing barium sulfate. Use liquid barium or paste barium sulfate mixed with food unless aspiration is anticipated. An experienced radiologist may be needed to differentiate cricopharyngeal achalasia from pharyngeal dysphagia. Affected animals will have several ineffectual attempts by the tongue to force the bolus from the pharynx and inadequate relaxation of the cricopharyngeal, prohibiting bolus entry into the proximal esophagus. In normal dogs the time between onset of swallowing and opening of the upper esophageal sphincter following a bolus of liquid barium is 0.09 ± 0.02 second, whereas opening in those with cricopharyngeal achalasia is delayed (0.31 ± 0.14 second) (Warnock et al, 2003). A thin stream of contrast may be seen passing through the sphincter. Some contrast may be seen refluxing into the nasopharynx or being aspirated into the airway. Patients with cricopharyngeal achalasia have adequate pharyngeal strength to push the food bolus into the esophagus, but the cricopharyngeal sphincter stays shut or opens at the wrong time during the swallowing reflex. Patients with pharyngeal dysphagia do not have adequate oropharyngeal strength or coordination of the pharyngeal muscles to properly push the food bolus into the esophagus. Positive contrast in the trachea or outlining airways indicates aspiration. Esophageal motility should be evaluated during fluoroscopic studies to identify concurrent problems because many animals with pharyngeal dysphagia have concurrent esophageal dysfunction, and for these patients cricopharyngeal surgery is absolutely contraindicated. Endoscopic examination of the pharynx and esophagus is normal.

Laboratory Findings

Laboratory findings are normal unless the patient is severely debilitated or has aspiration pneumonia. Then it may have a neutrophilia or hypoproteinemia.

DIFFERENTIAL DIAGNOSIS

Pharyngeal dysphagia caused by inadequate pharyngeal contraction is difficult to differentiate from cricopharyngeal achalasia. Pharyngeal dysphagia tends to occur in older dogs whereas cricopharyngeal dysfunction tends to occur in younger dogs, but age is an inadequate criterion to distinguish these two conditions. Sometimes more than one abnormality contributes to the dysphagia. Dental disease, oral masses, foreign bodies, trauma, stomatitis, cleft palate, hypoplastic palate, and other congenital and skeletal abnormalities should also be considered. Esophageal hypomotility and megaesophagus may also be associated with pharyngeal dysphagias. Other considerations include functional abnormalities resulting from rabies, central nervous system disease, peripheral neuropathies, neuromuscular disease, myopathies, and myositis.

SURGICAL TREATMENT

Cricopharyngeal myectomy is often curative for congenital cricopharyngeal achalasia. Surgery is not recommended for acquired cricopharyngeal achalasia. Some surgeons also resect a portion of the thyropharyngeus muscle. Cricopharyngeal myectomy for patients with other pharyngeal dysphagias can be disastrous because it allows food retained in the proximal esophagus to more easily reenter the pharynx and be aspirated.

Preoperative Management

Supportive care is important; patients should be well hydrated and nourished before surgery. Preoperative nutritional support should be provided with a gastrostomy tube if necessary (see p. 100). Oral feeding should include feeding food of a consistency (dry versus canned versus gruel) most successfully retained by the animal. Aspiration pneumonia should be treated with fluids, appropriate antibiotics, and expectorants. Perioperative antibiotics are recommended for debilitated patients.

Anesthesia

Anesthetic recommendations for esophageal surgery are provided on p. 374. Hypothermia and hypoglycemia are serious problems in young patients and should be prevented during anesthesia and surgery.

Surgical Anatomy

The cranial esophagus is located dorsal to the larynx and slightly to the left of midline. The cricopharyngeal muscle lies on the larynx and pharynx immediately caudal to the thyropharyngeal muscle (Fig. 19-55). It arises from the lateral surface of the cricoid cartilage and passes dorsally to insert on the median dorsal raphe. The cricopharyngeal muscle can be identified as a bundle of transverse muscle fibers converging on the dorsal midline and blending into the longitudinal muscle fibers of the cranial esophagus. The thyropharyngeal muscle can be difficult to differentiate from the cricopharyngeal muscles because their muscle fibers are both oriented transversely. The thyropharyngeal muscle lies cranial to the cricopharyngeal muscle and is separated from it by a thin septum of connective tissue. The separation is found dorsal to the attachment of the sternothyroideus muscle. The cricopharyngeal muscle controls most of the upper esophageal sphincter function. Branches of the glossopharyngeal and vagus nerves innervate it. Blood supply to the cricopharyngeal muscles is primarily from branches of the cranial thyroid arteries.

Positioning

The animal is positioned in dorsal recumbency with the legs positioned lateral to the thorax. The ventral neck (from the angle of the mandible to the manubrium) should be prepared for aseptic surgery. Alternatively the animal is positioned in lateral recumbency and a lateral incision is made.

SURGICAL TECHNIQUE

Make a ventral midline cervical incision beginning cranial to the larynx and extending caudally to the midcervical area. Separate and retract the sternohyoid muscles laterally to expose the trachea. Rotate the larynx and trachea laterally by using traction on the sternothyroid muscle to expose the cricopharyngeal musculature (Fig. 19-56, A). Place a suture through the lamina of the thyroid cartilage to maintain laryngeal rotation and exposure of the cricopharyngeal muscle and dorsal esophagus. Pass a gastric tube into the esophagus to aid identification of the esophageal wall. Identify the cricopharyngeal muscles. Incise the cricopharyngeus (and, if necessary, the thyropharyngeus) muscle on its midline (Fig. 19-56, B). Elevate the muscle fibers from the underlying esophageal submucosa with care to avoid perforating the esophageal wall. Resect the lateral portion of each cricopharyngeus (and the thyropharyngeus) muscle. Inspect the esophageal wall for damage, and lavage the area. Allow the larynx and trachea to return to their normal position. Appose the sternohyoid muscles with a continuous suture pattern. Close subcutaneous tissues and skin routinely.

POSTOPERATIVE CARE AND ASSESSMENT

Provide analgesia and treat aspiration pneumonia as necessary. Immediately following surgery, improvement in swallowing function is expected. When fully recovered from anesthesia, evaluate swallowing function by giving a small amount of soft food. A gruel or canned food should be fed for the first 1 to 2 days after surgery, then the food should gradually be returned to normal consistency over the next 3 to 4 days. If necessary, intravenous fluids should be continued to maintain hydration. Continue feeding through a

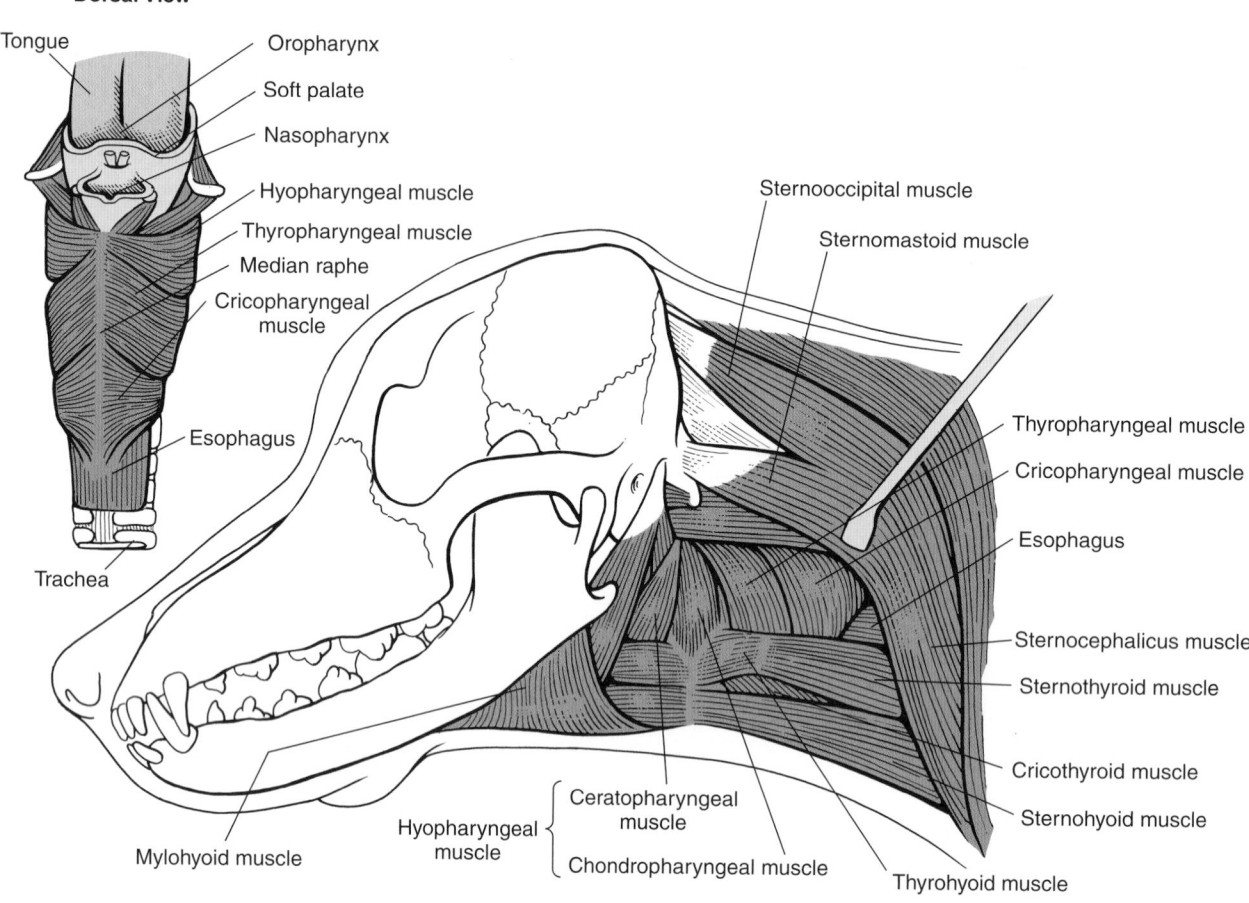

Dorsal View

Tongue
Oropharynx
Soft palate
Nasopharynx
Hyopharyngeal muscle
Thyropharyngeal muscle
Median raphe
Cricopharyngeal muscle
Esophagus
Trachea

Sternooccipital muscle
Sternomastoid muscle
Thyropharyngeal muscle
Cricopharyngeal muscle
Esophagus
Sternocephalicus muscle
Sternothyroid muscle
Cricothyroid muscle
Sternohyoid muscle
Thyrohyoid muscle

Mylohyoid muscle
Hyopharyngeal muscle
{ Ceratopharyngeal muscle
Chondropharyngeal muscle }

FIG. 19-55
Surgical anatomy of the cranial esophagus and neck.

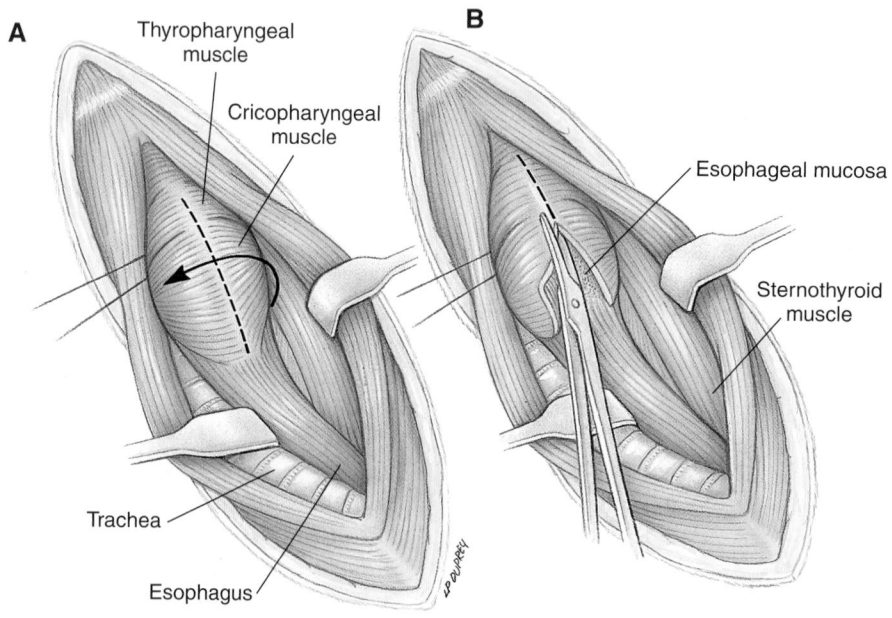

A
Thyropharyngeal muscle
Cricopharyngeal muscle
Trachea
Esophagus

B
Esophageal mucosa
Sternothyroid muscle

FIG. 19-56
Cricopharyngeal myectomy. **A,** Expose the cranial esophagus through a ventral midline cervical incision. Place a stay suture through the thyroid lamina and rotate the cricopharyngeal muscle into view. **B,** Resect the lateral portion of each cricopharyngeal muscle.

gastrostomy tube if necessary to improve body condition. Antibiotics should be continued if aspiration pneumonia is present. Inadequate or unilateral myectomy may not relieve signs of cricopharyngeal achalasia.

COMPLICATIONS

Recurrence of dysphagia because of fibrosis and constriction at the myectomy site can be prevented by adequate removal of muscle. If pharyngeal dysphagias or proximal esophageal dysfunction are present, then cricopharyngeal myectomy will worsen the patient's dysphagia and pneumonia. Aspiration pneumonia may continue to be a problem if esophageal hypomotility exists. Other potential complications include laryngeal paralysis, esophageal perforation, and pharyngocutaneous fistula.

PROGNOSIS

The prognosis is good if the only abnormality present is cricopharyngeal achalasia and guarded if other dysphagias or related conditions are present. Although complete resolution of signs is expected, some have only partial resolution and others have recurrence of clinical signs within 2 to 36 weeks (Warnock et al, 2003). Persistent regurgitation may result in aspiration pneumonia. The prognosis without surgery is guarded because it is difficult to effectively nourish the patient and control pneumonia.

Reference

Warnock JJ, Marks SL, Pollard R et al: Surgical management of cricopharyngeal dysphagia in dogs: 14 cases (1989-2001), *J Am Vet Med Assoc* 223:1462, 2003.

Suggested Reading

Davidson AP, Pollard RE, Bannasch DL et al: Inheritance of cricopharyngeal dysfunction in golden retrievers, *Am J Vet Res* 65:344, 2004.
Videofluoroscopy was performed on 117 dogs; 21 had abnormalities of the upper esophageal sphincter. Heritability was discovered and it is suggested that a single recessive allele of large effect contributed to expression of the disease.
Ladlow J, Hardie RJ: Cricopharyngeal achalasia in dogs, *Compend Contin Educ Pract Vet* 22:750, 2000.
This is a recent review with a case report and comparison to the disorder in humans.
Niles JD, Williams JM, Sullivan M et al: Resolution of dysphagia following cricopharyngeal myectomy in six young dogs, *J Small Anim Pract* 42:32, 2001.
A lateral approach to myotomy was used. Immediate and continued resolution of signs was seen for 2 to 8 years.

VASCULAR RING ANOMALIES

DEFINITION

Vascular ring anomalies are congenital malformations of the great vessels and their branches that cause constriction of the esophagus and signs of esophageal obstruction. Persistent right aortic arch, the most common type of vascular

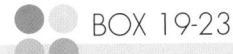

BOX 19-23

Vascular Ring Anomalies: Key Points

Regurgitation begins at weaning with introduction of solid food
Aspiration pneumonia is a concurrent risk
95% are persistent right aortic arch ± other aberrant vessels
Mostly diagnosed in German shepherds
Radiographic signs: esophageal dilation cranial to heart base and tracheal deviation to the left
Perform surgery early to prevent irreversible changes
Treat pneumonia and improve body condition before surgery
Identify, isolate, occlude, and divide offending vessels
Dissect constricting fibrous bands from around esophagus
Feed gruel while standing erect on hind legs; gradually increase food consistency
Most regurgitate less following surgery, some are clinically normal

ring anomaly, is also known as *PRAA* and *persistent fourth right aortic arch*.

GENERAL CONSIDERATIONS AND CLINICALLY RELEVANT PATHOPHYSIOLOGY

The most common type of vascular ring anomaly is a persistent fourth right aortic arch, right dorsal aortic root, and rudimentary left ligamentum arteriosum (left sixth arch). The left pulmonary artery and the descending aorta are connected by the ligamentum arteriosum. The esophagus is encircled by the ligamentum arteriosum (or patent ductus arteriosus) on the left, the base of the heart and pulmonary artery ventrally, and the aortic arch on the right. The esophagus is constricted by this vascular "ring" and begins to dilate cranially as food accumulates. Food that does not pass beyond the constriction is intermittently regurgitated. Chronic regurgitation predisposes the animal to aspiration pneumonia. Approximately 95% of animals diagnosed with vascular ring anomalies have a PRAA (Box 19-23).

Abnormal location of the great vessels mechanically interferes with functioning of the esophagus and sometimes the trachea and other adjacent structures. The severity of clinical signs and the degree of esophageal stricture depend on the vascular structures involved. In approximately 44% of those with PRAA, there is a coexisting compressive arterial anomaly. Other types of vascular ring anomalies include (1) PRAA with persistent left subclavian artery; (2) PRAA with persistent left ligamentum arteriosum and left subclavian artery (33%); (3) double aortic arch (12%); (4) normal left aortic arch with persistent right ligamentum arteriosum; (5) normal left aortic arch with persistent right subclavian artery; and (6) normal left aortic arch with persistent right ligamentum arteriosum and right subclavian artery (2%). A patent ductus arteriosus rather than the ligamentum arteriosum persists in approximately 12% to 16% of those with vascular ring anomalies. Additionally, persistent left vena cava in conjunction with PRAA occurs in about 12% to 40% of cases and a left hemiazygos vein in 6% of the cases (Buchanan et al, 2004).

Six pairs of aortic arches surround the esophagus and trachea during early fetal life. Normal maturation and selective regression of these arches form the adult vasculature. All vascular ring anomalies have resulted from abnormal development of arches three, four, and six. The mechanism of inheritance is complex and polygenic, probably involving multiple recessive genes. In the embryo, the first and second aortic arches disappear, and the fifth arches are incomplete and inconsistent. The third arch joins the dorsal aortic arch and continues anteriorly as the right and left internal carotid arteries. The third arch also forms the brachiocephalic trunk. The dorsal aortas disappear between the third and fourth arches. Normally the left fourth aortic arch and the dorsal aortic root persist to form the permanent aortic arch. The left sixth arch becomes the ductus arteriosus, and the right fourth arch contributes to the right subclavian artery.

DIAGNOSIS
Clinical Presentation

Signalment. Vascular ring anomalies occur in both dogs and cats, but are more common in dogs. German shepherds, Irish setters, and Boston terriers are the most commonly affected breeds. PRAA may be a hereditary condition in greyhounds (Gunby et al, 2004). Siamese and Persian cats have been diagnosed more often than other cat breeds. Males and females are equally affected. The condition may affect several animals in a litter. Vascular ring anomalies are present at birth. Clinical signs usually are evident at the time of weaning, most being diagnosed between 2 and 6 months of age; however, the condition may not be recognized until later in life if obstruction is partial and if signs are mild. Early diagnosis and treatment of PRAA may improve the prognosis.

History. The classic history is acute onset of regurgitation when solid or semisolid food is first fed. Regurgitation of undigested food occurs soon after eating early in the disease; later it may occur at variable times (minutes to hours). Affected animals may grow more slowly than litter mates and appear malnourished. They often have a voracious appetite; some immediately eat the regurgitated food. Coughing with respiratory distress may be a result of aspiration pneumonia or tracheal stenosis, which occurs secondary to a double aortic arch.

Physical Examination Findings

Affected animals are often thin and small. An enlarged esophagus may sometimes be palpated at the thoracic inlet and neck. The thoracic inlet and caudal neck area may bulge when the chest is compressed. Murmurs are rare; an occasional animal may have a continuous murmur associated with concurrent patent ductus arteriosus. Fever and auscultation of pulmonary crackles suggests pneumonia.

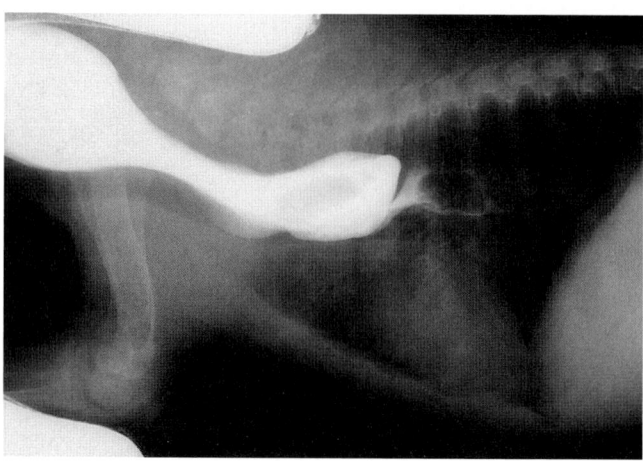

FIG. 19-57
Contrast esophagogram of a dog with a persistent right aortic arch. Note the esophageal narrowing at the base of the heart. The cranial esophagus is dilated.

Diagnostic Imaging

Thoracic radiographs may reveal a dilated esophagus cranial to the heart containing air, water, or food. Focal leftward deviation of the trachea near the cranial border of the heart on dorsoventral or ventrodorsal radiographs is a reliable sign of PRAA in symptomatic young dogs (Buchanan et al, 2004). The trachea may be displaced ventrally, and the esophagus may overlap it. Signs of pneumonia may be identified. Positive contrast radiography using a barium sulfate liquid mixed with food demonstrates esophageal constriction at the base of the heart with varying degrees of esophageal dilatation extending cranially (Fig. 19-57). The ratio of the area of maximal esophageal dilation after liquid barium sulfate (8 ml/kg body weight) to the narrowest height of the fifth thoracic vertebrae in normal dogs and cats is equal to 1 (Rallis et al, 2000). The animal is considered to have mild dilatation if the ratio is equal to 2.5, moderate with a ratio equal to 4, and severe with a ratio greater than 4 (Rallis et al, 2000). The caudal esophagus usually is normal in size, although it sometimes is dilated. Fluoroscopy is beneficial in evaluating esophageal motility. The dilated esophagus does not usually demonstrate normal peristaltic contractions. Although not routinely performed, angiography can be beneficial for identifying the type of vascular ring anomaly and other cardiac anomalies before surgery. MRI evaluation may be more helpful in identifying abnormal vasculature than angiography. Echocardiography may also be beneficial. Endoscopic examination of the esophagus helps rule out other causes of esophageal stricture or obstruction and may reveal esophageal ulceration. Sometimes a dilated esophagus proximal to the heart is due to focal esophageal weakness, but radiographically mimics PRAA. Esophagoscopy can determine if there is a stricture caused by a vascular ring or if there is no stricture (and therefore the dilated area is due to esophageal weakness). Tracheoscopy is not routinely performed, but may document narrowing of the tracheal lumen caused by external compression.

Laboratory Findings

Laboratory findings are expected to be normal (for the animal's age) unless debilitation is severe or pneumonia is present. In animals with pneumonia, neutrophilia may be present and debilitated animals may be hypoproteinemic.

DIFFERENTIAL DIAGNOSIS

The primary differential diagnoses are generalized megaesophagus and obstruction caused by a foreign body, stricture, mass, or hiatal hernia. It can be difficult to radiographically differentiate between esophageal dilatation caused by a vascular ring anomaly and a large outpouching cranial to the heart associated with megaesophagus.

MEDICAL MANAGEMENT

Patients with vascular ring anomalies are treated both medically and surgically. Surgery should be performed as soon after the onset of clinical signs as possible to reduce damage to the esophageal muscles and nerves. Clients should be informed that medical treatment without surgery is palliative at best and is not recommended. Medical management includes treating aspiration pneumonia (see p. 374) and improving the animal's nutritional status. An affected animal should be fed gruel while standing on its hind legs with the food dish elevated on a platform. The animal should be maintained in an upright position (standing on hind legs) for 5 to 10 minutes after eating to allow gravity to assist in emptying the dilated esophagus. Placement of a gastrostomy feeding tube may be beneficial for severely debilitated patients, particularly if aspiration is present and if surgery is being considered.

SURGICAL TREATMENT

Surgical treatment of PRAA is described below. Other types of vascular ring anomalies can be managed in a similar fashion. A persistent left vena cava often covers the left ventral area of the vascular ring. A persistent right ligamentum arteriosum and some aberrant right subclavians should be approached from the right side. Angiograms are helpful in patients with double aortic arches to determine which arch is dominant and if adequate circulation can be maintained after transection of the other arch. It may not be possible to relieve constrictions caused by a double aortic arch. If the animal is severely debilitated, a gastric feeding tube should be placed for several days before surgery.

Some surgeons attempt to reduce the size of the esophageal lumen if the esophagus is severely dilated and not expected to return to normal size. Placing a series of nonpenetrating "plication" or "gathering" sutures in the accessible lateral esophageal wall accomplishes this. As an alternative, a portion of the esophagus may be resected. These techniques are not recommended routinely because they increase the risk of complications.

Preoperative Management

Hydration, electrolyte, and acid-base abnormalities should be corrected before surgery if possible. If pneumonia is present or if the animal is severely debilitated, nutrition should be provided via a gastrostomy feeding tube (see p. 100) for several days to a week. Antibiotics are indicated for debilitated animals and for those with pneumonia (see p. 374).

Anesthesia

Anesthetic recommendations for animals undergoing thoracotomies are presented on p. 867. Pediatric patients must be kept warm and well hydrated during surgery and should be carefully monitored for hypoglycemia. Animals with pneumonia should be preoxygenated. Nitrous oxide should not be used in these patients.

Surgical Anatomy

The anatomy of the esophagus is provided on p. 375 and the anatomy of the heart on p. 777. See also the discussion under General Considerations and Clinically Relevant Pathophysiology on p. 405.

Positioning

Most patients with vascular ring anomalies should be positioned in right lateral recumbency for a left lateral thoracotomy (see p. 871); however, those with persistent right ligamentum arteriosum are positioned in left lateral recumbency. Positioning of animals with double aortic arches varies, depending on the dominant arch.

SURGICAL TECHNIQUE

Surgical transection of the constricting structure or structures is recommended before esophageal dilatation becomes severe. Transection is feasible with most vascular ring anomalies with the exception of some double aortic arches. Staples may be used rather than sutures to occlude vascular structures. Thoracoscopic assisted division of PRAA is an alternative approach.

Perform a lateral thoracotomy at the left fourth (fifth) intercostal space for patients with PRAA. Pack the cranial lung caudally to expose the mediastinum dorsal to the heart. Identify the aorta, pulmonary artery, ligamentum arteriosum, and vagal and phrenic nerves (see Figs. 27-3 and 19-37). Identify the anomalous structure or structures. If a persistent left cranial cava is present, dissect and retract the vena cava to improve visualization. If a prominent hemiazygos vein is also present, dissect, ligate, and divide it. If a constricting subclavian artery is identified, isolate, ligate, and transect it. If an atretic left aortic arch is present, isolate, ligate, and transect it. Incise the mediastinum, and dissect and elevate the ligamentum arteriosum. Double ligate the ligamentum arteriosum, and then transect it. If a large diameter patent ductus arteriosus is present rather than a ligamentum arteriosum, oversew both ends after transection. Pass a balloon catheter or large orogastric tube through the constricted esophagus to aid identification of constricting fibrous bands and to dilate the site. Dissect and transect these fibrous bands from the esophageal wall. Lavage the area, reposition the lung lobes, place a thoracostomy tube, and close the thorax routinely.

POSTOPERATIVE CARE AND ASSESSMENT

Postoperative analgesics should be provided as described on p. 868. The patient should be closely monitored for dyspnea and the chest tapped if necessary. Nasal oxygen may benefit dyspneic patients. If a thoracostomy tube has been placed, the thorax should be aspirated at regular intervals (initially every 15 to 30 minutes) and the volume of air and fluid collected at each interval noted. Thoracostomy tubes generally can be removed the day of surgery or by the next morning in these patients. Antibiotics should be continued in debilitated patients if thoracic contamination occurred or if pneumonia exists.

Pediatric patients should be closely monitored for hypoglycemia in the postoperative period. Oral intake can be resumed within 12 to 24 hours of surgery. Initially a canned food gruel should be fed with the animal in an upright posture. This stance should be maintained for 5 to 10 minutes after eating to help prevent distention of the dilated esophagus and help reestablish esophageal muscle tone and size. Owners may gradually reduce the amount of water in the food 2 to 4 weeks after surgery if minimal regurgitation has occurred with gruel feeding. Hopefully, addition of water ultimately can be eliminated without increased regurgitation. Animals who can eat solid food without regurgitation should be allowed to eat with the bowl on the floor while standing normally. This feeding practice is continued unless regurgitation recurs. Some animals eventually can be fed any type food from a normal stance, whereas others must continue eating gruel from an elevated stand.

If the patient is still having trouble, the esophagus should be reevaluated with an esophagogram 1 to 2 months after surgery to assess persistent dilatation and motility. Sometimes the esophagus returns to a normal size and function. Other times the esophagus remains severely dilated with poor motility. If esophageal stricture occurs at the surgery site, balloon dilation (see p. 391) may be beneficial. Owners should be advised against breeding affected animals because the condition is genetic.

COMPLICATIONS

Surgical complications are common because of the initial malnourished and debilitated condition of affected animals and concurrent aspiration pneumonia. Approximately 80% of patients are expected to survive the initial postoperative period. Persistent regurgitation is the most common postoperative problem. Preoperative client education must emphasize the high incidence of continued regurgitation and the need for prolonged dietary management. Aspiration pneumonia and death may occur if regurgitation persists. Esophageal resection or imbrication increases the risk of contamination and infection secondary to esophageal leakage or dehiscence.

PROGNOSIS

Most animals that survive surgery improve. Animals with severe esophageal dilatation (esophageal to the fifth thoracic vertebrae ratio >4) before surgery may have a worse long-term outcome than those with mild or moderate dilatation (Rallis et al, 2000). Persistence of esophageal dilatation, however, may not be associated with either continued regurgitation or an adverse long-term prognosis. Animals may not have completely normal esophageal function, but they generally regurgitate less and their body condition improves. If surgery is performed soon after signs appear, normal esophageal tone and function might return. The longer the delay before surgical correction, the more cautious the prognosis; some patients show little or no improvement. Megaesophagus often persists with mild to moderate improvement in motility, although most patients no longer have regurgitation. The prognosis is poor with esophageal dilatation caudal to the constriction because this area often is hypomotile and frequently does not regain normal size. Without surgery, regurgitation usually continues and worsens as the esophagus continues to dilate. Aspiration pneumonia is a continuous threat, and the animal may have difficulty maintaining adequate body condition.

References

Buchanan JW: Tracheal signs and associated vascular anomalies in dogs with persistent right aortic arch, *J Vet Intern Med* 18:510, 2004.

Gunby JM, Hardie RJ, Bjorling DE: Investigation of the potential heritability of persistent right aortic arch in Greyhounds, *J Am Vet Med Assoc* 224:1120, 2004.

Rallis T, Papazoglou LG, Patsikas MN et al: Persistent right aortic arch: does the degree of esophageal dilatation affect long-term outcome? A retrospective study in 10 dogs and 4 cats, *Eur J Comparative Gastroenterol* 5:29, 2000.

Suggested Reading

Holt D, Heldmann E, Michel K et al: Esophageal obstruction caused by a left aortic arch and an anomalous right patent ductus arteriosus in two German Shepherd littermates, *Vet Surg* 29:264-270, 2000.

Clinical signs were alleviated in these two dogs by dissection and division of the patent right ductus arteriosus.

Isakow K, Fowler D, Walsh P: Video-assisted thoracoscopic division of the ligamentum arteriosum in two dogs with persistent right aortic arch, *J Am Vet Med Assoc* 217:1333, 2000.

The technique is described in detail. The laparoscopic procedure took longer than thoracotomy, but the authors suggested that the decreased complications made it a desirable technique.

Lee KC, Lee HC, Jeong SM et al: Radiographic diagnosis of esophageal obstruction by persistent right aortic arch in a kitten, *J Vet Clin* 20:248, 2003.

This case report describes a 3 month old, male Persian kitten with PRAA.

Vianna ML, Krahwinkel DJ: Double aortic arch in a dog, *J Am Vet Med Assoc* 225(8):1222, 2004.

This is a case report of a dog that did well after surgery; however, most dogs die or are euthanized.

White RN, Burton CA, Hale JSH: Vascular ring anomaly with coarctation of the aorta in a cat, *J Small Anim Pract* 44:330, 2003.

This 1-month-old, male domestic short-hair cat had PRAA with a coexisting aberrant left subclavian artery, which was the primary cause of esophageal constriction. Following surgery, the cat was clinically normal.

Surgery of the Stomach

GENERAL PRINCIPLES AND TECHNIQUES

DEFINITIONS

Gastrotomy is an incision through the stomach wall into the lumen. **Partial gastrectomy** is a resection of a portion of the stomach, and **gastrostomy** is the creation of an artificial opening into the gastric lumen. **Gastropexy** permanently adheres the stomach to the body wall. Removal of the pylorus (**pylorectomy**) and attachment of the stomach to the duodenum (**gastroduodenostomy**) is a **Billroth I** procedure. Attachment of the jejunum to the stomach (**gastrojejunostomy**) after a partial gastrectomy (including pylorectomy) is a **Billroth II** procedure. In a **pyloromyotomy,** an incision is made through the serosa and muscularis layers of the pylorus only. For a **pyloroplasty,** a full-thickness incision and tissue reorientation are performed to increase the diameter of the gastric outflow tract.

PREOPERATIVE MANAGEMENT

Gastric surgery is commonly performed to remove foreign bodies (see p. 424) and to correct gastric dilatation-volvulus (see p. 427). Gastric ulceration or erosion (see p. 436), neoplasia (see p. 440), and benign gastric outflow obstruction (see p. 433) are less common indications. Gastric disease may cause vomiting (intermittent, or profuse and continuous) or just anorexia. Dehydration and hypokalemia are common in vomiting animals and should be corrected before induction of anesthesia. Alkalosis may occur secondary to gastric fluid loss; however, metabolic acidosis may also be seen. Hematemesis may indicate gastric erosion or ulceration, or coagulation abnormalities. Peritonitis arising from perforation of the stomach caused by necrosis or ulceration often is lethal if not treated promptly and aggressively (see p. 439). Aspiration pneumonia or esophagitis may also occur in vomiting animals. If possible, severe aspiration pneumonia (see p. 374) should be treated before induction of anesthesia for gastric surgery.

Mild esophagitis generally can be treated by withholding food for 24 to 48 hours (see p. 373) and treating with H_2-antagonists. However, severe esophagitis may necessitate withholding oral food for 7 to 10 days. A gastrostomy tube (see p. 100) placed during surgery may be considered if continued vomiting is not expected. If continued vomiting is likely, an enteral feeding tube is preferred (see p. 107). Treatment with H_2-antagonists (i.e., cimetidine, ranitidine, fa-motidine; see Box 19-15) or omeprazole is important. Orally administered sucralfate slurries may help, but should be given 1 hour after other medications (see p. 438). Administration of metoclopramide or cisapride will improve gastric emptying. Antibiotics effective against oral contaminants (e.g., ampicillin, amoxicillin, clindamycin, and cephalosporins) may be considered (see Box 19-16).

When possible, food should be withheld for at least 8 to 12 hours before surgery to ensure that the stomach is empty. If gastroscopy will be performed, it is best the patient fast for at least 18 and preferably 24 hours before the procedure. However, fasting for only 4 to 6 hours may help prevent hypoglycemia in pediatric patients (see the discussion on anesthetic and surgical management of pediatric patients below). Surgery for gastric obstruction, distention, malpositioning, or ulceration should be performed as soon as possible after the animal's condition has been stabilized.

ANESTHESIA

Numerous anesthetic protocols have been used in animals with gastric disorders (Boxes 19-24 and 19-25). Because vomiting, reflux, and aspiration are common, anticholinergics (i.e., atropine or glycopyrrolate) should be considered to reduce gastric secretion and damage to the esophageal mucosa or respiratory tract. Nitrous oxide should be avoided whenever gastric or intestinal distention is present (e.g., gastric dilatation-volvulus, intestinal volvulus, or torsion) because it rapidly diffuses into gas-filled areas, causing additional organ distention. Dogs may be premedicated with an anticholinergic and opioid (e.g., hydromorphone, butorphanol, and buprenorphine; see Table 13-4 on p. 133), and then induced with a thiobarbiturate or propofol or a combination of diazepam and ketamine (given slowly intravenously). A combination of hydromorphone and diazepam given intravenously may be sufficient for induction of severely depressed dogs. If additional drugs are needed for intubation, etomidate or a reduced dose of a thiobarbiturate or propofol may be administered intravenously. Rapid induction and immediate intubation are essential if vomiting is a concern; however, mask induction is acceptable if vomiting is not a concern. Isoflurane or sevoflurane is the inhalation agent of choice in arrhythmic patients.

Animals younger than 6 months of age should be anesthetized with care. Because hepatic glycogen stores are rapidly depleted during fasting in puppies and kittens, fasting longer than 4 to 6 hours is not generally recommended. If you are unable to monitor the blood glucose level, intravenous fluids containing balanced electrolytes in a 2.5% dextrose solution should be given for surgeries lasting longer than 1 hour or if anesthetic recovery is delayed. Hypothermia commonly develops in puppies and kittens during surgery because they have a higher surface area to body weight ratio, which causes greater heat loss by radiation and evaporation. Hypothermia may cause bradycardia, low cardiac output, and hypotension, which may prolong drug elimination and anesthetic recovery. Drugs that normally redistribute to muscle or fat have prolonged effects in puppies and kittens after repeated adminis-

BOX 19-24

Selected Anesthetic Protocols for Use in Stable Animals With Gastric Disorders

Premedication

Give atropine (0.02–0.04 mg/kg SC, IM) or glycopyrrolate (0.005–0.011 mg/kg SC, IM) plus hydromorphone (0.1–0.2 mg/kg SC, IM) or butorphanol (0.2–0.4 mg/kg SC, IM), or buprenorphine (5–15 μg/kg IM)

Induction

Thiopental (10–12 mg/kg IV) or propofol (4–6 mg/kg IV) or a combination of diazepam and ketamine (diazepam 0.27 mg/kg plus 5.5 mg/kg ketamine IV, titrated to effect)

Maintenance

Isoflurane or sevoflurane

SC, Subcutaneous; *IM,* intramuscular; *IV,* intravenous.

BOX 19-25

Selected Anesthetic Protocols for Use in Patients That Are Hypovolemic, Dehydrated, or Shocky*

Dogs

Induction

Hydromorphone (0.1 mg/kg IV) plus diazepam (0.2 mg/kg IV).
 Give in incremental dosages. Intubate if possible. If necessary give etomidate (0.5–1.5 mg/kg IV). As an alternative, give thiopental or propofol at extremely reduced dosages.

Maintenance

Isoflurane or sevoflurane.

Cats

Premedication

Butorphanol (0.2–0.4 mg/kg SC, IM) or buprenorphine (5–15 μg/kg IM) or hydromorphone (0.05–0.1 mg/kg SC, IM).

Induction

Diazepam (0.2 mg/kg IV) followed by etomidate (0.5–1.5 mg/kg IV). As an alternative, give thiopental or propofol at reduced dosages. If there are no contraindications to ketamine, reduced dosages of diazepam and ketamine may also be used.

Maintenance

Isoflurane or sevoflurane.

IV, Intravenous; *SC,* subcutaneous; *IM,* intramuscular.
*Anticholinergics may be administered if indicated.

tration. Reduced hepatorenal function may also prolong drug effects. Phenothiazine tranquilizers should be used with care in animals younger than 3 months of age because the drugs may cause prolonged central nervous system depression. If used, phenothiazines should be given at one fourth to one half the adult dose. Opioids can be used in young animals; however, they should be given at half the adult dose, and large or multiple doses should not be given.

ANTIBIOTICS

Perioperative antibiotics may be used if the gastric lumen will be entered; however, animals with normal immune function undergoing simple gastrotomy (i.e., proper aseptic technique and no spillage of gastric contents) rarely require them. If antibiotics are used (e.g., cefazolin; 22 mg/kg given intravenously at induction; repeat once or twice at 2- to 4-hour intervals), they should be given intravenously before induction of anesthesia and continued for up to 12 hours postoperatively. Except for *Helicobacter* organisms, bacteria are scarce in the stomach compared with other parts of the gastrointestinal tract because of the low gastric pH.

SURGICAL ANATOMY

The stomach can be divided into the cardia, fundus, body, pyloric antrum, pyloric canal, and pyloric ostium. The esophagus enters the stomach at the cardiac ostium. The fundus is dorsal to the cardiac ostium, and although relatively small in carnivores, it is easy to identify on radiographs because it typically is filled with gas. The body of the stomach (the middle one third) lies against the left lobes of the liver. The pyloric antrum is funnel shaped and opens into the pyloric canal. The pyloric ostium is the end of the pyloric canal that empties into the duodenum.

> NOTE: The gastric mucosa accounts for one half of the stomach's weight. You can easily separate the mucosa from the submucosa and serosa when raising flaps or making partial-thickness incisions during a gastropexy or pyloromyotomy.

The gastric (lesser curvature) and gastroepiploic (greater curvature) arteries supply the stomach and are derived from the celiac artery. The short gastric arteries arise from the splenic artery and supply the greater curvature. The portion of the lesser omentum that passes from the stomach to the liver is the hepatogastric ligament. The stomach of the beagle holds more than 500 ml of fluid when distended (a mature cat's stomach may hold 300 to 350 ml). When the stomach is highly distended, it can be palpated beyond the costal arch.

> NOTE: The short gastric vessels often are avulsed in animals with gastric dilatation-volvulus (GDV), which typically accounts for the intraabdominal hemorrhage seen in these cases (see also the discussion of GDV on p. 431).

SURGICAL TECHNIQUE

Gastric surgery often is performed in small animals. Generally, performing a gastrotomy is safer than performing an esophagotomy or enterotomy. Peritonitis is uncommon after gastrotomy if proper techniques are used. Stricture or obstruction is also rare. Billroth procedures are more difficult and may be associated with severe complications.

Gastroscopy

Endoscopic removal of foreign bodies is preferred over surgical removal, but requires appropriate endoscopic snares. Likewise, endoscopy is more sensitive than gastrotomy when looking for erosions, ulcers, *Physaloptera,* and other small lesions. However, it is imperative that the entire gastric mucosa be systematically examined, including the fundus and lower esophageal mucosa. Similarly, endoscopy is the preferred method for gastric mucosal biopsy because it allows one to obtain more tissue samples than surgery, which is important because gastric mucosal lesions can be very spotty. Scirrhous carcinomas, pythiosis, and submucosal lesions are the most important gastric lesions that cannot be reliably diagnosed with endoscopic biopsy. Rarely, intraoperative gastroscopy can be performed to help the surgeon find a mucosal lesion (e.g., ulcer) that is not obvious from the serosal surface.

Gastrotomy

The most common indication for gastrotomy in dogs and cats is removal of a foreign body (see p. 424).

Make a ventral midline abdominal incision from the xiphoid to the pubis. Use Balfour retractors to retract the abdominal wall and provide adequate exposure of the gastrointestinal tract. Inspect the entire abdominal contents before incising the stomach. To reduce contamination, isolate the stomach from remaining abdominal contents with moistened laparotomy sponges. Place stay sutures to assist in manipulation of the stomach and help prevent spillage of gastric contents. Make the gastric incision in a hypovascular area of the ventral aspect of the stomach, between the greater and lesser curvatures (Fig. 19-58). Make sure the incision is not near the pylorus, or closure of the incision may cause excessive tissue to be enfolded into the gastric lumen, resulting in outflow obstruction. Make a stab incision into the gastric lumen with a scalpel (Fig. 19-59, A), and enlarge the incision with Metzenbaum scissors (Fig. 19-59, B). Use suction to aspirate gastric contents and reduce spillage. Close the stomach with 2-0 or 3-0 absorbable suture material (e.g., polydioxanone, polyglyconate) in a two-layer inverting seromuscular pattern (Fig. 19-59, C). Include serosa, muscularis, and submucosa in the first layer using a Cushing or simple continuous pattern, then follow it with a Lembert or Cushing pattern that incorporates the serosal and muscularis layers (Fig. 19-59, D). As an alternative, close the mucosa in a simple continuous suture pattern as a separate layer to reduce postoperative bleeding. Before closing the abdominal incision, substitute sterile instruments and gloves for those contaminated by gastric contents. Whenever you remove a gastric foreign body, be sure to check the entire intestinal tract for additional material that could cause an intestinal obstruction.

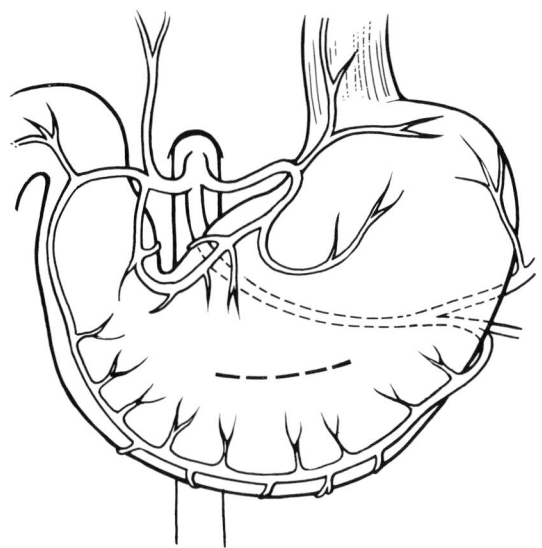

FIG. 19-58
Preferred location of gastrotomy incisions.

Partial Gastrectomy and Invagination of Gastric Tissue

Partial gastrectomy is indicated when necrosis, ulceration, or neoplasia involves the greater curvature, or middle portion, of the stomach. Necrosis of the greater curvature is primarily associated with GDV and may be treated by resection or invagination. Invagination does not require opening of the gastric lumen; however, obstruction from excessive intraluminal tissue and excessive bleeding are possible, although rare. The extent of necrosis is assessed by observing the serosal color, gastric wall texture, vascular patency, and bleeding on incision; however, in many cases it is difficult to determine tissue viability with these techniques (see p. 447 for a discussion of methods for determining tissue viability). Necrotic tissue may range in color from gray-green to black and often feels thin. A full-thickness incision can be made into the suspected necrotic tissue to assess arterial bleeding. Intravenous fluorescein dye has not proved to be an accurate method of determining gastric viability in dogs with GDV. Generally, if you question the viability of the gastric tissue, remove it or invaginate it. Failure to remove or invaginate necrotic tissue may result in perforation, peritonitis, and death. Melena is commonly observed for a few days after gastric invagination.

NOTE: Do not use mucosal color to predict gastric viability; the mucosa is commonly black in dogs with GDV because of vascular obstruction. Damage to the mucosa may predispose these animals to gastric ulceration.

To remove the greater curvature of the stomach, ligate branches of the left gastroepiploic vessels or short gastric vessels (or both) along the section of the stomach to be

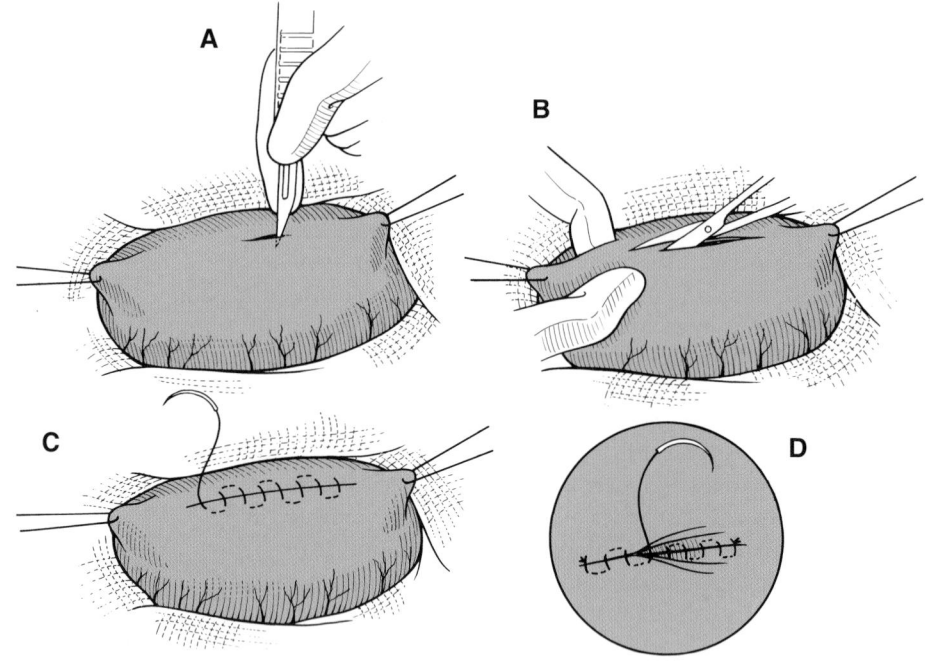

FIG. 19-59
Gastrotomy. **A,** Make a stab incision into the gastric lumen with a scalpel. **B,** Enlarge the incision with Metzenbaum scissors. **C** and **D,** Close the stomach with a two-layer inverting seromuscular suture pattern.

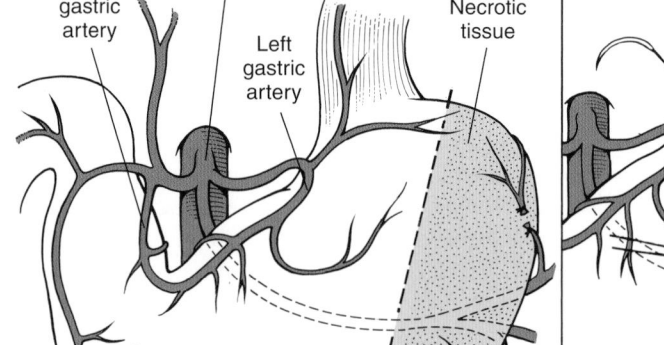

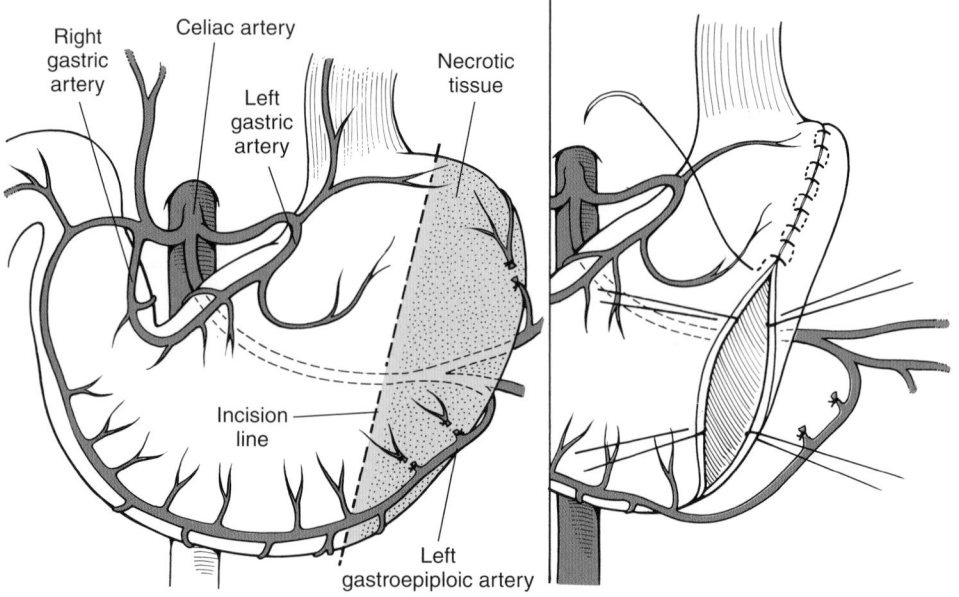

FIG. 19-60
To remove the greater curvature of the stomach, ligate branches of the left gastroepiploic vessels or short gastric vessels (or both) and excise the necrotic tissue. Close the stomach with a two-layer inverting suture pattern.

removed (Fig. 19-60). Excise the necrotic tissue, leaving a margin of normal, actively bleeding tissue to suture. Close the stomach in a two-layer inverting pattern using 2-0 or 3-0 absorbable suture (e.g., polydioxanone or polyglyconate). Incorporate the submucosa, muscularis, and serosal layers in a Cushing or simple continuous pattern in the first layer. Then use a Cushing or Lembert pattern to invert the serosa and muscularis over the first layer. As an alternative, you may use a TA stapling device to close the incision. To invaginate necrotic tissue, use a simple continuous suture pattern followed by an inverting pattern. Place sutures in healthy gastric tissue on both sides of the tissue that is to be invaginated, bringing the healthy tissue over the top of the

necrotic tissue. Make sure the sutures are placed in healthy tissue to prevent dehiscence.

Removal of neoplasia (see p. 442) or ulceration (see p. 439) of the greater or lesser curvature is similar to that described for necrotic tissue. Most neoplasms in the gastric body, except for leiomyomas and leiomyosarcomas, have metastasized by the time they are diagnosed. If the abnormal tissue involves the dorsal or ventral aspect of the stomach, an elliptic incision encompassing the lesion and some adjacent normal tissue is used. Closure is the same as for a simple gastrotomy. Occasionally the extent of the lesion requires resection of both the dorsal and ventral walls of the stomach.

In such cases, ligate branches of the right and left gastric artery and vein (lesser curvature) and left gastroepiploic artery and vein (greater curvature) and remove the omental attachments. After removal of the suspect tissue, perform a two-layer end-to-end anastomosis of the stomach. If the luminal circumferences are of disparate size, the larger circumference can be partly closed using a two-layer suture pattern (see Fig. 19-61, B). Close the mucosa and submucosa of the dorsal surface of the stomach in a simple continuous pattern using 2-0 or 3-0 absorbable suture (e.g., polydioxanone or polyglyconate). Then with the same suture close the ventral aspect. Suture the serosa and muscularis layers in an inverting pattern (e.g., Cushing or Lembert).

Temporary Gastrostomy

Temporary gastrostomy is used to decompress the stomach and occasionally is indicated in dogs with GDV until more definitive surgery can be performed, but is rarely done. For a description of the technique, see *Small Animal Surgery*, second edition.

Pylorectomy With Gastroduodenostomy (Billroth I)

Removal of the pylorus and gastroduodenostomy are indicated for neoplasia (see p. 440), outflow obstruction caused by pyloric muscular hypertrophy (see p. 433), or ulceration of the gastric outflow tract (see p. 436). If neoplasia is present, at least 1- to 2-cm margins of normal tissue should be removed with the abnormal tissue. The margins of the resected tissue should be evaluated histologically for evidence of neoplasia. If the common bile duct has been damaged, a cholecystoduodenostomy or cholecystojejunostomy may be required (see p. 564). If the pancreatic ducts are inadvertently ligated, supplementation with pancreatic enzymes may be necessary postoperatively.

> NOTE: Use extreme care when incising in the pyloric area to prevent damaging the common bile duct where it traverses the lesser omentum.

Identify the common bile duct and pancreatic ducts, then place stay sutures in the proximal duodenum and pyloric antrum. If increased caudoventral retraction of the pylorus is desired, identify and transect a portion of the hepatogastric ligament. Ligate branches of the right gastric and right gastroepiploic artery and vein to the affected tissue and remove the omental and mesenteric attachments (Fig. 19-61, A). Use noncrushing (Doyen) forceps or fingers to occlude the stomach and duodenum proximal and distal to the area to be resected. With Metzenbaum scissors or a scalpel blade, excise the area of pylorus to be removed and inspect the remaining edges to ensure that all abnormal tissue has been excised. If the gastric and duodenal lumens are notably different in size, incise the duodenum at an angle or partly close the antrum (Fig. 19-61, B). Perform a one- or two-layer end-to-end anastomosis of the pyloric antrum to the duodenum

using 2-0 or 3-0 absorbable suture material (polydioxanone, polyglyconate, or poliglecaprone 25) in a simple continuous, crushing, or simple interrupted pattern.

In one study, no difference was noted in the prevalence of postoperative leakage and incisional dehiscence between one-layer and two-layer closures.

Close the far (dorsal) aspect of the incision first (Fig. 19-61, C), followed by the near (ventral) aspect (Fig. 19-61, D). Prevent inverting excessive tissue, which might reduce the diameter of the gastric outflow tract.

Partial Gastrectomy With Gastrojejunostomy (Billroth II)

If the extent of the lesion precludes end-to-end anastomosis of the pyloric antrum to the duodenum, consider a Billroth II procedure. If only mucosal hypertrophy is present, a Y-U pyloroplasty (see p. 415) is easier to perform and is effective. Before undertaking this procedure, make sure that there is no gross evidence of metastasis (see p. 440 for information regarding gastric neoplasia). In most cases, a cholecystojejunostomy or cholecystoduodenostomy is required in addition to the gastrojejunostomy (see p. 564). Exocrine insufficiency may occur if the pancreatic ducts are damaged. Exocrine plus endocrine (i.e., diabetes mellitus) pancreatic insufficiency may occur as a result of pancreatic resection or severe damage to the pancreatic blood supply.

The procedure is similar to a Billroth I except that the distal stomach and proximal duodenum are closed after a pylorectomy, and the jejunum is attached with a side-to-side anastomosis to the diaphragmatic surface of the stomach.

Resect the pylorus, antrum, and proximal duodenum as described above, ligating appropriate branches of the right and left gastric and gastroepiploic vessels (Fig. 19-62, A). Close the duodenal and pyloric antral stumps in a two-layer pattern. For the first layer, incorporate the mucosa and submucosa in a simple interrupted or simple continuous pattern using 2-0 or 3-0 absorbable suture (Fig. 19-62, B). Then use an inverting suture pattern (e.g., Lembert) in the seromuscular layer. Identify an avascular area between the gastric incision and greater curvature. Bring a loop of proximal jejunum to the selected site, and attach it to the stomach with stay sutures. Suture the seromuscular layers of the stomach and intestine together using a simple continuous pattern with 2-0 or 3-0 absorbable suture (Fig. 19-62, C). Make full-thickness, longitudinal incisions into the stomach and intestinal lumens near the suture line (Fig. 19-62, D). Suture the mucosa and submucosa of the stomach to the intestine in a continuous pattern using 3-0 or 4-0 absorbable suture (Fig. 19-62, E). Next, place a continuous suture pattern in the serosa and muscularis.

Use of stapling devices has also been described for stump closure and creation of the gastrojejunostomy.

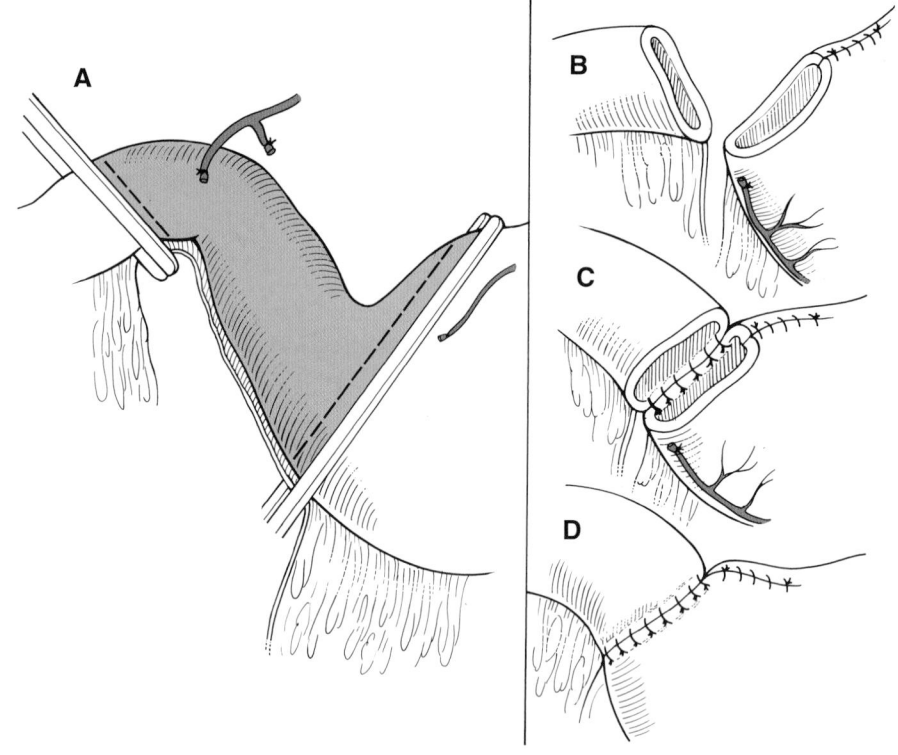

FIG. 19-61

Billroth I procedure. **A,** Ligate the vasculature, remove the omental and mesenteric attachments, and excise the area of the pylorus to be removed. **B,** If the gastric and duodenal lumens are greatly different in size, incise the duodenum at an angle or partly close the antrum. **C,** Close the far (dorsal) aspect of the incision first. **D,** Close the near (ventral) aspect.

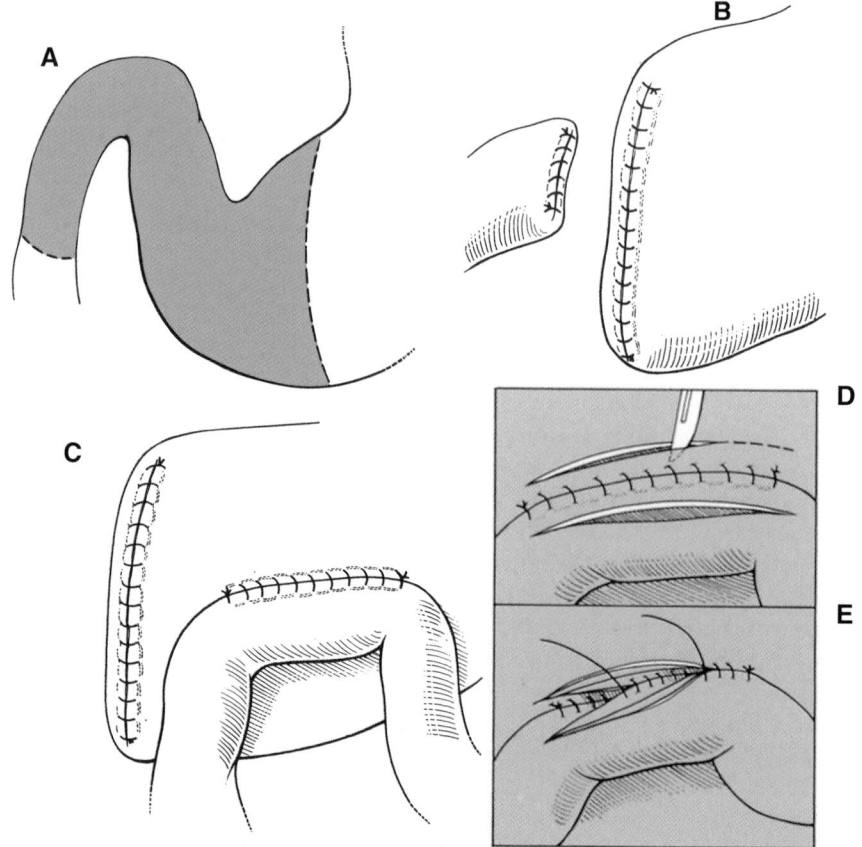

FIG. 19-62

Billroth II procedure. **A,** Resect the pylorus, antrum, and proximal duodenum. **B,** Close the duodenal and pyloric antral stumps with a two-layer suture pattern. **C,** Bring a loop of proximal jejunum to the stomach and suture the seromuscular layers of the stomach and intestine together. **D,** Make full-thickness, longitudinal incisions into the stomach and intestinal lumens. **E,** Suture the mucosa and submucosa of the stomach to the intestine with a continuous suture pattern.

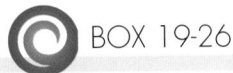

BOX 19-26

Prokinetic Drugs

Metoclopramide (Reglan)
0.25–0.5 mg/kg PO, IV, IM, or SC, qd to qid

Erythromycin
1–2 mg/kg qd to tid

Cisapride
Dogs: 0.1–0.5 mg/kg PO, qd to tid
Cats: 2.5 to 5 mg/cat PO, bid to tid

PO, Oral; *IV,* intravenous; *IM,* intramuscular; *SC,* subcutaneous; *qd,* once a day; *qid,* four times a day; *tid,* three times a day; *bid,* twice a day.

Pyloromyotomy and Pyloroplasty

Pyloromyotomy and pyloroplasty increase the diameter of the pylorus and are used to correct gastric outflow obstruction (i.e., chronic antral mucosal hypertrophy or pyloric stenosis).

These procedures must be done with care because they can be difficult to revise. However, they should not be performed routinely in dogs without evidence of pyloric dysfunction (e.g., most dogs with GDV) because they can slow gastric emptying. Gastric outflow procedures that increase the diameter of the pyloric lumen seem to favor early passage of viscous, nonhomogeneous, and hyperosmolar gastric contents into the duodenum. This early passage may overstimulate the enterogastric reflex, prematurely inhibiting antral motor activity and delaying gastric emptying. In addition, gastroduodenal reflux may occur if pyloric function is altered by surgery. Metoclopramide, cisapride, or low-dose erythromycin (Box 19-26) may stimulate gastric emptying.

Fredet-Ramstedt pyloromyotomy. Fredet-Ramstedt pyloromyotomy is the simplest and easiest of these procedures. It does not allow inspection or biopsy of the pyloric mucosa and probably provides only temporary benefit because healing may reduce the size of the lumen.

Hold the pylorus between the index finger and thumb in the nondominant hand. Select a hypovascular area of the ventral pylorus and make a longitudinal incision through the serosa and muscularis but not through the mucosa (Fig. 19-63). Make sure the muscularis layer is completely incised to allow the mucosa to bulge into the incision site. If the mucosa is inadvertently penetrated, close it with interrupted sutures of 2-0 or 3-0 absorbable suture material.

Heineke-Mikulicz pyloroplasty. Heineke-Mikulicz pyloroplasty allows limited exposure of the pyloric mucosa for biopsy and is easy to perform.

Make a full-thickness, longitudinal incision in the ventral surface of the pylorus (Fig. 19-64). Place traction sutures at

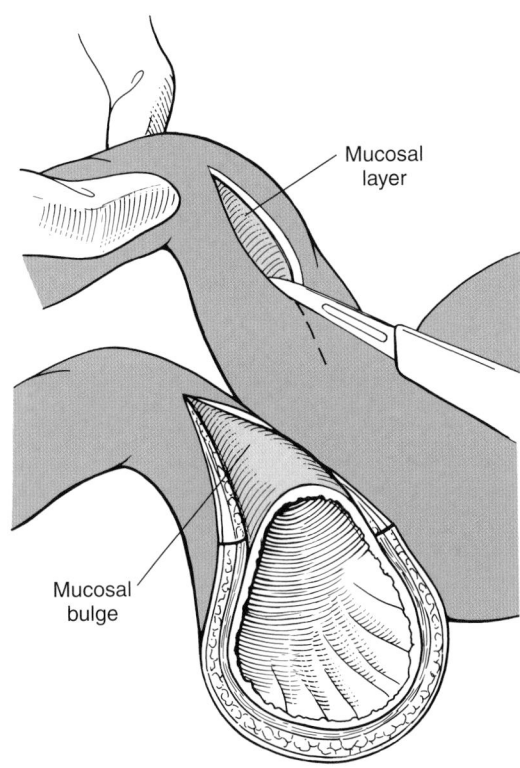

FIG. 19-63
Fredet-Ramstedt pyloromyotomy.

the center of the incision and orient the incision transversely. Suture the transverse incision in a one-layer pattern (simple interrupted or crushing) using 2-0 or 3-0 absorbable suture. Place the sutures carefully so that the incision edges are properly aligned and tissue inversion is prevented.

Y-U pyloroplasty. The Y-U pyloroplasty allows greater accessibility for resection of the pyloric mucosa in dogs with mucosal hypertrophy while simultaneously increasing the luminal diameter of the outflow tract.

Make a longitudinal incision (limb) in the serosa overlying the ventral pylorus, and extend it into the stomach by making two incisions (arms) that run parallel to the lesser and greater curvature of the stomach (creating a Y-shaped incision) (Fig. 19-65, A). Make sure the angle of the Y is not overly narrow, or necrosis may result. The limbs and arms of the Y-shaped incision should be approximately the same length. Make a full-thickness incision. Inspect the mucosa and resect it if necessary. If the mucosa is resected, appose the remaining mucosal edges in a continuous pattern using absorbable 3-0 to 4-0 suture before closing the Y incision. Suture the base of the antral flap to the distal end of the duodenal incision in a simple interrupted pattern using absorbable 2-0 or 3-0 suture, creating a U-shaped closure (Fig. 19-65, B). Close the remainder of the incision (the limbs) with simple interrupted sutures (Fig. 19-65, C). Make sure that tissue approximation is adequate to prevent leak-

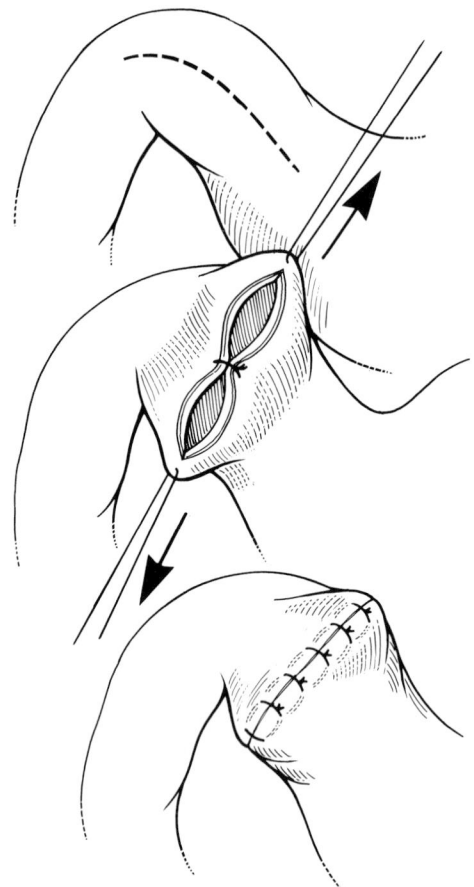

FIG. 19-64
Heineke-Mikulicz pyloroplasty.

age and that minimal tissue has been enfolded into the pyloric lumen.

> NOTE: To reduce necrosis of the pointed tip of the gastric tissue flap, you may wish to excise the point of the Y before suturing it.

Gastropexy

Gastropexy techniques are designed to permanently adhere the stomach to the body wall. The most common indications are GDV (pyloric antrum to right body wall) and hiatal herniation (fundus to left body wall). Numerous gastropexy techniques have been described. Although the strength and extent of adhesions created by these techniques differ, all of them (when properly performed) prevent movement of the stomach.

> NOTE: To create a permanent adhesion, the gastric muscle must be in contact with the muscle of the body wall; intact gastric serosa does not form permanent adhesions to an intact peritoneal surface.

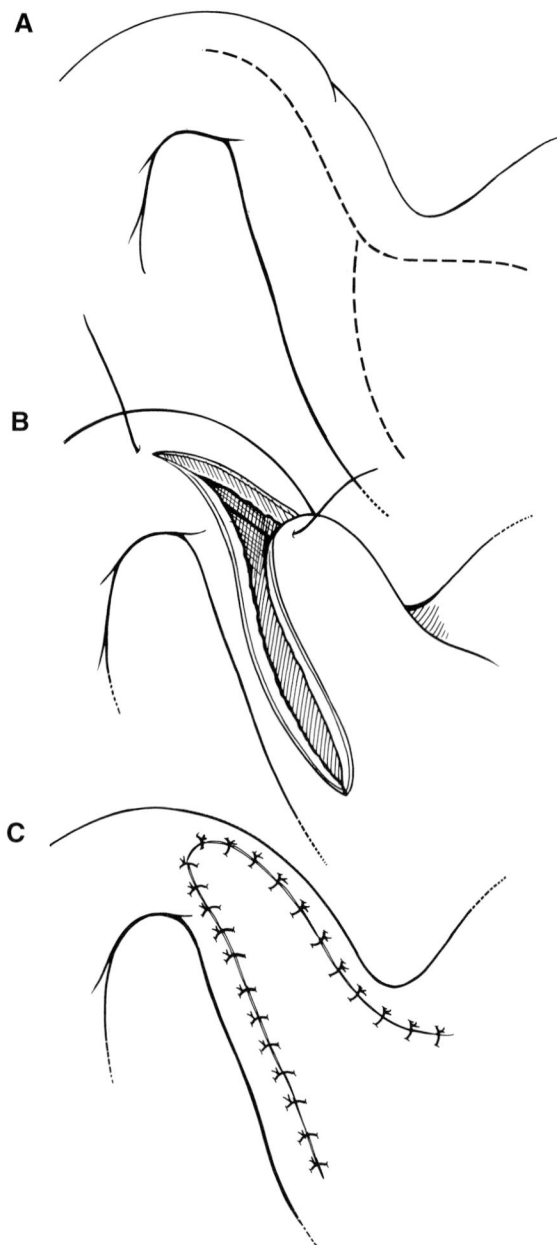

FIG. 19-65
Y-U pyloroplasty. **A,** Make a Y-shaped incision in the pylorus and pyloric antrum. **B,** Begin by suturing the base of the antral flap to the distal point of the duodenal incision. **C,** Close the remainder of the incision in a U shape.

A technique for gastropexy has been described in which the stomach is incorporated into the abdominal incision during closure. Although this technique is easy and quick, and reduces the recurrence of GDV, it results in the stomach being permanently adhered to the ventral body wall. The main advantage of the procedure is that it can be performed quickly. However, the subsequent abdominal exploration via a midline abdominal incision could perforate the stomach. Therefore, although this technique is preferable to not per-

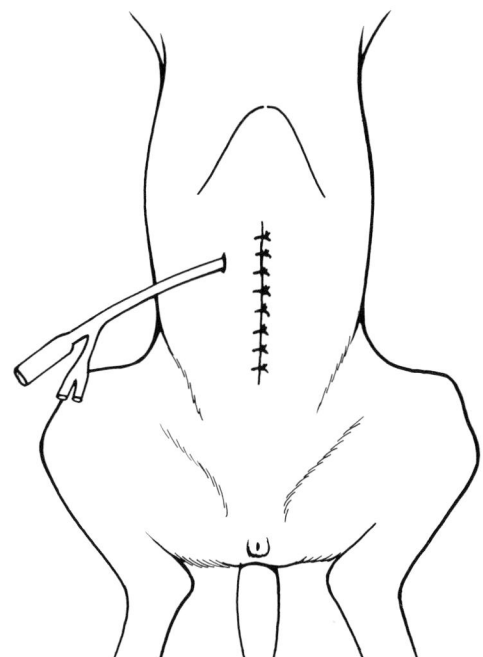

FIG. 19-66
Tube gastropexy.

forming any type of "pexy," it is not generally recommended. Surgeons should become familiar with one of the techniques described next.

Tube gastropexy. Tube gastropexy (gastrostomy) is quick and relatively simple (Fig. 19-66). Also, it allows postoperative gastric decompression and placement of medications directly into the stomach in inappetent animals. The tube should be left in place 7 to 10 days to form a permanent adhesion. Although this may lengthen the postoperative hospitalization period compared with other techniques, the tube can be capped and secured against the trunk and the patient sent home on oral feeding. The risk of leakage is minimal if proper technique is used; however, improper placement may result in peritonitis.

Make a stab incision into the right abdominal wall caudal to the last rib and 4 to 10 cm lateral to the midline. Place a Foley catheter (18 to 30 French) through the stab incision. Select a site in a hypovascular region of the seromuscular layer of the ventral surface of the pyloric antrum where the balloon of the catheter will not obstruct gastric outflow. Place a purse-string suture of 2-0 absorbable suture (e.g., polydioxanone or polyglyconate) at this site. Make a stab incision through the purse-string suture, and insert the Foley catheter tip into the gastric lumen (Fig. 19-67, A). (Note: The Foley catheter can be placed through the omentum before entry into the stomach so that the omentum is secured between the stomach and body wall, or the omentum can be wrapped around the site after the stomach has been secured to the body wall.) Inflate the bulb of the Foley catheter with

saline (not air), and secure the purse-string suture around the tube. Preplace three or four absorbable sutures between the pyloric antrum and the body wall where the tube exits (Fig. 19-67, B). Prevent penetrating the catheter or balloon when placing the sutures. Draw the stomach to the body wall by placing traction on the catheter, and tie the preplaced sutures (Fig. 19-67, C). Secure the tube to the skin with a Roman sandal suture pattern (see p. 900), but prevent penetrating it with a suture. Place a bandage around the dog's abdomen and over the tube to prevent premature removal (use an Elizabethan collar if necessary). Leave the tube in place 7 to 10 days, then deflate the balloon and remove it. Leave the skin incision open to facilitate drainage. Place a light bandage over the open wound if desired.

> NOTE: Cut the tip off the end of the Foley catheter if food or viscous fluids are to be injected through it. Inflate the balloon with saline, not air.

Circumcostal gastropexy. Circumcostal gastropexy forms a stronger adhesion than most other techniques, but is technically more challenging (Box 19-27). Because the lumen of the stomach is not entered, the risk of gastric leakage and abdominal contamination is diminished compared with tube gastropexy. Possible complications associated with circumcostal gastropexy include pneumothorax and rib fracture.

Make either a one- or two-layer hinged flap (approximately 5 to 6 cm long in large dogs) by incising through the seromuscular layer of the pyloric antrum (Fig. 19-68, A). Do not incise the gastric mucosa or enter the lumen (if this occurs, suture the mucosa with 3-0 absorbable suture). Elevate the flap by dissecting under the muscularis. If a one-hinged flap is made, place the hinge toward the lesser curvature. Make a 5- to 6-cm incision over the eleventh or twelfth rib at the level of the costochondral junction (Fig. 19-68, B). Make sure the incision does not penetrate the diaphragmatic attachments to the body wall, causing pneumothorax. Form a tunnel under the rib using a Carmalt clamp or hemostat (Fig. 19-68, C). Place stay sutures on the flap (if using a two-flap technique, place the sutures on the flap nearest the lesser curvature). Pass the gastric antral flap craniodorsal under the rib (Fig. 19-68, D), and suture it with 2-0 absorbable suture to the original gastric margin (one-flap technique; Fig. 19-69, A) or the other flap (two-flap technique; Fig. 19-69, B).

Muscular flap (incisional) gastropexy. Muscular flap (incisional) gastropexy is easier than circumcostal gastropexy and prevents the possible complications associated with tube gastropexy (Box 19-28).

Make an incision in the seromuscular layer of the gastric antrum. Then make an incision in the right ventrolateral

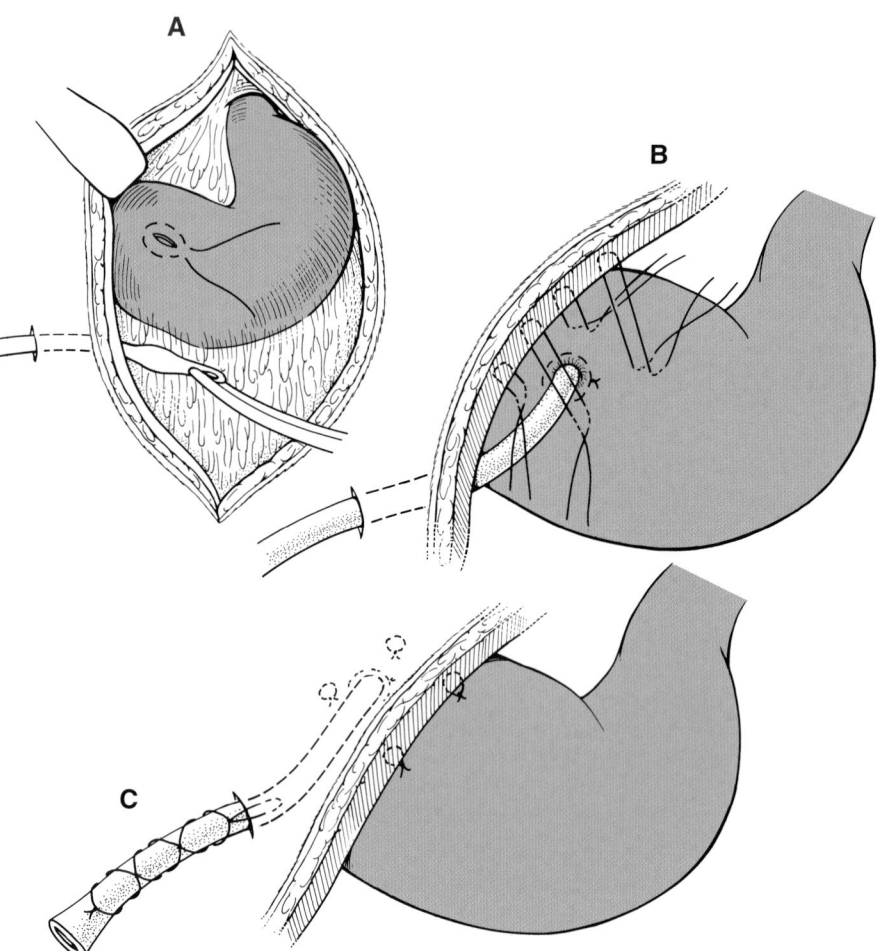

FIG. 19-67
Tube gastropexy. **A,** Insert the tip of a Foley catheter into the gastric lumen through a purse-string suture. **B,** Preplace three or four absorbable sutures between the pyloric antrum and the body wall where the tube exits. **C,** Draw the stomach to the body wall and tie the preplaced sutures. Secure the tube to the skin with a Roman sandal suture pattern.

 BOX 19-27

Advantages and Disadvantages of Circumcostal Gastropexy

Advantages
- Strong adhesion to body wall
- Gastric lumen not opened

Disadvantages
- More difficult to perform
- Risk of pneumothorax
- Possibility of rib fractures
- Does not provide direct access to gastric lumen if postoperative decompression is necessary

abdominal wall by incising the peritoneum and internal fascia of the rectus abdominis or transverse abdominis muscles (Fig. 19-70, A). Suture the edges of the incisions in a simple continuous pattern using 2-0 absorbable or nonabsorbable suture (Fig. 19-70, B). Make sure the muscularis layer of the stomach is in contact with the abdominal wall muscle (Fig. 19-70, C). Suture the cranial margin first, then the caudal margin. As an alternative, you may raise flaps in the stomach and body wall to increase the extent of muscle contact between these tissues.

Belt-loop gastropexy. A belt-loop gastropexy is similar to a muscle flap gastropexy except that a single flap is elevated and passed beneath a tunnel created in the abdominal wall. It is technically simple and seems to result in adequate adhesions.

Elevate a seromuscular flap in the gastric antrum (Figure 19-71, A). Make two transverse incisions in the ventrolateral abdominal wall by incising the peritoneum and abdominal musculature (Fig. 19-71, B). The incisions should be 2.5 to 4 cm apart and 3 to 5 cm long. Create a tunnel under the abdominal musculature with forceps. Place stay sutures in the edge of the antral flap and use them to pass the flap from cranial to caudal under the muscular flap (Fig. 19-71, C). Suture the flap to its original gastric margin in a simple continuous pattern using 2-0 absorbable or nonabsorbable suture (Fig. 19-71, D) or skin staples. You may wish to place additional sutures between the body wall and the stomach to reduce tension on the gastropexy.

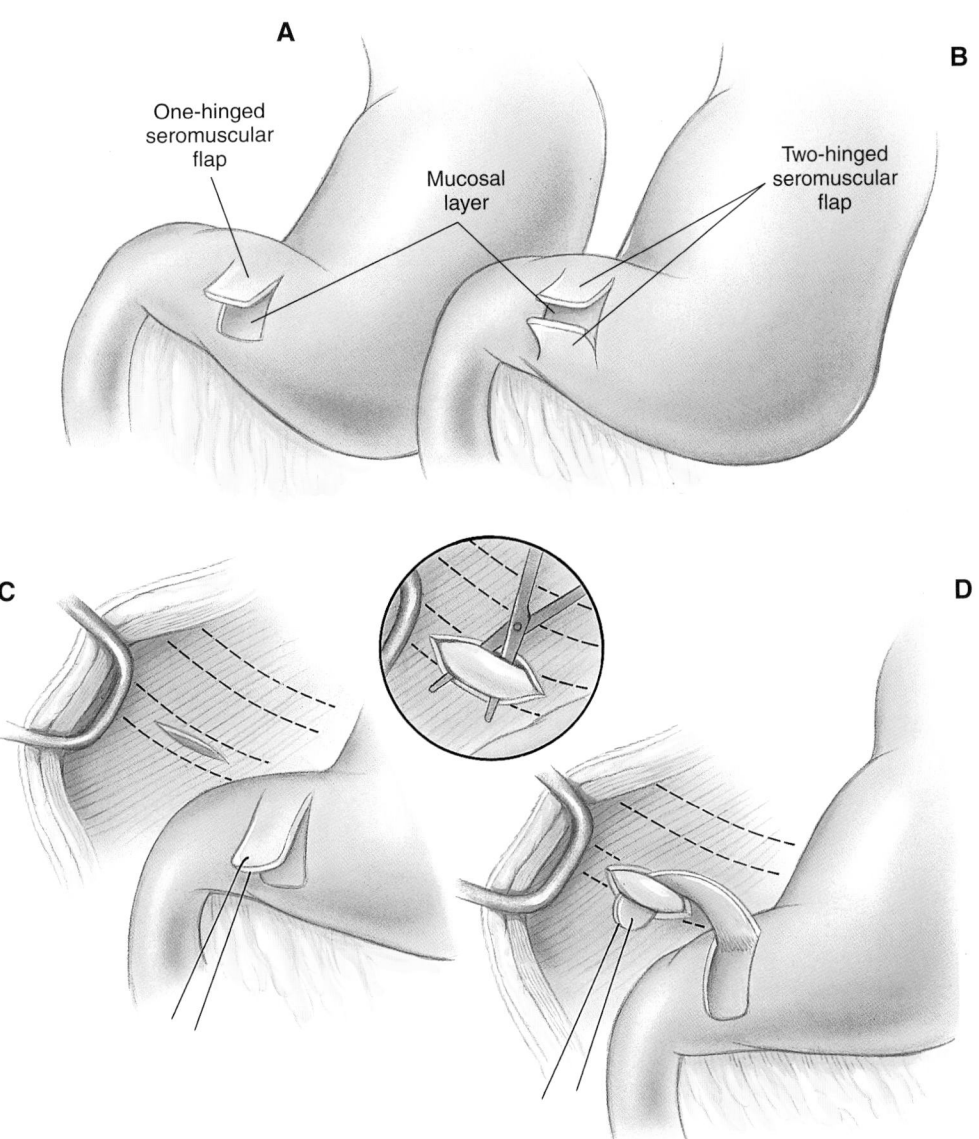

FIG. 19-68
Circumcostal gastropexy. **A,** Make a single- or double-layer hinged seromuscular flap in the pyloric antrum. **B,** Make an incision over the eleventh or twelfth rib at the level of the costochondral junction. **C,** Form a tunnel under the rib using a Carmalt clamp or hemostat. **D,** Pass the gastric antral flap craniodorsal under the rib and suture it to the original gastric margin or to the other flap (see Fig. 19-69).

Gastrocolopexy. Gastrocolopexy has also been described as a method of preventing recurrence of GDV. In this technique the greater curvature of the stomach is sutured to the transverse colon. This technique resulted in a recurrence rate of 20% in one study (Eggerstdottir et al, 2001).

Laparoscopic prophylactic gastropexy. This minimally invasive technique allows a rapid gastropexy.

With the dog in dorsal recumbency, place the first cannula just caudal to the umbilicus and place the second 10-mm cannula just right of midline, approximately 2 to 4 cm behind the last rib (make this incision parallel to the rib

([Fig. 19-72, A]). Use Babcock forceps to grasp the antrum, midway between the greater and lesser curvatures and 6 to 8 cm back from the pylorus. Pull this portion of the stomach up to the end of the cannula, and then pull the cannula, Babcock forceps, and stomach out of the abdomen as one unit until the stomach wall can be seen protruding from the peritoneal cavity (Fig. 19-72, B). Enlarge the incision through which the cannula was placed to 4 to 5 cm. Grasp the gastric wall with Allis tissue forceps or Babcock forceps, and place stay sutures between it and the body wall (Fig. 19-72, C). Release the endoscopic Babcock forceps. Perform the gastropexy as described above under muscular

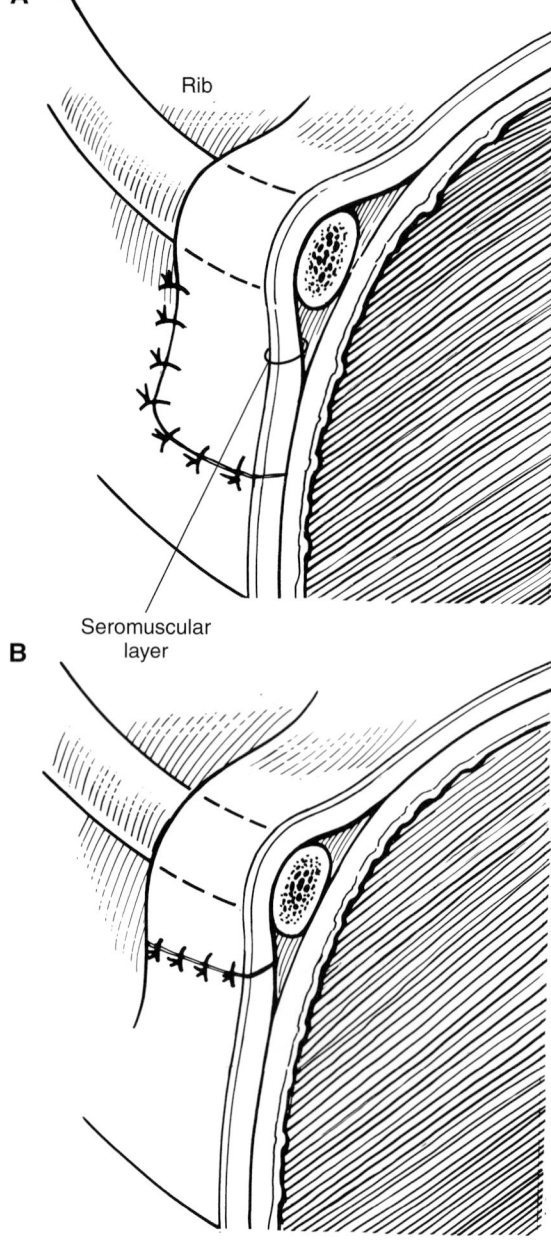

FIG. 19-69
A, For a single-flap technique, suture the circumcostal flap to the original gastric margin. **B,** For a double-flap technique, pass the seromuscular flap under the rib and suture it to the second flap.

flap gastropexy. Take care to not twist the antrum as it is brought up to and out the incision.

It is best to reexamine the stomach laparoscopically before final closure to ensure that malpositioning did not take place (Rawlings et al, 2001).

Minilaparotomy prophylactic gastropexy. *Place the dog in left lateral recumbency. Make a 6-cm vertical*

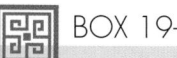 BOX 19-28

Advantages and Disadvantages of Muscular Flap and Belt-Loop Gastropexy

Advantages
- Easy and quick to perform
- Gastric lumen not opened

Disadvantages
- Less strong than circumcostal gastropexy
- Does not provide direct access to gastric lumen if postoperative decompression is necessary

skin incision just caudal and ventral to the thirteenth rib. Bluntly dissect through the external and internal abdominal obliques and transversus abdominis muscles. Enter the abdomen via blunt dissection and visualize the stomach. If the stomach cannot be visualized, palpate the duodenum and pylorus with two fingers and locate the antrum of the stomach. Grasp the stomach with Babcock intestinal forceps, and retract the gastric antrum into the surgical field (Fig. 19-73, A). Identify the stomach by palpating the pylorus and visualizing the omental attachments, right gastric vessels, and right gastroepiploic vessels. Place stay sutures at each end of the intended gastric incision to hold the stomach in the surgical field. Allow the gastric antrum to fall back into the abdomen (Fig. 19-73, B). Palpate the pylorus to ensure proper placement of the gastric incision. Make a 3-cm longitudinal incision through the serosa and muscularis layers of the gastric antrum approximately 5 cm orad to the pylorus (Fig. 19-73, C). Beginning at the dorsal edge, suture the edges of the incision to the abdominal muscles using a simple continuous suture pattern. Close the muscles, subcutaneous tissue, and skin routinely (Steelman-Szymeczek et al, 2003).

HEALING OF THE STOMACH

The extraordinarily rich blood supply, reduced bacterial numbers (as a result of gastric acidity), rapidly regenerating epithelium, and defense mechanisms provided by the omentum allow gastric incisions to heal quickly. Because the stomach has a thicker wall than the bowel, it can be difficult to find and stop bleeding vessels. Gentle pressure applied to the bleeding tissue usually is effective; crushing clamps or forceps and electrocautery should be avoided.

SUTURE MATERIALS AND SPECIAL INSTRUMENTS

Monofilament absorbable suture material (i.e., polydioxanone [PDS], polyglyconate [Maxon], or poliglecaprone 25 [Monocryl]) is preferred for gastrointestinal surgery. These sutures are strong, have minimal tissue drag, and maintain tensile strength for longer than 10 days. Chromic gut suture is rapidly removed by digestion and phagocytosis and should

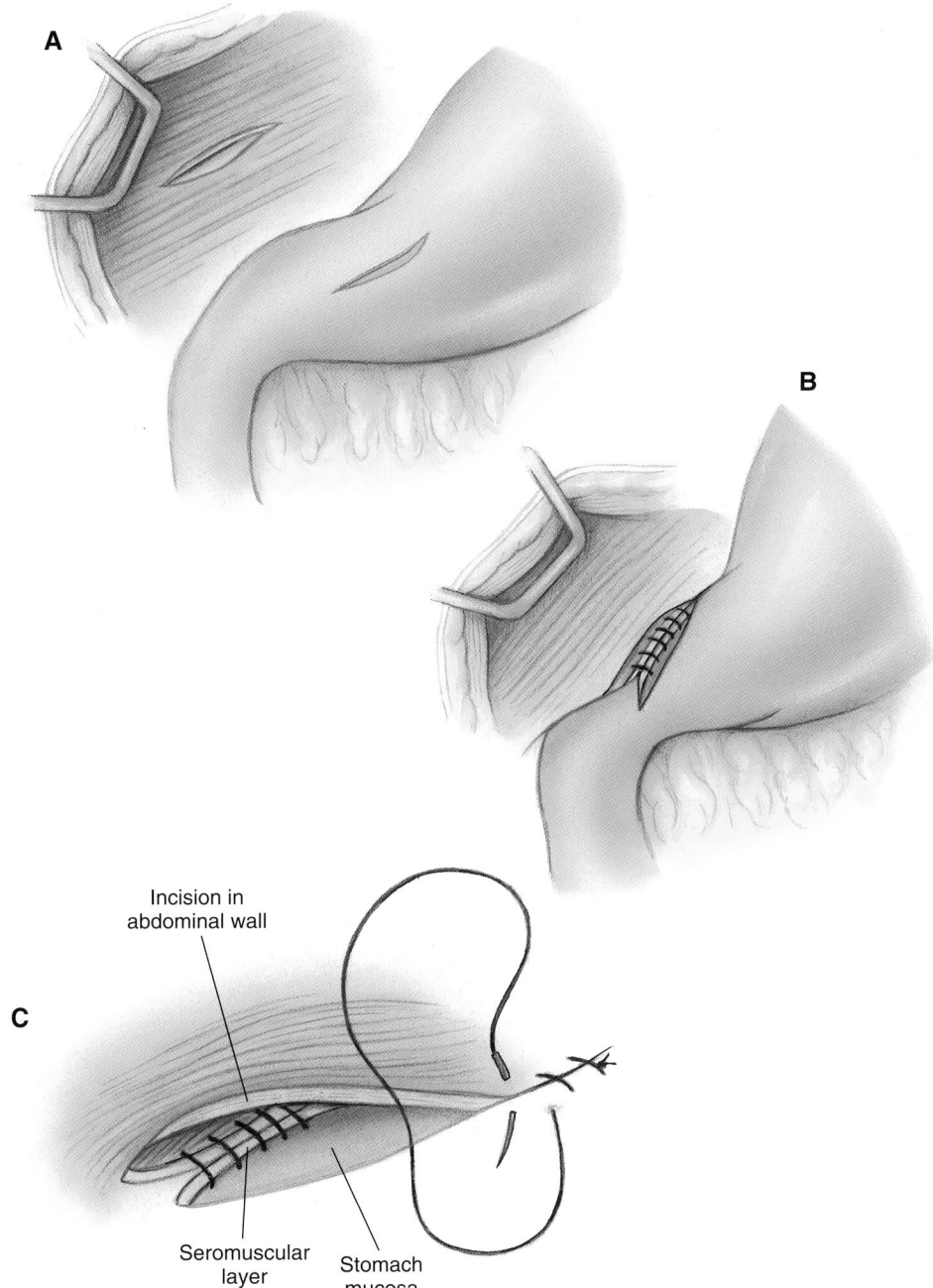

FIG. 19-70
Muscular flap gastropexy. **A,** Make an incision in the seromuscular layer of the gastric antrum and in the right ventrolateral abdominal wall. **B,** Suture the edge of the abdominal incision to the gastric incision using a simple continuous pattern. **C,** Make sure the muscularis layer of the stomach is in contact with the abdominal wall muscle.

be prevented. Nonabsorbable suture material that penetrates the lumen may cause gastric ulcers to form along the suture line if a continuous suture pattern is used; therefore nonabsorbable suture material should be avoided in the stomach. Small-diameter, swaged-on, taper point needles generally are preferred for gastrointestinal surgery. However, cutting needles are sometimes used because they more readily penetrate

submucosa and require less stabilization of tissue, which might result in less crushing.

Noncrushing forceps (e.g., Doyen forceps or some vascular clamps) are useful for occluding the gastric and duodenal stumps during gastroduodenostomy or gastrojejunostomy procedures (see p. 413). Pediatric Doyen forceps are the appropriate size for occluding the duodenal lumen. If non-

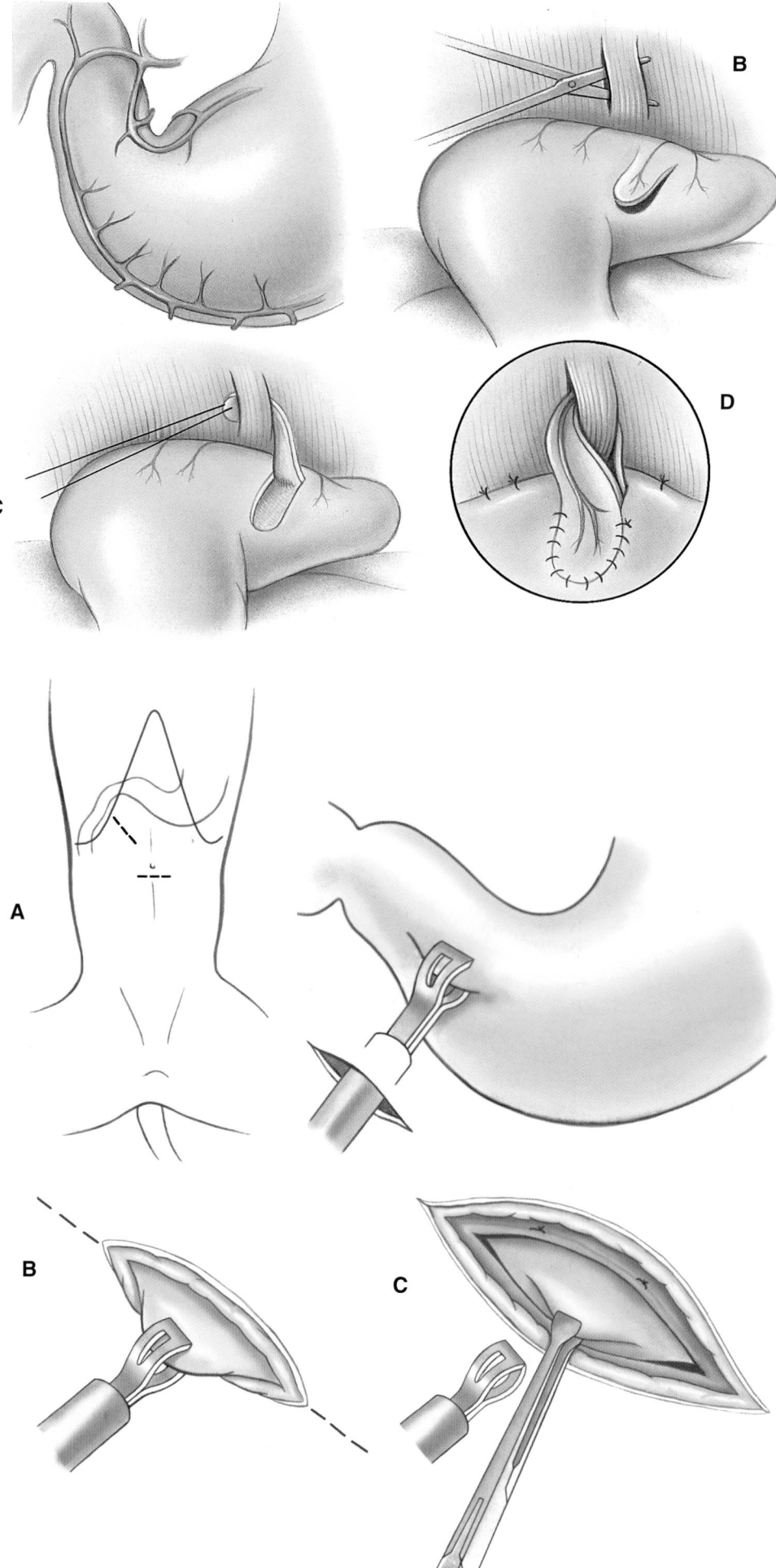

FIG. 19-71
Belt-loop gastropexy. **A** and **B,** Elevate a seromuscular flap in the gastric antrum. **B,** Make two transverse incisions in the ventro-lateral abdominal wall and create a tunnel under the abdominal musculature with forceps. **C,** Pass the flap from cranial to caudal under the muscular flap. **D,** Suture the flap to its original gastric margin.

FIG 19-72
For a laparoscopic gastropexy. **A,** Place the first cannula just caudal to the umbilicus, and place the second cannula just right of midline, approximately 2 to 4 cm behind the last rib (make this incision parallel to the rib). **B,** Pull the stomach out through the incision. **C,** Place stay sutures between it and the body wall. Perform a gastropexy as described in Fig. 19-70.

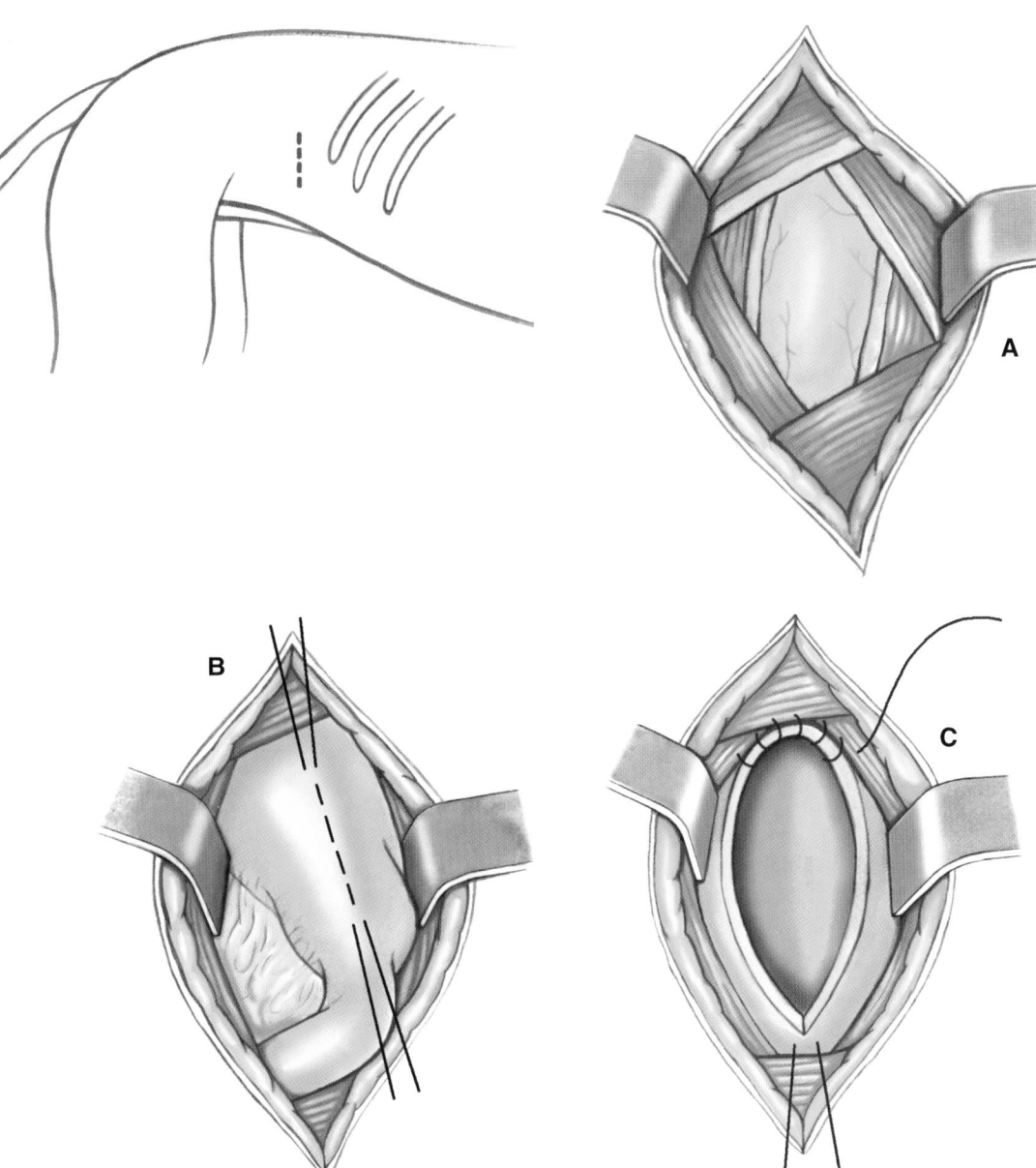

FIG 19-73
For a minilaparotomy. **A,** Make a 6-cm vertical skin incision just caudal and ventral to the thirteenth rib. Bluntly dissect through the muscles. Enter the abdomen and view the stomach. Grasp the stomach with Babcock intestinal forceps and retract the gastric antrum into the surgical field. **B,** Place stay sutures at each end of the intended gastric incision to hold the stomach in the surgical field. Allow the gastric antrum to fall back into the abdomen. Palpate the pylorus to ensure proper placement of the gastric incision. Make a 3-cm longitudinal incision through the serosa and muscularis layers of the gastric antrum approximately 5 cm orad to the pylorus. **C,** Beginning at the dorsal edge, suture the edges of the incision to the abdominal muscles using a simple continuous suture pattern.

crushing forceps are not available, the straight portion of an Allis tissue forceps can be wrapped with a moistened sponge. Crushing forceps, such as Carmalt or Allen forceps, are useful for occluding the portion of the gastrointestinal tract to be removed, but should not be placed on tissues that are not to be excised.

POSTOPERATIVE CARE AND ASSESSMENT

Electrolytes, especially potassium, should be monitored postoperatively. Analgesics should be provided as needed. Intravenous fluids are continued until the patient is drinking adequate amounts to maintain hydration. If prolonged vomiting or anorexia is anticipated, enteral hyperalimentation should be provided by means of a gastrostomy or enterostomy tube (see Chapter 11). With planning, feeding tubes can be placed during the initial surgery so as to avoid a second procedure. Food can be offered 12 hours postoperatively if there is no vomiting. ECGs should be monitored if arrhythmias were present before surgery or are anticipated postoperatively.

COMPLICATIONS

Complications associated with gastric surgery may include vomiting, anorexia, peritonitis secondary to intraoperative or postoperative leakage, ulceration at anastomotic sites, gastric outlet obstruction, and pancreatitis.

SPECIAL AGE CONSIDERATIONS

Young animals and those that are severely emaciated and have little or no body reserve should not have food withheld for longer than 4 to 6 hours before surgery and should be fed as soon as they are fully recovered from the anesthetic. If they cannot be fed, blood glucose concentrations should be monitored and, if necessary, maintained by adding glucose to the intravenous fluids (see the discussion of anesthesia on p. 409) Polydioxanone suture has been reported to cause calcinosis circumscripta in young dogs. Because the skin of puppies and kittens is delicate and elastic, skin sutures should be placed loosely. Geriatric animals may have delayed wound healing and may be immunosuppressed as a result of concurrent disease (e.g., diabetes mellitus and Cushing's disease). Strong absorbable or nonabsorbable suture material should be used in these patients and prophylactic antibiotic therapy should be initiated at induction of anesthesia.

References

Eggertsdottir AV, Stigen O, Lonaas L et al: Comparison of the recurrence rate of gastric dilation with or without volvulus in dogs after circumcostal gastropexy versus gastrocolopexy, *Vet Surg* 30P:546, 2001.

Rawlings CA, Foutz TL, Mahaffey MB et al: A rapid and strong laparoscopic-assisted gastropexy in dogs, *Am J Vet Res* 62:871, 2001.

Steelman-Szymeczek SM, Stebbins ME, Hardie EM: Clinical evaluation of a right-sided prophylactic gastropexy via a grid approach, *J Am Anim Hosp Assoc* 39:397, 2003.

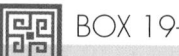 BOX 19-29

Important Considerations for Gastric Foreign Bodies

- Initial clinical signs may not alert the owner to seriousness of condition.
- Linear foreign objects must be resolved as soon as possible to prevent intestinal perforation and peritonitis.
- Not all animals with gastric foreign objects vomit.
- Finding a foreign object in the stomach does not mean that it is always the cause of vomiting.
- Linear foreign bodies are more common in cats; always check under the tongue (this often requires sedation).
- Most gastric foreign objects can be removed endoscopically.
- Complete exploration of the entire intestinal tract is mandatory.
- Always repeat the radiographs immediately before surgery to make sure that the object has not moved.

SPECIFIC DISEASES

GASTRIC FOREIGN BODIES

DEFINITIONS

A **gastric foreign body** is anything ingested by an animal that cannot be digested (e.g., rocks and plastic) or that is slowly digested (bones). **Linear foreign bodies** usually are pieces of string, yarn, thread, cloth, or dental floss.

GENERAL CONSIDERATIONS AND CLINICALLY RELEVANT PATHOPHYSIOLOGY

Gastric foreign bodies usually cause vomiting as a result of outflow obstruction, gastric distention, and/or mucosal irritation (Box 19-29). Occasionally, however, gastric foreign bodies are asymptomatic, incidental findings on abdominal radiographs. Dogs are indiscriminate eaters and often ingest rocks, plastic toys, cooking bags, and other objects. Cats more commonly ingest linear material (e.g., yarn or sewing thread attached to a needle). In cats, linear foreign bodies frequently are anchored under the tongue or at the pylorus and often cause intestinal plication (Fig. 19-74). Noxious stimuli or distention of the duodenum or pyloric antrum stimulates vomiting, whereas similar stimulation of the gastric body often does not. Therefore vomiting often is intermittent, occurring when the object is forced into the pyloric antrum.

Foreign bodies may occur in the stomach and small intestine concurrently, therefore the entire intestinal tract should be explored thoroughly whenever surgery is done to remove a gastric foreign body. If endoscopic removal is selected, examine the small intestine as far as possible and consider radiographing the patient before waking it up; the gas that has been insufflated will act as a negative contrast. Small, blunt foreign bodies may pass through the digestive system without causing harm; however, most should be removed when

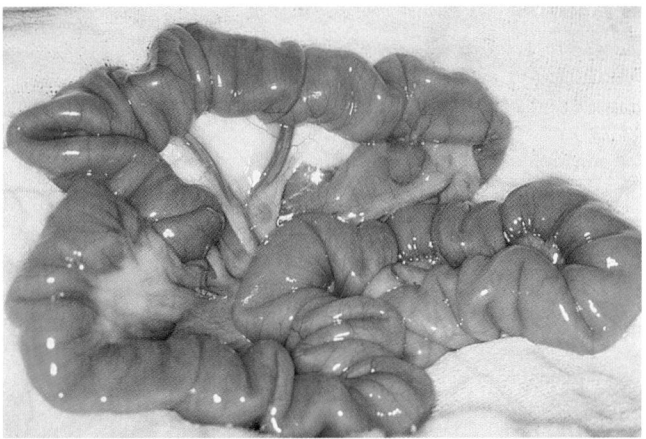

FIG. 19-74
Plication in the intestines of a cat caused by a string foreign body. (Courtesy Dr. J. Hauptman, Michigan State University.)

they are diagnosed because of the risk of obstruction and perforation. Repeat radiographs are indicated immediately before surgery, even if only a few hours have elapsed since the initial radiographs, because the object may exit the stomach and be located in either the small intestine or the colon. Foreign objects in the colon usually are eliminated without difficulty unless they have sharp edges that catch in the anus. There is seldom justification in surgically opening the colon; if a colonic foreign body must be removed, endoscopy is the preferred technique.

DIAGNOSIS
Clinical Presentation

Signalment. Young animals more commonly ingest foreign bodies than do older animals, and gastric or intestinal foreign bodies should be suspected in any puppy or kitten brought in for treatment of acute or persistent vomiting.

History. Most animals with gastric foreign bodies have vomiting, anorexia, and/or depression. Vomiting may be intermittent, and some animals may continue to eat and remain active. Vomiting often is absent if the foreign body is in the gastric fundus and does not obstruct the pylorus. Occasionally, abdominal pain is noted.

Physical Examination Findings

Physical examination often is unremarkable. The patient may be dehydrated; however, many animals with gastric foreign bodies continue to drink water. The object usually cannot be palpated because of the stomach's proximal location in the abdomen. Plicated intestines may be felt if a linear foreign object is present, and pain may be evident if gastric perforation has caused peritonitis or if the intestines are bunched together. A thorough examination of the mouth, especially the area ventral to the tongue, is mandatory in all cats suspected of having a linear foreign object. General anesthetic or sedation may be necessary to properly evaluate the base of the tongue.

> NOTE: Do not forget to check under the tongue in cats that may have a linear foreign object.

Diagnostic Imaging

Radiopaque foreign bodies may be diagnosed with survey radiographs, but many foreign bodies are relatively radiolucent. Some radiolucent foreign bodies can be identified ultrasonographically if the stomach is fluid filled and an appropriate acoustic window is obtained. A positive contrast gastrogram or double-contrast gastrogram can be used to delineate radiolucent foreign bodies, although in many tertiary care facilities, these studies have been replaced with endoscopy. If contrast studies are performed, it should be remembered that barium sulfate should not be used if gastrointestinal perforation is suspected (i.e., pneumoperitoneum and abdominal effusion); an iodinated, water-soluble contrast agent should be used in such cases. However, any effusion should be cytologically examined; evidence of sepsis is adequate to recommend surgery, and contrast radiographs are unnecessary. Likewise, spontaneous pneumoperitoneum is automatically assumed to indicate perforation and justifies exploratory surgery. Double-contrast studies using both air and a positive contrast agent (i.e., barium sulfate) are more sensitive than positive contrast procedures, but are more difficult to perform. Contrast procedures are especially useful if the foreign object absorbs or is coated by the contrast material. Radiographic findings in cats with linear foreign bodies include plication of the small bowel, increased intraluminal gas bubbles, and peritonitis secondary to bowel perforation (see p. 331).

Currently, radiographic contrast procedures are seldom performed to look for foreign objects. Gastroduodenoscopy is more sensitive than radiographs in finding foreign objects (unless the stomach is filled with food), and it offers the chance to remove it at the same time. In addition, one can find other gastric lesions and take a biopsy from them (see Chapter 14).

> NOTE: Do not do an upper gastrointestinal (GI) series using barium sulfate if you will perform endoscopy within 24 hours and do not use barium sulfate if perforation is likely.

Gastroduodenoscopy. Once the foreign body is located, the endoscopist should first examine and study it to determine the best retrieval device to use, and whether any special equipment (e.g., an overtube) is needed. If there are sharp edges or points, then consideration must be given to which end of the foreign body will be grasped. Endoscopic removal of linear foreign bodies should probably only be attempted when the linear foreign body has only been present for a relatively short time (e.g., less than 3 to 4 days) and the orad-most aspect is lodged at the pylorus. One may try to gently pull the foreign object out of the pylorus, but if it does not readily come out, this tack must be quickly abandoned. A better technique is as follows:

Insert the endoscope between the foreign object and the pylorus, and then advance the tip of the endoscope to as close to the end of the foreign object as possible. This can be tedious, so be patient. Then grasp the linear foreign object as close to the distal end as possible, and retrieve the foreign object by pulling the distal end out first. Take a plain abdominal radiograph afterwards to check for spontaneous pneumoperitoneum, a sign of perforation.

In rare cases, when the orad end of the linear foreign object is lodged at the pylorus, one may use the endoscope to push the orad end into the duodenum, thus relieving the point of fixation. This approach is similar to cutting a linear foreign body off the base of the tongue and seeing if it will then pass without incident. This may allow the entire foreign object to pass in the feces. In these cases, if the patient does not feel better within 9 to 12 hours, surgery is indicated to remove the foreign object.

Laboratory Findings

The laboratory findings depend on the severity and duration of the obstruction; they cannot be predicted. Laboratory parameters may be normal or may show only changes caused by dehydration (hemoconcentrations, increased serum albumin, and prerenal azotemia). If vomiting causes loss of gastric secretions, a hypochloremic, hypokalemic metabolic alkalosis with paradoxical aciduria may occur. Sometimes a metabolic acidosis occurs because of dehydration and subsequent lactic acidosis. A recent study found no difference in the electrolyte or acid-base derangements of dogs in regard to where their foreign body was located (Boag et al, 2005). Both proximal and distal gastrointestinal foreign bodies were associated with hypochloremic, hypokalemic metabolic acidosis.

DIFFERENTIAL DIAGNOSIS

Gastric neoplasms sometimes cause filling defects in the gastric lumen that could be confused with a foreign object. However, such lesions should remain in the same location when the animal is positioned for different radiographic views. Radiographs and endoscopy distinguish animals with gastric foreign objects from those with other causes of pyloric obstruction (e.g., chronic antral mucosal hypertrophy or pyloric stenosis; see p. 433) or gastric ulceration (see p. 436).

MEDICAL MANAGEMENT

If the object is small with rounded edges or is cloth, one can attempt to expel it by inducing vomiting with apomorphine (dogs) or xylazine (cats) (Box 19-30). However, this should be attempted only when the clinician is certain the object will be expelled without causing harm. Factors that must be considered include whether the esophagus is apt to be lacerated, the likelihood of the object lodging in the esophagus, and whether the object or gastric contents might be aspirated. Esophageal surgery carries more risk than gastric surgery because the esophagus does not heal as readily as the

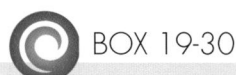 BOX 19-30

Induction of Vomition

Dogs
Apomorphine
0.02–0.04 mg/kg IV or IM; 0.1 mg/kg SC
Cats
Xylazine (Rompun)
0.05 mg/kg IV, IM or SC

IV, Intravenous; *IM,* intramuscular; *SC,* subcutaneous.

stomach (see p. 383). Indiscriminate use of antibiotics may mask clinical signs of peritonitis or pyothorax and delay treatment.

SURGICAL TREATMENT
Preoperative Management

If possible, metabolic and acid-base abnormalities should be identified and corrected, and food should be withheld for 12 hours. Radiographs should be taken immediately before surgery (especially before endoscopy) to verify the position of the object in the digestive tract. Perioperative antibiotics may be given at induction of anesthesia and continued for up to 12 hours postoperatively (see p. 410).

Anesthesia

See p. 409 for suggested anesthetic protocols in dogs with gastric disorders.

Surgical Anatomy

See p. 410 for the surgical anatomy of the stomach.

Positioning

The animal is placed in dorsal recumbency, and the abdomen is prepared for a ventral midline incision. The prepped area should extend from midthorax to the pubis to allow the entire digestive system to be explored for foreign objects.

SURGICAL TECHNIQUE

Most gastric foreign bodies can be easily removed via a gastrotomy incision (see p. 411).

Inspect the entire digestive system for material that could cause obstruction or perforation. If a linear foreign body is found in the pylorus and extends into the intestinal tract, do not try to pull it into the stomach unless it moves easily. Instead, make several incisions into the stomach and intestines to prevent causing further damage to the intestinal tract. Inspect the stomach for perforation or necrosis and, depending on the location, remove or patch abnormal tissue (see p. 457 for a description of a serosal patch). Close the gastric incision as described on p. 411.

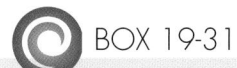 BOX 19-31

Treatment of Vomiting

Prochlorperazine (Compazine)
0.1–0.5 mg/kg IM or SC, tid to qid

Metoclopramide (Reglan)
0.25–0.5 mg/kg PO, IV, or SC, qd to qid or 1–2 mg/kg/day via continuous IV infusion

Dolasetron (Anzemet)
0.6–1.0 mg/kg IV or SC, qd

Ondansetron (Zofran)
0.5–1.0 mg/kg IV or PO, qd to bid

IM, Intramuscular; *SC,* subcutaneous; *tid,* three times a day; *qid,* four times a day; *PO,* oral; *IV,* intravenous; *qd,* once a day; *bid,* twice a day.

SUTURE MATERIALS AND SPECIAL INSTRUMENTS

Absorbable suture material (2-0 or 3-0) should be used to close the gastrotomy incision (see p. 420). Instruments helpful in performing gastric surgery are listed on p. 421.

POSTOPERATIVE CARE AND ASSESSMENT

The patient's fluid status should be monitored and hydration maintained with intravenous fluids postoperatively until the animal is drinking. Electrolyte abnormalities should be corrected. Hypokalemia is likely if the animal has been vomiting, and especially if it was also anorexic. A bland diet should be fed starting 12 to 24 hours after surgery if the patient is not vomiting. If vomiting continues, centrally acting antiemetics such as prochlorperazine, metoclopramide, or dolasetron (Box 19-31) may be administered, and oral food and water should be withheld. See p. 438 for treatment of ulcers that may occur secondary to foreign bodies.

PROGNOSIS

The prognosis is good if the stomach has not been perforated and the foreign body is removed. If perforation has occurred, the prognosis is guarded (see the discussion on peritonitis on p. 329).

Reference

Boag AK, Coe RJ, Martinez TA et al: Acid-base and electrolyte abnormalities in dogs with gastrointestinal foreign bodies, *J Vet Intern Med* 19:816, 2005.

Suggested Reading

Horstman CL, Eubig PA, Cornell KK et al: Gastric outflow obstruction after ingestion of wood glue in a dog, *J Am Anim Hosp* 39:47, 2003.
This is a description of a dog that had a large mass of solidified glue that essentially made a mold of the gastric lumen. It had to be removed surgically.

Hunt G, Worth A, Marchevsky A: Migration of wooden skewer foreign bodies from the gastrointestinal tract in eight dogs, *J Small Anim Pract* 45:362, 2004.

Radiographs found two of the foreign objects. Five had draining tracts, two had inflammatory disease in a body cavity, one had pneumothorax.

Kao LS, Nguye T, Dominitz J et al: Modification of a latex glove for the safe endoscopic removal of a sharp gastric foreign body, *Gastrointest Endoscop* 52:127, 2000.
This short report describes how to make a "hood" out of a rubber glove to protect the stomach and intestines when removing a sharp foreign object.

GASTRIC DILATATION-VOLVULUS

DEFINITIONS

Enlargement of the stomach associated with rotation on its mesenteric axis is referred to as **gastric dilatation-volvulus** (**GDV**). The term **simple dilatation** refers to a stomach that is engorged with air or froth but not malpositioned. **Dilatation** refers to a condition in which an organ or structure is stretched beyond its normal dimensions; **dilation** is the act of stretching a cavity or orifice. GDV is also called *gastric torsion or bloat.*

GENERAL CONSIDERATIONS AND CLINICALLY RELEVANT PATHOPHYSIOLOGY

Classically, GDV syndrome is an acute condition with a mortality rate of 20% to 45% in treated animals. The gastric enlargement is thought to be associated with a functional or mechanical gastric outflow obstruction. The initiating cause of the outflow obstruction is unknown; however, once the stomach dilates, normal physiologic means of removing air (i.e., eructation, vomiting, and pyloric emptying) are hindered because the esophageal and pyloric portals are obstructed.

The stomach becomes enlarged as gas or fluid or both accumulate in the lumen. The gas probably comes from aerophagia, although bacterial fermentation of carbohydrates, diffusion from the bloodstream, and metabolic reactions may contribute. Normal gastric secretion and transudation of fluids into the gastric lumen secondary to venous congestion contribute to fluid accumulation. The cause of GDV is unknown, but exercise after ingestion of large meals of highly processed food or water has been suggested to contribute to it. Epidemiologic studies have not supported a causal relationship between feeding soy-based or cereal-based dry dog food and GDV. However, Irish setters fed a single feed type appear to have an increased risk of GDV compared with those fed a mixture of feed types. Likewise, adding table food or canned food to the diet of large and giant breed dogs is associated with a decreased incidence of GDV. A recent study suggested that dogs fed a larger volume of food per meal were at significantly increased risk of GDV, regardless of the number of meals fed daily (Raghavan et al, 2004). In the aforementioned study, the risk of GDV was highest for dogs fed a larger volume of food once daily. Feeding dry dog foods in which one of the first four ingredients is oil or fat may also increase the risk of GDV (Raghavan et al, 2006). Other contributing causes

BOX 19-32

Recommendations for Clients

- Feed several small meals a day rather than one large meal.
- Avoid stress during feeding (if necessary, separate dogs in multiple-dog households during feeding).
- Restrict exercise before and after meals (of questionable benefit).
- Do not use an elevated feed bowl.
- Do not breed dogs with a first-degree relative that has a history of GDV.
- For high-risk dogs, consider prophylactic gastropexy.
- Seek veterinary care as soon as signs of bloat are noted.

include an anatomic predisposition, ileus, trauma, primary gastric motility disorders, vomiting, and stress. Recommendations for clients with animals at high risk are provided in Box 19-32. Male gender, increasing age, being underweight, being fed a large volume of food per meal, eating one meal (especially a large volume meal) per day, eating rapidly, having a raised feeding bowl, and having a fearful temperament are predisposing factors that may significantly increase a dog's risk of GDV (Glickman et al, 2000; Raghavan et al, 2004). Having a deeper and narrower thorax may change the anatomic relationship between the stomach and esophagus such that the dog's ability to eructate is impaired. Feeding dogs from a raised feed bowl may increase the risk of GDV because it may promote aerophagia. Finally, military working dogs were found to be more likely to develop GDV in November, December, and January, but the reasons for this were uncertain (Herbold et al, 2002).

> NOTE: Having a first-degree relative with a history of GDV is significantly associated with an increased risk of GDV (Glickman et al, 2000). Recommend that dogs with a first-degree relative that has had GDV not be used for breeding.

Generally, with GDV the stomach rotates in a clockwise direction when viewed from the surgeon's perspective (with the dog on its back and the clinician standing at the dog's side, facing cranially; Fig. 19-75). The rotation may be 90 to 360 degrees, but usually is 220 to 270 degrees. The duodenum and pylorus move ventrally and to the left of the midline and become displaced between the esophagus and stomach. The spleen usually is displaced to the right ventral side of the abdomen.

Caudal vena cava and portal vein compression by the distended stomach reduces venous return and cardiac output, causing myocardial ischemia. Central venous pressure, stroke volume, mean arterial pressures, and cardiac output are reduced. Obstructive shock and inadequate tissue perfusion affect multiple organs, including the kid-

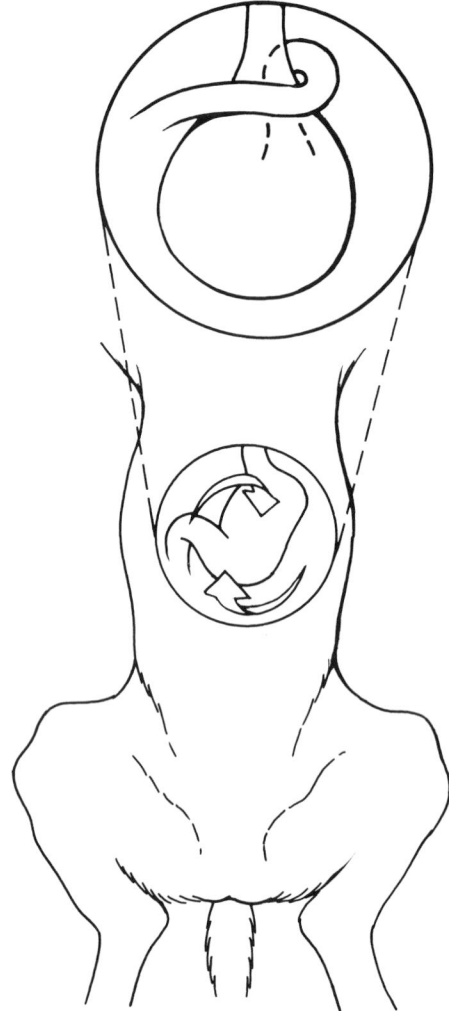

FIG. 19-75
Direction of gastric rotation in most dogs with GDV.

neys, heart, pancreas, stomach, and small intestine. Cardiac arrhythmias occur in many dogs with GDV, particularly those with gastric necrosis. Arrhythmias may contribute to mortality and require appropriate monitoring and treatment (see discussion under Postoperative Care and Assessment on p. 432). Myocardial depressant factor has also been recognized in affected dogs, and cardiac damage is common as seen by increased serum concentrations of troponin (Schober et al, 2002). Reperfusion injury has been implicated as causing much of the tissue damage that ultimately results in death after correction of GDV. Lazaroids (e.g., U74389G), which are radical-quenching antioxidants that inhibit oxygen-derived free radical production and lipid peroxidation, appear to reduce reperfusion injury and may eventually increase survival rates; however, further studies are needed.

Partial or chronic GDV may occur in dogs and usually is a progressive but non–life-threatening syndrome that may be associated with vomiting, anorexia, and/or weight loss.

These dogs may have chronic, intermittent signs and appear normal between episodes. Gastric malpositioning may be intermittent or chronic but without dilatation. Plain or contrast radiographs are diagnostic, but repeat radiographs may be necessary if the stomach is intermittently malpositioned.

DIAGNOSIS
Clinical Presentation

Signalment. GDV primarily occurs in large, deep-chested breeds (i.e., Great Dane, Weimaraner, Saint Bernard, German shepherd, Irish and Gordon setters, and Doberman pinscher), but has been reported in cats and small-breed dogs. Shar-Peis may have an increased incidence compared with other medium-sized breeds. Basset hounds may have a higher risk of GDV, despite their relatively small size. GDV may occur in a dog of any age, but is most common in middle-aged or older animals. The thoracic depth to width ratio appears to be highly correlated with the risk of bloat.

History. A dog with GDV may have a history of a progressively distending and tympanic abdomen, or the owner may simply find the animal recumbent and depressed with a distended abdomen. The dog may appear to be in pain and may have an arched back. Nonproductive retching, hypersalivation, and restlessness are common.

Physical Examination Findings

Abdominal palpation often reveals various degrees of abdominal tympany or enlargement; however, it may be difficult to feel gastric distention in heavily muscled large-breed or very obese dogs. Splenomegaly occasionally is palpated. Clinical signs associated with shock may be present, including weak peripheral pulses, tachycardia, prolonged capillary refill time, pale mucous membranes, and/or dyspnea.

Diagnostic Imaging

Radiographs are necessary to differentiate simple dilatation from dilatation plus volvulus. Affected animals should be decompressed before radiographs are taken. Right lateral and dorsoventral radiographic views are preferred to facilitate filling the abnormally displaced pylorus with air so that it can be easily identified. The pylorus is normally located ventral to the fundus on the lateral view and on the right side of the abdomen on the dorsoventral view. On a right lateral view of a dog with GDV, the pylorus lies cranial to the body of the stomach and is separated from the rest of the stomach by soft tissue (reverse C sign or double bubble) (Fig. 19-76). On the dorsoventral view, the pylorus appears as a gas-filled structure to the left of midline (Fig. 19-77). Free abdominal air suggests gastric rupture, and air within the wall of the stomach indicates necrosis, both of which warrant immediate surgery.

NOTE: Caution! Positioning these animals for a ventrodorsal view may lead to aspiration. Remember that the right lateral and dorsoventral views are preferred when attempting to diagnose GDV.

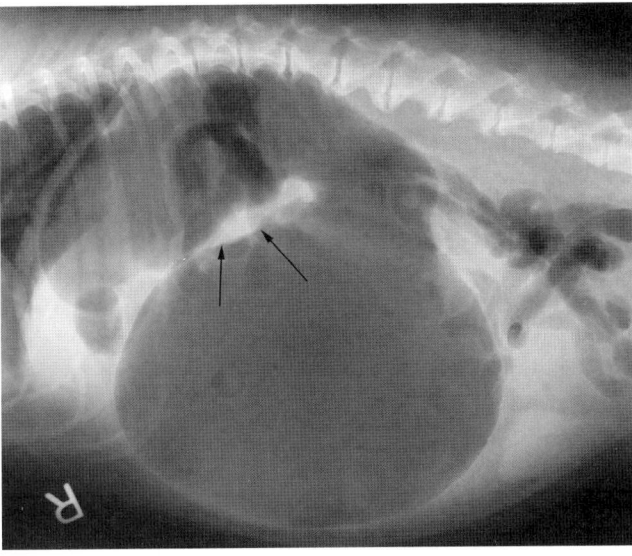

FIG. 19-76
Right lateral abdominal radiograph of a dog with GDV showing a distended, gas-filled stomach. Note the reverse C sign or double bubble caused by the shelf of soft tissue *(arrows)*. The pylorus is located dorsal to the shelf of tissue.

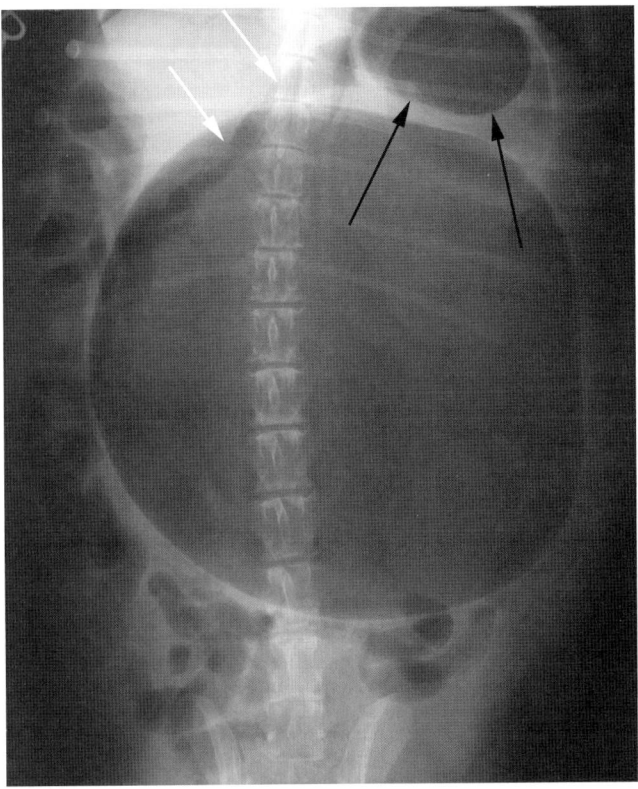

FIG. 19-77
Dorsoventral radiograph of a dog with GDV. The pylorus appears as a gas-filled structure to the left of the midline *(black arrows)*. Notice the duodenum coursing from the pylorus towards the right abdomen *(white arrows)*.

Laboratory Findings

The CBC is seldom helpful unless disseminated intravascular coagulation causes thrombocytopenia. Potassium concentration may be normal or elevated, but hypokalemia is more common. Vascular stasis may cause increased lactic acid and metabolic acidosis. However, metabolic alkalosis caused by sequestration of hydrogen ions in the gastric lumen can offset the metabolic acidosis, causing the blood pH to be normal (i.e., a mixed acid-base disorder). Respiratory acidosis may be caused by hypoventilation secondary to gastric impingement on the diaphragm and diminished ventilatory compliance. Therefore routine administration of sodium bicarbonate is inappropriate. Plasma lactate concentrations are prognostic, higher values being associated with gastric necrosis and a poor prognosis (de Papp et al, 1999).

DIFFERENTIAL DIAGNOSIS

Simple gastric dilatation occurs commonly in young puppies from overeating and seldom requires specific treatment. The stomach, although greatly enlarged with ingesta and gas, is not malpositioned. Small intestine volvulus is a differential diagnosis because it results in a tympanic and enlarged abdomen (see p. 476); however, dilatation of the intestinal tract is apparent on radiographs. Primary splenic torsion (see p. 629) often causes acute abdominal pain; however, abdominal distention is absent to mild. Diaphragmatic herniation may produce clinical signs similar to GDV, particularly if the stomach is herniated and outflow is obstructed (see p. 904). Ascites can cause abdominal distention, but a fluid wave should be felt during ballottement, which distinguishes it from the tympanic abdomen found in GDV.

> NOTE: You cannot differentiate GDV from gastric dilatation without volvulus simply because you are able to pass a stomach tube. Stomach tubes frequently can be passed in dogs with twisted stomachs.

MEDICAL MANAGEMENT

Stabilizing the patient's condition is the initial objective (Box 19-33). One or more large-bore intravenous catheters should be placed in either a jugular or both cephalic veins. Either isotonic fluids (90 ml/kg/hr), hypertonic 7% saline (4 to 5 ml/kg over 5 to 15 minutes), hetastarch (5 to 10 ml/kg over 10 to 15 minutes), or a mixture of 7.5% saline and hetastarch (dilute 23.4% saline with 6% hetastarch until you have a 7.5% solution; administer at 4 ml/kg over 5 minutes) is administered. If hypertonic saline or hetastarch is given, the rate of subsequent crystalloid administration must be adjusted. Blood should be drawn for blood gas analyses, a CBC, and a biochemical panel. Broad-spectrum antibiotics (e.g., cefazolin and ampicillin plus enrofloxacin) should be administered. If the animal is dyspneic, oxygen therapy may be given by nasal insufflation (see p. 27) or mask.

Gastric decompression should be performed while shock therapy is initiated. The stomach may be decom-

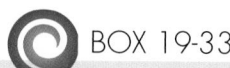 BOX 19-33

Medical Management of Gastric Dilatation-Volvulus

- Fluids (see text)
- Antibiotics such as cefazolin (22 mg/kg given intravenously [IV]) or a combination of enrofloxacin (Baytril), 7–15 mg/kg IV (give diluted and slowly, over 30 minutes) plus ampicillin at 22 mg/kg IV

pressed percutaneously with several large-bore intravenous catheters or a small trocar, or (preferably) a stomach tube may be passed. The stomach tube should be measured from the point of the nose to the xiphoid process and a piece of tape applied to the tube to mark the correct length. A roll of tape can be placed between the incisors and the tube passed through the center hole. Attempts should be made to pass the tube to the measured point. Placing the animal in different positions (i.e., sitting and reclining on a tilt table) may help if it is difficult to advance the tube into the stomach. Do not perforate the esophagus with overly rigorous attempts to pass the tube. If these attempts fail, percutaneous decompression of the stomach should be attempted. This may relieve pressure on the cardia and allow the tube to enter the stomach. Once the air has been removed, the stomach should be flushed with warm water. Failure to lavage the stomach usually results in rapid redilatation after the tube is withdrawn. If blood is seen in the fluid from the stomach, prompt surgical intervention is warranted because this may indicate gastric necrosis. If the stomach tube still cannot be passed and immediate surgical correction is not possible, temporary decompression may be achieved by performing a temporary gastrostomy (see p. 413). A Foley catheter should not be placed in the stomach percutaneously unless the stomach is simultaneously tacked to the body wall (see p. 417) because of the high risk of peritonitis if the stomach pulls away from the tube. The disadvantages of a temporary gastrostomy are that the stomach must be closed when the permanent gastropexy is performed, and there is a high risk of peritoneal contamination. However, a temporary gastrostomy maintains gastric decompression if the animal is being referred or if surgery is delayed. If immediate surgery is not possible in an animal in which a stomach tube was passed but that dilates rapidly after decompression, the stomach tube can be exteriorized through a pharyngostomy approach. This prevents the animal from chewing on the tube until definitive surgery can be performed. Radiographs may be taken after the patient has been decompressed and is stable.

SURGICAL TREATMENT

Surgery should be performed as soon as the animal's condition has been stabilized, even if the stomach has been decompressed. Rotation of an undistended stomach interferes with gastric blood flow and may potentiate gastric necrosis.

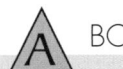

BOX 19-34

Selected Anesthetic Protocols for Dogs With Gastric Dilatation-Volvulus

Induction

Give hydromorphone (0.1 mg/kg given intravenously [IV]) plus diazepam (0.2 mg/kg IV). Give in incremental doses as necessary to intubate. If intubation is not possible, give etomidate (0.5–1.5 mg/kg IV) or thiopental or propofol (at reduced dosages) or (after diazepam and hydromorphone) use a combination of lidocaine and thiobarbiturates (see text).

Maintenance

Isoflurane or sevoflurane.

Preoperative Management

The animal should be given intravenous fluids and antibiotics before surgery (see discussion in Medical Management section). Significant electrolyte and acid-base abnormalities should be corrected. A greatly enlarged stomach may hinder respiration and make it difficult for the animal to ventilate during induction of anesthesia. An ECG should be monitored to detect cardiac arrhythmias, which should be treated with lidocaine before surgery if they are significant (i.e., long runs of ventricular tachycardia, which can decrease cardiac output).

Anesthesia

Numerous anesthetic protocols have been described for dogs with GDV. If the animal has been decompressed and its condition is stable without significant cardiac arrhythmias, then hydromorphone and diazepam may be given intravenously and the patient induced with etomidate, thiobarbiturates, or propofol (Box 19-34). If the animal is depressed, hydromorphone and diazepam alone or with etomidate may be used for induction. Etomidate is a good choice for induction if the animal's condition has not been well stabilized because it maintains cardiac output and is not arrhythmogenic. Lidocaine and thiobarbiturate may be used if arrhythmias are present; 9 mg/kg of each is drawn up, and half is given initially intravenously. Additional drug is given to effect to allow the dog to be intubated. Generally, no more than 6 mg/kg of lidocaine is given intravenously to prevent toxicity. If bradycardia occurs, anticholinergics (e.g., atropine or glycopyrrolate) may be given. Nitrous oxide should not be used in dogs with GDV (see p. 409). Isoflurane and sevoflurane are the inhalation agents of choice.

Surgical Anatomy

Normally, when viewed from the surgeon's perspective (i.e., with the animal in dorsal recumbency), the pylorus is located on the dog's right side, and the greater omentum arises from the greater curvature of the stomach and covers the intestines. The gastric (lesser curvature) and gastroepiploic (greater curvature) arteries supply the stomach and are derived from the celiac artery. The short gastric arteries arise from the splenic artery and supply the greater curvature. Rupture of the short gastric arteries in dogs with GDV is common and may contribute to blood loss and gastric infarction or necrosis. Eighty percent of the arterial flow is to the mucosa, and the remainder is to the muscularis and serosa; therefore observation of mucosal color is not a reliable indicator of gastric wall viability. The mucosa often appears darkened because of vascular compromise, even when full-thickness necrosis is not present.

Positioning

The dog is placed in dorsal recumbency, and the abdomen is prepared for a midline abdominal incision. The prepped area should extend from midthorax to the pubis. If a tube gastropexy is to be performed, the prepped area should be extended cranially and dorsally to allow the tube to be exteriorized behind the caudal right rib.

SURGICAL TECHNIQUE

The goals of surgical treatment are threefold: (1) to inspect the stomach and spleen so as to identify and remove damaged or necrotic tissue; (2) to decompress the stomach and correct any malpositioning; and (3) to adhere the stomach to the body wall to prevent subsequent malpositioning. Upon entering the abdominal cavity of a dog with GDV, the first structure noted is the greater omentum, which usually covers the dilated stomach.

Decompress the stomach before repositioning by using a large-bore needle (i.e., 14 or 16 gauge) attached to suction. If the needle becomes occluded with ingesta, have an assistant pass an orogastric stomach tube and perform gastric lavage.

Intraoperative manipulation of the cardia usually allows the tube to be passed into the stomach without difficulty. If adequate decompression is still not achieved or if an assistant is not available, a small gastrotomy incision can be performed to remove the gastric contents, although this should be avoided if possible.

For a clockwise rotation, once the stomach has been decompressed, rotate it counterclockwise by grasping the pylorus (usually found below the esophagus) with the right hand and the greater curvature with the left. Push the greater curvature, or fundus, of the stomach toward the table while simultaneously elevating the pylorus towards the incision. Check to make sure the spleen is normally positioned in the left abdominal quadrant. If there is splenic necrosis or significant infarction, perform a partial or complete splenectomy (see pp. 626-628). Remove or invaginate (see p. 411) necrotic gastric tissues. Avoid entering the gastric lumen if possible. If you are uncertain whether gastric tissue will remain viable, invaginate the abnormal tissue (see p. 412). Verify that the gastrosplenic ligament is not torsed, and before closure, palpate the intraabdominal esophagus to ensure that the stomach is derotated.

Perform a permanent gastropexy (see pp. 416-420). Gastropexy usually is curative for dogs with partial or chronic GDV.

> NOTE: To prevent recurrence of GDV, the stomach must be permanently adhered to the body wall. However, gastropexy does not guarantee that dilatation or volvulus will not recur; it simply makes it less likely (Eggertsdottir et al, 2001). Gastropexy should always be performed in conjunction with abdominal exploration and derotation of the stomach.

SUTURE MATERIALS AND SPECIAL INSTRUMENTS

Absorbable (polydioxanone or polyglyconate) or nonabsorbable (polypropylene) suture material may be used for the gastropexy (0 or 2-0). A Foley catheter is needed for a tube gastropexy. Balfour retractors, hand-held retractors (i.e., Army-Navy retractors or malleable retractors), and extra towel clamps (for placement on the rib when doing a circumcostal gastropexy) are helpful.

POSTOPERATIVE CARE AND ASSESSMENT

Electrolyte, fluid, and acid-basis status should be monitored closely postoperatively. Many dogs with GDV are hypokalemic postoperatively and require potassium supplementation (see Table 5-6 on p. 29). Small amounts of water and soft, low-fat food should be offered 12 to 24 hours after surgery and the patient observed for vomiting. Gastritis that occurs secondary to mucosal ischemia is common and may be associated with gastric hemorrhage or vomiting. If vomiting is severe or continuous, a centrally acting antiemetic may be given (see p. 427). Secondary gastric ulcers may occur and require treatment (see p. 436). H_2-receptor blockers (e.g., cimetidine, ranitidine, or famotidine; see Box 19-15) reduce gastric acidity and may be beneficial. Intravenous fluid therapy should be continued until the patient's oral fluid intake is adequate to maintain hydration. Patients should be monitored for hypoalbuminemia and anemia in the early postoperative period.

> NOTE: Lidocaine toxicity may be enhanced in patients given cimetidine concurrently.

Ventricular arrhythmias are common in dogs with GDV and usually begin 12 to 36 hours after surgery. Their cause is unknown, but myocardial depressant factor, reduced cardiac output, and myocardial ischemia may contribute. Treatment of cardiac arrhythmias includes maintenance of normal hydration and correction of electrolyte imbalances. Sometimes the arrhythmia can be corrected simply by correcting hypokalemia. Some antiarrhythmic drugs (i.e., lidocaine) are in-

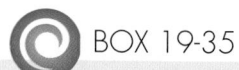

BOX 19-35

Antiarrhythmic Therapy in Dogs

Lidocaine (Xylocaine)

IV bolus (2 mg/kg increments up to total dose of 8 mg/kg) then IV drip at 50 µg/kg/minute (500 mg in 500 ml of fluid, administered at maintenance rate [66 ml/kg/day])

Procainamide (Pronestyl)

10–15 mg/kg slow IV bolus or 25–60 µg/kg/min as a continuous IV infusion or 15 mg/kg IM, PO, bid to qid

Sotalol (Betapace)

1–2 mg/kg PO, bid

IV, Intravenous; *IM,* intramuscular; *PO,* oral; *bid,* twice a day; *qid,* four times a day.
If seizures occur, you must stop the drug and consider using another antiarrhythmic agent.

effective when the animal is hypokalemic (see Table 5-6 on p. 29). If the arrhythmias interfere with cardiac output as noted by poor peripheral pulses; are multiform; have subsequent premature beats inscribed on the wave of the previous complex (R on T); or have a sustained ventricular rate above 160 beats per minute, they should be treated with intravenous drugs. A test bolus of lidocaine given intravenously (2 mg/kg bolus, up to 8 mg/kg total dose) can be used to determine responsiveness to this drug. If the arrhythmias diminish or stop, lidocaine should be given by a continuous intravenous infusion of 50 to 75 µg/kg/min (Box 19-35). Low doses should be used initially and increased only if necessary. Signs of lidocaine toxicity include muscle tremors, vomiting, and seizures; lidocaine therapy should be discontinued if these signs occur. Other possibly effective antiarrhythmic drugs are procainamide and sotalol. Procainamide may be given as an intravenous bolus, by continuous infusion, intramuscularly, or orally (see Box 19-35). Sotalol may be effective in animals that have not responded to lidocaine or procainamide.

COMPLICATIONS

Sepsis and peritonitis may be caused by gastric necrosis or perforation if devitalized tissue is not adequately removed. Diagnostic peritoneal lavage (see p. 335) may help diagnose peritonitis. Peritonitis requires immediate surgical intervention. Disseminated intravascular coagulation may occur in dogs with GDV or peritonitis. Assessment of clotting parameters and appropriate treatment with plasma, fluids, and heparin (see p. 625) may be necessary.

PROGNOSIS

With timely surgery the prognosis is fair; however, mortality rates of 45% and higher have been reported. Gastric dilatation without volvulus has a better prognosis than GDV. The prognosis is poor if gastric necrosis or perforation occurs or if surgery is delayed. Preoperative measurement of plasma lactate may be a good predictor of gastric necrosis and outcome for dogs with GDV (de Papp et al, 1999). Plasma lactate concentrations under 6 mmol/L suggest that gastric necrosis is not present, and thus a fair prognosis is warranted. In one study, dogs with gastric necrosis were 11 times more likely to die than those that did not have gastric necrosis (Glickman et al, 1998). Recurrence rates for GDV differ, depending on techniques used, but most have reported rates of less than 10%. Tube gastropexy has the highest reported recurrence rate, varying from 5% to 29%.

Some dogs with GDV respond to tube decompression and medical stabilization alone. Occasionally the stomach becomes normally positioned after the air is removed, or it was only partly rotated (less than 180 degrees) or merely dilated. However, these dogs still have a high likelihood of recurrence, and gastropexy should be recommended even when conservative management successfully alleviates the gastric malpositioning. The reported recurrence rates in dogs operated on for GDV in which the stomach was repositioned but gastropexy was not performed approaches 80%.

References

de Papp E, Drobatz KJ, Hughes D: Plasma lactate concentration as a predictor of gastric necrosis and survival among dogs with gastric dilatation-volvulus: 102 cases (1995-1998), *J Am Vet Med Assoc* 215:49, 1999.

Eggertsdottir AV, Stigen O, Lonaas L et al: Comparison of the recurrence rate of gastric dilatation with or without volvulus in dogs after circumcostal gastropexy versus gastrocolopexy, *Vet Surg* 30:546, 2001.

Elwood CM: Risk factors for gastric dilatation in Irish setter dogs, *J Small Anim Pract* 39:185, 1998.

Glickman LT, Glickman NW, Shellenberg DB et al: Incidence of and breed-related risk factors for gastric dilatation-volvulus in dogs, *J Am Vet Med Assoc* 216:40, 2000.

Glickman LT et al: Nondietary risk factors for gastric dilatation-volvulus in large- and giant-breed dogs, *J Am Vet Med Assoc* 217:1492, 2000.

Glickman LT et al: A prospective study of survival and recurrence following the acute gastric dilatation-volvulus syndrome in 136 dogs, *J Am Vet Med Assoc* 34:253, 1998.

Herbold JR, Moore GE, Gosch TL et al: Relationship between incidence of gastric dilatation-volvulus and bimeterologic events in a population of military working dogs, *Am J Vet Res* 63:47, 2002.

Raghavan M, Glickman NW, Glickman LT: The effect of ingredients in dry dog foods on the risk of gastric dilatation-volvulus in dogs, *J Am Anim Hosp Assoc* 42:28, 2006.

Raghavan M, Glickman N, McCabe G et al: Diet-related risk factors for gastric dilatation-volvulus in dogs of high-risk breeds, *J Am Anim Hosp Assoc* 40:192, 2004.

Schober KE, Cornand C, Kirbach B et al: Serum cardiac troponin I and cardiac troponin T concentrations in dogs with gastric dilatation-volvulus, *J Am Vet Med Assoc* 221:381, 2002.

Suggested Reading

Steelman-Szymeczek SM, Stebins ME, Hardie EM: Clinical evaluation of a right-sided prophylactic gastropexy via a grid approach, *J Am Anim Hosp* 39:397, 2003.
This technique is less invasive than a ventral midline approach.

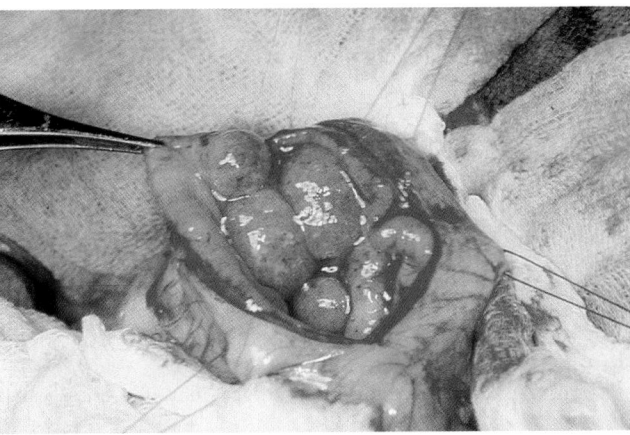

FIG. 19-78
Intraoperative photograph showing mucosal hypertrophy in a dog with chronic hypertrophic pyloric gastropathy.

Winkler KP, Greenfield CL, Schaeffer DJ: Bacteremia and bacterial translocation in the naturally occurring canine gastric dilatation-volvulus patient, *J Am Anim Hosp Assoc* 39:361, 2003.
The authors did not find evidence of bacterial translocation from the stomach, and survival was not influenced by the presence or absence of bacteria.

BENIGN GASTRIC OUTFLOW OBSTRUCTION

DEFINITIONS

Pyloric stenosis refers to benign muscular hypertrophy of the pylorus. **Chronic antral mucosal hypertrophy** refers to benign hypertrophy of the pyloric mucosa causing outflow obstruction (Fig. 19-78). **Chronic hypertrophic pyloric gastropathy (CHPG)** is a term that denotes pyloric hypertrophy without specifying whether the mucosa or the muscularis is involved. CHPG has been used specifically to refer to acquired mucosal hypertrophy by some authors and to either muscular (type I) or mucosal (types II and III) hypertrophy by others. **Polyps** are benign, adenomatous proliferations that can be single or multiple. Pyloric stenosis is also known as *benign antral muscular hypertrophy, congenital hypertrophic stenosis,* and *congenital pyloric muscle hypertrophy.* Chronic antral mucosal hypertrophy is also called *pyloric* or *gastric mucosal hypertrophy, chronic hypertrophic gastritis, multiple polyps of the gastric mucosa,* and *acquired hypertrophy.*

GENERAL CONSIDERATIONS AND CLINICALLY RELEVANT PATHOPHYSIOLOGY

Gastric outlet obstruction may be caused by pyloric abnormalities, disorders of gastric motility, or extrinsic lesions compressing the outflow tract (e.g., pancreatic, duodenal, or hepatic neoplasia; Box 19-36). Hypertrophy of the pyloric mucosa or muscle may be isolated or may occur in conjunction with other abnormalities. A syndrome of polycystic kidneys, hepatic disease, polyneuropathy, and hypertrophic gastropathy has been described in the Drentse patrijshond

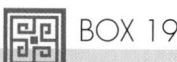

BOX 19-36

Important Considerations for Gastric Outlet Obstruction

- Not all older patients with proliferative masses causing outlet obstruction have malignancies.
- Not all obstructed patients have hypokalemic, hypochloremic, metabolic alkalosis.
- Not all animals with hypokalemic, hypochloremic, metabolic alkalosis have gastric outlet obstruction.
- Benign gastric outflow obstruction usually has a good prognosis with appropriate therapy.
- Gastroduodenoscopy is usually more appropriate than contrast radiographs; with endoscopy you can take a biopsy and often determine if malignancy is present and remove foreign objects.

breed. Hyperplastic pyloric polyps have been reported in French bulldogs with a history of chronic vomiting since weaning.

The cause of pyloric stenosis is unknown, but excessive production of gastrin has been suggested. Gastrin is the major regulator of gastric acid secretion and is trophic for gastric smooth muscle and mucosa. Congenital pyloric stenosis has been produced in puppies by administering gastrin to pregnant bitches. Neurogenic dysfunction may also play a role. Acute stress, inflammatory disease, or trauma might stimulate the sympathetic nervous system, reducing gastric motility and causing retention. Prolonged gastric distention may then lead to increased gastrin secretion and subsequent hypertrophy.

DIAGNOSIS
Clinical Presentation

Signalment. In dogs, pyloric stenosis is most commonly seen in brachycephalic breeds (i.e., boxers, bulldogs, and Boston terriers). Siamese cats have also been reported with this condition. Affected cats may have both vomiting (caused by gastric outlet obstruction) and regurgitation (caused by secondary esophagitis and esophageal dysfunction). Chronic antral mucosal hypertrophy occurs most commonly in small-breed dogs (less than 10 kg), particularly Lhasa apso, Shih Tzu, and Maltese breeds. Some dogs reported with chronic antral mucosal hypertrophy have been considered particularly excitable or vicious. Males may be more commonly affected than females. Pyloric stenosis is more common in young animals, although animals of any age may be affected. Chronic antral mucosal hypertrophy is more common in middle-aged or older dogs and may mimic neoplasia.

History. The clinical signs are caused by obstruction of gastric outflow. Vomiting is the most common sign, and may be intermittent or delayed hours after feeding or both. Cats commonly have regurgitation and vomiting. Liquids often pass through the pylorus, therefore severe dehydration is uncommon, and vomiting may occur for months to years before diagnosis. Animals with congenital pyloric stenosis often begin vomiting when they start eating solid food. The

frequency of vomiting varies from several times daily to once or twice a week.

Physical Examination Findings

The physical examination findings generally are nonspecific. They may include weight loss, anorexia, depression, and/or dehydration. Abdominal pain is rare. Aspiration pneumonia or reflux esophagitis (or both) may occur secondary to chronic vomiting.

Diagnostic Imaging

Survey abdominal radiographs and ultrasound may reveal gastric distention (usually filled with fluid) and are useful for eliminating extrinsic causes of pyloric obstruction. Ultrasonography usually reveals pyloric wall thickening, and it may detect extrinsic lesions (e.g., abscesses or neoplasms) that may obstruct gastric outflow and neoplastic metastases. Contrast radiographs may show delayed emptying, pyloric wall thickening, and/or a filling defect in the pylorus. However, normal elimination of liquid barium does not rule out gastric outflow obstruction, and it can be difficult to accurately interpret studies when barium is mixed with food. In general, contrast radiographs are infrequently used to detect gastric outflow obstruction because endoscopy is probably more sensitive and also allows a biopsy of any lesions that are found. Radiographs and ultrasound cannot accurately distinguish inflammation, hypertrophy, or neoplasia whereas endoscopy usually can distinguish between them, thereby avoiding unnecessary surgery.

> **NOTE:** Neoplastic pyloric disease and benign disease causing hypertrophy are often difficult to distinguish visually; a biopsy is imperative.

Laboratory Findings

The hematologic and biochemical changes in animals with benign gastric outlet obstruction usually are nonspecific. If vomiting has caused loss of gastric secretions, a hypochloremic, hypokalemic metabolic alkalosis may be present. Prerenal azotemia may occur, and mild hypoalbuminemia sometimes is seen in young dogs that are severely emaciated.

DIFFERENTIAL DIAGNOSIS

Any condition that causes vomiting is a differential diagnosis. Gastrointestinal foreign bodies, pythiosis, inflammation, neoplasia, and ulceration may cause gastric outlet obstruction. Other causes of vomiting that should be eliminated before surgery are uremia, hypoadrenocorticism, hypercalcemia, diabetic ketoacidosis, hepatic insufficiency, peritonitis, pancreatitis, feline hyperthyroidism, early right-sided heart failure in cats, gastritis, and inflammatory bowel disease.

MEDICAL MANAGEMENT

Dehydration, electrolyte, and acid-base abnormalities should be corrected before surgery or endoscopy (see p. 409). H_2-receptor blockers (i.e., cimetidine, ranitidine, and famoti-

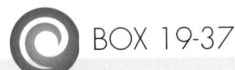

dine) or omeprazole may be used to treat esophagitis caused by frequent exposure of the esophagus to gastric acid (Box 19-37). Antibiotics may be indicated for esophagitis (see p. 373), ulceration (see p. 438), or aspiration (see p. 374). Gastric prokinetics (e.g., metoclopramide and cisapride) should not be used if outflow obstruction is suspected.

SURGICAL TREATMENT

Surgery is recommended for benign pyloric obstruction. The goal is to remove the obstruction and reestablish normal gastric emptying. A full-thickness biopsy should be submitted to ensure that the thickening is benign (Fig. 19-79). Benign polyps should be removed if they are obstructing gastric outflow or if they are bleeding.

Preoperative Management

Food should be withheld for 24 hours before surgery. Presurgical endoscopy can define the extent of the lesion and usually confirm its benign or malignant nature by histologic or cytologic examination. Intravenous prophylactic antibiotics (e.g., cefazolin; 22 mg/kg given intravenously at induction; repeat once or twice at 2- to 4-hour intervals) may be given at induction of anesthesia if antibiotic therapy has not already been initiated, but this is not essential.

Anesthesia

See p. 409 for suggested anesthetics to use in animals with gastric disorders.

Surgical Anatomy

See p. 410 for the surgical anatomy of the stomach.

Positioning

The animal is placed in dorsal recumbency, and the abdomen is prepared for a ventral midline incision. The prepped area should extend from midthorax to near the pubis.

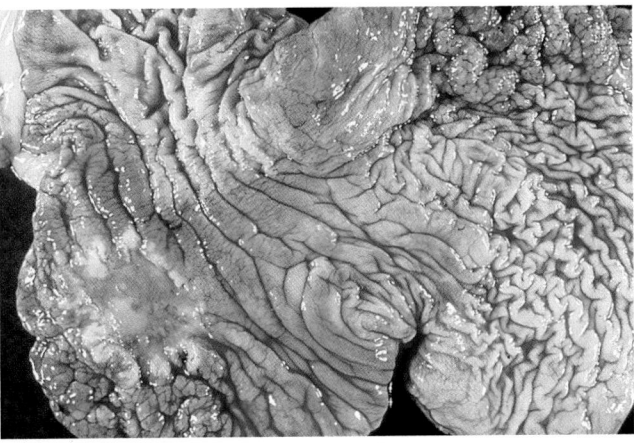

FIG. 19-79
Gastric ulceration associated with a gastric carcinoma.

ENDOSCOPIC REMOVAL OF POLYPS

Polyps with a narrow stalk can be removed by using an electrocautery snare. The area should be free of fluids and debris.

Carefully place the snare around the base of the polyp, and then pull tight. Do not touch the metallic part of the snare on other aspects of the stomach, and hold the polyp up such that it is not bent over and touching gastric mucosa. Keep the tip of the snare several centimeters away from the tip of the endoscope lest the current go back up the endoscope and damage the videoprocessor. Apply a mixed coagulation and/or cutting setting while gradually tightening the snare around the base of the polyp. Start at lower settings and gradually increase the current as necessary. If excessive current is applied, a severe electrical burn may occur that can cause anorexia and vomiting. Perform the process slowly to be sure that the vascular supply to the polyp is coagulated and will not cause hemorrhage.

This procedure should generally only be done by individuals trained in using endoscopic electrocautery. After the mass is cut off, it can be retrieved for histopathology.

SURGICAL TECHNIQUE

Surgical procedures to correct outlet obstruction caused by mucosal and/or muscular hypertrophy include pyloroplasty and Billroth I procedures. Pyloromyotomy (see p. 415) is often ineffective and is not recommended. If muscular hypertrophy without significant mucosal hypertrophy is present, a Heineke-Mikulicz pyloroplasty (see p. 415) is easy to perform. However, mucosal exposure is limited, and it does not allow adequate resection of hypertrophied mucosa. When mucosal hypertrophy is present, a Y-U pyloroplasty (see p. 415) or Billroth I procedure (see p. 413) is preferred. A Y-U pyloroplasty allows hypertrophied mucosa to be removed and the outflow tract widened (see Fig. 19-65). A Billroth I procedure is more difficult and carries additional risk of dehiscence or leakage, but has been successfully performed in numerous dogs with benign outflow obstruction. A Billroth I procedure, rather than a pyloroplasty, should be considered when the mucosa or muscular layers are so thickened as to be inflexible.

For mucosal hypertrophy, perform a Y-U pyloroplasty as described on p. 415. Be sure to perform a full-thickness biopsy and to resect the hypertrophied mucosa. Approximate incised edges of the mucosa in a continuous pattern with 3-0 absorbable suture before closing the pyloroplasty.

SUTURE MATERIALS AND SPECIAL INSTRUMENTS

If the animal is severely hypoproteinemic or debilitated, wound healing may be delayed. Strong absorbable suture (2-0 or 3-0) should be used and chromic gut suture avoided.

POSTOPERATIVE CARE AND ASSESSMENT

Small amounts of water should be given the day after surgery and the patient observed for vomiting. If vomiting does not occur, small amounts of moist food can be given 24 hours postoperatively. Fluid therapy should be continued until the animal is eating and drinking normally. Electrolyte abnormalities should be monitored postoperatively and corrected as necessary.

PROGNOSIS

The prognosis with surgical correction of these conditions is good. In one study of 39 dogs available for long-term evaluation, 85% had good or excellent outcomes. A poor outcome generally is the result of technical failures (i.e., dehiscence or leakage) or of using an inappropriate surgical technique for the lesion.

GASTRIC ULCERATION AND EROSION

DEFINITIONS

An **ulcer** is a mucosal defect extending through the muscularis mucosae into the submucosa or deeper layers of the stomach, whereas an **erosion** does not penetrate the muscularis mucosae. **Gastrinomas** are gastrin-secreting tumors of the alimentary tract. **Zollinger-Ellison syndrome** is a condition in which gastroduodenal ulceration occurs as a result of hypersecretion of gastrin from a gastrinoma of the pancreas. The terms gastrinoma and Zollinger-Ellison syndrome are often used interchangeably; however, gastrinomas can be located anywhere in the alimentary tract, whereas Zollinger-Ellison syndrome refers specifically to a gastrin-secreting tumor in the pancreas.

GENERAL CONSIDERATIONS AND CLINICALLY RELEVANT PATHOPHYSIOLOGY

Gastric ulceration/erosion (GUE) in small animals often is iatrogenic (i.e., nonsteroidal antiinflammatory drugs [NSAIDs]) or occurs secondary to an underlying disease process (e.g., mast cell disease, shock, tumor, and hepatic failure) (Box 19-38). The most common sites for nonneo-

 BOX 19-38

Important Considerations for Gastroduodenal Ulcers and Erosions

- Initial clinical signs (e.g., anorexia, depression) may not alert owner to seriousness of disease.
- Not all animals with ulcers vomit, and those that vomit may not vomit blood.
- NSAIDs are a very common cause, yet without careful questioning the history may not reveal their use.
- Look for underlying causes; do not just treat symptomatically.
- Anytime a patient with severe hepatic disease suddenly worsens, consider gastroduodenal ulceration even if there is no vomiting.
- Perforation may occur unexpectedly and cause potentially fatal peritonitis (see p. 329).
- Any patient with a spontaneous pneumoabdomen or septic peritonitis should be presumed to have a perforated ulcer and should be treated accordingly, regardless of a lack of historical findings suggestive of ulceration.
- Surgical resection should be considered for ulcers resistant to medical therapy and those causing the patient to hemorrhage vigorously.
- Intraoperative endoscopy may be helpful in locating ulcers.

plastic gastric ulcers are in the non–acid-producing parts (i.e., fundus and pyloric antrum).

NSAIDs (e.g., aspirin, phenylbutazone, naproxen, flunixin meglumine, piroxicam, and ibuprofen) are common causes of GUE in dogs. Newer NSAIDs, primarily inhibiting COX-2 (e.g., carprofen, etodolac, deracoxib, and meloxicam), are regarded as safer than the more traditional NSAIDs that inhibit COX-1. However, while these newer NSAIDs are safer and have fewer gastric complications, they can still cause GUE, especially if used improperly. The mechanism of ulcer formation secondary to NSAIDs is probably multifactorial, but inhibition of prostaglandin synthesis is important. Prostaglandins exert a protective effect on the mucosal barrier by stimulating mucus and bicarbonate production. Prostaglandin agonists (e.g., misoprostol) may help prevent NSAID-induced lesions.

Corticosteroids (particularly dexamethasone) may be ulcerogenic in dogs, especially when used at very high dosages. Prednisone, when administered at appropriate dosages (2.2 mg/kg/day or less), infrequently causes GUE unless the dog is hypoxic (e.g., immune mediated hemolytic anemia) or hypoperfused. Chronic steroid administration may reduce gastric mucus production, diminish the ability of mucosal cells to replicate, and increase exfoliation of mucosal cells into the gastric lumen. Concurrent use of steroids and NSAIDs clearly increases the likelihood of GUE.

Gastric ulceration may be caused by neoplasia (see Fig. 19-79), either as a direct effect or by paraneoplastic mechanisms. Gastric adenocarcinoma and lymphoma are probably the most common gastric tumors, but leiomyomas are especially prone to ulcerate and bleed. Paraneoplastic ulceration caused by mast cell tumors (common) or gastrinomas (rare) primarily occurs in the duodenum, just past the pylorus. Gastroduodenal ulceration is a common complication of mast cell disease because histamine is a potent stimulator of gastric acid secretion. The cytoplasmic granules of mast cell tumors contain vasoactive amines (e.g., histamine and serotonin) and heparin. Histamine also causes vasodilatation of gastric vessels and alters endothelial permeability, which promotes intravascular thrombosis and gastric necrosis.

Gastrin, which normally is secreted by the antral G cells in response to vagal stimulation and gastric distention, is a potent stimulator of gastric acid secretion. Zollinger-Ellison syndrome is a condition in which hypersecretion of gastrin is associated with neoplasia of the non-β pancreatic islet cells. Severe duodenal ulceration is seen with this disease, and removal of the pancreatic mass may be necessary to alleviate clinical signs (see p. 599). Because of the aggressive biologic behavior of this malignant neoplasm, the prognosis for long-term cure is poor; however, aggressive medical management with omeprazole (0.7 to 1.5 mg/kg given orally once a day) may be helpful.

Acute and chronic liver disease may be associated with GUE, with or without bleeding. Chronic hepatic disease causes gastric mucosal injury through a variety of mechanisms, which are poorly understood. Thrombosis associated with disseminated intravascular coagulation may reduce gastric blood flow and enhance ulcer formation.

Circulatory shock causing poor gastric perfusion is one cause of "stress" GUE. Ulcers and erosions may also form secondary to septic shock, extreme exertion, and intervertebral disk disease (IVDD). Administration of high doses of corticosteroids to dogs with severe neurologic disease probably contributes to the high prevalence of GUE in these patients. Other contributing factors in dogs with IVDD include alterations in mucosal blood flow, sympathetic and parasympathetic stimulation of the bowel, and the stress of major surgery and prolonged hospitalization. Colonic perforation of dogs with neurologic disease is associated with a high rate of mortality. Other conditions associated with GUE in small animals include gastroduodenal reflux of bile, major surgery, uremia, pythiosis, recurrent pancreatitis, and maybe inflammatory bowel disease.

> NOTE: Use steroids with caution in patients with neurologic disease.

The stomach has an enormous ability to increase local blood flow, which helps remove caustic substances from the gastric lumen. In addition, the rapid rate of cell turnover in the gastric mucosa helps heal minor erosions in 1 to 2 days, providing the cause is removed. Other normal defenses that help prevent the formation of ulcers include those properties that interfere with absorption of hydrogen ions (i.e., phospholipid membranes and tight junctional complexes), neutralization of acid by bicarbonate (secreted by the oxyntic, pyloric, and duodenal mucosae), and a thick, alkaline mucus coating that traps and neutralizes hydrogen ions. For mucosal damage to occur, the gastric pH usually (but not always) must be lower than 3 to 5. Deep ulcers do not heal rapidly, and they heal by the formation of scar tissue rather than by reepithelialization.

DIAGNOSIS
Clinical Presentation

Signalment. GUE occurs more commonly in dogs than in cats. Most noniatrogenic gastric ulcers in dogs occur in middle-aged or older dogs. The disorder shows no breed predisposition.

History. Although vomiting is a common clinical sign of GUE, some dogs are brought in for anorexia or anemia (or both) without vomiting, and sometimes GUE is an unexpected finding in dogs without clinical signs of disease. Vomitus may contain digested blood, fresh blood, or blood clots. Digested blood looks like "coffee grounds." Owners may report that the stools of dogs with ulcers are black (melena) and that the dog has a poor appetite.

Physical Examination Findings

Most patients have no abnormalities on physical examination unless they are anemic from blood loss. Some have abdominal pain when palpated. Rectal examination sometimes reveals melena. However, most of the time what people describe as "dark feces" is normal feces that is dark brown or dark green. Melena is pitch black feces that, when put upon white, absorbent paper will be seen to have red color diffuse out from it. Melena is only seen when there has been substantial hemorrhage over a short period of time; most dogs with gastric bleeding do not have melena.

Diagnostic Imaging

Radiography and ultrasonography will not detect erosions. Positive contrast radiographs or ultrasonography may detect ulceration, but the sensitivity of these tests is relatively low. Gastroduodenoscopy is the most sensitive test for finding GUE. However, the entire mucosal surface must be examined. The patient should not have received Carafate or barium for at least 24 hours before endoscopy lest the lesions be obscured. If there has been gastrointestinal bleeding, one must be prepared to flush and aspirate repeatedly until the debris is removed and the mucosa can be examined. Ulcers just inside the pylorus are particularly hard to visualize.

Laboratory Findings

A hemogram and serum biochemical profile should be performed in animals in which GUE is suspected to assess the severity of blood and protein loss and to identify underlying potential causes (e.g., hepatic or renal failure). Animals with GUE may be anemic or hypoproteinemic or both. Platelet counts and clotting profiles should be performed when a coagulopathy is suspected. Electrolyte and acid-base abnormalities may occur if vomiting has been severe (e.g., hypochloremic, hypokalemic metabolic alkalosis or a metabolic acidosis). Gastrinomas (see p. 436) are uncommon, but if no other underlying cause is identified, serum gastrin levels can be measured.

DIFFERENTIAL DIAGNOSIS

Coagulopathies may mimic GUE. Gastric neoplasia and gastritis are best distinguished from other causes of GUE by endoscopic biopsy. Exploratory gastrotomy is required if full-thickness biopsies are necessary because the lesion is submucosal or scirrhotic, and the flexible endoscope is unable to tear off a diagnostic piece. Coagulopathies from ingestion of toxins, disseminated intravascular coagulation, or inherent clotting abnormalities occasionally cause gastric bleeding. Coagulation profiles should be performed if a coagulopathy is suspected.

MEDICAL MANAGEMENT

Therapy depends on whether an underlying cause can be found, the severity of the bleeding, the depth of the ulcer, the likelihood of perforation, and the animal's status. Medical treatment is typically recommended to control bleeding if perforation seems unlikely and if the cause of the bleeding is known or strongly suspected. Symptomatic therapy (i.e., fluids, antibiotics, blood, and antiemetics) must be combined with trying to identify and remove the initiating cause (e.g., discontinue NSAIDs, reestablish mucosal perfusion, remove mast cell tumors or gastrinomas, and treat hepatic disease). Gastric foreign bodies will inhibit GUE healing, even if they are not the initiating cause. Therefore they should be removed promptly to allow the ulcer or erosion to heal.

Drugs used to treat GUE include those that lessen gastric acidity and those that protect the gastric mucosa from damage (Box 19-39). Cimetidine, ranitidine, and famotidine are H_2-receptor blockers that reduce gastric acid secretion, a key step in treating GUE. Famotidine is the most potent and has the fewest side effects. Omeprazole and other proton pump inhibitors are more potent inhibitors of gastric acid secretion than the H_2-receptor blockers, but they take 2 to 5 days to achieve their maximal effect. Proton pump inhibitors are seldom required except for severe esophagitis and for gastrinoma or mast cell tumor–induced GUE. Antacids (e.g., magnesium hydroxide) stimulate endogenous prostaglandin release, neutralize acids, and bind bile salts. Because they are most effective if administered frequently (i.e., up to six times a day), they are less useful in dogs and cats than in human beings. Misoprostol is a prostaglandin analog that helps prevent ulceration in dogs receiving NSAIDs, and it can be used to cure gastric ulcers.

Sucralfate forms a protective coating over the ulcer or erosion. However, its major drug actions that contribute to ulcer healing are related to stimulation of mucosal defense and

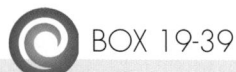 **BOX 19-39**

Medical Therapy of Animals With Gastric Ulceration

Sucralfate (Carafate)
0.5–1 g PO, tid to qid

Cimetidine (Tagamet)
5–10 mg/kg PO, IV, SC, tid to qid

Ranitidine (Zantac)
2.2 mg/kg PO, IV, IM, SC, bid to tid

Famotidine (Pepcid)
0.5–1.0 mg/kg PO, qd to bid

Omeprazole (Prilosec)
0.7–1.5 mg/kg PO, qd to bid

Misoprostol (Cytotec)
1–5 µg/kg PO, tid to qid

PO, Oral; *tid,* three times a day; *qid,* four times a day; *IV,* intravenous; *SC,* subcutaneous; *IM,* intramuscular; *bid,* twice a day; *qd,* once a day.

reparative mechanisms, and antipeptic effects, which are induced by both prostaglandin-dependent and prostaglandin-independent pathways. Sucralfate should be given 1 hour after administration of other oral medications because it may interfere with their absorption. Drugs that interact with sucralfate include fluoroquinolones, tetracycline, theophylline, aminophylline, and digoxin. The major disadvantage of sucralfate is that it must be administered orally, which can be problematic in vomiting animals.

ENDOSCOPIC TREATMENT

Endoscopic electrocautery may be used, usually to stop hemorrhage in emergency situations and allow surgery to occur at a more opportune time.

Once the bleeding lesion has been identified, advance an electrocautery probe with suction capability until the tip of the probe is in contact with the bleeding lesion. Keep the tip of the electrocautery probe several centimeters away from the tip of the endoscope. If there is fluid, blood, or debris, suction it away to allow for as dry a field as possible, and then apply a low coagulation current for 2 to 5 seconds. If that is not successful, aspirate the field again and use more current with a coagulation setting. Alternatively, grasp the bleeding site with electrocautery biopsy forceps and use them much like electrocautery applied to a hemostat. Again, keep the tip of the forceps away from the tip of the endoscope. Endoscopic electrocautery should only be done by individuals trained in its use, or damage to the scope and patient may occur. Alternatively, one may use sclerotherapy needles to inject alcohol or other such agents into bleeding lesions, but there are no reports of this being done in clinical veterinary medicine.

SURGICAL TREATMENT

Surgical resection of ulcers is indicated if medical therapy does not substantially alleviate clinical signs within 6 to 7 days, if bleeding is profuse and life threatening, or if perforation is believed imminent.

> NOTE: Gastric ulcers, even very deep ones, cannot be reliably detected from the serosal surface of the stomach. Preoperative (or intraoperative) endoscopy will allow accurate localization of all important gastric ulcers.

Preoperative Management

If possible, the animal's condition should be stabilized before surgery. Whole blood should be given if the animal is severely anemic (i.e., has a packed cell volume under 20%). If the animal has disseminated intravascular coagulation, one may administer plasma with or without heparin therapy. Electrolyte and acid-base abnormalities should be corrected and fluid therapy initiated.

Anesthesia

See p. 409 for anesthetic recommendations for animals undergoing gastric surgery.

Surgical Anatomy

See p. 410 for the surgical anatomy of the stomach.

Positioning

The dog is placed in dorsal recumbency, and the abdomen is prepared for a ventral midline incision. The prepped area should extend from midthorax to the pubis.

SURGICAL TECHNIQUE

If possible, remove the ulcer with a full-thickness gastric resection and submit tissue for histopathologic examination. Assess the regional lymph nodes and liver for evidence of metastatic neoplasia or pythiosis and take a biopsy from them if they appear abnormal. Check both limbs of the pancreas for masses.

Occasionally location of the ulcer near the pylorus makes full-thickness resection difficult.

If the ulcer is located at the pylorus and if perforation is present or imminent, perform a serosal patch (see p. 457) over the site to help prevent leakage and promote healing of the ulcer.

A serosal patch is simpler to perform than a pylorectomy and gastroduodenostomy (Billroth I; see p. 413). Occasionally an abscess will be noted where an ulcer has perforated and the omentum or other abdominal structures have walled off the site.

If this is the case, carefully drain the abscess and resect or patch the ulcer. Consider preoperative or intraoperative endoscopy to help locate ulcers that are difficult to discern from the serosal surface. If there is extensive disease secondary to a condition that may not resolve quickly (e.g., inflammatory bowel disease or hepatic failure), place an enterostomy feeding tube (see p. 107).

SUTURE MATERIALS AND SPECIAL INSTRUMENTS

If the animal is severely hypoproteinemic or anemic, wound healing may be delayed. Polydioxanone, polyglyconate, polyglycolic acid, or polyglactin 910 suture (2-0 or 3-0) is preferred to close the gastrotomy incision (see p. 420). Gut suture should be not be used for gastric surgery.

POSTOPERATIVE CARE AND ASSESSMENT

Small amounts of water should be given the day after surgery and the patient observed for vomiting. If vomiting does not occur, small amounts of food can be given 24 hours postoperatively. To aid gastric emptying, the diet should be low fat and contain moderate amounts of protein and carbohydrates. Moist diets usually are preferable to dry diets. Fluid therapy should be continued until the animal can maintain hydration with oral fluids.

PROGNOSIS

The prognosis depends on identification and treatment of underlying diseases and whether peritonitis is present. The prognosis is good if the ulcer is the result of treatable disease and if perforation has not occurred. If peritonitis is present, the prognosis is guarded (see the discussion of peritonitis on p. 329).

Suggested Reading

Bergh MS, Budsberg SC: The coxib NSAIDs: potential clinical and pharmacologic importance in veterinary medicine, *J Vet Intern Med* 19:633, 2005.
This is a detailed review of this class of drugs.

Boston SE, Moens NMM, Kruth SA et al: Endoscopic evaluation of the gastroduodenal mucosa to determine the safety of short-term concurrent administration of meloxicam and dexamethasone in healthy dogs, *Am J Vet Res* 64:1369, 2003.
The study showed that combining meloxicam and dexamethasone enhanced the potential for gastric erosions over using meloxicam alone.

Hinton LE, McLoughlin MA, Johnson SE et al: Spontaneous gastroduodenal perforation in 16 dogs and seven cats, *J Am Anim Hosp Assoc* 38:176, 2002.
Sixty-three percent of 16 dogs and 14% of 7 cats survived. The authors believe that many patients with gastroduodenal perforation have relatively mild signs initially and would be easy to miss.

Lascelles BDX, Blikslager AT, Fox SM et al: Gastrointestinal tract perforation in dogs treated with a selective cyclooxygenase-2 inhibitor: 29 cases (2002-2003), *J Am Vet Med Assoc* 227:1112, 2005.
This is a study of deracoxib-associated gastric perforation. Most of the dogs had received a higher-than-recommended dose or had received another NSAID or steroid in addition to deracoxib.

Liptak JM, Hunt GB, Baarrs VRD et al: Gastroduodenal ulceration in cats: eight cases and a review of the literature, *J Fel Med Surg* 4:27, 2002.

Five of the eight affected cats had neoplasia. These animals usually came in critical condition, and anemia was relatively common.

Neiger R, Gaschen F, Jaggy A: Gastric mucosal lesions in dogs with acute intervertebral disc disease, *J Vet Intern Med* 14:33, 2000.

Gastric lesions were common in affected dogs, and neither misoprostol nor omeprazole had a beneficial therapeutic or preventive effect that could be detected.

Nishihara K, Kikuchi H, Kanno T et al: Comparison of the upper gastrointestinal effects of etodolac and aspirin in healthy dogs, *J Vet Med Sci* 63:1131, 2001.

Etodolac had no effects on the stomach, whereas aspirin produced gastric lesions.

Peters R, Goldstein R, Erb H et al: Histopathologic features of canine uremic gastropathy: a retrospective study, *J Vet Intern Med* 19:315, 2005.

Only 1 of 28 dogs had ulceration. The authors conclude that unlike the situation in people, dogs generally do not have ulcers or erosions due to uremia.

Reimer ME, Johnston SA, Leib MS et al: The gastroduodenal effects of buffered aspirin, carprofen and etodolac in healthy dogs, *J Vet Intern Med* 13:472, 1999.

Etodolac and carprofen produced fewer gastrointestinal lesions than aspirin.

Rohrer CR, Hill RC, Fischer A et al: Gastric hemorrhage in dogs given high doses of methylprednisolone sodium succinate, *Am J Vet Res* 60:977, 1999.

High doses of methylprednisolone (30 mg/kg IV followed by 15 mg/kg IV) caused severe gastric hemorrhage.

GASTRIC NEOPLASIA AND INFILTRATIVE DISEASE

DEFINITIONS

Adenocarcinomas arise from glandular tissue or consist of tumor cells that form glandular structures. The term **lymphoma** denotes a malignant neoplasm arising from the lymphoid system. **Leiomyosarcomas** are malignant tumors, and **leiomyomas** are benign tumors that arise from smooth muscle. **Pythiosis** is a fungal infection caused by *Pythium insidiosum* that may cause a severe inflammatory and infiltrative lesion in the stomach. **Phycomycosis** is a more general term for mycoses caused by fungi of the group Phycomycetes. The terms *lymphoma* and *lymphosarcoma* are used synonymously to denote a malignant neoplasm of the lymphoid system.

GENERAL CONSIDERATIONS AND CLINICALLY RELEVANT PATHOPHYSIOLOGY

Benign gastric tumors are more commonly found in dogs than in cats; however, most gastric neoplasms are malignant (Box 19-40). Adenocarcinoma is the most common canine gastric tumor, accounting for 60% to 70% of reported cases. Adenocarcinomas tend to metastasize to the regional lymph nodes, the liver, or the lungs, or all three, and they may appear diffusely infiltrative or nodular. They usually occur in the pyloric antrum or lesser curvature.

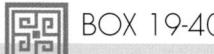

BOX 19-40

Important Considerations for Gastric Neoplasia

- Most gastric tumors are malignant.
- Anorexia, not vomiting, is the most common sign.
- Some patients are anemic.
- Most patients do not vomit until the neoplasm is well advanced or is causing gastric outflow obstruction.
- Neoplasia is a possible cause of ulceration in the dog and cat, but many neoplasms do not cause ulceration.
- Not all obstructed patients have hypokalemic, hypochloremic, metabolic alkalosis.
- Gastroduodenoscopy is usually more appropriate than contrast radiographs; with endoscopy, you can biopsy and often (not always) diagnose malignancy.

Infection with *Helicobacter pylori* has been linked with gastric carcinoma and gastric mucosa–associated lymphoma in human beings, but dogs and cats have other species of *Helicobacter* in their stomachs. Other reported malignant gastric tumors in dogs include leiomyosarcoma, lymphosarcoma, and fibrosarcoma.

Lymphoma is the most common gastric tumor in cats; adenocarcinomas are rare. Most affected cats test negative for feline leukemia virus (FeLV). Lymphoma may be solitary or diffuse in the stomach and may or may not simultaneously affect the intestine.

Leiomyomas are the most common benign canine gastric tumor. They tend to be slow growing, submucosal, and expansile. Clinical signs may not be apparent until the tumors are large. Leiomyomas usually occur at the cardia, and complete surgical excision may be possible because they often are pedunculated. Adenomatous polyps occasionally are found in dogs. They may be multiple and rarely cause clinical signs, but vomiting or anorexia (or both) may be seen if the polyps occur at the pylorus and cause obstruction. Other benign tumors rarely found in dogs include adenomas, lipomas, and fibromas.

Pythiosis is a fungal infection caused by *P. insidiosum*, which can affect any part of the alimentary tract and the skin. It is primarily found in the southeastern United States, particularly near the Gulf Coast. The fungus causes intensive submucosal infiltration of fibrous connective tissue and a profound inflammatory reaction in the mucosa (often with eosinophils) and deeper layers of the gastric wall (Fig. 19-80). The organism often is difficult to find histologically, and large tissue samples that include substantial submucosa should be submitted.

DIAGNOSIS
Clinical Presentation

Signalment. Belgian shepherd dogs and chow chows may have a higher than normal incidence of gastric carcinoma, whereas beagles appear to have a higher incidence of leiomyoma. Males appear to be more commonly affected than females. Adenocarcinoma is most common in dogs 7 to 10

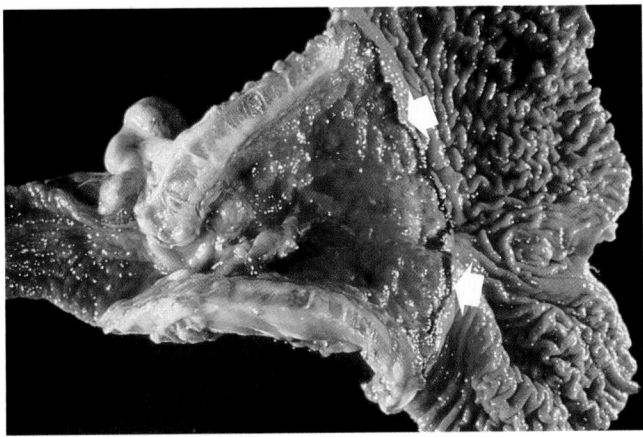

FIG. 19-80
Pythiosis affecting the pylorus and antrum of a dog's stomach. Note the sharp line of demarcation between normal and abnormal tissue *(arrows).*

years of age. Gastric adenocarcinoma is extremely rare in cats. Lymphoma affects primarily middle-aged and older dogs (average age, 6 years) and cats, but can occur at any age. Pythiosis may affect dogs of any age.

History. Animals with gastric neoplasia or other infiltrative disease usually have a history of anorexia. Vomiting, hematemesis, melena, lethargy, weight loss, and/or edema may also occur. Many animals are relatively asymptomatic until the tumor becomes large enough to affect gastric emptying or starts bleeding. Clinical signs with pythiosis generally are the result of gastric outflow obstruction and gastric stasis.

Physical Examination Findings

The physical examination findings in animals with gastric neoplasia or pythiosis often are nonspecific (e.g., weight loss, anemia, and/or edema). Weight loss may be caused by anorexia, chronic vomiting, or cancer cachexia. Occasionally a large mass may be palpated in the stomach; however, detailed palpation of the stomach usually is difficult. Abdominal pain may be present with ulceration or pancreatitis.

Diagnostic Imaging

Noncontrast (survey) radiographs generally are nondiagnostic. Survey thoracic radiographs should be taken to rule out pulmonary metastasis (rare). Contrast radiographs may reveal filling defects, delayed gastric emptying, ulceration, loss of normal rugal folds, mucosal thickening, or loss of gastric wall compliance; however, contrast radiographs are being done less frequently because of the advantages that ultrasound and endoscopy have over such procedures.

Ultrasonographically, gastric neoplasia is associated with mural thickening with loss of normal wall and diminished to absent local motility. An ultrasound-guided, fine-needle aspirate or core needle biopsy may provide a preoperative diagnosis in affected animals. Ultrasonography may also detect metastasis to the liver or regional lymph nodes and help define the gastric lesion.

Endoscopy. Endoscopy is the preferred test because it finds almost all gastric tumors and other mucosal diseases, plus it allows one to take a biopsy from the lesion. However, tumors may be difficult to to obtain a biopsy from if they are completely submucosal or if they are scirrhous. The gross appearance can be very suggestive of neoplasia and may help the client decide if surgery is appropriate. Finding a deep ulcer with a hard, dense, necrotic base surrounded by raised or distorted mucosa is very suggestive of scirrhous carcinoma. Scirrhous tumors are very dense, and it may be impossible to tear a diagnostic piece of tissue from the lesion. Leiomyomas and leiomyosarcomas are usually submucosal masses with or without ulcers. They are also hard to obtain a biopsy from with flexible endoscopic forceps, but a diagnostic sample can usually be obtained if the endoscopist is persistent. Pythiosis causes severe mucosal inflammation and necrosis; however, the organism is best found in the dense, hard fibrotic reaction under the diseased mucosa. This makes it difficult to obtain a diagnostic tissue sample.

Laboratory Findings

Clinical pathologic changes in animals with gastric neoplasia usually are nonspecific. A microcytic, hypochromic anemia or a normocytic, normochromic anemia may occur. The anemia may be the result of blood loss or chronic disease. If biliary drainage is obstructed, icterus ensues. If vomiting causes loss of gastric secretions, a hypochloremic, hypokalemic metabolic alkalosis with or without paradoxical aciduria may occur.

NOTE: If the animal is icteric, the lesion probably is near the pylorus. Be prepared to perform a cholecystoenterostomy (see p. 564).

DIFFERENTIAL DIAGNOSIS

Anorexia may be associated with many systemic diseases (e.g., uremia, hypoadrenocorticism, hepatic insufficiency, hypercalcemia, and inflammatory disease). Gastric outlet obstruction caused by nonneoplastic disease (i.e., mucosal hypertrophy and foreign object) may produce similar clinical signs (see p. 434). Cytologic or histologic examination of tissue (or both) is necessary to differentiate these conditions. Gastric foreign bodies can be differentiated from neoplasia with imaging or endoscopy. Pythiosis and neoplasia may be differentiated by cytology or histopathology (see Fig. 19-107 on p. 475).

MEDICAL MANAGEMENT

Medical management depends on the severity of the clinical signs. If possible, electrolyte, acid-base, hydration, and coagulation abnormalities should be corrected before surgery.

SURGICAL TREATMENT
Preoperative Management

Food should be withheld for 12 hours before surgery. Perioperative antibiotics may be given at induction of anesthesia and continued for up to 12 hours postoperatively.

Anesthesia

See p. 409 for suggested anesthetics to use in dogs with gastric disorders.

Surgical Anatomy

See p. 410 for the surgical anatomy of the stomach.

Positioning

The animal is placed in dorsal recumbency, and the abdomen is prepared for a ventral midline incision. The prepped area should extend from midthorax to the pubis.

SURGICAL TECHNIQUE

With the exception of lymphoma, surgery is the only potentially curative treatment for gastric neoplasia (Fig. 19-81). Unfortunately, most carcinomas are not diagnosed until they are so far advanced as to be unresectable.

Palpate the regional lymph nodes for evidence of metastasis. Inspect the liver and other abdominal structures for metastasis or thickening and take a biopsy from suspicious lesions. If the lesion appears localized to the stomach, consider gastric resection because it might be curative.

If wide excision and bypass procedures, such as gastrojejunostomy and cholecystojejunostomy (see p. 564) are necessary, then surgery is of dubious value because of the likelihood of tumor recurrence plus the likelihood of unacceptable morbidity from surgery. Solitary gastric lymphoma is rarely cured by surgery alone, and chemotherapy is only palliative for diffuse lymphoma. Likewise, wide surgical excision is currently the only potentially curative therapy available for pythiosis; however, obtaining wide surgical margins is difficult because of the extensive nature of the disease at diagnosis. Medical therapy of pythiosis is infrequently beneficial and almost never curative if the lesion cannot be resected.

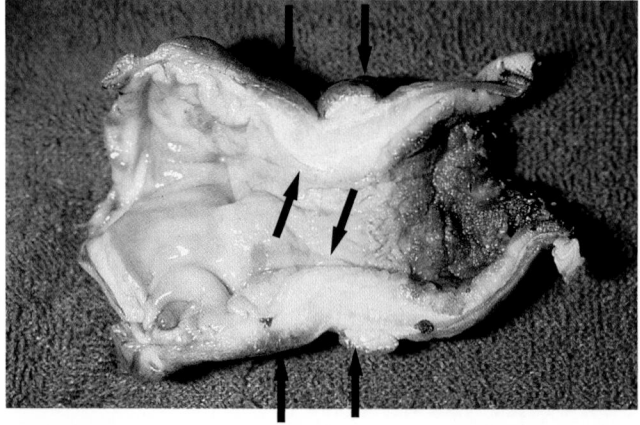

FIG. 19-81
A resected pylorus from a dog that had gastric outflow obstruction caused by a submucosal adenocarcinoma *(arrows),* which did not disrupt the mucosa.

If the lesion appears small enough that it can be resected without causing unacceptable morbidity, then wide surgical margins (including some normal tissue) should be obtained for both gastric malignancies and pythiosis. Cytologic examination of tissues submitted during the surgical procedure or frozen sections are helpful for determining the adequacy of the tissue margins. Surgical techniques for gastric resection are described on pp. 411 to 414.

SUTURE MATERIALS AND SPECIAL INSTRUMENTS

Absorbable suture materials, such as polydioxanone or polyglyconate (2-0 or 3-0), should be used. Chromic gut suture should be avoided.

POSTOPERATIVE CARE AND ASSESSMENT

The patient's electrolyte and fluid status should be monitored postoperatively and deficiencies corrected. The animal can be fed a low-fat, bland diet beginning 24 hours after surgery if vomiting does not occur. If vomiting continues, centrally acting antiemetics such as prochlorperazine, metoclopramide, or dolasetron (see Box 19-31 on p. 427) may be beneficial. An enterostomy feeding tube should be considered to help provide nutrition in the postoperative period.

PROGNOSIS

The prognosis is guarded for most gastric neoplasms because of their malignant characteristics and the fact that most are not diagnosed until they are advanced and have metastasized. A retrospective study of gastric adenocarcinomas and leiomyosarcoma found that although a Billroth I or gastrojejunostomy provided immediate relief of gastric outflow obstruction and clinical improvement in the early postoperative period, recurrence of clinical signs occurred within 3 days to 10 months and caused all owners to elect euthanasia (Swann and Holt, 2002). For animals with benign lesions, surgery may be curative. Pythiosis may be difficult to treat surgically because of its rapid growth rate and extensive nature, but surgical cures have been achieved.

Reference

Swann HM, Holt DE: Canine gastric adenocarcinoma and leiomyosarcoma: a retrospective study of 21 cases (1986-1999) and literature review, *J Am Anim Hosp Assoc* 38:157, 2002.

Suggested Reading

Easton S: A retrospective study into the effects of operator experience on the accuracy of ultrasound in the diagnosis of gastric neoplasia in dogs, *Vet Radiol Ultrasound* 42:47, 2001.
This paper documents how increased experience of the ultrasonographer increased sensitivity and specificity of diagnosing gastric neoplasia in dogs.
Graham JP, Newell SM, Roberts GD et al: Ultrasonographic features of canine gastrointestinal pythiosis, *Vet Radiol Ultrasound* 41:273, 2000.
Ultrasonographic findings do not allow one to distinguish between neoplasia and pythiosis.

Helman RG, Oliver J: Pythiosis of the digestive tract in dogs from Oklahoma, *J Am Anim Hosp* 35:111, 1999.

Pythiosis in 9 dogs is reported. Seven had a detectable mass; anorexia and weight loss were the most consistent clinical findings.

Liljebjelke KA, Abramson C, Brochku C et al: Duodenal obstruction caused by infection with *Pythium insidiosum* in a 12 week-old-puppy, *J Am Vet Med Assoc* 220:1188, 2002.

This is an example of how young affected animals can be.

Richter KP: Feline gastrointestinal lymphoma, *Vet Clin North Am* 33:1083, 2003.

This is a discussion of lymphosarcoma in the cat and includes a discussion of well-differentiated lymphoma that can be impossible to histologically distinguish from inflammatory bowel disease.

Surgery of the Small Intestine

GENERAL PRINCIPLES AND TECHNIQUES

DEFINITIONS

Enterotomy is an incision into the intestine, and **enterectomy** is removal of a segment of intestine. **Intestinal resection** and **anastomosis** is an enterectomy with reestablishment of continuity between the divided ends. **Enteroenteropexy**, or **intestinal plication**, is surgical fixation of one intestinal segment to another; **enteropexy** is fixation of an intestinal segment to the body wall or another loop of intestine.

PREOPERATIVE MANAGEMENT

Surgery of the small intestine is most often indicated for gastrointestinal obstruction (i.e., foreign bodies and masses). Other indications include trauma (i.e., perforation and ischemia), malpositioning, infection, and diagnostic or supportive procedures (i.e., biopsy, culture and cytologic tests, and feeding tubes).

Diagnosis of small intestinal disease is based on the history, clinical signs, physical examination, radiographs, ultrasound scans, laboratory data, endoscopy, and/or biopsy. Diet, medications, stressful events, and response to prior therapy should be ascertained from owners. Clinical signs of small intestinal disease vary and are nonspecific, although weight loss, diarrhea, vomiting, anorexia, and/or depression are the most common (Table 19-1). Pain and shock may result from trauma, vascular occlusion, or complete intestinal obstruction. Severe vomiting, shock, or an acute abdomen suggests intestinal malposition, ischemia, perforation, or upper intestinal obstruction. Visual examination provides information about the animal's mental state, temperament, nutritional state, and comfort. Abdominal palpation may identify pain, thickened intestine, abdominal masses, or malpositioned organs.

Hematologic and biochemical profiles should be performed on animals suspected of having small intestinal abnormalities to help identify concurrent systemic disease (e.g., renal disease, hepatic disease, hypoadrenocorticism, hypercalcemia, diabetes mellitus, and pancreatitis) and to direct preoperative therapy (Box 19-41). Dehydration, acid-base abnormalities, and electrolyte imbalances are common sequelae to vomiting, diarrhea, and fluid sequestration. These abnormalities should be corrected before induction of anesthesia if possible. Alleviating hypotension is important because it is associated with intense portal vasoconstriction, which causes the breakdown of the intestinal mucosal barrier, allowing increased endotoxin absorption. Profuse vomiting typically results in dehydration and may cause hypochloremia, hypokalemia, and/or hyponatremia. Duodenal vomitus may cause greater sodium, potassium, and water losses than gastric vomiting. Alkalosis generally occurs with loss of gastric fluid; however, metabolic acidosis may occur as a result of fluid depletion from vomiting, insensible water losses, lack of intake, and/or catabolism of body stores. Cross-matched whole blood or red cells should be administered when the packed cell volume drops below 20% or if the dog is weak or clinically hypoxic. Chronically ill, anemic patients should be given whole blood if hypovolemic and packed red blood cells if normovolemic. Clotting factor deficiencies should be corrected with whole fresh blood or fresh or fresh-frozen plasma. Platelet-rich plasma or platelet transfusions should be used if the animal is severely thrombocytopenic. Administration of plasma (5 to 20 ml/kg), whole blood transfusions, or hetastarch several hours before surgery should be considered if serum albumin concentrations are below 1.5 g/dl. If the patient has a severe protein-losing enteropathy, administration of plasma is seldom effective in raising the serum albumin concentration because most of the albumin is quickly lost into the gastrointestinal tract. Therefore hetastarch is usually preferred. There is some evidence that blood transfusions may impair intestinal healing and increase susceptibility to intraabdominal sepsis.

Plain radiographs may demonstrate abnormal gas-fluid patterns, masses, foreign bodies, abdominal fluid, or displaced viscera (Fig. 19-82). Both lateral recumbent views and a ventrodorsal projection should be taken. Contrast studies can demonstrate foreign bodies, obstructions, abnormal displacements, abnormal bowel wall thickness, irregular mucosal patterns, and distortion of the bowel wall. The positive contrast agent usually used for gastrointestinal radiology is micropulverized barium sulfate suspension; however, iodinated contrast or iohexol should be used when intestinal perforation is suspected but septic peritonitis cannot be demonstrated with abdominocentesis or diagnostic peritoneal lavage (see p. 335). Contrast studies are infrequently done now because of the availability of ultrasound and endoscopy.

> NOTE: Do not use barium sulfate for a gastrointestinal radiographic study if intestinal perforation is suspected. Instead document peritonitis by abdominocentesis, diagnostic peritoneal lavage, or exploratory surgery.

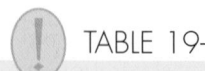

TABLE 19-1

Clinical Signs of Chronic Intestinal Disease

CLINICAL SIGN	SMALL INTESTINE	LARGE INTESTINE
Weight loss	Consistent	Infrequent
Appetite	Variable	Usually normal; variable
Vomiting	Occasional	Rare
Belching	Occasional	Rare
Flatulence and borborygmus	Occasional	Occasional
Distended abdomen	Variable	Rare
Defecation quantity	Normal to large	Small to normal
Defecation frequency	Normal to slightly increased	Normal to very frequent
Blood in feces	If present, usually dark, black (melena)	If present, usually red to red-brown (hematochezia)
Mucus in feces	Absent	Present or absent
Steatorrhea	Occasional	Absent
Fecalith	Absent	Sometimes
Urgency or tenesmus	Absent	Sometimes present
Dyschezia	Absent	Present with rectal disease
Rectal examination	Normal	May be normal or abnormal (blood, mucus, pain, mass)
Abdominal pain	Variable	Variable
Poor hair coat	Variable	Uncommon
Depression	Variable	Uncommon

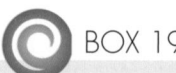

BOX 19-41

**Preoperative Management of Patients Undergoing
Intestinal Surgery**

- Obtain minimum data base: complete blood cell count, chemistry profile, urinalysis, coagulation profile (if possible) with or without an electrocardiogram.
- Localize the lesion with abdominal palpation, radiographs, ultrasonography, and/or endoscopy.
- Correct hydration, electrolyte, and acid-base abnormalities.
- Transfuse if the packed cell volume is less than 20% or if the animal is clinically weak or debilitated (see Table 5-4 on p. 26).
- Withhold food from mature animals for 12 to 18 hours and from pediatric patients 4 to 8 hours before induction.
- Administer prophylactic antibiotics if indicated.

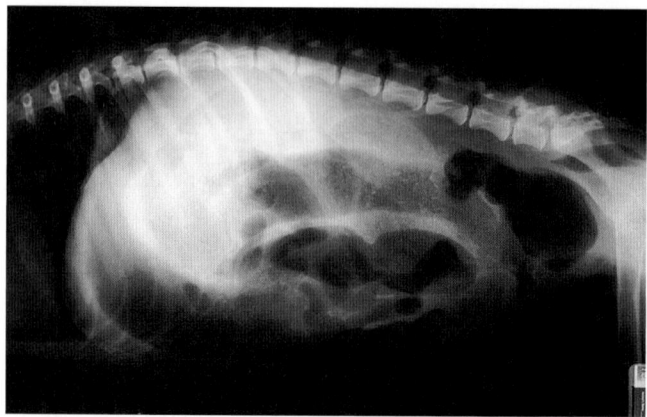

FIG. 19-82
Lateral radiograph of a depressed, anorectic, constipated, 2-year-old boxer with a "doughy" abdomen. Note the massive intestinal distention with gas and ingesta. A corncob was removed from the distal jejunum.

Ultrasonography can detect and define intestinal and other abdominal masses and evaluate intestinal wall thickness (a normal small intestinal wall is 2 to 3 mm thick), the appearance and symmetry of the various wall layers, the number of peristaltic contractions, the pattern of intestinal contents (gas hyperechoic, mucus echogenic without acoustic shadowing, fluid anechoic), the location of the lesion, and the extent of disease. Five layers are normally visible ultrasonographically in the intestinal wall: the hyperechoic mucosal surface, hypoechoic mucosa, hyperechoic submucosa, hypoechoic muscularis, and hyperechoic serosa. Ultrasound is very important in helping the clinician decide whether to

BOX 19-42

Emergency Surgery Indications

Explore Without Delay If:	**Consider Exploring Without Delay If:**
Penetrating abdominal injury	Peritoneal fluid has greater than or equal to 13,000 nucleated cells/μl
Effusion with intracellular bacteria	Peritoneal fluid pH less than 7.2
Blood-to-peritoneal fluid glucose difference greater than 20 mg/dl	Peritoneal fluid PCO_2 greater than 55 mm Hg
Peritoneal fluid lactate greater than 2.5 to 5.5 mmol/L	Peritoneal fluid PO_2 less than 50 mm Hg
Imaging reveals spontaneous extraluminal gas bubbles or volvulus	Peritoneal fluid glucose less than 50 mg/dl
Esophageal or gastric intussusception is identified	Blood-to-peritoneal fluid lactate is negative
Bacteria isolated from peritoneal fluid	Animal deteriorates despite aggressive medical management and complete obstruction, perforation, strangulation, necrosis or sepsis is suspected
Greater than 25,000 neutrophils/μl in abdominal fluid	

perform endoscopic or surgical biopsy of the intestines. If the intestine generally looks the same throughout all or most of its length, then endoscopic biopsy is usually appropriate. If ultrasound reveals that the only sections of bowel that appear involved are out of reach of the endoscope, then surgical biopsy is often preferred.

Gastroduodenoscopy allows visualization and a biopsy of the duodenum (and sometimes the upper jejunum), whereas colonoileoscopy allows visualization and biopsy of the ileum. Visualization of intestinal mucosa may detect ulcers, erosions, infiltrated mucosa, and/or lymphangiectasia that cannot be detected with radiographs or ultrasound. Endoscopy also allows multiple biopsies of the small intestine, and in particular allows one to direct the biopsy to obviously affected areas.

The benefits of stabilizing the animal's condition before surgery must be weighed against the risk of ischemic necrosis. Explore the animal without delay if one or more of the following is true. (1) The animal has received a penetrating abdominal injury; (2) large numbers of neutrophils (greater than 25,000/μl) or very toxic neutrophils are identified on cytology of the effusion; (3) bacteria are found in abdominal effusion; (4) the blood-to–peritoneal fluid glucose difference is greater than 20 mg/dl; (5) the peritoneal fluid lactate concentration is greater than 2.5 to 5.5 mmol/L; (6) extraluminal gas bubbles (i.e., spontaneous pneumoperitoneum) or volvulus are identified during imaging; (7) esophageal or gastric intussusception is identified during imaging; and (8) bacterial culture of the fluid is positive for pathogenic bacteria. Consider exploring the animal without delay if the above factors are not identified but an emergency is suspected and one or more of the following is true: (1) The peritoneal fluid has $\geq$ 13,000 nucleated cells/μl; (2) the peritoneal fluid pH is less than 7.2; (3) the peritoneal fluid PCO_2 is greater than 55 mm Hg; (4) the peritoneal fluid PO_2 is less than 50 mm Hg; (5) the peritoneal fluid glucose concentration is less than 50 mg/dl; (6) a negative blood-to-fluid lactate difference exists; and (7) the animal deteriorates clinically despite aggressive medical management, and complete obstruction, perforation, strangulation, necrosis, or sepsis is suspected (Box 19-42).

 BOX 19-43

Selected Anesthetic Protocols for Use in Stable Animals With Intestinal Disorders

Premedication

Give atropine (0.02–0.04 mg/kg SC or IM) or glycopyrrolate (0.005–0.011 mg/kg SC or IM) plus hydromorphone* 0.1–0.2 mg/kg SC or IM) or butorphanol (0.2–0.4 mg/kg SC or IM) or buprenorphine (5–15 μg/kg IM)

Induction

Thiopental (10–12 mg/kg IV) or propofol (4–6 mg/kg IV) or a combination of diazepam and ketamine (diazepam 0.27 mg/kg plus 5.5 mg/kg ketamine IV; titrated to effect)

Maintenance

Isoflurane or sevoflurane

SC, Subcutaneous; *IM*, intramuscular; *IV*, intravenous.
*May use 0.05 mg/kg in cats.

ANESTHESIA

Mature animals should fast for 12 to 18 hours before surgery, but pediatric patients should fast for only 4 to 8 hours. Special anesthetic considerations are needed for patients with bowel obstruction, ischemia, or perforation. Complications may arise because of uncorrected electrolyte, acid-base, and fluid imbalances. Enlarged viscera may compress the vena cava, causing circulatory and vascular compromise. Viscera displacing the diaphragm cranially may compromise respiration. Nitrous oxide increases the volume of air trapped in body viscera and therefore should be avoided in patients with intestinal obstruction. Visceral manipulation may induce bradycardia; however, atropine (0.02-0.04 mg/kg, SC, IM, IV) or glycopyrrolate (0.005-0.011 mg/kg SC, IM, IV) can resolve this. Water evaporates from exposed abdominal viscera at an increased rate; therefore IV fluid administration must be increased to replace this loss. Body heat is lost from exposed viscera and may cause hypothermia, which reduces the need for anesthesia. Care should be taken during surgery to try to main-

BOX 19-44

Prophylactic Antibiotics for Animals Undergoing Intestinal Surgery

Cefazolin (Ancef, Kefzol)

22 mg/kg given intravenously (IV)

Cefmetazole (Zefazone)

15 mg/kg IV

Cefoxitin (Mefoxin)

30 mg/kg IV

tain the patient's body temperature above 95° F (35° C). Selected anesthetic protocols for animals in stable condition undergoing small intestinal surgery are provided in Box 19-43. Sick or debilitated animals should be anesthetized with care. Selected anesthetic protocols for animals with peritonitis are provided on p. 318.

ANTIBIOTICS

Bacteria populate the gastrointestinal tract. Bacterial numbers are smaller in the duodenum and jejunum than in the ileum, colon, and rectum. The colon has the greatest number of bacteria (both aerobic and anaerobic). Normally, fewer potentially pathologic bacteria reside proximal to the ileocecal valve unless peristalsis is interrupted by ileus or obstruction. However, some patients have surprisingly large numbers of bacteria (i.e., $>10^8$/ml of intestinal fluid) in the upper small intestine, including potential pathogens, such as *Bacteroides*, *Clostridium*, *Enterococcus*, *Staphylococcus*, and enterics like *Escherichia coli*. Resident bacteria typically proliferate in diseased bowel because stagnant luminal contents and devitalized wall are excellent growth media. Six hours of abnormal conditions may allow bacterial numbers to increase from 10^2 to 10^4/ml of ingesta to 10^8 to 10^{11}/ml. Holding animals off food reduces bacterial numbers in the small intestine and stomach. Antibiotic therapy alters the normal intestinal flora and promotes resistant strains of bacteria. Nonetheless, antibiotics are indicated in animals with severe mucosal damage or acute gastrointestinal disease associated with fever, leukocytosis, leukopenia, and/or shock.

Surgical techniques that involve entering the intestinal lumen are classified as clean-contaminated or contaminated procedures, depending on the amount of spillage (see p. 84). The risk of infection in contaminated wounds increases with patient stress, the organism's pathogenicity, tissue susceptibility, and time. Pathogens that often cause peritonitis after intestinal surgery are *E. coli*, *Enterococcus* spp., and coagulase-positive *Staphylococcus aureus*. Although less frequently isolated, anaerobes are also common and may cause peritonitis (see p. 333). Prophylactic antibiotics are indicated in animals with intestinal obstruction because there is an increased risk of contamination associated with bacterial overgrowth. They are also indicated when devascularized and traumatized tissue is present, and when surgery is expected to last longer than 2 to 3 hours. First-generation cephalosporins (e.g., cefazolin; Box 19-44) should be administered before surgery on the upper and middle small intestine, whereas second-generation cephalosporins (e.g., cefmetazole or cefoxitin; see Box 19-44) or an extended spectrum penicillin (e.g., ticarcillin plus clavulanic acid; see Box 19-4) should be considered for procedures involving the distal small intestine and large intestine. Antibiotics should be redosed 2 hours after the initial dose.

SURGICAL ANATOMY

The intestines in dogs are approximately five times the body (crown to rump) length, with 80% being small intestine. Duodenum, jejunum, and ileum make up the small intestine. The duodenum is the most fixed portion, beginning at the pylorus to the right of midline and extending approximately 25 cm. It courses dorsocranially for a short distance, turns caudally at the cranial duodenal flexure, and continues on the right as the descending duodenum. The duodenum turns cranially at the caudal duodenal flexure where the duodenocolic ligament attaches. The ascending duodenum lies to the left of the mesenteric root. The common bile duct and pancreatic duct open in the first few centimeters of the duodenum at the *major duodenal papilla* in dogs. The accessory pancreatic duct enters caudal to this at the *minor duodenal papilla*.

The jejunum forms most of the small intestinal coils lying in the ventrocaudal abdomen. It is the longest and most mobile segment of the small intestine. It begins to the left of the mesenteric root where the ascending duodenum turns to the right at the duodenojejunal flexure. The ileum has an antimesenteric vessel and is approximately 15 cm long. It passes from the left to the right side in a transverse plane through the midlumbar region caudal to the root of the mesentery and joins the ascending colon on the right of the midline at the ileocolic orifice. The root of the mesentery attaches the jejunum and ileum to the dorsal body wall. Branches of the celiac and cranial mesenteric arteries supply the small intestine. Mesenteric lymph nodes lie along vessels in the mesentery.

The layers of the intestinal wall are the mucosa, submucosa, muscularis, and serosa. Mucosa is an important barrier that separates the luminal environment from that of the abdominal cavity. Mucosal health and the intestinal blood supply are important for normal intestinal secretion and absorption. The submucosal layer provides blood vessels, lymphatics, and nerves. It is the layer of greatest tensile strength. The muscularis is needed for normal motility. The serosa is important for forming a quick seal at a site of injury or incision.

NOTE: Because the submucosa is the intestinal layer that provides mechanical strength, it must be engaged when suturing intestine to provide a secure closure.

SURGICAL TECHNIQUE

Surgical correction of mechanical obstructions preferably is performed within 12 hours of diagnosis, allowing time for partial to complete correction of fluid, acid-base, and elec-

BOX 19-45

Principles of Intestinal Surgery

- Early diagnosis and good surgical technique prevent most complications.
- Perform surgery as soon as anesthesia is possible in patients with perforation, strangulation, or complete obstruction.
- Optimal healing requires a good blood supply, accurate mucosal apposition, and minimal surgical trauma.
- Systemic factors may delay healing and increase the risk of dehiscence, hypovolemia, shock, hypoproteinemia, debilitation, and infection.
- Use approximating suture patterns: simple interrupted, Gambee, crushing, or simple continuous. Stapling techniques are feasible.
- Engage submucosa in all sutures or staples.
- Select a monofilament, synthetic absorbable suture, such as polydioxanone, polyglyconate, or poliglecaprone 25, glycomer 631.
- Cover surgical sites with omentum or a serosal patch.
- Replace contaminated instruments and gloves before closing the abdomen.

trolyte abnormalities. The benefits of stabilizing the patient's condition must be weighed against the risk of ischemic necrosis caused by vascular disruption, which increases with time (Box 19-45). Perforation, loss of mucosal integrity, and systemic exposure to intestinal bacteria and toxins are life-threatening developments. Surgery for penetrating abdominal wounds, intestinal perforation, volvulus, or peritonitis should be performed as soon as the diagnosis is made.

Ischemic necrosis of the bowel wall may occur with obstruction (complete or partial), strangulation, and thrombosis. Routine criteria for assessing bowel viability include observation of intestinal color (pink to red rather than blue to black), wall texture, peristalsis, pulsation of arteries, and bleeding when incised. Because these factors are subjective, assessment of viability often is difficult. Bathing the involved segment in warm saline for a few minutes may improve color and peristalsis. However, a normal appearance does not guarantee that the bowel will heal after surgery; therefore bowel of questionable viability should be resected. A number of techniques have been proposed for increasing the accuracy of standard clinical criteria for viability assessment. Their most common error is that viable bowel would be resected. Viability assessment techniques include the use of electromyography, radioactive microspheres, microtemperature probes, and pH measurements. These techniques are technically cumbersome, expensive, and not generally suited for clinical use. Doppler ultrasonic flow probes have been used to detect pulsatile mural blood flow with an accuracy of 80%. Pulse oximetry measures oxygen saturation via pulse probes and may be superior to Doppler ultrasound in determining intestinal viability. Pulse oximetry of the intestinal wall as compared with peripheral oxygen saturation has shown that normal intestine remains within 1 cm of a normal pulse oximetry reading. Pulse oximetry is a reliable, reproducible means of assessing arterial perfusion of ischemic intestine, exceeding the overall accuracy of either standard clinical criteria or Doppler ultrasound and is comparable to fluorescein dye. Pulse oximetry is not as sensitive as fluorescein dye in detecting viability in segments with combined arterial and venous occlusion.

Intravenous injection of various agents (primarily fluorescein dye) is practical but of limited accuracy (95% accurate in detecting nonviable bowel, less than 58% accurate in detecting viable bowel). Fluorescein dye is injected intravenously (15 to 25 mg/kg), allowed to equilibrate for 2 to 3 minutes, and then the intestine is viewed with a Wood's lamp in a darkened operating room. Viable intestine has fluorescing areas of a smooth, uniform, green-gold color or a finely mottled pattern with no areas of nonfluorescence larger than 3 mm in diameter. Fluorescein can be used only once in a 24-hour period. Dyes such as fluorescein assess only perfusion and not mucosal integrity, which is essential for maintaining the mucosal barrier. Although this technique is a test of vascularity, but not viability, it still can be a valuable adjunct in predicting viability.

Biopsy Techniques

Intestinal biopsy is indicated to diagnose intestinal diseases that have not been defined by other tests. A biopsy may be taken from the small intestine during endoscopy, ultrasonography, laparoscopy, or laparotomy. All biopsy techniques require general anesthesia or sedation.

Ultrasonographic biopsy. The main advantages of ultrasound-guided biopsy of the small intestine are (1) these procedures are applicable to the entire intestine; (2) they are generally safe and quick, and can be done on an outpatient basis; (3) they are likely to be very specific if a diagnosis of neoplasia or fungal infection is made; and (4) one may also obtain a biopsy from abdominal masses, if they are present. The main disadvantages are that (1) ultrasound is insensitive in detecting mucosal lesions; (2) it is very hard to examine the entire intestinal tract with ultrasound, meaning that it is easy for ultrasound to miss focal lesions of the intestines, and (3) there are no data on how diagnostic these samples are for inflammatory lesions of the intestines. Ultrasound-guided biopsy would appear to be the biopsy method of choice for intestinal masses, with surgery being indicated if the ultrasound-guided technique failed to diagnose a tumor. Fine-needle aspiration biopsy, microcore biopsy, or automated microcore biopsy may be performed during ultrasonographic examination of intestinal lesions; however, they may be difficult to perform if mild or moderate infiltration is present. For fine-needle aspiration of lesions smaller than 2 cm in diameter, a 23- to 25-gauge, 2½-inch spinal needle or a Westcott biopsy needle may be used. If aspirated samples are nondiagnostic and if the lesion is larger than 2 cm in diameter, an automated microcore biopsy may be performed (Bard Biopty-Cut biopsy needle). As an alternative, a microcore biopsy may be performed using a 20- or 22-gauge needle, which is passed repeatedly through the lesion. A syringe with a small amount of air is then attached to the needle, and the cells are blown out onto a slide. Possible complications include peritonitis, hematoma, tumor seeding, and trauma to adjacent organs.

Localize the lesion with the transducer, and aseptically pre-pare the skin over this site. Tense the skin and puncture with the needle. Using ultrasound guidance, direct the needle into the lesion but not through the mucosa. For aspiration biopsies, remove the stylet and apply suction with a 6-ml syringe three to six times. After releasing suction, remove the needle and syringe. Collect two to four samples and evaluate the cytologic preparations. For a microcore biopsy, select a site as far from the intestinal lumen as possible. Using the TruCut biopsy instrument with ultrasound guid-ance, collect one or two biopsies. Transfer the samples to biopsy traps and place in 10% formalin. After sampling, observe the biopsy site with ultrasound for fluid collection suggestive of leakage or hemorrhage. Abdominal radiog-raphy may be used to look for pneumoperitoneum. Monitor the mucous membrane color, capillary refill time, pulse, and respiratory rate during recovery.

Flexible endoscopic biopsy. The main advantages of flexible endoscopic biopsy are (1) it is the least invasive tech-nique available and it can be done as an outpatient proce-dure; (2) it allows visualization of the mucosa and biopsy of focal lesions not visible with imaging or laparotomy; and (3) it allows multiple biopsies of each organ, which is important because lesions can be very spotty, even in very ill animals. The main disadvantages of flexible endoscopy are (1) the jejunum is generally out of reach, except in small patients; (2) only a limited amount of submucosa and no muscular tunic is included in these biopsies; and most importantly (3) it is easy to obtain poor quality, nondiagnostic tissue samples with this method. Unless careful attention is paid to tech-nique, endoscopic biopsy of duodenal mucosa often results in artifact-ridden, twisted, nonoriented biopsies that are dif-ficult to impossible to meaningfully evaluate. See Chapter 14 for one technique for obtaining flexible endoscopic biopsies of the duodenum.

Laparoscopic biopsy of the small intestine. The main advantages of laparoscopic biopsy of the small intes-tine are (1) it is relatively noninvasive and can be performed as an outpatient procedure; (2) it can be performed at the same time as hepatic and pancreatic biopsies; (3) one may biopsy the jejunum, which is usually out of reach of flexible endoscopes; and (4) one obtains a full-thickness biopsy. The main disadvantages of laparoscopic biopsy of the small in-testine are (1) one cannot readily access the duodenum or ileum; (2) one is limited in the number of biopsies that may be taken; and (3) one cannot see mucosal lesions and direct the biopsy to affected spots.

Perform a routine, double puncture laparoscopy. At the end of the procedure, use Babcock forceps to gently grasp a sec-tion of jejunum and bring it up to the cannula. Then pull the cannula, Babcock forceps, and intestine from the abdomen as a single unit.

It helps if the cannula used is a 10-mm cannula (if neces-sary, a 5-mm adapter may be placed over the top to accom-modate smaller diameter instruments).

If necessary, enlarge the skin incision to make it easier to exteriorize that portion of the small intestine. Place stay sutures in the intestine and remove the cannula and Babcock forceps. Next, perform an incisional biopsy as described in the Enterotomy section.

There are variations on this technique (Rawlings et al, 2002).

Enterotomy

The main advantages of laparotomy and enterotomy are that (1) it allows access to the entire gastrointestinal tract; (2) it provides full-thickness biopsies, which are important in sub-mucosal masses; and (3) one can examine and sample the rest of the abdomen at the same time. The main disadvan-tages of laparotomy are that (1) it is the most expensive and most invasive technique (i.e., it is not an outpatient proce-dure); (2) it does not allow one to detect mucosal lesions; (3) it does not allow one to obtain as many mucosal samples as flexible endoscopy; and (4) it is possible to take nondiagnos-tic tissue samples if proper technique is not followed. Lapa-rotomy should be performed if other techniques are not possible, or if other techniques have been or are likely to be nondiagnostic.

Longitudinal or transverse enterotomy incisions can be made to collect biopsy samples. Multiple biopsies should be performed, and the samples should be reasonably large (4 to 5 mm in diameter) and should contain adequate amounts of mucosa. The entire abdomen should be explored thoroughly before biopsies are performed. Samples should be collected from the lymph nodes, liver, kidneys, or other tissues before gastric or intestinal procedures to prevent cross-contamination. Other indications for enterotomy include removal of foreign bodies and luminal examination.

Exteriorize and isolate the diseased or desired intestine from the abdomen by packing with towels or laparotomy sponges. Gently milk chyme (intestinal contents) from the lumen of the identified intestinal segment. To minimize spillage of chyme, occlude the lumen at both ends of the isolated segment by having an assistant use a scissorlike grip with the index and middle fingers 4 to 6 cm on each side of the proposed enter-otomy site (Fig. 19-83, A). If an assistant is not available, use noncrushing intestinal forceps (Doyen) or a Penrose drain tourniquet to occlude the intestinal lumen. Make a full-thickness stab incision into the intestinal lumen on the antimesenteric border with a No. 11 scalpel blade. Obtain full-thickness biopsy samples 4 to 5 mm wide, either by mak-ing a second longitudinal incision parallel to the first with the scalpel blade or by removing an ellipse of intestinal wall at one margin of the first incision with Metzenbaum scissors (Figs. 19-83, B and C).

Transverse enterotomy incisions can be made or a skin biopsy punch used to obtain biopsies.

Place the biopsy serosal side down on a heavy piece of sterile paper to help prevent curling of the specimen. Close

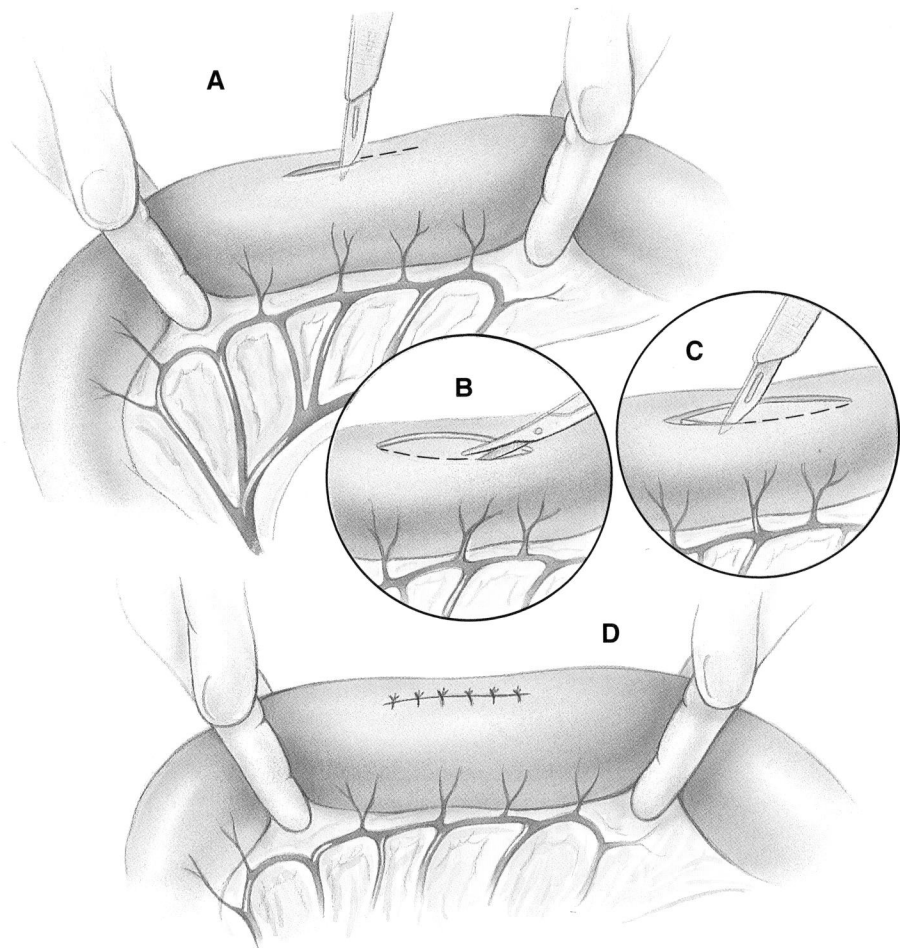

FIG. 19-83
Intestinal biopsy. **A,** Occlude the lumen then make a stab incision into the lumen with a No. 11 blade. **B,** Remove a 2- to 3-mm ellipse of tissue with Metzenbaum scissors, or **(C)** make a second incision approximately parallel to the first with a scalpel. **D,** Close the incision with simple interrupted sutures.

the incision as described below with simple interrupted sutures (Fig. 19-83, D).

Simple continuous or crushing sutures may also be used to close the enterotomy. Successful use of skin staples has also been described for intestinal closure.

If a foreign body is present, make the incision in healthy-appearing tissue distal to the foreign body (Fig. 19-84). Lengthen the incision along the intestine's long axis with Metzenbaum scissors or scalpel as necessary to allow removal of the foreign body without tearing the intestine.

After biopsy or removal of the foreign body, prepare the incision for closure by trimming everted mucosa so that its edge is even with the serosal edge (if necessary). Suction the isolated lumen. Close the incision with gentle apposi-tional force in a longitudinal or transverse direction using simple interrupted sutures (Fig. 19-85). Place sutures through all layers of the intestinal wall 2 mm from the edge and 2 to 3 mm apart with extraluminal knots. Angle the

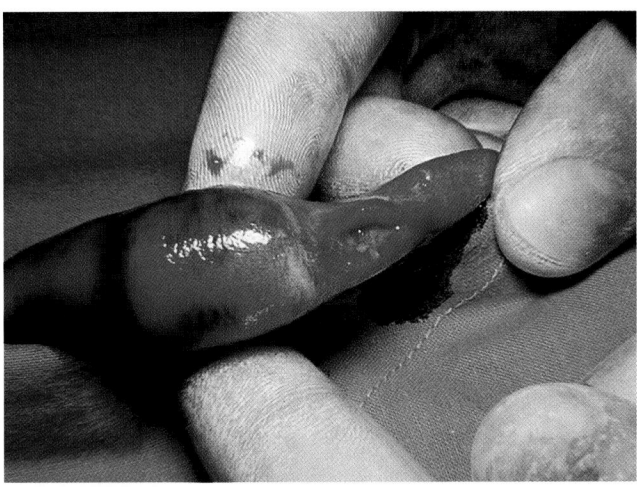

FIG. 19-84
Intestinal segment with a foreign body that was removed via an enterotomy. Note the dilated proximal intestine with some ischemic areas. The incision was made in the healthier distal intestine.

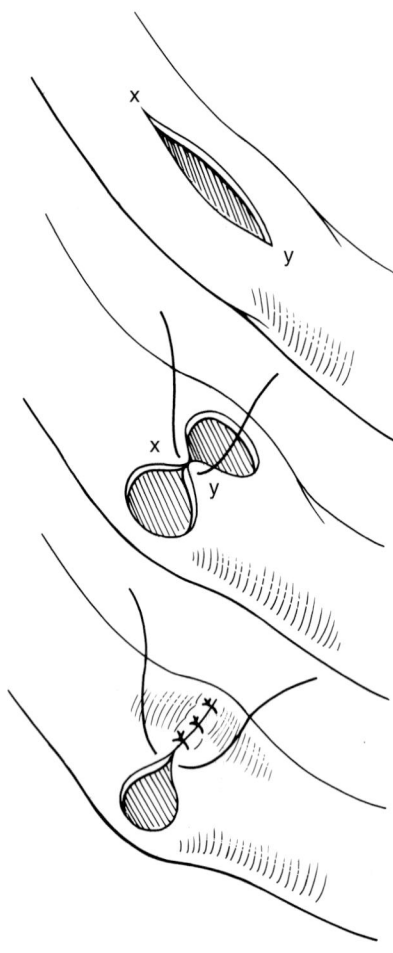

FIG. 19-85
Enterotomy incisions may be closed transversely if the intestinal lumen is small. Join the extremes (*x* and *y*) of the longitudinal incision with a simple interrupted suture to transpose the incision to a transverse orientation. Place remaining sutures 2 to 3 mm apart.

needle so that the serosa is engaged slightly farther from the edge than the mucosa (Fig. 19-86) to help reposition everting mucosa within the lumen. Tie each suture carefully without cutting through layers of the intestinal wall to gently appose all intestinal layers without crushing the tissue. Use a monofilament, absorbable suture material (4-0 or 3-0 polydioxanone, polyglyconate, or poliglecaprone 25) with a swaged-on taper or tapercut point needle. Consider a monofilament, nonabsorbable suture (4-0 or 3-0 polypropylene, nylon, or polybutester) if the patient has an albumin level of 2 g/dl or lower. While maintaining luminal occlusion near the enterotomy site, moderately distend the lumen with sterile saline, apply gentle digital pressure, and observe for leakage between sutures or through needle holes. Place additional sutures if leakage occurs between sutures. Lavage the isolated intestine and the entire abdomen if contamination has occurred. Place omentum over the suture line before closing the abdomen. Use a serosal patch (see p. 457) rather than omentum if intestinal integrity is questionable or if leakage occurs from needle holes.

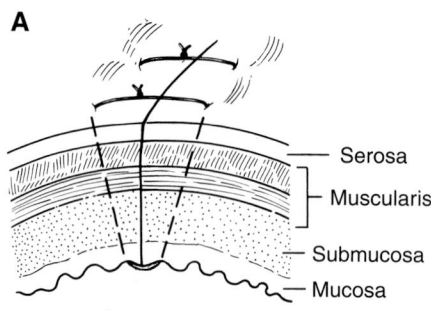

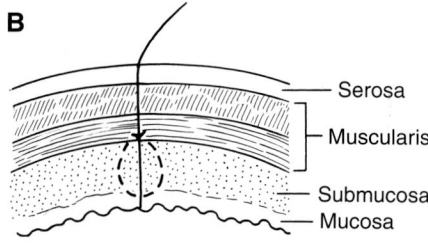

FIG. 19-86
A, For an approximating suture closure of the intestine, place simple interrupted sutures 2 mm from the edge and 2 to 3 mm apart. Engage slightly more serosa than mucosa to force everted mucosa back into the lumen. **B,** Place crushing sutures similarly, but pull them tight to cut through all layers except the submucosa when tying.

Replace contaminated instruments and gloves before closing the abdomen.

Intestinal Resection and Anastomosis

Intestinal resection and anastomosis is recommended for removing ischemic, necrotic, neoplastic, or fungus-infected segments of intestine. Irreducible intussusceptions are also managed by resection and anastomosis. End-to-end anastomoses are recommended.

Sutured anastomoses. *Make an abdominal incision long enough to allow exploration of the abdomen. Thoroughly explore the abdomen and collect any nonintestinal specimens; then exteriorize and isolate the diseased intestine from the abdomen by packing with towels or laparotomy sponges. Assess intestinal viability and determine the amount of intestine needing resection. Occlude (double ligate, staple, or heat seal) and transect the arcadial mesenteric vessels from the cranial mesenteric artery that supplies this segment of intestine (Fig. 19-87). Occlude (double ligate, staple, or heat seal) the terminal arcade vessels and vasa recta vessels within the mesenteric fat at the points of proposed intestinal transection. Gently milk chyme (intestinal contents) from the lumen of the identified intestinal segment. Use fingers or intestinal forceps to occlude the lumen at both ends of the segment to minimize spillage of chyme (see previous discussion). Place forceps across each end of the diseased bowel segment (these forceps may be either crushing or noncrushing because this segment of the intestine will be excised). Transect the intestine with either a scalpel blade or Metzen-*

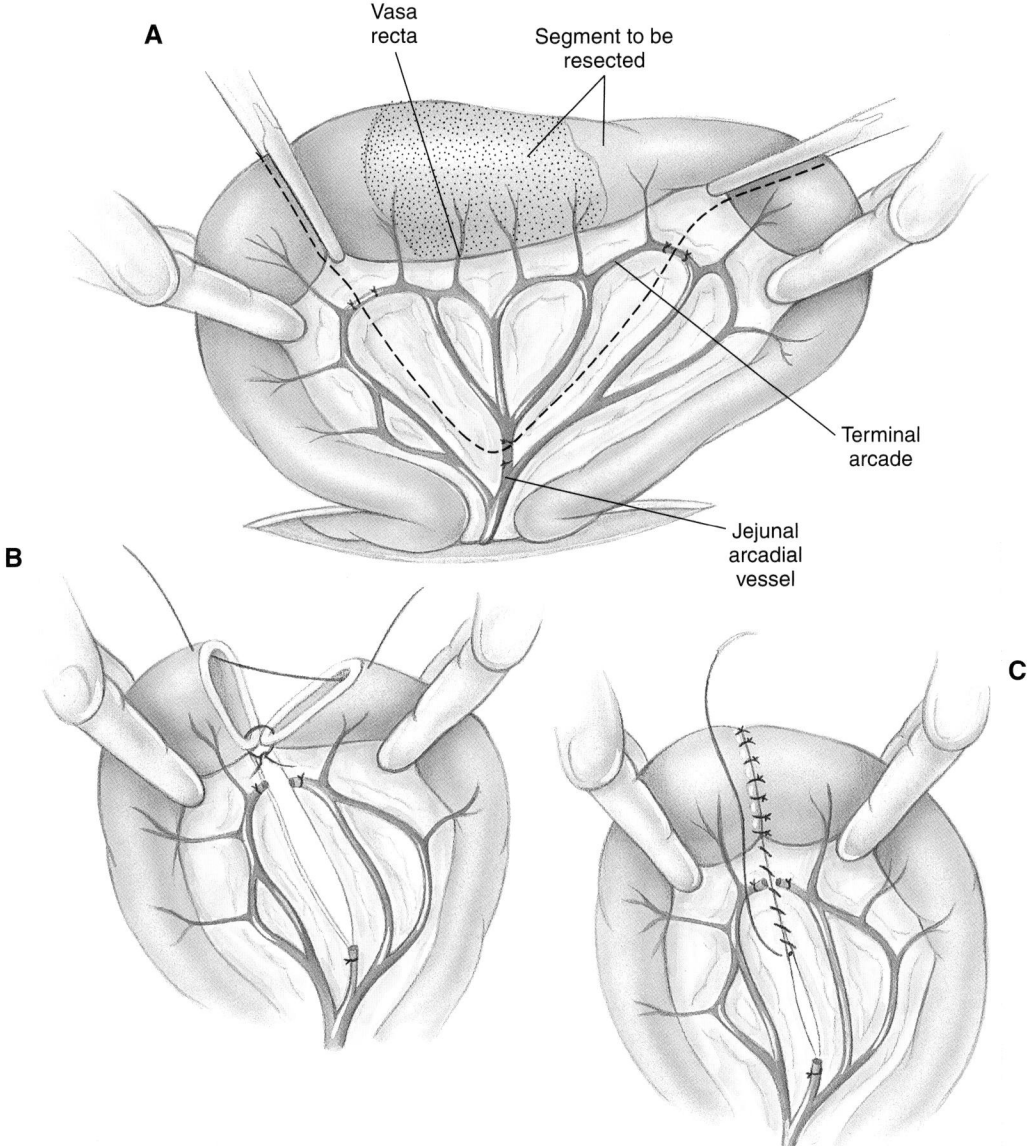

Vasa recta

Segment to be resected

Terminal arcade

Jejunal arcadial vessel

A

B

C

FIG. 19-87
For small intestinal resection and anastomosis, place forceps transversely across the dilated proximal intestine and obliquely across the distal intestine **(A).** Ligate vessels as indicated. Occlude the lumen of the normal intestine, then transect the intestine and mesentery where the dashed lines indicate. **B,** Place the first suture at the mesenteric border and the second at the antimesenteric border. **C,** Place additional simple interrupted sutures to complete the anastomosis. Appose the mesentery in a simple continuous pattern.

baum scissors along the outside of the forceps. Make the incision either perpendicular or oblique to the long axis. Use a perpendicular incision (75- to 90-degree angle) at each end if the luminal diameters are the same. When the luminal sizes of the intestinal ends are expected to be unequal, use a perpendicular incision across the intestine with the larger luminal diameter and an oblique incision (45- to 60-degree angle) across the intestine with the smaller luminal diameter to help correct size disparity (Fig. 19-88). Make the oblique incision such that the antimesenteric border is shorter than the mesenteric border. If further correction for size disparity is needed, space sutures around the larger lumen slightly

farther apart than around the smaller lumen or remove a wedge from the antimesenteric border of the smaller segment (Fig. 19-89). Suction the intestinal ends and remove any debris clinging to the cut edges with a moistened gauze sponge. Trim everting mucosa with Metzenbaum scissors just before beginning the end-to-end anastomosis.

Use 3-0 or 4-0 monofilament, absorbable suture (polydioxanone, polyglyconate, or poliglecaprone 25) with a swaged-on taper or tapercut point needle. In peritonitis cases, monofilament, nonabsorbable suture (3-0 or 4-0 polypropylene, polybutester, or nylon) is sometimes used. Place simple interrupted sutures through all layers of the intestinal wall. Angle

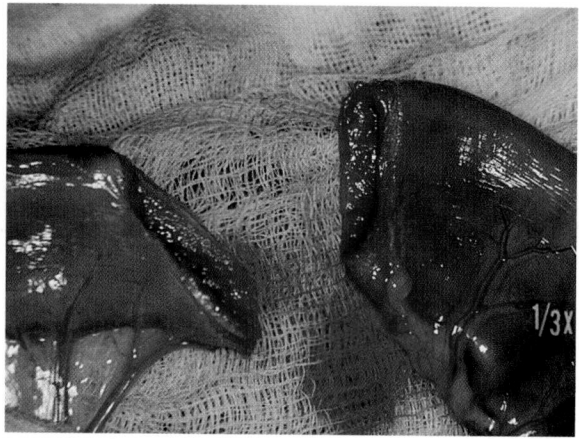

FIG. 19-88
To perform an end-to-end anastomosis when the intestinal segments are of disparate size, transect the dilated intestine at a right angle and the smaller segment at an oblique angle (45 to 60 degrees).

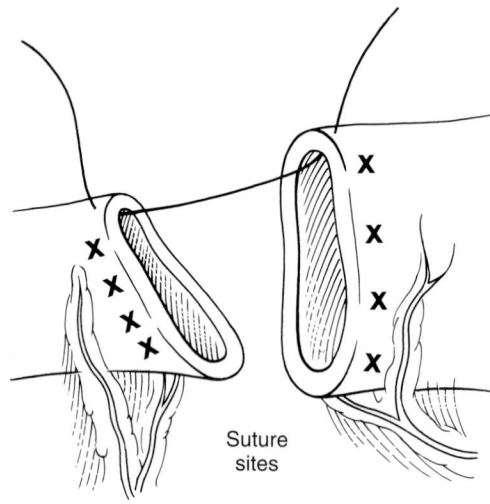

FIG. 19-89
In addition to angling the incisions (see Fig. 19-88), further correct for size disparity by spacing sutures around the larger lumen slightly farther apart than around the smaller lumen.

the needle so that the serosa is engaged slightly farther from the edge than the mucosa (see Fig. 19-86, A). This helps reposition everting mucosa within the lumen. Tie each suture carefully to gently appose the edges of the intestine with the knots positioned extraluminally.

Tying sutures roughly or with too much tension causes the suture to cut through the serosa, muscularis, and mucosa, creating a crushing suture (see Fig. 19-86, *B*). Some surgeons prefer this suture, but most prefer a simple interrupted or simple continuous pattern. Pulling continuous sutures too tight has a purse-string effect, and significant stenosis may occur. A continuous pattern around the intestine may limit dilation at the anastomotic site and cause a partial obstruc-

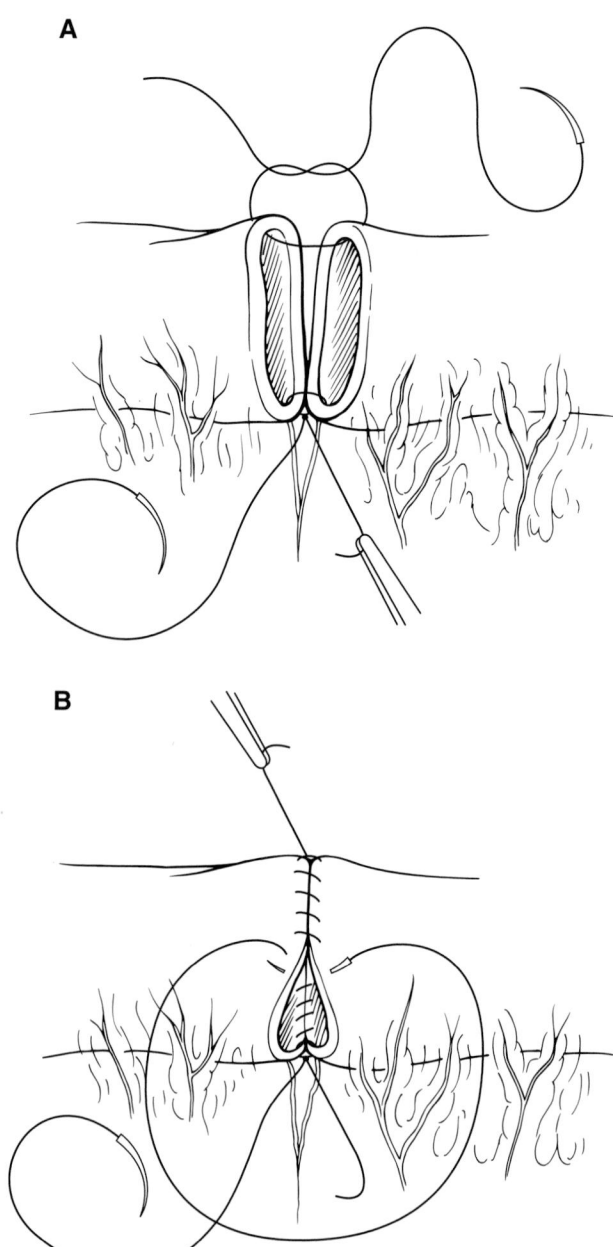

FIG. 19-90
End-to-end anastomosis using a modified simple continuous pattern. **A,** Place and tie appositional sutures at the mesenteric and antimesenteric borders, leaving the needles attached. **B,** Using the suture tags as stay sutures to maintain tension, place a continuous suture pattern between the antimesenteric and mesenteric sutures. Reposition the intestine and begin a second continuous suture line on the opposite side.

tion. Therefore a divided, modified simple continuous suture pattern is used to prevent these effects (Fig. 19-90) (Weisman et al, 1999). Two stay sutures are placed at the mesenteric and antimesenteric borders, then one simple continuous suture is placed between the sutures on each side. Experimentally, skin staplers have been used successfully in lieu of interrupted sutures (Coolman et al, 2000).

Appose the intestinal ends by first placing a simple interrupted suture at the mesenteric border (see Fig. 19-87) and then placing a second suture at the antimesenteric border approximately 180 degrees from the first (this divides the suture line into equal halves and allows determination of whether the ends are of approximately equal diameter).

The mesenteric suture is the most difficult suture to place in the anastomosis because of mesenteric fat. It is also the most common site of leakage.

If the ends are of equal diameter, space additional sutures between the first two sutures approximately 2 mm from the edge and 2 to 3 mm apart (see Fig. 19-87, C). If minor disparity still exists between lumen sizes, space the sutures around the larger lumen slightly farther apart than the sutures in the intestine with the smaller lumen (see Fig. 19-89). To correct luminal disparity that cannot be accommodated by the angle of the incisions or by suture spacing, resect a small wedge (1 to 2 cm long and 1 to 3 mm wide) from the antimesenteric border of the intestine with the smaller lumen (Fig. 19-91). This enlarges the perimeter of the stoma, giving it an oval shape. Do not suture together the edges of the intestine with the larger lumen in an attempt to reduce luminal size to that of the smaller intestine.

Narrowing the larger lumen is not recommended because there is greater tendency for stricture at the anastomotic site when the dilated intestine contracts to a normal size.

After suture placement, inspect the anastomosis and check for leakage. While maintaining luminal occlusion adjacent to the anastomotic site, moderately distend the lumen with sterile saline, apply gentle digital pressure, and observe for leakage between sutures or through needle holes.

This is a subjective test because all anastomoses can be made to leak if enough pressure is applied.

Place additional sutures if leakage occurs between sutures. Close the mesenteric defect in a simple continuous or interrupted pattern using 4-0 monofilament absorbable suture, taking care not to penetrate or traumatize arcadial vessels near the defect. Lavage the isolated intestine and the entire abdomen if abdominal contamination has occurred. Wrap the anastomotic site with omentum before closing the abdomen or use a serosal patch (see p. 457) if intestinal integrity is questionable and leakage is likely.

Stapled anastomoses. Resection may also be accomplished with staples. Three stapled anastomotic techniques are available: (1) triangulating end-to-end, (2) inverting end-to-end, and (3) side-to-side or functional end-to-end anastomoses. The small size of the intestine (less than 20 mm) often precludes the use of everting triangulating and inverting stapling techniques. A functional end-to-end anastomosis creates a larger stoma than the original intesti-

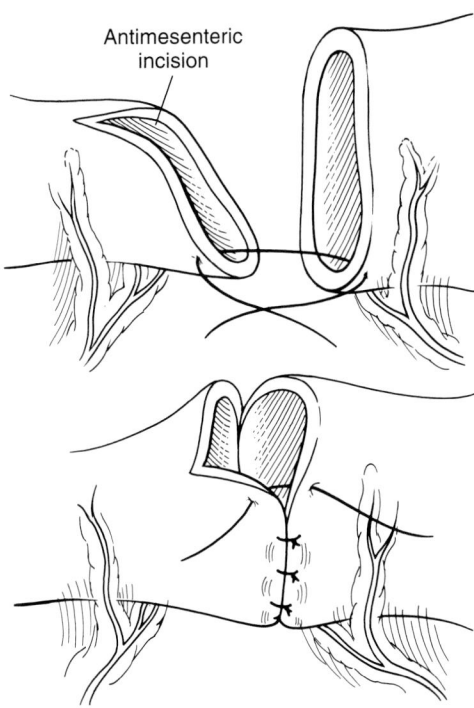

Antimesenteric incision

FIG. 19-91
If incision angling and suture spacing do not totally accommodate the luminal size differences, remove a wedge from the antimesenteric border of the distal intestine.

nal lumen and is the preferred technique because the other two stapling techniques may reduce the size of the lumen. Stapled anastomoses have a higher tensile strength than sutured anastomoses after 7 days. They heal by primary intention with minimal inflammation. Thick, inflamed, and edematous tissue may prevent proper firing of the stapler by preventing complete penetration and formation of the staples into a B-shaped configuration. Dilation causes thinning of the visceral walls and may make tissue too thin for the staples to be effective.

> NOTE: Staple cartridges are expensive; weigh the cost against the value of your time and the patient's condition when determining which technique to use.

A triangulating end-to-end anastomosis is performed with a transverse (TA) stapling instrument or a disposable skin stapler. This technique is very expensive as it requires three staple cartridges. The skin stapler is more economical and allows rapid application of individual 4.8 mm × 3.4 mm rectangular staples (Coolman et al, 2000 a and b).

Remove the diseased intestine, then place three stay sutures to divide the stoma into three equal segments and appose the divided intestinal ends. Apply the TA stapler across each segment, partly overlapping the previous staple line (Fig. 19-92). Trim protruding tissue before removing the instrument.

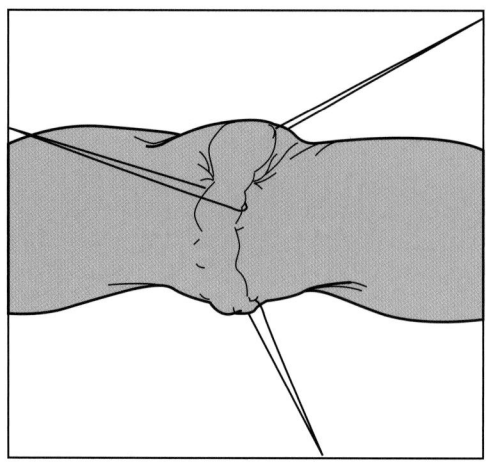

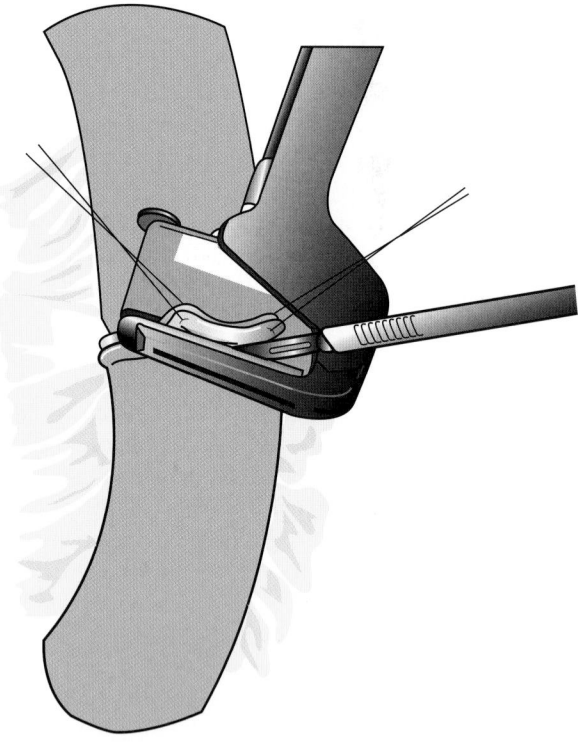

FIG. 19-92
End-to-end anastomosis using a triangulation technique and linear stapler. Place three stay sutures, which appose the ends of the intestine and divide the circumference into three equal parts *(inset)*. Apply tension between two of the sutures, and fire the stapler, leaving a double staggered row of sutures. Trim protruding tissue before removing the stapler. Apply tension between the next two sutures, and position the stapler so it overlies the end of the first row of staples and fire again. These steps are repeated a third time to complete the anastomosis.

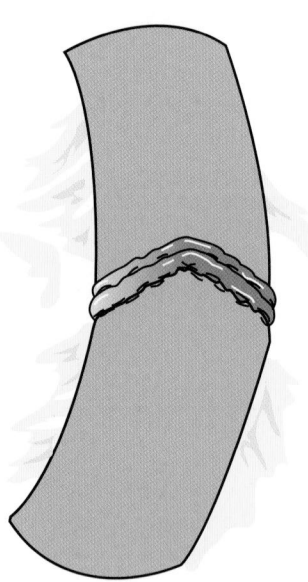

Each application of the stapler applies a double staggered row of staples. This technique everts the edges.

Inspect the anastomosis for leakage and lavage. Appose the mesentery in a continuous suture pattern.

Using the disposable skin stapler, apply tension between two of the triangulation sutures to appose the serosa and compress the mucosa into the lumen with a moistened sponge. Then position the center of the stapler over the junction of the two edges, apply firm pressure, and fire the instrument (Fig 19-93). Space staples 2 to 3 mm apart between the triangulation sutures. Edges of the intestinal wall will be slightly everted.

An end-to-end anastomosis is performed using a circular, inverting, end-to-end anastomosis stapler (EEA, Premium CEEA, or ILP staplers). These instruments consist of a staple cartridge with a circular blade attached to a dome-shaped anvil and rod (Fig. 19-94). They are available in several sizes that create anastomotic stomas approximately 10 mm smaller than their cartridge size (EEA, 31 mm, 28 mm, 25 mm, and 21 mm; ILP, 33 mm, 29 mm, 25 mm, and 21 mm). The intestinal lumen should be 0.6 mm larger in diameter than the stapler. Activation applies a circular double row of staples and simultaneously resects a doughnut of intestinal wall at the anastomotic site. End-to-end staplers are used less often

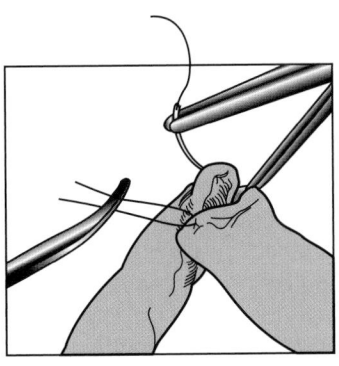
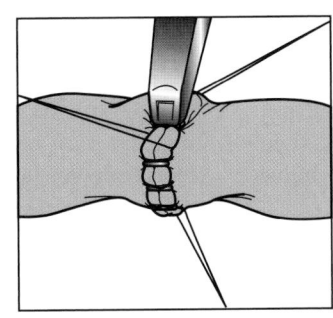
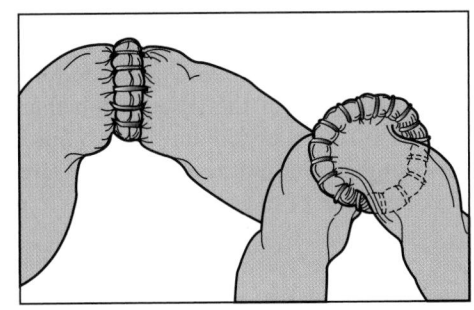

FIG. 19-93
End-to-end anastomosis using a triangulation technique and a skin stapler. Place three stay sutures to appose the ends of the intestine and divide the circumference into three equal parts. Apply tension between two sutures. Center the skin stapler between the two segments, then apply staples with gentle pressure approximately 2 to 3 mm apart. Apposed edges of the intestinal wall be slightly eveced.

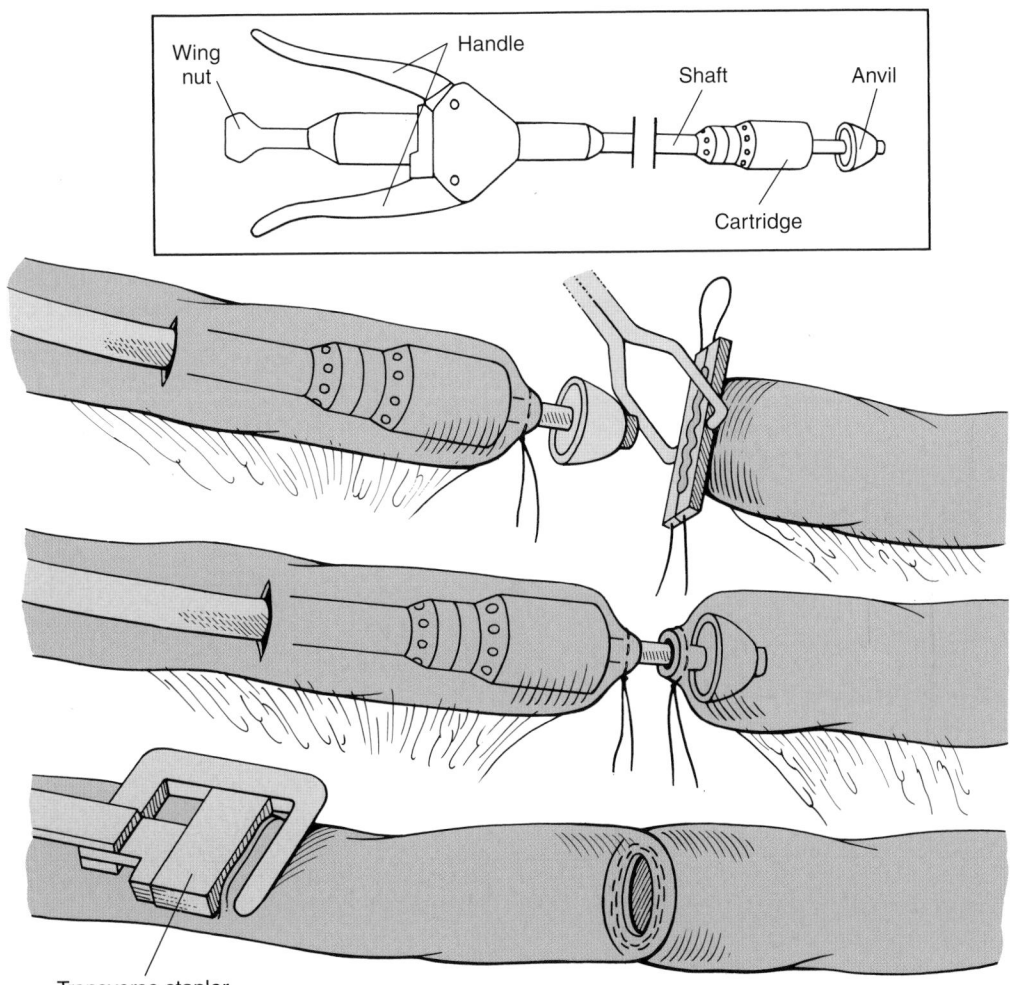

FIG. 19-94
For an inverting end-to-end anastomosis, use an EEA stapler and a transverse stapler. Insert the stapler cartridge into the intestinal lumen through an enterotomy 3 to 4 cm from the transection site. Insert the anvil into the other intestinal end. Tie purse-string sutures securely around the shaft of the stapler. After completing the anastomosis, close the enterotomy with sutures or a transverse stapler.

in the small intestine than in other areas of the gastrointestinal tract because of the small lumen size of the small intestine. End-to-end staplers are commonly used during Billroth I, esophageal, and large bowel anastomotic procedures. Do not use the stapler if the tissue is too thick (i.e., will not compress to 2 mm) or too thin (i.e., compresses to less than 2 mm) and only if sufficient tissue is available to allow proper inversion of tissue edges.

Ligate and divide vessels to the diseased intestine as usual. Dissect the mesentery away from each intestinal segment (31-mm cartridge, 1.5 cm; 28-mm cartridge, 1 cm; 25- or 21-mm cartridge, 0.5 cm) because these tissues or ligatures may interfere with closing of the instrument. Place the purse-string instrument around the proximal intestine at the point of desired transection. Place the purse-string suture and transect the intestine using the purse-string instrument as the cutting guide. Place a purse-string suture and make the distal transection using the same technique. Insert a lubricated ovoid sizer through an enterotomy to determine the appropriate staple cartridge size and to dilate the intestine. Insert the stapler cartridge into the intestinal lumen through an enterotomy 3 to 4 cm from the transection site.

Insert the anvil into the other intestinal end. Facilitate placement by placing three or four stay sutures at the edge of the intestine. Using the stay sutures, first pull the mesenteric border of the intestine over the anvil and then over the antimesenteric border. If it appears that the lumen of the intestine will not easily accommodate the anvil or the sizer of the desired diameter, insert a well-lubricated, 26 to 30 French Foley catheter

with a 30-ml balloon. Slowly inflate the balloon with sterile water to dilate the intestine adequately. After dilation, insert the stapler components. Tie both purse-string sutures securely around the shaft of the stapler (see Fig. 19-94). Twist the wing nut to compress the intestinal segments between the cartridge and the anvil until the unit is aligned. Examine the anastomotic site for evidence of intestinal slippage. Release the safety and activate the instrument by squeezing the handles. Partly separate the anvil and cartridge by loosening the wing nut and remove the stapling instrument. Facilitate removal of the instrument by placing a traction suture around the staple line and lift the edge of the staple line over the anvil while gently rotating the instrument. Inspect the severed, inverted intestinal segment; to prevent leakage, make sure all tissue layers are present. Inspect the anastomotic site for hemorrhage and integrity. Close the enterotomy with sutures or a transverse stapler. Close the mesenteric defect in a continuous pattern. Lavage the surgical site and place an omental or a serosal patch (see p. 457) before closing the abdomen.

A side-to-side anastomosis or a functional end-to-end anastomosis is created using a linear cutting stapler (GIA stapler) and a transverse anastomotic stapler (TA or RU 60). This is the preferred technique for small intestinal anastomosis because the resulting stoma is larger than the original, and disparity in luminal size is easily accommodated.

Resect diseased intestine and use the linear cutting stapler to join the bowel segments at their antimesenteric borders, creating an antiperistaltic side-to-side anastomosis. Fully insert

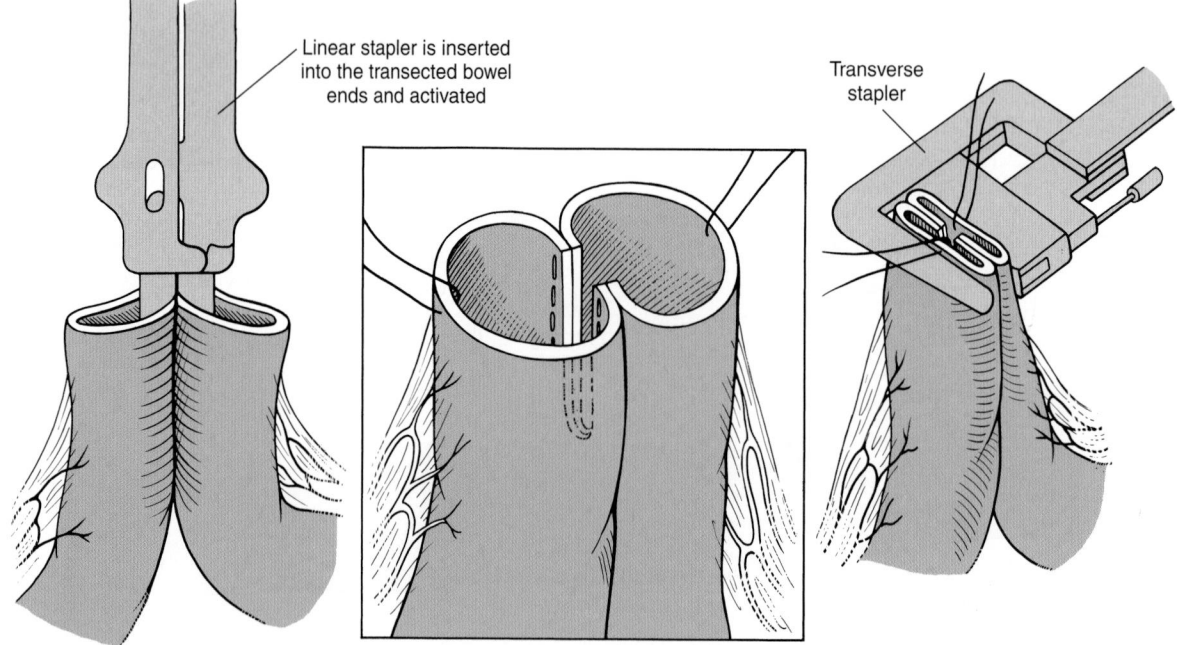

Linear stapler is inserted into the transected bowel ends and activated

Transverse stapler

FIG. 19-95
For a functional end-to-end anastomosis, use a linear cutting stapler and a transverse stapler. Fully insert (50 mm) the linear cutting stapler into the stomas of each intestinal loop and activate it. Separate the stapled suture line and apply the transverse stapling instrument to close the anastomosis.

(50 mm) the linear cutting stapler into the stomas of each intestinal loop and activate it (Fig. 19-95).

Activation results in the placement of two double staggered staple lines that join the intestinal loops as the knife simultaneously incises between them.

Separate the stapled suture line and apply the transverse stapling instrument to close the anastomosis. The transverse stapler places a double staggered row of staples but has no cutting action. Transect protruding intestinal wall flush with the stapler. Remove the stapler and place an anchoring suture at the base of the staple line, where tension is greatest, to discourage staple pullout. Close the mesenteric defect in a continuous pattern before lavaging, patching, and closing the abdomen.

A similar stapling method, the closed, one-stage functional end-to-end anastomosis, involves creating the side-to-side anastomosis with the linear cutting stapler by inserting it through small antimesenteric stab incisions before resection of the diseased bowel.

Transect the diseased bowel after application of the transverse stapler.

Serosal Patching

Serosal patching consists of putting the antimesenteric border of a loop of small intestine over a suture line or organ defect and securing it with sutures (Fig. 19-96). Serosal patching provides support, a fibrin seal, increased resistance to leakage, and blood supply to the damaged area plus it may prevent intussusception. Patches are commonly used after intestinal surgery when closure integrity is questioned or when dehiscence is repaired. Patches that span visceral defects are covered with mucosal epithelium within 8 weeks. Most commonly, jejunum adjacent to the defect or area of questionable viability is used for the serosal patch. Other

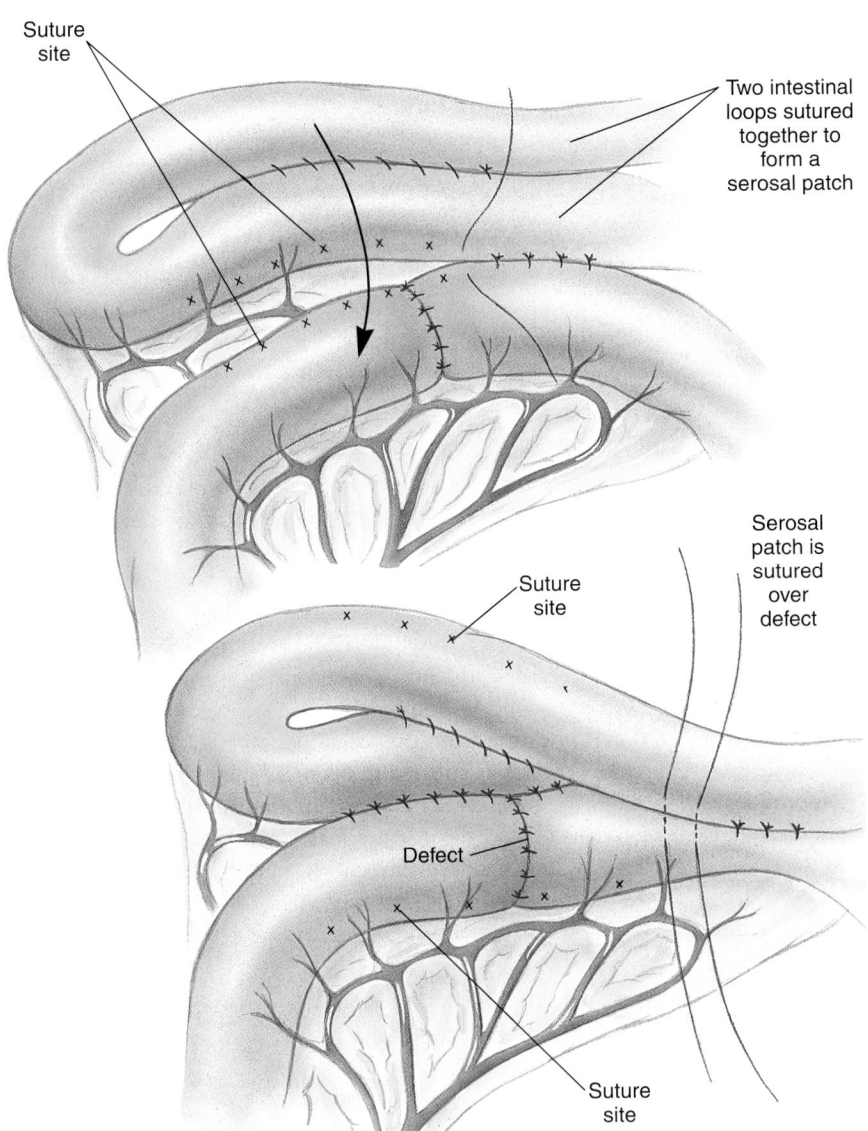

FIG. 19-96
Create a serosal patch by suturing adjacent intestinal loops together with simple continuous or interrupted sutures. Suture the patch over the defect or suture line.

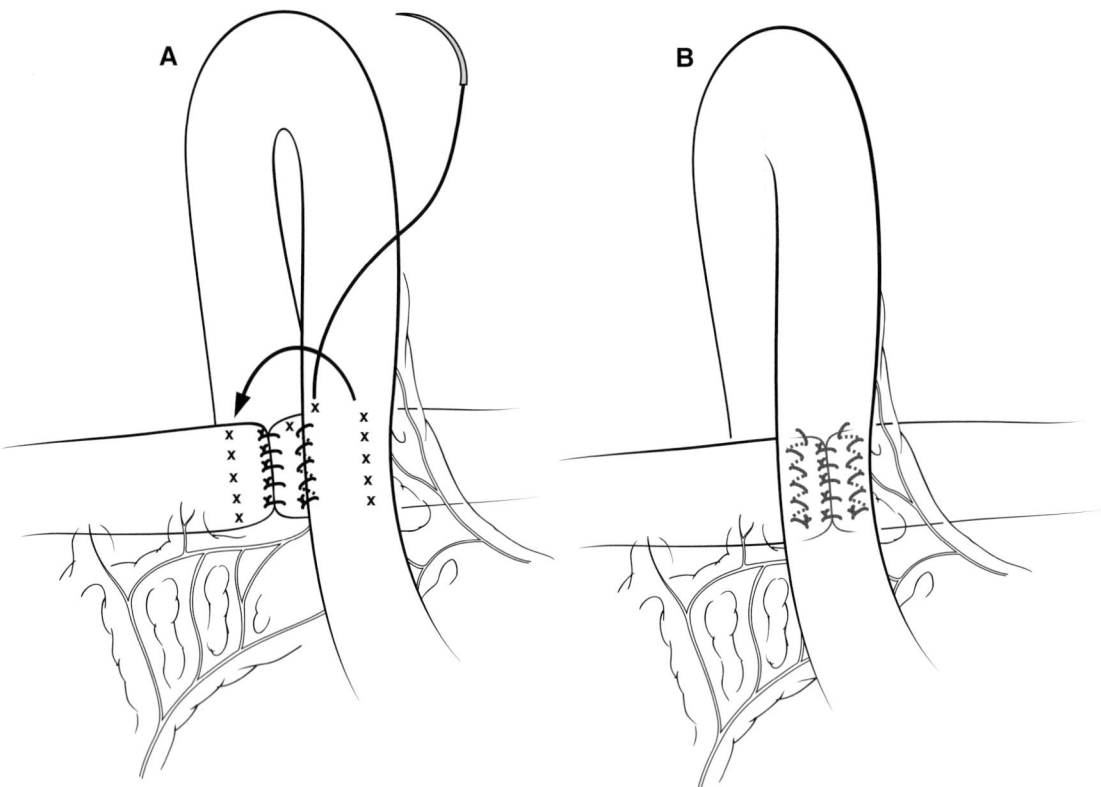

FIG. 19-97
To patch over an anastomosis, **(A)** use a piece of normal intestine and loop it perpendicular to the area to be patched. Be sure that the loop is gentle so as not to cause obstruction. Using a simple continuous suture pattern, suture between the looped piece of normal intestine starting at the mesenteric border and continuing up to the antimesenteric border. **B,** Then suture across the anastomosis and back down to the mesenteric border on the same side. Repeat the process on the opposite side of the anastomosis. Be careful not to compromise the vasculature at the mesenteric border with your sutures.

sources could include the stomach, other intestinal segments, or the urinary bladder.

Use one or more loops of intestine to form the patch. Use gentle loops to avoid stretching, twisting, or kinking the intestine and mesenteric vessels. If using more than one loop of intestine, suture these loops together before securing the patch to the damaged area (see Fig. 19-96).

Place interrupted or continuous sutures in healthy tissue to secure the patch and isolate the damaged area. All sutures used to create or secure the patch engage the submucosa, muscularis, and serosa; they should not penetrate the intestinal lumen.

Alternatively, to patch over an anastomosis, use a piece of normal intestine and loop it perpendicular to the area to be patched (Fig. 19-97, A). Be sure that the loop is gentle so as not to cause obstruction. Using a simple continuous suture pattern, suture between the looped piece of normal intestine starting at the mesenteric border and continuing up to the antimesenteric border. Then suture across the anastomosis and back down to the mesenteric border on

the same side (Fig 19-97, B). Repeat the process on the opposite side of the anastomosis. Be careful not to compromise the vasculature at the mesenteric border with your sutures.

Bowel Plication

Enteroenteropexy, or bowel plication, is performed to prevent recurrence of intussusception. Suturing together adjacent loops of intestine forms serosa-to-serosa adhesions. The small intestine from the duodenocolic ligament to the ileocolic junction is sutured to decrease the potential for intestinal strangulation. The bends in the intestine are gentle to prevent obstruction, and plication sutures are placed at intervals that will prevent entrapment and strangulation of other intestinal segments.

NOTE: Although one study suggested that enteroplication was not helpful in preventing recurrence, it is our belief that this technique is an important tool for preventing reintussusception. It must, however, be performed properly to prevent complications (see p. 474).

Place small intestinal loops side by side to form a series of gentle loops from the distal duodenum to the distal ileum. Secure the loops by placing sutures that engage the submucosa, muscularis, and serosa 6 to 10 cm apart. Use 3-0 or 4-0 monofilament, absorbable or nonabsorbable sutures with a swaged-on taper point needle. Avoid positioning the intestinal loops at acute angles, or intestinal obstruction may occur. Entering the lumen with pexy sutures may increase the risk of leakage and abdominal contamination.

HEALING OF THE SMALL INTESTINE

Optimal intestinal healing depends on a good blood supply, accurate mucosal apposition, and minimal surgical trauma. Approximating suture patterns facilitate rapid healing. Everting and inverting suture patterns retard intestinal healing and may cause greater stricture formation. Healing is facilitated by adjacent serosal surfaces and omentum, which help seal wounds and contribute to the blood supply. The intestine generally heals rapidly, but healing can be delayed by local and systemic factors. Systemic factors such as hypovolemia, shock, hypoproteinemia, debilitation, and concurrent infections may delay healing and increase the risk of incisional breakdown. Tension on the repair caused by accumulated ingesta, fluid, gas, or poor mobilization of the bowel increases the risk of intestinal suture breakdown. Serosal and peritoneal adhesions occur as a result of trauma from excess handling or rough technique, foreign material, and drying during surgery. Administration of corticosteroids or nonsteroidal antiinflammatory drugs can inhibit the housekeeping prostaglandins and may render the gastrointestinal tract more susceptible to injury.

The three overlapping phases of healing are the lag phase, the proliferative phase, and the maturation phase. The *lag phase* occurs during days 0 to 4 and is associated with inflammation and edema of the healing intestine. A fibrin seal forms during the first few hours. Although the fibrin clot contributes to wound strength, during this phase most of the wound strength is attributed to sutures. During the lag phase, macrophages are important in wound débridement and the production of growth factors that modulate fibroplasia and angiogenesis (transforming growth factor-β, platelet-derived growth factor, epidermal growth factor, cytokines). Healing is functionally weakest at the end of the lag phase because of fibrinolysis and collagen deposition, therefore dehiscence most commonly occurs 3 to 5 days after intestinal surgery. Inflammation is more severe and healing time is slower with inverting patterns than with approximating patterns. Everted intestinal anastomoses have reduced tensile and bursting strength during the lag phase and therefore have a greater tendency to leak. The *proliferative phase* occurs between days 3 and 14. Fibrous repair occurs, accompanied by a rapid gain in wound strength. The strength of the repair site approximates that of normal intestine 10 to 17 days after surgery. The *maturation phase* occurs between 10 and 180 days. Collagen is reorganized and remodeled during this phase.

SUTURE MATERIALS AND SPECIAL INSTRUMENTS

Instruments recommended to facilitate intestinal surgery include self-retaining abdominal retractors, malleable retractors, Doyen noncrushing forceps, Babcock forceps, Metzenbaum scissors, No. 11 scalpel blade, Penrose drains, and suction. Although most absorbable suture materials can be used, 3-0 or 4-0 monofilament polydioxanone, polyglyconate, or poliglecaprone 25 is preferred. Long-lasting monofilament, absorbable suture (polydioxanone, polyglyconate, poliglecaprone 25, glycomer 631) or nonabsorbable suture (nylon, polybutester, or polypropylene) should be selected for patients with low albumin levels. Patching techniques should also be considered in these patients to reinforce and facilitate healing of the surgical site. As an alternative, surgical stapling equipment can be used for some procedures (i.e., transverse stapling instrument, EEA stapler, linear stapler, ligate-and-divide instrument, and skin stapler). Other instruments useful for diagnosis of digestive disorders are Westcott biopsy needles and Bard Biopty-Cut needles.

POSTOPERATIVE CARE AND ASSESSMENT

Postoperative care must be individualized to each patient and its problems. The animal should be monitored closely for vomiting during recovery. Analgesics (i.e., hydromorphone, butorphanol, or buprenorphine; see Table 13-4 on p. 133) should be provided as needed. Hydration should be maintained with intravenous fluids, and electrolyte and acid-base abnormalities monitored and corrected. Small amounts of water may be offered 8 to 12 hours after surgery. If no vomiting occurs, small amounts of food may be offered 12 to 24 hours after surgery. Early feeding is important as it preserves or increases gastrointestinal blood flow, prevents ulceration, increases IgA concentrations, stimulates other immune system defenses, and stimulates wound repair (Ralphs et al, 2003). Animals should be fed a bland, low-fat food (e.g., i/d [Hill's Pet Products] or boiled rice, potatoes, and pasta combined with boiled, skinless chicken, yogurt, or low-fat cottage cheese) three or four times daily. The normal diet should be reintroduced gradually, beginning 48 to 72 hours after surgery. Debilitated patients may require feeding tubes or parenteral nutrition. Antibiotics should be discontinued within 2 to 6 hours of surgery unless peritonitis is suspected. Early ambulation and feeding should be encouraged to minimize ileus.

After intestinal surgery, clinical signs (e.g., depression, high fever, excessive abdominal tenderness, vomiting, and/or ileus) and response to abdominal palpation should be monitored for evidence of leakage and subsequent peritonitis or abscess formation. If peritonitis is suspected, an abdominocentesis, chemistry profile, and CBC should be performed. Abdominal fluid should be submitted for culture and sensitivity testing, and antibiotics (e.g., cefazolin, cefmetazole, cefoxitin, enrofloxacin plus ampicillin, clindamycin plus enrofloxacin, and ticarcillin plus clavulanic acid; Box 19-46) and fluid therapy should be initiated. Continuation of anti-

BOX 19-46

Antibiotic Therapy for Treatment of Postoperative Peritonitis

Cefazolin (Ancef, Kefzol)

22 mg/kg IV, tid

Cefmetazole (Zefazone)

15 mg/kg IV, tid-qid

Cefoxitin (Mefoxin)

30–40 mg/kg IV, qid

Enrofloxacin (Baytril)

10–20 mg/kg IV, qd; give diluted in IV fluids slowly over 30 minutes

Ampicillin

22 mg/kg IV or IM, tid to qid

Amikacin (Amiglyde-V)

20–25 mg/kg IV, qd

Clindamycin (Anterobe)

11 mg/kg PO or IV, tid

Ticarcillin Plus Clavulanic Acid (Timentin)

50 mg/kg IV, tid to qid

IV, Intravenous; *IM,* intramuscular; *qd,* once a day; *bid,* twice a day; *tid,* three times a day; *qid,* four times a day.

 BOX 19-47

Perioperative Factors Contributing to the Risk of Leakage or Dehiscence

Peritonitis
Intestinal foreign body
Hypoalbuminemia less than 2.0–2.5 g/dl
Malnutrition
Preoperative weight loss (greater than 4.5 kg in humans)
Sepsis, concurrent infection
Bowel obstruction
Increased age
Systemic disease: diabetes, heart failure, malignancy
High blood urea nitrogen
Neutrophilia
Preoperative corticosteroids
Blood transfusions
Supplemental nutrition

Poor blood supply or perfusion
Tension
Poor apposition
Sutures placed in nonviable tissue
Traumatic tissue handling
Long operative time
Contaminated or dirty surgery
Intraabdominal drains
Colonic resection
Increased anesthetic risks
Prolonged hospitalization
Emergency surgery
Hypovolemia, hypotension, shock

 BOX 19-48

Common Errors in Treating Animals With Small Intestinal Disorders

- Failure to diagnose and treat the condition before ischemia and necrosis occur
- Failure to prevent abdominal contamination
- Failure to prevent intestinal leakage
- Failure to maintain hydration and nutritional homeostasis

biotics should be based on the results of culture and susceptibility testing. The abdomen should be explored if toxic neutrophils with engulfed bacteria or intestinal debris are present. Aggressive treatment of generalized peritonitis by open peritoneal drainage may be necessary (see p. 336). The small intestinal dehiscence rate approaches 7% to 16%, with 74% to 85% of those patients dying (Ralphs et al, 2003). There is a high risk for developing leakage if two or more of the following factors are identified: preoperative peritonitis, intestinal foreign body, or serum albumin concentration less than or equal to 2.5 g/dl (Ralphs et al, 2003). Other factors may also contribute to dehiscence, especially those indicating general debility and malnourishment (Box 19-47).

COMPLICATIONS

Shock, leakage, ileus, dehiscence, perforation, peritonitis, stenosis, short bowel syndrome, recurrence, and death are possible complications of intestinal surgery (Box 19-48). Hypoalbuminemic dogs have the same postoperative complication rate as dogs with normal plasma albumin levels in some studies, but a higher risk in others. Clinically significant strictures are rare unless inverting or everting suture patterns are used or excessive tension exists at the resection site. Recurrent intestinal obstruction has been reported after using polypropylene suture in a continuous pattern for closure (Milovancev et al, 2004).

Resection of excessively long sections of bowel puts the patient at risk for short bowel syndrome (SBS). SBS has been defined many different ways. It is not simply resection of a long section of intestine; rather, it is resection of so much intestine that the body cannot compensate without parenteral/enteral nutritional therapy. There will be considerable variation between patients, but SBS usually does not occur unless more than 70% to 80% of the small intestine is resected. Weight loss, diarrhea, and malnutrition are the predominant clinical signs. Treatment is based on the severity of clinical signs and must be planned individually and modified as necessary. The goal of treatment is to provide nutritional support until intestinal adaptation occurs (1 to 2 months) and diarrhea is controlled. Acute signs should be treated by correcting hydration and electrolyte imbalances, providing adequate nutrition (i.e., enteral and/or total parenteral nutrition), and controlling diarrhea. H$_2$-antagonists (cimetidine, ranitidine, or famotidine) may be useful in reducing gastric hypersecretion, which contributes to diarrhea and damages duodenal mucosa. Opiate antidiarrheals (e.g., loperamide; Box 19-49) may help decrease intestinal secretion and augment intestinal absorption. Intestinal bacterial overgrowth should be controlled with antibiotics (e.g., tylo-

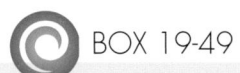 BOX 19-49

Selected Drugs Used to Treat Short Bowel Syndrome

Loperamide (Imodium)
Dogs: 0.1 mg/kg PO, bid to tid
Cats: 0.08–0.16 mg/kg PO, bid

Famotidine (Pepcid)
0.5–1.0 mg/kg PO, qd to bid

Omeprazole (Prilosec)
0.7–1.5 mg/kg PO, qd to bid

PO, Oral; *bid,* twice a day; *tid,* three times a day; *qd,* once a day.

sin and metronidazole plus enrofloxacin). Growth factors given immediately after resection of large segments of intestine may facilitate intestinal adaptation and minimize clinical signs (Johnson et al, 2000).

However, the most important aspect of treating SBS is to provide nutritional support. By definition, SBS requires more than just a highly digestible diet (e.g., i/d or k/d [Hill's Pet Products]). Enteral and parenteral nutrition are discussed in Chapter 11. Most patients with SBS will require elemental enteral diets, at least initially. It is critical that enteral nutrition be included, even if the patient requires total parenteral nutrition. The clinician must be prepared to treat for 1 to 2 months to allow the intestines to adapt. If the patient responds and is able to be taken off parenteral and elemental enteral diets, then they should be fed several times daily when traditional oral feeding begins. Daily vitamin-mineral supplements should be given. Surgical attempts to control SBS should be made only when medical and dietary therapy fails.

The prognosis for SBS depends on the extent and site of resection, the degree of intestinal adaptation, the preoperative condition, and the postoperative care, but it is guarded at best. Because of the guarded prognosis and the difficulty and cost involved, it is better to proactively try to avoid SBS. If faced with a patient with extensive disease and a potentially long section of bowel to resect, it may be preferable to resect a short section and then do a "second look" procedure 2 to 3 days later in hopes that some bowel can be preserved. Preservation of the ileocolic valve helps prevent colonic bacteria from easily gaining access to the upper small intestine.

SPECIAL AGE CONSIDERATIONS

Young animals more frequently have gastrointestinal parasitic infestations or garbage- or foreign body–induced gastroenteritis and intussusceptions. Young animals can quickly become hypothermic and hypoglycemic during surgery and require special care. Healing may be delayed in old animals because of concurrent problems.

References

Coolman BR, Ehrhart N, Pijanowski G et al: Comparison of skin staples with sutures for anastomosis of the small intestine in dogs, *Vet Surg* 29:293, 2000.

Coolman BR, Ehrhart N, Manfra Marretta S: Use of skin staples for rapid closure of gastrointestinal incisions in the treatment of canine linear foreign bodies, *J Am Anim Hosp Assoc* 36:542, 2000.

Johnson WF et al: Keratinocyte growth factor enhances early gut adaptation in a rat model of short bowel syndrome, *Vet Surg* 29:17, 2000.

Miovancev M, Weisman DL, Palmisano MP: Foreign body attachment to polypropylene suture material extruded into the small intestinal lumen after enteric closure in three dogs, *J Am Vet Med Assoc* 225:1713, 2004.

Ralphs SC, Jessen CR, Lipowitz AJ: Risk factors for leakage following intestinal anastomosis in dogs and cats: 115 cases (1991-2000), *J Am Vet Med Assoc* 223:73, 2003.

Rawlings CA, Howerth EW, Bement S et al: Laparoscopic-assisted enterostomy tube placement and full-thickness biopsy of the jejunum with serosal patching in dogs, *Am J Vet Res* 63:1313, 2002.

Weisman DL et al: Comparison of a continuous suture pattern with a simple interrupted pattern for enteric closure in dogs and cats: 83 cases (1991-1997), *J Am Vet Med Assoc* 214:1507, 1999.

Suggested Reading

Agrodnia M, Hauptman J, Walshaw R: Use of atropine to reduce mucosal eversion during intestinal resection and anastomosis in the dog, *Vet Surg* 32:365, 2003.
This two-part study showed no reduction in mucosal eversion after systemic atropine injection, whereas there was a reduction after jejunal intraarterial injection.

Bonczynski JJ, Ludwig LL, Barton LJ et al: Comparison of peritoneal fluid and peripheral blood pH, bicarbonate, glucose, and lactate concentration as a diagnostic tool for septic peritonitis in dogs and cats, *Vet Surg* 32:161, 2003.
This study evaluated parameters that may be predictive of septic peritonitis.

Coolman BR, Ehrhart N, Manfra Marretta S: Healing of intestinal anastomoses, *Compend Cont Educ Pract Vet* 22:363, 2000.
This is an up-to-date review of intestinal healing. It reviews different anastomosis methods.

Keats MM, Weeren R, Greenlee P et al: Investigation of Keyes skin biopsy instrument for intestinal biopsy versus a standard biopsy technique, *J Am Anim Hosp Assoc* 40:405, 2004.
In this prospective study using 12 dogs, there were no differences between techniques; the skin punch biopsy technique was safe, rapid, and diagnostic.

Kim JS, Jeong SW, Kim JY et al: A comparison of three suture techniques on adhesion in end-to-end intestinal anastomosis in dogs, *J Vet Clin* 20:12, 2003.
This study showed no statistical difference when comparing adhesions after simple continuous, simple interrupted, and continuous Connell closures with omental wrapping and intraperitoneal sodium carboxymethylcellulose administration.

Kirpensteijn J, Maarschalkerweed RJ, van der Gaag I et al: Comparison of three closure methods and two absorbable suture materials for closure of jejunal enterotomy incisions in healthy dogs, *Vet Quart* 23:67, 2001.
In this study, monofilament suture caused more fibrous reaction in the intestine than multifilament, and an appositional single-layer method was the best for closing the enterotomy.

Lanz OI, Ellison GW, Bellah JR et al: Surgical treatment of septic peritonitis without abdominal drainage in 28 dogs, *J Am Anim Assoc* 37:87, 2001.

Twenty-eight dogs were studied, and the mortality rate was comparable with that reported for open-abdominal drainage.

Levin GM, Bonczynski JJ, Ludwig LL et al: Lactate as a diagnostic test for septic peritoneal effusions in dogs and cats, *J Am Anim Hosp Assoc* 40:364, 2004.

The test was not accurate in detecting septic peritoneal effusions in cats.

Mueller MG, Ludwig LL, Barton LJ: Use of closed-suction drains to treat generalized peritonitis in dogs and cats: 40 cases (1997-1999), *J Am Vet Med Assoc* 219:789, 2001.

Thirty dogs and 10 cats were studied. The study suggested that this was an effective technique.

Rumbaugh ML, Burba DJ, Natalini C et al: Evaluation of a vessel-sealing device for small intestinal resection and anastomosis in normal horses, *Vet Surg* 32:574, 2003.

A vessel sealing device (LigaSure) was found to be a safe and rapid method for occluding vessels less than 7 mm.

Shales CJ, Warren J, Anderson SM et al: Complications following full-thickness small intestinal biopsy in 66 dogs: a retrospective study, *J Small Anim Pract* 46:317, 2005.

The authors could not find any consistent predictors of intestinal dehiscence.

Tomlinson J, Blikslager A: Role of nonsteroidal anti-inflammatory drugs in gastrointestinal tract injury and repair, *J Am Vet Med Assoc* 222:946, 2003.

This is a detailed review of the effects of NSAIDs on the gastrointestinal tract.

SPECIFIC DISEASES

INTESTINAL FOREIGN BODIES

DEFINITION

Intestinal foreign bodies are ingested objects that may cause complete or partial intraluminal obstruction.

GENERAL CONSIDERATIONS AND CLINICALLY RELEVANT PATHOPHYSIOLOGY

The oropharyngeal opening is larger than any other orifice in the gastrointestinal tract. Foreign bodies that traverse the esophagus and stomach may lodge in the smaller diameter intestine (Box 19-50). Common intestinal foreign bodies include bones, balls, toys, rocks, corncobs, cloth, metal objects (e.g., fish hooks and needles), peach pits, acorns, pecans, hairballs, tampons, and linear objects (i.e., string, thread, fabric, pantyhose, plastic, cassette tape, or ribbon). Some foreign bodies continue to move slowly through the intestine, whereas others become lodged in an intestinal segment, where they cause complete or partial obstruction.

Partial or incomplete obstruction allows limited passage of fluid or gas, whereas complete obstruction does not allow fluid or gas to advance past the obstruction (Fig. 19-98). The clinical course and signs are more severe in animals with complete intraluminal obstruction, particularly a "higher" obstruction, than in those with a partial obstruction. With complete intraluminal obstruction, the intestine orad to the lesion distends with gas and fluid. The gas is a combination of swallowed air, carbon dioxide formed in the lumen by

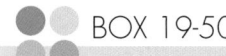

BOX 19-50

Intestinal Foreign Bodies: Key Points

Many different objects can cause obstruction
Signs vary with location and degree of obstruction
Dilation occurs proximal to the obstruction
Imaging detects most foreign bodies
Explore for multiple objects and evidence of peritonitis
Incise through healthy tissue distal to the object for removal
Assess bowel viability after removal of object
Resect devitalized intestine and anastomose if necessary
Lavage thoroughly
Place omentum or create a serosal patch at the site

bicarbonate neutralization, and organic gases from fermentation. Fluid accumulation is caused both by retention of ingested fluid in the intestinal lumen and by secretion (i.e., salivary, biliary, gastric, intestinal, and pancreatic glands). Secretion increases and absorption diminishes (secretions normally are reabsorbed in the lower jejunum and ileum) during obstruction. Absorption is reduced because of lymphatic and venous congestion, increased intraluminal osmolality, and decreased enterocyte turnover rate. After 24 hours of complete obstruction, the distended bowel may lose its ability to absorb fluids, and local hypersecretion occurs. The major mechanisms of hypersecretion and decreased absorption are believed to originate from four sources (Papazoglou et al, 2003): (1) Hypersecretion mediated by enteric bacterial toxins secreted by noninvasive pathogenic bacteria that bind specific enterocyte receptors and stimulate salt and water production via the messenger cyclic adenosine monophosphate (cAMP) or cyclic guanosine monophosphate pathways (cGMP); (2) increased concentrations of bile and fatty acids and products of tissue ischemia at the obstruction site; (3) increased blood flow in the proximal parts of the obstructed intestine that may stimulate secretory activity; and (4) release of serotonin (5-hydroxytryptamine) by entero-endocrine cells that may be stimulated by increased luminal distention, which activates reflex pathways that increase chloride ion secretion. Other sources include chemical mediators of the enteric nervous system (acetylcholine, vasoactive intestinal polypeptide, substance P) that activate chloride ion–rich fluid secretion.

Intraluminal pressure proximal to the obstruction gradually increases because of the accumulation of fluid and gas. Lymphatic and capillary stasis occurs when intraluminal pressures reach 30 mm Hg (normal is 2 to 4 mm Hg with peristaltic pressures of 15 to 25 mm Hg); venous drainage is prevented when pressures reach 50 mm Hg. The arterial supply is not affected, and hydrostatic pressure increases at the capillary bed, producing a net shift of fluid into the interstitium and causing intestinal wall edema. Eventually fluid shifts not only into the lumen but also from the serosa into the peritoneal cavity. At a pressure of 44 mm Hg, the intestinal segment may be so compromised that blood is shunted away from the intestinal capillaries and into arteriovenous

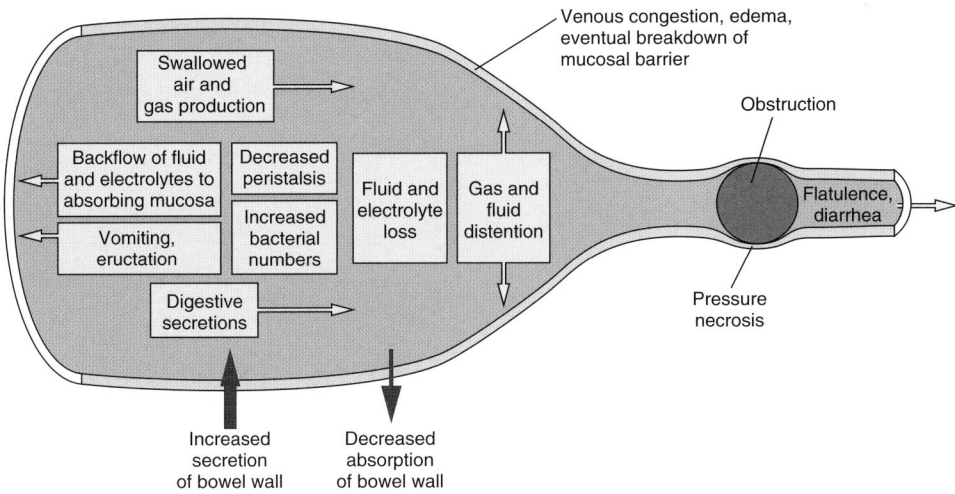

FIG. 19-98
Pathophysiologic events associated with mechanical obstruction of the intestinal lumen.

anastomoses. Circulation in the mucosa and submucosa is impaired, oxygen consumption declines, arteriovenous shunting occurs, and the mucosa becomes ischemic. Full-thickness wall necrosis may occur at the obstruction site. Small intestinal stasis leads to luminal bacterial overgrowth. If the normal mucosal barrier is impaired by distention and ischemia, permeability may increase, with bacterial migration and absorption of toxins into the systemic circulation or peritoneal cavity or both.

Intestinal luminal distention causes increased myoelectrical activity proximal to the obstruction and decreased activity distally. The clusters of intense myoelectrical activity that migrate distally are interrupted by periods of absent motor activity as the duration of obstruction increases. The increased myoelectric activity proximal to the obstruction may be cholinergically mediated, whereas the distal inhibition of spike bursts is thought to be caused by noncholinergic noradrenergic pathways.

Large foreign bodies apply pressure to the intestinal wall. This may cause venous stasis and edema followed by arterial flow compromise, ulceration, necrosis, and perforation.

More proximal and complete obstructions cause more acute and severe signs, with increased likelihood of dehydration, electrolyte imbalance, and shock. Proximal or high obstructions (i.e., duodenum or proximal jejunum) cause persistent vomiting, loss of gastric secretions, electrolyte imbalances, and dehydration. Large volumes of secretions and ingested fluid do not establish contact with jejunal and ileal mucosa for reabsorption. The major cause of mortality from upper small intestinal obstruction is severe, rapid hypovolemia. Untreated dogs with high, complete obstructions usually die within 3 to 4 days. Distal or low obstructions (i.e., distal jejunum, ileum, or ileocecal junction) cause varying degrees of metabolic acidosis. Clinical signs of distal and incomplete obstructions may be insidious, with vague, intermittent anorexia; lethargy; diarrhea; and occasional vomiting spanning several days or weeks. Signs are associated with maldigestion and malabsorption of nutrients. Diarrhea may be attributed to combined osmotic effects of unabsorbed substances in the intestinal lumen and to secretory activity

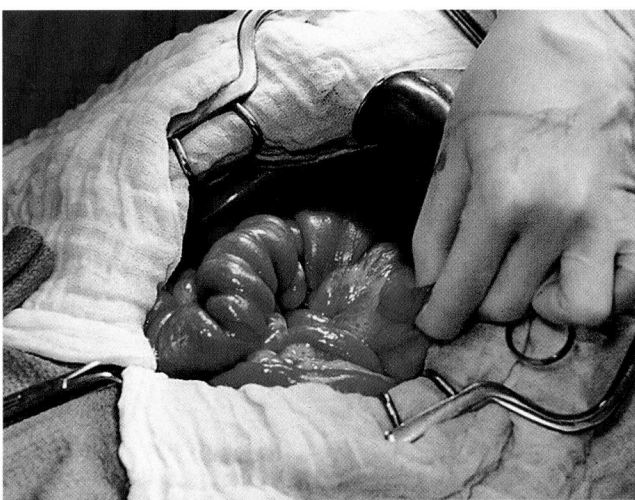

FIG. 19-99
Intraoperative appearance of bunched intestines that resulted secondary to a towel "string" foreign body.

of enterocytes. These animals usually lose weight, but may live for more than 3 weeks if water is available. Causes of death associated with complete distal obstruction are fluid loss and toxemia related to bacterial proliferation.

A number of objects can assume a linear configuration, including string, thread, dental floss, nylon stockings, cloth, sacks, ribbon, plastic, and cassette tapes. Part of the object lodges, usually at the base of the tongue (cats) or pylorus (dogs), and the remainder advances into the intestine. As peristaltic waves attempt to advance the object, the intestine gathers around it, causing partial or complete obstruction (Fig. 19-99). Linear foreign bodies can cause similar signs. Initially, they produce partial or complete intestinal obstruction but the clinical presentation may change. Continued peristalsis may cause the object to become taut, cut into the mucosa, and then lacerate the mesenteric border of the intestine, causing peritonitis. Multiple perforations may occur, and this is associated with high mortality. Some animals with linear foreign bodies have concurrent intussusceptions.

> NOTE: Linear foreign bodies typically perforate at the mesenteric border of the small intestine.

DIAGNOSIS
Clinical Presentation

Signalment. There is no breed or gender predisposition; however, cats more commonly ingest linear foreign bodies than do dogs. Most dogs and cats with linear foreign bodies are under 4 years of age (for dogs, the mean age is 4.5 years and the median age is 2 years; for cats, the mean age is 2.7 years and the median age is 1 year). Other types of foreign bodies are more commonly found in dogs. Playful young animals seem more prone to foreign body ingestion.

History. The presentation and clinical signs depend on the location, completeness, and duration of the obstruction and the vascular integrity of the involved segment. Acute onset of vomiting and anorexia are the most common presenting complaints. Depression, diarrhea, and abdominal pain are sometimes noted. Occasionally the animal is seen swallowing the object. Profuse vomiting may be seen with complete proximal obstruction; vomiting with partial distal obstructions is usually intermittent. Defecation may be absent or decreased in frequency, and the stool is occasionally bloody. Diarrhea is more common in animals with partial obstruction.

Physical Examination Findings

The physical examination may reveal abdominal distention, diarrhea, abdominal pain, abnormal posture, and/or shock. Animals with high obstructions may be severely dehydrated; those with low obstructions may be thin. Abdominal palpation may identify a corrugated-feeling loop of bowel or an abnormal mass of bunched intestines, or may elicit pain. Linear foreign bodies may sometimes be visualized around the base of the tongue, but sedation/anesthesia is often required to visualize this area well enough to detect thin strings or thread. Abdominal pain is common if linear foreign bodies have caused bunching of the intestines. Abdominal auscultation may detect noise from peristaltic activity or silence associated with ileus.

Diagnostic Imaging

Survey radiography often reveals intestinal ileus as a result of complete or almost complete obstruction and may allow identification of the cause, especially if radiopaque foreign bodies are present. Radiolucent foreign objects are sometimes seen if surrounded by gas. Obstructed intestinal loops often become distended with air, fluid, and/or ingesta (Figs. 19-100 and 19-101). "Stacking" of distended intestines and sharp bends or turns in the dilated intestine suggest anatomic ileus as opposed to physiologic ileus. Assessment of intestinal distention can be performed by one of two methods. The maximum intestinal diameter is compared with the height of the body of the fifth lumbar ver-

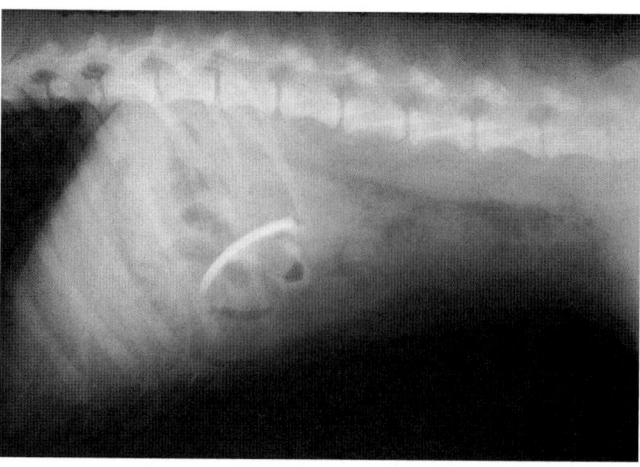

FIG. 19-100
Lateral abdominal radiograph of a 3-year-old female Labrador retriever. Note the radiopaque foreign body in the proximal small intestine. The multiple, well-circumscribed, soft tissue masses visible throughout the caudal abdomen are fetuses in the uterus. One fourth of a tennis ball was removed from the proximal duodenum.

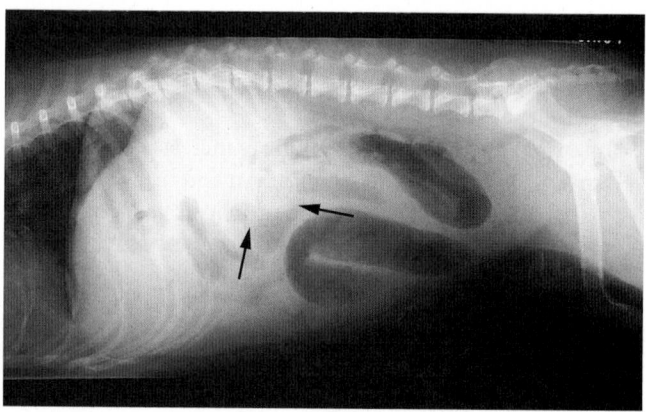

FIG. 19-101
Lateral abdominal radiograph of a dog with segmental ileus. Note the gas and fluid accumulation and the midabdominal, 2.5-cm circular, radiopaque foreign body *(arrows)*. A hazelnut was removed from the jejunum.

tebra at its narrowest point. A ratio higher than 1.6 indicates distention and those greater than 2 indicate a high probability of obstruction (Graham et al, 1999). Another method is to compare the intestinal diameter to the width of a rib; normal is less than 2. Linear foreign bodies may cause the intestines to appear bunched or pleated together, with small gas bubbles in the lumen (comma shaped) and without gas-distended intestinal loops (plication). However, some patients (especially cats) with linear foreign bodies have no obvious lesions on plain radiographs.

Contrast studies can often differentiate anatomic from physiologic ileus although in general, anatomic or mechanical ileus is often focal, whereas physiologic or functional ileus is usually generalized. These two categories may be difficult to differentiate in cases of a distal obstruction. Contrast may delineate the foreign body, reveal luminal-filling defects, or demonstrate delayed transit time or displacement of intestinal loops. Prolonged transit time or complete stasis characterizes simple obstruction. However, patients with severe ileus due to low jejunal/ileal obstruction may be more difficult to accurately define with contrast studies because the contrast may or may not be able to reach the lesion. In general, radiographic contrast studies are infrequently done for this purpose.

Ultrasonography may identify foreign objects that cannot be seen radiographically, especially those with a hyperechoic margin with or without fluid accumulation. However, if there are large amounts of intestinal gas, a negative ultrasound examination should be viewed with skepticism. Finding loops of hypermotile bowel filled with fluid is very suggestive of obstruction. However, it is difficult to examine the entire intestinal tract ultrasonographically, and some foreign objects will not be revealed with ultrasound. Ultrasound also allows assessment of motility.

Endoscopy. Endoscopy rarely diagnoses intestinal foreign bodies that were not detected radiographically or with ultrasound. This is because the scope seldom can be advanced beyond the descending duodenum. However, endoscopy is useful in removing high duodenal foreign bodies. In addition, endoscopy can find linear foreign bodies lodged at the pylorus; such foreign bodies can sometimes be removed endoscopically.

> NOTE: Be sure to repeat radiographs of animals with gastrointestinal foreign bodies immediately before surgery to ensure that the foreign body is still in the stomach or small intestine. Most foreign bodies that enter the large intestine are eliminated in the feces.

Laboratory Findings

Fluid, electrolyte, and acid-base abnormalities often are identified on CBC and biochemistry profiles. Packed cell volume and total protein are sometimes increased in dehydrated patients. However, hypoalbuminemia may occur as a result of gastrointestinal losses. Leukocytosis with a left shift or degenerative leukopenia accompanied by septic abdominal effusion indicates intestinal ischemia or perforation with peritonitis. Vomiting as a result of high duodenal obstruction may cause a hypochloremic hypokalemic metabolic alkalosis. Vomiting associated with duodenal and proximal jejunal obstructions may be associated with mild metabolic acidosis and dehydration. Distal obstructions are more commonly associated with hypokalemia and metabolic acidosis. A slight increase in alanine aminotransferase, alkaline phosphatase, blood urea nitrogen, and creatinine may be seen with intestinal obstruction.

DIFFERENTIAL DIAGNOSIS

The differential diagnosis includes all other causes of intestinal obstruction: intussusception, intestinal volvulus or torsion, intestinal incarceration, adhesions, strictures, abscesses, granulomas, hematomas, neoplasia, or congenital malformations. Physiologic ileus may be due to inflammatory diseases (e.g., parvovirus, peritonitis, and pancreatitis).

MEDICAL MANAGEMENT

Some foreign bodies pass through the intestine without requiring therapy. Foreign body advancement may be monitored radiographically unless vomiting is severe, debilitation occurs, or evidence of peritonitis is seen (i.e., abdominal pain, fever, or neutrophilia; see also p. 329). Radiographs should always be repeated shortly before surgery, even if previous ones were taken several hours before, because the foreign body may have moved into the colon or passed in the feces. Hairballs in cats are treated by administration of semisolid petrolatum-based laxatives for lubrication and a commercial hairball diet. Linear foreign bodies lodged at the base of the tongue in cats that are presented within 1 to 3 days after ingestion may be cut and then monitored for passage, depending upon how ill the cat appears. If the cat does not obviously feel better within 12 to 18 hours of cutting the foreign body off the tongue, it should be taken to surgery.

SURGICAL TREATMENT

In cases of partial obstruction, failure to radiographically demonstrate foreign body movement within the intestine over an 8-hour period or failure to pass the object within approximately 36 hours indicates the need for surgery. Surgery should not be delayed to observe for passage of the object through the intestinal tract if abdominal pain, fever, vomiting, or lethargy is apparent. Most foreign bodies can be removed by enterotomy rather than resection and anastomosis unless intestinal necrosis or perforation is present. If a linear object has been present a long time, it may become embedded in the mucosa, requiring intestinal resection. Multiple enterotomies (two to four) often are necessary to remove linear foreign bodies. Iatrogenic laceration of the mesenteric border may occur if excessive tension causes the object to saw through the wall before or during extraction.

Preoperative Management

Fluid, electrolyte, and acid-base deficits should be corrected before surgery if possible. Prophylactic antibiotics should be administered according to the recommendations on p. 446.

Anesthesia

Anesthetic recommendations for animals undergoing intestinal surgery are provided on p. 445. Nitrous oxide should be avoided in animals with obstructions to prevent further gas accumulation in the intestinal tract.

Surgical Anatomy

The surgical anatomy of the small intestine is described on p. 446.

Positioning

The patient should be positioned in dorsal recumbency for a ventral midline celiotomy. The surgically prepared area should extend from the midthorax to the perineum.

ENDOSCOPIC TECHNIQUE

The endoscopic technique of removal of duodenal foreign bodies consists of advancing the scope until the foreign body is visualized and studying it before attempting to grasp it. Consideration must be given to which foreign body retrieval device (e.g., four wire basket, snare, alligator jaws, W-type coin forceps, etc.) should be used. It can sometimes be hard to pull the foreign body out of the pylorus. Administering ketamine as a preanesthetic may relax the pylorus and lower the esophageal sphincter, making it easier to retrieve the object after it has been snared. The endoscopic technique for removing linear foreign bodies is given on p. 425 under the Gastric Foreign Bodies section.

SURGICAL TECHNIQUE

Make an incision through the linea alba that is sufficient to allow complete exploration of the abdomen. Explore the entire abdomen and gastrointestinal tract to prevent overlooking concurrent abnormalities or multiple foreign bodies. Once the foreign body has been located, isolate this loop of intestine from the remainder of the abdominal cavity with laparotomy pads or sterile towels. Complete obstructions may cause the bowel to be severely distended and appear cyanotic; however, reserve determination of intestinal viability until the bowel has been decompressed and the foreign body has been removed by enterotomy. Bathe the intestine in warm saline for a few minutes to help improve its color and peristalsis. Normally the appearance of the intestine improves rapidly after decompression. If the intestinal segment is determined to be viable, close the enterotomy with simple interrupted or continuous sutures as described on p. 449. Resect nonviable or questionable intestine and reestablish bowel continuity by end-to-end anastomosis (see p. 450). After removing the foreign body, carefully examine the intestine for evidence of perforation that might require resection of the involved segment or segments. Create a serosal patch (see p. 457) when the intestinal wall is contused to prevent leakage.

Removal of linear foreign bodies may require gastrotomy and multiple enterotomies.

Release the foreign body from where it is lodged. Cut the thread that is embedded sublingually or perform a gastrotomy. Attach a hemostat to the distal end of the object when the mass is removed from the pylorus. Pull gently on the hemostat and identify the next more distal point of attachment. Perform an enterotomy, and withdraw the more proximal foreign body. Again attach a hemostat distally, transect the foreign body, apply gentle tension on the remaining intraluminal foreign body, and identify the next point of attachment. Repeat until the entire linear foreign body is removed. Avoid excess tension on the foreign body as this may lead to full-thickness laceration of the mesenteric border. Close the enterotomies (see p. 449), and inspect the mesenteric border for evidence of perforation.

A single-enterotomy catheter technique has been described for removing linear foreign bodies. It is most successful when foreign bodies have not penetrated the mucosa. This technique may not be successful if the condition is chronic and the foreign body is embedded in the mesenteric border.

Make an incision into the stomach or intestine at the site where the object is fixed. Suture the linear object to a soft catheter, and then completely advance the catheter into the distal intestine. Close the enterotomy site and milk the catheter and foreign body through the intestinal tract and out through the anus. This technique reduces the number of enterotomies and may thereby reduce the risk of leakage and dehiscence.

SUTURE MATERIALS AND SPECIAL INSTRUMENTS

Instruments for enterotomy or intestinal resection and anastomosis are discussed on p. 459. Polydioxanone, poliglecaprone 25, polyglyconate, and glycomer 631 (3-0 or 4-0) are the preferred suture materials for these procedures; however, nonabsorbable suture (nylon or polypropylene) sometimes is used in hypoalbuminemic animals.

POSTOPERATIVE CARE AND ASSESSMENT

Postoperative treatment includes further correction of fluid, electrolyte, and acid-base deficits. Analgesics should be given as necessary to control pain (see Table 13-4 on p. 133). Antibiotics should be continued if peritonitis was diagnosed or if gross abdominal contamination occurred. If no vomiting has occurred, water can be offered 8 to 12 hours after surgery, and food can be given 12 to 24 hours after surgery. These patients should be monitored for signs of leakage and peritonitis (see p. 329).

COMPLICATIONS

Early diagnosis of intestinal foreign bodies and good surgical technique are necessary to prevent complications (e.g., intestinal necrosis, perforation, leakage, dehiscence, peritonitis, endotoxic shock, and stenosis). The risk of anastomotic leakage is greater when associated with a foreign body, debilitation, and hypoalbuminemia (Ralphs et al, 2003). The risk of peritonitis and death is much higher if free gas is present on preoperative radiographs. Resecting large segments of intestine may result in a patient with SBS (see p. 460) and a guarded prognosis.

PROGNOSIS

The prognosis is good if peritonitis and extensive resections are avoided. The prognosis without surgery is guarded because animals may die from hypovolemic or endotoxic shock, septicemia, peritonitis, or starvation.

Reference

Graham JB, Lord PF, Harrison JM: Quantitative estimation of intestinal dilation as a predictor of obstruction in the dog, *J Small Anim* Pract 39:521, 1998.

Papazoglou LG, Patskas MN, Rallis T: Intestinal foreign bodies in dogs and cats, *Compend Cont Educ Pract Vet* 25:830, 2003.

Ralphs SC, Jessen CR, Lipowitz AJ: Risk factors for leakage following intestinal anastomosis in dogs and cats: 115 cases (1991-2000), *J Am Vet Med Assoc* 223:73, 2003.

Suggested Reading

Capak D, Simpraga M, Maticic D et al: Incidence of foreign-body-induced ileus in dogs, *Berl Munch Tierarztl Wochenschr* 114:290, 2001.

One hundred and three cases were studied. Dogs younger than 2 years of age had a better prognosis, and the jejunum was the most commonly affected site.

Coolman BR, Ehrhart N, Manfra Marretta S: Use of skin staples for rapid closure of gastrointestinal incisions in the treatment of canine linear foreign bodies, *J Am Anim Hosp Assoc* 36:542, 2000.

This is a report of three cases where skin staples were used successfully for gastrotomy and enterotomy closure.

Evans KL, Smeak DD, Biller DS: Gastrointestinal linear foreign bodies in 32 dogs: a retrospective evaluation and feline comparison, *J Am Anim Hosp Assoc* 30:445, 1994.

Most linear foreign bodies in dogs are not found under the tongue, and intussusceptions were found in 25% of the dogs. Dogs had a higher risk of peritonitis and death compared with cats with linear foreign bodies.

Milovancev M, Weisman DL, Palmisano MP: Foreign body attachment to polypropylene suture material extruding into the small intestine lumen after enteric closure in 3 dogs, *J Am Vet Med Assoc* 225:1713, 2004.

The authors suggested that absorbable suture was better since it would not act as a nidus for foreign body formation.

Penninck D, Mitchell SL: Ultrasonographic detection of ingested and perforating wooden foreign objects in four dogs, *J Am Vet Med Assoc* 223:206, 2003.

The ultrasonographic appearance of wooden foreign bodies is discussed and shown.

INTESINAL NEOPLASIA

DEFINITION

Intestinal neoplasia is a condition in which tumors arise from one of the layers of the intestinal wall, its glands, or associated cells or lymphatics.

GENERAL CONSIDERATIONS AND CLINICALLY RELEVANT PATHOPHYSIOLOGY

Intestinal tumors most often occur in the canine rectum or colon, and the feline small intestine (Box 19-51). Most intestinal tumors are malignant. Intestinal tumors may cause intramural or intraluminal mechanical obstruction. They most commonly invade the muscular layer of the intestinal wall where they compromise the lumen diameter and reduce distensibility. The proximal bowel distends with fluid and gas, and its function is compromised as with foreign body obstruction. The disease usually is advanced at the time of diagnosis, and most malignant tumors have metastasized. Malignant tumors spread by local invasion (e.g.,

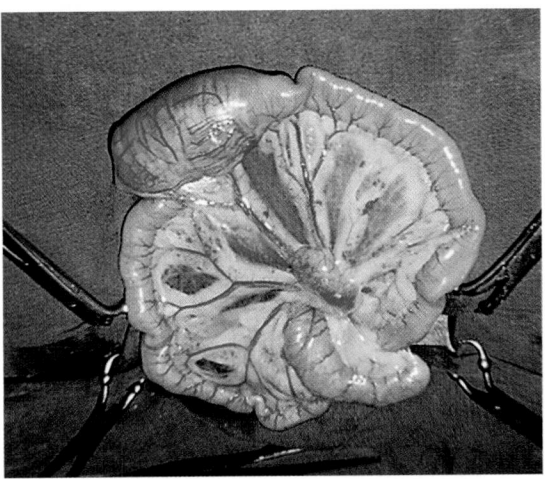

FIG. 19-102
Intraoperative photograph of an adenocarcinoma that was partly obstructing the jejunum of a 15-year-old cat.

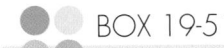 BOX 19-51

Intestinal Neoplasia: Key Points

Most are malignant; most common adenocarcinoma, lymphosarcomas, leiomyosarcomas
Cause intramural or intraluminal mechanical obstruction
Resect with 4- to 8-cm margins of normal appearing intestine
Prognosis varies with tumor type

serosa, mesentery, omentum, and local lymph nodes) and distant metastasis (i.e., lungs, liver, and spleen). The most common small intestinal malignancies are adenocarcinomas (Fig. 19-102) and lymphosarcomas. Other small intestinal neoplasms are leiomyomas, leiomyosarcomas, fibrosarcomas, mast cell tumors, hemangiosarcomas, anaplastic sarcomas, carcinoids, plasmacytomas, neurolemmomas, adenomas, and adenomatous polyps.

Adenocarcinomas are locally invasive and slow growing. They most commonly arise in the duodenum and colon of dogs, but the distal jejunum and ileum of cats. These tumors have three main morphologic forms: (1) infiltrative adenocarcinomas cause a thickened stenotic area that obstructs the intestinal lumen; (2) ulcerative adenocarcinomas have a deep indurated mucosal ulcer with raised edges; and (3) proliferative adenocarcinomas are lobulated, expanding intraluminal masses. Mucosal ulceration may cause melena and iron deficiency anemia. The tumors spread to adjacent serosal surfaces, mesentery, omentum, and regional lymph nodes by local invasion and may metastasize distally to the lungs and liver. Mucinous intestinal adenocarcinomas extend transmurally to the mesentery with accumulation of variable amounts of mucin.

Lymphosarcomas (lymphomas) are neoplastic proliferations of lymphocytes. In cats they may be caused by feline leukemia virus (FeLV) or feline immunodeficiency virus (FIV), but most are caused by unknown mechanisms. The cause in dogs is unknown. Affected animals may have multicentric disease. Lymphomas have two intestinal types: diffuse and nodular. Diffuse infiltration of the lamina propria and submucosa with neoplastic lymphocytes causes malabsorption and occasional deep ulceration. Nodular lymphoma is an expanding intestinal mass that causes obstruction, usually in the ileocecocolic area. Involvement of regional lymph nodes and other organs is common.

Intestinal leiomyosarcomas are slow growing, malignant smooth muscle tumors of older dogs that usually occur in the cecum and jejunum. Neoplastic spread is by local invasion, and metastasis is slow. Metastasis occurs in the mesentery, mesenteric lymph nodes, peritoneum, and liver. Median survival of approximately 21 months is expected after resection of a localized lesion, with 75% survival at 1 year and 66% survival at 2 years (Cohen et al, 2003). This is true of those with metastasis at the time of surgery as well.

Intestinal leiomyomas are slow growing, benign, smooth muscle tumors. Adenomatous polyps are found in the feline duodenum and canine rectum. Recurrence after complete resection is not expected.

DIAGNOSIS
Clinical Presentation

Signalment. Adenocarcinomas are more common in dogs than in cats. In dogs, adenocarcinomas are the most common intestinal tumor, and leiomyosarcomas are the most common sarcoma. Boxers, collies, and German shepherds may be predisposed to intestinal tumors. In cats, lymphosarcomas are most commonly followed by adenocarcinomas and mast cell tumors. Siamese cats may be predisposed to small intestinal adenocarcinomas. Intestinal tumors generally occur in older animals. Carcinomas are seen at a mean age of 9 years in dogs and 10 years in cats. Leiomyosarcomas occur at a mean age of 11 years in dogs. Lymphosarcomas occur in dogs and cats at a mean age of 10.6 years. The mean age for cats with intestinal mast cell tumors is 13 years.

History. Patients initially have vague clinical signs of depression, anorexia, and lethargy, which may progress to diarrhea and/or vomiting. Weight loss is progressive. Other clinical signs may include dehydration, melena, hematemesis, anemia, fever, icterus, polyuria, polydipsia, and/or abdominal effusion. Signs of intestinal obstruction, abscessation, and malabsorption may also occur. Lymphatic obstruction may cause steatorrhea from lymphangiectasia. Signs involving other organs may develop secondary to metastasis.

Physical Examination Findings

The animal may be in poor body condition. Abdominal palpation may reveal a firm abdominal mass, thickened intestinal loops, or mesenteric lymphadenomegaly.

Diagnostic Imaging

Masses, abnormal gas and fluid patterns, visceral displacement, and abdominal fluid may be seen on survey abdominal radiographs. Contrast radiographs can be helpful for delineating regions of mucosal irregularity, luminal narrowing, and intramural infiltration, thickening, or nodularity; but they are seldom necessary if ultrasound is available. If neoplasia is suspected, thoracic radiographs should be taken.

Abdominal ultrasonography often delineates the mass, finds evidence of metastasis, and may facilitate percutaneous biopsy. Intestinal tumors produce a broad spectrum of ultrasonic patterns. Ultrasonographic findings may include intestinal wall thickening and loss of discrete wall layers, but lymphosarcoma may be present despite a normal appearing intestine. Smooth muscle tumors may appear as eccentric, poorly echogenic masses with anechoic cavities. Ileus, fluid accumulation, and lymphadenomegaly may be recognized.

Endoscopy. Flexible endoscopic evaluation of intestinal tumors beyond the duodenum may be difficult. Mucosal irregularity, inflammation, ulceration, and a narrowed duodenal or high jejunal lumen may be detected, or the intestine may appear normal. Mucosal biopsies can be diagnostic if the tumor involves the mucosa.

> NOTE: Ultrasonography is preferable to contrast radiography in affected animals.

Laboratory Findings

Hematologic and biochemical profiles often are normal. Laboratory evaluation may reveal blood loss anemia, neutrophilic leukocytosis with left shift, hypoalbuminemia, hypoglycemia, and/or elevated serum hepatic enzyme concentrations. A definitive diagnosis of intestinal neoplasia can only be made by cytology or histopathology.

DIFFERENTIAL DIAGNOSIS

The differential diagnosis includes all other causes of intestinal obstruction (i.e., foreign bodies, intussusception, intestinal volvulus or torsion, adhesions, strictures, abscesses, granulomas, hematomas, or congenital malformation). Another cause might be physiologic ileus that occurs secondary to severe inflammation (e.g., parvovirus or peritonitis).

MEDICAL MANAGEMENT

Lymphosarcoma may respond to chemotherapy. (Refer to an oncology text for additional information and chemotherapeutic protocols.) The response of other tumor types to chemotherapy is unknown or poor. Radiation therapy is used primarily for tumors in the distal half of the rectum and anal canal.

SURGICAL TREATMENT

Surgical resection is the treatment of choice for intestinal tumors; however, many tumors are too advanced to allow complete resection by the time they are diagnosed. If metastasis has occurred, surgical resection may be palliative. However, if resection is attempted, it is important to suture healthy tissue to healthy tissue; suturing tumor-containing tissue to healthy tissue makes dehiscence likely.

Preoperative Management

Fluid, electrolyte, and acid-base deficits should be corrected before surgery if possible. Transfusions should be considered if the packed cell volume is below 20%. Prophylactic antibiotics should be given according to the recommendations on p. 446. Debilitated animals or those that are likely to remain anorectic or have continued vomiting should have enteral feeding tubes placed at the time of surgery (see p. 107).

Anesthesia

General anesthetic recommendations for animals undergoing intestinal surgery are provided on p. 445. Many tumor patients are debilitated, therefore balanced anesthesia using injectable agents (i.e., opioids) and isoflurane or sevoflurane is recommended.

Surgical Anatomy

The surgical anatomy of the small intestine is presented on p. 446.

Positioning

Patients should be positioned in dorsal recumbency for a ventral midline celiotomy. The entire abdomen and caudal thorax should be clipped and prepared for aseptic surgery.

SURGICAL TECHNIQUE

Make an incision through the linea alba from the xiphoid process to the pubis to allow complete exploration of the abdomen. Explore the entire abdomen and gastrointestinal tract to avoid overlooking concurrent abnormalities. Take a biopsy from the mesenteric lymph nodes and other organs as needed before incising the intestine. Resect the mass with 4- to 8-cm margins of grossly normal tissue, and perform an end-to-end anastomosis (see p. 450). Pay special attention to surgical technique because these patients often are debilitated. Submit tissue for histopathologic evaluation and tumor staging. Change gloves, and use uncontaminated instruments and suture for abdominal closure.

SUTURE MATERIALS AND SPECIAL INSTRUMENTS

Instruments for enterotomy or intestinal resection and anastomosis are discussed on p. 459. Polydioxanone, poliglecaprone 25, polyglyconate, and glycomer 631 (3-0 or 4-0) are the preferred suture materials for these procedures; however, nonabsorbable suture (nylon, polypropylene, or polybutester) may be used in hypoalbuminemic animals.

POSTOPERATIVE CARE AND ASSESSMENT

Postoperative care should be individualized according to the patient's status and concurrent diseases. Fluid support should be maintained until the animal is drinking enough to maintain hydration. Electrolyte and acid-base deficits

should be corrected. Analgesics should be provided as necessary (see Table 13-4 on p. 133). If peritonitis, abdominal contamination, or severe debilitation occurs, therapeutic antibiotics should be given. Nutritional support should be provided by enterostomy tube if vomiting or anorexia persists (see p. 107). Adjuvant chemotherapy has been recommended for some malignant intestinal tumors, but its efficacy is unproven (see previous section on Medical Management) except for lymphoma. However, chemotherapy of intestinal lymphoma is often associated with morbidity directly or indirectly related to the drugs and destruction of malignant cells in the intestinal wall. Second-look laparotomy or laparoscopy is helpful in evaluating disease progression or response to adjuvant therapy and allows further biopsy or further resection if indicated.

COMPLICATIONS

Leakage, dehiscence, and peritonitis are possible complications and may occur more frequently in debilitated patients. Stenosis after surgical resection or tumor recurrence may cause recurrent signs of obstruction. SBS (see p. 460) is a possible complication if large portions of the bowel are resected.

PROGNOSIS

The prognosis is excellent when benign tumors or polyps are completely excised. The prognosis is good for patients with a localized intestinal adenocarcinoma or leiomyosarcoma if complete resection is possible. The median survival time is 10 months; the 1-year survival rate is 40.5%, and the 2-year survival rate is 33% for dogs with an adenocarcinoma or a leiomyosarcoma (Crawshaw et al, 1998). Cats with an intestinal adenocarcinoma may live longer than 2 years after surgery. The prognosis for solitary nodular lymphoma is better than that for diffuse lymphoma, which carries a poor prognosis. The prognosis for leiomyosarcoma is good even with metastasis at the time of resection, with a median survival of 21.3 months, 75% survival at 1 year, and 66% survival at 2 years (Cohen et al, 2003). A guarded to poor prognosis should be given if nonresectable tumors are present because other modes of therapy are ineffective, of questionable value, or not advised because of severe side effects.

References

Cohen M, Post GS, Wright JC: Gastrointestinal leiomyosarcoma in 14 dogs, *J Vet Intern Med* 17:107, 2003.
Crawshaw J, Berg J, Sardinas JC et al: Prognosis for dogs with non-lymphomatous, small intestinal tumors treated by surgical excision, *J Am Anim Hosp Assoc* 34:451, 1998.

Suggested Reading

Bertazzolo W, Roccabianca P, Crippa L et al: Clinicopathological evidence of pseudomyxoma peritonei in a dog with intestinal mucinous adenocarcinoma. *J Am Anim Hosp Assoc* 39:72, 2003.
This is thought to be the first case report of "gelatinous ascites" (pseudomyxoma peritonei) associated with a mucin-producing jejunal adenocarcinoma in a dog.

McEntee MR, Cates JM, Neilsen N: Cyclooxygenase-2 expression in spontaneous intestinal neoplasia of domestic dogs, *Vet Path* 39:428, 2002.

Thirteen out of 20 canine colorectal adenocarcinomas had Cox-2 expression.

Miura T, Maruyama H, Saka M et al: Endoscopic findings on alimentary lymphoma in 7 cats, *J Vet Med Science* 66:577, 2004.

Four cats had a cobblestone appearance to the duodenal mucosa, and endoscopic ultrasound revealed thickened intestinal wall in 2 cases that were examined.

Penninck D, Smyers B, Webster CRL et al: Diagnostic value of ultrasonography in differentiating enteritis from intestinal neoplasia in dogs, *Vet Radiol Ultrasound* 44:570, 2003.

This retrospective study reviews 155 dogs with enteritis or intestinal neoplasia. Findings include thicker intestinal walls (1.5 cm versus 0.6 cm), loss of wall layering (99% versus 12%), and thicker lymph nodes (1.9 cm versus 1.0 cm) with neoplasia compared with enteritis.

Stanclift RM, Gilson SD: Use of cisplatin, 5-fluorouracil, and second-look laparotomy for the management of gastrointestinal adenocarcinoma in three dogs, *J Am Vet Med Assoc* 225:1412, 2004.

Favorable results were obtained with this chemotherapeutic regimen. Second-look laparotomy was important in determining response and the need for continued therapy.

INTUSSUSCEPTION

DEFINITIONS

Intussusception is the telescoping or invagination of one intestinal segment (**intussusceptum**) into the lumen of an adjacent segment (**intussuscipiens**) (Fig. 19-103, *A*).

GENERAL CONSIDERATIONS AND CLINICALLY RELEVANT PATHOPHYSIOLOGY

Gastrointestinal tract intussusceptions may occur anywhere; however, ileocolic and jejunojejunal intussusceptions are most common (Box 19-52). Intussusceptions often are associated with enteritis (i.e., parasitism, viral or bacterial infection, dietary indiscretion or change, foreign bodies, and masses) or systemic illness; however, the cause of most intussusceptions is unknown. They have also been reported after environmental change and surgery. Intussusceptions after surgery may be associated with ileus, adhesions, or anastomotic malfunction. Intestinal irritation that results in hypermotility may cause one intestinal loop to invaginate into another. The direction of the intussusception can be from proximal to distal or vice versa. The intussusceptum is more commonly a proximal intestinal segment and the intussus-

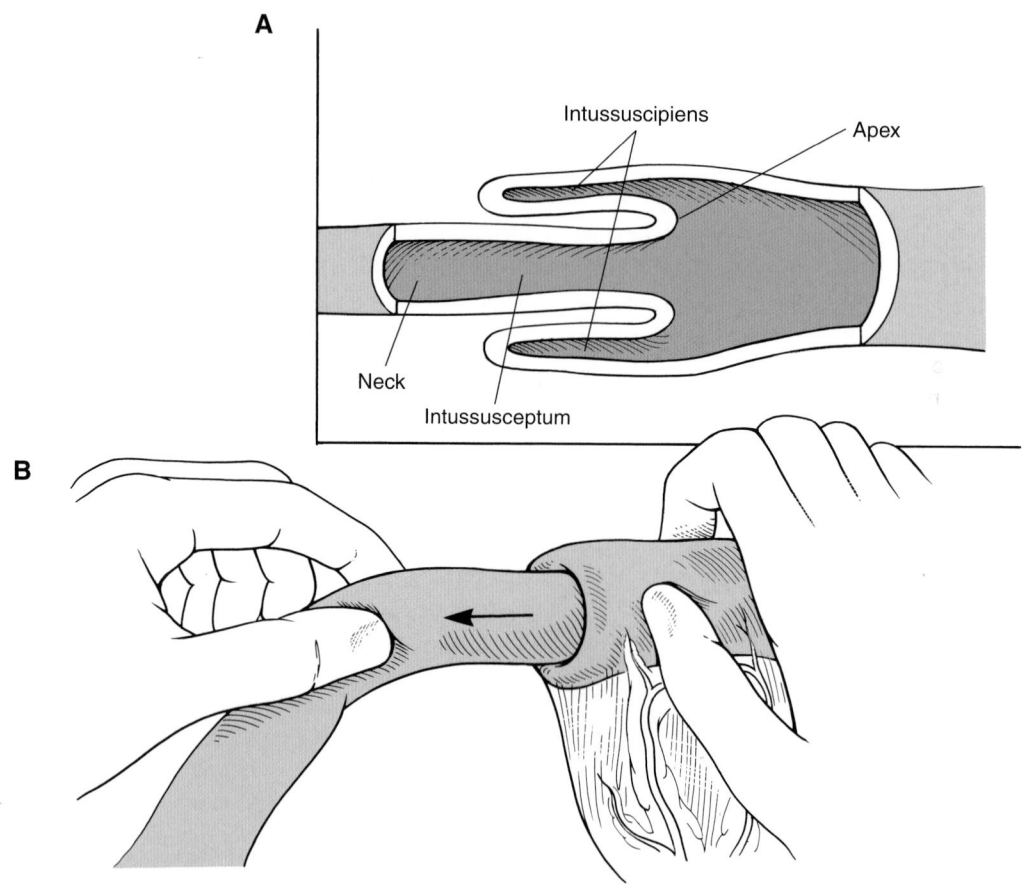

FIG. 19-103
A, Configuration of an intussusception: neck, intussusceptum, apex, intussuscipiens. **B,** To reduce an intussusception, place traction on the neck as you milk the apex out of the intussuscipiens.

cipiens a more distal segment (i.e., the intussusception occurs in the direction of normal peristalsis; direct or normograde intussusception). Intussusceptions can occur at more than one site and are sometimes double (two invaginations at same site). Reverse peristalsis may increase the length of intestine involved in the intussusception. The amount of available mesentery limits the extent of intestinal involvement and the degree of vascular compromise.

The formation of an intussusception is thought to be a result of nonhomogeneity of the wall caused by any abnormality within the wall that alters local intestinal motility or pliability. As the intussusception is formed, longitudinal and circular contractions of normal intestine in an adjacent area cause displacement of the intestine and a fold in the intestine is formed. The fold is propagated circumferentially and longitudinal muscle contraction completes the invagination.

Initially, invagination causes partial intestinal obstruction, which may progress to complete obstruction. Vessels attached to the intussusceptum collapse because of increased intraluminal pressure or kinking, and those vessels may avulse. The wall becomes edematous, ischemic, and turgid. Blood extravasates into the lumen, and the serosa fissures. Fibrin seals the layers of the intestine together and may help localize peritonitis as wall necrosis occurs. Eventually intestinal devitalization occurs, with subsequent contamination of the abdominal cavity. Intussusceptions may occur as agonal events (i.e., are incidental findings and not the cause of death). Agonal intussusceptions are easily reduced and are associated with minimal inflammation; intestinal walls are not edematous, and fibrin does not seal the layers of intestine together.

DIAGNOSIS
Clinical Presentation

Signalment. Intussusceptions occur more commonly in dogs. German shepherd dogs and Siamese cats may be more commonly affected than other breeds. Intussusceptions appear to be more common in immature animals (75% younger than 1 year). Parasitism or enteritis should be suspected as a cause for intussusception in young dogs, and intestinal thickening or masses should be suspected in adults.

History. Most animals have been ill, have changed environments, or have had recent surgery before signs of intussusception begin. The severity and type of clinical signs depend on the location, completeness, vascular integrity, and duration of the intestinal obstruction. Scant, bloody diarrhea, vomiting, abdominal pain, and a palpable mass may occur with intussusceptions. Acute intussusceptions must be considered in puppies with parvoviral enteritis that suddenly become worse or that persists much longer than expected. In particular, a diagnosis of "chronic parvoviral enteritis" is very suggestive of intussusception. Chronic cases can have less notable clinical signs. Patients with chronic intussusception often have intractable, intermittent diarrhea, and hypoalbuminemia; intussusceptions and parasites are the two major causes of chronic protein-losing enteropathy in dogs less than 8 to 12 months of age. Other clinical signs include depression, anorexia, and emaciation.

> NOTE: Consider chronic intussusception as a possible reason why a puppy with an apparently acute episode of enteritis (e.g., parvovirus) has persistent diarrhea.

Physical Examination Findings

A presumptive diagnosis of intussusception can be made when an elongated, thickened intestinal loop (sausage-shaped mass) is palpated. Jejunojejunal intussusceptions are easier to palpate than ileocolic intussusceptions because they are usually more caudal and ventral in the abdomen. Some intussusceptions slide in and out of the colon and can be missed during palpation. Others may protrude from the rectum and can be mistaken for a rectal prolapse. To distinguish rectal prolapse from protruding intussusception, the area around the protruding tissue should be palpated; the existence of a fornix indicates rectal prolapse rather than intussusception.

Diagnostic Imaging

Survey radiographs of patients with intussusception may reveal obstruction; however, intussusceptions causing partial obstruction may be missed if little gas has accumulated. Jejunojejunal intussusception more often results in an obstructive pattern than does ileocolic intussusception (Figs. 19-104 and 19-105). A tubular soft tissue mass may be identified. If sufficient gas accumulates in the distal intestinal segment, the apex of the intussusception may be outlined. A barium enema or upper gastrointestinal tract study can localize the obstruction. A ribbon of contrast material may be seen in the intussusceptum aborad to a dilated intestinal segment. A large "coiled-spring" appearing filling defect may be present when barium within the lumen surrounds the intussusceptum. Occasionally, contrast material accumulates in the lumen between the intussusceptum and the intussuscipiens.

 BOX 19-52

Intussusception: Key Points

Young animals most often affected, especially postparvoviral enteritis
This and parasites are major causes of protein-losing enteropathies in young dogs
Older animals with intussusceptions often have masses
Associated with enteritis or systemic illness
Signs progress from partial to complete obstruction
Clinical course may span several weeks
Invagination usually normograde but occasionally retrograde
Ultrasound reveals "target" or "bull's eye" (concentric intestinal layers)
Manually reduce or resect and anastomose
Enteroenteropexy prevents recurrence

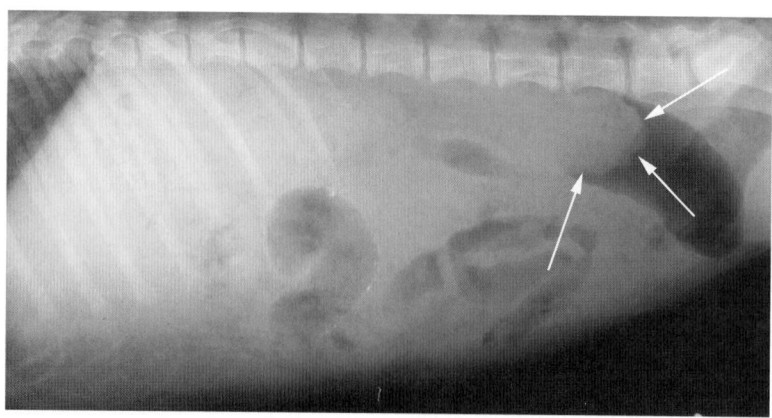

FIG. 19-104
Lateral radiograph of a dog with an ileocolic intussusception. Notice the soft tissue mass within the air-filled colon *(arrows)*.

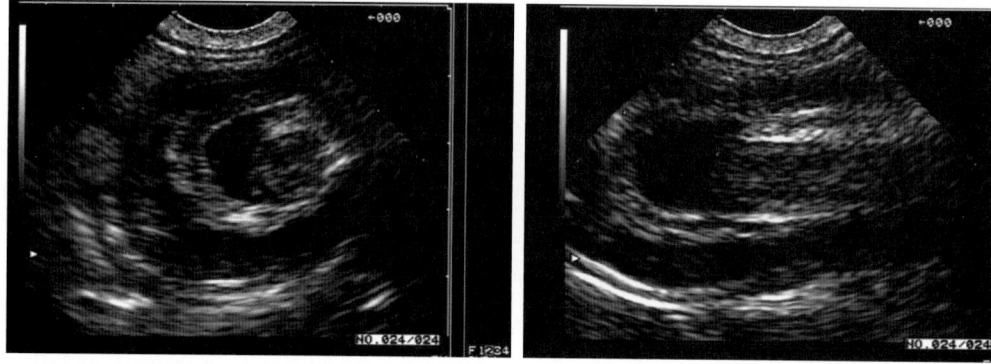

FIG. 19-105
Transverse *(left)* and sagittal *(right)* images of an intussusception. Notice the target-like appearance on the transverse view

Ultrasonography is considered the most useful method for detecting intussusceptions. The ultrasonographic appearance of an intussusception in the transverse plane is that of a multilayered, targetlike lesion (concentric hyperechoic and hypoechoic rings with an overall width greater than 8 to 9 mm) with associated proximal fluid accumulation and diminished intestinal motility. The juxtaposition of the wall layers of the intussusceptum and intussuscipiens creates more than the normal 10 hyperechoic and hypoechoic concentric rings, although these layers may be indistinct. Longitudinal scans demonstrate a layered appearance with alternating parallel hyperechoic and hypoechoic lines. Identification of distinct layers on ultrasound examination is an indication that the intussusception may be reducible. Multiplane imaging; the presence of an eccentric, semilunar or G-shaped hyperechoic center (mesenteric fat); and visualization of the inner intussusceptum are helpful in differentiating an intussusception from similar conditions where targetlike lesions may also be identified. Ultrasonography may identify concurrent abdominal abnormalities, such as lymphadenopathy or infiltrative intestinal lesions.

Colonoscopy. Colonoscopy may identify invaginated intestine protruding into the colon in patients with ileocolic or cecocolic intussusception. In such cases, colonoscopy can usually be performed with little more than manual restraint, if the endoscopist is gentle and careful.

Laboratory Findings

Abnormal laboratory findings may include dehydration, stress leukograms, anemia, and electrolyte and acid-base abnormalities. Chronic intussusception may cause hypoalbuminemia because of protein loss from congested mucosa. Fecal examination sometimes reveals parasitic infestation.

DIFFERENTIAL DIAGNOSIS

The differential diagnoses include all other causes of intestinal obstruction (i.e., foreign bodies, intestinal volvulus or torsion, intestinal incarceration, adhesions, strictures, abscesses, granulomas, hematomas, tumors, or congenital malformations). Another cause might be physiologic ileus that occurs secondary to inflammation (i.e., parvovirus or peritonitis).

MEDICAL MANAGEMENT

Occasionally percutaneous manual reduction of the intussusception is successful, and the intussusception does not recur. In rare cases, intussusceptions self-correct by forming adhesions and sloughing the intussusceptum. However, most intussusceptions require surgical reduction and ancillary procedures to prevent recurrence. Medical therapy should be aimed at correcting fluid and electrolyte imbalances and determining the underlying cause of the intussusception (i.e., enteritis and parasitism).

SURGICAL TREATMENT

Because recurrence is common, intussusceptions should be treated surgically even if they can be manually reduced. Biopsying the intestine at the time of surgical correction may help identify the cause of the intussusception. The tip of the intussusceptum should be evaluated for masses.

Preoperative Management

Hydration, electrolyte, and acid-base deficits should be corrected before surgery if possible. Pediatric patients should not fast for longer than 4 to 8 hours to reduce the chances of hypoglycemia. Prophylactic antibiotics should be given according to the recommendations on p. 446.

Anesthesia

General anesthetic recommendations for animals undergoing intestinal surgery are provided on p. 445. Nitrous oxide should not be used if ileus is present. Care must be taken to prevent hypothermia, especially in pediatric patients. Blood glucose concentrations should be monitored during and after surgery in young patients.

Surgical Anatomy

The surgical anatomy of the small intestine is presented on p. 446.

Positioning

Animals should be positioned in dorsal recumbency for a ventral midline celiotomy. The entire abdomen and caudal thorax should be clipped and prepared for aseptic surgery.

SURGICAL TECHNIQUE

Explore the abdomen, collect specimens, and isolate the involved intestine with laparotomy pads (Fig. 19-106). Reduce intussusceptions manually if possible by gently applying traction on the neck of the intussusceptum while milking its apex (leading edge) out of the intussuscipiens (see Fig. 19-103, B). Avoid excessive traction because this may tear the compromised intestine. Push on the intussusceptions more than pull on the intussusceptum. Manual reduction is successful only if fibrin has not formed firm serosal adhesions. Evaluate the reduced intestine for viability and perforation. Carefully palpate the leading edge of the intussusceptum to detect mass lesions. Perform a resection and anastomosis if a mass is detected, manual reduction is impossible, tissue is devitalized, or mesenteric vessels have been avulsed from a portion of the involved intestine. Submit biopsies of the involved intestine to help identify the cause of the intussusception.

NOTE: Consider performing an enteroenteropexy (see p. 458) on these patients to help prevent recurrence.

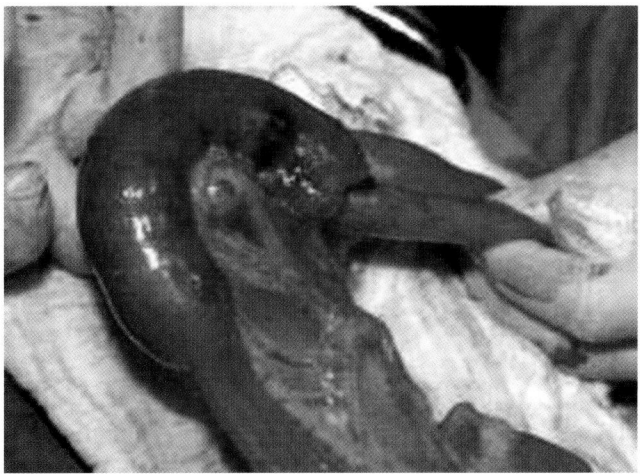

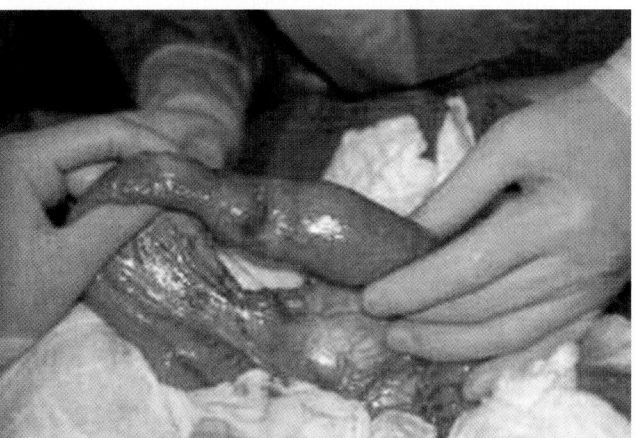

FIG. 19-106
A, Intraoperative appearance of an intussusception.
B, Following partial manual reduction of this intussusception, serosal and mesenteric tearing are noted.

SUTURE MATERIALS AND SPECIAL INSTRUMENTS

Instruments for enterotomy or intestinal resection and anastomosis are discussed on p. 459. Polydioxanone, poliglecaprone 25, polyglyconate, and glycomer 631 (3-0 or 4-0) are the preferred suture materials for these procedures; however, nonabsorbable suture (nylon, polybutester, or polypropylene) may be used in hypoalbuminemic animals. Chromic gut suture should be avoided in young animals and those that are debilitated because the suture may be rapidly catabolized and weakened.

POSTOPERATIVE CARE AND ASSESSMENT

Postoperative management should be individualized according to the patient's status and concurrent diseases. Hydration, electrolyte, and acid-base abnormalities should continue to be corrected postoperatively until the animal resumes adequate oral intake. Analgesics should be provided according to the recommendations in Chapter 13. Administration of butorphanol tartrate or other opioids may reduce recurrence. Therapeutic antibiotics are appropriate if peritonitis, abdominal contamination, or severe debilitation is present. Nutritional support via an enterostomy tube (see p. 107) may be necessary if the patient is debilitated or vomiting or remains anorectic. Monitor for recurrence and peritonitis.

COMPLICATIONS

Complications following treatment of intussusceptions include recurrence, intestinal obstruction, ileus, anastomotic dehiscence, peritonitis, and SBS. Leakage, dehiscence, peritonitis, and death are possible complications that occur more frequently in debilitated patients. Stenosis and SBS may occur if large segments of the bowel are removed (see p. 460). Complications of enteroenteropexy include intestinal obstruction and strangulation of intestine between enteroplication sutures (Applewhite et al, 2002); however these complications are avoidable with meticulous technique.

PROGNOSIS

Prognosis depends on the cause, location, completeness, and duration of the intussusception. Animals with untreated intestinal intussusceptions may die within 3 or 4 days or may live for several weeks. Those that die acutely usually have high obstructions or enterotoxemia; death is due to hypovolemia and electrolyte and acid-base imbalances. Animals with an intussusception may live for several weeks if the obstruction is partial or distal, the vasculature is functional, and an adequate fluid intake is maintained. Prognosis worsens with perforation of the intestine and peritonitis. In rare cases, an animal self-cures if the neck of the intussusception seals, a firm adhesion forms to the intussuscipiens, and the intussusceptum sloughs, reestablishing luminal patency. The prognosis with surgery is good with aggressive supportive care and early surgical intervention, assuming recurrence is prevented and extensive resections are avoided. Without enteroenteropexy, recurrence may be expected in approximately one third of affected animals.

Reference

Applewhite AA, Hawthorne JC, Cornell KK: Complications of enteroplication for the prevention of intussusception recurrence in dogs: 35 cases (1989-1999), *J Am Vet Med Assoc* 219:1415, 2001.

Suggested Reading

Applewhite AA, Cornell KK, Selcer BA: Diagnosis and treatment of intussusceptions in dogs, *Compend Contin Educ* 24:110, 2002.
This review is nicely illustrated, which enhances understanding of the condition.
Doherty D, Welsh EM, Kirby BM: Intestinal intussusception in five postparturient queens, *Vet Rec* 146:614, 2000.
There was no obvious reason for the intussusceptions. All cats were 2 years old or younger.
Patsikas MN, Jakovljevic S, Moustrardas N et al: Ultrasonographic signs of intestinal intussusception associated with acute enteritis or gastroenteritis in 19 young dogs, *J Am Anim Hosp Assoc* 39:57, 2003.
Consistent hypoechoic and hyperechoic patterns were found during imaging of animals with intussusceptions.
Patsikas MN, Papazoglou LG, Papaioannou NG et al: Normal and abnormal ultrasonographic findings that mimic small intestinal intussusception in the dog, *J Am Anim Hosp Assoc* 40:147, 2004.
Multiplane imaging is important to determine the cause of target-like lesions. Causes other than intussusceptions include bowel wall thickening from inflammation, neoplasia, edema, parasites, foreign bodies, or uterine involution.

PYTHIOSIS

DEFINITION

Enteritis is inflammation of the intestine. Organisms or syndromes that cause chronic enteritis may cause obstruction, diarrhea, or vomiting, or all of these.

GENERAL CONSIDERATIONS AND CLINICALLY RELEVANT PATHOPHYSIOLOGY

A regionally common inflammatory lesion of the intestine that requires surgery for diagnosis and treatment is pythiosis. *Pythium* spp. are ubiquitous, being found in water, soil, vegetable matter, and feces. *Pythium insidiosum* is an aquatic organism (oomycete) to which animals in contact with swamp water are commonly exposed. High water temperatures may enhance the growth of *Pythium* organisms and asexual reproduction (motile, biflagellated zoospores), predisposing animals to infection during the summer and fall months. *Pythium* lesions are slow growing and commonly involve the stomach, small and large intestine, rectum, mesentery, skin, and mesenteric lymph nodes. *Pythium* spp. may invade traumatized tissue (devitalized, necrotic, or ulcerated), but the motile spores may also penetrate intact mucosa. Fungal hyphae invade the intestinal wall, causing infarction, necrosis, and a granulomatous tissue reaction. The intestinal wall thickens, and signs of partial intestinal obstruction or malabsorption occur. Invasion by extension occurs along blood vessels, nerves, lymphatics, and fascial planes to other areas and organs. Invasion into blood vessels can cause thrombosis and visceral infarction.

Other causes of intestinal inflammation include inflammatory bowel disease (IBD), such as lymphocytic-plasmacytic enteritis, eosinophilic gastroenterocolitis, and granulomatous enteritis; intestinal lymphangiectasia; antibiotic responsive enteropathy (which used to be called intestinal bacterial overgrowth); and other fungal infections such as *Histoplasma capsulatum*. IBD is a syndrome in which there is persistent or recurrent inflammatory intestinal disease of undetermined cause. These diseases are classified according to the predominant inflammatory cell present and the area of intestine affected. The most common form is lymphocytic-plasmacytic enteritis. Lymphangiectasia is the dilation of lymph vessels in the intestine and is a major cause of protein-losing enteropathy. Laparotomy findings in animals with lymphangiectasia may include thickened small intestine, lipogranulomas in or on the wall of the intestine, dilated lymphatics, lymphadenomegaly, and/or adhesions. Gastroduodenoscopy may be as or more sensitive than laparotomy in diagnosing lymphangiectasia. Intestinal biopsy is important in the diagnosis of IBD, but IBD is not just a histologic diagnosis. IBD is a diagnosis of exclusion, meaning that all other causes of intestinal disease (i.e., parasites, diet, bacteria, cancer, fungi, and exocrine pancreatic insufficiency) and other causes of diarrhea (i.e., hyperthyroidism, feline infectious peritonitis, and hypoadrenocorticism) must be eliminated. Refer to a medicine text for a discussion of these conditions.

DIAGNOSIS
Clinical Presentation
Signalment. Pythiosis most commonly occurs in large-breed male dogs living in the southern Gulf states, but has been reported in the Midwestern states. The disease is rare in cats, but may cause ulcerative gastroenteritis. Young dogs (1 to 3 years of age) are most frequently affected.

History. Diarrhea and weight loss are the most common complaints. Clinical signs include diarrhea, vomiting, anorexia, depression, and/or progressive weight loss. Intestinal ulceration and necrosis may cause bloody diarrhea.

Physical Examination Findings
Affected animals frequently are thin. An abdominal mass or notable regional intestinal thickening may be detected on abdominal palpation or rectal examination. Sometimes there may be fistula near the rectum, mimicking perianal fistulae.

Diagnostic Imaging
An abdominal mass, thickened intestine, and/or signs of partial obstruction may be visualized on survey radiographs; however, severe weight loss and loss of abdominal fat may cause poor radiographic contrast. Contrast radiography may delineate thickened, stenotic areas. Intestinal thickening and abnormal wall layering are common findings on ultrasonography. Ultrasonography or fluoroscopy may show a lack of motility in the involved segment.

Endoscopy. A narrowed, nondistensible gastric or intestinal lumen with or without mucosal necrosis and/or ulceration may be seen endoscopically. Rigid endoscopic biopsies are more likely to be diagnostic than flexible endoscopic mucosal biopsies because the former allows one to obtain a more generous amount of fibrous submucosa, where hyphae are typically found.

Laboratory Findings
A CBC may reveal mild to moderate nonregenerative anemia and mild neutrophilia with or without a left shift. Definitive diagnosis depends on identification of broad-branching, nonseptate, or sparsely septate hyphae in tissues (Fig. 19-107). Hyphae are most easily found in necrotic granulomas of the submucosa and muscularis. Biopsies of enlarged mesenteric lymph nodes generally reveal granulomatous inflammation. The intestinal lesion should be cultured to identify the fungal organism more specifically. An enzyme-linked immunosorbent assay (ELISA) is available for the detection of anti-*Phythium insidiosum* antibodies in

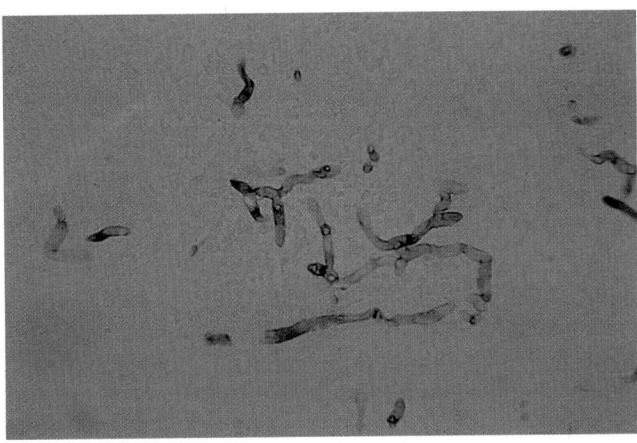

FIG. 19-107
Photomicrograph of *Pythium* hyphae that are broad-branching, nonseptate, or sparsely septate.

canine serum, which shows high sensitivity and specificity for diagnosis and monitoring treatment response (Grooters et al, 2002).

DIFFERENTIAL DIAGNOSIS
Pythiosis must be differentiated from other causes of partial intestinal obstruction (especially intussusception), neoplasia, other fungal lesions, and regional enteritis. In the perineum, pythiosis may cause lesions similar to perianal fistulae.

MEDICAL MANAGEMENT
Antifungal agents have not proved consistently efficacious, therefore radical surgical excision is required for possible cure. However, the extensive nature of many of the lesions limits complete resection.

SURGICAL TREATMENT
Preoperative Management
Fluid, electrolyte, and acid-base abnormalities should be corrected before surgery. Prophylactic antibiotics should be given based on the recommendations provided on p. 446.

Anesthesia
General anesthetic recommendations are provided on p. 445. Because most affected animals are debilitated, balanced anesthesia using injectable agents (i.e., opioids) and isoflurane or sevoflurane is recommended.

Surgical Anatomy
The surgical anatomy of the small intestine is discussed on p. 446.

Positioning
The animal should be positioned in dorsal recumbency for exploratory celiotomy. The ventral abdomen and caudal thorax should be clipped and prepared for aseptic surgery.

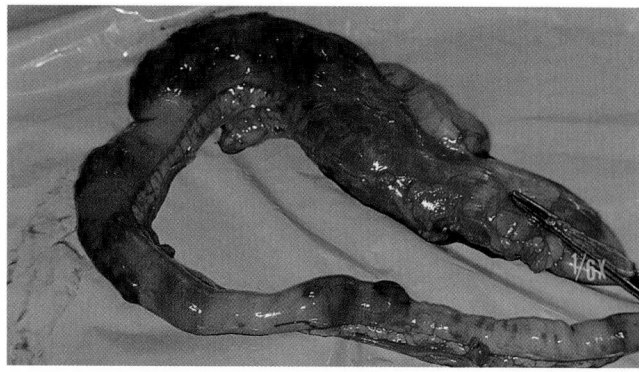

FIG. 19-108
Multiple small, firm masses causing partial intestinal obstruction associated with pythiosis in a dog.

SURGICAL TECHNIQUE

Expose the abdomen from the xiphoid process to the pubis. Explore the abdomen; the intestinal lesion may be extensive or multicentric, and the mesenteric lymph nodes generally are enlarged. Intestinal lesions are firm, granulomatous masses with mural thickening (Fig. 19-108). Take a biopsy from the lymph nodes and any other abnormal tissue. Resect the entire intestinal lesion with 4 to 8 cm of grossly normal intestine surrounding it because fungal hyphae have been found to extend several centimeters into normal-appearing tissue. Reappose intestinal ends with an end-to-end anastomosis (see p. 450).

SUTURE MATERIALS AND SPECIAL INSTRUMENTS

Instruments for enterotomy or intestinal resection and anastomosis are discussed on p. 459. Polydioxanone, poliglecaprone 25, polyglyconate, and glycomer 631 (3-0 or 4-0) are the preferred suture materials for these procedures. Nonabsorbable suture (i.e., nylon, polybutester, or polypropylene) generally should be avoided in infected sites. Chromic gut suture should be avoided when infection is present in young animals and in those that are debilitated.

POSTOPERATIVE CARE AND ASSESSMENT

Fluid, electrolyte, and acid-base abnormalities should be monitored and corrected after surgery. Analgesics should be provided as needed (see Table 13-4 on p. 133). Therapeutic antibiotics should be given if the animal has evidence of peritonitis, if abdominal contamination occurs during surgery, or if severe debilitation is present. Nutritional support via an enteral feeding tube or parenteral hyperalimentation may be necessary postoperatively if the patient is debilitated or unlikely to eat (see Chapter 11). Adjuvant antifungal therapy (e.g., itraconazole, liposomal amphotericin-B, and terbinafine) has been tried, but the results have not been encouraging. Vaccines made from fungal cultures have been used as adjuvant therapy with transient benefit. Leakage, dehiscence, peritonitis, stenosis, and SBS are possible complications of surgery. Signs of pythiosis may recur if tissue margins are not free of fungal hyphae.

PROGNOSIS

The prognosis with complete resection is fair to good. Some dogs have recurrence, and others are clinically normal without adjuvant therapy. The prognosis is guarded if the disease is advanced and if mesenteric vessels have thrombosed or adjacent structures have been invaded. The prognosis for nonresectable lesions is poor to guarded because current antifungal drugs are of questionable efficacy.

Reference

Grooters AM, Leise BS, Lopez MK et al: Development and evaluation of an enzyme-linked immunosorbent assay for the serodiagnosis of pythiosis in dogs, *J Vet Intern Med* 16:142, 2002.

Suggested Reading

Baez JL, Hendrick MJ, Walker LM et al: Radiographic, ultrasonographic, and endoscopic findings in cats with inflammatory bowel disease of the stomach and intestine: 39 cases (1990-1997), *J Am Vet Med Assoc* 215:349, 1999.
Ultrasonography appeared to predict histologic grade of feline IBD better than gross endoscopic appearance or radiographs.
German AJ, Hall EJ, Day MJ: Chronic intestinal inflammation and intestinal disease in dogs, *J Vet Intern Med* 17:8, 2003.
This review article of inflammatory bowel disease includes discussion of lymphocytic-plasmacytic enteritis, ulcerative colitis, idiopathic small intestinal overgrowth and other conditions.
Grooters AM, Gee MK: Development of a nested polymerase chain reaction assay for the detection and identification of *Pythium insidiosum*, *J Vet Intern Med* 16:147, 2002.
The authors have developed a test that appears to be useful in diagnosing infection with *Pythium insidiosum*.
Jergens AE, Schreine CA, Frank DE et al: A scoring index for disease activity in canine inflammatory bowel disease, *J Vet Intern Med* 17:291, 2003.
A system has been developed to allow objective assessment of improvement or decline in dogs being treated for IBD. The system was applied to 58 dogs and appeared to be clinically useful.
Kull PA, Hess RS, Craig LE et al: Clinical, clinicopathologic, radiographic and ultrasonographic characteristics of intestinal lymphangiectasia in dogs: 17 cases (1996-1998), *J Am Vet Med Assoc* 219:197, 2001.
This retrospective study reports mean age as 8.3 years; common clinical signs, including diarrhea, anorexia, lethargy, vomiting, and weight loss; and notable clinicopathologic signs of low serum ionized calcium concentration and hypoalbuminemia.

INTESTINAL VOLVULUS AND TORSION

DEFINITIONS

Intestinal volvulus is twisting of the intestine that causes obstruction. **Intestinal torsion** is twisting of the intestines about the root of the mesentery. The terms torsion and volvulus often are used interchangeably. The terms *mesenteric volvulus* and *mesenteric torsion* may also be used for these conditions.

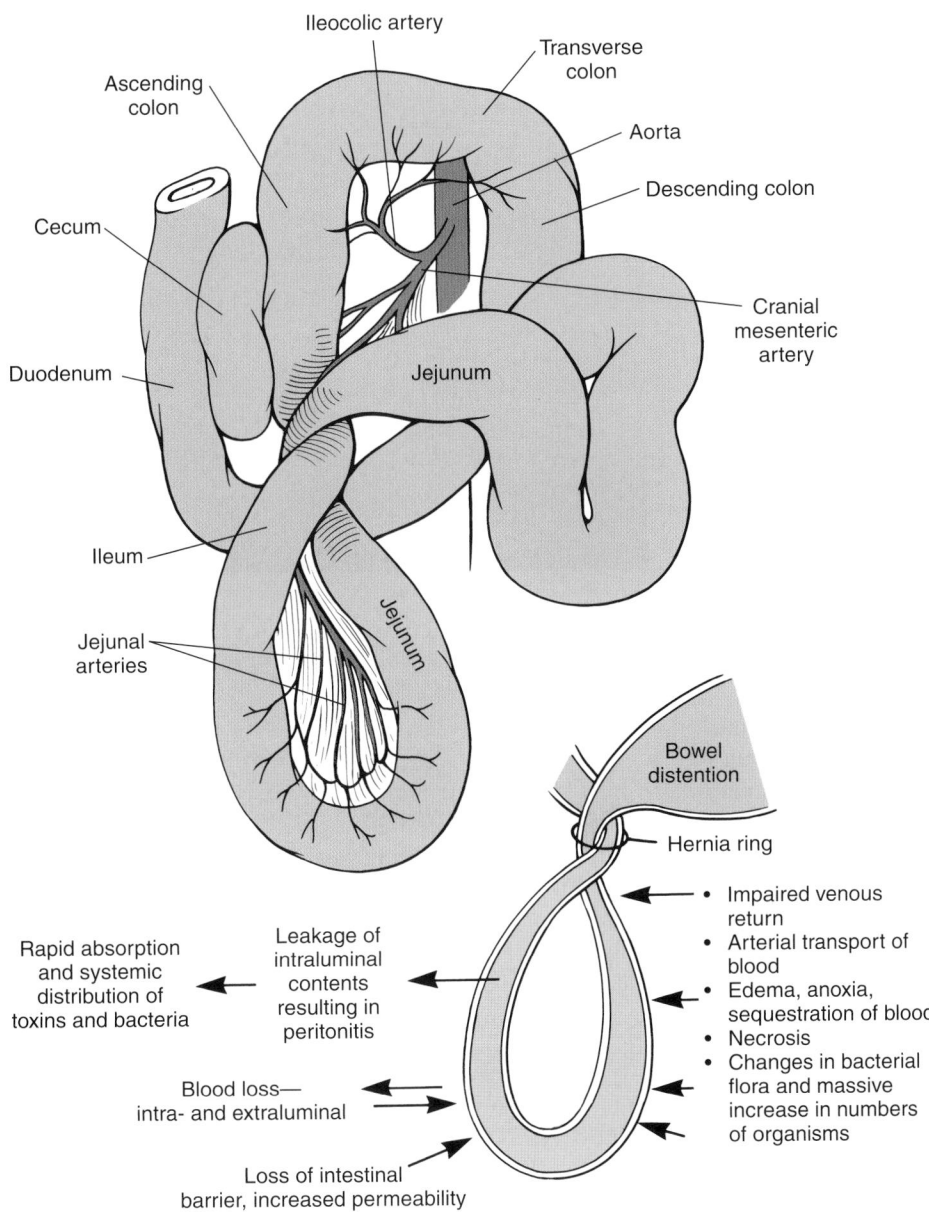

Ileocolic artery

Transverse colon

Ascending colon

Aorta

Descending colon

Cecum

Cranial mesenteric artery

Duodenum

Jejunum

Ileum

Jejunum

Jejunal arteries

Jejunum

FIG. 19-109
Pathophysiologic events associated with strangulating intestinal obstructions.

Bowel distention

Hernia ring

Rapid absorption and systemic distribution of toxins and bacteria

Leakage of intraluminal contents resulting in peritonitis

- Impaired venous return
- Arterial transport of blood
- Edema, anoxia, sequestration of blood
- Necrosis
- Changes in bacterial flora and massive increase in numbers of organisms

Blood loss— intra- and extraluminal

Loss of intestinal barrier, increased permeability

GENERAL CONSIDERATIONS AND CLINICALLY RELEVANT PATHOPHYSIOLOGY

Intestinal volvulus and torsion is uncommon in small animals because they have short mesenteric attachments. When it does occur, the jejunum is most commonly involved. Intestinal volvulus causes both mechanical and strangulation obstruction, a medical and surgical emergency (Fig. 19-109). Areas of the intestines that are not fixed in location by attachments to parietal peritoneum or adjacent viscera are suspended by mesentery, which provides greater freedom of movement. Movement and physiologic twisting or turning of suspended intestine occurs during physical activity and normal peristalsis. Twisting occurs around the mesenteric axis, or root. If mesenteric attachments fail to prevent excessive rotation, then vascular compromise, tissue ischemia, and luminal obstruction oc-

cur. Rotation may exceed 360 degrees in either a clockwise or counterclockwise direction. Predisposing factors in humans include an absence of mesenteric fat, a narrow mesenteric root, excessive mesenteric length, and an increased bowel length.

Twisting compromises the cranial mesenteric artery and all its branches, compromising blood flow to the distal duodenum, jejunum, ileum, cecum, ascending colon, transverse colon, and proximal descending colon. The ensuing rapid cascade of vascular obstruction, intestinal anoxia, circulatory shock, endotoxemia, and cardiovascular failure results in death if the condition is not corrected immediately. Mesenteric twisting reduces venous return and arterial perfusion. The arteries and veins may thrombose. Edema and congestion of the intestinal wall lead to anoxia. Blood is lost into both the intestinal lumen and the abdominal cavity.

Motility is disrupted, and the normal bacterial flora proliferates rapidly both proximal to and within the strangulated intestine. Small intestinal bacterial concentrations may increase to 10^8 to 10^{11}/ml within 6 hours of strangulation. Endotoxins (primarily from *E. coli*) and exotoxins from *Clostridium* spp. are produced. These toxins and bacteria escape into the abdomen through the damaged mucosal barrier and are absorbed into the systemic circulation. Death from strangulation obstruction usually results in a combination of hypovolemic shock, sepsis, and products of tissue necrosis. Reperfusion injury caused by oxygen-derived free radicals after derotation and tissue reoxygenation may be severe and may contribute to mortality.

DIAGNOSIS
Clinical Presentation

Signalment. Male, medium-to-large, sporting or working breeds have most commonly been diagnosed with intestinal volvulus and torsion. German shepherds (with pancreatic insufficiency) and English pointers appear to be predisposed to the condition. Young adult dogs (2 to 4 years of age) are most commonly affected.

History. Vigorous activity, dietary indiscretion, or trauma often precedes volvulus. Other factors that might be associated with intestinal volvulus include recent gastrointestinal surgery, enteritis, parvoviral infection, parasitism, foreign bodies, intussusception, obstructive masses, exocrine pancreatic insufficiency, and concurrent GDV. Some animals have been ill for several days and then suddenly deteriorate. Others progress from appearing normal to near death in less than 6 hours. Clinical signs range from peracute to acute and are commonly associated with partial obstruction and ischemia. Dogs with colonic volvulus rather than small intestinal volvulus may have a less acute progression of clinical signs (Bentley et al, 2005). Signs include acute pain, shock (tachycardia, pale to injected mucous membranes, prolonged capillary refill, weak pulses), and mild abdominal enlargement. There is an acute onset of nausea, retching, vomiting, hematochezia, depression, weakness, or recumbency, or all of these.

Physical Examination Findings

Affected animals usually are in shock with an acute abdomen. Pain and dilated loops of intestine may be detected by abdominal palpation. Occasionally, abdominal fluid is found, the amount varying with the duration of clinical signs.

Diagnostic Imaging

Survey radiographs often are diagnostic, with the entire intestinal tract uniformly distended with gas (Fig. 19-110). The intestines are often severely distended with gas and the loops lie parallel to each other. These findings combined with the physical presentation and history are often highly suggestive of intestinal volvulus. Intestinal fluid, free abdominal fluid, and generalized loss of serosal detail are expected. Definitive diagnosis of intestinal volvulus and torsion is made at surgery or necropsy.

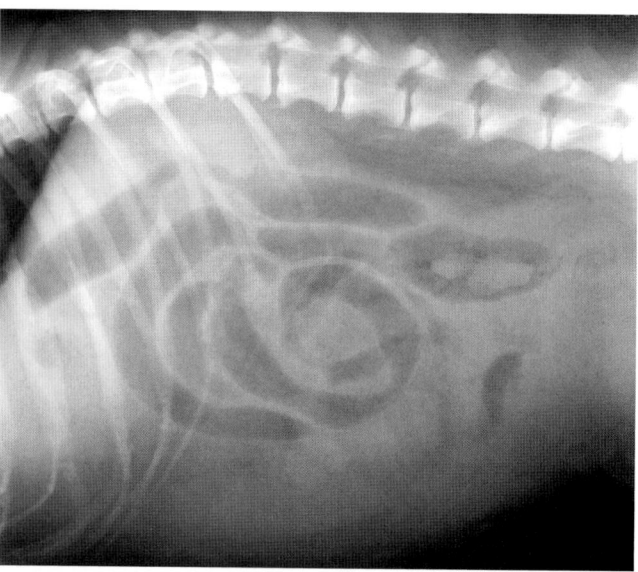

FIG. 19-110
Lateral radiograph of a dog with a mesenteric torsion. Notice the dilated small intestines and decreased visceral detail consistent with effusion.

Laboratory Findings

Common laboratory findings are a normal packed cell volume, leukocytosis, hypoproteinemia, hypoalbuminemia, and hypokalemia. Serosanguineous fluid or an exudate may be collected on abdominocentesis. The fluid is initially a transudate from serosal vessel leakage secondary to lymphatic and venous congestion, but once the mucosal barrier becomes incompetent, bacteria (intracellular and extracellular) and degenerative neutrophils will be found.

DIFFERENTIAL DIAGNOSIS

Any systemic or mechanical cause of acute abdomen should be included in the differential diagnosis. Surgical differential diagnoses include GDV, cecocolic volvulus, splenic torsion and rupture, physiologic ileus, mechanical obstruction, abdominal trauma, and peritonitis. Systemic illnesses may include hemorrhagic gastroenteritis, viral enteritis, and pancreatitis.

MEDICAL MANAGEMENT

Shock therapy (fluids and antibiotics, with or without corticosteroids; see later discussion) is essential but not curative. Immediate diagnosis and surgery are necessary if the patient is to survive.

SURGICAL TREATMENT
Preoperative Management

Initial treatment consists of aggressive shock therapy and correction of electrolyte and acid-base abnormalities. Shock doses of fluids (i.e., 90 ml/kg/hr) should be administered rapidly; however, central venous pressure should be monitored if possible to avoid volume overload. As an alternative, hypertonic saline or hetastarch may be given (see p. 29). Broad-spectrum antibiotic therapy and possibly an NSAID should be administered. Blood transfusions may be warranted if massive blood loss has occurred. Drugs that block formation of or that scavenge oxygen free radicals (e.g., superoxide dismutase, allopurinol, dimethylsulfoxide, corticosteroids, and gold compounds) may prove beneficial in the future.

Anesthesia

These patients are extreme anesthetic risks. A balanced anesthetic protocol should be used (e.g., opioids plus isoflurane). Selected anesthetic protocols for use in dogs with intestinal volvulus and torsion are provided in Box 19-53. They should be preoxygenated before surgery. Placing two venous catheters before surgery (i.e., two cephalic catheters or a cephalic and a jugular catheter) is recommended to allow fluids, blood, pressors, or other agents to be given simultaneously if needed. Hypotension should be corrected before and prevented during and after surgery. If the serum albumin concentration is less than 1.5 g/dl, perioperative administration of colloids may be indicated. Hetastarch may be given preoperatively, intraoperatively, and/or postoperatively for a total dose of 20 ml/kg/day (Box 19-54). If colloids are given during surgery, acute intraoperative hypotension should be treated with crystalloids. Dobutamine (2 to 10 µg/kg/min given intravenously) or dopamine (2 to 10 µg/kg/minute given intravenously) may be administered during surgery for inotropic support. Dobutamine is less arrhythmogenic and chronotropic than dopamine and is preferred if the patient is hypotensive and anuric. If the patient is anuric and normotensive, low-dose dopamine (0.5 to 1.5 µg/kg/min given intravenously) plus furosemide (0.2 mg/kg given intravenously) may be preferable. These patients should be monitored for arrhythmias or tachycardia. An electrocardiogram, a pulse oximeter, and direct and indirect blood pressure measurements should be monitored throughout surgery. Nitrous oxide is contraindicated.

Surgical Anatomy

The surgical anatomy of the small intestine is provided on p. 446. The cranial mesenteric artery branches to form the caudal pancreaticoduodenal, jejunal, ileocolic, right colic, and middle colic arteries.

Positioning

The patient should be positioned in dorsal recumbency for a ventral midline celiotomy. The caudal thorax and entire abdomen should be prepared for aseptic surgery.

SURGICAL TECHNIQUE

Quickly explore the abdomen to confirm the diagnosis and determine the direction of twisting. The intestine will appear dilated, edematous, and discolored, with the serosal surfaces ranging from red to black. Decompress the intestine if necessary to allow derotation and reposition the intestines. Allow the intestine to reperfuse and stabilize while the abdomen is

BOX 19-53

Selected Anesthetic Protocols for Use in Dogs With Intestinal Volvulus and Torsion

Induction

Hydromorphone (0.1 mg/kg given intravenously [IV]) plus diazepam (0.2 mg/kg IV). Give in incremental doses. Intubate if possible. If necessary, give etomidate (0.5–1.5 mg/kg IV). As an alternative, give thiopental or propofol at reduced dosages.

Maintenance

Isoflurane or sevoflurane.

BOX 19-54

Colloid Administration (Hetastarch, Dextrans)

Total daily dose:
Dogs: 10–20 ml/kg/day
Cats: 10–15 ml/kg/day

more thoroughly explored. Evaluate intestinal viability and resect devitalized tissue. Thoroughly lavage the abdomen with warm physiologic saline or a balanced electrolyte solution. Perform open peritoneal drainage (see p. 336) if intestinal necrosis and peritonitis are identified.

Some have recommended concurrent right-sided gastropexy, gastrocolopexy, and colopexy of the descending colon when the colonic torsion is discovered.

SUTURE MATERIALS AND SPECIAL INSTRUMENTS

Suction is useful for decompressing the intestine before derotation and repositioning. Suture material for small intestinal surgery is discussed on p. 459.

POSTOPERATIVE CARE AND ASSESSMENT

Fluid, electrolyte, and acid-base abnormalities should continue to be corrected after surgery. These patients may benefit from nasal oxygen postoperatively, and they should be monitored for signs of continued abdominal discomfort. Analgesics should be used if necessary (see Table 13-4 on p. 133). Continuation of perioperative antibiotics is reasonable, particularly if full-thickness necrosis of the intestine was present. Nutritional support should be provided by parenteral hyperalimentation if the animal is likely to be anorectic or to continue to vomit.

PROGNOSIS

Mortality approaches 100%, although one report had a 40% survival (5 of 12) (Junius et al, 2004). Vomiting, diarrhea, shock, intestinal necrosis, dehiscence, and peritonitis are common. Patients that survive may develop SBS after massive intestinal resection (see p. 460). Most animals that have survived were incidentally diagnosed during celiotomy for another problem, had rotation limited to 180 degrees, and were operated on within a few hours of occurrence.

References

Bentley AM, O'Toole TE, Kowaleski MP et al: Volvulus of the colon in four dogs, *J Am Vet Med Assoc* 227:253, 2005.

Junius G, Appeldoorn AM, Schrauwen E: Mesenteric volvulus in the dog: a retrospective study of 12 cases, *J Small Anim Pract* 45:104, 2004.

Suggested Reading

Jasani S, House AK, Brockman DJ: Localised mid-jejunal volvulus following intussusception and enteroplication in a dog, *J Small Anim Pract* 46:398, 2005.

The dog, an 11-month-old German shepherd, was successfully treated.

Milner HR, Newington AN: Longitudinal colonic torsion as a cause of tenesmus in an adult Irish water spaniel, *N Z Vet J* 52:40, 2004.

This dog was diagnosed with the aid of a barium enema and treated by untwisting the descending colon and colopexy.

Surgery of the Large Intestine

GENERAL PRINCIPLES AND TECHNIQUES

DEFINITIONS

Colopexy is surgical fixation of the colon. **Colectomy** is partial or complete resection of the colon, and **typhlectomy** is resection of the cecum. **Colostomy** is surgical creation of an opening between the colon and the surface of the body. **Tenesmus** is straining to defecate, and **dyschezia** is pain or discomfort on defecation. **Hematochezia** is passage of stools that contain red blood, and **melena** is passage of tarry stools (i.e., digested blood).

PREOPERATIVE MANAGEMENT

Surgery of the large intestine is indicated for lesions that cause obstruction, perforation, colonic inertia, or chronic inflammation. The most common causes of obstruction are tumors, intussusceptions, and granulomatous masses. Foreign bodies that reach the colon generally are expelled with the feces unless the distal colon or rectum is obstructed or the object has sharp points.

Differentiation of large bowel disease from small intestinal disorders usually is based on the history and physical examination (see Table 19-1). However, imaging (especially ultrasonography) and/or endoscopic biopsy (or all of these) may be necessary. Differentiation of the various causes of large intestinal disorders is based on the history, physical examination, fecal examination, endoscopy and biopsy, therapeutic trials, and/or bacterial culture. Most patients with large bowel disease do not have significant weight loss except those with histoplasmosis, pythiosis, protothecosis, histiocytic ulcerative colitis, megacolon, or tumors. Affected patients may have diarrhea or be constipated. Tenesmus, dyschezia, fresh fecal blood, and/or fecal mucus may or may not be present. Other clinical signs may include diarrhea, vomiting, anorexia, abdominal enlargement, abdominal pain, fecaliths, abnormal fecal shape, rectal prolapse, depression, and/or poor hair coat (see Table19-1).

The physical examination findings vary, depending on the disease and its location in the large bowel (see Table 19-1). The colon is usually palpable in the dorsocaudal abdomen, except in obese animals. Feces often can be differentiated from masses (e.g., tumor) by applying gentle pressure; normal feces deform whereas animals with constipation or obstipation have hard, dry feces. Sublumbar lymph node enlargement sometimes can be detected by palpation of the caudal abdomen or occasionally on rectal examination; lymphadenomegaly is suggestive of metastatic neoplasia. Rectal examination should be done in all patients with large bowel disease. Rectal exam evaluates the shape and symmetry of the pelvis and mucosal thickness. It may also detect masses in the pelvic canal, intraluminal masses, and distal strictures. The anus and anal sacs should be checked for thickening, enlargement, and pain. The feces should be examined for the presence of blood or mucus, and then examined for parasites.

Most animals with large bowel disease have no laboratory abnormalities. Rarely, dehydration, electrolyte changes, anemia, or hypoalbuminemia is seen (see Table 19-1). Although nonspecific, elevation of the serum alkaline phosphatase, creatine phosphokinase, lactic dehydrogenase, and serum glutamic oxaloacetic transaminase may be seen in animals with intestinal ischemia.

Survey colonic radiographs rarely contribute in animals with diarrhea, but may help in those with megacolon. Withholding food (24 hours) and evacuating the colon improve visualization. Luminal masses may be identified if the colon contains gas. A "coiled-spring" appearance when the colon is filled with air (or barium) indicates a possible cecal inversion or intussusception. Contrast barium enemas may identify dilatations, constrictions, wall thickening, filling defects, infiltrative disease, extraluminal compression, intraluminal masses, intussusceptions, volvulus, or cecal inversion. However, barium enemas are labor intensive procedures and have been almost totally replaced by colonoscopy. Ultrasonography is the preferred imaging modality; it gives information about large bowel wall thickness, wall layers, wall symmetry, peristalsis, and echogenicity of intestinal contents. Biopsies may be obtained with ultrasound guidance. CT and MRI are beneficial in some cases, but these diagnostic techniques often are unavailable. Colonoscopy is safe and more sensitive than radiography for diagnosing masses, ulcers, infiltrates, and intussusceptions. It allows for direct visualization of the

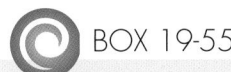

BOX 19-55

Bowel Preparation for Large Intestinal and Rectal Surgery

Polyethylene Glycol Electrolyte Solution (Colyte or GoLytely)

25–30 ml/kg; PO via stomach tube twice the afternoon before the procedure, approximately 4 to 6 hours apart (repeat early the next morning if necessary)

Bisacodyl (Dulcolax)

Dogs: 5 mg/dog PO, qd or bid
Cats: 2.5–5 mg/cat PO, qd to bid

PO, Oral; *qd,* once a day; *bid,* twice a day.

NOTE: Be careful; enemas can cause further deterioration of debilitated, anorectic patients and in rare cases can cause colonic perforation. They may be ineffective in cats with megacolon. Never give hypertonic phosphate enemas to small or constipated patients or cats.

---

lumen, fecal/mucosal culture, mucosal cytology, and mucosal biopsy.

If the patient is not rapidly deteriorating, hydration, acid-base, and electrolyte deficits should be corrected before induction of anesthesia. Cross-matched whole blood should be administered when the packed cell volume drops below 20% or the patient is clinically weak from the anemia. Anemic patients should be given whole blood if hypovolemic and packed red blood cells if normovolemic. Clotting factor deficiencies should be corrected with fresh whole blood (Box 5-1 on p. 25) or fresh or fresh-frozen plasma. Administration of plasma (5 to 20 ml/kg), whole blood (10-22 ml/kg), or preferably hetastarch (5 to 20 ml/kg/day) should be considered if albumin levels are below 1.5 g/dl. There is some evidence that blood transfusions may impair intestinal healing and increase susceptibility to intraabdominal sepsis.

The colon contains more bacteria (i.e., more than 10^{10}/g of feces) than the rest of the gastrointestinal tract. Preoperative colonic emptying and cleansing are indicated to reduce bacterial numbers unless the colon is perforated or obstructed. Feeding an elemental diet that requires no digestion (e.g., glucose and amino acids) reduces colonic bacterial numbers to 10^3/g of feces. If possible, an elemental diet or a low-residue diet of hamburger and white rice should be fed for 2 to 3 days before surgery. Holding animals off food also reduces bacterial numbers in the colon. Food should be withheld 24 hours before surgery, but free access to water should be allowed. Laxatives, cathartics, and warm water enemas should be given 24 hours before surgery. Colon electrolyte solutions (i.e., Colyte or GoLytely; Box 19-55) more effectively cleanse the colon than enemas; the only contraindication to their use is obstruction. Bisacodyl, a stimulant laxative, may be administered to facilitate colonic evacuation. Although colonic electrolyte solutions work well alone, enemas facilitate complete cleansing. A warm water enema should be given the day before surgery, and a 10% povidone-iodine enema should be given 3 hours before surgery. Enemas given any closer to surgery than 3 hours are contraindicated because they liquefy intestinal contents and may add to dissemination of contaminated material during surgery.

ANESTHESIA

Anesthetic complications may arise because of uncorrected hydration, electrolyte, or acid-base abnormalities. Large masses or visceral displacement may impair circulation and respiration. Nitrous oxide increases the volume of air trapped in hollow viscera and should be avoided in patients with intestinal obstruction. Atropine (0.02 to 0.04 mg/kg, SC, IM, IV) or glycopyrrolate (0.005 to 0.011 mg/kg SC, IM, IV) may prevent bradycardia induced by visceral manipulation. Water evaporates from exposed abdominal viscera at an increased rate; therefore fluid administration must be increased to replace this loss. Body heat is lost because of vasodilation and visceral exposure, which cause hypothermia, reducing the need for anesthesia. Patients should be kept dry to minimize the effects of hypothermia. Selected protocols for animals in stable condition undergoing large intestinal surgery are provided in Box 19-43 (see p. 445).

ANTIBIOTICS

The risk of infection after colorectal surgery is high. Although controversial, the use of antibiotics with colorectal surgery reduces morbidity and mortality associated with infection. Systemic perioperative antibiotics effective against anaerobes and gram-negative aerobes should be given (Box 19-56). Recommended drugs include the second-generation cephalosporins (i.e., cefmetazole, cefoxitin, and cefotetan), which are given at the time of induction. Third-generation cephalosporins effective against gram-positive and gram-negative aerobes and some anaerobes are available but expensive. Amikacin plus clindamycin can be given intravenously at induction of anesthesia. Aminoglycosides (i.e., neomycin and kanamycin) and metronidazole can be given orally in combination beginning 24 hours before surgery. Metronidazole is absorbed from the gastrointestinal tract and is effective against anaerobes. Aminoglycosides are effective only against aerobic bacteria. Gastrointestinal absorption of aminoglycosides is minimal in normal patients, but can be substantial if the bowel is eroded or inflamed. The use of such nonabsorbable antibiotics has been linked with the emergence of resistant infections. A combination of oral neomycin and erythromycin can be given beginning 24 hours before surgery to rapidly reduce the number of aerobes and anaerobes. Metronidazole combined with first-generation cephalosporins (cefazolin) or aminoglycosides is also useful.

SURGICAL ANATOMY

The cecum, ascending colon, transverse colon, descending colon, and rectum are segments of the large bowel. The ascending colon and cecum are located at the termination of

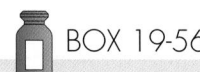 BOX 19-56

Prophylactic Antibiotic Use in Animals Undergoing Perineal, Rectal, or Colonic Surgery

Cefmetazole (Zefazone)

15 mg/kg IV; repeat every 1½ to 2 hours for 2 or 3 doses

Cefoxitin (Mefoxin)

15–30 mg/kg IV; repeat every 1½ to 2 hours for 2 or 3 doses

Cefotetan (Cefotan)

30 mg/kg IV; repeat every 8 hours for 24 hours

Neomycin (Biosol)

10–15 mg/kg PO, tid

Metronidazole (Flagyl)

10 mg/kg IV (give slowly over 20 min) or PO, tid

Erythromycin*

11–22 mg/kg PO, bid to tid

Amikacin (Amiglyde-V)

20–25 mg/kg IV, qd

Ampicillin (Omnipen, Principen, others)

22 mg/kg IV, tid to qid

IV, Intravenous; *qd,* once a day; *PO,* oral; *tid,* three times a day; *bid,* twice a day: *IM,* intramuscular.
*Vomiting and diarrhea are common side effects due to the prokinetic activity of the drug.

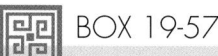 BOX 19-57

Approximate Lengths of Colonic Segments

Ascending Colon

Dogs: 3–9 cm
Cats: 1–2 cm

Transverse Colon

Dogs: 6–8 cm
Cats: 2–4 cm

Descending Colon

10–16 cm; varies with size of animal

---

the ileum. In dogs, the *cecum* is an S-shaped, blind pouch located to the right of the mesenteric root; in cats, it is a short, straight, blind pouch. The cecum is ventral to the right kidney, dorsal to the small intestine, and medial to the descending duodenum. A short antimesenteric vessel helps identify the ascending colon lying to the right of the mesenteric root. The *ascending colon* communicates with the ileum via the ileocolic orifice and with the cecum via the cecocolic orifice (approximately 1 cm caudal to the ileocolic orifice). The short ascending colon turns from right to left at the right colic flexure (hepatic flexure) and becomes the *transverse colon,* traveling cranial to the mesenteric root. The colon turns caudally at the left colic flexure (splenic flexure) and becomes the descending colon. The *descending colon* is the longest segment of colon (Box 19-57). It begins on the left, where it is dorsal to the small intestine, and continues caudally to the pelvic inlet. The large bowel continues through the pelvic canal to the anus as the *rectum.* The colorectal junction is difficult to identify. Landmarks include the pubic brim, pelvic inlet, seventh lumbar vertebra, and seromuscular point of penetration of the cranial rectal artery. The *mesocolon* is the short mesenteric attachment of the colon to the body wall. The layers of the large intestinal wall are the same as the layers of the small intestinal wall (mucosa, submucosa, muscularis, and serosa).

The blood supply to the large bowel is from the ileocolic artery, a branch of the cranial mesenteric artery, and the caudal mesenteric artery. These major branches run parallel to the intestine, giving off short vasa recta vessels, which penetrate the intestinal wall. Branches of the ileocolic and left colic artery anastomose. The ileocolic artery supplies the ileum, cecum, and ascending and transverse colon. It gives rise to the middle colic and right colic arteries. The right colic artery supplies the cecum, the ascending colon, and part of the transverse colon. The middle colic artery supplies part of the transverse colon and half of the descending colon; it anastomoses with the left colic artery, which supplies the distal half of the descending colon. The left colic and cranial rectal arteries originate from the caudal mesenteric artery. The cranial rectal artery primarily supplies the cranial rectum, but also sends several vasa recta to a short segment of the terminal colon. The internal iliac artery supplies branches to the rectum via prostatic or vaginal artery branches. Venous drainage essentially mirrors arterial supply. The caudal mesenteric vein is short and enters the portal vein. The vagus and pelvic nerves supply the colon with parasympathetic innervation. Sympathetic innervation is supplied from the paravertebral sympathetic trunk via the sympathetic ganglia.

SURGICAL TECHNIQUE

The surgical principles for large intestinal surgery are similar to those for small intestinal surgery (Box 19-58), but dehiscence of large bowel incisions is more likely than small bowel incisions. Bowel viability can be difficult to assess, but it is important that necrotic or avascular areas of the colon be removed at surgery and that unnecessary resection be avoided. Because of the short mesocolon, avulsion of the colonic blood supply is less common than avulsion of the mesenteric blood supply. Techniques for assessing bowel viability are presented on p. 447.

Resection and anastomosis may be performed using sutures or staples. The four stapled anastomosis techniques are the (1) triangulating end-to-end anastomosis, (2) inverting end-to-end anastomosis, (3) side-to-side or functional end-to-end anastomosis, and (4) end-to-side anastomosis. End-to-end anastomoses (see p. 450) are most commonly performed

BOX 19-58

Principles of Large Intestinal Surgery

- Reduce colonic bacterial numbers by eliminating oral intake, preparing the colon, and giving antibiotics.
- Early diagnosis and good surgical technique prevent most complications.
- Perform surgery as soon as anesthesia permits in patients with perforation, strangulation, or complete obstruction.
- Optimal healing requires a good blood supply, accurate mucosal apposition, and minimal surgical trauma.
- Systemic factors (e.g., hypovolemia, shock, hypoproteinemia, debilitation, infection) may delay healing and increase the risk of dehiscence.
- Dehiscence is more likely with large bowel surgery than with small bowel surgery.
- Use approximating suture patterns: simple interrupted, Gambee, crushing, or simple continuous.
- Engage submucosa in all sutures.
- Select a monofilament, synthetic absorbable suture: polydioxanone, polyglyconate, or poliglecaprone 25, glycomer 631.
- Cover surgical sites with omentum or a serosal patch.
- Replace contaminated instruments and gloves before closing the abdomen.

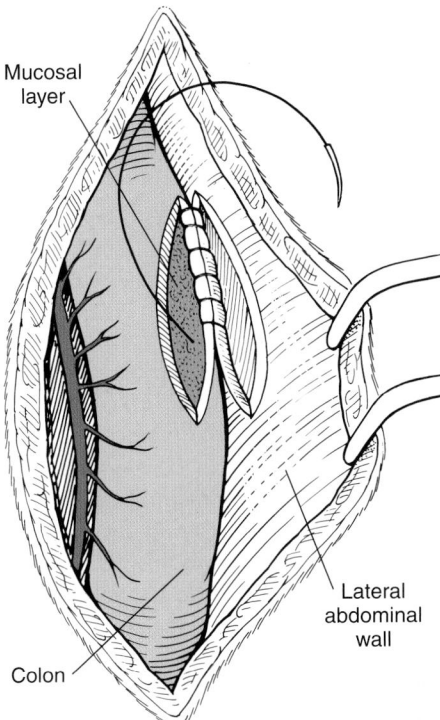

FIG. 19-111
To pexy the colon to the abdominal wall, make a 3- to 5-cm seromuscular incision along the antimesenteric border of the colon. Make a similar incision 2 to 3 cm lateral to the linea alba through the peritoneum and the underlying muscle of the left abdominal wall. Appose the edges of the seromuscular incision to the edges of the abdominal wall incision with two simple continuous suture lines.

during colonic anastomosis. Although more expensive, stapled anastomoses show less tissue reaction, more mature fibrous connective tissue, greater tensile strength, fewer mucoceles and necrotic areas, and less luminal stenosis than suture techniques. The staples in the cartridge are bent against the anvil into a **B** shape when fired, providing a degree of hemostasis without collapsing the microcirculation. Thick, inflamed, and edematous tissues may prevent proper firing of the stapler by preventing complete penetration and formation of the staples into the **B** shape. Dilatation causes thinning of the visceral walls and may result in tissues that are too thin for the staples to be effective. In such cases a suture anastomosis should be performed. Circular, inverting, end-to-end staplers often are used to anastomose the colon. It is easier to use end-to-end staplers in the colon than in other areas of the gastrointestinal tract because the instrument can be introduced through the anus rather than through a separate enterotomy or gastrotomy incision. The colon of most adult animals can accommodate the size of available staplers. Transanal introduction of the stapler may not be possible in all cats and small dogs because of the small anus and narrow pelvic canal.

Biopsy Techniques

Intestinal biopsy is indicated to establish a diagnosis for intestinal diseases that have not been diagnosed by other means. A biopsy may be taken from the large intestine during endoscopy, ultrasonography, or laparotomy. Full-thickness colonic biopsy should be avoided unless absolutely necessary. Colonoscopy is the preferred method for colonic mucosal biopsy; rigid endoscopes routinely allow biopsies with generous amounts of submucosa to be obtained. Flexible endoscopic

biopsies also routinely include the mucosa, but are not as large as those obtained with rigid scopes. Rigid proctoscopes permit diagnostic biopsies of dense, submucosal rectal lesions.

Colopexy

Colopexy is performed to create permanent adhesions between the serosal surfaces of the colon and the abdominal wall to prevent caudal movement of the colon and rectum (Fig. 19-111). Colopexy is used most often to prevent recurring rectal prolapse. Incisional and nonincisional techniques have been described and are equally effective. Colopexy can be performed laparoscopically using similar techniques. A possible complication is infection resulting from suture penetration of the colonic lumen.

Expose and explore the abdomen. Locate the descending colon and isolate it from the remainder of the abdomen. Pull the descending colon cranially to reduce the prolapse. Verify reduction of the prolapse by having a nonsterile assistant inspect the anus visually and perform a rectal examination. Make a 3- to 5-cm longitudinal incision along the antimesenteric border of the distal descending colon through only the serosal and muscularis layers. Make a similar incision on the left abdominal wall several centimeters (2.5 cm or more) lateral to the linea alba through the peritoneum and underlying muscle. Appose each edge of the colonic and abdominal wall incisions with two simple continuous or simple interrupted rows of sutures using 2-0 or 3-0 monofilament, absorbable suture (e.g., polydioxanone, polyglyconate, or poliglecaprone 25) or nonabsorbable suture (nylon, polybutester, or polypropylene) (see Fig. 19-111). Engage the submucosa as each suture is placed. Lavage the surgical site and surround it with omentum before closing the abdomen. As an alternative, scarify an 8- to 10-cm antimesenteric segment of the descending colon by scraping the serosa with a scalpel blade or rubbing it with a gauze sponge. On the left abdominal wall opposite the prepared colon, scarify the peritoneum in the same manner. Preplace and then tie six to eight horizontal mattress sutures between the two scarified surfaces. Roll the colon toward the midline and place a second row of six to eight sutures using 2-0 or 3-0 monofilament, absorbable or nonabsorbable suture. Engage the submucosa with the sutures, but do not penetrate the colonic mucosa. Tie the sutures apposing the scarified surfaces.

Colon Resection and Anastomosis

Colectomy and resection are primarily performed to excise colonic masses or to treat megacolon. Other surgical indications include trauma, perforation, intussusception, and cecal inversion. The procedure is much the same as for small intestinal resection and anastomosis (see p. 450) with the exception of vascular ligation.

> NOTE: Up to 70% of the colon can be resected in animals without adverse side effects; cats tolerate colonic resection better than dogs. Subtotal colectomy (i.e., removal of 90% to 95% of the colon) is often done in cats, but should be avoided in dogs. Warn owners that after subtotal colectomy, the cat probably will defecate frequently and have soft stools.

Explore the entire abdomen through a ventral midline celiotomy. Collect nonintestinal specimens before entering the bowel lumen. Carefully isolate the diseased bowel with laparotomy pads or sterile towels. Assess intestinal viability and determine the resection sites. Double ligate all the vasa recta vessels to the diseased segment (Fig. 19-112), but do not ligate the major colic vessels running parallel to the mesenteric border of the bowel unless performing a subtotal colectomy. Gently milk fecal material from the lumen of the isolated bowel. Occlude the lumen at both ends to minimize fecal contamination by having an assistant use a scissorlike grip with the index and middle fingers positioned 4 to 6 cm from the diseased tissue on the colonic wall. Noncrushing intestinal forceps (Doyen) or a Penrose drain tourniquet can also be used to occlude the intestinal lumen.

Place another pair of forceps (either crushing [Carmalt] or noncrushing [Doyen]) across each end of the diseased bowel segment. Transect through healthy colon using a scalpel blade or Metzenbaum scissors along the outside of the

crushing forceps (see Fig. 19-87 on p. 451). If the lumen sizes are about equal, make the incision perpendicular to the long axis. When the lumen sizes are expected to be unequal, use an oblique incision (45- to 60-degree angle) across the smaller intestinal segment. Angle the incision such that the antimesenteric border is shorter than the mesenteric border. Suction the intestinal ends and remove any debris clinging to the cut edges with a moistened gauze sponge. Trim everting mucosa with Metzenbaum scissors just before beginning the anastomosis, if necessary.

Sutured anastomoses. *Reappose the intestinal ends with a one- or two-layer suture closure. Use 3-0 or 4-0 monofilament, absorbable suture (polydioxanone, polyglyconate, poliglecaprone 25) or nonabsorbable suture (nylon, polypropylene, polybutester) with a taper or tapercut, swaged-on needle. Place simple interrupted sutures through all layers of the wall and position knots extraluminally when a one-layer closure is used. Angle the needle such that slightly more serosa than mucosa is engaged with each bite to help prevent the mucosa from protruding between sutures (see Fig. 19-86 on p. 450).*

Begin by placing one suture at the mesenteric border and one at the antimesenteric border. If the intestinal ends are of equal diameter, space additional sutures between the first two sutures approximately 2 mm from the edge and 2 to 3 mm apart. Gently appose the tissue edges when tying knots to prevent tissue strangulation and disruption of the blood supply. If minor disparity still exists between the lumen sizes, space sutures around the larger lumen slightly farther apart than the sutures in the intestinal segment with the smaller lumen (see Fig. 19-89 on p. 452).

Luminal disparity that cannot be accommodated by the angle of the incisions or suture spacing usually is correctable by resecting a small wedge (1 to 2 cm long, 1 to 3 mm wide) from the antimesenteric border of the intestine with the smaller lumen (see Fig. 19-91 on p. 453). This enlarges the stomal perimeter and gives it an oval shape.

After completing the anastomosis, check for leakage by moderately distending the lumen with saline and applying gentle digital pressure. Look for leakage between sutures or through suture holes. Place additional sutures if leakage occurs between sutures. Close the mesenteric defect. Lavage the isolated intestine thoroughly without allowing the fluid to seep into the abdominal cavity. Remove the laparotomy pads and change gloves and instruments. Lavage the abdomen with sterile, warm saline, then use suction to remove the fluid. Wrap the anastomotic site with omentum or create a serosal patch (see p. 457).

A two-layer anastomosis occasionally is recommended if there is tension at the anastomotic site. A two-layer anastomosis is performed in the same manner as a one-layer closure except that the serosa and muscularis are apposed in a separate layer. All sutures engage the submucosa. The first layer of

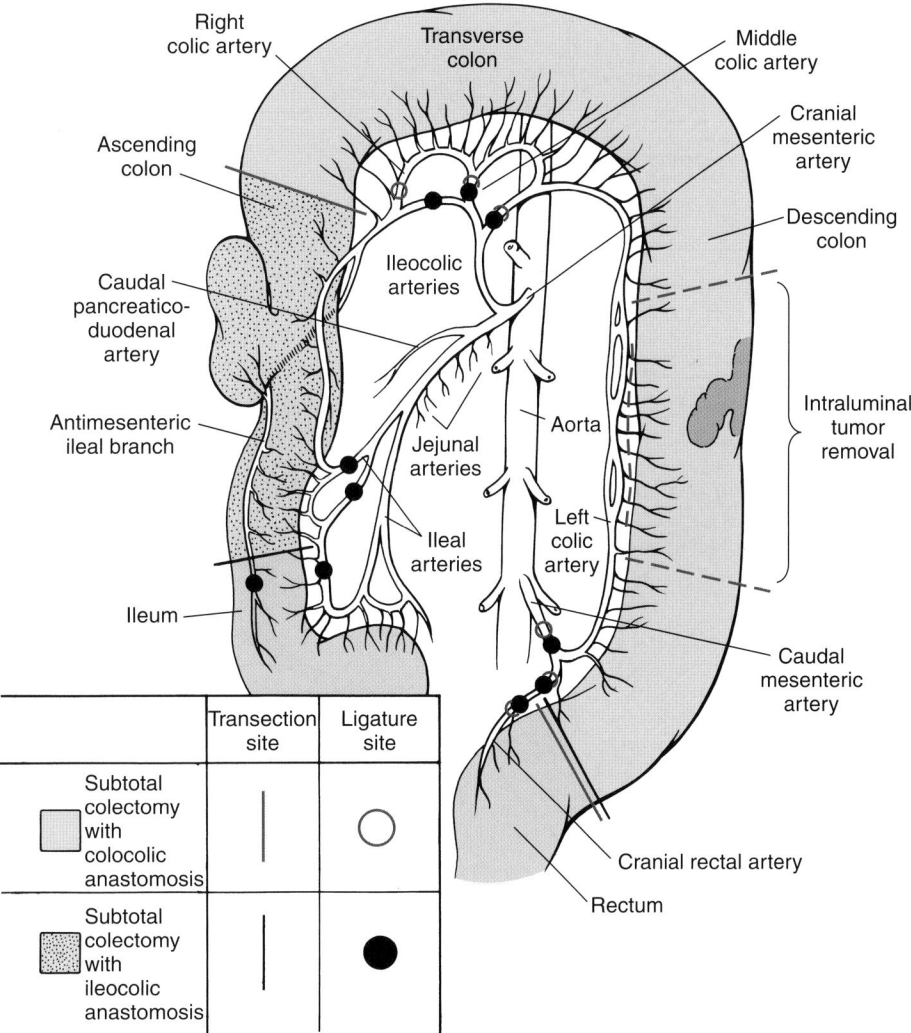

FIG. 19-112
For a partial colectomy *(dashed lines)*, double ligate the vasa recta vessels; preserve the major colonic vessels. Perform a subtotal colectomy, preserving the ileocolic junction by double ligating the paired arteries and veins *(open red circles)*. Perform a subtotal colectomy and ileocolic anastomosis by double ligating the paired arteries and veins *(shaded dark circles)*. Transection sites are identified by the corresponding symbol. *In dogs, do not ligate the cranial rectal artery; ligate the left colic and vasa recta from the cranial rectal artery.*

simple interrupted sutures is placed to appose the mucosa and submucosa, and the knots are tied within the lumen. The second layer of interrupted sutures apposes the muscularis and serosa, and the knots are positioned extraluminally.

Stapled anastomoses. The distal colon may be anastomosed to the ileum or jejunum using skin staples, inverting end-to-end, functional end-to-end, or end-to-side stapling techniques. The inverting end-to-end and functional end-to-end techniques are performed in the same way as for small intestinal anastomoses (see p. 453).

For an end-to-side technique, first insert the end-to-end stapling instrument (without anvil) through the open transected end of the colon. Advance the center rod through an antimesenteric stab wound surrounded by a purse-string

suture. Tie the suture and place the anvil on the center rod. Introduce the anvil into the lumen of the ileum. Tie the ileal purse-string suture, close the instrument, and fire the staples. Gently rotate and remove the instrument. Inspect the anastomotic site for hemostasis and integrity. Close the transected colon with a transverse stapler. Lavage the surgical sites, and place an omental or serosal patch (see p. 457).

Typhlectomy

Typhlectomy, or cecal resection, is performed when the cecum becomes impacted, inverted, perforated, or neoplastic, or is severely inflamed.

Begin typhlectomy for a noninverted cecum by double ligating the cecal branches of the ileocecal artery in the ileocecal

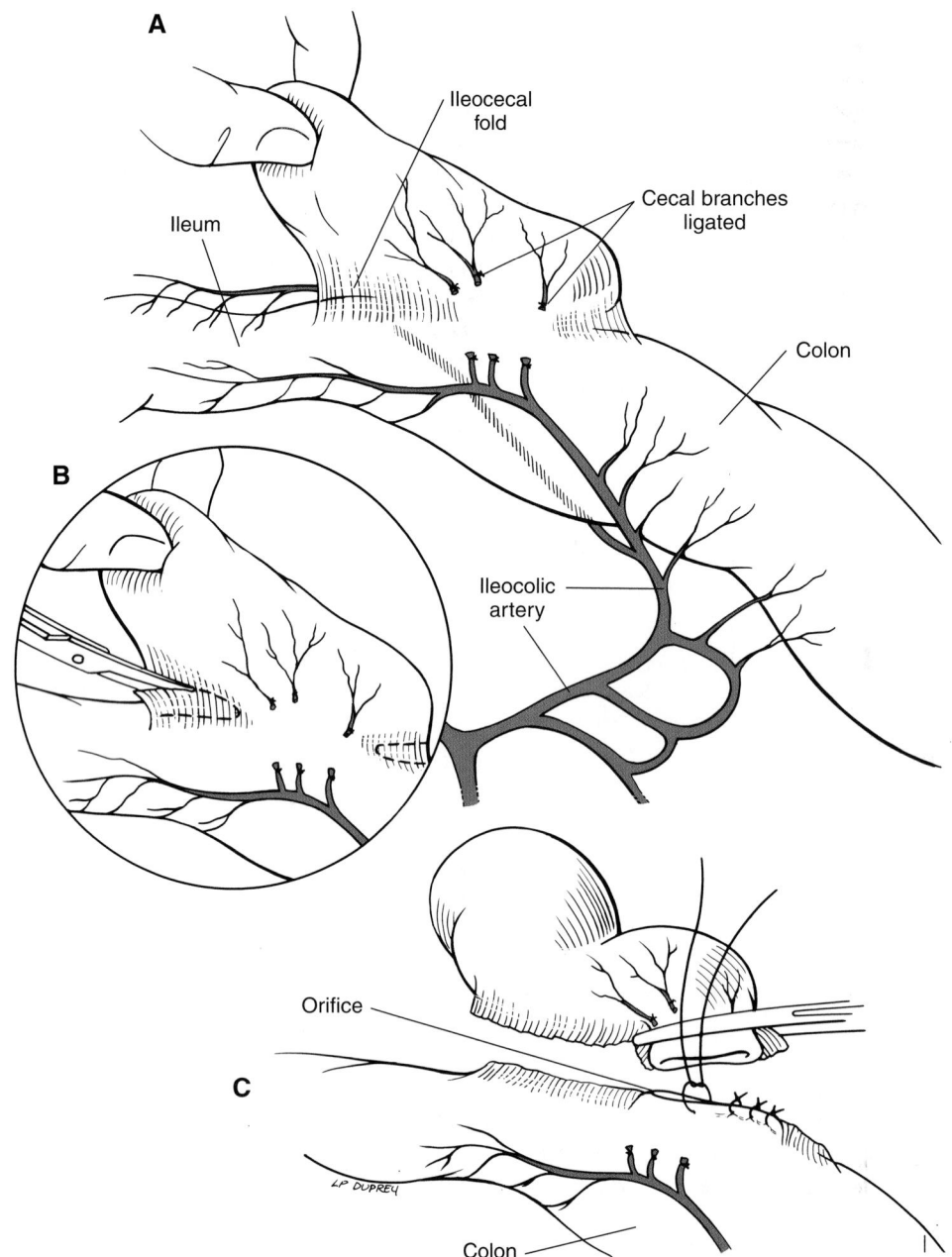

FIG. 19-113
Typhlectomy. **A,** Double ligate the cecal branches of the ileocolic vessels. **B,** Dissect the ileocecal fold of the mesentery. **C,** Place a clamp across the base of the cecum near the cecocolic orifice and transect. Close the colonic defect with simple interrupted sutures.

mesenteric attachment (ileocecal fold) (Fig. 19-113, A). Dissect the ileocecal fold, freeing the cecum from the ileum and colon (Fig. 19-113, B). Place a clamp across the base of the cecum (Fig. 19-113, C). Milk intestinal contents from the ascending colon and ileum adjacent to the cecocolic orifice and occlude the lumen. Transect the cecum where it joins the ascending colon. Close the defect with simple interrupted sutures. As an alternative, place a transverse or linear cutting stapling instrument across the base of the cecum. Activate the stapler. Transect the cecum before removing the

transverse stapling instrument. Lavage, then cover the surgical site with an omental or serosal patch (see p. 457).

The cecum may be difficult to locate if it is inverted, but its location may be identified by a small indentation where it can be palpated within the colonic lumen (Fig. 19-114).

If possible, manually reduce the cecum before resection. If it cannot be reduced manually, perform an antimesenteric colotomy and exteriorize the cecum (Fig. 19-115). Resect the

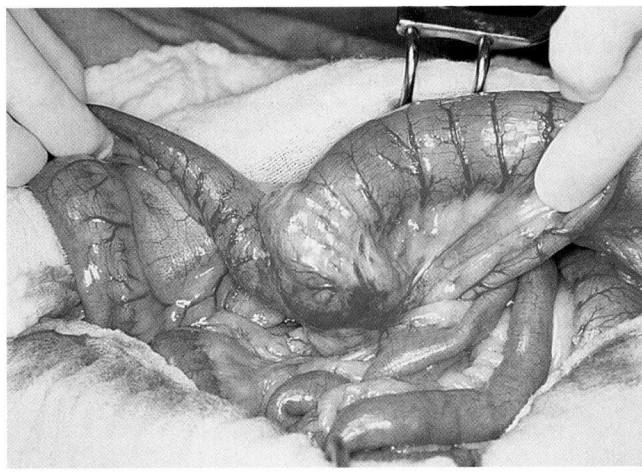

FIG. 19-114
Cecum that is inverted into the colonic lumen.

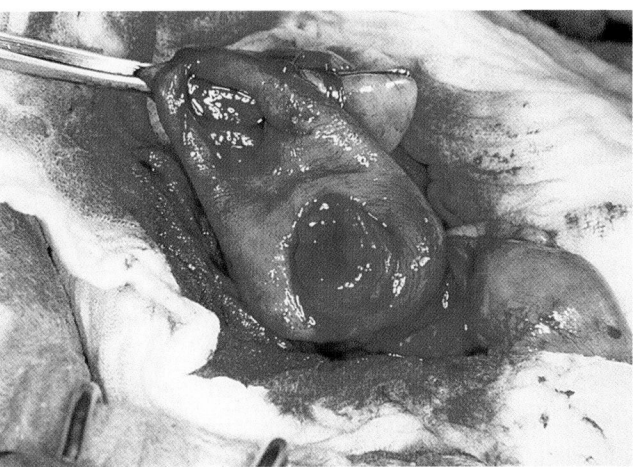

FIG. 19-116
The inverted cecum in Fig. 19-115 has been excised, allowing visualization of the ileal and colonic lumens.

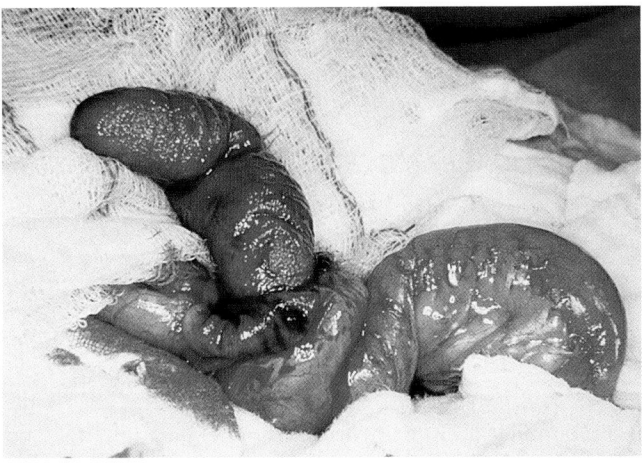

FIG. 19-115
During typhlectomy, an incision is made on either side of the cecal dimple and the inverted cecum is exteriorized.

cecum and close the cecocolic orifice with sutures or staples as described above (Fig. 19-116).

Colostomy

Colostomies are seldom indicated in animals, but may be performed as radical surgical treatment of obstructive colorectal neoplasia or strictures or for trauma with fecal leakage. However, the fecal incontinence that results from the procedure makes animal management difficult, and client acceptance often is poor. Many of the techniques for end-on or loop colostomies have been developed in animals for use in humans. Loop colostomies usually are temporary; in such cases the distal colon is intact and allows for closure of the colostomy after resolution of the initial problem. An end-on colostomy is performed after removing the distal colon and temporarily closing the ventral midline incision

and rotating the animal into a right lateral oblique recumbent position.

Excise a 2-cm circular segment of skin from a flat area of the left flank. Make a dorsoventrally oriented incision (4 cm) through the lateral abdominal musculature (external abdominal oblique, internal abdominal oblique, and transversus abdominis muscles) and enter the abdominal cavity. Exteriorize the proximal colon by passing it through the flank incision. Suture the circumference of the serosal surface of the colon to the abdominal musculature using 3-0 monofilament, absorbable suture (polydioxanone, polyglyconate, poliglecaprone 25). Complete the stoma by suturing the full thickness of the transected colon wall to the incised skin edge using 3-0 or 4-0 monofilament, absorbable suture. Then, through the ventral midline incision, perform a colopexy near the stoma to prevent bowel herniation. Attach a colostomy flange and bag to the stoma to collect feces. Replace the colostomy bags and flanges as needed, and perform colonic irrigation as desired.

Perform a diverting loop colostomy after aseptically preparing the left flank. In an area free of skin folds, make a circular incision 4 cm in diameter. Remove the circle of skin. Separate the muscle fibers to allow entry into the abdomen. Grasp the descending colon and exteriorize it through the skin incision. Place a straight plastic loop ostomy rod (90-mm loop ostomy rod*) through the colonic mesentery at right angles to the long axis of the bowel. Create subcutaneous pockets dorsal and ventral to the skin incision. Place the ends of the rod in these pockets and suture the rod to the subcutaneous tissue and muscle fascia. Using a simple continuous pattern, suture the seromuscular layers of the colon to the subcutaneous tissue at the border of the skin incision. Create a stoma by making a longitudinal incision into the lumen of the colon and then placing simple continuous sutures to appose the seromuscular layers of the colon to the incised skin edge. Apply an adhe-

*Convatec, Squibb Co, Princeton, NJ.

BOX 19-59

Colonic Bacteria

Anaerobes	Aerobes
• *Bacteroides* spp.	**Gram Negative**
• *Bifidobacterium* spp.	• *Escherichia coli*
• *Lactobacillus* spp.	• *Klebsiella* spp.
• *Clostridium* spp.	• *Proteus* spp.
• *Fusobacterium* spp.	
• Anaerobic *Streptococcus* spp.	**Gram Positive**
	• *Staphylococcus* spp.
	• *Corynebacterium* spp.
	• *Enterococcus* spp.

sive, 45-mm plastic flange (Surfit Flexible*) to the surrounding skin and attach a colostomy bag* to the flange. Place a bandage to hold the collection bag against the flank. Close the colostomy when fecal diversion is no longer necessary.

HEALING OF THE LARGE INTESTINE

Colonic healing is similar to that of the small intestine (see p. 459), but delayed. Wound tensile strength lags behind return of strength in the small intestine, and dehiscence is more likely. Optimal healing depends on a good blood supply, accurate mucosal apposition, minimal surgical trauma, and a tension-free closure. A number of factors may delay healing. Collateral circulation to the large intestine is poor compared with the small intestine, and large numbers of anaerobic and aerobic intraluminal bacteria compose up to 10% of the dry fecal weight. Normal colon bacterial counts range from 10^{10} to 10^{11} bacteria/g of feces. More anaerobes (Box 19-59) than aerobes populate the colon. Also, high intraluminal pressure develops during passage of a solid fecal bolus. This mechanical stress on the suture line may lead to dehiscence. The risk of dehiscence is high during the first 3 to 4 days because collagen lysis exceeds synthesis. Using antibiotics and placing sutures that do not strangulate tissue may improve healing.

Stapled anastomoses have a higher bursting pressure during the early lag phase of healing and a higher tensile strength after 7 days than hand-sutured anastomoses. Minimal inflammation and a double row of staples increase wound strength. The B-shaped staples provide hemostasis without collapsing the microcirculation, and their alignment ensures equal tension around the circumference of the anastomosis. However, unhealthy tissue should not be stapled.

SUTURE MATERIALS AND SPECIAL INSTRUMENTS

The instruments and suture materials for large intestinal surgery are the same as those for small intestinal surgery (see p. 459).

POSTOPERATIVE CARE AND ASSESSMENT

Postoperative care should be individualized for each patient. Patients should be closely monitored for vomiting or regurgitation during recovery to prevent aspiration pneu-

*Convatec, Squibb Co, Princeton, NJ.

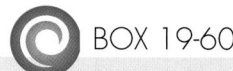 BOX 19-60

Stool Softeners and Laxatives

Dioctyl Sodium Sulfosuccinate or Docusate Sodium (Colace)
Dogs: 50–200 mg PO, bid to tid
Cats: 50 mg PO, qd to bid

Bisacodyl (Dulcolax)
Dogs: 5 mg/kg PO, qd to bid
Cats: 2.5–5 mg/cat PO, qd to bid

Lactulose (Chronulac)
Dogs: start with 1 ml/4.5 kg PO, qd to tid; titrate to obtain soft, formed feces
Cats: start with 5 ml/cat PO, tid; titrate to obtain soft, formed feces

Psyllium (Metamucil)
Dogs: 1 teaspoon/5–10 kg bid in food; titrate to obtain desired effect
Cats: 1 teaspoon/cat bid in food, titrate to obtain desired effect

Magnesium Hydroxide (Milk of Magnesia) (Cathartic Dose)
Dogs: 15–50 ml/dog PO, qd
Cats: 2–6 ml PO, qd

Canned Pumpkin
Cats: 1–4 tablespoons PO, qd

Coarse Wheat Bran
Dogs: 1–4 tablespoons PO, qd

PO, Oral; bid, twice a day; tid, three times a day; qd, once a day.

monia. Analgesics (i.e., hydromorphone, butorphanol, and buprenorphine; see Table 13-4 on p. 133) should be given as needed. Hydration, electrolyte, and acid-base abnormalities should be monitored and corrected. Intravenous fluid therapy should be continued until the animal is eating and drinking normally. Antibiotics may be discontinued 2 to 4 hours after surgery unless peritonitis is present. Small amounts of water may be offered 8 to 12 hours after surgery. If vomiting does not occur, small amounts of food can be given beginning 12 to 24 hours after surgery. A bland, low-fat diet (i/d by Hill's Pet Products or boiled rice, potatoes, and pasta combined with boiled, skinless chicken, yogurt, or low-fat cottage cheese) may be fed three or four times daily. The animal's normal diet can be gradually reintroduced beginning 48 to 72 hours after surgery. Debilitated patients may require enteral or parenteral nutrition (see Chapter 11). Stool softeners or laxatives (or both) should be administered when oral intake begins (Box 19-60). They may be given orally as a supplement (e.g., dioctyl sulfosuccinate-docusate sodium, bisacodyl, lactulose, and magnesium salts) or added to food (e.g., psyllium, pumpkin, bran cereal, and coarse wheat bran). In some cats the appetite can be stimulated by oral cyproheptadine (Box 19-61). Cyproheptadine is preferred as a feline appetite stimulant over diazepam.

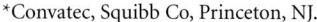

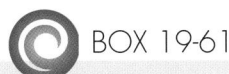 BOX 19-61

Appetite Stimulants in Cats

Cyproheptadine (Periactin) (preferred)
2 mg/cat PO, bid

Megestrol Acetate*
0.25–0.5 mg/kg PO; or, 2.5–5 mg/cat for 1-5 days

Oxazepam (Serax)
Cats: 2.5 mg/cat PO

PO, Oral; *bid,* twice a day.
*Megestrol is a very strong appetite stimulant; however, it can cause diabetes mellitus, pyometra, and mammary problems; therefore it should only be used in extreme cases and with owner consent.

Abdominal palpation and measurement of body temperature should be performed postoperatively to monitor for peritonitis or abscess formation. Depression, high fever, excessive abdominal tenderness, vomiting, and ileus may indicate peritonitis. If peritonitis is suspected, abdominocentesis or a diagnostic peritoneal lavage should be performed (see p. 335). Early ambulation and oral intake should be encouraged to reduce postoperative ileus. The presence or absence of fecal blood (and its color and consistency, if present) should be noted after surgery. Tenesmus and hematochezia may be observed.

In cats, subtotal colectomy generally increases the frequency of defecation 30% to 50%. Stools frequently remain loose for days to weeks and then become more semiformed. After colostomy, the parastomal area must be kept clean and treated as necessary for irritation. Although colonic irrigation is not necessary after colostomy, it reduces fecal production and makes management more practical and cost-effective (Williams et al, 1999).

COMPLICATIONS

Hemorrhage and fecal contamination of the abdomen are the most common complications of large intestinal surgery. Other possible complications are shock, leakage, dehiscence, perforation, peritonitis, stenosis, incontinence, or death. Fecal contamination can be prevented by preoperative colon preparation or by manually displacing the contents of the colon away from the resection sites, properly using atraumatic intestinal forceps, and performing copious lavage before closure. The frequency of leakage at the anastomotic site is similar for staple and suture techniques. Leakage may be minimized by placing a serosal patch around the anastomosis (see p. 457). In human beings, long-term use of corticosteroids is associated with a high incidence of abscess formation after colonic anastomosis and may predispose to dehiscence. Hemorrhage can be prevented with proper ligature placement and careful inspection of the anastomosis.

Postoperative strictures are rare unless inverting or everting suture patterns are used or excessive tension exists at the resection site. Strictures may be managed by incision with an electrosurgical tip or laser ablation. Dilating strictures by balloon or bougienage may also be effective (see p. 391). If these techniques do not alleviate signs of obstruction, surgical resection may be required.

Incontinence is rarely associated with colectomy. Complications associated with colostomy include prolapse of the stoma and skin irritation.

SPECIAL AGE CONSIDERATIONS

Young animals more often have rectal prolapse or intussusception as a result of parasite infestation, or garbage or foreign body ingestion. They are prone to hypoglycemia and hypothermia during surgery. Neoplasia is more common in older animals.

Reference

Williams FA et al: The use of colonic irrigation to control fecal incontinence in dogs with colostomies, *Vet Surg* 28:348, 1999.

Suggested Reading

Kumagai D, Shimada T, Yamate J: Use of an incontinent end-on colostomy in a dog with annular rectal adenocarcinoma. *J Small Anim Pract* 44:363, 2003.
This dog was managed for 4 months with a colostomy after removing the terminal rectum, anus, and perineum. Minor peristomal dermatitis, bags, and flanges were easily managed.

SPECIFIC DISEASES

NEOPLASIA

DEFINITIONS

Tumors that occur in the colon or rectum are called **colorectal neoplasms. Polyps** are grossly visible protrusions from the mucosal surface of either neoplastic or nonneoplastic cells.

GENERAL CONSIDERATIONS AND CLINICALLY RELEVANT PATHOPHYSIOLOGY

Intestinal tumors occur most often in the rectum or colon of dogs and in the small intestine of cats. Adenomatous polyps and adenocarcinomas are the most common colorectal neoplasms. Other reported tumors include lymphosarcomas, leiomyomas, leiomyosarcomas, plasmacytomas, mast cell tumors, and carcinoids. Intestinal wall tumors usually invade the muscular layer of the intestines, causing obstruction through luminal compromise or interference with peristalsis (or both). Feces, fluid, and/or gas may distend the proximal bowel, which compromises its function. Clinical signs of tenesmus, dyschezia, and hematochezia can be attributed to the presence of a friable luminal mass that bleeds when abraded by the passage of feces. In some animals, tenesmus and dyschezia are caused by partial luminal obstruction by a full-thickness annular mass. Physical examination (especially digital rectal examination), endoscopy, ultrasonography, CT, and MRI are the principal means of assessing abdominal and pelvic structures for neoplasia.

The cause of colorectal polyps is unknown. Most polyps occur in the dog's rectum, near the anorectal junction, although they occasionally may be found in the colon. Most appear dark red or pink, soft, friable, and hemorrhagic. They usually are sessile or slightly pedunculated and may be single or multiple. Single masses may be so large as to suggest a broad-based mass when in fact they have a small stalk. Most polyps are hyperplastic or adenomatous, and epithelial changes do not cross the lamina muscularis; however, some have atypia and are considered carcinoma *in situ*.

Adenocarcinomas of the colon and rectum are rare in cats; they are more common, although still relatively rare, in dogs. In human beings, most of these tumors are believed to rise from preexisting adenomatous polyps. Most adenocarcinomas of the large intestine are located in the canine and feline rectum (more than 50% are midrectum). They may be annular (intramural) or intraluminal. Intraluminal masses may be multiple, pedunculated, nodular, and/or ulcerated. Annular masses typically infiltrate all layers of the intestinal wall, causing circumferential narrowing. These tumors are firm, grayish white, and often ulcerated. Tumors of the large intestine usually grow slowly and spread to adjacent serosal surfaces, mesentery, omentum, and regional lymph nodes by local invasion. Distant metastases may occur to the lymph nodes, lungs, liver, spleen, pancreas, adrenals, and peritoneal surfaces.

Leiomyomas are benign neoplasms of smooth muscle that occur sporadically in the large intestine. They are well encapsulated, circumscribed, and light in color with a smooth, glistening, cut surface. Clinical signs (i.e., tenesmus) may not be seen until the mass reaches an appreciable size. Because the mucosa usually is not involved, melena or hematochezia is uncommon. They usually are removed by blunt dissection from the colorectal wall via an anal, perineal, or abdominal approach. Recurrence is uncommon, and long-term survival is expected.

Leiomyosarcomas are invasive, malignant, smooth muscle tumors that usually are slow to metastasize. Most reported cecal tumors are leiomyosarcomas. Cecal leiomyosarcomas occur most commonly in old, larger breed dogs of either gender. Some patients are presented for treatment of cecal rupture and peritonitis, others because of vomiting, diarrhea, polyuria, polydipsia, lethargy, and anorexia. Metastasis to the mesentery, mesenteric lymph nodes, peritoneum, and liver occurs in approximately 50% of those affected. The prognosis for long-term survival is good with early complete resection. Reported median survival (with or without metastasis) is about 21 months, with a 1-year survival rate of 75% and a 2-year survival rate of 66% (Cohen et al, 2003).

DIAGNOSIS
Clinical Presentation

Signalment. Colorectal tumors are more common in dogs than in cats. The incidence of polyps is equal in males and females, with an increased prevalence suggested in poodles, Airedale terriers, German shepherds, and collies. Colonic carcinomas are two to three times more common in males than in females. Mixed breed dogs, poodles, German shep-

herds, collies, West Highland white terriers, Airedales, and Lhasa apsos appear to be most commonly affected. Leiomyomas and leiomyosarcomas occur more frequently in medium to large breeds, with no particular breed or gender predilection. Most large intestinal tumors occur in middle-aged and old dogs; however, dogs as young as 2 years of age have been affected. Mean ages for colorectal tumors are 7 years for polyps, 11 years for leiomyomas and leiomyosarcomas, and 8 to 9 years for carcinomas.

History. Most dogs are presented for treatment because the owners noticed blood and mucus in the feces. Common clinical signs include constipation, straining to defecate, passage of blood and mucus with feces, painful defecation, and passage of ribbonlike feces. Vomiting, anorexia, weight loss, depression, septic peritonitis, and/or malabsorption occur occasionally. Some animals are asymptomatic, and masses are found during a routine physical examination. Tenesmus often is present and can cause prolapse of the mass or rectum. Sometimes the only sign is prolapse of a mass during defecation. Signs involving other organ systems may develop secondary to metastasis and paraneoplastic syndromes.

Physical Examination Findings

Animals with colorectal neoplasia may be thin. Colorectal masses often are identified during abdominal or rectal palpation. More than 60% of anal and rectal canal masses are diagnosed during rectal palpation. Masses may bleed and fragment during palpation, and they may be pedunculated, sessile, nodular, firm, soft, or friable. Prolapse of the mass often is possible, which allows visual inspection. During the rectal examination, it should be determined whether the mass is fixed or movable and whether the sublumbar lymph nodes are enlarged.

Diagnostic Imaging

Thoracic and abdominal radiographs should be obtained to evaluate the extent of disease. The rectum and anus are difficult to evaluate on survey radiographs; however, a mass may be identified protruding into the lumen if it is surrounded by intraluminal gas. Sublumbar lymphadenomegaly often indicates metastasis. A barium enema may help delineate a mass, but ultrasound is usually more valuable. In human beings, intrarectal ultrasonography appears to be the most accurate imaging technique for staging rectal cancers. Intrarectal ultrasonography helps predict the degree of tumor invasion, allowing for better treatment planning. CT or MRI imaging is helpful to determine tumor extent and invasiveness if radical resection or radiation therapy is anticipated.

Proctoscopy/colonoscopy. Proctoscopy or colonoscopy should be performed to identify diffuse or multiple lesions and to localize lesions. The size, location, distribution, and multiplicity of lesions should be determined. Examination may reveal a pedunculated or sessile mass, irregular luminal narrowing, and/or ulceration. A biopsy should be taken of all lesions, and the submucosa should be included in biopsy samples with obvious, deep, infiltrating disease. Presurgical biopsies are useful prognostic tools, which can help avoid unnecessary surgery in patients with a poor prognosis. Endoscopic snare polypectomy is often performed in human beings with sessile masses smaller than 15 mm and pedunculated masses smaller than 35 mm; the procedure occasionally can be performed in dogs.

Laboratory Findings

The results of CBC and biochemical profiles are nonspecific for colorectal tumors. In rare cases, anemia and hypoproteinemia are present if chronic bleeding has occurred from an ulcerated mass.

DIFFERENTIAL DIAGNOSIS

The differential diagnoses include all other causes of large bowel obstruction or irritation, including intussusception, constipation, obstipation, colitis, perforation, benign stricture, congenital stricture, granulomas, hematomas, or congenital malformation.

MEDICAL MANAGEMENT

Lymphosarcomas may respond to chemotherapy. Rectal tubulopapillary polyps may respond to piroxicam treatment. The response of most other tumors to chemotherapy is unpredictable. Radiation therapy is restricted to masses smaller than 3 cm that are confined to the rectal wall and located in the distal half of the rectum and anal canal.

SURGICAL TREATMENT

Surgical resection is the treatment of choice for intestinal tumors. Unfortunately, many tumors are too advanced for successful resection when diagnosed. Incontinence may occur after resection.

Preoperative Management

Hydration, electrolyte, and acid-base abnormalities should be corrected before surgery. Transfusion should be performed if the patient's packed cell volume is below 20% (see p. 25). If the animal has no obstruction, bacterial numbers may be reduced by evacuating the colon with oral cathartics, enemas, and fasting (see p. 481). Manual evacuation of the rectum is recommended when obstructed. Antibiotics effective against aerobic and anaerobic intestinal bacteria flora should be given (see p. 481).

Anesthesia

General anesthetic recommendations for animals undergoing large intestinal surgery are provided on p. 481. Because patients with tumors may be debilitated, balanced anesthesia using injectable agents and isoflurane or sevoflurane is recommended. Epidural anesthesia may be advantageous (see Chapter 13).

Surgical Anatomy

The surgical anatomy of the large intestine is presented on p. 481.

Positioning

Tumors of the cecum and colon are approached via a ventral celiotomy with the patient in dorsal recumbency. Rectal tumors may be approached using either a ventral midline celiotomy with pelvic osteotomy, anal eversion, or perineal dissection. Tumors of the cranial to middle rectum are approached with the patient in dorsal recumbency using a ventral celiotomy and pelvic osteotomy. Tumors of the caudal rectum and anal canal are approached with the patient in ventral recumbency using DePage's position and anal eversion or a dorsal (see p. 504) or lateral (see p. 505) perineal approach. For DePage's position, tilting the table, padding the hindquarters, and securing the tail over the back elevate the perineum.

ENDOSCOPIC BIOPSY

The most common mistake made when taking a biopsy of submucosal rectal masses is obtaining a sample of mucosa without adequate submucosa attached. Rigid endoscopy can reliably obtain large amounts of submucosa, if done correctly. Rigid biopsy forceps that open widely and have a large jaw are preferred. It is often best to remove the proctoscope and guide the biopsy forceps to the lesion digitally.

Once the rigid forceps have been directed to an obviously thickened area (take time and be sure of the placement of the biopsy forceps), forcefully push it into the mass while at the same time closing the jaws of the forceps.

This maneuver typically results in an audible "crunch" sound. When the tissue is retrieved, one should be able to clearly see mucosa and underlying submucosa.

SURGICAL TECHNIQUE

Surgical resection is the most common treatment for large intestinal neoplasia. Margins of 4 to 8 cm are recommended for partial colectomy (see p. 484) for malignant tumors. Noninvasive anal or rectal masses often are everted through the anus and excised with limited normal tissue margins. In human beings, local excision is performed when rectal tumors are: limited to the submucosa or muscularis, mobile, 3 cm or smaller, and well or moderately differentiated. Full-thickness resection of the involved colon or rectum is required for large, sessile masses. Tumors invading the serosa or perirectal tissue that are fixed, 3 cm in diameter or larger, poorly differentiated, or atypical should be excised by means of an abdominal incision, rectal pull-through (see p. 501), or perineal resection (see p. 501) with lymph node excision. Abdominal resection may require a pelvic osteotomy to remove a pubic bone flap (see p. 670).

Dilate and retract the anus to allow visualization of the mass. Place stay sutures in the rectal mucosa near the mass to facilitate eversion through the anus (see Fig. 19-119 on p. 502). Use an electrosurgical electrode, laser, or scalpel blade to incise the mucosa and submucosa surrounding the mass. Remove the mass and appose the mucosa and submucosa with simple interrupted 4-0 absorbable suture (polydioxanone, polyglyconate, poliglecaprone 25, or glycomer 631).

Colostomy may be indicated to allow more aggressive resection or therapy.

SUTURE MATERIALS AND SPECIAL INSTRUMENTS

Absorbable suture (i.e., polydioxanone, polyglyconate, or poliglecaprone 25) is preferred when removing masses from the rectum. Absorbable or nonabsorbable suture may be used for colectomy (see p. 484), but absorbable suture is preferred.

POSTOPERATIVE CARE AND ASSESSMENT

Care and management after surgery should be individualized. Hydration and electrolyte balance are maintained with fluid therapy. Analgesics should be provided as necessary. Therapeutic antibiotics are appropriate when contamination, peritonitis, or severe debilitation is present. Nutritional support (see Chapter 11) may be necessary if the patient is debilitated and refuses to eat. Adjuvant chemotherapy has been recommended for malignant tumors, but its efficacy is unknown.

COMPLICATIONS

Leakage, dehiscence, and peritonitis are possible complications. Tenesmus, dyschezia, and hematochezia are expected after colorectal surgery. Incontinence may be seen in animals after rectal pull-through procedures. Stricture or tumor recurrence may cause signs of intestinal obstruction.

PROGNOSIS

The prognosis is poor for animals with nonresectable tumors because other modes of therapy are ineffective, of questionable value, or unusable because of severe side effects. In some cases lymphosarcoma responds well to chemotherapy. The prognosis for patients with benign masses generally is good to excellent if excision is complete; however, recurrence and malignant transformation are possible when polyp excision is incomplete. Unlike people, most canine colorectal polyps do not have carcinoma *in situ*. The prognosis for patients with malignant tumors is fair to guarded, depending on the tumor's type, location, stage, and resectability. Excision is expected to be curative for leiomyoma. Leiomyosarcoma patients live approximately 21 months before signs of recurrence or metastasis. Complete surgical excision of colorectal adenocarcinomas is curative; however, the prognosis is poor because most cannot be completely excised as a result of local infiltration, the spread to lymph nodes, and the pelvic canal location. Dogs with colorectal adenocarcinomas usually are euthanized because of failure to control dyschezia and hematochezia. Dogs with single, pedunculated, polypoid masses typically survive longer than those with nodular masses. Animals with annular masses that cause stricture survived for only a few months. Adjuvant chemotherapy or radiation therapy (or both) is suggested for patients with adenocarcinoma and leiomyosarcoma, but the efficacy of this treatment is unproven.

Reference

Cohen M, Post GS, Wright JC: Gastrointestinal leiomyosarcoma in 14 dogs, *J Vet Intern Med* 17:107, 2003.

Suggested Reading

Knottenbelt CM, Simpson JW, Tasker S et al: Preliminary clinical observations on the use of piroxicam in the management of rectal tubulopapillary polyps, *J Small Animal Pract* 41:393-397, 2000.
Cases with and without evidence of inflammation responded with good or excellent clinical improvement (7/8).
Kupanoff PA, Popovitch CA, Goldschmidt MH: Colorectal plasmacytomas: a retrospective study of nine dogs, *J Am Anim Hosp Assoc* 42:37, 2006.
These tumors progressed slowly and did not recur with complete excision.

COLITIS

DEFINITIONS

Colitis is inflammation of the colon caused by a variety of organisms, diets, and syndromes. **Inflammatory bowel disease (IBD)** is idiopathic inflammation of the bowel. Although the terms colitis, acute colitis, chronic colitis, ulcerative colitis, and IBD often are used interchangeably, they are different.

GENERAL CONSIDERATIONS AND CLINICALLY RELEVANT PATHOPHYSIOLOGY

The underlying causes of acute infectious and inflammatory conditions of the large intestine often are not diagnosed because they are self-limiting. However, with chronic diseases, the cause often must be determined to resolve the condition. A variety of factors may cause colitis, including bacteria, fungi, parasites, and diet. The mucosa may be infiltrated by various inflammatory cells (lymphocytes, plasma cells, eosinophils, neutrophils, or macrophages). Lymphocytic-plasmacytic colitis is the most common cause of IBD of the feline colon; IBD is less common in the canine colon. Another cause of colitis is the late effects of pelvic irradiation. Giving smaller doses per fraction and avoiding systemic radiation potentiators minimize radiation effects on the colon.

Colonic inflammation disrupts the normal secretory and absorptive functions of the colon such that net secretion is increased and absorption of sodium, chloride, and water is diminished. Colonic motility patterns change so that segmental contractions, which provide resistance to the flow of feces, are reduced, whereas peristaltic contractions are normal or diminished. The colon usually is hypomotile, and diarrhea results from diminished resistance to flow, accelerated transit, increased secretion of water and electrolytes, and accentuated reflux urge to defecate as a result of mucosal irritation. Mucosal ulceration and smooth muscle spasms may be present, and microbial populations are altered.

DIAGNOSIS
Clinical Presentation

Signalment. Boxers and French bulldogs are predisposed to histiocytic ulcerative colitis, although this currently is an uncommon diagnosis. Young and middle-aged dogs are most likely to be affected by infiltrative fungal disease.

History. Patients usually are presented for treatment with a history of constant or intermittent large intestinal diarrhea. They sometimes void small amounts frequently, have a sense of urgency to defecate, or have accidents in the house (or all three). Hematochezia, fecal mucus, and tenesmus are common but inconsistent findings. Other less common signs include vomiting, depression, weight loss (rare except for fungal infections and neoplasia), dyschezia, and constipation. The animal's diet should be investigated.

Physical Examination Findings

The physical examination findings often are normal. Rectal examination findings may be normal or abnormal (e.g., painful and roughened mucosa).

Diagnostic Imaging

Survey radiographs, contrast studies, and ultrasonography sometimes show intestinal wall thickening, but are seldom performed in these patients. Colonoscopy with mucosal biopsy provides a definitive diagnosis for fungal infections and neoplasia.

Laboratory Findings

A positive result may be seen on fecal examination for parasites (e.g., whipworms and *Tritrichomonas*). CBC and serum biochemical profiles usually are normal. Hemograms may reflect chronic inflammation, stress, or anemia. Hypoalbuminemia may be seen in some patients with histoplasmosis or pythiosis.

DIFFERENTIAL DIAGNOSIS

Food allergy or intolerance, neoplasia, whipworms, *Tritrichomonas*, histoplasmosis, prototheosis, pythiosis, clostridial colitis, FIV, FeLV, irritable bowel syndrome (i.e., fiber-responsive disease), and ileocolic or cecocolic intussusception are important differential diagnoses.

MEDICAL MANAGEMENT

Therapy for acute colitis initially is symptomatic. Food should be withheld for 24 to 48 hours, and then a bland, easily digested, low-fat, and nonallergenic diet should be introduced (e.g., i/d [Hill's Pet Products], or homemade rice, potatoes, and lean meat, cottage cheese, or eggs). Anthelmintics are appropriate if parasites are present or suspected. Clostridial colitis is reasonably common and typically responds promptly to tylosin or amoxicillin therapy. Motility modifiers sometimes are used on a short-term basis.

Patients with chronic colonic disease that have normal serum albumin concentrations and have not lost weight may first be given therapeutic trials of anthelmintics, hypoallergenic diets, fiber-supplemented diets, metronidazole, and/or antibiotics effective against *Clostridium* spp (tylosin or

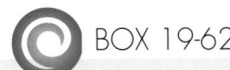 BOX 19-62

Medical Management of Colitis

Metronidazole
10–15 mg/kg PO, qd

Prednisolone
1.1–2.2 mg/kg qd

Azathioprine (Imuran)
Dogs: 2.2 mg/kg qd to qod
Cats: do not administer this drug to cats

Chlorambucil (Leukeran)
Cats <3 kg: 1 mg twice a week
Cats >3 kg: 2 mg twice a week

Sulfasalazine (Azulfidine)
Dogs: 10–25 mg/kg PO, bid to tid
Cats: 5–12.5 mg/kg PO, tid

Mesalamine (Asacol, Pentasa, and Rowasa are other trade names)*
10 mg/kg PO, bid to tid

Olsalazine (Dipentum)*
10 mg/kg PO, bid to tid

PO, Oral; *bid*, twice a day; *qd*, once a day; *qod*, every other day; *tid*, three times a day.
*This drug is not approved for use in dogs or cats.

amoxicillin). Corticosteroids and antimetabolites (azathioprine, chlorambucil; Box 19-62), are typically only given if a histopathology has been done. NSAIDs (sulfasalazine, mesalamine, olsalazine) are typically given after biopsy, but can be given without a histologic diagnosis. Colonic resection is rarely needed or considered in dogs with colonic inflammatory disease. However, partial or complete colectomy may be required in very severe cases (mucosal sloughing) when medical therapy has not or is not expected to stop severe protein losses.

SURGICAL TREATMENT

Biopsy and colectomy may be indicated in affected animals.

Preoperative Management

Preoperative care should be provided as discussed on p. 480. Fluids and transfusions should be given before surgery if indicated. Prophylactic antibiotics should be given before surgery. If surgery is indicated, antibiotics effective against colonic aerobes and anaerobes should be given (see p. 481).

Anesthesia

General anesthetic recommendations for large intestinal surgery are provided on p. 481.

Surgical Anatomy

The surgical anatomy of the large intestine is described on p. 481.

Positioning

If colectomy is to be performed, patients should be positioned in dorsal recumbency for a ventral midline celiotomy. The entire ventral abdomen should be clipped and prepared for aseptic surgery.

COLONOSCOPIC BIOPSY

Biopsy samples should be obtained by colonoscopy. The techniques for large intestinal biopsy with a flexible scope are similar to those for the small intestine (see pp. 445 and 448). Rigid colonoscopic biopsy provides a better tissue sample, and care must be taken to not perforate the colon.

Deflate the colon and move the scope back and forth to throw up folds of mucosa. Partially open the rigid biopsy forceps, and advance it to gently grasp a fold of mucosa such that the tip of the biopsy cup (NOT the entire cup) is filled with mucosa. Before closing the forceps completely and cutting off the tissue, gently move the tip back and forth. If just the mucosa moves, then the forceps has been properly placed around a fold of mucosa; completely close the forceps and retrieve the biopsy. However, if the colonic wall moves, then you have grasped too deep a bite and must let go lest you perforate the colon. Then, without reinflating the colon, withdraw the endoscope a few centimeters and repeat the process. The exception is when taking a biopsy from dense, submucosal lesions; in that case do not forcefully but very carefully push the biopsy forceps into the lesion while closing the jaws to obtain submucosa in addition to mucosa.

If there is any doubt, it is better to take a conservative biopsy at first and then gradually increase the force used to push into the mass if the first biopsy was inadequate. In general, one should obtain 6 to 8 biopsies of the colon, but only 2 to 3 of a dense, focal, submucosal lesion.

SURGICAL TECHNIQUE

Surgical biopsy may be required to establish the appropriate medical therapy; however, colonic biopsy during exploratory laparotomy is seldom indicated. Colectomy is described on p. 484.

SUTURE MATERIALS AND SPECIAL INSTRUMENTS

See p. 459 for instruments for intestinal surgery. Polydioxanone or polyglyconate suture (3-0 or 4-0) is preferred for colectomy or colonic biopsy; however, nonabsorbable suture (e.g., nylon or polypropylene) may be used in hypoalbuminemic animals. Chromic gut suture should be avoided in young or debilitated animals because the suture may be rapidly catabolized and weakened.

POSTOPERATIVE CARE AND ASSESSMENT

Severely affected patients may benefit from enteral or parenteral nutritional support after surgery. Analgesics, antibiotics, and fluids should be given as necessary. After surgery, patients should be monitored for evidence of peritonitis (see p. 329).

COMPLICATIONS

Colonic perforation is a rare complication of colonoscopic or ultrasonographic biopsy, and leakage may occur from colotomy biopsy or colectomy sites. Strictures may occur after partial colectomy.

PROGNOSIS

Signs of acute colitis often are alleviated by a 24- to 36-hour fast (see discussion in Medical Management section on p. 493). The prognosis for chronic colitis depends on the underlying cause; it is poor for prototothecosis, nonresectable pythiosis, and nonresectable malignancy. Lifetime treatment may be necessary for some patients with chronic colitis. The prognosis for recovery after surgical biopsy of the large intestine is good if appropriate surgical principles are followed. The patient may require lifetime medical treatment for the underlying cause of colitis.

Suggested Reading

Anderson CR, McNiel EA, Gillette EL et al: Late complications of pelvic irradiation in 16 dogs, *Vet Radiol Ultrasound* 43(2):187, 2002.
The major late side effect following pelvic irradiation was colitis, which occurred in 56% (9/16).
Hostutleer R, Luria B, Johnson S et al: Antibiotic-responsive histiocytic ulcerative colitis in 9 dogs, *J Vet Intern Med* 18:499, 2003.
This paper documents that histiocytic ulcerative colitis, a disease that formerly had a poor prognosis, is curable with antibiotics.
Leib MS, Baechtel MS, Monroe WE: Complications associated with 355 flexible colonoscopic procedures in dogs, *J Vet Intern Med* 18:642, 2004.
Major complications occurred in 0.85% of dogs that had colonoscopy. This is a safe procedure.
Willard MD: Colonoscopy, proctoscopy, and ileoscopy, *Vet Clin North Am* 31:657, 2001.
This is a more detailed review of equipment and techniques.

MEGACOLON

DEFINITIONS

Megacolon is a descriptive term for persistent increased large intestinal diameter and hypomotility associated with severe constipation. A diagnosis of **idiopathic megacolon** is made if mechanical, neurologic, or endocrine causes cannot be identified. **Constipation** is difficult or infrequent defecation with passage of unduly hard, dry fecal material; **obstipation** is extreme constipation (no feces may be passed).

GENERAL CONSIDERATIONS AND CLINICALLY RELEVANT PATHOPHYSIOLOGY

Megacolon is most often diagnosed in cats (Box 19-63). It is not a specific disease, but a clinical sign associated with failure to normally void feces. It may be congenital or ac-

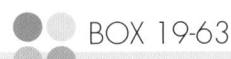

quired, occurring secondary to colonic inertia and outlet obstruction. Causes of colonic inertia may be prolonged distention, neurologic trauma, congenital dysfunction, endocrine disease, metabolic disease, or behavioral abnormalities, or the condition may be idiopathic. Pelvic fracture malunion, large intestinal strictures or neoplasia, anal atresia or stricture, compressive extraluminal masses, foreign bodies, or improper diet can cause outlet obstruction. Idiopathic megacolon may be associated with other disease processes, such as active colonic inflammation, dysautonomia, and metabolic disorders, including hypokalemia, hypercalcemia, and hypothyroidism. Idiopathic megacolon in cats associated with colonic inertia is thought to be the result of an abnormality of either the intrinsic or extrinsic innervation to the lower large intestine. Recently, however, cats with idiopathic megacolon have been characterized with generalized dysfunction of colonic smooth muscle that involves the activation of smooth muscle myofilaments.

Feces retained in the colon for prolonged periods dehydrate and solidify because of continued water absorption. Fecal concretions are produced that are difficult and painful to eliminate. The fecal mass may become so large and hard that passage through the pelvic canal is impossible. Prolonged, severe colonic distention eventually causes irreversible changes in colonic smooth muscle and nerves, causing inertia. Absorption of bacterial toxins from the retained feces may cause depression, anorexia, and weakness. Vomiting occurs secondary to prolonged obstruction, absorbed toxins. and/or vagal stimulation. Liquid may pass around fecal concretions and cause diarrhea. Blood and mucus from mucosal irritation may be seen in the feces.

Feline longitudinal colonic smooth muscle contraction is calcium-, calmodulin-, and myosin light chain kinase–dependent (Washabau et al, 2002). Myosin light chain phosphorylation is necessary for the initiation of contraction in feline longitudinal colonic smooth muscle. These facts may be important in feline colonic motility disorders.

DIAGNOSIS
Clinical Presentation

Signalment. Idiopathic megacolon is primarily seen in cats but in rare cases occurs in dogs. There is no gender predisposition, but Manx cats may be predisposed. Megacolon that occurs secondary to neurologic, obstructive, or medical disease may be seen in any animal. Middle-aged or older cats are most commonly diagnosed with idiopathic megacolon (range, 1 to 16 years; mean age, approximately 5 to 7½ years).

History. Affected animals are brought in for evaluation of constipation or obstipation. They may be depressed and anorexic and have tenesmus, weakness, lethargy, poor hair coat, vomiting, weight loss, and occasionally watery, mucoid, or bloody diarrhea. The clinical signs often are severe and chronic because many clients pay little attention to their pet's elimination habits.

Physical Examination Findings

A lean body condition and poor hair coat may be evident on physical examination. Some animals are depressed and dehydrated. Abdominal palpation reveals a distended colon. Rectal examination reveals hard feces at the pelvic inlet.

Diagnostic Imaging

Abdominal radiographs demonstrate a distended colon impacted with fecal material. Enlargement of colon diameter beyond 1.5 times the length of the body of the seventh lumbar vertebra is considered a megacolon. Radiographs should be obtained to rule out obstructive diseases (i.e., pelvic fracture malunions, sacrocaudal spinal trauma or deformities, and intramural or mural colonic or rectoanal obstructive lesions; Fig. 19-117).

Laboratory Findings

Nonspecific changes in the CBC and biochemistry profile may be evident. Histologic examination of colons removed from most cats with idiopathic megacolon usually reveals normal colonic wall ganglion cells.

DIFFERENTIAL DIAGNOSIS

Idiopathic megacolon must be differentiated from congenital, obstructive, neurologic, and systemic causes of megacolon. Causes of obstipation/megacolon are considered idiopathic (62%) or associated with pelvic canal stenosis (23%), nerve injuries (6%), or Manx cat sacral spinal cord deformity (5%). Causes of constipation include drugs (e.g., opiates, anticholinergics, Carafate, and barium), severe dehydration, environmental changes, perianal pain (e.g., from perianal fistulae), inappropriate diet, perineal hernia, colorectal masses or strictures, hypercalcemia, hypokalemia, hypothyroidism, and spinal cord or nerve damage.

MEDICAL MANAGEMENT

Constipation is difficult to treat once megacolon develops; however, medical management should be attempted before colectomy. Initial management includes correction of hydration, electrolyte, and acid-base abnormalities in se-

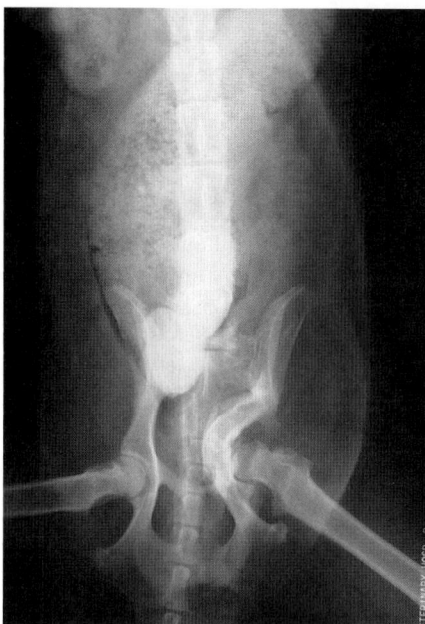

FIG. 19-117
Radiograph of a dog with megacolon, which occurred as a result of malunion of pelvic fractures and narrowing of the pelvic canal.

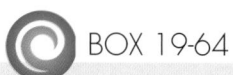 BOX 19-64

Drugs Used for Constipation in Dogs and Cats

Lactulose (Chronulac)

Dogs: Start at 1 ml/4.5 kg PO, qd to tid: adjust the dose so that the stools are soft but not watery
Cats: Start at 5 ml/cat PO, tid, adjust the dose so that the stools are soft but not watery

PO, Oral; qd, once a day; tid, three times a day.

verely affected animals. The colon should be evacuated with stool softeners, enemas, and/or digital evacuation. General anesthesia typically is required for digital evacuation. Because mucosal damage may occur with digital evacuation, antibiotics may be indicated to protect against systemic absorption of bacteria and toxins. To control constipation, long-term use of high-fiber diets, stool softeners, bulk laxatives, and/or enemas may be necessary. Osmotic laxatives (e.g., lactulose; ice cream or milk in some cats; Box 19-64) and prokinetic drugs (cisapride) may help prevent recurrence once the colon has been evacuated by enemas. If recurrent obstipation requires frequent fecal extraction, surgery may be indicated. Some owners find medical therapy intolerable and opt for euthanasia if surgery is not available. However, it must be clear to the owners that dogs do not adapt to colectomy, and not all cats with a colectomy do well.

SURGICAL TREATMENT

Surgery for megacolon entails removing the entire colon except a short distal segment necessary to reestablish intestinal continuity. Megacolon that occurs secondary to pelvic fracture malunion should be treated with subtotal colectomy, pelvic reconstruction, or both. Pelvic reconstruction involves partial pelvectomy and bone repositioning to widen the pelvic canal. Pelvic reconstruction is recommended before irreversible myoneural damage has occurred secondary to chronic colonic distention. Reconstruction should be performed as soon as pelvic narrowing and constipation or obstipation are diagnosed. Signs of obstruction generally are eliminated if the pelvic canal is widened within 6 months of the injury; however, reconstruction alone may not alleviate clinical signs if megacolon is severe. A subtotal colectomy in addition to a pelvectomy may be necessary to alleviate signs in these patients. Care should be taken during pelvectomy to protect adjacent soft tissue structures (i.e., the urethra, rectum, blood vessels, and nerves). After colectomy, the small intestine adapts by increasing stool capacity and water absorption.

Preoperative Management

Preoperative intestinal preparation using multiple enemas to evacuate the large colon is ineffective and unnecessary. Prophylactic antibiotics effective against aerobic and anaerobic colonic bacteria should be given (see p. 481).

Anesthesia

General anesthetic recommendations for large intestinal surgery are given on p. 481.

Surgical Anatomy

The surgical anatomy of the large intestine is described on p. 481.

Positioning

The animal should be positioned in dorsal recumbency with the entire ventral abdomen clipped and prepared for aseptic surgery. The prepared area should extend caudal to the pubic brim.

SURGICAL TECHNIQUE
Subtotal Colectomy

Controversy over whether to remove or preserve the ileocolic junction exists. Removal is thought to allow colonic microorganisms easy access to the small intestine with subsequent malabsorption and be associated with more severe diarrhea. Preservation is thought to minimize postoperative diarrhea but potentially allow recurrence of constipation.

Explore the abdomen, and biopsy abnormal tissue. Isolate the distal small intestine, cecum, and colon from the remainder of the abdomen with several moistened laparotomy pads. Identify resection sites at the distal jejunum or proximal ileum and the distal 1 to 2 cm of the colon. Choose sites that will allow apposition without tension. Ligate and transect branches of the ileal artery and vein, ileocolic artery and vein, caudal mesenteric artery and vein, and cranial rectal artery (see Fig. 19-112).

As an alternative, the ileocolic sphincter can be preserved; however, a tension-free apposition is more difficult to achieve if this is done. Ileocolic anastomosis is technically easier and allows removal of more colon.

If the ileocolic valve is preserved, ligate the right colic, middle colic, and caudal mesenteric vessels. If the ileum is partly or completely removed, also ligate the ileocolic and terminal ileal arcadial vessels.

> NOTE: Do not ligate the cranial rectal artery in dogs. Instead, ligate the left colic artery and the vasa recta from the cranial rectal artery.

Milk feces into the dilated colon, which will be resected. Place intestinal forceps proximal and distal to the planned resection site. Resect the dilated colon at its junction with the small intestine or just distal to the cecum. Perform an end-to-end anastomosis with either a circular stapler or sutures. Correct for luminal size disparity when performing a suture anastomosis by altering the angle of transection (oblique angles on small lumens and perpendicular angles on large lumens), using unequal suture spacing (farther apart on the large lumen), and/or resecting an antimesenteric wedge from the intestine (see p 453).

If a stapling technique is used, place purse-string sutures at each colonic end before resection. Insert the stapler into the colon transanally or through an antimesenteric incision in the cecum or colon. Lavage the anastomotic site and close the mesenteric defect. Remove the laparotomy pads, lavage the abdomen, and place omentum over the surgical site.

> NOTE: Transanal introduction of the stapler may not be possible in all cats because of the small anus and narrow pelvic canal.

SUTURE MATERIALS AND SPECIAL INSTRUMENTS

Instruments for large intestinal surgery are discussed on p. 459. Absorbable suture (polydioxanone, poliglecaprone 25, polyglyconate, or glycomer 631) (3-0 or 4-0) is preferred for colectomy; however, nonabsorbable suture (nylon, polybutester, or polypropylene) may be used in debilitated or hypoalbuminemic animals.

POSTOPERATIVE CARE AND ASSESSMENT

Hydration should be maintained with intravenous or subcutaneous fluids for 1 to 3 days after surgery, and analgesics should be given as necessary. Prophylactic antibiotics should be continued if gross abdominal contamination occurred or if the patient is extremely debilitated. Patients should be monitored frequently for signs of anastomotic leakage or signs of peritonitis from intraoperative contamination with anaerobic and aerobic bacteria. Food may be offered within 24 hours of surgery, although anorexia may persist for 5 days or longer. Cyproheptadine (see Box 19-61) may be used to stimulate eating in some cats. It may be necessary to keep animals on a low-volume, high-calorie diet for 10 to 14 days. Liquid, tarry feces and tenesmus should be expected immediately after surgery. The character of the feces changes gradually from diarrhea to soft, formed stool in 80% of cats by 6 weeks after surgery. Semiformed stools and, in rare cases, diarrhea persist in some cats. The frequency of defecation usually increases 30% to 50% compared with normal cats; however, most cats are continent. The litter pan should be kept clean to encourage defecation.

COMPLICATIONS

Leakage, dehiscence, peritonitis, ischemic necrosis, stricture, and abscess formation are possible complications of a subtotal colectomy. In some cases diarrhea persists, and in other cases constipation recurs. Persistent diarrhea may be the result of antibiotic-responsive diarrhea therapy or hypersecretion in the small intestine, or it may be bile salt and fatty acid mediated. Treatment for persistent diarrhea includes antidiarrheal agents, a low-fat diet, oral antibiotics, and/or bile salt–binding agents. Constipation after subtotal colectomy often is controlled by dietary management and stool softeners, and occasionally by manual extraction. Cats with resistant postoperative constipation may benefit from a repeat colectomy, but others are euthanized.

PROGNOSIS

The long-term results of subtotal colectomy for idiopathic megacolon in cats usually are good to excellent. The prognosis is fair to guarded without surgery. Medical management of chronic constipation is possible; however, the frequency of enemas and the need for manual evacuation often become intolerable, prompting euthanasia. Dogs do not do as well with subtotal colectomy as cats.

Reference

Washabau RJ, Holt DE, Brockman DJ: Mediation of acetylcholine and substance P induced contractions by myosin light chain phosphorylation in feline colonic smooth muscle, *Am J Vet Res* 63:695, 2002.

Suggested Reading

Demetriou JL, Welsh EM: Colonic obstruction in an adult cat following open castration, *Vet Rec* 147:165, 2000.
This is a case report of an unusual iatrogenic cause of colonic obstruction in a cat.
Freeman CB, Adin CA, Lewis DD et al: Intrapelvic granuloma formation six years after total hip arthroplasty in a dog, *J Am Vet Med Assoc* 223:1446, 2003.
This is a case report of an unusual cause of colonic obstruction in a dog.

Washabau RJ: Gastrointestinal motility disorders and gastrointestinal prokinetc therapy, *Vet Clin North Am* 33:1007, 2003.

This is an excellent review that discusses newer prokinetics, which may benefit patients with motility disorders of the colon and other gastrointestinal sites.

White RN: Surgical management of constipation, *J Feline Med Surg* 4:129-138, 2002.

This is a review article that summarizes findings from research and clinical studies.

BOX 19-65

Possible Indications for Rectal, Anal, or Perineal Surgery

- Diagnostic biopsy
- Anal sac disease
- Colonic obstruction
- Perineal hernia
- Rectal perforation
- Perianal fistulae
- Rectal ischemia
- Rectal prolapse
- Neoplasia
- Fecal incontinence

Surgery of the Perineum, Rectum, and Anus

GENERAL PRINCIPLES AND TECHNIQUES

DEFINITIONS

Rectal resection is removal of a portion of the terminal large intestine. **Rectal pull-through** is resection of the terminal colon or midrectum (or both) using an anal approach, with or without an abdominal approach. **Anal sacculectomy** is removal of one or both of the anal sacs.

PREOPERATIVE MANAGEMENT

Rectal surgery usually is performed to resect masses or nonfunctional bowel and to repair rectal prolapse, perforation, or fistula (Box 19-65). Perineal surgery is most often performed to treat perineal hernias, perianal fistulae, anal sac disease, tumors, rectovaginal or rectourethral fistulae, and other traumatic or congenital anomalies (e.g., atresia ani and anovaginal cleft). Scooting, anal licking, constipation, tenesmus, and dyschezia are typical presenting complaints associated with perineal and rectal disease (Table 19-2). Fresh blood may be seen in the feces or perianal region. Perianal tumors and perineal fistulae often cause perianal thickening and ulceration, whereas perineal swelling usually is associated with perineal hernias. Pelvic sacroiliac fractures and separations occasionally cause rectal perforation (fewer than 1% of cases). Fresh blood and omentum may be found during rectal examination in animals with rectal laceration or perforation.

Diagnosis of rectal, perianal, or perineal disease is primarily based on the history, clinical signs, physical examination, imaging (i.e., radiology, ultrasonography, CT, and MRI), endoscopy, and histopathologic examination. If impaired anorectal innervation is suspected, myelographic, manometric, and electrodiagnostic evaluations are required. Many conditions can be diagnosed on physical examination, and a thorough rectal examination is crucial (Box 19-66). Anesthesia may be required for adequate rectal examination of painful animals. Visual inspection of the perineum may reveal unilateral or bilateral swelling, perianal masses, ulceration, fistulae, fecal soiling, or prolapsed mucosa.

The results of CBC and serum biochemistry tests are nonspecific. Neoplastic masses may be associated with hypercalcemia, anemia, and other paraneoplastic syndromes. Azotemia with or without hyperkalemia may occur with bladder entrapment caused by perineal hernia. Hypercalce-mia is common with some anal sac tumors (see p. 507) and may be reduced preoperatively with fluids and diuretics (see p. 509).

Rectal and perineal radiographs may confirm the physical examination findings. If possible, the colon and rectum should be evacuated with enemas, laxatives, and/or cathartics before radiographic studies. The rectum should be evaluated for size, location, and masses. Sublumbar lymphadenomegaly suggests metastasis. The prostate may be enlarged and malpositioned. The urinary bladder may be identified within a perineal hernia. A perforated rectum may allow gas into the perineal, intrapelvic, or caudal retroperitoneal soft tissues or into the peritoneal cavity. Gastrointestinal barium studies (enema or oral), urethrograms, and cystograms sometimes help evaluate patients with perineal hernias. Proctoscopy and/or biopsy helps define rectal disease, but should often be combined with colonoscopy because tumors and inflammatory disease may also affect the colon (see p. 490). Samples should be collected for culture, cytology, and histopathology. A biopsy of normal tissue should be taken in addition to thickened folds, masses, strictures, or ulcers. Perforation is an uncommon complication of proctoscopy.

Preoperative patient preparation is similar to that used before colon surgery (see p. 480). Warm compresses should be applied to inflamed or infected areas two or three times a day, and stool softeners should be used if surgery is delayed (see Box 19-60). The locations of fistulae and tumors should be mapped before surgery. Unless the colon is perforated or obstructed, mechanical emptying and cleansing help reduce bacterial numbers. Rectal perforation should be corrected as soon as it is diagnosed. Minimally the terminal rectum should be evacuated digitally after anesthetic induction but just before surgery in all patients. Some surgeries (e.g., extensive rectal resection) require more complete patient preparation. If possible, an elemental diet or a low-residue diet (e.g., hamburger and white rice) should be fed for 2 to 3 days before surgery. Food should be withheld 24 hours before surgery in adult patients (4 to 8 hours in pediatric patients), but free access to water should be allowed. Bisacodyl, a stimulant laxative, facilitates colonic evacuation (see Box 19-60). Laxatives, cathartics, and warm water enemas should be given 24 hours before surgery (see Box 19-60). Colyte or GoLytely should be administered orally by stomach tube 24 hours and 18 to 20 hours before surgery if the animal is not obstructed (see Box 19-55). Although these colonic lavage solutions work well, enemas facilitate complete cleansing. A warm water enema

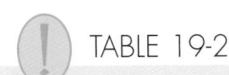 TABLE 19-2

Clinical Signs of Rectal, Anal, and Perineal Disease

	ANAL TUMOR	ANAL SACCULITIS	PERINEAL HERNIA	PERIANAL FISTULA	RECTAL PROLAPSE	FECAL INCONTINENCE
Anal biting or scooting	±	+	−	±	±	−
Anal licking	±	+	−	+	±	−
Tenesmus	+	+	+	+	+	±
Thickening or swelling	+	+	+	+	−	±
Constipation or obstipation	±	±	+	±	±	−
Diarrhea	−	±	−	±	±	±
Hemorrhage or hematochezia	±	±	−	±	±	−
Mass	+	±	+	−	+	−
Pain or dyschezia	+	+	+	+	+	−
Ulceration or fistula	±	±	−	+	+	−
Pelvic diaphragm weakness	−	−	+	−	±	±
Diminished anal tone	−	−	−	±	±	±
Fecal incontinence	−	−	±	±	±	+
Stricture	±	−	−	±	−	±
Abnormal discharge	−	±	−	±	−	−
Febrile	−	±	−	±	−	−
Inflammation	±	+	±	+	±	±
Rectal prolapse	−	−	±	−	+	−
Other	± Hypercalcemia	Dermatitis, odor, tail chasing	Shock, uremia, stranguria, vomiting, bulging of perianal area	Odor, weight, ? appetite, lethargy, poor		Self-trauma, hyperesthesia or paresthesia hair coat

+, Present; −, absent; ±, may be present or absent.

should be given the day before surgery, and a 10% povidone-iodine enema should be given 3 hours before surgery. Patients with perianal disease may be in too much pain to allow preoperative enemas. Furthermore, enemas may cause perforation or trauma, further deteriorating debilitated, anorexic patients. Enemas given any closer to surgery than 3 hours are contraindicated because they liquefy intestinal contents and may promote dissemination of contaminated material during surgery. After large bowel evacuation using laxatives, cathartics, and/or enemas, feces may remain in a deviated or dilated rectal area, necessitating manual removal.

After induction of anesthesia, a urinary catheter should be placed to aid intraoperative identification of the urethra;

 BOX 19-66

Abnormalities That May Be Noted During Rectal Examination

- Masses
- Strictures
- Perianal thickening
- Anal sac enlargement
- Pain
- Reduced sphincter tone
- Pelvic diaphragm weakness
- Rectal deviation or sacculation
- Sublumbar lymph node enlargement
- Prostatomegaly
- Pelvic canal distortion
- Thickening or irregularity of rectal mucosa

the rectum should be manually cleaned if necessary; and the anal sacs should be expressed. The entire perineum, from dorsal to the tail head and including the ventral tail, should be clipped and aseptically prepared for surgery. If a celiotomy is planned, the ventral abdomen should also be clipped and prepared for aseptic surgery.

ANESTHESIA

Anesthetic complications may arise from uncorrected hydration, electrolyte, or acid-base abnormalities. Nitrous oxide increases the volume of air trapped in body viscera and should be avoided in patients with intestinal obstruction. Atropine or glycopyrrolate (Box 19-67) may prevent bradycardia induced by visceral manipulation. Water evaporates more quickly from exposed abdominal viscera, therefore fluid administration should be increased to replace this loss. Hypothermia occurs because of vasodilatation and visceral exposure, reducing the need for anesthetics. These patients should be kept dry and warm. Opioid premedicants (e.g., butorphanol, hydromorphone, or buprenorphine; see Table 13-4 on p. 133) may also provide preoperative and postoperative analgesia. Ketamine gives poor visceral analgesia and should not be used alone for surgical procedures. It is also contraindicated in cats with renal dysfunction.

BOX 19-67

Selected Anesthetic Protocols for Use in Animals Undergoing Perineal, Rectal, or Anal Surgery

Dogs

Premedication

Atropine (0.02–0.04 mg/kg IV, IM, SC) or glycopyrrolate (0.005–0.011 mg/kg IV, IM, SC) plus butorphanol (0.2–0.4 mg/kg SC or IM) or buprenorphine (5–15 µg/kg IM) or hydromorphone (0.1–0.2 mg/kg SC or IM)

Induction

Thiopental (10–12 mg/kg) or propofol (4–6 mg/kg) administered IV to effect

Maintenance

Isoflurane or sevoflurane

Cats

Premedication

Atropine (0.02–0.04 mg/kg IV, IM, SC) or glycopyrrolate (0.005–0.011 mg/kg IV, IM, SC) plus ketamine (5 mg/kg IM) plus butorphanol (0.2–0.4 mg/kg SC, IM)

Induction

Diazepam (0.27 mg/kg) plus ketamine (5.5 mg/kg) combined and administered IV to effect or thiopental (10–12 mg/kg) or propofol (4–6 mg/kg) administered IV to effect or use mask or chamber induction

Maintenance

Isoflurane or sevoflurane

IV, Intravenous; *IM*, intramuscular; *SC*, subcutaneous.

If there are no contraindications (e.g., sepsis, bleeding diatheses, and hypovolemia [for epidurals using local anesthetics]), epidurals (see Chapter 13) may be used in dogs to supplement general anesthetic. Epidural anesthesia alone rarely is sufficient for surgery. If general anesthesia is not used, heavy sedation (i.e., hydromorphone) is necessary. Epidural doses should be reduced if cerebrospinal fluid is encountered when using local anesthetics, if the patient is pregnant or obese, or if there are space-occupying vertebral canal lesions. Opioids may be preferred over local anesthetics in epidurals because opioids cause sensory loss without motor block and do not promote hypotension. Because local anesthetics in epidurals may cause hypotension, dehydration should be corrected before performing the procedure.

ANTIBIOTICS

The risk of infection after colorectal surgery is high. Although controversial, the use of antibiotics in colorectal surgery reduces morbidity and mortality associated with infection. Systemic perioperative antibiotics effective against anaerobes and gram-negative aerobes should be given (see Box 19-56 on p. 482). Recommended drugs include second-generation cephalosporins (i.e., cefmetazole, cefoxitin, and cefotetan) given at the time of induction. Third-generation cephalosporins effective against gram-positive and gram-negative aerobes and some anaerobes are available but expensive. Amikacin plus either ampicillin or clindamycin can be given intravenously at induction. Aminoglycosides (i.e., neomycin and kanamycin) and metronidazole can be given orally in combination beginning 24 hours before surgery.

Metronidazole is absorbed from the gastrointestinal tract and is effective against anaerobes. Aminoglycosides are effective only against aerobic bacteria. Gastrointestinal absorption of aminoglycosides is minimal in normal patients, but can be substantial if the bowel is eroded or inflamed. The use of such nonabsorbable antibiotics has been linked with the emergence of resistant infections. A combination of neomycin and erythromycin can be given beginning 24 hours before surgery to rapidly reduce aerobes and anaerobes. Metronidazole combined with first-generation cephalosporins (cefazolin) or an aminoglycoside (see Box 19-56) is usually effective.

SURGICAL ANATOMY

The rectum is the segment of large intestine coursing through the pelvic canal and ending at the anus. The colorectal junction is difficult to identify. Landmarks used to estimate the location of the colorectal junction include the pubic brim, pelvic inlet, seventh lumbar vertebra, and seromuscular penetration point of the cranial rectal artery. The cranial rectum is attached to the sacrum by the mesorectum. The mesorectum does not cover the entire rectum; the terminal rectum is retroperitoneal. At the level of the second caudal vertebra, the mesorectum reflects onto the sides of the pelvis as parietal peritoneum, forming a pararectal fossa on each side. The peritoneal reflection is cranial to the rectococcygeus muscles and contains the autonomic nerve fibers of the pelvic plexus that innervate the rectum. The pelvic plexus is paired, composed of parasympathetic pelvic and sympathetic hypogastric nerves, and lies dorsal to the prostate in males (see p. 708). The caudal part of the rectum is supported by the levator ani muscles medially and coccygeus muscles laterally. The external anal sphincter muscle demarcates the caudal limit of the rectum.

The anal canal is a continuation of the rectum to the anus and is only 1 to 2 cm long. It is divided into three zones: the columnar zone, the intermediate zone, and the cutaneous zone. The innermost (columnar) zone has a series of longitudinal mucosal and submucosal ridges called anal columns or pillars. The pockets between these columns are the anal sinuses, which extend caudally and end in blind pouches under the anocutaneous line. The columnar zone varies from 3 to 25 mm in length. The intermediate zone usually is less than 1 to 2 mm wide, but forms a distinct, raised, circumferential ridge called the anocutaneous line. Anal glands are found in the columnar and intermediate zones. The outermost (cutaneous) zone has very fine hairs, but appears as hairless skin. Sebaceous, circumanal, and apocrine sweat glands are found only in the cutaneous zone. The anus is the external opening of the anal canal.

The cranial rectal artery is a branch of the caudal mesenteric artery and is the major blood supply to the rectum. Blood supply from the middle rectal artery (from the internal pudendal branch of the internal iliac artery) and caudal rectal artery (from the middle caudal branch of the median sacral artery or from the internal pudendal branch of the internal iliac artery) varies and is relatively insignificant. To ensure an adequate anastomotic blood supply, the cranial rectal artery in dogs should be preserved unless the intrapelvic rectum is resected. Lymphatics from the anal canal and rectum drain cranially into the medial iliac lymph node.

The internal and external anal sphincter muscles surround the terminal rectum and anal canal to control defecation. The anal sacs lie between these two muscles on each side of the anus (see p. 513). The internal anal sphincter is a caudal thickening of the circular smooth muscle lining the anal canal. It is an involuntary smooth muscle that works with other muscles of defecation to prevent indiscriminate defecation. It is innervated by the parasympathetic branches of the pelvic nerve (S1-S3), which are inhibitory. Motor fibers from the hypogastric nerves are sympathetic to the internal anal sphincter. The external anal sphincter is a large, circumferential band of skeletal (striated) muscle chiefly responsible for fecal continence. It is wider dorsally than ventrally where its fibers decussate and spread to insert on the urethra and bulbospongiosus muscle. The only voluntary nerve supply to the external anal sphincter comes from the caudal rectal branches of the pudendal nerves. The blood supply to the external anal sphincter is from the perineal arteries. See p. 517 for the surgical anatomy of the pelvic diaphragm.

> NOTE: Fecal incontinence usually occurs if more than 4 cm or the final 1.5 cm of the terminal rectum is resected, if the perineal nerves are damaged, or if more than half the external anal sphincter is damaged.

SURGICAL TECHNIQUE
Rectal Resection

The primary indication for rectal resection is to excise a neoplastic, necrotic, traumatized (e.g., prolapse, fistula, or diverticulum), or strictured segment of rectum. Other indications include congenital anomalies and perforations or lacerations. The rectum may be exposed using a ventral, dorsal, rectal pull-through, lateral, or anal approach. The diseased rectum is resected, and the remaining rectum is reapposed to the rectum, colon, or ileum using the techniques described for colectomy on p. 484.

Ventral approach. Lesions at the colorectal junction are resected using this approach. A ventral approach to the rectum must be accompanied by a pubic symphysiotomy or pubic osteotomy (Fig. 19-118; also see p. 670) to gain access to the pelvic canal. Pubic symphysiotomy provides more limited exposure than pubic osteotomy.

For pubic symphysiotomy, incise the entire length of the adductor aponeurosis. Divide the pubis and the ischium on the midline with an osteotome and mallet or an oscillating saw. Separate the pubis and the ischium with a self-retaining retractor (e.g., pediatric Finochietto).

Anal approach. An anal approach is suitable for excision of small, noninvasive, pedunculated polyps, and broad-based rectal masses that can be exteriorized through the anus. Lesions involving the caudal rectum or anal canal can be exteriorized using this approach. Perforations of the terminal rectum may be apposed through this approach, although a lateral approach (see p. 505) allows lavage and drainage of contaminated adjacent tissue. The mucocutaneous junction and skin must be resected if they are diseased, but fecal incontinence is a common sequela.

With the patient in ventral recumbency, dilate the anus with three or four stay sutures placed through the mucocutaneous junction (Fig. 19-119, A and B). Evert the rectal wall by placing stay sutures (e.g., 3-0 nylon or other monofilament suture) in the rectal mucosa cranial or caudal to the mass or lesion and applying caudal traction. Place additional stay sutures to further retract the mass or lesion if necessary (Fig. 19-119, C). Use electrosurgery, laser, or scalpel incisions to remove masses. Make a partial-thickness or full-thickness incision, depending on malignancy and the need for wide borders. Appose cut edges with simple interrupted sutures (e.g., 3-0 or 4-0 polydioxanone, polyglyconate, poliglecaprone 25, or glycomer 631; Fig. 19-119, D). Remove the stay sutures and allow the surgical site to retract within the pelvic canal.

AP **Rectal pull-through approach.** The primary indication for a rectal pull-through is to resect a distal colonic or midrectal lesion not approachable through the abdomen and too large or cranial for an anal approach. When circumferential or near-circumferential lesions are resected using this technique, postoperative stricture is a major concern.

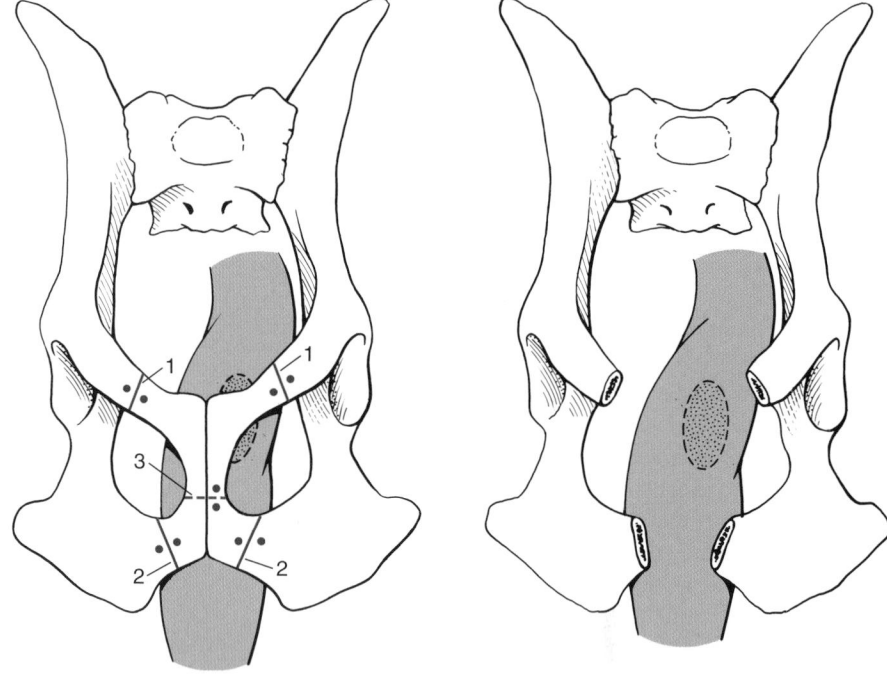

FIG. 19-118
For a ventral rectal approach, extend the ventral celiotomy incision over the symphysis of the pelvis. Incise and elevate the aponeurosis of the adductor and gracilis muscles. Predrill holes on each side of the proposed osteotomy sites. Perform a pubic osteotomy at sites 1 and 2 to expose the entire intrapelvic rectum. Perform an osteotomy at sites 1 and 3 if exposure of the caudal intrapelvic rectum is unnecessary.

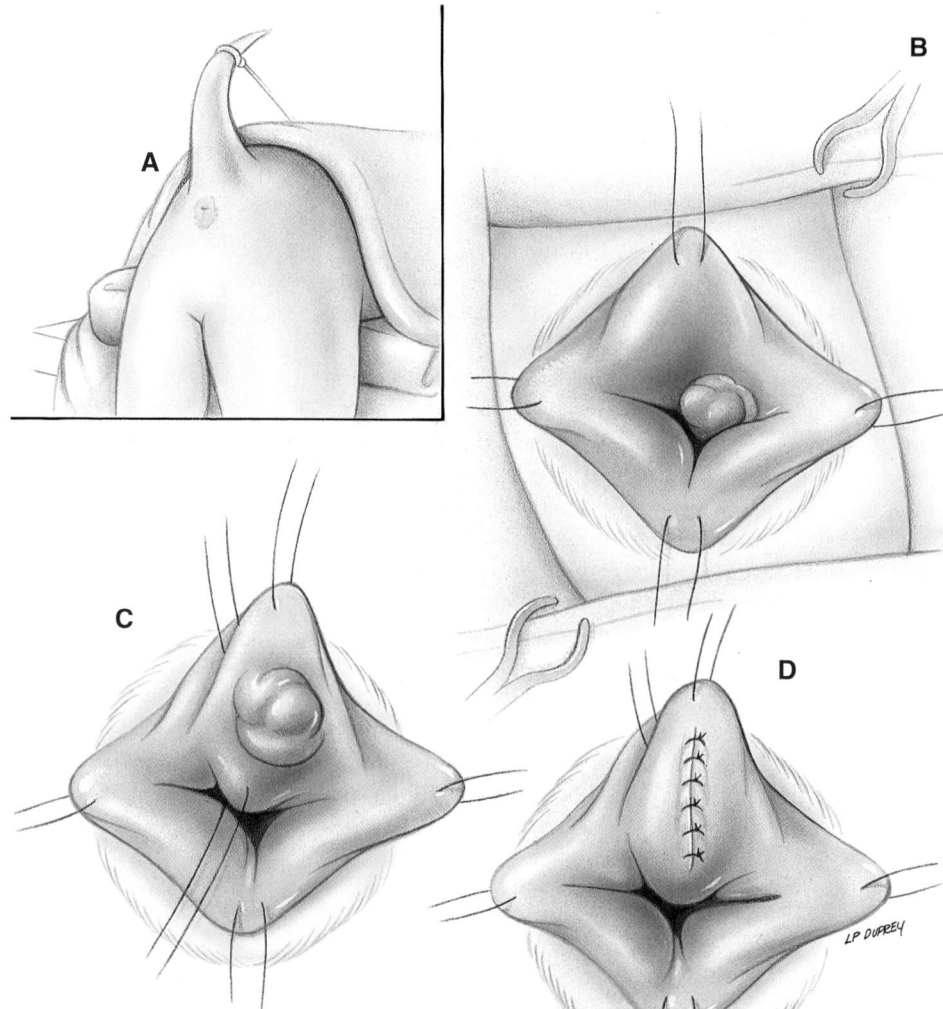

FIG. 19-119
Anal approach to the rectum.
A, Place the patient in a perineal position. **B,** Place stay sutures around the anus to dilate it and expose the lesion. **C,** Place additional stay sutures near the lesion, and apply caudal traction to exteriorize it. **D,** Resect the mass and suture the defect.

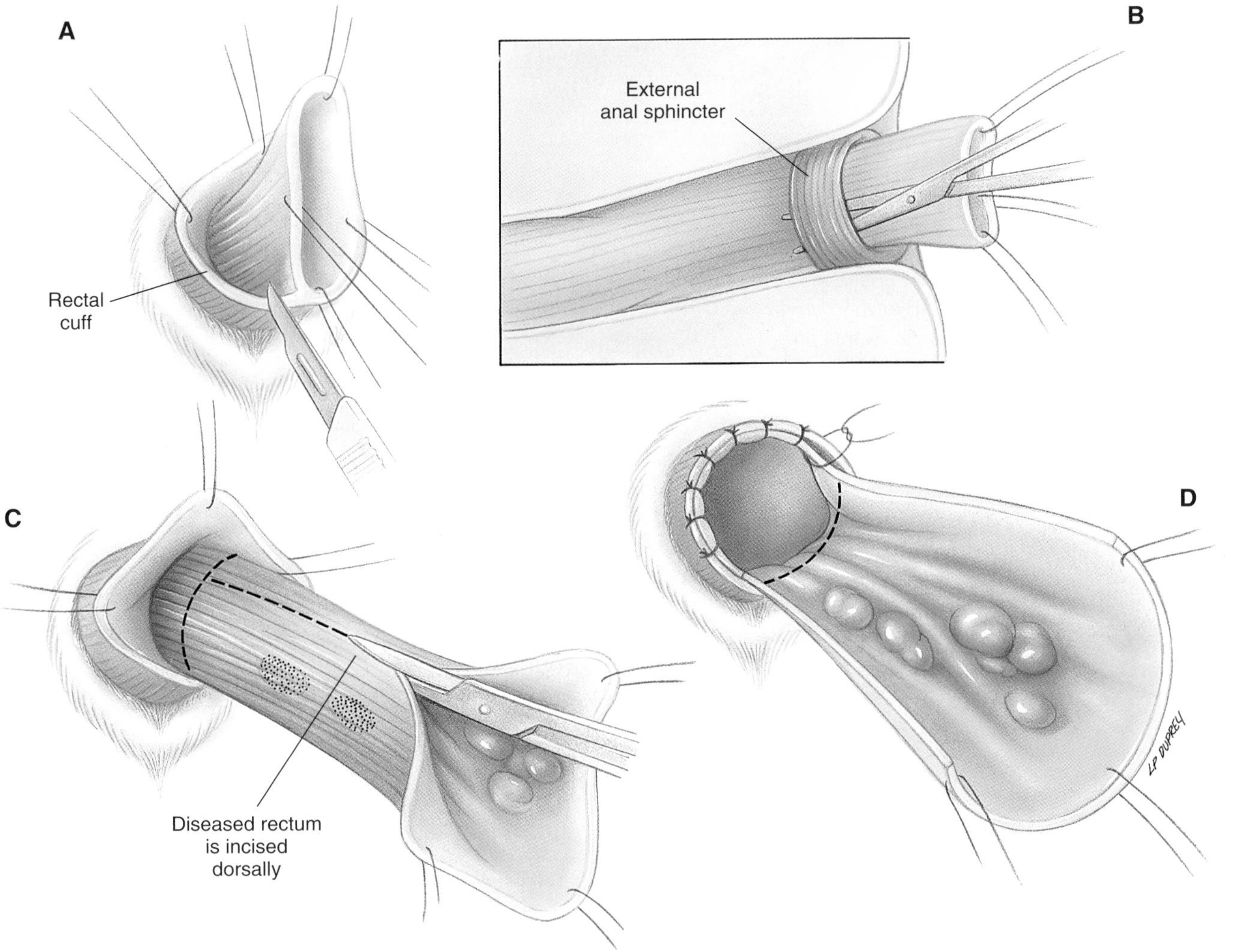

A

Rectal
cuff

B

External
anal sphincter

C

Diseased rectum
is incised
dorsally

D

LP DUPREY

FIG. 19-120
Rectal pull-through procedure. **A,** Evert the rectal wall through the anus with stay sutures. Make a full-thickness incision through the rectal wall, preserving a 1.5-cm cuff of distal rectum. **B,** Mobilize the rectum by dissecting directly against the rectal wall to separate it from the external anal sphincter and surrounding tissue. **C,** Pull the mobilized rectum caudally and incise longitudinally to normal tissue. **D,** Appose the cut edge of the normal cranial rectum to the preserved rectal cuff with simple interrupted sutures.

Position the animal in ventral recumbency with the hindquarters elevated. Evert the rectum with stay sutures placed cranial to the mucocutaneous junction (1.5 cm or more if possible; Fig. 19-120. A). Using the stay sutures, apply caudal traction to the cranial rectum. Begin a full-thickness, 360-degree incision through the rectum, leaving a 1.5-cm cuff of nondiseased rectal wall attached to the anus if possible. Place three or four stay sutures in the rectal cuff. Mobilize the rectum by bluntly dissecting along the external wall (Fig. 19-120, B). Continue dissection as far cranially as the cranial rectal artery if necessary.

If dissection occurs cranial to the second caudal vertebra, the peritoneal cavity will be entered.

Ligate or coagulate rectal vessels as they are encountered. If the lesion is diffuse, split the rectum longitudinally until normal tissue is identified (Fig. 19-120, C). Transect the diseased rectum in stages with 1 to 2 cm of normal tissue at each end. Transect one fourth to one third of the circumference and then appose the cranial end of the rectum to the caudal rectal cuff with simple interrupted sutures (e.g., 3-0 or 4-0 polydioxanone, polyglyconate, poliglecaprone 25, or glycomer 631; Fig. 19-120, D). Continue transecting and apposing until all diseased tissue has been excised.

> NOTE: Some surgeons prefer a two-layer closure; first appose the seromuscular layer and then the mucosal-submucosal layer.

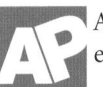 A Swenson's pull-through is performed when disease extends into the colon.

For this procedure, position the patient in dorsal recumbency so that both a ventral abdominal and an anal approach may be used. Transect the colon proximal to the mass. Oversew the ends of the colon and rectum.

Linear cutting or transverse stapling instruments may be used to reappose the colon and rectum.

Ligate the vessels supplying the distal colon and rectum (see p. 484). Place stay sutures through the end of the remaining colon or ileum and rectum. Grasp the sutures with transanally placed forceps and evert the rectum through the anus. Advance the colon or ileum through the pelvic canal with stay sutures. Resect the lesion and anastomose the end of the colon or ileum to the terminal rectum as described above. Gently replace the intestine into the pelvic canal.

Dorsal approach. A dorsal approach is used if the lesion involves the caudal or middle rectum and not the anal canal.

Position the patient in ventral recumbency with the pelvis elevated and the tail fixed over the back. Pad the cranial aspect of the hind limbs to prevent pressure on the femoral nerves. Make a curvilinear incision from one ischiatic tuberosity to the other, curving dorsal to the anus (Fig. 19-121, A). Incise the subcutaneous fat and perineal fascia. Locate the rectum, external anal sphincter, levator ani, and coccygeus muscles laterally and the rectococcygeus muscles dorsally. Transect the paired rectococcygeus muscles near their origin on the rectal wall or their insertion on the caudal vertebrae (Fig. 19-121, B). Elevate the external anal sphincter and caudal edge of the levator ani to the level of the caudal rectal nerve. For more cranial rectal resections, partly transect the levator ani muscles if necessary. Position a self-retaining retractor (i.e., Gelpi or Weitlaner) to improve visualization if necessary. Gently retract the rectum caudally and mobilize the rectum cranially to the normal bowel. Repair the lacerated rectum or resect the diseased bowel. Ligate or cauterize vessels to the diseased bowel. Place stay sutures in the cranial bowel before transection.

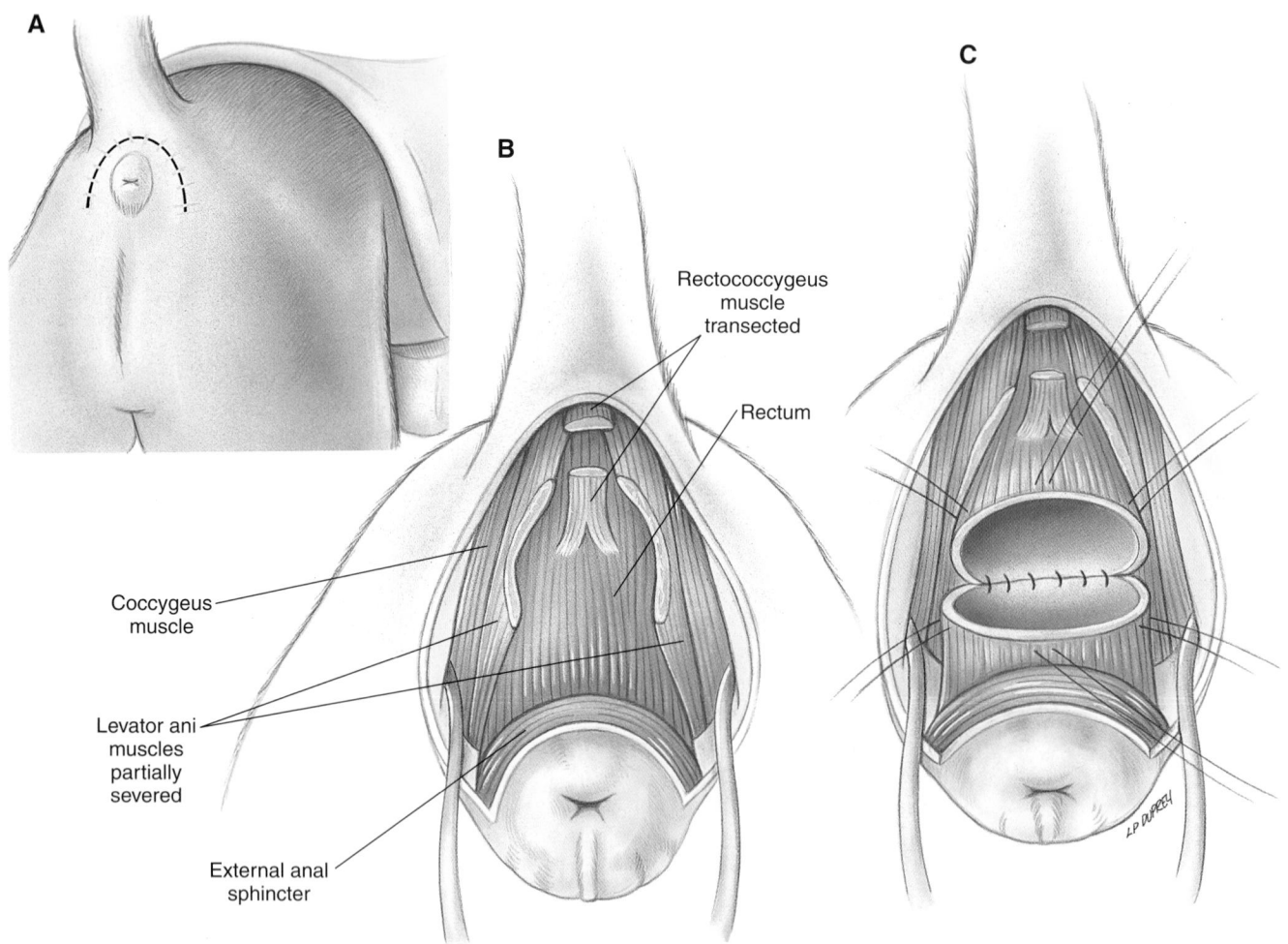

FIG. 19-121
Dorsal rectal approach. **A,** Make a curvilinear incision from one ischial tuberosity to the other, curving dorsally to the anus. **B,** Identify the rectococcygeus, levator ani, and coccygeus muscles. Transect the rectococcygeus muscle and partly incise the levator ani. **C,** Resect the diseased rectum, and appose the ends with a suture triangulation technique or end-to-end stapling instrument.

Appose the bowel ends with interrupted appositional sutures (e.g., 3-0 or 4-0 polydioxanone, polyglyconate, poliglecaprone 25, or glycomer 631; Fig. 19-121, C) or with an end-to-end stapling device (see p. 453). Reappose the transected levator ani muscle with appositional cruciate or mattress sutures.

Some surgeons reattach the rectococcygeus muscles and external anal sphincter to the rectal wall.

Thoroughly lavage the area, and place drains if significant contamination has occurred.

Placement of a drain against the anastomotic site may cause dehiscence.

Separately appose the subcutaneous tissue and skin with continuous or interrupted sutures of 3-0 or 4-0 polydioxanone and 3-0 or 4-0 nylon or polypropylene, respectively.

Lateral approach. The lateral approach limits exposure to one side of the rectum and may be suitable for repair of lacerations or resection of a diverticulum.

Make a curvilinear incision 1 to 3 cm lateral to the anus, beginning dorsal to the tail head and extending ventral to the anus (Fig. 19-122, A). Incise the subcutaneous tissue

to expose the pelvic diaphragm. Separate the fascia between the external anal sphincter and the levator ani muscle. Preserve the caudal rectal nerve to the external anal sphincter (Fig. 19-122, B). Repair the laceration with a one- or two-layer closure using simple interrupted sutures (e.g., 3-0 or 4-0 polydioxanone, polyglyconate, poliglecaprone 25, or glycomer 631). Thoroughly lavage the area, and place a closed suction drain if soft tissues were contaminated with feces. Resect diverticula with a linear stapling device. Reappose the external anal sphincter and levator ani muscles with interrupted appositional sutures. Place additional sutures between the external anal sphincter and internal obturator muscle if this fascial plane is disrupted. Close the subcutaneous tissue and skin routinely.

Anal Sacculectomy

Anal sacculectomy is performed to remove chronically infected or impacted anal sacs, anal sac fistulae, or neoplasia. Meticulous dissection is required to prevent fecal incontinence by preserving the anal sphincter muscles and nerves. A closed or open technique may be used. The closed technique is preferred because the external anal sphincter muscle is not transected, and the lumen of the anal sac remains closed, preventing contact between secretions and adjacent tissues. See p. 513 for a description of open and closed anal sacculectomy techniques.

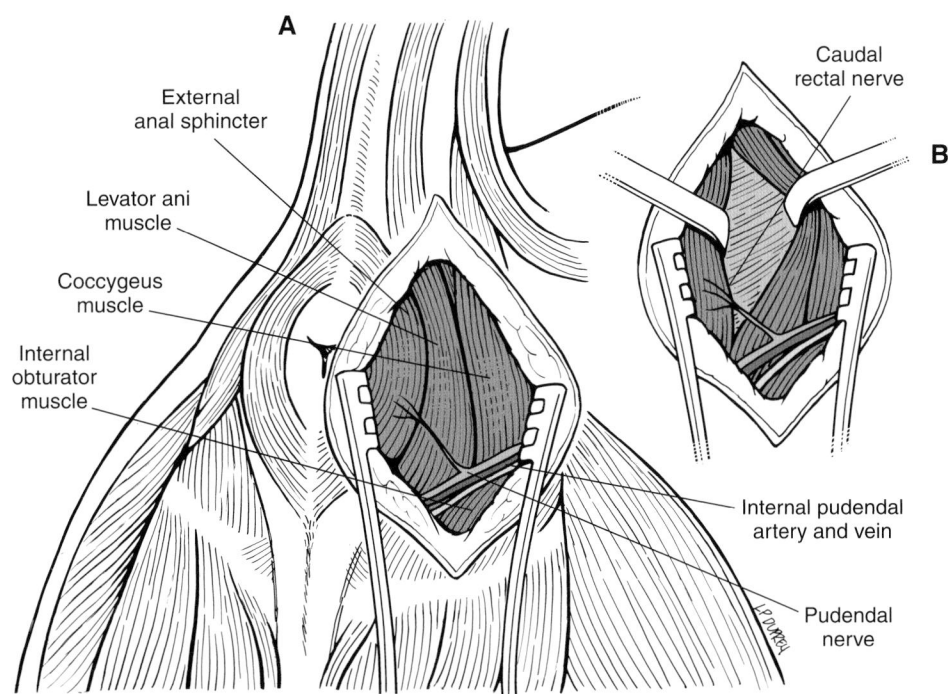

FIG. 19-122
Lateral rectal approach. **A,** Make an incision 1 to 3 cm lateral to the anus. Identify the internal pudendal artery and vein and the pudendal nerve crossing the internal obturator muscle. **B,** Note the caudal rectal nerve to the external anal sphincter. Separate the fascia between the external anal sphincter and levator ani muscles to expose the lateral aspect of the rectum.

NOTE: Perform a histopathologic examination to rule out anal sac tumors.

HEALING OF THE RECTUM

Rectal healing is affected by the same factors that affect colonic healing (see p. 488). Optimal healing requires a good blood supply, accurate mucosal apposition, and minimal surgical trauma. Systemic factors that may delay healing and increase the risk of dehiscence include hypovolemia, shock, hypoproteinemia, debilitation, and infection.

SUTURE MATERIALS AND SPECIAL INSTRUMENTS

In addition to a general pack, abdominal (i.e., Balfour), perineal (e.g., Gelpi), and pelvic (e.g., Finochietto) retractors are recommended to aid in exposing the surgical field. Doyen, Babcock, and Carmalt forceps may be needed to occlude or retract the intestine. Metzenbaum and iris scissors are indicated for dissection. Closed suction drains are used in contaminated areas. Other special instruments or equipment that may be necessary for rectal or perianal surgery include a probe or groove director, fulguration unit, laser unit, silicone elastomer, and surgical stapling equipment.

For optimal healing, a monofilament, synthetic absorbable suture (e.g., polydioxanone or polyglyconate) and approximating suture patterns (i.e., simple interrupted, Gambee, crushing, or simple continuous) should be used for rectoanal surgery. A monofilament, nonabsorbable suture (e.g., polypropylene, polybutester, or nylon) or absorbable suture material (e.g., polydioxanone, polyglyconate, or poliglecaprone 25) may be used for herniorrhaphy.

POSTOPERATIVE CARE AND ASSESSMENT

Postoperative care is individualized for the patient. The animal should be observed closely during recovery for vomiting. Analgesics (see Table 13-4 on p. 133) should be given as necessary. Hydration should be maintained with intravenous fluids until the patient is eating and drinking normally, and electrolyte and acid-base abnormalities have been corrected. Encouraging early ambulation and eating may minimize ileus. An Elizabethan collar, bucket, or sidebars should be used to protect the surgical site. Purse-string sutures should be removed immediately or within 2 to 3 days after surgery. Prophylactic antibiotics generally can be discontinued 2 to 4 hours postoperatively; however, they should be continued if contamination has occurred (see previous discussion under Antibiotics).

If vomiting does not occur, water should be offered 8 to 12 hours postoperatively. A stool softener should be given when oral intake begins (see Box 19-60) and should be continued for 2 weeks or as needed. After rectal surgery, a bland, low-fat food (i/d [Hill's Pet Products] or boiled rice, potatoes, and pasta combined with boiled, skinless chicken, yogurt, or low-fat cottage cheese) should be fed three or four times daily. The animal's normal diet should be gradually reintroduced beginning 48 to 72 hours after surgery. Ani-

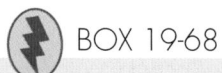

BOX 19-68

Possible Complications of Perianal and Rectal Surgery

- Infection
- Dehiscence
- Tenesmus
- Rectal prolapse
- Dyschezia
- Hematochezia
- Temporary or permanent incontinence
- Anal stricture
- Flatulence
- Hemorrhage
- Recurrence
- Metastasis
- Nerve damage (pudendal, sciatic, femoral)
- Urethral obstruction
- Stranguria
- Dysuria
- Urinary incontinence
- Bladder atony
- Death

mals having perineal surgery may resume their normal diet with the first feeding. Debilitated animals may require enteral or parenteral nutrition.

Initially, cold compresses are applied to reduce residual bleeding and inflammation; later, warm compresses should be applied. Apply compresses two or three times daily for 15 to 20 minutes to minimize postoperative swelling after perianal or perineal surgery. Redness and pain at the incisional site may indicate early infection. Anal sphincter function, continence, perineal swelling, and drainage should be assessed daily. The presence or absence of fecal blood (and its color and consistency, if present) should be noted. Increased frequency of defecation may occur after major colorectal resections. Perianal and perineal area surgeries are predisposed to infection because of the high bacterial numbers in these areas. Depression, high fever, abdominal tenderness, vomiting, ileus, or perineal inflammation may indicate infection or peritonitis. If peritonitis is suspected, abdominocentesis or diagnostic peritoneal lavage (see p. 335), a chemistry profile, and a CBC should be performed and antibiotic and fluid therapy initiated. If toxic neutrophils, bacteria, or intestinal debris are present in abdominal fluid or lavage solution, the abdomen should be explored. Aggressive treatment of generalized peritonitis by open peritoneal drainage (see p. 336) may be necessary.

COMPLICATIONS

Numerous complications are possible after rectoanal, perianal, and perineal surgery (Box 19-68). Postoperative tenesmus, hematochezia, and fecal incontinence are common. Postoperative tenesmus and hematochezia should resolve in most animals after suture removal or absorption. Incontinence with extensive rectal resection results from loss of rectal afferent nerves or from disruption of the pelvic plexus at the peritoneal reflection. Removal of the distal 1.5 cm of rectum may cause fecal incontinence even if the external anal sphincter is preserved. Fecal incontinence is uncommon when 4 cm or less of the rectum is resected, preserving the terminal rectal cuff. Longer rectal resections (6 cm or longer) disrupt the peritoneal reflection and frequently result in incontinence. Other possible complications are rectal prolapse, perirectal abscesses, dehiscence, and stenosis.

Significant strictures occur more commonly after rectal resection than colonic resection, probably because of excessive tension at the resection site. These strictures usually can be managed by incision with an electrosurgical tip or laser or by balloon dilation. If these techniques do not alleviate obstruction, surgical resection may be required. Anal stricture is a complication of anal sac disease, perianal fistula, neoplasia, and surgical or nonsurgical trauma. It may be treated by anoplasty; balloon dilation; incision with electrosurgery, laser, or scalpel; or resection.

SPECIAL AGE CONSIDERATIONS

Young animals may have a congenital abnormality, such as anal atresia or imperforate anus. Neoplasia is more common in older animals.

SPECIFIC DISEASES

ANAL NEOPLASIA

DEFINITION

Perianal glands are modified sebaceous glands. Perianal gland adenomas are also called *circumanal tumors* and *hepatoid tumors;* anal sac tumors are also known as *apocrine gland tumors.*

GENERAL CONSIDERATIONS AND CLINICALLY RELEVANT PATHOPHYSIOLOGY

The most common perianal tumors are adenomas and carcinomas of the perianal and apocrine glands. Apocrine gland tumors usually involve the anal sacs. Perianal glands are located primarily around the anus and base of the tail; however, they are also found in the thigh, prepuce, and dorsal and ventral midline from the base of the skull to the umbilicus. Perianal tumors may occur at any of these locations. Androgen and estrogen hormone receptors and growth hormone have been identified in both perianal gland adenomas and adenocarcinomas (Petterino et al, 2004). The most common malignant tumors are perianal gland adenocarcinomas and apocrine gland adenocarcinomas. Other common tumors are listed in Box 19-69.

Perianal adenomas are the most common canine perianal tumors (80%). They are the third most frequent tumor in male dogs. They occur 12 times more often in intact males than in intact females and are more common in ovariohysterectomized females than in intact females. They are hormone dependent and usually diminish in size after castration. They may be single or multiple and usually are small, raised, firm, and well circumscribed; however, some are large and ulcerated. Many dogs with perianal adenomas also have testicular interstitial cell tumors (see p. 759).

Perianal gland adenocarcinomas cannot be grossly differentiated from adenomas. They usually are solitary, ulcer-

BOX 19-69

Common Tumors of the Perianal Region

- Perianal gland adenoma
- Perianal gland adenocarcinoma
- Apocrine gland adenocarcinoma
- Lipoma
- Leiomyoma
- Squamous cell carcinoma
- Melanoma
- Lymphoma
- Mast cell tumor
- Miscellaneous skin tumors

ated, and locally invasive and can be confused with perianal fistulae or anal sacs that have ruptured or are impacted. These tumors are not hormone responsive. Both primary and metastatic sites grow more slowly than many other malignancies. They usually metastasize to the intrapelvic and sublumbar lymph nodes. Other metastatic sites include the liver, lungs, kidneys, spleen, bone, and abdominal lymph nodes.

Anal sac apocrine gland adenocarcinomas (anal sac adenocarcinoma, apocrine gland adenocarcinoma) arising in the anal sac account for approximately 2% of skin tumors in dogs. Most patients have unilateral tumors. These tumors can cause hypercalcemia of malignancy with subsequent polyuria, polydipsia, poor appetite, and/or vomiting. Anal sac adenocarcinomas initially grow slowly and are confined to the anal sac; however, invasion into surrounding tissue, the rectum, and the pelvic canal occurs with continued growth. Most show evidence of stromal and lymphatic invasion. Metastasis to the iliac, sacral, and sublumbar lymph nodes may occur. Distant metastasis may occur anywhere, but lungs, liver, and spleen are the most common sites.

NOTE: Suspect perianal gland adenomas in male dogs. Suspect anal sac adenocarcinomas if the dog is hypercalcemic.

Anal SCCs arise from the anocutaneous line. They are typically malignant and metastasize quickly. Extensive fistulae or mucosal-cutaneous, ulcerlike lesions occur and often are covered with mucus. Anal function is impaired, and pain, tenesmus, and hemorrhage are typical. The prognosis is grave because of their malignant nature. Treatment often is discouraged.

DIAGNOSIS
Clinical Presentation

Signalment. Perianal tumors are common in middle-aged or older male dogs, but rare in females. The median age for anal sac apocrine gland adenocarcinoma is 10 years (range 5 to 15 years) (Williams et al, 2003). Adenomas are more prevalent in cocker spaniels, beagles, bulldogs, and Samoyeds. Cats do not have perianal or circumanal glands. Apocrine gland adenocarcinomas usually occur in older dogs. In

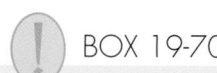

BOX 19-70

Signs of Hypercalcemia

- Anorexia
- Weight loss
- Vomiting
- Polyuria

- Polydipsia
- Muscle weakness
- Constipation

the past, old ovariohysterectomized females were reported to be most often affected; however, recent publications report no gender predisposition (Bennett et al, 2004; Williams et al, 2003).

History. Tumors in the perianal region cause irritation with subsequent licking, scooting, and tenesmus. Continued growth of the tumor or excoriation of the thin perianal skin causes mild hemorrhage, which may be noted in the feces or where the animal sits. Constipation, obstipation, and dyschezia may occur with large, invasive tumors. Some tumors are asymptomatic and found incidentally on a physical examination. Benign tumors usually are slow growing and painless. Malignant tumors usually are fast growing, firm, and invasive and are commonly ulcerated. Perianal tumors in castrated males should be considered malignant until proven otherwise. Paraneoplastic hypercalcemia is common with anal sac adenocarcinomas (Box 19-70); polyuria, polydipsia, anorexia, and/or vomiting secondary to renal failure may be seen, depending upon the magnitude of the hypercalcemia. Fecal incontinence may occur with aggressive tumors. Other signs that may be associated with metastatic lesions are chronic cough, limb edema, and urethral and rectal obstruction. Some anal sac adenocarcinomas are asymptomatic, being found incidentally during routine examinations.

Physical Examination Findings

Multiple perianal masses often are identified around the circumference of the anus in the hairless area. They may vary in size and may be covered with epithelium or be ulcerated, friable, and broad-based (Fig. 19-123). Most adenomas are well circumscribed, whereas carcinomas are invasive. Careful palpation of the perianal tissue during rectal examination often identifies masses that are difficult to visually differentiate from normal perianal tissue. Anal sac tumors are not always obvious when the anal sacs are palpated.

NOTE: Check the sublumbar and other regional lymph nodes for enlargement and asymmetry.

Diagnostic Imaging

Radiographs of the abdomen and thorax are used to help stage the disease. Enlarged sublumbar lymph nodes suggest metastasis. Abdominal ultrasonography allows evaluation of lymph nodes. CT can be used to help determine tumor size and invasiveness.

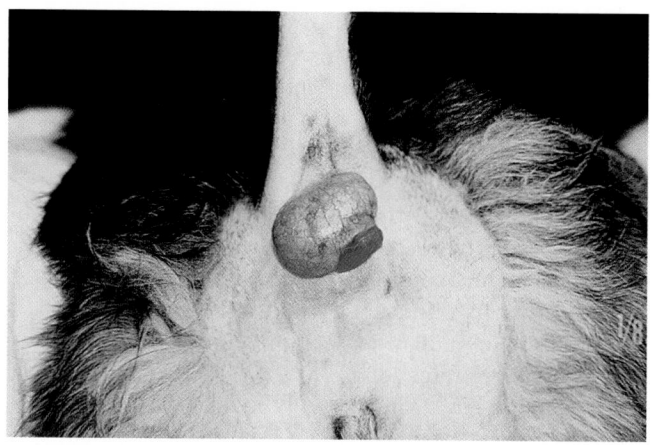

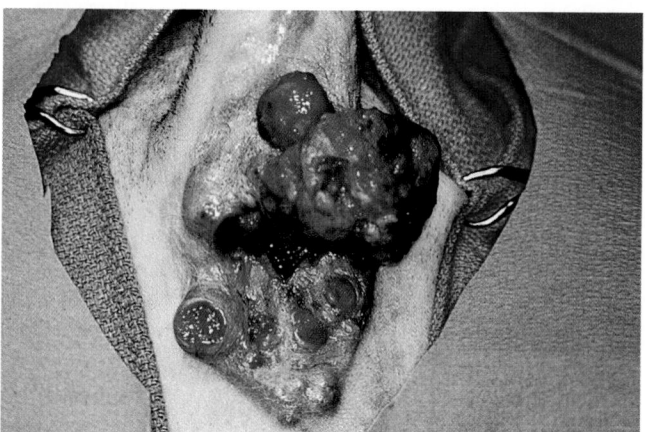

FIG. 19-123
Perianal tumors. **A,** A single tumor with partially intact epithelium. **B,** Multiple ulcerated perianal tumors.

Laboratory Findings

Cytologic studies help, but histologic examination is necessary to differentiate perianal adenomas from carcinomas. However, it can be difficult to distinguish between benign and malignant tumors, even with histopathologic examination. Anal sac tumors often cause hypercalcemia (27% to 51%) and renal dysfunction. The total serum calcium concentration is affected by the serum total protein and serum albumin concentrations. Although there are formulae to correct the total serum calcium concentration for changes in the serum albumin concentration, it is preferable to measure ionized serum calcium. Renal dysfunction is common, and it is important to measure serum creatinine and perform a urinalysis on urine obtained before fluid therapy. Some hypercalcemic patients are also hypophosphatemic.

DIFFERENTIAL DIAGNOSIS

Differential diagnoses of anal and perianal irritation include anal sacculitis, dermatitis, endoparasites, perianal fistula, fungal infection, or tumors. Differential diagnoses for perianal swelling include perineal hernia, perianal neoplasia, perianal gland hyperplasia, anal sacculitis, anal sac neoplasia, atresia ani, rectal pythiosis, and vaginal tumors. Differential diagnoses for dyschezia include rectal foreign body, perineal hernia, perianal fistula, anal stricture, rectal stricture, anal sac abscess, rectal or anal neoplasia, anal trauma, anal dermatitis, anorectal prolapse, IBD, histoplasmosis, and pythiosis.

MEDICAL MANAGEMENT

Some perianal tumors respond to chemotherapy or radiation therapy, but reports documenting the effectiveness of these treatments are lacking. Perianal gland adenomas may shrink after a short course of diethylstilbestrol (0.5 to 1 mg daily for 1 to 2 weeks). Radiation therapy or chemotherapy is recommended for nonresectable malignancies. Vincristine, doxorubicin, and cyclophosphamide (VAC) or melphalan, mitoxantrone, carboplatin, or cisplatin have also been recommended. Radiation therapy or chemotherapy may convert a marginally operable tumor to an operable tumor.

SURGICAL TREATMENT

Surgical excision is the treatment of choice for perianal tumors. Generally, perianal masses that do not involve the anal sacs are perianal adenomas; therefore castration and resection of small masses or biopsy of multiple or large masses is recommended. Patients should be reevaluated 4 to 6 weeks after castration and biopsy. Adenomas will be smaller at this time and generally can be resected with less trauma to the external anal sphincter. Some adenomas regress completely after castration. Prompt, wide resection of malignancies is recommended.

Preoperative Management

Fluid, electrolyte, and acid-base abnormalities should be corrected before surgery. Mildly to moderately hypercalcemic animals should first be rehydrated and given diuretics with physiologic saline solution and furosemide. Hypercalcemia causes renal dysfunction. Although the renal dysfunction is initially mild and reversible, it can become severe, oliguric, and irreversible if therapy is delayed. Therefore it is important to be sure the patient is not oliguric. Prednisolone may also be given (Box 19-71) to help lower the serum calcium. Severely affected animals (total serum calcium concentration greater than 16 mg/dl) may also be treated with alkalinizing agents (e.g., sodium bicarbonate) and bone resorption inhibitors (i.e., pamidronate disodium). Pamidronate disodium (1 to 2 mg/kg IV) has been used in dogs that were hypercalcemic from different causes, and it quickly lowered serum calcium concentrations. However, at the time of this writing, pamidronate is very expensive. Peritoneal dialysis may be performed in oliguric patients, but is of uncertain value. Perioperative antibiotics are indicated in old or debilitated patients. The antibiotics should be given intravenously at induction of anesthesia and discontinued within 12 to 24 hours of surgery. Enemas should not be administered on the day of surgery because they may increase contamination of the surgical site. Remaining feces may be removed manually after induction but before preparing the animal for aseptic surgery.

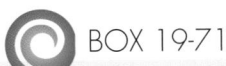

BOX 19-71

Treatment of Hypercalcemia

Furosemide (Lasix)
2–4 mg/kg IV, PO, SC, bid to tid or can give it as CRI (load with 0.66 mg/kg bolus, and then give 0.66 mg/kg/hr for 4 to 5 hours; alternatively, can estimate the IV or PO dose to be given over the course of the next 24 hours and then give that amount as a CRI over the next 24 hours); be sure patient is volume replenished before administering

Prednisone
1.1–2.2 mg/kg IV, PO, SC, bid

Sodium Bicarbonate
0.5–1.0 mEq/kg given in IV fluids (check blood gas first)

Pamidronate Disodium†
1–2 mg/kg IV over 2 hours, once weekly

Clodronate†
20–25 mg/kg IV over 4 hours

Etidronate Disodium (Didronel)†
Dogs: 15 mg/kg/day PO

Salmon Calcitonin†
4 U/kg IV; then 4–6 U/kg SC, qd to tid

Mithramycin*†
25 µg/kg IV over 4 hours, once every 2–4 weeks

IV, Intravenous; *PO*, oral; *SC*, subcutaneous; *bid*, twice a day; *tid*, three times a day; *qd*, once a day.
*This drug has many potential side effects; a medical text should be consulted before administering it.
†Not approved for use in dogs.

Anesthesia

Patients with perianal tumors may be old and debilitated and may have other serious medical problems requiring special care during anesthesia. Anesthetic recommendations for animals undergoing perianal surgery are given on p. 500. Antihistamines (e.g., diphenhydramine [Benadryl], 0.5 mg/kg given intravenously; famotidine [Pepcid], 0.5 mg/kg given intravenously, twice daily) should be administered to patients with mast cell tumors before surgery to reduce the effects of tumor histamine release. Benadryl may be given intravenously immediately before surgery, but should be administered extremely slowly to prevent hypotension. As an alternative, it may be administered intramuscularly 30 minutes before induction of anesthesia.

Surgical Anatomy

The anatomy of the rectum and perianal region is presented on p. 500. Cats do not have perianal or circumanal glands.

Positioning

Position the patient in ventral (preferred) or dorsal recumbency to allow access to the tumors and scrotal region. Fix the tail over the back, elevate the pelvis, and pad the hind legs when using a perineal position.

SURGICAL TECHNIQUE

Removal of one half of the anal sphincter is possible, with some return of fecal continence within a few weeks. Resection of metastatic sites (e.g., lymph nodes) from patients with anal sac adenocarcinomas may help control hypercalcemia.

Begin by performing a prescrotal or perineal castration on intact male dogs with perianal adenomas (see p. 714). Incise the perianal skin surrounding perianal adenomas with minimal margins of normal tissue. Dissect the tumor from the subcutaneous tissue and the external anal sphincter with minimal trauma. Thoroughly lavage the area. Close dead space with monofilament, absorbable suture (e.g., 3-0 or 4-0 polydioxanone, polyglyconate, or poliglecaprone 25) and close the skin with interrupted appositional sutures (e.g., monofilament, 3-0 or 4-0 nylon, polybutester, or polypropylene). Submit the excised masses and testicles for histologic evaluation.

Resect malignant tumors with a minimum of 1 cm of normal tissue on all borders (Fig. 19-124). This includes partial resection of the external anal sphincter, anal canal, and anal sacs in some cases. Appose the epithelial edges to prevent anal stricture.

POSTOPERATIVE CARE AND ASSESSMENT

Give systemic analgesics (see Table 13-4 on p. 133) as necessary for pain. The serum calcium concentration should be monitored at least daily for the first 2 days. Hypercalcemia should be treated until the serum calcium level is normal. Most animals become normocalcemic within 24 hours of primary tumor resection; however, some become hypocalcemic and require calcium supplementation to prevent tetany. If necessary, administer 10% calcium gluconate (0.5 to 1.5 ml/kg of 10% calcium gluconate IV over 10 to 20 minutes and monitor the heart; then add 10 ml of 10% calcium gluconate to 250 ml of lactated Ringer's solution and drip at maintenance rate; or give the IV dose diluted in an equal volume of saline solution, subcutaneously). The perianal area should be kept clean, and an Elizabethan collar or similar restraint device should be used to prevent the patient from licking at surgical sites. Animals that are not vomiting may receive water and food within 8 to 12 hours after surgery. A stool softener may be added to the food for 2 to 3 weeks (see Box 19-60). Chemotherapy may slow recurrence and metastatic tumor growth, but its efficacy is unknown. The rectum and perianal area should be palpated for evidence of stricture or tumor recurrence when the sutures are removed at 7 to 10 days. Patients with malignancies should be reevaluated for recurrence or metastasis at 2, 4, and 6 months and then yearly. Rectal palpation, measurement of serum calcium values, and imaging (e.g., abdominal radiog-

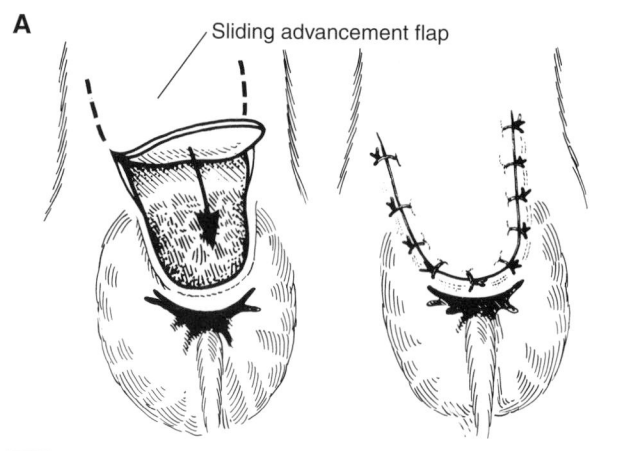

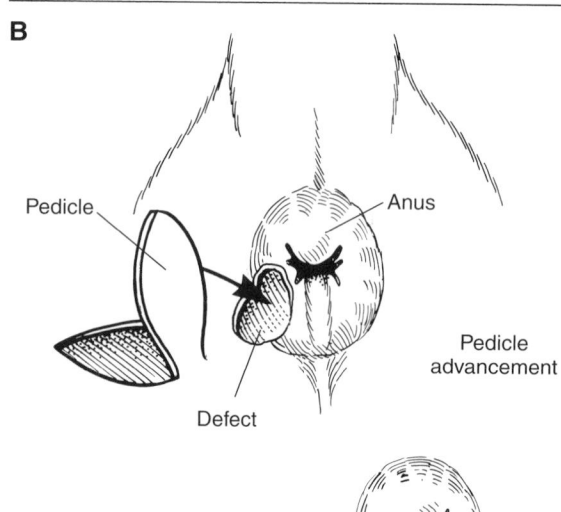

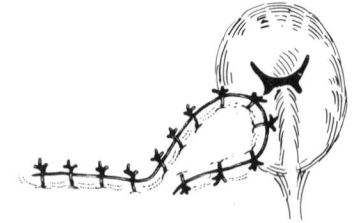

FIG. 19-124
Resect perianal masses with involved muscle. To help prevent anal stenosis, close large defects in the sphincter with **(A)** a sliding advancement flap or **(B)** a local pedicle flap.

raphy, CT, or ultrasonography) are indicated during reevaluation. Recurrence of malignant tumors often is detected by 3 months after surgery. Possible complications of perianal surgery are listed in Box 19-72.

> NOTE: Always administer calcium gluconate to hypocalcemic animals; NEVER administer calcium chloride.

PROGNOSIS

Prolonged estrogen therapy is not recommended because of its myelotoxic effects and it only temporarily reduces tumor size. Radiation therapy is an option, but surgery is less expensive, faster, and safer. The prognosis after surgery is good

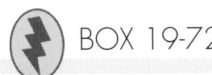

BOX 19-72

Possible Complications of Surgery for Perianal Tumors

- Infection
- Dehiscence
- Tenesmus
- Rectal prolapse
- Dyschezia
- Hematochezia
- Temporary or permanent incontinence
- Anal stricture
- Tumor recurrence
- Metastasis

---

for benign perianal tumors, but guarded to poor for malignant tumors, although some malignant tumors may be slow growing and late to metastasize. Palliation for nonresectable malignant tumors may involve partial resection, cryosurgery, chemotherapy, or radiation therapy. The prognosis for perianal gland adenomas is good to excellent after castration. Adenomas occasionally recur (fewer than 10%) and a new biopsy should be taken. Early, complete excision of perianal gland adenocarcinomas can be curative, but most carcinomas are invasive or metastasize to lymph nodes. Recurrence is common, although it may take many months; therefore the prognosis is poor.

Anal sac adenocarcinomas in dogs warrant a poor prognosis because they frequently have metastasized by the time of diagnosis. Recurrent hypercalcemia suggests recurrence or metastasis. If metastasis is present, survival of less than a year can be expected, whereas dogs that do not have detectable metastasis before surgery have an expected mean survival of approximately 16-18 months. In a recent study (Williams et al, 2003), median survival of affected dogs was 544 days (18 months; range 0 to 1873 days). In this study, dogs treated with chemotherapy alone survived a median 212 days; without surgery, they survived a median 402 days. In addition, dogs with tumors less than 10 cm^2 survived longer than those with tumors greater than 10 cm^2 (median, 292 days). The prognosis for anal SCC is grave with or without surgery.

References

Bennett PF, DeNicola DB, Bonney P et al: Canine anal sac adenocarcinomas: clinical presentation and response to therapy, *J Vet Intern Med* 16:100, 2004.

Petterino C, Martini M, Castagnaro M: Immunohistochemical detection of growth hormone (GH) in canine hepatoid gland tumors, *J Vet Med Sci* 66:569, 2004.

Williams LE, Gliatto JM, Dodge RK et al: Carcinoma of the apocrine glands of the anal sac in dogs: 113 cases (1985-1995), *J Am Vet Med Assoc* 223:825, 2003.

Suggested Reading

Hoelzler MG, Bellah JR, Donofro MC: Omentalization of cystic sublumbar lymph node metastases for long-term palliation of tenesmus and dysuria in a dog with anal sac adenocarcinoma, *J Am Vet Med Assoc* 219:1729, 2001.
Clinical signs were palliated for 18 months after omentalization.

Hostutler RA, Chew DJ, Jaeger JQ et al: Uses and effectiveness of pamidronate disodium for treatment of dogs and cats with hypercalcemia, *J Vet Intern Med* 19:29, 2005.
The drug effectively decreased serum calcium, which was increased as a result of various causes without toxic side effects.

Kadar R, Rush JE, Wetmore L et al: Electrolyte disturbances and cardiac arrhythmias in a dog following pamidronate, calcitonin and furosemide administration for hypercalcemia of malignancy, *J Am Anim Hosp Assoc* 40:75, 2004.
This is a case report of a dog with anal sac carcinoma that had cardiac arrhythmias believed to be a result of hypomagnesemia.

Kim DY, Mauldin GE, Hosgood G et al: Perianal malignant melanoma in a dog, *J Vet Intern Med* 19:610, 2005.
A 10-year-old poodle diagnosed, treated by excision and chemotherapy died 8 weeks after surgery with metastasis.

Milner RJ, Farese J, Henry CG et al: Bisphosphonates and cancer, *J Vet Intern Med* 18:597, 2004.
This is a detailed review of these drugs and their use in hypercalcemic animals.

Turek MM, Adams LJ, Adams WM et al: Postoperative radiotherapy and mitoxantrone for anal sac adenocarcinoma in the dog: 15 cases (1991-2001), *Vet Comparative Oncol* 1:94, 2003.
This retrospective study reports findings similar to others and reports acute and chronic adverse effects.

ANAL SAC INFECTION AND IMPACTION

DEFINITION

Anal sac impaction is an abnormal accumulation of anal sac secretions that occurs secondary to inflammation (*anal sacculitis*), infection (*anal sac abscess*), or obstruction of the duct. Anal sacs sometimes are erroneously referred to as anal glands.

GENERAL CONSIDERATIONS AND CLINICALLY RELEVANT PATHOPHYSIOLOGY

Anal sac diseases include impaction, infection, abscessation, and neoplasia. The anal sacs are a modified adnexal skin structure. They are paired, lying between the fibers of the anal sphincter, and are lined by squamous epithelium with modified apocrine and sebaceous glands. They serve as reservoirs for their malodorous, pastelike secretions. The excretions are expelled through the ducts during normal defecation and extreme excitement. Forceful contractions of the sphincter are necessary for anal sac emptying.

Anal sacculitis affects approximately 10% of dogs and usually is caused by infection or duct obstruction. Ductal obstruction leads to infection and inflammation. Inflammation enhances secretions, which serve as an ideal medium for bacterial growth. Secretions continue to accumulate despite ductal obstruction, and the sacs become impacted and eventually rupture. Distention causes pain. Chronic fistulation may result if infection or duct obstruction persists. Anal sacculitis also occurs without duct obstruction. In these cases hypersecretion occurs, and the sac is easy to express. Secretions are more liquid than normal, with yellowish-white granules. Factors that may cause chronic hypersecretion include infectious, endocrine, allergic, behavioral, and idiopathic mechanisms. Malfunction of the anal sphincter mechanism secondary to chronic diarrhea, anal laxity, constipation, and obesity may contribute to retention of anal sac secretions and the development of anal sacculitis.

DIAGNOSIS
Clinical Presentation

Signalment. Anal sacculitis may occur in an animal of any age, breed, or gender; however, it is most common in small and toy breed dogs and rare in cats. In some animals, anal sacculitis may be associated with seborrheic dermatitis or other dermatoses.

History. Many animals have a history of recent diarrhea (1 to 3 weeks), soft stools, or estrus. They usually evidence anal irritation (e.g., scooting, licking, and biting at the tail head or anus). Other complaints include tail chasing, malodorous perianal discharge, pain or tenderness, and behavioral change. Tenesmus, dyschezia, constipation, and hematochezia occasionally occur. Generalized dermatitis or dermatitis at a secondary site sometimes is recognized.

Physical Examination Findings

The anal sac region may appear swollen and inflamed. Abscesses or impaction may cause the anal sac to rupture and create a draining lesion at the 4 o'clock or 7 o'clock position. Fever may occur with abscesses or severe sacculitis. Palpation of the perianal tissue during rectal examination may identify an enlarged, firm, and sometimes painful anal sac. Digital expression of the anal sac may expel normal secretions (serous, slightly viscid, granular, pale yellow liquid) or abnormal secretions (whitish gray, brown, yellow, or green, bloody, purulent, gritty, turbid, opaque). It may be impossible to express material from diseased sacs. Animals with untreated anal sac abscesses may be debilitated, may have other perianal or rectal abscesses, or may develop anal stricture. Perineal fistulae occasionally occur.

> NOTE: Routine palpation and expression of the anal sacs during physical examination may allow early detection of anal sac disease.

Impaction is diagnosed when the sac is distended and mildly painful and cannot be readily expressed. Anal sacculitis is diagnosed when moderate or severe pain is elicited on palpation, and secretions are liquid, yellowish, blood-tinged, or purulent. The diagnosis of anal sac abscessation is made when there is notable distention of the sac with a purulent exudate, cellulitis of surrounding tissue, erythema of overlying skin, pain, and fever. An anal sac rupture is diagnosed by finding a draining tract associated with the anal sac.

Diagnostic Imaging

Survey radiographs, CT, or MRI are recommended if neoplasia is suspected (see p. 508). A fistulogram may help determine whether a draining tract is associated with the anal sac region or some other perineal location.

Laboratory Findings

Hematologic and serum biochemistry changes are nonspecific. Leukocytosis with a left shift may be noted with anal sac contents abscesses. Cytologic studies from diseased anal sac secretions reveal cellular debris, large numbers of leukocytes, and numerous bacteria. Culture and antibiotic sensitivity of the anal sac is recommended. The normal bacterial flora of anal sacs contents include micrococci, *E. coli*, *Streptococcus faecalis*, and *Staphylococcus* spp. Bacteria typically cultured from diseased anal sacs include *S. faecalis*, *Clostridium perfringens*, *E. coli*, *Proteus* spp., *Staphylococcus* spp., micrococci, and diphtheroids.

DIFFERENTIAL DIAGNOSIS

The primary differential diagnoses for anal sacculitis are flea allergy (from licking and biting), perianal tumor (caused by swelling and ulceration), perianal fistulae, or tail fold pyoderma (resulting in abscessation and draining tracts). Differential diagnoses for anal or perianal irritation include anal sacculitis, dermatitis, endoparasites, perianal fistulae, vaginitis, or tumors. Differential diagnoses for perianal swelling include perianal hernia, perianal neoplasia, perianal gland hyperplasia, anal sacculitis, anal sac neoplasia, atresia ani, rectal pythiosis, and vaginal tumors. Differential diagnoses for dyschezia include rectal foreign body, perineal hernia, perianal fistulae, anal stricture, rectal stricture, anal sac abscess, rectal neoplasia, anal neoplasia, anal trauma, anal dermatitis, rectal pythiosis, and anorectal prolapse.

MEDICAL MANAGEMENT

Treatment depends on the stage of infection. Manual expression, lavage, topical antibiotics, and dietary change effectively manage most anal sac problems. Treatment of concomitant dermatoses facilitates treatment of anal sacculitis. Mild sacculitis or impaction is treated by expressing, lavaging (with saline), and infusing the glands with an antibiotic-corticosteroid preparation. Dry secretions may be softened by lavaging with saline or infusing a ceruminolytic agent. If the anal sacs are infected, 0.5% chlorhexidine or 10% povidone-iodine may be added to saline flushes. Adding fiber (e.g., w/d Hill's Pet Products, pumpkin, bran, or psyllium) to the diet makes the feces bulky, which may stretch the anus during defecation, causing the anal sacs to be compressed and emptied. In more severe cases, weekly evaluation, expression, and lavage with a dilute antiseptic solution or saline may be required. Chronic cases may require antibiotics as determined by sensitivity results. Anal sac abscesses should be lanced, drained, and flushed. Hot compresses, applied two or three times daily for 15 to 20 minutes each, are beneficial for abscesses. Appropriate oral antibiotics should be administered to patients with anal sac abscesses. Chemical cauterization is not recommended because severe perineal sloughing may result (Fig. 19-125).

SURGICAL TREATMENT

Failure of medical therapy and suspicion of neoplasia are indications for anal sacculectomy. If a draining tract persists after anal sac rupture, surgery should be delayed until inflam-

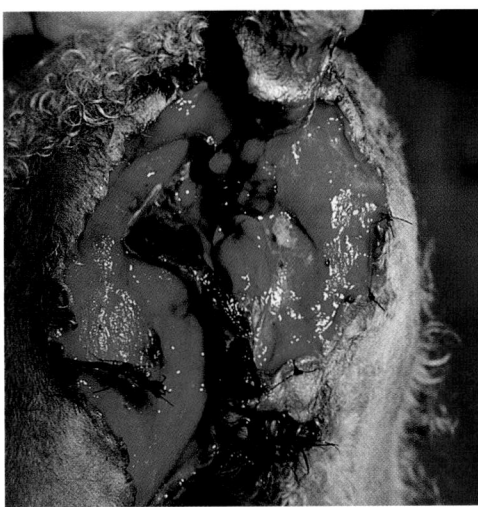

FIG. 19-125
Note the extensive perineal sloughing that occurred after chemical cauterization to treat anal sacculitis. This dog was euthanized because of deep vascular erosion and hemorrhage. Chemical cauterization is not recommended for treatment of anal sacculitis.

mation is controlled. Both anal sacs should be removed, even if only one is obviously involved. Either an open or closed technique may be used; however, the open technique carries a greater risk of fecal incontinence and local infection.

> NOTE: Warn owners of the risk of incontinence after anal sacculectomy.

Preoperative Management

Anal sacculitis, abscessation, or fistulation should be treated for several days as described above to reduce inflammation before surgery. Inflammation and fibrosis present at the time of surgery increase the risk of damage to the anal sphincter. Temporary or permanent fecal incontinence may result secondary to sphincter damage.

Anesthesia

Anesthetic recommendations for animals undergoing perianal surgery are given on p. 500.

Surgical Anatomy

One anal sac lies on each side of the anus between the internal and external anal sphincters. The anal sac is a cutaneous diverticulum lined by microscopic glands. Secretions of these sebaceous and apocrine glands accumulate in the anal sac and are normally expelled through the ducts during defecation or contraction of the anal sphincter. The ducts of the anal sacs open in the cutaneous zone at approximately the 4 o'clock to 5 o'clock and 7 o'clock to 8 o'clock positions. The duct opening in cats is more lateral to the anocutaneous line than in dogs. They are visible lateral to the anus in the normal contracted state.

Positioning

Position the patient in ventral recumbency with the tail fixed dorsally over the back. Elevate the pelvis and pad the hind legs when using a perineal position.

SURGICAL TECHNIQUE

Palpate the anal sacs to determine their location and extent by placing the index or middle finger in the rectum and the thumb over the sac. Manually evacuate feces from the rectum if present. Prepare the perineal area for surgery.

Closed technique. *Insert a small probe, hemostat, or balloon-tip catheter into the orifice of the anal sac duct (Fig. 19-126, A). Advance the instrument or inflate the balloon with saline until the lateral extent of the sac is identified.*

As an alternative, wax or synthetic resin may be infused to distend the sac before resection.

Make a curvilinear incision over the anal sac. Dissecting directly against the anal sac, separate the internal and external anal sphincter muscle fibers from the sac's exterior with small Metzenbaum or iris scissors. Avoid excising or traumatizing the muscles or the caudal rectal artery medial to the duct. Continue dissecting to free the sac and duct to its mucocutaneous junction at the anal canal (Fig. 19-126, B). Perforation of the sac may occur during dissection, and tissue may be contaminated with secretions. Place a ligature around the duct at the mucocutaneous junction using 4-0 monofilament absorbable suture (Fig. 19-126, C). Excise the anal sac and duct, then inspect for completeness of removal. Control hemorrhage with ligatures, electrocoagulation, or pressure. Lavage the tissue thoroughly. Appose subcutaneous tissue with 4-0 interrupted, monofilament, absorbable sutures (polydioxanone, polyglyconate, or poliglecaprone 25) and appose the skin with 3-0 or 4-0 monofilament, nonabsorbable (nylon, polypropylene, or polybutester) sutures.

Open technique. *Place a scissors blade or groove director into the duct of the anal sac (Fig. 19-127, A). Apply medial traction on the duct while incising through the skin, subcutaneous tissue, external anal sphincter, duct, and sac. Continue the incision to the lateral extent of the anal sac. Elevate the cut edge of the sac and use small Metzenbaum or iris scissors to dissect the sac free of its attachments to muscle and surrounding tissue (Fig. 19-127, B). Complete the procedure the same as for a closed sacculectomy (Fig. 19-127, C).*

> NOTE: The lining of the anal sac is grayish and glistening; it is easily distinguished from surrounding tissue.

POSTOPERATIVE CARE AND ASSESSMENT

Systemic analgesics (see Table 13-4 on p. 133) should be given as necessary. The perianal area should be kept clean, and an Elizabethan collar or similar restraint device should

Closed technique

A

B

C

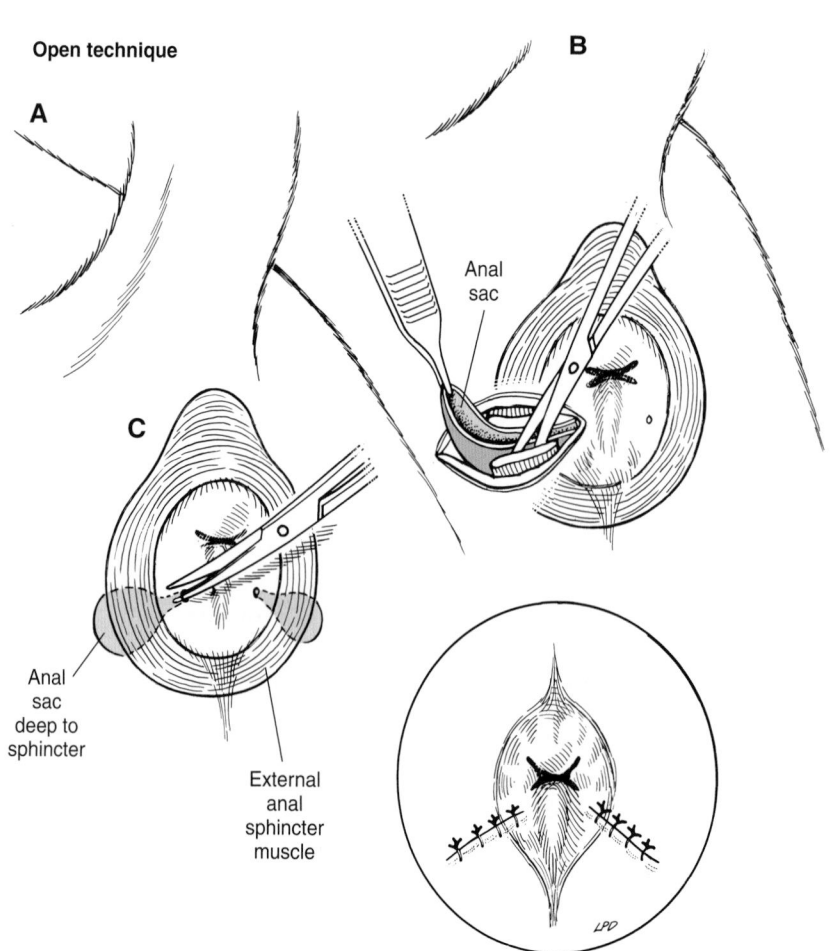

FIG. 19-126
Closed technique for anal sacculectomy.
A, Locate the anal sacs at the 4 o'clock to 5 o'clock and 7 o'clock to 8 o'clock positions between the internal and external anal sphincter muscles. Insert a small probe, hemostat, or balloon-tip catheter into the anal sac. Dashed line indicates incision location. **B,** Make an incision at the lateral aspect of the anal sac and carefully dissect the sac from the sphincter muscle fibers. **C,** Ligate the duct near the orifice.

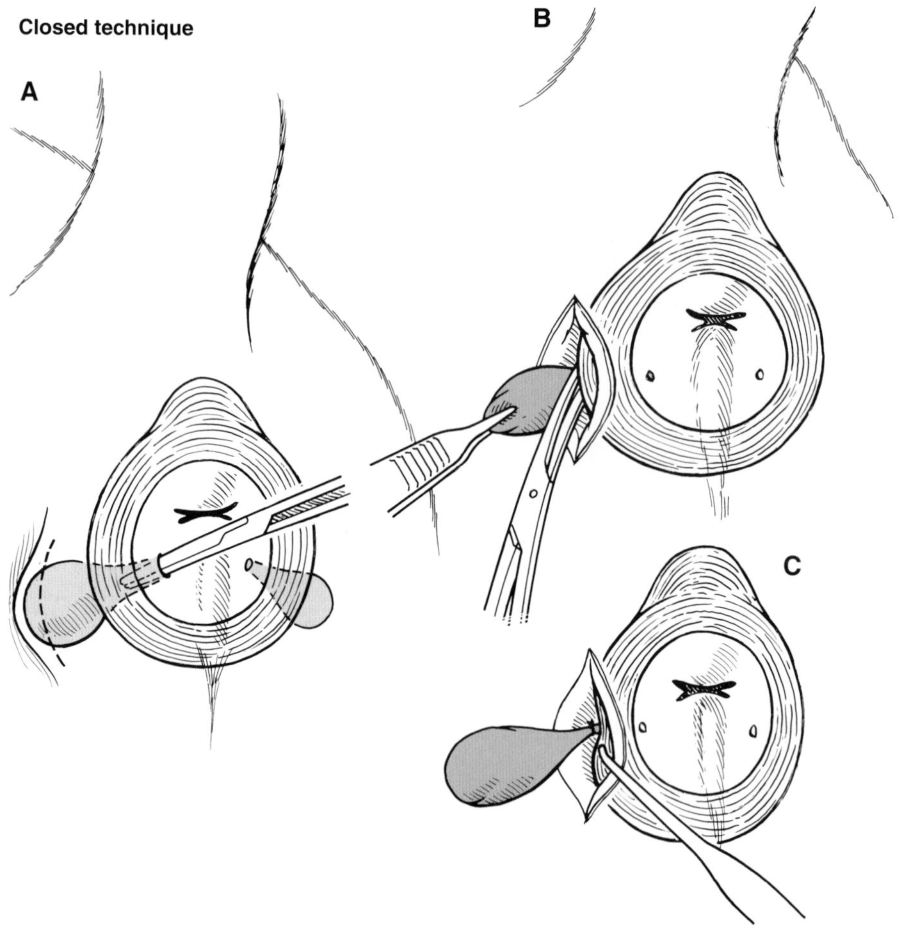

Open technique

A

B

Anal
sac

C

Anal
sac
deep to
sphincter

External
anal
sphincter
muscle

FIG. 19-127
Open technique for anal sacculectomy.
A, Insert the blade of the scissors into the sac and incise through the skin, subcutaneous tissue, external anal sphincter, and anal sac. **B,** Elevate the cut edge of the sac, and dissect it from the anal sphincter. **C,** Appose the sphincter, subcutaneous tissue, and skin.

be used to prevent the animal from licking the sites. Food and water may be offered 8 to 12 hours postoperatively if no vomiting has been noted. A stool softener may be added to the food for 2 to 3 weeks (see Box 19-60). The surgical site should be monitored for signs of infection or drainage, and the rectum and perianal area should be palpated for evidence of stricture when sutures are removed at 7 to 10 days. Fecal continence may be impaired during the healing process, but usually returns to normal within several weeks.

COMPLICATIONS

Short-term complications (within 14 days) may include excessive drainage, scooting, inflammation, and seroma formation. Long-term complications include continued licking of the surgical site, fecal incontinence, fistulation, and stricture formation. Fecal incontinence after anal sacculectomy may be temporary or permanent. A draining tract after surgery suggests that a piece of anal sac was left at the surgical site. This occurs more commonly with inexperienced surgeons or with inflamed and fibrotic tissue. Surgical excision is necessary, or drainage will continue. Other complications include infection, dehiscence, tenesmus, rectal prolapse, dyschezia, and hematochezia.

PROGNOSIS

The prognosis for nonneoplastic anal sac disease is good if it is not associated with perianal fistulae. Most cases of anal sacculitis can be treated medically if they are recognized early, treated appropriately, and not associated with neoplasia or perianal fistulae.

Suggested Reading

Hill LN, Smeak DD: Open versus closed bilateral anal sacculectomy for treatment of non-neoplastic anal sac disease in dogs: 95 cases (1969-1994), *J Am Vet Med Assoc* 221(5):662, 2002.
Closed procedures were associated with fewer complications than standard open procedures. Overall, short-term complications occurred in approximately 3% and long-term complications in 15%. Of those with long-term complications, 78% (11 of 14) occurred following open procedures.

PERINEAL HERNIA

DEFINITIONS

Perineal hernias occur when the perineal muscles separate, allowing rectal, pelvic, and/or abdominal contents to displace perineal skin. Depending on their location, they may be referred to as a *caudal hernia, sciatic hernia, dorsal hernia,* or *ventral hernia.*

GENERAL CONSIDERATIONS AND CLINICALLY RELEVANT PATHOPHYSIOLOGY

Perineal hernia occurs when pelvic diaphragm muscles fail to support the rectal wall, allowing persistent rectal distention and impaired defecation. The cause of pelvic diaphragm weakening is poorly understood, but is believed to

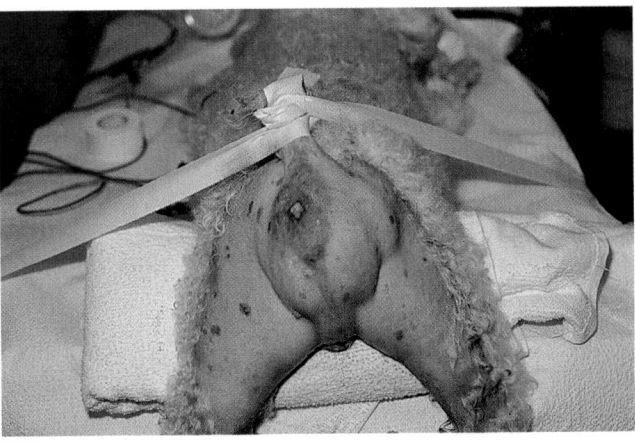

FIG. 19-128
Bilateral perineal hernias in a dog.

  BOX 19-73

Conditions That Cause Straining and May Predispose to Perineal Herniation

- Prostatitis
- Cystitis
- Urinary tract obstruction
- Colorectal obstruction
- Rectal deviation or dilation
- Perianal inflammation
- Anal sacculitis
- Diarrhea
- Constipation

be associated with male hormones, straining, and congenital or acquired muscle weakness or atrophy. The pelvic diaphragm is stronger in female dogs than in males. Atrophy of the pelvic diaphragm muscles, possibly of neurologic origin, has been identified in some animals with hernias. Any condition that causes straining may stress the pelvic diaphragm (Box 19-73).

Herniation may be unilateral or bilateral (Fig. 19-128). Most herniations occur between the levator ani, external anal sphincter, and internal obturator muscles (caudal hernia); however, some occur between the sacrotuberous ligament and coccygeus muscle (sciatic hernia), levator ani and coccygeus muscles (dorsal hernia), or ischiourethralis, bulbocavernosus, and ischiocavernosus muscles (ventral hernia). Hernial contents are surrounded by a thin layer of perineal fascia (hernial sac), subcutaneous tissue, and skin. The hernial sac may contain pelvic or retroperitoneal fat, serous fluid, a deviated or dilated rectum, a rectal diverticulum, prostate, urinary bladder, or small intestine (Fig. 19-129). Cats usually have only rectum within the hernial sac. Organs displaced into the hernia may become obstructed and strangulated. Visceral obstruction or strangulation is associated with rapid deterioration unless the obstruction or entrapment is corrected.

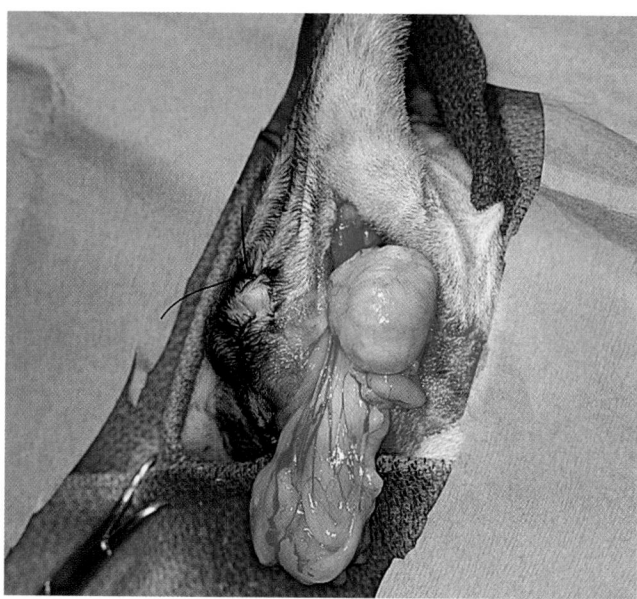

FIG. 19-129
Perineal hernia in a dog. Note the urinary bladder and pelvic fat occupying this hernial sac.

DIAGNOSIS
Clinical Presentation

Signalment. Perineal hernias are common in dogs and rare in cats. They occur almost exclusively in intact male dogs (93%). Perineal hernias in female dogs are often related to trauma. Feline perineal hernias usually occur in neutered males; however, female cats are more prone to perineal hernias than female dogs. Dogs with short tails may be predisposed to herniation. Breeds most commonly affected are Boston terriers, boxers, Welsh corgis, Pekingese, collies, poodles, kelpies, dachshunds, Old English sheepdogs, and mongrels. Most perineal hernias occur in dogs over 5 years of age. The median age is approximately 10 years in both dogs and cats. The risk of occurrence increases with age until 14 years in intact male dogs.

History. Affected animals usually are presented for treatment because of difficulty defecating. Some owners notice a swelling lateral to the anus. Occasionally, animals are presented as emergencies because of postrenal uremia associated with bladder entrapment or shock associated with intestinal strangulation. Clinical signs may include perineal swelling, constipation, obstipation, dyschezia, tenesmus, rectal prolapse, stranguria, anuria, vomiting, flatulence, and/or fecal incontinence.

Physical Examination Findings

The diagnosis is based on finding a weakened pelvic diaphragm during digital rectal examination, with or without a perineal swelling lateral to the anus (see Fig. 19-128). Not all dogs with perineal hernias have perineal swelling. When present, the swelling may appear to surround the anus and cause it to bulge. A rectal deviation often contains impacted feces. Some reports indicate a right-sided predominance. Cats typically have bilateral hernias, which seldom cause obvious perineal swelling. The prostate sometimes is found in the hernia. Severe straining can cause rectal prolapse. Some animals are systemically ill and shocky because of visceral strangulation. If ballottement suggests that liquid is present and the animal is dysuric, ultrasound or peritoneocentesis should be performed to determine if fluid (i.e., urine) is present. A hernia filled with a full bladder may have a tight, resilient feel when palpated, instead of a fluid wave. Concurrent inguinal hernias have been identified in some dogs with perineal hernia.

> NOTE: A fluctuant swelling in the perineal region may indicate that the bladder is entrapped in the hernia. Prompt therapy may be necessary to relieve urinary obstruction in these animals.

Diagnostic Imaging

Survey radiographs are seldom needed for diagnosis; however, they are useful in ascertaining whether the urinary bladder, prostate, or small intestines are in the hernia (Figs. 19-130 and 19-131). Radiographically documenting retroflexion of the urinary bladder often requires a urethrogram, cystogram, or both or the use of ultrasonography. Administration of oral or rectal barium demonstrates the position of the colon and rectum. Most dogs have rectal deviation and some also have rectal dilatation. Diverticula are typically not documented radiographically or at surgery.

Laboratory Findings

Patients with bladder retroflexion often have azotemia, hyperkalemia, hyperphosphatemia, and neutrophilic leukocytosis.

DIFFERENTIAL DIAGNOSIS

Differential diagnoses for perianal swelling include perineal hernia, perianal neoplasia, perianal gland hyperplasia, anal sacculitis, anal sac neoplasia, atresia ani, and vaginal tumors. Differential diagnoses for dyschezia include rectal foreign body, perineal hernia, perianal fistula, anal stricture, rectal stricture, anal sac abscess, rectal neoplasia, anal neoplasia, anal trauma, anal dermatitis, rectal pythiosis, and anorectal prolapse.

MEDICAL MANAGEMENT

The goal of treatment is to relieve and prevent constipation, dysuria, and organ strangulation. Causative factors (i.e., urinary tract obstruction or infection, megacolon, and prostatitis) should be corrected. Normal defecation sometimes can be maintained using laxatives, stool softeners, dietary changes, periodic enemas, and/or manual rectal evacuation. The urinary bladder can be decompressed by centesis or catheterization. However, long-term use of these treatments is contraindicated because life-threatening visceral entrapment and strangulation may occur.

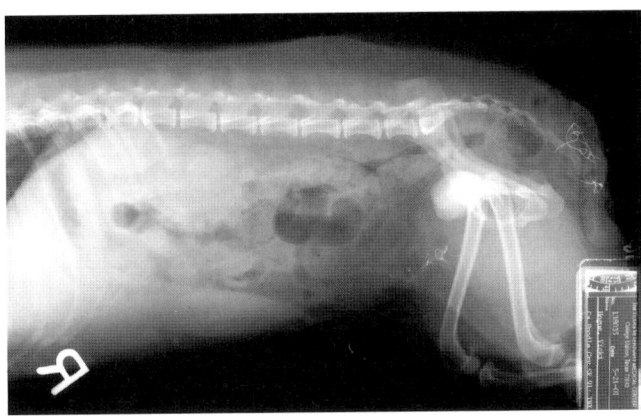

FIG. 19-130
Lateral radiograph of a dog with a perineal hernia. Note the nonstrangulated intestines in the hernial sac.

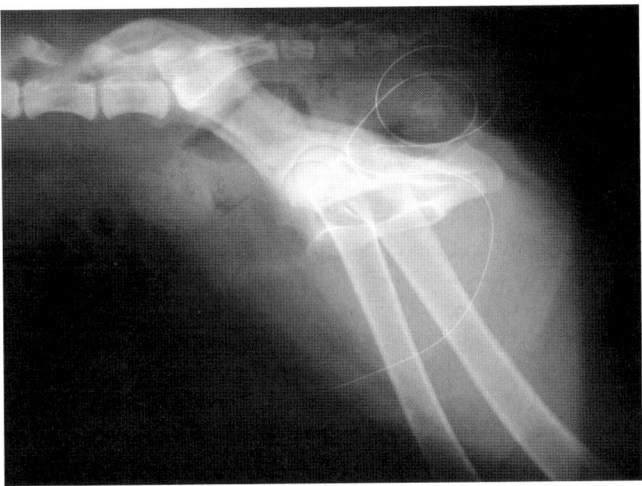

FIG. 19-131
Lateral radiograph of a dog with its bladder retroflexed into the hernia. Note the urinary catheter in the bladder.

SURGICAL TREATMENT

Herniorrhaphy should always be recommended. Retroflexion of the urinary bladder and visceral entrapment require emergency surgery. Castration, although controversial, is recommended during herniorrhaphy because it has been reported to reduce recurrence. Noncastrated dogs have a recurrence rate 2.7 times greater than castrated dogs.

The two most commonly used techniques are (1) the traditional, or anatomic reapposition; and (2) the internal obturator roll-up, or transposition technique. It is more difficult to close the ventral aspect of the hernia using the traditional technique. Temporary deformity of the anus occurs and is especially pronounced after bilateral herniorrhaphy. Postoperative tenesmus and rectal prolapse may be more common in these cases. The internal obturator transposition technique is more difficult, especially if internal obturator

muscle atrophy is severe. However, it causes less tension on sutures and less deformity of the anus, and creates a ventral patch or sling for the defect. Other herniorrhaphy techniques have included using the superficial gluteal, semitendinosus, or semimembranosus muscles, fascia lata, placement of synthetic mesh, small intestinal submucosa, or dermal collagen, or a combination of techniques. Bilateral herniorrhaphy is possible, but postoperative discomfort and tenesmus may be greater than after unilateral procedures. If accessible, a biopsy should be taken from an enlarged prostate. Either a perineal or prescrotal castration may be performed (see p. 714). Rectal imbrication or sacculectomy is rarely indicated and significantly increases the risk of postoperative infection. Colopexy may help prevent recurrent rectal prolapse after herniorrhaphy. Fixation of the ductus deferens may help prevent recurrence when the bladder or prostate has been displaced into perineal hernias. Cystopexy has also been performed, but is not routinely recommended as retention cystitis may occur.

> **NOTE:** Some surgeons prefer waiting 4 to 6 weeks before performing the second herniorrhaphy in dogs with bilateral disease.

Preoperative Management

Stool softeners (see Box 19-60) should be given 2 to 3 days before surgery. The large intestine should be evacuated with laxatives, cathartics, enemas, and manual extraction (see p. 481). Prophylactic antibiotics effective against gram-negative and anaerobic organisms (see Box 19-56) should be given intravenously after induction of anesthesia. If the urinary bladder is retroflexed into the hernia, a urinary catheter should be placed or cystocentesis performed via the perineum to relieve distress and prevent further physiologic deterioration.

Anesthesia

Anesthetic recommendations for animals undergoing perineal surgery are given on p. 500. Epidural analgesia may reduce the occurrence of postoperative rectal prolapse. Many affected animals are geriatric and have concurrent abnormalities that may influence drug selection.

Surgical Anatomy

The pelvic diaphragm is composed of the paired medial coccygeal and levator ani muscles. The paired levator ani muscle originates from the floor of the pelvis and medial shaft of the ilium, fans out around the sides of the rectum, and then narrows and inserts ventrally on the seventh caudal vertebra. The paired coccygeus muscle is a thick muscle lying lateral to the thin levator ani. The coccygeus originates from the ischiatic spine on the pelvic floor and inserts ventrally on caudal vertebrae two through five.

The paired rectococcygeus muscle arises from the external longitudinal musculature of the rectum caudal to the levator and coccygeus muscles and inserts on the ventral surface of the fifth to sixth caudal vertebrae. The rectococcygeus muscle shortens the rectum when the tail is raised during defecation. The peritoneal reflection is cranial to the rectococcygeus muscles. The sacrotuberous ligament in the dog is a fibrous band running from the transverse process of the last sacral and first caudal vertebrae to the lateral angle of the ischiatic tuberosity rostral to the pelvic diaphragm. Cats do not have a sacrotuberous ligament. The sciatic nerve lies just cranial and lateral to the sacrotuberous ligament. The internal obturator muscle is a fan-shaped muscle covering the dorsal surface of the ischium. It originates from the dorsal surface of the ischium and pelvic symphysis. Its tendon of insertion passes over the lesser ischiatic notch, ventral to the sacrotuberous ligament. The internal pudendal artery and vein and the pudendal nerve run caudomedially through the pelvic canal on the dorsal surface of the internal obturator muscle, lateral to the coccygeus and levator ani muscles. The pudendal nerve is dorsal to the vessels and divides into the caudal rectal and perineal nerves. The obturator nerve passes through the ventral aspect of the levator ani in a caudolateral direction.

> NOTE: Perineal vessels and nerves may be displaced from their normal anatomic location by the hernial contents. Careful observation and dissection is required to preserve these structures.

Positioning

Clip and aseptically prepare the perineum for surgery. The prepared area should extend 10 to 15 cm cranial to the tail base, laterally beyond the ischial tuberosity, and ventrally to include the scrotum. The animal should be positioned in ventral recumbency with the tail fixed over the back, the pelvis elevated, and the hind legs padded. As an alternative, a well-padded perineal stand may be used.

SURGICAL TECHNIQUE
Approach

Make a curvilinear incision beginning cranial to the coccygeus muscles, curving over the hernial bulge 1 to 2 cm lateral to the anus, and extending 2 to 3 cm ventral to the pelvic floor (Fig. 19-132). Incise the subcutaneous tissue and hernial sac. Identify and reduce the hernial contents by dissecting subcutaneous and fibrous attachments. Biopsy any abnormal structures within the hernia (e.g., prostate and masses). Maintain hernial reduction by packing the defect with a moistened, tagged sponge. Identify the muscles involved in the hernia, the internal pudendal artery and vein, the pudendal nerve, the caudal rectal vessels and nerve, and the sacrotuberous ligament. Repair the hernia with one of the described techniques. After herniorrhaphy, perform a caudal castration through a median perineal incision (see p. 714).

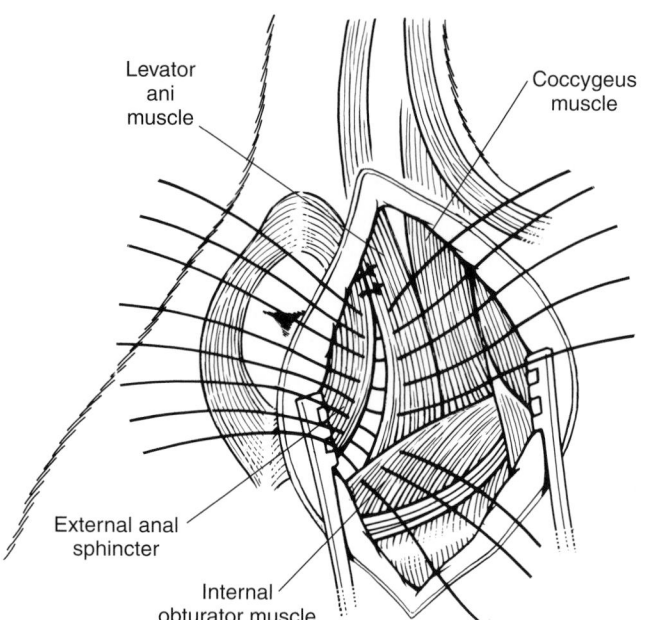

Levator ani muscle

Coccygeus muscle

External anal sphincter

Internal obturator muscle

FIG. 19-132
For perineal hernia repair using the traditional technique, make a curvilinear incision 1 to 2 cm lateral to the anus from dorsal to the tail head to ventral to the anus. Appose the external anal sphincter to the combined levator ani and coccygeus muscles (with or without the sacrotuberous ligament) laterally and the external anal sphincter and internal obturator muscles ventrally.

> NOTE: Do not mistake the prostate for a mass and attempt to excise it.

Traditional (Anatomic) Herniorrhaphy

Preplace simple interrupted 0 or 2-0 monofilament sutures using a large, curved needle (see Fig. 19-132). Begin suture placement between the external anal sphincter and the levator ani, coccygeus, or both muscles. Space sutures less than 1 cm apart. As placement progresses ventrally and laterally, incorporate the sacrotuberous ligament for a secure repair if necessary.

To avoid entrapping the sciatic nerve, place sutures *through* rather than around the sacrotuberous ligament.

Direct ventral sutures between the external anal sphincter and the internal obturator muscle. Be cognizant of the pudendal vessels and nerves at all times to prevent traumatizing these structures. Tie sutures beginning dorsally and progressing ventrally. Remove the sponge used to maintain reduction before tying the last few sutures. Evaluate the repair; place additional sutures if weaknesses or defects persist. Lavage the area. Close the subcutaneous tissue in an interrupted or continuous appositional pattern with 3-0 or 4-0 monofilament absorbable suture (polydioxanone, poly-

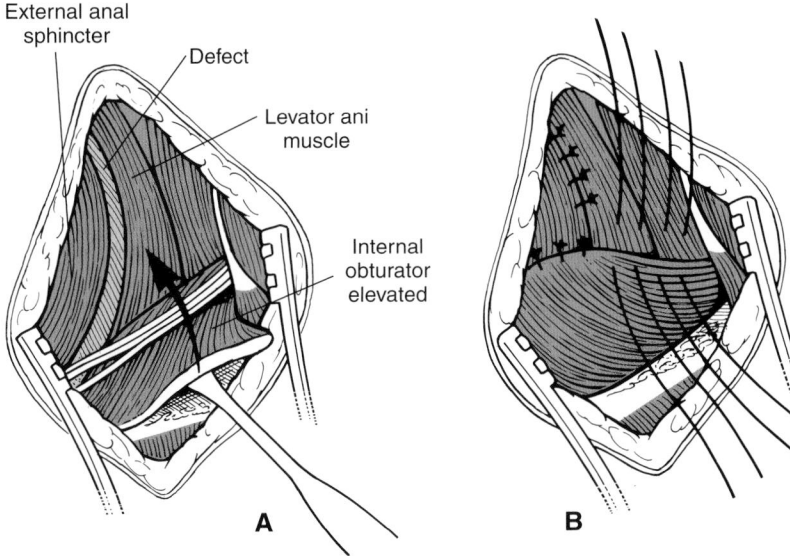

External anal sphincter

Defect

Levator ani muscle

Internal obturator elevated

A

B

FIG. 19-133
Internal obturator transposition technique. **A,** Elevate the internal obturator muscle from the ischium. **B,** Appose the external anal sphincter muscle and combined levator ani and coccygeus muscles dorsally. Transpose the internal obturator muscle dorsomedially to fill the ventral defect, and suture it to the external anal sphincter muscle medially and the coccygeus muscle and sacrotuberous ligament laterally.

glyconate, poliglecaprone 25, or glycomer 631) and close the skin in an appositional interrupted pattern with nonabsorbable suture (e.g., 3-0 or 4-0 nylon).

Internal Obturator Transposition Herniorrhaphy

Incise the fascia and periosteum along the caudal border of the ischium and origin of the internal obturator muscle. Using a periosteal elevator, elevate the periosteum and internal obturator muscle from the ischium (Fig. 19-133, A). Transpose dorsomedially or roll up the muscle into the defect to allow apposition between the coccygeus, levator ani, and external anal sphincter. Transect the internal obturator tendon of insertion, if necessary, to get adequate coverage of the defect. The internal obturator tendon often is difficult to visualize, making transection difficult. Take care to prevent transection of the caudal gluteal vessels and perineal nerve. Preplace simple interrupted sutures the same as with the traditional technique. Begin by apposing the combined levator ani and coccygeus muscles with the external anal sphincter muscle dorsally. Then place sutures between the internal obturator and external anal sphincter medially and the levator ani and coccygeus muscles laterally (Fig. 19-133, B).

Ductus Deferopexy

After castration and herniorrhaphy in dogs with bladder or prostate retroflexion, the ductus deferens can be secured to the abdominal wall to prevent recurrent caudal organ displacement.

Approach the abdomen through a caudal ventral midline incision. Retroflex the urinary bladder caudally through the incision to expose the ductus deferens. Separate the ligated ductus deferens from the testicular artery and vein, and gently pull it through the inguinal ring. Dissect each ductus def-

erens from its peritoneal attachments to the level of the prostate. Pull the urinary bladder and prostate forward by applying moderate traction on the ductus deferens. At an adjacent site on the ventrolateral abdominal wall, make two incisions (1.5 to 2 cm apart) through the peritoneum and transversus abdominis muscle. Tunnel between these incisions and draw the ductus deferens through the tunnel. Suture the ductus deferens to itself and the abdominal wall with three or four 3-0 monofilament sutures. Repeat the procedure on the opposite side to fix the bladder and prostate in a more cranial position.

POSTOPERATIVE CARE AND ASSESSMENT

Analgesics (see Table 13-4 on p. 133) should be given as necessary to minimize straining and rectal prolapse. If rectal prolapse occurs, a purse-string suture should be placed. Recurrent rectal prolapse may be prevented by performing a colopexy. Fluid therapy should be continued in uremic patients. Cold compresses applied immediately after surgery and two to three times daily for 15 to 20 minutes during the first 48 to 72 hours minimize hemorrhage and inflammation. After 48 to 72 hours, warm compresses applied to the surgical site two or three times daily for 15 to 20 minutes reduce swelling and perianal irritation. Antibiotics may be discontinued within 12 hours of surgery unless ischemic, necrotic, or contaminated tissue was present before surgery or the patient is debilitated. After herniorrhaphy, patients should be monitored for signs of wound infection (i.e., redness, pain, swelling, or discharge). Stool softeners (see Box 19-60) should be continued for 1 to 2 months. The animal should be fed a canned diet high in fiber.

COMPLICATIONS

Most postoperative complications can be prevented by meticulous surgical technique. Hernia recurrence or contralateral herniation is believed to be reduced by castration during

BOX 19-74

Possible Complications of Perineal Herniorrhaphy

- Hemorrhage
- Depression
- Anorexia
- Tenesmus
- Dyschezia
- Flatulence
- Hematochezia
- Rectal prolapse
- Anal sacculitis
- Fecal incontinence
- Urethral damage
- Dysuria
- Stranguria
- Bladder atony
- Bladder necrosis
- Urinary incontinence
- Intestinal necrosis
- Rectocutaneous or perineal fistula

herniorrhaphy. Recurrence is related to the expertise of the surgeon; inexperienced surgeons have higher recurrence rates. Infection and dehiscence usually can be prevented by appropriate antibiotic prophylaxis and surgical technique. Notable pain, non–weight-bearing lameness, and knuckling after surgery suggest sciatic nerve entrapment. If this is suspected, the offending suture should be removed immediately via a caudolateral approach to the hip. Other possible complications are listed in Box 19-74.

PROGNOSIS

Defecation in affected patients is facilitated by medical and dietary management. The danger of prolonged medical therapy is that the bladder, intestine, or prostate will become trapped in the hernia, causing life-threatening consequences. The prognosis is fair to good when surgery is performed by an experienced surgeon. Patients with bladder retroflexion have the poorest prognosis. Preexisting neurologic abnormalities (i.e., anal sphincter incompetence or compromised urinary bladder innervation) are not corrected by the herniorrhaphy.

Suggested Reading

Bongartz A, Carofiglio F, Balligand M et al: Use of autogenous fascia lata graft for perineal herniorrhaphy in dogs, *Vet Surg* 34:405, 2005.

This prospective clinical study involving 12 dogs demonstrated the effective use of the ipsilateral fascia lata as an augmentation procedure when the internal obturator muscle is thin or friable or when the hernia recurs.

Brissot HN, Dupre GP, Bouvy BM: Use of laparotomy in a staged approach for resolution of bilateral or complicated perineal hernia in 41 dogs, *Vet Surg* 33:412, 2004.

This retrospective study describes laparotomy to perform colopexy (41 dogs), ductus deferopexy (32), cystopexy (6), and/or prostatic omentalization (9) a median of 6 days before herniorrhaphy. Herniorrhaphy was successful in 90%; however, wound complications (17%), urine dribbling (37%), and tenesmus occurred.

Head LL, Francis DA: Mineralized paraprostatic cyst as a potential contributing factor in the development of perineal hernias in a dog, *J Am Vet Med Assoc* 221:533, 2002.

This case report describes a dog whose paraprostatic cyst caused tenesmus by compressing the colon and urinary bladder.

Merchav R, Feuermann Y, Shamay A et al: The expression of relaxin receptor LRG7, canine relaxin, and relaxin-like factor in the pelvic diaphragm musculature of dogs with and without perineal hernia, European College of Veterinary Surgeons Proceedings 2005, pp. 261-264.

Fifteen dogs with perineal hernia were evaluated and found to have up-regulation of relaxin receptors in pelvic diaphragm muscles.

Stoll MR, Cook JL, Pope ER et al: The use of porcine small intestinal submucosa as a biomaterial for perineal herniorrhaphy in the dog, *Vet Surg* 31:379, 2002.

This experimental study in 12 dogs found that small intestinal submucosa compared favorably to internal obturator muscle transposition technique in failure characteristics and histologic evaluation.

PERIANAL FISTULAE

DEFINITION

Perianal fistulae are chronically relapsing suppurative, progressive, deep ulcerating tracts in the perianal tissue. They have also been referred to as *perianal sinuses, perineal fistulae, perianal fissures, furunculoses, pararectal fistulae, anusitis, fistulae-in-ano,* and *anorectal abscesses.*

GENERAL CONSIDERATIONS AND CLINICALLY RELEVANT PATHOPHYSIOLOGY

The cause of perianal fistulae is unknown. The current theory is a multifactorial immune-mediated disease process. Other theories include poor conformation, crypt fecalith impaction and abscessation, and spread of infection from anal sacs or trauma. The combination of infection and abscessation of glands and hair follicles around the anus, moist contaminated anal environment, and a broad-based low-set tail conformation is believed to contribute to the formation of perianal fistulae. Colitis and enteral triggers such as dietary antigens, bacterial antigens, or superantigens may initiate the condition (Patterson and Campbell, 2005). German shepherd dogs have a greater density of apocrine glands in the cutaneous zone of the anal canal, which may predispose them to perianal fistulae. Bacterial infection may occur after development of cutaneous lesions. Endocrine studies have found no abnormalities in affected dogs.

Fistulae first appear as small, draining holes in perianal skin that is inflamed and hyperpigmented. As the disease progresses, these punctate holes enlarge and coalesce, forming large areas of ulceration and granulation. Tracts may extend into the deep perirectal tissue and anal sacs. These tracts are typically lined by squamous epithelium and are infiltrated with a mixture of lymphocytes, plasma cells, macrophages, neutrophils, and eosinophils. Hidradenitis, chronic necrotizing pyogranulomatous inflammation of the skin and hair follicles, cellulitis, dilated and inflamed lymphatics, necrosis, and fibrosis occur. Partial rectal stricture caused by inflammatory infiltrates may occur.

DIAGNOSIS

The diagnosis is based on history, physical examination findings, and ruling out other differentials primarily by histopathologic findings.

Clinical Presentation

Signalment. Perianal fistulae occur most commonly in German shepherd dogs, but Irish setters also are predisposed. Various other breeds have been diagnosed with this condition, including collies, Border collies, Old English sheepdogs, Labrador retrievers, English bulldogs, beagles, Bouvier des Flandres, spaniels, and mixed breeds. The disease appears to be more common in males than in females (approximately 2:1) with a predominance in intact animals, but not all studies have identified a gender predilection. Perianal fistulae are extremely rare in cats. Perianal fistulae may occur at any age; however, the mean age of affected dogs is approximately 5 years.

History. Dogs with perianal fistulae usually are presented for treatment because of anal discomfort, constipation, diarrhea, odor, licking, scooting, tenesmus, dyschezia, ulceration, and/or purulent perianal discharge. Clinical signs of discomfort, licking, and scooting may be present before the fistulae are evident externally. Many owners have noticed perianal ulcers or tracts. Pain may cause dogs to become vicious when the tail or perineum is examined or manipulated. Weight loss, diminished appetite, and lethargy may occur.

Physical Examination Findings

Dogs with perianal fistulae often appear normal; however, some are thin with a poor hair coat (Box 19-75). The perianal area should be examined for fistulae that are recognized as dissecting ulcerative tracts usually with a malodorous mucopurulent discharge. The perineum often is painful, and affected dogs may snap, bite, or cry when the tail is lifted. Sedation or general anesthesia is often required for thorough perineal examination. Tracts may be single, but typically are multiple, of varying depths, and epithelium-lined (Fig. 19-134). Fistulae can be difficult to identify if there are only a few punctate lesions and minimal ulceration. The condition becomes more evident as tracts coalesce and as swelling and inflammation develop. In severe cases the entire circumference of the anus may be ulcerated. Previously unidentified tracts often become obvious when the dog is anesthetized and clipped. A rectal examination should determine the depth of involvement, the degree of fibrosis, and the relationship of the anal sacs to fistulae. The tracts should be probed with a sterile instrument to determine their extent. Cannulating and flushing the anal sacs with sterile saline may demonstrate communication with adjacent fistulae. Anal stenosis and rectocutaneous fistulae may be identified during rectal examination.

> NOTE: Examination of the perineal area establishes the tentative diagnosis; however, histologic examination is necessary to rule out squamous cell carcinoma, pythiosis, and other erosive conditions.

Diagnostic Imaging

Imaging is generally not necessary unless there is a suspicion of neoplastic involvement.

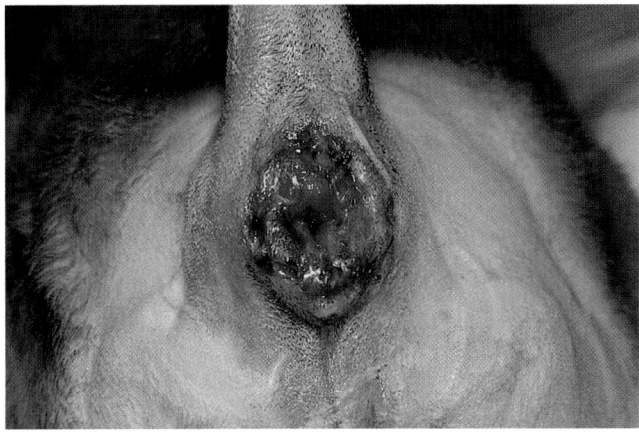

FIG. 19-134
Coalescing ulcers that characterize moderately severe perianal fistulae.

 BOX 19-75

Clinical Signs of Perianal Fistulae

Tenesmus	Perianal discharge—purulent,
Dyschezia	hemorrhagic
Hematochezia	Offensive odor
Constipation or	Perianal licking
obstipation	Perianal pain
Ribbonlike stool	Scooting
Increased defecation	Self-mutilation
frequency	Low tail carriage
Weight loss	

Laboratory Findings

Laboratory findings are nonspecific. Cytology reveals pyogranulomatous inflammation with a mixed bacterial population. Commonly isolated bacteria from deep, intraoperative perianal fistulae samples are *E. coli, Staphylococcus aureus,* α-hemolytic streptococci, and *Proteus mirabilis.* Bacterial contamination is believed to occur after ulceration. Tissue biopsy rules out neoplasia. Acute and chronic inflammation with fibrosis and granulation tissue are expected. Some tracts have an epithelial lining, whereas others involve the anal crypts and rectal mucosa. Histopathologic diagnosis of mild to moderate colitis may be identified if biopsy is taken from the colon. A restrictive diet trial helps rule out adverse food reactions. Other diagnostics that may be performed are fecal parasite exams, fungal culture, and ELISA testing for pythiosis.

DIFFERENTIAL DIAGNOSIS

The early stages of anal SCC may resemble perianal fistulae. Other important differential diagnoses include perianal tumors, anal sac or rectal tumors, anal sac fistulae, atypical bacterial infections, pythiosis, lagenidiosis, and fistulae associated with tail fold pyoderma.

MEDICAL MANAGEMENT

Medical management includes immunosuppression, hygiene, and dietary therapy. Management of perianal fistulae requires diligence, is frustrating for veterinarians and clients, and is uncomfortable for patients. Stool softeners may reduce dyschezia. Regular perianal cleansing and antibiotic therapy reduce inflammation, but seldom allow the fistulae to heal and may allow the disease to progress. However, administration of immunosuppressives (e.g., tacrolimus, prednisolone, cyclosporine, ketoconazole, azathioprine, and metronidazole) and antibiotics can effectively treat perianal fistulae. Initial treatment is necessary for several months, and lifelong treatment may be required. If one drug combination is not achieving the treatment goal, then another drug protocol can be initiated (Boxes 19-76 and 19-77). Medical treatment can be expensive; however, continence is maintained. Treatment of concurrent diseases (e.g., hypothyroidism and IBD) facilitates treatment of perianal fistulae. Dogs with perianal fistulae and concomitant infiltrative bowel disease or colitis may improve with initial high-dose prednisolone therapy (i.e., 2 mg/kg PO given once a day for 2 weeks). The prednisolone dose then is reduced (1 mg/kg PO given once a day) and continued for 4 weeks. Prednisolone therapy directed at fistulae is at a higher dose and usually combined with azathioprine or metronidazole (see Box 19-77).

Cyclosporine is effective in most dogs. The drug affects the immune response by blocking proliferation of activated T lymphocytes (T-helper cells). Adverse side effects have included vomiting, diarrhea, gingival hyperplasia, papilloma-like skin lesions, hypertrichosis, and increased hair shedding. Microemulsion formulations of cyclosporine are recommended because they are more bioavailable (Atopia, Neoral; Novartis); however, absorption is erratic between dogs, and

---

 BOX 19-76

Perianal Fistula Treatment Goals

Goal 1: Alleviate signs of tenesmus, dyschezia, hematochezia, constipation, diarrhea, and pain. Reduce defecation frequency. Obtained by induction phase treatment lasting 8 to 20 weeks.
Goal 2: Reduce diameter, depth, extent, and recurrence of fistulae. Obtained by maintenance therapy at the lowest effective dose every 24–72 hours; may be required for life.

 BOX 19-77

Management of Perianal Fistulae in Dogs

Immunosuppressive/Immunomodulatory Therapy

Cyclosporine (Atopica, Neoral)* [± ketoconazole]

3–5 mg/kg (initial dose) PO 2 hours before or after feeding, bid. Adjust this dose based upon therapeutic drug monitoring to achieve a whole blood cyclosporine trough measurement of 400–600 ng/ml

Ketoconazole (Nizoral)

3–10 mg/kg PO, qd (In this case, ketoconazole is being used to inhibit metabolism of cyclosporine and thereby increase blood levels. It is very important to measure trough blood levels of cyclosporine to determine further adjustments to dose of cyclosporine and ketoconazole).

Azathioprine (Imuran) [plus metronidazole]

2.2 mg/kg/day PO, qod†

Metronidazole (Flagyl) [plus azathioprine]

10–15 mg/kg PO bid

Glucocorticoids [± azathioprine ± metronidazole]

2 mg/kg PO qd for 2 weeks, 1 mg/kg PO qd for 4 weeks, then 1 mg/kg PO q48h maintenance

Tacrolimus 0.1%

Topical, thin film bid for induction, then every 24 to 72 hours for maintenance; apply with gloved hand

Hygiene Therapy

Clipping and cleaning
  Keep area free of hair
  Lavage once or twice daily and dry
Antimicrobial therapy
  Oral—pending sensitivity use amoxicillin-clavulanic acid or metronidazole
  Topical—mupirocin

Dietary Therapy

Stool Softener

Trial diets with alternative protein source
  Lamb and rice
  Fish and potato
  Kangaroo and oats
  Vegetarian

Surgical Therapy

Deroof and fulgurate or laser ablate
Excise persistent fistulae
Remove involved anal sacs

PO, Oral; *bid,* twice a day; *qd,* once a day; *qod,* every other day; *q48h,* every 48 hours.
*Do not use Sandimmune.
†Giving the drug every other day is safer than giving it every day, but it will take longer to see beneficial effects.

therapeutic drug monitoring is essential (especially in dogs that do not respond to therapy). The recommended initial cyclosporine dosage is shown in Box 19-77. Trough blood cyclosporine concentrations should be measured 7 to 12 days after initiating therapy. Treatment is continued for at least 16 weeks or 2 weeks beyond resolution of fistulae. The dosage and cost of cyclosporine can be reduced by oral administration of ketoconazole (see Box 19-77), which alters hepatic metabolism of cyclosporine. Therapeutic drug monitoring becomes even more important when combining ketoconazole and cyclosporine.

Combination therapy using azathioprine and metronidazole (see Box 19-77) reduces perianal irritation and the severity and extent of lesions. Azathioprine suppresses both humoral and cell-mediated immunity. Side effects include gastrointestinal upset, bone marrow suppression, hepatotoxicity, and pancreatitis. Metronidazole has immunomodulating effects, reduces fecal bacterial colonization, and is antiprotozoal. Its potential side effects include anorexia, gastrointestinal upset, and central vestibular signs. Surgery is recommended if improvement plateaus after 4 to 6 weeks of therapy. Azathioprine and metronidazole are continued for 3 to 6 weeks after surgery.

Topical tacrolimus is initially co-administered with other drugs unless the animal has a very mild case of perianal fistula. Tacrolimus is a calcineurin inhibitor with pharmacologic actions similar to but 10 to 100 times more potent than cyclosporine. Potential side effects are stinging and burning. Application is initially twice daily, but then is reduced to the lowest frequency that controls inflammation (see Box 19-77).

Monitoring medical therapy requires reevaluation every 3 to 5 weeks. Monitoring signs and mapping fistulae help to assess the effectiveness of treatments and dosages. Dosages are modified according to the response noted. Hematologic and biochemical monitoring may be required, depending on the drugs used.

SURGICAL TREATMENT

Perianal fistulae were once considered a surgical disease, but now medical management is the initial treatment of choice. Surgery is recommended for fistulae resistant to medical therapy and those associated with the anal sacs. The goals of surgery are to eliminate necrotic or unhealthy tissue and stimulate healing by secondary intention without causing fecal incontinence or anal stenosis. Numerous surgical procedures have been used to treat perianal fistulae, including superficial or radical excision, cryotherapy, fulguration, laser ablation, chemical cautery, and tail amputation. Staged procedures may be necessary during the initial months of treatment and may need to be repeated intermittently for life. Dogs with mild to moderate disease usually respond better to treatment than do those with severe disease.

Radical resection is the excision of all diseased skin, subcutaneous tissue, muscle, and fascia. The rectum is apposed to remaining skin with widely spaced interrupted sutures. The remainder of the defect is allowed to heal by secondary

intention. Fecal incontinence is a common postoperative problem. Superficial resection (i.e., excision of all skin involved in the inflammatory process) is recommended with severe or unresponsive perianal fistulae. Débridement and fulguration of fistulae are less likely to cause fecal incontinence than extensive resection, but tend to be ineffective in severe cases. Some surgeons recommend concurrent tail amputation. Anal sacculectomy (see p. 513) is necessary when fistulae involve the anal sacs. Débridement and chemical cauterization (resection of epithelium overlying coalescing fistulous tracts followed by application of an irritant chemical to the underlying granulation tissue) may be performed using a strong iodine solution (Box 19-78). This technique is less effective than débridement and fulguration or ablation, but may be selected for patients with mild disease, when healing begins to lag, or when small fistulae are identified after débridement and fulguration or ablation. Use of chemical cauterization at this time may eliminate the need for general anesthesia and reoperation.

Cryotherapy of perianal fistulae involves the application of a cryogen to destroy diseased tissue. Tissue that has been frozen necroses and then sloughs off during the subsequent 1 to 2 weeks. The wounds heal by secondary intention. Appropriately controlling the freeze by using thermocouples is helpful. However, cryosurgery is not recommended because it is very difficult to control the freeze; muscles and nerves often are inadvertently destroyed. Up to one half of the patients have severe anal stenosis after cryosurgery. Other complications include flatulence, tenesmus, incontinence, diarrhea, and constipation.

Preoperative Management

Initiate medical management and only operate on persistent fistulae. Owners should be told the expected results of treatment, and their important postoperative role should be thoroughly explained. Owners must make a firm commitment of ability and willingness to provide long-term postoperative care. Fistula location should be mapped on a chart of the perianal region. Administration of stool softeners should be initiated several days before surgery (see Box 19-60). The colon should be evacuated, and food withheld the day before surgery. Hot compresses should be applied to the perineum to help remove exudate and debris. Analgesics may be necessary if the patient objects to perianal manipulations. Prophylactic antibiotics effective against gram-negative and anaerobic bacteria should be given during induction of anesthesia.

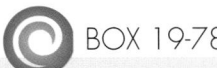

BOX 19-78

Chemical Cauterizing Agents

- Silver nitrate
- 4.5%–5.0% phenol
- 7% iodine

Anesthesia

Anesthetic recommendations for animals undergoing perianal surgery are given on p. 500.

Surgical Anatomy

The surgical anatomy of the perianal region is presented on p. 500.

Positioning

The patient should be positioned in ventral recumbency with the hind legs over the end of the table. The pelvis should be elevated with padding and the tail secured over the back. The end of the table should be padded to prevent pressure on the femoral nerves. As an alternative, a padded perineal stand may be used.

SURGICAL TECHNIQUE

Surgery is seldom indicated for treatment of perianal fistulae. The reader is referred to *Small Animal Surgery*, second edition or the e-dition for a description of "débridement with fulguration or laser ablation" and concurrent "tail amputation."

POSTOPERATIVE CARE AND ASSESSMENT

Systemic (see Table 13-4 on p. 133) or epidural analgesics (see Table 13-6 on p. 134) should be used as needed. The perineum should be cleaned three or four times daily, especially after defecation, with warm saline (water) or a dilute antiseptic solution. Using a hose and warm tap water is a convenient and acceptable method of cleaning. An Elizabethan collar, bucket, or sidebars should be used to prevent self-mutilation, and stool softeners should be given to facilitate fecal passage during the first 3 to 4 weeks (see Box 19-60). The stool softener should make the stool soft, but not sticky or pasty. A low-bulk diet should be fed. Giving antibiotics effective against gram-negative and anaerobic bacteria is helpful although not essential. The size of the débrided areas should be mapped immediately after surgery and at each reevaluation to allow accurate monitoring. The patient should be reevaluated every 2 to 4 weeks, and nonhealing or new fistulae should be treated as needed. After the fistulae have resolved, owners should keep the perineum clipped and clean. They should check for new fistulae monthly.

COMPLICATIONS

Fecal incontinence, anal stenosis, and recurrence sometimes precipitate euthanasia. These are common complications with some surgical techniques. Flatulence, tenesmus, constipation, and diarrhea may also occur. Complications are more common and severe after radical resection (Box 19-79) than after superficial resection or fulguration and ablation. Hair loss and lameness may occur with cyclosporine therapy, but these resolve when therapy is discontinued. Recurrence often may be controlled with a 7- to 14-day course of cyclosporine.

PROGNOSIS

Medical therapy with cyclosporine and tacrolimus or other immunomodulating drugs is effective in resolving most fistulae and reducing the severity of others. Mild perianal fistulae may be controlled if owners are diligent about daily perianal care. The area must be kept clean and dry to prevent progression of the disease. The prognosis after surgery alone is fair to poor, depending on the severity of the disease at the time of surgery and the owner's postoperative compliance. Early diagnosis and preoperative medical therapy allow less radical surgical procedures with fewer postoperative complications. Recurrence is common with either medical or surgical therapy. Many animals are euthanized because of pain, lack of response to treatment, recurrence, and/or client frustration.

Reference

Patterson AP, Campbell KL: Managing anal furunculosis in dogs, *Compend Cont Educ Pract Vet* 27:339, 2005.

Suggested Reading

Hardie RJ, Gregory SP, Tomlin J et al: Cyclosporine treatment of anal furunculosis in 26 dogs, *J Small Anim Pract* 46:3, 2005.
Approximately 4 mg/kg bid was administered with complete resolution in 69% and improvement in 27% after a mean of 8.8 weeks (range 4 to 24).

Jamieson PM, Simpson JW, Kirby BM et al: Association between anal furunculosis and colitis in the dog: preliminary observations, *J Small Anim Pract* 43:109, 2002.
Eighteen dogs with anal furunculosis had colon biopsies, and 50% were found to have colitis.

Misseghers BS, Binnington AG, Mathews KA: Clinical observations of the treatment of canine perianal fistulas with topical tacrolimus in 10 dogs, *Can Vet J* 41:623, 2000.
Improvement was noted in 90%, and 50% were completely healed after 16 weeks of application.

O'Neill R, Edwards G, Holloway S: Efficacy of combined cyclosporine A and ketoconazole treatment of anal furunculosis, *J Small Anim Pract* 45:238, 2004.
Using combined medications, lesions in 19 dogs were resolved in 3 to 10 weeks with remissions of 1 to 6 months.

 BOX 19-79

Possible Complications of Wide Resection of Fistulae

- Fecal incontinence
- Flatulence
- Diarrhea
- Tenesmus
- Dyschezia
- Constipation
- Anal stenosis
- Recurrence

RECTAL PROLAPSE

DEFINITION

Rectal prolapse *(anal prolapse)* is a protrusion or eversion of the rectal mucosa from the anus.

GENERAL CONSIDERATIONS AND CLINICALLY RELEVANT PATHOPHYSIOLOGY

Rectal prolapse is principally associated with endoparasitism or enteritis in young animals, and tumors or perineal hernias in middle-aged and older animals. However, any condition that causes tenesmus may result in rectal prolapse (Box 19-80). Weakness of perirectal and perianal connective tissues or muscles, uncoordinated peristaltic contractions, and inflammation or edema of rectal mucous membranes predispose patients to rectal prolapse.

Rectal prolapse may be complete or incomplete. Incomplete prolapse involves only mucosa. Any part of the entire anorectal circumference may be affected. Complete prolapse involves all layers of the rectal wall and the entire circumference. The amount of eversion increases with continued straining, varying from a few millimeters to many centimeters. Everted tissue becomes edematous, preventing spontaneous retraction into the pelvic canal. Continued exposure causes excoriation, bleeding, desiccation, and necrosis.

DIAGNOSIS
Clinical Presentation

Signalment. Rectal prolapse occurs in dogs and cats, with no documented breed predisposition. However, it may occur more often in Manx cats because of their anal laxity. It may occur at any age, but is more common in young animals.

History. Straining or recent perineal surgery is common. Constipation, diarrhea, prostatitis, urinary tract infections, dyspnea, and dystocia may produce tenesmus. Perineal or perianal irritation from trauma or surgery may also cause straining and rectal prolapse.

Physical Examination Findings

The patient's physical status is unpredictable because of the numerous possible causes of rectal prolapse. Protrusion of anorectal mucosa is obvious on physical examination. The degree of prolapse may vary from a few millimeters to several centimeters (Fig. 19-135). Rectal prolapse must be differentiated from an ileocolic intussusception that is protruding from the anus (see later discussion).

Diagnostic Imaging

Imaging may help identify the cause of the prolapse.

Laboratory Findings

Laboratory tests are nonspecific for rectal prolapse, but may identify the cause and define the patient's physiologic status. Parasites and acute enteritis are common in young animals.

DIFFERENTIAL DIAGNOSIS

The primary differential diagnosis for rectal prolapse is intussusception. Insertion of a finger (preferred) or probe (i.e., thermometer or smooth tube) alongside the prolapsed mass

is possible with an intussusception, but not with a rectal prolapse.

> NOTE: Be sure to differentiate prolapse from intussusception. Palpation of the outer surface of the prolapse identifies a fornix.

MEDICAL MANAGEMENT

The treatment and prognosis depend on the cause, degree of prolapse, chronicity, and whether it is a recurrent prolapse. Acute rectal prolapse is easily treated, but chronic disease may require resection. Manual reduction and placement of a purse-string suture around the anus are recommended for acute prolapses with minimal tissue damage and edema (Fig. 19-136, *A* and *B*). Warm saline lavages, massage, and lubrication (e.g., with a water-soluble gel) should be applied to the everted tissue before digital reduction. Giving a retention enema of several milliliters of Kaopectate will help alleviate further straining. A purse-string suture tight enough to maintain prolapse reduction without interfering with passage of soft stool should be placed. Epidural anesthesia may also help prevent additional straining and reprolapse. Most rectal prolapse patients respond well to manual reduction when the cause is treated and resolved.

SURGICAL TREATMENT

Nonreducible or severely traumatized prolapses require amputation. Colopexy should be performed when rectal prolapse repeatedly recurs after manual reduction or amputation (see pp. 483, 501, and 526).

> NOTE: Be sure to identify potential underlying causes of the prolapse and treat them.

Preoperative Management

Surgery should be prompt to prevent further trauma to the everted tissue. Extensive colorectal preparation is unnecessary. Prophylactic antibiotics effective against gram-negative

 BOX 19-80

Conditions Associated With Rectal Prolapse

- Endoparasitism
- Enteritis
- Intestinal foreign bodies
- Dystocia
- Urolithiasis
- Constipation
- Congenital defects
- Sphincter laxity
- Prostatic disease
- Perineal surgery

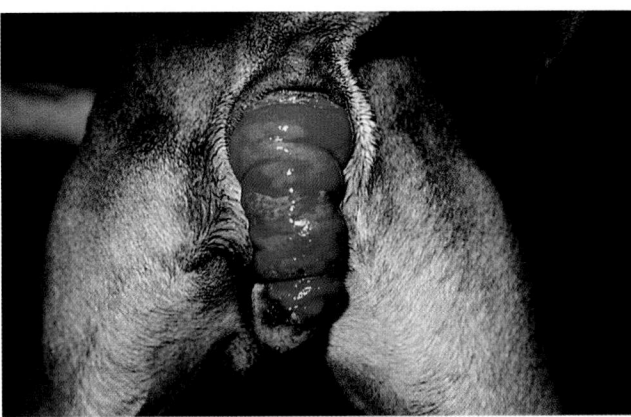

FIG. 19-135
Rectal prolapse. Note the large amount of everted rectum that must be differentiated from an intussusception.

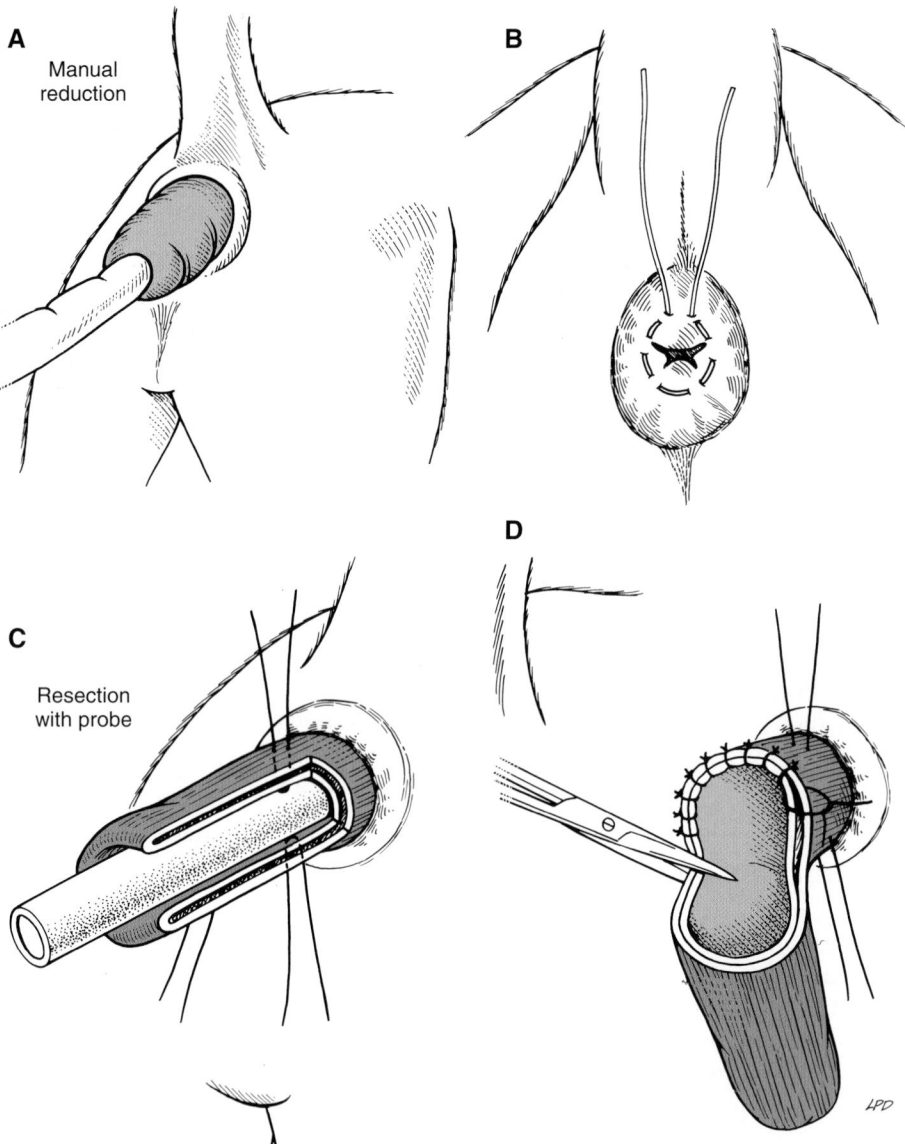

FIG. 19-136
A, Digitally reduce small prolapses with healthy mucosa and place a purse-string suture around the rectum. **B,** Resect irreducible or traumatized prolapses. **C,** Place a probe in the rectal lumen and three or four stay sutures in the rectal wall. **D,** Make a full-thickness incision through the prolapsed tissue one third to one half the distance around the circumference. Appose the edges with simple interrupted sutures. Then complete the resection.

and anaerobic bacteria (see Box 19-56) should be given at induction of anesthesia. The exposed tissue should be lavaged with warm sterile saline and lubricated with a water-soluble gel.

Anesthesia

Anesthetic recommendations for animals undergoing rectal and perineal surgery are given on p. 500.

Surgical Anatomy

The surgical anatomy of the rectum and perineum is presented on p. 500.

Positioning

After the perianal area has been clipped and aseptically prepared for surgery, the everted tissue should again be lavaged and lubricated. The patient should be positioned in ventral recumbency with the hind legs over the end of the table. The pelvis should be elevated with padding and the tail secured over the back. The end of the table should be padded to prevent pressure on the femoral nerves. As an alternative, a perineal stand may be used.

SURGICAL TECHNIQUE

Place a probe into the rectal lumen to serve as a guide (Fig. 19-136, C). Place three horizontal mattress stay sutures (at the 12 o'clock, 5 o'clock, and 8 o'clock positions) through all layers of the prolapse just cranial to the proposed transection site. These sutures should enter the rectal lumen with the needle being deflected by the probe before being passed through the rectal tissue again. Transect the traumatized tissue in stages caudal to the stay sutures. After each stage of the resection, anatomically appose the transected edges with simple interrupted sutures (e.g., 3-0 or 4-0 monofilament, absorbable [Figure 19-136, D]). Space the sutures approximately 2 mm apart and 2 mm from the cut edge. Inspect the anastomosis for gaps between sutures. Remove the stay sutures and gently replace the anastomotic site in the pelvic or anal canal. Place a purse-string suture around the anus if postoperative tenesmus is expected.

POSTOPERATIVE CARE AND ASSESSMENT

The cause of the prolapse must be treated to prevent recurrence. Retention enemas of Kaopectate or epidural opioids may eliminate postoperative tenesmus for several hours (see p. 525). Systemic analgesics should be given if necessary (see Table 13-4 on p. 133). A low-fiber diet should be fed while the purse-string suture is in place. The purse-string suture generally can be removed 3 to 5 days after manual reduction and 1 to 2 days after resection. Stool softeners should be given for 2 to 3 weeks after resection (see Box 19-60). Amputees must be monitored for leakage from the surgical site.

COMPLICATIONS

Possible complications of manual reduction of rectal prolapses are tenesmus, dyschezia, hematochezia, and recurrence. Additional complications of resection include hemorrhage, leakage, anal stenosis, infection, dehiscence, and fecal incontinence.

PROGNOSIS

Incomplete prolapses that occur during defecation may reduce spontaneously. The prognosis for chronic rectal prolapse without manual reduction or surgery is poor. Chronically exposed rectal mucosa is traumatized by licking, sitting, and environmental exposure, ultimately becoming necrotic with secondary sepsis. The prognosis for most animals treated surgically is good provided the primary cause of tenesmus or irritation is appropriately treated.

FECAL INCONTINENCE

DEFINITIONS

Fecal incontinence is the inability to voluntarily control defecation. **Reservoir incontinence** results from a failure of the large bowel to adapt to and contain the colorectal contents. **Sphincter incontinence** is a failure of the sphincter mechanism to resist propulsive forces in the rectum, so that feces are involuntarily passed.

GENERAL CONSIDERATIONS AND CLINICALLY RELEVANT PATHOPHYSIOLOGY

Fecal incontinence is uncommon in dogs and cats. Fecal continence depends on maintenance of colonic reservoir function and anal sphincter control. Muscles involved in fecal continence include the internal anal sphincter, external anal sphincter, rectococcygeus, levator ani, and coccygeus muscles. As fecal material is propelled distally into the terminal rectum, the rectum distends and the internal anal sphincter dilates whereas the external anal sphincter and

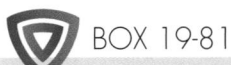 BOX 19-81

Causes of Fecal Incontinence

Reservoir Incontinence
- Diffuse colonic disease resulting in decreased distensibility
- Reduced colonic length after resection (e.g., two thirds or more)

Sphincter Incontinence
- Rectal resection (more than 4 cm of terminal rectum)
- Inadequate cuff of terminal rectal mucosa (less than approximately 1.5 cm)
- Damage to the caudal rectal nerves
- Sacral spinal cord lesions of S1–S3 cord segments (L5 vertebral level in dogs and L6 in cats)
- Peripheral pudendal nerve damage
- Physical disruption of the external anal sphincter after:
  - Anorectal trauma
  - Rectal prolapse
  - Severe perianal disease (e.g., inflammation, tumors)
  - Surgical resection
- Resection of more than half the external anal sphincter

caudal portion of the levator ani muscles contract. Subsequently, propulsive contractions diminish, and normal resting tone is restored in 2 to 3 minutes. Thus the rectum distends and adapts with each new bolus to increase its storage capacity, and a resting anorectal high-pressure zone is created by the internal anal sphincter, external anal sphincter, and caudal portion of the levator ani muscles. The internal anal sphincter contributes 50% to 80% of the resting tone in the high-pressure zone. The external anal sphincter is tonically active, but contributes minimally to the resting tone; its short contractions resist peristaltic waves. The role of the levator ani is uncertain. Animals posture and increase abdominal pressure by closing the glottis, fixing the diaphragm, and contracting the abdominal wall when defecation is appropriate. This causes the external anal sphincter to relax and the rectococcygeus, levator ani, and coccygeus muscles to contract.

Reservoir incontinence (Box 19-81) usually is characterized by frequent, conscious defecation. Loss of reservoir continence results in abnormally soft, unformed, or liquefied feces. Loss of reservoir continence may be caused by diffuse colonic disease resulting in diminished distensibility, or it may occur secondary to reduced colonic length after resection (e.g., two thirds or more). The small intestine increases water absorption and capacity after subtotal colectomy, therefore many animals regain reservoir continence.

Sphincter incontinence (see Box 19-81) may be neurogenic or nonneurogenic. Partial fecal incontinence may occur if only one muscle group malfunctions. Loss of sensory receptors and the afferent limb of the continence mechanism can be secondary to rectal resection. An adequate cuff of rectal muscularis must be preserved to maintain sphincter continence. Efferent neural control is lost when caudal rectal nerves are damaged. Sacral spinal cord lesions of the S1-S3 cord segments (L5 vertebral level in dogs and L6 in cats) damage the cell bodies of the pudendal nerve. Peripheral pudendal nerve damage can occur anywhere from the cauda equina distally. Unilateral pudendal nerve damage causes fecal incontinence for only 3 to 4 weeks because of cross-innervation and muscle fiber decussation. Bilateral pudendal nerve damage causes permanent incontinence. Nonneurogenic sphincter incontinence occurs secondary to physical disruption of the external anal sphincter after anorectal trauma, rectal prolapse, severe perianal disease (inflammation, tumors), or surgical resection. The incidence of incontinence increases as external anal sphincter resection approaches 180 degrees. Resection of more than half of the external anal sphincter usually results in fecal incontinence.

DIAGNOSIS
Clinical Presentation

Signalment. Any breed or gender of dog or cat may have fecal incontinence. Manx cats may be predisposed because of anal laxity resulting from abnormal innervation. Dogs with perianal fistulae (see p. 520) and those with surgery of the anal region (e.g., anal sac ablation) may develop fecal incontinence. Fecal incontinence may occur in any age animal, although 50% of affected animals are 11 years or older.

History. The history is important for differentiating reservoir incontinence from sphincter incontinence and for determining possible causes. Animals are presented for treatment because of inappropriate defecation. Some affected animals posture and void normally despite having inappropriate defecation. A fecal bolus may be voided when barking, coughing, or rising from a recumbent position without posturing or recognition of the event. It is important to find out if the onset of incontinence is associated with recent colorectal or perineal surgery, trauma, perianal disease, or neurologic disease. Signs of incontinence vary from occasional incontinence to perineal soiling and fecal dribbling. Reservoir incontinence may be associated with frequent defecation, tenesmus, hematochezia, and mucoid stools.

Physical Examination Findings

Patients with fecal incontinence often appear normal. Rectal and perineal examination may reveal colorectal or perianal disease. Anal sphincter tone may be diminished, the anus dilated, and/or the rectal mucosa prolapsed. The abdomen should be palpated to determine the size of the colon and bladder tone and how difficult it is to express the urinary bladder. A thorough neurologic examination should be performed. Self-inflicted skin trauma suggests paresthesia. Hyperesthesia may be detected in the lumbosacral area. Hind limb paresthesia, urinary incontinence, and hyperesthesia suggest cauda equina syndrome. A Foley catheter can be inflated in the rectum to determine if the dog has a normal anal reflex.

Diagnostic Imaging

Survey radiographs should be evaluated for colorectal or pelvic canal masses, vertebral abnormalities (e.g., lumbosacral stenosis or fracture), or pelvic fractures. Myelography, epidurography, CT, or MRI helps diagnose spinal cord or cauda equina lesions. In human beings, endoanal ultrasonography is used to help evaluate anal sphincter morphology and localize weak areas. A defect of the external anal sphincter muscle is identified as either a hypoechogenic or hyperechogenic wedge-shaped area. An internal sphincter defect is identified as a loss of continuity of the normal hypoechoic ring. Endoscopic biopsy of the colon and anus is indicated if reservoir incontinence is suspected.

Laboratory Findings

A hemogram, serum biochemistry profile, urinalysis, and fecal examination are recommended. Hematologic and serum biochemistry values may suggest the cause. Electromyography and manometry help assess the anorectal sphincter complex in some cases. These examinations help differentiate reservoir incontinence from sphincter incontinence and neurogenic incontinence from nonneurogenic incontinence. Electromyography can reveal denervation or myopathy. Manometry gives anal and colorectal pressure profiles and evaluates the degree of impairment of anorectal tone and internal and external anal sphincter function. The presence of an intact reflex arch may be determined more simply by inflating a Foley catheter in the rectum and observing the response.

DIFFERENTIAL DIAGNOSIS

Differential diagnoses and possible causes of fecal incontinence include anal disease (e.g., anal sacculitis, dermatitis, endoparasites, perianal fistulae, or tumors), colorectal disease (e.g., colitis and neoplasia), poor diet, trauma to or denervation of the muscles of continence, damage to somatic peripheral nerves (i.e., pudendal or S2-S3-Cd1 spinal nerves), damage to autonomic peripheral nerves (i.e., pelvic plexus or pelvic nerves), cauda equina syndrome, central nervous system injury (e.g., sacral spinal segments, spinothalamic tracts, and frontal cortex), and behavioral abnormalities. Fecal incontinence must also be differentiated from partial or type 3 atresia ani and congenital or traumatic rectovaginal or rectourethral fistula. With these conditions, feces may mix with urine, causing perineal soiling and inappropriate passage of feces.

MEDICAL MANAGEMENT

The causative disease or condition should be treated if possible. Owner acceptance may require that the pet be kept outdoors. Many patients are euthanized because owners are unable or unwilling to tolerate incontinence. The goals of medical management are to reduce fecal water content and fecal bulk, slow transit time, and increase anal sphincter tone. Symptomatic medical management includes dietary

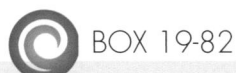 BOX 19-82

Opioids That Slow Bowel Transit Time

Diphenoxylate Hydrochloride (Lomotil)
Dogs: 0.1–0.2 mg/kg PO, bid to tid
Cats: 0.05–0.1 mg/kg PO, bid

Loperamide Hydrochloride (Imodium)
Dogs: 0.1 mg/kg PO, bid to tid
Cats: 0.08–0.16 mg/kg PO, bid

PO, Oral; *bid,* twice a day; *tid,* three times a day.

change, pharmacologic therapy, and induced defecation. A low-residue diet (i.e., cottage cheese and rice) reduces fecal volume by up to 85% and lessens the frequency of defecation. Opioids (Box 19-82) promote segmental contractions, slowing bowel transit time and increasing water absorption. Enemas and rectal stimulation can promote colonic evacuation at appropriate times and help prevent inappropriate defecation.

SURGICAL TREATMENT

Sphincter-enhancing procedures for treating fecal incontinence in animals have been inadequately investigated; described surgical techniques must be considered investigational. Anal sphincter function has been enhanced by using a fascial sling, silicone elastomer (Silastic sheeting #501-3), or dynamic myoplasty.

Preoperative Management

The colon should be evacuated with laxatives, oral cathartics, and/or enemas, and any remaining fecal material should be manually evacuated after induction of anesthesia. Antibiotics effective against gram-negative and anaerobic bacteria (see Box 19-56) should be given after induction.

Anesthesia

General anesthetic is recommended. Anesthetic recommendations for animals undergoing rectal and perineal surgery are given on p. 500.

Surgical Anatomy

The surgical anatomy of the rectum and perineum is presented on p. 500.

Positioning

Clip and aseptically prepare the perineum or ventral abdomen. The patient should be positioned in ventral recumbency with the hind legs over the end of the table. The pelvis should be elevated with padding, and the tail should be secured over the back. The end of the table should be padded to prevent pressure on the femoral nerves. As an alternative, a perineal stand may be used.

SURGICAL TECHNIQUE
Fascial Sling

Harvest two strips of tensor fasciae latae (6 cm × 0.5 cm) from the lateral thigh, suture them together, and transfer to the anus. Close the fascial defect, and appose the subcutaneous tissue and skin. Make a 3- to 4-cm incision on each side of the anus just lateral to the tail base. Connect the two incisions by undermining the tissue ventral to the anus with a curved hemostat. Direct the fascial strip around the ventral anus using curved hemostats. Suture the fascia to the coccygeus muscle at the base of the tail on one side, pull it snug, and suture it to the tail base on the opposite side using 2-0 or 3-0 monofilament, nonabsorbable suture (nylon, polybutester, or polypropylene). As an alternative, secure one end to the coccygeus muscle and direct the other end of the fascial strip over the base of the tail, pull it snug, and suture it to itself at the tail base. Lavage the area and reappose the subcutaneous tissue and skin.

Implantation of a Silicone Elastomer

Make two incisions lateral to the anus as described above (Fig. 19-137, A). Make a tunnel ventral and dorsal to the anus with curved hemostats. Insert the implant through the tunnels (Fig. 19-137, B). Overlap the implant ends and pull it snug around the anus. To prevent overtightening, place a 1-cm probe in the rectum while the implant is tightened (Fig. 19-137, C). Suture the overlapping ends of the implant together with nonabsorbable, monofilament suture (e.g., 2-0 or 3-0 nylon, polybutester, or polypropylene). Lavage the area and reappose the subcutaneous tissue and skin.

POSTOPERATIVE CARE AND ASSESSMENT

Analgesics should be given as needed, and antibiotics should be continued for several days to minimize the risk of implant infection. Stool softeners should be administered (see Box 19-60), and a low-residue diet fed. The animal should be monitored for infection and effectiveness of the procedure. Tenesmus is expected for several days.

COMPLICATIONS

The major complications associated with these procedures are failure or recurrence of incontinence. Slings often loosen slightly after implantation. Correction of incontinence may be only partial, and some signs may persist. Infection, dehiscence, and sloughing of the implant are risks. Persistent tenesmus and obstruction may occur if the sling is too snug.

PROGNOSIS

The prognosis depends on the type and extent of the incontinence. Complete lower motor neuron incontinence is incurable. Improved sphincter function is expected after surgery, although signs may worsen with loosening of the implant. Muscle trauma or irritation often causes partial or temporary incontinence, which improves as the muscles heal.

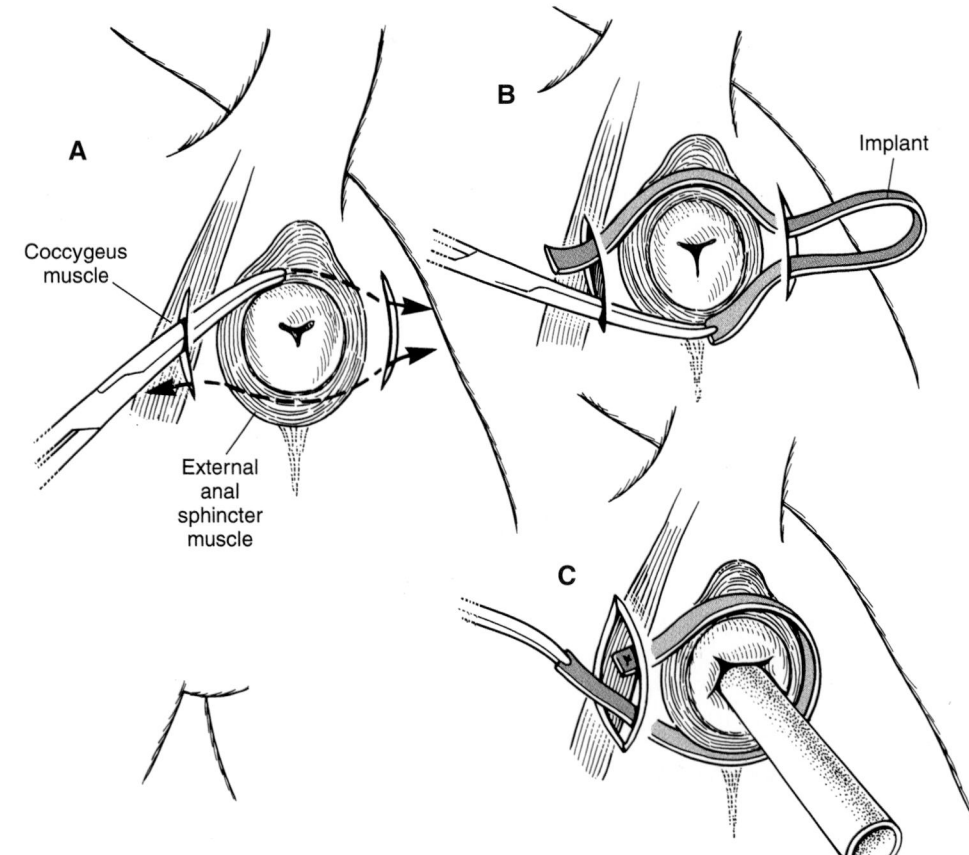

FIG. 19-137
Fecal continence may be improved by enhancing the function of the anal sphincter with an implant. **A,** Make 3- to 4-cm incisions on each side of the anus. Connect the incisions with a tunnel dorsal and ventral to the anus. **B,** Direct the implant through the tunnels. **C,** Secure the implant to the coccygeus muscle, pull it snug around a probe, and secure it to itself.

Suggested Reading

Mahler S, Williams G: Preservation of the fistula for reconstruction of the anal canal and the anus in atresia ani and rectovestibular fistula in 2 dogs, *Vet Surg* 34:148, 2005.
This case report describes an episiotomy approach combined with a dorsal perineal incision to separate and reposition the rectal fistula.

Vianna ML, Tobias KM: Atresia ani in the dog: a retrospective study, *J Am Anim Hosp Assoc* 41:317, 2005.
This study reviews the types of atresia ani and reports findings from 119 dogs.

CHAPTER 20
Surgery of the Liver

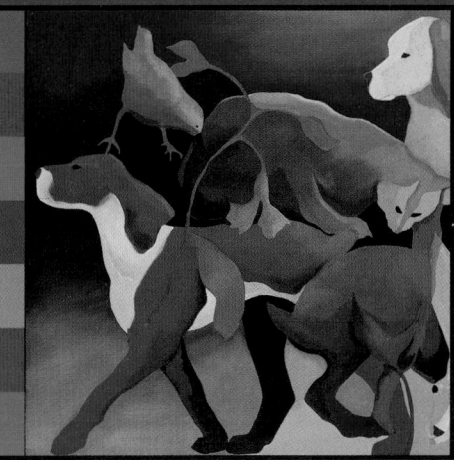

DEFINITIONS

Hepatectomy refers to removal either of the entire liver (**total hepatectomy**) or of a portion of the liver (**partial hepatectomy**).

PREOPERATIVE MANAGEMENT

The liver is the largest gland in the body. It is the primary site of the metabolism (detoxification) of many substances and plays a central role in the metabolism of protein, fat, and carbohydrates. Unfortunately, clinical signs of hepatic disease may not be apparent until the disease is advanced and dysfunction is irreversible. Hepatic failure may affect many other organ systems, including the central nervous system (CNS), kidneys, intestines, and heart.

The liver produces most of the plasma proteins, including albumin, α-globulins and β-globulins, fibrinogen, and prothrombin. Hypoalbuminemia is common in patients with advanced hepatic disease. Fluid therapy may further dilute the serum albumin; plasma or colloid infusions should be considered in these patients, in addition to electrolyte solutions. Albumin levels below 2 g/dl may be associated with delayed wound healing. Electrolyte abnormalities are common in patients with hepatic disease but except for potassium alterations are seldom severe. Coagulopathies may occur because of diminished synthesis of clotting factors or consumption. Preoperative evaluation of clotting function, especially the mucosal bleeding time, is warranted; transfusions with fresh whole blood may reduce intraoperative hemorrhage in selected patients. Some patients with hepatic disease are anemic because of nutritional deficiencies, coagulation abnormalities, or gastrointestinal hemorrhage. Animals with a hematocrit below 20% or anemic animals that are clinically hypoxic or weak should be given preoperative blood transfusions (see Box 5-1 on p. 25). Many patients with liver disease are anorexic and may require nutritional supplementation before surgery (see Chapter 11). Hypoglycemia sometimes occurs with severe hepatic insufficiency; monitoring of blood glucose levels and supplementation of fluids with glucose may be needed. Patients with massive ascites may have ventilatory disturbances as a result of diaphragmatic displacement and restriction of lung expansion. In such patients, removing some abdominal fluid before induction of anesthesia may help prevent hypoventilation. Patients with severe hepatic encephalopathy should be treated with dietary therapy, appropriate antibiotics, enemas, fluids, and other medications (see p. 543) to diminish or eliminate clinical signs before surgery.

> NOTE: The cranial location of the liver may make hepatic biopsy somewhat difficult, particularly in large, deep-chested breeds or when the liver is abnormally small. In these animals, extend the incision as far cranially as necessary to facilitate hepatic exposure.

ANESTHESIA

In animals with hepatic dysfunction, the ability to metabolize and inactivate some drugs may be impaired because of decreased hepatic metabolism, hepatic blood flow, volume of distribution (i.e., of drugs that are highly protein bound), and extraction efficiency. Consequently, drugs commonly used to anesthetize veterinary patients may have a prolonged duration of action or altered function. Acetylpromazine is believed to lower the seizure threshold and should not be used in patients with severe hepatic insufficiency and/or encephalopathy. It also lowers systemic vascular resistance and blood pressure and may alter the metabolism of some drugs (i.e., procaine and succinylcholine).

Diazepam (Box 20-1) is useful as a premedicant or induction agent in patients with hepatic dysfunction because it causes mild, dose-related CNS depression, does not depress the cardiopulmonary system, raises the seizure threshold, and can be antagonized with flumazenil. Diazepam is best used in conjunction with an opioid because it may disinhibit some behaviors when used alone. It should be used with caution in hypoalbuminemic patients. Most opioids have little or no adverse effect on the liver; however, intravenous morphine should be avoided in dogs with hepatic dysfunc-

BOX 20-1

Selected Anesthetic Agents for Animals With Hepatic Disease Causing Hepatic Insufficiency*

Premedication

Give atropine (0.02–0.04 mg/kg SC or IM) or glycopyrrolate (0.005–0.011 mg/kg SC or IM) plus hydromorphone (0.1–0.2 mg/kg SC or IM)† or butorphanol (0.2–0.4 mg/kg SC or IM) or buprenorphine (5–15 μg/kg IM)

Induction

Diazepam (0.2 mg/kg IV) plus etomidate (0.5–1.5 mg/kg IV) or propofol (4 mg/kg IV to effect); as an alternative, if the patient is not vomiting, use mask induction or give thiopental at reduced doses

Maintenance

Isoflurane or sevoflurane

SC, Subcutaneous; *IM,* intramuscular; *IV,* intravenous.
*See p. 545 for recommendations for patients with portosystemic shunts.
†Use 0.01 mg/kg in cats.

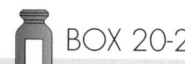 BOX 20-2

Antibiotics in Animals With Hepatocellular Compromise

Ampicillin

22 mg/kg IV, IM, or SC, tid to qid

Metronidazole (Flagyl)

10–15 mg/kg PO, tid

Cefazolin (Ancef, Kefzol)

22 mg/kg IV or IM, tid to qid

Clindamycin (Antirobe)

11 mg/kg IV or PO, bid to tid

IV, Intravenous; *IM,* intramuscular; *SC,* subcutaneous; *tid,* three times a day; *qid,* four times a day; *PO,* oral; *bid,* twice a day.

tion because it may cause hepatic congestion through histamine release and hepatic vein spasm. Although some opioid analgesics may have prolonged action when hepatic function is reduced, their effects can be antagonized.

Barbiturates (e.g., thiopental) should be used cautiously or avoided in patients with significant hepatic disease because these drugs may have a prolonged duration of action; however, propofol (at reduced doses) has been used successfully in patients with hepatic dysfunction. Ketamine is metabolized in the liver of dogs (it is excreted largely unchanged in the urine of cats), and its central stimulant action may precipitate seizures in encephalopathic patients. Therefore ketamine should be administered at reduced dosages to dogs with mild hepatic dysfunction and avoided in patients with severe dysfunction. See recommendations on p. 545 for anesthetic management of animals with portosystemic shunts.

Inhalation anesthetics are the preferred method of maintaining anesthesia in patients undergoing hepatic surgery. The heart rate and rhythm, respiratory rate, and urine output should be monitored. Hyperventilation may cause a significant decrease in portal blood flow. Isoflurane causes decreases in portal blood flow, but hepatic arterial blood flow tends to increase during isoflurane anesthesia, preserving hepatic oxygenation. Isoflurane and sevoflurane have not been associated with postoperative hepatic dysfunction; therefore they are the inhalation agents of choice for patients with severe hepatic disease. Monitoring of the blood gases, blood pressure, blood glucose concentration, hematocrit, and total protein is advantageous in these patients.

ANTIBIOTICS

Aerobic and anaerobic bacteria normally reside in the liver, but may proliferate with hepatic ischemia or hypoxia. Therefore prophylactic antibiotics are warranted in patients

with severe hepatic disease that are undergoing hepatic surgery. The pharmacokinetics of antibiotics may be altered in these patients by depressed hepatic metabolism, alterations in hepatic arterial or portal blood flow, hypoalbuminemia, or reductions in biliary excretion. Antibiotics are specifically indicated in the treatment of hepatic encephalopathy (see p. 544), bacterial hepatitis, and hepatic abscesses. Broad-spectrum antibiotics effective against anaerobes (i.e., penicillin derivatives, metronidazole, and clindamycin) are appropriate and relatively safe in patients with hepatocellular compromise (Box 20-2). Potentially hepatotoxic antibiotics (e.g., chloramphenicol, chlortetracycline, or erythromycin) should be avoided if possible.

NOTE: Metronidazole, when administered at doses above 50 mg/kg of body weight per day, can cause severe neurologic signs (e.g., central vestibular signs including ataxia, nystagmus, head tilt, and seizures) in some dogs.

SURGICAL ANATOMY

The diaphragmatic surface (parietal surface) of the liver is convex and lies mainly in touch with the diaphragm. The visceral surface faces caudoventrally and to the left, and contacts the stomach, duodenum, pancreas, and right kidney. There are six hepatic lobes (Fig. 20-1). The borders of the liver are normally sharp, but appear more rounded in young animals and in those with infiltrated, congested, or scarred livers. The liver has two afferent blood supplies, a low-pressure portal system and a high-pressure arterial system. The portal vein drains the stomach, intestines, pancreas, and spleen and supplies four fifths of the blood that enters the liver. The remainder of the afferent blood supply is from the proper hepatic arteries. These arteries are branches of the common hepatic artery and may number between two and five. The efferent drainage of the liver is through the hepatic veins. In the fetal pup, the ductus venosus shunts blood from

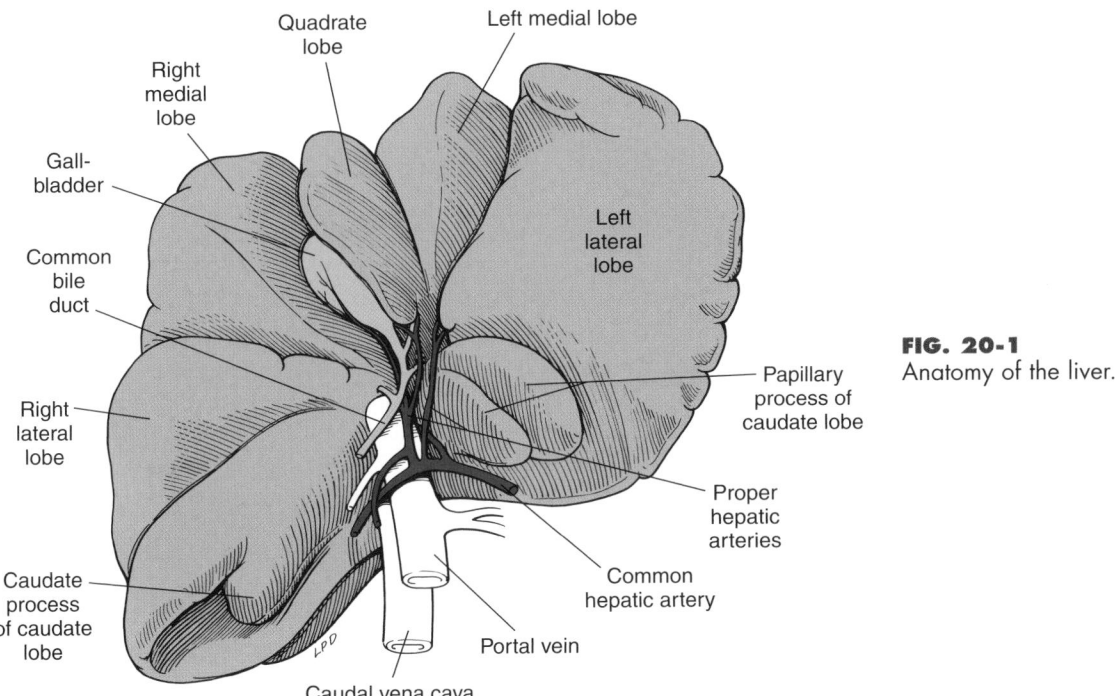

FIG. 20-1
Anatomy of the liver.

the umbilical vein to the hepatic venous system. The ductus venosus becomes fibrotic after birth and is known as the ligamentum venosum. Bile, formed in the liver, is discharged into bile canaliculi lying between the hepatocytes. These canaliculi unite to form interlobular ducts that ultimately merge to form lobar or bile ducts (see p. 561). The portal vein, bile ducts, hepatic artery, lymphatics, and nerves are contained in the lacelike and nonsupporting portion of the lesser omentum known as the hepatoduodenal ligament.

> NOTE: Use caution when dissecting around the pylorus to prevent damaging the common bile duct.

SURGICAL TECHNIQUE

Surgery of the liver is complicated by the fact that hepatic tissue is friable. Because of the sparsity of fibrous protein in the liver, sharp dissection is difficult and results in retraction of blood vessels and bile ducts in the friable stroma. Ligation of structures (i.e., blood vessels and bile ducts) after they have been cut is extremely difficult. Packing the liver firmly enough to obtain hemostasis may cause compressed cells to become ischemic and necrotic. Maintaining hepatic blood supply is important because the liver normally harbors pathogenic anaerobes. For these reasons, surgery of the liver requires techniques different from those used in surgery on most other abdominal organs.

Hepatic biopsies are commonly indicated in patients known to have or suspected of having hepatic disease. The biopsies may be obtained percutaneously, with laparoscopy (see p. 535), or at surgery. Partial hepatectomies are less commonly performed, but may be indicated for focal neo-

plasms or trauma. The standard approach for hepatic surgery is a cranial ventral midline abdominal incision. The caudal aspect of the sternum can be split if additional exposure is needed.

> NOTE: Be sure to obtain a liver biopsy in all patients with clinical signs or laboratory abnormalities consistent with hepatic disease, or whenever the liver appears grossly abnormal.

Percutaneous Liver Biopsy

Percutaneous core biopsies or fine-needle aspirations are relatively inexpensive, easy techniques that can be sensitive and specific for focal lesions (i.e., tumors such as carcinomas and lymphosarcoma) when used with ultrasound guidance. However, with the exception of feline hepatic lipidosis, these percutaneous techniques are very insensitive and unreliable in patients with diffuse hepatic disease (i.e., inflammation, fibrosis, cirrhosis, and necrosis) and those that may have congenital vascular shunts, and are not recommended in these cases. Animals with clinical bleeding, severe thrombocytopenia (i.e., fewer than 20,000 platelets/μl), cavitary lesions, a prolonged mucosal bleeding time, or highly vascular lesions (determined with ultrasound) generally should not have percutaneous core biopsies because of the risk of uncontrollable hemorrhage or abdominal infection. Caution is also recommended with fine-needle aspiration in these patients.

Tissue core biopsies may be obtained with a TruCut biopsy (Fig. 20-2), a large-bore needle, or an automated biopsy device (e.g., Bard Biopty Instrument). For histopathologic

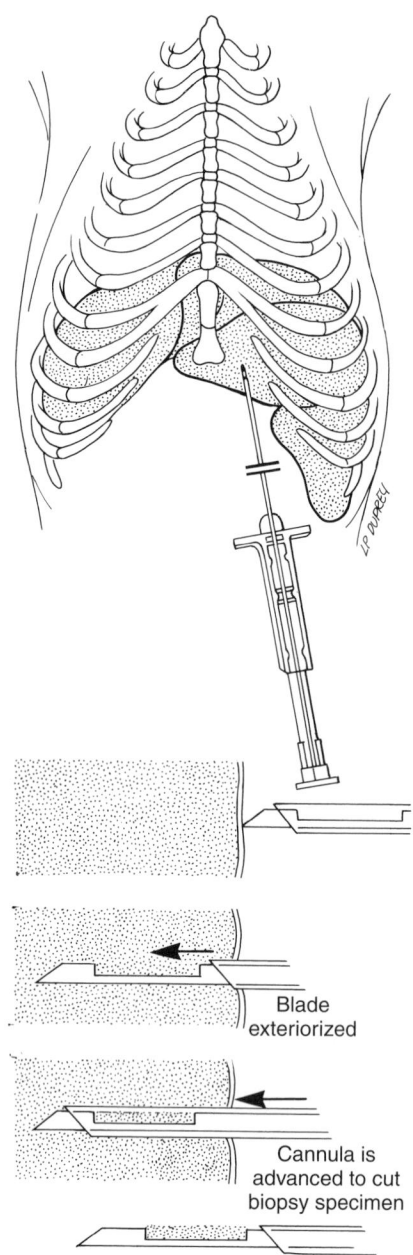

FIG. 20-2
Tissue core biopsy.

Blade
exteriorized

Cannula is
advanced to cut
biopsy specimen

the liver and lacerate structures (e.g., veins, stomach, intestines, diaphragm, lungs, and heart) under the hepatic lobe from which a biopsy is being taken.

Fine-needle aspirates may be obtained using two different techniques. First, a hand-held syringe or an aspiration gun with a syringe may be attached to a 20- to 25-gauge, 1- to 3-inch needle. A syringe with a small amount of air is then attached to the needle, and the cells are blown out onto a slide. In the second technique, the needle is repeatedly passed through the liver without any suction being applied. After several passes, the needle is attached to a syringe and the contents are blown out onto a slide. Fine-needle aspiration is most likely to be diagnostic in patients with diffuse hepatic neoplasia (e.g., lymphosarcoma) or feline idiopathic hepatic lipidosis. However, inability to diagnose these conditions on a fine-needle aspirate does not preclude disease, and even if one of these conditions is found, there could be other, undiagnosed diseases present. This latter possibility is particularly important in cats because almost all sick, anorexic cats will have some fat vacuoles in the hepatocytes (Willard et al, 1999). However, before clinical illness due to hepatic lipidosis can be diagnosed, one must determine that there is sufficient fat in the hepatocytes to be causing hepatic dysfunction. Furthermore, diagnosing hepatic lipidosis does not guarantee that there is not other hepatic disease present that was not found by the fine needle technique. Cytologic evaluation of ultrasound-guided, fine-needle aspirates is most likely to agree with histopathologic findings when the animal has vacuolar hepatopathy; however, this condition was commonly misdiagnosed by cytology. In a recent study, overall agreement between cytology and histopathology in dogs and cats was 30.3% and 51.2%, respectively (Wang et al, 2004). In another study, in which morphologic diagnoses were made by use of an 18-gauge needle, concurrence with wedge biopsy specimens was approximately 50% in both dogs and cats (Cole et al, 2002). The substantial limitations of diagnosing hepatic disease in dogs and cats by percutaneous techniques should be recognized by clinicians (Cohen et al, 2003).

NOTE: Percutaneous biopsies may be obtained under tranquilization or heavy sedation using a transthoracic or transabdominal approach, although the former should only be used if the latter is not possible to prevent laceration of the liver during respiration. The latter is described here.

Percutaneous blind biopsy. *With the animal in dorsal recumbency, clip the hair from the area surrounding the xiphoid process and prepare it for aseptic surgery. Make a small incision in the skin on the left side between the costal arch and the xiphoid process. Insert the biopsy needle through the skin incision in a craniodorsal direction, angling it slightly toward the left of midline. Advance the needle until ultrasound guidance shows the needle to be positioned at the surface of the liver. Advance the biopsy needle into the hepatic tissue and obtain the biopsy sample (see Fig. 20-2).*

specimens, the TruCut needle should be removed from the syringe or gun and placed in formalin. Once the sample has been fixed, it should be removed from the needle for processing. A core biopsy should use the largest gauge needle that may safely be used in the patient, typically a 14-gauge needle. If core biopsies are performed, at least two or three (2 cm long) samples should be obtained. Core biopsies are generally only taken from one liver lobe (i.e., the left liver lobe so as to minimize the chance of lacerating the bile ducts or gallbladder, which are on the right side). However, this is a significant limitation because hepatic lesions may not be present in all liver lobes. Finally, extreme care must be taken to ensure that the core biopsy needle will not pass through

Percutaneous ultrasound-guided biopsy. There are three ultrasound-guided methods that can be used to biopsy or aspirate hepatic structures or lesions. Any of these techniques may be used when obtaining samples of the liver. If diffuse disease is suspected, the left liver should be sampled to avoid the main biliary structures. The first technique is called the *indirect guidance method* and is not generally recommended. It entails using ultrasound to find the structure of interest and then the ultrasound probe is removed. The needle is passed blindly in the area of interest. This technique is only applicable when the target is extremely large and direct visualization of the needle is not required as it is passed into the structure for biopsy or aspiration.

The other two techniques allow direct visualization of the needle as it is passed into the liver. It is critical that the needle pass at an oblique angle to the ultrasound beam for it to be seen on the image. A needle that passes parallel to the beam will not create useful echoes. The second technique is the *freehand technique*. This method requires good hand-eye coordination and takes practice to master it. Many sonographers prefer this technique because it allows the operator more choices in approaching the structure.

Handle the ultrasound probe with one hand (usually the nondominant hand) and the needle with the opposite hand. Use the probe to visualize the structure of interest and then pass the needle into it and obtain the biopsy.

The last technique is the *needle guide technique*. Many ultrasound machines have a manufactured needle guide, which fits onto the transducer. This equipment will guide the needle in a preset angle and maintain the orientation to the transducer. Software on the machine will project the needle path onto the screen, which allows accurate placement of the needle. One problem with this approach is that the needle guide is often bulky and thus the choice of approaches may be limited, particularly in small animals. Because the needle is passed through the needle guide, sterile technique is essential.

Sterilize the guide before use. Apply a sterile covering to the transducer (a sterile surgical glove works well). Place coupling gel into the glove, and then fit it over the transducer. Then attach the guide. Pass the needle through the needle guide, and obtain the biopsy.

Laparoscopic Liver Biopsy

Laparoscopy (see Chapter 14) offers the clinician several advantages over other hepatic biopsy techniques. First, laparoscopy not uncommonly finds lesions missed by ultrasound, allowing the clinician to take a biopsy from clearly abnormal areas that would have been missed if using a percutaneous technique (Cardi et al, 1997). Second, laparoscopy allows one to obtain better tissue samples than is possible with percutaneous techniques (sufficient hepatic tissue can readily be obtained for histopathology, mineral analysis, and culture), and it allows biopsies from multiple liver lobes (as

opposed to just one lobe, as commonly occurs with core needle techniques). At the same time, the endoscopist can quickly look around the abdomen and examine the peritoneum, omentum, stomach, pancreas, intestines, and/or kidneys to see if there is any other unsuspected disease. Finally, laparoscopy can be done quickly (i.e., <20 minutes), and the patient routinely is able to be discharged within hours of completion of the procedure. Coagulopathies are not an absolute contraindication unless they are severe; electrocautery and coagulation-enhancing materials can be used, but are seldom needed.

Hepatic biopsy is obtained by using "double spoon" type forceps.

If no focal abnormalities are found, open the forceps and place them around the edge of the liver lobe. Then push the forceps into the lobe until the entire cup of the biopsy forceps is filled with hepatic tissue. Tightly close the jaws, and pull the sample off the lobe. If a biopsy of a different area of the liver lobe is desired, open the forceps and thrust the lower jaw into the liver lobe at the desired spot. Once the lower jaw is thrust as far as desired into the liver lobe, close the upper jaw over the lower jaw, and retrieve the tissue sample.

> NOTE: Hemorrhage routinely occurs when the sample is torn off the liver; but remember that the laparoscope will magnify any hemorrhage that occurs. Typically, there is less than 1 to 5 ml of blood lost with a biopsy.

Surgical Liver Biopsy

Biopsies of the liver should be routinely done during exploratory laparotomy in animals known to have or suspected of having liver disease. Surgical biopsy allows the entire liver to be thoroughly inspected and palpated, and biopsies taken of focal lesions for histopathologic examination, culture, or copper analysis. Furthermore, hemorrhage from the biopsy site can be readily identified and controlled with proper technique. If generalized hepatic disease is present, the sample can be taken from the most accessible site (marginal biopsy samples). With focal disease, the entire liver should be carefully palpated for intraparenchymal nodules or cavities and representative samples obtained. The information gained from histologic examination of the patient's liver may prove beneficial in determining the prognosis, diagnosis, and long-term management of hepatic dysfunction.

A biopsy of the hepatic margin may be obtained by the "guillotine" method.

Place a loop of suture around the protruding margin of a liver lobe. Pull the ligature tight, and allow it to crush through the hepatic parenchyma before tying it (Fig. 20-3, A). As the suture tears through the soft hepatic tissue, vessels and biliary ducts are ligated. Hold the liver gently between the fingers and, using a sharp blade, cut the hepatic tissue approximately 5 mm distal to the ligature (allowing the

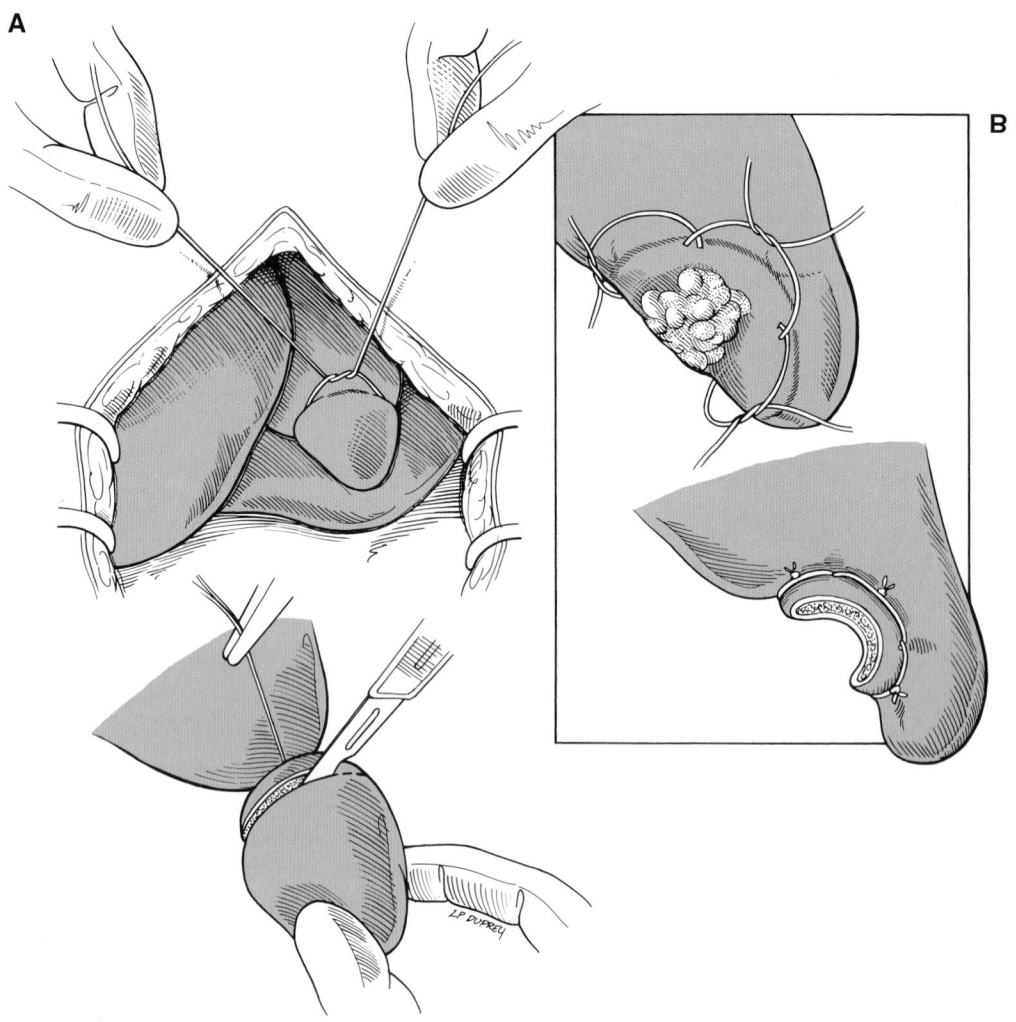

FIG. 20-3
Biopsy of the hepatic margin by the "guillotine" method. **A,** Place a loop of suture around the protruding margin of a liver lobe. Pull the ligature tight and allow it to crush through the hepatic parenchyma before tying it. Using a sharp blade, cut the hepatic tissue approximately 5 mm distal to the ligature. **B,** As an alternative, place several overlapping guillotine sutures around the margin of the lesion and excise it.

stump of crushed tissue to remain with the ligature). To prevent crushing the biopsy sample and causing artifacts, do not handle it with tissue forceps. Place a portion of the sample in formalin for histologic examination; reserve the remainder for culture and cytologic study. Check the biopsy site for hemorrhage. If hemorrhage continues, place a pledget of absorbable gelatin foam over the site. As an alternative, if a biopsy of a focal (nonmarginal) area of the liver is to be taken, use a punch biopsy or TruCut biopsy (see Fig. 20-2), or place several overlapping guillotine sutures around the margin of the lesion and excise it (Fig. 20-3, B).

Biopsies may also be obtained using a biopsy punch. The punch is used to excise a small portion of the liver, and a pledget of absorbable gelatin sponge is placed into the defect until bleeding stops.

Use caution with a punch biopsy to avoid penetrating more than half the thickness of the liver with each biopsy. Apply pressure to the site until bleeding stops. If hemorrhage continues, place a pledget of absorbable gelatin sponge over the site.

Partial Lobectomy

Partial lobectomy may be indicated in some cases when the disease involves only a portion of a liver lobe (e.g., peripheral hepatic arteriovenous [A-V] fistulae, focal neoplasia, hepatic abscesses, or trauma). Partial lobectomy may be challenging because of the difficulty in obtaining hemostasis and should be done with extreme caution in animals with bleeding disorders. Stapling instruments have been used for both partial and complete lobectomies, but discretion should be exercised in their use because hemorrhage may occur if the staples do not adequately compress hepatic tissue.

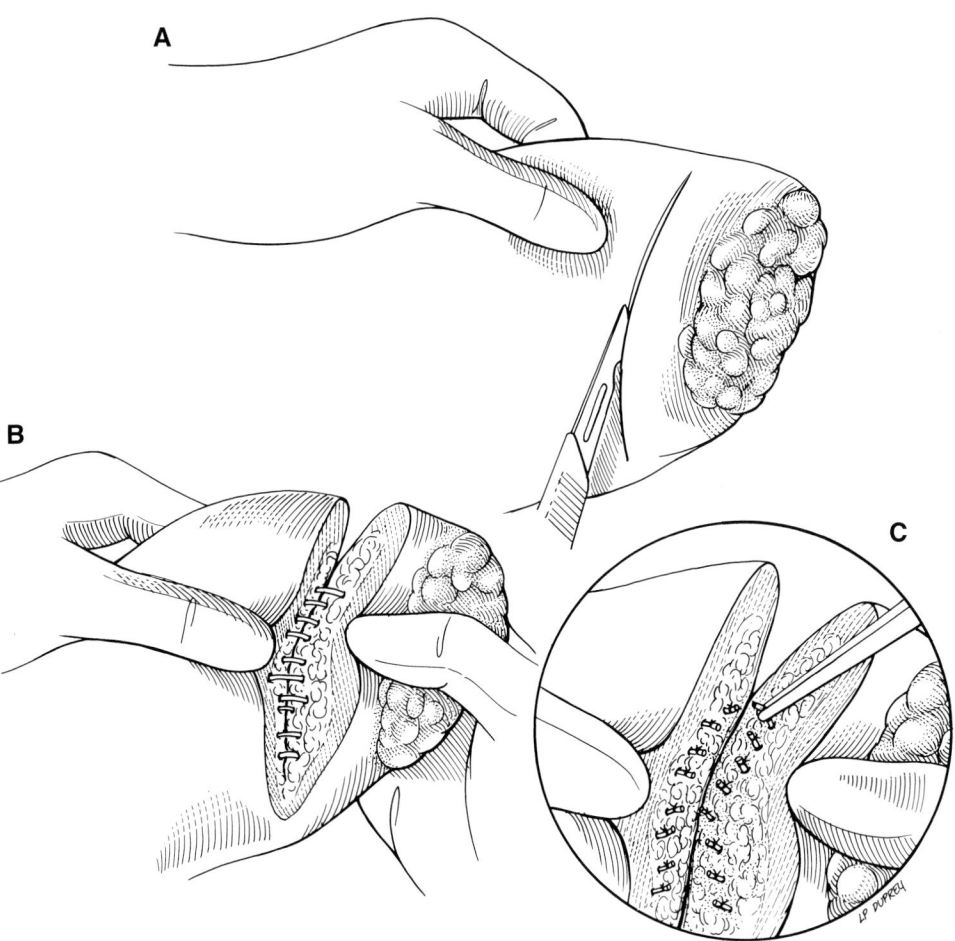

FIG. 20-4
Partial lobectomy. **A,** Determine the line of separation between normal hepatic parenchyma and that to be removed, and sharply incise the liver capsule along the selected site. **B,** Bluntly fracture the liver and expose the parenchymal vessels. **C,** Ligate large vessels and electrocoagulate small bleeders.

Determine the line of separation between normal hepatic parenchyma and that to be removed, and sharply incise the liver capsule along the selected site (Fig. 20-4, A). Bluntly fracture the liver with the fingers (Fig. 20-4, B) or the blunt end of a Bard-Parker scalpel handle, and expose the parenchymal vessels. Ligate large vessels (hemoclips may be used), and electrocoagulate small bleeders encountered during the dissection (Fig. 20-4, C). As an alternative, place a stapling device (Autosuture TA 90, 55, or 30) across the base of the lobe and deploy the staples. Excise the hepatic parenchyma distal to the ligatures or staples. Before closing the abdomen, make sure the raw surface of the liver is dry and free of hemorrhage. In small dogs and cats, several overlapping guillotine sutures (as described previously) may be placed along the entire line of demarcation (Fig. 20-5). Be sure the entire width of the hepatic parenchyma is included in the sutures. After tightening the sutures securely, use a sharp blade to cut the hepatic tissue distal to the ligature, allowing a stump of crushed tissue to remain with the ligature.

Complete Lobectomy

Complete lobectomy may be indicated for some focal lesions involving one or two hepatic lobes (e.g., traumatic lacerations of the liver or hepatic A-V fistulae). The left lobes of the liver (i.e., left lateral and left medial lobes) maintain their separation near the hilus more than do the other lobes; therefore the left lobes often can be removed in small dogs and cats by placing a single encircling ligature around the base of the lobe.

For the right lateral and caudate lobes, careful dissection around the hepatic caudal vena cava usually is necessary. Before performing the dissection, pass umbilical tape around the portal vein, celiac artery, cranial mesenteric arteries, and caudal vena cava in front of and behind the liver. The tape is passed through rubber tubing, which can be used to occlude the hepatic blood supply if uncontrollable hemorrhage occurs.

For the left lobes in small dogs and cats, crush the parenchyma near the hilus with the fingers or a forceps. Place an encircling ligature around the crushed area and tie. For the left lobes in larger dogs and for the right and caudate lobes, carefully dissect, if necessary, the lobe from the caudal vena cava. Isolate the blood vessels and biliary ducts near the hilus and ligate them. Double ligate or oversew the ends of large vessels. Resect the parenchymal tissue, leaving a stump of tissue distal to the ligatures to prevent retraction of the hepatic tissue from the ligatures and subsequent hemorrhage.

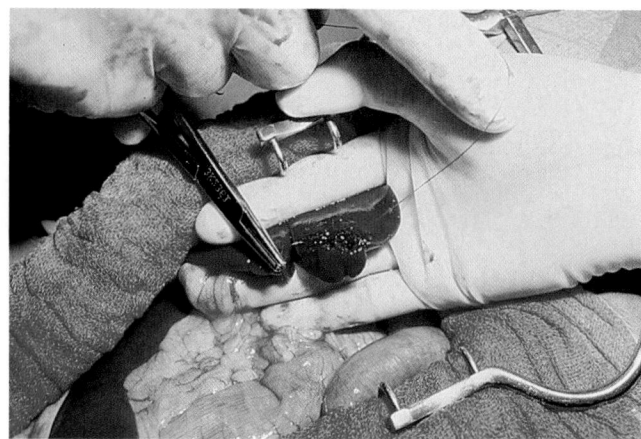

FIG. 20-5
In small dogs and cats, partial hepatectomy may be performed by placing several overlapping guillotine sutures proximal to the tissue to be excised.

HEALING OF THE LIVER

The liver is unique among the visceral organs in its healing properties. It has relatively little connective tissue stroma, is highly susceptible to small changes in blood flow, and has an enormous regenerative capacity. With regeneration, adequate liver function is possible in patients even after 80% of the organ has been removed or destroyed. Lacerations of the liver should be closed only when bleeding is profuse. If lacerations are sutured, they should be closed in a manner that does not create an internal pocket of bile or blood or cause ischemia of the surrounding cells. The proper hepatic artery can be ligated as an emergency measure to control hemorrhage from extensive liver lacerations. Complex fractures or severe contusions should be treated by hepatic lobectomy if ligation of the hepatic artery does not result in hemostasis.

SUTURE MATERIALS AND SPECIAL INSTRUMENTS

Guillotine biopsies often are performed with large (0 or 2-0) chromic gut suture or polyglactin 910. Suture with good knot security (e.g., silk suture) may facilitate partial hepatectomy. Polydioxanone or polyglyconate suture may also be used for vessel ligation in complete and partial lobectomies.

POSTOPERATIVE CARE AND ASSESSMENT

Recovery from anesthesia should be closely monitored in animals with severe hepatic dysfunction. Because of the increased half-life of some drugs in patients with hepatic dysfunction, recovery may be prolonged. Intravenous fluids should be provided until the patient is able to maintain hydration, but care must be taken not to overhydrate hypoalbuminemic patients. Blood glucose levels should be monitored; transient hypoglycemia is common after removal of large portions of the liver. Albumin levels should be monitored. If the patient becomes severely hypoalbuminemic (i.e., less than 2 g/dl) or has substantial worsening of third

space fluid accumulation, one should consider administering plasma, whole blood, or synthetic colloids (e.g., hetastarch). Clotting times may be assessed if hemorrhage or petechiation occurs. Antibiotics given during surgery should be continued for 2 to 3 days if partial hepatectomy has been performed. Nutritional supplementation may be necessary in some patients during the early postoperative period, particularly if the animal is anorexic or has severe vomiting or diarrhea (see Chapter 11).

Analgesics (e.g., hydromorphone, butorphanol, and buprenorphine) should be provided to patients after surgery (see Table 13-4 on p. 133). For severe pain, a fentanyl-lidocaine-ketamine combination given as a continuous rate infusion (CRI) may be indicated (see Box 13-1 on p. 136).

COMPLICATIONS

Biopsy samples may be useless for diagnosis if the tissue sample is crushed, fragmented, or too small or if the specimen contains predominantly blood or necrotic portions of mass lesions. Bile peritonitis may occur if the gallbladder or bile ducts are inadvertently penetrated. One study found the complication rate in 246 animals undergoing ultrasound-guided biopsy of abdominal structures to be 1.2%. The most important complication may be the propensity for an incorrect diagnosis when this technique is used (see previous discussion).

The most common and serious complication of hepatic surgery is hemorrhage. This may result from ligatures slipping off friable hepatic tissue. Care should be taken to ensure that a stump of tissue remains distal to the ligature when encircling sutures are used for biopsy or partial hepatectomy. With hepatic trauma anaerobic bacteria may proliferate in hypoxic portions of the liver and cause sepsis; therefore broad-spectrum antibiotics should be used in patients with severe hepatic trauma and in those undergoing hepatic surgery. Complications after major hepatic resection may include portal hypertension, ascites, fever, hemorrhage, or persistent bile drainage.

SPECIAL AGE CONSIDERATIONS

Portosystemic shunt ligation (see p. 544) often is performed in young animals, which are particularly prone to hypoglycemia. Serum glucose concentrations should be carefully monitored. Hypothermia, also a particular problem in young patients, reduces the minimum alveolar concentration (MAC) of inhalants used for anesthetic maintenance.

References

Cardi M, Muttillo IA, Amaderi L et al: Superiority of laparoscopy compared to ultrasonography in diagnosis of widespread liver disease, *Dig Dis Sci* 42:546, 1997.

Cohen M, Wright JC, Welles EA et al: Evaluation of sensitivity and specificity of cytologic examination: 269 cases (1999-2000), *J Am Vet Med Assoc* 222:964, 2003.

Cole TL, Center SA, Flood SN et al: Diagnostic comparison of needle and wedge biopsy specimens of the liver in dogs and cats, *J Am Vet Med Assoc* 220:1483, 2002.

Wang KY, Panciera DL, Al-Rukibat RK et al: Accuracy of ultrasound-guided fine-needle aspiration of liver and cytologic findings in dogs and cats: 97 cases (1990-2000), *J Am Vet Med Assoc* 224:75, 2004.

Willard MD, Weeks BR, Johnson M: Fine needle aspirate cytology suggesting hepatic lipidosis in 4 cats with infiltrative hepatic diseases, *J Fel Med Surg* 1:215, 1999.

Suggested Reading

Niza MMRE, Ferreira AJA, Peleteiro MC et al: Bacteriologic study of the liver in dogs, *J Small Anim Pract* 45:401, 2004.
This study showed that the normal liver of healthy dogs harbors different bacterial species. The types of bacteria seen are reviewed along with histologic findings.

SPECIFIC DISEASES

PORTOSYSTEMIC VASCULAR ANOMALIES

DEFINITIONS

Portosystemic vascular anomalies (PSVA) or **portosystemic shunts (PSS)** are anomalous vessels that allow normal portal blood to drain from the stomach, intestines, pancreas, and spleen and pass directly into the systemic circulation without first passing through the liver. The term portacaval shunt is frequently used; however, this term technically refers to a specific type of vascular anomaly (i.e., portal vein to caudal vena cava). **Extrahepatic shunts** are vascular anomalies located outside the hepatic parenchyma; **intrahepatic portosystemic shunts (IHPSS)** are located in the liver. The term "**hepatic microvascular dysplasia**" seems to be in the process of being replaced with "**portal vein hypoplasia**." Portal vein hypoplasia appears to be a condition characterized by small or absent intrahepatic portal vessels and portal arteriolar hyperplasia that is associated with microscopic shunting of blood through the liver without a macroscopic portosystemic shunt.

GENERAL CONSIDERATIONS AND CLINICALLY RELEVANT PATHOPHYSIOLOGY

When portal blood bypasses the liver, many substances that are normally metabolized or excreted in the liver enter the systemic circulation. Also, important hepatotropic substances from the pancreas (e.g., insulin) and intestines do not reach the liver, resulting in hepatic atrophy or failure of the liver to attain normal size. Hepatic insufficiency or hepatic encephalopathy frequently occurs. Hepatic encephalopathy is a clinical syndrome of altered CNS function resulting from hepatic insufficiency. A variety of substances (i.e., ammonia, methionine/mercaptans, short-chain fatty acids, alterations in the ratio between circulating levels of branched-chain and aromatic amino acids, and γ-aminobutyric acid) have been incriminated in the resulting elaboration of false neurotransmitters.

Portosystemic shunts may be broadly categorized as intrahepatic or extrahepatic. Extrahepatic shunts may be congenital or acquired. Congenital extrahepatic shunts usually are

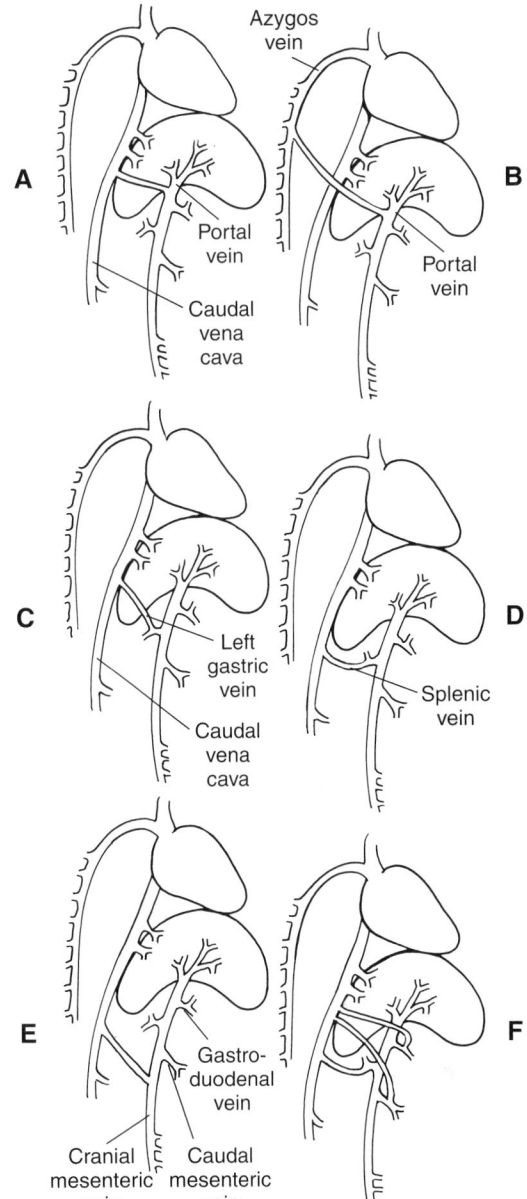

FIG. 20-6
Portosystemic shunts described in dogs and cats. **A,** Portal vein to caudal vena cava. **B,** Portal vein to azygos vein. **C,** Left gastric vein to caudal vena cava. **D,** Splenic vein to caudal vena cava. **E,** Left gastric, cranial mesenteric, caudal mesenteric, or gastroduodenal vein to caudal vena cava. **F,** Combinations of the above.

single anomalous vessels that allow abnormal blood flow from the portal vein to the systemic circulation. Extrahepatic PSS account for nearly 63% of single shunts in dogs; they also occur in cats. Many different types of PSS have been described in dogs, including (1) portal vein to caudal vena cava; (2) portal vein to azygos vein; (3) left gastric vein to caudal vena cava; (4) splenic vein to caudal vena cava; (5) left gastric, cranial mesenteric, caudal mesenteric, or gastroduodenal vein to caudal vena cava; and (6) combinations of the above (Fig. 20-6). Cats most commonly have a large single vessel that empties

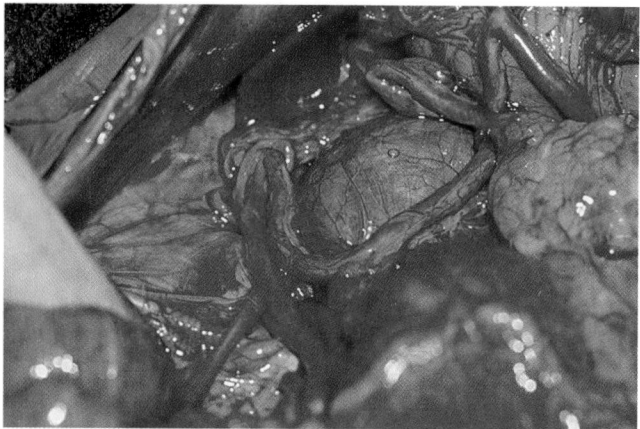

FIG. 20-7
Multiple shunts near the left kidney in a dog with hepatic disease and portal hypertension.

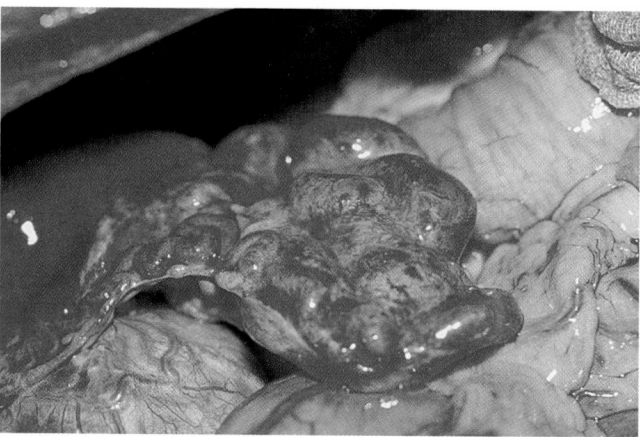

FIG. 20-8
Hepatic arteriovenous fistula in a 1-year-old Labrador. Note the dilated vessels in the hepatic parenchyma. The fistula was found during surgery for a gastric foreign body.

directly into the prehepatic vena cava; however, they may have atypical PSS connections and the shunt may flow into any systemic vessel including the renal, phrenicoabdominal, azygos, or internal thoracic veins. Intrahepatic shunts usually are congenital, singular shunts, which occur because the ductus venosus fails to close after birth, or they may arise when other portal to hepatic vein or caudal vena cava anastomoses exist. Congenital IHPSS constitute about 35% of single shunts in dogs and approximately 10% in cats.

Acquired extrahepatic shunts typically are multiple and represent about 20% of all canine PSS. They are thought to arise partly because of increased resistance to portal blood flow and subsequent portal hypertension. This hypertension causes normal, nonfunctional microvascular connections, which are present at birth, between portal and systemic veins to become functional. Multiple shunts are most commonly associated with chronic, severe hepatic disease (i.e., cirrhosis), but have been reported secondary to hepatoportal fibrosis in young dogs. Venoocclusive hepatic disease has been reported as a cause of multiple PSS in young cocker spaniels. Multiple shunts most commonly occur in the left renal area and the root of the mesentery (Fig. 20-7), and connections to the caudal vena cava or azygos veins usually are seen.

Our knowledge of hepatic microvascular dysplasia (i.e., portal vein hypoplasia [PVH]) is currently being redefined, and it may be different by the time this chapter is published. Current thought is that PVH is a congenital condition characterized by small or absent intrahepatic portal vessels and portal arteriolar hyperplasia, which allows an abnormal communication between the portal and systemic circulations. This condition is sometimes difficult to differentiate from congenital PSS because both may have similarly increased serum bile acid concentrations. Furthermore, the histologic lesions of PSS and PVH are identical, and PVH is common in some breeds that are at increased risk for PSS. In general, most dogs with PVH are asymptomatic and do not have ob-

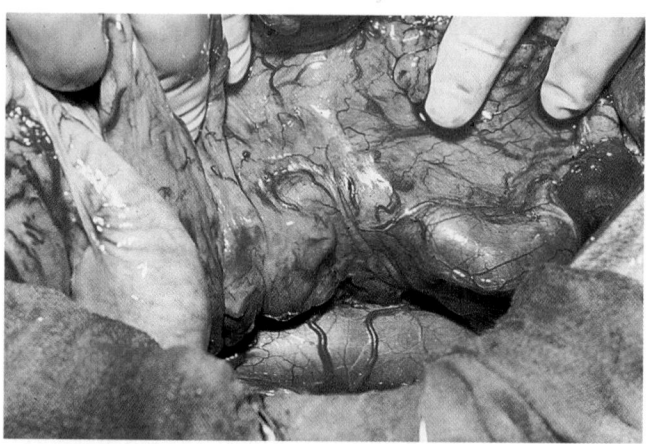

FIG. 20-9
Multiple collateral shunting vessels in the dog in Fig. 20-8.

vious microhepatica, but exceptions exist. In particular, there is concern that PVH can progress and result in noncirrhotic portal hypertension and/or hepatoportal fibrosis in some patients. Currently, PVH is diagnosed by hepatic histology plus elimination of PSS. Mesenteric portograms and nuclear scintigraphy in dogs with PVH should be normal.

A-V fistulae account for about 2% of single shunts and may be congenital or acquired. Acquired A-V fistulae occur secondary to trauma, tumors, surgical procedures, or degenerative processes that cause arteries to rupture into adjacent veins. The fistulae typically are macroscopic communications that form between branches of the hepatic artery and portal vein; however, microscopic hepatic A-V fistulae have also been suspected. As congenital lesions, they are believed to develop as a result of failure of the common embryologic capillary plexus to differentiate into an artery or a vein. Affected animals usually develop portal hypertension and multiple collateral shunting vessels, resulting in an acute onset of low protein transudative ascites between the ages of 2 and 18 months (Figs. 20-8 and 20-9). In contrast, dogs with congenital PSS rarely have ascites.

DIAGNOSIS
Clinical Presentation

Signalment. Purebred dogs are at increased risk for PSS and PVH. Domestic shorthair cats are most commonly affected, although these aberrations also occur in purebred cats (i.e., Himalayan). Single PSS usually are congenital and are most commonly diagnosed in animals under 1 year of age, although dogs as old as 13 years have been diagnosed. Extrahepatic shunts have been most frequently diagnosed in miniature and toy-breed dogs (e.g., Yorkshire terriers, Maltese, Silky terriers, miniature schnauzers, poodles, Lhasa apso, Bichon Frise, Jack Russell Terriers, Shih Tzu, and Pekingese). They are clearly hereditary in Yorkshire terriers (Tobias, 2003; Tobias and Rorbach, 2003) and may be genetic in other breeds as well. Intrahepatic PSS are more commonly diagnosed in large-breed dogs (e.g., German shepherds, golden retrievers, Doberman pinschers, Labrador retrievers, Irish setters, Samoyeds, and Irish wolfhounds). Small-breed dogs most likely to have IHPSS are toy and miniature poodles. There may be a hereditary basis for IHPSS in Irish wolfhounds. Congenital extrahepatic and IHPSS have been reported in cats. There is no convincing gender predisposition for these anomalies in either species.

> NOTE: In general, small-breed dogs are more likely to have extrahepatic shunts, and large-breed dogs are more likely to have IHPSS.

Multiple shunts are most commonly diagnosed in animals between 1 and 7 years of age; however, multiple acquired PSS that occur secondary to hepatoportal fibrosis have been reported in dogs as young as 4 months of age. Breeds most commonly affected include the German shepherd, Doberman pinscher, and cocker spaniel. Multiple acquired shunts have been described in cats.

Most dogs with hepatic A-V fistulae have been young (i.e., under 1½ years of age) at the time of diagnosis. Congenital hepatic A-V fistulae have rarely been reported in cats.

History. The presenting history for animals with PSS varies considerably. Affected animals usually are evaluated because of failure to grow, small body stature, or weight loss. Other common abnormalities include intermittent anorexia, depression, vomiting, polydipsia or polyuria, ptyalism (especially in cats), pica, amaurosis, and behavioral changes. Some animals are presented for evaluation of urinary dysfunction (i.e., hematuria, dysuria, pollakiuria, stranguria, and urethral obstruction) associated with urate urolithiasis (see p. 542). Signs of hepatic encephalopathy can vary tremendously from those that are extremely mild and hard to identify as a significant abnormality (e.g., lethargy, being "tired," being "slow") to severe changes (e.g., ataxia, weakness, stupor, head pressing, circling, amaurosis, pacing, sei-

zures, or coma). These signs may be constant or intermittent and sometimes, but not invariably, worsen after eating (especially a high-protein diet composed of animal protein). Hepatic encephalopathy may also worsen after gastrointestinal hemorrhage (e.g., caused by parasites or ulceration). In a recent study, 82% of dogs had CNS signs, 76% had gastrointestinal signs, and 39% had urinary signs (Mehl et al, 2005). In addition to ptyalism, affected cats typically show episodic central blindness.

> NOTE: Consider PSS in any young animal with a prolonged response to anesthetic agents or tranquilizers that require hepatic metabolism for clearance. These may be the first abnormalities you note in some affected animals.

The most common presenting sign in dogs with hepatic A-V fistulae is sudden onset of depression, ascites, and vomiting. Despite the chronic nature of this condition, the animal often has an acute onset of gastrointestinal or neurologic signs. The ascites typically is a pure transudate despite a serum albumin greater than 1.8 g/dl.

> NOTE: Animals with hepatic A-V fistulae may be presented for evaluation of gastrointestinal foreign bodies. Presumably gastric irritation causes pica in these animals.

Physical Examination Findings

Most animals with PSS have microhepatica, and the kidneys may feel prominent or plump. A golden or copper color to the iris has been observed in many cats with PSS. Neurologic abnormalities may be noted (see previous discussion). Ptyalism is a common finding in cats, but rare in dogs. Animals with hepatic A-V fistulae may have a palpably enlarged liver (rare) or ascites. An audible bruit sometimes can be auscultated in the cranial abdomen of affected animals.

Diagnostic Imaging

Survey abdominal radiographs are an important part of screening for congenital PSS. Microhepatica is expected in affected patients and may vary from mild to marked. It is extremely rare to find a dog with PSS that does not have some degree of microhepatica, and failure to find this change is an indication to look for diseases other than congenital PSS. Plain abdominal radiographs are more sensitive in finding microhepatica than abdominal ultrasound.

Definitive diagnosis of PSS is made by surgical identification of the shunt, intraoperative positive contrast portography, ultrasound identification of the shunt, or nuclear hepatic scintigraphy. Various positive contrast techniques have been described, including splenoportography, cranial mesenteric arterial portography, celiac arteriography, transsplenic portal catheterization, and jejunal vein portography. Jejunal vein portography is the simplest and most effective

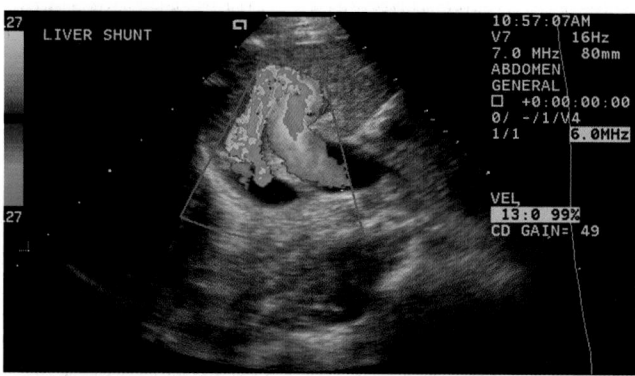

FIG 20-10
Ultrasound image with color Doppler showing a large, tortuous intrahepatic shunt.

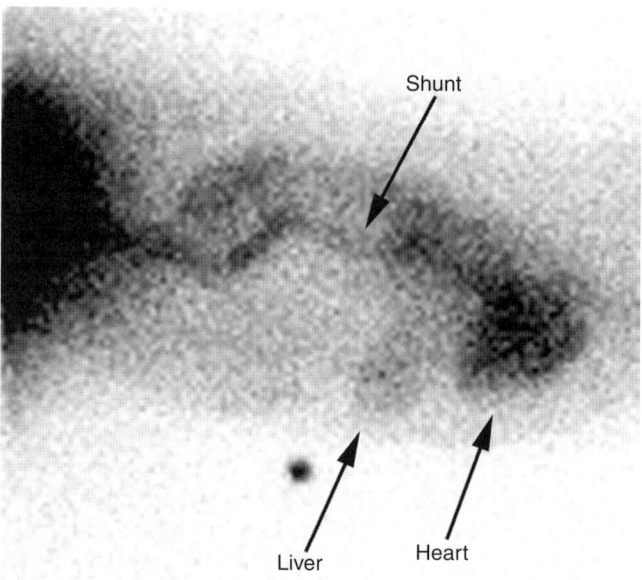

FIG 20-11
Composite image of transrectal portal scintigraphy. The dog's head is to the right of the image. Notice the severe lack of uptake by the liver, which supports the diagnosis of portosystemic shunting. The shunt vessel can be identified in this study.

portographic technique (see p. 548). Ultrasound-guided splenoportography can also be performed in large- breed dogs. The most consistent finding on survey abdominal radiographs is microhepatica.

Ultrasound has become the diagnostic tool of choice for imaging PSS. Both intrahepatic and extrahepatic shunts have been identified with this technique; however, an inconclusive ultrasound examination does not rule out PSS. Ultrasound diagnosis of PSS is dependent upon operator experience and the time allotted to examine the patient. Occasionally a dilated intrahepatic vessel or the communication of an intrahepatic shunt with the caudal vena cava is noted (Fig. 20-10). With extrahepatic shunts, overlying bowel may obscure the shunt, but a small liver with few detectable hepatic or portal veins may be noted. Increased hepatic arterial detection using Doppler is also a common finding. The bladder and renal pelves should be assessed for calculi because urate stones usually are radiolucent and difficult to see on survey abdominal radiographs. Ultrasound scanning is also useful to identify the anechoic, tortuous vessels seen with hepatic A-V fistulae. Pulsed wave Doppler ultrasound may assist in making a diagnosis of hepatic A-V fistulae. Visualization of retrograde (hepatofugal), pulsatile flow in the abnormal portal vein branch and the main portal vein may allow one to discern the involved liver lobe and resect it.

Nuclear scintigraphy is a rapid, noninvasive method of documenting abnormal hepatic blood flow. Sodium pertechnetate technetium 99m (99mTc) is typically used in scintigraphic studies to detect PSS. After colonic administration of 99mTc, the time when activity in the region of the liver is first noted is compared with the time when activity appears in the region of the heart (Fig. 20-11). Animals with liver-to-heart intervals longer than 12 seconds are generally considered clinically normal. Sometimes studies in very small animals can be difficult to interpret because of the close proximity of the liver and heart, and occasional studies must be repeated if the 99mTc is not rapidly absorbed from the colon. If a study must be repeated, it must be done the following day to allow the body to eliminate the technetium from the invalid study. False positive results have not been reported; however, false negative results may occur if a small shunt involves only a peripheral portion of the portal system. PVH will have a normal scintigraphic study, which distinguishes it from PSS. Computed tomography (CT) angiography appears to be a useful technique for identifying PSS, including multiple acquired shunts; however, there are too few studies to know the accuracy of this technique. A new scintigraphic technique has recently been reported (Cole et al, 2005; Morandi et al, 2005)—transsplenic portal scintigraphy. This technique is unique in that it uses ultrasound guidance to inject a small amount of 99mTc into the parenchyma of the spleen. Dynamic phase imaging of the splenic vein drainage yields a nuclear angiogram of the portal system and is useful for detecting the presence of either single or multiple extrahepatic shunts. An advantage of this technique is that a very small amount of radioactivity is used, thus the animal can be released from radiation isolation shortly after the procedure, depending on the state's release criteria. Furthermore, the authors have found that transsplenic portal scintigraphy yields higher quality images than transrectal scintigraphy.

> NOTE: Nuclear scintigraphy is a useful, noninvasive screening tool for diagnosing congenital or acquired shunts, and distinguishes them from PVH.

Laboratory Findings

Hematologic, serum biochemical, and urine analysis of animals with PSS may disclose various abnormalities, but dogs can have a congenital PSS without any abnormalities on complete blood count (CBC) or serum biochemistry panel. Hematologic abnormalities may include microcytosis with normochromic erythrocytes, mild nonregenerative anemia, target cell formation, or poikilocytosis. Low serum iron concentrations appear to be related to the development of microcytosis in dogs with PSS. Biochemical tests often reveal a reduction in the serum albumin, cholesterol, and/or blood urea nitrogen (BUN) concentrations. Low serum albumin is a common finding in dogs; however, some dogs (and most cats) with PSS have normal albumin levels. Low BUN results from reduced conversion of ammonia to urea in the hepatic urea cycle, but the polyuria-polydipsia seen in many patients may contribute. Other abnormalities occasionally include mild to major increases in serum alanine aminotransferase, aspartate aminotransferase, and alkaline phosphatase. The serum bilirubin concentration usually is normal. Fasting hypoglycemia rarely occurs. Functional measurements of coagulation (i.e., prothrombin time, activated partial thromboplastin time, and activated coagulation time) usually are normal. Routine urinalysis may disclose dilute urine or ammonium biurate crystals. Hyperuricemia and hyperammonemia lead to increased urinary excretion of urate and ammonia, promoting urinary precipitation of ammonium biurate crystals. Hematuria, pyuria, and proteinuria may occur if urate calculi form. The hematologic and biochemical profiles of canine hepatic A-V fistulae can be similar to those of dogs with single or multiple PSS.

Hepatic function tests are important in screening for congenital PSS. Serum bile acids have been the standard hepatic function test in dogs and cats for years, but it is now recognized that they have some major limitations. First, it is critical to measure both preprandial and postprandial serum bile acid concentrations; approximately 20% of dogs have a higher preprandial value. Second, some dogs with very high serum bile acid concentrations (>150 μmol/L) do not have clinically significant hepatic disease, whereas some dogs with congenital PSS have serum bile acid concentrations that are only moderately increased (e.g., 50 to 60 μmol/L, normal <30 μmol/L). Third, unlike what is expected for most biochemical determinations, there can be substantial variation in bile acid concentrations from day to day (as much as or greater than 100%). Currently, urinary bile acids (Balkman et al, 2003; Trainor et al, 2003) appear to be about as useful as serum bile acids, but may have the advantage of being easier to collect (i.e., the owner can bring in a urine sample as opposed to bringing in the patient), especially in cats.

Hyperammonemia is very specific for hepatic insufficiency, but simply measuring resting blood ammonia is very insensitive, even in patients experiencing hepatic encephalopathy. The ammonia tolerance test (ATT) is a very sensitive test, but performing the test is difficult (many animals vomit or defecate the ammonia chloride that is administered). Measuring 6- to 8-hour postprandial blood ammonia concentrations appears to be more sensitive than measuring fasting blood ammonia (Walker et al, 2001), but is probably less sensitive than the ATT. The biggest disadvantage of measuring blood ammonia is that it is easy to obtain artifactual values if instructions in collecting, storing, and preparing the blood are not followed exactly. This test must be run in-house; it cannot be sent to an outside lab.

DIFFERENTIAL DIAGNOSIS

PSS must be differentiated from other diseases that cause hepatic insufficiency (e.g., cirrhosis) or neurologic abnormalities (e.g., hydrocephalus and epilepsy) in dogs and cats. Performing survey abdominal radiographs (to look for microhepatica) and a hepatic function test (usually preprandial and postprandial serum bile acids) are the typical means of screening for congenital PSS. If either of these tests is normal, then congenital PSS is unlikely, and other diseases must be seriously considered.

MEDICAL MANAGEMENT

Surgery is the treatment of choice for most animals with PSS because hepatic function may continue to deteriorate as long as most of the blood is shunted away from the liver. The life expectancy of animals that are managed medically generally is reported to be 2 months to 2 years; however, one study suggested that the older a dog is when presented for treatment, the better its prognosis on conservative treatment (Watson and Heritage, 1998). In particular, medical management must be considered in asymptomatic dogs that have been fortuitously diagnosed and dogs older than 7 years old that have minimal clinical signs. In these patients, one must weigh the reported 7% mortality associated with corrective surgery versus the likelihood of substantial deterioration if surgery is not done. Although not proven, intuitively it appears that the patients described above, if they have only modest changes on serum biochemistry panel and only modest to moderate microhepatica on abdominal radiographs, may be the best candidates for medical management. If there are histologic changes (e.g., bridging hepatic fibrosis or bridging biliary hyperplasia) that would seem to make postsurgical complications (e.g., portal hypertension) more likely, then medical management should probably be chosen over surgery. However, surgery is desirable in that restoration of hepatotropic factors in the liver postoperatively should promote hepatic regeneration. Medical management should be initiated before surgical intervention in animals with substantial signs of hepatic encephalopathy (some argue this should be routine; see later discussion in the Preoperative Management section).

The goals of medical therapy are to identify and correct factors predisposing to hepatic encephalopathy (i.e., reduce absorption of toxins produced by intestinal bacteria, diminish the interaction between enteric bacteria and nitrogenous substances, and avoid drugs that predispose to encephalopathy), and to decrease oxidative damage to hepatocytes. Precipitating factors for hepatic encephalopathy include high-protein meals (especially meat), bacterial infections, gastrointestinal bleeding, blood transfusions, inappropriate drug therapy, and electrolyte and acid-base abnormalities. General supportive care of the patient with hepatic encephalopathy should include fluid therapy (0.9% sodium chloride

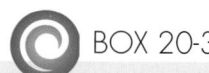

BOX 20-3

Drugs Used in the Management of Portosystemic Shunts

Neomycin (Biosol)
10–15 mg/kg PO, bid to tid

Metronidazole (Flagyl)
10 mg/kg PO, tid

Ampicillin
22 mg/kg IV, IM, or SC, tid to qid

Lactulose (Cephalac, Chronulac)
Dogs: start with 1 ml/4.5 kg PO, qd to tid, titrate to obtain soft, formed feces
Cats: start with 5 ml/cat PO, tid, titrate to obtain soft, formed feces

PO, Oral; *bid*, twice a day; *tid*, three times a day; *IV*, intravenous; *IM*, intramuscular; *SC*, subcutaneous; *qid*, four times a day; *qd*, every day.

[NaCl] or 0.45% NaCl and 2.5% dextrose), normalization of acid-base disturbances, and supplementation of potassium as needed. A highly digestible diet in which the primary source of calories is carbohydrates should be fed. For long-term dietary management, feed the lowest-protein diet (preferentially vegetable protein or cottage cheese) the animal will tolerate. Moderately protein-restricted diets (i.e., k/d or in some animals u/d; Hill's Pet Products) that contain high levels of branched-chain amino acids and arginine are often used, but there is no good evidence that preferentially feeding branched-chain as opposed to aromatic amino acids benefits dogs with PSS. Antibiotics (Box 20-3) are used to reduce the enteric flora that produce many of the toxins (i.e., ammonia) thought to cause hepatic encephalopathy. Oral neomycin frequently is used for this purpose, but it should be avoided in animals that are azotemic. Metronidazole or ampicillin (either oral or parenteral) also reduces intestinal ammonia concentrations. Lactulose is a synthetic disaccharide that acidifies colonic contents and traps ammonium ions in the lumen (see Box 20-3). It is also an osmotic cathartic that shortens the intestinal transit time and reduces the production and absorption of ammonia. Lactulose may be given orally or as a retention enema. Side effects of lactulose administration may include diarrhea, vomiting, anorexia, and increased gastrointestinal loss of potassium and water. Treatment of animals that are presented for therapy in hepatic coma must be prompt and aggressive; cleansing enemas (warm water) and retention enemas with neomycin or lactulose (or both) should be given. Acid-base and electrolyte abnormalities and hypoglycemia must be identified and corrected. Diazepam is often ineffective in encephalopathic dogs having seizures; phenobarbital may be more effective, and some patients must be anesthetized with propofol. A medical text should be consulted for additional recommendations on the management of coma that occurs secondary to hepatic insufficiency.

It is now recognized that dogs with PSS experience oxidative damage to the hepatocytes. Antioxidants help protect the hepatocyte membrane, especially in those patients that will not have surgery. Vitamin E (be sure to use d-alpha-tocopherol), s-adenosyl-L-methionine, and vitamin C are commonly used and appear effective. Ursodeoxycholic acid helps protect the hepatocyte. Consult a medical text for further details on hepatosupportive therapy with such drugs.

SURGICAL TREATMENT

The goal of surgery is to identify and occlude or attenuate the abnormal vessel. Ameroid constrictors (Fig. 20-12) or cellophane bands are now commonly used in animals with extrahepatic shunts to slowly occlude the shunt vessel. With an ameroid constrictor, initial shunt constriction is effected by swelling of the hygroscopic material that makes up the inner portion of the device (see Fig. 20-12); additional shunt occlusion occurs as fibrosis develops around the vessel. Importantly, the rate of vascular occlusion may affect the animal's propensity to develop acquired shunts after occlusion. Plasma protein concentration may affect the rate of closure of ameroid constrictors, and applying silicone to the ameroid may slow its rate of closure (Monnet and Rosenberg, 2005). Complete occlusion of the vessel may not occur; 8 of 14 cats had persistent shunting 8 to 10 weeks after ameroid constrictor placement in one study (Kyles et al, 2002). Approximately 21% of animals have persistent shunting 6 to 10 weeks after placement of an ameroid (Mehl et al, 2005). Vascular occlusion may occur as a result of thrombus formation in some dogs.

Cellophane banding causes an initial acute inflammatory response followed by a chronic low-grade foreign body tissue reaction. Vascular attenuation may be slower and less complete with cellophane bands than with ameroid constrictors. In a recent study of 106 dogs and 5 cats in which cellophane bands were placed, clinical signs attributed to PSS resolved or were substantially attenuated in all survivors (Hunt et al, 2004). Multiple acquired shunts occurring post PSS ligation were documented in only two animals in the aforementioned study.

When the shunt or shunts are identified during abdominal exploration, positive contrast portography examination generally is unnecessary. However, if a shunt is not identified visually, mesenteric portography or retrograde portography may be used to help identify its location and nature. Sometimes placing a catheter through the shunt during retrograde portography (see p. 549) and leaving it there will allow the surgeon to find some shunts that are especially difficult to find.

Preoperative Management

Encephalopathic patients should be stabilized before surgery. There is currently debate as to the value of pretreating surgical candidates with potassium bromide (dogs) or phenobarbital (cats) to attempt to lessen the incidence of postoperative seizures. The high incidence of postligation sei-

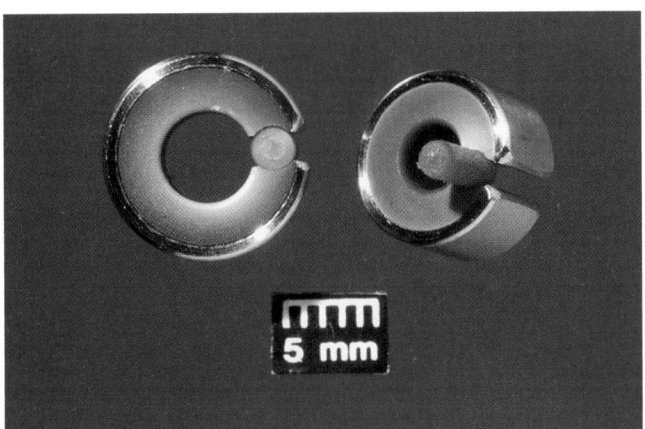

FIG. 20-12
An ameroid constrictor.

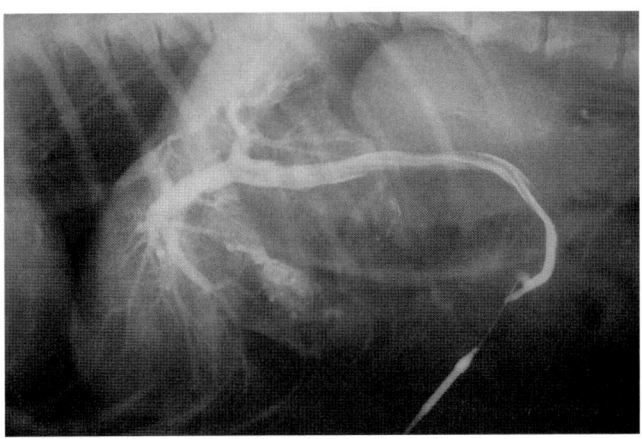

FIG. 20-13
Mesenteric portogram in a dog with a normal portal system. The portal system originates at the level of the first lumbar vertebra. Note the hepatic vasculature.

zures in cats makes this approach seem reasonable in that species. Fluid and electrolyte imbalances should be corrected preoperatively. Perioperative antibiotics (e.g., cephalosporins) are recommended for patients with PSS. See the previous section on Medical Management for other recommendations.

Anesthesia

Extreme care must be exercised when anesthetizing an animal having PSS. Because of the reduced liver function and abnormal hepatic blood flow, drug absorption, metabolism, and clearance are notably reduced. In addition, drugs that are highly protein bound are affected by the low albumin concentrations that may accompany PSS (i.e., resulting in increased levels of circulating, unbound drugs). Therefore drugs that are metabolized by the liver (e.g., phenothiazine tranquilizers) and those that are highly protein bound (e.g., diazepam) should be avoided. Benzodiazepines may also negatively affect neurologic function in hepatoencephalopathic patients. A reversible opioid may be administered with an anticholinergic, followed by mask or chamber induction with isoflurane or sevoflurane and oxygen and endotracheal intubation (Box 20-4). Propofol, a noncumulative, nonbarbiturate hypnotic, has been used successfully at reduced doses for induction of patients with PSS (Box 20-4). Blood glucose levels should be monitored because patients with PSS may have reduced hepatic glycogen stores. Care should be taken to prevent hypothermia. Inotropic support (i.e., dobutamine [2 to 10 μg/kg/minute IV] or dopamine [2 to 10 μg/kg/minute IV]) may be necessary in some patients. These patients should be monitored for arrhythmias or tachycardia.

Surgical Anatomy

The canine portal vein varies from 3 to 8 cm long, depending on the animal's size. On a radiographic contrast study of the normal portal system, the portal system usually originates at the level of the first lumbar vertebra (Fig. 20-13). Knowledge

 BOX 20-4

Selected Anesthetic Protocols for Animals With Portosystemic Shunts

Dogs

Premedication

Give atropine (0.02–0.04 mg/kg SC or IM) or glycopyrrolate (0.005–0.011 mg/kg SC or IM) plus hydromorphone (0.1–0.2 mg/kg SC or IM)

Induction

Mask induce with isoflurane or sevoflurane or administer propofol (4 mg/kg IV to effect)

Maintenance

Isoflurane or sevoflurane

Cats

Premedication

Give atropine (0.02–0.04 mg/kg SC or IM) or glycopyrrolate (0.005–0.011 mg/kg SC or IM) plus butorphanol (0.2–0.4 mg/kg SC or IM) or buprenorphine (5–15 μg/kg IM) or hydromorphone (0.05 mg/kg SC or IM)

Induction

Chamber induce with isoflurane or sevoflurane or administer propofol (4 mg/kg IV to effect)

Maintenance

Isoflurane or sevoflurane

SC, Subcutaneous; *IM*, intramuscular; *IV*, intravenous.

of the anatomy of the portal and hepatic venous systems is imperative to locate shunts, particularly intrahepatic shunts (Fig. 20-14). The portal vein is formed by the confluence of the cranial and caudal mesenteric veins and the splenic vein. The splenic vein enters the portal vein at the level of the thoracolumbar junction. The phrenicoabdominal veins ter-

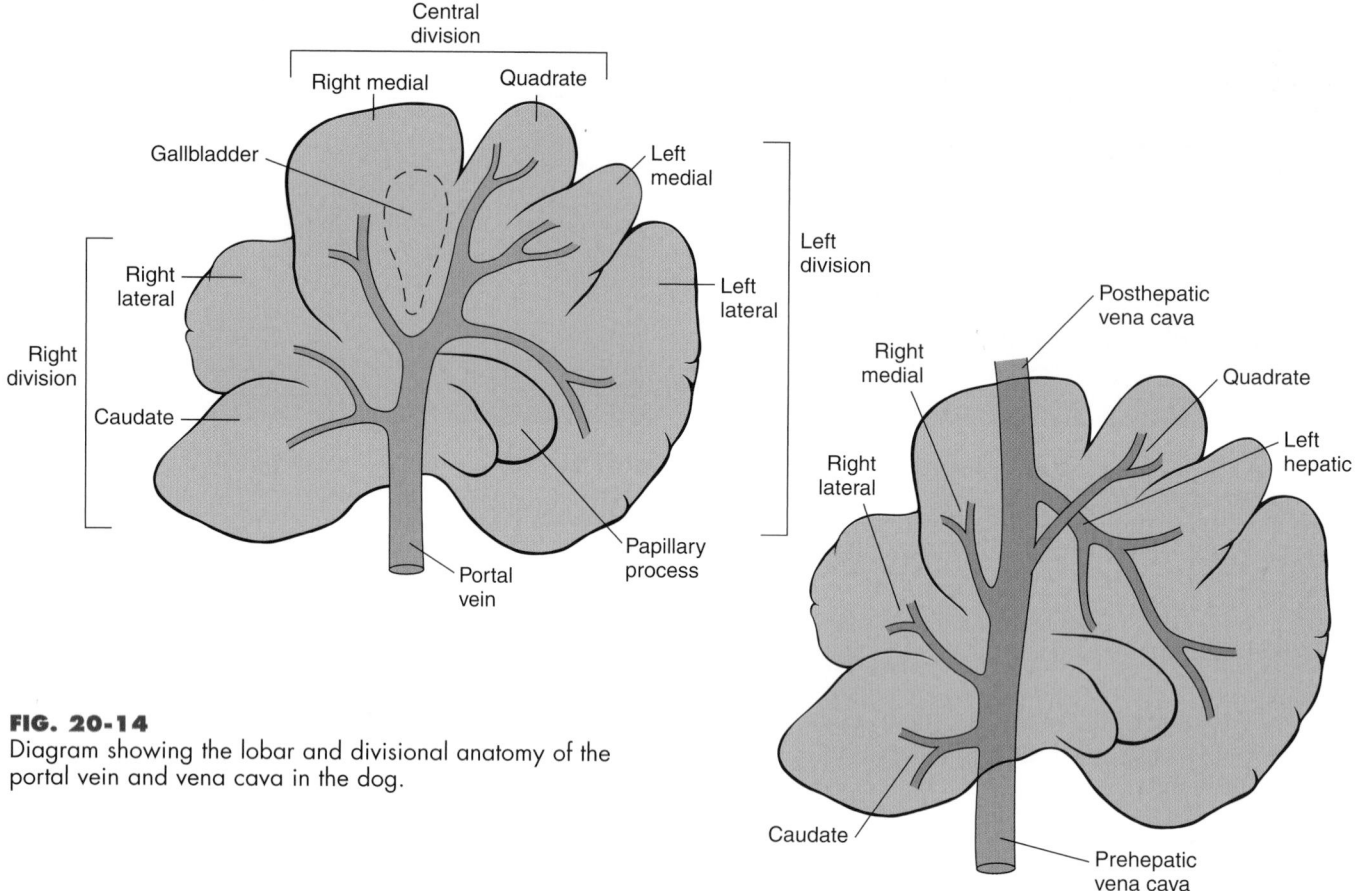

FIG. 20-14
Diagram showing the lobar and divisional anatomy of the portal vein and vena cava in the dog.

minate in the caudal vena cava about 1 cm cranial to the renal veins. Any vein that enters the caudal vena cava cranial to the phrenicoabdominal veins (before the hepatic veins) may be considered an anomalous structure.

> NOTE: Examine the caudal vena cava carefully. The only vessels that should enter the caudal vena cava between the renal veins and the hepatic veins are the small phrenicoabdominal veins.

Positioning

A standard ventral midline celiotomy is performed from the xiphoid cartilage caudally, and the portal system is examined. For IHPSS and A-V fistulae, the incision may need to extend cranially through the xiphoid process and caudal sternebrae.

SURGICAL TECHNIQUE

Single extrahepatic shunts generally are treated by placing an ameroid constrictor or cellophane band on the vessel. Because the vessel slowly becomes occluded, portal hypertension is rare and most surgeons no longer evaluate portal pressures in conjunction with this surgery. When compared with surgical ligation, surgical time is shortened and intraoperative and postoperative complications are decreased with ameroid constrictors (Murphy et al, 2001). In rare

cases, animals with IHPSS may have an ameroid constrictor or cellophane band placed on the vessel; however, IHPSS generally requires ligation. Two additional techniques, intravascular coil occlusion and placement of a portacaval venograft using the jugular vein (with an ameroid constrictor placed on it) with complete ligation of the intrahepatic shunt, have also been used for intrahepatic shunt occlusion. With the latter technique, an unacceptably high incidence of multiple, extrahepatic acquired shunts was noted at long-term follow-up (Kyles et al, 2001).

Animals with congenital PSS should generally have a liver biopsy performed when the shunt is attenuated. However, if the gross appearance of the liver is abnormal (especially if it is rough or irregular), a biopsy of the liver should be taken and the histology report received before attenuating the shunt. PSS patients with chronic fibrotic or biliary hyperplastic changes may be at increased risk for portal hypertension following shunt attenuation.

Animals with multiple hepatic shunts secondary to acquired hepatic disease often benefit from medical management directed at the cause of the hepatic disease (e.g., antiinflammatories, antifibrotic drugs, antioxidants), and subsequent ascites and encephalopathy (e.g., dietary restriction of protein and salt, diuretics). Good medical care may result in long-term survival and a good quality of life; noncirrhotic portal hypertension in particular may respond

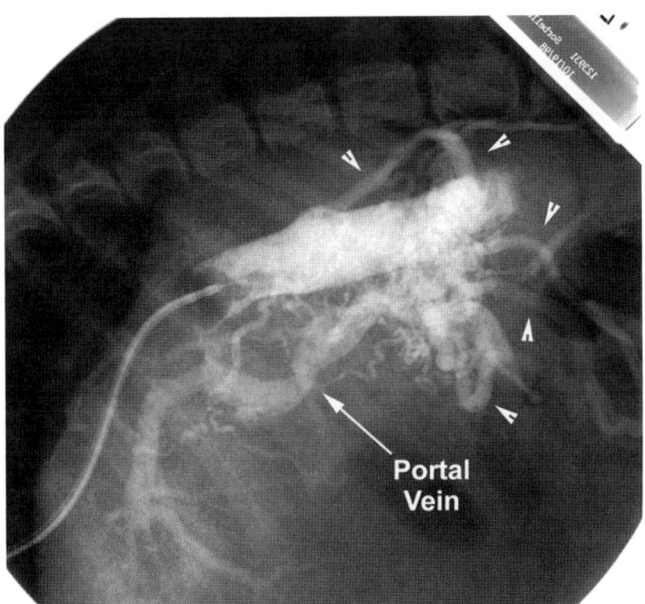

FIG. 20-15
Transvenous retrograde portogram in a dog with multiple acquired shunts.

well. Caudal vena cava banding has been suggested to raise the systemic venous pressure in the abdomen to or slightly above that of the portal venous system, but this technique is of questionable value and is seldom performed. Multiple extrahepatic PSS usually are evident upon exploratory laparotomy in these patients. Findings that may be noted include enlarged mesenteric veins, a larger than normal portal vein, and anomalous connections between the portal venous system and the systemic venous circulation. The most common location for multiple PSS is the area of the left kidney; however, anomalous venous connections between the mesenteric circulation and the caudal vena cava or its tributaries may be noted throughout the abdomen (Fig. 20-15). Portoazygos connections have also been observed in clinical cases. Care should be taken when incising the abdominal wall in patients suspected of having multiple PSS because large, dilated vessels may be present in the falciform ligament or the greater omentum or both. Trauma to these vessels upon abdominal entry may cause significant hemorrhage. Dissection of the falciform ligament usually requires ligation or cauterization of multiple vessels. Because many patients with multiple extrahepatic PSS have ascites, suction should be available upon entry into the abdomen to evacuate ascitic fluid.

NOTE: If you find multiple shunts in an animal, be sure a biopsy is taken from the liver.

A-V fistulae are treated by removing the affected liver lobe or in rare cases by ligating the fistulae directly. Portal pressure should be measured in conjunction with occlusion of IHPSS or vena cava banding. The normal portal pressure

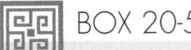 BOX 20-5

Normal Pressures in Dogs

Portal Pressures	Systemic Venous Pressures
8–13 cm H_2O	0–6 cm H_2O
6–10 mm Hg	0–4 mm Hg

in dogs is 8 to 13 cm H_2O, which is 7 to 8 cm H_2O higher than the systemic venous pressure (Box 20-5). However, in animals with single PSS, the resting portal pressure often is closer to the systemic venous pressure. Excessive portal venous pressure can result in splanchnic congestion, portal hypertension, and death.

Ameroid Constrictor Placement on Extrahepatic Shunts

Perform a midline abdominal incision. Identify the portal vein by retracting the duodenum to the left and ventrally. Locate the caudal vena cava, renal veins, phrenicoabdominal veins, and portal vein (ventral to the caudal vena cava at the most dorsal aspect of the mesoduodenum). Note any veins entering the caudal vena cava proximal to the phrenicoabdominal veins. If the shunt has not been identified, open the omental bursa and retract the stomach cranially, the duodenum to the right and ventrally, and the left lobe of the pancreas caudally. Identify shunts that communicate with the caudal vena cava through the epiploic foramen by observing abnormal tributaries of the portal vein, left gastric vein, or splenic vein. Once the shunt has been identified, select the appropriately sized ameroid constrictor. Generally, use a 3.5- or 5-mm ameroid in most small dogs with extrahepatic shunts. Dissect around the shunt vessel to allow placement of the device, but avoid dissecting a large area next to the vessel.

Excessive dissection may allow movement of the ameroid on the vessel and predispose to premature kinking of the vessel.

Place the vessel in the opening of the ameroid so that it sits in the inner circular space of the device. If necessary, place several loops of small (2-0) multifilament suture around the vessel, and use these sutures to flatten the vessel and facilitate manipulation of the vessel into the opening of the ameroid. Once the vessel has been positioned in the ameroid, insert the key in the slit of the device. Evaluate the intestines for evidence of congestion (rare), and close the abdominal incision routinely.

NOTE: The ameroid should fit on the vessel without compromising the lumen; however, avoid using an ameroid that is too large because the weight of the device may cause the vessel to kink, obstructing flow prematurely.

Cellophane Banding of Extrahepatic Shunts

Fold a 10 cm long × 1.2 cm wide strip of cellophane (purchased from a store and sterilized, or use MS 350 grade cellophane [Cello Paper Pty]) longitudinally to form a three-layer strip that is approximately 4 mm wide.

The cellophane may be attached in either of two ways: (1) causing partial obstruction of the shunt at the time of placement (Hunt et al, 2004), or (2) where the cellophane causes no shunt occlusion initially. The second technique is easier to perform, eliminates the need for monitoring portal pressures, and may result in a more favorable outcome than the first technique (H. Seim, personal communication).

For the first technique, pass the cellophane around the shunt and a pin of predetermined size, and place a titanium clip on the strip. To determine pin size in dogs less than 10 kg (which will determine the diameter of the cellophane band), evaluate changes in heart rate, arterial pressure, intestinal color and motility, and pancreatic color when the shunt is totally occluded, or measure portal pressures (see later discussion). If elevations in heart rate are minimal (less than 10 beats/min) and if arterial systolic pressure does not decrease more than 10 mm Hg, use a 2-mm pin to determine the final diameter of the band. If changes are moderate, use a 2.5-mm pin; and if they appear to be severe, use a 3-mm pin. Secure the cellophane band with two titanium ligaclips (Autosuture, Ethicon).

For the second technique, prepare the cellophane as described above, and place it around the vessel without causing any occlusion of the shunt. Secure the cellophane with a hemoclip(s).

Ligation of Single Extrahepatic Shunts

If placement of an ameroid constrictor or cellophane band is not possible, the vessel may be ligated or attenuated; however, extreme care must be taken to prevent causing portal hypertension.

Identify the anomalous vessel, isolate it, and pass 2-0 silk suture around the vessel (Fig. 20-16). If jejunal portography was not performed (see later discussion), exteriorize a segment of jejunum and insert a 20- to 22-gauge over-the-needle catheter (Angiocath, Abbocath) into a jejunal vein. Do not damage the corresponding jejunal artery. Obtain baseline portal pressures. Temporarily occlude the shunt, and observe portal pressures during this manipulation.

Occlusion of the shunt should result in a rapid increase in portal pressure, which aids in confirmation that it is an anomalous vessel.

Check portal pressures carefully before and during shunt ligation. If you are unsure whether complete ligation should be attempted, err on the conservative side and attenuate the shunt. If you are uncertain whether the vessel you have occluded is the shunt, perform jejunal portography.

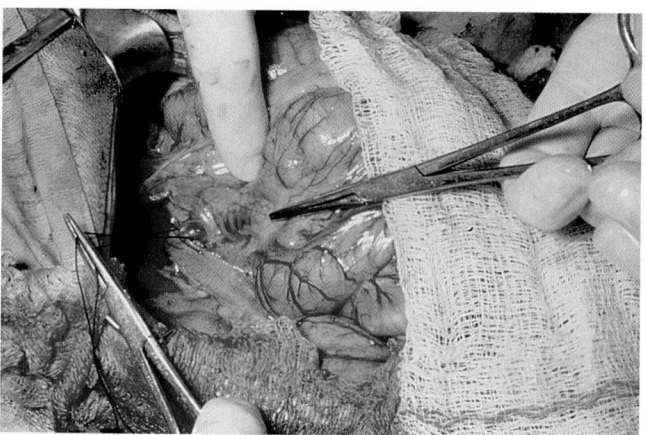

FIG. 20-16
To identify the portal vein, retract the duodenum to the left and ventrally. Note any vessels entering the caudal vena cava proximal to the phrenicoabdominal veins (hemostat). The suture is around a portocaval shunt.

Once you have positively identified the shunt, slowly tighten the ligature while monitoring the portal pressure. If possible, completely occlude the shunting vessel, but do not allow postligation portal pressures to exceed 10 cm H_2O (8 mm Hg) above baseline pressures or 20 to 23 cm H_2O (15 to 18 mm Hg). If intraoperative Doppler ultrasound is available, once hepatopetal flow is established in the cranial portal vein and shunt, do not occlude the shunt further (Szatmari et al, 2004). You may be able only to attenuate the vessel. Observe the viscera for evidence of splanchnic congestion for 5 to 10 minutes. If excessive splanchnic congestion is noted, loosen the suture. Remove the jejunal vein catheter and ligate the vein. Examine the kidneys and bladder for calculi. If cystic calculi are present and if the patient is in stable condition, remove the calculi during the shunt ligation surgery. If operative time has been lengthy or if renal calculi are present, it may be best to schedule a second surgery. Obtain a liver biopsy (see p. 535) before closing the abdomen.

Jejunal Portography

Positive contrast radiographs can determine if the shunt is extrahepatic or intrahepatic. If the caudal extent of the PSS is cranial to T13, the shunt is probably intrahepatic. If the caudal extent of the shunt is caudal to T13, it probably is extrahepatic. Sensitivity of this procedure may be less in dorsal and right lateral recumbency than in left lateral recumbency (Scrivani et al, 2001).

Exteriorize a loop of jejunum. Identify a jejunal vein near the mesenteric border of the intestine and place one or two sutures around the vessel. Insert a 20- to 22-gauge over-the-needle catheter into the vessel (Fig. 20-17), and use the preplaced sutures to secure it to the vessel. Attach a heparinized extension set and three-way stopcock to the catheter.

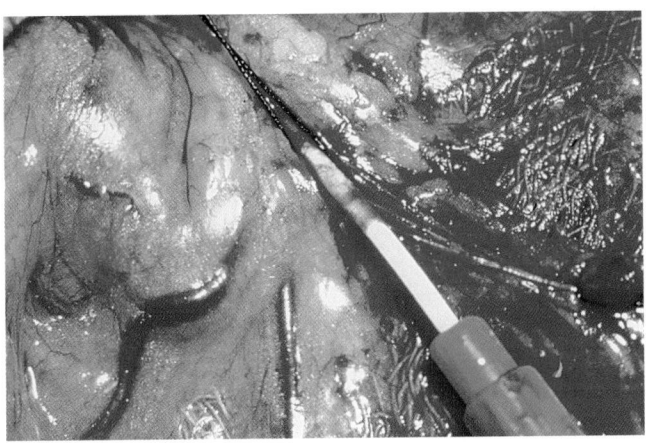

FIG. 20-17
To catheterize a jejunal vein, place one or two sutures around the selected vessel. Insert a 20- to 22-gauge over-the-needle catheter into the vein and use the preplaced sutures to secure it to the vessel.

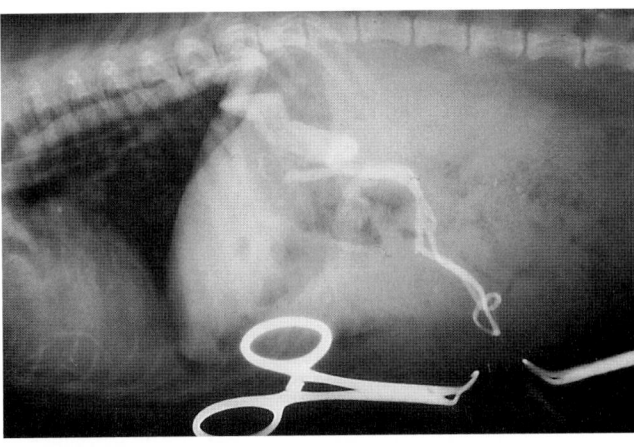

FIG. 20-18
Portogram in a dog with a portoazygos shunt. Notice the lack of contrast filling in the hepatic portal system. Instead, it flows through a tortuous shunting vessel into the azygos vein.

Inject a water-soluble contrast agent (e.g., Renovist) (2 ml/ kg of body weight) as a bolus into the catheter, and make an exposure while the last milliliter is injected. If necessary, make both lateral and ventrodorsal projections to help fully define the location of the shunt (Fig. 20-18). The catheter can also be used for pressure measurement.

With multiple hepatic shunts, radiographic confirmation of the shunts is rarely necessary. The technique of intraoperative mesenteric portography in these patients is the same as for single PSS, except that exposures should be delayed approximately 3 or 4 seconds after the start of injection of the contrast material to allow filling of the shunting vessels.

Transvenous Retrograde Portography

Transvenous retrograde portography provides a method of identifying and characterizing shunts without the need for abdominal surgery (Miller et al, 2002). This technique may be particularly useful in dogs in which the presence of a shunt is questioned because of an atypical history (e.g., a much older patient), discordant findings between nuclear scintigraphy and ultrasonography, or when surgical identification of a shunt was unsuccessful in an animal in which one was strongly suspected preoperatively.

Place the patient in left lateral recumbency, and aseptically prepare the right jugular furrow. In patients that weigh less than 10 kg, catheterize the jugular vein using a percutaneous technique. If the patient weighs more than 10 kg, perform a jugular venous cutdown to facilitate insertion of a large catheter into the vein.

The large catheter is required in big dogs to totally occlude the caudal vena cava.

> NOTE: In patients weighing less than 10 kg, use a 7.5 French dual-lumen flow balloon (Swan-Ganz) catheter; in patients that weigh more than 10 kg, use variably sized balloon dilation catheters to facilitate occlusion of the caudal vena cava.

Following insertion into the introducer or venotomy site, direct the occluding catheter down the cranial vena cava and then in a dorsal direction into the azygos vein. Advance the catheter into the azygos vein as far as is possible without resistance. Inflate the balloon only enough to occlude the vein.

Occasionally, when larger balloon catheters are used, inflation of the balloon is unnecessary because the catheter itself may occlude the lumen sufficiently to allow for retrograde filling of the azygos vein. This seems to be especially true when the azygos vein is normal.

Make a vigorous hand injection of contrast (1 to 2 ml/kg) during fluoroscopic evaluation.

This injection normally results in retrograde filling of the intercostal and vertebral vessels. It is common to see the contrast flow in retrograde fashion into the abdominal cava.

Record the entire injection on videotape. If necessary, make an additional injection if hard copy of the study is required. Make initial images in the lateral projection; perform ventrodorsal or oblique views when indicated.
After the initial injection into the azygos vein, withdraw the catheter into the right atrium and then advance it caudally through the right atrium and into the caudal vena cava. Advance the catheter to a position immediately cranial to the

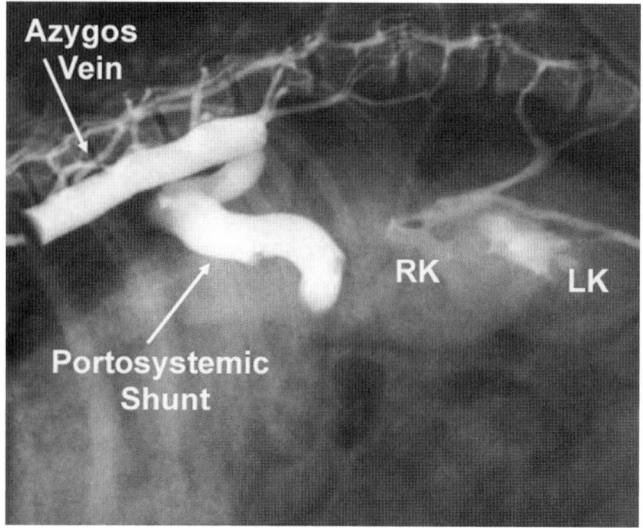

FIG. 20-19
Transvenous retrograde portogram *(lateral view)* in a dog with a portoazygos shunt. *RK,* Right kidney; *LK,* left kidney.

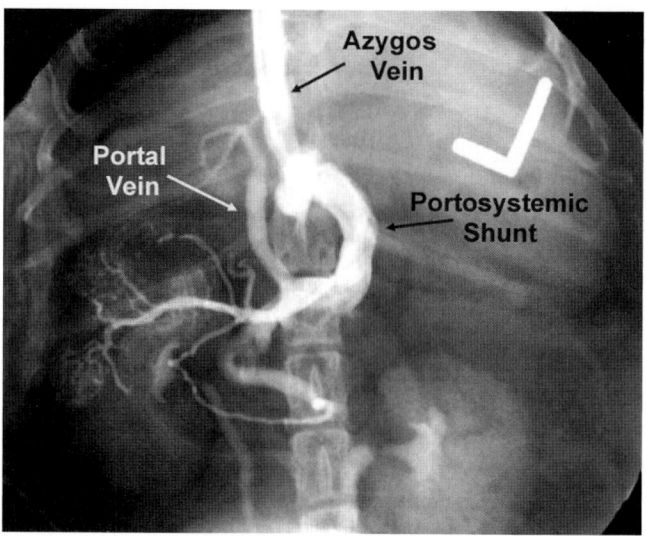

FIG. 20-20
Transvenous retrograde portogram *(ventrodorsal view)* in a dog with a portoazygos shunt.

diaphragm. Once the catheter is in position, inflate the balloon enough to completely occlude the caudal vena cava. Once the caudal vena cava has been occluded, make a vigorous hand injection of contrast (1 to 2 ml/kg) during fluoroscopic evaluation (Figs. 20-19 and 20-20). Occlusion of the caudal vena cava results in retrograde filling of the abdominal cava and the shunt.

In some cases the retrograde filling of the shunt is suboptimal. In those cases, positive pressure ventilation (20 cm H_2O for 5 to 8 seconds) during the injection usually results in improved retrograde filling of the shunt.

> NOTE: It is imperative that the occlusion of the caudal vena cava and subsequent contrast injection be made immediately cranial to the diaphragm. If the occluding balloon is placed at the level of or caudal to the diaphragm, the ostia of shunts that arise in a cranial position may be occluded by the balloon, resulting in a false negative study.

Once the shunt has been identified, attempt selective catheterization of the shunt.

Selective catheterization with a flow-directed balloon allows for more specific opacification of the shunt, providing more detailed anatomic information. In addition, the configuration of the flow-directed balloon catheter allows for measurement of portal pressure both when the shunt is open and when it is occluded by the inflated balloon. Furthermore, selective catheterization of the shunt provides the opportunity to leave the catheter in the shunt lumen, facilitating intraoperative identification of the anomalous vessel.

Remove the catheter after the vessel has been identified and isolated. Remove the introducer and apply local pressure or sacrifice (ligate) the jugular vein and close the skin routinely.

The timing of removal of the introducer and catheters depends on whether the surgeon desires the catheter to be left in the lumen of the shunt during surgery.

Ligation or Attenuation of Intrahepatic Shunts

Both intravascular and extravascular methods have been described for ligation of IHPSS. Ligation of IHPSS can be extremely challenging because the vessel often is difficult to locate. Occasionally the shunt can be identified as a palpable depression or soft spot in a liver lobe, or it may be seen entering the caudal vena cava if it is not completely encircled by hepatic parenchymal tissue. Intraoperative ultrasound scans have been used to help identify the shunt in hepatic tissue, but this technique is not always successful. Intrahepatic shunts are classified as left, central, or right sided. Left and central divisional shunts account for a majority of shunts (see Fig. 20-14). Left sided IHPSS (patent ductus venosus) are typically located in the left lateral or medial hepatic lobes. Ligation or attenuation of the left hepatic vein may be performed in these animals. Central shunts are generally found in the right medial lobe, whereas right shunts are typically located in the right lateral or caudate lobes. An intravascular technique involving temporary hepatic vascular occlusion in conjunction with caudal caval venotomy was described by Breznock for intrahepatic shunt occlusion; however, because this procedure is technically difficult and surgery time is prolonged, many surgeons prefer extravascular techniques. Isolation and obstruction of the specific branch of the portal vein supplying the IHPSS have been described. Indirect passage of suture for ligation of right sided intrahepatic PSS was recently reported (Tobias et al, 2004). The ligature should encircle the right portal branch approximately 4 mm lateral to its bifurcation from the parent vein (see later discussion).

> NOTE: Warn owners that ligation of IHPSS is difficult because the shunts are often hard to identify at surgery.

Isolation and Ligation of IHPSS Involving the Left Medial or Lateral Liver Lobes

Many shunts can be found cranial to the liver.

AP *Extend the abdominal incision proximally into the caudal sternebrae. Incise the diaphragm if necessary. Incise the left triangular ligament, and free the left lateral liver lobe so that it can be retracted to the right. Use a combination of sharp and blunt dissection to isolate the anomalous vessel at its junction with the hepatic vein. Place a single silk ligature around the vessel and attenuate flow while measuring portal pressure. Alternately, ligate or attenuate the left hepatic artery as it enters the liver while measuring portal pressure.*

Isolation and Ligation of Right Sided IHPSS

AP *If necessary, ligate the right hepatic duct. Pass a Carmalt forceps from the dog's right to left over the dorsal surface of the main portal vein, just caudal to its bifurcation, but cranial to the termination of the gastroduodenal vein (Fig. 20-21). Grasp one end of a 2-0 silk suture, and pull it back over the portal vein. Then pass the forceps from the dog's right to left, dorsal to the left portal vein and within 5 mm of its bifurcation from the main portal vein. Grasp the opposite end of the suture, and pull it back over the vein.*

Partial Hepatectomy for Removal of Hepatic Arteriovenous Fistula

Treatment of a hepatic A-V fistula involves removal of the affected lobes and abnormal vascular structures. This has been done with or without temporary hepatic vascular occlusion. If temporary vascular occlusion is used, the vascular clamps and occlusive ligatures should be released within 15 minutes.

Extend the abdominal incision cranially through the caudal sternebrae, and incise the diaphragm down to and partly around the hiatus of the caudal vena cava. Place moistened umbilical tapes around the thoracic portion of the caudal vena cava, the abdominal portion of the caudal vena cava (between the liver and renal veins), and the portal vein (just proximal to the first hepatic branch). Pass the umbilical tapes through a piece of rubber tubing (Rumel tourniquet). Identify, isolate, and ligate the phrenicoabdominal veins, and isolate the celiac and cranial mesenteric arteries. Place a purse-string suture in the portal vein or a splenic tributary, and pass a 3.5 or 5

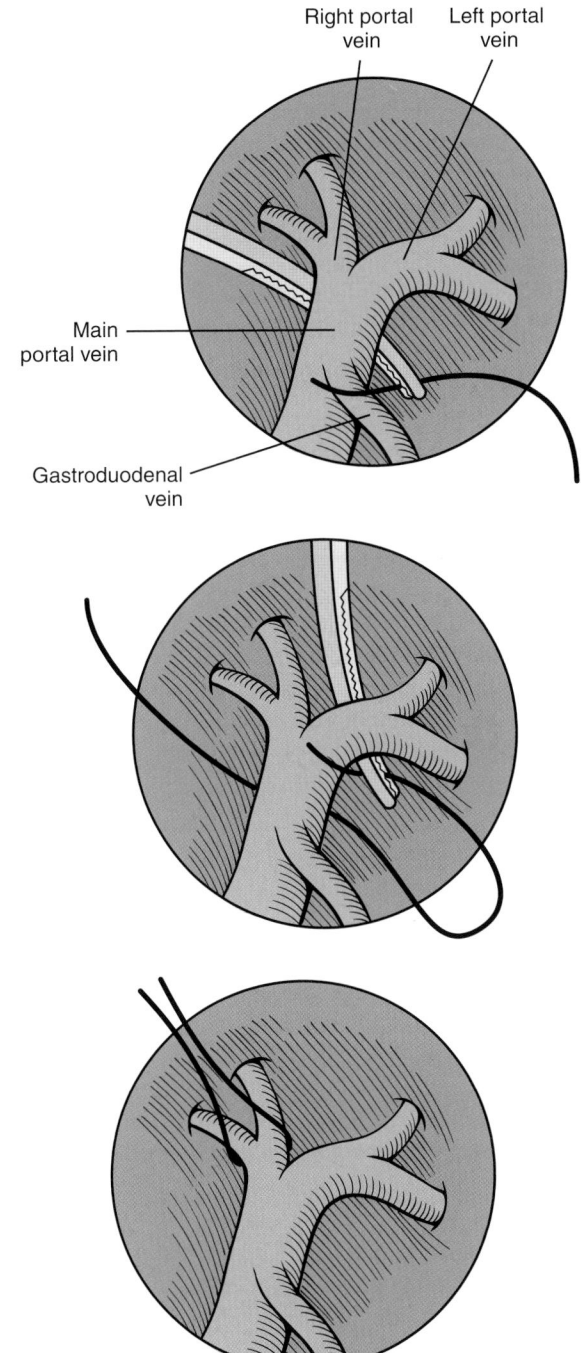

FIG. 20-21
Illustration showing isolation and ligation of right sided IHPSS.

French catheter into the vessel to monitor portal pressure. Monitor blood pressure carefully during surgery; manipulation and ligation of the fistula may cause sudden, severe fluctuations. Isolate the affected lobes by dissection of the triangular, coronary, and hepatorenal ligaments and the ligaments of the lesser omentum. Identify the hepatic arterial branch supplying the affected lobe and temporarily occlude it to see if pressure in the fistula diminishes. Double ligate the arterial supply of the fistula with nonabsorbable suture (e.g., 2-0 silk). Isolate the portal branch and biliary ducts to the affected lobe and double ligate them. Temporarily occlude the vasculature by tightening the preplaced umbilical tape ligatures and by placing vascular clamps on the celiac and cranial mesenteric arteries. Sharply dissect the liver parenchyma to resect the affected lobe. Ligate any vascular structures not already occluded and control hemorrhage by packing the area for several minutes.

Sometimes the affected portion of the liver can be removed by partial hepatectomy without performing vascular occlusion as described here.

SUTURE MATERIALS AND SPECIAL INSTRUMENTS

Generally 3.5- and 5-mm ameroid constrictors are used for occlusion of single extrahepatic shunts. Blunt-tipped, right-angled, or Mixter forceps are useful for dissecting around venous structures. Shunt ligation usually is performed with silk suture because of the relative knot security this suture affords. Delayed wound healing may be a problem if the patient is hypoproteinemic. To prevent dehiscence, a long-lasting absorbable suture material, such as polydioxanone or a nonabsorbable suture material, should be used to close the linea alba.

> NOTE: Ameroid constrictors are available through Research Instruments Northwest, 1369 N. 47th Ave., Sweet Home, OR 97386 (541-753-2018).

Right-angled forceps (e.g., Mixter, gallbladder or gall duct, or thoracic forceps) are widely available from many instrument manufacturers or suppliers, including Weck, Miltex, V. Mueller, Scanlan, and Codman.

POSTOPERATIVE CARE AND ASSESSMENT

Generally, animals can be sent home the day after placement of an ameroid constrictor. Continuing medical management and feeding a low-protein diet may be necessary until the shunt vessel occludes and the hepatic parenchyma regenerates. The patient should be reevaluated 2 to 3 months after surgery and tested for evidence of improved hepatic function (i.e., normal serum albumin). The animal may be weaned off medications and returned to a normal diet when hepatic function is determined to be reasonable.

When shunt ligation or attenuation is performed, intensive care management and close observation of the patient are extremely important because portal hypertension may develop several hours after the procedure. Hypertension and splanchnic congestion may be evidenced as a painful abdomen, hemorrhagic diarrhea, endotoxic shock, and death. Many shunt patients have a painful abdomen during the early postoperative period, which makes it difficult to recognize life-threatening portal hypertension. However, should signs of endotoxic shock or hemorrhagic diarrhea or other signs of

a deteriorating condition occur, emergency surgery to remove or loosen the ligature around the shunting vessel is advisable. Portal vein thrombosis may occur in single PSS cases in which the shunt has been partly ligated; it is a potentially life-threatening complication. If a shunt is only partly ligated, some authors recommend a single anticoagulant dose of regular heparin at the time of shunt attenuation. Ascites may occur after single shunt ligation; it is usually self-limiting, resolving in 1 to 3 weeks. Diuretics may be used if drainage occurs from the incision site or if the animal experiences dyspnea or discomfort from abdominal distention.

Status epilepticus after PSS ligation has been reported. These seizures generally are first noted 2 to 3 days after shunt ligation; their cause is unknown. This complication seems more common in cats, so much so that some recommend routine pretreatment of cats undergoing surgery for PSS with phenobarbital (not potassium bromide, which can cause respiratory problems in cats). Diazepam is not recommended for these patients; constant rate infusion of propofol seems to be the most effective therapy (Heldman et al, 1999). The patient is anesthetized for 24 hours and then awakened. If seizures recur, then the patient is reanesthetized and awakened in another 24 hours. This cycle is repeated until control is achieved. Long-term anticonvulsant therapy may be required. Owners should be counseled that permanent neurologic abnormalities, such as blindness, may occur (especially in cats). Medical management of hepatic encephalopathy should be continued postoperatively until the hepatic parenchyma regenerates; this may take several months. If the clinical signs have not improved within 2 to 3 months, nuclear scintigraphy or jejunal portography should be repeated.

PROGNOSIS

Overall mortality in a recent study was 8.7% for extrahepatic shunts and 20% for IHPSS (Winkler et al, 2003). Most dogs have an excellent or good outcome after placement of an ameroid constrictor. The complication rate for ameroid constrictors in the aforementioned study was 15.4%. Complications occurred in approximately 10% of dogs, and the mortality rate was 7.1% in another study (Mehl et al, 2005). Potential complications include hemorrhage, ascites, seizures, and/or coagulopathies. Portal hypertension may be secondary to kinking of the shunt; limiting dissection around the vessel may reduce this complication. The cause of seizures in these patients is not well understood (see previous discussion), but animals that have grand mal seizures after surgery are more likely to die than those that have partial seizures characterized by disorientation, hyperesthesia, vocalization, salivation, and/or jaw clenching. In one study, 12% of dogs developed neurologic signs within 6 days of surgical attenuation of congenital extrahepatic shunts (Tisdall et al, 2000). Prophylactic treatment with phenobarbital did not significantly reduce the incidence of neurologic sequelae, but it may have made the seizures less severe. In addition, development of multiple acquired shunts may occur after placement of an ameroid constrictor (see p. 544). With ligation, the surgical mortality is relatively high, a fact that reflects the many variables and unknown factors that exist in relation to portal physiology and dynamics.

Patients that only tolerate partial shunt occlusion and have persistence of clinical signs postoperatively require dietary and medical management. In such animals, reoperation and total shunt occlusion are recommended. Dogs that tolerate complete ligation of their shunt tend to have fewer clinical signs than those that tolerate only partial occlusion at surgery. Factors that appear to be significant predictors of continued portosystemic shunting include low preoperative albumin concentrations, high portal pressure during complete temporary occlusion of the PSS, and high portal pressure difference (Mehl et al, 2005). Predictors of an unsuccessful long-term outcome include lower preoperative albumin concentration, high WBC count, high portal pressure measured during complete temporary occlusion of the PSS, postoperative seizures, and continued shunting detected via portal scintigraphy. Outcome after placement of cellophane bands seems to be similar to that after placement of ameroid constrictors.

Hemorrhage, hypotension, and acute hepatic congestion are possible complications during surgical correction of IHPSS in dogs. Packed cell volume and total protein may be positive prognostic indicators for long-term survival in dogs with IHPSS, whereas low body weight (less than 15 kg) and low total protein, albumin, and BUN may be negative prognostic factors (Papazoglou et al, 2002). The long-term prognosis is good for dogs with hepatic A-V fistulae that survive surgery.

References

Balkman CE, Center SA, Randolph JF et al: Evaluation of urine sulfated and nonsulfated bile acids as a diagnostic test for liver disease in dogs, *J Am Vet Med Assoc* 222:1368, 2003.

Cole RC, Morandi F, Avenell J et al: Trans-splenic portal scintigraphy in normal dogs, *Vet Radiol Ultrasound* 46:146, 2005.

Heldman E, Holt DE, Brockman DJ et al: Use of propofol to manage seizure activity after surgical treatment of portosystemic shunts, *J Small Anim Pract* 40:590, 1999.

Hunt GB, Kummeling A, Tisdall PLC et al: Outcomes of cellophane banding for congenital portosystemic shunts in 106 dogs and 5 cats, *Vet Surg* 33:25, 2004.

Kyles AE, Gregory CR, Jackson J et al: Evaluation of portocaval venograft and ameroid ring for the occlusion of intrahepatic portocaval shunts in dogs, *Vet Surg* 30:161, 2001.

Kyles AE, Hardie EM, Mehl M et al: Evaluation of ameroid ring constrictors for the management of single extrahepatic portosystemic shunts in cats: 23 cases (1996-2001), *J Am Vet Med Assoc* 220:1341, 2002.

Mehl ML, Kyles AE, Adin CA et al: Evaluation of ameroid ring constrictors for extrahepatic portosystemic shunts in 168 cases (1996-2001), *J Am Vet Med Assoc* 226:2020, 2005.

Miller MW, Fossum TW, Bahr AM: Transvenous retrograde portography for identification and characterization of portosystemic shunts in dogs, *J Am Vet Med Assoc* 221:1586, 2002.

Monnet E, Rosenberg A: Effect of protein concentration on rate of closure of ameroid constrictors in vitro, *Am J Vet Res* 66:1337, 2005.

Morandi F, Cole RC, Tobias KM et al: Use of 99mTCO4(-) trans-splenic portal scintigraphy for diagnosis of portosystemic shunts in 28 dogs, *Vet Radiol Ultrasound* 46:153, 2005.

Murphy ST, Ellison GW, Long M et al: A comparison of the ameroid constrictor versus ligation in the surgical management of single extrahepatic portosystemic shunts, *J Am Anim Hosp Assoc* 37:390, 2001.

Papazoglou LG, Monnet E, Seim HB: Survival and prognostic indicators for dogs with intrahepatic portosystemic shunts: 32 cases (1990-2000), *Vet Surg* 31:561, 2002.

Samii VF, Kyles AE, Long CD: Evaluation of interoperator variance in shunt fraction calculation after transcolonic scintigraphy for diagnosis of portosystemic shunts in dogs and cats, *J Am Vet Med Assoc* 218:116, 2001.

Scrivani PV, Yeager AE, Dykes NL et al: Influence of patient positioning on sensitivity of mesenteric portography for detecting an anomalous portosystemic blood vessel in dogs: 34 cases (1997-2000), *J Am Vet Med Assoc* 219:1251, 2001.

Szatmari V, van Sluijs FJ, Rothuizen J et al: Ultrasonographic assessment of hemodynamic changes in the portal vein during surgical attenuation of congenital extrahepatic portosystemic shunts in dogs, *J Am Vet Med Assoc* 224:395, 2004.

Tisdall PLC, Hunt GB, Youmans KR et al: Neurologic dysfunction in dogs following attenuation of congenital extrahepatic portosystemic shunts, *J Small Anim Pract* 41:539, 2000.

Tobias KM: Determination of inheritance of single congenital portosystemic shunts in Yorkshire terriers, *J Am Anim Hosp Assoc* 39:355, 2003.

Tobias KM, Byarlay JM, Henry RW: A new dissection technique for approach to right-sided intrahepatic portosystemic shunts: anatomic study and use in three dogs, *Vet Surg* 33:32, 2004.

Tobias KM, Rohrbach BW: Association of breed with the diagnosis of congenital portosystemic shunts in dogs: 2,400 cases (1980-2002), *J Am Vet Med Assoc* 223:1636, 2003.

Trainor D, Center SA, Randolph JF et al: Urine sulfated and nonsulfated bile acids as a diagnostic test for liver disease in cats, *J Vet Intern Med* 17:145, 2003.

Walker MC, Hill RC, Guilford WG et al: Postprandial venous ammonia concentrations in the diagnosis of hepatobiliary disease in dogs, *J Vet Intern Med* 15:463, 2001.

Winkler JT, Bohling MW, Tillson DM et al: Portosystemic shunts: diagnosis, prognosis and treatment of 64 cases (1993-2001), *J Am Anim Hosp Assoc* 39:168, 2003.

Suggested Reading

Havig M, Tobias KM: Outcome of ameroid constrictor occlusion of single congenital extrahepatic portosystemic shunts in cats: 12 cases (1993-2000), *J Am Vet Med Assoc* 220:337, 2002.

Results of this study suggest that long-term outcome of ameroid constrictor occlusion of PSS in cats is poor.

Hunt GB: Effect of breed on anatomy of portosystemic shunts resulting from congenital diseases in dogs and cats: a review of 242 cases, *Aust Vet J* 82:746, 2004.

This retrospective study of 233 dogs and 9 cats with PSS affirmed that breed has a significant influence on shunt anatomy in dogs. Unusual or inoperable shunts are more likely to occur in breeds that are not predisposed to congenital PSS.

CAVITARY HEPATIC LESIONS

DEFINITIONS

Cavitary hepatic lesions usually are cysts or abscesses, although occasionally large neoplastic lesions, such as hemangiomas and adenomas, cavitate. **Hepatic abscesses** are localized collections of pus in the hepatic parenchyma. **Hepatic cysts** are closed, fluid-filled sacs lined by secretory epithelium.

GENERAL CONSIDERATIONS AND CLINICALLY RELEVANT PATHOPHYSIOLOGY

Hepatic abscesses are rare in dogs and cats and usually are associated with extrahepatic infection (i.e., ascending biliary tract infections, hematogenous infection via the portal vein or hepatic artery, or direct extension from areas adjacent to the liver), hepatic trauma (i.e., surgical biopsy, penetrating wounds, or blunt trauma), or neoplasia. Despite the normal presence of bacteria in the liver of dogs, hepatic abscesses seldom occur. This may be related to a well-developed local defense system provided by the liver's rich blood supply and the phagocytic ability of reticuloendothelial cells.

Hepatic abscesses are most often recognized as a complication of omphalophlebitis in puppies and usually are diagnosed at necropsy. Diabetes mellitus has been associated with hepatic abscesses. The organisms most often isolated from hepatic abscesses in dogs include *Escherichia coli* and *Clostridium* spp. Small abscesses may not cause clinical signs and may resorb without therapy.

Hepatic cysts usually are incidental findings, although in rare cases they become large enough to interfere with the function of adjacent organs. A single hepatic cyst may be noted, or several cysts may be present in the same or different lobes. Concurrent polycystic renal disease has been reported in cats. If hepatic cysts are present in an animal with clinical evidence of hepatic dysfunction, liver biopsy often is warranted to determine the cause.

DIAGNOSIS

Clinical Presentation

Signalment. No gender or breed predisposition has been reported for hepatic abscesses or cysts.

History. Clinical signs of hepatic abscessation vary and may include anorexia, lethargy, weight loss, vomiting, and intermittent abdominal pain. Most animals with hepatic cysts are asymptomatic; however, some cysts cause abdominal distention. Secondary infections of hepatic cysts may cause clinical signs similar to those of hepatic abscesses.

Physical Examination Findings

Physical examination findings in patients with hepatic abscessation typically include persistent fever, hepatomegaly, and abdominal enlargement. Palpation of a firm abdominal mass and notable abdominal distention may be noted in some animals with hepatic cysts. In a recent study of hepatic abscesses in 14 cats, clinical signs were vague and included anorexia, lethargy, and weight loss. Fever was present in only 23% of the cats, whereas 31% were hypothermic (Sergeeff et

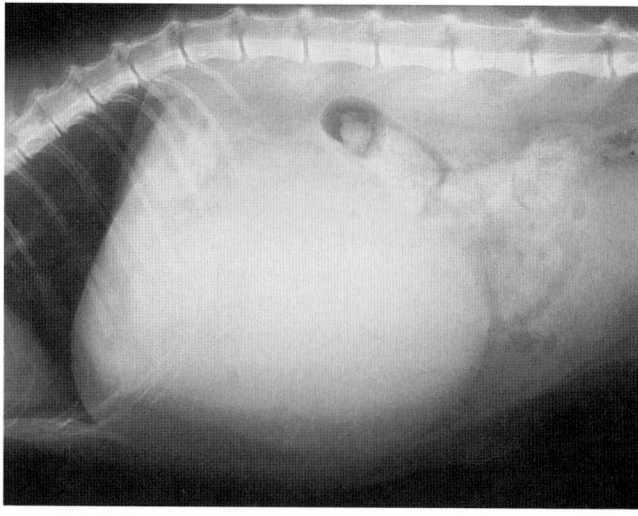

FIG. 20-22
Lateral abdominal radiograph of a 2-year-old cat with a large hepatic cyst. The cat was asymptomatic. Radiographically, a large, soft tissue mass arising from the liver can be seen. The diagnosis of a cyst would require ultrasound examination.

al, 2004). Clinical signs of sepsis are common in cats with small multifocal abscesses and in those with microabscesses.

Diagnostic Imaging

Small hepatic cysts often are incidental radiographic and sonographic findings. Large hepatic cysts usually are well-defined, radiopaque structures in the cranial abdomen (Fig. 20-22). Abdominal radiographs may demonstrate hepatomegaly in animals with hepatic abscesses, but a well-defined hepatic mass is seldom evident. Occasionally, gas is noted in the hepatic parenchyma, which strongly suggests abscessation caused by gas-forming bacteria. Ultrasonography is the most useful diagnostic test for defining hepatic abscesses and cysts in dogs and cats. Hepatic abscesses appear as hypoechoic or anechoic structures that may contain mixed echogenicities, depending on the cellularity. The abscesses may appear solitary, multifocal, and small, or they may be microabscesses. Scintigraphy, CT, and magnetic resonance imaging (MRI) also are highly sensitive in diagnosing hepatic lesions, but these techniques are used less often than ultrasonography. Ultrasound-guided fine-needle aspirations of hepatic abscesses can be performed before surgery; however, there is a risk that the abscess will rupture or drain into the abdomen and cause diffuse peritonitis. Fluid removed from cysts during fine-needle aspiration usually is transudative.

> NOTE: Evaluate the kidneys for cystic disease in cats with hepatic cysts. Both conditions may be present.

Laboratory Findings

Laboratory abnormalities are seldom present with hepatic cysts. They are variable in animals with hepatic abscesses, but may include an inflammatory leukogram and nonregenerative anemia. Serum biochemical abnormalities may include hypoalbuminemia, hypokalemia, hyperglycemia, and elevated hepatic enzymes; however, elevation of alanine transaminase activity is not a consistent finding. *E. coli* is the organism most commonly isolated from cats with hepatic abscesses (Sergeeff et al, 2004).

DIFFERENTIAL DIAGNOSIS

Hepatic cysts, abscesses, neoplasms, and parasitic lesions must be differentiated. Hepatic abscesses often are difficult to diagnose because they produce nonspecific signs that may be masked by associated disease processes. Large neoplastic hepatic lesions may necrose and become secondarily infected. Infection of hepatic cysts is also possible. Therefore, histologic evaluation of surgically resected tissue is important.

MEDICAL MANAGEMENT

Medical management of hepatic abscesses entails administration of fluid/electrolyte/acid-base therapy plus appropriate antibiotic therapy. Percutaneous ultrasound-assisted drainage and alcoholization using 95% ethanol has been reported for treatment of focal abscesses in 5 dogs and a cat (Zatelli et al, 2005).

To perform this technique, position a spinal needle attached to extension tubing and a syringe into the abscess using ultrasound guidance and drain the fluid. Use a syringe that is twice the volume of the estimated amount of exudate in the lesion. Before removing the spinal needle, inject a volume of alcohol equal to half the volume of exudate removed. Leave the ethanol in the abscess cavity for 3 minutes, and then gently remove it. Submit the exudate for culture and susceptibility testing. Continue appropriate antibiotic therapy for an additional 30 days.

If surgery is elected, resection of hepatic abscesses is indicated as soon as the animal is an acceptable anesthetic risk. Preoperative antibiotic therapy may be based on culture and sensitivity results if fine-needle aspiration has been performed, or antibiotics with bactericidal activity against anaerobes and gram-negative bacteria (e.g., ticarcillin/clavulanic acid plus enrofloxacin, or cefoxitin; or clindamycin plus enrofloxacin, or ticarcillin/clavulanic acid plus amikacin [Box 20-6]) may be given empirically. Parenteral antibiotics are indicated in the perioperative period. Combination therapy may be necessary, particularly if multiple organisms are isolated. Percutaneous drainage of hepatic cysts and sclerosis of the cyst lining have not been reported in dogs or cats.

SURGICAL TREATMENT

Whether hepatic cysts should be removed when diagnosed in asymptomatic animals is not clear. Although these cysts could enlarge or become infected and cause clinical signs, little information is available about the long-term follow-up of large hepatic cysts that are not surgically resected in dogs or cats. Hepatic cysts associated with clinical signs and hepatic abscesses should be promptly resected.

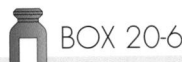 BOX 20-6

Antibiotics Used to Treat Hepatic Abscesses

Amoxicillin plus clavulanate (Clavamax)
Dogs: 12.5–25 mg/kg PO, bid
Cats: 62.5 mg PO, bid

Enrofloxacin (Baytril)*
7–20 mg/kg PO or IV (must give diluted and slowly over 30 minutes), qd

Cefoxitin (Mefoxin)
30 mg/kg IV, tid to qid

Cefazolin (Ancef, Kefzol)
22 mg/kg IV or IM, tid to qid

Clindamycin (Antirobe)
11 mg/kg IV or PO, tid

Metronidazole (Flagyl)
10–15 mg/kg IV (must be given diluted and slowly) or PO, tid

Ticarcillin plus clavulanic acid (Timentin)
50 mg/kg IV, tid to qid

Amikacin
25 mg/kg IV, qd

PO, Oral; *qd,* once a day; *bid,* twice a day; *IV,* intravenous; *tid,* three times a day; *qid,* four times a day; *IM,* intramuscular.
*Doses greater than 5 mg/kg may be associated with blindness in cats.

Preoperative Management

Symptomatic animals should be in stable condition before surgery. Antibiotics may be initiated before surgery, or in some animals they may be administered after intraoperative cultures have been taken.

Anesthesia

See p. 531 for the anesthetic management of animals with hepatic disease.

Surgical Anatomy

See p. 532 for the surgical anatomy of the liver.

Positioning

The animal is positioned in dorsal recumbency for a midline abdominal incision. The prepped area should extend from midthorax to the pubis.

SURGICAL TECHNIQUE

Hepatic abscesses and cysts generally are treated by partial hepatectomy (see pp. 536-537). If hepatectomy cannot safely be performed and the cyst completely removed, it may be omentalized (Friend et al, 2001). Although there is less concern about spillage of cystic contents into the abdomen, it is wise to try to remove the cyst without entering the lumen. Culture of hepatic cysts may be optional if the fluid does not appear infected cytologically; however, some cysts can develop secondary bacterial infections.

Pack the area surrounding the liver with moistened laparotomy sponges to diminish intraoperative contamination if the lumen of the abscess or cyst is entered. If possible, resect the affected portion of the liver without entering the lesion. Culture the lesion, and submit it for histologic examination. Palpate the remainder of the liver parenchyma for other nodules, and explore the abdominal cavity for associated infection or disease.

For omentalization, identify a segment of the omentum that will extend into the cyst cavity. Remove as much of the wall of the cyst as possible, and spread the omentum over the remaining cyst and adjacent liver. Tack it gently in place to the remaining cyst capsule.

SUTURE MATERIALS AND SPECIAL INSTRUMENTS

See p. 538 for recommendations for suture choices during partial hepatectomy.

POSTOPERATIVE CARE AND ASSESSMENT

Fluid therapy for animals with hepatic abscesses should be continued until the animal is drinking normally. Antibiotic therapy should be continued for 7 to 10 days. The animal should be monitored for peritonitis (i.e., leukocytosis, fever, abdominal fluid, abdominal pain) if abdominal contamination occurred. Minimal postoperative care is needed for most animals with hepatic cysts.

PROGNOSIS

The prognosis for animals with hepatic abscesses depends on the rapidity with which the abscess is diagnosed, whether concurrent peritonitis is present, and the animal's overall health. The overall mortality rate in a recent report of 14 cats with hepatic abscesses was 70% (Sergeeff et al, 2004). The prognosis for animals with hepatic cysts (with or without surgery) is good unless concurrent hepatic or renal disease exists.

References

Friend EJ, Niles JD, Williams JM: Omentalisation of congenital liver cysts in a cat, *Vet Rec* 149:275, 2001.

Sergeeff JS, Armstrong PJ, Bunch SE: Hepatic abscesses in cats: 14 cases (1985-2002), *J Vet Intern Med* 18:295, 2004.

Zatelli A, Bonfanti U, Zini E et al: Percutaneous drainage and alcoholization of hepatic abscesses in five dogs and a cat, *J Am Anim Hosp Assoc* 41:34, 2005.

HEPATOBILIARY NEOPLASIA

DEFINITIONS

Hepatocellular tumors arise from hepatocytes; **cholangiocellular neoplasms** arise from intrahepatic or extrahepatic bile duct epithelium. The term *hepatoma* has been used to refer both to hepatocellular carcinomas and to hepatocellu-

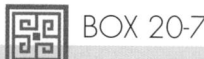 **BOX 20-7**

Primary Hepatic Neoplasia in Dogs and Cats

Epithelial
- Hepatocellular carcinoma
- Hepatocellular adenoma
- Cholangiocellular carcinoma
- Cholangiocellular adenoma
- Hepatic carcinoids

Mesenchymal
- Hemangiosarcoma
- Fibrosarcoma
- Extraskeletal osteosarcoma
- Leiomyosarcoma

lar adenomas. Cholangiocellular carcinomas are also known as *bile duct carcinomas*.

GENERAL CONSIDERATIONS AND CLINICALLY RELEVANT PATHOPHYSIOLOGY

Primary hepatic neoplasms are uncommon in dogs and cats. They may be of epithelial or mesenchymal origin (Box 20-7). Hepatocellular carcinomas and cholangiocellular carcinomas are the most commonly diagnosed primary hepatic malignancies in dogs. Hepatocellular carcinomas may involve a single liver lobe or may be nodular or diffuse, involving multiple lobes. In cats, cholangiocellular adenomas are the most common primary tumor. Hepatic carcinoids are rare tumors that arise from neuroectodermal cells in the liver. Biliary cystadenomas are uncommon benign liver tumors of older cats that may occur as focal or multifocal cystic lesions. Benign hepatic masses (i.e., adenomas or cysts) often are incidental findings at necropsy. They may be more common than malignant tumors in both species, but often go undiagnosed because they seldom cause clinical signs. Cholangiocellular carcinomas arise primarily from intrahepatic bile duct epithelium; neoplasms of the extrahepatic bile duct and gallbladder are rare.

Malignant primary hepatic tumors have typically been considered to be highly metastatic; however, a median survival of greater than 1460 days and a metastatic rate of only 4.8% have been reported after lobectomy for hepatocellular carcinoma (Liptak et al, 2004). They may metastasize by direct extension to other liver lobes or adjacent organs, or they may spread distantly via lymphatics or blood. Epithelial tumors most often metastasize to the regional lymph nodes and lungs. Mesenchymal tumors most often metastasize to the spleen.

Metastatic neoplasia is more common in the liver than are primary tumors. The liver is a common site for metastasis because it acts as a filter between the abdominal organs and the systemic circulation. Lymphosarcoma is the most common secondary hepatic tumor. Other tumors that commonly metastasize to the liver are pancreatic adenocarcinomas, hemangiosarcomas, insulinomas, and tumors of the alimentary and urinary tracts.

DIAGNOSIS
Clinical Presentation

Signalment. Primary hepatic neoplasia usually is a disease of aged dogs and cats. There is no known breed predisposition. Hepatocellular carcinomas may be more common in male dogs, whereas cholangiocellular carcinomas may be more common in cats and female dogs. Dogs with metastatic liver cancer may be slightly younger (7.8 years of age) than those with primary hepatic malignancy (10 years of age).

History. Many animals with primary hepatic neoplasia are presented for treatment of signs associated with hepatic failure. The animal may be lethargic, weak, anorexic, losing weight, or vomiting or may have polyuria or polydipsia. The clinical signs associated with metastatic hepatic neoplasia vary considerably. Primary hepatic tumors and metastatic hemangiosarcomas may rupture and bleed, causing signs of shock.

Physical Examination Findings

The most significant finding on physical examination of most primary hepatic tumors is an enlarged liver; however, hepatic carcinoids may not cause significant hepatomegaly. Additional findings may include jaundice and ascites. Hemangiosarcomas and hepatocellular adenomas may rupture and cause hemoperitoneum, shock, and pale oral mucous membranes. Notable hepatomegaly is less common with metastatic neoplasia; however, lymphosarcoma often causes diffuse hepatic enlargement.

Diagnostic Imaging

Survey radiographs help localize the mass to the liver (Fig. 20-23) and may reveal extrahepatic metastasis. Thoracic radiographs are indicated whenever hepatic neoplasia is suspected because pulmonary metastasis is common. Ultrasonography often localizes and defines the extent of disease. Ultrasound-guided biopsies may allow presurgical diagnosis (see p. 535), but these tumors are often highly vascular and can bleed profusely. Although conventional ultrasound may detect lymph node enlargement and therefore help define metastasis in dogs with hepatic neoplasia, Doppler and contrast-enhanced ultrasound may prove to be even more sensitive diagnostic aids (Nyman et al, 2004).

> NOTE: Ultrasonography is particularly useful in animals with ascites. Radiographs often show little abdominal detail when ascites is present.

Laboratory Findings

Neutrophilia and biochemical abnormalities compatible with hepatic disease (elevated serum alanine transaminase, aspartate transaminase, and serum alkaline phosphatase) are expected but often absent in animals with hepatic neo-

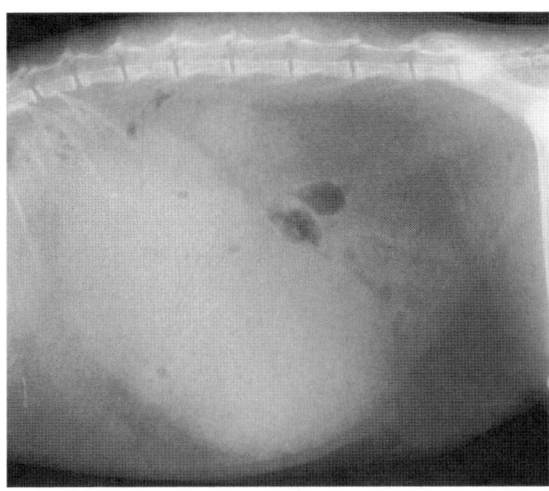

FIG. 20-23
Lateral abdominal radiograph of a dog with a large, malignant hepatic tumor. Note the similarities between the radiographic appearance of this tumor and the benign hepatic cyst in Fig. 20-22. Benign and malignant hepatic masses cannot be differentiated radiographically.

plasia. They are nonspecific, but recognition may prompt further evaluation of the hepatobiliary system. Mild to moderate anemia is less commonly associated with hepatic neoplasia. Serum bilirubin concentrations may be elevated, particularly if extrahepatic biliary obstruction occurs. Occasionally, hypoglycemia causes clinical signs. Albumin levels usually are normal in patients with primary hepatic neoplasia. Biochemical abnormalities seldom correlate with the extent of hepatic involvement with either primary or metastatic tumors.

> NOTE: Laboratory abnormalities often do not occur until the neoplasm is large enough to make surgical excision difficult.

DIFFERENTIAL DIAGNOSIS

Primary hepatobiliary tumors must be differentiated from regenerative nodules, abscesses, hematomas, and cysts. Histologic and/or cytologic evaluation of fine-needle aspirates or biopsy specimens is necessary to distinguish definitively between these lesions (see p. 533). Percutaneous biopsies should not be performed in animals with clinical bleeding disorders or if the lesions appear cavitary or highly vascular. Cytologic evaluation of abdominal fluid is seldom helpful in differentiating between these lesions.

MEDICAL MANAGEMENT

Surgical excision of primary malignant hepatic tumors is the treatment of choice. Unfortunately, these tumors often are not diagnosed until they are large and metastasis has occurred. Because they usually are diagnosed in older animals, concurrent cardiac, renal, or other metabolic problems are common. Medical therapy should aim at correcting fluid and electrolyte imbalances and providing nutrition to improve the chances of surviving surgery.

SURGICAL TREATMENT

If the tumor is localized to a single lobe or confined to the gallbladder, surgical resection may be curative. Partial hepatectomy and cholecystectomy are described on pp. 536 and 562, respectively. Ultrasound is often used to screen for metastasis, but it is not a particularly sensitive way to detect these lesions, particularly if the metastases are on serosal surfaces. Although not as sensitive as an exploratory laparotomy, laparoscopy is more sensitive than ultrasound for finding metastasis. One can first perform laparoscopy to look for gross evidence of metastasis before proceeding to surgery to resect a tumor.

Surgical biopsies should be performed on all animals with hepatomegaly or nodularity because differentiation of lesions requires histopathologic evaluation. Finding multiple hepatic masses does not diagnose metastatic disease; many benign lesions can present as multiple hepatic nodules (e.g., regenerative nodules associated with cirrhosis or lobular collapse) or even neoplasia because primary hepatic tumors may spread to other portions of the liver. Multiple benign masses may be seen in the liver. If neoplasia is suspected, the draining lymph nodes and surrounding organs should be carefully assessed for metastasis. Hepatocellular tumors are most commonly found in the left medial and left lateral liver lobes.

PREOPERATIVE MANAGEMENT

The animal's condition should be stabilized before surgery if possible. Fluid therapy should be initiated and electrolyte imbalances corrected. Blood transfusions (see Box 5-1 on p. 25) should be given to severely anemic animals (i.e., packed cell volume less than 20%), especially if bleeding tendencies are present (i.e., petechiation, ecchymosis, or hemorrhage). If the animal has clinical evidence of a significant coagulopathy on the mucosal bleeding time (i.e., bleeding time >5 to 7 minutes) or is severely thrombocytopenic (i.e., fewer than 20,000 platelets/μl), consider plasma or whole blood transfusions and ensure hemostasis at surgery. Many patients with a prolonged one-stage prothrombin time (OSPT or PT) and partial thromboplastin time (PTT) do not have bleeding problems at surgery, but they should be monitored for such before, during, and after surgery. If the patient has massive ascites, slow removal of some fluid before induction of anesthesia may help prevent hypoventilation associated with positioning the patient while it is prepared for surgery.

Anesthesia

Ventilation of patients with ascites requires support (i.e., intermittent positive-pressure ventilation [IPPV]). Compression of the caudal vena cava in patients with large hepatic masses or massive ascites may diminish venous return and reduce cardiac output. See pp. 531-532 for additional comments about the anesthetic management of patients with hepatic disease.

Surgical Anatomy

See p. 532 for the surgical anatomy of the liver.

Positioning

Exploration of the liver generally is performed through a cranial ventral midline abdominal incision (see p. 319). The incision may be extended paracostally to allow enhanced visualization and manipulation of large tumors. The prepped area should extend from midthorax to the pubis.

SURGICAL TECHNIQUE

See pp. 536 and 562 for a description of surgical techniques for partial hepatectomy or cholecystectomy, respectively.

SUTURE MATERIALS AND SPECIAL INSTRUMENTS

Absorbable suture material is used for hepatic biopsy (see p. 538). Ligation of the cystic duct for cholecystectomy generally is done with nonabsorbable suture material (see p. 566).

POSTOPERATIVE CARE AND ASSESSMENT

Postoperative nutritional support of patients with hepatic neoplasia often is necessary (see Chapter 11). Nonresectable primary hepatic tumors seldom respond to chemotherapy or radiation therapy. Chemotherapy may palliate hepatic lymphosarcoma. For other considerations in animals undergoing partial hepatectomy, see p. 538.

PROGNOSIS

The prognosis for dogs and cats with primary hepatobiliary malignancies often is poor; however, some dogs may live for a year or longer with aggressive therapy. In a recent report of cats with malignant, nonlymphomatous hepatobiliary disease that underwent surgery, the median length of the survival was 0.1 month (range, less than 1 day to 4 months). The high rate of metastasis and degree of invasion make surgical resection unlikely to be curative in most patients. Benign tumors may be surgically resected, and long-term survival of patients with benign hepatic tumors has been reported. Survival times in cats with hepatobiliary cystadenomas has ranged from 12 to 44 months after surgery.

References

Liptak JM, Dernell WS, Monnet E et al: Massive hepatocellular carcinoma in dogs, *J Am Vet Med Assoc* 225:1225, 2004.

Nyman HT, Kristensen AT, Flagstad A et al: A review of the sonographic assessment of tumor metastases in liver and superficial lymph nodes, *Vet Radiol Ultrasound* 45:438, 2004.

HEPATIC LOBE TORSION

DEFINITIONS

Hepatic lobe torsion occurs when a liver lobe twists around its axis.

GENERAL CONSIDERATIONS AND CLINICALLY RELEVANT PATHOPHYSIOLOGY

Liver lobe torsions are rare in dogs and cats. Torsion of the left lateral lobe is most common, presumably because it has greater mobility, is larger, and is relatively more separated from the adjacent lobes than are the other liver lobes. In most animals the cause is unknown, but congenital absence or traumatic rupture of hepatic ligaments is generally suspected. A ruptured hepatocellular carcinoma was diagnosed in one cat with torsion of the right medial liver lobe (Swann and Brown, 2001). When a liver lobe twists on its axis, it creates venous obstruction, causing increased hydrostatic pressure, ascites, and thrombosis. The liver lobe will eventually necrose.

Clinical Presentation

Signalment. No breed or sex predisposition has been identified for hepatic lobe torsions in dogs or cats. Most reported dogs have been middle-aged.

History. Clinical signs of hepatic lobe torsion are often nonspecific and may include depression, lethargy, anorexia, collapse, and/or abdominal enlargement of one to several days' duration. Acute death may occur.

Physical Examination Findings

Physical examination findings may include pain on abdominal palpation and the presence of ascites. The animal should be examined carefully for signs of trauma.

Diagnostic Imaging

Survey radiographs may show ascites and should be reviewed for signs of associated trauma (e.g., diaphragmatic hernia). Ultrasonography may help define the lesion and localize it to a defined area of the liver.

Laboratory Findings

Blood work abnormalities are nonspecific and are not helpful in identifying hepatic lobe torsion. Neutrophilia may be present and biochemical abnormalities compatible with hepatic disease (elevated serum alanine transaminase, aspartate transaminase, and serum alkaline phosphatase) are commonly seen.

DIFFERENTIAL DIAGNOSIS

Liver lobe torsion must be differentiated from nonsurgical diseases of the liver, such as hepatitis.

MEDICAL MANAGEMENT

Surgical excision of torsed hepatic lobes is warranted. The animal should be stabilized *before* surgery.

SURGICAL TREATMENT

Surgical resection of the devitalized lobe is warranted. The technique for hepatic lobectomy is described on p. 536.

Preoperative Management

The animal's condition should be stabilized before surgery if possible. Fluid therapy should be initiated and electrolyte imbalances corrected. If the patient has massive ascites, slow removal of some fluid before induction of anesthesia may help prevent hypoventilation associated with positioning the patient while it is prepared for surgery.

Anesthesia

Ventilation of patients with ascites may require support (i.e., IPPV). See pp. 531-532 for additional comments about the anesthetic management of patients with hepatic disease.

Surgical Anatomy

The liver lobe is supported by a series of ligaments, including the left and right lateral triangular ligaments, which extend from the left and right lateral hepatic lobes to the muscular portion of the diaphragm; left and right lateral coronary ligaments, which attach the right and left lobes to the central tendinous portion of the diaphragm; and the falciform ligament, which attaches to the liver, abdominal wall, and sternal portion of the diaphragm.

Positioning

Exploration of the liver generally is performed through a cranial ventral midline abdominal incision (see p. 533). The prepped area should extend from midthorax to the pubis.

SURGICAL TECHNIQUE

See pp. 536 for a description of the surgical technique for removal of a liver lobe. Histologic evaluation of the excised liver lobe is warranted, as the devitalized mass may be similar in appearance to a hepatic tumor.

SUTURE MATERIALS AND SPECIAL INSTRUMENTS

Absorbable suture material is used for liver lobectomy (see p. 538).

POSTOPERATIVE CARE AND ASSESSMENT

Instructions on postoperative care of the patient after liver lobe resection are provided on p. 538. Dogs with associated diaphragmatic hernias or other trauma should be carefully observed for evidence of respiratory distress after surgery. Fluid support should be continued until the animal is eating and drinking sufficiently on its own. Pain medication should be given postoperatively (see p. 538).

PROGNOSIS

The prognosis for dogs and cats with hepatic lobe torsion is good if the underlying disease can be effectively treated.

Reference

Swann HM, Brown DC: Hepatic lobe torsion in 3 dogs and a cat, *Vet Surg* 30:482, 2001.

CHAPTER 21
Surgery of the Extrahepatic Biliary System

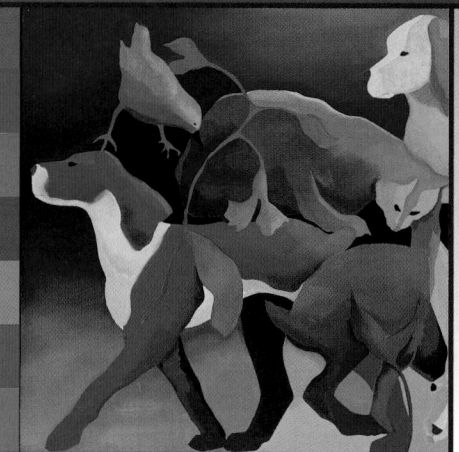

DEFINITIONS

Cholecystotomy is the creation of an opening into the gallbladder for drainage; **cholecystectomy** is removal of the gallbladder. **Choledochotomy** is incision of the common bile duct for exploration or removal of a calculus. **Choledochoduodenostomy** is a rarely indicated procedure in dogs and cats that involves surgical anastomosis of the common bile duct to the duodenum. **Cholecystoenterostomy** is a term used to describe biliary diversion in which the gallbladder is opened and sutured to a portion of the intestine. **Cholecystoduodenostomy** and **cholecystojejunostomy** are surgical anastomoses of the gallbladder to the duodenum or jejunum, respectively. Calculi may form in the gallbladder (**cholelithiasis**) or the common bile duct (**choledocholithiasis**).

PREOPERATIVE MANAGEMENT

Biliary disease may be caused by extrahepatic biliary tract obstruction (EHBO), neoplasia, infection, or trauma. Lesions that cause EHBO may be extraluminal or intraluminal. Extraluminal obstruction may be caused by pancreatitis, pancreatic neoplasia, duodenal or pyloric neoplasia, hepatic or biliary neoplasia, diaphragmatic hernias, congenital abnormalities, or pancreatic abscessation. Intraluminal obstruction is less common, but may occur in association with cholelithiasis, choledocholithiasis, inspissated bile, or liver flukes (cats). Pancreatic disease is the most common cause of EHBO in dogs and may have an increasing incidence in cats. Scar formation may occur in or around the duct, or the duct may be compressed by fibrotic or inflamed pancreatic tissue. Pancreatic abscesses and cysts may rarely cause biliary obstruction.

Animals with EHBO should have electrolyte and fluid abnormalities corrected before surgery. Prolonged EHBO may cause vitamin K malabsorption, resulting in deficiencies of factors VII, IX, and X. Animals with clinical evidence of bleeding or an increased mucosal bleeding time should receive vitamin K₁ (subcutaneously [SC], not intravenously [IV] or intramuscularly [IM]) for 24 to 48 hours before surgery (Box 21-1) or fresh whole blood (see p. 28). Partial or complete

---

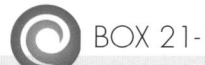 **BOX 21-1**

Dosage for Vitamin K$_1$ (AquaMephyton, Mephyton)

0.5–1 mg/kg/day SC, given in divided doses*

SC, Subcutaneous.
*Do not give intravenously or intramuscularly.

---

biliary obstruction may allow ascending aerobic and anaerobic infection and subsequent bacteremia, therefore perioperative antibiotic therapy is indicated (see Chapter 10).

Extrahepatic biliary injury may be caused by blunt or penetrating trauma. Common bile duct, gallbladder, cystic duct, or hepatic duct lacerations may cause bile peritonitis or, if the infection is "walled off," a localized inflammatory process with adherence to surrounding organs. Necrotizing cholecystitis occurs when bacteria damage the gallbladder wall, often resulting in peritoneal spillage of bile (Fig. 21-1). This frequently results in severe, generalized septic peritonitis. Sometimes bile becomes inspissated before the gallbladder ruptures, and spillage of the relatively thick, gelatinous mass into the cranial abdomen causes a localized peritonitis. Adhesions or fistulous tracts around the gallbladder occasionally occur. See p. 572 for a discussion of the preoperative management of animals with bile peritonitis.

Animals with EHBO should be differentiated from those with intrahepatic cholestasis causing partial obstruction because the former sometimes needs surgery, whereas the latter almost never requires surgical correction. The indications for exploratory surgery in animals with suspected extrahepatic biliary obstruction are not well defined. An increasing serum bilirubin level over 7 to 10 days in the apparent absence of defined hepatic disease or pancreatitis, combined with supportive radiography or ultrasonographic evidence of obstruction, is generally considered to be an indication for surgery. Dogs with EHBO due to pancreatitis almost never need surgery, although patients that do not respond to appropriate medical therapy sometimes require surgery. The reader is referred to medical texts for an in-depth discussion of the treatment of pancreatitis. Nuclear scintigraphy may

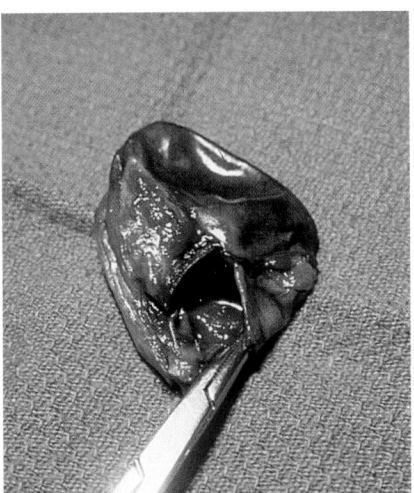

FIG. 21-1
Ruptured gallbladder in a dog with necrotizing cholecystitis.

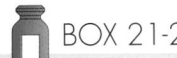 BOX 21-2

Antibiotics Commonly Used in the Treatment of Biliary Disease

Amoxicillin (Amoxi-Tabs, AmoxiDrops, Amoxi-inject)
20 mg/kg PO, IM or SC, bid or tid

Cefazolin (Ancef, Kefzol)
22 mg/kg IV or IM, tid or qid

Clindamycin (Antirobe)
11 mg/kg IV or PO, tid

Enrofloxacin (Baytril)*
7–20 mg/kg PO, IM, or IV (diluted and given slowly over 30 minutes), qd

Ticarcillin plus clavulanic acid (Timentin)
50 mg/kg IV, tid to qid

Amikacin (Amiglyde)
20–25 mg/kg IV, qd

PO, Oral; *IM*, intramuscular; *SC*, subcutaneous; *qd*, once a day; *bid*, twice a day; *tid*, three times a day; *IV*, intravenous; *qid*, four times a day.
*Doses greater than 5 mg/kg may be associated with blindness in cats.

aid in the diagnosis of complete extrahepatic biliary obstruction (see Diagnostic Imaging below).

ANESTHESIA

The anesthetic requirements and concerns for patients with biliary disease are similar to those for hepatic disease (see p. 531). An additional concern in patients with obstructive biliary disease relates to the effect of μ-agonists (e.g., hydromorphone, morphine) on smooth muscle tone. In human beings with biliary obstruction, these drugs increase both sphincter tone and pain. Mixed agonist-antagonists (e.g., butorphanol; see Table 13-4 on p. 133) may be preferable as premedicants and analgesics in these patients.

ANTIBIOTICS

Prophylactic antibiotics are recommended in patients undergoing biliary surgery because of the detrimental effects of bacterial infection on healing. Antibiotic therapy for biliary infections should be based on the results of culture and susceptibility testing of liver parenchyma or bile or both. The organisms most often isolated from biliary infections are *Escherichia coli, Klebsiella* spp., *Enterobacter* spp., *Proteus* spp., and *Pseudomonas* spp. Antibiotics that are excreted in active form in the bile and are commonly used to treat biliary disease include amoxicillin, cefazolin, and enrofloxacin (Box 21-2).

NOTE: Chloramphenicol is dependent on hepatic metabolism; do not use it in patients with severe hepatic dysfunction.

SURGICAL ANATOMY

The hepatic and cystic ducts, the bile duct (also known as the common bile duct), and the gallbladder constitute the extrahepatic biliary system (Fig. 21-2). Bile drains from the hepatic ducts into the bile duct and is stored and concentrated in the gallbladder. The gallbladder lies between the quadrate lobe of the liver medially and the right medial lobe laterally. It is a pear-shaped organ that, in medium-size dogs, holds approximately 15 ml of bile. The rounded end is the fundus. Between the neck of the gallbladder (i.e., the tapering end leading into the cystic duct) and the fundus is the body, or middle portion, of the gallbladder.

The cystic duct extends from the neck of the gallbladder to the junction with the first tributary from the liver. From this point to the opening of the biliary system into the duodenum, the duct is called the bile duct. The bile duct runs through the lesser omentum for approximately 5 cm and enters the mesenteric wall of the duodenum. The bile duct of dogs is generally approximately 3 mm in diameter, whereas that of cats is 2 to 2.5 mm. By contrast, the human bile duct is approximately 10 mm in diameter. The canine bile duct terminates in the duodenum near the opening of the minor pancreatic duct. This combined opening of the minor (accessory) pancreatic duct and the bile duct is the major duodenal papilla. The feline bile duct usually joins the major pancreatic duct before entering the duodenum. Thus cats with intestinal and hepatic disease may be at increased risk for pancreatitis as a result of ascending infection.

Diagnostic Imaging

Radiographic findings in patients with extrahepatic biliary obstruction are generally nonspecific. Hepatomegaly and gallbladder distention may be noted. Mineral opacities in the right cranial abdominal quadrant may be indicative of

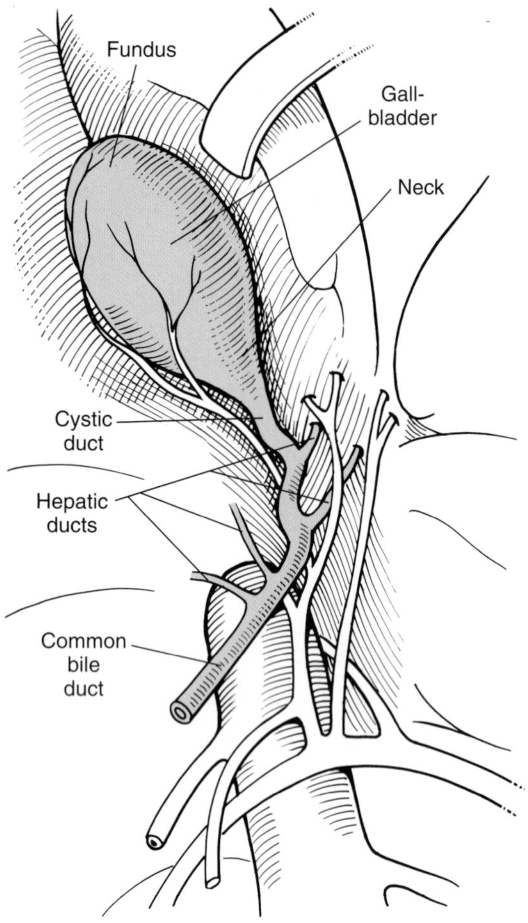

FIG. 21-2
Anatomy of the extrahepatic biliary system.

cholecystic calculi (see p. 567); however, these calculi may also be incidental findings in dogs and cats. Ultrasound evaluation may help distinguish intrahepatic causes of biliary obstruction from extrahepatic. Identification of severe pancreatitis or a mass in the region of the pancreas may raise suspicion of EHBO. With experimental bile duct ligation, the gallbladder becomes distended within 24 hours, whereas the extrahepatic bile ducts will distend within 48 to 72 hours. Intrahepatic ducts take longer to dilate (approximately a week). Remember that dilation from a previous obstructive episode may not resolve, and thus it may be difficult to discern if the present dilation is due to recent or past disease.

Hepatobiliary scintigraphy has been used to determine patency of the common bile duct. With ultrasound, it may be difficult to discern if dilation of the common bile duct in the absence of an obvious obstruction (i.e., calculus or mass) is associated with complete or partial biliary obstruction. A recent study evaluated the usefulness of serum biochemical values and scintigraphic studies for differentiating between animals that had complete EHBO and those that had partial obstruction (Head and Daniel, 2005). They determined that

animals that did not have intestinal radioactivity within 3 to 4 hours should have additional imaging performed (up to 24 hours) to determine if they had complete EHBO. Those that had partial obstructions had delayed arrival of the radioactivity and less radioactivity in the intestine. Reevaluating these animals at 24 hours may lead to greater specificity. Hepatobiliary scintigraphy appears to be an insensitive test for structural hepatobiliary disease (e.g., cholangiohepatitis) (Newell et al, 2001).

SURGICAL TECHNIQUE

Exploratory laparotomy should be performed when leakage of bile into the abdomen is suspected; when biliary obstruction appears to be caused by other than pancreatitis; and when neoplasia (biliary tract, intestinal, or pancreatic), biliary calculi, or parasitic disease is suspected. During exploration, the patency of the common bile duct must be ensured by manually expressing the gallbladder or by catheterization of the duct, either retrograde (i.e., from the duodenum; see p. 563) or in some cases normograde (i.e., from the gallbladder).

The treatment of animals with EHBO secondary to benign pancreatic disease initially consists of medical management of the pancreatitis. If clinical or laboratory improvement is not seen within 7 to 10 days of initiating appropriate therapy or if clinical deterioration occurs despite excellent medical therapy, cholecystoduodenostomy or cholecystojejunostomy may be considered. In extremely ill patients with biliary obstruction that cannot undergo surgical exploration, temporary decompression of the gallbladder may be warranted using ultrasound-guided aspiration, a Foley catheter, or a self-retaining accordion catheter.

Cholecystotomy

Cholecystotomy is rarely performed, but may be indicated to remove some choleliths (see p. 567) or when the gallbladder's contents are inspissated and cannot be aspirated into a syringe.

Pack the area surrounding the gallbladder with sterile, moistened laparotomy sponges. Place stay sutures in the gallbladder to facilitate manipulation and reduce spillage. Make an incision in the fundus of the gallbladder (Fig. 21-3). Remove the gallbladder contents and submit for culture. Lavage the gallbladder with warmed, sterile saline. Catheterize the common bile duct via the cystic duct with a 3.5 or 5 French (Fr) soft catheter, and flush it to ensure patency. Close the incision with a one- or two-layer inverting suture pattern using absorbable suture (3-0 to 5-0).

Cholecystectomy

Cholecystitis that is not responsive to or that relapses after antibiotics, spontaneous rupture, and cholelithiasis that is associated with disease (many are asymptomatic) is best treated by cholecystectomy (see p. 567). Cholecystectomy may also be indicated for primary neoplasia or traumatic rupture of the gallbladder.

Expose the gallbladder, and use Metzenbaum scissors to incise the visceral peritoneum along the junction of the gallbladder and the liver (Fig. 21-4, A). Apply gentle traction to the gallbladder, and use blunt dissection to free it from the liver. Free the cystic duct to its junction with the common bile duct. Be sure

to identify the common bile duct and avoid damaging it during the procedure. If necessary, identify the common bile duct by placing a 3.5 or 5 Fr soft catheter into the duct via the duodenal papilla. Make a small enterotomy in the proximal duodenum, locate the duodenal papilla, and place a small red rubber tube into the common bile duct (Fig. 21-4, B). Flush the duct to ensure its patency. Clamp and double ligate the cystic duct and cystic artery (Fig. 21-4, C) with nonabsorbable suture (2-0 to 4-0). Sever the duct distal to the ligatures, and remove the gallbladder. Submit a portion of the wall, plus bile, for culture if infection is suspected. Submit the remainder of the gallbladder for histologic analysis if indicated (for cholecystitis or neoplasia). Close the duodenal incision in a simple interrupted pattern with absorbable suture (i.e., 2-0 to 4-0).

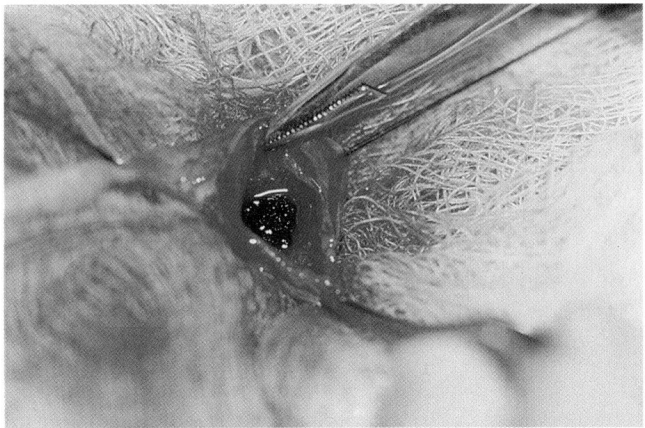

FIG. 21-3
Before cholecystotomy, place stay sutures in the gallbladder to facilitate manipulation and reduce spillage. Then make an incision in the fundus of the gallbladder.

> NOTE: Be sure that the common bile duct is patent before performing a cholecystectomy. The animal must have a pathway for biliary drainage into the intestinal tract.

Choledochotomy

Direct incision of the bile duct should be performed only in animals in which the duct is greatly dilated, such as with chronic obstruction, and when the obstruction can be re-

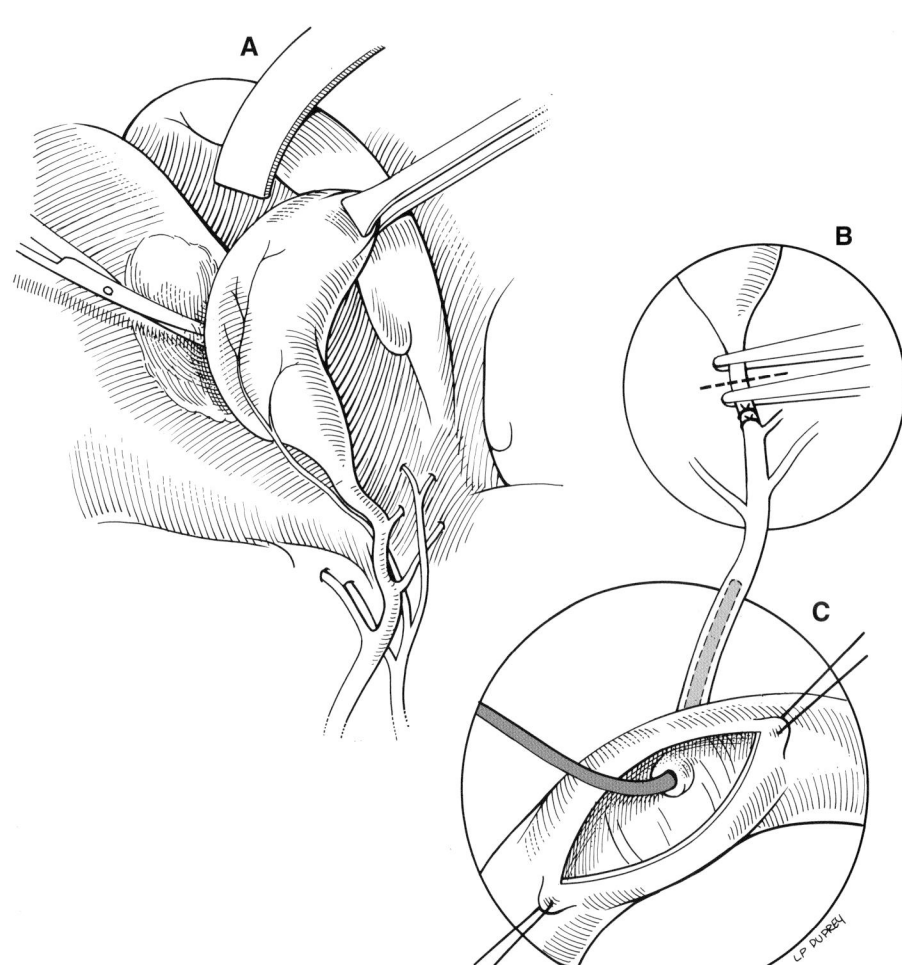

FIG. 21-4
Cholecystectomy. **A,** Expose the gallbladder and then use Metzenbaum scissors to incise the visceral peritoneum along the junction of the gallbladder and the liver. **B,** Identify the common bile duct; take care not to damage it during the procedure. If necessary, cannulate the duct via the duodenal papilla. **C,** Clamp and double ligate the cystic duct and cystic artery.

moved (i.e., choledocholithiasis and biliary sludge). An attempt should first be made to remove the obstruction by flushing the common bile duct using a catheter placed by means of an enterotomy or by cholecystotomy. Extraluminal obstruction or stricture of the duct is best treated with biliary diversion techniques (see later discussion).

Pack the area surrounding the common bile duct with sterile, moistened laparotomy sponges. Place traction sutures in the distended duct. Make a small incision in the duct, and remove the obstruction (Fig. 21-5). Flush the duct with copious amounts of warmed, sterile saline, and pass a 3.5 to 5 Fr soft catheter into the gallbladder and duodenum to ensure patency. Close the incision in a simple continuous or simple interrupted pattern with absorbable suture (4-0 or 5-0). If leakage is a concern, pass a catheter into the duct through an incision in the proximal duodenum (see p. 563). Small leaks may be treated by stenting the incision with a 3.5 to 5 Fr soft catheter (see discussion on repairing common bile duct injuries).

Bile Flow Diversion

Bile flow diversion is indicated if the common bile duct is obstructed or if the duct has been severely traumatized and the gallbladder is not directly involved in the disease process.

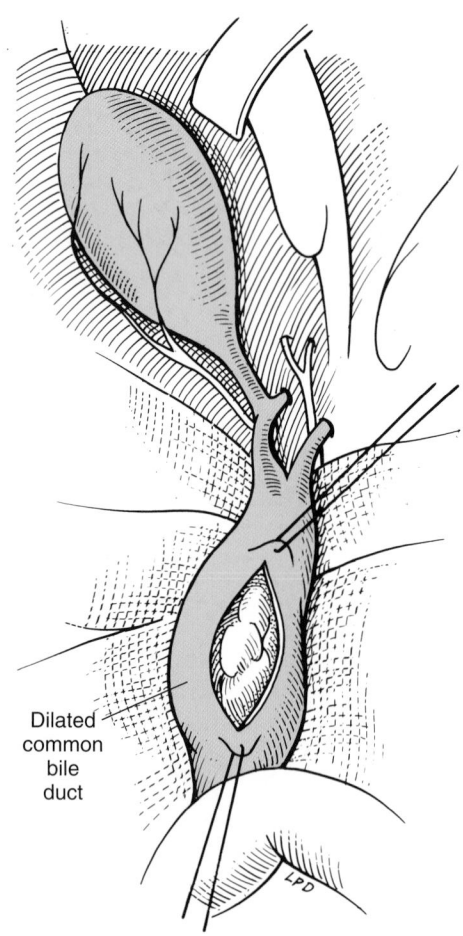

FIG. 21-5
Choledochotomy.

Cholecystoenterostomy (i.e., cholecystojejunostomy or cholecystoduodenostomy) is preferred over choledochoduodenostomy in dogs and cats because the small size of the common bile duct in these species often makes the latter procedure difficult to perform successfully. If cholecystojejunostomy is performed, the proximal jejunum should be used to reduce the incidence of postoperative maldigestion of lipids. In dogs, it has been recommended that the stoma between the bowel and the gallbladder be at least 2.5 cm long to minimize the potential for obstruction of bile flow or retention of bowel contents in the gallbladder. Making the stoma too small is more apt to result in ascending or chronic cholecystitis than making the stoma too large.

> NOTE: If possible, avoid biliary diversion in dogs with pancreatitis. Almost all affected animals improve with medical management, making the technique unnecessary.

Mobilize the gallbladder from the liver as described for cholecystectomy. Place stay sutures approximately 3 cm apart in the gallbladder. Bring the gallbladder into apposition with the antimesenteric surface of the descending duodenum so that little or no tension is exerted on the gallbladder or intestine. Pack the area surrounding the gallbladder and duodenum with sterile, moistened laparotomy sponges. Place a continuous suture of absorbable suture material (i.e., 2-0 to 4-0) between the serosa of the gallbladder and the serosa of the duodenum, near the mesentery (referred to as the original suture line; Fig. 21-6, A). Make the suture line 3 to 4 cm long. Leave the ends of the suture long, and use them to manipulate the intestine and gallbladder. Drain the gallbladder and make a 2.5- to 3-cm incision in it, parallel to the preplaced suture line (Fig. 21-6, B). Have an assistant occlude the duodenum proximal and distal to the proposed incision site. Make a similar parallel incision in the antimesenteric surface of the duodenum (Fig. 21-6, C). Place a continuous suture line of absorbable suture material (2-0 to 4-0) from the mucosa of the gallbladder to the mucosa of the duodenum, beginning with the edges closest to the original suture line (Fig. 21-6, D). Then use the same suture material to suture the mucosal edges of the stoma farthest from the original suture line (Fig. 21-6, E). Complete the stoma by suturing the serosal edges of the gallbladder and intestine over the near side of the stoma (i.e., the side farthest from the original suture line; Fig. 21-6, F).

> NOTE: If you cannot identify the mucosa of the gallbladder and suture it as a separate layer, perform a two-layer anastomosis of the far side, followed by a two-layer anastomosis of the near side.

Repair of Common Bile Duct Injuries

The surgical technique used to repair lacerations of the common bile duct depends on the location and severity of the lesion. Severely damaged ducts are difficult to repair, par-

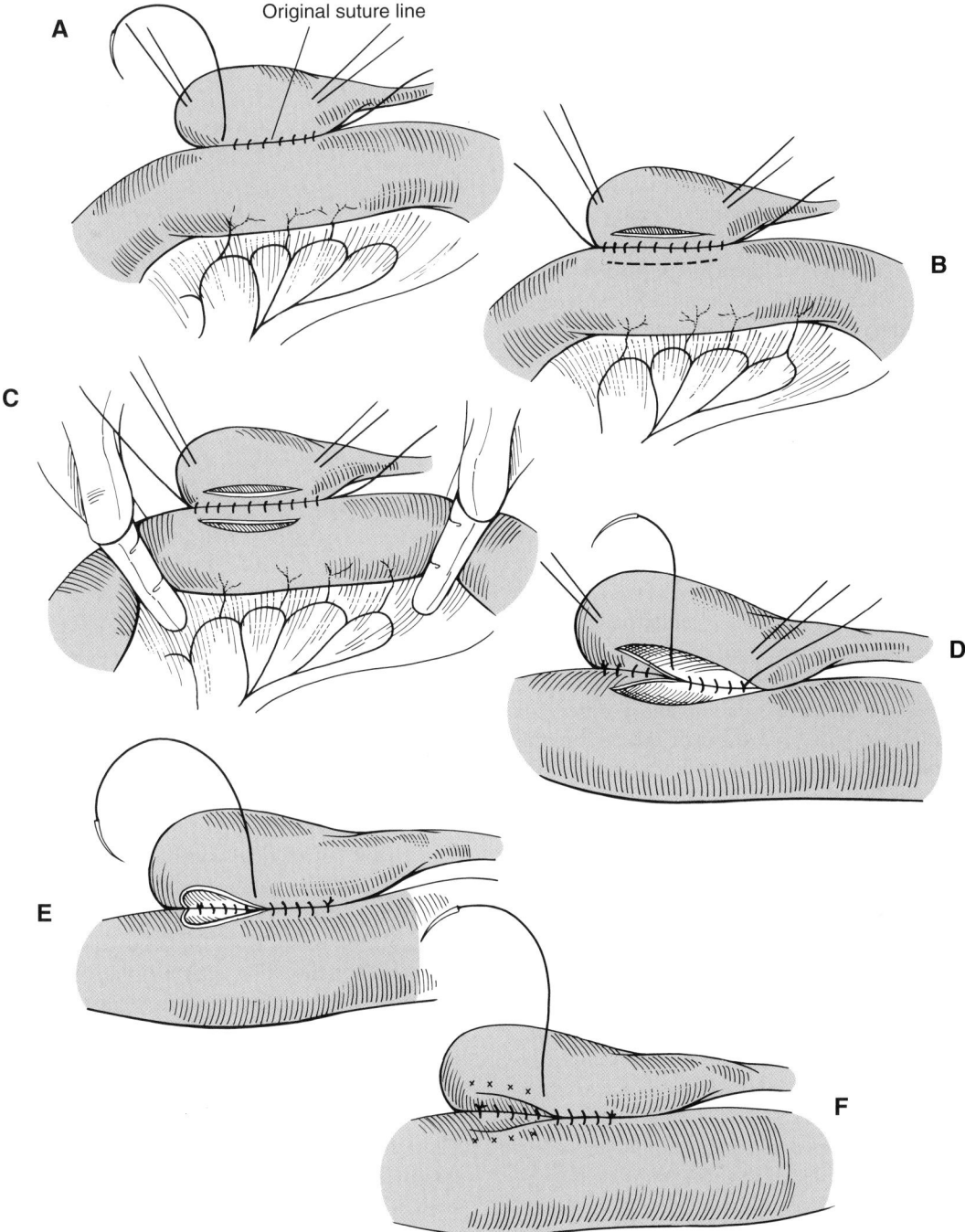

FIG. 21-6

For cholecystoduodenostomy (or cholecystojejunostomy), bring the gallbladder into apposition with the antimesenteric surface of the descending duodenum. **A,** Place a 3- to 4-cm continuous suture line between the serosa of the gallbladder and the serosa of the duodenum (original suture line). **B,** Drain the gallbladder and make a 2.5- to 3-cm incision in it, parallel to the preplaced suture line. **C,** Have an assistant occlude the duodenum proximal and distal to the proposed incision site and make a parallel incision in the antimesenteric surface of the duodenum. **D,** Place a continuous suture line from the mucosa of the gallbladder to the mucosa of the duodenum, beginning with the edges closest to the original suture line. **E,** Suture the mucosal edges of the stoma farthest from the original suture line. **F,** Complete the stoma by suturing the serosal edges of the gallbladder and intestine over the near side of the stoma.

ticularly with bile leakage or adhesion formation. Incisional dehiscence, leakage, and stricture formation are common. If the injury is distal to the entrance of the hepatic ducts, the common bile duct should be ligated proximal and distal to the injury and biliary diversion performed (i.e., cholecysto-duodenostomy or cholecystojejunostomy; see p. 564). If the duct has been cleanly severed and the luminal diameter is greater than 4 to 5 mm (which is seldom), primary suturing and anastomosis are possible. Similarly, proximal lacerations or perforations may be treated with primary suturing. The mucosa of the bile duct should be accurately reapposed. Small sutures should be used and tension on the suture line avoided.

The use of stenting catheters in the common bile duct is controversial, but temporary bile diversion may allow healing of bile duct injuries that otherwise would dehisce, leak, or form a stricture. The tube acts to decompress the biliary tree and minimizes bile leakage from the site during healing. Disadvantages of tubes placed in the bile duct include a greater risk of stricture formation because of the presence of a foreign body at the injury site, obstruction of the tube, and ascending infection. If the bile duct is stented, a soft tube that is smaller than the diameter of the duct should be used to minimize irritation to the duct wall. The use of rubber tubes or catheters that enter the duodenum and T-tubes that exit the duct and are exteriorized through the abdominal wall has been described in the veterinary literature. The use of a straight catheter (i.e., Sovereign feeding tube or Dover red rubber Robinson catheter) has been described here.

Identify the common bile duct. This may be facilitated by passing a catheter into the duct from the duodenum (see previous discussion of cholecystectomy).

Be careful not to interfere with the blood supply to the duct during manipulation. Carefully débride the transected ends of the duct, but be sure to leave adequate duct length to prevent tension on the suture line when the ends are reapposed. Reapprose the ends of the duct in a simple interrupted pattern using absorbable suture (4-0 to 6-0). Place a 3.5 to 5 Fr soft catheter in the duct from the duodenum to stent the suture line (Fig. 21-7). Suture the distal end of the catheter to the duodenal lumen with small chromic gut suture (3-0 or 4-0). As the suture dissolves, peristalsis will cause the catheter to enter the intestinal lumen, where it will pass in the feces.

Healing of the Biliary Tract

Studies have shown that if just a small strip of the common bile duct wall remains intact, the duct regenerates. However, longitudinal tension on the suture line of a repaired biliary duct causes severe stenosis. In addition to promoting stricture of the duct, there is some suggestion that intraluminal tubes may interfere with normal biliary drainage, thus promoting cholangitis. Because of uncertainties regarding healing of the duct in the presence of infection, leakage, or tension, drainage procedures such as cholecystojejunostomies are commonly performed rather than direct repair of the common bile duct (see p. 564).

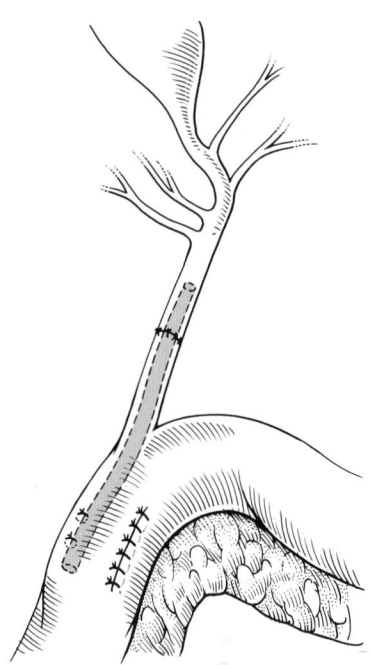

FIG. 21-7
Lacerations in the common bile duct may be sutured over a stent placed by means of a duodenotomy.

SUTURE MATERIALS AND SPECIAL INSTRUMENTS

Absorbable suture material should be used in the biliary tree because nonabsorbable suture may act as a nidus for stone formation. Biliary duct surgery is aided by the use of small instruments, such as those used for ophthalmic surgery. With biliary diversion surgery, the gallbladder should be emptied with a syringe and needle or a needle attached to suction before surgical manipulation to reduce spillage of bile during the procedure.

POSTOPERATIVE CARE AND ASSESSMENT

Fluid therapy should be continued until the animal is able to maintain hydration with oral fluids. Electrolytes and acid-base status should be assessed and corrected during the postoperative period. Many patients with bile peritonitis (see pp. 570-572) are debilitated before surgery, and nutritional supplementation may be beneficial (see Chapter 11). Antibiotic therapy should be continued for 7 to 10 days if cholecystitis was present or if bile leakage occurred before or during surgery. Open abdominal drainage may be considered in patients with generalized bile peritonitis. See Table 13-4 on p. 133 for postoperative analgesic recommendations in patients with bile peritonitis.

PROGNOSIS

The prognosis for cats with EHBO is guarded. In a recent study of 22 cats with this condition, biliary or pancreatic adenocarcinoma was diagnosed in 6 cats and 1 had an unidentified mass (Mayhew et al, 2002). All cats with neoplasia died or were euthanized. Mortality in cats with nonneoplastic disease was 40%.

Biliary diversion in cats may be associated with a high early mortality and surviving cats may have chronic vomiting and anorexia (Bacon and White, 2003). Vomiting is typically transient in nature and responsive to antibiotics. Thus biliary diversion should be avoided if possible in cats, but should be considered if no other viable alternatives exist. The prognosis after biliary diversion in dogs is unknown; there are few recent reports with long-term follow-up. However, bleeding at the stoma site and ascending infections are known to occur.

COMPLICATIONS

Surgery of the extrahepatic biliary tree requires technical competence, manual dexterity, and sound surgical judgment to prevent serious complications. Potential complications after cholecystectomy (particularly if perforation was present) include generalized peritonitis, shock, sepsis, hypoglycemia, hypoproteinemia, and hypokalemia. Stricture, bile leakage, and dehiscence may occur after surgery of the common bile duct. Ascending cholangiohepatitis may occur in some animals after biliary diversion, particularly if the stoma of the enteric-biliary anastomosis is too small and if intestinal contents remain in the gallbladder lumen for prolonged periods. Intermittent antibiotic therapy may be necessary in such animals. Long-term complications after biliary decompression include cholangiohepatitis, recurrence of obstruction, and chronic weight loss.

SPECIAL AGE CONSIDERATIONS

Trauma should be suspected in young animals with bile peritonitis. Obstruction that occurs secondary to pancreatitis or neoplasia is more common in middle-aged or older animals.

References

Bacon NJ, White RAS: Extrahepatic biliary tract surgery in the cat: a case series and review, *J Small Animal Pract* 44:231, 2003.

Head LL, Daniel GB: Correlation between hepatobiliary scintigraphy and surgery or postmortem examination findings in dogs and cats with extrahepatic biliary obstruction, partial obstruction, or patency of the biliary system: 18 cases (1995-2004), *J Am Vet Med Assoc* 227:1618, 2005

Mayhew PD, Holt DE, McLear RC et al: Pathogenesis and outcome of extrahepatic biliary obstruction in cats, *J Small Anim Pract* 43:247, 2002.

Newell SM, Graham JP, Roberts GD et al: Quantitative hepatobiliary scintigraphy in normal cats and in cats with experimental cholangiohepatitis, *Vet Radiol Ultrasound* 42:70, 2001.

CHOLELITHIASIS

DEFINITIONS

Calculi found in the gallbladder are **choleliths;** those found in the common bile duct are **choledocholiths**. Calculi are often called *gallstones.*

GENERAL CONSIDERATIONS AND CLINICALLY RELEVANT PATHOPHYSIOLOGY

Choleliths are often fortuitous findings at necropsy or during imaging with radiographs or ultrasound. They frequently are clinically silent; however, they may be associated with cholecystitis and/or cholangiohepatitis, vomiting, anorexia, icterus, fever, or abdominal pain. Whereas human beings usually develop dietary-induced cholesterol gallstones, cholesterol, bilirubin, and mixed stones have been reported in dogs and cats. The rarity of canine cholelithiasis may be due to (1) decreased concentrations of cholesterol in canine bile, (2) absorption of ionized calcium from the gallbladder, limiting the amount of free ionized calcium in bile, and (3) failure to recognize choleliths. Calcium salts are the major components of pigment gallstones, therefore the availability of ionized calcium may be important in gallstone formation in dogs. Pigment gallstones can be experimentally produced in dogs after 6 weeks of a methionine-deficient diet or with a high-cholesterol diet that is deficient in taurine. Calcium carbonate and mixed choleliths (calcium carbonate, calcium bilirubinate, and cholesterol) are also the most common types found in cats.

DIAGNOSIS

> NOTE: Most choleliths are asymptomatic; treatment is indicated only when the calculi are associated with clinical signs.

Clinical Presentation

Signalment. Aged female small-breed dogs appear to be at increased risk for the development of choleliths. Middle-aged to older male cats may be more commonly affected.

History. Most animals with choleliths are asymptomatic; however, they may be presented for treatment of fever, vomiting, icterus, or abdominal pain if cholecystitis or biliary obstruction occurs. Clinical signs may be mild and intermittent in some animals. The most common clinical signs in cats with cholelithiasis were progressive vomiting, dehydration, anorexia, icterus, and lethargy (Eich and Ludwig, 2002).

Physical Examination Findings

Icterus may be noted if the calculus causes biliary obstruction or ascending cholangitis. Abdominal pain and vomiting may also occur. In rare cases, choleliths have been associated with perforation of the gallbladder or common bile duct (see p. 571).

Diagnostic Imaging

Gallstones are seldom radiopaque (Fig. 21-8), but they are readily identified by ultrasound. A hyperechoic focus with acoustic shadowing originating from the lumen of the gallbladder may be noted (Fig. 21-9). If obstruction is present, dilation of the common bile duct or intrahepatic ducts may also be detected. Contrast radiographs of the biliary tree are rarely useful in icteric patients. Endoscopic retrograde pancreatography is difficult and rarely performed in dogs. Di-

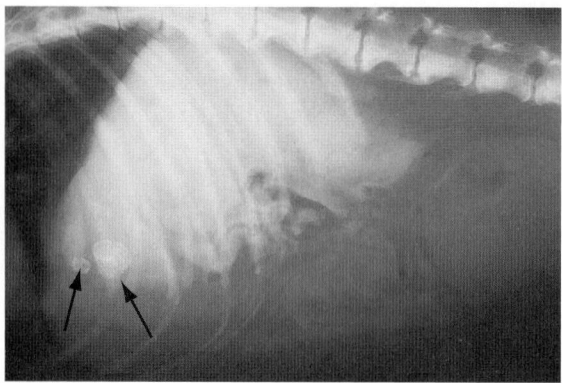

FIG. 21-8
Lateral abdominal radiograph in a dog with radiopaque choleliths *(arrows)*.

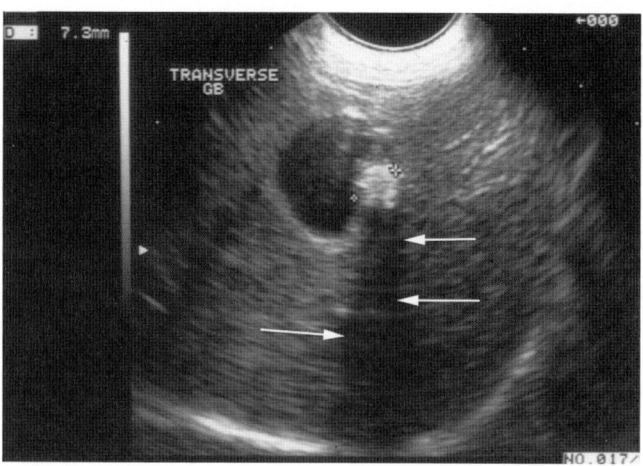

FIG. 21-9
Abdominal ultrasound showing a calculus in the lumen of the gallbladder. Notice that the calculus is hyperechoic and casts an acoustic shadow *(arrows)*.

rect injection of contrast into dilated bile ducts via transabdominal placement of a "slim" needle has been accomplished in people, but is seldom done in dogs.

Laboratory Findings

Abnormalities are uncommon; however, clinically ill animals typically have abnormalities compatible with EHBO. Dogs typically have a notable increase in serum alkaline phosphatase (SAP) and cholesterol, and some increase in alanine transferase (ALT). Hyperbilirubinemia is typical in partial or complete obstruction and when ascending cholangitis occurs. Coagulation profiles are typically normal. Cats are similar, but have lesser elevations of SAP than dogs and may have notable increases in ALT. Urinalysis may be especially helpful in cats because bilirubinuria is always abnormal in that species and occurs before hyperbilirubinemia.

DIFFERENTIAL DIAGNOSIS

Evidence of concurrent cholecystitis should be sought in symptomatic animals with choleliths. Sludge and true concretions may be difficult to differentiate in some animals before surgery. Ultrasonographic-guided, percutaneous cholecystocentesis (Savary-Bataille et al, 2003 ; Voros et al, 2002) with cytology and culture of bile appears to be a very sensitive test for cholecystitis.

MEDICAL MANAGEMENT

Medical dissolution of gallstones in dogs and cats has not been reported and is probably not feasible because of the expected content of most gallstones. Medical management of animals with biliary obstruction is discussed on p. 560. Concurrent cholecystitis should be treated with appropriate antibiotics.

SURGICAL TREATMENT

Because choleliths may be associated with cholecystitis and cause vomiting, anorexia, icterus, fever, or abdominal pain, they should be removed if they are found in a patient with biliary tract disease.

Preoperative Management

See p. 560 for the preoperative management of patients with biliary obstruction. The bacteria isolated from animals with choleliths are typically sensitive to aminoglycosides and fluoroquinolones.

Anesthesia

See pp. 531 and 561 for discussions of the anesthetic management of patients with hepatic or obstructive biliary disease, respectively.

Surgical Anatomy

The surgical anatomy of the biliary tract is described on p. 561.

Positioning

Choleliths generally are removed via a cranial midline abdominal incision.

SURGICAL TECHNIQUE

Cholecystectomy (see p. 562) is the surgical treatment of choice in dogs with clinical signs that occur secondary to cholelithiasis. If stones are also present in the common bile duct, the duct can be catheterized via the duodenum and the stones flushed into the gallbladder (see p. 563). As an alternative, if the bile duct is enlarged, the duct can be incised (choledochotomy) and the stones removed directly; however, care must be taken when suturing the common bile duct to prevent stricture formation (see p. 566). Clinical studies have found a greatly increased mortality in human patients with cholelithiasis when choledochotomy is performed rather than cholecystectomy. Cholecystoenterostomy (see p. 564) should be performed when ductal obstruction cannot be relieved. Bile should be cultured.

SUTURE MATERIALS AND SPECIAL INSTRUMENTS

The gallbladder and common bile duct should be sutured with absorbable suture material to reduce the likelihood of suture serving as a nidus for calculi formation.

POSTOPERATIVE CARE AND ASSESSMENT

See p. 566 for the postoperative management of patients with obstructive biliary disorders. For cholangitis or cholangiohepatitis, aggressive antibiotic therapy plus antioxidant therapy (i.e., vitamin E, vitamin C, s-adenosyl-L-methionine) is indicated. Ursodeoxycholic acid (15 mg/kg given orally once a day) will also help protect hepatocyte membranes, but should only be used if there is no obstruction.

Prognosis

The prognosis is excellent when ductal obstruction can be relieved and a cholecystectomy is performed.

References

Eich CS, Ludwig LL: The surgical treatment of cholelithiasis in cats: a study of nine cases, *J Am Anim Hosp Assoc* 38:290, 2002.

Savary-Bataille KCM, Bunch S, Spaulding KA et al: Percutaneous ultrasound-guided cholecystocentesis in healthy cats, *J Vet Intern Med* 17:298, 2003.

GALLBLADDER MUCOCELES

DEFINITIONS

A **gallbladder mucocele** is a mucus-filled dilation or distention of the gallbladder that is associated with dysfunction of mucus-secreting cells within the gallbladder mucosa. The gallbladder contents are so thick that they cannot be excreted out the bile duct.

GENERAL CONSIDERATIONS AND CLINICALLY RELEVANT PATHOPHYSIOLOGY

Gallbladder mucoceles are becoming an increasingly common cause of extrahepatic biliary obstruction in dogs (Pike et al, 2004); they are rarely reported in cats. They are characterized histologically by hyperplasia of mucus-secreting glands within the gallbladder mucosa, resulting in an abnormal accumulation of mucus within its lumen. They may be caused by obstruction of the common bile duct, or they may be associated with a functional obstruction because of the altered gallbladder wall contractility. EHBO may occur secondarily if mucus extends into the common bile ducts and/or cystic and hepatic ducts. Rupture of the gallbladder may occur, resulting in bile peritonitis (see p. 570) or a modified transudative effusion. Cholecystitis and necrotizing cholecystitis have been suspected as predisposing causes; however, histopathology typically does not indicate an inflammatory or bacterial origin in most animals.

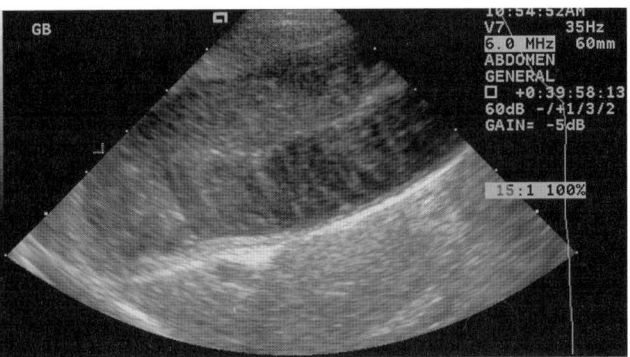

FIG. 21-10
Ultrasound image of a gallbladder mucocele. Notice the typical hyperechoic striations within the lumen of the gallbladder ("kiwi fruit" appearance).

DIAGNOSIS
Clinical Presentation

Signalment. Aged female and male dogs are most commonly affected. A sex or breed predisposition has not been identified, although 30% of dogs in one study were Cocker spaniels (Pike et al, 2004).

History. Some animals with gallbladder mucoceles are asymptomatic; however, they may be presented for signs of systemic illness of several days' to several weeks' duration. Clinical signs are nonspecific and may include vomiting, anorexia, lethargy, polyuria and polydipsia, diarrhea, and abdominal distention.

Physical Examination Findings

Physical examination findings include signs of abdominal discomfort on palpation, depression, icterus, tachypnea, fever, and/or tachycardia. If gallbladder rupture has occurred, abdominal distention may also be noted.

Diagnostic Imaging

Abdominal radiographs are not helpful in diagnosing gallbladder mucoceles; however, they may indicate the presence of abdominal fluid. Gallbladder mucoceles have a classic appearance on ultrasound. Typically, ultrasound reveals echogenic material within the lumen of the gallbladder, which is nongravity dependent and has a classic stellate or "kiwi fruit" appearance (Fig. 21-10). The gallbladder may or may not appear distended. Gallbladder rupture may be suspected on ultrasonography based on the finding of free abdominal fluid, lack of continuity of the gallbladder wall, and the presence of hyperechoic cranial abdominal fat. However, one study suggested that ultrasonography was not sensitive for detecting the severity of disease in affected animals, and focal peritonitis and adhesion may go undetected (Worley et al, 2004).

Laboratory Findings

Common abnormalities include elevated concentrations of ALT, alkaline phosphatase (ALP), aspartate aminotransferase (AST), and γ-glutamyltransferase (GGT). Serum total bilirubin is inconsistently elevated in affected animals. Leukocytosis, neutrophilia, and monocytosis may be seen on hematologic examination. Elevations of ALP, AST, GGT, and serum bilirubin are typically higher in dogs with gallbladder rupture than in those without. High venous lactate levels may also indicate biliary rupture.

DIFFERENTIAL DIAGNOSIS

Surgery may be required upon definitive documentation of a gallbladder mucocele. Other conditions causing partial or complete EHBO should be considered.

MEDICAL MANAGEMENT

Medical management may be considered in dogs that are asymptomatic; however, exploratory celiotomy and cholecystectomy are recommended. Because gallbladder rupture is common in affected animals, serial examinations should be performed in animals managed medically, and surgical intervention should be considered if there is evidence of biliary obstruction.

SURGICAL TREATMENT

Cholecystectomy or cholecystoenterostomy should be performed and cultures of the gallbladder and/or peritoneal fluid submitted for susceptibility testing.

Preoperative Management

See p. 560 for the preoperative management of patients with biliary obstruction. If gallbladder rupture is present, the animal may be debilitated; prompt and aggressive surgery is indicated. Perioperative antibiotics are indicated although they may be delayed in some cases until after cultures have been obtained. The most common bacteria isolated from the abdomen of dogs with gallbladder mucoceles are streptococci and *E. coli*; however, negative cultures are common.

Anesthesia

See pp. 531 and 561 for discussions of the anesthetic management of patients with hepatic or obstructive biliary disease, respectively.

Surgical Anatomy

The surgical anatomy of the biliary tract is described on p. 561.

Positioning

Cholecystectomy and cholecystoenterostomy are performed via a cranial midline abdominal incision.

SURGICAL TECHNIQUE

Cholecystectomy (see p. 562) is the surgical treatment of choice in animals with ruptured gallbladders, particularly when the gallbladder wall is nonviable. In animals with a viable gallbladder, cholecystoenterostomy may be considered. Surgery is indicated on an emergency basis in dogs with gallbladder rupture, whereas those with an intact gallbladder usually can have surgery performed on an elective basis. Hepatic biopsies (see p. 533) are indicated.

SUTURE MATERIALS AND SPECIAL INSTRUMENTS

Nonabsorbable monofilament suture should be used on the cystic duct during cholecystectomy (see p. 566)

POSTOPERATIVE CARE AND ASSESSMENT

See p. 566 for the postoperative management of patients with obstructive biliary disorders. For bile peritonitis see p. 572.

PROGNOSIS

The prognosis is excellent for animals that survive the postoperative period. These dogs typically have complete resolution of their clinical signs and no recurrence. Prompt surgical intervention in dogs with gallbladder rupture typically results in a good or excellent outcome; however, if bile peritonitis is severe, a high mortality can be expected (see p. 572).

References

Besso JG, Wrigley RH, Gliatto JM et al: Ultrasound appearance and clinical findings in 14 dogs with gallbladder mucocele, *Vet Rad Ultrasound* 41:261, 2000.

Pike FS, Berg J, King NV et al: Gallbladder mucocele in dogs: 30 cases (2000-2002), *J Am Vet Med Assoc* 224:1615, 2004.

Worley DR, Hottinger HA, Lawrence HJ: Surgical management of gallbladder mucoceles in dogs: 22 cases (1999-2003), *J Am Vet Med Assoc* 225:1418, 2004.

BILE PERITONITIS

DEFINITION

Bile peritonitis is an inflammation of the peritoneum caused by the leakage of bile into the abdomen. This condition has also been called *bilious ascites*.

GENERAL CONSIDERATIONS AND CLINICALLY RELEVANT PATHOPHYSIOLOGY

Acute abdomen (i.e., shock or pain or both caused by severe abdominal disease) may be caused by leakage of bile into the abdominal cavity, particularly with concurrent septic peritonitis. Leakage of bile into the abdominal cavity may occur with traumatic rupture of any portion of the extrahepatic biliary tree or may occur secondary to necrotizing cholecystitis or chronic obstruction (rare).

Untreated bile peritonitis often is lethal, therefore early diagnosis is imperative. If rupture is associated with biliary tract infection, clinical signs of bile peritonitis usually develop quickly. Dogs with sterile bile peritonitis (i.e., rupture caused by trauma) may only have ascites and icterus for weeks. Bile in the abdominal cavity causes chemical peritonitis, which may not be associated with overt clinical signs initially; however, changes in intestinal mucosal permeability may lead to secondary bacterial infection of the effusion. If diagnosis of a ruptured biliary tract is delayed, repair of the biliary tract is complicated by necrotic tissue and adhesions. Diagnostic peritoneal lavage (see p. 335) may assist in the early diagnosis of bile peritonitis (before the onset of clinical signs) in animals that have suffered abdominal trauma.

NOTE: Diagnose and repair ruptured gallbladders or common bile ducts as soon as possible. Delaying surgery means that the animal will be more debilitated, and fibrosis and adhesions in the area will make surgery more difficult.

Rupture of the extrahepatic biliary ducts or gallbladder may be due to blunt abdominal trauma, necrotizing cholecystitis, or obstruction that occurs secondary to calculi, neoplasia, or parasites. Trauma usually causes rupture of the common bile duct rather than the gallbladder. Ductal rupture probably occurs when a force is applied adjacent to the gallbladder sufficient to cause rapid emptying, combined with a shearing force on the duct. In human beings, biliary duct rupture has been reported in individuals who had previously undergone cholecystectomy, suggesting that shearing of the duct alone sometimes is sufficient. The most common site of ductal rupture appears to be the common bile duct just distal to the entrance of the last hepatic duct; however, rupture may occur in the distal common bile duct, cystic duct (rare), or hepatic ducts. Gallbladder rupture is principally caused by necrotizing cholecystitis or cholelithiasis, but has also been reported secondary to gunshot wounds. Many dogs with necrotizing cholecystitis have obstruction of the common bile duct; however, rupture can be caused by necrosis and perforation of only the gallbladder wall.

DIAGNOSIS
Clinical Presentation

Signalment. Traumatic rupture of the common bile duct or gallbladder may occur in animals of any age. Necrotizing cholecystitis is more common in middle-aged or older animals.

History. The animal may have sustained trauma several weeks before presentation. Clinical signs may be slowly progressive or acute if the bile becomes infected (see later discussion).

Physical Examination Findings

The clinical signs of bile peritonitis depend on the presence of bacteria and on whether the peritonitis is diffuse or localized. Animals with infected bile peritonitis generally are in shock and have acute abdominal pain, fever, vomiting, and anorexia. Animals that develop localized peritonitis secondary to inspissated bile tend not to be as sick as those with diffuse peritonitis. Pain sometimes can be localized to the anterior abdomen. Some animals are diagnosed before a diseased gallbladder ruptures, in which case signs are similar to those of localized peritonitis.

NOTE: Perform diagnostic peritoneal lavage before the onset of clinical signs to help identify bile peritonitis in dogs that have suffered trauma.

Diagnostic Imaging

Radiographs of animals with bile peritonitis may show a generalized loss of visceral detail if the peritonitis is diffuse, or a soft tissue ill-defined opacity in the cranial abdomen if the infection is localized. Survey radiographs may reveal radiopaque gallstones or air in the gallbladder wall or lumen. Ultrasonography may also delineate the location of mass lesions and evaluate the gallbladder and biliary ducts. Exploratory laparotomy is indicated in any patient with bile peritonitis and negates the need for extensive diagnostic workups.

Laboratory Findings

Comparing bilirubin concentrations in serum and abdominal fluid is 100% effective in diagnosing bile leakage. Bilious effusions have bilirubin concentrations greater (typically two times) than those found in serum. Neutrophilia often is noted if the peritonitis is generalized; however, the white blood cell count may be normal with localized infections. A normal or almost normal peripheral white blood cell count plus low numbers of immature neutrophils may be associated with improved survival. Serum biochemical abnormalities commonly found in dogs with bile peritonitis include hyperbilirubinemia, increased ALP, increased ALT, hypoalbuminemia, and hyponatremia. Other findings are inconsistent and depend on the severity of the peritonitis. With septic biliary effusion, multiple types of gram-negative bacteria are typically found on bacterial culture and susceptibility tests.

DIFFERENTIAL DIAGNOSIS

A bilious effusion is obvious because the fluid looks like bile; it is usually easy to distinguish from effusions of other causes that have been stained by bilirubin. However, simultaneous bilirubin concentrations in the serum and effusion should be compared (see previous discussion).

NOTE: To diagnose bile peritonitis, compare bilirubin concentrations in the fluid to those in serum. With bilious effusions, the bilirubin concentration generally is at least twice the bilirubin concentration of serum.

MEDICAL MANAGEMENT

Animals with bile peritonitis may be anemic, hypoproteinemic, or dehydrated or may have electrolyte imbalances. The irritating effects of bile on the peritoneum cause inflammation and fluid transudation into the abdominal cavity, and the animal may be brought in for treatment in hypovolemic or septic shock (or both). Aggressive fluid therapy may be necessary, and electrolyte imbalances should be corrected. Broad-spectrum antibiotics should be administered before, during, and after surgery. Whole-blood transfusions (see Box 5-1, on p. 25) may be indicated (i.e., hematocrit less than 20%). Administration of vitamin K_1 (see Box 21-1) or fresh frozen plasma should also be considered if there are no coagulation abnormalities (vitamin K malabsorption and disseminated intravascular coagulation [DIC] are potential complications).

SURGICAL TREATMENT

Surgical treatment options for common bile duct rupture include ductal repair or biliary diversion (see pp. 564-566). Repair is possible if the rupture is diagnosed early, but becomes difficult once adhesions develop. Cholecystoduodenostomy or cholecystojejunostomy usually is easier and safer. Rupture of a hepatic duct can be treated by ligation of the leaking duct. Gallbladder rupture that occurs secondary to infective processes should be treated by cholecystectomy (see p. 562).

Treatment of necrotizing cholecystitis includes early surgical exploration once the animal's condition has been stabilized. Treatment consists of cholecystectomy, antibiotics, and appropriate therapy for peritonitis. Generally, attempts to salvage the gallbladder by closing the defect are inappropriate because the wall usually is necrotic. Be sure that the common bile duct is not ligated when the gallbladder is removed. Delayed diagnosis probably contributes to the high mortality associated with necrotizing cholecystitis.

> NOTE: Animals with necrotizing cholecystitis have infected bile; therefore clinical signs often begin soon after the gallbladder ruptures. Unless diagnosis and surgical intervention are prompt, mortality is high.

Preoperative Management

Surgery should be performed as soon as the animal's condition has been stabilized. Electrolyte and fluid abnormalities should be corrected before surgery. See also previous discussion of medical management of patients with bile peritonitis.

Anesthesia

Hypovolemic, septic, or shocky dogs may be induced with hydromorphone plus diazepam IV (Box 21-3), given to effect. If intubation is not possible, etomidate may be given, or mask induction with isoflurane or sevoflurane may be used if the patient is not vomiting. For patients in stable condition, see p. 531 for the anesthetic management of patients with hepatobiliary disease.

Surgical Anatomy

See p. 561 for the surgical anatomy of the extrahepatic biliary system.

Positioning

The gallbladder generally is exposed via a cranial midline abdominal incision (see p. 319). The caudal thorax and entire abdomen should be prepared for aseptic surgery.

SURGICAL TECHNIQUE

Cholecystectomy is discussed on p. 562. Laceration or transection of the bile ducts may be treated by primary repair (see p. 564) or biliary diversion (p. 564). A damaged hepatic duct may be ligated because alternative routes for biliary drainage from a single liver lobe will develop. The abdominal fluid and site of rupture or perforation should be cultured during surgery.

 BOX 21-3

Selected Anesthetic Protocol for Dogs With Biliary Disease

Induction

Hydromorphone (0.1 mg/kg given intravenously [IV]) plus diazepam (0.2 mg/kg IV). Give in incremental dosages. Intubate if possible. If necessary, give etomidate (0.5–1.5 mg/kg IV) or propofol (4–6 mg/kg IV) to effect.

Maintenance

Isoflurane or sevoflurane.

Note: Give anticholinergics as needed.

Once the site of leakage has been identified and corrected, the abdomen should be flushed with copious amounts of warm, sterile fluids. Open abdominal drainage (OAD) (see p. 336) may be considered if generalized peritonitis is present.

SUTURE MATERIALS AND SPECIAL INSTRUMENTS

A Poole suction tip is useful for removing abdominal fluid and can help identify the site of leakage. It also is used to remove fluid instilled in the abdomen during lavage.

POSTOPERATIVE CARE AND ASSESSMENT

Fluid therapy should be continued until the animal is able to maintain hydration on its own. Electrolytes and acid-base status should be monitored. Many patients with bile peritonitis are extremely debilitated before surgery. Animals with bile peritonitis are in extreme pain. Postoperative analgesia may be provided with hydromorphone (see Table 13-4 on p. 133) or a fentanyl-lidocaine-ketamine continuous rate infusion (CRI) (see Box 13-1 on p. 136). Butorphanol is also effective, but the analgesia is of shorter duration than with hydromorphone. Nutritional supplementation via a needle-catheter jejunostomy or parenterally is beneficial in these patients (see Chapter 11). Antibiotic therapy based on culture of bile should be continued for at least 7 to 14 days after surgery.

PROGNOSIS

The prognosis for patients with diffuse, septic bile peritonitis is guarded. Without aggressive surgical management, most of these patients die. The prognosis is better if the condition is diagnosed and treated early and is better in animals with nonseptic biliary effusions. In one study of 24 dogs and 2 cats with bile peritonitis, only 27% of animals with septic biliary peritonitis survived, whereas 100% of those with nonseptic biliary peritonitis survived (Ludwig et al, 1997).

Reference

Ludwig LL, Shertel ER, Pratt JM et al: Surgical treatment of bile peritonitis in 24 dogs and 2 cats: a retrospective study (1987-1994), *Vet Surg* 26:90, 1997.

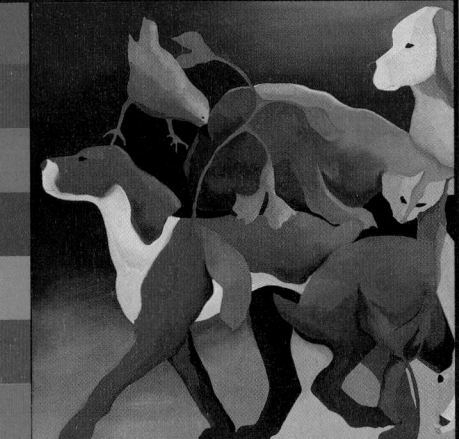

CHAPTER 22
Surgery of the Endocrine System

Surgery of the Adrenal and Pituitary Glands

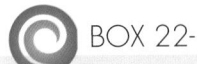

DEFINITIONS

Adrenalectomy is the removal of one or both adrenal glands. **Hypophysectomy** is removal of the pituitary gland (hypophysis). **Hyperadrenocorticism** (HAC) is a multisystemic disorder caused by an excess of glucocorticoids. **Cushing's disease** refers to HAC caused by a pituitary adenoma. **Addison's disease** is caused by a deficiency of glucocorticoids or mineralocorticoids or both.

PREOPERATIVE MANAGEMENT

Adrenocortical insufficiency may be primary, secondary to other diseases, or iatrogenic (i.e., due to administration of glucocorticoids, progestins, or adrenocorticolytic drugs [e.g., o,p'-DDD]). The history should include the dosages of corticosteroids or other drugs given, the type of corticosteroids, the duration of administration, and the time since the last dose. It is easier to inhibit secretion of glucocorticoids than mineralocorticoids (see the discussion of anatomy on p. 574). When glucocorticoid secretion is severely suppressed, the patient may experience depression, inappetence, lethargy, collapse, and/or weakness without electrolyte abnormalities. If mineralocorticoid secretion is suppressed, hyponatremia, hyperkalemia, acidosis, and/or azotemia may occur. Diminished ability to retain sodium results in volume depletion, diminished cardiac output, and reduced vascular tone, which may cause acute vascular collapse. Gastrointestinal disturbances and prolonged vomiting may contribute to electrolyte abnormalities and volume depletion. Electrolyte concentrations should be corrected before surgery. Some dogs with hypoadrenocorticism are hypoalbuminemic. A protective steroid release normally occurs during surgery that prevents circulatory collapse; however, animals with hypoadrenocorticism may be unable to respond to such stress and often re-

BOX 22-1

Protocol for Glucocorticoid Administration in Animals With Adrenocortical Insufficiency Undergoing Minor Elective Procedures

1. 1 hour before surgery give *one* of the following intravenously:

Prednisolone Sodium Succinate

1–2 mg/kg, or

Dexamethasone

0.1–0.2 mg/kg, or

Hydrocortisone Hemisuccinate or Hydrocortisone Phosphate

2 mg/kg

2. Repeat dose at recovery intravenously or intramuscularly.
3. Monitor patient and repeat steroid administration as needed.
4. Resume maintenance glucocorticoid therapy on first postoperative day if needed.

quire glucocorticoid supplementation before and during surgery. When minor elective surgery is performed in animals with adrenocortical insufficiency, glucocorticoid therapy may be given intravenously before induction of anesthesia (Box 22-1). The same dose can be given intravenously or intramuscularly after recovery from anesthesia, and the animal is returned to its oral maintenance glucocorticoid therapy the day after surgery. A similar protocol is used for major surgery, except that glucocorticoid therapy is continued at approximately five times the maintenance dose for 2 to 3 days (Box 22-2). Normal maintenance doses are then reinstituted. Once the animal is eating, medications can be given orally.

HAC is primarily found in dogs; it is very rare in cats. Iatrogenic HAC is the most common type. Spontaneous HAC usually is caused by excessive pituitary secretion of adrenocorticotropic hormone (ACTH), resulting in bilateral adrenocor-

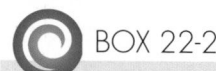

BOX 22-2

Protocol for Glucocorticoid Administration in Animals With Adrenocortical Insufficiency Undergoing Major Elective Procedures

1. Administer preoperative steroids as described in Box 22-1.
2. Repeat dose at recovery intravenously (IV) or intramuscularly (IM).
3. Days 1 and 2 postoperatively, administer *one* of the following IV or IM.

Prednisolone

0.5 mg/kg bid, or

Dexamethasone

0.1 mg/kg qd, or

Cortisone Acetate

2.5 mg/kg bid

4. Resume maintenance glucocorticoid therapy on third postoperative day unless complications arise.

tical hyperplasia or pituitary-dependent hyperadrenocorticism (PDH) (80% to 90% of noniatrogenic cases). Functional adrenocortical tumors (adrenal-dependent hyperadrenocorticism [ADH]) are less common (10% to 20% of noniatrogenic cases). Diagnosis and differentiation of PDH from ADH are potentially complex, and the reader is referred to a medical text for further information.

Patients with HAC are catabolic and are often protein depleted, which may adversely affect wound healing. They may have connective tissue abnormalities and muscle wasting resulting in a pot-bellied appearance, redistribution of fat, and thin, fragile skin. Pyodermas are common in affected dogs, meaning that postoperative suture line healing may be compromised. These dogs may pant because of their catabolic state, but intraabdominal fat deposition plus abdominal muscular weakness sometimes causes ventilatory abnormalities. Hypernatremia, hypokalemia, and alkalosis may be present; substantial abnormalities should be corrected before surgery. Concurrent abnormalities (e.g., congestive heart failure and diabetes mellitus) increase the anesthetic risk in these patients. Cardiovascular abnormalities may occur secondary to hypertension; a thorough preoperative cardiac examination, including blood pressure measurement, is appropriate. Animals with HAC are at increased risk for postoperative pulmonary thromboembolism. If hypercoagulability is suspected, preventive measures (e.g., low-dose heparin therapy) may be indicated before surgery. Many animals with HAC have clinically silent urinary tract infections; therefore a urine culture is indicated in all patients regardless of urinalysis findings.

ANESTHESIA

A variety of anesthetic protocols may be used in adrenocortical-insufficient or hyperadrenal animals. Etomidate causes transient adrenal suppression and should be avoided in patients with hypoadrenocorticism and those in which postoperative hypoadrenocorticism is anticipated perioperatively. Steroid replacement should be provided in animals showing signs of adrenal insufficiency. Maintenance of electrolyte and glucose levels is important. Glucocorticoid supplementation often is necessary in animals with adrenocortical insufficiency undergoing surgery (see previous discussion). Glucocorticoid therapy should be instituted before surgery in patients with HAC that are undergoing adrenalectomy. Because of the close association of the adrenals and the caudal vena cava, retraction of the caudal vena cava often is necessary for adrenalectomy. Vascular pressures should be closely monitored during surgery, and retraction should be done carefully to avoid obstructing venous return. Special anesthetic considerations are required for animals with pheochromocytomas to prevent complications associated with excessive secretion of catecholamines (see p. 583).

ANTIBIOTICS

Animals with HAC are at increased risk of developing postoperative infections as a result of high levels of circulating glucocorticoids and immunosuppression. Perioperative prophylactic antibiotics are recommended for these patients.

SURGICAL ANATOMY

The adrenal glands are near the craniomedial pole of the kidneys (Fig. 22-1). The left adrenal is slightly larger than the right. The left gland lies beneath the lateral process of the second lumbar vertebra; the right adrenal is more cranial, lying beneath the lateral process of the last thoracic vertebra. Because of the proximity of the right adrenal to the caudal vena cava, surgical removal of neoplastic glands can be difficult. The phrenicoabdominal (cranial abdominal) vessels cross the ventral surface of the adrenal. The adrenal glands are composed of two functionally and structurally different regions. The *outer cortex* produces mineralocorticoids (e.g., aldosterone), glucocorticoids, and small amounts of androgenic hormones. Mineralocorticoids regulate sodium and potassium concentrations. Aldosterone causes transport of sodium and potassium through the renal tubular walls and also causes hydrogen ion transport.

The adrenal *medulla* is functionally related to the sympathetic nervous system and secretes epinephrine and norepinephrine in response to sympathetic stimulation. Epinephrine and norepinephrine have almost the same effects as direct sympathetic stimulation (e.g., vascular constriction, resulting in increased arterial pressure; inhibition of the gastrointestinal tract; pupillary dilatation; increased rates of cellular metabolism throughout the body), except that their effects last significantly longer because they are removed from the circulation slowly.

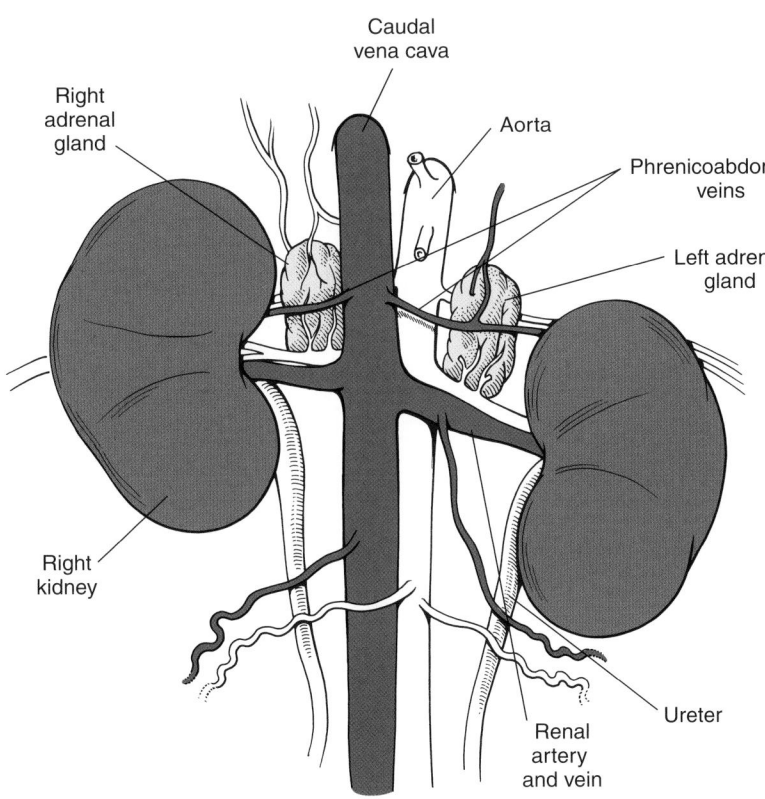

FIG. 22-1
Location of the adrenal glands.

SURGICAL TECHNIQUE

Adrenalectomy usually is performed for adrenal tumors. Bilateral adrenalectomy for canine PDH is controversial and uncommonly performed; but it has been effective for feline PDH. Two approaches may be used. A ventral midline approach allows the entire abdomen to be explored for metastasis and bilateral adrenalectomy to be performed with a single surgical incision if necessary. However, exposure and dissection of the adrenal may be difficult with this approach, particularly in large dogs. A paracostal incision provides better access to the adrenal gland, but does not allow evaluation of the liver or other organs for metastasis. It may be considered in animals with unilateral lesions that have no evidence of metastasis on ultrasound, computed tomography (CT), or magnetic resonance imaging (MRI). Concurrent diabetes mellitus might be a contraindication to bilateral adrenalectomy because lack of endogenous catecholamines may make it difficult to regulate the diabetes.

Adrenalectomy via a Midline Abdominal Approach

Prepare the entire ventral abdomen and caudal thorax for aseptic surgery. Make a ventral midline abdominal incision that extends from the xiphoid cartilage to near the pubis. Identify the enlarged adrenal, and carefully inspect the entire abdomen, including the other adrenal, for abnormalities or evidence of metastasis. Palpate the liver for evidence of nodularity and biopsy if indicated. Palpate the caudal vena cava near the adrenals for evidence of tumor invasion or thrombosis. If additional exposure is necessary for adrenal-

ectomy, extend the incision paracostally on the side of the affected gland by incising the fascia of the rectus abdominis muscle and the fibers of the external abdominal oblique, internal abdominal oblique, and transversus abdominis muscles, respectively. Use self-retaining retractors to improve visualization of the abdominal cavity. Retract the liver, spleen, and stomach cranially, the kidney caudally, and the vena cava medially to expose the entire gland. Identify the blood supply and ureter to the ipsilateral kidney and avoid these structures during dissection. Ligate the phrenicoabdominal vein, and divide it between sutures. Using a combination of sharp and blunt dissection, carefully dissect the adrenal gland from surrounding tissue (Fig. 22-2). Numerous vessels may be encountered. Obtain hemostasis with electrocautery if the vessels are small or with hemoclips if they are large. If possible, do not invade the adrenal capsule.

Removing the adrenal in one piece reduces the chances of leaving small pieces of neoplastic tissue in the abdominal cavity.

If tumor thrombosis is present in the caudal vena cava but extensive metastasis is not apparent, temporarily occlude the vena cava using Rumel tourniquets (see p. 551). Make a longitudinal incision in the vein and remove the thrombus. Close the vena cava in a continuous pattern with 5-0 or 6-0 vascular suture and close the abdomen routinely (see discussion of suture material on p. 576). If a paracostal incision was made, begin the closure by approximating the abdominal wall at the junction of the combined ventral and paracos-

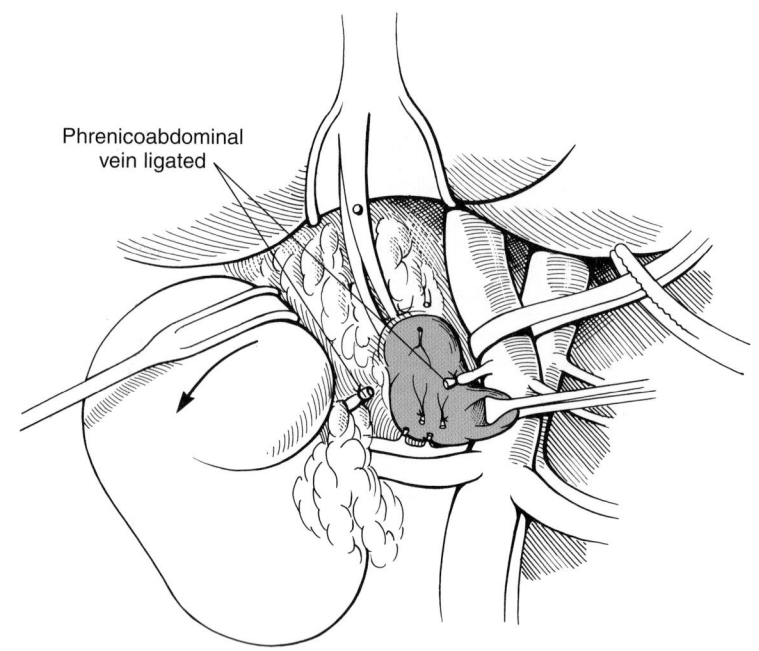

FIG. 22-2
To resect the right adrenal gland, retract the vena cava medially. Ligate the phrenicoabdominal vein and divide it between sutures. Carefully dissect the adrenal gland from surrounding tissue.

Phrenicoabdominal vein ligated

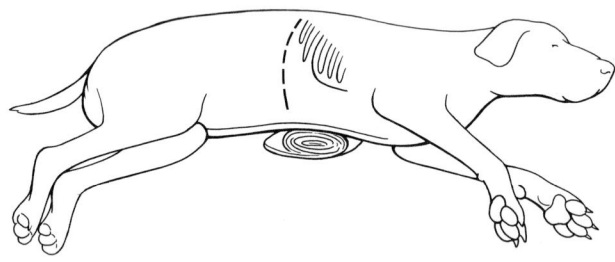

FIG. 22-3
Adrenalectomy may be performed via a paralumbar approach. Place the animal in lateral recumbency with a rolled towel or sandbag between the abdomen and the operating table. Make an incision just caudal to the thirteenth rib, extending it from the lateral vertebral processes to within 3 to 4 cm of the ventral midline.

tal incisions. After closing the linea alba, suture each muscle layer of the paracostal incision with a continuous pattern of synthetic absorbable sutures. Close the skin and subcutaneous tissue routinely.

Adrenalectomy via a Paralumbar Approach

Place the patient in lateral recumbency with a rolled towel or sandbag between the abdomen and the operating table. Prepare the caudal hemithorax and lateral abdomen for aseptic surgery. Make an incision just caudal to the thirteenth rib, extending it from the lateral vertebral processes to within 3 to 4 cm of the ventral midline (the incision will be approximately 10 to 14 cm long, depending on the animal's size [Fig. 22-3]). Incise the abdominal muscles individually, and identify the adrenal gland cranial to the kidney. Retract

the kidney ventrally, and ligate any vascular structures that cross its surface. Dissect the gland free from surrounding tissue (Fig. 22-4). Suture each muscle layer of the paracostal incision in a continuous suture pattern of synthetic absorbable (i.e., 2-0 or 3-0) material. Close the skin and subcutaneous tissues routinely.

HEALING OF THE ADRENAL AND PITUITARY GLANDS

Because adrenal or pituitary biopsies are rarely performed, little information is available about the healing of these glands after surgery.

SUTURE MATERIALS AND SPECIAL INSTRUMENTS

HAC may cause delayed wound healing; therefore abdominal closure should be performed with strong, slowly absorbed, or nonabsorbable suture material (e.g., polydioxanone, polyglyconate, polypropylene, or nylon). Self-retaining retractors, such as Balfour abdominal retractors, are recommended to improve abdominal visualization. Malleable retractors covered with moistened sponges are used to retract viscera from the adrenal glands. Hemostasis is easier to achieve with electrocautery and hemoclips than with suture ligation of vessels.

POSTOPERATIVE CARE AND ASSESSMENT

After adrenalectomy the patient's hydration status and electrolyte balance should be monitored carefully and corrected as necessary. Bilateral adrenalectomy causes permanent adrenal insufficiency, and these animals require lifelong glucocorticoid (prednisone or prednisolone) and/or mineralocorticoid (deoxycorticosterone or fludrocorti-

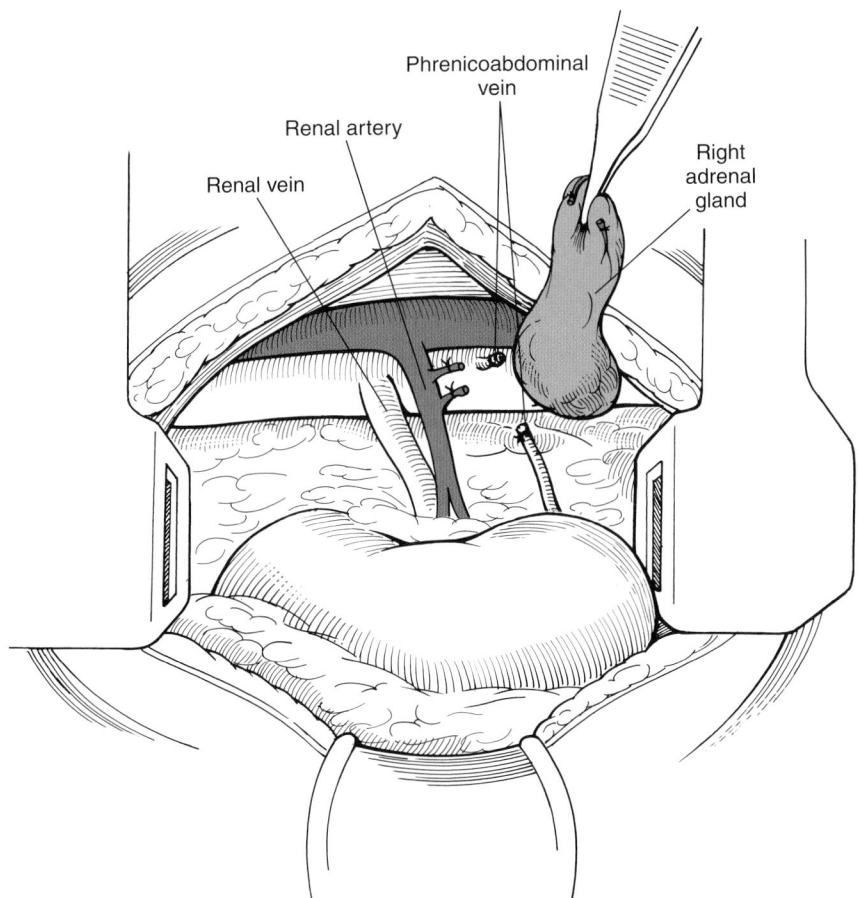

FIG. 22-4
To expose the adrenal gland via a para-lumbar approach, retract the kidney ventrally and ligate any vascular structures that cross its surface.

Labels in figure: Phrenicoabdominal vein; Renal artery; Renal vein; Right adrenal gland

sone) replacement (Box 22-3). These animals should be closely monitored for hypoadrenocortical collapse. They are most likely to have an Addisonian crisis after they have been released to the owner's care. Owners must be advised to watch for malaise, inappetence, vomiting, weakness, and other clinical signs suggesting decompensation. Temporary adrenal insufficiency occurs after unilateral removal of functional adrenal tumors because the tumor has suppressed the opposite adrenal's function. Glucocorticoids should be supplemented postoperatively (see Box 22-3), but may be discontinued when the remaining adrenal begins to function normally, as determined by the results of an ACTH stimulation test.

Pulmonary thromboembolism is a potentially life-threatening complication of adrenal surgery, particularly in dogs with adrenal neoplasia. Sudden, severe, postoperative respiratory distress may indicate pulmonary thromboembolism. Lung perfusion scans may help identify lung regions that are underperfused. Treatment with strict cage rest, oxygen, anticoagulants (e.g., heparin), and thrombolytic agents (e.g., streptokinase) may be beneficial (see Box 22-3). Animals treated for pulmonary thromboembolism should be assessed frequently for signs of hemorrhage, and the hematocrit should be checked every 2 hours. If the packed cell volume (PCV) drops or if hemorrhage is noted, the streptokinase infusion should be discontinued.

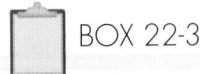 BOX 22-3

Postoperative Drug Therapy After Adrenalectomy in Dogs

Fludrocortisone Acetate (Florinef)*
0.01 mg/kg PO, bid

Prednisolone
0.5 mg/kg bid for 7–14 days, then 0.2 mg/kg qd, or

Cortisone
2.5 mg/kg bid for 7–14 days, then 0.5 mg/kg bid

Heparin (Unfractionated)
Add 35 U/kg to the total amount of plasma required before and during surgery, then give 25 U/kg SC tid the day after surgery†

Streptokinase
Loading dose: 5000 IU/kg IV over 30 minutes; then 2000 IU/kg/hr IV over 24 hours (constant-rate infusion)

PO, Oral; *qd*, once a day; *bid*, twice a day; *SC*, subcutaneous; *tid*, three times a day; *IV*, intravenous.
*Fludrocortisone is much less reliable than desoxycorticosterone pivalate for normalizing serum electrolyte concentrations; however, fludrocortisone's effects only last a day, whereas one injection of desoxycorticosterone acetate lasts 28 days.
†The total amount of plasma to be given will depend on the amount required to replace ATIII or treat hypoalbumenia.

COMPLICATIONS

The main complications of adrenalectomy are hemorrhage, fluid and electrolyte imbalances, pancreatitis, wound infections, delayed wound healing, and thromboembolism. Postoperative hemorrhage usually is associated with incomplete occlusion of small vessels surrounding an enlarged, highly vascular tumor. Judicious use of electrocautery and hemoclips helps prevent this complication. For prevention of thromboembolism, animals may be started on heparin during surgery and continued on it postoperatively (see Box 22-3). Delayed wound healing often is encountered in animals with HAC because of the adverse effect of steroids on wound healing; therefore care should be taken with abdominal closure in these animals (see previous discussion). Strong monofilament absorbable (i.e., polydioxanone or polyglyconate) or nonabsorbable (i.e., polypropylene) suture should be used.

SPECIAL AGE CONSIDERATIONS

Animals with adrenal neoplasia usually are old and often have concurrent abnormalities, such as hypertension or cardiovascular abnormalities; therefore extreme care should be exercised during anesthesia. These animals also require extensive postoperative monitoring. If the animal is debilitated, anorexic, or vomiting, placement of an enteral feeding tube during surgery (see p. 107) or parenteral nutrition is advised.

SPECIFIC DISEASES

ADRENAL NEOPLASIA

DEFINITIONS

Adrenal carcinomas are autonomously functioning, malignant tumors of the adrenal cortex; **adrenal adenomas** are benign adrenocortical tumors. **Pheochromocytomas** are catecholamine-secreting tumors of the chromaffin tissue, which usually arise in adrenal medullary tissue. Pheochromocytomas are also known as *paragangliomas*.

GENERAL CONSIDERATIONS AND CLINICALLY RELEVANT PATHOPHYSIOLOGY

The most common tumors of the canine adrenal glands are adrenal adenomas, carcinomas, and pheochromocytomas. Most adrenal tumors are nonfunctional, in which case clinical signs are caused by local invasion of the tumor into surrounding tissue, distant metastases, or both. Functional tumors secrete excessive amounts of cortisol, which inhibits pituitary ACTH secretion and causes atrophy of the contralateral adrenal. Adrenocortical adenomas and carcinomas appear to occur with equal frequency. They usually are unilateral, although bilateral adrenocortical neoplasia rarely occurs. History, physical examination, and laboratory findings do not differentiate between bilateral and unilateral adrenal neoplasia. Ultrasonographic evaluation of the adrenals often identifies adrenomegaly on one side and adrenal atrophy on the other, which localizes the tumor. Colonic perforation is a rare sequela of excessive glucocorticoid secretion. Corticosteroids may inhibit collagen synthesis and increase collagen breakdown. They also may cause breakdown of the mucosal barrier and inhibit normal immune responses.

> NOTE: Most animals with HAC have pituitary (rather than adrenal) tumors.

Pheochromocytomas are tumors of the adrenal medulla that secrete excessive amounts of catecholamines (primarily norepinephrine, but also epinephrine and dopamine) and other vasoactive peptides (i.e., vasoactive intestinal polypeptide, somatostatin, enkephalin, and corticotropin). Excessive catecholamine and vasoactive peptide levels may manifest as cardiovascular, respiratory, or central nervous system (CNS) disease. Although these tumors classically have been reported as benign, recent reports suggest that regional invasion and distant metastases (liver, regional lymph nodes, lungs, spleen, ovaries, diaphragm, and vertebrae) occur in as many as 50% of affected dogs. Invasion of the caudal vena cava, phrenicoabdominal (cranial abdominal) artery or vein, renal artery or vein, or hepatic vein may cause signs of ascites, edema, or venous distention. Pheochromocytomas usually are unilateral, although bilateral tumors occur. These masses are usually reddish tan, multilobulated, firm or friable, and may be completely or partly encapsulated. Occasionally, pheochromocytomas may be associated with neoplastic transformation of multiple endocrine tissues of neuroectoderm origin (e.g., pituitary, adrenocortical, or thyroid adenomas or pancreatic islet cell tumors). Extraadrenal pheochromocytomas have been reported in dogs and cats. Other tumors rarely arising from the adrenal medulla include neuroblastomas and ganglioneuromas.

DIAGNOSIS
Clinical Presentation

Signalment. Adrenocortical tumors usually occur in older, large-breed dogs and appear to be diagnosed more commonly in females. A definitive breed predisposition has not been identified. Pheochromocytomas usually occur in older dogs, but have been reported in dogs as young as 1 year of age. Both genders appear to be equally affected, and boxers may be predisposed to this tumor. Adrenal tumors are rarely diagnosed in cats.

History. Functional adrenocortical tumors commonly cause HAC (i.e., polyuria, polydipsia, polyphagia, pendulous abdomen [i.e., "pot belly"]), endocrine alopecia, muscle wasting, weakness, lethargy, panting, and/or hyperpigmentation). Vomiting has been associated with intestinal perforation in a dog with adrenocortical adenoma, but this is rare. High circulating levels of glucocorticoids may make diagnosis of intestinal perforation difficult, because signs of peritonitis (abdominal discomfort, restlessness, panting, weakness, and/or dyspnea) initially are obscured. Occasionally, dogs are asymptomatic, and the adrenal mass is a fortuitous finding at surgery or necropsy.

Pheochromocytomas may cause vague, intermittent signs of weakness or panting as a result of episodic hypertension and tachycardia. Many times they are often incidental findings of ultrasonography or necropsy. Signs of nonfunctional adrenocortical tumors may include anorexia, abdominal enlargement, abdominal pain, diarrhea, vomiting, and lethargy; however, they too may be incidental findings of ultrasonography or necropsy.

Physical Examination Findings

Clinical findings in animals with adrenocortical tumors depend on whether the tumors are functional. Dogs with ADH usually have obvious signs of HAC (see previous discussion), whereas ascites, abdominal pain, edema, diarrhea, and/or vomiting are common with nonfunctional tumors.

Clinical findings in animals with pheochromocytomas may include tachycardia or cardiac arrhythmias, acute collapse, polypnea, panting, cough, lethargy, anorexia, dyspnea, weakness, abdominal distention, congestive heart failure, ataxia, incoordination, polyuria-polydipsia, and alopecia. Hypertension (paroxysmal or sustained) also is frequently present. However, pheochromocytomas are often incidental findings in dogs that have no clinical signs associated with the tumor.

Diagnostic Imaging

Adrenal tumors are difficult to detect radiographically unless they are associated with significant adrenal enlargement (20 mm or larger) or calcification. Food should be withheld for 24 hours before radiography to allow the gastrointestinal tract to empty. In some dogs, mineralization of tissue cranial to the kidney may be seen on survey radiographs and may or may not be associated with obvious adrenal enlargement. This finding is suggestive of adrenocortical neoplasia (adenoma or carcinoma). The incidence of nonneoplastic mineralization of adrenal glands is low in dogs; however, bilateral adrenal calcification may occur with PDH. Conversely, adrenal gland mineralization is considered an incidental finding in cats (Fig. 22-5). Hepatomegaly, calcinosis cutis, or osteoporosis may be seen with PDH and ADH. Enhanced abdominal contrast caused by increased abdominal fat may occur. Dogs with HAC are more likely to have calcium-containing uroliths than are dogs with no clinical evidence of HAC. Although pheochromocytomas may be detected radiographically if sufficiently enlarged, ultrasonography is more sensitive.

> **NOTE:** If you note mineralization of an adrenal gland radiographically in a dog, consider the possibility of neoplasia.

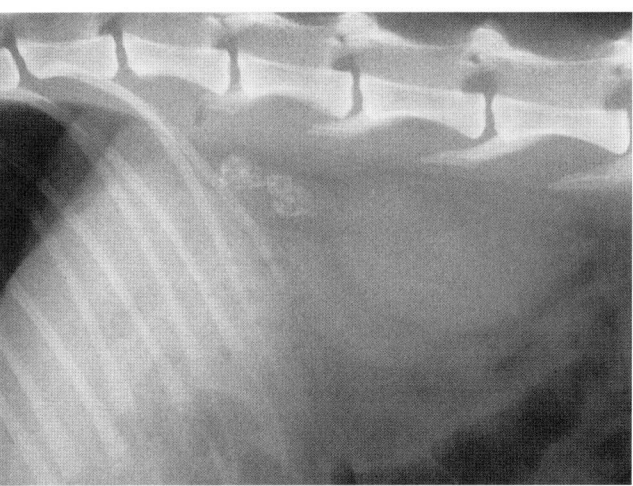

FIG. 22-5
Lateral abdominal radiograph of a cat with a mineralized adrenal gland. (Courtesy L. Homco, Ithaca, N.Y.)

Ultrasonography is useful for assessing the adrenal gland's size, echogenicity, and shape and whether there is invasion of an adrenal mass into adjacent structures. The normal canine adrenal gland size in mature dogs is dependent upon body size. There are several methods that can be used to assess the size of the adrenal gland on ultrasound. One method is to compare the maximal width versus the length of the gland, which should be less than approximately 30%. Alternatively the width of the gland should not be larger in diameter than the diameter of the adjacent aorta. Absolute measurements have also been reported (i.e., the canine adrenal should be less than 7.4 mm; the feline adrenal should be less than 4.3 mm).

Both adrenals should be routinely imaged in dogs with HAC because one normal adrenal gland does not exclude the existence of a contralateral functional adrenocortical tumor. Bilateral adrenocortical tumors are very rare, but do occur. Pheochromocytomas have been reported to have mixed echo patterns and cannot be definitively differentiated from adrenocortical tumors. Although bilateral adrenal enlargement is suggestive of PDH, atrophy of the contralateral adrenal gland in dogs with functional adrenocortical tumors may not be apparent ultrasonographically. Adrenal metastasis may be diagnosed ultrasonographically.

> **NOTE:** It is not possible to differentiate definitively between benign and malignant adrenal lesions using ultrasonographic criteria alone.

CT and MRI allow accurate localization of adrenal neoplasia, but they do not allow differentiation of adrenal adenomas, carcinomas, and pheochromocytomas. Adrenal carcinomas may appear as well-demarcated, homogeneous masses, or they may be poorly demarcated, with irregular

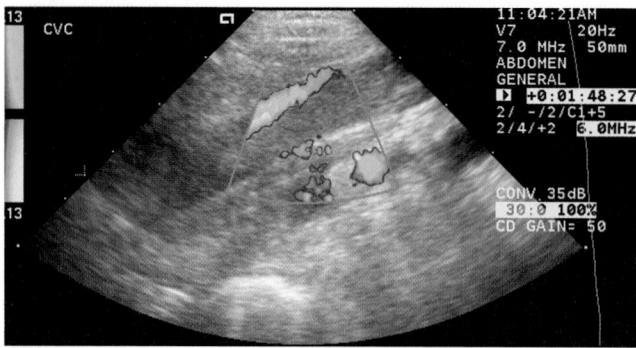

FIG. 22-6
Color Doppler evaluation of the caudal vena cava. There is a hyperechoic mass within the lumen of the cava from invasion of an adrenal tumor. Notice the disruption of the blood flow around the mass (blue).

 BOX 22-4

ACTH Stimulation Test in Dogs

1. Obtain serum to determine pretest adrenocorticotropic hormone (ACTH) level.
2. Administer 0.25 mg synthetic ACTH (Cortosyn) intramuscularly.
3. Obtain serum for testing 1 hour after ACTH administration.

 BOX 22-5

Patterns of ACTH Stimulation Tests (Post-ACTH Cortisol)*

More than 24 µg/dl: Suggestive of hyperadrenocorticism†
19–24 µg/dl: Equivocal for hyperadrenocorticism
8–18 µg/dl: Normal
Less than 4 µg/dl: Potentially consistent with iatrogenic Cushing's disease
Less than 1 µg/dl: Consistent with hypoadrenocorticism, either spontaneous or iatrogenic

*There may be substantial variation between laboratories. To convert µg/dl to nmol/L, multiply µg/dl × 27.59.
†Severe nonadrenal disease can be associated with stress causing values this high or higher; hyperadrenocorticism is not diagnosed simply by performing an adrenal function test.

texture and contrast enhancement. Masses that are poorly demarcated, irregularly shaped, and nonhomogeneous with mineralization usually are carcinomas. Determination of caudal vena cava invasion is best evaluated using contrast-enhanced CT. However, administration of a contrast agent in patients with pheochromocytomas may result in severe hypertension; thus it should be done with caution (Rosenstein, 2000). If contrast-enhanced CT is not performed, caudal vena caval angiography (note precautions in previous discussion) or color Doppler ultrasonography may be considered before surgery if caudal vena caval thrombosis is suspected (Fig. 22-6). Excretory urography may help identify tumor invasion requiring nephrectomy (i.e., ureteral obstruction or renal invasion).

NOTE: CT and MRI do not differentiate adrenal adenomas, carcinomas, or pheochromocytomas. Concurrent clinical signs, biochemical evidence, and a tissue sample are necessary for a definitive diagnosis.

Laboratory Findings

There are no consistent changes in animals with HAC; however, common laboratory abnormalities include substantially increased serum alkaline phosphatase, neutrophilic leukocytosis, lymphopenia, eosinopenia, mild polycythemia, modestly increased alanine aminotransferase, and hypercholesterolemia. Urinary tract abnormalities may include hyposthenuria (urine specific gravity below 1.007) or isosthenuria (1.008 to 1.012). Urinary tract infections are common, even when bacteriuria and pyuria are absent.

Diagnosis of HAC requires assessment of the history, physical examination, imaging, routine clinical pathology tests, and adrenal function tests. The ACTH stimulation test (Box 22-4) and the low-dose dexamethasone suppression (LDDS) test are the primary adrenal function tests used. The ACTH stimulation test is easy sand quick to perform, and is the best test to look for iatrogenic HAC (Box 22-5). How-

ever, the ACTH stimulation test has some disadvantages. Dogs with ADH can have almost any response (i.e., normal, exaggerated, or diminished) to ACTH, and many dogs without HAC have exaggerated test results that mimic HAC. Classically, one measures cortisol concentrations before and after administration of ACTH, but one may also measure sex steroids (e.g., 17-hydroxyprogesterone [Ristic et al, 2002]). However, the sensitivity and specificity of measuring sex steroids are still being determined at the time of this writing, and there is some evidence that increased 17-hydroxyprogesterone concentrations post–ACTH administration may not be as specific for HAC as was originally thought (Behrend et al, 2005). The LDDS test requires 8 hours to perform, but is often a better test to look for spontaneous HAC. Furthermore the LDDS test often permits differentiation of PDH and ADH.

It is critically important to note that HAC cannot be diagnosed simply by performing an adrenal function test; these tests may be substantially altered by nonadrenal disease or drugs. For example, exaggerated test results often occur in chronically stressed or ill dogs. In particular, animals with abnormal adrenal function tests but normal-sized adrenal glands should be carefully scrutinized before beginning therapy. PDH and ADH very rarely coexist. Because of the complexity in diagnosing HAC and differentiating PDH from ADH, readers are referred to a medical text for further information.

Laboratory abnormalities are inconsistent and nonspecific in animals with pheochromocytomas.

DIFFERENTIAL DIAGNOSIS

Pheochromocytomas and adrenocortical tumors must be differentiated because the operative management of these cases is different. Generally, clinical signs and laboratory analysis allow preoperative differentiation (see previous discussion). At surgery, pheochromocytomas may be identified grossly by application of Zenker's solution (potassium dichromate or iodate), which results in oxidation of catecholamines, forming a dark brown pigment within 10 to 20 minutes after application to the surface of a freshly sectioned tumor. Although adrenal carcinomas are apt to be large and invasive, differentiation of adenomas and carcinomas is impossible without histopathologic evaluation. Apparent metastatic lesions in the liver or draining lymph nodes may suggest malignancy, but care should be taken to differentiate benign hepatic nodules from neoplastic disease.

> NOTE: Be sure to submit the adrenal gland for histologic examination. Definitive diagnosis of adrenal tumors requires histopathologic evaluation.

MEDICAL MANAGEMENT

Adrenergic blockage (i.e., phenoxybenzamine, phentolamine, or prazosin) is used to control blood pressure in patients with pheochromocytomas. These drugs are also used preoperatively and intraoperatively (see discussions of Preoperative Management and Anesthesia on p. 582 and 583, respectively). If tachycardia or cardiac arrhythmias are present, β-adrenergic blockade may also be used; however, unopposed β-blockade may cause severe hypertension.

Medical therapy of HAC is potentially complex and can have significant side effects. Therefore the reader is referred to a current medical text for a more complete discussion. Mitotane (o,p′-DDD) destroys the adrenal cortex in a dose-dependent fashion. It has been the major drug used for canine HAC (Behrend et al, 1999). Mitotane can often control clinical signs in animals with ADH; however, tumors are more resistant to mitotane's adrenocorticolytic effects than are normal or hyperplastic adrenal cortices. Larger doses (Box 22-6) are often required to obtain and maintain control in ADH dogs than in PDH dogs, and stronger side effects (i.e., gastric irritation and vomiting) can be expected. The major advantages of mitotane are: (1) it is effective; and (2) after an induction therapy (usually 4 to 14 days), maintenance therapy consists of one to two treatments per week. The major disadvantages of mitotane are: (1) it can destroy the entire adrenal gland, resulting in temporary or permanent hypoadrenocorticism (or death); (2) some dogs are resistant to its effects; and (3) some dogs are very sensitive to its effects. The last two disadvantages mean that there is substantial variation in how patients respond. Some patients

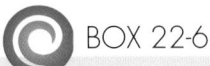

BOX 22-6

Mitotane (Lysodren) Treatment for Adrenal Tumors

- Administer 50–75 mg/kg/day for 14 days.
- If needed, increase dose to 100 mg/kg and treat for another 25–35 days.
- Repeat this increment every 14 days until the disease is controlled or the animal does not tolerate this drug.

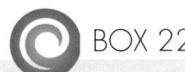

BOX 22-7

Ketoconazole Treatment for Adrenal Tumors

1. Administer 5 mg/kg with food bid for 7 days.
2. Increase dosage to 10 mg/kg bid for 7–14 days.
3. Perform ACTH stimulation test 2 to 4 hours after giving ketoconazole dose.
4. If no adrenocortical response to ACTH is seen and if clinical improvement occurs without causing illness, continue same dosage.
5. If a response to ACTH occurs or if no clinical improvement is seen, increase the dosage to 15 mg/kg bid, assuming that the patient tolerates the ketoconazole.

bid, Twice a day; *ACTH,* adrenocorticotropic hormone.

respond well and are easy to treat, whereas others are extremely difficult to control using this drug. This has led to investigation into other drugs for treating this disease.

Ketoconazole causes reversible inhibition of adrenal steroid production and has little effect on mineralocorticoid production. Therefore ketoconazole (Box 22-7) may be used (1) in dogs with ADH who are not surgical candidates; (2) before surgery to reduce anesthetic and surgical risks in animals with uncontrolled HAC; and (3) as a diagnostic trial in dogs in which equivocal test results make the diagnosis of HAC difficult. If used for diagnostic purposes, the drug should be given for a minimum of 4 to 8 weeks. The major advantages of ketoconazole are: (1) it is relatively safe (i.e., if signs of hypoadrenocorticism occur, all you have to do is stop the drug and allow time for the blood levels of ketoconazole to decrease); and (2) it is very effective. The major disadvantages of using ketoconazole are: (1) it only works while there are blood levels of the drugs, meaning that it must be given for the duration of the animal's life; (2) it is relatively expensive; and (3) it is so effective at decreasing the cortisol concentrations that it is easy to make patients feel sick when first starting the drug. Furthermore, adverse reactions to ketoconazole (i.e., anorexia, depression, vomiting, diarrhea, icterus) are not that rare and may necessitate stopping the drug or reducing the dosage. If an overdose is suspected of causing acute illness or collapse, administer glucocorticoids and stop the ketoconazole. Rechecks (including the ACTH stimulation test) are recommended every 3 to 6 months.

Trilostane inhibits one of the synthetic enzymes, thus blocking production of cortisol and other adrenal steroids. It is effective in most dogs and relatively safe (Niger et al, 2004). It is currently not sold in the United States (as of January 2006), but can be imported for use in a specific patient. Small animal veterinary medicine currently has less than 5 years experience with this drug, so there is much that is not yet known. At this time, the major advantages of trilostane appear to be that (1) it is generally safer than the other two drugs, and (2) it is effective in most patients. The major disadvantages are: (1) it must be given daily; (2) it has occasional side effects (Chapman et al, 2004); and (3) it is currently not readily available in the United States.

SURGICAL TREATMENT

The animal's overall health, the presence of unresectable metastases, and apparent invasiveness of the tumor (i.e., evidence of caudal vena cava thrombosis on CT or ultrasound) should be considered when determining the appropriateness of surgery for adrenal tumors. Long-term survival (i.e., longer than 1 year) may be possible, even in dogs with widespread metastatic lesions. If the tumor appears invasive, a midline abdominal approach is preferred to allow evaluation of the caudal vena cava and other abdominal structures. Thrombus removal may require that the midline incision be extended into the caudal thorax through a caudal median sternotomy approach (see p. 874). Thrombi more commonly occur because of intraluminal extension via the adrenal or renal vein and less commonly by direct invasion. In one study, caval thrombi were detected in 25% of dogs with adrenal gland tumors (Kyles et al, 2003). They are more common with pheochromocytomas than with adrenocortical tumors, but may occur with either. Venotomy may be used to remove tumors extending into the caudal vena cava. If venotomy cannot be performed, gradual occlusion of the caudal vena cava may allow removal of adrenal gland tumors with vascular invasion that would otherwise be difficult or impossible to resect (Peacock et al, 2003). En bloc resection of the caudal vena cava during removal of a pheochromocytoma was recently reported in a dog (Louvet et al, 2005). Small tumors or those that do not appear invasive may be removed through a paralumbar approach (see p. 576).

Preoperative Management

Renal function should be determined before surgery in case ipsilateral nephrectomy is necessary. Substantial electrolyte or acid-base abnormalities, blood glucose concentrations greater than 200 mg/dl, and hypertension should be corrected before surgery if possible. Fluid therapy should be initiated before induction of anesthesia. Animals with HAC are at increased risk of postoperative pulmonary thromboembolism. Low-dose heparin therapy may be indicated in patients with disseminated intravascular coagulation (DIC) (Box 22-8) or in patients with adrenocortical tumors to prevent thromboembolism (see Box 22-3). Heparin (75 to 100 U/kg) may be added to plasma during surgery, with the animal continuing to take heparin for 3 to 4 days. Low molecular weight heparin (150 U/kg) may be more effective than unfractionated heparin, but it requires different monitoring than unfractionated heparin. Perioperative antibiotics

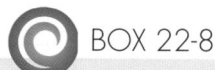 **BOX 22-8**

Heparin Therapy for Disseminated Intravascular Coagulation

Plasma (fresh frozen)

10–20 ml/kg, then re-assess the plasma ATIII activity. Repeat as needed to increase the ATIII to near-normal concentrations.

Heparin (unfractionated)*

50–100 U/kg SC, bid or tid

Heparin-Activated Plasma

Place the first heparin dose (50–100 U/kg) into the plasma and incubate for 30 minutes before administration. Once ATIII levels are above 60%, continue the heparin subcutaneously. If additional plasma is needed, incubation with heparin is not necessary.
  Note: Adequate levels of ATIII are critical in these patients.

Low Molecular Weight Heparin (Dalteparin)˙

100–150 U/kg SC, qd to bid

ATIII, Antithrombin III; *SC,* subcutaneous; *bid,* twice a day; *tid,* three times a day.
*Low molecular weight (LMW) heparin is more effective than unfractionated heparin. There are substantial differences between the two forms, and the reader is referred to a medical text for a more complete discussion including the differences in monitoring the effectiveness of therapy. As more becomes kown regarding LMW heparin, this dosage recommendation may change.

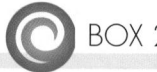 **BOX 22-9**

Drugs Used During Perioperative Management of Animals With Pheochromocytomas

Phenoxybenzamine (Dibenzyline)

0.25 mg/kg up to a maximum of 2.5 mg/kg PO, bid, for at least 2 weeks before surgery*

Esmolol (Brevibloc)

0.05–0.1 mg/kg slow IV boluses every 5 minutes to total cumulative dose of 0.5 mg/kg or 50–70 μg/kg/min CRI

Phentolamine (Regitine)

0.02–0.1 mg/kg IV, follow by CRI of 1–2 μg/kg/min

Sodium Nitroprusside (Nipride)

0.5–5 μg/kg/min IV

PO, Oral; *IV,* intravenous; *CRI,* constant rate infusion.
*Slowly and gradually increase the dose until signs of hypotension occur.

should be administered and continued postoperatively in hyperadrenal animals.

Particular emphasis should be placed on preoperative examination of the cardiovascular system for evidence of arrhythmias or congestive heart failure in animals with pheochromocytomas. A dosage of 2.5 mg/kg of phenoxybenzamine administered every 12 hours PO for at least 2 weeks before surgery may reduce the incidence of severe hypertension at surgery and reduce mortality (Box 22-9).

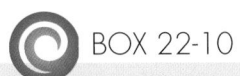 BOX 22-10

Lidocaine Administration

Dogs: Give intravenously (IV) (2 mg/kg bolus, up to 8 mg/kg total dose) to determine responsiveness to this drug. If the arrhythmias decrease or stop, lidocaine should be given by a continuous (IV) infusion (CRI) of 50–75 μg/kg/min (for 50 μg/kg/min, place 500 mg lidocaine in 500 ml of fluids and administer at maintenance rate [66 ml/kg/day]).
Cats: Give IV (1 mg/kg bolus, up to 4 mg/kg total dose); if necessary administer 25–50 μg/kg/min by CRI.

IV, Intravenous; *CRI,* constant rate infusion.

Anesthesia

Anesthetic complications are common during adrenalectomy for pheochromocytomas, and wide fluctuations in heart rate and blood pressure are typical. The cardiac rhythm, arterial blood pressure, and pulse oximetry should be closely monitored. Treatment for several weeks before surgery with an α-adrenergic blocker (i.e., phenoxybenzamine; see Box 22-9) is recommended. The dose of phenoxybenzamine is increased until blood pressure is within the normal range. The heart rate can be controlled with a β-blocker (i.e., propranolol or esmolol); however, it should not be initiated until adequate α-blockade has been established (i.e., normal blood pressure). Intraoperative β-blockade with esmolol (see Box 22-9) is preferred because of its short half-life. Cardiac arrhythmias may be treated with lidocaine (Box 22-10). Hypertension may result from tumor manipulation and can be minimized by isolating the tumor's blood supply before manipulating the tumor. Hypertension may be treated with phentolamine given as an intravenous bolus (see Box 22-9). Sodium nitroprusside may also be infused to maintain blood pressure. Hypotension frequently occurs after tumor removal, and high doses of crystalloids may be necessary to maintain perfusion. If hypotension persists, dobutamine should be administered (2 to 10 μg/kg/min IV). These tumors tend to be highly vascular, and significant intraoperative hemorrhage may require blood transfusions, particularly if caudal vena cava venotomy is performed to remove a thrombus.

Atropine, xylazine, and ketamine should not be used in patients suspected of having pheochromocytomas. Atropine potentiates the chronotropic effects of epinephrine and lowers its arrhythmogenic threshold. Xylazine (an α₂-agonist) may cause transient hypertension followed by hypotension, may increase the sensitivity of the myocardium to catecholamines, and may potentiate cardiac arrhythmias. Ketamine increases the heart rate, blood pressure, and circulating levels of catecholamines. If etomidate is used in patients with arrhythmia, the need for perioperative steroid replacement should be anticipated. When using etomidate, the advantages of cardiovascular stability should be weighed against the possibility of transient adrenal suppression that may occur in patients undergoing unilateral adrenalectomy. Isoflurane or sevoflurane is the inhalation agent of choice because they do not sensitize the myocardium to epinephrine-induced arrhythmias.

Surgical Anatomy

See p. 574 for the discussion of the surgical anatomy of the adrenal gland.

Positioning

The animal is positioned either in dorsal recumbency or in lateral recumbency with the affected side up, depending on the operative approach chosen. With large or invasive tumors, a generous area should be clipped and prepared for surgery to allow a caudal thoracotomy (median sternotomy) to be performed if necessary.

SURGICAL TECHNIQUE

Adrenalectomy via either a midline abdominal or a paralumbar approach is described on pp. 575 to 576. Concurrent nephrectomy may be necessary in some patients with invasive tumors. Surgical resection of adrenal tumors should be aggressive to ensure complete tumor removal. *En bloc* resection should be performed if possible to prevent leaving small fragments of neoplastic tissue. The vascular supply to pheochromocytomas should be isolated before tumor manipulation to reduce catecholamine release and help prevent shedding of tumor cells. Venotomy may be required to remove tumor thrombi. The entire abdomen should be explored, with special attention paid to the bladder, pelvic canal, kidneys, and aorta near the junction of the caudal mesenteric artery, where extraadrenal neoplasia is reported to occur.

SUTURE MATERIALS AND SPECIAL INSTRUMENTS

Delayed wound healing may occur in any debilitated animal (see p. 162). Self-retaining retractors (e.g., Balfour abdominal retractors) and malleable retractors are useful for improving visualization of the adrenal glands. With vascular tumors, electrocautery and hemoclips obtain hemostasis more easily than does suture ligation of vessels.

POSTOPERATIVE CARE AND ASSESSMENT

Animals with HAC caused by ADH often develop hypoadrenocorticism postoperatively as a result of atrophy of the contralateral gland. These animals require glucocorticoid therapy postoperatively (see discussion of postoperative care on p. 576). If HAC continues postoperatively, medical therapy should be considered. Fluid therapy should be continued until the animal is able to maintain hydration. The blood pressure, heart rate, and heart rhythm should be carefully monitored after surgery. Blood transfusions may be required intraoperatively or postoperatively in some patients. Dogs should be reevaluated periodically for tumor recurrence. The most common complications after adrenal tumor removal include dyspnea, hemoperitoneum, ventricular arrhythmias, anuric acute renal failure, and coagulopathies. Dogs with adrenocortical tumors are at increased risk to develop thromboembolism (see p. 577).

PROGNOSIS

Prognosis for dogs with adrenocortical carcinomas depends on the tumor's size and invasiveness. Long-term survival of 778 days was reported in dogs with adrenocortical carcinomas (Anderson et al, 2001). Fifteen of 17 dogs that survived the perioperative period had long-term resolution of their clinical signs. In another study, the overall mortality of dogs with pheochromocytomas and adrenocortical tumors was 22% (Kyle et al, 2003). In the aforementioned study, there were no significant differences in perioperative morbidity or mortality between dogs that had tumors extending into the caudal vena cava (tumor thrombi) and those that did not. Prolonged survivals (1 to 2 years) are possible in dogs with invasive, metastatic pheochromocytomas after aggressive surgical resection. Recurrence of clinical signs is likely if there are tumor thrombi or if the tumor is incompletely removed.

> NOTE: Warn owners that animals with pheochromocytomas may die suddenly as a result of arrhythmias and hypertension.

References

Behrend EN, Kemppainen RJ, Clark TP et al: Treatment of hyperadrenocorticism in dogs: a survey of internists and dermatologists, *J Am Vet Med Assoc* 215:938, 1999.

Behrend EN, Kemppainen RJ, Boozer AL et al: Serum 17-hydroxyprogesterone and corticosterone concentrations in dogs with nonadrenal neoplasia and dogs with suspected hyperadrenocorticism, *J Am Vet Med Assoc* 227:1762, 2005.

Chapman P, Kelly D, Archer J et al: Adrenal necrosis in a dog receiving trilostane for the treatment of hyperadrenocorticism, *J Small Anim Pract* 45:307, 2004.

Kyles AE, Feldman ED, DeCock HEV et al: Surgical management of adrenal gland tumors with and without associated tumor thrombi in dogs: 40 cases (1994-2001), *J Am Vet Med Assoc* 223:654, 2003.

Neiger R, Ramsey, I, O'Connor J et al: Trilostane treatment of 78 dogs with pituitary-dependent hyperadrenocorticism, *Vet Rec* 150:799, 2004.

Peacock JT, Fossum TW, Bahr AM et al: Evaluation of gradual occlusion of the caudal vena cava in clinically normal dogs, *Am J Vet Res* 64:1347, 2003.

Ristic JME, Ramsey IK, Heath FM et al: The use of 17-hydroxyprogesterone in the diagnosis of canine hyperadrenocorticism, *J Vet Intern Med* 16:433, 2002.

Rosenstein DS: Diagnostic imaging in canine pheochromocytoma, *Vet Radiol Ultrasound* 41:499, 2000.

PITUITARY NEOPLASIA

DEFINITIONS

Pituitary tumors arise from the hypophysis in the **sella turcica**. **Hypophysectomy** is the surgical removal of the pituitary gland. The pituitary gland is also called the *hypophysis*.

GENERAL CONSIDERATIONS AND CLINICALLY RELEVANT PATHOPHYSIOLOGY

Pituitary tumors are the most common cause of canine HAC. They may be functional (60%) or nonfunctional (40%). Clinical signs are usually caused by hypersecretion of ACTH from tumors in the pars distalis (adenohypophysis) or pars intermedia. Large pituitary tumors often grow dorsally into the brain because the diaphragm of the sella is incomplete. Such tumors may cause clinical signs by impinging on adjacent brain tissue (i.e., optic chiasm, hypothalamus, thalamus, infundibular recess, and third ventricle). The tumor's size and the development of neurologic signs do not always correlate. Adenomas and carcinomas may arise from pituitary tissue; however, carcinomas represent less than 3% of all pituitary neoplasms. Adenomas usually are classified as microadenomas (less than 1 cm in diameter) or macroadenomas (greater than 1 cm in diameter). Microadenomas are most common, accounting for nearly 70% of all pituitary tumors.

DIAGNOSIS
Clinical Presentation

Signalment. Poodles, dachshunds, and boxers may be predisposed to PDH. Middle-aged and older dogs are most commonly affected; however, young dogs occasionally may develop pituitary tumors.

History. Most dogs are presented for evaluation of typical signs of HAC (i.e., polyuria, polydipsia, polyphagia, abdominal enlargement, endocrine alopecia, muscle wasting, weakness, lethargy, panting, and/or hyperpigmentation). Concurrent neurologic signs may also be noted (seizures, visual deficits, ataxia, incoordination, facial hemiplegia, head tilt, somnolence, compulsive walking, depression). The diversity of neurologic signs in dogs with pituitary tumors probably is a result of impingement on various parts of the brain responsible for differing functions. Mental depression and stupor were reported as the most common abnormalities in two studies describing dogs with large pituitary tumors. In animals with nonfunctional macroadenomas or carcinomas, neurologic signs may be the only presenting abnormality, and some owners only report anorexia without any obvious CNS abnormalities.

> NOTE: Large, nonfunctional pituitary tumors may cause neurologic abnormalities. Functional tumors usually cause hyperadrenocorticism, but may also cause neurologic signs.

Physical Examination Findings

Typical signs of HAC (see previous discussion) are expected in animals with functional pituitary tumors. Neurologic abnormalities (e.g., papillary edema, ataxia, and incoordination) or poor appetite occasionally occur as the only signs.

Diagnostic Imaging

Diagnosis of pituitary neoplasia is best made with CT or MRI (Fig. 22-7). Pituitary adenomas and carcinomas cannot be differentiated with CT; however, animals with microadenomas, which might benefit from hypophysectomy, can be differentiated from animals with macroadenomas. The latter seldom benefit from surgery. Bilateral adrenal enlargement usually is indicative of PDH.

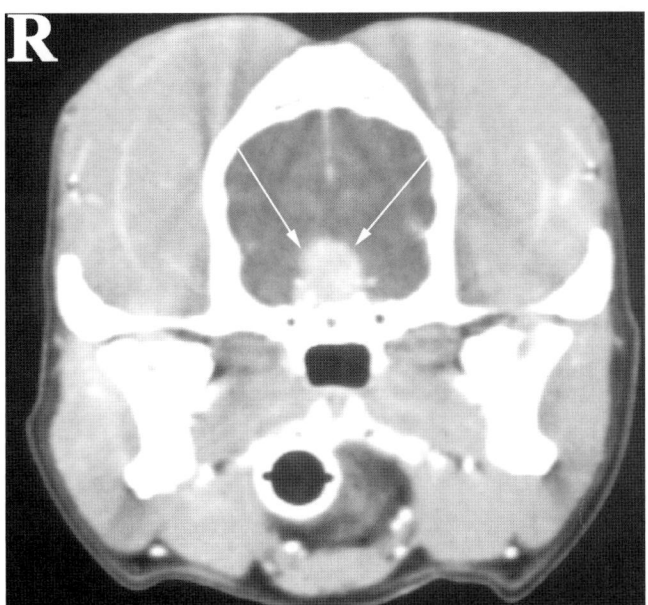

FIG. 22-7
Contrast enhanced CT image of a dog with a macroadenoma of the pituitary gland *(arrows)*.

Laboratory Findings

Laboratory abnormalities generally are consistent with HAC. Small, nonfunctional pituitary tumors seldom cause laboratory abnormalities. Large tumors may cause increased intracranial pressure, measured on a cerebrospinal fluid (CSF) tap. See p. 580 for differentiation of PDH from ADH.

DIFFERENTIAL DIAGNOSIS

Animals with PDH must be differentiated from those with iatrogenic HAC or ADH (see p. 580). Once a diagnosis of pituitary dysfunction has been made, pituitary neoplasms must be differentiated from other lesions that may arise in the pituitary (i.e., cysts, abscesses, and craniopharyngiomas); however, such lesions are extremely rare.

MEDICAL MANAGEMENT

Clinical signs of HAC may be treated medically (see p. 581). External beam radiation therapy appears to be an effective treatment for large pituitary tumors when combined with concurrent adrenal-suppressive treatment (mitotane, trilostane, or ketoconazole). Long-term survival may be possible with radiation therapy.

SURGICAL TREATMENT

Hypophysectomy can be performed in animals with pituitary microadenomas and functional adenohypophyseal hyperplasia (rare); however, it is seldom performed by veterinary surgeons. Advocates of this procedure suggest that most dogs with PDH are surgical candidates for hypophysectomy and that this technique is preferable to long-term medical management. There is evidence that dogs with nonenlarged pituitary glands have fewer postoperative com-

plications than dogs with enlarged pituitary glands (Hanson et al, 2005). However, if concurrent neurologic signs are present or if the tumor has extended intracranially or transsphenoidally, hypophysectomy is not indicated. Hypophysectomy should not be considered in animals intended for breeding purposes because it renders them infertile. There are no clinical or experimental data suggesting that hypophysectomy is safe and effective in cats. Hypophysectomy is described in *Small Animal Surgery*, second edition or in the e-dition.

> NOTE: Hypophysectomy should be performed only by surgeons familiar with the regional anatomy and experienced in the technique.

Preoperative Management

If surgery is considered for a pituitary neoplasm, extensive preoperative work-up is indicated to confirm and localize the lesion. A CT or MRI of the pituitary fossa (including a contrast-enhanced image) is used to determine the height and width of the pituitary gland and to localize pertinent landmarks. Animals with HAC are at increased risk of developing postoperative infections because of the high levels of circulating glucocorticoids. Perioperative prophylactic antibiotics are recommended. See p. 582 for additional comments on the preoperative management of animals with HAC.

Anesthesia

Most animals with pituitary tumors do not require special anesthetic consideration; however, patients with large masses that increase intracranial pressure need special precautions. Fluid therapy should be restricted to the volume required to maintain adequate circulation. Isoflurane and sevoflurane are the inhalants of choice because they interfere less with autoregulation of cerebral blood flow than does halothane. The faster recovery that sevoflurane offers provides some advantage over isoflurane. Although most injectable anesthetics reduce cerebral metabolic oxygen requirements, cerebral blood flow, and intracranial pressure, ketamine does not. Therefore ketamine should not be used in patients with intracranial masses and other conditions in which increased intracranial pressures may occur as a result of surgery. Patients with increased intracranial pressure should be modestly hyperventilated (end tidal CO_2 approximately 28 to 32 mm Hg) during surgery.

Surgical Anatomy

The pituitary is a small appendage of the diencephalon (Fig. 22-8). It occupies a shallow, oval recess in the basisphenoid bone called the sella turcica. The gland varies greatly in size among breeds of dogs and within the same breed, but it usually is approximately 1 cm long. The pituitary is composed of the adenohypophysis and the neurohypophysis, and the adenohypophysis is further subdivided into the pars proximalis, pars intermedia, and pars distalis. The arterial supply of the pituitary arises from the internal carotid arteries and caudal communicating arteries.

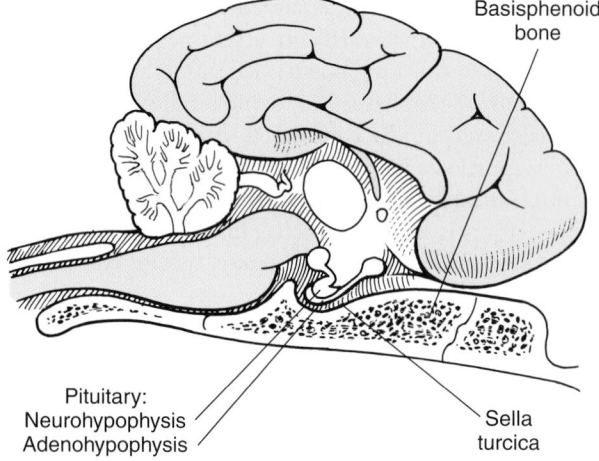

FIG. 22-8
Location of the pituitary gland.

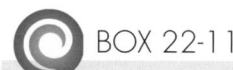 **BOX 22-11**

Postoperative Drug Therapy After Hypophysectomy

Desmopressin Acetate

Nasal preparation: give 1–4 drops of 100 µg/ml intranasal or in conjunctiva qd to bid
Parenteral form: give 0.5–2 µg/dog SC qd or bid
Tablets: give 0.1 mg tid and adjust dose as needed

Hydrocortisone (Solu-Cortef)

1 mg/kg IV, qid

Prednisolone

0.2 mg/kg qd

Thyroid Hormone (Soloxine, Thyrotabs, Synthroid)

22 µg/kg PO, bid

qd, Once a day; *bid*, twice a day; *SC*, subcutaneous; *tid*, three times a day; *IV*, intravenous; *qid*, four times a day; *PO*, oral.

Positioning

For a description of hypophysectomy, see *Small Animal Surgery*, second edition, or the e-dition.

 SURGICAL TECHNIQUE

Transsphenoidal, intracranial, and peripharyngeal approaches have been described for hypophysectomy. For a description of the transsphenoidal approach see *Small Animal Surgery*, second edition, or the e-dition.

SUTURE MATERIALS AND SPECIAL INSTRUMENTS

Delayed wound healing may occur in animals with HAC; therefore incisions should be closed with strong, slowly absorbed or nonabsorbable suture material (e.g., polydioxanone, polyglyconate, polypropylene, or nylon).

POSTOPERATIVE CARE AND ASSESSMENT

For a discussion of the postoperative care of patients after hypophysectomy, see *Small Animal Surgery*, second edition, or the e-dition. See also Box 22-11.

COMPLICATIONS

See *Small Animal Surgery*, second edition, or the e-dition.

PROGNOSIS

Long-term survival is possible after hypophysectomy, radiation therapy plus chemotherapy, or chemotherapy alone in dogs with PDH caused by microadenomas. Long-term survival has also been reported in dogs with large, functional tumors after radiation therapy. In one study, 43 of 52 dogs went into remission after hypophysectomy; hyperadrenocorticism subsequently recurred in five (Meij et al, 1998). In this study, postoperative CT findings did not correlate well with remission or subsequent recurrence of HAC. In a more recent study, 4-year estimated relapse-free fraction was 58% (Hanson et al, 2005).

References

Hanson JM, van't Hoofd MM, Voorhout G et al: Efficacy of transsphenoidal hypophysectomy in treatment of dogs with pituitary-dependent hyperadrenocorticism, *J Vet Intern Med* 19:687, 2005.

Meij BP et al: Results of transsphenoidal hypophysectomy in 52 dogs with pituitary-dependent hyperadrenocorticism, *Vet Surg* 27:246, 1998.

Surgery of the Pancreas

GENERAL PRINCIPLES AND TECHNIQUES

DEFINITIONS

Pancreatectomy is surgical removal of all or part of the pancreas. **Insulinoma** is a functional tumor of pancreatic β-islet cells; excessive insulin production commonly causes hypoglycemia in affected animals (see p. 595). **Zollinger-Ellison** syndrome is a condition caused by non–β-islet islet cell tumors in which excess gastrin is secreted (see p. 599).

PREOPERATIVE MANAGEMENT

Although an acute onset of anorexia, vomiting, and anterior abdominal pain have been considered the hallmarks of canine pancreatitis, affected dogs may have a wide range of clinical signs ranging from peracute to chronic and including ascites, shock, dyspnea, and melena. Cats are even more variable, with the primary signs being lethargy, poor appetite, and dehydration; vomiting is much less common or much less noticeable in affected cats. It is important to try to diagnose pancreatitis before surgery because (1) these animals often neither require nor benefit from surgery if pancreatitis is the major problem (dogs with abscesses may be different—see later discussion), and (2) poor visceral perfusion due to anesthesia and/or unnecessary manipulation of the pancreas during surgery can cause exacerbation and acute worsening of the disease. Abdominal ultrasonography has been one of the best tools to diagnose pancreatitis; however, the canine pancreatic lipase immunoreactivity (cPLI) test has recently become available and seems to have the best sensitivity and specificity for canine pancreatitis (Steiner et al, 2003). The reader is referred to a medical text for a more detailed discussion of the diagnosis of pancreatitis.

Vomiting animals often require correction of fluid, electrolyte, and acid-base abnormalities before surgery. Diabetic animals may be prone to pancreatitis and are often anesthetized for elective and nonelective procedures. Diabetics should be carefully evaluated before surgery, including a complete blood count (CBC), serum biochemical panel (including fasting blood glucose, blood urea nitrogen, and creatinine), urinalysis, and urine culture. Severe hyperglycemia (more than 300 mg/dl), ketoacidosis, major electrolyte abnormalities (e.g., hypokalemia and hypophosphatemia), and urinary tract infections should be corrected before surgery. Animals with pancreatic tumors may have a wide variety of metabolic disorders.

ANESTHESIA

Many protocols have been described for anesthetic management of diabetic animals. Blood glucose concentrations ideally should be maintained between 100 and 300 mg/dl during surgery. Hypoglycemia may occur if animals are given their regular insulin dose and if food is withheld before surgery; however, the stress of surgery usually results in hyperglycemia. Animals should be fed their normal diet the day before surgery, and their regular dose of insulin should be administered. Food should be withheld 12 hours before surgery or a small meal given after the morning insulin. Surgery should be performed in the morning. Blood glucose concentrations should be measured the morning of surgery. One to 2 hours before surgery, if the blood glucose concentration is between 150 and 300 mg/dl, the animal should receive one half of its usual morning dose of insulin subcutaneously. Blood glucose should be checked at induction and hourly thereafter. If the blood glucose level is low, administer 0.45% saline and 2.5% dextrose (5 ml/kg for the first hour and then 2.5 ml/kg thereafter). If the blood glucose level is normal, administer lactated Ringer's solution (at the same rate). Fluids should be changed to 5% dextrose and an additional small dose of regular insulin given if the blood glucose concentration is more than 300 mg/dl.

> NOTE: Be sure to maintain excellent perfusion during surgery to help prevent postoperative pancreatitis.

Selected anesthetic protocols for animals with pancreatic disease that are in stable condition are provided in Box

BOX 22-12

Selected Anesthetic Protocols for Use in Stable Dogs and Cats With Pancreatic Disease

Premedication

Give atropine (0.02–0.04 mg/kg SC or IM), or glycopyrrolate (0.005–0.011 mg/kg SC or IM) plus hydromorphone* (0.05–0.1 mg/kg SC or IM), or butorphanol (0.2–0.4 mg/kg SC or IM), or buprenorphine (5–15 μg/kg IM)

Induction

Thiopental (10–12 mg/kg IV) or propofol (4–6 mg/kg IV)

Maintenance

Isoflurane or sevoflurane

SC, Subcutaneous; *IM*, intramuscular; *IV*, intravenous.
*Use 0.05 mg/kg in cats.

BOX 22-13

Selected Anesthetic Protocols for Use in Hypovolemic, Dehydrated, or Shocky Animals With Pancreatic Disease

Dogs

Induction

Hydromorphone (0.1 mg/kg IV) plus diazepam (0.2 mg/kg IV). Give in incremental doses. Intubate if possible. If necessary, give etomidate (0.5–1.5 mg/kg IV). (See text also.)

Maintenance

Isoflurane or sevoflurane.

Cats

Premedication

Butorphanol (0.2–0.4 mg/kg SC or IM), or buprenorphine (5–15 μg/kg IM), or hydromorphone (0.05 mg/kg SC or IM).

Induction

Diazepam (0.2 mg/kg IV) followed by etomidate (0.5–1.5 mg/kg IV). (See text also.)

Maintenance

Isoflurane or sevoflurane.

IV, Intravenous; *SC*, subcutaneous; *IM*, intramuscular.

22-12. These animals may be premedicated with an anticholinergic and opioid, induced with thiopental or propofol, and maintained on isoflurane or sevoflurane inhalants. If the animal is shocky, dehydrated, or hypovolemic, anesthesia must be induced and maintained with greater care. Suggested anesthetic protocols are provided in Box 22-13. As an alternative, animals that are not vomiting may be induced with a mask or placed in a chamber, or they may be given thiopental or propofol at reduced dosages. If ketamine is not contraindicated, reduced dosages of diazepam and ketamine may also be used in cats.

> NOTE: It is important to realize that dehydration is often not appreciated or is underestimated, especially in obese animals.

ANTIBIOTICS

Antibiotics have not been shown to benefit dogs with pancreatitis, which is almost exclusively a nonseptic disease. They often are administered in an effort to prevent secondary infections in necrotic pancreatic and peripancreatic tissue, but there is no evidence that they benefit the patient. Nonetheless, prophylactic antibiotic therapy is often administered in animals undergoing pancreatic biopsy or partial pancreatectomy to prevent pancreatic abscessation (e.g., cefazolin, 22 mg/kg IV). Treatment with imipenem or ciprofloxacin has been shown to reduce early and late septic pancreatic complications and improve survival in experimental pancreatitis in rats; however, there is no evidence that these drugs benefit dogs or cats with pancreatitis. Antibiotic therapy should be based on the results of culture and sensitivity testing of infected tissue in animals with pancreatic abscessation.

SURGICAL ANATOMY

The pancreas of dogs and cats is composed of a right and left limb and a small central body (Fig. 22-9). The right limb of the pancreas lies within the mesoduodenum and is closely associated with the duodenum, particularly at its cranial aspect. The dorsal aspect of the right pancreatic lobe is visualized by retracting the duodenum ventrally and toward the midline; the ventral aspect of the right pancreatic lobe is examined by retracting the duodenum laterally. The pancreatic body (angle) lies in the bend formed by the pylorus and the duodenum. The left pancreatic lobe is viewed within the deep leaf of the greater omentum by retracting the stomach cranially and the transverse colon caudally.

> NOTE: Visualize the left lobe of the pancreas by looking in the deep leaf of the greater omentum while retracting the stomach cranially.

The main blood supply to the left pancreatic lobe is via branches of the splenic artery; however, branches from the common hepatic and gastroduodenal arteries also supply portions of it. The main vessels of the right lobe of the pancreas are the pancreatic branches of the cranial and caudal pancreaticoduodenal arteries that anastomose in the gland.

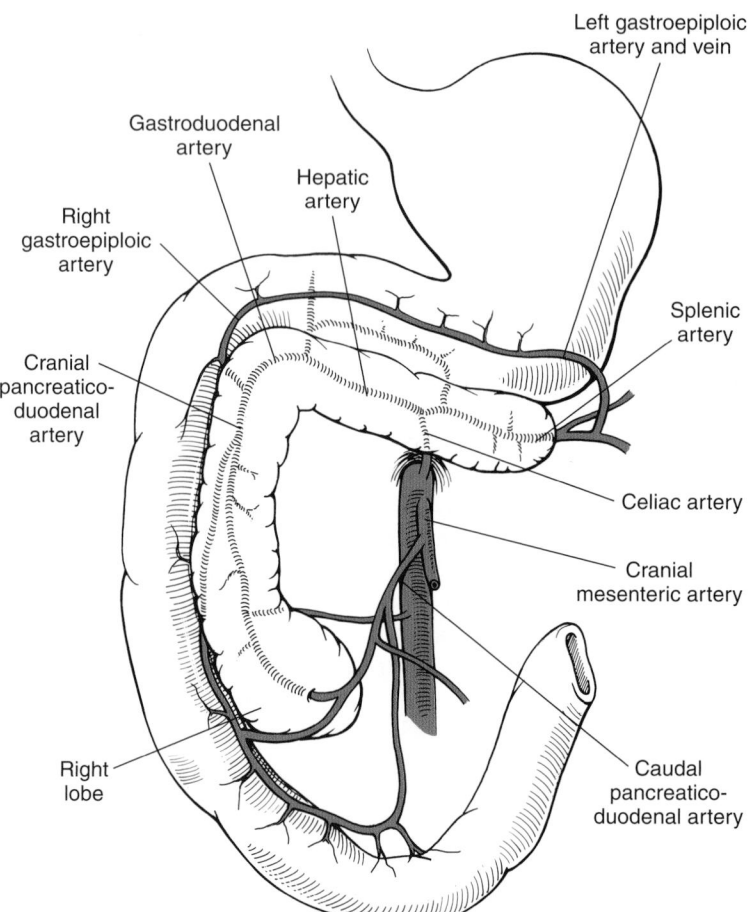

FIG. 22-9
Vascular supply to the pancreas.

The cranial pancreaticoduodenal artery is a terminal branch of the hepatic artery; the caudal pancreaticoduodenal arises from the cranial mesenteric vessel. These vessels also provide branches that supply the duodenum. Because they are closely associated with the proximal portion of the right lobe of the pancreas, care must be taken not to damage these vessels during pancreatic surgery, or devitalization of the duodenum may occur.

> NOTE: The proximity and shared blood supply of the pancreas and duodenum make duodenal resection difficult if pancreatic function is to be maintained.

The pancreas has both endocrine (insulin) and exocrine (digestive secretions) functions. Digestive secretions enter the duodenum via one of two ducts. These ducts may communicate within the gland or may cross each other. When the two ducts do not communicate, the *pancreatic duct* drains the right lobe and the *accessory pancreatic duct* drains the left lobe. The accessory pancreatic duct is the largest excretory pancreatic duct in dogs. It opens into the duodenum at the *minor duodenal papilla.* The smaller pancreatic duct is occasionally absent. The latter usually enters the duodenum on the *major duodenal papilla,* adjacent to the common bile duct. The pancreatic duct is the principal and oftentimes only duct in cats.

> NOTE: Extrahepatic biliary obstruction may occur secondary to pancreatic swelling or masses because of impingement of the common bile duct as it enters the major duodenal papilla. Attempting to resect such masses may cause laceration and/or rupture of the bile duct.

SURGICAL TECHNIQUE

A ventral midline abdominal incision is made that extends from the xiphoid cartilage caudal to the umbilicus, and the pancreas is examined using a combination of gentle palpation and visual inspection. The free portion of the greater omentum is retracted cranially and covered with moist sponges. The omental leaf overlying the pancreas can be bluntly separated to allow direct visualization of the left pancreas. When neoplasia is suspected, lymph nodes that lie along the splenic vessels and portal vein and those at the hilus of the liver and head of the pancreas should be examined for evidence of metastasis.

> NOTE: Handle the pancreas gently to avoid causing pancreatitis.

Pancreatic biopsy and partial pancreatectomy are performed in dogs and cats. Because of the difficulty in diagnosing feline pancreatitis, biopsy may be indicated more often than currently performed. Laparoscopic biopsy of the canine and feline pancreas is generally well tolerated. Pancreatic biopsy occasionally is performed in dogs to differentiate benign pancreatic conditions (e.g., pancreatitis or pancreatic fibrosis) from neoplastic disease. Although ultrasound-guided biopsies of large pancreatic lesions may be possible, exploratory laparotomy and direct visualization of pancreatic tissue usually are indicated. Partial pancreatectomy is indicated in animals with insulin-secreting or gastrin-secreting tumors, and pancreatic adenocarcinoma (see p. 600). Total pancreatectomy is infrequently performed in veterinary patients. Removal of the pancreas without duodenectomy requires that pancreatic tissue be bluntly dissected from the pancreaticoduodenal vessels without damaging branches supplying the duodenum. This is difficult in animals with pancreatic disease because of adhesions, fibrosis, and edema. Therefore total pancreatectomy usually is performed in conjunction with resection and anastomosis of the proximal duodenum, ligation of the common bile duct, and cholecystojejunostomy (i.e., Billroth II procedure; see p. 413) and is associated with high rates of morbidity and mortality. Pancreatic drainage or omentalization is indicated in some conditions (e.g., large abscesses or cysts) in which pancreatectomy is not feasible.

> NOTE: Total pancreatectomy is difficult because it usually necessitates cholecystoenterostomy and removal of the duodenum.

Laparoscopic Pancreatic Biopsy

This is generally performed during double puncture laparoscopy. Diagnosing pancreatitis in cats can be more difficult than in dogs; therefore pancreatic biopsy is more commonly done in cats.

Use a punch type of biopsy forceps (as opposed to "double spoon" forceps). Obtain biopsies from the edge of the pancreas, and take care to examine both sides (a large vein typically runs under the pancreas, near the edge). If you see obviously diseased pancreatic tissue, take a biopsy; however, some cats with pancreatitis do not have grossly diseased pancreatic tissue. Because canine pancreatitis can be a focal or multifocal lesion (Newman et al, 2004), take multiple biopsies from such animals.

Surgical Pancreatic Biopsy

If obvious, diffuse pancreatic disease is present, a biopsy is best obtained by removing a small portion of the caudal aspect of the right pancreatic limb (see the discussion of Partial Pancreatectomy in the next section). Focal lesions near the extremity of the pancreas may be removed in a similar fashion. If there is no obviously diseased tissue, then multiple biopsies should be taken because pancreatitis can be a localized or a multifocal disease (Newman et al, 2004).

For focal lesions within the pancreatic parenchyma, use a TruCut or Vim-Silverman needle (see p. 534), or shave off a portion of the lesion with a scalpel to obtain a small sample of pancreatic tissue. Take care not to damage adjacent blood vessels or pancreatic ducts.

Partial Pancreatectomy

Focal lesions near the extremity of the pancreas can be removed by the suture fracture technique.

Incise the mesoduodenum or omentum on each side of the pancreas. Pass nonabsorbable (i.e., 2-0 to 3-0) suture material from one side of the pancreas to the other, through the incisions, so that the suture is just proximal to the lesion to be excised. Tighten the suture, and allow it to crush through the parenchyma, which ligates vessels and ducts (Fig. 22-10). Excise the specimen distal to the ligature. Close any holes in the mesoduodenum with absorbable suture material.

Blunt separation of pancreatic lobules and ligation of ducts can be performed for lesions anywhere in the pancreas. With small lesions it may be possible to identify and preserve the pancreatic ducts. Identify the lesion to be removed, and gently incise the mesoduodenum or omentum overlying it (Fig. 22-11, A). For lesions involving the pancreatic body or proximal aspect of the right lobe, use gauze sponges to bluntly dissect pancreatic tissue from the pancreaticoduodenal vessels. Ligate or cauterize small pancreatic vessels but take care not to damage the pancreaticoduodenal vessels. Using sterile Q-tips or Halsted mosquito hemostats, separate the affected lobules from adjoining tissue by blunt dissection (Fig. 22-11, B). Identify the blood vessels and ducts supplying the portion of the pancreas to be removed and ligate them (Fig. 22-11, C). Excise the affected pancreatic tissue, and close any holes in the mesoduodenum.

> NOTE: Ligate the pancreatic ducts with nonabsorbable suture. If there is or may be substantial pancreatitis, it is often a wise idea to put in a jejunostomy feeding tube (see p. 107) during the procedure.

HEALING OF THE PANCREAS

The fibrous stroma of the pancreas allows healing to occur by protein synthesis, epithelialization, and fibrin polymerization. Obstruction of the pancreatic duct is seldom caused by wound contraction; rather, parenchymal edema or obstruction at the duodenal papilla usually is the cause. The main concern associated with pancreatic healing after surgery is the effect of healing on the flow and drainage of pancreatic secretions. If the duct to the remaining portion is left intact, as much as 80% of the pancreas can be removed without causing deleterious decreases in exocrine or endocrine function.

SUTURE MATERIALS AND SPECIAL INSTRUMENTS

Duct ligation is performed with nonabsorbable suture material (i.e., polypropylene or nylon) in animals with inflammatory, aseptic, or neoplastic conditions. In septic conditions of the pancreas, monofilament absorbable suture material (e.g., polydioxanone or polyglyconate) may be used; braided suture material should be avoided. Chromic gut suture should be not be used because it may be rapidly digested by pancreatic enzymes.

POSTOPERATIVE CARE AND ASSESSMENT

Medical treatment of canine and feline pancreatitis is replete with opinions, but almost no controlled studies have been performed. The following recommendations are, rightly or wrongly, generally agreed upon, but the reader is referred to a current medical text for a more complete discussion. Oral feedings should be delayed for 2 to 5 days after extensive pancreatic surgery or if pancreatitis is present. Hydration and electrolytes (especially potassium) should be maintained with IV fluid therapy since pancreatic perfusion is probably paramount in healing the diseased pancreas. Remember that visceral perfusion may be inadequate in animals that subjectively appear normally hydrated; dehydration is often missed by clinicians. Plasma oncotic pressure should be maintained by administering plasma or hetastarch if hypoalbuminemia (i.e., serum albumin less than 2 gm/dl) occurs. DIC should be treated by maintaining perfusion and administering clotting factors by plasma transfusions; heparin therapy may be given in addition. Antiemetics, H_2-receptor antagonists, and analgesics may be administered, as needed. Feeding should be initiated first with water to observe whether vomiting occurs. If the animal does not vomit, small amounts of ultra low-fat (less than 2% fat on a dry matter basis), bland food (e.g., rice and defatted white chicken or white turkey without the skin) may be given. Animals with severe or prolonged pancreatitis appear to benefit from parenteral nutrition (partial or peripheral is much easier than total; see Chapter 11) or from feeding through the jejunostomy postoperatively (see p. 107). If sepsis is identified, then appropriate antibiotic therapy generally should be continued for 10 to 14 days after surgery, but this is exceedingly rare in dogs.

COMPLICATIONS

The most common complication of pancreatic surgery is pancreatitis; this can be minimized by gentle tissue handling. Octreotide (1 to 2 μg/kg given subcutaneously before surgery) may be useful in preventing postoperative pancreatitis.

Severe, acute pancreatitis is associated with a high rate of mortality from multiorgan failure. Exocrine pancreatic insufficiency (EPI) may occur if pancreatic drainage is completely obstructed. EPI is treated with pancreatic supplements of commercial pancreatic extract (e.g., pancrelipase; Box 22-14); feeding low-fat, highly digestible meals; and administration of antibiotics for associated antibiotic-responsive enteropathy. Endocrine pancreatic insufficiency (diabetes mellitus) may result when more than 80% to 90% of the pancreatic tissue is removed. Supplementation with insulin may be necessary.

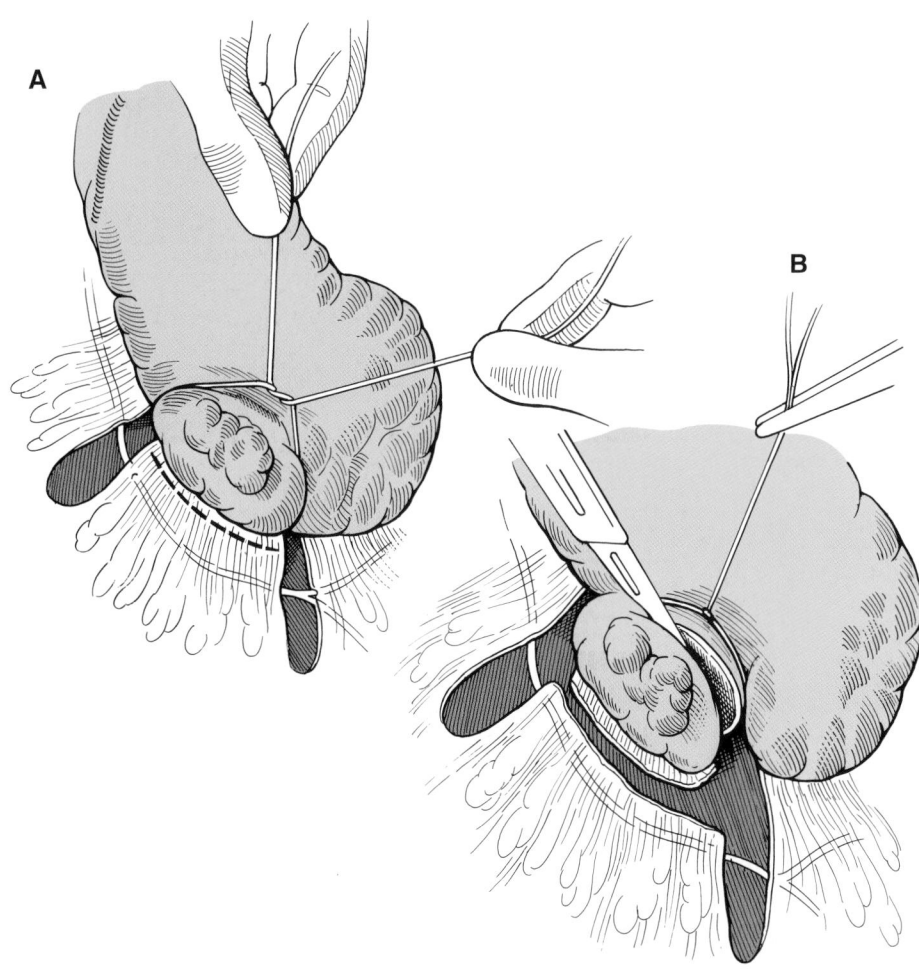

FIG. 22-10
Focal lesions near the extremity of the pancreas can be removed by the suture fracture technique. Incise the mesoduodenum or omentum *(dotted line)* and pass nonabsorbable suture from one side of the pancreas to the other through the incisions. Tighten the suture and allow it to crush through the parenchyma.

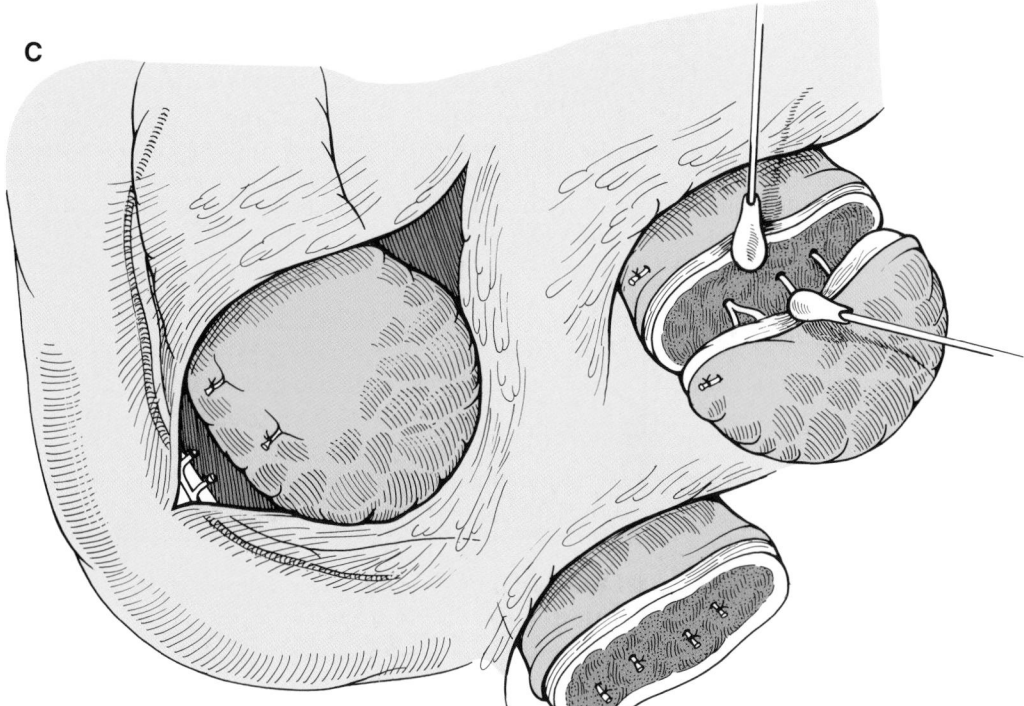

FIG. 22-11
Blunt separation of pancreatic lobules and ligation of ducts can be performed for lesions anywhere in the pancreas. **A,** Identify the lesion to be removed and gently incise the mesoduodenum or omentum overlying it. **B,** Separate the affected lobules from adjoining tissue by blunt dissection using sterile Q-tips or Halsted mosquito hemostats. **C,** Ligate the blood vessels and ducts supplying the portion of the pancreas to be removed.

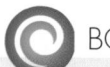

BOX 22-14

Pancreatic Enzyme Treatment of Exocrine Pancreatic Insufficiency

Pancreazyme

Up to 2 teaspoons in each meal

Viokase

1 to 2 teaspoons in each meal

If oral lesions (stomatitis, glossitis) occur, stop the preparation for 3–5 days and then start back at half the dose.

SPECIAL AGE CONSIDERATIONS

Pancreatic disease usually is found in middle-aged or older animals. Special care must be taken to meet the nutritional and metabolic needs of geriatric patients, particularly when disease may have caused inappetence or chronic vomiting. Parenteral hyperalimentation may be necessary before and after surgery in these patients.

References

Newman S, Steiner J, Woosley K et al: Localization of pancreatic inflammation and necrosis in dogs, *J Vet Intern Med* 18:488, 2004.

Steiner JM, Williams DA: Development and validation of a radio-immunoassay for the measurement of canine pancreatic lipase immunoreactivity in serum of dogs, *Am J Vet Res* 64:1237, 2003.

Suggested Reading

Harmoinen J, Saari S, Rinkinen M et al: Evaluation of pancreatic forceps biopsy by laparoscopy in healthy beagles, *Vet Ther* 3:31, 2002.

Biopsies were taken from four healthy beagles laparoscopically with double spoon type of forceps without any problems. Description of the technique is included.

SPECIFIC DISEASES

PANCREATIC ABSCESSES AND PSEUDOCYSTS

DEFINITIONS

Pancreatic abscesses are a collection of purulent material and necrotic tissue within and extending from the pancreatic parenchyma. **Pancreatic pseudocysts** are collections of pancreatic secretions and cellular debris enclosed within a wall of granulation tissue or fibrous sac that lacks an epithelial wall. Pancreatic pseudocysts have also been called *pancreatic cysts.*

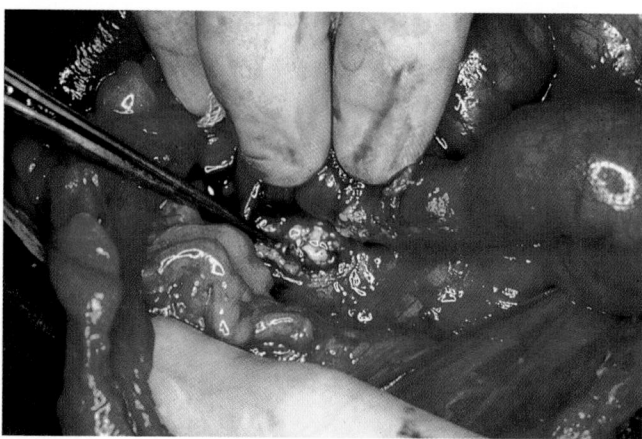

FIG. 22-12
Pancreatic abscess in a dog.

GENERAL CONSIDERATIONS AND CLINICALLY RELEVANT PATHOPHYSIOLOGY

Pancreatic abscesses (Fig. 22-12) are pancreatic or peripancreatic collections of purulent, necrotic, and hemorrhagic tissue that usually occur as a consequence of acute pancreatitis. Pancreatic abscesses may also occur in human beings as a consequence of chronic ductal obstruction. Bacteria probably gain entrance to the pancreas hematogenously or from enteric reflux.

Pancreatic pseudocysts (Fig. 22-13) are a common complication of acute pancreatitis in human beings, but are only rarely diagnosed in small animals. They may be associated with recurrent bouts of pancreatitis or trauma. The fluid in the cysts is a combination of blood, pancreatic fluids, and enzymes. These are not true cysts because the fluid is thought to leak from damaged pancreatic ducts and vessels rather than being secreted by the lining of the cyst. Pancreatic pseudocysts may be incidental findings or may be associated with nonspecific abdominal signs, such as pain and vomiting. In human beings, complications—such as infection, rupture, or acute hemorrhage—may occur and are associated with a high mortality rate.

> NOTE: Large pancreatic masses in symptomatic or asymptomatic animals may be pseudocysts or sterile abscesses; cancer is a much less common cause. Do not recommend euthanasia solely on the basis of a radiographic finding of an abdominal mass.

DIAGNOSIS
Clinical Presentation

Signalment. Pancreatic abscesses probably arise after acute pancreatitis; therefore the signalment of animals with pancreatic abscesses closely parallels that of animals diagnosed with acute pancreatitis (see p. 586). Most animals are mid-

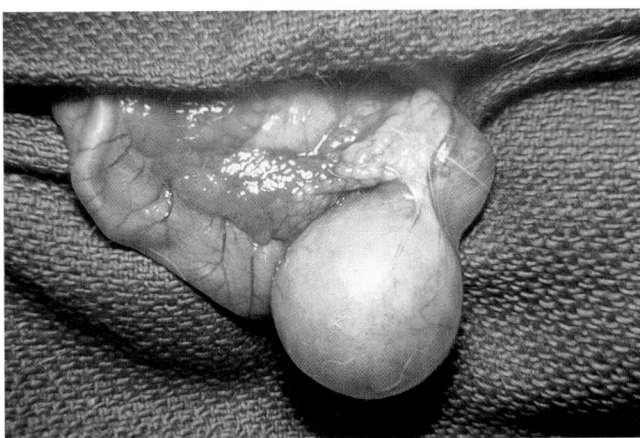

FIG. 22-13
Pancreatic pseudocyst. (Courtesy H.P. Hobson, Texas A&M University.)

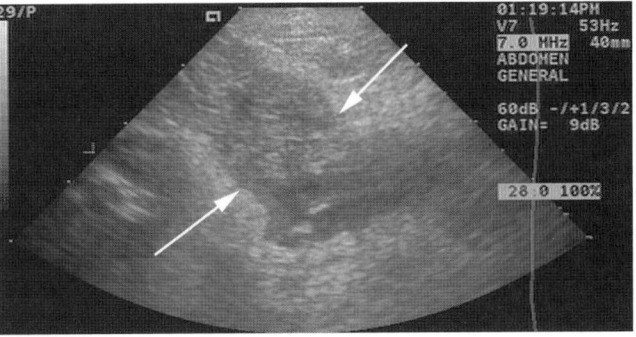

FIG. 22-14
Ultrasound parasagittal image of the pancreas. It is hypoechoic *(arrows)*, enlarged, and surrounded by hyperechoic fat consistent with pancreatitis.

dle-aged or older, and dogs are more commonly affected than cats.

History. Animals with pancreatic abscesses may have a previous history of acute onset of anorexia, depression, diarrhea, or vomiting, and some have previously been treated for gastroenteritis that probably was pancreatitis. Other clinical findings may include ataxia, anorexia, abdominal pain, or pyrexia. These patients may have dramatic acute signs or vague, smoldering, chronic signs of disease. Animals with pancreatic cysts may be asymptomatic or may show vague signs of abdominal discomfort, anorexia, and/or vomiting.

Physical Examination Findings

Typical findings with pancreatic abscesses may include pain during abdominal palpation, depression, icterus, pyrexia, palpable cranial abdominal mass, or abdominal distention. However, the animal may have none of these findings. Some animals may be weak and reluctant to stand. Pyrexia is an uncommon finding.

Diagnostic Imaging

The most consistent finding with pancreatic abscesses on survey abdominal radiographs is an ill-defined increase in soft tissue density in the right cranial abdominal quadrant. If peritonitis is present, a generalized increase in soft tissue opacity and loss of visceral detail in the right quadrant or throughout the abdomen may be observed. Abdominal ultrasonography is more sensitive and usually reveals a mass in the area of the pancreas. Gallbladder and bile duct distention may also be noted. Ultrasonography may also identify pancreatitis (Fig. 22-14). Gastric outflow obstruction is rarely observed on contrast studies of the upper gastrointestinal tract. Ultrasound examination is the best tool for identifying pancreatic abscesses and pseudocysts; however, differentiation of pseudocysts from other fluid-filled masses is not possible without evaluation of the

fluid. Percutaneous fine-needle aspiration of masses is reasonable in dogs because of the extremely low incidence of septic pancreatitis in that species. This risk must be weighed against the advantage of a preoperative diagnosis. Resolution of pancreatic pseudocysts after percutaneous, ultrasound-guided drainage is possible (Smith and Biller, 1998).

> NOTE: Fine-needle aspiration of cavitary pancreatic masses is not without some risk. Perform with caution and use care.

Laboratory Findings

Hematologic and serum biochemical findings with pancreatic abscesses are inconsistent, but may include leukocytosis, neutrophilia with or without a left shift, lymphopenia, or monocytosis. Serum biochemical abnormalities may include hyperbilirubinemia and high serum alkaline phosphatase caused by extrahepatic cholestasis, high alanine aminotransferase, hypocholesterolemia, hyponatremia, hypochloremia, and hypokalemia. Serum lipase and serum amylase are insensitive and nonspecific; they should not be performed. Bilirubinuria often is present. Blood test values in animals with pseudocysts may be consistent with those for pancreatitis or may be normal.

> NOTE: The absence of neutrophilia does not exclude pancreatic abscessation.

DIFFERENTIAL DIAGNOSIS

Pancreatic abscesses must be differentiated from other causes of vomiting and cranial abdominal pain (e.g., pancreatitis, gastric foreign bodies, intestinal foreign bodies, gastritis, cholecystitis, pancreatic neoplasia, and gastrointestinal neoplasia). Ultrasound evaluation of the pancreas is the most useful test for differentiating these abnormalities preoperatively; however, exploratory surgery may be required in some animals to make a definitive diagnosis. Pancreatic pseudocysts must be differentiated from pancreatic abscesses or neoplasia based on gross appearance, culture results, and histopathologic examination.

MEDICAL MANAGEMENT

Pancreatic abscesses have classically been considered surgical diseases. However, since these are almost invariably sterile in dogs, the place of ultrasound-guided, percutaneous aspiration is being explored, especially in dogs with less severe clinical signs. The mortality rate in human beings with pancreatic abscesses is nearly 100% when medical therapy without drainage is used; with surgical treatment, mortality has been reduced. Similar studies have not been reported in dogs or cats. Small pancreatic pseudocysts may resolve spontaneously without therapy.

SURGICAL TREATMENT

Dogs that clearly have fluid-filled structures probably benefit from drainage procedures; however, many dogs with pancreatitis have hypoechoic areas in the pancreas that do not represent fluid accumulations that can be drained. Generalized, sterile peritonitis is present in some dogs with pancreatic abscesses (if septic peritonitis or pancreatitis is present, a thorough search should be made for a primary cause, such as a perforated duodenum). On opening the abdomen, a mass is observed originating from the pancreas in the cranial portion of the abdomen. The mass may be firm and fibrotic or friable. Multiple adhesions to omentum and adjacent loops of small or large intestine often are present. These lesions can look malignant; however, the vast majority of pancreatic lesions and masses are inflammatory without malignancy, no matter how bad they appear. Adhesions may be present with pseudocysts if the cyst has ruptured and re-formed; however, fewer adhesions are expected than with pancreatic abscesses. Omentalization of the pancreatic lesion is preferred over external drainage (see later discussion). Pseudocysts may be drained at surgery or by fine-needle aspiration.

Preoperative Management

If clinically apparent pancreatitis is present, medical management should be initiated before surgery. See the discussion on p. 590 for treatment of pancreatitis. A broad-spectrum antibiotic can be administered intravenously before surgery if sepsis is believed to be present, but is seldom necessary. If infection is found by cytology or culture, then antibiotics should be used for at least 10 to 14 days postoperatively.

Anesthesia

See the discussion of the anesthetic management of animals with pancreatic disease on p. 587.

Surgical Anatomy

See the discussion of the surgical anatomy of the pancreas on pp. 588 to 589.

Positioning

The animal is positioned in dorsal recumbency, and the caudal thorax and entire abdomen are prepared for aseptic surgery.

SURGICAL TECHNIQUE
Pancreatic Abscesses

Perform a midline abdominal laparotomy that extends from the xiphoid cartilage caudally to distal to the umbilicus. Gently explore the abdomen. Locate the pancreatic mass and obtain cultures of infected tissue. Gently break down adhesions in the intestine and omentum as needed to visualize the lesion. Preserve the pancreatic ducts, common bile ducts, and adjacent vascular structures during dissection. Débride necrotic or purulent areas of the pancreas using a combination of sharp and blunt dissection. Resect as much of the necrotic pancreas as possible without damaging adjacent blood vessels or tissue. Once the lesion has been débrided, place a piece of omentum in it and secure it with sutures. If possible, loop the omentum through a tunnel in the pancreatic tissue and suture it back to itself. Determine common bile duct patency by gently expressing the gallbladder. If the common bile duct is not patent, catheterize the duct and try to obtain flow or perform a cholecystoenterostomy (see p. 564). Make sure you do not ligate the common bile duct. If generalized peritonitis is present, lavage the abdomen thoroughly with warm, sterile saline or lactated Ringer's solution. The abdomen may be closed or left open for drainage if peritonitis is present (see p. 336).

Pancreatic Pseudocysts

Explore the abdominal cavity as described previously. Locate the pancreatic mass and obtain cultures of the cystic fluid. Gently break down any adhesions. Resect as much of the fibrous wall surrounding the pseudocyst as possible. If the mass is not resectable, aspirate the fluid. Place omentum in the cavity and suture it in place. Close the abdomen routinely.

SUTURE MATERIALS AND SPECIAL INSTRUMENTS

Absorbable suture material should be used for partial pancreatectomy in animals with pancreatic abscesses. Aerobic and anaerobic culture swabs should be available. Copious amounts of warmed fluids should be available for abdominal flushing; suction allows complete removal of instilled fluid and facilitates dilution of infected fluids in the abdominal cavity.

POSTOPERATIVE CARE AND ASSESSMENT

The patient should be treated for pancreatitis, as described previously. Antibiotic therapy should be continued if infection is found. Animals should be monitored postoperatively for signs of worsening inflammation. The clinical assessment of these patients (i.e., presence or absence of fever, abdominal pain, anorexia, vomiting, and icterus) is more important than the CBC or ultrasonographic appearance. Repeat operations may occasionally be required. Blood cultures are warranted if bacteremia is suspected. Pancreatitis is a potential complication of any surgery involving the pancreas (see p. 590).

NOTE: Warn owners that repeat surgery may be necessary in some animals with pancreatic abscesses.

PROGNOSIS

The prognosis in animals with pancreatic abscesses is guarded. The prognosis for pancreatic pseudocysts is good; many resolve spontaneously. Pancreatic masses caused by inflammation, even those causing biliary tract obstruction, often respond well to medical management, and surgical resection is seldom required.

References

Smith SA, Biller DS: Resolution of a pancreatic pseudocyst in a dog following percutaneous ultrasonographic-guided drainage, *J Am Anim Hosp Assoc* 34:515, 1998.

Suggested Reading

Bailiff NL, Norris CR, Seguin B et al: Pancreatolithiasis and pancreatic pseudobladder associated with pancreatitis in a cat, *J Am Anim Hosp Assoc* 40:69, 2004.
This is a case report of a cat with a congenital defect causing a structure resembling a gallbladder arising from the pancreas.
VanEnkevort BA, O'Brien RT, Young KM: Pancreatic pseudocysts in 4 dogs and 2 cats: ultrasonographic and clinicopathologic findings, *J Vet Intern Med* 13:309, 1999.
Pancreatic pseudocysts were found in four dogs and two cats; five were in the left pancreatic limb. All were aspirated without problems.

INSULINOMAS

DEFINITION

Insulinomas are functional tumors of the β-cells of the islets of Langerhans. These tumors secrete insulin despite the presence of hypoglycemia. They have also been called *pancreatic β-cell tumors, adenomas,* or *adenocarcinomas of the pancreatic islets.*

GENERAL CONSIDERATIONS AND CLINICALLY RELEVANT PATHOPHYSIOLOGY

Insulinomas are pancreatic islet cell tumors that secrete excessive amounts of insulin, causing hypoglycemia. They are more commonly recognized in dogs than in cats. Unlike human beings, in whom up to 90% of insulinomas are benign, malignant tumors predominate in dogs. They typically metastasize to the regional lymph nodes, liver, and omentum. Occasionally nodules may be found in the lung. They are slow growing tumors that compress adjacent pancreatic parenchyma. Because they are typically sharply de-

lineated and encapsulated, palliative surgical excision often prolongs survival. Tumor state may correlate with survival time following surgery and medical management (see Prognosis section).

NOTE: More than 90% of canine insulinomas are malignant. They nearly always metastasize even though they may lack histologic criteria of malignancy.

DIAGNOSIS
Clinical Presentation

Signalment. Insulinomas generally occur in middle-aged or older dogs, and there is no gender predisposition. Medium- to large-breed dogs (e.g., Irish setters, German shepherds, Labrador retrievers, standard poodles, and boxers) appear to be more commonly affected.

History. The clinical signs, which are attributable to hypoglycemia, include muscle tremors, muscle weakness, ataxia, mental dullness, disorientation, collapse, and/or convulsions. Dogs may be easily agitated and may have intermittent periods of excitability and restlessness. These clinical signs suggest hypoglycemia of any cause, not just insulinoma. Owners may notice clinical signs for months before presenting the animals for evaluation. The clinical signs often are intermittent initially, but occur more frequently as the disease progresses. Owners often report that clinical signs diminish or resolve with feeding. Animals sometimes are treated for seizures with anticonvulsant agents before the diagnosis is made.

NOTE: Warn owners that chronic, severe hypoglycemia may cause permanent neurologic abnormalities.

Physical Examination Findings

Physical examination findings may reveal a normal or ataxic animal, muscle weakness (usually seen as shaking or collapse in the rear), mental dullness, or disorientation. Affected dogs are usually normal between hypoglycemic episodes, a fact that may help differentiate insulinoma from other causes of hypoglycemia. Withholding food before and during the evaluation may precipitate seizures in affected animals. Neuronal demyelination and axonal degeneration may result from chronic hypoglycemia. Although the cause is not known for certain, direct toxic effects of hypoglycemia on peripheral nerves or a paraneoplastic neuropathy have been postulated. Signs of peripheral polyneuropathy, such as ataxia and weakness, may continue despite appropriate therapy.

Diagnostic Imaging

Thoracic and abdominal radiographs do not contribute to the diagnosis; however, the location of the tumor in the pancreas sometimes can be determined using ultrasound. Unfortunately tumor masses are often so small that they are difficult to identify. Ultrasonography may also reveal metastasis to the liver and regional lymph nodes in some affected animals. Thoracic radiographs are indicated to look for metastasis, although pulmonary metastasis is rare. In one study of 14 insulinomas, 5 tumors were detected by ultrasound and 10 by CT. CT also identified 2 of 5 lymph node metastases, but found 28 false-positive lesions. Intraoperative inspection and palpation of the pancreas was the superior test (Robben et al, 2005). Somatostatin receptor scintigraphy, using single-photon emission computed tomography (SPECT) (with [111In-DTPA-D-Phe1]-octreotide) was reported to be no more effective than ultrasound or CT in identifying canine insulinomas (Robbins et al, 2005).

LABORATORY FINDINGS

A tentative diagnosis of insulinoma is based on demonstration of Whipple's triad (Box 22-15). Fasting or nonfasting blood glucose concentrations often are below 70 mg/dl. If blood glucose concentrations initially are within the normal range, most affected dogs can be made hypoglycemic by fasting for 12 to 24 hours. Blood glucose measurements should be determined every 2 to 3 hours in these animals until hypoglycemia is detected. Serum fructosamine may be useful for diagnosing chronic, occult hypoglycemia (Mellanby et al, 2002).

Once hypoglycemia has been confirmed, blood for serum insulin measurement should be obtained immediately. If food has been withheld from the animal to induce hypoglycemia, serum insulin concentrations should be measured on the first hypoglycemic sample (i.e., below 55 mg/dl). Normal fasting serum immunoreactive insulin concentrations range from 5 to 26 μU/ml, whereas insulin levels in affected animals often exceed 70 μU/ml. If insulin levels fall within the normal range, an amended insulin/glucose ratio can be determined; however, false-positive results are possible (Box 22-16). Evaluating the absolute insulin concentration when the patient is hypoglycemic while considering the history, physical examination, and other clinical pathology data is the best approach. In some cases, definitive diagnosis of insulinoma may require exploratory surgery.

DIFFERENTIAL DIAGNOSIS

Insulinomas should be considered a differential diagnosis in any dog with persistent and progressive seizures. Once hypoglycemia has been verified, these tumors must be differentiated from other causes of hypoglycemia, including extrapancreatic neoplasms, hunting dog hypoglycemia, sepsis, hepatic failure, hypoadrenocorticism, glycogen storage disorders (very rare), and hypopituitarism.

MEDICAL MANAGEMENT

Dogs with insulinomas should be fed frequent, small meals. Three to six meals a day of a diet high in protein and complex carbohydrates but low in refined sugar reduces clinical signs. Exercise restriction may also help alleviate clinical signs. Glucocorticoid therapy (Box 22-17) may also help prevent hypoglycemia caused by islet cell tumors by increasing hepatic glucose production and decreasing cellular glucose uptake. The lowest possible dose that controls hypoglycemia should be used to prevent iatrogenic HAC (e.g., polyphagia, polydipsia, bilateral symmetric alopecia, and thin epidermis). If clinical signs of HAC occur, glucocorticoid therapy may be reduced and alternate drugs used; however, HAC may be preferable to hypoglycemia. Diazoxide (see Box 22-17) is an oral hyperglycemic agent that inhibits pancreatic insulin secretion and glucose uptake by tissue. It raises blood glucose concentrations in some dogs with insulinomas; however, side effects may occur, such as anorexia, vomiting, aplastic anemia, cataracts, bone marrow suppression, thrombocytopenia, anorexia, diarrhea, tachycardia, and fluid retention. Diazoxide should be used cautiously in animals with hepatic dysfunction. If hypoglycemia is severe and unresponsive, intravenous administration of 5% or 10% dextrose may be necessary to maintain blood glucose concentrations in the normal range until surgery can be performed. Alloxan and a somatostatin ana-

BOX 22-16

Amended Insulin/Glucose Ratio (μU/mg)

$$\frac{\text{Serum insulin } (\mu U/ml) \times 100}{\text{Plasma glucose } (mg/dl) - 30*}$$

*If the blood glucose concentration is 30 mg/dl or lower, use 1 for the denominator.

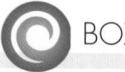

BOX 22-17

Oral Hyperglycemic Agents

Prednisolone
0.25–2 mg/kg bid

Diazoxide (Proglycem)
Start with 5 mg/kg bid with meals; may gradually increase to 60 mg/kg divided bid; concurrent administration of hydrochlorothiazide may enhance effects of diazoxide

bid, Twice a day.

BOX 22-15

Whipple's Triad

- Clinical signs associated with hypoglycemia (usually neurologic abnormalities)
- Fasting blood glucose concentrations of 40 mg/dl or lower
- Relief of neurologic signs with feeding or glucose administration

log (octreotide) have been used in a few dogs with insulinomas; however, too little information is available at this time to recommend their use.

Streptozotocin may be efficacious in dogs with insulinomas that have metastatic disease. A recent study suggested that it can be given safely to dogs at a dosage of 500 mg/m², IV, every 3 weeks when combined with a protocol for induction of diuresis (Moore et al, 2002). Give 0.9% NaCl administered at a rate of 18.3 ml/kg/hr, IV for 3 hours before streptozotocin administration. Dilute the streptozotocin to an appropriate volume and give over 2 hours at the same rate as the fluid administration. Then give 0.9% NaCl for an additional 2 hours. To reduce vomiting, butorphanol or other antiemetics may be given IM immediately after streptozotocin administration; however, these drugs are usually ineffective. Repeat the treatment every 3 weeks until there is evidence of tumor progression (i.e., the tumor increases significantly in size), there is recurrence of hypoglycemia, or toxicity (e.g., renal, hepatic) is noted that is unresponsive to supportive care. Other abnormalities that may occur in association with streptozotocin administration include neutropenia, thrombocytopenia, anorexia, diarrhea, and diabetes mellitus.

SURGICAL TREATMENT
Preoperative Management
Fluid therapy with 5% glucose should be initiated 12 to 24 hours before surgery. Food is withheld 12 hours before surgery. Blood glucose concentrations should be measured immediately before surgery and additional glucose given if the concentration is below 75 to 100 mg/dl.

Anesthesia
The goal of surgery is to maintain blood glucose concentrations above 75 to 100 mg/dl. Thiopental, propofol, or etomidate may be used for induction of anesthesia because they reduce cerebral glucose metabolism. After intubation, anesthesia should be maintained with isoflurane or sevoflurane. Isoflurane and sevoflurane reduce the cerebral metabolic rate

more than does halothane. Blood glucose concentrations should be monitored regularly during surgery (i.e., every 20 to 40 minutes) to prevent intraoperative hypoglycemia.

Surgical Anatomy
See the discussion of the surgical anatomy of the pancreas on pp. 588 to 589.

Positioning
The animal is positioned in dorsal recumbency, and the caudoventral thorax and entire abdomen are prepared for aseptic surgery.

SURGICAL TECHNIQUE
Explore the cranial abdominal cavity thoroughly for evidence of neoplasia. Carefully and gently palpate the entire pancreas for evidence of tumor nodules.

Most dogs have solitary nodules (Fig. 22-15). Tumors are found with equal frequency in the left and right lobes of the pancreas and in the body. Metastasis is noted in approximately 50% of cases at the time of surgery. Metastasis usually occurs to the regional lymph nodes and liver; however, duodenal, mesenteric, and omental metastasis may also occur.

Perform a partial pancreatectomy (see p. 590), removing tumor nodules with as wide a margin of normal tissue as possible. Submit excised lesions for histopathologic examination. Excise metastatic nodules if possible.

If the tumor cannot be identified, methylene blue may be administered intravenously (Box 22-18). Methylene blue may stain neoplastic islet cells, helping to differentiate them from surrounding normal tissue. Maximum staining occurs within 30 minutes. A common side effect of methylene blue administration is hemolytic anemia resulting from the formation of Heinz bodies.

> NOTE: Fatal Heinz body anemia in dogs has been reported with the use of methylene blue.

SUTURE MATERIALS AND SPECIAL INSTRUMENTS
Balfour abdominal retractors are useful for abdominal exploration. Sterile Q-tips or fine hemostats are useful for separating pancreatic tissue during partial pancreatectomy.

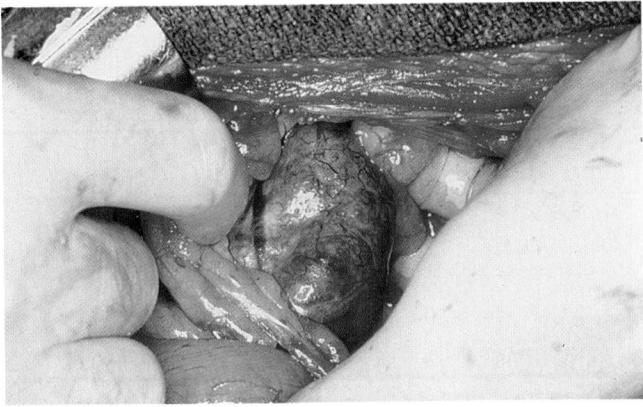

FIG. 22-15
Functional islet cell adenocarcinoma in a dog.

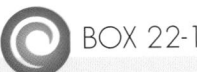 BOX 22-18

Methylene Blue Administration

Dilute 3 mg/kg of 1% methylene blue in 250 ml of 0.9% sterile saline and give intravenously over 30–40 minutes.

Duct ligation is performed using 3-0 or 4-0 nonabsorbable suture material (see p. 590). Methylene blue may be given intravenously to help identify primary and metastatic nodules (see previous discussion).

POSTOPERATIVE CARE AND ASSESSMENT

Blood glucose concentrations should be measured frequently during the first 24 hours after surgery. Pancreatitis may result from surgical manipulation of the pancreas and should be treated aggressively, as described on p. 590. Small amounts of water may be administered the day after surgery, and if vomiting does not occur, feeding of small, frequent meals may be initiated. Once the blood glucose concentration stabilizes at 75 to 100 mg/dl or higher, the glucose infusion can be discontinued (Box 22-19). If persistent hypoglycemia continues, medical therapy (glucocorticoids, diazoxide; see Box 22-17) should be initiated. Prolonged hypoglycemia may cause cerebral laminar necrosis. Neurologic signs (i.e., ataxia, bizarre behavior, coma, and seizures) may persist in such animals despite normoglycemia. Transient hyperglycemia occasionally occurs and may persist for years after surgery. Insulin therapy may be indicated if blood glucose concentrations above 180 mg/dl persist for longer than 3 to 5 days.

COMPLICATIONS

Complications of surgery in animals with insulinomas include persistent hypoglycemia, pancreatitis, diabetes mellitus, epilepsy, and diffuse polyneuropathy. The most common causes of postoperative hypoglycemia are unrecognized or unresectable metastases or multiple or incompletely resected primary tumors. Persistent hyperglycemia occurs in up to one third of dogs undergoing surgical removal of insulinomas and is thought to be a result of suppression of normal β-cells by tumor insulin, resulting in loss of insulin production.

PROGNOSIS

The long-term survival and duration of normoglycemia in animals with insulinomas after surgery depends on the clinical stage of the tumor at the time of surgery. If the tumor is confined to the pancreas (Stage I), or if metastasis is present but confined to the regional lymph nodes (Stage II), a median survival time of approximately 18 months can be expected. Dogs with distant metastases (Stage III) have a median survival time of less than 6 months (Moore et al, 2002). Tumor stage may have its greatest effect on the period in which the animal remains normoglycemic after surgery. Dogs with Stage I disease typically are normoglycemic for a median of 14 months, while those that are Stage II or III have significantly shorter periods of normoglycemia (Table 22-1). Long-term disease-free periods can be obtained in some dogs with multiple surgeries to remove hepatic nodules as clinical signs occur. Young dogs may have a poorer prognosis than older dogs.

NOTE: If metastasis is not apparent at surgery, survival of longer than 1 year may occur, even though cures are unlikely.

References

Mellanby RJ, Herrtage ME: Insulinoma in a normoglyceaemic dog with low fructosamine, *J Small Anim Pract* 43:506, 2002.

Moore AS, Nelson RW, Henry CJ et al: Streptozotocin for treatment of pancreatic islet cell tumors in dogs: 17 cases (1989-1999), *J Am Vet Med Assoc* 221:811, 2002.

Robben J, Pollak Y, Kirpensteijn J et al: Comparison of ultrasonography, computed tomography, and single-photo emission computed tomography for the detection and localization of canine insulinoma, *J Vet Intern Med* 19:15, 2005.

 BOX 22-19

Postoperative Recommendations for Maintaining Glucose Concentrations

- Initially monitor blood glucose every 2–3 hours.
- Continue providing glucose-containing fluids until the blood glucose concentration is more than 75 mg/dl.
- If hypoglycemia persists, administer steroids or diazoxide.

 TABLE 22-1

Prognosis for Insulinomas

STAGE OF DISEASE	CRITERIA	MEDIAN SURVIVAL TIMES	MEDIAN NORMOGLYCEMIA TIME
I	Tumor is confined to the pancreas	18 mo	14 mo
II	Metastasis is confined to the regional lymph nodes	18 mo	1 mo
III	Distal metastasis is present	Less than 6 mo	1 mo

From Moore AS, Nelson RW, Henry CJ et al: Streptozocin for treatment of pancreatic cell tumors in dogs: 17 cases (1989-1999), *J Am Vet Med Assoc* 221:911, 2002.

GASTRINOMAS

DEFINITIONS

Gastrinomas are tumors that secrete excessive gastrin. **Zollinger-Ellison syndrome** is a term used to describe a syndrome of gastric acid hypersecretion, gastrointestinal ulceration, and non–β-cell pancreatic tumors. Gastrinomas are also called *non–β-cell tumors* and *gastrin-secreting tumors*. The terms gastrinoma and Zollinger-Ellison syndrome often are used interchangeably; however, gastrinomas can arise in other parts of the alimentary tract. Zollinger-Ellison syndrome refers specifically to gastrinomas arising in the pancreas.

GENERAL CONSIDERATIONS AND CLINICALLY RELEVANT PATHOPHYSIOLOGY

Gastrinomas are rare tumors in dogs and cats. They are derived from ectopic amine precursor uptake decarboxylase (APUD) cells in the pancreas and produce an excess of the hormone gastrin. Gastrin normally is secreted by cells of the antral and duodenal mucosa in response to antral distention and stimulation by amino acids. Excess gastrin causes hyperacidity, which produces multiple duodenal ulcerations and/or erosions. Pancreatic gastrin-secreting tumors usually are locally invasive into adjacent parenchyma and frequently metastasize to regional lymph nodes or the liver or both.

DIAGNOSIS
Clinical Presentation

Signalment. Dogs and cats may be affected. Too few cases have been reported to determine breed or gender predisposition. Affected animals usually are middle-aged.

History. Most animals have clinical signs of anorexia, vomiting (which occasionally is blood tinged), regurgitation, intermittent diarrhea, weight loss, and/or dehydration. Clinical signs may be present for several days or months before diagnosis. Animals may have been treated for gastric ulcers for months with poor response.

Physical Examination Findings

Clinical findings are nonspecific and may include dehydration, diarrhea, melena, hematemesis (coffee-ground appearance), steatorrhea, and/or weight loss. Abdominal pain is inconsistent. Gastric ulcer perforation may cause generalized peritonitis (see p. 436).

Diagnostic Imaging

Radiographs and ultrasonography are nondiagnostic for gastrinomas because pancreatic masses generally are too small to be visualized. Endoscopy is the most useful technique for diagnosing esophagitis, gastric mucosal hypertrophy, or duodenal ulceration in dogs with suggestive clinical signs. Ulcers are most commonly located in the proximal duodenum.

Endoscopy. On endoscopy, patients typically have esophagitis (because of profuse vomiting of acid) and duodenal ulcers or erosions. Duodenal biopsies typically have minimal inflammation. Gastric ulceration is much less common, but erosions and/or mucosal hypertrophy may be seen.

Laboratory Findings

Nonspecific laboratory abnormalities noted in animals with gastrinomas include anemia, hypoproteinemia, elevated serum alkaline phosphatase activity, and/or leukocytosis. Electrolyte and acid-base abnormalities may occur if vomiting has been severe (e.g., hypochloremia, hypokalemia, metabolic alkalosis, or metabolic acidosis). Preoperative diagnosis of gastrinoma is based on demonstration of hypergastrinemia. Blood samples for serum gastrin analysis should be obtained after a 12-hour fast and before treatment with any antacid drug. Serum gastrin levels of animals with Zollinger-Ellison syndrome may exceed 1000 pg/ml.

DIFFERENTIAL DIAGNOSIS

Gastrinomas must be differentiated from other causes of peptic ulceration, including nonsteroidal antiinflammatory drugs (NSAIDs), corticosteroids, gastric neoplasia, infiltrative disease, mast cell tumors, DIC, hepatic disease, circulatory shock, and septic shock (see also p. 438). Other causes of hypergastrinemia include renal failure, gastric outflow obstruction, chronic gastritis, and current H_2-blocker therapy.

MEDICAL MANAGEMENT

Because of the aggressive biologic behavior of this malignant neoplasm, the prognosis for long-term cure is poor; however, aggressive medical management with proton pump inhibitors (Box 22-20) or high dose H_2-receptor antagonists may be helpful. Proton pump inhibitors (e.g., omeprazole and lansoprazole) are the most potent inhibitors of gastric-acid secretion known. Other agents that may be used to help treat ulcers in dogs with gastrinomas include those that

---

 BOX 22-20

Medical Therapy for Animals With Gastrinoma

Omeprazole (Prilosec)*

Dogs: 0.7–1.5 mg/kg PO, qd to bid (preferred)
Cats: Not recommended

Sucralfate (Carafate)

Dogs: 0.5–1 g/dog PO, tid to qid
Cats: 0.25 g/cat PO, bid to tid

Famotidine (Pepcid)†

0.5–1 mg/kg PO, IM, or SC, qd to bid

PO, Oral; *qd*, once a day; *bid*, twice a day; *tid*, three times a day; *qid*, four times a day.
*Will take 2–5 days to achieve maximal effect. Best if given 30 minutes before meals.
†Give if must use parenteral instead of oral therapy, or if omeprazole is inadequate to control signs.

lessen gastric acidity and those that protect the gastric mucosa from damage (see Box 22-20). However, the effectiveness of these drugs in animals with gastrinomas often is limited, and beneficial effects may be short-lived.

Sucralfate forms a protective coating over the ulcer or erosion. Cimetidine, ranitidine, and famotidine are H_2-receptor blockers that reduce acid secretion, but they tend to be much less effective than omeprazole (see Box 22-20).

SURGICAL TREATMENT

Exploratory laparotomy often is required to confirm the diagnosis. Surgical resection of the pancreatic mass may provide a cure if metastasis is not present. If metastasis is present, surgical debulking of the mass and removal of operable metastatic lesions may improve the efficacy of medical therapy and prolong survival. The gastrointestinal tract should be closely inspected during surgery for evidence of ulcerations that may perforate. Any such lesions should be removed or should have a serosal patch (see p. 457). Total gastrectomy has been recommended for animals in which the condition is unresponsive to medical therapy; however, because of long-term complications (i.e., malnutrition, dysphagia, or bile reflux), this procedure is seldom performed.

Preoperative Management

If possible, the animal's condition should be stabilized before surgery. Whole blood should be given if the animal is severely anemic (i.e., PCV below 20% [see Box 5-1 on p. 25]), and anemic animals should be oxygenated before induction of anesthesia. Electrolyte and acid-base abnormalities should be corrected and fluid therapy initiated before surgery.

Anesthesia

See p. 587 for anesthetic recommendations for animals undergoing pancreatic surgery. Inotropic therapy may be necessary.

Surgical Anatomy

See pp. 588 to 589 for discussion of the surgical anatomy of the pancreas and p. 410 for discussion of the surgical anatomy of the stomach.

Positioning

The animal is placed in dorsal recumbency, and the abdomen is prepared for a ventral midline incision. The caudal thorax and entire ventral abdomen should be prepared for aseptic surgery.

SURGICAL TECHNIQUE

Perform a thorough abdominal exploration. Inspect the draining lymph nodes, liver, duodenum, and mesentery for evidence of metastasis. Inspect the entire pancreas for a mass lesion. Perform a partial pancreatectomy (see p. 590) and resect metastatic lesions that are accessible. Submit excised tissues for histopathologic examination.

SUTURE MATERIALS AND SPECIAL INSTRUMENTS

If the animal is severely hypoproteinemic or anemic, wound healing may be delayed. In such cases, polydioxanone or polyglyconate suture (2-0 or 3-0) is preferred to close gastrotomy and abdominal incisions (see p. 63). These sutures may also be used to perform a serosal patch.

POSTOPERATIVE CARE AND ASSESSMENT

Anemic animals benefit from nasal oxygen postoperatively. The patient must be monitored, and if signs suggestive of pancreatitis are seen, aggressive therapy is indicated (see p. 590 for treatment of pancreatitis). Small amounts of water should be given the day after surgery and the patient observed for vomiting. If vomiting does not occur, small amounts of food can be given 24 hours postoperatively. The diet should be low in fat and fiber, and contain moderate amounts of protein and carbohydrates to aid gastric emptying. Fluid therapy should be continued until the animal is eating and drinking. Medical therapy for ulcers should be continued until clinical signs resolve. Long-term medical therapy may be necessary to control gastric hypersecretion caused by hypergastrinemia and to reduce the incidence and severity of ulcers.

PROGNOSIS

Because of the malignant nature of this tumor, the long-term prognosis generally is grave. In one study, 3 of 4 dogs had evidence of metastatic disease in the lymphatic system at the time of surgery (Green and Gartrell, 1997).

Reference

Green RA, Gartrell CL: Gastrinoma: a retrospective study of four cases (1985-1995), *J Am Anim Hosp Assoc* 33:524, 1997.

EXOCRINE PANCREATIC NEOPLASIA

DEFINITION

Exocrine pancreatic carcinomas are malignant tumors that arise from either acinar or ductular epithelial cells. They are also called *pancreatic adenocarcinomas*.

GENERAL CONSIDERATIONS AND CLINICALLY RELEVANT PATHOPHYSIOLOGY

Exocrine pancreatic tumors are slightly more common than tumors of the pancreatic islet cells in dogs and cats. Pancreatic tumors are more common in human beings than in dogs and are associated with an extremely high mortality rate (approximately 90% within 1 year of diagnosis). Most pancreatic tumors are malignant (adenocarcinoma); they are aggressive tumors that invade locally and metastasize readily. The most common sites for metastasis are the liver, lungs, peritoneum, and regional lymph nodes. Metastatic pancreatic carcinoma was diagnosed in one dog that was presented for evaluation of diabetes insipidus. Benign pancreatic tumors (i.e., adenomas) are extremely rare.

NOTE: Most pancreatic masses are caused by pancreatitis, not neoplasia. Never euthanize a patient with a pancreatic mass without a histologic diagnosis, no matter how "bad" the mass looks grossly.

DIAGNOSIS
Clinical Presentation

Signalment. Pancreatic adenocarcinomas occur more commonly in older animals, and Airedale terriers and boxers have been reported to have higher risk for this tumor. A gender predisposition has not been proved in dogs, although pancreatic carcinoma seems to be more common in males.

NOTE: You cannot differentiate pancreatic adenocarcinoma from benign pancreatic disease on the basis of clinical signs or gross appearance.

History. Animals with pancreatic adenocarcinoma may have vomiting, abdominal pain, anorexia, weight loss, lethargy, abdominal distention, and/or diarrhea. The history may be acute or chronic. Adenomas usually are incidental findings at surgery or at necropsy and are not associated with clinical signs.

Physical Examination Findings

Physical examination findings for exocrine pancreatic carcinoma may include abdominal pain on palpation and/or ascites occurring secondary to compression of the portal vein or other vessels or because of widespread abdominal metastasis. Some animals may have a palpable abdominal mass, but some have icterus secondary to common bile duct obstruction. Extremely high lipase values may suggest pancreatic carcinoma.

Diagnostic Imaging

An ill-defined increase in soft tissue opacity in the right cranial abdominal quadrant may be noted on survey abdominal radiographs. If ascites is present, a loss of visceral detail throughout the abdomen may be observed. Abdominal ultrasonography often reveals a mass in the area of the pancreas, but it is not necessarily easy to distinguish from pancreatitis (Bennett et al, 2001). Distention of the gallbladder and bile ducts may be noted with obstruction of the extrahepatic biliary tract. Obstruction of gastric outflow may be seen on contrast studies of the upper gastrointestinal tract.

Laboratory Findings

Laboratory abnormalities have not been well defined in animals with exocrine pancreatic neoplasia. Abnormalities consistent with extrahepatic cholestasis (i.e., elevated alkaline phosphatase and hyperbilirubinemia) often are present. Some animals may show mild leukocytosis, dehydration, and hemoconcentration.

DIFFERENTIAL DIAGNOSIS

Exocrine pancreatic carcinoma must be differentiated from benign and metastatic pancreatic disease. Nodular pancreatic hyperplasia, a condition seen in older animals, is characterized by multiple small, white lesions that protrude minimally from the pancreatic surface. Adenomas usually are small masses that may contain cysts. These conditions are not associated with clinical signs. Pancreatic carcinomas are usually well advanced at the time of diagnosis, and it may be difficult to determine grossly the site of origin for neoplastic masses.

MEDICAL MANAGEMENT

Although numerous treatments have been used in human beings in an attempt to improve the survival of patients with pancreatic adenocarcinoma, only those with resectable lesions at the time of laparotomy have a fair prognosis. Chemotherapeutic agents have not prolonged the life of people or animals with this tumor.

SURGICAL TREATMENT

Surgical resection is the treatment of choice; however, many animals are presented with advanced disease, and surgical resection is not possible.

Preoperative Management

The animal's condition should be stabilized before surgery with administration of intravenous fluids and correction of acid-base and electrolyte abnormalities.

Anesthesia

See the discussion of anesthetic management of animals with pancreatic disease on p. 587.

Surgical Anatomy

The surgical anatomy of the pancreas is described on pp. 588 to 589.

Positioning

The animal is prepared for a ventral midline exploratory procedure. The entire abdomen and caudal thorax should be prepared for aseptic surgery.

SURGICAL TECHNIQUE

Make an abdominal incision that extends from the xiphoid cartilage as far caudally as necessary to allow complete exploration of the abdominal cavity. After identifying the pancreatic mass (Fig. 22-16), explore the abdominal organs, peritoneum, and regional nodes for evidence of metastasis.

Euthanasia should be considered in animals with widespread metastasis.

Perform a partial pancreatectomy if possible. Confirm the patency of the common bile duct before closing the abdomen.

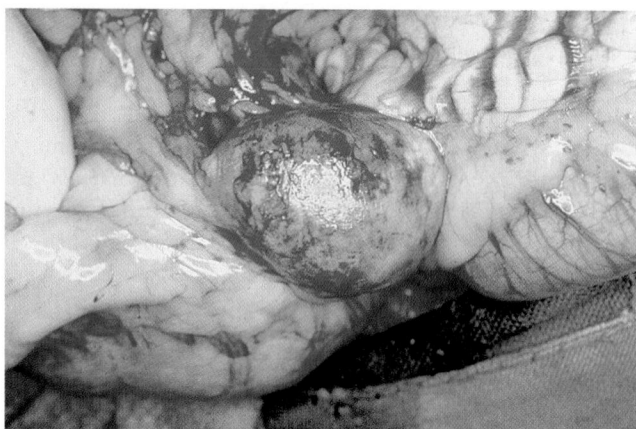

FIG. 22-16
Pancreatic carcinoma in a dog.

SUTURE MATERIALS AND SPECIAL INSTRUMENTS

A standard soft tissue pack or general surgery pack usually is all that is required. See p. 590 for requirements for partial pancreatectomy.

POSTOPERATIVE CARE AND ASSESSMENT

These animals may have pancreatitis secondary to the tumor at the time of diagnosis, and this may require therapy (see p. 590). Animals presented for treatment that have pancreatic carcinomas often are debilitated and require special attention to ensure that their nutritional needs are met postoperatively. Enteral or parenteral hyperalimentation should be considered. See also p. 590 for postoperative care of patients with pancreatic disease.

PROGNOSIS

The prognosis is extremely poor for animals with pancreatic carcinomas. Most have widespread disease at the time of diagnosis, and many are euthanized at surgery. Survival of less than 3 months should be expected for most of the remaining animals.

Reference

Bennett PF, Hahn KA, Toal RL et al: Ultrasonographic and cytopathological diagnosis of exocrine pancreatic carcinoma in the dog and cat, *J Am Anim Hosp Assoc* 37:466, 2001.

Surgery of the Thyroid and Parathyroid Glands

GENERAL PRINCIPLES AND TECHNIQUES

DEFINITIONS

Thyroidectomy is removal of a thyroid gland. **Hypothyroidism** is deficient secretion of thyroxine. **Goitrous hypothyroidism** is caused by an abnormal iodine uptake or by defects in iodine uptake, organification, or thyroglobulin formation. **Nongoitrous hypothyroidism** is spontaneous hypothyroidism that may be immune mediated (i.e., lymphocytic thyroiditis) or a result of idiopathic atrophy. **Hyperthyroidism** is excessive secretion of thyroxine. **Primary hyperparathyroidism** is excessive secretion of parathyroid hormone (PTH) by one or more abnormal parathyroid glands.

PREOPERATIVE MANAGEMENT

Hypothyroidism is a common endocrinopathy in dogs. It usually is due to thyroid dysfunction (primary hypothyroidism), although pituitary and hypothalamic causes occasionally are diagnosed. Three weeks of administration of trimethoprim-sulfamethoxazole (14.1 to 16 mg/kg PO, bid) will depress total thyroxine and free thyroxine and elevate canine thyroid-stimulating hormone concentrations, conditions compatible with a diagnosis of hypothyroidism (Frank et al, 2005). Thyroid function tests should also be interpreted carefully in dogs that are receiving glucocorticoids, phenobarbital, and carprofen (Daminet and Ferguson, 2003). Secretion of thyroid hormones triiodothyronine (T_3) and thyroxine (T_4) from the thyroid is controlled by a feedback mechanism between the hypothalamus, pituitary, and thyroid glands. Thyrotropin (thyroid-stimulating hormone [TSH]) is produced in the pars distalis of the pituitary gland. It stimulates the synthesis and release of thyroglobulin, a precursor of T_3 and T_4, as well as T_3 and T_4. Release of thyrotropin is controlled by a neuropeptide produced in the hypothalamus, thyrotropin-releasing hormone (TRH). TRH secretion is inhibited by high circulating levels of glucocorticoids (e.g., HAC) or thyroid hormone. Primary hypothyroidism usually is caused by idiopathic follicular atrophy or lymphocytic thyroiditis. Dogs with lymphocytic thyroiditis often have circulating thyroglobulin antibodies that form antigen-antibody complexes in the gland, causing functional glandular tissue to be replaced by fibrous tissue. Hypothyroidism in cats usually is caused by surgical removal of the thyroid glands or damage to their blood supply during thyroidectomy (see p. 610); however, congenital hypothyroidism in a family of Abyssinian cats has been reported (Jones et al, 1992). The disease was inherited as an autosomal recessive trait and appeared to be the result of a defect of iodide organification. Congenital hypothyroidism also has been reported in dogs.

Hypothyroidism may be manifested as lethargy, exercise intolerance, weight gain, constipation, nonpruritic symmetric alopecia, peripheral neuropathies (i.e., laryngeal paralysis, vestibular deficits, and megaesophagus), reproductive problems, cardiovascular changes (i.e., bradycardia and weak apex beat), and/or coagulopathies. Hypothyroidism may also result in diminished activity of factor VIII or of factor VIII–related antigen, which may predispose animals with von Willebrand disease to spontaneous bleeding or serious hemorrhage during surgery. The mean von Willebrand factor/antigen concentration in hypothyroid dogs has been found to be significantly reduced compared with that in euthyroid dogs. It appears that reduced concentrations of plasma von Willebrand factor/antigen can be found in dogs in associa-

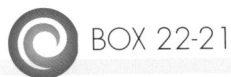

BOX 22-21

Treatment of Canine Hypothyroidism

Maintenance

Levothyroxine (Soloxine) 22 μg/kg PO, bid

Before surgery (if not on maintenance therapy, which is preferred)
1. Oral: liothyronine (T_3; Cytobin or Cytomel) 4–6 μg/kg PO, tid or qid, or
2. Intravenous: L-thyroxine 20–40 μg/kg (1 dose) (use with caution)

PO, Oral; *bid,* twice a day; *tid,* three times a day; *qid,* four times a day.

tion with congenital von Willebrand disease or with von Willebrand disease acquired through hypothyroidism. Animals with untreated severe hypothyroidism and bleeding tendencies undergoing emergency procedures should be given oral L-triiodothyronine (Box 22-21) three or four times a day or a single intravenous dose of L-thyroxine. Elective procedures should be postponed until replacement therapy has been maintained for a minimum of 2 weeks. If excessive bleeding is noted despite thyroid supplementation, whole blood, plasma, or cryoprecipitate should be given (see Box 5-1 on p. 25).

> NOTE: See p. 601 for preoperative concerns in animals with hypothyroidism.

> NOTE: Hypothyroid animals may bleed excessively during surgery. Monitor hemostasis carefully.

Animals with hyperparathyroidism often are brought in because of signs caused by hypercalcemia. Parathyroid hormone is synthesized by chief cells of the parathyroid glands. PTH stimulates renal reabsorption of calcium, mobilizes calcium from bone, and promotes intestinal calcium reabsorption. PTH also controls hydroxylation of 25-hydroxyvitamin D_3 to 1,25 dihydroxyvitamin D_3 in the proximal renal tubules. 1,25-Dihydroxyvitamin D_3 regulates PTH secretion through a negative feedback mechanism. PTH is synthesized and secreted in response to decreases in circulating calcium levels. Functional parathyroid neoplasms (primary hyperparathyroidism; see p. 611) cause hypercalcemia through excessive secretion of PTH, which causes increased renal reabsorption of calcium and increased renal excretion of phosphorus, increased release of calcium and phosphorus from bone, and increased intestinal absorption of calcium and phosphorus. The preoperative management of animals with functional parathyroid tumors is described on p. 613. Primary hypoparathyroidism is a rare cause of hypocalcemia in dogs and cats. It has been reported to affect primarily middle-aged female dogs, occurring secondary to lympho-

cytic parathyroiditis. Most affected animals have a history of neurologic disease (particularly seizures) or neuromuscular disease.

Cystic thyroid and parathyroid lesions have been reported in older cats, but are uncommon (Phillips et al, 2003). These lesions may be benign (thyroid cysts or cystadenomas) or malignant (parathyroid adenocarcinomas). Surgical resection may be curative and the long-term survival is excellent. Differentials for a cystic ventral cervical mass should include branchial cyst, thyroglossal cyst, thyroid cyst, thyroid cystadenoma, parathyroid cyst, parathyroid cystadenoma, thyroid carcinoma, salivary mucocele, and abscess.

ANESTHESIA

Hypothyroidism may prolong recovery from anesthesia. Dosages of premedications and anesthetics may need to be reduced in moderately or severely affected animals. The blood pressure, cardiac function, and hematocrit should be closely monitored during anesthesia and in the early postoperative period. Blood should be available in case excessive bleeding occurs intraoperatively. Hypothermia may be of greater concern in these patients because of their inability to regulate body temperature normally; care should be taken to maintain body temperature during surgery and to rewarm these patients after surgery. See pp. 608 and 615 for anesthetic recommendations for animals undergoing thyroidectomy.

> NOTE: Anesthetize hypothyroid animals with care; these patients may require reduced dosages of anesthetics.

ANTIBIOTICS

Guidelines for appropriate use of perioperative antibiotics should be followed in hypothyroid patients (see Chapter 10). Prophylactic antibiotic therapy should be considered in animals that are debilitated or obese or have pyoderma or that have concurrent HAC.

SURGICAL ANATOMY

The thyroid gland (with two lobes) is a dark red, elongated structure attached to the outer surface of the proximal portion of the trachea (Fig. 22-17). The lobes usually are positioned laterally and slightly ventral to the fifth to eighth cartilage rings. The left lobe usually is located one to three tracheal rings caudal to the right lobe. In adult dogs they are approximately 5 cm long and 1.5 cm wide; in cats they are 2 cm long and 0.3 cm wide. Occasionally the right and left lobes are connected by a ventral isthmus. Unlike most glandular organs, they often can be palpated when enlarged. Thyroid secretions (i.e., T_4, T_3, and calcitonin) exert a major effect on metabolism. Thyroid hormone is synthesized by follicular cells, stored intercellularly, and released into the circulation. In adults it causes an increase in the overall metabolic rate; in juveniles it stimulates growth. Calcitonin (formed by parafollicular C cells) lowers blood calcium by stimulating calcium uptake. Functional accessory thyroid tissue is common along the trachea, thoracic inlet, mediasti-

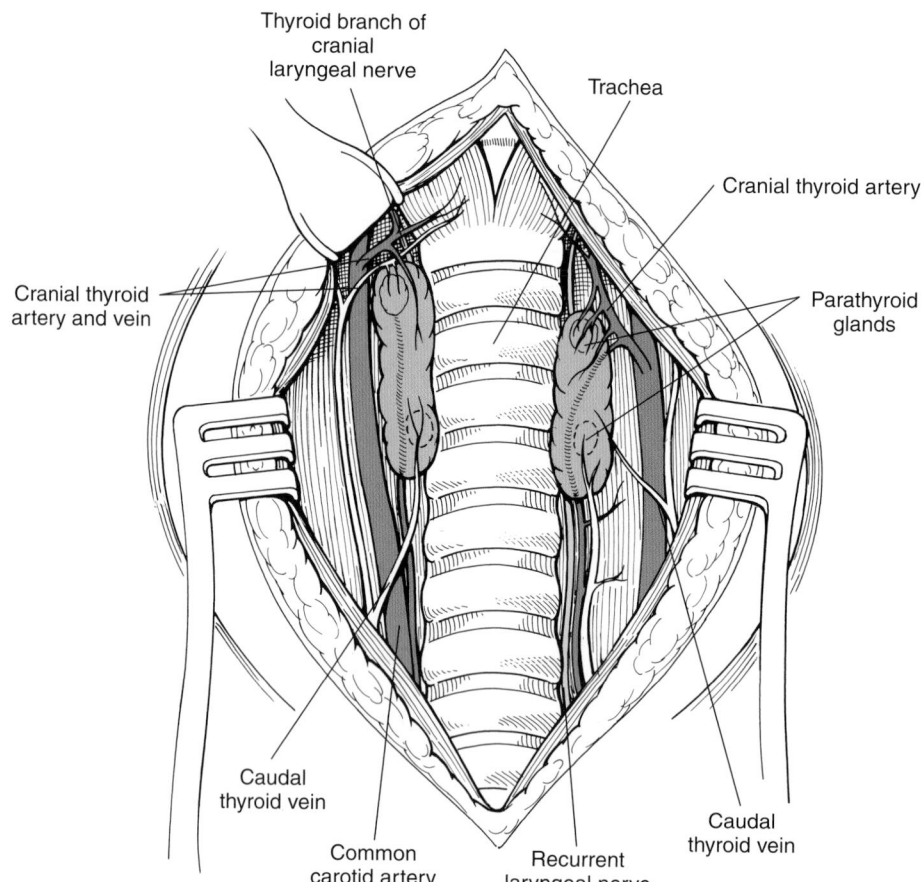

FIG. 22-17
The thyroid gland is lateral and slightly ventral to the fifth to eighth cartilage rings.

Labels on figure:
Thyroid branch of cranial laryngeal nerve
Trachea
Cranial thyroid artery
Parathyroid glands
Cranial thyroid artery and vein
Caudal thyroid vein
Common carotid artery
Recurrent laryngeal nerve
Caudal thyroid vein

num, and thoracic portion of the descending aorta. Thyroid follicular cells arise from a midline outpouching known as the thyroid diverticulum on the ventral pharyngeal floor. The diverticulum's pharyngeal connections usually separate completely; however, a persistent connection that has functional glandular epithelium and cysts along its course may remain *(thyroglossal duct)*.

The cranial and caudal thyroid arteries are the thyroid's principal blood supply. The cranial thyroid artery arises from the common carotid artery; the caudal thyroid artery typically arises from the brachiocephalic artery. The cranial and caudal thyroid arteries anastomose on the dorsal surface of the gland, where they send numerous vessels that supply the gland. The cranial thyroid artery in dogs usually sends a branch that supplies the external parathyroid gland before entering the thyroid parenchyma. In cats, the branch that supplies the external parathyroid gland may arise from the cranial thyroid artery after it has perforated the capsule. Caudal thyroid arteries may not be present in cats. Innervation to the thyroid is via the thyroid nerve, which is formed from the cranial ganglion and cranial laryngeal nerve.

The parathyroid glands are small, ellipsoid disks that usually occur as four structurally independent glands in close association with the thyroid glands. The external parathyroid glands (so named because they lie outside the thyroid capsule) normally are found on the cranial dorsolateral surface of the respective thyroid. The internal parathyroid

glands are embedded within the thyroid parenchyma, usually at the caudomedial pole.

SURGICAL TECHNIQUE

Thyroidectomy may be performed via an intracapsular or extracapsular approach. The extracapsular approach is used in dogs with malignant thyroid tumors (e.g., carcinomas; see p. 615), and no attempt is made to spare the ipsilateral parathyroid glands. Intracapsular and modified extracapsular approaches have been described for thyroidectomy in cats (see pp. 608 to 609). These techniques spare the external parathyroid glands in an attempt to prevent complications associated with hypoparathyroidism. A modification of the original intracapsular approach, developed to reduce the incidence of postthyroidectomy hyperthyroidism, involves excising most of the thyroid capsule once the thyroid tissue has been removed. Recurrence of hyperthyroidism in cats after thyroidectomy is thought to be the result of hypertrophy of small nests of functional thyroid tissue attached to the capsule and not removed.

HEALING OF THE THYROID AND PARATHYROID GLANDS

Abnormal thyroid tissue (i.e., adenomatous tissue) appears to regenerate and hypertrophy after incomplete feline thyroidectomy. Parathyroid tissue may be able to revascularize and regain function even if it has been totally separated from its blood supply. Therefore most surgeons recommend implanting an inadvertently excised parathyroid gland into surrounding muscle rather than discarding it. Ectopic parathyroid tissue may also hypertrophy after removal of the parathyroid glands, resulting in normal parathyroid function.

SUTURE MATERIALS AND SPECIAL INSTRUMENTS

Delayed wound healing may occur in animals with hypothyroidism, and care should be used in closing surgical wounds in these patients. See pp. 610 and 613 for a discussion of the instruments for thyroidectomy and parathyroidectomy, respectively.

POSTOPERATIVE CARE AND ASSESSMENT

The postoperative care and assessment of animals undergoing thyroidectomy for hyperthyroidism or neoplasia are provided on p. 610 and p. 615, respectively.

References

Daminet S, Ferguson DC: Influence of drugs on thyroid function in dogs, *J Vet Intern Med* 17:463, 2003.

Frank LA, Hnilica KA, May ER et al: Effects of sulfamethoxazole-trimethoprim on thyroid function in dogs, *Am J Vet Res* 66:256, 2005.

Phillips DE, Radlinsky MG, Fisher JR et al: Cystic thyroid and parathyroid lesions in cats, *J Am Anim Hosp Assoc* 39:349, 2003.

SPECIFIC DISEASES

FELINE HYPERTHYROIDISM

DEFINITIONS

Hyperthyroidism is a multisystemic disease that results from excessive production and secretion of T_4. *Goiter* is an enlargement of the thyroid gland. *Graves' disease* describes an autoimmune disorder of human beings in which circulating autoantibodies stimulate thyroid tissue. It is the most common cause of human hyperthyroidism.

GENERAL CONSIDERATIONS AND CLINICALLY RELEVANT PATHOPHYSIOLOGY

Hyperthyroidism may occur in dogs or cats; however, it is much more common in cats, in which it is generally associated with adenomatous hyperplasia of one or both thyroid glands. Approximately 80% of affected cats have bilateral thyroid lobe involvement, although the enlargement usually is asymmetric. In approximately 5% of cats, the thyroid mass is ectopic (i.e., at the thoracic inlet or in the cranial mediastinum). Feline hyperthyroidism that occurs secondary to malignant thyroid carcinomas is rare. The cause of feline hyperthyroidism is unknown. Suggested causes have included circulating thyroid-stimulating immunoglobulins, serum thyroid growth-stimulating immunoglobulins, dietary goitrogens, and viral causes. A recent study found that

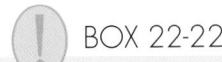

BOX 22-22

Neurologic Abnormalities in Hypokalemic, Hyperthyroid Cats

- Generalized weakness
- Neck ventroflexion
- Fatigue
- Muscle tremors
- Ataxia
- Incoordination
- Inability to jump
- Muscle atrophy
- Breathlessness
- Collapse

cats that preferred fish or liver and giblet flavors of canned food appeared to be at increased risk for the development of hyperthyroidism, possibly because these diets contain a relatively high concentration of iodine (Martin et al, 2000). Exposure to fertilizers, herbicides, plant pesticides, flea products, and smoke did not seem to be associated with an increased risk of this disease in the aforementioned study.

Excessive circulating T_4 causes multisystemic organ dysfunction. Thyrotoxicosis increases the metabolic rate and sensitivity to catecholamines and causes significant cardiovascular and metabolic abnormalities. Up to 80% of affected cats may have thyrotoxic heart disease, and approximately 20% of these may have congestive heart failure. Hypertension is sometimes identified, but does not appear to be as common as cardiac disease. Multifactorial mechanisms may cause neuromuscular and CNS dysfunction in some hyperthyroid cats. Neurologic signs associated with feline hyperthyroidism are listed in Box 22-22. T_4 and T_3 bind to receptor sites in the sarcoplasm that increase skeletal muscle heat production and mitochondrial oxygen consumption. The hyperthyroid state may reduce muscle contraction by uncoupling oxidative phosphorylation. Thyroid hormones may lower the threshold for cerebral tissue activation, alter the activity of some brain enzymes, and interact with catecholamines to alter the mental state of some affected animals. Abnormalities of the CNS may include hyperexcitability, irritability, aggression, seizures, confusion, and stupor.

DIAGNOSIS
Clinical Presentation

Signalment. Hyperthyroidism generally affects cats older than 8 years of age (mean age, 13 years); however, it has been reported in an 8-month old cat (Gordon et al, 2003). There is no gender predisposition. Siamese and Himalayan cats may be at decreased risk to develop hyperthyroidism. Cats fed primarily canned food and those using cat litter may have an increased risk. Cats that prefer to eat canned cat food of fish or liver and giblet flavor may have an increased risk of developing this condition (Martin et al, 2000).

History. Most affected cats are presented for treatment because of weight loss despite a normal or voracious appetite, restlessness, and/or hyperactivity. Occasionally, a small mass is noted in the ventral cervical region. Vomiting, diarrhea, polyuria, polydipsia, aggression, and/or a rough hair coat may also occur. There is sometimes an increased frequency of defecation. Body temperature may be slightly elevated. Approximately 10% of hyperthyroid cats are depressed, lethargic, inappetent, and/or weak (i.e., "apathetic" hyperthyroidism).

Physical Examination Findings

A palpable cervical mass is present in most affected cats. The weight of the enlarged gland often causes it to gravitate ventrally because the thyroid is loosely attached to tracheal fascia. Occasionally the gland may descend into the thoracic inlet, where it can no longer be palpated. Additional physical examination findings may include emaciation, a thin and/or roughened hair coat, and cardiac abnormalities (e.g., tachycardia, gallop rhythms, murmurs, left anterior fascicular block, and/or atrial and ventricular tachyarrhythmias). Electrocardiographic abnormalities may include tachycardia, prolonged QRS duration, increased R-wave amplitudes in lead II, and ventricular preexcitation.

Diagnostic Imaging

An enlarged heart, consistent with hypertrophic cardiomyopathy, often is found on thoracic radiographs and echocardiography. If the cat is in congestive heart failure, pleural effusion or pulmonary edema (or both) may occur. Ectopic thyroid tissue is rarely visible radiographically. Thyroid scintigraphy is the optimal diagnostic test as it can both definitively identify that the animal is hyperthyroid and confirm the presence of functional ectopic thyroid tissue. With this procedure, technetium 99m is administered intravenously or intramuscularly. The radionuclide is trapped in functional thyroid tissue, but not organified. Delayed phase imaging of the body using a gamma camera provided functional and rudimentary anatomic locations of the hyperfunctioning thyroid tissue (Figs. 22-18 and 22-19). A ratio of the uptake in the thyroid tissue compared with the salivary glands of greater than 2 is diagnostic of hyperthyroidism.

> NOTE: Before anesthetizing animals for a thyroidectomy, take thoracic radiographs and/or perform echocardiography to identify thyrotoxic heart disease.

Laboratory Findings

Most affected cats have high serum total T_4 (TT4) and free T_4 (fT4) by equilibrium dialysis concentrations. However, the diagnosis of hyperthyroidism cannot be excluded based on a normal TT4 concentration, and cats without hyperthyroidism may have increased fT4 concentrations. In general, the fT4 test is only measured if a cat that is suspicious for hyperthyroidism has a normal TT4 (Peterson et al, 2001). Other abnormalities may include mild elevations in red blood cell numbers, increased PCV, neutrophilic leukocytosis, eosinopenia, lymphopenia, and elevated alanine aminotransferase and alkaline phosphatase. Serum creatinine and blood ionized calcium concentrations are often decreased, and serum phosphorus concentrations are often increased

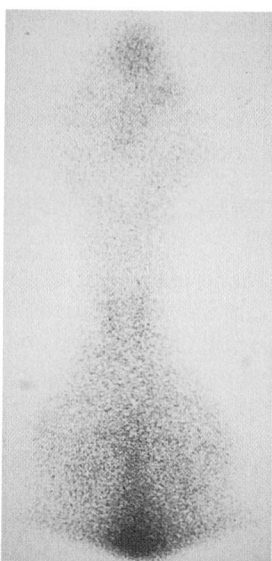

FIG. 22-18
Thyroid scintigraphy may be used to identify functional thyroid tissue. Compare this normal ventral view of the cervical region in this cat with that of the hyperthyroid cat in Fig. 22-19.

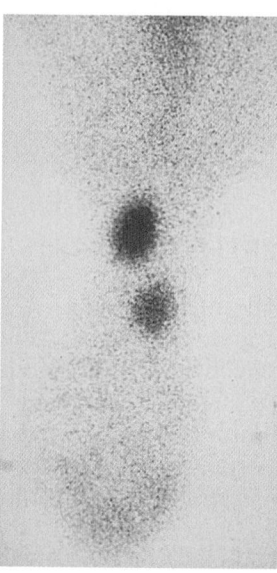

FIG. 22-19
Thyroid scintigraphy of a cat with bilateral thyroid adenomas.

because of hyperparathyroidism secondary to the low ionized calcium concentrations.

If baseline serum thyroid hormone concentrations are normal in a cat with appropriate clinical signs or if there is a palpable ventral cervical mass, the serum TT4 and fT4 concentration should be remeasured in 3 to 4 weeks, or nuclear scintigraphy should be performed. As an alternative, a T_3 suppression test (Box 22-23) or a TRH stimulation test may be performed. In normal cats, the serum T_4 concentration

BOX 22-23

T_3 Suppression Test

Day 1

Obtain morning baseline serum T_4 and T_3 concentrations.

Days 1 and 2

Give sodium liothyronine (Cytobin), 25 µg/cat PO, tid for 2 days.

Morning of Day 3

Administer sodium liothyronine, wait 2–4 hours, then measure serum T_4 and T_3.

T_3, Triiodothyronine; T_4, thyroxine; *PO*, oral; *tid*, three times a day.

 BOX 22-24

Possible Side Effects of Methimazole Therapy*

- Anorexia
- Vomiting
- Pruritus
- Lethargy
- Development of serum antinuclear antibodies
- Hepatopathy
- Thrombocytopenia with or without bleeding
- Agranulocytosis
- Leukopenia
- Positive Coombs' test result

*Also see text.

should decline by more than 50% after administration of sodium liothyronine (i.e., below 1.5 mg/dl), whereas in hyperthyroid cats a minimal decrease in the serum T_4 concentration is seen. The T_3 concentration should increase in both hyperthyroid and euthyroid cats if the medication was given appropriately. For the TRH test, the serum T_3 and T_4 concentrations are measured before and 4 hours after intravenous administration of TRH (0.1 mg/kg). Hyperthyroid cats usually have a relative increase of T_4 of less than 50%; normal cats have a relative increase of greater than 50%. As an alternative, the response to oral antithyroid drugs may be used to help confirm the diagnosis.

> NOTE: If Total T_4 fails to diagnose hyperthyroidism, then measurement of free T_4 should be requested.

Cats with hyperthyroidism have been shown to have an increased glomerular filtration rate (GFR) compared with normal cats; treatment with methimazole has resulted in a reduced GFR in affected cats (Becker et al, 2000). The authors of the aforementioned study recommended that a trial course of methimazole be given when treating hyperthyroid cats suspected of having renal dysfunction, with follow-up serum biochemical analyses and urinalyses before electing bilateral thyroidectomy or radioactive iodine therapy. This is based on the fact that methimazole's effects are reversible, whereas surgery and radioactive iodine are not. For cats that develop overt renal failure after establishment of euthyroidism, the withdrawal of therapy may result in improved renal function.

DIFFERENTIAL DIAGNOSIS

Cats presented for treatment with weight loss or vomiting caused by hyperthyroidism must be differentiated from those with intestinal lymphoma or inflammatory bowel disease. Those with neurologic signs must be differentiated from cats with primary CNS abnormalities. Cardiac dysfunction that occurs secondary to hyperthyroidism should be differentiated from that resulting from other acquired or congenital causes.

MEDICAL MANAGEMENT

Treatment of feline hyperthyroidism may include long-term administration of antithyroid drugs (see Preoperative Management below), iodine-131 (^{131}I), or surgical removal of the affected glands. The choice of treatment for the individual cat depends on the animal's age and condition (i.e., presence of cardiovascular or renal disease) and the therapies available to the practitioner.

Long-term administration of antithyroid drugs (e.g., methimazole or carbimazole) can cause remission; however, clinical signs return once the drug is discontinued. Methimazole inhibits several steps in thyroid hormone synthesis and is effective in restoring a euthyroid status to most cats; however, up to 20% of cats experience gastrointestinal upset during treatment (Box 22-24). In rare cases, drug-induced hepatopathy, thrombocytopenia, and agranulocytosis occur with chronic therapy. Although in general the drug is well tolerated and many side effects resolve with continued therapy, administration of an oral compound may be difficult in fractious cats or those with impaired or elderly owners. A pluronic organogel formulation for transdermal application has recently been offered. The incidence of adverse gastrointestinal signs is less with the transdermal application; however, efficacy of this route of administration does not appear to be as high as with the oral route (Sartor et al, 2004). If thyroid carcinoma is suspected, medical therapy with antithyroid drugs may palliate clinical signs while allowing tumor growth. Propylthiouracil (PTU) is an effective oral antithyroid drug in cats; however, it is not recommended because of severe side effects (i.e., autoimmune hemolytic anemia and immune-mediated thrombocytopenia).

^{131}I is a safe and effective method of treating hyperthyroidism; however, it requires facilities to safely handle the isotope. The cat must be confined days to weeks (depending upon specific state laws), during which time it is a human health hazard. It is important to detect other diseases before treating with ^{131}I so that minimal contact with the cat is required during treatment. Radioactive iodine is trapped in the thyroid gland and causes tissue destruction. However, normal thyroid tissue is spared as it is suppressed and thus does not uptake the radioactive iodine. In the past, the effect of recent administration of antithyroid medications has been proposed to decrease the efficacy of radioactive iodine treatment because of decreased uptake. A recent study in normal cats, however, showed that methimazole may cause an increase in uptake because of up-regulation of TSH (Nieckarz, 2001). A definitive conclusion will require evaluation in hyperthyroid cats. If carcinoma is present, larger doses of ^{131}I may be necessary, requiring longer isolation periods.

Percutaneous ethanol ablation of bilateral thyroid nodules (Goldstein et al, 2001) is not recommended as a treatment for hyperthyroidism in cats. A recent study found that the longest period of euthyroidism in 7 cats was 27 weeks and complications, such as Horner's syndrome, dysphonia, and laryngeal paralysis, were noted (Wells et al, 2001).

SURGICAL TREATMENT

Surgical treatment of hyperthyroidism involves thyroidectomy. The major complication of bilateral thyroidectomy is hypoparathyroidism that occurs secondary to removal or damage of the parathyroid glands. The procedure must be performed carefully to prevent this complication. If the parathyroid gland is inadvertently removed, it should be transferred to a nearby muscle belly (e.g., sternohyoideus muscle) so that the gland may revascularize and become functional again (parathyroid gland autotransplantation). To prevent the complication of hypocalcemia, some surgeons recommend a two-stage procedure in which one thyroid lobe is removed and its associated parathyroid is reimplanted into adjacent musculature during the first surgery. Two to three weeks later, the other thyroid lobe is removed and its associated parathyroid is similarly reimplanted. Although this may reduce the risk of postoperative hypocalcemia, there is the added risk of a second anesthetic event.

Preoperative Management

Metabolic and cardiovascular abnormalities associated with hyperthyroidism make anesthesia risky, therefore cats should be made euthyroid preoperatively by administering methimazole (Tapazole) (Box 22-25). Generally, administration for 1 to 3 weeks before surgery is sufficient; however, measurement of the TT4 concentration should be repeated to ensure that it is within the normal range before surgery is performed (see comment on side effects above). If preoperative therapy with methimazole is not tolerated, propranolol may be given for 1 to 2 weeks before surgery (see Box 22-25) to reduce the heart rate. Propranolol should be discontinued 24 to 48 hours before surgery because of its β-blocking effects, which may interfere with treatment of hypotension.

Because cardiac abnormalities are common, an ECG, chest radiographs, and/or echocardiogram should be performed before surgery. Many hyperthyroid cats have concurrent renal disease, hypokalemia, and/or azotemia. These cats should be given fluids before, during, and after surgery, and care should be taken to ensure that uremia does not occur during surgery (see the discussion of anesthetic management of animals with

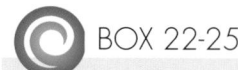

Preoperative Drug Therapy for Cats With Hyperthyroidism

Methimazole (Tapazole)

2.5–5 mg/cat PO, qd, and adjust the dose as needed*
Transdermal application (to the hairless skin of the pinna) is also available†

Carbimazole

5 mg/cat PO, tid, and then adjust as needed

Propranolol (Inderal)‡

2.5–5 mg/cat (0.4–1.2 mg/kg) PO, bid or tid

PO, Oral; *qd*, every day; *tid*, three times a day; *bid*, twice a day; T_4, thyroxine.
*If long-term administration is considered, this dose should be adjusted to maintain the T_4 concentration within the normal range.
†The overall efficacy of transdermal methimazole may not be as high as orally administered drug; however, it is associated with fewer gastrointestinal adverse effects.
‡Propranolol should be used with care in hyperthyroid cats. Administration of propranolol to hypokalemic cats may cause sudden death.

renal disease on p. 636) or after surgery, when cardiac output drops because the cat becomes euthyroid. Fluid therapy should be adjusted if the cat is in congestive heart failure.

Anesthesia

Inhalants that sensitize the heart to arrhythmias should be avoided (e.g., halothane). Cats with cardiomyopathy may be premedicated with butorphanol (0.2 mg/kg given intramuscularly or subcutaneously) and induced with diazepam (0.2 mg/kg given intravenously) followed by etomidate (1 to 3 mg/kg given intravenously). Maintenance on isoflurane or sevoflurane in oxygen should be used. If the cat does not have thyrotoxic heart disease, a variety of anesthetic protocols can be used (e.g., premedicate similarly and chamber induce with isoflurane or sevoflurane in oxygen). If arrhythmias occur during surgery that are not caused by hypoxemia or the anesthetic, lidocaine may be given as an intravenous bolus (see Box 22-10 on p. 583).

Surgical Anatomy

See p. 603 for a description of the surgical anatomy of the thyroid gland.

Positioning

The animal is placed in dorsal recumbency with the neck slightly hyperextended and the forelimbs pulled caudally. The entire ventral neck and cranioventral thorax should be prepared for aseptic surgery.

SURGICAL TECHNIQUE
Intracapsular Thyroidectomy

Make a skin incision from the larynx to a point cranial to the manubrium. Bluntly separate the sternohyoid and sternothyroid muscles. Use a self-retaining (e.g., Gelpi) retractor to

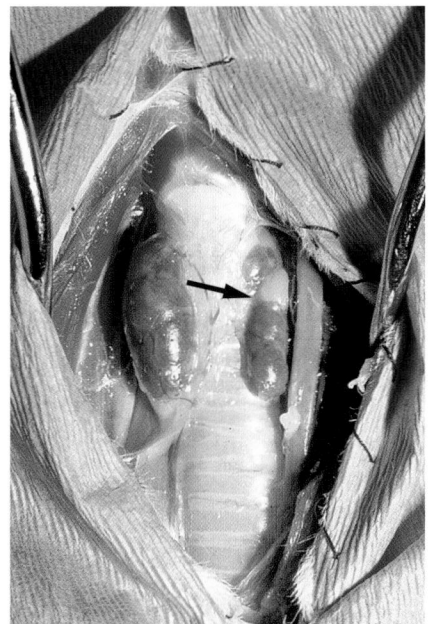

FIG. 22-20
Thyroid enlargement in a cat. Note the parathyroid gland at the cranial pole of the left thyroid gland *(arrow)*.

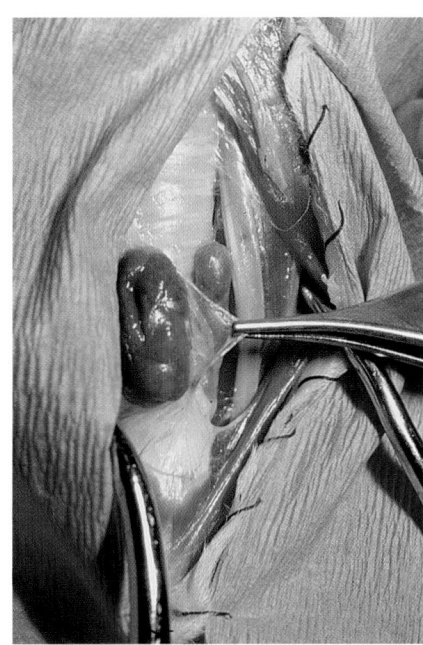

FIG. 22-21
For intracapsular thyroidectomy, make an incision on the caudoventral surface of the gland in an avascular area and extend it cranially with small scissors (e.g., iris scissors). Using a combination of blunt and sharp dissection, carefully remove the thyroid tissue from the capsule.

maintain exposure. Identify the enlarged thyroid gland and external parathyroid gland (Fig. 22-20). Make an incision on the caudoventral surface of the gland in an avascular area (Fig. 22-21), and extend it cranially with small scissors (e.g., iris scissors). Using a combination of blunt and sharp dissection, carefully remove the thyroid tissue from the capsule. Perform the dissection carefully to prevent damaging the parathyroid gland or its blood supply. Use bipolar cautery to achieve hemostasis but avoid damaging the gland's blood supply. After the thyroid parenchyma has been removed, excise most of the thyroid capsule; however, do not excise the capsule that is intimately associated with the external parathyroid gland. If the parathyroid gland is inadvertently excised or if its blood supply is damaged, transplant the gland to a nearby muscle belly (see p. 608). Close subcutaneous tissue in a simple continuous suture pattern (i.e., 3-0 or 4-0 absorbable). Close the skin in either a simple continuous or simple interrupted suture (i.e., 3-0 nonabsorbable) pattern.

NOTE: Sterile Q-tips are useful to help separate the gland from the capsule.

Modified Extracapsular Approach for Thyroidectomy

Position the animal as previously described. Locate the thyroid gland as described before, and ligate or cauterize the caudal thyroid vein. Using fine-tipped, bipolar cautery

forceps (Fig. 22-22, A), cauterize the thyroid capsule approximately 2 mm from the external parathyroid gland. With small, fine scissors, cut the gland at the cauterized area, and use sharp and blunt dissection to remove the gland from the parathyroid gland (Fig. 22-22, B). Carefully dissect all thyroid gland from the surrounding tissue and parathyroid gland (Fig. 22-22, C). Do not damage the cranial thyroid artery or its branches to the external parathyroid gland. If the parathyroid gland is inadvertently excised or if its blood supply is damaged, transplant the gland to a nearby muscle belly (see p. 608). Close as described above.

NOTE: To prevent hypocalcemia, take special care to avoid damaging the cranial thyroid artery.

Modified Intracapsular Approach for Thyroidectomy

Position the animal as described previously. Locate the thyroid gland and remove the gland as described above under the Intracapsular Thyroidectomy section. Using a No. 15 scalpel blade or fine scissors, create a peninsula of capsular tissue containing only the parathyroid gland and its blood vessel. Excise the remainder of the capsule. If the parathyroid gland is inadvertently excised or if its blood supply is damaged, transplant the gland to a nearby muscle belly (see p. 608). Close as described above.

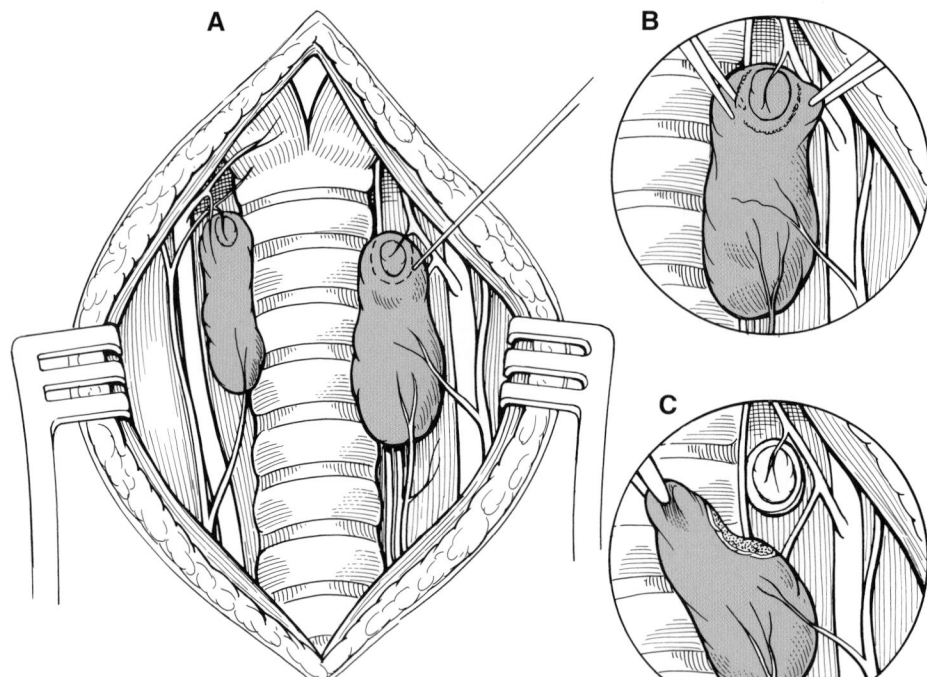

FIG. 22-22
Modified extracapsular thyroidectomy. **A,** Using fine-tipped bipolar cautery forceps, cauterize the thyroid capsule approximately 2 mm from the external parathyroid gland. **B,** With small, fine scissors, cut the gland at the cauterized area and remove from the parathyroid gland. **C,** Carefully dissect all of the thyroid gland from the surrounding tissue and parathyroid gland.

SUTURE MATERIALS AND SPECIAL INSTRUMENTS

Small, fine instruments, such as iris scissors and Bishop-Harmon thumb forceps, facilitate removal of the thyroid glands. Bipolar cautery forceps are advantageous for providing hemostasis because they allow finer control of coagulation than do unipolar forceps. Sterile Q-tips are useful for dissecting the thyroid glands from the parathyroid glands.

POSTOPERATIVE CARE AND ASSESSMENT

Complications may include hypocalcemia, hypothyroidism, recurrence of hyperthyroidism, worsening of renal disease, Horner's syndrome, and/or laryngeal paralysis. Hypocalcemia (serum calcium level less than 9 mg/dl in adult dogs and less than 8.5 mg/dl in adult cats) is the most important, acute, life-threatening complication of thyroidectomy. Most animals do not develop clinical signs until the serum calcium level is below 7.5 mg/dl, depending upon the acid-base status. Animals should be closely observed for signs of hypocalcemia (i.e., panting, nervousness, facial rubbing, muscle twitching, ataxia, and seizures) for 2 to 4 days. In cats, early signs may include lethargy, anorexia, panting, and facial rubbing. Clinical signs usually are noted within 24 to 96 hours, although delayed signs have been reported up to 5 to 6 days later. Acute signs of hypocalcemia may be treated with intravenous 10% calcium gluconate; never administer calcium chloride. The 10% calcium gluconate should be given slowly intravenously (Box 22-26), and the cardiac rate and rhythm should be monitored during administration. Calcium administration should be discontinued if bradycardia develops. Calcium gluconate can also be added to the fluids, or the intravenous dose can be diluted in an equal volume of saline (or for

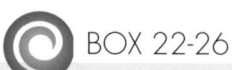 BOX 22-26

Treatment of Hypocalcemia Following Thyroidectomy

Management of Acute Signs

Give 0.5–1.5 ml/kg of 10% calcium gluconate slowly IV (over 10–20 minutes) and monitor the heart; then add 10 ml of 10% calcium gluconate to 250 ml of lactated Ringer's solution and drip at maintenance rate or give IV dose diluted in saline (1:3–1:4) SC (in multiple sites). Monitor serum calcium frequently (two or three times a day if necessary).

Maintenance Therapy

Give calcium lactate 0.2–3.0 gm/cat/day in divided doses PO

Give vitamin D, EITHER*:
1. Dihydrotachysterol at 0.02–0.03 mg/kg/day PO for 3–5 days; then 0.02 mg/kg/day for 4 days; then 0.005 mg/kg/day for 1–4 months; **OR** give
2. Calcitriol at 2.5 to 10 ng/kg/day (usually 0.25 µg/cat every 48 hours)

IV, Intravenous; *SC,* subcutaneous; *PO,* oral.
*It is important to give EITHER dihydrotachysterol OR calcitriol, but NOT BOTH.

greater safety, dilute 1:3 or 1:4) and given subcutaneously every 6 to 8 hours (see Box 22-26) until the animal is eating and able to be given oral medications. Administration of undilute calcium gluconate may be associated with abscess formation. Subcutaneous or intravenous administration of calcium should be discontinued when the serum calcium level is above 8 mg/dl. Maintenance therapy consists of oral calcium and vitamin D administration (see Box 22-26). The form of vitamin D most commonly used is dihydrotachysterol. It does not accumulate in fat and has a more rapid onset of action than vitamin D_3. Serum calcium levels should be monitored weekly and the dosage of calcium changed accordingly. Vitamin D supplementation often can be discontinued once the parathyroid gland revascularizes. Some animals must be maintained on vitamin D for months before the dose can be reduced; others require lifelong therapy.

> NOTE: Do not give calcium chloride intravenously; you can overdose the animal too easily.

PROGNOSIS

Hypocalcemia caused by hypoparathyroidism may be permanent or temporary. It has been reported to occur in between 15% and 36% of patients undergoing an intracapsular approach, in 33% of patients after a modified intracapsular approach, in 82% of patients after an extracapsular approach, in 23% of cats after a modified extracapsular approach, and in 11% of cats after a staged intracapsular approach (Padgett, 2002). Persistent hypocalcemia may occur if all four parathyroid glands are removed or if their blood supply is irreversibly damaged. Temporary hypocalcemia usually is caused by disruption of the parathyroid blood supply. Hypocalcemia should not occur after unilateral thyroidectomy. Recurrent hyperthyroidism may result from hypertrophy of adenomatous tissue not removed during thyroidectomy or from adenomatous changes in ectopic thyroid tissue. Hyperthyroidism has been reported within 2 to 3 years in 5% to 11% of cats having bilateral thyroidectomy. If possible, a thyroid scan should be performed to localize hyperfunctioning tissue in these animals before repeating surgery.

> NOTE: Hypocalcemia is extremely rare after unilateral thyroidectomy for feline hyperthyroidism.

In one study of 231 cats treated with radioactive iodine, only age at diagnosis and gender were found to affect survival (Slater et al, 2001). Increasing age and being male increased the likelihood of death. Cats with renal disease or cancer were more likely not to survive.

References

Becker TJ et al: Effects of methimazole on renal function in cats with hyperthyroidism, *J Am Anim Hosp Assoc* 36:215, 2000.

Goldstein MR, Long C, Swift NC et al: Percutaneous ethanol injection for treatment of unilateral hyperplastic thyroid nodules in cats, *J Am Vet Med Assoc* 218:1298, 2001.

Gordon JM, Ehrhart EJ, Sisson DD et al: Juvenile hyperthyroidism in a cat, *J Am Anim Hosp Assoc* 39:67, 2003.

Martin KM et al: Evaluation of dietary and environmental risk factors for hyperthyroidism in cats, *J Am Vet Med Assoc* 217:853, 2000.

Nieckarz JA, Daniel GB: The effect of methimazole on thyroid uptake of pertechnetate and radioiodine in normal cats, *Vet Radiol Ultrasound* 42:448, 2001.

Padgett S: Feline thyroid surgery, *Vet Clin Small Anim* 32:851, 2002.

Peterson ME, Melian C, Nichols R: Measurement of serum concentrations of free thyroxine, total thyroxine, and total triiodothyronine in cats with hyperthyroidism and cats with nonthyroidal disease, *J Am Vet Med Assoc* 218:529, 2001.

Sartor LL, Trepanier LA, Kroll MM et al: Efficacy and safety of transdermal methimazole in the treatment of cats with hyperthyroidism, *J Vet Intern Med* 18:651, 2004.

Slater MR, Geller S, Rogers K: Long-term health and predictors of survival for hyperthyroid cats treated with iodine 131, *J Vet Intern Med* 15:47, 2001.

Wells AL, Long CD, Hornof WJ et al: Use of percutaneous ethanol injection for treatment of bilateral hyperplastic nodules in cats, *J Am Vet Med Assoc* 218:1293, 2001.

HYPERPARATHYROIDISM

DEFINITION

Primary hyperparathyroidism is a disorder resulting from excessive secretion of PTH by the parathyroid gland or glands.

GENERAL CONSIDERATIONS AND CLINICALLY RELEVANT PATHOPHYSIOLOGY

Primary hyperparathyroidism is uncommon in dogs and rare in cats. It usually is caused by parathyroid adenomas, although parathyroid carcinomas and parathyroid hyperplasia have also been reported. Parathyroid adenomas are typically small, well-encapsulated tumors that appear brown or red and are located near the thyroid glands; however, ectopic adenomas may be located near the thoracic inlet or in the cranial mediastinum. Clinical signs are caused by PTH increasing calcium absorption and phosphorus excretion in the kidneys and enhancing bone resorption. The net result is an increase in serum calcium levels and a decrease in serum phosphorus levels. Clinical abnormalities caused by hypercalcemia may include dystrophic calcification, impaired renal tubular concentrating ability, and calcium oxalate nephrolithiasis and urolithiasis.

DIAGNOSIS
Clinical Presentation

Signalment. Parathyroid tumors usually occur in older dogs. There is no gender predisposition. Keeshonden (and possibly German shepherds and Norwegian elkhounds) may be predisposed to the disorder. Primary gland hyperplasia has been reported in young dogs.

History. Dogs may be asymptomatic or may be presented for treatment of nonspecific signs (e.g., polyuria, polydipsia, vomiting, weakness, constipation, lethargy, and/or inappetence). Clinical signs may be insidious at onset. The most common clinical signs in cats with primary hyperparathyroidism are anorexia, lethargy, vomiting, weakness, and weight loss; polyuria and polydipsia are less common in cats than in dogs. Occasionally, bone and joint pain and pathologic fractures may occur secondary to skeletal demineralization. Cystic calculi may occur secondary to hypercalcemia.

> NOTE: Consider primary hyperparathyroidism as a differential diagnosis in animals with hypercalcemia, dystrophic calcification, calcium oxalate urolithiasis, and/or nephrolithiasis.

Physical Examination Findings

The physical examination findings usually are nonspecific. The enlarged parathyroid gland can seldom be palpated in dogs; however, a cervical mass may be palpated in some cats.

Diagnostic Imaging

Cervical radiographs seldom identify the neoplasm; however, ultrasonographic evaluation of the cervical region may reveal a parathyroid mass. Evaluation of the parathyroid gland requires use of a high-frequency transducer. Notable demineralization of the skeleton, nephrolithiasis, and/or nephrocalcinosis may be seen radiographically. Ultrasonography may also be used to evaluate the parathyroid glands. Ultrasonographic detection of a parathyroid gland exceeding 4 mm in diameter is highly suspicious for parathyroid adenoma or carcinoma. Parathyroid scintigraphy has not proved to be a sensitive or specific indicator for definitive identification of abnormal parathyroid glands in dogs with hypercalcemia (Matwichuk et al, 2000).

Laboratory Findings

Serum biochemical abnormalities in dogs with primary hyperparathyroidism include hypercalcemia and hypophosphatemia. Hypercalcemia is the most consistent finding in affected cats. Measurement of PTH in animals with normal renal function is a sensitive test. High normal or increased serum concentrations of PTH in hypercalcemic animals with normal renal function are strongly suggestive of hyperparathyroidism. Other causes of hypercalcemia (see later discussion) usually are associated with low or low normal levels of PTH. Renal dysfunction, which may occur secondary to hypercalcemia or may be a primary disorder, may also elevate serum concentrations of PTH. If renal function is abnormal, serum PTH concentrations should be evaluated in conjunction with the serum ionized calcium concentration. Serum ionized calcium levels are increased with hyperparathyroidism, but usually low to low normal with renal failure (Table 22-2). Definitive diagnosis of primary hyperparathyroidism requires surgical exploration of the parathyroid glands.

Careful physical examination, including rectal examination, thoracic and abdominal radiographs, abdominal ultrasonography, skeletal radiographs, routine blood work, and/or lymph node aspirations should be performed in animals with hypercalcemia to identify neoplastic causes of hypercalcemia of malignancy (e.g., lymphosarcoma and apocrine gland ad-

 Table 22-2

Serum Parathyroid (PTH) and Calcium (Ca²⁺) Levels With Primary Hyperparathyroidism (HPTH) and Renal Disease

	PTH	Ca²⁺*
HPTH	↑	↑
Renal failure	↑	↓

*Serum ionized calcium.

enocarcinoma) before pursuing a diagnosis of hyperparathyroidism. Other causes of hypercalcemia include granulomatous diseases, chronic renal failure, hypoadrenocorticism, and hypervitaminosis D. Thyroglossal cysts (formed when the embryonic thyroglossal duct fills with fluid) may be confused with parathyroid masses on palpation.

> NOTE: Paraneoplastic hypercalcemia of malignancy is a more common cause of hypercalcemia than primary hyperparathyroidism. Hypercalcemia of malignancy can rapidly cause renal failure if diagnosis and therapy are delayed, but hypercalcemia caused by hyperparathyroidism is often not as high as that seen in primary hyperparathyroidism.

MEDICAL MANAGEMENT

Hypercalcemia may be treated by diuresis (see the later discussion of Preoperative Management). Surgical removal of the neoplastic parathyroid tissue is the definitive treatment for primary hyperparathyroidism. Glucocorticoid therapy usually is transiently effective in lowering the serum calcium concentration in animals with lymphosarcoma and may also lower the calcium concentration in animals with other disorders.

SURGICAL TREATMENT

Parathyroidectomy is the treatment of choice for hyperparathyroidism caused by parathyroid neoplasia and primary hyperplasia. If the parathyroid glands are uniformly enlarged, secondary hyperparathyroidism should be suspected and other diagnostic tests performed to identify the cause (e.g., renal secondary hyperparathyroidism); however, enlargement of all four glands may occur with primary hyperplasia. If one or several glands are slightly enlarged, parathyroid adenomas or primary hyperplasia should be suspected. Most dogs with primary hyperparathyroidism have a single parathyroid adenoma. If the parathyroid glands appear normal, ectopic parathyroid tissue may be located adjacent to the thyroid or as far caudal as the base of the heart. Percutaneous ultrasound-guided chemical parathyroid ablation (Gear et al, 2005) and radiofrequency heat ablation have been reported for treatment of hyperparathyroidism in dogs (Pollard et al, 2001).

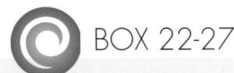

BOX 22-27

Diuresis of Hypercalcemic Dogs

0.9% Physiologic Saline Solution
90 ml/kg/day IV

Furosemide (Lasix)
2–4 mg/kg IV, bid or tid or can give it as CRI (load with 0.66 mg/kg bolus, and then give 0.66 mg/kg/hr for 4–5 hours; alternatively, can estimate the IV or PO dose to be given over the course of the next 24 hours and then give that amount as a CRI over 24 hours) (be sure patient is volume replenished before administering), or give total daily dose as a CRI

CRI, Constant rate infusion; *PO,* oral.

NOTE: If you cannot find any other cause of hypercalcemia and if the parathyroid glands appear normal, look for ectopic parathyroid tissue.

Preoperative Management

Before induction of anesthesia, diuresis should be instituted with physiologic saline solution to help lower serum calcium levels (Box 22-27). In severe hypercalcemia, salmon calcitonin can be used to lower the serum calcium. Fluids should be used with caution in animals with severe renal dysfunction. Once the animal has been appropriately hydrated, furosemide administration may promote further calciuresis. Electrolytes should be monitored to prevent iatrogenic hypokalemia.

Anesthesia

Theoretically, notable hypercalcemia may cause bradycardia, peripheral vasoconstriction, and hypertension. Hypotension may occur during anesthesia associated with relaxation of peripheral vascular tone. Hypercalcemia also may predispose to cardiac arrhythmias. Anesthetic agents that potentiate arrhythmias (i.e., thiobarbiturates and halothane) should be avoided.

Surgical Anatomy

A discussion of the anatomy of the parathyroid glands is provided on p. 604.

Positioning

The animal is placed in dorsal recumbency with the neck slightly hyperextended and forelimbs pulled caudally. The entire ventral neck and cranioventral thorax should be prepared for aseptic surgery.

SURGICAL TECHNIQUE

All four parathyroid glands should be carefully inspected. If the external parathyroid gland is involved, the gland can be removed without removing the thyroid gland; however, removal of the internal parathyroid gland requires that thyroidectomy be performed (see p. 604). The external parathyroid gland should be spared when the internal parathyroid gland is neoplastic if possible. Visualization of the abnormal parathyroid gland may be facilitated with infusion of intravenous methylene blue in saline solution (see Box 22-18). Abnormal parathyroid tissue may stain dark blue with this procedure. A common side effect of methylene blue administration is hemolytic anemia caused by Heinz body formation. Severe and occasionally fatal Heinz body anemia has been reported after the use of methylene blue. If carcinoma is suspected based on the apparent invasiveness of the tumor, complete thyroidectomy and removal of draining lymph nodes are indicated.

SUTURE MATERIALS AND SPECIAL INSTRUMENTS

Small, fine instruments, such as iris scissors and Bishop-Harmon thumb forceps, facilitate removal of the parathyroid glands. Bipolar cautery forceps are advantageous for providing hemostasis because they allow finer control of coagulation than do unipolar forceps. Sterile Q-tips are useful for dissecting the parathyroid glands from the thyroid glands.

POSTOPERATIVE CARE AND ASSESSMENT

Hypocalcemia is the most common postoperative complication in dogs; it may be less common in cats. Hypocalcemia may occur after removal of a single parathyroid adenoma because negative feedback from high circulating levels of PTH suppresses function in the other normal glands. PTH has a functional half-life of 20 minutes, therefore PTH levels fall rapidly once neoplastic tissue has been removed. Hypocalcemia may be most pronounced in animals with higher preoperative serum calcium levels and those with notable skeletal demineralization. The treatment of hypocalcemia is presented in Box 22-26; treatment should not be necessary for prolonged periods in these patients. Renal function should be monitored postoperatively in patients with hypercalcemia. The prognosis for long-term survival after parathyroidectomy for hyperparathyroidism secondary to adenomas or hyperplasia is excellent if severe renal damage has not occurred.

References

Gear R, Neiger R, Skelly B et al: Primary hyperparathyroidism in 29 dogs: diagnosis, treatment, outcome and associated renal failure, *J Small Anim Pract* 46:10, 2005.

Matwichuk CL, Taylor SM, Daniel GB et al: Double-phase parathyroid scintigraphy in dogs using technetium-99m-sestamibi, *Vet Radiol Ultrasound* 41:461, 2000.

Pollard RE, Long CD, Nelson RW et al: Percutaneous ultrasonographically guided radiofrequency heat ablation for treatment of primary hyperparathyroidism in dogs, *J Am Vet Med Assoc* 218:1106, 2001.

Suggested Reading

Barber PJ: Disorders of the parathyroid glands, *J Fel Med Surg* 6:259, 2004
This is a comprehensive review of the function of parathyroid hormones and pathophysiology of disease associated with the parathyroid glands.

THYROID CARCINOMAS IN DOGS

DEFINITIONS

Thyroid neoplasms may be carcinomas (malignant) or adenomas (benign). **Carcinomas** may arise from follicular cells and may be classified as follicular, compact, papillary, or mixed, or they may arise from parafollicular or C cells (medullary thyroid carcinomas).

GENERAL CONSIDERATIONS AND CLINICALLY RELEVANT PATHOPHYSIOLOGY

Thyroid neoplasms make up 1% to 4% of all canine tumors. Canine thyroid carcinomas are more common than adenomas (63% to 87% of canine thyroid tumors are carcinomas), whereas functional adenomas prevail in cats (see the discussion of feline hyperthyroidism on p. 605). Adenocarcinomas generally are rapidly growing, highly invasive tumors that frequently metastasize to the draining lymph nodes and lungs. Reportedly, large tumors (i.e., those larger than 100 cm^3) are always associated with pulmonary metastasis. Although histologic classification of thyroid tumors based on the predominant microscopic pattern has been done (e.g., compact cellular or solid, follicular, mixed solid follicular, or anaplastic), the histologic pattern has been thought to correlate poorly with prognosis. However, medullary thyroid carcinomas are more apt to be well circumscribed and resectable and to have gross and histologic characteristics of a less malignant nature than are other thyroid carcinomas. Ectopic thyroid tumors have been reported at the heart base, caudal mediastinum, and tongue.

> NOTE: Warn owners that surgical excision of canine thyroid tumors usually is difficult because of the tumors' invasiveness and the tendency to have substantial hemorrhage.

Tumors arising in cystic remnants of the thyroglossal duct are rarely reported in dogs. They are usually well circumscribed, fluctuant, movable enlargements in the ventral midline cervical region. Histologically they usually are well-differentiated papillary carcinomas.

DIAGNOSIS
Clinical Presentation

Signalment. Thyroid neoplasia is most common in medium- to large-breed dogs; boxers, beagles, and golden retrievers may be predisposed to the condition. Most affected dogs are middle-aged or older (mean age, 9 years). A gender predisposition is not apparent.

History. Affected animals often are presented for evaluation of a palpable cervical enlargement, dysphagia, dyspnea, coughing, voice change, and/or exercise intolerance. Respiratory abnormalities may be the result of tracheal compression or pulmonary metastasis, and regurgitation may be caused by compression and/or invasion of the esophagus. In rare cases, hyperthyroidism (i.e., polydipsia, polyuria, weakness, restlessness, and a propensity to seek cool places) is caused by canine thyroid carcinomas.

Physical Examination Findings

A ventral cervical mass often is palpable. Carcinomas usually appear firm and poorly encapsulated; adenomas typically are small and freely movable. Abnormal lung sounds may occur secondary to pulmonary metastasis. Bilateral ptosis and prolapse of the nictitating membrane may be associated with paralysis of the extraocular and intraocular muscles secondary to thyroid adenocarcinoma invasion of the cavernous sinuses in dogs.

Diagnostic Imaging

Cervical radiographs or ultrasonography may reveal diffuse cervical edema and soft tissue swelling caudal to the mandible and surrounding the trachea. The mass may be partly mineralized. Thoracic radiographs should be taken to identify pulmonary metastasis. Thyroid imaging (see p. 606) may reveal abnormal thyroid gland uptake (heterogeneous uptake with "hot" and "cold" regions compared with normal thyroid or salivary gland uptake) and focal accumulations of the radiopharmaceutical in the lungs, indicative of pulmonary metastasis.

Laboratory Findings

Cytologic evaluation of a fine-needle aspirate of the cervical mass may reveal bizarre, pleomorphic cells consistent with neoplasia. Nondiagnostic samples may be obtained if the sample is contaminated with blood or is hypocellular. Additionally, neoplastic follicular epithelial cells are fragile and often are broken during sample preparation. Hyperthyroidism and hypothyroidism occasionally are associated with thyroid carcinomas; therefore measurement of serum fT4 and endogenous canine thyroid-stimulating hormone (cTSH) concentrations is warranted. Hematologic and serum biochemical results often are normal. Hypocalcemia has been reported in a dog with a thyroid medullary carcinoma.

DIFFERENTIAL DIAGNOSIS

Cervical swelling caused by thyroid neoplasia must be differentiated from abscesses, lymphadenopathy, or sialadenopathy. This usually can be done by cytologic evaluation of fine-needle aspirates.

MEDICAL MANAGEMENT

Dogs with thyroid carcinomas, particularly if hyperthyroid, may be palliated with radioactive iodine (^{131}I); however, much larger doses of ^{131}I appear to be necessary in dogs than in cats with thyroid adenomas, and this option is not routinely used. These large doses require lengthy hospital stays and make this treatment prohibitively expensive for many owners. Chemotherapy with doxorubicin may benefit animals in which complete excision is not possible. External beam radiation therapy appears beneficial for reducing tumor volume in animals after debulking procedures; however, large doses are required. In a recent study, fractionated, definitive radiation therapy using multiple, moderate doses of

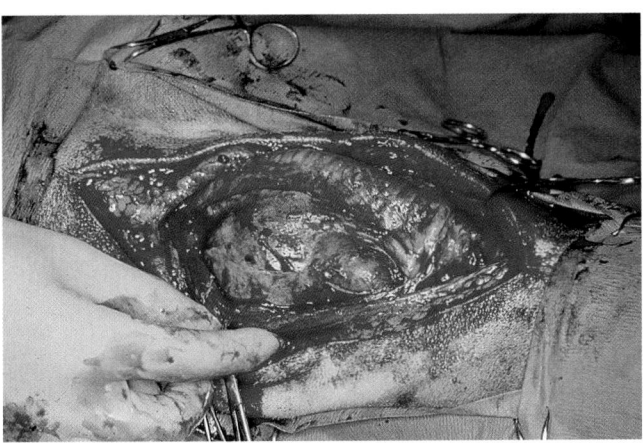

FIG. 22-23
Thyroid carcinoma in a dog. Note the invasiveness of the tumor.

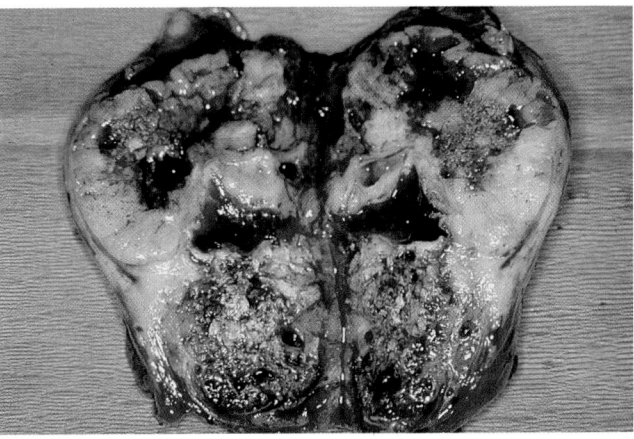

FIG. 22-24
A well-encapsulated thyroid carcinoma in a dog. Note the areas of necrosis in the gland.

radiation was effective in providing local control of invasive thyroid carcinoma in dogs (Pack et al, 2001). All dogs in this study had a reduction in tumor size to a clinically undetectable level on follow-up examination and the median survival time was 24.5 months. Linear accelerators are replacing cobalt therapy for treatment of these tumors.

SURGICAL TREATMENT

Surgical excision of thyroid adenomas is the treatment of choice. Surgical removal of thyroid carcinomas often is difficult because of their invasive nature (Slensky et al, 2003) and pronounced vascularity (Fig. 22-23), but should be considered if metastasis is not evident and if the lesion is localized. Marginal excision (i.e., just outside the tumor pseudocapsule) in tumors that are freely movable results in fewer complications than more extensive resection and does not appear to affect the local recurrence rate. Adjunctive radiation therapy or chemotherapy may be warranted if complete surgical excision is not possible. Chemotherapy may be indicated if debulking is done in animals with metastasis.

> NOTE: Have blood or purified bovine hemoglobin available during surgery because hemorrhage is often excessive.

Preoperative Management

Substantial electrolyte and acid-base abnormalities should be corrected before surgery. Fluid therapy should be initiated before surgery in geriatric patients with reduced renal function and in those that are dehydrated.

Anesthesia

In human beings, life-threatening thyroid storms are reported intraoperatively and postoperatively for thyroid tumors. Clinical signs of tachycardia or arrhythmias may occur because of catecholamine release, and treatment should be

anticipated. It may be wise to avoid drugs that are arrhythmogenic (e.g., barbiturates and halothane) in these patients.

Surgical Anatomy

The surgical anatomy of the thyroid glands is discussed on p. 603. Important structures that may adhere to or surround the tumor include the carotid artery, internal jugular vein, recurrent laryngeal nerve, and esophagus. These structures should be identified and preserved, if possible, during the dissection.

Positioning

The animal is placed in dorsal recumbency with the neck slightly hyperextended. The front limbs should be tied back, away from the neck. The entire neck, cranial thorax, and caudal intermandibular space should be clipped and prepared for aseptic surgery.

SURGICAL TECHNIQUE

Make a ventral midline incision over the thyroid glands. Identify the neoplastic mass and adjacent structures. If necessary, ligate the carotid artery and jugular vein. Remove the mass (thyroid and parathyroid glands) by a combination of sharp and blunt dissection. Identify and remove abnormal cervical lymph nodes. Use electrocautery and ligation to provide hemostasis. Inspect the contralateral thyroid and biopsy or remove if indicated. Close the incision routinely. Submit tissue for histologic evaluation (Fig. 22-24).

SUTURE MATERIALS AND SPECIAL INSTRUMENTS

These tumors frequently are very vascular, and electrocautery is useful for obtaining hemostasis.

POSTOPERATIVE CARE AND ASSESSMENT

A light pressure wrap may be used postoperatively to help reduce hemorrhage and swelling; however, it should be placed with care and monitored to prevent airway obstruction. The hematocrit should be monitored postoperatively and transfusions given as necessary. If unilateral thyroparathyroidectomy is performed, the animal should be observed for hypocalcemia or hypothyroidism, but supplementation usually is not necessary. If bilateral thyroparathyroidectomy is performed, vitamin D, calcium, and thyroid supplementation should be initiated postoperatively (see p. 603).

PROGNOSIS

The prognosis is guarded for thyroid carcinomas and depends on the tumor's size and resectability, and on whether metastasis has occurred. Surgical excision alone of freely movable tumors that do not have evidence of metastasis may result in survival of approximately 18 to 22 months or longer. Chemotherapy (e.g., cisplatin) may result in survival of several hundred days in dogs with large tumors, whereas radiation therapy resulted in survival of 24.5 months in one study (see the Medical Management section). In another study, the progression-free survival times for dogs with large, nonresectable thyroid carcinomas treated with megavoltage irradiation was 80% at 1 year and 72% at 3 years (Theon et al, 2000). The prognosis for thyroid adenomas is excellent.

References

Pack L, Roberts RR, Dawson SD et al: Definitive radiation therapy for infiltrative thyroid carcinoma in dogs, *Vet Radiol Ultrasound* 42:471, 2001.

Slensky KA, Volk SW, Schwarz T et al: Acute severe hemorrhage secondary to arterial invasion in a dog with thyroid carcinoma, *J Am Vet Med Assoc* 223:649, 2003.

Theon AP et al: Prognostic factors and patterns of treatment failure in dogs with unresectable differentiated thyroid carcinomas treated with megavoltage irradiation, *J Am Vet Med Assoc* 216:1775, 2000.

CHAPTER 23
Surgery of the Hemolymphatic System

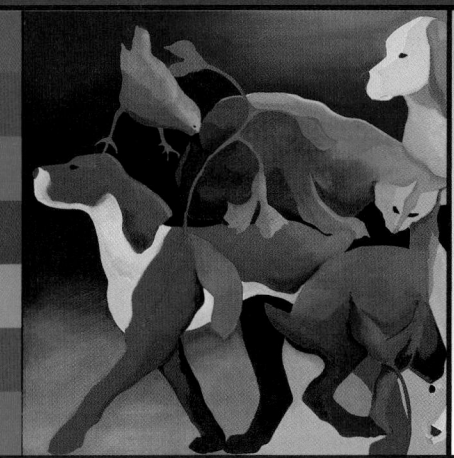

Surgery of the Lymphatic System

GENERAL PRINCIPLES AND TECHNIQUES

DEFINITIONS

Tissue for histopathologic examination of lymph nodes may be obtained by removing the entire node (**lymphadenectomy**) or by excising a portion of it. **Lymphangiomas** are benign tumors of peripheral lymphatics, and **lymphangiosarcomas** are malignant tumors of peripheral lymphatics.

PREOPERATIVE MANAGEMENT

Lymphadenomegaly is one of the more common lymphatic abnormalities of dogs and cats and may be caused by infection, inflammation, neoplasia (metastatic or primary), or systemic disease. It is important to distinguish generalized lymphadenomegaly from localized (regional) disease. With localized lymphadenopathy, areas drained by the node should be examined for evidence of infection, inflammation, or neoplasia. Conversely, one must remember that lymph node size does not necessarily correlate with disease, and neoplastic cells may be retrieved from normal-sized lymph nodes. In a recent study of dogs with oral malignant melanoma, although a significant relationship was identified between lymph node size and metastasis to the lymph node, the association was not clinically relevant (Williams and Packer, 2003). Although cytology of lymph node and splenic aspirates is very *specific* for neoplastic and fungal diseases (i.e., you can trust the diagnosis if you find such cells), it is not *sensitive* (i.e., not finding cancer or organisms never eliminates such disease because fine-needle aspirates of lymph nodes and spleens can easily miss the cells or organisms). Nonetheless, fine-needle aspirates and/or fine-needle core biopsies should be done before lymph node and sometimes splenic biopsy, because finding neoplasia or fungal elements by these less invasive techniques will make more invasive techniques unnecessary. The

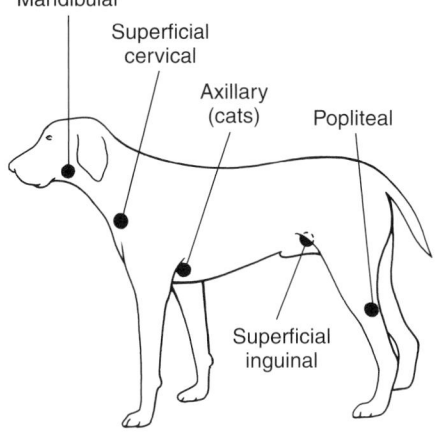

FIG. 23-1
Location of palpable lymph nodes.

reader is referred to a medicinal text for an in-depth discussion of lymph node cytology.

> NOTE: If several lymph nodes are enlarged, do not take a biopsy of the submandibular node because this node tends to be more reactive.

The mandibular, superficial cervical (prescapular), superficial inguinal, and popliteal lymph nodes are palpable in most animals (Fig. 23-1). The tonsils may be visualized in the oral cavity, and facial lymph nodes may be found in some normal animals. In dogs, the maxillary, accessory axillary, cervical, femoral, and retropharyngeal lymph nodes usually are palpable only when enlarged; however, the axillary node may be located readily in cats, even when it is only moderately enlarged. Unless the animal is extremely thin or cachectic, sublumbar and mesenteric lymph nodes must be at least moderately enlarged to be detected on rectal or abdominal palpation. The texture of the enlarged node and sensitivity to pressure or manipulation should be noted. Acute enlargement (i.e., suppurative lymphadenitis) can be

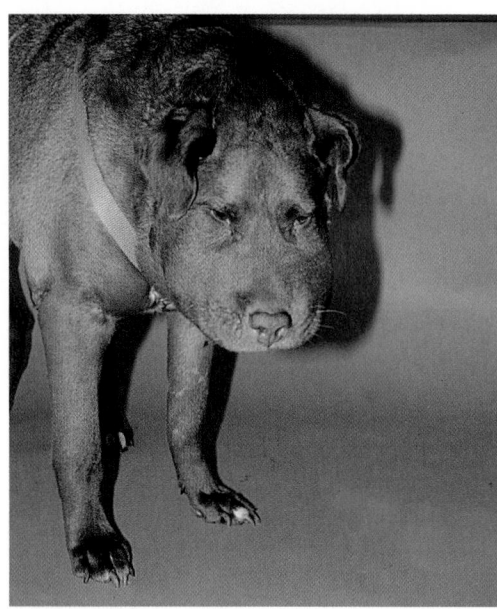

FIG. 23-2
Massive head and neck swelling in a dog with diffuse lymphangiosarcoma.

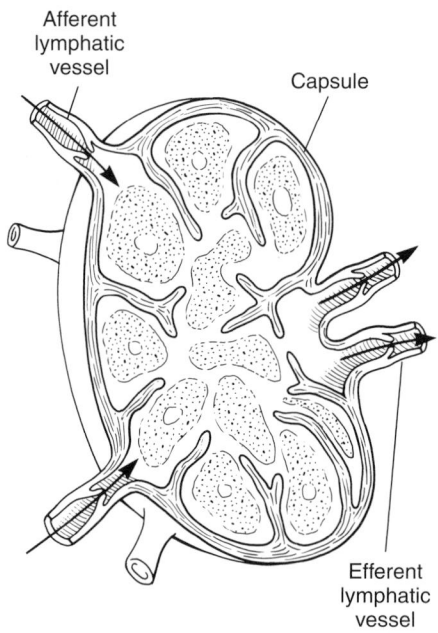

FIG. 23-3
Structure of a lymph node, showing afferent and efferent drainage.

associated with pain, but lymphoid neoplasia usually causes painless enlargement. Metastatic neoplasia and fungal infections sometimes cause nodes to become fixed to surrounding tissue. Clinical signs may result from lymphadenomegaly (e.g., coughing because of tracheal compression by enlarged hilar lymph nodes or constipation as a result of sublumbar lymphadenopathy).

Lymphangiomas are rare, benign neoplasms originating from lymphatic capillaries. They are believed to be developmental anomalies associated with failure of primitive lymphatic sacs to establish venous communication. These endothelial sprouts continue to grow, infiltrate surrounding tissue, cause pressure and subsequent necrosis, and form cystic structures. They typically manifest as large, fluctuant swellings that are noticed incidentally or because of interference with normal structures as a result of expansive growth. They have been identified arising from subcutaneous tissue, the nasopharynx, and the retroperitoneal space of dogs. Affected dogs usually are middle-aged or older; however, lymphangiomas may occur in young dogs. Treatment for lymphangioma is complete surgical excision or marsupialization. *Lymphangiosarcomas* (Fig. 23-2) are malignant tumors that arise from lymphatic capillaries. They are locally aggressive, and metastasis has been reported to regional lymph nodes, lungs, spleen, kidneys, and bone marrow. Even without metastasis, the local invasiveness of this tumor often calls for euthanasia. Surgical management may be considered; however, cures are unlikely. Histologically, lymphangiomas and lymphangiosarcomas are composed of vascular spaces lined by endothelial cells and focal lymphoid aggregates divided by connective tissue

stroma. Unlike hemangiomas, the cystic spaces of these tumors are not filled with blood.

ANESTHESIA

Superficial (e.g., popliteal) nodes can be excised using local anesthetic and sedation if necessary; however, short-duration general anesthesia usually facilitates extirpation.

ANTIBIOTICS

Perioperative antibiotics are seldom indicated in animals undergoing lymph node biopsy or removal.

SURGICAL ANATOMY

Lymph nodes are bean-shaped structures with a convex surface and a small flat or concave hilus (Fig. 23-3). They usually are found encased in fat at flexor angles or joints, in the mediastinum and mesentery, and in the angle formed by the origin of larger blood vessels.

DIAGNOSTIC IMAGING

Survey radiographs may detect internal lymphadenomegaly. Thoracic films should be examined for evidence of mediastinal, hilar, and sternal lymphadenomegaly; abdominal radiographs may reveal ventral deviation of the descending colon caused by sublumbar lymphadenomegaly or ill-defined mass effects in the midabdomen caused by mesenteric lymphadenopathy.

Ultrasound is useful in detecting mesenteric, gastric, and hepatic lymphadenomegaly. Doppler ultrasound, and to a lesser extent contrast ultrasound, has been used to determine the angioarchitecture of lymph nodes as a criterion for

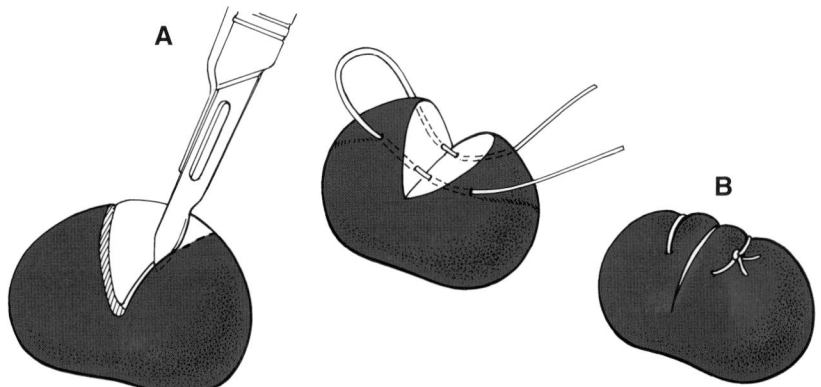

FIG. 23-4
A, Incisional (wedge) biopsy of lymph nodes occasionally is performed. Use a No. 15 scalpel blade to remove a wedge-shaped section of the parenchyma. **B,** Place a horizontal mattress suture of absorbable suture material to close the incision.

the diagnosis of malignancy in humans. A recent study determined that the vascular characteristics of malignancy in lymph nodes of dogs is similar to that of humans (Salwei et al, 2005). In the aforementioned study, power Doppler was found to be superior for examination of pericapsular vessels, whereas the contrast tissue harmonic mode was superior for depicting angioarchitecture and demonstrating the presence of malignant vascular patterns within lymph nodes.

SURGICAL TECHNIQUE

Lymph node biopsy is easy and relatively inexpensive, and it provides valuable information. There are no absolute contraindications to lymph node biopsy. Significant hemostatic disorders should be corrected preoperatively if possible, and care must be taken to ligate blood vessels properly.

The selection of a lymph node for a biopsy is based on the clinical findings. With generalized lymphadenopathy, the popliteal, inguinal, and prescapular lymph nodes are the preferred sites; a biopsy should be obtained from at least two nodes. The mandibular lymph node and nodes draining the gastrointestinal tract are undesirable because their morphologic appearance often is distorted by reactive hyperplasia caused by constant antigenic exposure.

Fine-Needle Aspiration

There are two main techniques.

The first is to attach a 23- to 25-gauge needle to a 6- or 12-ml syringe. Insert the needle into the lymph node and briefly pull back the plunger to 5 or 10 ml of negative pressure several times (stop if blood is seen in the hub of the needle). Then blow the contents of the barrel of the needle out onto a clean glass slide. Make both horizontal and vertical pull-apart preparations.

The second technique is to stick a 23- to 25-gauge needle repeatedly through a lymph node. Then attach the lymph node to a syringe and blow the contents out onto a clean glass slide.

This technique is less likely to have blood contamination and should be done if the first technique is unsuccessful. It is also the preferred technique for aspiration of splenic masses.

Both techniques may need to be modified, depending on the patient and the tissue. Some lymphosarcomas are very fragile, and the cells will readily rupture. Being less aggressive in aspirating or passing a needle through the node, and/or being more gentle and careful in making the cytology smear, may allow one to obtain a diagnostic smear with a 20-gauge needle.

TruCut Biopsy

If the lymph node is large enough, a 14- to 16-gauge TruCut type needle can be used to obtain a core of tissue.

> NOTE: Be sure to consider how deep a core you will obtain and what is behind the lymph node, so that you do not traumatize or lacerate structures on the other side of the node.

Incisional Biopsy

Incisional (wedge) biopsy of lymph nodes is indicated when lymphadenectomy may be difficult because of a node's size or location (i.e., nodes that are located close to major vessels or nerves).

Use a No. 15 scalpel blade to remove a wedge-shaped section of the parenchyma (Fig. 23-4, A), and place the sample in a buffered formalin solution. To provide hemostasis, place a horizontal mattress suture of absorbable suture material (i.e., 3-0 chromic catgut) to close the incision (Fig. 23-4, B).

Lymphadenectomy

Prepare the skin overlying the lymph node for aseptic surgery. Immobilize the lymph node firmly in one hand, and make an incision in the overlying skin. Bluntly dissect the node from surrounding tissue. Generally a vessel near the hilus of the node requires ligation to prevent postoperative hemorrhage. Handle the node gently to prevent damage and distortion of the lymph node tissue. Section the node to provide samples for aerobic and anaerobic cultures, fungal cultures, and histopathologic and cytologic evaluations. Make impression smears by lightly blotting the cut edge of the node with absorbent paper and touching the sample lightly to a glass slide before placing it in formalin. Close dead space and suture the skin routinely.

HEALING OF THE LYMPHATIC SYSTEM

The lymphatics usually heal rapidly. Lymphedema is rare after lymphadenectomy because collateral pathways form. If lymphedema occurs, it usually is transient and seldom requires specific therapy. Frequently, prolonged obstruction of lymphatics may cause a lymphaticovenous anastomosis to open or form, providing an alternate pathway for lymph flow.

SUTURE MATERIALS AND SPECIAL INSTRUMENTS

Special instruments are not required for lymph node biopsy or removal. Absorbable suture should be used in the lymph node parenchyma.

POSTOPERATIVE CARE AND ASSESSMENT

After lymphadenectomy, the patient should be observed for swelling at the surgical site. Swelling usually is associated with hematoma formation as a result of inadequate hemostasis or with seroma formation if dead space was not obliterated.

COMPLICATIONS

Manipulation of a tumor during biopsy procedures may transiently increase the number of neoplastic cells present in the lymphatic and vascular systems; however, finding cancer cells in a lymph node typically means either that there is a diffuse neoplasia (i.e., lymphoma) or that metastasis has already occurred. Subsequent metastasis after lymph node biopsy has seldom been substantiated. A hematoma may develop if vessels are not ligated adequately.

SPECIAL AGE CONSIDERATIONS

The age and physical condition of animals with lymphadenopathy must be considered. Increased lymph node size may be expected in young animals as part of an appropriate immunologic response. As an animal ages, lymph nodes usually decrease in size, making nodes difficult to palpate. Loss of fat that normally surrounds the nodes in cachectic patients may make the nodes prominent.

References

Salwei RM, O'Brien RT, Matheson JS: Characterization of lymphomatous lymph nodes in dogs using contrast harmonic and power Doppler ultrasound, *Vet Radiol Ultrasound* 46:411, 2005.

Williams LE, Packer RA: Association between lymph node size and metastasis in dogs with oral malignant melanoma: 100 cases (1987-2001), *J Am Vet Med Assoc* 222:1234, 2003.

Suggested Reading

Langenbach A, McManus PM, Hendrick MJ et al: Sensitivity and specificity of methods of assessing the regional lymph nodes for evidence of metastasis in dogs and cats with solid tumors, *J Am Vet Med Assoc* 218:1424, 2001.

This study suggested that fine-needle aspiration was potentially a more sensitive method of evaluating regional lymph nodes in dogs and cats with solid tumors than was needle core biopsy.

SPECIFIC DISEASES

LYMPHEDEMA

DEFINITIONS

Lymphedema is an accumulation of fluid in the interstitial space. **Primary lymphedema** is caused by an abnormality or disease of lymph vessels or lymph nodes; **secondary lymphedema** occurs as a result of lymphatic obstruction of the nodes or vessels by neoplasia, filariasis, lymphoproliferative disorders, or surgery.

GENERAL CONSIDERATIONS AND CLINICALLY RELEVANT PATHOPHYSIOLOGY

Lymphedema results from a disturbance of the equilibrium between the amount of fluid in the interstitial space that needs to be cleared (capillary filtrate) and the capacity of the lymphatic and venous systems to remove this fluid. Possible causes include (1) overload of the lymphatic system, (2) inadequate collection by the lymphatic terminal buds, (3) abnormal lymphatic contractility, (4) insufficient lymphatics, (5) lymph node obstruction, and (6) central vessel (i.e., thoracic duct) defects. Regardless of the cause, edema results when capillary filtration exceeds the combined resorptive capabilities of the venous and lymphatic systems. This edema is relatively protein rich (2 to 5 g/dl). Because of the resultant high osmotic pressure, additional fluid is pulled into the interstitial space, worsening the edema. If the lymphatic system cannot adequately drain this interstitial fluid, collagen deposition and fibrosis may result. Hence, although the early stages are reversible, chronic edema is associated with thickening and fibrosis of tissue, making treatment difficult. The domestic species most commonly reported to have lymphedema is the dog.

Lymphedema may be a result of a primary defect in the lymphatic system or may occur secondary to other diseases or surgical procedures. Distinguishing between primary and secondary lymphedema often is difficult. Lymph node obstruction, although more commonly associated with secondary lymphedema, has been associated with primary lymphedema. Many of the dogs reported with primary lymphedema have had small or absent lymph nodes. Perhaps the initial defect in some dogs with lymphedema is fibrosis of the lymph nodes, which leads to secondary obstructive changes in the lymphatic vessels. As the vessels dilate, they lose contractility, and the lymphatic valves become permanently nonfunctional. Secondary lymphedema may be caused by conditions that increase the rate of interstitial fluid formation as a result of altered capillary permeability (e.g., trauma, heat, irradiation, or infection). Venous congestion (i.e., because of heart failure) may also cause lymphedema by reducing fluid resorption. Secondary lymphedema can result from neoplasia or infiltration of lymph nodes by filaria, such as *Wuchereria bancrofti* and *Brugia timori,* and from lymphoproliferative disorders.

NOTE: Lymphedema may be caused by primary lymphatic abnormalities or may occur secondary to other diseases or surgery. Distinguishing between primary and secondary lymphedema often is difficult. The age of onset of clinical signs does not help distinguish the two conditions in many cases because middle-aged animals may have acute signs of lymphedema that occur secondary to congenital lymphatic abnormalities.

DIAGNOSIS
Clinical Presentation

Signalment. Primary lymphedema usually is noted at birth or shortly thereafter; however, older animals may develop lymphedema associated with congenital abnormalities. The lymphatic system may function normally until a precipitating cause (e.g., infection, trauma, or surgery) overwhelms the marginal lymphatic system. Congenital, hereditary lymphedema has been reported in bulldogs and poodles. A gender predisposition is not evident.

NOTE: Congenital lymphatic abnormalities may not cause lymphedema until the animal is several years old. Clinical signs of primary lymphedema may be precipitated by infection, trauma, or surgery.

History. The age of onset; progression of disease; extent of involvement (unilateral or bilateral, pelvic limb or forelimb); and history of previous surgery, trauma, or exposure to infectious agents should be ascertained. Lymphedema typically manifests as a spontaneous, painless swelling of the extremities with pitting edema. The onset may be insidious. The rear limbs are more commonly affected, and the swelling may be unilateral. Lymphedema usually begins in the distal extremity and progresses proximally. In severely affected animals, all four limbs and the trunk may be edematous. Although the patient may be less active than normal because of the weight of the limb or may carry the limb when ambulating, lameness and pain are uncommon without massive enlargement or cellulitis.

Physical Examination Findings

The diagnosis of lymphedema usually is made on the basis of clinical signs (Fig. 23-5). The limb generally is not excessively warm or cool. Although the condition often is bilateral, the degree of swelling frequently is greater in one limb. Occasionally the swelling may be precipitated by minor trauma or superficial skin infections. Fibrosis occurs as the edema becomes chronic, and the edema tends to progressively pit less until pitting is absent. With chronic edema, massage and rest do not appreciably reduce the size of the limb.

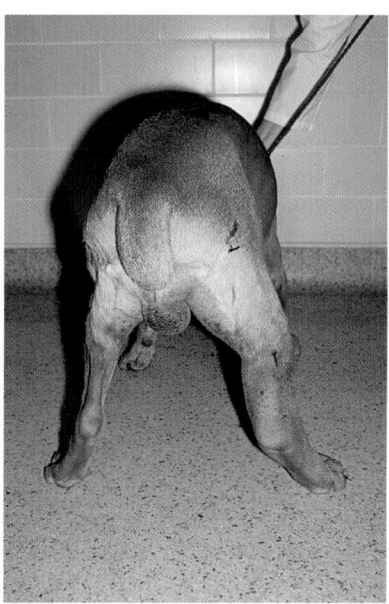

FIG. 23-5
A 2-year-old boxer with lymphedema. Note the massive swelling of the right rear limb.

Laboratory Findings

No specific laboratory abnormalities are found with lymphedema. Importantly, these animals are not hypoalbuminemic; hypoalbuminemia is always an important differential for edema, even localized edema.

DIFFERENTIAL DIAGNOSIS

The key differential diagnosis is abnormality of the venous system, such as venous stasis or arteriovenous fistula. The clinical signs usually are adequate to differentiate lymphedema from edema caused by venous obstruction. Typical changes with edema caused by venous obstruction include varices, stasis hyperpigmentation, and cutaneous ulceration. Arteriovenous fistulae are vascular abnormalities in which a direct communication exists between an adjacent artery and vein. They may be congenital or acquired (e.g., after trauma, neoplasia, infection, or iatrogenic ligation of an artery and vein together). Clinical signs with arteriovenous fistulae vary depending on the location; however, palpation of strong pulsatile vessels, often of a fremitus or thrill, and auscultation of a machinery murmur (i.e., bruit) are classic findings. Angiography is necessary to confirm the diagnosis and determine the size, extent, and location of the fistula. The physical examination should eliminate systemic causes of bilateral edema, including heart failure, renal failure, cirrhosis, and hypoproteinemia. Other differential diagnoses include trauma, neoplasia, and foreign bodies.

MEDICAL MANAGEMENT

In the early stages of lymphedema, before the development of fibrosis, nonsurgical therapy may reduce the swelling and make the patient more comfortable. Nonsurgical therapy

consists of heavy bandages or splints that exert pressure on
the limb, meticulous care of the skin to prevent infection,
weight control, and appropriate use of antibiotics to treat
and prevent cellulitis and lymphangitis. Drugs that have
been used to treat human patients with lymphedema include
steroids, diuretics, anticoagulants, and fibrinolysin inhibitors. For the most part, the proposed benefits of these pharmaceuticals have not been substantiated. Long-term treatment of lymphedema with diuretics is contraindicated.
Diuretics act by removing fluid from the tissue; proteins that
are not reabsorbed become increasingly concentrated, further damaging tissues.

> NOTE: Medical therapy often is ineffective in sub-
> stantially reducing swelling caused by lymphedema;
> however, medical management has received little
> attention in veterinary medicine. Amputation is a
> reasonable alternative for unilateral lymphedema,
> particularly when it interferes with limb function and
> when initial medical management is ineffective.

The benzopyrones are a group of drugs that have been
used to successfully treat experimental lymphedema in dogs
and spontaneous lymphedema in human beings. All the
drugs in this group appear to reduce high-protein edema.
Their main action appears to be stimulation of macrophages, which promotes proteolysis. Protein fragments can
then be reabsorbed into the blood. These drugs are active
orally and topically, are inexpensive, and are relatively free of
side effects. Included in this category of drugs are coumarin
(5,6 benzo-[a]-pyrone), O-(β-hydroxy-ethyl)-rutosides, di-
osmin, and rutin. Recommended dosages for human beings
are 440 mg/day of coumarin and 3 g/day for rutosides, dios-
min, and rutin (Box 23-1). Although these drugs (e.g., rutin)
are being investigated for spontaneous lymphedema in dogs,
their efficacy currently is uncertain.

Lymphography and Lymphoscintigraphy

The classic diagnostic tool has been direct lymphography
(see p. 123 for a description of the technique). Oil-based
contrast media are contraindicated in patients with primary
lymphedema because the high volume of contrast medium
necessary to visualize the lymphatics and the propensity for
extravasation may further damage existing lymphatics. Lym-

phoscintigraphy, an alternative method of imaging the peripheral lymphatics, involves intradermal injection of high
molecular weight, radiolabeled colloids. A gamma camera is
used to obtain images of the affected limb over time to observe the progression of radioactivity through the lymphatics. Primary lymphedema typically shows slow absorption of
the radiopharmaceutical, reduced visualization of lymphatic
vessels and lymph nodes, and no interstitial activity. Secondary lymphedema typically shows poorly visualized primary
lymph vessels and dilated secondary lymph vessels. There is
also significant interstitial activity.

SURGICAL TREATMENT

Except for amputation, no current surgical treatment offers
a cure for lymphedema. Numerous therapies have been described in human patients, including lymphangioplasty,
bridging procedures, lymphaticovenous shunts, omental
transposition, superficial to deep anastomosis, and excision
(with or without skin grafting). These techniques have not
been adequately evaluated in dogs with spontaneous lymphedema. Lymphangiography rarely provides information that
helps manage animals with spontaneous lymphedema, but it
occasionally defines the underlying lymphatic abnormality
(i.e., hypoplasia, aplasia, or hyperplasia of lymphatics). It is
a tool that must be correlated with other historical and
physical findings. Biopsy samples of affected tissues should
be submitted because lymphangiosarcoma, a highly malignant neoplasm, has been reported to occur in human beings
with long-standing lymphedema. The technique for lymphangiography is described on p. 623.

> NOTE: Biopsies should be performed in lymph-
> edematous animals to rule out neoplasia. Neoplastic
> transformation of chronically edematous tissue may
> occur.

Preoperative Management

Perioperative antibiotics are indicated in patients undergoing lymphangiography because the risk of subsequent lymphangitis is high. Before other preoperative procedures, inject 1 ml of 3% Evans blue dye between the second and third,
or third and fourth, digits to aid in the visualization and cannulation of lymphatics.

Anesthesia

General anesthesia is required for direct lymphangiography.

Surgical Anatomy

The lymphatic system of the extremities can be divided into
two parts: the superficial lymphatics and the deep (i.e., muscular) lymphatics. The superficial system appears to be the
one most commonly involved in lymphedema. This is the
system of lymphatics observed during pedal lymphangiography (Fig. 23-6). These lymphatics empty into a valved
group of vessels found at the junction of the dermis and
subcutaneous tissue. Lymph then drains into afferent lym-

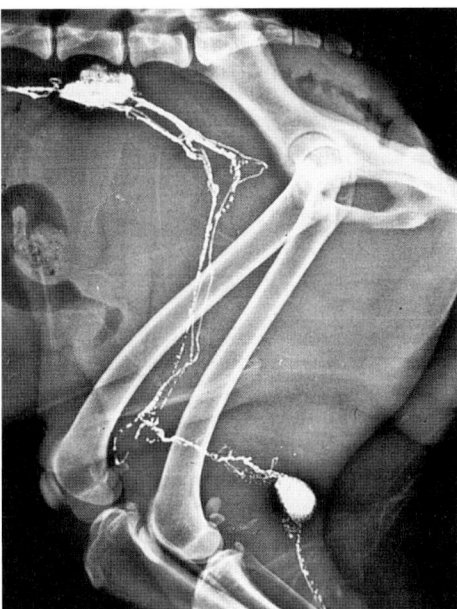

FIG. 23-6
Pedal lymphangiogram in a dog. The superficial lymphatic system is filled with contrast.

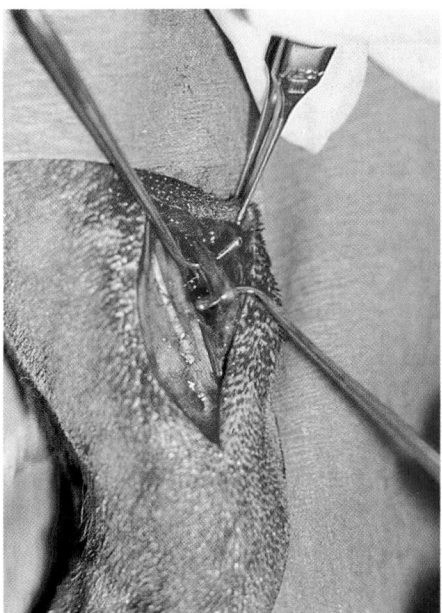

FIG. 23-7
Pedal lymphangiography. Evans blue dye is injected interdigitally before pedal lymphangiography. A 5-cm longitudinal incision is made on the dorsomedial aspect of the metatarsus, and a combination of sharp and blunt dissection is used to identify the blue-stained superficial metatarsal lymphatic vessel. Use small, blunt probes to meticulously clear the lymphatic of all subcutaneous tissue.

phatics in the subcutaneous fat. The superficial lymphatics of the pelvic limb consist of a larger medial group and a smaller lateral group. Lymphatics follow the branches of the medial saphenous vein and drain into the superficial inguinal lymph nodes. Efferent lymphatics from the lymph nodes drain into the larger lymphatic ducts. The deeper lymphatics drain the fascial planes surrounding skeletal muscles (lymphatics are not found in skeletal muscle bundles), joints, and synovium. Deep lymphatic collector vessels accompany the main blood vessels of the extremities. Controversy exists as to whether the two lymphatic systems (superficial and deep) communicate; however, communications usually appear to be a result of a lymphatic pathologic condition or a response to abnormal lymph flow. The lumbar lymph trunks receive vessels from the pelvic limbs, the abdominal lymph nodes, and the intestines before uniting to form the cisterna chyli.

Positioning

Position the animal on the radiology table in lateral recumbency with the affected limb down and the opposite limb retracted from the radiographic field. Prepare and drape the dorsomedial aspect of the metatarsus for aseptic surgery.

SURGICAL TECHNIQUE
Direct Lymphangiography

Make a 5-cm skin incision over the middorsomedial metatarsal region. Use sharp and blunt dissection until a blue-stained, superficial metatarsal lymphatic vessel is identified (Fig. 23-7). Meticulously dissect the lymphatic free from surrounding tissue with fine, blunt dissection probes and cannulate the lymphatic using a lymph duct cannulator or a 27- or 30-gauge over-the-needle catheter. Inject a small

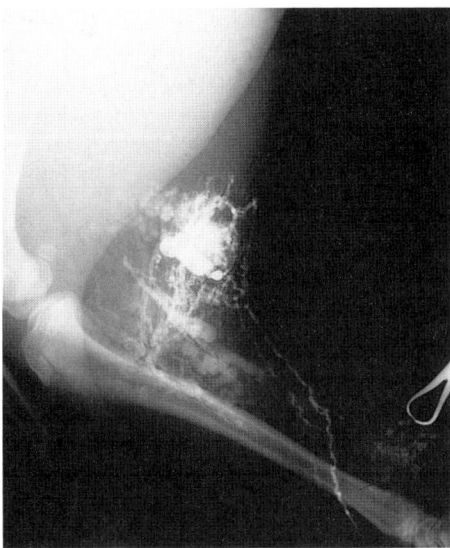

FIG. 23-8
Lymphangiogram of a dog with lymphedema. Note the dilated, tortuous lymphatics. Compare this to the lymphangiogram of a normal dog in Fig. 23-6.

amount of sterile saline into the catheter or cannulator to verify patency. Then manually infuse an aqueous-based radiographic contrast agent into the lymphatic vessel. Take radiographs immediately after the injection (Fig. 23-8); additional radiographs may be made, depending on the rate of lymphatic transport of the contrast agent, which varies from patient to patient. Upon completion of the lymphangiogram, withdraw the cannulator, ligate the lymphatic vessel, and close the incision in a routine fashion.

SUTURE MATERIALS AND SPECIAL INSTRUMENTS

A commercial lymphatic duct cannulator, such as a Tegtmeyer lymph duct cannulator, may facilitate cannulation of the lymphatic vessel.

POSTOPERATIVE CARE AND ASSESSMENT

If the lymphatics appear abnormal in character or quantity or if an obvious obstruction is not noted on the lymphangiogram, medical therapy or amputation should be considered. The patient should be observed for swelling or worsening of the edema after the procedure.

PROGNOSIS

Primary lymphedema seldom resolves spontaneously. Neoplastic change in chronic lymphedematous tissue has been reported in dogs (Webb et al, 2004).

Reference

Webb, JA, Boston SE, Armstrong J et al: Lymphangiosarcoma associated with primary lymphedema in a Bouvier des Flandres, *J Vet Intern Med* 18:122, 2004.

Suggested Reading

Fossum TW, King LA, Miller MW et al: Lymphedema. II. Clinical signs, diagnosis, and treatment, *J Vet Intern Med* 6:312, 1992.
This manuscript is a concise review of the various causes of lymphedema and its treatment in dogs.

Surgery of the Spleen

GENERAL PRINCIPLES AND TECHNIQUES

DEFINITIONS

Splenomegaly is enlargement of the spleen arising from any cause. **Splenectomy** is surgical removal of the spleen. **Splenosis** is the congenital or traumatic presence of multiple nodules of normal splenic tissue in the abdomen. **Siderotic plaques** are brown or rust-colored deposits of iron and calcium that may be found on the splenic surface (Fig. 23-9).

PREOPERATIVE MANAGEMENT

Animals with surgical diseases of the spleen often have either diffuse or focal splenomegaly. Diffuse (symmetric) splenomegaly may be attributed to congestion (e.g., splenic torsion, right-sided heart failure, gastric dilatation-volvulus [GDV], and drugs) or infiltration due to infection (e.g., fungal, bacterial, and rickettsial), immune-mediated disease (e.g., immune-

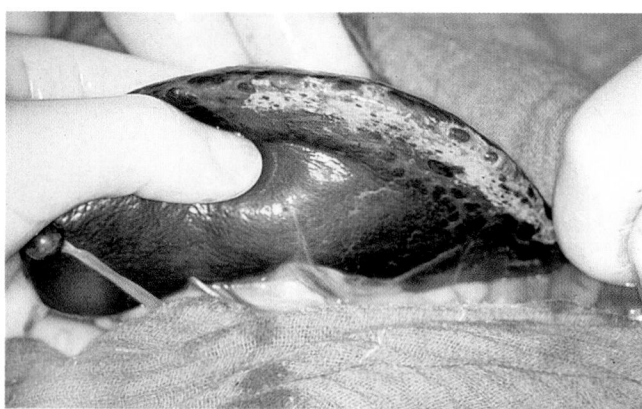

FIG. 23-9
Siderotic plaques on the splenic surface.

mediated thrombocytopenia and immune-mediated hemolytic anemia), or neoplasia (e.g., lymphosarcoma or feline mastocytosis). Focal (asymmetric) splenomegaly may be caused by benign processes (e.g., nodular regeneration, hematoma [see p. 633], or trauma) or neoplastic processes (e.g., hemangiosarcoma [see p. 631]). Infiltrative splenomegaly resulting from neoplasia is one of the most common causes of spontaneous (noniatrogenic) splenomegaly in dogs and cats.

Anemia may be present because of acute hemorrhage associated with splenic trauma, rupture of a hematoma, or hemorrhage from an underlying disease (i.e., chronic infection, immune-mediated disease, or disseminated intravascular coagulation [DIC]). Coagulation profiles should be done in animals with bleeding that is not thought to be the result of trauma. Normally hydrated animals with a packed cell volume (PCV) below 20% or a hemoglobin level under 5 to 7 g/dl may benefit from preoperative blood transfusions or administration of purified hemoglobin (oxyglobin) (see Box 5-1 and Table 5-5 on p. 25 and p. 28, respectively). If DIC is suspected, administration of plasma with or without heparin therapy may be helpful (Box 23-2). Intravenous fluids should be administered to dehydrated animals before surgery.

ANESTHESIA

Anemic patients should be given oxygen before induction of anesthesia and during recovery. Anticholinergic drugs may be used to prevent bradycardia. Barbiturates that cause splenic congestion should be avoided. Acetylpromazine should also be avoided in these patients because of the possibility of red blood cell sequestration, hypotension, and impact on platelet function. A hypotensive episode may occur as a result of volume depletion after splenectomy, and the arterial blood pressure should be monitored carefully during surgery.

ANTIBIOTICS

Antibiotic use in animals with splenic disease is dictated by the nature of the underlying disease. The merit of perioperative prophylactic antibiotics for splenectomy in dogs is largely unknown and depends on the animal's age, concur-

Therapy for Disseminated Intravascular Coagulation

Plasma (fresh frozen)

10–20 ml/kg, then re-assess the plasma ATIII activity. Repeat as needed to increase the ATIII to near-normal concentrations.

Heparin (unfractionated)*

50–100 U/kg SC, bid or tid

Heparin-Activated Plasma

Place the first heparin dose (50–100 U/kg) into the plasma and incubate for 30 minutes before administration. Once ATIII levels are above 60%, continue the heparin subcutaneously. If additional plasma is needed, incubation with heparin is not necessary.

Note: Adequate levels of ATIII are critical in these patients.

Low Molecular Weight Heparin (Dalteparin)

100–150 U/kg SC, qd to bid

ATIII, Antithrombin III; *SC,* subcutaneous; *bid,* twice a day; *tid,* three times a day.
*Low molecular weight (LMW) heparin is more effective than unfractionated heparin. There are substantial differences between the two forms, and the reader is referred to a medical text for a more complete discussion including the differences in monitoring the effectiveness of therapy. As more becomes known regarding LMW heparin, this dosage recommendation may change.

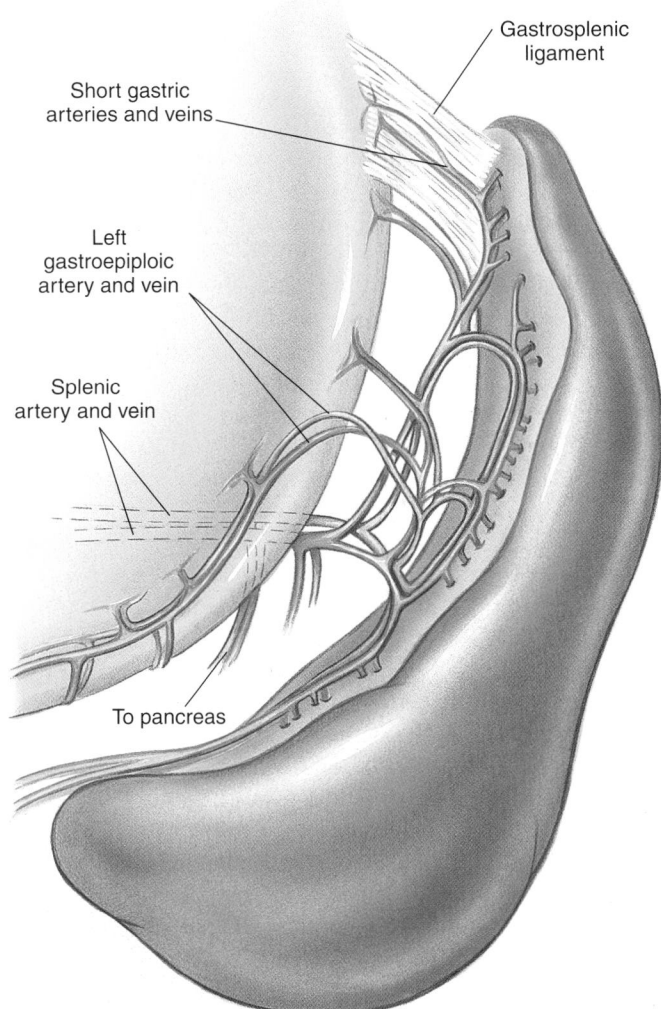

FIG. 23-10
Splenic vasculature. Note the short gastric arteries, which often are avulsed in dogs with gastric dilatation-volvulus.

rent disease, and the length of surgery. Perioperative antibiotics in healthy animals usually are unnecessary, but may be given at induction of anesthesia and discontinued within 24 hours. Longer term antibiotic therapy may be warranted in immunosuppressed or severely debilitated animals. A case of multiple abscessation, septicemia, and death associated with splenectomy performed in conjunction with dental cleaning and extraction has been reported.

SURGICAL ANATOMY

The spleen is situated in the left cranial abdominal quadrant. It usually lies parallel to the greater curvature of the stomach; however, its exact location depends on its size and the position of other abdominal organs. When the stomach is contracted, the spleen usually lies in the rib cage. However, with massive gastric enlargement, it may be in the caudal abdomen. The splenic capsule is composed of elastic and smooth muscle fibers. The parenchyma consists of a white pulp (i.e., lymphoid tissue) and red pulp (i.e., venous sinuses and cellular tissue filling the intravascular spaces). Large numbers of α-adrenergic receptors are responsible for splenic contraction. When the spleen is contracted, it feels firm in consistency. The spleen normally is red, but siderotic plaques or fibrin deposits may change its appearance.

The arterial supply of the spleen usually is the splenic artery, a branch of the celiac artery. The splenic artery generally is more than 2 mm in diameter and gives off three to five long primary branches as it courses in the greater omentum toward the ventral third of the spleen. The first branch usually is to the pancreas and is the main supply of the left limb of that organ. The two remaining branches run toward the proximal half of the spleen, where they send 20 to 30 splenic branches that enter the parenchyma. The branches then continue in the gastrosplenic ligament to the great curvature of the stomach, where they form the short gastric arteries (which supply the fundus) and left gastroepiploic artery (which supplies the greater curvature of the stomach) (Fig. 23-10). Other branches supply the splenocolic ligament and greater omentum. Venous drainage is via the splenic vein into the gastrosplenic vein, which empties into the portal vein.

SURGICAL TECHNIQUE

The spleen is approached via a ventral midline abdominal incision that extends from the xiphoid to a point caudal to the umbilicus. The incision may need to be lengthened for large lesions or to allow complete abdominal exploration.

Complete abdominal exploration should be performed in any animal suspected of having neoplasia.

Splenic Biopsy

Splenic biopsies are indicated to ascertain the cause of clinically significant splenomegaly or suspected metastatic lesions to the spleen. They may be obtained percutaneously (i.e., fine-needle aspiration or core biopsy) or at surgery. Ultrasound-guided biopsies improve the likelihood of obtaining diagnostic samples percutaneously. Percutaneous biopsies often are diagnostic for diffuse lesions (e.g., mastocytosis or lymphosarcoma); however, focal or nodular lesions may be missed. Fine-needle aspiration is potentially specific (if cancer cells are found), but very insensitive for differentiating hemangiosarcoma and hematoma (see p. 633). When cavitary lesions are identified with ultrasound scans, fine-needle aspiration should be performed with care or not at all. Cavitary lesions may rupture during aspiration, which could be fatal, especially in animals with coagulopathies.

Larger tissue samples should be placed in 10 volumes of formalin to 1 part tissue for routine histopathologic examination. Special preservatives may be required if additional staining techniques are desired (e.g., Bouin's fixative is preferred for identification of viral inclusions). Samples larger than 5 cm should be scored (cut into) before placement in formalin to allow the sample to fix properly. Large splenic masses should be scored at several sites, but left intact to allow orientation of the entire lesion by the pathologist. If this is not possible, several representative samples should be submitted from diverse sites, including the margin of the abnormal- and normal-appearing tissue. If the lesion is cavitary (i.e., splenic mass, cyst, or abscess), it should be ruptured before being placed in formalin.

Splenic aspiration. *Place the animal in right lateral or dorsal recumbency using manual restraint or mild sedation. Avoid using phenothiazine tranquilizers or barbiturates because the resultant splenic congestion may result in a nondiagnostic sample as a result of blood dilution. Surgically prepare a small area on the left side of the abdomen and isolate the spleen. Penetrate the abdominal wall with a small needle (23 or 25 gauge, 1 to 1½ inches) and pass the needle into the spleen several times, being careful not to lacerate splenic arteries. If you start to see blood in the hub of the needle, stop. Remove the needle from the abdomen, and blow out the contents of the needle onto a clean glass slide.*

Although uncommon, major hemorrhage can occur after needle aspiration of the spleen (not only splenic hemangiosarcomas but also spleens with diffuse lymphosarcoma). Ultrasound can be used to guide the placement of the needle (see p. 633).

Surgical biopsy. During celiotomy, biopsies of focal lesions may be taken by fine-needle aspiration or with a Tru-Cut (see p. 619), Jamshidi, modified Franklin-Silverman, or punch biopsy.

To remove focal lesions near the center of the spleen, make a rectangular or oval incision through the capsule and into the parenchyma to sufficient depth to remove the lesion. Close the defect by placing simple interrupted or mattress sutures of absorbable material (3-0 or 4-0) in the splenic capsule.

Partial splenectomy may be performed if more diffuse lesions are present (see later discussion).

Repair of Lacerations

Splenorrhaphy is indicated to provide hemostasis in superficial traumatic lesions of the splenic capsule.

Explore the lesion and ligate any large traumatized vessels. Place simple interrupted or mattress sutures of absorbable material (3-0 or 4-0) in the splenic capsule. Apply gentle pressure to the area for several minutes. If bleeding continues, ligate the splenic branches supplying the lesion as close to the hilus of the spleen as possible.

Small areas of ischemia revascularize as a result of collateralization.

Partial Splenectomy

Partial splenectomy is indicated in animals with traumatic or focal lesions of the spleen to preserve splenic function.

Define the area of the spleen to be removed and double ligate and incise the hilar vessels supplying the area (Fig. 23-11, A). Note the extent of ischemia that develops, and use this as a guideline for the resection. Squeeze the splenic tissue at this line between a thumb and forefinger, and milk the splenic pulp toward the ischemic area. Place forceps on the flattened portion, and divide the spleen between the forceps (Fig. 23-11, B). Close the cut surface of the spleen adjacent to the forceps in a continuous pattern using absorbable suture (3-0 or 4-0) (Fig. 23-11, C). As an alternative, place two rows of mattress sutures in a continuous overlapping fashion at the line of demarcation. If hemorrhage continues, oversew the end of the spleen with a continuous suture of absorbable suture material.

Automated stapling devices (e.g., TIA staplers) may also be used for partial splenectomy; however, there is some risk that if the staples are not secured in sufficient tissue, they will loosen and allow hemorrhage to occur from the splenic stump. Either 3.5- or 4.8-size stainless steel staples are recommended. When properly performed, surgical stapling for partial splenectomy significantly reduces surgical time and omental adhesion to the spleen.

Total Splenectomy

Total splenectomy is most commonly performed in animals with splenic neoplasia, torsion (stomach or spleen), or severe trauma that is causing life-threatening hemorrhage that cannot be stopped. Splenectomy previously was advocated for

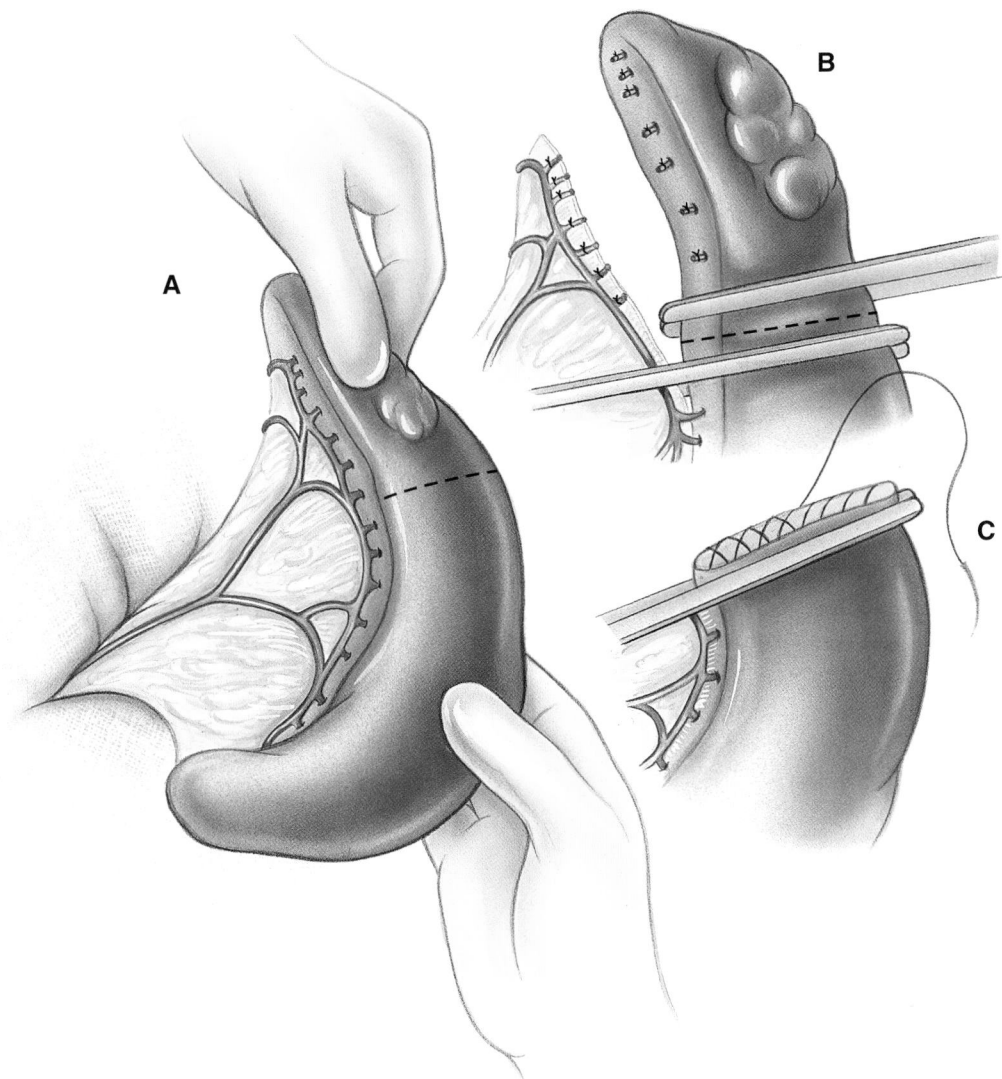

FIG. 23-11
Partial splenectomy preserves splenic function in animals with traumatic or focal lesions.
A, Define the area of the spleen to be removed and double ligate and incise the hilar vessels supplying the area. **B,** Transect the spleen between forceps. **C,** Close the cut surface in a continuous suture pattern.

immune-mediated hematologic disorders refractory to medical therapy (e.g., thrombocytopenia or hemolytic anemia). Immunosuppressive drugs (e.g., cyclosporine or azathioprine) and corticosteroids have reduced the need for splenectomy; however, splenectomy is reasonable if drug therapy is unsuccessful or if it causes unacceptable side effects. Although life-threatening sepsis has occurred in splenectomized people, this has not been recognized in dogs. Nevertheless, partial splenectomy is preferred over total splenectomy when possible. The spleen normally contains a reservoir of red blood cells (RBCs), has hematopoietic capabilities, has important phagocytic functions, and is helpful in maintaining immunocompetence; total splenectomy eliminates these beneficial actions. Elective splenectomy is sometimes performed in dogs to be used as blood donors so that subclinical infections with *Ehrlichia, Mycoplasma* (formerly *Haemobartonella*), or *Babesia* will become obvious and the dog can be eliminated from the program. Splenectomy is contraindicated in patients with bone marrow hypoplasia in which the spleen is a main site of hematopoiesis.

After exploring the abdomen, exteriorize the spleen and place moistened abdominal sponges or laparotomy pads around the incision under the spleen. Double ligate and transect all vessels at the splenic hilus with absorbable (preferred) or nonabsorbable suture material (Fig. 23-12). If possible, preserve the short gastric branches supplying the gastric fundus.

As an alternative, open the omental bursa and isolate the splenic artery. Identify the branch or branches supplying the left limb of the pancreas. Double ligate and transect the splenic artery distal to this vessel (or these vessels).

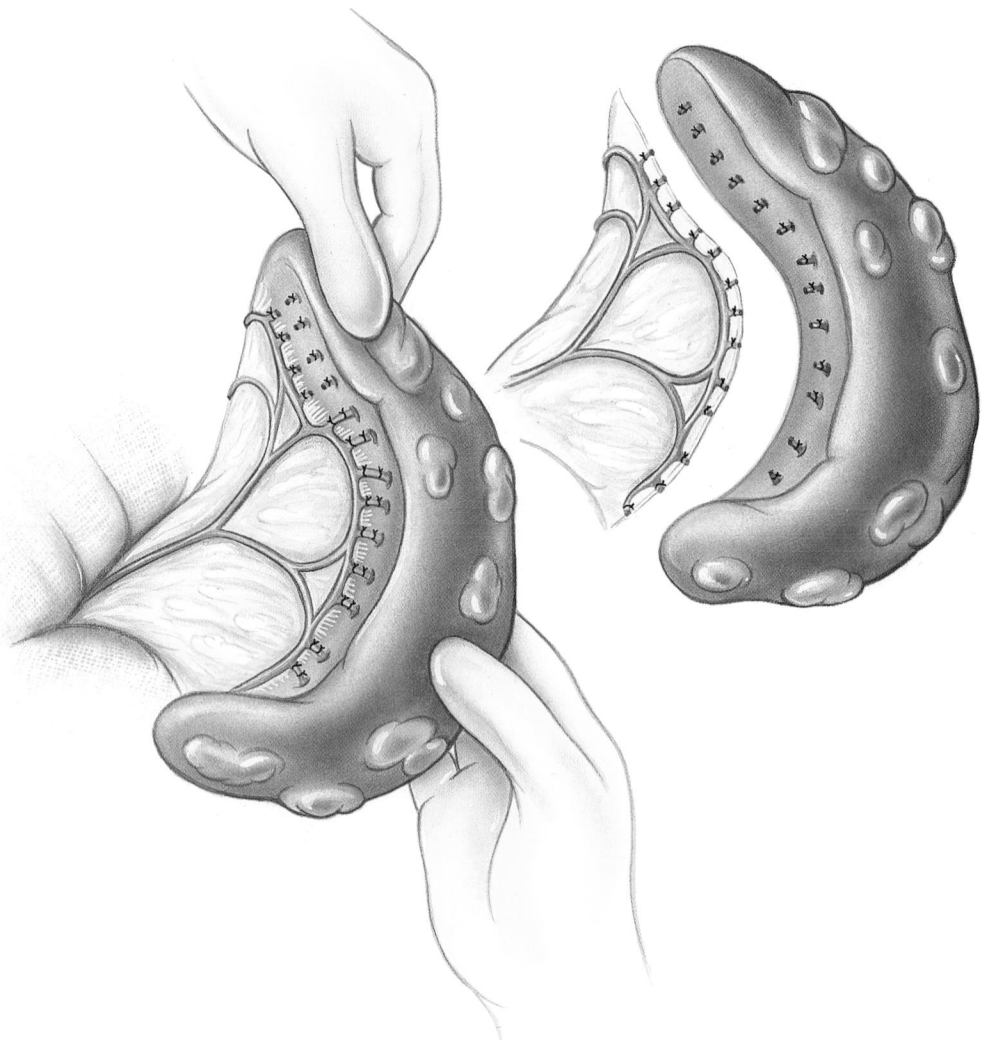

FIG. 23-12
For total splenectomy, double ligate and transect all vessels at the splenic hilus. If possible, preserve the short gastric branches supplying the gastric fundus.

NOTE: Gastropexy may be performed after splenectomy to reduce the incidence of GDV after removal of large splenic tumors or after splenic torsion; however, the frequency of occurrence of GDV after splenectomy is unknown and the need for this procedure is currently uncertain.

Interference with blood flow through the pancreatic branch of the splenic artery may cause pancreatic ischemia and peritonitis. An ultrasonically activated scalpel has been used for splenectomy in dogs with minimal need for vascular ligation (Royals et al, 2005).

SUTURE MATERIALS AND SPECIAL INSTRUMENTS

Other than a general soft tissue pack, special instruments are not required; however, a large number of clamps should be available for splenectomy. Absorbable suture material generally is used for splenic surgery. If generalized peritonitis is present, monofilament, synthetic absorbable suture (e.g.,

polydioxanone or polyglyconate) should be used to ligate vessels.

POSTOPERATIVE CARE AND ASSESSMENT

After splenic biopsy or splenectomy, the animal should be closely observed for 24 hours for evidence of hemorrhage. The hematocrit should be evaluated every few hours until the animal is stable. Nasal oxygen should be administered to anemic patients and analgesics given if necessary (see Chapter 13 [for opioid analgesics see Table 13-4; for NSAIDS see Tables 13-7 and 13-8; and for adjunctive drug therapy see Table 13-9]). Hemorrhage may indicate technical failures or DIC (which can be associated with neoplastic lesions or torsed spleens). Fluid therapy should be continued until the animal is able to maintain its own hydration, and electrolyte and acid-base abnormalities should be corrected. Mild postoperative leukocytosis may occur after splenectomy in dogs because the spleen influences bone marrow leukocyte production; however, steep or prolonged elevations may indicate infection (i.e., splenic abscess or peritonitis). An increase in the number of Howell-Jolly bodies, nucleated erythrocytes, target cells, and/or platelets may also be found after splenectomy.

COMPLICATIONS

The major complication of splenic surgery is hemorrhage. This is more of a problem with splenic biopsy or partial splenectomy than with total splenectomy, providing proper technique is used for vessel ligation. Reported complications of splenectomy in dogs include abscessation, traumatic pancreatitis, and gastric fistulation due to impairment of gastric blood flow. The risk of septic complications after splenectomy appears to be significant only in animals that are immunosuppressed before surgery (e.g., those undergoing immunosuppressive therapy for immune-mediated hemolytic anemia). Previous subclinical infections with hemoparasites (e.g., *Babesia, Ehrlichia, Mycoplasma* [formerly *Haemobartonella*] may become obvious after splenectomy.

SPECIAL AGE CONSIDERATIONS

Splenic surgery is most commonly performed in middle-aged or older animals. Special care must be taken to meet the metabolic and nutritional needs of these patients. Physical examinations and laboratory analyses must be thorough to determine if concurrent disease exists that may influence the surgery or postoperative care.

Reference

Royals SR, Ellison GW, Adin CA et al: Use of an ultrasonically activated scalpel for splenectomy in 10 dogs with naturally occurring splenic disease, *Vet Surg* 34:174, 2005.

Suggested Reading

Cuccovillo A, Lamb CR: Cellular features of sonographic target lesions of the liver and spleen in 21 dogs and a cat, *Vet Radiol Ultrasound* 43:275, 2002.
Hanson JA, Papageorges M, Girard E et al. Ultrasonographic appearance of splenic disease in 101 cats, *Vet Radiol Ultrasound* 42:441, 2001.

SPECIFIC DISEASES

SPLENIC TORSION

DEFINITION

Splenic torsion is the twisting of the spleen on its vascular pedicle.

GENERAL CONSIDERATIONS AND CLINICALLY RELEVANT PATHOPHYSIOLOGY

Splenic torsion most often occurs in association with GDV; isolated splenic torsion occurs rarely in dogs (Fig. 23-13). Typically the thin-walled splenic vein is occluded, although the splenic artery remains partly patent, resulting in congestive splenomegaly. Vascular thrombosis (particularly of the

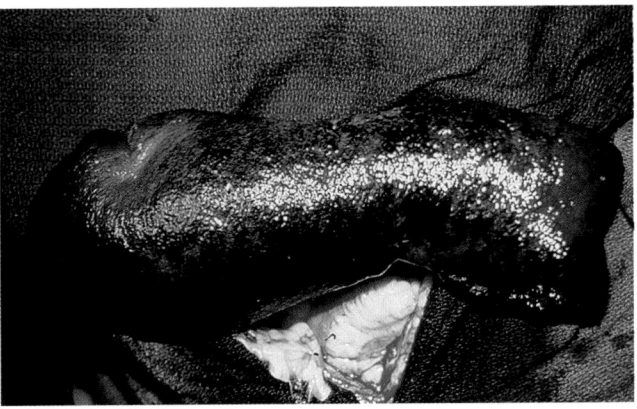

FIG. 23-13
Torsed spleen in a dog with acute cardiovascular collapse and shock. Note the dark, congested appearance of the spleen.

splenic vein) may occur. In some dogs the clinical signs are acute; in others the torsion presumably is intermittent, and abnormalities are noted weeks before diagnosis.

The cause of isolated splenic torsion is unclear. It may be related to congenital abnormalities or traumatic disruption of the gastrosplenic or splenocolic ligaments. It also has been hypothesized that splenic torsion may occur after partial gastric torsion (i.e., an intermittently malpositioned stomach), in which case the spleen remains torsed despite repositioning of the stomach. Primary splenic torsion may be acute or chronic. The chronic form is difficult to diagnose because clinical signs are sometimes vague and typically intermittent.

Splenic infarction may be associated with other disease, such as liver disease, renal disease, hyperadrenocorticism, neoplasia, or thrombosis associated with cardiovascular disease. In these cases splenic infarction appears to be a sign of altered blood flow and coagulation rather than of the primary disease. In such patients splenectomy should be reserved for animals with life-threatening complications, such as hemoabdomen or sepsis.

> **NOTE:** Splenic torsion can be acute and life threatening, requiring prompt diagnosis and treatment.

DIAGNOSIS
Clinical Presentation

Signalment. Splenic torsion usually occurs in large-breed dogs (e.g., Great Danes) and shows no age or gender predilection.

History. Most animals are presented for treatment because of some combination of vomiting, weakness or depression, icterus, hematuria or hemoglobinuria, abdominal pain, and/or diarrhea. Clinical signs may be acute or chronic. Some owners have reported chronic intermittent signs up to 3 weeks before evaluation. In one dog, torsion was thought to be associated with a diaphragmatic hernia that occurred 2 years previously (Weber, 2000). Acute torsion may cause signs of cardiovascular collapse and shock.

Physical Examination Findings

The most prominent physical examination finding is splenic enlargement or a midabdominal mass. Abdominal pain, fever, dehydration, pale mucous membranes, or icterus (or all of these) sometimes are found. Dogs with cardiovascular collapse and shock have tachycardia, pale mucous membranes, prolonged capillary refill times, and/or weak peripheral pulses.

Diagnostic Imaging

The most common radiographic findings are diminished visceral detail associated with peritoneal effusion and displacement of the small intestine by an enlarged spleen. The splenic outline often is difficult to discern. Sometimes, obvious splenomegaly is seen. If the dorsal extremity (head) or body of the spleen is not observed in its normal position, splenic torsion is suggested. Occasionally, gas bubbles are present within the splenic parenchyma, presumably formed by gas-producing bacteria (e.g., *Clostridium* spp.) in devitalized spleen.

Ultrasonographically the splenic parenchyma may be normal, hypoechoic, or anechoic with interspersed linear echoes. Ultrasonography may reveal a notably enlarged spleen that is diffusely hypoechoic, with linear echoes separating large, anechoic areas (Fig. 23-14). This pattern may be unique to splenic torsion. Enlargement of hilar splenic vessels may also suggest this condition. B-mode evaluation of the splenic veins for intraluminal echoes and spectral or color Doppler evaluation for absent velocity flow may be important assessments to make in dogs with splenic torsion and/or infarction. Visible splenic vein intraluminal echogenicities compatible with thrombi may be seen in dogs with splenic torsion on ultrasound associated with vascular congestion and compression and thrombosis of the splenic vein. Spectral Doppler and color Doppler imaging of the splenic vein will show an absence of flow in affected dogs.

Laboratory Findings

Laboratory analysis may reveal anemia, leukocytosis, hemoglobinuria, elevated serum alkaline phosphatase activity, and/or elevated alanine transaminase activity.

DIFFERENTIAL DIAGNOSIS

Differential diagnoses include other causes of splenomegaly (i.e., neoplasia, trauma, hematoma, abscess, or immune-mediated disease), peritoneal effusion (i.e., peritonitis or ascites), other midabdominal masses (e.g., gastrointestinal, pancreatic, renal, or lymph node enlargement), and GDV.

MEDICAL MANAGEMENT

Splenic torsion is a surgical disease; medical management usually is limited to stabilizing the animal for surgery (see later discussion in the Preoperative Management section). If the animal is shocky, intravenous fluids and antibiotic therapy should be initiated.

SURGICAL TREATMENT

The timing of surgical therapy is influenced by the animal's status at presentation. An animal presented for treatment with signs of shock should be operated on as quickly as possible after its condition has been stabilized. Surgery may be reasonably delayed for a short period in animals with chronic disease; however, prompt surgical intervention is recommended. Because GDV may occur in dogs after splenic torsion and stretching of the gastric ligaments, prophylactic gastropexy (see p. 416) may be warranted at the time of splenectomy.

Preoperative Management

If possible, fluid deficits and electrolyte and acid-base abnormalities should be corrected before surgery. Whole blood administration is warranted in animals with a hematocrit below 20% (see Box 5-1 on p. 25). Perioperative antibiotic therapy (e.g., cefazolin, 22 mg/kg IV) is recommended because vascular occlusion and necrosis may allow proliferation of bacteria in the spleen. Electrocardiograms are warranted to determine if cardiac arrhythmias are present that may require therapy before induction of anesthesia or during surgery. Blood transfusion products should be available because the enlarged and congested spleen may rupture with handling, causing abdominal hemorrhage.

Anesthesia

See GDV on p. 431 for anesthetic recommendations. Avoid barbiturates or other drugs that cause splenic congestion.

Surgical Anatomy

See p. 625 for the surgical anatomy of the spleen.

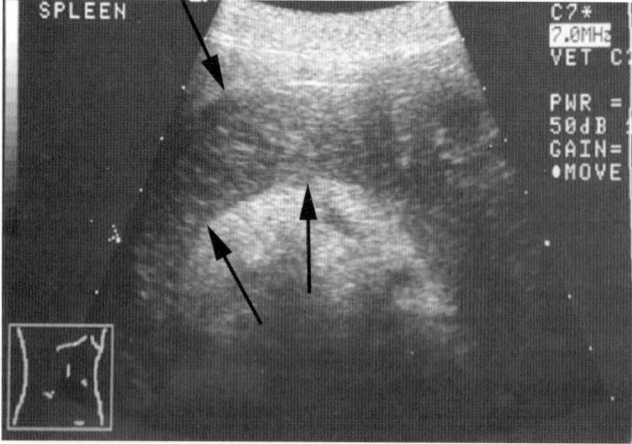

FIG. 23-14
Ultrasound image of the spleen in a dog with splenic torsion. Notice the hypoechoic appearance of the splenic parenchyma with hyperechoic lines throughout *(arrows)*.

Positioning

The animal is positioned in dorsal recumbency, and the entire ventral abdomen is prepared for aseptic surgery. The ventral incision should extend from the xiphoid and should be long enough to allow the enlarged spleen to be manipulated and exteriorized.

SURGICAL TECHNIQUE

Splenectomy (see p. 626) is the treatment of choice in dogs with acute splenic torsion because there is no good way to secure the spleen in its normal position, and torsion may recur. Furthermore, derotating the spleen may allow necrotic debris to enter the systemic circulation. Splenectomy is the only viable option in animals with chronic torsion in which the vascular pedicle cannot be untwisted because of fibrosis, splenic rupture, or vascular thrombosis. Gastropexy may be performed concurrently (see previous discussion on splenectomy).

SUTURE MATERIALS AND SPECIAL INSTRUMENTS

See p. 628 for the suture materials and special instruments used for splenectomy.

POSTOPERATIVE CARE AND ASSESSMENT

Most animals recover quickly after repositioning or removal of the torsed spleen. Intravenous fluid therapy should be continued until the animal is able to maintain its own hydration. Vomiting may occur postoperatively, associated with pancreatic ischemia and pancreatitis. The blood supply to the left limb of the pancreas arises from the splenic artery, and the vascular obstruction may extend to this pancreatic branch. Previously subclinical infections with hemoparasites (e.g., *Babesia, Ehrlichia, Mycoplasma* [formerly *Haemobartonella*]) may become obvious after splenectomy.

PROGNOSIS

The prognosis generally is good after surgical management of splenic torsion. Delayed diagnosis may result in splenic necrosis, sepsis, peritonitis, and/or DIC.

References

Janthur M: Splenic torsion in the dog with special emphasis on B mode and color Doppler imaging, *Berl Munch Tierarztl Wochenschr* 110:272, 1997.

Neath PJ, Brockman DJ, Saunders HM: Retrospective analysis of 19 cases of isolated torsion of the splenic pedicle in dogs, *J Small Anim Pract* 38:387, 1997.

Szatmari V, Pentek G, Voros K: Spontaneous resolution of splenic torsion in a dog, *Vet Rec* 147:247, 2000.

Weber NA: Chronic primary splenic torsion with peritoneal adhesions in a dog: case report and literature review, *J Am Anim Hosp Assoc* 36:390, 2000.

SPLENIC NEOPLASIA

DEFINITIONS

Hemangiosarcomas (HSA) are malignant neoplasms that arise from blood vessels; **hemangiomas** are benign tumors of dilated blood vessels. A **hematoma** is a swelling or mass of blood (usually clotted) confined to an organ, tissue, or space that is caused by seepage from any reason. Hemangiosarcoma is also known as *angiosarcoma* and *hemangioendothelioma*.

GENERAL CONSIDERATIONS AND CLINICALLY RELEVANT PATHOPHYSIOLOGY

The spleen is composed of a variety of tissues, and splenic neoplasia may arise from blood vessels, lymphoid tissue, smooth muscle, or the connective tissue that makes up the fibrous stroma. The most common tumor in dogs is HSA. Other malignant and benign (Box 23-3) neoplasms may also occur (Fig. 23-15). The most frequently recognized nonneoplastic lesions of the spleen are nodular hyperplasia, hemangioma, and hematoma (Fig. 23-16).

Canine splenic HSA is more common than all other types of malignant splenic tumors; it accounts for approximately half of all splenic malignancies identified. In a recent study, HSA was diagnosed in 70% of dogs presenting with acute nontraumatic hemoabdomen (Pintar et al, 2003). Because HSA arise from blood vessels, they may form in several different sites in the body (e.g., spleen, right atrium, subcutaneous tissue, and liver). As many as 25% of dogs with splenic HSA may have concurrent right atrial HSA. Splenic HSA are aggressive tumors that frequently metastasize to the liver, omentum, mesentery, and brain. A majority of dogs with HSA have gross evidence of metastatic disease on initial presentation.

Splenic hematomas vary in size and are encapsulated, blood- and fibrin-filled masses that often are grossly indistinguishable from HSA. Histologically, the cavities are surrounded by congestion, fibrosis, and areas of necrosis. They

BOX 23-3

Differential Diagnoses for Splenic Enlargement, Nodules, or Masses (in alphabetical order)

Neoplastic Disease	Nonneoplastic Disease
Benign	Abscessation
Fibroma	Extramedullary hematopoiesis
Hemangioma	Hematoma
Lipoma	Thrombosis/infarction
Myelolipoma	Torsion
Malignant	
Chondrosarcoma	
Fibrosarcoma	
Hemangiosarcoma	
Histiocytosis	
Liposarcoma	
Lymphosarcoma	
Mast cell tumor	
Mesenchymoma	
Metastatic neoplasia	
Myxosarcoma	
Osteosarcoma	
Rhabdomyosarcoma	
Undifferentiated/anaplastic sarcoma	

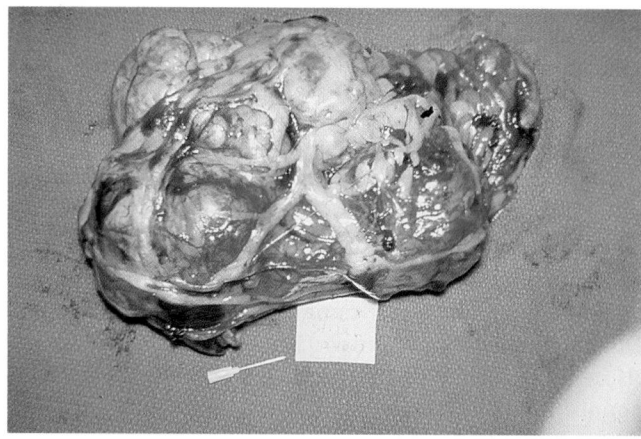

FIG. 23-15
Splenic leiomyosarcoma in a 6-year-old mixed-breed dog.

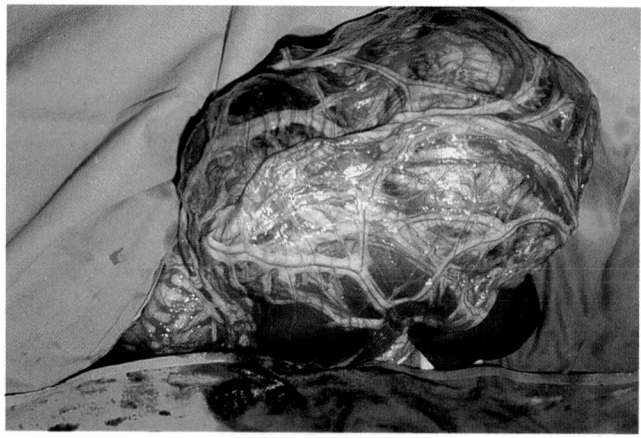

FIG. 23-16
Splenic hematoma in a 10-year-old Labrador retriever. Note the similar appearance of this benign mass to the malignant tumor in Fig. 23-15.

may result from trauma, may occur spontaneously, or may develop secondary to other diseases (e.g., nodular hyperplasia). Hemangiomas and HSA may be difficult to distinguish histologically, but because the prognosis for these lesions is very different (see later discussion), it is important that they be accurately differentiated. Splenic masses with evidence of malignant neoplastic endothelial cell proliferation can be easily identified as HSA. However, multiple sections of a malignant mass may be studied without obvious malignancy being seen. More important, proliferation of plump endothelial cells that resemble neoplastic endothelium, but do not have evidence of mitotic activity, may be misdiagnosed as HSA. Splenic hematoma and hemangioma account for 20% to 34% of splenic masses, whereas HSA accounts for 10% to 20% of all splenic samples submitted to veterinary pathology laboratories. However, this 10% to 20% underestimates the true incidence of HSA in dogs with large splenic masses because many such masses are not submitted for pathologic examination, especially if apparent metastasis is seen at surgery. Hyperplastic nodules are an even more common finding at necropsy than HSA.

Mastocytoma, lymphosarcoma, myeloproliferative disease, and HSA are the most common neoplasms of the feline spleen. Splenic involvement is a consistent finding in cats with noncutaneous systemic mastocytosis. It is not associated with the feline leukemia virus (FeLV) and is primarily a disease of older cats. Mast cell infiltrates may also be recognized in other organs (i.e., the liver, lymph nodes, and bone marrow), and circulating mastocytosis may be present in 50% of affected cats. Splenomegaly is one of the most common gross findings in feline mast cell disease, which usually is diagnosed by finding neoplastic cells in the circulation or on bone marrow examination. Splenic HSA is less commonly recognized in cats than in dogs. Extraabdominal metastasis of mast cell tumors, particularly to the myocardium, appears to be common.

DIAGNOSIS
Clinical Presentation

Signalment. Splenic tumors, including hematomas, usually occur in medium to large dogs. German shepherds are at increased risk for HSA and hemangioma. Some authors have reported that spayed female dogs have an increased risk, although others have reported this tumor to occur more often in male dogs. No breed or sex predisposition has been reported in cats with HSA, and no obvious breed or gender predilection has been observed in dogs with nonangiogenic and nonlymphomatous splenic sarcomas. The mean age of occurrence of HSA in dogs is 8 to 13 years and from 8 to 10.5 years in the cat.

History. Dogs with HSA may be presented because of abdominal enlargement, anorexia, lethargy, depression, and/or vomiting; or they may have acute signs of weakness, depression, anorexia, and hypovolemic shock caused by splenic rupture and hemorrhage. The clinical signs of splenic hematoma are similar, except that rupture leading to collapse and anorexia are less common because large masses frequently become apparent before rupture occurs. The most common clinical signs of disease with other types of sarcomas are diminished appetite, abdominal distention (as a result of peritoneal effusion or tumor mass or both), polydipsia, vomiting, and/or lethargy. In contrast to dogs with HSA, splenic rupture and hemorrhage are uncommon in dogs with nonangiogenic and nonlymphomatous splenic tumors.

Physical Examination Findings

The physical examination findings include lethargy, weakness, abdominal distention, and possibly splenomegaly or a splenic mass. If a splenic mass is palpated, it should be handled gently to prevent iatrogenic rupture. If abdominal effusion is present, it is not always possible to palpate the enlarged spleen. If rupture occurs, the animal may have signs of hypovolemic shock (tachycardia, pale mucous membranes, and weak peripheral pulses). Hemoabdomen is more commonly associated with HSA than with hemangioma or

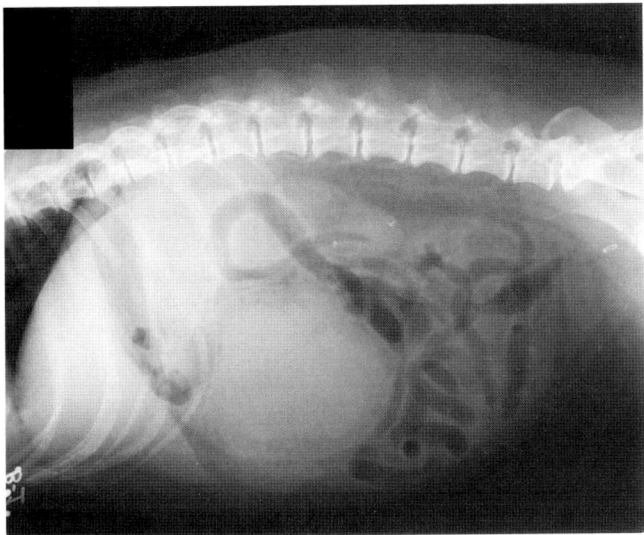

FIG. 23-17
Lateral radiograph of a dog with a large, soft tissue mass in the cranial ventral abdomen. This mass arose from the tail of the spleen.

hematoma. Some dogs with HSA will have cutaneous metastasis (dark reddish-purple mass). Sometimes a murmur is heard in patients with HSA in the right atrium; or pericardial effusion due to such an HSA may cause muffled heart sounds or a jugular pulse.

Diagnostic Imaging

Abdominal masses usually are detected radiographically in dogs with HSA and nonangiogenic and nonlymphomatous sarcomas; however, peritoneal fluid may make locating the lesion in the spleen difficult. Masses involving the tail of the spleen are typically identified in the cranial ventral abdomen on the lateral radiographic projection (Fig. 23-17). Thoracic radiographs should be taken in animals with splenic masses to detect pulmonary or thoracic neoplasia.

Ultrasonography is more definitive in locating lesions in the spleen and detecting abdominal metastases than radiography; however, differentiation of hematomas from neoplastic lesions is unreliable. Finding internal septation and encapsulation or apparent metastasis may help differentiate hematomas from HSA. A recent study suggested that there were significant differences in imaging characteristics between malignant and nonmalignant masses with contrast-enhanced computed tomography (CT), and thus it may be a useful diagnostic imaging modality for evaluation of focal canine splenic masses (Fife et al, 2004). Magnetic resonance imaging (MRI) may also be a useful tool for differentiating benign and malignant splenic lesions in dogs (Clifford et al, 2004).

NOTE: Before surgery, it may be wise to obtain an echocardiogram of the heart to look for right atrial HSA in dogs with splenic masses.

Laboratory Findings

Neutrophilic leukocytosis may be present in some dogs. Mild or moderate anemia associated with chronic disease or hemoperitoneum also is common. Other hematologic abnormalities caused by HSA may include numerous nucleated RBCs (inappropriate numbers for the degree of anemia), Howell-Jolly bodies, poikilocytosis, acanthocytosis, schistocytosis, and/or thrombocytopenia. Hemostatic disorders, particularly thrombocytopenia caused by DIC, are common in dogs with splenic tumors. Abdominal effusion generally is serosanguineous or hemorrhagic. Cytologic analysis of abdominal fluid rarely reveals tumor cells.

DIFFERENTIAL DIAGNOSIS

Splenic hematoma and hemangioma must be differentiated from HSA and other neoplastic diseases of the spleen (see comments above and Box 23-3). If cavitary lesions are identified ultrasonographically, fine-needle aspiration should be performed cautiously or not at all. Diagnosis of HSA is difficult with fine-needle aspirates because the cells exfoliate poorly. In addition, cytologic differentiation of hematomas and HSA with samples obtained by fine-needle aspiration often is impossible because large numbers of neoplastic cells frequently are necessary to make an accurate diagnosis. Furthermore, cavitary lesions may rupture during aspiration, which could be fatal. Exploratory surgery usually is indicated; however, it is difficult to differentiate these lesions by direct visualization. Although the presence of hepatic nodules may indicate metastasis and malignancy in dogs with splenic masses, the hepatic nodules may also represent extramedullary hematopoiesis or nodular hyperplasia in animals with benign or malignant tumors. If desired, one may perform laparoscopy first to see if there is apparent metastasis to liver, omentum, or peritoneum before deciding whether or not to do surgery. This is a potentially specific technique for finding metastatic disease undetectable by imaging, but its sensitivity is dependent upon the size of the metastatic lesions. Other causes of hemoperitoneum include hepatocellular carcinoma, rodenticide poisoning, and trauma.

NOTE: Histologic diagnosis of splenic HSA may require review of several sections of the mass.

MEDICAL MANAGEMENT

Surgical resection is the mainstay of therapy in dogs with splenic HSA; however, postoperative chemotherapy or immunotherapy may prolong survival. Readers are referred to an oncology text for discussion of protocols and treatment regimens used in dogs with HSA.

SURGICAL TREATMENT

Splenectomy is the treatment of choice for animals with splenic hematoma and hemangioma. It is also the treatment of choice for animals with HSA in which evidence of extensive metastasis or other organ failure does not preclude the short-term benefits of removing the enlarged or ruptured spleen. Laparoscopy is a more sensitive method of detecting visceral HSA metastasis than imaging and can be done before surgery to decide if surgery is appropriate for a given patient. Splenectomy may not be warranted in dogs with concurrent right atrial tumors, therefore careful preoperative examination (e.g., echocardiogram) of patients is necessary. Dogs with splenic lymphoma and clinical signs associated with massive splenomegaly, splenic rupture, and hemoperitoneum may also benefit from splenectomy. Gastropexy may be performed concurrently (see previous discussion on splenectomy).

Preoperative Management

Anemic animals may require blood transfusions (see Box 5-1 on p. 25) or purified hemoglobin (oxyglobin; see Table 5-5 on p. 28) before surgery, and they should be preoxygenated. An electrocardiogram should be performed to determine if ventricular arrhythmias requiring preoperative or intraoperative therapy are present. Ventricular arrhythmias are present in some dogs with splenic masses, and anemia and hemoabdomen may be strongly associated with arrhythmia development. Hydration, electrolyte, and acid-base abnormalities should be corrected before induction of anesthesia, but it must be remembered that fluid therapy may result in previously mild anemia being made worse; the hematocrit must be reexamined shortly before anesthesia. Perioperative antibiotics (e.g., cefazolin, 22 mg/kg IV) may be indicated in some animals undergoing splenectomy (see p. 624).

Anesthesia

See GDV (p. 431) for recommendations on anesthesia. Avoid barbiturates or other drugs that cause splenic congestion.

Surgical Anatomy

See p. 625 for the surgical anatomy of the spleen.

Positioning

The animal is placed in dorsal recumbency for a ventral midline celiotomy (see p. 319).

SURGICAL TECHNIQUE

Splenectomy is described on p. 626. Total splenectomy, rather than partial splenectomy, is warranted in animals with malignant tumors or large benign masses.

> NOTE: It is difficult to differentiate HSAs and hematomas. You must submit several samples of the mass for histopathologic evaluation.

SUTURE MATERIALS AND SPECIAL INSTRUMENTS

Surgical instruments for diseases of the spleen are described on p. 628. Patients with neoplasia (particularly debilitated animals) may heal poorly, therefore care should be taken in closing abdominal incisions, and strong, monofilament absorbable or nonabsorbable suture should be used.

POSTOPERATIVE CARE AND ASSESSMENT

Animals with splenic HSA should be closely observed for DIC after splenectomy. Fluid therapy should be continued until the animal can maintain its own hydration. The hematocrit should be monitored and blood transfusions provided if the PCV falls below 20%. Septic complications after splenectomy appear to be rare, and antibiotic therapy can be discontinued within 24 hours in most animals.

> NOTE: Be prepared to treat cardiac arrhythmias, particularly if hemoabdomen or anemia (or both) are present.

PROGNOSIS

Survival of dogs with HSA is typically not influenced by signalment, presenting signs, stage of disease, or clinicopathologic findings, although dogs with hemoperitoneum at the time of diagnosis may have a shortened survival. The median survival time of dogs with splenic HSA treated by splenectomy alone has varied from 19 to 86 days. Less than 10% of affected dogs will be alive at 1 year. Adjuvant chemotherapy may be prolong survival in some dogs. Because most tumors of the spleen cannot be differentiated on gross inspection alone and survival of dogs with hematomas is much longer than dogs with HSA-associated lesions, surgery should not be denied dogs in which a definitive diagnosis of HSA has not been made.

References

Clifford CA, Pretorius ES, Weisse C et al: Magnetic resonance imaging of focal splenic and hepatic lesions in the dog, *J Vet Intern Med* 28:330, 2004

Fife WD, Samii VF, Drost WT et al: Comparison between malignant and nonmalignant splenic masses in dogs using contrast-enhanced computed tomography, *Vet Radiol Ultrasound* 45:289, 2004.

Pintar J, Breitschwerdt EB, Hardie EM et al: Acute nontraumatic hemoabdomen in the dog: a retrospective analysis of 39 cases (1987-2001), *J Am Anim Hosp Assoc* 39:518, 2003.

Suggested Reading

Clifford CA, Mackin AJ, Henry CJ: Treatment of canine hemangiosarcoma: 2000 and beyond. *J Vet Intern Med* 14:479, 2000.
This manuscript reviews the use of multimodality therapy for treating HSA in dogs.

Smith AN: Hemangiosarcoma in dogs and cats, *Vet Clin Small Anim* 33:533, 2003.
A detailed review of HSA is given including information regarding chemotherapeutic protocols.

Wood CA, Moore AS, Gliatto JM et al: Prognosis for dogs with stage I or II splenic hemangiosarcoma treated by splenectomy alone: 32 cases (1991-1993). *J Am Anim Hosp Assoc* 34:417, 1998.

CHAPTER 24

Surgery of the Kidney and Ureter

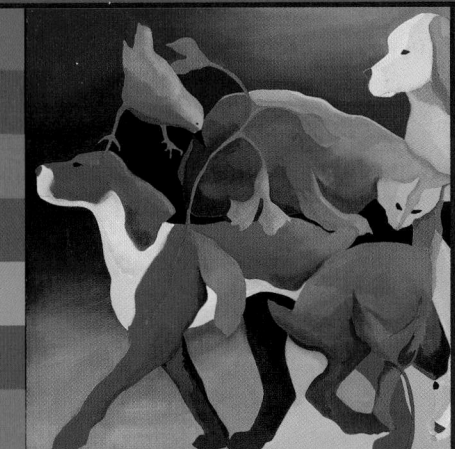

DEFINITIONS

Nephrectomy is excision of the kidney; **nephrotomy** is a surgical incision into the kidney. **Nephrostomy** is creation of a permanent fistula leading into the pelvis of the kidney; temporary nephrostomy tubes (**nephropyelostomy**) are occasionally used to divert urine when obstructive uropathy occurs or when the proximal ureter has been avulsed from the kidney. **Pyelolithotomy** is an incision into the renal pelvis and proximal ureter; a **ureterotomy** is an incision into the ureter; both are generally used to remove calculi. **Neo-ureterostomy** is a surgical procedure performed to correct intramural ectopic ureters; **ureteroneocystostomy** involves implantation of a resected ureter into the bladder. **Chronic renal disease** (CRD) refers to patients with azotemia or concentration deficits or excessive urinary protein loss that are clinically normal because they are able to compensate. **Renal failure** refers to patients that are unable to compensate for their renal disease and have clinical manifestations due to the abnormality. **Chronic renal failure** (CRF) refers to patients with CRD that are no longer able to compensate. They typically are anemic, polyuric-polydipsic, and/or have so much glomerular protein loss that signs associated with hypoalbuminemia ensue. **Acute renal failure** (ARF) refers to patients that have developed renal disease within the last 2 weeks and are in failure because of the recently acquired renal disease. Sometimes this becomes confusing; animals with CRF or CRD can become acutely worse if mild ARF is superimposed upon the chronic condition.

PREOPERATIVE MANAGEMENT

Renal, ureteral, or urethral disease may cause ARF or CRF, or disease in these organs may be associated with ARF or CRF from other causes. The minimum database for patients with urinary dysfunction includes measurement of the hematocrit, blood urea nitrogen (BUN), phosphorus, calcium, creatinine, total protein, albumin, magnesium, electrolytes (especially potassium), total carbon dioxide levels, urinalysis, blood pressure, and an electrocardiogram if electrolyte values

are not readily available. Renal patients may have significant metabolic derangements besides azotemia. CRF and especially ARF may be associated with varying degrees of dehydration. Oliguria may be present in ARF or in severe CRF; however, both ARF and CRF may be associated with polyuria. Preoperative intravenous (IV) fluid therapy is necessary to restore circulating blood volume and urine production; however, fluids must be administered judiciously to prevent overloading these patients. Diuretics may also be helpful for enhancing urine production in animals that are adequately hydrated. The urine production of hydrated animals on maintenance fluids that do not have abnormal extrarenal losses should be at least 50 ml/kg/day or more than 2 ml/kg/hr.

Various electrolyte and acid-base abnormalities may occur, depending on the severity and duration of the renal, urethral, or ureteral disease. Hyperkalemia often is present in ARF due to obstructive disorders, uroabdomen, parenchymal dysfunction, and very severe CRF. Hypokalemia may occur with CRD and diuretic therapy. Hyperkalemia and hypokalemia predispose the patient to cardiac arrhythmias and should be corrected before surgery. Hypermagnesemia and hypomagnesemia can likewise cause cardiac conduction disturbances and central nervous system (CNS) aberrations, if severe. Clinically important hypocalcemia occasionally is associated with ARF. Metabolic acidosis may also be present in animals with ARF or CRF, but tends to be worse with ARF.

NOTE: Abnormalities in the serum potassium level may lead to cardiac arrhythmias and death; correct these abnormalities before surgery.

Animals with CRF are typically anemic, assuming that dehydration has not masked the anemia. Diminished erythropoietin production by the kidneys is responsible. Elevated circulating parathormone concentrations may also have a negative effect on erythropoietin concentrations. Gastric ulceration, bleeding, or increased red cell fragility may occur in uremic patients. Coagulation profiles are warranted in animals with severe ARF or CRF. Normally hydrated animals with a packed cell volume (PCV) below 20% or a hemoglobin level below 5 g/dl may benefit from preoperative blood transfusions (see Box 5-1 on p. 25).

ANESTHETIC CONSIDERATIONS

Severely anemic patients should be transfused before induction of anesthesia and may benefit from oxygen before, during, and after anesthesia. Anticholinergic drugs are used to prevent bradycardia. Systemic arterial blood pressure should be monitored in severely ill patients, and urine output should be monitored during surgery. Because of intrinsic properties of the kidney, renal blood flow tends to remain constant despite variations in the systemic arterial pressure between 75 and 160 mm Hg, a phenomenon called autoregulation. However, hypotension during surgery may cause renal vasoconstriction, diminished blood flow, and subsequent renal damage. Hypotensive drugs (e.g., acetylpromazine) should not be used in animals with renal impairment. If the animal is oliguric but normotensive, low-dose dopamine (1 to 2 mg/kg/min given IV) with or without furosemide (2.0 mg/kg given IV or a constant rate infusion of 0.6 mg/kg/hr) can be tried. As an alternative, mannitol (0.25 to 0.5 g/kg given IV) may be used in cats. If both oliguria and hypotension are present, dopamine (2 to 10 μg/kg/min given IV) or dobutamine (2 to 10 μg/kg/min given IV) may be administered. Once oliguria is established, dopamine is minimally effective at creating a polyuric state. Thiobarbiturates should be avoided if arrhythmias are present. Isoflurane and sevoflurane are the inhalation agents of choice in arrhythmic patients. If nephrectomy is to be performed, function in the remaining kidney should be protected by ensuring adequate blood flow during and after surgery.

The following general anesthetic principles should be considered in animals with renal disease. The patient may be premedicated with an anticholinergic (i.e., atropine or glycopyrrolate; Box 24-1) and hydromorphone, butorphanol, or buprenorphine (Boxes 24-1 and 24-2). If the animal has minimal renal compromise, a thiobarbiturate, propofol, or a mask can be used for induction. Ketamine should be avoided in cats with renal compromise. If a dog is severely depressed, hydromorphone plus diazepam (see Box 24-2) may allow intubation. If additional drugs are needed, etomidate (see Box 24-2) or a reduced dose of thiobarbiturate or propofol may be administered IV, or mask induction may be used if the animal is not vomiting. Urine output should be monitored during and after surgery.

The use of IV fluids in healthy dogs undergoing elective procedures is controversial. IV fluids have typically been recommended in this population of animals to offset the myocardial depression and vasodilation associated with inhalant anesthetics that may result in decreased cardiac output and lowered blood pressure with subsequent decreased renal perfusion. However, one study did not detect clinically relevant signs of renal dysfunction in a group of healthy dogs undergoing elective surgery (Lobetti and Lambrechts, 2000). The authors suggested that IV administration of flu-

BOX 24-1

Selected Anesthetic Protocols for Use in Stable Dogs and Cats With Renal Disease

Premedication

Give atropine (0.02–0.04 mg/kg SC or IM) or glycopyrrolate (0.005-0.011 mg/kg SC or IM) plus hydromorphone* (0.1–0.2 mg/kg SC or IM); or butorphanol (0.2–0.4 mg/kg SC or IM); or buprenorphine (5–15 μg/kg IM)

Induction

Thiopental (10–12 mg/kg IV) or propofol (4–6 mg/kg IV) (see text also)

Maintenance

Isoflurane or sevoflurane

SC, Subcutaneous; *IM,* intramuscular; *IV,* intravenous.
*Use 0.05 mg/kg in cats.

BOX 24-2

Selected Anesthetic Protocols for Use in Decompensated Patients in Renal Failure or in Hypovolemic, Dehydrated, or Shocky Animals

Dogs
Premedication and induction

Hydromorphone (0.1 mg/kg IV) plus diazepam (0.2 mg/kg IV), give in incremental doses. Intubate if possible. If necessary, give etomidate (0.5–1.5 mg/kg IV)

Maintenance

Isoflurane or sevoflurane

Cats
Premedication

Butorphanol (0.2–0.4 mg/kg SC or IM) or buprenorphine (5–15 μg/kg IM) or hydromorphone (0.05 mg/kg SC or IM)

Induction

Diazepam (0.2 mg/kg IV) followed by etomidate (0.5–1.5 mg/kg IV) (see text also)

Maintenance

Isoflurane or sevoflurane

IV, Intravenous; *SC,* subcutaneous; *IM,* intramuscular.

ids to healthy dogs undergoing elective surgery (not those undergoing renal surgery) may not be necessary for maintenance of renal homeostasis. IV fluids should be given to dogs with renal disease. Potentially nephrotoxic drugs (e.g., aminoglycosides and nonsteroidal antiinflammatory drugs [NSAIDs]) should be avoided, if possible. NSAIDs are often well tolerated by healthy dogs undergoing anesthesia, but

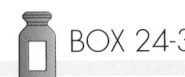 BOX 24-3

Selected Antibiotics of Use in Animals With Renal Disease

Ampicillin
22 mg/kg IV, IM, SC, tid

Amoxicillin plus Clavulanate (Clavamox)
Dogs: 12.5–25 mg/kg PO, bid
Cats: 62.5 mg PO, bid

Cefazolin (Ancef, Kefzol)
22 mg/kg IV or IM, bid to tid

Cephalexin
22 mg/kg PO, tid

Enrofloxacin (Baytril)
2.5 mg/kg PO or IV, bid for simple UTI
7–20 mg/kg PO or IV, qd for pyelonephritis

IV, Intravenous; *IM,* intramuscular; *SC,* subcutaneous; *tid,* three times a day; *PO,* oral; *bid,* twice a day; *qid,* four times a day; *qd,* once a day; *UTI,* urinary tract infection.

when combined with other nephrotoxic drugs or given to dogs with CRD, NSAIDs may cause ARF.

ANTIBIOTICS

Animals with renal calculi, ectopic ureters, or urinary tract obstruction may have concurrent infections and should be given appropriate antibiotics based on urine culture and susceptibility testing; or antibiotics can be withheld until appropriate intraoperative cultures have been taken. Potentially nephrotoxic antibiotics (i.e., aminoglycosides, tetracycline [except doxycycline], and sulfonamides) should be avoided, if possible. Penicillins and cephalosporins (e.g., ampicillin, amoxicillin, cefazolin, cephalexin; Box 24-3) are highly concentrated in urine. They are effective against most gram-positive organisms, and cephalosporins also have an enhanced gram-negative spectrum. Fluoroquinolones (e.g., enrofloxacin; see Box 24-3) have broad activity against aerobic gram-negative bacteria. Drug doses or dosing frequency should be altered as required by the degree of renal compromise.

SURGICAL ANATOMY

The kidneys lie in the retroperitoneal space lateral to the aorta and caudal vena cava. They have a fibrous capsule and are held in position by subperitoneal connective tissue. The cranial pole of the right kidney lies at the level of the thirteenth rib. In an average-sized dog, the cranial pole of the left kidney lies about 5 cm caudal to the upper third of the last rib. The renal pelvis is the funnel-shaped structure that receives urine and directs it into the ureter. Generally, five or six diverticula curve outward from the renal pelvis. The renal artery normally bifurcates into dorsal and ventral branches; however, variations are common. The ureter begins at the renal pelvis and enters the dorsal surface of the bladder obliquely by means of two slitlike orifices. The blood supply

to the ureter is from the cranial ureteral artery (from the renal artery) and the caudal ureteral artery (from the prostatic or vaginal artery).

> NOTE: The anatomy of the renal vasculature varies considerably, so use care when ligating these vessels during nephrectomy.

SURGICAL TECHNIQUE

For the kidney, a ventral midline abdominal incision is performed from the xiphoid to caudal to the umbilicus. If the distal ureter must be transected (i.e., for nephrectomy) or if a cystotomy is necessary, the incision should extend to the pubis. Balfour retractors are used to retract the abdominal wall and expose the kidney. The entire abdominal contents should be inspected before exploring the urinary tract. The right kidney is exposed by elevating the duodenum and displacing the other loops of intestine toward the animal's left side. Similarly the left kidney is exposed by elevating the mesocolon so that the small intestine is retracted to the animal's right side. The kidney can be isolated from the remaining abdominal contents with moistened laparotomy sponges.

Renal Biopsy

Renal biopsy may be indicated to diagnose the cause of ARF, renal infiltrative disease, hematuria (rare), and sometimes proteinuria. It may be performed at surgery or it may be done percutaneously by ultrasonography, laparoscopy, or digitally using a keyhole abdominal incision. Ultrasound-guided and laparoscopic biopsies are the preferable percutaneous techniques. Percutaneous biopsy should be avoided in patients with bleeding disorders, large intrarenal cysts, perirenal abscesses, and obstructive uropathy. Giving fluids before, during, and shortly after biopsy to initiate and maintain a mild diuresis may reduce the formation of blood clots in the renal pelvis that could cause hydronephrosis. Spring-loaded biopsy needles, biopsy guns, or manual devices—such as a TruCut device—may be used. Advantages of the spring-loaded devices are that they can be manipulated with one hand. In healthy dogs, serial ultrasound-guided renal biopsies were not found to induce functional changes in the kidneys or histologic changes that might be confused with progressive renal disease (Groman et al, 2004).

> NOTE: For patients with glomerular disease, obtain at least two quality samples; for patients with acute renal failure, one quality sample may suffice. It is critical that the sample primarily consist of renal cortex; medullary tissue samples are of minimal value in most cases. Obtaining multiple biopsies of the kidney does not appear to produce more damage than a biopsy with only a single pass, provided that the biopsy needle remains in cortical tissue (Vaden, 2004).

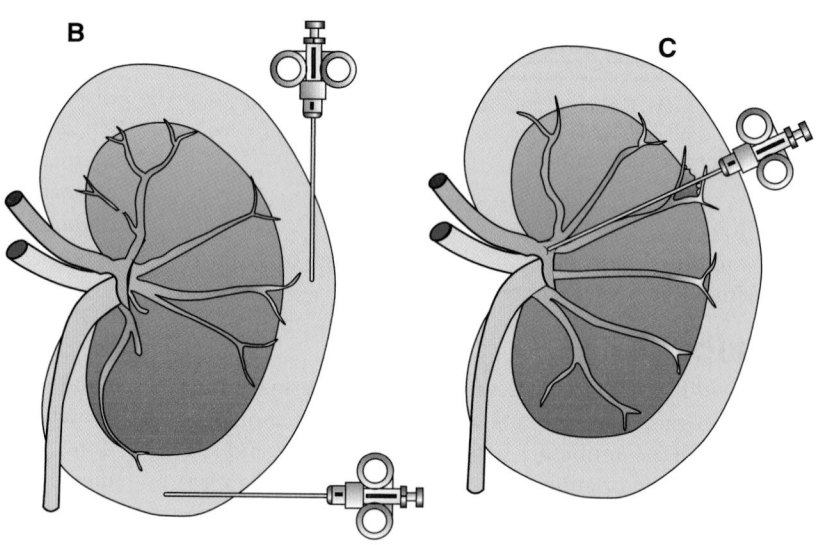

FIG. 24-1
A, Monopty biopsy needle with biopsy guide attached. **B,** To obtain a biopsy of the kidney, advance the biopsy instrument until it penetrates the capsule. Position the biopsy needle to take a biopsy of the renal cortex. **C,** Do not advance too deeply to avoid transecting the large arcuate vessel.

Ultrasound-guided percutaneous biopsy. Ultrasound-guided percutaneous biopsies require heavy sedation or preferably general anesthetic. Place the patient in ventrodorsal recumbency. If generalized disease is suspected such as occurs with glomerular disease, the right kidney is the preferred side for a biopsy because it is technically easier. However, either kidney may be sampled from this position.

*Clip the hair over the biopsy site and aseptically prepare it. Place a sterile sleeve over the ultrasound probe. Using sterile ultrasound coupling gel, identify and examine the kidney. Once the site of entry for the biopsy has been determined (the safest location is to pass the biopsy instrument through the most lateral aspect of the kidney cortex; this is the furthest area away from the major vasculature, which should be avoided), make a small stab incision in the skin using a No. 15 Bard-Parker scalpel blade. Insert the biopsy device (e.g., an 18- or 16-gauge, single spring-fired biopsy core needle [E-Z Core Single Action Biopsy Device, Products Group International, Lyons Colo.] or an automatic spring-loaded biopsy gun [e.g., Bard Biopty or Monopty single-use spring-*loaded disposable biopsy instrument, C. R. Bard, Murray Hill, N.J.]) through the nick in the skin, and advance it until it just penetrates the kidney capsule (Fig 24-1, A). Position the biopsy needle such that a biopsy is taken of the glomerular tissue in the renal cortex, rather than medullary tissue (Fig. 24-1, B). Place the tip of the needle through the renal capsule before activating it to prevent sliding of the needle along the capsule and to avoid tearing the capsule. Fire the biopsy device, and retract the needle through the skin. Gently manipulate the sample from the biopsy needle and place it into 10% formalin solution for light microscopy; into glutaraldehyde for electron microscopy; freeze it for immunofluorescence; or place it into other preservatives for special tests.*

NOTE: Do not place the biopsy needle too deeply or you may end up with too few glomeruli in your sample. You could also transect the large arcuate vessels (Fig. 24-1, C) by placing the biopsy needle too deeply.

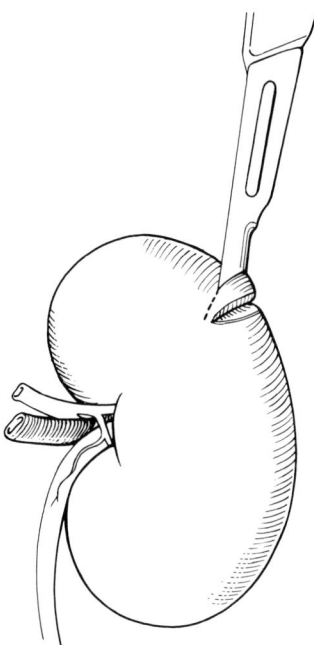

FIG. 24-2
Wedge biopsies provide larger samples than needle biopsies.

Laparoscopic-guided biopsy. Laparoscopy for renal biopsy requires general anesthetic. In general, renal biopsy is only done laparoscopically when other biopsies (e.g., hepatic and pancreatic) are required and are the primary indication for laparoscopy. If the primary purpose of the procedure is to obtain renal biopsies, ultrasound is the preferred technique. Double puncture or single puncture laparoscopy will suffice for renal biopsy.

Using a No. 15 Bard-Parker scalpel blade, make a third small opening for penetration of a 14-gauge core biopsy needle. Use the manipulation instrument to position and secure the kidney, and place a double spring-fired biopsy needle against the renal capsule and direct it tangentially before discharge. After the biopsy, withdraw the needle and apply pressure via the manipulating instruments. Process the sample as described previously.

Surgical biopsy. Surgical biopsies may be performed using an automatic biopsy instrument (see previous discussion) or a manual device, such as a TruCut or Franklin modified Vim-Silverman biopsy needle), or a wedge resection can be performed using a scalpel blade (Fig. 24-2). Spring-loaded devices are easier to use than manual devices and can be manipulated with one hand. Wedge resection allows a larger sample to be obtained than do needles or guns. With either technique, it is important to ensure that adequate amounts of cortical tissue are obtained.

Needle biopsy. *Perform a needle biopsy with a Tru-Cut type instrument by placing the tip of the instrument on*

the kidney capsule with the obturator specimen rod fully retracted within the outer cannula. Position the biopsy needle as described previously (see Fig. 24-1). Push the specimen rod into the lesion by advancing the plastic handle or by triggering the firing mechanism. With manual devices, advance the outer sheath of the needle into the tissue to sever the biopsy sample. Withdraw the needle with the outer sheath over the specimen rod. Apply digital pressure to the site to control hemorrhage. Be sure the sample is primarily cortical tissue. Process the sample as described previously.

NOTE: Avoid taking a biopsy near the renal pelvis to prevent extravasation of urine. To make sure that you get a diagnostic sample, position the biopsy device across the cortex, as indicated previously.

Wedge biopsy. *For a wedge biopsy, make an incision into the renal parenchyma with a No. 15 scalpel blade. Make another incision at an angle to the first incision to remove a wedged-shaped piece of parenchyma (see Fig. 24-2). Be sure to include cortex in the sample. Close the incision with a mattress suture of 3-0 absorbable suture material.*

Nephrectomy

Nephrectomy (ureteronephrectomy) is indicated for renal neoplasia, severe trauma resulting in uncontrollable hemorrhage or urine leakage, pyelonephritis resistant to medical therapy (e.g., associated with nephroliths), hydronephrosis, and ureteral abnormalities that defy surgical repair (i.e., avulsion, stricture, rupture, or obstruction due to calculi). Traumatic ureteral rupture was recently reported in 10 animals (Weisse et al, 2002). Nephrectomy was performed in six animals and ureteroneocystostomy was performed in two. The two animals that did not receive nephrectomies died of ARF postoperatively, suggesting that in animals with normal renal function in the contralateral kidney nephrectomy may be the best option to treat ureteral rupture. Before nephrectomy, renal function in the opposite kidney should be assessed by determining its glomerular filtration rate (GFR) if possible. Excretory urograms are not innocuous and can cause anuric or oliguric renal failure in animals with previously mild or moderate renal disease. If excretory urograms are done, avoid large doses of contrast material and maintain good renal perfusion during and after the procedure. Bilateral renal dysfunction may warrant a guarded prognosis. If renal neoplasia is suspected, radiography (thoracic and abdominal) and ultrasonography should be used to help rule out metastasis, including to the opposite kidney. To avoid unintentional transection, the opposite ureter should always be identified; this is particularly important when removing large neoplasms.

Grasp the peritoneum over the kidney and incise it. Using a combination of blunt and sharp dissection, free the kidney from its sublumbar attachments. Elevate the kidney and retract it medially to locate the renal artery and vein on the

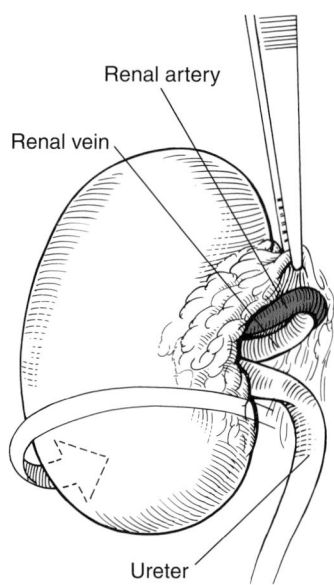

Renal artery

Renal vein

Ureter

FIG. 24-3
During nephrectomy, elevate the kidney and retract it medially to locate the renal artery and vein on the dorsal surface of the renal hilus.

dorsal surface of the renal hilus (Fig. 24-3). Identify any branches of the renal artery. Double ligate the renal artery with absorbable suture (e.g., polydioxanone, polyglyconate, or poliglecaprone 25) or nonabsorbable suture (e.g., cardiovascular silk) close to the abdominal aorta to ensure that all branches have been ligated. Identify the renal vein and ligate it similarly.

The left ovarian and testicular veins drain into the renal vein and should not be ligated in intact dogs. Avoid ligating the renal artery and vein together to prevent the formation of an arteriovenous fistula.

Ligate the ureter near the bladder. Remove the kidney and ureter and after procuring appropriate culture specimens, submit them for histologic examination.

Partial Nephrectomy

Partial nephrectomy occasionally is warranted for focal renal lesions, particularly if optimal preservation of renal function is necessary because of bilateral renal dysfunction. However, in most cases total nephrectomy is usually easier and carries less risk of postoperative hemorrhage. If partial nephrectomy is performed, electrocoagulation of bleeding vessels should be avoided because it causes excessive parenchymal damage. Avoid partial nephrectomy in animals with clinically significant coagulopathies; excessive blood loss may occur after this procedure.

If possible, strip the renal capsule from the area of the kidney to be excised. Use absorbable suture (No. 0 or 1) with two long, straight needles attached. Thread the needles into the

kidney at the proposed resection site (Fig. 24-4, A and B). Tie the thread into three separate ligatures but avoid damaging the renal vessels or ureter (Fig. 24-4, C). Excise the renal tissue distal to these ligatures. Ligate any bleeders and suture the exposed diverticula with absorbable suture (2-0 or 3-0). Approximate the capsule over the end of the kidney (Fig. 24-4, D) and anchor it to the sublumbar tissues to prevent rotation of the kidney. As an alternative, clamp the renal vessels with vascular forceps and excise the kidney parenchyma. Ligate the parenchymal vessels and close the renal pelvis and diverticula. Suture the capsule as described previously and remove the clamps from the renal vessels.

Nephrotomy

Nephrotomy usually is performed to remove calculi (see p. 654) lodged in the renal pelvis, but it may also be performed to explore the renal pelvis for neoplasia or hematuria. Nephrotomy should be avoided in patients with severe hydronephrosis because ample parenchyma may not be available to prevent postoperative urine leakage. In addition, nephrotomy may temporarily diminish renal function by 25% to 50%. Although bilateral nephrotomies can be performed, this could precipitate ARF if renal function is sufficiently compromised preoperatively. Staged procedures are indicated in such patients. Nephrotomy may be done by bisecting the kidney or by using an intersegmental approach where the plane of dissection follows the terminal branches of the posterior and anterior renal arteries. The interlobar arteries are not transected, which theoretically minimizes nephron destruction. A recent study found that neither technique affected GFR in dogs; thus, because the bisection approach requires less surgical manipulation and time, it is preferred (Stone et al, 2002).

Nephrotomy incisions may be closed without sutures or with transparenchymal horizontal mattress sutures. The latter may cause increased vascular strangulation, pressure necrosis, infarction, and postoperative hemorrhage. Cyanoacrylate adhesive provides rapid hemostasis; however, if the adhesive enters the renal diverticula, calculi may form.

Locate the renal vessels and temporarily occlude them with vascular forceps, a tourniquet, or an assistant's fingers. Mobilize the kidney to expose the convex lateral surface. Make a sharp incision along the midline of the convex border of the kidney capsule, then bluntly dissect through the renal parenchyma, ligating renal vessels as necessary (Fig. 24-5). Culture the renal pelvis. Remove the calculi and flush the kidney with warm saline or lactated Ringer's solution. Assess the ureter for patency by placing a 3.5 French soft rubber catheter down the ureter and flushing it with warm fluids. Close the nephrotomy by apposing the cut tissues and applying digital pressure for approximately 5 minutes while restoring blood flow through the renal vessels (sutureless technique). As an alternative, appose the capsule with a continuous pattern of absorbable suture material (see Fig. 24-5). If adequate hemostasis is not achieved or if urine leakage is a concern, place absorbable sutures through the cortex in a horizontal mattress fashion (see previous com-

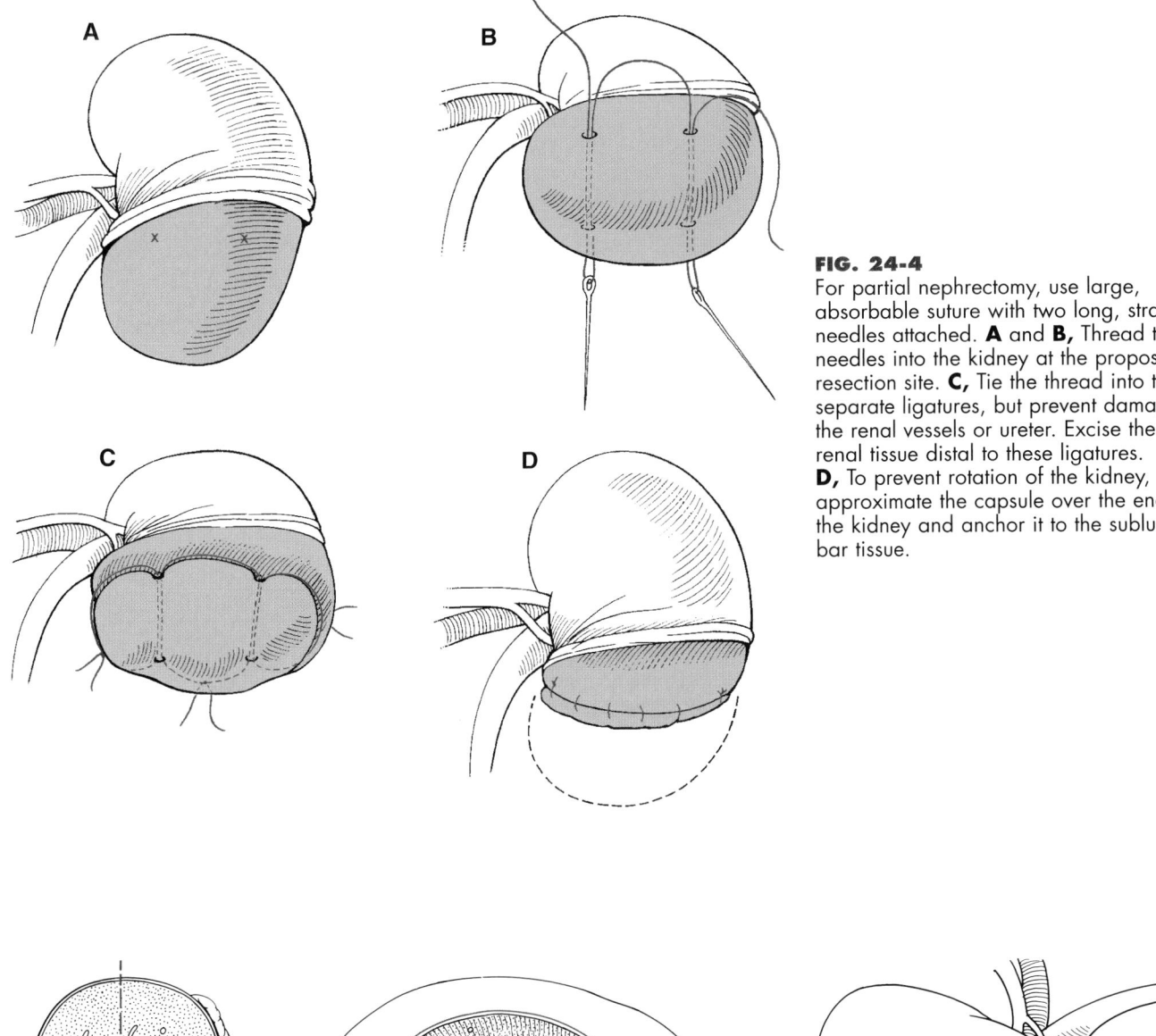

FIG. 24-4
For partial nephrectomy, use large, absorbable suture with two long, straight needles attached. **A** and **B,** Thread the needles into the kidney at the proposed resection site. **C,** Tie the thread into three separate ligatures, but prevent damaging the renal vessels or ureter. Excise the renal tissue distal to these ligatures. **D,** To prevent rotation of the kidney, approximate the capsule over the end of the kidney and anchor it to the sublumbar tissue.

FIG. 24-5
Nephrotomy usually is performed to remove calculi lodged in the renal pelvis. Make a sharp incision along the capsule of the convex border of the kidney, and bluntly dissect the renal parenchyma to the renal pelvis. Remove the calculi and close the nephrotomy by apposing the cut tissue and suturing the capsule in a continuous pattern with absorbable suture material (see text for sutureless technique). If adequate hemostasis is not achieved or if urine leakage is a concern, place absorbable sutures through the cortex in a horizontal mattress fashion. Then suture the capsule in a continuous pattern with absorbable suture material.

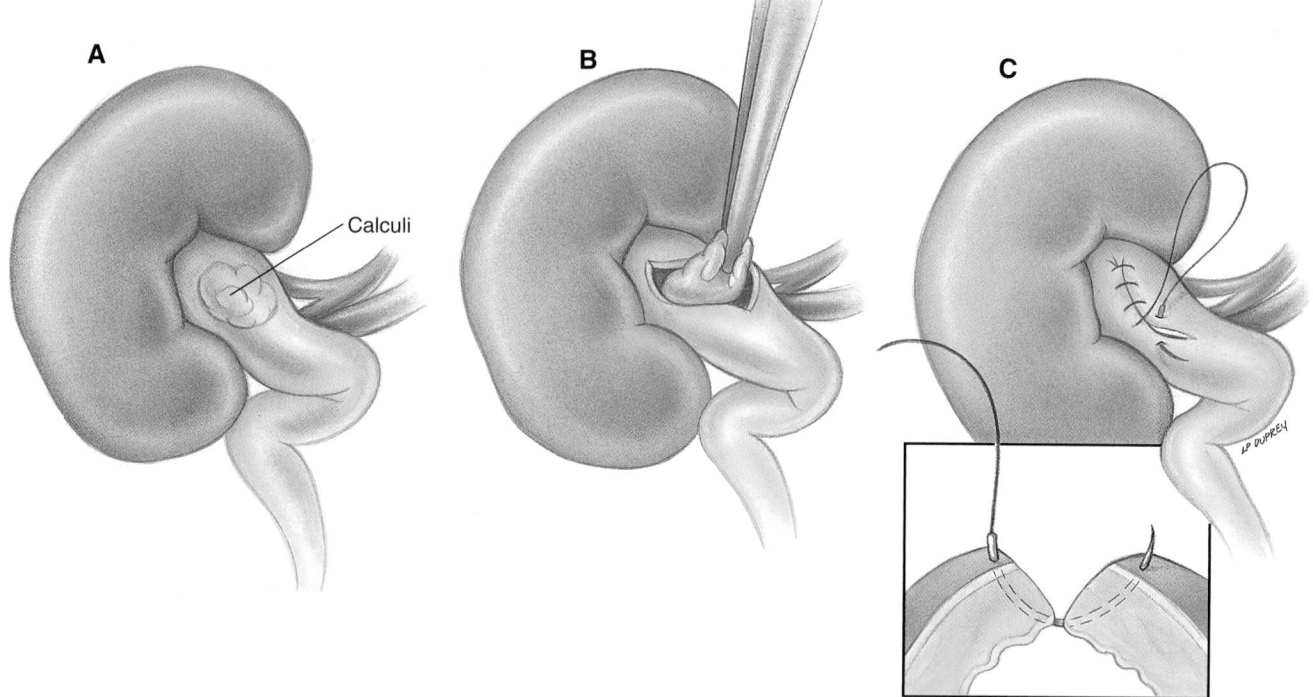

FIG. 24-6
Pyelolithotomy may be performed when the proximal ureter is dilated. **A,** Expose the dorsal surface of the kidney, and identify the ureter and renal vessels. **B,** Make an incision over the dilated pelvis and proximal ureter and remove the calculi. **C,** Close the incision in a continuous pattern with absorbable suture.

ments and Fig. 24-5). Then suture the capsule in a continuous pattern with absorbable suture. Replace the kidney in its original location. Sutures may be placed in the peritoneum where the kidney was elevated to help stabilize it.

Pyelolithotomy

Pyelolithotomy may be performed to remove renal calculi if the proximal ureter and renal pelvis are sufficiently dilated. This procedure prevents trauma to the renal parenchyma associated with nephrotomy. Pyelolithotomy is extremely difficult if the ureter is not dilated.

Dissect the kidney from its sublumbar attachments, and expose the dorsal surface. Identify the ureter and renal vessels (Fig. 24-6, A). Make an incision over the dilated pelvis and proximal ureter, and remove the calculi (Fig. 24-6, B). Flush the renal pelvis and diverticula with warm saline to remove small debris. Next, flush the ureter to ensure its patency. Close the incision in a continuous pattern with 5-0 or 6-0 absorbable suture (Fig. 24-6, C).

Ureterotomy

Ureterotomy occasionally is performed to remove obstructive calculi. The procedure carries the risk of postoperative leakage and stricture formation and should be performed with care. If obstruction is not present, dietary dissolution of struvite calculi may be attempted. However, removal of calculi is indicated if obstruction occurs or seems likely (e.g.,

hydroureter or hydronephrosis). Depending on the animal's size, removal of the stones with a ureteroscope may be possible. Some stones in the distal ureter may be flushed or pulled into the bladder through a cystotomy, making a ureterotomy unnecessary. Although ureteral mucosa regenerates over a stent if the mucosa has not been completely disrupted, the use of stenting catheters is controversial because they may promote stricture formation and infection. If stents are used, they should be smaller than the diameter of the ureter. In some animals, ureteral stents may be placed so that they exit the urethral orifice and are sutured to the exterior. Transverse or longitudinal incisions may be made in the ureter; however, there may be less tension on transverse ureterotomies, which therefore may heal more readily.

Make a transverse or longitudinal incision in the dilated ureter proximal to the calculi and remove them (Fig. 24-7, A). Place a small, soft rubber catheter into the ureter proximal and distal to the incision, and flush the ureter with warm fluid. Make sure that all calculi have been removed and that the ureter is patent. Close the incision in a simple interrupted pattern with 5-0 to 7-0 absorbable suture (Fig. 24-7, B). As an alternative, if the ureter is not dilated and if stricture formation seems likely, make a longitudinal incision over the calculi and close the incision in a transverse fashion (Fig. 24-7, C). If the ureter has been damaged, perform a resection and anastomosis (see next section) or proximal urinary diversion via a nephropyelostomy tube (see p. 643).

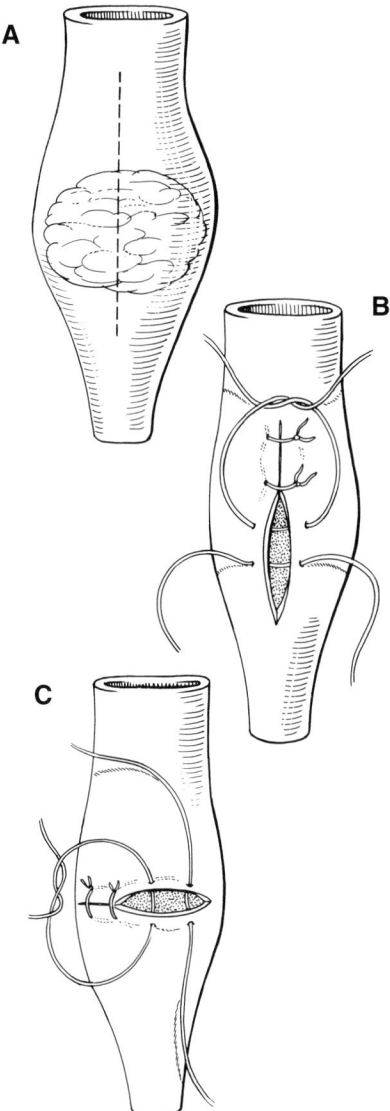

FIG. 24-7
Ureterotomy occasionally is performed to remove obstructive calculi. **A,** Make a transverse or longitudinal incision in the dilated ureter proximal to the calculi and remove them. **B,** Close the incision in a simple interrupted pattern with absorbable suture. **C,** As an alternative, make a longitudinal incision over the calculi, and close the incision in a transverse fashion with absorbable suture.

NOTE: Ureterotomy and ureteral anastomosis are greatly facilitated by wearing loupes for magnification.

Ureteral Anastomosis

Ureteral anastomosis is technically difficult in small patients (i.e., small dogs and cats) and has a high rate of postoperative obstruction. If the ureter is transected or damaged near the bladder, ureteroneocystostomy may be performed (see p. 650). If the ureter is avulsed from the renal pelvis, urinary drainage can be performed by placing a catheter through the renal parenchyma into the ureter (Fig. 24-8); however, nephrectomy appears to result in less morbidity and death than ureteral repair if the contralateral kidney is normal (see previous discussion in the Nephrectomy section). If function is adequate in the opposite kidney, nephrectomy may also be considered to prevent leakage, stricture, or infection. The end of the catheter is exteriorized through the body wall. Minimal dissection should be done around the ureter to prevent compromising its blood supply. To prevent damaging the ureter, stay sutures should be placed for manipulation and traumatic forceps should be avoided. The amount of tension that can be placed on the ureter without causing stricture formation is unknown; therefore tension across the anastomotic site should be avoided. Various synthetic materials have been used to replace the ureter, but most are unacceptable because they promote fibrosis, calculus formation, and/or infection. A bladder-flap ureteroplasty has been described for ureteral trauma near the bladder (Fig. 24-9). With this technique, a flap is elevated from the ventral surface of the bladder, and the ureter reimplanted into the flap. The flap is then closed as a tube. As with ureterotomy, stenting catheters should be used with caution because they may promote stricture formation.

For ureteral anastomosis, suture the ureter directly or spatulate it by making a longitudinal incision on opposite sides of each end of the ureter (Fig. 24-10, A). Preplace absorbable monofilament sutures (6-0 to 8-0) at the apex of the spatulated incisions and align the ureteral ends (Fig. 24-10, B). Appose the ureteral ends in a simple interrupted pattern using the preplaced sutures. Close the remainder of the ureter with simple interrupted sutures (Fig. 24-10, C). Ensure that the ends of the ureter are not twisted and that sufficient sutures have been placed to prevent leakage (Fig. 24-10, D).

Tension on the anastomosis can be relieved by freeing up the kidney from its peritoneal attachments and repositioning it more caudally. The kidney is then pexied to the body wall to prevent renal torsion. Alternately the apex of the bladder can be moved cranially and laterally toward the kidney and sutured to the psoas muscle dorsally. If necessary, place a nephropyelostomy tube.

Nephropyelostomy Tube Placement

Nephrostomy tubes may be placed percutaneously (see p. 656) or at surgery. Nephrostomy tubes are prone to poor drainage, tube dislodgement, and urine leakage; thus their use should be reserved for cases in which urine leakage is considered highly likely after ureterotomy or ureteral anastomosis. A tube specifically designed for use as a nephrostomy tube that has a flanged or pigtail end will likely stay in the renal pelvis better than a red rubber tube (Percutaneous Malecot Nephrostomy Set or Percutaneous Pigtail Nephrostomy Set; Cook Urological, Spencer, Ind.).

After proximal ureterotomy, insert a 20-gauge over-the-needle IV catheter through the ureterotomy incision, and advance

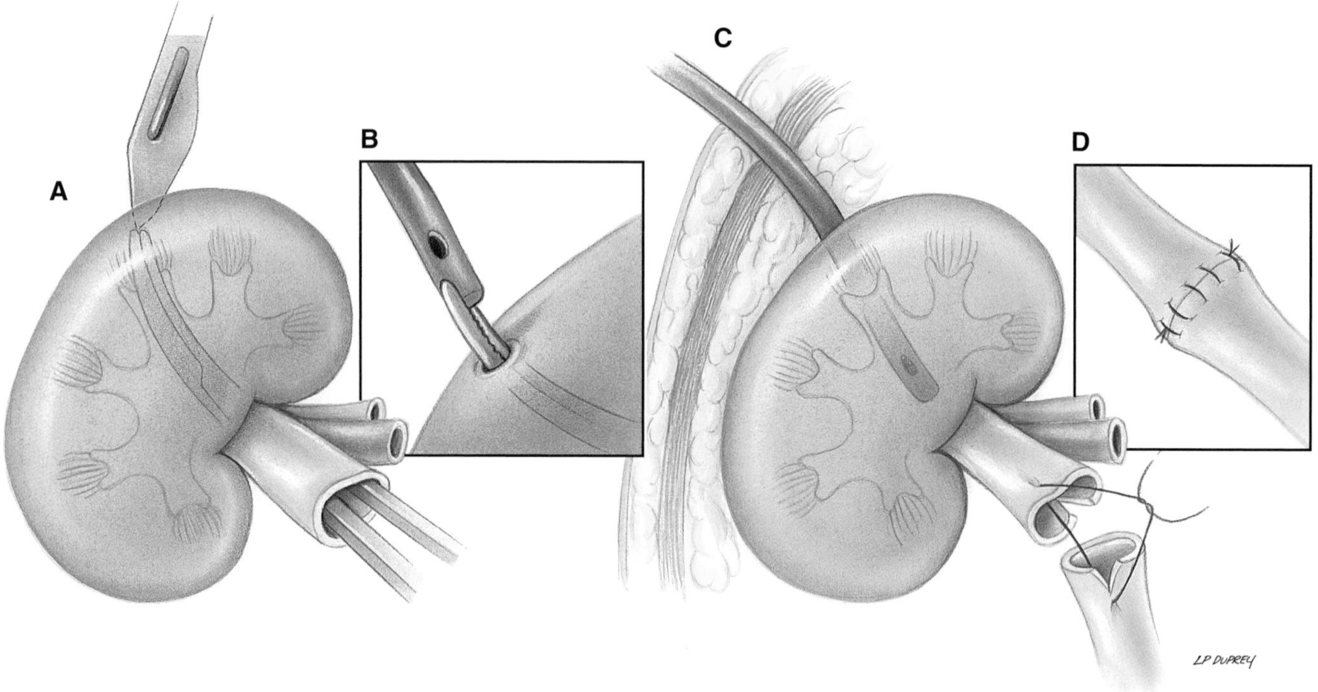

FIG. 24-8
Urinary drainage can be performed by placing a catheter through the renal parenchyma into the renal pelvis. **A,** Place a hemostat into the renal pelvis via the ureter, and incise over its tip with a scalpel blade. **B,** Grasp a catheter with the hemostat. **C,** Pull the catheter into the renal pelvis. **D,** Anastomose the torn ureteral ends.

FIG. 24-9
A bladder-flap ureteroplasty may be performed when ureteral trauma occurs near the bladder. **A,** Elevate a flap from the ventral surface of the bladder. **B,** Reimplant the ureter into the flap. **C,** Close the flap as a tube.

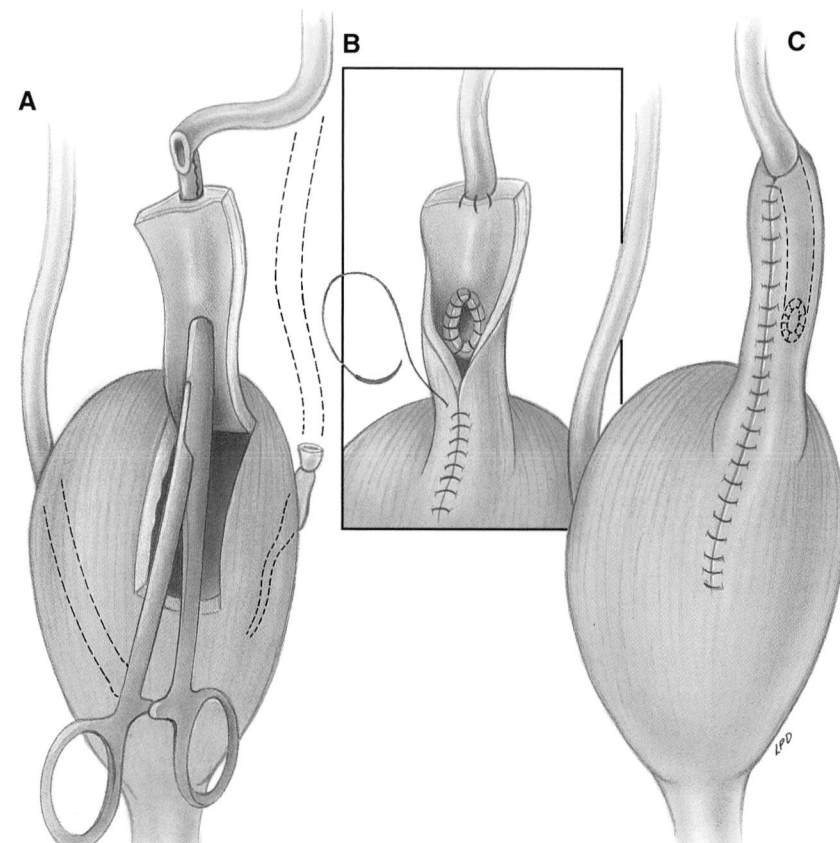

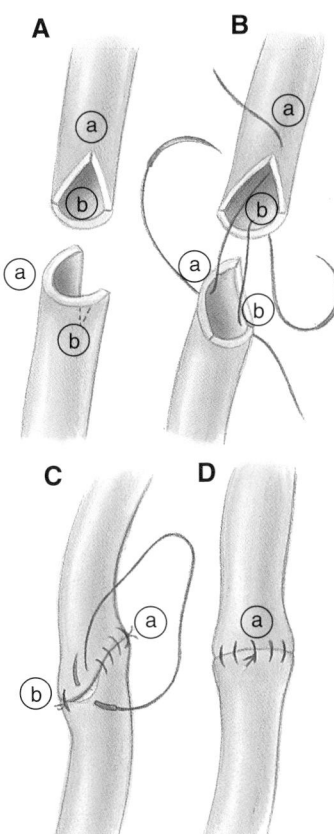

FIG. 24-10
For ureteral anastomosis, suture the ureter directly or **(A)** spatulate it by making a longitudinal incision on opposite sides of each end of the ureter. **B,** Preplace absorbable sutures at the apex of the spatulated incisions and align the ureteral ends. Appose the ureteral ends with simple interrupted absorbable sutures using the preplaced sutures. **C** and **D,** Close the remainder of the ureter with simple interrupted sutures.

it through the renal pelvis. Exit it through the renal cortex. Tie a length of suture material to a 5 French red rubber or Foley catheter, and pass the other end of the suture through the IV catheter. Slowly withdraw the catheter and suture, pulling the tip of the nephrostomy tube into the ureterotomy incision. Cut the suture and position the tip of the catheter in the renal pelvis. Perform a nephropexy by placing sutures between the renal capsule and the body wall where the tube exits. Secure the tube to the skin and underlying musculature, and connect it to a closed drainage system.

Alternately, use a nephrostomy tube with a flanged or pigtail end (see previous discussion). Place the catheter using the dilator and stylet supplied in the kit. Secure as described previously.

Neoureterostomy

Neoureterostomy (see p. 650) is performed for intramural ectopic ureters. Although some ectopic ureters completely bypass the bladder, most travel under the bladder mucosa before exiting and opening into the urethra or vagina.

Ureteroneocystostomy

Ureteroneocystostomy is performed for extraluminal ectopic ureters and to repair ureters that are damaged near the bladder. The ureter is resected or débrided and reimplanted into the bladder lumen (see p. 650).

HEALING OF THE KIDNEY AND URETER

Mild contusions or fractures of the kidney parenchyma heal primarily by synthesis of fibrous connective tissue. Although scar production occurs and may obliterate some functional nephrons, wound contraction usually is minimal. However, renal pelvis and collecting ducts experience wound contraction and scar tissue formation, resulting in strictures. Uroepithelium has enormous proliferative potential and may seal a damaged area within 48 hours. If at least 50% of the ureteral circumference remains, the ureter will heal by epithelialization, fibrous connective tissue synthesis, and longitudinal rather than circumferential wound contraction. Peristalsis is absent in the distal segment of a transected ureter for at least 10 days after repair. This may promote hydroureter in the proximal segment and subsequent hydronephrosis. Immobilizing the ureter to surrounding structures also inhibits peristalsis and diminishes urine flow. Five centimeter ureteral defects will heal over a stent; however, the ureter is typically narrow, and the wall is composed of fibrous tissue.

> NOTE: The uroepithelium has enormous regenerative capacity, but improper technique may result in strictures.

SUTURE MATERIALS AND SPECIAL INSTRUMENTS

Absorbable suture material, such as polyglactin 910 (Vicryl), polyglycolic acid (Dexon), polydioxanone (PDS), polyglyconate (Maxon), or poliglecaprone 25 (Monocryl) should be used in the kidney, ureter, and bladder. Nonabsorbable suture material may promote calculus formation and infection. Although PDS and Maxon maintain tensile strength and are more slowly absorbed than is desirable for most urinary surgery, they have less tissue drag than Dexon or Vicryl. The use of pediatric or ophthalmic instruments facilitates surgery of the ureter. These instruments tend to be smaller and more delicate and may cause less tissue trauma than larger instruments.

POSTOPERATIVE CARE AND ASSESSMENT

The hematocrit should be monitored postoperatively and ultrasound-guided abdominocentesis performed if hemorrhage or leakage is suspected. Significant hemorrhage may require blood transfusions (see Box 5-1 on p. 25) or repeat surgery. Severely anemic animals should have nasal oxygen during the anesthetic recovery period. Central venous pressure and urine output may be monitored to evaluate hydration postoperatively. Indwelling urinary catheters allow measurement of urine output. Patients (particularly young ones) should be closely monitored for urethral obstruction after repair of ectopic ureters. Ureteral obstruction as a result of surgical swelling or stomal stenosis may occur; however, unless the surgery was performed bilaterally, this typically goes undetected unless abdominal radiographs or ultrasonography document significant hydroureter or hydronephrosis. Urinary leakage may be diagnosed by abdominocentesis and comparison of fluid and serum creatinine levels (not BUN). With uroperitoneum, the creatinine level in the abdominal fluid is higher than the serum creatinine level (see p. 678). Electrolyte and acid-base abnormalities should be monitored and corrected postoperatively. Postoperative analgesics should be given as necessary (see Table 13-4 on p. 133).

COMPLICATIONS

The major complications of surgery of the kidney are renal failure, hemorrhage, and urinary leakage. Urinary leakage or obstruction due to stenosis or stricture is common after ureteral surgery. Complications of renal biopsy are typically not life threatening, but have varied in frequency from 1% to 18% (Vaden, 2004). In a recent study, 13% to 18% of dogs and cats, respectively, had a complication from renal biopsy, of which severe hemorrhage was the most common (Vaden et al, 2005). Older patients, patients less than 5 kg, and patients with severe azotemia may be more likely to have complications. Reported complications include microscopic hematuria, gross hematuria, arteriovenous fistula formation, cyst formation, perirenal hematoma, intrarenal hematoma, lacerated renal artery or vein, intraabdominal hemorrhage caused by laceration of an organ or vessel, infarction or thrombosis, infection, scar formation and fibrosis, or hydronephrosis that occurs secondary to the formation of blood clots in the renal pelvis. Severe hemorrhage requiring blood transfusion may occur in some animals. In one study, microscopic hematuria was reported in 20% to 70% of dogs and cats after renal biopsy, whereas macroscopic hematuria occurred in 1% to 4% (Vaden, 2004).

SPECIAL AGE CONSIDERATIONS

Older animals often have some degree of renal compromise and require careful monitoring during any surgical procedure. Hypotension should be avoided during surgery and the postoperative period to prevent further renal damage. If cardiac disease is also present, fluids should be used judiciously to prevent overhydration while maintaining renal blood flow.

References

Groman RP, Bahr A, Berridge BR et al: Effects of serial ultrasound-guided renal biopsies on kidneys of healthy adolescent dogs, *Vet Radiol Ultrasound* 45:62, 2004.

Lobetti R, Labrechts N: Effects of general anesthesia and surgery on renal function in healthy dogs, *Am J Vet Res* 61:121, 2000.

Stone EA, Robertson JL, Metcalf MR: The effect of nephrotomy on renal function and morphology in dogs, *Vet Surg* 31:391, 2002.

Vaden SL: Renal biopsy: methods and interpretation, *Vet Clin Small Anim* 34:887, 2004.

Vaden SL, Levin JF, Lees GE et al: Renal biopsy: a retrospective study of methods and complications in 283 dogs and 65 cats, *J Vet Intern Med* 19:794, 2005.

Weisse C, Aronson LR, Drobatz K: Traumatic rupture of the ureter: 10 cases, *J Am Anim Hosp Assoc* 38:188, 2002.

Suggested Reading

Bostrom I, Nyman G, Kampa N et al: Effects of acepromazine on renal function in anesthetized dogs, *Am J Vet Res* 64:590, 2003.

Acepromazine was administered to six healthy beagles, and it was found to possibly protect renal function despite lowering blood pressure.

Crandell DE, Mathews KA, Dyson DH: Effect of meloxicam and carprofen on renal function when administered to healthy dogs prior to anesthesia and painful stimulation, *Am J Vet Res* 65:1384, 2004.

The authors concluded that these two NSAIDs did not compromise renal function in six healthy dogs undergoing anesthesia.

Lobetti RG, Joubert KE: Effect of administration of nonsteroidal anti-inflammatory drugs before surgery on renal function in clinically normal dogs, *Am J Vet Res* 61:1501, 2000.

The authors concluded that ketorolac and ketoprofen and carprofen were not contraindicated in healthy dogs undergoing anesthesia, and carprofen had the least effect on renal function.

Rawlings CA, Howerth EW: Obtaining quality biopsies of the liver and kidney, *J Am Anim Hosp Assoc* 40:352, 2004.

This is a comprehensive review describing techniques for obtaining liver and hepatic biopsies in dogs.

SPECIFIC DISEASES

ECTOPIC URETER

DEFINITIONS

Ectopic ureter, or *ureteral ectopia,* is a congenital anomaly in which one or both ureters empty outside the bladder. **Extraluminal ectopic ureters** are those that completely bypass the bladder; **intraluminal ectopic ureters** course submucosally in the bladder to open in the urethra or vagina.

GENERAL CONSIDERATIONS AND CLINICALLY RELEVANT PATHOPHYSIOLOGY

The ureter normally enters the dorsolateral caudal surface of the bladder and empties into the trigone after a short intramural course (Fig. 24-11). Ectopic ureters are the most common congenital cause of urinary incontinence in dogs. They result from an abnormal development of the metanephric ducts in utero. Abnormalities in embryogenesis of the urinary system may also cause associated abnormalities (i.e., urethral sphincter incompetence, bladder hypoplasia, vestibulovaginal abnormalities, and/or ureteroceles; Fig. 24-12). Ureteroceles are focal dilations of the distal ureter that may be ectopic or intravesical. Surgical correction of ureteral ectopia is recommended; however, the presence of other abnormalities increases the likelihood of postoperative incontinence.

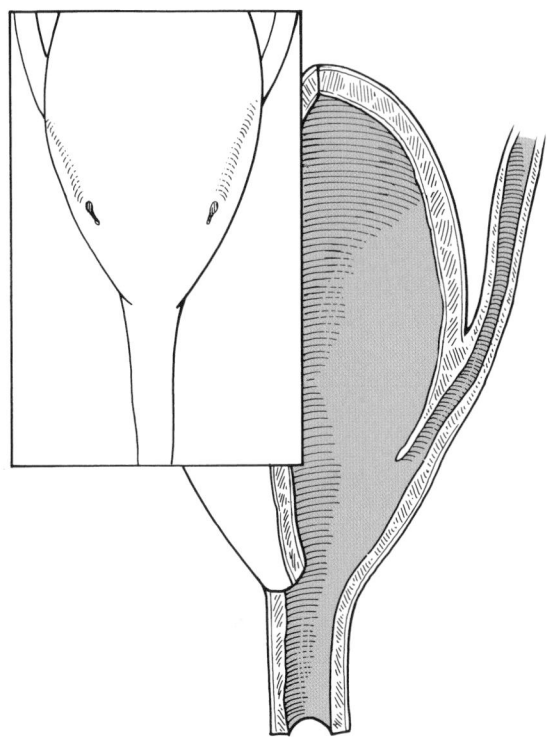

FIG. 24-11
The ureters normally enter the dorsolateral caudal surface of the bladder and empty into the trigone after a short intramural course.

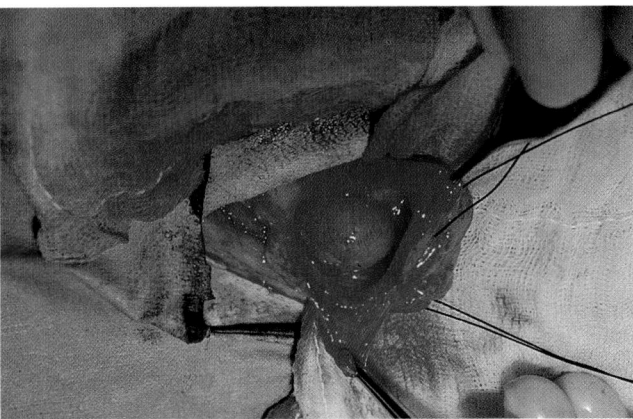

FIG. 24-12
A ureterocele in the bladder of a dog. The contralateral ureter was ectopic.

The most common location for termination of ectopic ureters is in the urethra, although termination in the uterus and vagina can occur. Ectopic ureters are classified as being *intramural* (they enter the bladder wall at a normal anatomic position, but a portion of the ureter extends submucosally within the bladder wall before it enters the urethral lumen) or *extramural* (the ureter bypasses the bladder to enter the urethral lumen). Approximately 70% to 80% of affected dogs have unilateral intramural (Fig. 24-13, *A*) or extramural (Fig. 24-13, *B*) ectopia. Of these, intramural lesions are more common. Other abnormalities noted in some dogs include double ureteral openings (i.e., where the ureter opens in the bladder plus more distally; Fig. 24-13, *C*) or ureteral troughs (Fig. 24-13, *D*). Although ureteral ectopia is less common in cats, bilateral ectopia may occur more frequently in cats than in dogs. Diagnosis of ureteral ectopia is important because it can be corrected surgically.

Upper and lower urinary tract infections are common in dogs with ureteral ectopia. Small kidneys may be caused by end-stage pyelonephritis, congenital dysplasia, or congenital cystic disease. Hydronephrosis may be caused by chronic pyelonephritis or ureteral obstruction (e.g., stenosis or absence of a functional opening). Hydroureter, the most common urogenital abnormality in dogs with ureteral ectopia, may be caused by chronic infection, obstructed urine outflow, or a primary lack of ureteral peristalsis. Hypoplastic bladders or intrapelvic bladders may be congenital or may

occur secondary to a lack of normal filling of the bladder. With unilateral ectopia, hydroureter and hydronephrosis may occur in the contralateral ureter as a result of chronic ascending urinary tract infections.

DIAGNOSIS
Clinical Presentation

Signalment. Ectopic ureters are more commonly diagnosed in female dogs than males. Male dogs are also affected, but may be less commonly diagnosed because the opening of the ectopic ureter is closer to the bladder than to the tip of the penis; distal urethral pressures may prevent urine dribbling. Female dogs are typically diagnosed at a young age (median age, 10 months); however, males with ectopic ureter tend to be older at the time of diagnosis (12 to 24 months). Siberian huskies have an increased incidence of ureteral ectopia. Golden retrievers, Labrador retrievers, Newfoundlands, bulldogs, miniature poodles, and some terrier breeds may also have a higher than expected incidence. Ureteral ectopia should be suspected in any young animal that has a history of incontinence (intermittent or continuous) since birth or weaning; however, this condition should also be included as a differential in older animals with lifelong urinary incontinence. Ectopic ureteroceles also cause urinary incontinence and have been reported in dogs and a cat.

NOTE: Ectopic ureters should not be excluded as a possible diagnosis even if urinary incontinence is intermittent or if the animal seems to urinate normal volumes. Affected dogs with ectopic ureters opening near the sphincter may have some response to medical management, mimicking dogs with acquired urinary incontinence.

History. Urinary incontinence may have an apparent, partial response to drugs and usually is constant, but may be

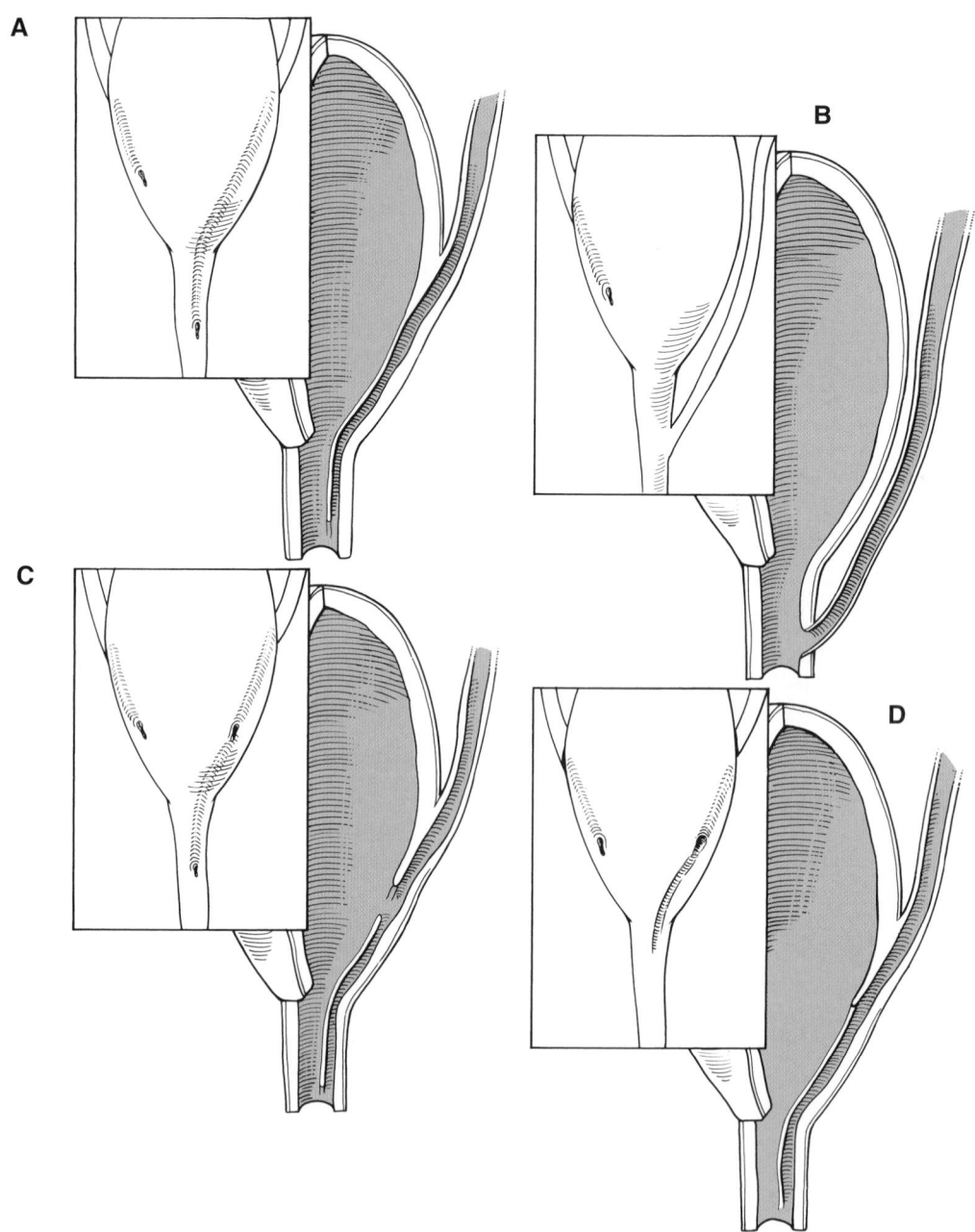

FIG. 24-13
The different types of ureteral ectopia. **A,** Intramural. **B,** Extramural. **C,** Double ureteral openings. **D,** Ureteral troughs.

intermittent. Many affected animals are able to urinate normally, particularly if the condition is unilateral. The ureters open near the trigone and retrograde filling of the bladder occurs, or the bladder is of sufficient size to act as a reservoir. Even animals with bilateral ectopia may have normal voiding associated with intermittent urine dribbling. Dogs with ectopic ureteroceles typically have a history that is similar to those with ectopic ureters. Dogs with intravesicular ureteroceles may have incontinence, dysuria, hematuria, chronic urinary tract infections, and complete or partial urinary obstruction, or there may be incidental findings in animals with no clinical signs.

NOTE: Ectopic ureters have been diagnosed in older animals that have no evidence of incontinence (Steffey and Brockman, 2004). Thus congenital ectopic ureters should be considered a differential diagnosis in animals with hydronephrosis, even if there is no urinary incontinence.

Physical Examination Findings

Physical examination findings include wetness of perivulvar hair, odor, and irritation or urine scalding of surrounding skin. Some dogs may have a persistent hymen that is de-

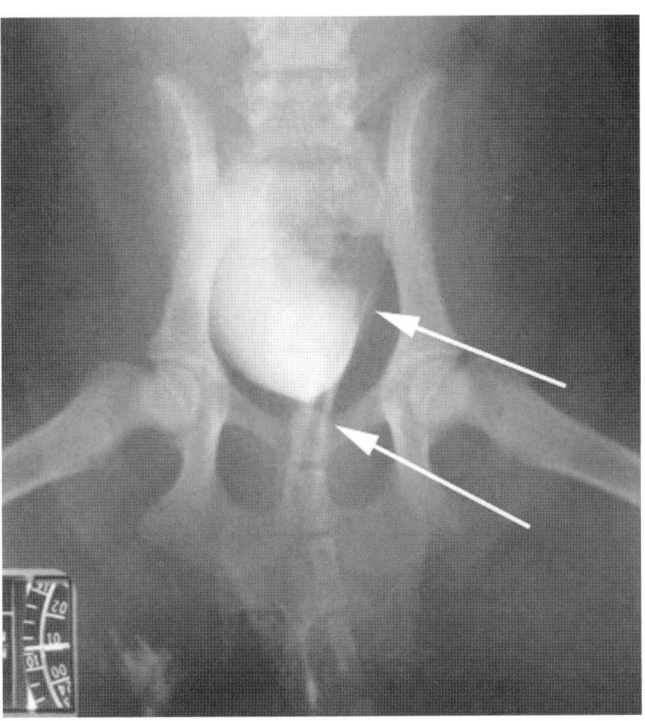

FIG. 24-14
Excretory urogram in a dog with an ectopic ureter. Note the ureter filled with contrast adjacent to the neck of the bladder and extending past the trigone *(arrows)*. This is the ectopic ureter.

tected digitally or with vaginoscopy. Other findings are unremarkable unless pyelonephritis is present.

Diagnostic Imaging

The size and shape of the kidneys, bladder, and prostate should be assessed with survey abdominal radiographs. Excretory urography is the most commonly used method for confirming ectopic ureters (Fig. 24-14) and defining associated urogenital abnormalities (i.e., hydronephrosis, hydroureter, hypoplastic bladder, and ureteroceles; see Fig. 24-12). Radiographs should be made both early and late after contrast administration because extramural ectopia is best identified before the bladder completely fills with contrast (alternatively, a pneumocystogram may be performed before excretory urography to facilitate visualization of the ureters when they are filled with positive contrast). However, contrast radiography does not accurately identify all ectopic ureters and often fails to differentiate between intramural and extramural lesions. The colon should be emptied to enhance visualization of the ureters and their site of termination. Retrograde cystography, pneumocystography (with the animal in the dorsoventral position to allow gas contrast to rise adjacent to ureters), and vaginoscopy may help correctly define ectopic ureter morphology. Cystoscopy probably is the most reliable method for diagnosing ectopic ureters in females. Ultrasonography is useful for defining ectopic ureters in dogs, and it may allow more accurate determination of normal ure-

teral anatomy than excretory urography. Cystoscopy is the most sensitive and specific method for diagnosing ectopic ureters in females. Contrast-enhanced computed tomography (CT) has also been used to evaluate the presence of ectopic ureters. Renal technetium scintigraphy (Tc 99m diethylenetriamine pentaacetic acid; ^{99m}Tc-DTPA) may be useful in dogs after neoureterostomy to diagnose partial obstruction of the operated ureter (Barthez et al, 2000).

> NOTE: Excretory urography is not as sensitive as cystoscopy and does not accurately differentiate all intramural and extramural lesions.

Laboratory Findings

A complete blood cell count, serum chemistry profile, and urinalysis (with microbial culture) should be performed. Concomitant urinary tract infection is common. Renal failure may be present because of chronic pyelonephritis, obstructive uropathy, or concurrent congenital abnormalities (see p. 635).

DIFFERENTIAL DIAGNOSIS

Ureteral ectopia should be considered likely in any young animal presented for treatment of incontinence. Behavioral incontinence is also common in young animals because of exaggerated submissiveness. Other causes of incontinence include urge incontinence (associated with inflammation or infection), neurogenic disorders (i.e., lower- and upper-motor neuron disorders or reflex dyssynergia), anatomic outflow obstruction (i.e., paradoxical incontinence), and urethral sphincter incontinence (i.e., hormone-responsive incontinence). Behavioral, urge, neurogenic, and hormone-responsive incontinence should be eliminated before considering tests for ectopia in older animals.

MEDICAL MANAGEMENT

Incontinence may persist after surgical correction if concomitant urethral sphincter incompetence is a factor. Urethral pressure profilometry can detect sphincter incompetence before surgery. α-Adrenergic agonists (i.e., phenylpropanolamine or ephedrine; Box 24-4), imipramine, or diethylstilbestrol may be used to increase urethral sphincter tone. See also Chapter 25.

SURGICAL TREATMENT

Surgical correction is the treatment of choice for ectopic ureters even if marginal improvement occurs with medical management. Surgery should be performed as soon as possible to prevent secondary abnormalities (i.e., hydroureter and hydronephrosis) caused by ascending urinary tract infections or outflow obstruction. Neoureterostomy is performed for intramural ectopic ureters. Although some ectopic ureters completely bypass the bladder, most travel under the bladder mucosa before exiting and opening into the urethra or vagina. If the ureter is extraluminal, the ureter must be resected and reimplanted into the bladder lumen.

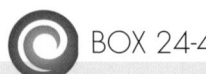

Preoperative Management

Hydration, acid-base, and electrolyte abnormalities should be corrected before surgery (see p. 635). Appropriate antibiotics should be administered as indicated by urine culture and susceptibility testing. If antibiotic therapy has not been initiated before surgery, antibiotics (e.g., cefazolin) should be administered after intraoperative cultures have been taken. Renal function should be determined before surgery if hydronephrosis or renal fibrosis is present. Nonfunctional kidneys should be removed (see later discussion).

> NOTE: Be sure to determine the function of each kidney before surgery, even when one kidney appears to be obviously nonfunctional.

Anesthesia

If renal impairment is not present, many different anesthetic regimens can be used safely. If renal impairment is present, see p. 636 for suggested anesthetic protocols.

Surgical Anatomy

The surgical anatomy of the kidney and ureter is described on p. 637.

Positioning

The animal is placed in dorsal recumbency, and the abdomen is prepared for a ventral midline incision. The prepared area should extend from above the xiphoid to below the pubis.

SURGICAL TECHNIQUE

The entire urinary system should be explored before the ureter is repaired. Nonfunctional kidneys and their ureter should be removed; otherwise, the ureter and kidney should be preserved. If nephrectomy is considered, bilateral ectopia should first be ruled out. If nephrectomy is done, the end of the ectopic ureter should be ligated as close as possible to its termination.

Neoureterostomy

Handle the bladder tissue with extreme care, and use stay sutures whenever possible. Once the bladder has been emptied of urine, use sterile, cotton-tipped swabs rather than a sponge to absorb urine to prevent abrading the mucosal surface.

Using pediatric instruments may help reduce tissue trauma. Swelling or hyperemia makes the ureters difficult to locate beneath the mucosa.

Make an incision into the ventral bladder near the urethra (Fig. 24-15, A). Place stay sutures to facilitate retraction of the bladder wall edges. Inspect the trigone for ureteral openings. Identify a submucosal swelling or ridge within the bladder wall; this may be facilitated by digitally occluding the urethra to cause ureteral dilation. Use a No. 15 scalpel blade to make a 3- to 5-mm longitudinal incision through the bladder mucosa into the ureteral lumen. Using 5-0 to 7-0 absorbable suture material, suture the ureteral mucosa to the bladder in a simple interrupted pattern (Fig. 24-15, B). Place a 3.5 or 5 French catheter into the distal ureter (Fig. 24-15, C). Just distal to the new stoma, pass one or two nonabsorbable sutures (3-0 or 4-0) from the serosal surface circumferentially around the tube, staying beneath the mucosa (Fig. 24-15, D). Be sure the suture does not penetrate the bladder lumen. Use this suture to ligate the distal ureter after removing the catheter. Close the proximal urethra with simple interrupted or simple continuous sutures (single or double layer), but ensure that the urethral diameter is not compromised. Close the bladder in such a manner as to ensure a watertight seal (i.e., simple continuous or inverting suture pattern, see p. 666).

Ureteroneocystostomy

If the ureter is extraluminal, it must be resected and reimplanted into the bladder lumen. In dogs, the ureter may be implanted into the bladder using a simple transverse pull-through or an intramural tunnel (3:1 tunnel length to ureteral orifice diameter). The latter technique may cause less fibrosis and quicker return of normal ureteral function.

The diameter of the feline ureter is approximately 0.4 mm at the level of the bladder, and standard ureteroneocystostomy techniques often cause ureteral obstruction. Microsurgical techniques may be necessary to prevent ureteral obstruction in cats, particularly when the ureter is not dilated due to disease (e.g., renal transplantation). A "drop-in" technique was originally described for ureteroneocystostomy of cats undergoing renal transplantation; however, granuloma formation and hemorrhage were common. Extravesical

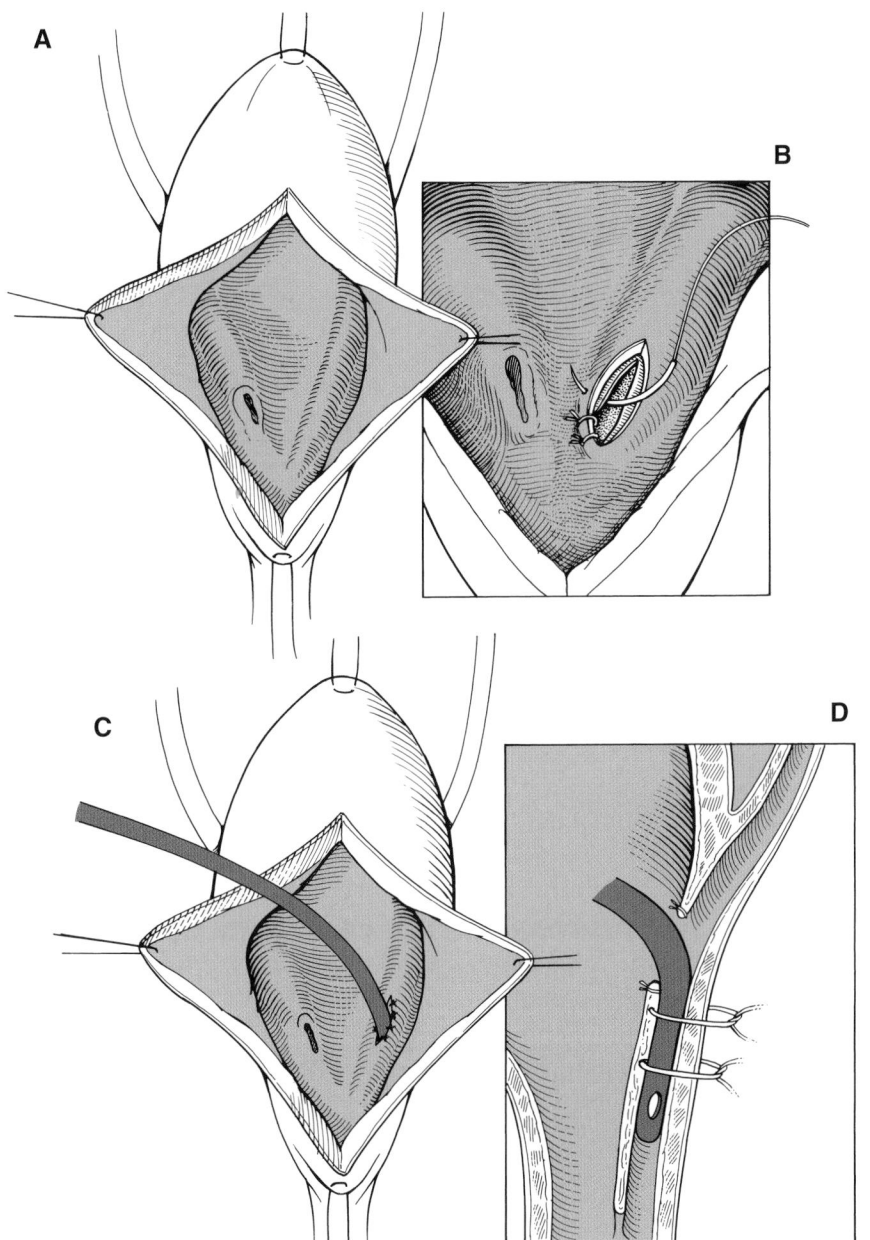

FIG. 24-15
Neoureterostomy is performed for intramural ectopic ureters. **A,** Perform a cystotomy and make a 3- to 5-mm longitudinal incision through the bladder mucosa into the ureteral lumen. **B,** Using absorbable suture material, suture the ureteral mucosa to the bladder in a simple interrupted pattern. **C,** Place a 3.5 or 5 French catheter into the distal ureter. **D,** Just distal to the new stoma, pass one or two nonabsorbable sutures from the serosal surface circumferentially around the tube, staying beneath the mucosa.

techniques have largely replaced intravesical techniques in humans. A recent study in cats suggested that extravesical technique using a simple interrupted suture pattern was preferred over an extravesical technique using a continuous suture pattern or an intravesical mucosal apposition technique (Mehl et al, 2005). Although all three techniques resulted in renal pelvis dilation, the dilation resolved more rapidly with the extravesical technique using a simple interrupted pattern, and this technique was associated with consistently lower serum creatinine concentrations for the first week after surgery.

Perform a ventral cystotomy as described previously for neoureterostomy. Ligate the ureter and transect it, preserving as much length as possible (Fig. 24-16). Place a stay suture on

the proximal end of the transected ureter. Incise the bladder mucosa, and create a short, oblique submucosal tunnel in the bladder wall. Use the stay suture to draw the ureter into the bladder lumen to prevent damaging the ureter. Make a 1- to 2-mm longitudinal incision in the ureter end (i.e., spatulate it), and suture it to the bladder mucosa with absorbable suture (e.g., polyglycolic acid or polyglactin 910).

To perform an extravesical simple interrupted suture pattern technique, make a partial-thickness incision through the muscularis and submucosa of the ventral aspect of the apex of the urinary bladder to expose the mucosa (Fig. 24-17, A). Spatulate the distal end of the ureter, and make an incision equal in length to the spatulation incision in the ureter through the bladder mucosa in the caudal aspect of the muscularis incision. Place a simple interrupted suture

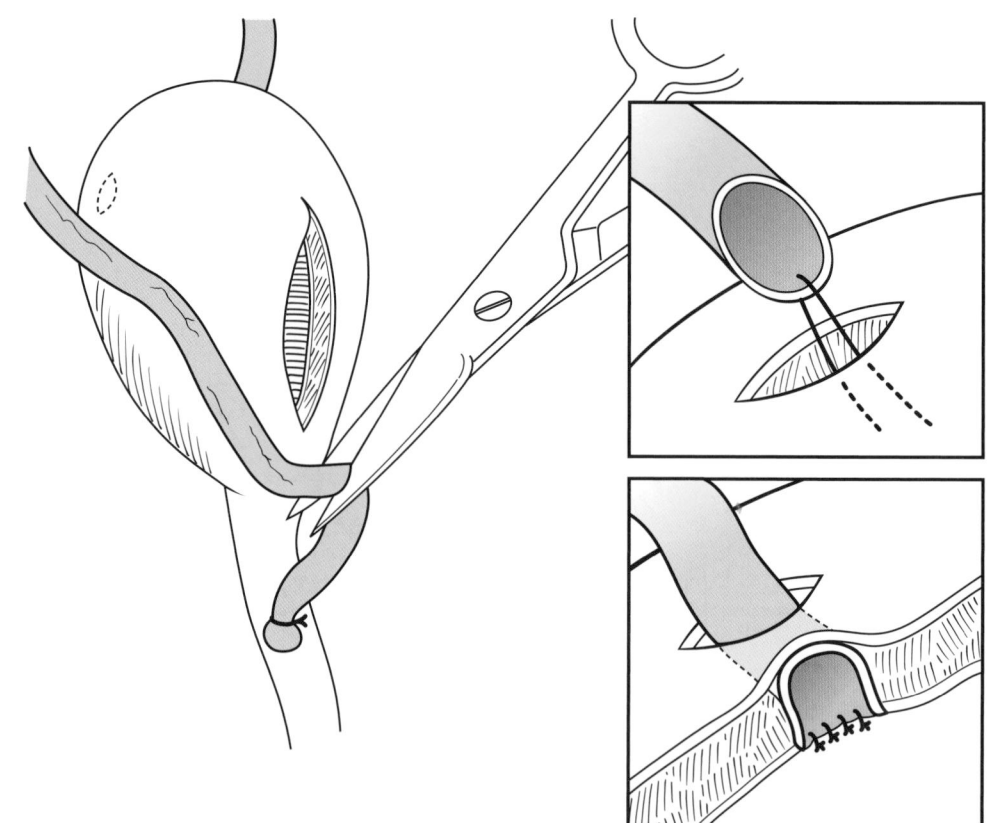

FIG. 24-16
Ureteroneocystostomy is performed when the ureter is extraluminal. Ligate the ureter and transect it. Place a stay suture on the proximal end of the transected ureter. Incise the bladder mucosa and create a short, oblique, submucosal tunnel in the bladder wall. Spatulate the ureter end and suture it to the bladder mucosa with absorbable suture.

(7-0 or 8-0 nylon) between the proximal ureter at the end of the spatulation and the cranial aspect of the bladder mucosal incision and a second interrupted suture between the distal end of the ureter and the caudal aspect of the bladder mucosal incision (Fig. 24-17, B). Place a 4-0 polypropylene stent into the lumen of the ureter to ensure patency. Place the stent after the first two sutures are tied, and remove it before tying the final sutures of the mucosal layer. Place two additional interrupted sutures between the ureteral and bladder mucosa on one side of the incision (Fig. 24-17, C).

SUTURE MATERIALS AND SPECIAL INSTRUMENTS

Absorbable suture material, such as polyglactin 910 (Vicryl), polyglycolic acid (Dexon), polydioxanone (PDS), polyglyconate (Maxon), or poliglecaprone 25 (Monocryl), should be used in the bladder because nonabsorbable suture materials may promote calculus formation or infection. Keep in mind that polyglycolic acid and polyglactin 910 may be rapidly degraded in infected urine; however, polydioxanone and polyglyconate maintain tensile strength when in contact with urine and thus may be preferable for closing a cystotomy. Small suture (i.e., 4-0 or 5-0) is preferred to suture the ureter to the bladder mucosa. The distal ureter should be ligated with nonabsorbable suture because incontinence may recur as a result of recanalization of the distal ureter if absorbable suture is used.

POSTOPERATIVE CARE AND ASSESSMENT

The animal should be observed closely after surgery for signs of urinary obstruction or leakage. If urethral obstruction occurs because of postoperative swelling, an indwelling urinary catheter should be placed for 3 to 4 days until normal voiding occurs. If bilateral ectopia is corrected during the same surgery (or if significant renal impairment exists in the contralateral kidney with unilateral surgery), the animal should be monitored for renal failure due to ureteral swelling and subsequent obstruction. ^{99m}Tc-DTPA may be a useful aid for evaluating ureteral function in dogs after ureteroneocystostomy (Barthez et al, 2000). If incontinence continues for longer than 2 to 3 months postoperatively, an excretory urogram or cystoscopy should be performed to evaluate the ureters. Occasionally the distal end (i.e., ligated end) is patent or a bilateral ectopia was missed initially.

NOTE: Ureteral stoma swelling is probably common after this surgery and may cause some obstruction to ureteral flow, but it usually goes undetected and resolves without therapy.

PROGNOSIS

As many as 30% to 55% of patients continue to show some degree of incontinence postoperatively. Many dogs with ectopic ureters have functional abnormalities of the urinary

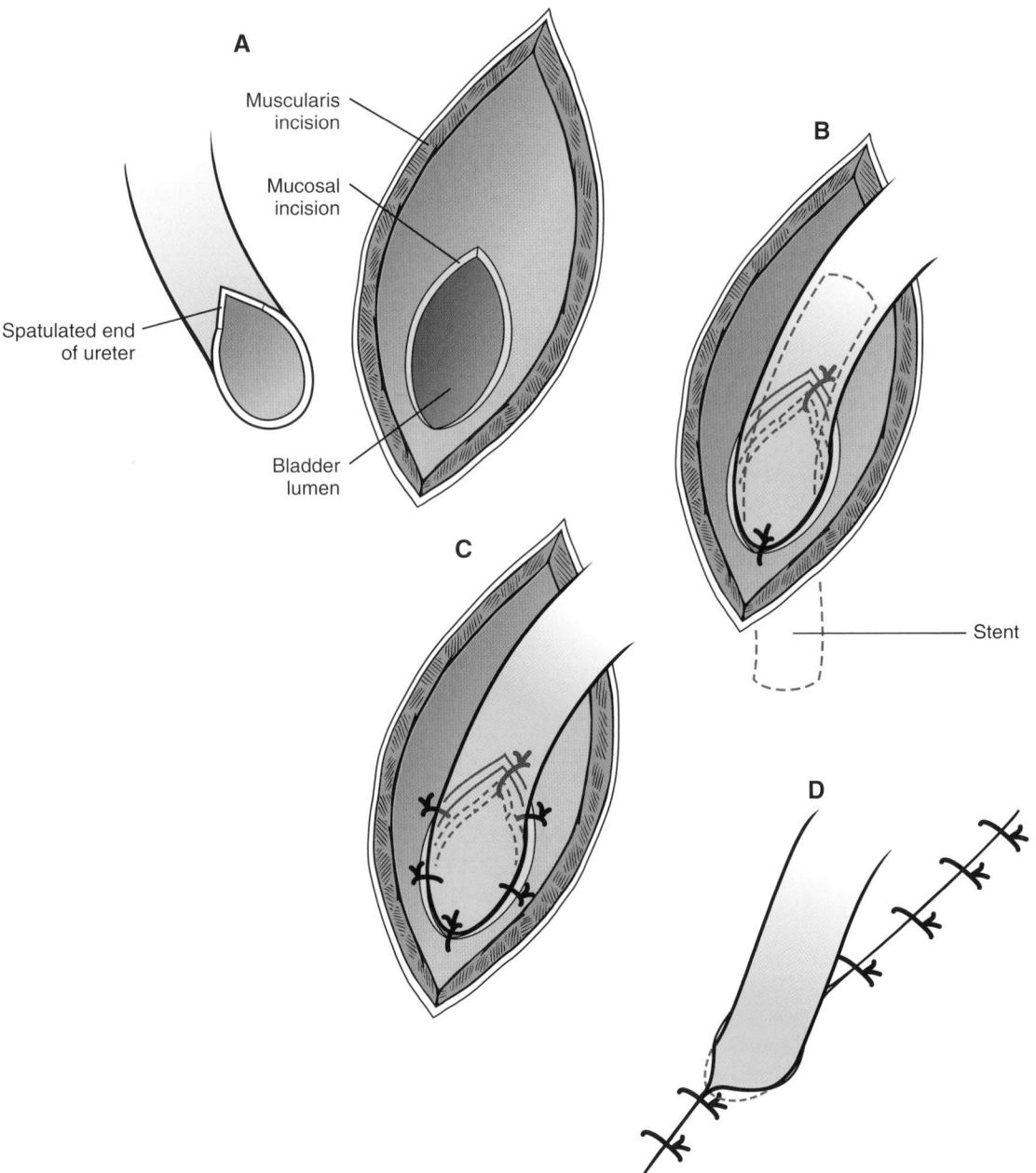

FIG. 24-17

To perform an extravesical simple interrupted suture pattern technique: **A,** make a partial thickness incision through the muscularis and submucosa of the ventral aspect of the apex of the urinary bladder to expose the mucosa. Spatulate the distal end of the ureter and make an incision equal in length to the spatulation incision in the ureter through the bladder mucosa in the caudal aspect of the muscularis incision. **B,** Place a simple interrupted suture (7-0 or 8-0 nylon) between the proximal ureter at the end of the spatulation and the cranial aspect of the bladder mucosal incision and a second interrupted suture between the distal end of the ureter and the caudal aspect of the bladder mucosal incision. Place a 4-0 polypropylene stent into the lumen of the ureter to ensure patency. Place the stent after the first two sutures are tied and remove it before tying the final sutures of the mucosal layer. **C,** Place two additional interrupted sutures between the ureteral and bladder mucosa on one side of the incision. **D,** Close the seromuscular incision.

bladder or urethra. Obtaining urethral pressure measurements before surgery and after initiating phenylpropanolamine therapy (see p. 649) has been instituted may help predict the likelihood of continence after surgery. Siberian huskies are particularly prone to postoperative incontinence because of a high incidence of urethral sphincter incompetence. These dogs may respond to α-adrenergic agonists. If bladder hypoplasia is present, incontinence may continue until the bladder enlarges and properly functions as a reservoir. Dogs with ureteral troughs may have a poorer prognosis than dogs with nondistended intramural ectopic ureters. Failure to resect a ureterocele may result in continued incontinence and urinary tract infection.

References

Barthez PY et al: Ureteral obstruction after ureteroneocystostomy in dogs assessed by technetium (Tc 99m) diethylenetriamine pentaacetic acid (DTPA) scintigraphy, *Vet Surg* 29:499, 2000.

Cannizzo KL, McLoughlin MA, Mattoon JS et al: Evaluation of transurethral cystoscopy and excretory urography for diagnosis of ectopic ureters in female dogs: 25 cases (1992-2000), *J Am Vet Med Assoc* 223:475, 2003.

Mehl ML, Kyles AE, Pollard R et al: Comparison of 3 techniques for ureteroneocystostomy in cats, *Vet Surg* 34:114, 2005.

Samii VF, McLoughlin MA, Mattoon JS et al: Digital fluoroscopic excretory urography, digital fluoroscopic urethrography, helical computed tomography, and cystoscopy in 24 dogs with suspected ureteral ectopia, *J Vet Intern Med* 18:271, 2004.

Steffye MA, Brockman DJ: Congenital ectopic ureters in a continent male dog and cat, *J Am Vet Med Assoc* 224:1067, 2004.

Suggested Reading

Sutherland-Smith J, Jerram RM, Walker AM et al: Ectopic ureters and ureteroceles in dogs: presentation, cause, and diagnosis, *Compend* 26:303, 2004.

This article reviews embryogenesis of the urinary tract and malformations that may lead to ureteral ectopia or ureteroceles.

RENAL AND URETERAL CALCULI

DEFINITIONS

Urolithiasis refers to the condition of having urinary calculi or uroliths (kidney, ureter, bladder, or urethra). The condition of having renal or ureteral calculi (i.e., **nephroliths** or **ureteroliths**) is **nephrolithiasis** or **ureterolithiasis**, respectively. **Nephrolithotomy** is performed to remove renal calculi from the renal pelvis by incising through kidney parenchyma; **pyelolithotomy** is an incision into the renal pelvis and proximal ureter. **Ureterolithotomy** is the removal of calculi from the ureter by incision (**ureterotomy**). A **staghorn calculus** is one that occurs in the renal pelvis and extends into the diverticula. Nephrolithotomy is also known as *lithonephrotomy*.

GENERAL CONSIDERATIONS AND CLINICALLY RELEVANT PATHOPHYSIOLOGY

Only 5% to 10% of canine uroliths are in the kidney and ureter. The prevalence in cats is unknown; however, the incidence of feline calcium oxalate ureterolithiasis appears to be increasing (Kyles et al, 2005). Uroliths are named according

to their mineral content and location. Nephroliths pose a unique diagnostic and therapeutic challenge because they may be clinically silent or affected animals may have pain, fever, and/or renal failure attributable to urinary outflow obstruction, fibrosis, or infection. Clinical signs of ureteroliths may be nonspecific (see p. 655). Renal and ureteral calculi may be unilateral or bilateral. Bilateral ureteral calculi may be present in as many as 25% of affected cats. Less than 10% of these cats typically have associated cystic calculi.

Struvite (magnesium ammonium phosphate) and calcium oxalate uroliths are the most common types in dogs, but other types include calcium oxalate, urate, silicate, cystine, and mixed stones. Calcium oxalate nephroliths and ureteroliths are the most common types in cats (Kyles et al, 2005). The pathogenesis of calcium oxalate uroliths is poorly understood. Some disease processes (i.e., portosystemic shunts) are associated with a high rate of urolithiasis (see p. 542). Certain breeds (i.e., Dalmatians and dachshunds) also have a high incidence of urolithiasis because of metabolic abnormalities (see p. 683).

Whether all renal or ureteral stones should be removed is controversial. If they are associated with infection, they should be removed; however, removal of uninfected stones from the renal pelvis may cause more renal damage than the stone. Other facts to be considered include the effectiveness of medical therapy in dissolving the stone, renal function in the affected and contralateral kidney, the animal's overall health, and the presence of obstructive uropathy (i.e., hydronephrosis, hydroureter, or renal failure). Ureteral calculi often cause obstruction and require prompt surgical removal.

Although nonsurgical removal of renal calculi is common in human beings (i.e., lithotripsy), these techniques are less available to pets and may be less effective. While lithotripsy has been used to fragment ureteroliths in dogs, it is not recommended in cats because the feline kidney is more sensitive to shock wave–induced injury. Medical dissolution may be effective with some stones, but calcium oxalate nephroliths and ureteroliths are not generally amenable to dissolution (Bollinger et al, 2005). Any stone that is surgically removed should be submitted for analysis (Fig. 24-18). Knowledge of the stone's mineral composition directs the appropriate treatment to prevent recurrence. Because of the relationship between infection and calculi, microbial cultures of urine (and calculi, if available) are mandatory for patients with uroliths. Factors contributing to the formation of uroliths include a favorable urine pH, infection, a high concentration of crystalloids in the urine, and a diminished concentration of urine crystallization inhibitors (see p. 682 for a more detailed discussion of stone formation and treatment). In general, it is difficult or impossible to eliminate urinary tract infections if calculi are present.

DIAGNOSIS
Clinical Presentation

Signalment. Some breeds have a higher incidence of urolithiasis because of metabolic abnormalities or underlying disease processes (see p. 683). Breeds at highest risk for developing calculi are miniature schnauzers, Shih Tzus, Lhasa

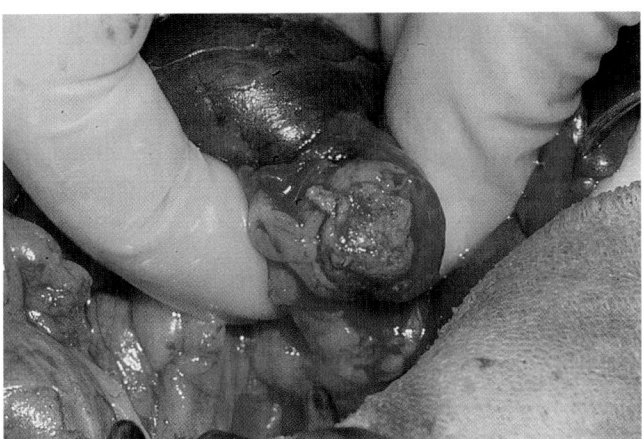

FIG. 24-18
Intraoperative photograph of a renal calculus in a dog.

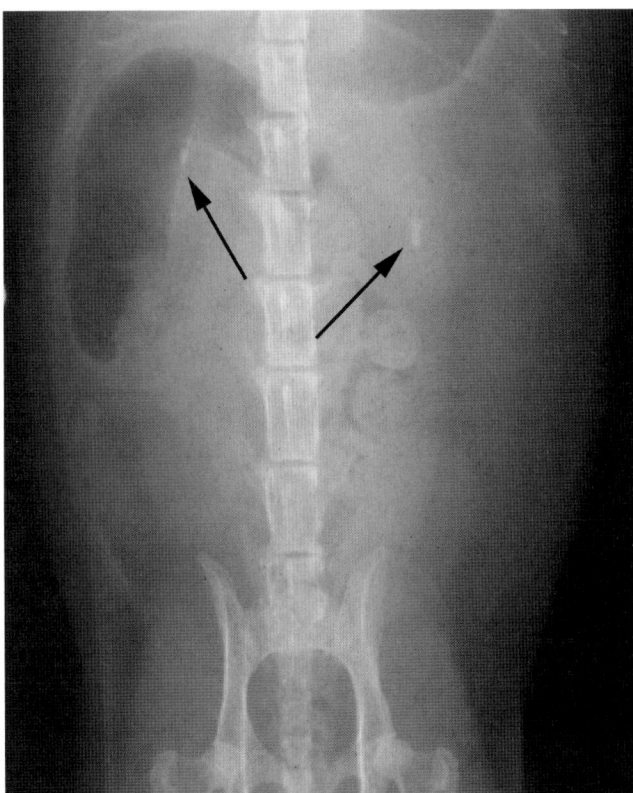

FIG. 24-19
Radiopaque renal calculi in a cat *(arrows).*

apsos, Yorkshire terriers, and female pugs. Also at high risk are male dalmatians and male basset hounds. Among small breed dogs, females generally are at higher risk of developing renal calculi than males. Middle-aged to older animals have a higher rate of urolithiasis than young animals. However, some calculi occur in young animals (i.e., urate calculi associated with portosystemic shunts and struvite calculi in schnauzers). Ureteroliths tend to form in middle-aged to older cats, but young cats may be affected. There is no sex predisposition in cats.

History. The history varies, depending on whether the stone has caused obstruction or whether concurrent infection is present. Clinical signs may be intermittent, particularly if the animal has been treated with antibiotics. Stranguria, hematuria, and/or pollakiuria are relatively common signs. A previous history of urolithiasis is common if stone analysis was not performed or appropriate therapy not instituted after previous surgery. The most common clinical signs in cats with ureteral calculi are nonspecific (e.g., anorexia or inappetence, vomiting, weight loss, polyuria, and polydipsia). Other less common clinical signs may include stranguria, hematuria, pollakiuria, signs of abdominal pain, and hypersalivation.

> NOTE: Because clinical signs in cats with ureteroliths are typically nonspecific, it may be wise to perform survey radiographs in all cats with ill-defined disease, regardless of whether they have evidence of ARF or CRF.

Physical Examination Findings

Renal calculi may be asymptomatic, or they may be associated with hematuria, signs of urinary tract infection (e.g., pollakiuria and stranguria), signs of CRF or ARF (anorexia, depression, vomiting, polyuria-polydipsia), flank pain, and/or renomegaly. Hematuria often is the clinical sign noted in cats with nephrolithiasis; these cats may be erroneously diagnosed as having feline lower urinary tract disease

(FLUTD). Polyuria-polydipsia, lethargy, depression, fever, and/or anorexia are consistent with pyelonephritis. Infection may cause substantial renal destruction and uremia (i.e., anorexic, depressed, dehydrated, and vomiting). Dysuria or stranguria may occur with concurrent lower urinary tract infection. Signs associated with ureteral calculi usually are caused by concurrent pyelonephritis or obstructive uropathy (i.e., uremia). Physical examination findings in cats with ureteral calculi may be nonspecific (i.e., pain on abdominal palpation and weight loss), or urinary tract abnormalities may be noted (e.g., hematuria, stranguria, and pollakiuria).

Diagnostic Imaging

Renal and ureteral calculi may be incidental radiographic or ultrasonographic findings. Most renal and ureteral calculi are radiopaque and appear as increased opacities in the renal pelvis or ureter (Fig. 24-19). The ureters, bladder, and urethra should also be examined carefully for calculi anytime nephroliths are found. Associated abnormalities (i.e., hydronephrosis or hydroureter) may be assessed by ultrasonography (preferred) or excretory urography (see p. 649). Most cats with ureteral calculi also have renal calculi, and some have cystic calculi. The most sensitive test for identifying ureterolithiasis is survey radiography; however, a combination of survey radiographs and ultrasonography is recommended. Most cats with ureteral calculi have ureteral obstruction (i.e., dilation of the ureter and/or renal pelvis) on ultrasonographic evaluation.

Antegrade pyelography may also be useful for evaluating ureteral obstruction in cats (Adin et al, 2003).

Stabilize the kidney by applying firm pressure on the ultra-sound transducer. Insert a 25-gauge 2.5-inch spinal needle into the renal cortex perpendicular to the capsule, and advance it into the renal pelvis using ultrasonographic guid-ance. Remove the stylet of the spinal needle, and attach a small volume extension set. Aspirate 1 to 2 ml of urine from the renal pelvis for culture and cytology. Then, in multiple small boluses, inject an equal volume of ionic or nonionic iodinated contrast material into the renal pelvis during fluo-roscopic imaging. Repeat bolus injections of contrast mate-rial until adequate ureteral opacification is achieved as determined with fluoroscopy. Withdraw the needle and image the kidney with fluoroscopy. Take abdominal radio-graphs and repeat fluoroscopy as needed over the next 10 to 15 minutes. Lastly, evaluate the kidney for perirenal fluid indicating hemorrhage or leakage of contrast material or urine.

Laboratory Findings

A complete blood cell count, serum chemistry profile, uri-nalysis, and urine culture should be performed. Concomi-tant urinary tract infection is common. Renal failure may be caused by chronic pyelonephritis or obstructive uropathy (see p. 698). Evidence of hepatic disease (low blood urea nitrogen, hypocholesterolemia, hypoalbuminemia, increased serum bile acids) may be present in some animals with urate calculi (see p. 683). Feline ureterolithiasis is commonly as-sociated with azotemia, hyperphosphatemia, anemia, and hyperkalemia (Kyles et al, 2005). Occasionally, hypercalce-mia is found, but hypocalcemia is more common. Unilateral ureterolithiasis is often associated with azotemia and hyper-phosphatemia in cats, suggesting impairment of renal func-tion in the contralateral kidney.

DIFFERENTIAL DIAGNOSIS

Uroliths are possible in any animal presented for CRF, ARF, uroabdomen, urinary tract infection, hematuria, stranguria, or pollakiuria.

MEDICAL MANAGEMENT

Possible underlying causes of renal or ureteral calculi should be identified and treated (e.g., infection, portosystemic shunts, or metabolic abnormalities). Some stones can be managed with dietary therapy or pharmacologic agents (see the discussion on bladder calculi, p. 682). Fluid diuresis alone or in combination with diuretic drugs may resolve intraluminal causes of obstruction. In cats, it has been sug-gested that glucagon (0.1 mg/cat, IV, bid) may cause relax-ation of the ureteral smooth muscle and promote passage of ureteral calculi (Hardie and Kyles, 2004). If dietary therapy is used to dissolve renal calculi, there is a risk that the stones will become small enough to enter the ureter and cause ob-

struction; these animals should be monitored carefully for evidence of ureteral obstruction during such therapy. In se-verely ill cats with ureteral obstruction, percutaneous place-ment of a nephropyelostomy tube may allow treatment of azotemia before surgery. This technique may also help deter-mine if the obstructed kidney has any remaining function before surgery.

Using ultrasound guidance, place a 16-gauge over-the-needle catheter through the body wall from lateral to medial adjacent to the kidney, and pass it through the kidney into the renal pelvis. Cut the tip off of a 3.5 French red rubber catheter and pass it down the IV catheter. Position the tip in the renal pelvis. Withdraw the IV catheter, and seat it onto the hub of the red rubber catheter. Secure the nephrostomy tube with a deep suture that incorporates skin and underly-ing musculature to minimize dislodgement. Attach the cath-eter to a closed drainage system.

SURGICAL TREATMENT

Surgical removal of renal and ureteral calculi should be con-sidered when they are infected or cause obstruction. To prevent irreversible renal damage, surgery should be per-formed as soon as possible once the animal's condition has been stabilized. However, some animals with pyelonephritis due to nephrolithiasis have CRF and are such poor anes-thetic and surgical risks that chronic, palliative medical management is safer.

Preoperative Management

If possible, hydration, acid-base, and electrolyte abnormali-ties should be corrected before surgery. Appropriate antibi-otics should be administered as indicated by urine culture and susceptibility testing. If antibiotic therapy has not been initiated before surgery, antibiotics (e.g., cefazolin) should be administered after intraoperative cultures have been taken. Renal function of both kidneys should be determined before surgery. Nephrectomy, rather than stone removal, is indicated in nonfunctional kidneys; otherwise, the kidney and ureter should be preserved.

> NOTE: Make sure you determine how functional each kidney is before surgery. Sometimes a kidney that grossly appears to be end-stage is the kidney with most of the remaining function.

Anesthesia

If renal impairment is not present, many anesthetic regi-mens can be used safely. If substantial renal impairment is present, see p. 636 for suggested anesthetic protocols. Pre-vent hypotension to protect blood flow to the remaining kidney during nephrectomy.

Surgical Anatomy

The surgical anatomy of the kidney and ureter is discussed on p. 637.

Positioning

The animal is placed in dorsal recumbency, and the abdomen is prepared for a ventral midline incision. The prepared area should extend from above the xiphoid to caudal to the pubis. If nephrectomy is performed, the incision must be extended caudally to allow the ureter to be ligated near the bladder.

SURGICAL TECHNIQUE

The entire urinary system, including the contralateral kidney and ureter, should be explored before the calculi are removed. Occasionally, multiple ureteral and renal calculi are found. Stones also may be found in the bladder or urethra. Renal calculi can be removed via a nephrotomy (see p. 640) or pyelolithotomy (see p. 642). If the renal pelvis and proximal ureter are sufficiently dilated, a pyelolithotomy is preferred because it avoids renal parenchymal incision and subsequent damage. However, if the stone is large and involves the diverticula and the pelvis, nephrotomy usually is necessary. Occasionally soft stones can be crushed and removed through the renal pelvis, but care is necessary to prevent ureteral damage that may cause subsequent stricture formation.

> NOTE: *Always* submit the stones for analysis and culture.

Bilateral nephrotomy puts the patient at increased risk for postoperative renal failure. If possible, staged procedures should be considered. The renal pelvis or ureter should be cultured. The stones should be submitted for analysis and culture. Fungal elements are rarely seen on cytologic analysis of material (grit, exudate) found in the renal pelvis, but when present, they suggest systemic aspergillosis, a generally fatal disease.

Ureterotomy may be performed in animals with ureteral calculi; however, a combination of microsurgical techniques and intensive postoperative care is necessary to minimize morbidity. If stones are located in the distal ureter, they may be removed by partial ureterectomy and ureteroneocystostomy (see p. 650). If they are located in the proximal third of the ureter, they may be removed by ureterotomy plus nephrostomy tube drainage if indicated.

SUTURE MATERIALS AND SPECIAL INSTRUMENTS

Absorbable suture material, such as polyglactin 910 (Vicryl), polyglycolic acid (Dexon), polydioxanone (PDS), polyglyconate (Maxon), or poliglecaprone 25 (Monocryl) should be used in the kidney and ureter. Pediatric or ophthalmic instruments may facilitate ureteral surgery.

POSTOPERATIVE CARE AND ASSESSMENT

The animal should be observed closely after surgery for signs of urinary obstruction or leakage. Renal failure may occur if bilateral nephrotomy was performed or if significant renal impairment was present in the contralateral kidney before surgery. See p. 645 for postoperative care of patients with renal disease.

COMPLICATIONS

The major complications of renal surgery are renal failure, hemorrhage, and urinary leakage. Urinary leakage or obstruction caused by stenosis or stricture is common with ureteral surgery. Nephrotomy is infrequently associated with urine leakage, persistent hematuria, renal pelvis dilation, renal mineralization, nephrolithiasis, suppurative pyelitis, bacterial urinary tract infection, and/or hydronephrosis.

SPECIAL AGE CONSIDERATIONS

Many animals (especially those more than 5 years old) have some degree of renal disease and require careful monitoring during any anesthetic procedure. Hypotension should be prevented during and after surgery to avoid further renal damage. If cardiac disease is also present, fluids should be used judiciously to prevent overhydration while maintaining renal blood flow.

PROGNOSIS

Most uroliths recur if the underlying disease, infection, or metabolic abnormality is not treated, often within a few months but sometimes within weeks. The effect of nephrotomy on renal function is unclear. Nephrotomy may decrease renal function as a result of a combination of direct nephron damage plus changes caused by vascular occlusion (i.e., inflammation, edema, scar formation, and ischemic damage). As much as a 50% reduction in the GFR has occurred after nephrotomy in dogs, whereas other studies have not found an adverse effect of nephrotomy on the GFR. A modest relative reduction in renal function after nephrotomy (10% to 20%) occurred in normal cats, but there was little effect on total GFR (Bolliger et al, 2005). However, the effect of nephrotomy on cats with renal disease is unknown.

Surgical treatment of ureteral calculi in cats may afford a better prognosis than does medical treatment. In a recent study, 12-month survival rates after treatment were 66% for cats treated medically and 91% for those treated surgically (Kyles et al, 2005). Many of the deaths were related to urinary tract disorders, including ureteral calculus recurrence and worsening of CRF. Return of renal concentrating ability can be expected after complete unilateral ureteral obstruction, if the obstruction is resolved less than 1 week after onset. The damage is permanent after 4 weeks of obstruction (Hardie and Kyle, 2004).

References

Adams LG, Senior DR: Electrohydraulic and extracorporeal shock-wave lithotripsy, *Vet Clin North Am Small Anim Pract* 29:293, 1999.

Adin CA, Herrgesell EJ, Nyland TG et al: Antegrade pyelography for suspected ureteral obstruction in cats: 11 cases (1995-2001), *J Am Vet Med Assoc* 222:1576, 2003.

Bolliger C, Walshaw R, Kruger JM et al: Evaluation of the effects of nephrotomy on renal function in clinically normal cats, *Am J Vet Res* 66:1400, 2005.

Davidson E, Ritchey J, Higbee R et al: Laser lithotripsy for treatment of canine uroliths, *Vet Surg* 33:56, 2004.

Hardie EM, Kyles AE: Management of ureteral obstruction, *Vet Clin North Am Small Anim Pract* 34:989, 2004.

Kyles AE, Hardie EM, Wooden BG et al: Clinical, clinicopathologic, radiographic, and ultrasonographic abnormalities in cats with ureteral calculi: 163 cases (1984-2002), *J Am Vet Med Assoc* 226:932, 2005.

Kyles AE, Hardie EM, Wooden BG et al: Management and outcome of cats with ureteral calculi: 153 cases (1984-2002), *J Am Vet Med Assoc* 226:937, 2005.

RENAL AND URETERAL NEOPLASIA

DEFINITION

Nephroblastomas are rapidly developing, malignant mixed tumors that arise from embryonal elements of the kidney. They are also called *embryonal adenomyosarcoma, nephroma,* and *Wilms' tumor.*

GENERAL CONSIDERATIONS AND CLINICALLY RELEVANT PATHOPHYSIOLOGY

Primary renal tumors are uncommon in dogs and cats. Approximately 85% of renal tumors are malignant, and thoracic metastatic disease is common. Renal tumors are of four distinct origins (types): renal tubular, transitional cell, nephroblastic, and nonepithelial. In dogs, carcinomas (also known as renal tubular carcinoma and renal tubular adenocarcinoma) are most common (Box 24-5). Lymphoma is the most common renal neoplasm in cats and may be primary or metastatic (i.e., associated with the alimentary form). Nearly 10% of cats develop malignant tumors (especially lymphoma) after renal transplantation and immunosuppression (Wooldridge et al, 2002). Generalized nodular dermatofibrosis, a skin disorder seen in German shepherds, is associated with renal cystadenocarcinomas and other neoplasms. Nephroblastomas are rare tumors of juvenile and adult dogs that are associated with hypertrophic osteopathy (see p. 1333). Most are malignant, and these tumors are thought to arise from embryonic tissue or metanephric blastema (tissue that forms the proximal components of the nephron from the glomerulus to the distal convoluted tubule) that has persisted in a primitive state without fully differentiating into functional tissue.

Bilateral renal involvement occurs in nearly 30% of dogs with primary renal neoplasia. Metastasis to the liver, adrenal glands, lungs, lymph nodes, bone, and brain is common with renal tumors. Pulmonary metastasis is detected radiographically in nearly half of dogs with renal carcinoma. Pulmonary metastasis occurs with some nephroblastomas, but is infrequent for transitional cell tumors. Renal metastasis of other primary abdominal tumors is common. Renal neoplasia may cause local signs or systemic manifestations of renal failure. Tumors arising from the renal pelvis are more apt to cause hematuria or hydronephrosis than signs of renal fail-

BOX 24-5

Types of Canine Renal Tumors

Malignant
- Carcinomas
- Hemangiosarcomas
- Fibrosarcomas
- Transitional cell carcinomas
- Nephroblastomas
- Squamous cell carcinomas
- Undifferentiated carcinomas

Benign
- Adenomas
- Hemangiomas
- Teratoma

ure. If the contralateral kidney is normal, unilateral renal damage may not cause renal failure even if it becomes nonfunctional. Large renal neoplasms may compress or invade the caudal vena cava, causing vascular obstruction. Collateral circulation usually develops in such cases, preventing clinical signs (i.e., rear limb edema or ascites).

> NOTE: Primary renal neoplasia may occur bilaterally.

DIAGNOSIS

Clinical Presentation

Signalment. Renal carcinomas occur more commonly in males than in females and may be hormonally induced. Renal cystadenocarcinomas in German shepherds are associated with generalized nodular dermatofibrosis. This syndrome occurs most commonly in middle-aged dogs of either gender and appears to be inherited as an autosomal dominant trait. Renal neoplasia most commonly occurs in middle-aged or older animals. Nephroblastomas and undifferentiated renal sarcomas occur most commonly in young dogs and cats; however, they may also occur in older animals. Teratomas may occur in the kidneys of young dogs.

History. Animals with primary renal tumors often have vague, nonspecific signs. Although the owner may report intermittent or chronic signs associated with the urinary tract or systemic signs of renal failure, the most common signs are anorexia, depression, and weight loss. Abdominal enlargement due to a renal mass may be the only sign. Renal failure is seen primarily with bilateral involvement (e.g., lymphoma in cats). Dyspnea related to pulmonary metastasis occasionally is noted. With some benign neoplasms (i.e., hemangioma), intermittent or constant hematuria is common.

Physical Examination Findings

An abdominal mass often is palpated in dogs and cats with renal neoplasia. The kidney may feel enlarged, firm, or nodular. Other findings are often nonspecific and may include weight loss, anorexia, depression, anemia, dyspnea, and pyrexia. Lameness has been associated with bony metastasis and hypertrophic osteopathy.

Diagnostic Imaging

Renal enlargement may be identified on survey abdominal radiographs; however, ultrasonography is more sensitive and specific. Excretory urography may localize the neoplasm and define parenchymal involvement. If vascular involvement is suspected, selective angiography can detect intravascular or extravascular (compressive) lesions. Cross-sectional imaging (i.e., CT, magnetic resonance imaging [MRI]) may also be employed to evaluate renal masses. Thoracic radiographs should be taken to detect pulmonary metastasis.

Laboratory Findings

Laboratory findings often are nonspecific; however, anemia and azotemia are common. A complete blood cell count (including a platelet count), serum chemistry profile, and urinalysis are indicated. Polycythemia is rarely found. Gross hematuria may occur with mesenchymal tumors (i.e., anaplastic sarcomas, fibromas, hemangiosarcomas, and lymphosarcoma) and transitional cell tumors; however, microscopic hematuria is more common. Proteinuria may be noted.

DIFFERENTIAL DIAGNOSIS

Renal neoplasia must be differentiated from other causes of renomegaly (i.e., hydronephrosis, polycystic disease, and abscess) or abdominal enlargement (e.g., splenic or hepatic neoplasia). Abdominal ultrasonography is the most useful diagnostic tool. Ultrasound-guided biopsy can be performed if the kidney does not appear fluid filled; however, the biopsy may cause peritonitis or uncontrollable hemorrhage, or it may seed the abdomen with tumor cells.

Perirenal pseudocysts have been reported in cats and are formed when fluid accumulates between the parenchyma of the kidney and the renal capsule as a result of underlying parenchymal disease (Beck et al, 2000; Ochoa et al, 1999). Resection of the pseudocyst wall is effective in eliminating signs, but does not stop the progression of renal disease. The prognosis for cats with pseudocysts is related to the degree of renal dysfunction at the time of diagnosis.

MEDICAL MANAGEMENT

Preoperative medical management of animals with renal neoplasia is necessary if renal failure is present or if anemia is severe (i.e., the PCV is below 20%). Medical management of animals with renal failure is discussed on p. 635.

SURGICAL TREATMENT

Nephrectomy is indicated for malignant renal tumors if they are unilateral and without evident metastasis (Fig. 24-20). Dogs with renal carcinoma occasionally live for years after removal of the affected kidney. However, metastasis typically is present at the time of diagnosis because of the late onset of clinical signs. Adjuvant chemotherapy or radiation ther-

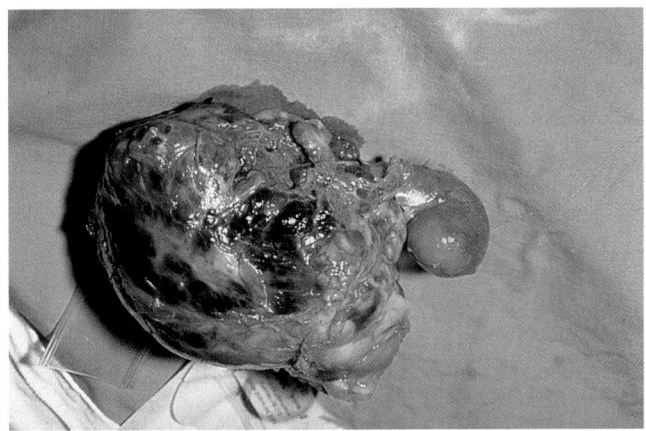

FIG. 24-20
Renal hemangioendothelioma in a 6-year-old dog.

apy may prolong the lives of dogs and cats with malignant renal neoplasia, but few data are available on which to base recommendations. Cats with renal lymphoma may respond to chemotherapy for variable time periods.

Preoperative Management

Hydration, acid-base, and electrolyte abnormalities should be corrected before surgery, if possible. Perioperative antibiotic therapy is indicated in some patients (i.e., large neoplasms that may be secondarily infected, or the patient may be immunosuppressed or chronically debilitated). Animals with preexisting urinary tract infections should be treated preoperatively with antibiotics. If the patient is substantially anemic, preoxygenation is beneficial. Preoperative blood transfusions should be considered in moderately to severely anemic patients, and blood should be available for intraoperative and postoperative transfusions if needed.

Anesthesia

If renal impairment is not present, many anesthetic regimens can be used safely. If renal impairment is present, see p. 636 for suggested anesthetic protocols.

Surgical Anatomy

The surgical anatomy of the kidney and ureter is discussed on p. 637.

Positioning

The animal is placed in dorsal recumbency and the abdomen prepared for a ventral midline incision. The prepared area should extend from above the xiphoid to below the pubis.

SURGICAL TECHNIQUE

The entire abdomen should be explored for metastasis before performing a nephrectomy (see p. 639). The other kidney should be palpated and biopsies performed if bilateral involvement is suspected. Intraoperative cytology or examination of frozen sections is helpful for determining if the tumor is malignant. The adjacent ureter should be located to ensure that it is not inadvertently ligated. Occasionally the tumor will invade surrounding tissue (e.g., sublumbar musculature or the caudal vena cava), making complete removal difficult. The entire ureter should be removed with the kidney. Careful handling of the neoplastic kidney and ligation of the renal vein may help prevent seeding of neoplastic cells via the vasculature or directly into adjacent tissue.

SUTURE MATERIALS AND SPECIAL INSTRUMENTS

Absorbable suture material, such as polyglactin 910 (Vicryl), polyglycolic acid (Dexon), polydioxanone (PDS), polyglyconate (Maxon), or poliglecaprone 25 (Monocryl), or nonabsorbable cardiovascular silk, can be used to ligate the renal vessels and ureter.

POSTOPERATIVE CARE AND ASSESSMENT

See p. 645 for postoperative care of patients with renal disease.

COMPLICATIONS

The major complications of nephrectomy are hemorrhage and urinary leakage. If the animal had preexisting CRD, ARF may occur postoperatively. With large renal tumors, inadvertent ligation of the opposite ureter is possible if care is not taken to determine its location intraoperatively.

SPECIAL AGE CONSIDERATIONS

Older animals often have some degree of CRD in the contralateral kidney and require careful monitoring during the surgical procedure. Also, many animals have bilateral renal neoplasia. Renal neoplasia should not be excluded as a possible diagnosis in young animals with renomegaly.

PROGNOSIS

Because most renal tumors are aggressively malignant, they are seldom diagnosed before they have metastasized, making for a poor prognosis. However, if nephrectomy is performed before metastasis, long-term survival is possible. Long-term survival (i.e., greater than 2 years) with nephroblastoma is possible (Seaman and Patton, 2003). Adjunctive chemotherapy may prolong the disease-free survival interval. With benign neoplasia, nephrectomy usually is curative.

References

Beck JA, Bellenger CR, Lamb WA et al: Perirenal pseudocysts in 26 cats, *Aust Vet J* 78:166, 2000.

Ochoa VB, DiBartola SP, Chew D et al: Perinephric pseudocysts in the cat: a retrospective study and review of the literature, *J Vet Intern Med* 13:47, 1999.

Seaman RL, Patton CS: Treatment of nephroblastoma in an adult dog, *J Am Anim Hosp Assoc* 39:76, 2004.

Wooldridge JD, Gregory CR, Mathews KG et al: The prevalence of malignant neoplasia in feline renal-transplant recipients, *Vet Surg* 31:94, 2002.

Suggested Reading

Castellano MC et al: Generalized nodular dermatofibrosis and cystic renal disease in five German shepherd dogs, *Canine Pract* 25:18, 2000.

The author reviews the clinical findings and outcome of five German shepherd dogs with generalized nodular dermatofibrosis and cystic renal disease.

Henry CJ, Turnquist SE, Smith A et al: Primary renal tumours in cats: 19 cases (1992-1998), *J Fel Med Surg* 1:165, 1999.

Signalment, history, and outcome of 19 cats with renal tumors are described.

RENAL AND PERIRENAL ABSCESSES

DEFINITIONS

Perirenal, or *perinephric*, abscesses are abscesses located outside the renal capsule in the perinephric fascia. These infections often result from the extension of an intrarenal abscess. **Renal**, or *intrarenal*, abscesses occur within the renal parenchyma.

GENERAL CONSIDERATIONS AND CLINICALLY RELEVANT PATHOPHYSIOLOGY

Focal renal infections are classified as intrarenal or perirenal. Intrarenal abscesses are further divided into renal cortical abscesses and renal corticomedullary abscesses. The incidence of intrarenal and perirenal abscesses in humans ranges from 1 to 10 cases per 10,000 hospital admissions. The incidence of perirenal abscesses in dogs and cats is unknown, but seems rare (Agut et al, 2004). Before the advent of antibiotics, most cases of renal abscesses in humans resulted from hematogenous seeding of the kidney from a distant focus of infection. Young males without an antecedent history of renal disease were predominantly affected. However, males and females today are equally affected, and most cases are a complication of urinary tract obstruction. Although few cases have been reported in dogs, they have been associated with pyelonephritis, hyperadrenocorticism, diabetes mellitus, and renal biopsy (Hess and Ilan, 2003). Most renal cortical abscesses are unilateral, and *Staphylococcus aureus* is the most commonly isolated etiologic agent. Some renal cortical abscesses rupture through the renal capsule, thereby forming a perinephric abscess. Renal corticomedullary abscesses generally result from bacteriuria and an ascending infection in patients with underlying urinary tract abnormalities. Enteric aerobic gram-negative bacilli (i.e., *Escherichia coli*, *Proteus* spp., and *Klebsiella* spp.) seem most common.

DIAGNOSIS
Clinical Presentation

Signalment. No breed or sex predisposition has been identified in dogs or cats for either condition. Dogs and cats of any age may be affected.

History. The history of animals with renal or perirenal abscesses varies from an acute pain and fever to chronic, mild, intermittent nonspecific signs. Occasionally the only abnormality noted is abdominal enlargement associated with a renal mass.

Physical Examination Findings

Animals with renal or perirenal abscesses typically demonstrate pain on abdominal palpation. The kidney may feel enlarged, soft, and fluctuant. Other findings are often nonspecific and may include weight loss, anorexia, and pyrexia. Physical examination findings cannot differentiate renal from perirenal abscessation.

Diagnostic Imaging

Renal enlargement may be identified on survey abdominal radiographs; however, ultrasonography is more sensitive and specific for detection of focal masses. Ultrasound and CT may differentiate between renal and perirenal abscesses. Perirenal pseudocysts and subcapsular hematomas can also typically be differentiated with advanced imaging modalities.

Laboratory Findings

Laboratory findings often are nonspecific; however, leukocytosis and renal azotemia may be found. A complete blood cell count (including a platelet count), serum chemistry profile, urinalysis, and urine culture should be performed. Urinary tract infection is common with renal abscesses.

DIFFERENTIAL DIAGNOSIS

Perirenal and intrarenal abscesses must be differentiated from renal neoplasia and other causes of renomegaly (i.e., hydronephrosis and polycystic disease; see p. 659).

MEDICAL MANAGEMENT

The treatment of renal and perirenal abscesses traditionally required surgical intervention. In people, some entities (i.e., renal cortical abscesses and acute focal bacterial nephritis) are now recognized as treatable with antibiotics alone and generally do not require drainage procedures. Thus it may be reasonable to try an intensive trial of appropriate antibiotic therapy before considering surgical drainage or nephrectomy for lesions localized to the renal parenchyma. By contrast, resolution of acute multifocal bacterial nephritis generally requires some form of drainage procedure for patients with large abscesses or for those who respond slowly to antibiotics alone. Percutaneous drainage, rather than open surgical drainage, may be possible in some patients, but should be done with care to prevent peritonitis. Ultrasound-guided percutaneous drainage of pyonephrosis (suppurative destruction of the kidney parenchyma with complete or nearly complete loss of renal function) has been reported in dogs (Szatmari et al, 2001). Early surgical drainage of perinephric abscesses is imperative because antibiotic therapy alone is inadequate and should be viewed as adjunctive treatment to drainage. In human patients, perinephric abscesses have been drained by percutaneous tube placement, aspiration of pus, and antibiotic irrigation before definitive surgery (nephrectomy), but nephrectomy is typically indicated. Patients with a renal or perirenal abscess require prolonged courses of antibiotic therapy, generally lasting 4 to 6 weeks.

SURGICAL TREATMENT

Surgical drainage may be indicated in some patients with reduced function in the contralateral kidney; however, renal and perirenal abscesses generally require nephrectomy (see previous discussion in the Medical Management section).

Preoperative Management

If possible, hydration, acid-base, and electrolyte abnormalities should be corrected before surgery. Perioperative antibiotic therapy is indicated in most patients. If the patient is substantially anemic, preoxygenation is beneficial.

Anesthesia

See p. 636 for suggested anesthetic protocols for animals with renal impairment.

Surgical Anatomy

The surgical anatomy of the kidney and ureter is discussed on p. 637.

Positioning

The animal is placed in dorsal recumbency, and the abdomen is prepared for a ventral midline incision. The prepared area should extend from above the xiphoid to below the pubis.

SURGICAL TECHNIQUE

Nephrectomy (see p. 639) may be performed for renal and perirenal abscesses if the other kidney is sufficiently normal to sustain renal function after surgery. The entire abdomen should be explored for other evidence of infection, and the contralateral kidney should be palpated and determined to be normal before removal of the diseased kidney. The ureters should be palpated for evidence of obstructive disease (e.g., ureteroliths) that might have been predisposed to the infection. Renal tissue should be cultured and submitted for histopathology. A urine sample should be submitted for culture at the time of surgery.

SUTURE MATERIALS AND SPECIAL INSTRUMENTS

Absorbable suture material, such as polyglactin 910 (Vicryl), polyglycolic acid (Dexon), polydioxanone (PDS), polyglyconate (Maxon), or poliglecaprone 25 (Monocryl), or nonabsorbable cardiovascular silk, can be used to ligate the renal vessels and ureter.

POSTOPERATIVE CARE AND ASSESSMENT

See p. 645 for postoperative care of patients with renal disease.

COMPLICATIONS

Major complications of nephrectomy are hemorrhage and urinary leakage. If the animal had preexisting renal dysfunction, ARF may occur postoperatively. With percutaneous drainage, peritonitis is a possible and serious complication.

SPECIAL AGE CONSIDERATIONS

Older animals may have some degree of CRD in the contralateral kidney and require careful monitoring during the surgical procedure.

PROGNOSIS

Perinephric abscesses are associated with significant mortality despite aggressive drainage of the abscess, surgical intervention, and antibiotics, possibly because the diagnosis is often delayed. Prompt diagnosis with nephrectomy of the abscessed kidney may lead to a positive outcome.

References

Agut A, Lardo FG, Belda E et al: Left perinephric abscess associated with nephrolithiasis and bladder calculi in a bitch, *Vet Rec* 154:562, 2004.

Hess RS, Ilan I: Renal abscess in a dog with transient diabetes mellitus, *J Small Anim Pract* 44:13, 2003.

Szatmari V, Osi Z, Manczur F: Ultrasound-guided percutaneous drainage for treatment of pyonephrosis in two dogs, *J Am Vet Med Assoc* 218:1796, 2001.

Zatelli A, D'Ippolito P: Bilateral perirenal abscesses in a domestic neutered shorthair cat, *J Vet Intern Med* 18:902, 2004.

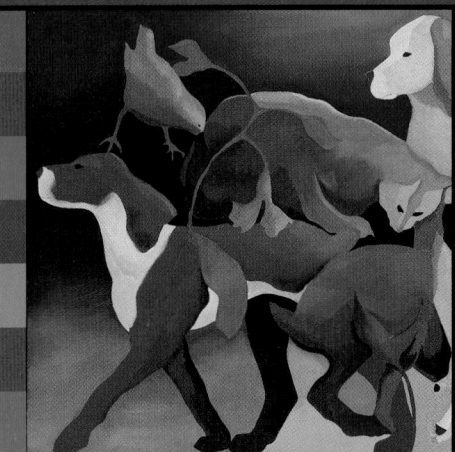

CHAPTER 25
Surgery of the Bladder and Urethra

GENERAL PRINCIPLES AND TECHNIQUES

DEFINITIONS

Cystotomy is surgical incision into the urinary bladder, whereas **urethrotomy** is an incision into the urethra. **Cystectomy** is removal of a portion of the urinary bladder. **Cystolithiasis** and **cystolithectomy** refer to the development of urinary bladder calculi and their removal, respectively. The **trigone** of the bladder is a smooth triangular portion of the mucous membrane at the base of the bladder (i.e., near the urethra) where the ureters empty. **Cystostomy** is the creation of an opening into the bladder; **prepubic catheterization** (temporary cystostomy) is usually performed to provide cutaneous urinary diversion in animals with urethral obstruction or trauma. **Uroabdomen** is the presence of urine in the abdominal cavity; the urine may be leaking from the kidneys, ureters, bladder, or urethra. **Urethrostomy** is the creation of a permanent fistula into the urethra and is generally performed for irreparable or recurrent urethral stricture, or to prevent repeated obstruction (i.e., with feline urologic syndrome or sterile cystitis).

PREOPERATIVE MANAGEMENT

Cystolithiasis, neoplasia, and rupture are the most common abnormalities of the urinary bladder in small animals. Urinary obstruction may occur if calculi become lodged in the urethra or if a tumor obstructs the proximal urethra or trigone. Male cats with sterile cystitis may develop penile urethral obstruction (see p. 698). Obstruction to urinary flow may cause a distended urinary bladder, postrenal uremia, and hyperkalemia. Bladder rupture primarily occurs after motor vehicular trauma, but may also be caused by necrotic bladders (e.g., following damage to its blood supply or prolonged partial urethral obstruction) or as a complication of bladder surgery (Fig. 25-1). Urinary leakage into the abdominal cavity causes uremia, dehydration, hypovolemia, hyperkalemia, and death if undiagnosed or untreated. Urinary obstruction and uroperitoneum are medical emergencies, not surgical emergencies. Hyperkalemia associated with these conditions makes the animal prone to cardiac arrhyth-

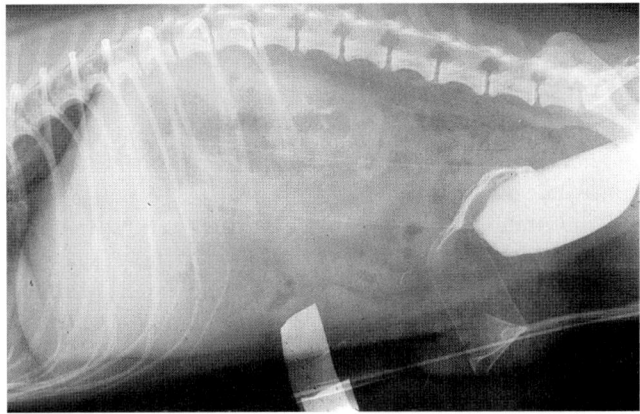

FIG. 25-1
Positive contrast cystourethrogram in a dog 3 days after a cystotomy was performed. Note contrast leaking from the incision at the dorsal aspect of the bladder.

mias; therefore fluid and electrolyte abnormalities should be corrected before anesthesia (see p. 635).

Hyperkalemia causes bradycardia, absent or flattened P waves, prolongation of the P-R interval, widened QRS complexes, and/or "tented" or spiked T waves in addition to predisposing to cardiac arrhythmias. Potassium concentrations greater than 7 mEq/L may cause irregular idioventricular rhythms, and potassium concentrations exceeding 9 mEq/L commonly cause atrial standstill. Mild or moderate hyperkalemia may be treated with intravenous (IV) fluids (i.e., 0.9% saline for dilution; Box 25-1). If the animal has concurrent hyponatremia, 5% dextrose solutions (i.e., D5W) and half-strength saline should be avoided.

Hyperkalemia from uroabdomen responds well to abdominal drainage plus intravenous fluid therapy. Hyperkalemia caused by urethral obstruction responds well to intravenous fluids plus elimination of the obstruction. Although seldom required, life-threatening hyperkalemia may be treated with sodium bicarbonate. Bicarbonate therapy drives potassium into cells in exchange for hydrogen ions. Alternatively, life-threatening hyperkalemia can be treated with in-

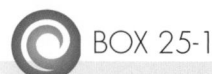

BOX 25-1

Treatment of Hyperkalemia in Cats

1. Dilute by giving physiologic saline solution (i.e., 0.9%) IV.
2. If necessary, give sodium bicarbonate (see Box 5-1 on p. 25) or insulin 0.2–0.4 U/kg regular insulin IV) plus dextrose (2 g/U of insulin).
3. If hyperkalemia is life threatening, may give 10% calcium gluconate (0.2–1.5 ml/kg) for transient cardiac protection. Give slowly (over 5–10 minutes) while monitoring the patient's ECG.

IV, Intravenous.

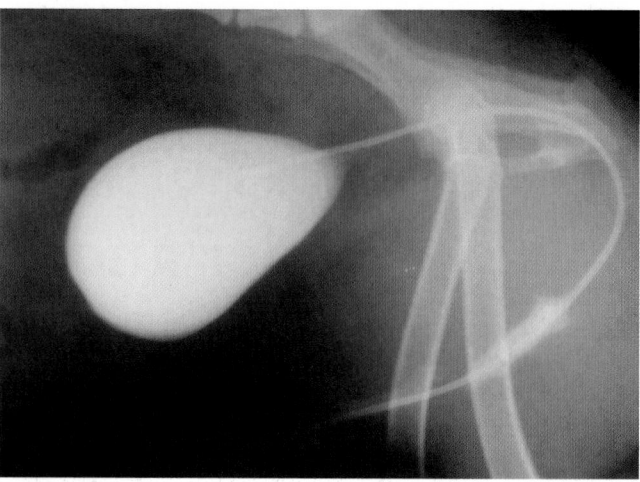

FIG. 25-2
Radiograph of a dog with spontaneous urethral rupture associated with a urinary tract infection. Note the leakage of contrast into the tissue just proximal to the os penis.

sulin and dextrose administration (see Box 25-1). Insulin facilitates cellular uptake of potassium, whereas dextrose prevents hypoglycemia following insulin administration. If the hyperkalemia appears immediately life threatening, 10% calcium gluconate given slowly intravenously may protect the heart until other therapy lowers the plasma potassium concentration.

Preventing reabsorption of electrolytes and waste products by abdominal drainage plus IV fluid therapy (i.e., dilution) is the best way to treat hyperkalemia and azotemia in animals with uroperitoneum. Penrose drains are ineffective for abdominal drainage of more than 12 to 24 hours because they are quickly isolated from the abdominal cavity by omentum and fibrin; closed systems (e.g., peritoneal lavage catheters and sump drains) are more appropriate for abdominal drainage. Peritoneal lavage catheters are preferred over Penrose drains because they can be attached to an empty fluid bag, allowing for a closed system. The goal of abdominal drainage in these patients is to normalize serum electrolytes and decrease azotemia, making the animal a better candidate for anesthesia. Fluid therapy plus abdominal drainage for 6 to 12 hours is often adequate for this purpose. Peritoneal dialysis may be useful when treating patients with concurrent renal dysfunction.

Urethral trauma (e.g., gunshot or bite wounds, rupture caused by vehicular trauma, and obstruction with stones) or neoplasia may result in urinary obstruction. If the prostatic or penile urethra is torn, subcutaneous urine leakage may occur. Spontaneous rupture of the urethra may also occur in some dogs (Fig. 25-2). Initial signs of subcutaneous urine leakage are bruising and/or swelling, especially of the inguinal tissue of male dogs. The skin and subcutaneous tissue can necrose if left untreated. Management of patients with urethral rupture before surgery may necessitate placement of an indwelling urinary catheter and/or cutaneous urinary diversion (tube cystostomy; see p. 667).

ANESTHESIA

Electrolyte (i.e., hyperkalemia) abnormalities and acidosis in patients with urinary obstruction or leakage should be corrected before anesthetic induction (see previous discussion and pp. 636 and 699). Fluids are given intravenously to restore hydration and combat postobstruction diuresis; relief of obstruction without appropriate parenteral fluids commonly causes hypovolemia and possibly death. An electrocardiogram (ECG) should be monitored before, during, and after surgery for cardiac arrhythmias. If the animal is hyperkalemic, 0.9% saline should be used for fluid therapy. If the serum potassium is normal, a balanced electrolyte solution should be administered.

Anticholinergics are not routinely recommended for trauma patients because they may increase heart rate and oxygen consumption, and cause a predisposition to cardiac arrhythmias. If analgesia is needed, butorphanol, hydromorphone, or buprenorphine may be given in small, incremental doses (see Table 13-4 on p. 133). Acetylpromazine should only be used if volume replacement has been adequate, and if shock or severe blood loss is unlikely. Thiobarbiturates are arrhythmogenic and should be used cautiously in animals with preexisting arrhythmias. Combinations of opioids and benzodiazepines (e.g., diazepam) do not cause severe vasodilation or myocardial depression and are useful for inducing anesthesia despite hypovolemia (Boxes 25-2 and 25-3). Etomidate may be used for induction since it maintains cardiovascular stability and is not arrhythmogenic. Alternatively, mask or chamber induction is acceptable if the patient is not vomiting, or thiopental or propofol may be administered at reduced dosages. Cats may be premedicated using low doses of butorphanol, buprenorphine, or hydromorphone and induced with etomidate. Because cats excrete the active form of ketamine in their urine, it should be avoided or used very cautiously if urinary obstruction or renal dysfunction is present. Isoflurane and sevoflurane in oxygen are the least cardiodepressant inhalation anesthetics and may be used for anesthetic maintenance.

BOX 25-2

Selected Anesthetic Protocols for Use in Stable Dogs and Cats With Urinary Abnormalities

Premedication

Hydromorphone* (0.1–0.2 mg/kg SC or IM) or butorphanol (0.2–0.4 mg/kg SC or IM) or buprenorphine (5–15 μg/kg IM)

Induction

Thiopental (10–12 mg/kg IV) or propofol (4–6 mg/kg IV) (see text also)

Maintenance

Isoflurane or sevoflurane

SC, Subcutaneoous; *IM,* intramuscular; *IV,* intravenous.
*Use 0.05 mg/kg in cats.

 BOX 25-3

Selected Anesthetic Protocols for Use in Decompensated Patients in Renal Failure or Hypovolemic, Dehydrated, or Shocky Animals With Urinary Abnormalities

Dogs

Premedication and induction

Hydromorphone (0.1 mg/kg IV) plus diazepam (0.2 mg/kg IV). Give in incremental doses. Intubate if possible. If necessary, give etomidate (0.5–1.5 mg/kg IV). (See text also.)

Maintenance

Isoflurane or sevoflurane.

Cats

Premedication

Butorphanol (0.2–0.4 mg/kg SC or IM) or buprenorphine (5–15 μg/kg IM) or hydromorphone (0.05–0.1 mg/kg SC or IM).

Induction

Diazepam (0.2 mg/kg IV) followed by etomidate (0.5–1.5 mg/kg IV). (See text also.)

Maintenance

Isoflurane or sevoflurane.

IV, Intravenous *SC;* subcutaneoous; *IM,* intramuscular.

ANTIBIOTICS

Perioperative antibiotic therapy should be considered in animals with urinary obstruction or leakage because infection prolongs healing and promotes stricture formation. Animals with cystic or urethral calculi often have concurrent infections and should be treated with appropriate antibiotics based on urine culture and susceptibility, or antibiotics can be withheld until intraoperative cultures are taken. When culture of urine obtained by cystocentesis is negative, aerobic cultures of a bladder mucosal biopsy should be obtained. In a recent study, *Escherichia coli* was the most common isolate from 383 dogs with recurrent or persistent urinary tract infections; however, 58% of the female and 55% of the male dogs had mixed bacterial infections (Norris et al, 2000). Potentially nephrotoxic antibiotics (i.e., aminoglycosides and tetracycline) should be avoided in patients with obstructions (see p. 637).

> NOTE: Organisms may be cultured from the bladder mucosa or a urolith in dogs with urolithiasis from which a negative urine culture was previously obtained; therefore all animals undergoing cystotomy should have cultures of bladder mucosa and uroliths submitted.

SURGICAL ANATOMY

The bladder location varies depending on the amount of urine it currently contains; when empty it lies entirely, or almost entirely, within the pelvic cavity. In a 12-kg dog, it holds up to 120 ml of urine without becoming overly distended. The bladder is divided into a neck, which connects it to the urethra, and a body. The bladder receives its blood supply from the cranial and caudal vesical arteries, which are branches of the umbilical and urogenital arteries, respectively. Sympathetic innervation is from the hypogastric nerves, whereas parasympathetic innervation is via the pelvic nerve. The pudendal nerve supplies somatic innervation to the external bladder sphincter and striated musculature of the urethra. The urethra in male dogs is divided into prostatic membranous and penile portions (see p. 666).

SURGICAL TECHNIQUE

For the bladder, an incision is made from the umbilicus caudal to the pubis (Fig. 25-3). The proximal urethra (i.e., prostatic urethra) can be reached by this approach; however, pelvic osteotomy or symphysiotomy is required for adequate exposure of the membranous urethra (i.e., from the caudal edge of the prostate to the ischial arch; Figs. 25-4 and 25-5). The penile urethra begins at the ischial arch and extends to the external urethral penile orifice. The penile urethra may be approached in the perineal (perineal urethrotomy) or scrotal (scrotal urethrotomy) regions, or between the scrotum and the external urethral orifice (prescrotal urethrotomy). The skin overlying the site is prepared for aseptic surgery in the standard fashion before using either approach.

Cystotomy

Cystotomy may be performed for removal of cystic and urethral calculi (see p. 682), identification and biopsy of masses (see p. 689), repair of ectopic ureters (see p. 646), or evaluation of urinary tract infection resistant to treatment. The incision is generally made on the dorsal or ventral surface of

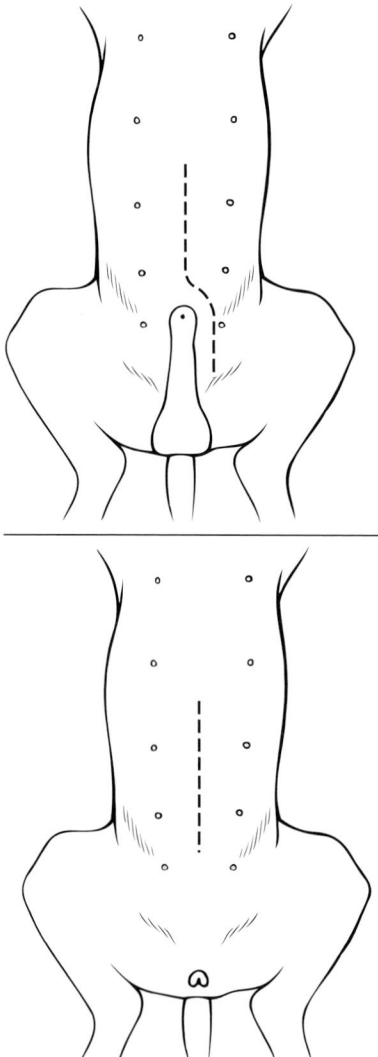

FIG. 25-3
To expose the bladder, make an incision from the umbilicus to the pubis.

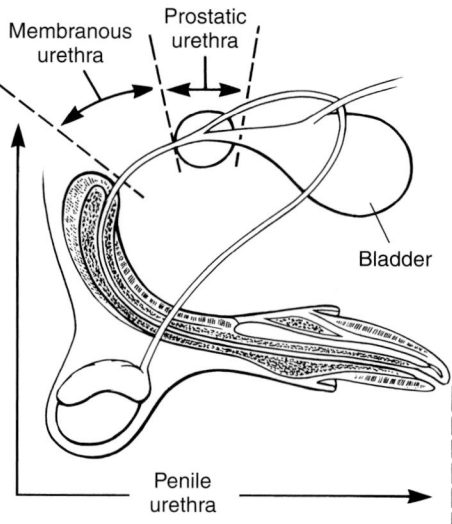

FIG. 25-4
The urethra of male dogs is composed of prostatic, membranous, and penile portions.

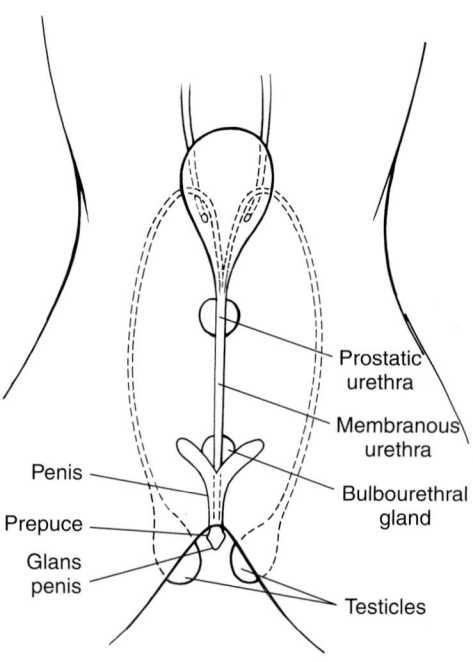

FIG. 25-5
Anatomy of the bladder, urethra, and reproductive system in male cats.

the bladder, away from the urethra; however, ventral exposure is performed if identification and/or catheterization of ureteral openings is necessary. The goal of cystotomy closure is to obtain a watertight seal that will not promote formation of calculi. This has traditionally been accomplished using a single- or double-layer appositional pattern or by inverting suture patterns using absorbable suture material. A single-layer appositional closure is always sufficient if the bladder wall is thick. Even in normal bladders, a single-layer appositional suture pattern (simple continuous) is typically adequate. Luminal penetration is common in thin-walled bladders, but this is not associated with calculus formation if absorbable monofilament suture is used. If hemorrhage is expected to be severe, suturing the bladder mucosa as a separate layer (in a simple continuous suture pattern) may decrease postoperative bleeding (see p. 677 for a discussion of suture materials).

Isolate the bladder from the rest of the abdominal cavity by placing moistened laparotomy pads beneath it. Place stay sutures on the bladder apex to facilitate manipulation (Fig. 25-6, A). Make the incision in the dorsal or ventral aspect of the bladder, away from the ureters and urethra and between major blood vessels. Remove urine by suction (perform intra-

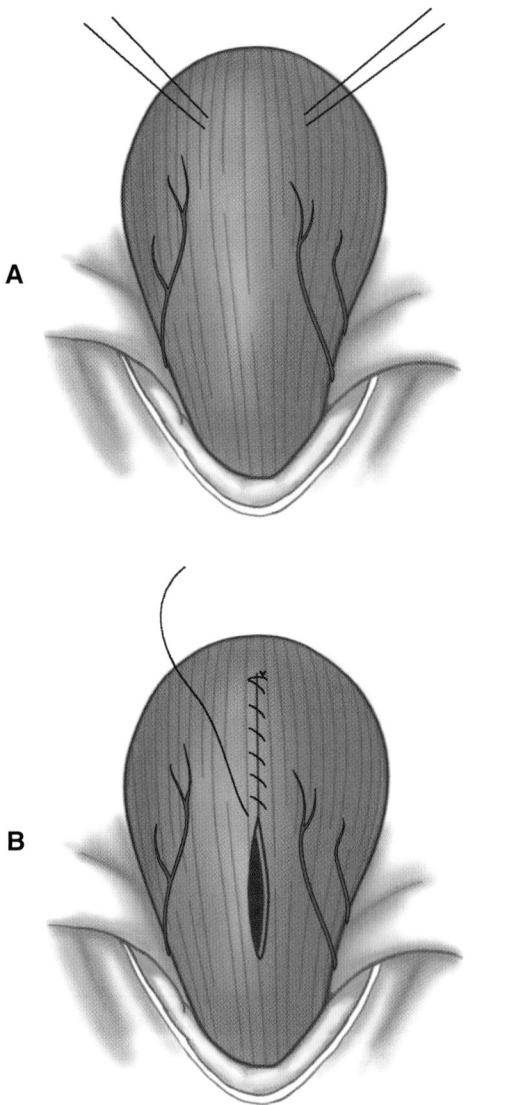

FIG. 25-6
Cystotomy is indicated to remove calculi, repair trauma, resect or biopsy neoplasms, or correct congenital abnormalities. **A,** Isolate the bladder and place stay sutures in it to facilitate manipulation. Make the incision in the dorsal or ventral aspect of the bladder. **B,** Use a simple continuous suture to close the incision. If the bladder is thin and if leakage occurs, a two-layer closure can be used, but this is seldom necessary.

operative cystocentesis before cystotomy if suction is not available). Excise a small section of the bladder wall adjacent to the incision, and submit it for culture. Check the bladder apex for a diverticulum, and remove it if necessary. Examine the mucosa for defects, and pass a catheter down the urethra to check for patency. Close the bladder in a single layer using a continuous suture pattern with absorbable suture material (see previous discussion). For a two-layer closure, suture the seromuscular layers with two continuous inverting suture lines (i.e., Cushing, followed by Lembert;

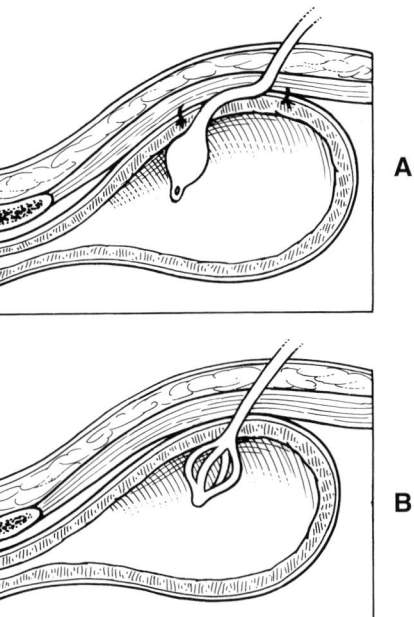

FIG. 25-7
Temporary cystostomy or prepubic catheterization may be performed by placing a Foley catheter **(A)** or a Stamey Malecot catheter **(B)** into the bladder.

Fig. 25-6, B). If the dog has severe bleeding tendencies, suture the mucosa as a separate layer with a simple continuous suture pattern (optional).

> NOTE: When removing cystic calculi, be sure to catheterize the urethra and flush until you are certain that the urethra is free of calculi. Leaving stones in the urethra is a common error.

Cystostomy (Prepubic Catheterization)

Temporary cystostomy or prepubic catheterization is performed to provide cutaneous urinary diversion in animals with urinary obstruction, or with traumatized or surgically repaired urethras. It may also be advisable for animals with bladder atony secondary to neurologic disease or to prevent overdistention of the bladder after surgery. Cystostomy may be performed by placing a Foley catheter (6 to 12 French) via a small abdominal incision, or percutaneously by placing a Stamey Malecot catheter (10 to 14 French) into the bladder (Fig. 25-7). Premature removal of the Stamey Malecot catheter may occur; therefore surgically placed Foley catheters may be preferred for long-term catheterization in ambulatory patients. Use of low-profile gastrostomy tubes was recently reported in dogs and cats for cystostomy (Stiffler et al, 2003) and appears to be well tolerated. Regular gastrostomy tubes have also been used for prepubic catheters. The catheters can generally be placed under local anesthesia (augmented by chemical restraint or mask inhalation anesthesia,

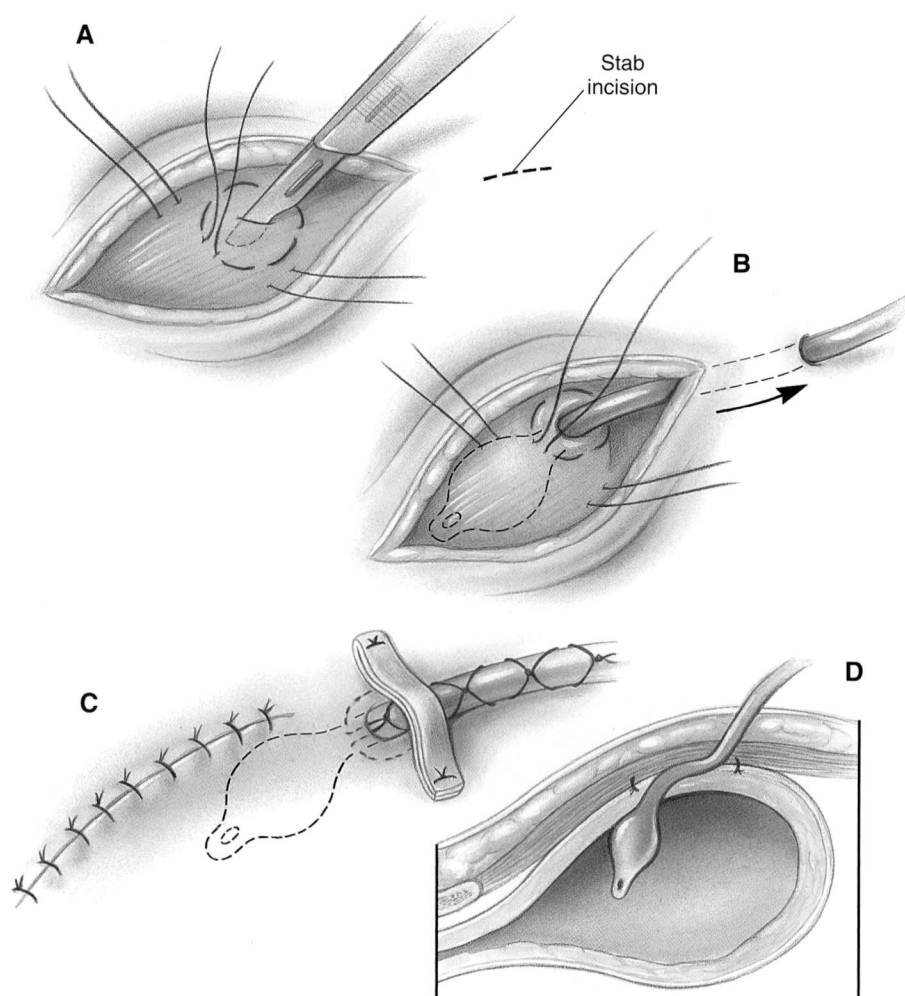

FIG. 25-8
A, To place a Foley catheter, make a small incision and locate the bladder. Place stay sutures and a purse-string suture in the bladder. Place the tip of the Foley catheter into the abdominal cavity through a separate stab incision in the abdominal wall. **B**, Make a small stab incision into the bladder, and place the Foley catheter into the bladder lumen. **C**, Inflate the balloon with saline, and secure the catheter within the lumen by tying the purse-string suture around it with a Roman sandal suture (see p. 901). **D**, Tack the bladder to the body wall with several absorbable sutures.

if necessary). They can also be placed during exploratory laparotomy. Removal of the Stamey catheter can be performed by gentle traction within 3 or 4 days after placement without risk of urinary leakage; however, it is recommended that a Foley catheter be left in 5 to 7 days.

To place a Foley catheter, make a small midline incision caudal to the umbilicus in females or adjacent to the prepuce in males. Locate the bladder, and place stay sutures and a purse-string suture into it (Fig. 25-8, A). Place the tip of the Foley catheter into the abdominal cavity through a separate stab incision in the abdominal wall (Fig. 25-8, B). Make a small stab incision into the bladder (within the purse-string suture), and place the Foley catheter into the bladder lumen. Inflate the balloon with saline, and secure the catheter within the lumen by tying the purse-string suture around it with a Roman sandal suture (see p. 901 and Fig. 25-8, C). Tack the bladder to the body wall with several absorbable sutures (Fig. 25-8, D). Close the initial incision, and tack the catheter to the skin by placing sutures through a piece of tape attached to the catheter.

For a Stamey catheter (see Fig. 25-7), place the dog in right- or left-lateral recumbency and prep the ventrolateral

aspect of the caudal abdominal wall. Do not evacuate the bladder before catheter placement. Make a small skin incision over the bladder and with the stylet securely fixed within the catheter (with the Malecot wings twisted flat), direct it through the stab incision. Thrust the catheter into the bladder lumen, making sure that the entire flanged portion of the catheter is within the bladder lumen (once urine is obtained, advance the catheter 1 cm farther). Release the Luer-Lok to open the Malecot wings, and remove the obturator. Secure the catheter to the skin.

INTRAPELVIC URETHRAL ANASTOMOSIS

The intrapelvic urethra may be torn secondarily to pelvic fractures or other trauma, or it may be damaged during surgery. Primary suture repair of a completely transected urethra is indicated whenever possible. Dependent on size, small lacerations or partial ruptures may heal if urine is diverted through a urethral catheter or tube cystostomy for 7 to 21 days.

Perform a caudal ventral midline abdominal incision and, if necessary, a pubic symphysiotomy or bilateral pubic and ischial osteotomy (see p. 669). Locate the transected ends of

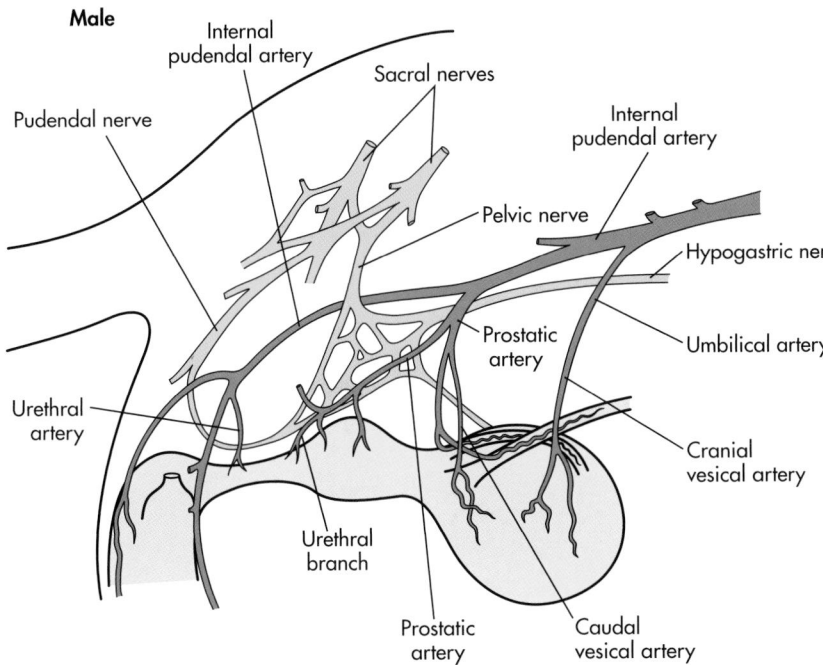

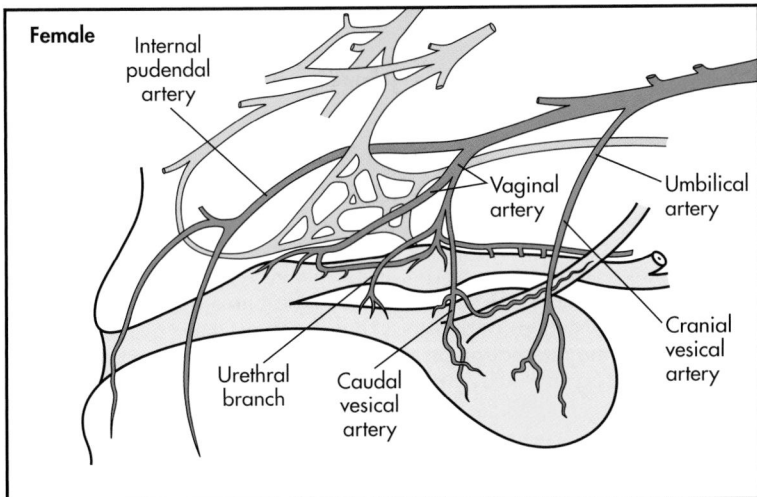

FIG. 25-9
Vascular and nerve supply to the bladder and urethra.

the urethra and débride them. Minimize dissection around the urethra and bladder to prevent damaging the vascular or nerve supply to these structures (Fig. 25-9). Suture the ends with six to eight absorbable interrupted sutures over a transurethral catheter (preferably a Foley catheter or other soft catheter). Leave the catheter in place for 7 to 10 days.

If the urethral tissues do not hold suture because of prolonged urine extravasation and subsequent tissue devitalization, delayed repair is indicated.

Place a transurethral catheter to divert urine flow for 5 to 7 days. If a catheter cannot be placed from the penile orifice into the bladder, pass a catheter from the bladder into the traumatized tissue, tie it to a catheter placed from the penile urethral orifice, and use it to pull the penile catheter into the bladder. If the urethra does not heal completely in

7 to 10 days or if stricture occurs, resect the urethral ends and suture them over a catheter as described for primary repair.

Tube cystostomy can also be used to provide urinary diversion while the urethra is healing, but one must ensure that bladder distention is not allowed, or urethral flow of urine will occur.

Adequate urethral exposure can be obtained in some dogs by splitting the symphysis on the midline. In other dogs, the cranial aspect of the pubis must be removed. Bilateral pubic and ischial osteotomy allows exposure of the entire urogenital tract in female dogs.

Make a ventral midline incision from the umbilicus to the vulva. Perform a celiotomy from the umbilicus to the pubis, then sharply separate the adductor muscles on the midline of

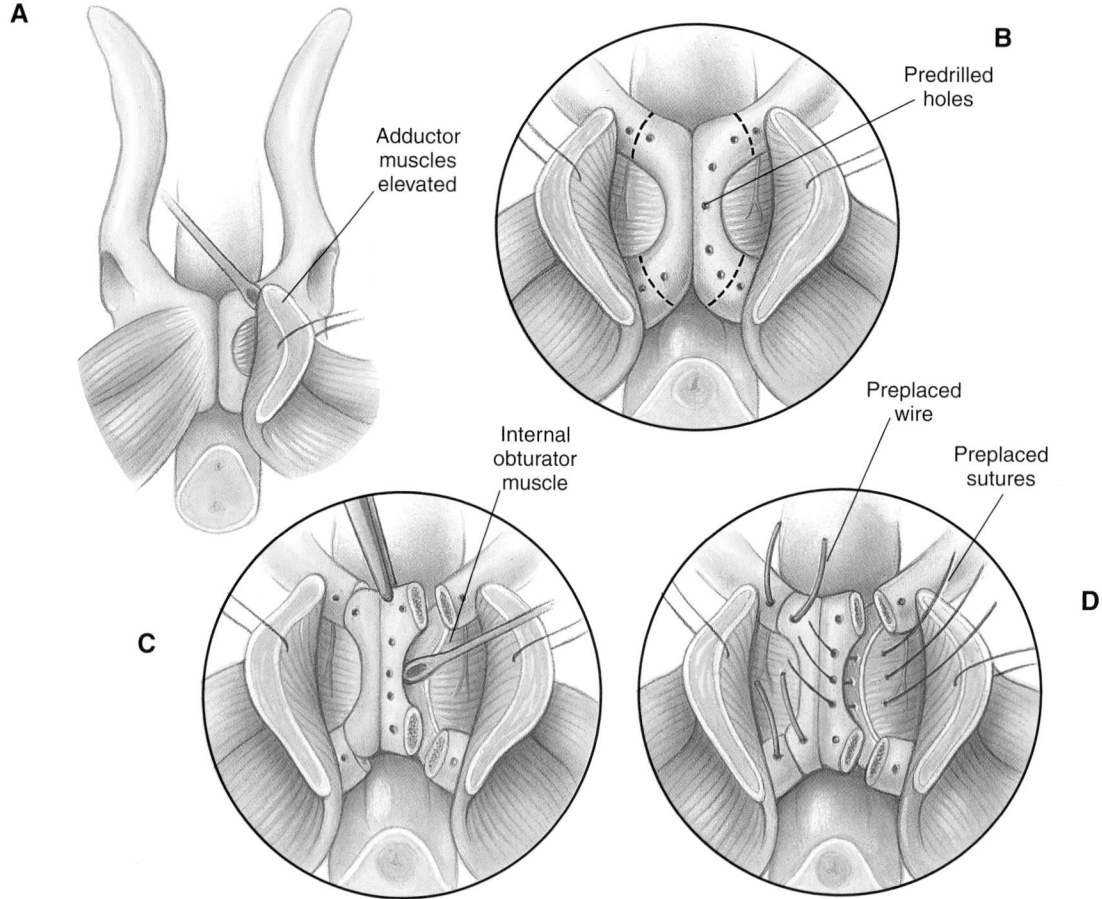

FIG. 25-10
A, For bilateral pubic and ischial osteotomy, elevate the adductor muscles until the obturator nerves and half of the obturator foramen are exposed. **B**, Predrill holes in the pubis and ischium on both sides of the four proposed osteotomy sites and craniocaudally along the left pubis. **C**, Osteotomize the pubis and elevate the internal obturator muscle from the left pubis and ischium, allowing reflection of the entire central bony plate. **D**, Close the osteotomy with orthopedic wire.

the pubis and ischium. Subperiosteally elevate the adductor muscles until the obturator nerves and half of the obturator foramen are exposed (Fig. 25-10, A). Transect the prepubic tendon along the left pubis to the proposed pubic osteotomy site. Predrill holes in the pubis and ischium on both sides of the four proposed osteotomy sites and craniocaudally along the left pubis (Fig. 25-10, B). Osteotomize the pubis, and elevate the internal obturator muscle from the left pubis and ischium, allowing reflection of the entire central bony plate to the right (Fig. 25-10, C). To close the osteotomy sites, preplace orthopedic wire through the previously drilled holes on the right side. Then, before replacing the bone plate, place sutures through the line of holes in the left pubis and ischium, through the left internal obturator muscle, and back through the adjacent holes in the pubis or ischium. Place orthopedic wire through the left osteotomy sites, then secure the preplaced wires and sutures (Fig. 25-10, D). Reappose the adductor muscles and prepubic tendon before closing the linea alba.

Urethrotomy

Urethrotomy is performed in male dogs to remove urethral calculi that cannot be retrohydropropulsed into the bladder (see p. 684) and to facilitate placement of catheters into the bladder. Occasionally, urethrotomy is performed for a biopsy of obstructive lesions (i.e., strictures, scar tissue, and neoplasms). Prescrotal or perineal urethrotomy may be performed. To prevent possible postoperative urethral stricture, cystotomy is preferred over urethrotomy if calculi can be dislodged into the bladder by urohydropropulsion.

Prescrotal urethrotomy. Prescrotal urethrotomy (Fig. 25-11) is used to remove calculi from the distal penile urethra or to place Foley catheters into the urinary bladder if the catheter is of sufficient length and if the obstruction is distal to the proposed urethrotomy incision. Occasionally, urethrotomy can be performed under local anesthesia with opioid sedation in severely depressed or uremic patients. Prescrotal urethrotomies can be left to heal by secondary intention; however, hemorrhage should be expected from

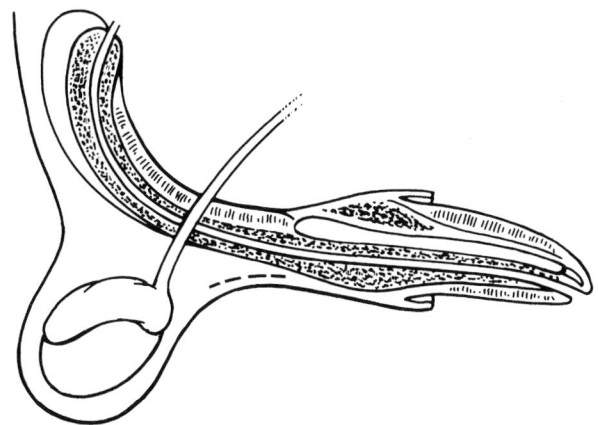

FIG. 25-11
Prescrotal urethrotomy.

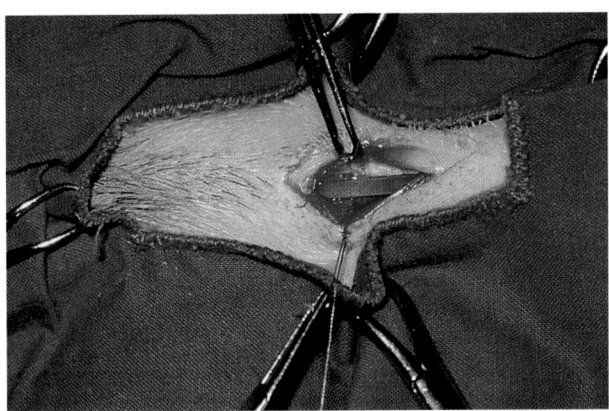

FIG. 25-13
Perineal urethrotomy.

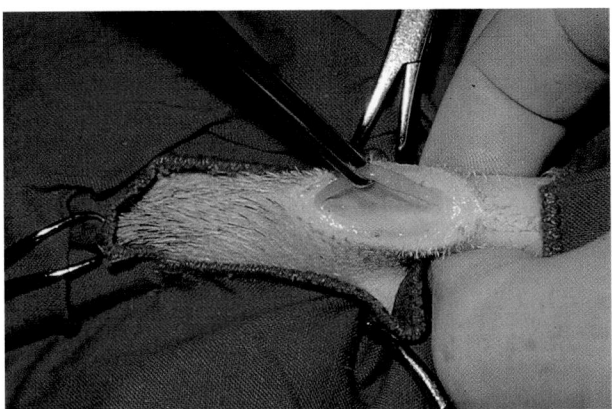

FIG. 25-12
For prescrotal urethrotomy, make a ventral midline incision through the skin and subcutaneous tissues, between the caudal aspect of the os penis and scrotum. Identify, mobilize, and retract the retractor penis muscle laterally to expose the urethra.

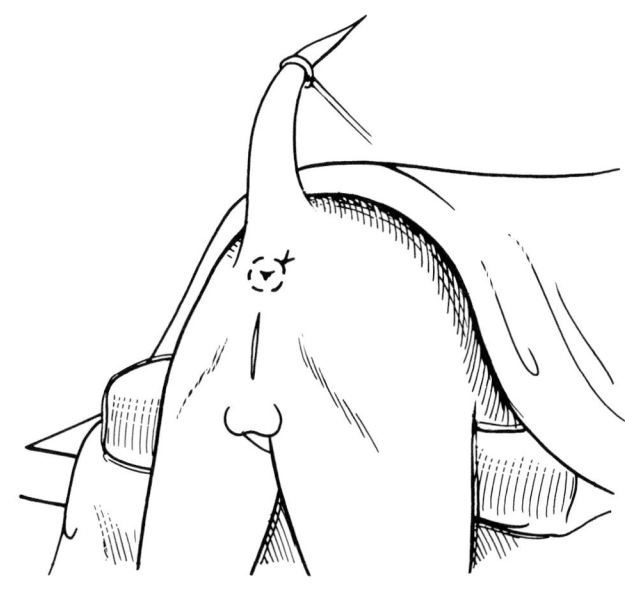

FIG. 25-14
Use a No. 15 scalpel blade to make an incision into the urethral lumen over the catheter (see Fig. 25-15).

the surgical site for 3 to 5 days (particularly during urination). Primary closure is preferred if the mucosa is healthy and if adequate apposition of the urethral mucosa can be achieved because it decreases postoperative bleeding.

With the dog in dorsal recumbency, place a sterile catheter into the penile urethra to the scrotum or to the obstruction. Make a ventral midline incision through the skin and subcutaneous tissue between the caudal aspect of the os penis and scrotum. Identify, mobilize, and retract the retractor penis muscle laterally to expose the urethra (Fig. 25-12). Using a No. 15 scalpel blade, make an incision into the urethral lumen over the catheter (Fig. 25-13). Use iris scissors to extend the incision, if necessary. Remove calculi with forceps, and gently flush the urethra with warm saline. Leave the incision to heal by secondary intention, or close the urethra with simple interrupted absorbable sutures (4-0 or 5-0). Place the

first layer in the urethral mucosa and corpus spongiosum, then appose subcutaneous tissue and skin with simple interrupted sutures or a continuous subcuticular suture pattern.

Some surgeons prefer a continuous suture pattern in the urethra to promote hemostasis.

Remove the urinary catheter following surgery, regardless of whether the urethra is sutured or not.

Perineal urethrotomy. Perineal urethrotomy (Fig. 25-14) is occasionally used to remove calculi lodged at the ischial arch and to place catheters into the bladder of large male dogs. Perineal urethrotomy is less commonly indi-

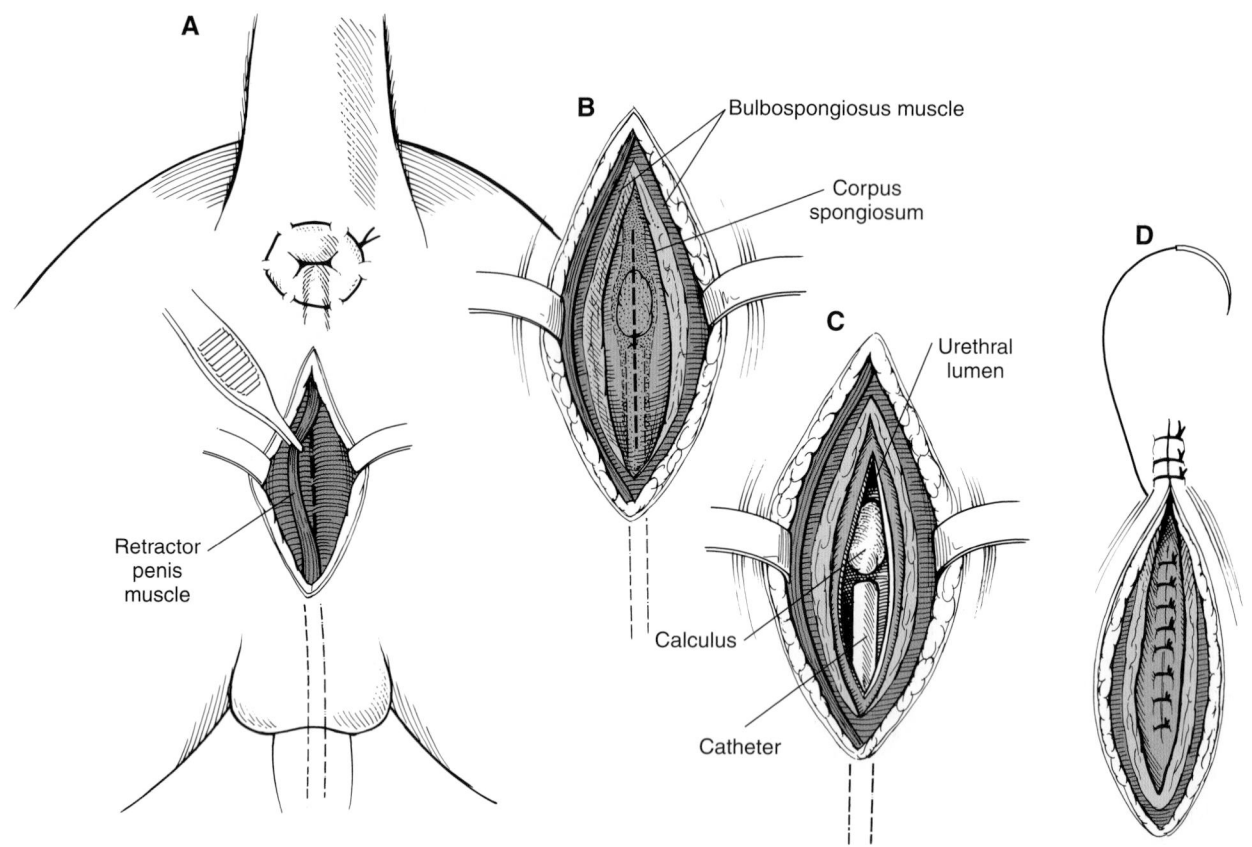

FIG. 25-15
For perineal urethrotomy, make a midline incision over the urethra, midway between the scrotum and anus. **A,** Identify the retractor penis muscle, elevate it, and retract it. **B,** Separate the paired bulbospongiosus muscles at their raphe to expose the corpus spongiosum, **C,** then incise the corpus spongiosum to enter the urethral lumen. **D,** Close the urethra with simple interrupted absorbable sutures. Place the first layer in the urethral mucosa and corpus spongiosum, then appose subcutaneous tissue and skin with simple interrupted sutures or a continuous subcuticular suture pattern.

cated than urethrotomy at other sites. They should be closed to prevent potential subcutaneous urine leakage.

Place a purse-string suture in the anus. Place a sterile catheter into the urethra to the level of the bladder or the site of the obstruction. With the dog in sternal recumbency and the rear limbs hanging over the edge of the table, make a midline incision over the urethra, midway between the scrotum and anus. Identify the retractor penis muscle, elevate it, and retract it (Fig. 25-15, A). Separate the paired bulbospongiosus muscles at their raphe to expose the corpus spongiosum, then incise the corpus spongiosum to enter the urethral lumen (Fig. 25-15, B and C). Close the incision as just described for prescrotal urethrotomy (Fig. 25-15, D).

Urethrostomy

Urethrostomy is indicated for (1) recurrent, obstructive calculi that cannot be managed medically; (2) calculi that cannot be removed by retrohydropropulsion or urethrotomy; (3) urethral stricture; (4) urethral or penile neoplasia or severe trauma; and (5) preputial neoplasia requiring penile

amputation. Depending on the site of the lesion, ureterostomy can be prescrotal, scrotal, perineal, or prepubic in dogs. Scrotal urethrostomy is preferred if castration is an option and if the lesion is distal to the scrotum. Perineal urethrostomy is routinely performed in cats; however, prepubic and subpubic urethrostomy are also described.

Prescrotal urethrostomy. Prescrotal urethrostomy is performed similarly to prescrotal urethrotomy except that the urethral mucosa is sutured to the skin.

Make a 3- to 4-cm incision in the urethral mucosa as described on p. 671. The length of the urethral incision should be 6 to 8 times its luminal diameter. Periurethral sutures can be placed to the subcutaneous tissue using a simple continuous suture pattern of absorbable suture material. Place simple interrupted absorbable sutures (3-0 to 5-0) from the urethral mucosa to the skin beginning at the caudal aspect of the incision. Suture the remainder of the urethral mucosa to the skin with simple interrupted sutures (Fig. 25-16). Suture skin at either end of the incision with simple interrupted sutures.

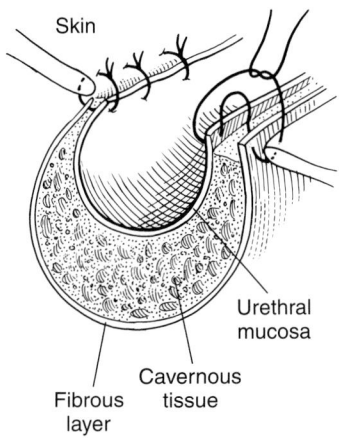

FIG. 25-16
For urethrostomy, place simple interrupted absorbable sutures from the urethral mucosa to skin. To improve hemostasis, avoid incorporating cavernous tissue in the sutures.

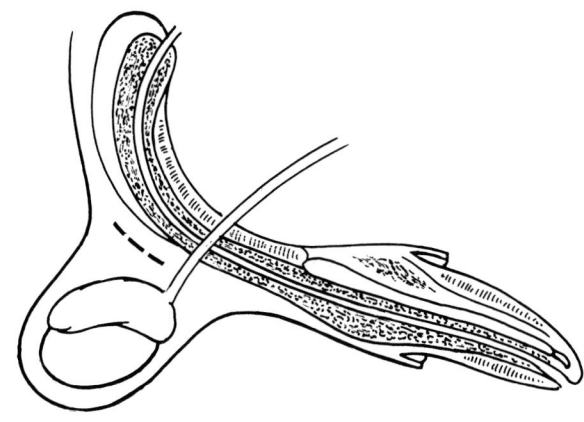

FIG. 25-17
Scrotal urethrostomy.

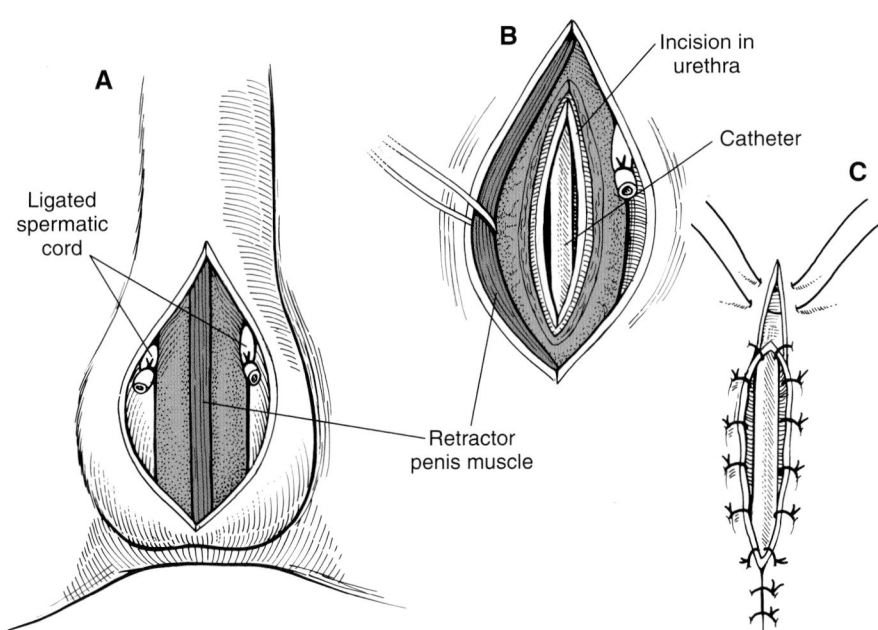

FIG. 25-18
Scrotal urethrostomy is preferred over other sites because there is less hemorrhage. Perform a scrotal ablation.
A, Make a midline incision over the urethra through the subcutaneous tissue. Identify the retractor penis muscle and mobilize and retract it laterally to expose the urethra. **B,** Using a No. 15 scalpel blade, make a 3- to 4-cm incision into the urethral lumen over the catheter. **C,** Suture urethral mucosa to skin with simple interrupted sutures.

Scrotal urethrostomy. Scrotal urethrostomy (Fig. 25-17) is preferred over perineal or prepubic urethrostomy because the urethra is wider, more superficial, and surrounded by less cavernous tissue here than at other sites. Therefore postoperative hemorrhage is often less than with other techniques, and stricture is less likely.

If the dog is intact, castrate him and excise the scrotum; otherwise, perform a scrotal ablation (Fig. 25-18, A). Place a sterile catheter into the urethra to the level of the ischial arch or beyond. Make a midline incision over the urethra through the subcutaneous tissue. Identify the retractor penis muscle, mobilize it, and retract it laterally to expose the urethra. Using a No. 15 scalpel blade, make a 3- to 4-cm incision into the urethral lumen over the catheter (Fig. 25-18, B).

Suture the urethra as described on p. 671 for prescrotal urethrostomy (Fig. 25-18, C).

Canine perineal urethrostomy. Perineal urethrostomy often causes unacceptable urine scalding and is only used in dogs that have urinary problems that a scrotal or prescrotal urethrostomy will not solve. The surrounding cavernous tissue is large at this location, and hemorrhage can be profuse. Furthermore, the urethra is less superficial here, and mobilizing it can result in excessive suture-line tension, causing dehiscence.

Make a 4- to 6-cm incision in skin and overlying tissue, and incise the perineal urethra as described for perineal urethrotomy. The urethral incision should be 1.5 to 2 cm in

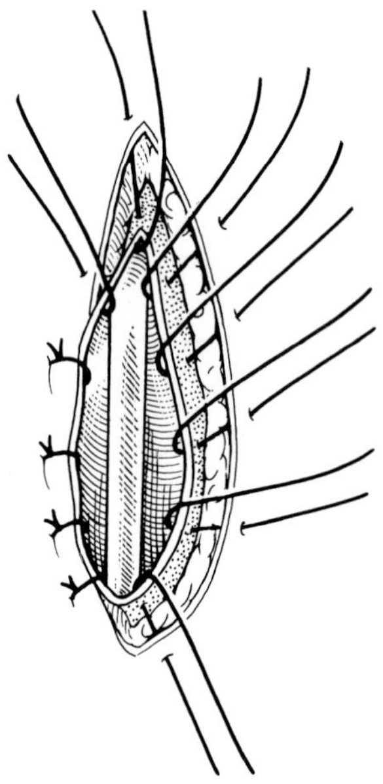

FIG. 25-19
For urethrostomy, place simple interrupted absorbable sutures from the urethral mucosa to skin beginning at the caudal aspect of the incision. Suture the remainder of the urethral mucosa to skin with simple interrupted sutures. Suture skin at either end of the incision with simple interrupted sutures.

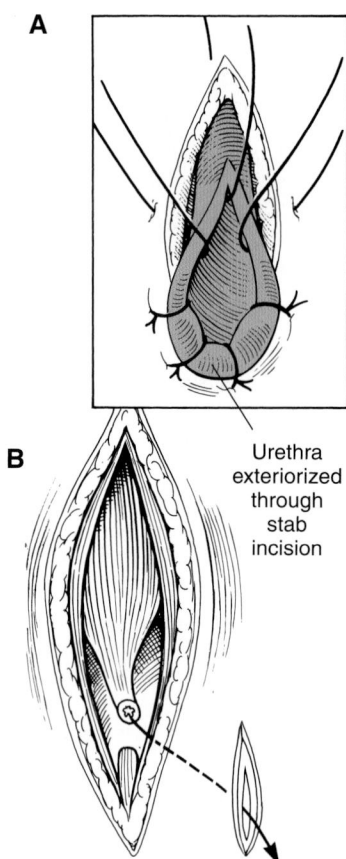

FIG. 25-20
Prepubic urethrostomy may be performed when distal urethral lesions are present. **A**, Sever the distal aspect of the intrapelvic urethra and exteriorize it through a small stab incision 2 to 3 cm lateral to the linea alba. **B**, Spatulate the distal end of the urethra to increase the luminal diameter, and suture the urethral mucosa to skin with interrupted sutures.

length. Suture the urethral mucosa to the skin as described for prescrotal urethrostomy (Fig. 25-19).

Prepubic urethrostomy.   Prepubic (antepubic) urethrostomy is a salvage procedure performed when damage to the membranous or penile urethra is irreparable (this is rare), or when removal of these tissues is necessary (i.e., neoplasia). Unless nerve damage occurs (this is most likely with prostatectomy), most animals are continent following this procedure.

Make a ventral midline incision from the umbilicus to the pubis. Free the intrapelvic urethra from the pelvic floor using blunt dissection. Be sure to preserve the urethral artery and its branches. Sever the distal aspect of the intrapelvic urethra. It may be necessary to carefully dissect the prostate from the urethra to ensure that there is ample urethra to exteriorize in some male dogs. Preserve the blood supply to the neck of the bladder. In male dogs, exteriorize the urethra through a small stab incision 2 to 3 cm lateral to the prepuce or within the prepuce. In females, exteriorize the urethra through the ventral midline incision or 2 to 3 cm lateral to the linea alba (Fig. 25-20, A). Spatulate the distal end of the urethra to increase the luminal diameter (Fig. 25-20, B), then suture the urethral mucosa to skin with interrupted sutures of absorbable (e.g., polyglyconate, polydioxanone, or poliglecaprone 25 suture) or nonabsorbable (e.g., nylon or polypropylene) suture. Be sure that there is little tension on the urethrostomy site and that the urethra is not bent sharply.

A Foley catheter can be placed into the bladder through the urethrostomy to divert urine during initial healing (i.e., 24 to 48 hours).

Subpubic urethrostomy.   Subpubic urethrostomy is similar to prepubic urethrostomy except that the urethra is exteriorized caudal to the brim of the pubis. In cats, this procedure may be less likely to cause postoperative stricture, recurrent urinary tract infection, or chronic urine-scald dermatitis. It is indicated when repeated stricture occurs after perineal urethrostomy.

Perform this procedure similarly to the one described above, but retract the skin caudally past the brim of the pubis. Expose the medial boundary of the obturator foramen by elevating the adductor muscle and cranial portion of the gracilis muscle from the periosteum of the pubis. Partially incise the prepubic tendon, and reflect it laterally to expose the pubic rami (Fig. 25-21). Osteotomize the pubic rami 1.5 cm lateral to the pubic symphysis. Make a transverse incision through the body of the pubic bone and across the pubic

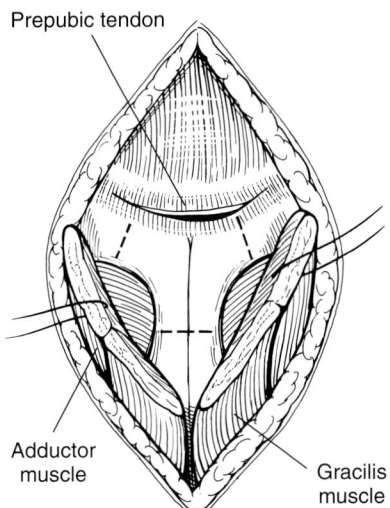

FIG. 25-21
For pubic osteotomy, partially incise the prepubic tendon
and reflect it laterally to expose the pubic rami. Osteotomize
the pubic rami 1.5 cm lateral to the pubic symphysis. Make
a transverse incision through the body of the pubic bone
and across the pubic symphysis.

*symphysis. Rotate the pubic flap ventrally to visualize the
intrapelvic urethra. Transect the urethra cranial to the lesion
(i.e., stricture and replace the pubic flap (Fig. 25-22, A).
Reappose the muscular aponeuroses of the gracilis and
adductor muscles with interrupted or horizontal mattress
sutures. Make a 1-cm stab incision 3 cm distal to the caudal
extent of the abdominal incision. Tunnel through the subcutaneous tissue and exteriorize the urethra (Fig. 25-22, B).
Spatulate the urethral end, and suture it to the skin with 4-0
suture material. Close the abdominal incision but leave the
caudal 1 cm of the linea alba open to prevent crimping the
urethra as it passes over the pubic flap. Resect the tissues at
the perineal urethrostomy site, and either close them or leave
them open to heal by secondary intention.*

Transpelvic urethrostomy. This technique was recently described as an alternative to prepubic and subpubic
urethrostomy in male cats (Bernadre and Viguier, 2004*).*

*Position the cat in dorsal recumbency with the feet secured to
the surgical table in a cranial position. Make a small caudal
ventral median celiotomy, and expose the urinary bladder 2
cm cranial to the cranial pubic margin. Make a small incision into the bladder, aspirate urine from it, and lavage the
bladder with sterile saline. Pass a 6 French urinary catheter
into the bladder, and advance it into the proximal urethra to
the obstruction site. Secure the catheter to the bladder wall
with a temporary purse-string suture. Excise the scrotum and
prepuce using an elliptical skin incision that extends to the
cranial margin of the pubis. Extend the penis caudally, and
denude its ventral surface. Remove fat to expose the caudal
and ventral aspects of the pubic symphysis. Elevate muscles*

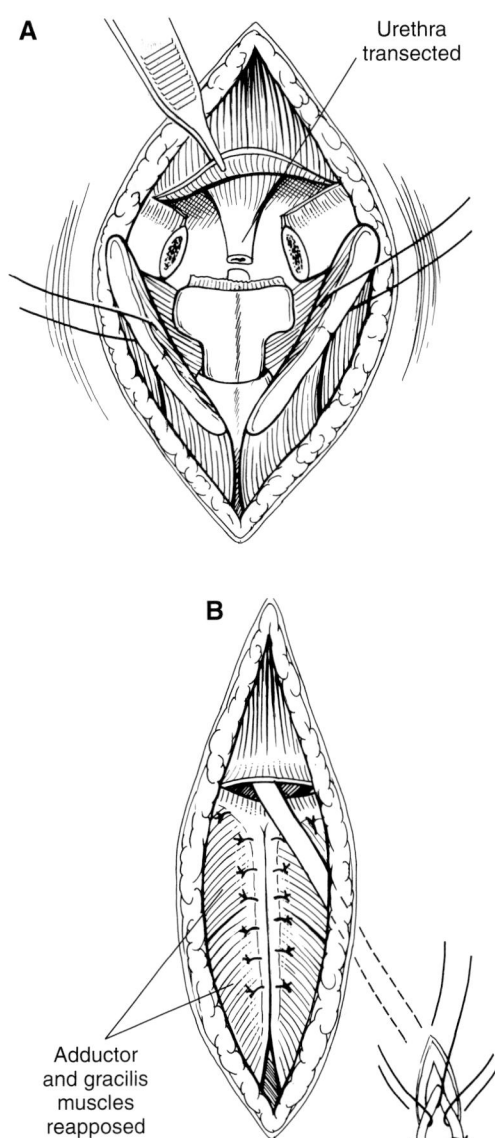

FIG. 25-22
For subpubic urethrostomy, perform a pubic osteotomy (see
Fig. 25-21) and rotate the pubic flap ventrally to visualize
the intrapelvic urethra. **A,** Transect the urethra cranial to the
lesion and replace the pubic flap. **B,** Exteriorize the urethra
through a stab incision, spatulate the urethral end, and
suture it to skin.

*medial to lateral on both sides of the ischium to expose its
ventral aspect (approximately 1.5 cm wide and 1.5 cm
long). Use bone rongeurs to remove the ischium in a caudocranial direction until an ostectomy area of approximately
10 mm wide and 12 mm long has been created. Take care
to avoid damaging underlying soft tissue. Palpate the
indwelling urethral catheter, and make a ventral longitudinal
urethral incision over the catheter from the bulbourethral
glands to a point 2 to 3 mm from the cranial margin of the
ostectomy. Place simple interrupted 4-0 monofilament sutures*

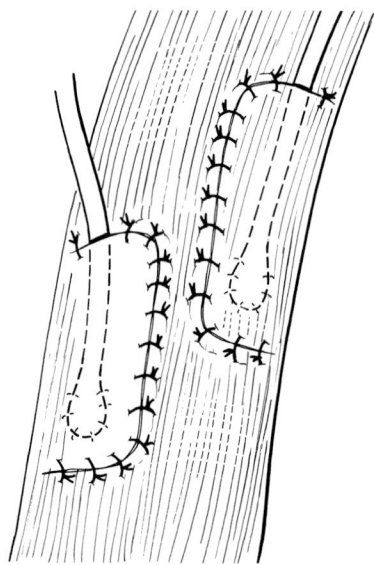

FIG. 25-23
Permanent urinary diversion may be performed by anastomosing the ureters into the intact colon, jejunum, or ileum.

from the urethral mucosa to the skin margins. Amputate the portion of the penis distal to the bulbourethral glands. Place additional skin sutures to close the remaining wound. Remove the urinary catheter, and pass it into the urethrostomy to ensure patency. Close the cystotomy and celiotomy incisions routinely.

Feline perineal urethrostomy. Perineal urethrostomy (see p. 699) is indicated to prevent recurrence of obstruction in male cats or to treat obstruction that cannot be eliminated by catheterization. It is also useful when treating strictures secondary to urethral obstruction and catheterization.

Urinary Diversion

Permanent urinary diversion may be indicated when neoplasia involves the bladder trigone. After cystectomy, the ureters may be anastomosed to an isolated bowel conduit or reservoir, or into the intact colon, jejunum, or ileum (Fig. 25-23). Complications associated with ureteral anastomosis in the bowel include reabsorption of electrolytes and nitrogenous waste products, upper urinary tract infection, and neurologic

FIG. 25-24
For colonic urinary diversion: **A,** make a three-sided seromuscular flap for each ureter; **B,** then create a 4-mm circular defect in the colonic mucosa with tenotomy scissors. Transect the end of the ureter, spatulate it, and tunnel the ureters through the seromuscular flap into the colonic lumen. **C,** Suture the ureter to colonic mucosa with simple interrupted sutures. **D,** Close the flap over the ureter, but avoid compromising the ureteral lumen.

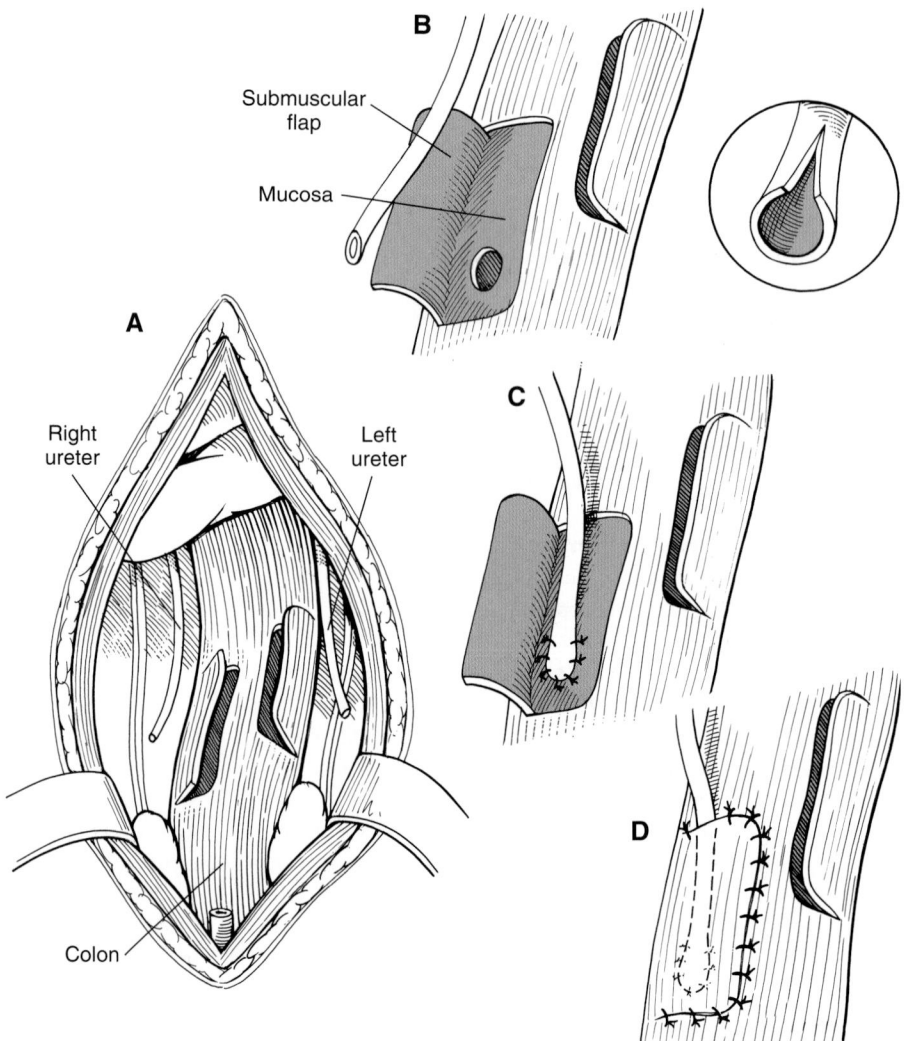

dysfunction. Azotemia, hyperammonemia, hyperchloremia, and metabolic acidosis are common after these procedures. Because it is a salvage procedure commonly associated with life-threatening complications, clients should be carefully counseled when considering this surgery. Ureterocolonic anastomosis is the most commonly performed technique for permanent urinary diversion. The patient should fast for 48 hours and saline enemas should be given 12 to 24 hours before surgery. Prophylactic antibiotics are given and should be continued for at least 8 weeks after surgery.

Excise the bladder and proximal urethra (1 to 2 cm distal to the suspected area of neoplasia), and ligate and transect the ureters. Dissect the ureters from their retroperitoneal attachments. Determine the length of the ureters, and choose a site for each to be implanted into the colon. Stagger the sites for anastomosis of the right and left ureters so that they are at different sites in the colon. Express feces from the proposed site of ureteral anastomoses, and place atraumatic forceps on the colon. Make a three-sided seromuscular colonic flap for each ureter (Fig. 25-24, A), then create a 4-mm circular defect in the colonic mucosa with tenotomy scissors (Fig. 25-24, B). Transect the end of the ureter, spatulate it, and tunnel the ureters through the seromuscular flap into the colonic lumen. Suture the ureter to the colonic mucosa with simple interrupted sutures (5-0 or 6-0 absorbable suture material; Fig. 25-24, C). Close the flap over the ureter, but be sure to avoid compromising the ureteral lumen (Fig. 25-24, D).

HEALING OF THE BLADDER AND URETHRA

Compared with other organs, the urinary bladder heals quickly, regaining 100% of normal tissue strength in 14 to 21 days. Complete reepithelialization of the bladder occurs in 30 days. Substantial portions of the bladder can be safely resected. As long as the trigone is undamaged, the bladder will expand (due to epithelial regeneration, scar tissue formation and remodeling, hypertrophy, and proliferation of smooth muscle) until it again functions as an effective reservoir. Use of reconstructed small intestine submucosa may allow replacement of large portions of the bladder, urethra, and ureters (Xie et al, 2000).

If urethral continuity is not completely disrupted, the urethra can heal by regeneration of urethral mucosa in as little as 7 days. Urine extravasation (particularly if infected) delays wound healing and promotes periurethral fibrosis and stricture. Urinary diversion via a urethral catheter or tube cystostomy is therefore indicated for small urethral lacerations. Differences are typically not noted when either an indwelling transurethral catheter, a cystostomy catheter, or a combination of the two is used for urinary diversion after transection and anastomosis of the intrapelvic urethra. When complete transection of the urethra occurs, fibrous tissue proliferation occurs in the gaps between the severed ends. Contraction of the fibrous tissue often leads to stricture and urinary obstruction. Primary anastomosis over an indwelling catheter (or proximal urinary diversion) should

be performed to decrease the likelihood of stricture formation. The catheter should be left in place for 3 to 5 days.

SUTURE MATERIALS AND SPECIAL INSTRUMENTS

Absorbable suture material (e.g., polydioxanone [PDS], polyglyconate [Maxon], polyglycolic acid [Dexon], polyglactin-910 [Vicryl], or poliglecaprone 25 [Monocryl]) is preferred for bladder and urethral surgery. Most sutures appear to lose tensile strength faster in alkaline urine (such as that seen with *Proteus* infections) than in infected, acidic urine or sterile urine. Polyglycolic acid, polyglactin 910, and poliglecaprone 25 are rapidly degraded in infected urine; polydioxanone, polyglyconate, and glycomer 631 are acceptable for use in sterile bladders and those infected with *E. coli*. However, use of any suture that is degraded via hydrolysis may be risky when the bladder is infected with *Proteus* spp. (see also p. 61). A recent study found that all monofilament absorbable sutures degraded within 7 days in *Proteus mirabilis*–inoculated urine (Greenberg et al, 2004). Nonabsorbable sutures should be avoided in the urinary bladder or urethra because they promote formation of calculi.

POSTOPERATIVE CARE AND ASSESSMENT

Urination should be closely monitored in patients after urethral surgery to detect obstruction caused by tissue swelling, fibrosis, or necrosis. Following removal of the urinary obstruction, intravenous fluid therapy should be maintained until postobstructive diuresis ceases. Electrolytes should be monitored (particularly potassium) because hypokalemia may occur secondary to diuresis or medical therapy of hyperkalemia. Patients should be monitored for postoperative pain, and analgesics provided as necessary (see Chapter 13). Elizabethan collars should be used in patients with indwelling urinary catheters, urethrotomies, or urethrostomies to prevent early catheter removal or self-mutilation. Patients with urethrotomies should be observed for postoperative hemorrhage. Digital pressure on the surgical site may be necessary to stop bleeding immediately after surgery or after urination (for 3 to 5 days). Bladder atony may occur in as little as 12 hours if the animal is sedated or given narcotic analgesics postoperatively, or does not void because of pain. The bladder should be kept decompressed by manually expressing it or by catheterization until the patient is urinating normally.

In cats with urethrostomies, paper instead of gravel litter should be used until the wound is healed, and urine cultures should be performed to check for urinary tract infection. An indwelling catheter may promote stricture formation and urinary tract infection in cats following surgery; therefore their use is not recommended. Animals with ureterocolonic anastomoses should be checked regularly for pyelonephritis. Inappetence in patients with ureterocolonic anastomoses may cause increased absorption of urine because of a lack of fecal bulk; therefore animals should be encouraged to eat as soon as possible after surgery. Excretory urography (e.g., presence of hydroureter and/or hydronephrosis) may help determine the long-term need for antibiotics in these patients.

COMPLICATIONS

The most common complications of urethral wound repair are stricture formation and urinary leakage. Indwelling catheters may allow ascending bacterial infection or cause fibrosis and stricture. Oversized stents (those that distend the urethra) should be avoided. Complications of prepubic catheterization (temporary cystostomy) may include bowel perforation from improper percutaneous placement, urinary tract infection, transient hematuria, uroabdomen, premature catheter removal, and breakage or incomplete removal of the catheter. Stricture formation in cats following perineal urethrostomy is generally a result of making the stoma too small (i.e., making the stoma in the proximal penile urethra instead of the distal pelvic urethra), or postoperative subcutaneous urine leakage and subsequent granulation tissue formation (see p. 701). Urinary and fecal incontinence may occur if the nerves are damaged during dissection around the pelvic urethra. Perineal urethrostomy is associated with a high prevalence of postoperative urinary tract infection. Rectal prolapse has also been reported following perineal urethrostomy in cats. Pyelonephritis, renal failure caused by end-stage kidney disease, neurologic dysfunction, hyperchloremic metabolic acidosis, and diarrhea with subsequent perineal irritation are possible complications of ureterocolonic urinary diversion (see p. 676).

Prepubic urethrostomy should be considered a salvage procedure only. In a recent study, the mean survival time in cats in which this procedure was performed was 13 months (Baines et al, 2001). Complications included lower urinary tract disease, peristomal skin irritation or necrosis, and urinary incontinence.

SPECIAL AGE CONSIDERATIONS

Older animals may have preexisting cardiac or renal dysfunction and should be monitored closely. Young animals may have very small urethras, making surgical repair of complete transections difficult.

References

Baines SJ, Rennie S, White RAS: Prepubic urethrostomy: a long term study in 16 cats, *Vet Surg* 30:107, 2001.

Bernarde A, Viguier E: Transpelvic urethrostomy in 11 cats using an ischial ostectomy, *Vet Surg* 33:246, 2004.

Greenberg CB, Davidson EB, Bellmer DD et al: Evaluation of the tensile strengths of four monofilament absorbable sutures after immersion in canine urine with or without bacteria, *Am J Vet Res* 65:847, 2004.

Norris CR, Williams BJ, Ling GV et al: Recurrent and persistent urinary tract infections in dogs: 383 cases (1969-1995), *J Am Anim Hosp Assoc* 36:484, 2000.

Stiffler KS, McCrackin Stevenson MA, Cornell K et al: Clinical use of low-profile cystostomy tubes in four dogs and a cat, *J Am Vet Med Assoc* 223:325, 2003.

Xie H, Shaffer BS, Wadia Y: Use of reconstructed small intestine submucosa for urinary tract replacement, *ASAIO J* 46:268, 2000.

Suggested Reading

Seguin MA, Vaden SL, Altier C et al: Persistent urinary tract infections and reinfections in 100 dogs (1989-1999), *J Vet Intern Med* 17:622, 2003.

More than half the dogs were asymptomatic the first time, and 29% of organisms isolated were resistant to orally administered antibiotics commonly used for urinary tract infection. Dogs with abnormal micturition were more likely to have resistant organisms cultured from their urine.

SPECIFIC DISEASES

UROABDOMEN

DEFINITIONS

Uroabdomen or *uroperitoneum* is an accumulation of urine in the peritoneal cavity. Urine may leak from the kidney, ureter, bladder, and/or proximal urethra.

GENERAL CONSIDERATIONS AND CLINICALLY RELEVANT PATHOPHYSIOLOGY

Bladder rupture is the most common cause of uroabdomen in dogs and cats. It may occur spontaneously (associated with tumor, severe cystitis, or urethral obstruction), be caused by blunt or penetrating abdominal trauma, or be iatrogenic following cystocentesis or bladder catheterization or manual expression of the bladder. Urinary tract leakage may also be a complication of surgery. Any animal brought in after a vehicular trauma should be assessed for possible urinary tract trauma. The impact of the collision may cause the bladder, urethra, or ureter to rupture or necrose. The sharp ends of pelvic fractures may sever or lacerate the urethra. Diagnosis is usually delayed because clinical signs are rarely present at initial examination (see p. 679).

Immediate surgery is contraindicated in animals with uroabdomen that are hyperkalemic or uremic. They should first be treated medically to normalize electrolytes and acid base, and to decrease circulating nitrogenous waste products. IV fluids should be given and abdominal drainage performed (see p. 664). Penrose drains or a peritoneal dialysis catheter (preferred because it can be made into a closed system) can be placed in the ventral abdomen under local anesthesia (sedate if necessary) to allow drainage for 6 to 12 hours. This will stabilize most animals with previously normal renal function.

When urine leaks into the abdominal cavity, some nitrogenous waste products and electrolytes are reabsorbed across the peritoneal membrane and reenter the circulation. Whether molecules are reabsorbed depends on their size. Urea rapidly equilibrates across the peritoneal surface, whereas some larger molecules (e.g., creatinine) cannot pass back into the bloodstream and remain concentrated in the abdominal fluid. Abdominal fluid creatinine concentrations must substantially exceed serum concentrations to diagnose uroabdomen. Because urea rapidly equilibrates across the peritoneum, blood urea nitrogen (BUN) may be approximately the same in both abdominal fluid and serum, regardless of the cause of the abdominal effusion. Potassium may also help diagnose uroabdomen. A potassium abdominal fluid to blood ratio of greater than 1 to 1.4 is definitive for uroabdomen.

> NOTE: Creatinine does not equilibrate across the peritoneal surface; BUN does. Compare creatinine or potassium concentrations (not BUN) in the fluid and serum.

DIAGNOSIS
Clinical Presentation

Signalment. Urinary bladder rupture has been suggested as being more frequent in male versus female dogs because their long, narrow urethras cannot dilate rapidly; however, ruptured bladders are common in females that have sustained vehicular trauma. Traumatic urethral rupture in female dogs is uncommon. Male dogs and cats with obstruction due to calculi or sterile cystitis (FUS) have a high risk of bladder rupture if the obstruction is not alleviated promptly (see pp. 684 and 698).

History. Clinical signs of urinary tract trauma are often vague and may be masked by other signs of trauma. In one study of dogs with pelvic trauma and concurrent urinary tract trauma, urinary trauma went clinically undetected in one third of the dogs. The animal may have azotemia (i.e., vomiting, anorexia, depression, and lethargy), or hematuria, dysuria, abdominal pain, and/or abdominal swelling or herniation may be noted. Abdominal and perineal bruising are common with vehicular trauma, particularly if there are pelvic fractures. Bruising in this region, however, may also indicate subcutaneous urine leakage. Further evaluation of the urinary tract is therefore warranted in such patients. In female dogs, there may be a history of previous catheterization using a rigid catheter. Rupture of the urethra is most frequently associated with pelvic fractures in male dogs. Urinary tract rupture is often overlooked in the initial workup of traumatized patients, and the diagnosis is not made until the animal shows signs of azotemia. It is important to remember that animals with ruptured bladders or unilateral ureteral trauma may urinate normal volumes, without evidence of hematuria. If the rupture is located dorsally or is small, leakage may only occur when the bladder becomes distended. Similarly, the ability to retrieve fluid while performing bladder catheterization does not preclude a diagnosis of a ruptured bladder.

> NOTE: Do not rule out bladder rupture in animals that urinate normal volumes.

Physical Examination Findings

Abdominal palpation should be performed to determine the size and shape of the bladder. The animal should be closely examined for abdominal swelling or fluid accumulation. Urine quantity and character (i.e., hematuria and dysuria),

and bruising on the ventral abdomen or perineum should be monitored.

Diagnostic Imaging

Survey radiographs may show reduced size or absence of the urinary bladder, decreased visceral detail, and increased size of the retroperitoneal space. If a ruptured bladder is suspected, a positive contrast cystogram should be performed; however, leakage of contrast medium into the peritoneal space during cystography does not necessarily mean that the animal needs exploratory surgery. If there is no clinical evidence of uroabdomen, conservative management of the patient may be appropriate. To perform cystography, a balloon-tipped catheter is placed into the urinary bladder; to perform a cystourethrogram in a male dog, the catheter is placed into the distal urethra (just past the os penis), and the balloon is inflated. While palpating the bladder for distention, approximately 2.2 ml/kg of diluted (1 part contrast medium to 2 parts sterile saline) aqueous organic iodide contrast medium is injected into the catheter. A radiograph is obtained while the last few milliliters of contrast are being injected. Fluoroscopy is advantageous to determine when the bladder is distended. It is critical to adequately distend the urinary bladder before determining that the study is normal because small lesions may not leak when the bladder wall is flaccid. Also, care should be taken not to completely occlude the neck of the urinary bladder with the bulb of the catheter as this may prevent leakage from a rupture in this area. Obtaining a radiograph while the contrast agent is being injected may show a "jet" lesion of contrast agent from the bladder (Fig. 25-25). Free contrast agent in the abdominal cavity will coat and highlight abdominal organs. If a lesion is not identified in the bladder after adequate distention of the urethra and if the animal is well hydrated, an excretory urogram can be performed (see p. 649). Contrast leak-

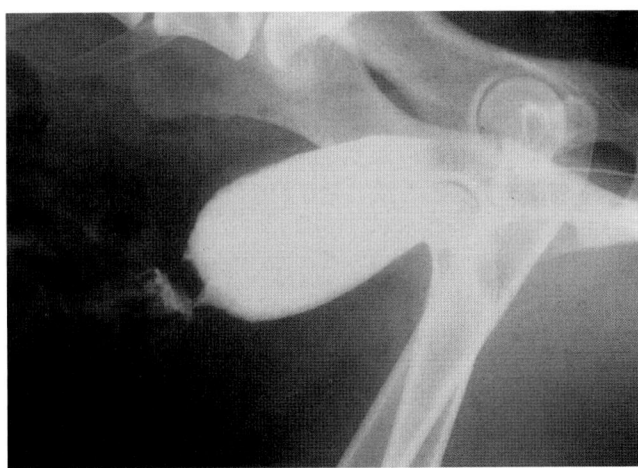

FIG. 25-25
Positive contrast cystourethrogram in a dog with a ruptured bladder. The radiograph was taken while the contrast agent was being injected and shows a "jet" lesion of contrast agent from the bladder.

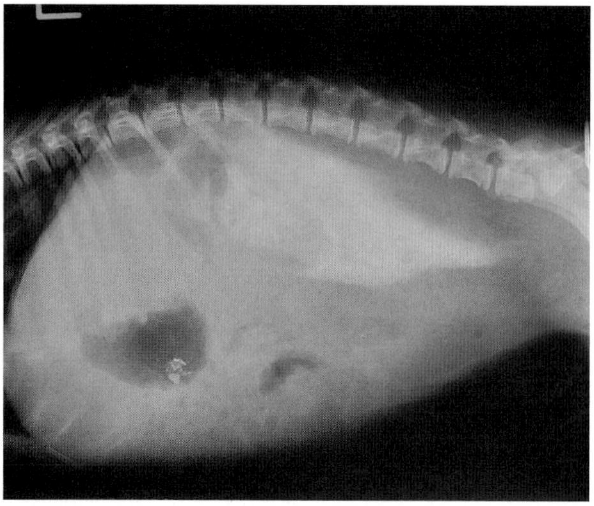

FIG. 25-26
Excretory urogram in a dog with a ruptured ureter. Note the accumulation of contrast in the retroperitoneal space. The contralateral ureter was avulsed from its blood supply.

age into the retroperitoneal space (for proximal lesions) or abdomen (for distal lesions) occurs with ureteral rupture or laceration (Fig. 25-26). If periureteral fibrosis has occurred, obstruction rather than leakage may be noted. Leakage of contrast from the renal capsule may be noted with renal parenchymal trauma. Parenchymal trauma of the right kidney should be suspected in dogs with uroabdomen and fractures of the thirteenth right rib.

Laboratory Findings

A complete blood count (CBC) and serum biochemical profile with electrolytes should be performed. Hyperkalemia and azotemia may be noted. Analysis of abdominal fluid should be performed if urinary tract rupture is suspected. With uroabdomen, creatinine levels of the abdominal fluid will be greater than those in the blood (see p. 678). Renal failure may be present if obstruction preceded the rupture (see p. 635). Bladder rupture secondary to urinary tract infection causes septic peritonitis (see p. 329).

DIFFERENTIAL DIAGNOSIS

Other causes of abdominal effusion or azotemia should be considered. Peritonitis may cause vomiting, dehydration, and prerenal azotemia. Vomiting may be caused by pancreatic, peritoneal, renal, splenic, hepatobiliary, or gastrointestinal abnormalities. In animals with abdominal effusion subsequent to trauma, uroabdomen, bile peritonitis, and septic peritonitis should be considered.

MEDICAL MANAGEMENT

If the animal is not hyperkalemic or azotemic (e.g., uroabdomen is diagnosed within 12 to 18 hours after rupture), it should be rehydrated with 0.9% saline, and immediate sur-

gical repair should be considered. Occasionally, concurrent trauma (e.g., traumatic myocarditis and pulmonary contusions) will delay surgery. In such patients, abdominal drainage and/or urinary diversion (i.e., urethral catheter and/or tube cystostomy; see p. 667) may be necessary until the animal is stable. With delayed diagnosis, correction of electrolytes, hydration, and acid-base balance should be performed before surgery (see pp. 663 and 699). Antibiotics may be administered based on culture results or upon bacterial morphology if a urinary tract infection is present, or prophylactically if abdominal drains are placed.

> NOTE: Animals with acid-base and electrolyte abnormalities are poor anesthetic candidates. Correct these abnormalities before surgery.

SURGICAL TREATMENT

Urethral trauma may be repaired by primary anastomosis (immediate or delayed) or the urethra may be allowed to heal over a urinary catheter if it is not completely transected. Ureteral rupture may be repaired by anastomosis or reimplantation into the bladder, depending on location of the damage (see p. 650). Bladder rupture generally occurs near the apex. Although small ruptures may heal if the bladder is kept decompressed, surgical exploration and repair are indicated in most patients. The entire abdomen should be explored to determine the reason for rupture and/or identify concurrent trauma. If bladder rupture is secondary to severe cystitis, tumor, or obstruction, the bladder may be extremely friable or large areas may be necrotic, making excision and primary closure of the rent difficult. In such cases, prolonged urinary diversion (see p. 676) may be beneficial. If cystitis or tumor is present, a biopsy of the bladder mucosa should be submitted for culture and histologic examination. In animals with rupture caused by obstruction from calculi, the urethra should be carefully checked for calculi and its patency verified before repairing the bladder defect.

Preoperative Management

An ECG should be evaluated for arrhythmias. If possible, hydration, acid-base, and electrolyte abnormalities should be corrected before surgery (see pp. 663 and 699). If antibiotic therapy has not been initiated before surgery, perioperative antibiotics (e.g., cefazolin) may be administered at induction.

Anesthesia

If renal impairment is not present, many different anesthetic regimens may be used safely. If renal impairment is present, see p. 636 for suggested anesthetic protocols. If the animal is vomiting, avoid mask or chamber induction.

Surgical Anatomy

Refer to p. 665 for surgical anatomy of the bladder and urethra.

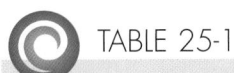 TABLE 25-1

Drugs Used to Improve Urination

DRUG	MECHANISM OF ACTION	CONTRAINDICATIONS/PRECAUTIONS
Phenoxybenzamine (Dibenzyline) Dogs: 0.25 mg/kg PO, bid-tid* Cats: 0.5 mg/kg PO, bid (may cause hypotension)—typically 1.25–7.5 mg/cat	Blocks the α_1 receptor on smooth muscle, causing relaxation; potent vasodilator	May cause prolonged hypotension in animals; use with caution in animals with cardiovascular compromise
Diazepam (Valium) Dogs: 2–10 mg/dog PO, tid Cats: 1–2.5 mg/cat PO, tid (duration of action is 1 to 2 hr when given orally)	CNS depressant	Idiopathic fatal hepatic necrosis reported in cats
Bethanechol (Urecholine)† Dogs: 5–15 mg/dog PO, bid-tid‡ Cats: 1.25–5 mg/cat PO, bid-tid‡	Muscarinic, cholinergic agonist; used to increase contraction of urinary bladder	There must be no obstructions in either the urinary or gastrointestinal tract, or the drug may cause severe pain or even rupture; should not be used in hyperthyroid animals; the drug may cause vomiting, ptyalism, and/or abdominal discomfort; can cause circulatory depression in sensitive animals

PO, Oral; *CNS*, central nervous system.
*Can try giving 0.5 mg/kg once daily; but it is better to start with 0.25 mg/kg bid to see if the drug will be effective.
†Be sure that there is no resistance to urinary or fecal outflow before using this drug.
‡Because this is a powerful stimulant, it is best to start at a low dose, observe the effects, and slowly increase the dose over several days, if necessary. Higher doses may be tried but should be used with caution.

Positioning

The animal is placed in dorsal recumbency, and the abdomen is prepared for a ventral midline incision. For bladder rupture, the entire ventral abdomen should be prepped to allow complete exploration of the abdomen.

SURGICAL TECHNIQUE

Cystotomy is described on p. 665.

Excise devitalized or necrotic bladder tissue, and suture the rent with a one- or two-layer continuous suture pattern. If the bladder is notably thickened, perform a single-layer anastomosing pattern; otherwise, use a two-layer inverting pattern. If tissues are friable and if a watertight seal is not achieved, perform a serosal patch over the incision line (see p. 457).

SUTURE MATERIALS AND SPECIAL INSTRUMENTS

Absorbable suture material (e.g., polydioxanone [PDS], polyglyconate [Maxon], polyglycolic acid [Dexon], polyglactin-910 [Vicryl], or poliglecaprone 25 [Monocryl]) is preferred for bladder and urethral surgery (see p. 677).

POSTOPERATIVE CARE AND ASSESSMENT

Intravenous fluids should be given until the animal is able to drink adequate fluids to maintain hydration. The patient should be observed closely after surgery for signs of urinary obstruction or peritonitis. If bladder atony is present, the bladder should be kept decompressed by intermittent urinary catheterization or by manual expression once the bladder incision has healed. Urinary tract infection is common with indwelling or repeated catheterization. An α-blocker (e.g., phenoxybenzamine; Table 25-1) and/or a somatic muscle relaxant (e.g., diazepam) can help decrease urethral sphincter tone. Bethanechol is a cholinergic that increases detrusor contractility and may aid voiding. Manual expression of the bladder should be done with care following surgery (particularly in patients with friable bladders secondary to infection or obstruction) to avoid disrupting the suture line.

> NOTE: Be sure that there is no excessive resistance to urinary or fecal outflow before using bethanechol. Use care when expressing a bladder in which you have recently performed a cystotomy.

COMPLICATIONS

The major complication of bladder surgery is urinary leakage, especially if a watertight seal is not achieved or if devitalized tissues are sutured and subsequently dehisce. Occasionally, peritonitis may occur from infected urine or secondary to surgically induced contamination.

PROGNOSIS

The prognosis is excellent for animals with traumatic bladder rupture. Occasionally, rupture secondary to obstruction may have a guarded prognosis if the majority of the bladder is necrotic.

BLADDER AND URETHRAL CALCULI

DEFINITIONS

When urine becomes supersaturated with dissolved salts, the salts may precipitate to form crystals (**crystalluria**). If the crystals are not excreted, they may aggregate into solid concretions known as *calculi*. **Urolithiasis** is a term that refers to having urinary calculi or uroliths (kidney, ureter, bladder, or urethra). **Cystolithiasis** and **cystolithectomy** refer to the development of urinary bladder calculi and their removal, respectively. **Cystotomy** is a surgical incision into the urinary bladder, whereas **urethrotomy** is an incision into the urethra.

GENERAL CONSIDERATIONS AND CLINICALLY RELEVANT PATHOPHYSIOLOGY

The large majority of canine uroliths are found in the bladder or urethra. Struvite (i.e., magnesium ammonium phosphate) and oxalate calculi are the most common canine uroliths, followed by urate, silicate, cystine, and mixed types. There appears to have been a long-term increase in the proportion of canine urinary calculi that contain calcium oxalate and a long-term decrease in the proportion of calculi that contain struvite for both male and female dogs (Ling et al, 2003).

Urinary tract infections with urease-producing bacteria are an important cause of struvite calculi in dogs. These bacteria split urea to ammonia and carbon dioxide. Hydrolysis of ammonia forms ammonium ions and hydroxyl ions, which alkalinize the urine and decrease struvite solubility. Bacterial cystitis also increases organic debris, which can serve as a nidus for crystallization. Feline struvite formation usually occurs without urinary tract infection.

Calcium oxalate calculi occur most commonly in dogs with transient, postprandial hypercalcemia and hypercalciuria. Many affected dogs have low-to-normal serum parathormone concentrations. Although rare, they may also occur in dogs with defective tubular resorption of calcium, primary hyperparathyroidism, lymphoma, vitamin D intoxication, decreased urine concentrations of citrate, or increased dietary oxalate. Concurrent urinary tract infection is rare. Acidic urine favors calcium oxalate crystal formation. Dogs eating canned diets with a high amount of carbohydrate were found to be at increased risk of calcium oxalate urolith formation (Lekcharoensuk et al, 2002A). Similarly, dogs fed dry diets formulated to contain high concentrations of protein, calcium, phosphorus, magnesium, sodium, potassium, and chloride appeared to have fewer calcium oxalate calculi (Lekcharoensuk et al, 2002B).

> NOTE: Struvite calculi are frequently associated with infection; be sure you culture the urine, bladder wall, and/or stone.

Urate calculi are usually composed of ammonium acid urate derived from metabolic degradation of endogenous

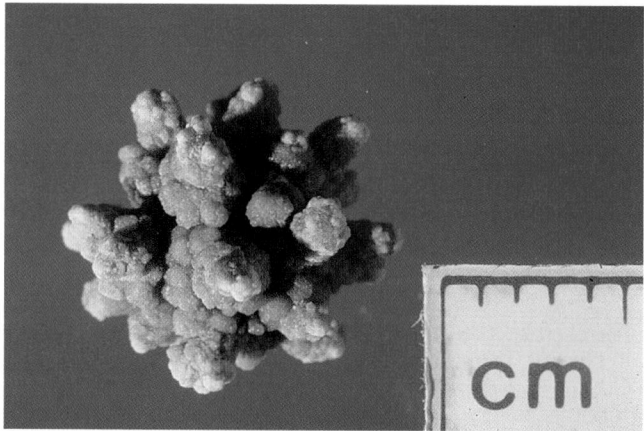

FIG. 25-27
Silicate urolith from a 12-year-old cat with chronic hematuria.

purine ribonucleotides and dietary nucleic acids. Dalmatians have defective hepatic transport of uric acid, resulting in decreased production of allantoin and increased urinary excretion of uric acid. Dalmatians also have decreased proximal tubular resorption and distal tubular secretion of uric acid, making urate urolithiasis common in this breed. Dogs with hepatic insufficiency (e.g., congenital portosystemic shunts) may form ammonium acid urate stones caused by increased renal excretion of ammonium urates. Secondary urinary tract infection may occur as a result of mucosal irritation. Silicate uroliths are often jack-shaped and are probably related to increased dietary intake of silicates, silicic acid, or magnesium silicate (Fig. 25-27). Male German shepherd dogs and old English sheepdogs are at increased risk for formation of silica-containing urinary calculi. Cystine uroliths occur because of an inherited disorder of renal tubular transport. Cystine stones usually occur in acid urine.

Although dissolution of some stones is possible, surgical removal is often necessary initially to allow a diagnosis of stone type. Appropriate medical management may help decrease the recurrence of canine uroliths (Table 25-2). Supersaturation of urine with salts appears to be the primary factor favoring calculi formation. Other factors (i.e., presence of a nidus on which the stone can form and decreased concentrations of urine crystallization inhibitors) also appear to contribute to stone formation.

> NOTE: It is necessary to remove and analyze stones to determine type; subsequent medical management is important to prevent recurrence.

DIAGNOSIS
Clinical Presentation

Signalment. Struvite calculi are more common in female dogs than in males because females more commonly have urinary tract infection; however, urethral obstruction from stones is more common in males (Box 25-4). Uroliths may

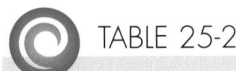 TABLE 25-2

Treatment and Prevention of Canine Urolithiasis

UROLITH TYPE	TREATMENT OPTIONS	PREVENTION
Struvite	Surgical removal (control infection first, if possible) Dissolve stones feeding Hill's s/d diet Voiding hydropropulsion, if stones are small enough	Feed Hill's c/d diet or Waltham Canine S/O Lower Urinary Support Diet Monitor urine pH and urine sediment, **MUST PREVENT** urinary tract infection and eliminate any that occur as quickly as possible Keep urine pH <6.5, BUN <10 mg/dl, and urine specific gravity <1.020
Calcium oxalate	Surgical removal Voiding hydropropulsion if stones are small enough	Feed Waltham Canine S/O Lower Urinary Support Diet, Hill's u/d diet, or Hill's w/d diet; with w/d, will probably need to administer potassium citrate to achieve urine pH ≥7.0; do not supplement vitamins C or D Increase water consumption
Urate	Surgical removal Voiding hydropropulsion if stones are small enough Dissolve stones using alkalinization with sodium bicarbonate or potassium citrate; feed Hill's u/d diet; administer allopurinol	Feed Hill's u/d diet Allopurinol if necessary
Silicate	Surgical removal	Feed Hill's u/d diet Prevent consumption of dirt
Cystine	Surgical removal Dissolve stones by feeding Hill's u/d diet and administering either D-penicillamine or N-(2-mercaptopropionyl)-glycine (MPG)	Feed Hill's u/d diet Administer thiol-containing drugs if necessary

 BOX 25-4

Breed, Sex, and Age Predispositions for Urinary Calculi

Struvite
- Miniature schnauzers, bichon frises, cocker spaniels, Shih Tzus, miniature poodles, Lhasa apsos
- Females more than males, middle-aged dogs
- Urinary tract infection

Calcium Oxalate
- Miniature schnauzers, Lhasa apsos, Yorkshire terriers, bichon frises, Shih Tzus, Cairn terriers, Pomeranians, Maltese, miniature poodles
- Males, neutered males more than intact males, middle-aged to older dogs, obese dogs

Calcium Phosphate
- Yorkshire terriers

Urate
- Dalmations
- Dogs with portosystemic shunts

Silicate
- German shepherds, Old English sheepdogs
- Males, middle-aged dogs

Cystine
- Dachshunds, English bulldogs, Chihuahuas, Mastiffs, Australian cattle dogs, Newfoundlands
- Males, middle-aged dogs

occur in dogs of any age, but they are most frequently observed in middle-aged dogs. Calculi in dogs less than 1 year of age are often struvite because of urinary tract infection. Calcium oxalate uroliths are more common in male dogs, particularly miniature schnauzers, miniature poodles, Yorkshire terriers, Lhasa apsos, and Shih Tzus. Middle-aged to older dogs are most commonly affected. In cats, calcium oxalate uroliths now occur nearly as frequently as struvite uroliths. Approximately one third of cats with calcium oxalate uroliths also have increased total serum calcium concentrations. Sixty percent of urate uroliths occur in dalmatians; most of the remainder are seen in breeds that commonly have portosystemic shunts (i.e., Yorkshire terriers, schnauzers, Pekingese, Lhasa apsos). Urate urolithiasis is more common in male dalmatians than in female dalmatians. Middle-aged, male German shepherds seem to be at increased risk for silicate urolithiasis. Cystine uroliths most frequently occur in middle-aged, male dachshunds. Other breeds that appear to be at increased risk for cystine urolithiasis include basset hounds, English bulldogs, Yorkshire terriers, Irish terriers, and Chihuahuas.

History. Clinical signs of urinary tract infection (i.e., hematuria, pollakiuria, and stranguria) are common in dogs with cystic or urethral calculi. Small stones lodging in the urethra of male dogs may cause partial or complete obstruction. Bladder distention, abdominal pain, stranguria, paradoxical incontinence, and/or signs of postrenal azotemia (i.e., anorexia, vomiting, and depression) may develop. Occasionally the bladder ruptures and causes uroabdomen (see p. 678).

Physical Examination Findings

The bladder wall is often thickened, and the stones themselves are occasionally palpable. Signs consistent with urinary tract infection may be noted. Abdominal pain, anorexia, vomiting, and/or depression may be noted if urinary tract obstruction occurs.

Diagnostic Imaging

Survey abdominal radiographs and/or ultrasonography are indicated in any animal with urolithiasis. In addition to defining the number and location of bladder and urethral calculi, the procedures may indicate the presence of calculi in the kidney and/or ureter. Calcium-containing uroliths (i.e., calcium phosphate and calcium oxalate) are the most radiopaque, whereas cystine and urate uroliths are the least radiopaque. Struvite calculi are normally radiopaque and are usually observed with survey radiography (Fig. 25-28). Double contrast cystography and/or retrograde urethrography may help identify radiolucent stones in the bladder or urethra. Size and number of the stones are best evaluated on radiographic studies; however, ultrasonography may be used to identify calculi and evaluate the kidneys and ureters for concurrent abnormalities.

> NOTE: Double contrast cystography/urethrography is probably the most sensitive method for finding stones (even better than ultrasound).

Laboratory Findings

A CBC, serum chemistry profile (including electrolytes), urinalysis, and urine culture should be performed. Urinary tract infection is common, even if pyuria, hematuria, proteinuria, and/or bacteriuria are absent. Renal failure may be due to chronic pyelonephritis or obstructive uropathy (see p. 635). Findings suggestive of hepatic insufficiency (e.g., low BUN, hypocholesterolemia, hypoalbuminemia, and increased serum bile acids) may be present in some animals with urate calculi.

> NOTE: Always identify and treat concurrent urinary tract infections.

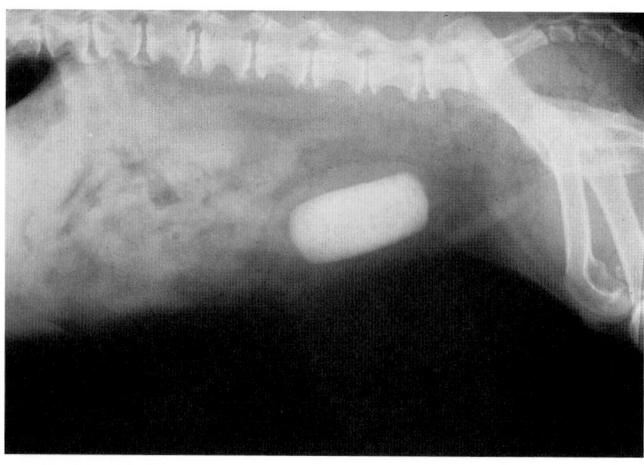

FIG. 25-28
A large radiopaque struvite calculus in the bladder of a dog with chronic cystitis.

DIFFERENTIAL DIAGNOSIS

Uroliths should be considered in any animal presenting for chronic urinary tract infection, hematuria, stranguria, pollakiuria, obstructive uropathy, or urinary incontinence. Other differentials include neoplasia and granulomatous inflammation.

MEDICAL MANAGEMENT

Urethral obstruction should be relieved and/or bladder decompression performed if necessary. Using a finger inserted in the rectum and massaging a urethral urolith toward the vagina may dislodge uroliths in female dogs. Urohydropropulsion may be used to propel urethral stones back into the bladder in both male and female dogs (Fig. 25-29, A). Voiding urohydropropulsion may remove small cystoliths. A catheter is placed in the urethra distal to the stone, and sterile saline or a combination of sterile saline and a 1:1 mixture of aqueous lubricant (e.g., Lubafax surgical lubricant) is injected while the urethra between the stone and bladder is occluded by a finger in the rectum (or vagina in females) (Fig. 25-29, B). Once the urethra is dilated, the finger should be removed, allowing the stone to be flushed into the bladder (Fig. 25-29, C). Stones lodged within the urethra causing obstruction that cannot be hydropropulsed into the bladder can be removed via urethrotomy (see p. 670).

> NOTE: Always try to flush urethral calculi into the bladder so that cystotomy (rather than urethrotomy) can be performed.

SURGICAL TREATMENT

Surgery should be considered if there are concurrent or predisposing anatomic abnormalities (e.g., urachal diverticula), if medical dissolution is not possible or is inadvisable, if a bladder mucosal culture is required, or if the stones

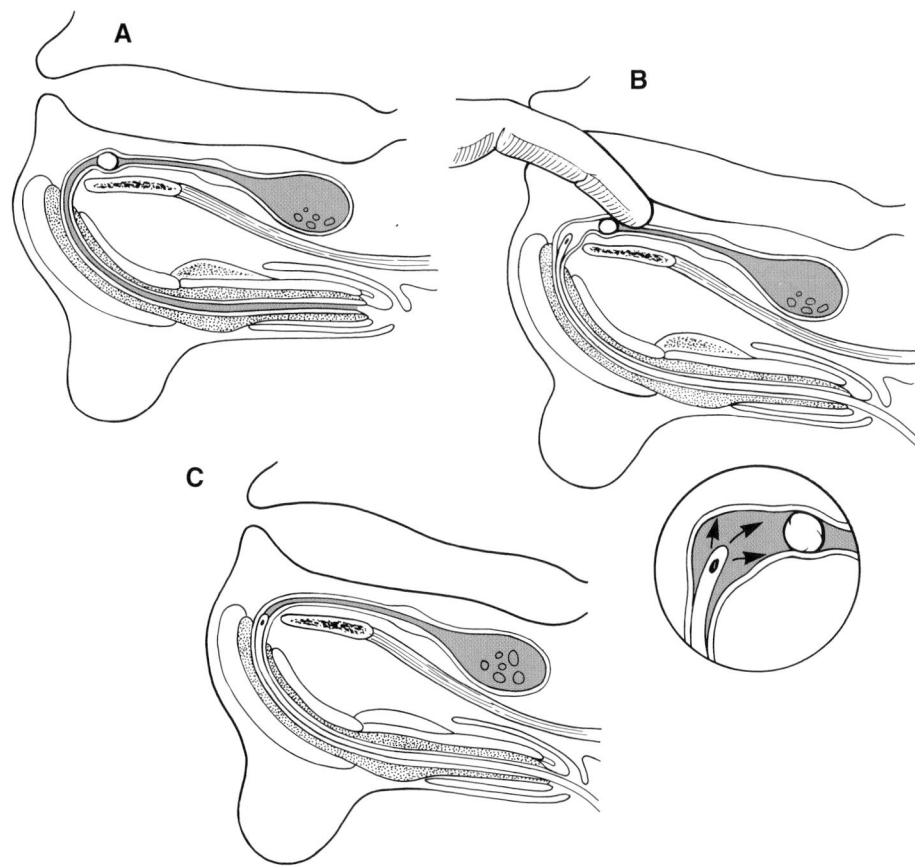

FIG. 25-29
A, Urohydropropulsion may be used to propel urethral stones back into the bladder. **B,** Place a catheter in the urethra distal to the stone, and inject sterile saline while the urethra is occluded by a finger in the rectum (or vagina in females). **C,** Once the urethra is dilated, remove the finger, allowing the stone to be flushed into the bladder.

are large enough that attempting voiding hydropropulsion is likely to cause urethral obstruction. Although medical dissolution of struvite, urate, and cystine calculi is possible, surgical removal of calcium oxalate, calcium phosphate, and silicate stones is necessary. Disadvantages of medical dissolution may include cost, necessity of frequent rechecks, possible urethral obstruction in males, and poor owner compliance with maintaining a suitable dietary regimen. Cystotomy should be performed preferentially over urethrotomy if the stones can be flushed into the bladder either preoperatively or intraoperatively. Cystotomy plus scrotal urethrostomy may be the most effective treatment in preventing recurrence of clinical signs in dalmatians with urate calculi. Recurrence is common when a cystotomy alone is performed.

> NOTE: Calculi should be submitted for stone analysis (and possibly culture) to guide postoperative management and help prevent recurrence. One cannot diagnose the type of stone based upon crystals found in the urine (e.g., it is possible to have a core of oxalate with a struvite shell because of secondary urinary tract infection with struvite crystalluria).

Lithotripsy. There are different techniques for lithotripsy, which can permit nonsurgical removal of bladder stones. Lithotripsy is seldom used, but can be useful if the equipment and expertise are available (Davidson et al, 2004).

Cystoscopy. Pecutaneous, transabdominal cystoscopy can be performed to remove bladder stones. The reader is referred to appropriate medical sources for more information (Rawlings et al, 2003).

Preoperative Management

Postrenal azotemia and hyperkalemia should be treated before surgery (see p. 663). Fluid therapy should be initiated to promote diuresis. An ECG should be evaluated for arrhythmias. Urinary tract infection should be controlled before surgery, and perioperative antibiotics should be considered if the animal is not already receiving antibiotics. Prophylactic antibiotics, however, may be withheld until after bladder mucosa has been excised for culture in animals with negative urine cultures.

> NOTE: If possible, eradicate concurrent UTI before surgery. Otherwise culture bladder mucosa and stones.

Anesthesia

If renal impairment is not present, many different anesthetic regimens may be used safely. If renal impairment is present, see p. 636 for suggested anesthetic protocols. Avoid mask or chamber induction if the patient is vomiting.

Surgical Anatomy

Refer to p. 665 for surgical anatomy of the bladder and urethra.

Positioning

The animal is placed in dorsal recumbency, and the abdomen is prepared for a ventral midline incision. The prepped area should extend from below the pubis proximally to the thorax.

SURGICAL TECHNIQUE

Bladder calculi are removed via cystotomy (see p. 665). Perform a cystotomy and incise a small piece of bladder at the incision for culture and possible histologic examination.

Remove the bladder stones, and carefully check the urethra for additional calculi. In male dogs, place a catheter into the urethra from the penile orifice, and occlude the vesicourethral opening with a finger from within the bladder lumen. Have an assistant gently occlude the penile urethra around the catheter with fingers to minimize fluid leakage. Flush the catheter with sterile saline to maximally dilate the urethra (i.e., when additional saline cannot be flushed into the catheter). While fluid is still being flushed into the catheter, remove the finger at the vesicourethral opening. Repeat this procedure until it is certain that no stones remain in the urethral lumen. Check the bladder for urachal diverticula, and excise if necessary. Submit the stones for mineral analysis and possibly for microbial culture.

SUTURE MATERIALS AND SPECIAL INSTRUMENTS

Absorbable suture material (e.g., polydioxanone [PDS], polyglyconate [Maxon], polyglycolic acid [Dexon], or polyglactin-910 [Vicryl]) is preferred for bladder and urethral surgery (see p. 677).

POSTOPERATIVE CARE AND ASSESSMENT

The animal should be closely monitored for urinary obstruction or leakage following surgery. Urine sediment and pH should be monitored regularly and urinary tract infection treated promptly. Therapy specific to the stone type should be implemented to help prevent stone recurrence (Box 25-5). D-penicillamine may inhibit wound healing and should not be initiated earlier than 2 weeks after surgery. Readers are referred to other sources for specific recommendations regarding medical treatment and prevention of urolithiasis.

COMPLICATIONS

Complications associated with cystotomy are uncommon; however, urine leakage is possible. The main complication of urethrotomy is hemorrhage, which may persist up to 7 days postoperatively. Urethral stricture is uncommon.

PROGNOSIS

The recurrence rate for calculi formation may be as high as 12% to 25%. Recurrence is more common in dogs with cystine and urate stones than in those with phosphate stones. Appropriate medical management (i.e., prevention of uri-

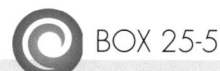 BOX 25-5

Drugs Used in the Treatment of Urinary Calculi

Allopurinol (Zyloprim)*

Dogs: To prevent reformation of stones: 7–10 mg/kg PO, qd-tid†
To dissolve urate calculi: 15 mg/kg PO, bid

D-Penicillamine (Cuprimine)

10–15 mg/kg PO, bid‡

N-(2-Mercaptopropionyl)-glycine (MPG) (Tiopronin)

To dissolve stones: 15–20 mg/kg PO, bid‡

PO, Oral; *qd,* every day; *tid,* three times a day; *bid,* twice a day.
*Use with caution in dogs with renal insufficiency. Also, the drug can cause xanthine uroliths if used with a nonpurine-restricted diet.
†Dosage should be adjusted based upon uric acid excretion.
‡Many side effects have been reported. Reader is referred to medical text for more information.

nary tract infection) is necessary to decrease the recurrence of struvite calculi.

References

Davidson E, Ritchey J, Higbee R et al: Laser lithotripsy for treatment of canine uroliths, *Vet Surg* 33:56, 2004.

Lekcharoensuk C, Osborne CA, Lulich JP: Associations between dietary factors in canned food and formation of calcium oxalate uroliths in dogs, *Am J Vet Res* 63:163, 2002. (A)

Lekcharoensuk C, Osborne CA, Lulich JP: Associations between dry dietary factors and canine calcium oxalate uroliths, *Am J Vet Res* 63:330, 2002. (B)

Ling GV, Thurmond MC, Choi YK et al: Changes in proportion of canine urinary calculi composed of calcium oxalate or struvite in specimens analyzed from 1981 through 2001, *J Vet Intern Med* 17:817, 2003.

Rawlings CA, Mahaffey MB, Barsanti JA et al: Use of laparoscopic-assisted cystoscopy for removal of urinary calculi in dogs, *J Am Vet Med Assoc* 222:759, 2003.

Suggested Reading

Houston DM, Moore AE, Favrin MG et al: Canine urolithiasis: a look at over 16,000 urolith submissions to the Canadian Veterinary Urolith Centre from February 1998 to April 2003, *Can Vet J* 34:225, 2004.

The purpose of this paper was to report on the age, sex, breed, and mineral composition of 16,647 uroliths submitted to the Canadian Veterinary Urolith Centre. The authors reviewed risk factors for various uroliths, along with recommendations for treatment and prevention.

Reimer SB, Kyles AE, Schulz KS et al: Unusual urethral calculi in two male dogs, *J Am Anim Hosp Assoc* 40:157, 2004.

This manuscript details the clinical presentation of large urethral calculi in the region of the ischial arch in two dogs. Surgical intervention failed to restore urinary continence in one dog that was managed medically for 2½ years before referral.

Seaman R, Bartges JW: Canine struvite urolithiasis, *Compend Cont Educ* 23:407, 2001.

This is a good review of struvite stones in dogs.

URETHRAL PROLAPSE

DEFINITIONS

Urethral prolapse is a protrusion of the urethral mucosa beyond the end of the penis.

GENERAL CONSIDERATIONS AND CLINICALLY RELEVANT PATHOPHYSIOLOGY

Urethral prolapse is uncommon. It may occur after excessive sexual excitement or masturbation, or it may be associated with genitourinary infections.

DIAGNOSIS
Clinical Presentation

Signalment. Young English bulldogs are most commonly affected, but it has also been reported in a Boston terrier and a Yorkshire terrier.

History. The owner may notice a reddened protrusion at the tip of the penis and/or intermittent penile bleeding, which may worsen when the dog becomes excited. Prolapse may be intermittent, occurring only when the dog has an erection. Some affected dogs lick at the preputial orifice and may traumatize the exposed urethral mucosa.

> NOTE: Penile bleeding may be intermittent (e.g., during erection).

Physical Examination Findings

A small, reddened mass may be visible protruding from the tip of the penis when the penis is extruded from the preputial orifice (Fig. 25-30). Penile erection may cause the protrusion to enlarge. Necrosis of the prolapsed urethra may occur secondary to drying or self-inflicted trauma. The prepuce should be checked for balanoposthitis or neoplasia.

Laboratory Findings

Anemia may occur in dogs with intermittent or chronic bleeding. Urinalysis or urine culture should be performed to exclude urinary tract infection. Exclusion of a coagulopathy in dogs with intermittent prolapse may be indicated.

DIFFERENTIAL DIAGNOSIS

Urethral prolapse may be differentiated from other causes of preputial bleeding by extruding the penis and examining the urethral orifice. Urethritis, fractures of the os penis, urethral calculi, and urethral stricture may be associated with hematuria and/or preputial bleeding. Other possible causes of penile bleeding include preputial, penile, or urethral neoplasia and prostatic lesions.

MEDICAL MANAGEMENT

Concurrent infection of the genitourinary tract should be treated. If the urethral mucosa is not necrotic, the prolapse can occasionally be reduced by gently manipulating it with a sterile cotton swab or by placing a lubricated catheter into the urethral orifice. A purse-string suture of 5-0 or 6-0 su-

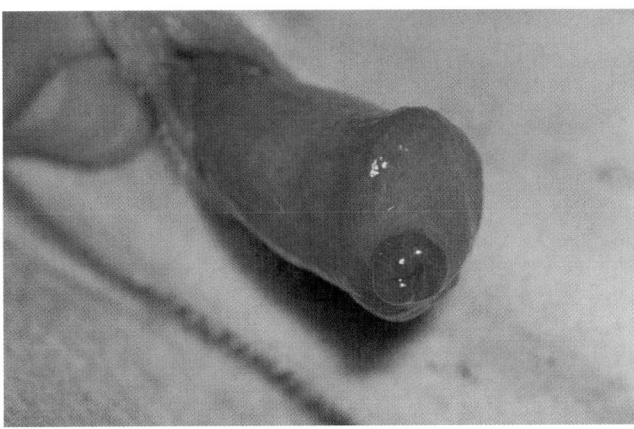

FIG. 25-30
Urethral prolapse in a dog. Note the small, reddened mass (urethra) protruding from the tip of the penis. (Courtesy H.P. Hobson, Texas A&M University.)

ture material can be placed in the penis around the orifice and tightened to prevent the prolapse from recurring without obstructing urination. The suture should be removed after 5 days and the patient monitored for recurrence. Spontaneous recovery has not been reported.

SURGICAL TREATMENT

Surgical resection of the prolapsed urethra is usually the treatment of choice. If the prolapse can be reduced, placing several mattress sutures from the urethral lumen and tying them on the external penile surface may cause fibrosis and prevent recurrence. The sutures should be left in place for 2 to 3 weeks. Bilateral orchiectomy should be performed, particularly in dogs that have prolapse associated with erection or sexual excitement.

Preoperative Management

The animal should be kept from traumatizing the urethra before surgery.

Anesthesia

Many different anesthetic regimens may be used safely if the animal is otherwise healthy.

Surgical Anatomy

Surgical anatomy of the urethra is discussed on p. 665.

Positioning

The animal is placed in dorsal or lateral recumbency and the penis extruded and gently cleaned with dilute chlorhexidine solution. Clipping of preputial hair is not necessary and may contribute to postoperative irritation.

SURGICAL TECHNIQUE

Prolapsed urethras may be treated by resecting the prolapsed tissue or by performing a urethropexy (Kirsch et al, 2002).

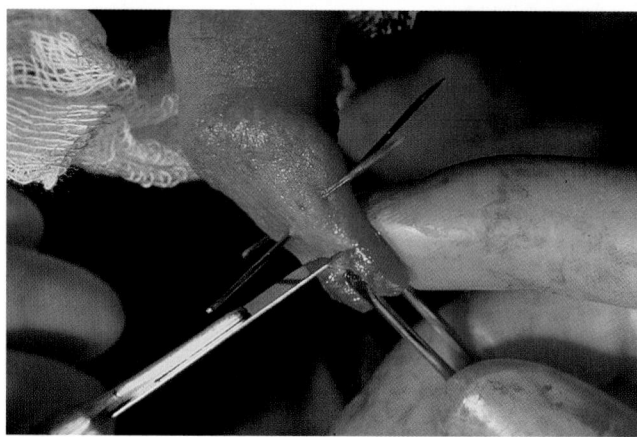

FIG. 25-31
To resect a urethral prolapse, place stay sutures in the urethral mucosa and apply gentle traction to straighten the prolapsed tissue. Place one or two straight needles through the penile tissue to prevent the urethra from retracting within the penis and circumferentially transect the urethra. (Courtesy H.P. Hobson, Texas A&M University.)

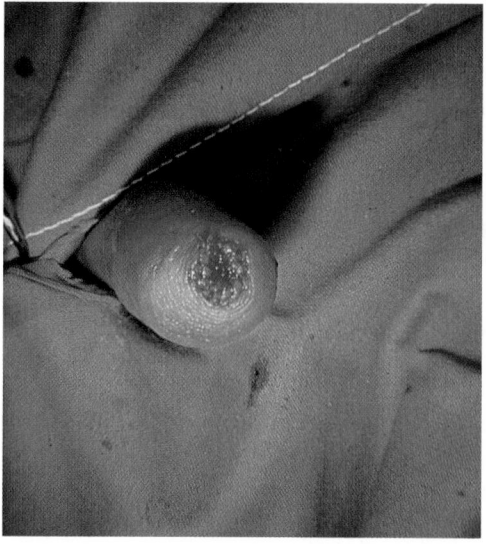

FIG. 25-32
After resecting the prolapsed urethra, suture the urethral mucosa to the penis with simple interrupted sutures. (Courtesy H.P. Hobson, Texas A&M University.)

Resection. *Place stay sutures in the urethral mucosa, and apply gentle traction to straighten the prolapsed tissue. Place one or two straight needles through the penile tissue (Fig. 25-31) or use stay sutures in the urethral mucosa distal to the proposed site of transection to prevent the urethra from retracting within the penis. Transect the urethra along its circumference, and suture it to the penis with 4-0 to 6-0 simple interrupted sutures of monofilament absorbable or nonabsorbable suture (Fig. 25-32). Alternately, make an incision on the ventral surface of the penis through both penile and urethral mucosa, extending halfway around the circumference of the urethra. Suture the urethral mucosa to the penile mucosa, then incise the dorsal surface of the urethral mucosa and suture it to the penis. This prevents retraction and the need for stay sutures.*

Concurrent excision of the distal end of the penis may be necessary in some dogs.

Urethropexy. *Manually extend the penis, and place a grooved director into the urethral orifice to reduce the prolapsed urethral mucosa. Pass the director to the distal aspect of the os penis. If this fails to achieve reduction of all urethral mucosa, have an assistant grasp the penis at its base and apply distal traction to invert the mucosa (Fig. 25-33, A and B). Using 2-0 or 3-0 monofilament absorbable suture on a large radius swaged-on taper-point needle, pass the suture full thickness through the penis from the external surface as far proximally on the penis as the needle curvature will allow. From the intraluminal surface, direct the needle distally out the urethral orifice (Fig. 25-33, C). Use the grooved director as a receiving surface for the needle to prevent penetration of the opposite wall of the urethral lumen. Then pass the needle in reverse fashion from the urethral orifice to the external surface of the penis and exit 0.5 cm distal to the initial needle*

entry site (Fig. 25-33, D). Tie the suture so that it creates a slight depression in the surrounding tissue (Fig. 25-33, E). Place 2 to 4 equally spaced sutures. Pass an 8 or 10 French urinary catheter to ensure urethral patency. Do not remove the sutures.

SUTURE MATERIALS AND SPECIAL INSTRUMENTS

Monofilament, nonreactive suture material, such as polydioxanone, polyglyconate, poliglecaprone 25, or glycomer 631 may be used.

POSTOPERATIVE CARE AND ASSESSMENT

An Elizabethan collar or sidebar should be used postoperatively to prevent the dog from licking. Tranquilizers may be helpful to prevent postoperative hemorrhage, but should only be used in patients in which pain has been appropriately managed. Nonabsorbable sutures should be removed in 7 to 10 days.

COMPLICATIONS

Hemorrhage from the surgical site may occur for 7 to 14 days. The dog should be prevented from becoming excited during the early postoperative period.

PROGNOSIS

Without surgery, the prolapse will not spontaneously resolve. Recurrence is uncommon following surgical resection, however.

Reference

Kirsch JA, Hauptman JG, Walshaw R: A urethropexy technique for surgical treatment of urethral prolapse in the male dog, *J Am Anim Hosp Assoc* 38:381, 2002.

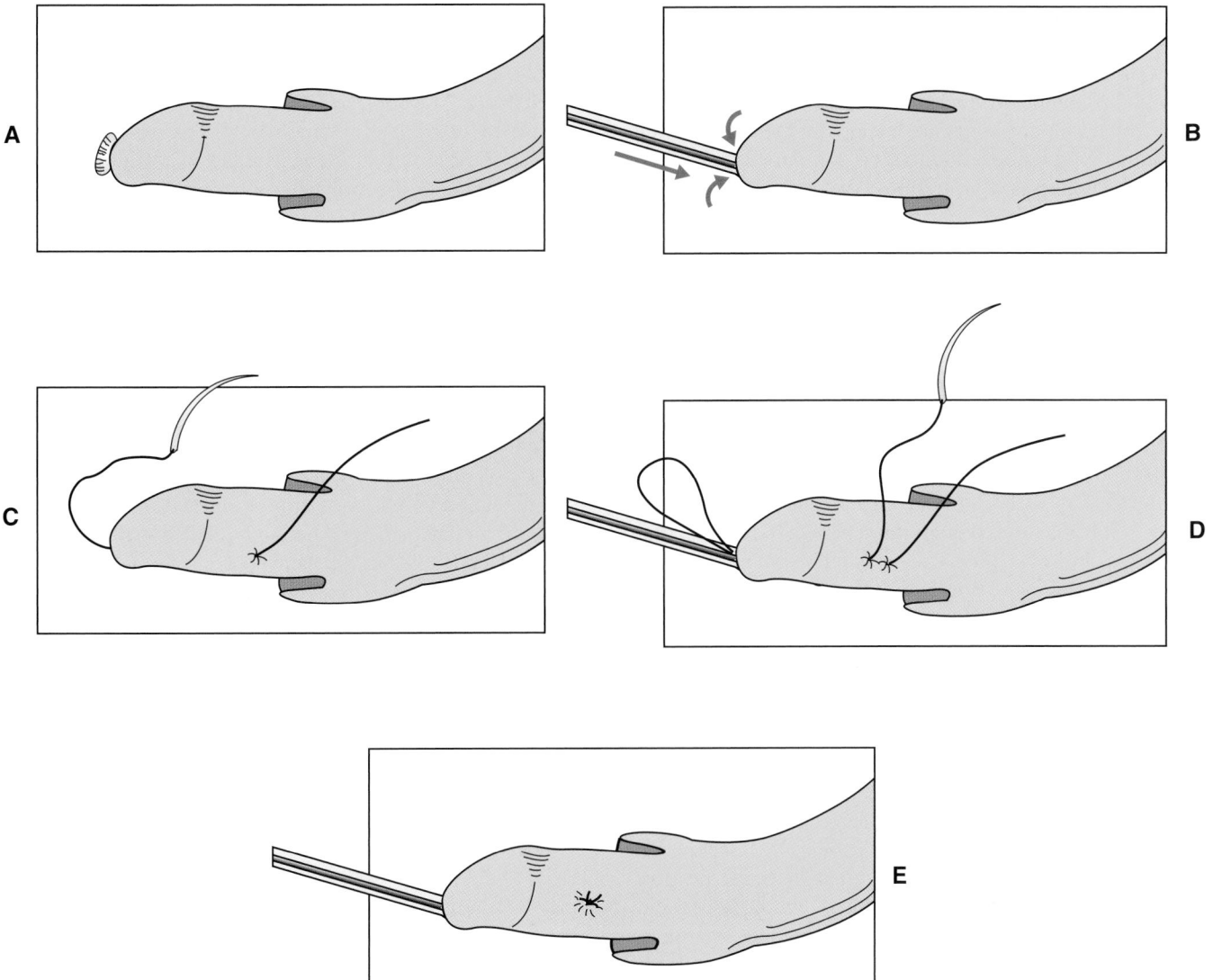

FIG. 25-33
A, Urethropexy for urethral prolapse. **B,** Pass a grooved director to the distal aspect of the os penis. **C,** Using 2-0 or 3-0 monofilament absorbable suture on a large radius swaged-on taper-point needle, pass the suture full thickness through the penis from the external surface, as far proximally on the penis as the needle curvature will allow. Direct the needle distally out the urethral orifice. Use the grooved director as a receiving surface for the needle to prevent penetration of the opposite wall of the urethral lumen. **D,** Then pass the needle in reverse fashion from the urethral orifice to the external surface of the penis and exit 0.5 cm distal to the initial needle entry site. **E,** Tie the suture so that it creates a slight depression in the surrounding tissue. Place 2 to 4 equally spaced sutures. Pass an 8 or 10 French urinary catheter to ensure urethral patency.

BLADDER AND URETHRAL NEOPLASIA

DEFINITIONS

Transitional cell carcinomas (TCC) are malignant tumors arising from a transitional type of stratified epithelium that usually affect the urinary bladder. **Rhabdomyosarcomas** are highly malignant tumors of striated muscle that may develop from pluripotent stem cells of the primitive urogenital ridge, which are remnants of the müllerian or wolffian ducts.

GENERAL CONSIDERATIONS AND CLINICALLY RELEVANT PATHOPHYSIOLOGY

Bladder neoplasia occurs more frequently than neoplasia of the remainder of the urinary system in dogs. In cats, renal lymphosarcoma is more common than bladder neoplasia. It has been hypothesized that the prevailing variation of bladder tumors between dogs and cats is because of differences in metabolism of tryptophan and its carcinogenic intermediary metabolites. Although dogs excrete aromatic amine metabolites of tryptophan in appreciable quantities into their urine, feline urine is almost devoid of them. Prolonged contact of the bladder mucosa with such carcinogenic substances may be important in the development of tumors. Cyclophosphamide may also cause bladder neoplasia in dogs. Most bladder tumors are malignant; metastasis to the sublumbar lymph nodes and lungs is common. Local extension to the ureters and/or urethra is common.

TCC are the most common tumors in canine and feline bladders; other malignant bladder tumors include squamous cell carcinoma, adenocarcinoma, fibrosarcoma, leiomyosarcoma, neurofibrosarcoma, rhabdomyosarcomas, and hemangiosarcoma. Fibromas, leiomyomas, hemangiomas, rhabdomyomas, myxomas, and neurofibromas are benign bladder tumors. Inflammatory cystic polyps are occasionally found. Metastasis of other tumors to the bladder is uncommon, although extension of prostatic or urethral tumors may occur. Dogs with bladder tumors commonly have other concurrent, primary tumors elsewhere. Fibromas are benign mesenchymal tumors that may occur in the bladder. They may be incidental findings or may cause clinical signs similar to those of urinary tract infection. Frequently, they are pedunculated; single or multiple-surgical excision is often curative. Single or multiple bladder papillomas may occur in older dogs and cause hematuria when ulcerated.

TCC are the most common canine urethral neoplasm; urethral tumors are exceedingly rare in cats. Other urethral tumors include squamous cell carcinoma and adenocarcinoma. These tumors may be primary urethral masses, or they may be extensions of prostatic or bladder neoplasia. Malignant urethral tumors are frequently locally invasive and may metastasize to the sublumbar lymph nodes and lungs. Proliferative urethritis and granulomatous inflammation of the urethra in female dogs may cause clinical signs similar to those of urethral neoplasia (i.e., stranguria, hematuria, pollakiuria, vaginal discharge, and/or urinary obstruction). Neoplasia and granulomatous inflammation may be differentiated by cytologic evaluation of urethral aspirates or surgical biopsies. The cause of granulomatous urethritis is unknown. Affected dogs may respond favorably to immunosuppressive therapy (i.e., prednisone or prednisone plus cyclophosphamide) plus antibiotics.

> NOTE: Granulomatous inflammation may cause clinical signs similar to those of urethral tumors. These lesions must be differentiated.

DIAGNOSIS
Clinical Presentation

Signalment. Bladder tumors are more common in dogs than in cats. Older dogs weighing more than 10 kg are most commonly affected; however, botryoid rhabdomyosarcoma (a rare tumor) may occur in young large-breed dogs and young cats. Female dogs and male cats have a higher risk for developing bladder cancer. Shetland sheepdogs, beagles, collies, and various terrier breeds (especially Scottish terriers)

seem to be predisposed to TCC. The average age of affected dogs and cats is approximately 10 years. Urethral tumors are more common in older female dogs.

History. Most dogs with bladder or urethral tumors are examined because of hematuria, pollakiuria, stranguria, and/or dysuria. Other signs include incontinence (especially paradoxical), polyuria-polydipsia, lameness, and dyspnea. Lameness may be due to bone metastasis or hypertrophic osteopathy. The most common clinical sign in cats is intermittent or persistent hematuria. If the tumor causes urethral or bladder obstruction, signs of uremia (i.e., vomiting, anorexia, and depression) may occur. Rectal prolapse has rarely been associated with TCC of the feline bladder.

Physical Examination Findings

The most common physical exam findings include a urethral or caudal abdominal mass, prostatomegaly, bladder distention, abdominal pain, weakness, lymphadenopathy, cough or dyspnea, and/or lameness. Lameness may be associated with hypertrophic osteopathy paraneoplastic syndrome in dogs with TCC. Urethral and prostatic involvement is common in dogs with TCC of the bladder; therefore in addition to careful abdominal palpation, rectal examination should be performed. Urethral masses in females may be palpated rectally or by digital examination of the vagina. Physical examination findings are normal in nearly one third of dogs with bladder neoplasia.

Diagnostic Imaging

Survey abdominal radiographs are rarely diagnostic, but may help exclude prostatic disease or urolithiasis. The sublumbar lymph nodes, pelvis, and vertebrae should be examined for metastasis. Diffuse thickening or calcification of the bladder wall is occasionally noted. Double contrast cystography or positive contrast urethrography and ultrasonography are the most useful tools for diagnosing urethral or bladder neoplasia (Fig. 25-34). Ultrasound is limited by the accessible acoustic window. Excretory urography may show hydroureter and/or hydronephrosis, and irregular filling defects in the bladder. Double contrast cystography is most effective for delineating bladder wall and luminal masses. Retrograde urethrography (see p. 684) can be performed in dogs with suspected urethral neoplasia to determine the tumor's extent and check for evidence of trigonal involvement. Thoracic radiographs should be performed to identify pulmonary metastasis. Ultrasonography is useful to look for abdominal metastasis. Although fine-needle aspirates of the mass may provide a presurgical diagnosis, they may cause seeding of the tumor along the needle tract.

Retrograde cystoscopy. Depending upon the patient's size and sex, either rigid or flexible scopes can be used. It is important in either case to be able to flush sterile saline ahead of the tip of the scope to facilitate visualization. However, it is seldom necessary to employ endoscopy for diagnosis because various catheter biopsy techniques work so well (see p. 691).

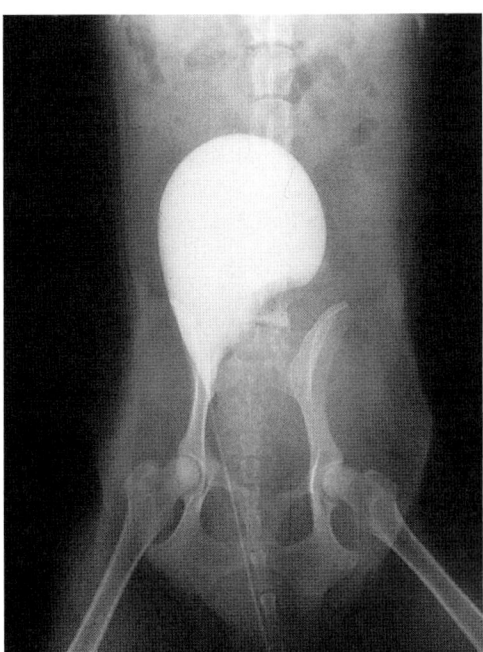

FIG. 25-34
Cystourethrogram in a dog with a large TCC. Note the filling defect near the bladder trigone.

Laboratory Findings

A CBC, serum biochemical profile, urinalysis, and urine culture should be performed in animals with bladder tumors. Hematologic and biochemical parameters are usually normal; however, elevations in serum creatinine and BUN may occur with partial obstruction of the lower urinary tract or ureter. Anemia is common in cats with bladder tumors. Hypereosinophilia has been reported in a cat with TCC of the bladder. Hematuria, pyuria, proteinuria, and/or bacteriuria are common. Although malignant cells may be found in the urine sediment of some dogs with bladder or urethral tumors, they are not detected in most cats with bladder neoplasia. Care should be taken to avoid confusing neoplastic and dysplastic cells; atypical transitional cells are common in animals with cystitis. Also, prolonged exposure to urine may make interpretation of abnormal cells difficult. Emptying the bladder and performing cytologic evaluation of a saline wash may be helpful in some animals.

Transurethral biopsy. Transurethral biopsy using a sterile urinary catheter is typically diagnostic.

First insert a finger into the rectum. Then, advance the largest urinary catheter that easily passes through the urethra until the tip is digitally felt to advance just to the point where the thickening or mass is palpated. At that point, apply negative pressure. If urine is obtained, empty the bladder. After the bladder is emptied, or if there is negative pressure to begin with, establish 8 to 12 ml of negative pressure with a syringe that has 10 ml of sterile saline in it, while pulling the catheter tip back out through the thickened area. Once the catheter tip is clearly out of the affected area, remove the catheter

from the urethra, place the tip in a clot tube, and blow the tissue fragments in the tip out by forcing saline out through the catheter. Examine the fluid, and retrieve tissue fragments and use them to make squash cytology preparations. In the case of female dogs with severe obstruction of the distal urethra, the most that may be possible is to insert a small, stiff polypropylene catheter a few millimeters into the urethra (which is as far as is possible in many cases), apply suction, and then blow the tissue fragments out, as described above.

A veterinary version of rapid latex agglutination urine dipstick test (bladder tumor antigen test) has been screened for use in dogs with TCC of the lower urinary tract (Henry et al, 2003). Test sensitivities were 88%, 87%, and 85% for all dogs with suspected and confirmed TCC, dogs with confirmed TCC at any site, and dogs with confirmed TCC of the urinary bladder, respectively. The test performed slightly better on centrifuged urine samples than on uncentrifuged urine samples.

DIFFERENTIAL DIAGNOSIS

Other causes of hematuria and/or bacteriuria (e.g., urolithiasis, prostatic disease, and polypoid cystitis) should be excluded. Many cats with lower urinary tract neoplasia are treated presumptively for sterile cystitis with antibiotics, urinary acidifiers, and/or dietary changes for months before diagnosis. Nonneoplastic (granulomatous) infiltrative urethral disease should be differentiated from neoplasia by cytology and/or histopathology. Polypoid cystitis is a rare urinary bladder disease in dogs, characterized by inflammation, epithelial proliferation, and development of a polypoid mass or masses without histologic evidence of neoplasia. These lesions must be differentiated from neoplastic masses. A mass is not seen in some animals with polypoid cystitis, and diffuse thickening of the bladder is noted. Most affected dogs are females, which are typically presented for hematuria or recurrent urinary tract infections (Martinez et al, 2003). *Proteus* spp., *E. coli*, *Staphylococcus*, and *Enterococcus* are commonly isolated. Most of the masses are located cranioventrally in the bladder rather than at the bladder neck or trigone. Surgery and removal of all polyps is typically effective.

MEDICAL MANAGEMENT

If partial or complete urinary obstruction is present, the animal should be stabilized before surgery with fluids and cutaneous urinary diversion (urethral catheter or tube cystostomy). Electrolyte and acid-base abnormalities should be corrected, and concurrent urinary tract infection treated with appropriate antibiotics. An ECG should be evaluated for arrhythmias. Treatment of malignant bladder tumors with excision and/or adjuvant chemotherapy has also been reported. Piroxicam (Box 25-6) has been used to treat nonresectable TCC of the urinary bladder in dogs. Complete remission may occur in some dogs, whereas others have a subjectively improved quality of life despite the lack of tumor remission. The exact mechanism of piroxicam antitumor activity is un-

Medical Treatment of Canine Cystic Transitional Cell Carcinoma

Piroxicam (Feldene)

0.3 mg/kg PO, qod to qd*

Misoprostol (Cytotec)†

1–5 μg/kg PO, tid

PO, Oral; *qod*, every other day; *qd*, once a day; *tid*, three times a day.

*Start with eod administration and observe response; qd administration may be associated with gastrointestinal ulceration. Do not use with any other NSAIDs or any steroids.

†Can cause diarrhea and/or abdominal discomfort. These signs usually subside after a few days. Note: this drug probably helps prevent GI problems in dogs receiving NSAIDs, but it cannot be relied upon to prevent ulceration/erosion. Misoprostol is only used in patients that appear to require it because of signs associated with piroxicam administration. The patient must still be observed closely to ensure that toxicity from piroxicam does not occur.

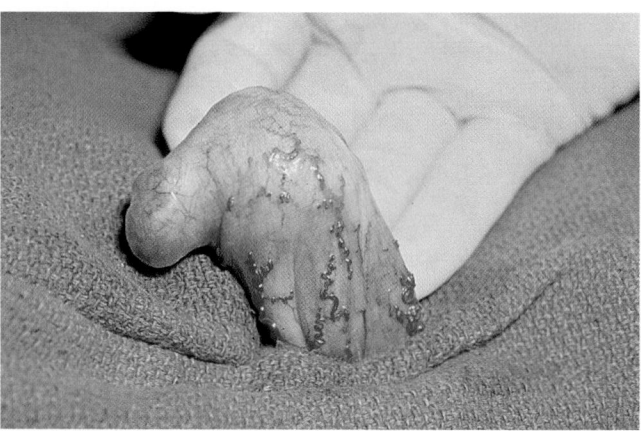

FIG. 25-35
Leiomyoma of the bladder. Surgical excision of benign tumors or those located at the bladder apex may be curative.

known; however, COX-2 is highly expressed in TCC cells, and it has been suggested that this isoform may be involved in tumor cell growth. Thus inhibition of COX-2 may be the mechanism by which nonsteroidal antiinflammatory drugs (NSAIDs) exert their antineoplastic effects (Nasir et al, 2000). Antiinflammatory activity might also be important. The most common side effect of piroxicam administration is gastrointestinal irritation (i.e., anorexia, melena, and/or vomiting). Concurrent use of misoprostol may be beneficial in selected cases (see Box 25-6).

SURGICAL TREATMENT

Surgical therapy is difficult because the most common site for urinary bladder neoplasia is the trigone. Although the ureters can be transected and implanted into the apex of the bladder following partial cystectomy, incontinence typically occurs if the trigone is removed. Similarly, implantation of the ureters at a distant site (i.e., the colon) following complete cystectomy typically causes pyelonephritis and/or incontinence (see p. 676). Tumor spread beyond the primary site is also common. Transplantation of TCC to the subcutaneous tissue of the surgical incision has been reported in dogs; therefore the same instruments should not be used on other tissues used for a biopsy of, or to resect, bladder tumors. Cystostomy catheter placement may also be considered (see p. 667). Surgical excision of neoplastic lesions may be curative if the tumor is benign (Fig. 25-35).

Resection of focal lesions of the urethra is possible with a transpubic surgical approach and urethral resection and anastomosis (see p. 675). Prepubic urethrostomy (see p. 674) with resection of neoplastic tissues may be performed if the distal urethra is involved. Urethral tumors that involve the entire length of the urethra or the bladder trigone are generally inoperable.

Preoperative Management

See the discussion on medical management on p. 691.

Anesthesia

If renal impairment is not present, many different anesthetic regimens may be used safely. If renal impairment is present, see p. 636 for suggested anesthetic protocols.

Surgical Anatomy

Refer to p. 665 for the surgical anatomy of the bladder and urethra.

Positioning

The animal is placed in dorsal recumbency, and the abdomen is prepared for a ventral midline incision. For bladder neoplasia, the incision should extend from above the umbilicus to the brim of the pelvis. With urethral neoplasia, the incision should be extended caudally to allow a pubic osteotomy to be performed.

SURGICAL TECHNIQUE

Examine the sublumbar lymph nodes, ureters, and other abdominal organs for evidence of tumor extension or metastasis. For bladder neoplasia, locate the entrance of the ureters into the trigone, and excise the tumor, removing at least 1 cm of normal tissue. Be sure to avoid damaging the ureters. If a large portion of the bladder has been removed, place a urinary catheter and suture the bladder with a continuous appositional suture pattern.

Otherwise a two-layer inverting pattern can be used (see p. 666).

If the bladder trigone is involved, consider ureterocolonic urinary diversion (see p. 676), chemotherapy, or euthanasia.

For urethral neoplasia, check the trigone, ureters, sublumbar lymph nodes, and other abdominal tissue for evidence of neoplasia. Perform a pelvic osteotomy, and carefully examine the entire urethra. If the tumor does not involve the entire urethra or trigone, perform a urethral resection and anastomosis (see p. 668). If only the distal urethra is involved and if neoplastic tissue can be resected, consider a prepubic urethrostomy (see p. 674).

In rare instances, a benign, pedunculated urethral tumor may be removed through a urethrotomy incision (see p. 670).

SUTURE MATERIALS AND SPECIAL INSTRUMENTS

Absorbable suture material (e.g., polydioxanone [PDS], polyglyconate [Maxon], polyglycolic acid [Dexon], polyglactin-910 [Vicryl], or poliglecaprone 25 [Monocryl] is preferred for bladder and urethral surgery (see p. 677).

POSTOPERATIVE CARE AND ASSESSMENT

The animal should be observed for urinary leakage or obstruction following surgery. With ureterocolonic anastomosis, intravenous fluids should be continued for 24 to 72 hours to ensure diuresis. The animal should be encouraged to eat the day following surgery (see p. 677). Kidneys should be monitored for function and postoperative infection. If neurologic dysfunction occurs, blood ammonia levels should be measured and the animal treated appropriately (see p. 635). Following this procedure, the addition of 0.5 to 2 g of sodium bicarbonate to the food twice daily may improve clinical signs associated with hyperchloremia and metabolic acidosis. Placement of Vaseline on the perineum may help prevent urine scalding.

COMPLICATIONS

The most common complications of bladder and urethral surgery are urinary leakage or obstruction (see p. 678). Pyelonephritis, renal failure, neurologic dysfunction, electrolyte abnormalities, metabolic acidosis, and diarrhea with subsequent perineal irritation are possible complications of ureterocolonic urinary diversion (see p. 676). Urinary tract infection is a common complication of cystostomy tube placement.

PROGNOSIS

Because of the malignant nature of most lower urinary tract tumors, the prognosis is guarded. Median survival times reported for prospective clinical trials have never exceeded 1 year, regardless of the treatment modality. With aggressive surgery, urethral tumors may have a better prognosis than bladder tumors. Chemotherapy may allow dogs with bladder tumors to survive for significantly longer periods than if they undergo surgery. In a recent study of 25 dogs with unresectable urinary bladder carcinoma treated with chemotherapy, the overall median survival time was 251 days (Rocha et al, 2000). Spayed females survived significantly longer than castrated males, and dogs that received either doxorubicin or mitoxantrone in addition to a platinum-based chemotherapeutic lived significantly longer than those that received only a platinum compound. For most owners, piroxicam as monotherapy or in conjunction with other agents may be the most appropriate medical therapy. The benefits of radiation and photodynamic therapy in dogs are still being evaluated. Cystostomy tube placement in dogs with known or suspected TCC typically resolves the stranguria, and most owners are satisfied with the procedure. Urinary tract infections are a common complication. Recently TCC of the bladder was treated with a combination of once-weekly coarse fraction radiation therapy, mitoxantrone chemotherapy, and piroxicam (Poirier et al, 2004). Although only two dogs achieved a measurable partial response, 90% had amelioration of their urinary clinical signs. The median survival time for all dogs was 326 days. Survival was no better than protocols using mitoxantrone and piroxicam without radiation therapy.

The results of ureterocolonic anastomosis in a large number of dogs have not been reported, but with improved techniques and the prevention of the deleterious effects of pyelonephritis on renal function, long-term survival might be possible. Newer treatment methods, such as photodynamic therapy, may improve the prognosis of animals with bladder tumors in the future.

References

Henry CJ, Tyler JW, McEntree MC et al: Evaluation of a bladder tumor antigen test as a screening test for transitional cell carcinoma of the lower urinary tract in dogs, *Am J Vet Res* 64:1017, 2003.

Martinez I, Maldoon JS, Eaton KA et al: Polypoid cystitis in 17 dogs (1978-2001), *J Vet Intern Med* 17:499, 2003.

Nasir K et al: Expression of cyclooxygenase-2 in transitional cell carcinoma of the urinary bladder in dogs, *Am J Vet Res* 61:478, 2000.

Prorier VJ, Forrest LJ, Adams WM et al: Piroxicam, mitoxantrone, and coarse fraction radiotherapy for the treatment of transitional cell carcinoma of the bladder in 10 dogs: a pilot study, *J Am Anim Hosp Assoc* 40:131, 2004.

Rocha TA, Mauldin GN, Patnaik AK et al: Prognostic factors in dogs with urinary bladder carcinoma, *J Vet Intern Med* 14:486, 2000.

Suggested Reading

Liptak JM, Brutscher SP, Monnet E et al: Transurethral resection in the management of urethral and prostatic neoplasia in 6 dogs, *Vet Surg* 33:505, 2004.

This procedure was useful in palliating male dogs with prostatic tumors, but was not advantageous in female dogs with urethral tumors.

Mutsaers AJ, Widmer WR, Knapp DW: Canine transitional cell carcinoma, *J Vet Med* 17:136, 2003.

This is a good review of this tumor in the dog.

Raghavan M, Knapp D, Bonney PL et al: Evaluation of the effect of dietary vegetable consumption on reducing risk of transitional cell carcinoma of the urinary bladder in Scottish Terriers, *J Am Vet Med Assoc* 227:94, 2005.

Eating certain vegetables may slow or prevent TCC in Scottish terriers.

Raghavan M, Knapp D, Dawson M et al: Topical flea and tick pesticides and the risk of transitional cell carcinoma of the urinary bladder in Scottish terriers, *J Am Vet Med Assoc* 225:389, 2004.

Use of topical tick and flea products was not associated with increased risk for TCC.

Takiguchi M, Mutsumi I: Diagnostic ultrasound of polypoid cystitis in dogs, *J Vet Med Sci* 67:57, 2005.

Inflammatory polyps can be found in the cranioventral and the craniodorsal bladder.

URINARY INCONTINENCE

DEFINITIONS

Urinary incontinence is due to failure of voluntary control of the vesical and urethral sphincters with constant or frequent involuntary passage of urine. Incontinence may be caused by neurogenic abnormalities or anatomic outflow obstruction (paradoxical or overflow incontinence), may be hormone responsive (urethral sphincter mechanism incontinence), or may be due to inflammation (urge incontinence), congenital abnormalities (e.g., ectopic ureters), or behavioral problems.

GENERAL CONSIDERATIONS AND CLINICALLY RELEVANT PATHOPHYSIOLOGY

Urinary incontinence is reported to occur in approximately 20% of spayed dogs. No true bladder sphincter exists in the bitch, so continence is maintained by multiple, interacting factors. Poor urethral tone, marked urethral hypoplasia, "pelvic" bladders, ovariohysterectomy, obesity, and congenital abnormalities have all been implicated as potential causes of urinary sphincter mechanism incontinence in female dogs. Congenital urethral sphincter mechanism incontinence has also been described in cats. Some animals respond to estrogen supplementation or sympathomimetic drugs, particularly α-adrenergic stimulants (e.g., ephedrine, phenylpropanolamine, and imipramine) that increase urethral sphincter tone. Surgical alternatives to improve urethral resistance include urethral slings, artificial sphincters, urethral lengthening procedures, periurethral injections of polytetrafluoroethylene, colposuspension, and cystourethropexy. Because these techniques are not uniformly successful, or because success has not been well documented in a large number of animals with urinary incontinence, surgical treatment (other than for congenital abnormalities, such as ectopic ureters; see p. 646) should be reserved for animals that do not respond to medical management (see later discussion), or when the owners refuse to consider long-term drug therapy.

> NOTE: Consider ectopic ureters (see p. 646) as a differential in any animal that develops urinary incontinence at a young age, including those that respond to medical therapy.

Estrogens probably exert their beneficial effect by improving smooth muscle contractility and sensitivity to α-adrenergic innervation. Bladder neck position may affect continence; increases in intraabdominal pressure are transmitted to both the bladder and proximal urethra in bitches with an intraabdominal bladder neck. Dogs, however, with more caudal (pelvic) bladders have this pressure transmitted to the bladder, but not the urethra. Experimentally a rise in intraabdominal pressure leads to shortening of the functional urethral length, which might increase the adverse effect of bladder neck position in these dogs, thereby worsening incontinence.

DIAGNOSIS
Clinical Presentation

Signalment. Medium-sized and large-breed dogs seem to be at increased risk, particularly Doberman pinschers, old English sheepdogs, and springer spaniels. Among small-breed dogs, miniature poodles may be at increased risk. Incontinence may be first noted at any age, depending on the cause.

History. Animals may have a lifelong history of urinary incontinence, or it may occur after ovariohysterectomy. The incontinence may be continuous, may be intermittent, or may only occur when the animal is excited or asleep. A history of "bed wetting" is probably one of the most important historic findings that suggest incontinence. The only reasons dogs will urinate on themselves while asleep are incontinence and either weakness or pain that makes them unable and/or unwilling to get up when they have to urinate.

Physical Examination Findings

Physical examination findings are usually unremarkable. Occasionally the bladder is caudally displaced in the abdominal cavity. Signs of concurrent urinary tract infection (i.e., hematuria, dysuria, and stranguria) may be noticed. In cats with urethral hypoplasia, vaginal aplasia is common, with the uterine horns emptying into the caudal part of the dorsal wall of the bladder.

Diagnostic Imaging

Excretory urography can be performed to identify the termination of the ureters into the bladder. The vesicourethral junction may appear blunted and abnormally dilated, or the urethra may seem abnormally short. In cats with vaginal aplasia, radiographic evidence of a communication between the lumen of the uterus and the bladder may be noted.

Cystoscopy. Retrograde cystoscopy is currently the most sensitive and specific minimally invasive way to diagnose and define ectopic ureters (Figs. 25-36 and 25-37). In one study, transurethral cystoscopy diagnosed ectopic ureters in 96% of affected dogs (Cannizzo et al, 2003). Contrast-enhanced computed tomography (CT) can also be used to evaluate ectopic ureters. Most female dogs with ectopic ureters have vestibulovaginal abnormalities, which can be so pronounced as to make it difficult to find the urethral orifice. Most ectopic ureters are easily identified as one advances up the urethra while infusing saline; however, some

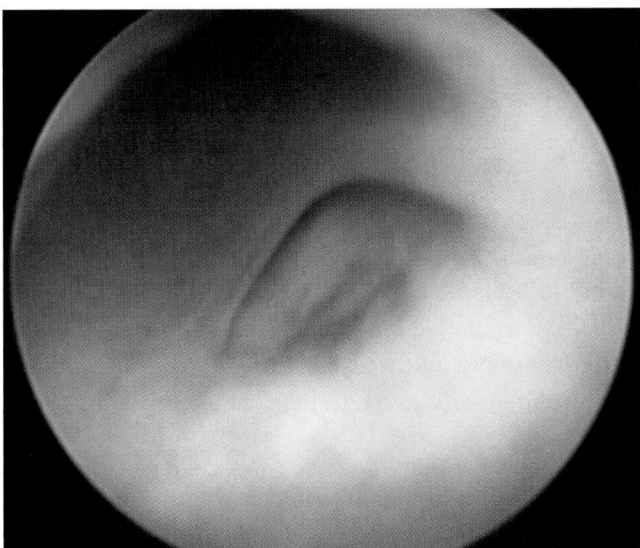

FIG. 25-36
Cystoscopic view of an ectopic ureter opening into the ure-thra, near the trigone.

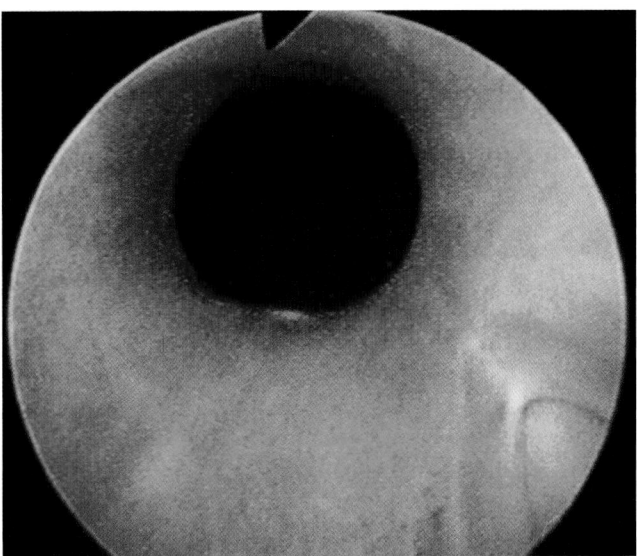

FIG. 25-37
Cystoscopic view of an ectopic ureter (lower right hand cor-ner) opening into the distal urethra, near the urethral orifice.

are located just at the junction of the urethra and bladder, making them difficult to see. If you are not sure if a slit or a fold is a ureter, observing it for a few minutes will often allow you to see a "puff" of yellow urine exit from it.

Laboratory Findings

Other than findings consistent with upper or lower urinary tract infection in some animals, laboratory findings are un-remarkable. Urine cultures should be performed in all ani-mals with incontinence, even if the urinalysis is not sugges-tive of a urinary tract infection.

DIFFERENTIAL DIAGNOSIS

The various causes of urinary incontinence must be differ-entiated. Urge incontinence secondary to cystic or urethral infection and/or inflammation should be excluded (e.g., re-sponse with appropriate antibiotics). Ectopic ureters should be detected and corrected surgically (see p. 649). Paradoxical incontinence (e.g., partial obstruction due to urethral cal-culi, neoplasia, or strictures) and neurogenic incontinence should be differentiated from urethral sphincter mechanism incompetence based on radiographic findings, neurologic examination, and/or catheterization. Urethral sphincter pro-filometry and cystometry can determine urethral sphincter tone and bladder emptying pressures, but these tests are seldom required.

MEDICAL MANAGEMENT

Dogs with suspected urethral sphincter mechanism incom-petence should be treated with estrogens and/or sympatho-mimetic drugs initially, and concurrent urinary tract infec-tions should be treated. Diethylstilbestrol (DES) and/or α-adrenergic agonists (i.e., phenylpropanolamine or ephed-rine; Box 25-7) may be used to increase urethral sphincter

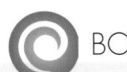 **BOX 25-7**

Drugs Used in the Treatment of Urinary Incontinence

Phenylpropanolamine*

Dogs: 1.5–2 mg/kg PO, bid to tid†
Cats: 1.5 mg/kg PO, tid

Ephedrine

Dogs: Start at 0.4 mg/kg and gradually increase to 4 mg/kg PO, bid to tid‡
Cats: 2–4 mg/cat PO, bid to tid

Diethylstilbestrol (DES)

Dogs: 0.1–0.2 mg/kg (maximum of 1 mg) PO, qd for 3–5 days, then same dose once every 3–7 days as needed, with maximum of 0.2 mg/kg/week§

Estriol

2 mg PO qd for 7 days, then reduced to lowest effective dose (0.5–2 mg/dog qd to qod)

Testosterone Cypionate (Depotestosterone)

Dogs: 1.1–2.2 mg/kg IM, once every 30 days

Imipramine (Tofranil)

Dogs: 2–4 mg/kg, PO, qd to bid

PO, Oral; *bid*, twice a day; *tid*, three times a day; *qid*, four times a day; *qd*, once a day; *qod*, every other day.
*Although this drug has been withdrawn from the human market, it is generally available from veterinary pharmacies that compound drugs.
†Best to start at low end of dose and gradually increase, if needed.
‡Toxicity typically starts at 5 mg/kg, and death can readily occur at 10 mg/kg.
§If benefit is not noted after 5 days of daily therapy, then it is unlikely that further administration will benefit the patient, and other drugs should be used.

tone. If the animal responds to DES (usually within 5 to 7 days), the frequency of administration should be decreased to the lowest effective dosage (usually 1 mg given 1 to 3 times per week). DES is a relatively safe estrogen, seldom causing problems when used appropriately. High doses of DES may cause estruslike signs, bone marrow toxicity, and/or alopecia; therefore frequent administration and/or dosages greater than 1 mg daily should be avoided, and other drugs used instead. Use of α-adrenergic agonists with DES may allow lower dosages to be used. Phenylpropanolamine is used more frequently than ephedrine because it has fewer side effects (i.e., hyperexcitability, panting, and/or anorexia) and greater efficacy over time. In a recent study, 85.7% of dogs treated with phenylpropanolamine had no episodes of unconscious urination compared with 33.3 % of placebo-treated dogs (Scott et al, 2002). The biggest disadvantage of phenylpropanolamine is that it must be given two to three times per day (versus one to two times per week with DES).

Some male dogs with urinary incontinence may be managed by parenteral testosterone. This is very uncommon, and other causes of incontinence should be sought before making such a diagnosis. Phenylpropanolamine or ephedrine should be used if possible. If they fail, then repositol testosterone (i.e., cypionate; see Box 25-7) may be used. If prostatic enlargement or perianal adenomas are present (or occur during therapy), testosterone therapy should be stopped.

SURGICAL TREATMENT

There is presently no single surgical procedure that will cure incontinence in all female dogs with urethral sphincter mechanism incontinence. Colposuspension has been performed on a large number of patients, with approximately half becoming continent after surgery. Cystourethropexy results in continence in most bitches immediately following surgery; however, incontinence recurs in a majority of treated dogs. A laparoscopy-assisted technique for cystopexy in dogs has been reported (Rawlings et al, 2002). The latter may be more useful in dogs with perineal hernias than in those with incontinence. In animals with notable urethral hypoplasia, reconstruction of the bladder neck may eliminate or decrease incontinence (see later discussion). A sling procedure using a polyester ribbon passed through the obturator foramen, around the urethra, and fixed outside the pelvis resulted in less than 25% of dogs becoming continent. This procedure was recommended for dogs weighing more than 20 kg. For the sling procedure to be beneficial, it must increase urethral pressure close to, or within, the normal range.

Injection of Teflon (e.g., polytef) into the submucosa of the proximal urethra has been used in dogs, but rejection of the Teflon resulted in recurrence of incontinence in most dogs. Recently collagen has been endoscopically injected into the urethral submucosa of dogs. Continence was achieved in 68% of treated dogs for 1 to 64 months (mean, 17 months) (Barth et al, 2005). In 6 of 10 partial responders, administration of additional medication was successful in achieving full continence. Only 3 of 40 treated dogs did not respond. Return of incontinence may be caused by flattening of the collagen deposits; they do not appear to be resorbed. Urinary retention was not observed in the aforementioned study.

> NOTE: Rule out other causes of incontinence and determine efficacy of medical management before attempting surgical correction. Urinary tract infection can cause medical therapy that would otherwise work to be ineffective.

Preoperative Management

Concurrent urinary tract infections should be treated before surgery.

Anesthesia

If renal impairment is not present, many different anesthetic regimens may be used safely. If renal impairment is present, see p. 636 for suggested anesthetic protocols.

Surgical Anatomy

See p. 665.

Positioning

The animal is placed in dorsal recumbency, and the abdomen is prepared for a ventral midline incision. The prepped area should be sufficient to allow the incision to extend from the pubis proximally to the umbilicus.

SURGICAL TECHNIQUE

Although numerous techniques have been described to correct urethral sphincter mechanism incontinence, only bladder flap reconstruction for treatment of hypoplastic urethras, and collagen injection are described here. Colposuspension and a transpelvic sling procedure are described in *Small Animal Surgery*, second edition or in the e-dition.

Bladder Flap Reconstruction of a Hypoplastic Urethra

Perform a ventral cystotomy that extends into the proximal aspect of the hypoplastic urethra. Identify the ureteral openings. In addition to an allowance for suturing, make two stab incisions into the bladder wall caudal and lateral to the ureteral stoma, with the distance between the stab incisions representing the desired circumference of the new urethral tube (Fig. 25-38). A 3.5 or 5 French (cats) or 8 French (dogs) catheter should pass easily into the newly created urethral tube. Use scissors to extend the incision towards the urethra, creating two full-thickness flaps. Reflect the flaps cranially (Fig. 25-39, A). Suture the defect from the urethral end cranially to form the urethral tube (Fig. 25-39, B) with a two-layer simple continuous suture pattern or a simple continuous suture pattern and a Cushing pattern. Use absorbable suture material (2-0 to 4-0). If the urethral lumen is compromised by placing two layers of sutures, suture the urethral tube with a single-layer appositional pattern, using care to ensure sufficient apposition of sutures such that urine leakage will not occur. Suture the flaps together. Perform

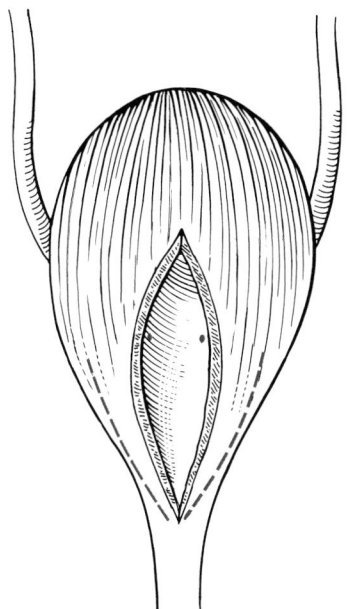

FIG. 25-38
For bladder flap reconstruction of a hypoplastic urethra, make two stab incisions into the bladder wall caudal and lateral to the ureteral stoma. Then make two full-thickness flaps (see Fig. 25-39).

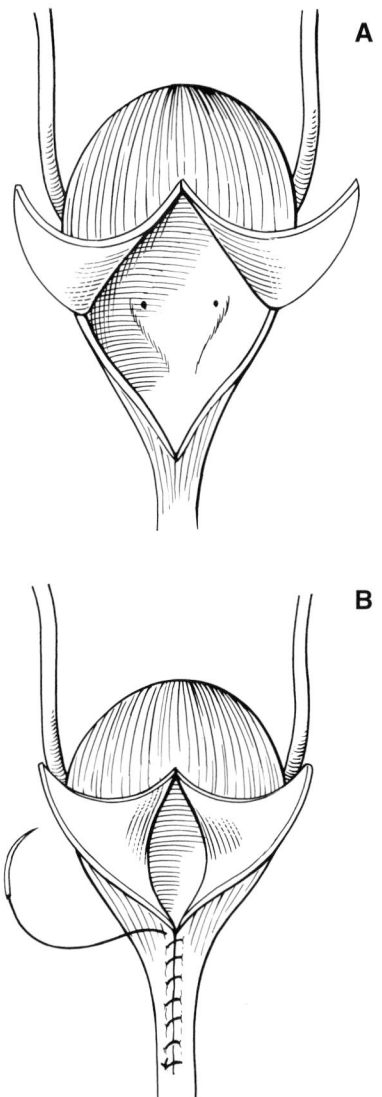

FIG. 25-39
A, Use scissors to extend the incisions illustrated in Fig. 25-38 towards the urethra, creating two full-thickness flaps. **B,** Reflect the flaps cranially and suture the defect from the urethral end cranially to form a urethral tube.

ovariohysterectomy in intact cats in which the uterine horns empty into the bladder.

Endoscopic Collagen Injection

Position the dog in dorsal recumbency with the limbs extended cranially. Pass a cystoscope into the urethra via the external orifice. Inject collagen (approximately 2 ml/dog) at the 2, 6, and 10 o'clock positions (three injections) approximately 1.5 cm caudal to the neck of the bladder until the lumen of the urethra appears to be closed by the collagen deposits.

If bleeding hinders the view through the cystoscope, a laparotomy can be performed and the collagen injected under direct visualization, although this is seldom necessary.

SUTURE MATERIALS AND SPECIAL INSTRUMENTS

Absorbable suture material (e.g., polydioxanone [PDS], polyglyconate [Maxon], polyglycolic acid [Dexon], or polyglactin-910 [Vicryl]) is preferred for bladder and urethral surgery (see p. 677). Bovine origin collagen may be used for the collagen injections (e.g., Zyplast, Inamed, Santa Barbara, Calif.).

POSTOPERATIVE CARE AND ASSESSMENT

The animal should be closely monitored for urinary obstruction or leakage following surgery. If urinary obstruction occurs, an indwelling urinary catheter should be placed and maintained for 3 to 5 days. Animals should be monitored for urinary tract infections periodically after surgery.

COMPLICATIONS

If the urethral lumen is of insufficient width or if swelling is excessive, urinary obstruction may occur. Other complications include return of incontinence and urinary leakage.

PROGNOSIS

Urinary continence or decreased frequency and volume of urine dribbling appear to occur in most animals with urethral hypoplasia following bladder flap reconstruction.

References

Barth A, Riechler IM, Hubler M et al: Evaluation of the long-term effects of endoscopic injection of collagen into the urethral submucosa for treatment of urethral sphincter incompetence in female dogs: 40 dogs (1993-2000), *J Am Vet Med Assoc* 226:73, 2005.

Cannizzo KL, McLoughlin MA, Mattoon JS et al: Evaluation of transurethral cystoscopy and excretory urography for diagnosis of ectopic ureters in female dogs: 25 cases (1992-2000), *J Am Vet Med Assoc* 223:475, 2003.

Rawlings CA, Howerth EW, Mahaffey MB et al: Laparoscopic-associated cystopexy in dogs, *Am J Vet Res* 63:1226, 2002.

Scott L, Leddy M, Bernay F et al: Evaluation of phenylpropanolamine in the treatment of urethral sphincter mechanism incompetence in the bitch, *J Small Anim Pract* 43:493, 2002.

Suggested Reading

Crawford JT, Adams WM: Influence of vestibulovaginal stenosis, pelvic bladder, and recessed vulva on response to treatment for clinical signs of lower urinary tract disease in dogs: 38 cases (1990-1999), *J Am Vet Med Assoc* 221:995, 2002.

Based on their findings, the authors recommend vaginectomy or resection and anastomosis in dogs with severe vestibulovaginal stenosis and signs of lower urinary tract disease.

Hostutler RA, Chew DJ, Eaton KA et al: Cystoscopic appearance of proliferative urethritis in 2 dogs before and after treatment, *J Vet Intern Med* 18:113, 2004.

These lesions seem consistent with chronic bacterial infection or immune-mediated disease. There are good endoscopic photographs of the lesions.

Rawlings CA: Colposuspension as a treatment for urinary incontinence in spayed dogs, *J Am Anim Hosp Assoc* 38:107, 2002.

This is a well illustrated description of colposuspension.

Samii VF, McLoughlin MA, Mattoon JS et al: Digital fluoroscopic excretory urography, digital fluoroscopic urethrography, helical computed tomography, and cystoscopy in 24 dogs with suspected ureteral ectopia, *J Vet Intern Med* 18:271, 2004.

Cystoscopy was 100% sensitive for diagnosing ectopic ureters, and had a positive predictive value of 97% and a negative predictive value of 100%. CT had a 100% positive predictive value, but a 57% negative predictive value.

Steffey MA, Brockman DJ: Congenital ectopic ureters in a continent male dog and cat, *J Am Vet Med Assoc* 224:1607, 2004.

Ectopic ureters should be considered in hydronephrotic animals, even if they are not incontinent.

FELINE UROLOGIC SYNDROME (STERILE CYSTITIS)

DEFINITIONS

Feline urologic syndrome (FUS) is a term once used to describe an idiopathic inflammatory process of the feline lower urinary tract that sometimes results in partial or complete urethral obstruction. The current accepted terminology is **feline lower urinary tract disease (FLUTD)**. *Feline idiopathic cystitis (FIC), interstitial cystitis, feline obstructive uropathy,* and *"blocked Tom cat"* are commonly used synonyms.

GENERAL CONSIDERATIONS AND CLINICALLY RELEVANT PATHOPHYSIOLOGY

Cats with FLUTD may account for as many as 10% of all feline admissions to veterinary hospitals. Most cats with FLUTD have FIC or interstitial cystitis; however, urolithiasis, bacterial urinary tract infection, anatomic malformations, neoplasia, behavioral disorders, and neurologic problems (e.g., reflex dyssynergia) may also occur. Struvite crystals and/or calculi may be found in some cats without signs of sterile cystitis. Urinary tract infection is uncommon in obstructed cats. Dietary factors (i.e., high dietary magnesium or ash content, and feeding dry food), obesity, urine alkalinity, urinary tract infection, decreased urine volume and decreased frequency of urination, viruses (e.g., feline calicivirus, bovine herpesvirus 4, and feline syncytia-forming virus), vesicourachal diverticula, and decreased glycosaminoglycan excretion have all been implicated as causes of feline interstitial cystitis; however, the cause is undefined and probably multifactorial. FIC may include multiple complex abnormalities of the endocrine and nervous systems that likely affect more than just the urinary bladder (Westropp and Buffington, 2004).

> NOTE: Struvite crystals are not always associated with signs of sterile cystitis, and some cats with sterile cystitis do not have struvite crystals or calculi.

DIAGNOSIS
Clinical Presentation

Signalment. Overweight cats may be predisposed to sterile cystitis. Males and females are equally affected; however, male cats are more likely to be obstructed because of the small diameter of their urethras. Middle-aged cats are more commonly affected, and indoor cats may be at increased risk.

History. Unobstructed cats usually are brought in for evaluation of pollakiuria, stranguria, hematuria, and/or inappropriate urination. Cats with obstruction may appear uncomfortable or anxious, restless, may attempt to urinate frequently, lick their genitalia, and may have abdominal pain. If obstruction has been present for more than 36 to 48 hours, anorexia, dehydration, vomiting, collapse, stupor, hypothermia, and/or bradycardia may be noted (see p. 663).

Physical Examination Findings

If the cat is obstructed, the bladder will feel distended and firm (unless it has ruptured) and cannot be expressed. Abdominal palpation may elicit pain. Care should be taken when palpating the bladder of obstructed cats to prevent iatrogenic rupture.

Laboratory Findings

Laboratory findings may be normal or may show evidence of uremia, metabolic acidosis, and/or hyperkalemia.

DIFFERENTIAL DIAGNOSIS

Other causes of urethral obstruction (e.g., neoplasia and trauma) should be excluded based on clinical signs, physical examination findings, and history.

MEDICAL MANAGEMENT

For obstructed cats, fluid therapy should begin before laboratory data are returned. Fluids should be given intravenously to restore normal hydration and treat hyperkalemia (see p. 663). Physiologic saline solution should be used in case the cat is hyperkalemic. In all but the very sickest cats, this will be adequate to dilute hyperkalemia and reverse cardiotoxicity. If serum potassium is later found to be normal, a balanced electrolyte solution should be administered. Obstruction should be promptly relieved by urethral catheterization or gentle penile massage, if possible. If the cat is severely depressed, minimal restraint may be necessary. In other cats, general anesthesia may be required (see later discussion). Sterile isotonic fluid should be used to flush plugs or calculi into the bladder. Nonmetal, smooth, well-lubricated catheters are preferred to minimize urethral trauma. If the catheter cannot be advanced, cystocentesis may be helpful. If a normal stream is not present following catheterization or if detrusor atony is present, an indwelling, soft urinary catheter may be sewn in place; however, this predisposes to urinary tract infection. The cat should be stabilized before performing a perineal urethrostomy.

SURGICAL TREATMENT

Perineal urethrostomy is indicated to prevent recurrence of obstruction in male cats or to treat obstruction that cannot be eliminated by catheterization. It is also useful to treat strictures that occur following urethral obstruction and catheterization. With appropriate nonsurgical treatment of obstructed cats, this procedure is less commonly indicated than previously. There is a high incidence of postoperative bacterial urinary tract infection after urethrostomy due to anatomic alterations of the urethral meatus, compromised intrinsic defense mechanisms, and the underlying uropathy. Many cats have a permanent loss of striated urethral sphincter function after this procedure, although incontinence is rare. A modified technique using preputial mucosa has been reported and may give a more cosmetic appearance (Yeh and Chin, 2000).

Preoperative Management

Electrolyte (i.e., hyperkalemia) and acid-base abnormalities should be corrected before anesthetic induction (see p. 663). Fluids should be given intravenously to restore normal hydration and combat postobstruction diuresis. Cats that were initially severely uremic will often have a substantial postobstruction diuresis during which they require large volumes (i.e., sometimes greater than two to three times maintenance requirements) of intravenous fluids to prevent severe hypovolemia. Serum potassium concentrations must be monitored to prevent hypokalemia.

 BOX 25-8

Selected Anesthetic Protocols for Use in Shocky, Dehydrated, or Hypovolemic Cats With FLUTD

Premedication

Anticholinergics*
Butorphanol (0.2–0.4 mg/kg SC or IM) or buprenorphine (5–15 µg/kg IM) or hydromorphone (0.05–0.1 mg/kg SC or IM)

Induction

Diazepam (0.2 mg/kg IV) followed by etomidate (0.5–1.5 mg/kg IV)

Maintenance

Isoflurane or sevoflurane

SC, Subcutaneous, *IM*, intramuscular; *IV*, intravenous.
*Anticholinergics may be given as needed if the animal is bradycardic.

Anesthesia

An ECG should be monitored before, during, and after surgery for cardiac arrhythmias. If the cat has been adequately stabilized (i.e., hydration and potassium are normal), diazepam followed by ultrashort-acting thiobarbiturates (thiopental sodium), or propofol, or mask induction may be used if the cat is not vomiting (after premedicating with an opioid; Box 25-8). Thiobarbiturates are arrhythmogenic and should therefore be avoided or used cautiously in animals with preexisting arrhythmias. Isoflurane and sevoflurane in oxygen are the least cardiodepressant inhalation anesthetics and should be used for maintenance. Shocky, dehydrated, or hypovolemic patients should be induced with diazepam followed by etomidate, after premedicating with an opioid. Because ketamine is renally excreted in active form, it should be avoided or used very cautiously and at low doses in cats with urinary obstruction. Mask induction should not be used if the cat is vomiting.

Surgical Anatomy

For a description of the surgical anatomy of the urethra, refer to p. 665.

Positioning

The cat is placed in sternal recumbency with the perineal region elevated slightly. Ventilation may need to be assisted when the cat is positioned in this manner.

SURGICAL TECHNIQUE
Perineal Urethrostomy

Place a purse-string suture in the anus, and catheterize the penis if possible. Make an elliptical incision around the scrotum and prepuce, and excise them. Place an Allis tissue forceps on the end of the prepuce or around the catheter to help manipulate the penis. Reflect the penis dorsolaterally, and sharply dissect the surrounding loose tissue on either

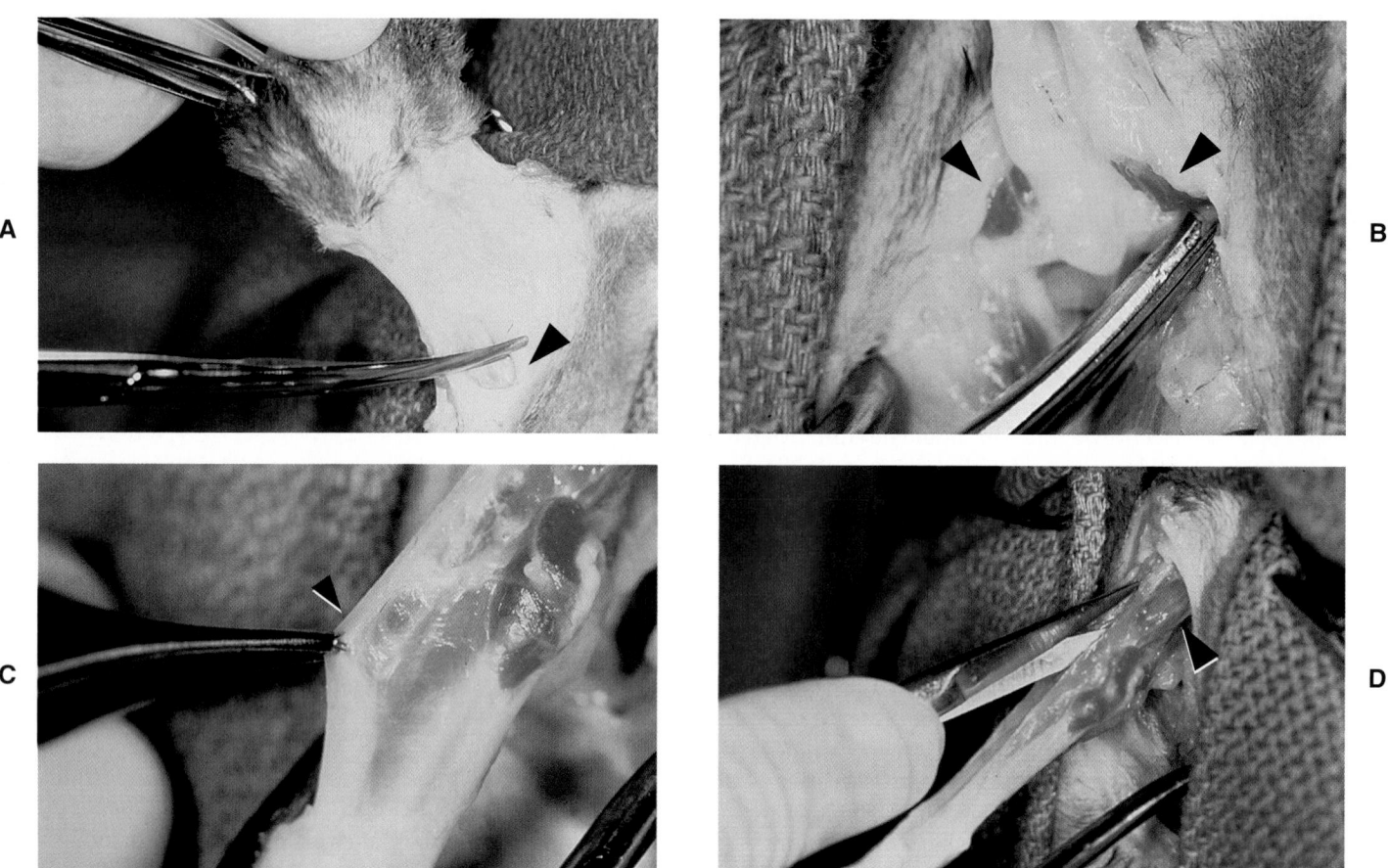

FIG. 25-40
Perineal urethrostomy may be performed in male cats with urinary obstruction. **A,** Reflect the penis dorsolaterally and sharply dissect surrounding loose tissue on either side. **B,** Transect the ischiocavernosus muscles and ischiourethralis muscles at their insertion on the ischium to avoid damaging branches of the pudendal nerves and to minimize hemorrhage. **C,** Elevate and remove the retractor penis muscle over the urethra, before making a longitudinal incision in the penile urethra. **D,** To ensure that the urethral width is adequate, extend the urethral incision approximately 1 cm beyond the level of the bulbourethral glands. (From Hosgood G, Hedlund CS: Perineal urethrostomy in cats, *Compend Contin Educ Pract Vet* 14:1195, 1992.)

side (Fig. 25-40, A). *Extend the dissection ventrally and laterally toward the penile attachments at the ischial arch. Elevate the penis dorsally and sharply sever the ventral penile ligament. Then, transect the ischiocavernosus muscles and ischiourethralis muscles at their insertion on the ischium to avoid damaging branches of the pudendal nerves and to minimize hemorrhage (Fig. 25-40, B). Reflect the penis ventrally to expose the dorsal surface. Expose the bulbourethral glands proximal and dorsal to the bulbospongiosus muscle and cranial to the severed ischiocavernosus and ischiourethralis muscles. Avoid excessive dorsal dissection to prevent damaging the nerves and vessels supplying the urethral muscle. Elevate and remove the retractor penis muscle over the urethra (Fig. 25-40, C), and longitudinally incise the penile urethra using a No. 11 blade or sharp tenotomy scissors. Continue the urethral incision proximal to the pelvic urethra approximately 1 cm beyond the level of the bulbo-*

urethral glands (Fig. 25-40, D). Pass a closed Halsted mosquito hemostat up the urethra to ensure that the urethral width is adequate.

The hemostat should be able to be passed to the level of the boxlocks without resistance.

Suture the urethral mucosa to the skin using 4-0 or 5-0 absorbable (polydioxanone or polyglyconate) or nonabsorbable (nylon or polypropylene) suture on a taper-cut, swaged-on needle using a simple interrupted or simple continuous suture pattern. Be sure to suture the urethral mucosa to skin (it is sometimes difficult to identify mucosa). Place the most proximal sutures at a 45-degree angle to the skin first, then place the remainder. Suture the proximal two thirds of the penile urethra to the skin, and amputate the distal end by placing a horizontal mattress suture through the skin and

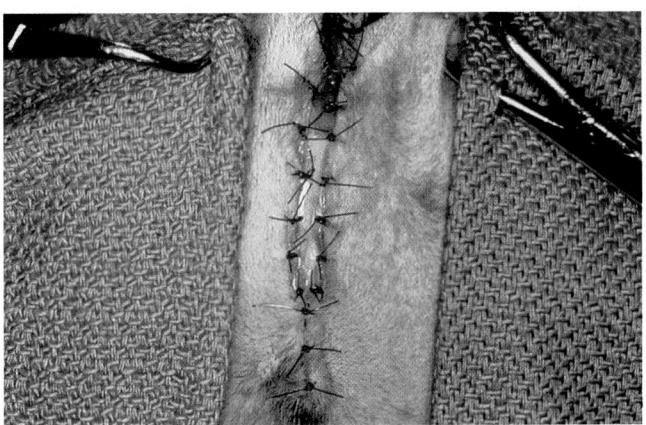

FIG. 25-41
Appearance of a completed perineal urethrostomy in a cat. (From Hosgood G, Hedlund CS: Perineal urethrostomy in cats, *Compend Contin Educ Pract Vet* 14:1195, 1992.)

penile tissues and severing the penis distal to this ligature. Close the remaining skin with simple interrupted sutures (Fig. 25-41).

SUTURE MATERIALS AND SPECIAL INSTRUMENTS

A urinary catheter is placed in the urethra to help locate it during the operation. Monofilament absorbable (polydioxanone, polyglyconate, or poliglecaprone 25) or nonabsorbable (polypropylene or nylon) suture is preferred. If nonabsorbable suture is used, the sutures should be removed 10 to 14 days after the surgery. A recent study showed no difference in the complication rate when a continuous suture pattern using absorbable sutures that were not removed was compared with nonabsorbable sutures that were removed (Agrodnia et al, 2004). Tenotomy scissors and small, atraumatic forceps are useful.

POSTOPERATIVE CARE AND ASSESSMENT

Paper, instead of gravel litter, should be used until the wound is healed. Urinary cultures should be performed periodically to check for urinary tract infection. Indwelling catheters should not be routinely used following surgery because they promote stricture formation and/or urinary tract infection.

NOTE: Stricture formation following perineal urethrostomy is usually due to making the stoma too small.

COMPLICATIONS

The most serious complication of perineal urethrostomy is stricture formation. Stricture formation in cats following perineal urethrostomy is generally a result of making the stoma too small (i.e., making the stoma in the proximal penile urethra instead of the distal pelvic urethra), or a result of postoperative subcutaneous urine leakage and subsequent granulation tissue formation (see p. 678). Urinary and fecal incontinence may occur if nerves are damaged during dissection around the pelvic urethra (see Surgical Technique section). Perineal urethrostomy is associated with a high prevalence of urinary tract infection postoperatively because of anatomic alterations of the urethral meatus, compromised intrinsic defense mechanisms, and the underlying uropathy. Indwelling catheters may allow ascending bacterial infection and/or cause fibrosis and stricture. Although incontinence is rare, many cats have a permanent loss of striated urethral sphincter function after this procedure. Rectal prolapse has been reported following perineal urethrostomy in cats.

NOTE: Evaluate these cats periodically for urinary tract infection

PROGNOSIS

The mortality rate of obstructed cats may exceed 35%. This high rate is often due to the financial constraints of owners reluctant to finance multiple or prolonged hospitalizations. Recurrence of obstruction is uncommon if perineal urethrostomy is performed properly; however, the cat should be monitored periodically for urinary tract infection for the remainder of its life.

References

Agrodnia MD, Hauptman JG, Stanley BJ et al: A simple continuous pattern using absorbable suture for perineal urethrostomy in the cat: 18 cases (2000-2002), *J Am Anim Hosp Assoc* 30:479, 2004.

Westropp JL, Buffington CAT: Feline idiopathic cystitis: current understanding of pathophysiology and management, *Vet Clin North Am Small Anim Pract* 34:1043, 2004.

Yeh L-S, Chin S-C: Modified perineal urethrostomy using preputial mucosa in cats, *J Am Vet Med Assoc* 216:1092, 2000.

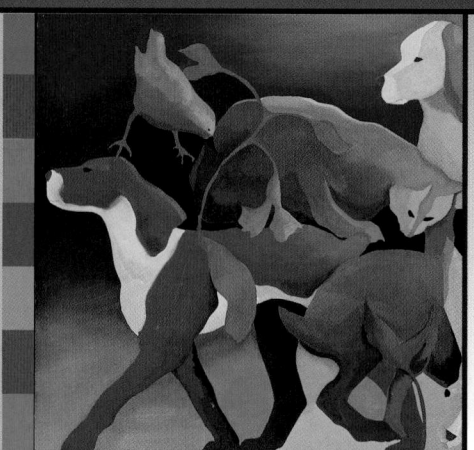

CHAPTER 26
Surgery of the Reproductive and Genital Systems

DEFINITIONS

Neuter, or **castration**, refers to either **ovariohysterectomy (OHE)** (surgical removal of the ovaries and uterus) or **orchiectomy** (surgical removal of the testicles). **Mastectomy** is excision of one or more mammary glands or mammary tissue. **Episiotomy** is incision of the vulvar orifice to expose the vulva and vagina, whereas **episioplasty** is reconstruction of the vulva. **Prostatectomy** is removal of all or a portion of the prostate gland. **Hysterotomy** is a surgical incision into the uterus (e.g., cesarean section).

PREOPERATIVE MANAGEMENT

Reproductive surgery encompasses a variety of techniques designed to alter the animal's ability to reproduce, aid parturition, and/or treat or prevent disease of the reproductive organs (Box 26-1). The primary indication for reproductive tract surgery is to limit reproduction, but it may also be done to relieve dystocia, prevent or treat tumors influenced by reproductive hormones (e.g., mammary tumors, testicular tumors, and perianal adenomas), help control certain diseases of the reproductive tract (e.g., pyometra, metritis, prostatitis, and prostatic abscessation), and help stabilize systemic disease (e.g., diabetes and epilepsy). Neutering is performed in some animals to prevent or alter behavioral abnormalities and to reconstruct traumatized, diseased, or malformed tissue. Diagnosis of reproductive tract disease is based on history, clinical signs, physical examination, diagnostic imaging (e.g., radiographs, ultrasound, computed tomography [CT], magnetic resonance imaging [MRI], and bone scan), endoscopy, cytology, microbiology, hormonal assay, hematology, serum biochemistry profile, urinalysis, and/or other laboratory results.

History. History and clinical signs of animals needing reproductive surgery depend on the gender and disease. Most animals brought in for elective reproductive surgery (i.e., castration or OHE) are healthy. Asymptomatic animals with neoplasia may have a mass found incidentally by the owner. Those with genital tract infections may be severely ill and have fever, toxemia, incontinence, and/or obstruction. Prostatic disease is common in male dogs; clinical signs may be nonspecific (i.e., fever, malaise, vomiting, dehydration, caudal abdominal pain, and/or gait abnormalities). Hematuria caused by reflux of blood from the prostatic urethra into the bladder and/or concurrent urinary tract infection may occur. Urethral discharge (preputial/urethral drip) is caused by passive release of blood, pus, or prostatic fluid into the prostatic urethra. Stranguria occurs when the prostate compresses or obstructs the urethra, or there is inflammation caused by urinary tract infection. Urinary incontinence (see p. 694) may be caused by prostatic impingement on the pelvic nerves. Prostatic enlargement compressing the rectum can cause tenesmus or smaller stool diameter. Constipation may occur secondary to obstruction or pain during defecation.

Females

Physical examination. Physical examination should include inspection and palpation of the abdomen, vulva, and mammary glands. Abdominal palpation may reveal an enlarged uterus, mass, visceral displacement, and/or pain. Abnormal vulvar skin folds, conformation, discharge, or enlargement may be noted. During estrus and proestrus, the vulva is swollen to two or three times its normal size, appears turgid, and has a hemorrhagic to straw-colored discharge.

 BOX 26-1

Surgical Procedures of the Reproductive Tract

- Ovariohysterectomy
- Castration
- Cesarean section
- Cryptorchid castration
- Mastectomy
- Scrotal ablation
- Episiotomy
- Vasectomy
- Episioplasty
- Prostatic drainage:
  Drains
  Omentalization
  Marsupialization
- Prostatectomy
- Penile amputation
- Preputial reconstruction
- Phallopexy
- Biopsy

The swelling and turgidity diminish during estrus and diestrus. A vaginal examination is recommended when vaginal discharge or enlargement is detected. The vestibule and vagina should be visualized and digitally palpated. If the vagina is too small to allow vaginal examination, then a rectal examination may allow the clinician to palpate abnormalities otherwise inaccessible during physical examination. Mammary glands should be inspected for symmetry, texture, size, mobility, discharge, and the presence of masses.

Clinical pathology. If masses are identified, cytology of aspirates or discharges may help differentiate inflammation from neoplasia. Vaginal, uterine, or mammary gland cultures are recommended if infection is suspected. Vaginal cytology should be consistent with the bitch's estrus cycle. The normal vaginal flora includes numerous aerobic and anaerobic bacteria (Box 26-2). Pure growth of bacteria from vaginal specimens can be normal unless accompanied by signs of reproductive tract disease. Persistent vaginal discharge is an indication for brucellosis testing.

Hormone concentrations. Assessment of hormone levels is occasionally helpful. In female dogs, estradiol levels are ≤ 10 pg/ml during late anestrus, ≥ 10 pg/ml at onset of proestrus, and 50 to 100 pg/ml at late proestrus. Progesterone levels are 0.5 to 1 ng/ml during anestrus and proestrus, 2 to 5 ng/ml at ovulation, peak at 15 to 90 ng/ml after the luteinizing hormone (LH) peaks, and remain elevated during gestation (Table 26-1). A drop in progesterone levels to less than 1 to 2 ng/ml for 2 consecutive days indicates pregnancy termination. For mean serum concentrations of LH and follicle-stimulating hormone (FHS), see Table 26-2. Measuring LH helps distinguish between neutered and intact bitches; measuring a single low LH test result indicates a sexually intact bitch. Knowing the time of the LH surge (greater than 1 ng/ml) is helpful in determining ideal breeding times, predicting parturition, and administering drugs for mismating. Predicting the LH surge may be possible by measuring an approximately 15% reduction in horizontal dimensions of the vulva (Nishiyama et al, 2000).

In queens, behavioral estrus occurs during peak follicular growth, with elevations in plasma estradiol to greater than 70 pmol/L and vaginal cornification. Mean serum progesterone concentration is 14.09 nmol/L in ovulating, 1.24 nmol/L in nonovulating, and 0.75 nmol/L in ovariohysterectomized queens. Serum progesterone concentration 2 weeks after ovulation induction with gonadotropin-releasing hormone (25 μg per cat IM) or human chorionic gonadotropin (250 IU per cat IM) is expected to exceed 6.4 nmol/L in cats with functional ovarian tissue. Serum progesterone concentration at parturition has been reported as 7 to 15.9 nmol/L and less than 3.18 nmol/L immediately after parturition.

Diagnostic imaging. Positive contrast vaginography may help evaluate vaginal anomalies, masses, or injuries if digital examination does not adequately define the problem. Positive contrast vaginography using a Foley catheter and a water-soluble iodinated contrast agent is easily performed. Endoscopy of the vagina is the best technique for direct visualization if performed properly. An otoscope or vaginal speculum allows visual inspection of the vestibule

 TABLE 26-1

Methods to Determine Pregnancy Risk After Mating

TEST	RESULT
Vaginal cytology within 48 hr • Saline moisten swab in vagina for 1 min • Incubate swab in test tube with 0.5 ml saline for 10 min • Compress swab against tube and centrifuge at 2000 rpm for 10 min • Extend sediment on slide and diff-Quik stain	Detect spermatozoa
Progesterone levels	Low risk with levels less than 2 ng/ml High risk with levels greater than 10 ng/ml

 **BOX 26-2**

Normal Vaginal Flora: Common Organisms

- α- and β-hemolytic *Streptococcus* spp.
- *Staphylococcus* spp.
- *Proteus* spp.
- *Escherichia* coli
- *Bacillus* spp.
- *Bacteroides* spp.
- *Pasteurella* spp.
- Anaerobic enterococci
- *Mycoplasma*

 TABLE 26-2

Serum Hormone Concentrations in Female Dogs (ng/ml)

	INTACT	NEUTERED
LH	1.2 (±0.9)	28.7 (±25.8)
FSH	98 (±49)	1219 (±763)

From Olson PN, Mulinix JA, Nett TM: Concentrations of luteinizing hormone and follicle-stimulating hormone in the serum of sexually intact and neutered dogs, *Am J Vet Res* 53:762, 1992.

TABLE 26-3

Methods of Pregnancy Determination

Abdominal palpation	Perform 26–28 days, but before 30 days, after mating to detect uterine swellings about 3 to 5 cm in diameter
Transabdominal ultrasonography	**Canine** Detect embryonic vesicles 19–20 days after LH peak Detect embryo at day 23–25 after LH peak Detect heartbeat by day 23–25 after LH peak
Relaxin ELISA test	Positive 21 days after breeding
Abdominal radiography	Detect enlarged canine uterus at 31 to 38 days after LH peak Detect canine fetal mineralization at 45 days after LH peak Detect enlarged feline uterus 25–35 days after LH peak Detect general feline fetal mineralization 25–29 days before parturition; or 25–35 days after LH peak; first evidence of mineralization is seen in the spinal column 22–27 days, skull 21–27 days, ribs 20–25 days, scapula 17–24 days, humerus 20–24 days, femur 19–23 days, radius 15–22 days, tibia 15–21 days, ulna 5–21 days, pelvis 8–20 days, fibula 0–17 days, tail 8–16 days, metatarsals and metacarpals 3–14 days, phalanges 0–11 days, calcaneus 0–10 days, and teeth 1–6 days before parturition

ELISA, Enzyme-linked immunosorbent assay; *LH,* luteinizing hormone.

and caudal vagina; however, an endoscope is needed to evaluate the cranial vagina and cervix. The vagina must be insufflated with air to distend mucosal folds and allow thorough evaluation.

Thoracic and abdominal radiographs and ultrasound, CT, or MRI images may be needed if reproductive tract tumors are suspected. The normal nongravid uterus is rarely identified by survey radiographs. Radiographically, an enlarged gravid uterus can be detected within 31 to 38 days and fetal skeletal mineralization by 45 days after the LH peak (within a mean of 0.5 day of onset of estrus) (Table 26-3). In cats it is difficult to know when the LH peak has occurred because behavioral estrus is variable (1 to 21 days); therefore fetal skeletal mineralization, which is first detected at 25 to 29 days before parturition, is used to predict when parturition will occur. Ovarian masses and follicular changes can be detected in the periovulatory period using ultrasonography. The normal, nongravid uterus can be identified using a high-frequency (>10 MHz) transducer. Using a fluid-distended urinary bladder as an acoustic window may reveal fluid-distended horns and a thickened uterine wall. Pregnancy and fetal viability can be detected ultrasonographically as early as 20 to 25 days after the LH surge in dogs (see Table 26-3) (Nyland and Mattoon, 2002). Ultrasonographic signs of abortion or lack of fetal viability include changes in fetal anatomy, placental detachment, and/or fetal resorption; however, serial evaluations may be necessary. Ultrasonography can also detect uterine cysts, masses, or fluid; premature placental separation; and a thickened uterine wall.

Other tests. Cystometrograms and urethral pressure profiles may rarely help assess urinary incontinence (see Chapter 25). Histologic evaluation is necessary to confirm the diagnosis and allow a more accurate prognosis with most conditions.

Males

Physical examination. Thorough abdominal and rectal palpation is needed to evaluate prostatic size, symmetry, texture, and mobility, and sublumbar lymph node size. Prostatic palpation sometimes elicits pain in animals with prostatitis. The scrotum should be examined for size, symmetry, thickening, masses, sensitivity, and scrotal adhesions. Testicles should be palpated for size, consistency, contour, symmetry, and sensitivity. The prepuce and penis are observed for signs of trauma, wounds, masses, irritation, and congenital abnormalities. The penis should be completely extruded from the prepuce for thorough examination.

Clinical pathology. Cytology of prostatic fluid is one of the most informative tests. Prostatic fluid is best obtained by ejaculation, but a prostatic wash or fine-needle aspirate is often acceptable. Prostatic massage or ejaculation fluid in normal dogs has few transitional cells, rare neutrophils, and varying numbers of erythrocytes. Fine-needle aspiration cytology is more likely to demonstrate neoplastic cells, increased neutrophils, bacteria, and other debris. Urine and prostatic fluid should be cultured to detect bacterial infections. Cytologic evaluation should be performed on all accessible masses. A biopsy is necessary to definitively diagnose prostatic, testicular, penile, preputial, or scrotal masses.

Hormone concentrations. Measurement of serum hormone concentrations may aid in determining whether a male dog has been neutered or has a hormone-producing tumor; however, episodic release of gonadotropins makes interpretation of hormone assays difficult, and reference values vary between laboratories. Expected serum concentrations of LH and FSH in intact and castrated male dogs are provided in Table 26-4. In intact male dogs, serum testosterone concentrations range between 0.5 and 9 ng/ml, whereas serum estrogen concentrations are generally less than 15 pg/ml. Finding testosterone levels less than 100 pcg/ml in

TABLE 26-4

Serum Hormone Concentrations in Male Dogs (ng/ml)

	INTACT	NEUTERED
LH	6.0 (±5.2)	17.1 (±9.9)
FSH	89 (+28)	858 (+674)
Estrogen	Less than 0.015	
Testosterone	0.5–9 ng/ml Cryptorchid: 0.1–0.5 ng/ml	Less than 0.1

LH, Luteinizing hormone; *FSH,* follicle-stimulating hormone.

dogs indicates that they have been neutered. In toms, testosterone secretion is episodic without diurnal rhythm. In normal toms, resting serum testosterone concentrations range from nondetectable to 1 to 6 ng/ml (81.5 nmol/L) and in castrated toms are less than 0.5 ng/ml.

Diagnostic imaging. Abdominal radiographs define prostatic size, shape, and location. Radiographically the normal prostate may be near the cranial brim of the pubis and should not displace the colon or bladder. Its contour should be smooth and symmetrical. Abnormal prostates may be asymmetric, irregular, and/or displace adjacent viscera. Sublumbar lymph nodes, lumbar vertebrae, and the bony pelvis should be evaluated for evidence of metastases. A positive contrast cystourethrogram helps evaluate prostatic position in relation to the bladder, urethral size, mucosal contour, and prostatic reflux. Ultrasonography defines parenchymal homogeneity, contour, disease distribution, and urethral diameter. Cytology and biopsy specimens can be collected with ultrasound guidance. A bone scan and thoracic radiographs may help stage prostatic neoplasia. Occasionally, radiography may help evaluate os penis fractures and urethral extension of disease. Ultrasonography may be used to evaluate scrotal swelling and detect testicular abnormalities including cryptorchidism, testicular torsion, and neoplasia. The normal testicular architecture is coarse but homogeneous, with the mediastinum testis represented as a central hyperechoic band. The epididymis is anechoic to hypoechoic, relative to the testicular parenchyma.

Other tests. Evaluating urinary incontinence with a cystometrogram and urethral pressure profile is rarely helpful.

ANESTHESIA

General anesthesia is recommended for elective surgeries involving the reproductive tract. Careful preoperative screening of animals undergoing elective surgery is important; anesthetic complications in apparently healthy animals may arise because of uncorrected hydration or electrolyte or acid-base abnormalities. Anesthetic equipment that does not function correctly may also result in anesthetic morbidity or mortality. Numerous anesthetic protocols may be used for elective surgery in healthy animals; suggested anesthetic

BOX 26-3

Selected Anesthetic Protocols for Elective Surgery in Healthy Animals Older Than 6 Months of Age

Dogs

Premedication

Atropine (0.02–0.04 mg/kg SC or IM) or glycopyrrolate (0.005–0.011 mg/kg SC, IM) plus acepromazine (0.05 mg/kg SC or IM; not to exceed 1 mg) and butorphanol* (0.2–0.4 mg/kg SC, IM)

Induction

Thiopental (10–12 mg/kg) or propofol (2.5–8 mg/kg) administered IV to effect, or diazepam (0.27 mg/kg IM) plus ketamine (5.5 mg/kg IM)

Maintenance

Isoflurane or sevoflurane

Cats

Premedication

Atropine (0.02–0.04 mg/kg SC or IM) or glycopyrrolate (0.005–0.011 mg/kg SC, IM) plus ketamine (5 mg/kg IM) and butorphanol (0.2–0.4 mg/kg SC, IM)

Induction

Diazepam (0.27 mg/kg) plus ketamine (5.5 mg/kg) combined and administered IV to effect or thiopental (10–12 mg/kg) administered IV to effect or propofol (2.5–8 mg/kg) IV to effect or mask or chamber induction

Maintenance

Isoflurane or sevoflurane

SC, Subcutaneous; *IM,* intramuscular; *IV,* intravenous.
*Other opioids may be substituted for butorphanol (see text).

protocols are provided in Box 26-3. Atropine or glycopyrrolate may prevent bradycardia induced by visceral manipulation. Opioid premedicants (e.g., butorphanol, hydromorphone, and buprenorphine) may also provide preoperative and postoperative analgesia. Ketamine provides poor visceral analgesia and should not be used alone for surgical procedures. During abdominal surgery, water evaporates from exposed viscera at an increased rate; therefore fluid administration must be increased to replace this loss. Body heat loss due to vasodilation and visceral exposure causes hypothermia, which reduces the anesthetic requirement. Be careful to maintain body temperature during surgery, and rewarm the patient postoperatively.

Neutering has traditionally been recommended at 5 to 7 months of age. Early neutering (i.e., 6 to 16 weeks) produces good results if precautions are taken to prevent hypoglycemia, hypothermia, and hemorrhage. Animals less than 6 months of age should be premedicated with an anticholinergic. If tranquilization is necessary in dogs in addition to analgesia, hydromorphone should be used but acepromazine avoided. Butorphanol may be used as a premedicant in young cats, but it provides little sedation. Mask or chamber

TABLE 26-5

Epidural Anesthesia in Dogs

DRUG	DOSE	ONSET OF ACTION	DURATION OF ACTION
Lidocaine 2%*	1 ml/3.4 kg (T5) 1 ml/4.5 kg (T13–L1)†	10 min	1 to 1.5 hr
Bupivacaine 0.25% or 0.5%* (preservative free)	1 ml/4.5 kg	20 to 30 min	4.5 to 6 hr
Fentanyl	0.001 mg/kg	4 to 10 min	6 hr
Hydromorphone	0.03–0.04 mg/kg	15 min	10 hr
Morphine (preservative free)	0.1 mg/kg‡	23 min to 1 hr	20 hr
Buprenorphine	0.005 mg/kg	30 min	12 to 18 hr

*Avoid head-down position after epidural.
†A block to T1 leads to intercostal nerve paralysis; a block to C7–C5 leads to phrenic nerve paralysis.
‡The dose for epidural morphine in cats is 0.1 mg/kg.

inductions may be useful for fractious animals. Depending on the animal's tractability, reduced dosages of thiopental or propofol—or a combination of diazepam and ketamine—may be used for intravenous induction. Isoflurane or sevoflurane is preferred for maintenance of anesthesia.

If there are no contraindications (e.g., sepsis, bleeding diatheses, or hypovolemia [for epidurals using local anesthetics]), epidurals may be used in dogs and cats to supplement general anesthetic (Table 26-5). Epidural anesthesia alone is rarely sufficient for surgery in dogs and is impractical in domestic cats. If general anesthesia is not used, heavy sedation (i.e., an opioid plus a benzodiazepine) is necessary. Epidural doses should be decreased if a spinal has been inadvertently performed, the patient is pregnant or obese, or there are space-occupying vertebral canal lesions. Opioids may be more useful than local anesthetic drugs in epidurals because opioids cause sensory loss without motor block, and they do not promote hypotension. Because local anesthetics in epidurals may cause hypotension, dehydration should be corrected before performing the procedure.

Patients requiring cesarean section are often greater anesthetic risks because of hypovolemia, hypoglycemia, hypocalcemia, and/or toxemia. A distended uterus may decrease tidal volume. Drugs that depress the mother also depress the fetus. The rate of placental transfer is directly related to lipid solubility and concentration of an un-ionized drug. Anesthetic time should be kept to a minimum, and return to consciousness should be rapid. Ideally, inhalation agents should be used only after the neonates are removed and at minimal concentrations. Nitrous oxide crosses the placental barrier, but lower levels are found in the fetus than in the mother. Nitrous oxide may also promote hypoxemia. Epidural anesthesia is safe for the fetus, but must be used with other drugs and may induce maternal hypovolemia (see previous discussion). Before making the skin incision, a lidocaine line block may be used in cats (at reduced dosages) and dogs. Suggested anesthetic protocols for cesarean sec-

tion are provided in Box 26-4. See pp. 718-720 for techniques for cesarean section and neonate care.

ANTIBIOTICS

Perioperative antibiotics are not necessary for elective OHE or castration. Antibiotic choice should be based on culture and susceptibility or on expected pathogens in patients with pyometra, metritis, or bacterial prostatitis. Until culture results are available, antibiotics used to treat pyometra should be efficacious against *Escherichia coli* because this is the most common pathogen. Aminoglycosides are nephrotoxic and should be avoided when possible because of the renal dysfunction seen in pyometra. Choice of prophylactic antibiotics for surgery involving tumors or trauma depends on the patient's condition and surgeon's preference (see Chapter 10).

Antibiotic selection for prostatic diseases should be based on culture results and expected blood-prostate barrier penetration. Antibiotics should be lipid-soluble (usually nonionized), nonprotein bound, and have a high pKa (degree of drug ionization; high pKa = more basic). Those with a high degree of lipid solubility are best at crossing the blood-prostate barrier. Antibiotics with a high pKa are less ionized at physiologic conditions and concentrate in the prostate. Prostatic infections produce acidic prostatic fluid that helps trap antibiotics in the fluid. Basic antibiotics that concentrate in the prostate include erythromycin, clindamycin, and trimethoprim (Box 26-5). Enrofloxacin and doxycycline achieve high prostatic fluid concentrations and are effective against some resistant gram-negative urogenital pathogens.

SURGICAL ANATOMY
Female Reproductive Tract

The female reproductive tract includes the ovaries, oviduct, uterus, vagina, vulva, and mammary glands. The ovaries are located within a thin-walled peritoneal sac; the ovarian bursa is located just caudal to the pole of each kidney. The uterine tube or oviduct courses through the wall of the ovarian bursa.

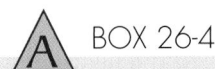 BOX 26-4

Selected Anesthetic Protocols for Cesarean Section*

General Principles

1. Place an IV catheter
2. Immediately begin volume replacement with IV crystalloids (10–20 ml/kg)
3. Preoxygenate before induction

Dogs

Premedication

Glycopyrrolate (0.005–0.011 mg/kg SC, IM)

Induction

Hydromorphone (0.05–0.2 mg/kg IV or IM) or butorphanol (0.2–0.4 mg/kg IV) plus diazepam (0.2 mg/kg IV) *and* etomidate (0.5–1.5 mg/kg IV) or propofol (4–6 mg/kg IV). Alternatively, small doses of thiopental may be used.

Maintenance

Isoflurane or sevoflurane

Cats

Premedication

Glycopyrrolate (0.005–0.011 mg/kg SC, IM) and butorphanol (0.2–0.4 mg/kg SC, IM)

Induction

Diazepam (0.2 mg/kg IV) followed by etomidate (0.5–1.5 mg/kg IV) or propofol (4–6 mg/kg IV). Alternately, a combination of diazepam (0.27 mg/kg) plus ketamine (5.5 mg/kg) may be administered IV to effect or reduced doses of thiopental may be used.

Maintenance

Isoflurane or sevoflurane

IV, Intravenous; *SC*, subcutaneous; *IM*, intramuscular.
*Addition of a lidocaine line block (see text) will facilitate anesthetic maintenance at a lower anesthetic concentration.

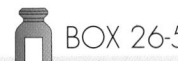 BOX 26-5

Antibiotics for Treatment of Reproductive Disorders

Cefazolin (Ancef, Kefzol)
22 mg/kg IV, IM, tid

Cefoxitin (Mefoxin)
30 mg/kg IV, tid

Amoxicillin plus Clavulanate (Clavamax)
Dogs: 12.5–25 mg/kg PO, bid
Cats: 62.5 mg/cat PO, bid

Ampicillin
22 mg/kg IV, IM, or SC, tid to qid

Erythromycin
10–20 mg/kg PO, bid to tid

Clindamycin (Antirobe)
11–22 mg/kg PO, bid to tid

Doxycycline (Vibramycin)
5 mg/kg PO, bid

Enrofloxacin (Baytril)
7–20 mg/kg PO or IV, qd (given dilute and slowly over 30 minutes if given IV)

Carbenicillin (Geocillin)*
22–33 mg/kg PO, tid for UTI
22–33 mg/kg IV, tid to qid for systemic infections

IV, Intravenous; *IM*, intramuscular; *tid*, three times a day; *qid*, four times a day; *PO*, oral; *bid*, twice a day; *SC*, subcutaneous; *qd*, once a day; *UTI*, urinary tract infection.
*The only indication for oral carbenicillin is urinary tract infection. If the infection involves soft tissue parenchyma, a different antibiotic should be used.

The right ovary lies further cranially than the left. The right ovary lies dorsal to the descending duodenum, and the left ovary lies dorsal to the descending colon and lateral to the spleen. Medial retraction of the mesoduodenum or mesocolon exposes the ovary on each side. Each ovary is attached by the proper ligament to the uterine horn and via the suspensory ligament to the transversalis fascia medial to the last one or two ribs. The ovarian pedicle (mesovarium) includes the suspensory ligament with its artery and vein, ovarian artery and vein, and variable amounts of fat and connective tissue. Canine ovarian pedicles contain more fat than feline ovarian pedicles, making it more difficult to visualize the vasculature. The ovarian vessels take a tortuous path within the pedicle. Ovarian arteries originate from the aorta. The left ovarian vein drains into the left renal vein; the right vein drains into the caudal vena cava. The suspensory ligament is a tough, whitish band of tissue that diverges as it travels from the ovary to attach to the last two ribs. The broad ligament (mesometrium) is the peritoneal fold that suspends the uterus.

The round ligament travels in the free edge of the broad ligament from the ovary through the inguinal canal with the vaginal process. The uterus has a short body and long narrow horns. The uterine arteries and veins supply blood to the uterus. The cervix is the constricted caudal part of the uterus and is thicker than the uterine body and vagina. It is oriented in a nearly vertical position with the uterine opening dorsally. The vagina is long and connects with the vaginal vestibule at the urethral entrance. The clitoris is broad, flat, vascular, infiltrated with fat, and lies on the floor of the vestibule near the vulva. The clitoral fossa is a depression on the floor of the vestibule that is sometimes mistaken for the urethral orifice. The vulva is the external opening of the genital tract. The vulvar lips are thick and form a pointed commissure. The constrictor vulvae and constrictor vestibule muscles encircle the vulva and vestibule. See p. 732 for a description of the anatomy of the mammary glands.

NOTE: If the broad ligament contains an excessive amount of fat, you may need to ligate the vessels in it.

Male Reproductive Tract

The major components of the male genital tract are the testicles, penis, and prostate. The prostate gland completely surrounds the neck of the bladder and beginning of the urethra. In dogs less than 4 years of age, the prostate is usually located in the pelvic cavity at the brim of the pubis. The prostate begins to enlarge at puberty, becoming intraabdominal in location. It varies greatly in size at maturity. The prostate is encapsulated by fibromuscular tissue and is bilobate with a prominent middorsal sulcus. The dorsal sulcus continues into the prostatic parenchyma as the median septum. The ventrolateral surfaces of the prostate are covered by a fat pad. The parenchyma is lobulated with tubuloalveolar glands that empty through small ducts (12 to 20) into the prostatic urethra. The ductus deferens enters the craniodorsal surface of the prostate and courses caudoventrally to enter the urethra at the colliculus seminalis. The blood and nerve supply (pelvic and hypogastric nerves) are located in the lateral pedicles (peritoneal reflection), entering the prostate at the 10 o'clock and 2 o'clock positions when viewed in a transverse plane. The prostatic arteries originate from the urogenital artery (branch of internal iliac artery) and supply branches to the ductus deferens, urethra, urinary bladder, ureters, and rectum. The hypogastric (sympathetic) and pelvic (parasympathetic) nerves follow the vasculature and are essential for micturition and continence (Fig. 26-1). The pudendal nerve sends branches along the ventral surface of the urethra extending to the bladder neck. The pudendal nerve innervates the skeletal muscle of the external urethral sphincter. The iliac lymph nodes drain the prostate. In cats, bulbourethral glands are found caudal to the prostate at the ischial arch.

> NOTE: Scottish terriers generally have larger prostates than other similarly sized breeds.

The penis has a root, body, and glans. The root of the penis is formed by the right and left crura, which originate from the ischiatic tuberosity. Each crus is composed of corpus cavernosum penis surrounded by tunica albuginea. The two corpora extend side by side, separated by a median septum, along the length of the penile body to the os penis in the glans penis. The distal end of the penis or glans penis is covered by the prepuce, a mucosa-lined fold of integument. The distal end of the dog's penis is directed cranially and located ventral to the abdominal wall. The distal end of the cat's penis is directed caudal and ventral in the perineum. The glans of the feline penis is covered with caudally directed cornified spines, which are more prominent in intact males and regress within 6 weeks of castration. The feline os penis is very small, whereas in dogs it is a long, grooved, rough bone. The urethra travels through the ventral groove in the os penis and penis. The corpus spongiosum surrounds the urethra. The ischiocavernosus muscle arises from the ischiatic tuberosity and inserts on the crus. The retractor penis muscles originate from the ventral surface of the sacrum or the first two caudal vertebrae and extend distally on the ventral surface of the penis to insert at the level of the glans. The retractor and external anal sphincter muscles share muscle fibers. The bulbospongiosus muscle bulges between the ischiocavernosus muscles ventral to the external anal sphincter.

> NOTE: Surgery of the penis is often associated with significant hemorrhage because of the vascular nature of the cavernosus tissue.

The scrotum is located between the inguinal region and anus. In dogs, scrotal skin is thin and sparsely haired. The feline scrotum is more dorsal and densely haired than the canine scrotum. The scrotum is a membranous pouch with a midline septum that houses the testes, epididymis, and distal spermatic cords. The testis, epididymis, ductus deferens, and associated vessels and nerves are covered by visceral and parietal vaginal tunic and spermatic fascia. The testes are relatively small and ovoid. The epididymis is

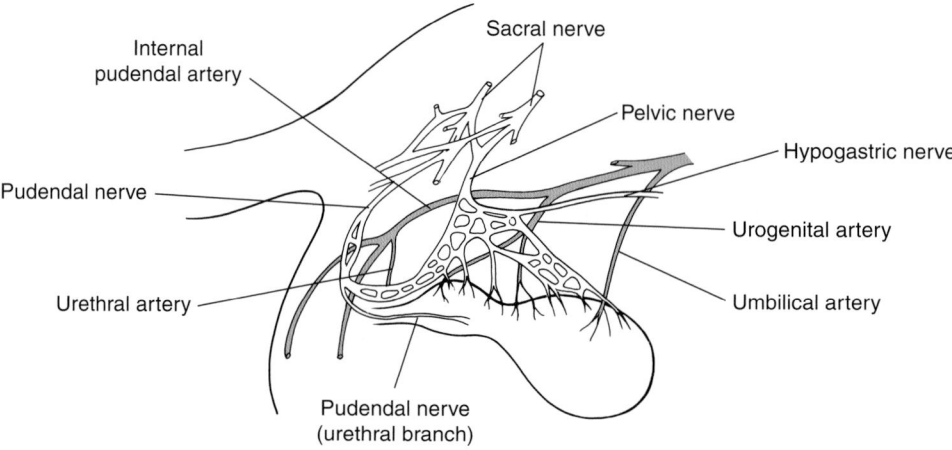

FIG. 26-1
Innervation to the prostate and bladder.

large, convoluted, and attached to the lateral side of the testis. The head of the epididymis communicates with the testis, and the caudal extremity or tail is continuous with the ductus deferens. The tail is attached to the testis by the proper ligament of the testis. The ligament of the tail of the epididymis attaches the epididymis to the vaginal tunic and the spermatic fascia. The ductus deferens loops around the ureter as it travels from the inguinal ring, enters the dorsal prostate, and terminates in the prostatic urethra. The ureter is dorsal to the ductus deferens. The spermatic cord begins at the inguinal ring where the testicular artery, testicular veins (pampiniform plexus), lymphatics, testicular autonomic nerve plexus, ductus deferens and its artery and vein, smooth muscle, and visceral layer of the vaginal tunic come together. The cremaster muscle travels along the external surface of the parietal tunic. The cremaster is a thin, flat extension of the internal abdominal oblique muscle.

> NOTE: You may be able to palpate the epididymis in dogs with epididymitis.

SURGICAL TECHNIQUE

Before elective surgeries, food should be withheld from adults for 12 to 18 hours and from pediatric patients for 4 to 8 hours. The ventral abdomen should be clipped and aseptically prepared for any procedure requiring celiotomy. The urinary bladder should be expressed if the patient has not voided immediately before induction. In dogs, the pre-scrotal area should be clipped and prepared for aseptic surgery; however, trauma to the scrotum (i.e., with clippers, antiseptic soaps, or solutions) must be avoided. Canine scrotal skin is sensitive and swells with minimal trauma or irritation. In cats, hair can be plucked or pulled from the scrotum. The prepuce or vestibule should be flushed with dilute antiseptic solutions before procedures involving these areas. For some procedures that involve the perineum, prostate, or penis, placement of a urethral catheter helps identify the urethra.

> NOTE: Many techniques are used for ovariohysterectomy and castration; however, the goals are the same—to remove the ovaries, in addition to the uterine horns and body, or testes, with secure ligature placement.

Pediatric tissues are more fragile than adult tissues and must be handled gently. In young animals, 3-0 to 5-0 ligatures should be used. Early neutering delays growth plate closure by an average of 8 to 9 weeks, resulting in increased bone length in male and female dogs and cats. Infantile vulva and mammary glands or penis, prepuce, and os penis persist following early neutering. Bitches are at a greater risk to develop urinary incontinence if OHE is performed before

3 months of age (Box 26-6). Early neutering affects weight gain, daily food consumption, and activity level to the same degree as neutering after puberty.

Ovariohysterectomy

The most common reason to perform OHE is to prevent estrus and unwanted offspring. Alternative methods of inhibiting reproduction are listed in Box 26-7. Other reasons for OHE include prevention of mammary tumors or congenital anomalies; prevention and treatment of pyometra, metritis, neoplasia (i.e., ovarian, uterine, or vaginal), cysts (Fig. 26-2 and 26-3), trauma, uterine torsion, uterine pro-

BOX 26-6

Early-Age Gonadectomy Expectations

Early gonadectomy is safe
Cat's and male dog's gonadectomy should not be delayed past 5 months of age because of concerns about long-term health or behavior
Female dogs are at greater risk of urinary incontinence if OHE is performed before 3 months of age
Is associated with increased bone length
Penis, prepuce, and vulva may appear small and infantile if neutered at 6 to 8 weeks
Not associated with increased obesity, lower urinary tract disease, long-bone fractures, arthritis, immune suppression, or small urethra

Pros

After 7 weeks, anesthesia recovery is more rapid than in older animals
Fewer perioperative complications are observed
Few adverse medical consequences

Dogs

Decreased: obesity, separation anxiety, escaping behaviors, inappropriate escaping behaviors when frightened, relinquishment of owners
• Males: decreased roaming

Cats

Decreased: asthma, gingivitis, and hyperactivity
• ± Lower urinary tract disease (varying reports)
• Males: decreased occurrence of abscesses, aggression toward veterinarians, sexual behaviors, and urine spraying

Cons

Dogs

Increased: hip dysplasia, noise phobias, and sexual behaviors
• Females: increased urinary incontinence, therefore, delay OHE until after 3 mos
Increased cystitis

Cats

Increased: shyness around strangers
• Males: may tend to hide more

OHE, Ovariohysterectomy.

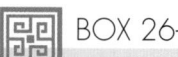

BOX 26-7

Options for Pregnancy Prevention or Termination

Surgical Prevention or Termination

Ovariohysterectomy
Ovariectomy
Castration (prevention only)

Medical Prevention

Chlormadinone acetate 10 mg/kg SC implant, every 2 years*

Medical Termination During Preossification Period (days 20 to 22 through 40 to 42 after LH peak)†:

$PGF_{2\alpha}$ 0.1–0.25mg/kg SC, bid for 4 to 6 days‡
Cloprostenol 1–2.5 μg/kg SC, qd to q48h for 5 days‡§
Cabergoline 5 μg/kg PO, qd for 5 days plus cloprostenol 1 μg/kg SC, q 48h
Bromocriptine 30 μg/kg PO, tid plus two doses cloprostenol 1 μg/kg SC on days 28 and 32 after LH peak
Bromocriptine 10 μg/kg PO, tid plus $PGF_{2\alpha}$ 100 μg/kg SC tid
Aglepristone 10 mg/kg SC, qd for 2 days (only available in Europe)

Medical Termination During Preattachment Period (fertilization to days 20 to 22 after LH peak):

Aglepristone 10 mg/kg SC, qd for 2 days (available in some European countries)
Estradiol benzoate 5–10 μg/kg (max. 1 mg) SC, divided into 2 to 3 injections given q 48h, begin 2 to 4 days after mating‖
Cloprostenol 1–2.5 μg/kg SC, bid to qid for 5 days beginning of day 5 of diestrus‡§
Natural $PGF_{2\alpha}$ 10–250 μg/kg bid to qid, days 5 to 11 of diestrus‡

SC, Subcutaneous; *LH,* luteinizing hormone; *$PGF_{2\alpha}$,* prostaglandin $F_{2\alpha}$; *bid,* twice a day; *qd,* once a day; *PO,* oral; *tid,* three times a day.
*Effectively prevents estrus, but inhibits fertility after implant removal; results in uterine cystic glandular hyperplasia, pyometra, and hydrometra.
†Recommended techniques. Ideally begin drugs on day 25 after the LH peak or 20 to 28 days after first mating. Monitor abortion by ultrasound or by measuring plasma progesterone level. Progesterone levels less than 1–2 ng/ml for 2 consecutive days indicate pregnancy termination.
‡Side effects may include excessive salivation, vomiting, defecation, urination, and papillary dilation followed by constriction.
§Estrumate® (cloprostenol 250 μg/ml; Schering-Plough Animal Health) must be diluted in saline at a ratio of 1 ml to 9 ml saline solution. Do not reuse solution.
‖Not recommended due to dangerous side effects of medullary aplasia, metritis, pyometra, ovarian cysts, estrus-like behavior, and irreversible infertility. Other estrogens are more potent and toxic.

lapse, subinvolution of placental sites, vaginal prolapse, and vaginal hyperplasia; and control of some endocrine abnormalities (i.e., diabetes and epilepsy) and dermatoses (e.g., generalized demodex). Many technical variations of OHE have been described, including flank and laparoscopic approaches and the use of stapling equipment, ultrasonic scalpel, vessel sealing devices, transfixation ligatures, or Miller's knots (Fig. 26-4). Only one technique is described here.

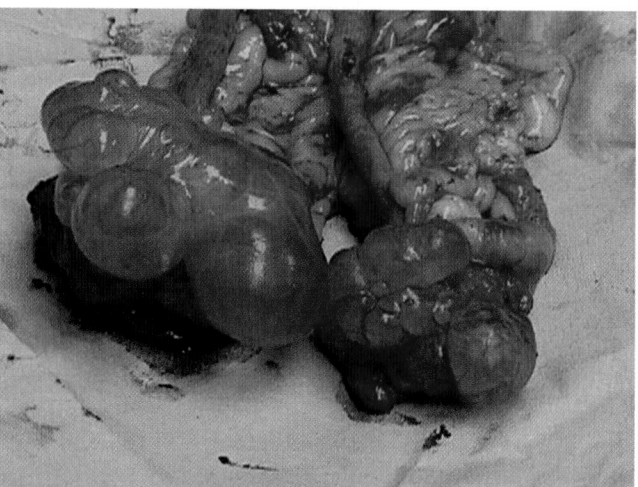

FIG. 26-2
These ovarian cysts were identified during an elective OHE.

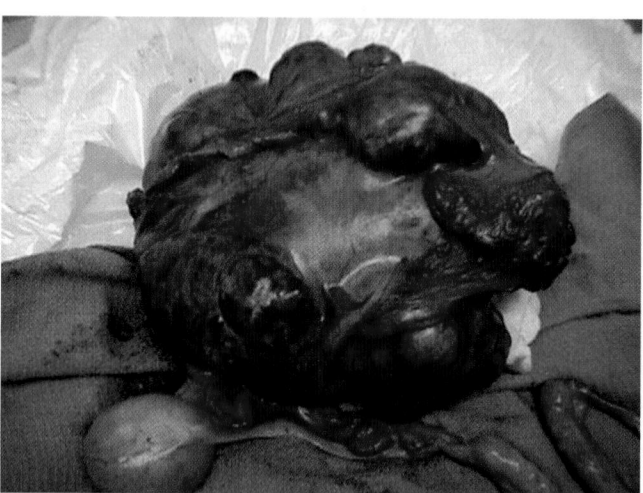

FIG. 26-3
Appearance of a large ovarian cystadenocarcinoma.

> **NOTE:** In dogs, make the incision immediately caudal to the umbilicus to facilitate ligation of the ovarian pedicles. Make the incision more caudal in cats to facilitate ligation of the uterine body.

Clip and surgically prepare the ventral abdomen from the xiphoid to the pubis. Identify the umbilicus and visually divide the caudal abdomen into thirds. In dogs, make the incision just caudal to the umbilicus in the cranial third of the caudal abdomen. More caudal incisions make it difficult to exteriorize canine ovaries. In deep-chested dogs or in those with an enlarged uterus, extend the incision cranially or caudally to allow exteriorization of the tract without

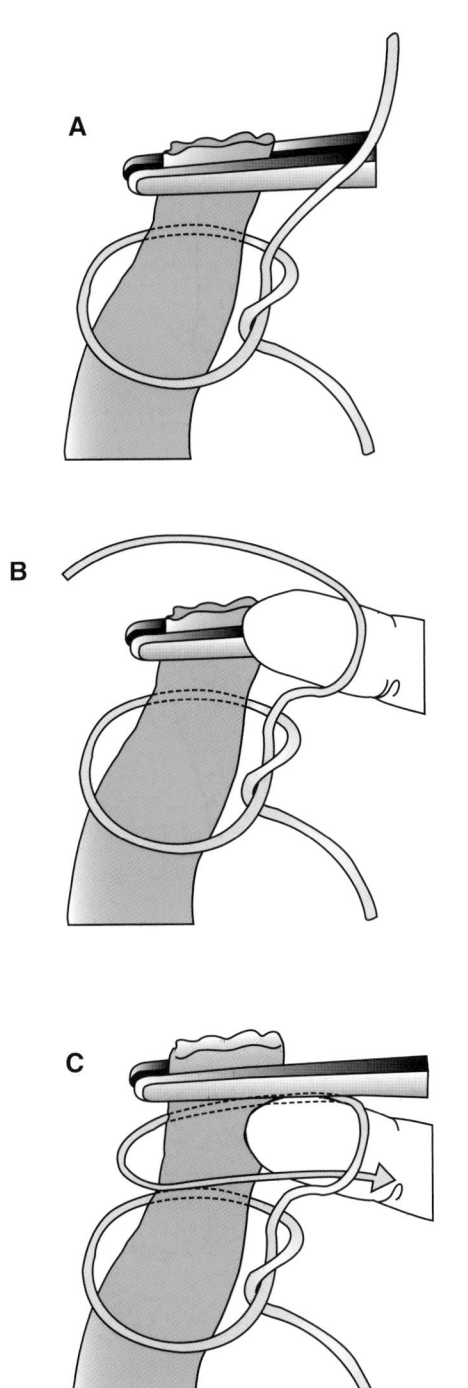

FIG. 26-4
A Miller's knot or clove hitch is preferred by some surgeons to occlude the pedicles. **A,** Place a ligature on the pedicle and secure with a half hitch. Have one end of the suture be relatively short and the other long. **B,** Position your finger between the long end of the suture and the ligature (palm up). Grab the long end of the suture with a needle holder and bring it around the pedicle a second time. **C,** Insert the end through the space reserved by your finger. Add two square knots to finish the ligature.

excessive traction. In prepubertal puppies, making the incision in the middle third of the caudal abdomen facilitates uterine body ligation. In cats, the body of the uterus is more caudal and difficult to exteriorize; therefore make the incision in the middle third of the caudal abdomen. Make a 4- to 8-cm incision through skin and subcutaneous tissue to expose the linea alba. Grasp the linea alba or ventral rectus sheath, tent it outward, and make a stab incision into the abdominal cavity. Extend the linea incision cranial and caudal to the stab with Mayo scissors. Elevate the left abdominal wall by grasping the linea or external rectus sheath with thumb forceps. Slide the ovariectomy hook (e.g., Covault or Snook) with the hook against the abdominal wall, 2 to 3 cm caudal to the kidney (Fig. 26-5, A). Turn the hook medially to ensnare the uterine horn, broad ligament, or round ligament, and gently elevate it from the abdomen. Anatomically confirm the identification of the uterine horn by following it to either the uterine bifurcation or ovary. If the uterine horn cannot be located with the hook, retroflex the bladder through the incision and locate the uterine body and horns between the colon and bladder. With caudal and medial traction on the uterine horn, identify the suspensory ligament by palpation as the taut fibrous band at the proximal edge of the ovarian pedicle (Fig. 26-5, B). Stretch or break the suspensory ligament near the kidney without tearing the ovarian vessels, to allow exteriorization of the ovary. To achieve this, use the index finger to apply caudolateral traction on the suspensory ligament while maintaining caudomedial traction on the uterine horn (Fig. 26-5, C).

Make a hole in the broad ligament caudal to the ovarian pedicle. Place one or two Rochester-Carmalt forceps across the ovarian pedicle proximal (deep) to the ovary and one across the proper ligament of the ovary (Fig. 26-5, D).

The proximal (deep) clamp serves as a groove for the ligature, the middle clamp holds the pedicle for ligation, and the distal clamp prevents backflow of blood after transection. When using two clamps, the ovarian pedicle clamp serves both to hold the pedicle and to make a groove for the ligature.

Place a figure-eight ligature proximal to (below) the ovarian pedicle clamps (Fig. 26-5, E). Choose an absorbable suture material for ligatures (i.e., 2-0 or 3-0 chromic catgut, polydioxanone, polyglyconate, poliglecaprone 25, or polyglactin 910). Begin by directing the blunt end of the needle through the middle of the pedicle, loop the suture around one side of the pedicle, then redirect the needle through the original hole from the same direction and loop the ligature around the other half of the pedicle. Securely tie the ligature. Remove one clamp or "flash" a single clamp while tightening the ligature to allow pedicle compression. Place a second circumferential ligature proximal to (below) the first to control hemorrhage that may occur from puncturing a vessel as the needle is passed through the pedicle.

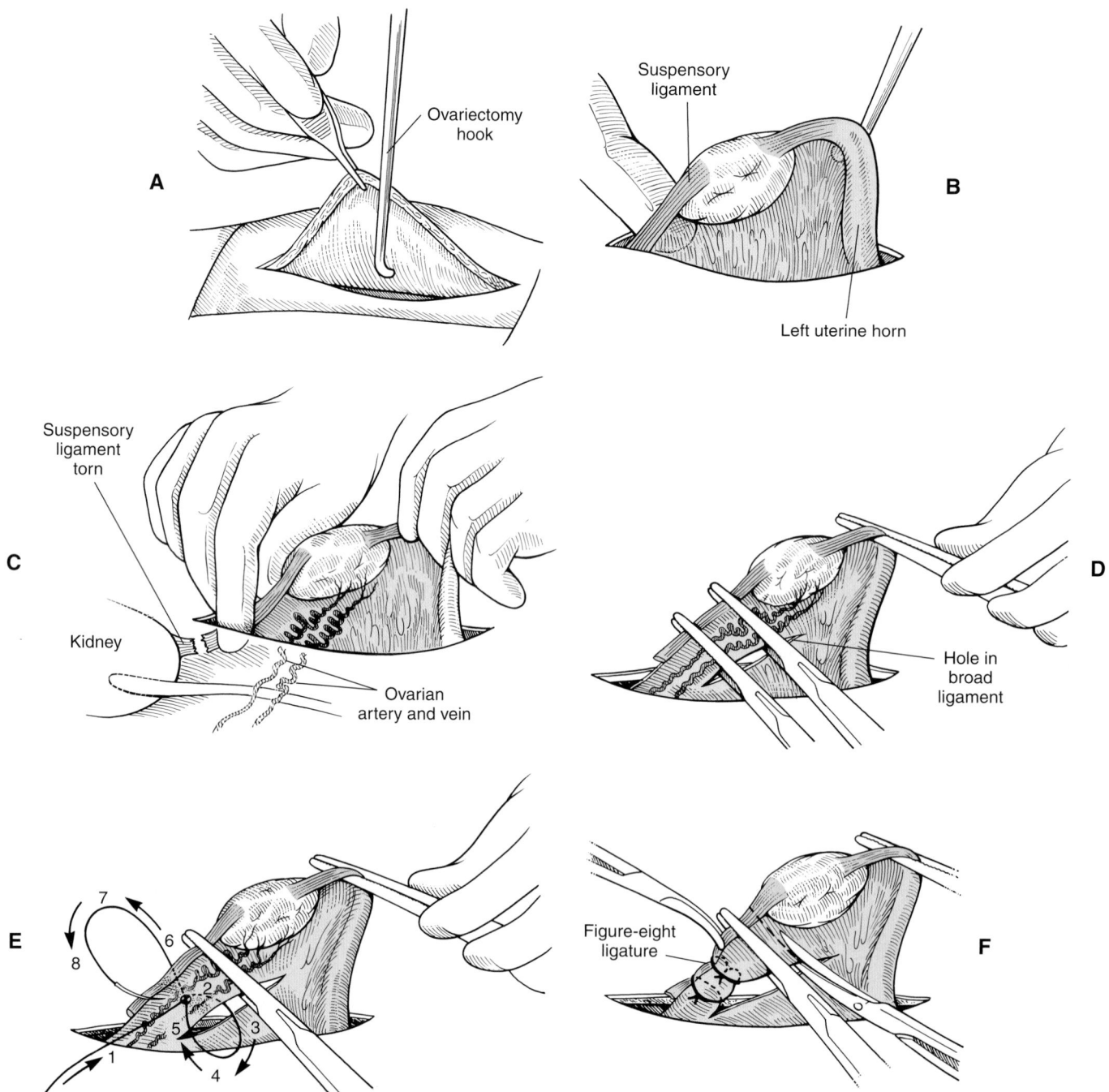

FIG. 26-5

A, For ovariohysterectomy, elevate the abdominal wall with thumb forceps and slide the ovariectomy hook against the abdominal wall, 2 to 3 cm caudal to the kidney. **B,** Exteriorize the uterine horn with the hook and identify the suspensory ligament at the cranial edge of the ovarian pedicle. **C,** Stretch or tear the suspensory ligament to allow exteriorization of the ovary using the index finger to apply caudolateral traction on the suspensory ligament while maintaining caudomedial traction on the uterine horn. **D,** Place two Carmalt forceps across the ovarian pedicle proximal to the ovary and one across the proper ligament (or place three forceps proximal to the ovary). Remove the most proximal clamp and place a figure-eight ligature at this site. **E,** Direct the blunt end of the needle through the middle of the pedicle (*1* to *2*), loop the suture around one side of the pedicle (*3* to *4*), then redirect the needle through the original hole from the same direction (*5* to *6*), and loop the ligature around the other half of the pedicle (*7* to *8*). Securely tie the ligature (*1* and *8*). **F,** Place a circumferential ligature proximal to the first ligature, then place a hemostat on the suspensory ligament near the ovary. Transect the ovarian pedicle distal to the clamp across the ovarian pedicle.

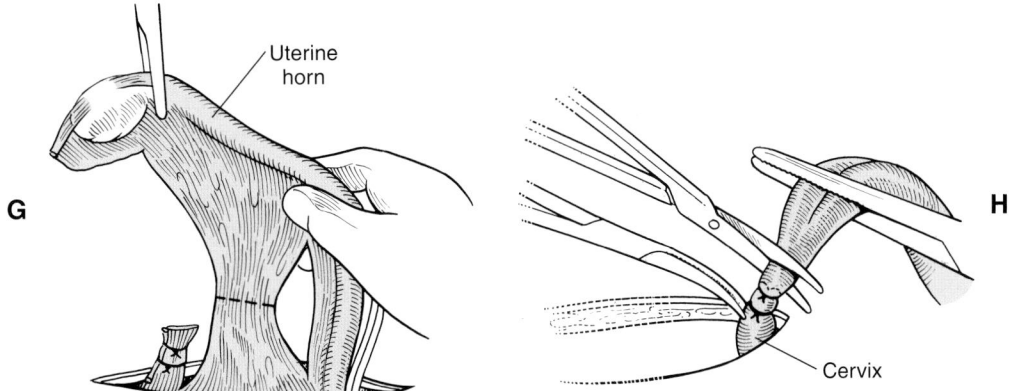

FIG. 26-5, cont'd
G, Separate the broad ligament from the uterine horn. Clamp and ligate the broad ligament *(dashed line)* if it appears vascular. **H,** To ligate the uterus, place a figure-eight suture through the uterine body near the cervix. Place a second circumferential ligature closer to the cervix, place a Carmalt forceps distal to the ligatures, and transect between the Carmalt forceps and ligatures. Inspect the uterine stump for hemorrhage (use a mosquito hemostat attached to the uterine wall to prevent retraction of the uterus into the abdomen).

Some surgeons prefer to place the circumferential ligature or Miller's knot (see Fig. 26-4) before the transfixing ligature to eliminate hemorrhage if a vessel is punctured during transfixation.

Place a mosquito hemostat on the suspensory ligament near the ovary (Fig. 26-5, F). Transect the ovarian pedicle between the Carmalt and ovary. Open the ovarian bursa and examine the ovary to be certain that it has been removed in its entirety. Remove the Carmalt from the ovarian pedicle and observe for hemorrhage. Replace the Carmalt and religate the pedicle if hemorrhage is noted.

Trace the uterine horn to the uterine body. Grasp the other uterine horn, and follow it to the opposite ovary. Place clamps and ligatures as just described. Make a window in the broad ligament adjacent to the uterine body and uterine artery and vein. Place a Carmalt across the broad ligament on each side and transect (Fig. 26-5, G). Apply a ligature around the broad ligament if the patient is in estrus or pregnant, or if the broad ligament is heavily infiltrated with vessels or fat. Apply cranial traction on the uterus, and ligate the uterine body cranial to the cervix.

Place a figure-eight suture through the body using the point of the needle and encircling the uterine vessels on each side. Place a circumferential ligature nearer the cervix (Fig. 26-5, H). Place a Carmalt across the uterine body cranial to the ligatures. Grasp the uterine wall with forceps or mosquito hemostats cranial to the ligatures. Transect the uterine body, and observe for hemorrhage. Religate if hemorrhage is observed.

Some surgeons place one to three Carmalts across the uterine body before ligation. In cats, clamps may cut rather than crush a friable or engorged uterus and cause transection before ligature placement. An alternative to ligatures is to use an ultrasonic scalpel, vascular sealer, or staples.

Replace the uterine stump into the abdomen before releasing the hemostats or forceps. Close the abdominal wall in three layers (fascia/linea alba, subcutaneous tissue, and skin).

Laparoscopic-Assisted Ovariohysterectomy

Different techniques and modifications of each technique have been reported. Two previously published techniques will be described here. The reader is referred to the references for additional detail.

Briefly, with the patient in dorsal recumbency, place an observation port at the umbilicus, and place two operating ports in the inguinal folds, on each side of the midline. Use Babcock forceps in the left operating port to retract the intestines medially, and grasp the ligament of the right ovary with forceps placed through the right operating port and lift so that traction is placed on the suspensory ligament. Transect this ligament, the broad ligament of the uterus, and the ovarian vascular pedicle after first applying coagulation via electrocautery or a suture. Continue the transection to the uterus, and transect the uterus and uterine arteries from left to right. Cut the uterus and seal it 1 cm proximal to the cervix, then coagulate and cut the right uterine artery. Lift the left uterine horn so that it can be visualized all the way to the ovary. Coagulate the ligament and pedicles, and transect them in reverse order as was done for the right side. Once the uterus and ovaries have been cut from all attachments, enlarge the left operating port as necessary to allow the uterus and ovaries to be withdrawn through this incision.

Observe the ovarian pedicles and uterine stump for several minutes, and if no excess bleeding is seen, remove the trocars and close the incisions (Austin et al, 2003).

This technique has been modified (Devitt et al, 2005):

Briefly, rotate the dog to the right and left as necessary to make retraction of the intestines and exposure of the ovary easier. Grasp the left ovary and bring it to the body wall. Then, using transabdominal illumination and direct laparoscopic observation, direct a transabdominal suspension suture with a large taper needle percutaneously through the ovary and out the abdominal wall. Tie this suture, thus maintaining exposure of the vasculature of the ovary. If necessary, use several sutures on one ovary. Next, progressively cauterize the ligament and vasculature using bipolar grasping forceps. Transect both ovaries. Enlarge a caudal operating port, and exteriorize both uterine horns and the body of the uterus. Transect the body of the uterus and uterine arteries, and replace the uterine stump into the abdomen. Close the incisions.

Orchiectomy

Castration reduces overpopulation by inhibiting male fertility and decreases male aggressiveness, roaming, and undesirable urination behavior. It helps prevent androgen-related diseases, including prostatic diseases, perianal adenomas, and perineal hernias. Other indications for castration include congenital abnormalities, testicular or epididymal abnormalities, scrotal neoplasia, trauma or abscesses, inguinal-scrotal herniorrhaphy, scrotal urethrostomy, epilepsy control, and control of endocrine abnormalities.

Canine castration. Either a prescrotal or perineal approach may be used for castration. A prescrotal approach is most common and more easily performed. The testicles are more difficult to exteriorize with a perineal approach, but this may be selected to avoid repositioning and aseptically preparing a second surgical site when the patient is in a perineal position for another surgical procedure (e.g., perineal hernia repair). Scrotal incision(s) are sometimes used when castrating prepubertal puppies.

Open prescrotal castration. *Position the patient in dorsal recumbency. Verify the presence of both testicles in the scrotum. Clip and aseptically prepare the caudal abdomen and medial thighs. Avoid irritating the scrotum with clippers or antiseptics. Drape the surgical area to exclude the scrotum from the field. Apply pressure on the scrotum to advance one testicle as far as possible into the prescrotal area. Incise skin and subcutaneous tissue along the median raphe over the displaced testicle (Fig. 26-6, A). Continue the incision through spermatic fascia to exteriorize the testicle. Incise the parietal vaginal tunic over the testicle (Fig. 26-6, B). Do not incise the tunica albuginea because this would expose the testicular parenchyma. Place a hemostat across the vaginal tunic where it attaches to the epididymis. Digitally separate the ligament of the tail of the epididymis from the tunic while applying trac-*

tion with the hemostat on the tunic (Fig. 26-6, C). Further exteriorize the testicle by applying caudal and outward traction.

Identify the structures of the spermatic cord. Individually ligate the vascular cord and ductus deferens, then place an encircling ligature around both. Many surgeons ligate the ductus deferens and pampiniform plexus together. Use 2-0 or 3-0 absorbable suture (e.g., chromic catgut, polyglactin 910, polydioxanone, poliglecaprone 25, or polyglyconate) for ligatures. Alternatively, use hemostatic staples. Place a hemostat across the cord near the testicle. Grasp the ductus deferens with thumb forceps above the ligature, and transect both the ductus deferens and vascular cord between the hemostat and ligatures (Fig. 26-6, D). Inspect the cord for hemorrhage, and replace the cord within the tunic. Encircle the cremaster muscle and tunic with a ligature. Advance the second testicle into the incision, incise the fascial covering, and remove the testicle as described. Appose the incised dense fascia on either side of the penis with interrupted or continuous sutures. Close subcutaneous tissue with a continuous pattern. Appose skin with an intradermal, subcuticular, or simple interrupted suture pattern.

> NOTE: Although the risk of ligature slippage and loosening may be slightly greater with closed than open techniques, removal of the tunics may reduce postoperative swelling.

Closed prescrotal castration. "Closed" castration is performed similarly to the "open" technique just described, except that the parietal vaginal tunics are not incised.

Maximally exteriorize the spermatic cord by reflecting fat and fascia from the parietal tunic with a gauze sponge. Place traction on the testicle while the fibrous attachments between the spermatic cord tunic and scrotum are torn. Place mass ligatures (e.g., 2-0 or 3-0 absorbable) around the entire spermatic cord and tunics. Pass the needle through the cremaster muscle if a transfixation ligature is desired. Hemostatic staples may also be used.

Perineal castration. Perineal castration is performed using the same techniques as for an open prescrotal castration. It is more difficult to displace the testicles into a caudal incision than into a prescrotal incision. An "open" technique must be used.

Make a midline skin and subcutaneous tissue incision dorsal to the scrotum in the perineum ventral to the anus. Advance one testicle to the incision, and incise the spermatic fascia and tunic. Exteriorize the testicle, and ligate the spermatic cord as described for an open prescrotal castration.

Scrotal ablation. Scrotal ablation is necessary for neoplastic scrotal diseases and for castration performed in conjunction with scrotal urethrostomy in dogs and perineal urethrostomy in cats. Other indications include severe scro-

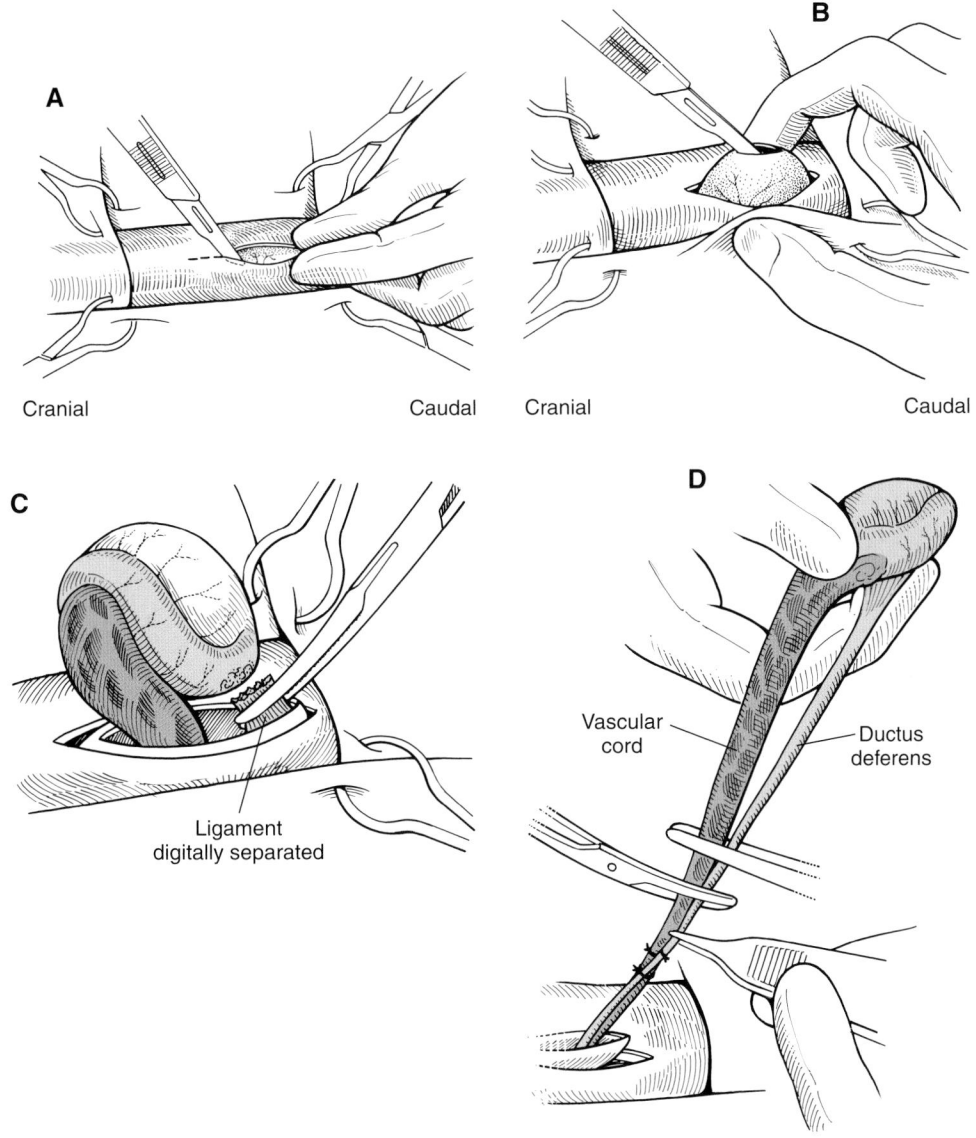

FIG. 26-6
A, To perform an open canine castration, advance one testicle into the prescrotal area by applying pressure over the scrotum. Make an incision over the testicle. **B,** Incise the spermatic fascia and parietal vaginal tunic. **C,** Place a hemostat across the tunic where it attaches to the epididymis and digitally separate the ligament of the tail of the epididymis from the tunic. **D,** Ligate the ductus deferens and vascular cord individually, and then encircle both with a proximal circumferential ligature. Apply a Carmalt forceps distal to the ligatures and transect between the clamp and ligatures.

tal trauma, abscesses, or ischemia. Scrotal ablation may improve the postcastration appearance of dogs if they have a pendulous scrotum. Surgical time is somewhat longer when scrotal ablation is performed.

Elevate the scrotum and testicles from the body wall. Make an elliptical skin incision at the base of the scrotum, being careful not to excise too much skin. Control hemorrhage with electrocoagulation, ligation, or pressure. Incise the vaginal tunics, and remove the testicles as described for open castration. Remove the scrotum after incising its median septum. Appose subcutaneous tissues with a simple continuous suture pattern (e.g., 3-0 absorbable suture). Appose skin edges with approximating interrupted sutures (e.g., 3-0 or 4-0 nonabsorbable suture).

Feline castration. Pluck hair from the scrotum rather than clipping (Fig. 26-7, *A*). In kittens less than 16 to 20

weeks of age, plucking scrotal hair may be difficult. Use clippers to gently remove scrotal hair in these animals.

Position the cat in dorsal or lateral recumbency with the hind legs pulled cranially. Mobilize a testicle in the scrotum by applying pressure with the thumb and index finger at the base of the scrotum. Make a 1-cm incision over each testicle at the end of the scrotum from cranial to caudal (Fig. 26-7, B). Incise the parietal vaginal tunic over the testicle and exteriorize the testicle. Digitally separate the attachment of the ligament of the tail of the epididymis to the vaginal tunic (Fig. 26-7, C). Double ligate the spermatic cord with absorbable suture (e.g., 3-0 chromic catgut) or hemoclips, or remove the ductus deferens from the testicle and tie it with the vessels (see p. 716). Alternatively, use a figure-eight knot (see p. 716). Transect the cord, inspect for bleeding, and replace it within the tunic. Excise the second testicle in a similar fashion. Resect any tags of

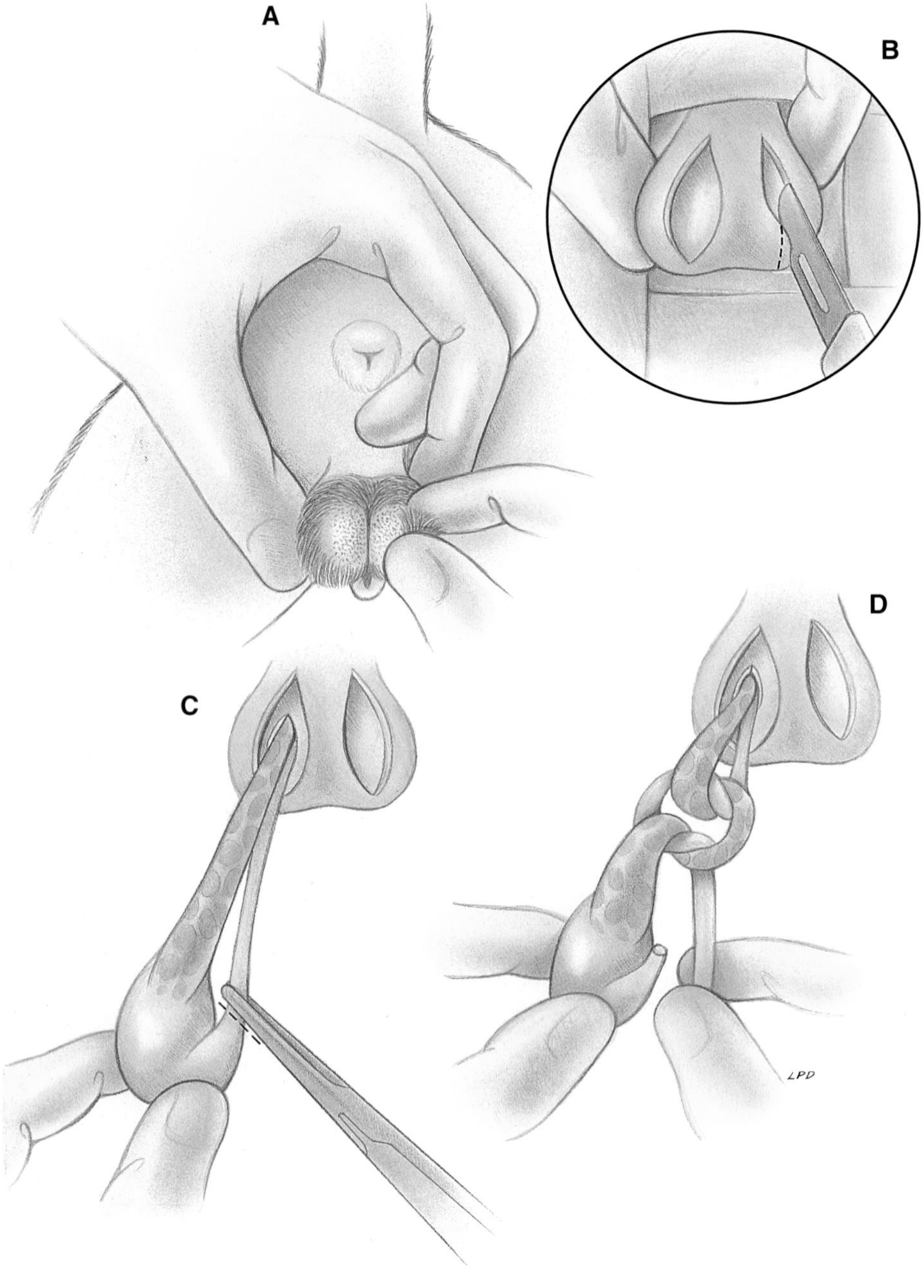

FIG. 26-7
A, For feline castration, pluck hair from the scrotum and aseptically prepare the scrotum for surgery. **B,** Make cranial to caudal skin incisions over each testicle. **C,** Incise and separate the parietal tunic from the testicle, then transect the ductus deferens near the testicle. **D,** Tie two to three square knots with the ductus deferens and the spermatic vessels.

tissue protruding from the scrotum. Allow the scrotal incision to heal by secondary intention.

To ligate the ductus deferens with the vessels, separate the ductus deferens from the testicle. Using the remainder of the spermatic cord (testicular vessels and testicle) as one strand and the ductus deferens as the other, tie two to three square knots (five to six throws) (Fig. 26-7, D). Sever the vessels with attached testicle and ductus deferens distal to the knot. Inspect for hemorrhage.

For an overhand or figure-eight knot, the spermatic cord is tied on itself with the aid of a curved mosquito hemostat. Preferably the parietal vaginal tunic is separated from the epididymis before tying the knot.

Place the hemostat on top of the cord (Fig. 26-8, A). Wrap the distal (testicle) end of the cord over the hemostat once (Fig. 26-8, B). Direct the wrapped hemostat ventral to the cord while holding the testicle in the opposite hand (Fig. 26-8, C).

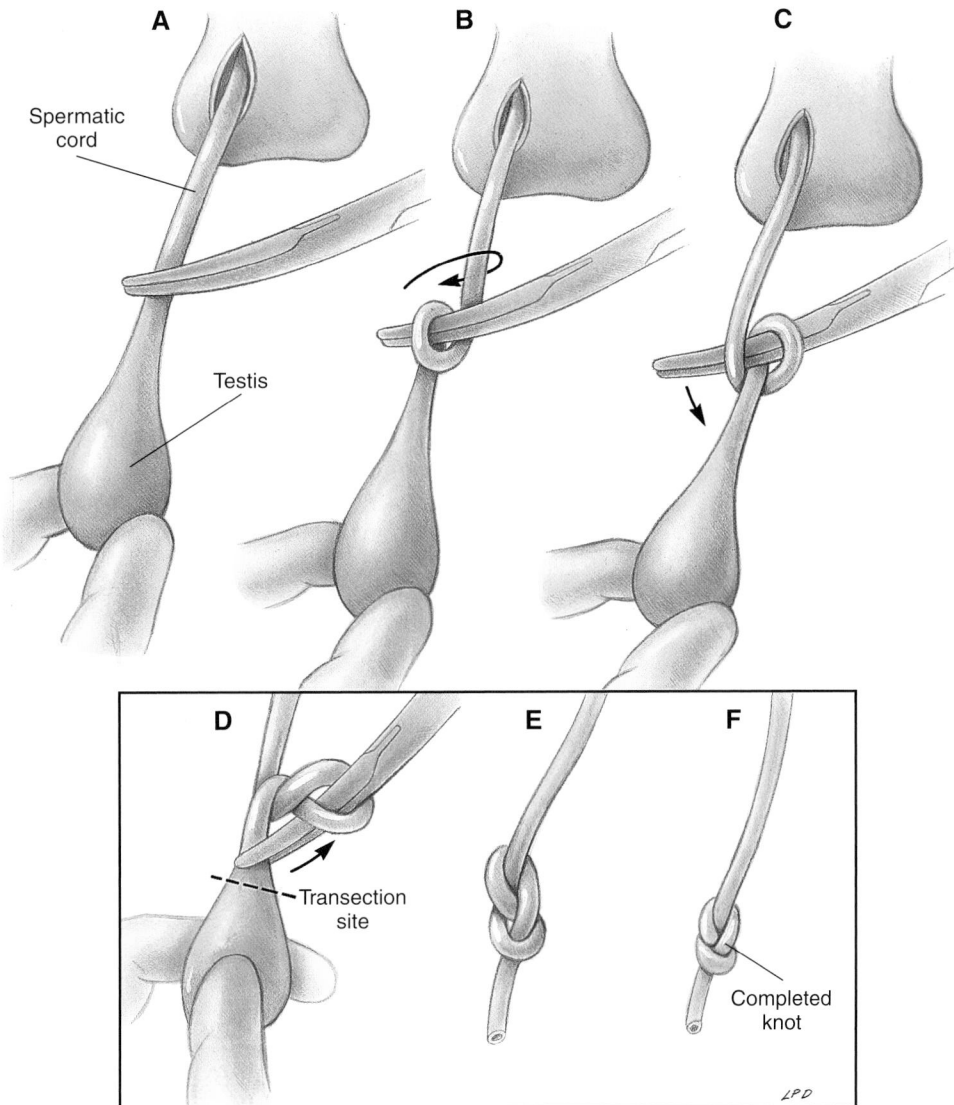

FIG. 26-8
An overhand technique may be used for feline castration. **A,** Place a curved hemostat on top of the cord and wrap the spermatic cord over it. Direct the hemostat's tip dorsally **(B)** and then ventrally **(C)** around the cord opposite the testicle. **D,** Next, grasp the cord near the testicle. **E,** Transect the testicle and pull the end of the cord through the wrap. **F,** Digitally snug the knot.

Open the tips of the hemostat, and grasp the distal end of the cord (Fig. 26-8, D). Transect the spermatic cord near the testicle, and manipulate the severed end of the cord through the loops around the hemostat (Fig. 26-8, E). Snug the knot, resect excess cord, inspect for bleeding, and replace the cord within the tunic before releasing (Fig. 26-8, F).

Cryptorchid Castration

Cryptorchidism is a congenital failure of the testicle(s) to descend into the scrotum. Testes normally are pulled into the scrotum soon after birth by fibrosis and contraction of the gubernaculum. There is little hope of further testicular descent after 2 months of age. One or both testicles may be in an abnormal position, although unilateral cryptorchidism is most common. Testicular agenesis (failure of testis development [one, monorchism; two, anorchism]) is rare. Cryptorchid testes are frequently small, soft, and proportionally misshapen. They may be in the inguinal area or abdominal cavity. Bilateral castration is recommended for cryptorchid animals because the condition is believed to be a sex-linked autosomal recessive trait in dogs. Retained canine testes are predisposed to neoplasia (seminomas and Sertoli cell tumors). If the testicle is in the inguinal region, it can often be palpated between the inguinal ring and scrotum once the animal is anesthetized; however, large inguinal fat pads may obscure testes in this area.

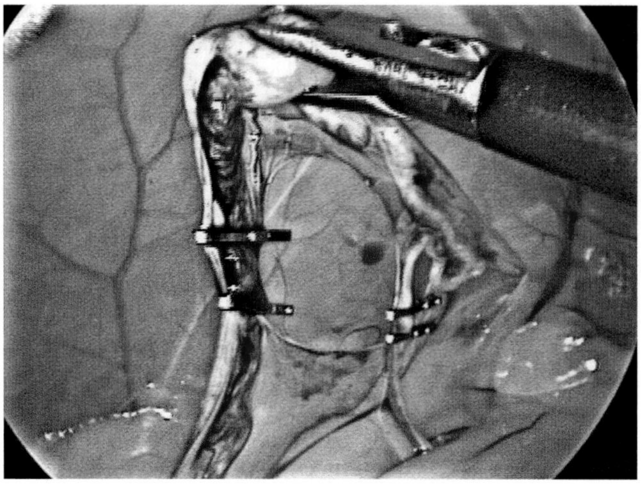

FIG. 26-9
This small, soft cryptorchid testicle is being removed laparoscopically. Note staples on the testicular vessels and ductus deferens.

Advance unilateral, mobile inguinal testicles to the prescrotal incision and remove. Remove nonmobile testicles by making an incision over the inguinal ring. Dissect through subcutaneous fat, and mobilize and remove the testicle. Submit the testicles for histologic examination to verify removal of testicular tissue and to rule out neoplasia.

Nonpalpable testes must be located via exploratory laparotomy or laparoscopy (Fig. 26-9).

Make a ventral midline incision from the umbilicus to the pubis or a paramedian incision adjacent to the prepuce when an exploratory laparotomy is performed. Find the testicle(s) by retroflexing the bladder, locating the ductus deferens dorsal to the neck of the bladder, and following the ductus deferens to the testicle. If the ductus deferens travels into the inguinal ring and the testicle cannot be manipulated into the abdomen, perform an inguinal incision. Avulse the ligament of the tail of the epididymis. Double ligate the testicular artery and vein, and ductus deferens separately. Transect and remove the testicle. Inspect for hemorrhage and close the abdomen in three layers.

> NOTE: Cryptorchid castration may also be performed laparoscopically or as a laparoscopic-assisted procedure.

Vasectomy

Vasectomy inhibits male fertility while maintaining male behavioral patterns. Androgens continue to be produced because Leydig cells are not significantly altered. The technique is rarely recommended because roaming, aggression, and urine marking persist while reduction of hormonally associated diseases does not occur. Most dogs become azo-ospermic by 1 week following vas occlusion (Schiff et al, 2003); however, spermatozoa may persist in canine ejaculates for 3 weeks and feline ejaculates for 7 weeks after vasectomy. In dogs, the time to azoospermia is shortened by flushing the ductus deferens at the time of vasectomy. Vasectomized males should be evaluated after the procedure to document azoospermic ejaculates before contact with intact bitches. This technique should be discouraged as a means of population control.

Make a 1- to 2-cm incision over the spermatic cord between the scrotum and inguinal ring (Fig. 26-10, A and B). Locate the spermatic cord, incise the vaginal tunic, and isolate the ductus deferens by blunt dissection (Fig. 26-10, B). Double ligate the ductus deferens and resect a 0.5-cm section of ductus between ligatures (Fig. 26-10, C). Repeat the procedure on the contralateral spermatic cord. Appose subcutaneous tissue and skin.

Cesarean Section

The goal of cesarean section (hysterotomy) is to remove all fetuses from the gravid uterus as quickly as possible. The primary indications for cesarean section are actual or potential dystocia (i.e., oversized, malpositioned, or maldeveloped fetuses; small pelvic canal size; uterine inertia) or fetal putrefaction. Elective cesareans are often scheduled for brachycephalic breeds and other animals with a history of dystocia or those with pelvic fracture malunion. Elective cesareans are most commonly performed on bulldogs, Labrador retrievers, mastiffs, golden retrievers, and Yorkshire terriers. Cesarean sections are more common in small dogs and brachycephalic breeds. Animals with dystocia often have fluid and electrolyte abnormalities that should be corrected before surgery. Although usually a postpartum problem, prepartum eclampsia causes hypocalcemia. Prophylactic antibiotics (e.g., cefazolin, 22 mg/kg intravenously) should be given if fetal death or uterine infection is suspected. Anesthetize these animals carefully (see p. 706); fetal depression and decreased viability are directly proportional to the degree of maternal depression.

OHE can be safely performed in conjunction with a cesarean section if the patient receives adequate fluid therapy. The cesarean section may be performed as described and followed by OHE, or an *en bloc* resection can be performed. *En bloc* OHE is performed before hysterotomy (uterine incision) and removal of the neonates. Neonatal survival with *en bloc* resection is similar to that for other techniques for managing dystocia. Changes in blood pressure and hematocrit are minimal following *en bloc* OHE, and mothering and lactation are normal following OHE. *En bloc* removal of the gravid uterus may be elective or necessary due to fetal death or questionable uterine integrity or health. Advantages of *en bloc* OHE of the gravid uterus include minimal anesthetic time, minimal potential for abdominal contamination, and population control without a second surgery. The disadvantage of this technique is that a second team is required to resuscitate the neonates.

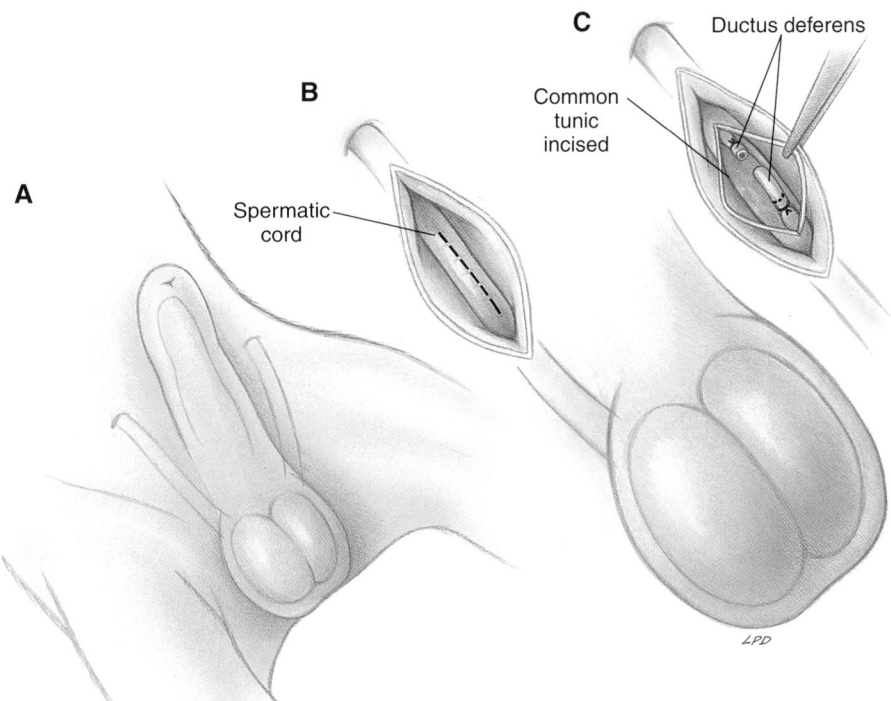

FIG. 26-10
Vasectomy. **A,** The ductus deferens are located lateral to the prepuce and penis between the inguinal rings and scrotum. **B,** Incise skin over the spermatic cord between the inguinal ring and scrotum. Dashed line indicates vaginal tunic incision site. **C,** Incise the vaginal tunic and isolate the ductus deferens. Ligate the ductus deferens and remove a small segment.

Cesarean without ovariohysterectomy. *Clip and perform a preliminary abdominal prep before anesthetic induction to minimize time from induction to delivery. Preoxygenate the bitch or queen if possible before induction. Anesthetize the animal using a general or regional protocol that is appropriate for the bitch or queen and minimizes neonatal depression (see the discussion on anesthesia on p. 706). Position the patient in dorsal recumbency. Apply a final aseptic scrub to the ventral abdomen. Make a ventral midline incision from just cranial to the umbilicus to near the pubis. Elevate the external rectus sheath before making a stab incision through the linea alba to prevent inadvertent laceration of the uterus. Exteriorize the gravid uterine horns by carefully lifting rather than pulling them out of the abdomen (Fig. 26-11) because uterine vessels are easily avulsed and the uterine wall readily tears. Isolate the uterus from the remainder of the abdomen with sterile towels or laparotomy pads. Tent and then incise the ventral uterine body to prevent lacerating the neonate. Extend the incision with Metzenbaum scissors.*

The incision should be long enough to prevent tearing during extraction of the fetus.

Empty each horn by gently squeezing (milking) cranial to each fetus to move it toward the incision, then grasping and gently pulling it from the uterus (Fig. 26-12). Rupture the amniotic sac and clamp the umbilical cord as each neonate is presented. Avoid contaminating the abdomen and surgical field with amniotic fluids. Aseptically pass each neonate to an assistant (see p. 720 for neonatal care). At term, the placenta

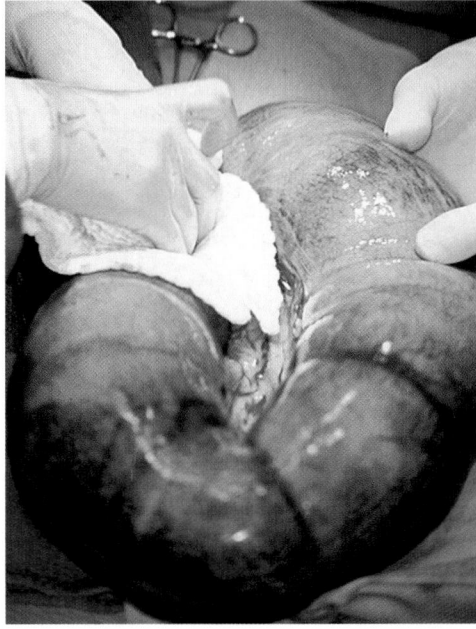

FIG. 26-11
Gravid horns should be carefully exteriorized from the abdomen to avoid tearing the uterine wall or vessels.

is often expelled with the neonate; however, if the placenta has not separated, gently pull it from the endometrium. Do not forcibly separate the placenta from the uterine wall, or severe hemorrhage may occur. Palpate the pelvic canal and remove any fetus from this location.

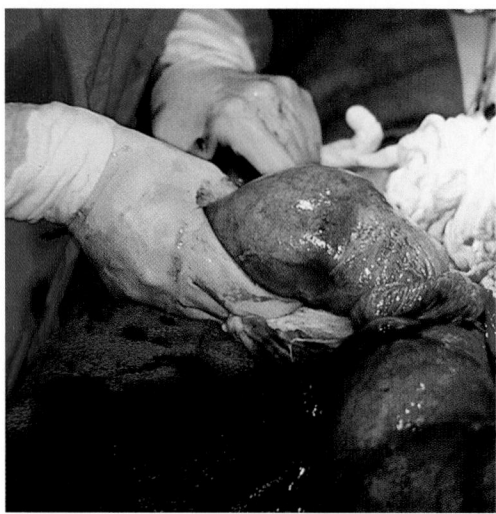

FIG. 26-12
Gently "milk" puppies toward the uterine incision by squeezing cranial to them.

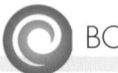 BOX 26-8

Drugs That Initiate Uterine Contraction

Oxytocin

Dogs: 2 units/kg up to 20 units IM
Cats: 2–4 units IV (repeat 20 min later after giving 1–2 ml
of 10% calcium gluconate; if this fails then give 2 ml of
50% dextrose IV only and repeat oxytocin a third and
last time)

IM, Intramuscular; *IV,* intravenous.

Uterine contraction usually begins when the fetuses are removed.

Administer oxytocin or ergonovine maleate (Box 26-8) if contraction has not occurred. Give oxytocin and compress the uterine walls if endometrial hemorrhage is severe. Lavage the external uterus to remove debris. Close the uterine incision with 3-0 or 4-0 absorbable sutures using an appositional pattern in a single layer simple continuous pattern, a double layer appositional closure (mucosa and submucosa followed by muscularis and serosa), or an appositional closure followed by a second layer inverting pattern (Cushing or Lembert). Lavage the surgical site and replace contaminated towels, sponges, instruments, and gloves. Inspect for uterine vessel avulsion and control hemorrhage. Lavage the abdomen if contamination or spillage of uterine contents has occurred. Cover the uterine incision with omentum. Appose the abdominal wall in three layers (rectus fascia, subcutaneous tissue, and skin). Use subcuticular or intradermal skin closure to eliminate suture ends that may

irritate neonates. Clean all antiseptics, blood, and debris from the ventral abdomen and mammae.

En bloc resection. *Perform en bloc OHE of the gravid uterus by first exteriorizing and isolating the ovarian pedicles and separating the broad ligament from the uterus to the point of the cervix. Manipulate fetuses in the vagina or cervix into the uterine body. Then double or triple clamp the ovarian pedicles and uterus just cranial to the cervix. Quickly transect between clamps, and remove the ovaries and uterus. Give the uterus to a team of assistants to open and resuscitate the neonates.*

The time from clamping the uterus to removal of the neonates should be 30 to 60 seconds.

Double ligate ovarian and uterine pedicles. Inspect for hemorrhage and close the abdomen.

Neonatal care. *Gently suction the nares and nasopharynx or firmly cradle the neonate and gently swing downward to help clear fluid from the upper airways. Briskly rub and dry each neonate to stimulate the respiratory drive. If necessary, antagonize opioids (place a drop of naloxone under the tongue) and give doxapram (place a drop under the tongue) to stimulate respiration.*

Stimulation of point GV (acupuncture point, governing point) 26 may stimulate respiration.

Use a 25-gauge, five-eighths-inch-long hypodermic needle, and place it 2 to 4 mm deep at the midline of the most dorsal aspect of the area between the upper lip and nose.
Ligate, transect, and disinfect the umbilical cord. Inspect each neonate for congenital or developmental anomalies (i.e., cleft palate, limb deformity, hernia, imperforate anus). Place neonates in a warm environment (32° C, 90° F) until their mother is able to care for them. Allow nursing as soon as possible to ensure colostrum intake. Closely observe the mother and her behavior toward the neonates during the first few hours; some mothers will reject or kill their neonates. Discharge the bitch or queen and neonates from the hospital as soon as possible to reduce stress and exposure to potential pathogens.

Mastectomy

Mastectomy or removal of the mammary gland(s) is usually performed to remove tumors. One gland (simple mastectomy), several glands (regional mastectomy), or an entire chain (complete unilateral mastectomy) may be excised and the defect closed. Simultaneous removal of both mammary chains (complete bilateral mastectomy) causes significant suture line tension and should be avoided if possible. Staged procedures are advised to facilitate defect closure and reduce patient discomfort when bilateral mastectomy is necessary. OHE during the same anesthesia is

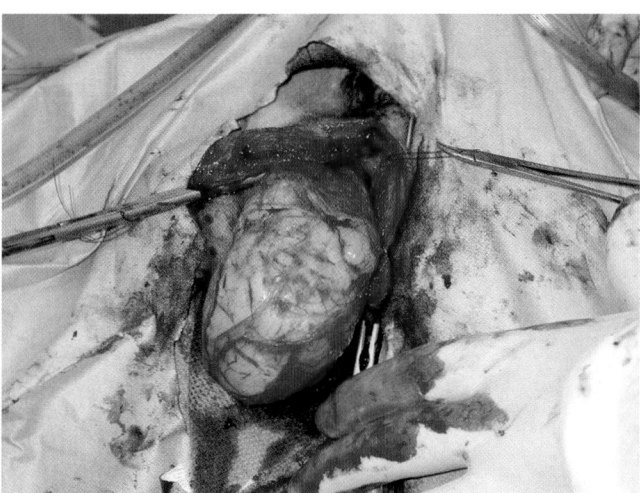

FIG. 26-13
Vaginal leiomyoma.

performed before mastectomy to prevent seeding the abdomen with tumor cells. If the tumor crosses the midline, however, it may be excised first. Clean instruments and gloves should be used for the OHE. The technique for mastectomy is described on p. 732.

Episiotomy

An episiotomy is an incision of the vulvar orifice to allow access to the vestibule and vagina. It is indicated to surgically explore the vagina, excise vaginal masses (Fig. 26-13), repair lacerations, modify congenital defects or strictures, expose the urethral papilla, and facilitate manual fetal extraction.

With the animal in a perineal position, place a noncrushing clamp (i.e., Doyen) with one shaft in the vagina on each side of the perineal midline (Fig. 26-14, A). Make a midline skin incision through the dorsal commissure of the vulvar lips to just distal to the external anal sphincter muscle with a scalpel blade. Continue the incision through the muscle and vaginal wall with Mayo scissors (see Fig. 26-14, A). Control hemorrhage with hemostats, electrocoagulation, and ligatures. Place two or three horizontal mattress stay sutures full-thickness through the skin and vaginal mucosa on each side of the incision to facilitate retraction and hemostasis. Then remove the Doyen clamps and position a self-retaining retractor (e.g., Gelpi) to improve exposure, if necessary. Evaluate the vagina and vestibule, and perform any needed procedures. Close the episiotomy incision in three layers. Preplace an interrupted suture to realign and reappose the dorsal vulvar commissure. First, reappose the vaginal mucosa with simple interrupted or continuous sutures (e.g., 3-0 or 4-0 polydioxanone or polyglyconate), tying the knots in the lumen (Fig. 26-14, B). Then reappose muscles and subcutaneous tissue in a continuous pattern (Fig. 26-14, C). Lastly, reappose skin with interrupted appositional sutures (e.g., 3-0 or 4-0 nylon or polypropylene). Place an Elizabethan collar, bucket, or

sidebars after surgery to prevent self-trauma. To reduce inflammation and edema, apply cold compresses immediately after surgery and for 2 to 3 days, then warm compresses for 2 to 3 days.

Episioplasty

Episioplasty (vulvoplasty) is a reconstructive procedure most commonly performed to excise excess skin folds around the vulva, which cause perivulvar dermatitis and recurrent urinary tract infections (see p. 251). Skin fold pyoderma should be treated medically before surgical reconstruction.

With the patient in a perineal position, assess the amount of skin to be excised by elevating the skin fold and evaluating expected tension (Fig. 26-15, A). Beginning near the ventral vulvar commissure, make a crescent-shaped incision encircling the vulva at the proposed lateral and dorsal borders of the resection. Make a second crescent-shaped incision medial and parallel to the first to outline the ellipse of skin to be removed (Fig. 26-15, B). Excise the outlined segment of skin and excess subcutaneous tissue (Fig. 26-15, C). Place interrupted sutures at the 3 o'clock, 9 o'clock, and 12 o'clock positions to assess the effectiveness of the resection (Fig. 26-15, D). Resect more skin along the outer margin if the vulva is still recessed or if skin folds persist. Bring the skin edges into approximation by first apposing the subcutaneous tissues using interrupted sutures with buried knots (e.g., 3-0 or 4-0 monofilament absorbable). Place the first sutures at the 12 o'clock, 3 o'clock, and 9 o'clock positions to symmetrically align the edges. Appose skin edges with simple interrupted sutures (e.g., 3-0 or 4-0 nylon, polybutester, or polypropylene; Fig. 26-15, E).

Place an Elizabethan collar or bucket over the head to prevent licking and chewing at the surgical site. Continue antibiotics if necessary to control the pyoderma.

Testicular Biopsy

Testicular biopsy may be performed in valuable breeding animals to help determine the cause of infertility or reduced fertility. Biopsies are obtained using a biopsy needle directed through the scrotal skin or by wedge resection. Ultrasound-guided percutaneous biopsy is warranted when a nonpalpable mass is identified deep within the parenchyma. A wedge of tissue is collected by making a prescrotal incision and then incising the spermatic fascia and tunics. Large blood vessels should be avoided to minimize hemorrhage.

Make a 1-cm incision through the tunica albuginea of one testicle with a sterile, thin razor blade or No. 11 scalpel blade. Excise a wedge of testicular parenchyma with the razor blade. Appose the tunica albuginea with 4-0 to 6-0 monofilament absorbable suture (i.e., polydioxanone, poliglecaprone 25, polyglyconate, or glycomer 631). Appose skin edges with intradermal (subcuticular) or simple interrupted sutures.

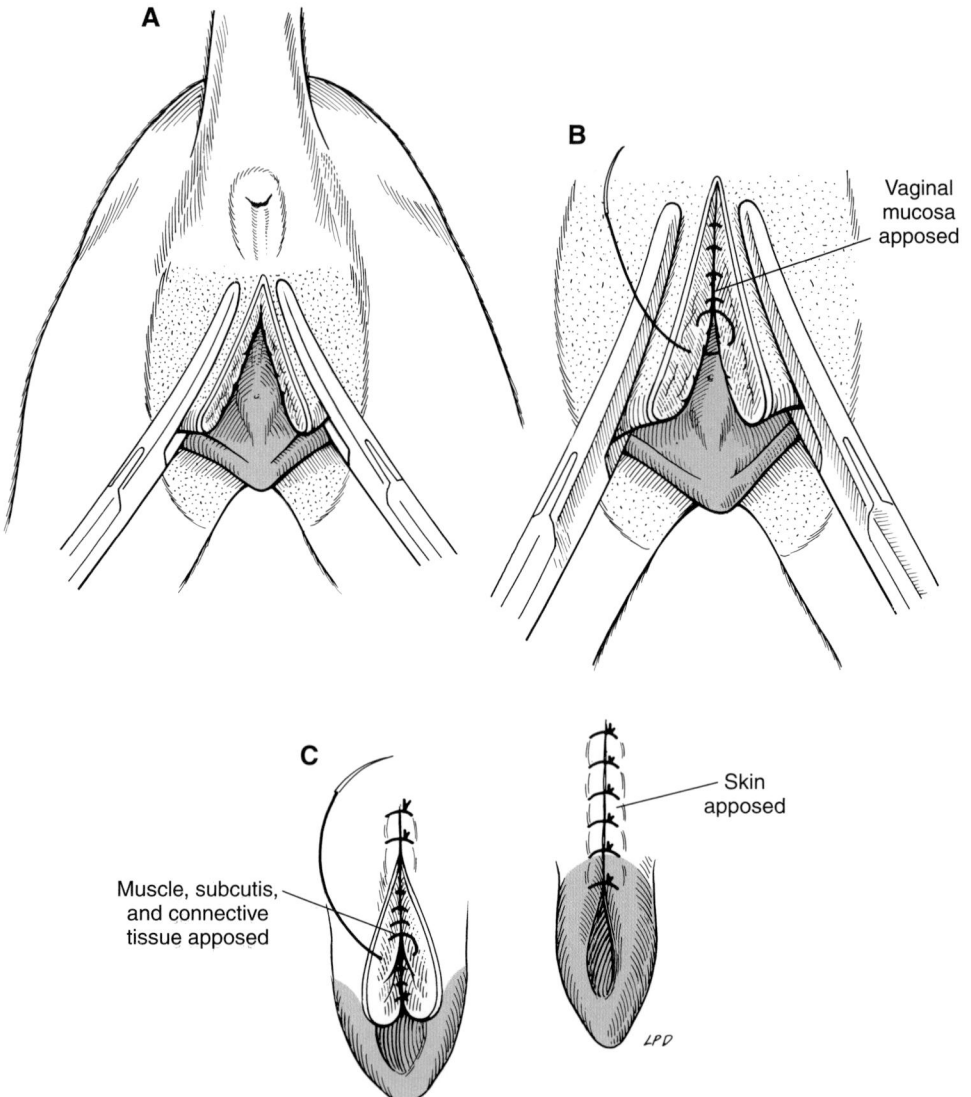

FIG. 26-14
A, For episiotomy, place non-crushing forceps on each side of the proposed incision site. Make a full-thickness incision from the dorsal vulvar commissure to near the external anal sphincter muscle. Explore the vagina and vestibule. **B,** Appose vaginal mucosa with a simple continuous suture pattern. **C,** Appose muscle, subcutis, and connective tissue with a second layer of sutures and skin with a third layer of appositional sutures.

Better preservation of architectural detail is obtained by placing the sample in Bouin's, Zenker's, or Stevie's fixative rather than formalin.

Prostatic Biopsy

Prostatic biopsy is needed to definitively diagnose some prostatic diseases. Percutaneous techniques are preferred because they are less invasive, less expensive, and cause less morbidity. However, operative techniques allow collection of larger samples from more specific sites. The prostatic urethra must not be damaged, and specimens should be submitted for both histologic and microbiologic evaluation. Percutaneous biopsies are performed using TruCut, Biopty needle, or Franklin-Silverman biopsy needles. They may be guided by palpation (blind) or with the aid of ultrasonography. The latter is preferred because it facilitates guiding the needle to abnormal areas. Biopsy should not be performed if abscesses or cysts are suspected.

Ultrasound-guided biopsy. *Position the patient in dorsal or lateral recumbency and ultrasonographically evaluate the prostate. Aseptically prepare the abdominal wall in the area in which the biopsy needle will be inserted. Nick the skin (3- to 5-mm incision) with a scalpel blade at the needle insertion site. Identify the desired biopsy site with ultrasound and visualize needle placement into the prostate. The needle must be parallel to the ultrasound beam to be visualized. Collect two to three biopsies with a Biopty needle/instrument. Observe the prostate for hemorrhage or fluid leakage with ultrasound.*

Palpation-guided biopsy. *Place the patient in a perineal position with the tail fixed over the back. Aseptically prepare the perineum around the anus. Mobilize and reposition the prostate in a more caudal position by having an assistant apply gentle dorsal and caudal pressure on the caudal abdomen. Make a nick incision (3 to 5 mm) slightly lateral to the midline, midway between the anus and ischial tuberosity.*

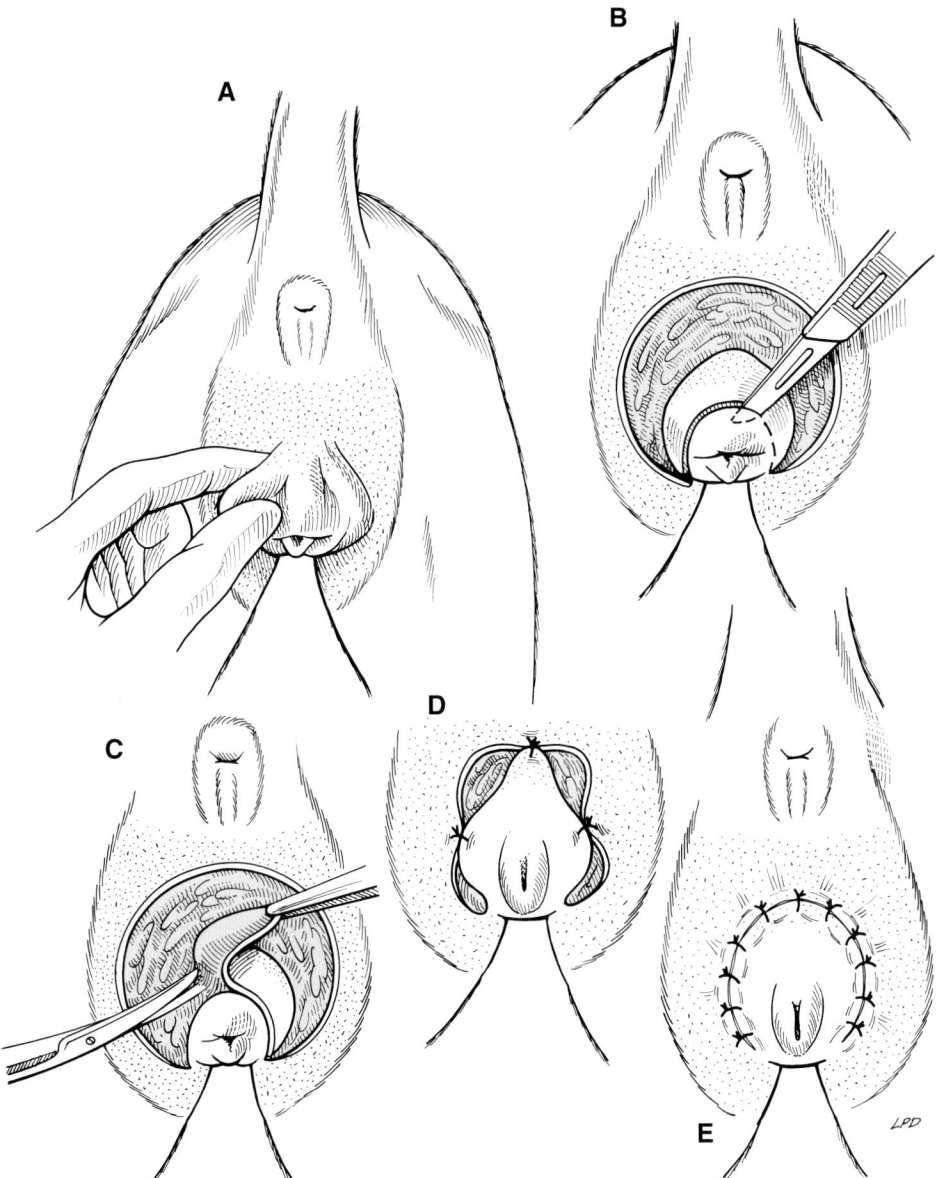

FIG. 26-15
A, Episioplasty is performed after assessing the amount of skin to be excised. **B,** Make two parallel crescent-shaped incisions encircling the vulva and excise the outlined segment of skin and underlying subcutaneous tissues **(C)**. **D,** Appose skin edges by placing the initial sutures at the 12 o'clock, 3 o'clock, and 9 o'clock positions. **E,** Appose remaining skin with simple interrupted sutures.

Confirm the location of the prostate by rectal examination. Insert the needle through the soft tissue ventral to the rectum. Guide the needle to the prostate digitally via rectal palpation. Penetrate the capsule at the caudal margin of the prostate with the needle in the closed position, then fully insert the inner cannula into the prostatic parenchyma. Quickly advance the outer cannula over the stationary inner cannula, or fire the trigger when using an automatic instrument to cut the specimen. Remove the needle from the prostate in the closed position. Evaluate the specimen size, and collect additional samples if necessary.

Transrectal fine-needle aspiration. *With the tip of a gloved digit covering the tip of the needle (the finger should be on the bevel of the needle to help prevent puncturing your finger), carefully insert the digit into the rectum until*

the prostate is felt at the tip of the finger. Carefully slide the needle down the finger, through the rectal wall, and into the prostate. Perform a fine-needle aspiration as with any other organ. There are devices that are designed to help do this, but they are not necessary.

Open biopsy. *Collect prostatic biopsies during exploratory laparotomy with a biopsy needle or wedge excision. Via a caudal midline abdominal incision, retract the urinary bladder cranially using stay sutures. Isolate the prostate from the remainder of the abdomen with sterile laparotomy pads. Palpate the prostate and select a biopsy site. Dissect periprostatic fat from the desired site. Excise a wedge of prostatic tissue using a No. 11 scalpel blade. Appose edges of the defect by placing cruciate or simple continuous monofilament absorbable sutures (e.g., 3-0 or 4-0 polydioxanone, poligle-*

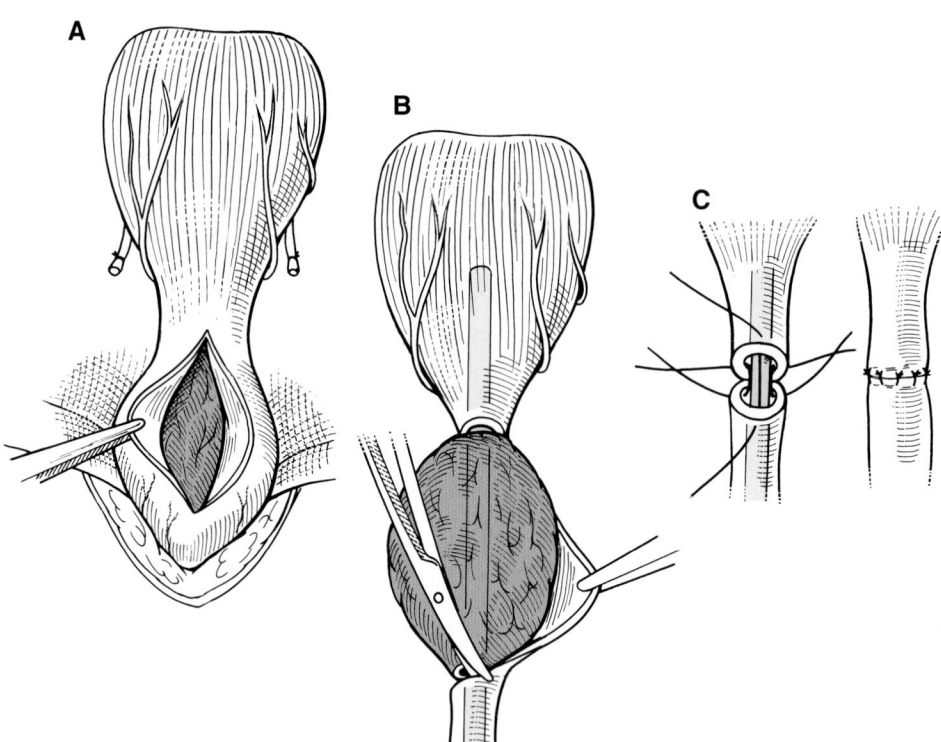

FIG. 26-16
A, To perform total prostatectomy, separate the fat, fascia, vessels, and nerves from the prostate by dissecting directly against the capsule. **B,** Then dissect the cranial and caudal edges of the prostate from the urethra and transect the urethra as close to the prostate as possible. **C,** Stent the urethra with a catheter and appose the ends with approximating sutures.

caprone 25, glycomer 631, or polyglyconate) in the prostatic capsule. Lavage the surgical site(s) and replace periprostatic fat. Close the abdomen in three layers.

AP **Prostatectomy**

Total prostatectomy. Total prostatectomy can be used for patients with tumors that have not metastasized; it is rarely performed for severe trauma or chronic prostatic disease that has been nonresponsive to other treatments. The procedure is infrequently performed because urinary incontinence commonly results.

Expose the prostate through a caudal ventral midline celiotomy and pubic osteotomy (see pp. 501 and 670). Place a urethral catheter. Retract the urinary bladder cranially with stay sutures. Dissect the lateral pedicles and periprostatic fat directly from the capsule without damaging the dorsal plexus of vessels and nerves (Fig. 26-16, A). Control hemostasis by ligation and electrocoagulation. Ligate and divide the prostatic vessels and ductus deferens as close to the prostate as possible. Dissect the prostate from the urinary bladder and extrapelvic urethra. Transect the urethra on both ends as close to the prostate as possible (Fig. 26-16, B). Avoid the trigone and neck of the bladder. Remove the prostate. Advance the urethral catheter into the urinary bladder. Approximate the urethral ends with simple interrupted sutures using 4-0 to 6-0 synthetic monofilament absorbable suture (i.e., polydioxanone, polyglyconate, poliglecaprone 25, glycomer 631) on a taper point swaged-on needle. Place the first two sutures at the 12 o'clock and 6 o'clock positions, leaving the ends long to aid rotation of the urethra

during suturing (Fig. 26-16, C). Place the dorsal suture first. Space sutures approximately 2 mm apart and 1.5 to 2 mm from the edge. Place a cystostomy tube (see p. 667) or transurethral Foley catheter to divert urine for 5 to 7 days. Take a biopsy of an iliac or sublumbar lymph node to evaluate for metastasis. Replace contaminated instruments and gloves. Lavage the surgical site and abdomen. Place omentum around the anastomosis. Wire the pubic segment into place. Perform a three-layer abdominal wall closure. Place an Elizabethan collar, bucket, or sidebars after surgery to prevent displacement of the catheter and surgical site trauma.

Subtotal prostatectomy. Subtotal prostatectomy is rarely indicated in valuable breeding dogs for benign prostatic hyperplasia in lieu of castration and in stable dogs with abscessation or cysts in lieu of drainage procedures. A urinary catheter should be placed to aid urethral identification. The prostate is approached and exposed as for total prostatectomy (see previous discussion). Alternatively, laparoscopic, transrectal, or transurethral approaches may be used. Submit excised tissue for histologic evaluation.

Subtotal prostatectomy with capsulectomy. *Isolate and ligate or cauterize all vessels as they enter the prostatic capsule when celiotomy is performed. Temporary occlusion of the aorta just cranial to its bifurcation into the external iliac arteries is sometimes recommended. Excise the prostate within 5 mm of the urethra using scissors, an electrosurgical unit, and an ultrasonic aspirator or laser (Fig. 26-17, A). Place a cystostomy tube if the urethral catheter is to be removed (see p. 667). Assess hemostasis and lavage the surgical site.*

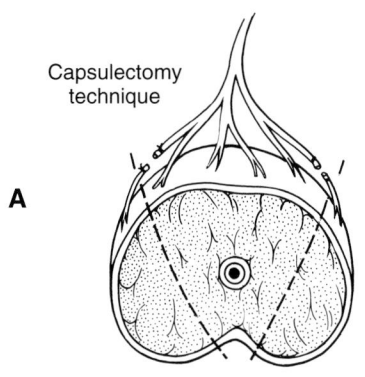

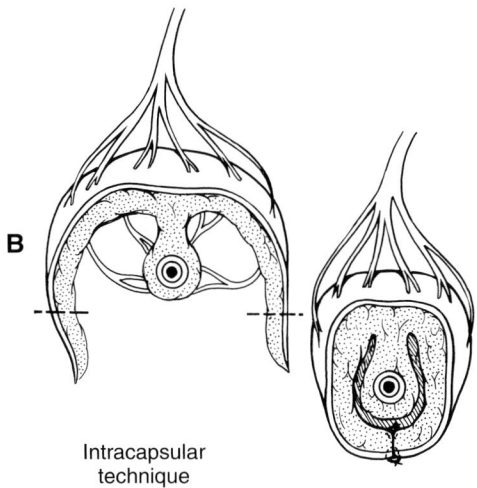

FIG. 26-17
Subtotal prostatectomy may be performed using capsulectomy
(A) or intracapsular techniques **(B)**.

*Surround the prostatic urethra with omentum or prostatic fat.
Close the abdomen routinely.*

   Intracapsular subtotal prostatectomy. *Incise the
ventral median septum with an electroscalpel. Continue the
incision through the parenchyma into the ventral urethra. Using the electroscalpel, resect all parenchyma except a 2- to
3-mm shell attached to the capsule (Fig. 26-17, B). Resect all
the urethra except a 3- to 5-mm dorsal strip. Lavage the prostatic shell, and close the capsule over a urethral catheter positioned in the urinary bladder. Use an approximating pattern
for the first layer and an inverting pattern for the second layer
of closure (e.g., 3-0 or 4-0 polydioxanone, poliglecaprone
25, glycomer 631, or polyglyconate). Maintain the catheter
for 10 days. Alternatively, use an ultrasonic surgical aspirator
or laser to remove parenchyma and preserve the urethra.*

HEALING OF THE REPRODUCTIVE AND GENITAL SYSTEMS

Reproductive organs heal like other visceral tissue. Incisions
into testicular parenchyma may cause an immunologic response and subsequent sperm granuloma. Scarring of the
uterus may inhibit placentation. To decrease uterine adhe-

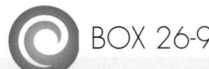 **BOX 26-9**

Suture Recommendations for Reproductive Suture

- Select a monofilament, synthetic, absorbable suture for
  visceral closure (i.e., polydioxanone, polyglyconate,
  poliglecaprone 25, or glycomer 631)
- Select an absorbable suture for ligatures (i.e., chromic
  catgut, polydioxanone, polyglyconate, polyglactin 910,
  poliglecaprone 25, or glycomer 631)

sions, omentum can be placed over incisions. Failure of
postpartum uterine involution may be caused by excessive
collagen breakdown as a result of uterine collagenase activity. Optimal healing requires a good blood supply, accurate
mucosal apposition, and minimal surgical trauma. Systemic
factors (i.e., hypovolemia, shock, hypoproteinemia, debilitation, and infection) may delay healing and increase the risk
of dehiscence.

SUTURE MATERIALS/SPECIAL INSTRUMENTS

Instruments needed for reproductive surgery include an
OHE hook (i.e., Covault, Snook), retractors (i.e., Balfour
[abdominal procedures], Gelpi or Weitlander [perineal pro-
cedures], Finochietto [pelvic procedures], vaginal speculum
or otoscope [vaginal procedures]), scissors (i.e., Metzenbaum, Mayo), forceps (i.e., Doyen, Carmalt, and curved
mosquito), biopsy instruments (Bard Biopty-cut Biopsy
Needle with a Bard Biopsy Instrument), and drains. Orthopedic instruments are needed if a pelvic osteotomy is performed. An electrosurgical unit, ultrasonic aspirator, laser
unit, ultrasonic scalpel, vascular sealer, and laparoscopic
equipment and instruments are sometimes beneficial.

   Monofilament absorbable and nonabsorbable sutures are
recommended for most reproductive tract procedures (i.e.,
2-0 to 6-0 polydioxanone, polyglyconate, poliglecaprone 25,
glycomer 631, polybutester, polypropylene, or nylon) (Box
26-9). Chromic catgut (2-0 to 0) or polyglactin-910 (Vicryl)
is preferred by some for ligatures. Stapling equipment (transverse, ligate and divide, and skin staplers) is sometimes
used.

POSTOPERATIVE CARE AND ASSESSMENT

Animals undergoing reproductive tract surgery should be
monitored postoperatively for pain, hemorrhage, and infection. Postoperative analgesics are indicated (see Chapter 13;
for dosages of opioids see Table 13-4 on p. 133). The incision
site should be assessed twice daily for redness, swelling, or
discharge. Activity should be limited to leash walks until
sutures are removed (generally 10 to 14 days). Water is usually offered 8 to 12 hours after surgery, unless vomiting occurs. If the animal does not vomit, food can be given 12 to
24 hours postoperatively.

   Nonelective procedures are often performed on sick animals with fluid, electrolyte, and acid-base abnormalities;

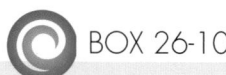 BOX 26-10

Stool Softeners

Dioctyl Sodium Sulfosuccinate or Docusate Sodium (Colace)
Dogs: 50 to 200 mg PO, bid to tid
Cats: 50 mg PO, qd to bid

Lactulose (Chronulac)
Dogs: Start with 1 ml/4.5 kg PO, tid and adjust so that stools are soft but not watery
Cats: Start with 5 ml/cat PO, tid and adjust to effect

Psyllium (Metamucil)
Dogs: Start with 1 teaspoon/5–10 kg bid in food and adjust until desired effect is obtained
Cats: Start with 1 teaspoon/cat bid and adjust until desired effect is obtained

PO, Oral; *bid,* twice a day; *tid,* three times a day; *qd,* once a day.

 BOX 26-11

Common Errors in Reproductive Surgery

- Failure to support septic or debilitated patients with fluids, antibiotics, and/or nutrition
- Failure to completely resect tumors
- Failure to obtain a histologic diagnosis
- Failure to prevent self-mutilation of the surgical site

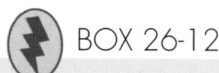 BOX 26-12

Potential Complications After Reproductive Surgery

Ovariohysterectomy
- Pain, hemorrhage, infection, dehiscence, urinary incontinence, ovarian remnant, ureteral ligation, fistula, adhesions

Castration
- Hemorrhage, scrotal hematoma, scrotal bruising, infection, dehiscence, urinary incontinence, behavior change, eunuchoid syndrome

Vasectomy
- Granuloma, scrotal swelling, incisional problems

Cesarean Section
- Hemorrhage, retained fetus, adhesions, uterine scarring, incisional problems, shock, hypothermia, hypocalcemia, agalactia, metritis, vomiting, anorexia

Mastectomy
- Pain, inflammation, hemorrhage, seroma formation, infection, ischemic necrosis, self-trauma, dehiscence, limb edema, tumor recurrence

Episiotomy
- Pain, swelling, inflammation, hemorrhage, infection, dehiscence, self-trauma

Episioplasty
- Inflammation, swelling, infection, dehiscence, recurrent perivulvar dermatitis

Testicular Biopsy
- Hemorrhage, infection, local hyperthermia, scarring, adhesions, immune-mediated orchitis, testicular atrophy, reduced sperm count (temporary)

Prostatic Biopsy
- Hemorrhage, hematuria, urine leakage, infection, tumor transplantation

Prostatectomy
- Hemorrhage, infection, incisional problems, urinary catheter displacement, urine leakage, dysuria, urethral stricture, urinary incontinence, tumor spread

these abnormalities require monitoring and continued treatment in the postoperative period. Therapeutic antibiotics should be continued in patients with preoperative infections. Surgical sites should be protected by using an Elizabethan collar, bucket, sidebars, or bandage to prevent self-trauma. Stool softeners may be administered after prostatic or perineal surgery to minimize discomfort during defecation (Box 26-10). Apply cold compresses two to three times daily for 2 or 3 days; then apply warm compresses for 2 or 3 additional days to minimize hemorrhage and swelling after perineal surgery.

COMPLICATIONS

Most complications associated with reproductive surgery can be prevented by using good surgical technique (i.e., gentle tissue handling, good hemostasis, and aseptic technique) (Boxes 26-11 and 26-12). OHE is difficult in larger dogs and is associated with more complications. Hemorrhage primarily occurs from the ovarian pedicles, uterine vessels, or uterine wall when ligatures are improperly placed; it rarely occurs from vessels that accompany the suspensory ligament or those within the broad ligament. Excessive hemorrhage may occur when OHE is performed during estrus. Ureter ligation or trauma may occur when ligating a dropped or hemorrhaging ovarian pedicle when exposure of the caudal renal pole is inadequate. The ureter may also be ligated if the urinary bladder is distended and the trigone and ureterovesical junction are displaced cranially. Hydronephrosis necessitating ureteronephrectomy results unless the offending ligature is promptly removed. Estrus may recur if ovarian tissue remains in the abdominal cavity. If this occurs, abdominal exploration during estrus may help identify the ovarian tissue. Fistulous tracts and granulomas may form if nonabsorbable multifilament suture material is used for ligations. These fistulae are usually located in the flank, but also occur along the medial thigh or inguinal region. They intermittently discharge blood-tinged fluid or mucopurulent exudate. Discharge may diminish during antibiotic therapy, but recurs when antibiotics are discontinued. These fistulae will not resolve until the suture material is removed. Caution must be exercised during dissection because there may be adhesions to the vena cava and other vital structures.

Urinary incontinence is uncommon after OHE (5%), but may occur soon after surgery or in geriatric bitches. A higher incidence of urinary incontinence is seen in females neutered before 3 months of age (approximately 13%) (Spain et al, 2004). Causes of urinary incontinence include low estrogen levels, uterine stump adhesions or granulomas to the urinary bladder, and vaginoureteral fistulae (see p. •••). Despite the belief that OHE causes obesity, properly fed and exercised neutered animals should not gain excessive weight. Neutered cats will often become obese if allowed free access to food (Harper et al, 2001; Nguyen et al, 2004). Juvenile behavior and external genitalia may persist in animals neutered at a very young age (6 to 12 weeks). Neutering may inhibit an animal's ability to slow cognitive impairment when it is present (Hart, 2001). Hypothermia, hypoglycemia, blood loss, and tissue handling problems occur more commonly with prepubertal OHE. Other possible complications of OHE include self-trauma, incisional swelling, seroma, infection, delayed healing, dehiscence, trauma to intestines or spleen, cervical pyometra, endocrine alopecia, colonic obstruction, behavioral change, and *eunuchoid syndrome* (having the characteristics of a castrated male; secondary sex characteristics do not develop).

Serious complications following properly performed castrations are rare but may include incisional problems (i.e., swelling, seroma formation, cellulitis, infection, self-trauma, and dehiscence), hemorrhage, scrotal hematoma, scrotal bruising, abscess, granuloma, urinary incontinence, endocrine alopecia, behavioral changes, eunuchoid syndrome, and constriction of the colon. Trauma to the penis and urethra may occur during dissection, especially with scrotal ablation. Although unlikely, an unwanted pregnancy may occur if a recently castrated male copulates with a female in estrus because spermatozoa persist in the ductus deferens up to 21 days in dogs and 49 days in cats. Inadvertent prostatectomy has occurred during cryptorchidectomy.

Complications of cesarean section, with or without OHE, include hemorrhage, hypovolemia, hypothermia, hypocalcemia, anorexia, anemia, agalactia, metritis, and vomiting. Severe hemorrhage may necessitate OHE. Calcium levels should be monitored if eclampsia is suspected; affected dogs usually have ionized calcium levels less than or equal to 6 mg/dl. Eclampsia more commonly occurs in small breed dogs with large litters. Eclampsia may occur anytime during the first postpartum month, and not all affected animals have typical signs (i.e., muscle tremors, tetany, and convulsions). An odorless, dark red-brown to serous uterine discharge or lochia is expected for 4 to 6 weeks postpartum. Incisional complications, such as swelling, infection, seroma, self-trauma, and/or dehiscence, may occur. Uterine scarring may prevent future placentation, and adhesions may interfere with uterine motility. Neonate mortality is most commonly associated with emergency surgery, large litters, brachycephalic bitches, and poor anesthetic choices.

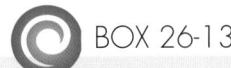

BOX 26-13

Treatment of Urinary Incontinence

Phenylpropanolamine*

Dogs: 1.5–2 mg/kg PO, bid to tid†
Cats: 1.5 mg/kg PO, tid

Ephedrine

Dogs: Start at 0.4 mg/kg, and gradually increase to 4 mg/kg PO, bid to tid‡
Cats: 2–4 mg/cat PO, bid to tid

Diethylstilbestrol (DES)

Dogs: 0.1–0.2 mg/kg (maximum of 1 mg) PO, qd for 3–5 days, then same dose once every 3–7 days as needed, with maximum of 0.2 mg/kg/week§

Estriol

2 mg PO qd for 7 days, then reduced to lowest effective dose (0.5–2 mg/dog qd to qod)

Testosterone Cypionate (Depotestosterone)

Dogs: 1.1–2.2 mg/kg IM, once every 30 days

Imipramine (Tofranil)

Dogs: 2–4 mg/kg PO, qd to bid

PO, Oral; *bid,* twice a day; *tid,* three times a day; *qd,* once a day; *qid,* four times a day; *qod,* every other day; *IM,* intramuscular.
*Although this drug has been withdrawn from the human market, it is generally available from veterinary pharmacies that compound drugs.
†Best to start at low end of dose and gradually increase, if needed.
‡Toxicity typically starts at 5 mg/kg, and death can readily occur at 10 mg/kg.
§If benefit is not noted after 5 days of daily therapy, then it is unlikely that further administration will benefit the patient, and other drugs should be used.

Although rare, complications can occur after mastectomy (see p. 734), episiotomy, episioplasty, testicular biopsy, and prostatic biopsy (see Box 26-12). Dehiscence after episioplasty may occur if skin resection causes excessive suture line tension, but perivulvar dermatitis will persist or recur if inadequate skin is excised.

Early postoperative complications of prostatectomy include hemorrhage, urine leakage, infection, and urethral catheter displacement; later complications include dehiscence, urethral stricture, and urinary incontinence. Urinary incontinence is expected (more than 85%) in dogs after prostatectomy, unless the prostate is of normal size and dissection does not traumatize trigonal innervation or vascularity. Incontinence caused by diminished urethral sphincter tone may be treated with α-adrenergic agonists (i.e., phenylpropanolamine, imipramine, or ephedrine) that increase urethral sphincter tone or with diethylstilbestrol (DES) (Box 26-13). Phenylpropanolamine is used more frequently than ephedrine because it has fewer side effects (i.e., hyperexcitability, panting, and/or anorexia) and greater efficacy over time (see also p. 695).

SPECIAL AGE CONSIDERATIONS

Elective neutering is most advantageous when the animal is less than 1 year old. Undesirable behaviors are usually not learned by this age, and some tumors (e.g., mammary adenocarcinoma) can be inhibited. Pediatric tissues are more fragile than adult tissues and must be handled gently. Long bone growth increases slightly following prepubertal gonadectomy. Tumors, pyometra, and prostatic infections are more common in geriatric patients.

References

Austin B, Lanz OI, Hamilton SM et al: Laparoscopic ovariohysterectomy in nine dogs, *J Am Anim Hosp Assoc* 39:391, 2003.

Devit DM, Cox RE, Hailey JJ: Duration, complications, stress, and pain of open ovariohysterectomy versus a simple method of laparoscopic-assisted ovariohysterectomy in dogs, *J Am Vet Med Assoc* 227:921, 2005.

Harper EJ, Stack DM, Watson TDG et al: Effects of feeding regimen on body weight, composition and condition score in cats following ovariohysterectomy, *J Small Anim Pract* 42:433-438, 2001.

Hart BJ: Effect of gonadectomy on subsequent development of age-related cognitive impairment in dogs, *J Am Vet Med Assoc* 219:51-56, 2001.

Nguyen PG, Dumon H, Siliart BS, et al: Effects of dietary fat and energy on body weight and composition after gonadectomy in cats, *Am J Vet Res* 65:1708, 2004.

Nishiyama T, Narita K, Tsumagari S et al: Shrinkage of the horizontal dimensions of the vulva (vulvar shrinkage) as an indicator of standing heat in the beagle, *J Am Anim Hosp Assoc* 36:556, 2000.

Schiff JD, Li PS, Schlegel PN et al: Rapid disappearance of spermatozoa after vassal occlusion in the dog, *J Anthrology* 24:361, 2003.

Spain CV, Scarlett JM, Houpt KA: Long-term risks and benefits of early-age gonadectomy in dogs, *J Am Vet Med Assoc* 224:380, 2004.

Suggested Reading

Austin B, Lanz OI, Hamilton SM et al: Laparoscopic ovariohysterectomy in nine dogs, *J Am Anim Hosp Assoc* 39:391, 2003.
This study used three triangulated ports and the harmonic scalpel to occlude and transect the ovarian pedicles, broad ligament, and uterine vessels and body, which took a median of 60 minutes to complete.

Davidson EB, Moll HD, Payton ME: Comparison of laparoscopic ovariohysterectomy and ovariohysterectomy in dogs, *Vet Surg* 33:62, 2004.
This comparison of techniques found laparoscopic ovariohysterectomy (n = 16) to be significantly longer and associated with more complications but less pain than a standard open ovariohysterectomy (n = 18).

DeNardo GA, Becker K, Brown NO et al: Ovarian remnant syndrome: revascularization of free-floating ovarian tissue in the feline abdominal cavity, *J Am Anim Hosp Assoc* 37:290, 2001.
Ovariohysterectomy was performed on nine cats, and a portion of ovary was sutured to the mesentery to determine that revitalization occurred.

Drobatz KJ, Casey KK: Eclampsia in dogs: 31 cases (1995-1998), *J Am Vet Med Assoc* 217:216, 2000.
Clinical characteristics of eclampsia were determined by comparing 31 dogs with eclampsia with 31 control dogs who had dystocia.

Gobello C, Castex G, Corrada Y: Use of cabergoline to treat primary and secondary anestrus in dogs, *J Am Vet Med Assoc* 220:1653, 2002.
This dopaminergic agonist was successful in inciting estrus to allow pregnancy.

Hancock RB, Lanz OI, Waldron DR, et al: Comparison of postoperative pain after ovariohysterectomy by harmonic scalpel-assisted laparoscopy compared with median celiotomy and ligation in dogs, *Vet Surg* 34:273, 2005.
The laparoscopic procedure was significantly longer but associated with less pain than the median celiotomy procedure.

Haney Dr, Levy JK, Newell SM et al: Use of fetal skeletal mineralization for prediction of parturition date in cats, *J Am Vet Med Assoc* 223:1614, 2003.
Mineralization times of specific bones are described and predictive of parturition within 3 days in 75% of cats.

Holst BS, Bergström A, Lagerstedt AS: Characterization of the bacterial population of the genital tract of adult cats, *J Am Vet Med Assoc* 64:963, 2003.
Evaluation of cultures taken during ovariohysterectomy or castration in 66 female and 29 male cats is reported; findings include a predominantly aerobic population in females, and both aerobic and anaerobic populations in males.

Hori T, Mukai K, Komoriya K et al: Fertility of bitches in which estrus was prevented with implantations of chlormadinone acetate for four years, *J Vet Med Sci* 67:151, 2005.
Evaluation in eight dogs demonstrated effectiveness in preventing pregnancy; however, following removal of implants, pregnancy rates were low, and the majority developed uterine disease including pyometra and hydrometra.

Howe LM, Slater MR, Boothe HW et al: Long-term outcome of gonadectomy performed at an early age or traditional age in cats, *J Am Vet Med Assoc* 217:1661, 2000.
This cohort study of 263 cats followed for a median 37 months after early age gonadectomy reports no increased incidence of physical or behavioral problems compared with standard age gonadectomy.

Löfstedt RM, VanLeeuwen JA: Evaluation of a commercially available luteinizing hormone test for its ability to distinguish between ovariectomized and sexually intact bitches, *J Am Vet Med Assoc* 220:1331, 2002.
Sexually intact (101) and ovariectomized (199) bitches were evaluated, finding the test to have excellent sensitivity (98%) and moderate specificity (78%). This means that finding a single low serum LH concentration was an excellent indication that the dog was intact, but finding a single high LH was not a reliable indicator of ovariectomy.

Luvoni GC, Grioni A: Determination of gestational age in medium and small size bitches using ultrasonographic fetal measurements, *J Small Anim Pract* 41:292, 2000.
Prediction of parturition date was possible and accurate using measurements from the gestational sac, uterine horn and placenta, and a derived equation.

McGrath H, Hardie RJ, Davis E: Lateral flank approach for ovariohysterectomy in small animals, *Compend Cont Educ Pract Vet* 26:922, 2004.
The technique is described and indications, contraindications, advantages, and disadvantages are reviewed.

Miller NA, Van Lue SJ, Rawlings CA: Use of laparoscopic-assisted cryptorchidectomy in dogs and cats. *J Am Vet Med Assoc* 224:875, 2004.

The technique is described using two ports, and results in 13 animals are presented.

Minami S, Okamoto Y, Eguchi H et al: Successful laparoscopy assisted ovariohysterectomy in two dogs with pyometra, *J Vet Med Sci* 59:845, 1997.

This case report described using 4 ports and an ultrasonic scalpel to transect the ovarian pedicles and broad ligament before exteriorizing and ligating the uterine body through an extended caudal portal incision.

Moon PF, Erb HN, Ludders JW et al: Perioperative risk factors for puppies delivered by cesarean section in the United States and Canada, *J Am Anim Hosp Assoc* 36:359, 2000.

Data from 807 cesarean-delivered litters are reviewed; findings include immediate survival of 92% compared with 86% for naturally born puppies. Perioperative risk factors included emergency surgery, brachycephalic breed, and more than four puppies in the litter.

Moon-Massat PF, Erb HN: Perioperative factors associated with puppy vigor after delivery by cesarean section, *J Am Anim Hosp Assoc* 38:90, 2002.

Data from 807 litters delivered by cesarean section are reviewed; conclusions included that anesthetic risk factors associated with increased puppy vigor included the use of isoflurane and avoidance of ketamine, thiamylal, and thiopental.

Olson PN, Root Kustritz MV, Johnston SD: Early-age neutering of dogs and cats in the United States (a review), *J Reprod Fertility Supplement* 57:223, 2001.

This review discusses early age neutering practices and includes a review of scientific studies that have evaluated this practice.

Peña FJ, Gil MC: Mismating and abortion in bitches: the preossification period, *Compend Cont Educ Pract Vet* 24:556, 2002.

Various drug protocols for terminating pregnancy are discussed.

Peña FJ, Gil MC: Mismating and abortion in bitches: the preattachment period, *Compend Cont Educ Pract Vet* 24:400, 2002.

Recent advances in managing canine mismating are discussed along with methods of early pregnancy detection.

Schaer M, Halling KB, Collins KE et al: Combined hyponatremia and hyperkalemia mimicking acute hypoadrenocorticism in three pregnant dogs, *J Am Vet Med Assoc* 218:897, 2001.

This case report describes weakness, inappetence, vomiting, and collapse in these three near-term greyhounds, which resolved with emergency treatment and surgical delivery of their puppies.

Spain CV, Scarlett JM, Cully SM: When to neuter dogs and cats: a survey of New York state veterinarians' practices and beliefs, *J Am Anim Hosp Assoc* 38:482, 2002.

Questionnaire responses from 616 veterinarians reported that most routinely recommend neutering and perceived both benefits and risks to early neutering.

Stornelli A, Arauz M, Baschard H et al: Unilateral and bilateral vasectomy in the dog: alkaline phosphatase as an indicator of tubular patency, *Reprod Dom Anim* 38:1, 2003.

Investigation concluded that alkaline phosphatase levels in semen can be used as an early indicator of unilateral or bilateral patency of epididymal and deferent ducts in dogs.

Syerek-Intas K, Wehrend A, Nak Y et al: Unilateral hysterectomy (cornuectomy) in the bitch and its effect on subsequent fertility, *Theriogenology* 61:1713, 2004.

The left uterine horn was removed from 18 bitches and 12 were later bred, with 10 pregnancies resulting. This technique is advocated for bitches with pathology in one horn.

Van Goethem BEBJ, Rosenveldt KW, Kirpenstein JN: Monopolar versus bipolar electrocoagulation in canine laparoscopic ovariectomy: a nonrandomized, prospective, clinical trial, *Vet Surg* 32:464, 2003.

Ovariectomy was performed on 103 dogs and found that using bipolar electrocautery decreased surgical time, intraoperative hemorrhage, and facilitated exteriorization of the ovaries.

Väisänen M, Lilius EM, Mustonen L et al: Effects of ovariohysterectomy on canine blood neutrophil respiratory burst: a chemiluminescence study, *Vet Surg* 33:551, 2004.

Data from 42 dogs having ovariohysterectomy performed showed no significant alteration of one of the immune functions.

Van Nimwegen SA, Van Swol CFP, Kirpenstein J: Neodymium: yttrium aluminum garnet surgical laser versus bipolar electrocoagulation for laparoscopic ovariectomy in dogs, *Vet Surg* 34:353, 2005.

Ovariectomy was performed on 72 dogs, and it was found that using bipolar electrocautery resulted in less intraoperative mesovarial bleeding when compared with using the laser.

Surgery of the Female Reproductive Tract

SPECIFIC DISEASES

MAMMARY NEOPLASIA

DEFINITIONS

Lumpectomy is removal of a mass or part of a mamma; **simple mastectomy** is excision of an entire gland, and **regional mastectomy** is excision of the involved gland and adjacent glands. **Unilateral mastectomy** is the removal of all mammary glands, subcutaneous tissue, and associated lymphatics on one side of the midline, whereas **bilateral mastectomy** is the simultaneous removal of both mammary chains.

GENERAL CONSIDERATIONS AND CLINICALLY RELEVANT PATHOPHYSIOLOGY

Mammary tumors are uncommon in male dogs, but the most common tumor of female dogs. They are less common in cats, but still account for nearly one third of all feline tumors. Approximately 35% to 50% of canine mammary tumors and 90% of feline mammary tumors are malignant. Canine mammary tumor types are listed in Box 26-14. Malignant mammary tumors spread via lymphatics and blood vessels to regional lymph nodes and lungs. Other less common metastatic sites include the adrenal glands, kidneys, heart, liver, bone, brain, and skin.

The cause of mammary gland neoplasia is unknown; however, many are hormone-dependent, and most can be prevented if OHE is performed before 1 year of age. The risk of mammary tumors for dogs spayed before their first estrus is 0.05%. This risk increases to 8% after one estrus cycle and

BOX 26-14

Canine Mammary Masses

- Benign mixed tumors
- Carcinomas
  Solid carcinomas
  Tubular adenocarcinomas
  Papillary adenocarcinomas
  Anaplastic carcinomas
- Hyperplasia
- Adenomas
- Malignant mixed tumors
- Sarcomas
- Myeloepitheliomas

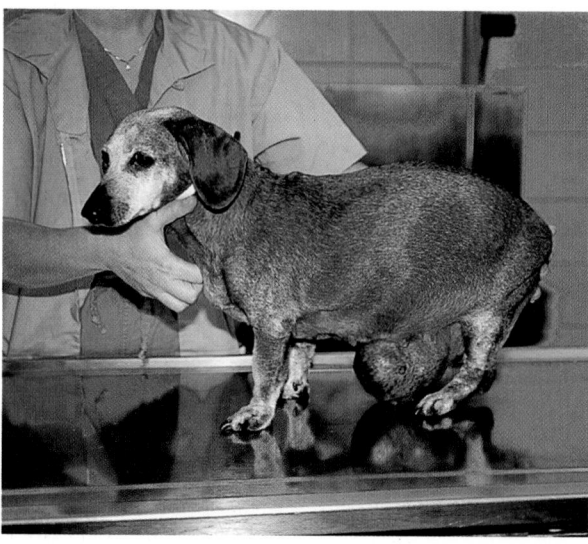

FIG. 26-18
Photograph of a large mammary tumor in a 13-year-old female dachshund.

26% after the second estrus. Cats ovariectomized before 6 months of age have a 9% risk, and those ovariectomized between 6 and 12 months have a 14% risk of developing mammary carcinomas compared with intact cats. Estrogen and/or progesterone receptors are found in 50% of malignant and 70% of benign canine mammary tumors. Dogs with tumors containing estrogen or progesterone receptors live longer than those without. Progesterone receptors are found in some feline mammary tumors. Progesterone administration may be associated with the development of malignant mammary tumors in cats and benign tumors in dogs. Dogs with benign mammary tumors have more than a threefold risk of developing malignant mammary tumors.

In dogs, benign tumors are usually classified as benign mixed tumors (fibroadenomas), adenomas, or benign mesenchymal tumors (Fig. 26-18). Most canine malignant mammary tumors are carcinomas (see Box 26-14); however, sarcomas (less than 5%) and carcinosarcomas (malignant mixed tumors) occur. Sarcomas metastasize more readily than carcinomas. Some "malignant" mammary tumors do not recur or spread after surgery. Papillary or tubular carcinomas have a better prognosis than solid or anaplastic carcinomas. Inflammatory carcinomas are poorly differentiated carcinomas with extensive mononuclear and polymorphonuclear cellular infiltrates. It may be difficult to differentiate mastitis from inflammatory carcinoma on physical examination or with cytology. These tumors grow rapidly, invading cutaneous lymphatics and causing marked edema, inflammation, and pain. Dogs are likely to be anorectic and weak, and experience weight loss. The tumors are poorly demarcated, firm, often ulcerated, and may involve both mammary chains. Some areas of involvement appear rashlike. Extensive lymphedema of the limbs may occur secondary to lymphatic occlusion or infiltration. Disseminated intravascular coagulation and thoracic metastasis are common with inflammatory carcinoma, and this tumor has a poor prognosis.

Most feline mammary tumors are adenocarcinomas (approximately 90%); however, other types of carcinomas and sarcomas occasionally occur (Box 26-15). Feline mammary tumors grow rapidly and metastasize to local lymph nodes

BOX 26-15

Mammary Tumors: Key Points

Most mammary tumors are prevented by OHE in the first year of life.
Male mammary tumors are rare but behave similar to those in females.
All mammary tumors should be evaluated when first identified.
Tumors in dogs are benign or malignant; 90% of those in cats are malignant.
Expectations are primarily dependent on histologic type.
Each mammary mass may be a different tumor, therefore remove them all.
Provided tumor-free margins are obtained, the tumor excision technique does not affect survival in dogs; perform a chain mastectomy in cats.
Do not excise inflammatory carcinomas; the prognosis is too poor.
Adjuvant therapy is not routinely recommended for malignant tumors.

and lungs early in the course of disease. Feline mammary tumors are not as well circumscribed as their canine counterparts; they are firm and often ulcerated. Mammary carcinomas in male cats behave similarly to those of females, but are less common. Feline mammary tumors must be differentiated from lobular hyperplasia and fibroepithelial hyperplasia. Hyperplasia is often associated with exogenous progesterone administration. A unilateral mastectomy is recommended to remove feline mammary tumors because local recurrence is common with less radical procedures. Cats with malignant mammary tumors generally survive less than 1 year.

DIAGNOSIS
Clinical Presentation

Signalment. Mammary tumors are common in female dogs and cats. The greatest frequency of mammary tumors is found in poodles, Boston terriers, fox terriers, Airedale terriers, dachshunds, Great Pyrenees, Samoyeds, keeshonden, and sporting breeds (pointers, retrievers, setters, and spaniels). Almost all feline mammary tumors (99%) occur in intact females. Most mammary tumors occur in middle-aged or older animals; they are rare in young animals. The incidence of mammary tumors increases greatly after 6 years of age. Dogs develop mammary tumors at a median age of 10 to 11 years, whereas feline carcinomas occur most often between 8 and 12 years of age.

History. Many mammary tumors are discovered during routine physical examination. Animals may be brought in because of a lump and/or abnormal discharge from the mammae. A delay of several months is common before a veterinarian evaluates the animal. Occasionally an animal with advanced disease is brought in because of dyspnea or lameness secondary to pulmonary or bone metastasis, respectively.

Physical Examination Findings

Mammary masses may be of various sizes (2 to 3 mm to 8 cm). The most common site for canine mammary tumors is the caudal mammary glands. Multiple masses may be found in one or both mammary chains. Most masses are easily movable, but occasionally are fixed to the underlying muscle or fascia. Masses may be sessile or pedunculated, solid or cystic, ulcerated or covered with skin and hair. Inflammatory carcinoma or mastitis should be suspected if the glands are diffusely swollen with poor demarcation between normal and abnormal tissue. Inflammatory carcinomas are often ulcerated. Axillary or inguinal lymph node enlargement may be palpable and sublumbar lymph node enlargement detected on rectal examination. Lameness or limb edema suggests metastasis. Weakness, anorexia, weight loss, and/or pain in the mammary region and limbs is common with inflammatory carcinoma.

Diagnostic Imaging

Thoracic radiographs (three views) should be evaluated for pulmonary metastasis. Thoracic metastasis occurs in 25% to 50% of dogs with malignant mammary tumors by the time of diagnosis. Pleural fluid may occur in cats with metastatic pulmonary disease. Abdominal radiographs should be evaluated for iliac lymph node enlargement with caudal tumors. Abdominal ultrasonography may detect abdominal metastasis. CT and MRI imaging may facilitate evaluation of invasive tumors and metastasis.

Laboratory Findings

Minimum data base (complete blood count [CBC], biochemistry profile, urinalysis) results are nonspecific for mammary neoplasia, but important in identifying concurrent geriatric problems or paraneoplastic syndromes. Aspiration or exfoliative cytology helps distinguish inflammatory, benign, and malignant masses. Detection of neoplastic cells in lymph node aspirates helps stage the disease. Pleural fluid should be evaluated cytologically. Bone scans help confirm bone metastasis. Definitive diagnosis is dependent on histopathology of biopsied or excised tissue. Each mass should be evaluated histologically because different tumor types may occur in the same individual. Immunohistochemical analysis of histologic specimens can provide useful prognostic information.

DIFFERENTIAL DIAGNOSIS

Mammary hypertrophy, mastitis, granulomas, duct ectasia, skin tumors, or foreign bodies (e.g., BB pellet or shot) are differential diagnoses. Mammary hypertrophy from endogenous or exogenous progesterone stimulation commonly occurs in young intact female cats 2 to 4 weeks after estrus (when progesterone concentrations are elevated). Hypertrophy can usually be ruled out based on history and cytologic findings. Mastitis occurs after estrus, parturition, or false pregnancy; the swelling is usually more localized than with inflammatory carcinoma.

MEDICAL MANAGEMENT

Reports on the efficacy of treatment modalities other than surgery are lacking. Chemotherapy may be beneficial in controlling some malignant tumors. Antiestrogens (tamoxifen; 0.4 to 0.8 mg/kg/d PO for 4 to 8 weeks), antiprogestins (aglepristone, Europe only), or antiprolactin drugs (cabergoline 5 μg/kg/day PO for 1 week before surgery) are advocated by some. Chemotherapy, radiation therapy, and hormonal therapy are not routinely recommended as an adjunct to surgery.

SURGICAL TREATMENT

Excision is the treatment of choice for all mammary tumors except inflammatory carcinomas. Excision allows histologic diagnosis and can be curative, improve quality of life, or modify disease progression. Inflammatory carcinomas are extremely aggressive, and surgery is of no value in controlling or palliating the disease. Selection of a surgical technique for removing the tumor and variable amounts of mammary tissue depends on tumor size, location and consistency, patient status, and surgeon preference. Survival is not influenced by technique unless incomplete resection is performed. However, local recurrence is decreased in cats when unilateral mastectomy is performed rather than lumpectomy. A combination of different techniques may be selected if an animal has several masses in both chains. All tumors should be excised because each mass may be a different tumor type. If complete excision is impossible with a single surgery, a second procedure should be delayed 3 to 4 weeks to allow healing and relaxation of stretched skin. OHE may be performed when the tumor is removed. OHE should be done before mastectomy to prevent seeding the abdominal cavity with tumor cells. Although OHE will not prevent further development of mammary tumors, it will prevent uterine disease (e.g., pyometra and metritis) and eliminate female hormonal influence on existing tumors.

Lumpectomy or *partial mammectomy* is the excision of a mass and a surrounding margin of grossly normal mammary tissue (greater than or equal to 1 cm). It is used when the mass is small (less than 5 mm), encapsulated, noninvasive, and at the periphery of the gland. Milk and lymph leakage from incised mammary tissue into the wound may cause postoperative inflammation and discomfort. *Simple mastectomy* is the excision of the entire gland containing the tumor. It is used when the tumor involves the central area of the gland or the majority of the gland. Removal of the entire gland may be easier than incising mammary tissue and prevents postoperative problems with milk and lymph leakage. *Regional mastectomy* involves excision of the involved and adjacent glands. This technique is selected when multiple tumors occur in adjacent glands in the chain or when the mass occurs between two glands. It is sometimes technically easier to remove the confluent caudal abdominal and inguinal glands than either gland alone. *Unilateral mastectomy* is performed when numerous tumors occur throughout the chain. A unilateral mastectomy may take less time and be less traumatic than multiple lumpectomies or mastectomies. *Bilateral mastectomy* can be performed when numerous masses occur in both chains; however, skin closure can be extremely difficult or impossible. Therefore it is not recommended. Instead, staged unilateral mastectomies are preferred.

> NOTE: Separate mammary masses on the same dog may be of different histologic types; therefore excise all masses and submit them for histologic examination. Be sure to mark them so that you can determine which mass originated from which site when the biopsy report returns.

Preoperative Management

A complete work-up to determine the stage of the disease and identify other problems that may alter the prognosis is important. Ulcerated, infected masses should be treated with warm compresses and antibiotics for several days before surgery to reduce inflammation and allow the gross tumor margins to be more accurately assessed. Preoperative antibiotics are necessary only in severely debilitated patients or those with evidence of infection. If renal disease (e.g., secondary to hypercalcemia or malignancy) is present, preoperative fluids should be administered. The entire ventral abdomen and caudal thorax should be clipped. Each mammary chain should be carefully palpated and the location of each mass mapped. Additional masses are frequently identified once the hair has been removed.

Anesthesia

A variety of anesthetic protocols can be used in animals with mammary masses. General anesthetic is usually less stressful to the patient than local anesthetic, even when

 BOX 26-16

Major Blood Vessels Supplying the Mammary Glands of Dogs and Cats

Mammary Glands 1 and 2
Ventral and lateral branches of the intercostal, internal thoracic, and lateral thoracic vessels

Mammary Glands 2 and 3
Cranial superficial epigastric vessels

Mammary Glands 4 and 5
Caudal superficial epigastric vessels

small lumps are resected. Consider administering an opioid epidural preoperatively or postoperatively if a large area of tissue is removed.

Surgical Anatomy

Dogs usually have five pairs of mammary glands; cats have four pairs. Mammary glands are compound, tubuloalveolar, apocrine glands. The caudal superficial epigastric arteries and veins supply the caudal glands (Box 26-16). The caudal superficial epigastric artery arises from the external pudendal artery near the superficial inguinal lymph node. Branches of the cranial and caudal superficial epigastric arteries anastomose. The cranial thoracic mammae are supplied by the fourth, fifth, and sixth ventral and lateral cutaneous vessels and nerves (from intercostals) and branches of the lateral thoracic vessels (from axillary artery). The caudal thoracic mammae are supplied by the sixth and seventh cutaneous nerves, and vessels and branches of the cranial superficial epigastric vessels. The cranial superficial epigastric vessels supply the cranial abdominal mamma and skin over the rectus abdominis muscle. The axillary lymph node drains the three cranial glands, and the inguinal lymph node drains the two caudal glands. However, there are lymphatic connections between glands and across the midline.

Positioning

Position the patient in dorsal recumbency with the thoracic limbs fixed cranially and the pelvic limbs fixed caudally in a relaxed position. The entire ventral abdomen, caudal thorax, and inguinal areas should be clipped and prepared for aseptic surgery.

SURGICAL TECHNIQUE

Make an elliptical incision around the involved mammary gland(s), a minimum of 1 cm from the tumor (Fig. 26-19, A). Continue the incision through subcutaneous tissue to the fascia of the external abdominal wall. Avoid incising mammary tissue; however, this is often impossible because mammary tissue may be confluent between adjacent glands. The midline separation between mammary chains is distinct.

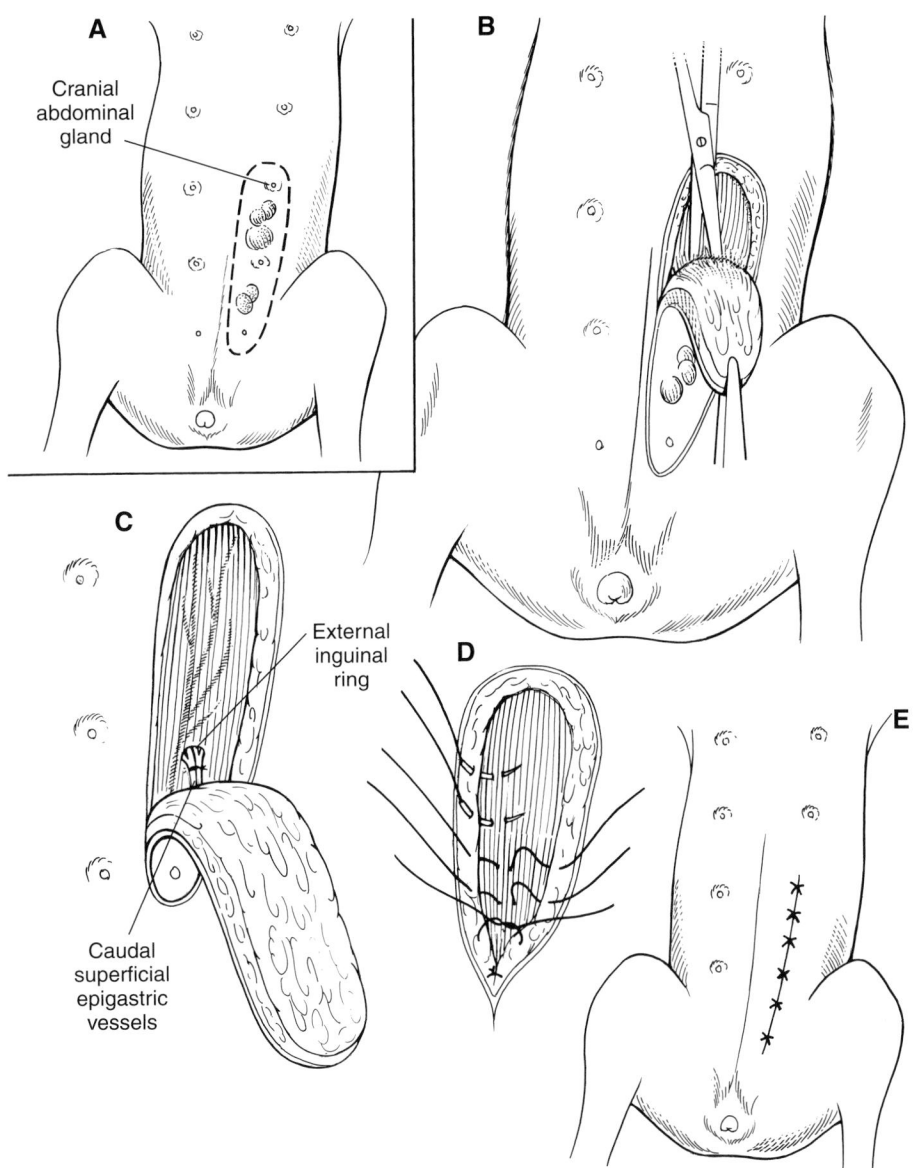

FIG. 26-19
A, For caudal mastectomy, make an elliptical incision around the glands to be excised.
B, Incise subcutaneous tissue to expose the abdominal fascia. Elevate the cranial edge of
the segment and separate subcutaneous tissue from the fascia by sliding sharp scissors
along the abdominal fascia. **C,** Ligate and divide the caudal superficial epigastric vessels
near the inguinal ring. **D,** Advance skin edges to the center of the defect with walking
sutures and subcuticular sutures. **E,** Appose skin edges with appositional sutures.

Control superficial hemorrhage with electrocoagulation, hemostats, and/or ligation. Perform an en bloc excision by elevating one edge of the incision and dissecting subcutaneous tissue from the pectoral and rectus fascia using a smooth gliding motion of the scissors (Fig. 26-19, B). Use traction on the elevated skin segment to facilitate dissection.

Abdominal and inguinal glands are loosely attached by fat and connective tissue and easily separated from rectus fascia. Thoracic glands adhere to the underlying pectoral muscles with little intervening fat or connective tissue.

Resect the inguinal fat pad and lymph node(s) with the inguinal mammary gland. The axillary lymph node is not included with en bloc resection of the thoracic glands. Excise fascia if the tumor has invaded subcutaneous tissue. Some neoplastic lesions will invade the abdominal musculature, and excision must include a portion of the abdominal wall.

Continue gliding scissor dissection until major vessels (i.e., cranial superficial epigastrics and caudal superficial epigastrics) to the gland are encountered. Isolate and ligate these vessels (Fig. 26-19, C). Ligate the cranial superficial epigastric vessel where it penetrates the rectus abdominis between the caudal thoracic and cranial abdominal (third) mammary glands (see Box 26-16). Ligate the caudal superficial epigastric vessel adjacent to the inguinal fat pad near the inguinal ring (see Box 26-16). Ligate branches supplying the first and second thoracic mammary glands (see Box 26-16) as they are encountered penetrating the pectoral muscles. Lavage the wound and evaluate for abnormal tissue. Undermine the wound edges, and advance skin toward the center of the defect with walking sutures (see Fig. 15-4). If dead space is extensive, place a closed suction or Penrose drain to help prevent fluid accumulation. Appose skin edges with a subcutaneous or subcuticular suture pattern (Fig. 26-19, E). Use 3-0 or 4-0 monofilament absorbable suture (polydioxanone, poliglecaprone 25, glycomer 631, or polyglyconate) on a swaged-on taper point needle in either an interrupted or continuous pattern.

Skin apposition is most difficult in the thoracic region because the skin is less mobile and the ribs make the area less compressible than the abdomen.

Use an axillary or flank fold skin flap to close the defect if tension is excessive (see pp. 207 and 208). Use appositional monofilament absorbable skin sutures (e.g., 3-0 or 4-0 nylon, polybutester, or polypropylene) or staples. Place a padded circumferential bandage to compress dead space, mobilize tissue, and support the wound.

POSTOPERATIVE CARE AND ASSESSMENT

Analgesics (see Chapter 13; for dosages of opioids see Table 13-4 on p. 133) and supportive care should be given as needed. An abdominal bandage should support the wound, compress dead space, and absorb fluid. Bandages are changed daily for the first 2 to 3 days, or as necessary to keep them dry. The wound should be inspected for inflammation, swelling, drainage, seroma, dehiscence, and necrosis. Any drains should be removed when drainage diminishes to a minimal amount (usually within 3 to 5 days). Bandages and sutures are generally removed 5 to 7 days and 7 to 10 days postoperatively, respectively. Patients with malignant tumors should be reevaluated for local recurrence and metastasis every 3 to 4 months.

COMPLICATIONS

Complications include pain, inflammation, hemorrhage, seroma formation, infection, ischemic necrosis, self-trauma, dehiscence, hind limb edema, and tumor recurrence. In dogs, local recurrence occurs within 2 years and varies from 20% to 73%.

PROGNOSIS

Significant prognostic factors in dogs are provided in Box 26-17. Significant prognostic factors in cats are tumor size, extent of surgery, and histologic grading. Risk of metastatic disease increases and survival time decreases with increasing primary tumor size. The prognosis for dogs with benign tumors is good with surgery. The prognosis for dogs with

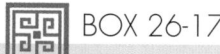

BOX 26-17

Significant Prognostic Factors for Mammary Tumors in Dogs

- Histologic type and immunohistochemical characteristics
- Degree of invasion
- Degree of nuclear differentiation and DNA ploidy
- Evidence of lymphoid cellular reactivity
- Tumor size
- Lymph node involvement
- Hormone receptor activity
- Presence of ulceration
- Fixation
- S-phase rate

DNA, Deoxyribonucleic acid.

malignant tumors is variable and depends on several factors, including tumor type and stage. Most dogs with malignant tumors without obvious metastasis at the time of surgery die or are euthanized for tumor-related problems within 1 to 2 years. Those with metastatic disease at the time of diagnosis have a shorter median survival (5 months versus 28 months) (Philbert et al, 2003). In dogs, tumors less than 3 cm have a better prognosis (35% recurrence at 2 years; 22 months survival) than tumors greater than 3 cm in diameter (80% recurrence at 2 years; 14 months survival). In cats, tumors less than 2 cm have less local recurrence than those greater than 2 to 3 cm. Cats with mammary carcinoma greater than 3 cm have a median survival of 6 months, whereas those with tumors less than 2 cm have a median survival of about 3 years. Queens with tumors less than or equal to 8 cm³ in volume have the longest disease-free interval and median survival times (4.5 years after surgery). Queens with local disease rather than vascular or lymphatic tumor invasion had longer survival (22 months versus 13 months, respectively). Likewise a low mitotic index had a better prognosis than a high one (22 months versus 12 months, respectively), and a low AgNOR index was more favorable than a high index (22 months versus 14 months, respectively) (Preziosi et al, 2002). The presence of multiple tumors does not affect the prognosis in dogs, but may decrease survival in cats.

Adenocarcinomas confined to the duct epithelium have a good prognosis after surgery. The prognosis worsens when neoplastic cells extend beyond the duct system and is poorest when neoplastic cells are found in blood or lymphatic vessels. Poorly differentiated adenocarcinomas have a 90% recurrence rate 2 years after surgery. The recurrence rate for moderately differentiated versus well-differentiated tumors is 68% versus 24%, respectively, 2 years after surgery. Median survival time for dogs with anaplastic carcinomas is 2.5 months compared with 21 months for adenocarcinoma, 16 months for solid carcinoma, and 14 months for other malignant tumors (Philbert et al, 2003). Mammary gland sarcoma and inflammatory carcinoma have a very poor prognosis.

OHE at the time of tumor removal improved survival in one study (Sorenmo et al, 2000), but in others it did not affect survival or recurrence. Treatment modalities other than surgery may slow tumor progression, but few data are available to accurately predict their effectiveness.

References

Philbert JC, Snyder PW, Glickman N et al: Influence of host factors on survival in dogs with malignant mammary gland tumors, *J Vet Intern Med* 17:102-106, 2003.

Preziosi R, Sarli G, Benassi L et al: Multiparametric survival analysis of histological stage and proliferative activity of feline mammary carcinomas, *Res Vet Sci* 73:53-60, 2002.

Sorenmo KU, Shofer FS, Goldschmidt MH: Effects of spaying and timing of spaying on survival of dogs with mammary carcinomas, *J Vet Intern Med* 14:266, 2000.

Suggested Reading

Alenza MDP, Peña L, Del Castillo N et al: Factors influencing the incidence and prognosis of canine mammary tumours, *J Small Anim Pract* 41:287, 2000.

This review article discusses risk factors influencing mammary tumors in dogs.

Alenza MDP, Tabanera E, Peña L: Inflammatory mammary carcinoma in dogs: 33 cases (1995-1999), *J Am Vet Med Assoc* 219:1110, 2001.

Dogs with inflammatory carcinoma were compared with 153 dogs with other types of malignant mammary tumors and described a hallmark for the pathologic diagnosis to be dermal lymphatic involvement.

Gobello C: Canine mammary tumors: an endocrine clinical approach, *Compend Cont Educ Pract Vet* 23:705, 2001.

This review article discusses the etiopathology and clinical aspects of the condition.

Miller AS, Kottler SJ, Cohn LA et al: Mammary duct ectasia in dogs: 51 cases (1992-1999), *J Am Vet Med Assoc* 218:1303, 2001.

Duct ectasia represented 2.8% of mammary biopsy specimens and was usually cured by mastectomy.

Overley B, Shofer FS, Goldschmidt MH et al: Association between ovariohysterectomy and feline mammary carcinoma, *J Vet Intern Med* 19:560, 2005.

Data were collated and compared from 308 cases and 400 controls; findings included an occurrence of mammary carcinoma of 9% if spayed before 6 months and 14% if spayed between 6 and 12 months.

Simon D, Knebel JW, Baumgärtner W et al: In vitro efficacy of chemotherapeutics as determined by 50% inhibitory concentrations in cell cultures of mammary gland tumors obtained from dogs, *Am J Vet Res* 62:1825, 2001.

This study used 30 tumors to establish cell cultures to investigate cell inhibition by doxorubicin, cisplatin, and carboplatin.

Skorupski KA, Overley B, Shofer FS et al: Clinical characteristics of mammary carcinoma in male cats, *J Vet Intern Med* 19:52-55, 2005.

Data collected from 39 affected male cats are reported; findings were similar to those for female cats.

Winston J, Craft DM, Scase TJ et al: Immunohistochemical detection of HER-2/neu expression in spontaneous feline mammary tumours, *Vet Comp Oncol* 3:8, 2005.

Data from 30 affected cats suggest that Her-2/neu is overexpressed in affected cats, which may serve as a model for human breast cancer.

Yazawa M, Okuda M, Setoguchi A et al: Telomere length and telomerase activity in canine mammary gland tumors, *Am J Vet Res* 62:1539, 2001.

This study investigated telomere length in 27 tumors and found that telomere length is maintained despite the dog's age and suggests that it may be useful for monitoring the effects of telomerase inhibitors.

Yazawa M, Setoguchi A, Hong SH et al: Effect of an adenoviral vector that expresses the canine p53 gene on cell growth of canine osteosarcoma and mammary adenocarcinoma cell lines, *Am J Vet Res* 64:880, 2003.

This study found that an adenoviral vector that expressed the canine p53 gene induced growth inhibition in a dose-dependent manner, which may be useful in gene treatment of dogs with tumors.

UTERINE NEOPLASIA

DEFINITIONS

Leiomyoma and **leiomyosarcoma** are benign and malignant smooth muscle tumors, respectively, that may occur in the uterus. **Uterine adenocarcinomas** are malignant tumors of the uterine glands.

GENERAL CONSIDERATIONS AND CLINICALLY RELEVANT PATHOPHYSIOLOGY

Uterine neoplasia is rare in dogs and cats; most tumors are incidental findings at necropsy or during abdominal exploration. Uterine tumors are more common in cats than other reproductive tract tumors. Tumors that may occur in the uterus are listed in Box 26-18. They may develop in the remnant of the uterine body following OHE and may have concurrent mammary tumors. Concurrent pathologic conditions may include cystic ovaries, cystic endometrial hyperplasia, and pyometra, suggesting a common hormonal influence.

Most uterine tumors are leiomyomas that arise from the myometrium. Leiomyomas are benign and generally noninvasive and slow growing. They may protrude into the uterine lumen on a stalk or cause the wall to bulge externally. German shepherd dogs have a syndrome characterized by multiple uterine leiomyomas, bilateral renal cystadenocarcinomas, and nodular dermatofibrosis. The most common malignant tumors of bitches and queens are leiomyosarcoma and endometrial adenocarcinoma, respectively. Leiomyosarcomas are grossly difficult to distinguish from leiomyomas. They are invasive tumors, usually slow to metastasize. Adenocarcinomas cause the endometrium to become thickened and nodular. The tumor may be solid or cystic, sessile, or polypoid, and may obliterate the uterine lumen. Multicentric adenocarcinoma has been reported. Metastasis is usually present at the time of diagnosis and may involve cerebrum, eyes, ovaries, adrenal glands, thyroid glands, lungs, liver, kidneys, bladder, intestines, pancreas, pericardium, myocardium, diaphragm, and/or regional lymph nodes.

BOX 26-18

Uterine Tumors

- Leiomyoma
- Leiomyosarcoma
- Adenocarcinoma
- Lipoma
- Fibroma
- Adenoma
- Fibrosarcoma

DIAGNOSIS
Clinical Presentation

Signalment. No breed predilections have been reported. Most affected animals are middle-aged or older.

History. Most uterine tumors are asymptomatic unless they are large and compress the gastrointestinal or urinary tracts. Animals may have abnormal estrus cycles and/or a mucoid or hemorrhagic vaginal discharge because of tumor irritation and vascular erosion. Uterine tumors may obstruct the cervix and cause pyometra; therefore presenting clinical signs may include a purulent vaginal discharge, pyrexia, anorexia, vomiting, polydipsia, and/or polyuria. Tumor growth may compress the colon, bladder, or urethra, causing straining or obstruction. Other signs may include abdominal distention, dysuria, hematuria, dyspnea, and/or loss of consciousness.

Physical Examination Findings

Physical examination is often normal, although large masses may be palpated. A hemorrhagic vaginal discharge may be noted. Some uterine masses are palpable during rectal examination. Enlarged, asymmetric sublumbar lymph nodes may be palpated if the tumor has metastasized. Digital vaginal examination is usually normal. Animals with pyometra may be depressed, febrile, and pain-sensitive on abdominal palpation, and may have a purulent vaginal discharge (see p. 738).

Diagnostic Imaging

Radiography and ultrasonography may show a mass in the uterine area. The echogenicity of uterine masses is variable. Ultrasound-guided biopsies may provide information regarding tumor type. Abdominal radiographs, CT, and MRI images should be evaluated for evidence of lymph node enlargement or visceral metastasis, and thoracic radiographs (three views) should be evaluated for metastasis.

Vaginoscopy. Vaginoscopy may reveal abnormal discharge. Neoplastic cells may be identified from specimens obtained by endoscopic transcervical uterine cannulation if the tumor invades or involves the endometrium.

Laboratory Findings

Hematologic and serum biochemical profile results are nonspecific. The patient may be anemic if a chronic hemorrhagic discharge or paraneoplastic syndrome is present.

Neoplastic cells are rarely identified on vaginal cytology. Definitive diagnosis requires histopathology.

DIFFERENTIAL DIAGNOSIS

Differential diagnoses for uterine masses include intestinal foreign bodies, tumor or fungal lesions, urinary tract masses, or lymph node enlargement secondary to neoplasia or inflammation. Differential diagnoses for vaginal discharge include estrus, parturition, abortion, placentitis, normal lochia, vaginitis, metritis, pyometra, placental subinvolution, mucometra, uterine torsion, or trauma.

MEDICAL MANAGEMENT

Effectiveness of chemotherapy and radiation therapy on uterine masses is unknown.

SURGICAL TREATMENT

OHE is the treatment of choice for uterine tumors.

Preoperative Management

Hydration, electrolyte, and acid-base abnormalities should be corrected before surgery. Patients with elevated blood urea nitrogen or creatinine concentrations should be given diuretics before surgery. If pyometra is present, antibiotic therapy should be initiated (see Box 26-5 on p. 707). Mature patients should fast for 12 to 18 hours before anesthetic induction.

Anesthesia

A variety of anesthetic protocols can be used in animals with uterine tumors if they are not debilitated and do not have concurrent pyometra. Anesthetic recommendations for animals with pyometra are provided on p. 741.

Surgical Anatomy

Surgical anatomy of the reproductive tract is discussed on p. 706.

Positioning

Patients are positioned in dorsal recumbency for a ventral midline celiotomy. The entire ventral abdomen and caudal thorax should be clipped and prepared for aseptic surgery.

SURGICAL TECHNIQUE

Perform a ventral midline celiotomy. Explore the abdomen for evidence of metastasis or other abnormalities. Take a biopsy or excise abnormal structures. Perform an OHE (see p. 709), removing the cervix if it is within 1 to 2 cm of the tumor. Culture the uterus if metritis or pyometra is suspected.

POSTOPERATIVE CARE AND ASSESSMENT

Fluid therapy should be continued if the patient was dehydrated or azotemic, and postoperative analgesics should be given as needed (see Chapter 13; for dosages of opioids see Table 13-4 on p. 133). Antibiotics are unnecessary unless a uterine infection was identified. Thoracic and abdominal radiographs should be evaluated periodically (e.g., 1 to 2 months, 6 months) if a malignant tumor was present. Complications of OHE are discussed on p. 726. The tumor may recur locally or metastasize.

PROGNOSIS

The prognosis for asymptomatic benign tumors without surgery is good unless the mass enlarges and impinges on gastrointestinal or urinary tracts. The prognosis following OHE is excellent for benign tumors and good for malignant tumors without evidence of metastasis or local infiltration. The prognosis for uterine adenocarcinomas is guarded because of its propensity to metastasize before diagnosis. The effectiveness of other treatment modalities for uterine tumors is unknown.

Suggested Reading

Miller MA, Ramos-Vara JA, Dickerson MF et al: Uterine neoplasia in 13 cats, *J Vet Diagn Invest* 15:575, 2003.
Clinical and pathologic findings are presented; in this group of cats, adenocarcinomas were more common than leiomyomas and leiomyosarcomas.

PYOMETRA

DEFINITIONS

Pyometra is an accumulation of purulent material within the uterus. Pyometra is sometimes referred to as *cystic endometrial hyperplasia-pyometra complex*. Uterine distention with sterile fluid is referred to as **hydrometra** (watery secretions) or **mucometra** (mucoid secretions), or **hematometra** (bloody secretions).

GENERAL CONSIDERATIONS AND CLINICALLY RELEVANT PATHOPHYSIOLOGY

Pyometra is a potentially life-threatening condition associated with cystic endometrial hyperplasia. Cystic endometrial hyperplasia and pyometra both develop during diestrus. Occasionally the diagnosis is delayed and unrecognized until anestrus. In dogs, the diestrual period of a normal, nongravid bitch lasts approximately 70 days. The uterus is influenced by progesterone produced by ovarian corpora lutea. Progesterone stimulates the growth and secretory activity of the endometrial glands and reduces myometrial activity. Cystic endometrial hyperplasia is an abnormal uterine response that develops during diestrus (luteal phase of cycle) when there is high or prolonged ovarian production of progesterone or exogenously administered progesterone. Excessive progesterone influence or an exaggerated progesterone response causes the uterine glandular tissue to become cystic, edematous, thickened, and infiltrated by lymphocytes and plasma cells. Fluid accumulates in endometrial glands and the uterine lumen with cystic endometrial hyperplasia. Uterine drainage is hindered by progesterone inhibition of myometrial contractility. This abnormal uterine environment allows bacterial colonization to cause pyometra. Administration of estrogen increases the risk of pyometra during diestrus. The risk of an intact bitch developing pyometra before 10 years of age is 23% to 25% (Egenvall et al, 2001).

 BOX 26-19

Organisms Most Commonly Cultured From Dogs With Pyometra

- *Escherichia coli*
- *Staphylococcus aureus**
- *Streptococcus* spp.*
- *Pseudomonas* spp.*
- *Proteus* spp.*
- *Pasteurella* spp.
- *Klebsiella* spp.
- *Haemophilus* spp.
- *Serratia* spp.
- *Moraxella* spp.

*Also found as normal vaginal flora.

Estrogen increases the number of uterine progesterone receptors, which may explain the increased incidence of pyometra after estrogens are administered to prevent pregnancy. Uterine tumors sometimes obstruct the outflow of uterine secretions and may contribute to development of pyometra. Feline pyometra is less frequent than canine pyometra because development of luteal tissue requires copulation or artificially induced ovulation; however, cats treated with progestins for skin disease have an increased incidence of pyometra.

Infection causes the morbidity and mortality associated with pyometra. Leukocyte response to bacteria is inhibited in a progesterone-primed uterus. *Escherichia coli* is the most common organism identified in canine and feline pyometra. *E. coli* has an affinity for the endometrium and myometrium. Bacterial invasion is thought to be opportunistic because the most commonly isolated organisms are also normal vaginal flora (Box 26-19). Bacterial virulence is associated with the serotype, presence of K antigen, and cytotoxin necrotizing factor. Ascension of fecal flora into the uterus is the primary route of infection based on biochemical fingerprinting of bacteria. Other bacterial sources include the urinary tract and transient bacteremia. Vaginal discharge occurs if the cervix is patent or "open." A closed cervix prevents discharge of infected fluid and causes more serious disease. Animals may become dehydrated and toxic. Septicemia and endotoxemia can develop if pyometra is untreated. Compression or overdistention of the uterus may allow infected uterine contents to leak out of the oviducts and cause peritonitis. Torsion of the distended uterus may also occur.

Concurrent abnormalities in animals with pyometra may include hypoglycemia, renal and hepatic dysfunction, anemia, and/or cardiac abnormalities (Box 26-20). Pyometra is often associated with systemic inflammatory response syndrome caused by production and release of inflammatory mediators with systemic effects (Box 26-21). Hypoglycemia is common in canine pyometra. Sepsis and systemic inflammatory response syndrome deplete glycogen stores, increase peripheral glucose use, and decrease gluconeogenesis. Transient hyperglycemia occasionally occurs because of excessive catecholamine and glucagon release. Progesterone-induced

BOX 26-20

Potential Abnormalities in Animals With Pyometra

• Hypoglycemia	• Anemia
• Renal dysfunction	• Cardiac arrhythmias
• Hepatic dysfunction	• Coagulation abnormalities

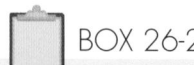 BOX 26-21

Criteria for Diagnosis of Systemic Inflammatory Response Syndrome*

Heart rate: Greater than 160 bpm
Temperature: Greater than 103.5° F or less than 100° F
Respiration: Rate greater than 20 breaths/min or partial pressure of CO_2 less than 32 mm Hg
White blood cell count: Greater than 12,000/μl, less than 4000/μl, or greater than 10% band neutrophils

*Diagnosis is made if two of the four criteria are present.

growth hormone production may cause persistent hyperglycemia and glucosuria. Judicious insulin treatment may be required in patients with persistent hyperglycemia (i.e. greater than 300 mg/dl) after appropriate medical and surgical treatment.

Patients with pyometra may have prerenal azotemia, primary glomerular disease, reduced tubular concentrating ability, tubular interstitial disease, reduced glomerular filtration, and/or concurrent renal disease unrelated to the pyometra. Prerenal azotemia is due to poor perfusion, dehydration, and shock. Primary glomerular disease occurs secondary to immune-complex glomerulonephritis. Bacterial antigens also interfere with renal tubular concentrating ability. Once the bacterial antigen is removed, these changes resolve and normal renal function returns. Reduced tubular concentrating ability is from inhibition of antidiuretic hormone at the level of the renal tubule by bacterial endotoxins, obligatory solute load from decreased glomerular filtration rate, and other unknown factors. Normal tubular concentrating ability usually returns 2 to 8 weeks after OHE. Hepatocellular injury may be secondary to intrahepatic cholestasis and retention of bile pigments, toxicity from sepsis and endotoxemia, and/or poor perfusion.

Anemia may be caused by chronic inflammation suppressing erythropoiesis, loss of red cells into the uterine lumen, hemodilution, or surgical blood loss. Nonregenerative anemia should spontaneously resolve a few weeks after OHE. Coagulation deficits infrequently occur secondary to concurrent metabolic imbalances. Cardiac arrhythmias result from toxic effects of pyometra, shock, acidosis, and electrolyte imbalance.

DIAGNOSIS
Clinical Presentation

Signalment. Pyometra affects intact dogs more commonly than cats. There is no breed predisposition in dogs although some reports (Egenvall et al 2001; Niskanen and Thrusfield, 1998) indicate a modestly increased risk in various breeds (golden retrievers, miniature schnauzers, Irish terrier, rough St. Bernard, leonberger, Airedale terrier, Cavalier King Charles spaniel, rough collie, rottweiler, Bernese Mountain dogs, and English cocker spaniels). Domestic shorthair and Siamese cats are affected more commonly than other breeds. Pyometra generally occurs in older (6 to 11 years, median 9 years) intact bitches and queens; however, it may occur in younger animals that have been given exogenous estrogen (dogs) or progestins (cats). Nulliparous bitches are at moderately greater risk for pyometra than are primiparous and multiparous bitches.

History. Pyometra usually occurs several weeks (i.e., in cats 1 to 4, in dogs 4 to 8) after estrus, or following mismating injections or exogenous administration of estrogens or progestins. The animal may have a purulent or bloody vaginal discharge. Others have obvious abdominal distention, fever, partial-to-complete anorexia, lethargy, polyuria, polydipsia, vomiting, diarrhea, and/or weight loss. Animals with closed pyometra more commonly have vomiting and diarrhea.

Physical Examination Findings

A purulent blood-tinged vaginal discharge may occur if the cervix is open. Uterine enlargement may be detected on abdominal palpation. Dehydration is frequent. Animals with endotoxemia or septicemia may be in shock, hypothermic, and/or moribund. Fever is infrequent.

Diagnostic Imaging

A fluid-filled uterus should be detected on abdominal radiographs (Fig. 26-20) and/or ultrasonography (Fig. 26-21). The enlarged uterus is located in the caudal abdomen and may displace intestines cranially and dorsally. Open pyometra or uterine rupture may cause enough drainage so that the uterus is not radiographically detected. Displacing the intestines with a wooden spoon or abdominal bandage may improve uterine visualization, but should be performed with caution if the uterus is significantly distended because it may induce rupture. Signs of uterine rupture and peritonitis (i.e., poor visceral detail) should be noted.

It is important to rule out pregnancy. Radiographic confirmation of pyometra may not be possible until 41 to 43 days after ovulation. Radiographically, fetal calcification can be identified after approximately 45 days of gestation. Ultrasonography can identify fetal structures (see Table 26-3), assess fetal viability, identify uterine fluid, and determine uterine wall thickness and irregularities. Pyometra, hydrometra, mucometra, or hematometra may appear similar ultrasonographically and radiographically. However, although mucometra and hydrometra typically are associated with

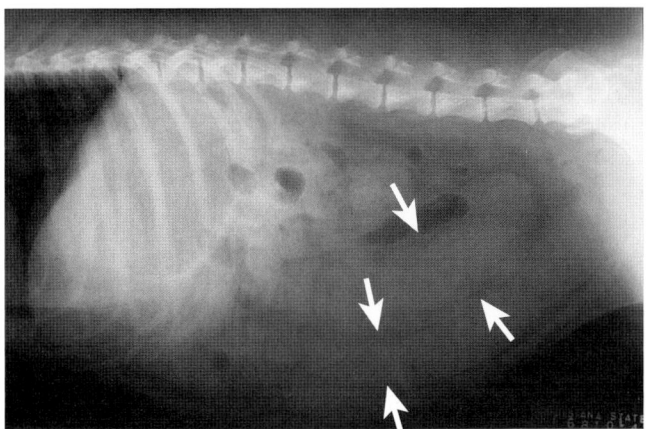

FIG. 26-20
Lateral abdominal radiograph of a dog with pyometra. Note the enlarged uterus *(arrows)* in the caudoventral abdomen displacing viscera cranially and dorsally.

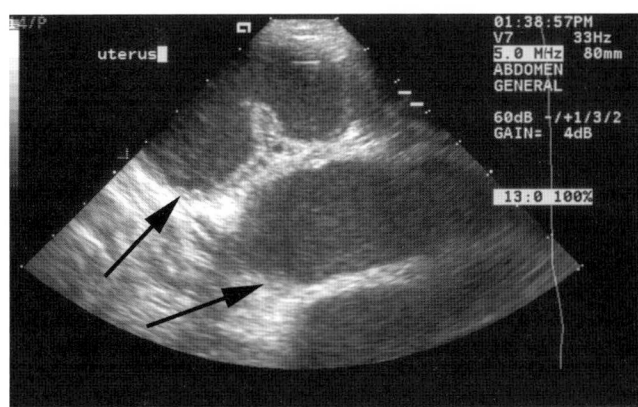

FIG. 26-21
Parasagittal ultrasound image of the caudal abdomen of a dog with pyometra. Note the enlarged, fluid-filled uterus *(arrows)*, which is convoluted. The fluid within the lumen of the uterus is mildly echogenic.

anechoic fluid within the uterine lumen on ultrasound, the fluid associated with pyometra is typically echogenic.

Laboratory Findings

Metabolic clinicopathologic abnormalities may occur. The most common hemogram findings are neutrophilia with a left shift, monocytosis, and white blood cell toxicity. White blood cell numbers usually exceed 30,000/μL with closed pyometras and may be as high as 100,000 to 200,000/μL. However, normal numbers of white blood cells are often seen with open pyometras. Leukopenia may indicate overwhelming infection and septicemia or uterine sequestration of neutrophils. Increased leukocyte count and decreased lymphocyte count are directly proportional to the disease severity. The high percentage of bands in most pyometras helps differentiate them from cystic endometrial hyperplasia with mucometra. Mild normocytic, normochromic, nonregenerative anemia or nonregenerative, microcytic, hypochromic anemia may occur. Clotting abnormalities and disseminated intravascular coagulation may occur in severely affected patients.

> NOTE: Do not rule out pyometra in animals with leukopenia or normal white cell counts. Sequestration of neutrophils in the enlarged uterus may cause neutropenia despite severe infection.

Common biochemical abnormalities include hyperproteinemia, hyperglobulinemia, and azotemia. Hyponatremia and hyperkalemia may occur with severe vomiting or diarrhea, mimicking hypoadrenocorticism. Less common abnormalities include increased alanine aminotransferase and alkaline phosphatase activities (secondary to toxemia-induced hepatocellular damage or dehydration). Hyperglycemia or hypoglycemia may be associated with concurrent diabetes or sepsis. Although C-reactive protein elevations help differentiate pyometra from cystic endometrial hyperplasia with mucometra, the test is not readily available. Urinalysis may reveal isosthenuria, proteinuria, and/or bacteriuria. To prevent uterine puncture and abdominal contamination, cystocentesis should not be performed if pyometra is suspected. Vaginal cytology confirms a septic exudate with open pyometra and is abnormal (i.e., predominantly neutrophils with some degenerative bacteria), even when the cervix is closed. Bacterial culture and susceptibility are essential for selection of appropriate antibiotics.

DIFFERENTIAL DIAGNOSIS

Differential diagnoses include mucometra, hydrometra, hematometra, hydrocolpos, pyovagina, pregnancy, metritis, placentitis, uterine torsion, and peritonitis (Figs. 26-22 and 26-23). A high percentage of band neutrophils, elevated C-reactive protein, elevated alkaline phosphatase, and evidence of clinical illness make pyometra more likely than mucometra.

MEDICAL MANAGEMENT

Medical evacuation of the uterus with prostaglandin therapy ($PGF_{2\alpha}$) is inappropriate for critically ill patients because evacuation is neither immediate nor complete.

Medical therapy with antibiotics for 2 to 3 weeks and with $PGF_{2\alpha}$ or preferably aglepristone (antiprogestin) combined with cloprostenol (synthetic PG) (Box 26-22) should be considered only for metabolically stable, valuable, breeding animals. Medical therapy is most appropriate for animals with an open pyometra. More than one series of prostaglandin injections may be necessary. Owners must be informed that $PGF_{2\alpha}$ therapy is not approved for use in dogs and cats,

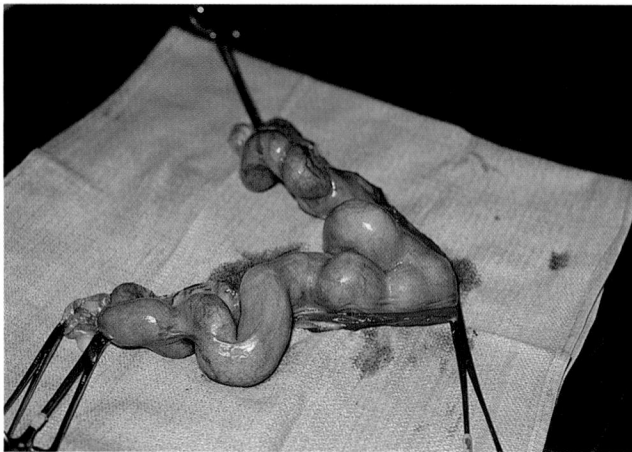

FIG. 26-22
An enlarged, friable uterus in an animal with pyometra. Compare this to the enlarged uterus in an animal with mucometra in Fig. 26-23. The two cannot be differentiated radiographically.

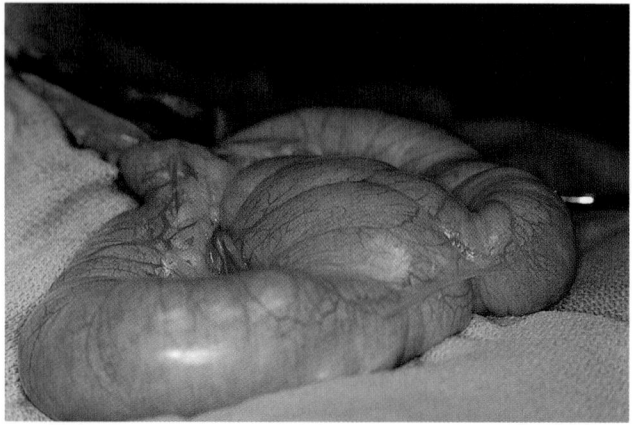

FIG. 26-23
Intraoperative appearance of the uterus in an animal with mucometra.

and serious complications (e.g., uterine rupture or leakage of intraluminal contents into the abdomen and sepsis) are possible. Short-term side effects (30 to 60 minutes) include panting, salivation, emesis, defecation, urination, mydriasis, nesting, tenesmus, lordosis, vocalization, and intensive grooming. High doses of prostaglandin may cause ataxia, collapse, hypovolemic shock, respiratory distress, or death. $PGF_{2\alpha}$ therapy may cause reduced fertility. Combination therapy of aglepristone and cloprostenol over 15 days has been reported safe and effective with few side effects (Gobello et al, 2003). Vulvar discharge increases and clinical signs begin to improve within 24 to 48 hours of initial aglepristone injection. Including an antilipopolysaccharide to reduce endotoxins may be beneficial. Mating should occur during the next estrus cycle. Expect pyometra to recur in 20% during subsequent estrus cycles.

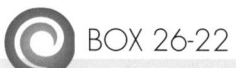

BOX 26-22

Medical Therapy of Pyometra*

Antibiotics for 2–3 weeks (see Box 26-23)
$PGF_{2\alpha}$ 0.1–0.25 mg/kg SC, qd or bid for 3–5 days

Or

$PGF_{2\alpha}$ 0.15 mg/kg administered intravaginally, raise hindquarters for 3–5 min.

Or

Aglepristone† (Alizine, Virbac, Carros, France)
   10 mg/kg SC, days 1, 3, 8 and 15 (if not cured based on ultrasonography)
With Cloprostenol (Estrumate, Schering Plough, Bs. As, Argentina)
   1 µg/kg SC, days 3 and 8, "far from feeding"; alternatively administer on days 3, 5, 8, 10, 12, and 15 (if not cured based on ultrasonography)

SC, Subcutaneous; *qd,* once a day; *bid,* twice a day.
*Dosages and efficacy of treatment are not definitively established.
†Available only in some European countries.
NOTE: Breeding should be attempted during the next estrus.

SURGICAL TREATMENT

Treatment (OHE) should not be delayed more than is absolutely necessary. Morbidity and mortality are associated with concurrent metabolic abnormalities and organ dysfunction (see previous discussion). Surgical drainage of the uterus without OHE is not recommended, but has been successful in a few cases. The corpus lutea are removed and each horn lavaged and suctioned. Indwelling drains are placed through the cervix to allow daily lavage with diluted antiseptics. Laparoscopic OHE for pyometra has been described.

Preoperative Management

Surgery should not be delayed more than a few hours while medical therapy (i.e., fluid therapy) is instituted, especially in patients with closed pyometra. Urine output, glucose, and arrhythmias should be monitored preoperatively. Hydration, electrolyte, and acid-base imbalances should be corrected before surgery, if possible (the prognosis is improved when azotemia is corrected before surgery). A broad-spectrum antibiotic effective against *E. coli* (e.g., cefazolin, cefoxitin, enrofloxacin, and ticarcillin plus clavulanate; Box 26-23) should be given IV while awaiting antibiotic susceptibility results. Aminoglycosides are nephrotoxic and not recommended because of the prevalence of renal dysfunction with pyometra. In addition to fluid volume replacement, severely endotoxic or septicemic patients may also be given corticosteroids (15 to 30 mg/kg prednisolone sodium succinate IV). Fluid input and urine output should be monitored to help assess renal function. Low-dose dopamine (0.5 to 1.5 µg/kg/min IV) may be used to improve renal function (see p. 742), or diuretics (e.g., furosemide, 2 to 4 mg/kg IV, IM, or SC or 20% dextrose IV) may be administered in volume-overloaded patients with reduced urine production. Administration of antiarrhythmics may occasionally be necessary.

CHAPTER 26 *Surgery of the Reproductive and Genital Systems* **741**

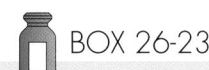 BOX 26-23

Selected Antibiotics of Use in Animals With Pyometra

Cefazolin (Ancef, Kefzol)

22 mg/kg IV or IM, tid

Cefoxitin (Mefoxin)

30 mg/kg IV, tid

Amoxicillin plus Clavulanate (Clavamox)

Dogs: 12.5–25 mg/kg PO, bid
Cats: 62.5 mg/cat PO, bid

Ampicillin

22 mg/kg IV, IM or SC, tid to qid

Ticarcillin plus Clavulanate (Timentin)

50 mg/kg IV, tid to qid

Enrofloxacin (Baytril)

7–20 mg/kg PO or IV, qd (give dilute and slowly over 30 minutes if given IV)

IV, Intravenous; *IM*, intramuscular; *tid*, three times a day; *qid*, four times a day; *PO*, oral; *bid*, twice a day; *SC*, subcutaneous; *qd*, once a day.

Anesthesia

Anesthetic protocols vary greatly depending on patient status. Animals that are systemically ill need to be closely monitored during anesthesia. They may be induced with an opioid plus a benzodiazepine, given in incremental doses as necessary to intubate (Box 26-24). If intubation is not possible, etomidate or reduced dosages of thiopental or propofol may be given. If etomidate is not available, arrhythmic dogs may be premedicated with hydromorphone and induced with thiopental and lidocaine. For the latter, 9 mg/kg of each is drawn up and half is given initially, IV. Additional drug is given to allow the dog to be intubated. To prevent toxicity, usually no more than 6 mg/kg of lidocaine is given IV. Isoflurane and sevoflurane are the inhalants of choice because they cause minimal cardiac depression, and induction and recovery are usually rapid. The anesthetic depth should be monitored closely in these patients. Anesthetic management of stable animals is described on p. 705.

Hypotension should be corrected before and prevented during and after surgery in animals with pyometra. The patient should be monitored for arrhythmias or tachycardia. Hypertonic saline with a colloid (e.g., dextran or hetastarch) improves hemodynamics and oxygenation in animals with septic shock (see Chapter 5 and Table 5-5 on p. 28). Animals with total protein less than 4 g/dl or albumin less than 1.5 g/dl may benefit from perioperative colloid (e.g., hetastarch) administration. Hetastarch may be given preoperatively, intraoperatively, and/or postoperatively for a total dose of 20 ml/kg/day in dogs and 10 to 15 ml/kg/day in cats. If colloids are given during surgery (7 to 10 mg/kg), acute intraoperative hypotension should be treated with crystalloids (see Chapter 5). Dobutamine (2 to 10 µg/kg/min IV) or dopamine (2 to 10 µg/kg/min IV) may be given

 BOX 26-24

Selected Anesthetic Protocols for Debilitated or Shocky Animals With Pyometra

Dogs
Premedication and Induction

Hydromorphone (0.05–0.2 mg/kg IV or IM) plus diazepam (0.2 mg/kg IV). Give in incremental doses. Intubate if possible. If necessary, give etomidate (0.5–1.5 mg/kg IV).
Alternatively, if not vomiting, mask induction can be used or give thiopental or propofol at reduced doses.

Maintenance

Isoflurane or sevoflurane.

Cats
Premedication

Butorphanol (0.2–0.4 mg/kg SC or IM) or buprenorphine (5–15 µg/kg IM) or hydromorphone (0.05–0.1 mg/kg SC or IM).

Induction

Diazepam (0.2 mg/kg IV) followed by etomidate (0.5–1.5 mg/kg IV). Alternatively, if not vomiting, mask or chamber induction can be used or give thiopental or propofol at reduced dosages. If there are no contraindications to ketamine (i.e., renal dysfunction), reduced dosages of diazepam and ketamine may also be used.

Maintenance

Isoflurane or sevoflurane.

IV, Intravenous; *IM*, intramuscular; *SC*, subcutaneous.

during surgery for inotropic support. Dobutamine is less arrhythmogenic and chronotropic than dopamine and is preferred if the patient is hypotensive and anuric. In dogs that are anuric and normotensive, low-dose dopamine (0.5 to 1.5 µg/kg/min IV) plus furosemide (0.2 mg/kg IV) may be preferable. In cats, mannitol (0.25 to 0.5 g/kg, IV slowly over 20 minutes) may be used for diuresis.

Positioning

Position the patient in dorsal recumbency for a ventral midline celiotomy. The entire ventral abdomen should be clipped and prepared for aseptic surgery.

Surgical Anatomy

Surgical anatomy of the reproductive tract is described on p. 706.

SURGICAL TECHNIQUE

Expose the abdomen through a ventral midline incision beginning 2 to 3 cm caudal to the xiphoid and extending to the pubis. Explore the abdomen and locate the distended uterus. Observe for evidence of peritonitis (i.e., serosal inflammation, increased abdominal fluid, and petechiation). Obtain abdominal fluid for culture, evacuate the urinary bladder by cystocentesis, and collect a urine specimen for culture and analysis if not previously submitted. Carefully exteriorize the uterus without applying pressure or excessive traction. A fluid-filled uterus is often friable; therefore lift rather than pull the uterus out of the abdomen.

Do not use a spay hook to locate and exteriorize the uterus because it may tear. Do not correct uterine torsion because this will release bacteria and toxins.

Isolate the uterus from the abdomen with laparotomy pads or sterile towels. Place clamps and ligatures as previously described for OHE except that the cervix may be resected in addition to ovaries, uterine horns, and uterine body. Ligate the pedicles with absorbable monofilament suture material (i.e., 2-0 or 3-0 polydioxanone or polyglyconate), and transect at the junction of the cervix and vagina. Thoroughly lavage the vaginal stump. Culture the contents of the uterus without contaminating the surgical field. Remove laparotomy pads and replace contaminated instruments, gloves, and drapes. Lavage the abdomen, and close the incision routinely unless peritonitis is present (p. 336). Submit the tract for pathologic evaluation.

POSTOPERATIVE CARE AND ASSESSMENT

Give analgesics as necessary (see Chapter 13; for dosages of opioids see Table 13-4 on p. 133). These patients should be monitored closely for 24 to 48 hours for sepsis and shock, dehydration, and electrolyte/acid-base imbalances. Severe hypoproteinemia or anemia may require plasma or blood transfusions, respectively. Fluid therapy should be continued postoperatively until the animal is eating and drinking normally. Antibiotic therapy based on culture and sensitivity results should be continued for 10 to 14 days. Low-dose dopamine (of questionable value) or diuretics (Box 26-25) may be given postoperatively if urine production is reduced. Evidence of abdominal discomfort, elevated temperature, or pain suggests peritonitis.

 BOX 26-25

Diuretic Therapy

Dopamine (Low-Dose)*
0.5–3.0 µg/kg/min IV

Mannitol†
0.25 mg/kg IV over 15 min

Furosemide (Lasix)*
2–4 mg/kg IV, PO, SC, bid to tid or can give it as CRI (load with 0.66 mg/kg bolus, and then give 0.66 mg/kg/hr for 4 to 5 hours; alternatively, can estimate the IV or PO dose to be given over the course of the next 24 hours and then give that amount as a CRI over the next 24 hours). Be sure patient is volume replenished before administering

IV, Intravenous; *PO,* oral; *SC,* subcutaneous; *bid,* twice a day; *tid,* three times a day; *CRI,* continuous rate infusion.
*Seldom effective once oliguria or anuria has developed. Dopamine has no propensity to improve renal function or alter outcome and can no longer be patently endorsed.
†This is a potentially dangerous drug because it is not metabolized if it is not excreted (consult an internist or medical text before using).

COMPLICATIONS

Complications associated with elective OHE may also occur following OHE for pyometra (see p. 726). Five to 8% of patients die despite appropriate therapy, especially after uterine rupture (57%). Septicemia, endotoxemia, peritonitis, and cervical or stump pyometra may occur. Stump pyometra may be associated with residual ovarian tissue. In these cases, the remaining stump should be excised and residual ovarian tissue removed. Other complications include anorexia, lethargy, anemia, pyrexia, vomiting, icterus, hepatic disease, renal disease, and thromboembolic disease. Most complications resolve within 2 weeks of surgery.

PROGNOSIS

Death usually occurs without surgical or medical therapy. A few animals spontaneously recover following corpus luteum regression and uterine drainage, but pyometra recurrence at subsequent diestrus is common. Pyometra commonly persists or recurs after prostaglandin therapy in dogs (77% of bitches at 27 months). However, 40% to 74% of bitches and 81% of queens produce at least one normal litter after prostaglandin therapy. Prognosis following surgery is good if abdominal contamination is avoided, shock and sepsis are controlled, and renal damage reversed by fluid therapy and bacterial antigen elimination. Death may occur when metabolic abnormalities are severe and unresponsive to appropriate therapy. Mortality rates after surgical treatment of pyometra are approximately 5% to 8%.

References

Egenvall A, Hagman R, Bonnett BN et al: Breed risk of pyometra in insured dogs in Sweden, *J Vet Intern Med* 15:530, 2001.

Gobello C, Castex G, Klima L et al: A study of two protocols combining aglepristone and cloprostenol to treat open cervix pyometra in the bitch, *Theriogenology* 60:901, 2003.

Niskanen M, Thrusfield MV: Associations between age, parity, hormonal therapy and breed, and pyometra in Finnish dogs, *Vet Rec* 143:493, 1998.

Suggested Reading

Bigliardi E, Parmigiani E, Cavirani S et al: Ultrasonography and cystic hyperplasia-pyometra complex in the bitch, *Reprod Dom Anim* 39:136, 2004.

Forty-five bitches were evaluated; results suggest that ultrasound is reliable for the diagnosis of cystic endometrial hypoplasia, mucometra, endometritis, and pyometra.

Campbell BG: Omentalization of a nonresectable uterine stump abscess in a dog, *J Am Vet Med Assoc* 224:1799, 2004.

This report describes management of a uterine stump abscess occurring following routine OHE in a 2-year-old Golden Retriever.

Dubey JP, Rosypal AC, Pierce V et al: Placentitis associated with leishmaniasis, *J Am Vet Med Assoc* 227:1266, 2005.

This case represents an unusual cause of vaginal discharge that could be confused with metritis or pyometra.

Faldyna M, Laznicka A, Toman M: Immunosuppression in bitches with pyometra, *J Small Anim Pract* 42:5, 2001.

Thirty-four affected bitches were studied; results of evaluated blood samples demonstrated notable suppression of immune system activity in addition to an inflammatory response.

Fransson BA, Ragle CA: Canine pyometra: an update on pathogenesis and treatment, *Compend Cont Educ Pract Vet* 25:602, 2003.
This is a good review of current concepts.

Fransson BA, Karlstam E, Bergstrom A et al: C-reactive protein in the differentiation of pyometra from cystic endometrial hyperplasia/mucometra in dogs, *J Am Anim Hosp Assoc* 40:391, 2004.
Data from 64 dogs were evaluated; findings of a high percentage of band neutrophils, elevated C-reactive protein, elevated alkaline phosphatase, and typical clinical signs were all predictive of pyometra rather than mucometra.

Gabor G, Siver L, Szenci O: Intravaginal prostaglandin F2 alpha for the treatment of metritis and pyometra in the bitch, *Acta Vet Hung* 47:103, 1999.
Data from 15 dogs treated intravaginally are presented; treatment was successful in 13 of 15, with no side effects.

Heine R, van Vonderen IK, Moe L et al: Vasopressin secretion in response to osmotic stimulation and effects of desmopressin on urinary concentrating capacity in dogs with pyometra, *Am J Vet Res* 65:404, 2004.
Six dogs were evaluated and found to have increased urine concentration in response to desmopressin and vasopressin; secretory ability was not reduced.

Misumi K, Fujiki M, Miura N et al: Uterine horn torsion in two non-gravid bitches, *J Small Anim Pract* 41:468, 2000.
Uterine horn torsion in these two dogs was associated with hematometra in one and pyometra in the other.

Trasch K, Wehrend A, Bostedt H: Follow-up examination of bitches after conservative therapy of pyometra with the anti-gestagen aglepristone, *J Vet Med* 50:375, 2003.
Forty-eight of fifty-two bitches were treated successfully; however, within 12 months, 20% had recurrence.

Troxel MT, Pastor KF, Hartzband LE et al: Severe hematometra in a dog with cystic endometrial hyperplasia/pyometra complex, *J Am Anim Hosp Assoc* 38:85, 2002.
A young German shepherd with a hemorrhagic vulvar discharge was discovered to have mildly dilated, fluid-filled uterine horns and a uterine wall with a cystic honeycombed appearance during ultrasonography.

Zaragoza C, Barrera R, Centeno F et al: Canine pyometra: a study of the urinary proteins by SDS-PAGE and Western Blot, *Theriogenology* 61:1259, 2004.
This report characterizes the electrophoretic pattern of urinary proteins and quantifies urinary excretion of IgG and IgA in bitches.

VAGINAL PROLAPSE/HYPERPLASIA/ TUMOR

DEFINITION

Vaginal prolapse/hyperplasia occurs during estrus or proestrus as a result of edematous enlargement of vaginal tissue. **Vaginal prolapse** involves the 360° protrusion of mucosa, whereas **vaginal hyperplasia** may originate from a stalk of mucosa on the floor of the vagina, both usually cranial to the urethral papilla. *Vaginal hypertrophy, vaginal edema, vaginal fold prolapse, estral eversion,* and *estral hypertrophy* have also been used to describe this condition.

GENERAL CONSIDERATIONS AND CLINICALLY RELEVANT PATHOPHYSIOLOGY

Vaginal hyperplasia/hypertrophy uncommonly occurs, usually during proestrus and estrus. The mucosa is not truly hyperplastic, but enlarges because of edema. Normal estrogenic stimulation causes vaginal mucosa to become hyperemic, edematous, and keratinized. These normal effects are accentuated with vaginal prolapse/hyperplasia, causing edematous mucosa to evert during proestrus and estrus and occasionally at the end of diestrus or near parturition. Prolapse may occur with hyperestrogenism or weakness of vaginal connective tissue. The amount of edema and eversion is extremely variable. Severe edema causes vaginal tissue to protrude from the vulva. Although the protruding mass may be large, the origin of the mass is usually small (approximately 1 cm) and located on the vaginal floor cranial to the urethral orifice. The width of the mass varies from stalklike to involving the entire vaginal floor. Prolapsing tissue promotes straining, which further increases the amount of prolapsed tissue. The edematous tissue mechanically obstructs and interferes with normal breeding. Tissue protruding from between the vulvar lips is often traumatized by abrasion, licking, or drying. Trauma results in ulceration and bleeding. The mass may compress surrounding structures, causing stranguria, hematuria, or tenesmus. Prepartum bitches may concurrently prolapse their urinary bladder. Although edema resolves spontaneously when the follicular phase of the cycle and ovarian production of estrogen have elapsed, prolapse may recur with each succeeding estrus cycle.

NOTE: Vaginal prolapse/hyperplasia appears to be familial. Affected animals should not be bred.

DIAGNOSIS
Clinical Presentation

Signalment. Although rare, vaginal prolapse/hyperplasia is most common in large-breed dogs. It most commonly occurs in young bitches (2 years or younger) during one of their first three estrus cycles. Vaginal prolapse/hyperplasia is extremely rare in cats.

History. Protrusion of a mass from the vulva, vulvar discharge, or bleeding is typical. Bitches refuse to allow intromission during breeding or have signs referable to fecal or urinary difficulties. The history should indicate if the animal is in estrus, proestrus, or gravid (rarely). Other signs of vaginal disease include frequent perineal licking, pollakiuria, dysuria, and perineal enlargement and swelling.

Physical Examination Findings

A mass may be seen protruding between the vulvar lips, or the perineum may bulge. Acute prolapse and nonprotruding prolapses are characterized by a glistening, edematous, pale pink mucosal surface. Chronic prolapses appear leathery (i.e., dry and dull), corrugated, and sometimes ulcerated or fissured. The mass should be examined carefully to determine origin, size at the base, locations of the vaginal lumen and urethral opening, and the extent of tissue damage. Vaginal palpation should identify a mass arising from the ventral vaginal floor. Vaginal areas other than those just cranial to the urethral orifice should feel normal. Vaginal cancers can cause severe pain, making vaginal examination impossible without chemical restraint.

Diagnostic Imaging

Radiographs are unnecessary unless neoplasia or visceral herniation is suspected. Concurrent herniation of the urinary bladder or intestines into the prolapsed tissue may require positive contrast studies for confirmation.

Laboratory Findings

Vaginal cytology should confirm estrogen stimulation (i.e., red blood cells in the absence of cornified vaginal epithelial cells). Aspiration cytology helps differentiate prolapse from neoplasia.

DIFFERENTIAL DIAGNOSIS

Uterine prolapse (see p. 745) and vaginal tumors are the most difficult to differentiate from vaginal prolapse/hyperplasia (Fig. 26-24; see also Fig. 26-13). The most common types of vulvar-vaginal tumors are fibroleiomyoma, lipoma, leiomyosarcoma, squamous cell carcinoma, and transmissible venereal tumor. Most vulvar-vaginal tumors occur in old (10 years or older), intact females. Benign vulvar-vaginal tumors are most common and respond to local excision and OHE. Fibroleiomyoma is the most common benign tumor. Fibroleiomyomas originate around the urethral papilla and are usually pedunculated, smooth, firm, and pale. The most common malignant tumors are transmissible venereal tumors. These tumors tend to be broad-based, irregular, friable, and bleed easily. Malignant vulvar-vaginal tumors are often locally invasive and metastasize early to local lymph nodes. Nonneoplastic differentials include vaginal cysts, hydrocolpos, and septa or congenital malformations.

MEDICAL MANAGEMENT

If protrusion is not circumferential, vaginal prolapse will spontaneously resolve when estrogen influence diminishes. Estrus may be shortened by administering gonadotropin releasing hormone (GnRH, 50 μg/40 lb) or human chorionic gonadotropin (HCG, 500-1000 IU, IM) to induce ovulation. Animals with vaginal prolapse/hyperplasia should not be used for breeding because the disease has a familial predisposition. Artificial insemination may be considered when a valuable bitch will not allow intromission and the owners insist on breeding. Transmissible venereal tumors (TVTs) can be treated with vincristine (0.025 mg/kg up to 1 mg or 0.5 mg/m² IV, weekly for 3 to 6 weeks) or combination chemotherapy. TVTs also respond to local excision, radiation therapy, and immunotherapy. TVTs sometimes regress spontaneously.

SURGICAL TREATMENT

OHE is recommended to prevent recurrence and injury to the everted mucosa. Large, protruding masses may require manual reduction via an episiotomy and vulvar sutures to prevent

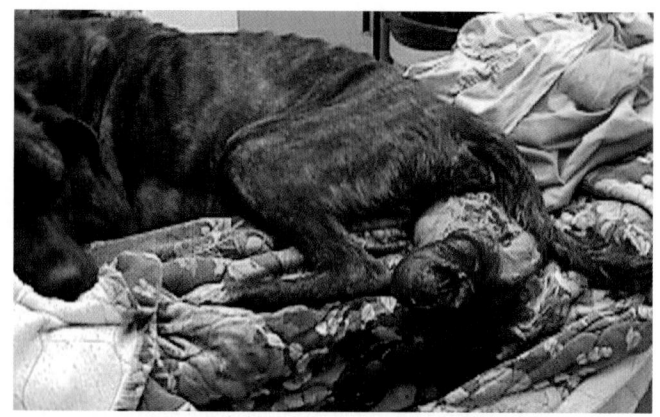

A

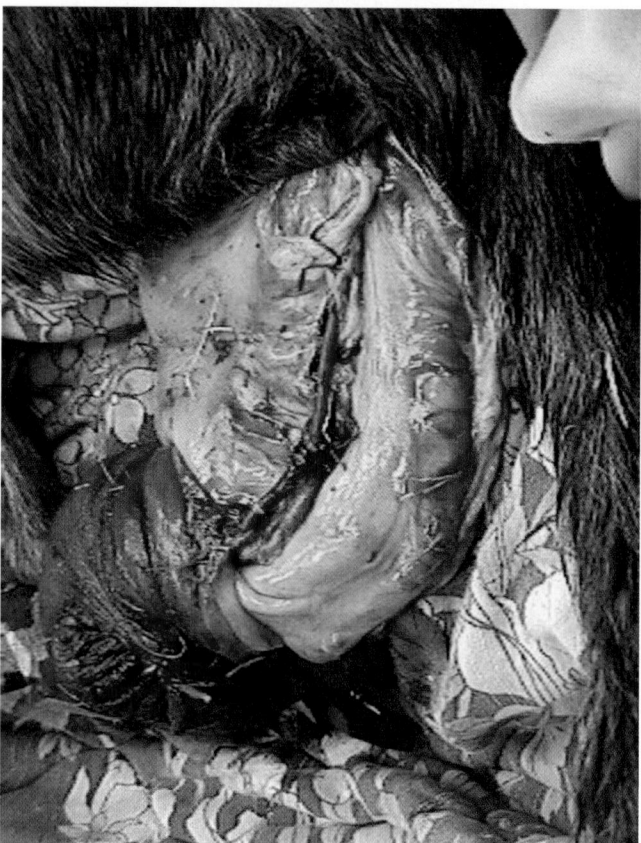

B

FIG. 26-24
A, Uterine prolapse and tearing following parturition.
B, Close-up of prolapse showing contamination and tearing.

re-prolapse until the edematous tissue shrinks. Resection of the protruding tissue without OHE is not recommended because the procedure is associated with significant hemorrhage and does not prevent recurrence during subsequent estrus cycles. Resection of protruding tissue is recommended when the tissue is severely damaged or necrotic. Reduction or resection without OHE may require hysteropexy, cystopexy, and/or colopexy to prevent recurrent prolapse and herniation, respectively. OHE and mass excision or biopsy is recommended for all vaginal tumors except TVTs. Many vaginal tumors are under hormonal influence and regress after OHE.

Preoperative Management

Protruding mucosa should be lavaged with warm saline or water to remove debris and necrotic tissue. An antibiotic or antibiotic/steroid ointment can be applied to the exposed tissue and the mass replaced within the vagina or vestibule, if possible. An Elizabethan collar, bucket, or sidebars are indicated to prevent self-trauma before surgery.

Anesthesia

Anesthetic recommendations for animals undergoing reproductive surgery are on p. 705.

Surgical Anatomy

Anatomy of the reproductive system is described on p. 706. Vaginal lymphatic drainage is to the internal iliac lymph nodes.

Positioning

The patient is positioned in dorsal recumbency for OHE. The entire ventral abdomen and perineum should be clipped and prepared for aseptic surgery. Episiotomy requires that they be repositioned in a perineal position (i.e., ventral recumbency, pelvic limbs over the edge of a padded table, and tail fixed dorsally over the back).

SURGICAL TECHNIQUE

Perform an OHE (see p. 709), and take a biopsy of the mass to rule out neoplasia. Perform an episiotomy if necessary to allow biopsy. Replace the protruding mass into the vagina or vestibule. Lavage, lubricate, and reduce the prolapsed tissue by digital manipulation. Maintain reduction by placing (take large bites) two to three horizontal mattress sutures (e.g., 2-0 nylon or polypropylene) between the vulvar lips.

If resection of necrotic or severely traumatized tissue is necessary, position the patient in a perineal position and perform an episiotomy to expose the mass. Place and maintain a urethral catheter during the procedure. In stages, incise the base of the edematous tissue. Control hemorrhage with pressure, ligatures, and electrocoagulation. Appose adjacent mucosal edges with interrupted or continuous approximating sutures (e.g., 3-0 or 4-0 polydioxanone, poliglecaprone 25, glycomer 631, or polyglyconate). Edema should resolve within 5 to 7 days of OHE.

POSTOPERATIVE CARE AND ASSESSMENT

Patients should be supported postoperatively with fluids and analgesics (see Chapter 13; for dosages of opioids see Table 13-4 on p. 133), as needed. Cold compresses should be applied immediately after episiotomy for 2 to 3 days, followed by warm compresses for 2 to 3 days to reduce inflammation and swelling. Self-trauma due to perineal discomfort associated with episiotomy and/or vulvar sutures may cause dehiscence; an Elizabethan collar, bucket, or sidebars should be used postoperatively. The vagina should be palpated 5 to 7 days after mass reduction and/or OHE, and vulvar sutures removed if tissue eversion has regressed with minimal threat of re-protrusion. Hemorrhage may occur following amputation of the protruding edematous

tissue, but is self-limiting if good surgical technique was employed.

PROGNOSIS

The prognosis is excellent following OHE; otherwise recurrence during subsequent estrus and difficult conception are common. Edema will resolve when estrogen levels diminish at the end of estrus. Offspring may be predisposed to the condition.

Suggested Reading

Markandeya NM, Patil AD, Bhikane AU: Pre-partum vaginal prolapse in a dog, *Indian Vet J* 81:449, 2004.
This short description of a 50-day pregnant dog with a prolapse, which was reduced, was managed successfully to parturition.
NamSoo K, JiHoon K, YoungJae P et al: Surgical treatment of the prolapse of bladder with vaginal prolapse in large breed dogs, *J Vet Clinics* 21:319, 2004.
This is a report of two term bitches that were managed with cesarean section, OHE, and prolapse reduction.
Viehoff RW, Sjollema BE: Hydrocolpos in dogs: surgical treatment in two cases, *J Small Anim Pract* 44:404-407, 2003.
Hydrocolpos (congenital obstruction of the vagina) is described; treatment included OHE, drainage, and then anastomosis of the vagina to the vestibule via an episiotomy.

UTERINE PROLAPSE

DEFINITIONS

Uterine prolapse (*uterine eversion*) is an eversion and protrusion of a portion of the uterus through the cervix into the vagina during or near parturition.

GENERAL CONSIDERATIONS AND CLINICALLY RELEVANT PATHOPHYSIOLOGY

Uterine prolapse is rare. It is similar to estrus-associated vaginal prolapse/hyperplasia (see p. 743); however, uterine prolapse is associated with parturition and involves the entire vaginal circumference. The cervix must be dilated for uterine prolapse to occur. One or both uterine horns may prolapse and reside in the cranial vagina or be everted through the vulva. Uterine prolapse usually occurs with prolonged labor. The everted tissue is doughnut-shaped and discolored from venous congestion, trauma, and debris. Uterine prolapse may tear the broad ligament and uterine artery. Hemorrhage may lead to hypovolemic shock unless controlled quickly.

DIAGNOSIS
Clinical Presentation

Signalment. The condition is rare but may occur near or at parturition. There is no recognized age predisposition. Although rare, the condition occurs more commonly in cats than in dogs.

History. Uterine prolapse is associated with excessive straining during parturition. A mucosal mass is generally noticed protruding from the vulva. Vague signs of abdominal distress and tenesmus may be noted. Signs of hemorrhagic shock may occur if the ovarian or uterine vessels have ruptured. Other signs may include restlessness, abnormal posture, pain, perineal bulging, licking, and dysuria.

Physical Examination Findings

Uterine prolapse is diagnosed on physical examination by digital examination of the vagina or visual observation (see Fig. 26-24). Perineal bulging may occur. Everted mucosa may protrude through the vulva or be digitally palpated in the vagina. A fornix will be identified by inserting a probe or finger along the protruding mass if it is a vaginal mass or prolapse, but not if it is a uterine prolapse. The animal may be stable or show signs of hemorrhagic shock (e.g., pale mucous membranes, tachycardia, and weak pulses).

Diagnostic Imaging

A gravid uterus or postpartum uterus may be identified on radiographs or ultrasound. Vaginoscopy may be used to confirm the diagnosis.

Laboratory Findings

Specific laboratory abnormalities are not seen. Anemia may be present if the uterine artery has ruptured.

DIFFERENTIAL DIAGNOSIS

Differential diagnoses include vaginal prolapse/hyperplasia (see p. 743), vaginal tumor (see p. 744), and uterine torsion.

MEDICAL MANAGEMENT

Medical treatment is rarely successful. Shock should be treated with fluids (plus or minus corticosteroids), and acid-base and electrolyte imbalances corrected. The protruding mass should be lavaged with warm saline and gently massaged to reduce edema. Lavaging with hypertonic dextrose solution may reduce swelling. The mass should be lubricated with a water-soluble gel and manually replaced by using external pressure and flushing sterile fluid under pressure into the uterine horn. After replacement, administration of oxytocin (5 to 10 U) promotes uterine involution and, together with closure of the cervix, helps prevent recurrence.

SURGICAL TREATMENT

The goals of treatment are to replace the uterus (see previous discussion under Medical Management) and prevent infection. Treatment options include manual reduction, manual reduction with immediate OHE, reduction during celiotomy, and amputation of the mass. OHE should be performed if tissue is devitalized or irreducible, or if broad ligament vessels have ruptured. Laparotomy may be necessary to facilitate manual reduction by placing cranial traction on the broad ligament or uterus. Occasionally, uterine amputation is necessary to allow reduction. Everted uterine tissue may be amputated similarly to that described for vaginal prolapse/ hyperplasia (see p. 745); however, the uterine arteries must be ligated. After uterine amputation, an OHE should be performed. Vaginapexy may be performed during cesarean section or celiotomy, or when the patient is stable.

> **NOTE:** Catheterize the urethra during uterine amputation to prevent traumatizing it or the urethral papilla.

Preoperative Management

Shocky patients should have surgery as soon as they are stabilized. Shock should be treated with fluids (plus or minus corticosteroids), and acid-base and electrolyte imbalances corrected. Prophylactic antibiotics are indicated when the prolapse is contaminated or traumatized. Hair should be clipped from the abdomen, perineum, and the areas prepared for aseptic surgery. Viability of the prolapsed tissue should be assessed, and if the tissue appears healthy, the mass should be lavaged and replaced. Use techniques described in the Medical Management section.

Anesthesia

Anesthetic recommendations for animals undergoing reproductive surgery are provided on p. 705. Animals in shock require special care during induction and anesthesia. Anesthetic protocols for debilitated and shocky patients are provided in Box 26-24, p. 741. Epidural anesthesia (see p. 706) may facilitate prolapse reduction and reduce postoperative straining. Local anesthetics should not be used for epidurals unless volume depletion has been corrected.

Positioning

Manual reduction may be accomplished with the patient in ventral, dorsal, or lateral recumbency. A perineal position is recommended for episiotomy and dorsal recumbency for celiotomy.

Surgical Anatomy

Surgical anatomy of the reproductive tract is provided on p. 706.

SURGICAL TECHNIQUE

Reduce acute prolapses manually. Lavage the protruding tissue with warm saline or water and diluted antiseptic. Hypertonic agents (e.g., sugar) may help reduce edema and facilitate reduction. Gently compress the mass to reduce edema while attempting to reduce the prolapse. If necessary, perform an episiotomy to assist reduction. Insert a urethral catheter. Place horizontal mattress sutures between the vulvar lips to maintain reduction and prevent recurrence. If necessary, perform celiotomy to facilitate reduction by cranial uterine traction, ensure proper alignment of the uterine horns, and assess integrity of the vasculature.

POSTOPERATIVE CARE AND ASSESSMENT

Shock, dehydration, and blood loss should be treated and analgesics given as necessary (see Chapter 13; for dosages of opioids see Table 13-4 on p. 133). Urination should be monitored because swelling and pain may cause urethral obstruction. If dysuria or anuria is anticipated, a urinary catheter should be placed. Antibiotics should be continued postoperatively if the uterus appeared moderately to severely traumatized and OHE was not performed. Complications include hemorrhage, shock, dehydration, infection, necrosis, urethral obstruction, recurrence, and death.

PROGNOSIS

Complete uterine prolapse will not regress spontaneously. Survival following successful manual reduction of uterine prolapses is common, but infertility and dystocia may occur with subsequent breeding. The prognosis following OHE is excellent if shock and hemorrhage are treated appropriately.

Suggested Reading

NamSoo K, JiHoon K, YoungJae P et al: Surgical treatment of the prolapse of bladder with vaginal prolapse in large breed dogs, *J Vet Clinics* 21:319, 2004.
This is a report of two term bitches that were managed with cesarean section, OHE, and prolapse reduction.

Surgery of the Male Reproductive Tract

SPECIFIC DISEASES

PROSTATIC HYPERPLASIA

DEFINITIONS

Prostatic hyperplasia is a benign enlargement of the prostate. Increased numbers of prostatic cells occur secondary to androgenic hormone stimulation.

GENERAL CONSIDERATIONS AND CLINICALLY RELEVANT PATHOPHYSIOLOGY

Benign prostatic hyperplasia (BPH) is the most common canine prostatic disorder; age-related, it occurs in 95% of male dogs by 9 years of age. Potential causes of BPH include an abnormal ratio of androgens to estrogens, increased number of androgen receptors, and increased tissue sensitivity to androgens. The primary androgen promoting hyperplasia is dihydrotestosterone, which is irreversibly converted from testosterone. Conversion occurs in the epithelial cells by the action of 5-alpha reductase. Dihydrotestosterone enhances growth in both prostatic stromal and glandular components. Testosterone declines with age, but estrogen levels remain the same and induce nuclear dihydrotestosterone receptors, which may increase the sensitivity of the prostate to dihydrotestosterone. Other hormones, including estrogen, prolactin, and growth hormone, are believed to be involved. BPH may be a normal aging change unassociated with clinical signs; however, substantial enlargement may cause constipation, tenesmus, altered stool shape, and/or dysuria. Prostatic enlargement rarely causes urinary obstruction; canine glands expand outward rather than inward as in humans. Pressure on the pelvic diaphragm may contribute to the development of a perineal hernia.

Hyperplasia may be glandular or complex. Glandular hyperplasia affects dogs as young as 1 year of age and peaks at 5 to 6 years. There is a uniform proliferation of secretory structures with glandular hyperplasia, and gland consistency is normal. Complex hyperplasia is seen in dogs as young as 2 years of age, but predominantly occurs between 8 and 9 years. Cystic dilated alveoli are present with heterogeneous epithelial cells varying from normal to nonfunctional cuboidal cells. Acini are filled with eosinophilic material, and plasma cells and lymphocytes are present in the hyperplastic stroma.

DIAGNOSIS
Clinical Presentation

Signalment. Sexually intact male dogs are affected. Doberman pinschers, Scottish terriers, Bouvier des Flandres, Bernese mountain dogs, and German pointers may be predisposed to BPH. The disease is found in most sexually intact male dogs over 6 years of age. Mean age at diagnosis is 8.9 years for most prostatic diseases.

History. Dogs may have tenesmus, hematuria, and/or urethral bleeding. Owners may observe ribbonlike stools.

Physical Examination Findings

Most dogs are asymptomatic, but tenesmus, hematuria, or urethral bleeding may occur. Rectal palpation reveals symmetric, nonpainful prostatic enlargement, which is soft and has a smooth contour. The median cleft is preserved. The prostate may be two to six times larger than normal.

Diagnostic Imaging

Radiographically the prostate appears symmetrically enlarged. The prostate is considered enlarged if it is greater than 70% of the distance between the sacral promontory and the pubis on lateral radiographs. The colon may be displaced dorsally and the urinary bladder cranially. Ultrasound is useful for evaluation of prostate size only when it is being used for serial comparisons in the same dog. Normal values are not available for ultrasound of the prostate. With hyperplasia, ultrasound may show diffuse, symmetric prostatic involvement, and small, multiple cysts are common. Overall glandular echogenicity is normal to increased. Small areas of decreased echogenicity may be seen if cystic hyperplasia is present.

> NOTE: Aspirates or core biopsies should be collected during ultrasonography to establish a tentative diagnosis of BPH.

Laboratory Findings

Ejaculate volume is reduced, but total sperm count and fertility are not affected. Ejaculate cytology reveals hemorrhage and mild inflammation without sepsis. Prostatic epithelial cells, erythrocytes, and a few leukocytes are identified. Urinalysis may identify blood. Definitive diagnosis requires histopathology.

DIFFERENTIAL DIAGNOSIS

Differential diagnoses include prostatic squamous metaplasia, prostatic cysts (see p. 754), periprostatic cysts (see p. 754), prostatitis (see p. 750), prostatic neoplasia (see p. 757), and prostatic abscesses (see p. 750) (Box 26-26 and Table 26-6). Prostatic aspiration or biopsy (see p. 722) is necessary to differentiate benign and malignant prostatic enlargement. Ultrasonography may differentiate parenchymal enlargement from cystic change.

MEDICAL MANAGEMENT

Estrogens, progestins, synthetic steroids, and antiestrogenic drugs have been used for their antiandrogenic effects, but relapses occur after therapy stops (Table 26-7). Finasteride is a synthetic steroid type II 5-alpha reductase inhibitor that significantly decreases dihydrotestosterone (~58%) without affecting serum testosterone or semen quality and reduces prostate diameter (~20%) and volume (~43%) (Sirinarumitr et al, 2001) (see Table 26-7); it is currently the drug of choice. Estrogen therapy will reduce prostatic size, but is not recommended because it causes infertility, squamous metaplasia, abscessation, and aplastic anemia. Medroxyprogesterone acetate alleviates signs of hyperplasia within 4 to 6 weeks in most (84%) dogs; however, they recur at an average of 13.6 months. Potential progestin side effects include increased appetite, weight gain, mammary neoplasia and dysplasia, and diabetes mellitus. Chlormadinone acetate (an antiandrogenic preparation) is being investigated.

SURGICAL TREATMENT

Asymptomatic animals do not require therapy. Castration is the best treatment for dogs with clinical disease. Castration permanently involutes the prostate within 3 to 12 weeks. Subtotal prostatectomy is an option for valuable breeding animals (see p. 724).

Preoperative Management

Constipation, tenesmus, and urine retention should be treated symptomatically. Stool softeners may facilitate defecation (see p. 726).

Anesthesia

Anesthetic recommendations for animals undergoing elective reproductive surgery are provided on p. 705.

Surgical Anatomy

Surgical anatomy of the prostate is provided on p. 708.

Positioning

The animal is positioned in dorsal recumbency for prescrotal castration (see p. 714) and a perineal position for perineal

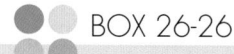 BOX 26-26

Prostatic Disease: Key Points

- Most dogs with prostatic disease present at approximately 8 years of age; those with tumors are usually 10 years old or older.
- Enlarged prostates can contribute to perineal hernia formation.
- Most geriatric intact male dogs have benign prostatic hyperplasia. Some are asymptomatic for life.
- Hyperplastic prostates are enlarged, nonpainful, and symmetric.
- Castration is the best treatment for benign prostatic hyperplasia, but valuable breeding dogs may respond to finasteride.
- Prostatic cysts may be associated with benign prostatic hyperplasia. Cysts are either within the parenchyma or outside the parenchyma (paraprostatic).
- Cystic prostates palpate similar to those with hyperplasia unless there are periprostatic cysts—these are enlarged, fluctuant, usually nonpainful, and asymmetric.
- Drain or excise prostatic cysts and castrate.
- Sertoli cell tumors predispose the prostate to squamous metaplasia, which can lead to prostatic cysts that can then abscess.
- *E. coli* is the most common organism isolated from abscessed prostates.
- Abscessed prostates are enlarged, fluctuant, usually painful, and asymmetric.
- Abscessed prostates may concurrently be neoplastic.
- Drain, administer appropriate antibiotics, and castrate dogs with prostatic abscesses.
- Castrated male dogs presenting with prostatic disease are at high risk for neoplasia.
- Prostatic carcinomas are the most common tumor; most originate from ductal/urothelial tissue and are nonandrogen sensitive.
- Neoplastic prostates may be normal size, but are often enlarged, asymmetric, nodular, firm, and fixed.
- Prostatic tumors are invasive and advanced at the time of diagnosis; therefore treatment is palliative. Survival time is longer if treated with NSAIDs (piroxicam, carprofen).
- Expect urinary incontinence if prostatectomy is performed.

NSAIDs, Nonsteroidal antiinflammatory drugs.

castration (see p. 714). See p. 714 for recommendations for clipping and surgically prepping for castration. Position the animal in dorsal recumbency for subtotal prostatectomy (see p. 724).

SURGICAL TECHNIQUE

Castration is described on p. 714. Subtotal prostatectomy is described on p. 724.

POSTOPERATIVE CARE AND ASSESSMENT

Analgesics should be provided for pain (see Chapter 13; for dosages of opioids see Table 13-4 on p. 133), if necessary. Symptomatic treatment for constipation, tenesmus, and urine retention may be necessary until involution diminishes clinical signs. Prostatic involution can be evaluated ul-

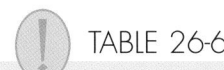 TABLE 26-6

Clinical Signs of Prostatic Disease

	DIAGNOSIS			
SIGNS	**HYPERPLASIA**	**INFECTION ABSCESS**	**CYST**	**NEOPLASIA**
Prostatomegaly	+	+	+	±
Symmetric prostatic enlargement	+	±	±	±
Pain on prostatic palpation	−	±	−	±
Fluctuant prostate	−	±	±	±
Lymphadenomegaly	−	±	−	±
Ultrasound	Normal, ↑ or ↓ echogenicity	Hypoechoic to anechoic cavities	Anechoic cavities	Heterogeneous irregular urethra
Cytology	Hemorrhage	Hemorrhage, inflammation, bacteria	Hemorrhage	Atypical cells ± inflammation and bacteria
Peripheral leukocytosis	−	±	±	±
Pyuria	Rare	+	Rare	±
Systemic signs	±	±	±	±

+, Present; −, absent; ±, variable.

 TABLE 26-7

Drugs Used for Medical Management of Benign Prostatic Enlargement

DRUG	**DOSAGE**	**EXPECTATIONS**
Finasteride (Proscar, Merck)	0.1–0.5 mg/kg PO, qd for 2–3 months* or 5.0 mg PO, qd for dogs weighing between 5–50 kg*	Decreases dihydrotestosterone, prostatic diameter, and volume No adverse effects on semen or testosterone levels Safe
Diethylstilbestrol†	0.2–1.0 mg PO, every 2–3 days for 3–4 weeks	Potentially causes infertility, myelosuppression (anemia, thrombocytopenia, pancytopenia) and prostatic squamous metaplasia leading to abscessation
Progestins: Medroxyprogesterone† acetate (DepoProvera) Megestrol acetate Cyproterone acetate Delmadinone acetate Chlormadinone acetate	 3 mg/kg (minimum dose of 50 mg) SC; repeat dose in 4–6 weeks if signs persist 2 mg/kg PO for 7 days 1.25–2.5 mg/kg PO, qd for 15 days 1–2 mg/kg SC every month 2 mg/kg PO qd for 3–4 weeks	53% have reduced prostate size Monitor for: weight gain, hypothyroidism, diabetes mellitus, mammary nodules; possible testes degeneration, and decreased serum testosterone and LH

PO, Oral; *qd,* once a day; *SC,* subcutaneous; *LH,* luteinizing hormone.
*The dose is uncertain; these are two dosages that have been suggested.
†Should not be used to treat dogs with prostatic disease.

trasonographically. A 50% reduction in prostatic size is expected within 3 weeks and 70% by 9 weeks after castration.

Complications

Complications of castration are found on p. 727. The most common complication of BPH is secondary bacterial infection causing prostatitis. Perineal hernias are less common complications. Complications of medical therapy are listed in Table 26-7.

PROGNOSIS

The prognosis following castration is excellent. Although symptomatic medical therapy alone may initially be helpful, clinical signs recur or worsen without castration.

References

Sirinarumitr K, Johnston SD, Kustritz MVR et al: Effects of finasteride on size of the prostate gland and semen quality of dogs with benign prostatic hypertrophy, *J Am Vet Med Assoc* 218:1275, 2001.

Suggested Reading

Gobello C, Corrada Y: Noninfectious prostatic disease in dogs, *Compend Cont Educ Pract* 24:99, 2002.
Benign prostatic hyperplasia, prostatic cysts, and prostatic neoplasia are reviewed.
Sirinarumitr K, Sirinarumitr T, Johnston SD et al: Finasteride-induced prostatic involution by apoptosis in dogs with benign prostatic hypertrophy, *Am J Vet Res* 63:495, 2002.
Nine dogs with naturally occurring benign prostatic hypertrophy were treated, and cells from prostatic fluid ejaculate were evaluated.
Teske E, Naan EC, Van Dijk EM et al: Canine prostate carcinoma: epidemiological evidence of an increased risk in castrated dogs, *Mol Cell Endocrinol* 197:251, 2002.
In this study from The Netherlands, 57% of the dogs having prostatic disease had benign prostatic hyperplasia, whereas 19% had prostatitis, 13% had prostatic carcinomas, and 11% had other conditions, including cysts, squamous metaplasia, and other tumor types.

PROSTATIC ABSCESSES

DEFINITIONS

Prostatic abscesses are localized accumulations of purulent material within the prostatic parenchyma. **Prostatitis** is an infection of the prostate gland, with or without abscess formation.

GENERAL CONSIDERATIONS AND CLINICALLY RELEVANT PATHOPHYSIOLOGY

Prostatitis is common in dogs, but rare in cats. Infection occurs when bacteria colonize the prostatic parenchyma. The prostatic epithelium creates a blood/prostate barrier because of its lipid bilayer. A high prostatic secretion concentration of zinc probably provides antibacterial activity and normal sperm function. Bacterial colonization of the prostate is reduced by normal defense mechanisms (Box 26-27). Ascending urethral infection is typical, but hematogenous infection is possible. Factors predisposing to infection include disruption of normal parenchymal architecture, urethral disease, urinary tract infections, altered urine flow, altered prostatic secretions, and reduced host immunity. Prostatic cystic hyperplasia, squamous metaplasia, and cysts increase risk of infection. Androgenic hormones are necessary for prostatic secretions; estrogenic hormones decrease secretory activity and may cause prostatic squamous metaplasia leading to cyst formation with subsequent abscessation. Microabscesses form and coalesce, causing large abscesses if not treated promptly. Prostatic enlargement compresses the colon (and rarely the urethra), causing obstruction. Abscess rupture may cause septicemia, peritonitis, and cardiovascular collapse.

BOX 26-27

Normal Prostatic Defense Mechanisms Against Infection

- Local production of IgA and IgG prostatic antibacterial factor
- Mechanical urethral flushing during urination
- Urethral high-pressure zone
- Urethral peristalsis
- Surface characteristics of the urethral mucosa

IgA, Immunoglobulin A; *IgG,* immunoglobulin G.

BOX 26-28

Frequency of Clinical Signs in 92 Dogs With Prostatic Abscesses

Depression/lethargy	85%
Straining to urinate or defecate	65%
Hematuria	54%
Vomiting	35%
Discomfort or pain	26%
Polyuria/polydipsia	18%

From Mullen HS, Matthiesen DT, Scavelli TD: Results of surgical and postoperative complications in 92 dogs treated for prostatic abscessation by a multiple drain technique. *J Am Anim Hosp Assoc* 26:369, 1990.

Pressure on the pelvic diaphragm associated with large prostatic abscesses or cysts may contribute to perineal hernia.

DIAGNOSIS
Clinical Presentation

Signalment. Abscesses primarily occur in older, sexually intact males with prostatitis, squamous metaplasia, or cysts. Although prostatic abscesses may occur in dogs as young as 2 years of age, most are older than 8 years. Feline prostatic infections are rare.

History. Dogs may have recurrent or nonresponsive urinary tract infections. Animals are usually brought in because of an acute onset of depression and/or lethargy, a tendency to strain when urinating or defecating, hematuria, vomiting, discomfort or pain, and polyuria or polydipsia (Box 26-28). Other clinical signs include fever, anorexia, diarrhea, and dehydration. Clinical signs result from compression of adjacent structures or infection.

Physical Examination Findings

Abscessed prostates are generally enlarged, painful, and asymmetric with fluctuant areas (Box 26-29; see also Table 26-6). Rectal palpation is often painful; caudal abdominal pain, lumbar pain, and/or pelvic limb stiffness may be seen. Peritonitis may cause abdominal distention. The scrotum and testicles should be palpated for masses, enlargement, or increased sensitivity. Some animals have perineal hernias, subcutaneous edema, and/or feminization. Depression, fever, anorexia, vomiting, diarrhea, and dehydration are asso-

BOX 26-29

Frequency of Physical Examination Findings on Rectal Palpation in 92 Dogs With Prostatic Abscesses

Prostatomegaly	93%
Pain	73%
Asymmetry with fluctuant areas	49%

 BOX 26-30

Radiographic Changes in 92 Dogs With Prostatic Abscesses

Prostatomegaly	85%
Indistinct prostatic borders	27%

 BOX 26-31

Most Commonly Isolated Bacterial Organisms in Animals With Prostatic Abscesses

- *Escherichia coli*
- *Pseudomonas* spp.
- *Staphylococcus* spp.
- *Streptococcus* spp.
- *Proteus* spp.

From Mullen HS, Matthiesen DT, Scavelli TD: Results of surgical and postoperative complications in 92 dogs treated for prostatic abscessation by a multiple drain technique. *J Am Anim Hosp Assoc* 26:369, 1990.

ciated with severe infections. Additionally, signs of tachycardia, pale or injected mucous membranes, delayed capillary refill, and/or weak pulses suggest sepsis and shock.

Diagnostic Imaging

Radiographic findings include prostatomegaly, indistinct borders, and occasional mineralization (Box 26-30). Prostatic emphysema is rare. Loss of abdominal visceral detail suggests peritonitis (see p. 329). Ultrasonographic evaluation may reveal alterations in echogenicity, and fluid-filled spaces with irregularly defined margins may be seen. Fluid within the lesion may have mixed echogenicity or a flocculent appearance.

> NOTE: Aspiration with ultrasound guidance usually establishes the diagnosis, but should be performed with caution as thin-walled abscesses may rupture secondary to aspiration.

Laboratory Findings

Neutrophilic leukocytosis with a left shift, toxic neutrophils, and monocytosis may occur. Additional abnormalities may include elevated serum alkaline phosphatase and alanine transaminase activities, azotemia, hyperglobulin-

emia, hypoglycemia, and hypokalemia. Hematuria, pyuria, and bacteriuria are common. Prostatic wash or fine-needle aspiration cytology yields highly cellular smears with large numbers of neutrophils and smaller numbers of macrophages and epithelial cells. Squamous metaplasia, hyperplasia, or normal epithelial cells may be detected. The most commonly isolated bacteria are listed in Box 26-31. Occasionally, anaerobic organisms or *Mycoplasma* are isolated. Urine culture, in addition to prostatic fluid culture, is indicated because concurrent infections are common. Antimicrobial sensitivity should be determined for all pathogens. Histologic evaluation may show localized or diffuse inflammation; glandular lumens are typically filled with neutrophils, bacteria, and necrotic debris. Fibrosis, atrophy, and stromal accumulations of lymphocytes and plasma cells are found with chronic prostatitis.

DIFFERENTIAL DIAGNOSIS

Differential diagnoses include prostatitis, prostatic cyst, periprostatic cyst, prostatic neoplasm, prostatic hyperplasia, rectal mass, and intrapelvic masses (see Table 26-6 and Box 26-26).

MEDICAL MANAGEMENT

Prostatitis and small prostatic abscesses are treated with antibiotics, fluid therapy, and nutritional support. If the animal is in septic shock (systemic inflammatory response syndrome), fluid replacement therapy should be initiated as soon as possible (see p. 27). If hypokalemia (see Table 5-6 on p. 29) and hyponatremia are present, intravenous supplementation is required. Hypoglycemia is common in systemic inflammatory response syndrome, and glucose supplementation may be needed (i.e., 2.5% to 5% dextrose-containing fluids) or given as a slow IV bolus (i.e., 10% dextrose) if rapid replacement is necessary. Corticosteroid administration in septic patients is controversial, and its use with flunixin meglumine greatly increases the risk of catastrophic gastrointestinal ulceration and/or perforation. Urine output should be monitored (normal urine output is more than 1 to 2 ml/kg/hr).

Broad-spectrum antibiotic therapy should be initiated as soon as the diagnosis is made. There are several combinations that are often effective (e.g., ampicillin plus enrofloxacin, amikacin plus clindamycin, enrofloxacin plus clindamycin, amikacin plus metronidazole [see p. 81]). A second-generation cephalosporin (e.g., cefoxitin sodium) may be used as a sole agent. If resistant bacterial infection is present in an animal with renal compromise, imipenem may be considered (see p. 81). Initial antibiotic therapy should be altered based on results of susceptibility testing.

Percutaneous prostatic drainage is most safely done with ultrasound guidance. Ultrasonographic drainage of abscesses is appropriate if the animal does not have signs of peritonitis. If necessary, have an assistant displace the prostate cranially via rectal digital manipulations.

After heavy sedation or during general anesthesia, insert a 22-gauge spinal needle with an attached extension set and

20-ml syringe into the fluid-filled cavity with ultrasound guidance. Completely evacuate the fluid, and submit samples for cytology, culture, and susceptibility evaluation. Following drainage. provide supportive care and monitor the animal closely for signs of leakage from the prostatic puncture or injury to adjacent structures for 24 to 48 hours. Two or three additional drainage procedures may be necessary, and castration should be performed.

SURGICAL TREATMENT

Acute bacterial prostatitis and prostatic abscesses are potentially life threatening. Shock therapy must be initiated promptly (see previous discussion). Large abscesses should be drained and castration performed when the patient is stable. Castration may reduce the duration of infection. Prostatic biopsy (see p. 722) should be performed during drainage or resection. Subtotal prostatectomy (see p. 724) is indicated in stable patients for recurrent abscessation or cysts that have not responded to drainage procedures. Rarely, total prostatectomy (see p. 724) is performed for recurrent prostatic infections.

Preoperative Management

The animal should be stabilized before surgery (see previous discussion). Place a urinary catheter before surgery to facilitate intraoperative identification of the urethra.

Anesthesia

Anesthetic recommendations for animals in shock are provided in Box 26-24 on p. 741. Anesthetic recommendations for animals undergoing reproductive surgery are provided on p. 705.

Surgical Anatomy

Surgical anatomy of the prostate is provided on p. 708.

Positioning

The ventral abdomen and medial thighs should be clipped and aseptically prepared for surgery and the prepuce flushed with 0.1% povidone iodine or a 1:40 dilution of 2% chlorhexidine solution. The patient is positioned in dorsal recumbency for a midline celiotomy.

SURGICAL TECHNIQUE

Large abscesses or cysts should be drained. Choice of drainage procedures depends on the size and location of the abscess and/or cyst. Marsupialization (see p. 756) is an option if the abscess and/or cyst can be mobilized to the ventral abdominal wall and if the capsule can hold sutures. It is more commonly used for cysts than abscesses. Prostatic omentalization may decrease postoperative care for patients with prostatic abscesses. Subtotal prostatectomy is an option if abscesses recur. Perform castration before performing the abdominal exploration.

Omentalization

Place a urethral catheter. Expose the prostate through a ventral midline celiotomy from the umbilicus to the pubis. Extend

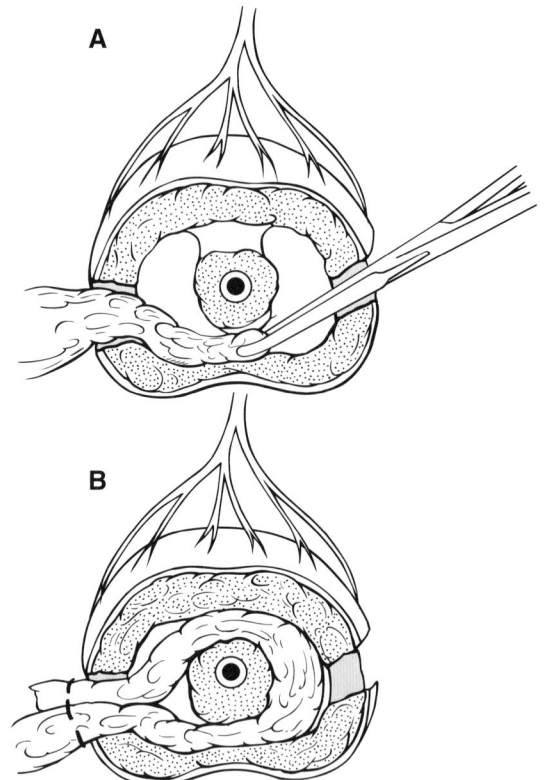

FIG. 26-25
Omentalization of a prostatic abscess. After making stab incisions bilaterally in the lateral aspects of the prostate gland—suctioning, exploring, and lavaging the abscess cavity—introduce omentum through one capsulotomy wound with forceps. The omentum is introduced through the contralateral wound **(A).** Then pass the omentum around the prostatic urethra, exit it through the entry incision, and anchor it to itself with absorbable mattress sutures **(B).**

the incision caudally, and perform a pubic osteotomy if necessary to adequately expose the prostate (see pp. 501, 670, and 675). Place Balfour retractors to facilitate exposure. Explore the abdomen and isolate the bladder and prostate with laparotomy sponges. Place traction sutures through the bladder wall to retract the prostate cranially. Make stab incisions bilaterally in the lateral aspects of the prostate gland and remove the purulent material by suction. Explore and digitally break down any loculated abscesses within the parenchyma. Identify the prostatic urethra by palpation of the previously placed urethral catheter. Place a Penrose drain around the prostatic urethra within the parenchyma to elevate the gland and facilitate irrigation of the abscess cavities with warm saline. Enlarge the stab incisions by resection of the lateral capsular tissue. Submit excised tissue for histopathologic examination. Introduce omentum through one capsulotomy wound with forceps introduced through the contralateral wound (Fig. 26-25). Pass the omentum around the prostatic urethra, exit it through the same incision, and anchor it to itself with absorbable mattress suture (see Fig. 26-25). Close the abdomen routinely.

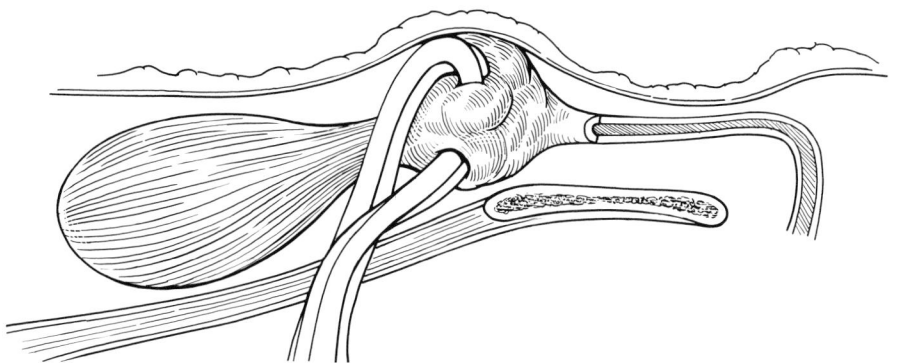

FIG. 26-26
Prostatic abscesses and cysts may be treated using multiple Penrose drains that exit the abdomen in the prepubic area.

Alternatively, omentum can be inserted through both capsular incisions.

Multiple Drain Technique

Expose, isolate, and culture the prostate as described for omentalization. Dissect the ventral fat pad from the prostatic capsule. Insert a large-gauge needle into the abscess and/or cyst, collect a sample for culture and susceptibility testing, and suction its contents. Avoiding vessels and nerves, incise the ventral aspect of the prostate over the abscess and/or cyst cavity. Digitally break down all trabecula and fibrous bands to connect adjacent abscesses and/or cysts, creating a common cavity. Suction and lavage the cavity to remove fluid accumulations. Débride necrotic tissue. Place two to four Penrose drains (½ inch) transversely across the ventrolateral aspect of both lobes of the prostate (Fig. 26-26). Periprostatic drains may also be placed. Alternatively, place a tube drain into the abscess and/or cyst cavity for continuous suction drainage. Exteriorize the end of the drain(s) 2 to 3 cm lateral to the abdominal incision and prepuce. Take a biopsy of the prostatic parenchyma. Secure the drains to the skin with cruciate sutures (e.g., 3-0 nylon). Lavage the surgical site and the entire abdomen if contamination has occurred. Surround the surgical site with omentum and periprostatic fat. Close the abdomen routinely. Remove drains in 1 to 3 weeks.

Postoperative Care and Assessment

Analgesics should be given as necessary (see Chapter 13; for dosages of opioids see Table 13-4 on p. 133) and the patient monitored for sepsis, shock, and anemia. Fluid and nutritional support should be provided until the patient is stable and able to eat. Appropriate antibiotics should be given for 2 to 3 weeks. Ideally, urine or prostatic fluid culture should be performed 3 to 5 days after starting antibiotics and 2 to 3 days after antibiotics are discontinued. The abdomen should be bandaged to protect drains or suction apparatus, and an Elizabethan collar, bucket, or sidebars used to prevent self-trauma and drain removal. Water-insoluble ointments applied around drains prevent skin scalding. Bandages should be changed daily or when "strike through" occurs. Drains may be removed when discharge becomes serosanguineous and diminishes in volume (1 to 3 weeks). Recurring or persistent infection should be identified by culturing prostatic fluid and performing ultrasonography every 3 to 4 months for 1 year.

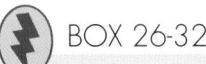

BOX 26-32

Short-Term Complications After Prostatic Drainage

- Hypoproteinemia
- Subcutaneous edema
- Hypoglycemia
- Anemia
- Sepsis
- Shock
- Hypokalemia
- Incisional infections
- Urine leakage
- Urinary incontinence

COMPLICATIONS

The most common short-term complications following drainage are listed in Box 26-32. Urine may be voided through the drains for a few days if urethral trauma or erosion occurs. Scalding around drains and subcutaneous edema may occur. Patients may prematurely remove drains. Subtotal prostatectomy may cause shock, urine leakage, and urinary incontinence. Death and urinary incontinence are more common following subtotal prostatectomy than after drainage procedures.

Long-term complications following drainage and resection include recurrent prostatitis, abscesses, urinary tract infections, urinary incontinence, urethrocutaneous fistula formation, and periprostatic cyst formation. Recurrence rates of 18% for prostatic disease, 33% for urinary tract infection, and 46% for urinary incontinence may occur following implantation of drains. Omentum encircling the urethra may compress it.

PROGNOSIS

Antibiotics and supportive therapy may resolve small abscesses. Large, untreated abscesses will eventually cause septicemia, toxemia, and death. Immediate postoperative mortality may approach 25%; if the prostatic abscess has ruptured, mortality approaches 50%. Fair to excellent results are expected if the patient survives 2 weeks after surgery. Peritonitis may occur after abscess rupture or surgical contamination. Prognosis after omentalization appears good if sufficient omentum is placed within the prostate. Subtotal prostatectomy using an ultrasonic aspirator has a good prognosis because it provides long-term disease resolution.

Reference

Mullen HS, Matthiesen DT, Scavelli TD: Results of surgical and postoperative complications in 92 dogs treated for prostatic abscessation by a multiple drain technique. *J Am Anim Hosp Assoc* 26:369, 1990.

Suggested Reading

Boland LE, Hardie RJ, Gregory SP et al: Ultrasound-guided percutaneous drainage as the primary treatment for prostatic abscesses and cysts in dogs, *J Am Anim Hosp Assoc* 39:151, 2003.

Diagnosis and drainage were possible in 13 diseased dogs without complications, although 1 to 4 procedures were necessary.

Jaegar GH, Law JM: Prostatic pythiosis in a dog, *J Vet Intern Med* 16:598, 2002.

This case report describes an unusual site of pythiosis infection and an unusual cause of prostatitis.

Rohleder JJ, Jones JC: Emphysematous prostatitis and carcinoma in a dog, *J Am Anim Hosp Assoc* 38:478, 2002.

This report describes an emphysematous prostatic abscess from which *E. coli* was isolated that was believed to be secondary to a poorly differentiated carcinoma.

Roura X, Camps-Palau MA, Lloret A et al: Bacterial prostatitis in a cat, *J Vet Intern Med* 16:593, 2002.

This may be the first report of bacterial prostatitis in a cat; the clinical findings and response are similar to those in dogs.

PROSTATIC CYSTS

DEFINITIONS

A **prostatic cyst** is a nonseptic, fluid-filled cavity within or attached to the prostate. Included are **parenchymal cysts** associated with prostatic hyperplasia or **periprostatic cysts,** which are attached to the prostate and may communicate with it.

GENERAL CONSIDERATIONS AND CLINICALLY RELEVANT PATHOPHYSIOLOGY

Parenchymal prostatic cysts occur within or have a physical communication with the prostatic parenchyma (Fig. 26-27). They are common in dogs and may be associated with BPH (see p. 747). Their etiology is unknown, but some are congenital. Sertoli cell tumors or exogenous estrogens may cause squamous metaplasia, which occludes ducts, causing secretory stasis with progressive acinar dilation. Cysts coalesce as they enlarge and are surrounded by dense collagen that can ossify. Small cysts often become confluent, forming larger cavities. Parenchymal cysts are typically found throughout the gland. Parenchymal prostatic cysts are lined by compressed epithelium (transitional, cuboidal, or squamous) and filled with secretory material and cellular debris.

Periprostatic (paraprostatic) cysts are rare compared with other types of prostatic disease. Periprostatic cysts are adjacent and attached to the prostate, but seldom communicate with the parenchyma. They may originate from the uterus masculinus, an embryonic structure derived from the müllerian duct

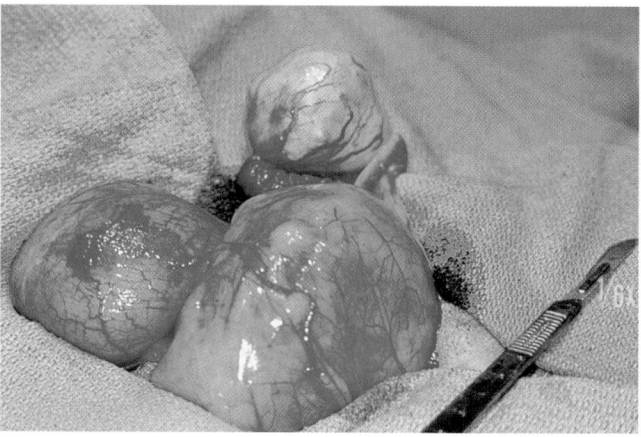

FIG. 26-27
Intraoperative appearance of a large prostatic cyst with squamous metaplasia. Note the enlarged, nodular cryptorchid testicle (dorsal) in which a Sertoli cell tumor was diagnosed histologically.

system and attached on the dorsal prostatic midline. These cysts are often large, extending into the perineal fossa or abdomen. They may displace and compromise adjacent viscera and its function. Periprostatic cysts are usually filled with pale yellow to orange fluid; hemorrhage changes it to brownish-red. Histologically the wall of a periprostatic cyst resembles the wall of a parenchymal cyst (compressed epithelium and dense collagen). Some walls are calcified. Prostatic cysts may become infected and abscess. Pressure on the pelvic diaphragm may contribute to the development of a perineal hernia.

DIAGNOSIS
Clinical Presentation

Signalment. Prostatic cysts are most common in older, intact male, large-breed dogs.

History. Dogs are often asymptomatic until the cysts become large enough to cause rectal, bladder, or urethral obstruction. Perineal bulge or abdominal distention may occur with large cysts. Presenting complaints include depression, inappetence, stranguria, dysuria, incontinence, tenesmus, and/or bloody penile discharge.

Physical Examination Findings

Clinical signs and examination findings due to prostatic cysts are similar to those caused by prostatic hyperplasia (see p. 747). However, periprostatic cysts are asymmetric, fluctuant, and sometimes cause abdominal distention. The most common physical finding is a palpable abdominal mass. Sterile prostatic cysts are not painful. The scrotum and testicles should be palpated for concurrent masses, enlargement, or increased sensitivity, all of which indicate a Sertoli cell tumor. The perineum is palpated to detect herniation.

Diagnostic Imaging

Prostatic cysts and periprostatic cysts may be difficult to differentiate from the urinary bladder without a cystourethrogram. Prostate or cyst wall calcification may be detected on

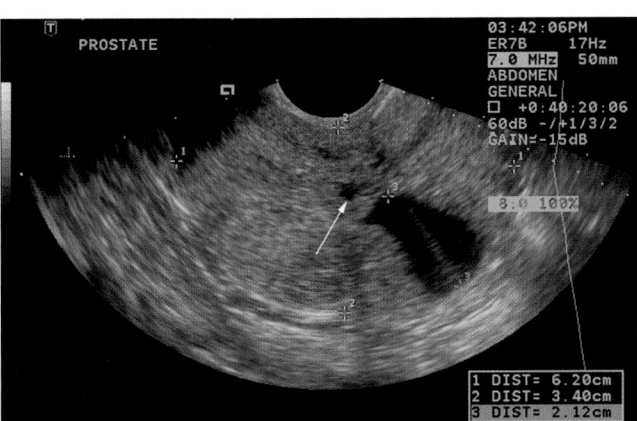

FIG. 26-28
Transrectal transverse ultrasound image of a dog's prostate, which is enlarged because of benign hypertrophy. Note the urethra in the center *(arrow)*. There is a 2-cm-diameter cyst within the left lobe of the prostate (anechoic region). This cyst is typical of prostatomegaly due to benign hypertrophy.

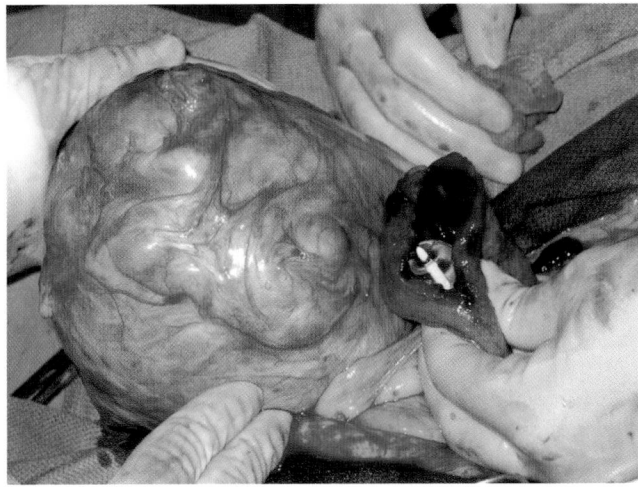

FIG. 26-29
This large periprostatic cyst originated from the dorsolateral aspect of the prostate and caused urethral obstruction and rupture of the urinary bladder.

survey radiographs. Ultrasonography helps detect and define cavitary changes (Fig. 26-28). Prostatic cysts typically appear as anechoic cavitary lesions with more regularly defined margins than abscesses. However, this finding is not 100% specific and cytology of the fluid is necessary for a definitive diagnosis. Periprostatic cysts are usually large anechoic structures with internal septa. Some communicate with large anechoic cavities within the prostatic parenchyma.

> NOTE: Ultrasound-guided aspirates can be obtained; however, be careful to prevent iatrogenic peritonitis if infection is likely.

Laboratory Findings

Specific laboratory abnormalities are rare. Aspiration of a sterile, yellow to serosanguineous fluid with minimal inflammation suggests a periprostatic cyst. Cytologic evaluation reveals prostatic epithelial cells and few leukocytes, but more erythrocytes and hemosiderophages than with prostatic hyperplasia. Numerous squamous epithelial cells suggest squamous metaplasia.

DIFFERENTIAL DIAGNOSIS

Differential diagnoses include prostatic abscess, squamous metaplasia, neoplasia, or hyperplasia (see Box 26-29).

MEDICAL MANAGEMENT

Medical therapy includes treatment of constipation and urine retention. Stool softeners (see p. 726) may be given and the bladder drained by centesis or catheterization as needed. Percutaneous drainage by centesis is palliative, but may cause abscessation (see p. 751).

Surgical Treatment

Treatment for small parenchymal cysts is castration. Dogs with large cysts should be castrated and the cyst drained, resected, or debulked. Incomplete resection may be necessary to prevent incontinence.

Preoperative Management

Animals with prostatic cysts are generally stable. Perioperative antibiotics are reasonable if marsupialization or prolonged surgery is anticipated.

Anesthesia

Anesthetic recommendations for animals undergoing reproductive surgery are provided on p. 705.

Positioning

The ventral abdomen, ventral perineum, and medial thighs are clipped and prepared for aseptic surgery. The dog is positioned in dorsal recumbency for a midline celiotomy.

SURGICAL TECHNIQUE

Castration should be performed and large cysts resected or drained (Fig. 26-29). Cystic fluid should be cultured and a biopsy taken from the prostate (see p. 723). Nonresectable cysts may be drained by omentalization (Fig. 26-30) or with multiple drains (see p. 752). Subtotal prostatectomy (see p. 724) or marsupialization (p. 756) may be appropriate for recurring cysts.

Omentalization

Omentalization of a large parenchymal prostatic cyst is performed similar to omentalization of an abscess. Omentalization of a periprostatic cyst differs somewhat from omentalization of an abscess (see p. 752).

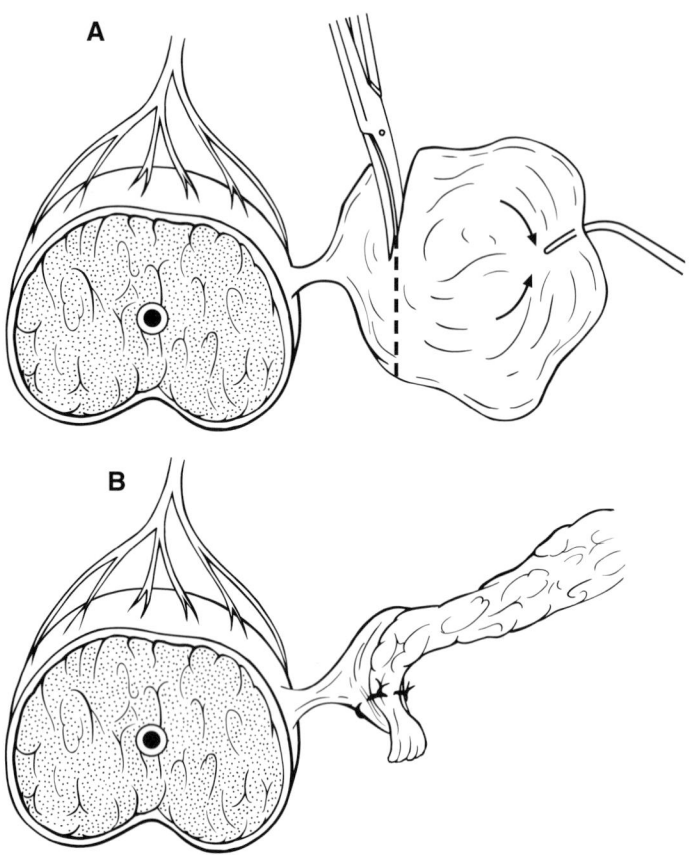

FIG. 26-30
Omentalization of a periprostatic cyst. **A,** After exposing the cyst, make a single stab incision into the cyst and aspirate its contents. Take samples for culture, cytology, and histopathology. Dissect and resect the cyst wall without damaging innervation or vasculature to the prostate and urinary bladder. **B,** Pack omentum into the cystic remnant and secure it with absorbable horizontal mattress sutures.

Expose the prostate through a caudal abdominal celiotomy. Identify the cyst, and make a single stab incision into the cyst and aspirate its contents. Take samples for culture, cytology, and histopathology. Dissect and resect the cyst wall without damaging innervation or vasculature to the prostate and urinary bladder (see Fig. 26-30). Pack omentum into the cystic remnant, and secure it with absorbable horizontal mattress sutures (see Fig. 26-30). Lavage and close the abdomen routinely.

Marsupialization

Expose and isolate the prostate as described on p. 752 for omentalization. Make a second incision (5 to 8 cm) through the abdominal wall lateral to the prepuce over the abscess and/or cyst cavity (Fig. 26-31, A). Excise 0.5 to 1 cm of abdominal muscle (Fig. 26-31, B). Suture the capsule or the cyst wall to the external rectus fascia (Fig. 26-31, C). Use continuous or interrupted 3-0 to 4-0 monofilament absorbable (polydioxanone, poliglecaprone 25, glycomer 631, or polyglyconate) sutures. Facilitate suturing by having an assis-

tant elevate the prostate toward the abdominal wall. Incise the abscess and/or cyst wall and suction the contents. Place a second layer of simple continuous or interrupted sutures (e.g., 3-0 or 4-0 nylon or polypropylene) between the skin edge and capsule and/or cyst edge (Fig. 26-31, D and E). Take a biopsy of the prostatic parenchyma. Digitally break down trabeculae and fibrous bands to create a confluent cavity. Lavage the cavity and surgical site, place omentum around the marsupialization, and close the abdomen in three layers.

An alternative technique is to incise the ventrolateral aspect of the cyst and/or abscess wall and suction the cavity before suturing it to the rectus fascia. The capsule and/or cyst wall is then sutured 5 mm from the incised edge of the cavity to the rectus fascia. This variation has a higher risk of abdominal contamination.

POSTOPERATIVE CARE AND ASSESSMENT

Analgesics (see Chapter 13; for dosages of opioids see Table 13-4 on p. 133) and supportive care (e.g., fluids and electrolytes) should be given as necessary. Monitor closely for shock and infection. Medical therapy may manage urine retention, constipation, and discomfort. See p. 753 for postoperative care and potential complications following prostatic or cystic drain placement. Drains should be left in place for 1 to 3 weeks. Marsupialization may cause a permanent fistula or may close prematurely. Urine may be voided through the marsupialization for a few days if urethral erosion is present. Adhesions following omentalization are minimized if exposed parenchyma within the prostatic capsule is oversewn and covered with omentum.

PROGNOSIS

The prognosis is good to fair after castration and surgical drainage. Some prostatic and periprostatic cysts recur and require repeated drainage, but this is rare if the dog is castrated. Recurrence following subtotal prostatectomy or omentalization is uncommon. Overzealous resection may cause detrusor atony, incontinence, or bladder ischemia. Infection of the cyst may occur following marsupialization.

Suggested Reading

Boland LE, Hardie RJ, Gregory SP et al: Ultrasound-guided percutaneous drainage as the primary treatment for prostatic abscesses and cysts in dogs, *J Am Anim Hosp Assoc* 39:151, 2003.
Diagnosis and drainage were possible in 13 diseased dogs without complications although 1 to 4 procedures were necessary.
Gobello C, Corrada Y: Noninfectious prostatic disease in dogs, *Compend Cont Educ Pract* 24:99, 2002.
Benign prostatic hyperplasia, prostatic cysts, and prostatic neoplasia are reviewed.
Welsh EM, Kirby BM, Simpson JW et al: Surgical management of perineal paraprostatic cysts in three dogs, *J Small Anim Pract* 41:358, 2000.
This report reviews the clinical course, management, and outcome following resection and omentalization.

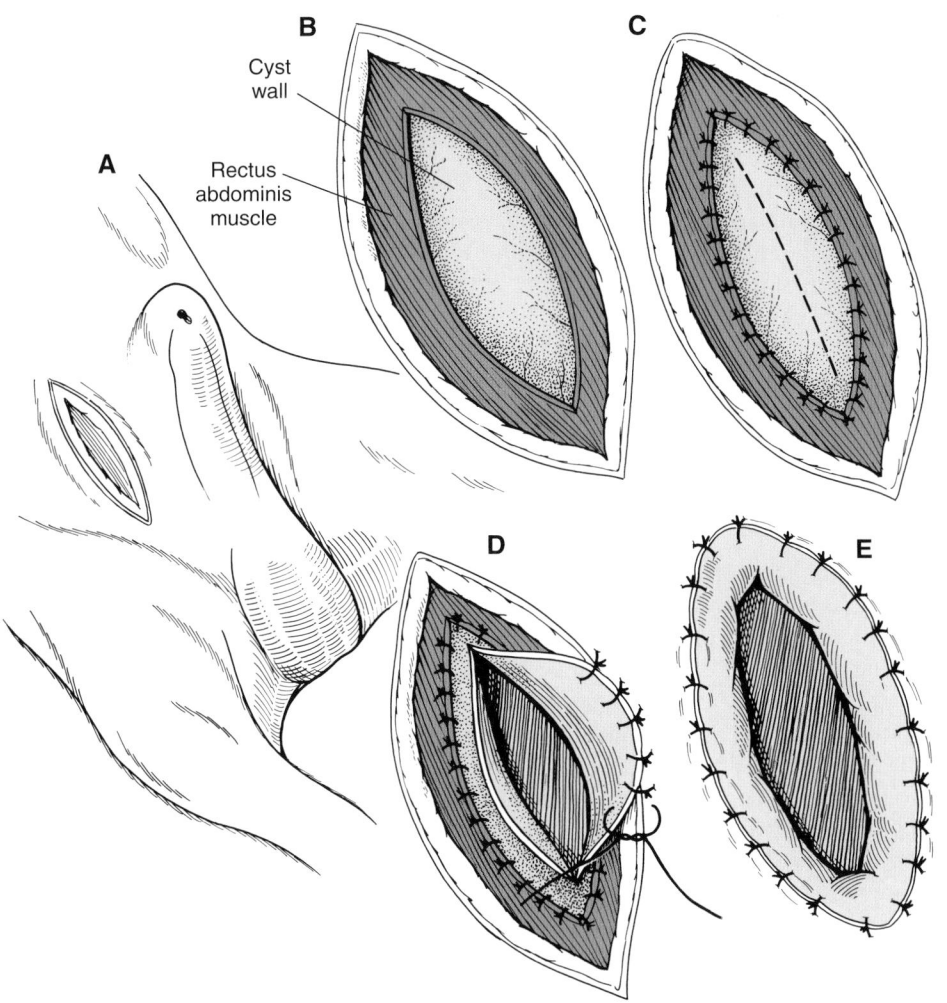

Cyst wall

Rectus abdominis muscle

FIG. 26-31
A, To marsupialize a prostatic cyst or abscess, make a longitudinal incision lateral to the prepuce over the enlarged mass. **B,** Excise an ellipse of abdominal muscle. **C,** Suture the prostatic capsule to the external rectus sheath. Make an incision through the prostatic capsule and suture the edge of the capsule to skin **(D** and **E)**.

PROSTATIC NEOPLASIA

DEFINITIONS

Prostatic tumors may originate from epithelial tissue (**carcinomas**), smooth muscle tissue (**leiomyosarcoma**), or vascular structures (**hemangiosarcoma**).

GENERAL CONSIDERATIONS AND CLINICALLY RELEVANT PATHOPHYSIOLOGY

Although prostatic neoplasia is the most common prostatic disease in neutered male dogs, it is still uncommon in dogs (0.2 to 0.6%) and rare in cats. Castration does not initiate the development of prostatic carcinoma in the dog, but does favor tumor progression (Sorenmo et al, 2003; Teske et al, 2002). Testicular hormones are not believed to cause prostatic tumors, but adrenal and pituitary hormones may be influential. Most prostatic tumors originate from ductal and/or urothelial, androgen-independent structures and are adenocarcinomas (Box 26-33). Well-differentiated adenocarcinomas are found more frequently in sexually intact dogs, whereas histologic types with more anaplasia are more common in castrated dogs. Dogs castrated before 2 years of

 BOX 26-33

Prostatic Tumor Types

Carcinomas
- Adenocarcinoma
- Transitional cell carcinoma
- Squamous cell carcinoma
- Undifferentiated

Leiomyosarcomas

Hemangiosarcomas

age are more likely to have tumors of ductal and/or urothelial origin (Sorenmo et al, 2003). Cyclooxygenase-1 (COX-1) expression is present in 94.1% and cyclooxygenase-2 (COX-2) expression in 88.2% of dogs with prostatic carcinomas (Sorenmo et al, 2004). Since COX-2 is not expressed in normal prostate glands, it may be involved in the pathogenesis of canine prostatic carcinoma. Prostatic carcinomas are locally invasive and metastasize early to regional lymph nodes (iliac, pelvic, and sublumbar), lung, and bone. They frequently invade bone, bladder, colon, and surrounding tissue by direct extension. Other metastatic sites include the liver, spleen, kidney, heart, adrenal glands, skeletal muscle, and subcutaneous tissue. Bone involvement may cause pain or pathologic fractures. Hypertrophic osteopathy has occasionally been associated with prostatic tumors. Prostatic enlargement causes compression and partial obstruction of the colon, rectum, and sometimes urethra. Pitting edema of the pelvic limbs may occur secondary to lymphatic invasion. Most tumors involve the trigone and urethra and have metastasized at the time of diagnosis. The behavior of feline prostatic tumors is unknown.

DIAGNOSIS
Clinical Presentation
Signalment. Prostatic neoplasia occurs in both intact and neutered males. Medium to large-breed dogs are overrepresented; the Bouvier des Flandres has an increased risk of prostatic carcinoma (Teske et al, 2002). The average age of occurrence is 10 years (Sorenmo et al, 2003; Teske et al, 2002). It is very rare in cats.

History. Signs may include weight loss; pelvic limb lameness or weakness; tenesmus; dyschezia; urine retention or incontinence; stranguria; dysuria; polyuria; polydipsia; hematuria; pelvic limb edema; and abdominal, pelvic, or lumbar pain. Prostatic neoplasia may cause substantial emaciation and debility. Metastasis may produce other signs (e.g., dyspnea). Castrated dogs presenting with prostatic disease are more likely to have neoplasia than other types of prostatic disease. The interval between castration and onset of disease is highly variable.

Physical Examination Findings
The animal may be debilitated and weak. Lymph node infiltration and lymphatic obstruction can cause pelvic limb edema. The prostate may be normal sized, but it is often asymmetrically enlarged. Pain, firmness, fixation, and nodular irregularity are characteristic of prostatic neoplasia. Sublumbar lymph node enlargement may be detected during rectal examination. Skeletal palpation sometimes elicits pain secondary to bone metastasis.

Diagnostic Imaging
Thoracic radiographs should be evaluated for metastasis. Abdominal and pelvic radiographs should be evaluated for prostatic size and mineralization, lymph node enlargement, colonic displacement, and osteolytic or proliferative vertebral or pelvic lesions. Retrograde urethrocystography may determine urethral size and mucosal smoothness, and prostatic symmetry. Most prostatic tumors involve the urethra and trigone of the urinary bladder. Ultrasonography may define the prostatic mass as cystic or solid and can be used to evaluate abdominal lymph nodes for metastasis. Prostatic aspiration and biopsy are facilitated by ultrasound guidance.

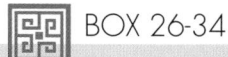 BOX 26-34

Additional Cytologic Criteria of Malignancy

- Variation in nuclear and nucleolar size
- Variable and increased nuclear cytoplasmic ratio
- Nuclear molding
- Abnormal mitotic figures
- Coarsely clumped chromatin

Scintigraphy may be used to locate metastatic sites involving bone.

Laboratory Findings
Hematology, serum biochemistry profile, urinalysis, urine culture, and electrocardiography are indicated. Results are nonspecific for prostatic neoplasia, although paraneoplastic syndromes and concurrent problems may be identified. Anemia, hematuria, and/or pyuria may be detected. Elevated concentrations of total acid phosphatase (TAP; approximately 21.4 ± 18.9 U/L) and prostatic acid phosphatase (PAP; approximately 11.9 ± 2.8 U/L) may indicate prostatic cancer.

Cytology or histopathology is needed for definitive diagnosis. Fine-needle aspiration of prostatic neoplasia may yield a moderately cellular sample with abnormal epithelial cells. Neoplastic-appearing epithelial cells have large, prominent, multiple nuclei with multiple nucleoli and cytoplasmic vacuolation. Additional cytologic criteria for malignancy are provided in Box 26-34. Prostatic washes are less reliable in obtaining neoplastic cells. Transurethral biopsy may be diagnostic if the tumor has invaded the urethra.

DIFFERENTIAL DIAGNOSIS
Differential diagnoses include prostatic hyperplasia, abscesses, cysts, periprostatic cysts, prostatitis, rectal masses, or pelvic masses. It can be difficult to differentiate cancer from prostatic hyperplasia associated with prostatitis (see Table 26-6).

MEDICAL MANAGEMENT
Efficacy of chemotherapy and radiation therapy for prostatic tumors is unreported. Ketoconazole and luteinizing hormone-releasing hormone agonists have been suggested. Ketoconazole inhibits testicular and adrenal testosterone synthesis. Luteinizing hormone-releasing hormone agonists ultimately decrease FSH, LH, and testosterone release. Recently, piroxicam and carprofen have been shown to improve survival in dogs with prostatic carcinomas, probably because of their binding to COX receptors. Treated dogs lived significantly longer than untreated dogs, 6.9 versus 0.7 months (Sorenmo et al, 2004). The dose of piroxicam was 0.3 mg/kg PO, qd and that of carprofen 2.2 mg/kg PO, bid in this study.

SURGICAL TREATMENT

Treatment is rarely successful. Treatment protocols combining surgery, chemotherapy, and radiation therapy are being investigated, but their efficacy is presently unknown.

PREOPERATIVE MANAGEMENT

Clip and aseptically prepare the ventral abdomen, ventral perineum, and medial thighs.

Anesthesia

Anesthetic recommendations for animals undergoing reproductive surgery are provided on p. 705.

Surgical Anatomy

Surgical anatomy of the male reproductive tract is provided on p. 708.

Positioning

The patient is positioned in dorsal recumbency for a midline celiotomy. The entire ventral abdomen and inguinal area should be clipped and prepared for aseptic surgery.

SURGICAL TECHNIQUE

Castration may temporarily slow tumor growth. Prostatectomy may be curative if the tumor is diagnosed early. Unfortunately, most tumors are advanced when diagnosed, making preservation of trigonal innervation impossible. Such dogs often are unacceptable pets after prostatectomy because of urinary incontinence. Palliation of clinical signs may occur following transurethral or subtotal prostatectomy; but this is not recommended because of the high risk of spreading tumor to surrounding tissue and the short-term benefits.

POSTOPERATIVE CARE AND ASSESSMENT

Analgesics (see Chapter 13; for dosages of opioids see Table 13-4 on p. 133) and fluids should be given as necessary. The bladder should be decompressed and urine diverted for 4 to 5 days with a urinary catheter or cystostomy tube after prostatectomy (see p. 667). Patients should be monitored for urine leakage, incontinence, and/or infection. Reevaluation at frequent intervals for local recurrence and metastasis is recommended. Complications and treatment of animals following prostatectomy are described on p. 727.

PROGNOSIS

The prognosis is poor because of metastasis, recurrence, and poor quality of life associated with urinary incontinence. Hormonal therapy has not been useful in dogs. Most untreated dogs are euthanized within 1 to 3 months because of progressive clinical signs.

References

Sorenmo KU, Goldschmidt M, Shofer F: Immunohistochemical characterization of canine prostatic carcinoma and correlation with castration status and castration time, *Vet Comp Oncol* 1:48, 2003.

Sorenmo KU, Goldschmidt MH, Shofer FS et al: Evaluation of cyclooxygenase-1 and cyclooxygenase-2 expression and the effect of cyclooxygenase inhibitors in canine prostatic carcinoma, *Vet Comp Oncol* 2:13, 2004.

Teske E, Naan EC, Van Dijk EM et al: Canine prostate carcinoma: epidemiological evidence of an increased risk in castrated dogs, *Mol Cell Endocrinol* 197:251, 2002.

Suggested Reading

Gobello C, Corrada Y: Noninfectious prostatic disease in dogs, *Compend Cont Educ Pract* 24:99, 2002.

Benign prostatic hyperplasia, prostatic cysts, and prostatic neoplasia are reviewed.

Liptak JM, Brutscher SP, Monnet E et al: Transurethral resection in the management of urethral and prostatic neoplasia in 6 dogs, *Vet Surg* 33:505, 2004.

Transurethral resection via cystoscopy placed through a cystotomy and combined with radiation and chemotherapy provided short-term palliation of urination difficulties in dogs with prostatic carcinomas.

Lucroy MD, Bowles MH, Higbee RG et al: Photodynamic therapy for prostatic carcinoma in dogs, *J Vet Intern Med* 17:235, 2003.

The affected Dachshund was given 5-aminolevulinic acid to photosensitize the prostate before diode laser treatment, which resulted in control for 34 weeks when signs suddenly increased and the dog was then euthanized.

Rohleder JJ, Jones JC: Emphysematous prostatitis and carcinoma in a dog, *J Am Anim Hosp Assoc* 38:478, 2002.

This report describes an emphysematous prostatic abscess from which *E. coli* was isolated that was believed to be secondary to a poorly differentiated carcinoma.

TESTICULAR AND SCROTAL NEOPLASIA

DEFINITIONS

Sertoli cells are supporting elongated cells of seminiferous tubules that nourish spermatids. **Leydig cells** are interstitial tissue cells believed to be responsible for internal secretion of testosterone.

GENERAL CONSIDERATIONS AND CLINICALLY RELEVANT PATHOPHYSIOLOGY

Scrotal tumors are most commonly mast cell tumors (MCTs) or melanomas. Mast cells are normal immune system cells and are important in inflammatory responses to tissue trauma. Cytoplasmic granules in mast cells contain heparin, histamine, platelet-activating factor, and eosinophilic chemotactic factor. The number and type of granules in MCTs depend on the degree of tumor differentiation. Well-differentiated MCTs contain more heparin, whereas undifferentiated tumors have more histamine. The cause of MCTs is unknown, although chronically inflamed areas have been reported to be at increased risk for tumor development. In dogs, 50% of MCTs are malignant, especially those in the preputial, inguinal, and perineal areas. Regional lymph nodes, spleen, liver, and bone marrow are common metastatic sites. MCTs have no distinctive appearance. They may

BOX 26-35

Scrotal and Testicular Tumors

Scrotal Tumors	Testicular Tumors
• Mast cell tumors (MCTs)	• Sertoli cell
• Melanomas	• Interstitial cell
	• Seminoma
	• Embryonal carcinoma
	• Lipoma
	• Fibroma
	• Hemangioma
	• Chondroma
	• Teratoma

be raised, hairless, ulcerated, erythematous, well-defined, and/or diffuse skin thickenings. Manipulation of MCTs may cause degranulation, erythema, and wheal formation. Steroid administration may cause degranulation. Gastroduodenal ulcers occur in up to 80% of dogs with MCTs because of histamine release. Ulcers may cause anorexia, vomiting, diarrhea, and/or melena (see p. 436). Heparin and proteolytic enzyme release may prolong coagulation and delay wound healing after resection.

Melanomas originate from melanocytes and melanoblasts, cells of neuroectodermal origin. Masses may be brown to black or occasionally nonpigmented. Melanomas are more common in dogs than in cats. Tumors originating in the skin tend to be benign. Local recurrence and distant metastasis are common with malignant melanomas. Lymph node metastasis usually occurs first, and then to the lungs.

The most common testicular neoplasms (i.e., Sertoli cell tumors, interstitial [Leydig] cell tumors, and seminomas) occur with equal frequency. Other testicular tumors are rare (Box 26-35). Many old dogs have multiple tumors in one or both testicles. Tumors involving scrotal testes are usually benign, whereas those in cryptorchid testes may be malignant. Metastases are slow growing, but occasionally are detected in lumbar, deep inguinal, and external iliac lymph nodes. Visceral metastasis is rare. Testicular tumors interfere with testicular function, invading or compressing seminiferous tubules or producing excessive estrogen or testosterone. Interstitial cell tumor production of excess testosterone may contribute to perianal adenomas, perineal hernia, and BPH. Sertoli cell tumors producing excess estrogens may cause squamous metaplasia of the prostate, feminization, and/or myelotoxicity.

Sertoli cell tumors arise from sustentacular cells. Normal and neoplastic Sertoli cells produce estrogenic hormones. Sertoli cell tumors are usually solitary, but may be multiple and bilateral. Sertoli cell tumors are more common in cryptorchid than scrotal testes. Tumors are discrete, with expansile growth, compressing and destroying surrounding testicular tissue. Large tumors may cause distention or destruction of the tunic, and growth may extend along the spermatic cord. They are firm, multilobulated, and gray-white with areas of necrosis, hemorrhage, or cysts. Dogs with Sertoli cell tumors often have signs of hyperestrogenism (see Box 26-36), especially those with large tumors. Signs regress with castration and tumor removal. Persistence or recurrence of clinical signs suggests estrogen-producing metastasis. Sertoli cell tumors have a higher rate of metastasis than other testicular tumors.

Interstitial (Leydig) cell tumors occur in scrotal testes as multiple or solitary forms and frequently coexist with Sertoli cell tumors. Most interstitial cell tumors are benign, soft, encapsulated, and rarely exceed 1 to 2 cm in diameter. Interstitial cell tumors may cause testicular enlargement, but are difficult to palpate. On cut surfaces they are discrete, round, tan to yellow-orange masses with foci of hemorrhage or cystic spaces. Dogs with interstitial cell tumors may be infertile. These tumors produce androgens or contribute to androgenic hormone imbalance. Perineal hernia, perianal adenomas and hyperplasia, and prostatic disease have been associated with interstitial cell tumors.

Seminomas arise from testicular germ cells and occur commonly in cryptorchid and scrotal testicles. They are usually solitary, but may be multiple, bilateral, and coexist with other tumor types. Seminomas can be large, replacing most testicular tissue. They are softer than Sertoli cell tumors with a glistening, pinkish gray-tan, multilobulated, unencapsulated cut surface. Signs of feminization rarely occur. They rarely metastasize.

DIAGNOSIS
Clinical Presentation

Signalment. Scrotal and testicular tumors are more common in dogs than in cats. They usually occur in dogs older than 10 years; however, tumors in cryptorchid animals may occur earlier. Cryptorchidism predisposes to Sertoli cell tumors and seminomas. Cryptorchid dogs are 13.6 times more likely to develop testicular tumors than normal dogs. Dogs with inguinal hernias are 4.6 times more likely. A breed predisposition for developing testicular tumors has not been identified. Dogs predisposed to MCTs include English bulldogs, English bull terriers, boxers, and Boston terriers.

History. Affected, asymptomatic animals may be brought in for evaluation of a mass seen or felt in the scrotal or inguinal areas or for endocrine abnormalities (e.g., changes in hair coat, infertility, lethargy, feminization [Box 26-36], perianal tumors, or prostatic disease).

Physical Examination Findings

Scrotal skin should be examined for inflammation, nodules, masses, and ulceration. Scrotal skin should be of uniform thickness. Both testicles should be evaluated for symmetry, firmness, irregularity, scrotal adhesions, and sensitivity. Small or deep intraparenchymal testicular tumors are not detectable on palpation, but the testes may be firm and hard, or one testicle may be firm and the other atrophied. If the animal is cryptorchid, the inguinal area should be checked for a retained testicle and the abdomen for a mass. Sublumbar lymphadenomegaly and prostatomegaly may be detected

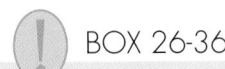

BOX 26-36

Signs of Hyperestrogenism

- Bilateral symmetrical alopecia
- Brittle hair
- Poor hair regrowth
- Thin skin
- Hyperpigmentation
- Nipple elongation
- Mammary enlargement
- Penile atrophy
- Preputial swelling and sagging
- Squatting micturition
- Reduced libido
- Male attraction
- Testicular atrophy
- Prostatic atrophy or cystic enlargement
- Anemia
- Thrombocytopenia or neutropenia

by rectal examination. The abdomen should be palpated for splenomegaly, hepatomegaly, lymph node enlargement, and signs of metastasis (i.e., with MCTs). Sertoli cell tumors and seminomas may cause feminization (see Box 26-36).

Diagnostic Imaging

Intraabdominal testicles may be seen radiographically as caudal abdominal masses. Radiographs also help identify intraabdominal lymphadenomegaly and organomegaly. Ultrasound may delineate scrotal and testicular neoplasia, abscesses, ischemia, testicular torsion, and scrotal hernias. Testicular tumors have variable echogenicity on ultrasound examination.

Laboratory Findings

Hematology, serum biochemistry panel, and urinalysis are indicated in animals with scrotal or testicular tumors. Nonregenerative anemia, leukopenia, and thrombocytopenia may be associated with hyperestrogenism and myelotoxicosis. Fine-needle aspirate cytology of scrotal and testicular lesions helps identify neoplastic cells, fungal elements, abnormal sperm, bacteria, and inflammation. Fine-needle aspiration of the testicle is rarely performed, but can help differentiate neoplasia from abscesses or granulomas. Cytology of the preputial mucosa may reveal cornification secondary to Sertoli cell tumor estrogen production. Fine-needle aspirate cytology is usually diagnostic for MCTs, but degranulated or poorly granular mast cells may be difficult for the novice cytologist. Although rare, buffy coat smears should be examined for mastocythemia. Microcytic hypochromic anemia, especially with hypoalbuminemia, suggests gastrointestinal hemorrhage. More than 10 mast cells per 1000 nucleated cells in the bone marrow is abnormal. Tumor histopathology is necessary to grade the tumor and determine prognosis. Cytology from melanomas usually reveals round to spindle-shaped cells,

frequently containing brown to black granules. It is easy to confuse amelanotic melanomas with fibrosarcoma on cytology.

Brucella canis infections may be diagnosed with serology or blood culture. Semen evaluation to determine fertility is rarely performed when neoplasia is diagnosed. Serum testosterone levels are sometimes elevated with interstitial cell tumors (see Table 26-4). Sertoli cell tumors and seminomas sometimes increase serum estradiol concentrations.

DIFFERENTIAL DIAGNOSIS

Other differentials for testicular masses include sperm granuloma, fibrosis, hematoma, spermatocele, varicocele, orchitis, and epididymitis. Other differential diagnoses for scrotal disease include dermatitis, self-trauma, chemical burn, and laceration. *B. canis* infection should be considered in animals having scrotal dermatitis, orchitis, reproductive failure, epididymitis, or testicular atrophy.

> NOTE: Be sure to test for *Brucella canis* infection in dogs with unexplained scrotal or testicular disease.

MEDICAL MANAGEMENT

MCTs may respond to chemotherapy or radiation therapy. The efficacy of chemotherapy or radiation therapy for other scrotal or testicular tumors is unknown. Cisplatin therapy may be beneficial in treating aggressive testicular tumors (Dhaliwal et al, 1999).

SURGICAL TREATMENT

Tumor excision gives the best chance for a good prognosis. Removal of both testicles is recommended for testicular neoplasia. Castration is described on p. 714. If the owner insists on preserving breeding potential, unilateral castration of the neoplastic testicle may be performed. The testicles should be submitted for histologic examination. Scrotal ablation (see p. 714) and castration are recommended to treat scrotal tumors and testicular tumors with scrotal adhesions. Even discrete MCTs may extend deep into surrounding tissue; therefore 3-cm margins on all sides are recommended.

Preoperative Management

Few patients with testicular tumors are debilitated, except those with myelosuppression, testicular torsion, or concurrent diseases (Fig. 26-32). Bone marrow suppression may necessitate blood transfusions and antibiotics. An antihistamine (e.g., diphenhydramine [Benadryl], 0.5 mg/kg IV, slowly) should be preoperatively administered to patients with MCTs to protect against histamine release. It may be given IV immediately before surgery, but should be given extremely slowly to avoid hypotension. Alternately, it may be administered IM 30 minutes before anesthetic induction. An H_2 receptor antagonist (i.e., ranitidine, cimetidine, or famotidine) or a proton pump inhibitor (i.e., omeprazole) reduces gastric acid secretion and the incidence and severity of gastrointestinal ulceration along with treating existing

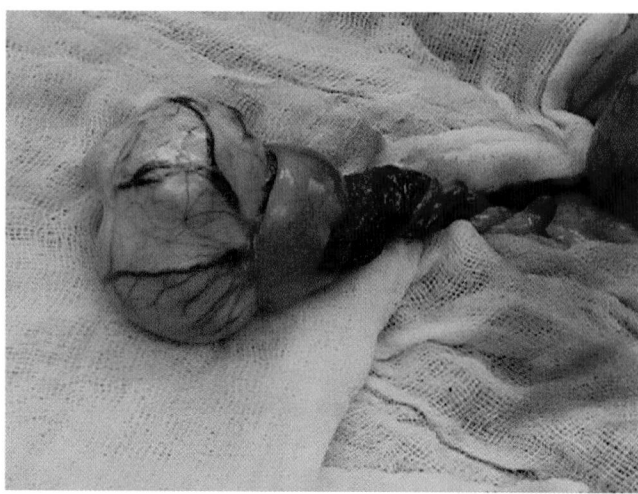

FIG. 26-32
Nodular, neoplastic cryptorchid testicle with testicular torsion. Note spermatic cord twisting.

ulcers. H_2 receptor antagonists are less effective than omeprazole, but they work quicker (i.e., it takes 2 to 5 days for omeprazole to have maximal effect). Sucralfate may be given for existing ulcers (see p. 438). Sucralfate should be given 1 hour after administration of other oral medications because it may interfere with their absorption.

Anesthesia

Anesthetic recommendations for animals undergoing reproductive surgery are provided on p. 705.

Positioning

Position the patient in dorsal recumbency for a prescrotal castration or an exploratory laparotomy. The entire ventral abdomen should be clipped and prepared for exploratory laparotomy; see p. 714 for surgical preparation recommendations for animals undergoing castration.

SURGICAL TECHNIQUE

Castration and scrotal ablation are described on p. 714.

POSTOPERATIVE CARE AND ASSESSMENT

Analgesics (see Chapter 13; for dosages of opioids see Table 13-4 on p. 133) and supportive care should be given as necessary. Patients with MCTs should be continued on an H_2 receptor antagonist, proton pump inhibitor, and/or protectant if gastrointestinal ulceration occurs (see p. 438). Adjunctive therapy for malignant tumors may prove beneficial. Patients with malignant tumors should be reevaluated every 3 to 4 months for recurrence or metastasis. Complications associated with paraneoplastic syndromes and metastasis may become evident or persist following castration.

PROGNOSIS

Surgery is curative for most testicular tumors. The prognosis for interstitial cell tumors, Sertoli cell tumors without metastasis or myelotoxicity, and seminomas without signs of hyperestrogenism is excellent. Myelotoxicity may be fatal despite appropriate therapy, but usually improves within 2 to 3 weeks of tumor removal. Chemotherapy can be instituted if Sertoli cell tumors or seminomas have metastasized. Low-grade MCTs are less likely to recur or metastasize. Nonresectable or incompletely resected MCTs may respond to radiation therapy or chemotherapy. Efficacy of nonsurgical treatment modalities for other tumors is unknown.

Reference

Dhaliwal RS, Kitchell BE, Knight BL et al: Treatment of aggressive testicular tumors in four dogs, *J Am Anim Hosp Assoc* 35:3113, 1999.

HYPOSPADIAS

DEFINITION

Hypospadias is a developmental anomaly in males in which the urethra opens ventral and caudal to the normal orifice.

GENERAL CONSIDERATIONS AND CLINICALLY RELEVANT PATHOPHYSIOLOGY

Hypospadias is rare, and many affected animals have other congenital or developmental anomalies. It occurs as a result of failure of the genital folds and genital swellings to fuse normally during fetal development. This causes abnormal development of the penile urethra, penis, prepuce, and/or scrotum. Hypospadias is accompanied by hypoplasia of the corpus cavernosum urethra. The urethra opens anywhere along its length at one or more locations. Hypospadias is classified based on the location of the urethral opening as glandular, penile, scrotal, perineal, or anal. The prepuce is similarly affected and ventrally incomplete. In some cases the penis may be underdeveloped and abnormal (ventral or caudal deviation and blunt) and the scrotum may be divided. Urine may pool within the prepuce, causing irritation and infection of the penis and preputial lining (balanoposthitis).

> NOTE: Do not use animals with hypospadias for breeding.

DIAGNOSIS
Clinical Presentation

Signalment. Breed predisposition has not been documented, but a familial predisposition has been suggested in Boston terriers. The defect is present at birth.

History. Small defects and those occurring in the glans may not cause problems. Some patients with hypospadias of the glans and abnormal preputial development may be evaluated because of a chronically exposed penis. Larger and more caudal urethral openings cause urine pooling within the prepuce or dermatitis as a result of urine contact. A pre-

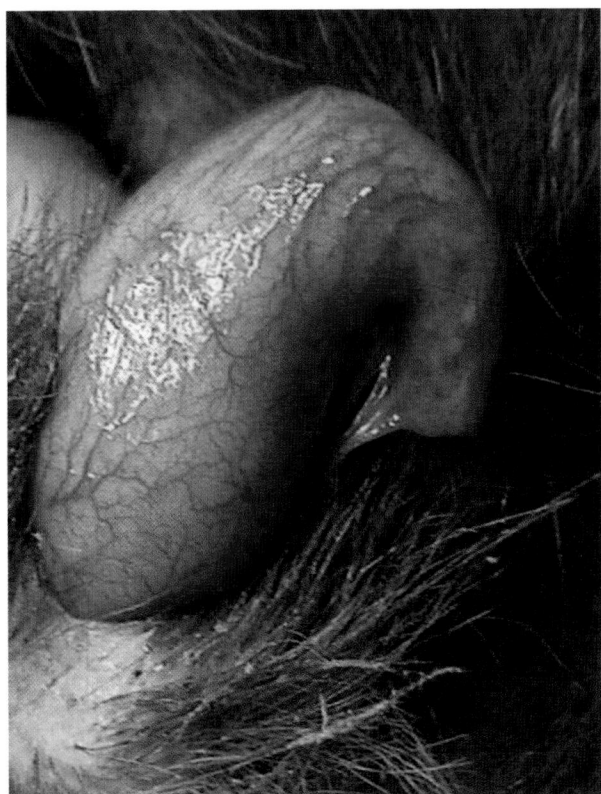

FIG. 26-33
A persistent frenulum is deviating the glans penis ventrally.
Note the thin band of fibrous tissue.

putial discharge may occur. There may be a history of urinary incontinence or infection.

Physical Examination Findings

Skin irritation or preputial inflammation may be identified. The preputial opening may be incompletely formed and the scrotum divided. The penis should be completely extruded from the prepuce and examined. A fibrous band may be noted running from the glans to the urethral opening and deviating the penis (persistent frenulum) (Fig. 26-33). The urethral opening is identified on the ventral aspect of the penis along the normal urethral path.

Diagnostic Imaging

Radiographs are unnecessary for diagnosis, but they occasionally identify other congenital anomalies.

Laboratory Findings

Urine culture may be positive. Other laboratory results are nonspecific.

DIFFERENTIAL DIAGNOSIS

Differential diagnoses include pseudohermaphrodite, true hermaphrodite, urethral fistula or trauma, persistent penile frenulum, and penile hypoplasia.

MEDICAL MANAGEMENT

Urine scalding should be treated with frequent bathing and application of water-impermeable ointments near the urethral opening. The penile mucosa should be kept moist with ointments. If urine pooling occurs, the prepuce should be flushed daily with physiologic saline solution.

SURGICAL TREATMENT

Abnormal urethral openings near the penile tip may not require surgery. In other cases, reconstruction (with or without penile amputation) is advised. Preputial reconstruction is needed in patients with an incompletely formed preputial orifice and hypospadias at the glans. Constant penile exposure is prevented by closing the preputial orifice to its normal extent. Excision of the external genitalia is recommended for major developmental defects involving the urethra, prepuce, and penis. Penile amputation is also indicated for severe trauma and neoplasia. Neutering affected animals is recommended.

Preoperative Management

A preoperatively placed urethral catheter facilitates urethral identification.

Anesthesia

Elective surgery on pediatric patients should be delayed until they are approximately 8 weeks old. Recommendations for anesthetic management of neonates for reproductive surgery are provided on p. 705.

Surgical Anatomy

Surgical anatomy of the penis is provided on p. 708.

Positioning

Dorsal recumbency is recommended unless the urethra opens in the perineal or anal regions, in which case a perineal position is preferred. The ventral abdomen, medial thighs, and ventral perineum should be clipped and prepared for aseptic surgery.

SURGICAL TECHNIQUE
Prepuce Reconstruction

Incise the mucocutaneous junction on the caudoventral aspect of the prepuce (Fig. 26-34). Separate mucosa from skin. Reappose the mucosa beginning at a more cranial location with simple interrupted monofilament absorbable sutures (e.g., 4-0 to 6-0 polydioxanone, poliglecaprone 25, glycomer 631, or polyglyconate). Appose skin with a second layer of simple interrupted sutures (e.g., 3-0 or 4-0 nylon, polybutester, or polypropylene). If this creates an orifice that is too small to allow penile extrusion, incise the dorsocranial aspect of the prepuce and suture the mucosa to the skin on each side with interrupted sutures (e.g., 4-0 nylon, polybutester, or polypropylene).

Urethral Reconstruction

Expose the defect by extrusion of the penis from the prepuce or by midline preputiotomy. Close small urethral defects by incising the margins of the defect and apposing the urethral

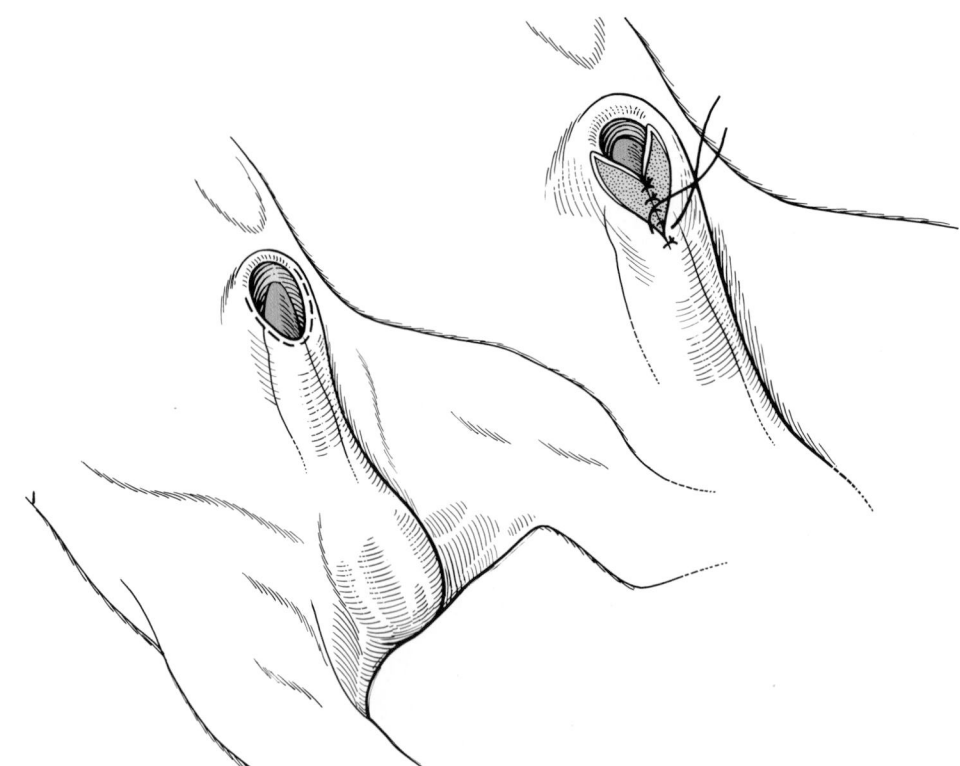

FIG. 26-34
Preputial reconstruction to narrow the orifice is accomplished by incising the mucocutaneous junction *(dashed line)* and reapposing the mucosa and skin in separate layers beginning at a more cranial location.

edges over a urethral catheter. Use 4-0 to 6-0 monofilament absorbable suture (e.g., polydioxanone, polyglyconate, poliglecaprone 25, or glycomer 631) in a simple interrupted or continuous pattern. Close skin over the urethral repair with 3-0 or 4-0 nonabsorbable suture (e.g., nylon or polypropylene) using an appositional pattern.

Subtotal Penile Amputation

Make an elliptical incision around the prepuce, penis, and scrotum, preserving adequate skin for closure (Fig. 26-35, A). Dissect the penis from the body wall from cranial to caudal (Fig. 26-35, B). Ligate or cauterize preputial vessels. Perform a castration as with scrotal ablation (see p. 714). Locate and ligate the dorsal penile vessels just caudal to the desired amputation site. Perform a urethrostomy; scrotal urethrostomy (see p. 673) is preferred. Reflect or transect the retractor penis muscle. Make a midline urethral incision over the catheter. Place a circumferential catgut ligature around the penis just caudal to the proposed amputation site and just cranial to the urethrostomy site. Amputate the penis in a wedge fashion (Fig. 26-35, C). Appose the tunica albuginea to close the end of the penis with 3-0 or 4-0 absorbable monofilament suture (e.g., polydioxanone, poliglecaprone 25, glycomer 631, or polyglyconate). Appose urethral mucosa to skin at the urethrostomy site with simple interrupted 4-0 to 6-0 monofilament absorbable or nonabsorbable sutures (e.g., polydioxanone, polyglyconate, poliglecaprone 25, glycomer 631, polybutester, polypropylene, or nylon) (Fig. 26-35, D). Close subcutaneous

tissue and skin cranial and caudal to the urethrostomy in two layers (Fig. 26-35, E).

POSTOPERATIVE CARE AND ASSESSMENT

Analgesics should be given as necessary (see Chapter 13; for dosages of opioids see Table 13-4 on p. 133) and urination monitored by observing for a nonrestricted urine stream. Hemorrhage may occur from cavernous tissue for days, especially during excitement or urination. Hemorrhage may be minimized by keeping the animal quiet and calm during the early postoperative period. An Elizabethan collar, bucket, or sidebars should be used to prevent self-trauma. Hemorrhage, urine leakage, infection, seroma, and dehiscence are potential incisional complications. Urethral or preputial reconstruction may cause stricture formation. Urethral stricture may interfere with urine flow and produce obstruction. Preputial stricture may prevent extrusion of the penis.

PROGNOSIS

Hypospadias is not life threatening; however, penile exposure and urine-induced dermatitis cause discomfort. Surgery usually salvages an animal as a pet, improves cosmesis, and reduces urine-induced dermatitis.

Suggested Reading

Papazoglou LG, Kazakos GM: Surgical conditions of the canine penis and prepuce, *Compend Cont Educ Pract* 24:204-218, 2002.

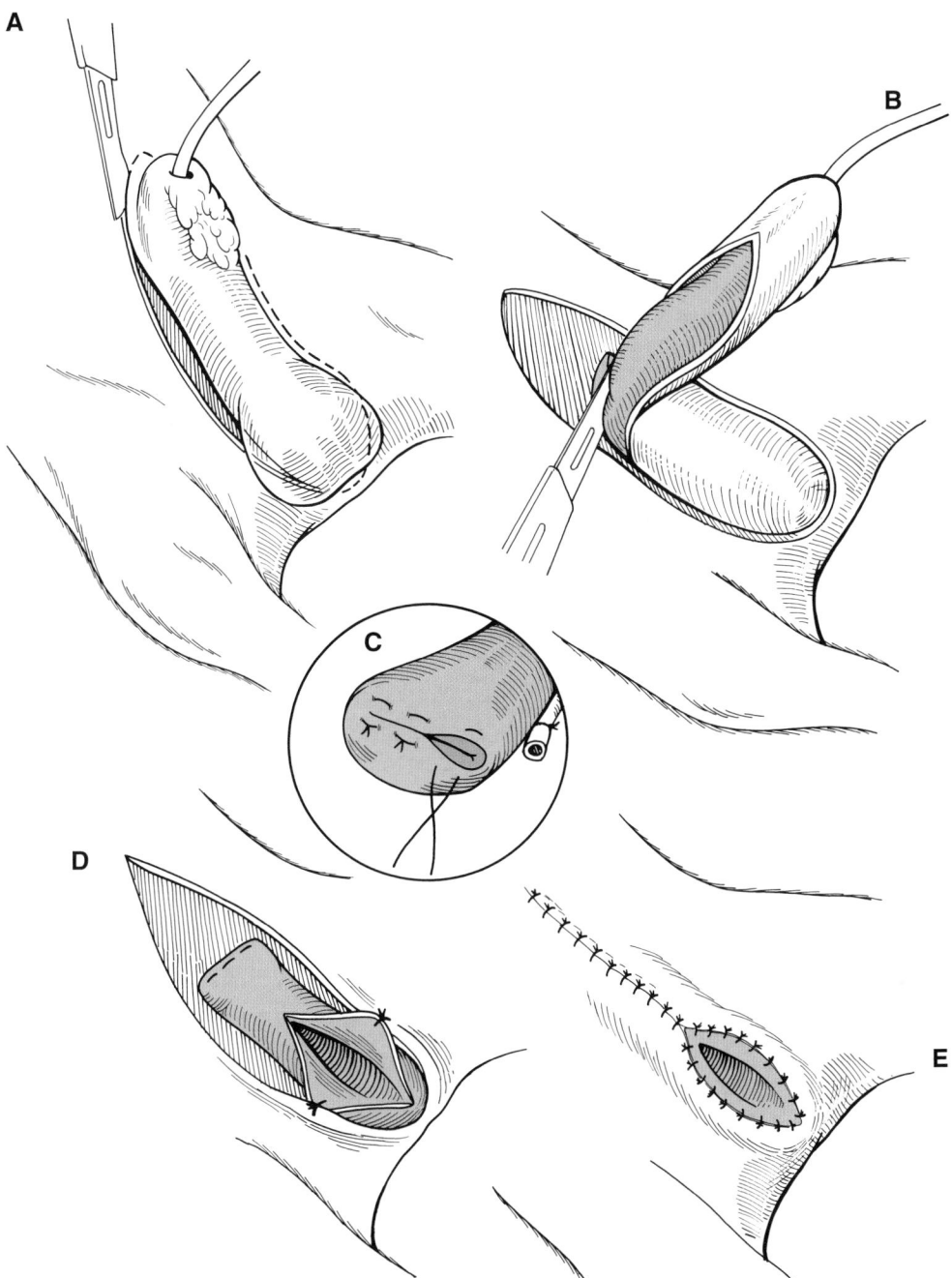

FIG. 26-35
Penile neoplasia, trauma, or congenital anomalies may be treated by subtotal penile amputation and scrotal urethrostomy. **A,** Make an elliptical incision around the base of the scrotum and prepuce and remove the testicles. **B,** Separate the penis from the external abdominal wall to just caudal to the os penis. **C,** Amputate the distal penis and appose the tunica albuginea over the cavernous tissue. **D** and **E,** Incise the urethra in the scrotal area and suture urethral mucosa to skin.

This review discusses and nicely illustrates common conditions affecting the penis and prepuce. Use of a buccal mucosal graft is described in this staged reconstruction.

PHIMOSIS

DEFINITION

Phimosis is the inability of the penis to protrude from the prepuce or sheath.

GENERAL CONSIDERATIONS AND CLINICALLY RELEVANT PATHOPHYSIOLOGY

Phimosis is rare. It is usually the result of a preputial opening that is too small or absent. Phimosis may be developmental or a result of trauma and preputial stenosis. It may also occur secondary to penile or preputial neoplasia or preputial cellulitis. Inability to extrude the penis causes preputial irritation and infection secondary to urine pooling within the prepuce. Balanoposthitis causes preputial discharge.

DIAGNOSIS
Clinical Presentation

Signalment. There is no known breed predisposition. Congenital phimosis is recognizable in neonates, but may go undetected for months. Congenital stenosis has been reported in Bouvier des Flandres, German shepherd dogs, Labradors, golden retrievers, and mixed breed dogs. Acquired phimosis may occur at any age.

History. Affected animals may retain urine, dribble urine, or be unable to copulate. Animals without a preputial opening cannot void urine appropriately and have preputial swelling. Acquired cases have a history of lacerations and scarring, sucking of a puppy's prepuce by littermates or licking by the bitch, or neoplasia.

Physical Examination Findings

Affected animals have a small or nonexistent preputial opening. There may be evidence of previous preputial trauma, and a purulent or hemorrhagic preputial discharge is common. The prepuce may be distended with urine, inflamed, and infected. Manual extrusion or palpation of the penis may reveal a mass preventing advancement of the penis.

Diagnostic Imaging

Imaging is unnecessary unless neoplasia is suspected.

Laboratory Findings

Results of laboratory tests are nonspecific. Preputial cytology may reveal inflammation and infection. Bacteria may be cultured from the prepuce.

DIFFERENTIAL DIAGNOSIS

Differential diagnoses include penile hypoplasia, persistent frenulum, and hermaphroditism.

MEDICAL MANAGEMENT

Phimosis caused by an inflammatory or infectious disease may be relieved by warm compresses, antibiotic therapy, and urine diversion with a catheter. The prepuce should be lavaged daily with physiologic saline solution to reduce urine scalding.

SURGICAL TREATMENT

Phimosis caused by a developmental anomaly or stricture is managed by reconstruction of the preputial orifice. The goal of surgery is to enlarge the preputial orifice and allow unrestricted movement of the penis in and out of the prepuce.

> NOTE: Recommend neutering animals with small preputial openings.

Preoperative Management

The prepuce should be lavaged with a dilute antiseptic solution before surgery and a urinary catheter placed to divert urine.

Anesthesia

Anesthetic recommendations for animals undergoing reproductive surgery are provided on p. 705.

Surgical Anatomy

Surgical anatomy of the male reproductive system is provided on p. 708.

Positioning

The patient is positioned in dorsal recumbency and the end of the prepuce clipped and prepared for aseptic surgery.

SURGICAL TECHNIQUE

Enlarge the preputial opening by making a full-thickness incision at the craniodorsal aspect of the prepuce. Determine the desired length and width of the preputial incision based on the severity of phimosis. Remove a small wedge (3 to 5 mm) of prepuce with the base at the mucocutaneous junction (Fig. 26-36, A). Appose mucosa to the ipsilateral skin edge on each side with a simple interrupted suture pattern (e.g., 4-0 to 6-0 polydioxanone, poliglecaprone 25, glycomer 631, or polyglyconate) (Fig. 26-36, B and C). Extrude the penis completely to examine for other developmental defects, injuries, or masses. Amputate the tip of the prepuce if stenosis is too long to be relieved by incision and if adequate preputial length can be maintained.

Amputation may cause a shortened prepuce, allowing chronic penile protrusion and exposure.

Identify the site of resection and amputate the preputial tip (Fig. 26-37, A). Circumferentially appose preputial mucosa to skin with a simple interrupted or continuous suture pattern (e.g., 4-0 to 6-0 polydioxanone, poliglecaprone 25, gly-

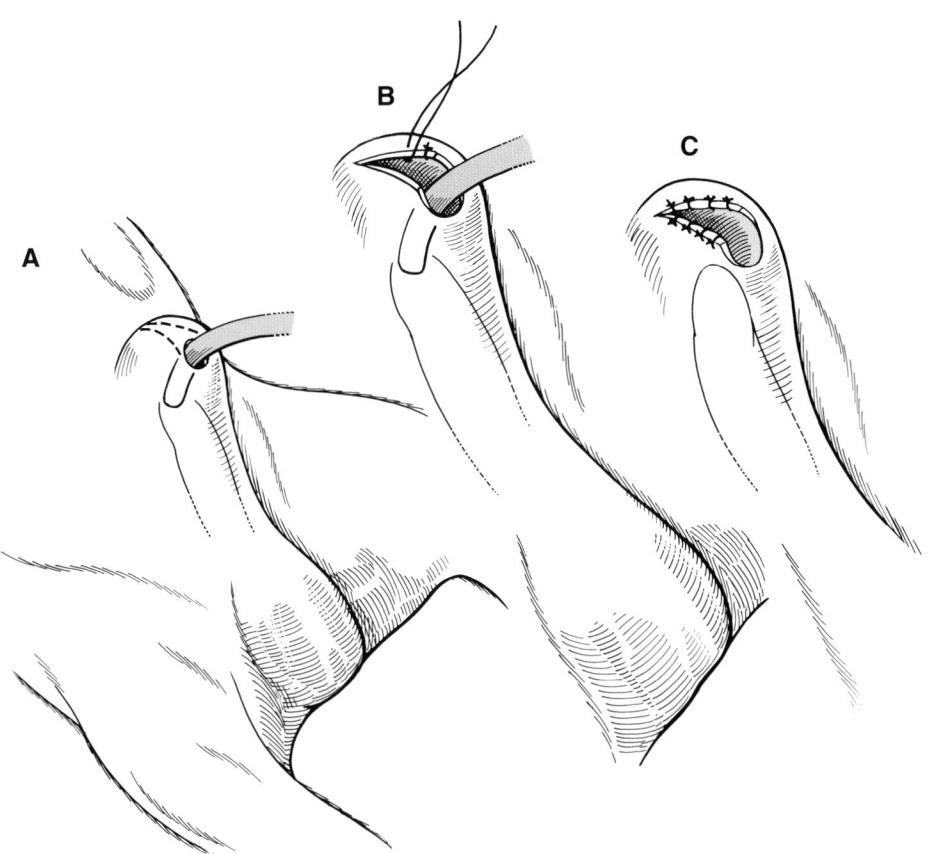

FIG. 26-36
A, For phimosis, enlarge the preputial orifice by resecting a full-thickness wedge from the craniodorsal aspect. **B** and **C,** Appose mucosa to the ipsilateral skin edge on each side.

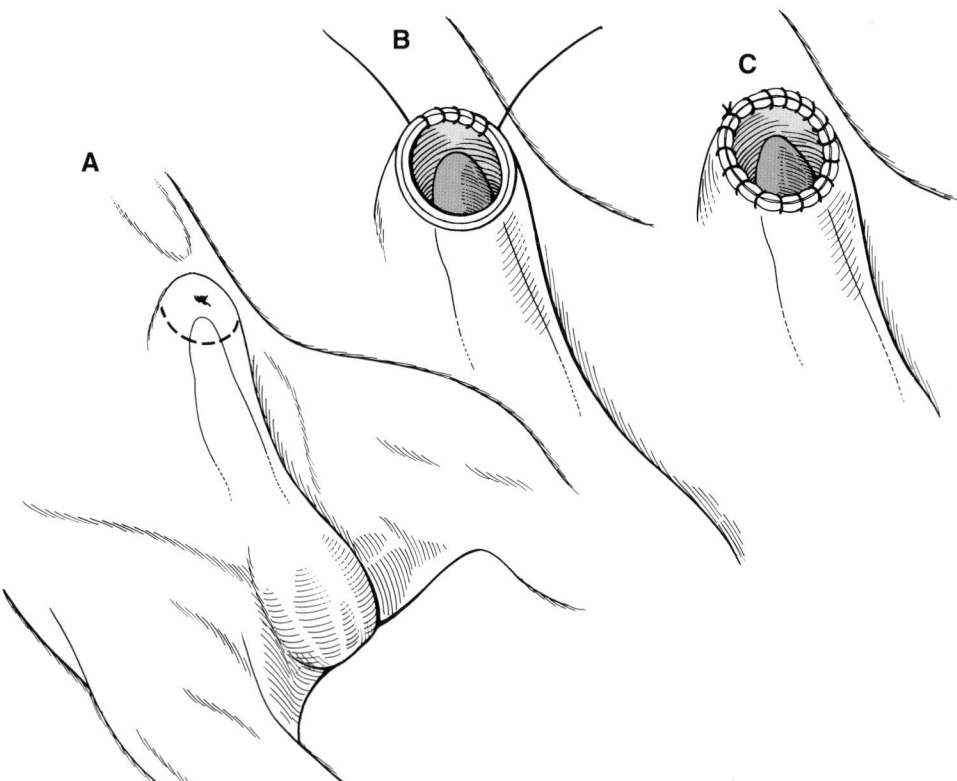

FIG. 26-37
A, To enlarge the preputial orifice, resect the tip of the prepuce and suture preputial mucosa to skin **(B** and **C).**

comer 631, or polyglyconate) (Fig. 26-37, B and C). Neuter affected animals.

POSTOPERATIVE CARE AND ASSESSMENT

Analgesics and supportive care should be given as needed. Warm compresses and antibiotics may be used to treat balanoposthitis. An Elizabethan collar, bucket, or sidebars should be used to prevent self-trauma. Phimosis may persist if the incision is not long enough. Persistent protrusion of the glans may occur if the ventrocaudal prepuce is incised. Self-trauma may cause dehiscence and stricture formation.

PROGNOSIS

Without surgery, balanoposthitis may become severe and cause discomfort. A second surgical procedure may be necessary after the animal matures.

Suggested Reading

Olsen D, Salwei R: Surgical correction of a congenital preputial and penile deformity in a dog, *J Am Anim Hosp Assoc* 37:187, 2001.

This report describes the correction for an extensive persistent frenulum and similar dorsal membrane with attachments to the prepuce, which caused accumulation of fluid within the prepuce.

Papazoglou LG, Kazakos GM: Surgical conditions of the canine penis and prepuce, *Compend Cont Educ Pract* 24:204, 2002.

This review discusses and nicely illustrates common conditions affecting the penis and prepuce.

PARAPHIMOSIS

DEFINITION

Paraphimosis is the inability to retract the penis into the sheath and/or prepuce. **Priapism** is persistent erection of the penis without sexual excitement. **Phallopexy** is a procedure to create a permanent adhesion between the penile shaft and preputial mucosa.

GENERAL CONSIDERATIONS AND CLINICALLY RELEVANT PATHOPHYSIOLOGY

Paraphimosis may be associated with copulation, masturbation, trauma, penile hematoma, neoplasia, foreign bodies, pseudohermaphroditism, neurologic deficits, or constriction by preputial hairs (Fig. 26-38). The penis may be unable to retract within the prepuce because the edges of the prepuce roll inward or the preputial orifice is too small to accommodate the swollen or engorged penis. Initially the penis appears normal. However, when the penis cannot be retracted, it is easily traumatized and circulation is impaired. Impaired circulation causes the penis to become edematous, which further compromises circulation (Fig. 26-39). Vascular engorgement may progress to thrombosis of the corpus spongiosum and necrosis. A moderately compromised, chronically protruded penis will become dry, fissured, and cornified.

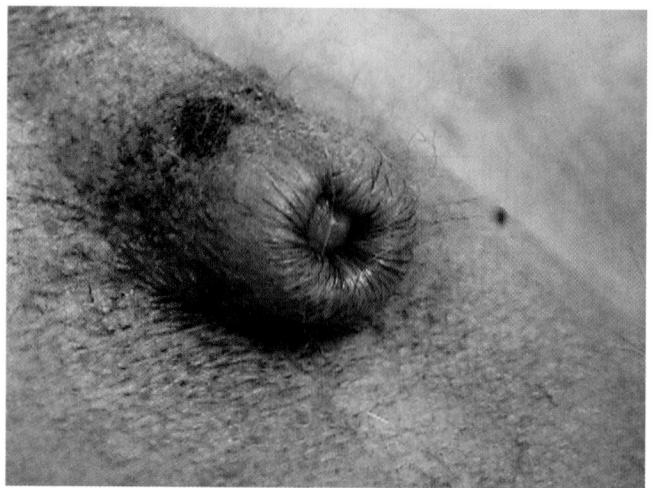

A

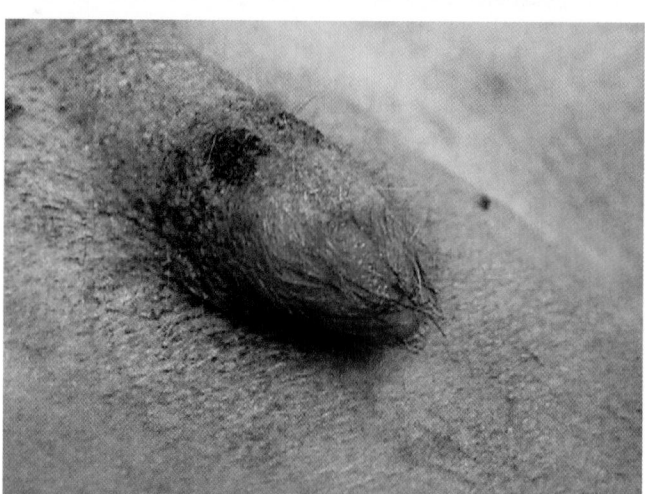

B

FIG. 26-38
Mild paraphimosis. **A,** The tip of the glans is protruding from the prepuce and unable to retract as a result of inversion of the skin. **B,** Reduction was accomplished by caudal traction on the prepuce to unroll the inverted skin.

DIAGNOSIS
Clinical Presentation

Signalment. The condition occurs more often in dogs than in cats. Sexual hyperactivity preceding paraphimosis may be noted in young dogs.

History. Paraphimosis can result from priapism, masturbation, or excessive sexual activity. Canine paraphimosis occurs most commonly after an erection. It may occur in long-haired cats if the penis becomes entangled in hairs. It may also be associated with posterior paralysis or the inability of preputial muscles to pull the prepuce over the penis after an erection.

Physical Examination Findings

Paraphimosis is diagnosed by visual inspection. The exposed, swollen, edematous penis is painful (see Fig. 26-39). The traumatized penis may be fissured, lacerated, and/or

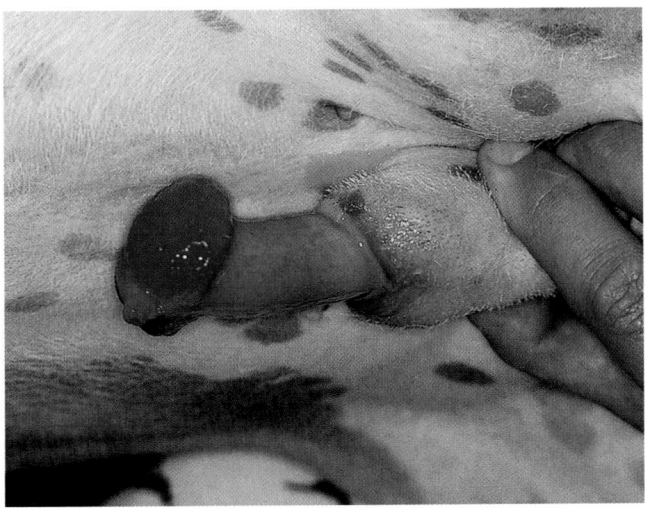

FIG. 26-39
Penile trauma, inflammation, and edema secondary to paraphimosis.

bleeding. The animal may require sedation or anesthesia before penile examination. The severity of penile trauma and vascular compromise should be determined. The prepuce should be evaluated to determine whether it is too short or whether the orifice is too small or too large. The retracted penis should normally be covered by at least 1 cm of prepuce cranial to its termination.

Diagnostic Imaging

Images are unnecessary unless urethral trauma is suspected.

Laboratory Findings

Laboratory findings are nonspecific.

DIFFERENTIAL DIAGNOSIS

Paraphimosis must be differentiated from priapism, vascular thrombosis, chronic urethritis, stretching or weakness of the retractor penis muscles, and hypoplastic or surgically damaged preputial muscles. Mechanical, vascular, or neural causes should be suspected when the penis is easily reduced.

MEDICAL MANAGEMENT

Initially, the prepuce should be pulled back until it unfolds and the preputial mucocutaneous junction is identified. This allows restoration of penile circulation and resolution of edema. The penis should be examined carefully for constricting foreign bodies and the protruded, edematous penis cleaned with warm physiologic saline solution or water. To reduce edema, gently massage the penis and apply a hypertonic or hygroscopic agent (e.g., sugar). Corticosteroids and diuretics may reduce edema after the constriction is relieved. When swelling has decreased, the prepuce should be flushed with a mild antiseptic soap or lubricant, and the preputial edges dilated or retracted, thus allowing the penis to retract within the prepuce.

SURGICAL TREATMENT

Patients with acute paraphimosis are often managed conservatively. Others may require preputial reconstruction, phallopexy, or penile amputation. A preputiotomy may be necessary to allow retraction of the penis into the prepuce if conservative measures fail. If the prepuce is of adequate length and the orifice too large, narrow it (see Fig. 26-34). Enlarge the preputial opening if the prepuce is of adequate length and the orifice too small (see Figs. 26-36 and 26-37). When the prepuce is too short, it may be lengthened or the penis may be amputated (see Fig. 26-35). Preputial deficiencies of less than 1 to 2 cm may be corrected by cranial advancement of the prepuce. Partial amputation of the penis is indicated for severe trauma or abnormalities of the penis or prepuce, neoplasia, recurring urethral prolapse, and recurring paraphimosis. Partial penile amputation is applicable when the site of transection is cranial to the caudal end of the os penis. Castration is recommended to prevent recurrence of paraphimosis because of sexual activity. Phallopexy is indicated for cases of recurrent paraphimosis or as the initial surgical treatment.

> NOTE: Castration may prevent recurrent paraphimosis caused by sexual activity.

Preoperative Management

See the discussion on medical treatment above.

Anesthesia

Anesthetic recommendations for animals with reproductive disorders are provided on p. 705.

Surgical Anatomy

The prepuce covers the nonerect penis in dogs and cats. The dog's prepuce should normally extend approximately 1 cm beyond the end of the penis.

Positioning

Position the patient in dorsal recumbency. Clip the prepuce and surrounding skin and prepare them for aseptic surgery.

SURGICAL TECHNIQUE
Preputiotomy

Make a full-thickness dorsal or ventral linear incision in the prepuce. If the preputial orifice is of normal size, anatomically reappose mucosa (e.g., 4-0 to 6-0 polydioxanone, poliglecaprone 25, or polyglyconate, approximating sutures) and skin (e.g., 3-0 or 4-0 nylon, polybutester, or polypropylene, approximating sutures) in separate layers.

Preputial Lengthening

Lengthen or translocate the prepuce cranially by resecting a crescent-shaped piece of skin from the body wall just cranial to the prepuce (Fig. 26-40, A). Preserve the preputial vessels. Identify the preputial muscles and shorten them by overlap-

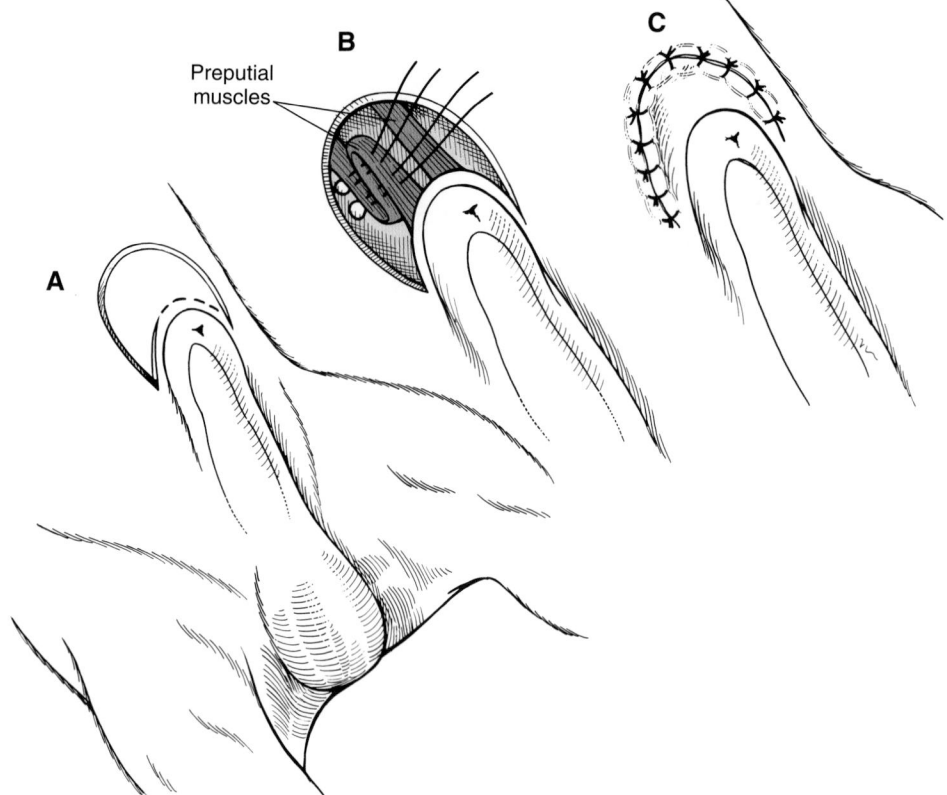

FIG. 26-40
A, Lengthen the prepuce by removing a crescent-shaped piece of skin cranial to the prepuce, shortening the preputial muscles **(B),** and advancing the prepuce cranially **(C).**

Preputial muscles

ping and suturing or by segmental excision and reapposition (Fig. 26-40, B). Close subcutaneous tissue and skin in two layers to further advance the skin cranially (Fig. 26-40, C).

Alternatively the prepuce can be lengthened with a two-stage procedure in which oral mucosa is transplanted cranial to the prepuce and later rolled into a tube to cover the end of the penis.

Partial Penile Amputation

Place a urethral catheter to facilitate orientation and prevent urethral trauma. Extrude the penis from the prepuce, and maintain this position by snugly closing the preputial orifice around the penis with a towel clamp. Place a Penrose drain tourniquet caudal to the proposed amputation site. Make a lateral "V" incision through the tunica albuginea and cavernous tissue on each side of the urethra and os penis (Fig. 26-41, A). Transect the os penis with bone cutters as far caudally as possible, being careful not to traumatize the urethra (Fig. 26-41, B). Transect the urethra 1 to 2 cm cranial to the penile transection, and spatulate the dorsal aspect. Identify and ligate the dorsal artery of the penis after loosening the tourniquet. Fold the spatulated urethra over the transected end of the penis (Fig. 26-41, C). Appose urethral mucosa to tunic albuginea; include some cavernous tissue with each bite (Fig. 26-41, D). Use 4-0 to 6-0 monofilament absorbable suture (i.e., polydioxanone, poliglecaprone 25, glycomer 631,

or polyglyconate) with a swaged-on, taper-point needle in a simple interrupted or continuous pattern. Shorten the prepuce if the new penile tip cannot be extruded from the prepuce; the prepuce should extend approximately 1 cm cranial to the retracted penis.

Resect an ellipse of prepuce approximately the same length as the amount of penis that was amputated (Fig. 26-41, E). Make an elliptical, transverse, full-thickness incision in the midportion of the prepuce (beginning approximately 2 cm caudal to the cranial junction of the prepuce and body wall). Remove this ventral skin and mucosal segment, reflect the penis caudally, and resect a similar segment of dorsal preputial mucosa. Close the defect by first apposing the dorsal and then ventral preputial mucosa with 4-0 or 5-0 monofilament absorbable suture (e.g., polydioxanone, poliglecaprone 25, glycomer 631, or polyglyconate) in a simple interrupted or continuous pattern. Then appose skin with approximating 3-0 or 4-0 nonabsorbable sutures (e.g., nylon, polypropylene, or polybutester).

Phallopexy

Phallopexy prevents complete exteriorization of the glans thus eliminating the risk of recurrent paraphimosis and subsequent penile trauma (Somerville and Anderson, 2001).

Perform a preputiotomy beginning 2.5 cm caudal to the preputial orifice by making a full-thickness incision into the

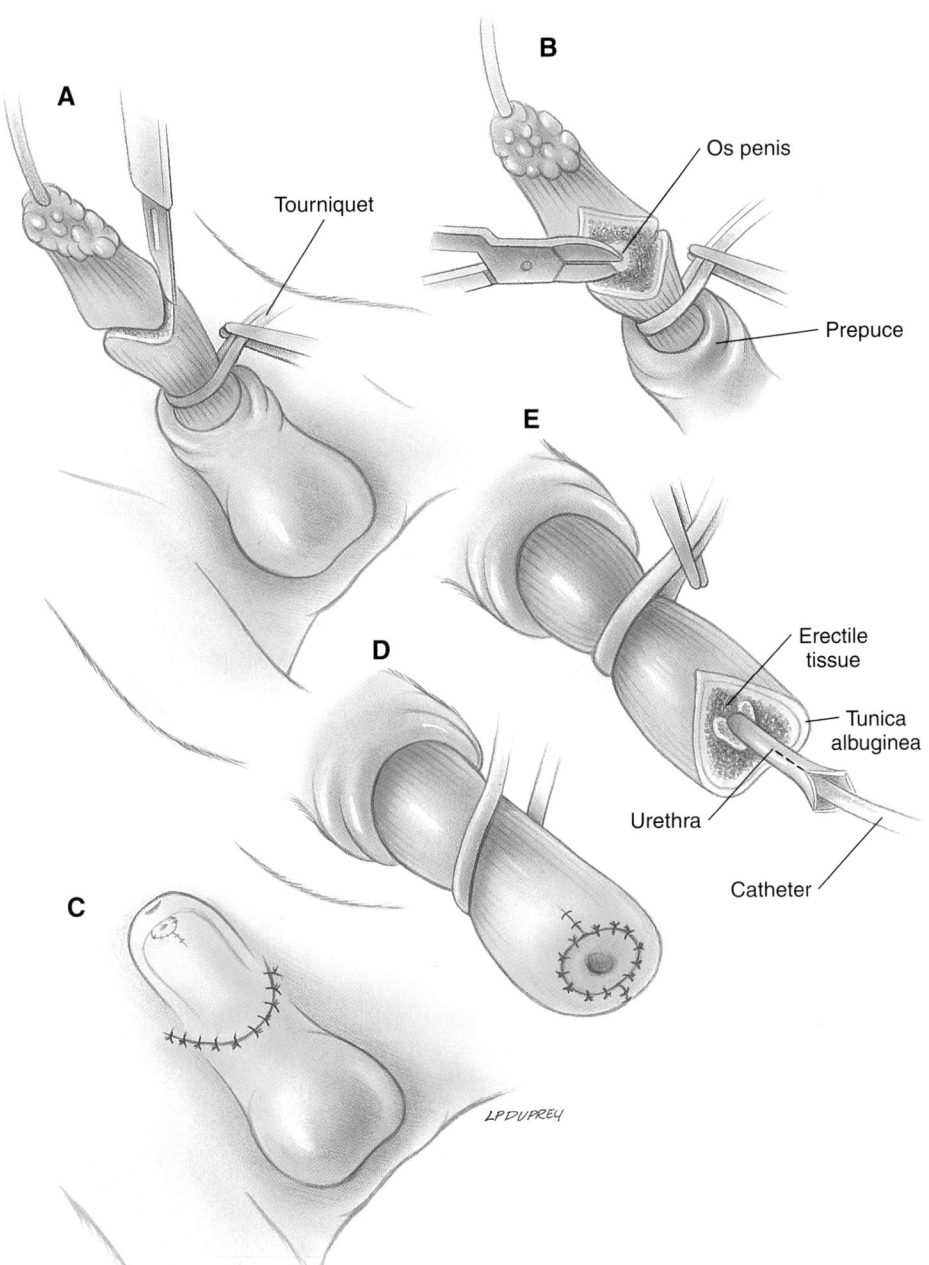

FIG. 26-41
A, During partial penile amputation, retract the prepuce, place a tourniquet around the penis, and make a lateral V incision through the tunica albuginea and cavernous tissue. **B,** Transect the os penis as far caudal as possible. **C,** Transect the urethra 1 to 2 cm cranial to the penile transection and spatulate the end. **D,** Appose urethral mucosa to the tunica albuginea. **E,** Shorten the prepuce to allow extrusion of the distal penis by removing a full-thickness segment from the midsection.

prepuce at the junction of the prepuce and body wall (Fig. 26-42, A). Extend the incision caudally 2 to 3 cm. Retract the penis laterally. Beginning 3 cm caudal to the preputial opening excise a strip of preputial mucosa 0.5 cm wide by 1.5 cm long from the dorsal midline of the preputial lumen. Then exteriorize the penile shaft through the preputial orifice and excise a strip of mucosa 0.5 cm wide and 1.5 cm long from the dorsal midline of the midportion of the glans penis beginning 2 cm caudal to the tip (Fig. 26-42, B). Care is taken to prevent incising the pars longa glandis. Replace the penis within the prepuce, and appose the penile and preputial incisions with simple interrupted 3-0 or 4-0 monofilament absorbable sutures. Place the most cranial sutures

first, then retract the prepuce caudally to determine if the glans can be exteriorized. If exteriorization is possible, remove the sutures, extend the preputial mucosal excision caudally, and begin suturing at a more caudal location. Complete the pexy by placing 6 to 8 sutures between the incised edges of the penile and preputial mucosa (Fig. 26-42, C). Close the preputiotomy incision in layers: preputial mucosa, subcutaneous tissue, and skin. Perform a castration (see p. 714).

POSTOPERATIVE CARE AND ASSESSMENT

Analgesics should be given as necessary; an Elizabethan collar, bucket, or sidebars should be used to prevent self-trauma.

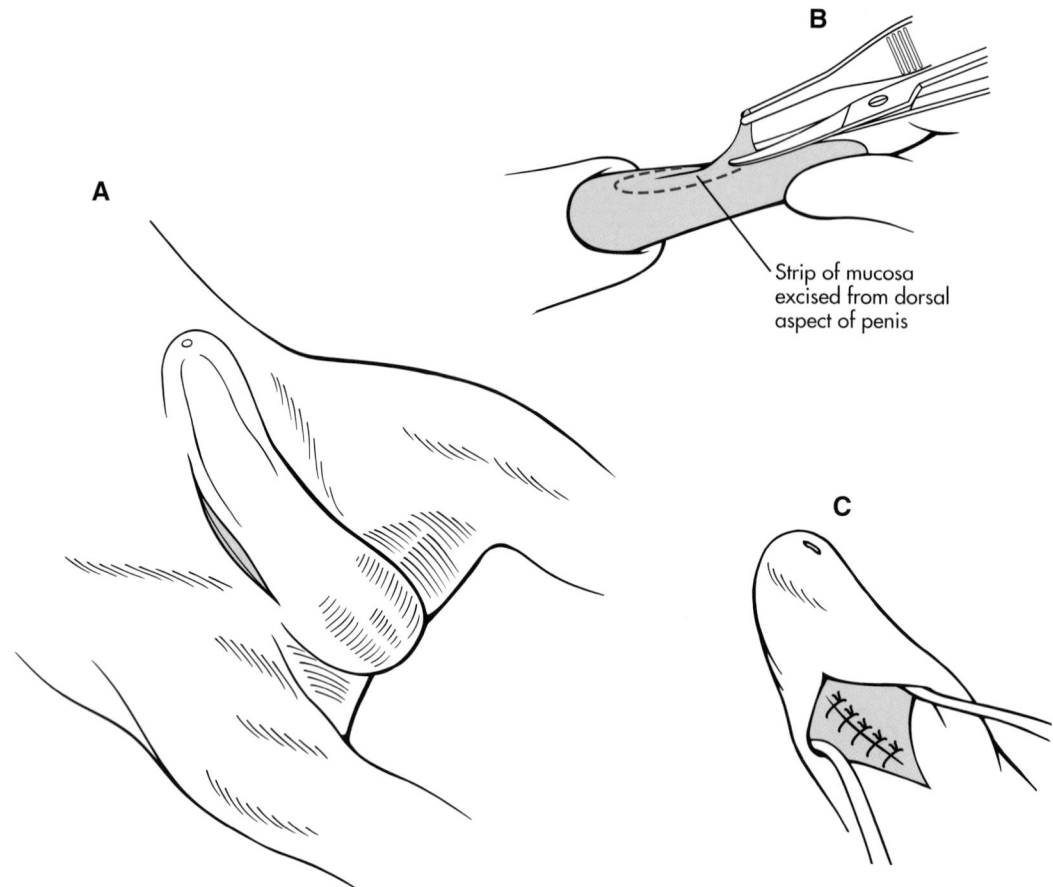

FIG. 26-42
Phallopexy. **A,** Perform a preputiotomy, beginning 2.5 cm caudal to the preputial orifice, by making a full-thickness incision into the prepuce at the junction of the prepuce and body wall. Extend the incision caudally 2 to 3 cm. **B,** After excising a strip of preputial mucosa from the dorsal midline of the preputial lumen, exteriorize the penile shaft through the preputial orifice and excise a strip of mucosa 0.5 cm wide and 1.5 cm long from the dorsal midline of the midportion of the glans penis beginning 2 cm caudal to the tip. **C,** Replace the penis within the prepuce and appose the penile and preputial incisions with simple interrupted 3-0 or 4-0 monofilament absorbable sutures.

Avoid exposure that will provoke excitement or sexual stimulation. Hemorrhage usually occurs during urination or excitement for several days after penile amputation. Persistent licking and signs of discomfort are not seen after phallopexies have healed, and balanoposthitis has not been reported following this procedure.

Complications

Dehiscence, stricture, infection, hemorrhage, urine retention, and recurrence are potential complications. Ventral preputial incisions may lead to chronic exposure of the glans penis. Preputial advancements may relax postoperatively, allowing the distal penis to be reexposed.

PROGNOSIS

The prognosis with manual reduction or reconstruction plus castration is good; however, recurrence is common if the animal is not castrated. Prognosis following phallopexy is good.

Reference

Somerville ME, Anderson SM: Phallopexy for the treatment of paraphimosis in the dog, *J Am Anim Hosp Assoc* 37:397, 2001.

Suggested Reading

Gunn-Moore DA, Brown PJ, Holt PE et al: Priapism in seven cats, *J Small Anim Pract* 36:262, 1995.

Clinical and pathologic features are reported; six cases were in Siamese cats and four of five were successfully treated with perineal urethrostomy.

Olsen D, Salwei R: Surgical correction of a congenital preputial and penile deformity in a dog, *J Am Anim Hosp Assoc* 37:187, 2001.

Paraphimosis occurring following correction of congenital preputial abnormalities was repaired by shortening the retractor penis muscle, preputial advancement, and wedge resection of the preputial ostium.

Papazoglou LG, Kazakos GM: Surgical conditions of the canine penis and prepuce, *Compend Cont Educ Pract* 24:204, 2002.

This review discusses and nicely illustrates common conditions affecting the penis and prepuce.

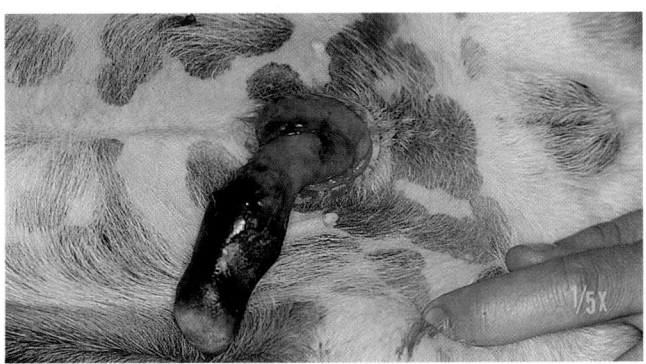

FIG. 26-43
Penile necrosis that occurred after trauma and necessitated partial penile amputation and preputial reconstruction.

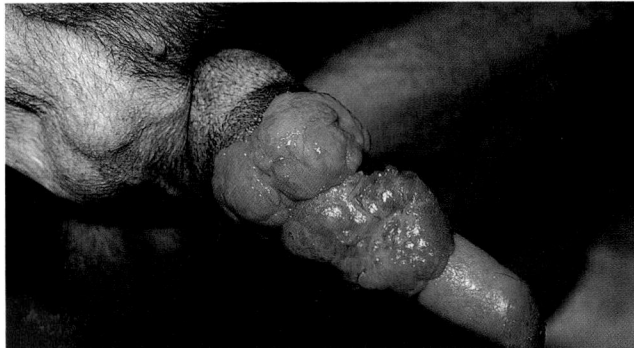

FIG. 26-44
Penile TVTs.

⌘ BOX 26-37

Preputial Tumors

Benign	Malignant
• Hemangiomas	• Melanomas
• Papillomas	• Mast cell tumors
• Histiocytomas	• Hemangiosarcomas
	• Squamous cell carcinomas

PENILE AND PREPUTIAL TRAUMA AND NEOPLASIA

DEFINITIONS

A penile hematoma is a localized collection of blood that accumulates secondary to laceration or puncture of the cavernous tissue.

GENERAL CONSIDERATIONS AND CLINICALLY RELEVANT PATHOPHYSIOLOGY

The prepuce and penis may be traumatized by animal bites, vehicular or other accidents, and human attacks (Fig. 26-43). Trauma may cause penile hematomas or os penis fracture. The hematoma swelling may cause the penis to protrude. Lacerations or punctures may bleed for days.

Neoplasms commonly found on skin occur on the prepuce (Box 26-37). Neoplasms of the penis and mucosal lining of the prepuce include transmissible venereal tumors (TVTs), squamous cell carcinoma, hemangiosarcoma, and papillomas. TVTs are contagious and are spread by sexual contact or licking. They are wartlike, friable, and bleed easily (Fig. 26-44).

DIAGNOSIS
Clinical Presentation

Signalment. Trauma and tumors are more common in intact males. Young animals are more commonly traumatized; old animals more commonly have tumors.

History. Signs of penile or preputial disease include serosanguineous, hemorrhagic, or purulent preputial discharge; inability or unwillingness to copulate; and/or pain. Some animals have phimosis (see p. 766) or paraphimosis (see p. 768). The urethra may be obstructed or lacerated, which causes dysuria, anuria, or urine extravasation. Many dogs are asymptomatic.

Physical Examination Findings

An injury or abnormal mass may be detected on physical examination. The prepuce may appear swollen, inflamed, nodular, lacerated, ischemic, and/or necrotic. There may be diffuse inguinal swelling due to leakage of urine from the urethra into surrounding tissue. Abnormalities involving preputial skin are usually apparent; preputial mucosal lesions may be detected only by palpation. It may be impossible to exteriorize the penis for examination if there is a mass within the prepuce or on the penis. In other cases, paraphimosis is present because of injury causing inflammation, edema, and engorgement (or a mass prevents penile retraction). Penile deviation may occur secondary to traumatic fractures of the os penis. Rectal palpation may reveal lymphadenomegaly.

Diagnostic Imaging

Abdominal and thoracic radiographs are indicated to stage tumors. Survey radiographs may reveal os penis fractures. An urethrogram may help assess urethral involvement with penile trauma or tumors. Ultrasonography may be useful to provide information if the penis cannot be exteriorized.

Laboratory Findings

Laboratory results are nonspecific for penile trauma or neoplasia. Cytology of preputial discharges may show toxic neutrophils, excess bacteria, fungi, or foreign material, but these findings can be found in normal animals. Cytology of preputial or penile masses may help identify tumor type. TVTs have large round cells with numerous mitotic figures.

DIFFERENTIAL DIAGNOSIS

Hematomas, abscesses, granulomas, and fungal infections may cause similar lesions.

MEDICAL MANAGEMENT

Some injuries heal spontaneously. Penile hematomas should be allowed to resolve spontaneously unless they cause persistent paraphimosis. TVTs are treated with vincristine (0.5 mg/m² IV or 0.025 mg/kg up to 1 mg IV) weekly for 3 to 6 weeks. Alternatively, radiation therapy is effective against TVTs resistant to chemotherapy and at metastatic sites.

SURGICAL TREATMENT

TVTs respond well to chemotherapy or radiation therapy; however, other tumors should be resected. Partial or complete penile amputation is necessary for severely traumatized, necrotic, or neoplastic lesions (see pp. 764 and 770). Hematomas causing persistent paraphimosis can be surgically exposed and evacuated; however, they may recur. Os penis fractures with minimal displacement require no surgery. Displaced fractures may be splinted with an indwelling polypropylene urethral catheter spanning the os penis and sutured to the tip of the urethra. More comminuted fractures may be stabilized with small plates, or the penis may be amputated.

Preoperative Management

The prepuce and penis should be lavaged with dilute antiseptic solutions. Antibiotics should be given if the penile or preputial tissue is severely damaged or necrotic.

Anesthesia

Anesthetic management of animals undergoing reproductive surgery is provided on p. 705.

Surgical Anatomy

Surgical anatomy of the male reproductive tract is provided on p. 708.

Positioning

Position the patient in dorsal recumbency. The ventral abdomen, ventral perineum, and medial thighs should be clipped and prepared for aseptic surgery.

SURGICAL TECHNIQUE
Preputial Lacerations

Débride, lavage, and appose preputial lacerations. Close full-thickness injuries in two layers, first apposing the preputial mucosa (e.g., 4-0 to 6-0 polydioxanone, poliglecaprone 25, glycomer 631, or polyglyconate), subcutaneous tissue (3-0 or 4-0 monofilament absorbable) and then skin (e.g., 3-0 or 4-0 nylon, polybutester, or polypropylene) with approximating sutures.

Hematomas that cause persistent paraphimosis can be surgically exposed and evacuated.

Incise the tunic albuginea over the hematoma. Remove blood clots and fibrin. Lavage the cavity and snugly appose the tunic albuginea. Take care to maintain an adequate preputial orifice and length when reconstructing preputial lacerations.

Penile Lacerations or Punctures

Suture the tunica albuginea to close penile lacerations or punctures, and minimize hemorrhage during excitement or urination. Use 4-0 to 6-0 monofilament absorbable (e.g., polyglyconate, poliglecaprone 25, glycomer 631, or polydioxanone), simple interrupted sutures on a swaged-on, taper-point needle.

Bleeding from small penile punctures or lacerations during penile engorgement is minimized by suturing the tunica albuginea.

POSTOPERATIVE CARE AND ASSESSMENT

Analgesics and antibiotics should be given as needed and the animal monitored for hemorrhage and/or urine leakage. Apply cold compresses following treatment of trauma or hematomas to reduce hemorrhage. An Elizabethan collar, bucket, or sidebars are used to prevent self-trauma. Reevaluation for tumor recurrence or metastasis should be performed every 3 to 4 months for 1 year. Hemorrhage, seroma, infection, urine leakage, dehiscence, stricture, recurrence, and metastasis are potential complications. Urethral obstruction may occur because of callus formation following os penis fractures.

Complications

Some injuries heal by secondary intention without complications; however, nonsutured preputial lacerations may fistulate. In other cases, persistent hemorrhage, urine extravasation, infection, and stricture may cause morbidity.

PROGNOSIS

The prognosis is good following appropriate surgical treatment for most injuries. The prognosis following tumor excision depends on the biologic behavior of the tumor and the tumor stage at presentation.

Suggested Reading

Papazoglou LG, Kazakos GM: Surgical conditions of the canine penis and prepuce, *Compend Cont Educ Pract* 24:204, 2002.
This review discusses and nicely illustrates common conditions affecting the penis and prepuce.

CHAPTER 27

Surgery of the Cardiovascular System

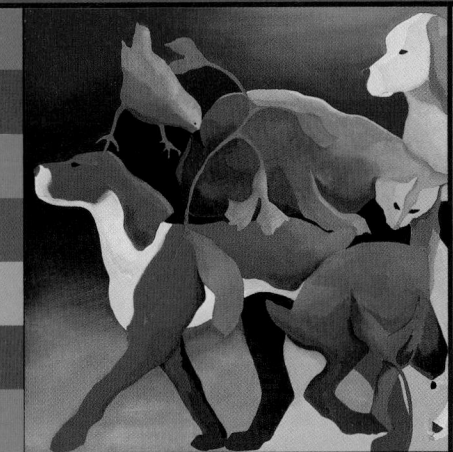

GENERAL PRINCIPLES AND TECHNIQUES

DEFINITIONS

Cardiac surgery includes procedures performed on the pericardium, cardiac ventricles, atria, venae cavae, aorta, and main pulmonary artery. **Closed cardiac procedures** (i.e., those that do not require opening major cardiac structures) are most commonly performed; however, some conditions require **open cardiac surgery** (i.e., a major cardiac structure must be opened to accomplish the repair). Open cardiac surgery necessitates that circulation be arrested during the procedure by inflow occlusion or cardiopulmonary bypass. **Venous inflow occlusion** provides brief circulatory arrest, allowing short procedures (under 5 minutes) to be performed. Longer open cardiac procedures require establishing an extracorporeal circulation by **cardiopulmonary bypass** to maintain organ perfusion during surgery.

PREOPERATIVE MANAGEMENT

Animals requiring cardiac surgery often have prior cardiovascular compromise that should be corrected or controlled medically when possible before anesthetic induction (Box 27-1). Congestive heart failure, particularly pulmonary edema, should be managed with diuretics (e.g., furosemide) and angiotensin-converting enzyme (ACE) inhibitors (e.g., enalapril, benazepril, and lisinopril) before surgery. Cardiac arrhythmias should be recognized and treated (see also later discussion in the Postoperative Care and Assessment section). Ventricular tachycardia should be suppressed before surgery with class I antiarrhythmic drugs (i.e., lidocaine and procainamide). Lidocaine is effective for management of ventricular tachyarrhythmias during and immediately after surgery. Supraventricular tachycardia may require digoxin, β-adrenergic blockers (e.g., esmolol, propranolol, and atenolol), or calcium channel blocking drugs (e.g., diltiazem) before surgery. Atrial fibrillation should be controlled before surgery with digoxin to lower the ventricular response rate below 140 bpm. This may require the addition of β-adrenergic blockade or calcium channel blocking drugs if digoxin alone does not decrease the ventricular rate sufficiently. Alterna-

tively, amiodarone may be used to control ventricular response rate and in some cases convert atrial fibrillation to normal sinus rhythm. Animals with bradycardia should undergo an atropine or glycopyrrolate response test before surgery. If bradycardia is not responsive to atropine or glycopyrrolate, temporary transvenous pacing or constant intravenous infusion of isoproterenol (see management of bradycardia on p. 813) may be required.

All animals should undergo a complete echocardiographic evaluation before cardiac surgery; an incomplete or inaccurate diagnosis can have devastating consequences. With the advent of Doppler echocardiography, cardiac catheterization is no longer routinely necessary before cardiac surgery.

ANESTHESIA

Preanesthetic medication is appropriate for most animals undergoing cardiac surgery (Boxes 27-2 and 27-3). Parenteral opioids (i.e., hydromorphone, butorphanol, buprenorphine, or fentanyl) induce sedation with minimal cardiovascular effects; however, all opioids can produce respiratory depression and/or bradycardia. In a recent study, fentanyl administration alone was not associated with a decrease in cardiac index; however, when co-administered with medetomidine, a significant decrease in cardiac index, heart rate, and oxygen delivery occurred (Grimm et al, 2005). Anticholinergics (i.e., atropine or glycopyrrolate) should be administered as needed to treat bradycardia when using an opioid. Benzodiazepines (i.e., diazepam, 0.2 mg/kg, or midazolam, 0.2 mg/kg) have minimal cardiopulmonary effects and enhance sedation when combined with opioids. Some patients may have an unpredictable behavioral response (e.g., excitation or aggressiveness) to benzodiazepine administration.

Induction of anesthesia should be undertaken with caution in animals with cardiopulmonary compromise. Thiobarbiturates should be avoided in patients with significant cardiac disease because they result in dose-dependent cardiac depression and are arrhythmogenic. Propofol (Diprivan or Rapinovet) produces rapid induction, but causes essentially the same cardiovascular compromise as thiobarbiturates. Ketamine combined with diazepam also is appropriate for induction of compromised patients, but should be

BOX 27-1

Selected Drugs Used in the Management of Animals With Cardiac Disease

Furosemide (Lasix)

2–4 mg/kg PO, IV, SC qd to qid as needed, or can give total daily dose as a constant rate infusion

Spironolactone

0.5–2 mg/kg PO qd to bid

Enalapril (Vasotec, Enacard)

0.25–0.5 mg/kg PO qd to bid

Benazepril (Lotensin)

0.25–0.5 mg/kg PO qd to bid

Lisinopril (Prinivil, Zestril)

Dogs: 0.25–0.5 mg/kg PO qd

Procainamide (Pronestyl)

Dogs: 10–15 mg/kg slow IV bolus or 25–60 µg/kg/min as a continuous IV infusion or 15 mg/kg IM, PO bid to qid

Lidocaine (Xylocaine)

Dogs: IV bolus (2 mg/kg increments up to total dose of 8 mg/kg/hr) then IV drip at 50–75 µg/kg/min (500 mg in 500 ml of fluid administered at maintenance rate [66 ml/kg/day] equals 50 µg/kg/min)

Amiodarone*

20 mg/kg PO qd for 5–7 days, then 10 mg/kg PO qd

Esmolol (Brevibloc)

100 µg/kg/min constant rate infusion or 0.05–0.1 mg/kg slow IV bolus every 5 min (up to 0.5 mg/kg total cumulative dose)

Propranolol (Inderal)

0.2–2 mg/kg PO bid to tid

Atenolol (Tenormin)

Dogs: 6.25–50 mg/dog PO qd to bid
Cats: 6.25–12.5 mg/cat PO qd to bid

Diltiazem (Cardizem)

1–1.5 mg/kg PO tid

Diltiazem (Dilacor)

Dogs: 3–5 mg/kg PO bid

Pimobendan (Vetmedin)

0.25–0.3 mg/kg PO bid

PO, Oral; *IV,* intravenous; *SC,* subcutaneous; *qd,* once a day; *qid,* four times a day; *bid,* twice a day; *IM,* intramuscular; *tid,* three times a day.
*Amiodarone can cause severe drug-induced hepatic disease in dogs; monitoring ALT and SAP in dogs treated with this drug is an important aspect of case management.

 BOX 27-2

Selected Anesthetic Protocols for Use in Stable Animals With Cardiovascular Disease

Premedication

Give atropine (0.02–0.04 mg/kg SC or IM) or glycopyrrolate (0.005–0.011 mg/kg SC or IM) if indicated plus hydromorphone* (0.1–0.2 mg/kg SC or IM) or butorphanol (0.2–0.4 mg/kg SC or IM) or buprenorphine (5–15 µg/kg IM)

Induction

Thiopental (10–12 mg/kg IV) or propofol (4–6 mg/kg IV)

Maintenance

Isoflurane or sevoflurane

SC, Subcutaneous; *IM,* intramuscular; *IV,* intravenous.
*Use 0.05 mg/kg in cats.

 BOX 27-3

Selected Anesthetic Protocols for Use in Animals With Heart Failure, Hypovolemia, Dehydration, and Those in Shock

Dogs

Premedication and induction

Hydromorphone (0.1 mg/kg IV) plus diazepam (0.2 mg/kg IV). Give in incremental dosages. Intubate if possible. If necessary, give etomidate (0.5–1.5 mg/kg IV). Alternately, give thiopental or propofol at reduced dosages. If there are no contraindications to ketamine, reduced dosages of diazepam and ketamine may also be used.

Maintenance

Isoflurane or sevoflurane

Cats

Premedication

Butorphanol (0.2–0.4 mg/kg SC or IM) or buprenorphine (5–15 µg/kg IM) or hydromorphone (0.05 mg/kg SC or IM)

Induction

Diazepam (0.2 mg/kg IV) followed by etomidate (0.5–1.5 mg/kg IV). Alternately, if not vomiting and there is no respiratory compromise, mask or chamber induction can be used or give thiopental or propofol at reduced dosages. If there are no contraindications to ketamine, reduced dosages of diazepam and ketamine may also be used.

Maintenance

Isoflurane or sevoflurane

IV, Intravenous; *SC,* subcutaneous; *IM,* intramuscular.

avoided in animals with mitral insufficiency because it increases regurgitant fraction. Diazepam has minimal cardiopulmonary effects sod helps offset the negative effects of ketamine (i.e., muscle rigidity and potential for seizures). Time to intubation is longer than with other agents, but is still considered relatively fast. Opioids can be used for induction of very sick and compromised dogs; however, opioids do not truly induce anesthesia, so intubation may be difficult in alert animals. Etomidate is not arrhythmogenic, maintains cardiac output, and offers rapid induction. Mask induction with isoflurane or sevoflurane is discouraged in

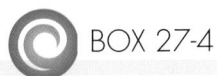

BOX 27-4

Drugs for Inflow Occlusion

Lidocaine (Xylocaine)
50–75 µg/kg/min IV infusion (see also Box 27-1)

Dobutamine (Dobutrex)
2–10 µg/kg/min IV

Epinephrine (Adrenaline, Generic)
0.1–0.4 µg/kg/min IV

Fentanyl Citrate (Sublimaze)
0.8 µg/kg/min IV

Atracurium Besylate (Tracrium)
0.1–0.2 mg/kg IV

Dexamethasone (Azium)
1 mg/kg IV

IV, Intravenous.

BOX 27-5

Anesthesia Protocol for Patients With Severe Cardiac Compromise That Will Not Tolerate Inhalant Anesthetic

Administer fentanyl citrate (0.8 µg/kg/min IV) plus midazolam (8 µg/kg/min IV)

IV, Intravenous.

patients with cardiopulmonary disorders because of the high inspired concentrations that are necessary and the time necessary to achieve intubation.

Anesthesia can be maintained with an inhalation agent in most cardiac patients. For compromised patients, isoflurane or sevoflurane in oxygen are the inhalation agents of choice. The insoluble nature of these inhalants allows rapid induction, recovery, and change in the depth of anesthesia. They depress contractility less than other inhalation agents and are less arrhythmogenic. Adjunct intravenous opioids decrease the levels of inhalant necessary to achieve adequate anesthesia. Opioids combined with low concentrations of isoflurane or sevoflurane may not produce adequate muscle relaxation, which may make administration of a nondepolarizing muscle relaxant desirable. Atracurium (Box 27-4) is a short-acting muscle relaxant that is not dependent on metabolism or excretion to terminate its action (it must be used with intermittent positive pressure ventilation [IPPV]).

For patients with compromised cardiac function, pericardial effusion, or cardiac compromise that do not tolerate inhalant anesthesia, fentanyl (Box 27-5) and midazolam (see Box 27-5) may be administered as an infusion. The dose will need to be adjusted to maintain adequate anesthesia. Oxygen

and IPPV must be provided due to the potent respiratory depression that occurs. In cases of pericardial effusion, once the pericardium is open, inhalant anesthesia may be instituted if cardiac function will tolerate the effects.

Thoracic surgery always requires controlled ventilation. Controlled ventilation can be achieved by manually squeezing the reservoir bag or by a mechanical ventilator attached to the anesthetic machine. Ideally, mechanical ventilation should achieve a tidal volume of 10 to 15 ml/kg of body weight at an inspiratory pressure of 20 cm of water. Assuring adequate ventilation is accomplished by optimizing tidal volume, inspiratory pressure, and respiratory rate to achieve ventilation with the least risk of causing pulmonary injury or cardiovascular compromise. Ultimately, the goal of mechanical ventilation is to maintain normocapnia. Ventilation can be monitored by measurement of end tidal CO_2 by capnography, or arterial CO_2 by blood gas analysis.

Successful inflow occlusion requires meticulous anesthesia. Balanced anesthetic techniques that minimize inhalation anesthetic agents are indicated (e.g., fentanyl citrate plus atracurium besylate combined with isoflurane [see Box 27-4] or fentanyl plus midazolam [see Box 27-5]). Administration of a single dose of dexamethasone (see Box 27-4) after induction may be beneficial in reducing cardiac damage (Yared et al, 2000). Animals should be hyperventilated for 5 minutes before inflow occlusion. Ventilation is discontinued during inflow occlusion and resumed immediately upon reestablishment of blood flow. Drugs and equipment for full cardiac resuscitation must be immediately available after inflow occlusion. Gentle cardiac massage may be necessary after inflow occlusion to reestablish cardiac function. Digital occlusion of the descending aorta during this period helps direct available cardiac output to the heart and brain. If ventricular fibrillation occurs, immediate internal defibrillation is necessary as soon as inflow occlusion is discontinued. Constant intravenous infusion of lidocaine (see Box 27-4) should be initiated before inflow occlusion and continued as necessary. Epinephrine, administered as a constant rate infusion, should be given as the animal is being weaned off inflow occlusion or a pump (see Box 27-4). If long-term inotropic support is necessary, dobutamine should be given (see Box 27-4).

ANTIBIOTICS

Perioperative antibiotics are indicated for cardiac procedures lasting more than 90 minutes. First-generation cephalosporins (e.g., cefazolin or cephapirin) can be administered intravenously at induction and repeated once or twice every 4 to 8 hours (Box 27-6). For cardiac procedures involving circulatory arrest or cardiopulmonary bypass, intravenous cefoxitin should be administered before surgery and continued for 24 to 48 hours after surgery (see Box 27-6).

SURGICAL ANATOMY

The heart is the largest mediastinal organ. It generally extends from the third rib to the caudal border of the sixth rib; however, variations exist among breeds and between individuals. The heart base (i.e., craniodorsal aspect that receives

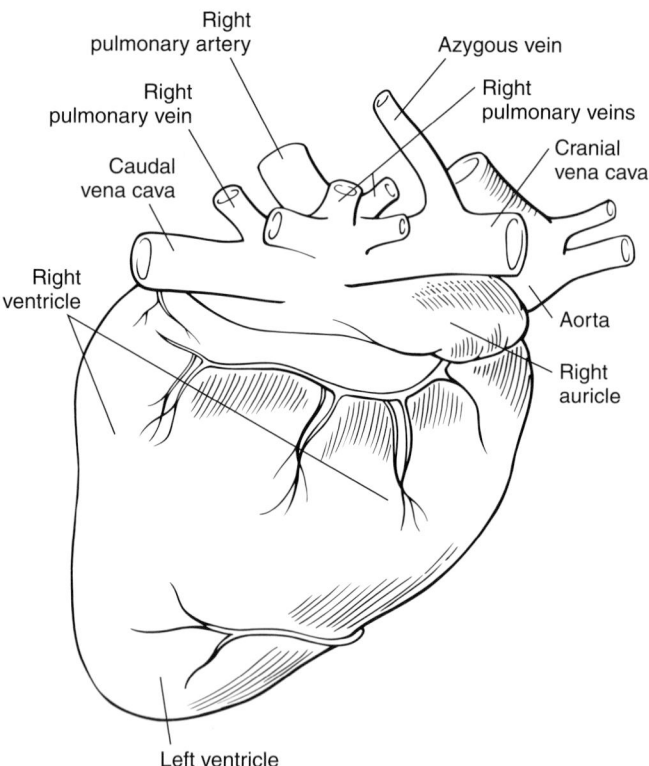

Right
pulmonary artery

Azygous vein

Right
pulmonary vein

Right
pulmonary veins

Caudal
vena cava

Cranial
vena cava

Right
ventricle

Aorta

Right
auricle

Left ventricle

FIG. 27-1
Cardiac anatomy as viewed from the right side.

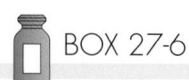 BOX 27-6

Prophylactic Antibiotics for Cardiac Surgery

Cefazolin (Ancef, Kefzol)

22 mg/kg IV at induction

Cephapirin (Cefadyl)

22 mg/kg IV at induction

Cefoxitin (Mefoxin)

30–40 mg/kg IV at induction

IV, Intravenous.

the great vessels) faces dorsocranially, whereas the apex (i.e., formed by muscles of the left ventricle) points caudoventrally. Except for a portion of the right side of the heart (cardiac notch), most of its surface is covered by lung. The right ventricular wall accounts for approximately 22% of the total heart weight; the left ventricular wall accounts for nearly 40%.

The right atrium receives blood from the systemic circulation. The coronary sinus enters the left caudal aspect of the atrium, ventral to the caudal vena cava. The caudal vena cava returns blood from the abdominal viscera, pelvic limbs, and a portion of the abdominal wall (Fig. 27-1). The cranial vena cava returns blood to the heart from the head, neck, thoracic

limbs, ventral thoracic wall, and a portion of the abdominal wall. The azygous vein usually enters in the cranial vena cava; it carries blood from the lumbar regions and caudal thoracic wall. The brachycephalic trunk is the first large artery from the aortic arch. The common carotid arteries usually arise from it as separate vessels. The left subclavian artery arises from the aortic arch distal to the brachycephalic trunk (the right subclavian is a branch of the brachycephalic trunk). The vertebral arteries, costocervical trunk, internal thoracic arteries, and axillary arteries branch from the subclavian vessels.

The pericardium is a thick, two-layered sac composed of outer fibrous and inner serous layers. The pericardial cavity is located between two layers (visceral and parietal) of serous pericardium and normally contains a small amount of fluid. The fibrous pericardium blends with the adventitia of the large vessels, and its apex forms the sternopericardiac ligament. Phrenic nerves lie in a narrow plica of pleura adjacent to the pericardium at the heart base. Complete pericardiectomy requires that these nerves be elevated to avoid incising them. The vagus nerves lie dorsal to the phrenic nerve. They divide to form dorsal and ventral branches that lie on the esophagus in the caudal thorax. The left recurrent laryngeal nerve leaves the vagus and loops around the arch distal to the ligamentum arteriosum to run cranially along the ventrolateral tracheal surface.

SURGICAL TECHNIQUE

Cardiac surgery is not fundamentally different from other types of general surgery, and similar principles of good surgical technique (i.e., atraumatic tissue handling, good hemostasis, and secure knot tying) apply. Consequences of poor surgical technique are often devastating. Cardiac surgery differs from other surgeries in that motion from ventilation and cardiac contractions adds to the technical difficulty of performing these procedures. Approaches that provide limited access to dorsal structures (e.g., median sternotomy; see p. 874) require that surgeons incise, suture, and/or ligate structures located deep within the thorax. Ligature placement using hand ties (see p. 70) is useful in such situations, and the ability to place hand-tied knots (versus instrument tying) should be considered a fundamental skill for cardiac surgeons. Secure knot tying is critically important to successful cardiac surgery. Hand tying knots is fast and produces tighter and more secure knots than instrument tying. The one-handed knot tie technique (see p. 72) is best suited to the fine sutures used in cardiac surgery. Tight knots are facilitated by throwing the first two or three throws in the same direction before finishing with square knots for security.

Closure of cardiovascular structures requires precise suturing techniques and good instrument handling skills to minimize hemorrhage. Using fine suture with swaged-on atraumatic needles (see discussion on suture materials on p. 780) and carefully following the needle contour when suturing (to minimize the size of needle tracts) are important. "Palming" of needle holders is a good skill for fast suturing,

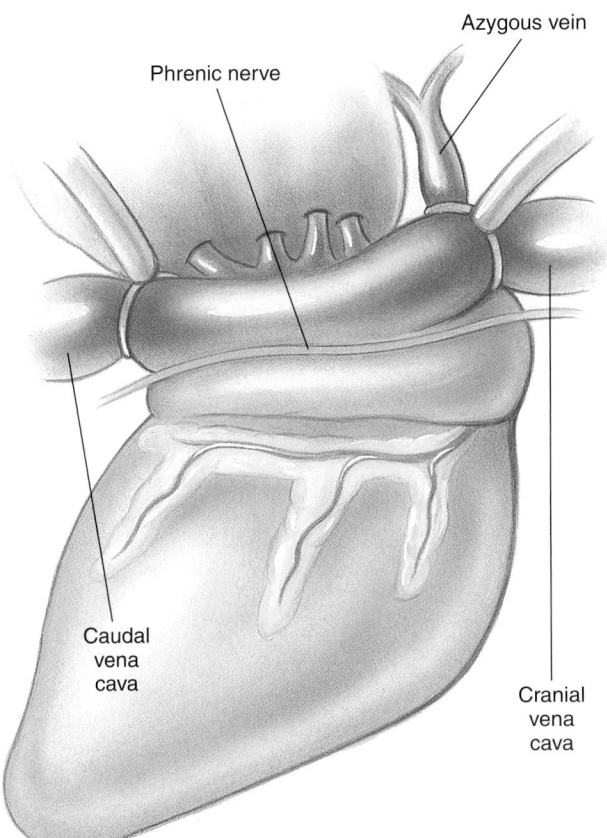

FIG. 27-2
To occlude cardiac inflow from the right side of the thorax, pass tapes around the caudal vena cava and the common drainage of the azygous veins and cranial vena cava. Fashion tourniquets as described in Fig. 27-3.

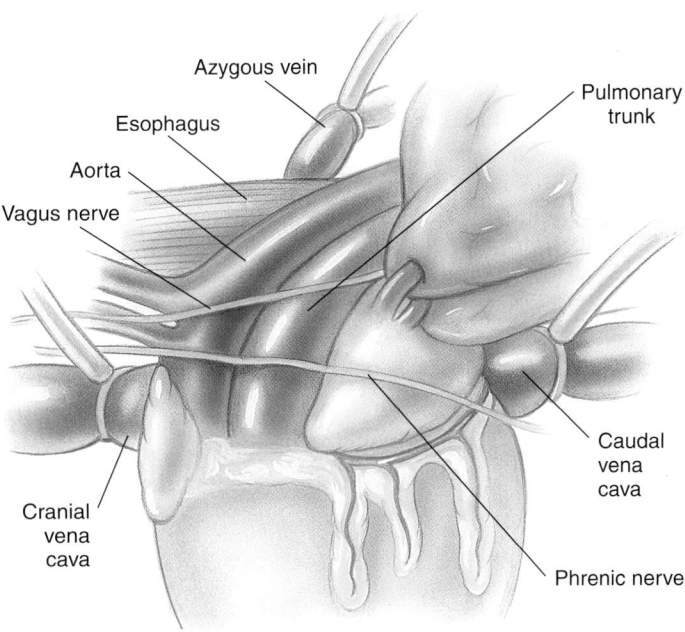

FIG. 27-3
During inflow occlusion from the left side of the thorax, pass tapes around the cranial and caudal vena cava and azygous vein. Fashion tourniquets for inflow occlusion by passing the tapes through rubber tubing.

but should be avoided when suturing inside the thoracic cavity. Finer control is gained by grasping instruments with fingers placed in the instrument rings.

Inflow Occlusion

Inflow occlusion is a technique used for open heart surgery in which all venous flow to the heart is temporarily interrupted. Because inflow occlusion results in complete circulatory arrest, it allows limited time to perform cardiac procedures. Ideally, circulatory arrest in a normothermic patient should be less than 2 minutes, but it can be extended to 4 minutes if necessary. Circulatory arrest time can be extended up to 6 minutes with mild, whole-body hypothermia (32° to 34° C). Temperatures below 32° C may predispose to fibrillation and should be avoided. The advantage of inflow occlusion is that it does not require specialized equipment; however, the limited time available to perform the surgery requires that the procedure be well planned and executed with speed and expertise.

Depending on the cardiac procedure being done, perform a left or right thoracotomy (see p. 871) or median sternotomy (see p. 874). With a right thoracotomy or median sternot- *omy, occlude the cranial and caudal vena cava and azygous vein with vascular clamps or Rumel tourniquets (Fig. 27-2). Make a Rumel tourniquet by passing umbilical tape around the vessel, then thread the umbilical tape through a piece of rubber tubing that is 1 to 3 inches long. When the umbilical tape has been adequately tightened to occlude the vessel, place a clamp above the rubber tubing to hold it securely in place. Take care to prevent injuring the right phrenic nerve during placement of the clamps or tourniquets. For left thoracotomies, pass separate tourniquets around the cranial and caudal venae cavae. Then, dissecting dorsal to the esophagus and aorta, occlude the azygous vein by placing a tourniquet around it (Fig. 27-3).*

Cardiopulmonary Bypass

Cardiopulmonary bypass is a procedure whereby an extracorporeal system provides flow of oxygenated blood to the patient while blood is diverted away from the heart and lungs. This greatly extends the time available for open cardiac surgery. Several advances (i.e., development of membrane oxygenators, improved methods of myocardial protection, increased availability of monitoring technologies, and improved veterinary critical care) have made cardiopulmonary bypass increasingly feasible in dogs. Cardiopulmonary bypass can be used to treat dogs with congenital or acquired cardiac defects. Readers are referred to a cardiovascular surgery text for details of performing cardiopulmonary bypass.

HEALING OF CARDIOVASCULAR STRUCTURES

Vascular structures heal quickly, forming a fibrin seal within minutes. Epithelialization and early endothelial regeneration occur in veins used for grafts. Thrombosis commonly occurs in small veins that have been traumatically occluded for short periods of time; however, thrombosis of large veins occluded during inflow occlusion or cardiac bypass procedures has not been a clinically recognized problem. To prevent thrombosis of vascular structures, they should be handled gently, as trauma may lead to the deposition of platelets, fibrin, and red cells on the intimal surface. If the torn intima is lifted upward, a flap may develop that partially or completely occludes the distal lumen. This in turn can lead to accumulation of blood within the vessel wall, vascular sludging, and thrombosis.

SUTURE MATERIALS AND SPECIAL INSTRUMENTS

Polypropylene and braided polyester suture are the standard sutures used for cardiovascular procedures. The most common sizes used are 3-0, 4-0, and 5-0, although small sizes may be used for vascular anastomoses. Sutures should be available with swaged-on taper-point cardiovascular needles in a variety of sizes. Some procedures require that the suture be double-armed (i.e., with needles at both ends). Teflon pledgets are useful for buttressing mattress sutures in ventricular myocardium or great vessels.

Successful cardiac surgery requires proper surgical instrumentation. Most of the basic instruments required for general surgery can be used for cardiac surgery; however, a few specialized instruments are desirable for thoracic surgery. The standard thoracic retractor is a Finochietto retractor (Fig. 27-4, *A*). It is helpful to have at least two sizes to accommodate different-sized animals. Self-retaining orthopedic retractors can substitute as thoracic retractors in small dogs and cats. The standard tissue forceps for thoracic surgery is a DeBakey tissue forceps (Fig. 27-4, *B*). At least two DeBakey forceps should be available, and it is helpful if one has a carbide inlay for grasping suture needles. Metzenbaum scissors are the standard operating scissors for cardiac surgery. Curved Metzenbaum scissors are more versatile than the straight design. Potts scissors (45-degree angle) are desirable for some cardiac surgery (Fig. 27-4, *B*). Needle holders should be long and available in different sizes to accommodate a variety of suture needle sizes. Mayo-Hegar, Crile-Wood, and Castroviejo needle holders represent a good selection of sizes for thoracic surgery in animals. Angled thoracic forceps are an important instrument for cardiac surgery and should be available in a variety of sizes (Fig. 27-4, *B*). Vascular clamps are noncrushing clamps used for temporary occlusion of cardiovascular and pulmonary structures. They come in a variety of sizes and shapes including straight, angled, curved, and tangential (Fig. 27-5). The most versatile shape for most cardiac surgery is a medium-width tangential clamp.

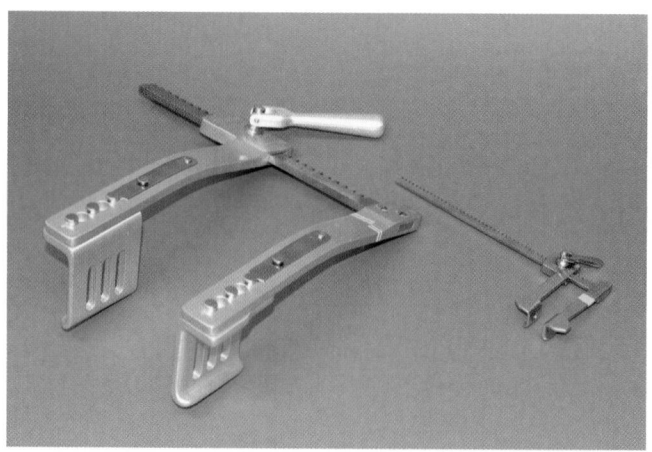

A

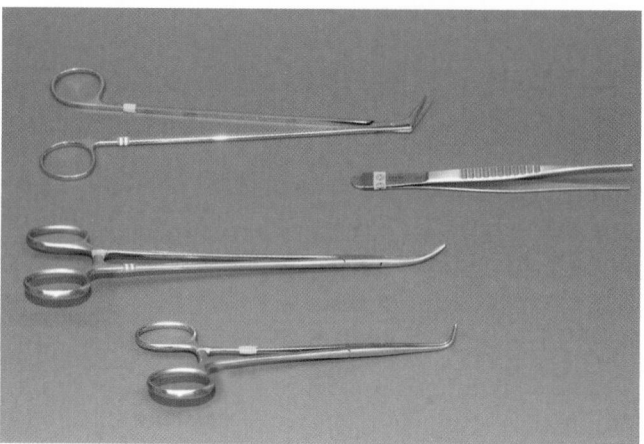

B

FIG. 27-4

Instruments for cardiovascular surgery: **A,** Large and small Finochietto retractors. **B,** (from top to bottom) Potts scissors, DeBakey tissue forceps, angled thoracic forceps (45 and 90 degree). The 90-degree forceps is also called a right angle or Mixter forceps; the 45-degree forceps is also called a Julian thoracic artery forceps or a Mixter forceps.

POSTOPERATIVE CARE AND ASSESSMENT

Patient monitoring and postoperative care are the cornerstones of successful cardiac surgery. The level of supportive care required for cardiac surgeries depends on the patient and on surgical procedure performed. A working knowledge of cardiopulmonary function and good patient observation skills are as important to successful patient management as advanced monitoring devices.

Evaluation of ventilation is important after any thoracic surgery. Poor ventilatory efforts may first be noted in the period after surgery when the influence of anesthetic drugs is still present but ventilatory support has been discontinued. Hypoventilation may also occur from uncontrolled pain. Total ventilation can be assessed directly by measuring the volume of expired gas with a respirometer. Tidal volume should be at least 10 ml per kg of body weight. Ultimately, the best measure of alveolar ventilation is arterial CO_2 tension ($PaCO_2$). Alveolar hypoventilation is pres-

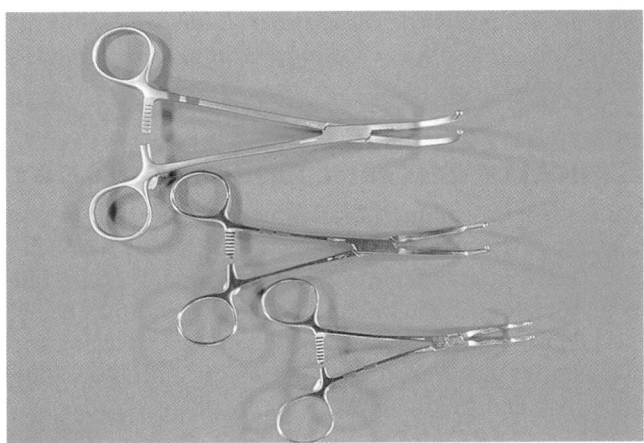

FIG. 27-5
Tangential (Satinsky) vascular clamps.

ent when $PaCO_2$ is increased above 40 mm Hg. Treatment of hypoventilation should be directed at correcting its underlying cause if possible. Drugs that are known to depress ventilation (i.e., opioids and muscle relaxants) should be used with caution in the perioperative period, and the risk of ventilatory depression weighed against the risk of hypoventilation due to pain (see p. 868 for analgesia after thoracotomy). Pleural air or fluid should be evacuated if present. Injury or dysfunction of the neuromuscular ventilatory apparatus should be corrected, if possible. If hypoventilation is severe and the cause is not immediately correctable, positive-pressure ventilation is indicated.

Under physiologic conditions, gas exchange between the alveolus and pulmonary capillary blood is efficient, and alveolar oxygen tension (PAO_2) and arterial oxygen tension (PaO_2) are nearly equal. In patients with impaired gas exchange, hypoxemia occurs because PAO_2 and PaO_2 are not equal. The most common causes of impaired pulmonary gas exchange in the postoperative setting are ventilation/perfusion (V_A/Q) mismatch and pulmonary shunts secondary to alveolar collapse. Impaired pulmonary gas exchange may or may not be responsive to supplemental oxygen therapy depending on its underlying cause. Therefore, response to supplemental oxygen therapy must be evaluated for each individual patient, preferably by blood gas analysis. The therapeutic goal of supplemental oxygen should be to keep PaO_2 above 80 mm Hg. Positive end-expiratory pressure (PEEP) therapy is indicated for patients with severe gas exchange impairment that is not responsive to supplemental oxygen therapy alone.

Maintaining an adequate PaO_2 in a patient is important because it is the major determinant of hemoglobin oxygen saturation (SaO_2). SaO_2 can be measured by pulse oximetry. The therapeutic goal should be to maintain SaO_2 at or above 90%. Oxygen content of the blood is a function of SaO_2 and hemoglobin concentration. Thus maintenance of an adequate oxygen content requires not only adequate pulmonary function (SaO_2 greater than 90%), but also an adequate hemoglobin concentration. Maintenance of the packed cell volume above 30% is an important therapeutic goal for ani-

mals undergoing cardiac surgery, especially if cardiopulmonary compromise is present.

Systemic blood pressure is directly proportional to cardiac output and systemic vascular resistance. Measurement of blood pressure provides a good assessment of cardiovascular function, especially during and immediately after surgery. Indirect techniques for measuring blood pressure include the oscillometric method, the basis of monitors such as the Dinamap, or Doppler method. Doppler technique provides only systolic pressure, but is useful for evaluating blood pressure trends during and after surgery. Indirect methods of blood pressure assessment are less invasive, but are also less accurate than direct measurements. Direct measurement of blood pressure requires placement of an arterial catheter. Arterial catheters have the additional advantage of providing access for arterial blood gas analysis. An arterial catheter can be placed percutaneously into a dorsal pedal artery. Direct blood pressure measurement also requires a pressure transducer and monitor, or a manometer. The therapeutic goal is to maintain a mean blood pressure above 65 mm Hg and systolic blood pressure above 90 mm Hg. Blood pressure can be elevated by increasing either cardiac output or systemic vascular resistance. In most instances, the more appropriate therapeutic strategy to correct hypotension is to improve cardiac output. Maintenance of adequate vascular volume is the most important aspect of maintaining adequate cardiac output. Central venous pressure should be maintained between 5 and 10 cm of water. Indications for arterial pressor therapy are rare. Inotropic and pressor support can be obtained by constant intravenous infusion of epinephrine (see Box 27-4). Long-term inotropic support is maintained by dobutamine (see Box 27-4).

Monitoring the electrocardiogram for disturbances in cardiac rhythm is important for animals undergoing cardiac surgery. Sinus tachycardia is the most common rhythm disturbance in surgery patients. Therapy for sinus tachycardia should be directed at correction of its underlying cause and improvement of cardiac output. Ventricular dysrhythmias, including premature ventricular complexes (PVCs) and nonsustained or sustained ventricular tachycardia, are frequently encountered during and after cardiac surgery. Frequent PVCs, particularly when they occur with a short coupling interval (i.e., R on T phenomena), and rapid ventricular tachycardia should be suppressed in the perioperative period. Continuous intravenous infusion of lidocaine is effective in most instances. Ventricular fibrillation is a form of cardiac arrest that requires immediate electrical defibrillation. If cardiac surgery is performed, equipment for defibrillation should be available. Recommendations for postoperative analgesics are provided in Chapter 13 (see Table 13-4 on p. 133).

COMPLICATIONS

The major complication associated with cardiac surgery is hemorrhage. Severe hemorrhage may be encountered intraoperatively or postoperatively. Materials for blood transfusion should be available (see Box 5-1 and Table 5-5 on pp. 25 and 28, respectively). Fresh whole blood should be collected as close as possible to the time that it is needed and should not be cooled because this may reduce platelet content. If possible, a compatible donor should be identified by cross-matching the patient before surgery. Cell Saver autologous blood recovery systems are available for collection and processing of blood in procedures in which there is rapid bleeding or high-volume blood loss. They can also be used to sequester platelets and plasma from a patient immediately before surgery, reducing the need for donor blood.

SPECIAL AGE CONSIDERATIONS

Most animals undergoing surgery for congenital cardiac defects are young. Special care must be given to these animals during and after surgery. Young animals should not have food withheld for greater than 4 to 6 hours before surgery and should be fed as soon as they are fully recovered from anesthesia. If they cannot be fed, blood glucose concentration should be maintained by adding glucose to intravenous fluids; blood glucose concentrations should be monitored intraoperatively. Hypothermia is common in young patients during thoracotomy and is protective during cardiac procedures. However, the temperature should be monitored closely, and they should be actively rewarmed postoperatively.

> NOTE: Remember, hypothermia decreases the minimum alveolar concentration (MAC) of inhalants used for maintenance.

References

Grimm KA, Tranquilli WJ, Gross DR et al: Cardiopulmonary effects of fentanyl in conscious dogs and dogs sedated with a continuous rate infusion of medetomidine, *Am J Vet Res* 66:1222, 2005.

Yared JP, Starr JN, Torres FK et al: Effects of single-dose, postinduction dexamethasone on recovery after cardiac surgery, *Ann Thorac Surg* 69:1420, 2000.

Suggested Reading

Meurs KM, Miller MW, Slater MR: Arterial blood pressure measurement in a population of healthy geriatric dogs, *J Am Anim Hosp Assoc* 36:497, 2000.

Thirty-three geriatric dogs were studied. Diastolic and mean blood pressures were lower in the geriatric group; systolic blood pressures were not significantly different.

SPECIFIC DISEASES

MITRAL REGURGITATION

DEFINITIONS

Mitral regurgitation (MR) occurs when blood leaks retrograde across the mitral valve into the left atrium during contraction of the left ventricle. Synonyms include *mitral valve disease* and *mitral insufficiency*. Endocardiosis of the mitral valve is also known as *myxomatous valvular degeneration* (MVD).

GENERAL CONSIDERATIONS AND CLINICALLY RELEVANT PATHOPHYSIOLOGY

MR is the most common form of acquired heart disease in dogs. Approximately 75% of dogs with chronic heart disease have MR attributable to MVD. It commonly occurs due to myxomatous degeneration of the valve and may be associated with one or more of the following: thickening and billowing of the leaflets, dilation of the mitral annulus, thickening and lengthening or rupture of the chordae tendineae, and flattening of the papillary muscles with left ventricular dilation. Morphologic changes associated with MVD in dogs are similar to those observed in humans with mitral valve prolapse (Corcoran et al, 2004). Tissue swelling occurs on the edge of valve leaflets, the chordae tendineae, and the chordal-papillary muscle junction. Damage to the valve complex endothelium is unevenly distributed. On rare occasions, annular dilation and MR occur without significant disease of the chordae or leaflets. Congenital valve dysplasia and dilated cardiomyopathy are other causes of mitral regurgitation.

Volume overload of the left ventricle is caused when blood regurgitates through the mitral valve, causing left atrial and left ventricular hypertrophy. As the mitral valve annulus dilates, MR typically becomes more severe, and left-sided congestive heart failure typically ensues. Atrial fibrillation may be associated with the left atrial dilation, especially in large and giant breeds of dogs with sufficient atrial mass to sustain the arrhythmia.

DIAGNOSIS
Clinical Presentation

Signalment. Myxomatous valve degeneration typically occurs in older small breed dogs, whereas congenital mitral valve dysplasia occurs most commonly in large and giant breeds of dogs, and also cats. King Charles Cavalier spaniels are a well-recognized, predisposed breed and typically develop MVD at a relatively young age (3 to 5 years old). Dilated cardiomyopathy may be associated with secondary mitral regurgitation as dilation of the valve annulus coupled with papillary muscle dysfunction causes valvular incompetence.

History. Affected animals may have a history of exercise intolerance, coughing, and/or shortness of breath. A murmur associated with MR may be picked up on physical examination in an asymptomatic animal.

Physical Examination Findings

Affected animals typically have a holosystolic murmur heard best at the left cardiac apex. Pulmonary crackles may be heard if pulmonary edema is present. Electrocardiographic evidence of left atrial and/or left ventricular enlargement may be manifested by a P wave duration greater than 0.04 second (P mitrale) or tall R waves (greater than 2 to 2.5 mV), respectively, in lead II.

Diagnostic Imaging

Left atrial and left ventricular enlargement may be evident on thoracic radiographs. When congestive heart failure develops, additional radiographic features include pulmonary venous congestion and pulmonary parenchymal infiltrate, typically with a perihilar or caudal and dorsal distribution.

Echocardiography. In addition to characteristic changes in the mitral valve (mild to moderate thickening and irregularity), echocardiographic findings also typically include left atrial dilation and left ventricular dilation. Initially, indices of systolic function (shortening fraction) are within normal limits. Echocardiographic evidence of myocardial systolic failure is indicative of advanced disease. Occasionally, echocardiography documents chordal rupture or pericardial effusion secondary to an atrial tear.

Laboratory Findings

Laboratory abnormalities are typically unremarkable unless cardiac output is reduced sufficiently to reduce organ perfusion (e.g., prerenal azotemia). Evidence of chronic renal disease may be noted in many affected animals. King Charles Cavalier Spaniels with mitral valve disease appear to have an increased plasma fibrinogen concentration and a low plasma von Willebrand factor (Tarnow et al, 2004). The latter is likely due to their destruction via shear stress to the blood. The importance of these changes on thromboembolic risk is unknown.

DIFFERENTIAL DIAGNOSIS

Other causes of heart failure and cardiac murmur in mature dogs include dilated cardiomyopathy and previously undiagnosed or unrepaired congenital heart disease (patent ductus arteriosus [PDA], ventricular septal defect [VSD], mitral dysplasia, subvalvular aortic stenosis [SAS]). Primary differentials include chronic bronchitis, heartworm disease, tracheal collapse, pneumonia, and primary or metastatic pulmonary neoplasia.

MEDICAL MANAGEMENT

There are few data to suggest that medical intervention before the onset of clinical signs of heart failure is beneficial. In fact, several placebo-controlled trials have demonstrated that therapy with ACE inhibitors has no effect on symptom-free interval (time to onset of heart failure) in asymptomatic patients. Once congestive heart failure is documented, treatment with diuretics (e.g., furosemide; see Box 27-1), ACE inhibitors (i.e., enalapril or benazepril; see Box 27-1), and inodilators (pimobendan, see Box 27-1), is indicated. Additional diuretics (e.g., spironolactone or hydrochlorothiazide) and vasodilators (e.g., hydralazine or amlodipine) should be considered in refractory cases. The role of β-blockers and adrenergic blockers has yet to be defined, but holds promise.

SURGICAL TREATMENT

Mitral valve replacement and repair have been reported in dogs. For mitral valve replacement, a mechanical or bioprosthetic heart valve is typically used. Disadvantages of these valves are that the animal must be placed on life-long anticoagulation therapy (mechanical), or early pannus formation and calcification may occur (bioprosthetic); their placement requires a cardiopulmonary bypass. Mitral valve repair may have advantages over valve replacement in that long-term anticoagulation is not required and myocardial function is better preserved. However, the results are variable and highly dependent on the surgeon's experience.

An option to mitral valve replacement has been reported in dogs without the use of a cardiopulmonary bypass (Buchanan and Sammarco, 1998). The authors described placement of a circumferential mitral purse-string suture to reduce the diameter of the mitral annulus. For a description and illustration of the procedure, see *Small Animal Surgery,* second edition or the e-dition. For description of placement of an artificial valve or valve repair with cardiopulmonary bypass, the reader is referred to a cardiac surgery textbook. Novel annuloplasty devices are being placed percutaneously via the coronary sinus and great cardiac run in human beings; however, there are no reports to date of their use in dogs with naturally occurring mitral valve disease.

> NOTE: Techniques for mitral valve repair that use cardiopulmonary bypass are probably safer than those that do not, particularly in animals with severe heart failure. However, bypass procedures are expensive and not readily available in veterinary medicine.

Preoperative Management

Preoperative arrhythmias should be controlled before surgery. Affected animals typically have signs of congestive heart failure, and treatment with positive inotropes (i.e., digoxin or pimobendan), vasodilators (i.e., hydralazine, enalapril, or amlodipine), and diuretics (i.e., furosemide or spironolactone) is indicated (see previously in Medical Management section).

Anesthesia

Refer to p. 775 for anesthetic recommendations for cardiac patients.

Surgical Anatomy

The right and left coronary vessels (Fig. 27-6) arise from the aortic bulb immediately distal to the aortic valve. The right coronary artery arises from the right sinus of the aorta and curves to the right and ventrocranially, lying in the fat of the coronary groove. Its initial part is bounded by the pulmonary trunk and the conus arteriosus craniolaterally; dorsally it is covered by the right auricle. The left coronary artery is a short trunk about 5 mm long and nearly as wide. It terminates in the circumflex and paraconal interventricular branches. The circumflex branch lies in the coronary groove as it extends to the left. On approaching the dorsal interventricular groove, it turns toward the apex of the heart and is known as the *subsinuosal interventricular branch*. The combined length of the circumflex and subsinual branch is approximately 8 cm in the dog. The paraconal interventricular branch is approximately 1.5 mm in width and 7 cm long. It winds obliquely and distally from left to right across the sternocostal surface of the heart in the paraconal interventricular groove.

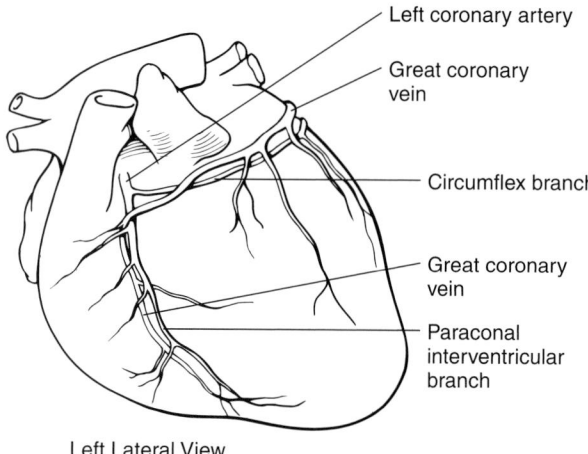

Left Lateral View

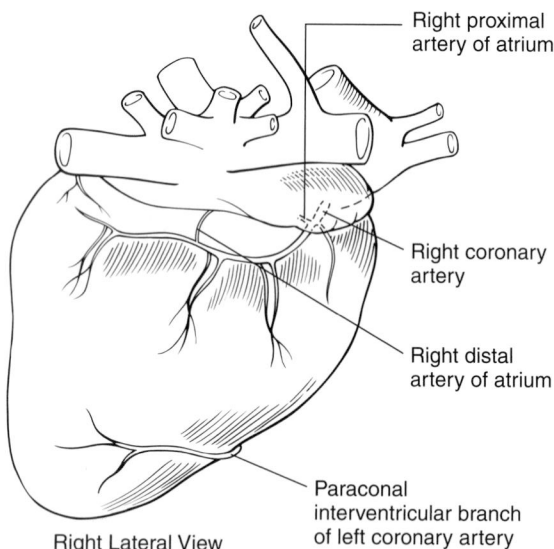

Right Lateral View

FIG. 27-6
Anatomy of the coronary vessels in a dog.

Positioning

Mitral valve repair or replacement may be done via right or left-sided thoracotomy. The entire thorax is prepped for aseptic surgery.

AP SURGICAL TECHNIQUE

For a description of a purse-string suture for mitral valve repair, see *Small Animal Surgery*, second edition or the e-dition. For a description of mitral valve repair or replacement, readers are referred to a cardiac surgery textbook.

SUTURE MATERIALS AND SPECIAL INSTRUMENTS

For a description of suture materials and special instruments used for a purse-string suture repair for mitral regurgitation, please see *Small Animal Surgery*, second edition or the e-dition.

POSTOPERATIVE CARE AND ASSESSMENT

Postoperative pain should be treated with systemic opioids and local anesthetic techniques (see p. 868 for postthoracotomy analgesia). Animals should be monitored for pulmonary edema after surgery. If pulmonary edema occurs, it should be treated with furosemide (see Box 27-1). Left ventricular failure should be treated as outlined in the Medical Management section.

PROGNOSIS

Circumferential suture of the mitral annulus has been reported in 15 dogs (Buchanan and Sammarco, 1998). Six dogs died during surgery because of hemorrhage, and three dogs died postoperatively because of coronary artery compression by the suture. Satisfactory suture placement was achieved in six dogs, three of which survived for between 6 and 26 months. However, the authors noted that the technique is difficult and requires practice. Mitral valve replacement with a mechanical valve prosthesis was recently reported in eight dogs with severe MR (Orton et al, 2005). Median survival after surgery was 4.5 months. Although most dogs survived the surgery, there was a high incidence of prosthetic valve thrombosis. Mitral valve repair (e.g., circumferential annuloplasty, placement of artificial chordae, chordal fenestration, papillary muscle splitting, and/or edge-to-edge repair) successfully resolved signs of congestive heart failure in 9 of 18 dogs for a median period of 1 year (range, 4 months to 3 years) after surgery (Griffiths et al, 2004).

References

Buchanan JW, Sammarco CD: Circumferential suture of the mitral annulus for correction of mitral regurgitation in dogs, *Vet Surg* 27:182, 1998.

Corcoran BM, Black A, Anderson H et al: Identification of surface morphologic changes in the mitral valve leaflets and chordae tendinae of dogs with myxomatous degeneration, *Am J Vet Res* 65:198, 2004.

Griffiths LG, Orton EC, Boon JA: Evaluation of techniques and outcomes of mitral valve repair in dogs, *J Am Vet Med Assoc* 15:224, 2004.

Orton EC, Hackett TB, Mama K et al: Technique and outcome of mitral valve replacement in dogs, *J Am Vet Med Assoc* 226:1508, 2005.

Tarnow I, Kristensen AT, Olsen LH et al: Assessment of changes in hemostatic markers in Cavalier King Charles Spaniels with myxomatous mitral valve disease, *Am J Vet Res* 65:1644, 2004.

PATENT DUCTUS ARTERIOSUS

DEFINITIONS

The **ductus arteriosus** is a fetal vessel that connects the main pulmonary artery and descending aorta. During development, it shunts blood away from the collapsed fetal lungs. Normally, it closes shortly after birth during the transition from fetal to extrauterine life. Continued patency of the ductus arteriosus for more than a few days after birth is called **patent ductus arteriosus (PDA)**.

GENERAL CONSIDERATIONS AND CLINICALLY RELEVANT PATHOPHYSIOLOGY

PDA is one of the most common congenital heart defects of dogs; it also occurs infrequently in cats. PDA typically causes a left-to-right shunt that results in volume overload of the left ventricle and produces left ventricular dilation. Progressive left ventricular dilation distends the mitral valve annulus, causing secondary regurgitation and additional ventricular overload. This severe volume overload leads to left-sided congestive heart failure and pulmonary edema, usually within the first year of life. Atrial fibrillation may occur as a late sequela because of notable left atrial dilation.

Rarely, dogs with PDA develop suprasystemic pulmonary hypertension that reverses the direction of flow through the shunt, causing severe hypoxemia and cyanosis (Eisenmenger's physiology). Right-to-left PDA can occur as a late sequela (6 months) to untreated PDA. When right-to-left PDA is noted in very young animals, it may be due to persistent pulmonary hypertension after birth. Reversal of PDA lessens the risk for developing progressive left-sided heart failure, but causes severe debilitating systemic hypoxemia, exercise intolerance, and progressive polycythemia.

> NOTE: Dogs with PDA should not be used for breeding, regardless of breed (Buchanan and Patterson, 2003).

DIAGNOSIS
Clinical Presentation

Signalment. PDA is seen more commonly in purebred female dogs. Maltese, Pomeranians, Shetland sheepdogs, English springer spaniels, keeshonden, bichon frises, miniature and toy poodles, and Yorkshire terriers are at an increased risk for developing PDA. A genetic basis has been established in poodles.

History. Most young animals with PDA are asymptomatic or have only mild exercise intolerance. The most common complaint in symptomatic animals with left-to-right shunts is cough or shortness of breath (or both) due to pulmonary edema. Animals with right-to-left or reverse PDA may be asymptomatic or may have exercise intolerance and hind limb collapse during exercise.

Physical Examination Findings

The most prominent physical finding associated with PDA is a characteristic continuous (machinery) murmur heard best at the high left heart base or left axillary region. The left apical cardiac impulse is prominent and displaced caudally, and a palpable cardiac "thrill" often is present. Femoral pulses are strong or hyperkinetic (water hammer pulse) due to a wide pulse pressure caused by diastolic runoff of blood through the ductus. Tall R waves (greater than 2.5 mV in lead II) or wide P waves on a lead II electrocardiogram are supportive of the diagnosis, but they are not always present. Atrial fibrillation or ventricular ectopy may occur in advanced cases.

The physical examination findings in animals with right-to-left or reverse PDA differ from those with left-to-right shunts. "Differential" cyanosis is typically present (i.e., cyanosis is most apparent in the caudal mucous membranes), but cyanosis may also be noted in the cranial half of the body in some animals. Cyanosis occurs because there is a mixture of nonoxygenated blood (from the pulmonary artery) with the oxygenated aortic blood. Femoral pulses are normal. A systolic cardiac murmur, rather than a machinery murmur, is often present. However, a murmur may not be auscultated if polycythemia is present (see later section on Laboratory Findings) or if left- and right-sided pressures are nearly equal and if shunting of blood through the ductus is minimal.

Diagnostic Imaging

Thoracic radiographs typically show left atrial and ventricular enlargement, pulmonary vasculature overcirculation, and a characteristic dilation of the descending aorta and sometimes the main pulmonary artery on the dorsoventral view. Quantitation of the left-to-right shunt can be obtained through the use of first pass nuclear scintigraphy (Bahr et al, 2002). With right-to-left PDA, thoracic radiographs show evidence of biventricular enlargement, notable dilation of the main pulmonary artery segment, and enlargement and tortuosity of lobar pulmonary arteries. Nuclear scintigraphy (^{99m}Tc-macroaggregated albumin) (Morandi et al, 2004) has also been used to diagnose right-to-left shunts.

Echocardiography. Echocardiography provides information that further confirms PDA and helps exclude concurrent cardiac defects, but it is not invariably required to establish the diagnosis. Echocardiographic findings that support a diagnosis of PDA include left atrial enlargement, left ventricular dilation, pulmonary artery dilation, increased transaortic and transmitral flow velocities, and a characteristic reverse turbulent Doppler flow pattern in the pulmonary artery. Echocardiographic features of right-to-left PDA typically include right ventricular dilation and thickening, dilation of the main pulmonary artery, and flattening of the interventricular septum. A right-to-left PDA can be documented by performing a saline microbubble contrast echocardiogram. Observing microbubbles in the descending aorta, but not in any left-sided cardiac chamber, is diagnostic.

Laboratory Findings

Laboratory abnormalities are uncommon in animals with left-to-right shunting PDA; however, animals with right-to-left shunts are commonly polycythemic. Polycythemia occurs in response to increased erythropoietin production due to chronic hypoxemia.

DIFFERENTIAL DIAGNOSIS

The characteristic physical examination findings (i.e., continuous murmur or bounding arterial pulses) make diagnosis of PDA straightforward in most affected animals. Rarely, a combination of aortic stenosis and/or aortic insufficiency (see p. 792), or VSD and/or aortic insufficiency (see p. 794) causes a to-and-fro murmur that may be difficult to differentiate from continuous PDA murmurs. In animals in which the diastolic component of the PDA murmur is difficult to detect, other differentials would include subaortic stenosis, pulmonic stenosis (PS), atrial septal defect (ASD), and VSD. Differentials for dogs with right-to-left PDA include tetralogy of Fallot, right-to-left shunting, ASD or VSD, or other complex forms of cyanotic heart disease (rare).

MEDICAL MANAGEMENT

Animals with pulmonary edema should be given furosemide (see Box 27-1) for 24 to 48 hours before surgery. If atrial fibrillation is present, the ventricular response rate should be controlled using digoxin (with or without β-adrenergic blockers or calcium channel blockers) or amiodarone before surgery. If hemodynamically significant arrhythmias are present, they must be controlled. Complete resolution of clinical signs of congestive heart failure may be difficult or impossible with medical management alone. Long-term medical management of dogs with right-to-left PDA with phlebotomy only has been reported (Cote and Ettinger, 2001).

SURGICAL TREATMENT

Surgical correction of PDA is accomplished by ligation of the ductus arteriosus. Ligation of PDA is considered curative and should be performed as soon as possible after diagnosis. Secondary MR usually regresses after surgery due to reduction in left ventricular dilation. Ligation may be performed using a standard dissection approach or the Jackson approach (see later discussion). The latter technique carries a higher risk of residual flow and should only be used when bleeding or rupture associated with the standard dissection precludes its use (Stanley et al, 2003). It has also been reported using a video-enhanced minithoracotomy incision and titanium ligating clips (Borenstein et al, 2004). Inadvertent ductal rupture during dissection is the most serious complication associated with PDA repair. The risk of this complication decreases with more experienced surgeons. Small ruptures, especially those on the back side of the ductus, often respond to gentle tamponade, but they may enlarge and worsen if dissection is continued. If bleeding occurs, sodium nitroprusside (5 to 25 μg/kg/min IV to effect) may be administered to lower the systemic mean arterial pressure to 50 to 65 mm Hg within 5 to 10 minutes such that ligation can be continued (Hunter et al, 2003). If bleeding is severe, vascular clamps may be needed to occlude the aorta while the ductus is ligated. Once bleeding is controlled, a decision must be made whether to continue surgery if the ductus was not ligated or to stop in favor of repair at a later time. Second surgeries are more difficult due to adhesions at the surgical site, so complete occlusion should be attempted during the initial procedure, if possible. Simple ductal ligation is often not possible after a rupture has occurred. In such instances, surgical alternatives include ductal closure with pledget-buttressed mattress sutures or ductal division and closure between vascular clamps. The divided ductal

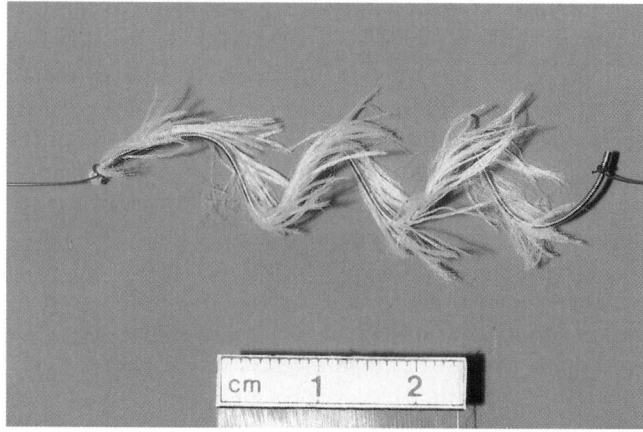

FIG. 27-7
Intravascular coil used to occlude a patent ductus arteriosus. (Courtesy Dr. M. Miller, Texas A&M University.)

ends are closed with a continuous mattress suture oversewn with a simple continuous pattern. Ductal closure without division is safer than surgical division, but recannulation of the ductus may occur. Because ductal division requires additional technical expertise, only experienced surgeons should perform this procedure.

Placement of hemoclips on the ductus to make medial dissection unnecessary has recently been reported (Corti et al, 2000). Hemorrhage occurred at the same rate as for ligation methods and was typically associated with dissection of the cranial aspect of the ductus. One dog out of the 20 reported had residual ductal flow identified 5 days after surgery; recanalization was not apparent in the remaining dogs. The aortic aneurysmal dilation seen in dogs with PDA persisted; however, a reduction in cardiac chamber size and resolution of mitral valve insufficiency was seen.

Intravascular coils and other occlusion devices are now used routinely for closure of patent ductus arteriosus (Fig. 27-7). These techniques have the advantage of not requiring a thoracotomy; percutaneous access to the femoral artery or a femoral artery cutdown is used. The coil or coils are placed in the ductus under fluoroscopic guidance, and complete occlusion is verified by injection of contrast agent into the aorta (Fig. 27-8).

Preoperative Management

Preoperative arrhythmias should be controlled before surgery. If the animal has signs of congestive heart failure, treatment with inodilators (i.e., pimobendan), vasodilators (i.e., hydralazine or enalapril), and diuretics (i.e., furosemide; see Box 27-1) should be initiated preoperatively. Excessive diuretics and/or vasodilators may cause hypotension and should be avoided.

Anesthesia

Bradycardia occasionally occurs during PDA ligation. An anticholinergic (i.e., atropine or glycopyrrolate) should be available and should be given if the heart rate drops below

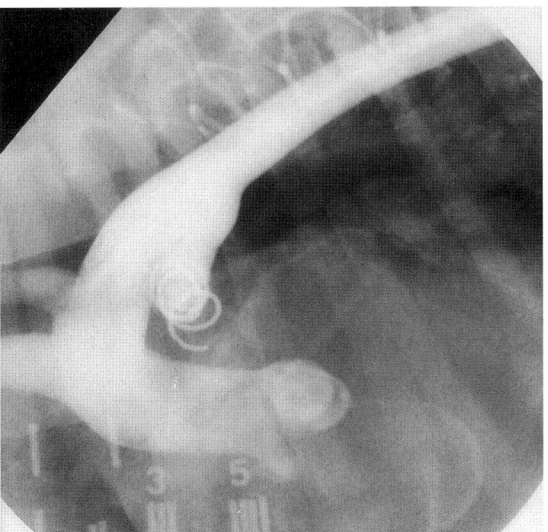

FIG. 27-8
Radiograph taken after deployment of a coil in a ductus. Contrast has been injected into the aorta at the site of coil deployment to verify complete occlusion of the ductus. (Courtesy Dr. M. Miller, Texas A&M University.)

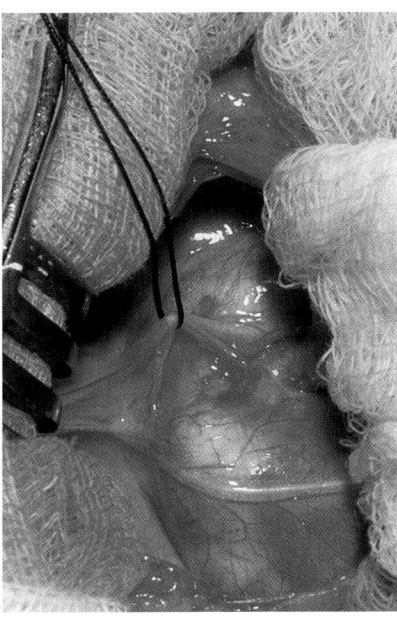

FIG. 27-9
During PDA ligation, elevate and retract the left vagus nerve to expose the ductus arteriosus. The left recurrent laryngeal nerve may be seen as it separates from the vagus nerve and courses caudally around the ductus arteriosus.

60 beats per minute in the dog. Blood should be available for transfusion if excessive hemorrhage occurs during the surgical procedure. Techniques for anesthetic management of cardiovascular patients are discussed on p. 775.

Surgical Anatomy

The ductus arteriosus in dogs and cats is usually wide (approximately 1 cm), but relatively short (less than 1 cm). It is located between the aorta and main pulmonary artery, caudal to the origin of the brachycephalic and left subclavian arteries. As a result, most mixing of oxygenated and nonoxygenated blood occurs in the descending aorta in dogs with reverse PDA. Thus normally oxygenated blood is supplied to the head and neck, whereas desaturated blood is presented to the caudal half of the body (see the comments in the Differential Diagnosis section on p. 785). The left vagus nerve always passes over the ductus arteriosus and must be identified and retracted during dissection. The left recurrent laryngeal nerve can often be identified as it loops around the ductus.

Positioning

The animal is positioned in right lateral recumbency, and the left thorax is prepared for aseptic surgery.

SURGICAL TECHNIQUE

Standard approach. *Perform a left fourth space intercostal thoracotomy (see p. 873). Identify the left vagus nerve as it courses over the ductus arteriosus, and isolate it using sharp dissection at the level of the ductus. Place a suture around the nerve and gently retract it (Fig. 27-9). Isolate the ductus arteriosus by bluntly dissecting around it without opening the pericardial sac. Pass a right-angle forceps be-*hind the ductus, parallel to its transverse plane, to isolate the caudal aspect of the ductus. Then dissect the cranial aspect of the ductus by angling the forceps caudally approximately 45 degrees (Fig. 27-10). Complete dissection of the ductus by passing forceps from medial to the ductus in a caudal to cranial direction. Grasp the suture with right-angle forceps. Slowly pull the suture beneath the ductus. If the suture does not slide easily around the ductus, do not force it. Regrasp the suture and repeat the process, being careful not to include surrounding soft tissue in the forceps. Pass a second suture using the same maneuver. Alternatively, the suture may be passed as a double loop and the suture cut so that the surgeon has two strands (Fig. 27-11). Slowly tighten the suture closest to the aorta first. Then tighten the remaining suture.*

Jackson approach. *Approach the ductus as described above. With scissors, incise the mediastinal pleura dorsal to the aorta from the origin of the left subclavian artery cranially to the origin of the first intercostal artery caudally. Bluntly dissect the loose areolar tissue on the medial aspect of the aorta. Insert a right-angled forceps immediately cranial to the ductus and pass it around the aorta from ventral to dorsal while gently elevating the aortic arch with a finger. Pass a loop of ligature from the dorsomedial aspect of the aorta to the cranial aspect of the ductus, ventral to the aorta. Then insert the right-angled forceps immediately caudal to the ductus and pass it around the aorta from ventral to dorsal to pick up the two free strands of the ligature. Draw the strands ventral around the ductus, and divide the loop to form two individual strands. Tie the ligature as described above.*

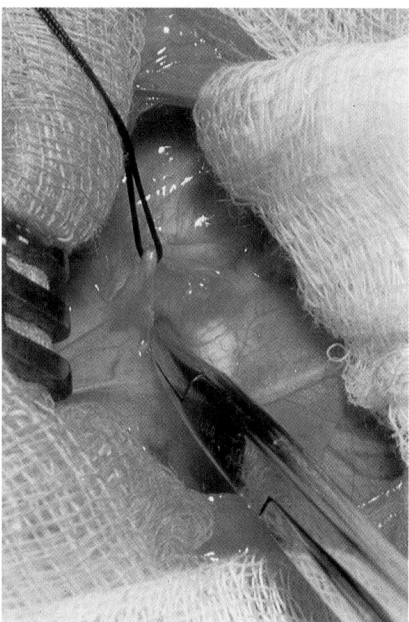

FIG. 27-10
Isolate the craniomedial aspect of the ductus arteriosus by bluntly dissecting with an angled forceps. The forceps should be directed at a 45-degree angle from the transverse plane.

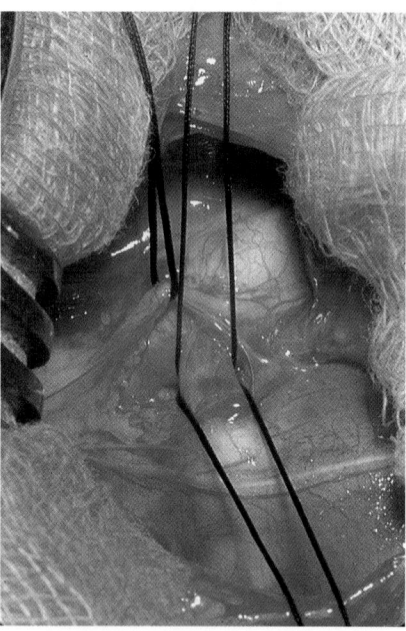

FIG. 27-11
Ligate the PDA by passing two ligatures around the ductus arteriosus. Tie the ligatures separately.

SUTURE MATERIALS AND SPECIAL INSTRUMENTS

Heavy silk (No. 1 or 0) or cotton tape is a suitable material for ductal ligation. Large hemoclips have also been used. Right-angle forceps are best suited for blunt dissection of the PDA and for passing ligatures. Angled or tangential vascular clamps are required for surgical division of PDA

or for repair of inadvertent ruptures. Polypropylene mattress sutures (4-0), buttressed with Teflon pledgets, are used for repair of ruptured PDA.

POSTOPERATIVE CARE AND ASSESSMENT

Postoperative pain should be treated with systemic opioids and local anesthetic techniques. Bupivacaine may be used intercostally or intrapleurally to supplement analgesia (see p. 868). Young animals should be fed as soon as they are fully recovered from surgery. Thoracostomy tubes are occasionally placed before thoracic closure (e.g., if intraoperative bleeding occurred). They can generally be removed within 12 to 24 hours after surgery.

COMPLICATIONS

The most serious complication of PDA ligation is rupture. In one study, ductal rupture occurred in 6.25% (4 out of 64 dogs); the mortality rate for PDA ligation was 1.6% (1 of 64 dogs) (Hunt et al, 2001). Residual shunting may also be a complication, but is more common with the Jackson approach than with standard dissection technique (see previous discussion). Pulmonary embolization of transcatheter coils or other devices used to embolize PDA occasionally occurs, but does not appear to cause short- or long-term complications.

PROGNOSIS

Dogs with untreated PDA usually develop progressive left-sided congestive heart failure and pulmonary edema. Seventy percent of dogs with untreated PDA die before 1 year of age, whereas the 1- and 2-year survival rates were 92% and 87%, respectively in a recent report of 52 dogs undergoing surgery for left-to-right shunting PDA (Bureau et al, 2005). Dogs with MR before surgery had similar survival times as dogs without MR; however, older animals and those with right atrial dilation on preoperative radiographs were less likely to survive. Dogs with PDA may also develop suprasystemic pulmonary hypertension that reverses the direction of the shunt, causing severe hypoxemia, cyanosis, and exercise intolerance. Ligation of a completely reversed PDA is contraindicated.

References

Bahr A, Miller MW, Gordon S: First pass nuclear angiocardiography in the evaluation of patent ductus arteriosus in dogs, *J Vet Intern Med* 16:74, 2002.

Borenstein N, Behr L, Chetboul V et al: Minimally invasive patent ductus arteriosus occlusion in 5 dogs, *Vet Surg* 33:309, 2004.

Buchanan JW, Patterson DF: Etiology of patent ductus arteriosus in dogs, *J Vet Intern Med* 17:167, 2003.

Bureau S, Monnet E, Orton EC: Evaluation of survival and prognostic indicators for surgical treatment of left-to-right patent ductus arteriosus in dogs: 52 cases (1995-2003), *J Am Vet Med Assoc* 227:1794, 2005.

Corti LB et al: Retrospective evaluation of occlusion of patent ductus arteriosus with hemoclips in 20 dogs, *J Am Anim Hosp Assoc* 36:548, 2000.

Cote E, Ettinger SJ: Long-term clinical management of right-to-left ("reversed") patent ductus arteriosus in 3 dogs, *J Vet Intern Med* 15:39, 2001.

Hunt GB et al: Intraoperative hemorrhage during patent ductus arteriosus ligation in dogs, *Vet Surg* 30:58, 2001.

Hunter SL, Culp LB, Muir WW et al: Sodium nitroprusside-induced deliberate hypotension to facilitate patent ductus arteriosus ligation in dogs, *Vet Surg* 32:336, 2003.

Morandi F, Daniel GB, Gompf RE et al: Diagnosis of congenital cardiac right-to-left shunts with ^{99m}Tc-macroaggregated albumin, *Vet Radiol Ultrasound* 45:97, 2004.

Saunders AB, Miller MW, Gordon SG et al: Pulmonary embolization of vascular occlusion coils in dogs with patent ductus arteriosus, *J Vet Intern Med* 18:663, 2004.

Stanley BJ, Luis-Fuentes V, Darke PGG: Comparison of the incidence of residual shunting between two surgical techniques used for ligation of patent ductus arteriosus in the dog, *Vet Surg* 32:231, 2003.

PULMONIC STENOSIS

DEFINITIONS

Pulmonic stenosis (PS) is a congenital narrowing of the pulmonic valve, pulmonary artery, or right ventricular outflow tract. Synonyms include *pulmonic valve dysplasia* and *right ventricular outflow tract obstruction*.

GENERAL CONSIDERATIONS AND CLINICALLY RELEVANT PATHOPHYSIOLOGY

PS is one of the most common congenital heart defects in dogs; it is uncommon in cats. In dogs, the condition is usually valvular, although supravalvular and subvalvular defects have been reported. Subvalvular stenosis can occur as a primary isolated defect, but more often occurs from infundibular hypertrophy secondary to a primary valvular stenosis. Valvular stenosis may be simple, consisting of incomplete separation of valve leaflets, or it may be due to valve dysplasia characterized by a hypoplastic valve annulus and thickened immobile valve leaflets. More than 80% of dogs with valvular PS have some degree of valve dysplasia. Based on their echocardiographic valvular anatomy and aortic:pulmonary annular ratio, affected dogs may be classified as having Type A PS (normal annulus diameter and aortic:pulmonary ratio less than or equal to 1.2) or Type B PS (pulmonary annulus hypoplasia and aortic:pulmonary ratio greater than 1.2) (Bussadori et al, 2001).

PS causes pressure overload and hypertrophy of the right ventricle. Right ventricular hypertrophy often compounds right ventricular outflow obstruction by narrowing the right ventricular outflow tract. Narrowing of the right ventricular outflow tract is greatest during systole, producing a dynamic obstruction that contributes to the fixed stenosis. Dynamic stenosis has important implications for surgical repair of PS. Dogs with mild to moderate obstructions may remain asymptomatic, whereas dogs with severe obstructions may show exercise intolerance, syncope, progressive right-sided congestive heart failure, or sudden death.

DIAGNOSIS
Clinical Presentation

Signalment. English bulldogs, beagles, miniature schnauzers, cocker spaniels, Samoyeds, mastiffs, and terrier breeds are at increased risk for developing PS. English bulldogs and boxers have a high concurrent incidence of aberrant left coronary artery (due to a single right coronary artery), which has important surgical implications. A hereditary form of pulmonary valve dysplasia has been found in the beagles and Boykin spaniels. Female English bulldogs and male bull mastiffs are more commonly affected; a sex predisposition has not been identified in other breeds.

History. Young animals with PS are often asymptomatic. Advanced cases may present with exercise intolerance, syncope, or abdominal distention from ascites.

Physical Examination Findings

The predominant physical finding is a systolic ejection murmur heard best at the left heart base. The electrocardiogram may show prominent S waves in leads I, II, III, and aVF indicative of a right axis shift and right ventricular hypertrophy.

Diagnostic Imaging

Thoracic radiographs show varying degrees of right ventricular enlargement and main pulmonary artery segment enlargement. Diagnosis of PS can be confirmed by echocardiography. Cardiac catheterization is usually only necessary if abnormal coronary anatomy is suspected or if an interventional procedure (e.g., percutaneous balloon valvuloplasty) is performed.

Echocardiography. Echocardiographic findings include right ventricular hypertrophy, poststenotic dilation of the main pulmonary artery, malformation and reduced mobility of the pulmonic valve, and a high pulmonary flow velocity. A systolic pressure gradient across the stenosis can be measured directly by right ventricular catheterization or calculated from the Doppler-derived peak systolic pulmonic flow velocity using the modified Bernoulli equation ($\Delta P = 4\ V^2$).

Laboratory Findings

Specific laboratory abnormalities are not found in animals with PS.

DIFFERENTIAL DIAGNOSIS

Differential diagnoses include SAS, VSD, ASD, and tetralogy of Fallot.

MEDICAL MANAGEMENT

There is no specific medical therapy for PS other than symptomatic treatment for congestive heart failure, if it occurs. Percutaneous balloon valvuloplasty is a nonsurgical alternative for correction of moderate to severe PS, if facilities and skilled personnel for cardiac catheterization are available. Simple valvular PS is more amenable to balloon valvuloplasty than severe pulmonic valve dysplasia or severe PS with dynamic obstruction. Balloon valvuloplasty is not recommended for patients with supravalvular PS, patients with coronary artery anomalies, or patients with substantial annular hypoplasia.

SURGICAL TREATMENT

Therapy for PS is based on its degree of severity and the type of lesion present. Severity is judged by the presence of signs, extent of right ventricular hypertrophy, and magnitude of systolic pressure gradient. Doppler-derived systolic pressure gradients measured in unsedated or unanesthetized animals are considered mild when they are less than 50 mm Hg, moderate when they are between 50 and 75 mm Hg, and severe when they are greater than 75 mm Hg. Animals with PS that have no signs, mild hypertrophy, and a pressure gradient less than 50 mm Hg generally do not require surgical intervention. If the pressure gradient is greater than 50 mm Hg and if right ventricular hypertrophy is significant, correction should be considered. Balloon valvuloplasty has become the treatment of choice for dogs with amenable lesions (valvular dysplasia). Dogs with Type A stenosis are most likely to benefit from balloon valvuloplasty (Bussardori et al, 2001).

English bulldogs with PS present a therapeutic dilemma because of the possibility of concurrent aberrant left coronary artery. In dogs with this defect, the left coronary artery courses across the right ventricular outflow tract and is at risk for injury during valve dilation. Sudden death due to rupture of the coronary artery has occurred during balloon valvuloplasty. Aberrant left coronary artery also precludes patch-graft valvuloplasty. A valved or nonvalved conduit placed between the right ventricle and pulmonary artery is a possible surgical option for this condition.

Preoperative Management

Right-sided congestive heart failure or cardiac arrhythmias should be managed medically before surgery. See preoperative management of animals with cardiovascular disease on p. 775.

Anesthesia

Refer to p. 775 for anesthetic management of cardiac patients.

Surgical Anatomy

The pulmonary valve is approached through a left fourth or fifth intercostal thoracotomy or median sternotomy. The valve consists of right, left, and intermediate semilunar cusps. Sounds associated with lesions of the pulmonary valve may be heard best at the fourth intercostal space, slightly below a line drawn through the point of the shoulder. See the comments about concurrent aberrant left coronary arteries above.

Positioning

Animals are positioned in right lateral recumbency, and the entire left hemithorax is prepared for aseptic surgery.

SURGICAL TECHNIQUE

Surgical options for correction of PS include valve dilation and patch-graft valvuloplasty. With the advent of balloon valvuloplasty, operative valve dilation is seldom indicated.

Animals with severe annular hypoplasia, dysplastic valve lesions, or severe hypertrophy are less likely to respond to valve dilation. In these animals, patch-graft valvuloplasty is indicated for severe PS, particularly if marked infundibular hypertrophy and dynamic stenosis are suspected. Patch-graft valvuloplasty also can be used effectively to relieve concurrent or isolated supravalvular PS. It may be performed "off pump" with or without inflow occlusion (with mild hypothermia; 32° C to 34° C) or during cardiopulmonary bypass. If inflow occlusion is used, circulatory arrest time should be less than 5 minutes.

Valve Dilation

For valve dilation, see *Small Animal Surgery*, second edition or the e-dition.

AP Open Patch-Graft Correction

With inflow occlusion. *Perform a left fifth intercostal thoracotomy. Pass tape tourniquets around the venae cavae and azygous vein (see Inflow Occlusion on p. 779). Make a partial-thickness incision in the right ventricular outflow tract (Fig. 27-12, A). Suture an autogenous pericardial or synthetic patch to the ventriculotomy incision and the cranial aspect of the pulmonary artery (Fig. 27-12, B). Initiate venous inflow occlusion and make full-thickness incisions into the pulmonary artery and right ventricle (Fig. 27-12, C). Incise or excise dysplastic pulmonic valve leaflets as necessary. Complete suturing of the pulmonary artery to the patch-graft and discontinue inflow occlusion (Fig. 27-12, D and E). Resuscitate the heart.*

It is important to remove air from the heart by discontinuing inflow occlusion just before tying the last suture.

SUTURE MATERIALS AND SPECIAL INSTRUMENTS

Polypropylene (3-0) suture buttressed with Teflon pledgets is suitable for transventricular valve dilation. Valve dilation can be accomplished with a Cooley or Tubbs valve-dilating instrument or with an appropriate size hemostatic forceps. Synthetic materials such as polytetrafluoroethylene (PTFE) or autogenous pericardium can be used for the patch-graft procedure. Polypropylene (4-0) suture is appropriate for suturing the patch graft.

POSTOPERATIVE CARE AND ASSESSMENT

Postoperative pain should be treated with systemic opioids and local anesthetic techniques (see p. 868 for postthoracotomy analgesia). Animals should be monitored postoperatively for complications associated with low output failure due to reduced function of the right ventricle.

PROGNOSIS

The prognosis for dogs with PS depends on its severity. Animals with systolic pressure gradients greater than 75 mm Hg are likely to experience heart failure or sudden death early in life. Balloon dilation is associated with mini-

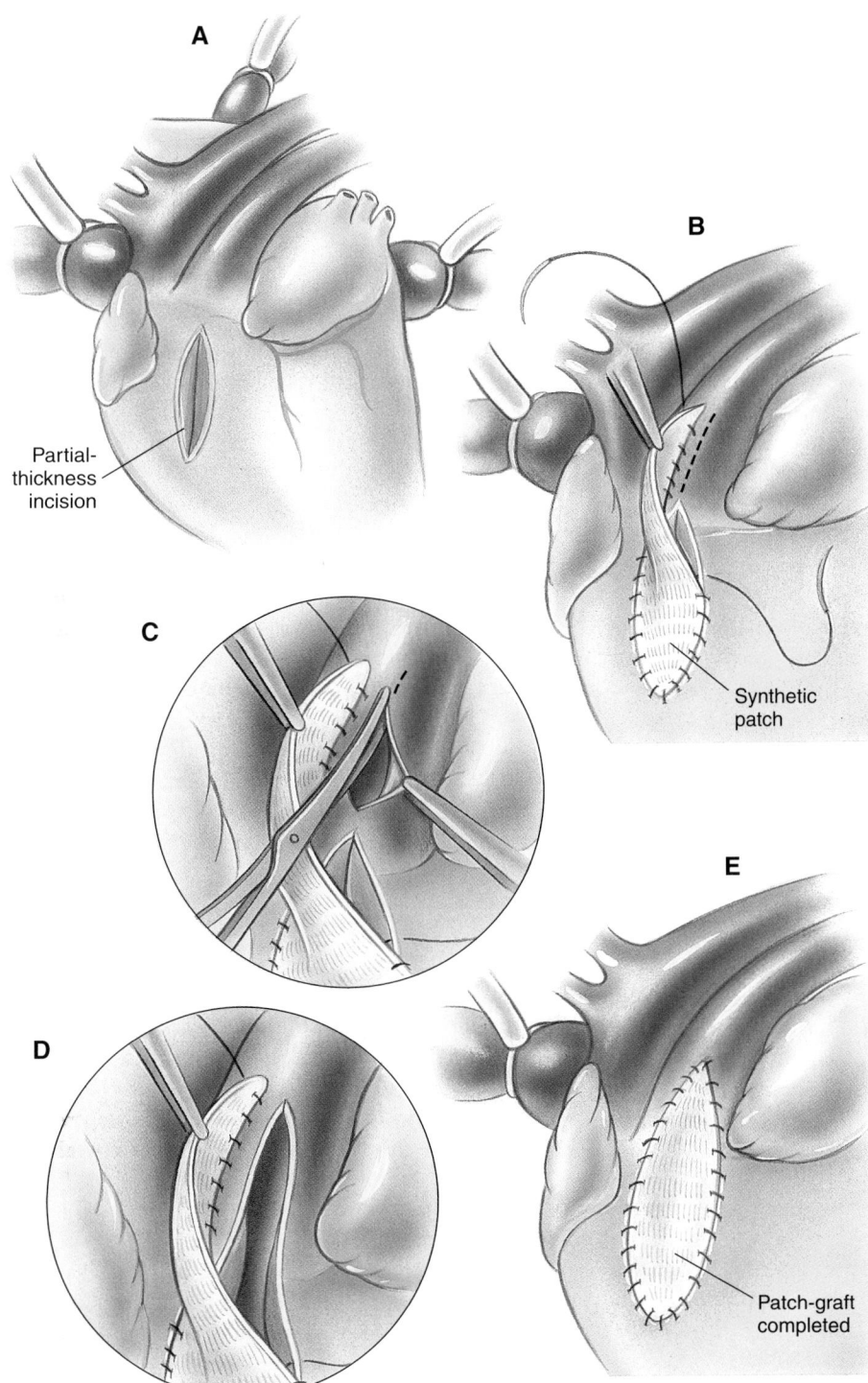

FIG. 27-12
To place a transvalvular patch for pulmonic stenosis, pass tapes for inflow occlusion as
described in Fig. 27-3. **A,** Partially incise the right ventricular outflow tract just ventral to
the pulmonic valve. **B,** Suture a synthetic or pericardial patch to the ventriculotomy and
cranial aspect of the pulmonary artery. **C,** Initiate inflow occlusion and incise the pulmonary artery, extending the incision across the pulmonary valve. **D,** Make the ventriculotomy
incision full thickness. **E,** Finish suturing the patch graft to the pulmonary artery.

mal risk of complications and carries a low operative mortality, but its effectiveness depends on the morphology of the defect. In one study, 100% of dogs with Type A lesions survived the procedure and had resolution of their clinical signs. Most remained free of clinical signs at 1 year. Conversely, 66.6% of dogs with Type B lesions survived the procedure and of these, resolution of clinical signs was only obtained in 50% at 1 year. In another study, balloon valvuloplasty resulted in a sustained clinical improvement in 80% of previously symptomatic cases (Johnson and Martin, 2004).

Patch grafting is effective in relieving severe PS, but is unforgiving of technical errors during surgery. Operative mortality for this procedure is approximately 15% to 20% in the hands of an experienced surgeon. The most common problem is inability to resuscitate the heart after inflow occlusion. Successful patch-graft valvuloplasty results in substantial pulmonic valve insufficiency, but this has minimal consequence as long as the tricuspid valve is competent and pulmonary hypertension is not present. If facilities are available, cardiopulmonary bypass may lead to a better outcome, particularly if the dog has evidence of right ventricular failure.

References

Bussadori C, DeMadron E, Santilli RA et al: Balloon valvuloplasty in 30 dogs with pulmonic stenosis: effect of valve morphology and annular size on initial and 1-year outcome, *J Vet Intern Med* 15:553, 2001.

Johnson MS, Martin M: Results of balloon valvuloplasty in 40 dogs with pulmonic stenosis, *J Small Anim Pract* 45:148, 2004.

Suggested Reading

Johnson MS, Martin M: Balloon valvuloplasty in a cat with pulmonic stenosis, *J Vet Intern Med* 17:928, 2003.
Successful balloon valvuloplasty was performed in a 7-month-old Rex.

AORTIC STENOSIS

DEFINITIONS

Aortic stenosis (AS) is a congenital narrowing of the aortic valve, aorta, or left ventricular outflow tract. The stenosis may be supravalvular, valvular, or subvalvular.

GENERAL CONSIDERATIONS AND CLINICALLY RELEVANT PATHOPHYSIOLOGY

SAS is the most common congenital heart defect affecting large-breed dogs. AS occurs uncommonly in cats. SAS accounts for greater than 90% of canine cases and occurs with widely disparate morphology and severity. The typical lesion is a discrete subvalvular fibrous ring that courses across the ventricular septum and reflects onto the anterior mitral valve leaflet. This lesion often is complicated by varying degrees of muscular septal hypertrophy and diffuse fibrosis of the outflow tract. The most severe lesions are associated with an immobile mitral valve leaflet that effectively results in a

tunnel-like stenosis. In most cases, SAS is associated with some degree of aortic insufficiency; however, this is usually mild. Concurrent mitral valve insufficiency also occurs.

SAS causes pressure overload of the left ventricle. Varying degrees of left ventricular concentric hypertrophy develop depending on severity. Dogs with moderate to severe SAS are at substantial risk for sudden death, presumably the result of myocardial ischemia and malignant ventricular arrhythmias. Dogs with SAS also may develop congestive heart failure, particularly if concurrent mitral insufficiency is present. Lastly, dogs with SAS are at increased risk for bacterial endocarditis of the aortic valve due to turbulent blood flow and resultant valvular damage.

DIAGNOSIS
Clinical Presentation

Signalment. Newfoundlands, golden retrievers, rottweilers, German shepherds, boxers, and Samoyeds are at increased risk for developing SAS. A genetic basis for SAS has been established in Newfoundland dogs. Phenotypic expression of SAS occurs a short time after birth. The defect may not be clinically apparent until several weeks of age. SAS should be considered a progressive lesion until maturity.

History. Dogs with SAS may be asymptomatic or may exhibit exercise intolerance, collapse, or syncope. Lack of clinical signs is not an appropriate reason to delay diagnostic evaluation because the first clinical evidence of SAS may be sudden death.

Physical Examination Findings

The predominant physical finding in animals with SAS is a systolic ejection murmur heard best at the left heart base. The murmur radiates well to the right base and thoracic inlet. In moderate to severe cases, femoral pulses are noticeably weak or hypokinetic, unless substantial concurrent aortic insufficiency is present. Electrocardiograms may show a left cranial axis shift or ventricular ectopy, but they are usually unremarkable.

Diagnostic Imaging

Thoracic radiographs may reveal a normal cardiac silhouette or mild left ventricular and left atrial enlargement. Enlargement of the ascending aorta frequently is evident.

Echocardiography. Definitive diagnosis of SAS is obtained by echocardiography. M-mode echocardiography demonstrates variable left ventricular free wall and septal thickening, depending on severity. With moderate to severe disease, left ventricular diameter is small unless substantial concurrent aortic or mitral insufficiency is present. Systolic anterior motion (SAM) of the mitral valve is indicative of a dynamic component to the obstruction and may cause mitral insufficiency. Early closure of the aortic valve suggests that dynamic obstruction may be present. Two-dimensional echocardiography provides direct visualization of the various morphologic components of the lesion. Doppler-measured aortic velocities are increased. The peak systolic pressure gradient across the aortic valve can be calculated from the peak aortic velocity ($\Delta P = 4V^2$). Systolic gradients obtained from the subxiphoid position of 25 to 50 mm Hg are mild, 50 to 75 mm Hg are moderate, and greater than 75 mm Hg are severe when measured in unsedated or unanesthetized animals.

Laboratory Findings

Dogs with SAS may have abnormalities in platelet function and von Willebrand factor multimer distribution (Tarnow et al, 2005). A form of platelet dysfunction detected at high shear rates was associated with mitral regurgitation and SAS in dogs; both are diseases in which turbulent high-velocity blood flows are seen. The clinical significance of this is unknown.

DIFFERENTIAL DIAGNOSIS

AS must be differentiated from other conditions that cause systolic murmurs (i.e., PS, VSD, and tetralogy of Fallot). Physiologic (flow/innocent) systolic murmurs are commonly detected in large-breed dogs, but are usually low grade (i.e., I or II/VI).

MEDICAL MANAGEMENT

β-adrenergic blockade therapy with propranolol or atenolol (Box 27-7) may reduce the risk for sudden death by decreasing myocardial oxygen requirements and suppressing ventricular arrhythmias during exercise. Symptomatic treatment (i.e., furosemide, enalapril; see Box 27-1)) for congestive heart failure is indicated if it occurs. Balloon valvuloplasty may be somewhat beneficial in animals with moderate SAS if facilities for cardiac catheterization are available; however, a recent study suggested that median survival times for dogs undergoing balloon valvuloplasty were not different from those receiving long-term atenolol therapy (55 versus 56 months).

SURGICAL TREATMENT

Surgical intervention should be considered for dogs with substantial left ventricular hypertrophy and systolic gradients above 75 mm Hg. If surgery is undertaken, it should be done early to minimize degenerative myocardial changes. Surgical options for dogs with SAS include valve dilation and open resection. Open resection during cardiopulmo-

nary bypass should be considered in dogs with severe SAS; however, long-term benefit of this procedure has not been established (see below under Prognosis). Direct visualization of the defect through an aortotomy, excision of the discrete fibrous ring, and septal myectomy can be performed (Fig. 27-13, *A*). Surgical correction of SAS via right ventriculotomy and septal resection (Fig. 27-13, *B*) has been described in one dog with long-term benefits (Nelson et al, 2004); however, too few dogs have been done to know the procedure's true benefit.

Preoperative Management

Arrhythmias should be controlled with appropriate antiarrhythmic drugs (i.e., atenolol, procainamide, amiodarone, and sotalol) before surgery (see p. 775). β-adrenergic blockade should be discontinued 24 hours before surgery by gradually tapering the dose over 3 to 5 days.

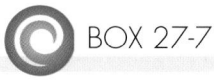

BOX 27-7

β-Adrenergic Blockers

Propranolol (Inderal)
0.2–2 mg/kg PO, bid to tid

Atenolol (Tenormin)
Dogs: 6.25–50 mg/dog PO, qd to bid
Cats: 6.25–12.5 mg/cat PO, qd to bid

PO, Oral; *bid,* twice a day; *tid,* three times a day; *qd,* once a day.

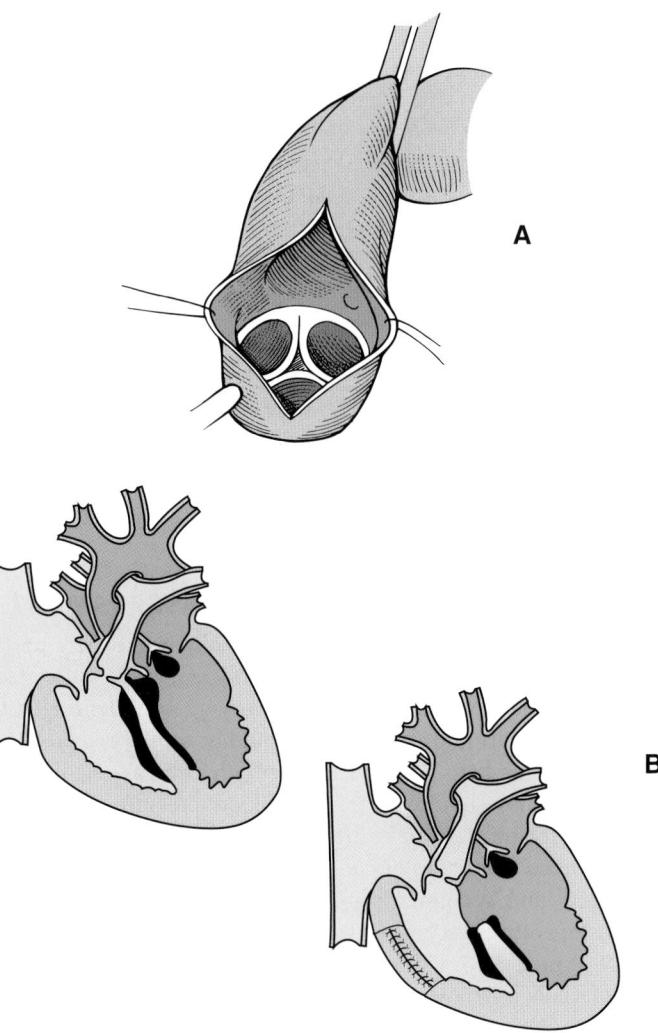

FIG. 27-13
Open resection for subvalvular aortic stenosis may be accomplished **(A)** through an aortotomy or **(B)** via a right ventriculotomy during cardiopulmonary bypass.

Anesthesia

Refer to p. 775 for anesthetic recommendations for cardiac patients.

Surgical Anatomy

The aortic valve consists of right, left, and noncoronary semilunar cusps. The three aortic sinuses are dilations of the aorta on the vessel side of the valve; the right and left coronary arteries leave the right and left sinuses. The aortic bulb is a widening of the base of the ascending aorta formed by the aortic sinuses. The sounds associated with lesions of the aortic valve may be heard best at the fourth intercostal space, slightly below a line drawn through the point of the shoulder.

SAS usually consists of a discrete fibrous ring located 1 to 3 mm below the aortic valve leaflets. The ring generally extends across the septum and reflects onto the anterior mitral valve leaflet. The conduction system (His bundle) courses through the septum at the juncture of the right and noncoronary aortic leaflets.

Positioning

Open resection of aortic stenosis is performed through a fourth right intercostal thoracotomy.

SURGICAL TECHNIQUE

The long-term benefits of surgical correction of SAS are unknown at this time. Cardiopulmonary bypass affords the best opportunity to resect the stenotic area. With additional experience, septal resection and patch grafting may prove beneficial in reducing transaortic pressures long term in affected dogs.

SUTURE MATERIALS AND SPECIAL INSTRUMENTS

Cardiopulmonary bypass is required for open repair of SAS. A glutaraldehyde fixed pericardial graft may be sutured into the defect caused by resecting the obstructing portion of the septum.

POSTOPERATIVE CARE AND ASSESSMENT

Ventilation should be monitored carefully in the early postoperative period. Poor ventilatory efforts may be associated with residual pneumothorax, hemorrhage, anesthetic agents, or pain. Heart rate and rhythm should be monitored postoperatively for 48 to 72 hours, and hemodynamically significant arrhythmias should be treated. Blood pressure should be measured by direct or indirect means until the animal is fully recovered from anesthesia. Analgesics (local anesthetic techniques and systemic opioids) should be given to decrease postoperative discomfort (see Table 13-4 on p. 133 and Box 29-2 on p. 868). Urine output should be monitored closely, especially if hypotension occurred during or after surgery.

PROGNOSIS

Dogs with systolic gradients above 75 mm Hg have a substantial risk for sudden death in the first several years of life. Valve dilation can be performed at an early age with low operative mortality and without cardiopulmonary bypass. However, there is little evidence that valve dilation results in sustained reduction in the systolic pressure gradient, and the long-term benefit of this procedure is questionable (see above under Medical Management). Modest gradient reduction (30% to 40%) has been achieved in approximately 33% of dogs that undergo valve dilation by balloon catheter. It is unclear if valve dilation reduces the risk for sudden death.

Open resection of SAS under cardiopulmonary bypass may result in a substantial reduction of the systolic pressure gradient that is sustained for at least several years after surgery. However, in a recent retrospective study of 44 dogs undergoing open surgical correction of subvalvular aortic stenosis, a positive benefit on survival was not found despite reducing the systolic pressure gradient (Orton et al, 2000). These dogs appear to remain at high risk for sudden death associated with either profound reflex vasodilation and bradycardia or fatal ventricular dysrhythmia. In a recent study, no clear benefit was seen in dogs with severe SAS that underwent balloon valvuloplasty, despite significantly decreasing the peak systolic pressure gradient (Meurs et al, 2005).

References

Meurs KM, Lehmkuhl LB, Bonagura JD: Survival times in dogs with severe subvalvular aortic stenosis treated with balloon valvuloplasty or atenolol, *J Am Vet Med Assoc* 227:420, 2005.

Nelson DA, Fossum TW, Gordon S et al: Surgical correction of subaortic stenosis via right ventriculotomy and septal resection in a dog, *J Am Vet Med Assoc* 225:705, 2004.

Orton EC et al: Influence of open surgical correction on intermediate-term outcome in dogs with subvalvular aortic stenosis: 44 cases (1991-1998), *J Am Vet Med Assoc* 216:364, 2000.

Tarnow I, Kristensen AT, Olsen LH et al: Dogs with heart diseases causing turbulent high-velocity blood flow have changes in platelet function and von Willebrand factor multimer distribution, *J Vet Intern Med* 19:515, 2005.

VENTRICULAR SEPTAL DEFECT

DEFINITIONS

Ventricular septal defect (VSD) is a congenital defect that results from failure or incomplete development of the membranous or muscular interventricular septum.

GENERAL CONSIDERATIONS AND CLINICALLY RELEVANT PATHOPHYSIOLOGY

VSD is the second most common congenital heart defect in cats and accounts for 5% to 10% of congenital heart defects seen in dogs. The cause of VSD is not completely understood, but is suspected to have a genetic component. VSD has been demonstrated to be a polygenic trait in keeshonden. Most VSDs in small animals occur in the membranous septum. Perimembranous defects are located in the membranous septum, medial to the septal tricuspid leaflet, and inferior to the crista supraventricularis. Infundibular or supracristal defects are located in the right outflow tract superior to the crista supraventricularis.

The pathophysiology of VSD depends on the size of the defect and pulmonary vascular resistance. VSD typically causes a left-to-right shunt. A typical VSD overloads the left ventricle and, depending on its size and location, may overload the right ventricle as well. A large VSD can progress to left-sided congestive heart failure. Chronic overcirculation of the lungs can cause progressive pulmonary vascular remodeling leading to severe pulmonary hypertension and right-to-left shunting of blood (Eisenmenger's physiology). Residence at altitude likely accelerates the development of pulmonary hypertension.

Aortic insufficiency is a fairly common secondary abnormality associated with VSD, particularly infundibular VSD. Aortic insufficiency results from prolapse of the right coronary aortic leaflet into the defect. This prolapse is due to the Venturi effect associated with VSD flow and loss of support of the aortic annulus. Aortic insufficiency adds to the left ventricular volume overload and is usually progressive.

DIAGNOSIS
Clinical Presentation

Signalment. No breed predisposition has been clearly determined for VSD; however, English bulldogs may have a higher than expected incidence.

History. Young animals with VSD often are asymptomatic at first presentation. Animals with large VSD may have signs of left-sided congestive heart failure (i.e., cough and shortness of breath).

Physical Examination Findings

The most prominent physical finding associated with VSD is a systolic murmur with the point of maximal intensity at the right sternum. The murmur is also heard well at the left heart base. When the defect is in the supracristal position, the murmur may actually be loudest at the left cardiac base. The murmur is ejection in quality if the defect is small, and regurgitant if the defect is large. A diastolic blowing murmur at the left heart base can give the murmur a continuous quality and suggests the presence of concurrent aortic insufficiency. Animals with right-to-left VSD may have no murmur due to polycythemia.

Diagnostic Imaging

Thoracic radiographs reveal varying degrees of left or biventricular enlargement depending on the size and position of the defect. The degree of pulmonary vascular enlargement from overcirculation also depends on the size of the defect and pulmonary vascular resistance.

Echocardiography. A VSD larger than 5 mm usually can be visualized directly on two-dimensional echocardiography. Color-flow Doppler is particularly useful for detecting small defects. The direction and velocity of shunt flow can be determined by spectral Doppler. A high velocity left-to-right shunt suggests that the VSD is "re-

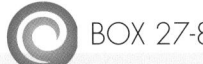

BOX 27-8

Medical Management of Congestive Heart Failure

Benazepril (Lotensin)
0.25–0.5 mg/kg PO qd

Enalapril (Vasotec)
0.25–0.5 mg/kg PO, qd to bid

Furosemide (Lasix)
2–4 mg/kg PO, IV, SC, qd to qid as needed

Pimobendan (Vetmedin)
0.25–0.3 mg/kg PO, bid

PO, Oral; *qd*, once a day; *bid*, twice a day; *IV*, intravenous; *SC*, subcutaneous; *qid*, four times a day.

strictive" or hemodynamically insignificant and warrants a good prognosis. Large defects are usually associated with lower shunt velocities and suggest that the animal is at risk for development of progressive heart failure or pulmonary hypertension. The pulmonary to systemic flow ratio can be calculated from Doppler analysis of aortic and pulmonary flows. Pulmonary to systemic flow ratios (Qp:Qs) greater than 2:1 are indicative of a hemodynamically significant VSD.

Laboratory Findings

Polycythemia may be present in dogs with right-to-left shunts.

DIFFERENTIAL DIAGNOSIS

Differential diagnoses include SAS, PS, tetralogy of Fallot, ASD, and atrioventricular septal defects.

MEDICAL MANAGEMENT

Medical management for VSD (Box 27-8) consists of symptomatic treatment for congestive heart failure. Useful drugs for congestive heart failure include ACE inhibitors (i.e., enalapril, benazepril, and lisinopril), diuretics (i.e., furosemide; see Box 27-1), and inodilators (i.e., pimobendan). There is no effective medical management for Eisenmenger's physiology. Vasodilator therapy generally causes increased right-to-left shunting due to preferential dilation of systemic vessels over remodeled pulmonary vessels. Periodic phlebotomy and replacement with crystalloid fluids may be necessary to keep the hematocrit below 60%. Low-dose aspirin therapy (e.g., 5 to 10 mg/kg, once or twice daily) is recommended to prevent thromboembolic complications.

SURGICAL TREATMENT

Surgical intervention should be considered for hemodynamically significant VSD. Concurrent aortic insufficiency usually is progressive and also is an indication for surgical intervention. Pulmonary artery banding has been used successfully to palliate dogs and cats with VSD. The goal of pulmonary artery banding is to increase right ventricular systolic pressure, thereby decreasing shunt flow.

Definitive patch closure of VSD can be accomplished with the aid of cardiopulmonary bypass in dogs over 4 kg in body weight. A perimembranous VSD is corrected from the right side via a right atriotomy approach. An infundibular VSD is corrected via a right ventriculotomy from a left thoracotomy or median sternotomy approach. Percutaneous transcatheter coil embolization of a VSD has been reported in a dog (Shimizu et al, 2005). Recent development of occlusion devices specifically designed for VSD closure holds promise for use in dogs with hemodynamically important VSD.

Preoperative Management

If heart failure is present, attempts should be made to control it medically. See also p. 775 for preoperative management of animals with cardiovascular disease.

Anesthesia

Anesthetic management of animals undergoing cardiac surgery is described on p. 775.

Surgical Anatomy

The interventricular septum is composed of a dorsal, thin, membranous part and a large, ventral, muscular part. The membranous part is formed by fusion of the atrioventricular cushions. When the cushions fail to fuse, a VSD arises. The AV node and its bundle are usually closely associated with the caudal margin of a perimembranous VSD.

Positioning

The animal is positioned in right lateral recumbency for pulmonary artery banding. The entire left thorax is prepared for aseptic surgery.

SURGICAL TECHNIQUE
Pulmonary Artery Banding

Perform a left fourth intercostal thoracotomy. Open the pericardium and suture it to the thoracotomy incision. Separate the pulmonary artery from the aorta using a combination of sharp and blunt dissection. Pass a large cotton or Teflon tape around the pulmonary artery just distal to the pulmonic valve (Fig. 27-14). Tighten the tape to reduce the circumference of the pulmonary artery. Place a purse-string suture in the pulmonary artery wall distal to the ligature, and insert a catheter into the pulmonary artery to measure pressures. Constrict the pulmonary artery until the pulmonary artery pressure distal to the band is less than 30 mm Hg. Also, monitor systemic artery pressures, which should increase during the banding.

Optimal banding occurs when the increase in systemic arterial pressures just reaches a plateau.

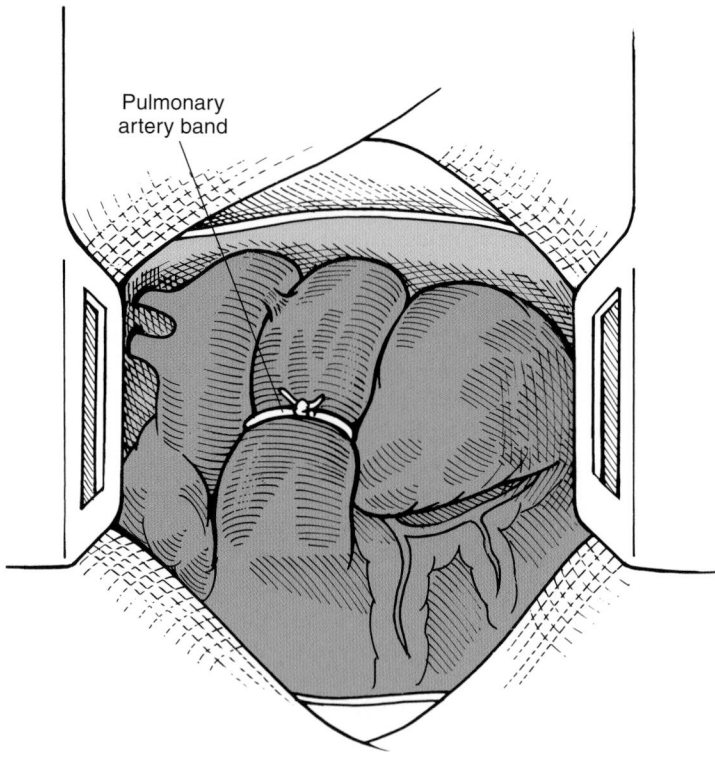

FIG. 27-14
For pulmonary artery banding, pass a tape around the main pulmonary artery. Tighten the tape until pulmonary artery pressure distal to the band is less than 30 mm Hg and systemic artery pressure increases and plateaus.

SUTURE MATERIALS AND SPECIAL INSTRUMENTS

Wide cotton or Teflon tape is used for pulmonary artery banding. A PTFE vascular graft is used for definitive closure of a VSD.

POSTOPERATIVE CARE AND ASSESSMENT

Animals should be closely observed for worsening of heart failure secondary to anesthesia, surgery, or arrhythmias. Hypoxemia or cyanosis suggests that the band may have been placed too tightly, potentially reversing the shunt. Postoperative pain should be treated with systemic opioids (see Table 13-4 on p. 133) and local anesthetic techniques (see p. 868).

PROGNOSIS

The prognosis for animals with VSD depends on the size of the defect. Spontaneous resolution of an isolated VSD was reported in a 5-month-old Maltese. Animals with small restrictive defects may tolerate the defect without ill effects. Large defects (i.e., Qp:Qs greater than 2:1) will likely result in the development of progressive heart failure or pulmonary hypertension. Pulmonary artery banding is a reasonably effective procedure for palliation of the consequences of a hemodynamically significant VSD in both dogs and cats.

Definitive closure of a VSD under cardiopulmonary bypass is considered curative. Dogs with uncorrected VSD are potentially at increased risk for development of bacterial endocarditis. Aortic insufficiency places an added volume load on the left ventricle and generally indicates a poor prognosis.

References

Rausch WP, Keene BW: Spontaneous resolution of an isolated ventricular septal defect in a dog, *J Am Vet Med Assoc* 223:219, 2003.

Shimizu M, Tanka R, Hirao H et al: Percutaneous transcatheter coil embolization of a ventricular septal defect in a dog, *J Am Vet Med Assoc* 226:69, 2005.

ATRIAL SEPTAL DEFECT

DEFINITIONS

Atrial septal defect (ASD) is a congenital defect that results from failure or incomplete development of the atrial septum.

GENERAL CONSIDERATIONS AND CLINICALLY RELEVANT PATHOPHYSIOLOGY

ASD is considered to be a rare congenital defect of dogs; however, it may be more common than previously considered, particularly in some breeds (e.g., standard poodles). The prevalence of feline ASD is unknown but it may be more common than in dogs, most notably as a portion of an atrioventricular canal or endocardial cushion defect. The cause of ASD is not completely understood, but is suspected to have a genetic component; therefore affected individuals and their parents should not be used for breeding. Siblings should be carefully screened via echocardiography to determine whether they are affected.

Four types of ASD are described according to the location of the septal defect. The most common type of ASD is an *ostium secundum,* which is dorsally located in the septum (region of the fossa ovalis) (Fig. 27-15). An *ostium primum* ASD is located in the lower part of the interatrial septum and originates from an altered fusion between the septum primum and the endocardial cushion. These defects are often large and may be associated with concurrent abnormalities resulting in a common atrioventricular channel between the left and right ventricular chambers. Rare defects include a sinus venosus and a coronary sinus defect. A *sinus venosus* ASD involves the dorsal part of the interatrial septum, close to the junction with the cranial vena cava, while a coronary sinus defect originates from a disruption in the formation of the wall between the coronary sinus and the left atrium.

The pathophysiology of ASD depends on the size of the defect and cardiac compliance. Because the right atrium typically has a higher compliance than the left atrium, ASDs normally result in a left-to-right shunt. Depending on the size of the defect, the shunt may overload the right side of the heart and eventually, if the defect is large, cause right-sided heart failure.

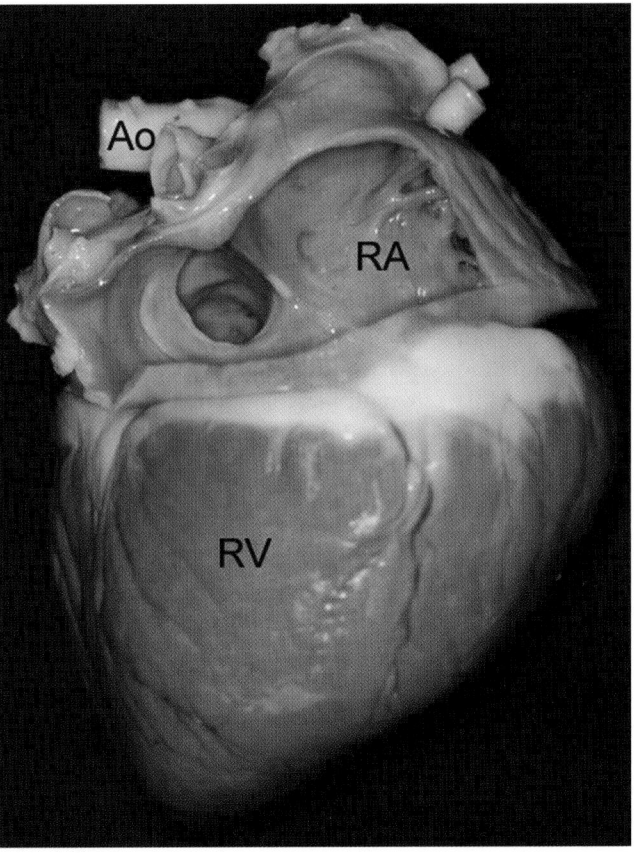

FIG. 27-15
The heart of a dog with a large secundum ASD. (Courtesy Dr. M. Miller, Texas A&M University.)

DIAGNOSIS
Clinical Presentation

Signalment. No breed predisposition has been clearly determined for ASD; however, standard poodles, boxers, Doberman pinschers, Samoyeds, and old English sheepdogs may be at increased risk.

History. Young animals with ASD often are asymptomatic at first presentation. Animals with large ASD may present with only exercise intolerance or they may have signs of congestive heart failure, depending on the size of their defect.

Physical Examination Findings

ASDs may be associated with a soft, midsystolic ejection murmur, which is loudest in the pulmonic area. There may be audible splitting of the second heart sound. Jugular distention and ascites may be noted in dogs with large defects and resultant right ventricular failure.

Diagnostic Imaging

Thoracic radiographs may be normal with small shunts. Right-sided cardiac enlargement and pulmonary overcirculation are common with larger shunts. The degree of pulmonary vascular enlargement from overcirculation depends on the size of the defect and pulmonary vascular resistance. An electrocardiogram may be normal, or it may show right ventricular and possibly right atrial enlargement. Deep S waves in leads I, II, III, and aVF; right axis deviation of the QRS; and delayed ventricular conduction are the main ECG findings in dogs with ASD. Partial or complete right bundle branch is common. Atrial fibrillation may occasionally be noted.

Echocardiography. An ASD larger than 5 mm usually can be visualized directly on two-dimensional echocardiography. Right atrial and ventricular dilation, enlargement of the main pulmonary artery, left atrial enlargement, and reduced or normal left ventricular and aortic size are suggestive of ASD on 2-D and M-mode echocardiography. Color-flow Doppler is particularly useful for detecting small defects. The direction and velocity of shunt flow can be determined by spectral Doppler. The pulmonary to systemic flow ratio can be calculated from Doppler analysis of aortic and pulmonary flows. Pulmonary to systemic flow ratios (Qp:Qs) greater than 2:1 are indicative of a hemodynamically significant ASD; ratios greater than 2.5:1 may indicate the need for surgery or catheter occlusion.

NOTE: The complex color-flow Doppler filling patterns of the left and right atria, coupled with false echo drop out of the interatrial septum in the area of the fossa ovalis, commonly result in an erroneous diagnosis of ASD by inexperienced echocardiographers.

Laboratory Findings

Laboratory abnormalities are typically not present.

DIFFERENTIAL DIAGNOSIS

Differential diagnoses include SAS, PS, tetralogy of Fallot, and atrioventricular septal defects.

MEDICAL MANAGEMENT

Medical management for ASD (see Box 27-8) consists of symptomatic treatment for congestive heart failure. Useful drugs for congestive heart failure include ACE inhibitors (i.e., enalapril), diuretics (i.e., furosemide; see Box 27-1), and inodilators (i.e., pimobendan).

SURGICAL TREATMENT

Surgical intervention should be considered for hemodynamically significant ASDs. Depending on the conformation of the defect (it must have a rim of tissue around the edge for the occluder to attach) a septal occluder device (e.g., Amplatzer Septal Occluder, AGA Medical Corp., Golden Valley, Minn.) may be used to close the defect (Figs. 27-16 and 27-17). If the defect does not have an appropriate rim of tissue for a septal occluder, definitive patch closure can be accomplished with the aid of cardiopulmonary bypass (Fig. 27-18). Surgical correction of an ASD is typically done from a right-sided thoracotomy via a right atriotomy incision.

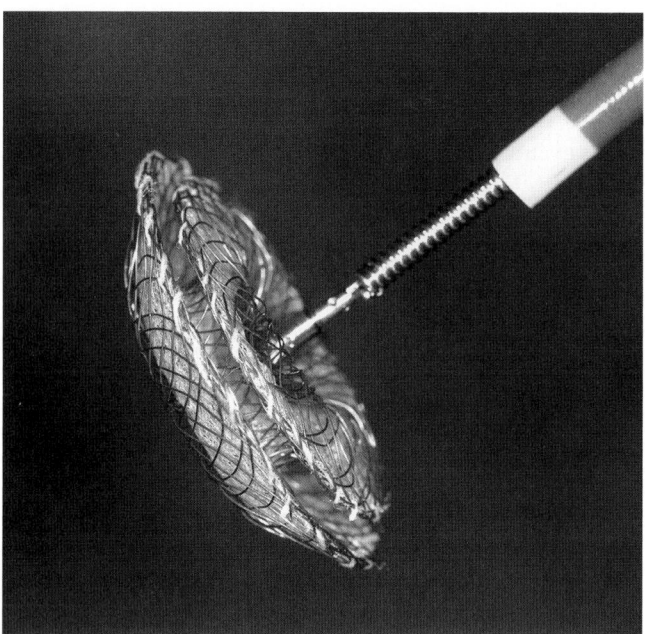

FIG. 27-16
Amplatzer device for transcatheter closure of an ASD. (Courtesy Dr. M. Miller, Texas A&M University.)

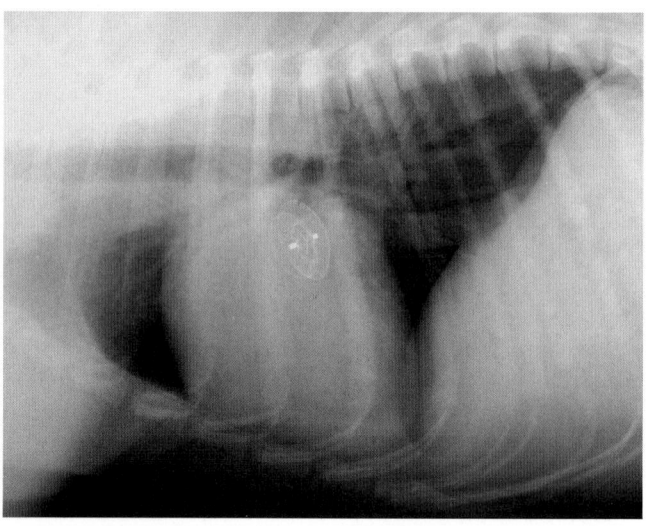

FIG. 27-17
Radiograph of a dog in which the device in Fig. 27-16 was placed to close a hemodynamically significant ASD. (Courtesy Dr. M. Miller, Texas A&M University.)

Preoperative Management

If significant heart failure is present, attempts should be made to control it medically. See also p. 775 for preoperative management of animals with cardiovascular disease.

Anesthesia

Anesthetic management of animals undergoing cardiac surgery is described on p. 775.

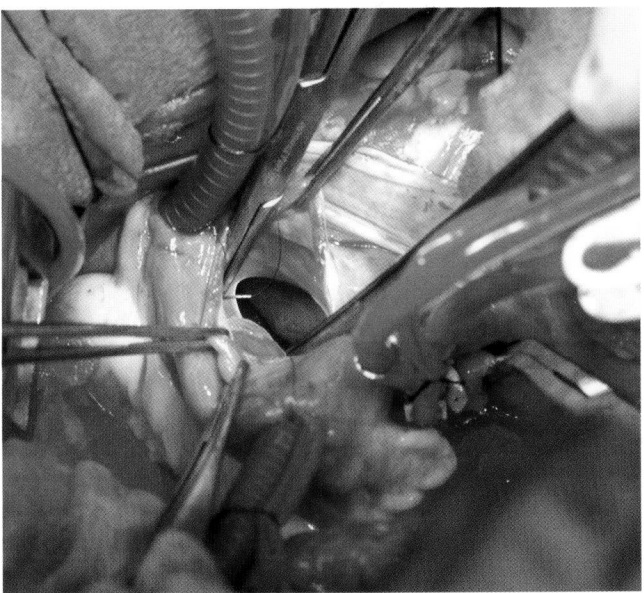

FIG. 27-18
Intraoperative photograph of sutures being placed in a pericardial graft to close a large ASD.

Surgical Anatomy

During cardiac development, the atria and ventricles are joined as a common chamber. The foramen ovale is a slitlike passage in the atrial septum that persists between the atria to permit right-to-left atrial shunting in the fetus. The foramen ovale closes in the neonate once left atrial pressure increases. Eventually, the lower portion of the atrial septum connects to the upper ventricular septum by differentiation of the endocardial cushion. The AV node lies adjacent to the anterior edge of the defect and must be avoided when sutures are placed to close the defect.

Positioning

The animal is positioned in left lateral recumbency for definitive closure of the defect via a right atriotomy. The entire right-sided thorax is prepared for aseptic surgery.

SURGICAL TECHNIQUE

Definitive patch closure of ASD can be accomplished with the aid of cardiopulmonary bypass in dogs more than 4 kg in body weight. A secundum ASD is corrected from the right side via a right atriotomy approach. Percutaneous transcatheter closure of an ASD has been reported in a dog (Sanders et al, 2005).

SUTURE MATERIALS AND SPECIAL INSTRUMENTS

A glutaraldehyde-fixed pericardial graft may be used to close the defect if it is too large for a direct suture technique. An Amplatzer Septal Occluder (AGA Medical Corp., Golden Valley, Minn.) may be used for transcatheter closure of the defect.

POSTOPERATIVE CARE AND ASSESSMENT

The postoperative care of these patients differs depending on the technique used for closure. After transcatheter closure, animals are generally released from the hospital within 24 hours of the procedure. Open surgical repair of the defect requires a longer postoperative recovery period. Animals should be closely observed for worsening of heart failure secondary to anesthesia, surgery, or arrhythmias. Postoperative pain should be treated with systemic opioids (see Table 13-4 on p. 133) and local anesthetic techniques (see p. 868).

PROGNOSIS

The prognosis for animals with ASD depends on the size of the defect. Animals with small restrictive defects typically tolerate the defect without ill effects. Large defects (i.e., Qp:Qs greater than 1.5-2:1) will likely result in the development of progressive heart failure or pulmonary hypertension. Definitive closure of an ASD under cardiopulmonary bypass or via transcatheter occlusion is considered curative.

Reference

Sanders RA, Hogan DF, Green HW et al: Transcatheter closure of an atrial septal defect in a dog, *J Am Vet Med Assoc* 227:430, 2005.

Suggested Reading

Guglielmini C, Diana A, Pietra M et al: Atrial septal defect in five dogs, *J Small Anim Pract* 43:317, 2002.
The clinical electrocardiographic, radiographic, and two-dimentional M-mode and Doppler echocardiographic findings are reported.

TETRALOGY OF FALLOT

DEFINITION

Tetralogy of Fallot is a complex congenital heart defect that consists of PS, VSD, a dextropositioned overriding aorta, and right ventricular hypertrophy.

GENERAL CONSIDERATIONS AND CLINICALLY RELEVANT PATHOPHYSIOLOGY

Tetralogy of Fallot is the most common congenital heart defect that causes cyanosis in small animals. It occurs in cats and a variety of canine breeds (see later discussion under Signalment). Tetralogy of Fallot can be simplified into two physiologically significant defects: PS and VSD. The pathophysiologic consequences of tetralogy depend on the relative magnitude of these two defects. If a large VSD and hemodynamically insignificant PS are present, the functional result is a left-to-right shunt and volume overload of the left ventricle similar to an isolated, large VSD. If severe PS, suprasystemic right ventricular pressures, and right-to-left shunt are present, the result is moderate to severe cyanosis, exercise intolerance, and progressive polycythemia. A shortened life span is expected in these animals because of complications of hyperviscosity (caused by polycythemia)-induced thromboembolism or sudden death. Animals that have PS and

VSD that are somewhat balanced are functionally similar to those that have a VSD and pulmonary artery banding performed (see p. 796). Animals with predominantly left-to-right shunt are termed *acyanotic or pink tetralogy* and may function reasonably well as long as the shunt flow is insufficient to cause left ventricular failure. Progression of PS due to infundibular hypertrophy is possible and may cause acyanotic animals to become cyanotic as they age.

DIAGNOSIS
Clinical Presentation

Signalment. Breeds most commonly reported to have tetralogy of Fallot include keeshonden, English bulldogs, poodles, schnauzers, terriers, collies, and shelties. In keeshonden, tetralogy is genetically transmitted as part of the spectrum of conotruncal defects.

History. Clinical findings at presentation for a typical tetralogy of Fallot include moderate to severe exercise intolerance, exertional tachypnea, collapse, and syncope.

Physical Examination Findings

Physical findings in animals with tetralogy of Fallot include cyanosis unresponsive to supplemental oxygen and systolic murmurs heard well at the left ventricular base and right sternum. If polycythemia is severe, a murmur may not be heard.

Diagnostic Imaging

Thoracic radiographs typically show evidence of right ventricular enlargement, usually without main pulmonary artery enlargement. Pulmonary vessels are usually small, suggesting pulmonary undercirculation. Electrocardiograms usually show a right axis shift in the frontal plane suggestive of right ventricular hypertrophy.

Echocardiography. Two-dimensional echocardiography demonstrates all the elements of tetralogy, including right ventricular hypertrophy, PS, VSD, and overriding aorta. Doppler interrogation of the pulmonic outflow tract and septal defect is useful in determining the direction and magnitude of the shunt.

Laboratory Findings

Polycythemia (i.e., packed cell volume greater than 55%) is often present because of chronic hypoxemia.

DIFFERENTIAL DIAGNOSIS

Differentials include right-to-left shunting VSD, ASD, atrioventricular septal defect, complex cyanotic cardiac disease, and PDA.

MEDICAL MANAGEMENT

Periodic phlebotomy with crystalloid fluid replacement may be necessary to maintain the hematocrit below 60% in animals with severe cyanosis and progressive polycythemia. Extreme caution must be taken during this procedure to avoid introducing intravenous air and causing air embolism. Low-dose aspirin therapy (e.g., 5 to 10 mg/kg, once or twice

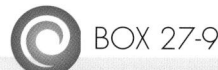 **BOX 27-9**

β-Adrenergic Therapy in Dogs

Propranolol (Inderal)
0.2–2 mg/kg PO, bid to tid, or titrate to control heart rate

Atenolol (Tenormin)
Dogs: 6.25–50 mg/dog, PO, qd to bid
Cats 6.25–12.5 mg/cat, PO, qd to bid

PO, Oral; *bid,* twice a day; *tid,* three times a day; *qd,* once a day.

daily) is also recommended to reduce the risk of thromboembolic complications.

β-adrenergic blockade therapy with propranolol or atenolol has been advocated as a palliative treatment for tetralogy of Fallot (Box 27-9). Possible beneficial effects include reduced dynamic outflow obstruction, decreased heart rate, increased systemic vascular resistance, and decreased myocardial oxygen demand.

SURGICAL TREATMENT

Surgery should be considered for severely cyanotic animals to lessen clinical signs and prolong life. Animals with a resting arterial oxygen saturation less than 70% should be considered candidates for surgery. Palliative surgeries for tetralogy include isolated correction of the PS or creation of a systemic-to-pulmonary shunt (e.g., Blalock-Taussig shunt; see later discussion). Correction of the PS risks overcorrection of the stenosis and an overwhelming left-to-right shunt. For this reason, valve dilation (see p. 790), either surgically or by balloon dilation, is preferred over a more definitive procedure, such as a patch graft (see p. 790). Definitive repair of tetralogy can be undertaken in medium- to large-breed dogs with cardiopulmonary bypass (Orton et al, 2001). Patch closure of the VSD and patch grafting of the pulmonary outflow tract are undertaken through a right ventriculotomy approach.

Preoperative Management

Although arrhythmias are uncommon, an ECG should be performed and hemodynamically significant arrhythmias controlled before surgery. Severe polycythemia should be corrected before surgery.

Anesthesia

Recommendations for anesthetic management of animals undergoing cardiac surgery are discussed on p. 775.

Surgical Anatomy

With tetralogy of Fallot, the parietal portion of the infundibular septum attaches more cranial and leftward than normal, resulting in a narrowing of the right ventricular outflow tract and dextropositioned overriding of the aorta.

The magnitude of this shift determines which type of physiology is associated with the defect. The VSD is usually located high in the infundibular septum, just at the level of the crista supraventricularis, although supracristal septal defects do occur.

Positioning

The animal should be positioned in right lateral recumbency for Blalock-Taussig shunt surgery. The entire left hemithorax is prepared for aseptic surgery.

AP SURGICAL TECHNIQUE

Several types of systemic-to-pulmonary shunts have been used to palliate tetralogy of Fallot. A modified Blalock-Taussig shunt is accomplished by harvesting the left subclavian artery as a free autogenous graft and placing it between the aorta and main pulmonary artery (Fig. 27-19).

Perform a left fourth intercostal thoracotomy. Harvest an autogenous arterial graft by ligating and dividing the proximal left subclavian artery. Open the pericardium and suture it to the thoracotomy incision. Place tangential vascular clamps on the pulmonary artery and ascending aorta. Make incisions into both vessels by making a longitudinal incision in the vessel wall held within the clamp. Interpose the graft between the aorta and pulmonary artery by end-to-side anastomoses, using simple continuous suture patterns. Be sure that the graft is not kinked. Release the clamps and verify hemostasis at the suture sites. The pulmonary artery clamp should be released first.

SUTURE MATERIALS AND SPECIAL INSTRUMENTS

Polypropylene (5-0) suture is used for the vascular anastomoses of the Blalock-Taussig shunt. Two tangential vascular clamps are required to control hemorrhage during the surgery.

POSTOPERATIVE CARE AND ASSESSMENT

Postoperative pain should be treated with systemic opioids (see Table 13-4 on p. 133) and local anesthetic techniques (see p. 868). Postoperative care of patients undergoing cardiac surgery is described on p. 780.

PROGNOSIS

Animals with reasonably balanced acyanotic tetralogy of Fallot should be monitored for progression, but otherwise generally do not require surgery. These animals have a reasonably good prognosis. The prognosis for animals with cyanotic tetralogy depends on the shunt fraction, magnitude of hypoxemia, and degree of polycythemia. Some animals may live several years without surgical therapy despite moderate to severe exercise intolerance. Animals with severe hypoxemia and progressive polycythemia will likely succumb to the effects of the disease or will experience sudden death early in life. Modified Blalock-Taussig shunts are reasonably

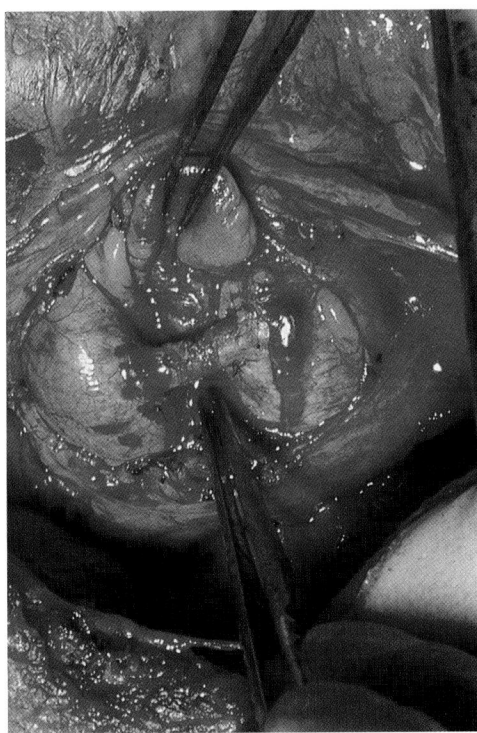

FIG. 27-19
Modified Blalock-Taussig shunt for tetralogy of Fallot.

effective at reducing the magnitude of hypoxemia and palliating the consequences of tetralogy of Fallot.

Reference

Orton EC, Mama K, Hellyer P et al: Open surgical repair of tetralogy of Fallot in dogs, *J Am Vet Med Assoc* 219:1089, 2001.

PERICARDIAL EFFUSION AND PERICARDIAL CONSTRICTION

DEFINITIONS

The **pericardium** is a fibroserous envelope that encompasses the heart and great vessels. **Pericardial effusion** is an abnormal accumulation of fluid within the pericardial sac. **Cardiac tamponade** refers to the decompensated phase of cardiac compression resulting from an unchecked rise in intrapericardiac fluid pressure. **Pericardial constriction** results from a restrictive fibrosis of the parietal and/or visceral pericardium that interferes with diastolic function of the heart. **Electrical alternans** is a beat-to-beat voltage variation of the QRS or ST-T complexes. *Pericardial tamponade* is a synonym for cardiac tamponade; pericardial constriction is a synonym for *constrictive pericarditis*.

GENERAL CONSIDERATIONS AND CLINICALLY RELEVANT PATHOPHYSIOLOGY

Diseases affecting primarily the pericardium account for approximately 1% of cardiovascular disease. Although primary pericardial disease represents a small percentage of the total number of cardiac diseases in small animals, it is an important cause of canine right-sided congestive heart failure. Pericardial diseases are uncommon in cats. Several types of primary and secondary pericardial diseases occur, the most common of which are those resulting in the accumulation of pericardial effusion. Pericardial effusion can be transudative, exudative (inflammatory), or sanguineous. Causes of pericardial transudation include right-sided congestive heart failure, hypoproteinemia, or incarceration of a liver lobe within the pericardial cavity (peritoneopericardial diaphragmatic hernia, see p. 906). Transudative pericardial effusions are usually subclinical.

Infectious pericarditis is an uncommon cause of pericardial effusion in dogs and cats, usually producing a purulent or fibrinous exudate. A variety of aerobic and anaerobic bacterial and fungal organisms have been associated with infectious pericarditis. Bacterial pericarditis can arise from bite wounds to the thorax, migrating foreign bodies, or hematogenous seeding. Coccidioidomycosis is an important cause of pericardial effusion in endemic regions. Feline infectious peritonitis and toxoplasmosis are potential causes of feline inflammatory effusions.

The most common causes of pericardial effusion in dogs are neoplasia and benign idiopathic effusion. Neoplasms that produce pericardial effusion in dogs include hemangiosarcoma, chemodectomas, mesothelioma, ectopic (heart base) thyroid carcinoma, lymphoma, and metastatic carcinoma to the heart. Hemangiosarcomas may be multicentric, with simultaneous splenic or hepatic involvement (see also p. 808). Aortic body tumors (chemodectoma, nonchromaffin paraganglioma) sometimes invade the heart base and cause pericardial effusion (see also p. 808). Lymphosarcoma, mesothelioma, and metastatic carcinoma have been implicated in cats with pericardial effusion. Neoplastic pericardial effusions usually are sanguineous.

Idiopathic (benign) pericardial effusions are common in dogs; this condition has not been reported in cats. The effusion usually appears sanguineous and must be differentiated from neoplastic effusions. Coagulopathies or left atrial rupture secondary to chronic mitral insufficiency are rare causes of acute pericardial hemorrhage.

Pathophysiologic alterations associated with pericardial effusion depend on the rate and volume of fluid accumulation and distensibility or compliance of the pericardium. If effusion accumulates slowly, the pericardium will expand to accommodate the fluid, intrapericardial pressure will not increase initially, and cardiac filling will not be compromised. Slow progressive accumulation of pericardial fluid allows compensation. First, the fibrous pericardium can stretch and remodel over time to accommodate an increased volume of fluid with only a modest increase in intrapericardial pressure. Second, neurohumoral mechanisms are evoked and lead to retention of vascular volume and increased intracardiac diastolic filling pressures. Although the later compensatory mechanism delays the onset of cardiac tamponade, it leads to progressive right-sided congestive heart failure, including jugular venous distention, ascites, peripheral edema, and pleural effusion. Cardiac tamponade eventually occurs despite compensatory mechanisms, leading to acute circulatory collapse.

Conversely, rapid or sudden accumulation of fluid (e.g., pericardial hemorrhage) causes acute cardiac tamponade. Rapid fluid accumulation in the pericardial space compresses the ventricles, restricts ventricular filling, and reduces cardiac output. Although significant volumes of fluid are usually required to raise pericardial pressure initially, additional small volumes may substantially increase intrapericardial pressure and greatly impede ventricular filling. Because of their thin walls and low pressures, the right atrium and ventricle are more vulnerable than the left to cardiac compression. Diastolic pressures (i.e., pulmonary wedge pressure, left and right ventricular end-diastolic pressures, and mean right atrial pressure) on both sides of the heart equilibrate.

Pericardial constriction occurs when visceral and/or parietal pericardial layers become fused, thickened, densely fibrotic, or inelastic and form a rigid case around the heart. The pericardial space may become totally obliterated or may contain small amounts of fluid (constrictive-effusive disease). Constrictive pericardial disease may develop asymmetrically so that one ventricle is more affected than the other; however, both ventricles are usually affected nearly equally. An audible "pericardial knock" may be heard during early diastolic filling and is attributed to vibrations produced by the sudden deceleration of blood as it strikes the encased nondistensible ventricular wall. As constriction worsens, cardiac output declines even though myocardial systolic function may be maintained. Fluid retention initiated by chronically reduced cardiac output further contributes to venous congestion, which is most commonly manifested as hepatomegaly and ascites accumulation.

DIAGNOSIS
Clinical Presentation

Signalment. Idiopathic benign and neoplastic pericardial effusions are more commonly observed in large- and giant-breed dogs. Right atrial hemangiosarcoma is especially common in German shepherds and golden retrievers (see also p. 808). Idiopathic pericardial effusion has been reported most commonly in golden retrievers, German shepherds, and other large-breed dogs. Aortic body tumors are most common in aged brachycephalic dogs. Medium- to large-breed, middle-age dogs are most commonly affected with constrictive pericardial disease; however, the condition is uncommon.

History. Presenting complaints associated with pericardial effusion include weakness, lethargy, exercise intolerance, and/or collapse. Patients often have right-sided congestion, ascites, and/or pleural effusion. The most common owner complaint with constrictive pericarditis is abdominal enlargement. Dyspnea, tachypnea, weakness, syncope, and/or weight loss are noted less frequently. Occasionally, there will be a previous history of idiopathic pericardial effusion.

Physical Examination Findings

Clinical findings are related to the consequences of cardiac tamponade and right-sided congestive heart failure. The classic triad of signs of cardiac tamponade (e.g., rapid and weak arterial pulse, distended jugular veins, and diminished heart sounds) is usually present. Jugular venous distention or a positive hepatojugular reflux will be present, but commonly overlooked. Measurement of central venous pressure will document systemic venous hypertension and frequently exceeds 10 cm H_2O (normal less than 5 to 6 cm H_2O). Lung sounds (especially ventrally) may be diminished if pleural effusion is present. Other auscultatory abnormalities (e.g., gallop rhythms, cardiac murmurs, and arrhythmias) are uncommon. Ascites, hepatomegaly, and/or peripheral edema may also be noted.

Although there are no pathognomonic electrocardiographic findings for pericardial disease, several abnormalities may occur. Electrical alternans may be recorded in as many as 50% of patients with pericardial effusion (Fig. 27-20). If present, electrical alternans is strongly suggestive of pericardial effusion. It is caused by swinging of the heart within large pericardial effusions rather than alterations in conduction within the heart, and is most likely to occur at heart rates between 90 and 144 beats per minute. Other findings supportive of pericardial effusion on electrocardiograms are diminished QRS voltages and ST segment depression. Sinus tachycardia is the predominant rhythm, although nonsustained ventricular tachycardia may occur.

Diagnostic Imaging

Thoracic radiography usually demonstrates varying degrees of globoid enlargement (i.e., the cardiac silhouette loses its angles and waists, and becomes globe-shaped) of the cardiac silhouette (Fig. 27-21). Radiographic evidence of pulmonary congestion or edema is not expected, which helps distinguish pericardial effusion from dilated cardiomyopathy. Pulmonary undercirculation is often noted. If right-sided congestion has developed, distention of the caudal vena cava, hepatomegaly, ascites, and pleural effusion are usually evident. Heart base tumors may deviate the trachea, typically cranial to the carina, producing a mass effect. Abnormal radiographic findings in animals with constrictive pericarditis are subtle; the cardiac silhouette may be rounded. Caudal vena cava dilation may be evident.

Fluoroscopy may demonstrate reduced cardiac motion in animals with pericardial effusion. Pneumopericardiography may help identify intrapericardial mass lesions, although this technique is no longer used with the advent of echocardiography. Angiography will usually show filling defects or tumor vascularity if neoplasia is causing the effusion; furthermore, angiography will show increased endocardial-pericardial distance typical of pericardial effusion. Although these modalities are reliable when properly used, echocardiography has supplanted most indications for their use.

Echocardiography. Definitive diagnosis of pericardial effusion is obtained readily by echocardiography. The fi-

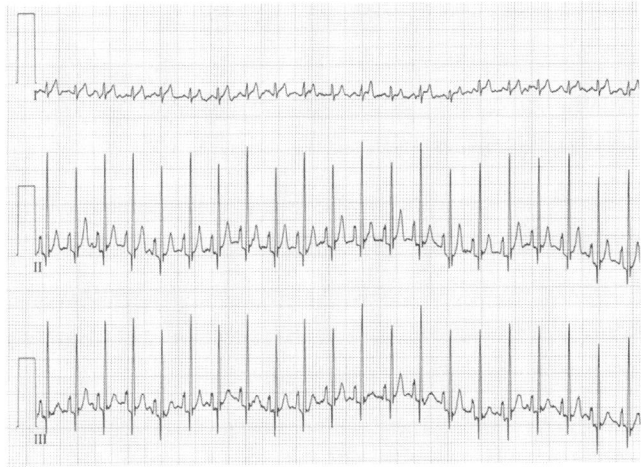

FIG. 27-20
Electrocardiogram of a dog with electrical alternans with pericardial effusion. Notice the overall small complex size and variable R-wave amplitude. (Courtesy Dr. M. Miller, Texas A&M University.)

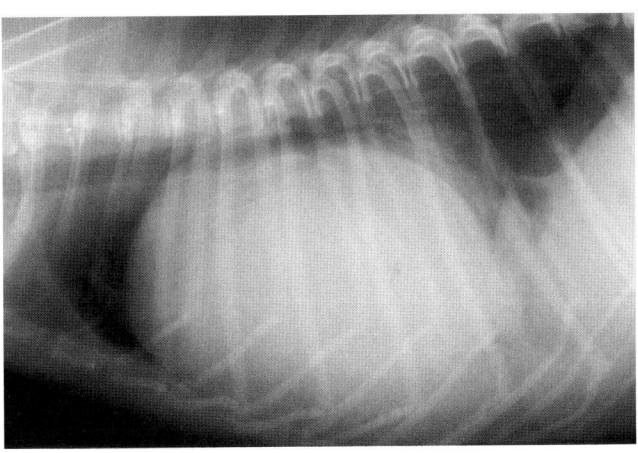

FIG. 27-21
Thoracic radiograph of a dog with pericardial effusion. Note the large, globoid heart.

brous pericardium is easily identified as a thin echo-dense structure, and any degree of separation or echo-free space between the pericardium and underlying cardiac structures on 2-D or M-mode echocardiography is diagnostic of pericardial effusion. Echocardiography is the most reliable procedure for identifying primary cardiac neoplasia, although failure to identify a mass does not rule out neoplasia. Flattening of the left ventricular endocardium during diastole, abnormal diastolic (early notch), and systolic septal motion are often noted in patients with constrictive pericarditis. Differentiation of constrictive pericardial disease and restrictive myopathy may be difficult with echocardiography.

Laboratory Findings

The complete blood count may reveal inflammation, and increased numbers of circulating nucleated red blood cells or large numbers of acanthocytes are suggestive of cardiac or splenic hemangiosarcoma. Cardiac enzymes may be elevated because of ischemia or myocardial invasion. Other abnormalities may be associated with the primary disease or with congestive heart failure. Serum fungal titers (coccidioidomycosis) or enzyme-linked immunosorbent assay tests for feline leukemia virus (cats) may be positive when pericarditis is related to these infections. Chronic systemic venous congestion associated with pericardial effusion or constriction can cause splenic dysfunction (functional hyposplenism) and protein-losing enteropathy (intestinal lymphangiectasia). Hyposplenism can cause increased numbers of circulating activated platelets, whereas protein-losing enteropathy may exacerbate the splenic dysfunction and reduce circulating antithrombin III levels. Both conditions promote a hypercoagulable state and may make affected animals prone to pulmonary thromboembolism (PTE). Aspirin (5 to 10 mg/kg, qd or bid) or low molecular weight heparin (dalteparin; 150 U/kg SC bid) may be useful for preventing PTE in dogs at risk.

> NOTE: Pulmonary thromboembolism should be considered likely in dogs with pericardial disease with effusion, particularly those with constriction, that exhibit severe, sudden respiratory distress.

Cytologic and microbiologic analysis should be performed on pericardial fluid. An inflammatory exudate on cytologic examination suggests infectious pericarditis. The causative organism may be visible on cytologic examination or identified by bacterial or fungal culture (NOTE: warn the lab if you suspect coccidioidomycosis because it is hazardous to attempt culture of this organism). Neoplastic effusions are usually sanguineous (i.e., characterized by large numbers of red blood cells and variable numbers of neutrophils and mononuclear cells). Cytology is unreliable in identifying neoplastic effusions because both false positives and false negatives occur. Idiopathic pericardial effusion produces a sanguineous effusion that is difficult to distinguish from neoplastic effusions on fluid analysis alone. Exploratory surgery or thoracoscopy and histopathology may be necessary to definitively differentiate between neoplastic and idiopathic pericardial effusion.

DIFFERENTIAL DIAGNOSIS

In addition to pericardial effusion, differentials for a globoid-appearing heart on thoracic radiographs include dilated cardiomyopathy and peritoneopericardial diaphragmatic hernia (see p. 906). The latter may be associated with pericardial effusion, particularly when the liver is herniated. Ultrasonography is used to detect incongruities in the diaphragmatic silhouette and identify abdominal contents within the pericardial sac. Echocardiography differentiates diffuse cardiac enlargement from pericardial effusion. If echocardiography is unavailable, nonselective angiography can be used.

MEDICAL MANAGEMENT

Pericardiocentesis is the treatment of choice for initial stabilization of dogs and cats with pericardial effusion and cardiac tamponade. When performed properly, pericardiocentesis is associated with minimal complications. It should be attempted in symptomatic animals with suspected pericardial effusion, even if echocardiography is not available to confirm the diagnosis.

> NOTE: If possible, monitor an electrocardiogram during pericardiocentesis because inadvertent cardiac contact usually produces premature ventricular complexes.

Shave and surgically prepare a large area of the right hemithorax (sternum to midthorax, third to eighth rib). Perform a local block with lidocaine and, if necessary, sedate the animal (e.g., hydromorphone or fentanyl; Box 27-10). Be sure to infiltrate the pleura with lidocaine because pleural penetration seems to cause significant discomfort. Place the animal in sternal or lateral recumbency, depending on its demeanor.

Pericardiocentesis can be accomplished in the standing animal, but adequate restraint is essential to prevent cardiac puncture or pulmonary laceration.

Determine the puncture site based on heart location on thoracic radiographs. This is most commonly between the fourth and fifth intercostal spaces at the costochondral junction.
Attach a 14- to 18-gauge needle or catheter to a three-way stopcock, extension tubing, and syringe to allow constant negative pressure to be applied during insertion and drainage. Once the catheter has been inserted through the skin, apply negative pressure. If pleural effusion is present, it will be obtained immediately upon entering the thoracic cavity. Pleural effusion associated with heart disease is usually a clear to pale yellow color. Advance the catheter until it contacts the pericardium and a scratching sensation is noticed. Then advance the catheter slightly to penetrate the pericardium. Stop advancing the catheter as soon as fluid is obtained. Withdraw the needle immediately if the epicardium is contacted and if cardiac motion is felt through the needle.

Ultrasound guidance is seldom necessary when performing pericardiocentesis unless the volume of fluid is small or it is compartmentalized.

Pericardiocentesis causes immediate clinical improvement in animals with cardiac tamponade. The pulse slows and strengthens as soon as an adequate volume of fluid has been removed. Pericardial effusion can usually be differentiated from peripheral blood in that it rarely clots and the

4

optimize

BOX 27-10

Sedation During Pericardiocentesis in Dogs

Hydromorphone
0.1–0.2 mg/kg SC, IM, or IV

Fentanyl (Sublimaze)
0.005 IV or 0.01 mg/kg SC, IM

SC, Subcutaneous; *IM*, intramuscular; *IV*, intravenous.

BOX 27-11

Oral Prednisolone Therapy for Dogs With Idiopathic Pericardial Effusion

Begin at a dose of 1 mg/kg PO every 12 hours; then gradually decrease the dosage over a 2- to 3-week period and discontinue.

PO, Oral.

packed cell volume is significantly lower than peripheral blood. Approximately 50% of dogs with idiopathic effusion are managed successfully by periodic pericardiocentesis, plus sometimes corticosteroids (oral prednisolone; Box 27-11), without pericardiectomy. In the remainder, repeat centesis is necessary to control clinical signs. Fluid may reaccumulate rapidly (within several days) or may not recur for months or even several years. In patients requiring more than two centeses within a few months, subphrenic pericardiectomy is usually indicated. Although antiinflammatory doses of prednisolone are commonly administered to dogs with idiopathic pericardial effusion, there are no controlled studies confirming the efficacy of this therapy. Subtotal pericardiectomy is usually curative in dogs with idiopathic pericardial effusion. Recurrent effusion and pericardial constriction are possible late sequelae of idiopathic effusions if pericardiectomy is not performed.

SURGICAL TREATMENT

Although temporary relief of cardiac tamponade is provided by pericardiocentesis, long-term palliation of pericardial effusion often requires pericardiectomy. Pericardiectomy can be performed through an intercostal thoracotomy (see p. 873) or median sternotomy (see p. 874), or it can be done with thoracoscopy (see p. 806). Concerns that removing only a small portion of the pericardium might allow the remaining pericardium to adhere to the heart and cause recurrence of pericardial effusion have not been borne out with thoracoscopic pericardiectomy. Nonetheless, a generous amount of the pericardium should be removed when pericardiectomy is done in conjunction with a thoracotomy.

For open thoracotomy, it is technically easier to perform a pericardiectomy through a median sternotomy because access to both sides of the heart and both phrenic nerves is provided by this approach. If right atrial hemangiosarcoma is suspected, either a right fifth intercostal thoracotomy or a median sternotomy should be used. Removal of right atrial tumors can be accomplished equally well from either approach (see p. 809). Chemodectomas can arise on either the left or right heart base. Pericardiectomy in these cases should be performed through a thoracotomy on the side where the bulk of the tumor is suspected to be. If cardiac neoplasia is not identified before surgery and if idiopathic pericardial effusion is suspected, then pericardiectomy should be performed through a right thoracotomy or medial sternotomy so that the right atrium can be examined and resected, if necessary. Although total pericardiectomy can be performed, subphrenic pericardiectomy is usually adequate for animals with pericardial effusion. Total pericardiectomy may be indicated in some animals with neoplasia or infectious processes of the pericardium. Total pericardiectomy is best performed from a median sternotomy approach.

Pericardiectomy is the therapy of choice for constrictive pericarditis. Complications associated with surgery include development of arrhythmias (most notably atrial fibrillation or ventricular tachycardia). The outcome with surgery depends on severity of the underlying disease. If the visceral pericardium (epicardium) is significantly involved, the surgical outcome is less favorable. Epicardial decortication may be necessary.

Preoperative Management

If hemodynamically significant quantities of pericardial effusion are present (i.e., cardiac tamponade as evidenced by jugular vein distention, ascites, and/or pleural effusion), the animal should have preoperative pericardiocentesis. Metabolic causes of pericardial effusion (e.g., hypoproteinemia) should be ruled out. Electrolyte and acid-base abnormalities (e.g., associated with high doses of diuretics) should be corrected before anesthetic induction.

Anesthesia

Refer to p. 775 for anesthetic management of cardiac patients. Care should be exercised when manipulating the heart because arrhythmias or hypotension may occur. Fentanyl and midazolam can be used to anesthetize patients with compromised cardiac function (see Box 27-5). Unilateral bronchial intubation (Kudnig et al, 2003) can be done for laparoscopic pericardiectomy; however, it is typically unnecessary.

Surgical Anatomy

The pericardium envelops the heart in a strong flask-shaped sac with extensions that enclose the origins of the ascending aorta, pulmonary artery, distal pulmonary veins, and venae cavae. The adventitia of the great arteries blends with fibrous tissue of the pericardium, forming strong attachments. The pericardium is firmly attached to the diaphragm via the pericardiophrenic ligament. Pericardium is composed of two layers: a fibrous outer layer and an inner serous membrane composed of a single layer of mesothelial cells. The inner serous layer forms the epicardium or visceral pericardium. It reflects back on itself to line the outer fibrous layer, and together they form the parietal pericardium.

The pericardial cavity is filled with a variable amount of pericardial fluid. This fluid is an ultrafiltrate of serum containing between 1.7 and 3.5 g/dl of protein and having a colloidal osmotic pressure approximately 25% that of serum. The volume of pericardial fluid present in normal dogs ranges from 1 to 15 ml. Lymphatic drainage of the pericardium is similar to that of the myocardium, with most drainage via epicardial lymphatics rather than from parietal pericardium. Functions ascribed to the pericardium include the ability to fix the heart anatomically and prevent excessive motion associated with changes in body position, reduction of friction between the heart and surrounding structures, and preventing extension of infection or malignancy from the pleural space.

Positioning

The animal should be placed either in lateral recumbency for an intercostal thoracotomy or in dorsal recumbency for median sternotomy. A sufficiently large area should be prepared to allow intraoperative placement of a thoracostomy tube.

SURGICAL TECHNIQUE

Regardless of the presence or absence of pericardial effusion at the time of surgery, dogs with aortic body tumors survive significantly longer if a pericardiectomy is done (median survival, 730 days) at the time of biopsy than if one is not done (median survival, 42 days) (Ehrhart et al, 2002). Dogs with pericardial effusion tend to survive substantially longer if pericardiectomy is done versus multiple pericardiocenteses.

Subphrenic (Subtotal) Pericardiectomy via Right Thoracotomy

After opening the chest, open the pericardium and submit fluid samples for microbiologic examination, fungal culture, and/or cytology, if indicated. Make a T-shaped incision in the pericardium from cardiac base to apex and across the cardiac base ventral to the phrenic nerve (Fig. 27-22, A). Extend the circumferential incision at the cardiac base around the venae cavae, taking care not to violate the vessel walls (Fig. 27-22, B). Have an assistant elevate the heart and retract it as the circumferential incision is extended to the opposite side (Fig. 27-22, C). Take care not to injure the contralateral phrenic nerve. Divide the pericardiophrenic ligament with cautery or between ligatures (Fig. 27-22, D). Check the remnants of the pericardium to ensure that there is no hemorrhage. Submit pericardium for histologic analyses. Place a thoracostomy tube before thoracic closure.

Total Pericardiectomy

Using blunt dissection, carefully elevate the phrenic nerves from the pericardial sac. Make a longitudinal incision in the pericardial sac and resect the pericardium as close to the base of the heart as possible. Place a thoracostomy tube before thoracic closure.

Thoracoscopic Pericardiectomy

Thoracoscopic pericardiectomy requires video and is best done with two people familiar with rigid endoscopy. There are different techniques (Dupre et al, 2001; Jackson et al, 1999).

Position the patient in dorsal recumbency, sometimes tilting 10 to 15 degrees to the left, or in left lateral recumbency, depending upon your preference. Typically, place the observation port substernally (paraxiphoid), entering the chest on the patient's right side. If the patient is large enough, placing an operating scope (i.e., a 10-mm-diameter scope with a 5-mm biopsy channel through it) in this position allows the port to simultaneously be used to observe and manipulate the pericardium. Usually place two ancillary ports on the right side, but one can place one on the right and one on the left (the latter requires making a large window in the mediastinum). It is helpful to place the ports at or above (from the perspective of the endoscopist) the level of the costochondral junction (i.e., ventral to the costochondral junction from the perspective of the dog) to minimize having the inflating lungs obscure vision. Place the ports around the sixth intercostal and ninth intercostal spaces (this can be varied based upon the needs in a particular animal). Use Babcock forceps, hemostats, and scissors (the latter two with electrocautery) to make a large opening in the mediastinum if necessary to enhance visualization, to grasp the pericardium, and to incise and resect a portion of pericardium. If possible, open the pericardium sufficiently so that you can visualize the right atrium and see previously undetected right atrial masses or diffuse intrapericardial proliferations. Take care to not cut the phrenic nerve. Either place a thoracostomy tube after the procedure or evacuate air with a needle and syringe.

SUTURE MATERIALS AND SPECIAL INSTRUMENTS

Electrocautery is useful for pericardiectomy to decrease intraoperative and postoperative hemorrhage. Inflamed pericardium often has an increased number of blood vessels, and significant hemorrhage can occur after pericardiectomy if they are not cauterized or ligated.

POSTOPERATIVE CARE AND ASSESSMENT

The thoracostomy tube should be aspirated every hour initially and the volume of pleural effusion quantitated. After 4 to 6 hours, frequency of drainage may be decreased to every 2 to 4 hours. Once the pleural effusion has decreased to levels consistent with those caused by the thoracostomy tube, the tube may be removed. If the patient develops acute respiratory distress without evidence of pleural effusion or significant pulmonary infiltrates suggestive of pulmonary edema, pulmonary thromboembolism should be suspected. Oxygen therapy may be beneficial in such cases. If pulmonary thromboembolism is diagnosed, thrombolytic agents may be used. Postoperative pain should be treated with systemic opioids (see Table 13-4 on p. 133) and local anesthetic techniques (see p. 868).

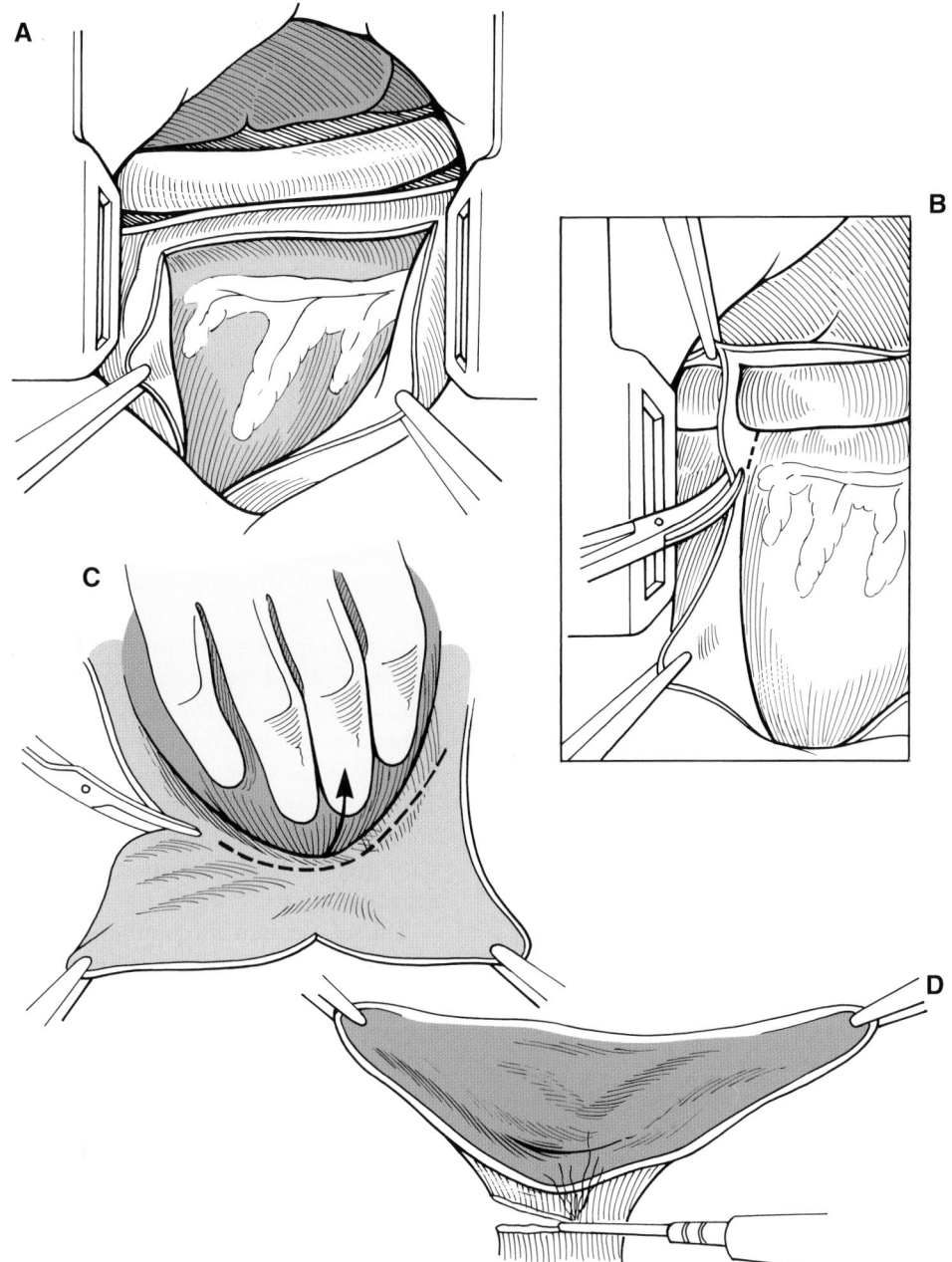

FIG. 27-22
For subtotal pericardiectomy via a right fifth intercostal thoracotomy, incise the epicardium vertically and horizontally ventral to the right phrenic nerve **(A)**. **B,** Carefully extend the incision around the vena cava, taking care to identify the vessel wall while making the incision. **C,** Gently retract the heart and extend the incision across the left side, ventral to the left phrenic nerve. **D,** Divide the pericardiophrenic ligament with cautery or between ligatures.

PROGNOSIS

Pericardiectomy is palliative for neoplastic pericardial effusion and curative for idiopathic pericardial effusion. Long-term palliation after pericardiectomy is possible for dogs with mesothelioma or chemodectoma. Intracavitary cisplatin has shown promise in achieving long-term remission in dogs with mesothelioma. Chemodectomas are slow-growing tumors, and long-term palliation with pericardiectomy and primary mass excision is possible. Median survival for dogs with cardiac hemangiosarcoma is approximately 4 months with pericardiectomy. A recent retrospective study of 143 dogs with pericardial effusion compared dogs in which a mass was seen on echocardiography (44 dogs) with those in which no mass was identified (99) (Stafford et al, 2004). Dogs with a mass had a median survival time of 26 days, whereas those that did not had a median survival time of

1068 days. Dogs presenting with collapse had significantly shorter survival than those that did not. Ascites was associated with a longer survival because dogs with a cardiac mass tended not to have ascites, whereas those that were echocardiographic negative for a mass typically had ascites. Dogs with aortic body tumors survive longer if a pericardiectomy is performed versus multiple pericardiocenteses.

References

Dupre GP, Corlouer JP, Bouvy B: Thoracoscopic pericardiectomy performed without pulmonary exclusion in 9 dogs. *Vet Surg* 30:21, 2001.

Ehrhart N, Ehrhart EJ, Willis J et al: Analysis of factors affecting survival in dogs with aortic body tumors, *Vet Surg* 31:44, 2002.

Jackson J, Richter KP, Launer DP: Thoracoscopic partial pericardiectomy in 13 dogs, *J Vet Intern Med* 13:529, 1999.

Johnson MS, Martin M, Binns S et al: A retrospective study of clinical findings, treatment and outcome in 143 dogs with pericardial effusion, *J Small Anim Pract* 45:546, 2004.

Kudnig ST, Monnet E, Riquelme M et al: Effect of one-lung ventilation on oxygen delivery in anesthetized dogs with an open thoracic cavity, *Am J Vet Res* 64:443, 2003.

Suggested Reading

De Laforcade AM, Freeman LM, Rozanski EA et al: Biochemical analysis of pericardial fluid and whole blood in dogs with pericardial effusion, *J Vet Intern Med* 19:833, 2005.

Differences between variable in dogs with neoplastic and nonneoplastic pericardial effusion were noted, but because of the degree of overlap between the 2 groups, clinical relevance was not found.

Fine DM, Tobias AH, Jacob KA: Use of pericardial fluid pH to distinguish between idiopathic and neoplastic effusions, *J Vet Intern Med* 17:525, 2003.

The authors found substantial overlap in the pH of idiopathic pericardial effusions and neoplastic effusions.

Macgregor JM, Faria MLE, Moore AS et al: Cardiac lymphoma and pericardial effusion in dogs: 12 cases (1994-2004), *J Am Vet Med Assoc* 227:1449, 2005.

Cardiac lymphoma is an uncommon cause of pericardial effusion in dogs, but it does not always warrant a grave prognosis.

Mellanby RJ, Merrtage ME: Long-term survival of 23 dogs with pericardial effusions, *Vet Rec* 156:568, 2005.

Three of 14 dogs with idiopathic pericardial effusions were treated with one pericardiocentesis, and 6 were treated by repeated pericardiocentesis. Five needed pericardiectomy.

Shubitz LF, Matz ME, Noon TH et al: Constrictive pericarditis secondary to *Coccidioides immitis* infection in a dog, *J Am Vet Med Assoc* 218:537, 2001.

This is a case report and a review of the literature. In a cited publication, 13 of 52 dogs with disseminated coccidioidomycosis had pericardial involvement.

Sims CS, Tobias AH, Hayden DW et al: Pericardial effusion due to primary cardiac lymphosarcoma in a dog, *J Vet Intern Med* 17:923, 2003.

This is a case report of a dog with T-cell lymphoma and a nonsanguinous pericardial effusion.

Stepien RL, Whitley NT, Dubielzig RR: Idiopathic or mesothelioma-related pericardial effusion: clinical findings and survival in 17 dogs studied retrospectively, *J Small Anim Pract* 41:342, 2000.

Clinical signs, physical examination findings, and results of noninvasive diagnostic testing did not differentiate effusion associated with mesothelioma from idiopathic pericardial effusion.

CARDIAC NEOPLASIA

DEFINITIONS

Cardiac neoplasia includes any neoplastic condition involving the heart, great vessels, or pericardium. Synonyms for hemangiosarcomas include *angiosarcomas* and *malignant hemangioendotheliomas*. Tumors arising from the chemoreceptor aortic bodies have also been called *chemodectomas, heart base tumors, aortic body adenomas* or *carcinomas,* or *nonchromaffin paragangliomas.*

GENERAL CONSIDERATIONS AND CLINICALLY RELEVANT PATHOPHYSIOLOGY

Cardiac neoplasia is relatively uncommon in small animals. The most important cardiac neoplasms in dogs are right atrial hemangiosarcoma and heart base chemodectoma. Hemangiosarcoma is the most common cardiac tumor, occurring nearly 10 times as frequently as the second most common tumor—aortic body tumor. A variety of primary intramural and intracavitary neoplasms have been reported in dogs including hemangiosarcoma, fibrosarcoma, chondrosarcoma, rhabdomyosarcoma, ectopic thyroid carcinoma, fibroma, and myxoma. Lymphosarcoma and metastatic neoplasia are the most frequent causes of cardiac neoplasia in cats.

The right atrium is a common primary site for hemangiosarcoma and accounts for 40% to 50% of canine cases of hemangiosarcoma. Other reported primary cardiac sites for hemangiosarcoma include the right ventricular free wall, interventricular septum, and main pulmonary artery. Primary cardiac hemangiosarcoma has not been described in cats, but metastasis of hemangiosarcoma to the heart is reported.

Chemodectomas can arise from the aortic body at the base of the heart (e.g., between aorta and pulmonary artery, between aorta and right atrium, or between pulmonary artery and left atrium) or from the carotid body in the neck. Aortic body chemodectomas account for approximately 80% of chemodectomas and occur in older dogs. Chemodectomas occur rarely in cats. Residence at altitude and chronic hypoxia probably increase the risk for developing these tumors. Chemodectomas can cause pericardial effusion, which probably accounts for the most common clinical presentation of this disease. However, chemodectomas are just as often an incidental finding in older dogs undergoing thoracic radiographs or echocardiography for other reasons. Ectopic thyroid adenomas and carcinomas account for approximately 5% to 10% of all heart base tumors in dogs.

DIAGNOSIS
Clinical Presentation

Signalment. German shepherds and golden retrievers have been identified as having an increased risk for developing hemangiosarcoma. Boxers, English bulldogs, and Boston terriers are the breeds most likely to develop chemodectomas.

History. Animals with cardiac neoplasia may be brought in for evaluation of dyspnea, cough, syncope, or congestive heart failure, or they may be asymptomatic.

Physical Examination Findings

The most common clinical presentation for right atrial hemangiosarcoma is acute or chronic cardiac tamponade resulting from intrapericardial hemorrhage (see the section on pericardial effusion, p. 801). Animals with chemodectomas may present for evaluation of congestive heart failure, signs of cardiac tamponade, or pleural effusion, or they may be asymptomatic.

Diagnostic Imaging

Thoracic radiographs of animals with chemodectomas may show dorsal elevation of the terminal trachea, pleural or pericardial effusion, pulmonary edema, or increased perihilar density. Selective angiography has identified canine chemodectomas. Suggestive findings on angiography include identifying tortuous, aberrant vessels at the base of the heart, displacement of the aortic arch, and/or filling defects in the left atria. Angiography is also useful for identifying intracardiac lesions; however, it is rarely performed with the advent of echocardiography. Echocardiography frequently is useful in identifying masses on the right atrial appendage or at the cardiac base.

Laboratory Findings

Specific laboratory abnormalities are not found with cardiac neoplasia. Cytologic analysis of the pericardial fluid does not reliably differentiate neoplastic from idiopathic pericardial effusion (see p. 804).

DIFFERENTIAL DIAGNOSIS

Cardiac neoplasia must be differentiated from other causes of pericardial effusion (see p. 804), congestive heart failure, or cardiac arrhythmias. Endomyocardial biopsy may be used to make a definitive diagnosis of intracardiac neoplasia. Differentials for radiographic masses near the heart base include hilar lymphadenopathy, left atrial enlargement, aberrant parathyroid or thyroid tissue, and fibrosing pleuritis or pericarditis.

MEDICAL MANAGEMENT

Various chemotherapeutic strategies can be used for cardiac neoplasia (as primary therapy or as an adjunct to surgery). Doxorubicin plus cyclophosphamide and vincristine have been used to palliate cardiac hemangiosarcoma with meager success.

SURGICAL TREATMENT

Pericardiectomy and excision of the right atrial tumor are palliative for atrial hemangiosarcoma (see later discussion in the Prognosis section). Chemodectomas are highly vascular, slow growing, and moderately locally invasive. Surgical exci-

sion of aortic body chemodectomas is possible depending on size, location, and degree of invasiveness of the tumor. However, many animals with chemodectomas and clinical signs associated with pericardial effusion benefit from pericardiectomy without tumor excision.

Surgical excision of intramural or intracavitary primary cardiac tumors has been attempted rarely in small animals. Surgical excision of well-defined primary cardiac tumors using inflow occlusion or cardiopulmonary bypass is possible in selected cases. However, because of the high incidence of malignancy of most primary cardiac tumors, echocardiographic, angiographic, and endomyocardial biopsy findings should be considered carefully when selecting appropriate cases for surgery.

Preoperative Management

Abdominal radiographs or ultrasonography should be performed before surgery to detect concurrent intraabdominal neoplasia (e.g., especially splenic hemangiosarcoma). If hemodynamically significant quantities of pericardial effusion are present (i.e., cardiac tamponade as evidenced by jugular vein distention, ascites, and/or pleural effusion), a pericardial tap should be performed before surgery.

Anesthesia

Refer to p. 775 for anesthetic management of cardiac patients.

Surgical Anatomy

Refer to p. 775 for surgical anatomy of the heart.

Positioning

The animal is positioned in dorsal recumbency for median sternotomy (see p. 874) or in lateral recumbency for intercostal thoracotomy (see p. 873). A sufficiently generous area should be prepped to allow a thoracostomy tube placement intraoperatively.

SURGICAL TECHNIQUE
Right Atrial Hemangiosarcoma

Perform a median sternotomy or right fourth space intercostal thoracotomy. Clamp the atrial appendage with a tangential vascular clamp and excise the appendage (Fig. 27-23). Close the atriotomy incision with a continuous mattress suture pattern. Remove the vascular clamp, and oversew the incision with a simple continuous suture pattern. Perform a pericardiectomy if pericardial effusion is present (see p. 806). Alternatively, the right atrial appendage may be excised with a TA stapling instrument (see p. 876).

Chemodectoma

The surgical approach for removing chemodectomas depends on the suspected location of the tumor.

Sharply dissect the tumor from the walls of the great vessels and atria. Use care to prevent rupturing these structures during dissection. Use electrocautery to decrease hemorrhage during excision of these highly vascular tumors.

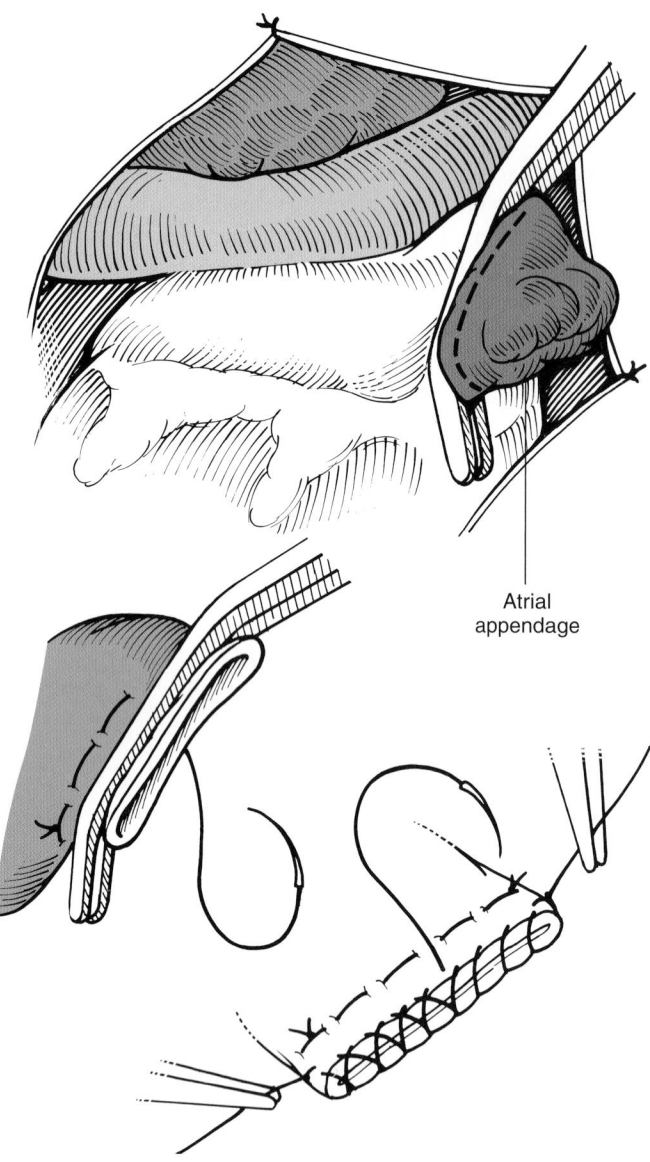

FIG. 27-23
To resect a right atrial hemangiosarcoma, place a tangential vascular clamp across the base of the right auricle and excise the tumor and auricle. Place a continuous horizontal mattress suture behind the vascular clamp. Remove the clamp, and oversew the incision with a simple continuous suture.

Atrial appendage

SUTURE MATERIALS AND SPECIAL INSTRUMENTS

A tangential vascular clamp is useful for excision of right atrial hemangiosarcoma. Closure of the right atrium can be accomplished with polypropylene (4-0) suture. Electrocautery is useful for excision of chemodectomas.

POSTOPERATIVE CARE AND ASSESSMENT

The animal should be monitored carefully for postoperative hemorrhage (pleural effusion). Arrhythmias are common, and electrocardiography should be monitored for 36 to 72 hours postoperatively. Postoperative pain should be treated with systemic opioids (see Table 13-4 on p. 133) and local anesthetic techniques (see p. 868).

PROGNOSIS

The prognosis for right atrial hemangiosarcoma is generally poor; however, surgery plus adjuvant chemotherapy has improved survival (Weisse et al, 2005). Micrometastasis is considered present in virtually all cases at the time of diagnosis. Pericardiectomy and excision of the right atrium are palliative. Median survival after surgery alone is approximately 4 months.

Long-term survival of up to several years is possible after surgical removal of an aortic body chemodectoma. In older animals with incidental asymptomatic chemodectoma, the risks of surgical excision should be weighed against the likelihood that the tumor will be slow growing and can remain asymptomatic for a long time.

Reference

Weisse C, Soares N, Beal MW et al: Survival times in dogs with right atrial hemangiosarcoma treated by means of surgical resection with or without adjuvant chemotherapy: 23 cases (1986-2000), *J Am Vet Med Assoc* 226:575, 2005.

Suggested Reading

Vicari E et al: Heart base tumors in dogs: a retrospective study of 25 cases, *Vet Surg* 29:478, 2000.
None of the variables examined, including initial complaints and results of physical examination, radiography, electrocardiography, and echocardiography were associated with survival time.

BRADYCARDIA

DEFINITIONS

Bradycardia is a heart rate that is slower than normal. Bradycardia can be physiologic (i.e., sinus bradycardia) or can result from a variety of pathologic disorders, including sick sinus syndrome, atrial standstill, or atrioventricular (AV) block with ventricular escape.

GENERAL CONSIDERATIONS AND CLINICALLY RELEVANT PATHOPHYSIOLOGY

Bradycardia can result from extrinsic causes, such as exaggerated vagal tone or electrolyte imbalance, or from intrinsic degenerative disorders of the heart. Sinus bradycardia results from a predominance of parasympathetic influence (sometimes associated with cranial or abdominal disease) and often is accompanied by other parasympathetically mediated rhythms (i.e., sinus arrhythmia, wandering pacemaker, or low-grade, second-degree AV block). It is generally considered a physiologic rather than pathologic rhythm.

Atrial standstill (Fig. 27-24, *A*) occurs when the atria fail to conduct an electrical impulse. The cardiac impulse may arise in the sinus node and be conducted to the AV node via internodal pathways in the atria (i.e., sinoventricular rhythm), or an escape rhythm may develop. Transient atrial

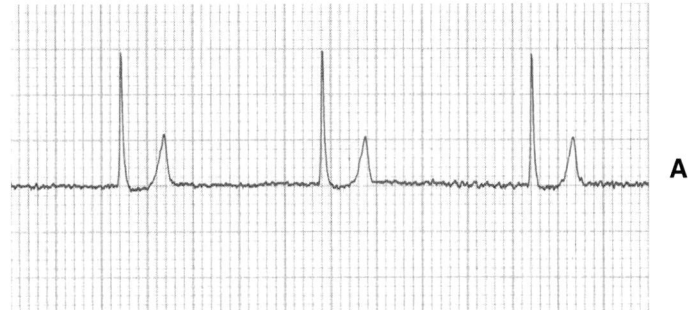

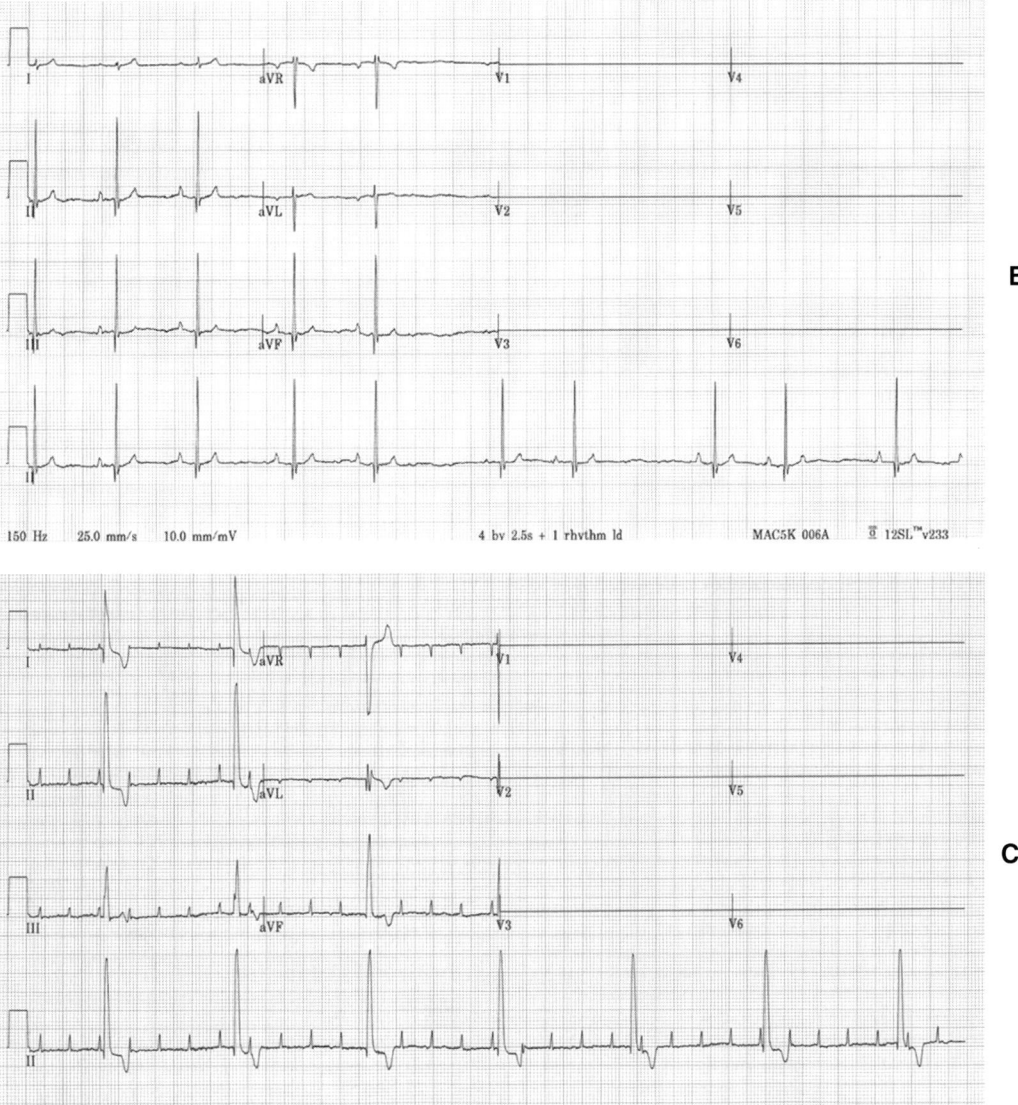

FIG. 27-24
Electrocardiograms from dogs with: **A,** atrial standstill; **B,** first-degree AV block; **C,** third-degree AV block.

Continued

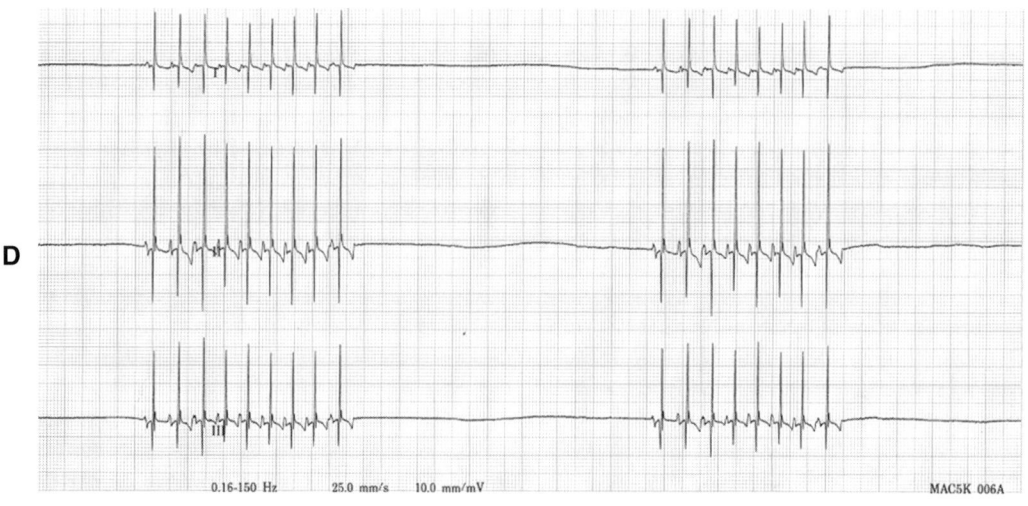

FIG. 27-24, cont'd
D, Bradycardia-tachycardia associated with sick sinus syndrome. (Courtesy Dr. M. Miller, Texas A&M University.)

standstill is caused by hyperkalemia. Persistent atrial standstill occurs due to a heritable muscular dystrophy syndrome involving the cardiac atria, ventricles, and scapulohumeral skeletal muscles.

AV block results when there is a delay or block of cardiac impulse conduction through the AV node. First-degree AV block is a prolongation of conduction through the AV node and usually results from exaggerated parasympathetic influence on the AV node (Fig. 25-24, *B*). Second-degree (incomplete) AV block is characterized by intermittent failure of impulse conduction through the AV node. Low-grade (infrequent) second-degree AV block usually results from exaggerated parasympathetic influence on the AV node. High-grade (frequent) second-degree AV block is more likely the result of intrinsic disease of the AV node. Third-degree (complete) AV block (Fig. 27-24, *C*) is a complete failure of conduction through the AV node and strongly implies intrinsic degenerative or infiltrative disease of the AV node. Third-degree AV block causes complete AV dissociation and development of a slow ventricular escape rhythm. The result is low and unresponsive cardiac output.

Frequent and long sinus pauses may result from degeneration and malfunction of the sinus node (Fig. 27-24, *D*). Sick sinus syndrome is the clinical result of sinus node malfunction and is characterized by frequent syncopal and near-syncopal episodes. Sick sinus syndrome may also be accompanied by frequent supraventricular tachycardia.

DIAGNOSIS
Clinical Presentation
Signalment. English springer spaniels and Siamese cats are predisposed to persistent atrial standstill. Small-breed dogs, particularly miniature schnauzers, are predisposed to sick sinus syndrome. Third-degree AV block occurs in all breeds.

History. Signs due to bradycardia include weakness, exercise intolerance, collapse, and syncope. The relatively short duration of syncopal episodes (usually only a few seconds) and lack of tonic-clonic motor activity or postictal signs can help distinguish syncope from neurologic seizures. However, sometimes syncopal and neurologic episodes are difficult to distinguish, sometimes requiring ambulatory ECG monitoring for definitive diagnosis.

Physical Examination Findings
Sinus bradycardia is recognized on the electrocardiogram as a normal but slow rhythm with normal P-QRS-T complexes. It is often accompanied by other vagal-mediated changes (i.e., sinus arrhythmia, wandering pacemaker, and low-grade, second-degree AV block). Sinus bradycardia is abolished by exercise or by administration of atropine or glycopyrrolate (Box 27-12).

Electrocardiography. Electrocardiographic abnormalities associated with transient atrial standstill are bradycardia, small or absent P waves, and shortening and widening of the QRS complexes (see Fig. 27-24, *A*). The major rule-outs for hyperkalemia are obstructive uropathy, acute renal failure, uroabdomen, adrenocortical insufficiency, diabetic ketoacidosis, and iatrogenic potassium intoxication. Electrocardiographic abnormalities associated with persistent atrial standstill are similar (e.g., an absence of P waves and a slow supraventricular or ventricular escape rhythm).

Electrocardiographic findings associated with sick sinus syndrome include intermittent severe bradycardia, sinus pauses that last several seconds, supraventricular escape complexes, and occasionally paroxysmal supraventricular tachycardia (see Fig. 27-24, *D*). Sick sinus syndrome causes frequent syncopal attacks but rarely causes sudden death. Sick sinus syndrome is usually not responsive to acute administration of atropine.

First-degree AV block (Box 27-13) is recognized by a prolongation of the P-R interval on an electrocardiogram (see

BOX 27-12

Atropine or Glycopyrrolate Response Test

Give 0.02–0.04 mg/kg atropine SC or IM; wait 15–20 minutes then recheck cardiac rhythm, or
  Give 0.01 mg/kg glycopyrrolate SC or IM; wait 15–20 minutes then recheck cardiac rhythm

SC, Subcutaneous; *IM,* intramuscular.

BOX 27-13

First-Degree AV Block

Dogs—PR interval >0.14 sec
Cats—PR interval >0.09 sec

Fig. 27-24, *B*). Second-degree AV block is intermittent failure of impulse conduction through the AV node. It is recognized on an electrocardiogram as a P wave that is not followed by a QRS-T complex. Low-grade, second-degree AV block is characterized by occasional "dropped complexes" after several normal complexes and usually is abolished by atropine. High-grade, second-degree AV is characterized by more dropped complexes than conducted complexes and usually does not respond to atropine. Third-degree AV block is recognized on an electrocardiogram by complete dissociation of the P waves and QRS-T complexes and by a slow ventricular escape rhythm (see Fig. 27-24, *C*). Third-degree AV block is not atropine-responsive.

Diagnostic Imaging

Thoracic radiographs are usually normal or show mild to moderate generalized cardiomegaly.

Echocardiography. With transient atrial standstill, echocardiography shows a lack of atrial motion and little or no flow through the mitral valve during the active atrial filling phase. Echocardiography is also used to rule out concurrent valvular or congenital abnormalities.

Laboratory Findings

Hyperkalemia may cause transient atrial standstill; however, with persistent atrial standstill, serum potassium levels are normal. Other specific laboratory abnormalities are not found.

DIFFERENTIAL DIAGNOSIS

Other causes of bradycardia (i.e., hyperkalemia, increased vagal tone from CNS disease [intracranial pressure] or abdominal disease) should be differentiated from intrinsic conduction system dysfunction.

MEDICAL MANAGEMENT

Therapy for atrial standstill secondary to hyperkalemia should be directed at immediately lowering serum potassium levels and correcting the underlying cause of hyperka-

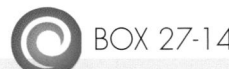

BOX 27-14

Therapy for Hyperkalemia

Physiologic Saline Solution (0.9%) IV
To dilute potassium

Sodium Bicarbonate*
1 to 2 mEq/kg IV (give over 10–20 min)

10% Calcium Gluconate†
0.5–1 ml/kg over 5–15 minutes, IV

IV, Intravenous.
*Used for moderate hyperkalemia.
†Temporary measure to sustain animal while other methods restore the potassium; monitor the ECG while administering this drug. If bradycardia occurs, stop infusion. Give only to patients that are critical and may die shortly from hyperkalemia.

BOX 27-15

Drugs Used to Increase Heart Rate in Animals With Unresponsive Bradycardia

Isoproterenol (Isuprel)
0.01 µg/kg/min IV

Propantheline Bromide (Pro-Banthine)
0.25–0.5 mg/kg PO, tid to qid

IV, Intravenous; *PO,* oral; *tid,* three times a day; *qid,* four times a day.

lemia. Intravenous fluid therapy should be initiated with physiologic saline solution. If the animal has concurrent hyponatremia, 5% dextrose solutions (i.e., D5W) and half-strength saline should be avoided. Very severe hyperkalemia rarely needs sodium bicarbonate therapy (Box 27-14). Bicarbonate therapy drives potassium into cells in exchange for hydrogen ions. Alternatively, insulin (0.5 to 1 unit/kg regular insulin intravenously) and dextrose (2 g per unit of insulin) can be administered. Insulin facilitates cellular uptake of potassium, whereas dextrose prevents hypoglycemia following insulin administration. If the hyperkalemia appears immediately life threatening, 10% calcium gluconate (NOTE: never give calcium chloride intravenously) given slowly intravenously may protect the heart until other therapy lowers the plasma potassium concentration.

Animals that have severe life-threatening bradycardia may require emergency therapy to increase their heart rate. Short-term anticholinergic therapy with atropine or glycopyrrolate may be attempted, but most clinically relevant bradycardias are not due to parasympathetic mechanisms and will not be responsive to these drugs. Intravenous adrenergic therapy with isoproterenol (Box 27-15) is sometimes effective as a short-term measure for the increasing heart rate associated with persistent atrial standstill or third-degree AV block.

The most reliable method for increasing heart rate in animals with unresponsive bradycardia is temporary transvenous pacing. This is accomplished by percutaneous jugular venous placement of a pacing electrode into the right side of the heart under sedation and local anesthetic (see later discussion under Anesthesia). The electrode is then connected to an external pulse generator. Long-term oral anticholinergic therapy with propantheline bromide (see Box 27-15) is sometimes advocated for various bradycardias. However, this drug is seldom effective for clinically relevant bradycardias and causes unpleasant side effects. Animals with sick sinus syndrome may require management of supraventricular tachycardia with digoxin, β-adrenergic blockade, or calcium channel blockade therapy after pacemaker implantation.

SURGICAL TREATMENT

Cardiac pacemaker therapy is indicated for bradycardias caused by intrinsic cardiac disease that is not responsive to atropine and that is causing clinical signs.

Preoperative Management

Most bradycardias are exacerbated by anesthetic drugs. Therefore some accommodation for maintaining an acceptable cardiac rhythm during permanent pacemaker implantation usually is necessary. Preanesthetic medication with an anticholinergic drug (e.g., atropine or glycopyrrolate) is indicated but rarely sufficient to prevent worsening of bradycardia during anesthesia. Temporary transvenous pacing is the most reliable method of maintaining an adequate heart rate during pacemaker implantation. Constant intravenous infusion of isoproterenol (see Box 27-15) is a less reliable means of maintaining heart rate during permanent pacemaker implantation. Perioperative antibiotic therapy (e.g., cefazolin) during pacemaker implantation is indicated to reduce the risk of implant-associated infections.

Anesthesia

Temporary pacemakers can be implanted in dogs under ketamine plus diazepam (Box 27-16) administered intravenously to effect for sedation; a local anesthetic is used to place the temporary pacemaker. Once the animal is paced, ketamine plus diazepam may be used for induction. Anesthesia should be maintained with isoflurane or sevoflurane and oxygen.

Surgical Anatomy

Refer to p. 777 for surgical anatomy of the heart.

> NOTE: If a unipolar system is used, the pulse generator does not begin to function until the generator casing is brought into contact with the patient to complete the electrical circuit.

Positioning

The animal is placed in dorsal recumbency for transdiaphragmatic pacemaker implantation. The entire abdomen and caudal thorax are prepared for aseptic surgery.

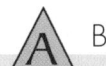 **BOX 27-16**

Anesthesia for Placement of a Temporary Pacemaker

Ketamine (5.5 mg/kg) plus diazepam (0.27 mg/kg)
Administer IV to effect for sedation
Use a local anesthetic at site of pacemaker insertion
Maintain anesthesia with isoflurane or sevoflurane and oxygen

IV, Intravenous.

SURGICAL TECHNIQUE

Epicardial pacemaker implantation in small animals is accomplished through a midline celiotomy diaphragmatic incision. The transdiaphragmatic approach has several advantages, including avoidance of a thoracotomy and abdominal placement of the generator.

Perform a celiotomy that extends cranially to the level of the xiphoid (Fig. 27-25, A). Make a vertical midline incision in the diaphragm, and expose the cardiac apex. Open the pericardium, and retract it gently with tissue forceps to expose the apex of the left ventricle (Fig. 27-25, B). Implant a screw-in electrode into the left ventricular apex by turning the electrode tip a specified number of rotations (see instruction sheet accompanying pacemaker; usually 2.5 turns) (Fig. 27-26). Bring the lead wire into the abdominal cavity through the diaphragmatic incision, and connect it to the pulse generator using the small screwdriver or locking mechanism provided by the manufacturer. Place the pulse generator in a pocket created between the transverse abdominis and internal abdominal oblique muscles (Fig. 27-25, C). Do not suture the pericardium. Close the diaphragm and abdomen in routine fashion (Fig. 27-25, D).

SUTURE MATERIALS AND SPECIAL INSTRUMENTS

Modern cardiac pulse generators are compact, have a long battery life, are programmable after implantation, and generally are capable of a variety of sophisticated pacing modes. A three-letter code identifies the intended site of cardiac sensing, intended site for cardiac pacing, and pacing mode. The most commonly used pacing mode in small animals is VVI, which stands for ventricular-sensing, ventricular-pacing, inhibited mode. This means that the pacemaker is intended to pace the cardiac ventricles, but it will sense naturally occurring ventricular impulses and inhibit its own output when they occur. This demand function prevents competitive rhythms between the heart and pacemaker should spontaneous intrinsic ventricular activity occur. Most recent model pulse generators are powered by lithium cells that have a life of 8 to 12 years. Pacemakers that have exceeded their shelf life for implantation in humans but still have several years of useful battery life left can often be obtained for a fraction of the cost of new pacemakers. Modern pacemakers are programmable by radiofrequency after implantation for several indices (i.e., pacing rate, stimulus volt-

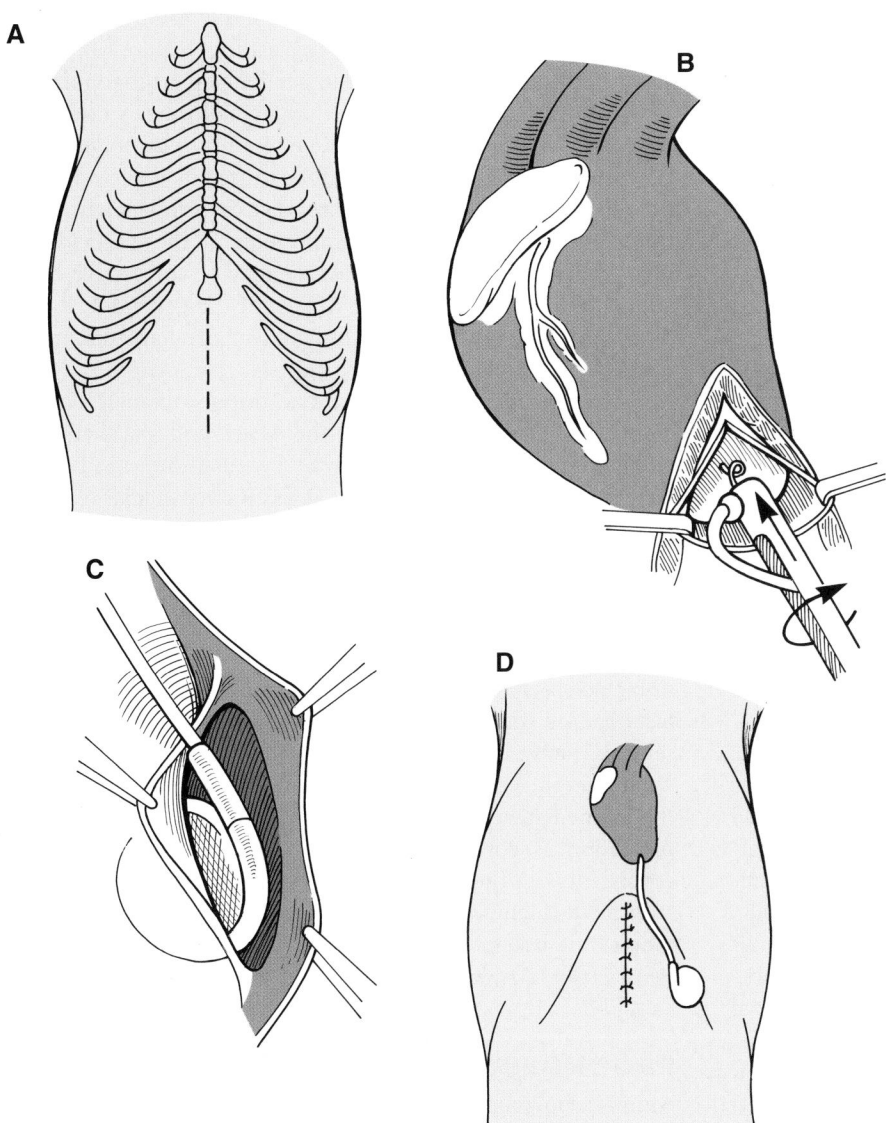

FIG. 27-25
A, Transdiaphragmatic pacemaker implantation may be performed via midline celiotomy. **B,** Incise the diaphragm on its midline and open and retract the pericardium to expose the cardiac apex. Implant a screw-in electrode into the left ventricular apex by turning the electrode the specified number of rotations. **C,** Bring the lead wire through the diaphragmatic incision and connect it to the pulse generator. Place the generator in a pocket created between the transverse abdominis and internal abdominal oblique muscles. **D,** Close the diaphragm and abdomen routinely.

age, and sensing voltage). Cardiologists or pacemaker technical representatives usually can provide appropriate programmers for setting pulse generator parameters before and after surgery. Dogs are paced at a rate of 70 to 110 beats per minute, depending on size and nature of the animal. Ideally, the stimulus voltage should be approximately two times the measured stimulus capture threshold. A voltage of 4 to 5 V is usually adequate.

Pacemaker electrodes are either endocardial (transvenous) or epicardial. Endocardial electrodes may be unipolar or bipolar and are intended for placement in the right ventricle via a jugular vein. Endocardial electrodes may be used for temporary or permanent cardiac pacing. Endocardial electrodes have the advantage of less invasive placement, but require facilities for cardiac catheterization and have a higher incidence of catheter dislodgement. Permanent endocardial electrode placement requires pulse generator implantation

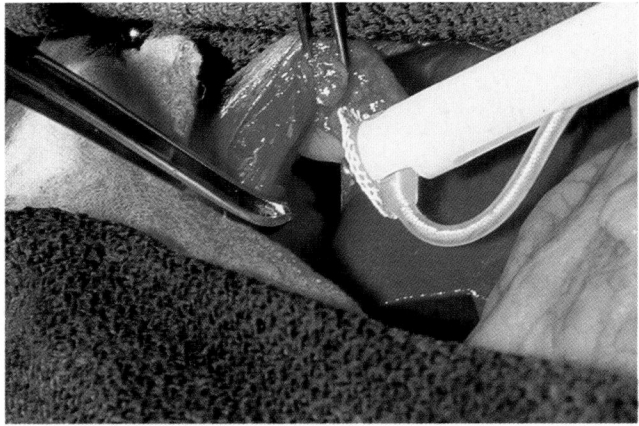

FIG. 27-26
Transdiaphragmatic pericardial electrode placement.

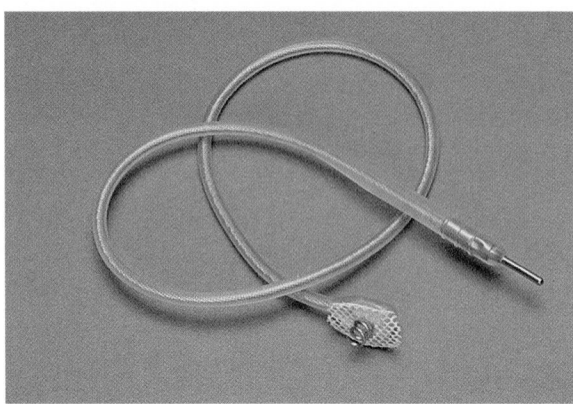

FIG. 27-27
Screw-in epicardial electrode.

in the neck. Epicardial leads are unipolar and require open thoracic surgery for implantation on the epicardial surface. The screw-in epicardial electrode has the advantage of not requiring epicardial sutures and allows a minimal thoracic approach for implantation (Fig. 27-27).

POSTOPERATIVE CARE AND ASSESSMENT

Pacemaker function should be monitored closely for the first 48 hours postoperatively, and thereafter every 3 to 6 months. Recognition of normal pacemaker function is an important aspect of pacemaker management after surgery. Demand (VVI) pacemakers should be monitored both for their ability to pace or capture the heart, and for their ability to sense intrinsic cardiac impulses and inhibit their output when intrinsic rhythms occur. Failure of either of these functions can cause serious problems for the patient. Paced beats are recognized on an electrocardiogram by the presence of a stimulus artifact just before the QRS-T. A stimulus artifact will be present on the electrocardiogram regardless of whether the stimulus captures the heart.

Failure to pace is recognized on an electrocardiogram by the presence of a stimulus artifact that is not followed by a QRS-T. Evaluation of paced beats for the presence of a T wave is important since artifacts that mimic the QRS complex may be present and can be misleading. Failure to pace also is recognized by its failure to generate an arterial pulse. Early failure to pace can be caused by an inadequate stimulus voltage or by a faulty connection between the electrode and generator. Late failure to pace can be caused by depletion of the generator battery, electrode breakage or dislodgement, or fibrosis leading to increased impedance at the electrode-myocardial interface. Failure to pace may be correctable by adjusting the pacing stimulus voltage of the generator. Radiographs are useful for evaluating for lead breakage, disconnection, or dislodgement.

Failure to sense intrinsic cardiac impulses can lead to competitive rhythms between the heart and pacemaker. Competitive rhythms are harmful because they result in tachycardia and place the patient at risk for ventricular fibrillation. Failure to sense is recognized on the electrocardiogram by the presence of an intrinsic cardiac impulse between two paced impulses with a normal pacing interval. Failure to sense may or may not be accompanied by failure to pace. Failure to sense can be caused by a failing generator battery or by increased impedance at the electrode-myocardial interface. Failure to sense may be correctable by adjusting the sensing voltage threshold of the generator.

Premature ventricular complexes are often observed in the immediate postoperative period after pacemaker implantation. The origin of the ventricular complexes is usually consistent with the site of electrode implantation. Ventricular ectopy usually is self-limiting and not a major problem as long as the pacemaker is sensing the premature complexes. Ventricular tachycardias that exceed 150 beats per minute should be suppressed with lidocaine therapy.

PROGNOSIS

Animals showing clinical signs of severe exercise intolerance or syncope as a result of bradycardia are at risk for sudden death or development of congestive heart failure. Pacemaker therapy is extremely effective in preventing these consequences and restoring reasonably normal activity to animals with clinically relevant bradycardia.

CHAPTER 28

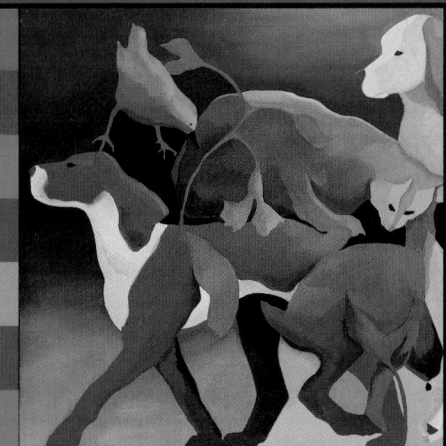

Surgery of the Upper Respiratory System

GENERAL PRINCIPLES AND TECHNIQUES

DEFINITIONS

Rhinotomy is an incision into the nasal cavity. **Tracheotomy** is an incision through the tracheal wall. **Tracheostomy** is creation of a temporary or permanent opening into the trachea to facilitate airflow. The permanent tracheostomy opening is called a **tracheostoma**. **Tracheal resection and anastomosis** is removal of a segment of trachea and reapposition of the divided tracheal ends. **Ventriculocordectomy** (*debarking* or *devocalization*) is resection of the vocal cords.

PREOPERATIVE MANAGEMENT

Upper airway procedures are performed to remove, repair, or bypass areas of obstruction, injury, or disease (Box 28-1). Affected animals may have mild to severe respiratory distress. Mild or moderately dyspneic patients initially should be examined from a distance to prevent exacerbating the condition. Open-mouth breathing, abducted forelimbs, labored breathing, and restlessness indicate moderate to severe respiratory distress that may require emergency therapy. Minimal restraint should be used with severely dyspneic patients, and they should be allowed to maintain the position in which they feel most comfortable. Supplemental oxygen may be given by means of nasal insufflation, tracheostomy tube or catheter, endotracheal intubation, mask (including an Elizabethan collar that has had plastic wrap put over it to form a "cage" over the head), or oxygen cage (see Chapter 5). Corticosteroids, sedation, or cooling (or all of these) may relieve distress. Sedation may be beneficial for anxious patients (especially those with upper airway obstruction) with moderate to severe respiratory distress. Combinations of intravenous drugs are commonly given; hydromorphone or butorphanol and either acepromazine or diazepam are frequently used in dogs (Box 28-2). As an alternative, fentanyl plus droperidol may be used. In cats, acepromazine or diazepam is recommended (Box 28-3). To cool dyspneic animals, a fan may be directed at the patient; ice packs may be applied to the head, axilla, inguinal area,

BOX 28-1

Indications for Upper Respiratory Tract Surgery

- Brachycephalic syndrome
- Devocalization
- Laryngeal collapse
- Laryngotracheal trauma
- Laryngeal paralysis
- Tracheal collapse
- Laryngeal masses
- Tracheal masses
- Nasal masses or infection
- Nasal trauma
- Foreign bodies
- Congenital abnormalities

BOX 28-2

Sedation of Severely Dyspneic Dogs

Hydromorphone
0.1–0.2 mg/kg IV, IM, or SC

Butorphanol (Torbutrol, Torbugesic)
0.2–0.4 mg/kg IV, IM, or SC

Acepromazine
0.02–0.05 mg/kg, max 1 mg IV, IM, or SC

Diazepam (Valium)
0.2 mg/kg IV

Fentanyl plus Droperidol (Innovar-Vet)
1 ml/20–40 kg IV or 1 ml/10–15 kg IM

IV, Intravenous; *IM,* intramuscular; *SC,* subcutaneous.

and extremities; and/or cooled fluids may be administered intravenously.

Diagnosis of upper respiratory disease is based on the history and clinical signs, physical examination findings, hematologic and serum biochemical parameters, radio-

BOX 28-3

Sedation of Severely Dyspneic Cats

Acepromazine
0.05 mg/kg, IV, IM, or SC

Diazepam (Valium)*
0.2 mg/kg IV

Butorphanol (Torbutrol, Torbugesic)
0.2–0.4 mg/kg IV, IM, or SC

IV, Intravenous; *IM,* intramuscular; *SC,* subcutaneous.
*Use with caution; may not reliably result in sedation.

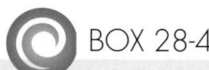

BOX 28-4

Premedicants for Laryngeal Examination in Dogs

Atropine
0.02–0.04 mg/kg IM or SC

Glycopyrrolate
0.005–0.011 mg/kg IM or SC

Hydromorphone (Dilaudid)
0.05–0.2 mg/kg IV or IM

Butorphanol (Torbutrol, Torbugesic)
0.2–0.4 mg/kg IM or SC

Buprenorphine (Buprenex)
5–15 µg/kg IM

IM, Intramuscular; *SC,* subcutaneous.

graphs, endoscopy, cytologic studies, culture, or biopsy, or all of these. The history and clinical signs may include abnormal respiratory noises (e.g., cough, inspiratory stridor, and wheeze), exercise intolerance, hyperthermia, tachypnea, dyspnea, cyanosis, restlessness, and/or collapse. Gagging and regurgitation of secretions are common with nasopharyngeal, laryngeal, and some tracheal abnormalities. Mucopurulent or bloody discharges are common with obstructive or infectious nasal disease. Voice change may occur with laryngeal paralysis, and dysphagia may be noted with supraglottic obstructions. Subcutaneous emphysema occurs with penetrating laryngotracheal or nasal injuries. Clinical signs may intensify or may be precipitated by excitement, stress, eating, drinking, or high ambient temperatures. Laboratory data should be evaluated to detect underlying metabolic disease and determine the advisability of general anesthesia. Tidal breathing flow volume loops are helpful in classifying obstructions as fixed or nonfixed. Pulmonary function tests, electromyography, and nerve conduction studies are ancillary tests that may indicate pulmonary or neuromuscular disease.

Animals with nasal neoplasia, fungal infection, or foreign bodies may be anemic as a result of profuse epistaxis. Affected animals should be carefully evaluated for clotting abnormalities by assessing platelet numbers, bleeding from venipuncture sites, or the presence of ecchymosis, petechiation, melena, hematuria, or retinal hemorrhage. If available, coagulative ability may be assessed by determining the activated clotting time, prothrombin time, partial thromboplastin time, and/or mucosal bleeding time. Blood transfusions or purified hemoglobin should be given before surgery if the packed-cell volume (PCV) is 20% or lower. Bleeding during rhinotomy may be severe, requiring intraoperative blood transfusion or carotid artery ligation, or both.

A preoperative antiinflammatory dose of a corticosteroid (dexamethasone [Azium], 0.5 to 2 mg/kg IV, IM, or SC; repeated administration of dexamethasone can cause gastrointestinal hemorrhage) may reduce nasopharyngeal and upper airway edema secondary to surgical or diagnostic manipulations. Corticosteroids are routinely given for nasopharyngeal and intraluminal laryngeal procedures.

ANESTHESIA

Patients with upper respiratory obstruction or disruption are extreme anesthetic risks. The periods of greatest danger are during induction of anesthesia and recovery (see p. 830 under Postoperative Care and Assessment). For laryngeal examination, care should be taken to avoid drugs that inhibit laryngeal function. If the animal has already been sedated (see previous discussion) an anticholinergic drug (atropine or glycopyrrolate; Box 28-4) should be given. An opioid (hydromorphone, butorphanol, or buprenorphine) may also be administered to unsedated animals. Propofol may be used for induction because it is noncumulative and may be given in small, incremental doses that maintain laryngeal function (Box 28-5). A combination of diazepam and ketamine is also useful for induction because these drugs maintain laryngeal function; however, exposure of the larynx in normal dogs is more readily accomplished with thiopental or propofol than with diazepam-ketamine (Gross et al, 2002). Oxygen should be supplemented during the examination, and oxygen saturation should be monitored with pulse oximetry (preferable) or by observation of mucous membrane color. Afterwards, the patient should be intubated and anesthesia maintained with inhalant drugs in oxygen for further diagnostics or surgery.

General anesthesia is preferred for most upper respiratory procedures because it ensures a patent airway, allows controlled ventilation, facilitates asepsis, and is less stressful for patients. Local anesthesia may allow placement of a tracheostomy tube when the patient is comatose or cannot tolerate general anesthesia. Dyspneic patients should be preoxygenated with a face mask if possible. Affected animals being anesthetized (see previous discussion for laryngeal examination) may be premedicated with an opioid, but continuous monitoring is necessary. Anticholinergics are indicated for bradycardia. Induction should be rapid (e.g., propofol, thiobarbiturate, or ketamine plus diazepam), and oxygen should be administered immediately. Mask induc-

BOX 28-5

Selected Anesthetic Protocols for Use in Animals Undergoing Upper Respiratory Tract Surgery

Preoxygenate 2–3 minutes before induction

For Dyspneic, Nonarrhythmic Animals

Premedication and induction*

Diazepam (0.2 mg/kg given IV) followed immediately with thiopental (10–12 mg/kg IV) or propofol (4–6 mg/kg IV) to effect. As an alternative, give diazepam (0.27 mg/kg IV) plus ketamine (5.5 mg/kg IV) titrated to effect.

Maintenance

Isoflurane or sevoflurane

For Very Sick or Arrhythmic Animals

Premedication and induction

Diazepam (0.2 mg/kg IV) followed by etomidate (1–3 mg/kg IV)

Maintenance

Isoflurane or sevoflurane

IV, Intravenous.
*For unsedated dogs, hydromorphone (0.1–0.2 mg/kg IV) may be given as part of the induction and the etomidate or barbiturate dose decreased. For unsedated cats, butorphanol (0.2–0.4 mg/kg IV) or buprenorphine (0.007–0.015 mg/kg IV) may be given as part of the induction and the etomidate or barbiturate dose decreased.

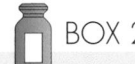 BOX 28-6

Antibiotic Choices for Upper Respiratory Infection

Ampicillin
22 mg/kg IV, IM, or SC, tid

Amoxicillin
22 mg/kg, PO, bid

Cefazolin (Ancef, Kefzol)
22 mg/kg IV or IM, tid

Amikacin (Amiglyde-V)
20–25 mg/kg IV, IM, or SC, qd

Enrofloxacin (Baytril)*
7–20 mg/kg PO or IV (administer dilute solution slowly, over 30 min) qd

Doxycycline
5 mg/kg PO or IV, bid†

Azithromycin (Zithromax)
Dogs: 5–10 mg/kg PO, qd or bid for 5 to 20 days
Cats: 5–15 mg/kg PO, qod to qd to bid for 3–5 days

IV, Intravenous; *IM,* intramuscular; *SC,* subcutaneous; *tid,* three times a day; *PO,* oral; *bid,* twice a day; *qd,* once a day; *qod,* every other day.
*Doses greater than 5 mg/kg may be associated with blindness in cats.
†Do not administer with milk products. Be sure to have the patient drink or eat after receiving the medication; if the pill sticks in the esophagus, it can cause severe esophagitis.

---

tion is not recommended. Anesthesia should be maintained with inhalant drugs in oxygen. Laryngeal or tracheal procedures may require temporary retraction of the endotracheal tube from the surgical site, placing an endotracheal tube distal to the surgical site through a tracheotomy, or using injectable anesthetic drugs. During surgery the animal should be sighed (given an extra large breath) every minute or two to renew surfactant. Oxygen saturation or blood gases (or both) should be monitored from induction until recovery and until abnormalities have been corrected. Selected anesthetic protocols are provided in Box 28-5.

ANTIBIOTICS

Because the respiratory tract has a normal bacterial flora, prophylactic antibiotics (e.g., cefazolin; Box 28-6) frequently are given before surgery. However, animals with normal immune function undergoing short procedures (e.g., nares resection, laryngeal saccule resection, and vocal cordectomy) do not need them. Streptococci, *Escherichia coli, Pseudomonas* spp., *Klebsiella* spp., and *Bordetella bronchiseptica* are most commonly isolated from normal dogs. A majority of tracheal cultures are sterile, whereas most pharyngeal cultures are not.

The gram-negative organisms that cause most canine respiratory tract infections are resistant to commonly used antibiotics. Antimicrobial drug selection is best based on cyto-

logic and culture results of tracheobronchial, pulmonary parenchymal, and/or pleural secretions. Bland aerosol therapy (e.g., sterile 0.9% saline) helps loosen secretions and facilitates their clearance in dogs with tracheostomies; addition of antibiotics to the aerosol generally is unnecessary. However, intratracheal or aerosolized antibiotics may be effective in some dogs with chronic respiratory infections. Lipid-soluble antibiotics that contain a benzene ring reach the highest levels in the normal trachea and bronchus; however, increased permeability associated with inflammation allows numerous antibiotics to achieve high levels during infection. Antibiotics commonly recommended for treatment of upper respiratory disease include ampicillin, fluoroquinolones, cephalosporins, aminoglycosides, doxycycline, azithromycin, and potentiated sulfonamides (see Box 28-6).

SURGICAL ANATOMY

The nasal cavity extends from the nostrils to the nasopharyngeal meatus and is separated into two halves by the *nasal septum* (Fig. 28-1). The septum is mostly cartilaginous, but also has bony and membranous portions. The *nasal conchae* develop from the lateral and dorsal walls of the nasal cavity. The air passages between the conchae are known as *meatus.* The *paranasal sinuses* include a maxillary recess, frontal si-

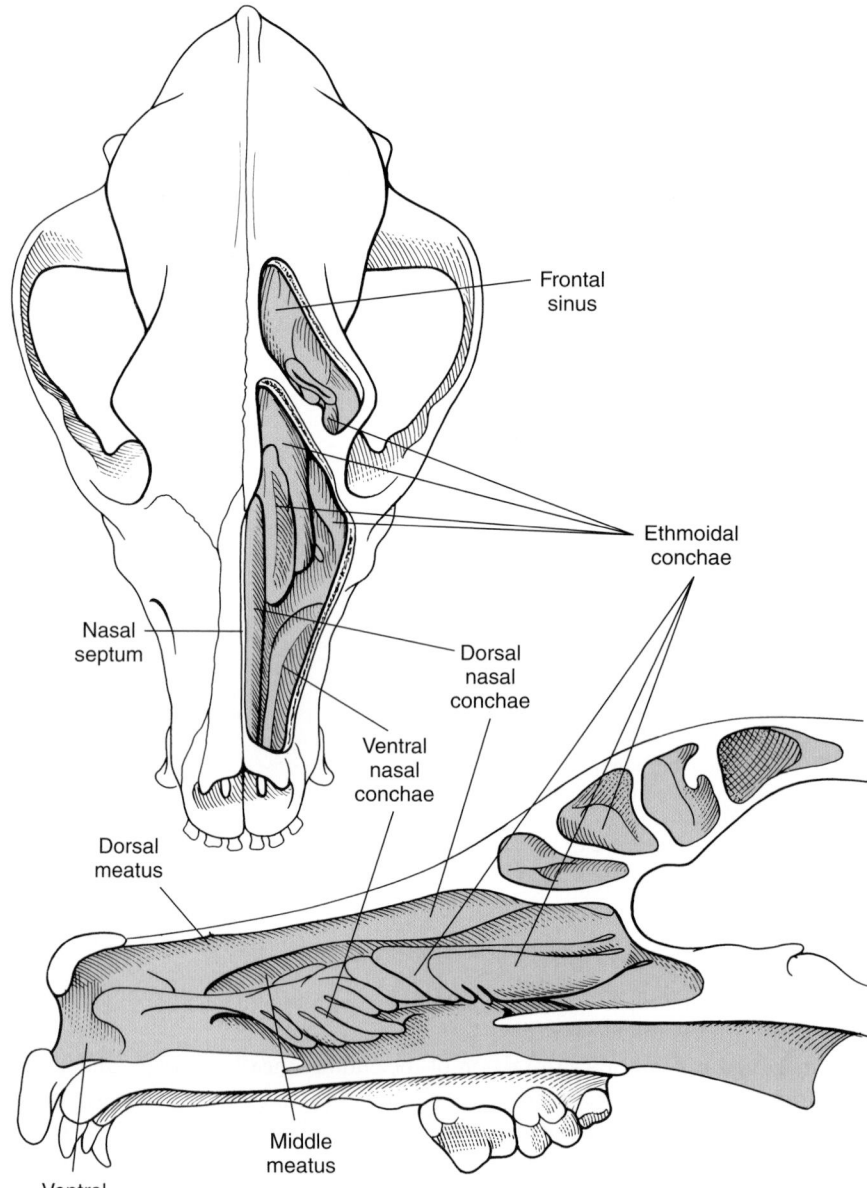

FIG. 28-1
Anatomy of the canine nasal cavity.

nus, and sphenoidal sinus. The *frontal sinus* occupies the supraorbital process of the frontal bone (see Fig 28-1). The two sides are separated by a median septum, and in dogs each side is divided into rostral, medial, and lateral compartments.

The *thyroid cartilage* forms the ventral and lateral walls of the larynx (Fig. 28-2). It surrounds the lateral aspect of the cricoid cartilage and articulates with the dorsolateral aspect of the cricoid cartilage (caudal) and thyrohyoid bones (cranial). Ventrally the cricothyroid ligament joins the caudal border of the thyroid cartilage to the cricoid cartilage. The *cricoid cartilage* is a complete ring that is five times wider dorsally than it is ventrally (see Fig. 28-2). It forms the dorsal wall of the larynx and cranially lies within the wings of thyroid cartilage. The cricoid cartilage articulates at its cra-

nial dorsolateral margin with the arytenoid cartilage, which is paired (see Fig. 28-2). At the entrance to the glottis (laryngeal inlet), the arytenoid cartilages have two *cuneiform processes* ventrally and two corniculate processes dorsally. The *vocal fold* attaches to the vocal process of the arytenoid at its ventral aspect. The muscular processes are dorsolateral at the caudal aspect of the arytenoid.

The *glottis* (laryngeal inlet) consists of the vocal folds, vocal processes of the arytenoid cartilages, and rima glottidis (see Fig. 28-2). The vocal folds extend dorsally from the vocal processes of the arytenoids to the thyroid cartilage ventrally. Rostral and lateral to the vocal folds are the laryngeal ventricles, or saccules. The laryngeal saccule is a mucosal diverticulum bounded laterally by the thyroid cartilage and medially by the arytenoid cartilage. The vestibular fold (false

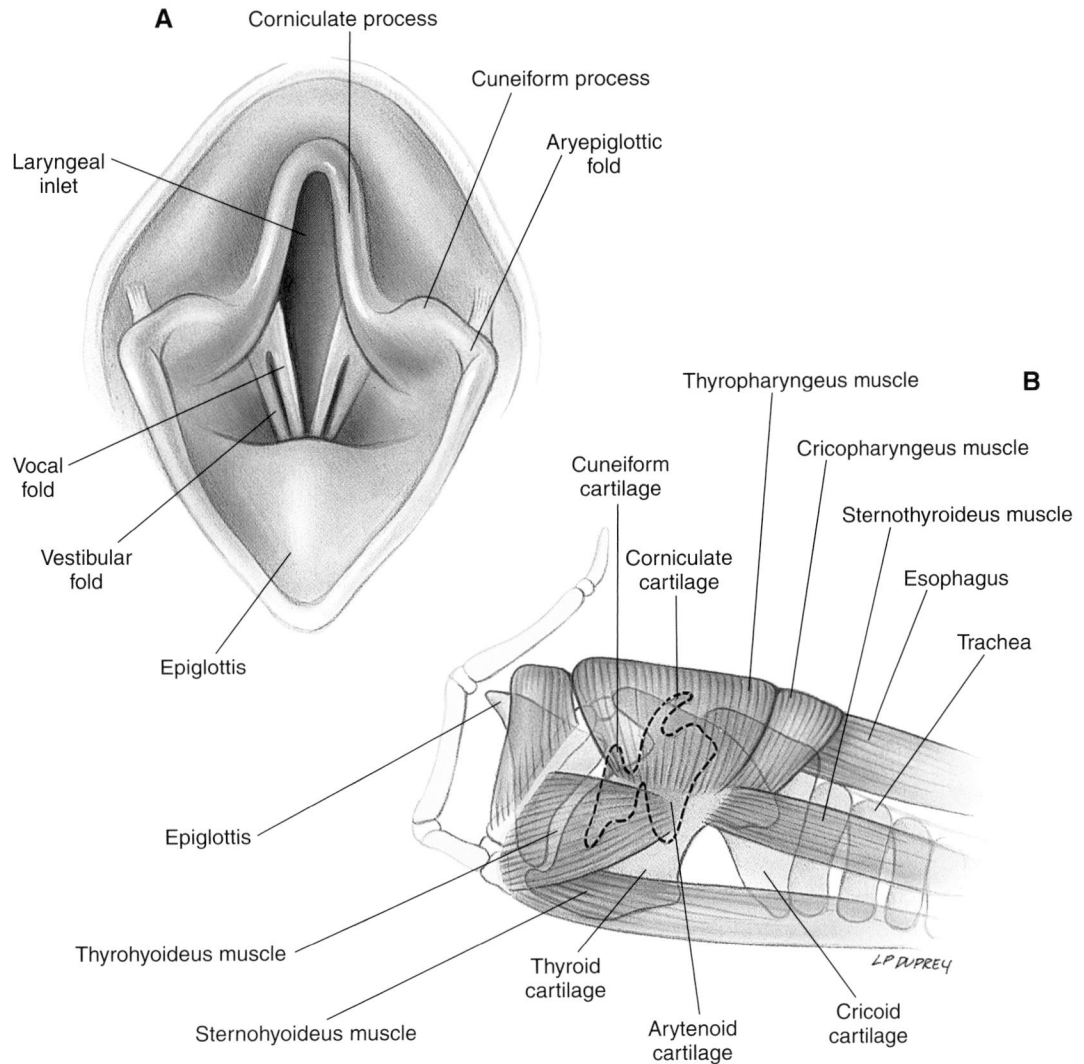

FIG. 28-2
Laryngeal anatomy. **A,** Oral view. **B,** Lateral view.

vocal cord) forms the rostral border of the laryngeal saccule and attaches to the cuneiform process.

The intrinsic muscles of the dog's larynx are innervated by somatic efferent axons from the vagus nerve. Some axons leave the vagus in the *cranial laryngeal nerve* to innervate the cricothyroid muscle; others provide sensory innervation to the mucosa. The *recurrent laryngeal nerve,* a branch of the vagus, terminates as the caudal laryngeal nerve, which innervates the remaining intrinsic muscles of the larynx. The *caudal laryngeal nerve* travels along the dorsolateral surface of the trachea and continues over the lateral surface of the cricoarytenoideus dorsalis before deviating to the medial surface of the thyroid cartilage lamina. The *cranial laryngeal artery,* a branch of the external carotid artery, travels with the cranial laryngeal nerve. It is the main blood supply to the larynx. The cranial laryngeal vein empties into the hyoid venous arch and then the external jugular vein. Lymphatics drain into the retropharyngeal lymph node.

The *trachea* is a semirigid, flexible tube extending from the cricoid cartilage to the mainstem bronchi at about the fourth or fifth thoracic vertebra. Thirty-five to 45 C-shaped hyaline cartilages, joined by annular ligaments ventrally and laterally and by trachealis muscle *(dorsal tracheal membrane)* dorsally, form the trachea. The tracheal vessels and nerves, which are found in the lateral pedicles, supply the trachea segmentally. Loose areolar connective tissue surrounds the trachea and forms the lateral pedicles. The cranial and caudal thyroid arteries and veins, bronchoesophageal arteries and veins, and internal jugular veins supply vascular branches to the trachea. Innervation is by the autonomic nervous system. Sympathetic fibers from the middle cervical ganglion and sympathetic trunk inhibit tracheal muscle contraction and glandular secretions, whereas parasympathetic fibers from the vagus and recurrent laryngeal nerves cause tracheal muscle contraction and glandular secretions.

SURGICAL TECHNIQUE

Surgical techniques for the management of animals with upper respiratory disease include rhinotomy (this page), tracheotomy (see page 825), tracheostomy (see page 825), tracheal resection and anastomosis (see p. 827), ventriculocordectomy (see p. 828), tracheoplasty (see p. 850), arytenoid cartilage lateralization (see p. 844), partial laryngectomy (see p. 845), and surgery for stenotic nares (see p. 832), elongated soft palate (see p. 835), and everted laryngeal saccules (see p. 838).

Rhinotomy

The nasal cavity may be approached through dorsal, ventral, or lateral approaches. The dorsal approach is most commonly used for exploration and biopsy; however, the ventral approach can be used to explore the region caudal to the ethmoid turbinates and the ventral aspect of the turbinates. Lateral approaches are limited to lesions in the rostral aspect of the nasal cavity.

Dorsal approach to the nasal cavity and paranasal sinuses. *With the animal in ventral recumbency, make a dorsal midline skin incision from the caudal aspect of the nasal planum to the medial canthus of the orbit. Either or both sides of the nasal cavity can be entered through a single midline skin incision. To explore the frontal sinus, extend the incision caudal to a line that connects the zygomatic processes of the frontal bone. Incise the subcutaneous tissue and periosteum on the midline. Elevate the periosteum and reflect it laterally on either or both sides of the nasal cavity. Use a bone saw to create and then elevate a flap of bone over the proposed site of entry into the nasal cavity (Fig. 28-3, A). Save the bone flap (if healthy) and replace it after the nasal cavity has been explored. As an alternative, drill a hole to one side of the nasal septum with a Steinmann pin. Use rongeurs to enlarge the hole and discard the bone fragments. If necessary, extend the bone removal bilaterally. Gently lavage the nasal passages and remove*

FIG. 28-3
Dorsal approach to the nasal cavity. **A,** Make a skin incision from the caudal aspect of the nasal planum to the medial canthus of the orbit (bold dashed line). Elevate a bone flap (dashed rectangle) or use rongeurs to remove bone. **B,** If a bone flap was made, suture it in place with wire or sutures placed through predrilled holes in the bone flap and adjacent bone. **C,** If rongeurs were used to remove bone, close the periosteum and subcutaneous tissue, leaving a stoma at the caudal aspect of the incision. Close the skin similarly, leaving a stoma.

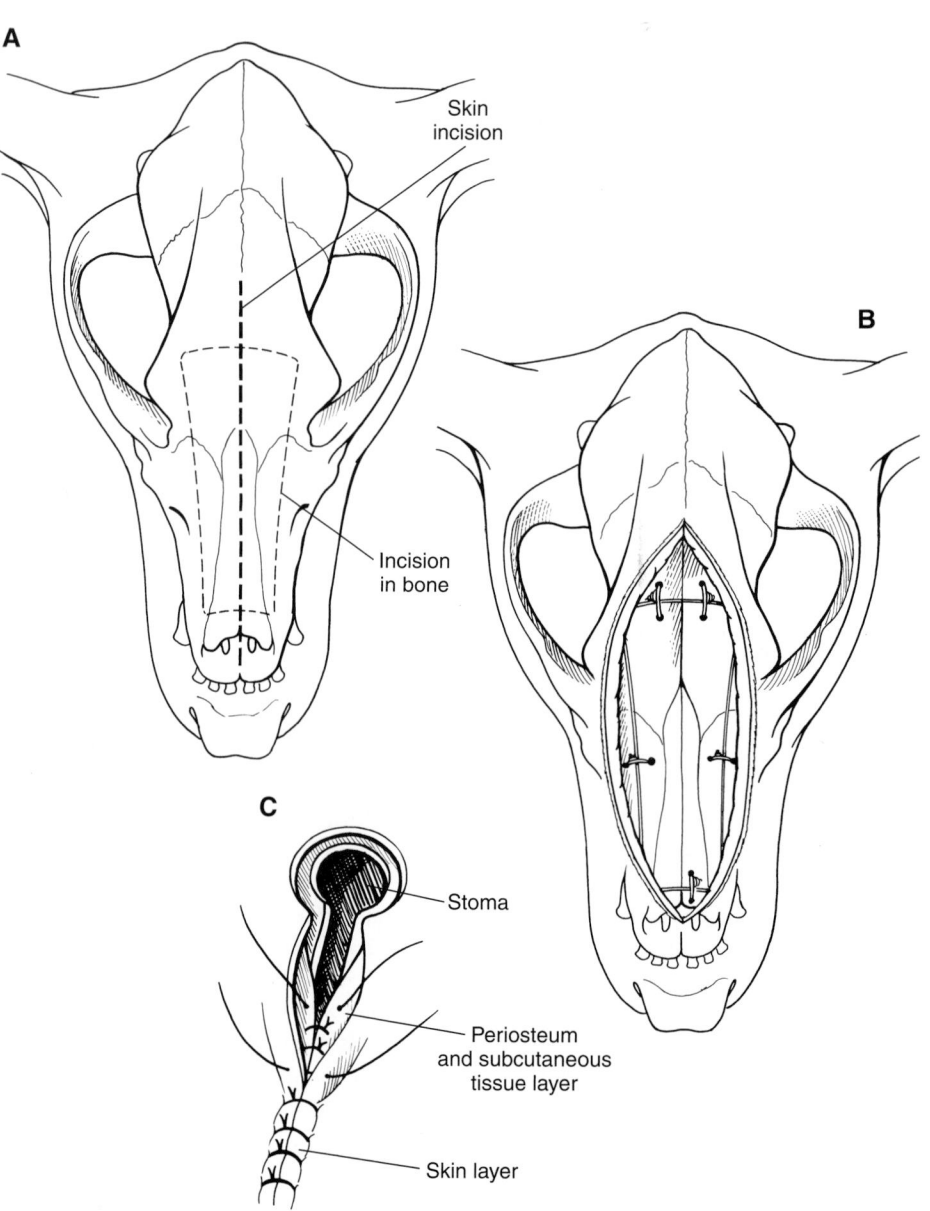

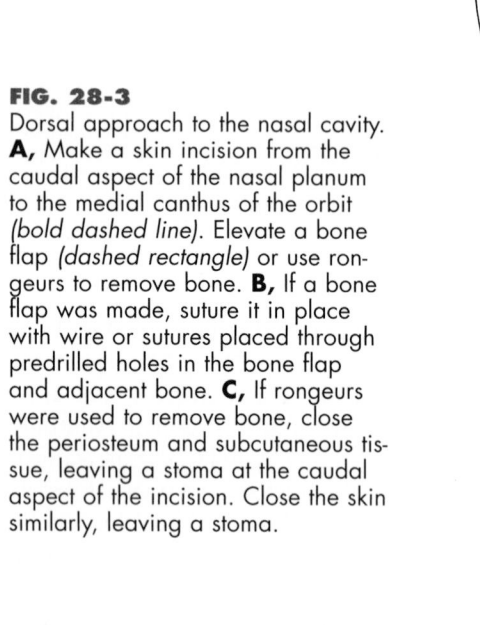

abnormal tissue. Submit tissues for histologic examination and culture. Use cautery, iced saline, or pressure (or all of these) to control hemorrhage. If continued hemorrhage is a problem, pack the nasal cavity with cotton gauze (see p. 862). If a bone flap was made, suture it in place with 3-0 or 4-0 wire (do not use wire to replace the bone flap if radiation therapy is planned) placed through predrilled holes in the bone flap and adjacent bone (Fig. 28-3, B). Close the periosteum and subcutaneous tissues with absorbable suture material in a simple continuous pattern. Close the skin routinely. If rongeurs were used, close the periosteum and subcutaneous tissues, leaving a stoma at the caudal aspect of the incision. Close the skin similarly, leaving a stoma (Fig. 28-3, C).

Ventral approach to the nasal cavity. *With the animal in dorsal recumbency (Fig. 28-4), make a midline incision in the hard palate. Elevate the mucoperiosteum of the hard palate laterally to the alveolar ridge. Be careful to spare the palatine nerves and vessels as they emerge from the major palatine foramen. Incise the mucoperiosteum and soft palate attachments to the caudal edge of the palatine bone and extend the incision as far caudally as necessary into the soft palate (full thickness). Retract the edges of the incision with stay sutures. Remove the palatine bone with a power-driven burr or rongeurs and discard it (Fig. 28-5, A). Explore the nasal cavity and remove abnormal tissues. Submit tissues for histologic examination and culture. Close the nasal mucosa of the soft palate with absorbable material in a simple continuous or simple interrupted pattern. Then close the submucosa-periosteum of the hard palate with absorbable suture in an interrupted pattern (Fig. 28-5, B).*

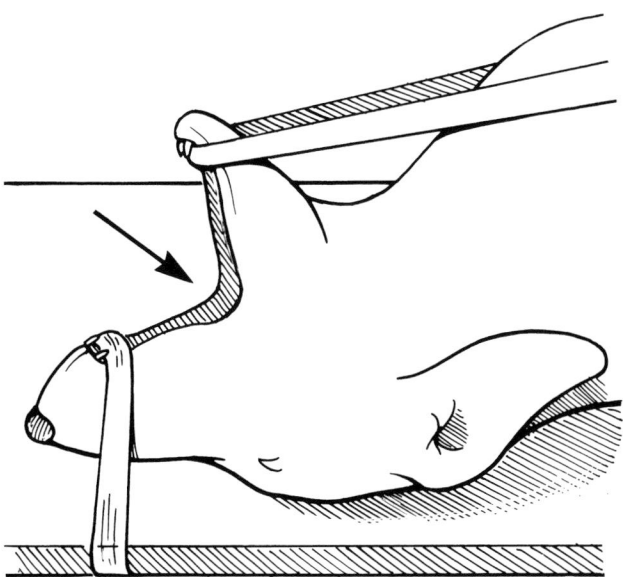

FIG. 28-4
Positioning for a ventral approach to the nasal cavity.

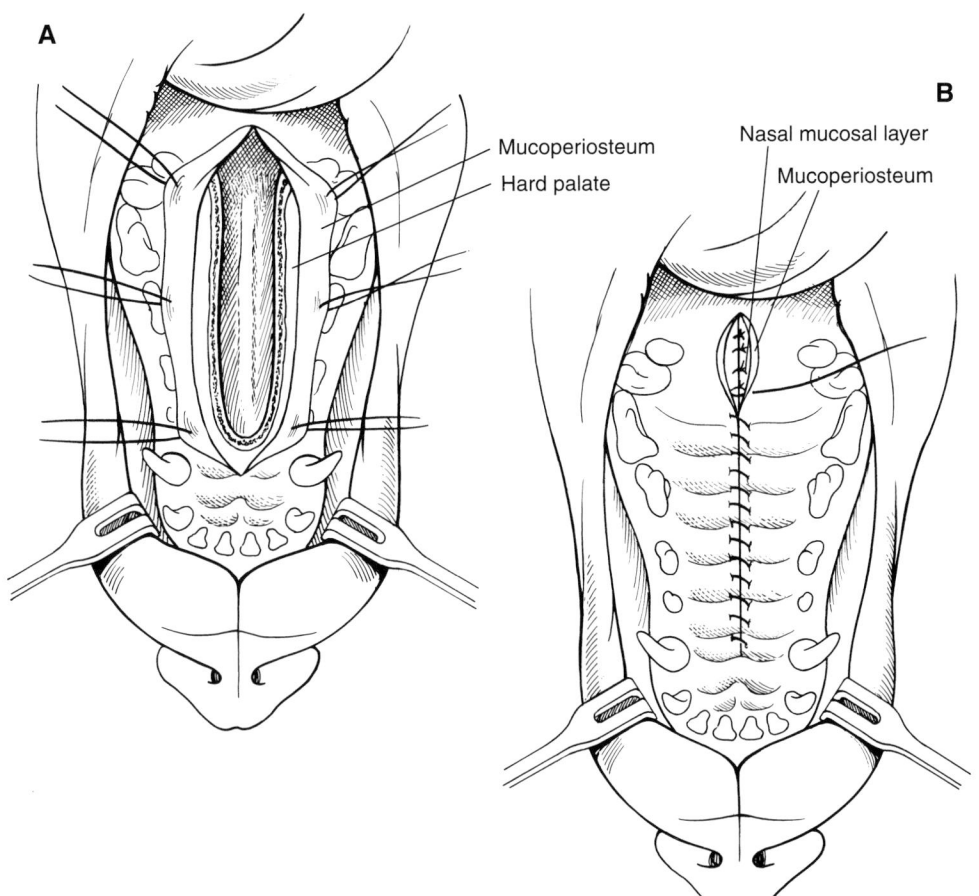

A

Mucoperiosteum
Hard palate

B

Nasal mucosal layer
Mucoperiosteum

FIG. 28-5
Ventral approach to the nasal cavity. **A,** Incise the mucoperiosteum of the hard palate. Remove the palatine bone with a power-driven burr or rongeurs and discard it. **B,** Close the nasal mucosa of the soft palate and submucosa-periosteum of the hard palate with absorbable suture in an interrupted or continuous pattern. Close the oral mucosa of the hard and soft palates with monofilament, nonabsorbable suture in a simple continuous pattern.

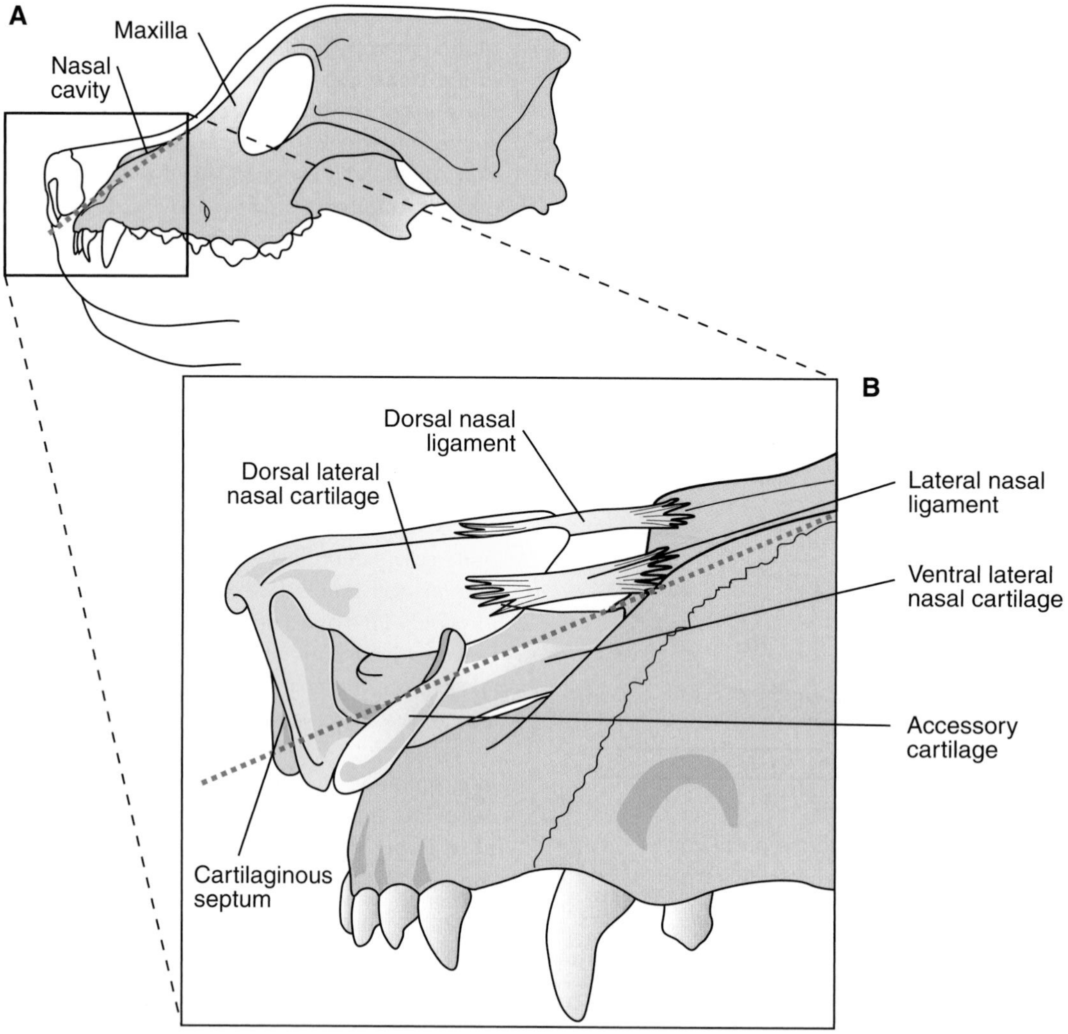

FIG. 28-6
Lateral approach to the rostral nasal cavity. **A,** Make the incision for lateral rhinotomy in a dorsocaudal direction from the nasal planum toward the nasomaxillary notch. **B,** Direct the incision between the dorsal lateral nasal cartilage and ventral lateral nasal cartilage. Transection of the accessory cartilage cannot be avoided.

Finally, close the oral mucosa of the hard and soft palates with monofilament nonabsorbable sutures in a simple continuous pattern.

Lateral approach to the rostral nasal cavity. This approach gives access to the nasal vestibule. Position the animal in lateral or dorsal recumbency.

Make an incision with a scalpel or Mayo scissors. When using scissors insert one blade into the nostril and position it so the incision will be made ventral to the nasal planum and dorsal lateral nasal cartilage (Fig. 28-6). Angle the incision in a dorsocaudal direction toward the nasomaxillary notch. Incise through all layers and retract the tissue dorsally to expose the vestibule. Explore and resect or biopsy abnormal tissue. Appose the nasal mucosa with 3-0 or 4-0 monofilament absorbable suture. Place 2 to 4

sutures in the musculocartilage layer (3-0 or 4-0 monofilament absorbable) and then reappose the skin (3-0 or 4-0 monofilament nonabsorbable).

Intraoral approach to the rostral nasal cavity. This approach has been used to remove foreign bodies (Priddy et al, 2001) and may be useful for removal or biopsy of rostral nasal masses, such as rhinosporidiosis.

Palpate the ridge along the rostrolateral aspect of the right (or left) nasal and incisive bone (Fig. 28-7). Incise the alveolar mucosa along this ridge from the nasal bone to the rostral end of the interincisive suture. Using a periosteal elevator, reflect the mucosa from these bones. Then retract the dorsal lateral nasal cartilage and the ventral lateral nasal cartilage medially. Penetrate the nasal mucosa and explore the rostral nasal cavity. Biopsy abnormal tissue and lavage the area.

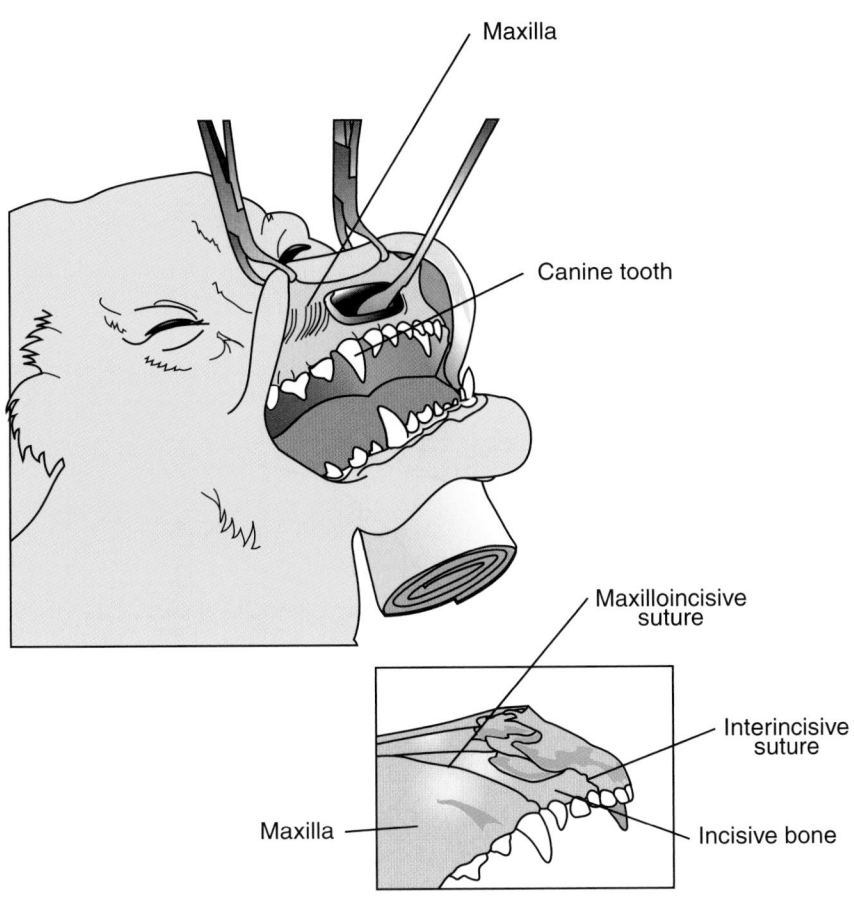

Maxilla

Canine tooth

Maxilloincisive
suture

Interincisive
suture

Maxilla

Incisive bone

FIG. 28-7
Oral approach to the rostral nasal cavity.
Elevate the lip and incise along the ridge at
the rostrolateral aspect of the right (or left)
nasal bone to the rostral end of the interincisive suture. Using a periosteal elevator,
reflect the mucosa from these bones. Retract
the dorsal lateral nasal cartilage and the
ventral lateral nasal cartilage medially.
Close the gingival and buccal mucosa with
3-0 or 4-0 monofilament absorbable suture.

*Close the gingival and buccal mucosa with 3-0 or 4-0 mono-
filament absorbable suture.*

Tracheotomy

Tracheotomy is performed to gain access to the tracheal lumen to remove obstructions, collect specimens, or facilitate
airflow. The tracheal incision may be closed or allowed to
heal by secondary intention. Position the patient as described on p. 850.

*Approach the cervical trachea through a ventral cervical
midline incision. Extend the incision from the larynx to the
sternum as needed to allow adequate exposure. Separate
the sternohyoid muscles along their midline and retract them
laterally (Fig. 28-8, A). Dissect the peritracheal connective
tissue from the ventral surface of the trachea at the proposed
tracheotomy site. Take care to prevent traumatizing the
recurrent laryngeal nerves, carotid artery, jugular vein, thyroid vessels, or esophagus. Immobilize the trachea between
the thumb and forefinger. Make a horizontal or vertical incision through the wall of the trachea (see Fig. 28-8, A). Place
cartilage-encircling sutures around adjacent cartilages to
separate the edges and allow lumen inspection or tube insertion. Suction blood, secretions, and debris from the tracheal
lumen. After completion of the procedure, appose the tracheal edges with simple interrupted 3-0 or 4-0 polypropylene sutures. To close the tracheal incision, place sutures*

*through the annular ligaments encircling adjacent cartilages
or through the annular ligaments only. Lavage the surgical
site with saline. Appose the sternohyoid muscles in a simple
continuous pattern with 3-0 or 4-0 absorbable suture (e.g.,
polydioxanone, polyglyconate, or polyglactin 910). Appose
the subcutaneous tissues and skin routinely.*

Tracheostomy

Tracheostomy allows air to enter the trachea distal to the
nose, mouth, nasopharynx, and larynx. A tracheotomy is
performed to insert a tube (temporary tracheostomy) or
create a stoma (permanent tracheostomy) to facilitate airflow. A nonreactive tube that is no larger than one half the
size of the trachea should be selected. Cuffed or cannulated
autoclavable silicone, silver, or nylon tubes are recommended. Polyvinyl chloride and red rubber tubes are irritating and should be avoided. If the animal is to be placed on a
respirator, a cuffed tube is necessary.

Temporary tracheostomy. A temporary tracheostomy is most commonly performed to provide an alternate
airflow route during surgery or as an emergency procedure
in severely dyspneic patients. Tube tracheostomies usually
are maintained for a short time.

*Make a ventral midline incision from the cricoid cartilage
extending 2 to 3 cm caudally. Separate the sternohyoid
muscles and make a horizontal (transverse) tracheotomy*

FIG. 28-8
Tube tracheostomy. **A,** Make a transverse incision through the annular ligament. Excise a small ellipse of cartilage from each tracheal cartilage adjacent to the tracheotomy incision to minimize tube irritation *(dotted line).* Facilitate tube placement by depressing the proximal cartilages with a hemostat **(B)** and elevating the distal cartilages with an encircling suture **(C).** Insert a tracheostomy tube that does not completely fill the lumen.

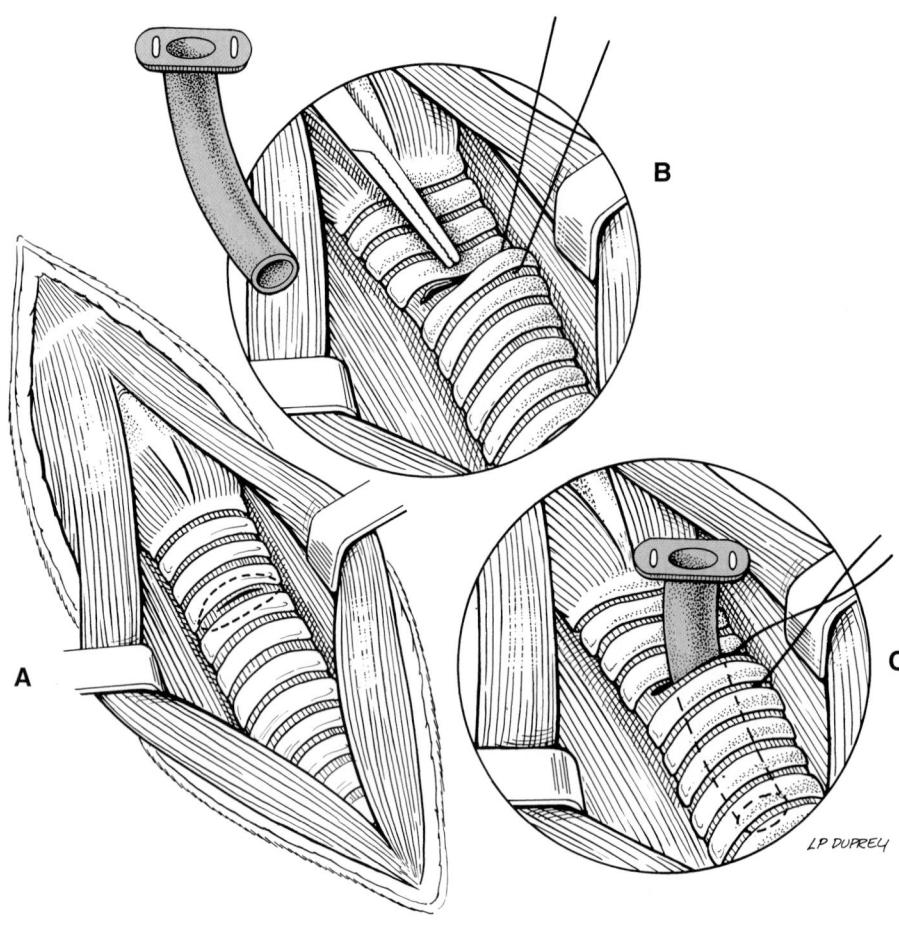

through the annular ligament between the third and fourth or fourth and fifth tracheal cartilages (see Fig. 28-8, A). Do not extend the incision around more than half the circumference of the trachea. As an alternative, make a vertical tracheotomy across the ventral midline of cartilages 3 through 5. Suction blood and mucus from the lumen, widen the incision, and insert the tracheostomy tube. Facilitate tube placement by opening a hemostat in the incision or depress the cartilages cranial to the horizontal incision (see Fig. 28-8, B). Place tension on this suture to open the incision. As an alternative, encircle a cartilage distal or lateral to the incision with a long stay suture (Fig. 28-8, C). Resect a small ellipse of cartilage if tube insertion is difficult. Appose the sternohyoid muscles, subcutaneous tissue, and skin cranial and caudal to the tube. Secure the tube by suturing it to the skin or tying it to gauze that is tied around the neck.

Permanent tracheostomy. Permanent tracheostomy is the creation of a stoma in the ventral tracheal wall by suturing tracheal mucosa to skin. Tracheostomas are maintained for life or until the stoma is surgically closed. Tracheostomy tubes are not needed to maintain lumen patency after this procedure. Permanent tracheostomies are recommended for animals with upper respiratory obstructions causing moderate to severe respiratory distress (e.g., laryn-

geal collapse and nasal neoplasia) that cannot be successfully treated by other methods. Owners should be warned that these animals must be restricted from swimming and that vocalization is diminished or absent after this procedure. Furthermore, ongoing care of the site to keep it clean will be necessary.

Expose the proximal cervical trachea with a ventral cervical midline incision. Create a tunnel dorsal to the trachea in the area of the third to sixth tracheal cartilages. Using this tunnel, appose the sternohyoid muscles dorsal to the trachea with horizontal mattress sutures to create a muscle sling to reduce tension on the mucosa-to-skin sutures (Fig. 28-9, A). Beginning with the second or third tracheal cartilages, outline a rectangular segment of tracheal wall three to four cartilage widths long and one third the circumference of the trachea in width. Incise the cartilage and annular ligaments to the depth of the tracheal mucosa (see Fig. 28-9, A). Elevate a cartilage edge with thumb forceps and dissect the cartilage segment from the mucosa. Place one or two prosthetic tracheal rings cranial and caudal to the stoma if the tracheal cartilages show any weakness or tendency to collapse (see p. 847). Excise a similar segment of skin adjacent to the stoma (excise larger segments of skin if the animal has loose skin folds or abundant subcutaneous fat). Suture the

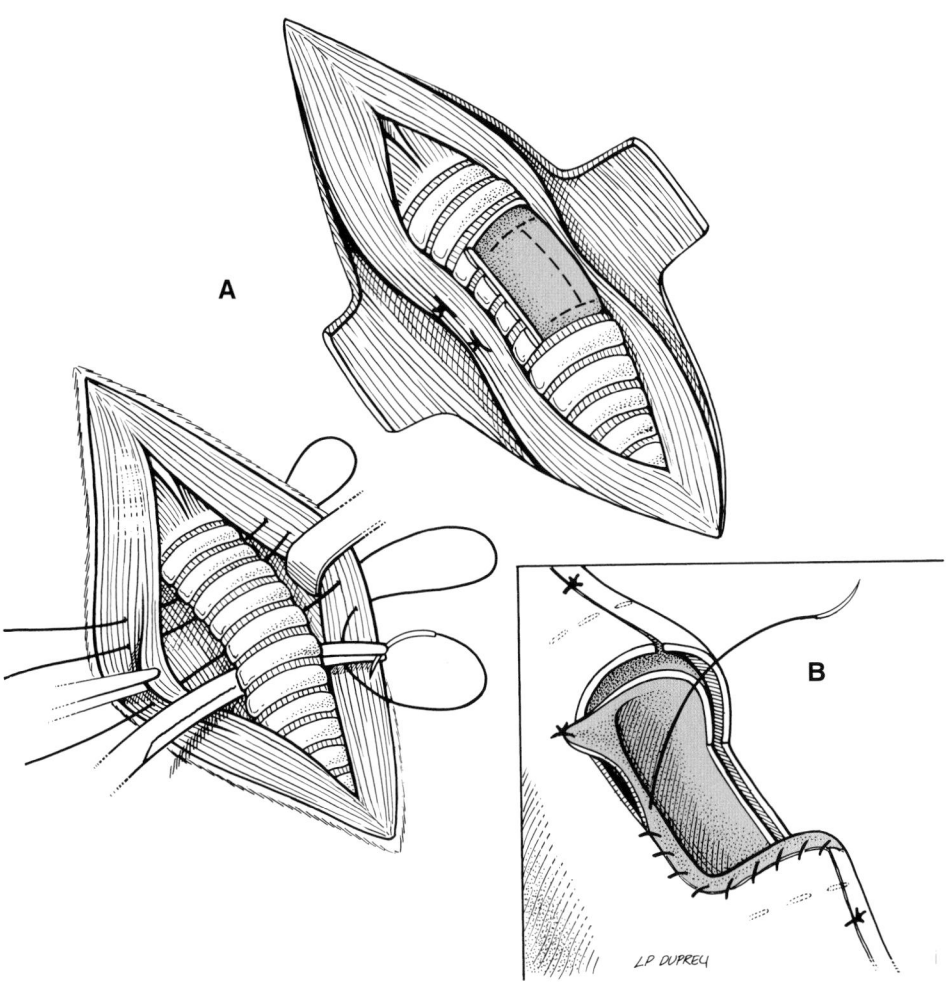

FIG. 28-9
Permanent tracheostomy.
A, Deviate the trachea ventrally by apposing the sternohyoid muscles with mattress sutures dorsal to the trachea. Excise a rectangular segment of ventral tracheal wall without penetrating the mucosa. Note the dotted line where the I-shaped incision is made after removing the cartilage segment. Excise loose skin adjacent to the stoma. **B,** Use intradermal sutures to appose the skin to the annular ligaments and peritracheal tissues (broken lines). Appose the tracheal mucosa to the skin with three or four interrupted sutures; complete the closure in a simple continuous pattern.

skin directly to the peritracheal fascia laterally and the annular ligaments proximal and distal to the stoma with a series of interrupted intradermal sutures (3-0 or 4-0 polydioxanone or polypropylene). Make an I- or H-shaped incision in the mucosa. Fold the mucosa over the cartilage edges and suture it to the edges of the skin with approximating sutures to complete the tracheostoma (Fig. 28-9, B). Use simple interrupted sutures at the corners and a simple continuous pattern to further appose skin and mucosa (using 4-0 polypropylene suture) (see Fig. 28-9, B).

Tracheal Resection and Anastomosis

Removal of a tracheal segment may be necessary to treat tracheal tumors, stenosis, or trauma. Depending on the extent of injury, tears in the tracheal wall that occur as a consequence of bite wounds or endotracheal intubation may be closed primarily, or they may be resected and the tracheal ends anastomosed. Depending on the degree of tracheal elasticity and tension, approximately 20% to 60% of the trachea may be resected and direct anastomosis achieved. The split cartilage technique is preferred because it is easier to perform and results in more precise anatomic alignment with less luminal stenosis than many other techniques. Diseased trachea that exceeds the limits of resection and anastomosis may be managed with permanent tracheostomy, intraluminal silicone tubes, grafts, or prostheses with variable success. Long-term successful repair of intrathoracic tracheal avulsion was recently reported in cats (White and Burton, 2000).

Expose the involved trachea through a ventral cervical midline incision, lateral thoracotomy (see p. 873), or median sternotomy (see p. 874). Mobilize only enough trachea to allow anastomosis without tension. Preserve as much of the segmental blood and nerve supply to the trachea as possible. Place stay sutures around cartilages cranial and caudal to the resection sites before transecting the trachea. Resect the diseased trachea by splitting a healthy cartilage circumferentially at each end or by incising annular ligaments adjacent to the intact cartilages (Fig. 28-10, A). Use a No. 11 blade to split the tracheal cartilages at their midpoint. Transect the dorsal tracheal membrane with Metzenbaum scissors. Preplace and then tie three or four simple interrupted sutures (3-0 or 4-0 polypropylene) in the dorsal tra-

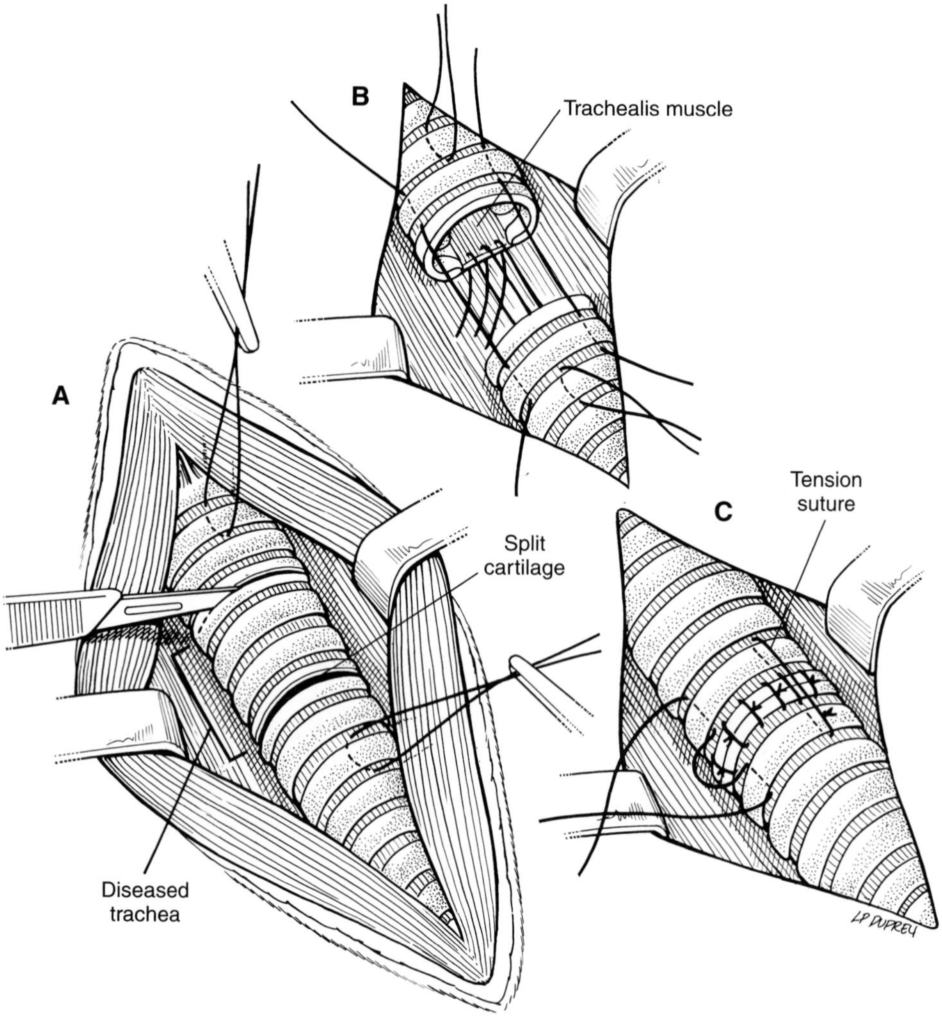

FIG. 28-10
Tracheal resection and anastomosis. **A,** Place stay sutures cranial and caudal to the resection sites. Split the cartilages with a No. 11 blade and transect the trachealis muscle with Metzenbaum scissors. **B,** Appose the trachealis muscle with three or four interrupted sutures, then approximate the split cartilages. **C,** Place three or four tension-relieving sutures around cartilages adjacent to the anastomosis.

cheal membrane (Fig. 28-10, B). Retract the endotracheal tube into the proximal trachea during resection and placement of sutures in the dorsal tracheal membrane. Remove blood clots and secretions from the lumen and advance the tube distal to the anastomosis after placing dorsal tracheal membrane sutures. Complete the anastomosis by apposing the split cartilage halves or adjacent intact cartilages with simple interrupted sutures beginning at the ventral midpoint of the trachea. Space additional sutures 2 to 3 mm apart. Place three or four retention sutures to help relieve tension on the anastomosis. Place and tie these sutures so that they encircle an intact cartilage cranial and caudal to the anastomosis, crossing external to the anastomotic site (Fig. 28-10, C). Lavage the area and appose the sternohyoid muscles in a simple continuous pattern. Close the subcutaneous tissues and skin routinely.

If tension-relieving sutures do not adequately relieve tension at the anastomosis, further mobilize the trachea, make partial-thickness incisions through annular ligaments proximal and distal to the anastomosis, or restrict head and neck movement after surgery. Prevent full extension of the neck by placing a suture from the chin to the manubrium or by fixing

a muzzle to a harness to maintain mild to moderate cervical flexion. Maintain the muzzle for 2 to 3 weeks.

Ventriculocordectomy

Ventriculocordectomy is removal of the vocal cords to alter vocalization, remove masses, or enlarge the ventral glottis. The procedure may be performed using an oral or ventral (laryngotomy) approach. Anesthesia is maintained by using a tube tracheostomy, manipulating the endotracheal tube to the contralateral side of the larynx, or using injectable anesthetic agents. Ventriculocordectomy performed to widen the ventral glottis requires that more vocal fold be resected than for debarking.

Oral approach. *Position the patient in ventral recumbency with the neck extended. Suspend the maxilla and pull the mandible ventrally to maximally open the mouth. Extend the tongue from the mouth to get maximum exposure of the glottis. Retract the cheeks laterally to improve visualization. Avoid placing padding or hands in the region of the larynx, because this may distort the nasopharynx. Remove the central margin of the vocal cord for debarking with a laryngeal*

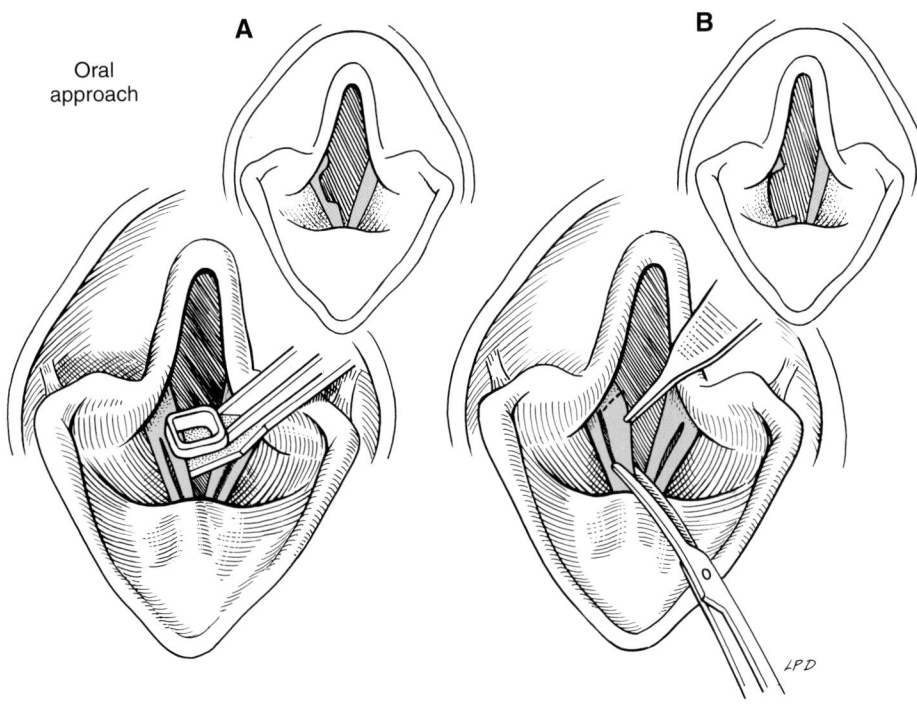

A Oral approach

B

FIG. 28-11
For ventriculocordectomy an oral approach may be used. **A,** Remove the central portion of the vocal fold with laryngeal cup forceps or uterine biopsy forceps. **B,** For laryngeal paralysis or devocalization, remove most of the vocal fold with Metzenbaum scissors. Dorsal and ventral commissures remain intact.

or uterine cup biopsy forceps (Fig. 28-11, A). To widen the glottis, use long-handled Metzenbaum scissors and remove as much of the vocal fold extending into the laryngeal lumen as possible (Fig. 28-11, B). With either technique maintain 1 to 2 mm of mucosa at the dorsal and ventral aspects of the vocal cord. Control hemorrhage with pressure. Remove blood clots and secretions with suction or sponges. Allow the incision to heal by secondary intention.

Laryngotomy approach. *Position the patient in dorsal recumbency with the neck extended over a rolled towel (Fig. 28-12). Expose the larynx using a ventral midline cervical approach, beginning rostral to the basihyoid bone and extending caudally to the proximal trachea. Separate and retract the paired sternohyoid muscles. Identify the midline of the thyroid cartilage. Ligate and divide the laryngeal impar vein if necessary. Incise the cricothyroid ligament with a No. 15 or No. 11 blade. Extend the incision along the midline of the thyroid cartilage as needed to expose the vocal folds. Excise the entire vocal fold from the arytenoid cartilage dorsally and the thyroid cartilage ventrally (see Fig. 28-12). Close the defect by apposing the mucosa in a simple continuous appositional pattern using 4-0 monofilament absorbable suture (see Fig. 28-12). Appose the cricothyroid ligament and thyroid cartilage with simple interrupted sutures. Appose the sternohyoid muscles in a simple continuous pattern with 3-0 or 4-0 monofilament absorbable suture. Close the subcutaneous tissues and skin routinely.*

HEALING OF THE RESPIRATORY TRACT

Laryngeal wounds heal by reepithelialization if mucosal edges are in apposition. Epithelial cells at the wound margins extend and spread over the wound until it is covered.

Constant motion associated with breathing and head movement inhibits primary healing. Laryngeal wounds with gaps heal by secondary intention, first filling with granulation tissue and then reepithelializing. Secondary-intention healing may cause scarring across the glottis. Restricting surgery to one side of the larynx and leaving epithelium at the dorsal and ventral commissures intact may prevent scarring.

Tracheal epithelium responds immediately to irritation or disease by increased mucus production. If the insult continues, cells desquamate and goblet cell hyperplasia occurs to increase the protective mucous layer. Superficial wounds heal by reepithelialization. Healing begins within 2 hours after slough of superficial cells. Intact ciliated columnar cells surrounding the defect flatten, lose their cilia, and migrate over the wound. Mitosis begins about 48 hours after injury in the ciliated columnar and basal epithelial cells. Organization and differentiation begin after 4 days. Squamous cells replace ciliated and goblet cells if injury recurs without healing. Full-thickness tracheal mucosal wounds with a gap between mucosal edges fill with granulation tissue before reepithelialization. Full-thickness wounds may heal with scar tissue protruding into the lumen. Scar tissue narrows the lumen and may interfere with mucus transport. A 20% reduction in lumen diameter may reduce mucociliary clearance by more than 50%.

SUTURE MATERIALS AND SPECIAL INSTRUMENTS

An assortment of long-handled instruments is beneficial. Skin hooks, laryngeal or uterine cup biopsy forceps, and tracheal prostheses (see p. 850) are needed for some procedures. Rhinotomy requires an oscillating saw, chisel and mallet, or rongeurs, and periosteal elevators and curettes.

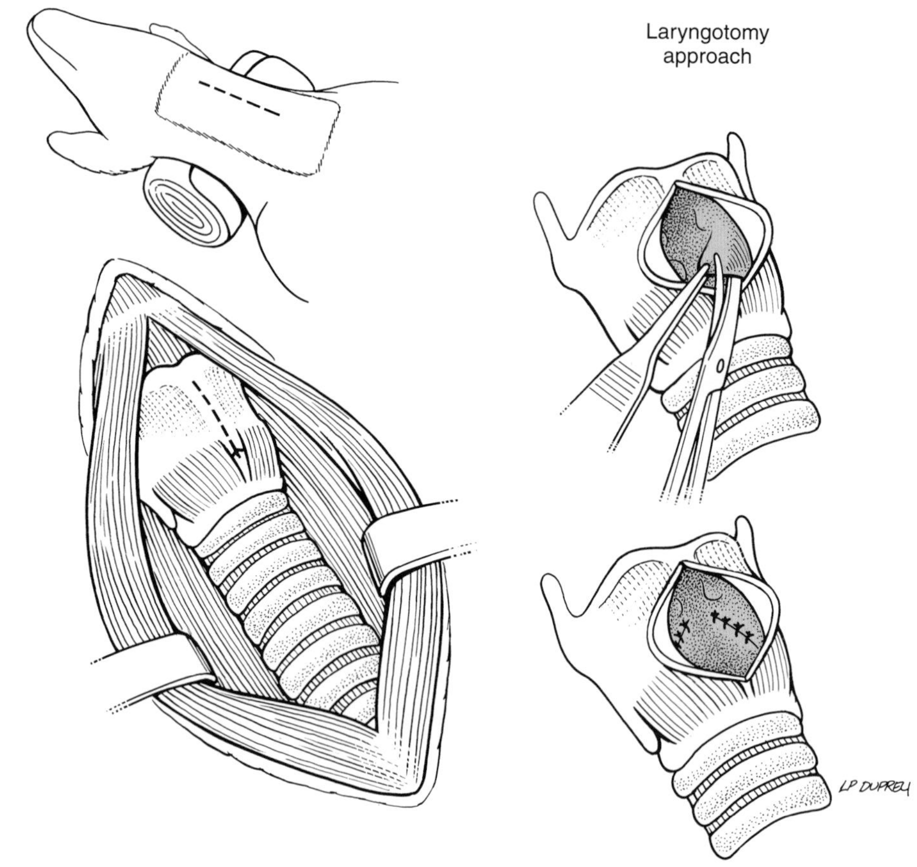

FIG. 28-12
For ventriculocordectomy by a laryngotomy approach, position the patient in dorsal recumbency with the neck extended over a rolled towel. Expose the larynx, identify the midline of the thyroid cartilage and the cricothyroid ligament, and then incise with a scalpel blade *(broken lines).* Expose the vocal folds and excise them. Close the defect by apposing the mucosa in a simple continuous appositional suture pattern.

Nonreactive, monofilament suture (e.g., polydioxanone or polypropylene) is recommended for surgery of the upper respiratory tract.

POSTOPERATIVE CARE AND ASSESSMENT

Patients must be closely monitored during anesthetic recovery for hemorrhage, coughing, gagging, or aspiration. They should be kept intubated as long as possible and reintubated or have a tracheostomy tube placed if respiratory distress occurs after extubation. Supplemental oxygen should be provided if necessary during recovery, and excitement and pain should be minimized by postoperative analgesics (see Table 13-4 on p. 133). Inserting a nasal oxygen catheter at the conclusion of surgery facilitates oxygen delivery (see Table 5-4 on p. 26). Alternatively the animal may be placed in an oxygen cage. Positioning the patient in sternal recumbency may facilitate respiration. Postoperative corticosteroids (dexamethasone [Azium], 0.5 to 2 mg/kg IV, IM, or SC; repeated administration of dexamethasone can cause gastrointestinal hemorrhage) may reduce mucosal swelling and edema. Prophylactic antibiotics can be discontinued immediately after surgery. Water may be offered 6 to 12 hours after surgery; soft food made into meatballs may be offered 18 to 24 hours postoperatively if gagging, regurgitation, or vomiting does not occur. Meatballs should be fed one at a time for 5 to 7 days after nasopharyngeal or laryngeal procedures to slow ingestion. Exercise should be restricted for 4 weeks. A harness rather than a collar should be used for 2 to 4 weeks to prevent incisional, tracheal, or laryngeal trauma.

After rhinotomy, animals should be recovered in a slightly head-down position, they should be kept quiet, and some sneezing should be expected. Breathing sounds are typically harsh and resonant after this procedure. Initially, nasal discharge is expected to be bloody, but it should gradually become serous and diminish in volume after the nasal cavity has reepithelialized (generally within a week). If bleeding continues after surgery, the nasal cavity can be packed with sterile gauze. If gauze strips are used (see p. 862), the end of the gauze can be exited from the nostril or a dorsal stoma and sutured to the side of the face. The packing is removed 1 or 2 days after surgery. A blood transfusion may be needed if hemorrhage is significant (see Box 5-1 on p. 25). Movement of the skin flap covering the bony defect is expected following dorsal rhinotomy, and subcutaneous emphysema may occur, but should be self-limiting. Subcutaneous air accumulates if the bone flap is not replaced adequately or if an adequate stoma is not left in the subcutaneous tissues and skin for air to exit. Subcutaneous air accumulation is generally not a problem if an adequate stoma is left. The stoma will contract and heal within 5 to 10 days. Do not allow the animal to chew on hard objects for a minimum of 3 to 4 weeks following ventral rhinotomy until the palate incision is healed. Animals may be depressed and unwilling to eat for several days; feed soft food for a minimum of 7 to 14 days following surgery.

Intensive postoperative care is required after tube tracheostomy. The animal must be observed closely to prevent asphyxiation secondary to tube obstruction or dislodgment. Mucus clearance is inhibited in these animals, and mucosal irritation leads to increased mucus production. Tube cleaning may be required every 15 minutes if the trachea is irritated. Sterile technique (i.e., gloves, instruments) should be used to clean tracheostomy tubes. Secretions may be removed by inserting a sterile suctioning cannula into the tube's lumen and distal trachea. When cannulated tubes are used, the inner cannula may be removed and cleaned while the outer tube is suctioned. Nebulization and injecting sterile saline (1 ml) into the tube a few minutes before suctioning help loosen secretions. A new tube should be used if these techniques do not adequately remove secretions. Tracheostomy tubes may be removed when an adequate airway and spontaneous ventilation have been established. Occasionally the tube should be occluded and the patient observed while breathing around the tube to determine if the tube can be removed. This should not be done in animals with cuffed tubes or in those that have large tubes that fill the tracheal lumen. After removal of the tube, the tracheostomy site should be allowed to heal by secondary intention.

Management of permanent tracheostomies usually is less demanding than that for tube tracheostomies. Initially the tracheostoma should be inspected for mucus accumulation every 1 to 3 hours. When mucus begins to occlude the tracheostoma or when respiratory effort increases, the site should be suctioned as described above for tube tracheostomies. Mucus at the stoma may be removed by aspiration or by gently wiping with a sponge or applicator stick. Only a moderate amount of mucus is expected to accumulate during the first 7 to 14 days after surgery unless the animal has severe tracheitis. By 7 days, the cleaning interval usually increases to every 4 to 6 hours, and after 30 days twice daily stomal cleaning usually is sufficient. However, smoke and other noxious stimuli increase mucus production and necessitate more frequent cleaning. Hair should be clipped as needed from around the stoma to prevent matting of the hair with mucus. Exercise and housing should be restricted to clean areas.

After tracheal resection and anastomosis, exercise and neck extension should be restricted for 2 to 4 weeks. Animals should be kept quiet and observed for signs of respiratory distress after ventriculocordectomy. Some animals gag and cough. Vocalization should be discouraged for 6 to 8 weeks.

COMPLICATIONS

Acute respiratory obstruction caused by mucosal swelling, edema, irritation, and increased mucus production and/or laryngeal or tracheal collapse may occur after upper respiratory surgery and must be relieved promptly (Box 28-7). Infection can be a problem because the nose, nasopharynx, larynx, and trachea have a resident bacterial flora. Using strict aseptic technique and lavaging contaminated tissues

 BOX 28-7

Common Errors in Managing Animals With Upper Respiratory Disease

- Failing to diagnose and treat upper respiratory disease before secondary problems develop (i.e., aspiration pneumonia)
- Failing to recognize laryngeal collapse
- Causing trauma to the recurrent laryngeal nerves
- Rough or over handling of tissue causing excessive swelling
- Failing to monitor the patient intensively after surgery

usually prevent infection. Injury to the recurrent laryngeal nerve may cause laryngeal spasms, paresis, or paralysis, leading to aspiration pneumonia. Mucostasis may occur after nerve damage. Gentle tissue handling, appropriate dissection, and careful tissue retraction prevent nerve damage.

Complications associated with rhinotomy include excessive blood loss, subcutaneous emphysema, gagging, coughing, and/or vomiting associated with aspiration of blood and exudates. Bone flaps that have been replaced following rhinotomy may sequester or harbor infectious organisms or tumor cells, leading to recurrence of disease. Caudal choanal stenosis may occur following severe rhinitis associated with infections or after extensive débridement of nasal epithelium. Signs include those of nasal obstruction with minimal nasal discharge and stridor. These stenotic lesions can be difficult to resolve; however, scar tissue may be perforated and then dilated with a balloon catheter or excised and covered with a mucosal flap.

Complications associated with tube tracheostomy include gagging, vomiting, coughing, tube obstruction, tube dislodgment, emphysema, tracheal stenosis, tracheal malacia, and tracheocutaneous or tracheoesophageal fistula. Some animals occlude the tracheostomy tube when the neck is flexed and when they sleep with bedding. The main complication of permanent tracheostomy is stomal occlusion from accumulated mucus, skin folds, or stenosis. Mucus accumulation, coughing, and gagging may also occur because of tracheal irritation. Tracheostomy tubes and endotracheal tubes that cause pressure necrosis of the tracheal mucosa or cartilages may cause strictures.

Complications after tracheal resection and anastomosis may include hemorrhage, voice change, fistula formation, and cartilage malacia. Malacia is uncommon, and the other complications are manageable. Dehiscence occurs after tracheal anastomosis if there is excessive postoperative tension or neck movement. Subcutaneous emphysema, acute respiratory distress, hemoptysis, and subcutaneous swelling suggest dehiscence. Excessive anastomotic tension and secondary-intention healing may cause tracheal stenosis. Excessive dissection may cause ischemic necrosis of the remaining trachea. Traumatizing the recurrent laryngeal nerves may cause laryngospasms, laryngeal paresis, or laryngeal paralysis.

After ventriculocordectomy, scar tissue may form within the larynx and trachea, causing obstruction weeks postoperatively. Clinical signs of obstruction are not usually apparent until luminal compromise approaches 50%. Scar tissue forms across the larynx from mucosal damage or with secondary-intention healing near the dorsal and ventral commissures. Other complications include edema, hemorrhage, cough, gag, stenosis, and altered vocalization. Mucosal edema may partly obstruct the glottis and can be reduced by pretreatment with corticosteroids. Stenosis may occur at the dorsal or ventral commissures of the glottis after ventriculocordectomy if intact mucosa is not preserved in these areas, and healing occurs by secondary intention. Approximating mucosa over the ventriculocordectomy sites also minimizes stenosis. Ventriculocordectomy is expected to alter the normal bark, making it lower pitched and harsher. Resumption of a near-normal bark may occur within months after removal of only the vocal fold margin and secondary-intention healing.

SPECIAL AGE CONSIDERATIONS

The tracheal and laryngeal cartilages of very young animals have a high water content, and these cartilages may not hold sutures well. Congenital abnormalities involving the respiratory tract should be treated early in the animal's life (within the first year) to prevent progressive respiratory distress and to improve the animal's quality of life. Old animals may have ossified, inelastic, brittle cartilages that are difficult to manipulate during surgery.

References

Gross ME, Dodam JR, Pope ER et al: A comparison of thiopental, propofol, and diazepam-ketamine anesthesia for evaluation of laryngeal function in dogs premedicated with butorphanol-glycopyrrolate, *J Am Anim Hosp Assoc* 38:503, 2002.

Priddy NH, Pope ER, Cohn LA et al: Alveolar mucosal approach to the canine nasal cavity, *J Am Anim Hosp Assoc* 37:179-182, 2001.

White RN, Burton CA: Surgical management of intrathoracic tracheal avulsion in cats: long-term results in nine consecutive cases, *Vet Surg* 29:430, 2000.

Suggested Reading

Boswood A, Lamb CR, Brockman DJ et al: Balloon dilatation of nasopharyngeal stenosis in a cat, *Vet Radiol Ultrasound* 44:53, 2003.

A balloon dilation technique using contrast and fluoroscopy is described.

Glaus TM, Tomsa K, Reusch CE: Balloon dilation for the treatment of chronic recurrent nasopharyngeal stenosis in a cat, *J Small Anim Pract* 43:88, 2002.

Stenosis followed an upper respiratory infection, which was initially treated by excision and later with three balloon dilations.

Griffon DJ, Tasker S: Use of a mucosal advancement flap for the treatment of nasopharyngeal stenosis in a cat, *J Small Anim Pract* 41:71, 2000.

This case report describes stenosis following an upper respiratory infection.

SPECIFIC DISEASES

STENOTIC NARES

DEFINITION

Stenotic nares are nostrils with abnormally narrow openings making the nostrils appear pinched together.

GENERAL CONSIDERATIONS AND CLINICALLY RELEVANT PATHOPHYSIOLOGY

Stenotic nares (congenital malformations of the nasal cartilages) are commonly seen in brachycephalic breeds. The cartilages lack normal rigidity and collapse medially, causing partial occlusion of the external nares. Airflow into the nasal cavity is restricted, and greater inspiratory effort is necessary, causing mild to severe dyspnea. Resistance to airflow through the nasal cavity in normal dogs is 76% to 80% of total resistance, depending on volume of airflow. As more and more negative pressure is exerted to breathe, intratracheal and intrapharyngeal pressures can become high enough to cause surrounding tissues to collapse. Concurrent soft palate elongation, everted laryngeal saccules, aryepiglottic collapse, corniculate collapse, tonsil eversion, pharyngeal collapse, or all of these often contribute to the severity of respiratory distress.

"Brachycephalic syndrome" refers to the combination of stenotic nares, soft palate elongation, and laryngeal saccule eversion that is commonly seen in brachycephalic dogs (Box 28-8). Concurrent tracheal hypoplasia or advanced laryngeal collapse often contributes to the respiratory distress. Brachycephalic animals exhibit signs of upper airway obstruction because of anatomic and functional abnormalities. They typically have a compressed face with poorly developed nares and a distorted nasopharynx. Their head shape is the result of an inherited developmental defect in the bones of the base of the skull. These bones grow to a normal width, but a reduced length. The soft tissues of the head are not proportionally reduced and often appear redundant.

DIAGNOSIS
Clinical Presentation

Signalment. Brachycephalic breeds (particularly English bulldogs, Boston terriers, pugs, and Pekingese) are preponderantly affected. Dogs are more commonly affected than cats (i.e., Himalayans and Persians). The condition can affect either gender. Stenotic nares are present at birth; however, many animals come for evaluation between 2 and 4 years of age.

History. Patients with upper airway obstruction usually have noisy (stridulous), difficult breathing. Some animals are brought in for evaluation because of frequent retching or gagging up of phlegm. Dogs may have trouble swallowing because the normal occlusion of the airway during deglutition compromises ventilation. Exercise intolerance, cyanosis, restless sleeping (sleep-disordered breathing), and collapse often are reported. Excitement, stress, and increased heat and humidity frequently make the clinical signs worse.

BOX 28-8

Breeds Commonly Affected With Brachycephalic Syndrome

- English bulldog
- Boston terrier
- Pug
- Pekingese
- Boxer
- Lhasa apso
- Shih Tzu
- Shar Pei

Physical Examination Findings

Stenotic nares are identified on physical examination. The nares may be mildly, moderately, or severely deviated medially. During inspiration the nares may be pulled medially or remain relatively stationary rather than abducting. Signs of increased inspiratory effort include retraction of lip commissures, open-mouth breathing or constant panting, forelimb abduction, and exaggerated use of abdominal muscles. Paradoxical movement of the thorax and abdomen, recruitment of accessory respiratory muscles, inward collapse of the intercostal spaces and thoracic inlet, and orthopneic posture (extended head and neck and reluctance to lie down) may be apparent. The mucous membranes are normal in color with mild or moderate dyspnea, but are pale or cyanotic with severe dyspnea. Affected animals often are restless and anxious, especially when restrained. Animals may be hyperthermic as a result of ineffective cooling. Careful thoracic auscultation is difficult because of referred upper airway noise. Gastrointestinal tract distention may occur secondary to aerophagia associated with open-mouth breathing.

Diagnostic Imaging

Thoracic radiographs should be evaluated to detect underlying cardiac abnormalities (i.e., cardiomegaly and heart failure) or pulmonary abnormalities (i.e., pulmonary edema and pneumonia). Lateral radiographs of the nasopharynx, larynx, and trachea sometimes detect concurrent airway abnormalities, such as tracheal collapse. The soft palate may be thickened and elongated. Nasopharyngeal, laryngeal, and tracheal masses may be identified. Determining the tracheal-to-thoracic inlet diameter ratios can help assess the tracheal size (see p. 847). If tracheal collapse is suspected, endoscopy should be performed.

Laboratory Findings

Hematologic and serum biochemistry findings usually are normal. In rare cases, blood gas evaluation may reveal hypoxemia and respiratory alkalosis. Oxygen saturation that acutely falls below 80% may cause syncope and collapse. Polycythemia may occur if hypoxia is chronic.

DIFFERENTIAL DIAGNOSIS

Stenotic nares generally occur in conjunction with the other respiratory abnormalities that comprise the brachycephalic syndrome (i.e., elongated soft palate and everted laryngeal saccules). Other abnormalities that may cause upper respiratory obstruction include aryepiglottic collapse; corniculate collapse; tracheal collapse; tracheal hypoplasia; laryngeal paralysis; masses obstructing the glottis, larynx, or trachea; and traumatic disruption of the airway.

MEDICAL MANAGEMENT

A weight-reduction program should be instituted for obese animals. Exercise restriction and elimination of precipitating causes may be beneficial when clinical signs are mild. Sedation (see Box 28-2), corticosteroids (dexamethasone [Azium], 0.5 to 2 mg/kg IV, IM, or SC; repeated administration of dexamethasone can cause gastrointestinal hemorrhage), supplemental oxygen (see Table 5-4 on p. 26), and cooling may be necessary for moderate to severe respiratory distress.

SURGICAL TREATMENT

Multiple procedures (e.g., stenotic nares resection, resection of elongated soft palate, and resection of everted laryngeal saccules) usually are required to alleviate signs of brachycephalic syndrome. Animals with upper respiratory obstruction are anesthetic and postoperative risks (see pp. 818 and 830). Stenotic nares resection should be performed as soon as the animal is old enough to be safely anesthetized and the animal's nasal tissues have matured enough to hold sutures (as early as 3 to 4 months of age).

Preoperative Management

These animals should be monitored carefully for decompensation and progressive respiratory distress. Emergency therapy (e.g., temporary tracheostomy; see p. 825) may be necessary if dyspnea worsens acutely. Animals undergoing concurrent laryngeal or nasopharyngeal procedures should be treated with antiinflammatory doses of corticosteroids (dexamethasone [Azium], 0.5 to 2 mg/kg IV, IM, or SC; repeated administration of dexamethasone can cause gastrointestinal hemorrhage).

Anesthesia

Anesthesia or sedation must be done carefully in these animals (see p. 818). Virtually all sedatives and anesthetic agents relax the upper airway dilating muscles while allowing the diaphragm to continue contracting. This allows the upper airway to collapse and reduces respiratory drive. Airway collapse is worsened by negative inspiratory pressure that draws the pharyngeal walls medially. Anesthetics also relax the muscles used by brachycephalic animals to facilitate breathing (e.g., the geniohyoid, genioglossus, and sternohyoid muscles). Oxygen saturation can drop rapidly during anesthesia or sedation; it should be monitored after premedication and during induction, oral examination, anesthesia, and anesthetic recovery. Preoxygenate these animals before induction. Anesthesia should be induced and the animal intubated as quickly as possible. General anesthetic recommendations and selected anesthetic protocols for animals with upper respiratory disease are given on p. 818.

Surgical Anatomy

The dorsal and ventral lateral nasal cartilages unite laterally to form a cartilage tube, the nostril (Fig. 28-13, *A* and *B*). The nostrils are supported medially and ventrally by the nasal septum and dorsally by the dorsal lateral nasal cartilages. The dorsal lateral cartilage also forms the lateral wall of the nostril. The lateral accessory cartilage contributes ventral support to the nostrils.

Positioning

Position the patient in sternal recumbency with the chin resting on a pad. Tape the head to the table to prevent rotation. The planum nasale should be scrubbed with antiseptic soap and solutions.

SURGICAL TECHNIQUE

Resection of a portion of the dorsolateral nasal cartilage may be performed to widen the nares (Fig. 28-13, *C*). Other techniques described include resection of horizontal or lateral tissue wedges.

Grasp the margin of the nares with a Brown-Adson thumb forceps. Maintaining this grip, make a V-shaped incision around the forceps with a No. 11 scalpel blade. Make the first incision medially and the second incision laterally. Remove the vertical wedge of tissue. Control hemorrhage with pressure and by reapposing the cut edges. Align the ventral margin of the nares and mucocutaneous junction and place three or four simple interrupted sutures (e.g., using 3-0 or 4-0 polydioxanone) to reappose the tissues. Repeat the procedure on the opposite side, being careful to excise the same size tissue wedge.

As an alternative, incisions can be made with an electrosurgical unit using a fine-tip incising blade. Oxygen combustion is a risk when using electrosurgery.

POSTOPERATIVE CARE AND ASSESSMENT

Patients require constant monitoring during recovery from anesthesia (see p. 830). Nasal insufflation of oxygen (see Table 5-4 on p. 26) may be beneficial. The animal should re-

FIG. 28-13
A, Normal and stenotic appearance of the nares. **B,** The dorsolateral, ventrolateral, and accessory nasal cartilages form the nostrils. **C,** To widen the nares, resect a portion of the dorsolateral nasal cartilages.

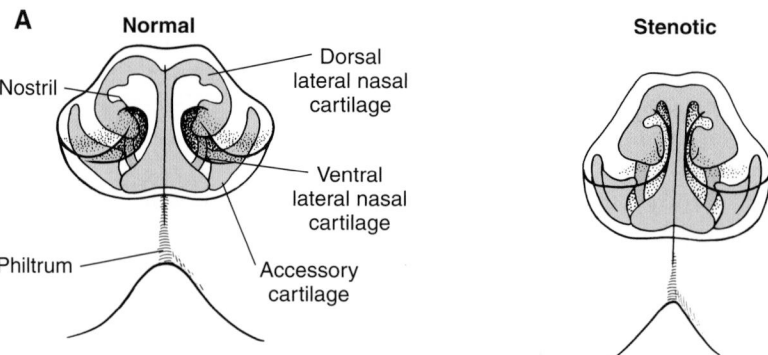

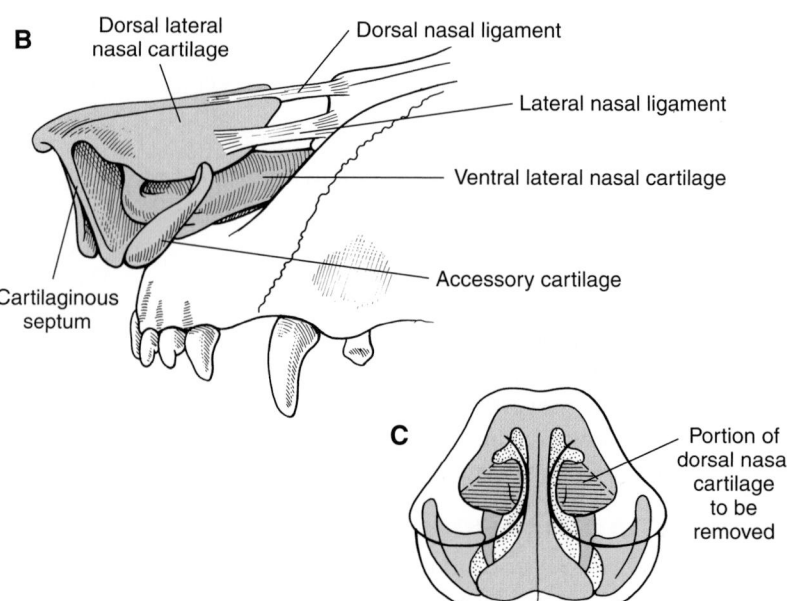

main intubated as long as possible; reintubation or placement of a tracheostomy tube may be necessary if respiratory obstruction or severe distress occurs. The surgical site should be cleaned and protected from the animal by using an Elizabethan collar if necessary. Slight hemorrhage may occur from the surgical sites.

COMPLICATIONS

If stenotic nares are the patient's only abnormality, complications are minimal. Dehiscence may occur if the patient frequently licks or rubs its nose; healing then occurs by secondary intention and may cause a pink scar. Respiratory distress may persist if other areas of the airway are obstructed.

PROGNOSIS

Animals with mild stenosis may do well without surgery; however, those with moderate or severe stenosis and other obstructive problems can develop severe respiratory distress. The prognosis after resection of stenotic nares in animals with brachycephalic syndrome is good if advanced laryngeal collapse is not present and if any palate or saccule abnormality is resected. Most animals have reduced inspiratory effort and increased exercise tolerance after surgery.

Suggested Reading

Ellison GW: Alapexy: an alternative technique for repair of stenotic nares in dogs, *J Am Anim Hosp Assoc* 40:484, 2004.
This technique is described to be useful when other techniques have failed or when the alar cartilage is flaccid.
Koch DA, Arnold S, Hubler M et al: Brachycephalic syndrome in dogs, *Compend Cont Educ Pract Vet* 25:48, 2003.
This review article discusses the syndrome and describes the craniofacial angles used to designate breeds as brachycephalic.

ELONGATED SOFT PALATE

DEFINITION

An **elongated soft palate** is one that extends more than 1 to 3 mm caudal to the tip of the epiglottis.

GENERAL CONSIDERATIONS AND CLINICALLY RELEVANT PATHOPHYSIOLOGY

Elongated soft palate is the most commonly diagnosed respiratory problem in brachycephalic dogs (Box 28-9). In addition to stenotic nares and laryngeal saccule eversion (see p. 838), it is part of the brachycephalic syndrome (see p. 832) The elongated soft palate, a congenital abnormality, is pulled caudally during inspiration, obstructing the dorsal aspect of the glottis. It is sometimes sucked between the corniculate processes of the arytenoid cartilages, which increases inspiratory effort and causes more turbulent airflow. The laryngeal mucosa becomes inflamed and edematous, further narrowing the airway. The tip of the soft palate is blown into the nasopharynx during expiration. Affected dogs may have trouble swallowing because normal occlusion of the airway during deglutition compromises ventilation. Dysfunctional

 BOX 28-9

Upper Airway Abnormalities Associated With Brachycephalic Breeds

Classic Components of Brachycephalic Syndrome
- Elongated soft palate
- Stenotic nares
- Everted laryngeal saccules

Common Concurrent Findings
- Hypoplastic trachea
- Aryepiglottic collapse

Other Findings
- Corniculate collapse
- Tracheal collapse
- Tonsil eversion
- Pharyngeal collapse
- Epiglottic collapse

swallowing may produce aspiration pneumonia. Some affected animals with concurrent gastrointestinal problems (e.g., esophagitis and hiatal hernia) have improved following surgical treatment of the brachycephalic syndrome (Lecoindre et al, 2004).

DIAGNOSIS
Clinical Presentation

Signalment. Elongated soft palate is uncommon except in brachycephalic breeds, especially English bulldogs, Boston terriers, pugs, and Pekingese. Cavalier King Charles spaniels and French bulldogs also commonly have an elongated soft palate. The condition, which can affect either gender, is present at birth, but many affected animals are not brought in for evaluation until 2 or 3 years of age. Older animals often have concurrent, advanced laryngeal collapse (see p. 840).

History. Patients with upper airway obstruction typically have a history of noisy (stridulous), difficult breathing (especially inspiratory). Some may retch or gag phlegm because they have trouble swallowing if normal occlusion of the airway during deglutition compromises ventilation. Exercise intolerance, cyanosis, and collapse are common and may be worsened by excitement, stress, heat, and humidity. Restlessness during sleeping (sleep-disordered breathing) may be noted. Some have regurgitation or vomiting.

Physical Examination Findings

Pharyngeal and laryngeal auscultation reveals prominent snoring (stertor) that obscures other respiratory sounds. Increased inspiratory effort may be apparent (i.e., retraction of lip commissures, open-mouth breathing or constant panting, forelimb abduction, exaggerated use of abdominal muscles, paradoxical movement of the thorax and abdomen, recruitment of accessory respiratory muscles, inward collapse

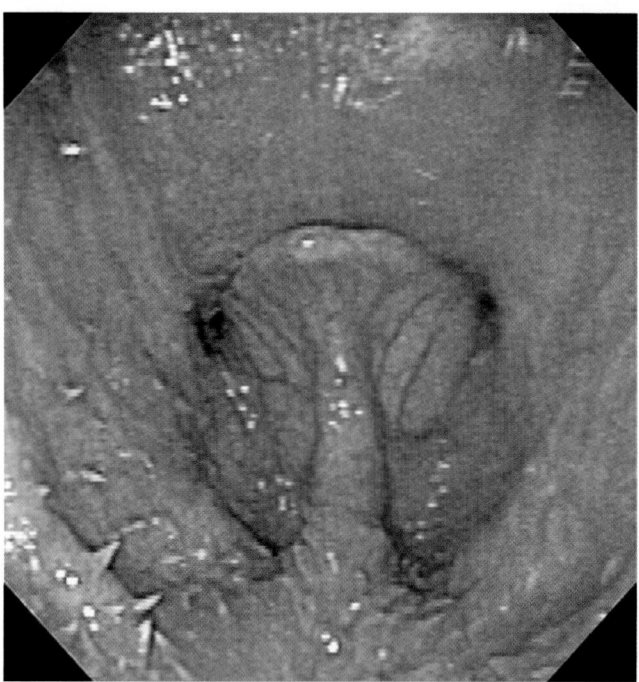

FIG. 28-14
Endoscopic view of an elongated soft palate. Note how the soft palate and the epiglottis overlap.

of the intercostal spaces and thoracic inlet, and orthopneic posture). Animals may be hyperthermic (see also p. 817). It is difficult to visualize the oropharynx and larynx in brachycephalic animals because their tongues are thick, and restraint may accentuate respiratory distress.

Diagnostic Imaging

Thoracic radiographs are needed to rule out concurrent diseases (i.e., hypoplastic trachea, cardiomegaly, and pneumonia). Pharyngeal radiographs may show an abnormally long, thickened soft palate.

Pharyngoscopy. Sedation or general anesthetic usually is necessary (see p. 818 for anesthesia for laryngeal examination). This endoscopy is best done with a rigid laryngoscope. An elongated soft palate overlies the epiglottis by more than a few millimeters (i.e., often more than 1 cm) (Fig. 28-14). The soft palate often is thickened and has a roughened, inflamed tip. Dorsally displacing the soft palate improves visualization of the arytenoid cartilages. The arytenoids frequently are inflamed and edematous. Tonsils may be inflamed and everted from their crypts.

Tracheoscopy. If there is any doubt about the trachea (i.e., the dog seems overly dyspneic for the lesions seen at pharyngoscopy), tracheoscopy can been done with a flexible scope (see p. 848). It is important to note that radiographs incorrectly diagnose some patients with severe tracheal collapse as normal.

Laboratory Findings

Laboratory abnormalities are uncommon (see also p. 833).

DIFFERENTIAL DIAGNOSIS

Concurrent abnormalities often are present (e.g., stenotic nares, laryngeal saccule eversion, aryepiglottic collapse, corniculate collapse, tracheal collapse). Concurrent tracheal hypoplasia (see p. 847) usually is diagnosed at a young age. Other causes of upper respiratory obstruction may include laryngeal paralysis; masses obstructing the glottis, larynx, or trachea; and traumatic disruption of the airway.

MEDICAL MANAGEMENT

Medical therapy is recommended to alleviate acute respiratory distress. A weight-reduction program should be instituted for obese animals. Exercise restriction and elimination of precipitating causes may be beneficial when clinical signs are mild. Sedation (see Box 28-2), corticosteroids (dexamethasone [Azium], 0.5 to 2 mg/kg IV, IM, or SC; repeated administration of dexamethasone can cause gastrointestinal hemorrhage), supplemental oxygen (see Table 5-4 on p. 26), and cooling may be necessary if the animal has moderate to severe respiratory distress. Prolonged medical therapy may allow progression of degenerative changes.

SURGICAL TREATMENT

Resection of elongated soft palates is best performed when the animal is young (i.e., 4 to 24 months old) before laryngeal cartilages degenerate and collapse.

Preoperative Management

Pretreatment with antiinflammatory doses of corticosteroids may reduce laryngeal swelling and postoperative obstruction (dexamethasone [Azium], 0.5 to 2 mg/kg IV, IM, or SC)). The oral cavity should be gently lavaged with dilute antiseptic solutions, and sponges should be placed around the endotracheal tube at the glottis to prevent fluids from entering the airway. To prevent irritation and edema, the mucosal surfaces should not be scrubbed. A tracheostomy tube may be placed before surgery; however, this usually is unnecessary unless other oral procedures are being done concurrently.

Anesthesia

Anesthesia of animals with brachycephalic syndrome is described on p. 833. General anesthetic recommendations for animals with upper respiratory disease are given on p. 818.

Surgical Anatomy

The soft palate is a fleshy piece of tissue extending from the hard palate to the tip of the epiglottis that separates the oropharynx from the nasopharynx. The palatine muscle, which is covered by mucosa and innervated by the pharyngeal plexus (cranial nerves IX and X), shortens the soft palate during contraction. Palatine glands keep the mucosa moist. Blood supply is via the palatine vessel (see p. 34). The epiglottis is a curved, triangular cartilage at the entrance to the larynx. The apex of the epiglottis points to the oropharynx and lies just dorsal to the soft palate (see Fig. 28-2). The lingual aspect of the base of the epiglottis is attached to the

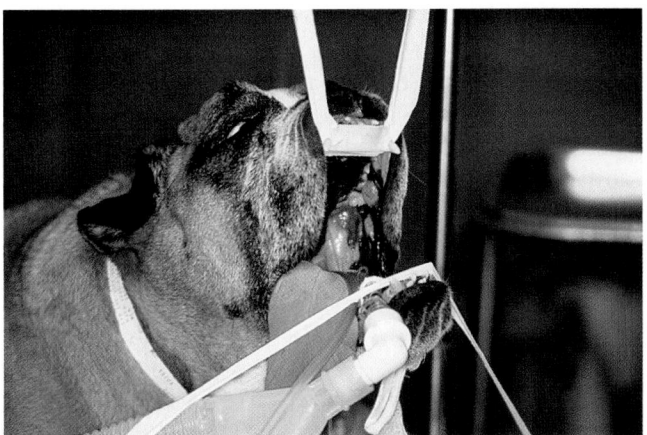

FIG. 28-15
For resection of an elongated soft palate, position the patient in ventral recumbency with the maxilla suspended and the mouth wide open.

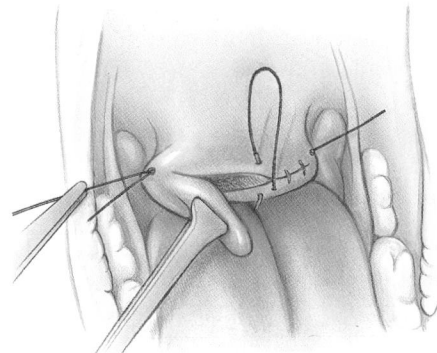

FIG. 28-16
To shorten the soft palate, place stay sutures at the proposed site of resection. Transect one third of the palate, then appose the mucosa with sutures. Continue alternating excision and suturing until the resection is complete.

basihyoid bone. Mucosa attaches the lateral aspects of the epiglottis to the cuneiform process of the arytenoid cartilage, forming the aryepiglottic fold (see Fig. 28-2). The epiglottis attaches to the body of the thyroid cartilage.

The end of the soft palate just covers the tip of the epiglottis in a normal dog. It generally extends no farther than the mid to caudal aspect of the tonsillar crypt. The distal end in a normal dog is concave; however, the distal end of an elongated soft palate frequently is sucked into the larynx, giving it a more pointed or pinched appearance.

Positioning

The patient is positioned in sternal recumbency with the mouth fully open. The maxilla should be suspended from a bar positioned several feet above the operating table and the mandible secured ventrally with tape. The chin should not be allowed to rest on the table or pads. For maximum visualization, the cheeks should be retracted laterally and the tongue pulled rostrally (Fig. 28-15).

SURGICAL TECHNIQUE

Resection may be done with scissors, carbon dioxide laser, or electrosurgery, although electrosurgery may increase postoperative swelling. Electrosurgery and lasers may ignite oxygen if proper safety precautions are not taken. Hemorrhage generally is mild to moderate after resection and can be controlled with gentle pressure. The caudal margin of the soft palate should be shortened so that it contacts the tip of the epiglottis and when pushed dorsally contacts the roof of the nasopharynx. Resection of too little soft palate does not optimally relieve respiratory distress, whereas resection of too much soft palate results in nasal regurgitation, rhinitis, and sinusitis.

Visually mark the site of proposed resection using the tip of the epiglottis and the caudal or midpoint of the tonsils as landmarks. Handle the soft palate gently and as little as possible to prevent excessive mucosal swelling. Grasp the tip of the soft palate with thumb forceps or Allis tissue forceps. Place stay sutures at the proposed site of resection on the right and left borders of the palate. Place hemostats on these sutures and have an assistant apply lateral traction. Transect across one third to one half of the width of the soft palate with curved Metzenbaum scissors. Begin a simple continuous suture pattern (4-0 absorbable monofilament suture) at the border of the palate, apposing the oropharyngeal and nasopharyngeal mucosa (Fig. 28-16). Continue transecting and suturing until the excess palate has been resected.

POSTOPERATIVE CARE AND ASSESSMENT

These patients should be closely monitored for respiratory distress postoperatively. Reduced respiratory noise is noted postoperatively in animals without advanced laryngeal collapse. Extubation should be delayed as long as possible, and the animal should be kept quiet. Oxygen may be administered by nasal insufflation (see Table 5-4 on p. 26). If severe dyspnea occurs, a tracheostomy tube should be placed (see p. 825). Corticosteroids may be administered postoperatively if swelling is severe and if respiratory obstruction persists. Intravenous fluids should be maintained until oral intake resumes. Hospital observation is recommended for 24 to 72 hours after surgery. Excessive mucosal swelling may cause asphyxiation. Postoperative coughing and gagging are common. Water may be offered when the animal is fully recovered from anesthesia (6 to 12 hours postoperatively); however, food should be withheld for 18 to 24 hours (see p. 830). Offering food soon after surgery may traumatize swollen tissues, causing swelling, airway obstruction, or aspiration, or all of these. Excising too little tissue does not optimally relieve clinical signs, and excising too much may result in nasal aspiration, rhinitis, and sinusitis.

PROGNOSIS

The prognosis without surgery is poor because laryngeal collapse and respiratory distress will worsen. The prognosis is good for young patients in which elongated soft palate is the primary problem; they breathe with less distress immediately after surgery. Older animals frequently do not respond as well because their laryngeal cartilages have begun to collapse. If advanced laryngeal collapse has developed, the prognosis is poor unless additional surgery is performed.

Reference

Lecoindre P, Richard S: Digestive disorders associated with the chronic obstructive respiratory syndrome of brachycephalic dogs: 30 cases (1999-2001), *Revue Med Vet* 155:141, 2004.

Suggested Reading

Davidson EB, Davis M, Campbell G et al: Evaluation of carbon dioxide laser and conventional techniques for resection of the soft palate in brachycephalic breeds, *J Am Vet Med Assoc* 219:776, 2001.

Clinical outcomes appear to be similar with the laser and incisional techniques. Regarding surgical time and ease, laser resection of the soft palate appears advantageous.

Dupre G, Findji L, Poncet C: The folded flap palatoplasty: a new technique for treatment of elongated soft palate in dogs, ECVS Proceedings 2005, pp. 265-267.

This technique reduces the thickness of the palate and pulls it rostrally by excising a partial-thickness segment of soft palate near its junction with the hard palate.

EVERTED LARYNGEAL SACCULES

DEFINITION

Prolapse of the mucosa lining the laryngeal crypts is known as **eversion of the laryngeal saccules**. It is also called *laryngeal saccule eversion, laryngeal ventricle eversion,* or *Stage I laryngeal collapse.*

GENERAL CONSIDERATIONS AND CLINICALLY RELEVANT PATHOPHYSIOLOGY

Laryngeal saccule eversion is a component of brachycephalic syndrome (see p. 832); however, it is diagnosed less often than either elongated soft palate or stenotic nares. Eversion of the laryngeal saccules is the first stage of laryngeal collapse. Increased airflow resistance and increased negative pressure generated to move air past obstructed areas (stenotic nares, dorsal glottis) pull the saccules from their crypts, causing them to swell. Once everted the saccules are continuously irritated by turbulent airflow and become increasingly edematous. They obstruct the ventral aspect of the glottis and further inhibit airflow. It may be difficult for an inexperienced examiner to differentiate everted laryngeal saccules from the vocal folds because of their close proximity. Everted saccules partly or completely obscure the vocal folds.

DIAGNOSIS
Clinical Presentation

Signalment. Brachycephalic dogs are most commonly diagnosed with everted laryngeal saccules; however, chronic barking may cause laryngeal saccule eversion in other breeds. Most brachycephalic dogs with laryngeal saccule eversion are diagnosed between 2 and 3 years of age, although it may occur at any age.

History. Affected animals have a history of stridulous breathing and respiratory distress, as described for animals with stenotic nares (see p. 832) and elongated soft palate (see p. 835). The stridor is most prominent during inspiration.

Physical Examination Findings

The animal may have mild to severe dyspnea. Increased inspiratory effort may be evident (i.e., retraction of lip commissures, open-mouth breathing or constant panting, forelimb abduction, exaggerated use of abdominal muscles, paradoxical movement of the thorax and abdomen, recruitment of accessory respiratory muscles, inward collapse of the intercostal spaces and thoracic inlet, and orthopneic posture; see also p. 833).

Diagnostic Imaging

Laryngeal saccule eversion is not diagnosed radiographically. Thoracic radiographs should be evaluated for evidence of cardiac or pulmonary abnormalities or concurrent disease (e.g., hypoplastic trachea, tracheal collapse, and pneumonia).

Pharyngoscopy and/or laryngoscopy. General anesthesia is necessary to evaluate the larynx (see p. 818 for general anesthetic during a laryngeal examination). A rigid laryngoscope is usually adequate, but soft palate elongation may make it difficult to visualize and evaluate the laryngeal saccules with a rigid scope. In that case a flexible bronchoscope may be necessary. When the saccules are everted, they cannot be visualized in their normal position between the vocal folds and the ventricular folds. Acutely everted saccules are whitish and glistening (Fig. 28-17). Chronically everted saccules are pink and fleshy.

If there is any doubt about the trachea (i.e., the dog seems too dyspneic for the lesions seen at pharyngoscopy and/or laryngoscopy), tracheoscopy can been done with a flexible scope (see p. 848). It is important to note that radiographs miss some patients with severe collapsing trachea.

Laboratory Findings

Laboratory abnormalities are uncommon (see also p. 833).

DIFFERENTIAL DIAGNOSIS

Stenotic nares and an elongated soft palate usually are present in animals with laryngeal saccule eversion. Advanced laryngeal collapse, laryngeal paralysis, tracheal collapse, and nasopharyngeal, laryngeal, or tracheal masses must be ruled out.

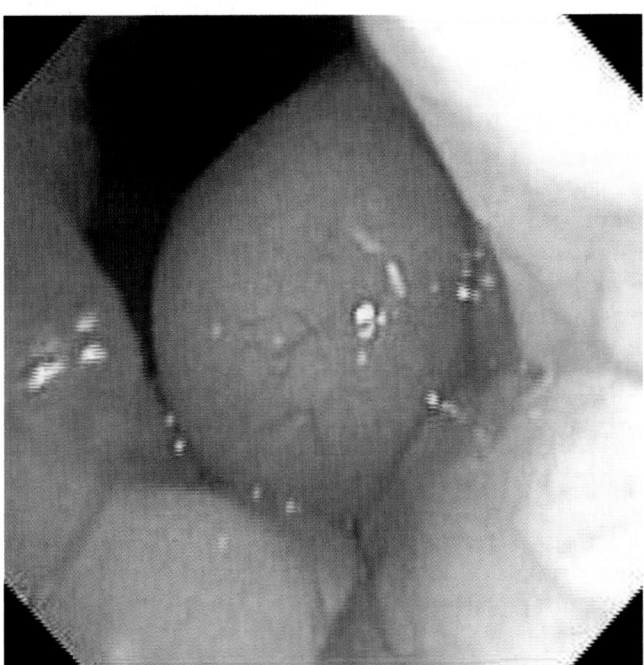

FIG. 28-17
Endoscopic view of an everted laryngeal saccule in a Bulldog. The everted saccule obscures the vocal fold.

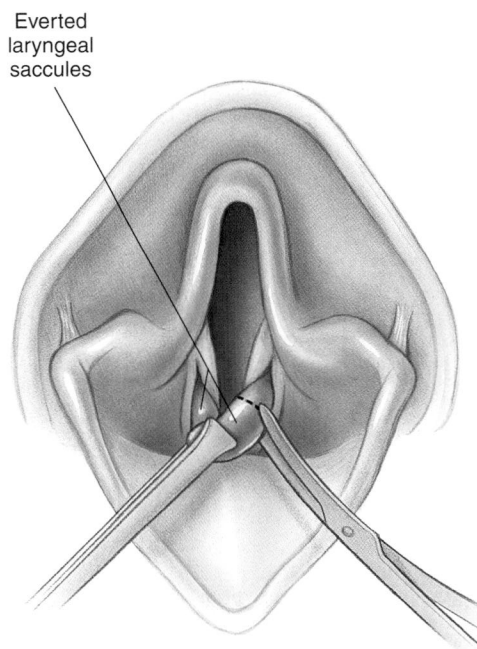

Everted laryngeal saccules

FIG. 28-18
To remove everted laryngeal saccules, grasp the protruding saccule and resect it with Metzenbaum scissors.

MEDICAL MANAGEMENT

Medical therapy is recommended to alleviate acute respiratory distress. A weight-reduction program should be instituted in obese animals. Exercise restriction and elimination of precipitating causes may be beneficial when clinical signs are mild. Sedation (see Box 28-2), corticosteroids (dexamethasone [Azium], 0.5 to 2 mg/kg IV, IM, or SC), supplemental oxygen (see Table 5-4 on p. 26), and cooling may be necessary if the animal has signs of moderate to severe respiratory distress. Prolonged medical therapy in place of surgery may allow progression of degenerative changes.

SURGICAL TREATMENT

Everted laryngeal saccules should be treated at the same time the stenotic nares and soft palate elongation are corrected (see pp. 832 and 835).

Preoperative Management

These patients should be monitored continuously before surgery because the respiratory distress may worsen.

Anesthesia

An antiinflammatory dose of corticosteroids should be given before induction of anesthesia (dexamethasone [Azium], 0.5 to 2 mg/kg IV, IM, or SC). If the endotracheal tube obscures visualization of the saccules, a smaller tube may be used or the tube may be placed via a tracheotomy (see p. 825). As an alternative, these patients can be maintained on injectable anesthetics (e.g., propofol [preferred], thiobarbiturates, or diazepam plus ketamine). Anesthesia of animals with brachycephalic syndrome is described on p. 833. General anesthetic recommendations for animals with upper respiratory disease are given on p. 818.

Surgical Anatomy

The laryngeal saccule is a slight dorsoventral depression between the vestibular and the vocal folds (see Fig. 28-2). The everted saccules lie just rostral to the vocal folds and should not be mistaken for the vocal cords. The surgical anatomy of the larynx is provided on p. 820.

Positioning

The patient is positioned in sternal recumbency with the mouth fully open. The maxilla should be suspended from a bar positioned several feet above the surgery table and the mandible secured ventrally with tape. The chin should not be allowed to rest on the table or pads. For maximal visualization, the cheeks should be retracted laterally and the tongue pulled rostrally (see Fig. 28-15).

SURGICAL TECHNIQUE

Retract the endotracheal tube dorsomedially so that the saccule on one side can be better visualized. Grasp the everted saccule with long-handled forceps or a tissue hook. Position the tip of a long-handled, curved Metzenbaum scissors at the base of the everted tissue and transect (Fig. 28-18). Biopsy forceps or laryngeal cup forceps may also be used. Control hemorrhage with gentle pressure. Repeat the procedure on the opposite side. Handle the tissues gently.

Excessive manipulation can cause local obstructive edema postoperatively. Use extreme care if laser or electrosurgical excision is used, to prevent trauma to surrounding tissues and igniting flammable gases.

POSTOPERATIVE CARE AND ASSESSMENT

These patients should be closely monitored for respiratory distress after surgery (see pp. 830 and 837). Mild hemorrhage from the resection sites may lead to coughing, gagging, and hematemesis. Postoperative swelling and edema may cause severe laryngeal obstruction, requiring temporary tracheostomy (see p. 825). Laryngeal stenosis may occur if excessive tissue is resected.

PROGNOSIS

Acute episodes of respiratory distress may be adequately managed with medical therapy alone. However, chronic medical management often allows laryngeal collapse to develop and/or worsen as a result of cartilage degeneration. Partial resection of the laryngeal saccules (in addition to the nares and soft palate when indicated) should relieve moderate to severe signs of respiratory distress in patients that do not have advanced laryngeal collapse. Animals breathe with less effort and noise and are more tolerant of exercise and excitement after surgery.

LARYNGEAL COLLAPSE

DEFINITIONS

Laryngeal collapse is a form of upper airway obstruction caused by loss of cartilage rigidity that allows medial deviation of the laryngeal cartilages. Collapse of the cuneiform process of the arytenoid cartilage is referred to as *aryepiglottic collapse* or *Stage 2 laryngeal collapse*. Collapse of the corniculate process of the arytenoid cartilage is referred to as corniculate collapse or *Stage 3 laryngeal collapse*.

GENERAL CONSIDERATIONS AND CLINICALLY RELEVANT PATHOPHYSIOLOGY

Laryngeal collapse occurs secondary to chronic upper airway obstruction or trauma. Trauma may fracture or disrupt the laryngeal cartilages and allow medial collapse. Laryngeal collapse most often is caused by chronic upper airway obstruction and cartilage fatigue or degeneration. The obstruction causes increased airway resistance, increased negative intraglottic luminal pressure, and increased air velocity. These forces displace laryngeal structures medially, with permanent cartilage deformation, and also fatigue the cartilages. Increased inspiratory effort irritates the mucosa, causing inflammation and edema. This further obstructs the airway, causing more airflow resistance and increasing the effort of breathing.

Laryngeal collapse is described in three stages. Stage 1 is commonly referred to as laryngeal saccule eversion (see p.

838); Stage 2 collapse is medial deviation of the cuneiform cartilage and aryepiglottic fold, or aryepiglottic collapse; Stage 3 collapse is medial deviation of the corniculate process of the arytenoid cartilages, or corniculate collapse. Stages 2 and 3 are advanced stages of laryngeal collapse.

The diagnosis of laryngeal collapse that occurs concurrently with other upper respiratory abnormalities (i.e., elongated soft palate [see p. 832] and stenotic nares [see p. 835]) is easily overlooked on oral examination. If the response to treatment is less than expected after appropriate surgery for these abnormalities, laryngeal collapse may be present.

DIAGNOSIS
Clinical Presentation

Signalment. Animals with brachycephalic syndrome (see p. 832) or laryngeal paralysis (see p. 842) are predisposed to laryngeal collapse. Advanced laryngeal collapse usually occurs in animals greater than 2 years of age; however, it may be seen in younger animals with severe upper airway obstruction.

History. Inspiratory stridor, stertor, and other signs of upper airway obstruction have usually been present in affected animals for years, but may have gradually or acutely worsened. Laryngeal collapse should be suspected in patients that had responded well to surgery for upper airway obstruction, but later relapsed with moderate to severe respiratory distress.

Physical Examination Findings

Stridulous, labored breathing is the most consistent finding. Animals with advanced laryngeal collapse (Stage 2 or Stage 3) usually have moderate to severe respiratory distress (i.e., retraction of lip commissures, open-mouth breathing or constant panting, forelimb abduction, exaggerated use of abdominal muscles, paradoxical movement of the thorax and abdomen, recruitment of accessory respiratory muscles, inward collapse of the intercostal spaces and thoracic inlet, and orthopneic posture). See also p. 817.

Diagnostic Imaging

The thorax and neck should be evaluated for evidence of concurrent abnormalities (see p. 836). A lateral radiograph of the pharynx may show cartilage ossification, cartilage fracture, or neoplasia.

Laryngoscopy. Laryngeal evaluation requires general anesthesia (see p. 833 for general anesthesia during laryngeal examination). A rigid laryngoscope is best suited for this examination. Patients with laryngeal collapse have a reduced glottic lumen aperture. Stage 1 laryngeal collapse (lateral saccule eversion) is recognized as prolapsed, edematous mucosa just rostral to the vocal cords at the ventral aspect of the glottis (see p. 838). Stage 2 laryngeal collapse is present when one or both aryepiglottic folds are deviated medially and obstruct the ventral aspect of the glottis (Fig. 28-19). Stage 3 laryngeal collapse occurs when the corniculate processes of the arytenoid cartilages deviate medially from their normal paramedian position and are not ade-

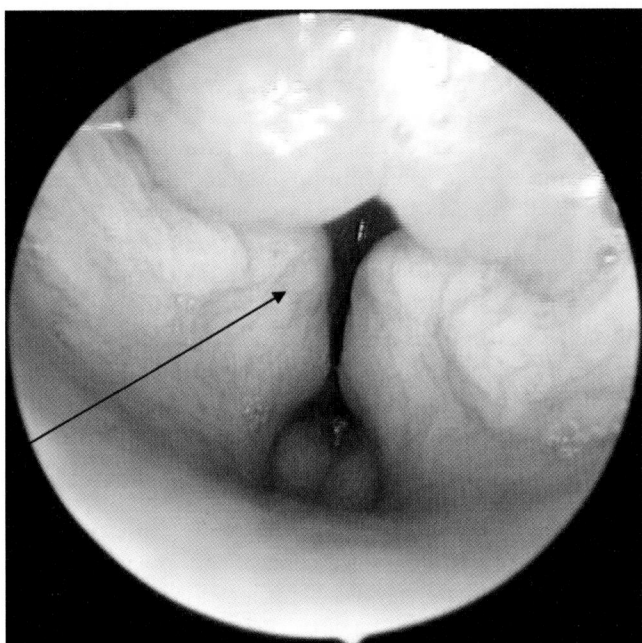

FIG. 28-19
Stage 2 laryngeal collapse is seen in this young English bulldog along with elongation of the soft palate and everted laryngeal saccules. The cuneiform processes in the aryepiglottic folds collapse medially with Stage 2 laryngeal collapse *(arrow)*.

quately abducted during inspiration. The cartilages often have a flaccid appearance.

If there is any doubt about the trachea (i.e., the dog seems too dyspneic for the lesions seen at laryngoscopy), tracheoscopy can been done with a flexible scope (see p. 848). It is important to note that radiographs miss some patients with severe collapsing trachea.

Laboratory Findings

Hematologic and serum biochemistry findings usually are normal (see also p. 833).

DIFFERENTIAL DIAGNOSIS

Differential diagnoses include laryngeal or tracheal obstruction caused by masses, paralysis, everted laryngeal saccules, elongated soft palate, and stenotic nares.

MEDICAL MANAGEMENT

Medical therapy is recommended to alleviate acute respiratory distress. A weight-reduction program should be instituted if the animal is obese. Exercise restriction and elimination of precipitating causes may be beneficial when clinical signs are mild. Sedation (see Box 28-1), corticosteroids (dexamethasone [Azium], 0.5 to 2 mg/kg IV, IM, or SC; repeated administration of dexamethasone can cause gastrointestinal hemorrhage), supplemental oxygen (see Table 5-4 on p. 26), and cooling may be necessary if the animal has signs of moderate to severe respiratory distress. Prolonged

medical therapy may allow progression of degenerative changes.

SURGICAL TREATMENT

In stable patients, the first step in treatment of laryngeal collapse is to treat concurrent abnormalities (e.g., resection of stenotic nares [see p. 832], elongated soft palate [see p. 835], and everted laryngeal saccules [see p. 838]). Resection of the aryepiglottic fold (see later discussion) may be performed in patients with mild to moderate Stage 2 laryngeal collapse, but is rarely needed. Permanent tracheostomy (see p. 826) is recommended for patients with advanced laryngeal collapse and moderate to severe respiratory distress that do not or are not expected to respond to resection. Partial laryngectomy or lateralization procedures are seldom beneficial because the weakened cartilages generally continue to collapse medially. Creation of a modified castellated laryngofissure that widens the ventral glottis is an alternative procedure advocated by some.

Preoperative Management

These patients should be stabilized before surgery (see preceding under Medical Management) and observed closely for worsening dyspnea. Pretreatment with corticosteroids (dexamethasone [Azium], 0.5 to 2 mg/kg IV, IM, or SC) is indicated for aryepiglottic fold resection (see later discussion).

Anesthesia

Anesthesia of animals with brachycephalic syndrome is described on p. 833. General anesthetic recommendations for animals with upper respiratory disease are given on p. 818. Recommended anesthetics for laryngeal examination are discussed on p. 818.

Surgical Anatomy

The surgical anatomy of the larynx is discussed on p. 820.

Positioning

For resection of the soft palate, laryngeal saccules, and aryepiglottic fold, the animal should be positioned in sternal recumbency with the maxilla suspended and the mouth wide open. Permanent tracheostomy is performed with the animal in dorsal recumbency (see p. 826).

SURGICAL TECHNIQUE

Aryepiglottic fold resection is accomplished through an oral approach. It is performed unilaterally in conjunction with resection of the nares, soft palate, and everted laryngeal saccules.

Grasp and stabilize the fold with forceps. Then transect the fold and cuneiform process with Mayo scissors or uterine biopsy forceps. Allow secondary-intention healing.

POSTOPERATIVE CARE AND ASSESSMENT

These patients should be monitored continuously during anesthetic recovery for signs of airway obstruction. Patients with advanced laryngeal collapse may develop acute respiratory obstruction after surgery. Tracheostomas should be managed as described on p. 831 to prevent occlusion of the stoma with mucus.

PROGNOSIS

Moderate to severe respiratory distress will persist without surgical intervention. Acute inflammation may cause cyanosis, collapse, and respiratory arrest. The prognosis for improvement with Stage 3 laryngeal collapse after surgery is poor if resection of the nares, soft palate, and laryngeal saccules is not done concurrently, but may be fair to good in animals with Stage 2 collapse. The prognosis in advanced laryngeal collapse (Stage 3) is fair to good if concurrent permanent tracheostomy is done.

LARYNGEAL PARALYSIS

DEFINITION

Laryngeal paralysis is complete or partial failure of the arytenoid cartilages and vocal folds to abduct during inspiration.

GENERAL CONSIDERATIONS AND CLINICALLY RELEVANT PATHOPHYSIOLOGY

Laryngeal paralysis causes upper respiratory obstruction and mild to severe dyspnea. It occurs because of dysfunction of the laryngeal muscles, recurrent laryngeal or vagus nerves, or cricoarytenoid ankylosis; acquired or congenital neurologic causes are most common. The intrinsic laryngeal abductor and adductor muscles are innervated by the recurrent laryngeal nerves (see p. 821). Subsequent atrophy of the cricoarytenoideus dorsalis muscle causes the cartilages to remain in a paramedian position during inspiration, preventing maximal air intake and increasing airflow resistance. The narrowed rima glottis increases resistance to airflow and creates turbulence, which gives rise to laryngeal stridor. To maintain the same flow rate through the paralyzed larynx as the remainder of the respiratory tract, the speed of airflow through the larynx must increase. Consequently, intraglottic pressure drops, and the arytenoid cartilages and vocal cords are sucked in medially, further increasing laryngeal obstruction. Ineffective laryngeal adduction and closure during swallowing predispose the patient to aspiration of food and secretions, resulting in subsequent aspiration pneumonia.

Congenital, inherited laryngeal paralysis occurs in the bouvier des Flandres, bull terrier, Siberian husky, Dalmatian, Rottweiler, and (white-coated) German shepherd breeds. Laryngeal paralysis in bouviers is due to degeneration of the nucleus ambiguus. Polyneuropathy associated with dying back of peripheral nerves causes laryngeal paralysis in Dalmatians. Acquired laryngeal paralysis usually is idiopathic, but may occur secondary to trauma or disease (e.g., polyneuropathy, myopathy, Chagas' disease [trypanosomiasis], hypothyroidism, and neoplasia), or it may be iatrogenic after surgery (e.g., tracheal collapse and thyroidectomy). It affects one or both sides of the larynx; however, unilateral paralysis often is asymptomatic.

DIAGNOSIS
Clinical Presentation

Signalment. Laryngeal paralysis is more common in large-breed than small-breed dogs. Males are affected two to four times more often than females. Acquired idiopathic laryngeal paralysis is most common in middle-aged or older Labrador retrievers, Afghan hounds, and Irish setters (median age, 11 years; mean age, 9½ to 10½ years; range, 4 to 13 years). In a study of 140 affected dogs, 34% were Labrador retrievers (MacPhail and Monnet, 2001). Laryngeal paralysis should be suspected in young (less than 1 year of age) bouviers, Siberian huskies, bull terriers, Dalmatians, Rottweilers, or white German shepherds with upper airway obstruction (see previous discussion). Laryngeal paralysis in cats is uncommon and has no breed or gender predilection (Schachter and Norris, 2000).

History. Laryngeal paralysis frequently causes progressive inspiratory stridor, voice change, and exercise intolerance. These animals may also have increased stridor, dyspnea, cyanosis, coughing, gagging, vomiting, restlessness, and anxiety. Some animals are asymptomatic at rest. Obesity, exercise, excitement, and high ambient temperatures may exacerbate the clinical signs. Laryngeal paralysis occurs in approximately one third of dogs with tracheal collapse. All animals with laryngeal paralysis are at risk for inhalation pneumonia from aspiration of food and saliva.

Physical Examination Findings

Physical examination findings are nonspecific for laryngeal paralysis. The animal may have labored breathing (from upper airway obstruction and/or pulmonary edema), continuous panting, and/or hyperthermia (from increased respiratory effort). Inspiratory stridor is often obvious. Patients with acquired laryngeal paralysis may have other neurologic signs and evidence of muscle wasting and weakness. Neurologic examinations should be performed to detect concurrent abnormalities. Coexistent cardiac, neurologic, gastrointestinal, and metabolic abnormalities may be recognized, making management more difficult.

Diagnostic Imaging

Lateral cervical and thoracic radiographs should be evaluated for abnormalities to rule out other causes of abnormal respiratory noises and dyspnea. Postobstruction pulmonary edema may occur in dogs and can be recognized as an interstitial pattern (sometimes coalescing to an alveolar pattern) on thoracic films. Laryngeal paralysis cannot be diagnosed radiographically. Animals with laryngeal paralysis are at risk for aspiration pneumonia. Ultrasound can also be used to evaluate laryngeal function.

Corrective surgery in animals with proximal esophageal dysfunction can cause devastating aspiration; therefore it is important to know preoperatively that the esophagus functions normally. Survey films of the esophagus may be adequate. However, dogs may have substantial esophageal dysfunction without any history of regurgitation or radiographic evidence of esophageal dilation. Therefore if there is any doubt whatsoever, contrast barium esophagrams (preferably done with fluoroscopy) should be strongly considered.

Laryngoscopy. Laryngoscopy requires light, general anesthetic (e.g., thiopental, propofol [preferred], and diazepam plus ketamine; see p. 818), but transnasal evaluation is possible in large, cooperative dogs using only sedation and topical lidocaine (Radlinsky et al, 2004). Laryngeal exposure may be best if done during recovery from propofol or thiopental anesthetic (Gross et al, 2002; Jackson et al, 2001). Apparent laryngeal motion must be compared with the phase of respiration for interpretation. Intubation should be delayed until the larynx has been examined, because placement of the endotracheal tube often obscures visualization.

The exam is usually best performed with a rigid laryngoscope, but can be done with flexible scopes as well. In affected dogs, the laryngeal cartilages are located in a paramedian position and do not abduct during inspiration. Fluttering of the vocal folds and arytenoid cartilages during turbulent airflow must not be mistaken for purposeful abduction. Paradoxical vocal fold movement may occur and may be confused with normal movement; however, a normal larynx maximally abducts during inspiration, not expiration. In questionable cases, give doxapram (1 mg/kg IV) to stimulate laryngeal motion if topical stimulation is unsuccessful in eliciting reflex activity (Jackson et al, 2001).

Laboratory Findings

Hematologic and serum biochemistry findings usually are normal (see p. 833). Hypothyroid neuropathy (see p. 602) should be excluded by evaluating serum free thyroxine (T_4) and endogenous canine thyroid-stimulating hormone (cTSH) concentrations. Acquired myasthenia gravis can be diagnosed by measuring circulating antibodies to acetylcholine receptors. Administration of edrophonium chloride may be diagnostic for myasthenia, but the test is not as sensitive or specific as measuring antibodies to acetylcholine receptors (Box 28-10). Finally, there are possible complications associated with using edrophonium (e.g., paralysis), and the clinician must be prepared.

Other tests are occasionally performed. Electromyography using bipolar concentric needle electrodes can detect denervation of the laryngeal muscles (dorsal cricoarytenoid, ventricular, and thyroarytenoid). Nerve conduction studies help rule out generalized neuromuscular disease. Tidal breathing flow volume loops show a reduction in the inspiratory flow rate. Histopathologic and histochemistry tests confirm neurogenic laryngeal muscle atrophy.

DIFFERENTIAL DIAGNOSIS

Other upper respiratory obstructions must be ruled out (e.g., brachycephalic syndrome, laryngeal collapse, tracheal collapse, and masses or trauma involving the upper airway).

MEDICAL MANAGEMENT

Animals with asymptomatic laryngeal paralysis often require no treatment if they maintain a sedentary lifestyle and avoid excess weight gain and stress. Small dogs are more successfully managed with medical therapy than large dogs. Medical therapy is recommended to alleviate acute respiratory distress. A weight-reduction program should be instituted for obese animals. Exercise restriction and elimination of precipitating causes may be beneficial when clinical signs are mild. Sedation (see Box 28-2), corticosteroids (dexamethasone [Azium], 0.5 to 2 mg/kg IV, IM, or SC; repeated administration of dexamethasone can cause gastrointestinal hemorrhage), supplemental oxygen (see Table 5-4 on p. 26), and cooling may be necessary if the animal has signs of moderate to severe respiratory distress. Affected animals should be maintained in a quiet, nonstressful environment. These patients can have postobstructional pulmonary edema, in which case furosemide may be helpful. Sometimes aspiration pneumonia is present, which necessitates aggressive antibiotic therapy (see Box 19-16 on p. 374).

SURGICAL TREATMENT

Surgical treatment is recommended for patients with laryngeal paralysis that have moderate to severe signs of respiratory distress. The goal of treatment is to enlarge the glottis without promoting aspiration of food or saliva. Many surgical techniques have been described to treat laryngeal paralysis, including partial laryngectomy, lateralization, castellated laryngofissures, and muscle-nerve pedicle transposition. Vocal fold excision (ventriculocordectomy; see p. 828) enlarges the ventral aspect of the glottis, is effective in mild to moderate cases, and is relatively easy to perform. However, glottic stenosis occurs in approximately 20% of these cases and is difficult to treat successfully. Partial arytenoidectomy (corniculate process) enlarges the dorsal aspect of the glottis. Its success depends on the skill of the surgeon. Serious complications and death occur in as many as 50% of cases after partial arytenoidectomy. The modified castellated laryngofissure technique is a combination of vocal fold excision, lateralization, and laryngofissure creation to enlarge the glottis. This technique is effective but technically difficult. Muscle-nerve pedicle transposition can successfully reinnervate the larynx and improve function, but the process takes 5 to 11 months before clinical improvement is seen. Arytenoid lateralization is recommended because it gives consistently good results with relatively few complications.

 BOX 28-10

Tensilon Test

Edrophonium Chloride (Tensilon)*

Dogs: 0.1–0.2 mg/kg IV
Cats: 0.2 mg/kg IV

IV, Intravenous.
*Use with caution. Have oxygen available in case of respiratory arrest. Some advocate pretreating with glycopyrrolate.

Preoperative Management

These patients should be observed closely before surgery for progressive respiratory distress. They should be kept cool, calm, and quiet. Pretreatment with an antiinflammatory dose of corticosteroids (dexamethasone [Azium], 0.5 to 2 mg/kg IV, IM, or SC) immediately before surgery is recommended.

Anesthesia

General anesthetic recommendations for animals with upper respiratory disease are given on p. 818. Intubation via a tracheotomy incision may be helpful when performing a partial laryngectomy, but is unnecessary for arytenoid cartilage lateralization. See p. 818 for anesthetic recommendations for laryngeal examination.

Surgical Anatomy

The cricoarytenoideus dorsalis is the abductor muscle of the larynx. It extends from the muscular process of the arytenoid cartilage in a dorsomedial direction to the cricoid cartilage. The surgical anatomy of the larynx is described on p. 820.

Positioning

For arytenoid cartilage lateralization, the animal should be positioned in lateral or dorsal recumbency with the neck over a rolled towel and rotated to elevate the ipsilateral mandible. The head is stabilized by taping it to the table. For partial laryngectomy via an oral approach, the patient is positioned in sternal recumbency with the head suspended by the maxilla and the mandible held open by an assistant or taped to the table. For partial laryngectomy via a ventral approach, the animal should be positioned in dorsal recumbency with the head extended and secured to the operating table. For arytenoid cartilage lateralization and partial laryngectomy via a ventral laryngotomy, the entire cervical area should be clipped and prepared for aseptic surgery.

SURGICAL TECHNIQUE

Unilateral Arytenoid Lateralization

Many technique variations have been described for this procedure including differences in the number and positioning of sutures, variations in the degree of disarticulation, and alterations in the amount of abduction. The outcome is generally the same unless abduction is excessive.

Make a skin incision just ventral to the jugular vein, beginning at the caudal angle of the mandible and extending over the dorsolateral aspect of the larynx to 1 to 2 cm caudal to the larynx (Fig. 28-20, A). Incise and retract the subcutaneous tissues, platysma, and parotidoauricularis muscles. Retract the sternocephalicus muscle and jugular vein dor-

FIG. 28-20
A, The larynx is exposed through a lateral cervical approach during arytenoid lateralization. Incise the skin and subcutaneous tissue ventral to the jugular vein. Then incise the thyropharyngeus muscle at the dorsal edge of the thyroid cartilage.
B, Separate the cricothyroid and cricoarytenoid articulations and transect the sesamoid band. **C,** Place a suture from the muscular process of the arytenoid to the dorsocaudal aspect of the cricoid or thyroid cartilage.

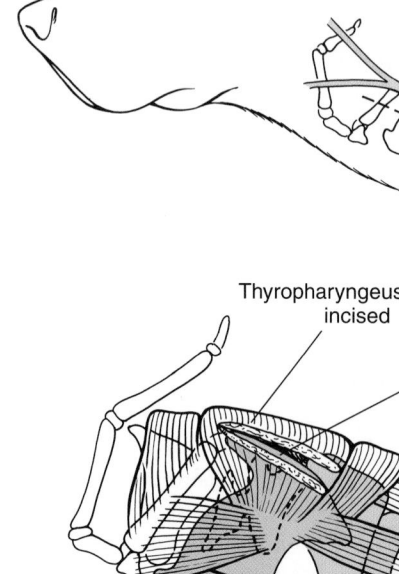

Thyropharyngeus muscle incised

Edge of thyroid cartilage

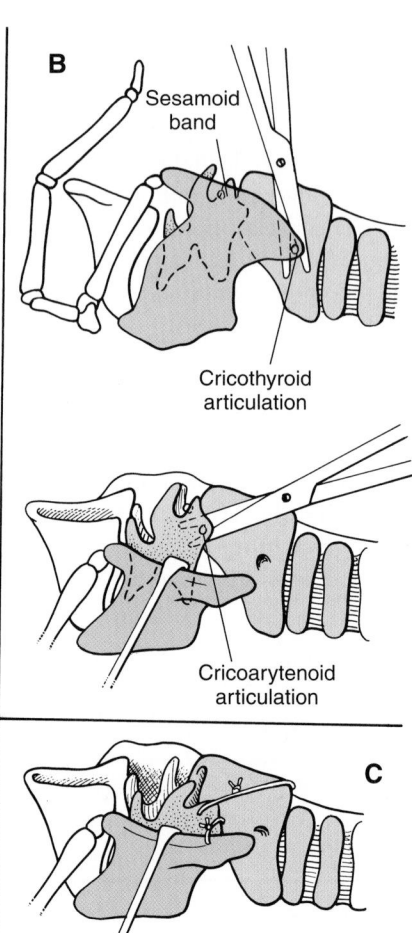

Sesamoid band

Cricothyroid articulation

Cricoarytenoid articulation

sally and the sternohyoid muscle ventrally to expose the laryngeal area. Palpate the dorsal margin of the thyroid cartilage. Incise the thyropharyngeus muscle along the dorsolateral margin of the thyroid cartilage lamina. Place a stay suture through the thyroid cartilage lamina to retract and rotate the larynx laterally. Identify the cricoarytenoideus dorsalis muscle. Disarticulate the cricothyroid articulation with a No. 11 blade or scissors (Fig. 28-20, B). Palpate, identify, and disarticulate the cricoarytenoid articulation at the muscular process. Using curved Metzenbaum scissors, transect the sesamoid band (interarytenoid ligament) between the two corniculate processes, taking care not to penetrate the laryngeal mucosa. Place a polypropylene suture (2-0 to 2) through the muscular process of the arytenoid cartilage and the caudal one third of the cricoid cartilage near the

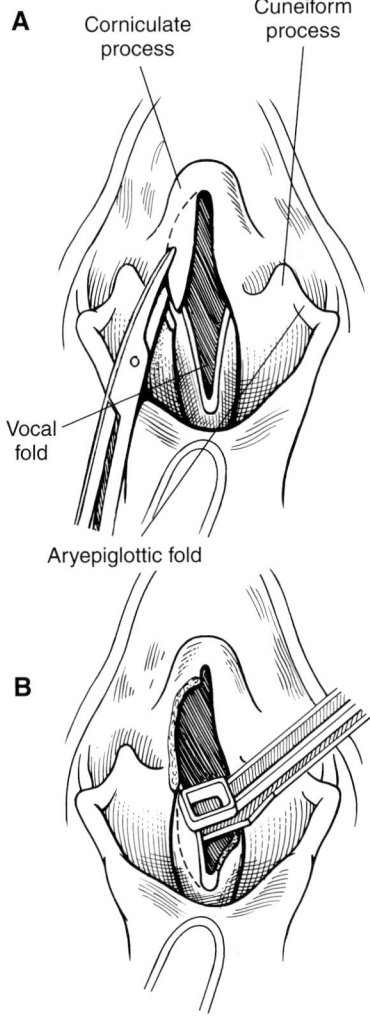

FIG. 28-21
A, For partial laryngectomy by an oral approach, use a long-handled scalpel or scissors to excise the corniculate process *(dashed line)* and the proximal half and base of the cuneiform process. Do not excise the aryepiglottic fold or the distal half of the cuneiform process. **B,** Remove the vocal fold, vocal process, and vocal muscle with biopsy forceps or Metzenbaum scissors (or both).

dorsal midline to mimic the direction of the cricoarytenoid muscle (Fig. 28-20, C). As an alternative, place the suture through the muscular process and the most caudodorsal aspect of the thyroid cartilage. Muscular process-to-thyroid cartilage sutures tend to pull the arytenoid laterally, whereas muscular process-to-cricoid cartilage sutures tend to rotate the arytenoid laterally. Tie the suture with enough tension to abduct the arytenoid cartilage moderately. Have an assistant verify abduction by intraoral visualization of the larynx. If abduction is insufficient, the suture can be repositioned to achieve better abduction. Lavage the surgical site. Appose the thyropharyngeus muscle in a cruciate or simple continuous pattern with 3-0 polydioxanone suture. Appose the subcutaneous tissues and skin routinely.

Partial Laryngectomy

Partial laryngectomy may be done by an oral approach or a ventral laryngotomy approach. Vocal fold resection and unilateral resection of the corniculate, cuneiform, and vocal processes of the arytenoid cartilage should be performed. Partial laryngectomy by an oral approach is extremely difficult in small dogs because of limited exposure.

Oral approach. Grasp the corniculate process and retract it medially with biopsy forceps. Use a long-handled scalpel or scissors to excise the corniculate process and the proximal half and base of the cuneiform process (Fig. 28-21, A). Do not excise the aryepiglottic fold or the distal half of the cuneiform process. Remove the vocal fold, vocal process, and vocal muscle with biopsy forceps or Metzenbaum scissors (or both) (Fig. 28-21, B). Leave the ventral aspect of the vocal cord intact. Control bleeding by applying pressure with gauze sponges. Limit resection to one side of the glottis.

Laryngotomy approach. Make a ventral midline incision over the larynx. Separate the sternohyoid muscles and incise the cricothyroid membrane and thyroid cartilage on the midline. Retract the edges of the thyroid cartilage with small Gelpi forceps. Visualize the arytenoid cartilages and vocal folds. Have an assistant visualize the larynx per os to help determine how much to remove. After incising the mucosa over the corniculate, cuneiform, and vocal processes of one arytenoid cartilage, excise them with scissors or a scalpel. Also excise the vocal fold on that side (if necessary, excise the vocal fold and process on the opposite side). Excise redundant mucosa and suture the defect with 4-0 to 6-0 monofilament absorbable suture material in a continuous pattern. Suture the thyroid cartilage with interrupted sutures that do not penetrate the laryngeal lumen. Close the subcutaneous tissues and skin routinely.

POSTOPERATIVE CARE AND ASSESSMENT

Postoperatively, these animals should be monitored closely for respiratory distress caused by airway obstruction. Analgesics should be given as necessary. Gagging and coughing may occur in the early postoperative period. Swallowing discomfort may occur, and impaired glottic function may persist. Intravenous fluids should be maintained until the animal is drinking. Soft food may be offered in 18 to 24 hours, but the animal should be observed for aspiration pneumonia. Exercise restriction should be enforced for 6 to 8 weeks and barking minimized. Occasional coughing occurs in most dogs. The bark is expected to be quiet and hoarse.

COMPLICATIONS

Early complications of suture lateralization include hematoma formation, suture avulsion, swallowing discomfort, temporary glottic impairment, and coughing after eating and drinking. These complications usually resolve within a few days unless aspiration occurs. Coughing and gagging after surgery may indicate mucosal irritation or aspiration. Although bilateral arytenoid lateralization enlarges the glottis more than unilateral lateralization, it is not routinely recommended because postoperative coughing, pneumonia, and death occur more often. Severe mucosal inflammation and swelling are rare after lateralization; therefore acute respiratory distress is unlikely. The cartilages of congenitally affected dogs may be insufficiently mineralized to retain sutures. Mineralized cartilages of older dogs may fracture or avulse the muscular process, causing failure of abduction and recurrence of clinical signs. If these events occur, the procedure may be repeated on the opposite side of the larynx. Bilateral lateralization is associated with a higher risk of aspiration pneumonia, but it is sometimes recommended in working dogs.

The most common complication after partial laryngectomy is aspiration pneumonia caused by resection of too much tissue, resulting in inadequate closure of the larynx during swallowing. Resection of too little tissue does not allow a functional airway. Other complications include intermittent coughing and production of excessive granulation tissue or a web of scar tissue at the surgery site.

Aspiration pneumonia occurs in approximately 26% of affected dogs (19% after unilateral lateralization) and is the most common complication after surgery for laryngeal paralysis (MacPhail and Monnet, 2001). It may occur shortly after surgery or many months later. In the aforementioned study, it was found that dogs with underlying neurologic disease were more than three times as likely to die of conditions related to laryngeal paralysis. Factors associated with a high risk of developing complications were increasing age, temporary tracheostomy, postoperative megaesophagus, esophageal disease, and concurrent neoplastic disease.

PROGNOSIS

Animals with mild or no clinical signs at rest do well without surgery; however, those with moderate to severe clinical signs may develop laryngeal collapse and acute respiratory obstruction. The prognosis after unilateral lateralization is good; more than 90% of patients have less respiratory distress and improved exercise tolerance. Up to 50% of animals undergoing partial arytenoidectomy develop fatal pneumonia and/or airway obstruction. However, with proper technique and experience with the procedure, the outcome can be excellent.

Overall median survival time after surgery has been reported as 1800 days (~5 years) (MacPhail and Monnet, 2001). Approximately 20% of dogs die of causes related to respiratory tract disease. A higher complication rate and more deaths occur in dogs following partial laryngectomy (40% complications and 30% mortality) and bilateral arytenoid lateralization (89% complications and 67% mortality) than those having unilateral arytenoid lateralization (28% complications and 14% die). Factors significantly associated with mortality were increasing age, tube tracheostomy, concurrent respiratory tract abnormalities, postoperative megaesophagus, and concurrent neurologic disease.

References

Gross ME, Dodam JR, Pope ER et al: A comparison of thiopental, propofol, and diazepam-ketamine anesthesia for evaluation of laryngeal function in dogs premedicated with butorphanol-glycopyrrolate, *J Am Anim Hosp Assoc* 38:503, 2002.

Jackson AM, Tobias K, Bartges J et al: Effect of doxapram HCl on normal laryngeal function, (abst.) *Vet Surg* 30:496, 2001.

MacPhail CM, Monnet E: Outcome of the postoperative complications in dogs undergoing surgical treatment of laryngeal paralysis: 140 cases (1985-1998), *J Am Vet Med Assoc* 218:1949, 2001.

Radlinsky MG, Mason DE, Hodgson D: Transnasal laryngoscopy for the diagnosis of laryngeal paralysis in dogs, *J Am Anim Hosp Assoc* 40:211, 2004.

Schachter S, Norris CR: Laryngeal paralysis in cats: 16 cases (1990-1999), *J Am Vet Med Assoc* 216:1100, 2000.

Suggested Reading

Bureau S, Monnet E: Effects of suture tension and surgical approach during unilateral arytenoid lateralization on the rima glottides in the canine larynx, *Vet Surg* 31:589, 2002.

This study of nine cadaver larynges found significantly worse epiglottic closure of the larynx when abduction was performed with high suture tension.

Demetriou JL, Kirby BM: The effect of two modifications of unilateral arytenoid lateralization on rima glottides area in dogs, *Vet Surg* 32:62, 2003.

This randomized clinical study included 20 dogs. Ten dogs received both cricoarytenoid and thyroarytenoid sutures and the other only a cricoarytenoid suture; no difference was found in outcome.

Griffiths LG, Sullivan M, Reid SWJ: A comparison of the effects of unilateral thyroarytenoid lateralization versus cricoarytenoid laryngoplasty on the area of the rima glottides and clinical outcome in dogs with laryngeal paralysis, *Vet Surg* 30:359, 2001.

This study compares change in glottic size, clinical status, and exercise tolerance before and after surgery in 20 dogs. Glottic size was greater after cricoarytenoid lateralization and operative time was longer, but no difference in clinical outcome was noted.

Jackson AM, Tobias K, Bartges J et al: Effects of anesthetic type and depth on laryngeal function of normal dogs, (abst.) *Vet Surg* 30:496, 2001.

Six anesthetic protocols were evaluated on six normal dogs to evaluate laryngeal motion. Evaluation immediately before recovery using thiopental was found to give the best assessment.

Ridyard AE, Corcoran BM, Tasker S et al: Spontaneous laryngeal paralysis in four white-coated German shepherd dogs, *J Small Anim Pract* 41:558, 2000.

This report describes another breed with probable congenital laryngeal paralysis.

Rudorf H, Barr F: Echolaryngography in cats, *Vet Radiol Ultrasound* 43:353, 2002.

Ultrasound technique for laryngeal evaluation is described.

Rudorf H, Barr FJ, Lane JG: The role of ultrasound in assessment of laryngeal paralysis in the dog, *Vet Radiol Ultrasound* 42:338, 2001.

This report describes the technique for ultrasound evaluation of the larynx.

TRACHEAL COLLAPSE

DEFINITION

Tracheal collapse is a form of tracheal obstruction caused by cartilage flaccidity and flattening. Tracheal collapse sometimes is erroneously referred to as congenital tracheal stenosis in older reports.

GENERAL CONSIDERATIONS AND CLINICALLY RELEVANT PATHOPHYSIOLOGY

The cause of tracheal collapse is unknown and probably multifactorial. Proposed causes include genetic factors, nutritional factors, allergens, neurologic deficiency, small airway disease, and cartilage matrices degeneration. Affected tracheal cartilages become hypocellular, and their matrices degenerate. Normal hyaline cartilage is replaced by fibrocartilage and collagen fibers, and the amounts of glycoprotein and glycosaminoglycans are diminished. The cartilages lose their rigidity and ability to maintain normal tracheal conformation during the respiratory cycle. They usually collapse in a dorsoventral direction. The cervical trachea collapses during inspiration, and the thoracic trachea collapses during expiration. Collapse reduces the lumen size and interferes with airflow to the lungs. Abnormal respiratory noises, exercise intolerance, gagging, and varying degrees of dyspnea occur with tracheal collapse. Chronic inflammation of the tracheal mucosa causes coughing, which exacerbates inflammation. Persistent inflammation leads to squamous metaplasia of the respiratory epithelium and interferes with mucociliary clearance; therefore coughing becomes an important tracheobronchial clearing mechanism.

Although the clinical signs may be similar, tracheal collapse should not be confused with tracheal stenosis. Tracheal stenosis is an abnormal narrowing of the tracheal lumen caused by congenital malformation or trauma. Trauma (e.g., penetrating or blunt wounds, foreign bodies, and indwelling tubes) or surgery may cause segmental tracheal stenosis when the wound heals by secondary intention, and excess fibrosis and scarring cause luminal narrowing, or tracheal cartilages heal with an abnormal shape. Traumatic stenosis is treated by balloon dilation or resection and anastomosis. Congenital stenosis occurs when tracheal cartilages are abnormally small, abnormally shaped, or malpositioned. Tracheal hypoplasia is a form of congenital tracheal stenosis. It

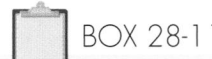

BOX 28-11

Radiographic Diagnosis of Hypoplastic Tracheas

- Ratio of tracheal lumen diameter at the thoracic inlet to the thoracic inlet diameter (TD/TI) less than 0.2
- Ratio of tracheal lumen diameter at the midpoint between the thoracic inlet and carina to width of the third rib (TT/3R) less than 3

is characterized by an abnormally narrow lumen along the entire length of the trachea, rigid tracheal cartilages that are apposed or overlap, and a dorsal tracheal membrane that is narrow or obscured. Tracheal hypoplasia primarily affects brachycephalic breeds, especially English bulldogs, which sometimes have other congenital abnormalities (e.g., stenotic nares, elongated soft palate, aortic stenosis, pulmonic stenosis, and megaesophagus). Tracheal hypoplasia can be associated with continuous respiratory distress, coughing, and recurrent tracheitis, but may be tolerated in the absence of concurrent respiratory or cardiovascular disease. Tracheal hypoplasia can be identified endoscopically or radiographically (Box 28-11). Treatment of tracheal hypoplasia is symptomatic medical therapy (i.e., antibiotics and cough suppressants) and correction of other airway obstructions (e.g., resection of nares, palate, and saccules).

DIAGNOSIS
Clinical Presentation

Signalment. Typically, tracheal collapse occurs in toy- and miniature-breed dogs, most commonly toy poodles, Yorkshire terriers, Pomeranians, Maltese, and Chihuahuas. Males and females are affected equally. Tracheal collapse in larger dogs usually is associated with trauma, deformity, or intraluminal or extraluminal masses and should not be equated with tracheal collapse in toy-breed dogs. Tracheal collapse is classically described as occurring in middle-aged or older toy breeds (average, 6 to 8 years). However, it frequently is diagnosed in dogs with respiratory problems between 1 and 5 years of age.

History. The onset of clinical signs often occurs before 1 year of age. Clinical signs often progress with age and include abnormal respiratory noise, dyspnea, exercise intolerance, cyanosis, and syncope. Some dogs never suffer respiratory distress, and others die of asphyxiation. Clinical signs are more severe in obese animals. Respiratory noises include wheezing, hacking, coughing, and stridulous breathing. Some dogs do not make abnormal respiratory noises. The cough may be productive or nonproductive but is classically a "goose honk" cough. Coughing often becomes cyclic and paroxysmal. Gagging after coughing may occur in as many as 50% of cases. Signs may be elicited or exacerbated by tracheal infections, tracheal compression, exercise, excitement, eating, drinking, or hot, humid weather. Noxious stimuli (i.e., smoke and other respiratory irritants) may also precipitate clinical signs.

Physical Examination Findings

Flaccid tracheal cartilages with prominent lateral borders occasionally are evident on palpation of the cervical trachea. Palpation may elicit paroxysmal coughing. Auscultation may localize abnormal respiratory noises and identify mitral valve disease. A soft end-expiratory snapping together of the tracheal wall may be auscultated in dogs with intrathoracic tracheal collapse. Abnormal heart sounds may be associated with concurrent cardiac disease. Hepatomegaly has been associated with this syndrome in some patients, and may result from venous congestion caused by cor pulmonale or fatty change.

Diagnostic Imaging

Inspiratory and expiratory lateral radiographs of the neck and thorax are diagnostic in approximately 60% of patients with severe tracheal collapse (greater than 50% of the lumen). The cervical trachea is expected to collapse on inspiration and the thoracic trachea on expiration. Thoracic radiographs often reveal cardiomegaly and pulmonary disease as well. Fluoroscopy facilitates evaluation of the dynamic movement of the trachea and mainstem bronchi through all phases of respiration and finds many cases missed by survey radiographs. However, fluoroscopy will miss collapse of the trachea in the lateral dimension; tracheoscopy is considered the optimal diagnostic test.

Laryngoscopy. Laryngoscopy (see pp. 840 and 843) should usually be done at the same time as tracheoscopy because laryngeal paralysis or collapse is present in approximately 30% of dogs with tracheal collapse. Approximately 50% of affected dogs have bronchial compression or collapse.

Tracheoscopy. Tracheoscopy is indicated in animals with diagnosed tracheal collapse that are about to undergo surgery and in patients in which tracheal collapse is an important differential but radiographs and fluoroscopy have failed to make a diagnosis. One should use a rigid or flexible bronchoscope with a small enough outer diameter to allow the patient to easily breathe around it, thus minimizing the likelihood of obstructing or traumatizing the trachea. If the patient is at risk for hypoxia or if the procedure will take more than a few minutes, one may attach a tube from the anesthetic machine to the biopsy port on the bronchoscope so that oxygen can be insufflated during the procedure. However, it is critical to use a judicious flow rate so as not to cause barotrauma. Alternatively, one may repeatedly insert and withdraw the scope until an adequate evaluation has been performed. Tracheal cultures and brushings taken during tracheoscopy are useful in selecting antibiotics. Tracheal cultures should be taken during the first insertion of the bronchoscope. A guarded cytology brush is useful for quickly obtaining a good mucosal sample for culture; the tip of the brush is aseptically cut off and allowed to fall into broth. If desired, cytology samples are obtained with a second cytology brush and may be taken at any time during the procedure.

Tracheal conformation should be evaluated to determine the location and severity of the collapse. It is often easier to

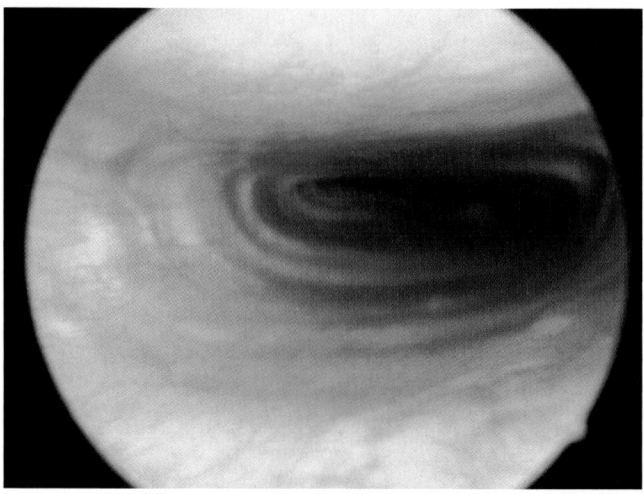

FIG. 28-22
Endoscopic view of a Grade III dorsoventral tracheal collapse.

insert the scope to the carina and then evaluate the trachea as it is withdrawn, but this may not be possible in critically ill patients. The entire trachea usually is collapsed; however, one area of the trachea often is more severely affected and is used for classification purposes. Grade I tracheal collapse is a 25% reduction in lumen diameter, with the trachealis muscle being slightly pendulous and the cartilages maintaining a somewhat circular shape. Grade II collapse is a 50% reduction in lumen diameter, with the trachealis muscle stretched and pendulous and the cartilages beginning to flatten. Grade III collapse is a 75% reduction in lumen diameter, with the trachealis more stretched and pendulous and the cartilages nearly flattened (Fig. 28-22). Grade IV collapse means the lumen is essentially obliterated, and the tracheal cartilages are completely flattened and may invert to contact the trachealis muscle.

Laboratory Findings

Hematologic and serum biochemistry findings are usually normal or insignificant unless concurrent systemic disease is present. Many dogs (especially when obese) have mild to moderate increases in serum alkaline phosphatase. Positive tracheobronchial cultures are found in more than 50% of animals with tracheal collapse (Johnson and Fales, 2001). Bacterial infection of the airways is generally accompanied by cytologic evidence of suppurative inflammation and detectable intracellular bacteria. Infection is also suggested by substantial growth of a single bacterial species in culture media. Electrocardiograms may reveal sinus arrhythmia, cor pulmonale, or left ventricular enlargement.

DIFFERENTIAL DIAGNOSIS

Other causes of chronic coughing or respiratory distress include brachycephalic syndrome, tonsillitis, laryngeal collapse, laryngeal paralysis, bronchitis, tracheobronchitis, allergies, heartworm disease, pulmonary disease, cardiac

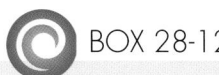

BOX 28-12

Drugs Used in Treatment of Tracheal Collapse

Butorphanol Tartrate (Torbutrol)
0.5–1 mg/kg PO bid to qid

Hydrocodone Bitartrate (Hycodan)
0.2 mg/kg PO tid to qid

Co-phenotrope (Lomotil) (2.5 mg diphenoxylate hydrochloride + 0.025 mg atropine per 5 ml)
0.2 to 0.5 mg/kg diphenoxylate PO bid

Ampicillin
22 mg/kg IV, IM, or SC tid

Amoxicillin
22 mg/kg PO bid

Cefazolin (Ancef, Kefzol)
22 mg/kg IV or IM tid

Clindamycin (Antirobe, Cleocin)
11 mg/kg PO, IV, or IM bid

Enrofloxacin (Baytril)
7–20 mg/kg PO or IV (given diluted and slowly over 30 min)

Aminophylline*
Dogs: 11 mg/kg PO, IM, or IV tid to qid (if given IV, give slowly over 5 min)
Cats: 5 mg/kg PO bid

Theophylline (Extended Release)
Dogs: 5–30 mg/kg PO qd to bid, depending upon the product
Cats: 10–25 mg/kg PO qd, depending upon the product

Propentofylline (Karsivan)
3 mg/kg PO bid

Dexamethasone (Azium)
0.2 mg/kg IV, IM, or SC bid; Can give up to 6 mg/kg for emergency treatment†

Prednisolone
1.1–2.2 mg/kg PO qd to bid

PO, Oral; *bid,* twice a day; *qid,* four times a day; *tid,* three times a day; *qd,* once a day; *IV,* intravenous; *IM,* intramuscular; *SC,* subcutaneous; *qd,* once a day.
*Do not give as a rapid IV bolus.
†Large doses can be associated with gastrointestinal hemorrhage.

disease (especially mitral valve insufficiency), hypoplastic trachea, tracheal stenosis, and tracheal neoplasia or mass.

MEDICAL MANAGEMENT

Medical therapy is recommended for all animals with mild clinical signs and for those with less than 50% collapse. Medical therapy for dogs with tracheal collapse includes antitussives (i.e., butorphanol tartrate, hydrocodone bitartrate, and diphenoxylate; Box 28-12), antibiotics (i.e., ampicillin, cefazolin, clindamycin, and enrofloxacin), bronchodilators (i.e., extended-release theophylline, aminophylline, albuterol, and terbutaline), and/or corticosteroids (i.e., dexamethasone and prednisolone). Sedation with acepromazine (0.05 to 0.2 mg/kg [maximum 1 mg] IV, IM, or SC tid) and/or diazepam (0.2 mg/kg IV bid) and supplemental oxygen (see Table 5-4 on p. 26) may be required in severely dyspneic patients. Pediatric metered dose inhalers used with spacers and face masks may be used in cooperative dogs to administer bronchodilators (i.e., albuterol) and corticosteroids (Padrid et al, 2000). Mucolytics and saline nebulization may benefit those with excess mucus production and infections. Weight reduction should be instituted for obese patients. Exercise restriction is recommended. Affected dogs should be maintained in an environment free of smoke and other respiratory irritants or allergens. Response to medical therapy is usually transient, and the disease typically progresses.

SURGICAL TREATMENT

Surgery is recommended for all dogs with moderate to severe clinical signs, a 50% or greater reduction of the tracheal lumen, or clinical signs refractory to medical therapy. Surgery should not be delayed until the animal is in severe respiratory distress. Tracheal collapse often is overlooked in young dogs, which allows degenerative changes to progress, clinical signs to worsen, and secondary problems to develop. Dogs brought in for treatment with laryngeal paralysis or collapse, generalized cardiomegaly, bronchial collapse, and chronic pulmonary disease are poor surgical candidates. Coughing and dyspnea caused by laryngeal, pulmonary, or cardiac disease are not expected to improve without appropriate therapy. Respiratory distress and death may occur in animals with severe laryngeal dysfunction or bronchopulmonary disease. Concurrent mainstem bronchial collapse is present in some dogs. There currently is no technique to support collapsed mainstem bronchi; cervical tracheoplasty may not be beneficial if mainstem bronchial collapse is severe.

The goal of surgery is to support the tracheal cartilages and trachealis muscle while preserving as much of the segmental blood and nerve supply to the trachea as possible. Many techniques have been described. Currently the only techniques that meet this goal are placement of extraluminal individual rings or modified spiral ring prostheses or intraluminal stents. Generally, only the cervical trachea and most proximal portion of the thoracic trachea are supported by extraluminal prostheses even when cervical and thoracic tracheal collapse are present. Intraluminal stent placement involves less risk of interrupting innervation and blood supply, but implants are expensive, require fluoroscopic or endoscopic placement, and are associated with serious complications. Currently, intraluminal stents are best used as a salvage procedure for severe, refractory tracheal collapse involving the thoracic trachea. Patients with concurrent laryngeal paralysis or laryngeal collapse may also require arytenoid lateralization (see p. 844) or permanent tracheostomy (see p. 826), respectively.

Preoperative Management

These patients should be observed closely for signs of progressive dyspnea after hospitalization. Prostheses should be placed immediately after endoscopy to prevent a second complicated anesthetic recovery. Prophylactic antibiotics (i.e., cefazolin; 22 mg/kg IV, repeated every 2 to 4 hours until completion of surgery) should be given at the time of induction. Corticosteroids may be given to dogs with very small tracheas (i.e., those weighing less than 2 to 4 kg) to minimize tracheal mucosal swelling.

Anesthesia

These patients should be preoxygenated, and they should be induced and intubated quickly. Manipulation of the endotracheal tube by an assistant is necessary during placement of each ring prosthesis to ensure that sutures have not been placed into the endotracheal tube or cuff. Extubation should be delayed as long as possible after surgery. Laryngeal paralysis may occur secondary to recurrent laryngeal nerve damage (see p. 842). Supplementation of oxygen via nasal insufflation (see Table 5-4 on p. 26) is beneficial, particularly if laryngeal paralysis or severe tracheal inflammation occurs. General anesthetic recommendations for animals with upper respiratory disease are given on p. 818.

Surgical Anatomy

The surgical anatomy of the trachea is discussed on p. 821. The segmental blood and nerve supply to the trachea travels in the lateral pedicles on each side of the trachea. Minimal mobilization of the trachea is necessary to maintain a good blood supply after surgery. The left recurrent laryngeal nerve is located in the lateral pedicle; the right is sometimes located within the carotid sheath.

Positioning

The animal should be positioned in dorsal recumbency with the neck extended and elevated over a pad (to deviate the trachea ventrally). The caudal mandibular area, ventral neck, and cranial thorax should be clipped and prepared for aseptic surgery.

SURGICAL TECHNIQUE

Extraluminal stents. Prosthetic tracheal rings or spirals are made by cutting 3-ml polypropylene syringe cases. To create individual rings, a pipe cutter can be used to divide a syringe case into cylinders 5 to 8 mm wide. Five or more staggered holes should be drilled through each ring for suture placement, and the ring should be split ventrally to allow placement. Rough edges of the rings can be smoothened by firing or trimming with a No. 11 blade or file. The rings should be autoclaved before implantation. Gas sterilization is possible, but the rings must be aerated at least 72 hours to prevent toxic tissue reactions and tracheal necro-

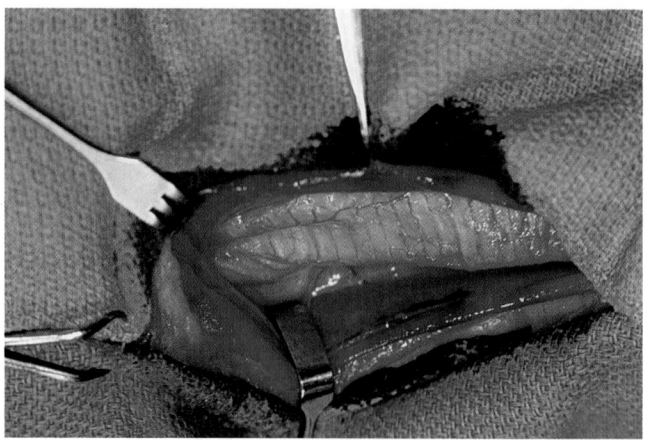

FIG. 28-23
Intraoperative appearance of a Grade IV tracheal collapse.

sis. Narrower notched rings of variable diameter are now commercially available (New Generation Devices, Franklin Lakes, N.J.).

Incise the skin and subcutaneous tissues along the ventral cervical midline from the larynx to the manubrium. Separate the sternohyoid and sternocephalicus muscles along their midline to expose the cervical trachea. Examine the trachea for evidence of collapse and deformity (Fig. 28-23). Identify and protect the recurrent laryngeal nerves. Place the first tracheal prosthesis one or two cartilages distal to the larynx. Dissect the peritracheal tissues and create a tunnel immediately around the trachea only in the areas of prosthetic ring placement. Guide and position a prosthetic ring through the tunnel and around the trachea with a long, curved hemostat (Fig. 28-24, A and B). Position the prosthetic ring with the split on the ventral aspect of the trachea. Chondrotomy occasionally is necessary to allow deformed, rigid cartilages to conform to the prosthesis. Secure the prosthesis with sutures ventrally, laterally, and dorsally (Fig. 28-24, C). Place three to six sutures (3-0 or 4-0 polypropylene) to secure each prosthesis. Direct sutures around rather than through cartilages and engage the trachealis muscle in at least one suture. Place four to six additional ring prostheses 5 to 8 mm apart along the trachea (Fig. 28-25). Cranial traction on the prostheses around the cervical trachea allows one or two rings to be placed at the thoracic inlet or beyond. Preserve the blood vessels and nerves between the rings. Manipulate the endotracheal tube or trachea after the placement of each prosthesis to be sure the tube cuff has not been engaged by a suture. Place a radiopaque marker on the last ring to radiographically identify its location postoperatively if desired. Lavage the surgical site with sterile saline. Appose the sternohyoid and sternocephalicus muscles with simple continuous sutures (3-0 or 4-0 polydioxanone) and appose the subcutaneous tissues and skin routinely.

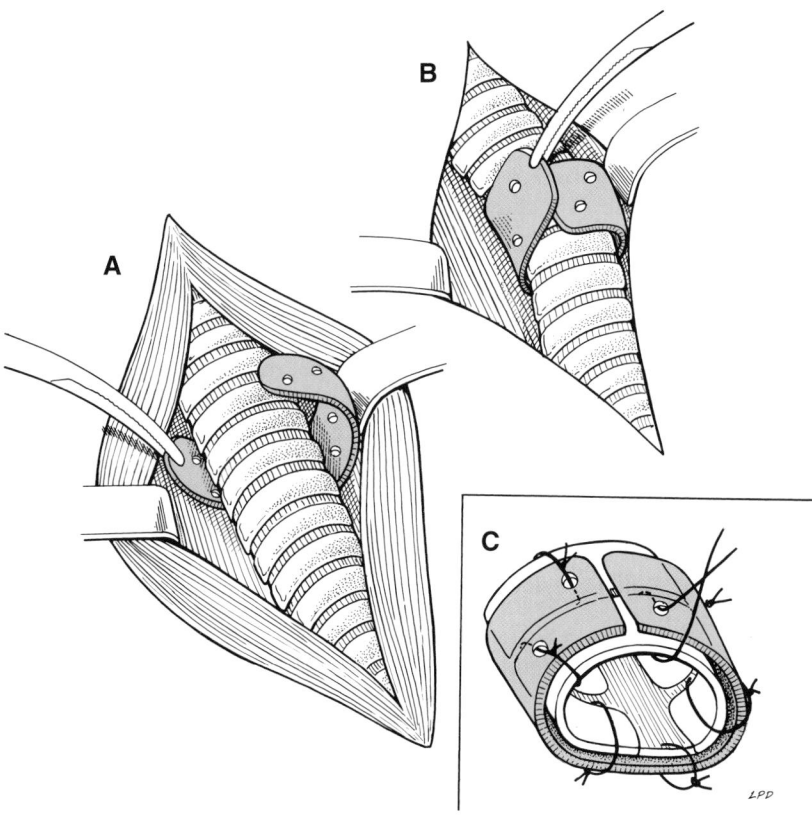

FIG. 28-24
A, To place prosthetic rings on the trachea, dissect a tunnel around the trachea at each implantation site and then guide the prosthesis through the tunnel. **B,** Rotate the prosthesis around the trachea. **C,** Secure the prosthesis with several sutures.

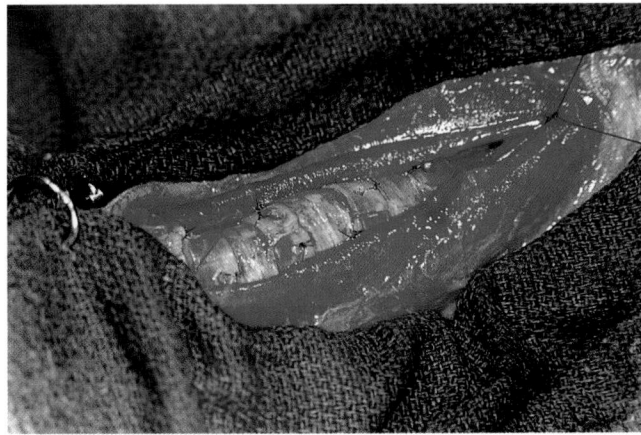

FIG. 28-25
Appearance of the trachea after placement of six tracheal ring prostheses.

Endoscopic placement of stents. The minimally invasive technique used for intraluminal prosthesis placement varies with the type of self-expanding elastic implant selected. Selection of implant size must be accurate and may be determined from measurements taken during tracheoscopy or imaging.

Place a metric radiopaque ruler beneath the patient to account for magnification error when taking measurements from radiographs.

The implant should remain about 10 mm from the larynx and the carina in most cases to prevent excess irritation and granulation. If the stent is near the thoracic inlet, constant movement at that point often leads to early fracture of the stent. Some have recommended measuring diameter from films captured while positive pressure airway insufflation to 10 mm Hg (20 cm H_2O) is applied with the end of the tube positioned at the end of the larynx. Open-looped or knitted implants are preferred because they promote coverage of the stent with tracheal epithelium.

After selection of the implant, anesthetize the dog, insert the implant, and deploy it according to manufacturer's instructions with the aid of fluoroscopy or endoscopic positioning. Place multiple stents if necessary. Repositioning stents is usually not possible after they have been deployed.

NOTE: Because intraluminal stents cannot be easily retrieved and there are many potential complications associated with their use, they are not generally recommended in the early management of tracheal collapse.

POSTOPERATIVE CARE AND ASSESSMENT

These animals should be continuously monitored during recovery. Acute respiratory distress may occur postoperatively secondary to inflammation, edema, and/or laryngeal paresis or paralysis. Animals with laryngeal paralysis may require surgery to widen the glottis (see p. 844), and those with collapse may require a permanent tracheostomy (see p. 826) within the first 24 hours to relieve respiratory distress. Nasal insufflation of oxygen and an antiinflammatory dose of corticosteroids may be beneficial in animals with edema and inflammation. Mucolytics and saline nebulization may be appropriate for those with severe inflammation. Antibiotics should be continued for 7 to 10 days if bacterial tracheitis is present. Antitussives, bronchodilators, analgesics, and sedatives may be given as necessary to control coughing and excitement (see Box 28-12). These animals should have strict exercise restriction (cage rest) for 3 to 7 days. Thereafter exercise may be increased gradually. A harness rather than a collar should be used for leash walking. Weight reduction is important in obese patients. Tracheoscopy is recommended 1 to 2 months after surgery and later if respiratory signs deteriorate.

Immediate improvement in clinical signs may be seen; however, coughing and lack of marked improvement in clinical signs should be expected for several weeks postoperatively because of tracheitis, peritracheal swelling, and suture irritation. However, clinical improvement (e.g., decreased respiratory noise, less respiratory effort, increased exercise tolerance, and fewer tracheobronchial infections) should be noted within 2 to 3 weeks of surgery. Some animals have nearly complete remission of clinical signs after surgery, whereas others continue to have episodes of coughing or other respiratory noises. The quality of life is improved for most patients, but neither surgery nor stents cures the condition.

COMPLICATIONS

Death may result if the trachea is obstructed by severe inflammation or damaged by severe infection or necrosis with either extraluminal or intraluminal prostheses. Coughing after surgery is expected until inflammation subsides. Infection is a possible problem because the trachea contains bacteria that may be harbored in implants.

Bruising and mild cervical swelling are expected postoperatively after placement of extraluminal prostheses. Recurrent laryngeal nerve damage may result in laryngospasms, laryngeal paresis, or paralysis. Tracheal necrosis may occur if too much dissection strips the blood supply away from the trachea or if improperly aerated prostheses (gas sterilized) are implanted.

Incorrect placement or sizing of intraluminal implants may result in death. Failure to stent the entire involved trachea typically results in collapse proximal and/or distal to the stent. A stent that is too narrow may migrate, whereas one that is too wide may cause pressure necrosis. Stents placed too close to the larynx may cause intractable laryngospasms. Tracheal obstruction caused by granuloma formation, which may be steroid responsive, occurs in about 20% to 30% of the cases. Other reported complications include cough, expectoration, tracheal hemorrhage, emphysema, pneumomediastinum, infection, mucous obstruction, tracheal rupture, squamous metaplasia and ulceration of the tracheal epithelium, implant shortening, implant fracture, and implant collapse or deformation.

PROGNOSIS

Clinical signs can sometimes be controlled medically if tracheal collapse is not severe, patients do not become obese, and a sedentary lifestyle is practiced. The prognosis is more dependent on concurrent respiratory problems, such as laryngeal paralysis or collapse and bronchial disease, than on the location or severity of tracheal collapse. Dogs with laryngeal and bronchial disease do not improve clinically as much as those with tracheal collapse alone. Approximately 80% to 90% of dogs with tracheal collapse improve clinically after tracheoplasty. Approximately 90% of dogs initially improve following stent implantation, but later complications worsen the prognosis (Moritz et al, 2004).

References

Johnson LR, Fales WH: Clinical and microbiologic findings in dogs with bronchoscopically diagnosed tracheal collapse: 37 cases (1990-1995), *J Am Vet Med Assoc* 219:1247, 2001.

Moritz A, Schneider M, Bauer N: Management of advanced tracheal collapse in dogs using intraluminal self-expanding biliary Wallstents, *J Vet Intern Med* 18:31, 2004.

Padrid P: Feline asthma: diagnosis and treatment, *Vet Clin North Am Small Anim Pract* 30:1279, 2000.

Suggested Reading

Gellasch KL, da Costa Gomez T, McAnulty JF et al: Use of intraluminal nitinol stents in the treatment of tracheal collapse in a dog, *J Am Vet Med Assoc* 221:1719, 2002.

This case report describes the placement of additional stents to treat complications following original stent placement.

Mittleman E, Weisse C, Mehler SJ et al: Fracture of an endoluminal nitinol stent used in the treatment of tracheal collapse in a dog, *J Am Vet Med Assoc* 225:1217, 2004.

This case report declares that because of complications, intraluminal stents should be viewed as a salvage procedure.

LARYNGEAL AND TRACHEAL TUMORS

DEFINITION

Oncocytomas arise from epithelial cells called oncocytes, small numbers of which are found in various organs, such as the larynx, thyroid, pituitary, and trachea.

GENERAL CONSIDERATIONS AND CLINICALLY RELEVANT PATHOPHYSIOLOGY

Laryngeal and tracheal tumors are rare; however, laryngeal tumors are more common than tracheal tumors in cats (Jakubiak et al, 2005). Various tumor types have been identified in the larynx of dogs (Box 28-13). In cats, lymphosarcoma is most common although squamous cell carcinoma and adenocarcinoma have also been reported. Rhabdomyomas and oncocytomas are laryngeal tumors that appear

BOX 28-13

Laryngeal Tumors

Malignant	Benign
• Squamous cell carcinoma	• Lipoma
• Lymphoma	• Oncocytoma
• Osteosarcoma	• Rhabdomyoma
• Fibrosarcoma	
• Rhabdomyosarcoma	
• Melanoma	
• Mast cell tumor	
• Other sarcomas	
• Granular cell myoblastoma	
• Adenocarcinoma	
• Undifferentiated carcinoma	

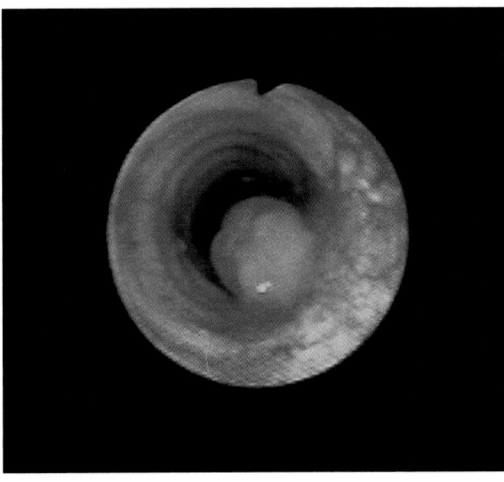

FIG. 28-26
Tracheal oncocytoma in a 7-year-old basset hound that was brought in for treatment of acute respiratory distress.

 BOX 28-14

Tracheal Tumors

Malignant	Benign
• Osteosarcoma	• Osteochondroma
• Chondrosarcoma	• Oncocytoma
• Lymphoma	• Leiomyoma
• Mast cell tumor	• Chondroma
• Adenocarcinoma	• Extramedullary
• Squamous cell carcinoma	plasmacytoma
• Rhabdomyosarcoma	• Polyp

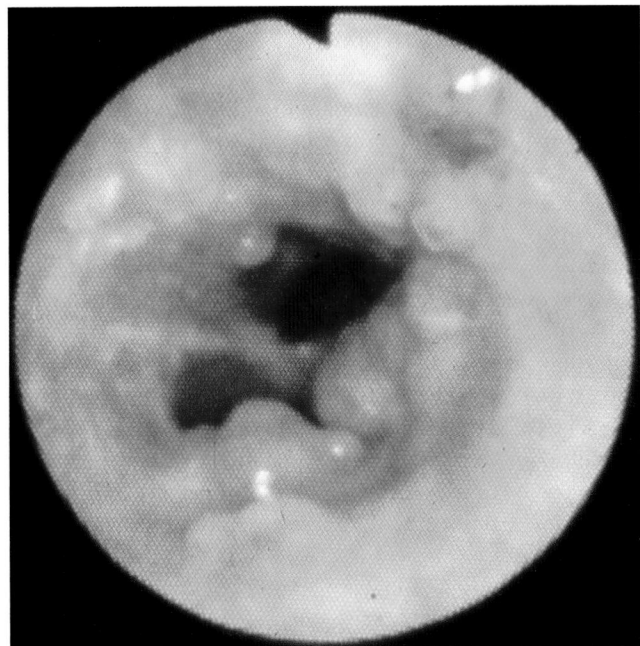

FIG. 28-27
Filaroides nodules at the carina of the trachea.

histologically similar with light microscopy; electron microscopy and immunocytochemistry are necessary to distinguish them. Oncocytomas have been reported in young dogs and warrant special consideration because long-term survival of patients without metastasis has been reported after surgical resection (Fig. 28-26).

Malignant and benign tracheal tumors have been reported (Box 28-14). Tracheal osteochondromas may occur in dogs younger than 1 year of age. These masses probably reflect a malfunction of osteogenesis and are benign. Their growth is expected to stop with skeletal maturity. In cats, tracheal squamous cell carcinomas, adenocarcinomas, and lymphosarcomas have been reported. Metastatic thyroid carcinomas, lymphomas, and pharyngeal rhabdomyosarcomas may also involve the larynx and trachea. The incidence of metastasis of laryngeal and tracheal tumors in dogs and cats is unknown.

Oslerus osleri (Filaroides osleri) is a nematode that forms neoplastic-appearing nodules in the canine trachea and mainstem bronchi (Figs. 28-27 and 28-28). Nonendoscopic diagnosis of filaroidosis (i.e., finding larvae by Baermann fecal examination) is difficult because larvae are intermittently shed in the feces. Diagnosis is best made by finding larvae or adults by tracheal cytology. Anthelmintic therapy

and surgical resection have met with varying success. Aberrant *Cuterebra* larvae and associated tissue trauma may obstruct the laryngeal or tracheal lumen. These lesions must be differentiated from neoplastic lesions.

Laryngeal and tracheal tumors cause luminal obstruction by occupying space or compressing the lumen externally. As lumen size decreases, signs of respiratory distress become apparent (see p. 856). Acute respiratory distress, cyanosis, or collapse (or all of these) may occur if excitement, stress, high temperatures, or infections cause mucosal swelling of an already compromised lumen.

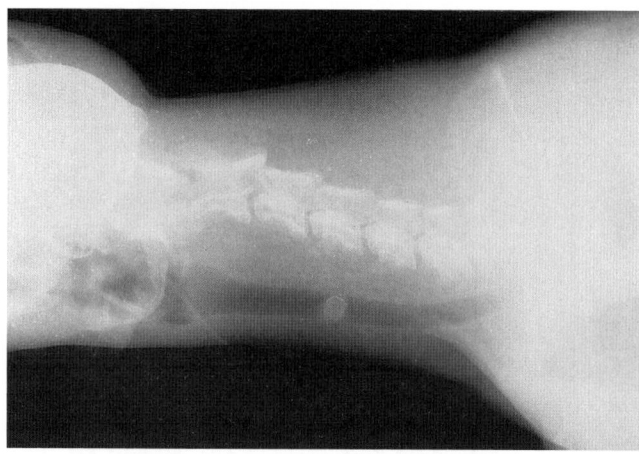

FIG. 28-28
Tracheal osteochondroma in a 6-month-old dog.

DIAGNOSIS
Clinical Presentation

Signalment. Laryngeal and tracheal tumors occur most often in middle-aged to older animals (i.e., 5 to 15 years) with a median age of 12 years for cats and 10 years for dogs with the exception of osteochondromas, which usually occur before 2 years. Tumors arising in older animals are more likely to be malignant; however, laryngeal oncocytomas and tracheal osteochondromas may occur in young animals. Benign tracheal osteocartilaginous tumors (osteochondromas) are most common in animals with active osteochondral ossification; they grow with the rest of the musculoskeletal system and may be recognized before 1 year of age. Siamese cats may be prone to lymphoma (Jakubiak et al, 2005).

History. Animals with laryngeal or tracheal tumors may have an acute or progressive history of upper airway obstruction. Signs may include dysphonia, stridor, dyspnea, cough, decreased exercise tolerance, voice change, hyperthermia, ptyalism, gagging, dysphagia, cyanosis, or syncope, or all of these. Weight loss and lethargy may also be reported. Development of a mass in the ventral neck may be reported.

Physical Examination Findings

The physical examination usually is normal unless concurrent diseases or abnormalities are present. Occasionally, extraluminal masses may be palpated along the ventral neck, and tracheal palpation may elicit coughing or increased dyspnea. A voice change may be noted in animals with laryngeal masses. Enlarged, accessible lymph nodes should be aspirated or a biopsy taken (see p. 619) to help stage the disease. The medial retropharyngeal lymph nodes drain the larynx and proximal trachea, but usually are inaccessible.

Diagnostic Imaging

Pharyngeal and cervical radiographs should be evaluated to determine the location and extent of the tumor. Laryngeal and tracheal masses may appear as soft tissue densities in the airway (see Fig. 28-28). Laryngeal distortion, decreased mar-gination of laryngeal structures, and decreased laryngeal space (stenosis) may also be seen. Extraluminal masses may compress the tracheal lumen.

Thoracic radiographs should be evaluated for metastasis and bronchopneumonia. In rare cases, the lungs may appear to be hyperinflated if a tracheal or bronchial mass is large enough to act as a one-way valve. Occasionally, contrast esophagrams or esophagoscopy are needed to rule out esophageal involvement. Computed tomography (CT) and magnetic resonance imaging (MRI) are expected to more precisely demonstrate the mass and its invasiveness.

Laryngoscopy. Laryngoscopy is preferred for examination and biopsy of pharyngeal and laryngeal masses. If a mass or abnormal structure is seen, it may be aspirated or brushed or a biopsy taken with punch-type biopsy forceps. Hemorrhage may be controlled with direct pressure or, in severe cases, with chemical cautery. However, care must be taken not to cause obstruction as a result of edema from such cautery.

Tracheoscopy. For tracheal masses, one should use a flexible bronchoscope with a small enough outer diameter to allow the patient to easily breathe around it, thus minimizing the likelihood of obstructing or traumatizing the trachea. If the patient is at risk for hypoxia or if the procedure will take more than a few minutes, one may attach a tube from the anesthetic machine to the biopsy port on the bronchoscope so that oxygen can be insufflated during the procedure. However, it is critical to use a judicious flow rate so as not to cause barotrauma. Alternatively, one may repeatedly insert and withdraw the scope until an adequate evaluation has been performed.

Most laryngeal and tracheal tumors are inflamed or edematous, pink, fleshy masses protruding into the lumen (Fig. 28-29); however, some laryngeal tumors appear as a diffuse thickening. The size and consistency of the tumor and the nature of its attachment to the tracheal wall should be noted. Biopsy may be performed using biopsy forceps or cytology brushes. It is usually advisable to first attempt brush cytology since that is faster and less risky. If cytology is not diagnostic, then one may take a biopsy of the mass; however, one should inspect the mass first and note the blood supply. If there are numerous vessels seen on the mass, then hemorrhage is a greater risk, and suction (usually through the endoscope) must be readily available.

Laboratory Findings

A complete blood count, serum biochemistry profile, and urinalysis are indicated to evaluate the patient's overall status and to look for paraneoplastic syndromes. If lymphoma is suspected, a bone marrow aspiration and (in cats) a feline leukemia virus (FeLV) test are warranted.

DIFFERENTIAL DIAGNOSIS

Differential diagnoses include obstruction of the larynx caused by elongated soft palate, laryngeal collapse, laryngeal paralysis, nasopharyngeal polyp, foreign bodies, inflammation, cysts, or granulomatous masses (*Oslerus osleri*). Inflammatory lesions include lymphoplasmacytic and

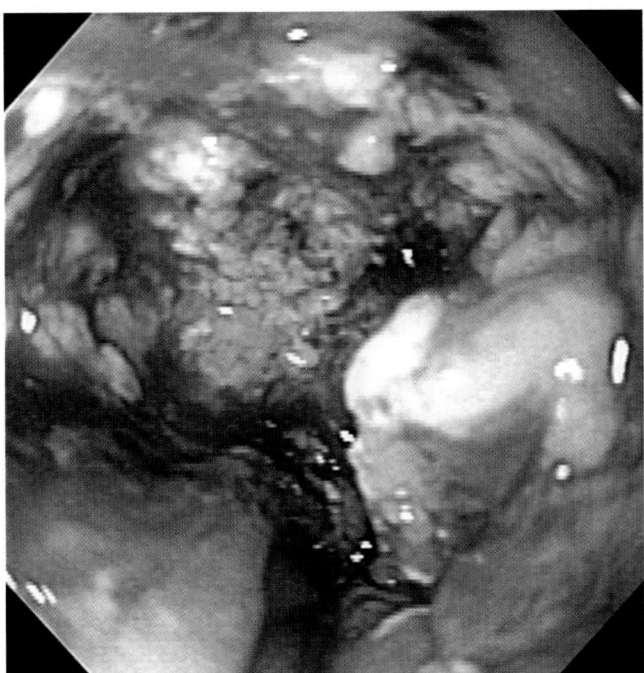

FIG. 28-29
Endoscopic view of a pharyngeal carcinoma in a cat. The mass is ulcerated and necrotic.

lymphoid hyperplastic masses. Other causes of tracheal obstruction include tracheal collapse or hypoplasia, foreign bodies, congenital malformations, cysts, inflammation, granulomatous masses, nodular amyloidosis, or excess respiratory secretions.

MEDICAL MANAGEMENT

Radiation therapy may help treat squamous cell carcinomas, mast cell tumors, and lymphomas, but little information is available. Some tumors respond to chemotherapy (e.g., lymphomas, mast cell tumors, and adenocarcinomas). Permanent tracheostomy can palliate signs of respiratory distress during medical therapy.

SURGICAL TREATMENT

Surgical excision may be curative if the tumor is benign, localized, and small. Complete excision of malignant tumors is rarely possible, but excision may palliate the dyspnea. Laryngeal tumors may be resected by partial or total laryngectomy. For removal of tracheal tumors, a tracheal resection and end-to-end anastomosis are required (see p. 827). Depending on its elasticity, 20% to 60% of the trachea (i.e., usually six to eight rings) may be resected. Resection of large tumors with a minimum of 1 cm of normal trachea on both sides of the mass is not always possible. When resection would be too extensive to achieve, end-to-end anastomosis, tracheal replacement, or prostheses may be considered, but are rarely successful. Resection of a segment of the tracheal wall without complete transection (i.e., wedge resection) and reapposition of the cut edges is not recommended because it narrows, or kinks, the trachea, which interferes with airflow and mucociliary transport.

Preoperative Management

The animal should be kept calm to prevent progressive dyspnea; sedation may be necessary in some animals (see p. 817). An antiinflammatory dose of corticosteroids may also be administered if dyspnea is severe (dexamethasone [Azium], 0.5 to 2 mg/kg IV, IM, or SC). Dyspneic animals should be oxygenated before surgery. An emergency tracheostomy may be necessary in severely dyspneic animals (see p. 825).

Anesthesia

Animals with laryngeal masses may require intubation via a pharyngostomy or tracheotomy incision (see p. 825). Intubation and ventilation of patients with intraluminal tracheal masses may require insertion of a small-diameter tube or tracheostomy distal to the obstruction. Specific anesthetic recommendations for animals with respiratory disease are given on p. 818.

Surgical Anatomy

The surgical anatomy of the larynx and trachea is discussed on p. 820.

Positioning

Patients requiring laryngotomy or cervical tracheal resection should be positioned in dorsal recumbency with the neck deviated ventrally with a dorsally placed pad or roll (see Fig. 28-12). The entire caudal mandibular area, ventral neck, and cranial thorax should be prepared for aseptic surgery. Partial laryngectomy may be performed with the patient in ventral recumbency with the head suspended and the mouth open widely or in dorsal recumbency. Total laryngectomy may be performed with the patient initially positioned in ventral recumbency for oropharyngeal mucosal incision and then repositioned in dorsal recumbency to allow removal of the larynx and permanent tracheostomy.

SURGICAL TECHNIQUE
Partial Laryngectomy

Partial laryngectomy is performed using either an oral or a laryngotomy approach (see p. 845). Mucosal closure after tumor resection helps prevent the formation of scar tissue and is more readily achieved when a laryngotomy approach is used.

Using sharp dissection, remove the mass with a margin of normal tissue. If possible, preserve the lateral margin of the corniculate process to allow appropriate epiglottic protection of the glottis. Avoid bilateral disruption of the dorsal and ventral laryngeal commissures to reduce the risk of postoperative glottic stenosis.

Complete or Total Laryngectomy

Total laryngectomy requires the creation of a permanent tracheostomy. It is a difficult procedure that is not often performed.

Expose the larynx by a ventral midline cervical incision. Transect the right and left sternohyoid muscles from their insertion on the basihyoid bone. Disarticulate the hyoid apparatus between the keratohyoid and basihyoid articulations with the thyrohyoid bones. Dissect dorsolaterally and excise the thyropharyngeus and cricopharyngeus muscles bilaterally from their insertion on the thyroid cartilage. Incise the pharyngeal mucosa at the base of the epiglottis, preserving as much mucosa as possible while keeping tumor-free margins. Free the larynx by transecting between the cricoid and first tracheal cartilage or between the first and second tracheal cartilages. Remove additional tissue as necessary to achieve an en bloc resection. Lavage the surgical field. Begin reconstruction by closing the pharyngeal submucosa in a continuous pattern with 3-0 polydioxanone suture.

This suture line will be under tension.

Attach the sternohyoid muscles to the basihyoid bone dorsal to the trachea. Place a closed suction or Penrose drain if dead space is not completely eliminated. As an alternative, incise and appose the pharyngeal mucosa through an oral approach.

The technique for permanent tracheostomy must be varied when a complete laryngectomy is performed. This procedure is rarely performed and may be challenging. Either close the end of the proximal trachea with a series of interrupted horizontal sutures and then perform a permanent tracheostomy as described on p. 826 or divert and incorporate the transected proximal trachea to create the tracheostoma.

To close the end of the proximal trachea, place a series of interrupted horizontal mattress sutures from the annular ligament or tracheal cartilage through the dorsal tracheal membrane. As an alternative, preserve a flap of dorsal tracheal membrane during resection, fold it over the end of the trachea, and secure it with interrupted sutures. To incorporate the proximal trachea in the tracheostoma, create the tracheostoma by first apposing the sternohyoid muscles dorsal to the trachea. Remove the ventral third of four to six tracheal cartilages, taking care to preserve the underlying tracheal mucosa. Elevate the dorsal tracheal membrane, apposing and suturing it directly to the skin proximally using 4-0 polypropylene suture. Excise excess skin surrounding the stoma and place intradermal sutures from the skin to peritracheal tissues to create adhesions and prevent skin flaps. Incise the mucosa and suture it laterally and distally to the skin in a simple continuous suture pattern.

SUTURE MATERIALS AND SPECIAL INSTRUMENTS

A laryngoscope, bronchoscope, alligator biopsy instrument, needle biopsy instruments, and endoscopic biopsy forceps are used for laryngeal and tracheal biopsy. Instruments and suture material for laryngeal and tracheal surgery are discussed on p. 829.

POSTOPERATIVE CARE AND ASSESSMENT

Postoperatively, these patients should be monitored carefully for signs of airway obstruction (see p. 830). Supplemental oxygen and corticosteroids may be given if needed. Water should be offered 6 to 12 hours postoperatively and food 18 to 24 hours after surgery if gagging, regurgitation, or vomiting does not occur. The animal should be kept quiet without exercise for 2 to 4 weeks. Endoscopic reevaluation is recommended at 4 to 8 weeks to identify tumor recurrence or stenosis. Stenosis of greater than 20% leads to mucostasis and infection, whereas approximately a 50% decrease in lumen size causes respiratory distress. Periodic physical and radiographic evaluation is recommended to check for metastasis or recurrence.

COMPLICATIONS

Dysphagia, gagging, and pharyngeal dehiscence may occur after complete laryngectomy. Some patients benefit from an esophageal or gastric feeding tube (see pp. 97 and 100, respectively). Vocalization is absent after laryngectomy. Tracheostomas must be monitored closely to maintain patency and prevent self-trauma (see p. 831). Other complications of laryngectomy include fistulas secondary to pharyngeal dehiscence, hypoparathyroidism secondary to ischemia, and tumor recurrence or metastasis.

Dehiscence may occur after tracheal anastomosis if tension is excessive and if head and neck motion are not restricted. To relieve tension, the neck should be kept mildly to moderately ventroflexed by attaching a muzzle to a harness with a lead or by placing a suture from the chin to the manubrium for 2 weeks. Subcutaneous emphysema may be evident with dehiscence or anastomotic leakage. Infection and fistula formation are possible. Mild stenosis (less than 20%) is expected with the split cartilage technique in which anastomotic tension is minimal.

PROGNOSIS

Although the prognosis undoubtedly is related to the tumor's histologic type, the prognosis is excellent with some tracheal tumors (e.g., oncocytomas and osteochondromas). Little information is available on the biologic behavior of laryngeal tumors; however, the long-term prognosis generally is poor. Without surgery, complete obstruction of the tracheal or laryngeal lumen and subsequent asphyxiation may occur. Radiation therapy may be a valuable adjuvant after surgery for patients with malignant tumors.

Reference

Jakubiak MJ, Siedlecki CT, Zenger E et al: Laryngeal, laryngotracheal, and tracheal masses in cats: 27 cases (1998-2003), *J Am Anim Hosp Assoc* 41:310, 2005.

Suggested Reading

Besancon MF, Stacy BA, Kyles AE et al: Nodular immunocyte-derived (AL) amyloidosis in the trachea of a dog, *J Am Vet Med Assoc* 224:1302, 2004.

This case was investigated and progressed to development of extramedullary plasmacytomas.

Brown MR, Rogers KS: Primary tracheal tumors in dogs and cats, *Compend Cont Educ Pract Vet* 25:854, 2003.

This review article tallies reported cases then describes expected clinical signs, tumor types, diagnostic methods, and treatment options.

Brown MR, Rogers KS, Mansell KJ et al: Primary intratracheal lymphosarcoma in four cats, *J Am Anim Hosp Assoc* 39:468, 2003.

These four cats treated with chemotherapy or radiation therapy had complete remission and long-term resolution of clinical signs. Four previously reported cases are also discussed and compared.

NASAL TUMORS

DEFINITIONS

Nasal tumors or sinonasal tumors are tumors that arise from the nasal cavity or paranasal sinuses. **Rhinotomy** is an incision into the nasal cavity.

GENERAL CONSIDERATIONS AND CLINICALLY RELEVANT PATHOPHYSIOLOGY

Neoplasms of the nasal cavity and paranasal sinuses are rare in most domestic species; the reported incidence varies from 0.3% to 2.4% of canine tumors. They occur more commonly in dogs than in cats. Sinonasal tumors may be classified histologically as epithelial, nonepithelial, or miscellaneous (Box 28-15). Neoplasms of epithelial origin are most common, with adenocarcinoma being the single most frequent histologic diagnosis in dogs. In cats, epithelial and lymphoproliferative tumors are most prevalent. In one study, 70% of cats with nasal tumors had lymphoma, whereas only 13% had adenocarcinomas (Henderson et al, 2004). Nonepithelial tumors of skeletal origin (i.e., chondrosarcoma and osteosarcoma) account for approximately one fifth of canine nasal tumors.

The metastatic rate of nasal tumors generally has traditionally been considered low, with metastasis occurring late in the natural course of these tumors; however, many dogs with sinonasal tumors have metastasis. The most common site of metastasis was the brain, followed in decreasing order of frequency by the lymph nodes, lungs, and liver. Esthesioneuroblastomas and neuroendocrine tumors of the nasal cavity are most likely to metastasize to the brain, whereas epithelial tumors usually metastasize to the regional lymph nodes and lungs. Osseous tumors in this region have a low incidence of metastasis. Prolonged survival rates in cats with lymphoreticular nasal tumors have been reported after radiotherapy, suggesting that metastasis of these tumors is slow.

DIAGNOSIS
Clinical Presentation

Signalment. Male dogs and cats seemingly have a higher incidence of sinonasal neoplasms than females, irrespective of histologic diagnosis. Intranasal tumors generally occur in older animals, with a median age of approximately 10 years in dogs and cats. However, the mean age varies according to

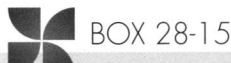

BOX 28-15

Histologic Classification of Sinonasal Neoplasms

Epithelial
- Squamous cell carcinoma
  Nonkeratinizing
  Keratinizing
- Adenocarcinoma

Nonepithelial
- Skeletal
  Chondrosarcoma
  Osteosarcoma
- Soft tissue
  Lymphosarcoma
  Fibrosarcoma
  Hemangiosarcoma
  Muscular origin
  Fibrous histiocytoma
  Malignant nerve sheath

Miscellaneous
Adenocarcinoid
Esthesioneuroblastoma
Carcinoid
Melanoma

Modified from Patnaik AK: Canine sinonasal neoplasms: clinicopathological study of 285 cases, *J Am Anim Hosp Assoc* 25:103, 1989.

the histologic diagnosis; the mean age of dogs with chondrosarcomas (7 years) is younger than that of dogs with other tumor types (9 years). In dogs 1 to 4 years of age, chondrosarcomas are more commonly diagnosed than all other tumor types. Soft tissue tumors involving the nasal cavity have even been reported in dogs as young as 1 year of age.

History. Most affected dogs are brought in for evaluation of nasal discharge, often with epistaxis. Tumors may cause paroxysmal sneezing (which is violent enough to produce epistaxis). Probably less than 10% of affected dogs do not have obvious nasal discharge or only have modest crusting at the nares. Clinical signs in cats are similar, with most evaluated for sneezing and nasal discharge and occasionally epistaxis. The duration of the clinical signs varies, but most animals have them for longer than 1 month and many for longer than 6 months before definitive diagnosis. Initially the clinical signs often are intermittent, gradually becoming persistent as the tumor progresses. Infections associated with nasal tumors often respond transiently to antibiotics and other drugs, delaying definitive diagnosis.

Physical Examination Findings

Clinical findings in dogs with nasal tumors include epistaxis, swelling of the facial region (including exophthalmos), nasal discharge, crust at the nares, sneezing or snuffling, dyspnea, ocular discharge, and/or bleeding from the oral cavity. Neurologic signs may be preponderant (seizures, behavior changes, obtundation, paresis, ataxia, circling, visual deficits, and/or proprioceptive deficits). Clinical signs may vary according to the tumor's histologic type. Seizures are more common in dogs with carcinoids and esthesioneuroblastomas than with tumors of epithelial origin, presumably because of differences in metastatic patterns. Dyspnea may be

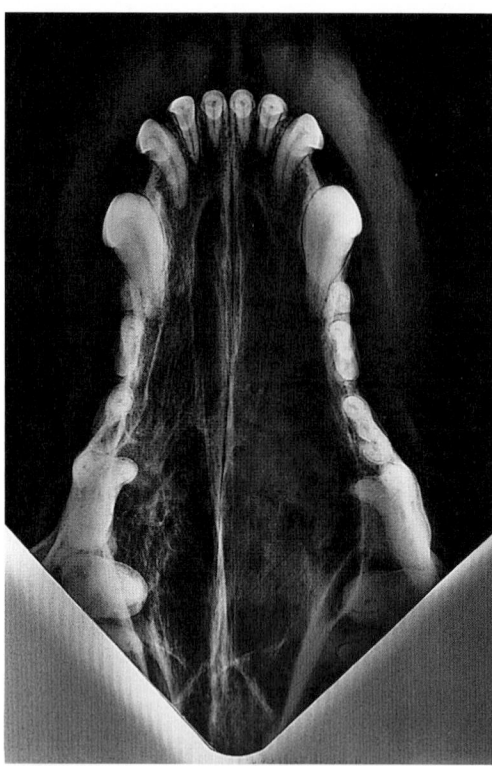

FIG. 28-30
Skull radiograph of an 8-year-old dog with a nasal adeno-carcinoma. Note the increased density and loss of turbinate detail in the left nasal cavity (right side of image).

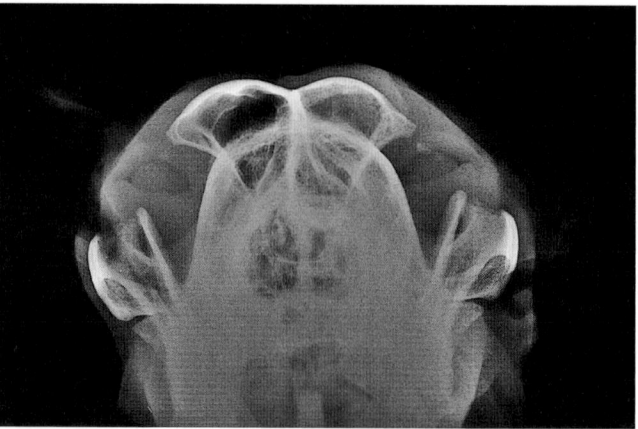

FIG. 28-31
Frontal sinus view of the dog in Fig. 28-30. Note the increased density of the frontal sinus on the right. This may represent neoplasia or fluid accumulation that has occurred secondary to obstruction of drainage caused by the nasal disease.

more typical with epithelial neoplasms, and sneezing has been reported most commonly with chondrosarcomas.

Diagnostic Imaging

Thoracic radiography should be performed to evaluate for metastasis. Skull imaging requires general anesthesia to obtain satisfactory positioning. Good quality nasal radiographs help define the extent and location of disease and should be performed before rhinoscopy (see endoscopy of the choana and nares, later, for the exception to this rule), nasal flushes, or surgical biopsies. Lateral, dorsoventral, open-mouth ventrodorsal, and frontal sinus views are suggested. Oblique views may be necessary occasionally to outline lesions that are masked by or superimposed over bony structures. The open-mouth ventrodorsal view consistently provides the most information by allowing visualization of the entire turbinate region and reducing superimposition of the mandibles. Radiographs should be evaluated for increased soft tissue opacity of the nasal cavity or frontal sinuses, bony lysis, destruction of the normal turbinate pattern, new bone formation, and foreign bodies (Figs. 28-30 and 28-31). Early nasal tumors often are difficult to recognize radiographically because of their similarity to inflammatory changes. Bone destruction usually suggests neoplasia, although severe fungal or bacterial infections may also be responsible. Increased soft tissue opacity may occur in both neoplastic and inflammatory diseases. Extension into

the frontal sinus or the contralateral nasal cavity and destruction of the hard palate indicate an aggressive process. Increased soft tissue opacity in the frontal sinus without bony erosion should not be interpreted as neoplastic extension into the frontal sinus because obstruction of outflow secondary to a nasal tumor often results in fluid accumulation there. Destruction of the cribriform plate may indicate extension into the brain and a poor prognosis.

CT or MRI is superior in evaluation of the extent of nasal disease in animals with nasal tumors, both for prognosis and for planning radiation therapy. CT scans provide good anatomic detail of the bony tissues (Fig. 28-32), and contrast-enhanced scans can give detail regarding the soft tissue abnormalities. MRI scans may be better for evaluating soft tissue structures (De Rycke et al, 2003; Dhaliwal et al, 2001). CT and MRI are also useful in patients with minimal neurologic signs, but with evidence of destruction of the rostral portion of the calvarium.

Endoscopy of the choana and nares. Endoscopy for possible nasal tumors includes examination of the choana and the anterior nares (Fig. 28-33, *A*). Although a relatively small percentage of nasal tumors extend caudally out into the nasopharynx, this is a very useful endoscopic procedure because it is exceedingly easy and quick (i.e., less than 2 minutes) to do. If the owners have decided that they will not attempt surgery or radiation if a neoplasm is diagnosed, then this technique is best performed before imaging is done since a positive diagnosis here will negate the need for more expensive imaging techniques. A retrospective study of 91 dogs and 27 cats that had undergone endoscopic examination of the choanae (Willard and Radlinsky, 1999) documented the technique's utility.

The patient must be under a deep plane of anesthesia because this technique will strongly stimulate the gag reflex. A strong mouth gag is mandatory.

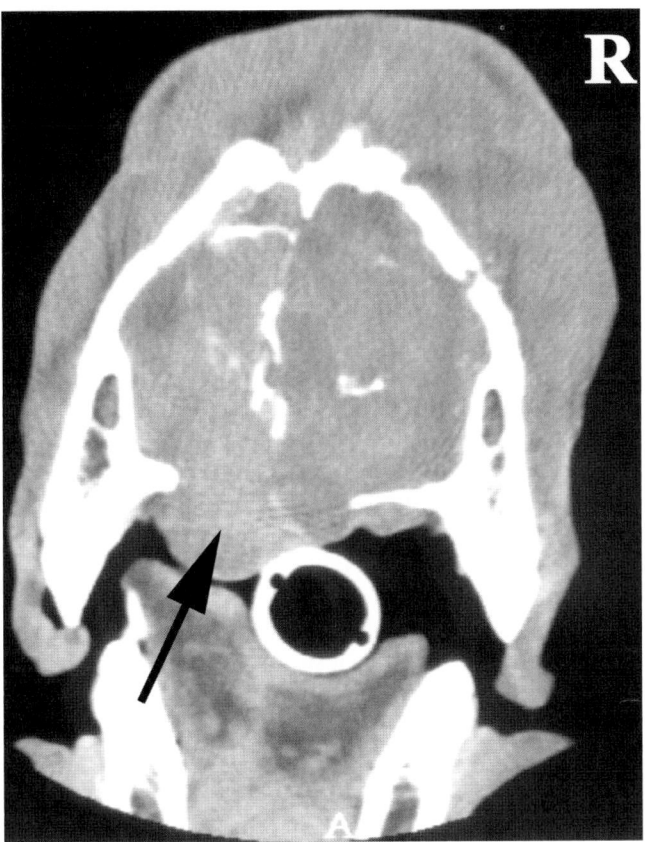

FIG. 28-32
Axial noncontrast CT image of the mid aspect of the nasal cavity in a dog with neoplasia. Notice the turbinate destruction in both nasal cavities and extension of the tumor mass through the hard palate *(arrow)*.

With the patient in sternal recumbency and the tongue pulled forward, advance the tip of a relatively small-diameter flexible scope a centimeter or more past the caudal edge of the soft palate. Then maximally flex the tip up (i.e., at least 180°) so that the tip is above the soft palate and looking cranially. The choana should be easily seen. If necessary push the scope caudally or cranially to obtain a better view. Use the smallest diameter scope that will work well since using a smaller diameter scope lessens the stimulation of the gag reflex and minimizes trauma (and subsequent bleeding) as the tip of the scope rubs against the dorsal pharynx as it is flexed. If a mass is seen protruding from the choana (Fig. 28-33, B), then carefully advance biopsy forceps through the scope and take a biopsy of the mass under direct vision. Be careful lest forcing the biopsy forceps through the maximally flexed channel ruptures it. If necessary preplace the biopsy forceps before flexing the scope up and over the soft palate. Alternatively, perform brush cytology of the mass (but biopsy is usually preferred).

Rarely the mass represents a tumor that has pushed up normal epithelium over it, and one cannot make a definitive diagnosis. However, most such masses can be definitively

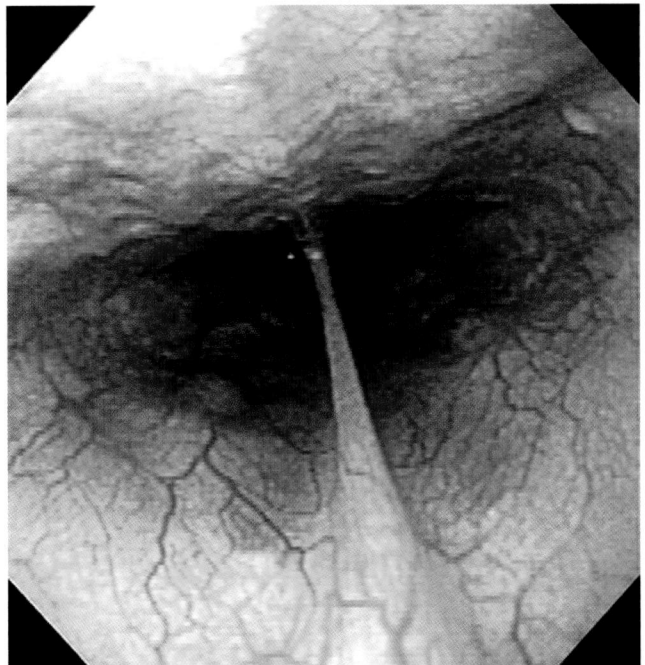

A

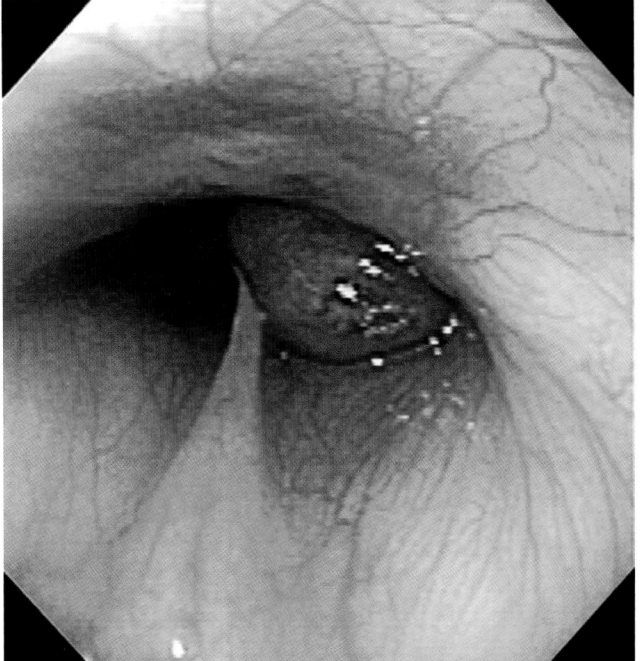

B

FIG. 28-33
A, Endoscopic view of normal choana and **B,** one with a nasal tumor protruding. The tumor was a carcinoma that was diagnosed with endoscopic biopsy.

identified. Finding a mass that is not fungal (e.g., cryptococcosis) is very strongly suggestive of neoplasia. Biopsies of these masses are sometimes associated with hemorrhage, and a cuffed endotracheal tube is mandatory. The bleeding typically stops within 5 minutes, but the back of the pharynx should be manually cleaned out before removing the endotracheal tube.

Rhinoscopy. Rhinoscopy sometimes locates nasal tumors, but many patients have substantial nasal discharge that makes it difficult to see the mass. Rhinoscopy is appropriate because it is an excellent method to diagnose nasal aspergillosis, a disease that closely mimics nasal malignancy. The patient must be under a deep plane of anesthesia or else the procedure may cause sneezing, which may traumatize the nose, causing hemorrhage that further obscures visualization. This procedure is more difficult and time consuming than examination of the choana; therefore it should be done after imaging studies.

Flexible and rigid scopes may be used. Rigid cystoscopes with outer cannulas allow one to flush away debris with cold saline during the procedure, improving visualization. One may attempt to do the same through the biopsy channel of a flexible scope.

Use care and methodically examine all passages. If the tip of the scope is pushed against the mucosa, hemorrhage typically results. If a mass is seen, take a biopsy. More often one cannot see a mass; therefore use imaging to help you blindly place punch-type biopsy forceps as close as possible to the lesion. Open the jaws and advance the forceps until resistance is felt (take care not to perforate the cribriform plate), and then close the jaws and retrieve the sample.

This technique is often successful, and sampling during rhinoscopy provides a definitive diagnosis in a majority of those evaluated. Keep in mind that biopsies may cause profuse hemorrhage, and a cuffed endotracheal tube is mandatory.

If the hemorrhage is worrisome, insert a nasal tampon into the affected nostril for 10 to 15 minutes. Be sure that hemorrhage has stopped before waking the patient and clean out the pharynx before removing the endotracheal tube.

Laboratory Findings

Laboratory abnormalities are uncommon. In rare cases, severe epistaxis may cause anemia and hypoalbuminemia. White cell counts are seldom increased even with a secondary bacterial infection. Coagulation should be assessed (e.g., platelet numbers, bleeding from venipuncture sites, presence of ecchymoses, petechiation, melena, hematuria, or retinal hemorrhages). Major, profuse epistaxis can cause thrombocytopenia, so care must be taken in deciding cause and effect. Cats should be evaluated for FeLV and feline immunodeficiency virus (FIV) infections. Imprint or brush cytologic studies of nasal lesions may help differentiate inflammation from tumor and assist in the identification of the tumor type. Cytology of nasal exudate seldom helps (most animals have neutrophils present caused by secondary bacterial infections), but *Cryptococcus* is occasionally identified. Finding fungal hyphae in nasal exudate is not diagnostic of aspergillosis because they are occasionally found in normal dogs. Fecal flotation may detect ova from nasal parasites. Serology may rule out rickettsial causes of thrombocytopenia and certain mycoses (i.e., cryptococcosis and possibly aspergillosis). Culturing the nose is seldom helpful. There is an abundant normal flora (e.g., *Escherichia coli*, *Streptococcus* spp., *Pasteurella* spp.), and most bacterial rhinitis is secondary to other causes (e.g., nasal tumor, aspergillosis, and foreign body).

DIFFERENTIAL DIAGNOSIS

Nasal tumors usually cause unilateral epistaxis or nasal discharge although some just cause relatively mild crusting, but with time bilateral discharge develops. Bacterial and fungal rhinitis also typically cause unilateral discharge initially; however, they are often not diagnosed until the discharge has become bilateral. Common nasal fungal diseases (i.e., aspergillosis, penicilliosis in dogs; cryptococcosis in cats) may be diagnosed by identifying fungal plaques and hyphae and/or yeast in tissues or by finding diagnostic titers. Foreign bodies, oronasal fistulae, tooth root abscesses, and bleeding diatheses may also be associated with unilateral nasal discharge. Nasal obstruction may also be caused by foreign bodies, nasopharyngeal polyps, or nasopharyngeal or caudal choanal stenosis. Nasal mites (*Pneumonyssoides caninum*) may cause rhinitis, sneezing, reverse sneeze, and an impaired sense of smell. They are diagnosed during rhinoscopy by seeing 1- to 1.5-mm light yellow mites in the nares or by the choana or by finding the mites exiting the nostrils during anesthesia. Other (rare) nasal parasites that cause rhinitis include nasal nematodes (*Capillaria aerophila*, *Eucoleus boehmi* [1.5 to 4 cm long]) and the arthropod *Linguatula serrata*. Other organisms that may cause epistaxis include *Cuterebra* and *Leishmania* (systemic protozoan). Hemostatic defects, ehrlichiosis, immune-mediated thrombocytopenia, lymphocytic-plasmacytic rhinitis, multiple myeloma, systemic hypertension, polycythemia vera, and hyperviscosity syndrome may cause epistaxis or nasal discharge and should be ruled out. Although rare, nasopharyngeal stenosis and choanal atresia cause nasal obstruction that mimics neoplasia. Facial deformity, which is sometimes seen with tumors, should be differentiated from a draining tract associated with a nasal dermoid sinus cyst.

MEDICAL MANAGEMENT

Therapy for nasal tumors is directed at control of local disease. Reported treatment options include surgical debulking, surgical debulking combined with radiation therapy, radiation therapy alone, iridium implants, chemotherapy (i.e., vincristine for transmissible venereal tumor [TVT]; combination chemotherapy for lymphosarcoma), immunotherapy, cryosurgery, and photodynamic therapy with laser ablation. Radiotherapy appears to be the most effective treatment for nasal carcinomas. Most studies have investigated orthovoltage irradiation (125 to 400 keV), although occasional studies have reported the use of megavoltage x-irradiation (more than 1 keV). The optimum dosage and method of delivery have not been determined. Radiotherapy of nasal tumors in cats may be as effective or more effective than in dogs. Whether radiation therapy should be combined with surgical debulking is controversial. One reason for doing so is to improve the clinical status of the dog before the radiation therapy. Prior surgery may reduce dyspnea from nasal cavity obstruction, nasal discharge, and epistaxis during radiation therapy. Cryosurgery or immunotherapy has not appreciably prolonged the survival times of dogs with nasal tumors. Administration of piroxicam may palliate some dogs with inoperable nasal tumors, but one must watch for gastric erosions and/or ulcers.

SURGICAL TREATMENT

Surgery as the sole treatment of dogs with nasal tumors has not prolonged survival time. The poor response of dogs with nasal tumors to surgery is due to the advanced nature of most tumors at the time of diagnosis, a propensity for these tumors to invade bones that are inaccessible or that cannot be surgically removed, and lack of appreciable encapsulation; each of these makes it almost impossible to completely remove the tumor. However, surgery may palliate clinical signs in some dogs by alleviating obstruction and epistaxis. Permanent tracheostomy (see p. 826) may benefit some dogs that have severe respiratory difficulties and in which other treatment options are not feasible.

Preoperative Management

Evaluate coagulation parameters and crossmatch animals before surgery in anticipation of needing a blood transfusion. Anemic animals may benefit from preoperative blood transfusions or purified oxyhemoglobin (see Preoperative Management, p. 817) and should be preoxygenated. Perioperative antibiotics may be given at induction of anesthesia and continued for 12 hours after surgery, but they generally are unnecessary and may inhibit bacterial growth from tissue obtained at surgery.

Anesthesia

Selected anesthetic protocols for animals undergoing nasal surgery are provided on p. 818. Biopsy and rhinotomy are performed under general anesthesia. A cuffed endotracheal tube is mandatory to prevent aspiration of blood or fluids into the airway. Blood, colloids, and/or hypertonic saline should be available in case severe hemorrhage occurs (see Chapter 5). Placement of two cephalic catheters allows simultaneous administration of blood and inotropes if necessary. Evaluation of arterial blood pressure during surgery is warranted, and acepromazine should be avoided. The animal should be extubated with the cuff slightly inflated to help remove partly aspirated blood and mucus.

Surgical Anatomy

See p. 819.

Positioning

For a dorsal approach to the nasal cavity, the animal is positioned in sternal recumbency with a rolled towel under the neck. The entire head and nasal area should be clipped and prepared for aseptic surgery. For a ventral approach to the nasal cavity, the animal is positioned in dorsal recumbency with the mouth tied open maximally (see Fig. 28-4). For an oral approach to the rostral nasal cavity, position the animal in lateral recumbency. The oral cavity is flushed with sterile saline, and the palate is swabbed with dilute Betadine or chlorhexidine solution.

SURGICAL TECHNIQUE

Nasal tumors may be diagnosed by blind biopsy with alligator forceps, by anterior rhinoscopy with biopsy, or by endoscopic examination of choanae and a biopsy of protruding masses.

Biopsy

Endoscopic biopsies are described previously under Diagnostic Imaging and Endoscopy of the Choana and Nares (see pp. 858-860).

Transnostril core biopsies. Transnostril core biopsies may be obtained using the outer protective shield of a Sovereign catheter with the end cut off at a sharp angle or an alligator forceps. To prevent inadvertent penetration of the cribriform plate, the catheter or forceps should be measured with the tip placed at the medial canthus of the eye; these instruments should not be advanced past this point. This technique is quite traumatic and is seldom done anymore.

Attach the catheter (with the metal stylet removed) to a 12-ml syringe. Discern the location of the lesion from the radiographs and advance the catheter through the tumor several times while applying negative pressure to the syringe. After withdrawing the catheter from the naris, remove the barrel of the syringe and add a small amount of air to the syringe. Use this air to propel the tissue sample forcefully from the syringe hub onto a microscopic slide or into a formalin-filled container. Repeat sampling at various angles until sufficient tissue is obtained.

When taking a biopsy of masses in the caudal nasal cavity, be sure to adjust the length of the catheter so as to prevent perforation of the cribriform plate.

Nasal flushes. Nasal flushes may be performed by using the same catheter as described for transnostril core biopsies. Hemorrhage may occur postprocedure, but is generally mild and transient.

To prevent inadvertent entry into the calvarium in patients with bony lysis of the cribriform plate, measure the distance from the medial canthus of the eye to the external naris and mark the catheter to correspond to this length. Place gauze sponges above the soft palate and below the external nares to collect fluid and tissues dislodged during flushing. Attach a 35-ml syringe to the catheter and flush 150 to 300 ml of saline into the nasal cavity. Evaluate the gauze sponges for the presence of tissue and debris. Examine the tissues cytologically and save samples for microbiologic examination, including fungal and bacterial cultures. If sufficient quantities are obtained, place samples in formalin for histopathologic examination.

Rhinotomy

When the aforementioned techniques do not allow diagnosis, surgical exploration and biopsy may be necessary. Generally, in such cases, the diagnostic and therapeutic procedures (rhinotomy and debulking) are combined. Intraoperative cytologic or frozen section examination of tissues (or both) is helpful. Although rhinotomy may not extend the life of patients with nasal tumors appreciably, it often makes them more comfortable. Some surgeons prefer to perform temporary carotid artery ligation before rhinotomy to lessen hemorrhage (see p. 342 for technique). Most nasal tumors are approached using a dorsal rhinotomy because greater exposure of the sinuses and caudal nasal cavity is possible (see p. 322). Ventral rhinotomy through the hard or soft palate or both is preferred for some lesions (see p. 323).

AP **Nasal planum resection.** This procedure is most commonly performed on cats with squamous cell carcinoma of the nasal planum. All or a portion of the nasal planum is excised. The procedure may be combined with rostral maxillectomy if the tumor invades or originates from the oral cavity (see p. 342). The basic technique is described later; other reconstructive techniques may be added to improve cosmesis (Pavletic et al, 1999).

NOTE: It is wise to show owners pictures of animals having had a similar procedure performed so they may fully appreciate its cosmetic effect. Not all owners will be accepting of this procedure (Fig. 28-34).

Position the animal in dorsal recumbency. Make an incision in the skin an acceptable distance from the lesion, continuing around or through the nasal planum (Fig. 28-35, A). Continue the incision through the nasal cartilages, bone, and turbinates. Control hemorrhage and inspect the rostral aspect of the nasal cavity for tumor invasion. If necessary, reconstruct the lip by creating a labial advancement flap from one or both sides of the defect. Appose the gingival and buccal mucosa with 3-0 to 4-0 monofilament absorbable suture. Anatomically align and suture the labial margin then appose the labial muscles and skin. Place a purse-string suture in the skin around the nasal opening and tighten to approximate the size of the defect (Fig. 28-35, B). Alternatively, create holes in the nasal bones surrounding the opening with a pin and pin chuck or drill and, using these holes, suture the skin to the bone.

SUTURE MATERIALS AND SPECIAL INSTRUMENTS

Vacuum suction devices and suction tips are extremely helpful during rhinotomy. Without suctioning devices, hemorrhage often is severe enough to preclude visualization of

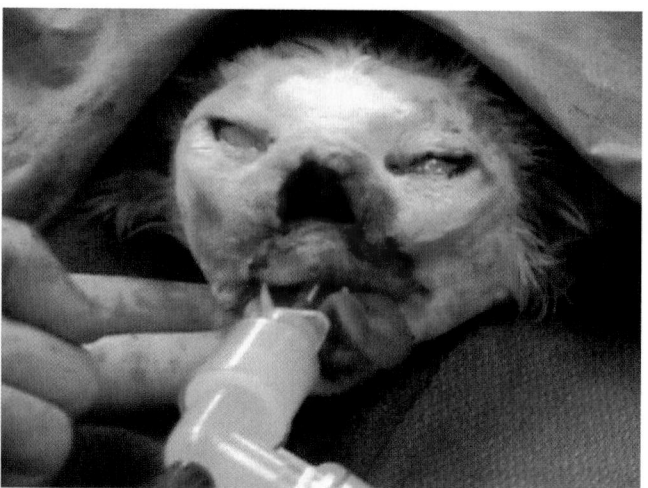

FIG. 28-34
Appearance of a cat following bilateral rostral maxillectomy and nasal planum resection with advancement of a full-thickness labial flap to reconstruct the lip.

abnormal tissues. An oscillating saw is preferred if a bone flap is to be removed, otherwise a Steinmann pin and rongeurs may be used. Sterile gauze packing (e.g., Plain Nu-Gauze packing strip, 2 inches by 3½ yards) may be used to pack the nose after completion of the procedure.

POSTOPERATIVE CARE AND ASSESSMENT

The airway should be suctioned to remove blood and fluid before extubation, and the patients should be recovered with their heads down to reduce aspiration of blood. These animals should be closely monitored for epistaxis after surgery or biopsy.

The hematocrit should be evaluated during and after surgery, and transfusions should be given if the PCV is below 20% (see Preoperative Management, p. 818). These patients should be prevented from banging their heads on the cage during recovery. If they appear to be excited or in pain during recovery, analgesics may be administered (see Table 13-4 on p. 133). Acepromazine (0.05 mg/kg IV or IM up to a *maximum* of 1 mg total dose; do not exceed 1 mg IV) may be given if the patient is normovolemic, is not hemorrhaging, does not have a history of seizures, and has been given adequate analgesics. Neurologic function should be assessed postoperatively.

Subcutaneous air may accumulate after a dorsal approach to the nasal cavity if the bone flap is not replaced adequately or if an adequate stoma is not left in the subcutaneous tissues and skin for air to exit. Generally, if an adequate stoma is left, subcutaneous air accumulation is not a problem. The stoma contracts and heals within 5 to 10 days. Soft food should be fed for several days after the ventral approach and the animal prevented from chewing on hard objects for 3 to 4 weeks until the palate incision is healed.

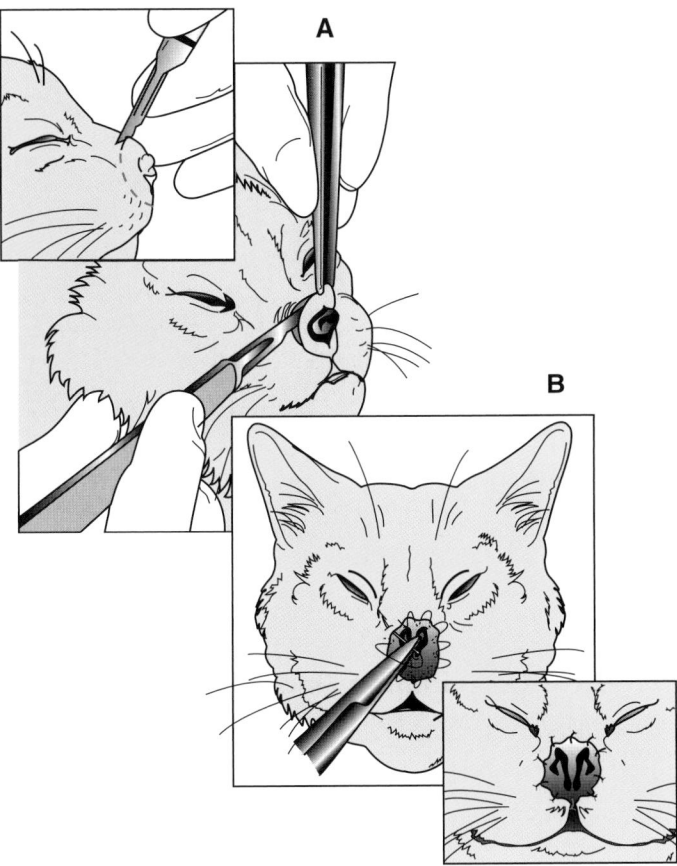

FIG. 28-35
Nasal planum resection. **A,** Make an incision around the nasal planum through the skin, nasal cartilages, and turbinates. **B,** Appose the skin to the nasal defect with a purse-string suture.

PROGNOSIS

The prognosis for dogs with nasal tumors generally is poor. In patients not treated and those treated with surgery, chemotherapy, immunotherapy, and cryosurgery, the mean survival time generally is 3 to 5 months. Improvement in this survival period has been accomplished with radiation therapy combined with surgical debulking (see previous discussion), with mean reported survival times of 8 to 25 months. Animals with lymph node or pulmonary metastasis have shortened median survival times. The prognosis for carcinomas is better than for sarcomas, and adenocarcinomas appear to have the best overall prognosis. It is unlikely that therapy will result in cure in most dogs, and more successful local control may lead to increased detection of metastasis. Conversely the prognosis for cats with lymphoid neoplasia of the nasal cavity appears good.

Intranasal TVT has a much better long-term prognosis than those tumors previously mentioned. Clinical signs associated with intranasal TVT are similar to other tumors of this location (epistaxis and sneezing), and the tumor may appear as a space-occupying mass in the nasal cavity. Some-

times it is multifocal with several masses evident. Occasionally, bony lysis may be noted. If the tumor is localized, radiation therapy may be curative. Chemotherapy with vincristine is also effective in treating localized or metastatic TVT.

References

De Rycke LM, Saunders JH, Gielen IM et al: Magnetic resonance imaging, computed tomography, and cross-sectional view of the anatomy of normal nasal cavities and paranasal sinuses in mesaticephalic dogs, *Am J Vet Res* 64:1093, 2003.

Dhaliwal RS, Kitchell BE, Losonsky JM et al: Subjective evaluation of computed tomography and magnetic resonance imaging for detecting intracalvarial changes in canine nasal neoplasia, *Intern J Appl Res Vet Med* 2:201, 2004.

Henderson SM, Bradley K, Day MJ et al: Investigation of nasal disease in the cat—a retrospective study of 77 cases, *J Feline Med Surg* 6:245, 2004.

Pavletic MM: Nasal reconstruction techniques. In *Atlas of Small Animal Reconstructive Surgery,* ed 2, Philadelphia, 1999, WB Saunders Co.

Willard MD, Radlinsky MA: Endoscopic examination of the choanae in dogs and cats: 118 cases (1988-1998), *J Am Vet Med Assoc* 215:1301, 1999.

Suggested Reading

Adams WM, Bjorling DE, McAnulty JF et al: Outcome of accelerated radiotherapy alone or accelerated radiotherapy followed by exenteration of the nasal cavity in dogs with intranasal neoplasia: 53 cases (1990-2002), *J Am Vet Med Assoc* 227:936, 2005.
Exenteration prolonged survival time, but increased the risk of complications.

Anderson DM, White RAS: Nasal dermoid sinus cysts in the dog, *Vet Surg* 31:303, 2002.
Six cases are reported with draining tracts on the bridge of the nose near the planum that resolved after complete surgical excision.

Correa SS, Mauldin GN, Mauldin GE et al: Efficacy of cobalt-60 radiation therapy for the treatment of nasal cavity nonkeratinizing squamous cell carcinoma in the dog, *J Am Anim Hosp Assoc* 39:86, 2003.
This report of six cases found poor response to radiotherapy.

de Vos JP, Burm AGO, Focker BP: Results from the treatment of advanced stage squamous cell carcinoma of the nasal planum in cats, using a combination of intralesional carboplatin and superficial radiotherapy: a pilot study, *Vet Comp Oncol* 2:75, 2004.
Six cats were treated; all tolerated treatment well with 100% response.

Gieger T, Northrup N: Clinical approach to patients with epistaxis, *Compend Cont Educ Pract Vet* 26:30, 2004.
This article reviews clinical presentation and diagnostics recommended to diagnose affected animals.

Hunt GB, Perkins MC, Foster SF et al: Nasopharyngeal disorders of dogs and cats: a review and retrospective study, *Compend Cont Educ Pract Vet* 24:184, 2002.
Findings from 38 dogs and 24 cats are reported; 54% of dogs had neoplastic lesions, whereas 71% of cats had inflammatory lesions.

Lascelles BDX, Henderson RA, Seguin B et al: Bilateral rostral maxillectomy and nasal planectomy for large rostral maxillofacial neoplasms in six dogs and one cat, *J Am Anim Hosp Assoc* 40:137, 2004.

This report documents amputation of the nasal planum and rostral maxilla between the first and second or second and third premolars.

Lucroy MD, Long KR, Blaik MA et al: Photodynamic therapy for the treatment of intranasal tumors in 3 dogs and 1 cat, *J Vet Intern Med* 17:727, 2003.

Use of photodynamic therapy and laser ablation of tumors resulted in temporary facial swelling and a decrease in clinical signs.

Northrup NC, Etue SM, Ruslander DM et al: Retrospective study of orthovoltage radiation therapy for nasal tumors in 42 dogs, *J Vet Intern Med* 15:183, 2001.

This study reports less effective control of nasal tumors in dogs treated with surgery and orthovoltage radiation therapy than previously reported. It also reports that dogs with facial deformity and those without resolution of clinical signs have a worse prognosis.

Strasser JL, Hawkins EC: Clinical features of epistaxis in dogs: a retrospective study of 35 cases (1999-2002), *J Am Anim Hosp Assoc* 41:179, 2005.

Epistaxis was caused by systemic disease in 7, neoplasia in 19, and other intranasal disease in 9 in this case series.

Weise C, Nicholson ME, Rollings C et al: Use of percutaneous arterial embolization for treatment of intractable epistaxis in three dogs, *J Am Vet Med Assoc* 224:1307, 2004.

This report describes embolization of the terminal branches of the maxillary artery.

NASAL ASPERGILLOSIS

DEFINITIONS

Nasal aspergillosis is characterized by destruction of the nasal turbinates by large colonies of fungal hyphae. Masses formed by the fungal hyphae are sometimes called **aspergillomas**.

GENERAL CONSIDERATIONS AND CLINICALLY RELEVANT PATHOPHYSIOLOGY

Nasal aspergillosis is a relatively common disease in dogs and clinically may mimic nasal neoplasia (Fig. 28-36). Nasal aspergillosis should not be confused with systemic aspergillosis; the latter is almost uniformly fatal. The nasal form usually remains confined to the nasal cavity or paranasal sinus where it causes marked turbinate destruction. Invasion of the cranial vault may also occur. Nasal aspergillosis usually occurs without concomitant malignant or immunosuppressive disease.

DIAGNOSIS
Clinical presentation

Signalment. Dogs with nasal aspergillosis tend to be younger than dogs with nasal neoplasia, but there is overlap. Aspergillosis is rare in brachycephalic breeds and cats. Male and female dogs are equally affected.

History. Affected dogs typically are brought in for treatment of chronic nasal discharge, often with epistaxis. The owners may also note ulceration of the external nares.

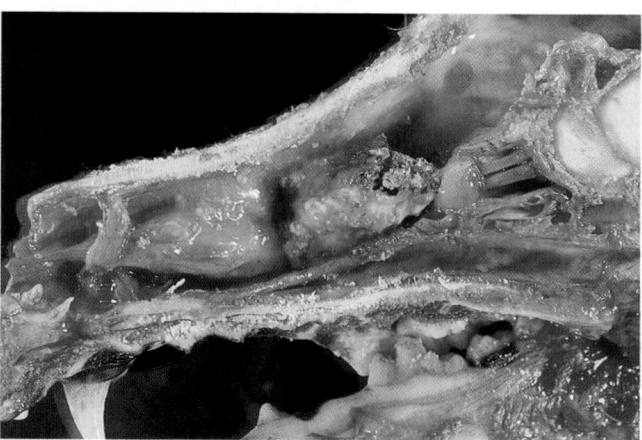

FIG. 28-36
Necropsy specimen of a dog with nasal aspergillosis. Note the large aspergilloma and associated destruction of turbinates.

Physical Examination Findings

Dogs may have erosion of the nasal planum associated with chronic nasal discharge. The nasal discharge may be unilateral or bilateral and may be sanguinopurulent, mucopurulent, or hemorrhagic. Although most dogs have profuse nasal discharge, a few have relatively sparse discharge.

Diagnostic Imaging

Affected dogs usually have obvious turbinate destruction plus areas of increased radiolucency, mimicking what may be seen in neoplasia. Frontal sinus osteomyelitis is commonly noted. CT and MRI are better than nasal radiographs at determining extent of the disease. CT images are best for detecting cortical bone lesions, whereas MRI is more useful for differentiating between thickened mucosa and secretions or fungal colonies (Saunders et al, 2004).

Rhinoscopy. On rhinoscopy cavernous areas caused by the marked destruction of turbinates often are present. Obvious mats of fungal hyphae (i.e., "fuzzy" plaques) or aspergillomas (e.g., looks like masses of inspissated mucus, but may have discoloration caused by the fungi) may be evident. Because aspergillosis causes marked turbinate destruction, there is usually much more space in the nose, typically making endoscopic diagnosis of aspergillosis relatively easy.

Laboratory Findings

False-positive and false-negative results occur with cytology, culture, and serology. Therefore it generally is recommended that at least two of the following criteria be met: (1) radiographic features typical of fungal rhinitis (see previous discussion); (2) fungal plaques on the nasal or sinus mucosa; (3) *Aspergillus* or *Penicillium* organisms on culture, cytologic, or histologic examination; and (4) a positive agar gel immunodiffusion, counterimmunoelectrophoresis, or enzyme-linked immunosorbent assay (ELISA). Different serologic tests vary as to their sensitivity and specificity.

Noticing fungal plaques on endoscopy in a dog with severe nasal turbinate destruction is highly suggestive of this disease. Cytologic examination of the exudate or fungal mats collected during rhinoscopy should reveal very large numbers of hyphae.

> NOTE: Finding a few hyphae or growing *Aspergillus* organisms from a nasal flush does not reliably indicate that the dog has clinical aspergillosis. A small number of hyphae may be found in dogs with clinical signs not associated with aspergillosis.

DIFFERENTIAL DIAGNOSIS

Tumors, allergic rhinitis, nasal foreign bodies, lymphocytic-plasmacytic rhinitis, and tooth root abscesses are other causes of chronic nasal discharge that must be differentiated from nasal aspergillosis. Most of these dogs will have secondary bacterial rhinitis, but primary bacterial rhinitis appears uncommon in dogs.

MEDICAL MANAGEMENT

Oral administration of azole antifungal agents is effective in only 43% to 70% of cases, requires months of therapy, and is costly. Conversely, clotrimazole can be infused into the nasal passages and frontal sinuses of dogs. In many patients, a single application is curative, but some dogs require repeated therapy. CT is necessary to ensure an intact cribriform plate before such therapy. Rhinoscopic débridement of fungal plaques followed by infusion of enilconazole is also described as effective in some animals, but enilconazole is more difficult to work with and is seldom used.

> NOTE: Infusion procedures should be performed with care because leakage of clotrimazole into the lungs can cause fatal pneumonitis.

SURGICAL TREATMENT

Rhinotomy and resection of the affected turbinates and associated soft tissues is seldom indicated and does not cure aspergillosis. Rhinostomas have been created to allow débridement and repeated topical treatment over many weeks; this treatment is traumatic to the animal, costly, and labor intensive. Canine nasal aspergillosis is most appropriately treated by topical clotrimazole (Lotrimin). Although placement of tubes through the dorsal aspect of the nasal bones has been described for instillation of antifungal drugs in the past, instillation through tubes placed through the oral cavity and nares has proved effective and eliminates the need for removal or trephination of bone. Placement through the oral cavity and nares is described here.

Preoperative Management

Complications and death may occur if the cribriform plate is not intact; therefore a CT scan should be done before administering clotrimazole therapy.

Anesthesia

The dog is placed under general anesthetic, and the cuff of the endotracheal tube is checked to make sure it is fully inflated, which prevents leakage of the infused solution into the trachea.

Surgical Anatomy

The surgical anatomy of the nasal cavity is described on p. 819.

SURGICAL TECHNIQUE
Technique for administering clotrimazole.

With the dog in lateral or dorsal recumbency, place a Foley catheter (24 French) into the mouth such that the tip of the catheter lies dorsal to the soft palate (Fig. 28-37).

This process may be aided by grasping the catheter tip with a pair of right-angle forceps or long-handled needle holders so that the catheter tip is directed rostrally.

If necessary, place a mouth gag and pull the tongue rostrally to improve visualization during placement of the catheter. Advance the catheter until the balloon is dorsal to the junction of the hard and soft palates. Inflate the balloon of the Foley catheter to occlude the nasopharynx. Palpate the balloon through the soft plate to confirm its position just caudal to the hard palate. Place moistened laparotomy sponges in the pharynx to prevent the catheter from migrating caudally and to absorb any infusion that might escape around the balloon. Remove the mouth gag and advance a polypropylene infusion catheter (10 French) through each nostril. Beginning dorsomedially, advance each catheter into the dorsal nasal meatus to the level of the medial canthus of the ipsilateral palpebral fissure. Then insert a Foley catheter (12 French) into each nostril and inflate the balloons so that they lie just caudal to and occlude the nostrils. With the dog in dorsal recumbency, place an additional laparotomy sponge just caudal to the upper incisors between the endotracheal tube and incisive papilla to control leakage of clotrimazole through the incisive ducts.

Evenly divide 1 g of clotrimazole in 100 ml of polyethylene glycol 200 (1% solution) between two 60-ml syringes. Infuse the clotrimazole slowly over 1 hour (50 ml per infusion catheter). Maintain the polypropylene catheters in a horizontal position, parallel to the table, throughout the infusion. Rotate the dog's head to ensure drug contact with all nasal surfaces. After 1 hour, place the dog in sternal recumbency and remove the catheters and sponges, allowing the clotrimazole to drain rostrally. Suction the pharynx and proximal esophagus and allow the dog to recover from the anesthesia.

POSTOPERATIVE CARE AND ASSESSMENT

The animal should be observed carefully after clotrimazole treatment for seizure or respiratory difficulty. Seizures and sometimes death occurs if the cribriform plate has been

FIG. 28-37
For placement of tubes for nasal instillation of clotrimazole, place a Foley catheter (24 French) into the mouth so that the tip of the catheter lies dorsal to the soft palate. Place moistened laparotomy sponges in the pharynx. Remove the mouth gag and advance a polypropylene infusion catheter (10 French) through each nostril. Then insert a Foley catheter (12 French) into each nostril and inflate the balloons so that they lie just caudal to and occlude the nostrils.

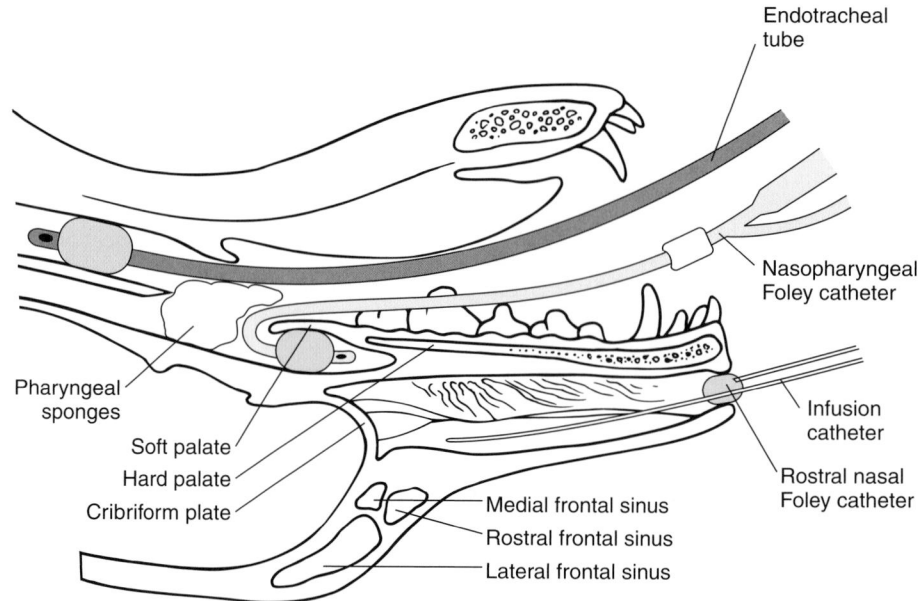

eroded. Pneumonia may occur if the antifungal agent is aspirated. Some dogs with advanced disease may require several 1-hour infusions. In most dogs, nasal pain and discharge resolve rapidly, and the nasal erosion heals quickly. Failure to cure the disease is a problem with some antifungal agents. Some animals with severe rhinitis may develop caudal choanal stenosis.

PROGNOSIS

Although the fungal disease can be eradicated, some dogs continue to have clinical signs associated with loss of normal turbinate structure. Owners should be warned that mild to moderate nasal discharge may continue in these dogs despite improvement in clinical signs. Bacterial rhinitis may occur in up to 25% of dogs after treatment, but it typically responds to appropriate antibiotic therapy. Relapse of aspergillosis does not appear to be a common problem.

Reference

Saunders JH, Clercx C, Snaps FR et al: Radiographic, magnetic resonance imaging, computed tomographic and rhinoscopic features of nasal aspergillosis in dogs, *J Am Vet Med Assoc* 225:1703, 2004.

Suggested Reading

Davidson AP, Mathews KG: CVT update: therapy for nasal aspergillosis. In *Current veterinary therapy XIII*, Philadelphia, 2000, WB Saunders.
Therapeutic recommendations are reviewed.
Gunnarsson LK, Zakrisson G, Christensson DA et al: Efficacy of selamectin in the treatment of nasal mite (*Pneumonyssoides caninum*) infection in dogs, *J Am Anim Hosp Assoc* 40:400, 2004.
Twelve beagles were infected with nasal mites; those treated were free of the parasite when evaluated 39 to 46 days after inoculation.

Gunnarsson LK, Zakrisson G, Egenvall A et al: Prevalence of *Pneumonyssoides caninum* infection in dogs in Sweden, *J Am Anim Hosp Assoc* 37:331, 2001.
This prospective necropsy study of 474 dogs and 145 cats and 66 red foxes found 20% of dogs only to be infested.
Johnson LR, Clarke HE, Bannasch MJ et al: Correlation of rhinoscopic signs of inflammation with histologic findings in nasal biopsy specimens of cats with or without upper respiratory tract disease, *J Am Vet Med Assoc* 225:395, 2004.
This prospective study showed weak or no correlation with inflammation severity between rhinoscopic and histologic findings.
Johnson LR, Foley JE, De Cock HE et al: Assessment of infectious organisms associated with chronic rhinosinusitis in cats, *J Am Vet Med Assoc* 227:579, 2005.
This prospective study of 10 affected and 7 unaffected cats evaluates nasal flush and biopsy specimens.
Moore AH: Use of topical povidone-iodine dressing in the management of mycotic rhinitis in three dogs, *J Small Anim Pract* 44:326, 2004.
Rhinostomas were created to allow insertion of sustained-release povidone-iodine dressings; these were changed every 48 to 72 hours until healthy granulation tissue covered the bone.
Windsor RC, Johnson LR, Herrgesell EJ et al: Idiopathic lymphoplasmacytic rhinitis in dogs: 37 cases (1997-2002), *J Am Vet Med Assoc* 224:1952, 2004.
This retrospective case series suggests that the disease is usually bilateral despite unilateral discharge.
Zonderland JL, Stork CK, Saunders JH et al: Intranasal infusion of enilconazole for treatment of sinonasal aspergillosis in dogs, *J Am Vet Med Assoc* 221:1421, 2002.
This study reports rhinoscopic débridement of fungal lesions followed by flushing with 1% or 2% enilconazole. One to three times was effective in resolving signs in most dogs.

CHAPTER 29

Surgery of the Lower Respiratory System: Lungs and Thoracic Wall

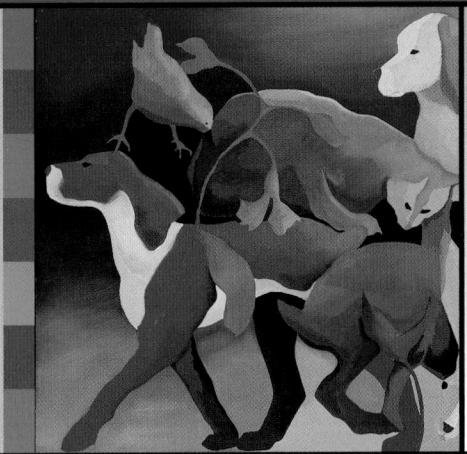

DEFINITIONS

Thoracotomy is surgical incision of the chest wall; it may be performed by incising between the ribs (**intercostal** or **lateral thoracotomy**) or by splitting the sternum (**median sternotomy**). Pulmonary **lobectomy** is removal of a lung lobe (**complete**) or a portion of a lung lobe (**partial**). **Pneumonectomy** is removal of all lung tissue on one side of the thoracic cavity.

PREOPERATIVE MANAGEMENT

Animals with traumatic lesions that impair respiration (e.g., flail chest) or those with acute respiratory impairment (i.e., ruptured bulla or ruptured pulmonary abscess) often require emergency stabilization (e.g., stabilization of rib segments, thoracentesis, and oxygen therapy) before surgery. Equipment for thoracentesis and chest tube placement should be readily available, and clinicians should be familiar with these techniques (see pp. 898 to 902). In a recent study, 58 percent of dogs brought in with blunt trauma had evidence of chest trauma on thoracic radiographs, and virtually all animals that had abdominal injuries showed concurrent chest abnormalities (Sigrsit et al, 2004).

> NOTE: Carefully auscultate the chest of all trauma patients. Most have pulmonary contusions, and finding abnormal sounds on chest auscultation typically correlates well with finding radiographic signs of thoracic trauma.

With large neoplastic lesions, positioning the animal in sternal recumbency or in lateral recumbency with the affected side down, and providing oxygen (i.e., nasal insufflation or oxygen cage) often is beneficial. Blood gas analysis or evaluation with pulse oximetry is warranted preoperatively in patients undergoing thoracic surgery to detect and define the severity of respiratory impairment. Unexplained abnormalities should be investigated because ventilatory impairment caused by nonsurgically correctable disease (i.e., diffuse micrometastasis) occasionally is identified. If possible, significant anemia should be corrected before surgery.

ANESTHESIA

Pulmonary neoplasia or other space-occupying lesions may prevent normal lung expansion and cause hypoxemia. Ventilation/perfusion disturbances are common with pneumonia or emphysematous lesions. In animals with respiratory dysfunction, oxygen may be administered by face mask or nasal insufflation (see Chapter 5) before induction of anesthesia to ensure that hemoglobin is optimally saturated and that hypoxemia does not occur during intubation. Sedation with acepromazine causes hypotension and should be avoided in severely affected patients. Anticholinergics can be used in bradycardic animals (i.e., a heart rate below 80 beats per minute in dogs or 110 beats per minute in cats). Nitrous oxide should be avoided in patients with respiratory compromise. Opioids may cause severe respiratory depression and should be administered only when oxygen can be provided (see Chapter 13). Endotracheal intubation in animals with respiratory dysfunction must be accomplished rapidly and anesthesia maintained with an inhalation anesthetics (i.e., isoflurane or sevoflurane; Box 29-1). Intubation of a bronchus rather than the trachea may be disastrous in compromised animals; therefore, both sides of the chest cavity should be auscultated to ensure proper placement of the endotracheal tube. It may be difficult to maintain an adequate depth of anesthesia in animals with severe pulmonary disease with inhalation anesthetics alone; supplemental opioids may be necessary.

All animals with open chest cavities require intermittent positive pressure ventilation (including those with diaphragmatic hernias). End-tidal CO_2 ($ETCO_2$) is the measurement of CO_2 in exhaled respiratory gases. $ETCO_2$ is measured by capnography and serves as an estimate of arterial CO_2. Thus capnography is a noninvasive method of measuring systemic

BOX 29-1

Selected Anesthetic Protocols for Animals With Respiratory Dysfunction

For Stable (Nonarrhythmic, Nondyspneic) Animals

Premedication

Hydromorphone* (0.1–0.2 mg/kg SC or IM)

Induction

Thiopental (10–12 mg/kg IV) or propofol (4–6 mg/kg IV); or give diazepam (0.27 mg/kg IV) and ketamine (5.5 mg/kg IV) combined and titrated to effect

Maintenance

Isoflurane or sevoflurane

For Dyspneic, Nonarrhythmic Animals

Induction†

Diazepam (0.2 mg/kg IV) followed immediately with thiopental (10–12 mg/kg/IV)† or propofol (4–6 mg/kg IV); or give diazepam (0.27 mg/kg IV) and ketamine (5.5 mg/kg IV) combined and titrated to effect

Maintenance

Isoflurane or sevoflurane

For Dyspneic, Arrhythmic Animals

Induction†

Diazepam (0.2 mg/kg IV) followed by etomidate (1–3 mg/kg IV)

Maintenance

Isoflurane or sevoflurane

SC, Subcutaneous; *IM,* intramuscular; *IV,* intravenous.
*Observe after premedication; use 0.05 mg/kg in cats.
†Can add hydromorphone (0.1–0.2 mg/kg IV) or butorphanol (0.2–0.4 mg/kg IV) in cats as part of the induction and reduce the induction drug dose.

metabolism, cardiac output, pulmonary perfusion, and ventilation; its measurement may be helpful in identifying potentially life-threatening situations (e.g., hypoventilation, airway obstruction, hypotension, ventilator malfunctions, or esophageal intubation). The normal arterial CO_2 in an awake healthy animal is 35 to 45 mm Hg. If ventilation and perfusion are well matched, $ETCO_2$ is generally 2 to 5 mm Hg less than that of the $PaCO_2$.

High ventilatory pressures should be avoided in patients with chronically collapsed lung lobes, pneumonia, or pulmonary bullae (see p. 908). For specific anesthetic recommendations for animals with flail chest or pectus excavatum, see pp. 881 and 892, respectively.

> **NOTE:** Do not use mask or chamber induction in animals with respiratory dysfunction. Use anesthetics that allow for rapid intubation and control of the patient's airway.

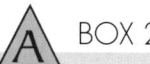 BOX 29-2

Local Anesthesia After Thoracotomy in Dogs*

- Interpleural bupivacaine (2 mg/kg)
OR
- Intercostal bupivacaine (2 mg/kg)
OR
- Dose may be split and half given interpleurally and half injected intercostally (see text)

*Bupivacaine has been used in a similar fashion for cats, but at reduced dosages (1 mg/kg, total dose).

Thoracoscopy is best done without insufflation; simply establishing a pneumothorax is sufficient for almost all cases. Should intrathoracic insufflation be done for thoracoscopy, it may have profound effects on cardiopulmonary parameters. In one study, cardiac output and systolic and diastolic arterial pressures significantly decreased at 3 mm Hg intrathoracic pressures (IP) (Daly et al, 2002). Heart rate decreased significantly at 5 to 6 mm Hg IP, but was not further decreased above 6 mm Hg IP. Because standard anesthetic monitoring variables, such as heart rate and arterial pressure measurements, may not accurately reflect the animal's cardiovascular status, insufflation-assisted thoracoscopy should be done with care using the lowest IP possible.

Thoracotomy procedures often cause substantial pain, and postoperative analgesic therapy is indicated (see also Chapter 13). Performing an intercostal nerve block before incision (inject dorsally in the intercostal space being incised and two intercostal spaces cranial and caudal to the incised space) or placing bupivacaine in the thoracic cavity after thoracic closure (interpleural) may reduce pain and improve ventilation in the postoperative period (Box 29-2). If both intercostal and interpleural blocks are performed, divide the bupivacaine dose between the two blocks. The bupivacaine may be diluted if necessary to cover the affected area. Patients given bupivacaine interpleurally should be placed with the affected side down for 20 minutes. Injectable analgesics may also be used (i.e., hydromorphone, butorphanol, or buprenorphine; see Table 13-4 on p. 133). Although opioids are respiratory depressants, their analgesic effects often outweigh their negative respiratory effects. If hypoventilation occurs after administration of these drugs, oxygen should be given by nasal insufflation (see Chapter 5). Epidural administration of morphine is an effective analgesic in patients undergoing thoracic procedures and should be considered where postoperative pain is likely to be intense (e.g., thoracic wall resections and sternal resections) (see Chapter 13). Epidural administration of morphine alone does not cause significant changes in cardiorespiratory measurements, but epidural administration of morphine and fentanyl may significantly decrease diastolic and mean arterial blood pressure and total peripheral resistance in dogs anesthetized with sevoflurane; this combination should be used with care (Naganobu et al, 2004).

NOTE: If a morphine epidural has been administered perioperatively, a μ-agonist (e.g., fentanyl, morphine, or hydromorphone) should be used postoperatively.

Pulmonary edema (reexpansion pulmonary edema; RPE) may develop in animals after reexpanding chronically collapsed lung lobes. Although the origin of RPE is unknown and probably multifactorial, it does not appear to be associated with cardiac failure. The patient typically develops progressively worsening dyspnea and tachypnea within a few hours after surgery. Hypoxemia develops and persists despite intense oxygen therapy. Contrary to the experience in human beings, in whom RPE usually is unilateral and therefore not life threatening, the condition can be rapidly fatal in animals. Reoxygenation of chronically collapsed lungs is thought to release superoxide radicals, which cannot be effectively scavenged, resulting in increased pulmonary capillary permeability and pulmonary edema. Chronically collapsed lung tissue may have decreased mitochondrial superoxide dismutase and cytochrome oxidase activity. Prophylaxis and therapy of patients with RPE are difficult and poorly understood. Reexpansion of chronically collapsed lung tissue should be accomplished slowly (i.e., the thorax may be closed with one or two lung lobes collapsed, allowing them to reexpand slowly), and high ventilation pressures (i.e., above 25 cm H_2O) should be avoided. Current recommendations for treating RPE include the use of positive end-expiratory pressure ventilation and drugs that stabilize pulmonary capillary membranes (i.e., methylprednisolone). A number of other pharmaceutical agents currently are under investigation, but conclusive evidence of their beneficial effects is not yet available.

NOTE: Avoid high ventilation pressures in patients with chronically collapsed lung lobes.

Obstruction of blood flow in the pulmonary vasculature by a thrombus or an embolus formed in the systemic venous system or right side of the heart is *pulmonary thromboembolism (PTE)*. It may occur as a complication of a number of diseases (e.g., neoplasia, cardiac disease, sepsis, immune-mediated hemolytic anemia, hyperadrenocorticism, and protein-losing nephropathy or enteropathy). It is difficult to diagnose antemortem because of the lack of specific signs. Clinical signs associated with feline PTE include lethargy, anorexia, weight loss, and difficulty breathing. In dogs, vomiting, melena, fever, labored breathing, and lethargy have been reported. Risk factors for PTE include administration of corticosteroids, chemotherapeutic agents, or blood; indwelling catheters; and recent surgery. PTE should be suspected in animals with thoracic radiographic changes suggestive of uneven distribution of blood flow between lung lobes or patchy interstitial densities; pulmonary perfusion scintigraphy or computed tomography (CT)

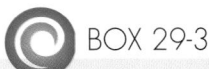

BOX 29-3

Drugs Used in Medical Management of Pulmonary Thromboembolism

Unfractionated Heparin

Dogs: Start with 250–300 U/kg SC every 6 hours*
Cats: Start with 175 U/kg SC every 6 hours*

Low-Molecular-Weight Heparin (Dalteparin)†

Dogs: 100–150 U/kg, SC qd to bid
Cats: 150–180 U/kg SC every 6 hr

Aspirin

Dogs: 0.5 mg/kg PO bid
Cats: 25 mg/kg PO twice weekly

Streptokinase‡

90,000 U given IV over 20–30 minutes, then 45,000 U given IV over 7–12 hours

Warfarin

Dogs: Start with 0.1–0.2 mg/kg PO qd§
Cats: Start with 0.25–0.5 mg PO qd§

SC, Subcutaneous; *qd,* once a day; *bid,* twice a day; *PO,* oral; *IV,* intravenous.
*Dose to be adjusted, based upon aPTT results (goal is to prolong it to 1.5–2 times baseline).
†These are doses currently thought to be appropriate; however, as of this writing, there has been minimal research published on the use of this product in diseased animals.
‡There is minimal experience with this drug in veterinary medicine, and serious side effects are possible.
§Dose to be adjusted, based upon PT results (goal is to prolong it to 1.5 times baseline; OR, attain international normalized ratio [INR] of 2.3). Reader is referred to a medical text for a discussion of INR. Attain adequate anticoagulation with heparin before starting Warfarin as animals are initially hypercoagulable.

angiography may help confirm the diagnosis. Treatment of PTE includes anticoagulant and thrombolytic therapies plus standard hemodynamic and respiratory support (Box 29-3). Heparin acts primarily to limit the conversion of fibrinogen to fibrin by accelerating the action of antithrombin III in inhibiting activated coagulation factors (II, IX, X, XI, and XII). Unfractionated heparin (UFH) has been most commonly used because of its widespread availability and low cost. It should be dosed to prolong the activated partial thromboplastin time (aPTT) 1.5 to 2 times that of baseline. Low molecular weight heparin (LMWH; enoxaparin, dalteparin) differs from UFH in that it more specifically acts on factor X and is likely more effective. It also requires different monitoring than UFH and is more expensive. Prolongation of the aPTT does not occur at therapeutic doses of LMWH, but patients may be monitored by following clinical signs and assessing for anti-Xa activity. Warfarin acts to prevent the formation of vitamin K–dependent coagulation factors (II, VII, IX, and X). It also inhibits production of protein C. With warfarin therapy, prothrombin time (PT) is measured and the desired end point is a PT of 1.5 to twice that of baseline. Low dose aspirin administration to inhibit platelet activity may be considered, but care must be taken to ensure that the aspirin does not cause renal or gastrointestinal complications, especially in patients receiving steroids or other nephrotoxic drugs.

ANTIBIOTICS

Animals with underlying pulmonary disease or trauma (i.e., pulmonary contusions) are at increased risk of developing pulmonary infections. These patients should be monitored carefully, and prophylactic antibiotics (e.g., cefazolin; 22 mg/kg IV at induction; repeat once or twice at 2- to 4-hour intervals) should be provided, or therapeutic antibiotics should be initiated at the earliest sign of infection (i.e., leukocytosis and/or fever). Until susceptibility tests become available, amikacin, ceftizoxime, and enrofloxacin are rational choices for treatment of suspected infectious lower respiratory tract diseases of dogs.

Appropriate use of prophylactic antibiotics depends on the length of surgery, the type of surgery being performed, the animal's immune status, and the underlying disease process. Debilitated animals undergoing thoracotomy for removal of large neoplastic lesions (which may contain focal areas of necrosis) are likely to benefit from prophylactic antibiotic therapy. Prophylactic antibiotics should be given intravenously at induction of anesthesia and generally discontinued within 12 to 24 hours (see Chapter 10).

SURGICAL ANATOMY

The thoracic cavities of dogs and cats are compressed laterally, therefore the greatest dimension is dorsoventral. The ribs, sternum, and vertebral column form the thoracic skeleton. The sternum is composed of eight unpaired bones and forms the floor of the thorax (Fig. 29-1). The first and last sternebrae are known as the manubrium and xiphoid, respectively. There are usually 13 pairs of ribs. The tenth, eleventh, and twelfth ribs do not articulate with the sternum, but instead form the costal arch bilaterally. The cartilaginous portion of the thirteenth rib terminates free in the musculature. The space between the ribs, known as the intercostal space, generally is two to three times as wide as the adjacent ribs. Blood supply to the thoracic wall is provided by the intercostal arteries, which lie caudal to the adjacent rib in conjunction with a satellite vein and nerve. A typical intercostal nerve begins where the dorsal branch of the thoracic nerve divides and runs distally among the fibers of the internal intercostal muscle. In most intercostal spaces, intercostal vessels and nerves are covered medially only by pleura.

The muscles of the thorax not only serve a structural function, but also are important in respiration. The deepest muscles of the thoracic wall are the intercostal muscles. The fibers of the *external intercostal muscle* arise on the caudal border of each rib and run caudoventrally to the cranial border of the next rib. This muscle is important primarily in inspiration. The *internal intercostal muscles,* on the other hand, run from the cranial border of one rib to the caudal border of the preceding rib, primarily functioning to aid expiration. Other inspiratory muscles are the scalenus, ser-

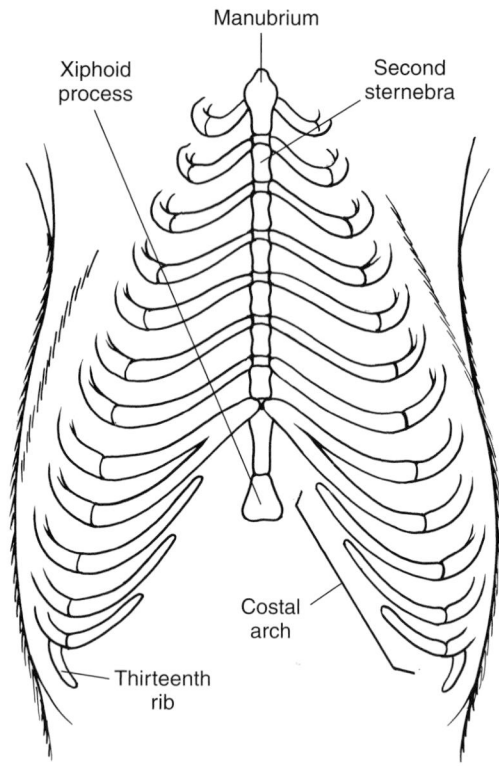

FIG. 29-1
Sternal anatomy.

ratus dorsalis cranialis, levatores costarum, and diaphragm. Additional expiratory muscles include the rectus abdominis, external abdominal oblique, internal abdominal oblique, transversus abdominis, serratus dorsalis caudalis, transversus costarum, and iliocostalis.

The lungs of dogs and cats have deep fissures that create distinct lobes, which allow the lungs to alter their shape in response to alterations in the shape of the thoracic cavity (i.e., that caused by diaphragmatic movement or flexion or extension of the spine). These fissures also allow individual lobes to be isolated and removed without compromising the integrity of the surrounding lobes. The left lung is divided into a cranial lobe, with a cranial and caudal part, and a caudal lobe (Fig. 29-2). The right lung is larger than the left and is divided into cranial, middle, caudal, and accessory lobes (see Fig. 29-2). The *cardiac notch* is a small area overlying the heart where lung tissue is not interposed between the heart and body wall. It usually is located at the ventral aspect of the fourth intercostal space and is larger on the right side.

The pulmonary arteries carry nonaerated blood from the right ventricle of the heart to the lungs, and the pulmonary veins return aerated blood from the lungs to the left atrium. The left pulmonary artery lies cranial to the left bronchus, whereas the left pulmonary veins are ventral to it. On the right side, the pulmonary artery lies dorsal and slightly caudal to the right bronchus, and the pulmonary veins lie craniodorsal and ventral to it.

Dorsal view

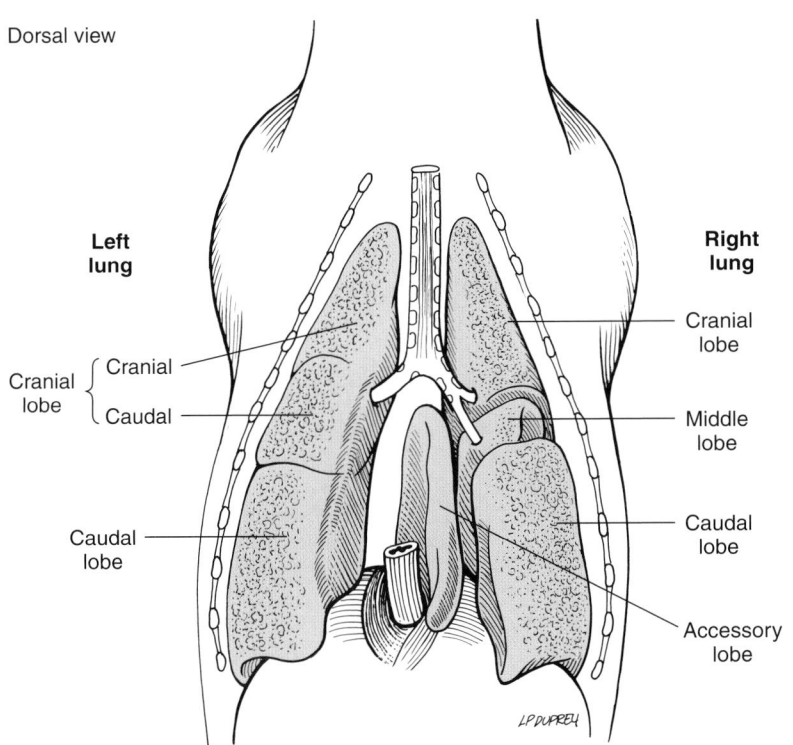

Left lung
Cranial lobe
{ Cranial
{ Caudal
Caudal lobe

Right lung
Cranial lobe
Middle lobe
Caudal lobe
Accessory lobe

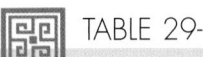

FIG. 29-2
Subdivisions of the canine and feline lung lobes.

SURGICAL TECHNIQUE
Thoracotomy

Thoracotomy may be performed by incising between the ribs or by splitting the sternum. The approach used depends on the exposure needed and underlying disease process. Regardless of the type of thoracotomy performed, a large area should be prepared for aseptic surgery to allow extension of the incision if needed. Depending on which left lobe is affected, a left lateral thoracotomy at the fourth, fifth, or sixth intercostal space provides adequate exposure for lobectomy (Table 29-1). A left fourth intercostal space thoracotomy allows exposure of the right ventricular outflow tract, main pulmonary artery, and ductus arteriosus. Bilateral removal of the pericardial sac can be difficult from this approach. A right intercostal thoracotomy provides exposure of the right side of the heart (auricle, atrium, and ventricle), cranial and caudal venae cavae, right lung lobes, and azygous vein. Median sternotomy affords exposure to both sides of the thoracic cavity. Bilateral, partial lobectomy is easily performed from a median sternotomy; however, complete lobectomy often is difficult. The caudal vena cava, main pulmonary artery, and both sides of the pericardial sac can be isolated and manipulated through this approach. A loose bandage should be placed on the thorax after surgery.

NOTE: Be sure to count your sponges at the start of the surgical procedure and before closure of the thoracic cavity. This helps to ensure that you do not leave a sponge in the thoracic cavity.

TABLE 29-1

Recommended Intercostal Spaces for Thoracotomy*

	LEFT	RIGHT
Heart	4,5	4,5
PDA	4(5)	
PRAA	4	
Pulmonic valve	4	
Lungs	4–6	4–6
Cranial lobe	4,5	4,5
Middle lobe		5
Caudal lobe	5(6)	5(6)
Esophagus		
Cranial	3,4	
Caudal	7–9	7–9
Cranial vena cava	(4)	4
Caudal vena cava	(6–7)	6–7

Modified from Orton EC: Thoracic wall. In Slatter D, editor: *Textbook of small animal surgery,* ed 2, Philadelphia, 1993, WB Saunders.
PDA, Patent ductus arteriosus; PRAA, persistent right aortic arch.
*Numbers in parentheses indicate alternative surgical sites.

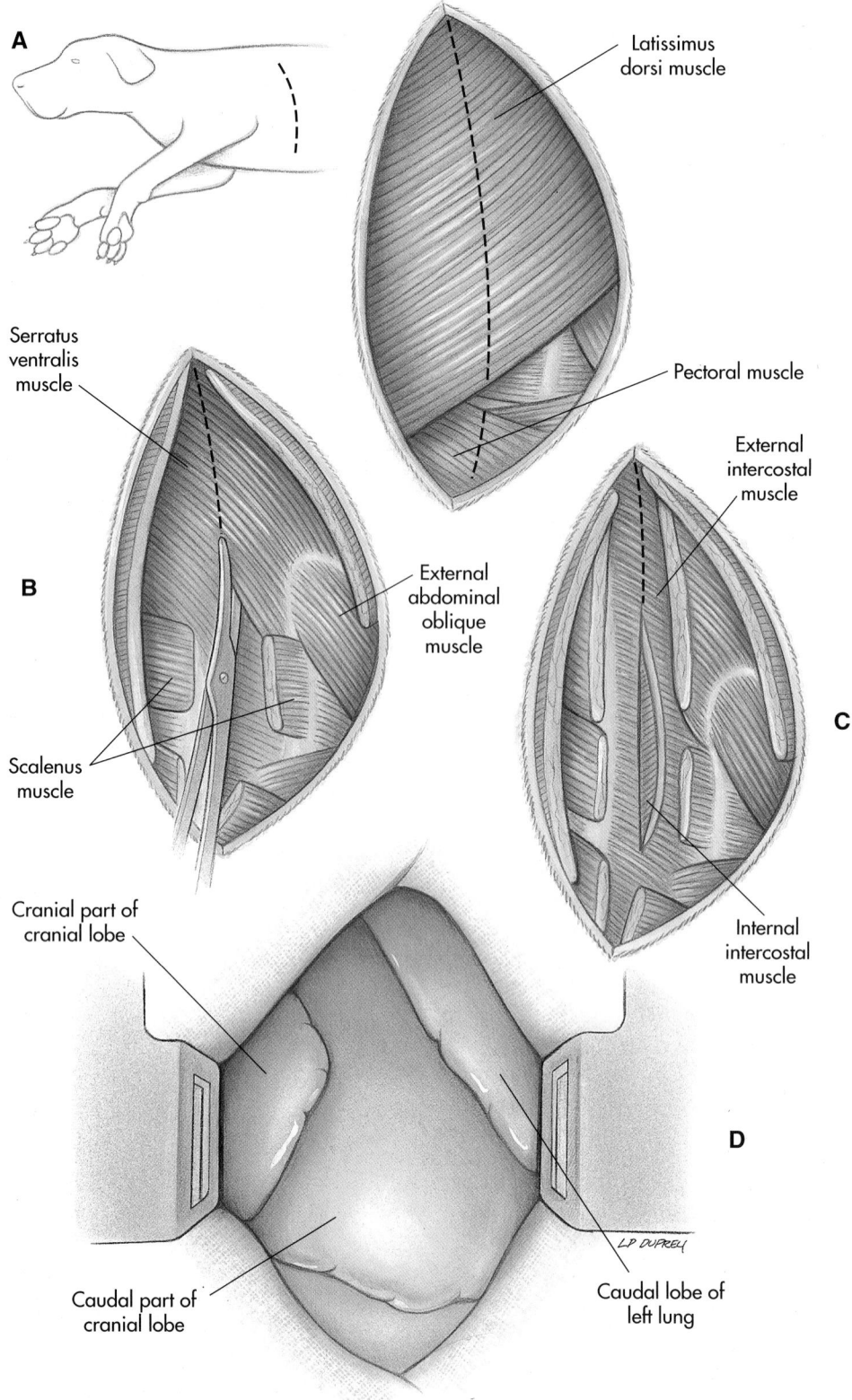

FIG. 29-3
Intercostal thoracotomy. **A,** Sharply incise the skin, subcutaneous tissues, and cutaneous trunci muscle. Deepen the incision through the latissimus dorsi muscle with scissors. **B** and **C,** Transect the scalenus, pectoral, serratus ventralis, and intercostal muscles. **D,** Use a Finochietto retractor to spread the ribs.

Intercostal thoracotomy. *With the dog in lateral recumbency, select the site for incision. Locate the approximate intercostal space, and sharply incise the skin, subcutaneous tissue, and cutaneous trunci muscle. The incision should extend from just below the vertebral bodies to near the sternum. Deepen the incision through the latissimus dorsi muscle with scissors (Fig. 29-3, A), then palpate the first rib by placing a hand cranially under the latissimus dorsi muscle. Count back from the first rib to verify the correct intercostal space.*

The ribs cranial to an intercostal incision are more easily retracted than the caudal ribs, therefore choose the more caudal space if you must choose between two adjacent intercostal spaces. Transect the scalenus and pectoral muscles with scissors perpendicular to their fibers, then separate the muscle fibers of the serratus ventralis muscle at the selected intercostal space (Fig. 29-3, B). Near the costochondral junction, place one scissor blade under the external intercostal muscle fibers, and push the scissors dorsally in the center of the intercostal space to incise the muscle (Fig. 29-3, C). Incise the internal intercostal muscle similarly. Notify the anesthetist that you are about to enter the thoracic cavity and, after identifying the lungs and pleura, use closed scissors or a blunt object to penetrate the pleura. This allows air to enter the thorax, causing the lungs to collapse away from the body wall. Extend the incision dorsally and ventrally to achieve the desired exposure. Identify and avoid incising the internal thoracic vessels as they course subpleurally near the sternum. Moisten laparotomy sponges and place them on the exposed edges of the chest incision. Use a Finochietto retractor to spread the ribs (Figs. 29-3, D and 29-4). If further exposure is necessary, a rib adjacent to the incision can be removed; however, this is seldom required. If a chest tube is to be placed, do so before closing the thorax. The tube should not exit from the incised intercostal space.

Close the thoracotomy by preplacing four to eight sutures of heavy monofilament absorbable or nonabsorbable suture (3-0 to No. 2, depending on the animal's size) around the ribs adjacent to the incision (Fig. 29-5, A). Approximate the ribs with a rib approximator or have an assistant cross two sutures to appose the ribs (Fig. 29-5, B), then tie the remain-

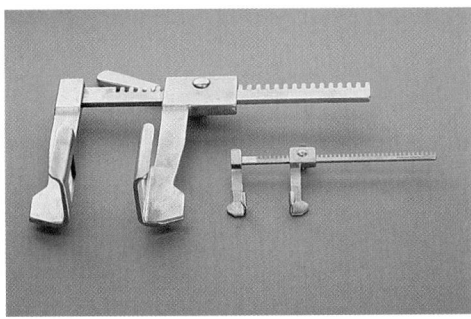

FIG. 29-4
Finochietto retractors.

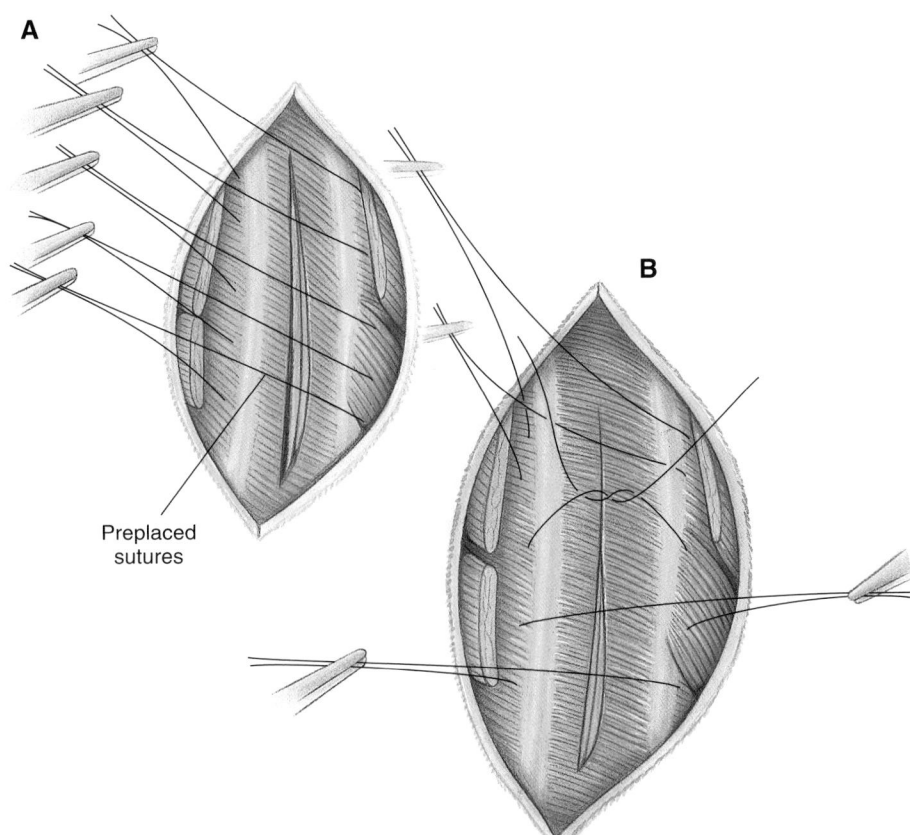

Preplaced sutures

FIG. 29-5
A, Close the thoracotomy by preplacing four to eight heavy monofilament sutures around the ribs adjacent to the incision. **B,** Approximate the ribs with a towel clamp or rib approximator or have an assistant cross two sutures to appose the ribs. Tie the remaining sutures.

ing sutures. Tie all the sutures before you remove the rib approximator. Suture the serratus ventralis, scalenus, and pectoralis muscles in a continuous pattern with absorbable suture material. Appose the edges of the latissimus dorsi muscle similarly. Remove residual air from the thoracic cavity using the preplaced chest tube or an over-the-needle catheter (see p. 898). Close the subcutaneous tissue and skin in a routine fashion.

A muscle-sparing technique may also be performed in cats and small dogs. Here, rather than incising the latissimus dorsi muscle, it is sharply separated along its ventral fascial attachments and elevated. Puppies may be more willing to ambulate shortly after thoracotomy if the latissimus dorsi muscle has not been cut; however, studies have not been done to compare lameness or other outcomes after various types of intercostal thoracotomy in dogs. Pain and physical function are similar after axillary, muscle-sparing versus posterolateral thoracotomy in human patients (Ochroch et al, 2005). Transcostal sutures have also been reported for closure of intercostal thoracotomies (Rooney et al, 2004). Here small holes are drilled in the ribs through which the suture is passed. The authors reported less pain associated with this closure method because nerve entrapment does not occur.

Median sternotomy. When performing median sternotomy, two or three sternebrae should be left intact cranially or caudally (depending on where the lesion is located) to reduce postoperative pain and prevent delayed healing caused by sternebral shifting. If exposure of the lungs or heart is necessary (i.e., in dogs with spontaneous pneumothorax or for pericardiectomy), the sternotomy should extend from the xiphoid cartilage cranially to the second or third sternebra. If exposure of the cranial mediastinum is desired, the sternotomy should extend from the manubrium caudally to the sixth or seventh sternebra.

With the dog in dorsal recumbency, incise the skin on the midline over the sternum. Expose the sternum by a combination of sharp incision and blunt dissection of the overlying musculature. Transect the sternebrae longitudinally on the midline with a sternal saw (Fig. 29-6), bone saw (Fig. 29-7), or chisel and osteotome. A sternal saw has a guide that sits under the sternum, making it much easier to cut the sternum without damaging the heart or lungs. In young animals, heavy scissors may be adequate; however, avoid crushing the bone. Splitting the sternebrae on the midline facilitates closure. If using a bone saw or chisel, take extra precaution to ensure that the underlying lung and heart are not damaged while completing the sternotomy. Place moistened laparotomy sponges on the incised edges of the sternebrae and retract the edges with a Finochietto rib retractor. If a chest tube is to be placed, do so before closing the sternotomy. Do not exit the tube from between the sternebrae; exit it from between the ribs or through the diaphragm. Close the sternotomy with wires (dogs larger than approximately 15 kg) or heavy suture (cats and dogs smaller than approximately

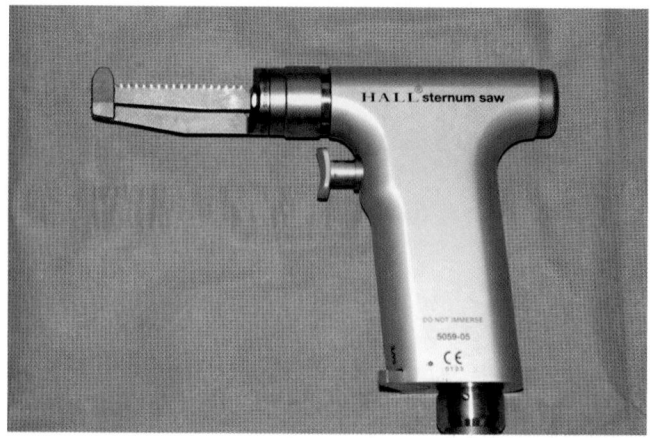

FIG. 29-6
Sternal saw for performing a median sternotomy.

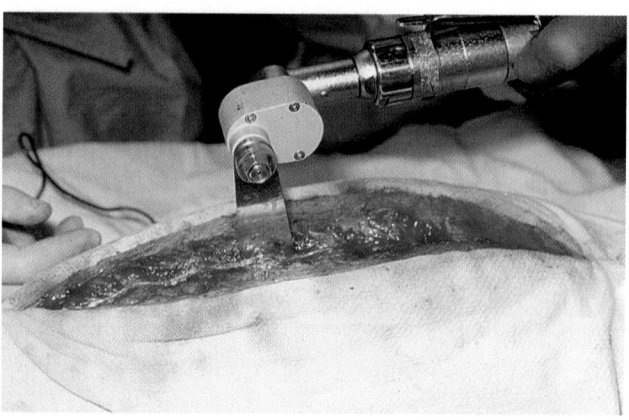

FIG. 29-7
When performing a median sternotomy, transect the sternebrae longitudinally on the midline with a bone saw, chisel and osteotome, or bone cutters.

15 kg) placed around the sternebrae (Fig. 29-8). Suture the subcutaneous tissue in a simple continuous pattern with absorbable suture. Remove residual air from the thoracic cavity and close the skin routinely.

Lung Biopsy

Fine-needle aspirate. This technique is best suited for nodular lesions that are close to the thoracic wall or diffuse pulmonary infiltrates. Fine needle aspiration may be performed blindly or be guided by ultrasound or fluoroscopy. Using ultrasound or fluoroscopy to direct the aspiration substantially increases the chances of accurate needle placement in focal lesions; it can be surprisingly easy to miss such lesions when determining needle placement from radiographs. Sometimes air in the lungs makes pulmonary lesions difficult to detect on ultrasound. In the case of nodules deep in the pulmonary parenchyma, one may anesthetize the patient and place it under a fluoroscopic unit so that respirations can be controlled and the needle accurately placed.

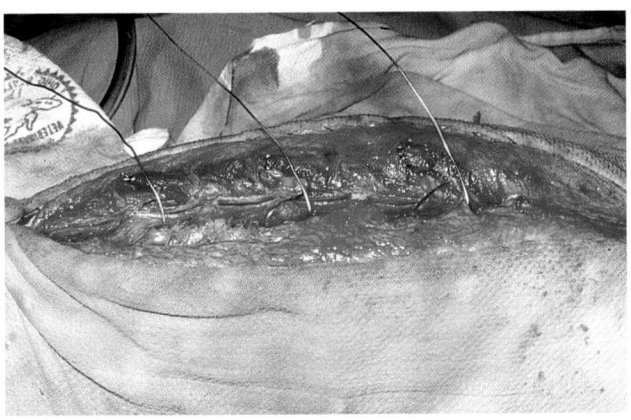

FIG. 29-8
Depending on the animal's size, close a sternotomy with wires or heavy suture placed around the sternebrae.

Radiographs may help determine the optimal site for needle placement if ultrasound or fluoroscopy is not available. In addition, CT-guided aspirates can be performed if this modality is available. In the case of diffuse lesions, it is usually best to aspirate the larger caudal lobes and stay away from the heart and major vessels. There is always the risk of pneumothorax after such a procedure. Despite the risk being small, patients have died from complications of aspirates, and clinicians must be prepared to place a chest tube and/or do a thoracotomy to stop air leakage.

After identifying the appropriate spot to puncture the thoracic wall, clip and prep the area.

If the patient will remain still, no sedation or anesthetic is required; however, anesthesia is generally recommended to ensure that the animal does not move during the procedure.

For superficial lesions, typically use a 25-gauge needle; for deep lesions, a 25-gauge spinal needle with a stylet is preferred. Once the needle is believed to be in the correct spot, apply several bursts of 5 to 8 ml of negative pressure, and then withdraw the needle without maintaining the negative pressure. Perform the procedure quickly so that respiratory movement does not cause pulmonary laceration. After performing the procedure, watch the patient carefully for the next 30 to 60 minutes to ensure that pneumothorax does not cause clinical compromise.

Keyhole biopsy. *Identify the appropriate intercostal space, and make a 3- to 7-cm keyhole intercostal thoracotomy approach (see previous discussion) to expose the lung. Place a small Finochietto rib retractor into the space to gain exposure to the thoracic cavity. Obtain a lung biopsy using a thoracoabdominal (TA) stapler (see p. 876). Inspect the stump that remains after biopsy for evidence of hemorrhage and evaluate it for air leakage by filling the thoracic cavity with warm sterile saline solution and examining for air*

bubbles. Evacuate the fluid using suction. Place a chest tube if necessary or close the chest routinely (see previous discussion), and aspirate air from the thoracic cavity with a needle or catheter (see p. 898).

Thoracoscopic biopsy. A paraxiphoid or substernal observation port is usually the best choice for this procedure, although a lateral port may work too (see p. 151). Examine the lung lobes thoroughly for abnormalities. These biopsies are usually done on the tips or margins of lung lobes. After identifying the site to be biopsied, there are two basic techniques:

Intrathoracic biopsy: Position a ligation loop of a commercially available ligature (e.g., 25/0 18-inch ligature, Endoloop, Ethicon, Overland Park, Kan.) in the intrapleural space and pass a forceps through the ligation loop. Grasp the margin of the affected portion of the lung, and pull the lung tissue into the ligation loop. Tighten the ligature around the base of the biopsy specimen or portion of lung to be removed. Once the ligature is secure, transect the pulmonary tissue, leaving the ligature on the lung.

Directed keyhole biopsy: Determine the optimal site for making a 1-inch incision into the chest.

This usually means making the incision 2 to 3 intercostal spaces cranial of where the tip of the lung extends during inspiration.

After making the incision, insert a Babcock forceps, grasp the tip of the lung lobe from which a biopsy will be taken, and pull it out of the chest. Place a ligature around the tip and resect it, leaving the ligature on the lung. Check the site for leakage, and then place the lung back in the chest.

Surgical biopsy. *Perform an intercostal thoracotomy and identify the affected lung lobe. Palpate each lung lobe for additional nodules and take a biopsy of the hilar lymph node for staging purposes. Perform a partial lobectomy (see later discussion) if the tumor is located at the peripheral margin of the lobe; otherwise, perform a complete lobectomy. Submit excised tissue for cytologic and histologic examination. If the lesion is cavitary or if there is evidence of preexisting pyothorax, submit cultures of the mass. Place a chest tube before closing the thorax if there is evidence of infection or if pneumothorax or hemorrhage seems likely postoperatively. Remove residual air from the pleural space after closure.*

Partial Lobectomy

Partial lobectomy may be performed to remove a focal lesion involving the peripheral one half to two thirds of the lung lobe or for biopsy. Partial lobectomy may be performed through a lateral fourth or fifth space intercostal thoracotomy or median sternotomy.

Identify the lung tissue to be removed, and place a pair of crushing forceps across the lobe proximal to the lesion (Fig.

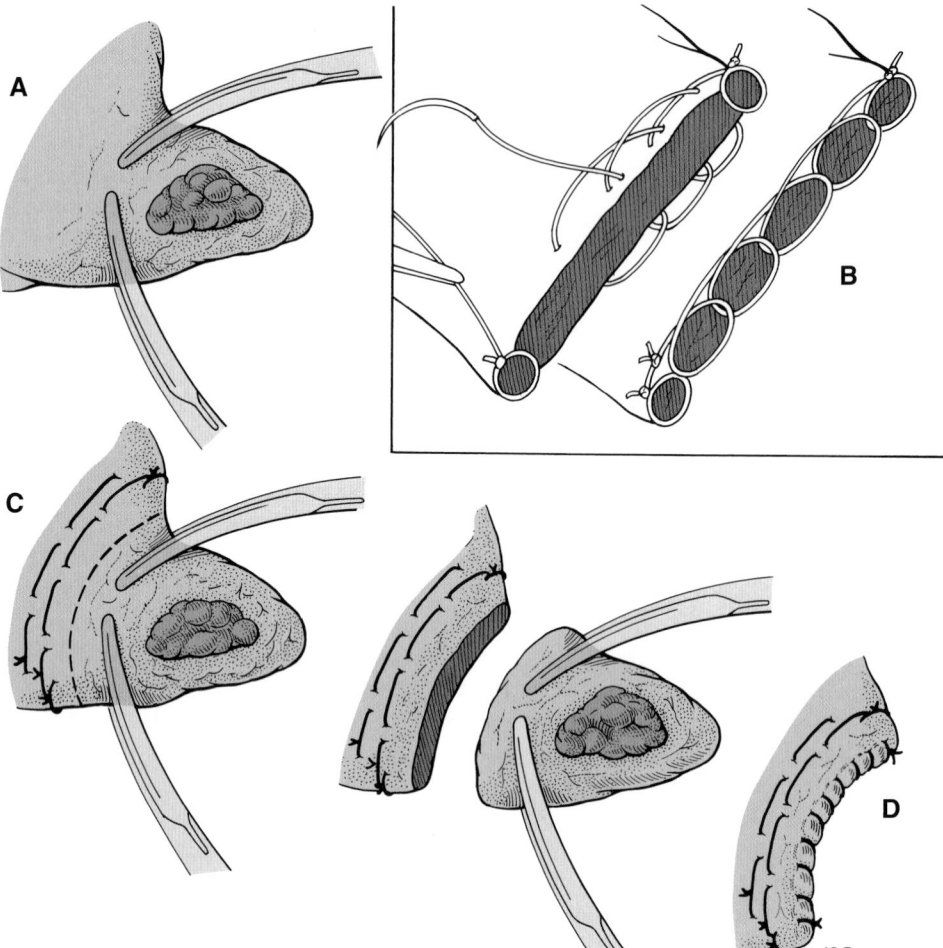

FIG. 29-9
Partial lobectomy may be performed through an intercostal thoracotomy or a median sternotomy. **A,** Identify the lung tissue to be removed and place a pair of crushing forceps proximal to the lesion. **B,** Place a continuous, overlapping suture pattern proximal to the forceps. **C,** Excise the lung between the suture lines and clamps. **D,** Oversew the lung in a simple continuous pattern with absorbable suture.

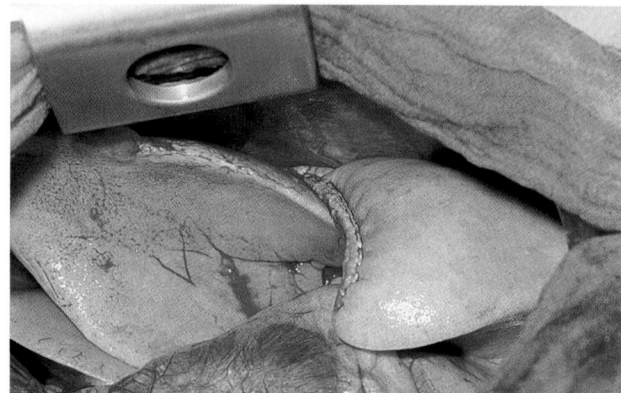

FIG. 29-10
Appearance of lung lobes after partial lobectomy using a stapling device.

29-9, A). Place a continuous, overlapping pattern of absorbable suture (2-0 to 4-0) 4 to 6 mm proximal to the forceps (Fig. 29-9, B). If necessary, place a second row of sutures in a similar manner. Excise the lung between the suture lines and clamps, leaving a 2- to 3-mm margin of tissue distal to the sutures (Fig. 29-9, C). Oversew the lung in a simple

continuous pattern with absorbable suture (3-0 to 5-0; Fig. 29-9, D). Replace the lung in the thoracic cavity and fill the chest cavity with warmed sterile saline solution. Inflate the lungs and check the bronchus for air leaks. Remove the fluid before closing the thorax.

Partial lobectomy may also be performed with stapling devices (e.g., TA stapler; Fig. 29-10). The stapling equipment comes in various sizes, which produce staple lines 30 mm, 55 mm, or 90 mm long. Select the staple size based on the width of the lung so that the staple line extends across the entire width of the lung to be removed, but does not extend beyond the edges. If air leaks or hemorrhage are noted, place a simple continuous pattern of absorbable suture along the lung margin. The stapling devices compress tissue to a thickness of 1.5 mm (3.5-mm staples) or 2 mm (4.8-mm staples). Avoid stapling excessively thick or fibrotic lung because this may result in large air leaks or hemorrhage. Check the lung for leaks and close as described above.

Complete Lobectomy

Complete lobectomy is best performed through a lateral thoracotomy. If the lung contains a large amount of purulent material, prevent excessive fluid from draining into the

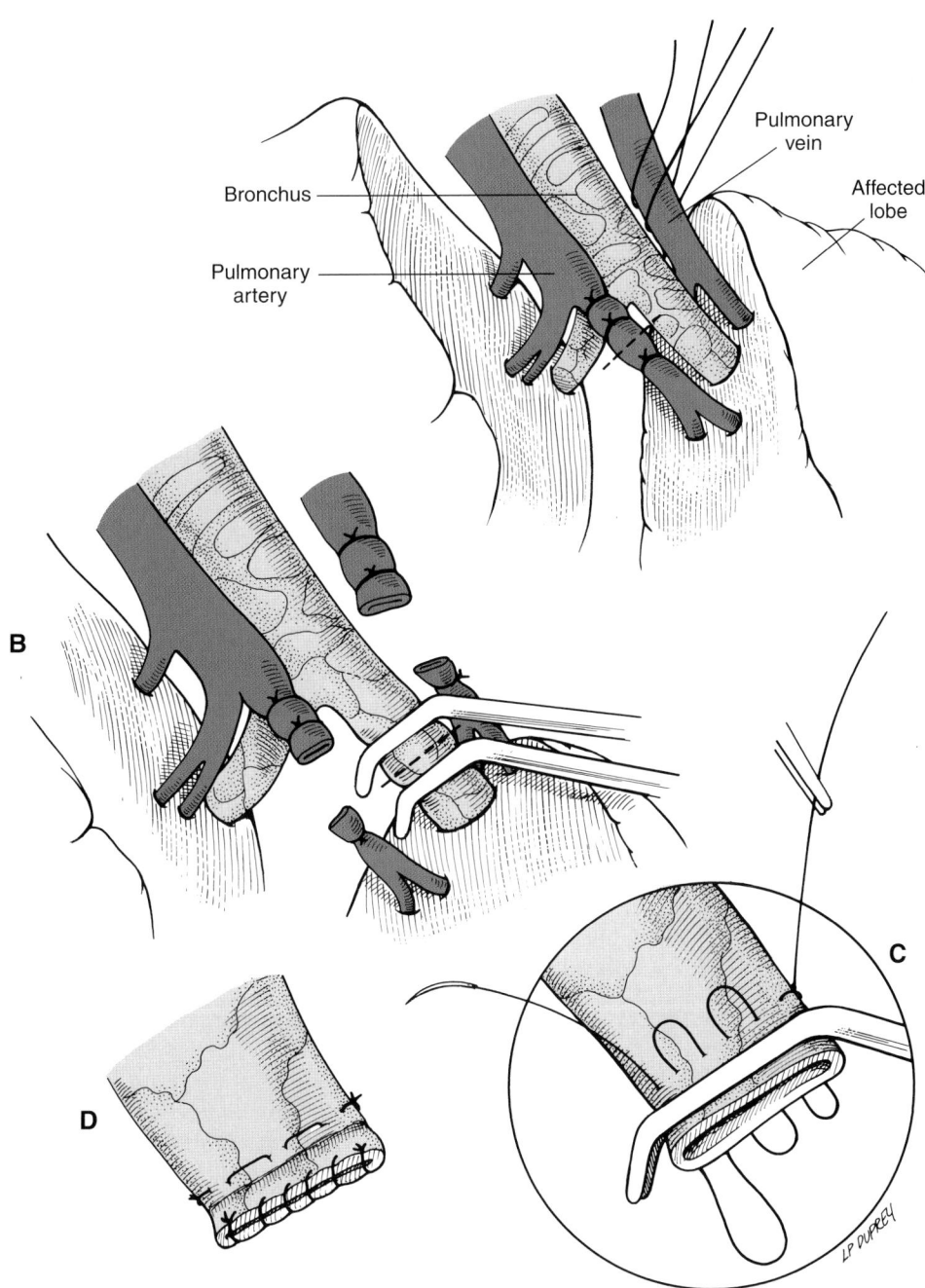

Bronchus

Pulmonary
artery

Pulmonary
vein

Affected
lobe

A

B

C

D

FIG. 29-11
Complete lobectomy. **A,** Ligate
and transect the vasculature to
the affected lobe. **B,** Clamp the
main bronchus with a pair of
Satinsky or crushing forceps;
sever the bronchus between the
clamps and remove the lung.
C, Suture the bronchus in a continuous horizontal mattress pattern. **D,** Oversew the end in a
simple continuous suture pattern.

LP DUPREY

proximal bronchi and trachea by clamping the bronchus near the hilus before manipulating the lobe. Similarly, torsed lung lobes should be removed without untwisting the pedicle (which would release necrotic material trapped in the lung) (see p. 887). Dogs can survive acute loss of up to 50 percent of their lung volume; however, transient respiratory acidosis and exercise intolerance may occur. In normal dogs, pneumonectomy causes compensatory changes in the contralateral lung and myocardium. Although residual lung volume, vital capacity, and maximal breathing capacity are substantially decreased initially, residual lung volume increases significantly after 3 months. Total lung capacity increases up to 37 percent more than expected for a normal, single lung (Liptak et al, 2004).

Identify the affected lobe or lobes and isolate them from the remaining lobes with moistened sponges (laparotomy or 4 × 4s, depending on the animal's size). Identify the vasculature and bronchus to the lobe (Fig. 29-11, A). Using blunt dissection, isolate the pulmonary artery supplying the affected lobe and pass a ligature of nonabsorbable or absorbable suture (2-0 or 3-0) around the proximal end of the vessel. Do not compromise the lumen of the parent vessel from which this vessel arises. Place a second ligature in a similar fashion distal to the site where the vessel is to be transected. A transfixing suture may be placed between these sutures proximal to the transection site to prevent the first suture from being inadvertently dislodged. Transect the artery between the distal two ligatures. Ligate the pulmonary vein in a similar fashion. Identify the main bronchus supplying the lobe and clamp it with a pair of Satinsky or crushing forceps proximal and distal to the selected transection site (Fig. 29-11, B). Sever the bronchus between the clamps and remove the lung. Suture the bronchus proximal to the remaining clamp in a continuous horizontal mattress pattern (Fig. 29-11, C) or, in cats and small dogs, place a transfixing ligature around the bronchus. Before removing the clamp, secure a suture in the bronchus distal to the clamp. After removing the clamp, over-sew the end of the bronchus in a simple continuous suture pattern (Fig. 29-11, D). Fill the chest cavity with warmed sterile saline solution. Inflate the lungs and check the bronchus for air leaks. Before closure, check lungs that have been "packed off" to make sure they reinflate and are not twisted. Remove the fluid and close the chest as described above.

A Miller's knot (see Fig. 26-4 on p. 711) or transfixation suture can be used successfully to ligate the vessels and bronchus in many animals. Stapling devices may also be used for complete lobectomy, but make sure the bronchus and vessels are adequately ligated by the staples.

HEALING OF THE LUNGS AND STERNUM

After multiple lobectomies or partial lobectomy of several lobes, expansion of the remaining lung may occur in an attempt to restore normal lung volume, therefore exercise intolerance may decline in some animals with time after pneumonectomy. The healing of median sternotomies has been a matter of concern; however, if several sternebrae are left intact and if the closure is performed properly, these incisions heal readily and without complication even in animals with pyothorax.

SUTURE MATERIALS AND SPECIAL INSTRUMENTS

Absorbable or nonabsorbable suture material can be used for complete lobectomy; however, braided, multifilament, nonabsorbable suture (e.g., silk) should be avoided if infection is present. Finochietto rib retractors, Satinsky clamps (for clamping the bronchus), and right-angled forceps (such as Mixter forceps [also known as gallbladder or gall duct forceps or thoracic forceps]) are useful when performing thoracic surgery (Fig. 29-12). A sternal saw or bone saw is recommended for median sternotomy, particularly in medium or large dogs. Vacuum suction devices facilitate removal of the fluid placed in the chest to identify air leaks. TA staplers are also useful for lobectomies.

POSTOPERATIVE CARE AND ASSESSMENT

Respiration should be monitored closely once the animal begins ventilating on its own. If respiratory excursions are inadequate, the chest should be evaluated to verify that residual air was removed after chest closure. If there is any doubt, thoracic radiographs should be examined for pneumothorax (see p. 908). Blood gas analysis can help evaluate the adequacy of ventilation; hypoxic animals should receive oxygen by nasal insufflation or oxygen cage (see Chapter 5).

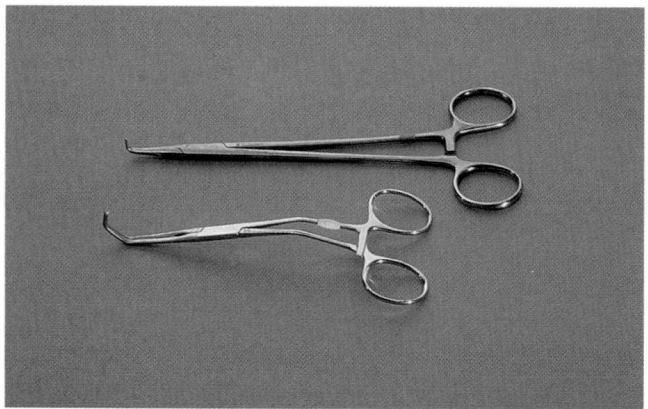

FIG. 29-12
Right-angled forceps *(upper)* and Satinsky clamp *(lower)*.

Animals with severe or progressive hypoxemia should be evaluated for pulmonary edema. Inadequate ventilation may be due to pain in some animals. Median sternotomy may cause decreased ventilation compared with that seen with intercostal thoracotomy. Analgesics are needed in all patients undergoing thoracotomy procedures (see p. 868). Hypothermia is common after thoracic surgery; warm water bottles and circulating water or warm air blankets should be used to rewarm these patients.

> NOTE: If the animal hypoventilates postoperatively, thoracic radiographs are indicated to rule out pneumothorax, hemothorax, and pulmonary edema.

COMPLICATIONS

The major complication of partial or complete lobectomy is air leakage or hemorrhage (or both). Minor air leaks usually seal, but massive air leaks or severe hemorrhage require reoperation. Subcutaneous fluid accumulation at the ventral aspect of the thoracotomy incision occasionally occurs, but can be avoided by carefully closing the distal musculature (i.e., serratus ventralis and pectoralis muscles). With median sternotomy, adequate closure and leaving several sternebrae intact prevents delayed healing or nonunion of the sternebrae. Postoperatively, lameness associated with pain and severing of the latissimus dorsi muscle is common, but usually resolves within 1 to 2 days.

> NOTE: Monitor these animals closely in the early postoperative period for pneumothorax or hemothorax or both.

SPECIAL AGE CONSIDERATIONS

Uptake of inhalation agents in pediatric patients (i.e., those younger than 12 weeks of age) may be more rapid than in adults, and the level of anesthesia fluctuates more readily in these patients; therefore extra care should be used when anesthetizing them. Young animals are particularly prone to hypothermia when the chest cavity is opened. Temperature regulation, blood glucose requirements, and fluid and electrolyte replacement should be aggressively managed in these patients. Geriatric patients with compromised pulmonary function and/or decreased cardiovascular capacity may also have abnormal uptake of inhalant anesthetics.

References

Daly CM, Swalec-Tobias K, Tobias AH et al: Cardiopulmonary effects of intrathoracic insufflation in dogs, *J Am Anim Hosp Assoc* 38:515, 2002.

Liptak JM, Monnet E, Dernell WS et al: Pneumonectomy: four cases and a comparative review, *J Small Anim Pract* 45:441, 2004.

Naganobu K, Maeda K, Miyamato T et al: Cardiorespiratory effects of epidural administration of morphine and fentanyl in dogs anesthetized with sevoflurane, *J Am Vet Med Assoc* 224:67, 2004.

Ochroch EA, Gottschalk A, Augoustides JG et al: Pain and physical function are similar following axillary, muscle-sparing vs posterolateral thoracotomy, *Chest* 128:2664, 2005.

Rooney MB, Mehl M, Monnet E: Intercostal thoracotomy closure: transcostal sutures as a less painful alternative to circumcostal suture placement, *Vet Surg* 33:209, 2004.

Sigrsit NE, Doherr MG, Spend DE: Clinical findings and diagnostic value of post-traumatic thoracic radiographs in dogs and cats with blunt trauma, *J Vet Emerg Crit Care* 14:259, 2004.

Suggested Reading

Alwood AJ, Downend AD, Simpson SA et al: Pharmacokinetics of dalteparin and enoxaparin in healthy cats (abstract), *Proceedings 11th International Veterinary Emergency Medicine Critical Care Society*, Atlanta, p. 1033, 2005.

A study on six healthy cats suggested that 180 U/kg every 6 hours was reasonable in cats.

Bauer TG: Lung biopsy, *Vet Clin North Am* 30:1207, 2000.

This is a good review of the techniques and indications.

Cantwell SI, Duke T, Walsh PJ et al: One-lung versus two-lung ventilation in the closed-chest anesthetized dog: a comparison of cardiopulmonary parameters, *Vet Surg* 29:365, 2000.

One lung ventilation was found to be a feasible procedure in anesthetized dogs.

Faunt KK, Jones BD, Turk JR et al: Evaluation of biopsy specimens obtained during thoracoscopy from lungs of normal dogs, *Am J Vet Res* 59:1499, 1998.

This paper has a detailed description of the technique, which was safely performed in six healthy dogs.

Johnson LR, Lappin MR, Baker DC: Pulmonary thromboembolism in 29 dogs: 1985-1995, *J Vet Intern Med* 13:338, 1999.

Diagnostically, there were no pathognomonic radiographic or clinicopathologic findings, and most cases were associated with neoplasia, immune-mediated hemolytic anemia, and systemic bacterial disease.

Mischke RH, Shutteret C, Grege SI: Anticoagulant effects of repeated subcutaneous injections of high doses of unfractionated heparin in healthy dogs, *Am J Vet Res* 62:1887, 2001.

The effects of high dose heparin on the coagulation system cannot be predicted; you must monitor the patient.

Norris CR, Griffey SM, Samii VF: Pulmonary thromboembolism in cats: 29 cases (1987-1997), *J Am Vet Med Assoc* 215:1650, 1999.

Radiographically, pulmonary vessel abnormalities, pleural effusion, and peripheral consolidations were the most common findings.

Norris CR, Griffey SM, Walsh P: Use of keyhole lung biopsy for diagnosis of interstitial lung diseases in dogs and cats: 13 cases (1998-2001), *J Am Vet Med Assoc* 221:1453, 2002.

This article describes the use of a keyhole biopsy and details the technique for diagnosing various interstitial lung diseases in dogs and cats.

Rozanski EA, Rondeau MP: Respiratory pharmacotherapy in emergency and critical care medicine, *Vet Clin Small Anim* 32:1073, 2002.

An excellent review of respiratory conditions and their treatment in dogs and cats.

Smith CE, Rozanski EA, Freeman LM et al: Use of low molecular weight heparin in cats: 57 cases (1999-2003). *J Am Vet Med Assoc* 225:1237, 2004.

Dalteparin was given to cats with aortic thromboembolism at 99 U/kg once or twice daily with minimal problems. The effectiveness of this therapy was uncertain.

SPECIFIC DISEASES

THORACIC WALL TRAUMA

DEFINITION

Flail chest occurs when several ribs on both sides of the point of impact are fractured, such that the fractured segment moves paradoxically with respiration.

GENERAL CONSIDERATIONS AND CLINICALLY RELEVANT PATHOPHYSIOLOGY

Thoracic wall injury may be due to blunt trauma (e.g., motor vehicle accidents or being kicked by a horse) or penetrating trauma. The most common causes of penetrating injuries of the thorax in dogs are bite wounds and gunshot injuries. Both blunt and penetrating trauma may cause extensive soft tissue damage of the thoracic wall (Fig. 29-13). Although soft tissue damage is rarely the cause of major morbidity or mortality, it may be the only external evidence of severe thoracic trauma in some animals. Pain associated with muscular tears may cause altered respiration because the animal is unwilling to breathe deeply. Unless associated with pulmonary parenchymal damage, hypoxia due to ventilatory alterations seldom occurs with chest wall trauma.

Subcutaneous emphysema may occur with both blunt and penetrating trauma, but usually is insignificant. This occurs when air is forced into subcutaneous tissue and dissects along muscular and fascial planes. The air may reach the subcutaneous tissue through a disruption of the pleura and intercostal muscles, by direct communication with an external wound, or as an extension of mediastinal emphysema. Treatment of subcutaneous air should be directed at its cause. Similarly, isolated rib fractures are seldom associated with major morbidity. Occasionally, rib fractures pro-

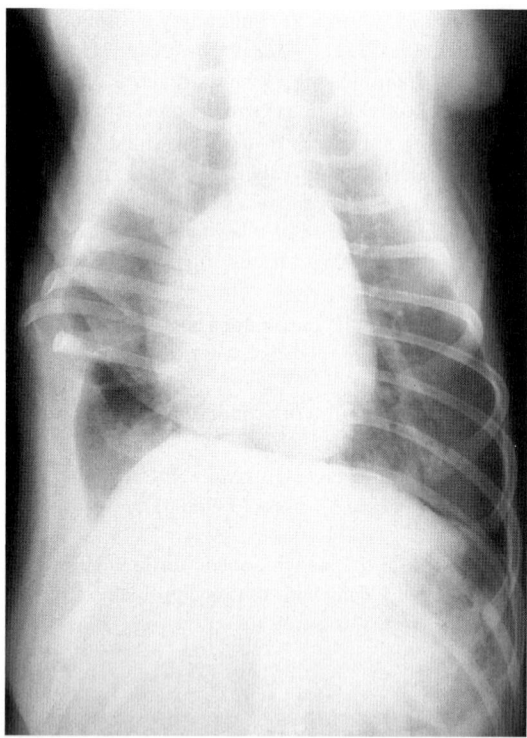

FIG. 29-13
Thoracic radiograph of a dog that was kicked by a horse. Note the large defect between the ribs on the right side of the thorax and the extrapleural sign (see text) created by the chest wall trauma.

duce sharp fragments that may injure a major vessel or lacerate the lung. Rib fractures may interfere with ventilation if the animal splints the thorax in an attempt to reduce pain by reducing motion of the fragments.

Flail chest occurs when several ribs on both sides of the point of impact are fractured such that the intervening rib segments lose their continuity with the remainder of the thorax (Fig. 29-14). Paradoxical movement of the chest wall occurs during respiration as a result of intrapleural pressure changes; the fractured segment moves inward during inspiration and outward during expiration. Respiratory abnormalities in patients with flail chest may be severe and may include decreased vital capacity, reduced functional residual capacity, hypoxemia, decreased compliance, increased airway resistance, and increased work to breathe. These abnormal respiratory parameters were once thought to be caused primarily by the movement of the flail segment; however, it is now believed that the underlying lung damage and hypoventilation from chest pain are more important factors in the development of respiratory insufficiency.

DIAGNOSIS
Clinical Presentation

Signalment. Thoracic wall trauma may occur in dogs or cats of any age, but is most common in young animals prone to trauma.

History. A history of trauma may or may not be obtained. The animal may be presented for evaluation of respiratory distress, reluctance to move because of pain, depression, lethargy, and/or anorexia.

Physical Examination Findings

Animals with thoracic trauma should be examined for delayed-onset cardiac arrhythmias. Cardiac arrhythmias, particularly premature ventricular contractions and ventricular tachycardia, may occur after either blunt or penetrating thoracic trauma; there is often little or no external evidence of chest injury. These arrhythmias may not begin until 12 to 72 hours after the trauma and may be associated with myocardial contusion, myocardial ischemia that occurs secondary to shock, or neurogenic injuries that result in sympathetic overstimulation. Cardiac contusions frequently are overlooked in injured patients because (1) attention is directed toward visually obvious injuries, (2) there is no external evidence of thoracic trauma, or (3) there is no evidence of thoracic trauma at the initial examination. Cardiac function, therefore, should be evaluated frequently in most trauma patients.

Diagnostic Imaging

Thoracic radiographs of animals with trauma should be carefully evaluated for pulmonary contusions or pneumothorax. Rib fractures are easily missed on thoracic radiographs if careful attention is not paid to the rib contour, particularly if the fractured segment is minimally displaced. Orthogonal radiographic views should be evaluated. Evidence of other bony trauma should be sought by carefully examining the vertebrae, scapulae, and proximal forelimbs.

> NOTE: Evaluate thoracic radiographs of dyspneic animals carefully to differentiate intraparenchymal damage (i.e., contusion) from pneumothorax.

Laboratory Findings

Laboratory findings are nonspecific. Blood gas analysis may show hypoxemia and respiratory acidosis (resulting from hypoventilation) or alkalosis (resulting from hyperventilation).

DIFFERENTIAL DIAGNOSIS

Rib fractures may occur secondary to neoplasia or infectious processes; however, these lesions generally are accompanied by lysis or proliferation of the adjacent bone.

MEDICAL MANAGEMENT

Most animals with thoracic wall trauma can be stabilized without surgery. Antibiotic therapy is indicated in patients with notable pulmonary contusion or hemorrhage. Concurrent pneumothorax should be identified and treated (see p. 908). If the animal is dyspneic, supplemental oxygen should be provided. With flail chest, the rib segment can initially be immobilized by positioning the patient with the affected side down. Mechanical ventilation rather than surgery is the treatment of choice in human beings with pulmonary con-

A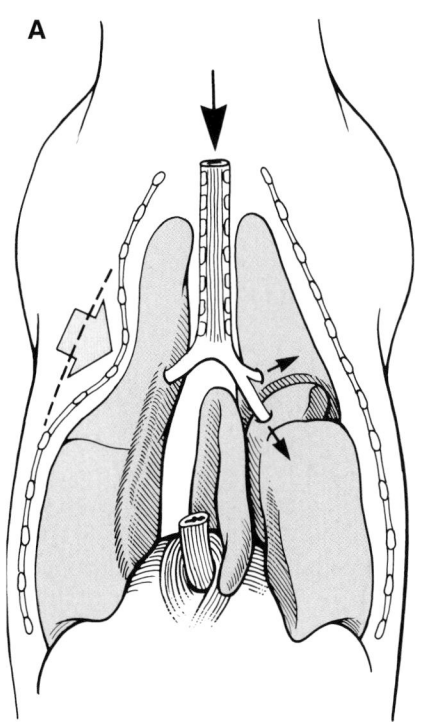

B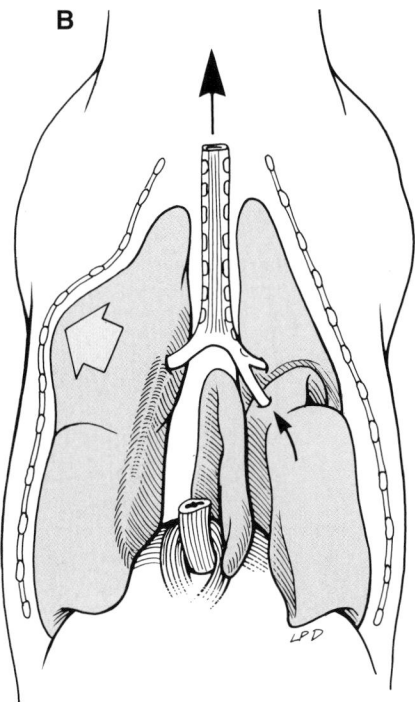

FIG. 29-14
With flail chest, paradoxical movement of the chest wall occurs during respiration because of intrapleural pressure changes; **(A)** the fractured segment moves inward during inspiration and **(B)** outward during expiration.

tusions and flail chest; however, long-term mechanical ventilation may not be possible or practical in many veterinary patients. Stabilization may prevent further damage to intrathoracic structures, improve pulmonary ventilation, and reduce pain associated with movement of fragments; however, its benefit is uncertain (see later in the Prognosis section).

SURGICAL TREATMENT

Rib fractures seldom require surgical treatment; however, multiple rib fractures may cause a defect in thoracic wall continuity (i.e., concavity) that warrants surgical repair. Also, open stabilization of rib fractures may be indicated if concurrent intrathoracic trauma requires surgery. Flail chest may be managed by placing an external splint over the thorax to stabilize the fractured segment (see later discussion).

Preoperative Management

If possible, animals with pulmonary contusions should be in stable condition before surgical repair of rib fractures. Shock treatment (i.e., fluids and antibiotics, with or without corticosteroids) should be initiated if necessary. Oxygen supplementation may be beneficial (see Chapter 5), and antibiotics are indicated if pulmonary contusions or hemorrhage are present. If a flail segment is present, placing the animal with the affected side down may be beneficial.

Anesthesia

A splint may be applied to the flail segment of some animals using an intercostal nerve block (see p. 868), rather than general anesthetic. See anesthetic recommendations on p. 867 for animals with respiratory disease. If general

anesthesia is required, refer to the anesthetic protocols and comments on p. 868.

Positioning

For rib fractures and flail chest, the lateral thorax encompassing the fractured ribs is clipped and prepared aseptically.

SURGICAL TECHNIQUE
Rib Fractures

Place a small intramuscular pin through the proximal fragment and into the marrow canal. Reduce the fracture and drive the pin into the distal fragment. Exit the pin through the cortex, and bend the ends slightly to help prevent migration. As an alternative, use cerclage wires or cross pins.

Flail Chest

Secure the affected ribs to a sheet of plastic splinting material (e.g., Orthoplast) that has been molded to conform to the thoracic wall (Fig. 29-15). Using a Steinmann pin, place holes in the splinting material large enough to pass the selected suture (see later discussion) through. Place sutures circumferentially around the affected ribs. Pass the suture ends through the predrilled holes and tie securely. As an alternative, aluminum rods or tongue depressors may be substituted for the plastic splinting material.

SUTURE MATERIALS AND SPECIAL INSTRUMENTS

For application of a splint in animals with flail chest, use large monofilament suture (2-0 to No. 2, depending on the animal's size) with an attached large, curved needle. A Steinmann pin

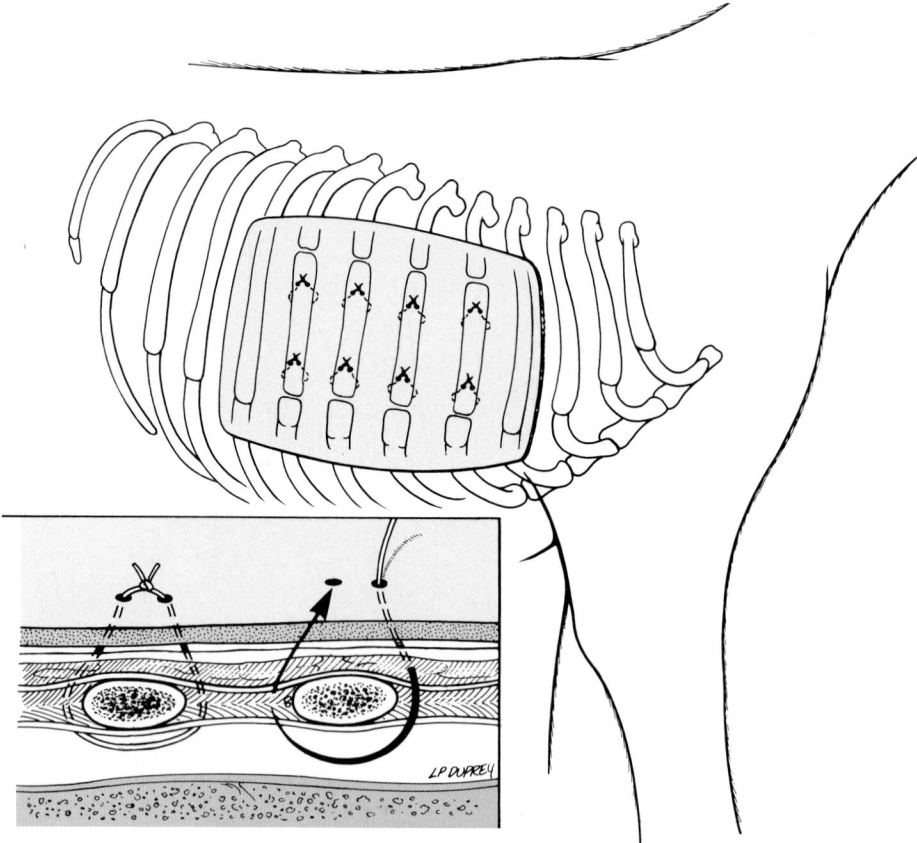

FIG. 29-15
To repair flail chest, secure the affected ribs to a sheet of plastic splinting material. Place sutures circumferentially around the affected ribs and through holes in the splinting material.

and pin chuck are also needed. For rib fracture repair, small intramedullary pins and cerclage wire are needed.

POSTOPERATIVE CARE AND ASSESSMENT

Animals with thoracic trauma should be monitored closely in the postoperative period for hypoventilation and pneumothorax. Analgesics are warranted in these animals (see p. 868). See p. 878 for additional comments on the postoperative management of animals with respiratory disorders.

PROGNOSIS

The prognosis for animals with thoracic wall trauma generally depends on the amount of concurrent pulmonary or cardiac trauma. Most rib fractures heal without surgery. A recent study showed no difference in outcomes when the flail segment was stabilized or not stabilized (Olsen et al, 2002). Cats with rib fractures secondary to trauma generally have a good outcome. The prognosis is worse if flail chest, pleural effusion, or diaphragmatic hernias are present (Kraje et al, 2000).

References

Kraje BJ, Kraje AC, Rohrbach BW: Intrathoracic and concurrent orthopedic injury associated with traumatic rib fractures in cats: 75 cases (1980-1998), *J Am Vet Med Assoc* 216:51, 2000.

Olsen D, Renberg W, Perrett J et al: Clinical management of flail chest in dogs and cats: a retrospective review of 24 cases (1989-1999), *J Am Anim Hosp Assoc* 38:315, 2002.

PULMONARY NEOPLASIA

DEFINITION

Primary pulmonary neoplasms originate in pulmonary tissue and may arise as a solitary mass or in rare cases may be multicentric.

GENERAL CONSIDERATIONS AND CLINICALLY RELEVANT PATHOPHYSIOLOGY

Primary pulmonary neoplasia is less common than metastatic neoplasia in dogs and cats. The diaphragmatic lobes are most frequently involved, with the right lung lobes more often affected than the left. Specific anatomic localization of tumor origin is not always possible, and more than one tumor type may be present; therefore classification of primary lung tumors usually is based on the predominant histologic pattern. Adenocarcinoma is the most common histologic type found in dogs and cats; squamous cell carcinoma and anaplastic carcinomas are less common. Primary pulmonary tumors of connective tissue origin (e.g., osteosarcoma, fibrosarcoma, and hemangiosarcoma) are rare. Although most pulmonary tumors are malignant, benign tumors (i.e., papillary adenoma, bronchial adenoma, fibroma, myxochondroma, and plasmacytoma) occur. Pulmonary neoplasms are highly aggressive and tend to metastasize early. Most anaplastic carcinomas and squamous cell carcinomas have metastasized at the time of diagnosis, whereas approximately half of adenocarcinomas have done so. Metastasis is often to the lung itself or to regional lymph nodes or both.

Metastatic pulmonary neoplasia is an important differential diagnosis for nodular lung disease. Tumors with a high likelihood of resulting in pulmonary metastasis include mammary carcinoma, thyroid carcinoma, hemangiosarcoma, osteosarcoma, transitional cell carcinoma, squamous cell carcinoma, and oral and digital melanoma.

DIAGNOSIS
Clinical Presentation

Signalment. The average age of dogs and cats with primary lung tumors is over 10 years. Anaplastic carcinomas tend to occur at a slightly younger age (8 to 9 years) than adenocarcinomas. There does not seem to be a gender or breed predilection, although boxers may be overrepresented.

History. Nearly 25 percent of dogs with pulmonary neoplasia are asymptomatic at the time of diagnosis (i.e., pulmonary neoplasia is an incidental finding when thoracic radiographs are evaluated for an unrelated problem). If clinical signs are present, the owner may report that they have been apparent for weeks to months.

Physical Examination Findings

The most common clinical finding in dogs with primary pulmonary neoplasia is a nonproductive cough; other signs include hemoptysis, fever, lethargy, exercise intolerance, weight loss, dysphagia, and anorexia. Lameness may be associated with metastasis to bone or skeletal muscle or with development of hypertrophic osteopathy. Weight loss, lethargy, and dyspnea are common clinical signs in cats with primary lung tumors; respiratory signs may be present in as few as one third of affected cats. In a recent study, 47 percent of cats hospitalized with a primary problem of respiratory distress that had pulmonary parenchymal disease on thoracic radiographs had neoplasia (Sauve et al, 2005).

Diagnostic Imaging

Thoracic radiographs should be obtained in animals suspected of having pulmonary neoplasia (Fig. 29-16). The most common finding with primary pulmonary neoplasia in dogs is a solitary nodular density in the periphery of a dorsocaudal lung lobe (Fig. 29-17). Multiple miliary lesions are less common (Fig. 29-18). The radiographic pattern may be classified as solitary nodular, multiple nodular, or disseminated-infiltrative. Multiple discrete lesions within a single lobe or multiple lobes usually represent metastatic neoplasia rather than multicentric primary neoplasia. Feline bronchoalveolar carcinoma may appear as a mixed bronchoalveolar pattern, an ill-defined alveolar mass, or a mass with cavitation (Ballegeer et al, 2002). Bronchial disease is typically seen in affected cats (i.e., bronchointerstitial pattern, peribronchial cuffing, or bronchiectasis) and may represent airway metastasis. Because radiographic signs of pulmonary neoplasia in cats are not specific (many inflammatory diseases will cause similar changes) lung fine-needle aspirates may be the most helpful diagnostic tool (Sauve et al, 2005).

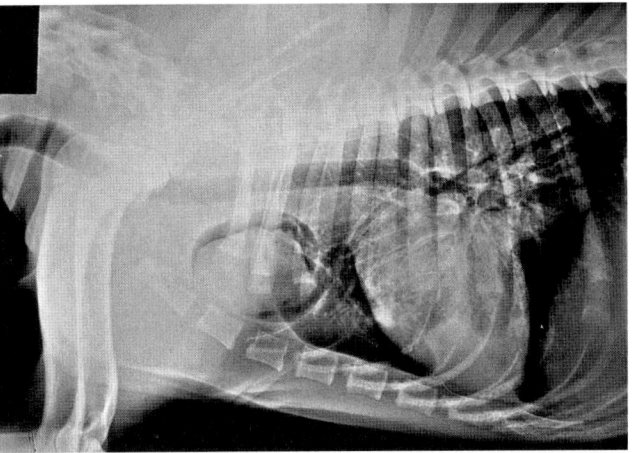

FIG. 29-16
Thoracic radiograph of a 1½-year-old German shepherd dog with a bronchogenic cyst in the left cranial lung lobe. Surgical excision was performed through a median sternotomy approach.

NOTE: Because of the lack of respiratory signs in many animals with lung tumors, take thoracic radiographs whenever you are presented with a cat or dog with unexplained clinical signs of long duration.

Thoracic evaluation should include a three-view radiographic study (opposite lateral views and an orthogonal view). Lung lesions may go undetected in recumbent lateral radiographs when the affected lung is dependent because of the recumbent atelectasis that occurs. Thoracic radiographs are relatively insensitive indicators of pulmonary neoplasia because nodules must be at approximately 0.5 to 1 cm in diameter to be reliably recognized. Radiographs should also be evaluated for sternal or hilar lymphadenopathy and/or pleural effusion. It may be difficult to differentiate metastatic pulmonary neoplasia from pulmonary metastasis of a primary pulmonary tumor. Compared with primary lesions, metastatic tumors generally are smaller and more well circumscribed and usually are located in the peripheral or middle portions of the lung. Multiple nodules associated with primary lung tumors often consist of one large mass and smaller secondary nodules. When multiple nodules are metastases, there are usually several large masses and a variety of smaller lesions. Contrast-enhanced CT is the most sensitive means for detecting pulmonary lesions.

NOTE: To improve the likelihood of diagnosing primary or metastatic pulmonary neoplasia, take a ventrodorsal and both lateral recumbent views. Always assess radiographs of animals with pulmonary neoplasia for multiple masses, lymphadenopathy, and/or pleural effusion.

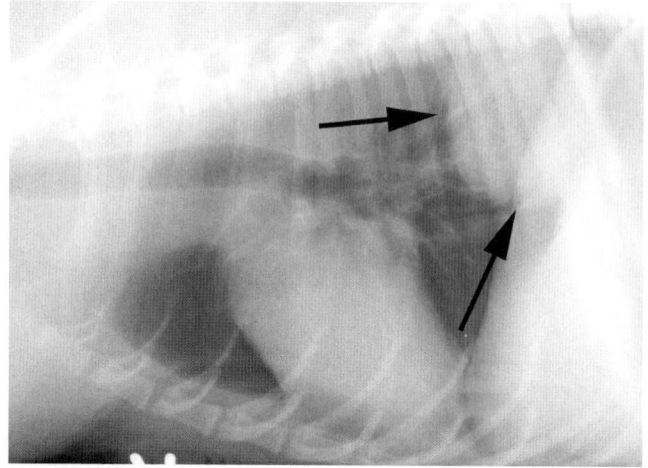

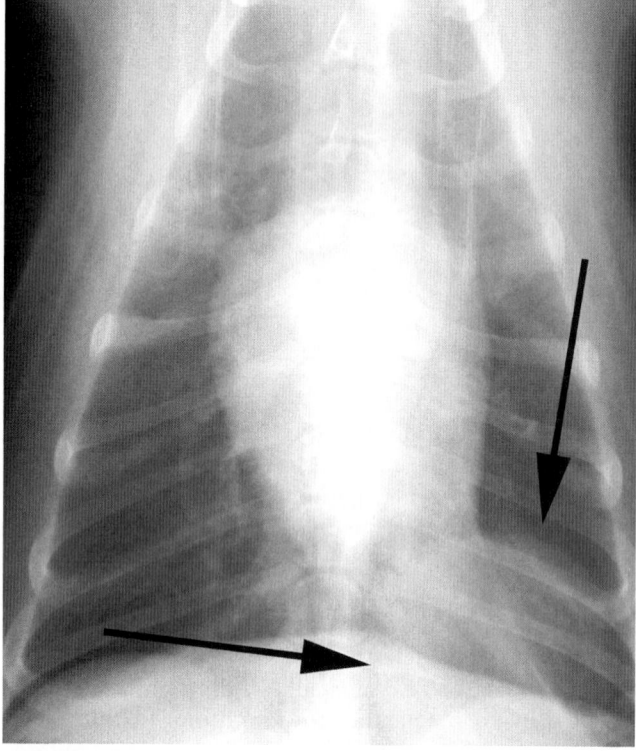

FIG. 29-17

A, Right lateral and **B,** ventrodorsal radiographs of a dog with a large mass in the left caudal lung lobe. Note the well-defined soft tissue mass *(arrows)*. The primary differential is a primary pulmonary neoplasm.

Ultrasound- and CT-guided aspirates of thoracic masses may be performed (see p. 874). Diagnoses obtained by fine-needle aspiration (ultrasound-guided and blind) cytopathology accurately reflected the diagnosis obtained on histopathologic examination in 82 percent of dogs and cats in one study (DeBerry et al, 2002). In another study, CT-guided intrathoracic fine-needle aspiration, core biopsies, or both were evaluated in animals with thoracic masses (Zekas et al, 2005). Diagnostic results were inconclusive in 35 percent using fine-needle aspiration and in 17 percent of biopsies. Overall accuracy for diagnosis in confirmed cases of neopla-

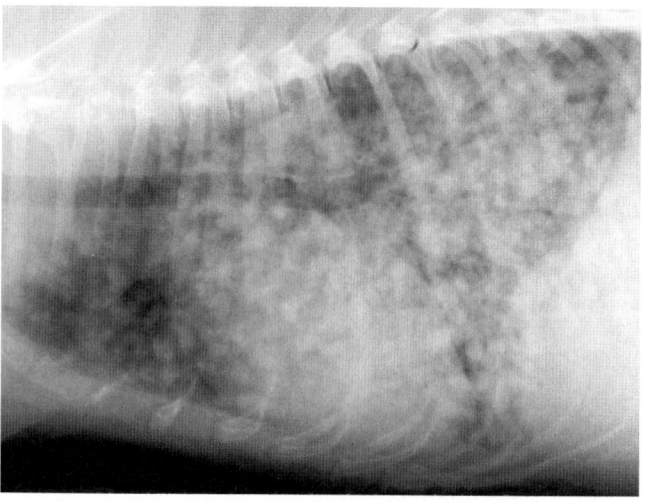

FIG. 29-18

Thoracic radiograph of a 7-year-old Siberian Husky with metastatic neoplasia. Notice the miliary nodular pattern in the lung. The other major differential for this pattern is fungal pneumonia.

sia in the aforementioned study was 92 percent for fine-needle aspiration and biopsy. Complications (e.g., pneumothorax, pulmonary hemorrhage, or both) were noted in 43 percent of patients; however, treatment was not required. Use of fine-gauge (25- or 27-gauge) needles may reduce complications.

Endoscopic ultrasonography may be a valuable tool in further evaluating radiographically detected intrathoracic lesions that do not lend themselves to routine ultrasonographic evaluation because of their location and superimposition of gas-filled structures. Ultrasound-guided tissue biopsies can be performed during the examination.

Laboratory Findings

Laboratory abnormalities are nonspecific, but may include nonregenerative anemia, leukocytosis, and hypercalcemia.

DIFFERENTIAL DIAGNOSIS

Pulmonary neoplasia must be differentiated from abscesses or granulomas (e.g., fungal and heartworm). Samples can be collected for cytologic examination by surgical biopsy, percutaneous fine-needle aspiration, transtracheal lavage, thoracoscopy, and/or bronchoscopy. Fine-needle aspiration cytology is a useful, noninvasive diagnostic tool if the needle can be directed into the nodule. Thoracoscopic lung biopsy can often obtain biopsy specimens in a safe and minimally invasive manner, depending upon the location of the lesion.

> NOTE: Distinguishing severe fungal disease from miliary neoplasia may be difficult radiographically.

MEDICAL MANAGEMENT

Surgical removal of primary pulmonary neoplasia is the treatment of choice in small animal patients. Chemotherapy is routinely used for some pulmonary neoplasms in human beings; adjunctive chemotherapy may be of benefit in veterinary patients. Readers are referred to an oncology text for information regarding chemotherapy for pulmonary neoplasia.

SURGICAL TREATMENT

Wide surgical resection is the treatment of choice for solitary nodules or multiple masses involving a single lobe if there is no evidence of distant metastasis or extrapleural involvement. Surgical resection occasionally is indicated for lung metastasis of a distant primary tumor (e.g., limb osteosarcoma). An intercostal thoracotomy is preferred over median sternotomy because it provides adequate exposure for lobectomy and lymph node biopsy. Partial lobectomy should be performed only when the tumor is located at the periphery of the lung lobe; otherwise, total lobectomy should be performed. Thoracoscopy can help determine whether pulmonary metastasis is present before a thoracotomy, particularly if the presence of metastasis is an important factor in determining whether resection of the pulmonary mass should be performed. Thoracoscopic removal of lung tumors in dogs has been reported (Lansdowne et al, 2005).

Preoperative Management

Preoperative management of patients with pulmonary neoplasia and dyspnea is similar to that for other animals with respiratory diseases (see p. 867). If the mass is large, positioning the animal with the affected side down may improve ventilation.

Anesthesia

See anesthetic management of patients with respiratory abnormalities, p. 867.

Surgical Anatomy

See the anatomic description of the lung lobes on p. 870.

Positioning

Because most neoplasms are removed through an intercostal thoracotomy, the lateral thorax should be prepared for aseptic surgery (see also p. 873).

NOTE: Be careful how you position dogs with large pulmonary masses during induction and preparation. They may not be able to ventilate if you place them in lateral recumbency with the normal (unaffected) lung down because the weight of the mass may prevent lung inflation. You may need to clip these patients in ventral or dorsal recumbency.

SURGICAL TECHNIQUE
Thoracoscopic Biopsy or Partial Lobectomy

The technique will depend upon the size and location of the mass.

Examine the lung lobes thoroughly for abnormalities. For small nodules at the periphery of a lobe, remove them as described above for lung biopsy (p. 875).

For larger masses requiring partial lobectomies, use thoracoscopy to determine the optimal position for making a minithoracotomy incision (the size of the incision will depend upon the size of the lung lobe to be exteriorized).

Grasp the affected lung lobe with Babcock forceps, and pull it out of the chest until a stapling device can be placed between the mass and the hilus. Staple and resect the affected portion. Check the incision site for leakage, and then reposition the lung in the chest.

Surgical Biopsy

See p. 875.

SUTURE MATERIALS AND SPECIAL INSTRUMENTS

Avoid nonabsorbable braided suture (e.g., silk) if there is evidence of infection (see also p. 61).

POSTOPERATIVE CARE AND ASSESSMENT

The animal should be monitored postoperatively for dyspnea. Oxygen should be available. Postoperative analgesics should be given (see p. 868). Evaluation of ventilation by analysis of blood gas parameters or pulse oximetry is useful. Sudden respiratory distress may be due to hemorrhage or pneumothorax.

COMPLICATIONS

The mortality associated with fine-needle aspiration of thoracic masses has varied depending on the study and type of needle used from 15% (Menghini needles) to 2.1% (Westcott 20-gauge needles). Mortality associated with 25- or 27-gauge needles is less common; however, fatal pneumothorax can occur even with small-gauge needles. The major complications of tumor removal in dogs are hemorrhage and pneumothorax associated with lobectomy (see p. 878).

PROGNOSIS

The prognosis is favorable for dogs with well-differentiated, nonmetastasized, primary lung tumors that do not have associated clinical signs. Dogs with tumors in the lung periphery or near the base of a lung have better survival times than those in which the tumor involves an entire lobe. The most important prognostic factor related to survival in dogs after surgery is whether lymph node metastasis has occurred. The prognosis for most cats with primary lung tumors is poor because of the advanced nature of the disease at the time of diagnosis and the tumors' aggressive metastatic behavior. As with dogs, cats with moderately well differentiated tumors have a significantly longer survival time than cats with poorly differentiated tumors.

References

Ballegeer EA, Forrest LJ, Stepien RL: Radiographic appearance of bronchoalveolar carcinoma in nine cats, *Vet Radiol Ultrasound* 43:267, 2002.

DeBerry JD, Norris CR, Samii VF et al: Correlation between fine-needle aspiration cytopathology and histopathology of the lung in dogs and cats, *J Am Anim Hosp Assoc* 38:327, 2002.

Lansdowne JL, Monnet E, Twedt DC et al: Thoracoscopic lung lobectomy for treatment of lung tumors in dogs, *Vet Surg* 34:530, 2005.

Sauve V, Drobatz KJ, Shokek AB et al: Clinical course, diagnostic findings and necropsy diagnosis in dyspneic cats with primary pulmonary parenchymal disease: 15 cats (1996-2002), *J Vet Emerg Crit Care* 15:38, 2005.

Zekas LJ, Crawford JT, O'Brien RT: Computed tomography-guided fine-needle aspirate and tissue-core biopsy of intrathoracic lesions in thirty dogs and cats, *Vet Radiol Ultrasound* 46:200, 2005.

Suggested Reading

Armbrust LJ, Hoskinson JJ, Biller DS et al: Comparison of digitized and direct viewed (analog) radiographic images for detection of pulmonary nodules, *Vet Radiol Ultrasound* 46:361, 2005.

This study determined that evaluation of original radiographs was the best method for detection of pulmonary nodules when compared with digitization of radiographs with a film scanner and seven digital cameras.

Gaschen L, Kircher P, Hoffman G et al: Endoscopic ultrasonography for the diagnosis of intrathoracic lesions in two dogs, *Vet Radiol Ultrasound* 44:292, 2003.

Endoscopic ultrasound was a useful tool in two dogs with caudal thoracic masses.

PULMONARY ABSCESSES

DEFINITION

A **pulmonary abscess** is a localized collection of pus that often causes cavitation in the lung.

GENERAL CONSIDERATIONS AND CLINICALLY RELEVANT PATHOPHYSIOLOGY

Pulmonary abscesses are rare, but may occur as a complication of foreign bodies, neoplasia, bacterial pneumonia, aspiration pneumonia, fungal infections, or parasites. Abscesses secondary to neoplasia may be sterile or infected. The most common organisms cultured from abscesses associated with necrotizing pneumonia in dogs are *Escherichia coli, Pseudomonas* spp., and *Klebsiella* spp. Rupture of pulmonary abscesses may result in pyothorax (see p. 922) or pneumothorax (see p. 908) or both. In some parts of the country, pulmonary abscesses often occur secondary to inhalation or thoracic penetration of plant material (e.g., foxtails) that migrate through the lung.

DIAGNOSIS
Clinical Presentation

Signalment. Pulmonary abscesses may occur in dogs or cats of any age, breed, or gender.

History. The animal may be brought in for treatment of a persistent low-grade fever, varying degrees of respiratory distress, weight loss, lethargy, and/or anemia. The duration of illness may vary from hours to days or even weeks. Rupture of the abscess often causes pneumothorax and dyspnea.

Physical Examination Findings

Physical examination findings vary depending on whether pneumothorax or pleural effusion (or both) is present (see pp. 908 and 912). Most animals are febrile, and inspiratory crackles may be heard over the mass.

Diagnostic Imaging

Pulmonary abscesses generally appear as nodular or cavitary radiopaque lesions on thoracic films. The walls of the abscess are usually poorly defined. If pleural effusion is present, thoracentesis may be necessary before a definitive diagnosis can be made. Ultrasound evaluation of thoracic masses may help differentiate noncavitary from cavitary lesions if an appropriate acoustic window is available.

Laboratory Findings

The leukogram may be normal or have leukocytosis with or without a degenerative left shift. If the infection is chronic, a nonregenerative anemia may be present.

DIFFERENTIAL DIAGNOSIS

Abscesses should be differentiated from other nodular or cavitary pulmonary lesions (i.e., granulomas, *Paragonimus* infection, and neoplasia) by cytologic and/or histologic examination of samples obtained by fine-needle aspiration or surgery. Preoperative aspiration of the mass may help distinguish between these lesions and provide samples for culture; however, care should be taken to prevent causing pyothorax. Ultrasound often is useful in locating the appropriate site for aspiration. Some nonneoplastic lesions can be managed without surgery (e.g., *Paragonimus* infection); however, a definitive diagnosis may require surgical biopsy.

MEDICAL MANAGEMENT

Initial therapy is aimed at stabilizing dyspneic animals. Thoracentesis should be performed if pleural fluid or air is present. A broad-spectrum antibiotic with a good anaerobic spectrum should be chosen (see p. 870) and later modified, based upon culture and susceptibility testing. Antibiotic therapy should be continued for 3 to 6 weeks. If pyothorax is present, chest tubes should be placed and the thorax lavaged (see Pyothorax on p. 924). Some animals respond to medical management and the abscess resolves. If after several days no improvement is seen in the clinical signs or lung expansion or if pleural fluid is loculated and does not resolve, surgical intervention is warranted.

SURGICAL TREATMENT

A solitary pulmonary abscess that does not resolve with medical therapy is best managed by partial or complete lobectomy of the diseased lung performed through an intercostal thoracotomy (see p. 873). A median sternotomy approach (see p. 874) is preferred if multiple opacities are present involving both sides of the thorax.

Preoperative Management

If the animal is dyspneic, thoracentesis should be performed before surgery. Antibiotic therapy should be initiated after the mass or pleural space (or both) have been cultured, if not before.

Anesthesia

Refer to comments and anesthetic protocols for animals with respiratory dysfunction on p. 867. See also specific comments regarding the anesthetic management of animals with pneumothorax on p. 912.

Surgical Anatomy

The surgical anatomy of the thorax is described on p. 870.

Positioning

See pp. 873 and 874 for positioning of animals for intercostal or median thoracotomy.

SURGICAL TECHNIQUE

Identify the diseased lobe and before handling it clamp the pedicle to prevent drainage of purulent material into dependent lung lobes. Perform a complete or partial lobectomy, depending on the size and location of the abscess. Submit the lung for bacterial or fungal cultures (or both) and for histologic examination. Explore the remainder of the chest cavity for the presence of foreign matter. Palpate all the lung lobes that can be reached to identify other pulmonary lesions. Free remaining lung lobes of adhesions so that all lobes are movable and remove loculated areas of exudate. Remove sheets of fibrin that cover the lung lobes. Place a chest tube before thoracic closure.

SUTURE MATERIALS AND SPECIAL INSTRUMENTS

Braided, multifilament, nonabsorbable suture (e.g., silk) should be avoided if infection is present.

POSTOPERATIVE CARE AND ASSESSMENT

Appropriate antibiotics should be continued for 3 to 6 weeks if infection is present. Pyothorax should be treated with thoracic lavage (see p. 924). Postoperative analgesics should be provided (see p. 868).

PROGNOSIS

The prognosis for animals with pulmonary abscesses depends on the underlying cause. With appropriate management, the prognosis for animals with abscesses associated with nonneoplastic disease is good.

LUNG LOBE TORSION

DEFINITION

Lung lobe torsion (LLT) is a rotation of the lung lobe along its long axis, with twisting of the bronchus and pulmonary vessels at the hilus.

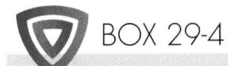 BOX 29-4

Possible Causes of Lung Lobe Torsion

Atelectasis associated with:
- Pneumonia
- Trauma
- Pneumothorax
- Pleural effusion
- Manipulation during surgery
Spontaneous
Surgical manipulation
Not replacing the lobe in its proper relationship after thoracic surgery

GENERAL CONSIDERATIONS AND CLINICALLY RELEVANT PATHOPHYSIOLOGY

Any mechanism that increases mobility of a lung lobe seems to favor torsion (Box 29-4). Partial collapse of the lung (i.e., with pulmonary disease or trauma) frees it from its normal spatial relationships with the thoracic wall, mediastinum, and adjacent lung lobes. This may enhance mobility. Pleural effusion or pneumothorax, along with subsequent atelectasis of lung lobes, can allow increased movement of a lobe, predisposing to torsion. Although LLT has been reported to cause chylothorax in dogs, it may be chylothorax that caused LLT. LLT has been reported secondary to previous thoracic surgery in which lung lobes are manipulated and remain partly collapsed after thoracic closure. LLT has typically been reported most commonly in the right middle lung lobe; however, in a recent study right middle lobe torsion was predominant in large dogs, whereas left cranial lobe torsion was more common in small dogs (D'Anjou et al, 2005). Underlying thoracic disease was found in only 5 of 15 dogs in the aforementioned study. Midlobar torsion of the right caudal lung lobe has been reported in a dog (Hofeling et al, 2004).

LLT causes venous congestion of the affected lobe; however, the arteries remain at least partly patent, allowing blood to enter. As fluid and blood enter the alveoli, lung consolidation occurs and the lobe becomes dark colored and firm, similar in shade to the liver. The shape of the affected lobe often is altered, and it may appear displaced from its normal location in the thorax radiographically. Pleural fluid usually accumulates because of continued venous congestion.

DIAGNOSIS
Clinical Presentation

Signalment. Deep-chested, large-breed dogs, especially Afghan hounds, are more commonly affected; however, 5 of 22 dogs with LLT in a recent study were toy breeds (Neath et al, 2000). Young male pugs appear to be predisposed to LLT (Murphy et al, 2005; Rooney et al, 2001). LLT in Afghan hounds may be associated with chylothorax (see p. 915). In large breed dogs and pugs, LLT frequently occurs spontaneously without previous history of disease or trauma. LLT in other small breeds is often secondary to primary pleural effusion, thoracic surgery, or trauma. LLT is rare in cats. Middle-aged dogs are more commonly affected, but LLT may occur in animals of any age.

History. In a recent study of 22 dogs with LLT, dyspnea was the most common reason for examination (Neath et al, 2000). Coughing and hemoptysis can also occur and may be chronic in nature. Some animals may be anorectic and depressed. There may be a previous history of pneumothorax, pneumonia, or trauma, or all three.

Physical Examination Findings

Pleural effusion is consistently present in animals with LLT, therefore findings often include muffled heart and lung sounds. Other findings may include depression, anorexia, coughing, fever, dyspnea, hemoptysis, hematemesis, and/or vomiting.

Diagnostic Imaging

Thoracic radiographic changes vary depending on the volume of pleural fluid, the presence or absence of preexisting disease, and the duration of the torsion. The most consistent finding is pleural effusion accompanied by an opacified lung lobe. Initially, air bronchograms are present in the torsed lobe and may be seen running in an abnormal direction. Air bronchograms eventually disappear as fluid and blood fill the bronchial lumen. The presence of a noninflated, radiopaque lung lobe that persists after removal of pleural fluid should increase suspicion for LLT (Fig. 29-19). Small dispersed air bubbles are often seen within the affected lobe. The lobar bronchi may be difficult to see but if located often appear irregular, focally narrowed or blunted, or displaced. Mediastinal shift, curved and dorsally displaced trachea, and axial rotation of the carina are also commonly seen (D'Anjou et al, 2005). Positional radiographs using horizontal beam x-rays (lateral decubitus or upright ventrodorsal) are often helpful. Pleural fluid that occurs secondary to LLT may persist around the affected lobe rather than fall to the dependent side. Failure of the lobe to reinflate in the "up" or nondependent hemithorax is a nonspecific indication of LLT.

Bronchoscopy. Bronchoscopy typically reveals a bronchus that is occluded and appears to be "twisted." Sometimes the tissue at the site seems edematous. There may or may not be blood in the bronchi (Fig. 29-20).

NOTE: Lung lobe torsion usually causes massive pleural effusion. You may not see the torsed lung on radiographs until you remove the fluid.

Laboratory Findings

Laboratory findings with LLT are variable. Fluid analysis may reveal a sterile, inflammatory effusion or chyle, or the fluid may be bloody. Pleural effusion of any etiology, however, can initiate a secondary LLT, making the results of

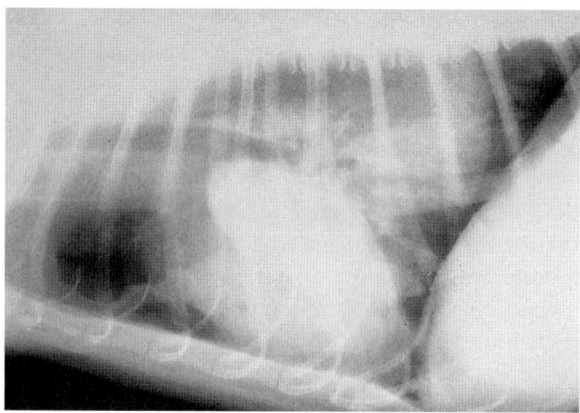

FIG. 29-19
Lateral thoracic radiograph of a dog with a torsion of the right middle lung lobe. Pleural fluid was removed before this radiograph was obtained. Notice the soft tissue mass overlying the cardiac silhouette.

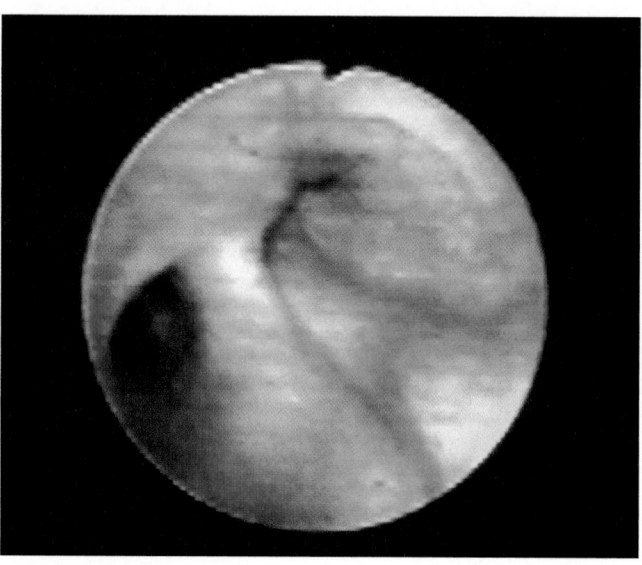

FIG. 29-20
Bronchoscopy of a dog with a torsed lung lobe. Note that the bronchus on the right is occluded, and hemorrhage is draining from it.

pleural fluid analysis variable and confusing. The appearance of blood in a previously nonhemorrhagic pleural fluid may indicate LLT. An inflammatory leukogram may be present; however, these changes may reflect the initial disease process rather than the LLT.

DIFFERENTIAL DIAGNOSIS

Pneumonia, pulmonary thromboembolism, contusion, neoplasia, atelectasis, hemothorax, diaphragmatic hernia, and pyothorax can mimic radiographic changes seen with

LLT. Demonstration of LLT at surgery provides the definitive diagnosis.

MEDICAL MANAGEMENT

Initial therapy is aimed at stabilizing the animal's condition and alleviating respiratory distress before surgery. Thoracentesis should remove pleural fluid (see p. 878), but persistent or massive pleural effusion may require a chest tube (see p. 899). Oxygen therapy given by oxygen cage or nasal insufflation is beneficial to some animals. Underlying diseases, such as pneumonia, should be identified and treated with appropriate antibiotic therapy. Intravenous fluid therapy is beneficial before and during surgery to maintain hydration.

NOTE: Spontaneous resolution of lung lobe torsion is extremely uncommon. This is a surgical condition.

SURGICAL TREATMENT

Spontaneous correction of a torsed lung lobe is uncommon because of swelling of the lobe and rapid formation of adhesions. The treatment of choice for LLT is lobectomy of the affected lobe. Unless LLT is diagnosed very quickly (i.e., immediately after a surgical procedure), damage to the pulmonary parenchyma generally is severe enough that attempts to salvage the lobe are not warranted. Recurrence has been reported after surgical correction where lobectomy was not performed.

Preoperative Management

Prophylactic antibiotics are warranted in animals with LLT. Pleural effusion should be removed before induction of anesthesia in animals that have compromised ventilation.

Anesthesia

See p. 867 for anesthetic management of animals with respiratory abnormalities.

Positioning

The affected lateral thorax should be prepared for an intercostal thoracotomy (see p. 873).

SURGICAL TECHNIQUE

Before attempting to derotate the affected pedicle, clamp it with a noncrushing forceps to prevent release of toxins into the bloodstream or fluids into the dependent lobes. Untwisting the lobe before its removal may help facilitate identification of the vascular structures and bronchus for ligation; however, in many cases the lobe cannot be easily returned to its normal position because of extensive adhesions. A transfixion suture or Miller's knot can often be used in such cases to ligate the vessels and bronchus. Check the remaining lobes for position and normal expansion. Culture the pulmonary parenchyma after removal of the lobe. Submit excised tissue for histologic examination to help determine underlying causes (i.e., pneumonia or neoplasia). Place a chest tube before closing the thoracic cavity.

SUTURE MATERIALS AND SPECIAL INSTRUMENTS

Avoid braided, multifilament suture because of the risk of infection. Large clamps, such as Satinsky clamps (see p. 878), are useful for clamping the bronchus.

POSTOPERATIVE CARE AND ASSESSMENT

Antibiotics should be continued if there is evidence of infection, and postoperative analgesics should be provided (see p. 868). The chest tube should be removed when the effusion diminishes to less than 2.2 ml/kg of body weight (see p. 901). Oxygen therapy may be warranted in some patients in the postoperative period, particularly if there is underlying lung disease, such as pneumonia. If dyspnea remains after surgery, thoracic radiographs are indicated to rule out recurrence of LLT (Spranklin et al, 2003).

PROGNOSIS

The prognosis is good for most animals with LLT if surgery is performed. Pleural effusion usually resolves within a few days of surgery unless the animal has concurrent chylothorax.

References

D'Anjou MA, Tidwell AS, Hecht S: Radiographic diagnosis of lung lobe torsion, *Vet Radiol Ultrasound* 46:478, 2005.

Hofeling AD, Jackson AH, Alsup JC et al: Spontaneous midlobar lung lobe torsion in a 2-year-old Newfoundland, *J Am Anim Hosp Assoc* 40:220, 2004.

Murphy KA, Brisson BA: Retrospective evaluation of lung lobe torsion in pugs: 7 cases (January 1991-November 2004), *Proceedings ACVS Veterinary Symposium*, 2005 (abstract).

Neath PJ, Brockman DJ, King LG: Lung lobe torsion in dogs: 22 cases (1981-1999), *J Am Vet Med Assoc* 217:1041, 2000.

Rooney MB, Lanz O, Monnet E: Spontaneous lung lobe torsion in two pugs, *J Am Anim Hosp Assoc* 37:128, 2001.

Spranklin DB, Gulikers KP, Lanz OI: Recurrence of spontaneous lung lobe torsion in a pug, *J Am Anim Hosp Assoc* 39:446, 2003.

PECTUS EXCAVATUM

DEFINITIONS

Pectus excavatum (PE) is a deformity of the sternum and costocartilages that results in a dorsal to ventral narrowing of the thorax. **Pectus carinatum** is a protrusion of the sternum, which occurs much less frequently than PE. Synonyms for pectus excavatum include *funnel chest, chondrosternal depression, chonechondrosternon, koilosternia*, and *trichterbust*.

GENERAL CONSIDERATIONS AND CLINICALLY RELEVANT PATHOPHYSIOLOGY

The cause or causes of PE in animals are unknown (Fig. 29-21). Theories proposed include shortening of the central tendon of the diaphragm, intrauterine pressure abnormalities, and congenital deficiency of the musculature in the cranial portion of the diaphragm. Abnormal respiratory gradients appear to play a role in the development of

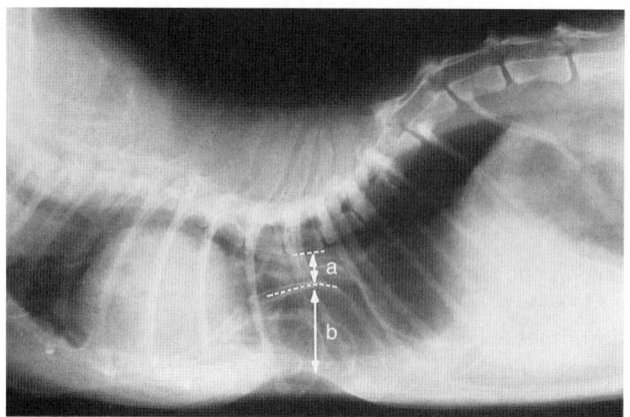

FIG. 29-21
Lateral thoracic radiograph of a cat with severe PE. The amount of depression is subjectively assessed based on the minimum distance between the vertebral column and the dorsal aspect of the sternum *(a)* or the depth of the concavity *(b)*. Note that in severe PE, costocartilages are also deformed. (From Fossum TW et al: Pectus excavatum in 8 dogs and 6 cats, *J Am Anim Hosp Assoc* 25:595, 1989.)

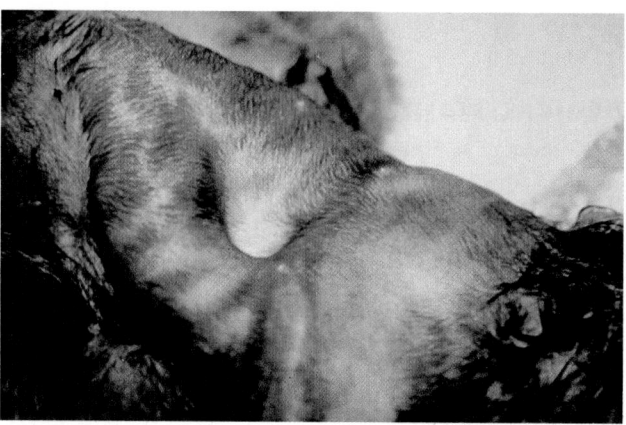

FIG. 29-22
PE in a cat. The head is pointed to the left, and a large depression is evident in the caudal sternum. (From Fossum TW et al: Pectus excavatum in 8 dogs and 6 cats, *J Am Anim Hosp Assoc* 25:595, 1989.)

this disease in some animals because brachycephalic dogs are most commonly affected, many of which have concurrent hypoplastic tracheas. Pectus excavatum may be associated with "swimmer's syndrome," which is a poorly characterized disease of neonatal dogs in which the limbs tend to splay laterally, impairing ambulation. Abnormalities of the joints of the limbs and the long bones may also occur.

Patients with PE may have abnormalities of both respiratory and cardiovascular function. Circulatory disorders in animals with PE may occur as a result of abnormal cardiac positioning, which causes kinking of the large veins and disturbance of venous return; compression of the heart, predisposing to arrhythmias (particularly the auricles); restriction of ventricular capacity; and diminished respiratory reserve. Cardiac abnormalities are also common (see later in Differential Diagnosis section).

DIAGNOSIS
Clinical Presentation

Signalment. Pectus excavatum is a congenital abnormality in dogs and cats. In symptomatic animals, clinical signs usually are present at birth or shortly thereafter. PE may occur in any breed, but brachycephalic dogs appear to be predisposed. A gender predisposition has not been identified.

History. Many animals with PE are asymptomatic; however, the defect often is palpable, and this may prompt owners to seek veterinary care despite lack of clinical signs (Fig. 29-22). Symptomatic animals may be presented for evaluation of exercise intolerance, weight loss, hyperpnea, recurrent pulmonary infections, cyanosis, vomiting, persistent and productive coughing, inappetence, and/or mild episodes of upper respiratory disease. A correlation between the severity of clinical signs and the severity of anatomic or physiologic abnormalities has not been observed.

> NOTE: Although the cause of PE is uncertain, multiple animals in some litters have been affected. Do not breed affected animals; neuter them.

Physical Examination Findings

The sternal deformity usually is palpable. Other physical examination findings may include cardiac murmurs and harsh lung sounds. Dyspnea is variable, but rapid, shallow respirations may be noted.

> NOTE: Do not assume that cardiac murmurs in animals with PE are due to heart disease. They may be due to abnormal positioning of the heart because of the sternal deformity.

Diagnostic Imaging

Thoracic radiographs show abnormal elevation of the sternum in the caudal thorax. Objective assessment of the deformity may be determined by measuring the frontosagittal and vertebral indices on thoracic radiographs (Box 29-5). The frontosagittal index is calculated by taking the ratio of the width of the chest at the tenth thoracic vertebra, measured on a dorsoventral or ventrodorsal radiograph, and the distance between the center of the ventral surface of the tenth thoracic vertebra and the nearest point on the sternum (Fig. 29-23). The vertebral index is calculated as the ratio of the distance between the center of the dorsal surface of the selected vertebral body to the nearest point on the sternum and the dorsoventral diameter of the center of the same vertebral body (see Fig. 29-23). The severity of PE may be characterized as mild, moderate, or severe based on the frontosagittal and vertebral indices (Table 29-2). Such de-

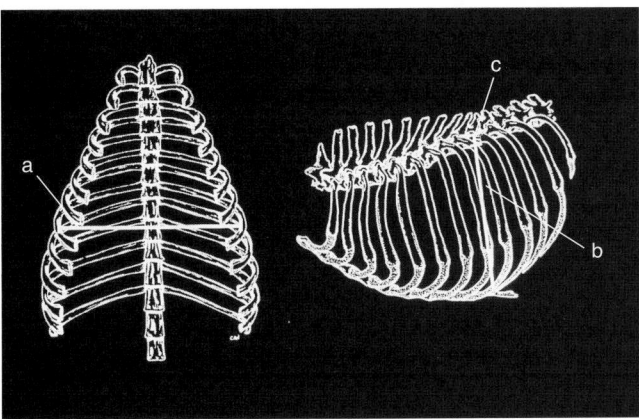

FIG. 29-23
The frontosagittal index is the ratio between the width of the chest at the tenth thoracic vertebra *(a)* and the distance between the center of the ventral surface of the tenth thoracic vertebral body and the nearest point on the sternum *(b)*. The vertebral index is the ratio between the distance from the center of the dorsal surface of the tenth vertebral body to the nearest point on the sternum *(b and c)* and the dorsoventral diameter of the vertebral body at the same level *(c)*. (From Fossum TW et al: Pectus excavatum in 8 dogs and 6 cats, *J Am Anim Hosp Assoc* 25:595, 1989.)

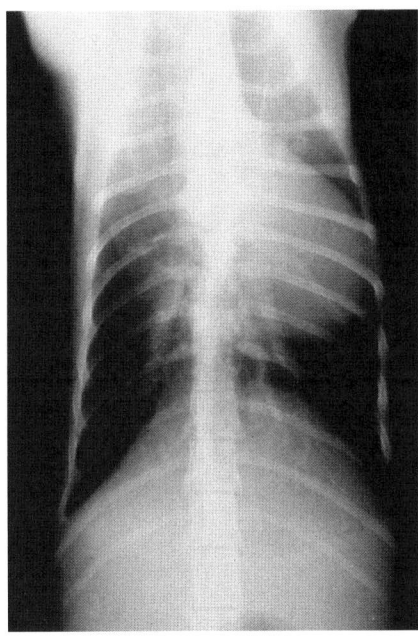

FIG. 29-24
Thoracic radiograph of a dog with PE. Note the displacement of the heart caused by the sternal abnormality. (From Fossum TW et al: Pectus excavatum in 8 dogs and 6 cats, *J Am Anim Hosp Assoc* 25:595, 1989.)

 BOX 29-5

Normal Frontosagittal and Vertebral Indices

Frontosagittal	Vertebral
Nonbrachycephalic dogs	**Nonbrachycephalic dogs**
0.8 to 1.4	11.8 to 19.6
Brachycephalic dogs	**Brachycephalic dogs**
1 to 1.5	12.5 to 16.5
Cats	**Cats**
0.7 to 1.3	12.6 to 18.8

 TABLE 29-2

Characterization of Pectus Excavatum in Dogs and Cats Based on Frontosagittal (FS) and Vertebral (Vert) Indices

PE	INDEX	
	FS	VERT
Mild	≤2	>9
Moderate	2–3	6–8.99
Severe	>3	<6

termination may aid in the objective assessment of improvement of thoracic diameters after surgery.

Thoracic radiographs should be evaluated for the evidence of concurrent abnormalities (i.e., tracheal hypoplasia, cardiac abnormalities, and pneumonia). Most animals with PE have abnormally positioned hearts (Fig. 29-24), which may cause the heart to appear enlarged radiographically; thus true cardiac enlargement cannot always be distinguished from apparent enlargement as a result of abnormal heart position.

Laboratory Findings

Laboratory abnormalities are uncommon.

DIFFERENTIAL DIAGNOSIS

Diagnosis of PE is straightforward; however, associated abnormalities may be more difficult to diagnose. Cardiac murmurs are common in patients with PE and appear to be as-

sociated with the cardiac malpositioning. These murmurs often disappear after surgical correction of the defect or a change in the patient's position. Systolic murmurs in some patients appear to be related to kinking of the pulmonary artery or to exaggeration of the artery's normal vibrations caused by its proximity to the chest wall. Animals with PE and innocent systolic murmurs must be differentiated from those that have underlying cardiac defects, such as pulmonic stenosis or atrial septal defects.

MEDICAL MANAGEMENT

Animals with merely a flat chest may contour to a normal or near normal configuration without surgical intervention. However, owners should be encouraged to regularly perform medial-to-lateral compression of the chest on these young

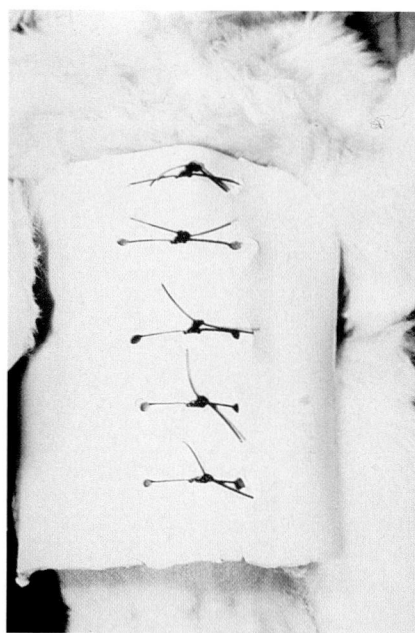

FIG. 29-25
Application of an external splint to the ventral aspect of the thorax in a young dog with PE. (From Fossum TW et al: Pectus excavatum in 8 dogs and 6 cats, *J Am Anim Hosp Assoc* 25:595, 1989.)

 BOX 29-6

Selected Anesthetic Protocols for Repair of Pectus Excavatum in Young Animals That Are Not Dyspneic*

Dogs

Premedication

Atropine (0.02–0.04 mg/kg SC or IM) or glycopyrrolate (0.005–0.011 mg/kg SC or IM) plus hydromorphone (0.1–0.2 mg/kg IM or SC) or butorphanol (0.2–0.4 mg/kg IM or SC)

Induction

Use mask induction with isoflurane or sevoflurane after 5 minutes of preoxygenation

Cats

Premedication

Atropine (0.02–0.04 mg/kg SC or IM) or glycopyrrolate (0.005–0.01 mg/kg SC or IM) plus butorphanol at dose above or buprenorphine (5–15 μg/kg IM or SC)

Induction

Use chamber induction with isoflurane or sevoflurane after preoxygenating for 5 minutes

SC, Subcutaneous; *IM*, intramuscular.
*See p. 868 if the animal is dyspneic.

animals. Animals with severe elevation of the sternum will not benefit from this technique or from splintage that simply provides medial-to-lateral compression and does not correct the malpositioned sternum. Other medical management includes treatment of respiratory tract infections and, if the animal is severely dyspneic, oxygen therapy.

SURGICAL TREATMENT

Application of an external splint to the ventral aspect of the thorax is the most common technique used to correct this defect in animals (Fig. 29-25). Definitive treatment of PE using external splintage is possible because of the young age of affected patients at the time of diagnosis. The costal cartilages and sternum are pliable in these young animals, and the thorax can be reshaped by applying traction to the sternum using sutures that are placed around the sternum and through a rigid splint. Soft tissues that might be abnormal and play a role in the development of this deformity probably are stretched or torn when the sternum is pulled ventrally. Whether surgical correction of the defect should be performed in asymptomatic patients with moderate or severe PE is unknown. Symptomatic patients that do not have associated cardiac abnormalities will benefit from surgery. Repair using an intrasternal pin and external splinting has been reported (Crigel and Moissonnier, 2005).

Preoperative Management

Respiratory infections should be treated before surgery. If the animal is severely dyspneic, oxygen should be provided by nasal insufflation or an oxygen cage until surgery is per-

formed. Prophylactic antibiotic therapy may be given; however, antibiotics are unlikely to prevent skin infections around the splint. Intrathoracic infection secondary to surgery is uncommon.

Anesthesia

Anesthetic management in these young animals should include attention to the airway, ventilation, body temperature, and blood glucose concentration. Animals should be intubated; ventilation should be assisted or controlled; a high inspired fraction of oxygen should be used; intravenously administered fluids should be warm; and fluids should contain glucose if serum glucose concentrations cannot be monitored (Box 29-6). Also the animal should be insulated from the cool surgical environment. The splint should be formed and fitted before anesthesia to reduce the duration of anesthesia. Do not use nitrous oxide in these patients because of the risk of pneumothorax. Postoperative analgesia should be provided in puppies with butorphanol, hydromorphone, or buprenorphine and in kittens with butorphanol or buprenorphine (see Box 29-6). Do not use chamber or mask induction if the animal is dyspneic.

Surgical Anatomy

The surgical anatomy of the thorax is described on p. 870.

Positioning

The patient is placed in dorsal recumbency, and the ventral thorax is prepared for aseptic surgery.

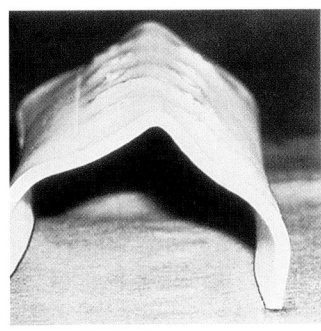
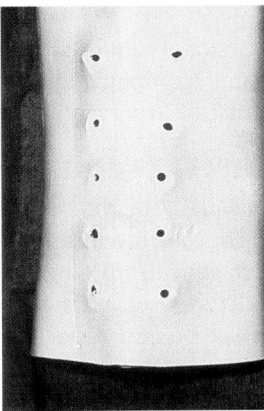

FIG. 29-26
External splint for correction of PE. Place two parallel rows of four to six holes in the splint with a small Steinmann pin. (From Fossum TW et al: Pectus excavatum in 8 dogs and 6 cats, *J Am Anim Hosp Assoc* 25:595, 1989.)

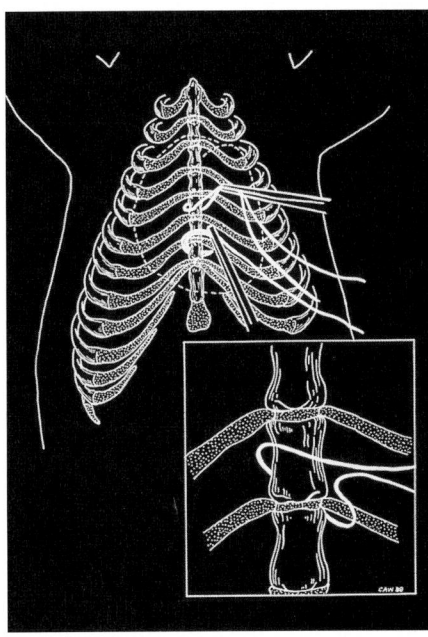

FIG. 29-27
Sutures placed around the sternebrae may be horizontal to the long axis or at a 45-degree angle. (From Fossum TW et al: Pectus excavatum in 8 dogs and 6 cats, *J Am Anim Hosp Assoc* 25:595, 1989.)

SURGICAL TECHNIQUE

Fashion a rectangular piece of moldable splinting material into a U shape (Fig. 29-26), and mold it to fit the ventral aspect of the thorax. Apply a small amount of adhesive padding to the cranial border and inner surface of the splint or, as an alternative, pad the splint with cast padding after it has been positioned. Place two parallel rows of four to six holes in the splint with a small Steinmann pin (see Fig. 29-26). Position the holes so that the distance between adjacent holes is slightly greater than the width of the sternum. Pass the selected suture (see later in the Suture Materials and Special Instruments section) around the sternum by maneuvering the needle blindly off the lateral edge of the sternum. As an alternative, pass the needle around the sternebra at a 45-degree angle to incorporate the costocartilage and possibly reduce the chance of the suture pulling through the soft sternebral bone (Fig. 29-27). Sutures must be placed around the sternum and not subcutaneously. Additionally, sutures must be placed in the area of the greatest concavity. If the sutures are placed proximal to the area with the greatest depression, the sternum cannot be pulled into a normal position, resulting in less than optimal correction of the defect. Keep the needle as close as possible to the dorsal aspect of the sternum to prevent piercing the heart or lungs. Leave the suture ends long and tag them. When all sutures have been placed, pass the ends through the predrilled holes in the splint and tie them securely on its ventral aspect (see Fig. 29-26). Two sutures may be placed and tied to themselves and then these sutures tied together so that the splint can be adjusted without replacement of sutures or use of anesthesia.

SUTURE MATERIALS AND SPECIAL INSTRUMENTS

A taper-point needle is recommended; if suture material with a large, swaged-on needle is not available, a large, eyed, taper-point needle should be selected (to prevent bending and possible breakage as it is passed around the sternum). Large (i.e., No. 0 to No. 2) monofilament absorbable or non-absorbable suture material is recommended (i.e., polydioxanone, polyglyconate, or nylon suture).

POSTOPERATIVE CARE AND ASSESSMENT

The animal should be evaluated in the early postoperative period for intrathoracic hemorrhage because piercing of the heart, lung, or internal thoracic vessels as the needle is passed around the sternum is possible. Positioning the animal in dorsal recumbency, paying close attention to the phase of respiration, and keeping the needle as close to the sternum as possible help prevent such complications. The splint should be left in place 10 to 21 days, if possible (although less time may be effective).

COMPLICATIONS

Suture abscesses, mild superficial dermatitis, and skin abrasions are common, but these usually are minor and heal quickly after removal of the splint. Adequate padding of the splint may help prevent abrasions. Fatal reexpansion pulmonary edema (see p. 869) has been reported in a kitten after correction of PE.

PROGNOSIS

The prognosis is excellent for animals without underlying disease in which surgery is performed at a young age. Older animals with a less pliable sternum may not respond as favorably to external splintage. Partial sternectomy may benefit such animals (see p. 895).

Reference

Crigel MH and Moissonnier P: Pectus excavatum surgically repaired using sternum realignment and splinting techniques in a young cat, *J Small Anim Pract* 46:352, 2005.

THORACIC WALL NEOPLASIA

DEFINITIONS

Thoracic wall neoplasia may arise from the ribs, musculature, or pleura. **Chondrosarcomas** are tumors that arise from cartilage, whereas **osteosarcomas** arise from bone.

GENERAL CONSIDERATIONS AND CLINICALLY RELEVANT PATHOPHYSIOLOGY

Primary tumors of the rib have a high metastatic rate and are uncommon in dogs or cats. Osteosarcomas are the most common neoplasm of the canine rib, followed by chondrosarcomas; the costochondral junction is the usual site of origin of these tumors. Metastatic and primary tumors of the sternum have rarely been reported in dogs. Primary sternal tumors of dogs include chondrosarcoma and osteosarcoma.

DIAGNOSIS
Clinical Presentation

Signalment. Primary rib tumors generally develop in young and middle-aged dogs. Rib tumors should be considered as a possible differential diagnosis for masses involving the thoracic wall, even in young dogs.

History. Animals with rib tumors may be brought in because of dyspnea or a painless thoracic wall mass. Animals with sternal neoplasia often are presented for evaluation of a palpable sternal mass.

Physical Examination Findings

Most rib tumors cause a localized swelling of the thoracic wall; however, pleural effusion without evidence of a thoracic mass occasionally occurs in dogs with small primary rib tumors and metastatic pulmonary lesions. Other clinical signs of rib tumors are weight loss and dyspnea. Sternal tumors usually cause a localized swelling, but may be associated with dyspnea if they metastasize to the lungs.

Diagnostic Imaging

Rib tumors generally are expansile masses that cause bone destruction and proliferation. They typically cause an extrapleural sign (protrusion of an infectious, neoplastic, or traumatic lesion medially from the thoracic wall causing a broad-based intrathoracic mass effect); moreover, it is not uncommon for the majority of the mass to be within the thoracic cavity. Sternal tumors may also produce lysis of sternebrae and adjacent ribs. Thoracic radiographs of animals with neoplasia of the ribs or sternum should be evaluated for pulmonary metastasis, lymph node involvement, and/or pleural effusion.

Laboratory Findings

Laboratory findings are nonspecific. Blood gas analysis may show hypoxemia and respiratory acidosis or alkalosis (because of hyperventilation).

DIFFERENTIAL DIAGNOSIS

Neoplasia of the sternum or ribs should be differentiated from osteomyelitis, fungal infections, or abscesses based on cytologic or histologic findings. A tentative diagnosis of the cell type usually can be made by fine-needle aspiration of the mass. Definitive diagnosis usually requires histologic examination of a biopsy specimen. Although pleural effusion is common in dogs with rib tumors, neoplastic cells are rarely found in the fluid.

MEDICAL MANAGEMENT

Medical management of animals with rib or sternal tumors (i.e., thoracentesis if pleural effusion exists and oxygen therapy for dyspnea) generally is palliative only. Pleuroperitoneal shunts are used in human beings with pleural effusion caused by terminal neoplasia; however, such use has not been reported in dogs or cats.

SURGICAL TREATMENT

Surgical resection of thoracic wall tumors is the treatment of choice. Full-thickness or *en bloc* resection of three or more ribs for thoracic wall neoplasia requires surgical reconstruction to reestablish thoracic wall continuity. Removal of more than six ribs is generally not recommended. With tumors of the caudal thorax, advancement of the diaphragm cranial to the resected ribs reduces the need for rigid fixation of the thoracic wall. Synthetic mesh may be used to fill other defects. A possible complication of polypropylene mesh is fistula formation secondary to adhesions; use of omentum over the implant may prevent this complication. Resection of large tumors may require a skin flap to close the resultant skin defect. Partial or complete sternectomy may be curative in dogs with primary sternal neoplasia. Although temporary instability of the thorax may occur after large sternal resections, this does not appear to cause any permanent or significant respiratory dysfunction.

Preoperative Management

Thoracentesis should be performed before induction of anesthesia in dogs with pleural effusion associated with thoracic wall neoplasia.

Anesthesia

See anesthesia recommendations for animals with respiratory disease on p. 867.

Positioning

With thoracic wall or sternal neoplasia, a generous area surrounding the tumor should be prepared for aseptic surgery.

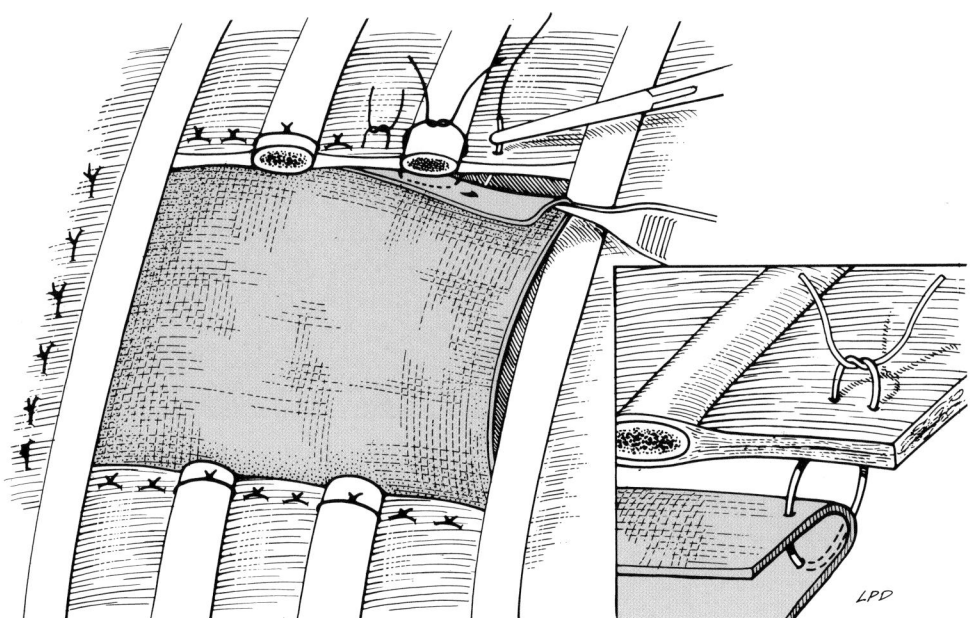

FIG. 29-28
Some thoracic tumors may be removed by *en bloc* resection of the thoracic wall. Remove the thoracic wall containing the neoplasm and a margin of normal tissue. Fold the edges of a piece of mesh over and suture the double thickness of mesh to the pleural side of the defect.

SURGICAL TECHNIQUE
En Bloc Resection of Thoracic Wall Neoplasia

Remove the thoracic wall containing the neoplasm and a margin of normal tissue, leaving a square or rectangular defect. Cut a piece of polypropylene mesh slightly larger than the defect. Fold over the edges of the mesh and suture the double thickness of mesh to the pleural side of the defect (Fig. 29-28). Draw the mesh tightly across the defect when suturing it to prevent it from moving paradoxically with respiration. If more than four or five ribs are removed, support the ribs with plastic spinal plates or rib grafts. Mobilize and advance the thoracic wall musculature over the defect or, if there is insufficient muscle, exteriorize an omental pedicle flap through a paracostal abdominal approach and tunnel it subcutaneously to the defect. As an alternative, exteriorize the omental flap through the diaphragm. Place the omental flap over the mesh and suture skin over the defect.

For caudal rib tumors, advancement of the diaphragm may be done after *en bloc* resection of the mass and surrounding tissue. Synthetic reconstruction of the rib cage is rarely necessary.

Partial Sternectomy

Partial sternectomy should be considered only for relatively small, localized sternal neoplasms that do not appear to have intrathoracic involvement.

Sternectomy has been used successfully for extensive sternal osteomyelitis. The entire sternum can be removed in small animals.

Incise through the skin overlying the neoplasm (if skin involvement is suspected, resect the skin). Identify the rib articulations on the sternum. Use rongeurs to remove the affected sternebrae and ribs. If possible, remove one sternebra caudal and one cranial to the lesion. Assess the thoracic cavity for involvement. Avoid lacerating the internal thoracic arteries; ligate them if necessary. Appose the ribs and intercostal muscles with a large (e.g., No. 1) monofilament suture in an interrupted or horizontal mattress pattern. Use a simple continuous suture pattern to appose remnants of the rectus abdominis muscle over the junction of the rib ends. Minimize dead space by apposing the skin and underlying tissue with walking sutures. Place a thoracostomy tube and evacuate air from the thoracic cavity. Place a light support wrap over the thorax to protect the incision and thoracostomy tube.

SUTURE MATERIALS AND SPECIAL INSTRUMENTS

Reconstruction of thoracic wall defects should be done with monofilament nonabsorbable suture (i.e., polypropylene or nylon). Polypropylene (Marlex) mesh may be used for thoracic wall reconstruction.

POSTOPERATIVE CARE AND ASSESSMENT

Animals with surgically created thoracic wall defects should be monitored closely in the postoperative period for hypoventilation or the development of pneumothorax (or both). Analgesic therapy is warranted in these animals (see Chapter 13; for dosages of opioids see Table 13-4 on p. 133). See p. 878 for additional comments on the postoperative management of animals with respiratory disorders.

PROGNOSIS

Because of the high rate of pulmonary metastasis, the prognosis for dogs with rib tumors is poor. Most dogs with rib tumors die or are euthanized within 6 months of the diagnosis. Too few sternal tumors have been reported to define the prognosis in affected animals.

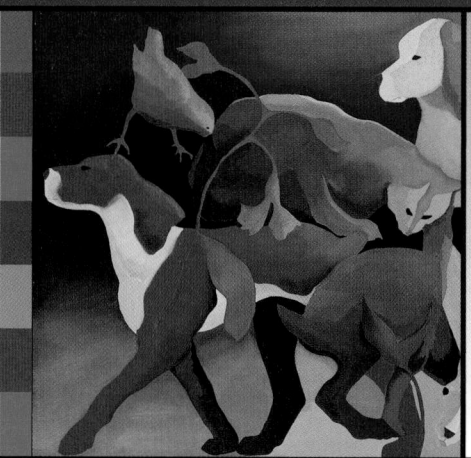

CHAPTER 30

Surgery of the Lower Respiratory System: Pleural Cavity and Diaphragm

GENERAL PRINCIPLES AND TECHNIQUES

DEFINITIONS

The **pleura** are the serous membranes that cover the lungs and line the thoracic cavity, completely enclosing a potential space known as the **pleural cavity**. The **parietal pleura** is the portion of the pleura that lines the walls of the thoracic cavity, whereas the **visceral**—or **pulmonary**—**pleura** invests the lungs and lines their fissures, completely separating the different lobes. **Thoracocentesis** (or **thoracentesis**) is a surgical puncture of the thoracic wall to remove air (**pneumothorax**) or fluid (**pleural effusion**) from the pleural space. **Pleurodesis** is the creation of adhesions between the visceral and parietal pleura by instilling irritating agents into the pleural cavity or by mechanically damaging the pleura at surgery.

PREOPERATIVE MANAGEMENT

Respiratory function should be carefully monitored in patients with pleural cavity or diaphragmatic abnormalities. Qualitative assessments of respiratory function include monitoring the respiratory rate and pattern and capillary refill time and color (Table 30-1 and Box 30-1). Animals with pleural cavity disease usually have a restrictive respiratory pattern (i.e., rapid and shallow respirations). Arterial blood gas analysis can augment qualitative information about the effectiveness of ventilation and gas exchange (Table 30-2). Pulse oximetry is a noninvasive tool that measures the hemoglobin saturation of blood and thus indirectly provides quantitative information about oxygenation. Cardiovascular parameters (i.e., heart rate and rhythm) should also be evaluated (see Table 30-1). An electrocardiogram (ECG) should be performed in all trauma patients to detect arrhythmias associated with traumatic myocarditis or ischemia. Intravenous fluids should be provided to dehydrated animals or those that are not drinking sufficient fluids to maintain hydration. Care should be taken to avoid causing overhydration and pulmonary edema, which further compromise respiration. Monitoring the central venous pressure may be useful in some patients.

 TABLE 30-1

Normal Heart Rate (HR) and Respiratory Rate (RR) in Conscious Dogs and Cats

	HR/MIN	RR/MIN
Dog	70–140	20–40
Cat	145–200	20–40

 BOX 30-1

Normal Capillary Refill Time

Less than 1–2 seconds

 TABLE 30-2

Normal pH and Blood Gas Values on Room Air

	VALUE	RANGE
pH	7.4	7.35–7.45
Pa_{O_2}	95 mm Hg	80–110
Pv_{O_2}	40 mm Hg	35–45
Pa_{CO_2}	40 mm Hg	35–45
Pv_{CO_2}	45 mm Hg	40–48
Hco_3^-	24 mEq/L	22–27

pH, Hydrogen ion concentration; *Pa_{O_2},* arterial oxygen concentration; *Pv_{O_2},* venous oxygen concentration; *Pa_{CO_2},* arterial carbon dioxide concentration; *Pv_{CO_2},* venous carbon dioxide concentration; *Hco_3^-,* bicarbonate.

Severely dyspneic animals strongly suspected of having pneumothorax or pleural effusion should have thoracentesis performed (see p. 898) before radiographs are made. If the patient is not severely dyspneic, it is safer to first obtain a dorsoventral thoracic radiograph because lung laceration during thoracocentesis will cause pneumothorax and worsen the dyspnea. Removal of even small amounts of pleural effusion or air may significantly improve ventilation, allowing safer manipulation of the patient for radiographic procedures. Most dyspneic animals allow thoracentesis to be performed with minimal restraint; general anesthetics should be avoided. The animal should be allowed to remain in sternal recumbency, and oxygen should be provided by face mask, flow-by, or nasal insufflation if the animal will tolerate it (see Chapter 5). A negative tap does not rule out pleural effusion (i.e., the fluid may be in pockets, there may be exudate plugging the needle, or the needle may be too short). If there is no evidence of third space disease or if removal of fluid or air from the chest does not help alleviate dyspnea, then underlying lung disease (i.e., pneumonia, pulmonary edema, pulmonary contusions, and pulmonary neoplasia) or severe fibrosing pleuritis should be suspected (see p. 902). Providing nasal oxygen or placing the animal in an oxygen cage may be beneficial while treatment of the pulmonary disease is initiated (see Chapter 5).

> NOTE: Do not attempt to place chest tubes or take radiographs in animals with pleural effusion that are extremely dyspneic; perform thoracentesis first.

Chest tube placement should not be attempted in an animal with severe respiratory distress. Generally, stabilization and improved ventilation can first be accomplished by removing some pleural air or fluid by means of needle thoracentesis. In critically ill patients, chest tubes occasionally can be placed without the use of general anesthetic; local anesthetic (i.e., local anesthetic infiltration or an intercostal nerve block) may be sufficient. However, this should be avoided if at all possible because animals with pleural cavity disease benefit from intermittent positive pressure ventilation and oxygen supplementation during tube placement. Control of the animal's airway (by means of endotracheal intubation and positive pressure ventilation) and oxygen therapy should be achieved rapidly (see later discussion). For preoperative concerns of patients with diaphragmatic herniation, see p. 905.

ANESTHESIA

Whenever possible, dogs and cats with respiratory insufficiency should be maintained with inhalation anesthetics (i.e., isoflurane or sevoflurane). Inhalation anesthesia is advantageous because it allows rapid recovery and more precise control of anesthetic depth than does maintaining anesthesia with intravenous anesthetics. Respiratory patients should be managed with extreme care until intubation has been accomplished and ventilation can be assisted. Oxygen can be provided by face mask in these patients until an airway has been secured (see Chapter 5). Intubation should be accomplished as rapidly as possible in patients with pleural effusion or pneumothorax; mask induction is not recommended. Endotracheal intubation and intermittent positive pressure ventilation allow maintenance of an adequate respi-

ratory volume in patients whose lungs may not expand normally because of pleural cavity or diaphragmatic abnormalities. Nitrous oxide should not be used in patients with pneumothorax or diaphragmatic hernias because it rapidly diffuses into air-filled spaces (i.e., pleural cavity or gas-filled organs), causing further lung compression or organ enlargement. Also, nitrous oxide is comparatively less soluble in plasma than are oxygen and other inhalation anesthetics; therefore, it rapidly diffuses into the alveoli when it is discontinued, resulting in diffusion hypoxia if the patient hypoventilates. For specific anesthetic recommendations for animals with pneumothorax (see p. 912) and diaphragmatic hernias (see pp. 905 and 908). See also Chapter 29.

> NOTE: Do not use mask or chamber induction in patients with respiratory distress; accomplish intubation as rapidly as possible using injectable anesthetic agents.

ANTIBIOTICS

Needle thoracentesis performed with proper aseptic technique is unlikely to induce infection in patients with normal immune function; therefore prophylactic antibiotics are not indicated. Prophylactic antibiotics in patients with chest tubes are controversial. Studies in human beings have not shown lower infection rates when patients with chest tubes are given prophylactic antibiotics. However, chest tubes must be maintained and handled with appropriate precautions (e.g., sterile gloves and syringes, and chest bandages) to reduce the potential for iatrogenic contamination. Gram-negative bacteria and anaerobes are common isolates in animals with respiratory disease. Therapy of pyothorax should be based on culture and sensitivity test results, if possible, because unpredictable antibiotic sensitivity is common with the microorganisms commonly encountered with this condition. For specific antibiotic recommendations for patients with pyothorax, see p. 924.

SURGICAL ANATOMY

Each pleural cavity is only a potential space unless air or fluid collects between the parietal and visceral pleurae, preventing normal lung expansion. In a normal animal, only a capillary film of fluid exists to moisten the mesothelial cells that line its pleural surface. Therefore, except for this capillary fluid, the visceral pleura is in contact with the pleural lining of the thoracic wall. The pleura of dogs contains smooth muscle fibers and a network of elastic fibers and is more delicate than in other domestic animals. The subserosa is composed of collagen and elastic fibers, which in the visceral pleura communicate with the underlying lung. Fluid secreted into the pleural cavity normally is reabsorbed by lymphatics underlying the parietal pleura. Thickening of the pleura (i.e., fibrosing pleuritis) may prevent reabsorption of fluid, resulting in pleural effusion.

Fibers of the diaphragm arise from attachments on the ventral surface of the lumbar vertebrae, ribs, and sternum

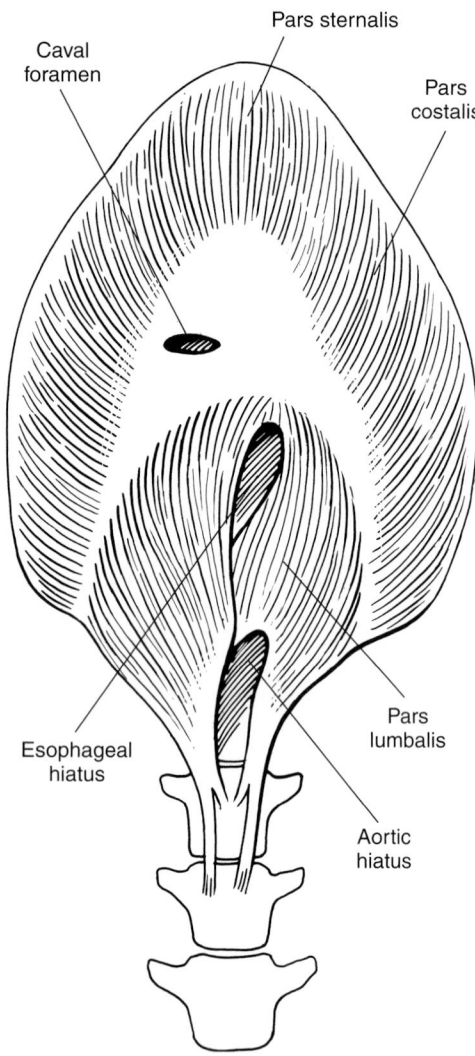

FIG. 30-1
Anatomy of the diaphragm.

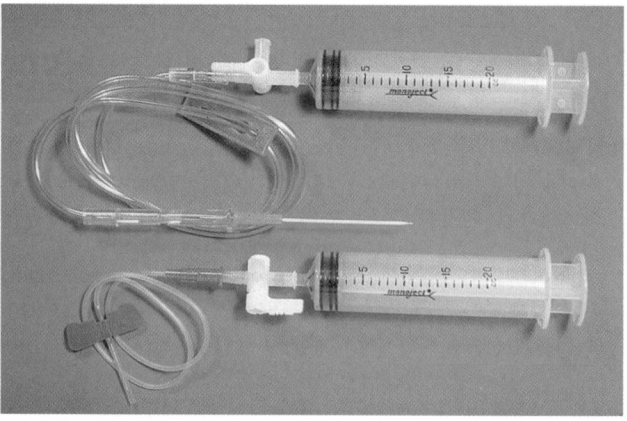

FIG. 30-2
A small-gauge butterfly needle *(lower)* or an over-the-needle catheter attached to extension tubing *(upper),* and a three-way stopcock and syringe are used for needle thoracentesis.

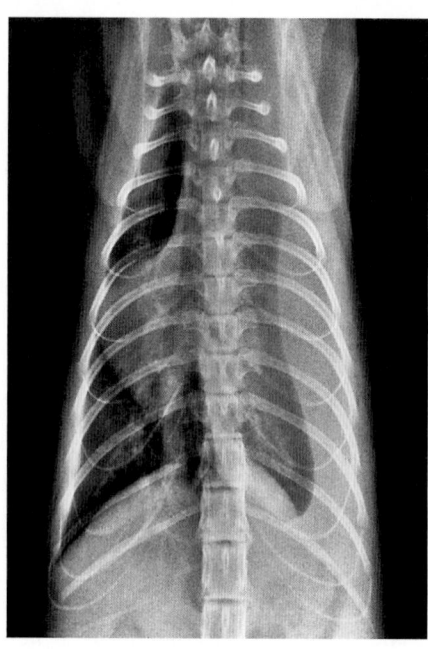

FIG. 30-3
Thoracic radiograph of a cat with unilateral pleural effusion that occurred secondary to chronic chylothorax. Notice the retraction of the left lung (right side of the image) away from the thoracic wall.

and radiate toward the tendinous center (Fig. 30-1). The diaphragm is composed of a central tendinous portion and an outer muscular portion. The costal part of the diaphragm attaches to the internal surface of the last few ribs, and the central portion extends cranially into the thoracic cavity.

SURGICAL TECHNIQUE

Treatment of pleural cavity disease varies, depending on the underlying cause. For traumatic pneumothorax (see p. 908), intermittent needle thoracentesis may be sufficient in some animals to prevent dyspnea while the lung heals, but chest tubes occasionally are required. With some types of pleural effusion (i.e., pyothorax; see p. 922), tube thoracentesis and thoracic lavage are mandatory in the primary treatment of most affected animals.

Needle Thoracentesis

Needle thoracentesis is performed with a small-gauge butterfly needle (No. 19 to No. 23) attached to a three-way stopcock and syringe, or an over-the-needle catheter attached to

an extension tubing, three-way stopcock, and syringe (Fig. 30-2). Be sure the needle is long enough to penetrate to the pleural space in large or obese animals. In such animals, a catheter rather than a butterfly needle may be needed. The appropriate site for thoracentesis should be selected based on the physical examination or, if available, radiographic findings. The mediastinum in dogs and cats is thin and permeable to fluids, and aspiration of one side of the thorax typically drains the contralateral hemithorax adequately. With some diseases, particularly chylothorax and pyothorax, unilateral effusions may occur as a result of thickening of the mediastinum associated with chronic inflammation (Fig. 30-3).

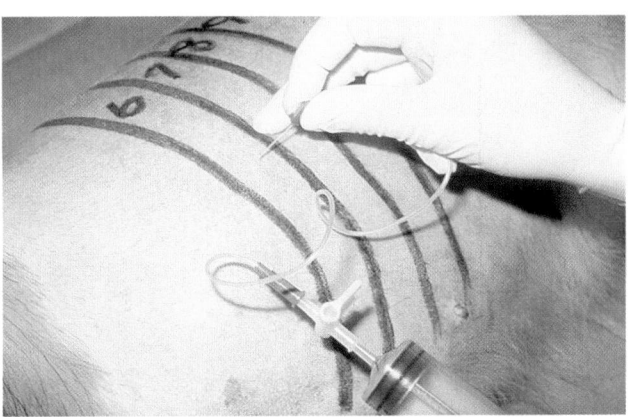

FIG. 30-4
Thoracentesis is performed at the sixth, seventh, or eighth intercostal space, near the level of the costochondral junction.

Perform thoracentesis at the sixth, seventh, or eighth intercostal space, near the level of the costochondral junction (Fig. 30-4). Clip the selected site, and perform a local anesthetic block if needed (this is rarely the case). Aseptically prepare the site, and introduce the needle into the middle of the selected intercostal space. Be careful to avoid the large vessels associated with the posterior aspect of the rib margins. Advance the needle into the pleural space. Aspirate fluid while the needle is being advanced to allow prompt recognition of the appropriate depth of needle placement. If you feel the heart beating or lungs rubbing across the tip of the needle, withdraw the needle and reassess the situation. With the bevel of the needle facing inward, orient the needle against the rib cage to prevent damage to the lung surface. Gently aspirate fluid, and place 5-ml samples in an ethylenediamine tetraacetic acid (EDTA) tube and a clot tube for a cell count and biochemical parameters, respectively. Also, make six to eight direct smears for cytologic evaluation. Submit samples for aerobic and anaerobic cultures.

Chest Tube Placement

Incorrectly placed or improperly managed chest tubes are extremely dangerous to animals. However, if precautions are taken to ensure that the animal cannot remove the tube prematurely or to prevent the animal from chewing on the tube, a pneumothorax should not occur. Chest tubes simplify the management of some animals with pleural effusion or pneumothorax. The choice of which side to place the chest tube is made by evaluating the radiographs. Occasionally, bilateral chest tubes may be necessary; however, in most dogs and cats the mediastinum is permeable to fluid or air, allowing drainage of both hemithoraxes through a single tube. The exception to this may be in chylothorax or pyothorax (see p. 898).

Equipment needed for a tube thoracostomy includes a chest tube, an apparatus to connect the tube to a syringe or to a continuous suction bottle, and a device to collect the drained material (syringe or collecting bottle). Commercially available tubes usually are made of polyvinyl chloride

 BOX 30-2

Guidelines for Estimating Chest Tube Size

Cats and Dogs Under 7 kg	**Dogs 16–30 kg**
14–16 French (Fr)	22–28 Fr
Dogs 7–15 kg	**Dogs Over 30 kg**
18–22 Fr	28–36 Fr

 BOX 30-3

Important Points When Placing a Chest Tube

- When placing additional holes in commercial tubes, make sure that the last hole is through the radiopaque line.
- Start the chest tube dorsally rather than midthorax to minimize fluid or air leakage around the tube.
- Firmly grasp the tube 1 to 2 cm above the body wall when inserting the tube.
- Clamp the tube before removing the stylet (trocar) to prevent pneumothorax.
- Securely fasten all connectors to the tube to prevent inadvertent dislodgment.

or silicone rubber and are less reactive than red rubber feeding tubes. Commercial tubes come with a metal stylet that simplifies tube placement, but may increase the risk of perforating lung tissue compared with red rubber feeding tubes. The red rubber feeding tubes usually are inserted using a large hemostat or Carmalt clamp. Commercial chest tubes come in various sizes ranging from 14 to 40 French. The size of the thoracostomy tube should approximate the diameter of the mainstem bronchus. Smaller tubes may be adequate for removing air, whereas larger tubes may be required with more viscous effusions (Box 30-2). If a commercial tube is used, attach it by means of a tube adapter (e.g., five-in-one connector or Christmas tree adapter) to either a three-way stopcock or the tubing from a continuous suction device. The ends of red rubber feeding tubes can be cut to accommodate a three-way stopcock. Attaching these tubes to a continuous suction device generally is not recommended because of their tendency to collapse (Box 30-3).

Clip and prepare the lateral thorax for aseptic surgery. To allow sufficient drainage, place additional holes in the tube by bending the tube and removing a notch with a pair of sterile scissors (Fig. 30-5). Make sure that the holes are no larger than one third the circumference of the tube. Be certain that all the holes will easily fit within the thoracic cavity. If using a commercial tube with a radiopaque line, place the last hole through the line to allow identification of its position on a thoracic radiograph. Make a small skin incision in the dorsal one third of the lateral thoracic wall at the level of the tenth or eleventh intercostal space. Advance the tube subcutaneously in a cranioventral direction for three to four

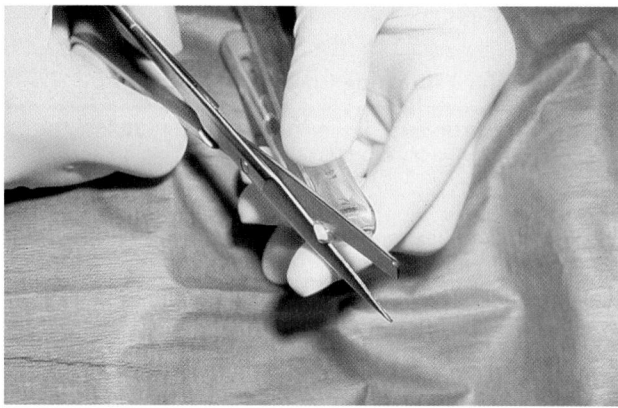

FIG. 30-5
For thoracostomy tube placement, make additional holes in the tube by bending it and removing a notch with a pair of sterile scissors.

intercostal spaces and introduce the tube through the muscle and pleura using the stylet or a large hemostat. When using a trocar tube, firmly grasp the tube 1 to 2 cm from the body wall with one hand while using the other hand to "pop" the tube through the intercostal musculature and pleura (Fig. 30-6). This prevents the tube from being inadvertently pushed farther into the thorax than anticipated, and thereby damaging the lung or other thoracic structures. Feed the tube in a cranioventral direction to a predetermined point. Before completely removing the trocar, clamp the tube with a hemostat. For added safety when the chest cavity is not being suctioned, clamp the tube where it exits the body wall with a hemostat or tube clamp device (Fig. 30-7).

The latter device is preferred as it will not damage the tube and is more comfortable for the patient than a hemostat.

Place a purse-string suture in the skin around the tube (do not enter the lumen of the tube), and leave both ends of the suture long. Use this suture to make a Chinese finger trap or Roman sandal suture (Fig. 30-8). Connect the chest tube to a three-way stopcock to increase the ease of thoracic drainage. Use a tube adapter or female Luer-Lok (with small tubes) between the tube and the three-way stopcock to ensure an airtight seal. Use suture to secure the tube to the connecting devices so that they are not inadvertently dislodged, resulting in a pneumothorax (Fig. 30-9). Verify appropriate placement of the chest drain radiographically (Fig. 30-10) before covering it with a loose bandage.

In selected cases (i.e., multiple adhesions or loculated fluid), it may be advantageous to place the chest tube under thoracoscopic guidance.

Drainage may be either intermittent or continuous. Generally, intermittent pleural drainage is adequate; however, in some situations continuous tissue suction is preferable (i.e., large volumes of air and pleurodesis). Heimlich valves should be

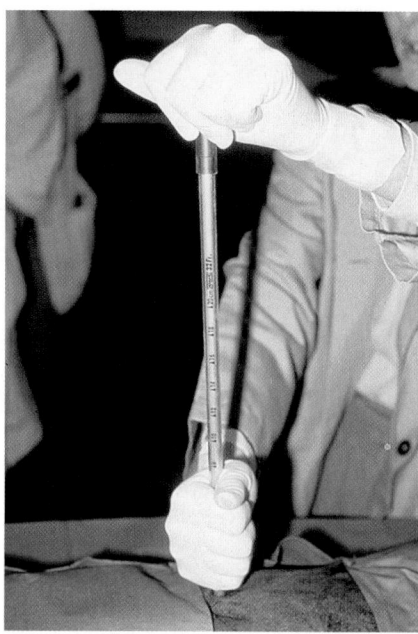

FIG. 30-6
When using a trocar tube, firmly grasp the tube 2 to 4 cm from the body wall with one hand while using the other hand to pop the tube through the intercostal musculature and pleura. Be sure that the hand holding the tube has a firm grasp on the tube as failing to do so may result in the tube inadvertently being pushed too far into the thoracic cavity and puncturing the lungs or heart.

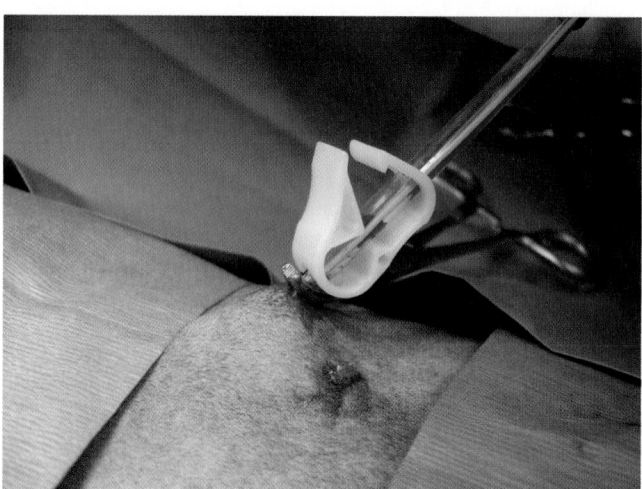

FIG. 30-7
For added safety when the chest cavity is not being suctioned, clamp the tube where it exits the body wall with a hemostat or tube clamp (preferred).

used only in medium to large dogs because small dogs and cats may not develop sufficient expiratory pressure for effective drainage. Also, these valves are prone to malfunction if fluid is aspirated into the apparatus. "Milking" or "stripping" of chest tubes to prevent obstruction of the tube by clots has been recommended in the veterinary literature; however,

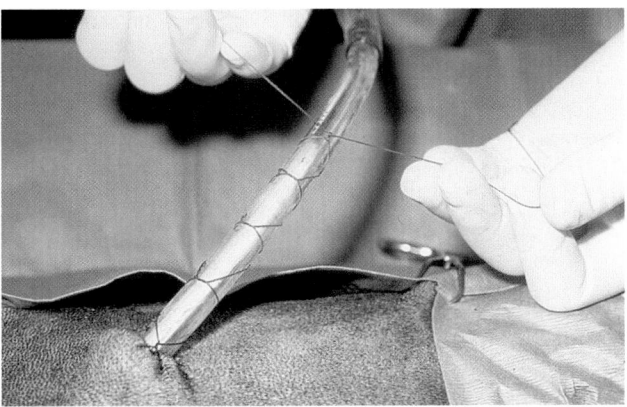

FIG. 30-8
Secure the tube with a Chinese finger trap or Roman sandal suture.

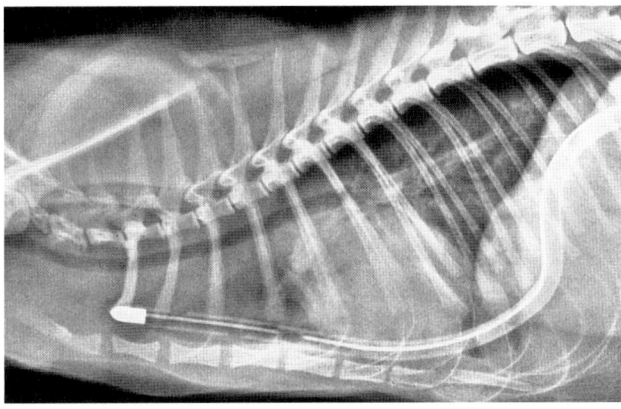

FIG. 30-10
Verify appropriate placement of the chest drain radiographically before covering it with a loose bandage.

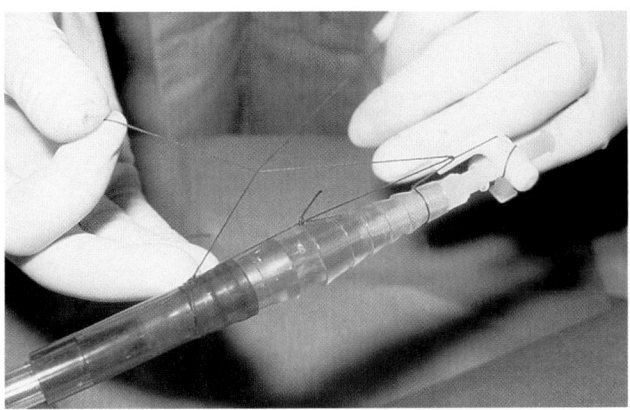

FIG. 30-9
Use suture to secure the tube to the connecting devices so that they are not inadvertently dislodged.

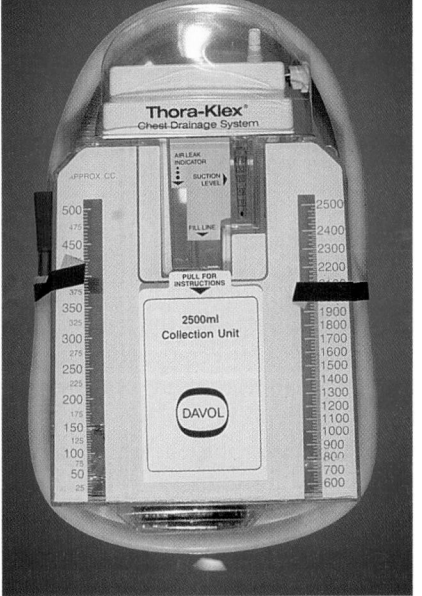

FIG. 30-11
Commercial continuous suction device.

these techniques generate high intrapleural pressures and may cause pulmonary damage.

Chest Tube Removal

With pleural effusion, the tube is removed when the drainage diminishes to a volume consistent with that caused by the presence of the tube itself (i.e., 2.2 ml/kg of body weight/day). The tube can be removed in patients with pneumothorax once negative pressure has been achieved for 12 to 24 hours. Culture the end of the tube after removal if the tube has been in place for several days or if the animal shows signs of infection. Close the skin incision with one or two simple interrupted sutures.

Continuous Thoracic Suction

If fluid accumulates so quickly that intermittent drainage is not practical, continuous suction may be used. It is also commonly used after open heart surgery to monitor tho-

racic bleeding. Two-bottle and three-bottle systems and commercial suction units are available for veterinary use and are economical and simple to use. A continuous 10- to 15-cm negative pressure on the thorax effectively aspirates pneumothorax, increasing the likelihood of spontaneous sealing of large pulmonary defects. Slightly higher pressures may be necessary (up to 20 cm H_2O) when viscous fluid is being drained.

Connect the chest tube to a commercial continuous suction device (Fig. 30-11). If a commercial continuous suction device is not available, use a three-bottle system. Connect

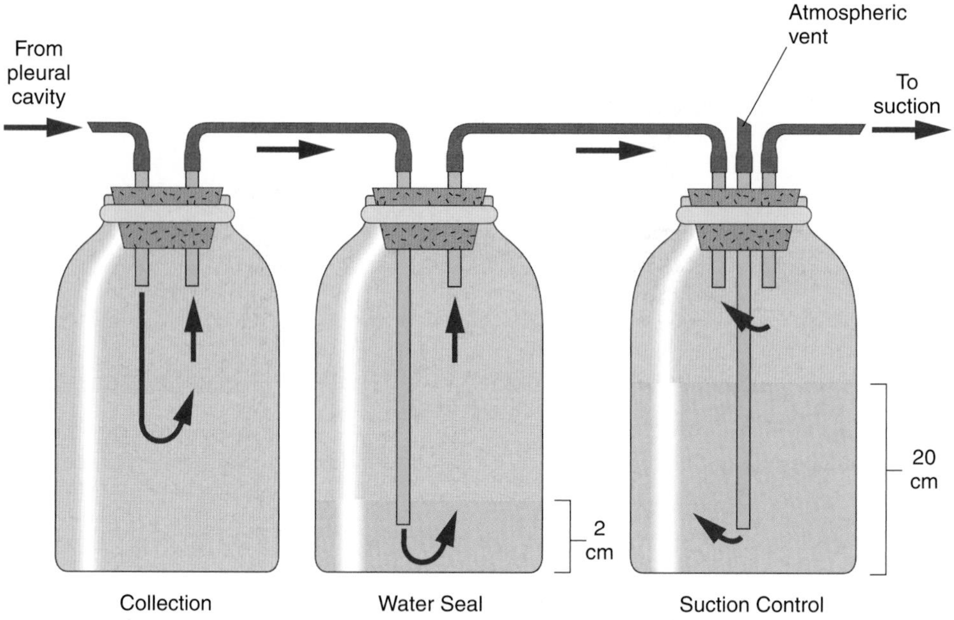

FIG. 30-12
Three-bottle system for continuous pleural drainage.

From pleural cavity

Atmospheric vent

To suction

Collection

Water Seal

Suction Control

2 cm

20 cm

the chest tube to a bottle that serves as an underwater seal (filled with 2 to 3 cm of sterile water), which in turn is connected to a suction bottle (also partly filled with water) attached to a suction device (Fig. 30-12). Vary the amount of suction by raising or lowering the level of water in the suction bottle.

A rigid plastic vent tube open to room air allows air to be aspirated into the bottle as the vacuum is applied. A third bottle interposed between the chest tube and the underwater seal bottle collects fluid and prevents the level from rising in the underwater seal bottle as fluid is drained from the chest. The third bottle is unnecessary in animals with pneumothorax.

HEALING OF THE PLEURA

Healing or damaged pleura is prone to adhesion formation in some species; however, dogs and cats seem resistant to chemical pleurodesis. They may have greater pleural fibrinolytic capacity than other species (e.g., rabbits or human beings). Fibrosing pleuritis has been reported in dogs and cats secondary to prolonged exudative or blood-stained effusions. In animals with fibrosis, the pleura is thickened by diffuse, fibrous tissue that restricts normal pulmonary expansion (the lungs do not adhere to the body wall in these patients; Fig. 30-13). Exudates are characterized by a high rate of fibrin formation and degradation because chronic inflammation induces changes in the morphologic features of mesothelial cells that cause increased permeability, desquamation of mesothelial cells, and triggering of both pathways of the coagulation cascade. The desquamated mesothelial cells have also been shown to produce type III collagen in cell culture, promoting fibrosis. Additionally, the chronic presence of pleural fluid might lead to impaired fibrin degradation.

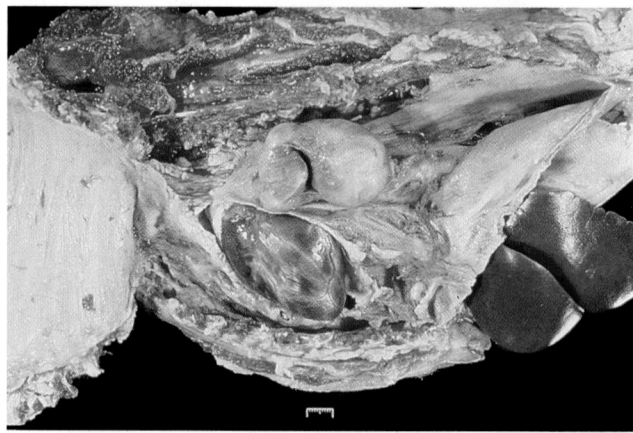

FIG. 30-13
Necropsy specimen of a dog with chronic chylothorax and severe fibrosing pleuritis. Note the small, consolidated lungs and thickened pleura.

SUTURE MATERIALS AND SPECIAL INSTRUMENTS

Trocar chest tubes (DekNatel thoracic trocar catheter, Argyle thoracic trocar catheter) and continuous suction devices (DekNatel Pleur-Evac chest drainage system, Thora-Seal III three-bottle underwater chest drainage system) (see Fig. 30-11) may be purchased from several commercial sources. Tubing clamps and tube adapters may be purchased from Global Veterinary Products (formerly Cook Veterinary Products) and other sources.

POSTOPERATIVE CARE AND ASSESSMENT

If dyspnea persists after needle thoracentesis or chest tube placement, oxygen therapy (nasal insufflation or oxygen cage) may be beneficial (see Chapter 5). Thoracic radiographs should be taken to assess fluid or air removal and/or to evaluate the position of the chest tube. Animals with chest tubes should be monitored continually to prevent iatrogenic dislodgment or damage to the tube or connectors, resulting in pneumothorax (see discussion below in Complications section). Care should be exercised when handling tubes to prevent thoracic contamination. Chest tubes should be aspirated gently so that lung tissue is not suctioned into the tube drainage ports.

COMPLICATIONS

Although lung penetration and damage are possible with needle thoracentesis, the risk is minimal if proper technique is used. The major complication associated with chest tubes is pneumothorax caused by damage to the tube by the patient (i.e., biting or scratching) or loosening of the connections of the tube to the adapters. The risk of these complications can be minimized by placing a clamp close to the tube's exit site (see Fig. 30-7) by securing the tube to the adapters (see Fig. 30-8) and by proper bandaging of the chest and tube. Constant surveillance of animals with chest tubes is recommended. Other complications associated with chest tube placement are rare, but include lung perforation, empyema, laceration of an intercostal vessel, and pulmonary injury caused by aspiration of a portion of lung into one of the tube drainage ports. The risk of lung perforation is related to the type of tube placed and underlying pleuropulmonary disease. If needle thoracentesis or ultrasonography suggests that the fluid is severely loculated or that extensive adhesions are present, surgical placement of the chest tube or placement under thoracoscopic guidance may be advisable.

SPECIAL AGE CONSIDERATIONS

Surgical correction of respiratory abnormalities in young animals requires special attention to their anesthetic requirements (see p. 892). Diaphragmatic hernia repair is commonly performed in young animals because they are prone to trauma producing such lesions. Peritoneopericardial diaphragmatic hernias usually are diagnosed at a young age (i.e., less than 1 year), and concurrent cardiac abnormalities may be present, complicating the anesthetic management of these patients (see p. 908). Geriatric animals may have severe, concurrent underlying pulmonary or cardiac conditions complicating management of pleural cavity disease, and careful monitoring is necessary.

SPECIFIC DISEASES

TRAUMATIC DIAPHRAGMATIC HERNIA

DEFINITION

A **diaphragmatic hernia** occurs when the continuity of the diaphragm is disrupted such that abdominal organs can migrate into the thoracic cavity.

GENERAL CONSIDERATIONS AND CLINICALLY RELEVANT PATHOPHYSIOLOGY

Diaphragmatic hernias are commonly recognized by small animal clinicians and may be congenital or may occur secondary to trauma. Congenital pleuroperitoneal hernias are seldom diagnosed in small animals because many affected animals die at birth or shortly thereafter. Most diaphragmatic hernias in dogs and cats are caused by trauma, particularly motor vehicle accidents. The abrupt increase in intraabdominal pressure accompanying forceful blows to the abdominal wall causes the lungs to rapidly deflate (if the glottis is open), producing a large pleuroperitoneal pressure gradient. Alternately, the pressure gradient that occurs between the thorax and the abdomen may cause the diaphragm to tear. The tears occur at the weakest points of the diaphragm, generally the muscular portions. Location and size of the tear or tears depend on the position of the animal at the time of impact and the location of the viscera. Traumatic diaphragmatic hernias are often associated with significant respiratory embarrassment; however, chronic diaphragmatic hernias in asymptomatic animals are not uncommon. Diaphragmatic hernias may also occur in animals with connective tissue disorders (Benitah et al, 2004).

DIAGNOSIS
Clinical Presentation

Signalment. There is no breed predisposition for traumatic diaphragmatic hernias. Young males were historically thought to be more commonly affected; however, a recent study of traumatic diaphragmatic hernias identified no sex predilection (Reimer et al, 2005).

History. The duration of a diaphragmatic hernia may range from a few hours to years. Many (15% to 25%) are diagnosed weeks after the injury. The animals may be presented in shock acutely after the trauma (see later discussion), or the hernia may be an incidental finding. Animals sustaining trauma often suffer from associated injuries (e.g., fractures). With a chronic diaphragmatic hernia, the clinical signs most often are referable to either the respiratory (i.e., dyspnea and exercise intolerance) or the gastrointestinal systems (i.e., anorexia, vomiting, diarrhea, weight loss, and pain after ingestion of food) or they may be nonspecific (e.g., depression). Many animals with chronic hernias are not dyspneic at the time of diagnosis.

Physical Examination Findings

Animals with recent traumatic diaphragmatic hernias frequently are in shock when presented for treatment; therefore, clinical signs may include pale or cyanotic mucous membranes, tachypnea, tachycardia, and/or oliguria. Cardiac arrhythmias are common and associated with significant morbidity. Other clinical signs depend on which organs have herniated and may be attributed to the gastrointestinal, respiratory, or cardiovascular system. The liver is the most commonly herniated organ, a condition that often is associated with hydrothorax caused by entrapment and venous occlusion.

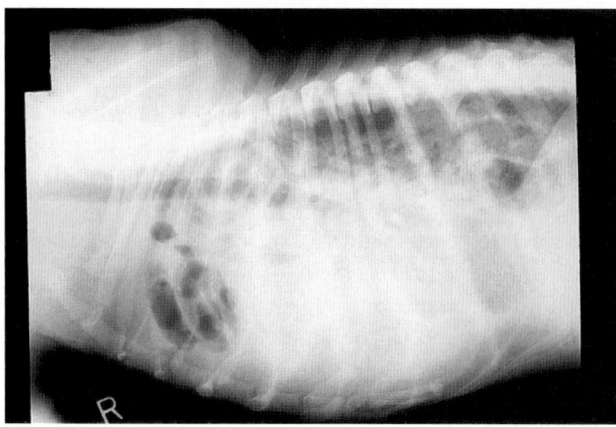

FIG. 30-14
Lateral thoracic radiograph of a dog with a diaphragmatic hernia. Note the air-filled intestinal loops in the thoracic cavity.

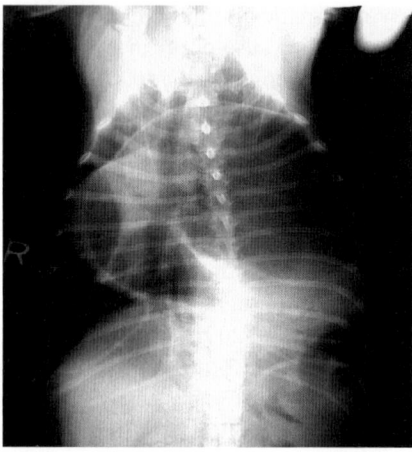

FIG. 30-15
Dorsoventral thoracic radiograph of a dog with a dilated, herniated stomach.

Diagnostic Imaging

Definitive diagnosis of pleuroperitoneal diaphragmatic hernia usually is made by radiography or ultrasonography. If significant pleural effusion is present, thoracentesis may be necessary for diagnostic radiographs. Radiographic signs of diaphragmatic hernia may include loss of the diaphragmatic line, loss of the cardiac silhouette, dorsal or lateral displacement of lung fields, presence of gas or a barium-filled stomach or intestines in the thoracic cavity, pleural effusion, and/or failure to observe the stomach or liver in the abdomen (Figs. 30-14 and 30-15). It may be difficult to diagnose diaphragmatic hernias radiographically if only a small portion of the liver is herniated. In a recent study, thoracic radiographs revealed evidence of diaphragmatic hernia in only 66% of affected animals (Minihan et al,

2004). Ultrasound examination of the diaphragmatic silhouette may help when herniation is not obvious radiographically (i.e., hepatic herniation and pleural effusion). Ultrasonography demonstrated the hernia in 9 of 10 cases in a recent study (Minihan et al, 2004) and was accurate in 23 of 25 cases (93%) in another study (Spattini et al, 2003). Ultrasonography may be particularly difficult if severe pulmonary contusions are present, which make the lung appear ultrasonographically similar to liver, if only omentum is herniated or if adhesions between the liver and lung are present. Also, care should be taken not to mistake a normal mirror-image artifact (usually seen as apparent liver parenchyma on the thoracic side of the diaphragmatic line) for herniated liver.

Positive contrast celiography occasionally may be helpful. Prewarmed water-soluble iodinated contrast agent is injected into the peritoneal cavity at a dosage of 1.1 ml/kg (the dose is doubled if ascites is present), the patient is gently rolled from side to side or the pelvis is elevated, and films are taken immediately after the injection and manipulation. Criteria used in evaluating these images should include the presence of contrast medium in the pleural cavity, absence of a normal liver lobe outline in the abdomen, and incomplete visualization of the abdominal surface of the diaphragm. Positive-contrast celiograms should be interpreted cautiously because omental and fibrous adhesions may seal the defect, resulting in false negative studies.

Laboratory Findings

Specific laboratory abnormalities are uncommon. Serum alanine aminotransferase and serum alkaline phosphatase values may be elevated in cases of liver herniation.

DIFFERENTIAL DIAGNOSIS

Any disorder causing respiratory abnormalities (e.g., pleural effusion, pneumothorax, and pneumonia) should be a differential diagnosis for traumatic diaphragmatic hernia. The concurrent presence of pleural effusion in many animals with liver herniation may make diagnosis of diaphragmatic hernia difficult (see previous discussion).

MEDICAL MANAGEMENT

If the animal is dyspneic, oxygen should be provided by face mask, nasal insufflation, or an oxygen cage (see Chapter 5). Positioning the animal in sternal recumbency with the forelimbs elevated may help ventilation. If moderate or severe pleural effusion is present, thoracentesis (see p. 898) should be performed. Fluid therapy and antibiotics should be given if the animal is in shock.

SURGICAL TREATMENT

Chronic diaphragmatic hernias may have a higher mortality rate than acute diaphragmatic hernias; however, the prognosis with both groups is good to excellent with surgery (see later discussion in the Prognosis section). If pulmonary contusions are severe, surgical repair of diaphragmatic hernias should be delayed until the patient's condition has been stabilized; however, herniorrhaphy should not be delayed unnecessarily. Animals with gastric herniation should be evaluated carefully for gastric distention and should be operated on as soon as they can safely be anesthetized because acute gastric distention within the thorax may cause rapid, fatal respiratory impairment.

> NOTE: Do not delay surgery unnecessarily in animals in stable condition. If the stomach has herniated into the thoracic cavity, perform surgery as soon as possible (i.e., on an emergency basis).

> NOTE: Be prepared to perform organ resection (i.e., partial lobectomy, intestinal resection, and anastomosis) if the hernia is chronic. Be aware that reexpansion pulmonary edema may occur in patients with chronic diaphragmatic hernias, but is rare.

Preoperative Management

Prophylactic antibiotics should be given before induction of anesthesia in animals with hepatic herniation. Massive release of toxins into the circulation may occur with hepatic strangulation or vascular compromise. Premedicating such patients with steroids may be beneficial. An ECG should be performed on all trauma patients before surgery.

Anesthesia

Chamber or mask induction should be avoided in animals with diaphragmatic hernia (see p. 897). Supplementing oxygen before induction improves myocardial oxygenation. Because of the animal's already compromised ventilation, drugs with minimal respiratory depressant effects should be used. Injectable anesthetics allowing rapid intubation are preferred (see also p. 867). Inhalation anesthetics should be used for maintenance of anesthesia. Intermittent positive pressure ventilation should be performed, and high inspiratory pressures should be avoided to help prevent reexpansion pulmonary edema (see p. 869). The lungs should be allowed to expand slowly after surgery. Nitrous oxide is contraindicated in patients with diaphragmatic hernia (see p. 897). Drugs such as methylprednisolone may be beneficial for preventing reexpansion pulmonary edema in animals with chronic diaphragmatic hernia. See Box 29-1, p. 868, for examples of selected anesthetic protocols that may be used in animals with diaphragmatic hernias.

Positioning

The animal is placed in dorsal recumbency for a midline abdominal incision. The entire abdomen and caudal one half to two thirds of the thoracic cavity should be prepared for aseptic surgery. Because acute ventilatory compromise may occur during positioning, these animals should be carefully monitored during this period.

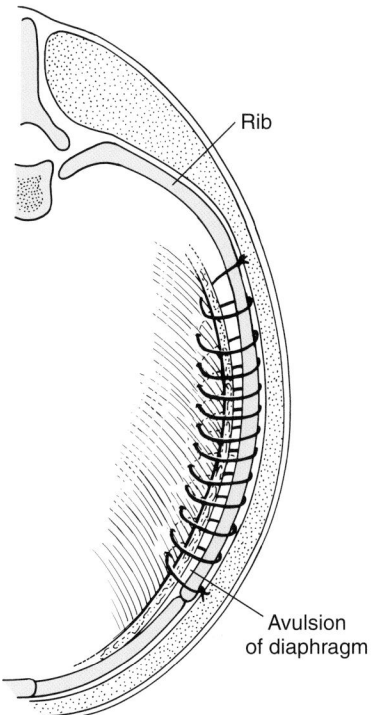

FIG. 30-16
To repair a diaphragm avulsed from the thoracic wall, incorporate a rib in the suture line.

> NOTE: Be sure to prep an adequate area so that the incision can be extended into the caudal sternum for thoracic access if necessary.

SURGICAL TECHNIQUE

Make a ventral midline abdominal incision; if greater exposure is needed, extend the incision cranially through the sternum. Replace the abdominal organs in the abdominal cavity (if necessary, enlarge the diaphragmatic defect). If adhesions are present, dissect the tissue gently from the thoracic structures to prevent pneumothorax or bleeding. With chronic hernias, débride the edge of the defect before closure. Close the diaphragmatic defect in a simple continuous suture pattern. If the diaphragm is avulsed from the ribs, incorporate a rib in the continuous suture for added strength (Fig. 30-16). Remove air from the pleural cavity after closing the defect. If continued pneumothorax or effusion is likely, place a chest tube (see p. 899). Explore the entire abdominal cavity for associated injury (i.e., compromise of the vasculature to the intestine or splenic, renal, or bladder trauma) and repair any defects.

> NOTE: If the diaphragmatic defect is particularly large, synthetic material such as Silastic sheeting can be used to close it; however, this is seldom necessary.

An abdominal flap graft has been reported for repair of chronic diaphragmatic hernia in dogs. The graft is obtained from the peritoneum and transverse abdominal muscle caudal to the diaphragm. The graft is elevated, placed over the defect, and sutured to the diaphragm.

SUTURE MATERIALS AND SPECIAL INSTRUMENTS

To close the diaphragm, use either a nonabsorbable (e.g., polypropylene) or an absorbable (e.g., polydioxanone or polyglyconate) suture.

POSTOPERATIVE CARE AND ASSESSMENT

Patients should be monitored postoperatively for hypoventilation, and oxygen should be provided if necessary. Reexpansion pulmonary edema (RPE) is a possible complication associated with rapid lung reexpansion after repair of a diaphragmatic hernia (see p. 869). Postoperative analgesics should be provided (see Chapter 13; for dosages of opioids see Table 13-4 on p. 133).

COMPLICATIONS

The most common complication after surgical repair of diaphragmatic hernias is pneumothorax, especially if the hernia is chronic and if adhesions are present. RPE may occur in lungs that have been chronically collapsed (see previous discussion).

PROGNOSIS

If the animal survives the early postoperative period (i.e., 12 to 24 hours), the prognosis is excellent, and recurrence is uncommon with proper technique. Reported mortality rates for animals with traumatic diaphragmatic hernia have varied from 12% to 48%. Perioperative survival in one study of 92 dogs and cats with traumatic diaphragmatic hernias was 89.1% (Gibson et al, 2005). A recent study of animals with *chronic* diaphragmatic hernias reported a mortality rate of 14% (Minihan et al, 2004). Older cats or those that had low to mildly increased respiratory rates and concurrent injuries were more likely to die after hernia repair (Schmiedt et al, 2003).

References

Benitah N, Matousek JL, Barnes RF et al: Diaphragmatic and perineal hernias associated with cutaneous asthenia in a cat, *J Am Vet Med Assoc* 224:706, 2004.

Gibson TWG, Brisson BA, Sears W: Perioperative survival rates after surgery for diaphragmatic hernia in dogs and cats, *J Am Vet Med Assoc* 227:105, 2005.

Minihan AC, Berg J, Evans KL: Chronic diaphragmatic hernia in 34 dogs and 16 cats, *J Am Anim Hosp Assoc* 40:51, 2004.

Schmiedt CW, Tobias KM, McCrackin Stevenson MA: Traumatic diaphragmatic hernia in cats: 334 cases (1991-2001), *J Am Vet Med Assoc* 222:1237, 2003.

Spattini G, Rossi F, Vignoli M et al: Use of ultrasound to diagnose diaphragmatic rupture in dogs and cats, *Vet Radiol Ultrasound* 44:226, 2003.

PERITONEOPERICARDIAL DIAPHRAGMATIC HERNIA

DEFINITION

A **peritoneopericardial diaphragmatic hernia (PPDH)** occurs when a congenital communication exists between the abdomen and the pericardial sac. Synonyms include *pericardial diaphragmatic hernia* and *congenital hernia*.

GENERAL CONSIDERATIONS AND CLINICALLY RELEVANT PATHOPHYSIOLOGY

PPDHs are less commonly recognized by small animal clinicians than traumatic diaphragmatic hernias. Although PPDH often is associated with respiratory embarrassment, asymptomatic PPDH is common. PPDHs may occur as a result of trauma in human beings (in whom the diaphragm forms one wall of the pericardial sac); however, these hernias are always congenital in dogs and cats in which no direct communication exists between the pericardial and peritoneal cavities after birth. The most widely accepted theory regarding the embryogenesis of this defect is that the hernia occurs because of faulty development or prenatal injury of the septum transversum. This could be a result of a teratogen, a genetic defect, or prenatal injury.

Cardiac abnormalities and sternal deformities often occur concomitantly with PPDH. The combination of congenital cranial abdominal wall, caudal sternal, diaphragmatic, and pericardial defects has been reported in dogs, and is often associated with ventricular septal defects or other intracardiac defects (Fig. 30-17). It is not known if this condition is heritable; however, several breed predispositions have been recognized (see later discussion). Polycystic kidneys have been reported in association with PPDH in cats.

> NOTE: If you identify a cranial abdominal wall defect in a young animal, consider that it may also have PPDH or a congenital cardiac abnormality, or both.

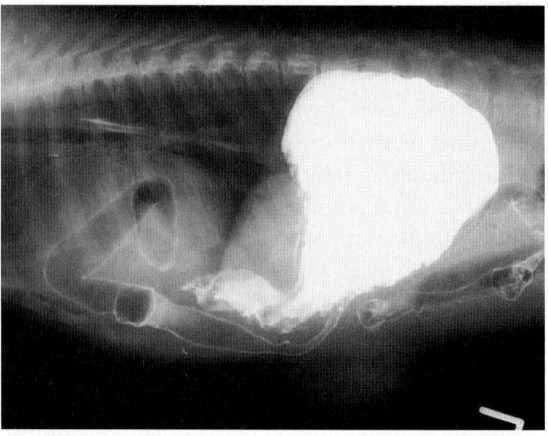

FIG. 30-17
Lateral thoracic radiograph of a dog with a PPDH. Note the cranial abdominal hernia.

DIAGNOSIS
Clinical Presentation

Signalment. Although PPDH is congenital, it is not uncommon for the diagnosis to be made when the animal is middle-aged or older because clinical signs vary and may be intermittent. Weimaraners and cocker spaniels may be at increased risk. Domestic longhair and Himalayan cats may be predisposed (Reimer et al, 2004).

History. The clinical signs may be referable to the gastrointestinal, cardiac, or respiratory systems and include anorexia, depression, vomiting, diarrhea, weight loss, wheezing, dyspnea, exercise intolerance, and/or pain after eating. Neurologic signs may occur as a result of hepatoencephalopathy.

Physical Examination Findings

Physical examination findings in animals with PPDH may include ascites, muffled heart sounds, murmurs caused either by displacement of the heart by visceral organs or by intracardiac defects, and concurrent ventral abdominal wall defects. The most commonly herniated organ is the liver, and associated pericardial effusion is common.

Diagnostic Imaging

A tentative diagnosis of PPDH may be made based on the history, clinical signs, and physical examination, but radiography or ultrasonography (or both) is essential for a definitive presurgical diagnosis. Box 30-4 lists the radiographic signs of PPDH (Fig. 30-18). Contrast studies (i.e., nonselective angiogram and barium contrast study) should be undertaken only if a definitive diagnosis cannot be made on survey films (Fig. 30-19) or with ultrasound. A distinct curvilinear radiopacity has been identified between the cardiac silhouette and the diaphragm on a lateral thoracic radiograph in cats with PPDH. This radiographic finding has been called the *dorsal peritoneopericardial mesothelial remnant*; however, it is not always apparent on radiographs of affected cats. Ultrasonography is useful because there often is discontinuity of the diaphragmatic outline and more importantly, abdominal organs may be visualized in the pericardial sac. Hepatic herniation usually is evident. Echocardiography should be performed in animals with murmurs.

BOX 30-4

Radiographic Signs of Peritoneopericardial Diaphragmatic Hernia

- Enlarged cardiac silhouette
- Dorsal elevation of the trachea
- Overlap of the heart and diaphragmatic borders
- Discontinuity of the diaphragm
- Gas-filled structures in the pericardial sac
- Sternal defects
- Dorsal peritoneopericardial mesothelial remnant

Laboratory Findings

Specific laboratory abnormalities are uncommon.

DIFFERENTIAL DIAGNOSIS

The most common differential diagnoses for PPDH are pericardial effusion and cardiomegaly. Ultrasound and echocardiography are useful for distinguishing these abnormalities from PPDH.

MEDICAL MANAGEMENT

If the animal is dyspneic, oxygen should be provided by face mask, nasal insufflation, or an oxygen cage (see Chapter 5). Positioning the animal in sternal recumbency with the forelimbs elevated may help ventilation.

SURGICAL TREATMENT

Surgical repair should be performed as early as possible (generally when the animal is between 8 and 16 weeks of age), when it is unlikely that adhesions will be present and

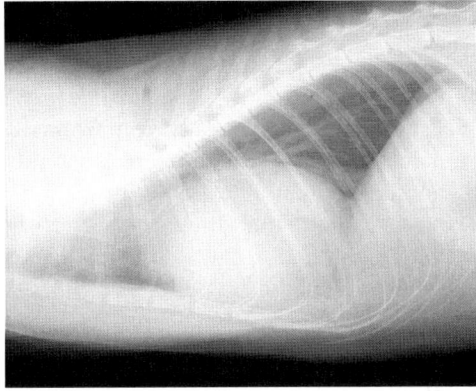

FIG. 30-18
Lateral thoracic radiograph of a cat with a PPDH. Note the large, globoid appearance of the cardiac silhouette.

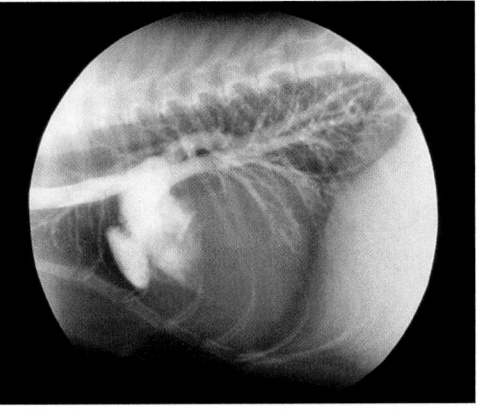

FIG. 30-19
Nonselective angiogram in a cat with a PPDH. Note the size of the heart in comparison to the cardiac silhouette. The liver is within the pericardial sac. (Courtesy M. Miller, Texas A&M University.)

the pliable nature of the skin, muscles, sternum, and rib cage facilitates closure of large defects. Early correction of PPDH may prevent acute decompensation and the possible development of acute postoperative pulmonary edema (see p. 867). If the hernia is not diagnosed until the animal is older, conservative or surgical management may be used; however, owner satisfaction was higher in operated animals than in animals managed conservatively in a recent study (Reimer et al, 2004). Some animals that are initially managed medically may have progression of clinical signs necessitating surgical intervention or resulting in death.

Preoperative Management

Prophylactic antibiotics should be given before induction of anesthesia in animals with hepatic herniation. In animals with hepatic strangulation or vascular compromise, repositioning of the liver into the abdominal cavity may cause a massive release of toxins into the bloodstream; premedicating such patients with steroids may be beneficial.

Anesthesia

Chamber or mask induction should be avoided in animals with PPDH (see p. 897). Before induction, supplementing the inspired oxygen improves myocardial oxygenation. If the animal's ventilation is already compromised, drugs with minimal respiratory depressant effects should be used. Injectable anesthetics that allow rapid intubation are preferred (see also p. 867). Inhalation anesthetics should be used for anesthetic maintenance. Intermittent positive pressure ventilation should be performed; however, high ventilatory pressures should be avoided to help prevent RPE (see p. 869). The lungs should be allowed to expand slowly after surgery. Nitrous oxide is contraindicated in patients with a diaphragmatic hernia (see p. 897). Drugs such as methylprednisolone may be beneficial in animals with chronic diaphragmatic hernias. See Box 29-1, p. 868, for examples of selected anesthetic protocols that may be used in animals with diaphragmatic hernias.

Positioning

The animal is placed in dorsal recumbency for a midline abdominal incision. The entire abdomen and caudal two thirds of the thoracic cavity should be prepared for aseptic surgery.

SURGICAL TECHNIQUE

Make a ventral midline abdominal incision. If greater exposure is needed, extend the incision cranially through the sternum. Enlarge the diaphragmatic defect if necessary and replace the abdominal organs in the abdominal cavity. If adhesions are present, gently dissect the tissue from the thoracic structures, resecting or débriding necrotic tissue as necessary. Débride the edges of the defect and close in a simple continuous suture pattern. Do not close the pericardial sac. Remove air from the pericardial sac or pleural cavity or both after closing the defect. If continued

pneumothorax or effusion is likely, place a chest tube (see p. 899). Repair concomitant sternal or abdominal wall defects.

SUTURE MATERIALS AND SPECIAL INSTRUMENTS

To close the diaphragm, use either nonabsorbable (e.g., polypropylene) or absorbable (e.g., polydioxanone or polyglyconate) suture.

POSTOPERATIVE CARE AND ASSESSMENT

These patients should be monitored postoperatively for hypoventilation, and oxygen should be provided if necessary. RPE is a possible complication associated with rapid lung reexpansion after diaphragmatic hernia repair (see p. 869). Patients with PPDH may also have pulmonary hypoplasia, which contributes to the development of high intrapleural pressures and RPE. Postoperative analgesics should be provided (see Chapter 13; for dosages of opioids see Table 13-4 on p. 133). Transient hyperthermia has been reported in cats following PPDH repair (Reimer et al, 2004).

PROGNOSIS

If the animal survives the early postoperative period (i.e., 12 to 24 hours), the prognosis is excellent, and recurrence is uncommon with proper technique. A postoperative mortality rate of 14% was recently reported in cats (Reimer et al, 2004). The prognosis is worse in patients with PPDH that have concurrent cardiac abnormalities.

Reference

Reimer SB, Kyles AE, Filipowicz DE et al: Long-term outcome of cat treated conservatively or surgically for peritoneopericardial diaphragmatic hernia: 66 cases (1987-2002), *J Am Vet Med Assoc* 224:728, 2004.

PNEUMOTHORAX

DEFINITIONS

Pneumothorax is an accumulation of air or gas in the pleural space. **Traumatic pneumothorax** may be classified as open or closed. An **open pneumothorax** is one in which there is free communication between the pleural space and the external environment. With a **closed pneumothorax**, air accumulates because of leakage from the pulmonary parenchyma, bronchial tree, or esophagus. A **tension pneumothorax** occurs when a flap of tissue acts as a one-way valve so that there is a continuous influx of air into the pleural cavity on inspiration that does not return to the lung on expiration. **Spontaneous pneumothorax** occurs as a result of air leakage from the lung, but without trauma as a precipitating cause. **Cysts** are closed cavities or sacs lined by epithelium that are usually filled with fluid or semisolid material. **Bullae** are nonepithelialized cavities produced by disruption of intraalveolar septa (Fig. 30-20). A **bleb** is a localized collection of air contained within the visceral pleura (see Fig. 30-20). For nontraumatic pneumothorax, the terms *spontaneous*

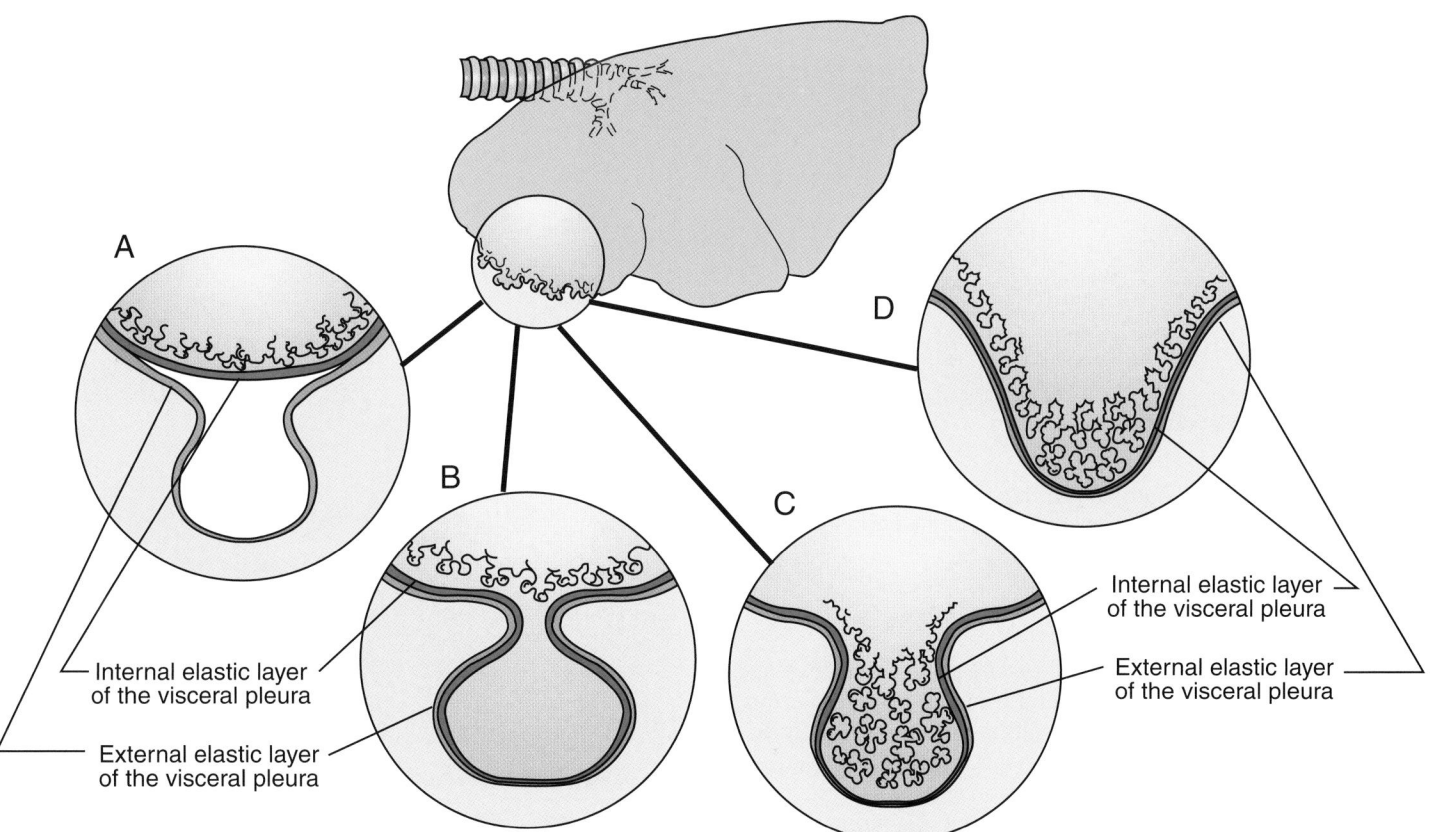

FIG. 30-20

Illustration showing the typical location and different forms of pulmonary blebs and bullae *(inset)*. **A,** Pulmonary bleb; **B,** a thin-walled bulla with a narrow connection to the pulmonary parenchyma; **C,** a subpleural bulla that is connected to the lung by a stalk of emphysematous tissue; and **D,** a large bulla that extends deep into the pulmonary parenchyma.

pneumothorax and *idiopathic pneumothorax* have been used interchangeably.

GENERAL CONSIDERATIONS AND CLINICALLY RELEVANT PATHOPHYSIOLOGY

Traumatic pneumothorax is the most common type of pneumothorax in dogs. It most often occurs as a result of blunt trauma (e.g., vehicular accidents or being kicked), which causes parenchymal pulmonary damage to the lung and a closed pneumothorax. When the thorax is forcefully compressed against a closed glottis, the lung or bronchial tree may rupture. In other cases, pulmonary parenchyma may be torn as a result of shearing forces on the lung. Pulmonary trauma occasionally results in the formation of subpleural blebs, similar to those seen with spontaneous pneumothorax (see later discussion; Fig. 30-21). Open pneumothorax is less common but is often caused by trauma (i.e., gunshot, bite or stab wounds, lacerations that occur secondary to rib fractures). Some penetrating injuries are called "sucking chest wounds" because large defects in the chest wall allow an influx of air into the pleural space when the animal inspires. These large, open chest wounds may allow enough air to enter the pleural space to cause lung collapse and notably reduced ventilation. Atmospheric and intrapleural pressures equilibrate rapidly through the defect, interfering with the normal mechanical function of the thoracic bellows, which normally provides the necessary pressure gradient for air exchange. Pneumomediastinum may be associated with pneumothorax or tracheal, bronchial, or esophageal defects, or it may be due to subcutaneous air migration along fascial planes at the thoracic inlet.

Tracheal rupture may occur due to trauma; it is especially associated with overinflation of the endotracheal tube cuff in cats. Tracheoscopy may be the method of choice for documenting tracheal rupture. The primary signs of tracheal rupture are pneumomediastinum and subcutaneous emphysema; pneumothorax is rare (Fig. 30-22). It is important to distinguish tracheal rupture without pneumothorax from that causing pneumothorax. Tracheal rupture without pneumothorax is best treated by cage rest; tracheoscopy is unnecessary. Tracheal rupture with pneumothorax may require surgery in which tracheoscopy is usually necessary, but it can be difficult to find the site of rupture at surgery or with endoscopy. Fortunately, many lesions heal spontaneously with medical management (Mitchell et al, 2000). A recent retrospective study evaluated the outcomes and complications in

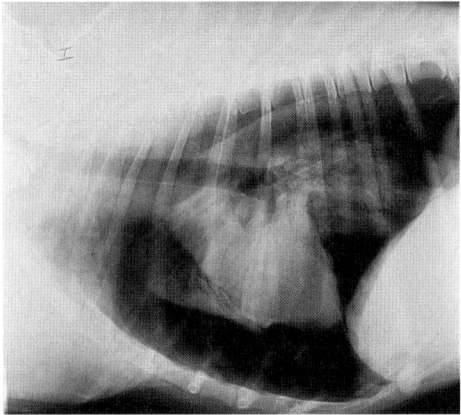

FIG. 30-21
Lateral thoracic radiograph of a dog with spontaneous pneumothorax. Note the apparent elevation of the heart from the sternum.

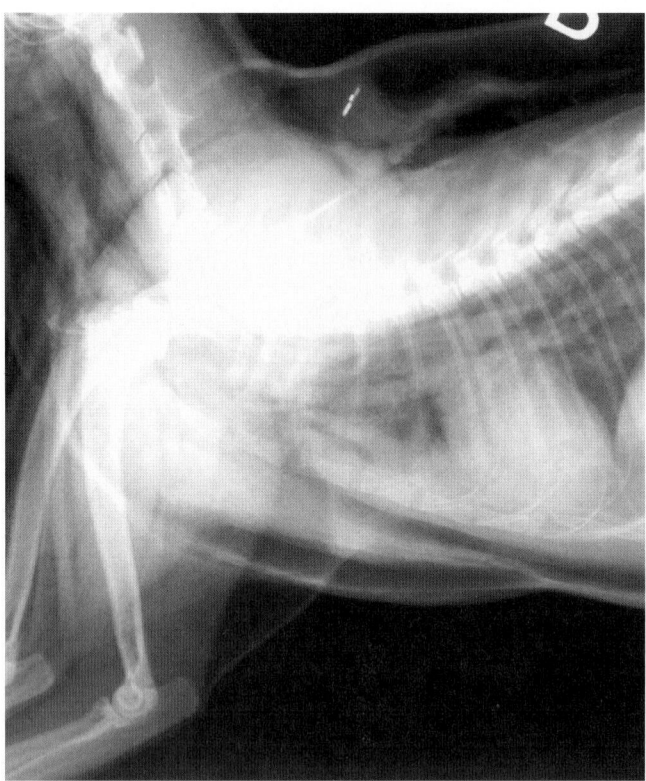

FIG. 30-22
Lateral thoracic radiograph of a cat with pneumomediastinum and subcutaneous emphysema associated with tracheal rupture.

a consecutive series of cats undergoing surgical repair of intrathoracic tracheal avulsion injuries. Long-term resolution of clinical signs was achieved in all cats after resection of the damaged trachea and tracheal repair by end-to-end anastomosis (White and Burton, 2000).

Spontaneous pneumothorax occurs in previously healthy animals without antecedent trauma and may be primary (without underlying pulmonary disease) or secondary (with underlying disease, such as pneumonia, pulmonary abscess, neoplasia, chronic granulomatous infection, or pulmonary parasitic infection, such as with *Paragonimus* spp.). Based on the histologic appearance of the pulmonary lesion, both cysts and bullae have been reported in dogs. Primary spontaneous pneumothorax in dogs may be due to rupture of subpleural blebs; remaining lung tissue may appear normal. These blebs are most commonly located in the apices of the lungs. Secondary spontaneous pneumothorax is more common in dogs than the primary form. In these animals, the subpleural blebs are associated with diffuse emphysema or other pulmonary lesions. It has been shown that volume strain from expansive pressure in the lung increases disproportionately at the apex as height increases. Most affected human beings are cigarette smokers, suggesting that the underlying pulmonary disease could be a result of interference with the normal function of α_1-proteinase inhibitor in inhibiting elastase. It is believed that α_1-proteinase inhibitor is inactivated in people who smoke, allowing increased elastase-induced destruction of pulmonary parenchyma. In a recent study of 12 dogs with spontaneous bullae and blebs, 10 had more than one lesion and 7 had bilateral lesions (Lipscomb et al, 2003).

NOTE: Be sure to differentiate traumatic and spontaneous pneumothorax because the former usually responds to medical management, whereas the latter requires surgery.

DIAGNOSIS
Clinical Presentation

Signalment. Traumatic pneumothorax is most common in young dogs because they are more likely to be hit by cars or to suffer other trauma resulting in pulmonary damage. For similar reasons, males may be more commonly affected than females. Traumatic pneumothorax is less common in cats. Spontaneous pneumothorax usually occurs in large and deep-chested breeds; however, it may occur in small dogs. Purebred dogs, particularly Siberian Huskies, may be more commonly affected than mixed breed dogs. Dogs of any age may develop spontaneous pneumothorax: in a recent study the mean age was 7.5 years (range, 3.5 to 12 years) (Lipscomb et al, 2003). Male and female dogs appear to be equally affected.

History. Pneumothorax due to trauma usually causes acute dyspnea. Trauma is often not reported, making differentiation between traumatic and spontaneous pneumothorax difficult. Although the history of dogs with spontaneous pneumothorax varies depending on underlying etiology, most animals have acute onset of dyspnea. Some dogs may have nonspecific signs (e.g., lethargy, anorexia, depression, coughing, or exercise intolerance), and respiratory signs may not be noted for several days until the pneumothorax worsens. Occasionally a chronic cough or fever may be noted.

Recurrence of dyspnea in an animal previously treated for pneumothorax suggests spontaneous rather than traumatic pneumothorax.

Physical Examination Findings

Most animals with pneumothorax have bilateral disease and are presented for treatment with an acute onset of severe dyspnea. Other evidence of trauma (i.e., rib fractures, limb fractures, traumatic myocarditis, or pulmonary contusions) may be evident in animals with trauma-induced pneumothorax. Most animals with pneumothorax show a restrictive respiratory pattern (i.e., rapid, shallow respirations). If hypoventilation causes hypoxemia, they may appear cyanotic, and the heart and lung sounds often are muffled dorsally. Dogs are able to tolerate massive pneumothorax by increasing their chest expansion. Respiration becomes ineffectual in animals with tension pneumothorax as the chest becomes barrel shaped and fixed in maximal extension. This condition is life threatening. Subcutaneous emphysema occasionally is noted in animals with pneumomediastinum and pneumothorax. The air may migrate from the mediastinal space to the thoracic inlet and be noticeable under the skin over the neck and trunk.

NOTE: Tension pneumothorax is a life-threatening condition. It must be recognized and treated promptly.

Diagnostic Imaging

Thoracic radiographs should be delayed until after thoracentesis in severely dyspneic animals (see p. 896) in which pneumothorax is strongly suspected. Pneumothorax usually occurs bilaterally in animals because air diffuses through the thin mediastinum. Pneumothorax causes large, air-filled spaces in the pleural cavity. On a recumbent lateral thoracic radiograph, the lungs collapse and retract from the chest wall, and the heart usually appears to be elevated from the sternum (see Fig. 30-21). This apparent elevation of the heart is not noticeable on a standing lateral radiograph. Partly collapsed, or atelectatic, lung lobes appear radiopaque compared with the air-filled pleural space. The vascular pattern does not extend to the chest wall as the lungs collapse. This may be particularly noticeable in the caudal thorax on a ventrodorsal view.

Radiographs should be carefully evaluated for underlying pulmonary disease (e.g., abscess and neoplasia) or associated trauma (e.g., rib fractures and pulmonary contusion). Pulmonary blebs found in some animals with spontaneous pneumothorax are seldom visible radiographically, although computed tomography (CT) is more sensitive for finding these lesions. This is probably because the large blebs have ruptured, causing the pneumothorax. CT may be useful in identifying bullae. If imaging does not identify the lesion, surgical or thoracoscopic identification of bullae is indicated. Air-filled bullae may be incidental findings on thoracic radiographs of some animals. Pneumomediastinum is characterized by the ability to visualize thoracic structures (i.e., aorta, thoracic trachea, vena cava, and esophagus) that are not usually apparent on thoracic radiographs.

NOTE: Remember that bullae may not be seen in dogs with pneumothorax because they often have already ruptured. Also, air in the thoracic cavity may make other (nonruptured) bullae difficult to visualize.

Laboratory Findings

Specific laboratory abnormalities are uncommon in animals with pneumothorax; however, blood gas derangements may occur.

DIFFERENTIAL DIAGNOSIS

Any abnormality causing respiratory distress (i.e., diaphragmatic hernia, pleural effusion, or pulmonary edema) is a differential diagnosis for pneumothorax. Because the management of animals with primary and spontaneous pneumothorax differs, once the animal's condition has been stabilized, the cause of the pneumothorax should be determined.

MEDICAL MANAGEMENT

Medical management of pneumothorax consists of initially relieving dyspnea by thoracentesis (see p. 898). If the pleural air accumulates quickly or cannot be managed effectively with needle thoracentesis, a chest tube should be placed (see p. 899). Tube thoracostomy typically is required in animals with spontaneous pneumothorax. Intermittent or continuous pleural drainage may be used, depending on the speed with which air accumulates. Continuous drainage may allow quicker resolution of pneumothorax in animals with large, traumatic defects. Providing an enriched oxygen environment may be beneficial, particularly in animals with concurrent pulmonary trauma (e.g., pulmonary contusion or hemorrhage). Providing analgesics to animals with fractured ribs or severe soft tissue damage may improve ventilation (see p. 868). Surgical intervention is seldom required in animals with traumatic pneumothorax. Thoracentesis should be performed as necessary to prevent dyspnea while the pulmonary lesion heals, usually within 3 to 5 days. Recurrence is uncommon. Conversely, animals with spontaneous pneumothorax commonly have recurrent pneumothorax if surgery is not performed.

An open chest wound should be covered immediately with any readily available material. A sterile occlusive dressing should be applied as soon as possible and intrapleural air evacuated by thoracentesis or tube thoracostomy.

SURGICAL TREATMENT

Surgical therapy of animals with traumatic pneumothorax is seldom necessary (see previous discussion). However, nonsurgical management of spontaneous pneumothorax usually results in an unsatisfactory outcome. Thoracoscopic treatment of bullous emphysema has been reported in dogs (Brissot et al, 2003). Mechanical pleurodesis of the lungs (see p. 912) may reduce the recurrence of pneumothorax in animals that undergo surgery for spontaneous pneumothorax. Mechanical pleurodesis damages the pleura, causing it to thicken.

Preoperative Management

An ECG and thoracentesis should be performed before induction of anesthesia. Preoxygenating these animals often is beneficial (see p. 867). Perioperative antibiotics seldom are warranted and may prevent culturing of bacteria from infected pulmonary tissue during surgery.

Anesthesia

Care should be used when anesthetizing and ventilating animals with pneumothorax and/or pulmonary bullae. Intermittent positive pressure ventilation (IPPV) may rupture intact bullae or accelerate air leakage from the damaged lung or bronchial tree. For these reasons, the inspiratory pressure should not exceed 10 to 12 cm H_2O in these animals until the chest cavity is opened. The adequacy of ventilatory pressures should then be reevaluated. Because IPPV may induce a tension pneumothorax, immediate treatment of this condition (i.e., needle thoracentesis or chest tube placement) may be necessary and should be anticipated. The use of nitrous oxide is contraindicated in patients with pneumothorax. See p. 867 for selected anesthetic protocols for use in animals with respiratory dysfunction.

Surgical Anatomy

See the discussion of the surgical anatomy of the pleural space on p. 897 and the anatomic description of the lungs in dogs and cats on p. 870.

Positioning

See intercostal thoracotomy, p. 873, or median sternotomy, p. 874.

SURGICAL TECHNIQUE

If an underlying pulmonary lesion is readily identified (i.e., pulmonary abscess or neoplasia) and can be localized to one hemithorax, an intercostal thoracotomy (see p. 873) allows lobectomy to be performed more readily than from a median sternotomy approach. However, dogs with spontaneous pneumothorax usually have diffuse, bilateral pulmonary disease with multiple bullae. A median sternotomy allows visualization of all lung lobes and partial resection of any diseased lobes (see p. 874). Mechanical pleurodesis might be of benefit in dogs with spontaneous pneumothorax to reduce recurrence (see later discussion).

Identify and remove diseased lung. If the source of the pleural air is not evident, fill the chest with warmed sterile saline and look for air bubbles when the anesthetist ventilates the animal. If multiple partial lobectomies are necessary, use an automatic stapling device to reduce operative time. Perform pleural abrasion using a dry gauze sponge. Gently abrade the entire surface of the lung. Before closure, fill the chest cavity with warmed fluid and look for air bubbles when the

animal is ventilated to ensure that no other air leaks are present. Place a chest tube and remove residual air before recovering the animal.

> NOTE: In animals with an open pneumothorax, definitive closure of large thoracic wall defects may require mobilization of adjacent muscles to provide an airtight closure.

SUTURE MATERIALS AND SPECIAL INSTRUMENTS

In animals with spontaneous pneumothorax (in which multiple pulmonary bullae may be present), stapling devices allow partial lobectomies to be performed rapidly (see p. 876). Continuous suction devices are available commercially, or three-bottle systems can be made (see p. 902).

POSTOPERATIVE CARE AND ASSESSMENT

The animal should be observed postoperatively for pain or hypoventilation or both. Nasal insufflation is beneficial in most patients, but is especially indicated in those with diffuse underlying pulmonary diseases or those in which significant portions of the lung were resected. Analgesic therapy should be considered for all animals undergoing thoracotomy (see p. 868).

PROGNOSIS

With appropriate monitoring and care, the prognosis is excellent for animals with traumatic pneumothorax in which therapy is initiated before extreme dyspnea or respiratory arrest. Most dogs with spontaneous pneumothorax that are treated with needle thoracentesis alone or thoracostomy tubes will have continued air leakage or recurrence of pneumothorax. In a recent study, no dogs undergoing thoracotomy and lobectomy for spontaneous pneumothorax suffered recurrences during a median follow-up time of 19 months (Lipscomb et al, 2003). In another study, recurrence occurred in one of 30 dogs that underwent surgery, while 6 of 12 dogs that were treated conservatively (thoracentesis or tube thoracostomy with or without cage rest) had a recurrence of pneumothorax (Puerto et al, 2002). Mortality was substantially higher (8 of 15 [53%] versus 4 of 33 [12%]) in the dogs managed conservatively.

References

Brissot HN, Dupre GP, Bouvy BM et al: Thoracoscopic treatment of bullous emphysema in 3 dogs, *Vet Surg* 32:524, 2003.

Lipscomb VJ, Hardie RJ, Dubielzig RR: Spontaneous pneumothorax caused by pulmonary blebs and bullae in 12 dogs, *J Am Anim Hosp Assoc* 39:435, 2003.

Mitchel SL et al: Tracheal rupture associated with intubation in cats: 20 cases (1996-1998), *J Am Vet Med Assoc* 216:1592-1595, 2000.

Puerto DA, Brockman DJ, Lindquist C et al: Surgical and nonsurgical management of and selected risk factors for spontaneous pneumothorax in dogs: 64 cases (1986-1999), *J Am Vet Med Assoc* 220:1670, 2002.

White RN, Burton CA: Surgical management of intrathoracic tracheal avulsion in cats: long-term results in nine consecutive cases, *Vet Surg* 29:430, 2000.

Suggested Reading

Sephens JA, Parnell NK, Clarke K et al: Subcutaneous emphysema, pneumomediastinum, and pulmonary emphysema in a young schipperke, *J Anim Hosp Assoc* 38:121, 2002.

The dog was believed to have a variation of congenital pulmonary emphysema, which was cured by resection of the right middle lung lobe.

White HL, Roxanski EA, Tidwell AS et al: Spontaneous pneumothorax in two cats with small airway disease, *J Am Vet Med Assoc* 222:1573, 2003.

The authors report and discuss two cases of pneumothorax secondary to airway disease; both were eventually cured with medical therapy.

PLEURAL EFFUSION

DEFINITIONS

Pleural effusion refers to excessive fluid in the potential space between the **visceral pleura** of the lung and the **parietal pleura** of the chest wall.

GENERAL CONSIDERATIONS AND CLINICALLY RELEVANT PATHOPHYSIOLOGY

Fluid may accumulate in the pleural space because of decreased oncotic pressure (i.e., pure transudate caused by hypoalbuminemia [serum albumin concentration usually less than 1.6 g/dl]), increased hydrostatic pressure (i.e., modified transudate caused by cardiac disease, diaphragmatic hernia, tumor, or lung lobe torsion), increased permeability (i.e., infection or tumor, lung lobe torsion), or hemorrhage (i.e., coagulopathy, tumor, or trauma). Chylothorax (see p. 915) and pyothorax (see p. 922) are discussed separately from effusion.

DIAGNOSIS
Clinical Presentation

Signalment. Any age, breed, or gender of dog or cat may be affected.

History. The history of affected animals typically depends on the underlying cause. Most owners note that the animal has exercise intolerance if not overt respiratory distress.

Physical Examination Findings

The most common physical examination finding in animals with pleural effusion is dyspnea. The dyspnea may be marked by a forceful inspiration with delayed expiration, making the animal appear to be holding its breath. This respiratory pattern is particularly noticeable in cats. Increased bronchovesicular sounds may be heard dorsally. Lung sounds may be absent ventrally (usually bilaterally, but occasionally unilaterally). Other physical examination findings in affected dogs may include muffled heart sounds and weight loss.

Diagnostic Imaging

If the animal is not severely dyspneic, thoracic radiographs should be obtained to confirm the diagnosis of pleural fluid. Taking dorsoventral (rather than ventrodorsal) and "standing lateral" radiographic views, minimizing handling, and supplementing oxygen by face mask during the radiographic procedures help prevent further compromise of respiration. If the animal is not dyspneic and if only small amounts of fluid are suspected, ventrodorsal and expiratory views may help delineate the effusion. Radiographic signs associated with pleural effusion include soft tissue opacity causing a silhouette sign with the heart and diaphragm, visualization of soft tissue interlobar fissure lines, rounding of lung margins at the costophrenic angles, widening of the mediastinum, separation of the lung borders from the thoracic wall by a soft tissue opacity, and scalloping of the lung margins at the sternal border (Figs. 30-23 and 30-24). The presence of pleural fluid often prevents satisfactory radiographic evaluation of the thoracic cavity. Adequate visualization of the entire thorax is necessary to rule out cranial mediastinal masses (e.g., lymphoma or thymoma); therefore radiographs should be repeated after removal of most of the pleural fluid. When available, ultrasound should be used to evaluate the mediastinum before removal of the pleural fluid as the fluid serves as an acoustic window. Ultrasonography may be used to evaluate cardiac function, valvular lesions and function, congenital cardiac abnormalities, the presence of pericardial effusion, and mediastinal masses.

> NOTE: Delay thoracic radiographs until after thoracentesis in animals with pleural effusion that are severely dyspneic.

Thoracoscopy. Thoracoscopy may be used to help determine the cause of pleural effusion. Histologic analysis of thoracoscopic biopsies of 18 dogs and cats with pleural effu-

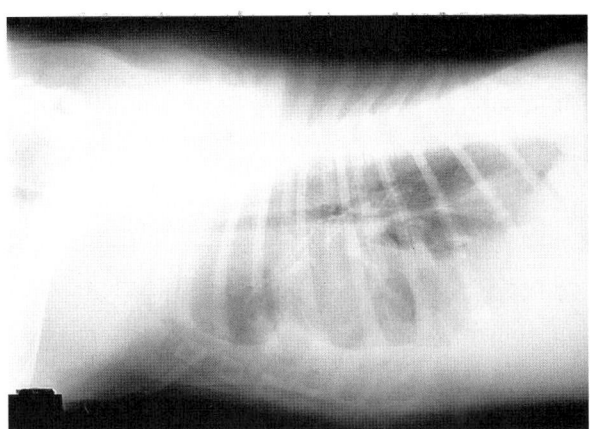

FIG. 30-23
Lateral thoracic radiograph of a dog with pleural effusion. Note the scalloped appearance of the ventral aspect of the lungs along the sternum.

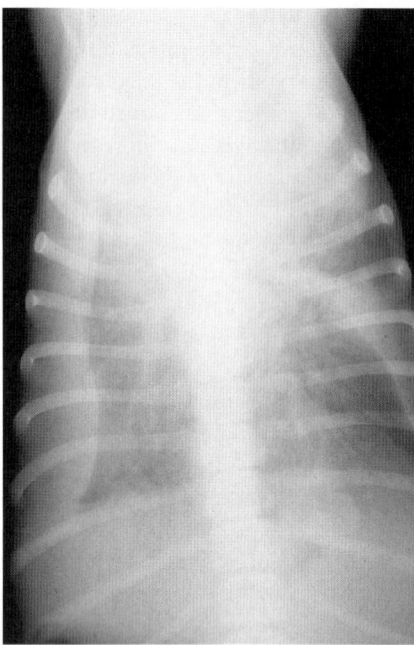

FIG. 30-24
Dorsoventral thoracic radiograph of a dog with pleural effusion. Note the interlobar fissure lines, the rounding of the lung margins at the costophrenic angles, and the separation of the lung margins from the thoracic wall.

sions determined that 8 animals had neoplasia; the remaining animals were determined to have nonneoplastic effusion (Kovak et al, 2002).

Laboratory Findings

Pleural fluid should be placed in a clot tube for biochemical studies and an EDTA tube for cytologic examination. Some should be saved in a sterile syringe for culture. It is important to analyze the fluid for protein concentration, nucleated cell count, and differential nucleated cell count. Pleural fluid may be cultured for mesothelioma cells by research laboratories. The serum albumin and electrolyte concentrations should be determined. Hyponatremia and/or hyperkalemia may be caused by pleural effusion.

DIFFERENTIAL DIAGNOSIS

Any cause of respiratory distress or coughing should be considered a differential diagnosis.

MEDICAL MANAGEMENT

For medical management of chylothorax and pyothorax, see pp. 917 and 924, respectively. Management of animals with lung lobe torsion is described on p. 889. For the medical management of the various other disorders causing pleural effusion, the reader is referred to a medical textbook. If the animal is severely hyperkalemic, symptomatic therapy with potassium-free fluids may be necessary until the effusion is controlled.

SURGICAL TREATMENT

If the cause of modified transudates or exudates cannot be found with routine laboratory testing, imaging, and/or thoracoscopy, then exploratory thoracotomy may be necessary. If the patient has a bicavitary effusion that is not due to hypoalbuminemia, then cardiac disease, neoplasia, and infectious diseases are the major differential diagnoses.

Preoperative Management

The preoperative management of animals undergoing thoracotomy is presented on p. 867.

Anesthesia

See p. 867 for selected anesthetic protocols for animals with respiratory disease. If the animal has moderate or severe pleural fluid, the chest should be tapped before induction of anesthesia.

Surgical Anatomy

The surgical anatomy of the thoracic cavity is presented on p. 870.

Positioning

See p. 871.

SURGICAL TECHNIQUE

Thoracotomy may be performed using a median sternotomy (see p. 874), if there is no discernible lesion and if the surgeon wishes to examine the entire thorax, or by using a lateral thoracotomy (see p. 873), if a lesion has been identified and if lung lobectomy is anticipated.

POSTOPERATIVE CARE AND ASSESSMENT

See p. 878 for the postoperative care of patients that have undergone thoracotomy.

PROGNOSIS

The prognosis for animals with pleural effusion depends on the underlying cause. See pp. 888, 922, and 925 for the prognosis in animals with lung lobe torsion, chylothorax, and pyothorax, respectively.

Reference

Kovak JR, Ludwig LL, Bergman PJ et al: Use of thoracoscopy to determine the etiology of pleural effusion in dogs and cats: 18 cases (1998-2001), *J Am Vet Med Assoc* 221:990, 2002.

Suggested Reading

Smeak DD, Birchard SJ, McLoughlin MA et al: Treatment of chronic pleural effusion with pleuroperitoneal shunts in dogs: 14 cases (1985-1999), *J Am Vet Med Assoc* 219:1590, 2001.
The authors concluded that they could manage intractable pleural effusions with these shunts, although numerous complications occurred.

CHYLOTHORAX

DEFINITIONS

Chyle is the term used to denote lymphatic fluid arising from the intestine and therefore containing a high quantity of fat. **Chylothorax** is a collection of chyle in the pleural space. Chylothorax is termed **idiopathic** when an underlying cause cannot be identified.

GENERAL CONSIDERATIONS AND CLINICALLY RELEVANT PATHOPHYSIOLOGY

In most animals, abnormal flow or pressures in the thoracic duct (TD) are thought to lead to exudation of chyle from intact but dilated thoracic lymphatic vessels (a condition known as thoracic lymphangiectasia; Fig. 30-25). These dilated lymphatic vessels may form in response to increased lymphatic flow (caused by increased hepatic lymph formation), decreased lymphatic drainage into the venous system as a result of high venous pressures, or both factors acting

 BOX 30-5

Abnormalities Associated With Chylothorax in Dogs and Cats

- Cardiomyopathy
- Mediastinal lymphosarcoma or thymoma
- Cranial vena cava thrombi
- Heartworm disease
- Fungal granulomas
- Pericardial effusion/heart base tumors
- Foreign objects
- Tetralogy of Fallot
- Tricuspid dysplasia
- Cor triatriatum dexter
- Congenital thoracic duct abnormalities
- Lymphangioleiomyomatosis

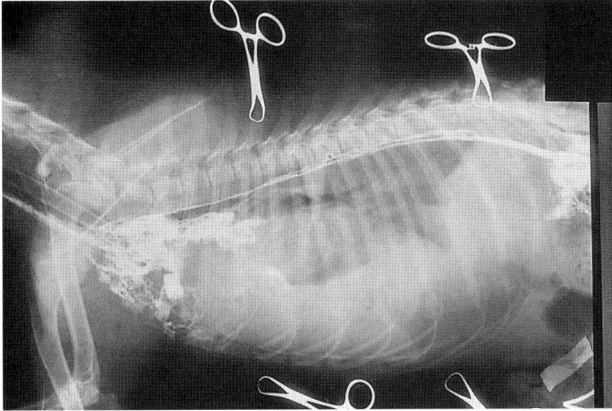

FIG. 30-25
Thoracic lymphangiectasia in a dog with idiopathic chylothorax. Note the dilated, tortuous lymphatics in the cranial mediastinum.

simultaneously to increase lymph flow and reduce drainage. Any disease or process that increases systemic venous pressures (i.e., right heart failure, mediastinal neoplasia, cranial vena cava thrombi, or granulomas) may cause chylothorax (Box 30-5). Trauma is an uncommonly recognized cause of chylothorax in dogs and cats because the TD heals rapidly after injury, and the effusion resolves within 1 to 2 weeks without treatment.

Possible causes of chylothorax include anterior mediastinal masses (mediastinal lymphoma, thymoma), heart disease (cardiomyopathy, pericardial effusion, heartworm infection, foreign objects, tetralogy of Fallot, tricuspid dysplasia, or cor triatriatum dexter), fungal granulomas, venous thrombi, and congenital abnormalities of the TD. It may occur in association with diffuse lymphatic abnormalities, including intestinal lymphangiectasia and generalized lymphangiectasia with subcutaneous chyle leakage. The underlying cause is undetermined in most animals (idiopathic chylothorax) despite extensive diagnostic work-ups. Because the treatment of this disease varies considerably depending on the underlying cause, it is imperative that clinicians identify concurrent disease processes before instituting definitive therapy.

DIAGNOSIS
Clinical Presentation

Signalment. Any breed of dog or cat may be affected; however, a breed predisposition has been suspected in the Afghan hound for a number of years. Recently, it has been suggested that the Shiba Inu breed may also be predisposed to this disease. Among cats, Oriental breeds (i.e., Siamese and Himalayan) appear to have an increased prevalence. Chylothorax may affect animals of any age; however, older cats may be more likely than young cats to develop it. This finding was believed to indicate an association between chylothorax and neoplasia. Afghan hounds appear to develop this disease in middle age, but affected Shiba Inus have been less than 1 year old. A gender predisposition has not been identified.

History. Coughing often is the first (and occasionally the only) abnormality until the animal becomes dyspneic. Many owners report that coughing began months before presenting the animal for care; therefore animals that cough and do not respond to standard treatment of nonspecific respiratory problems should be evaluated for chylothorax. Coughing may be due to irritation caused by the effusion or may be related to the underlying disease process (i.e., cardiomyopathy or thoracic neoplasia).

NOTE: Coughing may be the only clinical sign in animals with pleural effusion. Therefore chest radiographs are warranted in any animal with a chronic, nonresponsive cough.

Physical Examination Findings

Most animals with chylothorax have a normal body temperature unless they are extremely excited or severely depressed. Additional findings may include muffled heart sounds, de-

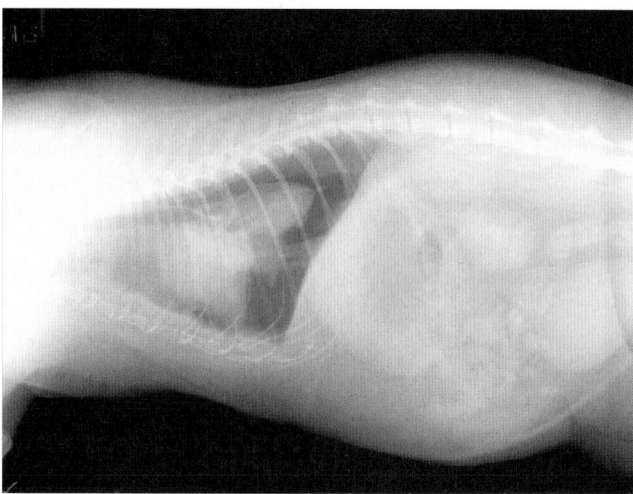

FIG. 30-26
Lateral radiograph of a cat with fibrosing pleuritis secondary to chronic chylothorax. Note the rounded margins of the lung lobes.

 TABLE 30-3

Characteristics of Chylous Effusions

CHARACTERISTIC	CATS	DOGS
Color	White or pink, (occasionally red)	Same
Clarity	Opaque, remains opaque when centrifuged	Same
SG	1.019–1.050	1.022–1.037
TP	2.6–10.3	2.5–6.2
WBC	Average: 7987	Average: 6167

SG, Specific gravity; *TP,* total protein (g/dl); *WBC,* total white cells/µl.

pression, anorexia, weight loss, pale mucous membranes, arrhythmias, murmurs, and pericardial effusion.

Diagnostic Imaging

The radiographic signs of pleural effusion are provided on p. 913. Animals that have collapsed lung lobes that do not appear to reexpand after removal of chyle or other pleural fluid should be suspected of having underlying pulmonary parenchymal or pleural disease, such as fibrosing pleuritis (Fig. 30-26). Although the cause of the fibrosis is unknown, it apparently can occur subsequent to any prolonged exudative or blood-stained effusion. Diagnosis of fibrosing pleuritis is difficult. The atelectatic lobes may be confused with metastatic or primary pulmonary neoplasia, lung lobe torsion, or hilar lymphadenopathy. Radiographic evidence of pulmonary parenchyma that fails to reexpand after removal of pleural fluid should be considered possible evidence of atelectasis with associated fibrosis. Fibrosing pleuritis should also be considered in animals with persistent dyspnea in the face of minimal pleural fluid.

> NOTE: Cats with fibrosing pleuritis are often mistaken as having postoperative pleural fluid based on radiographs. Perform an ultrasound exam on these cats before performing thoracentesis to ensure that fluid is present; thoracentesis in these cats often causes severe pneumothorax.

CT lymphangiography may be able to quantify branches of the TD more accurately than standard radiographic lymphangiography (Esterline et al, 2005). In a recent study, CT lymphangiography was performed by percutaneously injecting 1 to 2 ml of nonionic contrast material into the mesenteric lymph nodes of four dogs with chylothorax using ultrasound guidance (Johnson et al, 2005). Helical thoracic CT images were acquired before and after injection of the contrast media. The technique documented the location and character of the TD and its tributary lymphatics and may prove useful for surgical planning in animals with chylothorax.

Laboratory Findings

Fluid recovered by thoracentesis should be placed in an EDTA tube for cytologic examination. Placing the fluid in an EDTA tube rather than a clot tube allows cell counts to be performed. Although chylous effusions routinely are classified as exudates, the physical characteristics of the fluid may be consistent with a modified transudate (Table 30-3). The color varies depending on the dietary fat content and the presence of concurrent hemorrhage. The protein content is variable and often inaccurate because of interference with the refractive index by the high lipid content of the fluid. The total nucleated cell count usually is below 10,000/µl and consists primarily of small lymphocytes or neutrophils with lesser numbers of lipid-laden macrophages.

Chronic chylous effusions may contain low numbers of small lymphocytes because of the body's inability to compensate for continued lymphocyte loss. Nondegenerative neutrophils may predominate with prolonged loss of lymphocytes or if multiple therapeutic thoracenteses have induced inflammation. Degenerative neutrophils and sepsis are uncommon findings because of the bacteriostatic effect of fatty acids, but can occur iatrogenically as a result of repeated aspiration. To help determine if a pleural effusion is truly chylous, several tests can be performed, including comparison of fluid and serum triglyceride levels, Sudan III staining for lipid droplets, and the ether clearance test. The most diagnostic test is comparison of serum and fluid triglyceride levels (Box 30-6). Chylous effusions have a higher triglyceride concentration than simultaneously collected serum.

BOX 30-6

Other Characteristics of Chylous Effusions

- Triglyceride content higher than that of serum
- Cholesterol content less than or equal to that of serum
- Chylomicrons present
- Predominant cell type may be the lymphocyte or neutrophil
- Sudanophilic fat globules present
- Clears with ether

DIFFERENTIAL DIAGNOSIS

Once pleural effusion has been identified, differential diagnoses include diseases that cause exudative pleural effusion, such as pyothorax. Although chylous effusions have a characteristic appearance, the physical characteristics of chylous effusions and other exudative effusions may be similar. Also the appearance and cell populations of chylous effusions can be altered by diet and chronicity.

"Pseudochylous effusion" is a term that has been misused in the veterinary literature to describe effusions that look like chyle, but with which a ruptured TD is not found. Given the known causes of chylothorax in dogs and cats, this term should be reserved for effusions in which the pleural fluid cholesterol is greater than the serum cholesterol concentration and the pleural fluid triglyceride is less than or equal to the serum triglyceride. Pseudochylous effusions are extremely rare in veterinary patients, but may be associated with tuberculosis.

MEDICAL MANAGEMENT

If an underlying disease is diagnosed, it should be treated and the chylous effusion managed by intermittent thoracentesis. If the underlying disease is effectively treated, the effusion often resolves; however, complete resolution may take several months. Surgical intervention should be considered only in animals with idiopathic chylothorax or those that do not respond to medical management. Chest tubes should be placed only in animals suspected of having traumatic chylothorax (very rare) with rapid fluid accumulation, or occasionally after surgery. Electrolytes should be monitored; hyponatremia and hyperkalemia can occur in dogs with chylothorax undergoing multiple thoracentesis. A low-fat diet may reduce the amount of fat in the effusion, which may improve the animal's ability to resorb fluid from the thoracic cavity.

> NOTE: Animals with traumatic chylothorax heal and resolve the effusion within a few weeks; however, traumatic chylothorax is extremely rare.

Commercial low-fat diets are preferable to homemade diets; however, if commercial diets are refused, homemade diets are a reasonable alternative (Tables 30-4 and 30-5; the

 TABLE 30-4

Canine Homemade Low-fat Diet*

INGREDIENT	AMOUNT
Cooked white rice	2⅔ cups
Stewed chicken	⅓ pound
Dicalcium phosphate†	1¼ teaspoons
GNC Ca-Mg (250 mg calcium, 155 magnesium/tablet)‡	2 tablets
Morton Lite Salt	1 teaspoon
Zinc (50 mg zinc/tablet)§	½ tablet
Pet Tab	1 tablet
Radiant Valley Natural Selenium (100 µg Se/tablet)‖	1 tablet
GNC Copper (2 mg copper/tablet)‡	1 tablet

Directions: Cook rice without salt. Boil chicken and skim off fat. Crush tablets to a fine powder. Combine all ingredients and mix well. Refrigerate unused portions.
*Calculations based on the average published nutrient content of each ingredient indicate that this diet meets or exceeds the nutrient requirements for maintenance for adult dogs published by the Association of American Feed Control Officials. This recipe makes about 1½ lb of food that contains 910 kcals of metabolizable energy.
†Dicalcium phosphate 18.5% phosphorus, 22%–24% calcium, available at farm supply and feed stores.
‡Available at General Nutrition Centers (GNC).
§Available at most supermarkets.
‖Available at many supermarkets or health food stores.

fat content of these diets is about 6% on a dry basis). Medium-chain triglycerides (once thought to be absorbed directly into the portal system, bypassing the TD) are transported via the TD in dogs; therefore they may be less useful than previously believed. It is unlikely that dietary therapy will cure this disease, but it may help in the management of animals with chronic chylothorax. Clients should be informed that with the idiopathic form of this disease, the only surgical treatment that is likely to stop the effusion is TD ligation. However, the condition may resolve spontaneously in some animals after several weeks or months of medical management.

> NOTE: Do not expect low-fat diets to cure chylothorax; however, a lower fat chyle may be easier to resorb from the pleural space.

Benzopyrone drugs have been used for the treatment of lymphedema in human beings for years. Whether these drugs might be effective in reducing pleural effusion in animals with chylothorax is unknown; however, preliminary findings suggest that some animals treated with rutin

TABLE 30-5

Feline Homemade Low-fat Diet*

INGREDIENT	AMOUNT
Cooked white rice	3⅔ cups
Stewed chicken	½ pound
Dicalcium phosphate†	1½ teaspoons
GNC Ca-Mg (600 mg calcium/tablet)‡	1½ tablets
Morton Lite Salt	1 teaspoon
Taurine tablets (500 mg taurine/tablet)§	3 tablets
Zinc (50 mg zinc/tablet)‖	½ tablet
Feline Pet Tab	3 tablets
Radiant Valley Natural Selenium (100 μg Se/tablet)‖	½ tablet
Nature Made Balanced B-50 Complex‖	½ tablet
GNC Choline (250 mg choline/tablet)‡	1 tablet

Directions: Cook rice without salt. Boil chicken and skim off fat. Crush tablets to a fine powder. Combine all ingredients and mix well. Refrigerate unused portions.
*Calculations based on the average published nutrient content of each ingredient indicate that this diet meets or exceeds the nutrient requirements for maintenance for adult cats published by the Association of American Feed Control Officials. This recipe makes about 2¼ lb of food that contains 1293 kcals of metabolizable energy.
†Dicalcium phosphate 18.5% phosphorus, 22%–24% calcium, available at farm supply and feed stores.
‡Available at General Nutrition Centers (GNC).
§Taurine tablets can be purchased at most health food stores and cooperatives as 500-mg and 1000-mg tablets.
‖Available at many supermarkets.

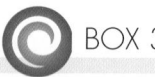 BOX 30-7

Benzopyrone for Treatment of Chylothorax*

Rutin† 50–100 mg/kg, given PO tid

PO, Oral; *tid*, three times a day.
*Efficacy is unproven at this time; clinical studies are needed.
†Obtained at health food stores.

(Box 30-7) have complete resolution of effusion 2 months after initiation of therapy. Whether the effusion resolves spontaneously in these animals or is associated with the drug therapy is unknown.

Somatostatin is a naturally occurring substance that has an extremely short half-life. It inhibits gastric, pancreatic, and biliary secretions (i.e., glucagon, insulin, gastric acid, amylase, lipase, and trypsin) and prolongs gastrointestinal transit time, decreases jejunal secretion, and stimulates gastrointestinal water absorption. In recent years, analogues of somatostatin have been used to successfully treat chylothorax in humans with traumatic or postoperative chylothorax. In these patients, reduced gastrointestinal secretions may aid healing of the TD by decreasing TD lymphatic flows. It has also been reported to result in early decreased drainage and early fistula closure in dogs with experimental transection of the TD. The mechanism by which nontraumatic chylothorax may benefit from this treatment is unclear; however, resolution of pleural fluid (chyle and postoperative serosanguineous effusion) in both dogs and cats has occurred after administration of octreotide. Octreotide (Sandostatin; 10 μg/kg subcutaneously three times a day for 2 to 3 weeks) is a synthetic analogue of somatostatin that has a prolonged half-life and minimal side effects. Soft stools that resolve after withdrawal of the drug may occur. Prolonged treatment should be discouraged because people treated for longer than 4 weeks are at risk for gallstones.

SURGICAL TREATMENT

Surgical intervention is warranted in animals that do not have underlying disease and in which medical management has become impractical or is ineffective. Surgical options include TD ligation plus pericardiectomy (with or without mesenteric lymphangiography), passive pleuroperitoneal shunting, active pleuroperitoneal or pleurovenous shunting, pericardiectomy, omental drainage, and pleurodesis. Only TD ligation, pericardiectomy, mesenteric lymphangiography, and active pleuroperitoneal shunting are recommended by the author and are described here. The mechanism by which TD ligation is purported to work is that after TD ligation, abdominal lymphaticovenous anastomoses form for transport of chyle to the venous system. Chyle bypasses the TD, and the effusion resolves. Properly performed, TD ligation results in more than 80% of dogs and cats resolving their effusion (Fossum et al, 2004). Formation of a nonchylous effusion (from pulmonary lymphatics) may occur in some animals after surgery.

Mesenteric lymphangiography may be particularly difficult to perform in cats. While mesenteric lymphangiography is not essential, catheterization of a mesenteric lymphatic and injection of methylene blue makes identification of the TD and its branches much easier. TD ligation has been performed using thoracoscopy (Radlinsky et al, 2002).

Many animals with chylothorax have either a thickened pericardium or thick tissue overlying the pericardium. This thickening is thought to be a result of the chronic irritation of chyle. It is believed that the thickened tissue might elevate systemic venous pressures, and these abnormal venous pressures may act to impede drainage of chyle into the cranial vena cava while increasing lymphatic flow through the TD. When the pericardium or overlying tissues are thickened or abnormal in animals with derangements in lymphatic flow (be it chylothorax or continued serosanguineous flow after TD ligation), pericardiectomy may act to lower right-sided venous pressures. Such normalization of venous pressures might be sufficient to allow the animal to route lymphatic fluid through normal channels. Pericardiectomy has been performed alone or in conjunction with TD ligation in a number of animals; in most of these animals the effusion has resolved (Fossum et al, 2004). Therefore pericardiectomy is recommended in conjunction with TD ligation.

> NOTE: Most failures of TD ligation are technical failures: complete ligation of the TD is not accomplished. This is particularly common in animals with severe restrictive pleuritis, and in cats in which the duct(s) is more difficult to visualize because of its small size.

Preoperative Management

Food is withheld 12 hours before surgery. Cream and/or oil may be fed before surgery (i.e., given every hour until induction of anesthesia starting 3 to 4 hours before surgery) to help visualize lymphatics. Methylene blue may be injected into a lymph node at surgery if absorption of the cream or oil is not sufficient.

Anesthesia

See p. 867 for selected anesthetic protocols for animals with respiratory disease.

Surgical Anatomy

The TD is the cranial continuation of the cisterna chyli and generally is said to begin between the crura of the diaphragm (Fig. 30-27). In cats the TD lies between the aorta and azygous vein on the left side of the mediastinum. In dogs it lies slightly on the right side of the mediastinum until it reaches the fifth or sixth vertebra and then crosses to the left side. The TD terminates in the venous system of the neck (left external jugular vein or jugulosubclavian angle).

Positioning

If a thoracic approach to the TD is used (see p. 920), the left side (cats) or right side (dogs) of the thorax and abdomen is prepared for aseptic surgery. If a transdiaphragmatic approach is used, the cranial abdomen and caudal chest are prepped.

SURGICAL TECHNIQUE
Mesenteric Lymphangiography

For a thoracic approach, make a paracostal incision (or for a transdiaphragmatic approach, make a cranial midline abdominal incision), exteriorize the cecum, and locate an adjacent lymph node.

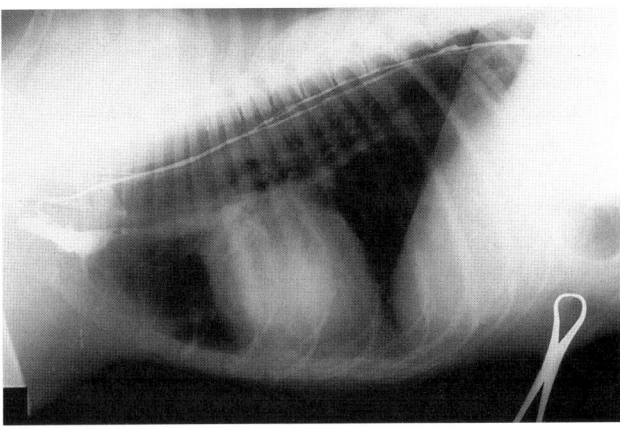

FIG. 30-27
Mesenteric lymphangiogram of a normal dog. Note the multiple branches of the TD.

> NOTE: The TD is difficult to approach transdiaphragmatically in deep-chested dogs. This approach may be used in small dogs and cats, but should be avoided in larger dogs. An intercostal approach to the TD is preferred in medium and large breeds and can be used in any animal.

If necessary, inject a small volume of dilute (1 part methylene blue to 5 to 10 parts saline) methylene blue (0.5 to 1 ml) into the lymph node to increase lymphatic visualization. Avoid repeated doses of methylene blue because of the risk of inducing a Heinz body anemia or renal failure. Find a lymphatic near the node to catheterize by gently dissecting the mesentery. Cannulate the lymphatic with a 20- to 25-gauge over-the-needle catheter and attach a three-way catheter and extension tubing (filled with heparinized saline) to the catheter with a suture (3-0 silk). Place an additional suture around the extension tubing and through a segment of intestine to prevent dislodgment of the catheter. Either inject a small amount of dilute methylene blue directly into the catheter or if a contrast radiograph is preferred, inject 1 ml/kg of a dilute (diluted 50% with sterile saline) water-soluble contrast agent (i.e., Renovist) into the catheter and take a lateral thoracic radiograph while the last milliliter is flushed into the catheter. Use the lymphangiogram to help identify the number and location of branches of the TD that need to be ligated. If desired, repeat the lymphangiogram after TD ligation (see later discussion) to identify branches that were not occluded.

> NOTE: I seldom perform contrast lymphangiography, but catheterization of a mesenteric lymphatic for injection of methylene blue is extremely helpful in localizing the ducts and ensuring their complete ligation.

Embolization of the TD with cyanoacrylate injected through a mesenteric lymphatic catheter has been reported in dogs. An advantage of TD embolization is that direct visualization of the TD is not required, which eliminates the need for a thoracotomy or diaphragmatic incision. Disadvantages of this procedure are the same as those for mesenteric lymphangiography and TD ligation (i.e., not all TD branches may fill with the cyanoacrylate mixture, and collateralization may occur past the obstruction).

Thoracic Duct Ligation

Perform an intercostal thoracotomy (right side for dogs, left side for cats) at the eighth, ninth, or tenth intercostal space or make an incision in the diaphragm (see p. 919). Locate the TD and use hemostatic clips and/or silk suture (2-0 or 3-0) to ligate it (see p. 921).

Visualization of the TD is greatly aided by injecting methylene blue into the lymphatic catheter (see previous discussion).

Perform a subtotal pericardiectomy by reaching forward under the rib cage.

NOTE: Wear magnification and use a headlight to help visualize the TD and its small branches.

Active Pleuroperitoneal or Pleurovenous Shunting

Commercially made shunt catheters (see later discussion for ordering information) are available and can be used to pump pleural fluid into the abdomen (Fig. 30-28) or into a vein (i.e., jugular, azygous, or caudal vena cava). Two types of shunts are available: a pleuroperitoneal shunt (Box 30-8) and an ascites (peritoneovenous) shunt (Box 30-9). The latter is meant to pump fluid from the abdomen into a vein and does not require manual pumping (i.e., it functions in an active fashion). This shunt can be placed from the pleural space into a vein (pleurovenous); when used in this manner, manual pumping is required (the shunt will not function in an active fashion). Close observation of these patients for several weeks after pleurovenous shunt placement is necessary, and preoperative heparinization and maintenance on heparin, aspirin, or other anticoagulants may be warranted. For other complications, see later discussion. Both types of catheters are placed under general anesthetic.

Place the pump chamber and tubing in a bowl of sterilized, heparinized saline. Prime the pump by compressing the valve repeatedly until the system is filled with fluid and flow is established. Expel any remaining air bubbles from the tubing or valve. Make a vertical incision over the middle of the sixth, seventh, or eighth rib. Bluntly insert the pleural end of the shunt catheter into the thoracic cavity. For a pleuro-

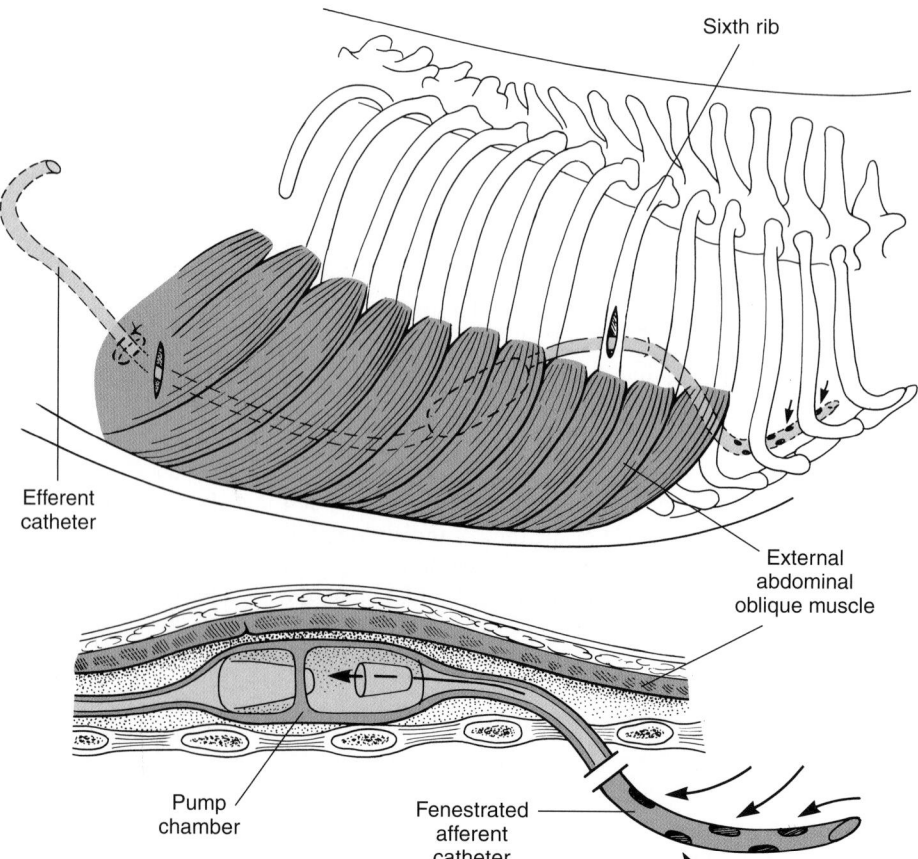

FIG. 30-28
To place a pleuroperitoneal shunt, put the afferent end of the catheter into the thoracic cavity and the efferent end into the abdominal cavity. Make sure the pump chamber overlies a rib so that the chamber can be compressed effectively.

Sixth rib

Efferent catheter

External abdominal oblique muscle

Pump chamber

Fenestrated afferent catheter

peritoneal shunt, use blunt dissection to create a tunnel under the external abdominal oblique muscle and pull the pump chamber through the tunnel. Place the efferent (peritoneal) end of the catheter into the abdominal cavity just caudal to the costal arch through a small skin incision and place a preplaced purse-string suture in the abdominal musculature. For a pleurovenous shunt, tunnel the efferent (venous) end of the catheter over the shoulder to the ventral cervical region. Make a small incision over the jugular vein, and insert the venous end of the catheter into the vein. Using fluoroscopy, place the distal end of the catheter at the caudal aspect of the cranial vena cava, just proximal to the right atrium (the venous end of the catheter may be shortened if necessary). As an alternative, the venous end of the catheter may be placed in the azygous or caudal vena cava through an abdominal incision. Make sure the pump chamber overlies a rib so that the chamber can be effectively compressed.

SUTURE MATERIALS AND SPECIAL INSTRUMENTS

The advantage of using hemoclips is that they can be used as a reference point on subsequent radiographs if further ligation is necessary. However, it is best to also ligate the duct with nonabsorbable suture (i.e., silk) if hemoclips are used. Shunts for active drainage include the Denver double-valve pleurovenous and pleuroperitoneal shunts (Denver Biomaterials, Inc. Denver).

POSTOPERATIVE CARE AND ASSESSMENT

If chylothorax resolves spontaneously or after surgery, periodic reevaluation for several years is warranted to detect recurrence. Fibrosing pleuritis is the most common serious complication of chronic chylothorax (see p. 902). Immunosuppression may occur in patients undergoing repeated and frequent thoracentesis because of lymphocyte depletion.

COMPLICATIONS

The most common complication of TD ligation is continued chylous or serosanguineous effusion. With proper technique, the incidence of continued chylous effusion is minimal. Unfortunately, when a serosanguineous effusion occurs after surgery, further surgery involving the TD is of no benefit. Somatostatin (see p. 918), pericardiectomy, or a pleuroperitoneal shunt should be considered.

The most common complication of pleurovenous shunt placement is shunt occlusion (Fig. 30-29). Conscientious pumping of the catheter multiple times a day may reduce this complication. It is also less likely to occur if the fluid is serosanguineous rather than chyle. If a clot occludes the pump, injection of streptokinase may help dissolve it. A possible complication of pleurovenous shunt placement is formation of a right atrial and/or ventricular thrombus. This complication may be life threatening; therefore pleuroperitoneal shunting is preferred if there is no reason to believe that the animal may not reabsorb the fluid from its abdominal cavity (e.g., presence of diffuse lymphatic disease or cardiac disease).

 BOX 30-8

Pleuroperitoneal Shunt Specifications

- 27-cm fenestrated pleural end
- Two one-way valves
- 49-cm fenestrated peritoneal catheter
- Each complete pump of the reservoir dome transferring 1.5 ml of fluid

From Denver Biomaterials, Inc., Denver.

 BOX 30-9

Pleurovenous (Peritoneovenous) Shunt Specifications*

- 27-cm fenestrated pleural end
- Single or double one-way valves
- 66-cm fenestrated venous catheter
- Double valve: comes in a standard flow rate (26–40 ml/min at 10-cm head of water) and a low flow rate (less than 26 ml/min at 10-cm head of water)

From Denver Biomaterials, Inc., Denver.
*This shunt comes in a single- and double-valve form; the double-valve catheter is indicated when the shunt is to be placed in a pleuro-venous fashion.

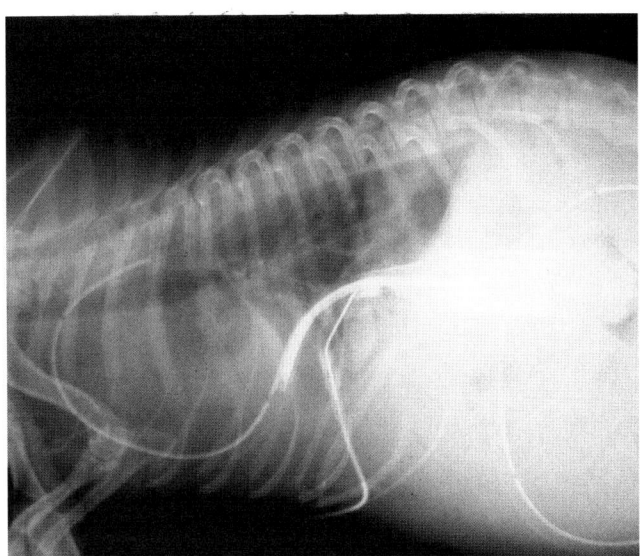

FIG. 30-29
Radiograph of a dog with a pleuroperitoneal shunt in which contrast has been injected into the catheter just proximal to the pump chamber. The inflow catheter has a large, occluding clot in it. (Courtesy Dr. Blaine Andrews.)

PROGNOSIS

This condition may resolve spontaneously or after surgery. Untreated or chronic chylothorax may cause severe fibrosing pleuritis and persistent dyspnea. Euthanasia frequently is performed in animals that do not respond to surgery or medical management. TD ligation plus pericardiectomy resolves pleural effusion in most animals if properly performed. In a recent study, clinical signs of pleural fluid accumulation resolved in 10 of 10 dogs and in 8 of 10 cats after surgery (Fossum et al, 2004). Continued chylous effusions are typically due to technical failures in completely ligating the duct and its branches. Postoperative serosanguineous fluid occurs in some dogs after surgery; octreotide may be beneficial in these animals. If octreotide is unsuccessful, a pleuroperitoneal shunt may be indicated.

References

Esterline ML, Radlinsky MG, Biller DS et al: Comparison of radiographic and computed tomography lymphangiography for identification of the canine thoracic duct, *Vet Radiol Ultrasound* 46:391, 2005.

Fossum TW, Mertens MM, Miller MW et al: Thoracic duct ligation and pericardiectomy for treatment of idiopathic chylothorax, *J Vet Intern Med* 18:307, 2004.

Johnson EG, Wisner ER, Marks SL et al: Contrast enhanced CT thoracic duct lymphography, ACVR Annual Scientific Conference, 2005 (abstract).

Radlinsky MG, Mason DE, Biller DS et al: Thoracoscopic visualization and ligation of the thoracic duct in dogs, *Vet Surg* 31:138, 2002.

Suggested Reading

Enwiller TM, Radlinsky MG, Mason DE et al: Popliteal and mesenteric lymph node injection with methylene blue for coloration of the thoracic duct in dogs, *Vet Surg* 32:359, 2003.

Thoracic duct coloration after mesenteric lymph node injection occurred within 10 minutes and persisted for 60 minutes.

Hayashi K, Sicard G, Gellasch K et al: Cisterna chyli ablation with thoracic duct ligation for chylothorax: results in eight dogs, *Vet Surg* 34:519, 2005.

Cisterna chyli ablation plus thoracic duct ligation resolved chylothorax in 88% of dogs.

Sicard GK, Waller KR, McAnulty JF: The effect of cisterna chyli ablation combined with thoracic duct ligation on abdominal lymphatic drainage, *Vet Surg* 34:64, 2005.

Cisterna chyli ablation plus thoracic duct ligation successfully rerouted chyle flow into abdominal veins in 5 of 6 dogs.

Smeak DD, Birchard J, McLoughlin MA et al: Treatment of chronic pleural effusion with pleuroperitoneal shunts in dogs: 14 cases (1985-1999), *J Am Vet Med Assoc* 219:1590, 2001.

Eight of 11 dogs with long-term follow-up developed complications; the overall mean survival time and the interval in which dogs remained free of clinical signs of pleural effusion were 27 months (range: 1 to 108 months) and 20 months (range: 0.5 to 108 months), respectively.

PYOTHORAX

DEFINITION

Pyothorax *(thoracic empyema)* is suppurative inflammation of the thoracic cavity with a resultant accumulation of pus.

GENERAL CONSIDERATIONS AND CLINICALLY RELEVANT PATHOPHYSIOLOGY

The route by which the thoracic cavity becomes infected usually is not evident (i.e., hematogenous spread; migrating foreign objects such as plant awns; penetrating wounds, particularly bite wounds; extension from discospondylitis; extension from pneumonia; pulmonary neoplasia or abscessation; pulmonary or thoracic wall trauma; esophageal perforation; and postoperative infection). Immunosuppressive diseases (e.g., feline leukemia virus [FeLV] and feline immunodeficiency virus [FIV]) should be excluded in animals with pyothorax, but there is no evidence that development of pyothorax requires debilitation or an increased susceptibility to infection. Thoracic puncture (e.g., bite wounds) may be a less common cause of pyothorax in cats than previously believed. Direct extension from pulmonary disease may be a cause in many animals.

A number of organisms often are cultured from animals with pyothorax; however, there is a high incidence of obligate anaerobes as sole pathogens (Table 30-6). Obligate anaerobic infections or gram-positive filamentous organisms (i.e., *Nocardia* and *Actinomyces* spp.) frequently are cultured from dogs with pyothorax (Fig. 30-30); obligate anaerobes and/or *Pasteurella* spp. are the most common feline isolates.

DIAGNOSIS
Clinical Presentation

Signalment. There is no breed predisposition, and pyothorax may occur in animals of any age. It has been widely held that young male cats that fight and receive chest wounds are at increased risk; however, in a recent study parapneumonic spread of infection after colonization and invasion of lung tissue by oropharyngeal flora was the most frequent cause of feline pyothorax (Barr et al, 2005). Cats from multi-cat households appear to be at increased risk. Adult large-breed dogs (particularly hunting dogs) may be more commonly affected because they often inhale plant foreign material and suffer penetrating thoracic wounds.

History. A delay of several weeks between the trauma that induced the pyothorax and the onset of clinical signs is not uncommon. Most animals are presented for evaluation of respiratory distress or anorexia or both. Coughing is a common presenting complaint in cats with pyothorax.

Physical Examination Findings

Affected animals usually have a restrictive respiratory pattern (i.e., rapid, shallow respirations), and many are febrile. Additional findings in patients with pyothorax may include depression, anorexia, weight loss, dehydration, muffled heart and lung sounds, and pale mucous membranes. The

TABLE 30-6

Morphologic Characteristics and Typical Antibiotic Susceptibilities of Bacteria Commonly Associated With Pyothorax in Small Animals

| | OXYGEN | | |
ORGANISM	REQUIREMENTS	GRAM'S STAIN	ANTIBIOTIC SENSITIVITY*
Actinomyces spp.	Facultative anaerobe to strict anaerobe	Gram positive	**Ampicillin, amoxicillin plus clavulanic acid, penicillin G,** clindamycin, chloramphenicol, erythromycin, minocycline
Bacteroides spp.	Obligate anaerobe	Gram negative	Most *Bacteroides* spp.: **ampicillin, amoxicillin plus clavulanic acid,** clindamycin, chloramphenicol, metronidazole *B. fragilis:* **amoxicillin plus clavulanic acid, clindamycin, metronidazole,** chloramphenicol
Clostridium spp.	Obligate anaerobe	Gram positive	Most *Clostridium* spp.: ampicillin, **amoxicillin plus clavulanic acid,** chloramphenicol, **metronidazole** *C. perfringens:* **ampicillin, amoxicillin plus clavulanic acid,** cefoxitin, clindamycin, chloramphenicol, metronidazole
Escherichia coli	Facultative anaerobe	Gram negative	**Amikacin, enrofloxacin,** ceftizoxime, cefotaxime, potentiated sulfa drugs
Fusobacterium spp.	Obligate anaerobe	Gram negative	**Ampicillin, amoxicillin plus clavulanic acid,** clindamycin, chloramphenicol, metronidazole
Klebsiella spp.	Facultative anaerobe	Gram negative	**Amikacin, ceftizoxime, cefotaxime, ceftriaxone,** enrofloxacin
Nocardia spp.	Aerobe	Gram positive (partly acid fast)	**Trimethoprim-sulfa, amikacin,** imipenem, cefotaxime, doxycycline, minocycline
Pasteurella spp.	Facultative anaerobe	Gram negative	**Ampicillin, amoxicillin plus clavulanic acid, cephalosporins,** aminoglycosides
Pseudomonas spp.	Aerobe	Gram negative	**Ticarcillin plus clavulanic acid, amikacin, enrofloxacin, ceftazidime**

*Drug names in boldface type are the typical drugs of choice.

chest wall may seem incompressible in cats with thoracic effusion.

Diagnostic Imaging

Thoracic radiographs usually reveal pleural effusion (see p. 913). The cause of the pyothorax is seldom apparent radiographically; however, increased opacity in the thoracic cavity after thoracentesis may indicate an abscess or foreign body. Consolidated lung lobes that do not reexpand after fluid removal may indicate fibrosing pleuritis (see p. 916) or lung lobe torsion (see p. 888).

Laboratory Findings

Neutrophilia (with or without a degenerative left shift) may be present on a complete blood cell count. Fluid analysis is necessary to differentiate pyothorax from other exudative effusions. The fluid can range from amber to red or white. The protein content usually is greater than 3.5 g/dl, and the fluid appears turbid or opaque because of the high nucleated

cell count. Nucleated cells consist primarily of degenerative neutrophils (Fig. 30-31), but nondegenerative neutrophils can predominate, depending on the causative agent and prior antibiotic therapy. Effusions associated with fungi and higher bacterial agents, such as *Actinomyces* and *Nocardia* spp., often are characterized cytologically by nondegenerative neutrophils and macrophages or may appear hemorrhagic. Macrophages and reactive mesothelial cells are present in purulent effusions in variable numbers, depending on the cause and the chronicity of the fluid. Bacteria are often found, and filamentous rods are suggestive of *Nocardia* spp. or *Actinomyces* spp. along with *Filifactor villosus.* Performing cytology of any "sulfur granules" in the fluid (yellow masses that resemble sulfur) increases the chance of finding *Nocardia* and *Actinomyces.* Occasionally, fungal elements may be noted in the pleural effusion of animals with fungal disease involving the pulmonary parenchyma. Positive culture results may not be obtained in all animals with pyothorax, particularly if anaerobic organisms are present. Hyponatre-

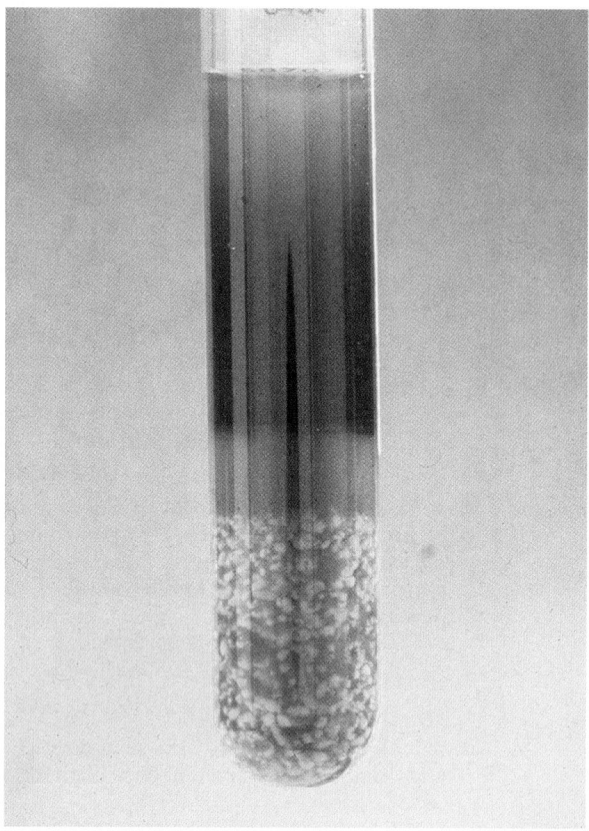

FIG. 30-30
Nocardial pleural effusion.

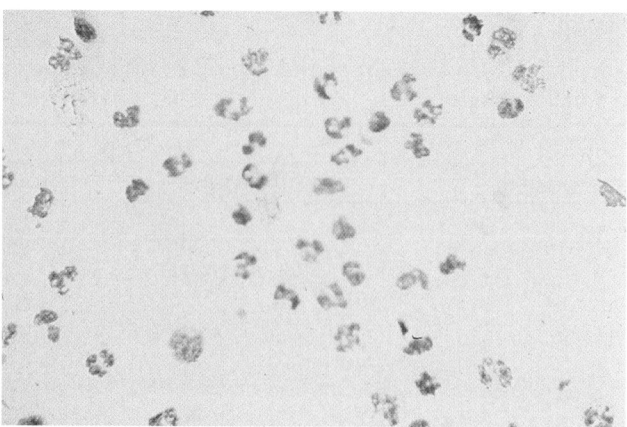

FIG. 30-31
Cytologic study of pleural fluid from a cat with pyothorax.
Note the predominance of degenerative neutrophils.

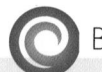 BOX 30-10

Management of Animals With Pyothorax

1. Perform Gram's stain and culture and sensitivity of fluid and initiate broad-spectrum antibiotic therapy (see text and Table 30-6).
2. Place one or more chest tubes and lavage thoracic cavity with 20 ml/kg body weight warmed, isotonic fluid with heparin added (1500 U heparin/100 ml lavage solution).*
3. Alter antibiotic therapy based on culture and sensitivity results (but treat for anaerobes even if none are grown in culture) and continue antibiotics for 4 to 6 weeks.

*Note: Although this dosage does not typically result in anticoagulation, monitor coagulation status and reduce dosage if necessary.

mia, hypochloremia, hypoalbuminemia, and increased serum total bilirubin concentrations and aminotransferase activity have been reported in cats with pyothorax (Waddell et al, 2002).

DIFFERENTIAL DIAGNOSIS

Any cause of dyspnea is a differential diagnosis (i.e., cardiac disease, pulmonary disease, mediastinal neoplasia, or diaphragmatic hernia). Once pleural effusion has been diagnosed, other causes of exudative effusion (i.e., chylothorax, feline infectious peritonitis [FIP]) or transudative effusion (i.e., hypoalbuminemia and congestive heart failure) must also be considered. Foul-smelling fluid suggests anaerobic bacteria.

MEDICAL MANAGEMENT

Although the cause of the effusion often is not discernible, attempts should be made to find and, if possible, correct underlying diseases. Management of these animals needs to be aggressive (Box 30-10). After diagnosis, a chest tube should be placed. If available, continuous suction devices can be used; however, most animals can be managed with intermittent aspiration. Lavage should be performed two or three times daily. Isotonic fluid, such as saline or lactated Ringer's solution (warmed to room temperature), should be used at a dosage of 20 ml/kg of body weight. The fluid remains in the thoracic cavity for 1 hour and is then re-

moved. Addition of antibiotics to the lavage fluid offers no advantage over the use of appropriate systemic antibiotics. If antibiotics are used in the lavage fluid, the systemic dose should be reduced to minimize toxicity. The use of proteolytic enzymes is controversial and is no longer recommended by most authors. However, the addition of heparin (1500 units/100 ml of lavage solution or administering 100 U/kg SC tid) appears beneficial. Lavage may be required for 5 to 7 days. Systemic antibiotic therapy should be based on the results of microbial culture and sensitivity testing (see Table 30-6). The prevalence of anaerobic infections is high (see previous discussion), and a combination of drugs that are active against obligate anaerobic bacteria (i.e., ampicillin, clindamycin, amoxicillin-clavulanic acid, or metronidazole) and facultative bacteria, especially *Escherichia coli* (e.g., amikacin, enrofloxacin, ceftizoxime, or potentiated sulfa drugs), should be used in dogs. In cats, *Pasteurella* spp. and anaerobes are commonly isolated, and penicillin and its derivatives (e.g., ampicillin and amoxicillin-clavulanic acid) may be indicated while awaiting results of culture and susceptibility testing. Antibiotics should be continued for a minimum of 4 to 6 weeks. Recommended antibiotics for

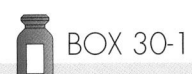

BOX 30-11

Selected Antibiotics for Use Against *Actinomyces* spp.* and *Nocardia* spp.

Actinomyces

Ampicillin†

22–44 mg/kg IM, SC, PO or IV qid

Nocardia

Potentiated sulfa drug‡

45 mg/kg PO bid or

Amikacin

20–25 mg/kg IV or SC qd§

IM, Intramuscular; *SC,* subcutaneous; *PO,* oral; *IV,* intravenous; *qid,* four times a day; *bid,* twice a day; *qd,* once a day.
*Treat for a minimum of 6 weeks.
†May not be effective against L-phase variants.
‡Observe for side effects (e.g., anemia, thrombocytopenia, hepatic disease, arthritis, vasculitis, and keratoconjunctivitis sicca).
§Monitor periodically for renal dysfunction. The dose used for *Nocardia* is much higher than is used for other infections.

Actinomyces and nocardial infections are provided in Box 30-11.

> NOTE: *Escherichia coli* isolates appear to be less sensitive to enrofloxacin than in the past; this should be considered when choosing antibiotics before receiving the results of culture and sensitivity testing.

SURGICAL TREATMENT

Surgery is indicated in animals that have underlying disease (i.e., lung abscess, lung lobe torsion, or foreign body) and in those that do not respond to medical management in 3 to 4 days. If pyothorax is chronic or localized, or if the patient remains dyspneic in the absence of significant volumes of pleural fluid, fibrosing pleuritis may be present (see p. 902). Surgical exploration of the thoracic cavity may be warranted in such patients.

Preoperative Management

Thoracentesis should be performed before induction of anesthesia if the animal is dyspneic. The animal should be normally hydrated, and significant electrolyte and acid-base abnormalities should be corrected before surgery.

Anesthesia

Refer to anesthetic management of animals with respiratory impairment, p. 867.

Surgical Anatomy

See p. 897 for a description of the pleural space and fluid movement in normal animals.

Positioning

See the description of thoracic procedures beginning on p. 871.

SURGICAL TECHNIQUE

Approach the thorax by an intercostal thoracotomy (see p. 873) if an abnormality can be localized to one hemithorax or by a median sternotomy (see p. 874) if localization is not possible. Explore the thoracic cavity for abscesses, foreign bodies, or other abnormalities, and remove affected tissue. If possible, remove fibrin covering the lung tissue. Submit appropriate samples for microbiologic examination and culture. Place a chest tube for postoperative lavage. Before closure, lavage the thoracic cavity with warmed, sterile saline solution.

SUTURE MATERIALS AND SPECIAL INSTRUMENTS

Braided, nonabsorbable, multifilament suture (e.g., silk) should not be used for lobectomy or partial lobectomy in these patients. Absorbable suture (i.e., polydioxanone or polyglyconate) is preferred if infection is present.

POSTOPERATIVE CARE AND ASSESSMENT

Thoracic lavage should be continued postoperatively until the infection resolves (see p. 924). Serum protein and electrolytes (i.e., potassium) should be monitored and fluid therapy continued until the animal is eating and drinking normally. Antibiotic therapy should be continued for at least 4 to 6 weeks (see p. 924). Refer to the postoperative management of animals undergoing thoracotomy procedures, p. 878, for additional recommendations.

PROGNOSIS

The prognosis for most animals with pyothorax is good if they are managed as described above. Recurrence is common in animals treated with antibiotics only (i.e., without thoracic lavage). Long-standing empyema may resorb, leaving a pleural "peel," which is a thick sheet of fibroblasts and inflammatory cells attached to the visceral pleura. This pleural peel may inhibit normal expansion of lung tissue (fibrosing pleuritis; see p. 902). If multiple lung lobes are fibrosed and cannot expand normally, the prognosis may be poor. The survival rate in a recent study of feline pyothorax was 66.1%; however, 28 of 80 cats were euthanized, the majority with no treatment (Waddell et al, 2002). Another study reported that 21 of 27 cats were successfully treated, 19 of which had tube thoracostomy drainage and lavage (Barrs et al, 2005). Hypersalivation, possibly associated with pain, was a common clinical finding in cats that did not survive in the aforementioned study. Interestingly, bradycardia was a negative predictor for survival, similar to what has been reported in cats with sepsis.

Reference

Wadell LS, Brady CA, Drobatz KJ: Risk factors, prognostic indicators, and outcome of pyothorax in cats: 80 cases (1986-1999), *J Am Vet Med Assoc* 221:819, 2002.

Suggested Reading

Demetriou JL, Foale RD, Ladlow J et al: Canine and feline pyothorax: a retrospective study of 50 cases in the UK and Ireland, *J Small Anim Pract* 43:398, 2002.

The authors suggested that lavage may decrease the duration of drainage in affected animals.

Rooney MB, Monnet E: Medical and surgical treatment of pyothorax in dogs: 26 cases (1991-2001), *J Am Vet Med Assoc* 221:86, 2002.

Nineteen dogs had thoracotomy with a median sternotomy; the authors concluded that surgical therapy was associated with a better outcome than medical therapy. The authors recommend surgery if *Actinomyces* is grown from the fluid, or if there are mediastinal or pulmonary lesions on radiographs.

Walker AL, Jang SS, Hirsh DC: Bacteria associated with pyothorax of dogs and cats: 98 cases (1989-1998), *J Am Vet Med Assoc* 216:359, 2000.

Bacteria were isolated from thoracic fluid in more than 92% of dogs and cats with pyothorax. Obligate anaerobes and facultative bacteria were most commonly isolated.

THYMOMAS, THYMIC BRANCHIAL CYSTS, AND MEDIASTINAL CYSTS

DEFINITIONS

Thymomas are tumors that arise from epithelial tissue of the thymus. **Thymic branchial cysts** develop from vestiges of the fetal branchial arch system. **Mediastinal cysts** are fluid-filled structures located in the cranial mediastinum that are typically benign.

GENERAL CONSIDERATIONS AND CLINICALLY RELEVANT PATHOPHYSIOLOGY

Masses in the mediastinum of dogs and cats are often neoplastic, although abscesses, granulomas, and cysts occasionally are found. A recent study reported 9 cats (mean age 13.6 years) that were diagnosed with cranial mediastinal cysts (Zekas and Adams, 2002). The majority of cats had no evidence of respiratory disease. The masses were all benign and the cats remained asymptomatic for 3 to 45 months after diagnosis. Thus many older cats having cystic mediastinal masses have benign lesions requiring no treatment. Although opacities in the cranial mediastinum on thoracic radiographs should be investigated with ultrasound, in asymptomatic cats with cystic lesions serial evaluation with radiography or ultrasound may be all that is warranted.

Lymphoma is the most common cranial mediastinal tumor in dogs and cats. Other tumors occasionally found here include thymomas, chemodectomas (aortic and carotid body tumors), and ectopic thyroid and parathyroid tumors. Thymomas are the most common surgically treatable neoplasm of the cranial mediastinum in dogs; most are benign. However, because the histologic appearance of the tumor correlates poorly with clinical behavior, the terms "invasive" or "noninvasive" are preferred. Stage I (i.e., noninvasive) thymomas are well circumscribed and do not extend beyond the thymic capsule (Table 30-7). Others may extend beyond

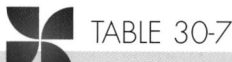 TABLE 30-7

Proposed Staging Scheme for Thymomas

STAGE	DESCRIPTION
I	Growth completely within intact thymic capsule
II	Pericapsular growth into mediastinal fat tissue, adjacent pleura, and/or pericardium
III	Invasion into surrounding organs and/or intrathoracic metastasis
IV	Extrathoracic metastasis

Paraneoplastic Syndromes

P_0	No evidence of paraneoplastic syndrome
P_1	Myasthenia gravis
P_2	Nonthymic malignant tumor

Modified from Aronson M: *Vet Clin North Am Small Anim Pract* 15:755, 1985.

the capsule locally or may invade surrounding organs and/or metastasize to other thoracic or extrathoracic structures.

The clinical signs associated with thymomas may be due to occupation of space and/or paraneoplastic syndrome. Thymomas may cause respiratory distress by compressing the lungs or trachea and/or by inducing pleural effusion as they enlarge. Effusions associated with thymomas may be serosanguineous or chylous. Paraneoplastic syndromes are distant effects of a tumor. Nearly 50% of dogs with thymoma have myasthenia gravis (Wood et al, 2001). Myasthenia gravis is an autoimmune neuromuscular disorder characterized by muscular weakness. The weakness is due to a deficiency of functional acetylcholine receptors in the neuromuscular postsynaptic membrane caused by autoantibodies that bind to and block the receptors. Another paraneoplastic syndrome associated with thymomas is polymyositis. As thymomas enlarge, they may compress the cranial vena cava and other cranial thoracic vessels, causing edema of the head, neck, and/or forelimbs (cranial vena cava syndrome). Thymic branchial cysts develop from vestiges of the branchial arch system of the fetus. They may be found in the subcutaneous tissues of the neck or in the thymus. Rupture of these cysts may result in a chronic inflammatory reaction and abscessation.

DIAGNOSIS
Clinical Presentation

Signalment. The average age of dogs with thymomas is 8 to 9 years; however, thymomas have been reported in dogs as young as 3 years old. Large-breed dogs, particularly German shepherds, golden retrievers, and Labrador retrievers, are more commonly affected than small dogs. A gender predisposition has not been identified. Most cats with thymomas have been older than 8 years of age. Thymic branchial cysts also occur most commonly in middle-aged and older animals; however, dogs as young as 18 months of age have been affected. Mediastinal cysts are found in older cats.

> NOTE: Even though the thymus involutes with age, both thymomas and thymic branchial cysts occur in middle-aged and older dogs.

History. Dogs with thymomas may be presented because of dyspnea, coughing, weight loss, lethargy, dysphagia, muscle weakness, vomiting and/or regurgitation, excessive salivation, and/or neck edema. Onset of clinical signs may be acute despite relatively slow tumor enlargement. Lethargy, anorexia, dyspnea, and pleural effusion are common in cats with thymoma. Occasionally thymomas are fortuitous findings on thoracic radiographs of asymptomatic animals. Clinical findings in dogs and cats with thymic branchial cysts are similar to those in animals with thymomas. Most are presented for evaluation of progressive dyspnea. Lameness and swelling of the head, neck, and forelimbs are also common.

Physical Examination Findings

Clinical findings in dogs with thymomas vary between patients. Respiratory abnormalities caused by pleural effusion or aspiration pneumonia may be the predominant finding. Other animals may be presented for evaluation of generalized exertional weakness without evidence of respiratory problems. Occasionally, localized forms of myasthenia are found in which the weakness is limited to the esophagus, larynx or pharynx, or facial musculature. The most common clinical findings in dogs and cats with thymic branchial cysts are dyspnea and pleural effusion.

> NOTE: Be sure to evaluate all dogs with thymomas for myasthenia gravis and megaesophagus.

Diagnostic Imaging

Animals with mediastinal masses may show dorsal elevation of the trachea and caudal displacement of the heart on lateral thoracic radiographs (Fig. 30-32). The mediastinum may appear widened on the ventrodorsal view, and the heart may be deviated laterally. Pleural effusion is commonly associated with invasive tumors, and pneumothorax is rare. Megaesophagus or secondary aspiration pneumonia (or both) may be noted on thoracic radiographs. Ultrasonography often is helpful in assessing mediastinal masses and in ruling out extrathoracic metastasis. Ultrasound-guided aspirates or biopsy may also be performed. Ultrasonographic evaluation of a mediastinal cyst usually reveals a thin-walled structure with anechoic fluid in the center.

Laboratory Findings

Specific laboratory abnormalities are not found with thymoma or branchial cysts. Leukocytosis may be present if the animal has aspiration pneumonia. Pleural effusion associ-

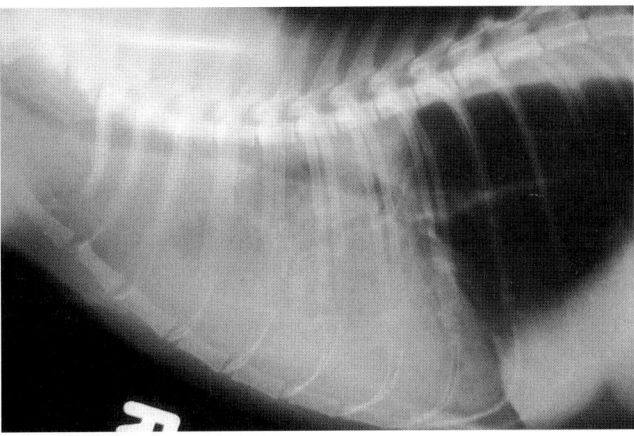

FIG. 30-32
Radiograph of a cat with a well-delineated thymoma. Note the dorsal elevation of the trachea, indicative of a mediastinal mass.

ated with thymoma or thymic branchial cysts may contain mature lymphocytes; however, immature lymphocytes indicate lymphoma. Both lymphoma and thymoma may cause chylous effusions (see p. 915).

DIFFERENTIAL DIAGNOSIS

Differential diagnoses for cranial mediastinal masses include both neoplastic and nonneoplastic disease (Box 30-12). The most important differential diagnosis is mediastinal lymphoma because treatment for lymphoma does not involve surgery. Therefore a definitive diagnosis should be made before surgery whenever possible. The presence of hypercalcemia suggests lymphoma, whereas myasthenia gravis or megaesophagus suggests thymoma. However, hypercalcemia has been reported in conjunction with thymoma in a dog (Harris et al, 1991). A definitive diagnosis of lymphoma may be made by fine-needle aspiration or transthoracic needle biopsy of the mass and/or by pleural fluid evaluation. Using ultrasound to pick the site for biopsies reduces risk of perforating the cranial vena cava or other vascular structures. If a definitive diagnosis cannot be made preoperatively, surgical biopsy with intraoperative cytology or analysis of frozen sections is indicated. The histologic appearance of thymomas does not correlate well with behavior, therefore exploratory thoracotomy often is required to determine if the tumor is invasive.

Acquired myasthenia gravis can be diagnosed by demonstrating circulating antibodies to acetylcholine receptors. As an alternative, clinical signs and the response to a cholinesterase inhibitor may help diagnose the disease. When edrophonium chloride is given intravenously, a dramatic but transient improvement in voluntary muscle function is expected in dogs with myasthenia gravis; however, the test gives false negative and sometimes gives false positive results. Furthermore, some dogs can have serious adverse side effects from excessive parasympathomimetic stimulation (e.g., bra-

BOX 30-12

Differential Diagnoses for Cranial Mediastinal Masses in Dogs and Cats

- Lymphoma
- Thymoma
- Chemodectoma
- Ectopic thyroid or parathyroid tumor
- Abscess
- Thymic branchial cyst
- Schwannoma
- Teratoma
- Thymic hyperplasia
- Granuloma

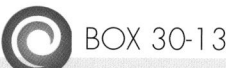 BOX 30-13

Drugs Used to Treat Acquired Myasthenia Gravis in Dogs

Pyridostigmine Bromide (Mestinon, Regonol)

0.02–0.04 mg/kg IV every 2 hours if condition is life-threatening, or start with 0.5 to 1 mg/kg and adjust dose up as needed, up to 3 mg/kg PO bid or tid to control signs.

Prednisolone

1.1–2.2 mg/kg/day

Azathioprine (Imuran)

2.2 mg/kg PO qd to every other day*

IV, Intravenous; *PO*, oral; *bid*, twice a day; *tid*, three times a day; *qd*, once a day.
*Watch for myelotoxicity, hepatitis, or pancreatitis. The onset of action is slower if treatment is initiated every other day, but the incidence of side effects is less.

dycardia and gastrointestinal signs). Pretreatment with glycopyrrolate or atropine is typically recommended, plus access to oxygen. The test is not useful for diagnosing megaesophagus due to localized myasthenia gravis.

> NOTE: Be aware of possible complications associated with the use of edrophonium (e.g., possible paralysis) and be prepared to deal with them.

MEDICAL MANAGEMENT

If aspiration pneumonia is present, the dog should be treated with appropriate antibiotics before surgery. Dogs with megaesophagus sometimes benefit from being fed in an upright position. Dyspneic animals should have pleural effusion removed by thoracentesis and an oxygen-enriched environment. Anticholinesterase (i.e., pyridostigmine bromide), corticosteroid, and/or cytotoxic (e.g., azathioprine) therapy may benefit dogs with clinical problems (e.g., megaesophagus and weakness) caused by myasthenia gravis (Box 30-13). Fluid therapy and correction of electrolyte abnormalities may be necessary in animals with severe or frequent regurgitation. Radiation therapy may reduce clinical signs in some animals with thymomas.

SURGICAL TREATMENT

Long-term survival without thymectomy has been reported in dogs with thymomas. However, surgical removal of stage I or stage II thymomas may be indicated. Concurrent myasthenia gravis makes therapy of thymoma more difficult. Thymectomy helps resolve myasthenia gravis in many people despite persistent serum antiacetylcholine receptor autoantibody titers. Too few dogs with both thymomas and myasthenia gravis have undergone surgery to predict the outcome in these patients. Surgical removal of thymic branchial cysts is indicated.

Preoperative Management

Aspiration pneumonia should be resolved before surgery, and severe muscle weakness should be treated (see previous discussion). Before induction of anesthesia, excess pleural fluid should be removed, and fluid and electrolyte abnormalities should be corrected.

Anesthesia

See p. 867 for recommendations for anesthetic management of patients undergoing thoracotomy procedures. Neuromuscular blocking agents (i.e., atracurium and pancuronium) should be avoided in patients with myasthenia gravis. Patients with megaesophagus should be intubated while positioned sternally rather than laterally, and the endotracheal cuff should be inflated immediately to protect the airway against aspiration.

Surgical Anatomy

The thymus is derived from the third and fourth pharyngeal pouches adjacent to the primordial cells of the thyroid gland and migrates caudally into the cranial mediastinum. It reaches maximum size in the dog at about 4 or 5 months. The thymus is bordered dorsally by the cranial vena cava and trachea. It is closely associated with many smaller blood vessels (e.g., branches of the brachycephalic trunk and internal thoracic arteries), which often require ligation during thymectomy. The phrenic nerve is closely associated with the dorsal border of the thymus.

Positioning

Depending on the surgical approach chosen (see later discussion), either the left thorax or the ventral thorax should be prepared for aseptic surgery.

SURGICAL TECHNIQUE

Thymectomy may be performed through a left third or fourth space intercostal thoracotomy if the tumor is small or through a cranial median sternotomy (see p. 874). If the mass is large, a median sternotomy approach allows better visualization of surrounding structures, such as the cranial vena cava. Small, encapsulated thymomas usually can be removed without difficulty, but cytoreduction often is all that is possible with large, invasive tumors. Thymomas often are friable and occasionally cystic, and they should be handled with care to prevent seeding the thoracic cavity with tumor cells. Thymic branchial cysts appear as multilobulated masses containing numerous cysts on transverse section.

> NOTE: If the tumor adheres to or closely surrounds the cranial vena cava, temporary occlusion of this vessel may facilitate surgery. Permanent ligation of the cranial vena cava may cause chylothorax.

Explore the thoracic cavity for evidence of metastasis. Identify the cranial vena cava and other associated vessels. Locate the phrenic nerve and preserve it if possible. Ligate small vessels, and bluntly dissect the mass and its capsule from surrounding tissue. Try to maintain the integrity of the thymic capsule. If complete removal of the mass is not possible, remove as much as can safely be excised. Submit tissue for histologic examination. Place a chest tube before thoracic closure.

SUTURE MATERIALS AND SPECIAL INSTRUMENTS

Electrocautery is useful when removing thymomas and other vascular neoplasms. See also recommendations for thoracotomy on p. 878.

POSTOPERATIVE CARE AND ASSESSMENT

Animals with thymomas are at great risk of aspiration during the postoperative period; positioning them with the head elevated may reduce the risk. Also, suctioning the pharynx before extubation, and extubating with the cuff slightly inflated, reduce the risk of aspiration if passive regurgitation has occurred during surgery. The animal should be observed for hemorrhage and pneumothorax postoperatively. Adjuvant radiation therapy may benefit animals with invasive tumors that cannot be completely excised. The animal should be closely observed for paraneoplastic disease after therapy. Analgesics should be provided postoperatively in these patients (see Chapter 13; for dosages of opioids see Table 13-4 on p. 133). With thymomas, the chest tube generally can be removed within 24 hours if hemorrhage or pneumothorax does not occur. Longer term tube thoracostomy may be necessary in animals with thymic branchial cysts if rupture of a cyst has caused pleuritis.

PROGNOSIS

The prognosis depends on the invasiveness of the tumor, its size at the time of diagnosis, and the presence or absence of paraneoplastic disease. The prognosis for thymic branchial cysts and noninvasive thymomas is good. If paraneoplastic syndromes are present, the prognosis is guarded.

References

Wood SL, Rosenstein DS, Bebchuk T: Myasthenia gravis and thymoma in a dog, *Vet Rec* 148:573, 2001.
Zekas LJ, Adams WM: Cranial mediastinal cysts in nine cats, *Vet Radiol Ultrasound* 43:413, 2002.

Suggested Reading

Holsworth I, Kyles A, Bailiff N et al: Use of a jugular vein autograft for reconstruction of the cranial vena cava in a dog with invasive thymoma and cranial vena cava syndrome, *J Am Vet Med Assoc* 225:1205, 2004.
This paper described the use of CT to evaluate a case and then used a vein graft to allow resection of the mass.

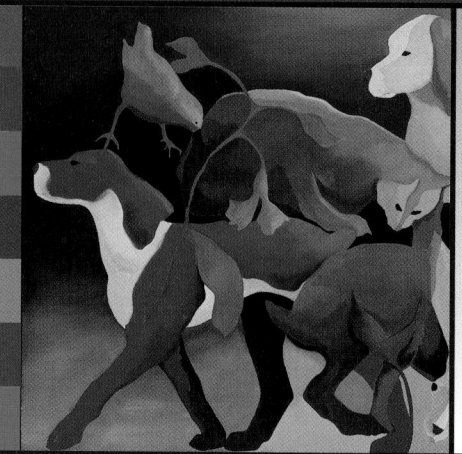

CHAPTER 31

Fundamentals of Orthopedic Surgery and Fracture Management

GENERAL PRINCIPLES AND TECHNIQUES

DEFINITIONS

Unique terms used in orthopedic surgery include descriptions of examination and reduction maneuvers, classification of fractures and fracture healing, types of grafting material, and surgical outcomes. A partial list of definitions is provided in Box 31-1. Other terms are described in the text of this chapter.

PROBLEM IDENTIFICATION

Orthopedic surgery includes procedures used to (1) stabilize fractured bones; (2) explore, débride, and stabilize injured joints; (3) replace damaged joints; (4) stabilize spinal column injuries; (5) decompress the spinal cord; (6) resect musculoskeletal tumors; and (7) repair tendon and ligament injuries. Patients with orthopedic problems represent a significant percentage of the general practice population. The most common complaints are associated with joint disease, and trauma is frequently noted. Before the most appropriate method for treating a problem can be selected, the orthopedic problem must be identified and assessed. Developing surgical skills and familiarity with specialized instrumentation is necessary for performing most orthopedic procedures. Veterinarians should be aware of their limitations and refer complicated cases when necessary. Knowledge of potential complications and pitfalls helps surgeons take the appropriate preventive steps.

Identifying a fracture as the cause of non–weight-bearing lameness is usually straightforward. The challenging problem is to assess the patient, classify the fracture, and develop plans for fixation that will allow predictable and consistent results. Occasionally, animals will have nondisplaced fractures that are difficult to detect and require special diagnostic techniques. Most orthopedic cases involve lameness and pain, but identifying the cause of the lameness may be difficult. Accurate historical information, thorough general examination, orthopedic examination,

and diagnostic imaging techniques are essential. It is important to realize that the most appropriate therapy is not always surgery.

DIFFERENTIAL DIAGNOSIS

A differential diagnosis is developed based on results of history, signalment, and physical examination. Other tests or procedures may be necessary to define the disease once the aforementioned findings have narrowed the diagnostic possibilities. Many orthopedic diseases are predictable within certain age groups and breeds (Table 31-1). Information on the animal's general condition includes anorexia, depression or fever, limb affected, multiple limb involvement, degree of pain or lameness, duration, intensity of onset, historical trauma, effect of exercise, time of day of greatest clinical signs, effect of rest, and changes in lameness associated with weather. Such information provides initial clues to form a differential list of potential causes. Additional questioning, physical examination, and radiographic examination will provide data to make a definitive diagnosis.

Physical Examination

The animal's general health should be assessed as part of the physical examination. Baseline examination includes obtaining the animal's temperature, pulse, and respiration. The animal's overall appearance should be noted (e.g., obesity) and thoracic auscultation and abdominal palpation performed. General health evaluation is important before anesthetizing any animal that has orthopedic disease. Traumatized animals brought in for fracture evaluation should have thoracic radiographs and serial electrocardiograms (ECGs) performed. Evaluation of the abdominal cavity is done initially with palpation and evaluation of serum chemistry tests. Abdominocentesis and radiographic evaluation of the urinary tract should be performed if clinical signs suggest injury (see p. 335). Traumatized animals with long bone fractures frequently have concurrent soft tissue injuries (e.g., pneumothorax, traumatic myocarditis, diaphragmatic hernia, and ruptured bladder or urethra). It is important to di-

BOX 31-1

Orthopedic Terms

Allograft—bone transplanted from one animal to another of the same species

Apophyseal osteotomies—procedures performed to enhance surgical exposure of a joint

Autograft—bone transplanted from one site to another in the same animal

Avulsion fracture—occurs when the insertion point of a tendon or ligament is fractured and distracted from the rest of the bone

Bridging plates—span a comminuted fracture

Cerclage wire—used to denote the use of orthopedic wire placed around the circumference of the bone and compressing an oblique fracture

Closed reduction—fracture repair performed without a surgical exposure

Compression plates—plates that act to compress the fracture

Corrective osteotomies—elective procedures in which the diaphysis or metaphysis of the bone is cut, realigned, and stabilized until union occurs

Cranial drawer—the abnormal movement elicited during a physical examination that is caused by the tibia sliding cranially in relationship to the femur in the absence of the cranial cruciate ligament

Crepitation—the "grating feel" or sound associated with manipulating a fractured bone or an arthritic joint

Delayed unions—fractures that heal more slowly than anticipated

Direct bone union—bone formed without evidence of callus

Endochondral bone formation—bone formed on a cartilaginous precursor

External coaptation—fracture fixation using casts or splints

External fixation—fracture fixation in which pins penetrate the bone and skin and are connected externally

Greenstick fracture—an incomplete fracture in which a portion of the cortex is intact

Hemicerclage wire or *interfragmentary wire*—denotes wire that is placed through predrilled holes in the bone

Indirect reduction—the process of restoring fragment and limb alignment by distracting the major bone segments

Internal fixation—fracture fixation using internal implants to secure the bone

Intramedullary pins—implants that are positioned in the medullary canal of long bones

Intramembranous bone formation—direct differentiation of mesenchymal stem cells into osteoblasts so bone forms without a cartilaginous precursor

Malunions—healed fractures in which anatomic bone alignment was not achieved or maintained during healing

Neutralization plates—support a reconstructed fracture

Nonunion—a fracture that has an arrested repair process that requires surgical intervention to create an environment conducive to bone healing

Normograde placement—the pin is started at one end of the bone, driven to the fracture area, and then seated at the other end of the bone

Open fracture—one in which the fracture is exposed to the external atmosphere

Open reduction—fracture repair performed after a surgical approach to the bone

Ortolani maneuver—the manipulation used to subluxate a dysplastic hip

Ostectomies—removal of a segment of bone

Osteomyelitis—an inflammatory condition of bone and the medullary canal

Osteotomies—procedures in which the bone is cut into two segments

Reduction—process of reconstructing or realigning a fractured bone

Retrograde placement—the pin is inserted at the fracture area, driven proximally to exit the bone, the fracture is reduced, and the pin is driven distally to seat at the end of the bone

Staged disassembly—process of modifying a fixation frame at approximately 6 wk after surgery to increase the loading on the healing fracture

---

agnose these injuries before the animal is anesthetized for fracture repair.

Orthopedic Examination

An orthopedic examination begins by observing the animal for signs of lameness while obtaining the history. This is necessary even if the owner has attributed the lameness to a particular limb because the correct limb may not have been identified. The animal should be allowed to walk around the examination room and is observed for obvious lameness and for more subtle signs, such as reducing the weight placed on the affected limb when standing or sitting. Other observations may include unilateral or bilateral muscle atrophy and abnormal muscle development. Dogs with bilateral hip dysplasia or chronic cruciate ligament rupture may appear underdeveloped or weak in the rear quarters and heavily muscled in the forequarters.

If the lameness has not been localized during the initial observation, the animal should be observed while walking and trotting. It may be necessary to take dogs outside to improve footing. To protect a sore limb, animals quickly shift their weight from the affected limb, making it appear that they are landing heavily on the opposite, or "good," limb. Animals with forelimb lameness will lift their heads after the lame limb strikes the ground in an attempt to remove weight from the affected limb. A short stride occurs when the animal has a decreased range of motion in a diseased joint (e.g., hip dysplasia). External swinging, or paddling, of the affected limb(s) occurs when the animal tries to advance a limb that cannot be adequately flexed. This is often observed in dogs with severe degenerative joint disease of the elbows. Animals with bilateral lameness may not limp, but often show more subtle signs, such as shifting their weight from limb to limb while standing, shortened stride, and bilateral muscle atrophy.

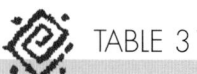 TABLE 31-1

Differential Diagnoses for Lameness

SIGNALMENT	HISTORY	DIFFERENTIAL DIAGNOSIS	SIGNALMENT	HISTORY	DIFFERENTIAL DIAGNOSIS
Immature, large dogs; front limb	Acute	Fractured physis*	Adult, large dogs; rear limb	Acute	Fractured bone*
		Fractured bone sprain*			Luxated hip*
	Chronic	OCD shoulder			Luxated stifle*
		OCD elbow			Cruciate and/or meniscus syndrome*
		UAP elbow			Ruptured Achilles tendon*
		FCP elbow			Luxated tarsus
		Premature closure of physes		Chronic	Degenerative joint disease caused by cruciate rupture*
		Elbow incongruity			
		Retained cartilage cores			Panosteitis
		Panosteitis			Patellar luxation*
		Hypertrophic osteodystrophy			Cruciate and/or meniscus syndrome*
Immature, large dogs; rear limb	Acute	Fractured physis*			Bone and/or soft tissue neoplasia*
		Fractured bone*			Lumbosacral syndrome
	Chronic	Hip dysplasia			Thoracolumbar disk disease
		OCD stifle			Inflammatory joint disease*
		Patellar luxation	Adult, small dogs; front limb	Acute	Fractured bone
		Avulsion of long digital extensor tendon			Luxated shoulder
		OCD hock			Luxated elbow
		Panosteitis		Chronic	Degenerative joint disease
		Hypertrophic osteodystrophy			Luxating shoulder
		Partial ACL rupture			Bone and/or soft tissue neoplasia
Immature, small dogs; front limb	Acute	Fractured physis			Inflammatory joint disease
		Fractured bone			Radius curvus and/or elbow incongruity
	Chronic	Congenital luxation, shoulder			Cervical disk disease
		Congenital luxation, elbow			
Immature, small dogs; rear limb	Acute	Premature closure of physes	Adult, small dogs; rear limb	Acute	Fractured bone
		Atlantoaxial instability			Luxated hip
		Fractured physis			Luxated stifle
		Fractured bone			Cruciate and/or meniscus syndrome
	Chronic	Avascular necrosis of femoral head			Luxated tarsus
		Patellar luxation*		Chronic	Degenerative joint disease
Adult, large dogs; front limb	Acute	Fractured bone*			Patellar luxation
		Luxated shoulder*			Cruciate and/or meniscus syndrome
		Luxated elbow*			Bone and/or soft tissue neoplasia
	Chronic	Degenerative joint disease caused by elbow dysplasia*			Lumbosacral syndrome
		Panosteitis			Thoracolumbar disk disease
		Bicipital tenosynovitis			Inflammatory joint disease
		Contracture of infraspinatus tendon			
		Radius curvus and/or elbow incongruity			
		Carpal hyperextension			
		Bone and/or soft tissue neoplasia*			
		Brachial plexus injury*			
		Cervical disk disease			
		Inflammatory joint disease*			

OCD, Osteochondritis dissecans; *UAP,* ununited anconeal process; *FCP,* fragmented coronoid process.
*Denotes potential differential diagnoses in cats.

TABLE 31-2

Sedation for Palpation and Radiographs of Dogs

DRUG/COMBINATION	DOSE	ROUTE	COMMENTS
Acepromazine* plus	0.05 mg/kg, maximum of 1 mg	IV, SC, IM	Acepromazine is not reversible. Animals will require restraint if used alone. It is contraindicated in patients with a history of seizure.
Oxymorphone or	0.05–0.1 mg/kg	IV, SC, IM	Oxymorphone can be reversed with 0.02 mg/kg of naloxone (Narcan) IV. Auditory hypersensitivity and panting occurs with this drug.
Butorphanol plus	0.2–0.4 mg/kg	IV, SC, IM	
Atropine or	0.02 mg/kg 0.04 mg/kg	IV SC, IM	
Glycopyrrolate	0.005–0.011 mg/kg	IV, SC, IM	
Xylazine plus	0.2 mg/kg	IV, IM	Xylazine can be reversed with 1–2 mg/kg tolazoline IV to effect or IM.
Butorphanol plus	0.2 mg/kg	IV, IM	Total dose of xylazine may vary with route of administration and weight of patient.
Atropine or	0.02 mg/kg 0.04 mg/kg	IV SC, IM	
Glycopyrrolate	0.005–0.011 mg/kg	IV, SC, IM	
Oxymorphone plus	0.05–0.1 mg/kg	IV, SC, IM	Oxymorphone can be reversed with 0.02 mg/kg of naloxone (Narcan) IV.
Diazepam plus	0.1–0.2 mg/kg	IV	
Atropine or Glycopyrrolate	0.02 mg/kg 0.04 mg/kg 0.005–0.011 mg/kg	IV SC, IM IV, SC, IM	Auditory hypersensitivity and panting may occur.
Butorphanol plus	0.2–0.4 mg/kg	IV, SC, IM	After administration of butorphanol and glycopyrrolate, wait 10 min before giving medetomidine.
Glycopyrrolate plus	0.005–0.011 mg/kg	IV, SC, IM	
Medetomidine	5–15 µg/kg	IV, SC, IM	

IV, Intravenous; *SC,* subcutaneous; *IM,* intramuscular.
*Acepromazine (0.05 mg/kg IM or SC; maximum of 2 mg) may be used alone for radiographs and palpation; however, it provides minimal restraint.

After the lame limb has been identified, the animal should be returned to the examination room. Limb palpation and an initial neurologic examination should be performed simultaneously. Optimally the first examination should be done without sedation to determine the animal's response to pain; however, this may not be possible in aggressive animals. The examiner should develop a consistent evaluation pattern. One technique is to start at the front of the animal and work toward the rear. Also, starting at the toes of each limb and progressing proximally is useful. It is preferable to begin examining a sound limb to identify the individual's normal response to manipulation and pressure. The initial examination should be done with the animal standing to assess muscular symmetry, joint enlargement, and proprioceptive responses. As each bone, joint, and soft tissue area is palpated, asymmetry (between limbs), response to pain, swelling, abnormalities in range of motion, instabil-

ity, and crepitation should be noted. Asymmetry should be assessed before and during individual limb palpation and may indicate tumor, abscess, atrophy, joint swelling, or greenstick fracture. Long bones should be palpated to determine if there is swelling (e.g., fracture or tumor), a response to pain while firm pressure is applied (e.g., panosteitis, fracture, or tumor), instability, or crepitation (e.g., fracture). Joints should be isolated and moved through a complete range of motion to detect crepitation, pain, or abnormalities in range of motion. Additional tests of shoulder, hip, and stifle instability should be performed if abnormalities are detected in these joints (see p. 935 [shoulder], p. 938 [hip], and p. 936 [stifle]). Muscles and tendons should be palpated to determine if they are normal and intact. After the initial orthopedic examination to localize pain, the animal may be sedated to facilitate closer examination and to obtain radiographs (Tables 31-2 and 31-3).

TABLE 31-3

Sedation for Palpation and Radiographs of Cats

DRUG/COMBINATION	DOSE	ROUTE*	COMMENTS
Acepromazine *plus*	0.05 mg/kg; maximum of 1 mg	IM	Acepromazine is not reversible.
Butorphanol *plus*	0.2 mg/kg	IM	Animal will require restraint if acepromazine is used alone.
Atropine *or*	0.04 mg/kg	IM	Acepromazine is contraindicated with seizure history.
Glycopyrrolate	0.005–0.011 mg/kg	IM	
Xylazine *plus*	0.2 mg/kg	IM	Xylazine can be reversed with 1–2 mg/kg of tolazoline IV to effect or IM.
Butorphanol *plus*	0.2 mg/kg	IM	
Atropine *or*	0.04 mg/kg	IM	
Glycopyrrolate	0.005–0.011 mg/kg	IM	
Ketamine	5 mg/kg	IM	Ketamine provides little to no muscle relaxation. It is often added to other sedatives or drugs (e.g., butorphanol, acepromazine, glypyrollate, or atropine).
Butorphanol *plus*	0.2 mg/kg	IM	Wait 10 min after administration of butorphanol and glycopyrrolate before giving medetomidine.
Glycopyrrolate *plus*	0.005–0.011 mg/kg	IM	
Medetomidine	10–20 µg/kg	IM	

IM, Intramuscular; *IV,* intravenous.
*Other routes of administration may be appropriate for some drugs (e.g., IV if a catheter is in place).

Forelimb

A complete orthopedic examination of the forelimb includes several manipulations.

Below the carpus. *Examine the paw closely to determine if there is any foreign material present. Spread the toes and nails apart and inspect the webbing and pads. Palpate each digit to determine if the bones are intact and if soft tissue swelling is present. Extend and flex the phalangeal joints, and palpate the corresponding extensor and flexor tendons to see if they relax and tighten appropriately. Test the lateral and medial stability of each joint in extension. Palpate the areas adjacent to the metacarpal pad and over the palmar sesamoids of metacarpophalangeal joints 2 and 5 for sensitivity to pressure. Palpate the metacarpal bones to determine if there is swelling or instability.*

Carpus. *Gently palpate the dorsal surface of the carpus to determine if fluctuant swelling is associated with joint effusion.*

This may be a subtle finding in the carpus and is more easily noted when the animal is standing because loading the joint forces the fluid peripherally.

Compare the affected limb with the opposite carpus.

Bilateral swelling may occur with some diseases, such as rheumatoid arthritis.

Extend and flex the carpus. Maximum extension of the carpus should be about 180 to 190 degrees; maximum flexion should be 35-45 degrees.

A decreased range of motion may indicate degenerative joint disease.

Note any crepitation. Extend and stress the carpus in the mediolateral plane to determine if there is joint instability.

Radius. *Palpate the radius for instability (fracture), swelling (fracture and tumor), and pain response to deep bone palpation (panosteitis).*

Elbow. *Palpate the elbow for fluctuant swelling in the space between the lateral condyle and olecranon and over the medial coronoid process.*

Fluctuant swelling indicates joint effusion, which results from several elbow diseases. Joint effusion may be more easily detected when the animal is standing. Firm, generalized swelling of the elbow often indicates degenerative joint disease.

Flex and extend the elbow (Figs. 31-1 and 31-2).

Normal extension and flexion are about 165 degrees and 40 to 50 degrees, respectively. The carpus should almost touch the shoulder when the elbow is flexed. Decreased range of motion caused by incomplete flexion of the elbow

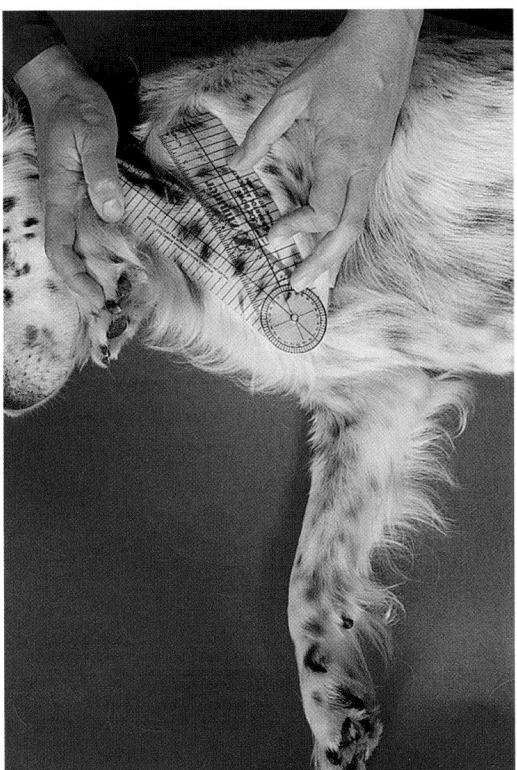

FIG. 31-1
Flex and extend the elbow. Notice the angle of greatest flexion of a normal elbow measured with a goniometer. The carpus should almost touch the shoulder. Compare this with the angle of flexion in an elbow with degenerative joint disease (Fig. 31-2).

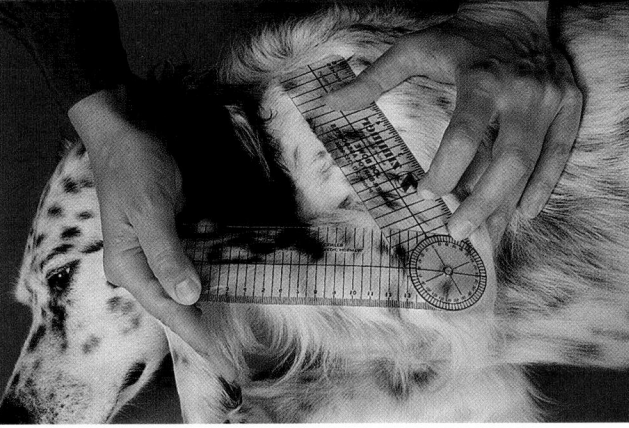

FIG. 31-2
Angle of greatest flexion of elbow in dog with degenerative joint disease. Compare this with the angle of flexion in a normal elbow (Fig. 31-1).

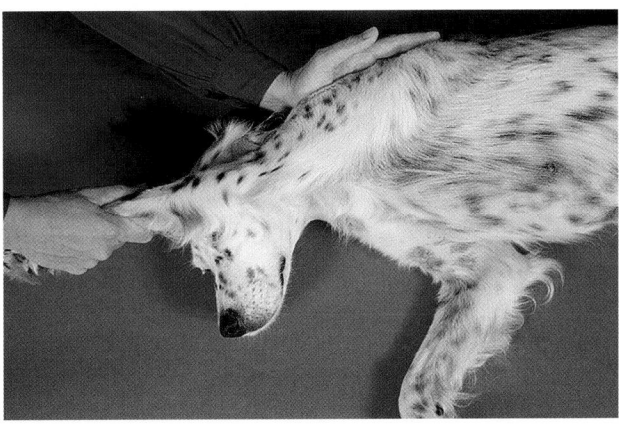

FIG. 31-3
Hyperextend the shoulder while stabilizing the scapula. Pain on hyperextension may indicate osteochondritis dissecans of the humeral head.

usually suggests degenerative joint disease, which may occur secondary to a fragmented coronoid process, an ununited anconeal process, or osteochondritis dissecans.

While the elbow is in extension, check the integrity of the collateral ligaments by applying medial and lateral force to the radius and ulna.

Humerus. *Palpate the humerus for instability (fracture), swelling (fracture or tumor), and pain response to deep palpation (panosteitis). Palpate the bone in areas where it is not covered by muscles to differentiate panosteitis from muscular pain.*

Shoulder. Swelling from joint effusion is difficult to detect in the shoulder because of the overlying muscles.

Move the shoulder through a range of motion, including hyperextension and hyperflexion, while stabilizing the scapula (Fig. 31-3).
Osteochondritis dissecans of the humeral head elicits a pain response when the shoulder is hyperextended.
Hold the acromial process stationary and mobilize the humeral head to detect luxation or subluxation.

Many shoulder joints pop or click without significance, but any translation of the humeral head in relationship to the acromion process is abnormal.

Palpate the biceps tendon and apply pressure; a painful response indicates tenosynovitis.

Scapula. *Palpate the scapula for instability (fracture) and swelling (fracture and tumor). Palpate the muscle over the scapula and compare it with the opposite side to determine atrophy secondary to disuse or nerve injury. Probe the axillary area for swellings and observe for signs of pain, which may indicate a nerve root tumor.*

Rear Limb

Complete orthopedic examination of the rear limb involves various manipulations.

Below tarsus. *Examine the paw closely to determine if there is any foreign material present. Spread the toes and nails apart and inspect the webbing and pads. Palpate each digit to determine if the bones are intact and if soft tissue swelling is present. Extend and flex the phalangeal joints, and palpate the corresponding extensor and flexor tendons to see if they relax and tighten appropriately. Test the lateral* *and medial stability of each joint in extension. Palpate the areas adjacent to the metatarsal pad and over the palmar sesamoids of metatarsophalangeal joints 2 and 5 for sensitivity to pressure. Palpate the metatarsal bones to determine if there is swelling or instability.*

Hock. *Palpate the tarsal joints for fluctuant swelling indicative of joint effusion.*

This may be a subtle finding in the hock and is more easily noted when the animal is standing because loading the joint forces the fluid peripherally. Firm swelling is suggestive of degenerative joint disease.

Extend and flex the hock.

Normal flexion should be about 40-45 degrees. Decreased flexion indicates degenerative joint disease, which may be secondary to osteochondritis dissecans. Pain on manipulation of the joint (especially coupled with soft tissue swelling) may indicate a fracture.

Extend, adduct, and abduct the hock and metatarsal bones to demonstrate instability of the collateral ligaments. With the stifle in extension and the hock stressed into flexion, palpate the Achilles tendon (Fig. 31-4).

Rupture of the entire tendon complex allows hock flexion while the stifle is extended. Rupture of the gastrocnemius tendon and common tendon of the biceps femoris, gracilis, and semitendinosus muscles, with preservation of the superficial digital flexor, allows partial flexion of the hock while the stifle is extended and causes simultaneous flexion of the digits.

Tibia. *Palpate the tibia for instability (fracture), swelling (fracture and tumor), and pain response to deep bone palpation (panosteitis).*

Stifle. *Perform the initial examination of the stifle with the animal standing. Simultaneously palpate both stifles to detect swelling.*

A swollen stifle usually indicates degenerative joint disease. The patellar ligament becomes less distinct with joint effusion, and the medial aspect of the stifle enlarges because of capsular thickening and osteophyte formation.

Patella. The remainder of the stifle examination is done with the animal in lateral recumbency.

Extend and flex the stifle while holding one hand over the cranial aspect of the joint to detect crepitation. Next examine the stability of the patella in relationship to the femur. Extend the stifle, internally rotate the foot, and apply digital pressure in an attempt to displace the patella medially (medial patellar luxation). Detect lateral patellar luxation by slightly flexing the stifle, externally rotating the foot, and applying digital pressure to attempt to displace the patella laterally (Fig. 31-5).

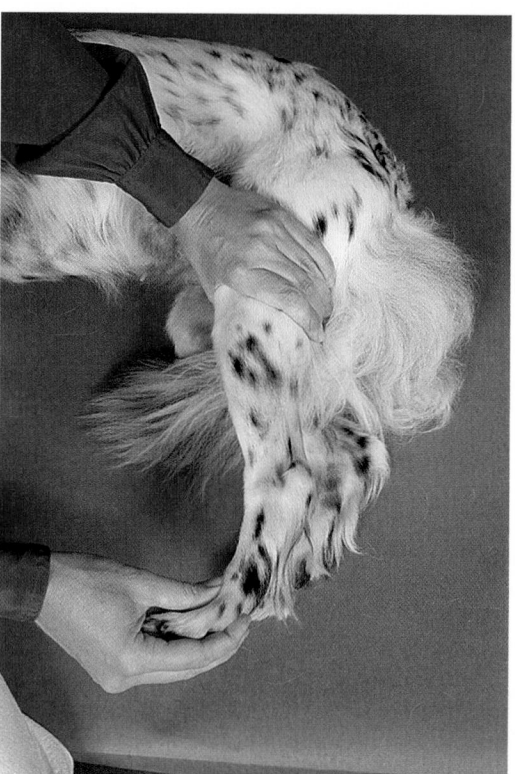

FIG. 31-4
To test integrity of the Achilles tendon complex, attempt to flex the hock with the stifle in extension.

The patella normally moves slightly medially and laterally, but is considered to be luxating when it leaves the trochlear groove.

Collateral ligaments. *Test the integrity of the collateral ligaments by holding the stifle in full extension and attempting to open the stifle on the medial and lateral aspects. Test the medial collateral ligament by using one hand to brace the femur while the other hand abducts the tibia.*

Normally the medial collateral ligament will not allow joint laxity.

Test the lateral collateral ligament by bracing the femur with one hand and using the other hand to adduct the tibia (Fig. 31-6).

An intact lateral collateral ligament will prevent joint laxity. If the stifle is allowed to flex while the tibia is adducted, it may feel as though there is lateral laxity of the joint. This is a result of anatomic location of the lateral collateral ligament and internal rotation of the tibia and is normal.

Cruciate ligaments. *Test the integrity of the cruciate ligaments by trying to elicit a cranial or caudal drawer motion or by performing a tibial compression test to elicit cranial tibial thrust.*

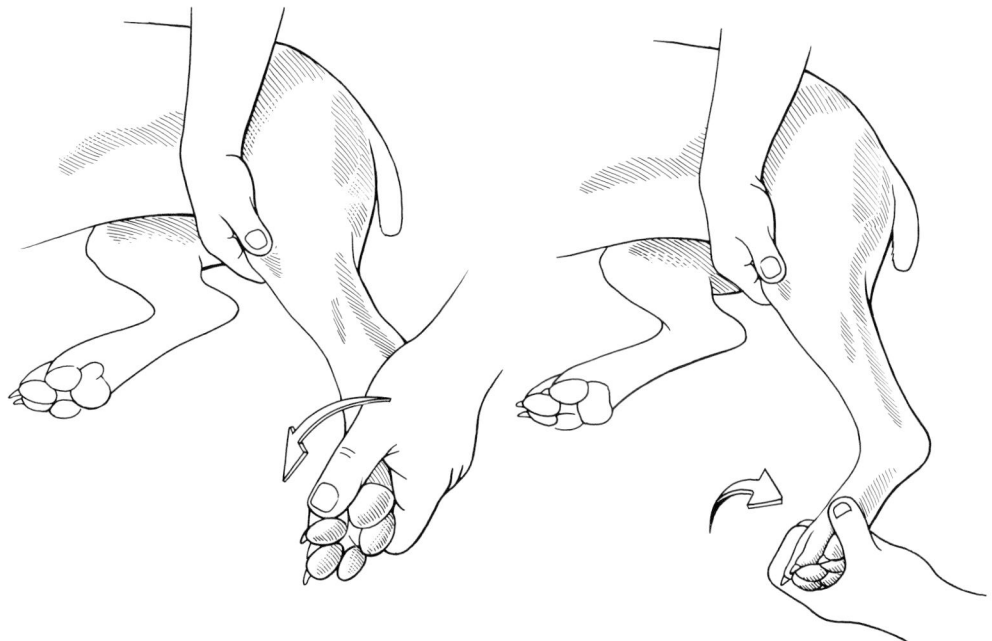

FIG. 31-5
To examine the stifle for medial patellar luxation, extend the stifle, internally rotate the foot, and apply medial pressure to the patella with the thumb. To examine the stifle for lateral patellar luxation, slightly flex the stifle, externally rotate the foot, and apply lateral pressure to the patella with the fingers.

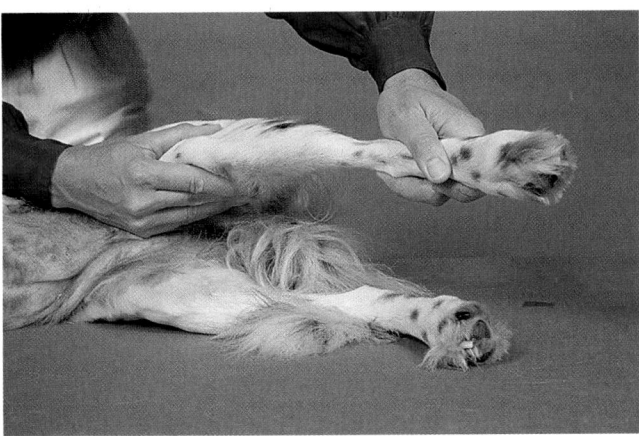

FIG. 31-6
To examine for collateral ligament injury, fully extend the stifle, stabilize the distal femur with one hand, and apply medial and lateral pressure to the tibia with the other hand.

prevent drawer motion. If tibial rotation occurs, gently flex and extend the stifle to relax the animal, and repeat the procedure. Test drawer motion with the femur flexed and extended (Fig. 31-7). Usually the greatest movement is felt with the stifle in flexion. If the patella is luxated, replace it in the trochlear groove before attempting the drawer motion.

Perform the **tibial compression test** to detect cranial tibial thrust. Detect forward motion of the tibia by placing the index finger along the patella and the tibial tuberosity. With the leg in a standing position, flex the hock to tense the gastrocnemius muscle (Fig. 31-8). This compresses the femur and tibia together, causing the tibia to move forward in a cranial cruciate-deficient stifle.

Drawer movement is caused by the tibia sliding cranially or caudally in relationship to the femur. This motion is not possible when the cruciate ligaments are intact in adult animals. Immature animals may have slight drawer motion, but it stops abruptly as the ligament tightens.

To elicit **direct drawer motion,** place the index finger and thumb of one hand over the patella and lateral fabellar regions, respectively. Place the index finger of the opposite hand on the tibial tuberosity and with the thumb positioned caudal to the fibular head, slightly flex the stifle. Stabilize the femur, and gently move the tibia cranial and distal to the femur. Do not allow tibial rotation. Tense muscles may

The presence and amount of *drawer motion* depend on the animal's age, size, state of relaxation, and the duration and type of cruciate pathology. There is minimal drawer motion in normal dogs and cats, although very young puppies may have a "lax" stifle. Eliciting drawer motion in larger animals or those that are tense is difficult; sedation or general anesthesia may be necessary. Minimal drawer motion may be noted with chronic cruciate pathology (especially in large dogs) because periarticular fibrosis restricts stifle motion. Minimal or partial drawer motion may also occur with incomplete tears or stretching of the cranial cruciate ligament. Drawer motion is evident with a torn caudal cruciate ligament.

To identify caudal drawer motion, start with the stifle in a neutral position.

Most caudal ligament ruptures are not discovered until exploration because they are mistaken for cranial ligament injuries.

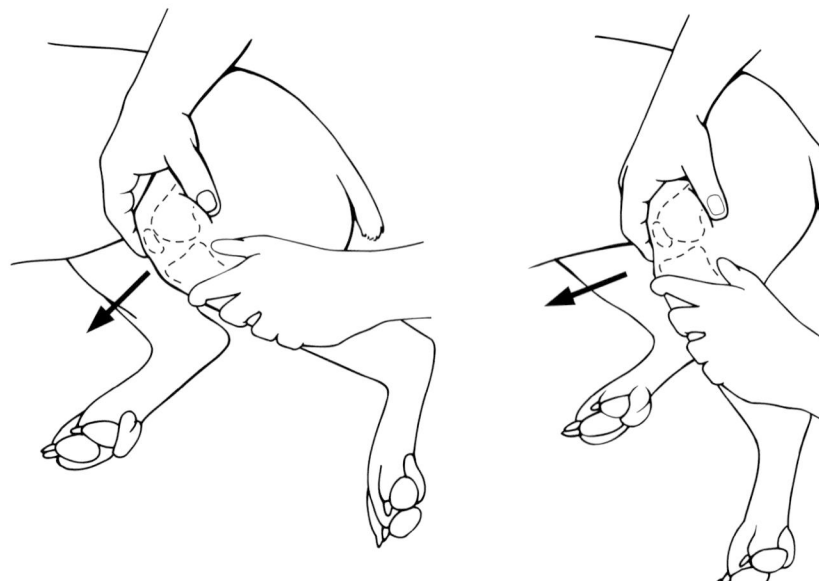

FIG. 31-7
To examine for cruciate ligament injury, place the thumb of one hand over the lateral fabella and the index finger over the patella. Stabilize the femur with this hand. Place the thumb of the opposite hand caudal to the fibular head with the index finger on the tibial tuberosity. With the stifle first flexed and then extended, attempt to move the tibia cranially and distally to the femur.

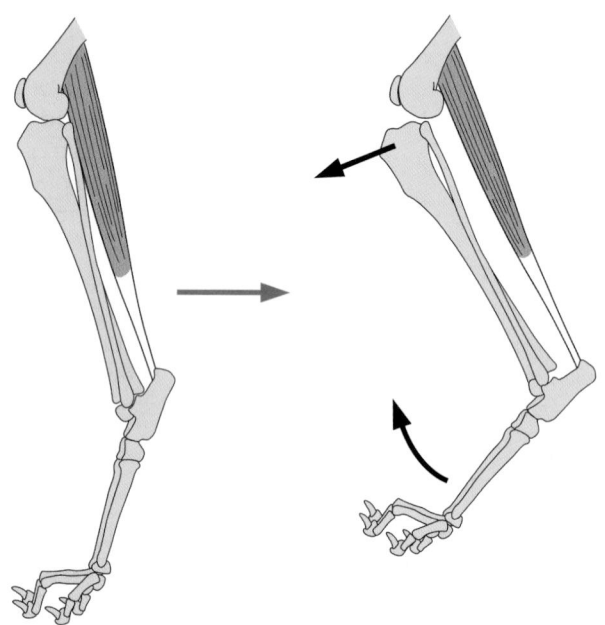

FIG. 31-8
Flexing the hock while the limb is in a standing position will tense the gastrocnemius muscle and force the proximal tibia forward if the cranial cruciate ligament is ruptured.

Meniscus. In most cases, meniscal tears are identified during exploratory arthrotomy or arthroscopic examination. A click or pop may be felt as the stifle is flexed and extended, causing the caudal horn of the medial meniscus to displace.

Femur. *Palpate the femur for instability (fracture), swelling (fracture and tumor), and pain response to deep bone palpation (panosteitis). Take care to isolate bone from muscle during deep palpation.*

Hip. *Extend and flex the hip while a hand is placed over the greater trochanter to detect crepitation.*

The femur should extend caudally to a position almost parallel to the pelvis without inducing pain in a normal hip. The stifle should approach the ilium with full flexion. Degenerative joint disease limits the range of motion and may induce pain.

Hip luxation. *To detect abnormalities of the hip, use the position of the greater trochanter in relationship to the tuber ischium as a landmark. In the standing animal, compare the distance from the greater trochanter with the tuber ischium bilaterally.*

A unilateral increase in the distance indicates hip luxation. Animals with acute hip luxations are nonweight bearing, and swelling over the greater trochanter may be noted.

Externally rotate the femur while placing the thumb in the space between the greater trochanter; displacement of the thumb should occur (Fig. 31-9, A and B).

With hip luxation, the trochanter rolls over the thumb (Fig. 31-9, *C* and *D*).

Hip laxity. Evaluation of hip laxity is best done under sedation.

With the animal in lateral recumbency, perform the Ortolani maneuver to detect hip laxity associated with hip dysplasia. Grasp the stifle with one hand and hold it parallel with the table surface. Place the other hand over the dorsal pelvis and adduct and push the stifle toward the pelvis.

With joint laxity, the hip will subluxate.

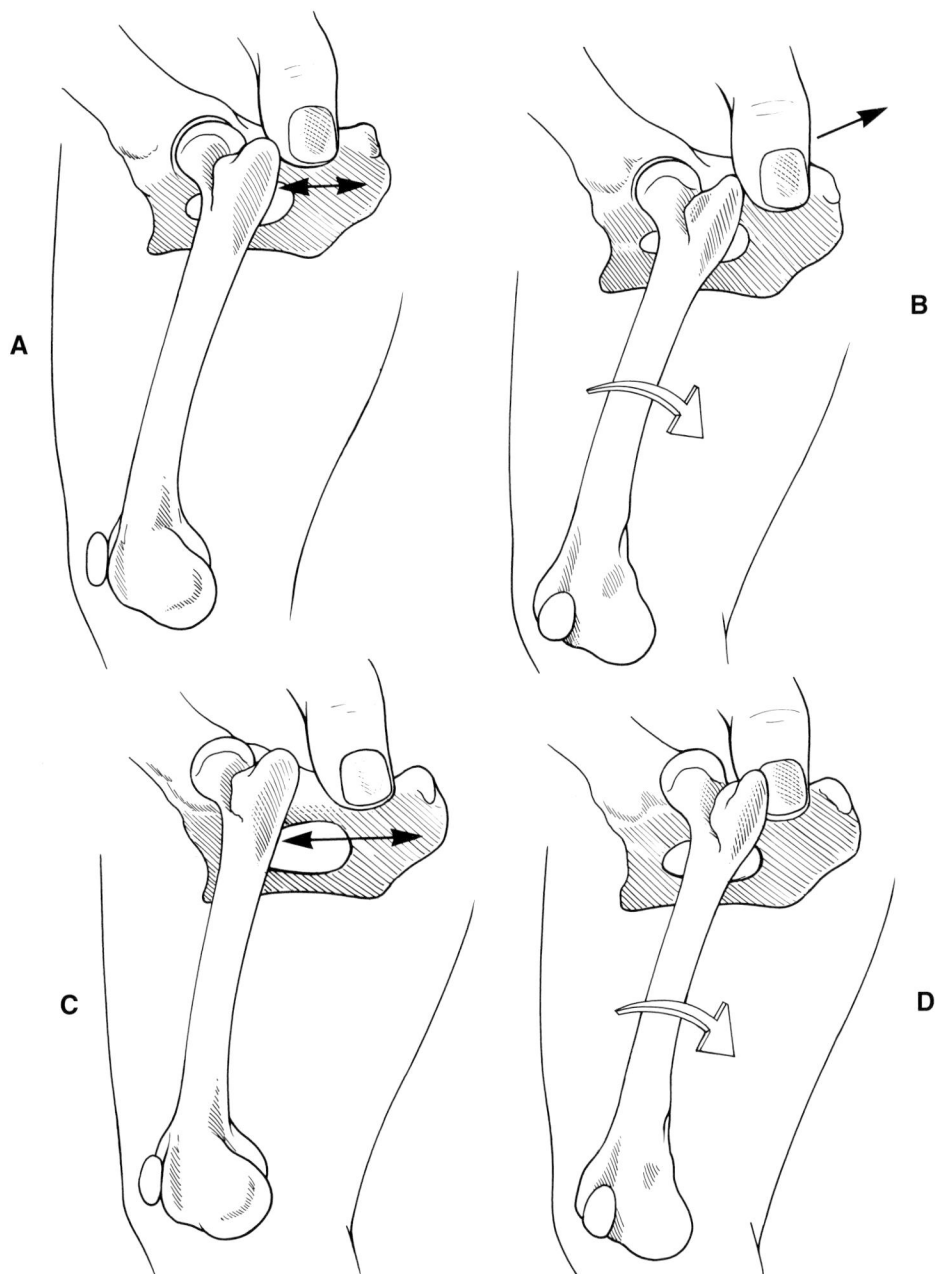

FIG. 31-9
A and B, To examine for hip luxation, place the thumb in the space caudal to the greater trochanter, and externally rotate the femur. If the coxofemoral joint is intact, the greater trochanter will displace the thumb. **C and D,** If the coxofemoral joint is luxated, the greater trochanter will roll over the thumb.

Maintain the pressure and abduct the stifle. As the femoral head returns to the acetabulum, use the hand stabilizing the pelvis to detect a click (Fig. 31-10).

The Ortolani maneuver can also be performed with the animal in dorsal recumbency, with the stifles held parallel to each other and perpendicular to the table.

Apply downward pressure on the stifle to subluxate the hip. Maintain pressure and abduct the stifle.

With laxity a click is noted as the femoral head returns to the acetabulum (Fig. 31-11). The *angle of subluxation* is the point at which the hip luxates, and the *angle of reduction* is the point at which the femoral head returns to the acetabulum.

Use these calculations to determine the feasibiliy of pelvic osteotomy (see p. 1238).

Pelvis. Examine the pelvic region for evidence of fracture, including asymmetry, instability, swelling, crepitation,

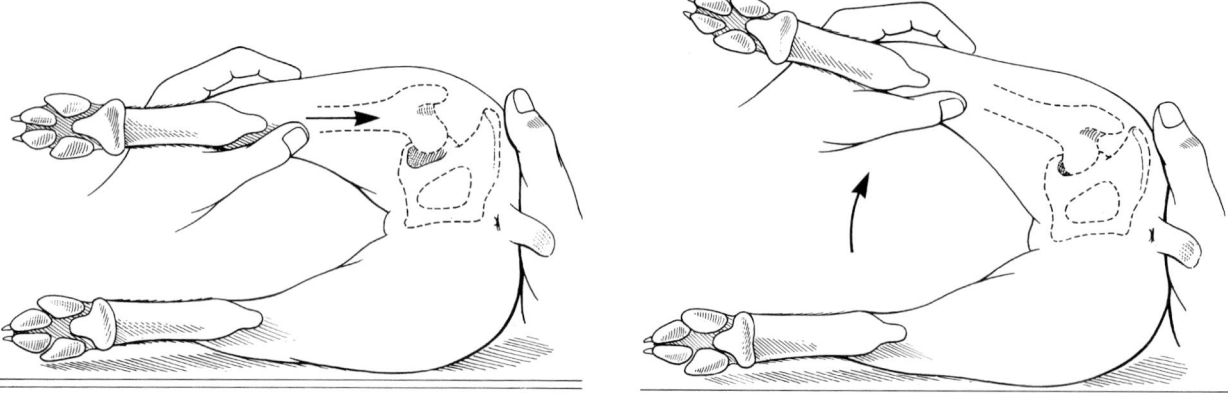

FIG. 31-10
To examine the hip for laxity with the animal positioned in lateral recumbency, place one hand over the back and grasp the stifle with the opposite hand. Hold the femur parallel to the table or in adduction and subluxate the femoral head by pushing the stifle toward the pelvis. While maintaining pressure, abduct the limb. As the femoral head returns to the acetabulum, a click will be felt.

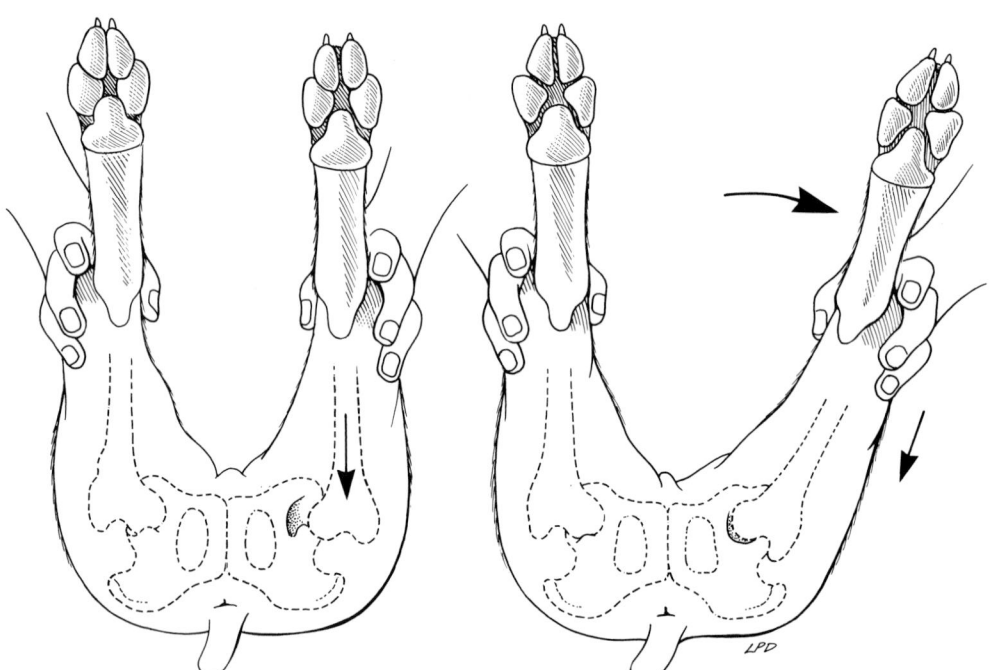

FIG. 31-11
To examine the hip for laxity with the animal positioned in dorsal recumbency, place the hands over the stifles. Hold the femurs parallel to each other and perpendicular to the table. Subluxate the femoral head by pushing the stifle toward the pelvis. While maintaining pressure, abduct the limb. As the femoral head returns to the acetabulum, a click will be felt.

bruising, and pain. To detect instability, manipulate the tuber ischia and wings of the ilium.

Radiographic evaluation is superior to physical manipulation for identifying fractures.

Perform a rectal examination, checking for pelvic canal stenosis, pelvic fractures, and prostate enlargement.

Rule Out Neurologic Disease

Because neurologic disorders may mimic orthopedic diseases or may occur concurrently, every orthopedic examination should include several neurologic examination maneuvers performed to rule out neurologic disease. If evidence of neurologic disease is discovered, a complete neurologic examination is indicated (see Chapter 36).

Evaluate conscious proprioception in all four limbs by gently supporting the animal and individually turning each paw until the dorsal surface of the paw contacts the ground.

Normal animals return the paw to the correct position almost immediately. Loss of conscious proprioception usually indicates neurologic disease; however, animals with fractured limbs may be reluctant to move the limb and therefore may appear to have conscious proprioception deficits.

Flex and extend the neck and bend it laterally in both directions. Apply direct pressure on the lateral processes of the sixth cervical vertebra.

Animals may exhibit a forelimb lameness associated with cervical nerve root pain (root signature sign) and it is important to rule out cervical disease or nerve root tumors.

Apply direct pressure on the thoracolumbar spine while supporting the abdomen.

A painful response, exhibited by vocalization, flinching, or tightening the abdominal musculature may indicate thoracolumbar spinal disease.

Apply direct pressure on the ventral lumbar musculature to isolate lumbosacral pain (Fig. 31-12).

It is important to differentiate lumbosacral and hip pain because many older dogs with radiographic signs of hip dysplasia have concurrent lumbosacral pain, which may cause lameness and reluctance to rise and move. Pressure on the dorsal lumbosacral area also pressures the hip, making it difficult to differentiate the source of the pain. Likewise, hip extension also pulls on the iliopsoas muscles, again making it difficult to pinpoint the source of the pain.

Apply pressure to digits of the affected limb to elicit a response to superficial and deep pain.

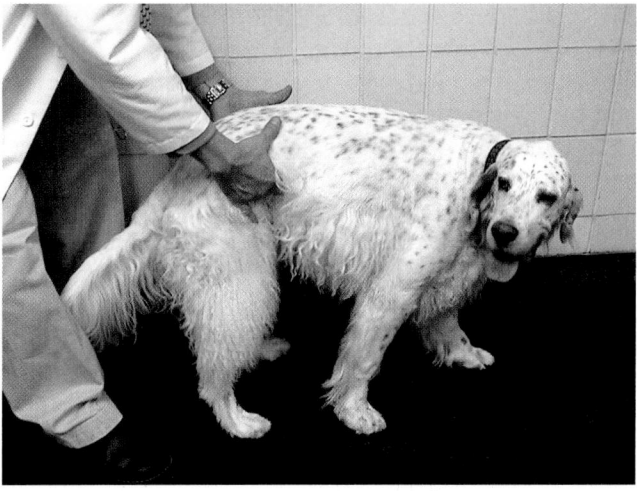

FIG. 31-12
To isolate lumbosacral pain, apply direct pressure to the ventral lumbar musculature.

Peripheral nerve damage may result concurrently with fractures of the middle to distal humerus (radial nerve) or sacrum (sciatic nerve). No response may indicate peripheral nerve damage.

ADDITIONAL DIAGNOSTIC TECHNIQUES

A differential diagnosis is developed based on results of history, signalment, and physical examination. Definitive diagnoses may require additional diagnostic tools including imaging, hematology, serum biochemistry, cytology, or electrodiagnostics. Diagnostic imaging is generally the first step toward definitive diagnosis. Joint taps are useful for differentiating degenerative and inflammatory disease (see p. 1145). Fine needle aspirates or biopsies are essential for diagnosing neoplastic disease (see p. 1341).

Diagnostic Imaging

Quality radiographs are essential for completing an orthopedic examination, refining the differential diagnosis, and arriving at a definitive diagnosis. Radiography is also used to evaluate fracture healing. Appropriate x-ray equipment (300 mA or greater) and processing capabilities are required to produce radiographs with sufficient contrast and detail. Correct patient positioning is important; chemical restraint is often necessary to allow proper patient manipulation, decrease radiographic study time, and minimize radiation exposure to the operator. Reversible drugs allow temporary patient immobilization (see Tables 31-2 and 31-3). Patient selection is important; some animals that are ill or in shock (e.g., after trauma) should not be sedated. To minimize magnification and loss of detail, the area of interest must be placed as close to the x-ray film as possible. Minimizing superimposition of structures overlying the area of interest requires careful patient positioning. For a given site, adequate evaluation usually requires that two views be made at 90 degrees to each other (orthogonal views). Additional views (e.g., oblique, flexed, and stress) may be needed to evaluate the problem accurately. To evaluate fractures and postoperative fracture repairs, radiographs of the long bones must include the joints above and below the bone of interest.

In addition to quality radiographs, detection, knowledge, and correlation of significant radiographic findings with clinical data are essential. Variations in anatomic structure and skeletal conformation among dog breeds may make it difficult to distinguish between normal and abnormal findings. Remember that animals usually have a normal "control" limb on the opposite side. Comparing radiographs of the affected and normal limbs helps determine whether the suspected abnormality is a normal structure. Subtle morphologic changes that are bilaterally symmetric are rare. Comparison radiographs are essential for evaluating physeal injuries in immature animals. Early changes in the function of a physis can be detected by measuring the length of the affected bone and comparing it with the length of the unaffected opposite bone. Always correlate the radiographic findings with clinical information.

Serial radiographs are necessary for correct interpretation of dynamic processes (e.g., fracture healing and inflammatory bone disease). This is especially important when interpreting the significance of bone reaction. Radiographs made 2 to 3 weeks apart may show rapidly accelerated growth with primary bone tumors or a reparative process with regression in nonneoplastic diseases.

Computed Tomography

Computed tomography (CT) provides a cross-sectional image of the area of interest. Advantages of CT over conventional radiographs include superior tissue density differentiation and no superimposition of overlying structures. CT also allows images to be reformatted in different planes including three dimensional reconstruction. CT is superior to conventional radiography for identifying neoplastic bone margins before tumor resection. CT is also used to identify stenosis of the spinal column and lesions of the spinal cord and surrounding soft tissue (particularly when used with myelography). CT can detect small fragments that may be obscured by surrounding bone on radiographs (e.g., fragmented coronoid processes and bone sequestra). CT also can identify bone bridging within the physis and facilitate early treatment of growth deformities. Three dimensional reconstruction is useful for assessment and treatment planning for complex comminuted fractures, particularly of the mandible and pelvis.

Magnetic Resonance Imaging

Magnetic resonance imaging (MRI) provides superior soft tissue definition. When the area of interest is placed within the magnetic field, hydrogen atoms align in a single plane. Pulsation of an external radiofrequency alters atom alignment, and realignment causes energy emission. The energy signal is picked up by a radiofrequency receiver, analyzed, and processed by a computer that reconstructs the image. The signal intensity is a complex combination of (1) hydrogen density in the various tissues, (2) the rate at which the hydrogen atoms realign along the magnetic field and lose synchronization with each other's spin, and (3) blood flow. The relative effect of each of these components is altered by varying the pulse sequence. The advantages of MRI include enhanced soft tissue contrast and absence of tissue superimposition over the area of interest. Contrast and definition between soft tissue structures, such as spinal cord, epidural fat, and disk material, are possible without using contrast materials. MRI does not provide cortical bone detail. Because bone does not contain hydrogen ions, it has a reduced signal compared with surrounding soft tissue. MRI is used to identify central nervous system changes, including spinal cord compression (especially in the cervical and lumbosacral spine) and soft tissue components of joints (e.g., cruciate ligament and menisci).

Ultrasonography

Ultrasonography is a diagnostic imaging procedure that uses high frequency sound waves (ultrasound) to produce dynamic visual images of organs, tissue, or blood flow inside the body. Ultrasonography is most useful in orthopedic evaluations of injured soft tissue structures, such as tendons, ligaments, and muscles. Additionally, ultrasonography may be used to monitor the healing process of these structures.

Bone Scintigraphy

Bone scintigraphy is used to evaluate the physiology or activity of bone. Bone-seeking radioisotopes, such as technetium 99m linked to methylene diphosphonate, are administered intravenously. This radiolabeled compound is gradually incorporated into actively metabolizing bone over hours; the distribution of the radiopharmaceutical can be visualized using gamma camera scanning. The images obtained represent the distribution of the bone tracer according to current rates of bone turnover and blood flow. Because increased bone turnover occurs before radiographic changes are visible, scintigraphy will identify bone abnormalities earlier than other imaging modalities.

Scintigraphy is the procedure of choice for obscure lameness in which the origin cannot be pinpointed with physical examination or identified with radiographs because the entire skeleton can be scanned relatively easily. Other indications for scintigraphy in small animals include identification of bone metastasis, acute osteomyelitis, and bone sequestration, and evaluation of bone activity in fracture nonunions. Scintigraphy and radiography complement each other because scintigraphy identifies areas of high bone turnover without specifying cause, whereas radiography often allows lesion interpretation. Therefore radiographs are usually performed after lesions have been identified with scintigraphy.

DEFINITIVE DIAGNOSIS OF ORTHOPEDIC DISEASE

Definitive diagnoses for orthopedic diseases generally include fractures (see Chapter 32), joint disease (see Chapter 33), muscle and tendon injuries (see Chapter 34), metabolic bone diseases (see Chapter 35), infectious disease (see Chapters 33 and 35) and neoplastic disease (see Chapter 35).

Suggested Reading

Brinker WO, Piermattei DL, Flo GL: *Handbook of small animal orthopedics and fracture treatment,* ed 3, Philadelphia, 1997, WB Saunders.

This textbook also provides an excellent step-by-step description of an orthopedic examination.

Kramer M, Gerwing M, Michele U et al: Ultrasonographic examination of injuries to the Achilles tendon in dogs and cats, *J Small Anim Pract* 42:531, 2001.

This study provides an evaluation of the usefulness of ultrasonography in examining Achilles tendon injuries. Identification and differentiation of tendon ruptures were possible. The healing process could also be monitored using this technique.

Kramer M, Gerwing M, Sheppard C et al: Ultrasonography for diagnosis of diseases of the tendon and tendon sheath of the biceps brachii muscle, *Vet Surg* 30:64, 2001.

This article provides information concerning the use of ultrasonography as a complementary imaging modality for diagnosis of disease processes of the tendon and tendon sheath of the biceps brachii muscle.

Thrall DE: *Textbook of veterinary diagnostic radiology,* Philadelphia, 2002, WB Saunders.

The preceding is a basic veterinary radiology textbook to be used as a reference for imaging and diagnosis of orthopedic disease.

PREOPERATIVE MANAGEMENT

Perioperative management of surgical patients is discussed in detail in Chapter 5. Orthopedic patients may be brought in for elective surgery (e.g., cranial cruciate ligament injury, hip dysplasia, and osteochondritis dissecans), nonelective surgery (e.g., bone fractures and joint luxations), or conditions that require emergency treatment (e.g., open fractures and open joint dislocations). When animals are brought in for elective surgery, there is ample time to perform an appropriate preoperative diagnostic evaluation. Younger patients (less than 2 years old) should have selected screening laboratory tests, including packed-cell volume (PCV), serum total solids, and urinalysis. Fecal analysis and heartworm tests may be indicated, depending on the history and the animal's geographic location. The need for further laboratory evaluation should be based on signalment, physical examination, and results of initial screening tests.

Older patients (2 years and older) with orthopedic disease must be assessed more carefully than younger patients. Just as the physiologic properties of the musculoskeletal system decline with age, other organ systems also deteriorate. Thorough physical examination remains the foundation of preoperative evaluation and should be supplemented with a complete blood count, chemistry profile, and urinalysis. Special diagnostic tests (e.g., coagulation profile) may be indicated, depending on the history, signalment, and physical findings.

Patients in need of immediate or emergency surgical care should have a thorough and complete physical evaluation. Serial examinations are important because serious or potentially lethal problems may not become evident for several hours or days after the injury. Although organ dysfunction may be evident (or suspected) on initial physical examination, repeated examinations may be necessary to define the severity of injury. Animals that have received an external blow severe enough to disrupt musculoskeletal integrity (e.g., fracture and luxation) often have concurrent external or internal organ system injury. Cardiovascular, pulmonary, urinary, and neurologic systems are most frequently injured. If abnormalities are found, a differential diagnosis and diagnostic plan for each problem should be developed and additional diagnostic tests completed. For example, cardiac arrhythmias and femoral pulse abnormalities may be found in patients with traumatic myocarditis, necessitating thoracic radiographs and an ECG to assess treatment options and anesthetic risk. Auscultation may detect pulmonary injury (e.g., lung contusion and pneumothorax), but physical changes may be subtle and missed on physical examination. Because one third or more of fracture patients have some degree of pulmonary injury, preoperative evaluation should include thoracic radiographs. Some abnormalities may necessitate that surgical repair of the orthopedic disease be delayed (e.g., uroabdomen), whereas others may alter the prognosis such that repairing the orthopedic condition is not justified (e.g., vertebral fracture with loss of deep pain sensation).

Because most orthopedic patients that need immediate or emergency surgical care have sustained trauma, laboratory evaluation is essential. A minimum database should include a complete blood count, chemistry profile, and urinalysis. Additional laboratory tests (e.g., coagulation profile, electrolytes, and acid-base balance) may be required to assess differential diagnoses developed on physical examination. Abnormal values should be assessed in light of physical findings, and the need for additional or serial tests should be determined. Serial tests are useful to validate abnormal findings and monitor patient progress. Delaying surgical intervention until abnormal organ function returns to normal is optimal; however, it is often not feasible.

PAIN MANAGEMENT AND ANESTHESIA

Trauma patients may benefit from preoperative analgesics, such as morphine or transdermal fentanyl (Box 31-2 and Table 31-4). The level of postoperative discomfort and the duration of discomfort should be assessed to determine choice of analgesic before surgery. Most orthopedic surgeries are considered moderately to severely painful. Clinical and experimental studies clearly indicate that analgesics are most effective when administered before painful stimuli; thus they should be administered initially as part of the preoperative medication (see Chapter 13).

Anesthetic protocols should be based on signalment, physical examination findings, and laboratory analysis. Patients who need correction of elective orthopedic problems (e.g., cruciate reconstruction) and who have no preoperative findings suggestive of major organ dysfunction can be managed using a variety of anesthetic techniques (Box 31-3; see also Chapter 13). Patients undergoing correction of acute

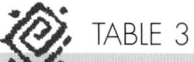 BOX 31-2

Orthopedic Pain Management in Dogs and Cats

Preoperative

- As dictated by current or anticipated pain
- Morphine: 0.4 mg/kg IV slowly, IM, or SC every 4–6 hr *or*
- Transdermal fentanyl patch: see Table 31-4, *or*
- Butorphanol* (Torbutrol, Torbugesic): 0.2–0.4 mg/kg IV, IM, or SC every 2–4 hr
- Oxymorphone* (Numorphan): 0.05–0.1 mg/kg IV, SC, or IM every 4 hr
- Buprenorphine* (Buprenex): 5–15 μg/kg IV or IM every 6 hr
- Hydromorphone (generic): 0.1–0.2 mg/kg, IV, SC, or IM every 4 hr

*Start with the lower dose when giving IV or administering to cats.

Intraoperative

- Balanced anesthesia, including epidural analgesia and CRI

Postoperative: First 24 hr

- Morphine: 0.4 mg/kg IV slowly, IM, or SC every 4–6 hr *or*
- Butorphanol (Torbutrol, Torbugesic): 0.2–0.4 mg/kg IV, IM, or SC every 2–4 hr (as needed) *or*
- Oxymorphone (Numorphan): 0.05–0.1 mg/kg IV or IM every 4 hr *or*
- Buprenorphine (Buprenex): 5–15 μg/kg IV, SC or IM every 6 hr *or*
- Hydromorphone: 0.1–0.2 mg/kg, IV, SC, or IM every 4 hr

Postoperative: After 24 hr*

- Carprofen (Rimadyl): 2.2 mg/kg PO bid for 3–7 days (dogs)
- Deracoxib: 1–2 mg/kg PO qd for 3–7 days (dogs)
- Meloxicam: 0.1–0.2 mg/kg SC once (cats)

IV, Intravenous; *IM,* intramuscular; *SC,* subcutaneous; *CRI,* continuous rate infusion; *PO,* oral; *bid,* twice a day; *qd,* once a day.
*Other NSAIDs are available, but are used off-label in this country. NSAIDs should be restricted to those with proven safety and efficacy in the target species. See label for side effects. These drugs are also labeled for preoperative use. See Chapter 13 for additional information on administration of these drugs.

 TABLE 31-4

Guidelines for Fentanyl Patch Dosing*

BODY WEIGHT (kg)	PATCH SIZE (μg/hr)
<3.2	12.5; not recommended†
3.2–6.8	25
6.8–18.2	50
18.2–27.3	75
>27.3	100

*Guidelines are not well established; generally, transdermal fentanyl patches should deliver 1–4 μg/kg/hr.
†A 25-μg/hr patch may deliver up to 7.8 μg/kg/hr in a 3.2-kg patient and is not recommended; it is unknown how covering a portion of the patch or cutting the patch affects delivery; a 12.5-μg patch is available but has not been tested in veterinary patients.

(A) BOX 31-3

Suggested Protocols for Anesthetic Management of Patients With Orthopedic Disease

For Stable Patients and Those Brought in for Elective Procedures

Premedication

Glycopyrrolate (0.005–0.011 mg/kg SC or IM) or atropine (0.02–0.04 mg/kg SC or IM) *plus* hydromorphone (0.1–0.2 mg/kg SC or IM) *or* butorphanol (0.2–0.4 mg/kg SC or IM) *or* buprenorphine (5–15 μg/kg IM) *and* acepromazine (0.05 mg/kg, not to exceed 1 mg SC or IM)

Induction

Thiopental (10–12 mg/kg IV) or propofol (4–6 mg/kg IV)

Maintenance

Isoflurane or sevoflurane

For Unstable Animals That Have Recently Had Trauma

Induction

Hydromorphone (0.1 mg/kg IV) *plus* diazepam (0.2 mg/kg IV). Give in incremental dosages. Intubate if possible. If necessary, give etomidate (0.5–1.5 mg/kg IV). Alternatively, mask induction or thiopental or propofol at extremely reduced dosages may be used.

Maintenance

Isoflurane or sevoflurane

SC, Subcutaneous; *IM,* intramuscular; *IV,* intravenous.

traumatic injuries or systemic disease should be anesthetized with care. ECG and thoracic radiographs should be performed and hypovolemia corrected before surgery.

Maintenance of fracture patients on inhalant anesthetics is preferred over barbiturate anesthesia because it provides better muscle relaxation for fracture reduction. Balanced anesthetic protocols that include analgesic agents supplemented with epidural analgesia are recommended to decrease intraoperative pain response and reduce the amount of anesthetic needed (Table 31-5). Epidural anesthesia (with lidocaine or bupivacaine) in combination with general anesthesia provides profound relaxation of rear limb muscles, easing fracture reduction of the pelvis, femur, and tibia (see Chapter 13). The duration of action depends on the drug used, but is usually 1 to 2 hours. Morphine can be added to the epidural injection, providing postoperative pain relief for up to 20 hours. A brachial plexus block using bupivacaine (see p. 137) may provide additional analgesia and muscle relaxation in some patients undergoing surgery of the forelimb.

Analgesics should be administered for 12 to 24 hours after surgery, depending on the procedure and results of serial patient evaluations (see Box 31-2). Butorphanol or buprenor-

TABLE 31-5

Epidural Anesthesia in the Dog

DRUG	DOSE	ONSET OF ACTION (MINUTES)	DURATION OF ACTION (HR)
Lidocaine 2%*	1 ml/3.4 kg (T5)† 1 ml/4.5 kg (T13–L1)†	10	1–1.5
Bupivacaine (0.25% or 0.5%)* (preservative free)	1 ml/4.5 kg	20–30	4.5–6
Fentanyl	0.001 mg/kg	4–10	6
Oxymorphone	0.1 mg/kg	15‡	10
Morphine (preservative free)	0.1 mg/kg§	23	20
Buprenorphine	0.003–0.005 mg/kg (diluted with saline)	30‡	12–18

*Avoid head-down position after epidural.
†A block to T1 leads to intercostal nerve paralysis; a block to C7-C5 leads to phrenic nerve paralysis.
‡Approximate onset of action.
§Same dose may be used in cats.

phine is recommended in patients undergoing procedures requiring minimal tissue manipulation. Buprenorphine provides longer postoperative relief (6 hours) compared with butorphanol (2 hours) and is more useful when redosing is inconvenient after surgery. In patients undergoing more painful procedures that require significant tissue manipulation (e.g., triple pelvic osteotomy) or in those with traumatic injuries, hydromorphone or morphine is recommended. In the latter patients, opioid epidural agents can be administered to supplement systemic opioid analgesia.

> NOTE: When using opioids preoperatively, be sure to adjust the systemic opioid dose to account for the dose given epidurally; calculate the total patient dose and divide between systemic and epidural administration.

Nonsteroidal antiinflammatory drugs (NSAIDs) are also advocated for pain control in orthopedic patients (see Box 31-2 and Table 31-6). They can be used alone or in combination with opioids. Opioids provide immediate relief, whereas the NSAIDs provide sustained relief. Both carprofen and deracoxib given before surgery are effective for postoperative pain relief in dogs. Meloxicam injection is approved for use in cats preoperatively (one dose only). Preemptive analgesia is important because even for healthy animals the anesthetic course cannot be predicted; however, it is prudent to reserve NSAIDs for postoperative administration. Opioids are preferred for use as preoperative analgesics because they have fewer cardiopulmonary effects than NSAIDs, and if hypotension does occur, its effects can be readily treated. Opioids are also less apt to potentiate hypotension than inhalants. Preemptive use of ketoprofen is contraindicated for surgical procedures in which noncompressible hemorrhage is antici-

 TABLE 31-6

Nonsteroidal Antiinflammatory Drugs Approved for Treating Dogs With Orthopedic Disease

Carprofen	2.2 mg/kg PO q 12 hr
Deracoxib	1–2 mg/kg PO q 24 hr*
Etodolac	10–15 mg/kg PO q 24 hr
Meloxicam	0.2 mg/kg q 24 hr for 1 day, followed by 0.1 mg/kg q 24 hr (in food)
Tepoxalin	10 mg/kg PO q 24 hr†
Firocoxib	5 mg/kg PO q 24 hr

PO, Oral.
*A higher dose (3–4 mg/kg/day) may be used short term for postoperative pain (do not confuse the two dosages).
†May give 20 mg/kg as the initial dose, followed by 10 mg/kg.

pated. NSAIDs can also be continued orally for several days after surgery to provide pain relief after the animal has been discharged from the hospital. See Chapter 33 (p. 1147) for additional information on NSAIDs.

ANTIBIOTICS

Antimicrobial agents are often used for prophylaxis and treatment of orthopedic infections. Debate continues over which patients should receive prophylactic antibiotics. Reviews of orthopedic patients have shown that those animals with severe soft tissue and bone trauma, multiple fractures, and traumatic surgical procedures are most likely to have postoperative wound infections develop. Therefore prophylactic antibiotics should be administered in contaminated cases (open injuries), patients with severe trauma (significant soft tissue bruising and swelling or multiple bone fractures), and cases requiring lengthy operative times (2 hours or longer). Prophylactic antibiotics are also effective in routine orthopedic surgery. Results of a recent clinical study showed that prophylactic antibiotics administered 30 minutes before clean orthopedic surgical procedures and repeated every 2 hours during surgery resulted in fewer postoperative infections than in control patients given a saline placebo (Whittem et al, 1999). Also, prophylactic antibiotics are recommended for elective procedures in which postoperative infection would be catastrophic (e.g., hip replacement). See Chapter 10 for general prophylactic antibiotic recommendations.

If prophylactic antibiotics are used, they must be used properly. Timing of antibiotic administration and rational selection of appropriate antibiotics must be considered. Effective antimicrobial use is based on two criteria: (1) which microorganisms are most likely to cause orthopedic wound infections and (2) which antibiotics are most likely to be effective against potential offending microorganisms. Coagulase-positive *Staphylococcus* species and *Escherichia coli* are the preponderant aerobic bacteria isolated from surgical wounds in small animal patients. Anaerobic bacteria (e.g., *Bacteroides*, *Fusobacterium*, and *Clostridium* spp.) are now also recognized as important pathogens in orthopedic patients. Knowledge of common offending microorganisms in correlation with results of periodic culture of surgical tables, instrument stands, and surgical lights provides insight into potential bacteria in the surgical environment.

At present *cefazolin* is the antibiotic of choice for prophylaxis in small animal orthopedic surgery. Adequate concentrations of cefazolin must be present within tissue at the time bacteria enter the wound to suppress bacterial growth effectively. Thus antibiotics must be administered before surgery rather than after completion of the procedure. However, there is no reason to begin prophylactic antibiotic administration long before surgery. Based on empiric and experimental evidence, antibiotics should be administered intravenously (IV) at the time of anesthetic induction, repeated every 2 to 4 hours, and discontinued at completion of surgery. Concentrations of the drug equal to or greater than the minimum inhibitory concentration (MIC) needed to prevent proliferation of known pathogens are desirable. The cefazolin MIC for coagulase-positive *Staphylococcus* species and *E. coli* is 4 mg/ml. Cefazolin, 22 mg/kg IV, administered 20 minutes before surgery and repeated every 2 to 4 hours, maintains drug concentrations at the surgery site above 4 mg/ml.

FRACTURE SUPPORT

Unstable injuries should be coapted to reduce further soft tissue injury and increase patient comfort. External splints can be used to provide temporary limb support or as a primary means of fracture stabilization. To prevent complications, external splints must be properly applied and carefully monitored. Most complications associated with external splints are minor (e.g., swelling of limb distal to splint, splint slippage, and skin abrasions), although serious complica-

tions may occur (e.g., fracture nonunion and loss of a limb from ischemic necrosis). Therefore the application of an external splint should not be considered a minor procedure or one that does not require careful observation. The most common temporary supports are Robert Jones bandages and lighter bandages supported with spoon splints or other coaptation materials (Table 31-7). Fractures or luxations below the elbow and stifle joint are best managed with a soft padded bandage, with or without additional support using fiberglass casting or metal splints. Fractures above the elbow or stifle joint are more difficult to coapt. A spica splint that crosses the body above the shoulder (or hip) provides the best external coaptation.

Bandages also serve many functions postoperatively, including wound protection, application of topical medication, soft tissue compression, increased patient comfort, and selective immobilization of soft tissue and joints. Bandages often used in veterinary orthopedics for postoperative comfort and soft tissue compression or limb immobilization include soft padded bandages, Ehmer slings, and Velpeau slings.

Robert Jones Bandages

Robert Jones bandages and their modifications are the external splints most often used in veterinary patients. These bulky, cotton-gauze wrappings are typically used before or after surgery for temporary limb splintage. The original Robert Jones bandage used commercially available, 12-inch, rolled cotton that was liberally applied to the limb to a thickness of 4 to 6 inches. Modified Robert Jones bandages use less cotton, but still provide compression (see Table 31-7). The thick cotton layer provides mild compression of soft tissue and immobilizes fractures without causing vascular compromise. Soft tissue and bone immobilization enhance patient comfort and prevent further soft tissue damage from sharp bone fragments. Additionally, Robert Jones bandages help eliminate dead space after surgery.

NOTE: Robert Jones bandages extend from the toes to the midfemur or midhumerus and are only useful when applied to injuries below the stifle or elbow joint.

Prepare the limb by clipping long hair from the midhumerus (midfemur) to the toes and treat any open wounds. Apply adhesive tape stirrups to cranial and caudal surfaces of the foot from carpus (tarsus) to 6 inches beyond the toes (Fig. 31-13, A). Wrap 3 to 6 inches of cotton padding (from a 12-inch roll or cast padding) around the limb from toes to midhumerus (midfemur) (Fig. 31-13, B). Ensure that the nails of the third and fourth digits are visible so that limb swelling can be detected. Then wrap elastic gauze firmly over the cotton to compress it (Fig. 31-13, C). Apply at least two to three layers of gauze to achieve smooth, even tension; sufficient compression will cause the bandage to sound like a ripe watermelon when tapped with a finger. Invert the tape

TABLE 31-7

Materials Needed for Application of Bandages, Splints, and Casts

ROBERT JONES BANDAGE	METAL SPOON SPLINT	SPICA SPLINT	CAST
Adhesive tape	Metal spoon splint	Adhesive tape	Cast material
Cotton padding	Adhesive tape	Cast padding	Stockinette
Gauze	Cast padding	Gauze	Adhesive tape
Elastic tape or Vetrap	Gauze	Elastic tape or Vetrap	Cast padding
	Elastic tape or Vetrap	Cast material	Gauze
			Elastic tape or Vetrap

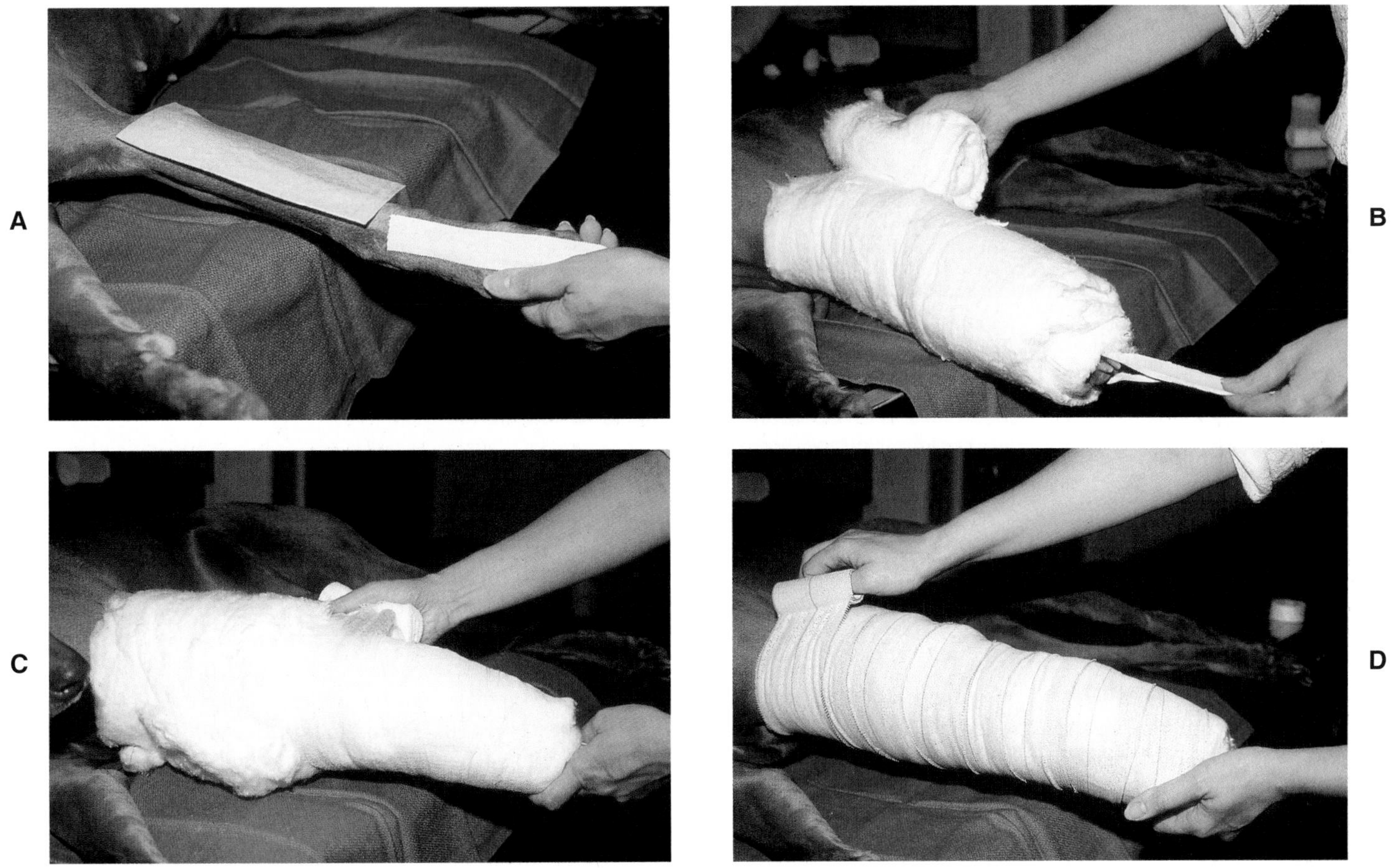

FIG. 31-13
A, When applying a Robert Jones bandage, place adhesive tape stirrups on the cranial and caudal surfaces of the foot from the carpus (tarsus) to 6 inches beyond the toes. Cover any wounds with a nonadhesive pad. **B,** Then wrap 3 to 6 inches of cotton padding around the limb. **C,** After applying tape stirrups and cotton padding on the limb, wrap elastic gauze firmly over the cotton to compress it. **D,** Then apply elastic tape to the outer surface of the bandage.

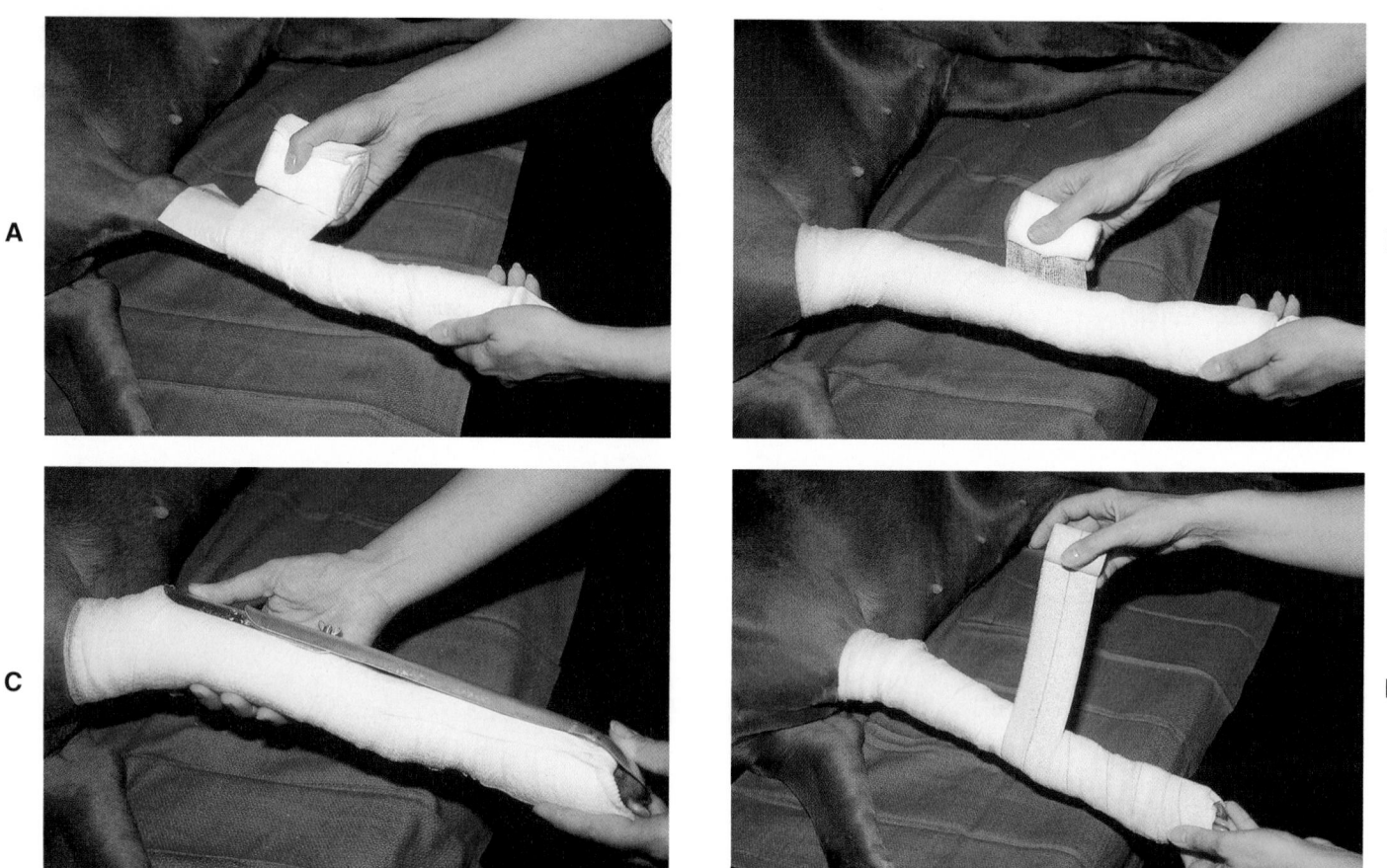

FIG. 31-14
A, When placing a spoon splint on a limb, firmly apply cast padding around the limb in a spiral fashion with a 50% overlap. **B,** Wrap elastic gauze firmly over the cast padding. **C,** Place the padded limb in an appropriate-sized splint. **D,** Secure the splint to the limb with Vetrap or elastic adhesive tape.

stirrups and stick them to the outer layer of gauze. Then apply elastic tape (e.g., Elasticon, Vetrap) to the outer surface of the bandage (Fig. 31-13, D).

Metal Spoon Splints

Metal spoon splints *(metasplints)* are used to provide support to injuries of the distal radius and ulna, carpus or tarsus, metacarpus or metatarsus, and phalanges. Metasplints are used for ancillary support of internal fixation devices or as a primary means of fixation when the patient fracture-assessment score (see p. 953) indicates minimal stress and rapid healing. Spoon splints are commercially available in aluminum or plastic in a variety of lengths and sizes (see Table 31-7).

Clip long hair and treat open wounds (see p. 163) before covering them with a sterile dressing. Apply adhesive tape stirrups from the carpus (tarsus) to toes, leaving the ends extending 6 inches beyond the toes. Firmly apply cast padding around the limb in a spiral fashion with a 50% overlap (Fig. 31-14, A). Begin the padding at the toes and extend it proximally 1 inch beyond the proximal aspect of the splint. Apply just enough cotton to prevent skin abrasions and pressure sores, but do not make the bandage so bulky that it will be awkward for the patient. Cover bony prominences with excess padding. Wrap elastic gauze over the cotton to compress it (Fig. 31-14, B). Place the padded limb in an appropriate-sized splint and secure it to the limb with Vetrap or elastic adhesive tape (Fig. 31-14, C and D). Invert and stick the stirrups to the final wrapping.

Soft Padded Bandages

Soft padded bandages are used when excessive compression of the tissue is not desired. The bandage is initially applied as described earlier for Mason metasplints. Instead of using the preformed metasplint, the bandage may be applied without a splint, or a lateral splint made of fiberglass casting material may be inserted to reinforce the bandage, as described next for spica splints. Reinforcing a padded bandage applied to the rear limb with a lateral splint also prevents the bandage from folding as the limb is used.

Spica Splints

Spica splints envelop the torso and affected limb and are often used as temporary splints to immobilize humeral or femoral fractures or as adjunctive stabilization after internal fixation (see Table 31-7). They are rarely used as a primary means of stabilization unless the fracture is nondisplaced and the fracture-assessment score indicates that rapid bone union will occur.

Clip long hair and treat open wounds (see p. 163) before covering them with a sterile dressing. Place adhesive tape stirrups on the cranial and caudal surfaces of the limb, and apply cotton cast padding to the limb and torso. Begin the padding at the paw and wrap it proximally in a spiral fashion, overlapping it 50%. When the inguinal or axillary region is reached, wrap the cotton padding around the animal's torso several times, alternating cranially and caudally to the affected limb. Then wrap elastic gauze over the cast padding (50% overlap). Wrap the gauze firmly around the limb for mild compression of the soft tissue. Reinforce the spica bandage with fiberglass casting material to provide additional stabilization of the fracture ends. Fold the casting tape onto itself to provide a lateral splint that is four to six layers thick, extending from toes to dorsal midline. Use Vetrap or elastic adhesive tape to hold the fiberglass cast to the limb and provide an outer covering for the splint (Fig. 31-15).

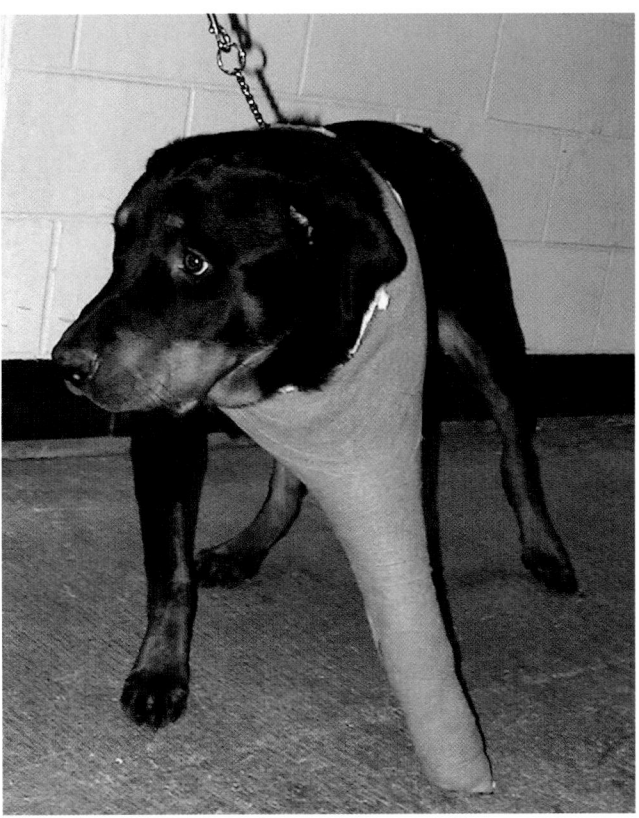

FIG. 31-15
Spica splint applied to the forelimb of a dog to temporarily immobilize the limb after fracture of the humerus.

Ehmer slings. Ehmer slings prevent weight bearing of the pelvic limb (Fig. 31-16). The most common use for Ehmer slings is to support closed or open reduction of hip luxations.

Place a thin layer of cast padding around the metatarsal area and wrap nonadherent gauze (e.g., Kling) multiple times over the padding. Maximally flex the stifle and wrap the gauze around the thigh by bringing it medially between the body wall and limb. Pull the gauze firmly and bring it over the front of the knee to maintain flexion. Then wrap the gauze over the lateral surface of the thigh and bring it distally medial to the tarsus and over the padded metatarsal area. Repeat the wrapping three or four times. Finish the bandage by applying elastic adhesive material in the same manner.

Velpeau slings. Velpeau slings prevent weight bearing and provide some stability to the proximal forelimb (Fig. 31-17). They are most often used to help maintain closed or open reduction of medial shoulder luxations and to support scapular fractures.

With the shoulder and elbow flexed and the limb adducted against the body wall, begin by placing two or three layers of padding around the torso and limb. Wrap layers cranial and caudal to the opposite limb to prevent slippage of the incorporated limb. Place an additional layer in a similar manner with gauze (e.g., Kling) to add mild compression. Place an outer layer of elastic tape or Vetrap to provide support.

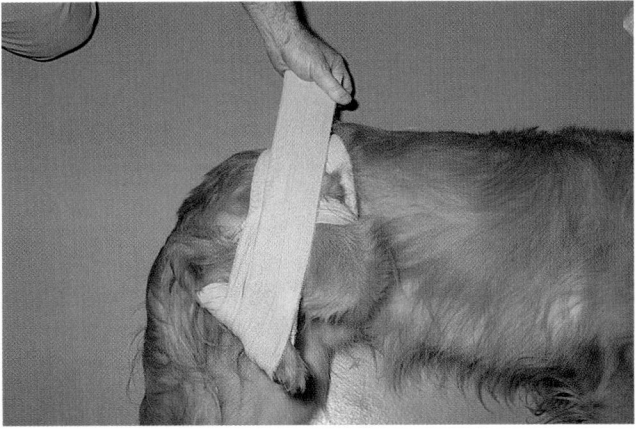

FIG. 31-16
Ehmer sling applied to rear limb of dog. These slings are used to prevent weight bearing (e.g., after hip luxation).

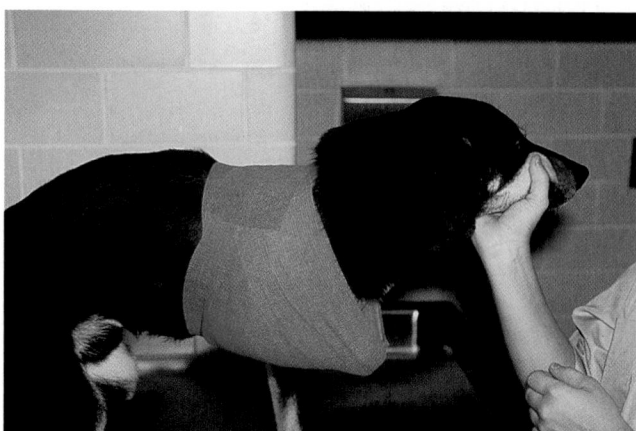

FIG. 31-17
Velpeau sling applied to forelimb of dog with scapular fracture.

POSTOPERATIVE CARE AND ASSESSMENT

Postoperative instructions for each orthopedic technique are presented in the discussions on various orthopedic conditions. Common to the success of all orthopedic procedures is adequate client communications concerning postoperative care, regular reevaluations, and the use of appropriate physical rehabilitation methods (see Chapter 12).

Adequate follow-up care for bandages and splints is essential for preventing complications After placing a Robert Jones bandage, soft padded bandage, metal spoon splint, lateral splint, spica splint or sling, the toes should be observed twice a day for swelling. The bandage or splint must be kept clean and dry. If it is wet outside, a plastic bag should be temporarily placed over the limb to cover the toes and bandage. The limb should be observed for signs of irritation or discharge, and the bandage or splint should be removed to inspect the limb if either is present. Velpeau and Ehmer slings should not be used for more than 2 weeks. Long-term limb immobilization in a flexed position makes rehabilitation difficult.

General postoperative instructions for fracture patients include postoperative radiographs made to document fracture reduction or alignment and implant position. After internal fixation, if possible, the limb is supported for a few days with a soft padded bandage to reduce swelling. Patient activity is generally restricted to leash walking and physical rehabilitation until the fracture has healed. Physical rehabilitation encourages controlled limb use and optimal limb function after fracture healing. Care must be taken to develop customized protocols for each patient depending on location of the fracture, stability and type of fracture fixation, potential for healing, abilities and attitudes of the patient, and willingness of the client (see Chapter 12 and specific fractures). Fracture fixation systems have specific follow-up care that is detailed in the discussions of each system and specific fractures. Establishing excellent client communications and a reevaluation schedule for each patient is paramount for successful fracture management (Box 31-4).

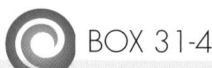 BOX 31-4

Postoperative Fracture Management: Evaluation Schedule

- 1 wk: Phone
- 2 wk: Suture removal and/or physical examination
- 4 wk: Phone
- 6 wk: Radiographic and physical examination
- Repeat phone contact and radiographic and/or physical examination every 6 wk until fracture is healed. Intervals and duration vary with fracture-assessment score.

Reference

Whittem T, Johnson AL, Smith CW et al: Effect of perioperative prophylactic antimicrobial treatment in dogs undergoing elective orthopedic surgery, *J Am Vet Med Assoc* 215:212, 1999.

Suggested Reading

Brinker WO, Piermattei DL, Flo GL: *Handbook of small animal orthopedics and fracture treatment,* ed 3, Philadelphia, 1997, WB Saunders.
This reference contains excellent step-by-step illustrations for bandage, splint, sling, and cast applications.

OPERATIVE PLANNING

CLASSIFICATION OF FRACTURES

Fractures are classified according to (1) displacement of the major bone segments and stability of the fracture; (2) the location, direction, and number of fracture lines; (3) whether the fracture fragments can be reconstructed to provide load bearing (reducible or nonreducible); and (4) whether the fracture is open to the environment. Fractures occur in the articular surface, the metaphysis, the physis, and the diaphysis. Fractures may be complete or incomplete. A *greenstick fracture,* occurring in immature animals, is an incomplete fracture in which a portion of the cortex is intact, thus stabilizing the bone to some extent. *Avulsion fractures* occur when the insertion point of a tendon or ligament is fractured and distracted from the rest of the bone. A fracture line perpendicular to the long axis of the bone is a *transverse* fracture. *Oblique* fracture lines run at an angle to the long axis of the bone; they are described as *short oblique* fractures if they are 45 degrees or less or *long oblique* fractures if they are greater than 45 degrees to the long axis of the bone. *Spiral* fractures are similar to long oblique fractures, but wrap around the long axis of the bone. *Comminuted* fractures have multiple fracture lines. They can range from three-piece fractures with a *butterfly fragment* (fragment with two oblique fracture lines resembling a butterfly's silhouette) to highly comminuted fractures with five or more pieces (Fig. 31-18). For operative planning, fractures should be mentally classified as *reducible* (usually single fracture line or fractures with no more than two large fragments) or *nonreducible* (fractures with multiple small fragments).

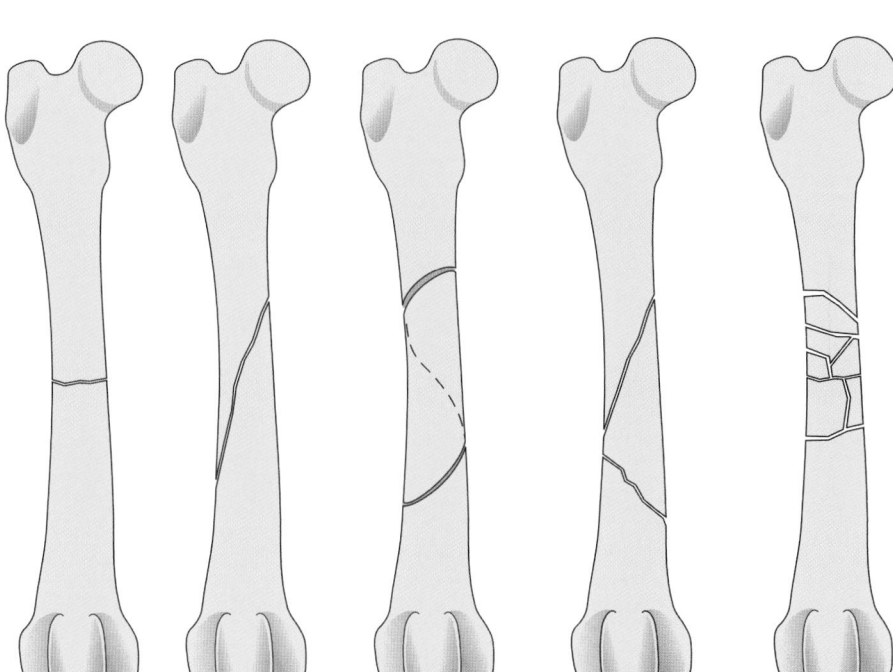

FIG. 31-18
Classification of fractures based on direction and number of fracture lines.

Transverse   Oblique   Spiral   Comminuted, reducible   Comminuted, nonreducible

Open Fractures

Open fractures are classified according to (1) the mechanism of puncture and (2) the severity of soft tissue injury. A *Grade I* open fracture has a small puncture hole located in the skin in the proximity of the fracture that was caused by the bone penetrating to the outside. The bone may or may not be visible in the wound. A *Grade II* open fracture has a variably sized skin wound associated with the fracture that resulted from external trauma. More damage to the soft tissue is generally associated with Grade II than with Grade I open fractures. Although the extent of the soft tissue damage may vary, the fracture is minimally comminuted. A *Grade III* open fracture has severe bone fragmentation associated with extensive soft tissue injury, with or without skin loss. These fractures are usually high-energy comminuted fractures, such as gunshot injuries or shearing type of injuries of the distal extremities.

Physeal Fractures

Physeal fractures are identified according to the Salter-Harris classification scheme, which identifies the location of the fracture line. *Salter-Harris Type I* fractures run through the physis. *Salter-Harris Type II* fractures run through the physis and a portion of the metaphysis. *Salter-Harris Type III* fractures run through the physis and the epiphysis and are generally articular fractures. *Salter-Harris Type IV* fractures are also articular fractures, running through the epiphysis, across the physis, and through the metaphysis. *Salter-Harris Type V* fractures are crushing injuries of the physis that are not visible radiographically, but that become evident several weeks

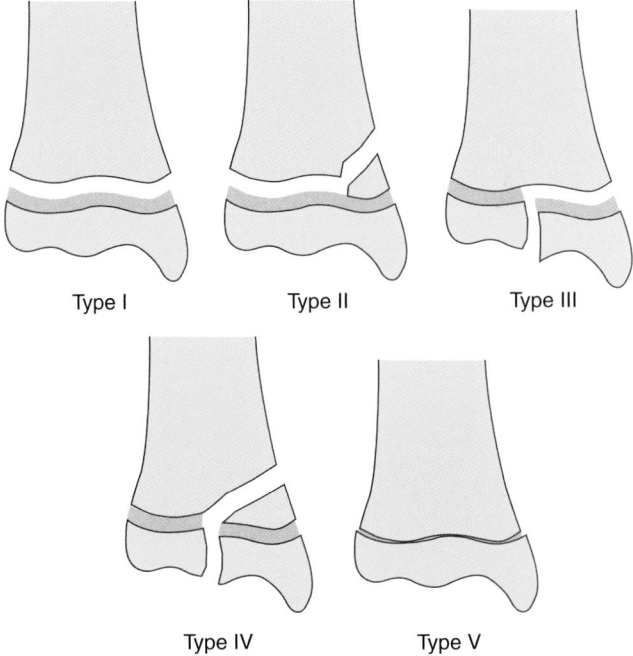

Type I   Type II   Type III

Type IV   Type V

FIG. 31-19
Salter-Harris classification of physeal fractures based on radiographic location of the fracture line.

later when physeal function ceases (Fig. 31-19). An additional Salter-Harris Type IV classification has been used to describe the partial physeal closures resulting from damage to a portion of the physis and causing asymmetric physeal closure.

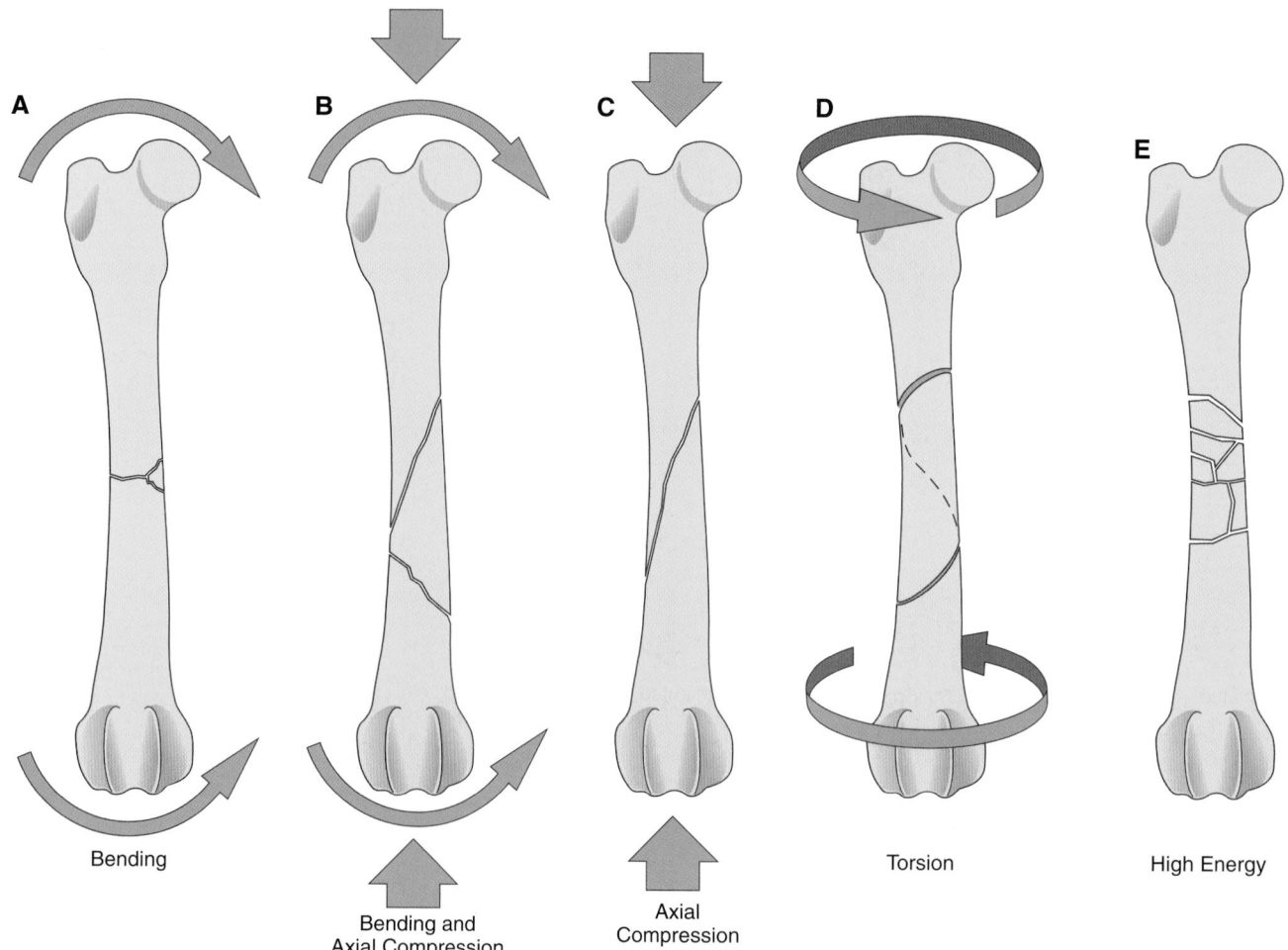

FIG. 31-20
Fracture lines created by forces applied to the bone. **A,** Bending causes a transverse fracture on the tension side and slight oblique fractures on the compression side of the bone. **B,** Axial load (compression) and bending cause oblique comminuted fractures. **C,** Axial load (compression) causes an oblique fracture. **D,** Torsion causes a spiral fracture. **E,** High energy causes a comminuted, nonreducible fracture.

BIOMECHANICS OF FRACTURE AND FRACTURE FIXATION

Fractures result from forces applied to the bone (Fig. 31-20). *Compressive forces* applied axially to the long bone result in oblique fractures. *Bending* of the long bone causes tensile forces on one side of the bone and compressive forces on the opposite side. Depending on the amount of axial load coinciding with the bending force, the fracture will begin as a transverse crack on the tensile side and propagate into oblique fractures on the compressive side. The two oblique fractures form a butterfly fragment of varying size. *Torsional forces* applied to the long bone result in a spiral fracture. *Tensile forces* applied to the bone result in a transverse fracture, most frequently as an avulsion fracture of a portion of bone where a strong tendon or ligament is attached.

The *velocity* of the force also determines the type of fracture and the amount of associated soft tissue injury. *Low velocity forces* or loading result in single fractures with little energy dissipated into the soft tissue. Conversely, *high veloc-*

ity forces result in comminuted fractures with the high energy dissipated through fracture propagation and surrounding soft tissue injury. Repetitive loading can result in *stress fractures*, in which the bone injury rate overcomes the response of bone production.

Stabilized bones and their implant systems are similarly subjected to compressive, bending, and torsional forces generated by weight bearing and adjacent muscular contraction (Fig. 31-21). It is imperative that the selected fixation be able to counteract the loads applied to the stabilized bone for successful outcomes in fracture treatment.

DECISION MAKING IN FRACTURE MANAGEMENT

The objectives in treating fractures, nonunions, or bone deformities are bone union and the patient's return to normal function. Appropriate decision-making processes to choose

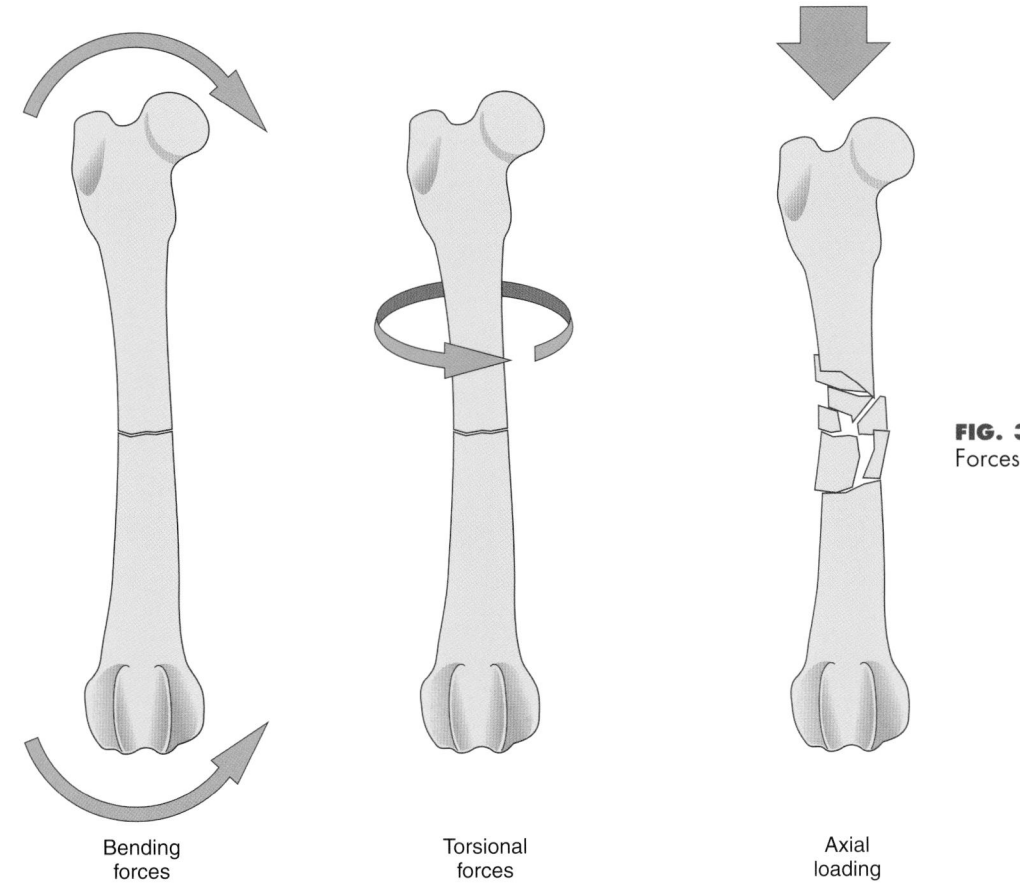

Bending forces

Torsional forces

Axial loading

FIG. 31-21
Forces acting on fractured bones.

implants and plan the procedure should produce consistent and predictable results. The surgeon must evaluate the fracture, the patient, and the client to identify which implants will achieve the necessary stability for the appropriate time to satisfy the objectives (i.e., develop a fracture-assessment score). It is also important to make a detailed plan for the entire surgical operation, including method of fracture reduction, sequence of implant application (i.e., fracture planning), and possibilities for bone grafting. Failure to plan the procedure results in prolonged operating times, excessive soft tissue trauma, and technical errors. The ultimate outcomes of improper planning are implant failure, delayed healing, infection, and nonunion.

FRACTURE-ASSESSMENT SCORE

After the patient has been thoroughly examined and life-threatening problems corrected, preoperative data must be analyzed to start the decision-making process. Preoperative data include patient information such as age, weight, general health, activity level, and presence of other orthopedic pathology; radiographs of the fractured and corresponding contralateral intact bones, which include the proximal and distal joints; and client information, such as their expectations and ability to perform postoperative care. These data can be summarized as a fracture-assessment score that re-

flects the mechanical, biologic, and clinical environment in which the implants must function and guides the types of implants chosen.

Mechanical Factors

An accurate mechanical evaluation gives an indication for how strong the fixation must be for the patient. Mechanical factors include the number of limbs injured, patient size and activity, and ability to achieve load-sharing fixation between the bony column and the implant (Fig. 31-22). Reducibility of the fracture must be determined. In general, two-piece fractures and fractures with large butterfly fragments that can be secured with cerclage wire or lag screws are considered *reducible,* allowing the reconstructed cortex to share the load of weight bearing with the implants. Fractures with multiple large fragments arranged like barrel staves or multiple small fragments that cannot be secured with implants are considered *nonreducible,* with the implants carrying the load of weight bearing until callus is formed. Because dogs and cats must bear weight with at least three limbs, weight bearing on the implant-bone construct cannot be prevented postoperatively when multiple limbs are injured or when preexisting lameness (e.g., degenerative joint disease of contralateral stifle secondary to cranial cruciate ligament injury) is present in another limb. Complications occur more fre-

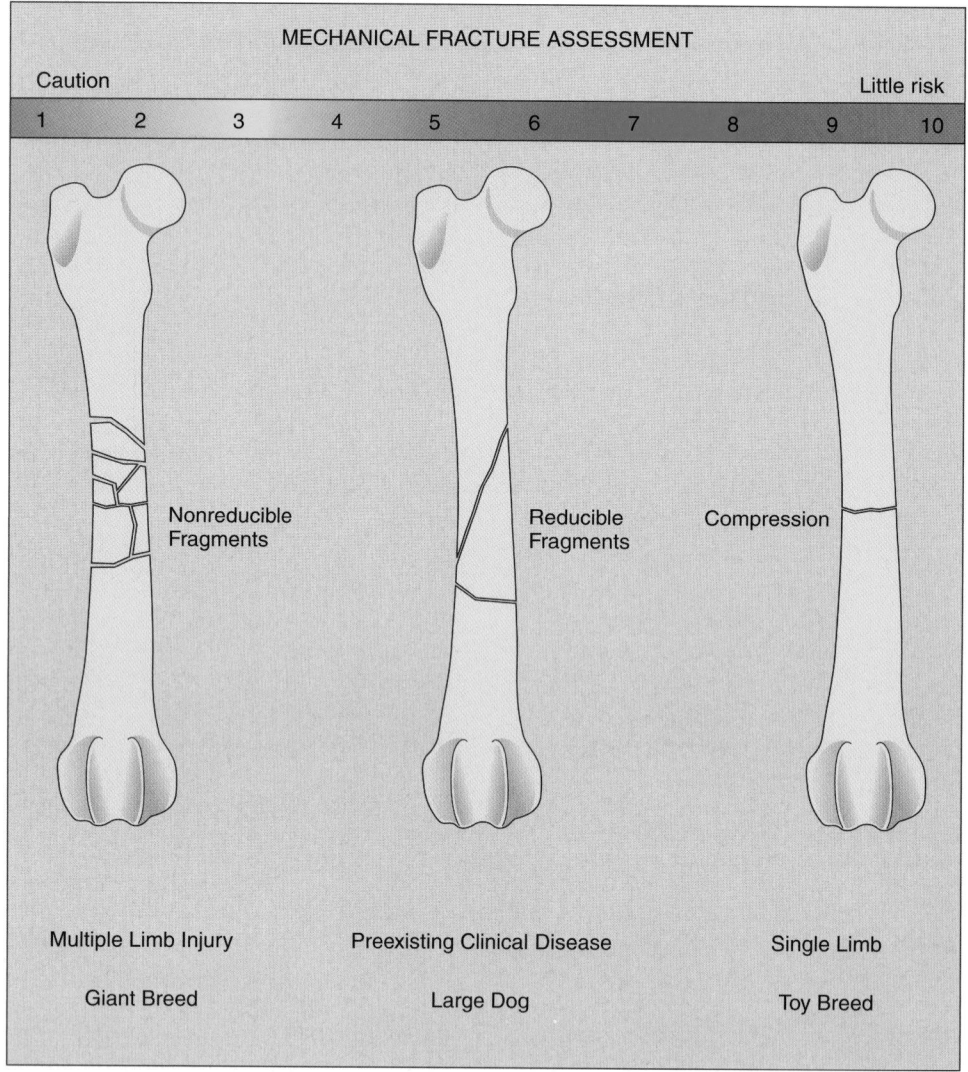

MECHANICAL FRACTURE ASSESSMENT

Caution   Little risk

| 1 | 2 | 3 | 4 | 5 | 6 | 7 | 8 | 9 | 10 |

Nonreducible
Fragments

Reducible
Fragments

Compression

Multiple Limb Injury   Preexisting Clinical Disease   Single Limb

Giant Breed   Large Dog   Toy Breed

FIG. 31-22
Mechanical factors to be considered when determining patient fracture assessment.
Conditions occurring on the left (e.g., buttress function and multiple limb injury) place maximum stress on an implant system and require thoughtful implant choice and application. In contrast, if conditions on the right are present, less stress is applied to the implant system, reducing the risk of complications.

quently when stresses are applied and implants are heavily loaded immediately after surgery. Large or active patients subject fixations to greater loads and are more prone to have implants loosen prematurely and fail.

The degree of load sharing between implants and the bony column also influences complication rates. Ideal load sharing occurs when a transverse or short oblique fracture is repaired because much of the force is transmitted axially through the limb. Loading of the implant is minimized, so loosening and fatigue failure are less likely. Conversely, when loads are transmitted from bone segment to bone segment through implants rather than through the bony column (e.g., highly comminuted fractures, such as gunshot wounds that cannot be anatomically reconstructed, segmental bone

resections, and limb-lengthening procedures), loosening and fatigue failure are more common.

Biologic Factors

An accurate biologic evaluation gives an indication of how fast callus may be formed, thus indirectly determining how long the implants need to function to support the bone. Many biologic factors influence the rate of bone healing (Fig. 31-23). The age and general health of the patient are important. A young (less than 6 months of age) healthy patient is a "healing machine" and requires functional fixation devices for only a limited time. Conversely the same fracture in an older animal will require stable fixation for a significantly longer time. Other biologic factors to consider are

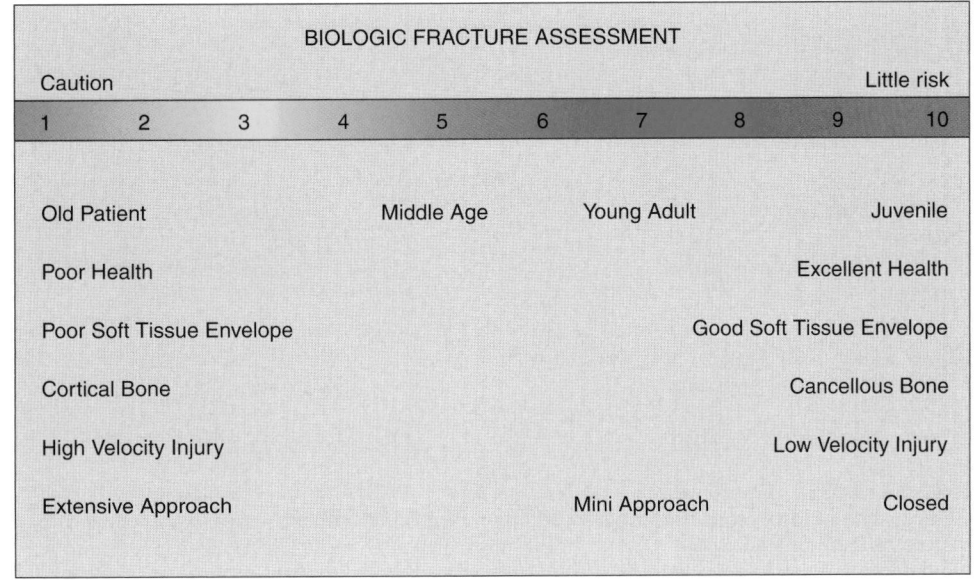

FIG. 31-23
Biologic factors to be considered when determining patient fracture assessment. Patient factors listed on the left do not favor rapid healing; thus the implant system must remain in place for prolonged periods. In contrast, patient factors on the right dictate rapid healing and necessitate that the implant function for a short time.

whether the fracture is open or closed and if it resulted from a low-energy or high-energy injury. A significant degree of soft tissue injury and bony comminution accompanies open, high-energy fractures (e.g., gunshot wounds). More time is required for bone union because soft tissue must heal first. The implant-bone construct must have high initial rigidity for neovascularization and healing of fragile tissue. It must also be rigid to function as a support until biologic callus is formed. With closed or low-energy fractures, less soft tissue damage is present, and bone union proceeds more rapidly.

Another factor influencing biologic assessment is whether open reduction is required. If the fracture must be opened, iatrogenic vascular damage occurs. A powerful biologic influence is the surgeon's skill in minimizing soft tissue envelope damage during open reduction. Obtaining desired reduction and stability with minimal soft tissue manipulation and operative time allows greater success than with longer surgeries in which reduction and stability are obtained at the expense of significant soft tissue manipulation. Preservation of the soft tissue envelope with open reduction is exceedingly important. This concept has led to a fracture management technique termed *bridging osteosynthesis,* in which minimal or no manipulation of the soft tissue envelope is done (see p. 959). For example, a comminuted fracture may be repaired through closed application of an external fixator or through open reduction and bridging of the fracture site with a bridging plate without manipulation of fracture fragments.

The bone injured and injury location influence biologic assessment because the soft tissue envelope surrounding various long bones differs. Distal radial or distal tibial di-

aphyseal fractures (i.e., locations with a sparse soft tissue envelope) have delayed unions or other complications more often than similar femoral or humeral fractures. Fractures occurring in cancellous metaphyseal or epiphyseal regions heal more rapidly than diaphyseal fractures because cancellous bone has a greater surface area for contact between fracture ends. Cancellous bone also has abundant osteoblasts and other biologic factors that favor bone union, which is fortunate because articular fractures require precise reduction for optimal outcome. The surgical manipulation required for reduction is balanced by the inherent healing potential of the region.

Clinical Factors

Clinical factors are patient and client factors that affect healing during the postoperative period and thus influence fracture-assessment score (Fig. 31-24). Factors include (1) the willingness and ability of clients to attend to their pet's postoperative needs, (2) anticipated patient cooperation after surgery, and (3) anticipated postoperative limb function. Unwilling clients or those unable to commit the time needed to care for stabilization systems requiring moderate or intensive postoperative maintenance (e.g., external coaptation and external skeletal fixations) should not be given this task. This is particularly valid if the biologic assessment dictates an extended time to bone union. Bone plates and screws would be more appropriate in this instance.

Patient cooperation is an important clinical factor after surgery. Very active, uncontrollable patients are not good candidates for external stabilization systems because high activity levels increase the likelihood of complications with

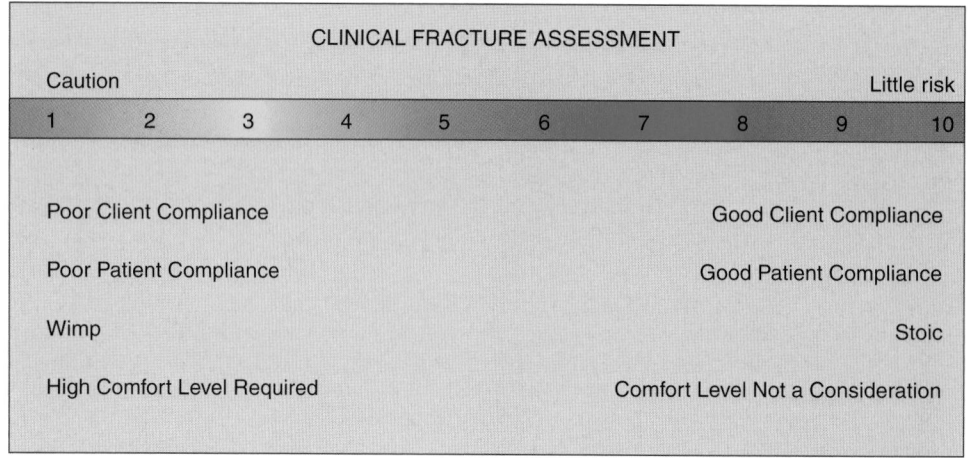

FIG. 31-24
Clinical factors to be considered when determining patient fracture assessment. Clinical factors on the left necessitate a comfortable implant system that requires little postoperative maintenance, whereas any implant system (regardless of postoperative maintenance) is appropriate with clinical factors on the right.

these systems. Hyperactive patients are not good candidates for external coaptation because casts or splints are difficult to maintain without shifting or sliding. Likewise, external skeletal fixators may be poor choices because these patients may continuously bump the external bar against objects, causing premature transfixation pin loosening.

Anticipated postoperative limb function must also be considered. Rapid return to normal limb function is a goal of fracture management. Therefore patient comfort during healing must be considered when selecting implants, including the patient's ability to cope with discomfort (i.e., a stoic animal) and estimated time to bone union. When early bone union is not anticipated (longer than 6 weeks), patient comfort that facilitates limb use and allows physical rehabilitation to be performed after surgery is essential. Implant systems vary in degree of comfort, depending on the involved bone and individual patient tolerance. As a general rule, bone plates provide the greatest level of postoperative comfort.

Interpretation of the Fracture-Assessment Score

Fracture-assessment scores are assigned on a scale of 1 to 10 (see Figs. 31-20 to 31-22). Fractures with high scores generally heal successfully with few complications, whereas fractures at the lower end of the scale are potentially less successful and have more complications. *Mechanical assessment* estimates the strength of implant necessary. *Biologic assessment* estimates the length of time implants must be functional (i.e., time to bone union). If the fracture-assessment score falls at the lower end of the scale, the implant will function as a buttress and must carry most, if not all, of the physiologic loads immediately after surgery. The implant must assume this function until bony callus

forms. This period will be prolonged for patients with low fracture-assessment scores because poor biologic factors prolong bony callus formation. Higher fracture-assessment scores mean less stress on the fixation system and less time required for bone healing. When the fracture-assessment score falls at the upper end of the scale, implants share the physiologic loads with the bone immediately after surgery, and bone union occurs relatively rapidly.

Low scores: 0 to 3. Generally, these are nonreducible fractures in older animals in which healing will be affected by other extenuating circumstances. Implants must bridge these fractures and therefore must have sufficient strength to prevent permanent bending or breakage for more than 6 weeks. Suggested implants (or combinations of implants) with sufficient strength and stiffness to function at the lower end of the fracture-assessment scale are lengthening bone plates (see p. 998), bone plate–intramedullary (IM) pin combinations (see p. 998), or Type II or Type III external skeletal fixators (see p. 973). Implants should purchase bone with raised threads to resist axial compression and tension (back-and-forth movement) at implant-bone interfaces. Bone plates and interlocking nails fulfill this requirement with the use of the bone screws, but the transfixation pins of external fixators may or may not have raised threads (see p. 969). Raised-threaded transfixation pins or a combination of smooth and raised-thread transfixation pins should be used with low fracture-assessment scores.

Moderate scores: 4 to 7. Overlapping biologic and mechanical factors affect healing and implant selection when the fracture-assessment score moves toward midscale. For example, in an older dog with a transverse fracture, the implant and bone share the load after surgery, and the implant will be subjected to less stress, but healing may be delayed. Alternatively, in an immature dog with a nonreducible fracture, the biologic assessment may indicate early callus formation, despite the implant being subjected to high initial loads as it functions to bridge the fracture. In both situations, less implant strength and endurance are required than in patients with low assessment scores because of either immediate load sharing or early callus formation. A fracture assessment toward the lower end of center means that the time to union will be long; therefore the implant should purchase the bone so as to preserve the implant-bone interface during the healing period. A fracture assessment toward the upper end of center means that the stress on the implant and the implant-bone interface will be high for a short duration; therefore the interface needs maximal stability until sufficient callus is formed to share the physiologic load. Suggested implants include bone plates, Type I or Type II external skeletal fixators, IM pin–external skeletal fixator combinations with or without a tie in, and interlocking nails. Connections at implant-bone interfaces should be a thread purchase or combination of thread and friction purchase, depending on assessment of stress at the interface and an estimation of endurance necessary at this site.

High scores: 8 to 10. When the fracture-assessment score is high, mechanical assessment indicates minimal implant stress caused by load sharing, and biologic assessment indicates enhanced healing potential. Immediate load sharing between the bone-implant construct and rapid bone union are expected. Therefore no need exists for the strength and stiffness of the implant to be extreme or for the implant to function for a long time. Suggested implants include Type I external skeletal fixators, IM pin–cerclage wires, and external coaptation. Implants that hold bone through frictional purchase (e.g., smooth pins and cerclage wire) provide adequate bone purchase.

FRACTURE REDUCTION

The method of reduction has an impact on the biology and mechanics of the fracture. Reduction is defined as the process of either reconstructing fractured bone fragments to their normal anatomic configuration or restoring normal limb alignment by reestablishing normal limb length and joint alignment while maintaining spatial orientation of the limb (Fig. 31-25). Techniques used to reduce fractures or align limbs must overcome the physiologic processes of muscle contraction and fracture fragment overriding.

The initial decision when planning fracture treatment is to determine whether to use closed or open reduction (Box 31-5). *Closed reduction* refers to reducing fractures or aligning limbs without surgically exposing fractured bones. Closed reduction enhances the biologic environment by (1) preserving soft tissue and blood supply, which speeds healing; (2) decreasing risk of infection; and (3) reducing operating time. The main disadvantage of closed reduction is the difficulty of gaining accurate reconstruction of reducible fractures. *Open reduction* refers to using a surgical approach to expose fractured bone segments and fragments so that they can be anatomically reconstructed and held in position

with implants. Open reduction is further classified as *limited open reduction* in which a small exposure is made to lever a transverse fracture into position, or secure an oblique fracture with lag screws or cerclage before placing an external fixator or interlocking nail, or *"open but do not touch" reduction* in which a lengthy exposure is made for realigning the bone and placing a plate, but the fracture fragments and hematoma are not manipulated. Advantages of open reduction include: (1) visualization and direct contact with bone fragments to facilitate anatomic fracture reconstruction; (2) direct placement of implants (e.g., cerclage wire, lag screws, and plates) is possible; (3) bone reconstruction allows bone and implants to share loads, which results in stronger fracture fixation (i.e., improving the mechanical environment); and (4) cancellous bone grafts can be used to enhance bone healing (see p. 962). Disadvantages of open reduction include increased surgical trauma to soft tissue and blood supply, diminishing the biologic environment, and greater opportunity to introduce bacterial contamination. The advantages and disadvantages of each method must be considered before selecting the reduction method.

CLOSED REDUCTION

Fractures that are appropriately treated with closed reduction include greenstick and nondisplaced fractures of bones distal to the elbow and stifle. These fractures may be managed with limb realignment and fracture immobilization with casts or external fixators (see pp. 967 and 969). Severely comminuted fractures (particularly tibial and radial fractures) that are difficult or impossible to reconstruct anatomically (i.e., those that are nonreducible) are also appropriately treated with closed reduction, limb alignment, and rigid stabilization with external fixators (see Box 31-5). When closed reduction is used, anatomic fracture reconstruction is seldom possible. Instead, goals for closed reduction are to restore bone length and limb alignment. Attention must focus on eliminating rotation and angular deformity of distal segments. True lateral and craniocaudal radiographic projections of proximal and distal joints allow the postoperative radiographs to be scrutinized to determine if joint surfaces above and below fractured bones are parallel to each other and in correct rotational alignment.

OPEN REDUCTION

Fractures that can be anatomically reconstructed (i.e., most simple displaced fractures, those with large fragments, and long oblique fracture lines classified as reducible fractures) or those that are displaced and involve joint surfaces are appropriately managed with open reduction. Bone columns and articular surfaces are restored and stabilized. Surgical approaches for exposing bones for fracture repair are found in subsequent chapters pertaining to individual bones. General principles of surgical approaches are to (1) follow normal separations between muscles, (2) obtain adequate exposure of fractured bones, (3) handle soft tissue gently and preserve soft tissue attachments to bone fragments, and (4) prevent trauma to major nerves and vessels.

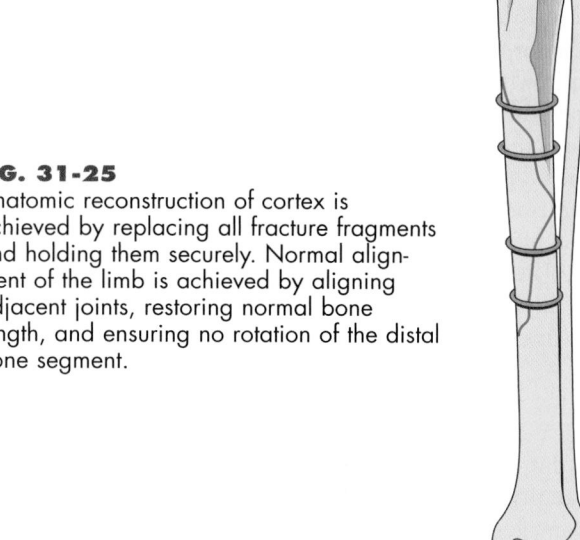

FIG. 31-25
Anatomic reconstruction of cortex is achieved by replacing all fracture fragments and holding them securely. Normal alignment of the limb is achieved by aligning adjacent joints, restoring normal bone length, and ensuring no rotation of the distal bone segment.

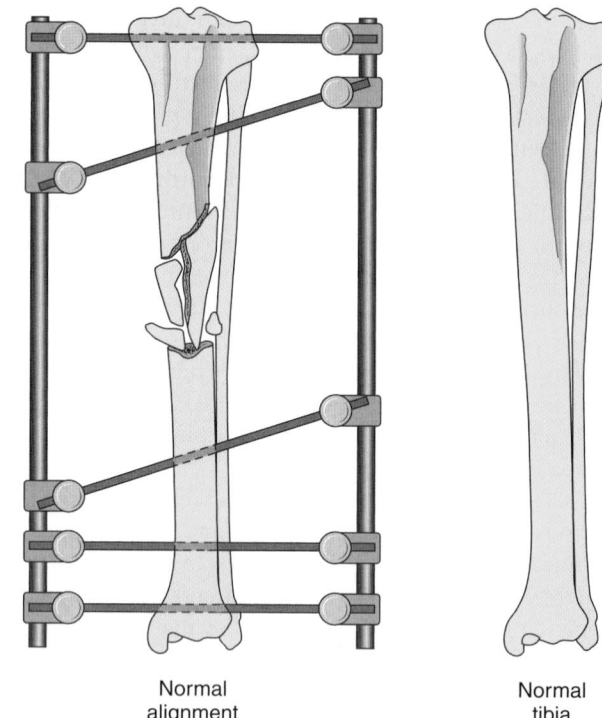

Anatomic reconstruction

Normal alignment

Normal tibia

 BOX 31-5

Indications for Open or Closed Reduction

Open Reduction
- Articular fractures
- Simple fractures that can be anatomically reconstructed
- Comminuted nonreducible diaphyseal fractures of long bones—"open, but do not touch"

Closed Reduction
- Greenstick and/or nondisplaced fractures of long bones below the elbow and stifle
- Comminuted nonreducible diaphyseal fractures of long bones treated with external fixators

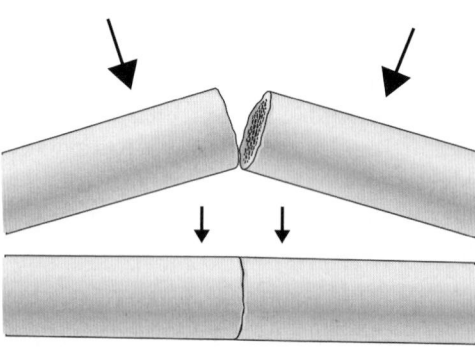

FIG. 31-26
To reduce a transverse fracture, lift the bone segments from surrounding soft tissue until the fracture surfaces are apposed. While maintaining contact, slowly replace the segments into a normal position.

SURGICAL TECHNIQUE
Direct Reduction

The major difficulty in achieving anatomic reduction is counteracting the muscle contraction that has caused bone segments to override. Slow, manual distraction of segments using bone-holding forceps will eventually fatigue muscles and allow reduction. Transverse fractures can be reduced by applying traction, countertraction, and bending forces. The bone ends should be lifted from the incision and brought into contact. Force is slowly applied to replace the bones in a normal position (Fig. 31-26). A lever can also be used to reduce transverse fractures (Fig. 31-27). In some cases fracture reduction is aided by applying a precontoured plate to one bone segment, reducing the fracture and maintaining reduc-

tion by securing the plate to the second bone segment. This technique is particularly useful for iliac body fractures and distal radial fractures. Long oblique fractures can be hard to reduce because the fracture line configuration makes bending or levering techniques difficult, and overriding may occur even after reduction. Two self-retaining reduction forceps can be used to force distraction of segments slowly until reduction is achieved (Fig. 31-28). Rough handling of bone with any of these techniques can cause additional fragmentation. The bone should be inspected for fissure fracture lines. Weak bone segments should be supported by cerclage wires before attempting reduction (Fig. 31-29). Fractures

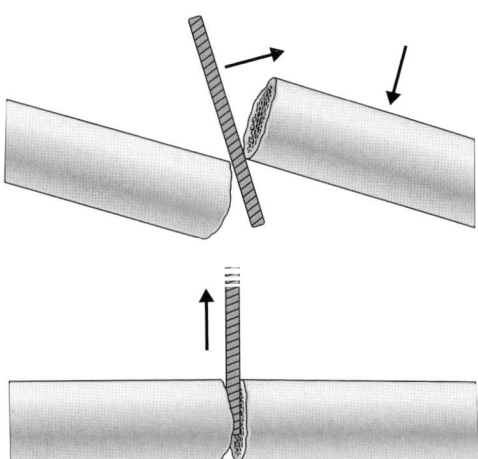

FIG. 31-27
To reduce overriding bone segments of a transverse fracture, carefully place a lever (small periosteal elevator or scalpel blade handle) between the overriding bone segments. Use the lever to apply pressure gently and help distract and reduce the bone segments.

with more than two pieces that can be completely reconstructed are first treated by securing loose fragments to one segment with lag screws or cerclage wire. The two-piece fracture is then carefully distracted and aligned for definitive fixation (Fig. 31-30).

Indirect Reduction

Nonreducible fractures are best managed with indirect reduction to preserve the biology and bridging fixations to provide the mechanical support. *Indirect reduction* is the process of restoring fragment and limb alignment by distracting the major bone segments. An IM pin can be used in this process. The pin is driven normograde through the proximal bone segment to the fracture site. It is then centered into the distal segment and driven distally until it engages metaphyseal bone. The proximal segment is steadied with bone-holding forceps while the pin is advanced distally until appropriate distraction is achieved (Fig. 31-31). Once the fractured bone is aligned, a bone plate or external fixator may be applied to bridge the fracture and maintain the reduction.

The animal's own weight can be used to advantage to achieve indirect reduction of tibial or radial fractures by suspending the fractured limb from a secure ceiling bolt. The animal is draped and the surgical procedure performed with the limb suspended. Temporarily lowering the operating table causes the animal's weight to distract the fracture. This method can be used during both closed and open reduction of fractures stabilized with external fixators or open reduction of fractures stabilized with plates. When the fracture is secured in the appropriate position, the operating table is raised to remove the traction force from the limb (Fig. 31-32).

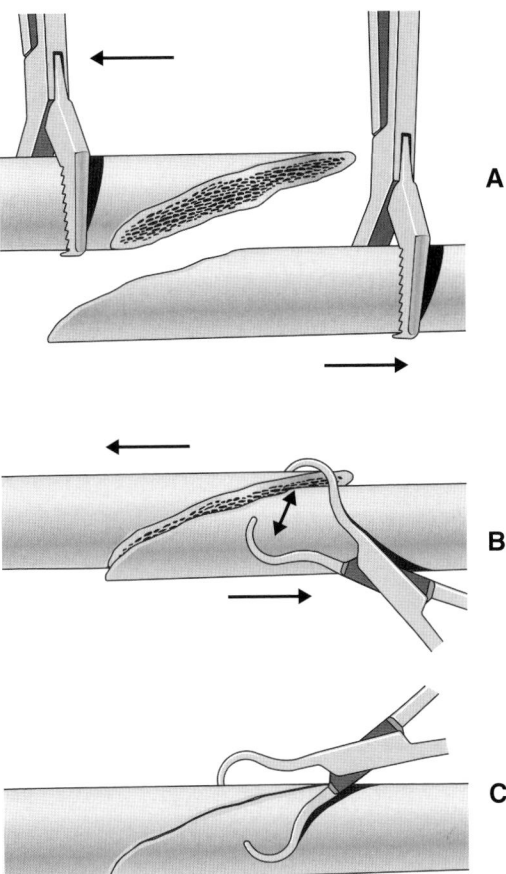

FIG. 31-28
A, Manually return the bone segments of a long oblique fracture to close approximation with bone-holding forceps. **B,** Place pointed reduction forceps at an angle to the fracture line. **C,** As the pointed reduction forceps are gently closed, the bone ends are distracted. The pointed reduction forceps should be manipulated to aid reduction and secured perpendicular to the fracture line. Multiple attempts may be necessary before reduction is achieved and held with pointed reduction forceps.

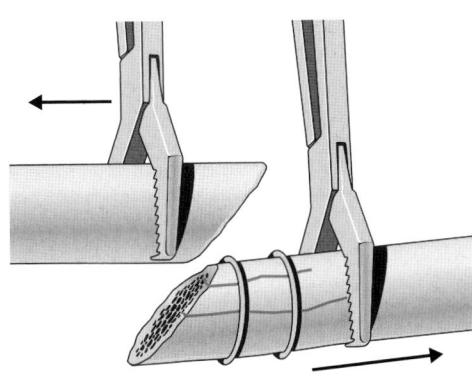

FIG. 31-29
Bone segment ends are secured with cerclage wire if fissure fractures are present.

Fracture distractors are instruments that can be attached to the proximal and distal metaphyses of fractured bones or to intact bones adjacent to the fracture by means of fixation pins. The distractor facilitates fragment distraction, and its offset position allows access to fractures for fragment recon-struction and plate application (Fig. 31-33). Distractors can also be used during closed reduction and fracture stabiliza-tion with external fixation. The fracture distractor is attached to proximal and distal fixation pins and used to lengthen the bone before the rest of the fixator frame is constructed.

FRACTURE TREATMENT PLANNING

Developing an appropriate plan for fracture treatment in-volves first determining a fracture-assessment score and choosing the appropriate implant system. Then the appro-priate technique for achieving fracture reduction should be selected and a detailed plan for applying the implants devel-oped. The decision to use a cancellous bone autograft is made. The surgical approach or approaches are selected and reviewed. It is important to check your implant and instru-ment inventory and precontour the plate if appropriate. Once these preparations are made, then the surgery is per-formed. After surgery it is important to critically evaluate the postoperative radiographs to determine if preoperative plan-ning goals were met or if remedial steps are necessary to ensure the desired outcome.

Suggested Reading

Aron DN, Johnson AL, Palmer R: Biologic strategies and a balanced concept for repair of highly comminuted long bone fractures, *Compend Cont Educ Pract Vet* 17:35, 1995.
This article provides a review of the concepts and application of biologic fracture fixation in small animals.
Johnson AL: Current concepts in fracture reduction, *Vet Comp Orthop Traumatol* 16:59, 2003.
This article provides a comprehensive overview of the various meth-ods of fracture reduction used in small animal orthopedics.

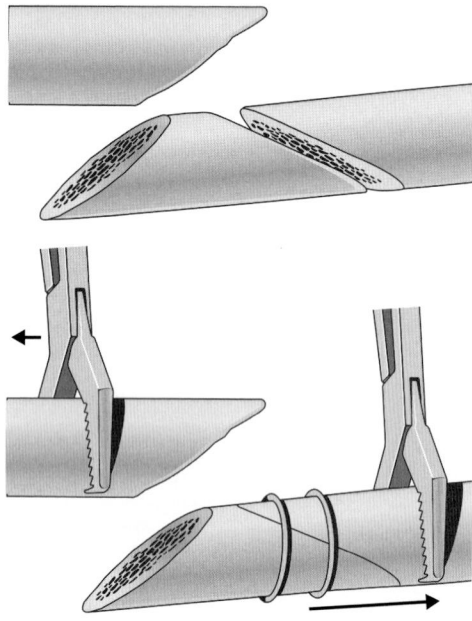

FIG. 31-30
Anatomic reconstruction of a fracture with a large butterfly fragment is achieved by first reducing the fragment and securing it to one segment of bone. This creates a two-piece fracture to be reduced and stabilized.

FIG. 31-31
When using an IM pin to distract fractures, stabi-lize the proximal segment with a bone-holding for-ceps and use an IM pin to push the distal segment of bone away from the proximal segment.

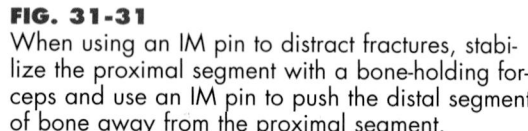
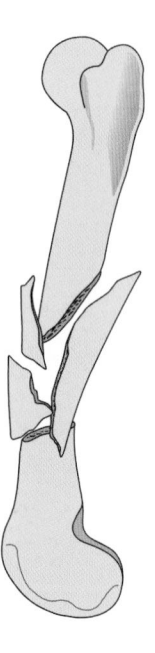
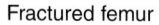
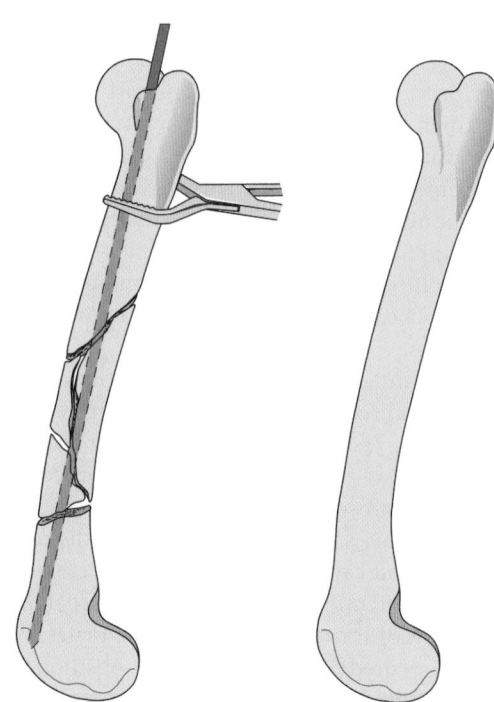
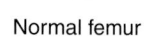

Fractured femur   IM pin distractor   Normal femur

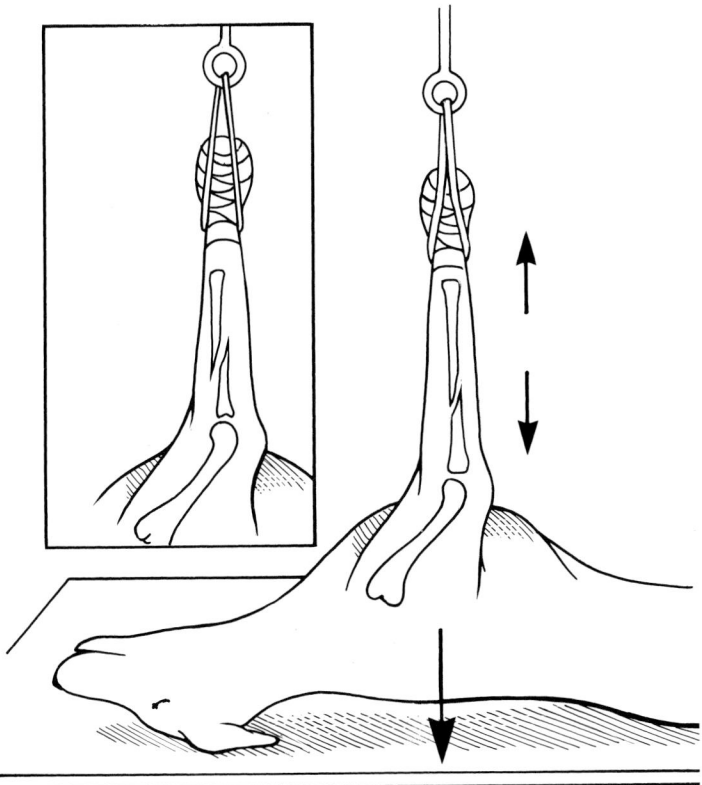

FIG. 31-32
Suspending the fractured limb from the ceiling allows the animal's weight to aid in fracture distraction.

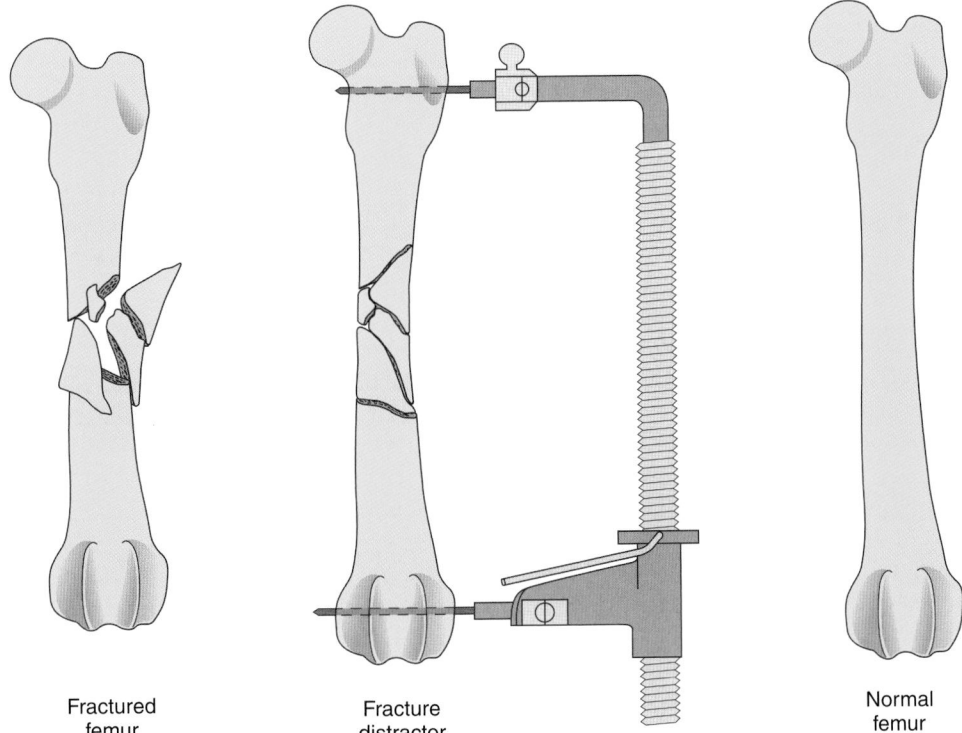

Fractured
femur

Fracture
distractor

Normal
femur

FIG. 31-33
When using a fracture distractor, attach the device to pins placed in the metaphyses perpendicular to the long bone. Engage the distractor by twisting the circular knob and distracting the distal arm of the distractor and distal segment.

BONE GRAFTS

Bone grafting, the technique of transplanting cancellous or cortical bone, has been used in veterinary medicine for many years. Bone grafts are named to indicate their structure and source. Autogenous cancellous bone grafting is a vital component of fracture management that helps fractures to heal before implants loosen or fail. Allogeneic cancellous bone or demineralized bone powder is available commercially and can be used to augment fracture repair. Cortical bone allografts are also available commercially and are occasionally used to treat long bone fractures with severe cortical bone loss or to replace bone removed in limb-sparing techniques. Corticocancellous grafts contain cortical and cancellous bone (e.g., rib or ilial wing); osteochondral grafts also contain articular cartilage (e.g., proximal femur). Vascularized grafts are harvested with their blood supply and implanted using microvascular anastomotic techniques that preserve the bone's blood supply.

Bones transplanted from one site to another in the same animal are *autografts*. Such grafts are histocompatible with host immune systems and will not initiate rejection responses. Bones transplanted from one animal to another of the same species are *allografts*. Cellular antigens of these grafts may be recognized as foreign by host immune systems, resulting in graft rejection. *Alloimplants* are bones treated by freezing, freeze-drying, autoclaving, chemical preservation, or irradiation so that they are devoid of cellular activity. Allografts reinforced with cancellous autografts are *composite grafts*. Bones transplanted from one animal to another of a different species are *xenografts*. Bone substitutes of tricalcium phosphate ceramics are available as extenders for cancellous bone grafts.

Bone grafts can be sources of osteoprogenitor cells (*osteogenesis*), either providing cells directly or inducing formation of osteoprogenitor cells from surrounding tissue (*osteoinduction*). Bone grafts provide varying degrees of mechanical support, ranging from forming space-occupying trellises for host bone invasion (*osteoconduction*) to supplying weight-bearing struts within fractures. The type of bone graft chosen to augment fracture repair is determined by the function required to optimize fracture healing. *Cancellous autografts* are highly cellular but mechanically weak. Therefore they provide superior osteogenic, osteoinductive, and osteoconductive capabilities, but do not provide substantial fracture support. In contrast, *cortical alloimplants* provide excellent mechanical support and are osteoconductive, but usually are acellular and stimulate little osteogenic response. *Allogeneic demineralized bone matrix* is revascularized quickly and is moderately osteoinductive, but provides no structural support. *Allogeneic cancellous bone grafts* provide limited mechanical support and are osteoconductive, but not osteoinductive because the matrix is mineralized.

The surgeon must make appropriate decisions to match the properties of the graft with the deficiencies anticipated in fracture healing. In general, autogenous cancellous bone grafts are most often used because of ease of harvest, availability, and osteogenic properties. Autogenous cancellous bone grafts are recommended when rapid bone formation is desired, to assist healing when optimal healing is not anticipated (e.g., cortical defects after fracture repair, adult and elderly animals with fractures, delayed unions, nonunions, osteotomies, joint arthrodesis, and cystic defects) or to promote bone formation in infected fractures.

CANCELLOUS BONE AUTOGRAFTS

Cancellous bone may be harvested from any long bone metaphysis; however, the proximal humerus, proximal tibia, and ilial wing are most often used because they are accessible and contain large amounts of cancellous bone. The graft is usually harvested after fracture stabilization; however, it may be harvested before the primary orthopedic procedure if the donor site could be contaminated with tumor cells or if infection is present at the recipient site. Alternately a separate surgical team and instrumentation may be used to harvest the graft. The graft site is selected because of accessibility when the animal is positioned for fracture repair.

Proximal Humerus

Prepare the graft site for aseptic surgery. Perform a craniolateral approach to the proximal humerus by incising through skin and subcutaneous tissue. Retract the acromial head of the deltoid muscle caudally and expose the flat aspect of the craniolateral metaphysis, just distal to the greater tubercle. Make a round hole in the bone cortex, using an IM pin or drill bit (Fig. 31-34, A). Ensure that the hole location is distal to the physis in the immature animal. A round hole is made through the cortex to minimize formation of a stress riser, which could contribute to fracture through the cortical defect. After penetrating bone cortex, insert a bone curette and harvest cancellous bone (Fig. 31-34, B). Place the cancellous bone directly into the recipient bed or store it in a blood-soaked sponge or stainless steel cup (Fig. 31-34, C and D). Add blood to the graft if it is placed in a cup to keep it moist.

The blood will clot and form a moldable composite with the graft, which facilitates handling.

Secure stored grafts on the instrument table to prevent inadvertent disposal. Flush the fracture site and loosely pack all defects and fracture lines with graft material. Try to fill the defect as much as possible for optimal osteogenesis. Close subcutaneous tissue around the grafts to hold them in position. Close subcutaneous tissue and skin of the graft site routinely.

Proximal Tibia

Make a craniomedial skin incision over the medial surface of the proximal tibia. After incising subcutaneous tissue, harvest cancellous bone as described above.

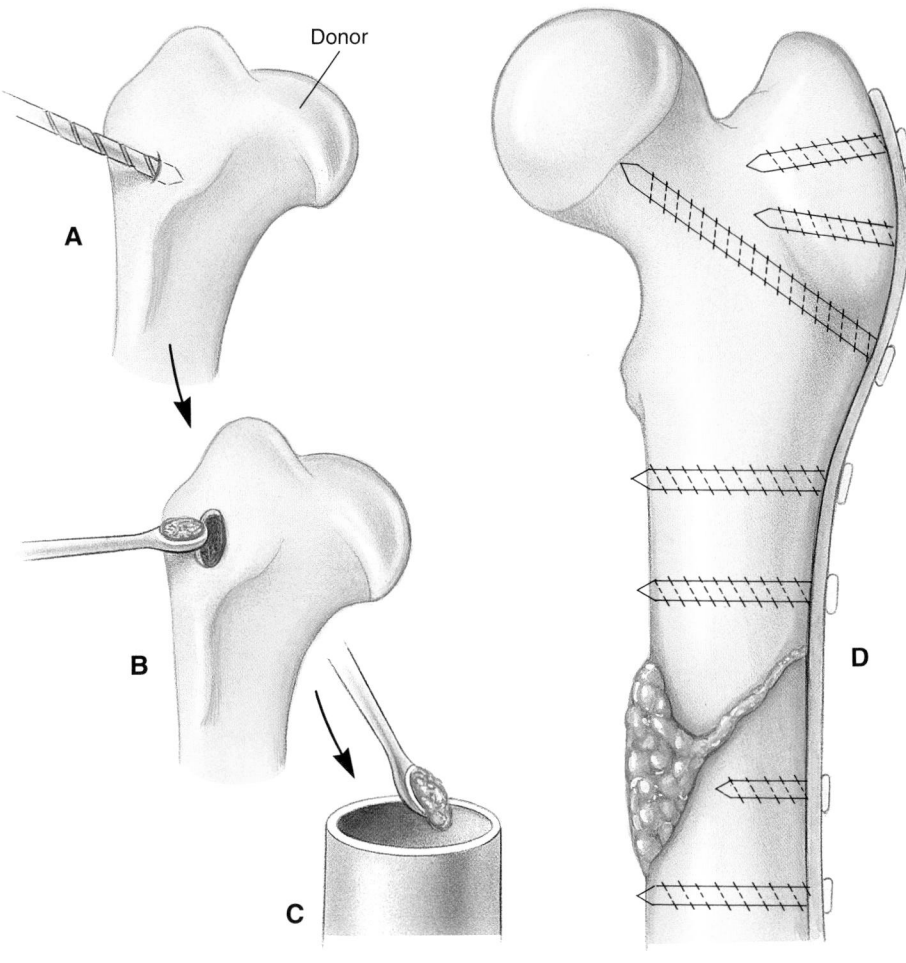

FIG. 31-34
A, To obtain cancellous bone from the humerus, make a round hole through the near cortex. **B,** Use a bone curette to harvest cancellous bone. **C,** Place the bone into a stainless steel cup with whole blood for short-term storage. **D,** Loosely pack the cancellous bone in the fracture gap or along fracture lines.

Ilial Wing

Make a skin incision over the craniodorsal iliac spine. Incise subcutaneous tissue and expose the dorsal surface of the ilial wing. Elevate gluteal musculature from the lateral surface and harvest cancellous bone as described above. Alternately, obtain a corticocancellous graft by using an osteotome to remove a cortical wedge from the ilial wing. Morselize the wedge with rongeurs (Fig. 31-35) and place it into the recipient site.

Revascularization of cancellous bone autografts begins as early as 2 days after grafting and is usually completed within 2 weeks (Fig. 31-36, *A* and *B*). Transplanted osteogenic cells or undifferentiated mesenchymal cells become active osteoblasts, secreting osteoid on transplanted trabecular bone (Fig. 31-36, *C*). This osteoid is mineralized and forms new host bone in fracture sites (Fig. 31-36, *D*). This new bone also incorporates the graft into host bone. Eventually the necrotic cores of trabecular bone are resorbed by osteoclasts, and grafts are totally replaced by host bone. Trabecular new bone is remodeled into cortical bone in response to the mechanical environment (Fig. 31-36, *E*). This healing response can be monitored radiographically by observing filling of

the defect with cancellous bone, followed by cortical reconstruction. The donor site is initially filled with hematoma, which is later replaced with fibrous connective tissue. Osteoblasts migrate to the area and deposit osteoid. Mineralization occurs, and new trabecular bone is formed within defects. This process takes approximately 12 weeks; additional cancellous bone should not be harvested from the same area before this time.

Few complications are associated with autogenous cancellous bone grafting techniques. Donor site pain is seldom clinically evident. Seroma formation or wound dehiscence may occur at donor sites. Infection or seeding of tumor to donor sites occurs rarely and can be prevented by proper sequencing of bone graft harvesting. Fractures through the donor site have been reported infrequently. Complications at the recipient site (e.g., failure of grafts to stimulate bone formation) are difficult to recognize.

BONE MARROW OSTEOGENESIS

Bone marrow is a source of osteoprogenitor cells. Autologous bone marrow can be aspirated and injected into a delayed union or nonunion site to stimulate bone production. However, the ability of marrow osteoprogenitor cells to

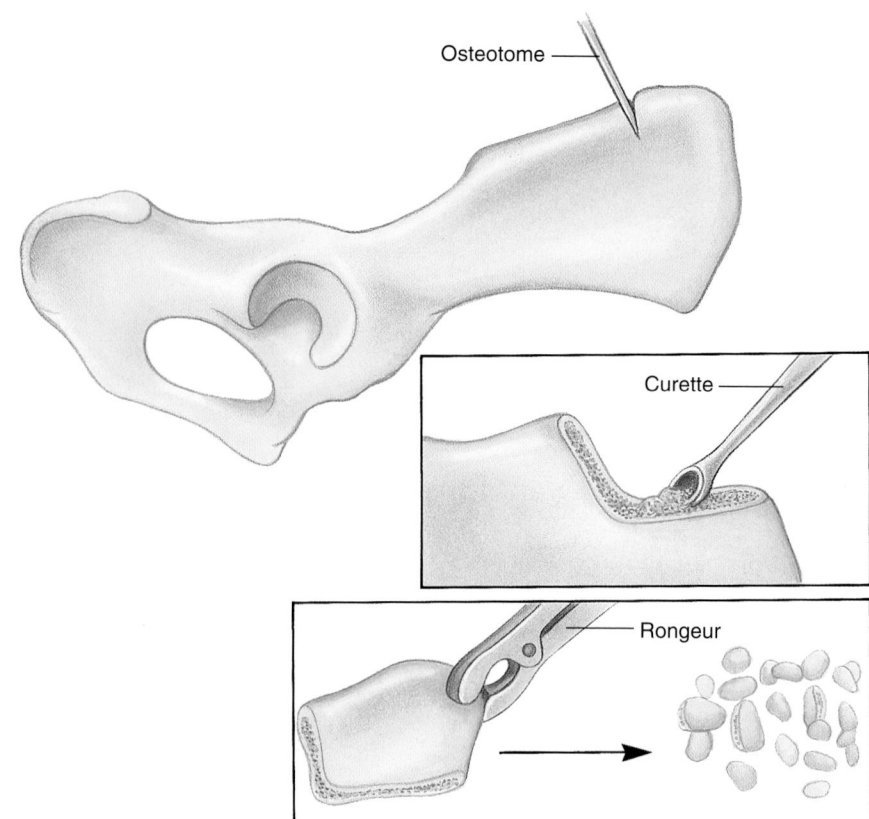

FIG. 31-35
To obtain cancellous bone from the wing of the ilium, use an osteotome to remove a wedge from the dorsocranial ilial wing. Use a bone curette to harvest cancellous bone. Use rongeurs to fragment the osteotomized wedge of corticocancellous bone.

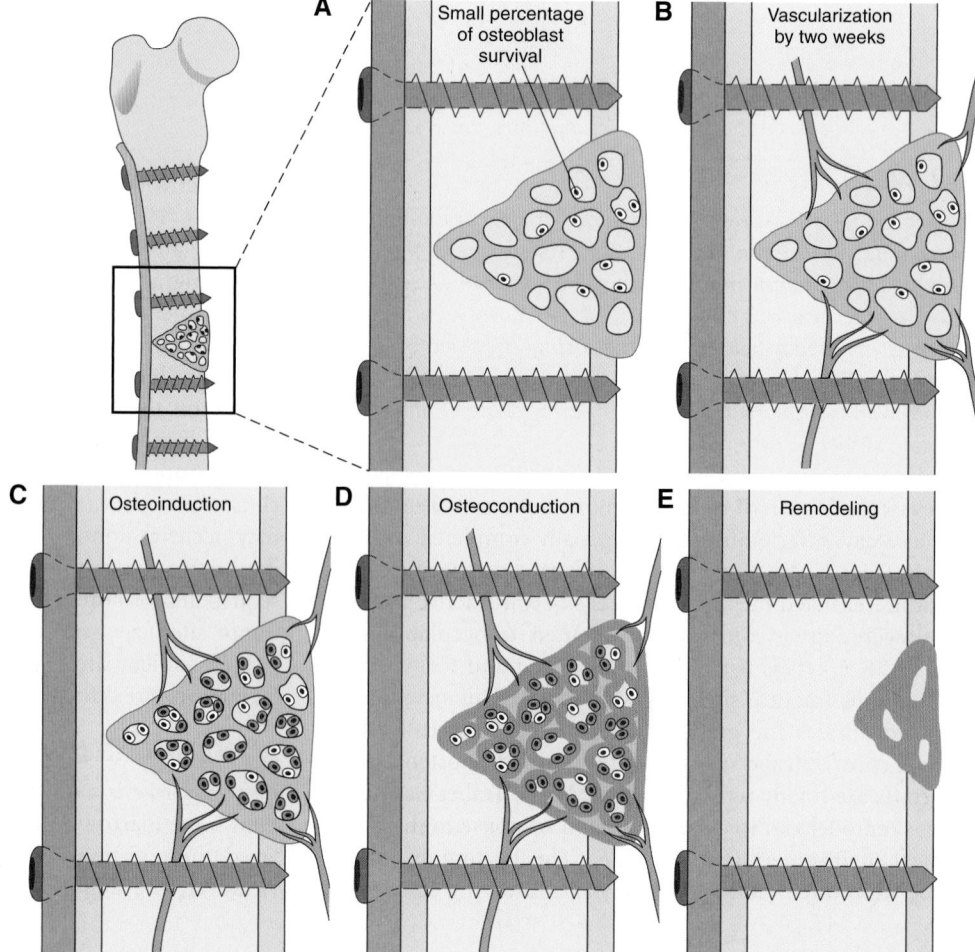

FIG. 31-36
Stages of cancellous bone incorporation into a healing fracture. **A,** Graft placement. **B,** Vascularization of the graft. **C,** Osteoinduction. **D,** Osteoconduction. **E,** Remodeling.

stimulate bone formation varies from individual to individual and between species.

CANCELLOUS BONE ALLOGRAFTS

Cancellous bone allografts are commercially available as frozen chips or as chips mixed with demineralized bone powder. Advantages to using prepared allografts are reduced operating time, availability of graft, and elimination of morbidity at a donor site. Disadvantages are the cost of the grafts and the lack of osteogenic properties in the cancellous bone chips. Allogeneic bone graft can be mixed to extend cancellous autograft to fill large defects or can be mixed with autologous marrow to increase the osteogenic properties.

The same stages of incorporation occur in cancellous allografts as in cancellous autografts. Autogenous graft is superior to allogeneic graft in promoting rapid new bone formation, but no difference exists in long-term outcome. Clinically, allogeneic graft has been used successfully in fracture repair.

CORTICAL BONE AUTOGRAFTS

Cortical autografts are harvested from areas where cortical bone can be removed without adversely affecting function (i.e., ribs, ilial wing, distal ulna, and fibula). The most common use of a cortical autograft is transplantation of a rib to form a segmental strut for mandibular fractures. Cortical autograft harvest is done during fracture repair, and the graft is incorporated into the fracture site as a *segmental graft* (placed between fracture segments) or as a *sliding onlay graft* (placed over the fracture site). Cortical autografts are usually held in place with the same implant used to stabilize the fracture.

CORTICAL BONE ALLOGRAFTS

Cortical bone can be harvested and transplanted immediately as a fresh allograft, or it can be harvested and banked to provide a ready source of cortical alloimplants. Harvesting must be done under aseptic conditions unless the bone is sterilized after collection. Frozen cortical allografts are available commercially.

With the advent of biologic fracture repair techniques (see p. 959) that incorporate fragments in comminuted fractures, cortical bone allografts are now used more often for limb-sparing procedures than for fracture repair. The principles of using cortical bone allografts are similar, regardless of their intended purpose. Plate and screw fixation is necessary to ensure stability of host-graft interfaces for prolonged periods while fractures heal and grafts remodel. Therefore adequate host bone must be present to allow placement of three bone screws proximal and distal to grafts. Radiographs of the contralateral matching bone are used to determine graft size and length and to serve as a model for precontouring plates. The required graft length is determined by measuring the lengths of intact segments of fractured bone on a lateral radiograph and subtracting this measurement from the length of the contralateral bone (Fig. 31-37).

Adherence to aseptic technique is essential for successful cortical allograft use.

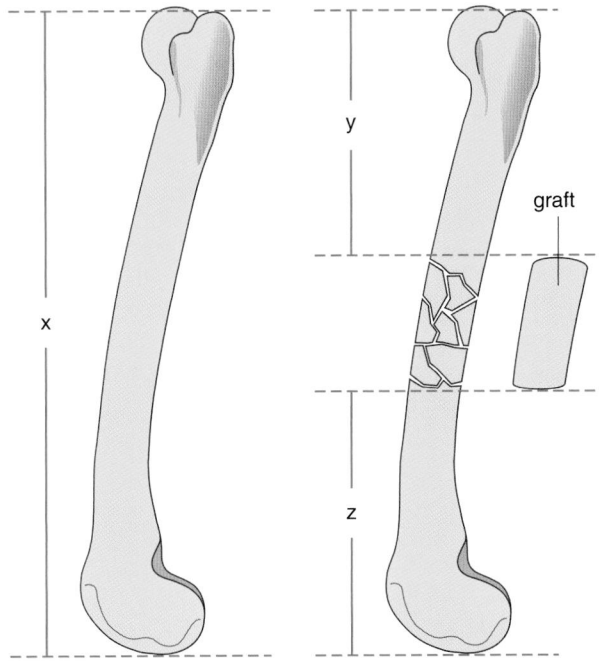

$$x - (y + z) = \text{Length of graft}$$

FIG. 31-37

To determine the proper length for the cortical allograft, measure the length of the normal bone from a lateral radiograph *(x)*. Measure the length of the intact proximal and distal segments of the fractured bone from a lateral radiograph *(y* and *z)*. Use the formula *x − (y + z)* to determine graft length.

Prepare the affected limb and a cancellous bone autograft donor site for aseptic surgery. Approach the fracture, remove fragments, and resect bone segments proximally and distally to uninjured bone. Use an oscillating bone saw to cut the bones perpendicular to their long axes. Cut the graft to an appropriate length in a similar manner (i.e., perpendicular to its long axis) to allow 360-degree contact of graft and host bone. Determine the appropriate number and length of cortical bone screws for the graft length, and secure the graft to the center of the precontoured plate. Place the graft-plate composite in the fracture gap, and reduce bone segments to the plate. Secure the plate to host bone segments using cortical bone screws. To achieve compression of host-graft interfaces, insert those screws that are immediately proximal and distal to the graft into the host bone in a loaded manner. Insert the remaining screws in a neutral position (Fig. 31-38). Flush the fracture with sterile saline. Then harvest a cancellous bone autograft and place it at host-graft interfaces. Obtain samples for microbiologic culture, and close the skin and subcutaneous tissue routinely. Document allograft and metal implant positioning with postoperative radiographs.

Fracture healing with cortical allografts or alloimplants consists of filling host-graft interfaces with bone, followed by graft vascularization, graft resorption, and graft replacement with host bone (Fig. 31-39). Host-graft interfaces heal within 1 to 3 months; however, graft remodeling takes months to years (depending on graft length) and may never

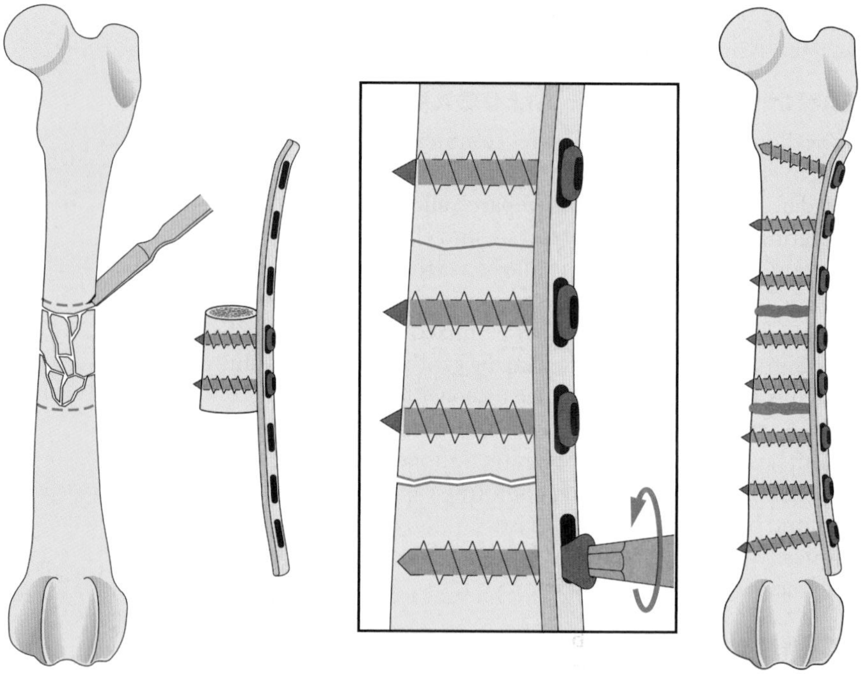

FIG. 31-38
To stabilize a cortical bone allograft, cut the bone segments perpendicular to the long axis of the bone and remove the fragments. Secure the graft to a precontoured plate. Reduce the graft plate segment into the fracture and compress the host-graft interfaces by loading the screws above and below the interfaces. Add cancellous bone autograft around the host-graft interfaces.

FIG. 31-39
Incorporation of cortical allografts or alloimplants into healing fracture. **A,** Host-graft interface is stabilized. **B,** Host-graft interface is filled with fibrous bone while bone remodeling units become active. **C,** The graft is vascularized, and portions of graft resorb and are replaced with host bone.

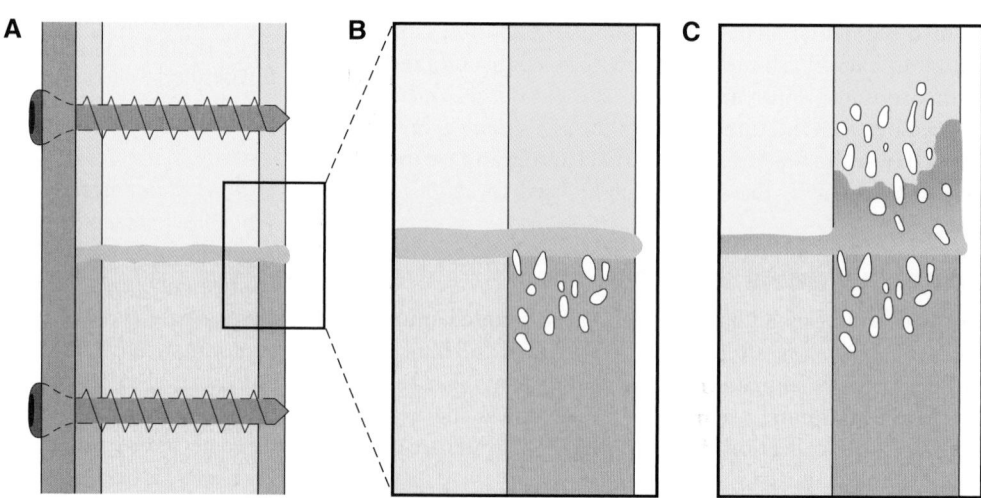

be completed. The process of remodeling can be monitored radiographically. Host-graft interfaces initially fill with the cancellous bone. As resorption and remodeling proceed from host-graft interfaces toward the graft center, grafts change from cortical structures to porous, cancellous bone. Eventually the cancellous bone remodels into cortical bone. It is often difficult to determine when plate removal should be done based on radiographic appearances because the amount of graft that has been remodeled may be difficult to ascertain. Because premature plate removal may predispose grafts to fracture, plate removal should not be done until definitive radiographic evidence of remodeling of the entire graft is noted. Generally, unless complications occur, plate removal is not recommended.

Complications associated with cortical allografts include infection, graft rejection, failure of fracture repair, and graft fracture. Graft infection usually results from graft or fracture site contamination, coupled with instability. This results in a large, sequestered piece of foreign material that must be débrided when fracture stabilization is performed. Cancellous bone autografts may be used to fill resultant fracture gaps. Signs of graft rejection (e.g., failure of graft and host bone to unite, graft resorption without replacement) are rarely noted clinically. Plate fracture may be observed when reduction and fixation of host-graft interfaces provide inadequate reconstruction of the bone column. Grafts may also fracture after plate removal.

Suggested Reading

Bauer TW, Muschler GF: Bone graft materials: an overview of the basic science, *Clin Orthop* 371:10, 2000.
This article provides an excellent review of the use of bone autograft, allograft, and synthetic bone graft substitute materials in reconstructive orthopedic surgery.

Connolly JF: Clinical use of marrow osteoprogenitor cells to stimulate osteogenesis, *Clin Orthop* 355S:257, 1998.
This article provides a review of 15 years of research into various methods and techniques of using marrow osteoprogenitor cells.

Fitch R, Kerwin S, Newman-Gage H et al: Bone autografts and allografts in dogs, *Compend Cont Educ Pract Vet* 19:558, 1997.
This article provides an overview of the use of bone autografts and allografts in small animal clinical practice.

Stevenson S: Enhancement of fracture healing with autogenous and allogeneic bone grafts, *Clin Orthop* 355S:239, 1998.
This article provides an excellent review of the optimal use of bone grafts to promote fracture healing. The information helps the clinician who performs a bone grafting procedure for the enhancement of fracture healing choose the right graft or combination of grafts for the biologic and mechanical environment into which the graft will be placed.

FRACTURE FIXATION SYSTEMS

EXTERNAL COAPTATION

External coaptation may be used to provide patient comfort before surgery and decrease soft tissue damage. It also may be used as the primary repair in some conditions. Bandages and splints for perioperative coaptation are described on pp. 946 to 949.

CASTS
Indications and Basic Principles

Full leg casts encircle the limb to stabilize a fracture. They can be used as a primary means of stabilization or as a supplement to internal fixation devices. As a primary stabilizer, full leg casts are most useful in stable fractures in which the fracture assessment (see p. 953) indicates rapid bone union. The functional period for a cast is short, usually no longer than 6 weeks before cast complications dictate removal. The classic casting material is plaster of paris, but with the development of synthetic casting materials, its use has declined. Synthetic casts made of fiberglass or polypropylene substrate impregnated with water-activated polyurethane resin have considerable advantages over plaster casts. Fiberglass bandages impregnated with polyurethane resin make the stiffest casts without being brittle when compared with other casting material. They are easy to apply, with maximal adhesiveness between layers, minimal wastage, and considerable durability. Fiberglass bandages interfere with radiographic observation of the healing fracture, however, because the weave pattern of the casting material is visible. Polypropylene substrates impregnated with polyurethane resin are more radiolucent with less distracting pattern (Langley-Hobbs et al, 1996).

BOX 31-6

Key Concepts in Applying Casts

Casts must span the joints above and below the fractured bone to be effective.
Apply the cast with the leg held in slight varus and flexion.
Excessive padding results in a loose cast after the padding compresses.
Extend the cast distally to encompass the toes, leaving only the toenails of the middle digits exposed.

Mechanically, a properly applied cast immobilizes the joints above and below the fractured bone, neutralizing bending and rotational forces on the fracture. A cast does not counteract axial forces applied to the fractured bone. The cast does not rigidly stabilize the fracture, resulting in indirect bone healing.

> NOTE: Full leg casts cannot be applied above the midhumerus or midfemur and therefore should only be used for fractures of the distal limb (radial and/or ulnar, tibial, and metacarpal and/or metatarsal fractures).

Application

General anesthesia is usually indicated for cast placement to allow closed fracture reduction (see p. 957). If the fractured bone ends cannot be reasonably reduced (i.e., varus-valgus and rotational alignment are maintained with at least 50% contact of major fragment ends), perform surgery. Most radial and tibial fractures are aligned in a valgus deformity because of the strong pull of the lateral musculature in the distal fragment. This deformity may be neutralized by holding the limb in a varus position during cast application. Applying the cast while the animal is in lateral recumbency with the affected limb down encourages the varus positioning of the limb (Box 31-6).

Clip long hair and apply tape stirrups to the distal limb. Avoid circumferential tape. Apply a single layer of cast stockinette onto the limb over the stirrups. Extend the stockinette from 2 inches distal to the toes to 2 inches above the estimated proximal extent of the cast. Fit the stockinette snugly against the limb. Have an assistant stretch the stockinette by pulling the ends during cast application to prevent folds or wrinkles in the material. Apply cast padding in a spiral fashion to the limb from the toes (i.e., exposing only the toenails of the middle digits) to the estimated proximal extent of the cast, overlapping the material 50%. Use sufficient cast padding to protect the limb from developing cast sores, but do not use excessive padding that would prevent the cast from resting snugly against and conforming to the limb (Fig. 31-40, A).

A   **B**

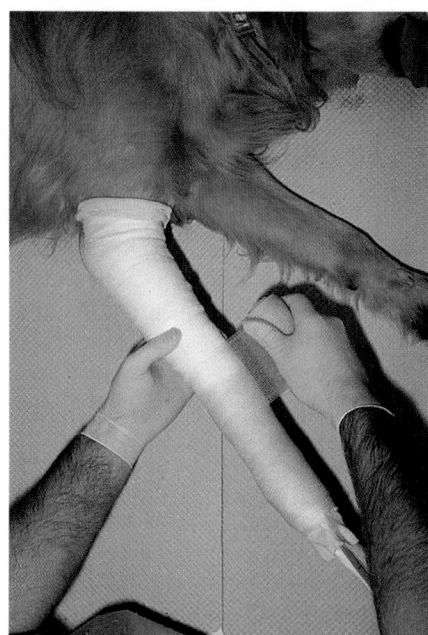

FIG. 31-40
A, When applying a fiberglass cast, place adhesive stirrups on the limb and cover them with a stockinette. Apply cast padding firmly over the stockinette using an overlapping pattern. **B,** Then place four to six layers of casting material on the limb, overlapping each layer 50%.

Generally, cast padding should be only two layers thick.

Immerse the casting tape into cold water, squeeze excess water gently from the roll, and apply it to the limb, beginning at the toes. Wrap the cast material in a similar fashion as the cast padding, with 50% overlap (Fig. 31-40, B). Encompass the toes, but leave the nails of the third and fourth phalanges exposed, to allow detection of limb swelling. As the cast tape is applied above the elbow or stifle, use firm pressure to compress the larger muscles and conform the cast to the limb. Use two layers of cast tape with 50% overlap (i.e., four layers on cross section) in small and medium-sized dogs and three layers (six on cross section) in larger dogs (more than 30 kg). **Apply the cast tape quickly because it will set in 4 to 6 minutes.** *Before the cast tape sets, roll the edges of the cast outward by pulling the proximal aspect of the stockinette over the end of the cast. Apply elastic adhesive or Vetrap around the cast, and stick the stirrups to this layer.*

An oscillating saw is required for cast removal. Sedation with oxymorphone, fentanyl, medetomidine, or acepromazine plus butorphanol (Box 31-7) generally facilitates cast removal because the vibration and noise generated by the saw often frighten the animal.

Cut the medial and lateral sides of the cast, separate the two halves, and remove it.

Frequent removal of a cast used for fracture stabilization is not desirable because fracture reduction may be lost. If skin abrasion or loosening of the cast occurs, replacement may be necessary.

 BOX 31-7

Drugs for Sedation During Cast Removal in Dogs

- Hydromorphone: 0.1–0.2 mg/kg IV, SC, or IM
- Oxymorphone (Numorphan): 0.05–0.1 mg/kg IV, IM, or SC
- Fentanyl (Sublimaze): 0.005–0.01 mg/kg IV, IM, or SC
- Acepromazine: 0.05 mg/kg IV, IM, or SC; not to exceed 1 mg total
- Butorphanol (Torbugesic, Torbutrol): 0.2–0.4 mg/kg IV, IM, or SC
- Medetomidine: 5–15 μg/kg IV or IM

IV, Intravenous; *IM,* intramuscular; *SC,* subcutaneous.

If frequent removal is anticipated, plan to use a bivalve cast. Slightly increase the amount of cast padding applied, place a layer of gauze over the cast padding, wrapping from the toes proximally, and bivalve the full cast on initial application. Use the oscillating saw to cut the medial and lateral walls. Separate the two halves, then tape them securely with three to four layers of adhesive tape. When the underlying skin needs to be treated or the cast needs modification, separate the halves by removing the adhesive tape. Apply new cast padding, replace the halves, and secure them with adhesive tape.

NOTE: A bivalve cast is used to supplement internal fixation devices, such as bone plate and screws in fractures of the carpus, tarsus, metacarpal and metatarsal bones and digits, and carpal or tarsal arthrodesis.

Cast care

Specific written instructions outlining proper at-home cast care should be provided for the client. Casts should be evaluated 24 hours after application and weekly thereafter. Clients should be instructed to observe the toes daily for evidence of swelling (spreading the exposed toenails), excessive chewing or licking at the cast, or a foul odor. Any of these signs requires that the animal be evaluated immediately. The cast should be kept clean and free of moisture. Instruct the client to place a plastic covering over the cast when the animal goes outside. In growing animals, the cast may need to be changed every 2 weeks; in adults the cast may last 4 to 6 weeks. Physical rehabilitation may be necessary after cast removal to encourage rapid return to normal function (see Chapter 12).

> NOTE: Be sure to have the owners check the toes daily and call immediately if any swelling or other abnormalities are noted.

EXTERNAL SKELETAL FIXATORS
Indications and Basic Principles

External skeletal fixators are a versatile and affordable treatment for long bone fractures, corrective osteotomies, joint arthrodesis, and temporary joint immobilization. They are not indicated for articular fractures and are rarely used for pelvic fractures. External fixators are well suited for stabilization after closed reduction of comminuted fractures. External fixators can be adjusted during and after surgery to improve fracture alignment. The functional period for external fixators varies depending on the frame constructed, but is related to the onset of pin loosening.

Fixation devices can be created to meet initial mechanical stabilization needs of the fracture and subsequently can be modified or destabilized to provide optimal stabilization throughout the healing period. Pin factors (type, size, number, location, and length), connecting bar material, and frame configuration (unilateral, bilateral, and biplanar) affect the stiffness of the fixator and its ability to resist the axial loading, bending, and rotation associated with weight bearing. Threaded pins have an interlocking hold with the bone and resist pullout and loosening. Increasing pin diameter increases pin stiffness, but should not exceed 25% of the bone diameter. The number of fixation pins in the proximal and distal major fragments influences the fixator's stiffness and affects the distribution of the physiologic loads among pins. The greater the number of fixation pins per fragment, the more effective is the device in stabilizing the fracture and maintaining pin-bone interface integrity. This is true for up to four pins per major proximal and distal fragment; beyond this number the increase in mechanical advantage is negligible. Locating pins both close to the fracture and at the ends of the bone increases the stiffness of the fixation and decreases the motion at the fracture site. Decreasing the distance between the bone and the fixation clamp increases the fixator's stiffness. Orienting the clamp so the pin clamping bolt is closest to the skin decreases the bone clamp distance.

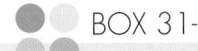
BOX 31-8

Key Concepts for Increasing Strength and Stiffness of an External Fixator

Predrill before inserting positive profile threaded pins.
Increase the pin numbers (up to four pins per bone segment).
Increase the pin size (up to 25% of bone diameter).
Locate pins near the joints and near the fracture.
Decrease the distance between the bone and the pin-clamp interface.
Increase the connecting bar size or use augmentation plates.
Increase the number and planes of connecting bars.
Tie the IM pin into the fixator frame.

Strength and stiffness increase as the size and number of external connecting bars increase. In addition, because bones are subject to bending in two planes (mediolateral and craniocaudal), biplanar fixators are more effective in resisting physiologic bending loads than are fixators with connecting bars aligned in a single plane (Box 31-8).

There has been much confusion in veterinary medicine about the naming of various external fixator configurations. Recently, efforts have been made to adopt a uniform and descriptive classification system that identifies the number of planes occupied by the frame and the number of sides of the limb from which the fixator protrudes. Using this system, common frames are unilateral-uniplanar (Type Ia), unilateral-biplanar (Type Ib), bilateral-uniplanar (Type II), and bilateral-biplanar (Type III) (Fig. 31-41). Because of an increasing number of bars and planes occupied by the different frame configurations, Type Ia, Type Ib, Type II, and Type III external fixators are successively stronger and stiffer. Type II frames are further divided into maximal Type II frames filled with full pins and minimal type II frames constructed with a minimum of two full pins. Combining external skeletal fixators with IM pins is an effective way to increase the rigidity of the fracture fixation in the humerus and femur. These systems are referred to as tie-in configurations (see Fig. 31-41). Type Ia frames are subject to bending when axial loads are applied. Adding a second connecting bar improves frame stiffness. Type Ib frames resist axial compression, bending, and rotation. Type II frames resist axial compression, bending in the same plane as the fixator, and rotation. Completely resisting out-of-plane bending requires a Type III fixator.

Equipment and Supplies

External fixation devices comprise three basic units: (1) fixation pins inserted into bone to hold major fragments, (2) external connectors to support fractured bone, and (3) linkage devices that attach the fixation pins and external connector. Several commercial external fixators are available for veterinary use.

Fixation pins. Fixation pins may be categorized by implantation method (e.g., half pin or full pin) or structural

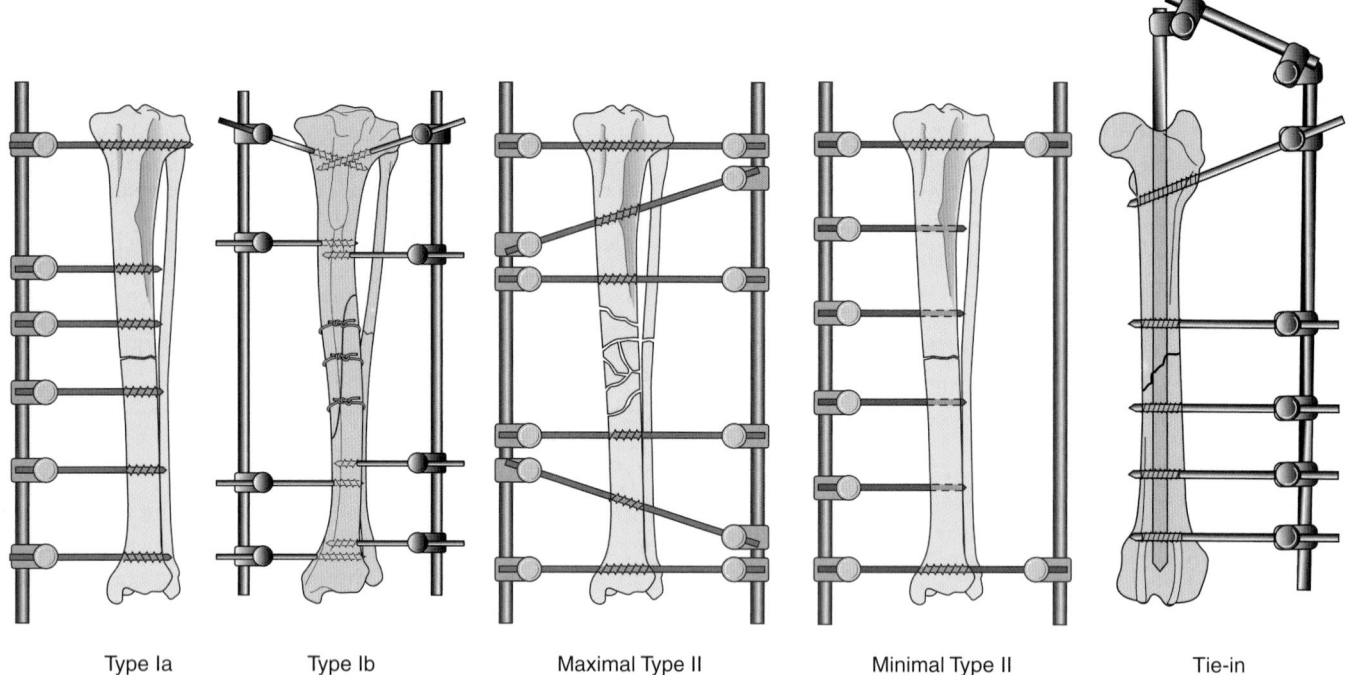

| Type Ia | Type Ib | Maximal Type II | Minimal Type II | Tie-in |

FIG. 31-41
Position of external bars and nomenclature for common external fixator frames. (Second and fourth images modified from Johnson AL, Dunning D: *Atlas of orthopedic surgical procedures of the dog and cat,* ed 1, St Louis, 2005, Saunders.)

FIG. 31-42
Placement of **A,** half pins, and **B,** full pins. Note that half pins are inserted so that they penetrate both cortices, but only one skin surface, whereas full pins penetrate both cortices and skin surfaces.

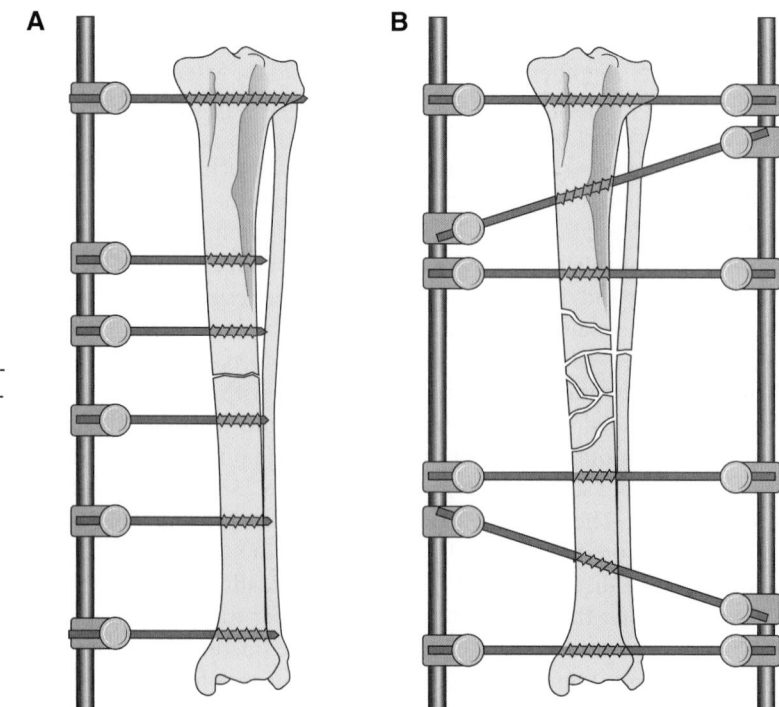

design (e.g., positive profile threaded or negative profile threaded). Half pins are inserted so that they penetrate both cortices, but only one skin surface (Fig. 31-42, *A*), whereas full pins penetrate both cortices and skin surfaces (Fig. 31-42, *B*). Fixation pins may be end-threaded or centrally

threaded. Centrally threaded pins are used as full pins with Type II or Type III external fixator frames (see later discussion). The central threads engage bone, and the smooth pin ends extend beyond the skin surface. End-threaded pins are often described according to the number of cortices to be

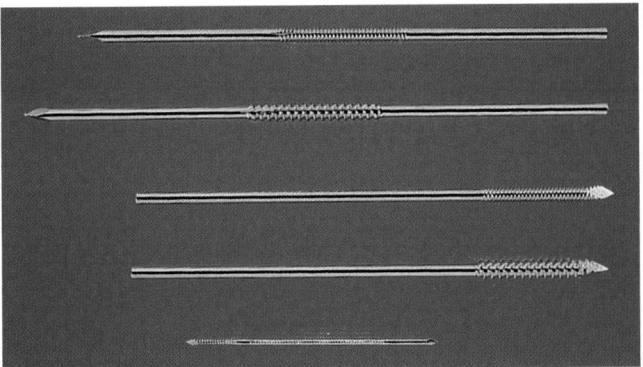

FIG. 31-43
Positive-profile fixation pins used with external skeletal fixation. *Top to bottom,* Centrally threaded cortical pin, centrally threaded cancellous pin, end-threaded cortical pin, end-threaded cancellous pin, and mandibular fixation pin.

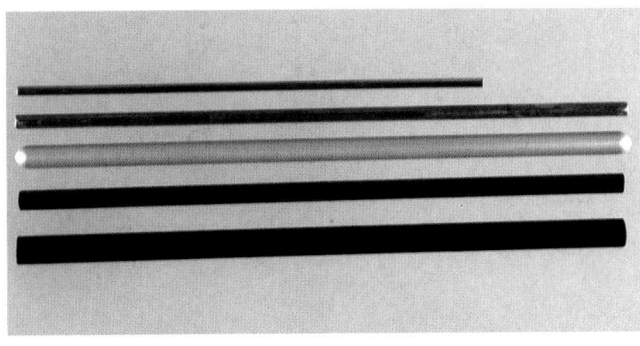

FIG. 31-44
Small, medium, and large external connectors (bars) used with external skeletal fixation are made of *(top to bottom)* stainless steel, titanium alloy, and carbon fiber.

engaged by the threads (i.e., one-cortex or two-cortex end-threaded pins). One-cortex end-threaded pins have threads near the pin tip; therefore although the pin itself penetrates both cortices, the threads engage only the far cortex. Two-cortex end-threaded pins have sufficient thread length to engage both cortices. Threaded pins can be further described according to thread profile (negative or positive). Centrally threaded and end-threaded pins in which the core diameter of the threaded section is smaller than the diameter of the smooth section have a negative thread profile. If the core diameter is consistent between smooth and threaded regions, the thread profile is positive. The thread height and thread pitch are specifically designed to engage dense cortical bone (threaded cortical pins) or spongy cancellous bone (threaded cancellous pins) (Fig. 31-43).

External connectors. External connectors are made of stainless steel, titanium alloy, carbon fiber, aluminum, or acrylic (Fig. 31-44). The carbon fiber rods are radiolucent, allowing radiographic visualization of the healing fracture. The different sizes of metal rods have correspondingly sized pin grippers (linkage devices; see below). The external fixator and linkage devices may be fashioned from acrylic using commercial kits for acrylic-pin external fixation (APEF) or from supplies designed to allow "homemade" acrylic splints to be applied (Fig. 31-45). The APEF system contains positive profile threaded fixation pins, prepackaged acrylic, and sterilized acrylic column-molding tubes. The application kit also contains reusable temporary alignment clamps. Homemade splints use individually purchased materials for construction of frames. The acrylic in homemade splints is polymethylmethacrylate and is derived from dental acrylic or hoof-repair acrylic. The fixation pins are purchased individually, and pediatric anesthesia tubing is used for the column-molding tubes.

Linkage devices. Advances in pin gripping clamp design have resulted in two commercially available clamps that enhance frame application and fracture fixation. The bar-

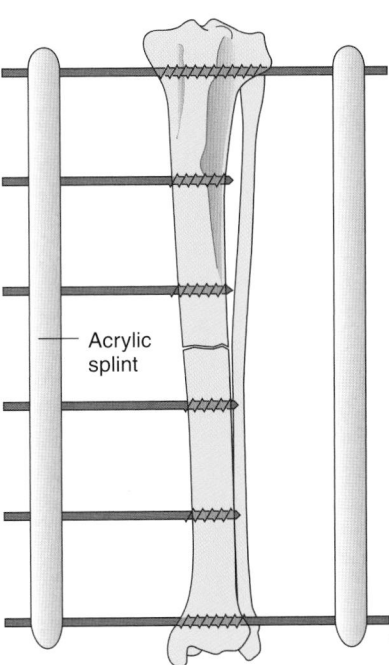

Acrylic splint

FIG. 31-45
Use of acrylic materials as external connectors rather than standard metal bars.

gripping portion of the SK™ clamp is separable to allow easy positioning on the connecting bar and is secured by two bolts. The hole in the bolt accepting the fixation pin is large enough to accept positive-profile threaded pins. Fixation pins are secured with a specially designed washer positioned on the pin fixation bolt. Double clamps (clamping connecting rod to connecting rod) are also available in this system. The Secur-U™ clamp has an altered U-shaped component that can be easily placed on the connecting bar. The head component of the clamp has a hole large enough to accept

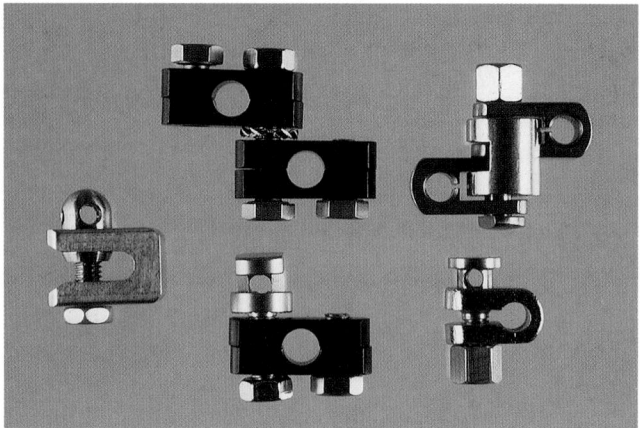

FIG. 31-46
Kirschner type of linkage devices for joining fixation pins to external connecting bars and external connecting bars to each other. Note the larger holes for the external connecting bars and smaller holes in the bolts for fixation pins. *Left to right,* Secur-U™, SK™ single and double clamps, and Kirschner single and double clamps.

positive-profile threaded pins. Securing the head with a bolt secures the fixation pin (Fig. 31-46).

Application

Preoperative planning for choosing the external fixator frame and the number and location of pins is essential for optimal outcome. The patient fracture-assessment score (see p. 953) must be considered when choosing an appropriate frame configuration. The lower the fracture-assessment score, the longer the fixator must remain in place and the stronger it must be (and vice versa). It is always better to err on the side of increased strength and stiffness rather than insufficient strength and stiffness. An insufficiently strong or durable frame will probably cause complications, whereas an overly rigid frame can be destabilized to a less rigid frame as healing progresses. Therefore it is important to understand the factors that significantly influence the strength and stiffness of the external fixator-bone combination, including frame configuration, pin number, size, placement, position, design, and bar placement (see Box 31-8).

A variety of frame configurations and pin designs are available, but certain principles of application are common for all external fixation devices. One of the most important principles is adherence to the practice of aseptic surgery. Proper aseptic technique, including patient preparation, gloving, gowning, draping, and instrument preparation, is just as important, if not more important, in the application of external fixators as for any other fixation method.

Suspend the injured limb from hooks in the ceiling (radius and tibia) or with an intravenous stand (humerus and femur). Scrub the liberally clipped area with an antiseptic soap. If the fixation is being applied to the radius or tibia, leave the limb suspended during application of the external fixator. If

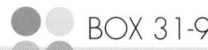

BOX 31-9

Key Concepts for Inserting Fixation Pins

Expose the pin insertion site.
Center the pin in the bone.
Predrill the pin hole.
Insert the pin with low RPM power.
Release the incision around the pin to prevent skin tension.

the fixation is being applied to the humerus or femur, release the limb from the suspension after it has been draped (see p. 36).

Once the number and size of pins have been selected, the method of placement and position of the pins relative to the fracture need to be considered. The most effective way to place a fixation pin is by using a miniapproach to expose the pin site and predrilling the hole before fixation pin insertion (Box 31-9).

Make a small (1-cm) longitudinal skin incision over the proposed pin site. Use a hemostat to dissect bluntly through the soft tissue from the skin surface to the bone to create a soft tissue tunnel that allows free gliding motion of surrounding muscles around the fixation pin. The tunnel also prevents the pain and discomfort that can result from impingement of soft tissue against fixation pins.

Create the soft tissue tunnel between large muscle bellies rather than through them, and avoid neurovascular structures. Protect the soft tissue in the walls of the tunnel from trauma using a drill sleeve, or retract and stabilize the tissue with a hemostat.

Predrill the bone using high RPM and a twist drill bit 0.1 mm smaller than the core diameter of the fixation pin. Place the fixation pin through the drilled hole with a hand chuck or a power drill, using low-RPM speed. Be sure the pin tip extends beyond the opposite cortex.

The site at which each fixation pin will be placed relative to the fracture is a factor that can positively influence the mechanical performance of external fixators. One pin should be placed 1 cm proximal and one pin 1 cm distal to the fracture. The closer these pins are placed on either side of the fracture, the shorter the distance between connecting clamps on the external bar. Therefore the length of the bar that must sustain the load is shortened, resulting in a stiffer external bar. Generally the most proximal and distal pins are placed in the respective metaphyses, and remaining pins are spaced evenly in the proximal and distal fragments.

NOTE: Each fixation pin should be drilled into the bone at the point of greatest cross-sectional diameter, and the trocar point should exit the far cortical surface for a distance of 2 to 3 mm.

The distance between the external bar and the body affects the length of the fixation pin from its attachment to the bolt on the clamp to its point of entrance into the bone. The shorter this distance, the less flexible is the fixation pin and the less micromovement at the pin-bone interface.

Once the fixation pins and external bar(s) are in place, adjust the position of the bar relative to the skin surface. Place the external fixation bar as close to the body as possible without allowing the clamps (pin grippers) or bar to impinge on the skin surface. Turn the pin-gripping clamps so the bolt is closest to the skin. As a rule of thumb, place the external bar so that one forefinger can be inserted between the clamps and the skin surface (approximately 1 cm).

Unilateral-uniplanar (Type Ia) fixators. Unilateral-uniplanar fixators (see Fig. 31-41) are usually applied to the cranial medial surface of the radius and tibia and the lateral surface of the femur or humerus. The fixation pins are referred to as half pins because they only penetrate the near skin surface and the bone.

Begin by placing a half pin in the metaphyses of the proximal and distal bone fragments. Place the pins in the center of the bone, perpendicular to its long axis and through both cortices. For efficiency, place an appropriate number of pin grippers on the bar to accommodate placement of subsequent pins. For example, if three pins are to be inserted in the proximal fragment and three pins in the distal fragment, then slide four empty pin grippers onto the external bar before connecting the pins initially placed in the proximal and distal metaphyses. Reduce the fracture (open or closed) and connect the two pins with an external bar. Place the additional half pins directly through the pin grippers. Once all the intermediate pins have been placed, tighten the pin grippers, and make a radiographic examination of the limb to assess fracture reduction and pin placement. Trim the fixation pins to prevent injury to the owners and immediate environment.

> NOTE: Either SK™ or Secur-U™ clamps can be easily added to an external connecting bar if an additional fixation pin is required.

Unilateral-biplanar (Type Ib) fixators. Unilateral-biplanar frame configurations (see Fig. 31-41) are applied most often to the radius and tibia. With the radius, one external bar is placed on the craniomedial surface of the bone and a second bar on the craniolateral surface. With the tibia, one external bar is placed on the craniomedial surface of the bone and a second bar on the craniolateral surface.

Apply a Type Ia frame to the cranial medial surface of the radius or tibia as described above. Then apply another Type Ia frame approximately 90 degrees to the first frame. Generally, plan to place four fixation pins per major bone

segment. Strengthen the frame for animals with low fracture-assessment scores by adding diagonal connecting bars, which span from the proximal lateral connecting bar to the distal cranial connecting bar and vice versa. Connect the diagonal bars to the existing connecting bars with double clamps or connect the diagonal bars to the existing pins with single clamps. Once all the intermediate pins have been placed, tighten the pin grippers, and make a radiographic examination of the limb to assess fracture reduction and pin placement. Trim the fixation pins to prevent injury to the owners and immediate environment.

A modified Type Ib fixator can be developed for the humerus by placing a full fixation pin through the condyles and constructing a unilateral frame on the lateral aspect of the humerus, coupled with a unilateral frame connecting the medial aspect of the full-fixation pin to half pins secured to the cranial aspect of the proximal humerus.

Bilateral-uniplanar (Type II) fixators. Because of the adjacent body trunk, bilateral configurations (Type II) (see Fig. 31-41) cannot be placed on the femur or humerus. They are applied only to the radius or tibia and are usually placed in a mediolateral plane. Minimal Type II frames are generally applied when using the SK™ equipment, but may be upgraded to a maximal Type II frame for animals with low fracture-assessment scores. Maximal Type II frames are generally applied when using Securos™ equipment because of the versatility of the aiming device.

First, place full pins in the proximal and distal metaphyses so that they lie in the same plane. Place the pins perpendicular to the bone surface and parallel to the adjacent joint line to facilitate restoring axial, varus-valgus, and rotational limb alignment. If necessary, use these pins to apply traction to the limb to aid in fracture reduction. Reduce the fracture, place the appropriate number of empty pin grippers on each external bar to accommodate placement of subsequent intermediate pins, and connect the proximal and distal full pins with a mediolateral connecting bar. Insert intermediate pins as half pins or full pins. Determine which pin type to use based on the fracture-assessment score.

Commercial aiming devices help direct the fixation pins used in maximal Type II frames to the contralateral clamp. A guide device can be constructed with an additional connecting bar and clamp.

Once all the intermediate pins are in place, tighten the pin grippers and take a radiograph of the limb to assess fracture reduction and pin placement. Trim the fixation pins to prevent injury to the owners and immediate environment.

Bilateral-biplanar (Type III) fixator. Bilateral-biplanar configurations (see Fig. 31-41) cannot be applied to the femur or humerus because of the position of the body wall. Type III frames are only indicated in very large dogs with low fracture-assessment scores.

To apply Type III fixators to the radius or tibia, place a bilateral-uniplanar frame (Type II) in a mediolateral plane, then place a unilateral-uniplanar (Type I) frame in a craniocaudal plane.

External skeletal fixators with intramedullary pins.

Humeral and femoral fractures are not usually stabilized with external skeletal fixators alone because the most stable frames (Type II and Type III) cannot be applied to these bones. To provide the strength and stiffness desired with complicated humeral or femoral fractures, a combination IM pin and Type Ia or Type Ib external fixator is often used (see Fig. 31-41). The fixation pin design and number of fixation pins are based on the fracture-assessment score, but normally the number of fixation pins is limited to two or three pins placed above and below the fracture. More fixation pins are not used because the greater the number of pins, the more intense the discomfort associated with pins placed through the large muscle groups.

Begin by reducing the fracture and inserting an IM pin that fills 60% to 75% of the medullary canal. Use cerclage wire to support long oblique fractures, spiral fractures, or comminuted fractures having one or two large fragments. If multiple fragments are present, bridge the comminuted section of bone with the IM pin and external fixator without disturbing soft tissue attachments to small bone fragments. Once the fracture is reduced and the IM pin has been placed, add the external fixator. Use the largest size fixation pin that does not exceed 25% of the diameter of the bone and will pass adjacent to the IM pin. If unsure about the track of the IM pin inside the bone relative to the chosen site for insertion of a fixation pin, drill the proposed fixation pin site with a small Kirschner wire. If the IM pin is encountered, select an alternative location; otherwise insert the fixation pin at this site. Insert the intermediate pins through preplaced pin grippers as described earlier. Connect the fixation pins to an external bar placed 1 cm from the skin surface.

Increasing the number of fixation pins strengthens the external fixator, but also increases postoperative discomfort. Two methods are used to strengthen external fixators without increasing the number of pins. One method is to add more external bars (the addition of a single external bar doubles the strength of the system), or add an augmentation plate. Additionally the IM pin may be left protruding above the skin surface at the exit point proximal to the greater trochanter. The IM pin is then "tied" into the external fixator by connecting the two with an additional short segment of external bar (see Fig. 31-41).

Acrylic splints.

Application of acrylic splints involves a one-stage or two-stage technique. The advantage of two-stage techniques is that pin placement and fracture reduction can be assessed before hardening of the acrylic. If the single-stage technique is used and if postoperative radiographs show fracture reduction or fixation pin placement to be unsatisfactory, a small section of the acrylic column

must be removed before corrective measures can be taken.

With either technique, insert the fixation pins in the bone fragments following the same principles and guidelines described for construction of standard external fixator frames. Place acrylic column-molding tubes over the ends of the fixation pins 2 cm from the skin surface. If using a single-stage technique, reduce the fracture and pour the acrylic into the columns. Place saline-moistened sponges or use a saline drip on the fixation pins to dissipate heat generated by the acrylic. Allow the acrylic to cure for 5 to 10 minutes. If using a two-stage technique, place the tubes over the ends of the fixation pins, but do not add the acrylic. Instead, reduce the fracture and apply a temporary alignment frame. Take radiographs to assess pin placement and fracture reduction; if satisfactory, pour acrylic into the columns and allow it to cure. If alignment needs to be changed after the acrylic has hardened, cut the acrylic column(s) at the fracture line with a saw. Once the appropriate adjustments are made, patch the acrylic column by adding new acrylic to fill the gap. Peel the plastic molding back from each end at the gap, and drill several holes in the remaining acrylic to provide a site of attachment for the old and new acrylic. Mold a small amount of new acrylic by hand and place it into the gap, then allow the acrylic to cure.

Postoperative Care

Postoperative analgesia should be provided (see p. 944). Immediately after surgery the pin-skin interface should be cleaned with antiseptic solution using cotton swabs. Incisions around the pins should be released or extended if there is skin tension around a pin during limb flexion and extension. Sterile gauze sponges should be placed around and between fixation pins and the limb wrapped with Vetrap or a similar bandage material. After surgery the pin-skin interface should be cleaned and the bandage changed daily. After approximately 1 week, gauze packing may be discontinued. A bandage may be applied to the fixator bars and pins to protect the frame and the animal's environment. The pin-skin interface should be cleaned daily until little or no serosanguineous transudate is noted at the surface. Once the interface seals, the daily observations should continue. Activity should be restricted to leash walking and physical rehabilitation until the fracture has healed. Physical rehabilitation encourages controlled limb use and optimal limb function after fracture healing (see Chapter 12). After the animal has been released from the hospital, postoperative examinations should be done at 2 and 6 weeks after surgery, then every 6 weeks. The pin-skin interface should be carefully examined and the clamp and skin observed for separation. If irritation or drainage is present, the involved skin surface should be cleaned and packed with gauze.

Staged disassembly is the process of modifying a fixation frame at approximately 6 weeks after surgery to increase the loading on the healing fracture. Increased loading on the fracture further stimulates bone healing and remodeling.

For example, Type Ib frames are destabilized to Type Ia frames by removing one frame. Type II frames are destabilized to Type Ia frames by removing a connecting bar. Frames may also be destabilized by removing fixation pins; however, a minimum of two pins on either side of the fracture must be maintained. Also, the increased load on the remaining pins will result in pin loosening. The fixator should be removed completely once the bone has healed. The patient should be sedated, the pin-gripper loosened, and the fixation pin removed with a hand chuck.

CIRCULAR EXTERNAL FIXATORS
Indications and Biomechanical Properties

Circular external fixators are used to stabilize fractures, compress or distract fractures or nonunions, transport bone segments, and dynamically correct bone angular and length deformities. The circular external fixator is uniquely suited for controlled distraction of bone segments, resulting in new bone formation in the trailing pathways called *distraction osteogenesis* (see p. 1004). Small-diameter tensioned wires provide adequate stability to bone segments, but allow controlled axial micromotion at the fracture site without compromising the fixator's stability. For optimal mechanical stability, the frame comprises four rings securing four pairs of wires that are placed as close to perpendicular as the soft tissue anatomy allows. The smallest ring diameter, allowing a minimum of 2 cm between skin and ring, provides the optimal mechanical performance. The most proximal and most distal rings are placed at their respective metaphyseal locations, and the inner two rings are placed close to the fracture.

Equipment and Supplies

Circular external fixators are composed of transosseous wires attached to rings or partial rings with wire fixation bolts. The rings are linked with threaded or telescopic rods, connecting plates, hinges and posts, and nuts and bolts to form a frame. A wire tensioner and various wrenches complete the set (Fig. 31-47). Although many specialized components can be used with the circular fixators, the main components of the system are described below.

Wires. Wires used for dogs and cats are generally 1.0, 1.2, or 1.5 mm in diameter. Wire strength and stiffness increase proportionally to the diameter of the wire squared. Cats and small dogs weighing up to 10 kg require 1.0-mm wires, dogs 10 to 20 kg require 1.2-mm wires, and dogs more than 20 kg require 1.5-mm wires. Wires with a bayonet point are preferred for drilling through cortical bone. Wires with a trocar point are reserved for drilling through cancellous bone. Wires with a bead positioned midway along the wire are called *olive wires* and are placed with the bead adjacent to the cortex to minimize bone translation along the wire. Appropriately placed, olive wires can provide interfragmentary compression and increase the stability of the frame construct.

Wires are placed so that one wire is adjacent to each surface of the ring for a total of two wires per ring. Additional

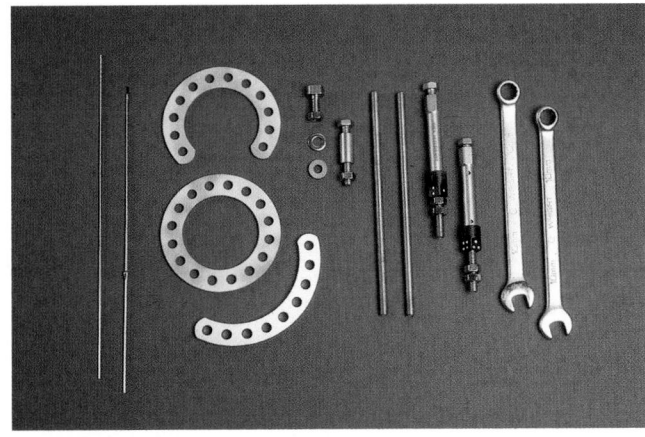

FIG. 31-47
Equipment used for circular external fixation includes wires with and without olives, rings, wire fixation bolts, threaded rods, nuts, and wrenches.

wires may be added to each ring with the addition of two posts to the ring to allow for a drop wire positioned at a distance from the ring surface. Increasing the number of fixation wires increases stability of the fixation. The angle of intersection of the wires and the positioning of the bone relative to the center of the ring affect the fixator's mechanical properties. Wires that intersect at 90 degrees maximize stability and minimize shearing forces. Often wires must intersect at less than 90 degrees to avoid vital neurovascular structures. Decreasing the angle of intersection results in a reduction of axial and bending rigidity. In general, wire angles less than 45 degrees should be avoided. Similarly, concentric placement of the bone within the ring is optimal. Often the soft tissue dictates that the bone is eccentrically placed, which decreases torsional stiffness and increases axial stiffness. Addition of olive wires increases the bending, axial, and torsional stiffness of the fixator. Increasing wire tension also increases the bending and axial stiffness, but decreases the torsional stiffness of the fixator.

Rings. Partial rings and full rings are selected based on size of the limb and location of the ring along the limb. *Fiveeighths rings or stretch rings* are used when full rings would limit joint motion in areas adjacent to the elbow and stifle. Judicious wire tensioning (50 kg or less) is used with partial rings to prevent ring deformation. Partial rings are versatile and can be used separately or bolted together to form full rings. *Full rings* have more available holes for rods and wires, but are less versatile. Ring diameter affects wire length and mechanical properties of the circular fixator. Increasing ring diameter decreases axial stiffness and to a lesser extent, torsional and bending stiffness. Ring size is dictated by the animal's size. The smallest ring that allows at least 2 cm in distance between skin and inner circumference of the ring at all points should be selected for frame construction.

Wire fixation bolts. Cannulated wire fixation bolts allow wire passage through a concentrically placed hole at the base of the bolt head. The fixation bolt is then tightened to the ring surface with a nut, securely clamping the wire. Slotted wire fixation bolts have an eccentric slot located under the bolt head and parallel to its long axis. Wires are fixed between the slot and the ring surface when the nut is tightened. Some slotted wire fixation bolts are also cannulated to accept wires in both positions. The wire must be fixed without deformation. Both slotted and simple washers are used to raise a wire fixation bolt to a wire not lying directly on the ring.

Frame construction. Threaded rods are used to connect the rings and form a frame. The rings are stabilized on each rod using one nut above and one nut below each ring. The nuts are tightened to clamp the ring securely. Compression or distraction of the fracture can be achieved by turning the nuts that fix the rods to the rings in the appropriate direction. Telescopic rods are hollow rods used as supports and connecting elements of the rings. These rods provide additional stability when relatively long distances must be spanned.

In general, frames are constructed so that one ring and its wires are placed at the proximal end of the long bone and another ring and wires are placed at the distal end of the long bone. Two additional rings are placed so that their wires penetrate the proximal and distal bone segments close to the fracture. This "far, near, near, far" construction provides optimal control and stabilization of the major bone segments.

Hinges are specialized posts that accept threaded rods and that can interface at an angle with each other when connected by a bolt and nut. Used in pairs, hinges connect proximal and distal ring frames and allow gradual reduction of an angular deformity.

Wire tensioner. The tensioner is an instrument used to tension the wires to an exact force (Fig. 31-48). Wire tension affects the overall rigidity of the fixator construct. The exact amount of tensioning needed depends on the animal's weight, the local bone quality, the treatment plan, and the frame construction. Cats and small dogs do not require tensioning of the wires. Dogs weighing 5 to 10 kg require 20 to 30 kg of tension in the wires. Dogs weighing 10 to 20 kg require 30 to 60 kg of tension in the wires. Dogs more than 20 kg require 60 to 90 kg of tension in the wires. Balanced tension, using two tensioners simultaneously to tension the wires for a single ring, is preferable. When using a tensioner that is not calibrated, tensioning the wire until the tensioner remains parallel with the ring without support is sufficient.

Wrenches. At least two appropriately sized crescent wrenches are necessary for tightening bolts and nuts simultaneously.

Application

Fracture treatment. Circular fixators are most applicable for fractures of the extremities below the elbow and stifle (Fig. 31-49). Modified circular fixators have been used for femoral and humeral fractures, but this application requires extensive use of arches and olive wires. Principles of frame construction and circular fixator application must be followed for optimal outcome in patients with all ranges of fracture-assessment score.

Radiographs are evaluated to determine fracture location and soft tissue diameter. The rings are selected to fit the soft tissue diameter while allowing 2 cm of distance between soft tissue and the rings. To expedite operating time, frames are generally preconstructed with four rings and three threaded rods. The rods are placed to form an equilateral triangle if possible. The rings are positioned on the rods in a "far, near, near, far" manner, with the proximal ring at the proximal metaphysis and the distal ring at the distal metaphysis. In most cases the proximal ring is a partial ring designed to limit interference with the stifle or elbow motion. The two

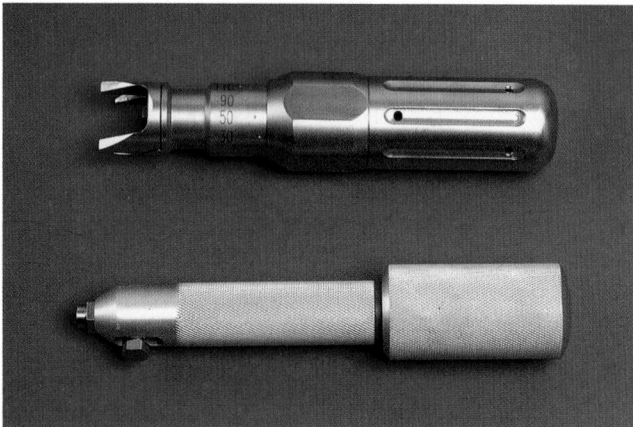

FIG. 31-48
Wire tensioners (calibrated and uncalibrated) used with circular fixators.

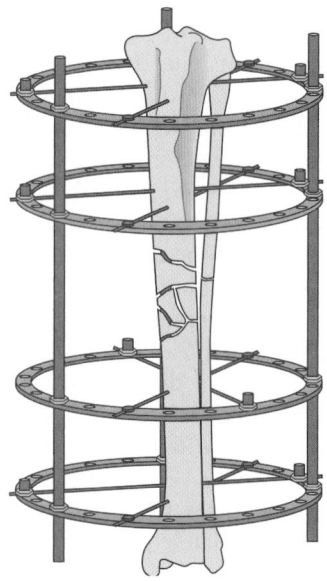

FIG. 31-49
Standard circular fixator frame for fracture management.

inner rings are positioned approximately 1 to 2 cm proximal and distal to the fracture line. The rings are stabilized in position on the threaded rods by tightening nuts placed adjacent to the top and bottom surfaces of the rings. Care is taken to secure the rings parallel to each other. Measuring the distance between rings on all three rods helps to ensure accurate placement. A short distal or proximal segment may limit the frame to three rings. The single ring will secure three wires placed in the short segment, two wires will be secured to the ring, and the third wire will be secured on posts arising from the ring.

Prepare the patient for aseptic surgery. Place the preconstructed frame around the limb.

If the limb is suspended for reduction purposes (see p. 959), it must detached, the frame positioned, and the limb reattached in suspension. Wire size is selected according to patient size.

Hold the frame in an approximate position, and select an appropriately sized wire to drive through the distal metaphysis of the bone, parallel to the distal joint surface, avoiding vital soft tissue structures. If necessary, as with a surgical approach disrupting normal skin position where the wire is to be located, hold the skin in approximately normal position while the wire is driven.

This precaution ensures minimal tension on the skin adjacent to the wire.

If the wire is penetrating muscle, position the limb to stretch the muscle maximally as the wire is driven. Manually push the wire through the skin and adjacent soft tissue until it centers on the bone, penetrating the periosteum. Then drive the wire through both cortices with a high-speed power drill. For optimal wire placement, hammer the wire out through the remaining soft tissue until it is centered in the bone. Secure the wire to the distal surface of the distal ring with slotted or cannulated bolts and nuts. Reposition the frame to ensure that the limb is centered in the frame and that the soft tissue is not compromised by the rings. Position a second wire adjacent to the proximal surface of the distal ring and drive it through the bone. Position the wire as close to 90 degrees (generally, 60 to 70 degrees is achieved) to the first wire as soft tissue constraints will allow.

Examine the position of the wire in relationship to the ring. If the wire lies immediately adjacent to the ring, secure it with a cannulated bolt if it passes over a hole or with a slotted bolt if it passes adjacent to a hole. If the wire is located above or below the ring surface, use washers to raise the surface to the wire, which is then secured as described earlier.

Pulling a wire to meet the ring causes undue forces on the wire that may cause pain, malalignment, and pin tract infection.

Reexamine the position of the frame, and place a second pair of wires through the proximal metaphysis, adjacent to the proximal ring, in a similar manner.

Circular fixators are unique in that fracture reduction can be controlled with the frame and wire application during a closed procedure. Fracture reduction can be achieved by distracting the proximal and distal rings to overcome fracture fragment overriding or using fixation with olive wires to bring fragments into contact. Alternately, using an arch wire technique involves placing a wire through the diaphysis of a bone segment and arching the wire before securing it to the ring. When the wire is tensioned, the arch is straightened and the bone segment drawn into alignment. Closed fracture reduction using the circular fixator is monitored with radiographic control.

Fill out the remainder of the frame with additional wires, using appropriate techniques to achieve fracture reduction and bone alignment as needed. Tension each pair of wires after they are placed, achieving appropriate tension for the patient's size. Optimally, tension each pair of wires simultaneously to prevent ring deformation. To tension the wire, tighten the nut securing one end of each wire. Apply the tensioner to the opposite end of the wire and tension. Secure the remaining end of the wire before removing the tensioner. After tensioning, cut the wires flush with the securing bolt or cut 2 to 3 cm from the bolt and curl the ends toward the ring. Examine the limb and the frame to ensure that (1) all rings clear the soft tissue, (2) all wire sites allow comfortable skin position, (3) all joints move freely, (4) all wires are tensioned, and (5) all nuts are tight. Make a radiographic assessment of the fracture alignment and fixation placement.

Arthrodesis. The circular external fixator can be used for carpal and tarsal arthrodesis. After articular cartilage removal and cancellous bone graft application, a preconstructed frame is placed and secured with two rings located proximally to the joint and two rings distally to the joint. Appropriate angulation of the frame to accommodate the joint angle can be achieved using hinges in place of threaded rods.

Bone lengthening. The ultimate advantages of the circular fixator over other forms of fracture fixation are its versatility and effectiveness in bone distraction or intercalary bone transport and the resultant distraction osteogenesis, or production of new bone in the trailing pathway (see pp. 1004). *Bone lengthening* is used to correct a shortened bone after premature physeal closure. *Bone transport* is used to fill a bone defect produced by traumatic bone loss or resection of a bone tumor. Successful application of this technique requires close attention to the details of appropriate osteotomy technique; preservation of marrow, periosteum, and extraosseous blood supply; application of a stable circular construct; and correct rate and rhythm of distraction.

Bone lengthening can be achieved unifocally or bifocally. *Unifocal* lengthening occurs when a single osteotomy is created in the bone. *Bifocal* bone lengthening occurs when two osteotomy sites are created in the bone, effectively doubling the rate of distraction. A preconstructed frame similar to the four-ring frame developed for fracture fixation is used for bone lengthening. Bifocal bone lengthening requires an additional ring to stabilize the center bone segment. The frame can be constructed using the threaded rods. However, telescoping rods or linear motors can be inserted for increased strength and ease of distraction.

Optimal osteotomy techniques for distraction osteogenesis have been the subject of extensive investigation. Ilizarov determined that a subperiosteal partial cortical osteotomy (called a *corticotomy* because the osteotome does not penetrate across the medullary canal) around three quarters of the bone's circumference, followed by osteoclasis or manually fracturing the remaining quarter of the bone, maximized preservation of endosteal and periosteal tissues and adjacent circulation (Stallings et al, 1998.) Other investigators have shown that osteotomy performed with an osteotome may be as effective as corticotomy and that preservation of periosteal tissue enhances the regenerative and reparative potential (Stallings et al, 1998). An oscillating saw cooled with saline can be used to perform the osteotomy, but may cause delayed consolidation. This concern may not be clinically relevant for young animals with greater osteogenic potential.

After frame application and osteotomy, a delay or latency period before initiation of distraction is recommended to allow local cellular and vascular responses to occur. Recommendations vary from 1 to 3 days for immature animals to 5 to 7 days for adult animals. Early distraction may cause diminished callus production. Delaying distraction may cause premature consolidation. In general, the animal's age and health, type and location of the osteotomy, and associated soft tissue trauma are considered when establishing a latency period (Box 31-10).

An optimum rate of 1 mm per day divided into a rhythm of four distractions per day (i.e., 0.25 mm per distraction) has been shown to favor regenerate bone formation without causing soft tissue discomfort and to be clinically achievable. Rate and rhythm of distraction can be varied slightly depending on the patient and on radiographic evidence of regenerate formation. Distraction is accomplished either by turning the nuts securing the rings to the threaded rods or by turning the cubes on the linear motors.

> NOTE: Take care to turn the nuts in the appropriate direction to cause distraction. Measure between the rings to ensure that distraction is achieved. Be sure the nuts are secured after distraction to restore frame stability.

Radiographs should be taken every 2 weeks to observe the appearance of the regenerate bone and adjust the rate of distraction accordingly. The regenerate bone should appear as definite columns of longitudinally oriented new bone extending from each osteotomy surface toward a central trans-

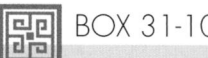

BOX 31-10

Factors Used to Determine Latency Period

Decrease Latency Period	Increase Latency Period
Immature animal	Adult animal
Excellent health	Compromised health
Subperiosteal corticotomy	Osteotomy with oscillating saw
Metaphyseal osteotomy	Diaphyseal osteotomy
Minimal soft tissue trauma	Massive soft tissue trauma

verse radiolucent area. Bone should also retain a constant diameter radiographically. An hourglass configuration of the regenerate bone indicates an overly rapid distraction rate. Inconsistent radiopacity, irregular bone columns, and focal failures of bone formation indicate instability or poor vascularity; the rate of distraction should be decreased until a normal regenerate is observed. A cross-sectional diameter of the regenerate bone exceeding the cortical diameter indicates a rapidly forming regenerate and the possibility of premature consolidation; the rate of distraction should be increased.

Bone transport. The principles and techniques described for bone lengthening are used when moving a segment of bone into a bone defect while stimulating new bone formation in the trailing pathway. The technique of bone transport is used to fill large bone column defects occurring after trauma or bone tumor resection (Fig. 31-50).

Preconstruct a frame with four stabilizing rings and a center transport ring. Apply the frame to the affected limb as described earlier. Approach and identify the osteotomy site. Secure the segment of bone to be transported to the center transport ring with two tensioned wires. Perform the osteotomy. Ensure that the osteotomy is complete and the bone segment movable. After the appropriate latent period, move the transport ring toward the defect at an appropriate rate and rhythm for the animal.

When the transported bone segment contacts the bone on the far side of the defect, called *docking*, compression is applied with the ring fixator to stimulate bone union. Occasionally, cancellous graft is necessary to achieve bone union.

Angular limb deformity correction. Circular fixators are indicated for dogs that have severe limb length discrepancy, when additional extensive growth is anticipated, and in dogs that have significant craniocaudal deformity. Circular fixators can be used to treat dogs with varus-valgus deformities, although techniques using the standard linear external fixator are also effective for treating this deformity. An advantage of circular fixators in treating angular deformities is that the flexibility of the system allows angular deformities and length discrepancies to be corrected simultaneously. Disadvantages of circular fixators for correcting

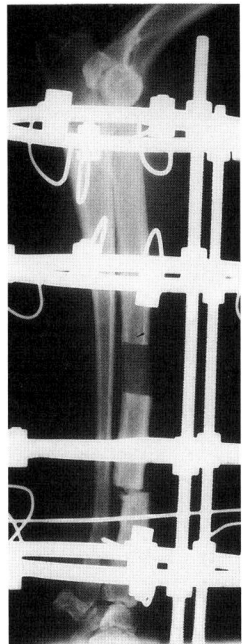

FIG. 31-50
Regenerated bone appears in the trailing pathway of a distracted bone segment in this dog treated with bone resection and distraction osteogenesis. (Courtesy Dr. Nicole Ehrhart.)

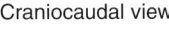

Craniocaudal view   Mediolateral view

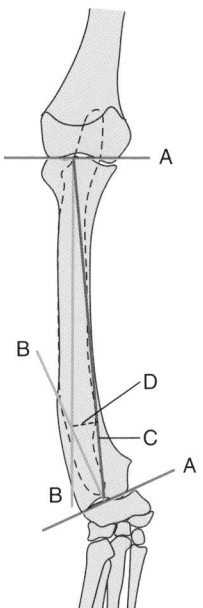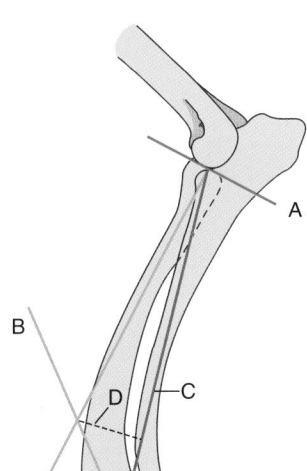

FIG. 31-51
Schematic for drawing the lines on tracings of the craniocaudal and lateral radiographs. Lines *A* parallel the joint surfaces. Lines *B* bisect the metaphyses and form the apex of the deformity. Lines *C* connect the intersections of the metaphyseal lines and the lines paralleling the articular surfaces. Lines *D*, connecting the apex of the deformity to line *C* and perpendicular to line *C*, are the vector components.

deformities include an intensive and often lengthy learning curve for surgeons, extensive preoperative planning, and intensive postoperative monitoring of the deformity correction process.

Initially, mediolateral and craniocaudal radiographs of the affected limb and the opposite control limb (if normal) are used to define the varus-valgus and craniocaudal components of the deformity. Length discrepancy is also determined by comparing lateral radiographs of the affected bone(s). Rotational deformity may be estimated from radiographs, although often it is best determined from physical examination. Rotational deformity is measured directly on the dog by comparing the planes of flexion and extension of the adjacent joints.

To determine the degree and plane of angular deformity and the optimal hinge and motor placement, trace the craniocaudal and mediolateral radiographic images of the affected bone. Draw two lines that bisect their respective metaphyses and are perpendicular to lines paralleling the adjacent articular surface on each tracing (Fig. 31-51).

The point of intersection of the two lines is the apex of the deformity.

To calculate the varus-valgus and craniocaudal components of the deformity, draw a line connecting the intersections of the metaphyseal lines and the lines paralleling the articular

surfaces on both radiographic views. Then draw a line from the point of intersection (i.e., apex of the deformity) to the line connecting the articular surface lines on each tracing (see Fig. 31-51).

These lines are perpendicular to the lines connecting the articular surface lines and represent the vector components of the deformity.

Draw the appropriately sized fixator ring with all holes represented. Identify and draw two lines within the circle connecting the craniocaudal and mediolateral aspects of the ring. The circle lines should intersect perpendicularly at the center of the circle. Plot a line the distance of the medial or lateral deformity (i.e., vector component), starting at the intersection of the circle lines and extending the appropriate distance and direction. Plot a second line the distance and direction of the cranial or caudal deformity, starting at the end of the mediolateral distance line and paralleling the craniocaudal circle lines. Drop a tangential line from the intersection of the circle lines, and terminate it at the end of the craniocaudal distance line; this line defines the plane of deformity. Place the motor on the ring in the plane of deformity and on the concave side of the deformity (Fig. 31-52) (Lewis et al, 1999).

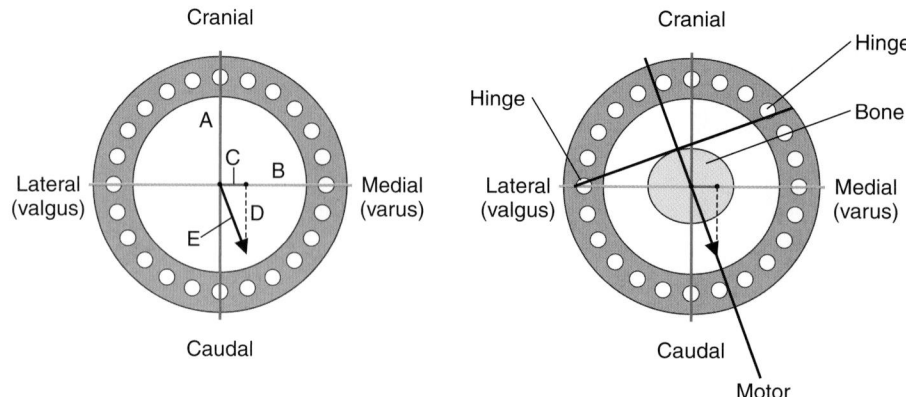

FIG. 31-52
Schematic of the ring drawing. Lines *A* and *B* connect the cranial and caudal aspects and the medial and lateral aspects of the ring and intersect perpendicularly in the center of the ring. Line *C* is the medial to lateral vector component (determined from the craniocaudal radiograph). Line *D* is the cranial to caudal vector component (determined from the lateral radiograph). Line *E* is the tangential line defining the plane of deformity. The motor is placed in the plane of deformity and on the concave side of the limb. The hinges are placed at the apex of the deformity.

> NOTE: The hinges are placed at the apex of the deformity. The positioning of the hinges is critical to the outcome. Hinges placed at the apex of the deformity and level with the convex surface of the bone will result in correction of the angular deformity, with an increase in length on the concave side of the bone equal to an opening wedge osteotomy. Hinges placed at the apex of the deformity and at a distance from the convex surface of the bone result in simultaneous opening of the wedge and an increase in the length of the convex surface of the bone.

The frame is constructed with the hinges and motor in the appropriate positions before the surgical procedure.

Following the protocol outlined above for application of a circular fixator in fracture fixation, place the preconstructed frame over the affected limb, and secure the proximal and distal rings with tensioned wires. Ensure that the tensioned wires are parallel to their respective articular surfaces. Place additional tensioned wires to fill out the frame. Approach the bone and perform an osteotomy at the apex of the deformity.

The osteotomy should parallel the closest articular surface. Rotational correction is usually performed acutely at surgery.

Close the incision. Ensure that the hinges and motor are appropriately placed, and secure all nuts in the frame (Fig. 31-53, A).

After an appropriate latency period, initiate the distraction with the motor.

The rhythm of distraction is two to four times per day. The rate of distraction will vary depending on the animal and on radiographic evaluation of the regenerate bone. Because the motor is offset from the deformity, calculations must be performed to ensure appropriate distraction at the motor to achieve 1 mm per day at the osteotomy site (Fig. 31-53, *B*).

Postoperative Care

Postoperative analgesia should be provided (see p. 944). Immediately after surgery the wire-skin interface should be cleaned with antiseptic solution using cotton swabs. Sterile gauze sponges should be placed around and between tensioned wires and the limb wrapped with Vetrap or a similar bandage material. Holes are cut in the bandage to allow access to the nuts involved in distraction. After surgery the wire-skin interface should be cleaned and the bandage changed daily or every 2 days. After approximately 1 week, gauze packing can be discontinued. The frame may still be protected with an external wrap. The wire-skin interface should be cleaned daily. Activity should be restricted to leash walking and physical rehabilitation until the fracture has healed. Physical rehabilitation encourages controlled limb use and optimal limb function after fracture healing.

If frame distraction is occurring, explicit instructions must be given to the owners to ensure proper rate and direction of distraction. After release from the hospital, the animal should be reevaluated weekly for the first 2 to 3 weeks postoperatively or during the distraction phase. The wire-skin interface should be carefully examined and the ring and

A   **B**

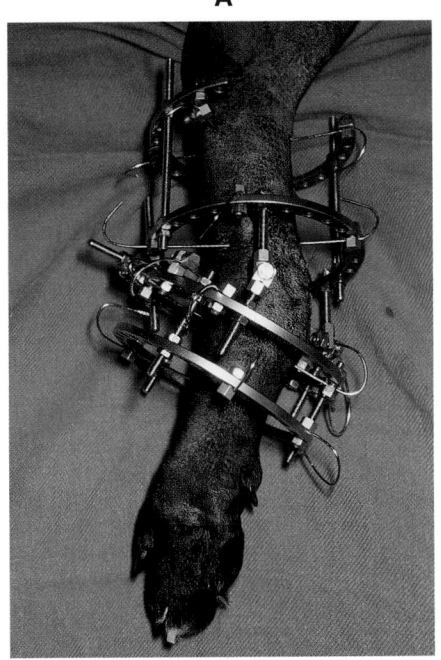
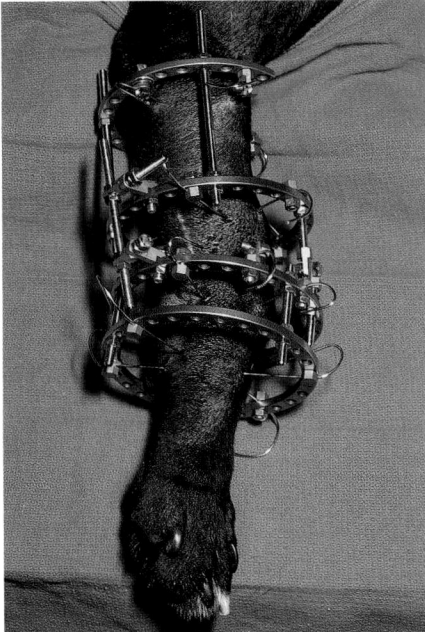

FIG. 31-53
Dog treated with circular fixator for angular deformity. **A,** Immediately after surgery. **B,** After the fixator had been distracted over 20 days, showing how the limb straightens as the proximal and distal rings begin to parallel each other.

skin observed for separation. If irritation or drainage is present, the involved skin surface should be cleaned and packed with gauze. Radiographs are made every 7 to 10 days during distraction and appropriate adjustments made to the rate of distraction. When the distraction is complete, the hinges are replaced with threaded rods, and the frame is stabilized by tightening all nuts. The fixation remains in place until radiographic evidence of bone consolidation. Occasionally, distraction will cause musculotendinous contracture, leading to flexural deformities or joint stiffness. Physical therapy and limb use are key to preventing this complication. The circular fixator is removed once the bone has healed. The appropriate time to take postoperative radiographs for healing depends on the estimated time to bone union and the patient fracture assessment. The patient should be sedated and the wires cut close to the bolts and removed with a hand chuck or vise grip. Smooth wires can be removed from either direction, whereas olive wires must be removed from the side of the olive.

HYBRID CIRCULAR EXTERNAL FIXATORS
Indications and Biomechanical Properties

Hybrid circular external fixators are a combination of a ring fixator and a linear fixator. Generally the frame consists of a ring with wires securing one segment of bone, and fixation pins and a connecting rod securing the other segment of bone. The connecting rod articulates with the ring to stabilize the fracture. Hybrid fixators are indicated for fractures with short juxtaarticular bone segments. The ring stabilizes

the short segment with two to three wires. Hybrid fixators may be applied to the radius, tibia, femur, and humerus. Hybrid fixators can also be used to stabilize corrective osteotomies for angular limb deformities.

The mechanical properties of the fixation frames are similar to those described for the circular and linear fixation systems.

Equipment and Supplies

See the sections on linear external fixators and circular external fixators for information on equipment and supplies. Additional frame components unique to the hybrid fixator frame are connecting bars that are threaded on one end. These bars are inserted into the ring and secured with paired nuts. Spherical nuts and washers are also available to some angular adjustment between the rod and the ring.

Application

Type Ia hybrid fixators. *Begin by placing the appropriately sized ring, with a connecting bar attached, around the juxtaarticular (short) bone segment. Hold the frame in an approximate position, and select an appropriately sized wire to drive through the metaphysis of the bone, parallel to the adjacent joint surface. Secure the wire. Add the appropriate number of pin gripping clamps to the connecting rod. Reduce the fracture and secure the proximal segment with a fixation pin inserted appropriately (see p. 972). Check alignment and secure the frame by clamping the fixation pin with the proximal pin gripping clamp. Check alignment then add the second wire to the ring and, if room permits, add a third wire (drop wire) secured to posts connected to the ring. Ten-*

sion and secure the wires. Place additional half pins directly through the pin grippers to achieve three to four pins in the long bone segment. Once all the intermediate pins have been placed, tighten the pin grippers, and make a radiographic examination of the limb to assess fracture reduction and pin and wire placement. Trim the fixation pins and wires to prevent injury to the owners and immediate environment.

Additional support may be added to the Type Ia hybrid frame by placing a second connecting bar, which is secured to the ring (opposite the first connecting bar) by a hinge created from two posts, and also to the proximal aspect of the connecting bar or the proximal pin.

Type Ib hybrid fixators. *Apply a Type Ia hybrid frame to the bone. Then secure another connecting bar to the ring at approximately 90 degrees to the first frame. Fill out the second connecting bar with fixation pins securing the long segment of bone. Once all the intermediate pins have been placed, tighten the pin grippers, and make a radiographic examination of the limb to assess fracture reduction and pin and wire placement. Trim the fixation pins and wires to prevent injury to the owners and immediate environment.*

Postoperative Care

Postoperative care including destabilization is similar to what is provided for linear external fixators (see p. 974).

INTERNAL FIXATION

INTRAMEDULLARY PINS AND KIRSCHNER WIRES

Indications and Biomechanical Properties

IM pins are most often used for diaphyseal fractures of the humerus, femur, tibia, ulna, and metacarpal and metatarsal bones. IM pins are contraindicated for the radius because the insertion point of the pin generally interferes with the carpus. The biomechanical advantage of IM pins is their resistance to applied bending loads (Fig. 31-54, *A*). In contrast to other implants (e.g., bone plates and external fixators), IM pins are equally resistant to bending loads applied from any direction because they are round. Biomechanical disadvantages of IM pins include poor resistance to axial (compressive) or rotational loads and lack of fixation (interlocking) with bone (Fig. 31-54, *B* and *C*). The only resistance to rotation or axial loads provided by an IM pin is friction generated between pin and bone. In general, this friction is not sufficient to prevent rotational movement or axial collapse of a fracture. Contact and friction between pin and epiphyseal cancellous bone vary with the amount of cancellous bone and accuracy of pin placement. The actual pin-bone contact is not substantial because the cross-sectional marrow cavity diameter varies, limiting the amount of friction created between these two surfaces. Because friction created between pin and bone is

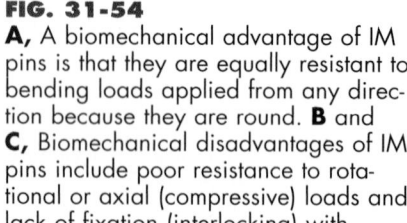

FIG. 31-54
A, A biomechanical advantage of IM pins is that they are equally resistant to bending loads applied from any direction because they are round. **B** and **C,** Biomechanical disadvantages of IM pins include poor resistance to rotational or axial (compressive) loads and lack of fixation (interlocking) with bone.

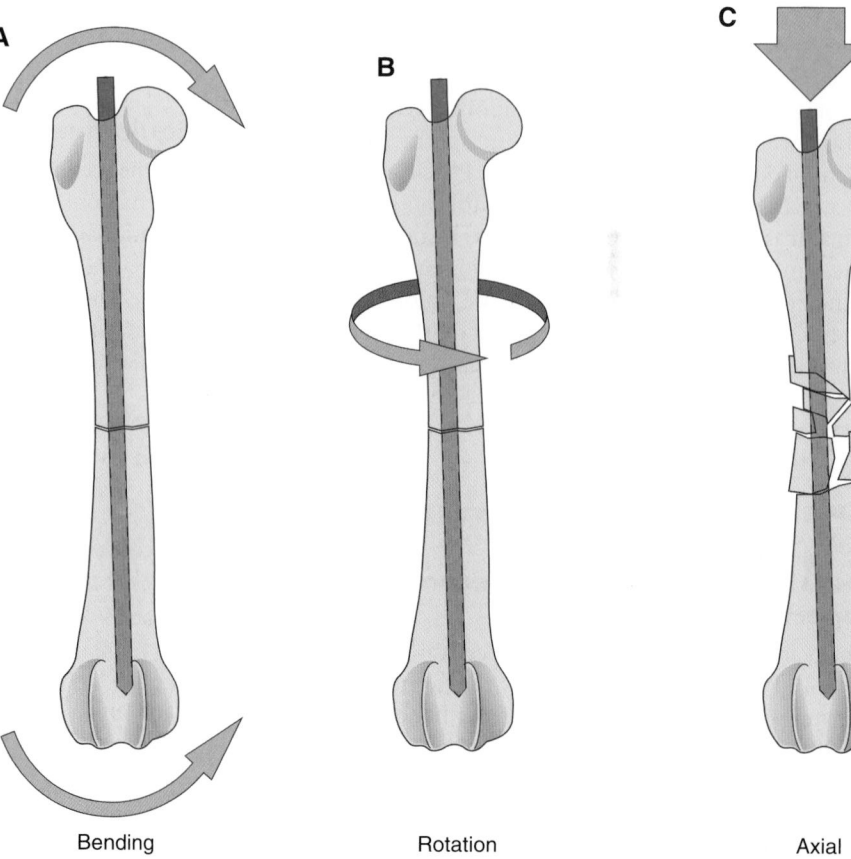

Bending
+++

Rotation
– – –

Axial
– – –

what prevents premature pin migration, stress associated with unstable fractures results in micromotion at the pin-bone interface, bone resorption, and pin migration. Because of these limitations in mechanical support afforded by single-pin or double-pin stabilization, IM pins should be supplemented with other implants (e.g., cerclage wire and external fixator or plate) to increase rotational and axial support.

Steinmann pins or Kirschner wires may be used as crossed pins (wires) or placed in a triangulated pattern to stabilize metaphyseal and physeal fractures in young animals. (See individual metaphyseal and physeal fractures in Chapter 32.) Kirschner wires are also used as IM pins in very small animals.

Equipment and Supplies

IM pins are smooth, round, 316L stainless steel rods that are inserted into the medullary cavity for fracture stabilization. The most common IM pins used in veterinary medicine are Steinmann pins. *Steinmann pins* are available in sizes ranging from $^1/_{16}$ to $^1/_4$ inch and come with a variety of point designs (Fig. 31-55). They can be *single armed* (one end with a point and one end blunt) or *double armed* (a point at each end). The most popular point designs are trocar points and chisel points. *Chisel points* have a two-sided cutting edge that is slightly more effective in cutting through dense cortical bone because it generates less heat than trocar points. *Trocar points* have a triple cutting edge and cut through cancellous bone easily. Because Steinmann pins are generally used as IM rods and are seated in proximal or distal epiphyseal cancellous bone, trocar points are most often used.

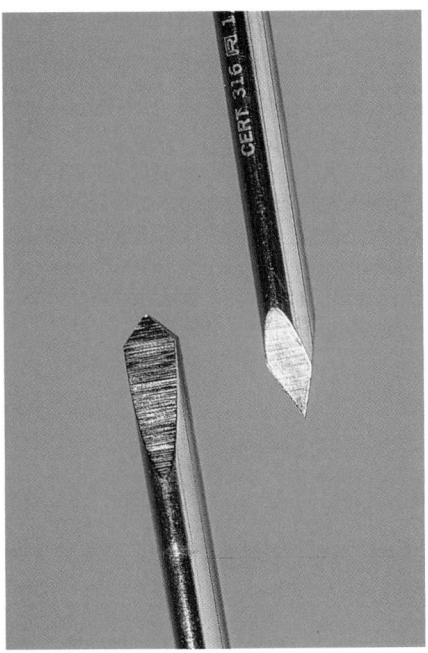

FIG. 31-55
IM pins with chisel *(left)* and trocar *(right)* points.

IM pins may be smooth or may have threads near the end of the pin. The end-threaded Steinmann pin was developed to increase the pin's holding power in cancellous bone. However, use of end-threaded pins is controversial. Threaded Steinmann pins have increased potential for premature failure compared with smooth Steinmann pins. In the manufacturing of the end-threaded Steinmann pin, threads are cut into the tip of a smooth Steinmann pin, causing the pin diameter to be greater in the nonthreaded section of the pin than in the threaded section. This difference in cross-sectional area acts as a stress concentrator that predisposes to premature pin bending or breakage.

Kirschner wires are small in diameter, ranging from 0.035 in to 0.062 in (see p. 1019 for conversion to metric), smooth pins, which generally have trocar points on each end.

Steinmann pins used as IM pins are generally driven with a Jacobs chuck. Steinmann pins and Kirschner wires used as crossed pins may be driven with a high-speed wire driver.

Application

Select an IM pin that equals 60% to 70% of the diameter of the marrow cavity at the isthmus of the bone when pairing the IM pin with cerclage wire. Choose a smaller diameter pin when pairing the pin with an external fixator or plate.

Although IM pins function most effectively if they fill the medullary canal, the curvature of most canine bones dictates that a smaller pin must be used if the fracture is to be reconstructed anatomically. Pin size determination is made after evaluating radiographs of the fracture. Appropriate size may be confirmed by comparing the pin with the medullary canal after the fracture is exposed.

Select two pins of the same length before starting the procedure.

The second pin serves as a guide pin when laid over the external surface of the limb. The guide pin is aligned with the bone so the operator can aim the IM pin in a similar direction.

An IM pin may be *normograded* or *retrograded* for placement in the femur or humerus. IM pins must be normograded in the canine tibia to prevent damage to the stifle.

To place a pin in a normograde fashion, start the pin at the appropriate location at one end of the long bone and drive it down the medullary canal to the fracture, reduce the fracture, and continue to drive the pin until it seats in metaphyseal bone (Fig. 31-56).

The advantages of normograde placement are that the pin can be placed more precisely and there is less manipulation of the fracture area. The disadvantage of normograde placement is that it may be difficult to identify the correct entry point into the bone if the insertion of the pin is done blindly.

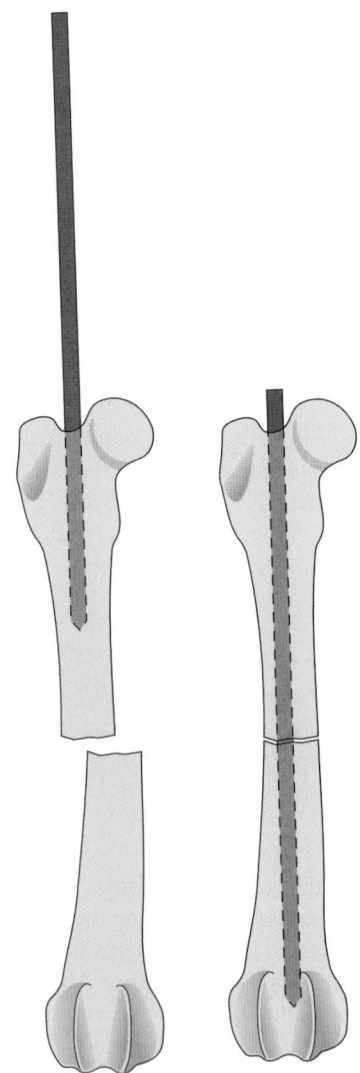

FIG. 31-56
For normograde placement of an IM pin in the femur, insert the pin so that it enters the bone proximally in the craniolateral trochanteric fossa. Direct it caudally to glide along the caudal cortex and seat it in the caudocentral aspect of the condyle.

To place a pin in a retrograde fashion, first expose the fracture and insert the pin into the medullary canal of the proximal bone segment. Drive the pin proximally to exit the proximal bone segment. Replace the pin chuck on the proximal portion of the pin, and withdraw it until the distal pin point is within the medullary canal. Reduce the fracture and drive the pin distally to seat in metaphyseal bone (Fig. 31-57). Check the pin insertion length by using the second pin as a reference. Approximate the position of the proximal tips of both pins and lay the reference pin over soft tissue outside the limb to determine the position of the distal tip of the IM pin. Check for pin interference in the distal joint by flexing and extending the joint.

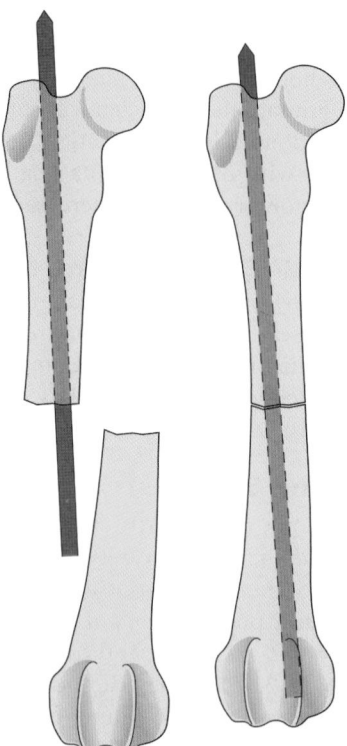

FIG. 31-57
For retrograde placement of an IM pin in the femur, insert the pin into the marrow cavity at the fracture surface. Force the shaft of the pin against the caudomedial cortex and drive the pin proximally. Reduce the fracture and drive the pin distally to seat in the caudocentral aspect of the femoral condyle.

Crepitation or decreased range of motion may indicate pin interference. Radiographs will confirm the presence of a pin in the joint.

Retract the pin so it is no longer interfering with the joint. Check the fracture for anatomic reduction or correct bone alignment and apply either cerclage wire (long oblique fractures in animals with high fracture-assessment scores), external fixators (frame construction depends on fracture-assessment score), or a bridging plate (animals with comminuted fractures and low fracture-assessment scores (Box 31-11) (see also pp. 974 and 998).

When satisfied with pin position, cut the excess pin by pushing down on the soft tissue and cutting the pin below the skin level with a pin cutter. Suture the soft tissue over the pin.

To apply Steinmann pins or Kirschner wires as crossed pins to secure a physeal or metaphyseal fracture, reduce the fracture and insert the pins on the lateral and medial surfaces on the epiphyseal segment. Drive the lateral pin across the fracture to exit on the medial surface of the metaphyseal segment. Drive the medial pin across the fracture to exit on the lateral surface of the metaphyseal segment (Fig. 31-58).

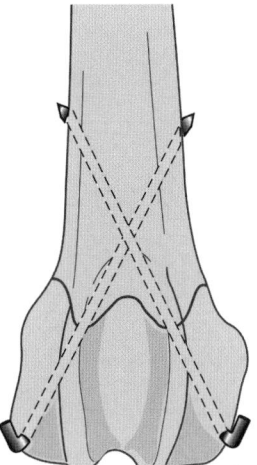

FIG. 31-58
Steinmann pins and Kirschner wires may be applied as crossed pins to secure juxtaarticular segments in animals with high fracture-assessment scores. (Modified from Johnson AL, Dunning D: *Atlas of orthopedic surgical procedures of the dog and cat*, ed 1, St Louis, 2005, Saunders.)

 BOX 31-11

Key Concepts in Applying Intramedullary Pins

Select a pin sized 60%–70% of the medullary canal width to pair with cerclage wire.
Select a pin sized 50%–60% of the medullary canal width to pair with an external fixator.
Select a pin sized 40%–50% of the medullary canal width to pair with a plate.
Span the length of the bone with the IM pin.
Use retrograde or normograde pin insertion in the humerus and femur.
Use normograde pin insertion in the tibia.
Check pin location with reference pin and by manipulating the joint.
Always use additional fixation to control rotation and axial loading.

The pins should exit sufficiently that the trocar tips are clear of the cortices, but should not be so long as to interfere with soft tissue.

Take care that the pins cross within the metaphyseal segment and not at the fracture. Check the fracture stability and pin position. With small diameter pins, bend the pin end and cut off the excess. With larger diameter pins, which resist bending, simply cut the excess pin.

Postoperative Care

Postoperative analgesia should be provided (see p. 944). Postoperative radiographs are made to evaluate implant location. Activity should be restricted to leash walking and physical rehabilitation until the fracture has healed. Physical rehabilitation encourages controlled limb use and optimal limb function after fracture healing (see Chapter 12). Radiographs should generally be repeated at 6-week intervals. The functional period of a Steinmann pin or Kirschner wire is short because of its reliance on frictional hold. IM pins supported with an external fixator or a plate have a longer functional period. Clients may become concerned about subcutaneous fluid swelling surrounding the pin end: this is a seroma caused by irritation of the pin moving in soft tissue. IM pins should be removed once bone union has occurred; if a seroma is present, it will resolve after pin removal. If the pin is easily palpable, then removal may be done with sedation and local anesthetic. If the pin is buried within soft tissue, then the patient must be anesthetized and taken to the operating room. Current radiographs are necessary for the surgeon to pinpoint the exact location of the pin. Kirschner wires and crossed pins are generally not removed unless they cause a problem.

To remove a pin, sedate or anesthetize the patient and clip and aseptically prepare the skin surface overlying the end of the pin. Instill a local anesthetic (if the patient is sedated) and make a small skin incision over the palpable end of the pin. Bluntly dissect soft tissue from the pin, grasp it with a pin remover, and extract it from the bone. Place a suture(s) in the skin wound.

INTERLOCKING NAILS
Indications and Biomechanical Properties

Interlocking nails are inserted in the medullary canal and locked in place with screws or cross-locking bolts placed through the proximal and distal fracture segments and the nail (Fig. 31-59). Interlocking nails resist all the forces acting on fractures. The nail provides bending support, whereas the locking bone screws or bolts provide axial and rotational support. Interlocking nails may be used effectively in animals with high and medium fracture-assessment scores.

The interlocking nail is used primarily for middiaphyseal humeral, femoral, or tibial fractures; it is contraindicated for the radius. The nails come in various sizes and lengths (see p. 986) and have holes in each end for screw insertion. The nails are indicated for both simple and comminuted middiaphyseal fractures. Ideally, normal cortex should be sufficient proximal and distal to the fracture to allow insertion of two screws in each segment, although this is not always possible in the humerus. Screws should be placed at least 2 cm from the fracture line to prevent excessive forces on the nail. Interlocking nails are weakest at the screw hole. Fatigue failure at the screw hole occurs when an inadequate-sized nail is used or when the nail hole is adjacent to the fracture line. Screws placed in the nail hole do not decrease the likelihood of nail failure if the nail is inappropriately placed. As newer nails were developed with smaller nail holes to protect the integrity of the nail, the subsequently smaller screws occasionally failed. Newly

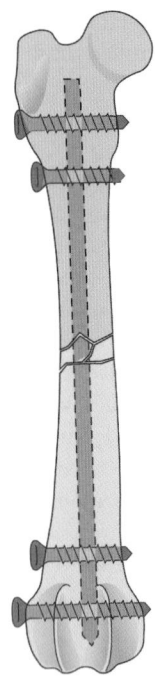

FIG. 31-59
Interlocking nail. The interlocking screws provide additional rotational and axial support.

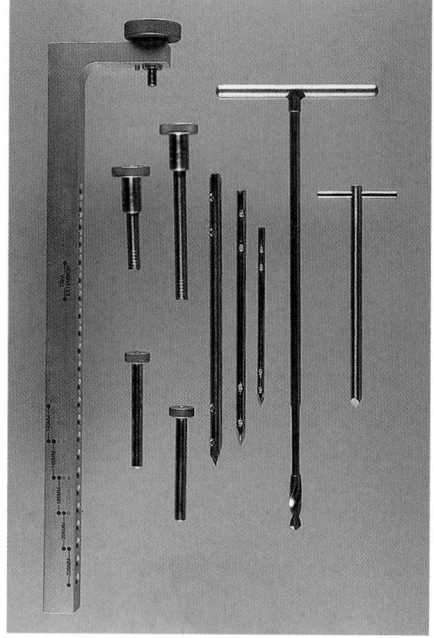

FIG. 31-60
Equipment used for interlocking nail fixation includes *(left to right)* drill-guide jig, drill guides, extension pieces, nails, reamer, and trocar.

developed locking bolts minimize the occurrence of locking screw failure.

Equipment and Supplies

Interlocking nails available for veterinary use are 4.0, 4.7, 6.0, 8.0, and 10.0 mm in diameter, with five or six lengths available in each size. Each nail has three or four screw holes (up to two in each end), and they may be 11 or 22 mm apart. The distal end may be a trocar or blunt point, and the proximal end has an internally threaded hole and two alignment tabs, to which an extension piece can be attached. An insertion tool is attached to the extension piece to insert the nail in a normograde direction. A drill-guide jig is then attached to the extension piece and used to align the drill bit with the holes in the nail (Fig. 31-60). The appropriate-sized cortex bone screws or locking bolts are needed for each size nail. The cross-locking bolts are solid bolts with self-tapping positive profile threads below the head of the bolt. The solid intersection provides greater resistance to failure. The bolts are cut to appropriate length before application.

Application

Select the largest nail that will fit into the bone. Be sure the nail is long enough to span the normal length of the fractured bone. Prepare the marrow cavity for nail placement by inserting a series of progressively larger Steinmann pins or a hand reamer, removing mainly medullary contents and metaphyseal cancellous bone. Attach the appropriate extension and the insertion tool to insert the appropriate-length nail. Remove the insertion tool, attach the drill-guide jig to the extension, and secure it in place. Drill a hole in the proximal fragment through the near cortex and the nail hole and exiting the far cortex. Prepare the hole and insert a bone screw to interlock with the nail.

The guide system is mandatory to ensure that the drilled hole intersects the bone at a site where a hole exists in the pin (Fig. 31-61).

Check rotational alignment and axial length before placing the distal screws and the remaining proximal screw (Box 31-12).

> NOTE: Drill the distal hole while maintaining a drill bit in the proximal hole to ensure that the drill-guide jig is aligned with the nail for the entire length of the bone.

When using locking bolts, drill a hole equal to the shaft diameter of the bolt. Measure to determine the bolt length necessary. Cut the bolt approximately 2 mm longer than the measured distance. Gently advance the bolt so the self-tapping threads engage the near cortex.

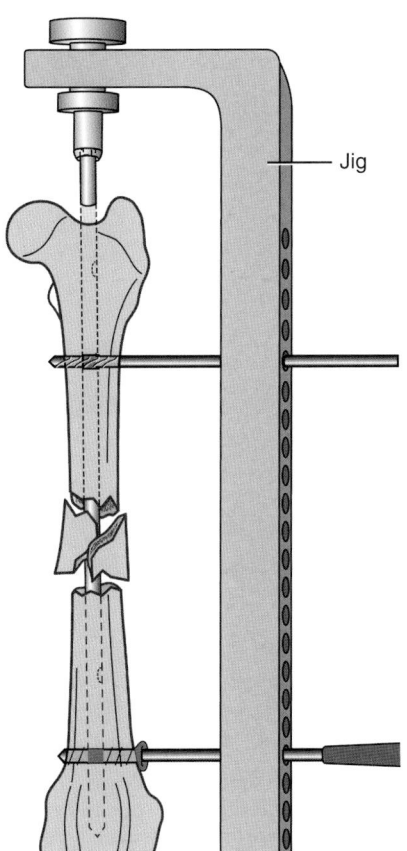

FIG. 31-61
Use of the jig to accurately position locking screws or bolts. (Modified from Johnson AL, Dunning D: *Atlas of orthopedic surgical procedures of the dog and cat,* ed 1, St Louis, 2005, Saunders.)

See pp 1105, 1038, and 1128 for instructions on placement of interlocking nails in the femur, humerus, and tibia, respectively.

Postoperative Care

Postoperative analgesia should be provided (see p. 944). Activity should be restricted to leash walking and physical rehabilitation until the fracture has healed. Physical rehabilitation encourages controlled limb use and optimal limb function after fracture healing (see Chapter 12). Generally, postoperative examinations should be done at 2 and 6 weeks after surgery and then every 6 weeks. The functional period of an interlocking nail is longer than that of a Steinmann pin or Kirschner wire because of the interlocking hold of the screws or bolts with the bone. Most interlocking nails are left in place after bone healing. The recessed end of the nail does not generally impinge on soft tissue. If a nail is removed, the patient must be placed under general anesthetic.

Clip and aseptically prepare the skin surface and make small skin incisions over the interlocking screws. Remove the

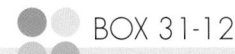 **BOX 31-12**

Key Concepts in Applying Interlocking Nails

Use the largest nail that fits in the bone.
Span the length of the bone with the nail.
Ream the medullary canal with a Steinmann pin or use the reamers.
Insert the nail in a normograde fashion.
Position the nail so the holes are 2 cm away from the fracture.
Secure the nail with four screws or fixation bolts for optimal fixation.

screws and make an incision over the end of the pin. Apply the distraction device and remove the pin.

ORTHOPEDIC WIRE

Orthopedic wire is often referred to as cerclage wire or hemicerclage wire. It is used in combination with other orthopedic implants to supplement axial, rotational, and bending support of fractures. The term *cerclage wire* is used to denote the use of orthopedic wire placed around the circumference of the bone. *Hemicerclage wire* or *interfragmentary wire* is the term used to denote wire that is placed through predrilled holes in the bone (see p. 1018). Cerclage wire can be combined with Kirschner wires to prevent wire slipping in areas where the bone diameter changes or to secure cerclage wires at an oblique angle to the long axis of the bone. Cerclage wire has two distinctions: it is the most commonly used implant and the most commonly misused implant in veterinary orthopedics. Misuse of cerclage wire causes a significant percentage of the postoperative complications seen in veterinary patients.

Indications and Biomechanical Properties

Cerclage wire is used to provide stability to anatomically reconstructed long oblique or spiral fractures (Fig. 31-62). To function as a stabilizer, wire must generate sufficient compression between fracture surfaces to prevent the fragments from moving or collapsing under weight-bearing loads. To accomplish this, three criteria must be met: (1) the length of the fracture line should be two to three times the diameter of the marrow cavity, (2) there should be a maximum of three (preferably only two) fracture fragments, and (3) the fracture must be anatomically reduced. When these criteria are met, cerclage wire can provide additional stability by generating sufficient compression between fragments to hold them in place during healing (Fig. 31-63). Cerclage wire is always supported by additional implants (e.g., IM pins, external fixators, and plates) that control the large weight-bearing (primarily bending) forces (Box 31-13).

If more than two or three fragments are present or if the fracture lines are not of sufficient length, cerclage wire can only be used to hold fragments in position; it cannot gener-

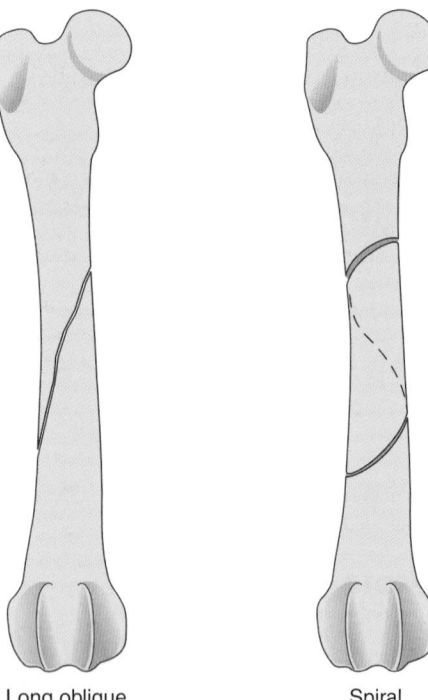

Long oblique   Spiral

FIG. 31-62
Fracture configurations in which cerclage wire is useful for providing mechanical support through interfragmentary compression.

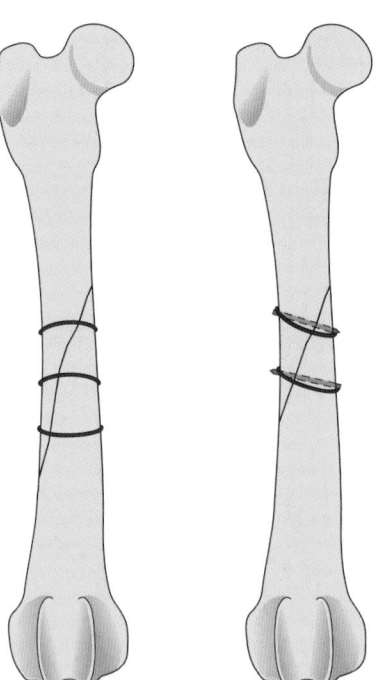

FIG. 31-63
Proper placement of cerclage wire. Wires are placed at least 5 mm from fracture ends and spaced one half to one times the diameter of the bone. Kirschner wires may be used to prevent cerclage wire slippage. (Modified from Johnson AL, Dunning D: *Atlas of orthopedic surgical procedures of the dog and cat,* ed 1, St Louis, 2005, Saunders.)

ate the compression needed to resist weight-bearing loads. The attempt to gain stability with cerclage wire in multifragmented fractures is the most common cause of cerclage wire failure. When multiple fragments are present, movement postoperatively may cause one of the pieces to shift in position, which would allow the entire segment of reconstructed bone to collapse. An analogy to the use of cerclage wire for stabilizing multiple bone fragments is the use of metal rings to hold slats in a wooden barrel. Collapse would occur if one slat (bone fragment) in the barrel were to loosen. When wire is misused, probable outcomes include collapse of the fracture, loss of stability, and wire loosening, which further delay healing.

Some mechanical variation in initial tension is generated by the wire and the resistance to load, depending on the method of tightening (loop versus twist) and the wire pattern (single-wrap versus double-wrap cerclage wires). In general, twist tightening generates less tension in the wire than loop tightening, and double-wrap patterns generate greater compression of the fragments with increased resistance to the load of weight bearing (Roe, 1997). Clinical performance of the two types of wire tightening and the single-wrap and double-wrap patterns appears similar as long as principles of wire application are followed.

Orthopedic wire fixation is generally not recommended for stabilizing short oblique (45 degrees) or transverse fracture lines and is contraindicated in dogs with fracture-

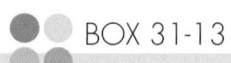 BOX 31-13

Key Concepts in Applying Cerclage Wire

Use only on anatomically reconstructed long oblique or spiral fractures.
Use 18-gauge wire for large dogs and 22-gauge or 20-gauge wire for cats and small dogs.
Place two to three cerclage wires per fracture line.
Place wires perpendicular to the long axis of the bone.
Space wires one half to one bone diameter apart.
Support cerclage wires with an IM pin, interlocking nail, external fixator, or plate.

assessment scores in the moderate to low ranges. Occasionally, wiring techniques are used to supplement IM pins stabilizing short oblique or metaphyseal fractures in animals with very high fracture-assessment scores. Use of a Kirschner wire crossing the fracture line, with a cerclage wire looped around the diaphysis of the bone and resting above and below the Kirschner wire, has been recommended for short oblique fractures, but is inferior to lag screw fixation (Smith et al, 1996).

Equipment and Supplies

Cerclage wire is made from a malleable form of 316L stainless steel. It may be purchased in a spool or as preformed loop wire and is available in sizes ranging from 22 gauge (0.64 mm) to 18 gauge (1.0 mm). The use of 22-gauge or 20-gauge wire is recommended for cats and small dogs, whereas 18-gauge wire is recommended for larger dogs. Hemicerclage wire should be 18-gauge or 20-gauge monofilament 316L stainless steel. A variety of instruments are available to secure the encircling wire to bone. Twist knots may be formed by using pliers or old needle holders. Cerclage wire with a preformed loop at one end is secured with a specially designed wire tightener.

Application

Cerclage wire. *Use a wire passer to place the wire around the bone without extensively reflecting soft tissue. Do not entrap tissue between the wire and periosteum. To prevent slippage and loosening of the wire, place the wires perpendicular to the bone surface. To tighten a wire with a twist knot, pull the wire tight to the bone and form the first three twists by hand. Grasp the twists with the pliers and pull the wire perpendicular to the long axis of the bone. Twist the wire while maintaining the tension. Once the wire is tight, either cut the wire near the third twist and leave it extended, or cut the wire near the fifth or sixth twist and bend it over in the direction of the twist while tightening (Fig. 31-64).*

A fibrous cap will rapidly form over the protruding end of the wire, providing protection from soft tissue irritation.

To tighten a cerclage wire with a preformed loop, pass the free end of the wire around the bone, through the loop, into the nose of the wire tightener and through the hole in the crank. Turn the crank until the wire is secure. Bend the wire tightener over so the free end of the wire folds on itself. Reverse the crank to expose more of the wire and complete the fold. Cut the excess wire, leaving about 0.5 to 1 cm in length and push the wire end to the bone (Fig. 31-65).

The instrument used for tightening the wire is not critical; however, the wire must be tight after securing the knot.

Ascertain the degree of tightness by touch and check it by attempting to move the wire with a pair of needle holders. Replace the wire if it is loose. When all the wires have been placed, recheck the tightness of each wire because loosening of the initial wires may occur with subsequent wire placement.

Cerclage wire used to stabilize shorter oblique fractures or in metaphyseal fractures must be perpendicular to the fracture to achieve compression, but the wire placed in this manner will slip.

To prevent slipping, place a Kirschner wire across the fracture and leave the ends of the Kirschner wire protruding 1 mm

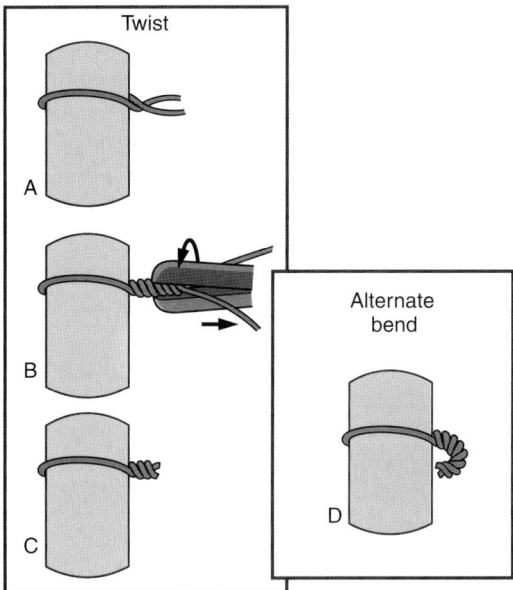

FIG. 31-64
A, For plain orthopedic wire, begin twisting the wire ends by hand. **B,** Place the wire twisting pliers or needle holders onto the twist and tighten the wire by pulling and twisting. **C,** When the wire is tight, cut the wire 3 mm from the start of the twist. **D,** Alternatively, cut the wire 5 to 7 mm from the twist and bend it over in the direction of the twist.

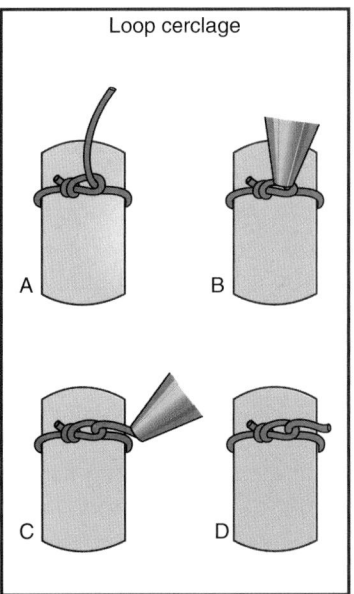

FIG. 31-65
A, For loop cerclage, tighten the wire by passing the plain end of the wire through the eye of the wire. **B,** Insert the wire into the wire tightener and crank the wire tight. **C,** Bend the wire over the eye. Retract the wire tightener and finish bending the wire. **D,** Cut the wire. (Modified from Johnson AL, Dunning D: *Atlas of orthopedic surgical procedures of the dog and cat,* ed 1, St Louis, 2005, Saunders.)

beyond the bone surface at both the near and far cortex. Place the cerclage wire around the bone such that the loop rests above the Kirschner pin at the far cortex and below the Kirschner pin at the near cortex (see Fig. 31-63). Alternatively, make a small notch in the bone surface with the point of a pin or small file. Place the wire loop within the notch to prevent slippage.

For a description of placing interfragmentary wires see application of wire to mandibular fractures on page 1018.

Postoperative Care

Postoperative analgesia should be provided (see p. 944). Wire used for fractures does not require special considerations postoperatively. Wire is generally not removed once the fracture has healed, unless it causes problems.

TENSION BANDS
Indications and Biomechanical Properties

Tension is the predominant force when avulsion fractures occur at a point where groups of muscles originate or insert in bone (e.g., greater trochanter, olecranon, and supraglenoid tuberosity of scapulae). Contraction of the muscle group at these sites generates tension that pulls the bony insertion or origin from its anatomic location. The most effective way to resist tension is through application of a tension band (Fig. 31-66). The purpose of a tension band is to convert distractive tensile forces into compressive forces.

Equipment and Supplies

Equipment needed for placement of a tension band includes small Steinmann pins or Kirschner wires and orthopedic wire. A high-speed wire driver is preferred for placing the Kirschner wires. The orthopedic wire is secured with a wire tightener (see previous discussion).

Application

When using pins and wire to apply a tension band, reduce the fracture first, then place two small pins or Kirschner wires across the fracture to maintain reduction. Place the pins perpendicular to the fracture line and parallel to each other. Try to seat the pins in the opposite cortex. Drill a small hole through the bone below the fracture at approximately the same distance present between the fracture and the insertion point of the pins. Locate the hole so the wire will rest on the bone's tension surface when tightened. In the femur, for example, drill the hole from cranial to caudal so that the wire will rest on the lateral, or tension, surface of the femur. Pass the wire through the drill hole and around the two small pins used to stabilize the fracture. Twist the ends to form a figure eight. The twist portion of the wire should be on top of the flat portion of the wire. Wind the twist knot to tighten the arms of the tension band. As the wire is tightened, tension is created that opposes that generated by muscle contraction. Bend the exposed ends of the Kirschner wires 90 degrees and turn the ends into the tendon (Box 31-14).

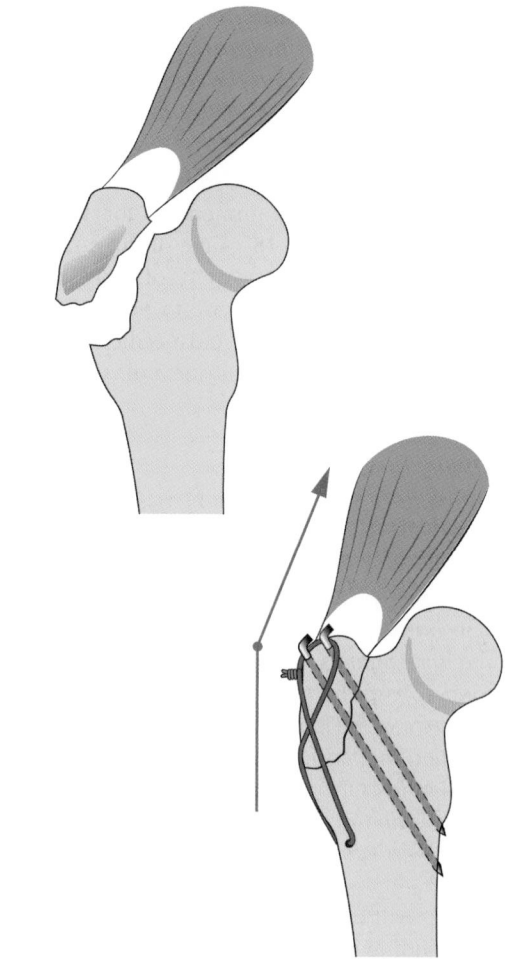

FIG. 31-66
Placement and mechanical principle of a tension band. Tightening the wire exerts a force that counters the force of muscle contraction and compresses the fracture surface.

 BOX 31-14

Key Concepts in Applying Tension Band Wires

Use two Kirschner wires or small Steinmann pins.
Place wires parallel to each other and perpendicular to the fracture.
Seat the wires in the opposite cortex.
Place the hole for the orthopedic wire the same distance below the fracture as the pins are inserted above the fracture.
Tighten the wire so it is in direct contact with the bone.

Postoperative Care

Postoperative analgesia should be provided (see p. 944). Special postoperative care is not required for tension bands. If the ends of the pins irritate soft tissue, the pins should be removed. Otherwise, tension bands are not removed once the fracture has healed.

BONE PLATES AND SCREWS

Stabilization of fractures with bone plates and screws is a popular method of fracture fixation. Modern plating technology began in the early 1960s when a group of Swiss surgeons formed an association for the study of fracture treatment in humans. This group, the Swiss Arbeitsgemeinschaft fur Osteosynthesefragen (AO), is referred to as the Association for the Study of Internal Fixation (ASIF) in the United States. The AO and/or ASIF developed and continues to develop recommendations for application of orthopedic devices, which have led to increased success and fewer complications associated with fracture management. In the 1970s an arm of the AO group, the AO-Vet, was established to document and address problems specifically associated with fracture management in animals. From this group's work, specialized instrumentation and bone plates were designed to treat animal injuries. To achieve consistent and predictable results with bone plating, a thorough understanding of the principles and techniques of application is essential. Although several companies are marketing varied designs of equipment, the AO-ASIF system is used to describe the principles of application in this text.

Indications and Biomechanical Properties

Bone plates and screws offer a versatile method of fracture stabilization and can stabilize any long bone fracture. They are often used for fractures of the axial skeleton and are imperative for fractures involving joint surfaces. Bone plates and screws are particularly useful when postoperative comfort and early limb use are desired (e.g., fractures involving joint surfaces and patients with fracture disease). Bone plates and screws are used to treat animals with high, medium, and low fracture-assessment scores, but are particularly useful for animals with low fracture-assessment scores.

Screws used as lag screws cause compression at the fracture, increasing the friction between fragments and resisting the forces acting on the fracture. Two or more screws must be used to counteract bending forces in the diaphysis, but are not sufficient to withstand the large loads generated by weight bearing without plate support. Screws may be used to reconstruct articular fractures without plate support in some cases. Screw resistance to bending load is determined by core diameter and increases by raising the radius to the fourth power. Screw-holding power increases in a linear relationship with increasing diameter of the threads.

Bone plates effectively resist the axial loading, bending, and torsional forces acting on fractured bones. Plates are susceptible to repeated bending stresses because of the plate's eccentric location in relationship to the long axis of the bone. Implant fatigue failure occurs when the opposite cortex is not reconstructed and fails to bridge with bone early enough to protect the plate. Plate holes concentrate stress, and failure generally occurs in this area. Increasing the plate size, using a broad lengthening plate, or using a plate-pin combination may strengthen the implant or reduce the stain sufficiently to reduce risk of fatigue failure.

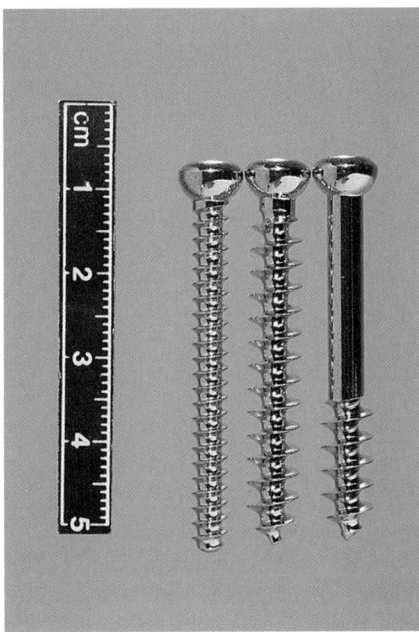

FIG. 31-67
Types of bone screws. *Left to right,* Cortical, fully threaded cancellous, partially threaded cancellous.

Locking screw plate systems, or internal fixators, have some mechanical advantages over conventional plate systems. The locking mechanism between the plate and the screw provides the stability; hence, frictional forces between the plate and bone are unnecessary. Additionally, the locking screw is not creating undue stress in the bone because it is in a neutral position. The result is an increase of the construct yield strength with the locking screws.

Equipment and Supplies

Bone plating sets are available that contain the instrumentation necessary to apply the implants. Drill guides and sleeves, taps, depth gauge, and screwdriver are used to insert screws. Bending and torquing irons are used to contour or shape the plates.

Cortical and cancellous bone screws are made of 316L stainless steel or titanium and may or may not be self-tapping. A non–self-tapping screw requires that threads be cut into bone with a tap; a self-tapping screw has a cutting tip to cut threads into bone and flutes to accept bone debris. Controversy surrounds which of these screws is best, but currently the most commonly used ASIF screws are non–self-tapping. Cortical screws are fully threaded and designed for use in compact cortical bone. The *pitch* (number of threads per inch) of the screw is greater than that of a cancellous screw (Fig. 31-67). This allows a greater number of threads to engage the matrix of the relatively narrow-diameter cortical bone. Cancellous screws are either completely or partially threaded and are used primarily in the epiphysis or metaphysis. The *thread height* (difference between the core diameter and outer screw diameter) of cancellous screws is greater than the thread height of cortical screws, which allows deep purchase into the soft, spongy epiphyseal or metaphyseal bone. Cortical and cancellous screws are named for the outside diameter; in 3.5-mm cortical screws, for example, the outer screw diameter is 3.5 mm. Cancellous and cortical screws are available in sizes ranging from 1.5 to 6.5 mm. *Locking head screws* are designed with threaded heads that screw or lock into specially designed plates with threaded plate holes, such as the locking compression plate. Locking head screws may be self-drilling and self-tapping and may be used monocortically or bicortically.

Bone screws are used either to anchor bone plates to bone or to hold bone fragments in place. When used to anchor a bone plate to bone, these screws are called *plate screws*. The screws used to hold bone fragments in anatomic position and prevent them from collapsing into the marrow cavity are called *position screws*. Position screws can be inserted through a plate hole or placed in bone independent of the plate. *Lag screws* (also termed *compression screws*) are used to apply compression between fragments.

Whether a screw is used as a plate screw, a position screw, or a lag screw, appropriate instrumentation must be used to implant the screw correctly. Specific drill guides are used for neutral and eccentric placement of plate screws and placement of screws independent of a bone plate. Each different screw size has a drill bit corresponding to the inner core diameter (shaft) of the screw, a drill bit corresponding to the outer diameter of the screw, and a tap corresponding to the threads of the screw. The manufacturer (ASIF) provides a chart to assist in choosing the appropriate instrumentation for each screw size. Additional instrumentation includes a depth gauge to measure the length of screw desired and a countersink to cut a circular groove in the cortex to accept the head of the screw. The countersink is used when a lag screw is inserted into the cortex independent of the bone plate.

ASIF bone plates are made of 316L stainless steel or titanium; however, because titanium plates and screws are more expensive than stainless steel plates, the latter are used more often. Bone plates are designated in several different ways, including plate length, screw size that the plate hole will accept, plate and screw hole configuration, and function. *Plate length* is designated by the number of plate holes. Each of the different plate sizes is available in a wide range of lengths. The 3.5 broad plates range in length from 4 to 22 holes and the 2.7 plates from 4 to 12 holes. *Plate size* is determined by the cortical screw that the plate holes will accept; in a 3.5 broad plate, for example, the plate holes will accept 3.5-mm cortical bone screws. Similarly, 2.7 bone plates accept 2.7-mm cortical bone screws, and 4.5 bone plates accept 4.5-mm bone screws (Fig. 31-68).

Plate hole configuration is also used to designate the type of plate. A plate hole can be round (e.g., veterinary cuttable plate) or oblong (e.g., dynamic compression plate). A bone plate with oblong holes is referred to as a *dynamic compression plate* (DCP) because compression can be applied to the bone through the dynamic action of the screw being tight-

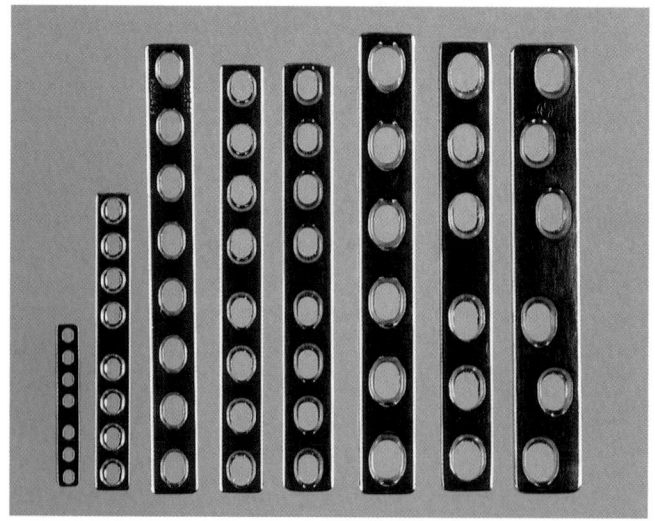

FIG. 31-68
Types of bone plates. *Left to right*, 2.0 DCP, 2.7 DCP, 3.5 LC-DCP, 3.5 narrow DCP, 3.5 broad DCP, 4.5 LC-DCP, 4.5 narrow DCP, and 4.5 broad DCP.

ened. The configuration of the oblong hole is based on a spherical gliding principle modeled after a ball rolling down an inclined plane. The conical shape of the screw head is representative of the ball, and the oblong plate hole is representative of the inclined plane. With the plate hole being inclined, the screw head will slide toward the center of the oblong hole as the screw is tightened. When the screw slides toward the center of the plate hole, horizontal movement of bone beneath the plate occurs. If this is done on each side of the fracture line, the bone is pushed together from both sides, resulting in compression at the fracture line. Proper screw placement is ensured by using drill guides that center the drill hole in either a loading or neutral position. In the loading position, approximately 1 mm of compression is achieved for each screw tightened, whereas in the neutral position approximately 0.1 mm of compression is achieved. The spherical gliding principle is implemented on both ends of each plate hole in the *limited-contact dynamic compression plate* (LC-DCP). Locking plates have threaded holes that accept and lock with the locking head screw. The *locking compression plate* (LCP) has a combination plate hole that can accept either conventional screws or locking head screws (Fig. 31-69).

In addition to plate hole design, *bone plate configuration* is also used to designate the plate type. The 3.5 and 4.5 bone plates are available as standard plates and broad plates. The broad plates are wider, which gives them increased strength and stiffness, an important feature when bone plates are used in large-breed and giant-breed dogs. Both titanium and stainless steel plates are designed as LC-DCPs. They are manufactured so that there is limited contact between the plate and bone to minimize interruption

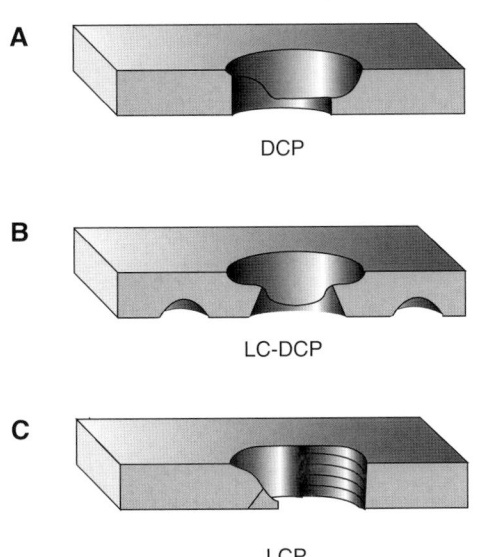

FIG. 31-69
A, Cross sections of plate hole in **A,** DCP, **B,** LC-DCP, and
C, LCP. (Modified from Fossum TW: *Small animal surgery,*
ed 2, St Louis, 2002, Mosby.)

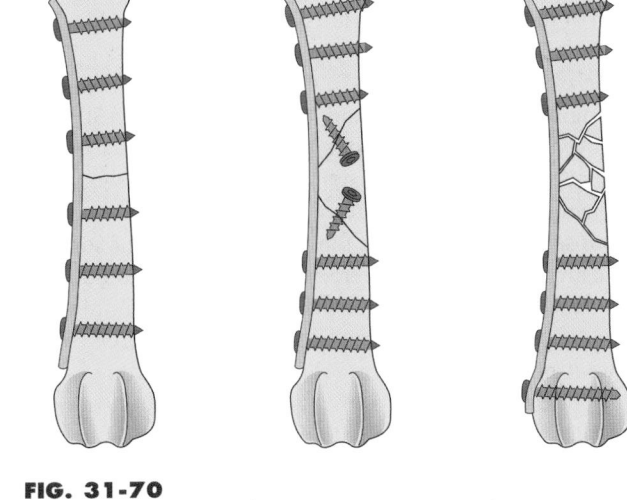

FIG. 31-70
Functions of a bone plate. **A,** Compression plate.
B, Neutralization plate. **C,** Buttress plate.

of blood flow. This is accomplished by undercutting the bottom surface of the plate between the screw holes. Undercutting the screw holes also evenly distributes the stress on the plate, eliminating the effect of the plate hole as a stress concentrator. The screw holes are based on the dynamic compression principle, but differ in that the oblong screw hole is inclined from both ends of the screw hole toward the center, allowing compression to be applied in either direction. Special drill guides are required. The undercutting also allows greater angulation (up to 40 degrees) of plate screws. Specialized bone plates (e.g., reconstruction plates, angled plates, and condylar screw plates) are available for selected orthopedic conditions.

Other plates useful in small animals include the reconstruction plate, veterinary cuttable plate, canine acetabular plate, and canine distal radial plate. These plates are advantageous for specific injuries. *Reconstruction plates* have deep indentations in the sides of the plate between plate holes. These plates may be contoured in three planes, making them especially useful for treating fractures of bones with complex 3-D geometry, such as the pelvis, the distal humerus and femur, or the mandible. *Veterinary cuttable plates* (VCPs) are available in two sizes, designated by the size screw that the plate hole will accept. The 2.0/2.7 VCP can be used with either a 2.0-mm or 2.7-mm cortical screw, whereas the 1.5/2.0 VCP can be used with either a 2.0-mm or a 1.5-mm cortical screw. The VCP is popular because it is available in varying lengths up to 50 screw holes (300 mm). The plate can be cut so that it has the desired number of holes. VCPs are often used in a stacked configuration to bridge comminuted fractures in smaller patients. Stacking two plates onto each other increases the strength and stiffness of the fixation compared

with using a single plate. The *canine acetabular plate* is manufactured to conform to the dorsolateral surface of the canine acetabulum and is available in two sizes. This plate is particularly useful in large and giant breeds because it is strong and stiff. The *canine distal radial plate* is made for distal radial and ulnar fractures in small breeds. Typically, this fracture has a very short distal segment, which makes it difficult to place an adequate number of plate screws. The canine distal radial plate has a T configuration, with the horizontal bar conforming to the epiphysis and/or metaphysis of the distal radius. The shape and size of the plate allow adequate plate screws to be placed in the short metaphyseal segment.

Although bone plates are designated as to their intended function (compression, neutralization, and bridging or buttress), depending on how they are applied to the bone, it is important to realize that the plate configuration (DCP plate, VCP, and broad plate) does not change. A 3.5 broad DCP may serve as a compression plate, neutralization plate, or buttress plate, depending on how it is applied to the bone (Fig. 31-70). A bone plate serves as a *compression plate* when compression is applied to the fracture line through proper application of the plate and screws. A DCP may only function as a compression plate if the fracture line is transverse or short oblique (no greater than 45 degrees). If the fracture line is greater than 45 degrees or is comminuted, the plate cannot be used to compress the fracture lines. A *neutralization plate* neutralizes physiologic forces acting on a section of bone that has been anatomically reconstructed and stabilized with screws and wire. Indications for a neutralization plate include reducible comminuted fractures and oblique fractures in which the fracture line exceeds 45 degrees. A *bridging plate* spans a fragmented section of bone and a *buttress plate* holds a collapsed epiphysis in position. The most common application of a bridging plate is with fragmented diaphyseal fractures in which surgical reduction and stabilization of the bone fragments are not technically feasible (i.e., nonreducible fractures).

The plate size (2.0, 2.7, 3.5, or 4.5) necessary varies depending on patient weight and bone dimensions. ASIF and AO have developed charts that can be used to select a suitable plate relative to body weight. The plate length should be sufficient to prevent premature loosening of plate screws and subsequent loosening of the plate from the bone surface. In most cases of diaphyseal fractures, the plate should span the bone length for optimal performance. The minimum length of plate should allow purchase of six cortices (three screws if both cortices are purchased by each screw) in the main bone fragment above the fracture and six cortices in the main fragment below the fracture. This number of screws will ensure adequate distribution of stress among the plate screws. However, the minimum of six cortices on each side of the fracture is often exceeded to ensure that the plate spans the diaphyseal length.

The surface on which the plate is located influences the degree of stability obtained. In general, all long bones are subject to bending forces because physiologic loads are applied eccentrically to the bone center. When a bone is subject to this type of loading, a bend will occur that causes compression on the concave surface of the bone and tension on the convex surface. This tension must be prevented because it will cause a fracture line to pull apart. This is accomplished by laying the plate on the tension surface and thereby allowing the plate to absorb the tensile stress that would separate the fracture.

Application

Screws. A precise order of maneuvers is followed when inserting a plate screw, position screw, or lag screw.

When inserting a plate screw in the diaphysis, drill a thread hole through the near (cis) and far (trans) cortices. Use the neutral drill guide to place the screw in the center of the plate hole. Use the load or eccentric drill guide with the arrow pointed toward the fracture line to place the screw eccentrically initially and cause compression at the fracture line when the screw is tightened (see compression plate application on p. 996). To insert a 3.5-mm plate screw, use a drill bit that corresponds to the inner core diameter (shaft) of the screw (2.5 mm) and a tap that corresponds to the outer thread diameter of the screw (3.5 mm). Determine the length of screw needed with the depth gauge placed through the plate hole and cut threads into the near and far cortices with a tap. Use a tap sleeve when cutting threads to maintain axial alignment relative to the thread hole and to prevent soft tissue from winding around the tap threads. Remove the tap, and flush the hole with sterile saline to eliminate bone debris and lubricate the hole. Insert a cortical screw and use fingers only on the screwdriver to tighten it (Fig. 31-71.) In spongy metaphyseal or epiphyseal bone, use a cancellous bone screw as a plate screw and place in a similar manner.

A lag screw functions to compress a fracture line between two bony fragments. It may be inserted through a plate hole or directly into bone, independent of the bone plate. The optimal position of a lag screw is perpendicular to the fracture line. On shorter oblique fractures, the lag screw is positioned to bisect the angle formed between a line perpendicu-

BOX 31-15

Key Concepts in Applying Lag Screws

Reduce and secure the fracture before placing the lag screw.
For optimal compression, place the screw perpendicular to the fracture.
Drill the near cortex with a bit equal to the screw thread diameter.
Drill the far cortex with a bit equal to the screw core diameter.
When using a partially threaded screw, be sure the threads do not cross the fracture.

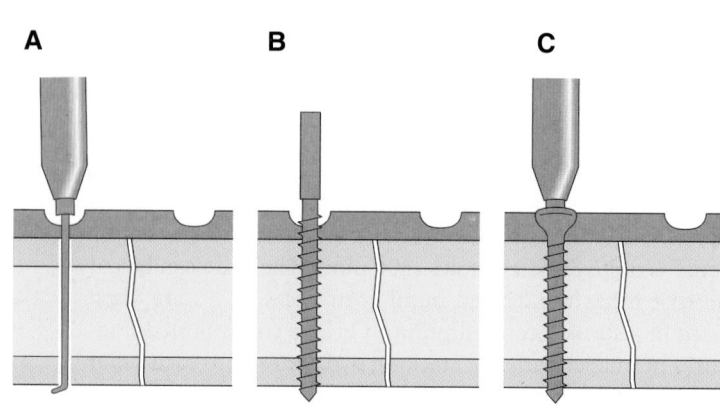

FIG. 31-71
To place a plate screw, drill the thread hole, then **A,** measure the screw length; **B,** tap threads in the near (cis) cortex and far (trans) cortex; and **C,** insert the screw.

lar to the fracture surface and one perpendicular to the long axis of the bone to prevent slipping of the fragments. The drill hole in the near cortex must be a *glide hole* (a hole equal in diameter to the outside diameter or thread diameter of the screw), whereas the drill hole in the far cortex must be a *thread hole* (a hole equal in diameter to the inner core diameter or shaft of the screw) (Box 31-15).

To insert a lag screw, use a drill bit that corresponds to the outer diameter of the screw or thread diameter to create a glide hole through which the screw will pass without purchasing bone. When creating the glide hole, drill the bone using a drill guide to maintain alignment and protect soft tissue. Insert a drill sleeve into the glide hole in preparation for creating the thread hole in the far cortex (the drill sleeve insert centers the thread hole in the far cortex relative to the glide hole, which prevents stripping the thread hole on screw insertion). After the glide hole and thread hole are made, use a countersink to prepare a site for the screw head in the cortex, and use a depth gauge to determine the appropriate-length screw to use. Tap the thread hole through a tap sleeve to maintain alignment and protect soft tissue. Insert the appropriate-length screw and tighten it with the fingers only on the screwdriver (Fig. 31-72).

The threads of the screw will glide through the hole in the near cortex (glide hole) and purchase the bone in the far cortex (thread hole). As the screw is tightened, the screw head contacts the near cortex. As the threads purchase the far cortex, the fracture line is compressed. A lag screw can be placed through a plate hole by following the same procedure. Because the screw head rests against the bone plate, however, it is not necessary to countersink the near cortex. Fully threaded cancellous screws can also be inserted as lag screws, either through the plate or independent of the plate, by following the same procedures. The only difference in placement is the instrumentation needed to match the screw size.

Partially threaded bone screws can also be used as lag screws.

With partially threaded screws, drill the near and far cortices as thread holes (Fig. 31-73). Use a depth gauge to

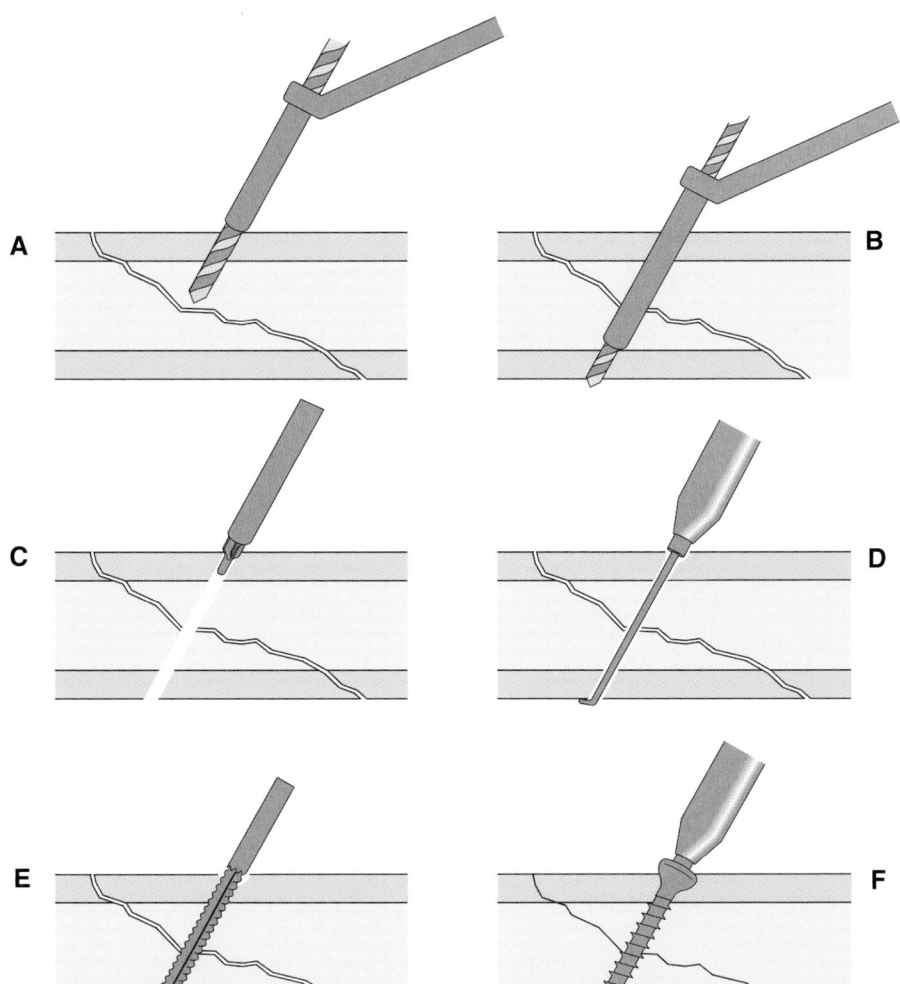

FIG. 31-72
A, To insert a cortex screw with lag function, drill a glide hole in the near bone segment with a drill bit that has the diameter of the outside screw thread. Use the drill guide to protect soft tissue and align the drill bit. **B,** Place an insert sleeve through the glide hole until the far bone segment is engaged. Drill a thread hole with a drill bit the same diameter as the core of the screw. The drill sleeve keeps the thread hole centered relative to the glide hole. **C,** Use a countersink to cut a bevel in the cortical bone at the entrance of the glide hole. This increases the contact area between the bone and screw and decreases the amount of the screw head exposed. This step is not needed if the lag screw is placed through a plate hole. **D,** Determine the length of screw to be inserted with a depth gauge. **E,** Use a tap to cut threads for the screw in the far bone segment. This step is unnecessary if self-tapping screws are used. **F,** Insert the screw and tighten it to create interfragmentary compression.

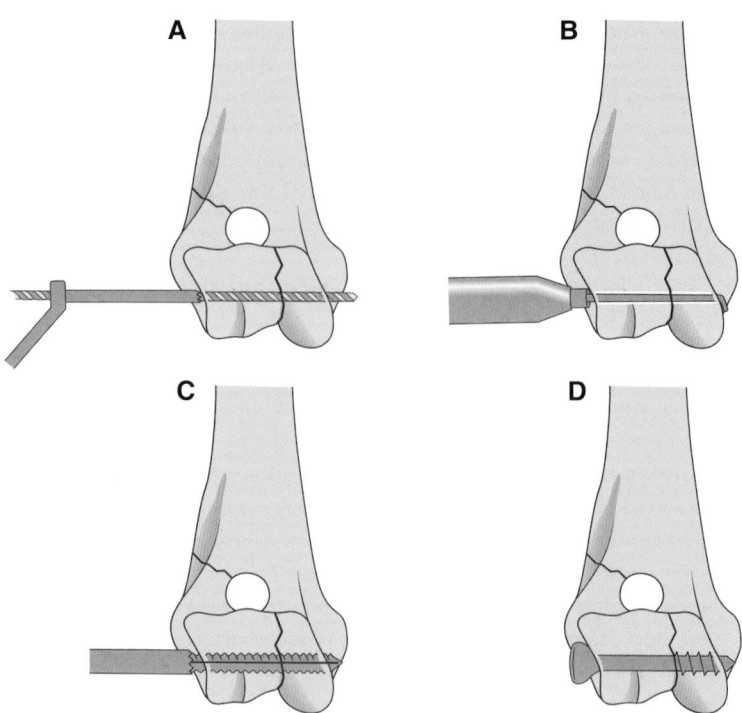

FIG. 31-73
A, To insert a partially threaded cancellous bone screw, drill the near and far cortices as threaded holes. **B,** Measure the depth of the hole. **C,** Tap the holes. **D,** Insert the screw to compress the fracture. For compression to occur, the threads must not be present at the fracture line. Note that the screw threads have crossed past the fracture line and that the smooth shaft of the screw lies within the fracture plane.

determine the appropriate-length screw and tap both cortices before inserting the screw.

Because the screw is only partially threaded, there are no threads to engage the bone on the near side of the fracture, and bone is purchased only in the far cortex. As the screw head contacts bone and the screw tightens, compression is achieved. It is critical that the smooth shaft of the screw crosses the fracture line; if threads are present at the fracture line, compression cannot be achieved.

> Warning: The 4.0-mm partially threaded cancellous screw is weaker than the 3.5-mm cortex screw when placed across the humeral condyle and may fail when used to treat dogs with incomplete ossification of the humeral condyle, which is slow to heal.

Either a cortical screw or a fully threaded cancellous screw can function as a position screw. A position screw is used to hold two bone fragments in anatomic alignment when compression would cause one fragment to collapse into the marrow cavity.

Hold the fragments in position with bone-holding forceps and drill a thread hole through the cortex of each fragment with a drill bit corresponding to the inner core diameter (shaft) of the screw. Use a depth gauge to determine the appropriate-length screw and cut threads in both cortices with the appropriate tap. Insert the screw, using bone-holding forceps to hold the

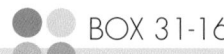 BOX 31-16

Key Concepts in Applying Bone Plates

Select the appropriate plate size.
Select a plate that spans the bone length for diaphyseal fractures.
Accurately contour the plate.
Place a minimum of three screws or secure six cortices above and below the fracture.
Use a longer and stronger plate as a bridging plate or augment it with an IM pin.

fragments in position and prevent distraction at the fracture line. Gently tighten the screws ("finger tight") until the screw head rests adjacent to the near cortex (or bone plate).

The screw holds the fragments in position while the bone-holding forceps is removed.

Plates (Box 31-16)

Compression plates. The compression plate is used to generate axial compression at the fracture. To achieve this function, it is important to contour the plate properly relative to the bone surface.

To apply a plate as a compression plate, contour it so that the plate remains slightly offset (1 to 2 mm) from the surface

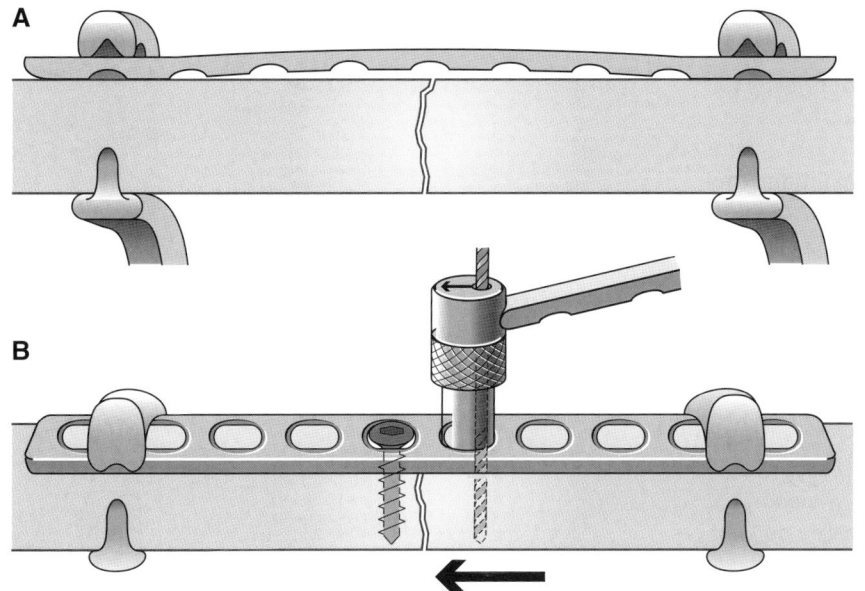

FIG. 31-74
To apply a DCP as a compression plate, prestress the plate by slightly overbending it at the fracture site during contouring. **A,** This creates a 1-mm to 2-mm gap between the plate and bone over the fracture. Secure the plate to the bone. **B,** Use the eccentric drill guide to locate a screw eccentrically through a plate hole over the unattached segment of bone. (**B,** Modified from Johnson AL, Dunning D: *Atlas of orthopedic surgical procedures of the dog and cat,*
ed 1, St Louis, 2005, Saunders.)

of the bone at the fracture line (Fig. 31-74). Secure the plate to the bone with plate-holding forceps, ensuring that the ends of the plate lie over the bone.

If the plate is contoured to conform accurately to the bone surface, asymmetric loading of the fracture line will occur. This occurs because the compression generated through the plate is applied to the bone eccentrically (it is greatest on the surface on which the plate rests). The net result is compression of the fracture line beneath the plate and widening of the fracture near the far cortex. Because a gap exists in the far cortex, the plate supports all the applied loads without any significant contribution from the bony column. The gap in the far cortex is prevented through prestressing the bone plate by overcontouring it relative to the bone surface so the center of the plate is lifted 1 to 2 mm above the bone surface. When the plate screws on each side of the fracture line are tightened, each main bone fragment is pulled up against the plate, compressing the far cortex.

Insert the two plate screws nearest the fracture first. Place both screws in a loaded position and tighten them to achieve compression of the fracture line.

Similar compression can be achieved by placing the first two screws in any of the plate holes as long as there is one screw on either side of the fracture.

Insert subsequent plate screws in holes in an alternating manner on either side of the fracture, working toward the plate ends. Adequate compression of the fracture is generally achieved with loading of the first two screws.

> NOTE: If you desire greater compression, place an additional screw on each side of the fracture in the loaded position (insert the remaining screws in a neutral position).

Neutralization plates. *First, reduce and stabilize the fracture with a series of lag screws, multiple cerclage wires, or a combination of both. Because the screws and wires are not sufficiently strong to resist physiologic forces generated by weight bearing, use a bone plate to bridge the area and to neutralize forces that would act to collapse the fracture. As with a compression plate, apply a neutralization plate to the tension surface of the bone, but contour it to the anatomic surface of the bone. Separation of the fracture line beneath the plate will not occur because the fracture lines have already been compressed with lag screws or cerclage wire (see Fig. 31-70).*

The neutralization plate protects the reconstructed bone from all torsional, bending, and shearing forces. The recommended number of cortices (six) engaged on each side of the fracture is the same as for a compression plate.

With a neutralization plate, insert all screws in the neutral position, beginning from the ends of the plate and working toward the center. If a plate screw cannot be inserted because it lies over a fracture line, leave the hole empty. If the plate hole lies over a lag screw placed through the bone, leave the hole empty, or insert a screw that purchases only the near cortex.

Bridging plates. *Precontour the plate to match the normal anatomic shape of the bone. Use a radiograph of the* *intact bone of the opposite leg as a template to help contour the plate if the affected bone is severely comminuted. Align the bone to restore length and correct rotational orientation before securing the plate (see Fig. 31-70).*

The bridging plate serves as a splint to maintain the spatial alignment of the bone during healing. All the applied loads will be carried by the plate and screws during the early postoperative period. This results in greater stress on the bone screws than with compression or neutralization plates, in which the applied loads are shared with the bone.

Therefore purchase a minimum of eight cortices rather than six. Similarly, use a stronger and stiffer plate because it also will be subject to substantial loads until bone is deposited within the fracture gap to form a bony column. For optimal strength and stiffness, use a broad plate, lengthening plate, or stacked VCP rather than a standard plate. Alternately, support the plate with ancillary implants (IM pins or external skeletal fixators) that share the applied loads during the early healing period. With a plate–IM pin combination, insert an IM pin approximately 50% of the diameter of the marrow cavity, being careful to maintain the rotational alignment and axial length of the bone. Contour a plate of appropriate length and apply it to the appropriate surface of the bone. Insert the most proximal and distal plate screws so that they avoid the IM pin and engage both near and far cortices. Insert the plate screws near the center of the plate so that they engage only the near cortex (monocortical screws) (Fig. 31-75).

Buttress Plates. *Apply a buttress plate to shore up a metaphyseal fracture or protect a screw repair of an intraarticular slab fracture.*

The buttress plate functions to prevent collapse of the adjacent articular surface.

To prevent any slipping of the plate and collapse of the articular surface, insert the screws in the juxtaarticular portion of the plate by first placing the drill guide adjacent to the part of the plate hole nearest the fracture. Butting the screw head to that portion of the plate during the initial screw insertion prevents sliding of the plate.

Postoperative Care

Bone plates and screws require minimal postoperative maintenance. Postoperative analgesia should be provided (see p. 944). Activity should be restricted to leash walking and physical rehabilitation until the fracture has healed. Physical rehabilitation encourages controlled limb use and optimal limb function after fracture healing (see Chapter 12). Generally, postoperative examinations should be done at 2 and 6 weeks after surgery and then every 6 weeks. The functional period of plates and screws is relatively long because of the

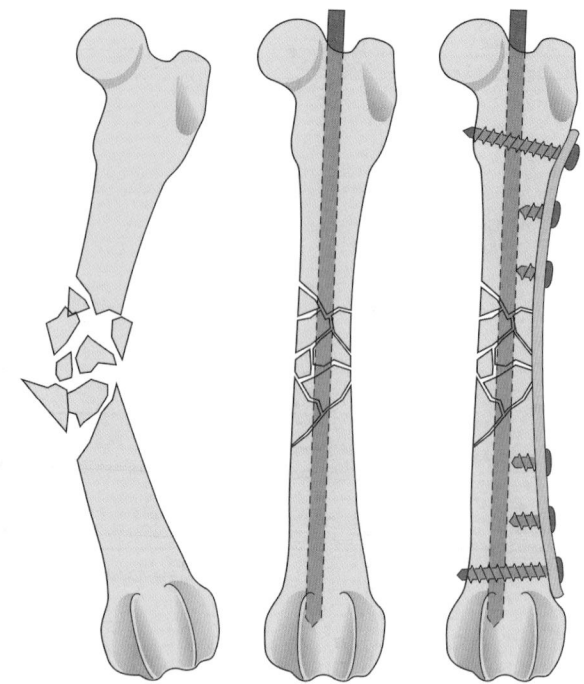

FIG. 31-75
Stabilization of a comminuted fracture with a plate-rod combination.

interlocking hold of the screws with the bone. Most interfragmentary screws are left in place after bone healing. If plates are removed, removal should be delayed until at least 3 to 4 months after radiographic bone union. When bone plates are applied to long bone fractures in younger patients, they should be removed. Removal is also recommended when plates have been applied in areas with limited soft tissue covering, such as the radius and tibia, because cold conduction may cause discomfort. Plate removal should be performed aseptically with the patient under general anesthetic.

Incise the skin overlying the plate screws and bluntly dissect through soft tissue to the head of the screw. Once all plate screws are removed, lift the plate from the bone surface at one end and extract it.

References

Lewis DD et al: Initial clinical experience with the IMEX circular external skeletal fixation system. Part II. Use in bone lengthening and correction of angular and rotational deformities, *Vet Comp Orthop Traumatol* 12:118, 1999.

Metelman LA et al: A mechanical evaluation of the resistance of various interfragmentary wire configurations to torsion, *Vet Surg* 25:213, 1996.

Roe SC: Mechanical characteristics and comparisons of cerclage wires: introduction of the double wrap and loop/twist tying methods, *Vet Surg* 26:310, 1997.

Smith BA et al: Mechanical comparison of two methods for interfragmentary fixation in a short oblique fracture model, *Vet Comp Orthop Traumatol* 9:145, 1996.

Stallings JT et al: An introduction to distraction osteogenesis and the principles of the Ilizarov method, *Vet Comp Orthop Traumatol* 11:59, 1998.

Suggested Reading

Anderson GM, Lewis DD, Radash RM et al: Circular external skeletal fixation stabilization of antebrachial and crural fractures in 25 dogs, *J Am Anim Hosp Assoc* 39:479, 2003.

This article provides a review of a series of fractures stabilized with circular external fixators. Surgical technique and fracture outcome are described.

Aper RL, Litsky AS, Roe SC et al: Effect of bone diameter and eccentric loading on fatigue life of cortical screws used with interlocking nails, *Am J Vet Res* 64:569, 2003.

This article provides results of investigative studies into the issues associated with screw failure in interlocking nail fracture fixation. The effects of bone diameter and eccentric loading on fatigue life of 2.7-mm-diameter cortical bone screws used for locking a 6-mm-diameter interlocking nail are described.

Cross AR, Lewis DD, Murphy ST et al: Effects of ring diameter and wire tension on the axial biomechanics of four-ring circular external fixator constructs, *Am J Vet Res* 62:1025, 2001.

This article provides results of mechanical studies investigating the effects of ring size and wire tension on the axial micromotion provided by a circular fixator.

Dueland RT et al: Interlocking nail treatment of diaphyseal long-bone fractures in dogs, *J Am Vet Med Assoc* 214:59, 1999.

This study provides the results of a large multicenter prospective study of the efficacy of interlocking nail for stabilizing diaphyseal fractures.

Emmerson TD, Muir P: Bone plate removal in dogs and cats, *Vet Comp Orthop Traumatol* 12:74, 1999.

This article provides a review of a series of 255 consecutive bone plate removals. Reasons for plate removal include instability, soft tissue irritation, infection, and chronic lameness.

Farese JP, Lewis DD, Cross AR et al: Use of IMEX SK-circular external fixator hybrid constructs for fracture stabilization in dogs and cats, *J Am Anim Hosp Assoc* 38:279, 2002.

This article provides a description of the use of SK-circular hybrids to stabilize long bone fractures (two femoral, one humeral, and three tibial fractures) with short distal bone segments in three dogs and three cats. Although three cases required surgical revision, animals ambulated well, and all fractures obtained union.

Horstman CL, Beale BS, Conzemius MG et al: Biological osteosynthesis versus traditional anatomic reconstruction of 20 long-bone fractures using an interlocking nail: 1994-2001, *Vet Surg* 33:232, 2004.

This article provides the results of a comparative clinical study designed to observe the differences in surgical and healing times and complication rates in dogs with a comminuted long bone fracture stabilized with an interlocking nail using either anatomic or biologic repair. Biologic osteosynthesis provided clinical advantages over anatomic reconstruction with respect to a reduction in surgical and healing time without increasing complication rates.

Koch D: Screws and plates, In Johnson AL, Houlton JEF, Vannini R, editors: *AO principles of fracture management in the dog and cat*, Thieme, NY, 2005, AO Publishing, pp 27-50.

This chapter provides a current and comprehensive overview of the types and the functions of bone plates and screws used in fracture stabilization in small animals.

Langley-Hobbs SJ, Abercromby RH, Pead MJ: Comparison and assessment of casting materials for use in small animals, *Vet Rec* 139:258, 1996.

This study provides the results of an investigation evaluating the properties and uses of the different casting materials available for small animals.

Marcellin-Little DJ, Ferretti A, Roe SC et al: Hinged Ilizarov external fixation for correction of antebrachial deformities, *Vet Surg* 27:231, 1998.

This article provides information on preoperative planning, surgical technique, and clinical outcome when hinged circular external fixation was used for correction of antebrachial deformities in six dogs. Despite complex preoperative planning, the placement of hinged circular external fixators was straightforward and allowed precise correction of complex antebrachial deformities with minimal tissue trauma.

Reems MR, Beale BS, Hulse DA: Use of a plate-rod construct and principles of biological osteosynthesis for repair of diaphyseal fractures in dogs and cats: 47 cases (1994-2001), *J Am Vet Med Assoc* 223:330, 2003.

This article provides a report of the application of the plate rod for technique stabilizing humeral, femoral, and tibial fractures. Clinical application and outcomes are discussed.

Roe SC: Evaluation of tension obtained by use of three knots for tying cerclage wires by surgeons of various abilities and experience, *J Am Vet Med Assoc* 220:334, 2002.

This paper provides results from an investigation into the compressive effects of three knots used to secure cerclage wire and the individual surgeon's ability to achieve compression with the cerclage wires. Cerclage applied with a twist knot did not compress fracture fragments as effectively as cerclage applied with single loop or double loop techniques. Experience and abilities of the surgeon were not associated with ability to tie cerclage wires tightly.

Roe SC: External fixators, pins, nails, and wires. In AO principles of fracture management in the dog and cat, Johnson AL, Houlton JEF and Vannini R editors, Thieme, NY, AO Publishing, p 53-70, 2005.

This chapter provides a current and comprehensive overview of external fixators, IM pins, interlocking nails, and orthopedic wire as used in fracture stabilization in small animals.

Tommasini-Degna M, Ehrhart N, Feretti A et al: Bone transport osteogenesis for limb salvage following resection of primary bone tumors: experience with 6 cases (1991-1996), *Vet Comp Orthop Traumatol* 13:18, 2000.

This article provides a description of the techniques and outcomes of using the circular fixator for bone transport after resection of a primary bone tumor.

BONE HEALING

Fracture healing is the biologic process after cartilage and bone disruption that restores tissue continuity necessary for function. The goals of fracture treatment are to (1) encourage healing, (2) restore function to affected bone and surrounding soft tissue, and (3) obtain a cosmetically acceptable appearance. Each goal should be kept in mind when selecting treatment regimens and fixation devices (see sections on decision making and fixation systems). Fracture healing varies depending on biologic factors (e.g., fracture location in cortical bone, cancellous bone, or physeal cartilage; cellular responses; circulation; and concurrent soft tissue injury) and mechanical factors (e.g., stability of bone segments and fragments after fixation device placement) that influence the sequence of cellular events in fracture healing.

All physiologic processes occurring within bone, including repair processes during fracture healing, are dependent on an adequate blood supply. Normal circulation to long bones consists of an afferent supply from the principal nutrient artery, proximal and distal metaphyseal arteries, and periosteal arteries that enter bone at areas of heavy fascial attachment. The direction of blood flow through the diaphysis is centrifugal, from medullary canal to periosteum. Under normal conditions, medullary pressure probably restricts periosteal blood flow to the outer third of the cortex (Fig. 31-76, *A*). In contrast to mature animals, immature animals have numerous arteries that perforate newly formed appositional bone running longitudinally over the periosteal surface. The metaphysis and epiphysis have separate blood supplies and generally do not communicate across the cartilaginous physis (Fig. 31-76, *B*). The epiphyseal blood supply nourishes the cartilaginous reserve cell zone and growing physeal cells. Interruption of this portion of the circulation results in death of growing cells and cessation of physeal function. Metaphyseal arteries supply cells involved with endochondral ossification; disruption of metaphyseal blood flow delays endochondral ossification, resulting in widening of the cartilaginous physis. When circulation is reestablished, endochondral ossification resumes. Flat bones with extensive muscle attachment (e.g., pelvis and scapula) have tremendous extraosseous blood supply in addition to that provided by nutrient arteries. Irregular bones (e.g., carpal and tarsal bones) generally have multiple nutrient arteries.

Medullary circulation is disrupted in most long bone fractures. Initially, existing components of the normal vasculature (i.e., metaphyseal vessels) are enhanced to supply the injured area. Additionally a transient extraosseous vascular supply develops in soft tissue and surrounding fractures to nourish the early periosteal callus (Fig. 31-76, *C*). As bone healing progresses and stability is restored, medullary blood supply is reestablished. Ultimately the extraosseous circulation diminishes, and normal medullary centrifugal flow dominates (Fig. 31-76, *D*). Closed fracture reduction with application of casts or external fixators causes the least disruption to surrounding soft tissue and newly formed extraosseous blood supply (Fig. 31-77, *A* and *B*), whereas open reduction disturbs developing extraosseous blood vessels and hinders reestablishment of medullary blood flow. Traumatic handling of surrounding soft tissue further impairs the extraosseous circulatory response. Insertion of any type of IM pin disrupts the medullary vasculature; pins that contact endosteal surfaces block medullary afferent flow. Stable implants allow new medullary circulation to develop, which supplies the adjacent endosteal surfaces (Fig. 31-77, *C*). Cerclage wire applied tightly to cortical surfaces does not significantly impair vasculature. Even in immature animals, circumferential wires seemingly do not significantly block periosteal blood flow. Although plate and screw application affords the greatest fracture stability and allows early reformation of medullary circulation, blood supply to outer cortical bone beneath plates may be impaired, causing affected cortices to remodel and become more porous. Newer plate designs (e.g., LC-DCPs) minimize this phenomenon (Fig. 31-77, *D*). Because adequate blood supply is essential for bone healing, any circulatory impairment may delay healing. The motion of loose implants, especially cerclage wires, disrupts developing vasculature; excessive fracture motion discourages reestablishment of medullary vasculature. Excessive medullary reaming interferes with circulation of the inner cortex, resulting in intense bone remodeling. Large bone fragments denuded of soft tissue (and thus blood supply) can be used to reconstruct fractures anatomically; however, these fragments must be rigidly immobilized to encourage early revascularization. It is preferable with multiple fracture fragments if the fracture is minimally disturbed and major bone segments are stabilized with a plate or external fixator. This "biologic treatment" consists of indirect reduction techniques to preserve the surrounding soft tissue and optimal stabilization to promote rapid callus formation. In these cases the fragments revascularize rapidly and incorporate into callus.

Immediately after fracture, an inflammatory phase of bone healing is initiated. The hematoma appears to signal molecules that have the capacity to initiate the inflammatory cascades of cellular responses critical to fracture healing. Inflammatory cells secreting cytokines, such as interleukin-1 and interleukin-6, may be important in regulating the early events in fracture healing. Platelets are likely to be the first source of platelet-derived growth factor (PDGF) and transforming growth factor-β1 (TGF-β1), both of which are important regulators of cell proliferation and differentiation. Inflammatory mediators, such as prostaglandins E1 and E2, may stimulate angiogenesis and may also be responsible for signaling early bone resorption by osteoclasts and proliferation of osteoprogenitor cells. Biologic techniques for fracture stabilization emphasize minimal manipulation of the fracture environment to preserve these inflammatory mediators.

The pathway of bone healing appears to be primarily influenced by the amount of interfragmentary movement caused by the load on the fracture and modulated by the stability of the fracture fixation. The pathways of bone formation include *endochondral* bone formation (bone formed

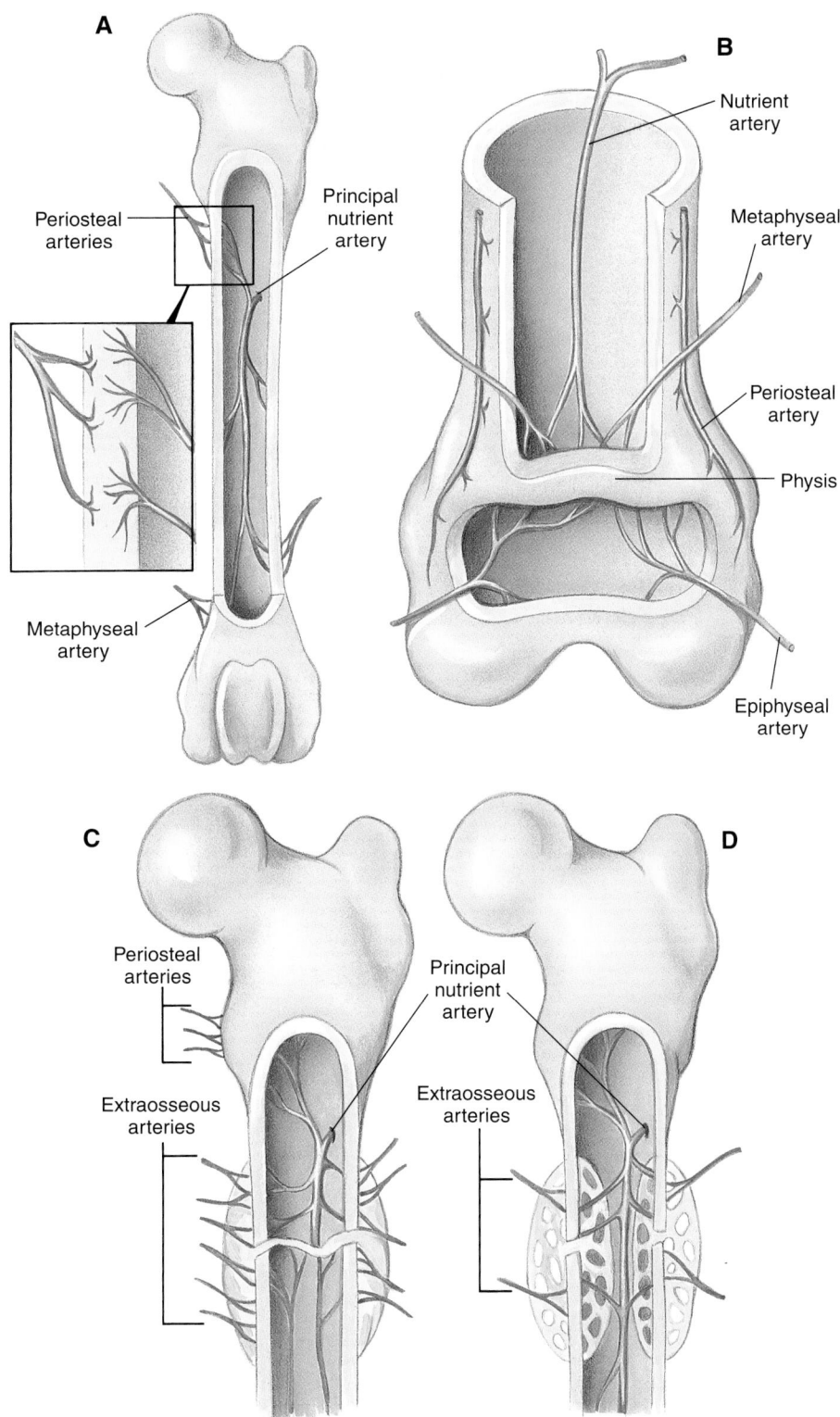

FIG. 31-76
Blood supply to **A,** normal bone; **B,** immature bone; **C,** fractured bone (extraosseous blood supply); and **D,** healing bone.

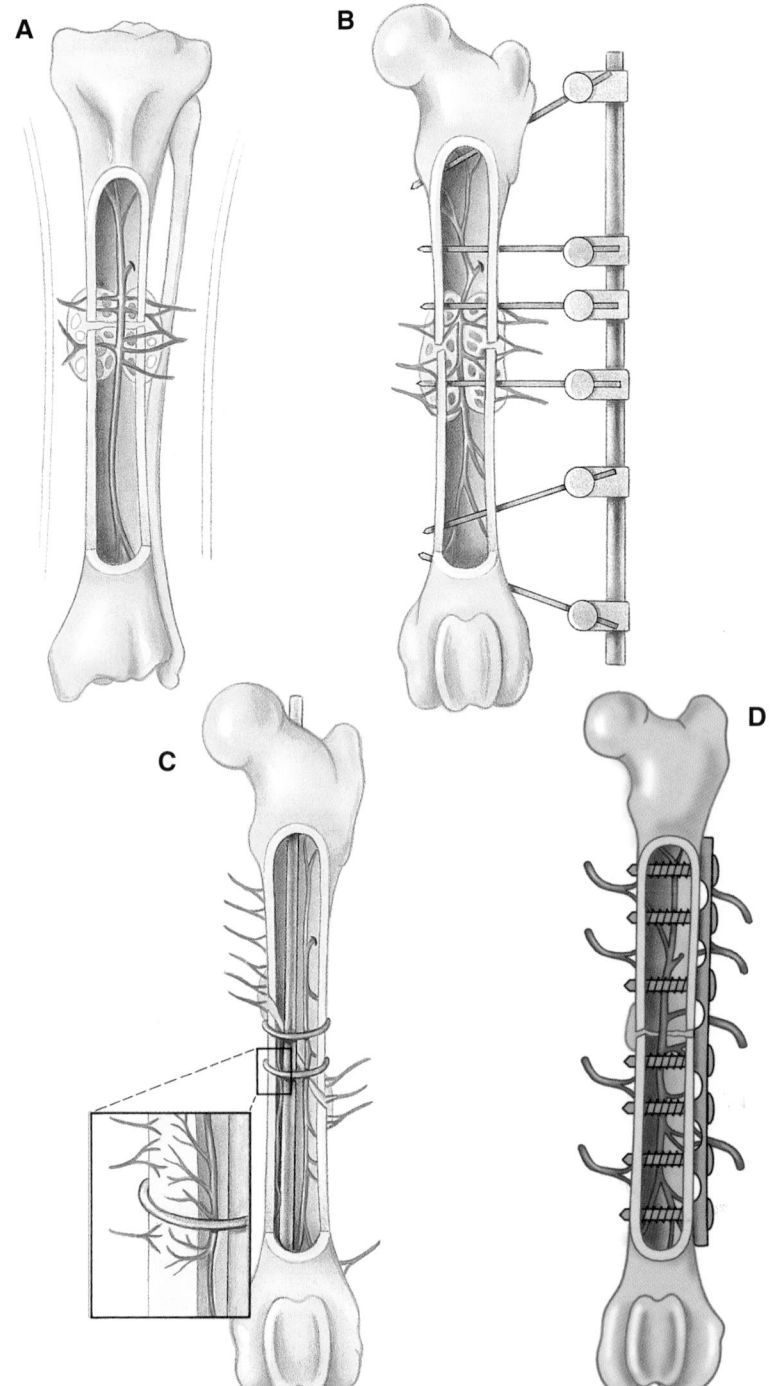

FIG. 31-77
Effect of fixation devices on circulation to fractured bone: **A,** cast; **B,** external fixator; **C,** IM pin and cerclage wires; **D,** plate and screws. Note that closed fracture reduction and application of casts or external fixators cause the least disruption to surrounding soft tissue and newly formed extraosseous blood supply. (Modified from Fossum TW: *Small animal surgery,* ed 2, St Louis, 2002, Mosby.)

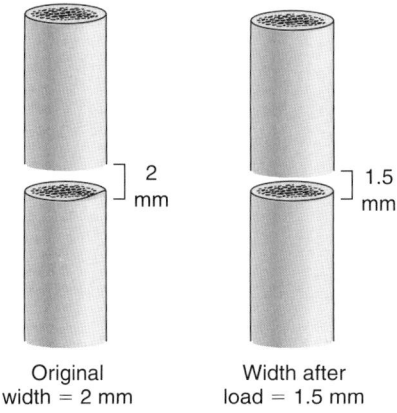

$$\text{Strain} = \cfrac{\text{Change in gap width (.5 mm)}}{\text{Original width (2 mm)}} = 25\%$$

FIG. 31-78
Ratio between the change in gap width to total gap width is called *strain.*

on a cartilaginous precursor), *direct bone union* (bone formed without evidence of callus, depends on the mechanical environment at the fracture), or *intramembranous bone formation* (direct differentiation of mesenchymal stem cells into osteoblasts so bone forms without a cartilaginous precursor).

Indirect bone healing is characterized by the formation of fibrous connective tissue and cartilage callus at the fracture site. This form of healing occurs in the unstable mechanical environment caused by motion of the bone segments. The amount of motion can range from the extremes of unrestricted motion of untreated fractures through the increasing levels of stability achieved with casts, IM pins, external fixators, interlocking nails, and bone plates. In general, as the motion at the fracture decreases, the amount of callus formation also decreases.

Motion at fracture sites affects the size of gaps between fragments. This motion is calculated as *strain,* which is the ratio between change in gap width to total gap width (Fig. 31-78). A given tissue will not proliferate under strain conditions that exceed that tissue's limits of deformation. Sequential formation of stiffer tissue in the fracture gap is a biologic method of decreasing the motion and subsequently the strain. Hematoma and granulation tissues have a high strain tolerance and can survive in an initially mobile fracture site with strains up to 100%. As the fracture site is infiltrated by these tissues, there is less motion, and consequently less strain in the gap. Also, resorption of bone occurs in excessive strain environments and results in widening of the fracture gap that in turn decreases the strain environment at the fracture site. The granulation tissue is gradually replaced by fibrous connective tissue and fibrocartilage that survive in

strains of 20% and 10%, respectively, and in turn continue to stabilize the fracture site. As the fracture stabilizes, mineralization of the cartilage begins at the fragment surfaces and continues toward the center of the gap. Local resorption of the mineralized tissue occurs followed by vascularization of the resorption cavity and the formation of lamellar bone within that cavity. Trabecular or cancellous bone is formed at the fracture site in this manner. Strain values of up to 10% may be tolerated by the three-dimensional configuration of woven bone. Formation of a wide cuff of periosteal callus increases the diameter of the bone at the fracture site. The stabilizing influence of a callus is a factor of its radius to the fourth power, thereby greatly increasing the ability of the bone to resist bending and torsional forces early in the fracture repair process. Formation and resorption of lamellar bone, which tolerates strain values up to 2%, result in remodeling of the callus to cortical bone (Fig. 31-79) (Rahn, 2002).

Direct bone healing (bone formation directly at fracture sites, without an intermediate cartilage stage or visible callus) occurs when fixation devices maintain absolute fragment stability. For this to occur, the mechanical environment must be such that fracture motion is negligible and the fragments are in contact or separated by only small (150- to 300-μm) gaps. Direct bone formation occurring in small gaps in the fracture line after rigid fixation is called *gap healing.* Initially, these gaps are filled with a network of fibrous bone, but within 7 to 8 weeks, this mechanically weak bone union begins to remodel (Fig. 31-80, *A*). The longitudinal reconstruction of fracture sites with haversian remodeling is the second stage of gap healing and provides a strong union between fracture fragments (Fig. 31-80, *B*). *Haversian remodeling* begins with osteoclastic resorption of bone and formation of resorption cavities that penetrate longitudinally through fragment ends and newly formed bone in fracture gaps. The osteoclasts are followed by vascular loops, mesenchymal cells, and osteoblast precursors. Osteoblasts line resorption cavities and secrete osteoid, which is mineralized to bone. This lamellar bone is arranged along the bone's long axis, through the fragment ends and fracture gaps, and results in a strong union of bone fragments. Where bone fragments are in contact under rigid fixation, there is simultaneous union and reconstruction with haversian remodeling (Fig. 31-80, *C*) (Rahn, 2002).

Intramembranous bone formation, a type of direct bone healing occurring where stability is optimal for direct differentiation of mesenchymal cells into osteoblasts, is possible in an environment of up to 5% strain. This type of bone formation is observed when bone is deposited directly on bone fragments at a distance from the fracture site or when bone bridging between comminuted bone fragments occurs to stabilize fragments after biologic fixation techniques. Intramembranous bone formation is generally combined to a varying extent with indirect bone healing responses. The resultant periosteal callus may be smaller in comminuted fractures stabilized with bridging fixation techniques, with

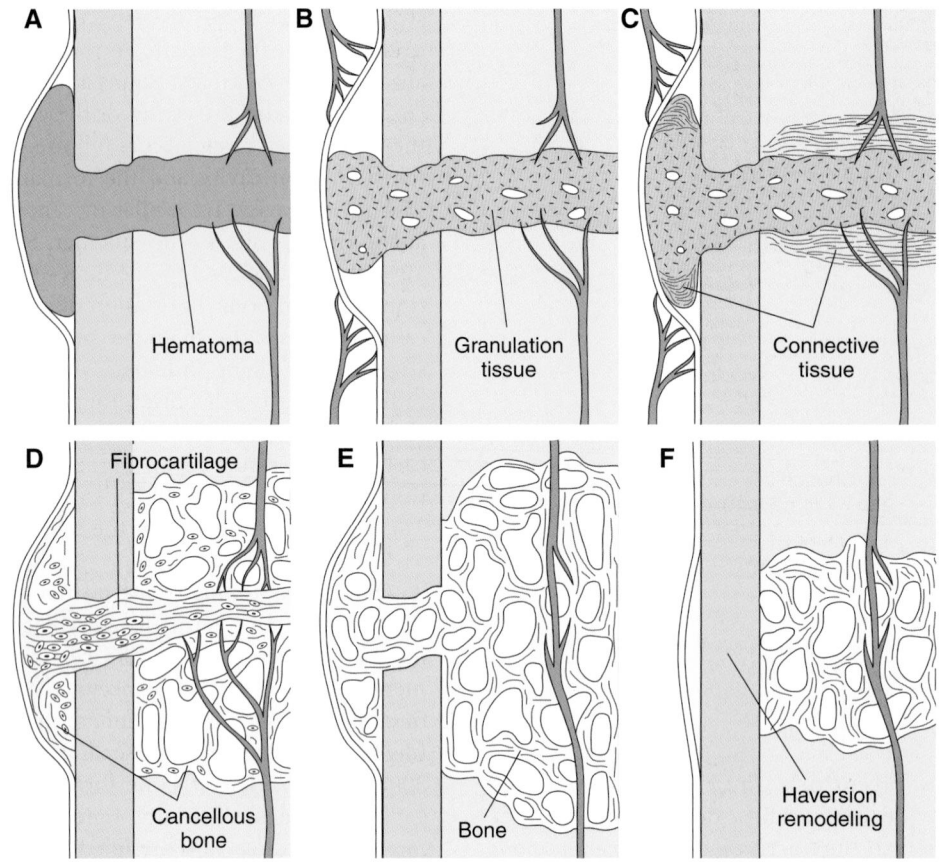

FIG. 31-79
Strain decreases with increased fracture rigidity as fractures are bridged first by more strain-tolerant tissue and later by less strain-tolerant tissue. **A,** Defect is first filled by a hematoma, which is then replaced by **B,** granulation tissue. **C,** Then connective tissue forms. **D,** Fibrocartilage is mineralized, forming cancellous bone and **E,** bone. **F,** Haversian remodeling occurs to eliminate the callus.

the endosteal and bridging callus supplying much of the fracture support. Again, resorption of woven bone and formation of lamellar bone at fracture sites result in remodeling of bony callus to cortical bone.

Distraction osteogenesis occurs when gradual traction is applied to cortical bone such that sufficient stress is created to stimulate and maintain formation of new bone. This concept is used in external fixation techniques for limb lengthening, treatment of angular deformities, and transportation of cortical bone. To achieve bone formation during slow distraction after corticotomy or osteotomy, medullary and periosteal blood supply must be preserved and major bone fragments optimally stabilized. The bone surface is covered with cells that may differentiate into osteoblasts or chondroblasts, depending on the cell's mechanical and biologic environment. Within 3 to 7 days after osteotomy, these cells organize and begin to proliferate. The ideal rate of distraction is 1 mm per day divided into two to four distraction periods. Osteoid is laid down in parallel columns that extend from osteotomy surfaces centrally. Nor-

mally, lamellar bone develops within these columns; if there is sufficient instability at the fracture site, however, formation of an intermediate cartilaginous phase or fibrous tissue formation may occur. After the desired limb length is achieved, the fixator remains in place to allow remodeling of new cortical bone (Fig. 31-81).

Metaphyseal fractures involving trabecular or cancellous bone heal differently than similar fractures through cortical bone (Fig. 31-82, *A*). Trabecular bone is inherently more stable than cortical bone and does not heal by periosteal callus formation unless there is significant instability. Increased osteoblastic activity occurs on either side of these fractures if they have been adequately immobilized (Fig. 31-82, *B*). New bone is deposited on existing trabeculae, and fracture gaps are filled with woven bone. Bridging between trabeculae occurs before union of the cortical shell (Fig. 31-82, *C*).

Physeal fractures generally occur because the physis is weaker than surrounding bone and ligaments (Fig. 31-83, *A*). The mechanically weak portion of the physis is the junc-

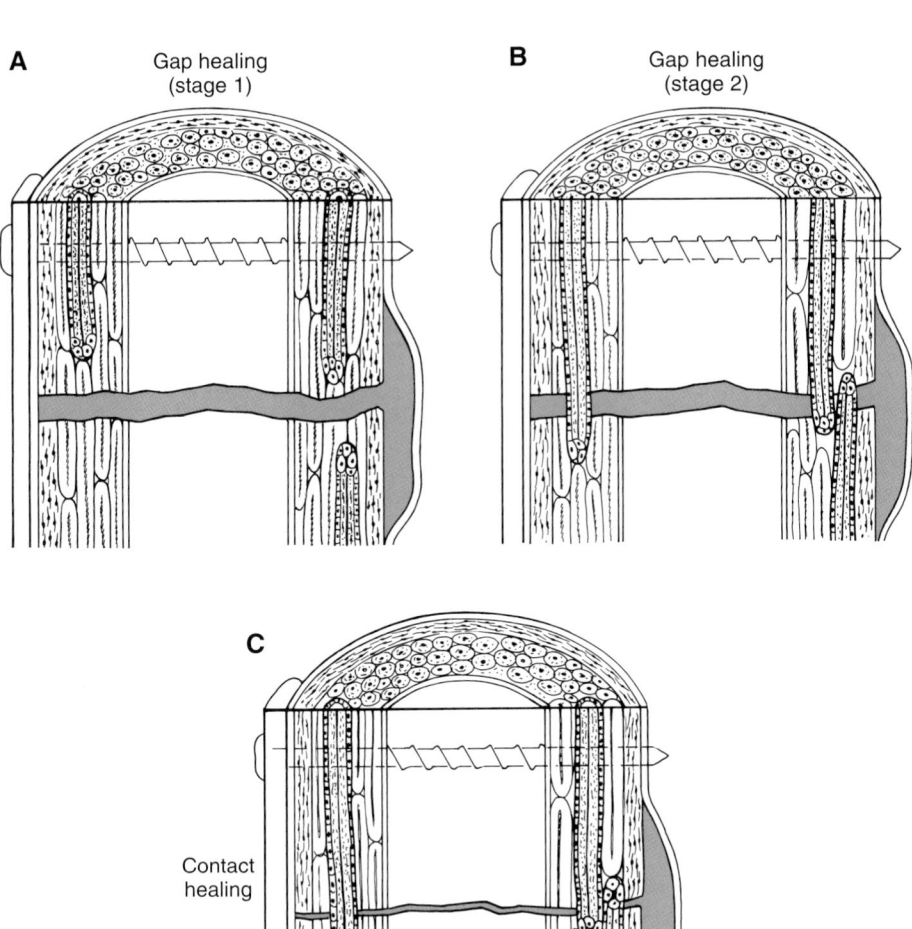

A Gap healing (stage 1)

B Gap healing (stage 2)

C Contact healing

FIG. 31-80
Sequence of events in direct bone healing. **A,** Stage 1: gap filled with fibrous bone (gap healing).**B,** Stage 2: longitudinal reconstruction of bone with haversian remodeling. **C,** Contact bone healing, with bone fragments in contact under rigid fixation; simultaneous union and reconstruction with haversian remodeling.

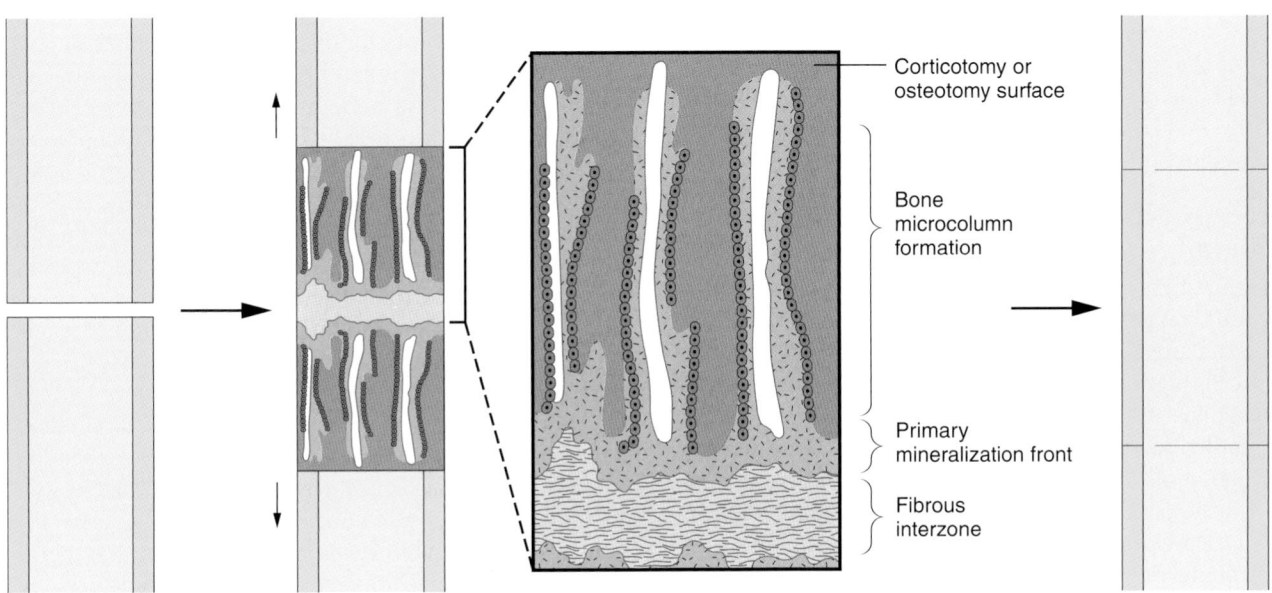

Corticotomy or osteotomy surface

Bone microcolumn formation

Primary mineralization front

Fibrous interzone

FIG. 31-81
During distraction osteogenesis, osteoid is laid down in parallel columns that extend from osteotomy surfaces centrally. Lamellar bone develops within these columns if the fracture is sufficiently stable.

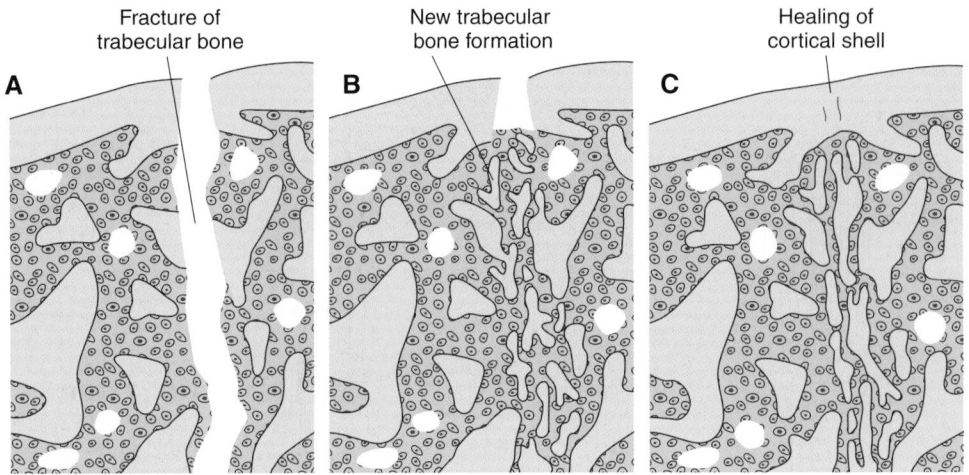

FIG. 31-82
A, Trabecular bone responds to fracture by increasing osteoblastic activity. **B,** New bone is deposited on existing trabeculae, and fracture gaps are filled with woven bone. **C,** Bridging between trabeculae occurs before union of the cortical shell.

tion of the hypertrophic zone where the cells are relatively large in comparison with the amount of matrix and the stronger zone of provisional calcification (Fig. 31-83, *B*). Avulsion or shearing forces can cause fractures through this zone that heal rapidly by continued growth of physeal cartilage and metaphyseal callus formation because the growing cells and adjacent vascularity are undamaged. Once fracture gaps are filled, normal endochondral ossification resumes and physeal function continues. If damage occurs to growing cells (reserve and proliferating zones), however, growth of physeal cartilage does not occur. Rather, endochondral ossification proceeds (Fig. 31-83, *C*), and bone formation in fracture gaps results in premature physeal closure. Malalignment of the fractured physis (where metaphyseal and epiphyseal bone are in contact) allows trabecular bone healing and physeal bridging. The bone bridge may prevent normal physeal function.

Radiographic Evaluation of Fracture Healing

Sequential radiographs allow evaluation of fracture healing. Generally, radiographs should be taken postoperatively to assess fracture alignment and implant position, and they should be repeated every 6 weeks during healing (see Box 31-4). Follow-up radiographs should be compared with earlier studies to determine the dynamics of bone healing. Fractures should be evaluated for evidence of bone formation, and implant position should be appraised to detect instability. Development of periosteal callus indicates that indirect bone formation is occurring (see p. 1003) (Fig. 31-84). Filling of stable fracture lines with bone without callus formation indicates direct bone healing (Fig. 31-85). Trabecular bone healing in metaphyseal fractures appears radiographi-

cally as the formation of one or two dense bands at the fracture site. Gradual bridging of these bands occurs until the cortical shell is completely spanned by bone. Periosteal callus is not usually evident in metaphyseal fractures unless there is instability of fracture fragments (Fig. 31-86). Physeal fractures most often heal with endochondral ossification, which is observed radiographically as filling of the physeal line with bone.

Deciding when to remove fixation devices may be difficult. This decision is usually made after evaluating radiographs of healing fractures. Knowledge of radiographic appearance of bone healing associated with various fixation systems is mandatory for informed decision making. In general, fixation systems can be removed when there is radiographic evidence of bone bridging the fractures. Fractures stabilized with casts heal by indirect bone formation; radiographically this appears as bridging periosteal and endosteal callus at fracture sites (see Fig. 31-84). The large amounts of callus that generally form with this type of fixation serve as an internal support for bone remodeling. An exception to this is with distal radial and ulnar fractures in toy-breed dogs, in which large amounts of callus may not be produced. The cast should be removed once the callus has bridged the fracture.

Bone healing with external fixators may be direct, indirect, or somewhere between these extremes, depending on fracture type, mechanical environment afforded by external fixators, and degree of bone reconstruction. In general, fractures stabilized with external fixators have less periosteal callus formation compared with similar fractures treated with casts. Also, fractures stabilized with external fixators develop more endosteal and bridging callus than periosteal callus. Radiographically, simple fractures that are anatomi-

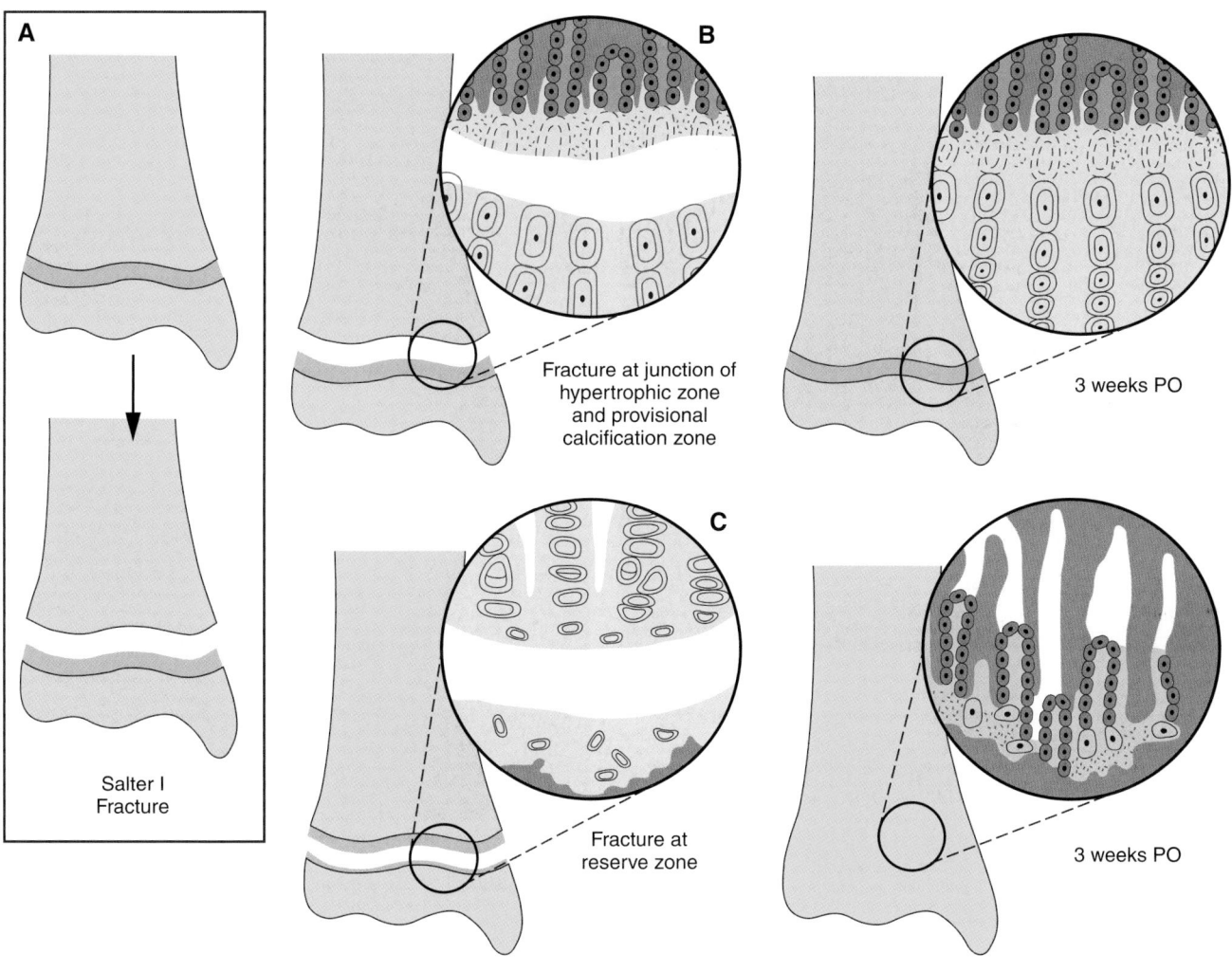

FIG. 31-83
Physeal cartilage healing. **A,** Salter-Harris Type I physeal fracture occurs through the hypertrophied zone of cartilage. **B,** If reduced accurately, these physeal fractures heal by continued formation of cartilage. **C,** If the fracture involves the reserve zone or if the germinal cells are damaged, healing occurs by endochondral ossification.

cally reduced and rigidly stabilized with external fixators (e.g., bilateral external fixators with multiple pins) heal with minimal periosteal or endosteal callus. This is radiographically similar to the direct bone union response observed in fractures treated with plates and screws. As fixator stiffness decreases, increased callus is usually evident. When simple fractures are not anatomically reduced (e.g., with closed reduction) and fixators are not rigid, resorption of bone at fracture lines and callus formation are often evident. This apparently occurs as a normal response of healing bone to high strain when the increased strain is concentrated in a single fracture line.

External fixators may be manipulated to provide optimal mechanical environment for bone formation and remodeling. In general, rigid fixation is recommended for the initial fixator to allow vascularization of the fracture and early bone formation. A window of opportunity appears to exist at about 6 weeks after surgery for destabilization of the external fixator frame to allow an increased load on the healing fracture and stimulate bone formation (Egger, 1993). Destabilization may be achieved by decreasing the planes of fixation, decreasing the strength of the connecting bars, or removing fixation pins (see p. 974). The external fixator is removed entirely when there is radiographic evidence of bone bridging all of the fracture lines.

The type of bone healing observed in comminuted fractures depends on how well the biologic environment is preserved and on the rigidity of the fixation. When anatomic reconstruction and rigid fixation of all fragments are difficult or impossible in severely comminuted fractures, preser-

A   **B**

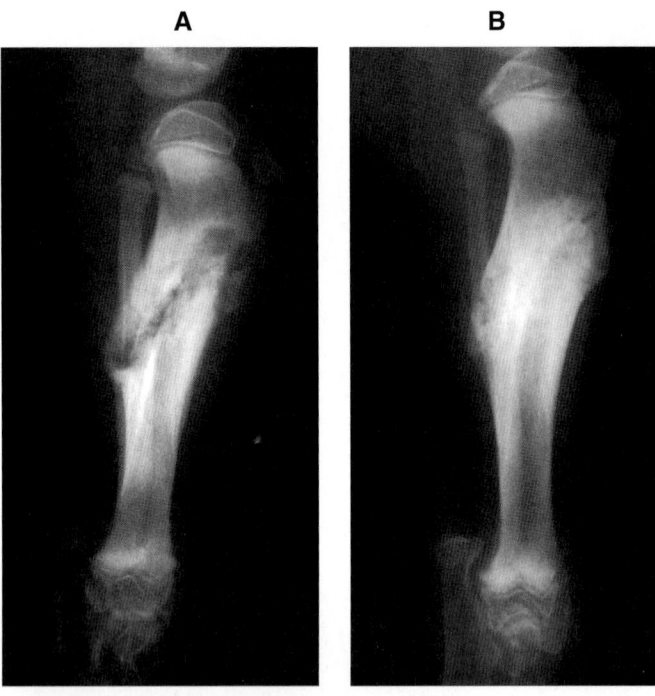

FIG. 31-84
Fracture healing of oblique tibial fracture in immature dog treated with a cast. **A,** Radiographic evidence of periosteal callus is seen 3 weeks after casting. **B,** Callus is remodeling into cortical bone 6 weeks after casting.

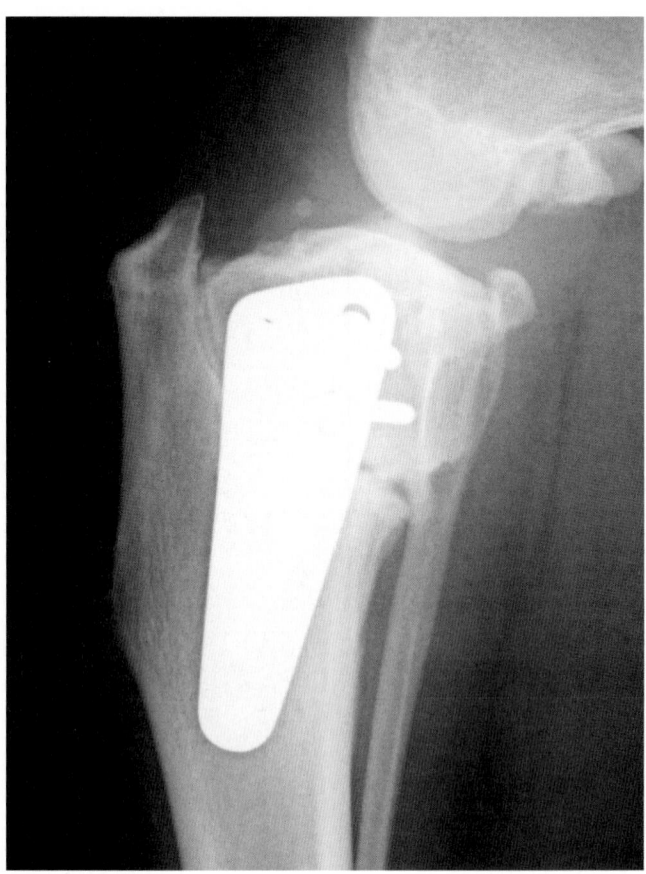

FIG. 31-86
Metaphyseal fracture healing after a tibial plateau leveling osteotomy, which is well stabilized showing trabecular bone healing.

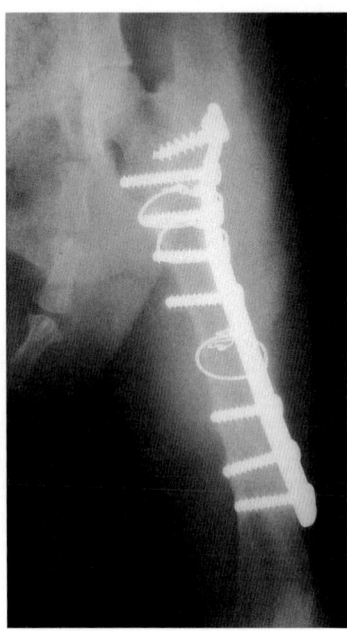

FIG. 31-85
Fracture healing in a transverse radial fracture in mature dog treated with bone plate. By 12 weeks after surgery, there is loss of visible fracture lines with no apparent callus, indicating primary bone union.

vation of the biologic environment is often best accomplished with closed reduction or limited exposure and rigid fixation (e.g., external fixators and bridging plates). Fractures treated by this method heal with endosteal bone formation and bone bridging between fragments. At 1 month, radiographs show increased mineral density throughout the fracture site with minimal formation of periosteal callus. In most patients, bone formation is evident within 2 months, and remodeling of callus is evident 3 months after fixation (Fig. 31-87). Computed tomography images show endosteal bone by 2 weeks and bridging endosteal and interfragmentary bone (which unites the bone fragments) by 12 weeks after fixation. There is minimal evidence of periosteal callus formation.

Fractures stabilized with pins and wires may heal by primary bone union if implants have rigidly stabilized fractures (e.g., long oblique fractures managed with IM pins and multiple, appropriately applied cerclage wires). However, in most cases, rigid fixation is not achieved with pins and wires, and callus formation will be evident radiographically. Pins should be removed once bone has bridged the fracture.

A   B   C

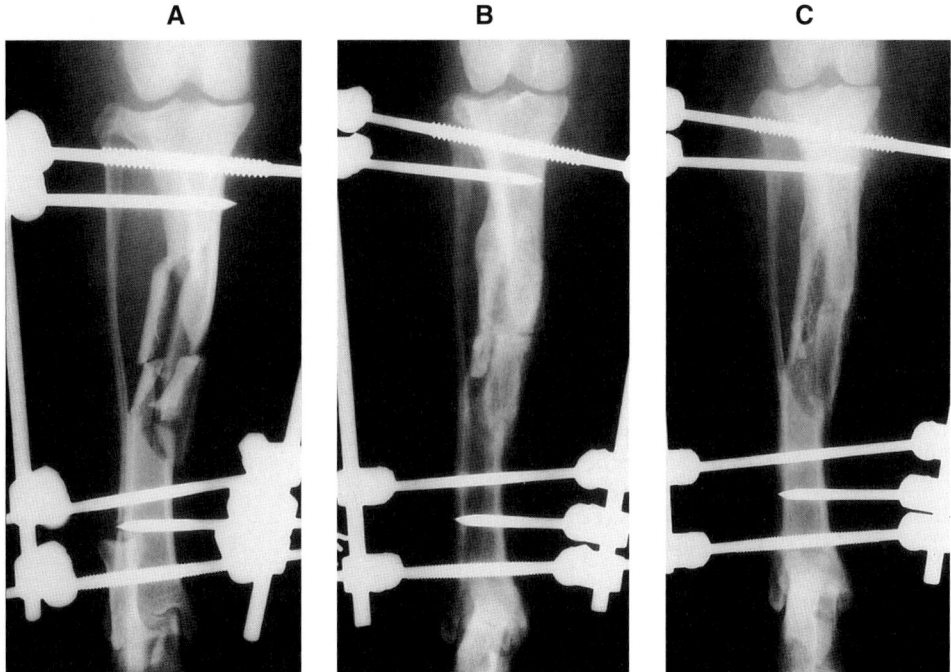

FIG. 31-87
Fracture healing in comminuted nonreducible tibial fracture in mature dog treated with closed reduction and external fixation. **A,** Immediate postoperative radiograph. **B,** Radiographic evidence of endosteal and bridging callus, with minimal periosteal callus, is seen 6 weeks after surgery. **C,** Callus is remodeling into cortical bone 12 weeks after surgery.

Wires are not removed unless they cause problems through migration or interference with fracture healing.

Fractures that are anatomically reconstructed and rigidly stabilized (e.g., with plates and screws) heal by direct bone union. With direct bone healing, fracture lines disappear, and fractures appear devoid of bridging periosteal and endosteal callus (see Fig. 31-85). Because the implant is acting as callus to support the fracture during haversian remodeling, implant removal should generally be delayed until 6 to 12 months after surgery to allow adequate time for bone remodeling.

References

Egger EL, Histand MB, Norrdin RW et al: Canine osteotomy healing when stabilized with decreasingly rigid fixation compared to constantly rigid fixation, *Vet Comp Orthop Traumatol* 6:182, 1993.

Rahn BA: Bone healing: histologic and physiologic concepts. In Sumner-Smith G (editor): *Bone in clinical orthopedics,* ed 2, Thieme, NY, AO Publishing, 2002, p 287.

Suggested Reading

Griffon DJ: Fracture healing. In Johnson AL, Houlton JEF, Vannini R, editors: *AO principles of fracture management in the dog and cat,* Thieme NY, 2005, AO Publishing, pp 73-97.

This chapter provides an excellent review of current concepts in fracture healing and methods of enhancing fracture healing, such as bone grafting.

Johnson AL, Egger EL, Eurell JC et al: Biomechanics and biology of fracture healing with external skeletal fixation, *Compend Cont Educ Pract Vet* 20:487, 1998.

This article provides information on the radiographic patterns of bone healing observed when external fixation is used clinically.

Wilson JW: Blood supply to developing, mature and healing bone. In Sumner-Smith G (editor): *Bone in clinical orthopedics,* ed 2, New York, 2002, AO Publishing, p 23.

This chapter provides a review of the research and clinical application of the concepts of vascular supply to normal and injured bone.

COMPLICATIONS
Delayed Union

Fractures that heal more slowly than anticipated are classified as *delayed unions.* Most long bone fractures have radiographic evidence of bone bridging the fracture lines by 12 weeks, with the surgeon confident that bone healing will occur. With delayed unions, signs of progressive bone activity are visible on sequential radiographs, and bone union is anticipated, but not ensured. Factors contributing to delayed unions include the systemic status of the patient (i.e., malnutrition and anemia), nature of the trauma (i.e., high-energy fractured diaphysis with extensive soft tissue injury and possibly open fractures), local host postinjury response (e.g., inadequate cellular response for healing), fracture management (i.e., poor decision making, large fracture gaps, unstable implants that are too rigid, cement in the fracture line, and radiation therapy), and pharmacologic factors (i.e., steroids and nonsteroidal antiinflammatory drugs) (Hayda, 1998).

As long as implants are adequate and remain intact, the animal should have strictly supervised activity (physical rehabilitation; see Chapter 12) with no need for additional surgery. Cancellous bone autografts (see p. 962) may be added to speed healing before implant failure occurs. Loose or migrating implants should be removed, fractures stabilized appropriately, and cancellous bone autografts applied. Stable implants promote weight bearing, which accelerates fracture healing and the strength of the union.

Nonunion

Fracture *nonunion* is defined as an arrested fracture repair process, which requires surgical intervention to create an environment conducive to bone healing. Most nonunions are a result of poor decision making and technical failure on the part of surgeons, rather than biologic failures attributable to the patient. Instability at the fracture site is the most common reason for nonunion. Common scenarios are distal radial diaphyseal fractures in toy-breed dogs stabilized with external coaptation, IM pins used with inadequate rotational and axial stability, external fixators of inadequate frame and pin size, loose cerclage wire that has migrated into the fracture site, and plates and screws that are inadequately sized for the patient. Poor biology at the fracture site, including fracture location, high-energy injury with extensive soft tissue destruction, and excessive surgical intervention, contributes to the development of nonunion. The risk factors for nonunion of fractures in cats are increased age, increased weight, open fracture, fracture of the proximal ulna and of the tibia, and the use of Type II external fixators to stabilize tibial fractures (Nolte et al, 2005).

Fracture nonunions are diagnosed when there is a lack of activity on sequential radiographs. A lucent line through fractures, representing cartilage and fibrous tissue, and ineffective callus formation at the fracture site are characteristic of the radiographic appearance of *vascular nonunions*. *Hypertrophic nonunions* are vascular nonunions with large amounts of nonbridging callus (Fig. 31-88). Hypertropic nonunions need stability to unite and are best treated by removal of loose implants and necrotic cortical bone pieces, joint alignment, and placement of a compression plate (see p. 996). Cancellous bone grafts may be used, although the hypertrophic callus usually provides adequate cancellous bone for healing. If sequestered bone is removed, the resultant defects are filled with cancellous bone autografts, which may be placed during the plating procedure or after 5 to 7 days of open wound management. This delay allows forma-

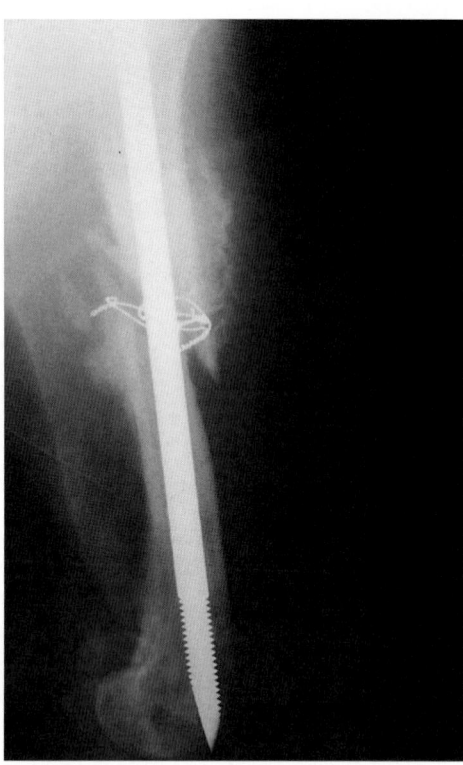

FIG. 31-88
Radiograph of dog with hypertrophic nonunion of femur. Notice formation of large periosteal callus that cannot bridge the fracture. The fracture was inadequately stabilized with an IM pin and cerclage wires.

tion of healthy granulation tissue beds before grafting. Swabs for bacterial culture and sensitivity should be obtained when nonunions are treated because concurrent osteomyelitis is common. If a radiographic or clinical diagnosis of osteomyelitis is made, treatment must include appropriate antimicrobial therapy. Plate removal is recommended after healing of infected nonunions because plates may serve as a nidus for continued infection.

Atrophic nonunions are biologically inactive pseudoarthroses. Radiographically, there is no evidence of bone reaction at fracture sites, and bone ends appear sclerotic (Fig. 31-89). Scintigraphy may confirm the lack of vascularity at the fracture. Histologically, fracture gaps are filled with fibrous tissue, necrotic bone, and cartilage. The medullary cavities are sealed with cortical bone. Atrophic nonunion requires surgery to remove fibrous tissue and open medullary canals. En bloc resection of the inactive bone and fracture site creates sufficient circumferential bony contact to allow excellent compression of the fracture with a bone plate (Blaeser et al, 2003). Plates and screws are generally the implants of choice to stabilize an atrophic nonunion, along with placement of autogenous cancellous bone graft. Swabs for bacterial culture and sensitivity should be obtained when

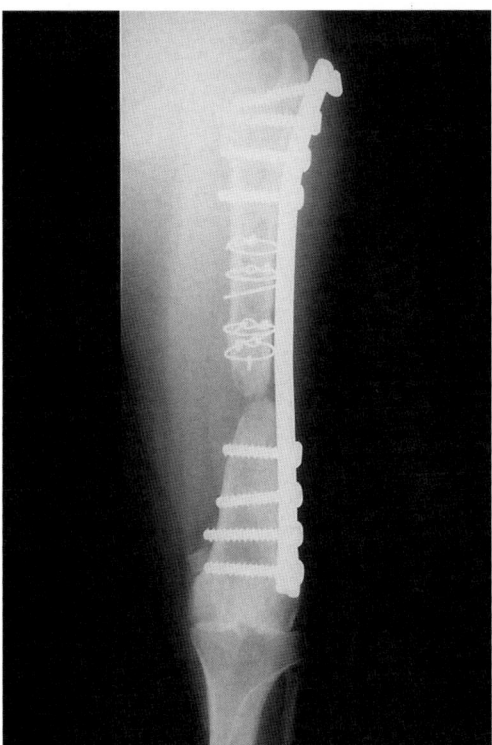

FIG. 31-89
Radiograph of dog with atrophic nonunion of femur. Notice lack of callus formation at the fracture site. The fracture eventually healed after surgical opening of the medullary canal, shortening of the femur to gain cortical contact, and application of an LC-DCP with a cancellous bone autograft.

atrophic nonunions are treated because concurrent osteomyelitis also occurs.

Osteomyelitis

Osteomyelitis is strictly defined as an inflammatory condition of bone and the medullary canal (see p. 1353). In posttraumatic osteomyelitis associated with delayed union and nonunion, the most common cause is bacterial infection, promoted by instability at the fracture and the bone implant interfaces. Open fractures provide increased opportunity for osteomyelitis, as does vascular compromise and tissue ischemia. Posttraumatic osteomyelitis occurs with microbial colonization of the implants and adjacent damaged tissue. Biofilms occur with the formation of a conditioning film on the implant surface, which encourages adhesion of microorganisms. Additionally, bacteria produce a glycocalyx, which also assists the cell in adhering to the implant. The biofilm (bacteria, glycocalyx, and implant surface) protects the microorganism from antimicrobials and host defenses. Radiographic and clinical evidence of osteomyelitis, coupled with a positive bacterial culture, provide the diagnosis. Treatment for posttraumatic osteomyelitis must include restoring a favorable fracture environment for healing (removal of loose implants and sequestered bone, disruption of the biofilm, and stabilization of the fracture) and appropriate antimicrobial therapy for at least 4 weeks.

Malunion

Malunions are healed fractures in which anatomic bone alignment was not achieved or maintained during healing. Malunions may have a deleterious effect on function. Angular deformities are characterized by loss of correct parallel relationships between joints above and below the fractured bone. Deformities may be classified as *valgus, varus, antecurvatum,* or *recurvatum* (Fig. 31-90, *A* to *D*). When severe, these deformities affect limb function and may precipitate osteoarthritis of adjacent joints. Translational and rotational deformities can also occur (Fig. 31-90, *E* to *F*). Rotation most often occurs with inadequately stabilized femoral fractures and may adversely affect hip and stifle function. Shortening of affected bones may also occur. A shortened bone in a single bone system (femur and humerus) can be compensated for by extension of adjacent joints; however, shortening of a single bone in a paired bone system (radius-ulna, tibia-fibula) causes incongruity in alignment of adjacent joints. Malunion should be treated with corrective osteotomy if it adversely affects the animal's ability to ambulate.

OSTEOTOMIES

Osteotomies are procedures in which the bone is cut into two segments. *Apophyseal osteotomies,* such as trochanteric or acromial osteotomies, are performed to enhance surgical exposure of a joint (see pp. 1100 and 1033). *Corrective osteotomies* are elective procedures in which the diaphysis or metaphysis of the bone is cut, realigned, and stabilized until union occurs. The indications for corrective osteotomies are to (1) correct angular deformities caused by physeal trauma or fracture malunion by realigning joint surfaces, (2) establish adequate bone length to shortened bones, (3) correct torsional deformities caused by physeal trauma or fracture malunion, and (4) improve articular configuration. *Ostectomies,* or removal of a bone segment, are generally performed in immature dogs to allow unimpeded growth of paired long bones where one of that pair has suffered early physeal closure. They may also be used to improve joint congruity (Table 31-8).

The objective in performing corrective osteotomy is to return a limb to normal function by restoring normal alignment to the bone or joint. Presurgical planning is a prerequisite for success. The surgeon must determine the correct location(s) to cut the bone, whether the soft tissue can tolerate the strain of repositioning the bone, and the appropriate fixation to maintain stability until bone union occurs. Currently, radiographs provide the most useful information for planning an osteotomy. Craniocaudal and mediolateral views of the affected bone, including the proximal and distal adjacent joints, are required to evaluate the deformity. Similar radiographs of the contralateral bone are used as a reference. Significant angular deformity in both views indicates

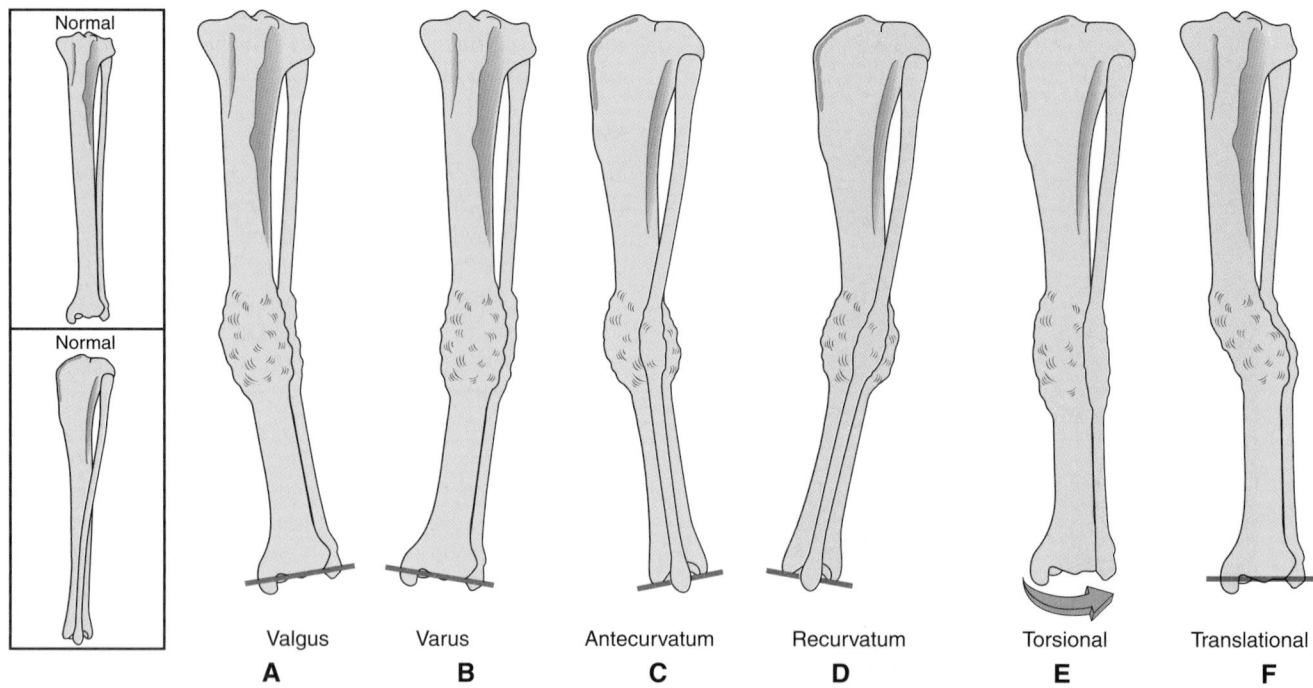

FIG. 31-90

Malalignment of bone. **A,** Valgus is lateral angulation of distal segment of bone. **B,** Varus is medial angulation. **C,** Antecurvatum is caudal angulation. **D,** Recurvatum is cranial angulation of distal segment of bone. **E,** Torsion is medial or lateral twisting of distal segment of bone. **F,** Translation is displacement of distal segment of bone with the joint surfaces parallel.

 TABLE 31-8

Indications for Corrective Osteotomy Procedures

DEFORMITY	OSTEOTOMY TECHNIQUE
Angular	Opening wedge Closing wedge Reverse wedge Dome
Shortening	Transverse lengthening Stair step Continuous distraction
Rotational	Derotational transverse
Angular, shortening, and rotational	Opening wedge Continuous distraction
Incongruent joint	Triple pelvic Intertrochanteric Tibial plateau leveling Transverse lengthening Stair step Ulnar osteotomy Continuous distraction

that the deformity lies in an oblique plane. Oblique views may be needed to determine the plane of the deformity. The degree of angular deformity and length discrepancy can be determined from radiographs. Rotational deformity may be estimated from radiographs, but is usually best determined from physical examination. Rotational deformity is measured directly on the dog by comparing the relationship of adjacent bones, such as the radius and metacarpal bones, during flexion and extension of the adjoining joint.

Outcomes of improper osteotomy planning are incomplete correction of the deformity, implant failure, delayed union, infection, and nonunion.

Corrective Osteotomy for Deformities

Deformities may result from growth abnormalities (usually premature physeal closure) or fracture malunion. Immature animals with premature closure of the physis in the radius or ulna may be treated with a segmental ostectomy to release the restraint of the affected bone to allow the unaffected bone to grow normally (see e-dition, premature physeal closure). Deformities in mature animals are treated with corrective osteotomy. Rotational deformities can be corrected with a *transverse osteotomy,* after which the distal segment is rotated to restore proper bone alignment (Fig. 31-91, *A*). Angular limb deformities are treated with *closing wedge* or

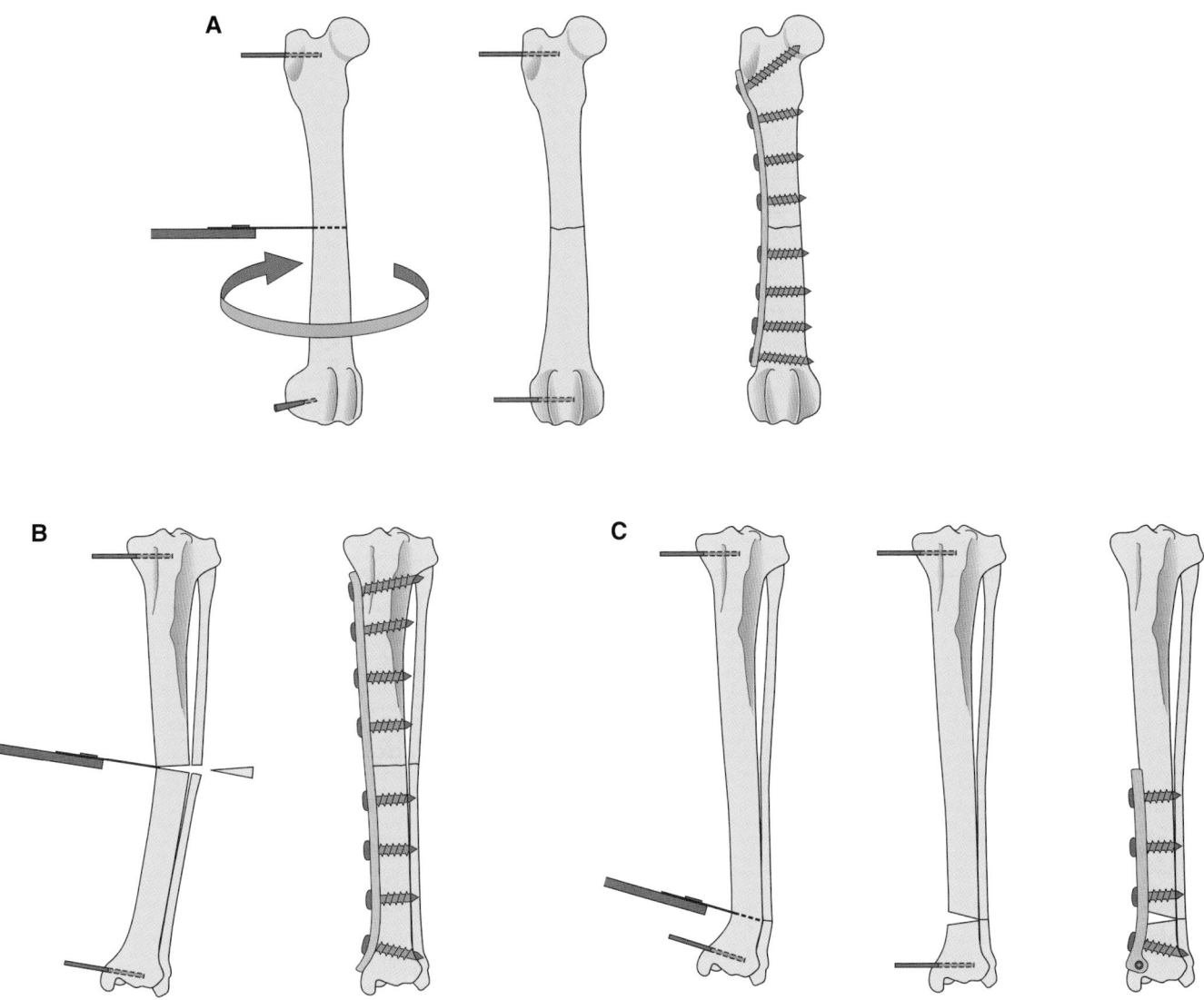

FIG. 31-91
Corrective osteotomies used to treat bone deformities. **A,** Derotational osteotomy. **B,** Closing wedge osteotomy. **C,** Opening wedge osteotomy.

opening wedge osteotomy to restore the proper alignment of the proximal and distal joint surfaces (Fig. 31-91, *B* and *C*). Opening wedge osteotomy preserves bone length, whereas closing wedge osteotomy provides a more stable fracture surface. These osteotomies may be stabilized with bone plates or external fixators.

Deformities with significant shortening of the affected bone require a lengthening procedure to restore limb function. *Lengthening osteotomies* may be acute or continuous. One-stage correction is often limited by the soft tissue, whereas *continuous distraction* overcomes this limitation and provides for new bone formation during distraction osteogenesis (see p. 978). Continuous distraction may also be used to treat growing dogs with complete physeal closure.

Corrective Osteotomy for Joint Incongruity

Most frequently performed corrective osteotomies provide for realignment of an incongruent joint. Dogs with early evidence of hip dysplasia are candidates for *triple pelvic osteotomy* designed to rotate the dorsal acetabular rim to provide additional stability to the hip joint (see p. 1241) (Fig. 31-92, *A*). *Release osteotomies* or *ostectomies* are performed when there is an incongruent elbow to allow the ulna to return to a more normal relationship with the distal humerus (Fig. 31-92, *B*). These procedures are also used to relieve the pressure on an ununited anconeal process (UAP) and/or fragmented coronoid process (FCP) (see pp. 1212 and 1204). If the incongruity is too great, a lengthening osteotomy may be indicated to restore elbow alignment.

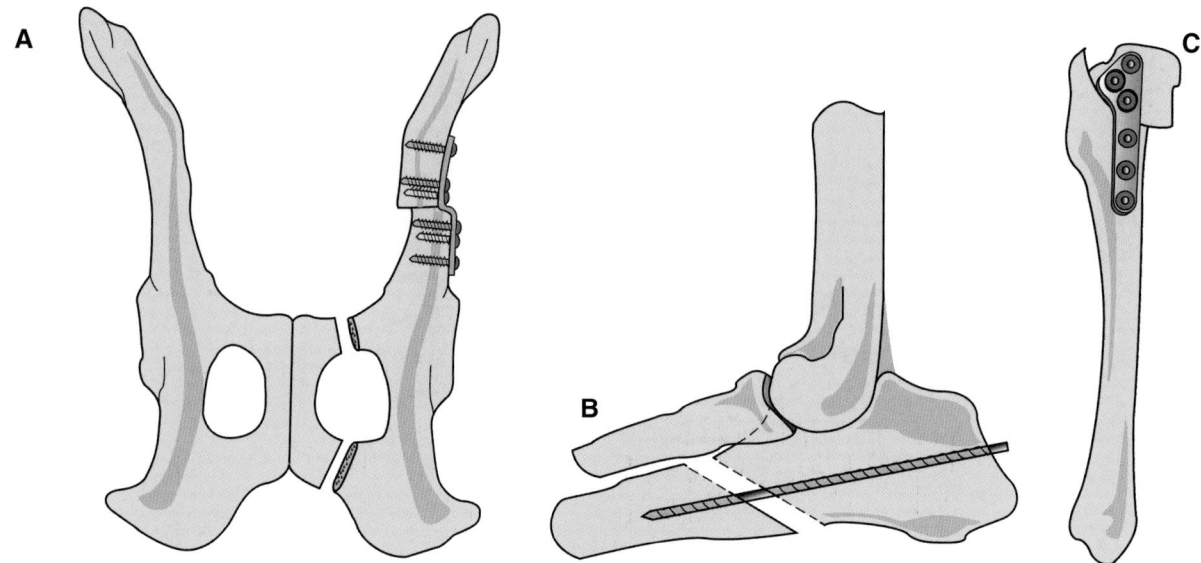

FIG. 31-92
Corrective osteotomies used to treat joint disease. **A,** Triple pelvic osteotomy. **B,** Dynamic ulnar osteotomy. **C,** Tibial plateau leveling osteotomy.

Dogs with cranial cruciate ligament rupture may be treated with a *tibial plateau leveling osteotomy* (TPLO) to improve the mechanics of the joint (Fig. 31-92, *C*). Occasionally, dogs with patellar luxation and associated femoral varus or valgus, or rotation, are treated with a corrective osteotomy to realign the femur.

References

Blaeser LL, Gallagher JG, Boudrieau RJ: Treatment of biologically inactive nonunions by a limited en bloc ostectomy and compression plate fixation: a review of 17 cases, *Vet Surg* 32:91, 2003.

Hayda RA, Brighton CT, Esterhai JL: Pathophysiology of delayed healing, *Clin Orthop* 355S:S31, 1998.

Nolte DM, Fusco JV, Peterson ME: Incidence of and predisposing factors for nonunion of fractures involving the appendicular skeleton in cats: 18 cases (1998-2002), *J Am Vet Med Assoc* 226:77, 2005.

Suggested Reading

Budsberg SC: Osteomyelitis, In Johnson AL, Houlton JEF, Vannini R, editors: *AO principles of fracture management in the dog and cat,* Thieme NY, 2005, AO Publishing.

This chapter provides a current and comprehensive review of the pathophysiology and treatment of osteomyelitis.

Johnson AL: Corrective osteotomies, In *AO principles of fracture management in the dog and cat,* Johnson AL, Houlton JEF and Vannini R editors, Thieme, NY, 2005, AO Publishing.

This chapter provides a current and comprehensive overview of corrective osteotomy procedures for small animal patients.

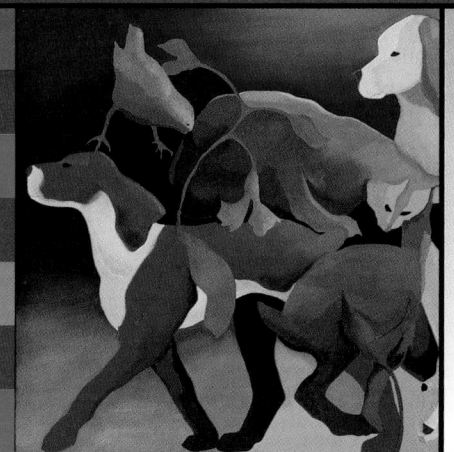

CHAPTER 32
Management of Specific Fractures

MAXILLARY AND MANDIBULAR FRACTURES

DEFINITIONS

Maxillary fractures and **mandibular fractures** may result from trauma, severe periodontitis, or neoplasia. **Periodontitis** is an inflammatory reaction of the tissue surrounding a tooth that usually results from the extension of gingival inflammation into the periodontium.

GENERAL CONSIDERATIONS AND CLINICALLY RELEVANT PATHOPHYSIOLOGY

Maxillary and mandibular fractures are usually caused by head trauma, and concurrent injuries are often present (i.e., upper airway obstruction, central nervous system trauma, pneumothorax, pulmonary contusions, and traumatic myocarditis). These abnormalities may be acutely life threatening and may require prompt diagnosis and treatment. Definitive fracture repair must often be delayed until the animal has

been appropriately stabilized. Mandibular fractures occasionally occur as a result of bone loss associated with severe periodontitis. Teeth extraction should be performed with care in older patients with severe periodontitis to prevent this complication. With severe periodontitis, bone healing may be impaired. Diseased teeth must be extracted before fracture stabilization in these patients. Pathologic fractures may also result from mandibular neoplasia (see p. 361). Histopathologic examination of bone from animals with mandibular fractures is warranted, unless fractures clearly are caused by trauma. Mandibular fractures associated with neoplasia are treated by mandibulectomy rather than definitive fracture repair (see p. 343).

The teeth occupy a large portion of the mandible and are integral components of normal mandibular structure (Fig. 32-1). Teeth involved in fractures should not be removed unless they are loose. This is especially important with fractures involving the caudal mandibular body because the large premolar and molar teeth occupy a substantial portion of this

FIG. 32-1
Skull anatomy. Note that the tooth roots occupy a large portion of the mandible. Normal relationships of the maxillary and mandibular dental arcades are illustrated.

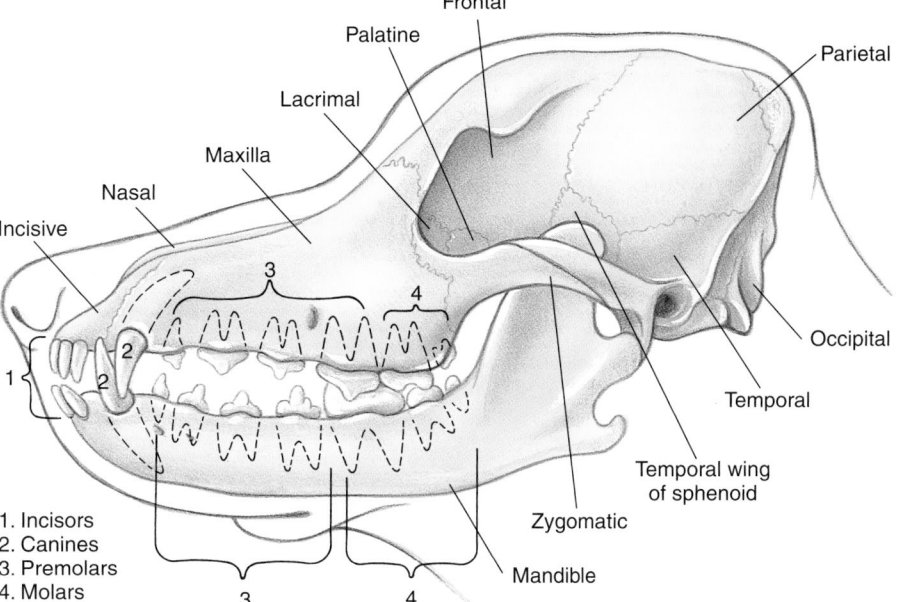

1. Incisors
2. Canines
3. Premolars
4. Molars

bone and are essential contributors to fracture stability. Fractures extending along the tooth root from the alveolar crest to the apex of the tooth are at risk for pulpal necrosis and periapical bone resorption. Temporary or permanent root canal therapy at the time of fracture stabilization may promote bone healing. If affected teeth are not treated at surgery, periodic evaluation for evidence of infection or loosening is necessary postoperatively to determine whether endodontic therapy or extraction is indicated. The anatomy and location of tooth roots must be considered when implants are applied to the mandible. Damage to tooth roots from pins, wires, drill bits, and screws may cause sufficient damage that extraction becomes necessary after fracture healing.

DIAGNOSIS
Clinical Presentation

Signalment. Although traumatic mandibular or maxillary fractures may occur in dogs at any age, young dogs are at greater risk. However, as the canine population reflects the increase in small and toy breeds and in urban leashed populations, the mean age of dogs with mandibular fractures has increased. Pathologic fractures of the mandible are particularly common in geriatric, small-breed, and toy-breed dogs (e.g., poodles) that have not had regular dental prophylaxis and are fed soft food and table scraps.

History. There is usually a history of trauma (e.g., stepped on, hit by car, or kicked by horse) in animals with traumatic oral fractures. Mandibular symphyseal fractures and fractures of the hard palate may occur in cats that fall from great heights ("high-rise syndrome"). Tooth extraction may be associated with pathologic fractures of dogs with severe periodontitis.

Physical Examination Findings

Animals with mandibular fractures may drool excessively, exhibit pain on opening of the mouth, and are often reluctant to eat. Saliva may be blood-tinged, but profuse bleeding is uncommon. Crepitation and instability can often be palpated during careful oral examination; however, thorough inspection of these structures for mucosal wounds and crepitation often requires general anesthetic. Mandibular symphyseal fractures allow one hemimandible to be moved separately from the other. Less instability is usually present with maxillary fractures than mandibular fractures. The teeth should be examined carefully for evidence of trauma. A biopsy should be taken of fractures associated with notable bony lysis or proliferation.

> NOTE: Use endodontic therapy to treat teeth fractured above the gumline; extract teeth that are fractured below the gumline.

Diagnostic Imaging

Radiographs of the mandible and maxilla generally require that animals be anesthetized. Thorough radiographic examination of the skull usually requires a minimum of four radiographic views: dorsoventral or ventrodorsal, lateral, and right and left lateral obliques. Because skull radiographs are often difficult to interpret because of the presence of multiple overlying structures, comparison with a normal skull is often helpful. Symmetry between the two sides is critical to interpretation and thus care in positioning is critical. Additional specialized views, such as intraoral views, may also be necessary for complete evaluation. Computed tomography (CT) can help identify fractures in the caudal mandibular body, vertical ramus, and mandibular condyle that may be difficult to detect radiographically. If CT is readily available, it is often more efficient for evaluating complex mandibular and maxillary fractures than survey radiography.

Laboratory Findings

Specific laboratory abnormalities are not present with mandibular or maxillary fractures from any cause. Traumatized animals should have sufficient blood work done to determine if contraindications to anesthesia exist.

DIFFERENTIAL DIAGNOSIS

Animals with mandibular or maxillary fractures should be evaluated to determine whether fractures are the result of trauma or underlying pathology (periodontitis, neoplasia, or metabolic disease; see previous discussion).

MEDICAL MANAGEMENT

A tape muzzle may be applied to support the mandible if there is minimal displacement of fracture fragments (usually fractures of the ramus), if dental occlusion is adequate, and if the fracture assessment score (see p. 953) is favorable and dictates early union. A muzzle can be made from two pieces of tape placed with the sticky sides together and fashioned into a circle that fits over the dog's nose. A similarly made piece of tape extends from the circle around the head and behind the ears (Fig. 32-2). The muzzle should allow the dog to open its mouth enough to lap water and eat gruel. To allow adequate healing, muzzles should remain in place for 6 weeks. Dogs with mandibular plus maxillary fractures may not tolerate tape muzzles because the muzzle may put pressure on the maxillary fracture. Because of the cat's short nose, tape muzzles are difficult to apply and maintain. Similarly, it may be difficult to maintain a tape muzzle in brachycephalic breeds.

INTERDENTAL STABILIZATION TECHNIQUES

Oral stabilization techniques incorporating wire ligatures and/or dental acrylics attached to the teeth allow closed reduction of mandibular and maxillary fractures, preserving the periosteal attachments and blood supply. These techniques are especially useful for fractures rostral to the first mandibular molars, and for comminuted fractures in which anatomic reduction may not be possible. Maxillomandibular fixation may also be used to stabilize temporomandibular joint luxations.

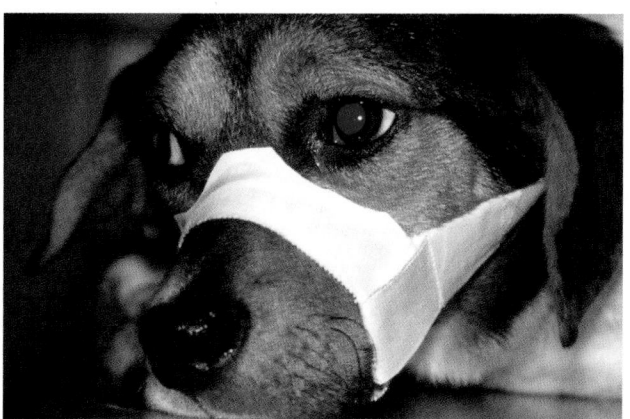

FIG. 32-2
Stabilization of a minimally displaced mandibular fracture with a tape muzzle. Tape muzzles can also be used preoperatively to support the mandible.

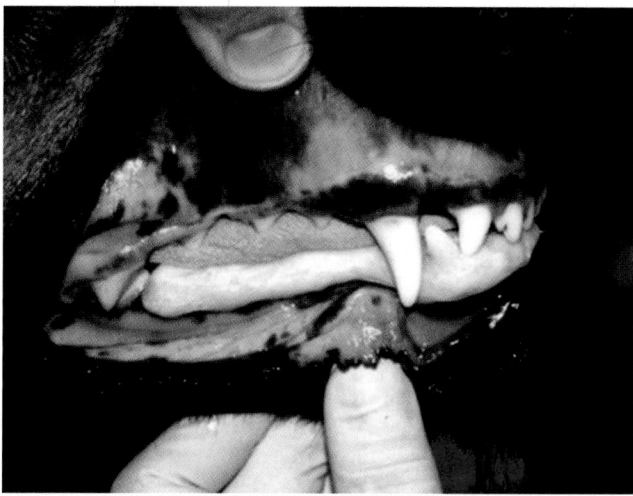

FIG. 32-3
Stabilization of a mandibular fracture in a dog with a wire reinforced acrylic splint. (Photo courtesy of Dr. Sandra Manfra Marretta and Dr. Robert Ulbricht.)

Application of Interdental Fixation

Interdental fixation is limited to use in mandibular and maxillary fractures occurring between intact canine and carnassial teeth. In dogs, interdental wire ligatures are combined with acrylic intraoral splints to provide stable fixation. In cats, acrylic intraoral splints may be used without metallic reinforcement. Acrylic materials with a low curing temperature are recommended for intraoral use.

The crowns of the mandibular teeth are cleaned, pumiced, and acid etched to improve acrylic resin bonding. The mandible is aligned using interdigitation of the teeth as a landmark for accurate reduction. Interdental wire ligatures (0.3 to 0.5 mm wire) are applied to initially stabilize the fracture(s). Dental acrylic is applied to the prepared teeth to stabilize the fracture (Fig. 32-3). The splints are removed when there is radiographic evidence of bone bridging the fracture by sectioning the splint interdentally and removing the splint in sections.

Application of Maxillomandibular Fixation

Bonding the maxillary and mandibular canine teeth together in anatomic alignment is an alternative to the tape muzzle for conservative fracture treatment. The canine teeth are cleaned, pumiced, acid etched, and aligned with dental composite, leaving the mouth open approximately 1 cm. Although simple, the technique requires that all four canine teeth be intact and healthy. This technique can be used in dogs and cats (Fig. 32-4).

NOTE: Warning: animals treated by limiting their ability to open their mouths are at risk for hyperthermia if placed in a warm environment and for aspiration pneumonia if vomiting occurs.

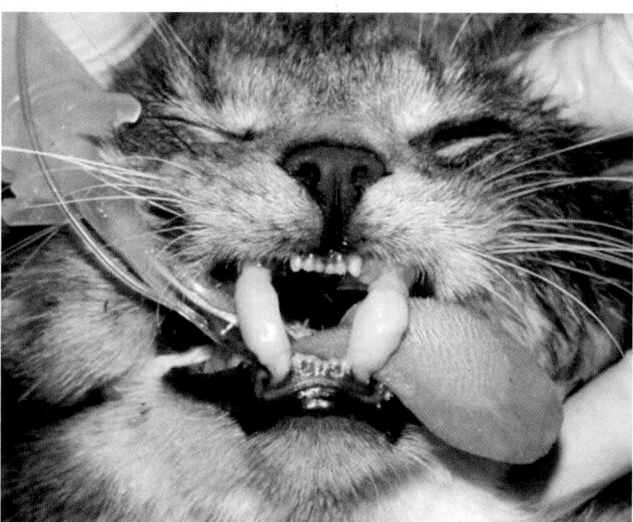

FIG. 32-4
Stabilization of a caudal mandibular fracture in a cat with acrylic bonding of the maxillary and mandibular canine teeth. (Photo courtesy of Dr. Sandra Manfra Marretta.)

SURGICAL TREATMENT

The appropriate method of treating mandibular and maxillary fractures is determined based on the fracture-assessment score (see p. 953) and fracture location. Conservative treatment with a tape muzzle or dental composite bonding may be appropriate for some fractures (see previous discussion). Internal fixation systems applicable for mandibular fractures are orthopedic wire, Kirschner wires, and plates and screws. Intramedullary (IM) pins are contraindicated as the mandibular canal contains the mandibular alveolar artery and

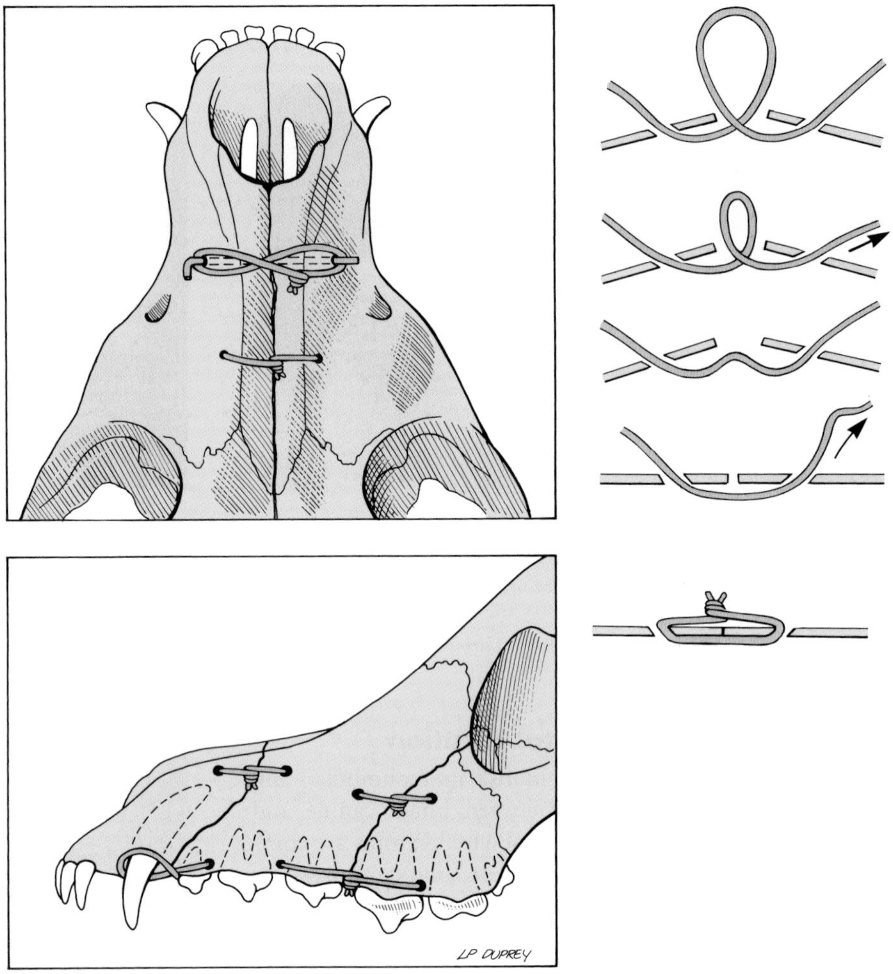

FIG. 32-5
Stabilization of maxillary fractures with Kirschner wire and orthopedic wire. Wires are applied perpendicular to the fracture and tightened to compress it. Kirschner wires are used to prevent collapse of fragments. Occasionally a canine tooth can be used to secure the wire. To facilitate passing cerclage wire, angle the drill holes toward the fracture. Loop a long piece of wire under the bone and through the second hole. Pull the wire until kinks caused by looping are beyond incorporation into the final cerclage, and tighten the wire.

inferior alveolar nerve. External fixators (both standard and acrylic frames) are very effective for nonreducible comminuted fractures. Many maxillary fractures are nondisplaced and require only conservative therapy; however, segmental maxillary fractures or depressed fracture lines may require repositioning and stabilization. Mandibular or maxillary fractures that alter normal occlusion should be reduced and stabilized. Maxillary fractures that result in nasal malpositioning or instability should be reduced and stabilized. Interfragmentary wires may be used to stabilize some maxillary fractures where only a few large bone fragments are involved and stable anatomic reduction is possible (Fig. 32-5), especially with Kirschner wires incorporated into the fixation to prevent overriding of the fragments. Maxillofacial miniplates are more effective for restoring anatomic contour to comminuted and depressed maxillary fractures involving thin portions of the skull.

Application of Interdental Wires

Interdental wires are placed around teeth adjacent to fracture lines. The wires must be positioned securely in the bone around the tooth's neck to prevent them from sliding off the crown. They are placed through guide holes that are drilled between the teeth and through the superficial cortical bone surface. The wire is passed through the guide holes, circling the teeth, and tightened. The ends of the wire should be bent into the mucosa (Fig. 32-6).

Application of Interfragmentary Wires

Interfragmentary wires are ideal for stabilizing relatively simple, reconstructible mandibular and maxillary fractures. Large-gauge wire (18 to 22 gauge), properly applied, provides adequate fracture support (Table 32-1); however, wires may be difficult to position and tighten unless certain application guidelines are followed. The largest gauge wire that can be manipulated should be used. Kirschner wires are used to drill holes in the bone, 5 to 10 mm from the fracture line (Fig. 32-7, *A*). These holes are positioned so that the wire will be perpendicular to the fracture line when it is tightened. The drill holes are sloped toward the fracture line because this results in obtuse angles on the bone side opposite to where the wire knot will be tightened. This positioning allows the wire to slide into position easily and enhances tightening efforts. Long segments of wire are used to facili-

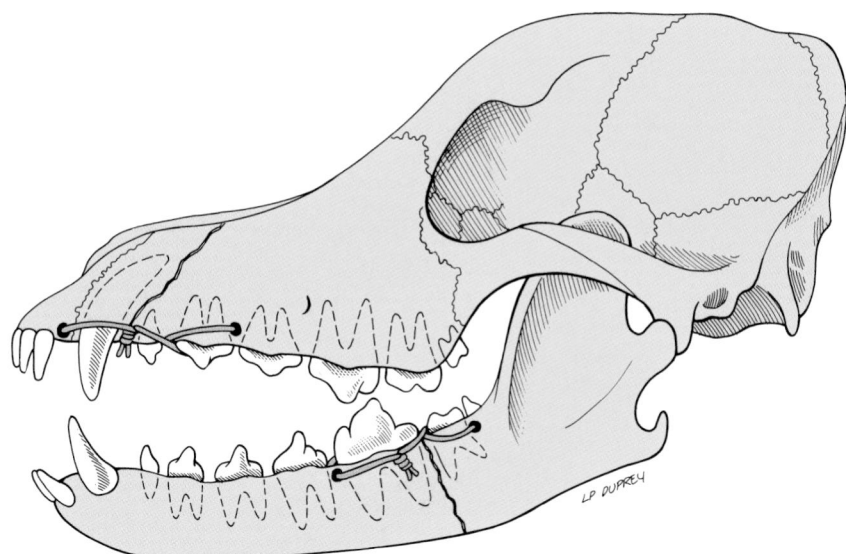

FIG. 32-6
Interdental wires may be placed through holes drilled in the maxillary or mandibular bone to prevent the wire from slipping.

 TABLE 32-1

Comparable Wire Sizes for Fracture Stabilization

GAUGE	MILLIMETER	INCH
16	1.25	.049
18	1.00	.040
20	0.80	.035
		.032
		.030
22	0.60	.028
24		.020

tate wire passage and allow manipulation of any wire kinks away from the area of wire that is to be tightened. The wire is tightened using either a twist knot or a tension loop (see p. 989). It is twisted in such a manner that equal tension is applied to both strands (Fig. 32-7, *B*). A periosteal elevator or large tissue forceps can be used to lever the orthopedic wire under the twist and eliminate slack (Fig. 32-7, *C*). When tightened, the wire is bent perpendicular to the wire surface and away from the gingival margin. The wire is cut and the ends twisted and bent into the bone surface (Fig. 32-7, *D*).

Optimally, wires should be located near the oral margin to neutralize forces that tend to disrupt fractures. Because this margin also contains the teeth, care must be used to position drill holes between teeth or tooth roots. When multiple wires are used, all holes should be drilled and wires positioned before any wires are tightened. Wires are tightened beginning at the caudal fracture line and working to-

ward the symphysis. If bending or slippage is encountered with oblique or transverse fractures, Kirschner wires with figure-eight-patterned orthopedic wire may be used. The Kirschner wire helps prevent sliding or bending while the orthopedic wire is tightened.

Application of Bone Plates and Screws

Bone plates can be used to stabilize single or comminuted mandibular fractures (see p. 991). Plates are applied to the ventrolateral mandibular surface. Care must be used to contour the plate correctly because the mandible aligns with the plate as the screws are tightened; malalignment results in malocclusion. Screws are positioned to avoid tooth roots. Maxillofacial miniplates may offer easier contouring and screw placement in mandibular and maxillary fractures and may be combined with standard straight plates and reconstruction plates (Fig. 32-8).

Application of External Skeletal Fixators

External fixators. External fixators (see p. 969) can be used to stabilize mandibular body fractures if there is sufficient bone to hold fixation pins. Fixation pins are placed percutaneously through the mandibular body, avoiding tooth roots. Type I fixators are applied to the ventrolateral mandibular surface with at least two pins inserted on either side of the fracture line. Positive-profile, end-threaded pins are used to increase the fixator's holding power. For bilateral mandibular body fractures, a Type II fixator may be constructed using bilateral and unilateral fixation pins. A connecting bar is placed on either side of the dog's jaw (Fig. 32-9).

Acrylic fixators. Dental acrylic, used to replace clamps and connecting bars, is a versatile rigid fixation for mandibular fractures, especially severely comminuted fractures. After pins have been placed in appropriate locations in the mandible (use fixation pins of appropriate size for the bone

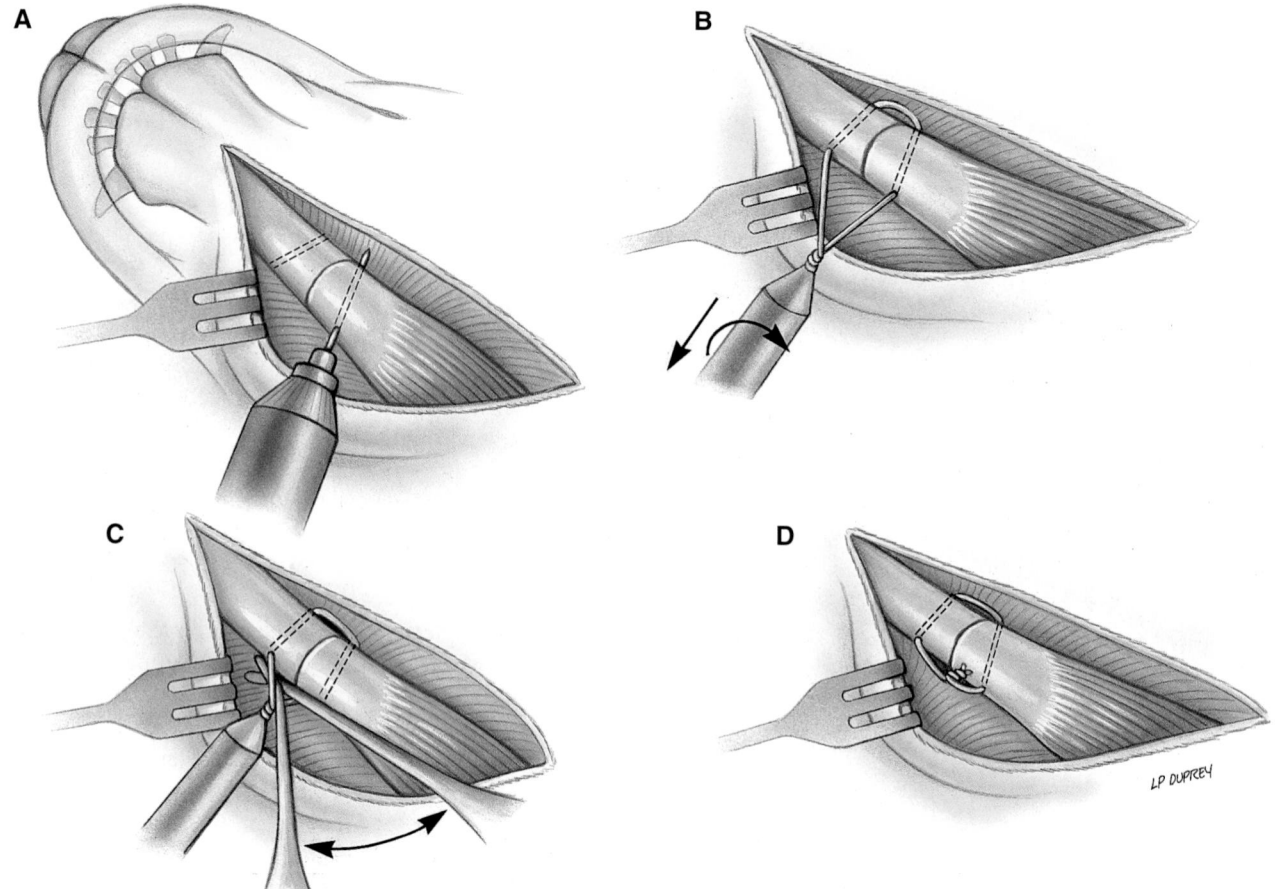

FIG. 32-7
A, To place an interfragmentary wire on the mandible, angle the drill holes toward the fracture. **B,** Place the wire and begin the twist while placing traction on the wire. **C,** To ensure that the wire is in contact with the far cortex, insert a forceps between the twist and the near cortex, and lever the wire away from the near cortex. **D,** Finish tightening the wire, cut the twist, and bend it into the bone.

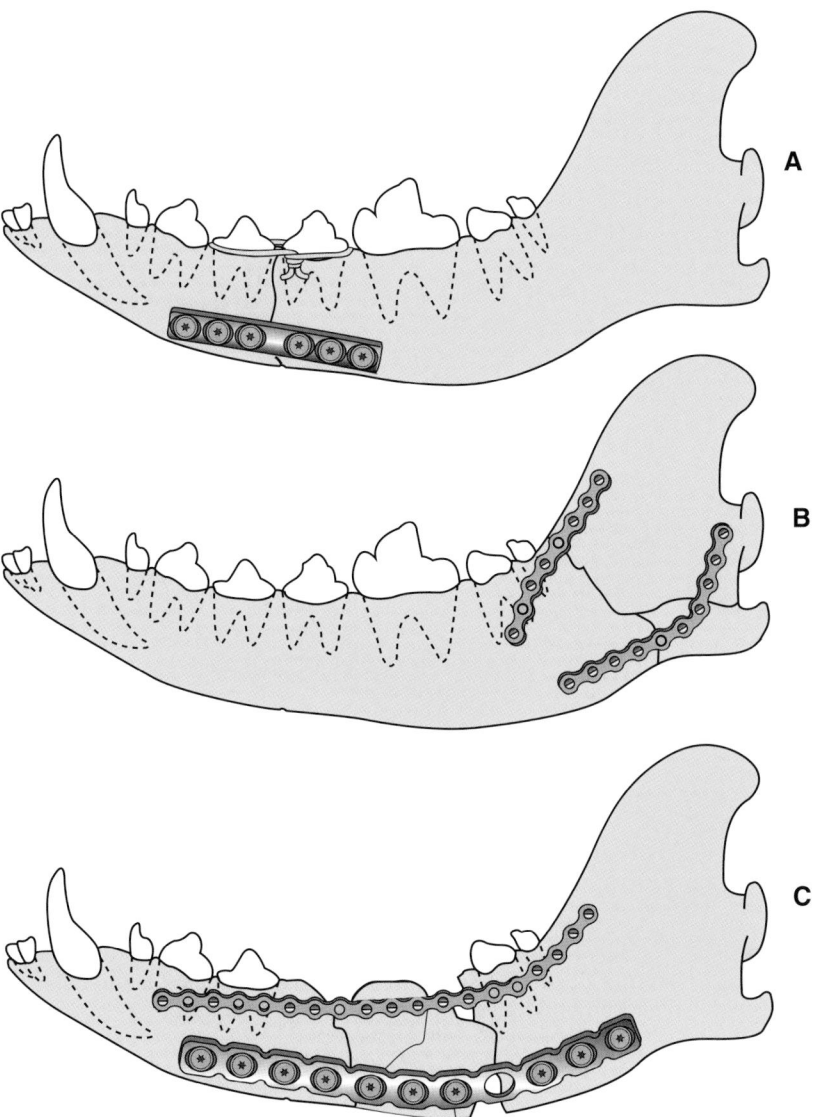

FIG. 32-8
A, Compression plates are applied to the lateral mandibular surface to stabilize transverse fractures. Avoid penetrating the tooth roots with screws. An interdental wire may function as an additional tension band fixation. **B,** Fractures of the vertical ramus may be stabilized with miniplates applied to the thicker rostral and ventral borders of the bone. **C,** Comminuted fractures of the mandible may be bridged with a reconstruction plate. Concurrent miniplate fixation adds stabilization to the tension surface of the mandible. (Modified from Johnson AL, Houlton JEF, Vannini R, editors: *AO principles of fracture management in the dog and cat,* Thieme, NY, 2005, AO Publishing.)

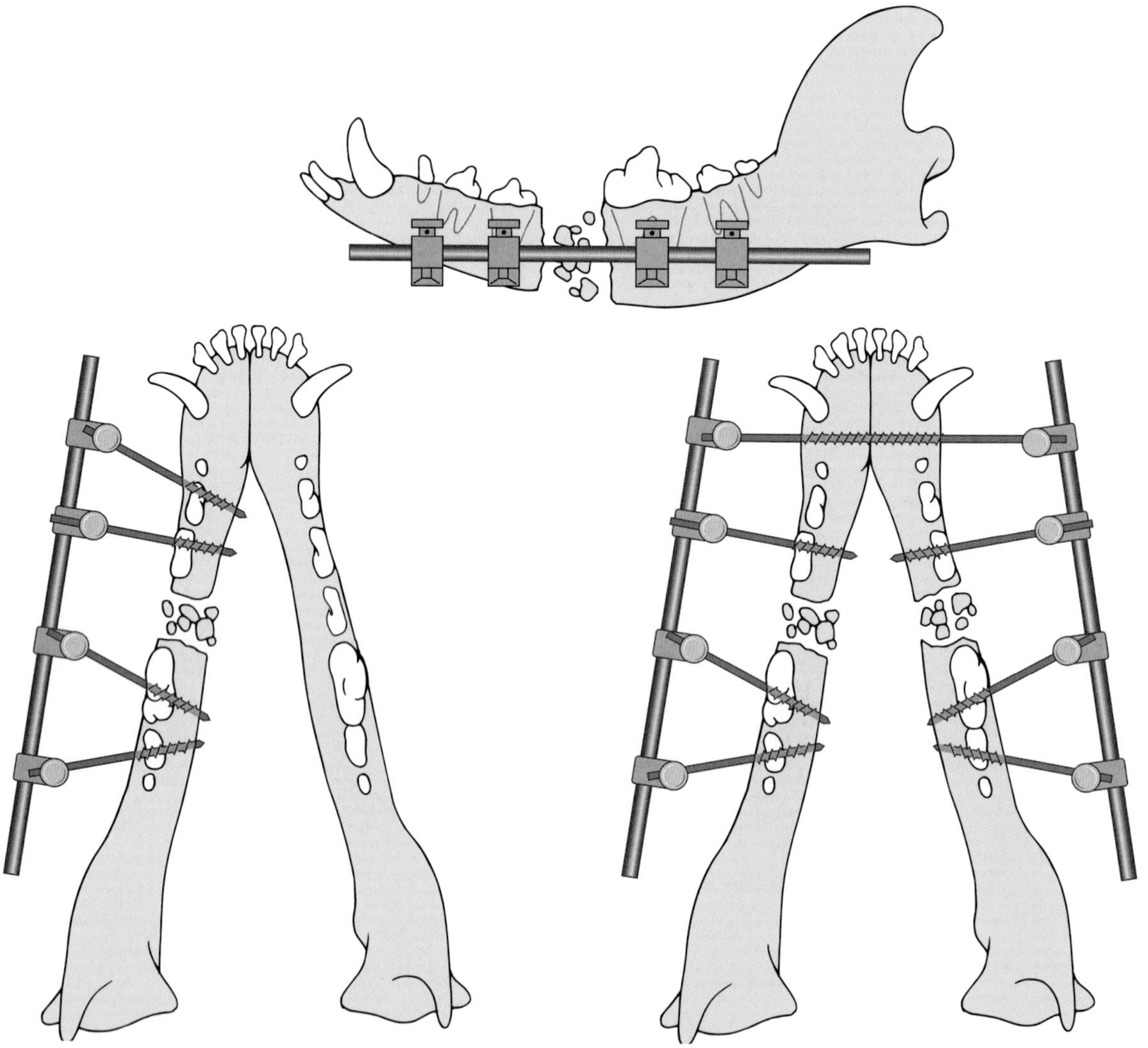

FIG. 32-9
When placing a Type I or II external fixator to stabilize comminuted mandibular fractures, use positive-profile, end-threaded pins if the fracture-assessment score indicates prolonged healing. Avoid penetrating tooth roots with fixation pins.

area), the ends are bent parallel to the skin (Fig. 32-10, *A*). To evaluate dental occlusion and reduce fractures, the animal's mouth is closed. If necessary, Kirschner clamps and a connecting bar can be placed to hold the fracture temporarily in reduction while the acrylic is being mixed and molded (Fig. 32-10, *B*). Soft tissue is protected by laying wet sponges beneath the pins. After the acrylic is mixed, it is molded over the bent pins to form a connecting bar (Fig. 32-10, *C*). Alternatively, plastic tubing may be impaled over the pins (do not bend them) and then used as a mold for the liquid-phase acrylic. The acrylic splint can be curved around the rostral portion of the mandible.

NOTE: Acrylic bars are versatile because they can accommodate various sizes of fixation pins placed in multiple planes.

Animals with mandibular fractures that have high fracture-assessment scores of 8 to 10 (e.g., simple fractures in young animals; see p. 953) may be treated with tape muzzles, interdental fixation, interdental wiring, or interfragmentary wiring techniques, depending on fracture location. Interfragmentary wire is usually sufficient to stabilize simple, bilateral, mandibular fractures if they can be anatomically reconstructed and if fracture-assessment scores indicate rapid healing (Box 32-1). It has the advantage of being internal fixation with minimal aftercare. With moderate fracture-assessment scores of 4 to 7 (e.g., larger or older dogs with longer healing times) and if bilateral fractures can be anatomically reconstructed, interfragmentary wires, interdental fixation, external fixation, or bone plates and screws may be used for fracture fixation. A cancellous bone autograft can be used to promote rapid bone union in these patients. With low fracture-assessment scores of 0 to 3 and comminution, bone

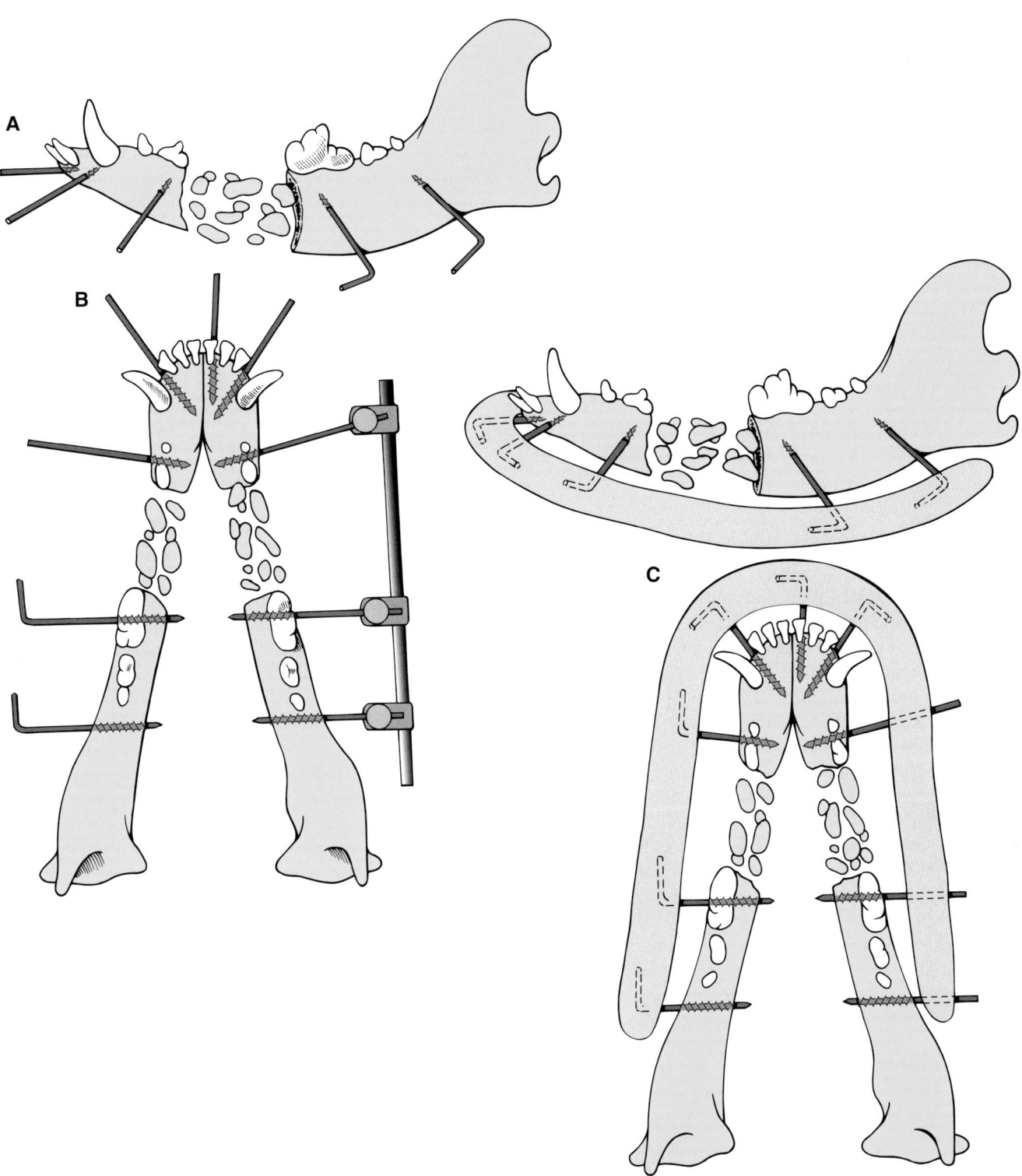

FIG. 32-10
Acrylic splints may be used to accommodate fixation pins of various sizes that are placed in multiple planes. **A,** Place the fixation pins where there is adequate bone. Use positive-profile, end-threaded pins when the fracture-assessment score indicates prolonged healing. **B,** Use a temporary fixation bar to maintain mandibular alignment. **C,** Bend the fixation pins, and apply the acrylic over them while it has a doughy consistency.

BOX 32-1

Implant Use for Maxillary and Mandibular Fractures According to Fracture-Assessment Score (FAS)

FAS 0 to 3
- Closed reduction and external skeletal fixation
- Bone plate and screws
- Maxillomandibular fixation for vertical ramus

FAS 4 to 7
- Interdental fixation techniques
- Bone plates and screws
- External skeletal fixation

FAS 8 to 10
- Tape muzzle
- Interdental fixation techniques
- Interfragmentary wiring
- Cerclage wires (symphyseal fractures)

loss, or severe soft tissue damage, mandibular fractures are best treated with closed reduction and external fixator application or bridging plate application. Closed reduction techniques preserve the biologic environment, but external fixators require intensive aftercare and the pin bone interface loosens over time. Mandibular alignment is determined by observing dental occlusion. Plate and screw fixation can be used to stabilize mandibular fractures with cortical bone loss; however, the plate must be carefully contoured to the normal shape of the fractured bone. If open reduction is performed in patients with low fracture-assessment scores, autogenous cancellous bone grafts can be used to facilitate healing.

Dogs with severely comminuted fractures of the vertical ramus may be treated with a tape muzzle, relying on the heavy masseter muscle to maintain fragment alignment. In some cases, maxillomandibular fixation can be used to maintain mandibular and maxillary alignment. Although most cats tolerate maxillomandibular fixation well, dogs may be more difficult to manage postoperatively.

Preoperative Management

After the status of the animal has been determined, mandibular fractures in most dogs may be gently reduced and temporarily held in position with a tape muzzle until a definitive stabilizing procedure can be performed (see Fig. 32-2). However, mandibular fractures in cats and brachycephalic dogs cannot be easily stabilized with tape muzzles and are often not treated until surgery. Because the oral cavity contains numerous bacteria, prophylactic antibiotics are recommended. Infections are rare, however, because the vasculature supplying this area is well developed and plentiful. If infection is likely and if open reduction is performed, bacterial cultures can be submitted during surgery. Analgesics should be provided to posttraumatic animals (see Box 31-2 on p. 944) and Chapter 13.

Anesthesia

Anatomic reconstruction or realignment of mandibular cortices is mandatory to provide proper dental occlusion in many patients. Simple mandibular fractures can be anatomically reconstructed using bone cortex as a guide. With complex fractures or cortical bone loss, however, dental occlusion must be used to guide mandibular realignment. Because mandibular and maxillary teeth closely interdigitate, precise alignment of upper and lower arcades is necessary. If precise dental occlusion cannot be determined with the endotracheal tube in place, it should be repositioned through a pharyngotomy incision (Fig. 32-11). This allows the mouth to be completely closed during surgery, which facilitates determination of adequate dental occlusion. After surgery, the endotracheal tube is removed, and the pharyngotomy incision is allowed to granulate closed.

Surgical Anatomy

The bones of the maxilla and mandibular body are easily palpated and surgically approached through skin and subcutaneous tissue (Fig. 32-12). The maxillary nerve (branch of the trigeminal nerve that innervates cutaneous muscles of the head, nasal, and oral cavities, and muscles of mastication) passes rostrally through the alar canal and can be injured with maxillary fractures. The mandibular alveolar nerve, which is sensory to the teeth of the mandible, passes through the mandibular canal along with the mandibular alveolar artery. These structures are frequently damaged with mandibular fractures, although clinical signs are seldom evident. Tooth roots must be avoided when placing implants in the maxilla or mandible. The approach to the ramus and temporomandibular joint involves dissection and elevation of the masseter muscle (Fig. 32-13). The parotid duct and gland and the facial nerve are dorsal and superficial to the masseter muscle and should be avoided.

> NOTE: The shape of the mandibular canal and the presence of major vessels and nerves preclude intramedullary pin fixation of mandibular fractures.

Positioning

Animals are positioned in ventral recumbency for treatment of maxillary fractures and dorsal recumbency for treatment of mandibular fractures. The surgical field, including the mouth, is aseptically prepared for surgery. If an autogenous cancellous bone graft is required, animals may be positioned in dorsal recumbency with forelimbs tied caudally. The skin over the proximal humerus is also prepared for aseptic surgery. This positioning allows simultaneous access to the proximal humeral metaphysis and oral cavity. Because this is an uncommon limb position for obtaining a bone graft, care must be taken to orient oneself before the procedure. Additionally, the graft should be harvested first to avoid bacterial contamination of the donor site. Draping may be performed to include access to the oral cavity.

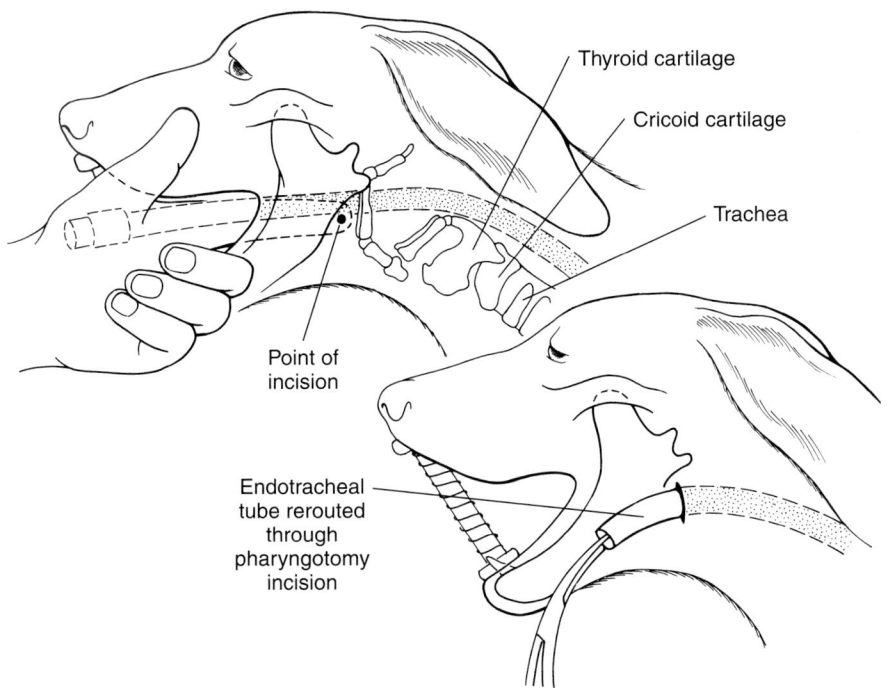

Thyroid cartilage

Cricoid cartilage

Trachea

Point of incision

Endotracheal tube rerouted through pharyngotomy incision

FIG. 32-11
To place an endotracheal tube through a pharyngotomy incision, insert an index finger into the oral cavity and locate the pharyngeal area immediately cranial to the hyoid bones. Incise skin, subcutaneous tissue, and mucous membrane to create a passage for the endotracheal tube. Place a forceps through the surgically created passage to grasp the endotracheal tube (with connector removed) and reroute it.

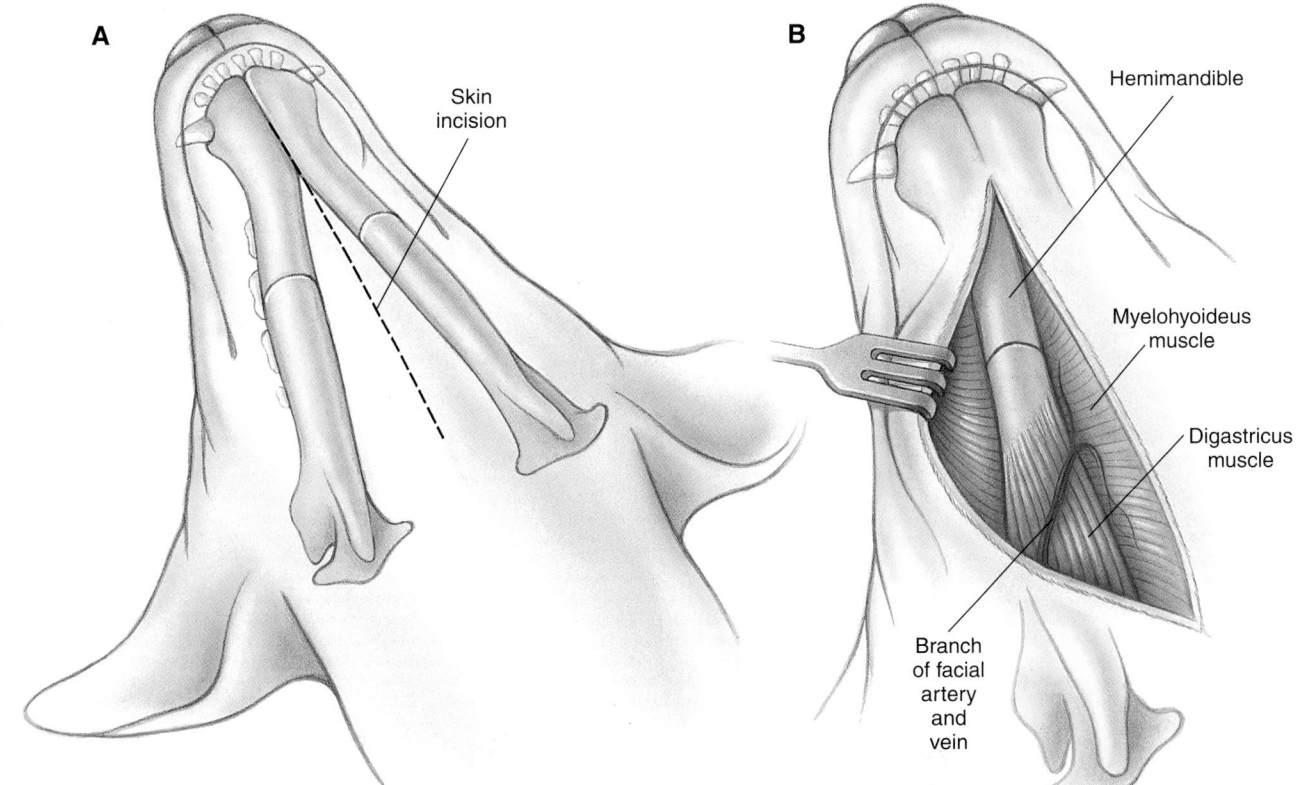

A

Skin incision

B

Hemimandible

Myelohyoideus muscle

Digastricus muscle

Branch of facial artery and vein

FIG. 32-12
A, For a ventral approach to the mandible, make a ventral midline incision in the skin between the mandibles. **B,** Elevate soft tissue from the mandibles to expose the fracture(s), but maintain the digastricus muscle attachment.

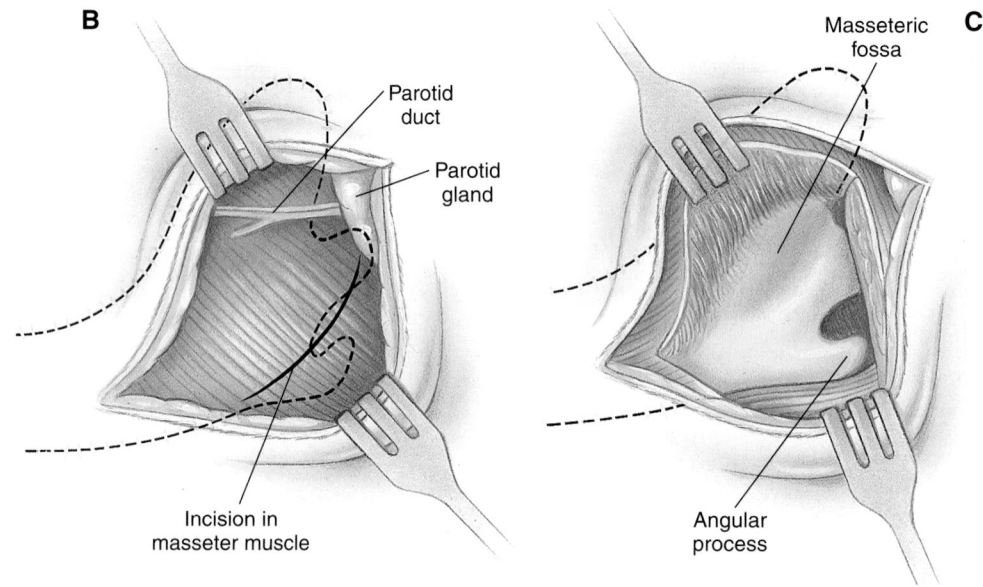

FIG. 32-13
A, For a lateral approach to the ramus of the mandible, make a skin incision over the ventrolateral border of the caudal mandibular body, and separate the platysma muscle to expose the masseter muscle. **B** and **C,** Incise and elevate the masseter muscle from the ramus to expose its lateral mandibular surface and angular and coronoid processes.

SURGICAL TECHNIQUE
Open Reduction of Mandibular Fractures

With bilateral mandibular fractures, make a ventral midline incision in the skin between the mandibles. Move this incision in either direction to expose both mandibles. If only one mandible is involved, make a ventral skin incision directly over that mandible. Elevate soft tissue from the mandibles to expose the fracture(s). Maintain the digastricus muscle attachment (see Fig. 32-12). Reduce and stabilize the fracture (see p. 1027). If there is a segmental fracture of the mandibular body, stabilize the caudal fracture first.

Because there is little musculature around the mandibular body, reduction usually is easily accomplished. Open reduction of the mandibular cortex will realign the teeth.

Evaluate the oral cavity for open wounds. If large wounds are present, close the mucosa partially to decrease their size. To allow postoperative drainage, do not completely close contaminated wounds. Place a Penrose drain if infection is present or likely. Close the surgical wound by suturing apposing layers.

Open Reduction of Fractures of the Vertical Ramus and Temporomandibular Joint

Make a skin incision over the ventrolateral border of the caudal mandibular body, and separate the platysma muscle to expose the digastricus muscle. Elevate the masseter muscle from the ramus to expose its lateral mandibular surface and angular and coronoid processes (see Fig. 32-13). Reduce the fracture and stabilize it (see p. 1027). Repair large, open wounds of the oral cavity as described

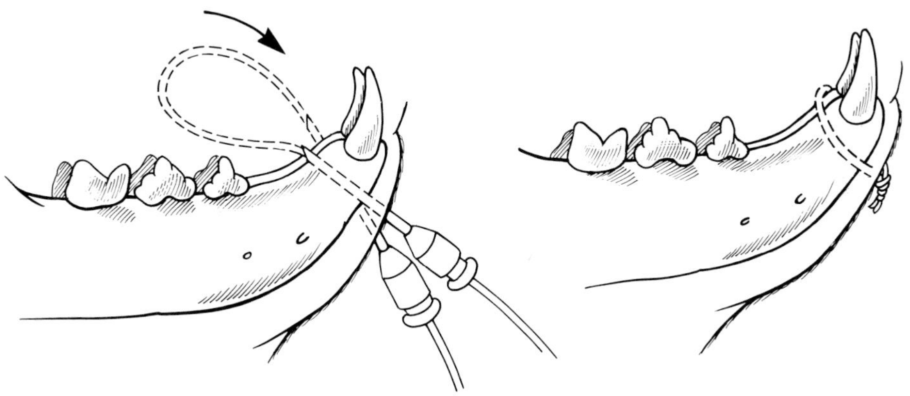

FIG. 32-14
To stabilize mandibular symphyseal fractures, use a 16-gauge or 18-gauge hypodermic needle to place the cerclage wire.

on p. 1026. Close the surgical wound by suturing apposing layers.

Open Reduction of Maxillary Fractures

Make a skin incision over the fracture(s), and gently elevate the soft tissue from the bone. Reduce the fracture and stabilize it. Repair large, open wounds to the oral cavity as described on p. 1026.

Stabilization of Mandibular Symphyseal Fractures

Symphyseal fractures are best treated with cerclage wire. A single wire is effective treatment for symphyseal fractures. Symphyseal cerclage wires encircle the mandible caudal to the canine teeth. The wire can be removed once the fracture has healed (generally 6 to 8 weeks) by cutting it with wire scissors, where it is exposed behind the canine teeth.

Make a small nick in the skin overlying the ventral aspect of the symphysis. Insert a 16-gauge or 18-gauge hypodermic needle through this nick and along one lateral mandibular surface (under the subcutaneous tissue). Exit the needle in the oral cavity caudal to the canine tooth, and thread an 18-gauge or 20-gauge wire through the needle. Reposition the needle on the opposite side of the mandible, curve the wire across and behind the canine teeth, and reinsert it through the hypodermic needle. Exit the wire from the skin incision at the original insertion point. Once the fracture is reduced, tighten the wire. Leave the ends of the wire exposed through the skin incision, and bend them to decrease the possibility of injury to the owner (Fig. 32-14).

Stabilization of Mandibular Transverse Fractures

Transverse fractures should be realigned and compressed.

Apply one or two interfragmentary wires perpendicular to the fracture line to achieve compression (Fig. 32-15, A to C). Alternatively, if the patient's fracture warrants more rigid fixation, use an external fixator or compression bone plate.

Stabilization of Oblique Fracture Lines

Oblique fractures may override when parallel wires are tightened so that alternative wire patterns may be required.

Stabilize caudal to rostral (or vice versa) oblique fracture lines with two wires placed at right angles to each other.

More than one wire may be placed through a single drill hole.

Stabilize medial to lateral (or vice versa) oblique fracture lines with two wires placed perpendicular to each other in two perpendicular planes.

In both cases the second wire prevents overriding of the fracture as the wires are tightened (Fig. 32-15, *D* to *F*).

Stabilization of Comminuted Fractures

Stabilize comminuted fractures that have long fracture lines and can be anatomically reconstructed with interfragmentary wires (Fig. 32-15, G). Support the reconstructed fracture with a bone plate or external fixator. Bridge comminuted fractures that cannot be reconstructed with a bone plate or external fixator. Pay careful attention to ensure that dental occlusion is appropriate.

SUTURE MATERIALS AND SPECIAL INSTRUMENTS

A low-rpm power drill is helpful for placing fixation pins. A pin chuck or power drill is used to drill holes in the bone for wires and to place Kirschner wires. Dental resin composite is needed for canine tooth bonding. Polymethylmethacrylate or dental acrylic may be used to form the acrylic splint. Bone-plating equipment is needed for plates.

POSTOPERATIVE CARE AND ASSESSMENT

Postoperative radiographs should be evaluated for implant position. Occlusion of the teeth, however, takes precedence over accurate fragment reduction. Dental occlusion is more readily determined on physical examination than with ra-

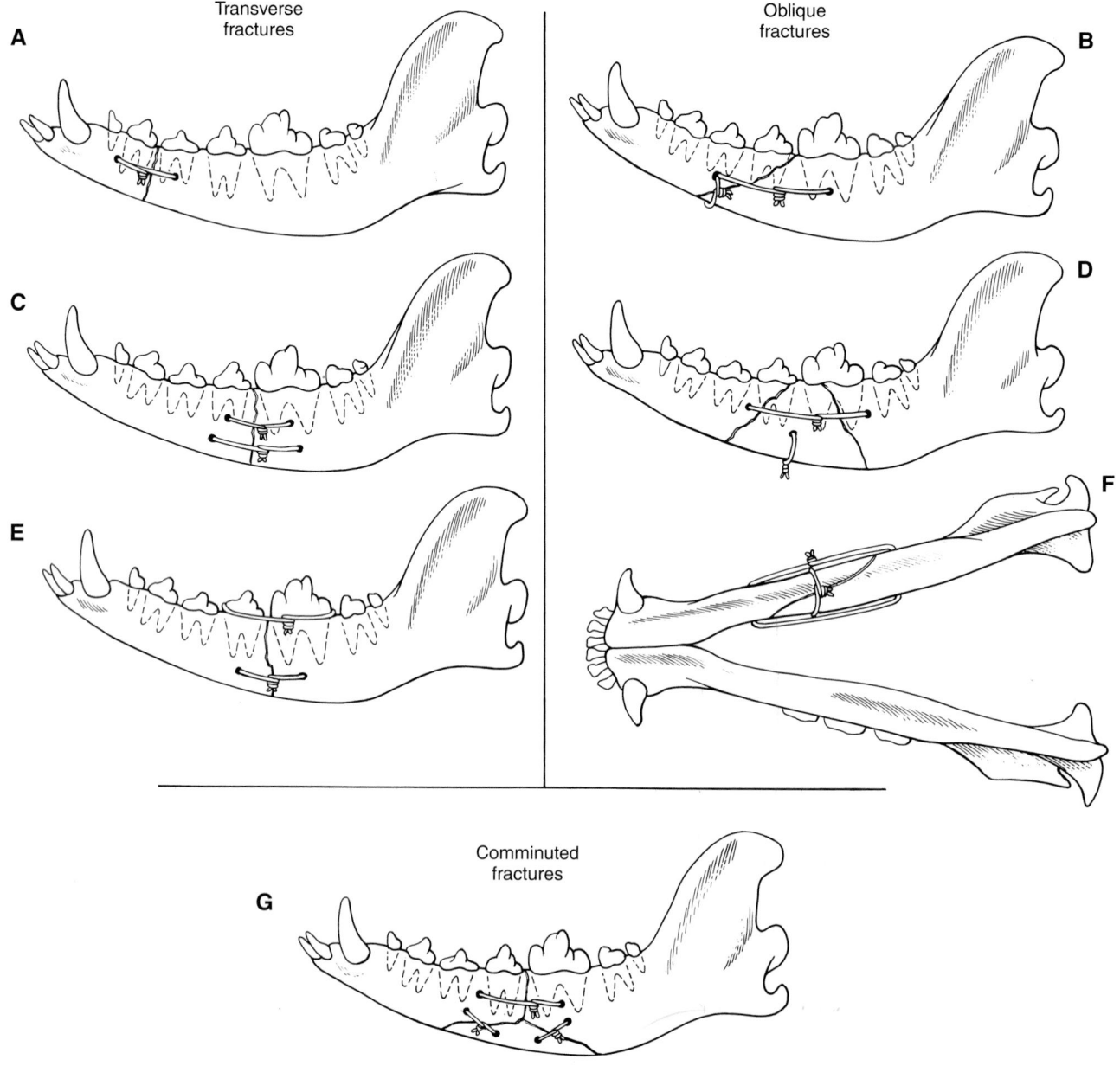

FIG. 32-15

Interfragmentary wire may be used to stabilize mandibular fractures. **A** to **C,** For transverse fractures, wires may be placed perpendicular to the fracture line. **D,** Stabilize caudorostral, long, oblique fracture lines with two wires placed at right angles to each other. Wire around the ventral mandibular border prevents the caudal segment from displacing rostrally when the interfragmentary wire is tightened. **E** and **F,** To stabilize long, oblique, slab fractures, place wire through both bone segments and around the ventral mandibular border to prevent overriding of bone segments. **G,** Secure large butterfly fragments with interfragmentary wires.

diographs. Occasionally a tape muzzle can be used postoperatively to support the fixation (see Fig. 32-2). When muzzles are used as primary fixation or support for internal fixation, the skin on the ventral surface of the mandible may become irritated. The skin should be carefully cleaned and treated with a soothing ointment. External fixators should be evaluated postoperatively to ensure that the clamps or acrylic are not too close to the skin.

The animal should be fed soft food until the fracture heals; chew toys should be avoided. Patients with maxillomandibu-

lar fixation who have difficulty with oral feeding may benefit from an esophageal feeding tube (see p. 97). Owners should be instructed not to allow the animal to chew on rocks or sticks or play tug-of-war. Clients should be instructed to clean the skin beneath a tape muzzle daily and to clean the area around external fixation pins. Oral chlorhexidine rinses are recommended twice daily for patients with interdental splints to minimize gingivitis associated with entrapped debris. The animal should be reevaluated 2 weeks postoperatively and sutures removed. Radiographs should be obtained after 6 weeks to evaluate healing and repeated every 6 weeks thereafter until healing is complete. Dental composite used for tooth bonding may break prematurely and require reapplication if healing is not complete. Dental composite, intraoral wires, and external fixators should be removed when fractures are healed; interfragmentary wires and bone plates and screws are not removed unless they cause problems. Sectioning the interdental splint and removing it segmentally helps avoid fracturing teeth during this maneuver.

COMPLICATIONS

The prognosis for healing of mandibular and maxillary fractures is generally excellent if proper techniques of fracture management are observed. However, complication rates have been reported as high as 34% in dogs and 24% in cats.[1,2] Common complications include malocclusion and osteomyelitis. Many animals learn to compensate for malocclusion; however, temporomandibular arthritis, impaired mastication, abnormal tooth wear, plaque and tartar accumulation, and periodontitis are possible sequelae.

PROGNOSIS

Mild malocclusion associated with interference of teeth can be treated by remodeling the involved teeth to allow clearance. Severe malocclusion may require tooth extraction or corrective osteotomy. Osteomyelitis (see p. 1353) and bone sequestration should be treated by sequestrectomy, removal of loose implants, mandibular stabilization (if necessary), cancellous bone autografts, culture/sensitivity, and appropriate antibiotics. Nonunions are treated with appropriate stabilization and cancellous bone autografts. Partial mandibulectomy (see p. 343) is an option for treatment of chronic nonunion of the mandible.

> NOTE: Mandibular and maxillary fractures generally heal without a large callus.

References

Umphlet RC, Johnson AL: Mandibular fractures in the cat: a retrospective study, *Vet Surg* 17:333, 1988.

Umphlet RC, Johnson AL: Mandibular fractures in the dog: a retrospective study of 157 cases, *Vet Surg* 17:272, 1988.

Suggested Reading

Bennett JW, Kapatkin AS, Manfra-Marretta S: Dental composite for the fixation of mandibular fractures and luxations in 11 cats and six dogs, *Vet Surg* 23:190, 1994.

This article provides an excellent description of the technique for dental composite stabilization achieved by bonding both pairs of canine teeth together. The technique was applied to stabilize 21 mandibular fractures in dogs and cats. All fractures healed with normal occlusion.

Boudrieau RJ: Fractures of the maxilla. In Johnson AL, Houlton JEF, Vannini R, editors: *AO principles of fracture management in the dog and cat,* Thieme, NY, 2005, AO Publishing.

This chapter provides an up-to-date collection of operative techniques for stabilizing maxillary fractures in small animals.

Detailed descriptions of procedures for wire application and miniplate application are included.

Boudrieau RJ: Fractures of the mandible. In Johnson AL, Houlton JEF, Vannini R, editors: *AO principles of fracture management in the dog and cat,* Thieme, NY, 2005, AO Publishing.

This chapter provides an up-to-date collection of operative techniques for stabilizing mandibular fractures in small animals. Detailed descriptions of procedures for wire application, plate application (including locking plate technology), and external fixation are included.

Owen MR, Langley Hobbs SJ, Moores AP et al: Mandibular fracture repair in dogs and cats using epoxy resin and acrylic external skeletal fixation, *Vet Comp Orthop Traumatol* 17:189, 2004.

A retrospective study detailing the patient tolerance and fracture healing associated with acrylic pin external fixator fixation of mandibular fractures. The study documents the results of mandibular fractures in 17 dogs and 8 cats.

SCAPULAR FRACTURES

DEFINITIONS

Scapular fractures may occur through the body, spine, acromion, neck, supraglenoid tuberosity, and glenoid cavity.

GENERAL CONSIDERATIONS AND CLINICALLY RELEVANT PATHOPHYSIOLOGY

Scapular fractures are relatively uncommon in dogs and cats (approximately 1.2% of canine fractures) because the large muscles surrounding the scapula protect it from direct injury (Cook et al, 1997). Common concurrent injuries include thoracic injuries (73%), such as pulmonary contusions, pneumothorax, rib fractures, and traumatic cardiomyopathy; and nerve injury (23%), such as brachial plexus and suprascapular nerve contusions (Cook et al, 1997). Thus cardiorespiratory parameters and neurologic function of the limb should be determined preoperatively in animals presenting with scapular fractures. It is difficult to determine the status of the suprascapular nerve preoperatively.

Scapular fractures are classified according to location (e.g., body, spine, acromion, neck, supraglenoid tubercle, and glenoid cavity), involvement of the articular surface, and stability. Scapular body and spine fractures may be minimally displaced and stable, requiring only conservative therapy. However, transverse fractures of the scapular body and spine may allow the scapula to fold on itself, resulting in a poor cosmetic appearance if the fractures are not reduced and stabilized. Similarly, comminuted fractures may be unstable and candidates for internal fixation. Avulsions of the supraglenoid tuberosity occur in immature dogs and are physeal separations subjected to the pull of the biceps muscle that should be stabilized with internal fixation methods.

> NOTE: Fractures of the scapular neck (if displaced and unstable) and glenoid cavity (intraarticular fractures) may affect scapulohumeral joint function and thus should be anatomically reduced and stabilized with internal fixation methods.

DIAGNOSIS
Clinical Presentation

Signalment. Although traumatic scapular fractures may occur in animals at any age, young large animals are at increased risk.

History. Affected animals usually have a history of trauma.

Physical Examination Findings

Most affected animals present with a non–weight-bearing lameness. Swelling may occur over the scapula, and crepitation may be obvious when this region is palpated.

Diagnostic Imaging

Radiographs of the scapula should include lateral and caudocranial views. Lateral views may be obtained by either placing the scapula dorsal to the vertebral column (preferred) or by superimposing the scapula over the cranial thorax. To avoid superimposing scapulae, the contralateral forelimb should be retracted away from the affected limb during the lateral projection. A distal-proximal or axial projection provides a skyline view of the scapular spine and cranial and caudal scapular borders. Because of the manipulation necessary for diagnostic radiographs, some animals may require sedation (see p. 933).

Laboratory Findings

Specific laboratory abnormalities are not present in animals with scapular fractures. Traumatized animals undergoing surgery should have sufficient blood work done to determine the optimal anesthetic regimen.

DIFFERENTIAL DIAGNOSIS

Animals with forelimb lameness attributable to scapular fractures should be carefully evaluated for concurrent nerve damage (brachial plexus, spinal cord trauma) before surgery. Fractures are generally evident radiographically. Special attention should also be given to identifying concurrent thoracic injuries.

MEDICAL MANAGEMENT

Conservative treatment with a Velpeau sling (see p. 949) and limited exercise are appropriate for most closed, minimally displaced fractures of the scapular body and spine in dogs that will heal rapidly. However, fractures of the articular surface must be treated with open reduction, anatomic alignment, and rigid fixation (see later discussion). Velpeau slings should be left on for no more than 2 to 3 weeks and care taken to prevent contracture of the carpus.

SURGICAL TREATMENT

Surgical treatment is indicated for unstable extraarticular fractures and for intraarticular fractures. Fixation systems applicable for scapular fractures are plates and screws, orthopedic wire, and Kirschner wires. The most appropriate fixation method should be determined based on fracture-assessment score and fracture location; however, bone

 BOX 32-2

Implant Use for Fractures of the Scapular Body and Spine According to Fracture-Assessment Score (FAS)

FAS 0 to 3
- Conservative therapy
- Bone plate and screws

FAS 4 to 7
- Conservative therapy
- Bone plate and screws

FAS 8 to 10
- Conservative therapy
- Interfragmentary wires
- Bone plate and screws

BOX 32-3

Implant Use for Scapular Articular Fractures According to Fracture-Assessment Score (FAS)

FAS 0 to 3
- Lag screws

FAS 4 to 7
- Lag screws

FAS 8 to 10
- Lag screws
- Tension band wire

plates and screws offer the most stable fixation (Boxes 32-2 and 32-3).

> NOTE: Plates and screw fixation is preferred to ensure optimal outcome for limb function.

Application of Orthopedic Wire

Orthopedic wire may be used as interfragmentary wire for fractures of the scapular spine and body (Figs. 32-16 and 32-17) or in conjunction with Kirschner wires as a tension band for avulsions of the supraglenoid tuberosity (Fig. 32-18) in animals with high fracture-assessment scores. Larger gauge (18 to 22) wire is used for interfragmentary fixation, whereas smaller gauge (20 to 24) wire is used in a figure-eight pattern (see Table 32-1). Large-gauge wire may be difficult to position and tighten unless application guidelines are followed (see p. 989).

> NOTE: Portions of the scapula are thin, and large-gauge wire may pull through when tightened.

Application of Kirschner Wires

Kirschner wires can be used as crossed pins to stabilize transverse fractures of the scapular neck (Fig. 32-19) in animals with high fracture-assessment scores (see p. 953). Kirschner wires with figure-eight orthopedic wire may also be used for tension band fixation of avulsion fractures or repair of acromial osteotomies (see Fig. 32-18).

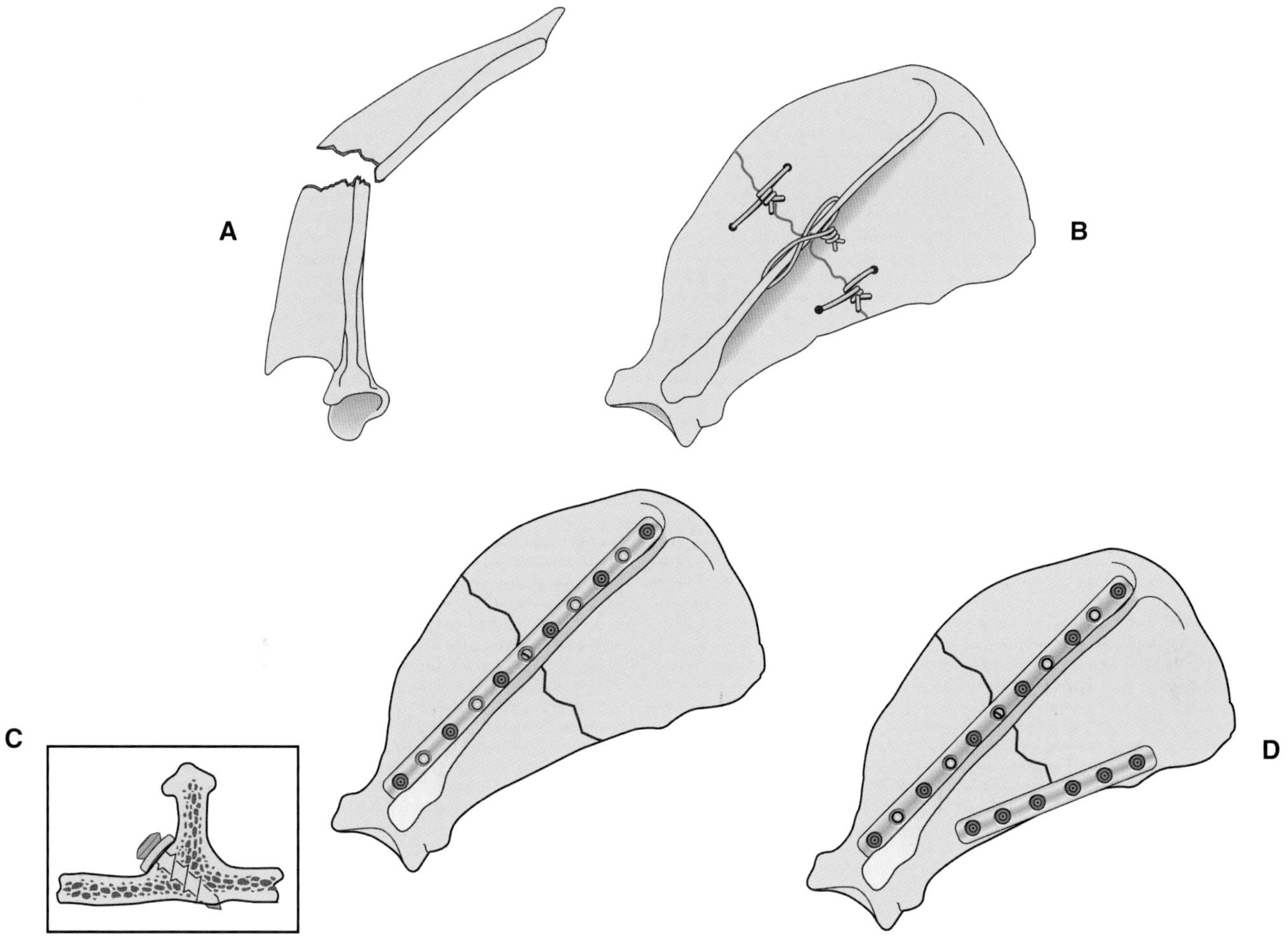

FIG. 32-16
A, Transverse fracture of the scapular body may cause unsightly folding deformities.
B, Orthopedic wire may be used to repair these fractures in some patients with a high fracture-assessment score. **C** and **D,** The same fracture in most patients should be stabilized with one or two veterinary cuttable plates. (Parts B, C, and D modified from Johnson AL, Dunning D: *Atlas of orthopedic surgical procedures of the dog and cat,* ed 1, St Louis, 2005, Saunders.)

Application of Bone Plates and Screws

Veterinary cuttable plates may be used to stabilize fractures of the scapular body and neck (see Fig. 32-16). Veterinary cuttable plates permit more screws per unit of plate length, making them particularly useful in scapular fractures. Plates applied to the body of the scapula must be secured with screws placed into the relatively thick bone that is under the spine. Additionally the caudal border of the scapula also offers thicker bone stock. Small (2.7- and 2.0-mm) angle and T plates may also be used to stabilize neck fractures (see Fig. 32-19). With neck fractures, plates are placed under the suprascapular nerve, and the nerve must be protected from trauma while the plate is positioned. Cancellous and cortical bone screws are used as lag screws for stabilizing avulsion fractures of the supraglenoid tuberosity and T fractures of the neck (see Figs. 32-18 and 32-19).

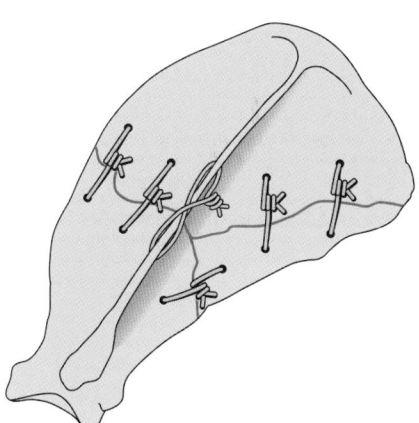

FIG. 32-17
Comminuted fractures of the scapular body can be reconstructed with orthopedic wire in patients with high fracture-assessment scores.

A   B   C

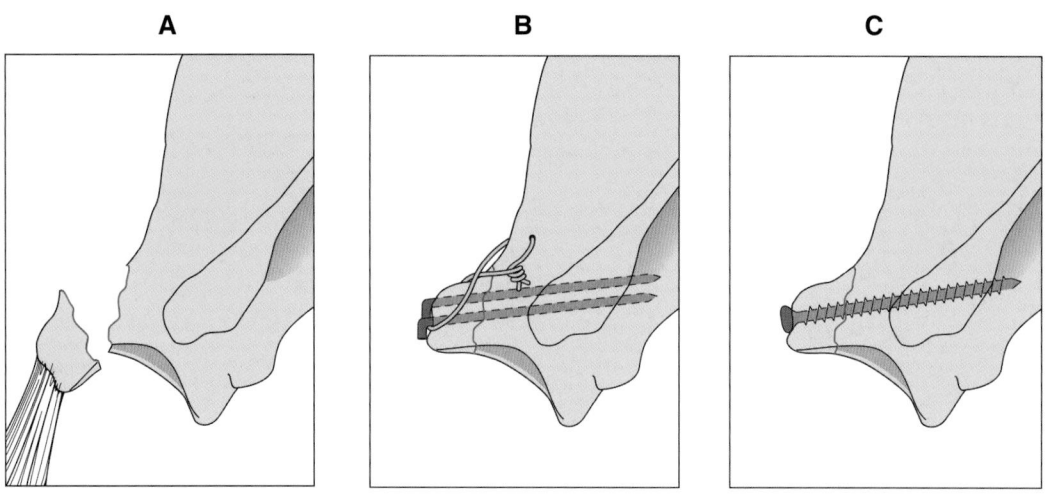

FIG. 32-18
To overcome the pull of the biceps brachii muscle **(A)**, avulsions of the supraglenoid tuber-osity are treated with a tension band wire **(B)** in patients with a high fracture-assessment score or a lag screw **(C)** in patients with a low fracture-assessment score.

A   B   C

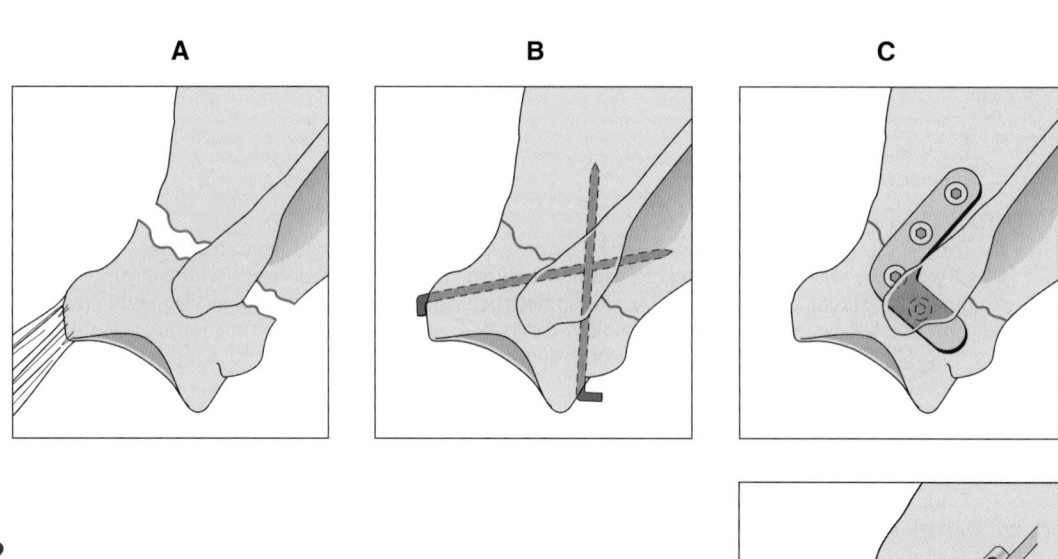

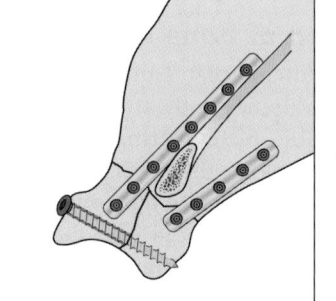

FIG. 32-19
A, Transverse fractures of the scapular neck are best treated with internal fixation. **B,** Crossed Kirschner wires may be used in some patients with high fracture-assessment scores. **C,** Angle plates may be used in those with low fracture-assessment scores. **D,** Articular fractures must be anatomically reconstructed and stabilized with a lag screw. The T fracture is then stabilized with a veterinary cuttable plate or plates. (Part D modified from Johnson AL, Dunning D: *Atlas of orthopedic surgical procedures of the dog and cat,* ed 1, St Louis, 2005, Saunders.)

D

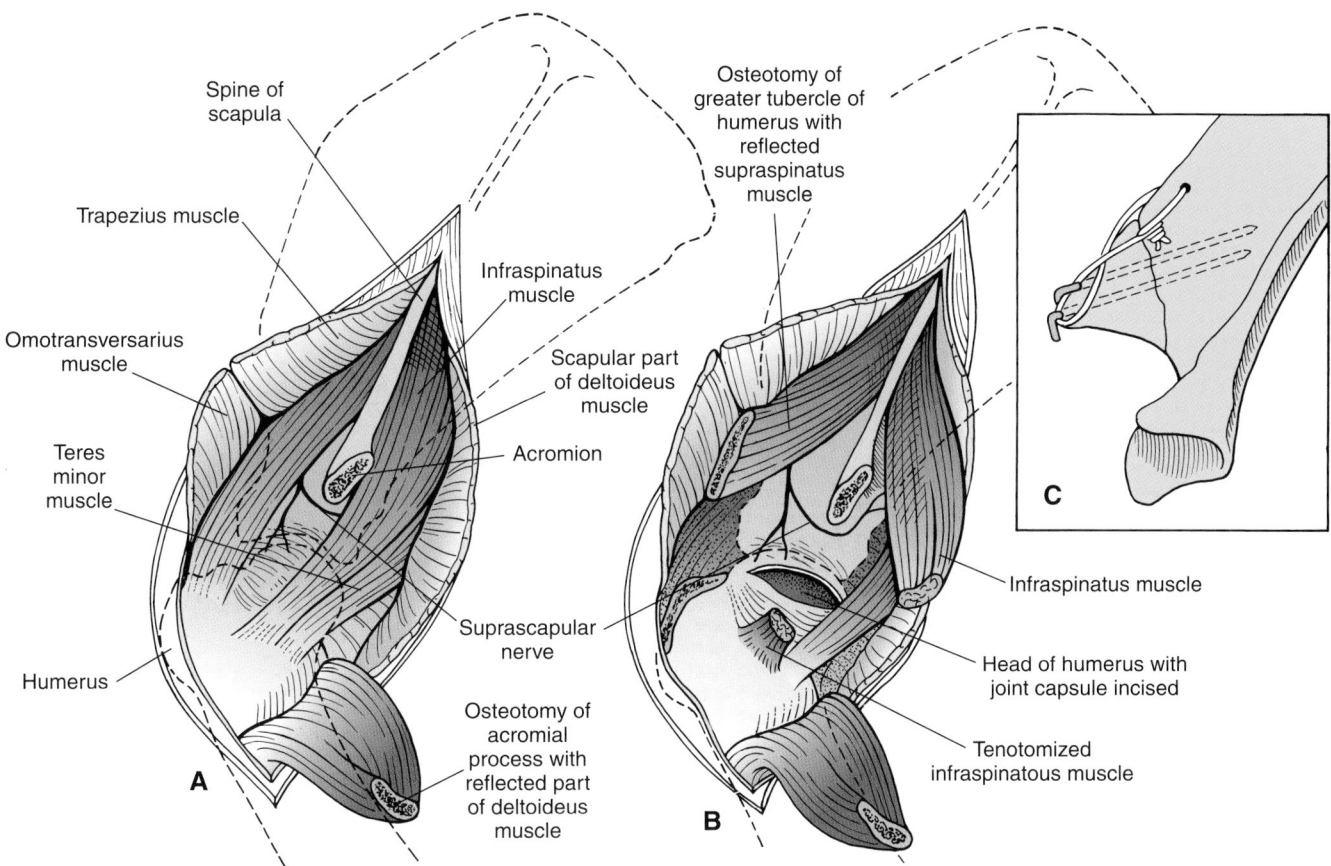

FIG. 32-20
A, For a lateral approach to the scapular neck, make a lateral skin incision from the midportion of the scapular spine distally to the shoulder joint. Incise scapular attachments of the omotransversarius and trapezius muscles and scapular head of the deltoid muscle. Osteotomize the acromial process and reflect it distally with the acromial head of the deltoid muscle. **B,** For additional exposure, tenotomize the infraspinatus muscle, and if necessary, osteotomize the greater tubercle of the humerus. Incise the joint capsule to observe the articular surface during reduction of fractures involving the glenoid cavity. **C,** Repair the osteotomy(ies) of the acromial process (and greater tubercle) with a tension band wire.

NOTE: Articular fractures are best treated with anatomic reconstruction and lag screw compression.

Preoperative Management

The overall health of the animal should be determined before surgery. Thoracic radiography and electrocardiographic analysis are warranted before anesthetic induction. Analgesics should be provided to posttraumatic animals (see Box 31-2 on page 944 and Chapter 13).

Anesthesia

Refer to p. 943 for anesthetic management of patients with fractures.

Surgical Anatomy

Palpable landmarks of the scapula are the spine, the acromial process, and the cranial, dorsal, and caudal borders. The body and spine of the scapula are easily approached with dissection and elevation of muscle. The neck of the scapula is surrounded by muscles and tendons that support the scapulohumeral joint (Fig. 32-20). Osteotomy of the acromial process allows reflection of a portion of the deltoideus muscle and visualization of the joint. The suprascapular nerve and artery course over the scapular notch and under the acromial process, and care should be taken to avoid these structures (see Fig. 32-20). The axillary artery and nerve are located immediately caudal to the joint, but are not usually visualized with routine approaches.

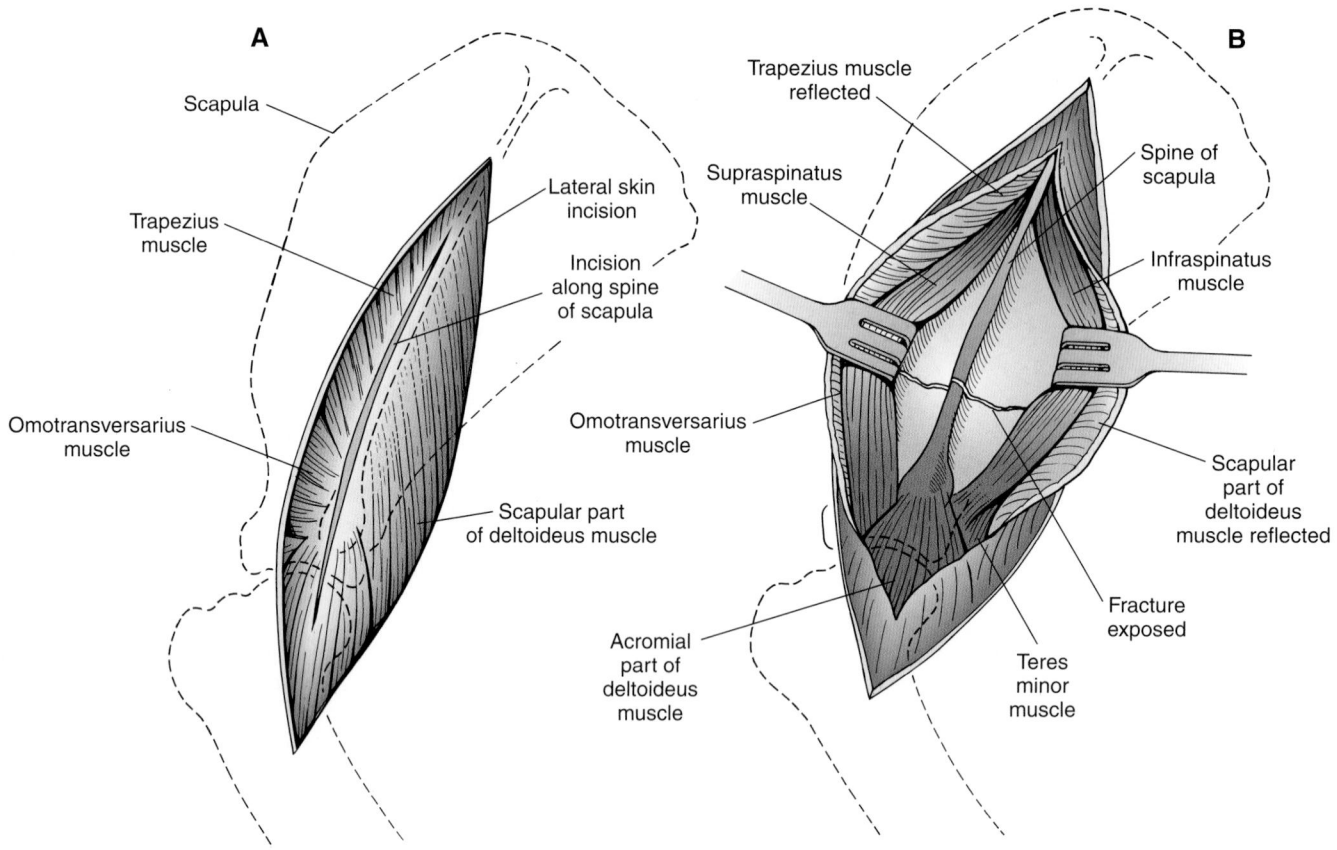

FIG. 32-21
A, For a lateral approach to the scapula, make a lateral skin incision extending the length of the spine distally to the shoulder joint. **B,** Incise the omotransversarius muscle, trapezius muscle, and scapular parts of the deltoid muscle from the spine. Elevate the supraspinatus and infraspinatus muscles from the scapular body to expose the fracture.

Positioning

The animal is placed in lateral recumbency with the affected side up. The entire scapular region should be prepared for aseptic surgery. For maximal maneuverability, drape out the forelimb. The most accessible site for a cancellous bone graft is the ipsilateral proximal humerus. If a bone graft is necessary (i.e., comminuted fractures with a fracture-assessment score less than 3), the prepped area should encompass the proximal humerus.

SURGICAL TECHNIQUE

Approaches to the scapulohumeral joint are described on pp. 1187 to 1189. Excision arthroplasty and shoulder arthrodesis are discussed on p. 1190.

Approach to the Scapular Spine and Body

Make a lateral skin incision extending the length of the spine distally to the shoulder joint (Fig. 32-21, A). Transect the omotransversarius muscle from the spine, and reflect it cranially. Incise trapezius and scapular parts of the deltoideus muscles from the spine and reflect them caudally. Incise the supraspinatus and infraspinatus muscular attachments to the

spine, and elevate these muscles from the scapular body (Fig. 32-21, B).

Approach to the Scapular Neck and Glenoid Cavity

Make a lateral skin incision from the middle portion of the scapular spine, and extend it distally to the shoulder joint. Expose the acromion process by incising attachments of the omotransversarius, trapezius, and scapular head of the deltoideus muscles to the scapula. Osteotomize the acromial process, and reflect it distally with the acromial head of the deltoideus muscle. Reflect the supraspinatus and infraspinatus muscles away from the scapular spine and neck. Take care to identify and protect the suprascapular nerve. If needed for complete joint exposure, tenotomize the infraspinatus muscle. Incise the joint capsule to observe the articular surface during reduction of fractures involving the glenoid cavity. For additional exposure, osteotomize the greater tubercle of the humerus and reflect the supraspinatus muscle. Close the joint capsule with interrupted sutures of 3-0 absorbable material. Reappose the infraspinatus tendon with a tendon suture (i.e., 3-loop pulley, Bunnell, or locking loop; see p. 1320) and support it with interrupted 0 or 2-0 nonabsorbable sutures. Repair the acromial osteotomy with a tension band wire (see Fig. 32-20, C). Repair the humeral osteotomy with lag screws. Suture deep fascia, subcutaneous tissue, and skin separately.

Stabilization of Scapular Body and Spine Fractures

If the patient fracture assessment (see p. 953) indicates rapid healing (score of 8 to 10), use conservative therapy for stable scapular body and spine fractures. If these fractures are grossly displaced or have resulted in folding of the body, consider open reduction and stabilization with veterinary cuttable plates or interfragmentary wiring (see Fig. 32-16). If the fracture-assessment score is 4 to 7 (e.g., older or larger dogs, in which healing may be delayed), treat displaced fractures of the scapular body and spine with open reduction and plate and screw fixation.

Fracture-assessment scores less than 3 indicate prolonged healing (see Box 32-2). If severe angulation of the joint is not present, treat severely comminuted fractures of the scapular body and spine that cannot be reconstructed in a conservative fashion. If the animal has multiple limb trauma or must bear weight on the limb, however, consider bridging the scapula with a bone plate or plates.

Stabilization of Avulsion Fractures of the Supraglenoid Tuberosity and Fractures of the Scapular Neck and Articular Surface

Treat avulsion fractures of the supraglenoid tuberosity with open reduction and placement of a lag screw or tension band wire. For simple fractures of the scapular neck, use open reduction and stabilization with crossed Kirschner wires, lag screws, or a small plate or plates to prevent malunion and subsequent malalignment of the articular surface. Reconstruct severely comminuted fractures involving the neck and buttress with a small plate or plates. Use cancellous bone autografts in conjunction with open reduction to promote healing in these patients.

Articular fractures must be anatomically reconstructed (see Box 32-3).

Stabilize fractures in animals with a patient fracture-assessment score of 8 to 10 with Kirschner wires or a tension band wire. Use plate or screw fixation in animals with lower patient fracture-assessment scores.

SUTURE MATERIALS AND SPECIAL INSTRUMENTS

Army-Navy, Myerding, and Hohmann retractors are useful for retracting muscles. A high-speed drill is necessary for application of a plate and can be used to drill holes for placement of orthopedic wire or Kirschner wires. Plating equipment is necessary for lag screw and plate placement.

POSTOPERATIVE CARE AND ASSESSMENT

Postoperative radiographs should be taken to evaluate fracture reduction and implant position. Radiographs should be repeated every 6 weeks until fractures are healed. If there is concern about implant stability during full weight bearing, a Velpeau sling (see p. 949) may be applied for a short time postoperatively; however, early return to function is preferred for joint fractures. Activity should be restricted to leash walking and physical rehabilitation until the fracture has healed. Physical rehabilitation (see Chapter 12) encourages controlled limb use and optimal limb function after fracture healing. Care must be taken to develop customized protocols for each patient depending on location of the fracture, stability and type of fracture fixation, potential for healing, abilities and attitudes of the patient, and willingness or ability of the client to participate in the animal's care (Tables 32-2 and 32-3). After fractures are healed, implant removal may be considered, but removal is usually unnecessary. If a Velpeau sling is applied, it should be kept clean and dry, and the owner should observe it daily for evidence of slippage or irritation.

COMPLICATIONS

Most scapular fractures heal without complication. Potential complications of scapular fracture repair include iatrogenic infection (with open reduction), malunion, delayed union, and secondary degenerative joint disease after articular fracture. Kirschner wires will migrate if the fracture is unstable.

PROGNOSIS

The prognosis for normal limb function is excellent unless malunion leads to scapulohumeral joint incongruity and secondary degenerative joint disease. Nonunions are uncommon after repair of scapular fractures because of the large muscle mass and good blood supply of this region.

Reference

Cook JL et al: Scapular fractures in dogs: epidemiology, classification, and concurrent injuries in 105 cases (1988-1994), *J Am Anim Hosp Assoc* 33:528, 1997.

Suggested Reading

Cabassu JP: Fractures of the scapula. In Johnson AL, Houlton JEF, Vannini R, editors: *AO principles of fracture management in the dog and cat,* Thieme, NY, 2005, AO Publishing.
This chapter provides an up-to-date collection of operative techniques for stabilizing scapular fractures in small animals. Detailed descriptions of tension band application and bone-plating procedures are included.
Jerram RM, Herron MR: Scapular fractures in dogs, *Comp Cont Educ Small Anim* 20:1254, 1998.
A review article providing a classification system for scapular fractures and a discussion of concurrent injuries, treatment options, and prognosis for scapular fractures.
Piermattei D, Johnson KA: *An atlas of surgical approaches to the bones and joints of the dog and cat,* ed 4, Philadelphia, 2004, WB Saunders.
An excellent reference for surgical approaches for repairing fractures of the scapula.

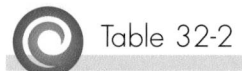 Table 32-2

Sample Physical Rehabilitation Protocol for Patients With Stable Scapular Body Fractures

ALL TREATMENTS BID	DAY 1 TO DAY 14	DAY 15 TO DAY 24	DAY 25 UNTIL HEALED	HEALED TO RETURN TO FUNCTION
Heat therapy		10 min	10 min	
Massage	5 min	5 min	5 min	
Passive range of motion (repetitions)	15*	15*		
Therapeutic exercise-total time	10 min	15 min	15 min	25–45 min
Walk/land treadmill	10 min	5 min	5 min	>10 min
Balancing	+	+	+	+
Obstacles	+	+	+	+
Weaving		+	+	+
Circles		+	+	+
Hills				+
Stairs				+
Jog/run				+
Underwater treadmill		10 min	10 min	>15 min
Swimming				5–10 min
Cryotherapy	15 min	15 min	15 min	PRN

BID, Twice a day; +, perform modality (see Chapter 12); PRN, as needed.
*Perform passive range of motion for all joints of the affected limb.

 Table 32-3

Sample Physical Rehabilitation Protocol for Patients With Stable Shoulder Fractures

ALL TREATMENTS BID	DAY 1 TO DAY 14	DAY 15 TO DAY 24	DAY 25 UNTIL HEALED	HEALED TO RETURN TO FUNCTION
Heat therapy		10 min	10 min	
Passive range of motion (repetitions)	20*	20*	10–15*	Stop-when ROM N
Therapeutic exercise-total time	10 min	15 min	15 min	25–45 min
Walk/land treadmill	10 min	5 min	5 min	>10 min
Balancing	+	+	+	
Obstacles	+	+	+	+
Weaving				+
Circles				+
Hills				+
Stairs				+
Jog/run				+
Underwater treadmill		10 min	10 min	>15 min
Swimming				5–10 min
Cryotherapy	15 min	15 min	15 min	PRN

BID, Twice a day; ROM, range of motion; N, normal; +, perform modality (see Chapter 12); PRN, as needed.
*Perform passive range of motion for all joints of the affected limb.

HUMERAL FRACTURES

HUMERAL DIAPHYSEAL AND SUPRACONDYLAR FRACTURES

DEFINITIONS

Humeral diaphyseal fractures result in disruption of the continuity of the diaphyseal cortical bone. An IM pin that is placed into the humerus in a **normograde** fashion is inserted from the greater tubercle across the fracture line and seated in the medial epicondyle. A pin that is placed in the humerus in a **retrograde** fashion is inserted at the fracture line, driven proximally to exit the greater tubercle, and after fracture reduction, driven across the fracture and into the distal fragment.

GENERAL CONSIDERATIONS AND CLINICALLY RELEVANT PATHOPHYSIOLOGY

High-velocity injuries (e.g., motor vehicle accidents, gunshot injuries, and blunt trauma) are a common cause of humeral fractures in veterinary patients. When evaluating a patient subjected to a high-velocity injury, it is important not to focus on the obvious fracture but to complete a thorough examination of all body systems to rule out any concurrent injury. Common injuries associated with fractures of the humerus include chest wall trauma, pneumothorax, and pulmonary contusion. Radiographs should be taken to assess the degree of thoracic injury before anesthesia. The radial nerve courses from medial to lateral in the musculospiral groove of the distal humerus. Radial nerve injury may occur with fractures involving the distal humerus; therefore a careful assessment of the animal's neurologic status is essential. Reflexes and proprioception may be difficult to assess due to muscle trauma and tissue swelling associated with the fracture. However, superficial pain sensation should be easily elicited on the dorsum of the paw if the radial nerve is functional.

DIAGNOSIS

Clinical Presentation

Signalment. Any age, sex, or breed of dog or cat may be affected.

History. Motor vehicle accidents cause the majority of humeral diaphyseal fractures. Other modes of injury include gunshots and falls.

Physical Examination Findings

Patients with humeral diaphyseal fractures are usually non–weight-bearing and exhibit varying degrees of limb swelling. Pain and crepitus may be elicited on limb manipulation. Affected animals often drag the limb when walking and may not lift the paw when proprioception is checked. This may cause the examiner to assume that neurologic injury is present. However, similar findings may occur because of the orthopedic injury alone if pain and swelling make the patient reluctant to move the limb when proprioception is evaluated.

Diagnostic Imaging

Most of these animals are painful and require sedation or general anesthesia for proper positioning to obtain quality radiographs (see p. 933). Caudocranial or craniocaudal and lateral views are necessary to assess the extent of bone and soft tissue injury. Radiographs can be taken under anesthesia just before surgery, but this decreases the time available for planning the surgical procedure. If the fracture is comminuted and if bone plate fixation is contemplated, radiographs of the contralateral limb are useful for assessment of bone length and shape. These radiographs assist in proper contouring of the bone plate.

Laboratory Findings

Complete blood count and serum chemistry evaluation should be done to assess the status of the animal for anesthesia. Consistent laboratory abnormalities are not present.

DIFFERENTIAL DIAGNOSIS

Differential diagnoses include shoulder or elbow luxation, severe soft tissue contusion, and pathologic fractures secondary to neoplasia.

MEDICAL MANAGEMENT

Medical or conservative management is not indicated. Casts or splints are not indicated for repair of humeral fractures because the scapulohumeral joint cannot be effectively immobilized.

SURGICAL TREATMENT

IM pins and orthopedic wire, interlocking nails, IM pins plus external skeletal fixation, external skeletal fixators alone, and bone plates may be used to repair humeral fractures. The implant system chosen should reflect the patient fracture-assessment score (Box 32-4). Factors that negatively affect healing include the presence of multiple inju-

 BOX 32-4

Implant Use for Fractures of the Humeral Diaphysis According to Fracture-Assessment Score (FAS)

FAS 0 to 3
- Bone plate and IM pin
- Bone plate and screws
- Interlocking nail
- Modified Type Ib external fixator with IM pin

FAS 4 to 7
- External skeletal fixation with or without IM pin
- Bone plate and screws
- Interlocking nail

FAS 8 to 10
- IM pin with cerclage wires or external fixator
- Flexible bone plate and screws

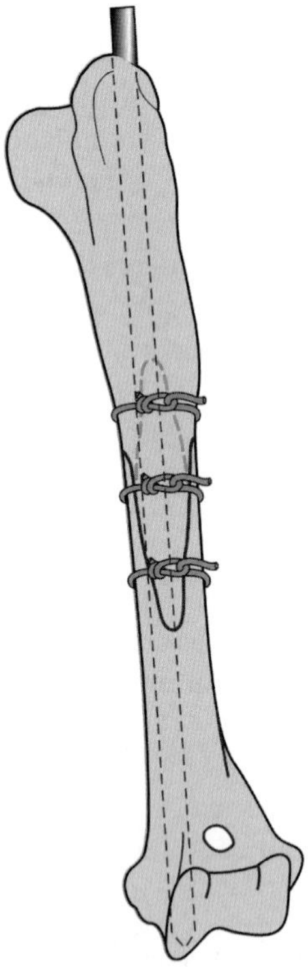

FIG. 32-22
Humeral fractures may be stabilized with an IM pin, which is either wedged into the most narrow part of the marrow cavity (isthmus) or guided through the epicondyloid ridge to seat into the medial epicondyle. Additional implants, such as cerclage wires, are needed to provide mechanical support. (Modified from Johnson AL, Dunning D: *Atlas of orthopedic surgical procedures of the dog and cat,* ed 1, St Louis, 2005, Saunders.)

ries, a large active patient, and the necessity for open reduction and tissue manipulation to reduce and apply interfragmentary compression. Implants that purchase bone are desirable if a long duration to healing is expected and if the implant needs to remain functional for 8 or more weeks. With shorter healing periods, implants that have frictional hold (smooth pins and wire) may be adequate.

Application of Intramedullary Pins

An IM pin can be used to stabilize humeral middiaphyseal fractures, providing excellent resistance to bending but not resistance to rotational forces or axial loading. Additional implants must be used to provide rotational and axial support for most fractures.

Two methods may be used to place an IM pin in the distal humerus: (1) wedging the pin into the narrowest part of the marrow cavity (isthmus) and (2) guiding the pin through the epicondyloid ridge to seat into the medial epicondyle (Fig. 32-22). Pin size depends on which method is chosen to seat the pin distally. If the pin is to be seated at the isthmus of the marrow cavity just proximal to the supracondylar foramen, a pin of the correct diameter to wedge into the isthmus can be determined at surgery or from the preoperative radiographs.

Similarly, if the pin is to be seated into the medial epicondyle, an estimation of space through the epicondyloid ridge can be made at surgery or by evaluating the preoperative radiograph. The medullary canal ends in the supracondylar area in many cats, and passage of the IM pin into the medial condyle is impossible (Langley-Hobbs and Straw, 2005). Pin placement is easier in cats because the marrow cavity has a uniform diameter, the bone has less curvature, and there is less of a soft tissue envelope covering the bone than in dogs. Care must be taken not to enter the supratrochlear foramen because the median nerve is in this area.

> NOTE: Estimate pin size from the preoperative radiograph.

An IM pin may be placed in a retrograde or normograde manner in the humerus (see p. 984). There are no advantages of one method over the other. Generally, if open reduction is performed, retrograde placement is used; if the fracture is to be stabilized through closed pinning, normograde placement is used. When retrograding an IM pin in the humerus, the pin is driven in a proximal direction from the fracture surface toward the shoulder joint. To ensure that the pin exits at the proper site proximally, the shaft of the pin is pressed against the medial and caudal surface of the marrow cavity. This forces the point of the pin to glide along the craniolateral cortex and exit craniolateral to the shoulder joint. This also "presets" the pin in the proximal fragment so that the distal pinpoint is directed toward the caudomedial cortex when the fracture is reduced and the pin is driven into the distal fragment. To place a pin in a normograde fashion, the pin is driven from proximal to distal starting at the craniolateral aspect of the greater tubercle and driven in line with the medullary canal to exit at the fracture. With either technique, the fracture is reduced and the pin driven distally. The depth of the pin into the distal fragment is estimated with a reference pin of equal length placed sagittal to the pin within the marrow cavity.

> NOTE: To align the pin properly with retrograde placement, press the shaft against the caudomedial cortex. This causes the pin to exit craniolateral to the shoulder joint.

Application of Interlocking Nails

Interlocking nails are used to stabilize both single and comminuted middiaphyseal humeral fractures (Fig. 32-23). The interlocking nail provides resistance to bending, rotational, and axial loading forces and can effectively bridge a nonreducible fracture. An open approach is used to reconstruct reducible fractures. An "open but don't touch" approach is used when major segment alignment is the goal. The size of nail selected should correspond to the width of the medullary canal at the isthmus of the bone. Although the medullary reaming may be normograde or retrograde, the inter-

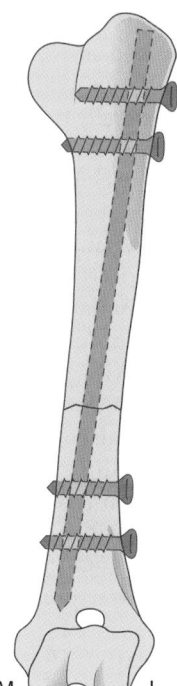

FIG. 32-23
Position of an interlocking nail in the humerus.

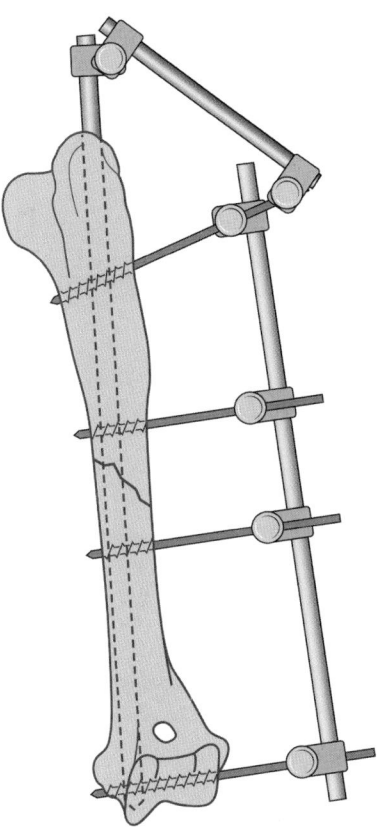

FIG. 32-24
To increase the strength of the fixation system, connect the IM pin to an external fixator frame to make a tie-in configuration. (Modified from Johnson AL Dunning D: *Atlas of orthopedic surgical procedures of the dog and cat,* ed 1, St Louis, 2005, Saunders.)

locking nail is inserted in a normograde manner starting on the ridge of the greater tubercle. A craniolateral approach (see p. 1052) is performed to expose the point of insertion. To facilitate nail insertion, the shoulder is flexed. The interlocking nail is "locked" with the application of bone screws. To avoid failures, two screws should be inserted in each major segment. In some cases, modified external fixator pins may be used to both lock the nail and be secured to an external connecting bar to provide additional support to unstable humeral fractures (Basinger and Suber, 2004).

Application of External Skeletal Fixation

Combining the bending support of an IM pin with axial and rotational support from an external fixator is useful to control all weight-bearing forces. An IM pin that occupies 50% to 60% of the medullary cavity is first inserted in a normograde or retrograde manner. An appropriate number of fixation pins and the external frame are then applied. The frame, number, and type of fixation pins vary with the rigidity of fixation desired and the length of time the fixator must remain in place (see p. 969). A single external bar with one fixation pin placed proximal to the fracture and one placed distal to the fracture is often added to support moderately stable fractures that are expected to heal in a relatively short time (less than 6 weeks). The proximal fixation pin is placed craniolaterally, just distal to the greater tubercle. A small Kirschner wire may be used as a "feeler" pin to identify the proper angle of insertion for the transfixation pin to avoid intersecting the IM pin (see p. 974). The condyle must be predrilled because this area is composed of dense cancellous

bone. The distal fixation pin is inserted laterally across the humeral condyle and centered within the condyle. The lateral epicondyle is palpated and the pin inserted 1 to 2 mm cranial and distal to the epicondylar prominence. The fixation pin is exited medially from the bone near the medial epicondylar prominence.

For unstable fractures, additional fixation pins may be added, but alternative strategies can also be used to enhance rigidity of the fixation while minimizing postoperative discomfort. Placing an additional external bar or connecting the IM pin to the external fixator frame to make a "tie-in" configuration increases the strength of the fixation system without adding to patient morbidity through placement of additional pins (Fig. 32-24). A modified Type Ib external skeletal fixator can be constructed by placing an additional fixation pin proximally at a 60-degree to 90-degree angle to the transfixation pin already in place and using a transfixation pin through the condyle that exits the skin on the medial aspect. An external bar connects the cranial pin to the medial aspect of the condylar transfixation pin (Fig. 32-25). The external bars are then connected with articulating external bars. Additional fixation pins can be added to the craniomedial or lateral external bars to achieve additional strength

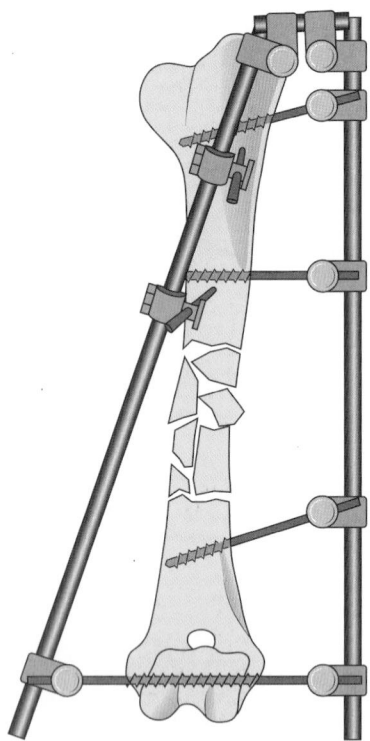

FIG. 32-25
External skeletal fixator (modified Type Ib shown here) may
be used with an IM pin or as the sole means of stabilizing a
comminuted fracture.

and stiffness. (Refer to p. 969 for guidelines on pin number,
design, and position.) If one or more fixation pins are placed
in the distal third of the humerus, care must be taken when
making the soft tissue tunnel and placing the fixation pins to
prevent radial nerve injury.

When external fixators are applied to the humerus as the
sole means of fixation, stress on fixation pins is high due to the
long distance from the external bar to their entrance into
the bone and the inability to use stronger bilateral frames.
Thoughtful preoperative planning and strict adherence to
principles of application are necessary to prevent fixator-
related complications and unacceptable patient morbidity.
"Open but don't touch" reduction may be necessary to achieve
adequate spatial alignment of the humerus. Achieving spatial
alignment can be assisted through placement of a temporary
IM pin through the intact proximal segment of intact bone,
across the area of comminution, and into the distal segment
of intact bone. In keeping with the concept of bridging osteosynthesis, bone fragments in the area of comminution should
not be reduced or manipulated. A modified Type Ib frame is
constructed as described above (see Fig. 32-25). The number
and type of fixation pins depend on the rigidity and duration
of function needed for the external skeletal fixator. It is better
to err on the side of being too rigid than to have a fixator that
is not rigid enough. The former can be destabilized as the
fracture heals, but the latter may result in premature fixation
failure and a high morbidity rate.

Application of Bone Plates and Screws

Bone plates provide needed stability and allow early return
to function when used for complex or stable humeral fractures. Bone plates are generally used when the time to bone
union will be lengthy or when postoperative comfort is desirable. Factors that influence plate size are its intended
function (i.e., compression, neutralization, or bridging plate)
and patient size. The plate may be placed on the cranial,
lateral, caudolateral, caudomedial, or medial surfaces of the
humerus (Fig. 32-26). Cranial plate application is easiest
with proximal and midshaft humeral fractures. Lateral plate
application is also easiest with proximal and midshaft fractures, but can be used with distal fractures. Medial, caudomedial, and caudolateral placement is easiest with distal
fractures. A minimum of three plate screws (six cortices)
proximal to the fracture and three plate screws distal to the
fracture is recommended with compression or neutralization plates. A minimum of four plate screws (eight cortices)
proximal and distal to the fracture is recommended for buttress plates.

Compression plates are used with transverse or short
oblique fractures. The plate is contoured to 1 mm offset
from the bone surface at the fracture site to achieve compression of the transcortex. **Neutralization plates** are used
with long oblique fractures or comminuted fractures in
which the bone fragments can be reduced and stabilized
with lag screws or cerclage wire. The plate is contoured to the
anatomic surface of the reconstructed bone. **Bridging plates**
are used with comminuted fractures in which bone fragments cannot be reduced anatomically or when attempted
reduction and stabilization of the fragments would cause
excessive soft tissue trauma. The plate is contoured to reflect
the anatomy of the humerus; this is most easily accomplished by contouring the plate to the appropriate radiographic view of the contralateral limb.

Spatial alignment of the bone is assisted by inserting an
IM pin. The pin is retrograded or normograded through the
proximal intact segment of bone, passed through the fragmented section of bone, and seated into the medial condyle.
When placing the pin into the medial condyle, do not prevent the fragment from displacing distally. This allows the
pin to distract the proximal and distal segments and helps to
regain humeral length. In keeping with the concept of bridging osteosynthesis, do not disturb the bone fragments in the
comminuted area. Once spatial alignment of the humerus is
achieved, the bone plate is attached to the bone with plate
screws. Leaving the alignment pin in place will provide a
plate-pin buttress of the fracture. The diameter of the alignment pin should equal approximately 40% to 50% of the
diameter of the marrow cavity to allow screws to be placed.
Bicortical screws (screws that engage both cortices) should
be used proximally and distally when possible and monocortical screws used centrally. The plate-pin combination increases the strength and fatigue life of the fixation and thus
protects the plate from premature breakage (Fig. 32-27). The
plate-pin system can be destabilized between 6 and 8 weeks
by removing the IM pin. Alternately, if the alignment pin is

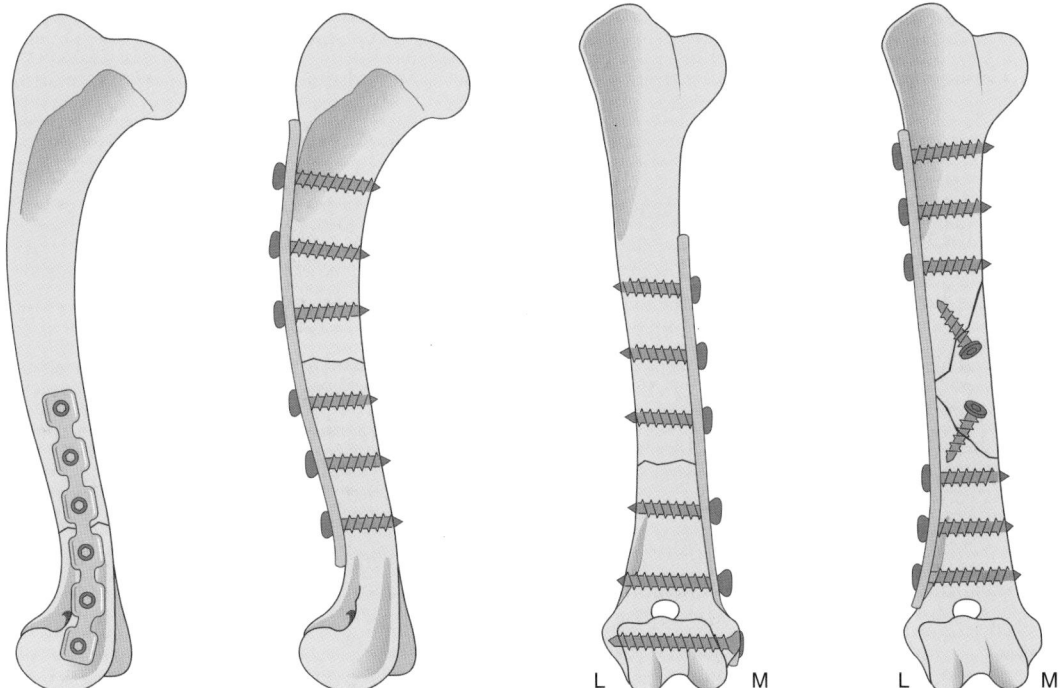

FIG. 32-26
Bone plates are applied as compression plates to the lateral cranial or medial humeral surface to stabilize transverse diaphyseal fractures. Oblique or comminuted reducible fractures are stabilized with lag screws and neutralization plates.

removed, bicortical plate screws may be used. A cancellous bone graft can be harvested and placed in the fracture zone if soft tissue is not excessively disrupted.

Preoperative Management

Before surgery, a spica splint (see p. 946) can be applied to increase patient comfort and protect soft tissue from further injury induced by bone fragments. Because these fractures result from trauma, all affected animals should be examined for concurrent injury and stabilized if necessary before surgery. Analgesics should be provided to posttraumatic animals (see Box 31-2 on p. 944 and Chapter 13).

Anesthesia

Anesthetic management of animals with fractures is discussed on p. 944.

Surgical Anatomy

Although the humerus may be approached from all four anatomic directions, most often a craniolateral exposure is used to approach the humeral diaphysis. The radial nerve must be identified and protected during fracture reduction and stabilization. The radial nerve lies superficial to the brachialis muscle and deep to the lateral head of the triceps. The canine humerus has a normal cranial to caudal curvature that positions the long axis of the marrow cavity cranial to the shoulder joint. This facilitates pin placement by ensuring that an IM pin will exit cranial to the joint. However, distally the su-

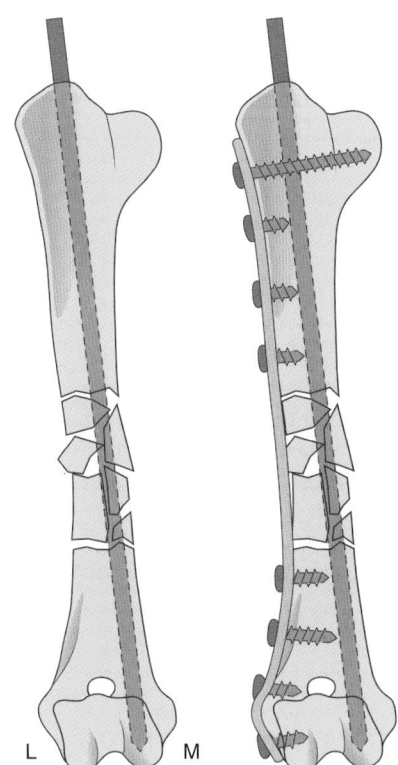

FIG. 32-27
Application of plate-pin combination for stabilization of comminuted humeral fracture. The intramedullary pin reduces cyclic bending stress in the bone plate.

pratrochlear foramen is in direct line with the long axis of the marrow cavity, which makes distal placement of the IM pin into the cancellous bone more difficult. The anatomy of the feline humerus is similar to that of the canine. However, there is less cranial to caudal curvature, and the diameter of the marrow cavity is more uniform. In many cats, the medullary canal ends at the level of the supratrochlear foramen. Care must be taken to avoid entering the supratrochlear foramen as a result of the presence of the median nerve. During the medial approach to the humerus, care must be taken to isolate and protect the median, musculocutaneous, and ulnar nerves and the brachial artery and vein.

> NOTE: Be sure to identify and protect the major nerves during surgical approaches to the humerus.

Positioning

For the craniolateral approach to the humerus, the animal is positioned in lateral recumbency with the affected leg up. For the medial approach to the humerus, the animal is positioned in dorsal recumbency. A hanging-leg preparation facilitates limb manipulation during surgery. The limb should be prepped from the dorsal midline to the carpus. If the fracture location permits, the proximal humerus may be used as a donor site for cancellous bone graft. If not, the ipsilateral iliac wing should be prepared for surgery.

SURGICAL TECHNIQUE
Surgical Approach to the Humeral Diaphysis

The proximal and central humeral diaphysis is most easily exposed through a craniolateral approach.

Make a skin incision from the cranial border of the tubercle of the humerus to the lateral epicondyle distally (Fig. 32-28, A). The incision should follow the normal curvature of the humerus. Incise the subcutaneous fat and brachial fascia along the same line, being careful to isolate and protect the cephalic vein (Fig. 32-28, B). The cephalic vein may be ligated if necessary to achieve the desired exposure. Incise the brachial fascia along the border of the brachiocephalicus muscle and the lateral head of the triceps. Use caution when incising the fascia along the cranial border of the triceps overlying the brachialis muscle until the radial nerve is visualized (Fig. 32-28, C). Once the nerve is isolated, reflect the brachiocephalicus and superficial pectoral muscles cranially and the brachialis muscle caudally to expose the proximal and central humeral shaft (Fig. 32-28, D). To gain further exposure of the distal humeral shaft, reflect the brachialis muscle cranially and the lateral triceps muscle caudally. Release the origin of the extensor carpi radialis muscle from the ridge of the lateral epicondyle for maximum exposure. To close, suture the brachiocephalicus muscle and superficial pectoral muscles to the fascia of the brachialis muscle. Suture the subcutaneous tissue and skin using standard methods.

The distal one half of the humerus is also accessible through a medial exposure and is the choice of some surgeons when a bone plate is used as the fixation method.

Make an incision from the greater tubercle proximally to the medial epicondyle distally. Incise the deep brachial fascia along the caudal border of the brachiocephalicus muscle (Fig. 32-29, A). Take care distally to preserve and isolate the neurovascular structures (i.e., median, musculocutaneous, and ulnar nerves and brachial artery and vein) (Fig. 32-29, B). Reflect the brachiocephalicus muscle cranially, and incise through the insertion of the superficial pectoral muscle. For exposure of the midportion of the humerus, reflect the superficial pectoral muscle cranially and the biceps brachii and neurovascular structures caudally (Fig. 32-29, C). For exposure of the distal humerus, reflect the biceps brachii, neurovascular structures, and superficial pectoral muscle cranially. To close, suture the superficial pectoral to the brachiocephalicus fascia. Suture the remaining deep fascia, subcutaneous tissue, and skin routinely.

Stabilization of Midshaft Transverse or Short Oblique Fractures

From a mechanical perspective, this fracture configuration allows load sharing between the bone and implant after surgery. Stabilization of a transverse or short oblique fracture requires rotational and bending support. This can be achieved with bone plates, an interlocking nail, an IM pin with an external fixator, or an external fixator alone.

Determine final implant choice based on fracture location and the patient's fracture-assessment score (Fig. 32-30).

Fixation systems that are useful with a low fracture-assessment score (0 to 3) include a bone plate and screws inserted to function as a compression plate, an interlocking nail, and a 6-pin Type Ib external skeletal fixator with raised-threaded transfixation pins "tied in" with an IM pin. With a moderate fracture-assessment score (4 to 7), a compression plate, an interlocking nail, or an IM pin tied in with a 3-pin Type Ib external skeletal fixator would be functional. Transverse or short oblique fractures are common in puppies and kittens because their owners often step on them. These patients have a high fracture-assessment score (8 to 10) and can be stabilized with an IM pin with a 2-pin Type Ia external skeletal fixator. Alternatively, flexible plating with a veterinary cuttable plate is an option in immature dogs (Fig. 32-31; see also p. 993).

Stabilization of Midshaft Long Oblique Fractures or Comminuted Fractures With Large Butterfly Fragment

From a mechanical perspective, these fractures can be reduced and interfragmentary compression applied with cerclage wire or lag screws. Once the interfragmentary fracture lines are reduced and compressed, the bone is able to share the loads with the implant postoperatively. Stabilization of

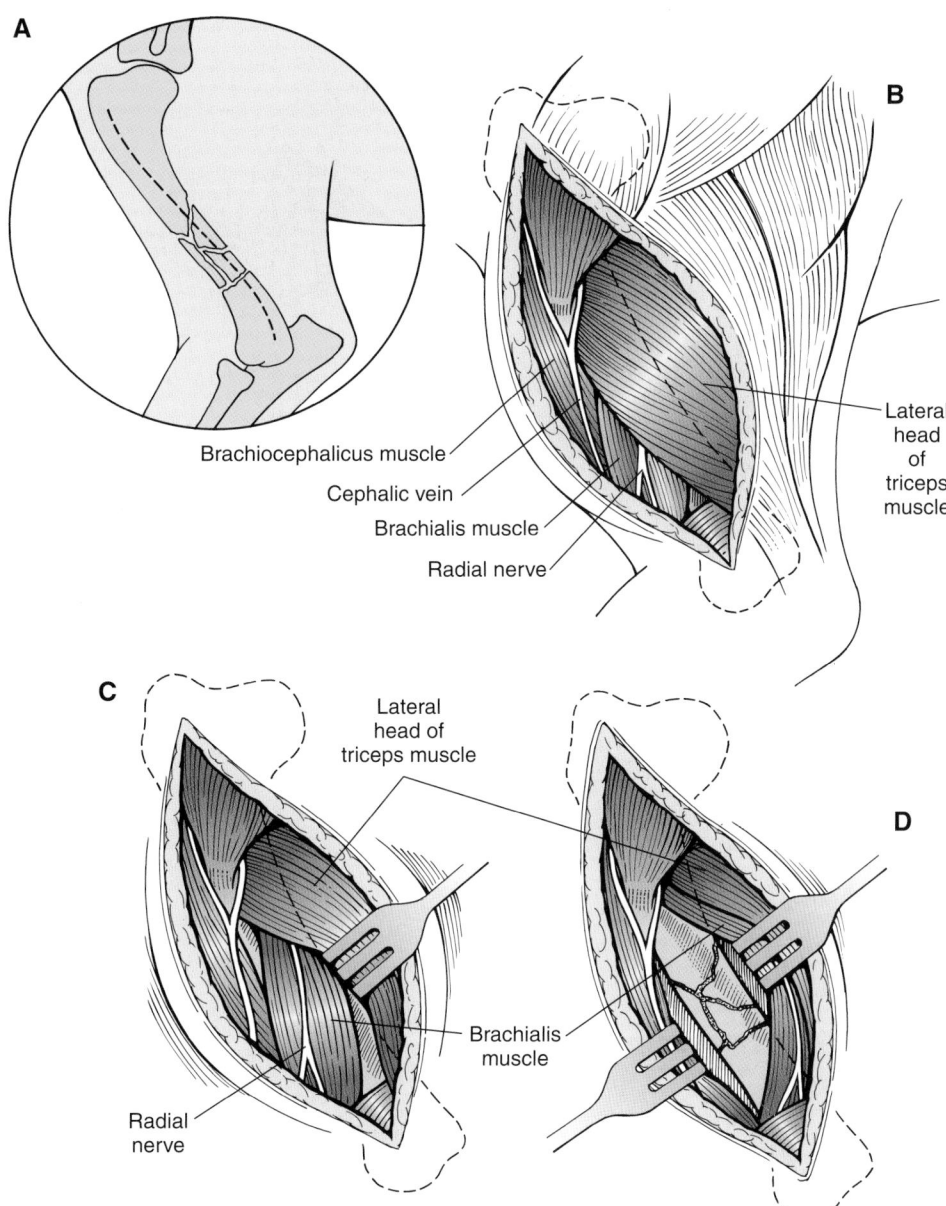

FIG. 32-28
A, To expose the midhumeral diaphysis, make a skin incision from the cranial border of the humeral tubercle to the lateral epicondyle distally. **B,** Incise subcutaneous fat and brachial fascia along the same line, being careful to isolate and protect the cephalic vein. **C,** Visualize the radial nerve when incising fascia along the cranial border of the triceps overlying the brachialis muscle. **D,** Retract the brachiocephalicus muscle cranially and the brachialis muscle caudally to expose the humerus.

this fracture configuration requires axial, rotational, and bending support. This can be achieved with lag screws and bone plates, IM pins/cerclage wire/external fixator combinations, and interlocking nail or IM pin and cerclage wire (Fig. 32-32). Fixation systems that are useful with a low fracture-assessment score (0 to 3) are neutralization plates, interlocking nails, and external fixators.

Achieve interfragmentary compression initially with cerclage wire or lag screws to reconstruct the cylinder of bone, and then bridge the area with a bone plate. Alternatively, use an interlocking nail or IM pin to support the reconstructed bone.

Additional support to the IM pin is then supplied by an external skeletal fixator, with or without a tie-in to the IM

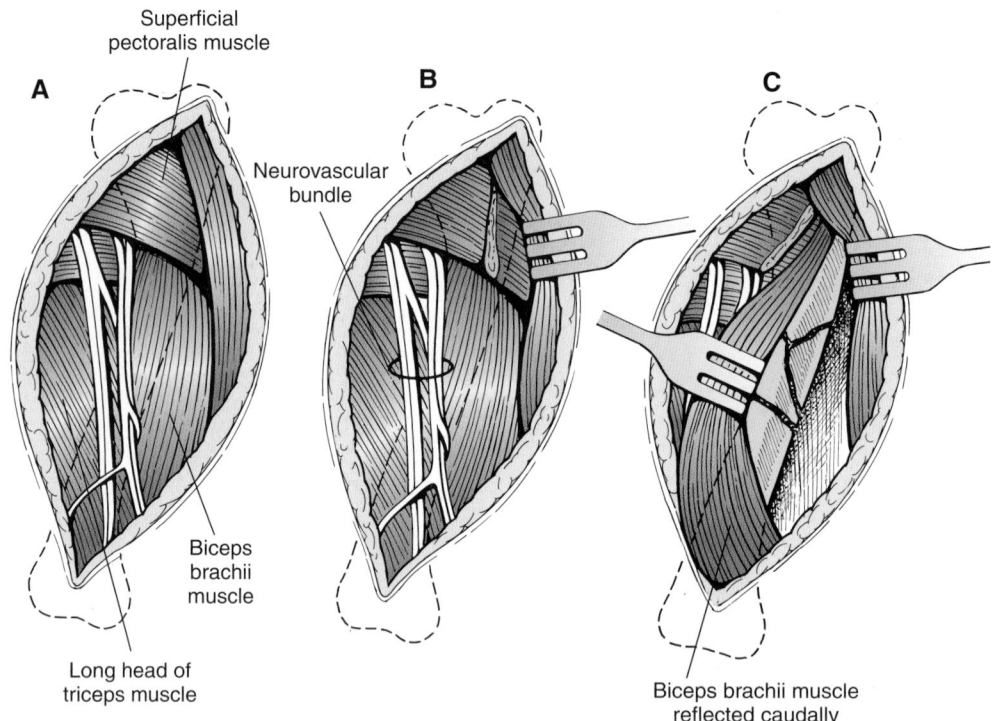

FIG. 32-29
A, To expose the medial surface of the distal third of the humerus, incise deep brachial fascia along the caudal border of the brachiocephalicus muscle. **B,** At the distal aspect, take care to preserve and isolate the median, musculocutaneous, and ulnar nerves and the brachial artery and vein. **C,** Reflect the biceps brachii and neurovascular structures caudally and the superficial pectoral muscle cranially.

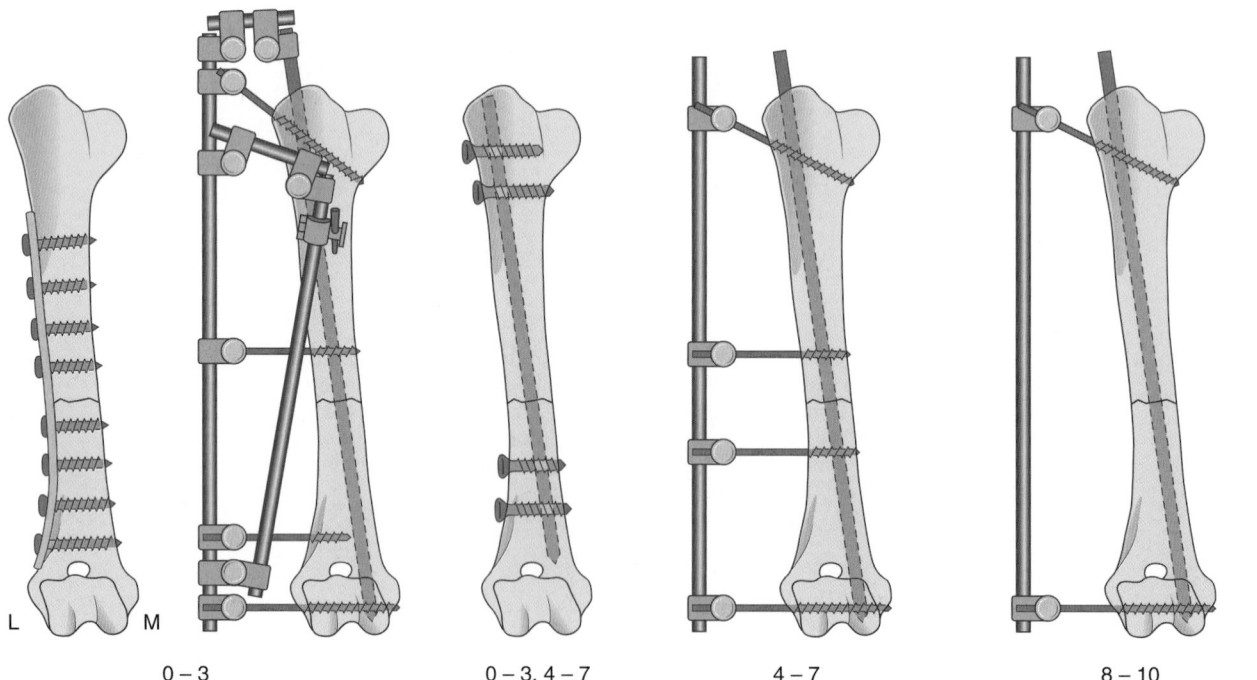

FIG. 32-30
Recommended methods of stabilizing transverse or short oblique humeral fractures based on fracture-assessment score. If the fracture-assessment score is 0 to 3, a compression plate, external skeletal fixator plus IM pin (tie-in configuration), or interlocking nail may be used. If the fracture-assessment score is 4 to 7, an interlocking nail or an external skeletal fixator with IM pin may be used. The IM pin may be tied in for extra stability. With fracture-assessment scores of 8 to 10, an external skeletal fixator plus IM pin provides necessary stability.

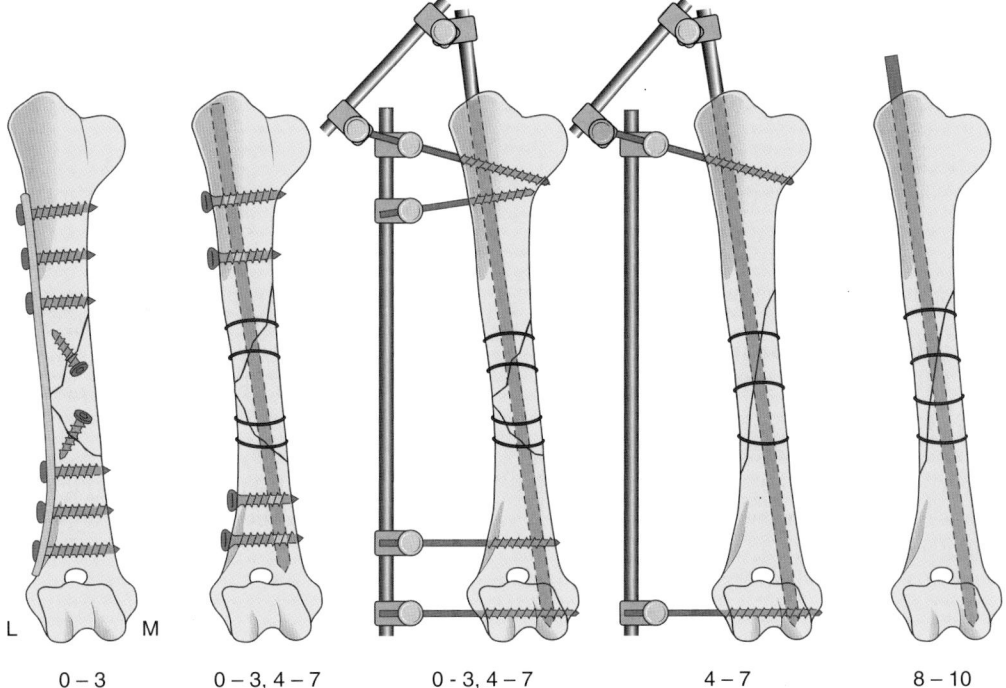

L   M

0 – 3   0 – 3, 4 – 7   0 - 3, 4 – 7   4 – 7   8 – 10

FIG. 32-31
Recommended methods for stabilizing long oblique or reducible comminuted humeral fractures (single large fragment) based on fracture-assessment score. If the fracture-assessment score is 0 to 3, a neutralization plate, interlocking nail, or 4-pin external skeletal fixator plus IM pin (tie-in configuration) and cerclage wires may be used. If the fracture-assessment score is 4 to 7, a 2-pin external skeletal fixator with IM pin (tie-in configuration) and cerclage wire may be used. With fracture-assessment scores of 8 to 10, an IM pin plus cerclage wire provides necessary stability. (Modified from Fossum TW: *Small animal surgery,* ed 2, St Louis, 2002, Mosby.)

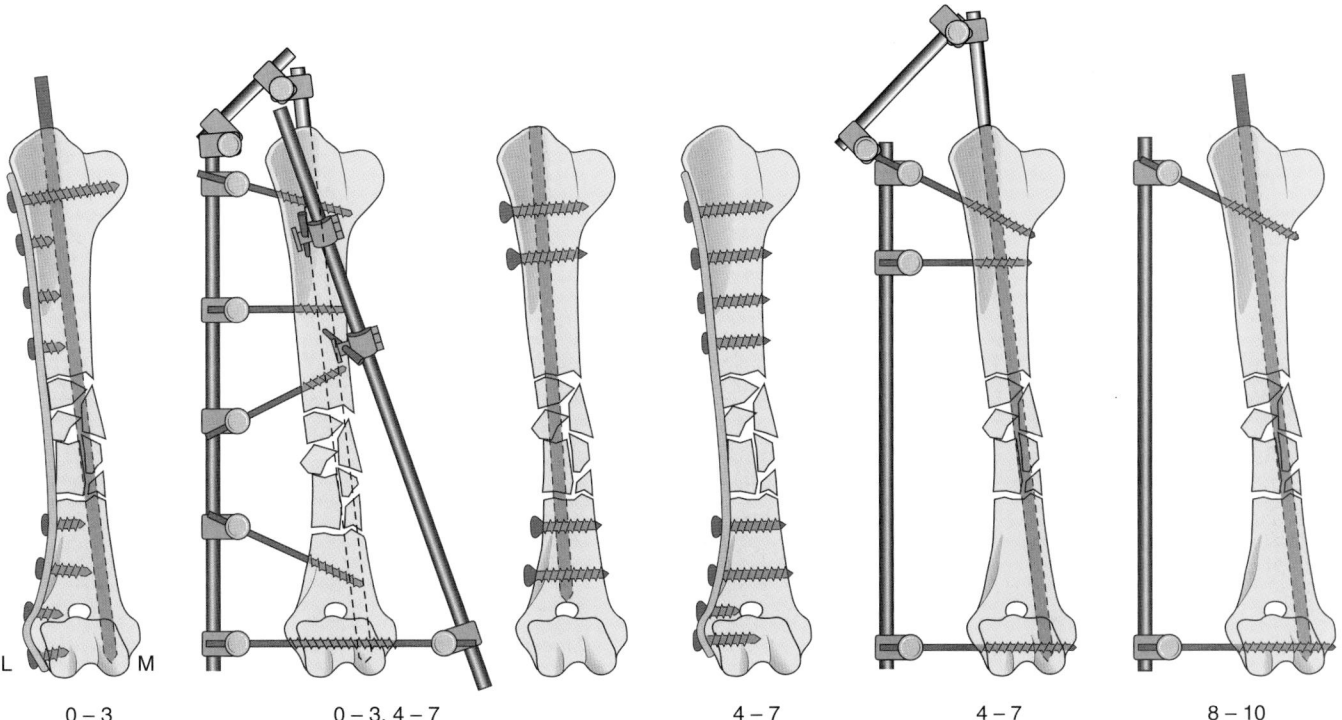

L   M

0 – 3   0 – 3, 4 – 7   4 – 7   4 – 7   8 – 10

FIG. 32-32
Recommended methods for stabilizing nonreducible comminuted humeral fractures (multiple fragments) based on fracture-assessment score. If the fracture-assessment score is 0 to 3, a plate-rod combination, interlocking nail, or 4-pin external skeletal fixator plus IM pin (tie-in configuration) may be used. If the fracture-assessment score is 4 to 7, a buttress plate or 3-pin external skeletal fixator with IM pin (tie-in configuration) may be used. With fracture assessment scores of 8 to 10, a 2-pin external skeletal fixator plus IM pin provides necessary stability.

pin. With a moderate fracture-assessment score (4 to 7), a neutralization plate, an interlocking nail, or an IM pin plus cerclage wire for interfragmentary compression combined with a 2-pin Type Ia external skeletal fixator may be used. With a high fracture-assessment score (8 to 10), an IM pin combined with cerclage wire for interfragmentary compression is a useful method to stabilize the fracture.

Stabilization of Midshaft Comminuted Fractures With Multiple Fragments

From a mechanical perspective, these fractures cannot be reduced without significant soft tissue manipulation, and no load sharing occurs between the implant and bone until biologic callus forms to provide support. These types of fractures need rigid axial, rotational, and bending support. Very high stresses will be imposed on the implant and its connection to the bone. If the biologic assessment is favorable, the imposed stresses will be of short duration, reducing the likelihood of implant failure. If the biologic assessment is not favorable, however, imposed stresses will act on the implant for an extended period, making implant failure more likely.

Enhance the biologic response by not attempting to reduce the fragments (bridging osteosynthesis), and insert an autogenous cancellous bone graft when appropriate.

Stabilization can be achieved with a bone plate–pin combination, a bone plate alone (lengthening plate, broad plate),

an interlocking nail (if the fracture is midshaft), or a Type Ib or Ia external skeletal fixator/pin tie-in combination (see Fig. 32-32).

Manage patients with a low fracture-assessment score (0 to 3) with a bone plate–pin combination, an interlocking nail, a rigid Type Ib external skeletal fixator tied in to an IM pin, or a modified Type Ib external skeletal fixator (Fig. 32-33). Use transfixation pins that have a raised thread, and apply at least three pins above and two pins below the area of comminution.

It is always better to err on the side of too much rigidity than too little rigidity since the fixator can be destabilized postoperatively.

Manage patients with a moderate fracture-assessment score (4 to 7) with a bone plate functioning as a buttress plate (lengthening plate or broad plate) or an interlocking nail. Apply the plate to the cranial, medial, or lateral surface, depending on the location of the fracture and your preference.

An external skeletal fixator, with or without a tie-in to the IM pin, or an interlocking nail may also be used. The choice of frame, the number of pins, and the pin design for the external skeletal fixator depend on the fracture-assessment score. A patient with this type of fracture would have a high fracture-assessment score (8 to 10) only when the biologic

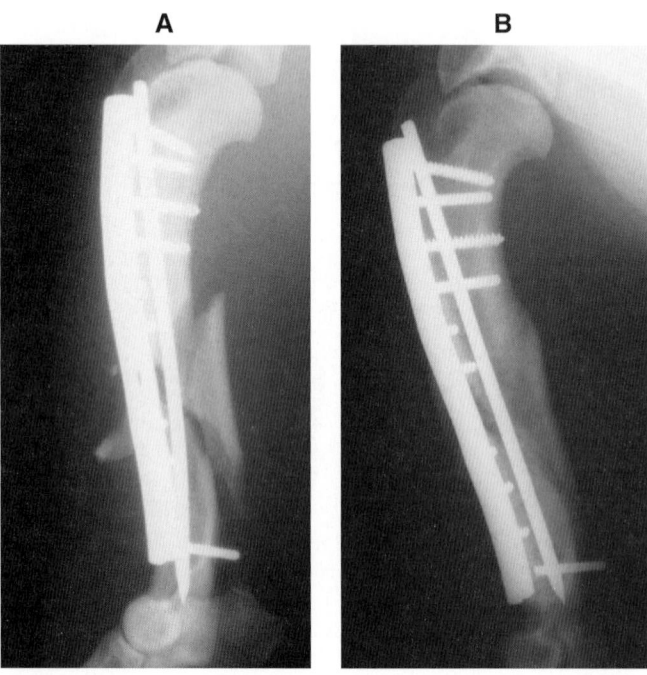

FIG. 32-33
Postoperative radiographs. **A,** Stabilization of comminuted fracture with IM pin and plate. **B,** Fracture healing 12 weeks later.

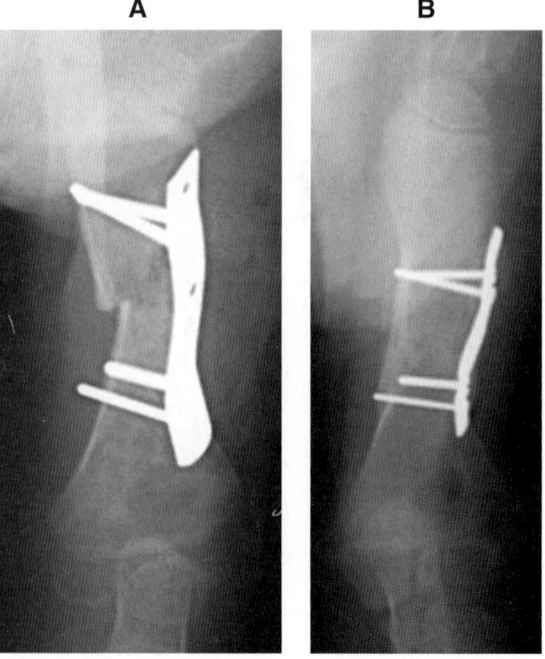

FIG. 32-34
A, Craniocaudal postoperative radiograph showing flexible plating for stabilizing a comminuted humeral fracture in a young dog. **B,** Rapid healing and remodeling of the fracture 4 weeks later.

assessment is extremely favorable (e.g., 4- to 5-month-old animal with a closed, single-limb injury).

Manage these animals using bridging osteosynthesis with an IM pin, with or without a tie-in to a Type Ia or Type Ib external skeletal fixator. Immature dogs may be treated with elastic plating techniques using a veterinary cuttable plate and screws (Fig. 32-34).

Stabilization of Supracondylar Fractures

Supracondylar fractures are usually transverse or short oblique fractures. Occasionally a comminuted fracture with multiple small fragments will be seen. When comminution is present, however, the length of bone involved is usually limited to a small area.

Bridge the fracture with an implant to serve as a buttress, or collapse the fracture to resemble a load-sharing transverse or short oblique fracture. If the zone of comminution is lengthy and if limb length must be preserved, reconstruct the bony column or bridge the area of comminution with an appropriate implant system serving as a buttress.

Stabilization of supracondylar fractures depends on the fracture configuration and patient fracture assessment (Fig. 32-35). Transverse or short oblique fractures require rotational and bending support, whereas comminuted fractures require axial, rotational, and bending support. In patients with a low fracture-assessment score (0 to 3), a caudolateral plate combined with a caudomedial plate or a caudolateral plate combined with a medial IM pin is preferred. The plate functions as a compression plate with transverse fractures and as a buttress plate with highly fragmented fractures. In patients with a moderate fracture-assessment score (4 to 7), a medial plate, a caudolateral plate, or an IM pin supported with an external skeletal fixator is suggested. The external skeletal fixator frame and number of pins depend on the fracture assessment. Closed reduction and application of a modified Type Ib external fixator can be used to preserve the biology of comminuted nonreducible fractures.

If an IM pin is used with an external fixator, tie it in with the external skeletal fixator to increase rigidity and reduce morbidity.

If the fracture is transverse and has a high assessment score (8 to 10), an IM pin seated into the medial portion of the condyle and a laterally positioned pin or Kirschner wire crossing the fracture provide the necessary stability to allow for fracture union.

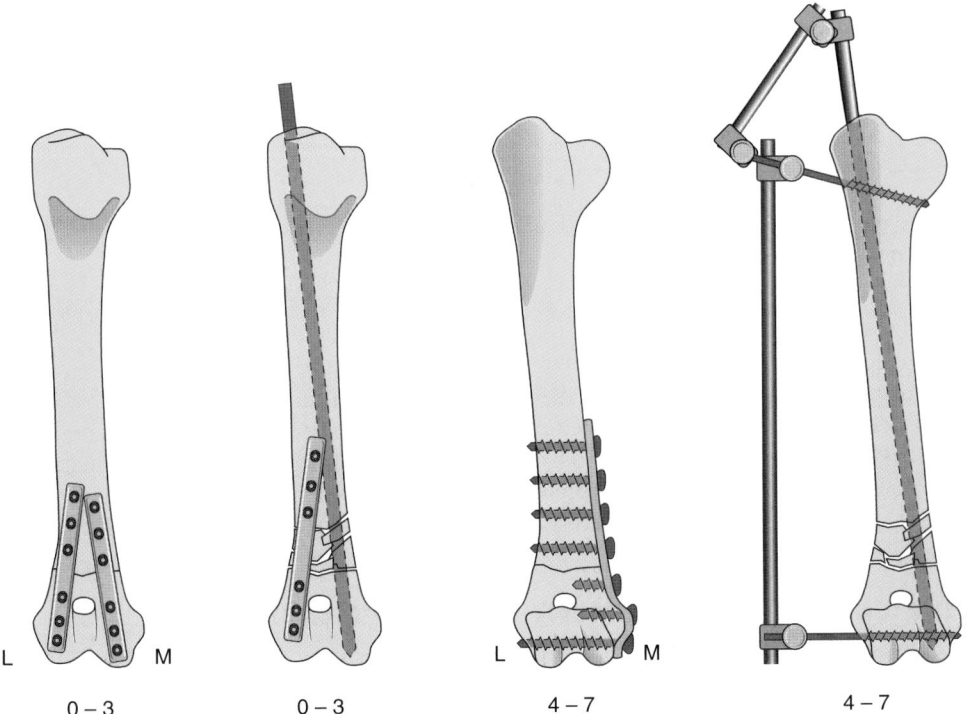

L M L M L M

0 – 3 0 – 3 4 – 7 4 – 7

FIG. 32-35
Recommended methods for stabilizing supracondylar fractures based on fracture-assessment score. If the fracture-assessment score is 0 to 3, two plates or a plate-rod combination may be used. If the fracture-assessment score is 4 to 7, a medial compression plate or 2-pin external skeletal fixator plus IM pin (tie-in configuration) may be used. With fracture-assessment scores of 8 to 10, an IM pin seated into the medial condyle and a laterally placed crossed pin may be used to stabilize a transverse fracture (not illustrated). (Modified from Fossum TW: *Small animal surgery,* ed 2, St Louis, 2002, Mosby.)

Table 32-4

Sample Physical Rehabilitation Protocol for Patients With Humeral or Femoral Diaphyseal Fractures Stabilized with Internal Fixation

ALL TREATMENTS BID	DAY 1 TO DAY 14	DAY 15 TO DAY 24	DAY 25 UNTIL HEALED	HEALED TO RETURN TO FUNCTION
Heat therapy		10 min	10 min	
Massage	5 min	5 min	5 min	
Passive range of motion (repetitions)	15*	15*		
Electrical stimulation†	10 min	10 min	10 min	>10 min
Therapeutic exercise-total time	10 min	15 min	15 min	25–45 min
Walk/land treadmill	10 min	5 min	5 min	10 min
Balancing	+	+	+	
Obstacles	+	+	+	+
Weaving				+
Circles				+
Hills				+
Stairs				+
Jog/run				+
Underwater treadmill		10 min	10 min	>15 min
Swimming				5–10 min
Cryotherapy	15 min	15 min	15 min	PRN

BID, Twice a day; +, perform modality; *PRN,* as needed.
*Perform passive range of motion for all joints of the affected limb.
†Electrical stimulation—to be performed on the biceps/triceps muscle groups for humeral fractures or semitendinosus/semimembrinosus for femur fractures in patients with muscle atrophy. See Chapter 12 for specifics.

SUTURE MATERIALS AND SPECIAL INSTRUMENTS

Equipment necessary for pin and wire placement includes retractors, bone-holding forceps, reduction forceps, a Jacobs pin chuck, IM pins, Kirschner wires, and orthopedic wire. Additional equipment needed for external fixation includes a low-rpm power drill and external fixation clamps and bars. The interlocking nail equipment is needed for nail application. Plating equipment and a high-speed drill are necessary for application of plates and screws.

POSTOPERATIVE CARE AND ASSESSMENT

Postoperative radiographs are made to evaluate fracture reduction and implant location. Activity should be restricted to leash walking and physical rehabilitation until the fracture has healed. Physical rehabilitation encourages controlled limb use and optimal limb function after fracture healing. Care must be taken to develop customized protocols for each patient depending on location of the fracture, stability and type of fracture fixation, potential for healing, abilities and attitudes of the patient, and willingness of the client (see Chapter 12) (Tables 32-4 and 32-5). External fixator man-

agement includes daily pin care and pin packing as needed. Radiographs should be evaluated in 6 weeks. External fixators may be destabilized at this time if healing is progressing satisfactorily. Radiographs should be repeated at 6-week intervals until fracture bridging is observed.

Time to bone union depends on the patient fracture assessment. IM pins and external skeletal fixations should be removed when healing occurs; interlocking nails and bone plates are not generally removed unless a problem is associated with their presence.

COMPLICATIONS

The prognosis depends on the fracture assessment; patients with poor assessment are more prone to complications. Poor implant choice relative to the fracture assessment is the most common reason for fixation failure. The most common complication seen in companion animals is premature loosening of the implant (i.e., loosening and migration of IM pins, external skeletal fixator fixation pins, and cerclage wires). Fatigue breakage of bone plates or plate screw pull-out can occur when principles of bone plating are not followed or when length of time to bone union is inaccurately assessed.

Table 32-5

Sample Physical Rehabilitation Protocol for Patients With Humeral or Femoral Diaphyseal Fractures Stabilized with External Fixators

ALL TREATMENTS BID	DAY 1 TO DAY 14	DAY 15 TO DAY 24	DAY 25 UNTIL HEALED	HEALED TO RETURN TO FUNCTION
Heat therapy		10 min	10 min	
Massage	5 min	5 min	5 min	
Passive range of motion (repetitions)	20*	20*	10–15*	Stop-when ROM N
Therapeutic exercise-total time	10 min	15 min	15 min	25–45 min
Walk/land treadmill	10 min	15 minn	15 min	>10 min
Balancing	+	+	+	
Obstacles	+	+	+	+
Weaving				+
Circles				+
Hills				+
Stairs				+
Jog/run				+
Underwater treadmill				>15 min
Swimming				5–10 min
Cryotherapy	15 min	15 min	15 min	PRN

BID, Twice a day; *ROM*, range of motion; *N*, normal; +, perform modality; *PRN*, as needed.
*Perform passive range of motion for all joints of the affected limb.

PROGNOSIS

If the initial implant system has failed, the recommended treatment is application of a bone plate serving as a compression plate or neutralization plate if the fracture configuration allows or application of a plate-rod construct if a zone of comminution must be bridged. These systems stabilize the fracture while providing patient comfort that allows limb use and early physical rehabilitation.

References

Basinger RR, Suber JT: Two techniques for supplementing interlocking nail repair of fractures of the humerus, femur, and tibia: results in 12 dogs and cats, *Vet Surg* 33:673, 2004.

Langley-Hobbs SJ, Straw M: The feline humerus: An anatomical study with relevance to external skeletal fixator and intramedullary pin placement, *Vet Comp Orthop Traumatol* 18:1, 2005.

Suggested Reading

Aron DN, Palmer RH, Johnson AL: Biologic strategies and a balanced concept for repair of highly comminuted long bone fractures, *Compend Cont Educ Pract Vet* 17:35, 1995.
This article provides a review of the concepts and application of biologic fracture fixation in small animals.

Cabassu JP: Elastic plate osteosynthesis of femoral shaft fractures in young dogs, *Vet Comp Orthop Traumatol* 14:40, 2001.
The authors describe a novel technique for fracture fixation in immature dogs that relies on the use of flexible veterinary cuttable plates and minimal numbers of screws to promote rapid callus formation. Although the article is limited to femoral fractures, the technique is applicable to humeral fractures.

Fearnside SM, Eaton-Wells RD, Mitchell RAS: Management of comminuted supracondylar fractures of the humerus with closed reduction and a hybrid type I-II external fixator, *Vet Comp Orthop Traumatol* 15:233, 2002.
The report of the technique and outcome of a series of comminuted supracondylar fractures treated biologically with closed reduction and an external fixator fabricated from pins and bars connected with dental acrylic is presented. Successful fracture healing was achieved in eight of nine patients.

Moses PA, Lewis DD, Lanz OI et al: Intramedullary interlocking nail stabilization of 21 humeral fractures in 19 dogs and one cat, *Aust Vet J* 80:336, 2002.
A case series of dogs and cats with humeral diaphyseal fractures stabilized with interlocking nails. The case series highlights the versatility of the interlocking nail for differing sizes of animals and complexity of the fracture. Eighteen of the 21 fractures healed.

Piermattei D, Johnson KA: *An atlas of surgical approaches to the bones and joints of the dog and cat*, ed 4, Philadelphia, 2004, WB Saunders.

This textbook is an excellent reference for surgical approaches for repairing fractures of the humerus.

Reems MR, Beale BS, Hulse DA: Use of a plate-rod construct and principles of biological osteosynthesis for repair of diaphyseal fractures in dogs and cats: 47 cases (1994-2001), *J Am Vet Med Assoc* 223:330, 2003.

This article provides a report of the application of the plate rod technique for stabilizing humeral, femoral, and tibial fractures. Clinical application and outcomes are discussed.

Turner TM: Fractures of the humerus. In Johnson AL, Houlton JEF, Vannini R, editors: *AO principles of fracture management in the dog and cat*, Thieme, NY, 2005, AO Publishing.

This chapter provides an up-to-date collection of operative techniques for stabilizing humeral diaphyseal fractures in small animals. Detailed descriptions of bone-plating procedures are included.

HUMERAL ARTICULAR, PHYSEAL, AND METAPHYSEAL FRACTURES

DEFINITIONS

Epiphyseal fractures and **metaphyseal fractures** occur at the proximal or distal ends of the humerus. **Physeal fractures** involve the growth plates in immature animals.

GENERAL CONSIDERATIONS AND CLINICALLY RELEVANT PATHOPHYSIOLOGY

Fractures of the proximal humeral metaphysis and epiphysis are uncommon, but occasionally occur through the proximal humeral physis in young animals. Fractures through the physis may result from minimal external force and exhibit only slight displacement. Careful scrutiny of the lateral radiograph and comparison to a radiograph of the contralateral limb may be necessary to correctly diagnose these fractures. Gunshot fractures can cause severe comminution of the proximal or distal humerus. Fractures of the distal humeral condyle (elbow) are common and include fractures of the lateral or medial portions of the condyle, or both, known as a T fracture or Y fracture of the condyle. These fractures can also occur with comminuted supracondylar fractures. Lateral condylar fractures predominate over medial condylar fractures for two reasons. First, the radial head articulates with the lateral portion of the condyle, transmitting weight-bearing forces primarily through the lateral portion of the condyle. Second, the anatomic position of the lateral portion of the condyle is eccentric to the bony column, causing weight-bearing forces to be transmitted through the weaker epicondyloid ridge to the humeral diaphysis. Fractures of the lateral portion of the condyle are frequently diagnosed in young, toy-breed dogs that fall or jump from furniture or the owner's arms with the elbow extended. When the animal lands, high loads are transmitted through the radial head–lateral condylar axis, resulting in separation of the lateral portion of the condyle. The fracture line passes between the lateral and medial portions of the condyle, crosses the physis, and exits through the metaphysis. Because the physis is involved, the fracture is classified as a Salter IV fracture (see

p. 951). Careful evaluation of the craniocaudal radiograph is essential since minimal displacement of the intercondylar fracture can occur. Adult animals also sustain lateral condylar fractures through the mechanism described above. In some breeds, particularly spaniels, incomplete ossification between the medial and lateral portions of the condyle predisposes to condylar fractures and may cause forelimb lameness. Incomplete ossification causing lameness (e.g., incomplete humeral condylar fractures) is best treated with preemptive placement of a large lag screw. Incomplete ossification often occurs bilaterally.

> NOTE: Evaluate radiographs carefully to avoid missing intercondylar fractures that are minimally displaced.

Isolated medial condylar fractures are not common, but do occur in both immature and mature patients. T or Y fractures of the elbow are more common and represent an intracondylar fracture combined with a transverse (T) or oblique (Y) fracture through both medial and lateral epicondyloid ridges.

DIAGNOSIS
Clinical Presentation

Signalment. Lateral condylar fractures are frequently diagnosed in young, toy-breed dogs; however, physeal fractures may occur in any juvenile dog or cat of any breed or sex that has open growth plates. Adult animals of any breed or sex may sustain a proximal epiphyseal or distal epiphyseal (elbow) fracture. Spaniel breeds appear to be predisposed to lateral condylar fractures (see previous discussion).

History. Physeal fractures usually result from a fall, but also may be caused by automobile accidents. Elbow fractures or proximal humeral fractures in adult animals are usually associated with vehicular trauma or gunshot wounds.

Physical Examination Findings

Most affected animals have a non–weight-bearing lameness. Swelling of the affected limb is usually obvious if the fracture is secondary to an automobile accident. Pain and crepitus can be elicited with limb manipulation.

Diagnostic Imaging

Craniocaudal and lateral radiographs are usually sufficient to make a diagnosis. In spaniels, if a fracture of the intercondylar articular surface or incomplete ossification is suspected but not evident, oblique radiographic views of both elbows are recommended. CT may be used to obtain definitive diagnosis of incomplete ossification.

Laboratory Findings

Complete blood count and serum chemistry evaluation should be done to assess the status of the animal sustaining trauma for anesthesia. Consistent laboratory abnormalities are not present.

DIFFERENTIAL DIAGNOSIS

Differential diagnoses include ligament injury of the shoulder or elbow, scapular fractures, and proximal radial or ulnar fractures.

MEDICAL MANAGEMENT

Fractures involving or close to the joint should not be managed with conservative treatment.

SURGICAL TREATMENT

Treatment of humeral metaphyseal and epiphyseal fractures depends on the animal's age, overall health, and fracture configuration. The fracture-assessment score (see p. 953) is used to help determine the rigidity of stabilization necessary for the fracture to heal. Surgical treatment of Salter I and II physeal fractures consists of anatomic reduction and stabilization with Kirschner wires or small pins that are smooth so as not to interfere with physeal function. Salter III fractures of the proximal humerus may also be treated with multiple Kirschner wires or small pins. Mechanically, the shape of the fractured physeal surfaces and the friction of cancellous bone resting on cancellous bone assist in preventing movement of the reduced proximal physeal fracture. These fractures heal rapidly because they occur in cancellous bone of young animals, so smooth implants are generally sufficient. In animals that are close to maturity, threaded implants may be used to compress the fractured physis. Anatomic reduction and rigid fixation with a lag screw are critical for optimal outcome with Salter IV fractures of the humeral condyle.

Preoperative Management

Patients that have sustained trauma should be stabilized before anesthesia and fracture treatment. Analgesics are indicated for posttraumatic patients (see Box 31-2 on p. 944 and Chapter 13).

Anesthesia

Anesthetic considerations for patients with fractures are discussed on p. 944.

Surgical Anatomy

Depending on the severity of injury, the normal anatomy and surgical landmarks of this region may be distorted by soft tissue bruising and swelling. Starting the surgical dissection in an area with less swelling or bruising and using bony landmarks are helpful. Proximally the greater tubercle and acromion of the scapula are readily palpable; distally the medial and lateral epicondyles are easy to identify. The cephalic vein courses within the subcutaneous tissue along the craniolateral surface of the limb. The radial nerve lies beneath the lateral head of the triceps near the distal third of the humerus. This nerve must be identified as it courses superficial to the brachialis muscle before the brachialis muscle is reflected from the humeral diaphysis. To visualize the nerve, dissection should be initiated adjacent to the cranial edge of the lateral head of the triceps, near the lateral epicondyle. The tissue plane between the brachiocephalicus and triceps muscles must be carefully dissected to prevent injury to this nerve. When performing an olecranon osteotomy, take care to avoid the ulnar nerve along the cranial edge of the medial head of the triceps muscle.

> NOTE: To make identification of landmarks easier, begin the surgical dissection proximal or distal to the area of bruising.

Positioning

The patient is positioned in lateral recumbency for all lateral approaches and for olecranon osteotomy. The patient is positioned in dorsal recumbency for medial or combined medial and lateral approaches to the elbow. A hanging-leg preparation will facilitate manipulation of the limb during surgery. The region from just dorsal to the scapula proximally to the carpus distally should be clipped and prepped for aseptic surgery.

SURGICAL TECHNIQUE
Surgical Approach to the Proximal Epiphysis

Make an incision over the craniolateral region of the proximal humerus (Fig. 32-36, A). Begin the incision 2 to 3 cm proximal to the greater tubercle and extend it distally to a point near the midshaft of the humerus. Incise through the subcutaneous tissue along the same line to expose deep fascia along the lateral border of the brachiocephalicus muscle and insertion of the deltoid muscle (Fig. 32-36, B). Elevate and reflect the brachiocephalicus muscle from the cranial surface of the bone. Elevate the deltoid muscle, and retract it caudally to expose the insertions of the teres minor and infraspinatus muscles. Make an incision through the insertions of these two muscles to expose the lateral surface of the proximal humerus (Fig. 32-36, C). If increased exposure of the craniomedial surface of the proximal humerus is needed, release the insertion of the superficial pectoral muscle deep to the brachiocephalicus muscle. To close, suture the tendons of the teres minor and infraspinatus muscles. Then suture the fascia of the superficial pectoral muscle to the fascia of the deltoid muscle. Appose the fascia of the brachiocephalicus muscle, then suture subcutaneous tissue and skin.

Surgical Approach to the Lateral Portion of the Humeral Condyle and Epicondyle

Make a lateral incision beginning over the distal third of the humerus and extending to a point 4 to 5 cm distal to the elbow overlying the ulna (Fig. 32-37, A). Incise the subcutaneous tissue to expose the deep brachial fascia. Incise the deep fascia along the cranial border of the lateral triceps muscle and continue this incision across the joint over the extensors (Fig. 32-37, B). Incise the intermuscular septum between the extensor carpi radialis and the common digital

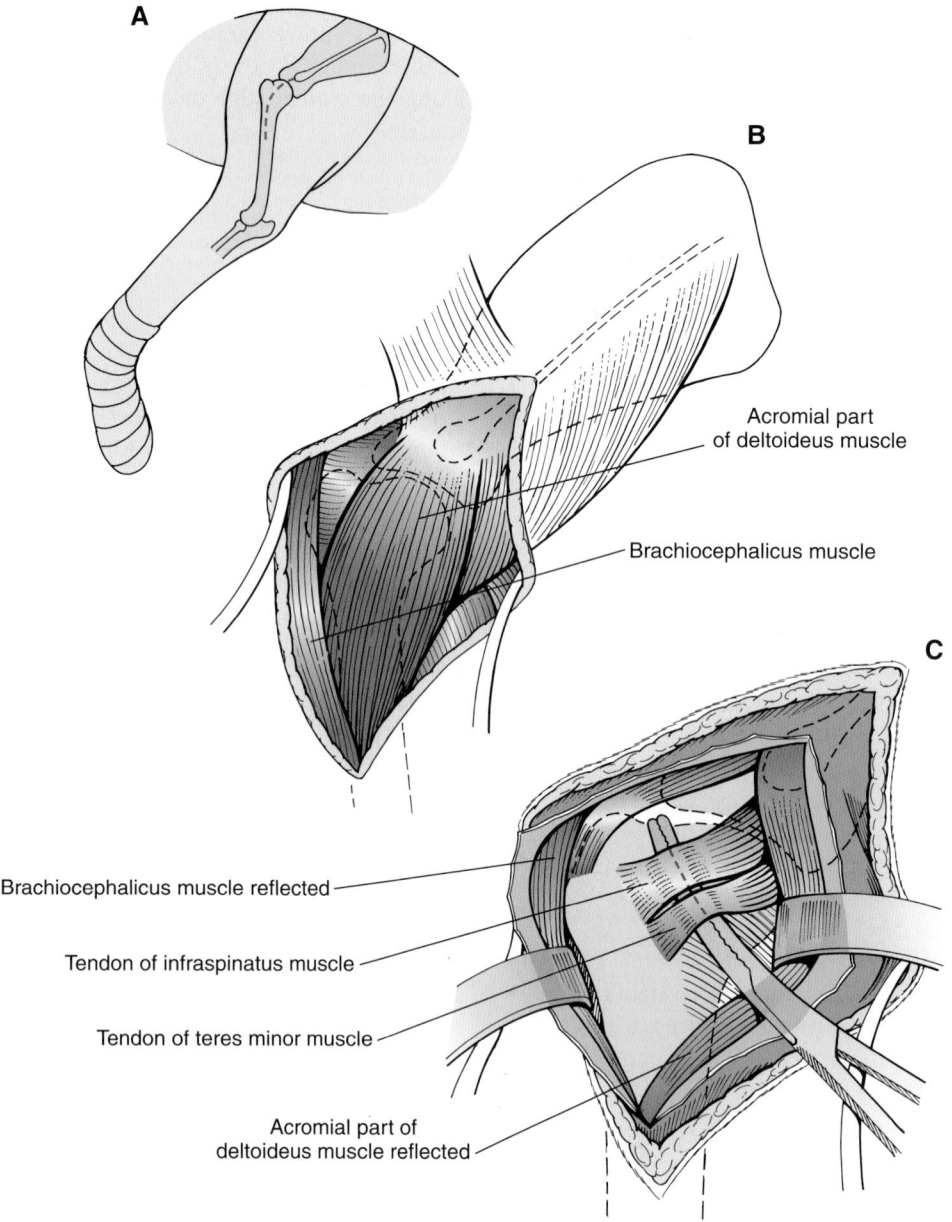

FIG. 32-36
A, To expose the proximal humerus, make an incision over its craniolateral region.
B, Expose deep fascia along the lateral border of the brachiocephalicus muscle and insertion of the deltoid muscle. **C,** Make an incision through the insertions of the infraspinatus and teres minor muscles to expose the lateral surface of the proximal humerus.

extensor muscle and continue the incision proximally through the periosteal origin of the extensor carpi radialis muscle (Fig. 32-37, C). Retract the muscle cranially to expose the joint capsule and underlying lateral condyle. For further exposure of the epicondyle, incise through the anconeus muscle at its origin on the epicondylar ridge (Fig. 32-37, D).

Incise the joint capsule with an L-shaped incision to visualize the humeral condyle. To close the incision, suture the joint capsule and close the intermuscular septum with interrupted sutures. Suture the origins of the external carpi radialis and anconeus muscles together with interrupted sutures, and then suture subcutaneous tissue and skin.

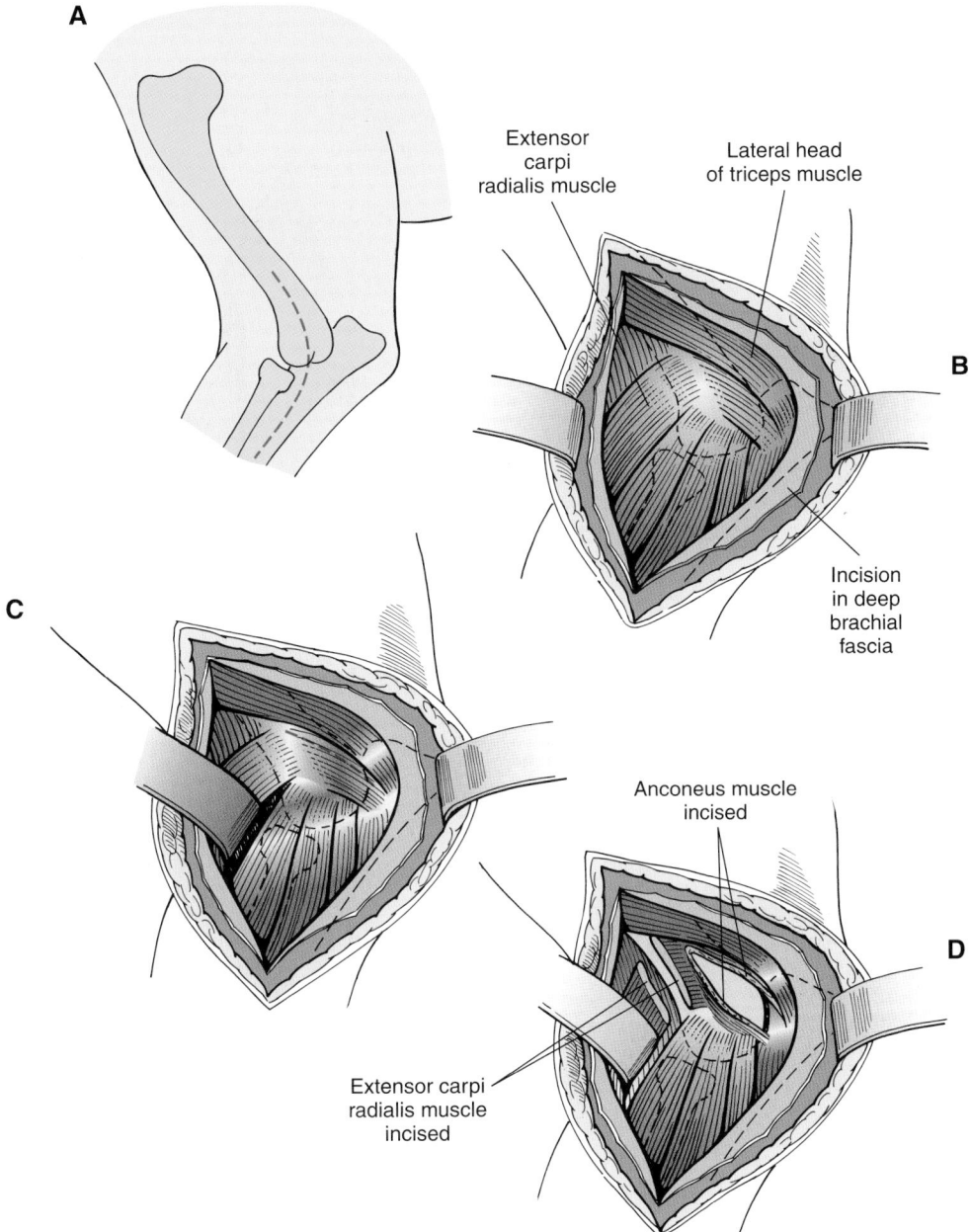

FIG. 32-37
A, To expose the distal humeral condyle, make a lateral incision over the distal third of the humerus, extending 4 to 5 cm distal to the elbow joint. **B,** Incise the deep fascia to expose the extensor muscles. **C,** Incise the intermuscular septum between the extensor carpi radialis and common digital extensor muscles. Continue the incision proximally through the periosteal origin of the extensor carpi radialis muscle. **D,** Retract the muscle cranially to expose the joint capsule and underlying humeral condyle. For further exposure of the epicondyle, incise through the anconeus muscle at its origin on the epicondylar ridge.

Surgical Approach to the Elbow via Olecranon Osteotomy

Make an incision from the distal third of the humerus to the proximal third of the ulna. Center the incision at the level of the olecranon process over the caudolateral region of the leg. Undermine the subcutaneous tissue such that the caudal skin margin can be reflected over the olecranon process to expose the medial epicondyle. Laterally, free the cranial border of the lateral head of the triceps near its tendinous insertion at the olecranon (Fig. 32-38, A).

Next, flex the elbow and palpate the ulnar nerve as it courses in the deep fascia along the cranial edge of the

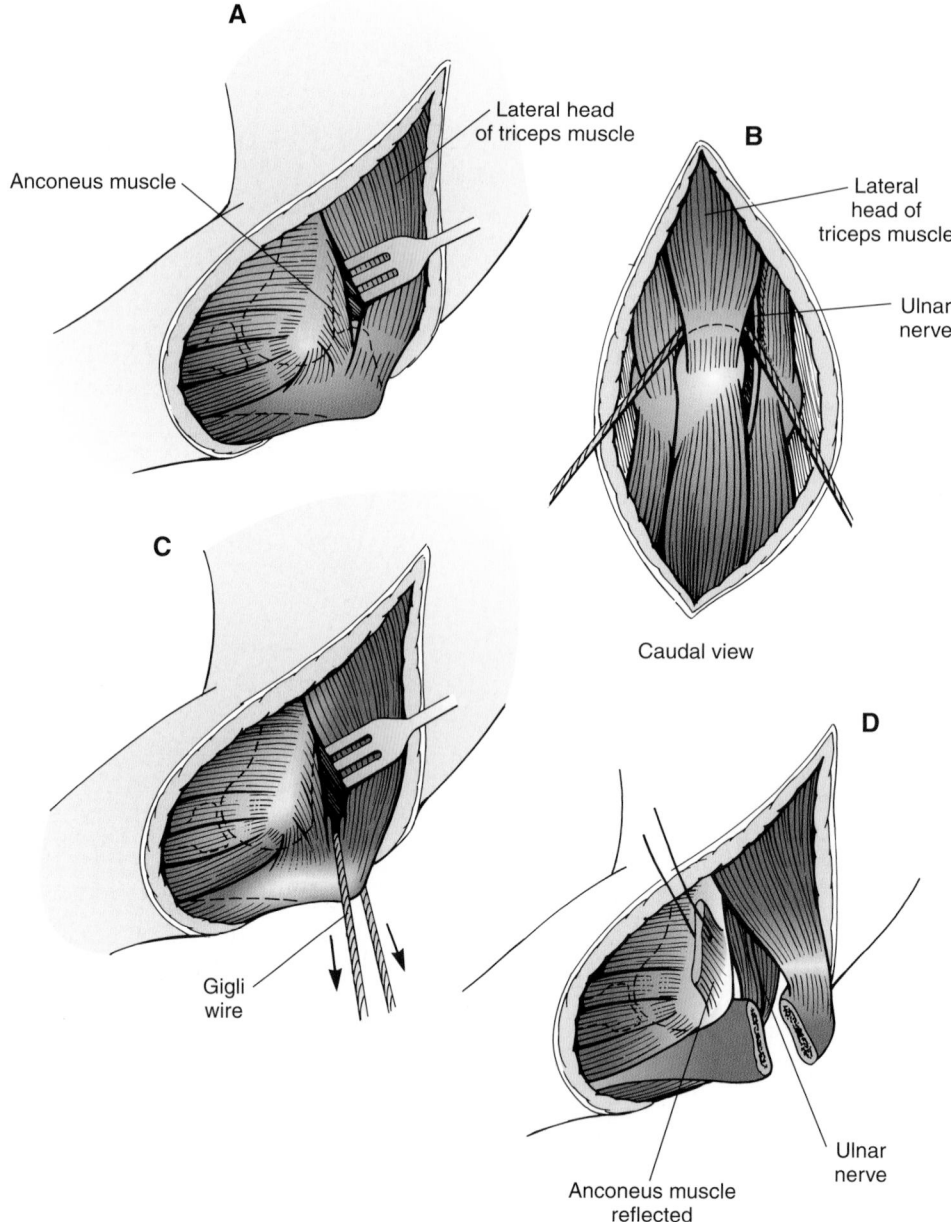

FIG. 32-38
A, For osteotomy of the olecranon, free the cranial border of the triceps lateral head near its tendinous insertion at the olecranon. **B,** Pass a Gigli wire through a lateral fascial incision to exit through a medial fascial incision. **C,** Pull the wire caudally next to the olecranon beneath the triceps tendon. **D,** Incise and retract the anconeus muscle from the lateral and medial epicondylar ridges.

medial head of the triceps. The nerve should be isolated and protected during the osteotomy procedure. Incise the fascia along the cranial border of the medial head of the triceps near its insertion at the olecranon. Pass a Gigli wire through the lateral fascial incision so that it exits through the medial fascial incision (Fig. 32-38, B). Pull the wire caudally next to the olecranon beneath the tendon of the triceps (Fig. 32-38, C). Make sure the ulnar nerve is free

from the wire and then osteotomize the olecranon process with the Gigli wire. Incise and retract the anconeus muscle from the lateral and medial epicondylar ridges (Fig. 32-38, D), then reflect the olecranon process and triceps muscle proximally to visualize the caudal surface of the elbow joint. For closure, reduce and stabilize the olecranon process with a tension band wire (see p. 990). Suture the border of the triceps to the deep fascia on the medial and

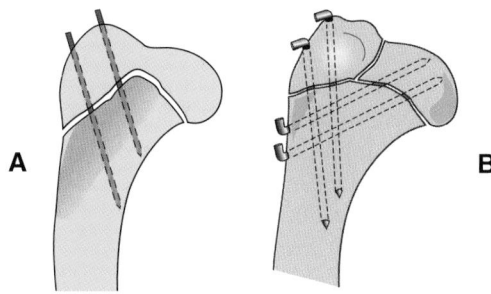

FIG. 32-39
A, Stabilize a proximal humeral Salter I fracture with two Kirschner wires or small Steinmann pins. **B,** Stabilize a proximal humeral Salter III fracture with multiple Kirschner wires or small Steinmann pins. (Part B modified from Johnson AL, Dunning D: *Atlas of orthopedic surgical procedures of the dog and cat,* ed 1, St Louis, 2005, Saunders.)

lateral sides of the leg and close the subcutaneous tissue and skin.

Stabilization of Proximal Epiphyseal and Metaphyseal Fractures

Patients with gunshot injuries or injuries resulting from high-velocity motor vehicle accidents generally have comminuted fractures and significant soft tissue injury.

In such patients with a low fracture-assessment score (0 to 3), consider using a buttress plate, or a buttress plate–rod construct. Repair comminuted fractures with a moderate fracture-assessment score (4 to 7) using a buttress plate or a modified Type Ib external skeletal fixator, with an IM pin tie-in. Treat patients with a low or moderate fracture-assessment score and a simple fracture pattern (i.e., transverse or oblique) using a compression plate or neutralization plate. Alternatively, use an IM pin combined with cerclage wire and Kirschner wire (in an oblique fracture) and supported with a Type Ia external skeletal fixator.

Stabilization of Proximal Physeal Fractures

Salter I physeal fractures of the proximal humerus may be closed reduced and stabilized with diverging Kirschner wires or small Steinmann pins if adequate reduction can be achieved.

Insert the pin into the bone proximally at the greater tubercle, and drive it distocaudally to cross the fracture line and seat in the caudal metaphysis. If closed reduction is not possible, perform open reduction and pin stabilization (Fig. 32-39, A).

Salter III fractures of the proximal physis are also stabilized with divergent Kirschner wires.

 BOX 32-5

Implant Use According to Fracture-Assessment Score (FAS) for Humeral Condylar Fractures

FAS 4 to 10
- Lag screw plus Kirschner wires
- Self-compressing pin

FAS 0 to 3
- Lag screw plus plate

Attach the humeral head to the proximal humerus with two Kirschner wires, then reduce the greater tubercle and secure it to the humerus with two Kirschner wires (Fig. 32-39, B).

Stabilization of Lateral or Medial Condylar Fractures

Condylar fractures are usually stabilized after open reduction and inspection of the joint reconstruction. Fluoroscopically guided closed reduction with internal fixation with screws and Kirschner wires or small pins is an alternative (Cook et al, 1999). In most cases, stabilization is best attained with an intercondylar lag screw or self-compressing pin combined with a Kirschner wire or small pin bridging the fracture of the epicondyloid crest.

In patients with suspected incomplete ossification and subsequently prolonged healing time, bridge the epicondyloid crest with a small plate to protect the lag screw from shearing forces (Box 32-5).
   Achieve intercondylar compression by placing a cortex screw as a lag screw using a glide hole drilled in the lateral condyle and a thread hole drilled in the medial condyle.
   Drill the glide hole before reducing the fracture.

The glide hole may be drilled from the fracture surface to exit at the lateral epicondyle or from the lateral epicondyle to exit at the fracture surface.

Reduce the fracture and hold it in position with bone-holding forceps and a Kirschner wire placed perpendicular to the fracture surface. Place an appropriately sized drill sleeve in the glide hole and drill, measure, then tap the thread hole to accept the appropriate screw (see Fig. 31-73 on p. 994). Achieve additional rotational support by placing a Kirschner wire, small pin, or caudal bone plate across the lateral epicondyloid crest.

Fracture assessment in immature toy-breed dogs with lateral condylar fractures is favorable for rapid bone union. Stabilization can be accomplished by intercondylar compression with a bone screw and a small pin crossing the epicondyloid crest for rotational support. Alternatively, stabilization can be accomplished with a small self-compressing pin across the condylar fracture coupled with a Kirschner wire crossing the epicondyloid crest.

Stabilization of T or Y Fractures of the Elbow

These elbow fractures most often result from motor vehicle accidents and falls from a significant height. Occasionally, these fractures occur after minimal trauma, as incomplete ossification of the condyle is the underlying pathology. The intercondylar fracture is accompanied by a transverse, oblique, or comminuted fracture through the medial and lateral epicondyloid crests. Open reduction is necessary for accurate alignment of the intercondylar fracture. A combined medial and lateral approach to the humeral condyle (see Figs. 32-29 and 32-37), or an osteotomy of the olecranon (see Fig. 32-38) may be used to expose the fracture. The method of stabilization depends on the patient's fracture-assessment score. Those with a low score (0 to 3) require an implant system rigid enough to resist major weight-bearing loads for an extended period.

Use a lag screw for the intercondylar fracture; affix the condyles to the humerus with a plate-rod combination or medial and lateral plates. When a plate-rod system is used, place the IM pin in the medial position and place the bone plate caudolaterally (see Fig. 32-35).

The condyles may also be affixed to the shaft of the humerus by using a plate applied to the caudomedial epicondyloid crest with a second plate applied to the caudolateral epicondyloid crest (see Fig. 32-35).

For elbow fractures in patients with an intermediate fracture-assessment score (4 to 7), use an intercondylar lag screw with the condyles affixed to the humeral diaphysis with a medially applied bone plate. For elbow fractures in patients with a favorable fracture-assessment score (8 to 10), use an intercondylar lag screw and two IM pins. Pass one pin through the medial epicondyloid crest, across the fracture plane, and into the proximal segment of the humerus; the pin will exit the bone near the greater tubercle. Place a second pin through the lateral epicondyloid crest and across the fracture to exit the metaphysis of the proximal segment of the humerus.

SUTURE MATERIALS AND SPECIAL INSTRUMENTS

Helpful instruments for fracture repair include a battery-powered or air-driven drill with a wire-driving attachment, self-retaining retractors, and pointed reduction forceps. A plating system is required for screws and bone plates.

 Table 32-6

Sample Physical Rehabilitation Protocol for Patients With Elbow or Carpal Fractures

ALL TREATMENTS BID	DAY 1 TO DAY 14	DAY 15 TO DAY 24	DAY 25 UNTIL HEALED	HEALED TO RETURN TO FUNCTION
Heat therapy		10 min	10 min	
Passive range of motion (repetitions)	20*	20*	10–15*	Stop-when ROM N
Therapeutic exercise-total time	10 min	15 min	15 min	25–45 min
Walk/land treadmill	10 min	5 min	5 min	>10 min
Balancing	+	+	+	
Obstacles	+	+	+	+
Weaving				+
Circles				+
Hills				+
Stairs				+
Jog/run				+
Underwater treadmill		10 min	10 min	>15 min
Swimming				5–10 min
Cryotherapy	15 min	15 min	15 min	PRN

BID, Twice a day; *ROM,* range of motion; *N,* normal; +, perform modality; *PRN,* as needed.
*Perform passive range of motion for all joints of the affected limb.

POSTOPERATIVE CARE AND ASSESSMENT

Postoperative radiographs are made to evaluate fracture reduction and implant location. Activity should be restricted to leash walking and physical rehabilitation until the fracture has healed. Physical rehabilitation encourages controlled limb use and optimal limb function after fracture healing and is particularly important fractures involving the joint. Care must be taken to develop customized protocols for each patient depending on location of the fracture, stability and type of fracture fixation, potential for healing, abilities and attitudes of the patient, and willingness of the client (see Chapter 12) (Table 32-6). External fixator management includes daily pin care and pin packing as needed. Radiographs should be evaluated in 6 weeks. External fixators may be destabilized at this time if healing is progressing satisfactorily. Radiographs should be repeated at 6-week intervals until fracture bridging is observed. IM pins and external fixators should be removed when the fracture is healed. Lag screws and plates are left in place unless they cause problems.

COMPLICATIONS

Proximal fractures of the humerus generally heal without complication. This is particularly true in young patients with physeal fractures because of their favorable healing potential. Kirschner wires and small pins may migrate. Intraartic-

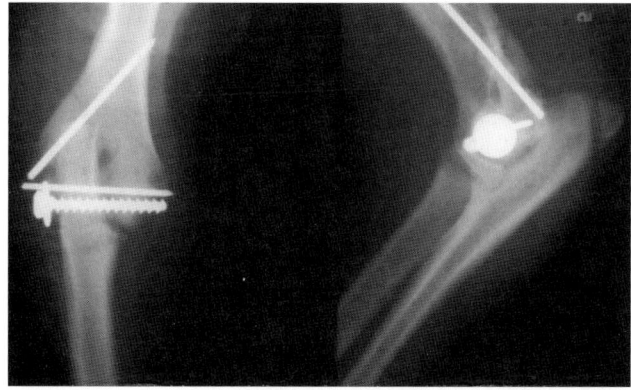
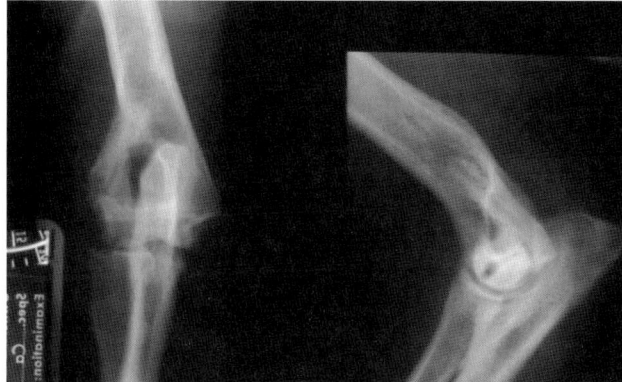

A

B

FIG. 32-40
Postoperative radiographs. **A,** Stabilization of a Salter IV fracture of the lateral portion of the humeral condyle with a lag screw and two Kirschner wires. **B,** Implants were removed 5 months later. Note the lack of callus and minimal degenerative joint disease.

ular fractures may result in postoperative degenerative joint disease, although this is minimized with careful reduction and rigid fixation (Fig. 32-40).

PROGNOSIS

Supracondylar and condylar fractures of the humerus may have prolonged healing periods, with the implant subjected to moderate stresses for extended periods. Bone resorption and implant loosening may eventually result. Fatigue breakage of implants can occur (Box 32-6). A high complication rate is associated with olecranon osteotomy repair. Distal condylar fractures generally heal quickly in immature dogs, but healing is often delayed in older dogs. Failure to reconstruct the joint surface anatomically will result in degenerative joint disease. A decreased range of motion of the elbow may occur after surgery.

Reference

Cook JL, Tomlinson JL, Reed AL: Fluoroscopically guided closed reduction and internal fixation of fractures of the lateral portion of the humeral condyle: prospective clinical study of the technique and results in ten dogs, *Vet Surg* 28:315, 1999.

Suggested Reading

Butterworth SJ, Innes JF: Incomplete humeral condylar fractures in the dog, *J Small Anim Pract* 42:394, 2001.
Eight dogs presenting with elbow pain associated with incomplete fracture (ossification) of the humeral condyle are reviewed. The dogs were treated with a transcondylar bone screw and six made a complete recovery.
Guille AE, Lewis DD, Anderson TP et al: Evaluation of surgical repair of humeral condylar fractures using self-compressing Orthofix pins in 23 dogs, *Vet Surg* 33:314, 2004.
A report of the short- and long-term clinical and radiographic outcomes achieved when dogs with humeral condylar fractures were treated with self-compressing Orthofix pins. Pins were used in place of lag screw fixation for the fractures.
Halling KB, Lewis DD, Cross AR et al: Complication rate and factors affecting outcome of olecranon osteotomies requiring pin and tension band fixation in dogs, *Can Vet J* 43:528, 2002.
Olecranon osteotomies performed to assist the surgical approach to distal humeral fractures were reviewed to determine a complication rate. Thirty-seven percent of the animals had complications related to the osteotomy, including osteomyelitis and implant-related failures.

 BOX 32-6

Common Errors in Humeral Condylar Fracture Fixation

- Failure to reduce a joint surface anatomically results in degenerative joint disease and loss of function.
- Failure to use a large lag screw and support the fracture with a plate can result in implant failure in mature animals with condylar fractures initiated by incomplete ossification.

McKee WM, Macais C, Innes JF: Bilateral fixation of Y-T humeral condylar fractures via medial and lateral approaches in 29 dogs, *J Small Anim Pract* 46:217, 2005.

A description of bilateral fixation of Y-T fractures of the humeral condyle via combined medial and lateral approaches. The technique's clinical and radiographic short-term outcomes are detailed. This technique avoids the complications associated with olecranon osteotomy.

Meyer-Lindenberg A, Heinen V, Fehr M et al: Incomplete ossification of the humeral condyle as the cause of lameness in dogs, *Vet Comp Orthop Traumatol* 15:187, 2002.

A retrospective and prospective study pursued over 6 years, which documents the diagnosis made by radiographs, CT, and arthroscopy. A good description of the arthroscopic lesions associated with the disease is presented and results of transcondylar lag screw treatment are detailed.

Turner TM: Fractures of the humerus. In Johnson AL, Houlton JEF, Vannini R, editors: *AO principles of fracture management in the dog and cat*, Thieme, NY, 2005, AO Publishing.

This chapter provides an up-to-date collection of operative techniques for stabilizing humeral fractures in small animals. Detailed descriptions of lag screw application and bone-plating procedures are included in radial and ulnar fractures.

RADIAL AND ULNAR DIAPHYSEAL FRACTURES

DEFINITIONS

Radial diaphyseal fractures and **ulnar diaphyseal fractures** are a result of trauma to the forelimb. Open fractures (wounds through the skin over the bone) may occur because of the sparse soft tissue coverage.

GENERAL CONSIDERATIONS AND CLINICALLY RELEVANT PATHOPHYSIOLOGY

Diaphyseal fractures usually involve the middle to distal diaphysis of both radius and ulna. Because these fractures are usually secondary to trauma, the animal should be closely evaluated to detect concurrent injuries (e.g., pulmonary contusions, pneumothorax, rib fractures, and traumatic myocarditis). The paucity of soft tissue increases the possibility of open fractures and potentially decreases the extraosseous blood supply, both of which can delay bone healing. Minimal soft tissue coverage of bone plates results in tissue irritation and cold hypersensitivity, but is advantageous for placing a bilateral external fixator.

Toy-breed dogs often fracture the radius and ulna after apparently minimal trauma of jumping or falling. These fractures are also associated with a high complication rate. Biomechanical instability related to the short oblique nature of these fractures, a paucity of distal diaphyseal vasculature compared with large-breed dogs, and limited surrounding soft tissue for the extraosseous vasculature may contribute to the high frequency of delayed unions and nonunions.

DIAGNOSIS

Clinical Presentation

Signalment. Any age, breed, or sex of dog or cat may be affected. Young animals sustain vehicular trauma more frequently.

History. Affected animals usually have a non–weight-bearing lameness after trauma. Toy-breed dogs are often brought in after apparently minimal trauma of jumping or falling.

Physical Examination Findings

Because of the traumatic nature of radial and ulnar fractures, the entire animal must be assessed to detect abnormalities of other body systems. Palpation of the limb reveals swelling, pain, and crepitation. The fracture may be open and there may or may not be substantial loss or damage of adjacent soft tissue. Affected animals often appear to have abnormal proprioceptive responses because they are reluctant to move the limb.

> NOTE: A careful neurologic examination will help differentiate between true neurologic injury and apparent neurologic injury associated with pain.

Diagnostic Imaging

Craniocaudal and lateral radiographs of the affected radius and ulna (which include the proximal and distal joints) are required to assess the extent of bone and soft tissue injury. Fractious or extremely painful animals may require sedation (see Tables 31-2 and 31-3 on pp. 933 and 934, respectively) or general anesthesia for radiography after it has been determined that no contraindications (i.e., shock, hypotension, or severe dyspnea) to administration of sedatives or anesthetics exist. Thoracic radiography should be performed to evaluate for thoracic trauma.

Laboratory Findings

Complete blood count and serum chemistry evaluation should be done to evaluate the status of the animal for anesthesia and to determine if concurrent injury or damage of the renal or hepatobiliary systems exists.

DIFFERENTIAL DIAGNOSIS

Animals having radial and ulnar fractures should be evaluated to determine whether the fractures result from trauma or underlying pathology (e.g., neoplasia and metabolic disease).

MEDICAL MANAGEMENT

Medical treatment of animals with radial and ulnar fractures includes analgesics for posttraumatic pain (see Box 31-2 on p. 944 and Chapter 13) and antibiotics to treat open fractures. Conservative management of radial and ulnar diaphyseal fractures consists of splints and casts and is reserved for closed nondisplaced or greenstick fractures in immature animals. Cast fixation is appropriate for these fractures because the joint above and below the fractured bone (elbow and carpus) can be immobilized, and they heal rapidly. Casts and splints are contraindicated for treatment of distal diaphyseal fractures in miniature and toy-breed dogs due to the high incidence of nonunion in these animals.

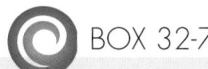 BOX 32-7

Decision Making for Open or Closed Reduction for Radial Diaphyseal Fractures

Open Reduction
- Displaced reducible fractures with plate application

Limited Open Reduction
- Displaced reducible fractures with external skeletal fixation
- Comminuted fractures for cancellous bone graft placement

Closed Reduction
- Nondisplaced fractures with external coaptation or external skeletal fixation
- Comminuted nonreducible fractures with external skeletal fixation

---

NOTE: Consider whether the animal will be able to bear weight on the other three limbs when choosing cast fixation.

SURGICAL TREATMENT

The decision to perform an open or a closed reduction of radial and ulnar diaphyseal fractures is made based on fracture configuration and fracture-assessment score (Box 32-7). Simple or moderately comminuted fractures with large fragments that can be anatomically reconstructed to establish the bone column are candidates for open reduction and stabilization with internal fixation, limited open reduction and external skeletal fixation, or a combination of techniques.

Severely comminuted fractures that cannot be completely reconstructed are candidates for closed reduction and external skeletal fixation or open reduction and application of a bridging plate and cancellous bone autograft (see p. 962). Whether the fracture is open or closed is less important than the potential of the fracture to be anatomically reconstructed. Advantages and disadvantages of open and closed reduction need to be weighed to determine the best approach for each individual fracture. The ulna is usually supported indirectly by radial stabilization; however, stabilization of the ulna is indicated when doing so will add support to a comminuted radial fracture, when additional support is needed for a large dog, and when anatomic reduction of the radius and ulna is essential to future performance of an athlete. Fixation systems applicable to fractures of the radial and ulnar diaphysis are casts, IM pins (ulna), external skeletal fixation, and plates and screws (Box 32-8).

Application of Casts

Casts can be applied as the sole method of fixation for stable fractures in young dogs or cats when the fracture will maintain adequate reduction and heal quickly (see p. 967). The

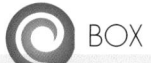 BOX 32-8

Implant Use for Fractures of the Radial Diaphysis According to Fracture-Assessment Score (FAS)

FAS 0 to 3
- Bone plate and screws
- Type II external skeletal fixation

FAS 4 to 7
- Type Ib or Type II external skeletal fixation
- Bone plate and screws

FAS 8 to 10
- Type Ia or Type Ib external skeletal fixation
- Cast

---

cast is applied so that it immobilizes the carpus and elbow. Although manipulation of the fracture is rarely possible during casting, the limb should be positioned with slight carpal flexion and varus angulation (Fig. 32-41). The cast can be applied over extra cast padding, cut longitudinally along the medial and lateral surfaces, and taped in position to form a "bivalve cast" that can be changed periodically. This type of cast does not offer as rigid a fixation as a cylinder cast, but it is easily changed to allow wound management.

NOTE: Warning: toy-breed dogs with radial fractures treated with casts and splints have a high complication rate; these fractures should be managed with plate fixation.

Application of Intramedullary Pins

IM pins are difficult to use in the radius because of the narrow configuration of the radial medullary canal and the necessity of invading the carpal joint to position the pin. Complications associated with IM pin placement in the radius include angulation, distraction, rotation, osteomyelitis, delayed union, nonunion, and degenerative joint disease of the elbow and carpus.

NOTE: IM pins and interlocking nails are contraindicated as a treatment for radial fractures because of the narrow configuration of the radial medullary canal and necessity of invading the carpal joint to position the pin.

An IM pin can be used to align the ulna, stabilize a simple ulnar fracture, and add support to the primary fixation of a comminuted radial fracture (i.e., external fixator or plate; see pp. 969 to 991). The IM pin should be introduced into the medullary canal from the proximal surface of the olecranon and driven in an antegrade manner to the fracture surface. Care should be taken to parallel the lateral cortex of the ulna to maintain the pin within the medullary

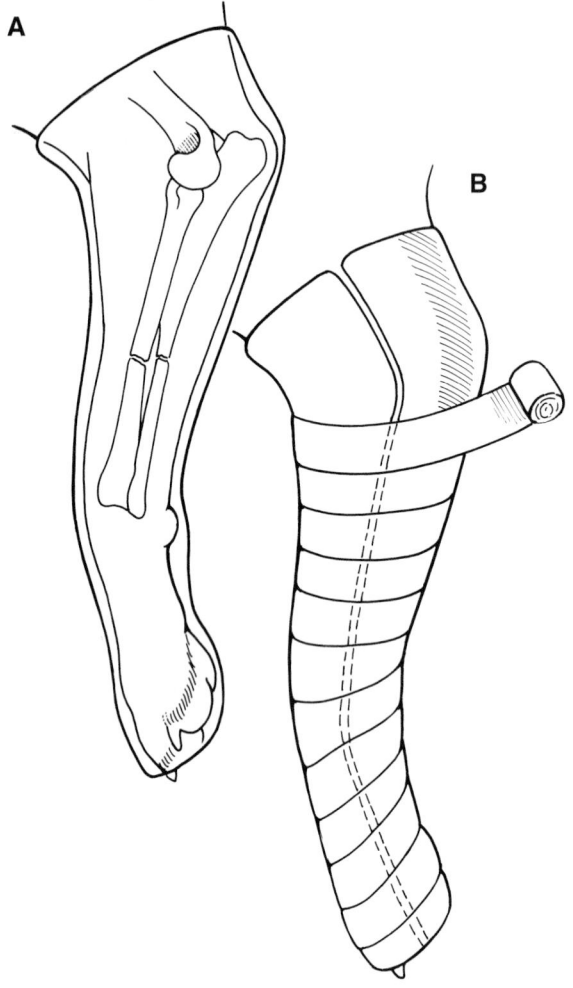

FIG. 32-41
Casts are used to stabilize closed, nondisplaced radial-ulnar fractures in patients with fracture-assessment scores of 8 to 10. **A,** Full cylinder cast, which immobilizes the elbow and carpus, is placed with the limb positioned in slight carpal flexion and varus angulation. **B,** Cast can be bivalved by placing the cast material over multiple layers of padding, cutting it on the lateral and medial aspects, and securing it with elastic tape.

canal. Once the fracture is aligned, the pin should be driven distally as far as possible without penetrating the cortex. The pin is cut below the level of the skin, over the proximal ulna.

Application of External Skeletal Fixators

Type Ia or Ib frames. External skeletal fixation (see p. 969) is particularly useful for treating a wide variety of radial diaphyseal fractures. The stiffness of the fixator can be increased in animals with low fracture-assessment scores by adding fixation pins and using bilateral and biplanar frames. Radial fractures are frequently open, making use of external fixation attractive for avoiding invasion of the fracture site with metal implants. With open fractures, implant removal is desirable after fracture healing and easily accomplished

with external fixation. A Type Ia (unilateral external fixation splint) is usually applied to the cranial medial surface of the radius (Fig. 32-42, *A* and *B*). Applying it to this location avoids penetration of the major muscle masses with the fixation pins and decreases the morbidity associated with the pins. When a Type Ib fixation splint is applied, every effort should be made to locate the fixation pins in areas of bone that have minimal muscle coverage, usually the cranial medial and cranial lateral surfaces (Fig. 32-42, *C*). Articulation and diagonal connecting bars may be added for additional stability.

> NOTE: Construct the fixator to suit the patient and the fracture. A lower fracture-assessment score requires a stiffer fixator.

Type II frames. Although penetration of major muscle masses is unavoidable with Type II or bilateral fixation splints, they are often used because of their increased stiffness and because the proximal and distal transfixation pins can be used as guide pins for limb alignment. The fixation splint should span the length of the bone, with the most proximal and distal pins placed in the metaphyses and the central pins placed about 1 to 2 cm from the fracture line. Additional pins can be placed when there is adequate bone. Some dogs have very thin radii when viewed from the lateral projection. If a Type II frame is applied to these dogs, use smaller fixation pins in the middle of the frame to avoid splitting the bone. Type II frames are placed in the following manner. The initial transfixation pins should be placed in the proximal and distal metaphyses of the radius. These pins should be centered in the bone on the medial to lateral plane and parallel to the respective joint surfaces.

Severely comminuted fractures are usually reduced in a closed manner. They are restored to length using the weight of the animal in the hanging-limb position, and realigned by maneuvering the transfixation pins parallel to each other. Open reduction through a limited approach may be used to facilitate reconstruction of the bone column in single fractures. The frame is filled out by placing at least two pins (preferably three) proximal and distal to the fracture (Fig. 32-43, *A*). Often the cranial curve of the radius precludes the placement of bilateral transfixation pins, and unilateral pins are used in the radial diaphysis (Fig. 32-43, *B*). Postoperative radiographs should be taken to ensure that appropriate fracture reduction, pin placement, and joint alignment were achieved. Residual valgus or varus deformities can be corrected by loosening the clamps and distracting the appropriate side of the limb (see p. 1130). Mild rotation can be corrected by reversing the position of the clamps on the appropriate side of the pins in the distal fragment. Every effort should be made to achieve correct alignment of the limb before the procedure is completed.

Acrylic pin external fixators. External fixation with fixation pins and methylmethacrylate connecting bars is a versatile alternative to the standard external fixation system

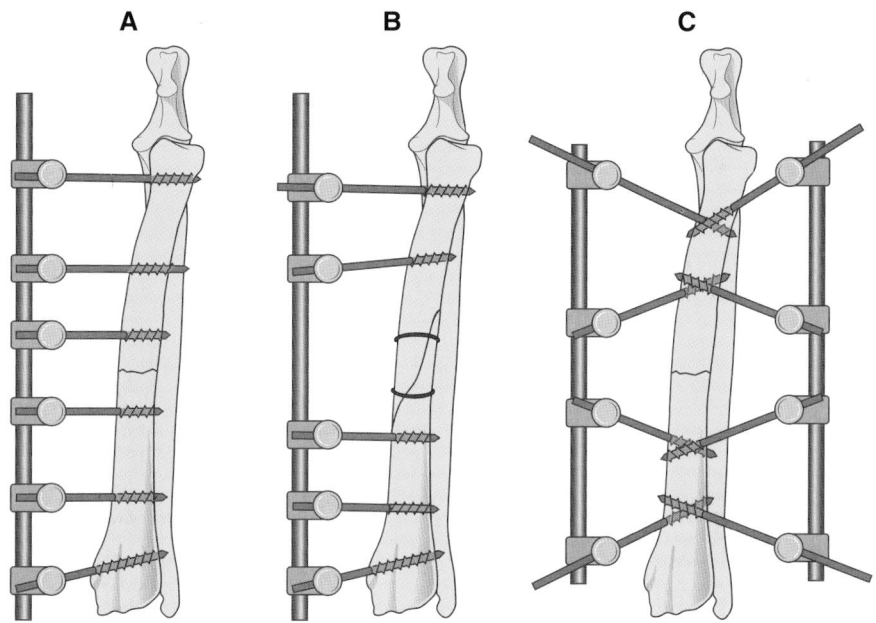

FIG. 32-42
Type Ia and Ib external fixators are used to treat radial fractures in patients with high and moderate fracture-assessment scores. **A,** A Type I external fixator is placed on the cranio-medial surface of the radius to stabilize a transverse fracture. **B,** Anatomic reconstruction of long oblique fracture with cerclage wire restores the bony column and allows load sharing with the external fixator. **C,** A Type Ib fixator is applied to patients with moderate fracture-assessment scores to provide additional stability.

(see p. 974). Fixation pins of any size can be directed at angles that optimize the purchase of good quality bone, without regard for clamp compatibility or uniplanar pin placement. This technique may be used to stabilize distal diaphyseal fractures in toy-breed dogs.

Circular and hybrid external fixators. Circular external fixators may be used effectively for radial diaphyseal fractures, especially comminuted nonreducible fractures treated with closed reduction. The fixation frame may be manipulated postoperatively to correct angular deformities in both cranial caudal and medial lateral planes. Circular fixators allow controlled axial micromotion of stabilized bone segments, promoting rapid bone union. However, circular fixators require considerable preoperative planning and frame construction to shorten surgical time, and optimal aftercare to minimize implant-related complications (see p. 967). Combining a distal ring and wires with a linear connecting rod and fixation pins placed proximally, a hybrid construct, is useful to stabilize complex radial fractures with short distal bone segments (see p. 981).

Application of Bone Plates and Screws

Bone plates are an excellent method of stabilizing radial and ulnar diaphyseal fractures. Plates are usually applied to the wide, flat, cranial surface of the radius; however, they are equally effective when applied to the medial surface of the

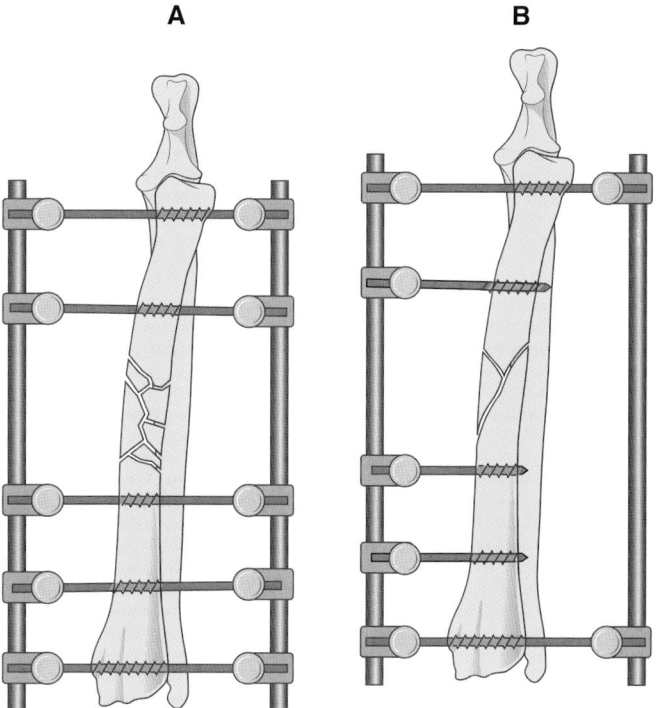

FIG. 32-43
A, A maximal Type II external fixator frame consists of all transfixation pins. **B,** Because of the cranial curve of the radius, a minimal Type II frame is constructed using unilateral fixation pins to fill out the frame.

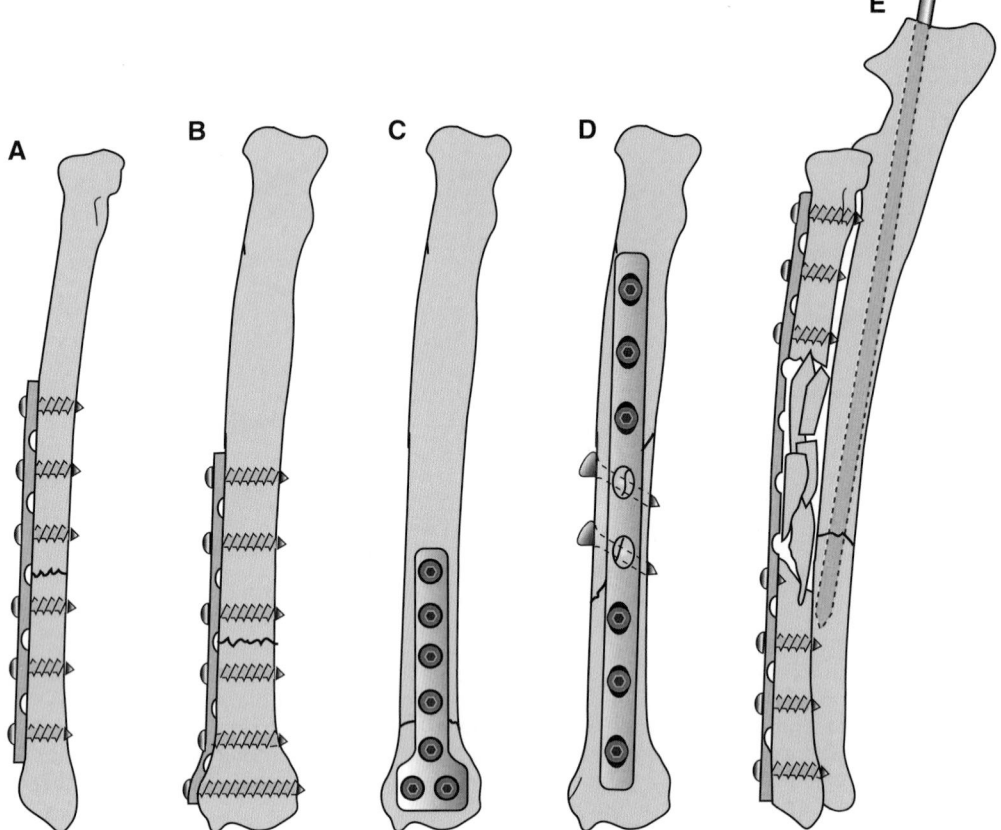

FIG. 32-44
A and **B,** A compression plate is used to stabilize transverse fractures of the radial diaphysis and can be applied to the cranial or medial surface of the bone. **C,** A T plate is used to stabilize distal radial diaphyseal fractures where there is a small distal bone segment.
D, Long oblique fractures may be stabilized with lag screws and a neutralization plate.
E, Comminuted nonreducible radial diaphyseal fractures are bridged with a plate. Additional support may be gained by supporting the ulna with an intramedullary pin. (Modified from Johnson AL, Dunning D: *Atlas of orthopedic surgical procedures of the dog and cat,* ed 1, St Louis, 2005, Saunders.)

distal radius (Fig. 32-44, *A* and *B*). A wide exposure of the fracture and intact bone is necessary for fracture reconstruction and plate application. Plates are applied as compression plates to transverse fractures. Transverse or short oblique fractures of the distal radial diaphysis can be treated with a T plate to achieve adequate screw purchase on the distal segment (Fig. 32-44, *C*). Mini T plates and veterinary cuttable plates are useful for stabilizing fractures in miniature and toy-breed dogs. Long oblique or spiral fractures should be reconstructed and the fracture lines compressed with lag screws. The reconstructed fracture is protected with a neutralization plate (Fig. 32-44, *D*). Comminuted diaphyseal fractures that cannot be reconstructed can be treated by distracting the fracture, realigning the limb, and bridging the fracture with a bone plate. An IM pin can be used in the ulna to support the radial repair (Fig. 32-44, *E*). If open reduction of the fractured radius is performed, consideration should be given to harvesting autogenous cancellous bone to en-

hance bone healing. The most accessible site for cancellous bone harvest is the ipsilateral proximal humerus (see p. 962). The ipsilateral ilium and tibia can also be prepared for cancellous bone harvest.

Preoperative Management

There may be extensive damage or loss of tissue in the area of the fracture. Open wounds should be managed initially by carefully clipping surrounding hair, cleaning the wound, and taking a swab for bacterial culture and susceptibility testing. The antebrachium should be temporarily stabilized with a Robert Jones bandage (see p. 946) to immobilize fragments, decrease or prevent soft tissue swelling, protect or prevent open wounds, and increase patient comfort until surgery can be performed. Perioperative pain management should also be instituted (see Box 31-2 on p. 944 and Chapter 13). Concurrent injuries should be managed before anesthetic induction for fracture fixation.

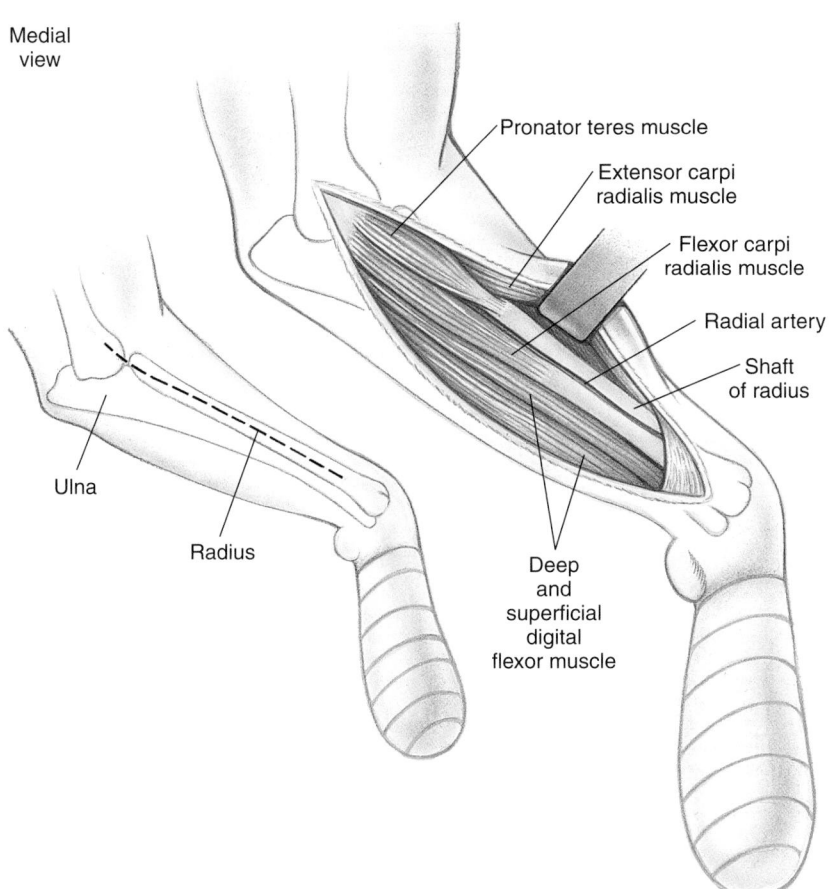

Medial view

Pronator teres muscle

Extensor carpi radialis muscle

Flexor carpi radialis muscle

Radial artery

Shaft of radius

Ulna

Radius

Deep and superficial digital flexor muscle

FIG. 32-45
For a craniomedial approach to the radial diaphysis, make an incision through skin and subcutaneous tissue to expose the radial diaphysis. Retract the extensor carpi radialis muscle laterally to expose the diaphysis.

Anesthesia

Anesthetic management of animals with fractures is discussed on p. 944.

Surgical Anatomy

The craniomedial surface of the radius and the caudal lateral surface of the ulna are not covered by muscle and can be easily palpated to serve as landmarks for location of the incision. Extensor muscles are located cranial to and flexor muscles caudal to the radius and can be retracted to expose the bone. The cephalic vein crosses the medial portion of the distal radius. The lateral radial head is palpable beneath the extensor muscles of the forearm.

Positioning

The limb should be clipped and prepped for aseptic surgery from the shoulder to carpus. If cancellous bone graft harvest is anticipated, a donor site (e.g., proximal humerus) should also be prepared. If closed reduction or limited open reduction with external skeletal fixation is chosen, positioning the animal with the affected leg suspended from the ceiling facilitates visualization of correct joint alignment (see p. 959). If open reduction with plate fixation is performed, the animal should also be positioned in dorsal recumbency and the limb draped out and pulled laterally to expose the craniomedial aspect of the radius.

SURGICAL TECHNIQUE
Craniomedial Approach to the Radius

Palpate the radius directly under the skin and subcutaneous tissue on the craniomedial surface of the limb. Make an incision through skin and subcutaneous tissue to expose the radial diaphysis. Extend the incision distally, and elevate the extensor tendons to expose the cranial surface of the distal metaphysis of the radius (Fig. 32-45).

Approach to the Proximal Ulna

Refer to p. 1070 for approach to the proximal ulna.

Stabilization of Midshaft Transverse or Short Oblique Radial Fractures

From a mechanical perspective, this fracture configuration allows load sharing between the bone and implant after surgery. Factors that negatively affect healing include multiple limb injuries, a miniature or toy-breed dog, or a large active patient. From a biologic perspective, patient fracture assessment dictates whether the time until union will be lengthy or short. With prolonged healing the implant needs to remain functional for 8 or more weeks (see p. 953). In these cases, implants that purchase bone with threads are desirable; frictional hold implants or casts are adequate for shorter healing periods.

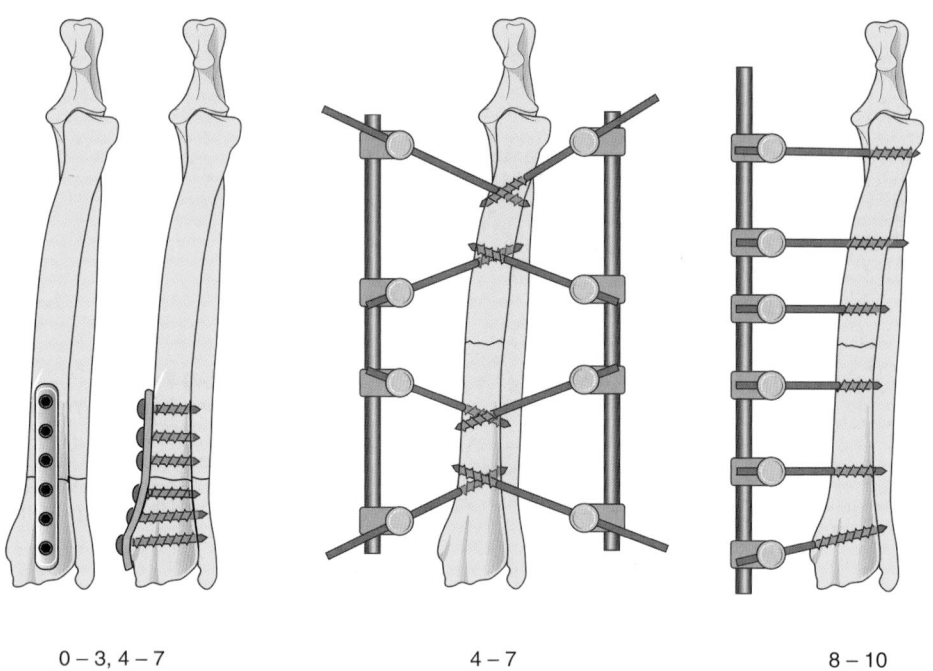

0 – 3, 4 – 7   4 – 7   8 – 10

FIG. 32-46
Recommended methods of stabilizing transverse or short oblique radial fractures based on fracture-assessment score. If fracture-assessment score is 0 to 3, a bone plate and screws are the implants of choice, but external fixators may be used. If fracture-assessment score is 4 to 7, a bone plate and screws or an external skeletal fixator may be used. With fracture-assessment scores of 8 to 10, an external skeletal fixator is preferred, or if the fracture is nondisplaced, a cast may be used.

Stabilization of a reduced transverse fracture requires only rotational and bending support; use bone plates, an external fixator, or a cast. Stabilization of a short oblique fracture requires some axial support as well to prevent shearing during load bearing. Use bone plates or external fixators for these fractures. Determine the final implant based on fracture location and patient fracture assessment.

Useful fixation systems in toy-breed dogs (in which the complication rate is high with these fractures) and in animals with a low fracture-assessment score (0 to 3) include a bone plate and screws inserted to function as a compression plate for transverse fractures, a neutralization plate for short oblique fractures, or a Type II acrylic pin external skeletal fixator.

With a moderate fracture-assessment score (4 to 7), use a compression plate, minimal Type II external skeletal fixator, or Type Ib external skeletal fixator. Stabilize transverse or short oblique fractures in patients with a high fracture-assessment score (8 to 10) with a 6-pin Type Ia external skeletal fixator or use a cast if the fracture is greenstick or nondisplaced (Fig. 32-46).

Stabilization of Midshaft Long Oblique Radial Fractures or Comminuted Fractures With Large Butterfly Fragment

From a mechanical perspective, these fractures can be reduced and interfragmentary compression applied with cerclage wire or lag screws. Once the interfragmentary fracture lines are reduced and compressed, the bone and implant can bear weight postoperatively. Factors that negatively affect healing include the presence of multiple injuries, a large active patient, and the necessity for open reduction and tissue manipulation to reduce and apply interfragmentary compression.

Stabilization of this fracture configuration requires axial, rotational, and bending support; achieve this with lag screws and bone plates or cerclage wire and/or external fixator combinations.

Fixation systems that are useful with a low fracture-assessment score (0 to 3) are lag screws to reconstruct the cylinder of bone and achieve interfragmentary compression, supported by neutralization plates or maximal Type II external skeletal fixation.

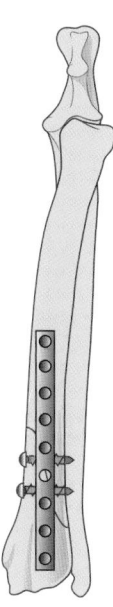
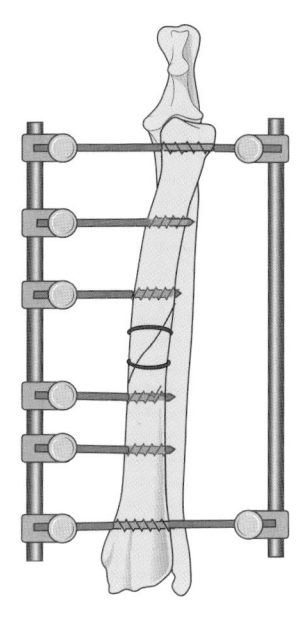
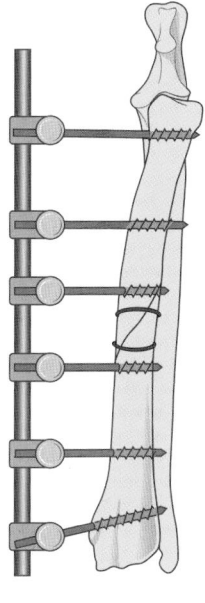

0 – 3   4 – 7   8 – 10

FIG. 32-47
Recommended methods for stabilizing long oblique or reducible comminuted radial fractures (single large fragment) based on fracture-assessment score. If fracture-assessment score is 0 to 3, a neutralization plate is preferred. If fracture-assessment score is 4 to 7, a Type II or Type Ib external fixator and cerclage wire may be used. With fracture-assessment scores of 8 to 10, a Type Ia external fixator plus cerclage wire provides necessary stability.

With a moderate fracture-assessment score (4 to 7), combine lag screws or cerclage wire for interfragmentary compression with a neutralization plate or minimal Type II or Ib external skeletal fixation. With a high fracture-assessment score (8 to 10), consider combining cerclage wire for interfragmentary compression with a Type Ia external skeletal fixator to stabilize the fracture (Fig. 32-47).

Stabilization of Midshaft Comminuted Radial Fractures With Multiple Fragments

From a mechanical perspective, these fractures cannot be reduced without significant soft tissue manipulation, and no load sharing between the implant and bone occurs until biologic callus forms to provide support. These types of fractures need rigid axial, rotational, and bending support provided by the implant. Very high stresses will be imposed on the implant and its connection to the bone. If the biologic assessment is favorable (see p. 953), the imposed stresses will be of short duration, reducing the likelihood of implant failure. If the biologic assessment is not favorable, however, imposed stresses will act on the implant for an extended period, and implant failure becomes more likely. Enhancing the biologic response by not attempting to reduce the fragments (closed reduction and bridging osteosynthesis) and by inserting an autogenous cancellous bone graft (when appropriate) is recommended.

Achieve stabilization in patients with low fracture-assessment scores (0 to 3) with a bone plate used in a bridging fashion or with maximal Type II external skeletal fixator.

At least three pins should be applied above and two pins below the area of comminution (or vice versa). It is always

better to err on the side of too much rigidity rather than too little since the fixator can be destabilized postoperatively.

Manage patients with a moderate fracture-assessment score (4 to 7) with a bone plate functioning as a bridging plate or a minimal Type II or Ib external skeletal fixator.

The choice of frame, number of pins, and pin design for the external skeletal fixator depend on the fracture assessment. A patient with this type of fracture would have a high fracture-assessment score (8 to 10) only when the biologic assessment is extremely favorable (e.g., 4- to 5-month-old animal with a low-velocity, closed, single-limb injury).

Consider managing such animals with indirect reduction and bridging of the fracture with a Type Ib external skeletal fixator (Fig. 32-48).

SUTURE MATERIALS AND SPECIAL INSTRUMENTS

Equipment necessary for pin and wire placement includes retractors, bone-holding forceps, reduction forceps, a Jacobs pin chuck, IM pins, Kirschner wires, and orthopedic wire. Additional equipment needed for external fixation includes a low-rpm power drill and external fixation clamps and bars or acrylic. Plating equipment and a high-speed drill are necessary for application of plates and screws.

POSTOPERATIVE CARE AND ASSESSMENT

Postoperative radiographs should be made to document fracture reduction or alignment and implant position. Activity should be restricted to leash walking and physical rehabilitation until the fracture has healed. Physical rehabilita-

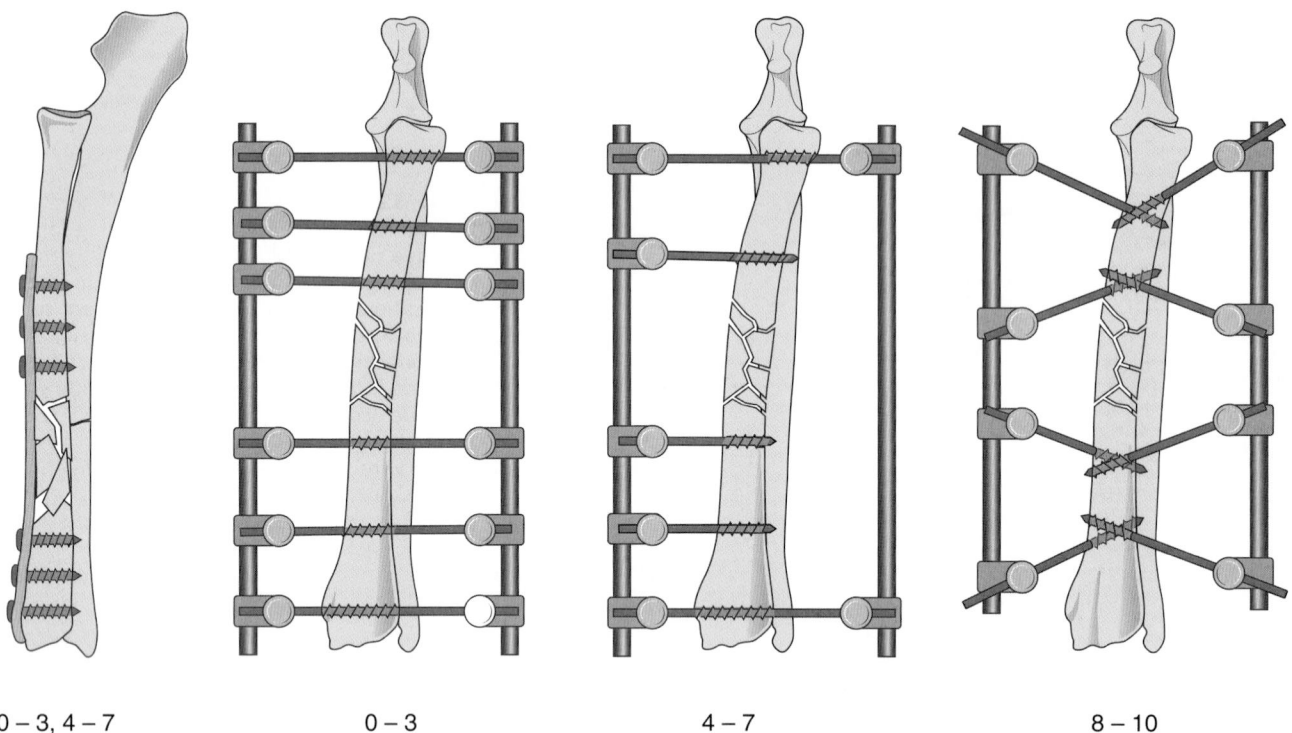

0 – 3, 4 – 7   0 – 3   4 – 7   8 – 10

FIG. 32-48
Recommended methods for stabilizing nonreducible comminuted radial fractures (multiple fragments) based on fracture-assessment score. If fracture-assessment score is 0 to 3, a bridging plate or maximal Type II external fixator may be used. If fracture-assessment score is 4 to 7, a bridging plate or minimal Type II may be used. With fracture assessment scores of 8 to 10, a Type Ib external fixator provides necessary stability. (Second and third images modified from Fossum TW: *Small animal surgery,* ed 2, St Louis, 2002, Mosby.)

tion (see Chapter 12) encourages controlled limb use and optimal limb function after fracture healing. Care must be taken to develop customized protocols for each patient depending on location of the fracture, stability and type of fracture fixation, potential for healing, abilities and attitudes of the patient, and willingness or ability of the client to participate in the animal's care (Tables 32-7 and 32-8).

Casts require intensive management by owners and frequent evaluations by the veterinarian. Abrasions and wounds often are caused by pressure from the cast. Management involves removal of the cast or replacement with a bivalve cast and wound treatment. Early destabilization of the fracture to treat wounds can cause delayed unions and nonunions.

After open reduction with external skeletal fixation, the incision should be covered, but the fixation splint may be left exposed. Alternatively, gauze sponges are opened and stuffed to fill the space between the fixation bar and the skin around the pins, then secured in place with a bandage around the fixator. Care should be taken to bandage the paw as well during the immediate postoperative period to prevent swelling. Open wounds should be treated daily with wet to dry dressings until a granulation bed has formed. Wounds are then covered with a nonadhesive pad and the bandage changed as needed. Daily hydrotherapy aids in cleaning open wounds,

reduces postoperative swelling, and cleans pin sites. The animal should be released to the owner with instructions to limit exercise and avoid fixator snares. If the external fixator bandage is maintained, it should be changed weekly. If a bandage is not used, daily hydrotherapy can be administered with a hand-held shower massage. Checkups should be scheduled at 2 weeks for suture removal and fixator evaluation and every 6 weeks for radiographic evaluation.

Although a rigidly stabilized fracture site is optimal for initial bone formation, subsequent bone remodeling is enhanced by increasing the load through the fractured bone. Removal of one half of a Type Ib external fixation splint (converting to a Type Ia frame) or removing selected transfixation pins from a Type I or Type II splint decreases rigidity of the fixator, allowing more load on the remodeling bone while still protecting the healing fracture. Destabilization is usually done at 6 weeks after surgery, depending on the fracture assessment. Early bone formation and bridging of the fracture site should be radiographically evident before destabilization is done. The external fixation splint can be removed completely when there is radiographic evidence of complete bone bridging of the fracture lines. A support bandage or a splint may be used to protect the healing bone for a few weeks after fixator removal.

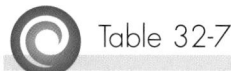 Table 32-7

Sample Physical Rehabilitation Protocol for Patients With Radial or Tibial Diaphyseal Fractures Stabilized with Internal Fixation

ALL TREATMENTS BID	DAY 1 TO DAY 14	DAY 15 TO DAY 24	DAY 25 UNTIL HEALED	HEALED TO RETURN TO FUNCTION
Heat therapy		10 min	10 min	
Massage	5 min	5 min	5 min	
Passive range of motion (repetitions)	15*	15*		
Electrical stimulation†	10 min	10 min	10 min	10 min
Therapeutic exercise-total time	10 min	15 min	15 min	25–45 min
Walk/land treadmill	10 min	5 min	5 min	>10 min
Balancing	+	+	+	
Obstacles	+	+	+	+
Weaving			+	+
Circles			+	+
Hills				+
Stairs				+
Jog/run				+
Underwater treadmill		10 min	10 min	>15 min
Swimming				5–10 min
Cryotherapy	15 min	15 min	15 min	PRN

BID, Twice a day; +, perform modality; PRN, as needed.
*Perform passive range of motion for all joints of the affected limb.
†Beneficial to strengthen flexors/extensors if nerve damage is present.

 Table 32-8

Sample Physical Rehabilitation Protocol for Patients With Radial or Tibial Diaphyseal Fractures Stabilized with External Fixators

ALL TREATMENTS BID	DAY 1 TO DAY 14	DAY 15 TO DAY 24	DAY 25 UNTIL HEALED	HEALED TO RETURN TO FUNCTION
Massage	5 min	5 min	5 min	
Passive range of motion (repetitions)	20*	20*	10–15*	Stop-when ROM N
Therapeutic exercise-total time	10 min	15 min	15 min	25–45 min
Walk/land treadmill	10 min	15 min	15 min	>10 min
Balancing	+	+	+	
Obstacles	+	+	+	+
Weaving				+
Circles				+
Hills				+
Stairs				+
Jog/run				+
Underwater treadmill				>15 min
Swimming				5–10 min
Cryotherapy	15 min	15 min	15 min	PRN

BID, Twice a day; ROM, range of motion; N, normal; +, perform modality; PRN, as needed.

BOX 32-9

Common Errors in Radial and Ulnar Diaphyseal Fracture Fixation

- IM pin placement through the carpus causes degenerative joint disease and loss of function.
- Inadequate rotational stabilization for transverse or short oblique fractures causes delayed union or nonunion, especially in toy-breed dogs.
- Premature removal of fixation from slowly healing distal radial fractures contributes to the formation of nonunions.
- Valgus deformities after comminuted fracture fixation occur because of malalignment with the external fixator.

After placement of a plate on a diaphyseal fracture, the limb should be supported for a few days with a soft padded bandage to reduce swelling. The animal will usually be fully weight bearing within 2 to 3 weeks. Confinement is recommended until there are radiographic signs of bone union. Although long-term plate application does not appear to have an effect on radial cortical bone density, plate removal is usually recommended after bone union because tissue irritation and cold sensitivity have been associated with minimal soft tissue coverage over the plate.

COMPLICATIONS

Complications with radial fractures include malunion, delayed union, and nonunion in animals treated with external coaptation (Box 32-9). These problems are common in toy-breed dogs sustaining fractures of the distal radial and ulnar diaphyses that have been inadequately stabilized. Complications are higher in toy dogs treated with external fixators compared with large dogs treated similarly. Complications after open reduction include osteomyelitis, implant migration and irritation of soft tissue, malunion, delayed union, and nonunion. Complications encountered with external fixation of the radius include pin loosening and pin or wire tract drainage; usually, neither problem is severe enough to warrant implant removal until the fracture has healed. Rarely, severe hemorrhage occurs from the medial exit hole of a proximal pin after the pin has eroded through an artery. Removal of the pin, with ligation of the vessel in some cases, is necessary to control hemorrhage.

PROGNOSIS

If none of the aforementioned complications occur, the prognosis is good. Treatment of nonunion involves open reduction and application of a bone plate and cancellous bone autograft.

Suggested Reading

Anderson GM, Lewis DD, Radasch RM et al: Circular external skeletal fixation stabilization of antebrachial and crural fractures in 25 dogs, *J Am Anim Hosp Assoc* 39:479, 2002.
Fracture stabilization using circular external skeletal fixation was evaluated in 14 dogs with antebrachial fractures and 11 dogs with crural fractures. Fractures in 23 dogs achieved radiographic union without additional surgery; two dogs required restabilization of their fractures with linear fixators.

Farese JP, Lewis DD, Cross AR et al: Use of IMEX SK-Circular external fixator hybrid for fracture stabilization in dogs and cats, *J Am Anim Hosp Assoc* 38:279, 2002.
This article provides a description of the use of SK-Circular hybrids to stabilize long-bone fractures (two femoral, one humeral, and three tibial fractures) with short distal bone segments in three dogs and three cats. Although three cases required surgical revision, animals ambulated well and all fractures obtained union.

Hamilton MH, Langley-Hobbs SJ: Use of the AO veterinary mini 'T'-plate for stabilization of distal radius and ulna fractures in toy breed dogs, *Vet Comp Orthop Traumatol* 18:18, 2005.
This article provides a description and evaluation of the use of the AO veterinary mini T plate to stabilize distal radial diaphyseal and metaphyseal fractures in toy-breed dogs.

Larsen LJ, Roush JK, McLaughlin RM: Bone plate fixation of distal radius and ulnar fractures in small- and miniature-breed dogs, *J Am Anim Hosp Assoc* 35:243, 1999.
Bone plate fixation is reviewed in 29 distal radial fractures of small- and miniature-breed dogs. Twenty-two fractures in 18 dogs were available for follow-up. A description of the incidence and types of complications associated with this procedure is included.

Toombs JP: Fractures of the radial diaphysis. In Johnson AL, Houlton JEF, Vannini R, editors: *AO principles of fracture management in the dog and cat,* Thieme, NY, 2005, AO Publishing.
This chapter provides an up-to-date collection of operative techniques for stabilizing radial diaphyseal fractures in small animals. Detailed descriptions of external fixator application and bone-plating procedures are included.

Sardinas JC, Montavon PM: Use of a medial bone plate for repair of radius and ulna fractures in dogs and cats: a report of 22 cases, *Vet Surg* 26:108, 1997.
This article provides a description of the technique of using a medially placed bone plate and screws to stabilize distal radial diaphyseal fractures. Medial plate application was considered technically easier by the authors, avoided the extensor tendons, and permitted the use of smaller plates for the fixation of distal radius fractures.

Welch JA, Boudrieau RJ, DeJardin LM et al: The intraosseous blood supply of the canine radius: implications for healing of distal fractures in small dogs, *Vet Surg* 26:57, 1997.
This article provides a description of the variation in radial interosseous vascular anatomy in large and small breed dogs. Small breed dogs have reduced vascularity in the distal radial diaphyseal area corresponding to the area frequently involved in delayed union and nonunions.

RADIAL AND ULNAR METAPHYSEAL AND ARTICULAR FRACTURES

DEFINITIONS

Metaphyseal fractures and **epiphyseal fractures** occur in trabecular bone. **Articular fractures** disrupt the joint surface. A **Monteggia fracture** is a fracture of the ulna coupled with a dislocation of the radial head.

GENERAL CONSIDERATIONS AND CLINICALLY RELEVANT PATHOPHYSIOLOGY

Fracture of the proximal ulna may occur singularly or in combination with luxation of the radial head (Monteggia's fracture). The fracture may involve the articular surface of the trochlear notch. The pull of the triceps muscle displaces the proximal segment of the ulna and must be neutralized by internal fixation to achieve bone union.

Fractures of the proximal radius are rare because the radial head is well protected by surrounding musculature. Fractures of the distal radius may be extraarticular or intraarticular. Intraarticular fractures usually disrupt the medial epicondyle and result in loss of ligamentous support for the carpus. The ligamentous attachment on the epicondyle causes displacement of the fragment that must be neutralized with internal fixation. Fractures of the styloid process of the ulna cause similar disruptions to the lateral aspect of the carpus.

DIAGNOSIS
Clinical Presentation
Signalment. Any age, breed, or sex of dog or cat may be affected. Young animals more frequently sustain vehicular trauma.

History. Affected animals usually present with a non–weight-bearing lameness after trauma. Owners may be unaware that trauma occurred.

Physical Examination Findings
Because of the traumatic nature of this injury, the entire animal must be assessed to detect abnormalities of other body systems. Palpation of the limb reveals swelling, pain, crepitation, and apparent instability of the adjacent joint. Degloving injuries of the carpus may be associated with fractures of the distal radius. Although there are no major nerves in the immediate area, dogs often have abnormal proprioceptive responses because they are reluctant to move the limb.

Diagnostic Imaging
Craniocaudal and lateral radiographs of the affected radius and ulna (which include the proximal and distal joints) are required to assess the extent of bone and soft tissue injury. Animals that are fractious or in extreme pain may require sedation (see Tables 31-2 and 31-3 on p. 933 and 934, respectively) or general anesthetic for radiography after it has been determined that no contraindications (i.e., shock, hypotension, or severe dyspnea) to administration of sedatives or anesthetics exist. Thoracic radiography should be performed to evaluate for thoracic trauma.

Laboratory Findings
Complete blood count and serum chemistry evaluation should be done to evaluate the advisability of anesthesia and to determine if concurrent injury or damage to the renal or hepatobiliary system is present.

DIFFERENTIAL DIAGNOSIS
Animals presenting with distal radial fractures should be evaluated to determine whether fractures are caused by trauma or underlying pathology (e.g., neoplasia and metabolic disease). Joint luxations can be differentiated from fractures radiographically.

MEDICAL MANAGEMENT
Medical treatment of animals with radial and ulnar metaphyseal and epiphyseal fractures includes analgesics for posttraumatic pain (see Box 31-2 on p. 944 and Chapter 13) and antibiotics to treat open fractures.

SURGICAL TREATMENT
Proximal ulnar fractures require implant systems that resist the pull of the triceps muscle. Appropriate implants include tension band wire techniques and plates and screws. Articular fractures require anatomic reduction and compression with a lag screw or plate. Radial and ulnar styloid fractures require tension band wire techniques to resist the pull of the collateral ligaments.

> NOTE: Failure to reduce a joint surface anatomically results in degenerative joint disease and loss of function.

Preoperative Management
There may be extensive damage or loss of tissue in the area of the fracture. Open wounds should be managed initially by carefully clipping surrounding hair, cleaning the wound, and sampling deep tissue for microbial culture and susceptibility testing. The antebrachium should be temporarily stabilized with a Robert Jones bandage (see p. 946) to immobilize fragments, decrease or prevent soft tissue swelling, protect or prevent open wounds, and increase patient comfort until surgery can be performed. Perioperative pain management should be instituted (see p. 944) and concurrent injuries managed before anesthetic induction for fracture fixation.

Anesthesia
Refer to p. 944 for anesthetic management of animals with fractures.

Surgical Anatomy
Landmarks for the approach to the proximal ulna are the olecranon and the palpable caudal border of the ulna. The articular surface of the trochlear notch can be exposed surgically by muscle elevation. The ulnar nerve courses over the medial aspect of the elbow, caudal to the medial epicondyle. The antebrachial carpal joint is supported by the short radial collateral ligaments, which arise from the medial styloid process of the radius, the dorsal radiocarpal ligament arising from the dorsal surface of the distal radius, and the short ulnar collateral and radioulnar ligaments arising from the ulnar styloid process. The extensor tendons lie cranial to the antebrachial carpal joint and may need to be retracted to expose the joint surface.

Positioning
The limb should be prepped from shoulder to carpus. If cancellous bone graft harvest is anticipated, a donor site should also be prepped. The animal is positioned in lateral recumbency and the limb draped out for proximal radial and ulnar

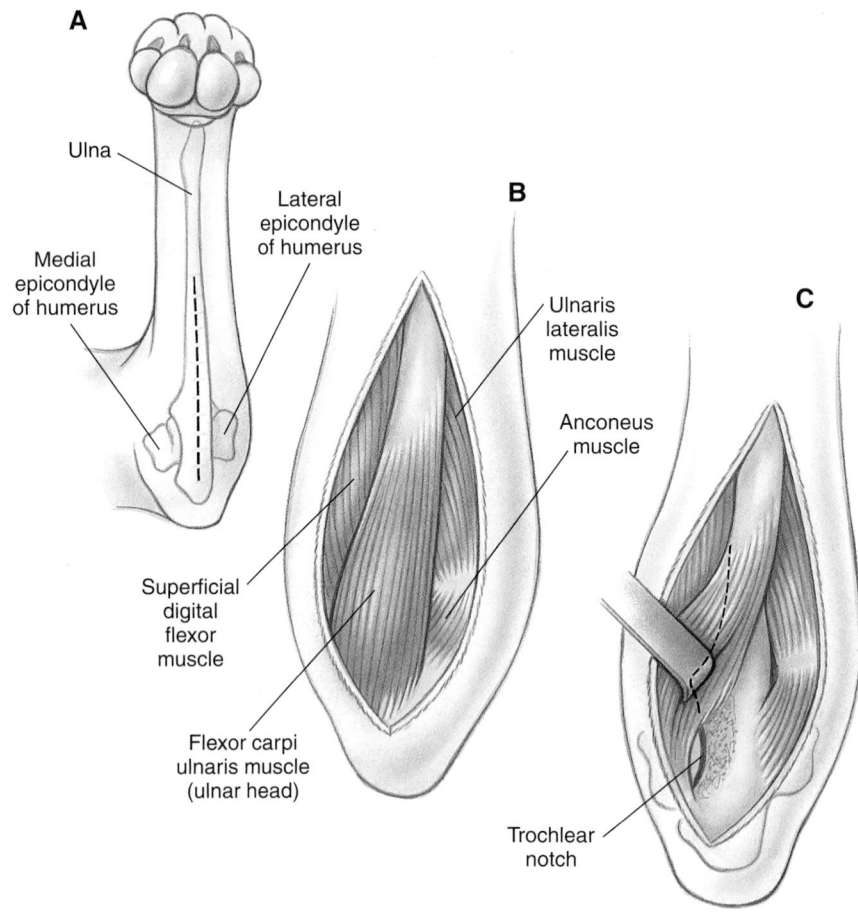

FIG. 32-49
A, For a caudal approach to the proximal ulna, make an incision through skin and subcutaneous tissue over the caudoproximal ulna. **B,** Elevate the flexor carpi ulnaris and deep digital flexor muscles to expose the bone surface. **C,** Reflect the origin of the flexor carpi ulnaris muscle to expose the trochlear notch.

fractures. Placing the animal in dorsal recumbency allows more flexibility in visualizing distal radial and ulnar fractures.

SURGICAL TECHNIQUE
Caudal Approach to the Ulna

Palpate the caudal border of the ulna directly under the skin and subcutaneous tissue on the caudal surface of the limb. Make an incision through skin and subcutaneous tissue along the ulnar diaphysis (Fig. 32-49, A). Elevate the flexor carpi ulnaris and deep digital flexor muscles medially and the ulnaris lateralis muscle laterally to expose the bone surface (Fig. 32-49, B). Reflect the origin of the flexor carpi ulnaris muscle to expose the trochlear notch (Fig. 32-49, C).

Approaches to the Proximal and Distal Radius and Ulna

Refer to p. 1047 under radial physeal fractures for approaches to the proximal radius and to p. 1232 for approaches to the carpus and extend the approach proximally.

Stabilization of Proximal Radial and Ulna Fractures

If the fracture-assessment score is 8 to 10, pins and wires are usually sufficient to stabilize the fracture. Extraarticular fractures of the proximal and distal radius can often be stabilized with crossed Kirschner wires or small IM pins in animals with fracture-assessment scores of 4 to 7. Severely comminuted, open fractures of the proximal ulna or fractures in dogs with anticipated prolonged healing times (fracture-assessment scores of 0 to 3) should be stabilized with plates and screws (buttress plate). Articular fractures must be anatomically reduced and stabilized with tension band wires, lag screws, or a compression plate (tension band plate) to restore joint continuity and function and to limit development of degenerative joint disease.

To place a tension band wire, reduce the fracture (proximal ulna, styloid process of ulna, medial epicondyle of radius) and start two Kirschner wires in the fragment.

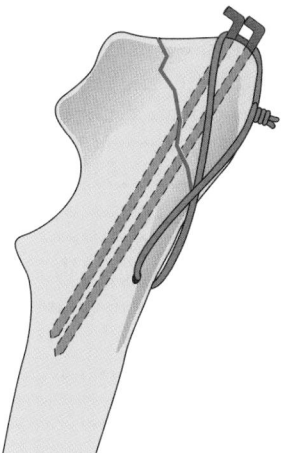

FIG. 32-50
Fractures (or osteotomies) of the olecranon can be treated with a tension band wire technique.

Although two Kirschner wires are recommended for tension band wire techniques, the ulna may only be large enough for one Kirschner wire in most dogs and cats.

Drive the wires across the fracture line to lodge in the major bone segment. Place a transverse drill hole in the major bone segment, pass a figure-eight wire through the hole and around the Kirschner wires, and tighten (Fig. 32-50).

Bone plates are an excellent method of stabilizing proximal ulnar fractures (see p. 991).

Apply the plate to the caudal surface to function as a tension band plate, compressing the fracture (Fig. 32-51, A). In some comminuted fractures, apply the plate to either the caudal or the lateral surface of the proximal ulna to function as a buttress plate (Fig. 32-51, B).

Stabilization of Distal Radial and Ulnar Fractures

Distal radial and ulnar fractures can be stabilized with a lag screw or tension band wire (Box 32-10 and Fig. 32-52, *A* and *B*).

To place a fully threaded cortical or cancellous lag screw, reduce the fracture and hold it in place with a Kirschner wire. Drill a gliding hole (equal to the diameter of the threads on the screw) in the epicondylar fragment (see p. 994). Insert a drill sleeve into the gliding hole, and drill a smaller hole (equal to the core diameter of the screw) across the radius. Measure and tap the hole, then select and place the appropriate length screw in it.

Compression of the fracture should occur. The Kirschner wire may be left to provide rotational stability.

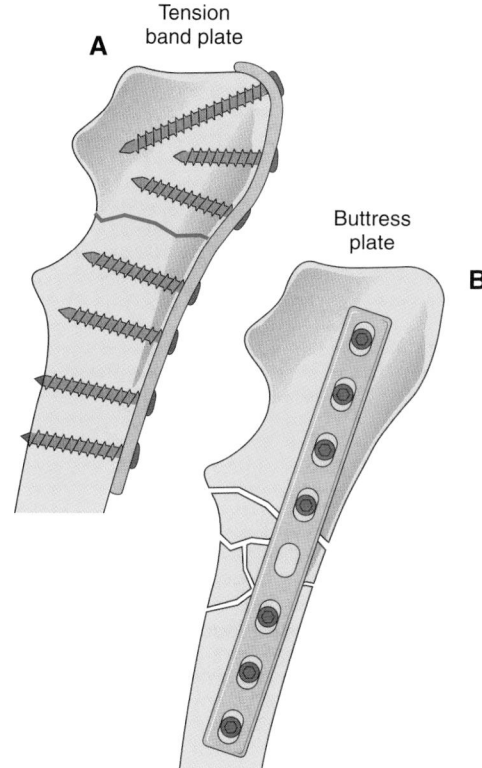

FIG. 32-51
A, Transverse articular fractures should be anatomically reduced and stabilized with a compression plate in patients with moderate or low fracture-assessment scores. **B,** Severely comminuted fractures are bridged with a buttress plate.

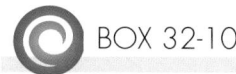 BOX 32-10

Implant Use for Distal Radial and Ulnar Fractures According to Fracture-Assessment Score (FAS)

FAS 0 to 3
• Lag screw

FAS 4 to 7
• Lag screw
• Tension band wire

FAS 8 to 10
• Tension band wire

SUTURE MATERIALS AND SPECIAL INSTRUMENTS

Plating equipment is necessary for plate and lag screws. Other equipment needed for the procedures described here includes a high-speed power drill, Kirschner wires, IM pins, orthopedic wire, and reduction forceps.

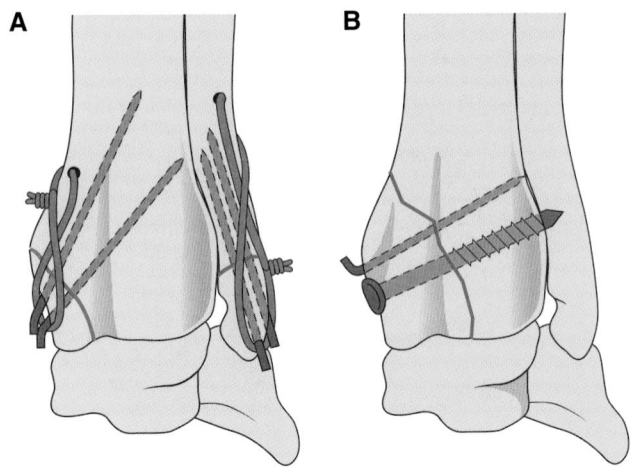

FIG. 32-52

A, Fractures of the styloid processes can be stabilized with tension band wire in patients with high and moderate fracture-assessment scores. Intraarticular fractures must be anatomically reduced and rigidly stabilized. **B,** Lag screws are used in patients with moderate and low fracture-assessment scores. Kirschner wire is used as an antirotational implant.

POSTOPERATIVE CARE AND ASSESSMENT

Postoperative radiographs should be made to document fracture reduction or alignment and implant position. Postoperative pain management may be indicated (see p. 994). After internal fixation a soft-padded bandage should be applied for a few days to control swelling and support soft tissue. Distal radial and ulnar fracture repairs are often supported by a splint for 6 weeks. Activity should be restricted to leash walking and physical rehabilitation until the fracture has healed.

Physical rehabilitation (see Chapter 12) encourages controlled limb use and optimal carpal function after fracture healing. Care must be taken to develop customized protocols for each patient depending on location of the fracture, stability and type of fracture fixation, potential for healing, abilities and attitudes of the patient, and willingness and ability of the client to participate in the animal's care (see Table 32-6). Physical rehabilitation for patients with fractures supported by splints for 6 weeks generally begins after the splint has been removed (Table 32-9). Open wounds are treated daily with wet to dry dressings until a granulation bed has formed. The wounds are then covered with a nonadhesive pad, and the bandage is

 Table 32-9

Sample Physical Rehabilitation Protocol for Patients With Fractures of the Distal Limbs

ALL TREATMENTS BID	DAY 1 TO DAY 14	DAY 15 TO DAY 24	DAY 25 UNTIL HEALED	HEALED TO RETURN TO FUNCTION
Heat therapy		10 min	10 min	
Massage	5 min	5 min	5 min	
Passive range of motion (repetitions)	15*	15*		
Electrical stimulation†	10 min	10 min	10 min	10 min
Therapeutic exercise-total time	10 min	15 min	15 min	25–45 min
Walk/land treadmill	10 min	5 min	5 min	>10 min
Balancing	+	+	+	
Obstacles	+	+	+	+
Weaving			+	+
Circles			+	+
Hills				+
Stairs				+
Jog/run				+
Underwater treadmill		10 min	10 min	>15 min
Swimming				5–10 min
Cryotherapy	15 min	15 min	15 min	PRN

BID, Twice a day; +, perform modality; *PRN,* as needed.
*Perform passive range of motion for all joints of the affected limb.
†Beneficial to strengthen flexors/extensors if nerve damage is present (see Chapter 12).

changed as necessary. Daily hydrotherapy aids in cleaning open wounds and reducing postoperative swelling. Rechecks should be scheduled at 2 weeks for suture removal and every 6 weeks for radiographic evaluation. Implant removal may be necessary after bone healing if the implants interfere with or irritate soft tissue.

COMPLICATIONS

Degenerative joint disease may occur after articular fractures and may be severe if anatomic reduction and rigid fracture fixation are not achieved. Degenerative joint disease is initially treated with conservative management, including rest, judicious exercise, and nonsteroidal antiinflammatory drugs (NSAIDs). Arthrodesis may be used to treat dogs with progressive instability, lameness, and pain that are unresponsive to medical management. Delayed union and nonunion can occur if the fracture is not adequately stabilized. The constant tensile stress exerted on the fracture line from the pull of the triceps muscle or collateral ligaments can cause nonunion. Treatment consists of rigid fixation with a tension band or lag screw and autogenous cancellous bone graft.

PROGNOSIS

The prognosis for bone healing depends on the mechanical and biologic factors present in each animal and the stability of the fixation. In general, trabecular bone heals quickly with minimal callus formation (see p. 1004), although comminuted proximal ulnar fractures may require long healing periods.

Suggested Reading

Autefage A: Fractures of the ulna. In Johnson AL, Houlton JEF, Vannini R, editors: *AO principles of fracture management in the dog and cat,* Thieme, NY, 2005, AO Publishing.

This chapter provides an up-to-date collection of operative techniques for stabilizing ulnar fractures in small animals. Detailed descriptions of tension band wire application and bone-plating procedures are included.

Muir P, Johnson KA: Fractures of the proximal ulna in dogs, *Vet Comp Orthop Traumatol* 9:88, 1996.

This article provides a description of the treatment and outcomes associated with a case series of proximal ulnar fractures. Fractures were frequently intraarticular and comminuted. Complications with tension band wires were common.

Toombs JP: Fractures of the proximal radius. In Johnson AL, Houlton JEF, Vannini R, editors: *AO principles of fracture management in the dog and cat,* Thieme, NY, 2005, AO Publishing.

This chapter provides an up-to-date collection of operative techniques for stabilizing proximal radial fractures in small animals. Detailed descriptions of lag screw application and bone-plating procedures are included.

Toombs JP: Fractures of the distal radius. In Johnson AL, Houlton JEF, Vannini R, editors: *AO principles of fracture management in the dog and cat,* Thieme, NY, 2005, AO Publishing.

This chapter provides an up-to-date collection of operative techniques for stabilizing distal radial fractures in small animals. Detailed descriptions of lag screw application and bone-plating procedures are included.

RADIAL AND ULNAR PHYSEAL FRACTURES

DEFINITIONS

Physeal fractures may occur through the cartilaginous growth plates of the proximal or distal radius or ulna in immature animals. Physeal fractures are also referred to as *epiphyseal plate fractures,* or *slipped physes.*

GENERAL CONSIDERATIONS AND CLINICALLY RELEVANT PATHOPHYSIOLOGY

The cartilaginous physis is weaker than surrounding bone and ligaments, making it more susceptible to injury. The weakest portion of the physis is the junction of the zone of hypertrophying cells with the zone of ossification (see Fig. 31-83 on p. 1007). The zone of hypertrophying cells has a large cell/matrix ratio, which results in a relatively weak structure. Additionally, stress concentration is created when two areas of different mechanical properties (weak hypertrophying zone and stronger zone of ossification) are located adjacent to each other. Consequently, when a physis is fractured, the separation should occur through the zone of hypertrophying cells. A fracture in this location does not affect proliferating cells and will not compromise potential growth. However, when severe trauma causes physeal fractures, the fracture line can occur anywhere within the physis and damage growing cells. Trauma resulting in compression of the zone of proliferating cells and destruction of the chondrocytes causes premature physeal closure. This often results from trauma to the V-shaped distal ulnar physis in dogs, and trauma that would normally result in physeal separation instead compresses the zone of growing cells.

Fractures of the proximal and distal radial physis are usually radiographically classified as Salter-Harris Types I and II (see p. 951). Occult Type V fractures of the radial physes can occur and are diagnosed after closure of the physis and alteration of forelimb growth have occurred. The most common fracture of the distal ulnar physis is the Salter-Harris Type V, which is caused by trauma and may be associated with a radial fracture. Because they are nondisplaced and confined to the cartilage, these fractures are not visible radiographically until 2 to 3 weeks after trauma when premature closure of the physis is observed (see p. 1007).

DIAGNOSIS
Clinical Presentation

Signalment. Radial and ulnar physeal fractures occur in immature dogs or cats with open physes.

History. Affected animals usually have a non–weight-bearing lameness after trauma. Owners may be unaware that trauma occurred.

Physical Examination Findings

Because of the traumatic nature of radial or ulnar physeal fracture, the entire animal must be assessed to detect abnormalities of other body systems. Palpation of the limb reveals swelling, pain, crepitation, and apparent instability of the adjacent joint. Dogs often appear to have abnormal proprioceptive responses because they are reluctant to move the limb.

Diagnostic Imaging

Craniocaudal and lateral radiographs of the affected radius and ulna (which include the proximal and distal joints) are required to diagnose Salter I to Salter IV fractures. Animals that are fractious or in extreme pain may require sedation (see Tables 31-2 and 31-3 on p. 933 and 934, respectively) or general anesthesia for radiography after it has been determined that no contraindications (i.e., shock, hypotension, or severe dyspnea) to administration of sedatives or anesthetics exist. Thoracic radiography should be performed to evaluate for thoracic trauma. Radiographs made at the time of injury do not give information about Salter V fractures (e.g., crushing injuries to physis) or damage to the physeal blood supply. It is therefore difficult to give an accurate prognosis for growth at the time of injury.

> NOTE: Compare radiographs of the contralateral bone to detect subtle changes in the physis.

Laboratory Findings

Complete blood count and serum chemistry evaluation should be done to evaluate the status of the animal for anesthesia and to determine if there is damage to the renal or hepatobiliary systems.

DIFFERENTIAL DIAGNOSIS

Physeal fractures can be differentiated from joint luxations or soft tissue trauma radiographically.

MEDICAL MANAGEMENT

Medical treatment of animals with radial and ulnar physeal fractures includes analgesics for posttraumatic pain (see p. 944) and antibiotics to treat open fractures.

SURGICAL TREATMENT

Most physeal fractures are classified as having assessment scores of 8 to 10 because affected animals are young and physeal fractures heal quickly (see p. 1004). Therefore the implant system chosen need not function for a long time. Nondisplaced radial physeal fractures may be adequately stabilized with a cast. Surgical treatment of displaced physeal fractures consists of anatomic reduction and stabilization with Kirschner wires or small pins that are smooth so as not to interfere with physeal function. In animals that are close to maturity, threaded implants may be used to compress the fractured physis.

> NOTE: Use smooth implants when crossing the physis.

Preoperative Management

The antebrachium should be temporarily stabilized with a Robert Jones bandage (see p. 946) to immobilize the fragments, decrease or prevent soft tissue swelling, protect or prevent open wounds, and increase patient comfort until surgery can be performed. Perioperative pain management should be instituted (see p. 944). Concurrent injuries should be managed before anesthetic induction for fracture fixation.

Anesthesia

Anesthetic management of animals with fractures is discussed on p. 943. Small dogs and cats may require pediatric anesthetic techniques.

Surgical Anatomy

The lateral radial head is palpable beneath the extensor muscles of the forearm. The radial nerve lies deep to the extensor carpi radialis muscle. The craniomedial surface of the distal radius can be easily palpated to serve as a landmark for location of the incision. Extensor tendons are located cranial to and flexor tendons caudal to the distal radius. The cephalic vein crosses the medial portion of the distal radius.

Positioning

The limb should be prepped from shoulder to carpus. The animal is positioned in lateral recumbency with the limb draped out for proximal radial physeal fractures. Placing the animal in dorsal recumbency allows more flexibility in visualizing distal radial and ulnar physeal fractures.

SURGICAL TECHNIQUE
Approach to the Proximal Radial Physis

Make a skin incision over the lateral humeral condyle, extending over the proximal third of the radius (Fig. 32-53, A). Continue the incision through subcutaneous tissue and brachial and antebrachial fascia (Fig. 32-53, B). Identify and separate the lateral digital extensor and ulnaris lateralis muscles to expose the proximal radius (Fig. 32-53, C). Close the wound by suturing fascia, subcutaneous tissue, and skin in separate layers.

Approach to the Distal Radial Physis

Use the craniomedial approach to the radius (see p. 1063) to expose the distal radial physis.

Approach to the Distal Ulnar Physis

Use the approach for ulnar ostectomy (see e-dition) to expose the distal ulnar physis.

Stabilization of Nondisplaced Physeal Fractures

Fractures of the radial physes and distal ulnar physis that are nondisplaced can be treated with a cast.

Cast the limb from the toes to above the elbow with the carpus held in slight flexion and varus (inward angulation) until the cast hardens (see pp. 967 and 1059).

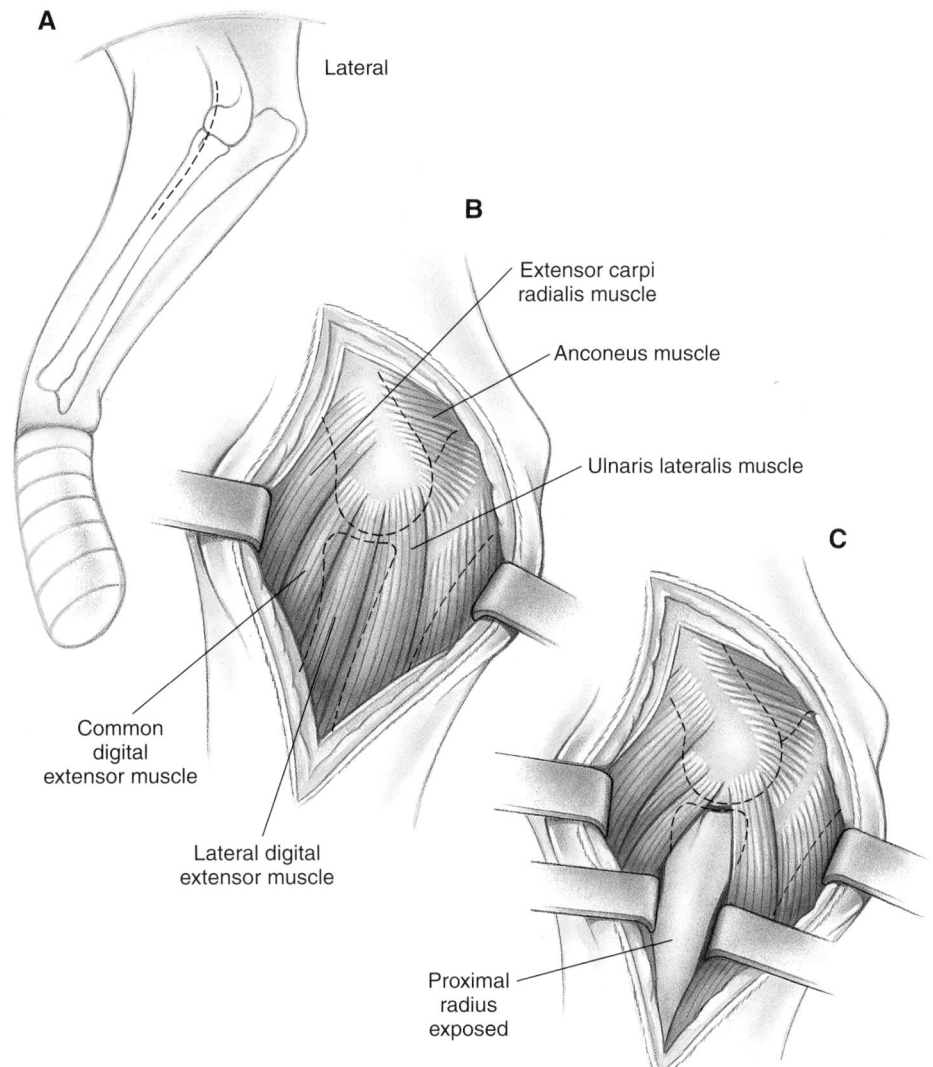

A

Lateral

B

Extensor carpi
radialis muscle

Anconeus muscle

Ulnaris lateralis muscle

C

Common
digital
extensor muscle

Lateral digital
extensor muscle

Proximal
radius
exposed

FIG. 32-53
A, For a lateral approach to the radial head, make a skin incision over the lateral humeral condyle and extend it over the proximal third of the radius. **B** and **C,** Identify and separate the lateral digital extensor and ulnaris lateralis muscles to expose the proximal radius.

Stabilization of Displaced Physeal Fractures With Crossed Kirschner Wires or Steinmann Pins

Physeal fractures should be reduced carefully so as to avoid crushing or injuring the physeal cartilage.

For proximal radial physeal fractures, drive a Kirschner wire from the lateral surface of the proximal radial epiphysis across the physis, into the radial metaphyses, and through the medial cortex. Then drive a second wire from the lateral proximal radial metaphysis across the fracture into the epiphysis (Fig. 32-54, A). Take care to avoid penetrating the articular surface. For distal physeal fractures, drive a Kirschner wire from the medial styloid process across the physis, into the radial metaphyses, and through the lateral cortex. Drive the second wire from the lateral aspect of the distal radial epiphysis, across the fracture into the metaphysis, and through the medial cortex (Fig. 32-54, B), avoiding the articular surface.

SUTURE MATERIALS AND SPECIAL INSTRUMENTS

Necessary equipment includes Kirschner wires, small IM pins, a Jacobs pin chuck, and reduction forceps.

POSTOPERATIVE CARE AND ASSESSMENT

Postoperative radiographs should be made to document fracture reduction and implant position. After internal fixation, a soft-padded bandage should be applied for a few days to control swelling and support soft tissue. Activity should be restricted to leash walking and physical rehabilitation until the fracture has healed. Physical rehabilitation (see Chapter 12)

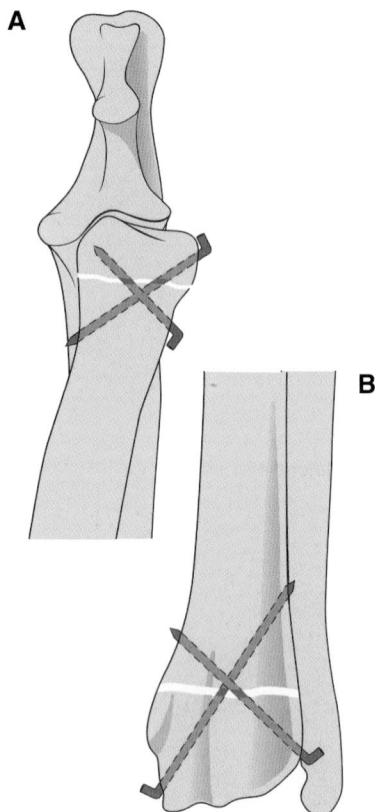

FIG. 32-54
A, For proximal radial physeal fractures, Kirschner wires can be driven from the lateral surface of the proximal radial epiphysis and from the lateral proximal radial metaphysis. **B,** For distal physeal fractures, Kirschner wires can be driven from the medial styloid process and from the lateral aspect of the distal radial epiphysis.

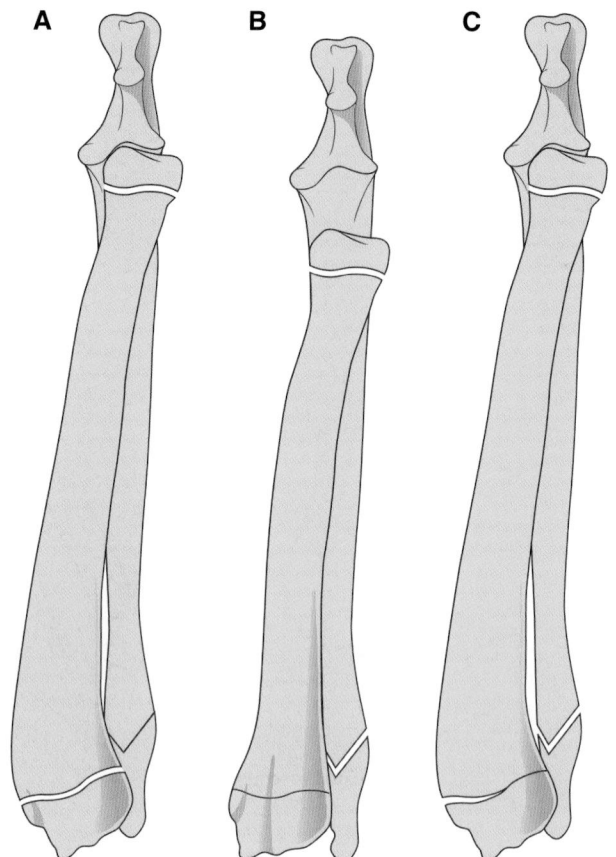

FIG. 32-55
A, Premature closure of the distal ulnar physis causes shortening, cranial bowing, external rotation, and valgus angulation of the radius. **B,** Complete premature closure of the distal (or proximal) radial physis causes shortening of the radius and subluxation of the radial humeral joint. **C,** Partial distal radial physeal closure causes angular deformity of the radius.

encourages controlled limb use and optimal joint function after fracture healing. Care must be taken to develop customized protocols for each patient depending on location of the fracture, stability and type of fracture fixation, potential for healing, abilities and attitudes of the patient, and willingness of the client (see Table 32-9; see also Table 32-6). Rechecks should be scheduled at 2 weeks for suture removal and at 4 to 6 weeks for radiographic evaluation of fracture healing. Radiographs of the injured bone and the contralateral bone can be made and compared for length as early as 2 to 3 weeks after the injury to determine physeal function. Cartilage physes that heal in a manner allowing continued function appear radiographically as a lucent line. Additionally, increased bone length should be apparent. If the physeal line appears as a bone density, endochondral ossification has occurred and continued physeal function is likely. Implant removal is indicated after physeal healing (4 weeks) to allow bone growth (if the physis is functional after the trauma).

COMPLICATIONS

The most common complication associated with radial and ulnar physeal fractures is premature physeal closure and resulting growth deformities. The severity of the deformity de-

pends on the animal's age when physeal closure occurs and the location and extent of the physeal closure. Younger animals with greater growth potential have more severe sequelae. Premature closure of the distal ulnar physis interferes with the normal development of the radius by acting as a restraint. This results not only in a shortened ulna but also in shortening, rotation, and angulation of the radius. Additionally, asynchronous growth of the paired bones results in incongruity of the elbow and carpal joints, leading to degenerative joint disease. Asymmetric or partial closure of the distal radial physis results in angular deformity of the bone and may affect the anatomy of adjacent joints, again resulting in degenerative joint disease (Fig. 32-55; see also p. 978 and Fossum, ed 2, Radial and ulnar growth deformities, on p. 955).

PROGNOSIS

Although the prognosis for fracture healing with physeal fractures is excellent, the prognosis for continued function or growth of the physis depends on the severity of damage sustained by the zone of proliferating cells. The prognosis is good for future physeal growth after a fracture that separates the cartilaginous physis at the zone of hypertrophying cells, whereas the prognosis is poor for future physeal growth after trauma that crushes the physis. Unfortunately, most traumatically induced physeal fractures sustain damage to the growing cells and have a guarded prognosis for growth. Bridging of bone across the physis may occur in fractures that cross the growth plate, causing abnormal bone growth. Damage to one physis of a paired bone system, such as the radius and ulna, can cause shortened limbs, angular deformities, rotational deformities, and disruption of normal joint anatomy, resulting in degenerative joint disease.

Suggested Reading

Johnson JM, Johnson AL, Eurell JA: Histological appearance of naturally occurring canine physeal fractures, *Vet Surg* 23:81, 1994.

This article provides a description of the histologic appearance of physeal fractures occurring after trauma. Despite the radiographic Salter-Harris classifications, the fracture lines involved all areas of the physis including the growing cells.

Toombs JP: Fractures of the proximal radius. In Johnson AL, Houlton JEF, Vannini R, editors: *AO principles of fracture management in the dog and cat,* Thieme, NY, 2005, AO Publishing.

This chapter provides an up-to-date collection of operative techniques for stabilizing proximal radial fractures in small animals. Detailed descriptions of physeal fracture fixation are included.

Toombs JP: Fractures of the distal radius. In Johnson AL, Houlton JEF, Vannini R, editors: *AO principles of fracture management in the dog and cat,* Thieme, NY, 2005, AO Publishing.

This chapter provides an up-to-date collection of operative techniques for stabilizing distal radial fractures in small animals. Detailed descriptions of physeal fracture fixation are included.

CARPAL AND TARSAL FRACTURES

DEFINITIONS

Carpal fractures and **tarsal fractures** may cause a loss of weight-bearing support if integrity of these bones is disrupted. A **plantigrade stance** occurs when the foot is positioned such that the plantar surface of the calcaneus contacts the ground. A **valgus position** of the foot is an outward deviation; a **varus position** is an inward deviation.

GENERAL CONSIDERATIONS AND CLINICALLY RELEVANT PATHOPHYSIOLOGY

Although carpal or tarsal fractures are rare in companion animals, such fractures are often disabling because the carpal and tarsal joints serve a major weight-bearing function. If injuries involving these joints are not treated, joint incongruity and subsequent development of osteoarthritis often lead to severe lameness. Fractures of the distal row of carpal bones may occur as compression fractures with carpal hyperextension injuries. Carpal fractures in racing dogs occur either as avulsion of bone fragments by ligamentous attachments or as compression, which results in slab or stress fractures. Carpal fractures in other breeds may have a different mechanism. Radial carpal bone fractures are the most frequently diagnosed injury involving fracture of the carpal bones in companion animals. Radial carpal bone fractures in these animals often involves a chronic lameness without his-

tory of trauma and may occur bilaterally. Three common fracture patterns occur, and there is speculation that the fractures are a result of an incomplete ossification of the radial carpal bone. Accessory carpal bone fractures occur in racing greyhounds and sled dogs, but are rare in other companion animals. Most accessory carpal bone fractures occur in the right leg because of the counterclockwise direction of racing. Accessory carpal bone fractures are considered avulsion injuries because they occur at tendinous or ligamentous insertions and are classified according to site of injury on the accessory carpal bone. Readers are referred to the Suggested Reading list for additional information about this injury in these breeds.

Fractures of the tarsus are seen regularly in working breeds of dogs, but are rare in companion animals with the exception of a fractured calcaneus. Because calcaneal fractures are distracted by the pull of the gastrocnemius muscle, preventing bone contact between fragments and interfering with healing, treatment methods must therefore resist the tensile forces. Talar neck fractures occur in cats and occasionally in dogs, and condylar fractures also occur. As with all articular fractures, anatomic reduction and rigid fixation are needed for optimal outcome. Reconstruction may be difficult due to the small size of the trochlea and degree of comminution. If reconstruction is not feasible, primary arthrodesis may be performed (see p. 1307).

Racing greyhounds often incur fractures of the central tarsal bone; however, this injury is rarely seen in companion animals. Central tarsal fractures are graded according to fracture type and degree of fragment displacement. Once the buttress effect of the central tarsal bone is lost, fractures of the fourth tarsal bone and calcaneus may occur. Repair requires accurate placement of one or more small lag screws. Readers are referred to the Suggested Reading list for detailed information on treatment methods.

DIAGNOSIS
Clinical Presentation

Signalment. Any age, breed, or sex of dog or cat may be affected. Racing greyhounds most often develop fractures of the central tarsal bone and accessory carpal bones. Boxers and sporting breeds most often develop chronic radial carpal bone fractures.

History. Affected animals usually have an acute onset of non–weight-bearing lameness after injury. Dogs with radial carpal bone fractures may have chronic thoracic limb lameness. If the calcaneus is fractured, it may be partially weight bearing with a plantigrade stance.

Physical Examination Findings

Patients with acute fractures of the carpus or tarsus usually have a non–weight-bearing lameness; attempts to place weight on the limb cause the carpus and/or tarsus to collapse in a plantigrade stance. Patients with chronic radial carpal bone fracture have a weight-bearing lameness (which may be intermittent), reduced carpal range of motion, and soft tissue swelling. If the calcaneus is fractured, the animal may walk plantigrade on the limb or may be nonweight bearing. Pain, swelling, and crepitus are present in the affected limb. Varus or valgus deviation of the foot is usually present.

Diagnostic Imaging

High detail radiographs using dorsopalmar (dorsoplantar), medial lateral, and oblique projections are usually sufficient to make the diagnosis. Bilateral carpal radiographs and/or CT may be helpful for diagnosing occult radial carpal bone fractures.

Laboratory Findings

Consistent laboratory abnormalities are not present. Traumatized animals undergoing surgery should have sufficient blood work done to assess the risk of anesthesia and surgery.

DIFFERENTIAL DIAGNOSIS

Fractures of the carpus and/or tarsus must be differentiated from ligamentous injury, which may occur concurrently with fractures. Standard radiographs are sufficient to make this observation. Calcaneal fractures must be differentiated from lacerations or rupture of the Achilles tendon. Acute lacerations have an open wound, and soft tissue swelling is limited to an area proximal to the calcaneal tuberosity. Fractures of the calcaneus exhibit swelling caudal to the tarsus, and crepitation may be elicited on palpation.

MEDICAL MANAGEMENT

Anatomic reduction and rigid fixation are necessary for optimal outcome in animals with intraarticular fractures of the carpus or tarsus; conservative treatment with casts or splints is not effective. External coaptation is also not appropriate for calcaneal fractures because bandaging or splint application is ineffective in countering tensile forces produced by the Achilles muscle-tendon unit.

SURGICAL TREATMENT

The radial carpal bone is a major weight-bearing structure. Congruity of the articular surface between it and the distal radius is necessary for optimal long-term function. Small chip fragments that cannot be stabilized should be removed; large fragments, however, should be anatomically reduced and rigidly stabilized with lag screws or a combination of lag screws and Kirschner wires. Dogs with chronic radial carpal bone fractures, severely comminuted fractures, osteoarthritis, luxation, bone loss, or infection are best treated with carpal arthrodesis (see p. 1228). With calcaneal fractures, the pull of the gastrocnemius muscle must be resisted with a tension band wire (see p. 990), lag screws, or a plate (Fig. 32-56). Articular fractures of the talus must be anatomically reduced and rigidly stabilized for optimal outcome; however, traction and immobilization with external skeletal fixation may be useful to treat talar neck fractures in cats. If preoperative assessment indicates that fracture repair is not feasible, arthrodesis of the tarsocrural joint should be considered (see p. 1308).

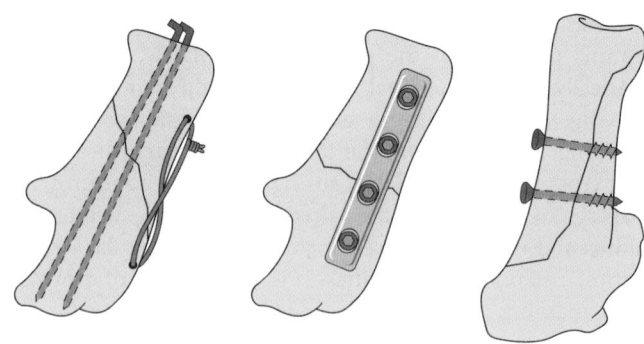

FIG. 32-56
Transverse calcaneal fractures can be stabilized with a tension band wire or plate. Oblique or slab fractures can be stabilized with lag screws.

Preoperative Management

Patients with comminuted fractures of the carpus and/or tarsus may be brought in with open wounds. These wounds should be cleaned and protected from further damage and contamination with a sterile bandage until surgery can be performed.

Anesthesia

See p. 944 for anesthetic management of animals with fractures. Racing greyhounds should be anesthetized with special care.

Surgical Anatomy

The carpus is composed of the proximal and distal row of carpal bones. The radial carpal bone articulates primarily with the radius and serves as the major weight-bearing area in the joint. The calcaneus is the largest of the tarsal bones. The distal half of the bone has two facets and two processes that articulate with the talus to form a stable joint. Proximally the tuber calcaneus forms a sturdy prominence to accommodate insertion of the Achilles tendon (see p. 1304). The talus is the second largest of the tarsal bones. It articulates proximally with the tibia and fibula and distally with the central tarsal bone. The body of the talus is divided into medial and lateral trochleae that articulate with the tibia and fibula proximally and a base that articulates with the central tarsal bone distally. The sides of the trochleae articulate with the medial and lateral malleoli.

Positioning

For carpal fractures, the animal is placed in dorsal recumbency. The limb should be clipped and prepared for aseptic surgery from the elbow to the digits. A hanging-limb preparation facilitates limb manipulation during surgery. Animals are placed in lateral recumbency with the affected limb uppermost for calcaneal fractures and in dorsal recumbency for fractures of the talus. With tarsal injuries, the limb should be clipped and surgically prepared from the stifle joint to the digits.

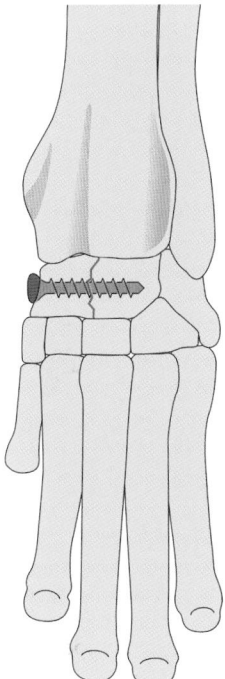

FIG. 32-57
Reduction of a radial carpal bone fracture with a lag screw.

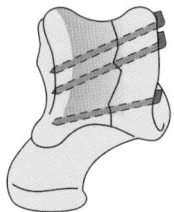 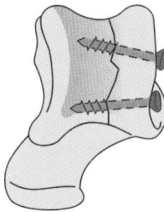

FIG. 32-58
Fractures of the articular surface of the talus may be stabilized with diverging Kirschner wires or lag screws.

SURGICAL TECHNIQUE
Stabilization of Radial Carpal Bone Fractures

Make a craniomedial incision beginning 3 to 4 cm proximal to the radiocarpal joint (see p. 1228). Extend the incision distally to the midmetacarpus, and incise subcutaneous tissue along the same line. Continue deep dissection medial to the extensor carpi radialis tendon to expose the joint capsule. Incise the capsule and identify the fracture plane through the radial carpal bone. Reduce the fracture and stabilize fragments with one or more lag screws (Fig. 32-57). Close the joint capsule and subcutaneous tissue with absorbable suture, and close skin with nonabsorbable suture.

Stabilization of Transverse Calcaneal Fractures

Make an incision along the lateral surface of the calcaneus. Begin the incision along the common calcaneal tendon, just proximal to the tuber calcanei. Continue the incision distally to the level of the tarsometatarsal joint. Incise superficial and deep fascia overlying the caudal border of the calcaneus. Identify the lateral aspect of the superficial digital flexor tendon, and make an incision parallel to this border. Retract the tendon medially to expose the caudal surface of the calcaneus. Reduce the fracture fragments, and place two small pins or Kirschner wires to maintain reduction. Drill a hole from lateral to medial in the distal fragment to accept orthopedic wire. Proximally, pass the wire around the ends of the pins or through a second predrilled hole positioned through the body of the calcaneus proximal to the fracture. Tighten

the wire to complete the tension band procedure. Alternatively, use a bone plate (see Fig. 32-56). Replace the superficial digital flexor tendon, and suture surrounding deep fascia with absorbable material to maintain the position of the tendon. Then suture superficial fascia and skin using standard techniques.

Stabilization of Talar Fractures

Exposure of the trochlea and visualization of the fracture are best accomplished with an osteotomy of the medial malleolus. To expose the lateral condyle of the talus, a distal fibula transverse osteotomy is performed.

Center the skin incision over the medial malleolus (see p. 1311). Begin 5 cm proximal to the malleolus, and carry the incision distally to the tarsometatarsal joint. Incise through superficial and deep fascia to identify the long component of the medial collateral ligament. Make a transverse caudal to cranial incision through the joint capsule overlying the distal tibia to allow visualization of landmarks for completion of an osteotomy of the medial malleolus. Make the osteotomy deep enough to include most of the origin of the collateral ligament, but do not interfere with the weight-bearing articular surface. Retract the malleolus and attached ligaments to expose the talus. Reduce fracture fragments and stabilize each with a lag screw or Kirschner wire (Fig. 32-58). Once fracture reduction and stabilization are satisfactory, reduce and stabilize the medial malleolus with a tension band (see pp. 990 and 1137). Suture superficial and deep fascia with absorbable suture, and close skin with nonabsorbable sutures.

A talar neck fracture may be stabilized with a lag screw angled from the caudal medial surface of the head of the talus into the trochlea of the talus, or alternatively the screw may be placed from the caudal medial base of the talus into the calcaneus. If reduction can be maintained with forceps, the screw may be placed as a position screw; if not, it should be placed as a lag screw (Fig. 32-59).

Incise skin, subcutaneous tissue, and deep fascia along the medial malleolus to the tarsometatarsal joint. Elevate the fascia to expose the talus. Reduce the distal fragment of the talus by manipulating it with pointed reduction forceps and stabilize the fracture. Suture superficial and deep fas-

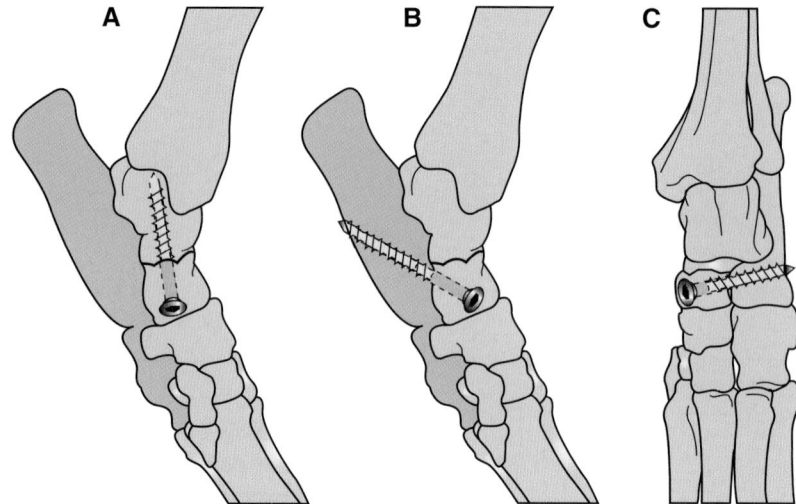

FIG. 32-59
Fractures of the neck of the talus may be stabilized with: **A,** a lag screw angled from the caudal medial surface of the head of the talus into the trochlea of the talus, or **B** and **C,** the screw may be placed from the caudal medial base of the talus into the calcaneus. (Modified from Johnson AL, Dunning D: *Atlas of orthopedic surgical procedures of the dog and cat,* ed 1, St Louis, 2005, Saunders.)

cia with absorbable suture, and close skin with nonabsorbable sutures.

SUTURE MATERIALS AND SPECIAL INSTRUMENTS

Necessary equipment includes Kirschner wire, small IM Steinmann pins, orthopedic wire, bone screws, and instrumentation for insertion of lag screws. An air-driven or battery-operated drill is helpful.

POSTOPERATIVE CARE AND ASSESSMENT

Coaptation with a soft padded bandage postoperatively controls bleeding and swelling. Postoperative pain management is indicated (see p. 943). Coaptation with a splint for up to 6 weeks may be indicated for active dogs. Controlled activity on a leash is mandatory until healing is complete. Short leash walks should be used initially to help maintain strength and joint mobility. The distance walked can be gradually increased. Passive flexion and extension of the carpus and/or tarsus can be performed to maintain joint motion, enhance patient comfort, and improve synovial nutrient presentation to the articular cartilage (see Table 32-9). Pins used in application of the tension band for stabilization of calcaneal fractures may irritate soft tissue and should be removed after healing. Screws used for reconstruction of the radial carpal bone and talus are not removed unless they cause a problem.

PROGNOSIS

Prognosis with calcaneal fractures is excellent for return to normal activity. Return to function with carpus and/or tarsus fractures is fair to good, depending on the degree of articular cartilage damage and whether the articular surface can be reconstructed.

Suggested Reading

Dee JF: Fractures of the tarsus. In Johnson AL, Houlton JEF, Vannini R, editors: *AO principles of fracture management in the dog and cat,* Thieme, NY, 2005, AO Publishing.
This chapter provides an up-to-date collection of operative techniques for stabilizing tarsal fractures in small animals. Detailed descriptions of tension band wire, lag screw, and plate application are included.

Gnudi G, Mortellaro CM, Bertoni G et al: Radial carpal bone fracture in 13 dogs, *Vet Comp Orthop Traumatol* 16:178, 2003.
This article provides a description of the techniques for diagnosing radial carpal bone fractures. Histologic examination of the fracture surface was suggestive of incomplete ossification of the radial carpal bone rather than a true fracture.

Johnson KA, Piras AP: Fractures of the carpus. In Johnson AL, Houlton JEF, Vannini R, editors: *AO principles of fracture management in the dog and cat,* Thieme, NY, 2005, AO Publishing.
This chapter provides an up-to-date collection of operative techniques for stabilizing carpal fractures in small animals. Detailed descriptions of tension band wire and lag screw application are included.

McCartney WT, Carmichael S: Talar neck fractures in 5 cats, *J Small Anim Pract* 41:204, 2000.
Talar neck fractures were treated with external skeletal fixation and lag screw application or traction of the fractured area. The fractures all healed.

Ost PC et al: Fractures of the calcaneus in racing greyhounds, *Vet Surg* 16:53, 1987.
Fifty-one calcaneus fractures associated with (41) or without (10) central tarsal bone (Tc) fractures in racing greyhounds were evaluated and categorized. Descriptions of the treatment techniques and outcomes are described.

Tomlin JL, Pead MJ, Langley-Hobbs SJ et al: Radial carpal bone fractures in dogs, *J Am Anim Hosp Assoc* 37:173, 2001.

This article provides a description of a retrospective study of the presenting clinical and radiographic signs of 11 radial carpal bone fractures in 9 dogs. Pancarpal arthrodesis was used to manage 55% of the radial carpal bone fractures in this report.

METACARPAL, METATARSAL, PHALANGEAL, AND SESAMOID FRACTURES AND LUXATIONS

DEFINITIONS

Sesamoid bones are small, round or oblong bones found adjacent to joints.

GENERAL CONSIDERATIONS AND CLINICALLY RELEVANT PATHOPHYSIOLOGY

Metacarpal and metatarsal bone fractures are common in dogs and cats. They may result from a direct blow or force to the paw or from hyperextension injuries. Complete metacarpal and metatarsal fractures in greyhounds occur as a result of either fatigue, or the relatively normal bone being loaded beyond its yield strain. Metacarpal and metatarsal fractures are classified according to location (e.g., base or proximal end of the bone, shaft, or diaphysis; head or distal end of the bone). Avulsion fractures of the base occur most often on the second and fifth bones because of their ligamentous insertions. Phalangeal fractures occur similarly in dogs and cats; however, fragments are often smaller and more difficult to secure. There are two palmar or plantar sesamoid bones per metacarpophalangeal or metatarsophalangeal joint, numbered one through eight beginning on the medial side. Sesamoid fractures occur after excessive tension on the digital flexor tendons; sesamoid bones two and seven of the forelimb are most often affected. Luxations of the metacarpophalangeal joints or interphalangeal joints typically occur in working dogs or racing greyhounds. Early surgical repair yields better results than closed reduction and splintage because chronic instability leads to degenerative joint disease and less than optimal function.

DIAGNOSIS
Clinical Presentation

Signalment. Any age, breed, or sex of dog or cat may be affected. Racing greyhounds develop stress fractures of the second metacarpal and third metatarsal bones of the right foot and luxations of the distal interphalangeal joints. Sesamoid fractures are most common in large-breed dogs.

History. There is generally a history of trauma. Dogs with sesamoid fractures may have a previous history of acute lameness that subsided but recurred with exercise.

Physical Examination Findings

Animals with metacarpal, metatarsal, or phalangeal fractures have a non–weight-bearing lameness of the affected limb. Soft tissue surrounding the fracture is swollen, crepitation can be palpated, and deformity of the paw may be noted. The animal will be in pain when the area is palpated. Dogs with sesamoid fractures, especially chronic fractures, usually have a weight-bearing lameness. Mild swelling may be evident, and affected animals have pain on deep palpation over the bone. Dogs with joint luxations have lameness, swelling over the affected joint, medial or lateral deviation of the digit, joint instability, and pain on palpation.

> NOTE: Most fractures in the paw cause non–weight-bearing lameness, but sesamoid fractures cause less obvious lameness.

Diagnostic Imaging

Detailed radiographs should include dorsopalmar/plantar and mediolateral views extending from the carpus or tarsus to the ends of the digits. Oblique views, with the digits spread, or a lateral view with the affected digit pulled cranially with tape or gauze may be necessary to isolate individual bones. Stress radiographs taken while the distal digit is displaced may be necessary to show joint instability.

Laboratory Findings

Specific laboratory abnormalities are not present with these fractures or luxations. Traumatized animals should have sufficient blood work done to assess the risk of anesthesia and surgery.

DIFFERENTIAL DIAGNOSIS

Animals presenting with fractures of the metacarpal, metatarsal, and phalangeal bones should be carefully evaluated for concurrent ligamentous injury in the carpus, tarsus, and distal joints of the paw. Radiographs help to differentiate between fractures and luxations caused by ligamentous injury.

MEDICAL MANAGEMENT

Conservative treatment with a fiberglass bivalve cast or metasplint (see p. 917) is appropriate for treating closed, nondisplaced metacarpal and metatarsal diaphyseal fractures affecting one or two bones, especially the second and fifth bones. This treatment is also appropriate for most phalangeal fractures and acute sesamoid bone fractures. The cast or splint should not be removed until there is radiographic evidence that the fracture has bridged with bone (usually 4 to 8 weeks).

Chronic sesamoid fractures causing lameness may not respond to conservative therapy. Acute luxations can be treated conservatively with a cast or splint, but are best treated surgically in working or racing dogs. Chronic luxations causing lameness do not respond to conservative care and are usually treated with arthrodesis or amputation.

SURGICAL TREATMENT

Metacarpal or metatarsal fractures occurring in athletic or racing dogs usually require anatomic reduction and rigid stabilization (plates and screws) for optimal return to racing form (Fig. 32-60). Large avulsed fragments from the base of the second and fifth metacarpals and metatarsals generally require open reduction and internal fixation be-

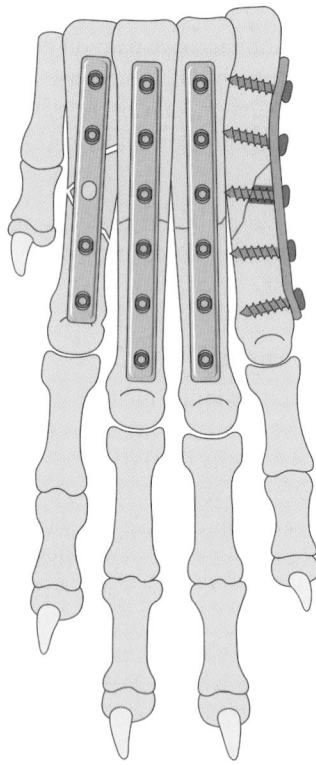

FIG. 32-60
Plate fixation of metacarpal/metatarsal fractures. Plate fixation is used when the fracture-assessment score is low or when athletic function is desired. A bridging buttress plate has been used to span and support a comminuted fracture (digit 2); compression plates have been applied to transverse fractures (digits 3 and 4); and lag screw compression of an oblique fracture line was protected by a neutralization plate (digit 5).

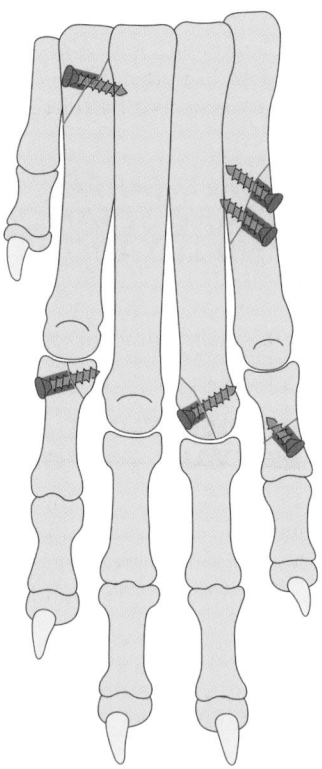

FIG. 32-61
Lag screw fixation for avulsion fractures. Lag screws are used to counteract the pull of adjacent ligaments or to compress oblique fractures.

cause their ligamentous insertions cause fragment distraction (Fig. 32-61). Fracture of the shaft of one or two metacarpal or metatarsal bones can be treated with external coaptation because the unaffected bones form an internal splint to prevent deformity (Box 32-11). Fractures affecting three or four metacarpal or metatarsal bones may require internal fixation for optimal alignment and outcome (Fig. 32-62; see also Fig. 32-60).

Fractures of the phalanges occur less frequently but are handled similarly to metacarpal and metatarsal bone fractures. Fractures of the proximal sesamoid bones of the metacarpophalangeal joints and metatarsophalangeal joints causing chronic lameness are generally treated by removing the fragments.

Acute luxations are treated surgically with open reduction and suturing of the joint capsule and collateral ligaments. Failure of the initial surgical stabilization and chronic joint luxations are best treated with amputation (second or fifth toe) or arthrodesis (middle weight-bearing third and fourth digits) (Box 32-12).

Fixation systems applicable for metacarpal, metatarsal, and phalangeal fractures include orthopedic wire, IM pins,

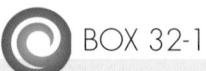 BOX 32-11

Treatment Considerations for Metacarpal/ Metatarsal Fractures

- Fractures of one or two metacarpal or metatarsal bones can be treated with a splint or cast.
- Fractures of three or four metacarpal or metatarsal bones should be treated with internal fixation.
- Large displaced avulsion fractures should be treated with a lag screw.
- A splint or bivalve cast should be applied after internal fixation until there is radiographic evidence of bone healing.

external fixation, and plates and screws. The most appropriate fixation method should be determined based on fracture-assessment score (see p. 953) and fracture location (Box 32-13). If the fracture assessment indicates rapid healing (score of 8 to 10), conservative therapy is indicated; however, if three or four bones are affected, resulting in gross displacement or

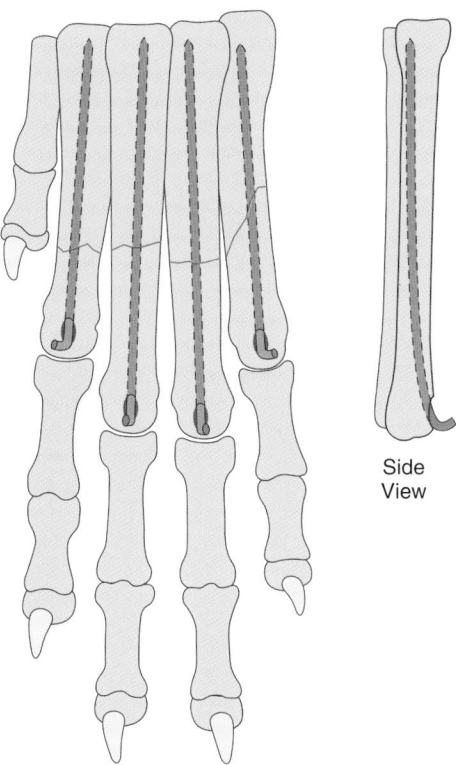

Side
View

FIG. 32-62
IM pinning technique used to treat multiple transverse or short oblique fractures in patients with high fracture-assessment scores. A slot is developed in the distal metaphysis, and the pin is directed through the slot (proximally across the fracture line) and is seated in the proximal metaphysis of the metacarpal or metatarsal bone.

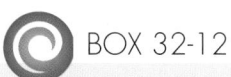 BOX 32-12

Treatment Considerations for Luxations

- Acute luxations in working or racing dogs are best treated with open reduction and suturing of the joint capsule and collateral ligaments.
- Chronic luxations of the second or fifth toe can be treated with amputation.
- Arthrodesis of metacarpophalangeal and interphalangeal joints can result in good function and pain relief.

folding of the paw, open reduction and stabilization with IM pins should be considered. If athletic function is desired, accurate reduction and plate and screw fixation should be considered. Nondisplaced avulsion fractures of the base or head of these bones can be treated with a splint or cast, but some displacement of the fracture usually occurs during the

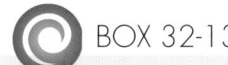 BOX 32-13

Implant Use for Metacarpal/Metatarsal/Phalangeal Fractures According to Fracture-Assessment Score (FAS)

FAS 0 to 3
- Bridging plates*
- External fixators*
- Lag screws for avulsion fractures

FAS 4 to 7
- Bone plates and screws*
- IM pins*
- Lag screws for avulsion fractures

FAS 8 to 10
- Splint or cast*
- IM pins*
- Tension band wire for avulsion fractures

*Choice depends on number of bones fractured, comminution, displacement, number of limbs injured, and desired function of animal (see pp. 1082-1083).

healing process. Open reduction and placement of a lag screw or tension band wire offer the best chance for return to normal function. If the fracture-assessment score is four to seven (e.g., older or larger dogs, in which healing may be delayed; displaced, comminuted diaphyseal fractures of three or four metacarpal or metatarsal bones; multiple limb fractures), treatment with open reduction and plate and screw fixations should be considered. Fracture-assessment scores less than 4 indicate prolonged healing. Severely comminuted fractures or open fractures with degloving injuries can be treated with bridging plates or external fixation with small pins and acrylic (Fig. 32-63). Cancellous bone autografts are indicated in conjunction with open reduction to promote healing in these patients.

Preoperative Management

The paw should be temporarily stabilized with a soft padded bandage and metasplint (see p. 946) to immobilize fragments, decrease or prevent soft tissue swelling, protect or prevent open wounds, and increase patient comfort until surgery can be performed. Open wounds should be initially managed by carefully clipping surrounding hair, cleaning the wound, obtaining a sample for microbial culture and sensitivity testing, and administering broad-spectrum bactericidal antibiotics. Concurrent injuries should be managed before anesthetic induction for fracture fixation. Pain management is indicated for posttraumatic patients (see Box 31-2 on p. 944 and Chapter 13).

Anesthesia

Refer to p. 944 for anesthetic management of patients with fractures. Greyhounds must be anesthetized with special care.

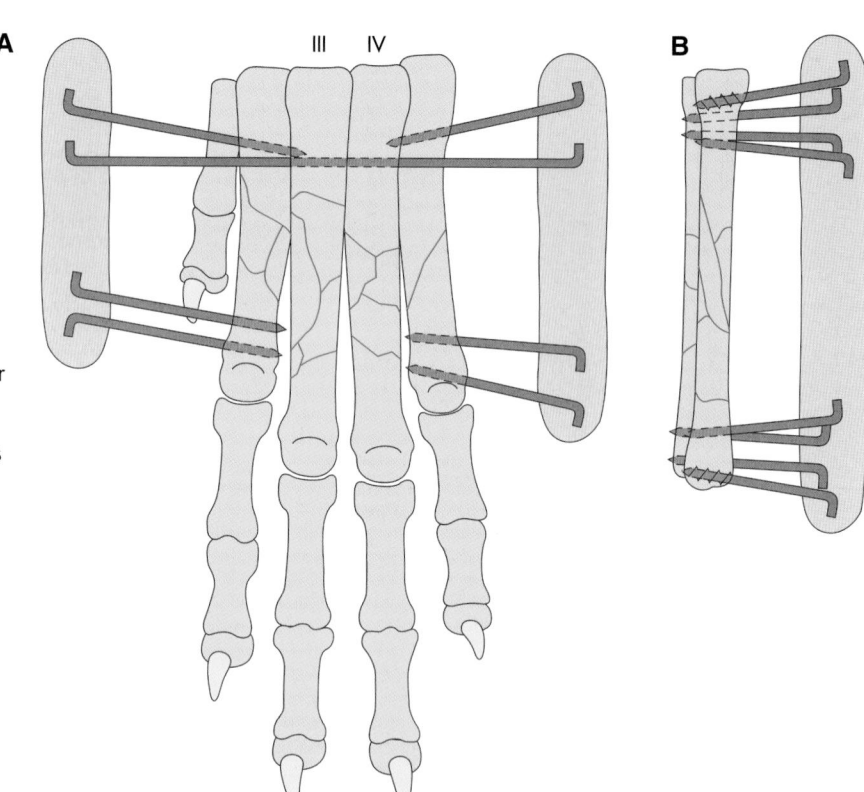

FIG. 32-63
A, Connect fixation pins with acrylic bars for rigid stabilization of comminuted fractures. This fixation does not interfere with open wound treatment. **B,** Alternatively, place pins in a Type Ib configuration and connect with acrylic.

Surgical Anatomy

The primary weight-bearing bones are the third and fourth digits. The superficial dorsal metacarpal or metatarsal artery courses over the dorsal aspect of the paw. The extensor tendons course down the dorsal aspect of each digit. The flexor tendons and superficial and deep metacarpal or metatarsal artery and vein lie on the palmar or plantar aspect of the digits. Each joint has a medial and lateral collateral ligament. The paired proximal sesamoid bones are located caudal to the metacarpophalangeal or metatarsophalangeal joints and have firm ligamentous attachments. With minimal soft tissue coverage, the bones and joints can be easily palpated. Skin incisions are generally made on the dorsal surface of the paw, directly over the fracture or luxation. The extensor tendons and ligaments of the dorsal surface of the paw need to be retracted to expose the bones or joints. Ventral approaches to the digits are made only to expose the proximal sesamoid bones.

> NOTE: A tourniquet is useful to control hemorrhage from the paw.

Positioning

The entire distal limb should be prepared for aseptic surgery. The animal is placed in dorsal recumbency with the affected paw isolated for draping. The most accessible site for harvesting a cancellous bone graft for the forelimb is the proximal humerus; for the hind limb, the site is the proximal tibia (see p. 962). These areas should be prepared and draped if a bone graft is needed (e.g., comminuted fractures with fracture-assessment score less than 4).

SURGICAL TECHNIQUE
Stabilization of Transverse Metacarpal or Metatarsal Fractures

Multiple, simple transverse (or very short oblique) metacarpal bone fractures in animals with fracture assessment scores of 8 to 10 and 4 to 7 may be repaired with IM pins. The medullary diameters of the second and fifth metacarpal and metatarsal bones are smaller than the third and fourth, affecting pin diameter selection.

Incise skin over the dorsal surface of the third and fourth bones. Incise subcutaneous tissue, and elevate and retract extensor tendons to expose the fractures. Introduce the pin into the distal, dorsal surface of the bone to avoid the joint (use a high-speed burr to develop a slot in the bone). Blunt the tip of the pin to prevent it from penetrating the intact opposite cortex. Drive the pin through the slot and proximally across the fracture line and seat it in the proximal bone segment. Bend the distal end of the pin to prevent migration and simplify removal. Repeat the procedure for at least the third and fourth metacarpal or metatarsal bone (and in some cases all four bones; see Fig. 32-62). Protect the fixation with a splint or cast for 4 to 6 weeks.

If more rigid fixation is required in animals with low fracture-assessment scores (e.g., large dogs with multiple-limb injury), veterinary cuttable plates or small dynamic compression plates are useful to stabilize the fracture (see Fig. 32-60).

Stabilization of Avulsion Fractures and Oblique Diaphyseal Fractures

The size, location, and degree of displacement of an avulsion fracture will dictate whether repair or removal is optimal. Small avulsed minimally displaced fragments associated with other fractures may not require stabilization. Basilar fractures with significant displacement require primary repair.

Repair avulsion fractures of the base or head and intraarticular fractures of the metacarpal, metatarsal, or phalangeal bones using lag screws (see p. 991). Place lag screws after anatomic reconstruction of these fractures to counteract the pull of attached ligaments (see Fig. 32-61). Use orthopedic wire with Kirschner wires as tension band wire (see p. 990) in avulsion fractures in animals with fracture-assessment scores of 8 to 10. Reconstruct simple oblique fractures of the diaphyses with lag screws, and support the repair with a splint or bivalve cast; the screws only minimally interfere with function. If diaphyseal fractures require additional support, consider applying veterinary cuttable plates as neutralization plates.

> NOTE: Use anatomic reconstruction with lag screws for best results in athletic dogs.

Stabilization of Comminuted Diaphyseal Fractures

Repair severely comminuted fractures of the diaphyses of the metacarpal and metatarsal bones with small, dynamic compression plates (2.7 or 2.0) or veterinary cuttable plates (see p. 991), which bridge the comminuted portions of the fracture (see Fig. 32-60). Leave fragments undisturbed, and attach the plate to the proximal and distal segments. Apply plates to two to four bones, depending on fracture configuration and number of bones fractured. Use a splint or cast to support the fixation after surgery. Alternatively, insert multiple Kirschner wires or IM pins through the proximal and distal segments of the bones and connect with acrylic to form an external fixator (see Fig. 32-63).

This type of fixation is also useful for treating open fractures.

> NOTE: Acrylic fixator bars are versatile; they can accommodate various sizes of pins placed in multiple locations.

Sesamoid Bone Excision

Incise the skin adjacent to the large central pad directly over the ventral aspect of the affected joint. Continue the incision through subcutaneous tissue, and identify the fractured sesamoid. Sharply dissect the sesamoid fragments from their ligamentous attachments. If the fragment is less than one third of the sesamoid bone, remove only the fragment. If the fragment is larger, remove the entire sesamoid bone. Suture subcutaneous tissue and skin separately.

Suture Repair of Luxations

Incise skin and subcutaneous tissue dorsally over the affected joint to expose the torn joint capsule and collateral ligaments. Use multiple absorbable horizontal mattress sutures to repair the joint capsule and ligament. Continue to imbricate (tighten the joint capsule with mattress sutures) the capsular tissue until the joint is stable. Repair the capsule bilaterally if necessary. Also, inspect the extensor tendon retinaculum for tears, and stabilize it with interrupted sutures. Suture subcutaneous tissue and skin.

Digit Amputation

Make an elliptic skin incision paralleling the long axis of and around the digit, starting proximodorsally and ending distally on the palmar or plantar surface (Fig. 32-64). Preserve the pad if amputating at the interphalangeal joints. Disarticulate the joint with sharp dissection. Remove the sesamoid bones (metacarpophalangeal or metatarsophalangeal joint amputation). Resect the distal end of the remaining proximal bone. Make a transverse osteotomy line for the interphalangeal joints and third and fourth metacarpal or metatarsal bones, but bevel the osteotomy distally toward the midline for the second and fifth metacarpal or metatarsal bones. Suture soft tissue and skin, taking care to obtain a cosmetic closure.

Arthrodesis

Expose the joint using the approach described for suturing joint luxations. Open the joint capsule, and remove the articular cartilage with rongeurs. Conform the surfaces to obtain good contact at a functional angle (determined by observing adjacent toes). Temporarily hold the bones in position by driving small Kirschner wires from the dorsal surface of each bone across the joint surface. Contour a small plate (2.0) to the dorsal surface of the bones. Attach the plate using at least one lag screw across the joint surface (Fig. 32-65, A). Alternatively, stabilize the arthrodesis with the small Kirschner wires and a tension band wire (Fig. 32-65, B) in small dogs or cats when rapid healing is anticipated.

SUTURE MATERIALS AND SPECIAL INSTRUMENTS

Equipment that should be available for management of fractures or luxations of the distal extremity includes IM pins, Kirschner wires, orthopedic wire, a Jacobs pin chuck, a wire tightener, plating equipment, hoof or dental acrylic, and

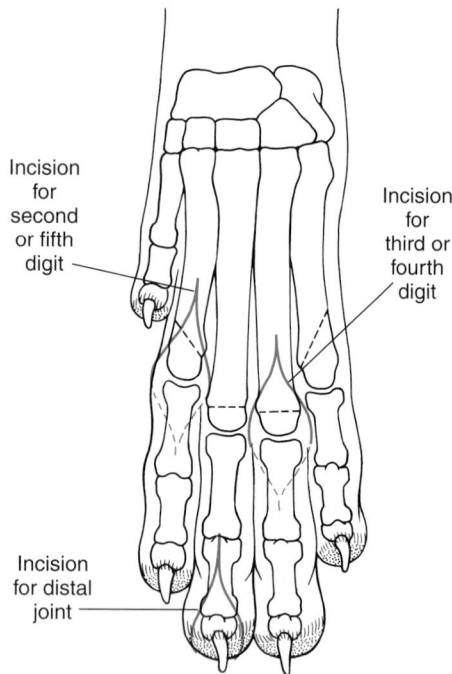

FIG. 32-64
Suggested skin incision lines and osteotomy lines for proximal and distal digit amputation.

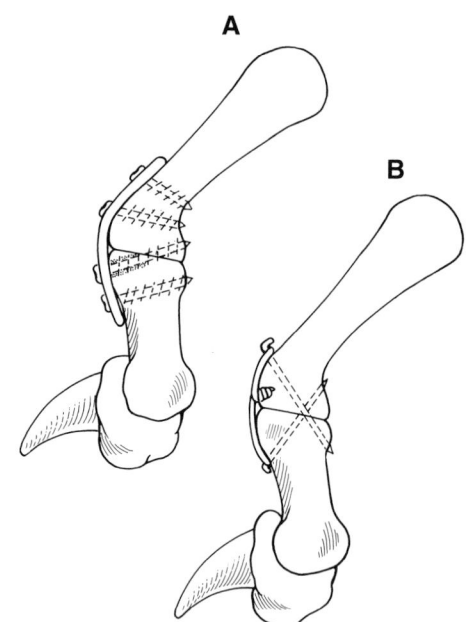

FIG. 32-65
Arthrodesis of proximal interphalangeal joint with plate and lag screw **(A)** or Kirschner wires and tension band wire **(B)**.

rongeurs, bone cutters, or an osteotome. A tourniquet applied to the distal limb is useful for controlling hemorrhage during surgery but should only be maintained for 1 hour.

POSTOPERATIVE CARE AND ASSESSMENT

Postoperative radiographs should be made to evaluate fracture reduction and implant position, reduction of luxations, and alignment of arthrodeses. Postoperative pain management may be indicated (see Box 31-2 on p. 944 and Chapter 13). Radiographs should be repeated every 6 weeks until the fracture(s) or the arthrodesis is healed. The foot should be supported in a splint or bivalve cast until there is radiographic evidence of bone healing (even after internal fixation). After digit amputation, the paw should be supported in a soft bandage for 1 to 2 weeks. After fracture healing, IM pins, plates, and external fixators should be removed, but orthopedic wire and screws may be left in place as long as no implant-associated complications arise. Limited activity is advised until there is radiographic evidence of fracture bridging with bone.

Physical rehabilitation (see Chapter 12) may be indicated to ensure optimal limb function after bone healing. Care must be taken to develop customized protocols for each patient depending on location of the fracture, stability and type of fracture fixation, potential for healing, abilities and attitudes of the patient, and willingness or ability of the client to provide for the animal's care. Physical rehabilitation for patients with fractures supported by splints for 6 weeks generally begins after the splint has been removed (see Table

32-9). Owners should be instructed to confine animals to a small area (preferably a cage). The cast or splint should be kept clean and dry, and the owner should observe it daily for evidence of slippage or irritation.

COMPLICATIONS

Most metacarpal and metatarsal fractures progress to healing. Fractures of the diaphyses of three or four metacarpal or metatarsal bones treated with a metasplint may develop delayed union or malunion and may become nonunions. Other potential complications include iatrogenic infection (with open reduction) and secondary degenerative joint disease after articular fracture.

PROGNOSIS

In most cases, the prognosis for normal limb function after fracture healing is good. Chronic lameness associated with sesamoid fragmentation may resolve or improve with conservative therapy. The prognosis after sesamoid removal is good for early resolution of the lameness, but degenerative joint disease progresses and lameness may recur with heavy use.

Prognosis for function after surgical repair of joint luxations depends on the stability of the repair. Unstable joints will develop progressive degenerative joint disease and cause lameness. Function after amputation of the second and fifth digit is usually good. The more distal the amputation, the better is the prognosis. Function after an arthrodesis procedure is generally good.

Suggested Reading

Dee JF: Fractures of the metacarpal and metatarsal bones. In Johnson AL, Houlton JEF, Vannini R, editors: *AO principles of fracture management in the dog and cat,* Thieme, NY, 2005, AO Publishing.

This chapter provides an up-to-date collection of operative techniques for stabilizing metacarpal and metatarsal bone fractures in small animals. Detailed descriptions of tension band wire, lag screw, and plate application are included.

Dee JF: Fractures of the digits. In Johnson AL, Houlton JEF, Vannini R, editors: *AO principles of fracture management in the dog and cat,* Thieme, NY, 2005, AO Publishing.

This chapter provides an up-to-date collection of operative techniques for stabilizing fractures of the digits in small animals. Detailed descriptions of tension band wire, lag screw, and plate application are included.

Mathews KG, Koblik PD, Whitehair JG et al: Fragmented palmar metacarpo-phalangeal sesamoids in dogs: a long-term evaluation, *Vet Comp Orthop Traumatol* 14:7, 2001.

This article provides an evaluation of the long-term clinical and radiographic response to surgical and conservative management of fragmented sesamoids in dogs. Conservative therapy was effective in resolving lameness in most cases. Surgical treatment resulted in significantly greater progression of degenerative joint disease.

Muir P, Norris JL: Metacarpal and metatarsal fractures in dogs, *J Small Anim Pract* 38:324, 1997.

Metacarpal fractures were more common than metatarsal fractures in this retrospective study of 37 dogs. Progressive fracture healing usually occurred irrespective of the stabilization method. Alignment issues are discussed.

PELVIC FRACTURES

DEFINITIONS

Sacroiliac luxation results when there is disruption of the articulation between the wing of the sacrum and the iliac wing. **Sacral fracture** may accompany sacroiliac luxation.

SACROILIAC LUXATIONS AND FRACTURES

GENERAL CONSIDERATIONS AND CLINICALLY RELEVANT PATHOPHYSIOLOGY

The sacroiliac joint is often injured when the pelvis is fractured. Displacement of the pelvic girdle after a fracture requires bilateral separation of the sacroiliac joints, fracture of the pelvic bones at three sites, or a combination of these injuries. One of these points of fracture may be a separation of the sacroiliac articulation. Displacement of the wing of the ilium is generally cranial and dorsal, with medial movement of the ilium to compromise the pelvic canal. The femoral and sciatic nerves are close to the sacroiliac joint, and concurrent nerve damage may occur. Preoperative attention to neurologic status is necessary before treatment. Neurologic deficits are common when sacral fractures traverse the spinal canal or sacral foramina (Anderson and Coughlin, 1997).

DIAGNOSIS

Clinical Presentation

Signalment. Any age, breed, or sex of dog or cat may be affected.

History. Sacroiliac luxations and fractures are most often caused by motor vehicle accidents.

Physical Examination Findings

Patients are usually non–weight-bearing or minimally weight bearing on the affected limb. If there is contralateral long bone or pelvic injury, however, the animal may be required to bear weight on the limb with sacroiliac luxation. Instability may be difficult to palpate. Animals with severe displacement of the ilium may have severe pain when movement occurs. When the patient is sedated, dorsoventral movement of the ilium may be detected.

Diagnostic Imaging

Ventrodorsal and lateral radiographs must be taken to assess the degree of injury to the hemipelvis and to delineate fracture planes. Sacroiliac luxation is diagnosed when there is a visible step at the sacroiliac joint and is usually identified on the ventrodorsal view. Care should be taken when positioning the animal to obtain as much symmetry as possible. Special attention should be paid to identifying sacral fractures because they are often missed. The width of the pelvic canal should be ascertained.

Laboratory Findings

Consistent laboratory abnormalities are not present. Traumatized animals undergoing surgery should have sufficient blood work done to assess the risk of anesthesia and surgery.

DIFFERENTIAL DIAGNOSIS

Differential diagnoses include fracture of the hemipelvis (i.e., ilium and acetabulum) and sacral fractures. These fractures can usually be differentiated with appropriate radiographs.

MEDICAL MANAGEMENT

Most patients function normally with asymmetric craniocaudal positioning of the hip joints. Conservative treatment is indicated with minimal patient discomfort and minimal displacement of the hemipelvis or when financial limitations preclude surgery. The majority of patients treated conservatively for a sacroiliac luxation regain normal function. However, lameness may persist for up to 12 weeks and malunion with pelvic narrowing can occur. Surgical reduction is indicated with significant narrowing of the pelvic outlet, which could lead to constipation or obstipation.

Conservative therapy should include enforced rest for the initial 3 weeks after injury. After 3 weeks, supervised activity

Table 32-10

Sample Physical Rehabilitation Protocol for Patients With Unstable Pelvic Fractures

ALL TREATMENTS BID	DAY 1 TO DAY 14	DAY 15 TO DAY 24	DAY 25 UNTIL HEALED	HEALED TO RETURN TO FUNCTION
Heat therapy		10 min	10 min	
Massage	5 min	5 min	5 min	
Passive range of motion (repetitions)		10*	20*	20*
Electrical stimulation†	10 min	10 min	10 min	10 min
Therapeutic exercise-total time	5 min	10 min	15 min	25–45
Walk/land treadmill		5 min	5 min	>10 min
Balancing	+	+	+	
Obstacles				+
Weaving				+
Circles				+
Hills				+
Stairs				+
Jog/run				+
Underwater treadmill		5 min	15 min	>15 min
Swimming				5–10 min
Cryotherapy	15 min	15 min	15 min	PRN

BID, Twice a day; +, perform modality; *PRN,* as needed.
*Perform passive range of motion for all joints of the affected limb.
†Apply to semimembranosus/semitendinosus muscles for patients with muscle atrophy (see Chapter 12).

on a leash should be encouraged for an additional 4 weeks, with the amount of exercise gradually increased. NSAIDs can be used to control inflammation and pain (see p. 945), but the animal must be observed for adverse side effects (i.e., vomiting or melena). The animal should be maintained on well-padded bedding that is changed frequently to prevent decubital ulcers and urine scalding. Bowel movements should be monitored and stool softeners given if necessary. Warm water sponge baths may be used to decrease odor and improve patient comfort. Physical rehabilitation should be performed to prevent joint and muscle contracture (Table 32-10).

SURGICAL TREATMENT

Surgical stabilization of a sacroiliac fracture-separation should be accomplished with bone screws. A transiliac bolt may be helpful to prevent undue forces on the bone screws and medial displacement of the ilium.

Preoperative Management

Patients with sacroiliac injuries should be adequately stabilized before fracture treatment. The animal's neurologic status must be determined preoperatively. Because urinary trauma may be associated with pelvic fractures, function of the lower urinary tract should be determined before surgical repair of the sacroiliac fracture. Pain management is indicated for posttraumatic patients (see Box 31-2 on p. 944 and Chapter 13).

Anesthesia

Refer to p. 944 for anesthetic considerations of patients with traumatic orthopedic disease.

Surgical Anatomy

The sacroiliac joint has two distinct components: a semilunar, crescent-shaped synovial joint and a fibrocartilaginous synchondrosis. The joint's strength is derived from dorsal and ventral ligaments, and the fibrocartilaginous synchondrosis (Fig. 32-66).

Positioning

The animal should be positioned in lateral recumbency with the dorsal midline raised 45 degrees from the table. The prepared area should extend from the dorsal midline to the stifle joint and from a point 10 cm cranial to the iliac crest to the tail head caudally.

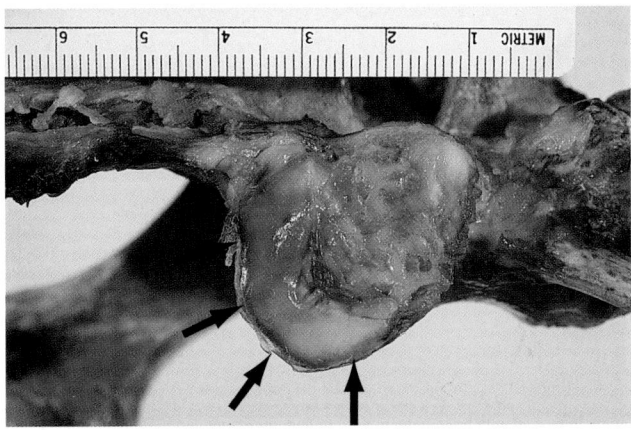

FIG. 32-66
Lateral surface of sacroiliac joint. Note C-shaped zone of articular cartilage *(arrows)*.

SURGICAL TECHNIQUE
Surgical Approach

Make a skin incision beginning over the dorsal iliac crest and continuing caudally, parallel to the spine to a point even with the hip joint (Fig. 32-67). Incise subcutaneous tissue and pelvic fat along the same line to expose the iliac crest. Incise through the periosteal origin of the middle gluteal muscle on the lateral ridge of the iliac crest. Make a second incision through the periosteal origin of the sacrospinalis muscle on the medial ridge of the iliac crest. The incisions merge caudally, where it may be necessary to incise through fibers of the superficial gluteal muscle.

The supporting ligamentous tissues between the sacrum and ilium are usually separated with the impact of the original trauma. Therefore incision of the lumbar fascia allows lateral reflection of the ilium and exposure of the sacroiliac joint.

Ventrally displace the ilium with a bone holding forceps, and remove the fibrous debris to obtain a clear view of the surface of the sacral wing. Elevate the middle gluteal muscle from the lateral surface of the ilium to expose the ilium further for placement of implants. To close the incision, suture fasciae of the middle gluteal and sacrospinalis muscles with an absorbable suture in an interrupted pattern. Then suture subcutaneous tissue and skin using standard methods.

Stabilization Using a Screw

Once the joint is exposed, position a blunt Hohmann retractor between the ilium and ventral bony shelf of the sacrum. Reflect the ilium ventrally with the retractor.

This maneuver exposes the crescent-shaped articular cartilage and fibrocartilaginous joint surfaces of the sacrum. To position a screw properly in the sacrum, direct visualization of the lateral surface of the sacral wing is preferred.

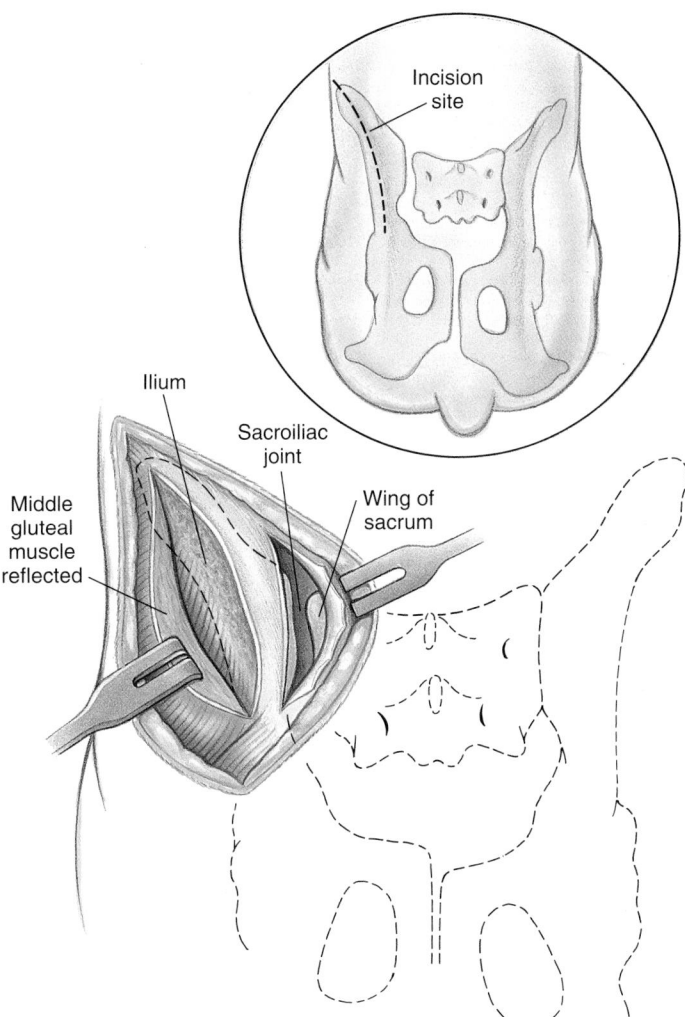

FIG. 32-67
To expose the sacroiliac joint through a dorsal exposure, make an incision over the iliac crest. Reflect the gluteal muscles laterally and the sacrococcygeus dorsalis lateralis muscle medially.

Use the appropriately sized drill bit to drill a thread hole 2 mm cranial and 2 mm proximal to the center of the crescent-shaped articular cartilage (Fig. 32-68, A). The depth of the thread hole in the sacral body should be such that the screw tip will extend to the midline of the sacral body. Determine the proper location of the glide hole in the ilium by palpating the articular prominence on the medial surface of the iliac wing. Drill the glide hole at the predetermined position with the appropriately sized drill bit. A glide hole is not needed if a partially threaded cancellous screw is used. Advance the proper-length screw through the glide hole until the tip appears on the medial surface of the ilium. Bring the ilium caudally in alignment with the articular surface of the sacroiliac joint. Visually guide the screw tip into the prepared thread hole in the sacrum, and tighten the screw (Fig. 32-68, B). Add a second screw placed immediately dorsal and

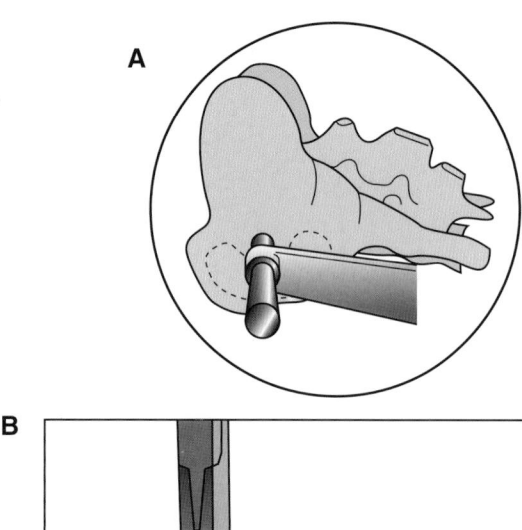

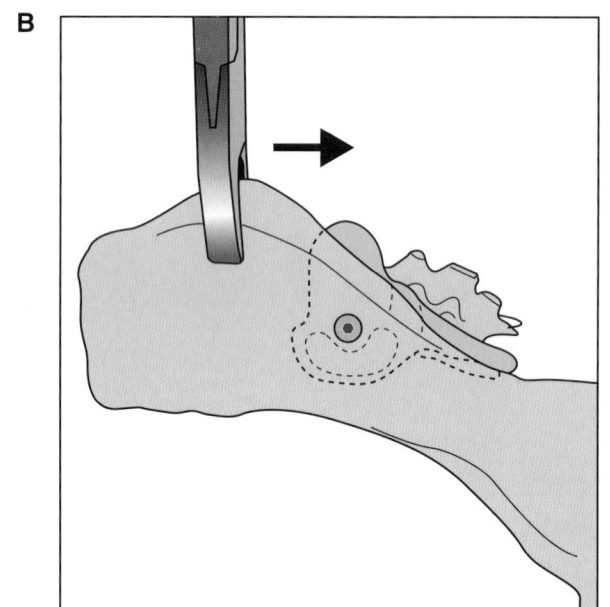

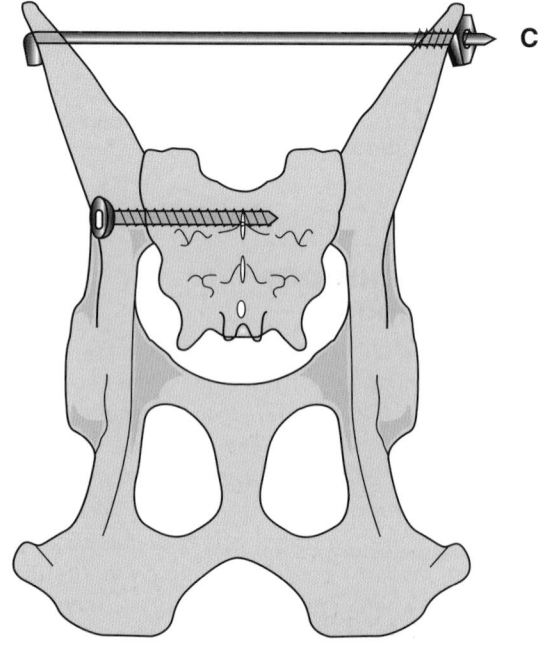

FIG. 32-68
To place a lag screw, lever the iliac body ventrally with a Hohmann retractor to expose the lateral surface of the sacroiliac joint. **A,** Drill the threaded hole in the sacrum directly. **B,** Then drill the glide hole in the iliac wing, reduce the fracture/luxation, and secure it with the lag screw. **C,** For additional stability, add a transiliac bolt. (Modified from Johnson AL, Dunning D: *Atlas of orthopedic surgical procedures of the dog and cat,* ed 1, St Louis, 2005, Saunders.)

cranial to the initial screw if space permits. This screw must be shorter to avoid the spinal canal.

Large or overweight dogs may benefit from the placement of a transiliac bolt. A small Steinmann pin may be placed through the iliac wings and over the dorsal surface of L7.

Bend the smooth end of the pin and place a nut on the threaded end to prevent migration (Fig. 32-68, C).

SUTURE MATERIALS AND SPECIAL INSTRUMENTS

Instruments required for placement of a lag screw are recommended. A Hohmann retractor and a drill sleeve facilitate implant insertion.

POSTOPERATIVE CARE AND ASSESSMENT

Postoperative radiographs are made to evaluate sacroiliac reduction and implant location. Activity should be restricted to leash walking and physical rehabilitation until the fracture has healed. Physical rehabilitation (see Chapter 12) encourages controlled limb use and optimal limb function after fracture healing. Care must be taken to develop customized protocols for each patient depending on location of the fracture, stability and type of fracture fixation, potential for healing, abilities and attitudes of the patient, and willingness and ability of the client to provide for the animal's care (Table 32-11). Radiographs should be evaluated in 6 weeks to ascertain pelvic width after healing. Implants do not need to be removed unless they cause a problem.

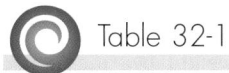 Table 32-11

Sample Physical Rehabilitation Protocol for Patients With Stable Pelvic Nonarticular Fractures

ALL TREATMENTS BID	DAY 1 TO DAY 14	DAY 15 TO DAY 24	DAY 25 UNTIL HEALED	HEALED TO RETURN TO FUNCTION
Heat therapy		10 min	10 min	
Massage	5 min	5 min	5 min	
Passive range of motion (repetitions)	15*	15*		
Electrical stimulation†	10 min	10 min	10 min	10 min
Therapeutic exercise-total time	10 min	20 min	20 min	25–45 min
Walk/land treadmill	5 min	5 min	5 min	>10 min
Balancing	5 min	5 min	5 min	N
Obstacles	+	+	+	+
Weaving				+
Circles				+
Hills				+
Stairs				+
Jog/run				+
Underwater treadmill		5 min	15 min	>15 min
Swimming				5–10 min
Cryotherapy	15 min	15 min	15 min	PRN

BID, Twice a day; *N,* normal; +, perform modality; *PRN,* as needed.
*Perform passive range of motion for all joints of the affected limb.
†Apply to semimembranosus/semitendinosus muscles for patients with muscle atrophy (see Chapter 12).

COMPLICATIONS

Pelvic canal narrowing may be present after sacroiliac luxation healing and is related to the preoperative width of the pelvic canal (Averill et al, 1997). Severe pelvic canal narrowing can result in pelvic canal stenosis, which can cause obstipation and dystocia.

PROGNOSIS

The prognosis for return to normal activity is excellent after surgical stabilization of sacroiliac luxations and fractures. Animals treated with surgical stabilization usually return to limb function within 6 weeks. Longer rehabilitation times can be expected without surgery. Factors that influence the prognosis include accuracy of implant placement and depth of the implant. Screws placed in the sacral body that in depth exceed 60% the width of the sacrum are less likely to have screw loosening than those that are placed more shallow.

References

Anderson A, Coughlin AR: Sacral fractures in dogs and cats: a classification scheme and review of 51 cases, *J Small Anim Pract* 38:404, 1997.

Averill SM, Johnson AL, Schaeffer DJ: Risk factors associated with development of pelvic canal stenosis secondary to sacroiliac separation: 84 cases (1985-1995), *J Am Vet Med Assoc* 211:75, 1997.

Suggested Reading

Burger M, Forterre F, Brunnberg L: Surgical anatomy of the feline sacroiliac joint for lag screw fixation of sacroiliac fracture-luxation, *Vet Comp Orthop Traumatol* 17:146, 2003.
This article provides a unique study detailing the surgical anatomy of the feline sacroiliac joint and the anatomic references for placing screws to stabilize a luxation.

DeCamp C: Fracture-luxation of the sacroiliac joint. In Johnson AL, Houlton JEF, Vannini R, editors: *AO principles of fracture management in the dog and cat,* Thieme, NY, 2005, AO Publishing.
This chapter provides an up-to-date description of the operative technique for stabilizing sacroiliac luxations in small animals. Detailed descriptions of lag screw application are included.

Piermattei D, Johnson KA: *An atlas of surgical approaches to the bones and joints of the dog and cat,* ed 4, Philadelphia, 2004, WB Saunders.
An excellent resource for surgical approaches to the pelvis.

ILIAC, ISCHIAL, AND PUBIC FRACTURES

DEFINITIONS

Fractures may occur through the body or wing of the ilium. Fractures of the ischium and pubis may occur through the ischial body, floor, or pubis.

GENERAL CONSIDERATIONS AND CLINICALLY RELEVANT PATHOPHYSIOLOGY

The pelvis is a boxlike structure, and generally the hemipelvis must be fractured at three different sites to displace bone fragments. Typically the ilium, ischium, and pubis are fractured simultaneously, resulting in loss of weight transfer from the affected limb to the spine, along with instability and pain. Iliac fractures are most often long oblique fractures of the body of the ilium. Transverse fractures and comminuted fractures also occur. The caudal fragment is usually displaced medially and cranially, compromising the pelvic canal. Because soft tissue injury may accompany obvious bony injury, careful patient assessment is necessary. Bladder and urethral rupture may occur concurrent with pelvic fractures, particularly if the bladder is full at the time of impact (see p. 663). Muscle separation or avulsion of the bony insertion of the rectus abdominis muscle and herniation of abdominal viscera may also occur (see p. 324). Herniation of abdominal viscera may result in strangulation and necrosis of tissue if early diagnosis and treatment are not initiated. Impaired sensory and motor functions of the lumbosacral plexus or sciatic nerve may result from an iliac fracture.

> NOTE: Because concurrent injuries (e.g., bladder and urethral tears, hernias, and peripheral nerve injuries) are common in patients with ischial, iliac, or pubic fractures, a complete physical examination should always be performed.

Isolated ischial or pubic fractures are rare. When ischial or pubic fractures occur in combination with other pelvic fractures, reduction and stabilization of the primary weight-bearing segment usually result in acceptable reduction and stabilization of the pubis and ischium. The most common reason for surgical intervention of a pubic or ischial fracture is associated soft tissue herniation. Herniation of abdominal viscera can result from separation of the pubis symphysis or from cranial pubic ligament avulsion; rarely, herniation may occur caudal to the acetabulum.

DIAGNOSIS
Clinical Presentation

Signalment. Any breed, age, or sex of dog or cat may be affected.

History. Vehicular accidents are the usual cause of iliac, ischial, and pubic bone injuries, but any type of blunt trauma may also result in these pelvic fractures.

Physical Examination Findings

Affected animals usually have non–weight-bearing lameness; with minimal displacement and soft tissue injury, however, they may be partially weight bearing. Bruising is common in patients sustaining pelvic fractures, but urethral trauma should be suspected if ventral abdominal bruising is severe or progresses. The integrity of abdominal musculature should be carefully assessed and the function of the sciatic nerve determined before surgery.

Diagnostic Imaging

Ventrodorsal and lateral radiographs should be taken to assess the degree of injury to the hemipelvis and to delineate fracture planes (Fig. 32-69). Additional diagnostic tests (e.g., cystogram and urethrogram) may be needed to confirm the presence or absence of soft tissue injury.

Laboratory Findings

Consistent laboratory abnormalities are not found. Bladder or urethral rupture may result in azotemia and hyperkalemia (see p. 663). Traumatized animals undergoing surgery should have sufficient blood work done to assess the risk of anesthesia and surgery.

DIFFERENTIAL DIAGNOSIS

Differential diagnoses include fracture and/or separation of the sacroiliac joint, acetabular fracture, and coxofemoral luxation.

MEDICAL MANAGEMENT

Conservative treatment is indicated with iliac fractures that are minimally displaced and relatively stable. Conservative treatment may also be considered in patients if the owners are unable to afford surgery (see p. 1087). The pelvic girdle is unstable when fractured, and excessive weight bearing may cause further medial displacement of the hemipelvis, resulting in continued pain, further compromise of the pelvic canal, and malunion of the ilium with malalignment of the coxofemoral joint. Conservative treatment is usually appropriate for isolated ischial and pubic fractures. If they occur in combination with other pelvic fractures, reduction and stabilization of the primary weight-bearing segment (i.e., ilium and acetabulum) results in acceptable reduction and stabilization of the pubis and ischium.

SURGICAL TREATMENT

Surgery is indicated to restore the weight-bearing arch of the pelvis when there is moderate to severe displacement and instability. Animals that have sustained bilateral pelvic limb injury benefit from surgery because they are able to walk more quickly and require less intensive postoperative care. Surgery is indicated for notably displaced ischial fractures and those associated with soft tissue herniation, or for reestablishment of integrity in the pelvic girdle of intact female dogs or cats that will be bred. Surgery is also

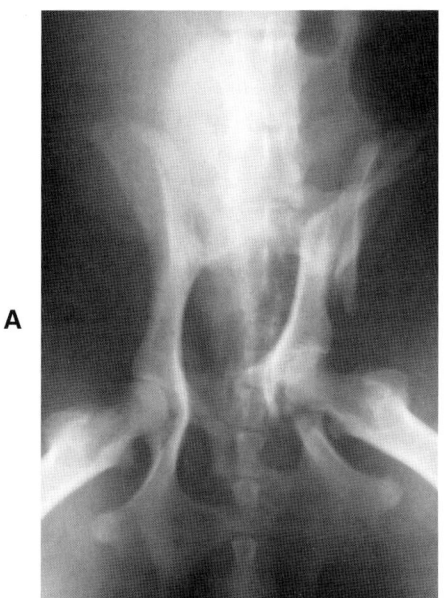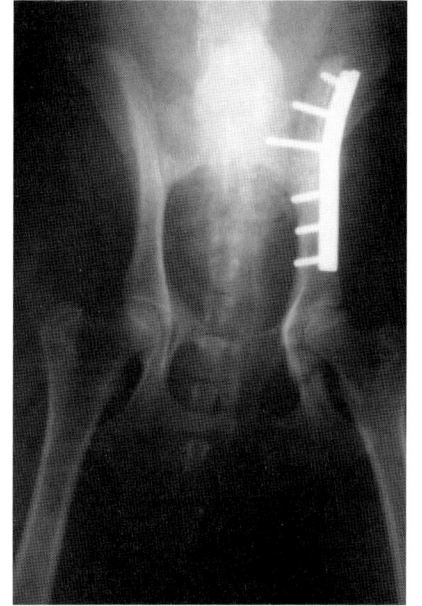

FIG. 32-69
A, Preoperative and postoperative radiographs **(B),** showing reduction and placement of a bone plate and screws to stabilize an iliac body fracture.

indicated for pubic fractures associated with soft issue herniation.

> NOTE: Inform owners that although many fractures heal adequately with conservative therapy, surgery will prevent malunion and shorten the rehabilitation time.

Application of Plates and Screws

Bone plates are the only implant that can be curved to mimic the shape of the lateral surface of the ilium and once applied will maintain the reduction of the ilium in that shape. Restoring the curve of the ilium prevents collapse of the pelvic canal. The dynamic compression plate is used most frequently (see Fig. 32-69). Reconstruction plates can be used when there are concurrent iliac body and ipsilateral acetabular fractures. Iliac fractures with a long oblique configuration may also be stabilized with lag screws. Combining a lateral plate with the application of a ventrally placed veterinary cuttable plate will gain additional screw purchase and support comminuted fractures, or fractures in large or obese dogs.

Preoperative Management

Urination and bowel movements should be monitored before surgery (see previous discussion). Respirations should be monitored, and chest radiographs are indicated. An electrocardiogram is useful to determine cardiac rhythm, particularly if peripheral pulses appear weak or irregular. Analgesics should be administered to posttraumatic patients (see Box 31-2 on p. 944 and Chapter 13).

Anesthesia

Refer to p. 944 for a discussion of anesthetic management of patients with orthopedic trauma.

Surgical Anatomy

The ilium is formed by the iliac wing and iliac body. The iliac wing is located cranially and is recognized by the palpable iliac crest dorsally. The bone curves medially to allow for the middle and deep gluteal muscles; the bone is thin in this area and may not hold implants well. The sacroiliac joint is located medially. The body of the ilium is rectangular and located between the wing of the ilium cranially and the acetabulum caudally. The iliac body holds implants well because of its cortical dimensions. The sciatic nerve is located medial to the body, along its dorsal longitudinal plane. Reestablishment of iliac integrity is required for weight transfer from the limb to the axial skeleton. With iliac fractures, the caudal fragment is often displaced medially and cranially to the wing of the ilium. For orientation purposes, it is often helpful to identify the ventral border of the iliac wing. The deep gluteal muscle is usually torn and lies between the two fragments. Because the sciatic nerve may be sandwiched between the dorsal borders of the two fragments, fragment manipulation should be done carefully.

> NOTE: Use caution when dissecting near the dorsal iliac border (or when placing bone-holding forceps over the dorsal border) to prevent injury to the sciatic nerve.

The ischium is formed by the lesser ischiatic notch cranially, ischial floor medially, and ischial tuberosity caudally. Caution must be exercised with surgical dissection of the ischial notch due to the presence of the sciatic nerve. Identification of the nerve is necessary for exposure and implant application. The sciatic nerve is protected once the insertion of the external rotators is incised and reflected.

Herniation of soft tissue is the most common indication for repair of pubic fractures. Often the surgical area is bruised and swollen, making identification of normal anatomic landmarks difficult. The key for surgical dissection is to begin cranial to the injury where the ventral midline is visible. Surgical dissection can be continued caudally along the midline to expose the fractured pubis. The obturator foramen is located caudal to the cranial pubic brim. Hernia repair is discussed on p. 324.

Positioning

For iliac and ischial fractures, the patient is positioned in lateral recumbency. The surgical site should be prepared from the dorsal midline to the stifle joint and from a point 10 cm cranial to the iliac crest to the tail head caudally. Animals with pubic fractures should be positioned in dorsal recumbency and the ventral midline prepped from the umbilicus to the perineal region.

SURGICAL TECHNIQUE
Approach to the Iliac Body

Make an incision from the cranial extent of the iliac crest to 1 to 2 cm beyond the greater trochanter caudally. Center the incision over the ventral third of the iliac wing. Incise subcutaneous tissue and gluteal fat along the same line to visualize the intermuscular septum lying between the middle gluteal muscle and long head of the tensor fasciae latae muscle (Fig. 32-70, A). Visualize the intermuscular septum between the superficial gluteal and short part of the tensor fasciae latae muscle caudally. Continue the incision to separate the tensor fasciae latae and middle gluteal muscles cranially and the tensor fasciae latae and superficial gluteal muscles caudally. Sharply dissect cranially to separate the middle gluteal muscle and long head of the tensor fasciae latae muscle (Fig. 32-70, B). Palpate the ventral border of the ilium, and make an incision at the ventral border of the middle gluteal muscle. Isolate and ligate the iliolumbar vessel, and reflect the deep and middle gluteal muscles from the lateral surface of the ilium (Fig. 32-70, C). If additional exposure is needed, incise the branch of the cranial gluteal nerve that innervates the tensor fasciae latae muscle. Also dissect the origin of the middle gluteal from the cranial wing of the ilium to achieve additional exposure and to ease reduction.

> NOTE: To increase exposure when inserting lag screws or applying a ventral plate, incise through the origin of the iliacus muscle along the ventral border of the iliac body.

Stabilization of the Ilium With a Bone Plate

Reduce the fracture by placing bone-holding forceps over the dorsal edge of the caudal iliac fragment and retracting it caudally and then laterally. Be careful not to injure the sciatic nerve when manipulating the fracture fragments. Contour a plate to fit the normal curvature of the lateral surface of the bone. Use a ventrodorsal radiograph of the opposite ilium as a guide for plate contouring. Attach the plate to the caudal fragment first to allow the contour of the plate to assist in reduction of the cranial fragment. Reduce the caudal fragment by aligning the fracture and lifting the caudal fragment laterally. Clamp the cranial portion of the plate to the cranial fragment of the ilium, then place screws in the cranial fragment (Fig. 32-71, A).

Caudal distraction of the iliac fragment is readily achieved, but lateral distraction of the caudal fragment can be difficult.

Use the contour of the plate to aid in mediolateral reduction of the fracture. The shape of the precontoured plate helps bring the caudal fragment into position. Place at least three plate screws in the cranial fragment and two in the caudal fragment. Secure the sacrum with a long screw through the cranial plate when possible (Fig. 32-71, B). For additional support, contour a veterinary cuttable plate to the ventral surface of the ilium and secure it with bone screws. To close the incision, place sutures between the fascia of the middle gluteal muscle and tensor fasciae latae muscle cranially and the superficial gluteal muscle and tensor fasciae latae muscle caudally. Approximate deep gluteal fat, subcutaneous tissue, and skin routinely.

Stabilization of the Ilium With Lag Screws

Reduce the fracture as described above, and temporarily stabilize it with bone-holding forceps. Rotate the hemipelvis to visualize the ventral surface of the body of the ilium, and insert two small Kirschner pins from ventral to proximal. To achieve additional stability, place two lag screws ventral to proximal (Fig. 32-72).

Approach to and Stabilization of Ischial Fractures

Make a skin incision adjacent to the caudal border of the greater trochanter. Reflect the biceps femoris muscle caudally to expose the sciatic nerve and external rotators as they insert into the trochanteric fossa (see previous discussion of surgical anatomy). Incise and reflect the insertions of the external rotators caudally to expose the ischial body. Reduce and stabilize the fragments with a small reconstruction bone plate and screws (Fig. 32-73).

Approach to and Stabilization of Pubic Fractures

Make a skin incision along the ventral midline (in the male dog adjacent to the penile sheath). Visualize the midline cranial to the pubic brim, and incise through the tissue

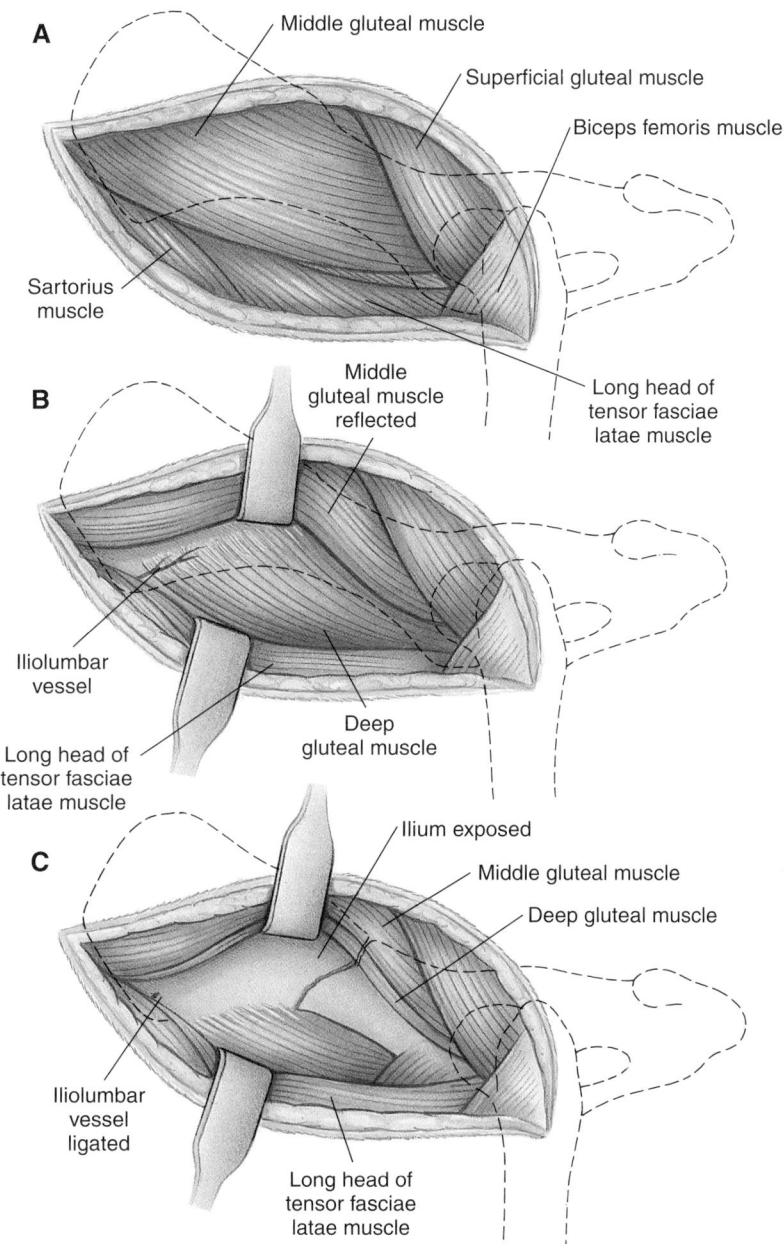

FIG. 32-70
A, To expose the ilium, dissect between the middle gluteal muscle and long head of the tensor fasciae latae muscle. **B,** Separate these muscles. **C,** Elevate the deep gluteal muscle to expose the fracture. Incise the insertion of the gluteal muscles from the iliac wing for additional exposure.

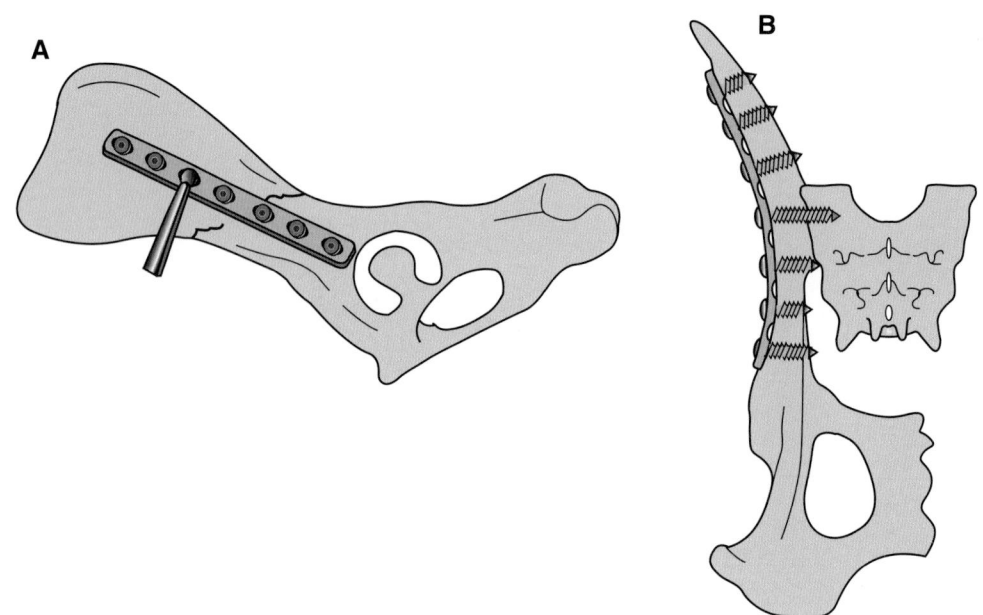

FIG. 32-71
Application of a bone plate and screws to the iliac wing. **A,** The fracture is reduced by clamping the cranial portion of the plate to the iliac wing before inserting the screws. **B,** The curve of the lateral plate restores the contour of the ilium. (Modified from Johnson AL, Dunning D: *Atlas of orthopedic surgical procedures of the dog and cat,* ed 1, St Louis, 2005, Saunders.)

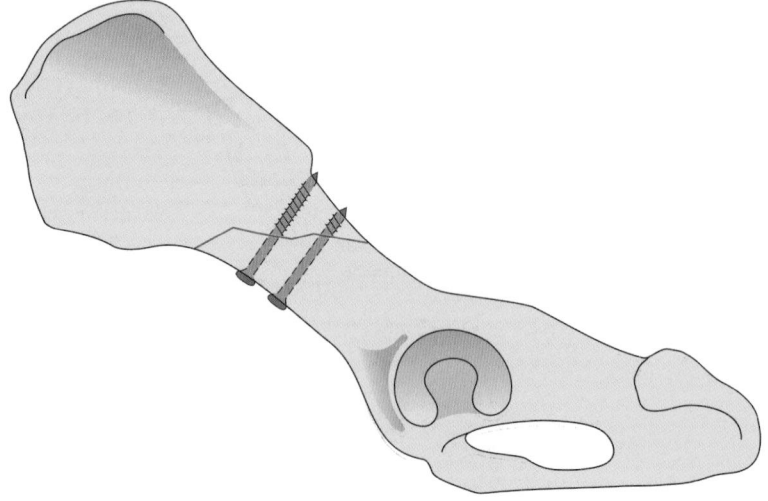

FIG. 32-72
Stabilization of oblique fracture of the iliac wing with lag screws. The screws have been inserted in a ventrodorsal direction, across the fracture line.

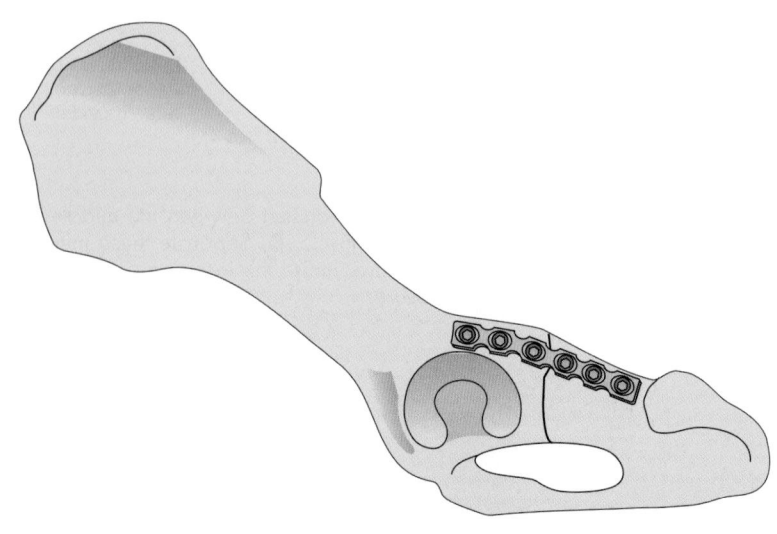

FIG. 32-73
Stabilization of ischial fracture with bone plate and screws. (Modified from Johnson AL, Houlton JEF, Vannini R, editors: *AO principles of fracture management in the dog and cat,* Thieme, NY, 2005, AO Publishing.)

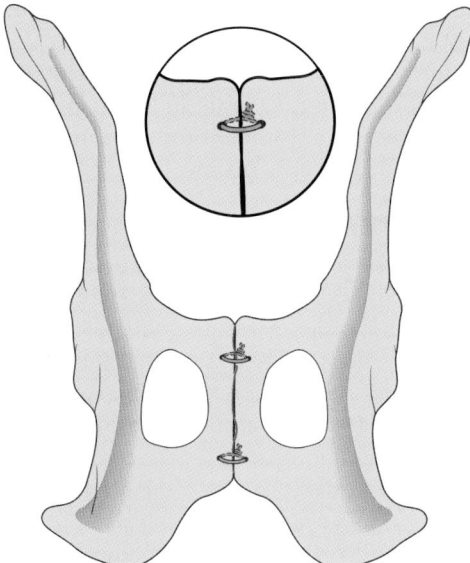

FIG. 32-74
Pubic fractures can be stabilized with orthopedic wire. The wire serves to align the bone fragments.

overlying the pubic symphysis. If herniated tissue is present, be careful to avoid inadvertently incising vital structures. Replace the herniated tissue into the abdominal cavity (see p. 324). Use a periosteal elevator to reflect adductor muscles from the pubis. Reduce the fragments and drill holes in adjacent fragments for placement of orthopedic wire (Fig. 32-74). Place and tighten the wire to stabilize the fragments.

SUTURE MATERIALS AND SPECIAL INSTRUMENTS

Instruments for implantation of bone plates and screws are needed. Bone-holding forceps and self-retaining retractors are beneficial. For pubic fractures, the symphysis can be stabilized with 20-gauge orthopedic wire in small and medium-sized dogs and 18-gauge wire in larger dogs.

POSTOPERATIVE CARE AND ASSESSMENT

Postoperative radiographs are made to evaluate fracture reduction and implant location. Activity should be restricted to leash walking and physical rehabilitation until the fracture has healed. Physical rehabilitation (see Chapter 12) encourages controlled limb use and optimal limb function after fracture healing. Care must be taken to develop customized protocols for each patient depending on location of the fracture, stability and type of fracture fixation, potential for healing, abilities and attitudes of the patient, and willingness and ability of the client to provide for the animal's care (see Tables 32-10 and 32-11 on pp. 1088 and 1091, respectively). Radiographs should be evaluated at 6-week intervals until healing has occurred. Implants do not need to be removed unless they cause a problem.

PROGNOSIS

The prognosis is excellent for return to normal function with most iliac fractures after surgery. Screw loosening is the most common implant-related complication and occasionally results in loss of fracture alignment with compromise of the pelvic canal. Factors that warrant a more guarded prognosis include ipsilateral acetabular fractures, with potential development of osteoarthrosis. The prognosis for isolated pubic and ischial fractures is excellent for return to normal function. If other pelvic fractures are present, the prognosis depends on how these fractures heal rather than the pubic or ischial fracture outcome.

Suggested Reading

Breshears LA, Fitch RB, Wallace LJ et al: Radiographic evaluation of repaired canine ilial fractures (69 cases), *Vet Comp Orthop Traumatol* 17:64, 2004.

This article provides a retrospective evaluation of the outcome of stabilized iliac body fractures. Radiographic complications were recognized in 24% of cases. A case is made for using ventral plate stabilization of these fractures to minimize implant loosening.

DeCamp C: Fractures of the ilium. In Johnson AL, Houlton JEF, Vannini R, editors: *AO principles of fracture management in the dog and cat,* Thieme, NY, 2005, AO Publishing.

This chapter provides an up-to-date collection of operative techniques for stabilizing fractures of the ilium in small animals. Detailed descriptions of plate and lag screw applications are included.

Matis U: Fractures of the ischium and pubis. In Johnson AL, Houlton JEF, Vannini R, editors: *AO principles of fracture management in the dog and cat,* Thieme, NY, 2005, AO Publishing.

This chapter provides an up-to-date collection of operative techniques for stabilizing fractures of the ischium and pubis in small animals. Detailed descriptions of plate application, pin and wire techniques, and lag screw applications are included.

Piermattei D, Johnson KA: *An atlas of surgical approaches to the bones and joints of the dog and cat,* ed 4, Philadelphia, 2004, WB Saunders.

This textbook is an excellent reference for surgical approaches to the pelvis.

ACETABULAR FRACTURES

DEFINITIONS

Acetabular fractures occur through the articular surface and medial fossa of the acetabulum.

GENERAL CONSIDERATIONS AND CLINICALLY RELEVANT PATHOPHYSIOLOGY

Acetabular fractures occur after blunt trauma, most often vehicular accidents, and are usually concomitant with other pelvic pathology. Recent studies give percentages of acetabular fractures as 12% of pelvic fractures in dogs and 7% of pelvic fractures in cats (Matis, 2005). Additionally, 24% of pelvic fractures studied involved either bilateral iliac body fractures, bilateral acetabular fractures, or acetabular fracture coupled with a contralateral iliac body fracture (Messmer and Montavon, 2004). The hip joint transfers weight from the rear limb through the pelvis to the spine. The sequelae to conservatively treated acetabular fractures are degenerative joint disease and loss of function. Occasionally the sciatic nerve may be injured in association with acetabular fractures.

Fractures of the acetabulum are classified as cranial, central, or caudal according to the location of involvement of the articular surface. The cranial and central portions of the acetabulum are the weight-bearing areas and fractures of these areas should be anatomically reduced and rigidly fixed for optimal function. Caudal fractures are less demanding but also may result in degenerative joint disease with conservative treatment.

DIAGNOSIS
Clinical Presentation
Signalment. Any age, breed, or sex of dog or cat may be affected.

History. Acetabular fractures usually result from motor vehicle accidents but may be associated with other forms of blunt trauma or falls.

Physical Examination Findings
Affected animals generally are brought in for evaluation of a non–weight-bearing lameness. Some patients bear weight on the affected limb if fracture displacement is minimal. Pain can generally be elicited on manipulation of the hip joint, but crepitation may or may not be present.

Diagnostic Imaging
Ventrodorsal and lateral radiographs should be taken to assess the pelvic fractures. Oblique radiographs made by positioning the animal in lateral recumbency and abducting the unaffected leg to expose the affected acetabulum often help delineate acetabular fractures. CT can be used to better delineate the fractures of the pelvis, particularly if the fractures involve the acetabulum. Reconstructed 2-D and 3-D CT images allow a better appreciation of the fracture appearance and facilitate fracture planning.

Laboratory Findings
Consistent laboratory abnormalities are not present. Traumatized animals undergoing surgery should have sufficient blood work done to determine the optimal anesthetic regimen.

DIFFERENTIAL DIAGNOSIS
Differential diagnoses include capital physeal fractures, coxofemoral luxations, proximal femoral fractures, and ipsilateral iliac or ischial fractures.

MEDICAL MANAGEMENT
To maintain joint congruity and the normal distribution of stress over the articular surface, reduction and stabilization of acetabular fractures are recommended in all cases. Occasionally, very young animals with stable fractures not involving the weight-bearing zone of the acetabulum or with nondisplaced physeal fractures may be treated with 10 to 14 days of a non–weight-bearing sling. Additionally, if the client cannot afford surgery, conservative treatment should be considered; however, it may result in less than optimal limb function. Conservative treatment for acetabular fractures is similar to that for sacroiliac luxations (see p. 1087).

SURGICAL TREATMENT
Anatomic reconstruction of the articular surface and rigid stabilization are mandatory to restore acetabular joint function and minimize degenerative joint disease. Plate and screw fixation is the preferred approach for acetabular reconstruction and stabilization regardless of the fracture-assessment score. However, accurate plate contouring is essential for maintaining anatomic reduction. As screws are tightened, the bone shifts to match the plate, often disrupting the reduction. Techniques such as plate luting and the use of screws and orthopedic wire reinforced with polymethylmethacrylate have been described to improve the accuracy of reduction (Anderson et al, 2002; Beaver et al, 2000). Dogs with irreparable acetabular fractures may be candidates for femoral head and neck ostectomy (see p. 1242), but the acetabulum should still be bridged and stabilized with a bone plate to decrease pain and to encourage early motion, which is paramount to a successful outcome.

Application of Bone Plates and Screws
Adequate exposure and manipulation of the caudal acetabular fragment are important components to anatomic reduction and plate application. Accurate plate contouring is essential for retaining anatomic reconstruction of the articular surface. A specially designed curved canine acetabular plate is easier to contour to the dorsal rim of the acetabulum than standard plates and is recommended for transverse or short oblique acetabular fractures. This plate does not require precontouring. Alternatively, reconstruction plates that can be contoured with specially designed bending pliers in the direction of both its long and short (width) axes can be used. It is helpful to precontour this plate to a similarly sized bone specimen before surgery. Smaller dogs and cats may require 2.7 or 2.0 T or L plates.

Acetabular fractures combined with iliac body fractures may be treated with two plates, a dynamic compression plate applied to the iliac body fracture and an acetabular plate applied to the acetabular fracture. Alternatively, a reconstruction plate can span the hemipelvis (Fig. 32-75). Comminuted acetabular fractures must be reconstructed with lag screws and supported with a reconstruction plate.

Preoperative Management
Urination and bowel movements should be monitored before surgery. Respirations should be monitored, and chest radiographs are indicated. An electrocardiogram is useful to determine cardiac rhythm, particularly if peripheral pulses appear weak or irregular. Analgesics should be administered to posttraumatic patients (see Box 31-2 on p. 944 and Chapter 13).

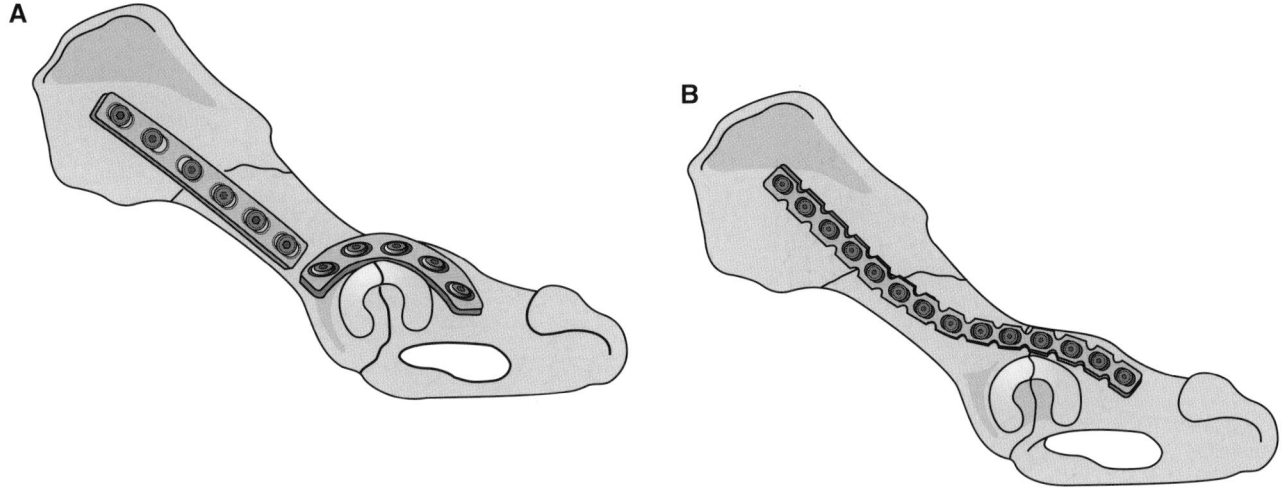

FIG. 32-75
Plate application for combined acetabular and iliac body fractures. **A,** Application of two plates: a dynamic compression plate applied to the iliac body fracture and an acetabular plate applied to the acetabular fracture. **B,** Alternatively, a reconstruction plate can span the hemipelvis. (Modified from Johnson AL, Houlton JEF, Vannini R, editors: *AO principles of fracture management in the dog and cat,* Thieme, NY, 2005, AO Publishing.)

Anesthesia

Special anesthetic considerations for patients with orthopedic disease are discussed on p. 944.

Surgical Anatomy

The hip joint is a ball-and-socket joint comprising the femoral head and acetabulum. The normal conformation, surrounding musculature, suctionlike effect of the synovial fluid, and ligament of the femoral head act to stabilize the joint. The articular surface is on the dorsolateral face of the acetabulum, and the medial face is occupied by the round ligament. The fibrous joint capsule originates from the lateral acetabular rim and inserts onto the femoral neck. Stabilizing musculature surrounding the hip includes the gluteal muscles, internal and external rotators, and the iliopsoas muscle medially.

The sciatic nerve courses dorsomedial to the acetabulum. Fractures cause the caudal acetabular segment to become displaced medial and cranial to the cranial segment. The sciatic nerve may be positioned directly dorsal or dorsolateral to the caudal acetabular segment. Caution must be exercised when exposing and reducing the caudal segment to avoid damaging this nerve. Soft tissue bruising and swelling often distort the normal anatomy. Dissection adjacent to the greater trochanter facilitates correct tissue identification and reflection. The insertion of the deep gluteal muscle at the greater trochanter can be used as a landmark for dissection.

Positioning

The animal is positioned in lateral recumbency with the dorsum raised 30 degrees from the operating table. The hip should be prepped from the dorsal midline to the tarsus. A hanging-leg preparation facilitates manipulation of the limb during surgery.

SURGICAL TECHNIQUE

Make a skin incision centered over the cranial border of the greater trochanter. Begin the incision 3 to 4 cm proximal to the dorsal ridge of the greater trochanter, and curve it distally 3 to 4 cm, following the cranial border of the femur. Incise the superficial leaf of the fascia lata at the cranial border of the biceps femoris muscle, and retract the muscle caudally (Fig. 32-76, A). Incise the deep leaf of the fascia lata, and carry the incision proximally through the insertion of the tensor fasciae latae muscle at the greater trochanter and along the cranial border of the superficial gluteal muscle. Incise through the insertion of the superficial gluteal muscle at the third trochanter. Reflect the superficial gluteal muscle proximally and the biceps femoris caudally to find and visualize the course of the sciatic nerve (Fig. 32-76, B). Perform an osteotomy of the greater trochanter with an osteotome and mallet or Gigli wire (Fig. 32-76, C). Position the osteotome just proximal to the insertion of the superficial gluteal muscle at the third trochanter. Angle the osteotome 45 degrees to the long axis of the femur to remove the trochanter with the insertions of the deep gluteal and middle gluteal muscles (Fig. 32-76, D). Reflect the gluteal muscles and greater trochanter from the joint capsule with a periosteal elevator. Visualize the insertions of the gemellus muscle and tendon of the internal obturator, and preplace a suture through the two insertions near the trochanteric fossa. Incise both structures together at the trochanteric fossa, and elevate the gemellus muscle from the caudolateral surface of the acetabulum with a periosteal elevator (Fig. 32-76, E). Use the suture to retract the muscle proximally and caudally. For additional exposure of the ilium, combine the lateral approach to the ilium (see p. 1095) with the approach to the acetabulum.

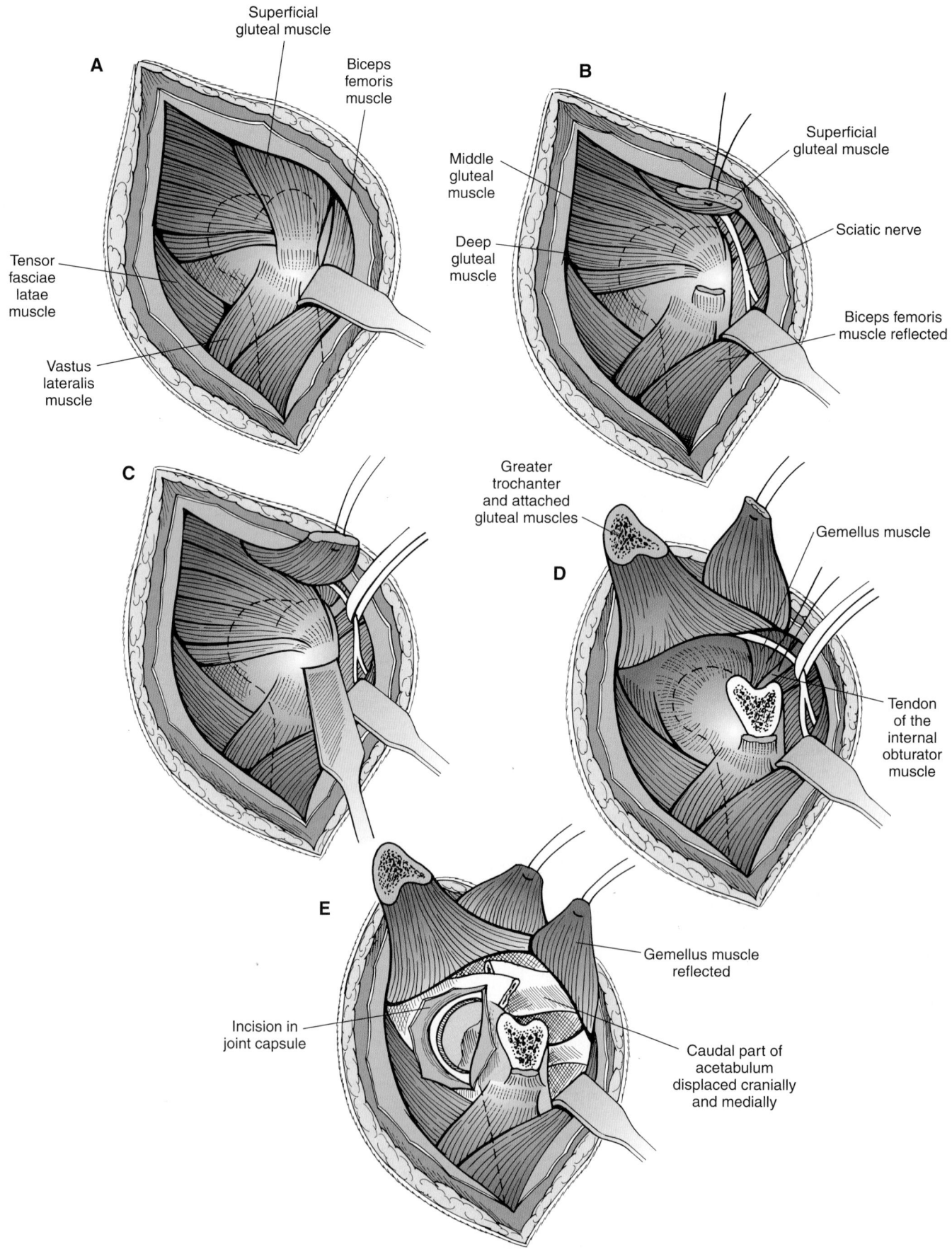

FIG. 32-76

A, To expose the hip joint through an osteotomy of the greater trochanter, retract the biceps femoris muscle caudally. **B,** Reflect the superficial gluteal muscle to expose the third trochanter. **C** and **D,** Osteotomize the greater trochanter, and reflect the attached musculature dorsally. **E,** Incise and reflect the gemellus and internal obturator muscles. Incise the joint capsule. Note that the caudal fragment of the fracture is displaced craniomedially.

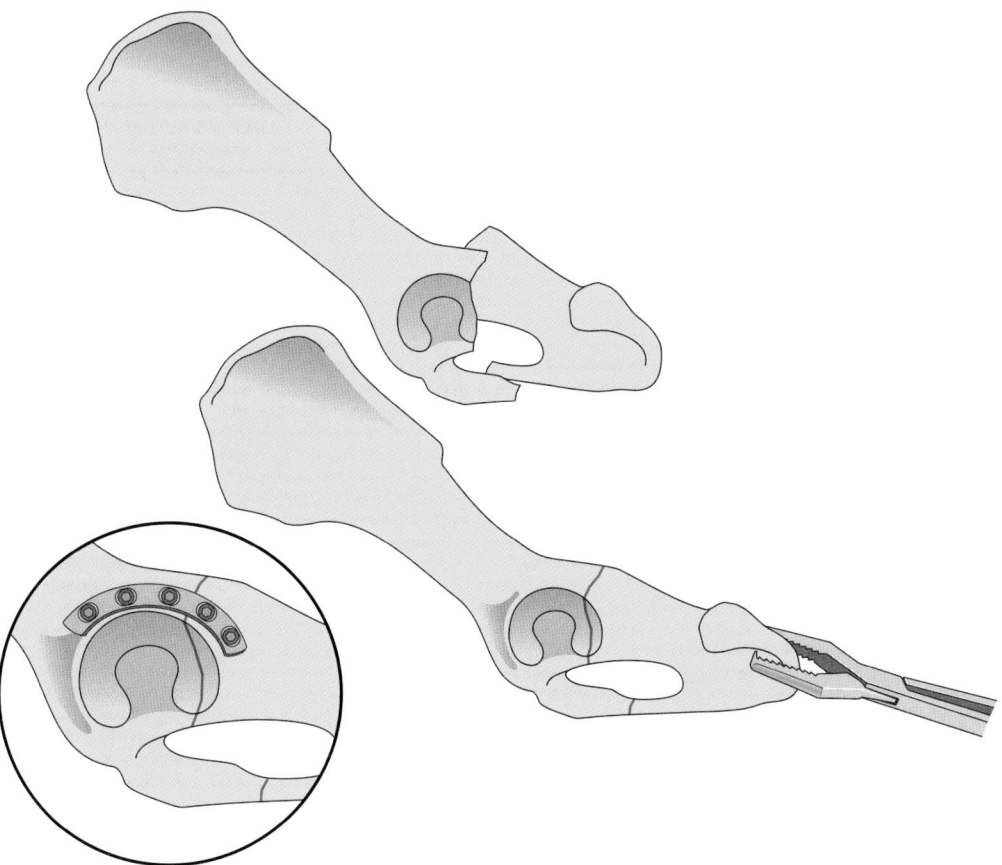

FIG. 32-77
Reduce the acetabular fracture by manipulating the caudal fragment with a bone-holding forceps secured to the ischium. Hold the fracture in reduction with bone-holding forceps placed across the lesser ischiatic notch, and stabilize it with a bone plate and screws.

If necessary for caudal fragment control, expose the tuber ischium and place a bone-holding forceps on it (Fig. 32-77). When reducing the fracture, pay particular attention to the alignment of the articular surface, which is facilitated by incising the joint capsule (see Fig. 32-76, E). Place plates on the dorsal rim of the acetabulum. Attempt to place at least two plate screws in the caudal fragment and three plate screws in the cranial fragment (see Fig. 32-77). After reduction and stabilization, suture the gemellus and internal obturator tendon to their points of insertion. Suture the joint capsule. Reduce and stabilize the greater trochanter with two Kirschner wires and a tension band wire (see p. 990). Place interrupted sutures in the insertion of the superficial gluteal muscle and a continuous suture in the insertion of the tensor fasciae latae muscle and deep leaf of the fascia lata. Use a continuous suture in the superficial leaf of the fascia lata and the subcutaneous tissue. Suture skin with an interrupted suture pattern.

SUTURE MATERIALS AND SPECIAL INSTRUMENTS

Equipment is needed for application of an acetabular bone plate or reconstruction plate. An osteotome and mallet or Gigli wire is necessary to perform a trochanteric osteotomy. Small pins and wire are used to stabilize the trochanteric osteotomy with a tension band.

POSTOPERATIVE CARE AND ASSESSMENT

Postoperative radiographs should be taken to assess fracture reduction, articular alignment, and implant position. Postoperative pain management is indicated (see Box 31-2 on p. 944 and Chapter 13). Activity should be restricted to leash walking and physical rehabilitation until the fracture has healed. Physical rehabilitation (see Chapter 12) encourages controlled limb use and optimal limb function after fracture healing. Care must be taken to develop customized protocols for each patient depending on location of the fracture, stability and type of fracture fixation, potential for healing, abilities and attitudes of the patient, and willingness or ability of the client to participate in the animal's care (Table 32-12). Radiographs should be evaluated at 6-week intervals until healing has occurred. Healing generally occurs between 6 and 12 weeks, depending on the biologic fracture assessment. Implants are not routinely removed. Occasionally the tension band wire and Kirschner wires need to be removed because of soft tissue irritation.

PROGNOSIS

The prognosis is good to excellent if the acetabular fracture is anatomically reduced and appropriately stabilized. Unsatisfactory limb function is associated with sciatic nerve injury and osteoarthrosis.

Table 32-12

Sample Physical Rehabilitation Protocol for Patients With Hip Fractures

ALL TREATMENTS BID	DAY 1 TO DAY 14	DAY 15 TO DAY 24	DAY 25 UNTIL HEALED	HEALED TO RETURN TO FUNCTION
Heat therapy		10 min	10 min	
Massage	5 min	5 min	5 min	
Passive range of motion (repetitions)	15*	15*	15*	
Electrical stimulation†	10 min	10 min	10 min	10 min
Therapeutic exercise-total time	15 min	25 min	20 min	25–45 min
Walk/land treadmill	10 min	10 min	10 min	>10 min
Balancing	5 min	5 min	5 min	+
Obstacles	+	+	+	+
Weaving			+	+
Circles				+
Hills				+
Stairs				+
Jog/run				+
Underwater treadmill		10 min	10 min	>15 min
Swimming				5–10 min
Cryotherapy	15 min	15 min	15 min	PRN

BID, Twice a day; +, perform modality; *PRN,* as needed.
*Perform passive range of motion for all joints of the affected limb.
†Apply to semimembranosus/semitendinosus muscles for patients with muscle atrophy (see Chapter 12).

References

Anderson GM, Cross AR, Lewis DD et al: The effect of plate luting on reduction accuracy and biomechanics of acetabular osteotomies stabilized with 2.7-mm reconstruction plates, *Vet Surg* 31: 3, 2002.

Beaver DP, Lewis DD, Lanz OI et al: Evaluation of four interfragmentary Kirschner wire configurations as a component of screw/wire/polymethacrylate fixation for acetabular fractures in dogs, *J Am Anim Hosp Assoc* 36:456, 2000.

Matis U: Fractures of the acetabulum. In Johnson AL, Houlton JEF, Vannini R, editors: *AO principles of fracture management in the dog and cat,* Thieme, NY, 2005, AO Publishing.

Messmer M, Montavon PM: Pelvic fractures in the dog and cat: a classification system and review of 556 cases, *Vet Comp Orthop Traumatol* 17:167, 2004.

Suggested Reading

Crawford JT, Manley PA, Adams WM: Comparison of computed tomography, tangential view radiography and conventional radiography in evaluation of canine pelvic fractures, *Vet Radiol Ultrasound* 44:619, 2003.
This article provides a comparison of imaging techniques to evaluate pelvic fractures. CT scanning is superior to survey radiography in assessing skeletal and soft tissue injuries in dogs with pelvic trauma, although all clinically significant surgical lesions were described accurately radiographically. Routine CT examination of dogs with pelvic trauma may not be justifiable for diagnosis, but may be advantageous for surgical planning.

Dyce J, Houlton JEF: Use of reconstruction plates for repair of acetabular fractures in 16 dogs, *J Small Anim Pract* 32:547, 1993.
This article provides a review of the technique and outcome when reconstruction plates are used to stabilize acetabular fractures.

Hardie RJ, Bertram JEA, Todhunter RJ et al: Biomechanical comparison of two plating techniques for fixation of acetabular osteotomies in dogs, *Vet Surg* 28:148, 1999.
This article provides a comparison of the failure properties of a 5-hole, 2.7-mm curved acetabular plate (AP) to a 5-hole, 3.5-mm reconstruction plate (RP) when applied to acetabular osteotomies. Both fixation techniques were comparable under the loading conditions of this study.

Roush JK, Manley PA: Mini plate failure after repair of ilial and acetabular fractures in nine small dogs and one cat, *J Am Anim Hosp Assoc* 28:112, 1992.
This article provides information based on a case series of the complications associated with miniplate use for stabilizing pelvic fractures in small animals.

Whitelock RG, Dyce J, Houlton JEF: Repair of femoral trochanteric osteotomy in the dog, *J Small Anim Pract* 38:195, 1997.
This article provides a retrospective evaluation of the radiographic and clinical outcome of 24 dogs that underwent femoral trochanteric osteotomy repair with either a pin and tension band wire or a lag screw technique. Femoral trochanteric osteotomy was not associated with significant clinical problems, despite a high incidence of abnormal radiographic findings.

FEMORAL FRACTURES

FEMORAL DIAPHYSEAL AND SUPRACONDYLAR FRACTURES

DEFINITIONS

The **femoral diaphysis** (shaft) is the midportion of the bone that curves craniocaudally in dogs and lies between the articular extremities. The condyle is the distal portion of the femur, which articulates with the tibia and the patella. An IM pin placed into the femur in a **normograde** fashion is inserted from the trochanteric fossa across the fracture line and seated in the femoral condyles. An IM pin placed in the femur in a **retrograde** fashion is inserted at the fracture line, driven proximally to exit the trochanteric fossa, and then (after fracture reduction) driven across the fracture and into the distal fragment.

GENERAL CONSIDERATIONS AND CLINICALLY RELEVANT PATHOPHYSIOLOGY

Femoral fractures are usually caused by trauma. Occasionally a patient will present with an acute femur fracture without discernible or historical trauma; fractures in these patients may be secondary to a preexisting bone pathologic condition. Primary or metastatic bone tumors are the most common cause of pathologic fractures. When preexisting disease is present, radiographs made at the time of injury show cortical lysis and new bone formation in the area of the fracture.

High-velocity injuries are the most common type of trauma that causes femoral fractures in veterinary patients. Most injuries result from automobile accidents, but gunshot injuries and blunt trauma are also common. A thorough physical examination is necessary to rule out concurrent injury (e.g., thoracic trauma, coxofemoral luxations, and pelvic girdle injuries). Careful thoracic auscultation and percussion help detect cardiac or airway abnormalities. Abnormal heart rhythm and pulse deficits suggest traumatic myocarditis, whereas lack of normal air movement on auscultation may indicate pulmonary contusion, pneumothorax, or diaphragmatic hernia. Thoracic radiographs and a lead II electrocardiogram are useful and should be done routinely as part of the anesthetic preoperative database for patients sustaining high-velocity injuries.

Coxofemoral luxations (see p. 1246) may occur concurrently with femoral fractures. Diagnosis is often made when radiographs are taken to evaluate the femur because swelling in the limb often precludes palpation of bony landmarks used for assessing femoral head position relative to the hip joint. Concurrent fractures or luxations must be considered when choosing the appropriate implant for fracture stabilization. Observation of pelvic girdle symmetry and gentle rectal palpation help determine the presence of pelvic fractures. Additional radiographs centered on the pelvis are indicated if abnormalities are found. If fractures of the pelvis are found, careful assessment of urinary tract integrity is recommended.

DIAGNOSIS
Clinical Presentation

Signalment. Any age, breed, or sex of dog or cat may be affected, but young male dogs are most likely to have trauma-induced femoral fractures.

History. Trauma may or may not have been observed. Motor vehicle accidents cause the majority of femoral diaphyseal fractures. Other modes of injury include gunshots and falls.

Physical Examination Findings

Patients with femoral diaphyseal fractures are usually nonweight bearing and have varying degrees of limb swelling. Pain and crepitus can often be elicited with limb manipulation. Proprioception may appear abnormal because the animal may not lift its paw when it is placed on its dorsum. The animal's reluctance to move the limb may be caused by pain.

Diagnostic Imaging

Both craniocaudal and lateral radiographs of the femur are necessary to assess the extent of bone and soft tissue injury. Most affected animals have pain on limb manipulation and require sedation (see Tables 31-2 and 31-3 on pp. 933 and 934, respectively) or general anesthetic for proper positioning to obtain quality radiographs. Alternatively, radiographs can be taken under anesthesia just before surgery; however, this reduces the amount of time available for planning surgical repair. Radiographs of the contralateral limb are useful to assess normal bone length and shape. These radiographs can be used to contour a bone plate more precisely before surgery, reducing operative time. Radiographs are also used as a reference to select appropriately sized implants.

Laboratory Findings

Consistent laboratory abnormalities are not present. Animals sustaining fractures secondary to trauma should have sufficient blood work done to determine appropriate anesthetic regimens and concurrent diseases.

DIFFERENTIAL DIAGNOSIS

Femoral fractures should be differentiated from muscle contusion, coxofemoral luxation, fractures of the pelvic girdle, and ligamentous injury to the stifle.

MEDICAL MANAGEMENT

The fracture must be stabilized to allow adequate healing. Casts or splints are not recommended for femoral fractures because adequate stabilization of the femur is difficult using these methods. However, animals that have stable or incomplete fractures and an excellent biologic assessment (see p. 953) may heal despite lack of rigid fixation.

SURGICAL TREATMENT

IM pins, interlocking nails, IM pins plus external skeletal fixation, external skeletal fixators alone, and bone plates may be used to repair femoral diaphyseal fractures. The implant system chosen should reflect the patient's fracture assess-

BOX 32-14

Implant Use for Fractures of the Femoral Diaphysis According to Fracture-Assessment Score (FAS)

FAS 0 to 3
- Bone plate and IM pin
- Bone plate and screws
- Interlocking nail

FAS 4 to 7
- External skeletal fixation with IM pin tie-in
- Bone plate and screws with or without IM pin
- Interlocking nail

FAS 8 to 10
- IM pin with cerclage wires or external fixator
- Flexible bone plate and screws

ment (Box 32-14). Factors that impair healing include multiple injuries, a large active patient, and the need for open reduction and tissue manipulation to reduce and apply interfragmentary compression. If a long duration of healing is expected, the implant needs to remain functional for 8 or more weeks; implants that purchase bone with threads are desirable. With shorter healing periods, implants that have frictional hold (smooth pins and wire) are adequate.

Application of Intramedullary Pins

An IM pin can be used to stabilize femoral middiaphyseal fractures, providing excellent resistance to bending but not resisting rotational forces or axial loading. Additional implants must be used to provide rotational and axial support for most fractures (Fig. 32-78).

Generally an IM pin should equal 70% to 80% of the diameter of the marrow cavity. The femoral diameter and curvature dictate the size of pin that can be used (see Surgical Anatomy section on p. 1106). An IM pin can be normograded or retrograded for placement in the femur (see p. 982). The advantage of normograde placement is that the pin can be placed laterally, adjacent to the greater trochanter. This positions the pin so that it passes through less soft tissue than when placed in a retrograde fashion and also ensures that the pin is positioned lateral to the sciatic nerve. The disadvantage of normograde placement is that it is difficult to identify the correct entry point into the bone because insertion of the pin into the trochanteric fossa is generally done blindly. To normograde an IM pin, a small skin incision is made at the point of pin entry over the bony prominence of the greater trochanter. Palpation of the greater trochanter may be difficult if the limb is swollen secondary to trauma of the soft tissue. Limited surgical exposure may be necessary to locate the greater trochanter prominence. After the greater trochanter is located using palpation or direct exposure, the point of the pin is pushed through soft tissue until it contacts the most proximal trochanteric ridge. The pinpoint is walked off the medial edge of the greater trochanter until it falls into

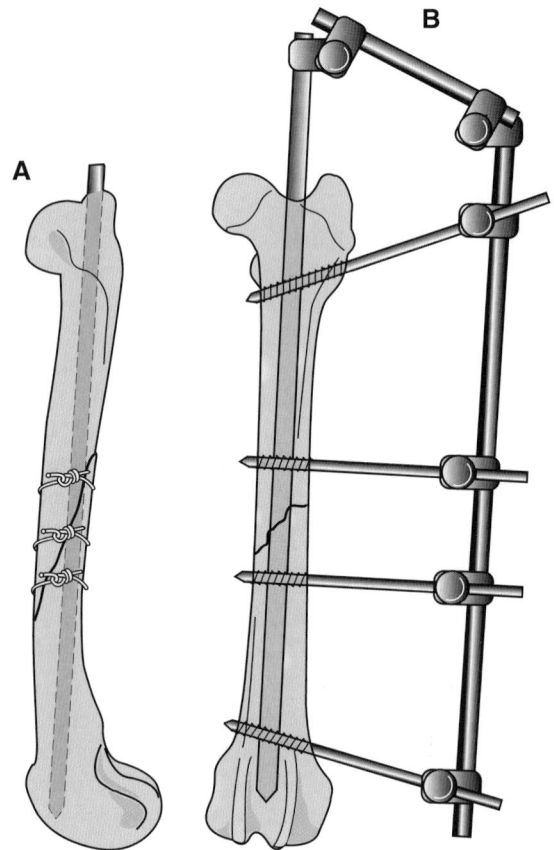

FIG. 32-78
Placement of an IM pin in the femur. Depending on fracture configuration the IM pin may be supported with **A**, cerclage wires or **B**, an external fixator, which may be tied into the IM pin. (Modified from Johnson AL, Dunning D: *Atlas of orthopedic surgical procedures of the dog and cat*, ed 1, St Louis, 2005, Saunders.)

the trochanteric fossa. From this point, the pin is driven through the proximal metaphyseal cancellous bone in a slightly caudomedial direction. As the pinpoint emerges from the marrow cavity at the fracture site, the fracture is reduced and the pin driven into the distal segment. To estimate the appropriate pin penetration into the distal bone segment, a second pin equal in length to that placed in the marrow cavity can be used for a point of reference.

> NOTE: Normograde placement of the pin is advantageous because it allows the pin to be inserted more laterally at the proximal aspect of the bone than can be done with retrograde placement. To help identify the correct entry point for the pin, consider a limited surgical exposure of the greater trochanter.

The advantage of retrograde pin placement in the femur is the ability to visualize the pin's site of insertion at the fracture. The disadvantage of retrograde placement is the difficulty in controlling the pin's site of exit at the trochanteric fossa because the pin may exit too far medially, causing soft tissue irritation and increasing the risk of sciatic palsy. Forcing the shaft of the pin against the caudomedial cortex of the proximal fragment will help ensure that the pin exits laterally in the fossa. It is important to hold the limb in a hip extended and adducted position while the pin exits the trochanteric fossa to prevent penetrating the sciatic nerve.

NOTE: Warning: failure to hold the femur adducted and the hip in extension when driving an IM pin retrograde through the trochanteric fossa may injure the sciatic nerve.

NOTE: Always have a reference pin available that is the same length as the IM pin being inserted.

Application of Interlocking Nails

Interlocking nails can be used to stabilize both single and comminuted middiaphyseal femoral fractures. The interlocking nail provides resistance to bending, rotational, and axial loading forces and can offer effective IM fixation to bridge a nonreducible fracture. An open approach is used to reconstruct reducible fractures. An "open but don't touch" approach is used when major segment alignment is the goal. The size of nail selected should correspond to the width of the medullary canal at the isthmus of the bone. Although the medullary reaming may be normograde or retrograde, the interlocking nail is inserted in a normograde manner starting at the trochanteric fossa. Slight overreduction of the distal femur may be necessary to insert the nail an appropriate distance into the distal segment (Fig. 32-79).

Application of External Skeletal Fixation

Combining the bending support of an IM pin with the axial and rotational support provided by an external fixator is useful to control physiologic forces acting on fractures during healing. An IM pin that occupies 50% to 60% of the medullary cavity is first inserted in a normograde or retrograde manner. An appropriate number of fixation pins and the external frame are then applied. The frame, number, and type of fixation pins vary with the rigidity of fixation desired and the length of time the fixator must remain in place (see p. 969). A single external bar with one fixation pin placed proximal to the fracture and one placed distal to the fracture may be used to support moderately stable fractures that are expected to heal in a relatively short time (less than 6 weeks). The proximal fixation pin is placed laterally at the level of the third trochanter. A small Kirschner wire is used as a "feeler" pin to identify a proper angle of insertion for the fixation pin that avoids intersecting the IM pin (see p. 974). The distal fixation pin is inserted laterally 2 to 3 cm proximal to the femoral condyles. The fabella is usually palpable and can be used as a landmark for this pin; a small Kirschner wire can be used as a feeler pin to avoid intersection with the IM pin. More often, two additional fixation pins are positioned to secure the diaphysis 1 cm from the fracture line proximally and distally for a more rigid frame. Connecting the IM pin to the external fixator frame to make a tie-in

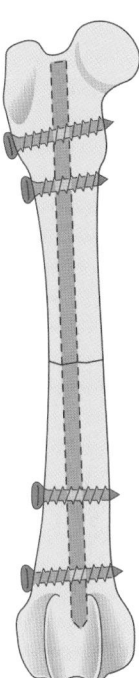

FIG. 32-79
Placement of interlocking nail in the femur.

configuration increases the fixation system strength without adding to patient morbidity through placement of additional fixation pins (see Fig. 32-78, *B*).

NOTE: Multiple transfixation pins increase morbidity and may reduce postoperative limb function.

Application of Bone Plates and Screws

Bone plates are ideally suited for complex or stable fractures of the femur when prolonged healing (bone union) is anticipated or when optimal postoperative limb function is desirable. Plate size depends on patient size and plate function. The plate may serve as a compression plate, neutralization plate, or bridging plate (Fig. 32-80). **Compression plates** are used with transverse or short oblique fractures. The plate is contoured to 1 mm offset from the bone surface at the fracture site to achieve compression of the transcortex. **Neutralization plates** are used with long oblique fractures or comminuted fractures in which the bone fragments can be reduced and stabilized with lag screws or cerclage wire. The plate is contoured to the anatomic surface of the reconstructed bone. **Bridging plates** are used with comminuted fractures in which bone fragments cannot be reduced anatomically or when attempted reduction and stabilization of the fragments would cause excessive soft tissue trauma. Regardless of function, the plate is placed on the lateral tension surface of the femur. A minimum of three plate screws (six cortices) proximal and three plate screws distal to the fracture is recommended with compression or neutralization plates. A minimum of four plate screws (eight cortices) proximal and distal to the fracture is recommended for bridging plates.

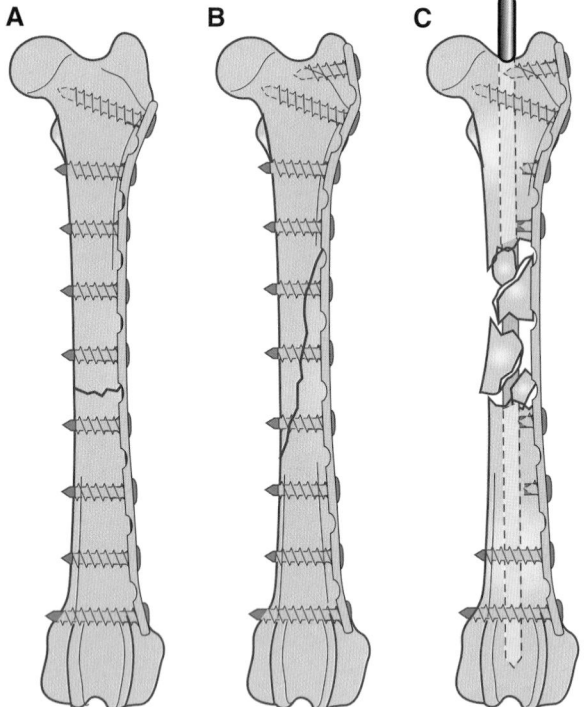

FIG. 32-80
A plate placed on the lateral surface of the femur may function as: **A,** a compression plate for transverse fractures; **B,** a neutralization plate to support long oblique fractures reconstructed with lag screws; or **C,** a bridging plate combined with an IM pin to span a nonreducible fracture. (Modified from Johnson A: *Atlas of orthopedic surgical procedures of the dog and cat,* ed 1, St Louis, 2005, Saunders.)

A bridging plate is contoured to reflect the femoral anatomy, most easily by contouring the plate to a craniocaudal radiograph of the contralateral limb. Spatial alignment of the bone is assisted by insertion of an IM pin. The pin may be retrograded or normograded through the proximal intact segment of bone, passed through the fragmented section of bone, and seated into the distal intact segment of bone. Passing the pin into the distal intact segment of bone without tightly restricting movement of the distal fragment allows the pin to distract the proximal and distal segments to regain femoral length. In keeping with the concept of bridging osteosynthesis, the bone fragments in the comminuted area are not disturbed.

Once spatial alignment of the femur is achieved, the bone plate is attached to the bone with plate screws at the most proximal and distal plate holes. If the alignment pin is removed, bicortical plate screws (screws that engage both cortices) are used. Alternatively, the alignment pin can be left in place to achieve a plate-pin bridging of the fracture. In this case, bicortical screws are used proximally and distally and monocortical screws centrally. The plate-pin combination increases the strength and fatigue life of the fixation and thus protects the plate from premature breakage. The plate-

pin system can be destabilized at 6 to 8 weeks by removing the IM pin. A cancellous bone graft (see p. 962) can be harvested and placed in the fracture zone.

Preoperative Management

Because these fractures result from trauma, all affected animals should be examined for concurrent injury and stabilized if necessary before surgery. Fractures of the femur are not usually immobilized preoperatively because of the difficulty in applying coaptation splints. Contraction of thigh muscles helps immobilize bone fragments, but patients should be confined to a small area until surgery. Analgesics should be provided to posttraumatic animals (see Box 31-2 on p. 944 and Chapter 13).

Anesthesia

Anesthetic management of patients with fractures is discussed on p. 944. Patients that have sustained significant soft tissue injury and bony comminution, or those requiring extensive exposure and soft tissue manipulation, will benefit from a preoperative epidural agent (see Box 31-2 on p. 944 and Chapter 13). An epidural anesthetic may make fracture reduction easier.

Surgical Anatomy

The shape of the femur dictates the pin size that can be used. The diameter of the femoral marrow cavity varies along its length and is narrower proximally than distally. The narrowest area of the marrow cavity is called the isthmus. In the femur, the isthmus is located within the proximal third of the bone, just distal to the third trochanter. When choosing an appropriate IM pin, the diameter of the marrow cavity at the isthmus must be considered and can be estimated from preoperative radiographs. Curvature of the femur also governs pin size. The canine femur is normally curved in a cranial to caudal direction; the curvature is most accentuated in the distal third of the femur. The amount of curvature varies between breeds, but the greater the curvature and more distal the fracture, the smaller the pin must be for proper seating within the femoral condyles. Proper implantation technique can compensate for the curvature of the femur to some extent, but the normal curvature remains a limiting factor when choosing the pin to be inserted. The cross-sectional diameter of the feline femur is uniform from proximal to distal.

> NOTE: The anatomy of the canine and feline femur differs. The cat femur is straighter, with little or no cranial to caudal bend.

Normal anatomy of the femur and surrounding tissue may be less apparent when fractures are present. Soft tissue swelling and bruising vary depending on the velocity of the injury. The vastus lateralis muscle often appears swollen and bruised when the fascia lata is incised. Cranial retraction of

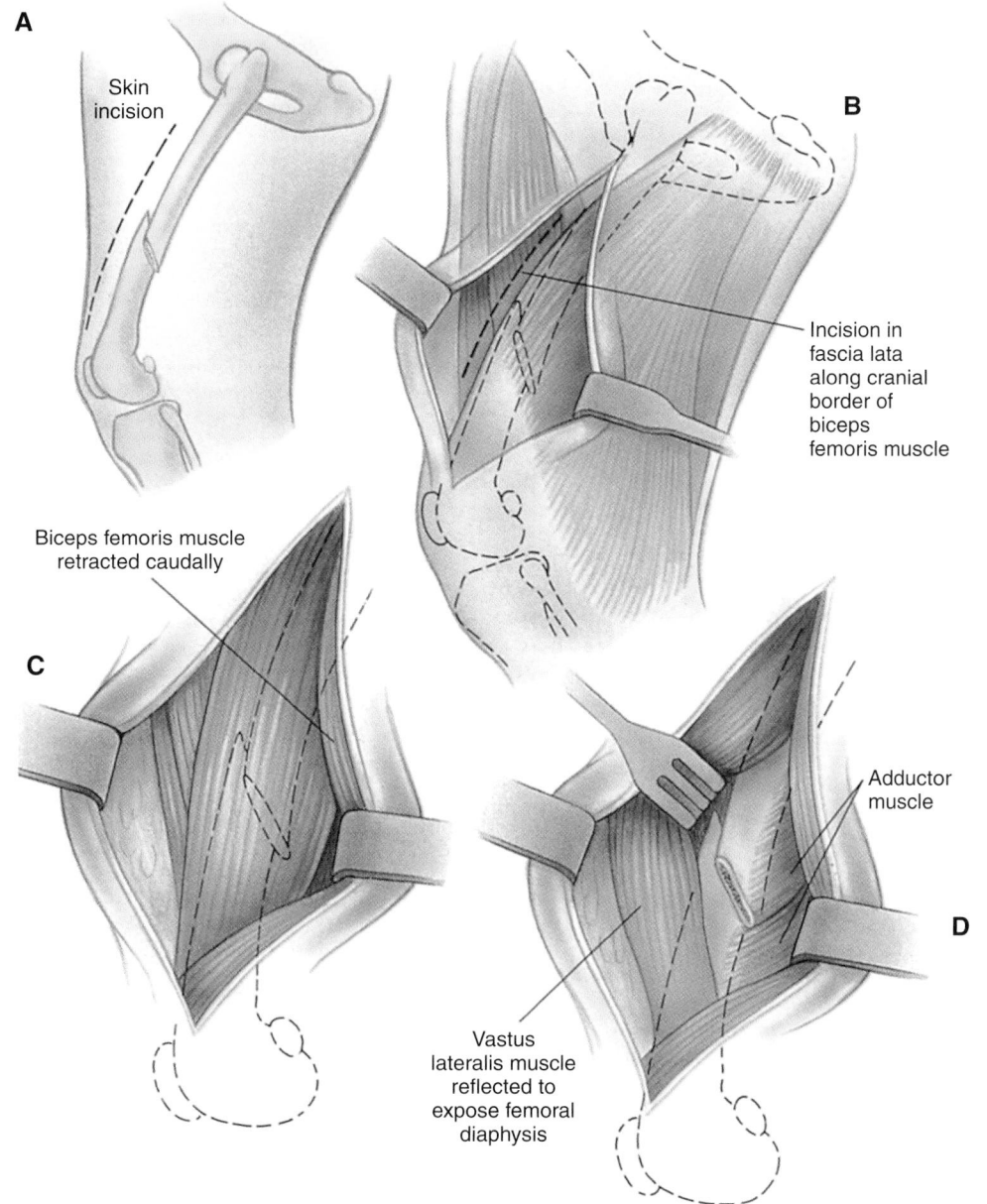

FIG. 32-81
A, To expose the femoral diaphysis, make an incision along the craniolateral border of the thigh. **B,** Incise the superficial leaf of the fascia lata along the cranial border of the biceps femoris muscle for the length of the incision. **C,** Retract the biceps femoris caudally to expose the vastus lateralis muscle. **D,** Reflect the vastus lateralis from the surface of the femur to expose the femoral diaphysis.

the vastus lateralis may be aided by releasing the muscle from the distal femoral caudolateral surface. Hematomas and serum are frequently encountered, which may make the fractured bones difficult to identify. Proximal and distal fracture segments can be identified using a combination of gentle retraction and probing. It is often useful to begin dissection proximal or distal to the fracture site in an area of more normal anatomy. The dissection is then carried into the fracture zone.

Rotational alignment is achieved in nonreducible comminuted fractures by (1) aligning the roughened caudal surface of the femur of the attachment of the adductor magnus muscle or (2) achieving the normal spatial relationship (generally 90 degrees) between the greater trochanter and the patella.

Positioning

The patient is positioned in lateral recumbency. The leg is prepped from the dorsal midline to the tarsal joint. It is advantageous to use a hanging-leg preparation to allow maximum manipulation of the limb during surgery. A donor site for cancellous bone graft harvest is prepared at the ipsilateral proximal humerus. Alternatively, the ipsilateral iliac wing or proximal tibia is used.

SURGICAL TECHNIQUE
Surgical Approach to the Femoral Diaphysis

Make an incision along the craniolateral border of the thigh (Fig. 32-81, A). Ensure that the incision is made slightly more cranial than lateral because the exposure plane will be at the cranial border of the biceps.

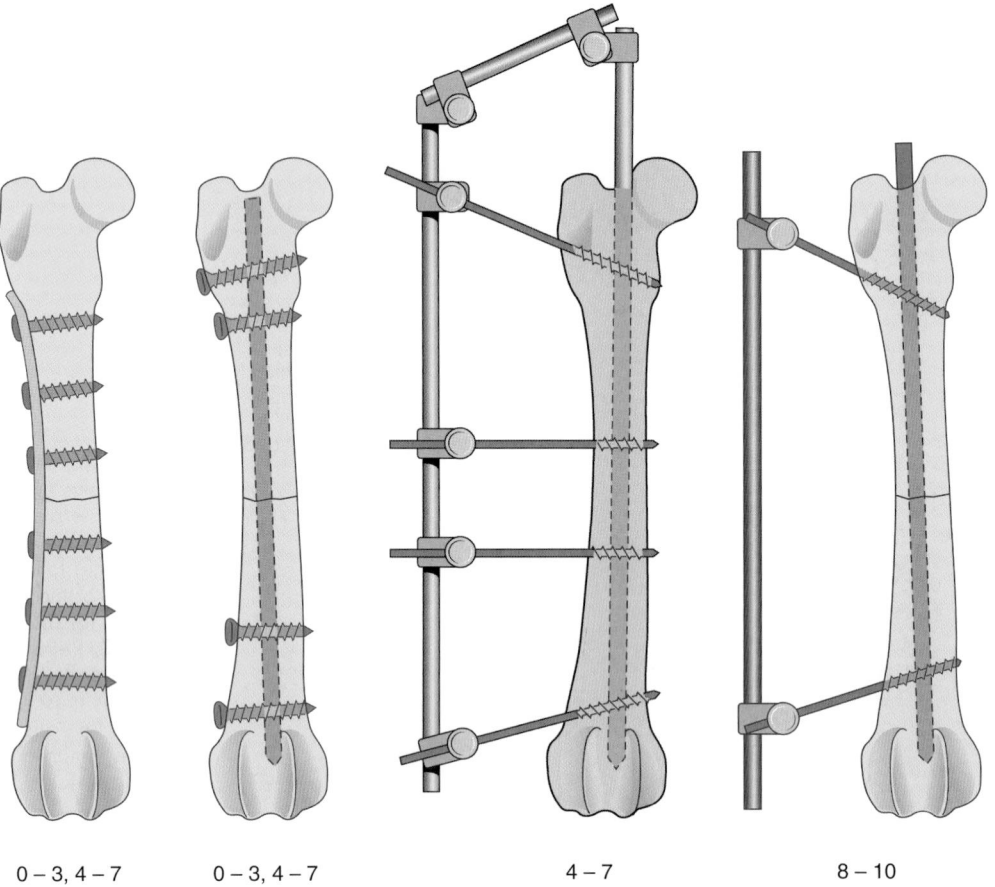

$$0-3, 4-7 \qquad 0-3, 4-7 \qquad 4-7 \qquad 8-10$$

FIG. 32-82
Recommended methods for stabilizing transverse or short oblique femoral fractures based on fracture-assessment score. If the fracture-assessment score is 0 to 3, a compression plate or interlocking nail may be used. If the fracture-assessment score is 4 to 7, a compression plate, an interlocking nail, or a 4-pin external skeletal fixator plus IM pin (tie-in configuration) may be used. With fracture-assessment scores of 8 to 10, an IM pin plus a 2-pin external skeletal fixator provides necessary stability. (Third figure modified from Johnson AL, Dunning D: *Atlas of orthopedic surgical procedures of the dog and cat,* ed 1, St Louis, 2005, Saunders.)

The length of the incision depends on the type of implant used for stabilization and fracture configuration. In general, bone plate insertion and comminuted fracture patterns require a longer incision.

Incise the superficial leaf of the fascia lata along the cranial border of the biceps femoris muscle for the length of the incision (Fig. 32-81, B). Retract the biceps femoris caudally to expose the vastus lateralis muscle (Fig. 32-81, C). Incise the fascial septum of the vastus lateralis as it inserts at the caudal lateral border of the femur. Reflect the vastus lateralis from the surface of the femur to expose the femoral diaphysis (Fig. 32-81, D). Carefully manipulate soft tissue and fracture hematoma to allow fracture reduction and application of a fixation system.

Stabilization of Midshaft Transverse or Short Oblique Fractures

From a mechanical perspective, midshaft fracture configuration allows load sharing between bone and implant after surgery. Stabilization of transverse or short oblique fractures requires rotational and bending support. This can be achieved with bone plates, interlocking nails, or an IM pin with an external fixator (Fig. 32-82).

Stabilize patients with a low fracture-assessment score (0 to 3) with a bone plate and screws (functioning as a compression plate) or an interlocking nail. Stabilize patients with a moderate fracture-assessment score (4 to 7) with a bone plate and screws, an interlocking nail, or an IM pin combined with or tied in to an external skeletal fixator. Stabilize

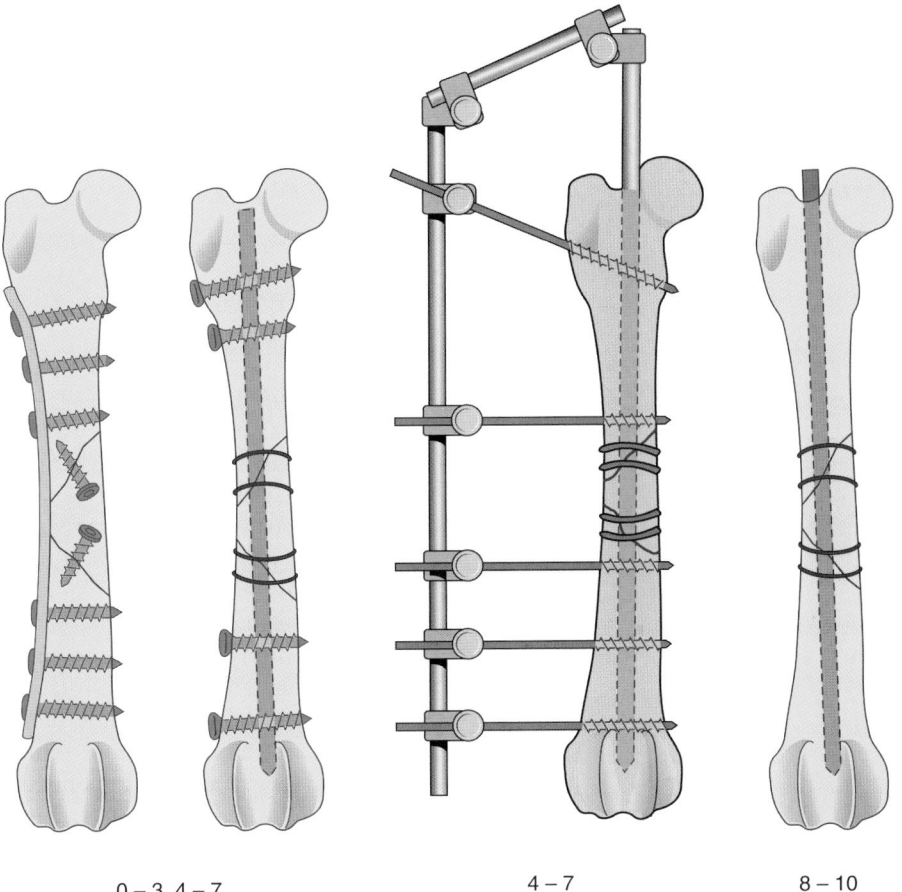

0 – 3, 4 – 7   4 – 7   8 – 10

FIG. 32-83
Recommended methods for stabilizing long oblique fractures or reducible comminuted femoral fractures (single large fragment) based on fracture-assessment score. If the fracture-assessment score is 0 to 3, a neutralization plate with lag screws or interlocking nail with cerclage wire may be used. If the fracture-assessment score is 4 to 7, a neutralization plate with lag screws, an interlocking nail with cerclage wire, or an external skeletal fixator plus IM pin (tie-in configuration) and cerclage wire may be used. With fracture-assessment scores of 8 to 10, an IM pin plus cerclage wire provides necessary stability. (Third figure modified from Johnson AL, Dunning D: *Atlas of orthopedic surgical procedures of the dog and cat,* ed 1, St Louis, 2005, Saunders.)

patients with a high fracture-assessment score (8 to 10) with an IM pin with a 2-pin external skeletal fixator.

Stabilization of Midshaft Long Oblique Fractures or Comminuted Fractures With One or Two Large Butterfly Fragments

From a mechanical perspective, these fractures can be reduced and interfragmentary compression applied with cerclage wire (used with IM fixation) or lag screws. Once the interfragmentary fracture lines are reduced and compressed, the bone is able to share loads with the implant postoperatively, removing undue stress on the implant and its attachment site. Stabilization of this type of fracture requires axial, rotational, and bending support. This can be achieved with

bone plates; interlocking nails; IM pins, cerclage wires, and external skeletal fixator combinations; or IM pins plus cerclage wires (Fig. 32-83).

Stabilize patients with a low fracture-assessment score (0 to 3) with lag screws combined with neutralization plates or interlocking nails to protect the reconstruction (Fig. 32-84). Stabilize patients with a moderate fracture-assessment score (4 to 7) with a neutralization plate combined with lag screws, an interlocking nail combined with cerclage wire, or an IM pin combined with cerclage wire and an external skeletal fixator. Stabilize patients with a high fracture-assessment score (8 to 10) with an IM pin combined with cerclage wire to compress the fracture.

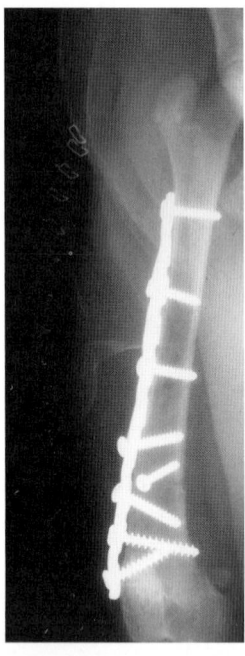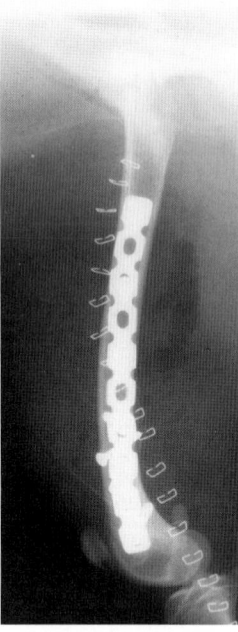

FIG. 32-84
Postoperative radiographs of a supracondylar femoral fracture repaired with an interfragmentary lag screw and a reconstruction plate functioning as a neutralization plate.

Stabilization of Midshaft Comminuted Fractures With Multiple Fragments

From a mechanical perspective, it is difficult to reduce and rigidly stabilize all small fragments in comminuted fractures. Even when reduction is attempted, it seldom can be accomplished without causing significant soft tissue disruption. The implant must carry the load until biologic callus forms to provide additional mechanical support, subjecting the implant to high stress levels. If the biologic assessment is favorable, the imposed stresses will be of short duration, and implant failure is less likely. If the biologic assessment is not favorable, however, stresses acting on the implant for extended periods will often cause implant failure. Enhancing the biologic response by applying the concept of bridging osteosynthesis (see pp. 997 and 959) and inserting an autogenous cancellous bone graft (see p. 962) is recommended.

From a mechanical perspective, these fractures need rigid axial, rotational, and bending support. This can be achieved with a bone plate–pin combination, a bone plate alone, an interlocking nail, or an external skeletal fixator and pin tie-in combination (Fig. 32-85).

Stabilize patients with a low fracture-assessment score (0 to 3) with a bone plate–IM pin combination that bridges the fracture (Fig. 32-86). Stabilize patients with a moderate fracture assessment using bone plates, interlocking nails, or IM pin and external fixator combinations.

A patient with this fracture and a high fracture-assessment score (8 to 10) must have an extremely favorable biologic assessment, such as young patients (4 to 5 months of age) with closed comminuted fractures and no other injuries.

Stabilize patients with high fracture-assessment scores with an IM pin and a 2-pin, Type Ia external skeletal fixator.

Immature dogs may also be treated with flexible plating techniques using a veterinary cuttable plate and screws (see p. 1046).

Stabilization of Supracondylar Fractures

Supracondylar fractures are usually transverse or short oblique fractures. Occasionally a comminuted fracture with multiple small fragments will be seen. When comminution is present, however, the length of bone involved is usually limited to a small area. Stabilization of supracondylar fractures depends on the fracture configuration and the patient's fracture assessment. Transverse or short oblique fractures require rotational and bending support, whereas comminuted fractures require axial, rotational, and bending support. The caudal curve of the femoral condyles and the likelihood of comminution contribute to the difficulty in stabilizing these fractures. In patients with low (0 to 3) and moderate (4 to 7) fracture-assessment scores, a compression plate is preferred for transverse fractures and a plate combined with an IM pin is preferred for comminuted fractures. A reconstruction plate is useful because it allows placement of additional screws in the distal segment (see Fig. 32-84). Locking plate technology is also useful for treating these fractures (see p. 993). If the fracture is transverse and has a high assessment score (8 to 10), crossed IM pins or Kirschner wires provide the needed stability to allow for fracture union.

SUTURE MATERIALS AND SPECIAL INSTRUMENTS

Equipment necessary for pin and wire placement includes retractors, bone-holding forceps, reduction forceps, a Jacobs pin chuck, IM pins, Kirschner wires, orthopedic wire, wire twisters, and wire cutters. Additional equipment needed for external fixation includes a low-rpm power drill and external fixation clamps and bars. The interlocking nail equipment is needed for nail application. Plating equipment and a high-speed drill are necessary for application of plates and screws.

POSTOPERATIVE CARE AND ASSESSMENT

Postoperative radiographs are made to evaluate fracture reduction and implant location. Activity should be restricted to leash walking and physical rehabilitation until the fracture has healed. Physical rehabilitation (see Chapter 12) encourages controlled limb use and optimal limb function after fracture healing. Care must be taken to develop customized protocols for each patient depending on location of the frac-

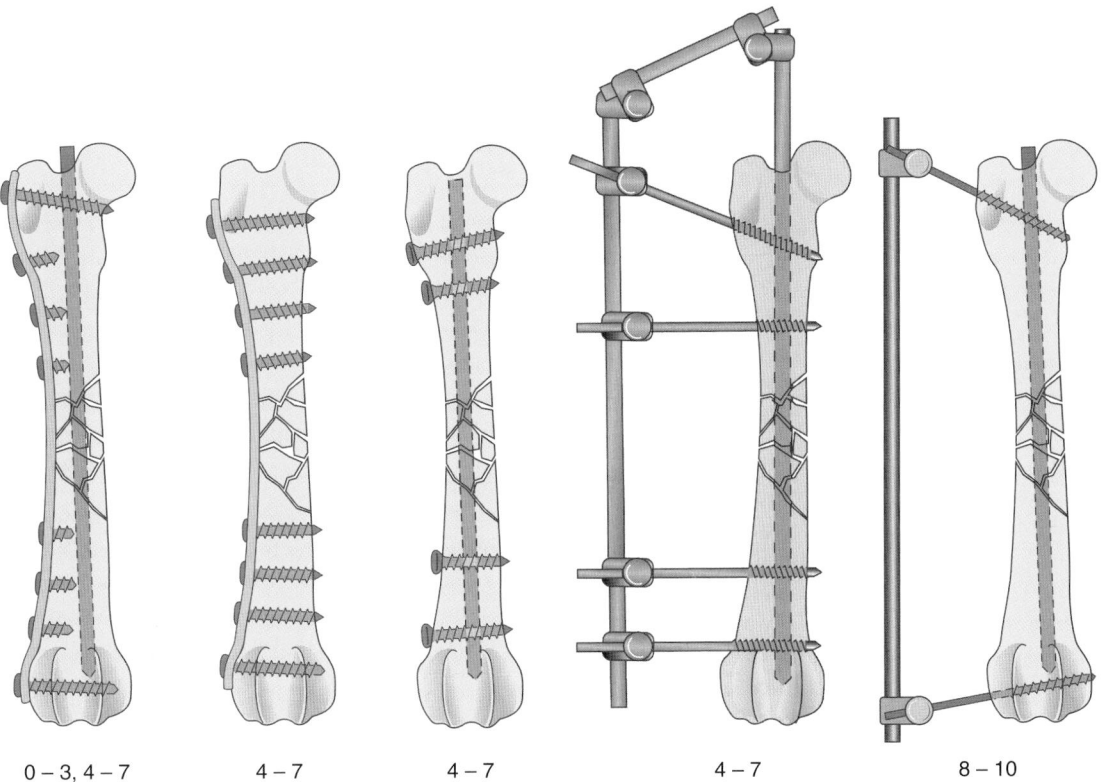

0 – 3, 4 – 7   4 – 7   4 – 7   4 – 7   8 – 10

FIG. 32-85
Recommended methods for stabilizing nonreducible comminuted femoral fractures (multiple fragments) based on fracture-assessment score. If the fracture-assessment score is 0 to 3, a plate-IM pin combination should be used. If the fracture-assessment score is 4 to 7, a plate-IM pin combination, a bridging plate, an interlocking nail, or an external skeletal fixator plus IM pin (tie-in configuration) may be used. With fracture-assessment scores of 8 to 10, an external skeletal fixator plus IM pin provides necessary stability. (Modified from Fossum TW: *Small animal surgery,* ed 2, St Louis, 2002, Mosby.)

A   **B**

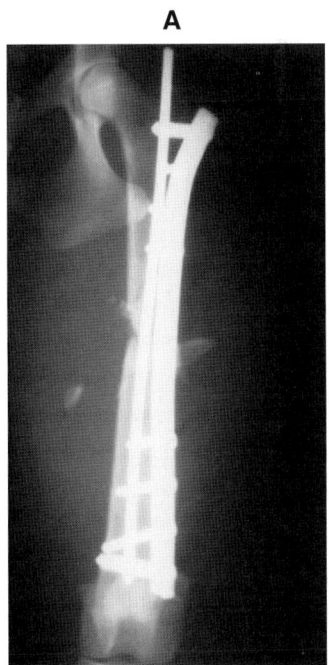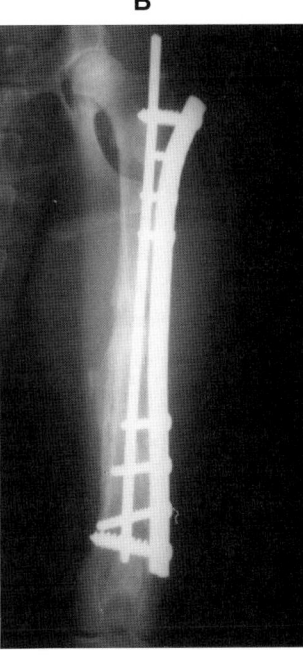

FIG. 32-86
Postoperative radiographs. **A,** Femoral fracture in a dog with a low fracture-assessment score stabilized with a plate-rod combination bridging the fracture. **B,** Healed fracture 12 weeks later.

BOX 32-15

Common Errors in Femoral Diaphyseal Fracture Fixation

- Failure to provide adequate rotational stability may lead to delayed union and nonunion, even in young animals.
- Using a single IM pin to stabilize a femoral diaphyseal fracture results in fracture instability and implant migration.
- Attempting to reconstruct nonreducible fractures destroys the biologic environment and delays healing, contributing to implant failure.

ture, stability and type of fracture fixation, potential for healing, abilities and attitudes of the patient, and willingness or ability of the client to provide for the animal's care (see Tables 32-4 and 32-5 on pp. 1048 and 1049, respectively). External fixator management includes daily pin care and pin packing as needed. Radiographs should be evaluated in 6 weeks. External fixators may be destabilized at this time if healing is progressing satisfactorily. Radiographs should be repeated at 6-week intervals until fracture bridging is observed. Time to bone union depends on the patient's fracture assessment. IM pins and external skeletal fixations should be removed when healing occurs; interlocking nails and bone plates are generally not removed unless a problem is associated with their presence.

COMPLICATIONS

Premature loosening and migration of IM pins, external skeletal fixator fixation pins, and cerclage wire often results from poor implant choice relative to the fracture assessment (Box 32-15). When inappropriate or improper implants or techniques are chosen, the implant and its bony connection are subjected to excessive stress, which promotes micromotion at the implant-bone interface. Alternatively, the stress may be moderate, but may occur over time, during which the implant may reasonably be expected to remain stable. In either case, bone resorption and eventual implant loosening result. Breakage of implants can occur through fatigue, most often with bone plates when reduction and stabilization of a zone of comminution with cerclage wire or lag screws are unsuccessful, causing devascularized bone fragments and small fracture gaps. The small gaps are unfavorable for healing and concentrate stress over a small section of the bone plate.

PROGNOSIS

Femoral fractures generally heal without complication unless the implant loosens prematurely. The result is delayed healing and long-term cyclic stress on the bone plate. If the initial implant system has failed, the recommended treatment is application of a bone plate. This system stabilizes the fracture and provides the patient comfort necessary to allow physical rehabilitation and optimal limb use.

Suggested Reading

Aron DN, Palmer RH, Johnson AL: Biologic strategies and a balanced concept for repair of highly comminuted long bone fractures, *Compend Cont Educ Pract Vet* 17:35, 1995.

This article provides a review of the concepts and application of biologic fracture fixation in small animals.

Cabassu JP: Elastic plate osteosynthesis of femoral shaft fractures in young dogs, *Vet Comp Orthop Traumatol* 14:40, 2001.

The authors describe a novel technique for fracture fixation in immature dogs, which relies on the use of flexible veterinary cuttable plates and minimal numbers of screws to promote rapid callus formation.

Hulse D, Kerwin S, Mertens D: Fractures of the femoral diaphysis. In Johnson AL, Houlton JEF, Vannini R, editors: *AO principles of fracture management in the dog and cat,* Thieme, NY, 2005, AO Publishing.

This chapter provides an up-to-date collection of operative techniques for stabilizing fractures of the femur in small animals. Plate application and screw application are emphasized.

Johnson AL, Smith CW, Schaeffer DJ: Fragment reconstruction and bone plate fixation compared with bridging plate fixation for treating highly comminuted femoral fractures in dogs: 35 cases (1987-1997), *J Am Vet Med Assoc* 213:1157, 1998.

This article provides a comparison of plating techniques for treating comminuted femoral fractures. Fractures treated with biologic bridging techniques healed faster than those fractures that were reconstructed and plated.

Larin A, Eich CS, Parker RB et al: Repair of diaphyseal femoral fractures in cats using interlocking intramedullary nails: 12 cases (1996-2000), *J Am Vet Med Assoc* 219:1098, 2001.

This article provides an overview of the technique and outcomes of using the 4.0 mm nail to stabilize femoral fractures in cats.

Lidbetter DA, Glyde MR: Supracondylar femoral fractures in adult animals, *Compendium* 22:1041, 2000.

This review article provides a perspective on the challenges of stabilizing supracondylar femoral fractures in adult animals. The authors emphasize the use of alternative fixation techniques, such as hybrid fixators and specialty plates.

Peirone B, Camuzzini D, Filippi D et al: Femoral and humeral fracture treatment with an intramedullary pin/external fixator tie in configuration in growing dogs and cats, *Vet Comp Orthop Traumatol* 15:85, 2002.

This article provides a retrospective study of the application of a simplified external fixator tie-in configuration to treat immature animals with diaphyseal fractures. Healing was rapid in all cases and functional recovery complete in 16 of 19 animals.

Piermattei D, Johnson KA: *An atlas of surgical approaches to the bones and joints of the dog and cat,* ed 4, Philadelphia, 2004, WB Saunders.

This textbook is an excellent reference for surgical approaches to the femur.

Reems MR, Beale BS, Hulse DA: Use of a plate-rod construct and principles of biological osteosynthesis for repair of diaphyseal fractures in dogs and cats: 47 cases (1994-2001), *J Am Vet Med Assoc* 223:330, 2003.

This article provides a report of the application of the plate rod technique for stabilizing humeral, femoral, and tibial fractures. Clinical application and outcomes are discussed.

Tomlinson J: Fractures of the distal femur. In Johnson AL, Houlton JEF, Vannini R, editors: *AO principles of fracture management in the dog and cat,* Thieme, NY, 2005, AO Publishing.
This chapter provides an up-to-date collection of operative techniques for stabilizing fractures of the distal femur in small animals. Detailed descriptions of plate application, pin techniques, and lag screw applications are included.

FEMORAL METAPHYSEAL AND ARTICULAR FRACTURES

DEFINITIONS

Femoral neck fractures occur at the base of the neck where it joins the metaphysis of the proximal femur. **Articular fractures** may occur through the femoral head or the femoral trochlea.

GENERAL CONSIDERATIONS AND CLINICALLY RELEVANT PATHOPHYSIOLOGY

Femoral neck fractures are generally single basilar fractures, but comminution of the femoral neck can occur. Mechanically, these are highly unstable fractures because (1) the length of the moment arm acting at the fracture is extensive (entire femoral neck) and (2) the plane of the fracture is along lines of maximal shear stress. Compression of the fracture surface is necessary to resist the high shear stress. The fracture plane is extracapsular, preserving blood flow to the fracture zone after injury. Femoral neck fractures may accompany comminuted proximal femoral fractures.

Articular fractures may occur through the femoral head or the femoral trochlea. Anatomic reconstruction and rigid internal fixation are essential to minimize degenerative joint disease and maximize function. Physical rehabilitation is also essential for restoring joint function.

DIAGNOSIS
Clinical Presentation

Signalment. Any age, breed, or sex of dog or cat may be affected. Femoral head and neck fractures occur more often in mature patients after the femoral capital physeal growth plate has closed. Trochlear fractures are uncommon.

History. Most injuries result from motor vehicle accidents, but some are caused by falls.

Physical Examination Findings

Most affected animals are brought in for evaluation of a non–weight-bearing lameness. Pain and crepitation are evident on manipulation of the hip joint or stifle. The stifle is swollen and unstable when a trochlear fracture is present.

Diagnostic Imaging

Femoral head and neck fractures do not require special radiographic views for detection. If only a lateral view of the hip joint is taken, however, the diagnosis may be missed. Femoral trochlear fractures are diagnosed with standard craniocaudal or caudocranial and lateral views of the femur.

Laboratory Findings

Complete blood count and serum chemistry evaluation should be done to assess anesthetic risk in an animal sustaining trauma. Consistent laboratory abnormalities are not present.

DIFFERENTIAL DIAGNOSIS

Differential diagnoses include coxofemoral luxation, acetabular fractures, proximal femoral fractures, and capital physeal fracture in young patients. Differential diagnosis for trochlear fractures includes deranged stifle and tumor.

MEDICAL MANAGEMENT

Medical or conservative management is not a treatment option. Surgical intervention is required.

SURGICAL TREATMENT

Femoral head and neck fractures with a single fracture plane are best treated with a lag screw and Kirschner wires. If irreparable comminution is present, total hip replacement and femoral head and neck ostectomy are treatment options. If financial restraints preclude fracture repair, a femoral head and neck ostectomy may be performed (see p. 1242). Trochlear fractures are reconstructed with lag screws and Steinmann pins. Comminuted fractures are supported with a buttress plate.

Preoperative Management

Because femoral head, neck, and trochlear fractures occur secondary to trauma, all affected animals should be examined for concurrent injury and stabilized if necessary before surgery. Pain management is indicated in posttraumatic animals (see Box 31-2 on p. 944 and Chapter 13).

Anesthesia

Anesthetic management of animals with orthopedic disease is discussed on p. 944.

Surgical Anatomy

The femoral neck, femoral shaft junction in the frontal plane is known as the *angle of inclination*. This angle is normally 135 degrees and should be approximated when surgical reduction is performed. The normal angle of anteversion is 15 to 20 degrees. This angle must also be taken into consideration when inserting screws or pins into the femoral neck.

Normal anatomy of the hip joint is described on p. 1099. A craniolateral approach is performed for exposure of these fractures (Fig. 32-87). Care must be taken to ensure adequate ventral reflection of the vastus lateralis muscle to visualize the fracture surface. The femoral shaft is located craniodorsal to the femoral head and neck, which remain in the acetabulum. Adequate longitudinal incision of the joint capsule is necessary for accurate reduction. A greater trochanteric osteotomy may be required (see Fig. 32-76) if visualization is not adequate for anatomic reduction and placement of implants.

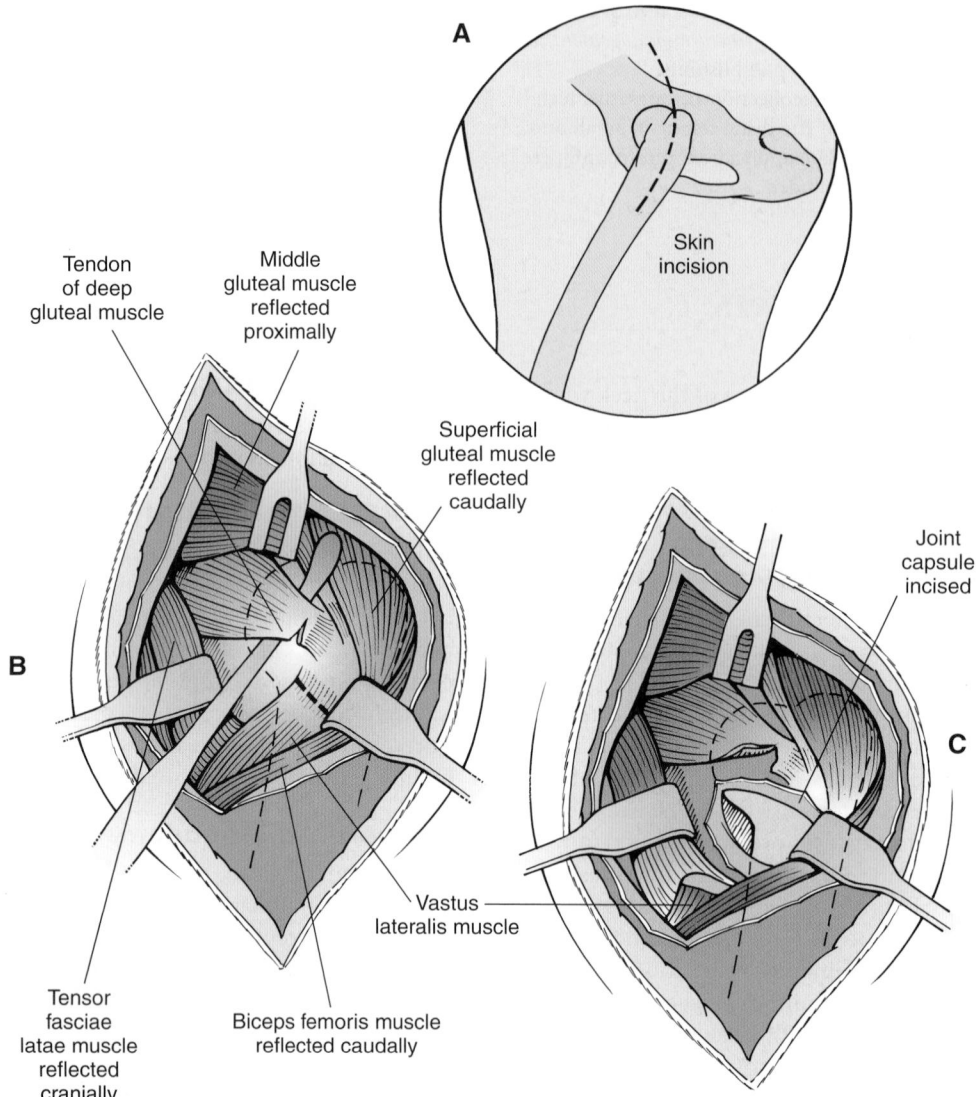

FIG. 32-87
A, To perform a craniolateral exposure of the hip joint, incise skin 5 cm proximal to the greater trochanter. Curve the incision distally adjacent to the cranial ridge of the trochanter, and extend it distally for 5 cm over the proximal femur. **B,** Reflect the tensor fasciae latae muscle cranially and the superficial gluteal and biceps femoris muscles caudally. Incise the deep gluteal tendon for one third to one half of its width at its point of insertion into the greater trochanter. **C,** Incise the joint capsule and the origin of the vastus lateralis muscle to expose the hip joint.

Surgical anatomy of the distal femur is described on p. 1262. A cranial lateral parapatellar approach is frequently used to expose the distal femur (Fig. 32-88). Fractures of the medial condyle should be approached medially and a tibial tuberosity osteotomy may be indicated for additional exposure of comminuted trochlear fractures.

Positioning

The animal is usually positioned in lateral recumbency with the affected leg up. A hanging-leg preparation will facilitate manipulation of the limb during surgery. Positioning the animal in dorsal recumbency facilitates exposure of the medial portion of the stifle.

SURGICAL TECHNIQUE
Femoral Head and Neck Fractures

A craniolateral approach to the hip joint (as for capital physeal fractures) is most often used (see Fig. 32-87). If alignment of the fracture is difficult, a trochanteric osteotomy can be performed to improve accessibility (see Fig. 32-76). Unless the biologic assessment is extremely favorable (allowing

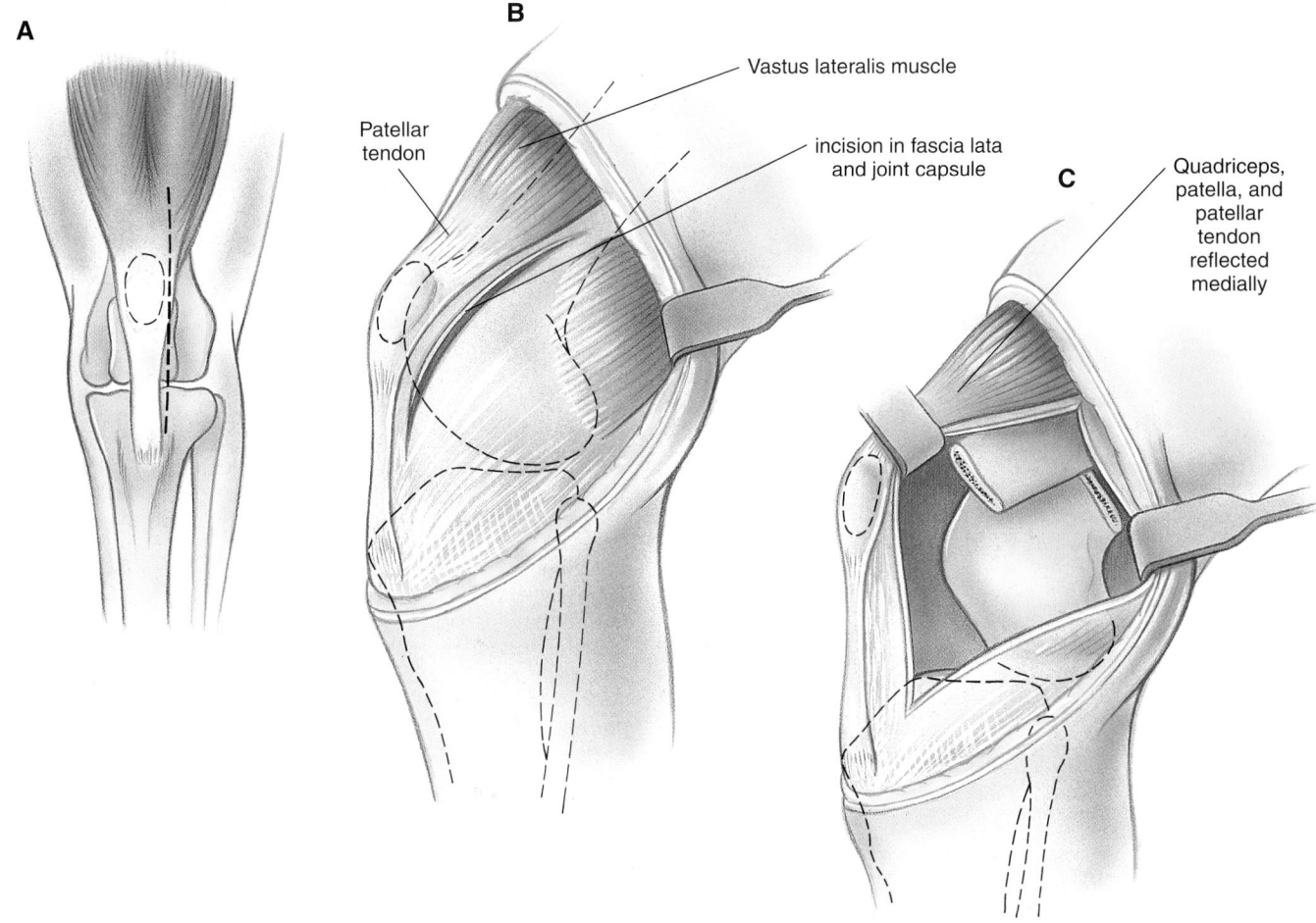

A

B

Patellar
tendon

Vastus lateralis muscle

incision in fascia lata
and joint capsule

C

Quadriceps,
patella, and
patellar
tendon
reflected
medially

FIG. 32-88
A, To expose the distal femur, make an incision on the craniolateral surface of the stifle joint centered over the palpable femoral shaft. **B,** Create a parapatellar arthrotomy through the distal fascia lata and joint capsule. **C,** Reflect the quadriceps muscles, patella, and patellar tendon medially to expose the articular surface of the femoral condyles.

Kirschner wires to be used), femoral head and neck fractures are best stabilized with lag screws.

Stabilization of an Avulsion Fracture of the Femoral Head Fracture With a Lag Screw

Visualize the fracture fragment and determine if it is large enough to repair. Reduce the fragment and maintain its position with pointed reduction forceps. Drill a glide hole through the near fragment. Drill a thread hole into the far fragment. Use the countersink to seat the screw head below the level of the articular cartilage. Measure, tap the thread hole, and insert the screw. If the fragment cannot be repaired, consider a femoral head and neck ostectomy.

Stabilization of a Femoral Neck Fracture With Partially Threaded Cancellous Lag Screw

Place two Kirschner wires so that they lie at the most proximal and distal level of the fracture surface (Fig. 32-89, A). Drive the wires from medial to lateral, beginning at the fracture surface or from the lateral surface medially to exit at the fracture surface. Reduce the fracture, and drive the Kirschner wires into the femoral epiphysis. Take care to avoid penetrating the articular surface. Drill a thread hole through the femoral epiphysis with the appropriate size drill bit parallel to and centered between the Kirschner wires. Measure the length of screw needed, and tap the thread hole. Insert a partially

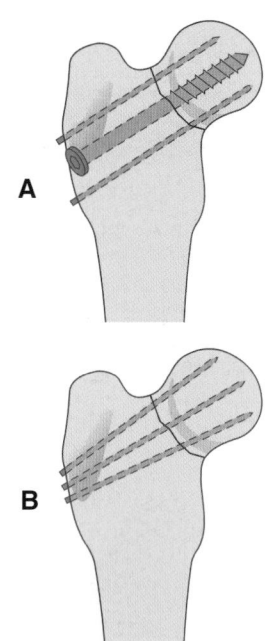

FIG. 32-89
Femoral neck fracture repair. **A,** A lag screw is centered between two Kirschner wires. **B,** Triangulated Kirschner wires.

threaded cancellous screw 2 mm shorter than the length measured so that all the threads cross the fracture plane and are seated into the femoral head. Leave one or both wires in place to serve as antirotational devices. To stabilize a femoral neck fracture with a cortex bone screw used as a lag screw, drill the glide hole through the femoral neck with a drill bit equal to the diameter of the threads of the screw.

Stabilization of a Femoral Neck Fracture With Triangulated Kirschner Wires

Insert three Kirschner wires from the fracture surface with the wires parallel to one another to form a triangle (Fig. 32-89, B). Retrograde the wires to exit the bone near the third trochanter. Alternatively, normograde the wires so that they enter the bone at the third trochanter and exit at the fracture site. Reduce the fracture, and drive the wires into the femoral epiphysis. Take care not to penetrate the articular surface.

Stabilization of Intertrochanteric Fractures

Intertrochanteric fractures are often complex and involve the femoral neck, greater trochanter, and proximal femoral metaphysis. The method of fixation depends on the fracture-assessment score (see p. 953), but includes lag screw stabilization of the femoral neck with some method of fixation applied to the proximal femur. The exception is the immature patient with a favorable biologic assessment, in whom multiple small pins can be used in the femoral neck and femoral metaphysis. In adult patients, IM pins are not used because the screw traverses the proximal metaphysis and does not allow placement of an IM pin. The preferred method of stabilization in adult patients is a bone plate. If the metaphyseal fracture is a transverse or short oblique fracture, the plate functions as a compression plate. If the

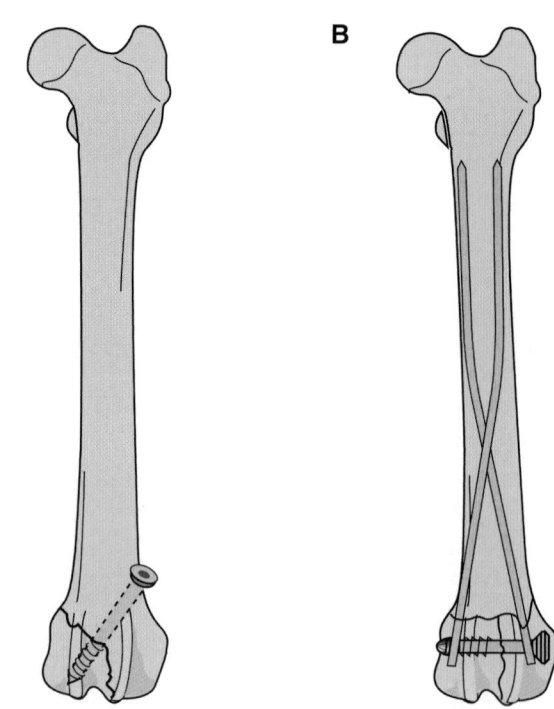

FIG. 32-90
A, Stabilization of a femoral unicondylar fracture may be done with a lag screw. **B,** Repairing a bicondylar fracture requires stabilization of the condyles with a lag screw. The condyles are then attached to the shaft of the femur with Steinmann pins or a bone plate. (Modified from Johnson AL, Houlton JEF, Vannini R, editors: *AO principles of fracture management in the dog and cat,* Thieme, NY, 2005, AO Publishing.)

area of comminution is reconstructed with cerclage wire and lag screws, the reconstruction can be protected with a neutralization plate. Alternatively, the area of comminution can be bridged with a buttress plate, without manipulating the fracture fragments. The lag screw used for stabilization of the femoral neck fracture can be placed through a plate hole or offset caudally to the plate.

Stabilization of a Unicondylar Fracture With a Lag Screw

Reduce the fracture and temporarily stabilize it with pointed reduction forceps and a Kirschner wire. Prepare for and insert a lag screw starting just proximal to the trochlear ridge on the same or opposite side of the femur depending on the fracture line orientation (Fig. 32-90, A). Orient the screw perpendicular to the fracture line for optimal compression and to prevent the fragment from shifting as the screw is tightened. The Kirschner wire may be removed or left in place for rotational stability.

Stabilization of a Bicondylar Fracture With a Lag Screw, and With Steinmann Pins or a Bone Plate

Reduce the femoral condyles, and apply compression with a lag screw placed across the fracture. After condylar reduction and stabilization, insert two small Steinmann pins as described for stabilization of Salter I and II fractures (Fig. 32-90, B; see

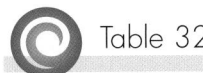 Table 32-13

Sample Physical Rehabilitation Protocol for Patients With Stifle or Tarsal Fractures

ALL TREATMENTS BID	DAY 1 TO DAY 14	DAY 15 TO DAY 24	DAY 25 UNTIL HEALED	HEALED TO RETURN TO FUNCTION
Heat therapy		10 min	10 min	
Therapeutic ultrasound	10 min†			
Massage	5 min	5 min	5 min	
Passive range of motion (repetitions)	20*	20*	10–15*	Stop-when ROM N
Electrical stimulation‡	10 min	10 min	10 min	10 min
Therapeutic exercise- total time	10 min	15 min	15 min	25–45 min
Walk/land treadmill	10 min	15 min	15 min	>10 min
Balancing	+	+	+	+
Obstacles	+	+	+	+
Weaving				+
Circles				+
Hills				+
Stairs				+
Jog/run				+
Underwater treadmill				>15 min
Swimming				5–10 min
Cryotherapy	15 min	15 min	15 min	PRN

BID, Twice a day; *ROM*, range of motion; *N*, normal; +, perform modality; *PRN*, as needed.
*Perform passive range of motion for all joints of the affected limb.
†Perform over quadriceps muscle and follow with stretching exercises QID for first 48–72 hours to decrease the risk of quadriceps contracture.
‡Apply to semimembranosus/semitendinosus muscles in patients with muscle atrophy (see Chapter 12).

also p. 1121). If the animal is approaching maturity, stabilize with a reconstruction plate on the lateral surface.

Stabilization of Comminuted Distal Femoral Physeal Fractures

Comminuted distal femoral physeal fractures often involve the trochlea and articular surface of the femoral condyles. Visualization of the fracture planes is necessary to achieve the anatomic reduction and rigid fixation required with articular fractures. Surgical exposure is best accomplished through a combination of the standard approach for osteotomy of the tibial crest and a medial arthrotomy. Proximal reflection of the patellar tendon, patella, and quadriceps muscle group allows excellent visualization.

Reconstruct the articular surface using a combination of lag screws and Kirschner wires. Once the articular fractures have been reconstructed, reduce the femoral condyles and stabilize them with a reconstruction plate. Contour the reconstruction plate to the lateral surface of the distal femur and femoral condyles.

SUTURE MATERIALS AND SPECIAL INSTRUMENTS

Appropriate surgical instrumentation for application of Kirschner pins or lag screws and plates is needed.

POSTOPERATIVE CARE AND ASSESSMENT

Postoperative radiographs are made to evaluate fracture reduction and implant location. Activity should be restricted to leash walking and physical rehabilitation until the fracture has healed. Physical rehabilitation (see Chapter 12) encourages controlled limb use and optimal limb function after fracture healing and is especially important after fractures affecting the stifle. Care must be taken to develop customized protocols for each patient depending on location of the fracture, stability and type of fracture fixation, potential for healing, abilities and attitudes of the patient, and willingness or ability of the client to provide for the animal's care (Table 32-13; see also Table 32-12). Radiographs should be repeated at 6-week intervals until fracture bridging is observed. Femoral metaphyseal and articular fractures may take 6 to 12 weeks to heal depending on biologic fracture assessment. Implants are generally not removed unless they cause a problem.

COMPLICATIONS

Inappropriate reduction and poor implant choice are the most common problems reported with femoral neck fractures. Significant bending and shear stress across the fracture plane place extreme bending loads on implants. The most common implant error is the use of Kirschner wires or small pins when the fracture assessment indicates prolonged healing. Micromotion at the pin-bone interface arising from the high physiologic stress may cause pins to loosen early. This problem can be avoided or treated by using a lag screw and antirotational pin except when the biologic assessment indicates rapid healing.

PROGNOSIS

The animal with a femoral neck fracture that fails to heal is usually treated with a femoral head and neck ostectomy. Intertrochlear fractures may be slow to heal. Femoral condylar fractures generally heal rapidly, as they are located in cancellous bone and generally occur in young animals. Comminuted trochlear fractures will usually result in degenerative joint disease, but most animals are functional on the limb.

Suggested Reading

Chico AC, Jont J, Marti JM: Trochlear femoral fractures in cats: results of seven cases, *Vet Comp Orthop Traumatol* 14:51, 2001.
This article provides a review of the techniques and outcomes of the treatment of intraarticular distal femoral fractures in cats. Six of the cats had a good functional outcome.

Hulse D, Kerwin S, Mertens D: Fractures of the proximal femur. In Johnson AL, Houlton JEF, Vannini R, editors: *AO principles of fracture management in the dog and cat,* Thieme, NY, 2005, AO Publishing.
This chapter provides an up-to-date collection of operative techniques for stabilizing proximal femoral fractures in small animals. Detailed descriptions of Kirschner wire techniques, lag screw application, and bone-plating procedures are included.

Tomlinson J: Fractures of the distal femur. In Johnson AL, Houlton JEF, Vannini R, editors: *AO principles of fracture management in the dog and cat,* Thieme, NY, 2005, AO Publishing.
This chapter provides an up-to-date collection of operative techniques for stabilizing fractures of the distal femur in small animals. Detailed descriptions of plate application, pin techniques, and lag screw applications are included.

FEMORAL PHYSEAL FRACTURES

GENERAL CONSIDERATIONS AND CLINICALLY RELEVANT PATHOPHYSIOLOGY

Because femoral physeal fracture occurs through cartilage of the growth plate, capital physeal injuries may occur without significant trauma. This is particularly true in young heavy male cats that have been neutered before 6 months of age. Delayed physeal closure and cartilage abnormalities may increase the susceptibility of these cats to physeal fracture (Fig. 32-91). The femoral neck is usually externally rotated and displaced craniodorsally such that it lies adjacent to the iliac wing. The physis of the greater trochanter may also be fractured, causing the femoral shaft to be displaced more dorsally than expected. Proximal physeal fractures are gener-

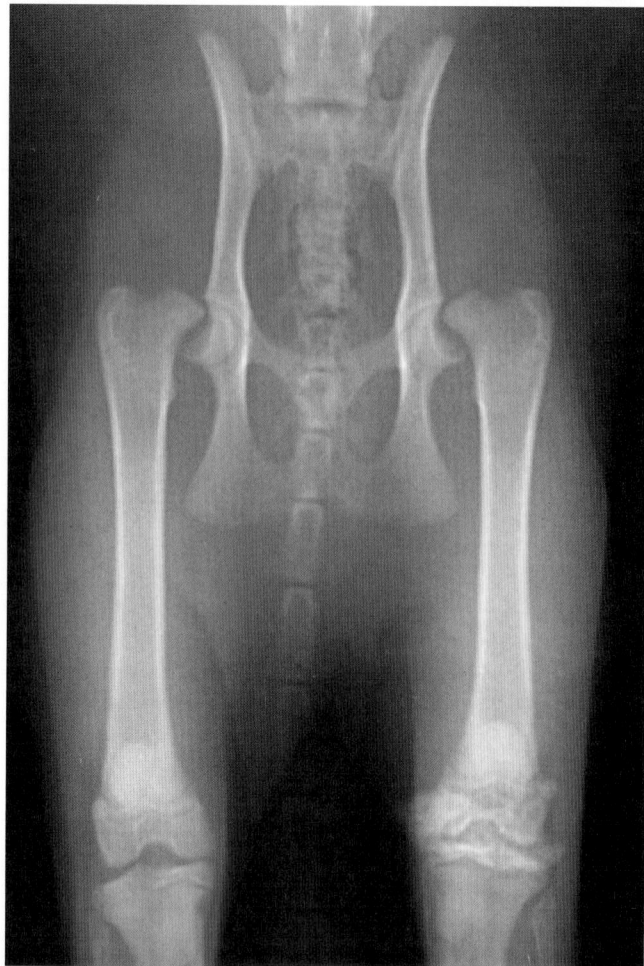

FIG. 32-91
Ventrodorsal radiograph of young cat with bilateral capital physeal fractures.

ally Salter I or Salter II fractures (see p. 951). Distal femoral physeal fractures are generally Salter II physeal fractures.

The capital physis functions to provide femoral neck length until the animal is approximately 8 months of age. The distal physis functions to provide the majority of femoral length. In most fractures, the growth cartilage is damaged either by the traumatic incident, in the posttraumatic period, or during surgery. Physeal fractures heal rapidly, but most of the time, the physis does not continue to function. The younger the animal, the more dramatic are the effects of premature closure of the injured physis.

DIAGNOSIS
Clinical Presentation

Signalment. Most affected animals are less than 10 months of age. Young male dogs are more likely to sustain trauma resulting in femoral physeal fracture, probably because of their tendency to roam. Young heavy male cats that have been neutered before 6 months of age are also at risk.

History. Most animals are presented for evaluation of an acute non–weight-bearing lameness. The trauma may or may not be witnessed by the owner. Femoral physeal fractures are often caused by motor vehicular accidents. However, minor trauma such as a fall may be sufficient to separate the growth plate.

Physical Examination Findings

Animals with proximal physeal fractures usually exhibit a non–weight-bearing lameness with pain and crepitation on manipulation of the hip joint. Some animals are weight bearing and do not have detectable crepitus referable to the hip joint. These animals usually have minimal displacement of the femoral head. Animals with distal femoral physeal fractures present with swelling, pain, and crepitus on manipulation of the stifle region.

Diagnostic Imaging

Standard ventrodorsal and mediolateral projections of the femur are required to confirm the diagnosis. Sedation is often required for proper positioning (see p. 933). A fractured capital physis with minimal displacement may be difficult to detect using an extended limb ventrodorsal radiographic projection. A ventrodorsal view with the limbs in "frog position" may help confirm the diagnosis in such cases. If a greater trochanteric physeal fracture is also present, the cap of the greater trochanter will be superimposed over the shaft of the femur and will appear as a half-moon radiodense object on a ventrodorsal radiograph. On a lateral projection, the cap of the trochanter will appear as a radiodense fragment caudal to the femur. With distal physeal fractures, the femoral shaft is displaced cranially and distally and may be superimposed over the femoral condyles. If the displacement is slight, the fracture may be missed when a single craniocaudal radiograph is taken. Additional oblique and skyline projections are useful to evaluate the articular surface of the trochlea and femoral condyles if fissures or fractures of these structures are suspected.

> NOTE: Superimposition may be such that the fracture could be missed with a single radiograph. Always take two orthogonal views.

Laboratory Findings

Complete blood count and serum chemistry evaluation should be done to evaluate the status of the animal for anesthesia and to determine if concurrent injury or damage to the renal or hepatobiliary systems exists. Consistent laboratory abnormalities are not present.

DIFFERENTIAL DIAGNOSIS

Differential diagnoses for proximal physeal fractures include coxofemoral joint luxation, femoral neck fracture, and acetabular fractures. For distal physeal fractures, the differential diagnosis includes diaphyseal fractures and ligamentous injury of the stifle.

MEDICAL MANAGEMENT

Surgical intervention is required to prevent severe degenerative joint disease and lameness.

SURGICAL TREATMENT

Surgical treatment of physeal fractures consists of anatomic reduction and stabilization with Kirschner wires or small pins that are smooth so as to not interfere with any residual physeal function. These fractures heal rapidly, and smooth implants are generally sufficient. In animals that are close to maturity, threaded implants may be used to increase the stability of the fixation. Anatomic reduction is critical for optimal outcome with capital physeal fractures. Mechanically, prevention of movement of the reduced capital physeal and distal physeal fractures is assisted by the shape of the fractured physeal surfaces. If separated, the physis of the greater trochanter must also be anatomically reduced and stabilized with a tension band to counteract the distractive forces of the gluteal muscles.

Preoperative Management

Because these fractures occur secondary to trauma, all affected animals should be examined for concurrent injury and stabilized if necessary before surgery. Analgesics should be administered to posttraumatic patients (see Box 31-2 on p. 944 and Chapter 13).

Anesthesia

Refer to p. 944 for a discussion of anesthetic management of animals with fractures.

Surgical Anatomy

The proximal capital physis lies between the femoral epiphysis and femoral neck and acts as a barrier for passage of blood vessels from the femoral neck to the femoral epiphysis. The blood supply to the femoral epiphysis involves a series of cervical ascending vessels lying outside the femoral neck that cross the physis and then penetrate the epiphysis. See p. 1099 for surgical anatomy of the hip.

The distal femoral growth plate is W shaped and lies at the joint capsule reflection. The configuration of the growth plate and cancellous bone surface provide a degree of inherent stability for the fracture. The position of the growth plate necessitates an arthrotomy incision to facilitate exposure (see p. 1262 for surgical anatomy of the stifle).

Positioning

The animal is positioned in lateral recumbency with the affected limb up. The limb should be clipped circumferentially from dorsal midline to distal tibia (distal physeal fractures) and draped from a hanging position to allow maximal manipulation during surgery.

SURGICAL TECHNIQUE
Surgical Approach to the Proximal Femur

Incise the skin 5 cm proximal to the greater trochanter. Curve the incision distally adjacent to the cranial ridge of the trochanter, and extend it distally for 5 cm over the proximal femur (see Fig. 32-87, A). Incise subcutaneous tissue and the juncture at the superficial leaf of the fascia lata and cranial border of the biceps femoris muscle. Incise the deep leaf of the tensor fascia lata between the tensor fasciae latae muscle

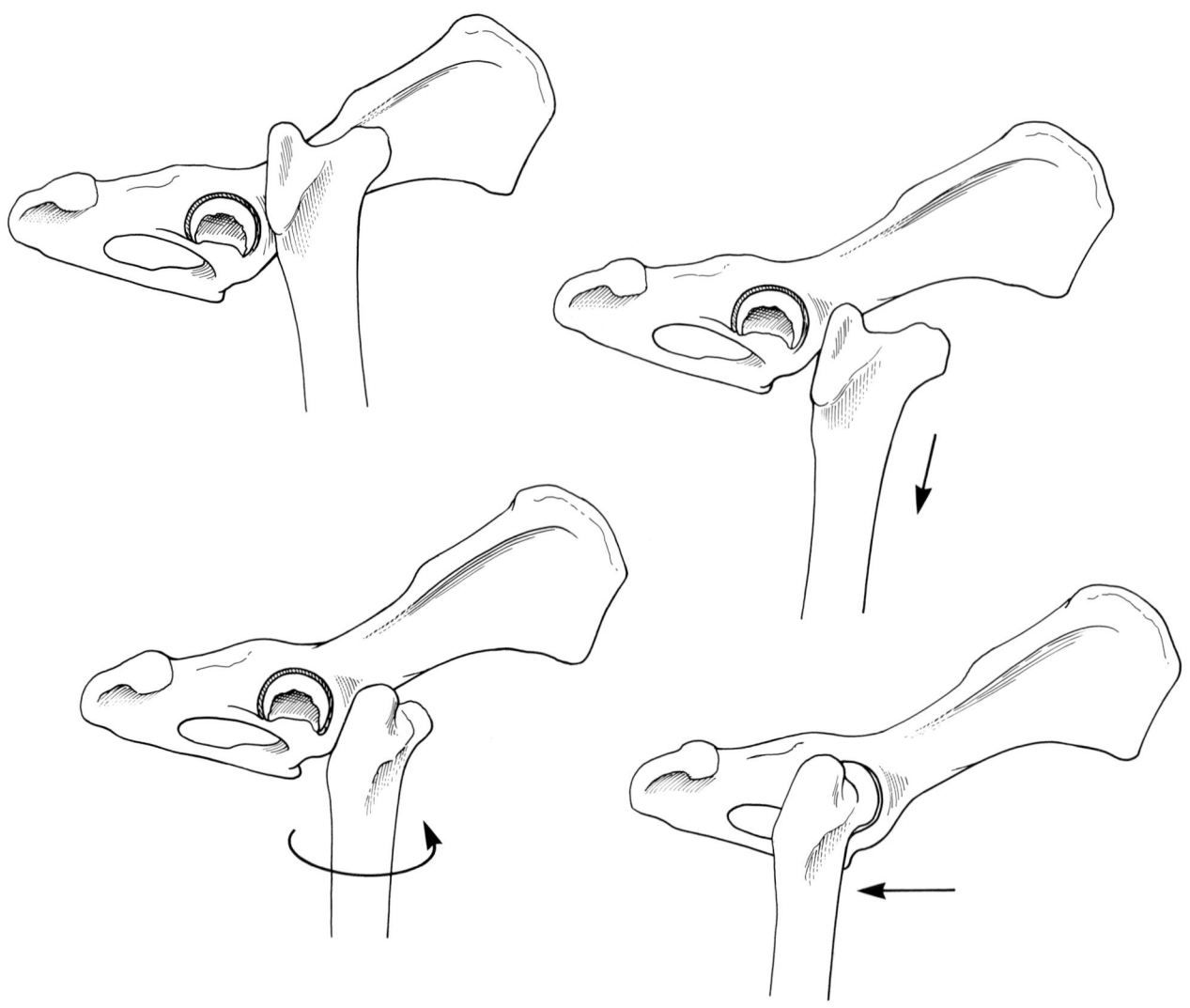

FIG. 32-92
To reduce a capital physeal fracture, bring the femoral neck ventral until it is level with the hip joint. Then derotate the femur and slide it caudally.

and deep border of the biceps femoris muscle and superficial gluteal muscle. Reflect the tensor fasciae latae muscle cranially and the superficial gluteal and biceps femoris muscles caudally (see Fig. 32-87, B). Visualize the tendinous insertion of the deep gluteal muscle by retracting the middle gluteal muscle proximally. Place a periosteal elevator beneath the deep gluteal muscle near its insertion, and separate the deep gluteal muscle from the joint capsule using a sweeping motion with the elevator. Incise the deep gluteal tendon for one third to one half of its width at its point of insertion onto the greater trochanter (Fig. 32-87, C). Leave 1 to 2 mm of tendon on the trochanter for closure, but make the incision through the tendon close to the bone. If the joint capsule is lacerated, exposing the fracture surface of the femoral neck, enlarge the opening in the joint capsule with an incision from the rim of the acetabulum laterally through the point of origin of the vastus lateralis muscle. If the joint capsule is intact, incise it parallel to the long axis of the femoral neck near its proximal ridge. Continue the joint

capsule incision laterally through the point of origin of the vastus lateralis muscle on the cranial face of the proximal femur. It is important to keep this cut at the proximal point of origin just under the cut edge of the deep gluteal tendon. Reflect the vastus lateralis distally to expose the hip joint. To reduce the proximal femoral physeal fracture, (1) bring the femoral neck distally so it lies cranial and level with the acetabulum, (2) derotate the femur to correct for the abnormal anteversion, and (3) slide the fracture surface of the femoral neck caudally into the matching surface of the femoral epiphysis (Fig. 32-92).

Surgical Approach to the Distal Femur

The most recognizable structure is often the palpable distal end of the femoral shaft, which serves as the center of the incision.

Make an incision on the craniolateral surface of the stifle joint centered over the palpable femoral shaft. Begin the

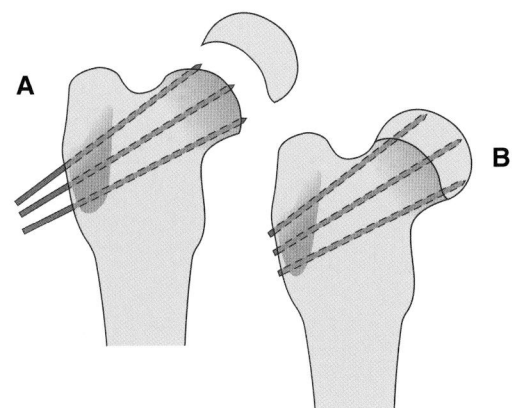

FIG. 32-93
A, To stabilize a femoral capital physeal fracture with Kirschner wires, place three wires through the femoral neck to the fracture surface. Triangulate the Kirschner wires. **B,** Reduce the fracture, and advance the wires into the epiphysis.

incision 4 to 5 cm proximal to the center point and extend it 4 to 5 cm distally (see Fig. 32-88, A). Incise the subcutaneous tissue along the line, and identify the fascia lata and patellar tendon. Create a parapatellar arthrotomy through the distal fascia lata and joint capsule (see Fig. 32-88, B). Make the incision along the caudal border of the vastus lateralis muscle through the intermuscular septum of the fascia lata.

Most often the distal femoral metaphysis lies cranial and lateral to the femoral condyles and is exposed while incising through the joint capsule and fascia lata (see Fig. 32-88, C).

Reflect the quadriceps muscles, patella, and patellar tendon medially to expose the articular surface of the femoral condyles. To reduce the distal femoral fracture, lever the condyles cranially and distally with a "spoon" Hohmann retractor placed between the fracture fragments.

Stabilization of Proximal Femoral Physeal Fracture With Triangulated Kirschner Wires

Place three Kirschner wires parallel to one another and positioned in the femoral neck so that they lie in a triangle. Two wires are sufficient in cats. Insert the wires from the lateral aspect of the femur paralleling the angle of the femoral neck; the points of the wires should be just visible at the fracture surface (Fig. 32-93, A). Reduce the fracture by holding the proximal femur in position, and drive the wires into the femoral epiphysis (Fig. 32-93, B).

A common problem with this technique is that the pins penetrating the articular cartilage are not visible to the surgeon at surgery. The exception is the feline femoral head, which may be distracted enough to view the articular cartilage. The femoral head is a dome structure, so the length of

pin placed in the periphery will be different from the length of pin placed in the center of the dome.

To determine the proper length of wires, place the first wire in the periphery of the femoral epiphysis so that it penetrates the articular cartilage where it is visible. Estimate the length of this wire that would not penetrate the articular cartilage, and use it as a gauge for the remaining wires. Drive the remaining wires into the femoral epiphysis, and place the joint through a normal range of motion after each wire to ensure that it has not penetrated the articular surface. Bend the wires at the lateral surface and cut off the excess. Close the incision routinely.

Stabilization of Proximal Femoral Physeal Fracture With Lag Screw

Initially, place two Kirschner wires in the femoral neck in a lateral to medial direction so that they lie parallel to one another. Position them so that one wire lies in the dorsal section of the femoral neck and one wire lies in the ventral section of the femoral neck. Drill a glide hole between the two wires to emerge at the center of the fracture surface (Fig. 32-94, A). Angle the Kirschner wires and glide hole to correct for normal anteversion of the femoral neck. Reduce the fracture, and drive the Kirschner wires into the femoral epiphysis. Place a drill insert into the glide hole for accurate drilling of the thread hole, into the femoral epiphysis (Fig. 32-94, B). Countersink the glide hole, and determine the appropriate screw length by measuring the distance from the lateral surface of the greater trochanter to the femoral epiphyseal articular surface. Choose a screw that is 2 mm shorter than that measured with the depth gauge. Tap the thread hole and insert the screw (Fig. 32-94, C). The wires may be left to provide additional rotational stability. Close the incision routinely.

Stabilization of Trochanteric Physeal Fracture With Tension Band Wire

Reduce the trochanter, and start two Kirschner wires in the fragment. Drive the wires across the physis to lodge in the proximal femur, and check the repair to see if stabilization is sufficient to prevent avulsion of the fracture. If not, use a tension band wire, even though it may prevent physeal growth. To place a tension band wire, (1) drill a transverse hole in the major bone segment, (2) pass a figure-eight wire through the hole and around the Kirschner wires, and (3) tighten the wire (see p. 990 for tension band wire techniques).

Stabilization of Salter I or II Distal Femoral Physeal Fractures With Steinmann Pins

With Salter I or Salter II fractures, Steinmann pins may be used alone or in combination with small Kirschner wires. The pins may be placed either in a Rush pin manner, as an IM pin, or as a crossed pin (Fig. 32-95).

*When using Steinmann pins in a **Rush pin** fashion, retrograde the pins from the fracture surface to exit at the trochanteric fossa. Position one pin in the lateral metaphysis*

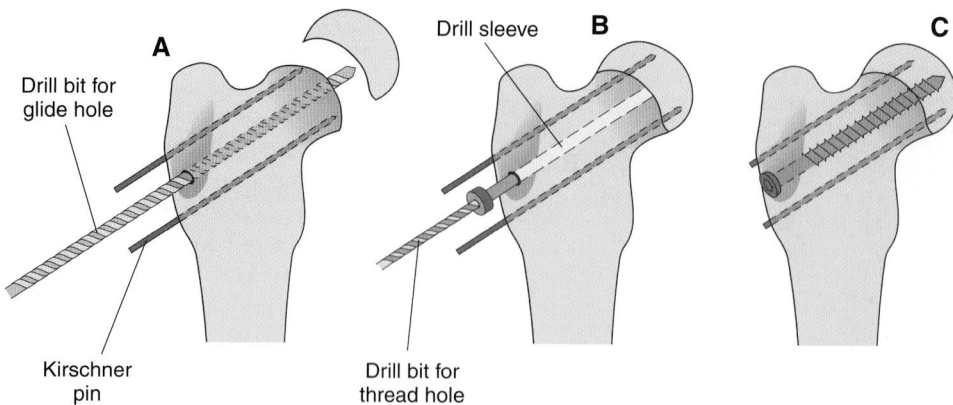

Drill bit for glide hole

Kirschner pin

Drill sleeve

Drill bit for thread hole

FIG. 32-94
A, To stabilize a femoral capital physeal fracture with a cortex bone screw used as a lag screw, place two Kirschner wires (one superior and one inferior) in the femoral neck, perpendicular to the fracture surface. Drill a glide hole between the Kirschner wires. **B,** Reduce the fracture, and advance the Kirschner wires into the femoral epiphysis. Drill the thread hole in the epiphysis, measure to determine screw length, and tap threads in the epiphysis. **C,** Insert the lag screw.

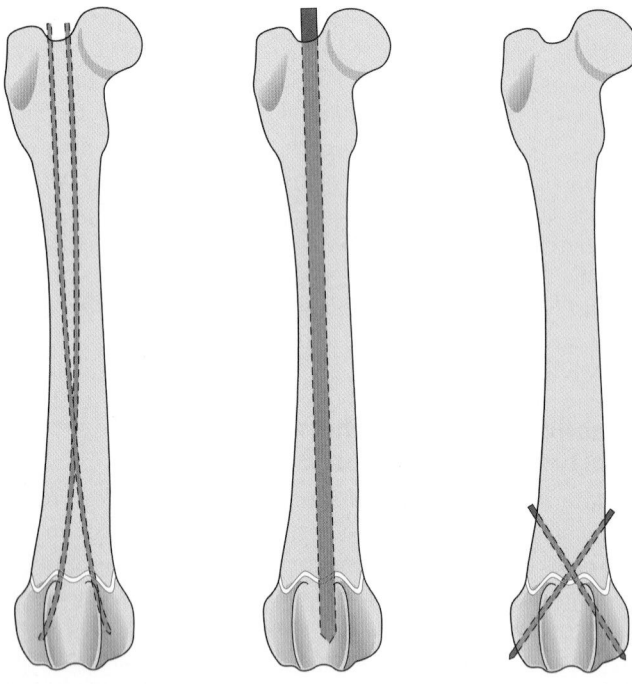

FIG. 32-95
Stabilization of distal femoral physeal fractures may be done with multiple pins placed in Rush fashion, a single IM pin, or crossed pins.

and one pin in the medial metaphysis. Use small-diameter pins so that they can bend with the curvature of the femur. With the pin tips withdrawn into the metaphysis, overreduce the fracture and drive the pins distally into the medial and lateral condyles. Cut the excess pin below the skin at the trochanteric fossa.

*When using a Steinmann pin as an **IM pin,** reduce the fracture and insert the pin through the articular cartilage cranial to the origin of the caudal cruciate ligament. Direct the pin in a normograde fashion across the fracture, proximally into the femur, to exit at the trochanteric fossa. Cut the distal part of the pin and countersink it below the level of the articular cartilage and cut any excessive pin off below the skin above the trochanteric fossa. Use a small diameter pin so it can bend with the curvature of the femoral canal as it passes proximally. Consider adding a small crossed pin at the fracture to establish rotational stability, as necessary (Fig. 32-96). When using Steinmann pins as crossed pins, position them so that they enter the epiphysis at a point cranial to the medial and lateral epicondyles, and drive them proximally to a point where they are just visible at the fracture surface. Overreduce the fracture, and drive the pins into the femoral metaphysis and through the cortices. Suture the joint capsule using an interrupted suture pattern. Close subcutaneous tissue and skin routinely.*

SUTURE MATERIALS AND SPECIAL INSTRUMENTS

A battery-operated or air-driven drill with a wire driver attachment is helpful for inserting Kirschner wires in proximal femoral physeal fractures. Instruments that facilitate fracture reduction include Hohmann retractors and pointed reduction forceps. Small IM Steinmann pins and an assortment of Kirschner wires are needed.

POSTOPERATIVE CARE AND ASSESSMENT

Postoperative radiographs are made to evaluate fracture reduction and implant location. Activity should be restricted to leash walking and physical rehabilitation until the fracture has healed. Physical rehabilitation (see Chapter 12) encourages controlled limb use and optimal limb function after fracture healing and is especially important

A   **B**

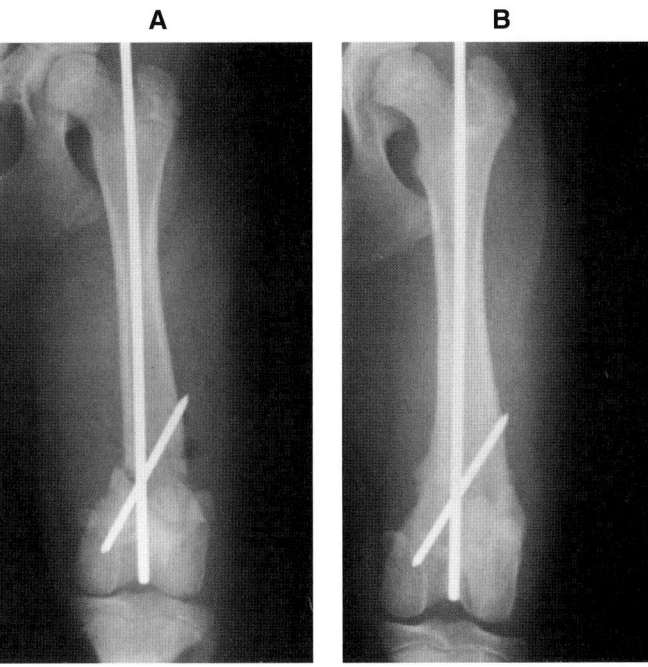

FIG. 32-96
Postoperative radiographs. **A,** Salter II fracture through the distal femoral physis stabilized with IM pin and crossed pin. **B,** Healed fracture 6 weeks later.

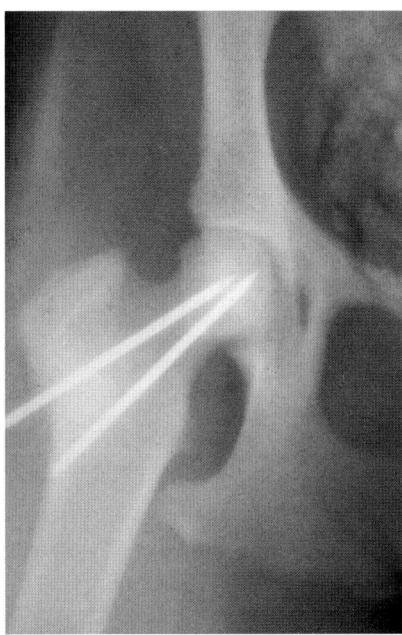

FIG. 32-97
Postoperative radiographs of a proximal femoral physeal fracture stabilized with Kirschner wires 6 weeks after surgery. Note the loss of bone density circumferentially on the femoral neck. This "apple coring" is a frequent postoperative observation, but rarely has clinical significance.

after fractures affecting the stifle. Care must be taken to develop customized protocols for each patient depending on location of the fracture, stability and type of fracture fixation, potential for healing, abilities and attitudes of the patient, and willingness or ability of the client to provide for the animal's care (see Tables 32-12 and 32-13). Radiographs should be repeated at 4 to 6 weeks (see Fig. 32-96). Kirschner wires and crossed pins are generally not removed unless they cause a problem. IM pins should be removed after the fracture has healed.

COMPLICATIONS

If a proximal physeal fracture is not appropriately reduced or if implants penetrate the articular cartilage, significant degenerative changes may develop, necessitating additional surgical treatment.

PROGNOSIS

The prognosis for long-term, pain-free function after proximal physeal fracture is good if the fracture is adequately reduced and appropriately stabilized (Fig. 32-97). In animals less than 5 months of age, however, a shortened femoral neck may result from closure of the capital physis, which may cause hip joint subluxation and may increase the risk of degenerative joint disease.

For distal physeal fractures, bone union occurs within 4 to 6 weeks. Although growth retardation or premature closure of the distal femoral growth plate is likely, the prognosis for normal limb use is excellent with Salter I or II fractures. The exception is if the injury occurs at 3 to 5 months of age in a large or giant breed dog, when considerable growth potential is still present.

Suggested Reading

Fischer HR, Norton J, Kobluk CN et al: Surgical reduction and stabilization of femoral capital physeal fractures in cats: 13 cases (1998-2002), *J Am Vet Med Assoc* 224:1478, 2004.
This article provides an evaluation of the outcome of surgical repair of proximal femoral physeal fractures in cats. Results suggested that surgical stabilization and repair of femoral capital physeal fractures facilitate a short recovery period and a good prognosis for return to normal function.

Hulse D, Kerwin S, Mertens D: Fractures of the proximal femur. In Johnson AL, Houlton JEF, Vannini R, editors: *AO principles of fracture management in the dog and cat,* Thieme, NY, 2005, AO Publishing.
This chapter provides an up-to-date collection of operative techniques for stabilizing proximal femoral fractures in small animals. Detailed descriptions of Kirschner wire techniques, lag screw application, and bone-plating procedures are included.

McNicholas WT, Wilkens BE, Blevins WE et al: Spontaneous femoral capital physeal fractures in adult cats: 26 cases (1996-2001), *J Am Vet Med Assoc* 221:1731, 2002.
This article provides an evaluation of the clinical, radiographic, and histologic abnormalities in adult cats >1 year old with spontaneous (i.e., nontraumatic) femoral capital physeal fractures. Results suggested that adult cats with spontaneous femoral capital physeal fractures were most likely to be heavier, neutered males with delayed physeal closure.

Stigen O: Supracondylar femoral fractures in 159 dogs and cats treated using a normograde intramedullary pinning technique, *J Small Anim Pract* 40:519, 1999.

This article provides a description of an intramedullary pinning technique used to stabilize supracondylar fractures, including physeal fractures, in dogs. Approximately 80% of the dogs and cats had an excellent long-term functional outcome.

Tomlinson J: Fractures of the distal femur. In Johnson AL, Houlton JEF, Vannini R, editors: *AO principles of fracture management in the dog and cat,* Thieme, NY, 2005, AO Publishing.

This chapter provides an up-to-date collection of operative techniques for stabilizing fractures of the distal femur in small animals. Detailed descriptions of plate application, pin techniques, and lag screw applications are included.

PATELLAR FRACTURES

DEFINITION

Patellar fractures result from loss of bony and articular continuity between the superior and inferior poles of the patella.

GENERAL CONSIDERATIONS AND CLINICALLY RELEVANT PATHOPHYSIOLOGY

Fractures of the patella may result from direct or indirect trauma but are uncommon. Direct trauma results from an external blow to the cranial surface of the patella. The resulting fracture may be a transverse separation midway between the proximal and distal poles, fragmentation of the proximal or distal pole, or comminution of the patellar body. Indirect trauma is caused by forceful contraction of the quadriceps muscle group, which causes excessive tensile forces to be applied across the body of the patella. These forces result in a transverse fracture midway between the superior and inferior poles. Tearing of the parapatellar fibrocartilage, quadriceps tendon, and straight patellar ligament may also occur. Transverse or comminuted fractures through the patellar body are disabling injuries because they cause loss of quadriceps function and resultant inability to bear weight on the affected limb. Without treatment, the proximal and distal fragments of the patella separate due to countering forces of the quadriceps muscle and patellar tendon. A fibrous union develops between the fragments and affords some stability, but the support is insufficient to allow normal function. Additionally, loss of articular surface congruity results in degenerative arthritis of the patellar-femoral articulation. Small fragments at the proximal or distal poles of the patella may not be disabling if integrity of the insertion of the quadriceps muscle group is maintained.

DIAGNOSIS
Clinical Presentation

Signalment. Any age, breed, or sex of dog may be affected. Breeds with congenital myotonia and sporting breeds are most prone to transverse fractures caused by forceful contraction of the quadriceps.

History. Animals with patellar fractures resulting from trauma are usually evaluated because of non–weight-bearing lameness. Owners seldom witness the trauma itself. Indirect trauma usually occurs when the animal is undergoing strenuous activity and acutely becomes non–weight bearing.

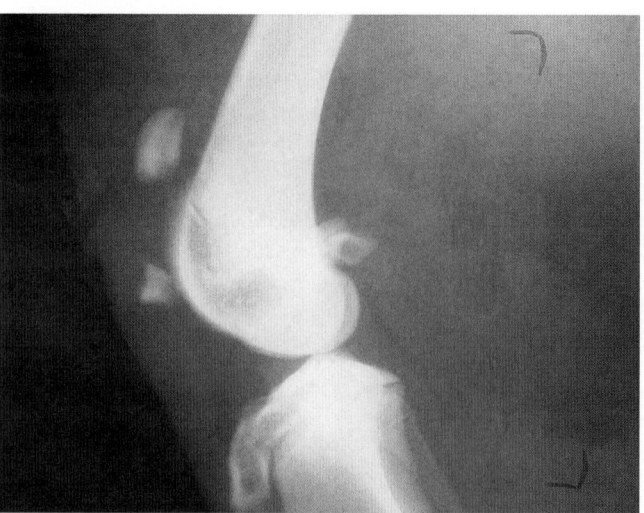

FIG. 32-98
Lateral radiograph of dog with transverse patellar fracture.

Physical Examination Findings

Animals are usually non–weight bearing on the affected limb. Palpation shows pain and swelling over the cranial surface of the stifle. Crepitation is usually not noted because the fragments separate. Palpation may detect a void in the quadriceps muscle–patellar tendon mechanism.

Diagnostic Imaging

Standard craniocaudal or caudocranial and mediolateral radiographs should be obtained (Fig. 32-98).

Laboratory Findings

Consistent laboratory abnormalities are not present.

DIFFERENTIAL DIAGNOSIS

Patellar fractures should be differentiated from lacerations or rupture of the patella tendon resulting in quadriceps insufficiency. This differentiation is made based on the radiographic appearance of the patella.

MEDICAL MANAGEMENT

Conservative management (i.e., rest or passive physical therapy) is not indicated if a transverse or comminuted fracture has separated the proximal and distal poles of the patella. Fibrous union may occur, but the stability afforded is insufficient to allow normal activity. Small fragments near the proximal or distal pole may be managed conservatively if they do not interfere with motion of the patellofemoral joint.

SURGICAL TREATMENT
Preoperative Management

The animal should be confined to a cage until surgery is performed. Analgesics should be administered to posttraumatic animals. A soft padded bandage with a lateral splint will help support the stifle.

Anesthesia

Refer to p. 944 for anesthetic management of animals with orthopedic disease.

Surgical Anatomy

The patella is the largest sesamoid in the body and is embedded within the tendons of the quadriceps muscle group. The undersurface tracks within the trochlear groove of the femur and is formed of hyaline articular cartilage. The function of the patella is twofold: (1) to maintain straight-line stability during contraction of the quadriceps muscle group and (2) to provide mechanical efficiency for the quadriceps muscle group. During surgery, care must be taken to preserve the insertions of the quadriceps tendon and patellar ligament.

Positioning

The patient is positioned in dorsal recumbency. The limb should be clipped and surgically prepped from the greater trochanter proximally to the tarsus distally. A hanging-leg preparation (see p. 34) facilitates manipulation of the limb during surgery.

SURGICAL TECHNIQUE

Make a craniolateral skin incision 1 cm lateral to the patella. Begin the incision 5 cm proximal to the patella and extend it distally to the tibial crest. Incise subcutaneous tissue overlying the patella and patellar tendon to expose the fragment ends. Place the limb in extension to reduce the fracture, then stabilize the fragments with a tension band placed over the cranial surface of the patella (Fig. 32-99). Since the patella is composed of very dense bone, predrill the holes to facilitate Kirschner wire placement.

In small dogs and cats, it may be possible to place only one Kirschner wire.

Place orthopedic wire around the Kirschner wire tips and tighten it. Visualize the articular surface of the patella to ensure anatomic reduction after tightening the wire.

Comminuted fractures are repaired with a tension band if there are two fragments large enough to stabilize. Small fragments are removed. The primary concern is restoring the integrity of the quadriceps mechanism.

SUTURE MATERIALS AND SPECIAL INSTRUMENTS

Self-retaining retractors are useful to reflect adjacent soft tissue. Orthopedic wire, small pins, a drill bit, and an air-driven or battery-operated drill are necessary for placement of the tension band.

POSTOPERATIVE CARE AND ASSESSMENT

Postoperative radiographs are made to evaluate fracture reduction and implant location. Activity should be restricted to leash walking and physical rehabilitation until the fracture has healed. Strict adherence to limited activity is mandatory

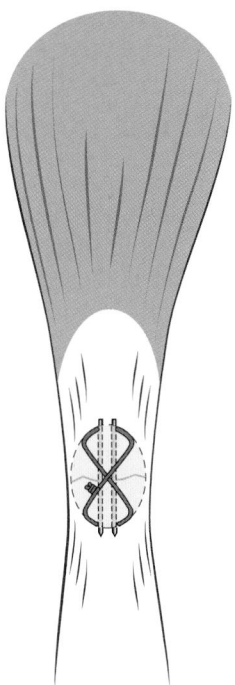

FIG. 32-99
Stabilization of transverse patellar fracture with a tension band wire. (Modified from Fossum TW: *Small animal surgery,* ed 2, St Louis, 2002, Mosby.)

because forceful contraction of the quadriceps will disrupt the repair. Physical rehabilitation encourages controlled limb use and optimal limb function after fracture healing and is especially important after fractures affecting the stifle. Care must be taken to develop customized protocols for each patient depending on location of the fracture, stability and type of fracture fixation, potential for healing, abilities and attitudes of the patient, and willingness or ability of the client to provide for the animal's care (see Chapter 12; see also Table 32-13 on p. 1117). Radiographs should be repeated at 6-week intervals until fracture healing is observed. Implants are generally not removed unless they cause a problem.

PROGNOSIS

Return to athletic function depends on adequate healing and reduction of the articular surface. Radiographic evidence of degenerative joint disease will usually develop. Functional prognosis is good to excellent if postoperative instructions are followed closely and if integrity of the patellofemoral joint is maintained.

Suggested Reading

Tomlinson J: Fractures of the patella. In Johnson AL, Houlton JEF, Vannini R, editors: *AO principles of fracture management in the dog and cat,* Thieme, NY, 2005, AO Publishing.
This chapter provides an up-to-date collection of operative techniques for stabilizing fractures of the patella in small animals. Detailed descriptions of tension band wiring techniques applicable to the patella are included.

TIBIAL AND FIBULAR DIAPHYSEAL FRACTURES

DEFINITIONS

Tibial diaphyseal fractures and **fibular diaphyseal fractures** occur as a result of trauma to the rear limb. Open fractures (with wounds through skin overlying the bone) may occur because of the sparse soft tissue coverage.

GENERAL CONSIDERATIONS AND CLINICALLY RELEVANT PATHOPHYSIOLOGY

Fractures of the tibia in dogs and cats are primarily the result of trauma, including motor vehicle trauma, gunshots, fights with other animals, and falls. Although the fibula is usually fractured as well, it is seldom stabilized unless stability of the stifle or hock is threatened. Underlying pathologic conditions (e.g., skeletal tumors) may predispose to fracture. The tibia is subject to several mechanical forces, and fractures can be avulsion fractures or transverse, oblique, spiral, comminuted, or severely comminuted. The paucity of soft tissue increases the possibility of open fractures and potentially decreases the extraosseous blood supply, both of which can delay bone healing. Minimal soft tissue coverage of bone plates results in tissue irritation and cold hypersensitivity, but is advantageous for placing a bilateral external fixator.

Because tibial fractures are most often caused by trauma, the entire animal must be evaluated to detect concurrent injuries, such as pulmonary contusions, pneumothorax, rib fractures, and traumatic myocarditis. Concurrent injuries to the limb may include extensive soft tissue damage or loss.

DIAGNOSIS
Clinical Presentation

Signalment. Any age, breed, or sex of dog or cat may be affected. Young animals more often sustain vehicular trauma.

History. Affected animals usually present with a non–weight-bearing lameness after trauma. Owners may be unaware that the trauma occurred.

Physical Examination Findings

Affected animals are usually non–weight bearing on the affected limb and have palpable swelling, crepitation, and pain at the fracture site. The fracture may be open, with or without soft tissue loss. Affected animals often appear to have abnormal proprioceptive responses because they are reluctant to move the limb.

Diagnostic Imaging

The extent of bone and soft tissue damage should be assessed on craniocaudal and lateral radiographs that include joints proximal and distal to the affected tibia. Fractious animals or those in extreme pain may require sedation (see Tables 31-2 and 31-3 on pp. 933 and 934, respectively) or general anesthetic for radiography after it has been determined that no contraindications (i.e., shock, hypotension, or severe dyspnea) to administration of sedatives or anesthetics exist. Thoracic radiography should be performed to evaluate for thoracic trauma. If bridging plate fixation is anticipated, a craniocaudal radiograph of the intact contralateral tibia is essential for accurate plate contouring.

Laboratory Findings

Complete blood count and serum chemistry evaluation should be done to evaluate the status of the animal for anesthesia and to determine if concurrent injury or damage to the renal or hepatobiliary systems exists.

DIFFERENTIAL DIAGNOSIS

Diagnosis of tibial fractures is based on physical and radiographic examination. Animals with tibial and fibular fractures should be evaluated to determine whether fractures are the result of trauma or an underlying pathologic condition (neoplasia or metabolic disease).

MEDICAL MANAGEMENT

Medical treatment of animals with tibial and fibular fractures may include analgesics (see Box 31-2 on p. 944 and Chapter 13) and antibiotics for open fractures. Conservative management of tibial and fibular diaphyseal fractures consists of splints and casts and is reserved for closed, nondisplaced, or greenstick fractures in immature animals. Cast fixation is appropriate for these fractures because the joint above and joint below the fractured bone (stifle and hock) can be immobilized and the fracture should heal rapidly.

> NOTE: Consider whether the animal will be able to bear weight on the other three limbs when choosing cast fixation.

SURGICAL TREATMENT

The decision to perform an open or a closed reduction of tibial diaphyseal fractures is made based on fracture configuration and fracture-assessment score (Box 32-16). Simple or moderately comminuted fractures with large fragments that can be anatomically reconstructed to establish the bone column are candidates for open reduction and stabilization with internal fixation, limited open reduction and external skeletal fixation, or a combination of techniques. Severely comminuted fractures that cannot be completely reconstructed are candidates for closed reduction and external skeletal fixation or open reduction and application of a bridging plate and cancellous bone autograft (see p. 962). Whether the fracture is open or closed is less important than the potential of the fracture to be anatomically reconstructed. Advantages and disadvantages of open and closed reduction need to be weighed to determine the best ap-

BOX 32-16

Decision Making for Open or Closed Reduction for Tibial Diaphyseal Fractures

Open Reduction
• Displaced reducible fractures with internal fixation

Limited Open Reduction
• Displaced reducible fractures with external skeletal fixation
• Comminuted fractures necessitating cancellous bone graft

Closed Reduction
• Nondisplaced fractures with external coaptation or external skeletal fixation
• Comminuted nonreducible fractures with external skeletal fixation

BOX 32-17

Implant Use for Fractures of the Tibial Diaphysis According to Fracture-Assessment Score (FAS)

FAS 0 to 3
• Bone plate and screws
• Bone plate and IM pin combination
• Type II external skeletal fixation
• Interlocking nail

FAS 4 to 7
• Type Ib or Type II external skeletal fixation
• Bone plate and screws
• Interlocking nail

FAS 8 to 10
• Type Ia external skeletal fixation
• IM pin and cerclage wire or external skeletal fixation
• Cast

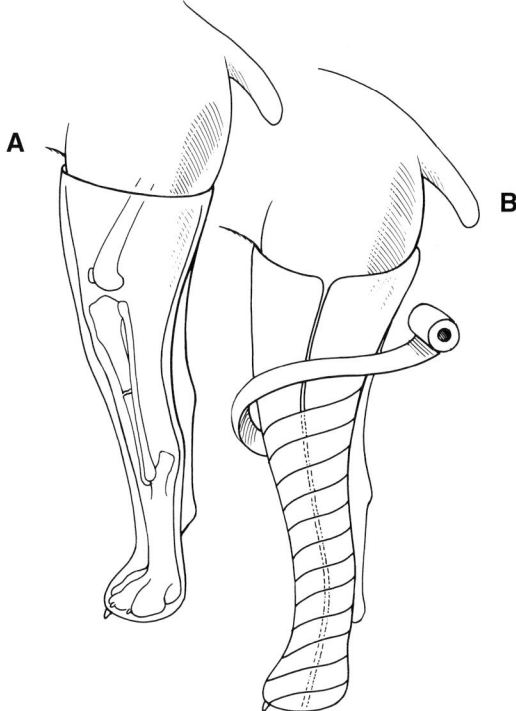

FIG. 32-100
Casts are used to stabilize closed, nondisplaced tibial-fibular fractures in patients with fracture-assessment scores of 8 to 10. **A,** Full cylinder cast, which immobilizes the stifle and hock, is placed with the limb in slight extension and varus angulation. **B,** Cast can be bivalved by placing cast material over multiple layers of padding, cutting it on the lateral and medial aspects, and securing the two halves around the limb with elastic tape.

as rigid a fixation as cylinder casts, but provide additional support with pin or plate fixation and are easily changed to allow wound treatment. The cast should be applied so that it immobilizes the stifle and hock (Fig. 32-100). Casts are applied with the limb positioned in slight extension with varus angulation.

NOTE: Be careful to avoid angular deformities when casting the limb. Placing the animal in lateral recumbency with the affected limb down during casting aids in attaining a varus position of the limb.

Application of Intramedullary Pins

IM pins can be used to stabilize tibial fractures (see p. 982). Transverse or short oblique fractures treated with an IM pin require a concurrent unilateral external fixation splint to control rotation (Fig. 32-101, *A*). Spiral or oblique fractures, in which the length of the fracture line is two to three times the diaphyseal diameter, can be treated with an IM pin and multiple cerclage wires (Fig. 32-101, *B*). Comminuted nonreducible fractures require an interlocking nail (Fig. 32-101, *C*). Correct placement of the IM pin is important to avoid

proach for each individual fracture. Fixation systems applicable to the tibial diaphysis include casts; IM pins with cerclage wire or external fixator support; interlocking nails; linear, circular, or hybrid external fixators; and bone plates (Box 32-17). The implant system chosen should reflect the fracture-assessment score (see p. 953).

Application of Casts

Casts can be applied as the sole method of fixation for stable fractures in young dogs or cats when the fracture will maintain adequate reduction and heal quickly. Greenstick or incomplete fractures of the tibia require minimal reduction. Casts that are applied over a padded bandage, cut on the lateral and medial sides, and taped together are occasionally used to support internal fixation. Bivalve casts do not offer

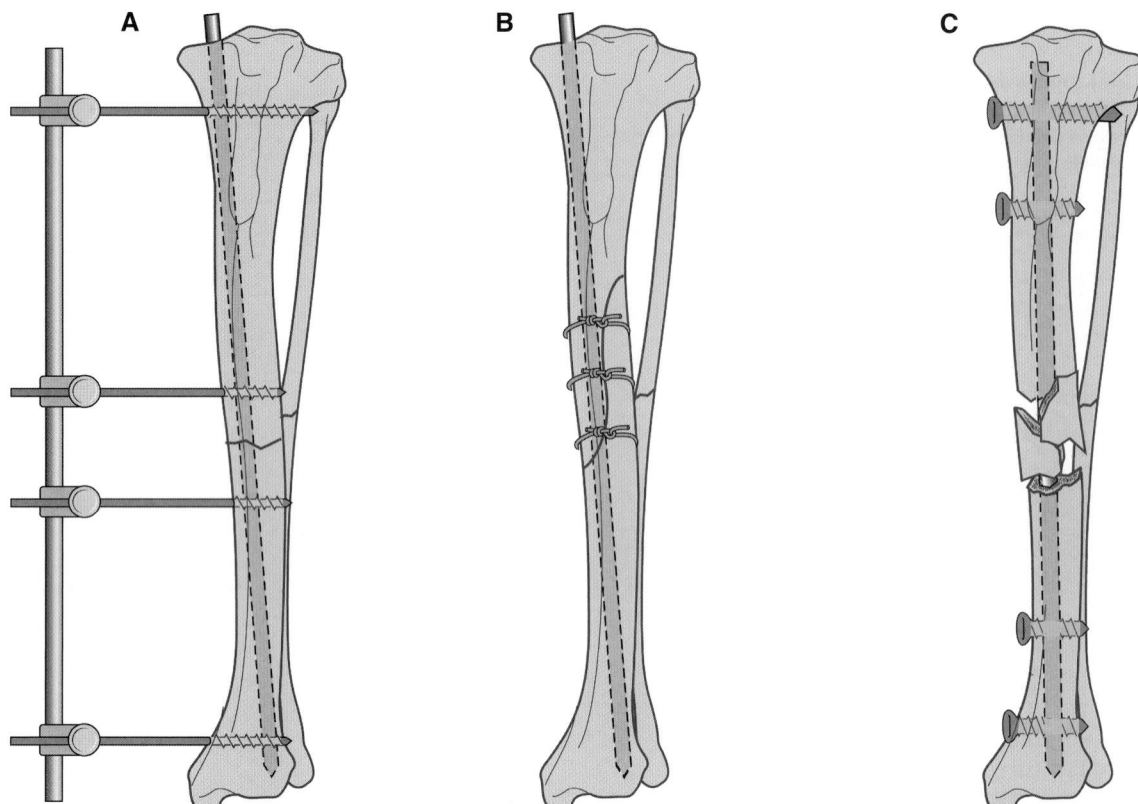

FIG. 32-101
A, Transverse or short oblique fractures may be stabilized with an IM pin and a unilateral external fixator. **B,** Spiral or oblique fractures may be treated with an IM pin and multiple cerclage wires. **C,** An interlocking nail may be used to support nonreducible fractures. (Modified from Johnson AL, Dunning D: *Atlas of orthopedic surgical procedures of the dog and cat,* ed 1, St Louis, 2005, Saunders.)

interfering with the stifle joint. Retrograde pinning techniques risk damage to intraarticular structures in dogs, and the patellar tendon in cats. The pin is inserted in a normograde manner through skin on the medial aspect of the proximal end of the tibia so that it penetrates the bone at a point midway between the tibial tubercle and the medial tibial condyle on the medial ridge of the tibial plateau (Fig. 32-102). The pin diameter should allow the pin to traverse the curve of the medullary canal without disrupting fracture reduction. To estimate the appropriate pin penetration into the distal bone segment, a second pin equal in length to that placed in the marrow cavity can be used for a point of reference. If an external skeletal fixator is used with the IM pin, the pin should be small enough so that fixation pins can be placed through the tibial diaphysis.

> NOTE: Pins must be placed in a normograde manner starting at the proximal tibia. Always manipulate the hock to ensure that the pin does not interfere with the joint.

Application of Interlocking Nails

Interlocking nails can be used to stabilize both single and comminuted tibial fractures (see p. 985). The interlocking nail provides resistance to bending, rotational, and axial loading forces and can effectively bridge a nonreducible fracture (see Fig. 32-101, *C*). An open approach is used to reconstruct reducible fractures. An "open, but don't touch" approach is used when major segment alignment is the goal. The size of nail selected should correspond to the width of the medullary canal at the isthmus of the bone. The interlocking nail is inserted in a normograde manner starting at the craniomedial aspect of the tibial plateau. A medial parapatellar approach (see p. 1263) is used to expose the point of insertion. Flexing the stifle 90 degrees facilitates nail insertion.

Application of External Skeletal Fixation

External skeletal fixation is particularly useful for treating a wide variety of tibial diaphyseal fractures. The stiffness of a fixator can be increased in animals with low fracture-assessment scores by adding fixation pins and using bilateral and biplanar frames (see p. 969). Because tibial fractures are frequently

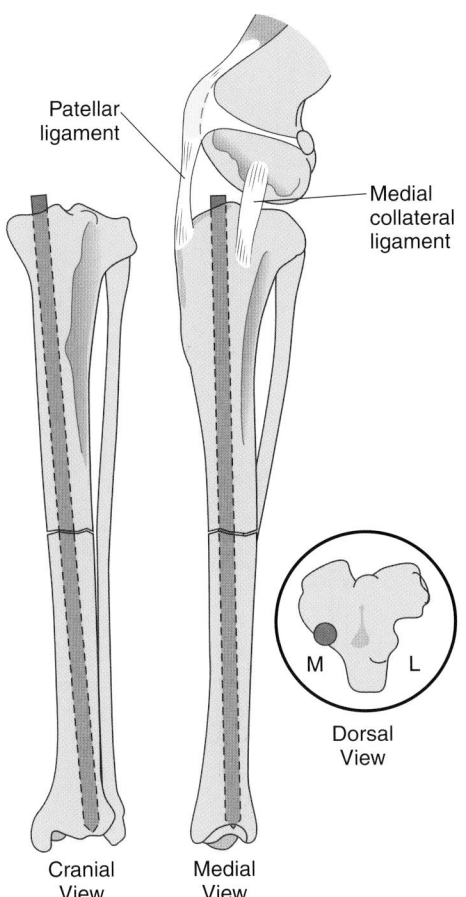

Patellar
ligament

Medial
collateral
ligament

M   L

Dorsal
View

Cranial
View

Medial
View

FIG. 32-102
Correct antegrade placement of IM pin in the tibia. Pin is inserted through skin on the medial aspect of the proximal tibia so that it penetrates bone at a point midway between the tibial tubercle and the medial tibial condyle on the medial ridge of the tibial plateau.

open, the use of external fixation is desirable to avoid invading the fracture site with metal implants. Another advantage is that removal of external fixation devices is easily accomplished. Implant removal is desirable because of the lack of soft tissue coverage and the frequency of open fractures.

Type Ia and Ib frames. For placement of Type Ia and Ib frames, the fracture is reduced using closed reduction to align nonreducible fractures or limited open reduction to accurately reduce transverse fractures and to apply cerclage wire to long oblique fractures. Type Ia external fixators are usually applied to the craniomedial surface of the tibia (Fig. 32-103, *A*). This location avoids penetration of the major muscle masses with fixation pins and thus decreases morbidity. Type Ib frames are placed cranially and medially on the tibia (Fig. 32-103, *B*). The fixator should span the length of the bone, with the most proximal and distal pins placed in the metaphyses and the central pins placed about 1 to 2 cm from the fracture line. Additional pins can be placed when there is adequate bone.

Type II frames. Penetration of major muscle masses is unavoidable with Type II external fixators, but they are often favored because of their increased stiffness and because the proximal and distal transfixation pins can be used as guide pins for limb alignment. The fixator should span the length of the bone, with the most proximal and distal pins placed in the metaphyses and the central pins placed about 1 to 2 cm from the fracture line. Additional pins can be placed when there is adequate bone.

Type II frames are placed in the following manner. The initial transfixation pins should be placed in the proximal and distal metaphyses of the tibia. These pins should be centered in the bone on the medial to lateral plane and parallel to the respective joint surfaces. Placing the proximal transfixation pin in the proximal diaphysis rather than the metaphysis will decrease pin morbidity. Severely comminuted fractures are usually reduced in a closed manner. They are restored to length using the weight of the animal in the hanging-limb position, and realigned by maneuvering the transfixation pins parallel to each other. Open reduction through a limited approach may be used to facilitate reconstruction of the bone column in single fractures. A minimal type II frame is filled out by placing at least two fixation pins (preferably three) proximal and distal to the fracture (Fig. 32-103, *C*). For the additional stiffness of a maximal Type II frame, transfixation pins that connect to both the medial and lateral bars may be placed using a guiding system (see p. 969). Postoperative radiographs should be taken to ensure that appropriate fracture reduction, pin placement, and joint alignment were achieved. Residual valgus or varus deformities can be corrected by loosening the clamps and distracting the appropriate side of the limb (Fig. 32-104). Mild rotation can be corrected by reversing the position of the clamps on the appropriate side of the pins in the distal fragment. Every effort should be made to achieve correct alignment of the limb before the procedure is completed.

Circular and hybrid external fixators. Circular external fixators may be used effectively for tibial diaphyseal fractures, especially comminuted nonreducible fractures treated with closed reduction. The fixation frame may be manipulated postoperatively to correct angular deformities in both craniocaudal and medial lateral planes. Circular fixators allow controlled axial micromotion of stabilized bone segments, promoting rapid bone union. However, circular fixators require considerable preoperative planning and frame construction to shorten surgical time, and optimal aftercare to minimize implant-related complications (see p. 975). Combining a distal ring and wires with a linear connecting rod and fixation pins placed proximally (a hybrid construct) is useful to stabilize complex tibial fractures with short distal bone segments (see p. 981).

NOTE: Do not manipulate the fragments at the comminuted fracture site.

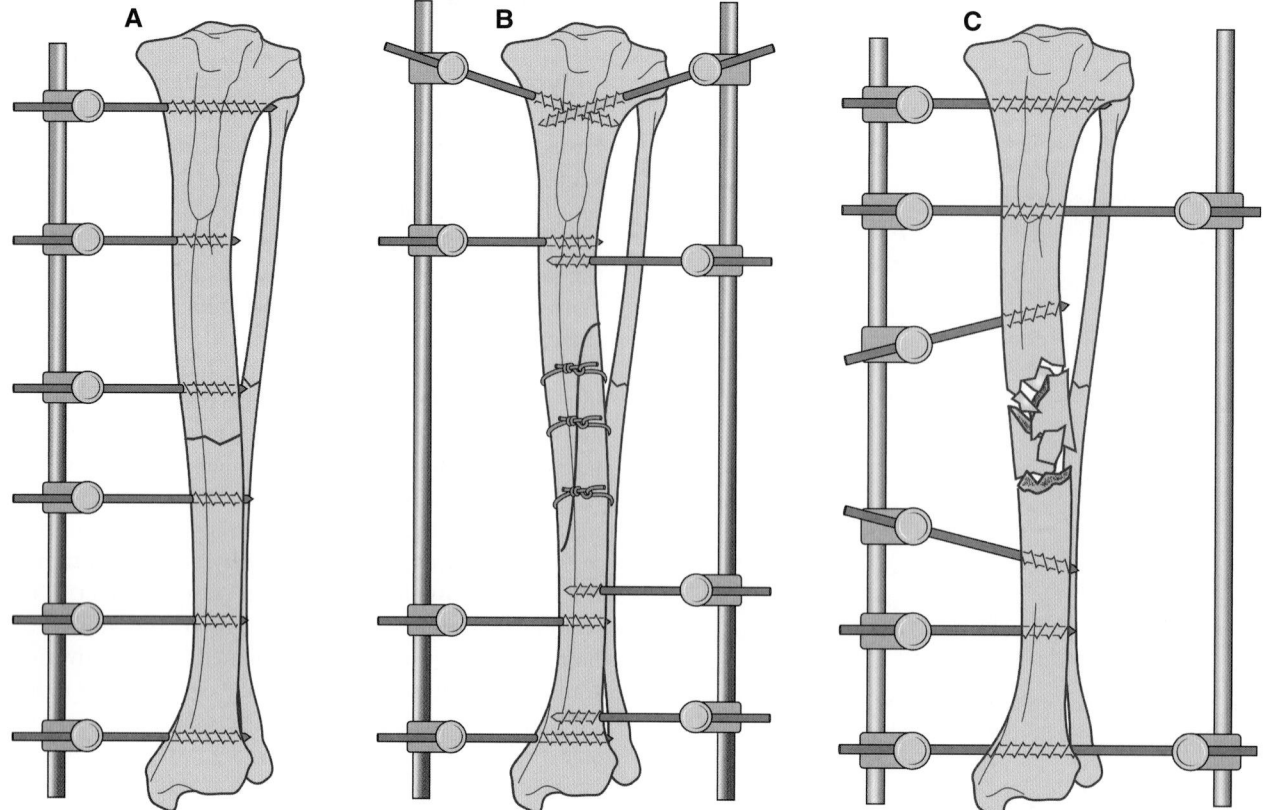

FIG. 32-103
Type Ia and Ib external fixators are used to treat tibial fractures in patients with high and moderate fracture-assessment scores. **A,** A Type I external fixator is placed on craniomedial surface of the tibia to stabilize a transverse fracture. **B,** Anatomic reconstruction of long oblique fracture with cerclage wire restores the bony column and allows load sharing with a Type Ib external fixator. **C,** Type II external fixators are used to treat patients with low fracture-assessment scores. A minimal Type II frame is constructed using unilateral fixation pins to fill out the frame. (Modified from Johnson AL, Dunning D: *Atlas of orthopedic surgical procedures of the dog and cat,* ed 1, St Louis, 2005, Saunders.)

FIG. 32-104
A, To correct a valgus angulation of the tibia, loosen the clamps distal to the fracture. Reposition the distal segment of bone by moving the clamps distally on the lateral bar and proximally on the medial bar until the joints are parallel. Reverse the procedure to correct a varus angulation. **B,** When the joints are aligned, tighten the clamps.

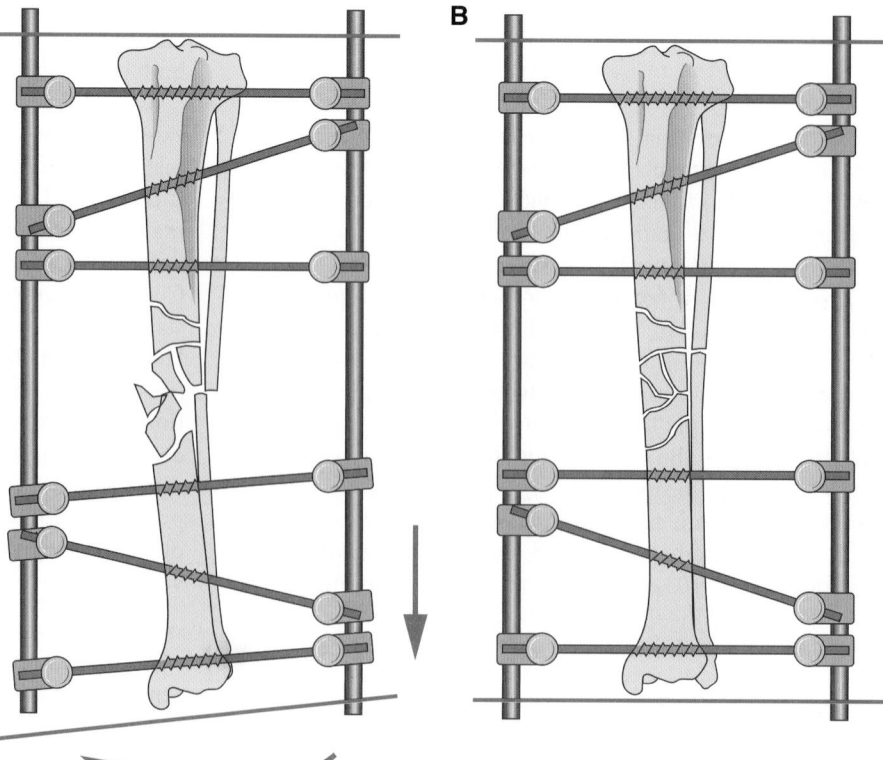

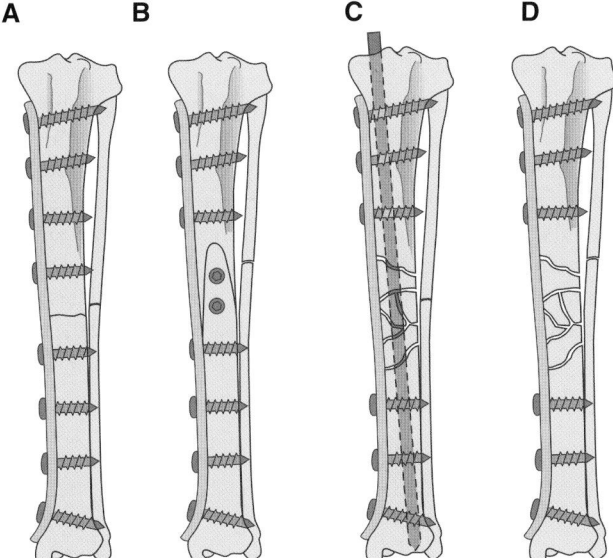

FIG. 32-105
A plate placed on the medial surface of the tibia may function as: **A,** A compression plate for transverse fractures; **B,** a neutralization plate to support long oblique fractures reconstructed with lag screws; or **C** and **D,** a bridging plate with or without an IM pin to span a nonreducible fracture.

Application of bone plates and screws. Bone plates are an excellent method of stabilizing tibial diaphyseal fractures. The plate is usually applied to the wide, flat, medial surface of the tibia. A wide exposure of the fracture and intact bone is needed for fracture reconstruction and plate application. Care must be taken to make the skin incision cranial to the position of the plate to avoid the implant irritating healing tissues. The plate is applied as a compression plate to transverse fractures. Long oblique or spiral fractures are reconstructed and the fracture lines compressed with lag screws. The reconstructed fracture is protected with a neutralization plate. Comminuted fractures that cannot be reconstructed may be treated by distracting the fracture, realigning the limb, and applying the plate in a bridging manner (attaching it to the intact bone without disturbing fragments). A plate-rod combination can also be used for comminuted fractures (Fig. 32-105). When planning the plate for a comminuted fracture, the plate should be contoured to match the craniocaudal radiographic view of the contralateral tibia.

> NOTE: Careful contouring of the plate to match the normal configuration of the tibia is essential. Failure to reproduce the normal curve of the tibia will result in valgus angulation of the limb.

If open reduction of the fractured tibia is performed, harvesting autogenous cancellous bone should be considered to enhance bone healing (see p. 962). The most accessible site for cancellous bone harvest is the ipsilateral proximal humerus. The ipsilateral ilium and tibia and the contralateral tibia can also be prepared for cancellous bone harvest.

Preoperative Management

Open wounds should be managed initially by carefully clipping surrounding hair, cleaning the wound, and obtaining a swab for bacterial culture and susceptibility testing. Cultures of open wounds should be obtained before administration of antibiotics. The limb should be temporarily stabilized with a Robert Jones bandage to immobilize the fragments, decrease or prevent soft tissue swelling, protect or prevent open wounds, and increase patient comfort until surgery can be performed (see p. 946). Analgesics should be administered to posttraumatic patients (see Box 31-2 on p. 944 and Chapter 13). Concurrent injuries should be managed before anesthetizing the animal for fracture fixation. Prophylactic antibiotics are indicated when open reduction is performed (see Chapter 10).

Anesthesia

Anesthetic management of animals with fractures is discussed on p. 944.

Surgical Anatomy

The tibial diaphysis is round in cross section and resembles an S-shaped curve when viewed from the cranial aspect. The craniomedial surface of the tibia is not covered by muscle and can be easily palpated to serve as a landmark for location of the incision. Extensor muscles on the lateral surface of the tibia and flexor muscles caudal to the tibia can be retracted to expose the bone. The medial saphenous vein crosses the medial portion of the distal tibia.

Positioning

The leg should be prepared from the hip to below the hock. If cancellous bone graft harvest is anticipated, a donor site should also be prepared. For closed reduction or limited open reduction and external skeletal fixation, the animal should be positioned with the affected leg suspended from the ceiling to improve visualization of correct joint alignment (see p. 959). If open reduction is performed, the animal should be positioned in dorsal recumbency and the limb draped out and released to expose the medial surface.

SURGICAL TECHNIQUE
Craniomedial Approach to the Tibia

Make a craniomedial skin incision parallel to the tibial crest, and extend it the entire length of the tibia (Fig. 32-106, A). Continue dissection through the fascia, avoiding the medial saphenous vein and nerve crossing the middle to distal third of the tibial diaphysis (Fig. 32-106, B).

Stabilization of Midshaft Transverse or Short Oblique Fractures

From a mechanical perspective, this fracture configuration allows load sharing between the bone and implant after surgery. Factors that negatively affect healing include multiple limb injuries and a large active patient. From a biologic per-

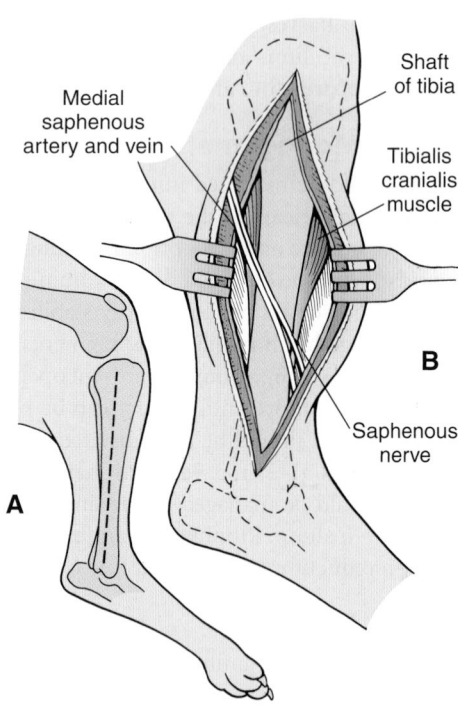

Medial
saphenous
artery and vein

Shaft
of tibia

Tibialis
cranialis
muscle

B

Saphenous
nerve

A

FIG. 32-106
A, To approach the craniomedial aspect of the tibia, make a craniomedial skin incision. Extend the incision the length of the tibia if a plate is being applied. **B,** Dissect through fascia, avoiding the medial saphenous vein and nerve crossing the middle to distal third of the tibial diaphysis.

spective, the patient's fracture-assessment score dictates whether the time until union will be lengthy or short. Older animals or those with open wounds and severe soft tissue loss will have prolonged healing requiring implants to remain functional for 8 or more weeks. In these cases, implants that purchase bone with threads are desirable; frictional-hold implants or casts are adequate for shorter healing periods. Stabilizing a reduced transverse fracture requires only rotational and bending support; bone plates, an external fixator with or without an IM pin, an interlocking nail, or a cast may be used. Stabilization of a short oblique fracture may require some axial support as well to prevent shearing during load bearing. Bone plates or external fixators should be used for these fractures. The final implant decision is based on fracture location and patient fracture assessment.

Stabilize transverse or short oblique fractures in patients with low fracture-assessment scores (0-3) with a compression plate or a maximal Type II external fixator. With a moderate fracture-assessment score (4 to 7), use a compression plate, interlocking nail, minimal Type II external skeletal fixator, or Type Ib external skeletal fixator. Stabilize transverse or short oblique fractures in patients with a high fracture-assessment score (8 to 10) with a 6-pin Type Ia external skeletal fixator, an IM pin, and a minimal Type Ia external fixator or use a cast if the fracture is greenstick or nondisplaced (Fig. 32-107).

Stabilization of Midshaft Long Oblique Fractures or Comminuted Fractures With Large Butterfly Fragment

From a mechanical perspective, these fractures can be reduced and interfragmentary compression applied with cerclage wire or lag screws. Once the interfragmentary fracture lines are reduced and compressed, the bone is able to share the loads with the implant postoperatively. Stabilization of this fracture configuration requires axial, rotational, and bending support. This can be achieved with bone plates and lag screws, interlocking nails and cerclage wire, cerclage wire or lag screw and external fixator combinations, and IM pin plus cerclage wires.

Stabilize long oblique fractures in patients with low fracture-assessment scores (0-3) by first achieving interfragmentary compression with cerclage wire or lag screws to reconstruct the cylinder of the bone; then bridge the area with a bone plate, interlocking nail, or Type II external fixator. With a moderate fracture-assessment score (4 to 7), use a neutralization plate or interlocking nail with lag screws or cerclage wire for interfragmentary compression combined with a Type II or Type Ib external fixator. Stabilize long oblique fractures in patients with a high fracture-assessment score (8 to 10) with an IM pin and cerclage wires or cerclage wires and a Type Ia external fixator (Fig. 32-108).

Stabilization of Midshaft Comminuted Fractures With Multiple Fragments

From a mechanical perspective, these fractures cannot be reduced without significant soft tissue manipulation, and there is no load sharing between the implant and bone until biologic callus forms to provide support. Therefore very high stresses will be imposed on the implant and its connection to the bone. If the biologic assessment is favorable, the imposed stresses will be of short duration, with less likelihood of implant failure. If the biologic assessment is not favorable, however, imposed stresses will act on the implant for an extended period, and implant failure is more likely. Enhancing the biologic response by indirectly reducing the fragments (closed reduction and bridging osteosynthesis) or by inserting an autogenous cancellous bone graft (with open reduction) is recommended. From a mechanical perspective, these types of fractures need rigid axial, rotational, and bending support. Stabilization can be achieved with a bridging plate and pin combination, a bridging plate, an interlocking nail, or a Type II or Type Ib external fixator.

Achieve stabilization in patients with low fracture-assessment scores (0 to 3) with a bone plate used in a bridging fashion, with or without an IM pin, an interlocking nail, or a maximal Type II external skeletal fixator. Manage patients with a moderate fracture-assessment score (4 to 7) with a bone plate functioning as a bridging plate, an interlocking nail, or a minimal Type external skeletal fixator.

A patient with this type of fracture would have a high fracture-assessment score (8 to 10) only when the biologic

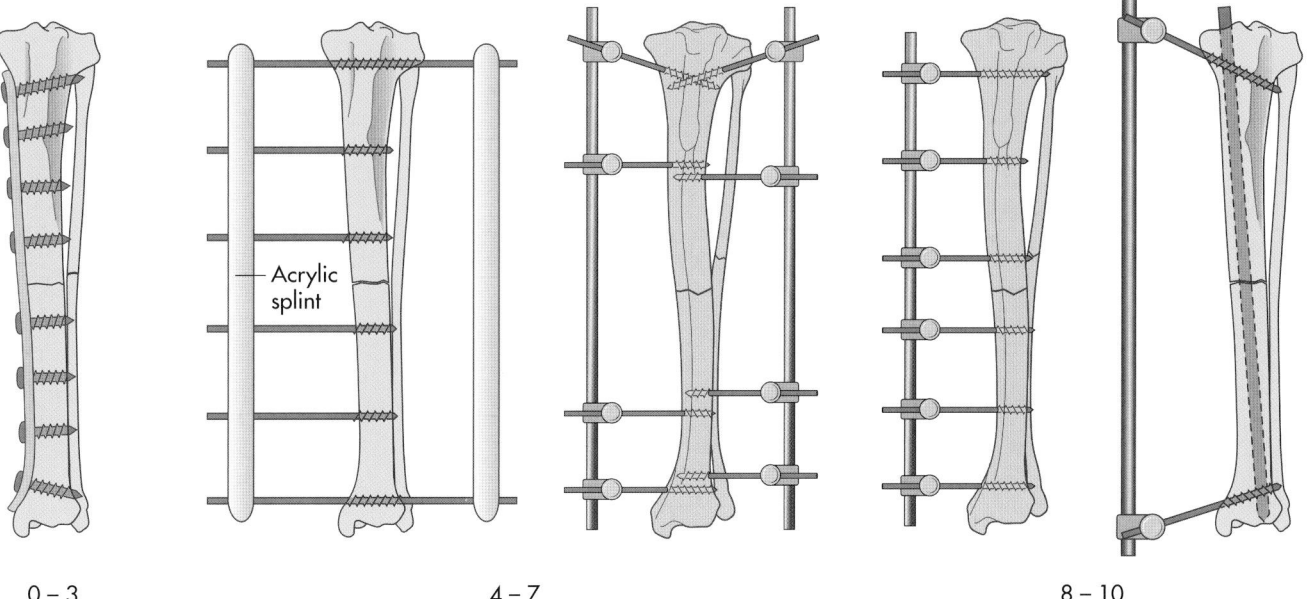

0 – 3   4 – 7   8 – 10

Acrylic
splint

FIG. 32-107
Suggested methods for stabilizing transverse or short oblique tibial fractures based on fracture-assessment score.

0 – 3   4 – 7   4 – 7   8 – 10

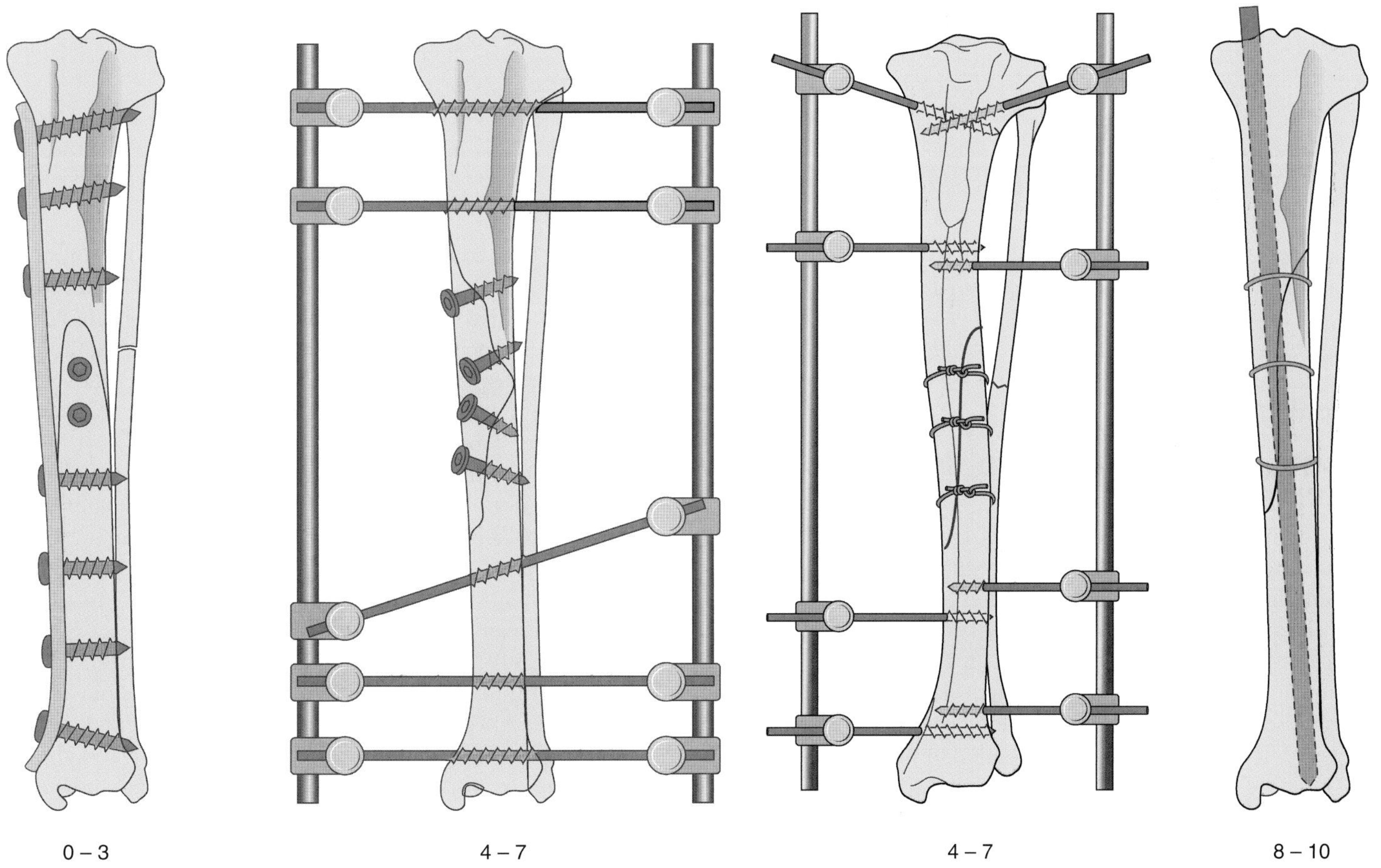

FIG. 32-108
Suggested methods for stabilizing long oblique or reducible comminuted tibial fractures based on fracture-assessment score.

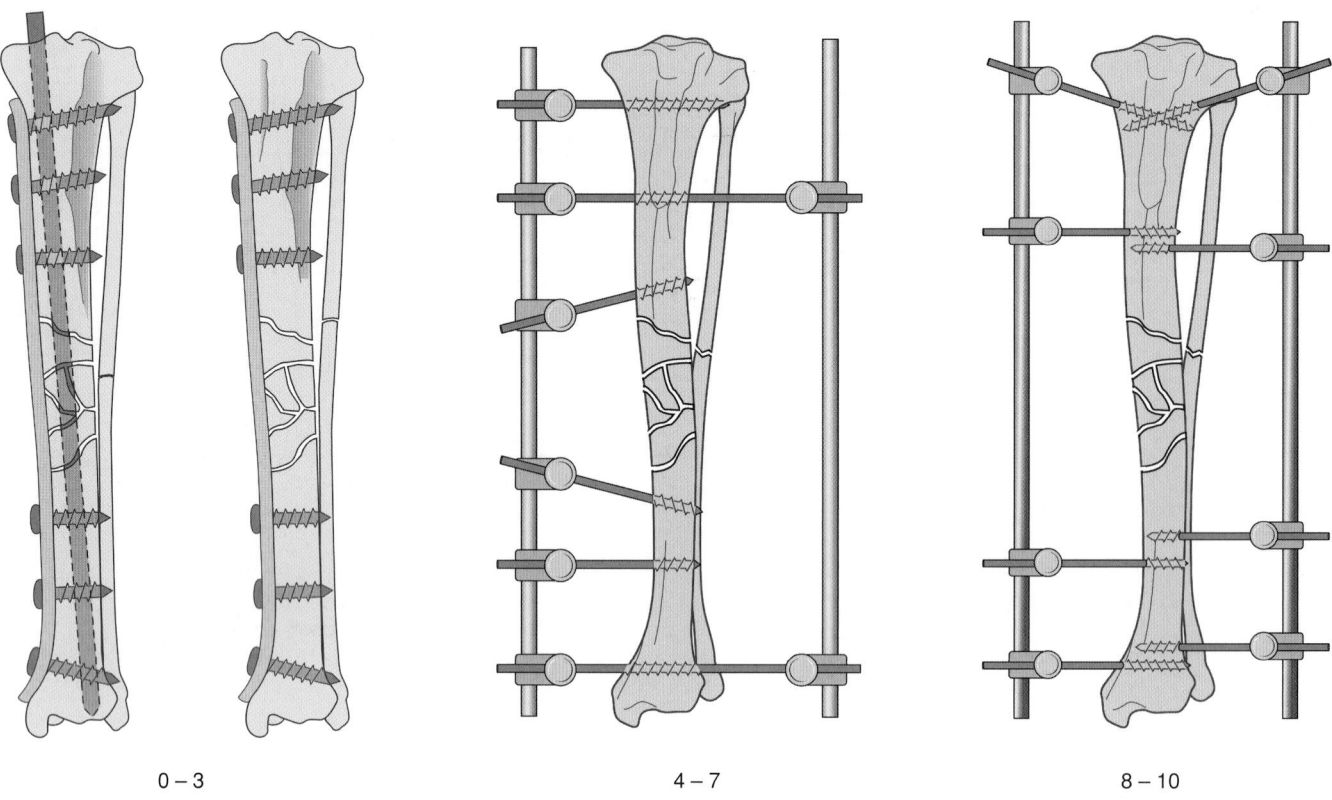

0 – 3   4 – 7   8 – 10

FIG. 32-109
Recommended methods for stabilizing nonreducible comminuted tibial fractures based on fracture-assessment score. (Modified from Fossum TW: *Small animal surgery,* ed 2, St Louis, 2002, Mosby.)

assessment is extremely favorable (e.g., 4- to 5-month-old animal with a low-velocity, closed, single-limb injury).

Consider managing such animals with indirect reduction and bridging of the fracture with a Type Ib external skeletal fixator (Fig. 32-109).

SUTURE MATERIALS AND SPECIAL INSTRUMENTS

Equipment necessary for pin and wire placement includes retractors, bone-holding forceps, reduction forceps, a Jacobs pin chuck, IM pins, Kirschner wires, orthopedic wire, wire twisters, and wire and pin cutters. Additional equipment needed for external fixation includes a low-rpm power drill and an external fixator system. Interlocking nail equipment is necessary for nail application. Plating equipment and a high-speed drill are required for application of plates and screws.

POSTOPERATIVE CARE AND ASSESSMENT

Postoperative radiographs should be made to document fracture reduction or alignment and implant position. Activity should be restricted to leash walking and physical rehabilitation until the fracture has healed. Physical rehabilitation (see Chapter 12) encourages controlled limb use and optimal limb function after fracture healing. Care must be taken to develop customized protocols for each patient depending on location of the fracture, stability and type of fracture fixation, potential for healing, abilities and attitudes of the patient, and willingness or ability of the client to provide for the animal's care (see Tables 32-7 and 32-8 on p. 1067).

Casts require intensive management by owners and frequent evaluations by the veterinarian. Abrasions and wounds often are caused by pressure from the cast. Management involves removal of the cast or replacement with a bivalve cast and wound treatment. Early destabilization of the fracture to treat wounds can delay healing.

After open reduction with external skeletal fixation, the incision should be covered, but the fixation splint may be left exposed. Alternatively, gauze sponges are opened and stuffed to fill the space between the fixation bar and the skin around the pins, then secured in place with a bandage around the fixator. Care should be taken to bandage the paw as well during the immediate postoperative period to prevent swelling. Open wounds should be treated daily with wet to dry dressings until a granulation bed has formed. Wounds are then covered with a nonadhesive pad and the bandage changed as necessary. Daily hydrotherapy aids in cleaning open wounds, reduces postoperative swelling, and cleans pin sites. The animal should be released to the owner with instructions to limit exercise and prevent fixator snares. If the external fixator bandage is maintained, it should be changed weekly. If a bandage is not used, daily hydrotherapy can be administered with a hand-held shower massage. Checkups should be scheduled at 2 weeks for suture removal and fixator evaluation and every 6 weeks for radiographic evaluation.

Although a rigidly stabilized fracture site is optimal for initial bone formation, subsequent bone remodeling is enhanced by increasing the load through the fractured bone. Removal of one half of a Type Ib external fixator (converting to a Type Ia frame) or removing selected transfixation pins from a Type I or Type II frame decreases rigidity of the fixator, allowing more load on the remodeling bone while still protecting the healing fracture. Destabilization is usually done at 6 weeks after surgery, depending on the fracture assessment. Early bone formation and bridging of the fracture site should be radiographically evident before destabilization is done. The external fixation splint can be removed completely when there is radiographic evidence of complete bone bridging of the fracture lines. A support bandage or a splint may be used to protect the healing bone for a few weeks after fixator removal.

After placement of a plate on a diaphyseal fracture, the limb should be supported for a few days with a soft padded bandage to reduce swelling. The animal will usually be fully weight bearing within 2 to 3 weeks. Confinement is recommended until there are radiographic signs of bone union. Plate removal may be necessary after bone union because tissue irritation and cold sensitivity have been associated with the minimal soft tissue coverage over the plate. IM pins are removed after the fracture has healed, but interlocking nails may be left in place unless implant-related complications occur.

COMPLICATIONS

Complications with tibial fractures after open reduction include osteomyelitis, implant migration resulting in soft tissue irritation, malunion, delayed union, and nonunion. Cats treated with rigid external fixators may be at risk for delayed healing or nonunion. Complications encountered with external fixation of the tibia include pin loosening and pin tract drainage.

PROGNOSIS

The prognosis is generally good after tibial fracture repairs. Occasionally, with external fixation, pin loosening and pin tract drainage are severe enough to warrant removal or replacement of the pin before fracture healing.

Suggested Reading

Dudley M, Johnson AL, Olmstead ML et al: Open reduction and bone plate stabilization compared with closed reduction and external fixation for treatment of comminuted tibial fractures: 47 cases (1980-1995), *J Am Vet Med Assoc* 211:1008, 1997.

This paper provides a comparison of the outcomes of open reductions and plate stabilization with the biologic technique of closed reduction and external fixator stabilization. Plate fixation resulted in more major complications, whereas external fixator application was faster and had more minor complications.

Dueland RT, Johnson KA, Roe SC et al: Interlocking nail treatment of diaphyseal long bone fractures in dogs, *J Am Vet Med Assoc* 214:59, 1999.

This paper provides the results of a multicenter prospective evaluation of a large population of animals with fractures treated with the interlocking nail. The high success rate and low complication rate suggest that the interlocking nail can be used to stabilize diaphyseal fractures in dogs. Good technique is necessary for optimal results.

Farese JP, Lewis DD, Cross AR et al: Use of IMEX SK-Circular external fixator hybrid for fracture stabilization in dogs and cats, *J Am Anim Hosp Assoc* 38:279, 2002.

This article provides a description of the use of SK-Circular hybrids to stabilize long-bone fractures (two femoral, one humeral, and three tibial fractures) with short distal bone segments in three dogs and three cats. Although three cases required surgical revision, animals ambulated well and all fractures obtained union.

Nolte DM, Fusco JV, Peterson ME: Incidence of and predisposing factors for nonunion of fractures involving the appendicular skeleton in cats: 18 cases (1998-2002), *J Am Vet Med Assoc* 226:77, 2005.

This article provides a unique overview of the most common sites of and possible predisposing factors for nonunions in cats. Results suggest that in cats, fractures involving the tibia and proximal portion of the ulna are more likely to develop nonunions. Use of excessively large and rigid type II external skeletal fixators may be associated with development of nonunions.

Payne J, McLaughlin R, Silvermnan E: Comparison of normograde and retrograde intramedullary pinning of feline tibias, *J Am Anim Hosp Assoc* 41:56, 2005.

This article provides an evaluation of the effects of two techniques for inserting pins into feline tibias on soft tissue structures of the stifle. Retrograde pin placement injured the patellar tendon.

Reems MR, Beale BS, Hulse DA: Use of a plate-rod construct and principles of biological osteosynthesis for repair of diaphyseal fractures in dogs and cats: 47 cases (1994-2001), *J Am Vet Med Assoc* 223:330, 2003.

This article provides a report of the application of the plate rod technique for stabilizing humeral, femoral, and tibial fractures. Clinical application and outcomes are discussed.

Schwarz G: Fractures of the tibial diaphysis. In Johnson AL, Houlton JEF, Vannini R, editors: *AO principles of fracture management in the dog and cat*, Thieme, NY, 2005, AO Publishing.

This chapter provides an up-to-date collection of operative techniques for stabilizing tibial fractures in small animals. Detailed descriptions of IM pin and wire techniques, external fixator application, and bone-plating procedures are included.

TIBIAL AND FIBULAR METAPHYSEAL AND ARTICULAR FRACTURES

DEFINITIONS

Metaphyseal fractures and **epiphyseal fractures** occur in trabecular bone. Articular fractures disrupt the joint surface.

GENERAL CONSIDERATIONS AND CLINICALLY RELEVANT PATHOPHYSIOLOGY

Fractures of the proximal tibial metaphysis and epiphysis occur infrequently in mature dogs and cats. These fractures are usually transverse or short oblique in nature, but may be comminuted as a result of severe trauma, such as a gunshot. Fractures of the distal tibia in mature animals usually involve the malleoli, either as fractures of the malleoli or as erosion injuries that remove the malleoli. Loss of malleolar stability results in loss of collateral ligament function and talocrural instability. Accurate alignment of the articular surface of malleolar fractures and rigid fixation of the fragment are necessary to achieve joint stability and decrease subsequent development of degenerative joint disease.

DIAGNOSIS

Clinical Presentation

Signalment. Any age, breed, or sex of dog or cat may be affected. Young animals more frequently sustain vehicular trauma.

History. Affected animals usually have a non–weight-bearing lameness after trauma.

Physical Examination Findings

Because of the traumatic nature of these tibial and fibular fractures, the entire animal must be assessed to detect abnormalities of other body systems. Palpation of the limb may reveal swelling, pain, crepitation, and instability of the adjacent joint. There may be a sharing injury of the tarsus (see p. 1302) associated with fracture of the distal tibia. Although no major nerves are in the immediate area, dogs often appear to have abnormal proprioceptive responses because they are reluctant to move the limb.

Diagnostic Imaging

The extent of bone and of soft tissue damage should be assessed on craniocaudal and lateral radiographs that include joints proximal and distal to the affected tibia. Stress radiographs may demonstrate abnormal laxity of the tarsal joints or motion of the proximal tibial epiphysis associated with the fracture. Fractious animals or those in extreme pain may require sedation (see Tables 31-2 and 31-3 on pp. 933 and 934, respectively) or general anesthesia after it has been determined that no contraindications (shock, hypotension, severe dyspnea) to administration of sedatives or anesthetics exist. Thoracic radiography should be performed to evaluate for thoracic trauma.

Laboratory Findings

Complete blood count and serum chemistry evaluation should be done to evaluate the status of the animal for anesthesia and to determine if concurrent injury to the renal or hepatobiliary systems exists.

DIFFERENTIAL DIAGNOSIS

Animals brought in with proximal or distal tibial fractures should be evaluated to determine whether the fractures are caused by trauma or by an underlying pathologic condition (neoplasia, metabolic disease). Joint luxations can be differentiated from fractures radiographically.

MEDICAL MANAGEMENT

Medical treatment of animals with tibial and fibular metaphyseal and epiphyseal fractures includes analgesics (see Box 31-2 on p. 944 and Chapter 13) and administration of antibiotics to treat open fractures (see p. 86). Nondisplaced proximal fractures may be treated with a cast.

SURGICAL TREATMENT

Simple proximal tibial metaphyseal ulnar fractures may be treated with IM pins and Steinmann pins or Kirschner wires placed as crossed pins. Comminuted tibial plateau fractures are best treated with buttress plate application. Cancellous bone autograft is used to augment the repair and speed healing. Articular fractures require anatomic reduction and stabilization with a lag screw or plate. Malleolar fractures require tension band wire techniques to resist the pull of the collateral ligaments. Animals with unstable degloving injuries to the hock are treated by reestablishing the stability to the hock with an external fixator or synthetic ligament and bivalve cast coupled with appropriate wound management (see p. 1163).

Preoperative Management

There may be extensive damage and loss of tissue in the area of the fracture. Open wounds should be managed initially by carefully clipping surrounding hair, cleaning the wound, and taking a culture for microbial sensitivity testing from deep tissue. The tibia should be temporarily stabilized with a Robert Jones bandage (see p. 946) to immobilize fragments, decrease or prevent soft tissue swelling, protect or prevent open wounds, and increase patient comfort until surgery can be performed. Concurrent injuries should be managed before anesthetic induction for fracture fixation.

Anesthesia

Anesthetic management of animals with fractures is discussed on p. 946.

Surgical Anatomy

The medial aspect of the proximal tibia is covered only with skin and subcutaneous tissue and can easily be palpated and approached. The saphenous nerve lies caudal to the medial surface of the proximal tibia. The lateral aspect of the tibia and fibula is covered by the cranial tibial muscle, and the tendon of the long digital extensor muscle is visible. The lateral collateral ligament attaches from the lateral femoral condyle to the fibular head and stabilizes the stifle. The peroneal nerve and popliteal artery lie caudal to the fibular head.

The medial malleolus of the distal tibia and lateral malleolus of the fibula extend distal to the articulating surfaces of the distal tibia and talus. The long and short parts of the medial collateral ligaments arise from the medial malleolus. The long and short parts of the lateral collateral ligaments arise from the lateral malleolus. These ligaments are essential for hock stability. Tendons of the cranial tibial and long digital extensor muscles cross the cranial surface of the distal tibia. The medial saphenous vein crosses the medial surface of the distal tibia.

Positioning

The limb should be prepared from the hip to below the hock. If cancellous bone graft harvest is anticipated, a donor site should be prepared (ipsilateral proximal tibia or proximal humerus). The animal should be positioned in lateral or dorsal recumbency and the limb draped out for proximal tibial and fibular fractures. The animal is positioned in dorsal recumbency for treatment of distal tibial and fibular fractures.

SURGICAL TECHNIQUE
Surgical Approach to the Proximal Tibia

The craniomedial approach to the tibia (see p. 1132) is extended proximally to include the metaphysis. The lateral approach to the stifle (see p. 1263) is used to expose the fibular head for stabilization.

Surgical Approach to the Distal Tibia

Extend the craniomedial approach to the tibia (see p. 1132) approach distally to expose the medial malleolus. The lateral malleolus via a lateral skin incision over the malleolus, with blunt and sharp dissection of surrounding tissue to expose the bone.

Stabilization of Proximal Tibial Fractures

Fractures of the proximal tibial metaphysis may be stabilized with a cast if the fracture can be reduced closed, is stable, and will heal rapidly (fracture-assessment score of 8 to 10).

Refer to p. 967 for general casting techniques and p. 1127 for application of a cast to the tibia. If open reduction is necessary, stabilize transverse or short oblique proximal tibial fractures with IM pins as described for diaphyseal fractures of the tibia (see p. 1127). If the fracture is not rotationally stable, angle a Kirschner wire across the fracture line. Place a figure-eight orthopedic wire around both ends of the Kirschner wire to provide compression to the fracture line (Fig. 32-110, A).

These fractures can also be stabilized with crossed pins.

Reduce the fracture and drive a Kirschner wire from the lateral surface of the tibial epiphysis across the fracture and into the tibial metaphysis, exiting the medial cortex. Drive a second wire from the medial tibial epiphysis across the fracture and into the metaphysis, exiting the lateral cortex. Take care to avoid penetrating the articular surface.

Alternatively, the Kirschner wires may be driven from the metaphysis to the epiphysis (Fig. 32-110, *B*). Additional external support may be required for dogs with moderate fracture-assessment scores.

Comminuted tibial plateau fractures must be supported to prevent collapse of the tibial plateau.

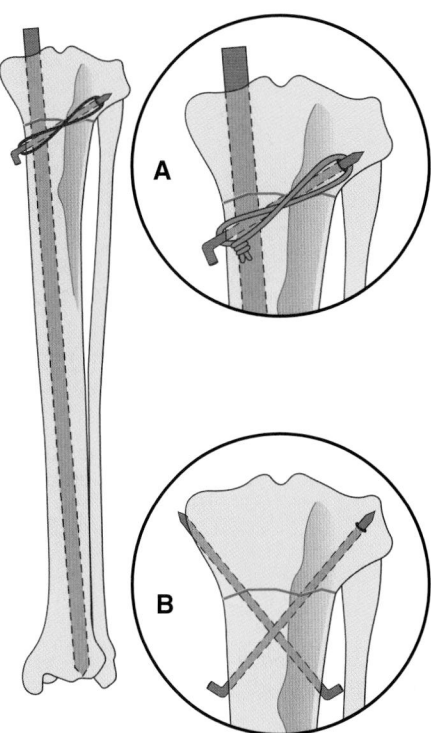

FIG. 32-110
Simple single fractures of the proximal tibial metaphysis in dogs with high fracture assessment scores can be stabilized with an IM pin. **A,** Kirschner wire and figure-eight orthopedic wire may be added for rotational stability. **B,** Crossed Kirschner wires may also be used.

Apply a bone plate functioning as a buttress plate to the medial side of the proximal tibia. If there is bone loss on the lateral side of the proximal tibia, consider adding a Type Ia external fixator to support the tibial plateau. Add cancellous bone autograft to any defects. Support the repair as necessary with a splint or a transarticular external fixator.

Stabilization of Malleolar Fractures

Fractures of the malleoli are usually treated with open reduction and internal fixation with a tension band wiring technique; however, a bone screw functioning as a lag screw can also be used if the fracture-assessment score is low and the fragment is large enough (Fig. 32-111, *A* and *B*). Additional external fixation or coaptation is used as necessary to support the internal fixation device.

Application of tension band. *Reduce the fracture (medial malleolus of tibia or lateral malleolus of fibula), and start two Kirschner wires in the fragment. Drive the wires across the fracture line to lodge in the major bone segment. Place a transverse drill hole in the major bone segment, pass a figure-eight wire through the hole and around the Kirschner wire, and tighten it (Fig 32-111, C).*

Application of lag screws. *For the medial malleolus, reduce the fracture and drill a gliding hole (equal to the di-*

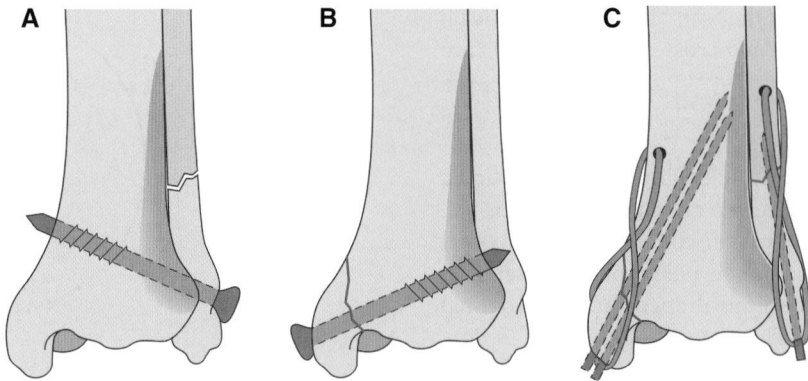

FIG. 32-111
A and **B,** Fractures of the tibial and fibular malleoli can be repaired with a lag screw.
C, Tension band wires can be used in patients with high fracture-assessment scores.

ameter of the threads on the screw) in the malleolar frag-
ment. Place an insert drill sleeve into the gliding hole, and
drill a smaller hole (equal to the core diameter of the screw)
across the tibia. Measure, tap, and select and place the
appropriate-length screw. Compression of the fracture should
occur (see Fig. 32-111, A and B and p. 994 for lag screw
techniques). When stabilizing the proximal or distal fibula
to the tibia, the fibula is treated as the fragment by drilling
the gliding hole through the fibula and the tapped hole in
the tibia.

SUTURE MATERIALS AND SPECIAL INSTRUMENTS

Instruments needed include a high-speed power drill, equipment for lag screws, Kirschner wires, IM pins, orthopedic wire, wire twisters, wire cutters, and reduction forceps. Bone-plating equipment is needed for buttress plate application.

POSTOPERATIVE CARE AND ASSESSMENT

Postoperative radiographs should be made to document fracture reduction or alignment and implant position. Postoperative pain management is indicated (see Box 31-2 on p. 944 and Chapter 13). After internal fixation, a soft padded bandage should be applied for a few days to control swelling and support soft tissue. Active dogs may require a splint for 3 to 6 weeks to protect distal tibial implants. Physical rehabilitation (see Chapter 12) encourages controlled limb use and optimal tarsal function after fracture healing. Care must be taken to develop customized protocols for each patient depending on location of the fracture, stability and type of fracture fixation, potential for healing, abilities and attitudes of the patient, and willingness and ability of the client to provide for the animal's care (see Table 32-13). Physical rehabilitation for patients with fractures supported by splints for 6 weeks generally begins after the splint has been removed (see Table 32-9). Open wounds are treated daily with wet to dry dressings until a granulation bed

has formed. The wounds are then covered with a nonadhesive pad, and the bandage is changed as needed. Daily hydrotherapy aids in cleaning open wounds and reducing postoperative swelling. Rechecks should be scheduled at 2 weeks for suture removal and every 6 weeks for radiographic evaluation. Implant removal may be necessary after bone healing if the implants interfere with or irritate soft tissue.

COMPLICATIONS

Possible complications include malunion, which may cause incongruities in joint and limb alignment. Fractures that involve the articular surface predispose the joint to development of degenerative joint disease. Malalignment of articular fractures routinely causes degenerative joint disease.

PROGNOSIS

Metaphyseal fractures usually heal quickly because of the large amounts of cancellous bone surrounding the fracture. In general, trabecular bone heals with minimal callus formation (see p. 1004).

Suggested Reading

Schwarz G: Fractures of the proximal tibia. In Johnson AL, Houlton JEF, Vannini R, editors: *AO principles of fracture management in the dog and cat,* Thieme, NY, 2005, AO Publishing.
This chapter provides an up-to-date collection of operative techniques for stabilizing fractures of the proximal tibia in small animals. Detailed descriptions of tension band wiring techniques, Kirschner wire application, and plating techniques are included.
Schwarz G: Fractures of the distal tibia and malleoli. In Johnson AL, Houlton JEF, Vannini R, editors: *AO principles of fracture management in the dog and cat,* Thieme, NY, 2005, AO Publishing.
This chapter provides an up-to-date collection of operative techniques for stabilizing fractures of the distal tibia in small animals. Detailed descriptions of tension band wiring techniques and Kirschner wire application are included.

TIBIAL AND FIBULAR PHYSEAL FRACTURES

DEFINITIONS

Physeal fractures may occur through the cartilaginous growth plate of the proximal or distal tibia or tibial tuberosity in immature animals. Physeal fractures are also called *epiphyseal plate fractures* or *slipped physes*.

GENERAL CONSIDERATIONS AND CLINICALLY RELEVANT PATHOPHYSIOLOGY

The cartilaginous physis is weaker than surrounding bone and ligaments, making it more susceptible to injury (see p. 1004). The Salter-Harris classification is used to categorize physeal fractures on the basis of radiographic and histologic appearance (see p. 951). Tibial physeal fractures may or may not be displaced. Proximal tibial physeal fractures are usually Salter I or II fractures, although rarely Salter III or IV fractures occur. With Salter I or II fractures and concurrent fracture of the fibula, the epiphysis may be displaced caudolateral to the tibial diaphysis, and additional injury to collateral ligaments may occur. Open reduction and internal fixation is usually required to restore normal anatomy. Distal tibial physeal fractures are also usually Salter I or II fractures.

DIAGNOSIS
Clinical Presentation

Signalment. These fractures occur in immature dogs or cats with open physes.

History. Affected animals usually have a non–weight-bearing lameness after trauma. Owners may be unaware that trauma occurred.

Physical Examination Findings

Because of the traumatic nature of physeal fractures, the entire animal must be assessed to detect abnormalities of other body systems. Palpation of the limb may reveal swelling, pain, crepitation, and instability of the adjacent joint. Dogs often appear to have abnormal proprioceptive responses because they are reluctant to move the limb.

Diagnostic Imaging

Craniocaudal and lateral radiographs of the affected tibia and fibula (which include the proximal and distal joints) are required to diagnose Salter I to Salter IV fractures. With minimally displaced fractures, it may be difficult to determine if the normally radiolucent physis is really fractured. Comparison radiographs of the opposite limb are often beneficial, particularly with tibial tuberosity avulsions. Fractious animals or those in extreme pain may require sedation (see Tables 31-2 and 31-3 on pp. 933 and 934, respectively) or general anesthetic for radiography after it has been determined that no contraindications (i.e., shock, hypotension, or severe dyspnea) to administration of sedatives or anesthetics exist. Thoracic radiography should be performed to evaluate for thoracic trauma.

> NOTE: Radiographs made at the time of injury do not provide information about crushing injuries to the physis or damage to the physeal blood supply. Therefore it is difficult to give an accurate prognosis for growth with these fractures at the time of injury.

Laboratory Findings

Complete blood count and serum chemistry evaluation should be done to evaluate the status of the animal for anesthesia and to determine if concurrent injury or damage of the renal or hepatobiliary systems exists.

DIFFERENTIAL DIAGNOSIS

Physeal fractures can be differentiated from joint luxations or soft tissue trauma radiographically.

MEDICAL MANAGEMENT

Medical treatment of animals with tibial physeal fractures may include analgesics (see Box 31-2 on p. 933 and Chapter 13) and antibiotics to treat open fractures (see p. 86). Nondisplaced or minimally displaced tibial physeal fractures may be adequately stabilized with a cast.

SURGICAL TREATMENT

Most physeal fractures are classified as having assessment scores of 8 to 10 because affected animals are young and physeal fractures heal quickly (see p. 953). Therefore the implant system chosen need not function for a long time. Surgical treatment of displaced physeal fractures consists of anatomic reduction and stabilization with Kirschner wires or small pins that are smooth so as not to interfere with physeal function. Pins placed perpendicular to the physis allow growth more readily than pins placed obliquely and anchored in cortical bone (cross-pinning technique). In animals that are close to maturity, threaded implants may be used to compress the fractured physis.

> NOTE: Use smooth implants when crossing the physis in animals with potential growth.

Preoperative Management

The rear limb should be temporarily stabilized with a Robert Jones bandage (see p. 946) to immobilize fragments, decrease or prevent soft tissue swelling, protect or prevent open wounds, and increase patient comfort until surgery can be performed. Concurrent injuries should be managed before anesthetic induction for fracture fixation. Analgesics are indicated for posttraumatic patients (see Box 31-2 on p. 933 and Chapter 13)

Anesthesia

Anesthetic management of animals with fractures is discussed on p. 944.

Surgical Anatomy

Surgical anatomy of the tibia and fibula is provided on p. 936.

Positioning

The limb should be prepped from hip to below the hock. The animal is positioned in dorsal recumbency and the limb draped out for physeal fractures of the tibia.

SURGICAL TECHNIQUE
Surgical Approach to the Craniomedial Tibia

Use a proximal extension of the craniomedial approach to the tibia (see p. 1131) for proximal tibial physeal fractures and tibial tuberosity avulsions.

Surgical Approach to the Distal Physis

Approach distal physeal fractures with a distal extension of the craniomedial approach to the tibia or with a cranial skin incision and retraction of the extensor tendons.

Stabilization of Nondisplaced Fractures

Treat nondisplaced physeal fractures with closed reduction and a cast that immobilizes the stifle and the hock (see Figs. 32-112 and 32-100).

Casts applied to the tibia should reach from the toes to above the stifle. The stifle should be extended to reduce proximal tibial physeal fractures during cast application. The limb should be held in slight extension with the hock in slight varus for distal tibial physeal fractures while the cast hardens.

Stabilization of Displaced Fractures

Displaced fractures require a surgical approach and gentle reduction to restore physeal alignment. Crossed Kirschner wires or Steinmann pins may be used to stabilize tibial physeal fractures.

To stabilize proximal tibial physeal fractures, drive one Kirschner wire from the lateral surface of the tibial epiphysis across the physis, into the tibial metaphysis, and through the medial cortex. Drive the second wire from the medial tibial epiphysis across the physis, into the metaphysis, and through the lateral cortex (Fig. 32-113).

A third wire may be driven from the tibial tuberosity into the metaphysis for additional stabilization.

To stabilize distal tibial physeal fractures, drive a Kirschner wire from the medial malleolus across the physis and into the lateral metaphysis. Drive the second wire from the lateral epiphysis or the lateral malleolus across the physis and into the metaphysis. Seat both pins in the cortex of the metaphysis (see Fig. 32-113).

Stabilization of Avulsion Fractures of the Tibial Tuberosity

Fractures through the physis of the tibial tuberosity result in proximal displacement of the tuberosity and must be reduced and stabilized to restore quadriceps muscle function and stifle extension. Occasionally, closed reduction through sufficiently extending the stifle realigns the tubercle. The

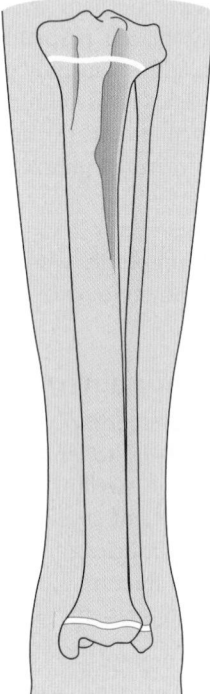

FIG. 32-112
Nondisplaced tibial physeal fractures can be stabilized with a cast.

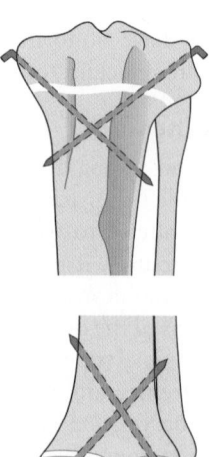

FIG. 32-113
Displaced tibial physeal fractures can be treated with open reduction and placement of crossed Kirschner wires.

limb can then be cast in extension for 2 to 3 weeks. If open reduction is necessary to reduce the tuberosity, then the fracture should be stabilized with Kirschner wires with or without a tension band wire.

Reduce the tibial tuberosity and drive two Kirschner wires across the physis to lodge in the proximal tibia. Check the repair to determine if stabilization is sufficient to prevent avulsion of the fracture; if not, place a tension band wire even though it may prevent physeal growth. To place a tension band wire, drill a transverse hole in the major bone segment, pass a figure-eight wire through the hole and around the Kirschner wire, and tighten the wire (Fig. 32-114; see p. 990).

SUTURE MATERIALS AND SPECIAL INSTRUMENTS

Kirschner wires, Steinmann pins, orthopedic wire, wire twisters, wire cutters, and reduction forceps are needed.

POSTOPERATIVE CARE AND ASSESSMENT

Postoperative radiographs should be made to document fracture reduction and implant position. After internal fixation, a soft padded bandage should be applied for a few days to control swelling and support soft tissue. Activity should be restricted to leash walking and physical rehabilitation until the fracture has healed. Physical rehabilitation (see Chapter 12) encourages controlled limb use and optimal joint function after fracture healing. Care must be taken to develop customized protocols for each patient depending on location of the fracture, stability and type of fracture fixation, potential for healing, abilities and attitudes of the patient, and willingness or ability of the client to provide for the animal's care (see Tables 32-9 and 32-13). Rechecks should be scheduled at 2 weeks for suture removal and at 4 to 6 weeks for radiographic evaluation of fracture healing. Radiographs of the injured bone and the contralateral bone can be made and compared for length as early as 2 to 3 weeks after the injury to determine physeal function. Cartilage physes that heal in a manner allowing continued function appear radiographically as a lucent line. Additionally, increased bone length should be apparent. If the physeal line appears as a bone density, endochondral ossification has occurred and continued physeal function is likely. Implant removal is indicated after physeal healing (4 weeks) to allow bone growth (if the physis is functional after the trauma). Three to 4 weeks postoperatively, the tension band wires used to stabilize the tibial tuberosity are removed to encourage physeal function and to prevent deformity.

PROGNOSIS

Although the prognosis for healing of a physeal fracture is excellent, the prognosis for continued function or growth of the physis depends on the amount of damage sustained by the zone of proliferating cells. The prognosis is good for future physeal growth after a fracture that separates the cartilaginous physis at the zone of hypertrophied cells. The prognosis is poor for future physeal growth after trauma that crushes the physis. Unfortunately, most trauma-induced physeal fractures sustain damage to the growing cells and have a guarded prognosis for growth. Although the tibia and fibula are a paired bone system, premature closure of the proximal or distal tibial physis usually results in a short but straight limb, for which the animal compensates by extending the stifle. Caudal malalignment of the proximal tibial epiphysis may result in increased tibial plateau angle. Premature closure of the tibial tuberosity physis can alter the conformation of the proximal tibia and result in impaired function and degenerative joint disease of the stifle.

Suggested Reading

Clements DM, Gemmill T, Corr SA et al: Fracture of the proximal tibial epiphysis and tuberosity in 10 dogs, *J Small Anim Pract* 44:355, 2003.

This article provides an evaluation of outcomes of conservative and operative treatment of fractures of the tibial tuberosity and proximal physis. All dogs regained full limb usage, regardless of the method of treatment chosen.

Johnson JM, Johnson AL, Eurell JA: Histological appearance of naturally occurring canine physeal fractures, *Vet Surg* 23:81, 1994.

This article provides a description of the histologic appearance of physeal fractures occurring after trauma. Despite the radiographic Salter Harris classifications, the fracture lines involved all areas of the physis including the growing cells.

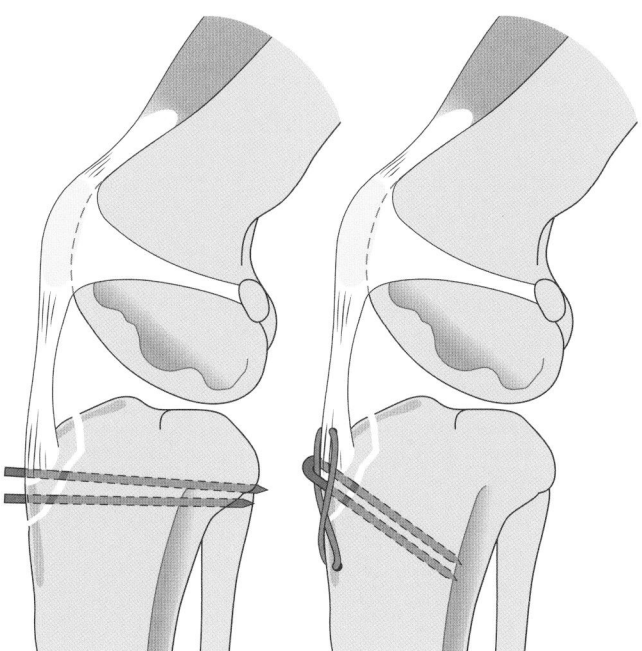

FIG. 32-114
Avulsions of the tibial tuberosity can be reduced and stabilized with two Kirschner wires. If displacement of the fragment occurs when the stifle is flexed, a figure-eight orthopedic wire may be added.

Schwarz G: Fractures of the proximal tibia. In Johnson AL, Houlton JEF, Vannini R, editors: *AO principles of fracture management in the dog and cat,* Thieme, NY, 2005, AO Publishing.
This chapter provides an up-to-date collection of operative techniques for stabilizing fractures of the proximal tibia in small animals. Detailed descriptions of tension band wiring techniques, Kirschner wire application, and plating techniques are included.

Schwarz G: Fractures of the distal tibia and malleoli. In Johnson AL, Houlton JEF, Vannini R, editors: *AO principles of fracture management in the dog and cat,* Thieme, NY, 2005, AO Publishing.
This chapter provides an up-to-date collection of operative techniques for stabilizing fractures of the distal tibia in small animals. Detailed descriptions of tension band wiring techniques and Kirschner wire application are included.

CHAPTER 33
Diseases of the Joints

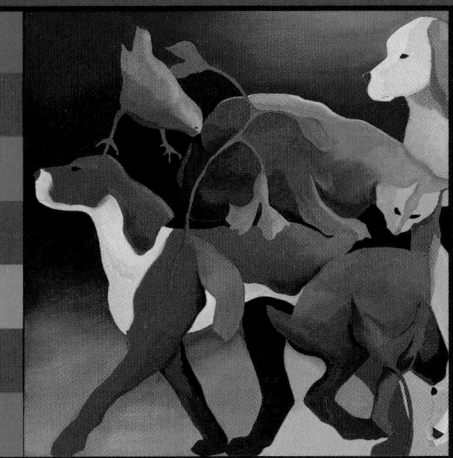

GENERAL PRINCIPLES AND TECHNIQUES

DEFINITIONS

Arthropathies are diseases that affect joints. **Arthritis** is the term used to denote inflammatory joint changes, whereas **arthrosis** denotes noninflammatory joint disease. **Polyarthritis** is inflammation that simultaneously affects several joints. **Osteoarthritis** or **osteoarthrosis** is a primarily noninflammatory degenerative joint disease (DJD) characterized by articular cartilage degeneration, marginal bone hypertrophy, and synovial membrane changes. **Ankylosis** is the end result of DJD or inflammatory diseases, in which the joint is fused after new bone production.

Synovial joints (e.g., shoulder joint, hip, or stifle) are lined with **synovial membrane** and allow for relatively free movement. Components of **fibrous** (i.e., skull and tooth sockets) and **cartilaginous** (i.e., mandibular symphysis and growth plates) **joints** are connected with fibrous tissue or cartilage, respectively; therefore these joints allow for little or no movement. **Arthroscopy** is the use of an endoscope to examine and treat joints. **Arthrotomy** is the surgical exposure of a joint. **Arthroplasty** is revision of a joint structure. **Arthrodesis** is surgical treatment leading to joint fusion.

GENERAL CONSIDERATIONS

Diagnosis and treatment of joint disorders are important aspects of veterinary orthopedic practice. Many joint diseases are managed medically rather than surgically, and a basic knowledge of nonsurgical joint diseases is necessary to differentiate surgical and nonsurgical joint disease and prescribe appropriate therapy. Knowledge of normal joint structure and function, the joint's response to injury, and treatment of joint diseases also is essential to selection of appropriate treatment regimens and accurate prognostication.

The common arthropathies of dogs and cats generally are categorized as inflammatory or noninflammatory (Box 33-1). Inflammatory arthropathies are further classified as infectious or noninfectious. Noninfectious arthropathies may be erosive or nonerosive. The common noninflammatory arthropathies in dogs and cats are DJD, which is often

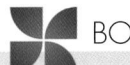 BOX 33-1

Classification of Arthropathies in Dogs and Cats

Inflammatory

Infectious

Bacteria
Rickettsiae
Spirochetes
Fungi
Mycoplasmas
Protozoa

Noninfectious

Erosive
Rheumatoid arthritis
Feline chronic progressive polyarthritis
Erosive polyarthritis of greyhounds
Periosteal proliferative arthropathy

Nonerosive
Idiopathic immune-mediated polyarthritis
Chronic inflammatory-induced polyarthritis
Plasmacytic-lymphocytic synovitis
Systemic lupus erythematosus

Noninflammatory

Dysplasia
Degenerative joint disease
Trauma
Neoplasia

due to dysplasia (e.g., hip or elbow dysplasia) or cranial cruciate ligament (CCL) rupture and those resulting from trauma or neoplasia. Numerous etiologic agents have been associated with infectious arthropathies in dogs and cats, including bacteria, spirochetes *(Borrelia burgdorferi)*, rickettsiae *(Ehrlichia* spp., *Rickettsia rickettsii)*, mycoplasmas, fungi, caliciviruses (cats), bacterial L-forms (cats), and protozoa. Nonerosive, noninfectious arthropathies include idiopathic immune-mediated nonerosive polyarthritis, chronic inflammatory-induced polyarthritis, plasmacytic-lymphocytic synovitis, and arthritis associated with systemic disease (i.e.,

1143

systemic lupus erythematosus [SLE]). Erosive, or deforming, arthropathies include rheumatoid arthritis, feline chronic progressive polyarthritis, erosive polyarthritis of greyhounds, and periosteal proliferative arthropathy. The pathophysiologies of the most commonly diagnosed arthropathies are discussed individually in this chapter (see later discussion). Further information about arthropathies may also be found in most medical texts.

DIAGNOSIS OF JOINT DISEASES
Clinical Presentation

History and clinical presentation of joint disease vary depending on the arthropathy (see sections on various arthropathies in this chapter). Dogs are typically presented with either acute or chronic histories of varying degrees of lameness. Joint disease affects dogs of all breeds, age, and size. Osteoarthritis, the most frequently diagnosed arthropathy, is estimated to affect 20% of dogs over 1 year of age. Cats are either affected less often or joint disease often goes unrecognized in this species. Importantly, there is growing evidence that feline osteoarthritis is much more common than previously reported.

Physical Examination Findings

Dogs show varying degrees of lameness associated with arthropathies. Muscular asymmetry (between limbs) and joint enlargement may be palpable. Abnormalities in range of motion, instability, pain, and crepitation during joint manipulations may be noted. For a more complete discussion of physical examination findings, see the sections on individual joints in this chapter.

Diagnostic Imaging

Survey radiography is an important and common method of screening affected joints; however, changes with many diseases may be similar and therefore radiography may be nonspecific. Radiographic findings in affected joints include proliferative or erosive bone lesions, increased joint fluid, and adjacent soft tissue changes. Radiographic findings help guide clinicians to a definitive diagnosis (Table 33-1); however, absence of radiographic changes does not ensure that the joint is normal. Radiography is particularly insensitive to mild to moderate disease affecting articular cartilage.

Cross-sectional imaging (i.e., computed tomography [CT] and magnetic resonance imaging [MRI]) is being more commonly used in evaluation of joint diseases. Both CT and MRI are superior to radiography because they enable visualization of joint structures without superimposition of overlying structures. CT is particularly useful for evaluating bony changes and is often helpful for identifying joint incongruities and fragmentation in osteoarthritic joints. MRI is widely used in the diagnosis of human joint disease and is increasingly being investigated for use in small animal joint disease. The primary indication for MRI is evaluation of soft tissue structures surrounding diseased joints. Cartilage of small animals is thin, which limits the usefulness of most MRI magnets for diagnosis of cartilage disease. Ultrasonography may also be used to evaluate intraarticular and extraarticular

 Table 33-1

Radiographic Findings of Arthropathies in Dogs and Cats

CATEGORIZATION*	RADIOGRAPHIC CHANGES
Inflammatory	
Infectious	Subchondral bone may be sclerotic or lytic ± periarticular bone formation ± joint space narrowing ± joint capsule distention and adjacent soft tissue swelling
Noninfectious	**Nonerosive** Soft tissue swelling and joint capsule distention without bony changes; multiple joints affected **Erosive** Joint space collapse; subchondral destruction; periosteal new bone formation along with soft tissue swelling; multiple joints affected
Noninflammatory	
Degenerative joint disease	Soft tissue swelling and intracapsular distention; diminished joint space, periarticular osteophytosis; subchondral bone plate, usually intact, but may be sclerotic
Trauma	Depends upon the trauma (i.e., fracture, luxation, etc). Ultimately, may lead to degenerative joint disease
Neoplasia	Soft tissue swelling and intracapsular distention; destruction of the subchondral bone plate (often on both sides of the joint) with aggressive bone proliferation

*Detection of these signs is dependent upon stage of the disease, type of disease, and joint(s) affected.

soft tissue structures, particularly in the canine shoulder. Bone scintigraphy (bone scan) has been used extensively in small animal orthopedics for localization of joint disease and screening for bone tumors. Although this technique is extremely sensitive in its detection of bone abnormalities, it is not specific.

Laboratory Findings

Synovial fluid often is evaluated to help differentiate between arthropathies. Cytologic findings range from normal to the presence of phagocytic mononuclear cells, nondegenerative neutrophils, or degenerative neutrophils plus organisms. Cytologic findings may help make a definitive diagnosis (Table 33-2) or may localize disease, but are typically nonspecific.

Synovial fluid collection. Joint taps to obtain synovial fluid are an essential technique for obtaining information to differentiate arthropathies. Sedation or general anesthesia is recommended, especially if the animal is fractious (see p. 933). Equipment needed includes sterile gloves, 25-gauge needles, 22-gauge 1½-inch needles (for shoulder, elbow, and stifle joints in larger dogs), 3-inch needles (for the hip joint), and 3-ml syringes. Only a small amount of fluid is needed to determine viscosity, estimated cell count, and differential cell count, and for culture.

Synovial fluid aspirates commonly show no bacterial growth when cultured directly on blood agar plates. More reliable results are obtained if the synovial fluid sample is incubated for 24 hours in a blood culture medium or specific enrichment broth before culturing onto blood agar plates.

Select the joint or joints that are swollen for initial taps. Clip the appropriate area over the joint, and prepare the site for *an aseptic procedure (Fig. 33-1). Use a gloved hand to palpate landmarks. Insert a needle attached to a syringe into the joint. Apply gentle suction to the syringe. After the fluid has been collected, release the negative pressure on the syringe and withdraw the needle. If blood appears in the syringe, withdraw the syringe immediately; contamination with blood can alter cell counts. If only a few drops of fluid are obtained (common in small dogs and cats), spray the material directly onto a slide and examine it cytologically. Estimate viscosity as the fluid drops from the needle to the slide.*

Normal joint fluid is viscous and forms a long string.

Place a drop of fluid on a slide and make a smear for an estimated complete cell count and a differential cell count. Culture fluid for bacterial and mycoplasmal growth. If you obtain an extremely small amount of fluid, spray the droplets from the needle onto a slide for cytology. Next, aseptically aspirate an appropriate culture broth (e.g., Trypticase soy broth from a blood culture vial) with the needle and syringe. Rinse the barrel of the syringe and hub of the needle with the culture medium, and then inject this culture medium into a blood culture vial with the same medium.

> NOTE: Not all joints with arthritis have large volumes of joint fluid. If you can only retrieve a very small amount of fluid, it is still important to do both cytology and culture. Spray the joint fluid onto a slide for cytologic evaluation and then rinse the syringe with bacterial culture medium and place the fluid in a blood culture vial for culture as described above.

DIFFERENTIAL DIAGNOSIS

Differential diagnoses include all of the noninflammatory and inflammatory arthropathies (see Box 33-1). The definitive diagnosis is made by evaluating the animal's history, clinical signs, radiographic findings (see Table 33-1), results of other imaging modalities, and joint cytology (see Table 33-2).

MEDICAL MANAGEMENT

Medical management of specific arthropathies is provided in the later discussion of specific diseases. Specific therapies may include antibiotics based on culture and susceptibility testing and immunosuppressive medications for immune-mediated joint disease. Regardless of cause, for virtually all joint diseases, there are five basic principles of medical management (Box 33-2).

Principle 1: Weight Management

All patients with joint disease except those with additional medical diseases that require specific dietary management can benefit significantly from proper body weight management. Excessive body weight places increased loads on joints and thereby exacerbates concurrent joint disease. Excessive

 Table 33-2

Cytologic Findings With Arthropathies in Dogs and Cats

SYNOVIAL FLUID FINDINGS	ARTHROPATHIES
Phagocytic mononuclear cells	Degenerative joint disease
Nondegenerative neutrophils	Systemic lupus erythematosus (SLE) Feline chronic progressive polyarthropathy Plasmacytic-lymphocytic synovitis Idiopathic immune-mediated nonerosive polyarthritis Chronic inflammatory-induced polyarthritis Rheumatoid arthritis Feline chronic progressive polyarthropathy
Degenerative neutrophils	Bacterial arthritis Rickettsial or spirochetal polyarthritis

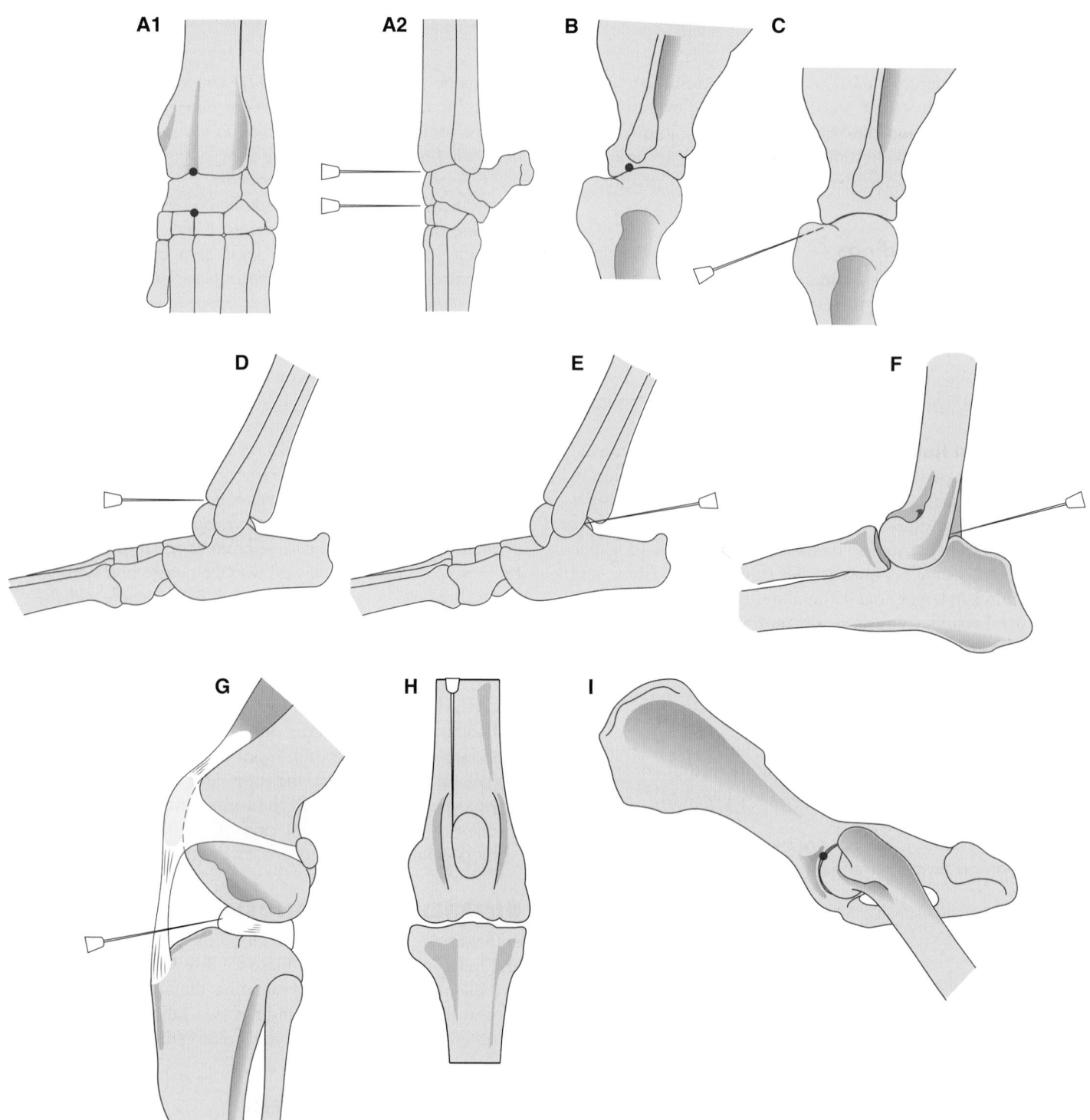

FIG. 33-1

Synovial fluid collection; recommended sites for arthrocentesis in dogs and cats. **A1** and **A2,** *Carpus:* Partly flex the joint. Palpate and enter the craniomedial aspect of the middle carpal or radiocarpal space. **B,** *Shoulder (lateral approach):* Insert the needle just distal to the acromion process. **C,** *Shoulder (cranial approach):* Insert the needle just medial to the greater tubercle and ventral to the supraglenoid tubercle of the scapula. **D,** *Hock (anterior approach):* Palpate the space between the tibia and tibiotarsal bone on the craniolateral surface of the hock; insert the needle in the shallow palpable space. **E,** *Hock (lateral approach):* Partly flex the joint and insert the needle under the lateral malleolus of the fibula. **F,** *Elbow:* Insert the needle just medial to the lateral epicondylar ridge, proximal to the olecranon process. Advance parallel to the olecranon process into the olecranon fossa. **G,** *Stifle (lateral approach):* Insert the needle just lateral to the straight patellar ligament and distal to the patella. **H,** *Stifle (dorsal approach):* Insert the needle just dorsal to the patella so it passes between the patella and trochlear groove of the femur. **I,** *Coxofemoral joint:* Abduct and medially rotate the limb. Insert the needle dorsal to the greater trochanter and angle ventrally and caudally.

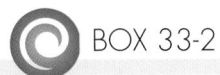 BOX 33-2

Five Principles of Medical Management of Osteoarthritis

Body weight management
Nutritional supplementation
Exercise moderation
Physical therapy
Antiinflammatory medication

body weight accelerates degeneration of joints with DJD and has been demonstrated to exacerbate clinical signs of osteoarthritis. Excessive body weight also exacerbates signs of dysplastic diseases (e.g., hip dysplasia). Current evidence suggests that proper body weight management can lessen and delay clinical signs of osteoarthritis and decrease the need for antiinflammatory medication and surgery (Kealy et al, 2002).

Recommended body condition scores (BCS) for dogs are 4.5 on a 1 to 9 scale (Table 33-3) and 2.5 on a 1 to 5 scale. Each BCS level above the target level of the 1 to 9 scale represents 10% excess body weight. Typical weight reduction programs aim to decrease body weight by 1% to 2% per week until the target BCS is attained. Simplified diet plans recommend feeding 80% to 100% of the caloric resting energy requirements (RER = 70 × [kg of body weight]$^{0.75}$) for the targeted body weight. When calculating the daily caloric intake, it is critical that all food, including treats, be included.

> NOTE: Although numerous diet programs are available for the reduction of body weight in cats and dogs, studies suggest that the most important element is repeated body weight evaluation and follow-up with a veterinarian. The importance of counseling and guiding owners in managing their pet's body weight cannot be overemphasized.

Principle 2: Nutritional Supplementation

Omega-3 fatty acids. Omega-3 fatty acids are nutritional supplements added to canine diets specifically for management of joint disease. They may be added to commercial foods or the owner may supplement them. They are antiinflammatory when given at the correct dosage and work by replacing arachidonic acid (AA) in cell walls with eicosapentaenoic acid (EPA). Replacing AA with EPA decreases pain and inflammation associated with joint injury or osteoarthritis. Omega-3 fatty acids may also help ease inflammation by blocking some of the genes that cause inflammation in osteoarthritic joints.

Studies in dogs suggest that omega-3 fatty acids can ease the pain of osteoarthritis. In one study, about 80% of the dogs studied showed improved function when they were fed diets that included omega-3 fatty acids (Cross et al, 2004). It has also been shown in both humans and dogs that including omega-3 fatty acids in the diet can decrease the need for non-

steroidal antiinflammatory drugs (NSAIDs) (Allen, 2004). Fatty-acid supplements rarely cause gastrointestinal problems, although sometimes dog owners claim that the supplement has given their dog "fishy-smelling breath." Omega-3 fatty acids appear to be safe.

Slow-acting, disease-modifying osteoarthritis agents. Alternative therapies for managing osteoarthritis focus on administering chondroprotective agents to slow cartilage degradation and promote cartilage matrix synthesis. Oral chondroprotective supplements are reported to provide supraphysiologic amounts of glucosamine and chondroitin sulfate to the joints to act as precursors for synthesis of hyaline cartilage matrix. These compounds appear to be safe; they cross the gastrointestinal-blood barrier intact when administered orally and may modify pain associated with osteoarthritis. Evidence regarding effectiveness of these products is anecdotal. Chondrotoin sulfate may provide a protective effect with chemically induced synovitis and cranial cruciate disease in dogs.

Pentosan polysulfate, isolated from beechwood hemicellulose, appears to provide protection against cartilage damage. When given once a week (3 mg/kg SC) it may relieve clinical signs associated with canine chronic osteoarthritis. Although not derived from animal sources, the compound preserves proteoglycan content and stimulates hyaluronic acid synthesis. Pentosan polysulfate may also increase bleeding times.

Principle 3: Exercise Moderation

Exercise moderation is critical to proper management of joint disease. The type and degree of exercise moderation depend upon the stage of the disease, time relative to surgery (if any), and function of the pet. Specific recommendations for exercise moderation for each disease are provided later in the discussion.

Principle 4: Physical Rehabilitation Therapy

Rehabilitation therapy can provide tremendous benefits in the management of small animal joint disease, particularly in dogs (see Chapter 12). The primary targets of physical therapy are strengthening, endurance, and range of motion. Specific recommendations for physical therapy are described in the section on the specific joint diseases.

> NOTE: The science of exercise moderation and rehabilitation therapy is expanding rapidly. Veterinarians are encouraged to consult with experts in the field and their publications for optimum therapy and rehabilitation of patients with joint disease.

Principle 5: Nonsteroidal Antiinflammatory Drug Therapy and Other Medical Therapies

NSAIDs. Medical management of DJD often includes therapy with NSAIDs. NSAIDs reduce pro-inflammatory mediators (e.g., thromboxanes, prostaglandins, prostacyclin, and oxygen radicals) by inhibiting cyclooxygenase 1 and 2 (COX-1 and COX-2) pathways. Inhibiting COX-1 inhibits normal

⌘ TABLE 33-3

Body Condition Score Table Using 1 Through 9 Categorization

▦ Nestlé PURINA
BODY CONDITION SYSTEM

TOO THIN

1 Ribs, lumbar vertebrae, pelvic bones and all bony prominences evident from a distance. No discernible body fat. Obvious loss of muscle mass.

2 Ribs, lumbar vertebrae and pelvic bones easily visible. No palpable fat. Some evidence of other bony prominence. Minimal loss of muscle mass.

3 Ribs easily palpated and may be visible with no palpable fat. Tops of lumbar vertebrae visible. Pelvic bones becoming prominent. Obvious waist and abdominal tuck.

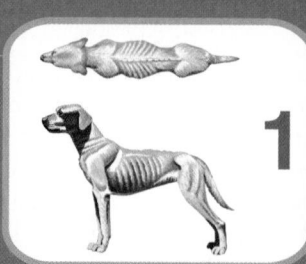

IDEAL

4 **Ribs easily palpable, with minimal fat covering. Waist easily noted, viewed from above. Abdominal tuck evident.**

5 **Ribs palpable without excess fat covering. Waist observed behind ribs when viewed from above. Abdomen tucked up when viewed from side.**

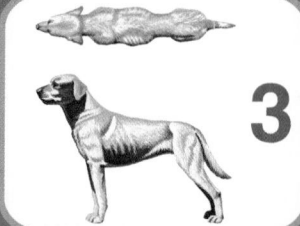

TOO HEAVY

6 Ribs palpable with slight excess fat covering. Waist is discernible viewed from above but is not prominent. Abdominal tuck apparent.

7 Ribs palpable with difficulty; heavy fat cover. Noticeable fat deposits over lumbar area and base of tail. Waist absent or barely visible. Abdominal tuck may be present.

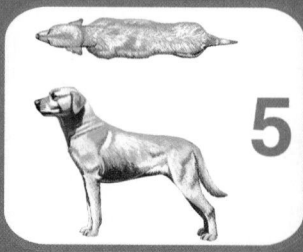

8 Ribs not palpable under very heavy fat cover, or palpable only with significant pressure. Heavy fat deposits over lumbar area and base of tail. Waist absent. No abdominal tuck. Obvious abdominal distention may be present.

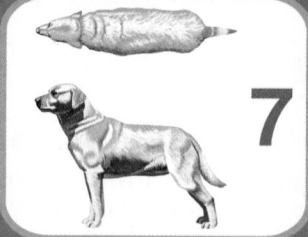

9 Massive fat deposits over thorax, spine and base of tail. Waist and abdominal tuck absent. Fat deposits on neck and limbs. Obvious abdominal distention.

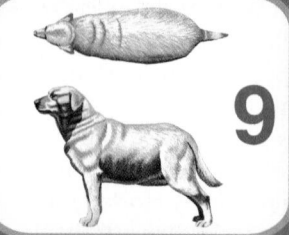

The **BODY CONDITION SYSTEM** was developed at the Nestlé Purina Pet Care Center and has been validated as documented in the following publications:

Mawby D, Bartges JW, Moyers T, et. al. *Comparison of body fat estimates by dual-energy x-ray absorptiometry and deuterium oxide dilution in client owned dogs. Compendium 2001; 23 (9A): 70*

Laflamme DP. *Development and Validation of a Body Condition Score System for Dogs. Canine Practice July/August 1997; 22:10-15*

Kealy, et. al. *Effects of Diet Restriction on Life Span and Age-Related Changes in Dogs. JAVMA 2002; 220:1315-1320*

Call 1-800-222-VETS (8387), weekdays, 8:00 a.m. to 4:30 p.m. CT

▦ Nestlé PURINA

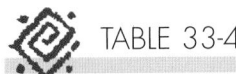

TABLE 33-4

Antiinflammatory Drugs for Treatment of Degenerative Joint Disease in Dogs

	RIMADYL	DERAMAXX	ETOGESIC	METACAM	ZUBRIN	PREVICOX
Generic name	Carprofen	Deracoxib	Etodolac	Meloxicam	Tepoxalin	Firocoxib
Source	Pfizer Animal Health	Novartis	Wyeth	Merial and Boehringer Ingelheim	Schering-Plough Animal Health	Merial
Mechanism of action	COX 2 > COX 1	COX 2 > COX 1	COX 2 > COX 1	COX 2 > COX 1	Dual pathway inhibitor	COX 2> COX 1
Dosage	2.2 mg/kg (1 mg/lb) bid or 4.4 mg/kg qd, or as needed for prevention or treatment of pain	3–4 mg/kg (1.5–2 mg/lb) qd for up to 7 days, 1–2 mg/kg (0.5–1 mg/lb) qd for chronic pain or as needed for prevention or treatment of pain	10–15 mg/kg (5–7.5 mg/lb) qd or as needed for prevention or treatment of pain	0.1 mg/kg (0.05 mg/lb) qd with food. A "loading dose" of 0.2 mg/kg (0.1 mg/lb) may be given on the first day	10 mg/kg (5 mg/lb) qd. A "loading dose" of 20 mg/kg (10 mg/lb) may be given on the first day	5 mg/kg (2.27 mg/lb) qd
Side effects	Gastric ulceration, vomiting, anorexia, liver disease, possible kidney effects	Gastric ulceration, vomiting, anorexia, possible kidney or liver disease; avoid in dogs with keratoconjunctivitis sicca	Gastric ulceration, vomiting, anorexia, possible colitis, possible kidney or liver disease	Gastric ulceration, vomiting, anorexia, possible colitis, possible kidney or liver disease	Gastric ulceration, vomiting, anorexia, possible colitis, possible kidney or liver disease	Vomiting, diarrhea, anorexia, lethargy, pain, somnolence, hyperactivity

Bid, Twice a day; *qd*, once a day.

physiologic responses in the gastrointestinal and renal systems. Use of NSAIDs that significantly inhibit COX-1 (e.g., aspirin, ibuprofen, and phenylbutazone) typically causes gastrointestinal ulceration and/or nephrotoxicity (see Fig. 33-2). Most contemporary veterinary NSAIDs (e.g., carprofen, deracoxib, meloxicam, and etodolac; Table 33-4) preferentially inhibit COX-2. It was initially believed that these drugs would provide clinical benefit without the risk of the older NSAIDs; however, the mechanisms of action and adverse effects of these drugs are not as clear as was initially postulated. Numerous studies have reported conflicting results regarding the COX-1:COX-2 ratios of these drugs. However, the method by which an NSAID is determined to affect COX-2 versus COX-1 involves *in vitro* tests that may or may not accurately reflect what happens *in vivo*. Presently, it is probably best to say that some drugs appear to be COX-1 sparing instead of COX-2 selective, and it may be more accurate to state that some of these drugs are "safer" as opposed to saying that they are "safe." Additionally, it appears that COX-2 can be beneficial in some situations. Finally,

some drugs (e.g., tepoxalin) significantly inhibit 5-lipoxygenase, an enzyme that is responsible for leukotriene production (another mediator of inflammation).

Side effects of the NSAIDs vary depending upon the specific drug and means of reporting adverse events. Owners should be cautioned that antiinflammatory medication may cause gastrointestinal, liver, or kidney disease (see Table 33-4). Aspirin is commonly used in dogs, but owners should be warned of its propensity to cause gastrointestinal toxicity. Concurrent administration of misoprostol may provide some degree of protection against NSAID-induced gastric lesions (Box 33-3), if needed.

> NOTE: Any NSAID can be dangerous in dogs, but some (e.g., naproxen and ibuprofen) are especially dangerous. Avoid using them! Also, if switching from one NSAID to another, it is important to allow 1 to 3 days for the first drug to "wash out" of the system before beginning the second NSAID.

BOX 33-3

Protectant Against NSAID-Induced Gastrointestinal Erosion

Misoprostol (Cytotec)
Dogs 2–5 µg/kg PO tid or qid

PO, Oral; *tid*, three times a day; *qid*, four times a day.

Other medical therapies. Compounds such as polysulfated glycosaminoglycans (PSGAGS) and hyaluronic acid (HA) enhance macromolecular synthesis by chondrocytes and hyaluron synthesis by synoviocytes, inhibit degradative enzymes or inflammatory mediators, and remove or prevent the formation of fibrin, thrombi, or plaques in synovia or subchondral blood vessels. Although there are anecdotal reports of positive results with both PSGAGS and HA, no controlled studies have been performed in dogs to establish their efficacy or safety.

Polysulfated glycosaminoglycans. PSGAGS are injectable, highly sulfated glycosaminoglycans marketed for treatment of osteoarthritis. They have a protective effect on cartilage homeostasis in models of osteoarthritis and inconsistently have shown anabolic effects on cartilage metabolism. PSGAGS have inconsistently decreased lameness caused by osteoarthritis in clinical trials. They have heparin-like activity and may increase bleeding times in dogs.

Hyaluronan. Hyaluronan is a large glycosaminoglycan found in joint fluid and cartilage. In joint fluid, it is a major contributor to viscoelasticity, whereas in cartilage it forms the backbone that links aggrecan molecules. Hyaluronan has been administered intraarticularly to help restore viscosity of joint fluid in arthritic joints. It also has antiinflammatory activity by interfering with oxygen-free radicals and inhibition of degradative enzymes. There is conflicting information regarding the value of hyaluronan administration in the management of canine osteoarthritis, although there is evidence that it may aid in pain relief of this condition (Hellstrom et al, 2003; Smith et al, 2005).

Antibiotics. Antibiotics should be administered for infectious arthritis (see p. 1158) and prophylactically for surgical procedures (see Chapter 10). In general, antibiotics should be selected for treatment of bacterial septic arthritis on the basis of identification of the organism and susceptibility testing. Broad-spectrum, bactericidal antibiotics should be administered until culture and susceptibility testing results are obtained and then adjusted as necessary (Table 33-5). Gram-positive bacteria are most commonly cultured from septic joints; therefore initial treatment with first generation cephalosporins is usually indicated before culture and bacterial susceptibility reports are received. If bacterial L-forms are suspected, doxycycline is the antibiotic of choice. Chloramphenicol and erythromycin might also be effective. Antibiotics should be administered for 4 to 6 weeks and at least 2 weeks after cessation of clinical signs.

 Table 33-5

Antibiotics for Septic Arthritis Before Culture Results

SUSPECTED TYPE	ANTIBIOTIC
Gram-positive	Cephalexin 22 mg/kg PO, IV bid to tid Amoxicillin-clavulanate 12.5–25 mg/kg PO bid
Borrelia, rickettsiae, *Mycoplasma*, bacterial L-forms	Tetracycline 22 mg/kg PO tid
Gram-negative	Baytril 7–20 mg/kg PO, IV* qd
Anaerobes	Metronidazole 10 mg/kg PO, IV* bid

PO, Oral; *IV*, intravenous; *bid*, twice a day; *tid*, three times a day; *qd*, once a day.
*Dilute and give slowly over 20 minutes.

Antibiotics may be administered initially when differentiation between immune-mediated and rickettsial infection has not been made; doxycycline is the antibiotic of choice (see Table 33-5). Doxycycline may be administered until tick titer results are available or as a trial to observe for resolution of clinical signs before initiating steroid therapy for presumptive nonerosive immune-mediated joint disease.

Antibiotics should be administered prophylactically to prevent surgical infections, especially in joint replacement procedures, but they are not a substitute for aseptic technique (see Chapters 3 to 7). A broad-spectrum, bactericidal antibiotic, such as cefazolin (22 mg/kg given IV), should be administered after an intraveous (IV) line has been placed and anesthesia induced. This dose can be repeated every 90 minutes to 3 hours during surgery. Antibiotics can be discontinued after surgery, or they may be continued until culture results are obtained. If culture results are negative, antibiotics should be discontinued; if results are positive, antibiotics may be continued or changed according to the results of susceptibility testing.

Corticosteroids. Corticosteroids effectively reduce synovial inflammation by inhibiting activity of phospholipase A (Fig. 33-2), reducing production of both cyclooxygenases and lipoxygenases. Corticosteroids may also protect cartilage matrix by reducing metalloproteinase activity; however, they depress chondrocyte metabolism and alter the matrix composition by diminishing proteoglycan and collagen synthesis. Because of the adverse systemic effects of long-term corticosteroid administration and their deleterious effects on cartilage, they are seldom indicated for treatment of cartilage injury or DJD. Corticosteroids often are used to treat inflammatory noninfectious arthropathies. When used long term, dosages should be titrated to the smallest amount that achieves an effect, and short-acting steroids (e.g., prednisolone) should be administered every other day if possible to prevent suppression of the hypothalamic-pituitary-adrenal axis.

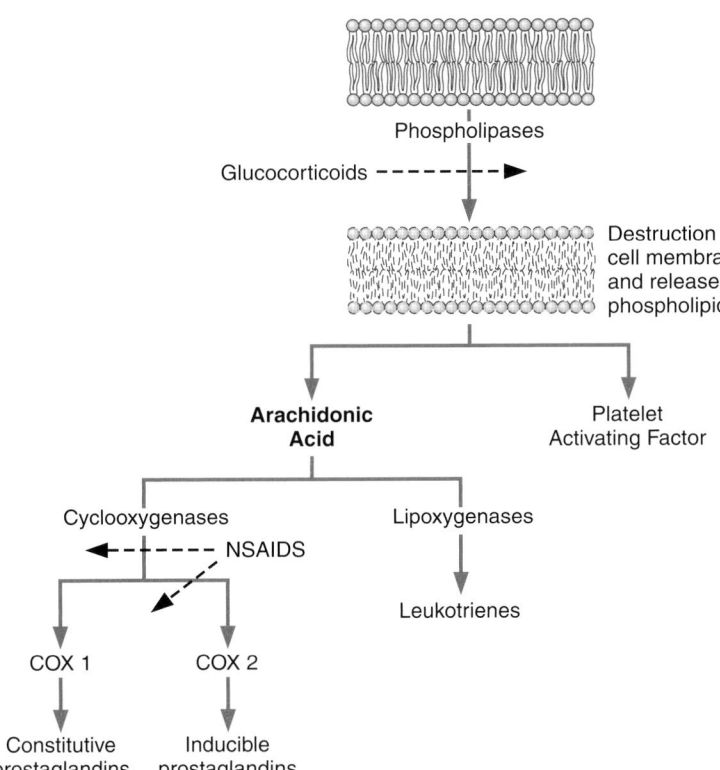

Phospholipases

Glucocorticoids ------->

Destruction of cell membrane and release of phospholipids

Arachidonic Acid

Platelet Activating Factor

Cyclooxygenases

Lipoxygenases

NSAIDS

Leukotrienes

COX 1

COX 2

Constitutive prostaglandins

Inducible prostaglandins

FIG. 33-2
Method of action of glucocorticoids and NSAIDs in inhibiting inflammatory pathways.

SURGICAL TREATMENT

See individual joints for specific surgical procedures.

SURGICAL ANATOMY

Synovial joints permit motion while providing stability for load transfer between bones (Box 33-4). Synovial joint cavities are surrounded by joint capsules made up of an outer layer of fibrous connective tissue lined with a synovial membrane. Nerves, blood vessels, and lymphatic vessels are located between the synovial membranes and the fibrous capsules. Synovial fluid is formed as a dialysate of plasma from the rich vascular supply of synovial membranes. This fluid filters through the vascular endothelium and synovial interstitium to lubricate the joint and provide nutrition for the articular cartilage. The synovial membrane is composed of synovial A and B cells and dendritic cells. Mucoproteins, such as hyaluronic acid, are added to the fluid by synovial B cells; synovial A cells function as phagocytes and secrete interleukin-1 and prostaglandin E. The articulating joint surfaces are covered with 1 to 5 mm of a dense, white connective tissue, usually hyaline cartilage. This articular cartilage facilitates the gliding motion of the joint, distributes mechanical loads, and prevents or minimizes injury to underlying subchondral bone. Some synovial joints (e.g., the stifle joint) also have intraarticular ligaments, menisci, and fat pads that further facilitate joint function and stress reduction during weight bearing (Fig. 33-3). External joint support is provided by surrounding ligaments and tendons.

 BOX 33-4

Joint Classification

Fibrous Joints

Syndesmosis (e.g., temporohyoid joints)
Sutures (e.g., skull)
Gomphosis (e.g., tooth sockets)

Cartilaginous Joints

Hyaline cartilage or synchondrosis (growth plates)
Fibrocartilage or amphiarthrosis (e.g., mandibular symphysis)

Synovial Joints

Articular hyaline cartilage (e.g., shoulder joint)

Loss of joint stability occurs after ligament rupture (i.e., ruptured cranial cruciate ligament [CCL]) or secondary to developmental or anatomic abnormalities (i.e., canine hip dysplasia). Abnormal joint motion places abnormal physiologic loads on portions of the articular cartilage. These loads can cause the cartilage matrix to fracture or fissure, disrupting the collagen fibril network and causing cell death. The tissue response to cartilage loss is similar to that which occurs during healing of cartilage defects (see p. 1153). Subchondral bone sclerosis, osteophyte formation, periarticular

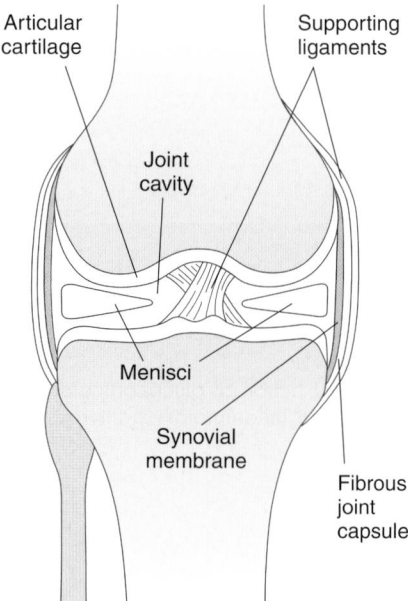

FIG. 33-3
Structure of a synovial joint.

soft tissue fibrosis, and synovial membrane inflammation are all definitive signs of DJD, and all are physiologic responses to joint instability.

Hyaline cartilage is a dense, white connective tissue made up of chondrocytes (10%) dispersed within an extracellular matrix (90%). Seventy percent of the weight of articular cartilage is fluid. Because articular cartilage is avascular and devoid of nerve endings, it relies on synovial fluid for nutrition. Chondrocytes produce matrix and are most numerous and active during cartilage formation; their numbers and metabolic activity decline with age. The noncellular matrix is composed of collagen, proteoglycans, and noncollagenous proteins. Collagen fibrils embedded in the matrix form a supporting scaffold for cartilage. Proteoglycans are primarily glycosaminoglycan chains (e.g., chondroitin sulfate, keratin sulfate, and HA) that repel each other and help to give form to the cartilage. Interaction between chondrocytes and a matrix is facilitated by the presence of noncollagenous proteins. This macromolecular conglomerate serves to organize and hold water in the extracellular matrix of articular cartilage.

Adult articular cartilage is categorized into four distinct zones based on cellular morphology and spatial arrangement. The *superficial zone* has a thin, cell-free matrix that provides the gliding surface of articular cartilage. Deep to this layer are thin, elongated chondrocytes oriented parallel to the articular surface. This *transitional zone* is wider than the superficial zone and is made of spherical chondrocytes and matrix with large collagen fibrils. The *deep zone* is the largest zone and contains small chondrocytes that are arranged in short columns perpendicular to the joint surface. The deep zone has the highest proteoglycan content and the least water of the cartilage zones. The zone of calcified cartilage is separated from the preceding zones by the "tidemark," which is visible when articular cartilage is stained with hematoxylin and eosin. The zone of calcified cartilage anchors cartilage to subchondral bone (Fig. 33-4).

Articular cartilage functions as a gliding surface to facilitate joint movement and as a shock absorber to buffer forces applied to long bones during locomotion. The dynamic fluid mechanics of cartilage provide these capabilities. Fluid movement through cartilage plays a fundamental role in (1) augmenting transport of nutrients into and waste products out of cartilage, (2) controlling cartilage deformation, and (3) lubricating joint surfaces during exudation and imbibition of fluid associated with cartilage deformation during weight bearing. Interstitial fluid containing water, metabolites, and small proteins is filtered from synovial fluid and absorbed into the cartilage matrix. This fluid nourishes cartilage cells and adds bulk and resilience to the matrix. As the cartilage deforms with weight bearing, some of this fluid is extruded into the joint, carrying waste products and lubricating joint surfaces. When the load is removed and the cartilage expands, interstitial fluid is resorbed by the matrix.

SURGICAL TECHNIQUE
Arthrotomy

An arthrotomy is an open surgical approach to a joint using traditional surgical instrumentation. Principles of arthrotomy are listed in Box 33-5. Arthrotomies should be based on a thorough knowledge of the local anatomy, particularly the local musculature and neurovascular structures. Standard approaches to the joints are typically recommended (Piermattie and Johnson, 2003).

Make the skin incision in a direction that permits easy retraction of the superficial musculature. When possible, reflect muscles by incising the adjacent fascia versus making an intramuscular incision. If you must incise through the muscles, make your incision parallel to the muscle fibers. Regardless of the technique, be sure that you have adequate exposure to provide proper visualization of the joint. Incise the joint capsule in such a way that it provides exposure while allowing it to be easily closed. At completion of the arthrotomy, close the joint capsule except in diseases in which release of the joint capsule and adjacent fascia may be necessary for proper alignment (i.e., patellar luxation). The joint capsule is not a holding layer; do not close it with tension.

Closure of the joint capsule does not need to result in a watertight seal because the joint capsule incision will seal with synovial tissue within days of the surgery. Similarly, if the joint capsule cannot be completely closed, a new capsule will form around the joint rapidly. The fascia surrounding the joint capsule is the holding layer and for most joints plays a role in the stability of the joint. Careful tissue layer apposition is important to joint stability and limb function.

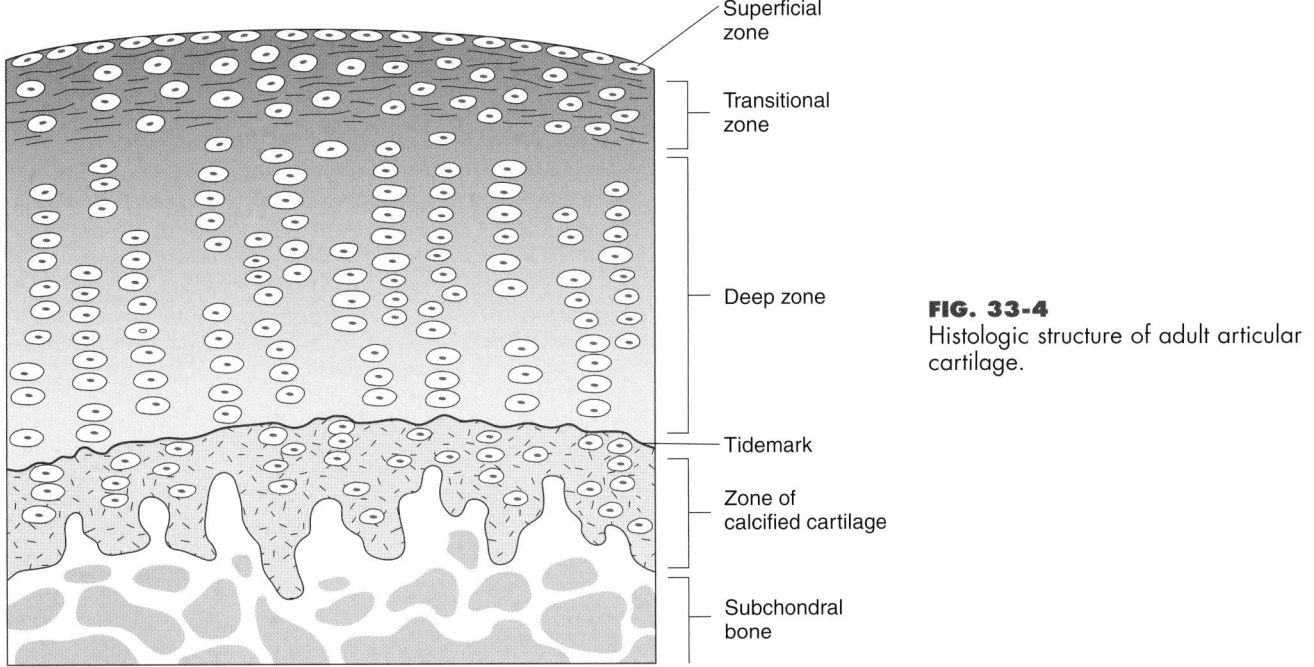

FIG. 33-4
Histologic structure of adult articular cartilage.

Labels: Superficial zone, Transitional zone, Deep zone, Tidemark, Zone of calcified cartilage, Subchondral bone

 BOX 33-5

Principles of Articular Surgery

- Surgical approaches to joints should be implemented so as to minimize damage to the supportive structures of the joints.
- Damage to the articular cartilage should always be avoided during surgery.
- While usually attempted, complete closure of joint capsule is not necessary as a synovial layer will rapidly reform, reestablishing the joint capsule.
- In suturing of the joint capsule, it is appropriate to prevent having a nonabsorbable suture within the joint where it may cause chronic irritation, contributing to osteoarthritis.
- Débridement of osteophytes has little value in alleviation of clinical signs of osteoarthritis.

Reappose muscles in individual layers to permit proper function, and minimize dead space and seroma formation. Close the remainder of the wound routinely.

Endoscopically Assisted Joint Surgery

General principles of arthroscopy are discussed in Chapter 14.

Closed Versus Open Joint Reduction

Closed reduction of luxated joints is generally preferred to open reduction whenever possible because it minimizes contamination, decreases soft tissue damage, and promotes rapid healing (Table 33-6). When determining if closed reduction and stabilization are appropriate, it is critical to de-

 Table 33-6

Reasons for Closed Reduction of Traumatic Joint Luxations

RULE	REASON
Closed reduction is generally preferred over open reduction of traumatic luxations of otherwise normal joints	• Closed reduction minimizes contamination • Closed reduction minimizes anesthetic time • Closed reduction lessens iatrogenic soft tissue trauma

termine if there are underlying diseases, such as hip dysplasia or congenital elbow luxation, that significantly decrease the chances of success with closed reduction. Other contraindications to closed reduction include fractures or significant soft tissue interposition.

HEALING OF CARTILAGE DEFECTS AND RESPONSE OF CARTILAGE TO TREATMENT

Loss of proteoglycans from matrix occurs with infection, inflammation, and joint immobilization; when cartilage is exposed during surgery; or as a result of traumatic disruption of synovial membranes. With reversible damage, chondrocytes may replace the lost matrix components after the insult is removed. However, irreversible damage may occur. Lacerations or abrasions of the cartilage surface destroy chondrocytes and disrupt the matrix. A standard inflammatory response does not occur with superficial lacerations

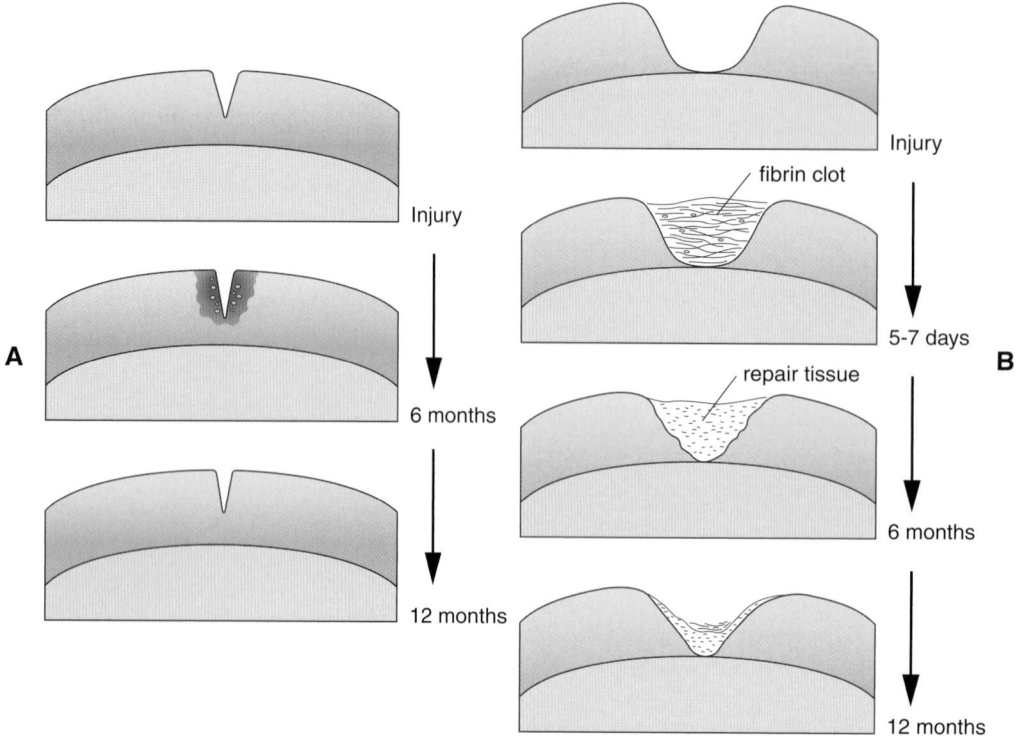

FIG. 33-5
Healing of superficial **(A)** and deep **(B)** lacerations of articular cartilage.

(those that do not penetrate to subchondral bone) because inflammatory cells from marrow and blood vessels cannot access the joint (Fig. 33-5, *A*). Chondrocytes near the injury respond by proliferating and synthesizing new matrix; however, this response usually is inadequate for healing. Although superficial lacerations do not heal, they seldom progress. When a full thickness cartilage defect occurs, marrow cells capable of participating in an inflammatory response gain access to the defect (Fig. 33-5, *B*). The size of the defect affects healing; small defects (1 mm in diameter) heal more completely than large defects. The defect initially is filled with a fibrin clot, which is replaced within 5 days by fibroblast-like cells and collagen fibers. Metaplasia of these fibroblast-like cells into chondrocytes occurs after 2 weeks. These chondrocytes do not function normally, as is indicated by lower concentrations of proteoglycans in the reparative tissue at 6 months after injury. The reparative tissue (fibrocartilage) is also thinner than articular cartilage and is prone to fibrillation and erosive changes.

Joint Stabilization

Joint stabilization that recreates normal anatomic relationships and permits normal joint function promotes cartilage repair in animals with acute joint instability (i.e., traumatic joint luxations and acute cruciate ligament injuries), if irreversible damage is not present and the cartilage was normal before injury. Dogs with CCL injuries are often presented for treatment after initial changes leading to DJD

have occurred. In addition, most surgical techniques for treatment of ruptured CCL injury do not restore normal anatomic relationships or allow normal joint function. Therefore many animals develop progressive DJD despite surgical treatment.

Joint Immobilization

Prolonged immobilization of synovial joints causes progressive proteoglycan loss and depression of proteoglycan synthesis, which leads to softening of the cartilage. When limited activity is allowed, cartilage is restored; however, forced activity after immobility may further damage softened cartilage. Rigid joint immobilization (i.e., that obtained with a transarticular external fixator) results in more severe cartilage degeneration than does less rigid immobilization (i.e., with a cast).

Continuous Passive Motion

Experimentally, early motion and weight bearing are beneficial for repair of full thickness cartilage defects. Continuous passive motion also appears to accelerate repair of full thickness cartilage defects, which results in repair tissue that more closely approximates hyaline cartilage. Although continuous passive motion is impractical in small animals, physical therapists can provide techniques or instruct owners on how to perform techniques that may have similar benefits. See Chapter 12 for additional information on physical rehabilitation.

POSTOPERATIVE CARE AND ASSESSMENT

Both medical and surgical management of animals with joint diseases must incorporate nutritional management, physical therapy, and rehabilitation.

Nutritional management. Nutritional management is important both in modifying developmental skeletal diseases (i.e., hip dysplasia and osteochondrosis) and in managing dogs with osteoarthritis. Avoiding excessive nutrition and obesity in growing and adult dogs with osteoarthritis will aid in managing their joint disease. Nutrient excesses are risk factors in development of skeletal abnormalities in fast-growing, large-breed dogs. Weight control can help reduce abnormal forces placed on joints and can prevent or delay the onset of symptomatic disease in predisposed patients or help alleviate symptoms in affected patients.

Physical rehabilitation. Physical rehabilitation is an important component of the treatment of joint diseases. Physical rehabilitation increases muscle strength, endurance, and joint range of motion; reduces muscle spasm and pain; and improves performance. Passive physical manipulation, heat, and cold are important considerations in rehabilitation of joint injuries. For additional information on general principles of physical rehabilitation, see Chapter 12. Supervised, regular short exercise periods of walking or swimming, when the animal is no longer showing signs of inflammation or after surgery to stabilize the joint, help strengthen supporting muscles. Exercise should be avoided when the animal shows signs of acute inflammation and should be limited to prevent discomfort. Effects of a physical rehabilitation program can be measured in terms of increases in muscle circumference, joint range of motion documented with a goniometer, and exercise endurance.

References

Allen TA: A multi-center practice-based study of a therapeutic food and a non-steroidal anti-inflammatory drug in dogs with osteoarthritis, unpublished data, Topeka, Kan, 2004, Hill's Pet Nutrition Center.

Cross AR, Roush JK, Renberg WC et al: Effects of feeding omega-3 fatty acids on clinical signs and force plate analysis in dogs with osteoarthritis, unpublished data, Topeka, Kan, 2004, Hill's Pet Nutrition Center.

Hellstrom LE, Carlsson C, Boucher JF et al: Intra-articular injections with high molecular weight sodium hyaluronate as a therapy for canine arthritis, *Vet Rec* 153:89, 2003.

Kealy RD, Lawler DF, Ballam JM et al: Effects of diet restriction on life span and age-related changes in dogs, *J Am Vet Med Assoc* 220:1315, 2002.

Piermattie D, Johnson K: *Atlas of surgical approaches to bones & joints of the dog & cat,* Philadelphia, 2003, Saunders.

Smith G, Myers SL, Brandt KG, et al: Effect of intraarticular hyaluronan injection on vertical ground reaction force and progression of osteoarthritis after anterior cruciate ligament transection, *J Rheumatol* 32:325, 2005.

Suggested Reading

Beale BS: Use of nutraceuticals and chondroprotectants in osteoarthritic dogs and cats, *Vet Clin North Am Small Anim Pract* 34:271, 2004.

This article is an excellent review of the mechanisms of action and use of nutraceuticals in dogs and cats.

Borer LR, Peel JE, Seewald W et al: Effect of carprofen, etodolac, meloxicam, or butorphanol in dogs with induced acute synovitis, *Am J Vet Res* 64:1429, 2003.

This study demonstrated that carprofen, etodolac, and meloxicam had greater efficacy than butorphanol in relief of acute pain.

MacWilliams PS, Friedrichs KR: Laboratory evaluation and interpretation of synovial fluid, *Vet Clin North Am Small Anim Pract* 33:153, 2003.

This article provides an excellent review of interpretation of joint fluid.

Millis D, Levine D, Taylor R: *Canine rehabilitation and physical therapy,* Philadelphia, 2004, Saunders.

This text contains a complete description of physical therapy for osteoarthritis in dogs.

Schulz KS, Beale B, Holsworth et al: The pet lovers guide to canine arthritis and joint problems, Philadelphia, 2005, Saunders.

This text is an excellent reference for veterinarians and clients on the management of the most common joint problems in dogs.

SELECTED NONSURGICAL DISEASES OF JOINTS

DEGENERATIVE JOINT DISEASE

DEFINITION

Degenerative joint disease (DJD), or *osteoarthritis*, is a noninflammatory, noninfectious degeneration of articular cartilage accompanied by bone formation at the synovial margins and by fibrosis of periarticular soft tissue. Although classified as noninflammatory, a low-grade, ongoing inflammatory process is associated with this condition.

GENERAL CONSIDERATIONS AND CLINICALLY RELEVANT PATHOPHYSIOLOGY

DJD may be classified as primary or secondary, depending on the cause. *Primary osteoarthritis* is a disorder of aging in which cartilage degeneration occurs for unknown reasons. *Secondary osteoarthritis* occurs in response to abnormalities that cause joint instability (e.g., CCL rupture) or abnormal loading of articular cartilage (i.e., developmental or anatomic abnormalities, such as hip dysplasia), or in response to other recognizable joint disease (e.g., infection and immune-mediated inflammation). Secondary osteoarthritis is more common than primary osteoarthritis in dogs and cats (see Box 33-1). Abnormal joint motion increases the physiologic loads placed on some portions of normal articular cartilage, initiating molecular changes that lead to osteoarthritis. Normal stress on abnormal cartilage (i.e., injured by genetic or metabolic cartilage disorders, inflammation, or immune responses) initiates identical changes. Initially, fibrillation of the superficial cartilage layer results in roughening of the articular surface, with fissures eventually extending to subchondral bone. Free cartilage fragments can initiate an inflammatory response from synovium with production of inflammatory mediators (i.e., cytokines and prostaglandins). Cartilage degradation results from altered chondrocytes, depletion of matrix proteoglycans, and damage to the collagen fibril network. Collagen breakdown is induced by cytokines (i.e., interleukin 1 [IL-1] and tumor necrosis factor [TNF]) and by up-regulation of the release of destructive enzymes (i.e., matrix metalloproteinases [MMPs] and aggrecanase) from chondrocytes, synoviocytes, and inflammatory cells. Affected cartilage is more susceptible to breakdown from the loads of weight bearing. The result is a vicious cycle of inflammation and cartilage destruction. Thus articular fibrillation, cartilage loss, subchondral bone sclerosis, osteophyte formation, periarticular soft tissue fibrosis, and synovial membrane inflammation cause pain and loss of function in osteoarthritis.

DIAGNOSIS
Clinical Presentation

Signalment. Osteoarthritis may affect any age or breed of dog or cat. Dysplastic diseases leading to osteoarthritis are often breed specific; however, osteoarthritis caused by trauma is not specific for age or breed.

History. The most common clinical sign of osteoarthritis is lameness, which may be acute or chronic and persistent or intermittent. Most animals have a history of exercise intolerance, particularly when multiple joints are affected (e.g., hip dysplasia). There may be a previous history of joint fractures, osteochondritis dissecans (OCD), congenital or chronic joint luxations, inflammatory joint disease, septic arthritis, and/or neuropathies. Other causes in the forelimbs include fragmented coronoid processes (FCP) (see p. 1197), ununited anconeal processes (UAP) (see p. 1209), and premature physeal closure (see p. 1218). In the rear limbs, hip dysplasia, aseptic necrosis of the femoral head, patellar luxation, and cruciate ligament rupture may also cause osteoarthritis.

Physical Examination Findings

Unilateral lameness usually is evident when affected animals stand or ambulate. Bilateral conditions (e.g., hip dysplasia) often appear as unilateral lameness if one joint is more severely affected than another. Acutely affected joints may be swollen because of joint effusion, but swelling is more commonly caused by periarticular fibrosis in chronic disease. Reduced range of motion, palpable crepitus during motion, and joint instability are common. Joint palpation may elicit pain.

Diagnostic Imaging

The severity of radiographic change depends on chronicity. Radiographic signs observed include subchondral bone sclerosis, articular and periarticular osteophyte formation, joint space narrowing, joint effusion, and greater prominence of periarticular soft tissue (Fig. 33-6). Because most radiographic changes are associated with chronic joint changes, osteoarthritis and significant cartilage damage may exist long before radiographic changes are apparent.

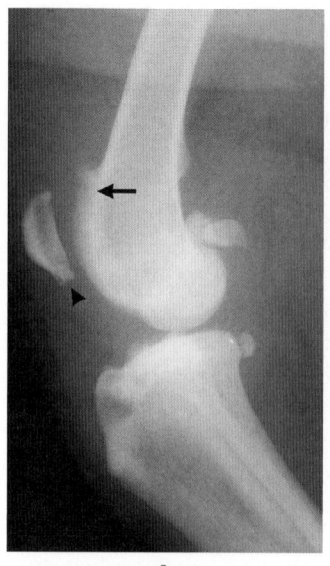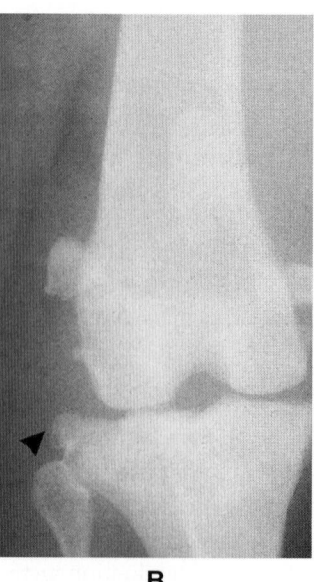

A   **B**

FIG. 33-6
A, Lateral radiograph of a canine stifle with DJD. Note the periarticular osteophytes along the trochlear ridges *(arrow)* and patella *(arrowhead).* Joint effusion is causing cranial displacement of the infrapatellar fat pad and caudal distention of the joint capsule. **B,** On a craniocaudal view, periarticular osteophytes *(arrowhead)* are evident off the lateral aspect of the tibial plateau and distal to the medial fabella. Increased prominence of periarticular soft tissue can be seen medially and laterally.

Arthroscopy. Arthroscopy typically allows early detection of osteoarthritis. Arthroscopic findings in osteoarthritis include varying grades of cartilage damage and synovial proliferation (Fig. 33-7).

Laboratory Findings

Laboratory abnormalities associated with systemic disease are seldom present with osteoarthritis. Rheumatoid factor, SLE preparations, and antinuclear antibody (ANA) test results are normal. Synovial fluid analysis may reveal decreased synovial fluid viscosity, increased synovial fluid volumes, and increased numbers of mononuclear phagocytic cells (6000 to 9000 white blood cells per microliter [WBC/μl]).

DIFFERENTIAL DIAGNOSIS

Differential diagnoses for osteoarthritis include septic arthritis, neoplasia, and joint trauma.

MEDICAL MANAGEMENT

Because osteoarthritis in small animals usually develops secondary to other orthopedic problems, the underlying problem should be corrected if possible. Surgical therapy plus medical treatment often is necessary to reduce or eliminate clinical signs. However, correction of the inciting problem, although necessary to reestablish function, does not usually eliminate or prevent progression of degenerative

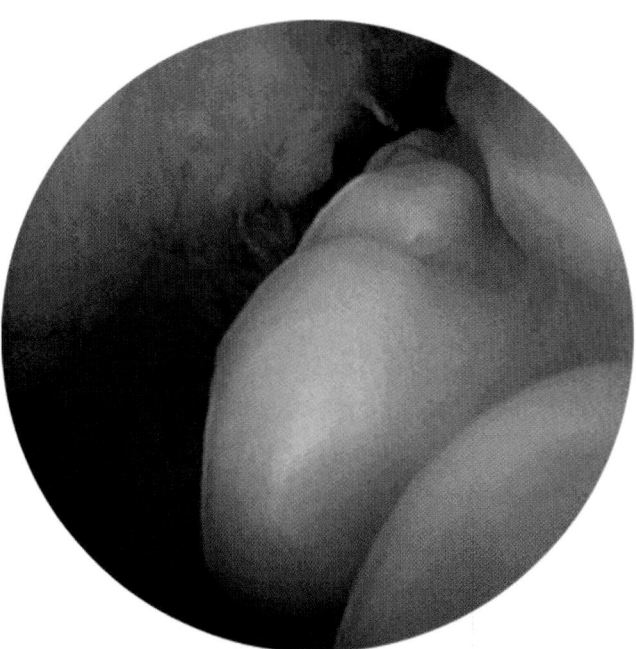

FIG. 33-7
Arthroscopic view of osteoarthritis. Note the osteophytes and synovial proliferation.

changes. Correction of the primary problem is not possible, or indicated, in some animals. Many animals with radiographic signs of osteoarthritis are asymptomatic and may or may not develop lameness as they age. Owners should be apprised of the animal's condition; however, they should be reassured that the animal may function normally with minimal or no treatment.

Inflammatory synovitis is often responsible for clinical signs of pain and lameness associated with osteoarthritis. Physical rehabilitation can play a key role in strengthening the periarticular structures, which will lead to improved comfort, stronger musculature to support compromised joints, and increased functional range of motion. These lifestyle changes can significantly improve comfort and quality of life for these patients (see also Chapter 12). Because excessive or uncontrolled exercise exacerbates and prolongs inflammation, cage confinement for 2 to 3 days plus judicious use of antiinflammatory drugs may be necessary to break the cycle and return the animal to controlled levels of activity.

> NOTE: Do not treat asymptomatic dogs just because they have radiographic signs of osteoarthritis.

Many dogs showing clinical signs of osteoarthritis are obese. Obesity may be a causative or inciting factor in the development of osteoarthritis, or it may be a response to chronic pain. Dogs that are reluctant to exercise may gain weight if food intake is not regulated. Weight loss or weight control for a dog with osteoarthritis should be stressed to the owners. Weight loss can be associated with diminished pain and increased function in animals with chronic osteoarthritis. Once the inflammatory phase of disease is under control, moderate regular exercise (not severe enough to cause lameness) is important to maintain joint mobility, muscle strength, and joint support. Swimming appears to maintain muscle strength without increasing joint loads.

Veterinary NSAIDs are effective for relieving pain associated with osteoarthritis and generally have few clinically obvious gastrointestinal side effects (see Table 33-4 on p. 1149); however, gastric ulceration, colitis, hepatocellular toxicosis, and renal disease may occur with any NSAID. Using NSAIDs designed for humans may be especially dangerous. Gastric mucosal sensitivity to NSAIDs and other side effects may be manifested by anorexia, vomiting, diarrhea, anemia, dyspnea, and/or melena. If any of these signs are noted, NSAID use should be discontinued to prevent worsening of the disease.

Corticosteroids have antiinflammatory effects on joint tissues. They depress chondrocyte metabolism and alter cartilage matrix, which causes decreased proteoglycan and collagen synthesis (see p. 1150). Because of this and the adverse systemic effects of long-term corticosteroid administration, they should be used in osteoarthritic animals only as a last resort. If they are used, they should be administered infrequently and the animal should be restricted from exercise for several weeks after treatment to protect the cartilage.

> NOTE: Always counsel owners about the side effects of NSAIDs and steroids. These drugs should **never** be given together, except in extreme and unique circumstances, and then only after warning the owner of potential risks.

SURGICAL TREATMENT

Surgical treatment of the underlying disease may be indicated to control signs of osteoarthritis (e.g., stabilization of stifles with CCL ruptures). Uncontrollable pain and loss of limb function associated with osteoarthritis warrant surgical intervention. Several surgical procedures are available to salvage limb function. Arthroplasty techniques, such as femoral head and neck ostectomy (see p. 1242) and glenoid cavity resection (see p. 1191) have been described in veterinary patients. After resection of bone, a fibrous tissue joint, or pseudoarthrosis, is allowed to form. Function varies after these procedures. Although the joint mechanics are not normal, in many cases limb function is satisfactory. Replacement of an arthritic joint with a prosthesis offers improved chances for normal limb function and superior pain relief. Currently, total hip replacement (THR) is the only joint replacement routinely available in small animal patients. Total elbow replacements have been developed, although they are not widely used. The biomechanical nature of the elbow joint makes successful design and placement of a prosthetic elbow joint significantly more complicated than a THR. Arthrodesis (surgical fusion of the joint) can relieve pain and allow good function of the limb when used to treat carpal or tarsal instability. Amputation is a salvage procedure that should be considered only in selected patients—those that are non–weight-bearing and have unilateral disease causing unrelenting pain that has been unresponsive to other therapies.

Preoperative Management

See previous Medical Management section. Specific preoperative treatment depends on the underlying disease.

Anesthesia

Anesthetic management of animals with orthopedic disease is provided on p. 944.

Surgical Anatomy

Surgical anatomy of the joints is provided under the specific procedures.

Positioning

Positioning depends on the procedure being performed (see later discussion).

SURGICAL TECHNIQUE

For arthroplasty techniques (i.e., femoral head and neck ostectomy and glenoid cavity resection), see pp. 1242 and 1191, respectively. For amputation see p. 1342 and for arthrodesis see p. 1228.

SUTURE MATERIALS AND SPECIAL INSTRUMENTS

Suture materials and special instruments required for joint surgery are listed under the specific procedures.

POSTOPERATIVE CARE AND ASSESSMENT

For postoperative care after joint surgery, see the specific procedures.

PROGNOSIS

Prognosis for patients with osteoarthritis varies tremendously depending upon severity of the disease, number of joints affected, and medical condition of the patient. In many cases of mild to moderate osteoarthritis, proper medical management can return the patient to near normal function. In more severe cases, particularly with multiple joint involvement, the prognosis for return to normal activity is guarded. However, in most cases, with the exception of severe end stage osteoarthritis, function as a house pet can be restored. Important considerations for management and prognosis of animals with osteoarthritis are listed in Box 33-6.

Suggested Reading

Johnston SA, Todhunter RJ: Osteoarthritis. In Slatter D, editor: *Textbook of small animal surgery,* Philadelphia, 2003, Saunders.
This chapter provides a detailed description of the mechanisms, diagnosis, and treatment of osteoarthritis.

 BOX 33-6

Important Considerations in Degenerative Joint Disease

- In most instances of degenerative joint disease (osteoarthritis) in dogs, a primary joint problem (e.g., hip dysplasia, fragmented coronoid process, or ruptured cruciate ligament) was the inciting cause. The underlying disease must be diagnosed and treated appropriately.
- Osteoarthritis is usually progressive, regardless of treatment.
- Diagnosis of osteoarthritis is based on radiographic evaluation, but treatment is based on clinical signs.
- Medical management of osteoarthritis includes weight control, exercise, or physical therapy to maintain joint mobility and muscle mass, rest during acute clinical signs, and medication.

SEPTIC (BACTERIAL) ARTHRITIS

DEFINITION

Septic arthritis *(infective arthritis, suppurative arthritis)* is joint infection caused by bacterial organisms.

GENERAL CONSIDERATIONS AND CLINICALLY RELEVANT PATHOPHYSIOLOGY

Septic arthritis may be initiated by hematogenous spread of infection from respiratory, digestive, urinary, umbilical, or valvular infections, but more often it is caused by direct bacterial inoculation of joints from penetrating trauma, surgical procedures, or intraarticular injections. Common organisms include staphylococci, streptococci, *Corynebacterium* spp., and coliforms. Bacterial contamination of synovium causes inflammation and promotes extravasation of fibrin, clotting factors, polymorphonuclear leukocytes, and proteinaceous serous fluid into the joint. Fibrin deposition on articular cartilage surfaces inhibits synovial fluid penetration. Leukocytes phagocytize bacteria and release lysosomal enzymes that break down cartilage matrix and expose collagen fibrils to further enzymatic destruction. Enzymatic destruction of matrix and collagen fibrils, loss of normal synovial fluid nutrition, and mechanical trauma on diseased cartilage cause loss of the cartilaginous joint surface. Eventually the infective process invades subchondral bone, causing bacterial osteomyelitis.

Severity of the pathologic changes in affected joints depends on the chronicity of infection. Early changes include hyperemia, edema, synovial inflammation, and a purulent-appearing joint fluid. Both hyperplasia and hypertrophy of synovial cells occur. Cartilage fibrillation and granulation tissue production within the joint soon ensue with loss of articular cartilage. The articular surface fills with granulation and fibrous tissue; eventually these tissues calcify, causing ankylosis. Diagnosis of septic arthritis is based on synovial fluid analysis (see Table 33-2 on p. 1145), radiographic changes (see Table 33-1 on p. 1144), and positive results on bacterial culture.

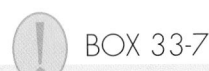

BOX 33-7

Clinical Signs of Septic Arthritis

Acute

Single-limb lameness
Severe lameness, may carry the limb
Joint swollen, painful, and warm

Chronic

Single-limb lameness or multiple-limb lameness with sub-acute endocarditis
Weight-bearing lameness
Joint swelling

DIAGNOSIS
Clinical Presentation

Signalment. Septic arthritis can be found in any aged dog, but males of larger breeds are more commonly affected.

History. Animals with septic arthritis after joint inoculation usually show a notable unilateral lameness (Box 33-7). Onset of clinical signs may be acute or gradual. Penetrating wounds, surgical intervention, or joint injection often are historical findings. Dogs with septic arthritis from septicemia (e.g., bacterial endocarditis) usually have multiple limb involvement and no history of joint intervention.

Physical Examination Findings

Animals with acute onset of signs often are severely lame or non–weight-bearing on the affected limb. The affected joint may be swollen, painful, warm, and crepitate; drain purulent material; and have reduced range of motion. Systemic signs (pyrexia, lethargy, and anorexia) occur in a small percentage of animals with septic arthritis. The signs may be more subtle (i.e., only lameness and joint swelling) with low-grade, chronic infections. Dogs with septic arthritis caused by bacterial endocarditis typically have multiple joint involvement, lameness, pyrexia, lethargy, anorexia, and/or cardiac murmurs.

Diagnostic Imaging

Early radiographic signs of septic arthritis are joint effusion and soft tissue swelling. Later changes include bone lysis, periosteal new bone formation, joint surface irregularities, subchondral bone sclerosis, and joint subluxation (Fig. 33-8). Echocardiography may demonstrate valvular lesions of bacterial endocarditis in dogs without heart murmurs; however, it is important to note that bacterial endocarditis can be associated with septic or nonseptic arthritis/polyarthritis.

Laboratory Findings

Complete blood counts (CBC) may indicate an inflammatory response in acute stages of septic arthritis. Chronic disease is essentially walled off within the joint and is seldom associated with significant changes in hemograms or serum

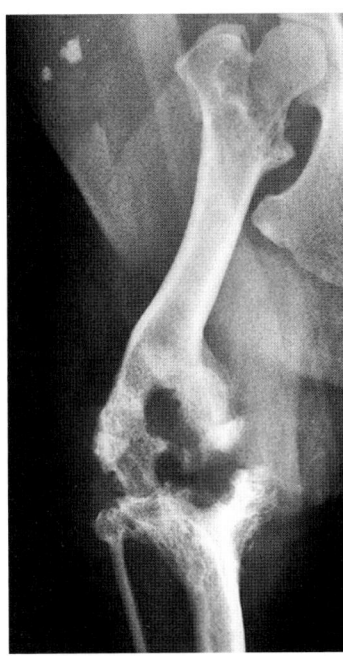

FIG. 33-8
Craniocaudal radiograph of a stifle joint with septic arthritis. There is extensive osteolysis of the femur and tibia. The subchondral margins of the joint surfaces are irregular and difficult to identify.

biochemistry profiles. Joint fluid obtained by means of arthrocentesis may provide a definitive diagnosis. Purulent joint fluid with an increased number of polymorphonuclear leukocytes (40,000 cells/μl to more than 100,000 cells/μl), especially if they are degenerative, and bacteria is indicative of a septic arthritis. However, septic joints do not always contain degenerative neutrophils. Positive bacterial culture and susceptibility results confirm the diagnosis and allow appropriate antibiotic selection. Results of bacterial culture of synovial fluid from septic joints vary, but positive results can be facilitated by securing a sample before antibiotics are administered and by using enrichment broth to facilitate bacterial growth from synovial fluid. Bacterial culture of surgically retrieved synovial samples may be necessary to identify bacterial agents. Blood and urine cultures sometimes grow the organism(s) when joint fluid does not.

> **NOTE:** Bacterial endocarditis may occur in dogs that do not have heart murmurs. Be sure to perform echocardiograms in these animals.

DIFFERENTIAL DIAGNOSIS

Other infectious agents causing arthropathies (e.g., spirochetes, rickettsiae, fungi, bacterial L-forms, mycoplasmas, and protozoa) must be differentiated from bacterial causes. Noninfectious causes of arthropathy, including osteoarthritis, also must be differentiated from infectious causes. Sam-

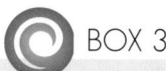 BOX 33-8

Treatment of Rickettsial Polyarthritis and Bacterial L Forms

Doxycycline

10 mg/kg PO qd*

Tetracycline

22 mg/kg PO bid†

Chloramphenicol

50 mg/kg PO tid (can rarely cause fatal aplastic anemia in people, therefore do not eat or drink while handling this product; do not touch eyes; wash hands after use; warn owners of same)

Enrofloxacin‡

3 mg/kg PO or IV qd

PO, Oral; *qd*, once a day; *bid*, twice a day; *tid*, three times a day.
*Must not be given with milk or milk products.
†Must not be given with food of any kind.
‡Not effective for Ehrlichiosis.

ples of joint fluid and synovium for bacterial culture and susceptibility testing should be obtained to identify causative organisms and determine appropriate antibiotic therapy.

MEDICAL MANAGEMENT

Treatment options for management of septic arthritis include administration of antimicrobials only, administration of antimicrobials plus surgical lavage, administration of antimicrobials plus arthroscopic lavage, administration of antimicrobials plus surgical or arthroscopic lavage and drain placement, or administration of antimicrobials and open joint management. Antibiotics should be administered immediately after samples for culture are obtained, and antibiotic therapy should be adjusted after microbial susceptibility tests are obtained. Because of the high incidence of gram positive infections, first generation cephalosporins are often recommended until susceptibility results are available (see Table 33-5 on p. 1150). If bacterial L-forms are considered likely, doxycycline is the drug of choice (Box 33-8). Antibiotics are administered for 4 to 6 weeks and for at least 2 weeks after clinical signs have resolved. It is important to remember that tetracycline drugs have some antiinflammatory activity, so care must be taken when ascribing cause-and-effect to an arthritic patient that improves after receiving doxycycline or tetracycline. NSAIDs are often necessary to alleviate pain in affected joints.

SURGICAL TREATMENT

Goals of surgical treatment are to control infections rapidly and remove purulent material and fibrin from joints to minimize cartilage destruction. Immediate joint exploration, including débridement of fibrin and granulation tissue and sterile saline lavage, is indicated for postoperative joint infections, septic joints for which treatment was delayed for 72 hours or longer, joints that have not responded

to 72 hours of appropriate medical therapy, and penetrating joint wounds. Surgery is not indicated in dogs with inflammatory joint disease that has occurred secondary to bacterial endocarditis.

Preoperative Management

The overall health of the animal should be determined before surgery. Most patients with septic arthritis are otherwise healthy; however, some patients may have secondary systemic effects, including dehydration and systemic inflammation. Antibiotics should not be administered until fluid has been obtained for culture and susceptibility testing.

Anesthesia

General anesthesia is required for exploration of the joint. Anesthetic protocols should be based on signalment, physical examination findings, and laboratory analysis. Patients who are brought in without preoperative findings suggestive of major organ dysfunction or systemic effects of joint infection can be managed using a variety of anesthetic techniques (see Box 31-3 on p. 944). Anesthetic management of animals with orthopedic disease is provided on p. 944.

Surgical Anatomy

Surgical anatomy of specific joints is provided elsewhere in this chapter.

Positioning

Positioning for arthroscopy or arthrotomy depends on the joint being evaluated (see sections on specific joints).

SURGICAL TECHNIQUE

Exploration of the joint may be performed either with a traditional arthrotomy or by arthroscopy (see sections on specific joints).

Aggressively lavage the joint and remove fibrin deposits. In severe cases, perform synovectomy.

When performing arthroscopic débridement, adequate lavage is provided by routine arthroscopic fluid lavage.

Perform débridement with a power shaver. After arthrotomy and joint lavage, install a system of ingress and egress drains, if necessary, so that joint lavage can be performed two or three times daily.

In most cases, only egress drains are required. Joint drains routinely clog with synovium and fibrin debris. Synovectomy may aid in preventing drain clogging. Use of a proper drain—such as a flat, multifenestrated, closed suction system—also aids in maintaining drainage.

Avoid use of Penrose drains because they may encourage retrograde contamination. In severe cases, leave the joint incision open for daily lavage; heavy sedation or general anesthesia is generally needed. Replace sterile bandages once or twice a day, as needed. Close the joint after 2 to 4 days of open drainage.

This type of management is extremely time-intensive, expensive, and rarely necessary.

When performing ingress-egress lavage, pay strict attention to sterile technique. For lavage fluid, use saline or a balanced electrolyte solution, either of which has minimal effects on joint tissue.

Povidone-iodine at a concentration of 0.1% has minimal adverse effects on synovium. However, stronger concentrations of povidone-iodine and chlorhexidine cause a chemical synovitis.

Perform ingress-egress flushing for 1 or 2 days. Maintain the egress drain until drainage is limited to that caused only by the presence of the drain itself, which usually amounts to a few milliliters per day.

NOTE: Acute septic arthritis is a surgical emergency.

SUTURE MATERIALS AND SPECIAL INSTRUMENTS

Absorbable sutures are recommended for closure of the joint capsule. Closed suction drains are valuable for drainage of septic joints.

POSTOPERATIVE CARE AND ASSESSMENT

Postoperative care for animals with septic arthritis consists of oral antibiotics, analgesics (see Chapter 13), daily wound management until joint drainage is no longer purulent, and passive range of motion. Oral antibiotics should be continued for 4 to 6 weeks. The limb should be protected in a bandage for 4 weeks to allow the cartilage to heal before allowing full-weight bearing. The animal can then be slowly returned to normal activity. Joint flushing and range of motion exercises are usually quite painful in septic osteoarthritis patients; therefore adequate pain management with opioids or NSAIDs is indicated.

PROGNOSIS

Prognosis for normal joint function varies and depends on the amount of cartilage that has been destroyed; however, most dogs with bacterial septic arthritis respond well to treatment and are free of clinical signs of the disease at follow-up. Salvage procedures for chronically painful joints include arthrodesis (see p. 1228) or amputation (see p. 1342). The prognosis for animals with bacterial endocarditis is poor if there is impending cardiac failure secondary to valvular dysfunction, especially aortic valvular insufficiency.

Suggested Reading

Clements DN, Owen MR, Mosley JR et al: Retrospective study of bacterial infective arthritis in 31 dogs, *J Small Anim Pract* 46:304, 2005.

This study provides a retrospective report of a large population of dogs with septic arthritis and discusses the causes and compares treatments.

Fitch RB, Hogan TC, Kudnig ST: Hematogenous septic arthritis in the dog: results of five patients treated nonsurgically with antibiotics, *J Am Anim Hosp Assoc* 39:563, 2003.

This study discusses nonsurgical management of septic arthritis in five dogs.

RICKETTSIAL POLYARTHRITIS

DEFINITION

Rickettsial polyarthritis is infection of the joints caused by small microorganisms that typically occur intracellularly in arthropods.

GENERAL CONSIDERATIONS AND CLINICALLY RELEVANT PATHOPHYSIOLOGY

Polyarthritis in dogs may be caused by *Rickettsia rickettsii* or *Ehrlichia* spp., *R. rickettsii*, the causative agent of Rocky Mountain spotted fever (RMSF), is transmitted by ticks of the *Dermacentor* genus and is endemic in wooded areas of the central and eastern United States.

Ehrlichia spp. have been observed in much of the United States, but especially in the southeastern portions. Strains that affect neutrophils (i.e., *Ehrlichia ewingii* and *Anaplasma phagocytophilum*) as opposed to mononuclear cells (i.e., *Ehrlichia canis*) appear more likely to cause arthritis. *Neorickettsia risticii* (ssp. atypicalis) (previously called *Ehrlichia risticii*) has also been implicated in canine polyarthritis.

DIAGNOSIS
Clinical Presentation

Signalment. Any breed dog of any age can be affected. Dogs that are exposed to ticks (e.g., hunting dogs) may be more likely to become infected.

History. RMSF is most commonly diagnosed from March through October in endemic areas. It typically causes an acute onset of symptoms, including multiple-limb lameness, joint pain, fever, petechial hemorrhages, lymphadenopathy, neurologic signs, facial edema, and edema of the extremities. Arthritis is typically just one aspect of a much larger picture of a dog with a serious systemic illness.

Ehrlichiosis can have a greater breadth of clinical findings than typically found with RMSF, ranging from acute to subclinical to chronic, and with signs varying from relatively mild (e.g., anorexia, depression, fever, or weight loss) to dramatic (e.g., epistaxis) to severe (e.g., seizures, hyperesthesia, and stupor).

Physical Examination Findings

Clinical signs associated with ehrlichiosis may be acute or chronic and can include fever, anorexia, lymphadenopathy, splenomegaly, hepatomegaly, weight loss, lameness, joint pain, petechiation, and/or neurologic signs. Clinical findings in RMSF classically include fever, cutaneous edema and/or hyperemia, scrotal edema, stiff gait, petechiation, and/or central nervous system (CNS) aberrations.

Diagnostic Imaging

Radiographic changes indicating rickettsial polyarthritis include joint effusion and periarticular soft tissue swelling. Surfaces of bones and cartilage usually appear normal. Occasionally a pulmonary interstitial pattern is noted. Splenomegaly and/or hepatomegaly can be seen.

Laboratory Findings

Thrombocytopenia is typically present in both RMSF and ehrlichiosis. Hyperglobulinemia is common in dogs with chronic ehrlichiosis caused by *E. canis*, but not *E. ewingii*. Anemia (often mild, but can be severe if bone marrow suppression has occurred) may be seen with both acute and chronic ehrlichiosis. Ehrlichiosis classically has normal to low neutrophil counts, whereas RMSF often causes substantial neutrophilic leukocytosis. A reactive lymphocytosis may occur with *E. ewingii*. Dogs that have been treated with steroids may have *E. ewingii* morula in circulating neutrophils. Joint fluid analysis usually reveals a neutrophilic synovitis and/or arthritis, and *E. ewingii* morula may be found in 1% to 7% of neutrophils from affected joints.

Diagnosis of rickettsial polyarthritis is usually based on serologic testing plus other evidence of the disease during historical, physical, and clinicopathologic evaluation. Titers to the causative agents may not increase for 2 to 3 weeks after exposure. Paired samples taken 3 to 4 weeks apart often are necessary for the diagnosis of RMSF because the first titer taken at the start of the illness is often negative. A four-fold increase in IgG titer or a positive IgM titer is considered diagnostic. Any titer to *Ehrlichia* organisms is significant. There is no serologic test specific for antibodies to *E. ewingii*; however, there is substantial cross-reactivity among *E. canis, E. ewingii,* and *E. chaffeensis*. If desired, polymerase chain reaction (PCR) for *E. ewingii* is possible. There is a serologic test for *N. risticii* (which has minimal cross-reactivity with *E. canis*), but it is an uncommon cause and is generally not requested until *E. ewingii* is first eliminated. It is important to note that ehrlichial titers may stay greatly increased for months or longer after effecting a clinical cure with doxycycline; therefore treatment should be based upon clinical disease and not just upon serology. Adding to the confusion is the fact that many animals infected with one tick-borne disease may harbor a second or a third, making interpretation of serology potentially difficult. The reader is referred to a medical text for a more complete discussion of diagnosis and serology of the various rickettsiae affecting dogs.

DIFFERENTIAL DIAGNOSIS

Differential diagnoses for rickettsial joint infections include bacterial infection and immune-mediated polyarthritis.

MEDICAL MANAGEMENT

Treatment of rickettsial polyarthritis usually involves administration of doxycycline or tetracycline for 3 weeks (see Box 33-8 on p. 1160). Enrofloxacin is effective for RMSF (see Box 33-8), but is not clearly effective against *E. canis* or *E. ewingii*. Imidocarb can treat ehrlichiosis, but is seldom needed because doxycycline is effective and has fewer side effects than imidocarb. Sometimes it is helpful to also administer short-term steroids to patients with severe ehrlichiosis because there may be an immune-mediated component to the disease in these animals. This is especially true in animals with thrombocytopenia. Limiting exposure to ticks by removing ticks daily from dogs is important in preventing future infections.

SURGICAL TREATMENT

Surgical therapy is not indicated for rickettsial polyarthritis.

PROGNOSIS

Prognosis for dogs with RMSF varies, depending on clinical signs and promptness of the diagnosis. Animals treated early in the disease process usually have a better prognosis. Dogs with RMSF that are not treated until late in the disease may develop generalized CNS signs, uveitis, necrosis of affected tissue, and chronic, progressive polyarthritis. Dogs treated for *Ehrlichia* infections generally respond well to appropriate medical therapy as long as treatment is initiated before severe, generalized bone marrow suppression occurs.

Suggested Reading

Neer TM, Breitschwerdt EB, Greene RT et al: Consensus statement on Ehrlichial disease of small animals from the infectious disease study group of the ACVIM, *J Vet Intern Med* 16:309, 2002.
This is an excellent paper dealing with 20 common questions about canine ehrlichiosis.

LYME DISEASE

DEFINITION

Lyme disease is a form of polyarthritis caused by *Borrelia burgdorferi*.

GENERAL CONSIDERATIONS AND CLINICALLY RELEVANT PATHOPHYSIOLOGY

B. burgdorferi infection should be suspected in dogs with transient or recurrent arthritis if they have been in an area endemic for borreliosis. The disease can be transmitted by larval, nymphal, and adult *Ixodes* ticks. Approximately 50 hours of feeding are necessary for the tick to transmit the spirochete. Septicemia then occurs, with spread to target organs. Any dog that has the potential for contact with vectors of the disease may be infected; however, joint signs may occur months after exposure. There is currently little evidence that cats develop disease from these agents. Although clinical disease may be transient, the pathologic joint condition may be progressive. Clinical signs may be intermittent, with animals appearing normal between acute exacerbations; episodes may include multiple-limb lameness, fever, lymphadenopathy, and anorexia. Glomerulonephritis, renal tubular damage, or cardiac abnormalities (atrioventricular block and myocarditis) may occur in chronically infected dogs.

DIAGNOSIS
Clinical Presentation

Signalment. Dogs of any age or breed may be affected. Dogs that are in endemic areas and are exposed to ticks are most likely to be infected.

History. Dogs with Lyme disease can have acute fever, shifting leg lameness, anorexia, and/or depression. A history of being exposed to ticks in an endemic area is important.

Physical Examination Findings

Although clinical disease may be transient, the pathologic joint condition may be progressive. Clinical signs may be intermittent, with animals appearing normal between acute exacerbations; episodes may include multiple-limb lameness, fever, lymphadenomegaly, and anorexia.

Diagnostic Imaging

Radiographs of affected joints may show effusion during the acute phase of the disease.

Laboratory Findings

There are no hematologic or serum biochemistry panel findings that are particularly useful in diagnosing borreliosis. Inflammatory changes in the cerebrospinal fluid (CSF) and/or urine and/or joint fluid are potentially consistent. Severe protein-losing nephropathy (azotemia, hypoalbuminemia) has been seen in some patients with borreliosis. Synovial fluid from affected joints is less viscous and contains an increased number of leukocytes (e.g., 5000 to 100,000/µl) compared with normal synovial fluid, most of which are nondegenerate neutrophils. Phase-contrast or dark-field microscopy may allow visualization of organisms in synovial fluid. Attempts to culture *B. burgdorferi* from synovial fluid usually are unsuccessful. Synovial biopsy typically shows invasion of the synovial lining with plasmacytes and lymphocytes.

Serology is potentially confusing in the diagnosis of canine borreliosis. Clinically normal animals from endemic areas can have high titers. Because of the complexity of the different serologic tests and PCR that are available for the diagnosis of borreliosis, the reader is referred to a medical text for a more complete explanation. In general, a very high titer or dramatic increase in a convalescent titer, coupled with clinical signs and a response to antibiotic therapy, suggests a diagnosis of Lyme borreliosis; however, it is very difficult to definitely diagnose borreliosis.

> NOTE: Positive serologic findings reflect exposure to the organism, not necessarily active infection.

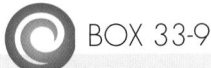 BOX 33-9

Treatment of Lyme Disease

Doxycycline (Vibramycin)
10 mg/kg PO bid

Amoxicillin
22 mg/kg PO bid

Chloramphenicol (Chloromycetin)
50 mg/kg PO tid (can rarely cause fatal aplastic anemia in people, therefore do not eat or drink while handling this product; do not touch eyes; wash hands after use; warn owners of same)

Azithromycin (Zithromax)
10 mg/kg PO bid for 5–7 days

Ceftriaxone (Rocephin)
50 mg/kg IM, SC, or IV bid

PO, Oral; *qd*, once a day; *bid*, twice a day; *tid*, three times a day; *IM*, intramuscular; *SC*, subcutaneous; *IV*, intravenous.

DIFFERENTIAL DIAGNOSIS

Differential diagnoses include other inflammatory, nonerosive, and erosive arthropathies (e.g., septic arthritis, rheumatoid arthritis, and osteoarthritis).

MEDICAL MANAGEMENT

Doxycycline generally is effective for treating Lyme disease (Box 33-9). Ceftriaxone, erythromycin, amoxicillin, azithromycin, and chloramphenicol also have been used (see Box 33-9).

SURGICAL TREATMENT

Surgery is not indicated for this disease.

PROGNOSIS

Dogs treated promptly for acute infections of *B. burgdorferi* probably have an excellent prognosis. The prognosis for dogs with chronic infections is uncertain. The spirochete apparently survives antibiotic treatment, and the disease can possibly be reactivated in immunosuppressed animals. Vaccination appears effective for protecting dogs against Lyme disease in endemic areas.

Suggested Reading

Fritz CL, Kjemtrup AM: Lyme borreliosis, *J Am Vet Med Assoc* 223:1261, 2003.
This article provides an excellent review of Lyme disease in dogs, including prevention, diagnosis, and treatment.

NONEROSIVE IDIOPATHIC IMMUNE-MEDIATED POLYARTHRITIS

DEFINITION

Nonerosive idiopathic immune-mediated polyarthritis is a noninfectious joint disease of unknown etiology. The term *canine idiopathic polyarthritis* is sometimes used for this condition.

GENERAL CONSIDERATIONS AND CLINICALLY RELEVANT PATHOPHYSIOLOGY

Idiopathic nonerosive inflammatory arthropathies have no identifiable cause and are diagnosed by ruling out all other causes of polyarthritis, septic arthritis, rickettsial arthritis, rheumatoid arthritis, other inflammatory nonerosive poly-arthropathies, and osteoarthritis. The cause is unknown, but presumed to be rooted in immune complex formation. The synovium is thickened, congested, and edematous and may contain fibrin deposits. Cartilage and bone are relatively unaffected; however, superficial fibrillation of the articular cartilage is an occasional finding.

Idiopathic immune-mediated nonerosive polyarthritis is diagnosed by synovial fluid analysis and culture, by joint radiographs that do not show erosive or proliferative bone lesions, and by eliminating other known causes. A therapeutic trial of antibiotics sometimes is used to help eliminate occult infectious causes, but it must be remembered that tetracyclines (which are commonly used) have antiinflammatory properties that can make it difficult to accurately decipher cause-and-effect in such cases.

DIAGNOSIS
Clinical Presentation

Signalment. All breeds and ages of dogs are susceptible to immune-mediated polyarthritis. Some studies have suggested breed predilections in German shepherds, Doberman pinchers, collies, spaniels, retrievers, terriers, and poodles. Females are more commonly affected (Davidson et al, 2003).

History. Stiffness, difficulty rising, pyrexia, anorexia, and/or lethargy may be present. Although more than one joint usually is involved, single-limb lameness is common. Affected animals may or may not have difficulty rising and walking. Some animals have a chronic fever of unknown origin.

Physical Examination Findings

Joint palpation may reveal pain, effusion, or loss of range of motion. It is important to note that joint effusion may be absent. Cervical pain and vertebral hypersensitivity may reflect intervertebral involvement. Other systemic abnormalities (dermatitis, glomerulonephritis, uveitis) may be found.

Diagnostic Imaging

Radiographs of affected joints usually reveal either no abnormalities or synovial fluid effusion and periarticular soft tissue swelling.

Laboratory Findings

Hematology often reveals a nonspecific neutrophilic leukocytosis, but it is not invariable. Synovial fluid is thin and turbid, and the mucin clot test usually is normal. Nucleated cell counts in joint fluid are notably elevated, with predominantly nondegenerative neutrophils. Most dogs test negative for or have insignificant titers of ANA and rheumatoid factor. Synovial biopsy usually reveals hypertrophy of the synovial lining plus polymorphonuclear or mononuclear cell infiltration. Microbial organisms are not observed, and bacterial cultures are negative.

DIFFERENTIAL DIAGNOSIS

Differential diagnoses for immune-mediated polyarthritis include all of the infectious arthritides.

MEDICAL MANAGEMENT

Glucocorticoids are the initial treatment of choice (Box 33-10). The dosage should be titrated to the lowest amount that prevents clinical signs; however, many animals require lifelong therapy. Azathioprine can be administered if clinical signs persist despite prednisone therapy (see Box 33-10), and cyclophosphamide can be used in difficult-to-control patients, although it is not recommended as it has a plethora of serious side effects. Cyclophosphamide and to a lesser extent azathioprine can cause myelosuppression, and a CBC and platelet count initially should be monitored every 2 weeks or whenever the patient seems unwell. Cyclophosphamide may also cause sterile cystitis, and azathioprine may cause hepatitis or pancreatitis. Use of cyclosporine requires therapeutic drug

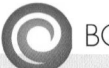 BOX 33-10

Treatment of Idiopathic Immune-Mediated Polyarthritis

Prednisone

2.2–4.4 mg/kg/day for 2 wk; then if clinical response is seen, can decrease to 1.1 to 2.2 mg/kg/day for 2 wk; if animal is clinically normal at this time and if synovial inflammation has subsided, reduce dosage to 1.1 mg/kg qod for 4 wk

Azathioprine (Imuran)

Dogs: 2 mg/kg/day given orally for 2 to 3 wk; then 2 mg/kg qod if clinical signs resolve; giving 2 mg/kg qod from the start will require longer to achieve remission, but may lessen the chance of hepatitis or pancreatitis

Cyclosporine

3–5 mg/kg PO bid with food; must do therapeutic drug monitoring to check trough levels and then adjust dose

Cyclophosphamide (Cytoxan)

50 mg/m²; give up to 4 consecutive days each week for up to 4 mo; this drug can have substantial and life-threatening side effects; it is best to use other drugs first and only use this drug if needed

---

qod, Every other day; *PO,* oral; *bid,* twice a day.

monitoring because absorption varies greatly between different products and different patients. Although the prognosis for achieving remission of clinical signs is good, adverse side effects may occur with long-term corticosteroid therapy.

SURGICAL TREATMENT

Surgery is not indicated.

PROGNOSIS

The prognosis for nonerosive immune-mediated polyarthritis varies. In most cases remission or cure can be achieved, but owners should be warned of the possibility of recurrence. A positive response to therapy should be based on arthrocentesis and cytology and not on clinical signs alone because medical therapy may result in clinical improvement but incomplete cessation of the inflammatory activity.

Reference

Davidson AP: Immune-mediated polyarthritis. In Slatter D, editor: *Textbook of small animal surgery,* ed 3, Philadelphia, 2003, Saunders.

Suggested Reading

Rondeau MP, Walton RM, Bissett S et al: Suppurative, nonseptic polyarthropathy in dogs, *J Vet Intern Med* 19:654, 2005.
This article reviews findings of a large case series of dogs with immune-mediated joint disease, and an excellent review of the literature on this subject.

CHRONIC INFLAMMATORY-INDUCED POLYARTHRITIS

Nonerosive inflammatory polyarthritis may occur secondary to any chronic inflammatory disorder or to persistent antigenic stimulus. Another disease (e.g., chronic infection, bacterial endocarditis, gastroenteritis, ulcerative colitis, or neoplasia) or drug therapy (e.g., sulfamethoxazole-trimethoprim or sulfadiazine-trimethoprim) incites formation of immune complexes, which mediate the arthritis. The synovium becomes thickened, congested, and edematous and may contain fibrin deposits. Occasionally, superficial fibrillation of articular cartilage may be seen, but cartilage and bone usually are unaffected.

It is crucial to differentiate this condition from septic arthritis, rheumatoid arthritis, idiopathic inflammatory nonerosive polyarthropathy, and DJD because antiinflammatory therapy in dogs with chronic infection can prove fatal. Diagnosis of chronic inflammatory-induced polyarthritis is based on synovial fluid analysis, identification of the inciting disease, and elimination of other diseases (see previous discussion).

DIAGNOSIS
Clinical Presentation

Signalment. Dogs and cats of any breed and age may be affected.

History. Affected animals may have a history of either acute or chronic lameness, stiffness, difficulty rising, pyrexia, anorexia, and/or lethargy. Other clinical signs may be associated with the inciting disease.

Physical Examination Findings

Joint palpation may elicit pain and detect effusion or diminished range of motion, but these findings are not obvious in all dogs.

Diagnostic Imaging

Radiographs of affected joints may reveal joint effusion and periarticular soft tissue swelling, or they may be normal. Thoracic and abdominal imaging should be done to look for the inciting disease.

Laboratory Findings

There are no characteristic hematology or serum biochemistry findings. Synovial fluid typically is thin and turbid, and the mucin clot test usually is normal. Nucleated cell counts are greatly elevated, and nondegenerative neutrophils are the preponderant cell type. Most dogs do not have significant titers to ANA or rheumatoid factor. Synovial biopsy reveals hypertrophy of the synovial lining with polymorphonuclear or mononuclear cell infiltration. Despite chronic infection elsewhere in the body, the joints usually are sterile.

DIFFERENTIAL DIAGNOSIS

Differential diagnoses include idiopathic immune-mediated joint disease and infectious polyarthritis.

MEDICAL MANAGEMENT

Treatment should be directed at eliminating the underlying disease. Antibiotics, selected after culture and susceptibility testing, are indicated for infections. Glucocorticoids, administered orally or by injection, may be given short term to control synovitis in severe cases, but only after making sure that there is no infection elsewhere in the body.

SURGICAL TREATMENT

Surgery is not indicated.

PROGNOSIS

Prognosis of chronic inflammatory-induced polyarthritis varies and depends greatly upon the underlying disease. If the underlying disease can be successfully treated, the polyarthritis may resolve or can usually be successfully treated.

PLASMACYTIC-LYMPHOCYTIC SYNOVITIS
DEFINITION

Plasmacytic-lymphocytic synovitis *(lymphoplasmacytic synovitis)* is an immune-mediated arthropathy associated with plasmacytic and lymphocytic infiltration of the synovium.

GENERAL CONSIDERATIONS AND CLINICALLY RELEVANT PATHOPHYSIOLOGY

Plasmacytic-lymphocytic synovitis often affects stifle joints, leading to cruciate ligament degeneration and rupture, joint instability, and osteoarthritis. The synovium is thickened, congested, and edematous and may contain fibrin deposits.

DIAGNOSIS
Clinical Presentation

Signalment. Plasmacytic-lymphocytic synovitis may affect younger dogs in association with CCL rupture. Purebred dogs, such as rottweilers, may be overrepresented (Pedersen et al, 2000).

History. Affected dogs generally have unilateral or bilateral rear limb lameness of either acute onset or chronic duration. The presenting history is similar to that for CCL rupture, and a cranial drawer sign usually is present once cruciate ligament rupture has occurred.

Physical Examination Findings

The stifles generally are enlarged because of joint effusion and chronic periarticular soft tissue fibrosis. Suspect joints should be biopsied during surgery for CCL rupture if plasmacytic-lymphocytic synovitis is suspected.

Diagnostic Imaging

Radiographs of the stifles reveal joint effusion and varying signs of osteoarthritis, depending on the chronicity of the CCL rupture.

Laboratory Findings

Hematology and serum biochemistry results usually are normal. The synovial fluid usually is thin and turbid with an increased nucleated cell count composed primarily of lymphocytes and plasma cells. Synovial biopsy reveals villous hyperplasia and infiltration of the synovium and cruciate ligament with lymphocytes and plasmacytes.

DIFFERENTIAL DIAGNOSIS

Cruciate ligament rupture in dogs with plasmacytic-lymphocytic synovitis must be differentiated from routine cruciate ruptures (see p. 1254).

MEDICAL MANAGEMENT

Medical treatment for plasmacytic-lymphocytic synovitis is the same as for idiopathic immune-mediated polyarthritis (see Box 33-10).

SURGICAL TREATMENT

Surgical therapy to stabilize the CCL is indicated in these patients.

Preoperative Management

Preoperative management of animals undergoing surgery for CCL rupture is described on p. 1262.

Anesthesia

Anesthetic management of animals with orthopedic disease is provided on p. 944.

Surgical Anatomy

Surgical anatomy of the stifle joint is provided on p. 1262.

Positioning

Positioning for cranial cruciate surgery is described on p. 1263. Positioning for subtotal synovectomy is described on p. 1263.

SURGICAL TECHNIQUE

For CCL surgery, see p. 1262.

SUTURE MATERIALS AND SPECIAL INSTRUMENTS

For suture materials and special instruments for cranial cruciate surgery see p. 1273.

PROGNOSIS

The prognosis generally is good for achieving remission of clinical signs.

Reference

Pedersen NC, Morgan JP, Vasseur PB: Joint diseases of dogs and cats. In Ettinger SJ, editor: *Textbook of veterinary internal medicine,* ed 5, Philadelphia, 2000, Saunders.

SYSTEMIC LUPUS ERYTHEMATOSUS–INDUCED POLYARTHRITIS

DEFINITION

SLE is a multisystemic disease caused by autoantibodies against tissue protein and DNA.

GENERAL CONSIDERATIONS AND CLINICALLY RELEVANT PATHOPHYSIOLOGY

In SLE, circulating immune complexes of antigen and autoantibodies pass through endothelial cell junctions and are trapped in basement membranes, causing inflammation and eventual organ dysfunction. The synovium typically is thickened and discolored, but cartilage and bone are relatively unaffected. A definitive diagnosis of SLE is established if a patient has two or more of the following criteria and tests positive for ANA: cutaneous lesions, oral ulcers, arthritis, serositis (pericarditis or pleuritis), renal disorders, neurologic disorders, lymphopenia, anemia and/or thrombocytopenia, antiphospholipids, and polymyositis or myocarditis (Stone, 2005).

DIAGNOSIS
Clinical Presentation

Signalment. Any breed or age of dog or cat may be affected.

History. Many drugs (e.g., allopurinol, griseofulvin, piroxicam, sulfonamides, and tetracycline) have been associated with causing SLE in human beings. Whether they do so in dogs is uncertain, but prior administration of these drugs must be considered while taking the history. Affected dogs may have skin lesions, lameness, malaise, anorexia, and any number of other signs, depending upon what organs are being affected (e.g., anemia, azotemia, etc).

Physical Examination Findings

Arthritis and fever are two of the most common findings in dogs with SLE.

Diagnostic Imaging

Radiographs of affected joints usually reveal either no abnormalities or synovial fluid effusion and periarticular soft tissue swelling.

Laboratory Findings

Hematology may reveal evidence of immune-mediated hemolytic anemia (e.g., spherocytes and autoagglutination) and/or immune-mediated thrombocytopenia. There may be protein-losing nephropathy (e.g., hypoalbuminemia, hypercholesterolemia, azotemia, or proteinuria despite a clean sediment) in some patients. Synovial fluid usually is thin and turbid, and the mucin clot test is normal. Joint fluid nucleated cell counts are greatly elevated and composed mostly of nondegenerative neutrophils. Lupus erythematosus (LE) cells are rarely present in the joint fluid. ANA test results should be strongly positive (ANA is a sensitive test for SLE), and rheumatoid factor usually is normal. However, ANA tests are nonspecific, and positive titers may be associated with diseases other than SLE. In such cases, the ANA titer tends to be lower than is seen in SLE, but that is subjective. LE cell preparations on peripheral blood are fraught with difficulties in interpretation and are not recommended.

Synovial biopsy typically reveals hypertrophy and hyperplasia of the synovial lining with an inflammatory infiltrate of polymorphonuclear cells, macrophages, lymphocytes, and plasma cells. Immunofluorescent studies may show IgG- and IgM-producing plasma cells. Microbial organisms are not observed histologically, and bacterial cultures are negative.

DIFFERENTIAL DIAGNOSIS

This condition must be differentiated from rheumatoid arthritis, idiopathic inflammatory nonerosive polyarthropathy, septic arthritis, and DJD.

MEDICAL MANAGEMENT

Glucocorticoids are the initial treatment of choice for SLE-induced polyarthritis (see Box 33-10 on p. 1164). The drugs may be stopped in some cases because of long periods of remission, but in other cases they must be maintained for the animal's entire life. Azathioprine can be administered with prednisolone to allow the clinician to use a lower dose of steroids. In rare cases, cyclophosphamide may be used, but it is not recommended because of the potential severity of its side effects. Cyclophosphamide and to a lesser extent azathioprine can cause myelosuppression; therefore a CBC and platelet count should be taken every 2 weeks initially. Cyclo-

phosphamide may also cause a sterile cystitis, and azathioprine may cause hepatitis or pancreatitis. Use of cyclosporine requires therapeutic drug monitoring because absorption varies greatly between different products and different patients. An alternative treatment of prednisone combined with levamisole (2 to 5 mg/kg to a maximum of 150 mg administered on alternate days) has met with some success. The prednisone is progressively reduced and eliminated over 1 to 2 months. Levamisole is continued for 4 months. Azathioprine is not recommended in cats. Chlorambucil (Leukeran) may be administered to cats at a dosage of 15 mg/m² (4 mg in most cats) orally, once a day for 4 days, and then repeated every 3 weeks. A CBC should be performed to evaluate for leukopenia (Stone, 2005).

SURGICAL TREATMENT

Surgical treatment is not indicated.

PROGNOSIS

Prognosis is generally good for control of the polyarthritis; however, abnormalities in other organs (e.g., glomerulonephritis) may progress. For resistant cases, newer immunosuppressive drugs (e.g., leflunomide and mycophenolate) may be tried.

Reference

Stone M: Systemic lupus erythematosus. In Ettinger SJ, Feldman EC, editors: *Textbook of veterinary internal medicine,* ed 6, Philadelphia, 2005, Saunders.

Suggested Reading

Chabanne L, Rigal D, Fournel C et al: Canine systemic lupus erythematosus. Part II, *Compend Cont Educ* 21:402, 1999.
This is a good review of current thoughts on diagnosis and therapy of canine SLE.
Smith BE, Tompkins MB, Breitschwerdt EB: Antinuclear antibodies can be detected in dog sera reactive to *Bartonella vinsonii* subsp *bekhoffii, Ehrlichia canis,* or *Leishmania infantum* antigens, *J Vet Intern Med* 18:47, 2004.
The authors show that ANA testing may be positive in dogs with infections by these organisms.

RHEUMATOID ARTHRITIS

DEFINITION

Rheumatoid arthritis is an erosive, noninfectious, inflammatory joint disease characterized by chronic, bilaterally symmetric, erosive destruction of the joints.

GENERAL CONSIDERATIONS AND CLINICALLY RELEVANT PATHOPHYSIOLOGY

The etiology of rheumatoid arthritis is unknown, but it is considered an immune-mediated arthropathy. The antigens are altered host immunoglobulins (IgG and IgM), which are known as "rheumatoid factors." Resultant immune complexes are deposited in the synovium, initiating an inflamma-

BOX 33-11

Characteristics of Rheumatoid Arthritis

- Stiffness after rest
- Pain in at least one joint
- Swelling in at least one joint
- Swelling of at least one other joint within 3 months
- Symmetric joint swelling
- Subcutaneous nodules over bony prominences or extensor surfaces, or in juxtaarticular regions
- Destructive radiographic lesions
- Positive rheumatoid factor
- Poor mucin precipitate from synovial fluid
- Characteristic histopathologic changes in the synovial membrane
- Characteristic histopathologic changes in subcutaneous nodules

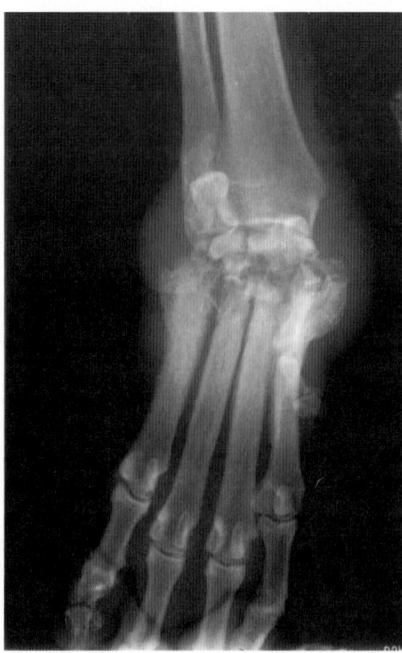

FIG. 33-9
Dorsopalmar radiograph of the canine carpus with advanced abnormalities associated with rheumatoid arthritis. Note the erosion of subchondral bone plates and the collapse of the joint space, suggesting erosion of the articular cartilage.

tory response followed by synovial cell proliferation, villous hypertrophy, pannus formation over the cartilage surface, cartilage and subchondral bone destruction, joint swelling, and rupture of the collateral ligaments. The outcome is a nonfunctional joint. The synovial membrane generally is discolored, edematous, congested, and thickened and may contain fibrin deposits. Pannus of granulation tissue originates at the periphery of the joint and covers portions of the articular cartilage, which may fibrillate and ulcerate.

Diagnosis of classic rheumatoid arthritis requires the presence of destructive lesions seen radiographically, a positive rheumatoid factor, characteristic histopathologic changes in the synovial membrane, and four additional criteria listed in Box 33-11. Rheumatoid arthritis usually is diagnosed when 7 of the 11 criteria are present and joint signs have been present for at least 6 weeks. Subcutaneous nodules are rare in dogs.

DIAGNOSIS
Clinical Presentation

Signalment. Rheumatoid arthritis can affect any breed of dog, but is primarily found in adults, usually greater than 5 years old.

History. Most affected dogs have a history of stiffness after rest, limping, or difficulty walking.

Physical Examination Findings

Joints are generally enlarged with periarticular soft tissue swelling and joint effusion. The distal joints (i.e., carpi and tarsi) may be unstable, with obvious deformity and angulation.

Diagnostic Imaging

Radiographs of the joints show a generalized loss of mineralization, radiolucent foci, and irregular joint margins. Bone proliferation may also be present. Soft tissue swelling and joint effusion may be evident (Fig. 33-9).

Laboratory Findings

Hematology may reveal anemia of chronic inflammation and a nonspecific leukocytosis. The synovial fluid often is yellow, turbid, and increased in volume. The mucin clot may be poor and friable. Joint fluid nucleated cell counts are greatly elevated with predominantly nondegenerative neutrophils. Between 20% and 70% of affected dogs show positive test results for rheumatoid factor; most show normal ANA levels. In the Rose-Waaler agglutination test for rheumatoid factor, a differential titer of 1:8 and above is positive. (Note: appropriate controls must be run with sheep red blood cells.) In latex agglutination tests, agglutination denotes a positive test result at serum dilutions specified by the producer of the test. However, dogs with no obvious evidence of rheumatoid arthritis may have positive titers; therefore care is warranted in interpreting tests for rheumatoid factor.

Synovial biopsy generally shows villous hypertrophy, proliferation of synovial cells, and lymphocyte and plasma cell infiltration. Immunofluorescent studies demonstrate complexes of IgG or IgM in synovial lining cells, blood vessel walls, and extracellular tissue. Microbial organisms are not observed on histologic samples, and bacterial cultures are negative.

DIFFERENTIAL DIAGNOSIS

Differential diagnoses include arthritis, inflammatory nonerosive polyarthropathies, and DJD.

MEDICAL MANAGEMENT

A combination of immunosuppressive drugs (prednisone, azathioprine, cyclosporine, cyclophosphamide, or gold salts) typically is necessary to achieve remission of clinical signs

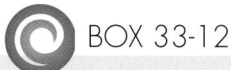 BOX 33-12

Therapy for Rheumatoid Arthritis

Prednisolone

2.2–4.4 mg/kg/day PO for 2 wk; then 1.1–2.2 mg/kg/day PO for 2 wk; then 1.1 mg/kg qod

Azathioprine (Imuran)

Dogs 2 mg/kg/day PO for 2 to 3 wk; then 2 mg/kg qod if clinical signs resolve; giving 2 mg/kg qod from the start will require longer to achieve remission, but may lessen the chance of hepatitis or pancreatitis

Cyclosporine

3–5 mg/kg PO bid with food; must do therapeutic drug monitoring to check trough levels and then adjust dose

Cyclophosphamide (Cytoxan)

50 mg/m²; give up to 4 consecutive days each week for up to 4 mo; this drug can have substantial and life-threatening side effects; it is best to use other drugs first and only use this drug if needed

Aurothioglucose (Gold Salts)*

Dogs <10 kg: 1 mg IM the first week, then 2 mg IM the second week, then 1 mg/kg/wk for 8 weeks or until remission occurs
Dogs >10 kg: 5 mg IM the first week, then 10 mg IM the second week, then 1 mg/kg/wk for 8 weeks or until remission occurs

PO, Oral; *qod,* every other day; *bid,* twice a day; *IM,* intramuscular.
*This drug may have adverse side effects and should only be used when absolutely necessary.

(Box 33-12). Therapy usually is initiated with prednisone, and then additional immunosuppressive drugs (e.g., azathioprine) are added. Cyclophosphamide should be avoided because it poses significant risks to the dog and the person administering the drug. Gold salts are rarely used now because of their side effects. After each month of treatment, the dog should be reevaluated and synovial fluid analyzed. The dose of steroid is gradually reduced with a goal of ultimately only needing 1 mg/kg every other day (plus either azathioprine or cyclosporine). If inflammation persists, gold salts may be added to the therapy. Gold salts can be toxic, and hematologic values should be monitored at least every 2 weeks. Joints that have lost all collateral ligament support may benefit from arthrodesis. However, the high concentrations of immunosuppressive drugs also inhibit body defenses against infection and may delay bone healing.

SURGICAL TREATMENT

Surgical treatment (other than possibly arthrodesis; see previous discussion) is not indicated.

PROGNOSIS

Rheumatoid arthritis is progressive, and dogs rarely, if ever, make a full recovery. Lameness and stiffness usually persist despite treatment.

FELINE CHRONIC PROGRESSIVE POLYARTHRITIS

DEFINITION

Feline chronic progressive polyarthritis is an immune-mediated disease of male cats and is associated with progressive periosteal-proliferative and erosive polyarthritis.

GENERAL CONSIDERATIONS AND CLINICALLY RELEVANT PATHOPHYSIOLOGY

The cause may involve exposure to the feline syncytium-forming virus (FeSFV) and feline leukemia virus (FeLV); however, the disease cannot be experimentally induced by these viruses. The periosteal-proliferative form of the disease results in osteoporosis and periosteal new bone formation around the joint. Periarticular erosions and collapse of the joint space with fibrous ankylosis occur with time. The erosive form of the disease causes joint changes similar to those seen in canine rheumatoid arthritis. The synovium is infiltrated with lymphocytes and plasma cells.

DIAGNOSIS
Clinical Presentation

Signalment. This condition affects only male cats; female cats are seemingly unaffected. Affected cats are generally between the ages of 1.5 and 4.5 years. Any breed of cat may be affected.

History. Most cats have a history of lameness, reluctance to move, depression, anorexia, weight loss, and occasionally deformity of affected joints.

Physical Examination Findings

Pyrexia, depression, lymphadenopathy, and multiple-joint involvement are common findings. Joint palpation causes pain. The joints sometimes are swollen and may be deformed in animals with the erosive form of the disease.

Diagnostic Imaging

Changes noted on radiographs of affected joints include proliferative new bone formation on the periphery of the joints, generalized loss of opacity of the subchondral bone, and loss of the joint space. Radiolucent foci in the subchondral bone and irregular joint margins may also occur. Periarticular soft tissue swelling and joint effusion may be noted (Fig. 33-10).

Laboratory Findings

FeSFV is identified in all cats with feline chronic progressive polyarthritis, and FeLV is identified in 60% of cats with the disease. Synovial fluid analysis demonstrates elevated neutrophil counts. Routine blood work may demonstrate leukocytosis.

DIFFERENTIAL DIAGNOSIS

Differential diagnoses include septic arthritis, DJD, and hypervitaminosis A.

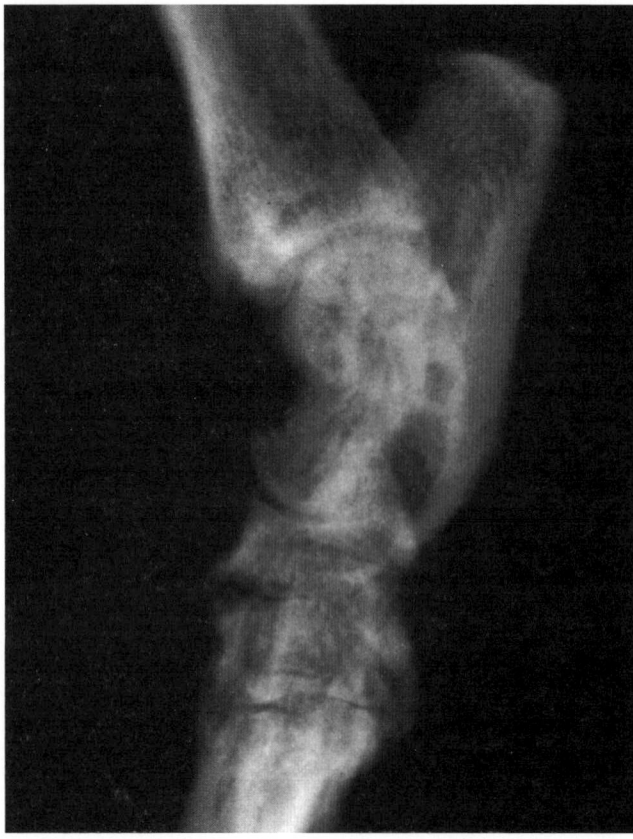

FIG. 33-10
Radiograph of the tarsus of a cat with the periosteal-prolifer-ative form of feline progressive arthritis. There is proliferative new bone formation on the periphery of the joints, general-ized loss of opacity of subchondral bone, and loss of the joint space. Radiolucent foci are visible throughout the tarsal bones. (From Olmstead ML: *Small animal orthopedics*, St Louis, 1995, Mosby.)

MEDICAL MANAGEMENT

Treatment involves immunosuppressive drugs and usually begins with prednisolone (Box 33-13). The cat often requires lifelong therapy. Chlorambucil may help control the signs. Cyclophosphamide and azathioprine are myelosuppressive in cats and should be avoided unless they are absolutely necessary.

> NOTE: If you lower the dose of medications too quickly in these patients, clinical signs often recur and are more resistant to therapy.

SURGICAL TREATMENT

Surgical therapy is not indicated.

PROGNOSIS

Prognosis is good for remission of signs, but guarded for complete control of the disease. Other FeLV-related disorders may occur in cats that test positive.

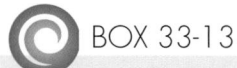

BOX 33-13

Treatment of Feline Chronic Progressive Polyarthritis

Prednisolone

4.4–6.6 mg/kg/day PO; if cat improves after 2 wk, reduce dosage to 2.2 mg/kg/day; then place on maintenance therapy (1.1–2.2 mg/kg qod)

Chlorambucil (Leukeran)

1 mg/cat PO twice weekly in cats <3.5 kg; 2 mg/cat PO twice weekly in cats >3.5 kg*

Cyclophosphamide (Cytoxan)

6.25–12.5 mg/cat PO given up to 4 consecutive days of each week for up to 4 mo; this drug can have substantial and life-threatening side effects; it is best to use other drugs first and only use this drug if needed*

PO, Oral; *qod*, every other day.
*Watch for neutropenia; do periodic CBCs to check.

TEMPOROMANDIBULAR JOINT

TEMPOROMANDIBULAR JOINT LUXATION

DEFINITION

Temporomandibular joint luxation or *dislocation* results when the mandibular condyles separate from articular surfaces of the temporal bone and mandibular fossae.

GENERAL CONSIDERATIONS AND CLINICALLY RELEVANT PATHOPHYSIOLOGY

Temporomandibular joint luxation occurs as a result of head trauma; however, luxation of this joint is uncommon because it is protected by the heavy temporal muscles. Luxation may occur unilaterally or bilaterally and may be associated with mandibular fractures. Although mandibular condyles can displace cranial or caudal to the mandibular fossa, craniodorsal displacement is most common.

DIAGNOSIS
Clinical Presentation

Signalment. The condition occurs in both dogs and cats. Animals of either gender and any age may be affected.

History. The animal usually has a history of recent trauma.

Physical Examination Findings

Animals usually have an open mouth, which they appear reluctant to close. Direction of the luxation often can be determined by evaluating the jaw position. A unilateral craniodorsal luxation causes the rostral aspect of the mandible to shift toward the opposite side of the mouth, whereas a bilateral craniodorsal luxation causes the entire mandible to protrude forward. Caudal condylar luxation causes the mandible to shift caudally and toward the side of the luxation.

With the patient under anesthesia and before closed reduction, the mandible and maxilla should be thoroughly inspected for oral wounds, visible fractures, and palpable crepitation of the caudal mandible. Radiographs are warranted when fracture is suspected.

Diagnostic Imaging

Definitive diagnosis is made from skull radiographs taken with the animal anesthetized or heavily sedated. Four radiographic views are standard for complete evaluation of the skull (see p. 1016). The most reliable radiographic finding is an increase in joint space width; this finding usually is most evident on a dorsoventral projection. Radiographs should be carefully assessed to determine if there are concurrent mandibular or maxillary fractures that warrant open reduction and stabilization. CT can also be used to assess the status of the temporomandibular joint.

Laboratory Findings

Specific laboratory abnormalities are not seen. Because this condition is caused by trauma, sufficient laboratory values should be obtained to evaluate the risk of anesthesia in affected animals.

DIFFERENTIAL DIAGNOSIS

Differential diagnoses include mandibular or maxillary fractures (see p. 1015) and temporomandibular joint dysplasia (see p. 1172), which may show similar clinical signs.

MEDICAL MANAGEMENT

The luxation usually can be reduced without surgical intervention, but general anesthesia is required. A wooden dowel rod is placed transversely between the mandibular and maxillary molars and used as a fulcrum to distract the condyles distally while the rostral mandible and maxilla are squeezed together. The mandible is manipulated cranially or caudally to move the condyle into place. After the joint has been reduced, it should be carefully palpated to determine its stability. Unstable joints can be supported with tape muzzles (see p. 1016), interarcade wiring (see p. 1017), or interarcade acrylic for 7 to 14 days until fibrosis occurs. If it is impossible to reduce the joint or to maintain joint reduction, open reduction and stabilization should be performed.

SURGICAL TREATMENT

Reduction of a temporomandibular joint luxation should be attempted as soon as the animal can undergo general anesthesia. Closed reduction (see previous discussion) frequently is successful and is the initial procedure of choice if concurrent fractures are not present; however, open reduction may be necessary if the luxation is unstable after closed reduction.

Preoperative Management

Animals should be evaluated for concurrent trauma and treated appropriately. Thoracic radiographs and electrocardiograms are indicated in animals that have sustained trauma.

Anesthesia

General anesthesia is necessary for closed or open reduction of a temporomandibular luxation (see p. 944). Endotracheal tubes may interfere with closed reduction techniques and with evaluation of occlusion. The endotracheal tube can be temporarily removed during closed reduction procedures or rerouted through a pharyngotomy incision (see p. 1025), or a tracheostomy (see p. 825) may be performed for longer procedures.

Surgical Anatomy

See p. 1015 for a description of the surgical anatomy of the mandible. Landmarks for approaching the temporomandibular joint are the ventral border of the zygomatic arch and the joint space (palpated while the mandible is manipulated). The masseter muscle is elevated off the zygomatic arch to expose the joint. The parotid duct and gland and facial nerve are located dorsal and superficial to the masseter muscle and should be avoided. The temporomandibular joint is composed of a mandibular condyle, articular disk (meniscus), mandibular fossa of the temporal bone, mandibular ligament, and joint capsule. The articular disk divides the joint into the dorsal (meniscotemporal) and ventral (meniscomandibular) compartments.

Positioning

The patient is positioned in lateral recumbency for a unilateral approach and in dorsal recumbency for bilateral approaches.

SURGICAL TECHNIQUE

Make a skin incision following the ventral border of the caudal zygomatic arch and centered over the temporomandibular joint. Be sure to avoid the parotid duct and gland and facial nerve. Elevate the caudal periosteal insertion of the masseter muscle from the zygomatic arch to expose the joint capsule. Incise the joint capsule and mandibular ligament to expose the articular surfaces. Irrigate the joint and remove any bone fragments or debris that may have interfered with reduction. Replace the mandibular condyle in the fossa. To hold the condyle in position, suture the joint capsule and mandibular ligament. Suture the masseter muscle to the fascia on the dorsal edge of the zygomatic arch. Close the platysma muscle and skin in separate layers.

SUTURE MATERIALS AND SPECIAL INSTRUMENTS

Joint capsule should be sutured with absorbable suture material (polydioxanone, polyglyconate). A periosteal elevator is needed to elevate the masseter muscle and expose the joint capsule. Gelpi retractors are useful for maintaining exposure.

POSTOPERATIVE CARE AND ASSESSMENT

Postoperative radiographs should be evaluated to document that the mandibular condyles are normally positioned. If the joints are stable, the animal should be allowed to eat only soft food for 2 to 3 weeks. Unstable joints in dogs can be supported with a tape muzzle (see p. 1016) for 1 to 2 weeks; muzzles are difficult to maintain on cats, and interarcade wiring or acrylic may be necessary (see p. 1016). Liquid diets should be fed to these animals until the muzzle or interarcade fixation is removed; then soft food is recommended for an additional 1 to 2 weeks.

> NOTE: Consider interarcade wiring or acrylic in cats if the joints appear unstable after reduction.

PROGNOSIS

The prognosis generally is good for normal function if the luxation can be reduced and the joints made stable. Complications include failure to reduce the joint, repeated luxation, and joint ankylosis. A mandibular condylectomy (see p. 1174) is recommended for joints that remain or become unstable, painful, fibrotic, or stiff after surgery.

Suggested Reading

Bennett JW, Kapatkin AS, Marretta SM: Dental composite for the fixation of mandibular fractures and luxations in 11 cats and 6 dogs, *Vet Surg* May-June;23(3):190-194, 1994.
This article provides an excellent description of the technique of interarcade acrylic for stabilization of the jaw.
Schwarz T, Weller R, Dickie AM et al: Imaging of the canine and feline temporomandibular joint: a review *Vet Radiol Ultrasound* March-Apr;43(2):85-97, 2002.
This article describes proper techniques for imaging of the temporomandibular joint in dogs and cats.

TEMPOROMANDIBULAR JOINT DYSPLASIA

DEFINITION

Temporomandibular joint dysplasia *(open-mouth jaw locking, temporomandibular subluxation, congenital temporomandibular luxation or subluxation)* is a disease characterized by locking of the jaws in an open position.

GENERAL CONSIDERATIONS AND CLINICALLY RELEVANT PATHOPHYSIOLOGY

Temporomandibular joint dysplasia is a disease of unknown etiology that affects young adult dogs. Deformation of the mandibular condyloid processes and mandibular fossa allows subluxation and recurrent locking of the mandible in an open-mouthed position. In some affected animals, the mandibular fossae are shallow and the condyloid processes more obliquely situated than normal. This combination allows joint subluxation. Joint instability leads to osteoarthrosis, pain, and locking of the jaw in an open position. Instability coupled with mandibular symphyseal laxity allows independent movement of the mandibles, which may result in malpositioning of coronoid processes lateral to the zygomatic arch, further promoting open-mouth locking. Open-mouth locking occurs in some dogs without evidence of coronoid process malpositioning.

DIAGNOSIS
Clinical Presentation

Signalment. The syndrome of open-mouth locking caused by coronoid process malpositioning has been reported in basset hounds, Irish setters, and a Saint Bernard. Pain and occasional open-mouth locking without malposition of the coronoid process occur in retriever and boxer breeds. Clinical signs usually are first noted when the dogs are young adults.

History. Owners usually describe repeated incidents of open-mouth locking after yawning. Usually the joints spontaneously reduce, but owners occasionally seek veterinary care because the jaws remain luxated. Some animals show pain on oral manipulation and are reluctant to eat. These animals have no history of trauma.

Physical Examination Findings

Animals are usually presented for treatment with the jaws locked in an open-mouth position. If the coronoid process is locked outside the zygomatic arch, a bulge in the subcutaneous tissue overlying the zygomatic arch on the affected side can be seen and palpated. Affected animals may show pain on palpation of the temporomandibular joint.

Diagnostic Imaging

A standard skull series with the mouth open and closed is used to evaluate the temporomandibular joints and the position of the coronoid process. This is often facilitated with the use of fluoroscopy to dynamically image the joints. Changes consistent with temporomandibular joint dysplasia include increased or irregular joint spaces on a lateral projection, shallow mandibular fossae, and secondary osteoarthritis. On ventral dorsal projections, the condyles may be more oblique than normal and the coronoid process may be positioned lateral to the zygomatic arch when the mouth is open.

> NOTE: Compare the radiographs with those of a normal animal if the diagnosis is in doubt.

Laboratory Findings

No specific laboratory abnormalities are seen.

DIFFERENTIAL DIAGNOSIS

Differential diagnoses include traumatic luxation of the temporomandibular joint, mandibular fractures, and lodged oral foreign bodies.

MEDICAL MANAGEMENT

Manual reduction may be possible by opening the mouth widely and manipulating the mandible away from the locked side. If the dog resists this manipulation, general anesthesia may be required.

SURGICAL TREATMENT

Repeated episodes can occur, and definitive treatment in such animals requires either partial resection of the zygomatic arch (if the coronoid process locks outside the zygomatic arch) or mandibular condylectomy (if displacement of the coronoid process does not occur outside the zygomatic arch).

Preoperative Management

These animals usually are young and healthy and require minimal preoperative care.

Anesthesia

A variety of anesthetic regimens can be used (see p. 944).

Surgical Anatomy

See the description of the surgical anatomy of the mandible on p. •••. Surgical anatomy of the temporomandibular joint is described on p. 1015.

Positioning

The patient is positioned in lateral recumbency with the affected side up for resection of the zygomatic arch and for mandibular condylectomy.

SURGICAL TECHNIQUE
Partial Resection of the Zygomatic Arch

Make an incision in the skin and subcutaneous tissue overlying the ventral border of the rostral portion of the zygomatic arch. Elevate the fascial attachments to the arch while preserving the dorsal buccal branch of the facial nerve. Open the mouth wide to induce coronoid process displacement to identify the portion of the arch that obstructs replacement of the process. Resect the obstructing portion of the arch with a rongeur or high-speed burr (Fig. 33-11). Before closure, ensure that the coronoid process is positioned normally. Close the subcutaneous tissue and skin separately.

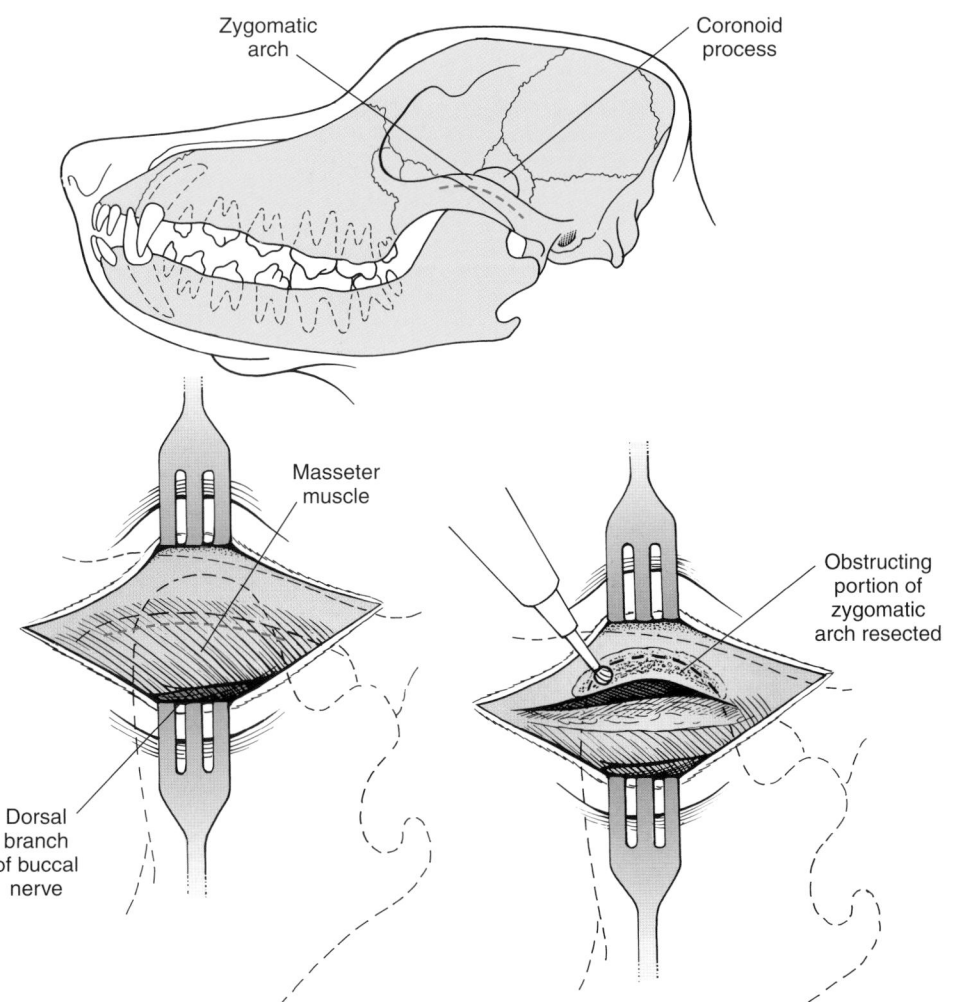

FIG. 33-11
To expose the zygomatic arch, make an incision in the skin and subcutaneous tissue overlying the ventral border of the rostral portion of the zygomatic arch. Elevate the fascial attachments to the arch and resect the obstructing portion of the arch with a rongeur or high-speed burr.

Mandibular Condylectomy

Make a skin incision along the ventral border of the caudal zygomatic arch, centered over the temporomandibular joint. Elevate the caudal periosteal insertion of the masseter muscle from the zygomatic arch to expose the joint capsule. Identify the joint by palpating it while an assistant moves the mandible. Incise the joint capsule between the meniscus and condyle, and elevate the capsule. Identify the condylectomy site at the base of the condylar neck (at the level of the mandibular notch) (Fig. 33-12). First, resect the lateral portion of the condyle with a rongeur, then make a cut along the osteotomy line with a high-speed burr. Fracture the remaining portion of the condyle with an osteotome, but leave the meniscus intact. Close the masseter fascia, subcutaneous tissue, and skin separately.

SUTURE MATERIALS AND SPECIAL INSTRUMENTS

A rongeur or high-speed burr is necessary for removal of the zygomatic arch. The fascial attachments of the masseter muscle should be elevated with a periosteal elevator. Instruments that facilitate mandibular condylectomy include a periosteal elevator and retractors. Rongeurs, high-speed burrs, and an osteotome and mallet are used to remove the condyle.

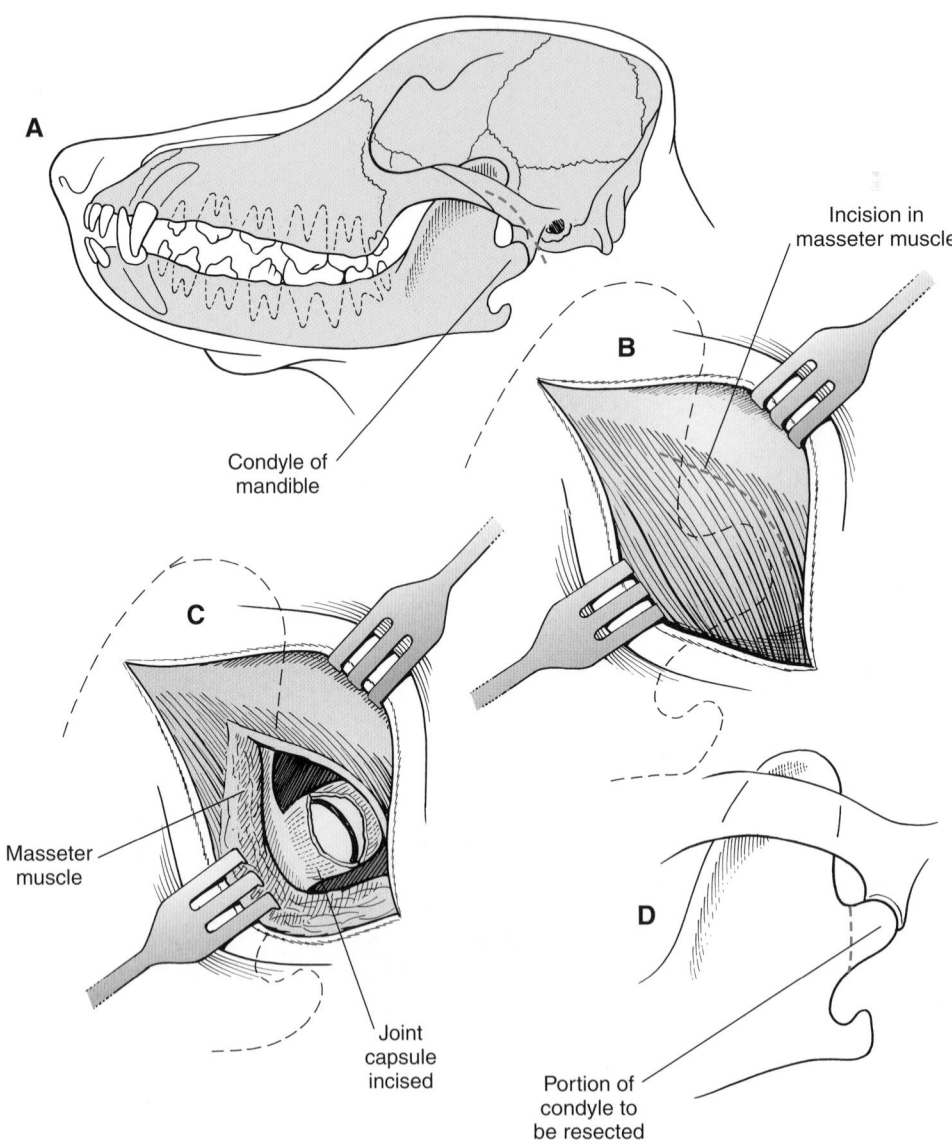

FIG. 33-12
Exposing the temporomandibular joint. **A** and **B,** Make a skin incision along the ventral border of the caudal zygomatic arch, centered over the temporomandibular joint. **C,** Elevate the caudal periosteal insertion of the masseter muscle from the zygomatic arch to expose the joint capsule. Incise the joint capsule between the meniscus and the condyle and elevate it. **D,** Identify the condylectomy site at the base of the condylar neck.

POSTOPERATIVE CARE AND ASSESSMENT

Dogs treated with zygomatic arch resection or condylectomy should be released to the owners with instructions to return for suture removal in 10 to 14 days. Limitation of exercise or dietary restriction is not necessary.

PROGNOSIS

If the opposite temporomandibular joint is affected, recurrence of jaw locking may be noted after unilateral mandibular condylectomy or zygomatic arch resection; however, most animals have normal jaw function after surgery. Possible complications of these procedures include seroma formation and iatrogenic infection.

SCAPULAR LUXATION

DEFINITION

Scapular luxation or *dislocation* is characterized by upward displacement of the scapula after rupture of supporting musculature.

GENERAL CONSIDERATIONS AND CLINICALLY RELEVANT PATHOPHYSIOLOGY

Scapular luxation is rare, but occasionally occurs with trauma that causes the serratus ventralis, rhomboideus, and trapezius muscular insertions to be torn from their scapular attachments. This allows upward displacement of the scapula during weight bearing. Concurrent injuries, such as rib fractures, pneumothorax, or pulmonary contusions, are common and may require immediate treatment.

DIAGNOSIS
Clinical Presentation

Signalment. Scapular luxation occurs more often in cats than dogs; animals of either gender or any age may be affected.

History. The animal typically has a recent history of trauma.

Physical Examination Findings

Notable dorsal displacement of the scapula is observed as the animal bears weight on the affected limb. Adduction of the limb induces lateral scapular displacement. The symmetry of scapular location and prominence should be compared with the normal limb.

Diagnostic Imaging

Survey radiographs of the thorax should be evaluated for signs of thoracic trauma, such as fractured ribs, pulmonary contusions, or pneumothorax. Usually the scapula is not fractured, but may appear displaced.

Laboratory Findings

Specific laboratory abnormalities are not seen. Traumatized animals undergoing surgery should have sufficient measurement of blood values to determine the optimum anesthetic regimen.

DIFFERENTIAL DIAGNOSIS

Scapular luxation must be differentiated from a scapular fracture (see p. 1029).

MEDICAL MANAGEMENT

Surgical stabilization of the scapula usually is required for a good cosmetic and functional result; however, closed reduction with placement of a Velpeau bandage (see p. 949) has been reported to be successful in cats with acute luxation.

SURGICAL TREATMENT

Although the torn muscles' bellies occasionally can be identified and reattached to the scapula, this repair usually is insufficient to allow weight bearing. Generally the scapula is held in its normal position by wire suture, which is placed around an adjacent rib and through holes drilled in the caudal scapular border.

Preoperative Management

Thoracic radiographs and electrocardiographic analysis are warranted to detect any concurrent thoracic or cardiovascular trauma in acute injuries. Prophylactic antibiotic therapy usually is unnecessary.

Anesthesia

If the animal is healthy and has no significant concurrent injuries, a number of anesthetic regimens can be used safely (see p. 944); however, if evidence of concurrent thoracic or cardiovascular injury is noted, anesthesia should be induced and monitored with care. Equipment should be available for ventilating the animal if the chest is opened inadvertently (see Chapter 29).

Surgical Anatomy

See p. 1033 for a detailed discussion of the anatomy of the scapula. Important landmarks for surgical repair of a scapular luxation are the dorsocaudal scapular border and the fifth, sixth, or seventh ribs.

Positioning

The animal is positioned in lateral recumbency with the affected side up. The entire scapular region from midcervical region to midthorax should be prepared for aseptic surgery.

SURGICAL TECHNIQUE

After returning the scapula to its normal position, incise through the skin and subcutaneous tissue along the dorsal caudal scapular margin to expose the caudal scapular border. If possible, identify the torn edges of the muscles. Elevate a small portion of the teres major muscle from the caudal scapular border, and identify the underlying rib. Elevate the periosteum from the rib surface, taking care to avoid penetrating the parietal pleura. Use a wire passer to position a piece of wire around the rib. Use 18- to 20-gauge wire to secure the scapula to the rib. Drill two holes in the caudal scapular border adjacent to the exposed rib, and pass the free ends of the wire through these holes in a medial to lat-

eral direction. Tighten the wire by twisting the ends to secure the scapula to the rib. If the torn muscle edges have been identified, reattach them before closing the subcutaneous tissue and skin.

SUTURE MATERIALS AND SPECIAL INSTRUMENTS

Necessary equipment includes 18- or 20-gauge wire, a wire passer, a periosteal elevator, Steinmann pins, and a hand chuck. Absorbable (polydioxanone or polyglyconate) or nonabsorbable (polypropylene or nylon) suture can be used to reattach the muscles to their scapular insertions.

POSTOPERATIVE CARE AND ASSESSMENT

The patient's respiratory rate and effort should be observed carefully postoperatively to determine if the animal is able to ventilate normally. Ventilatory difficulties may indicate a pneumothorax if the pleura was inadvertently penetrated during passage of the wire. Thoracic radiographs should be taken and thoracentesis performed in such patients. A spica splint (see p. 949) should be applied to immobilize the limb for 3 weeks after surgery (the bandage may need to be changed every 5 to 7 days). Owners should be instructed to confine the animal until the bandage is removed; normal exercise may be resumed at 6 weeks.

PROGNOSIS

Chronic luxation will not resolve without surgical intervention. Possible complications of surgery include fixation failure, iatrogenic infection, and eventual wire fatigue and breakage with migration; however, complications are rare. Most animals bear weight normally on affected limbs after surgery.

SCAPULOHUMERAL JOINT

OSTEOCHONDRITIS DISSECANS OF THE PROXIMAL HUMERUS

DEFINITIONS

Osteochondritis dissecans (OCD) in which a flap of cartilage is lifted from the articular surface is a manifestation of a general syndrome called **osteochondrosis**. **Osteochondrosis** is a disturbance in endochondral ossification that leads to cartilage retention. Detached pieces of articular cartilage are often referred to as **joint mice**.

GENERAL CONSIDERATIONS AND CLINICALLY RELEVANT PATHOPHYSIOLOGY

OCD commonly occurs in the shoulders, elbows, stifles, and hocks of immature large- and giant-breed dogs. Despite unilateral lameness, this condition often is bilateral. In the shoulder, it usually is evidenced as a cartilage flap found on the midline or lateral aspect of the dorsocaudal humeral head. In some cases, the subchondral bone defect occupies half the area of the humeral head. The abnormal cartilage may fissure and cause protrusion of a loose flap of cartilage into the joint, or the cartilage may completely detach from the underlying bone and become lodged in the caudoventral joint pouch or bicipital bursa.

> NOTE: OCD often is bilateral; radiograph and evaluate both shoulders even if the animal exhibits unilateral lameness.

OCD begins with a failure of endochondral ossification in either the physis or the articular epiphyseal complex that is responsible for long-bone epiphyseal formation. The cause of OCD is unknown, but is considered to be multifactorial, with management, genetic, and nutritional interactions occurring in young growing dogs. Risk factors for OCD include age, gender, breed (genetic), rapid growth, and nutrient excesses (primarily calcium). Failure of endochondral ossification leads to cartilage thickening (osteochondrosis). Because developing cartilage is nourished initially by synovial fluid and later by vascularization through subchondral bone, increased cartilage thickness may result in malnourished, necrotic chondrocytes. Loss of chondrocytes deep in the cartilage layer leads to formation of a cleft at the junction of calcified and noncalcified tissue. Subsequently, normal activity may lead to development of vertical fissures in the cartilage that eventually communicate with the joint, forming a cartilage flap (Fig. 33-13). This communication allows cartilage fragments and inflammatory mediators to reach the synovial fluid, induce joint inflammation, and initiate the cycle of DJD (see p. 1155). OCD does not apparently cause clinical signs until a cartilage flap forms. Free cartilage flaps can lodge in joints and may increase in size with calcification until they become radiographically visible joint mice. In some cases, the cartilage flaps are gradually resorbed. DJD often is the final outcome.

> NOTE: OCD has a hereditary component; counsel owners against breeding affected dogs.

DIAGNOSIS
Clinical Presentation

Signalment. Large- and giant-breed dogs are commonly affected; this disease is rarely diagnosed in cats or small dogs. Males are more commonly affected than females. Clinical signs often develop between 4 and 8 months of age; however, some dogs may not be presented for veterinary evaluation until they are mature or middle aged.

History. Affected animals usually are seen with unilateral forelimb lameness. Owners typically report a gradual onset of lameness that improves after rest and worsens after exercise. Owners occasionally may associate the onset of lameness with trauma.

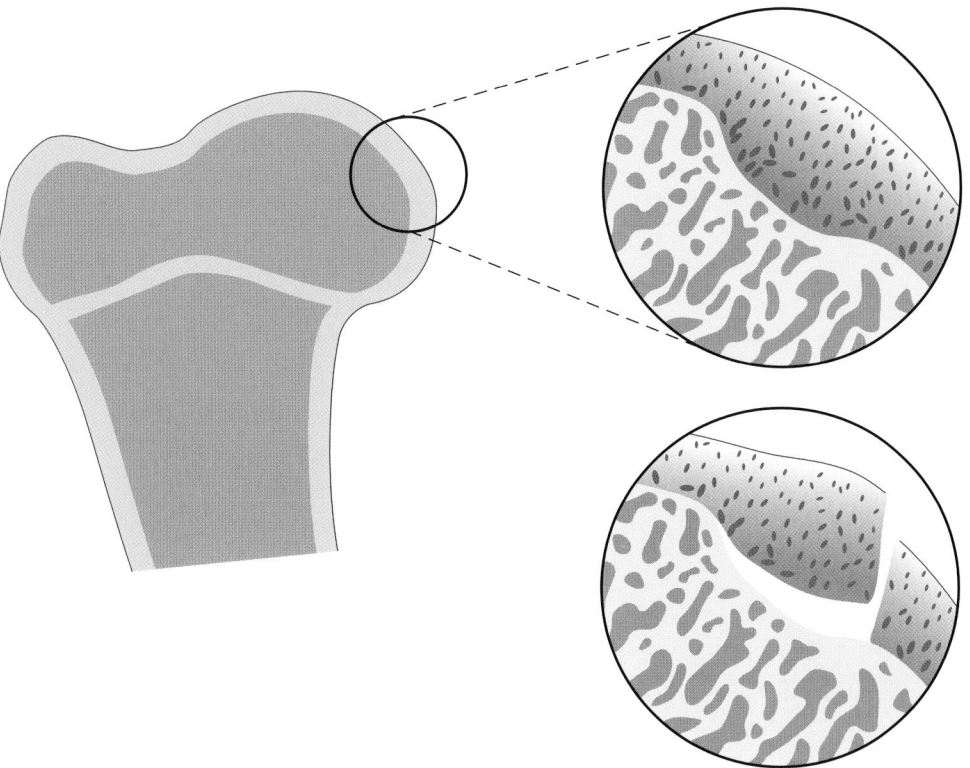

FIG. 33-13
Failure of endochondral ossification leads to cartilage thickening. Loss of chondrocytes deep in the cartilage layer produces a cleft and causes development of vertical fissures in the cartilage. These fissures eventually communicate with the joint, forming a cartilage flap.

Physical Examination Findings

The shoulder should be palpated and moved through a complete range of motion. Crepitation or palpable swelling of the joint is seldom evident, but affected animals usually show pain when the shoulder is moved into extreme extension (i.e., moving the humerus forward with one hand while the other hand is positioned as a fulcrum on the cranial aspect of the shoulder; see p. 935). Extreme flexion of the shoulder may also cause pain.

> NOTE: Be careful not to confuse elbow pain with shoulder pain when hyperextending the elbow to extend the shoulder.

Diagnostic Imaging

Diagnosis of OCD is based on typical radiographic findings evident on lateral projections of the scapulohumeral joints; craniocaudal projections do not contribute to the diagnosis, but may help identify the location of a joint mouse. Both shoulders should be imaged because this condition is often bilateral despite unilateral lameness. The dog should be positioned in lateral recumbency with the shoulder of interest dependent and the head elevated to prevent superimposition of the humeral head over the cervical spine (Fig. 33-14). The uppermost forelimb is retracted caudally and the dependent forelimb is extended cranially. Slight external rotation of the humerus may help silhouette the affected portion of the humeral head. Sedation may be required for quality radio-graphs (see Table 31-2 on p. 933). Multiple views made while the humerus is rotated (pronated and supinated) may be necessary to locate the lesion.

The earliest radiographic sign of OCD is flattening of the subchondral bone of the caudal humeral head. As the disease progresses, a saucer-shaped radiolucent area in the caudal humeral head may be visualized (Fig. 33-15). Calcification of the flap may allow visualization of the flap *in situ* or in the joint if it has detached from the underlying bone. In chronic cases, large calcified joint mice often are observed in the caudoventral joint pouch.

Contrast arthrography using 1.5 to 4 ml of a 25% solution of meglumine-sodium diatrizoate with an admixture of 0.2 mg of epinephrine can be used to determine the presence and location of cartilage flaps, although this is rarely performed, especially with the advent of CT and MRI. Most dogs with a cartilage flap overlying a subchondral bone defect are lame, whereas those identified with thick articular cartilage only typically are not lame.

Laboratory Findings

Analysis of synovial fluid in animals with OCD reflects underlying inflammation and the development of DJD. Other specific laboratory abnormalities are not present.

DIFFERENTIAL DIAGNOSIS

Forelimb lameness in large immature dogs can be caused by many diseases: OCD, ununited anconeal process (UAP), or fragmented coronoid process (FCP) of the elbow; panoste-

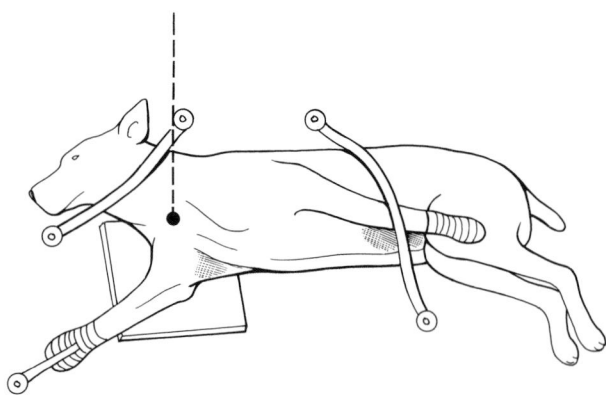

FIG. 33-14
Proper positioning of a dog to obtain a medial-lateral view of the scapulohumeral joint.

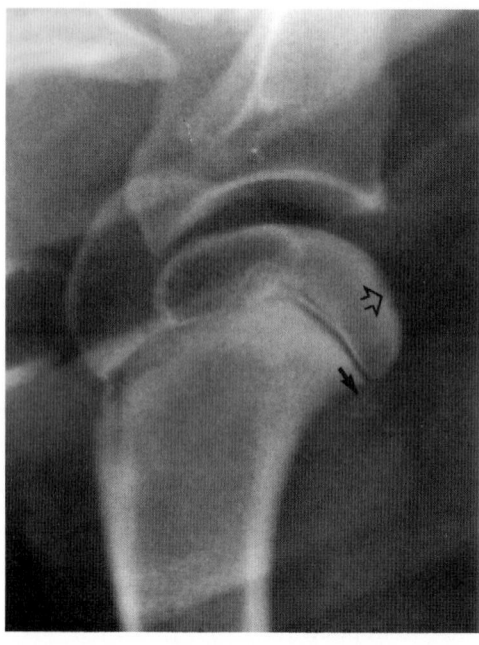

FIG. 33-15
Radiograph of a shoulder with OCD of the caudal humeral head. Note the flattening and irregularity of the subchondral bone of the caudal aspect of the humeral head *(open arrow)*. A portion of the cartilage flap is located in the caudal cul-de-sac of the joint, where it has become mineralized *(closed arrow)*. (From Olmstead ML: *Small animal orthopedics,* St Louis, 1995, Mosby.)

itis; premature closure of the physes; elbow incongruity; retained cartilage cores; and hypertrophic osteodystrophy. Forelimb lameness attributable to the shoulder or scapulohumeral joint must be differentiated from injuries associated with trauma or septic arthritis, usually by evaluation of the animal's history and the results of radiographic and synovial fluid analysis.

MEDICAL MANAGEMENT

Conservative therapy may benefit some dogs with OCD of the shoulder; however, long-term resolution of lameness usually requires arthroscopy or arthrotomy. A therapeutic trial of exercise restriction (brief leash walks only) can be attempted. NSAIDs may be administered to affected animals (see Table 33-4 on p. 1149). If lameness resolves, surgery may not be indicated; however, if lameness persists, the flap should be removed. If shoulder OCD has been definitively diagnosed, risks of medical or conservative management include prolonged lameness and muscle atrophy, migration of the flap and associated complications, and severe osteoarthritis.

SURGICAL TREATMENT
Preoperative Management

The overall health of the animal should be determined before surgery. A complete physical examination should be performed to determine if other joints are similarly affected.

Anesthesia

These animals usually are young and healthy, and a variety of anesthetic regimens can be used (see p. 944).

Arthroscopic Treatment of Shoulder OCD

Indications. Indications for shoulder arthroscopy include OCD, bicipital tenosynovitis, shoulder instability (i.e., joint capsule or ligament tears or both), and diagnostic examinations (e.g., biopsy of bone, cartilage, or the soft tissue envelope). Management of OCD is the most common indication. Arthroscopy provides outstanding exposure for visualization and treatment of OCD lesions; however, shoulder arthroscopy may be the most challenging of all of the routine small animal arthroscopy procedures.

Instrumentation. A 30-degree foreoblique arthroscope is commonly used in the shoulder joint. In most dogs, a 2.7-mm arthroscope can be easily inserted into the joint space. In small breeds of dogs, a 2.4-mm arthroscope is preferable to prevent iatrogenic cartilage damage during insertion or surgical manipulation. Shoulder arthroscopy in giant-breed dogs can be performed with a 4-mm arthroscope; the advantage of the larger scope is the superior viewing area and depth of focus. Use of a blunt obturator is always recommended over a sharp trocar.

> NOTE: Whichever size arthroscope is chosen, remember to consider the outside diameter of the arthroscope cannula because it, too, must enter the joint.

Shoulder arthroscopy requires an assortment of hand instruments (see Chapter 14). These include instruments to assist in the inspection of intraarticular structures (probes), grasping forceps for removal of free bodies, biopsy forceps, and instruments for surface abrasion. Instruments commonly used for abrasion arthroplasty are hand-held burrs, curettes, or a motorized shaver. Instruments can be inserted into the joint through an open instrument port, instrument cannulas, or a combination of the two. If the surgeon chooses to work through an instrument cannula, different-size cannulas and "switching sticks" are necessary.

Portal sites and technique. *Clip and prepare the area as if an open shoulder arthrotomy were to be performed so that the arthroscopy procedure can be aborted and an open arthrotomy performed if necessary.*

This occurs most often when the surgeon is beginning to learn arthroscopy. Use one of two methods for limb preparation, depending on the limb maneuverability desired.

For maximum maneuverability of the limb during surgery, use a hanging limb preparation. As you become more experienced and adept at shoulder arthroscopy, less maneuverability is needed, and you may wish to perform a lateral limb preparation for each limb. However, perform the lateral limb preparation such that an open procedure can be performed if needed. Use two or three portal sites for shoulder arthroscopy, depending on the purpose of arthroscopic intervention. If visual exploration of the shoulder joint is all that is required, use only an egress portal and an arthroscope portal. If tissue biopsy or treatment of a pathologic joint condition is undertaken, use an additional instrument portal.

Position the dog in lateral recumbency with the leg to be operated on uppermost. Remember to support the limb in neutral position to prevent excessive adduction that closes the joint line between the glenoid and humeral head. Establish the egress portal first. Use either a hypodermic needle (18-gauge, 1½-inch) or egress cannula (2.4 to 2.7 mm). (Note: most surgeons prefer a hypodermic needle.) Palpate the shoulder to locate the superior ridge of the greater tubercle, and insert the needle at the craniocaudal midpoint of the ridge. Direct the needle caudally and medially at an angle of 70 degrees from the perpendicular. To ensure placement within the joint, attach a syringe to the needle and aspirate synovial fluid.

In most cases, when the egress portal has been properly placed, synovial fluid is easily aspirated.

If synovial fluid is not aspirated and if you believe that the joint has been entered, instill fluid (lactated Ringer's solution) into the joint.

If the needle is located in the joint, fluid is easily instilled. Also, as one begins to fill the joint cavity with fluid, reverse pressure is felt on the syringe plunger from the instilled fluid. Cap off or remove the needle to maintain joint distention. If you are working with an assistant, have them maintain pressure on the syringe while you establish the scope portal. Alternatively, distend the joint at the site of the scope portal. This aids in determining the proper location for this portal.

Remove the needle after the joint is distended, and insert the arthroscope at an identical location.

Establish the arthroscope portal next. Insert the arthroscope cannula with the attached trocar pointed obturator or blunt obturator first.

A pointed blunt obturator is preferred.

For shoulder OCD, position the arthroscope portal just in front of and slightly distal to the acromion process of the scapula. Use a 20-gauge (1½-inch) needle to confirm the position for the arthroscope portal. Insert the needle perpendicular to the skin surface, and maintain this orientation through the soft tissue as the needle enters the joint.

Lactated Ringer's solution (previously used to distend the joint) will flow through the needle when the joint is entered, marking the point of entry for the arthroscope.

Use a No. 11 Bard-Parker blade to make a small entry wound through the skin and superficial soft tissue adjacent to the needle. Do not enter the joint with the scalpel blade because extravasation of fluid outside the joint cavity is more likely when this occurs. Remove the needle, and insert the arthroscope cannula with the attached pointed blunt obturator. Once in the joint, remove the obturator from the cannula.

Fluid will flow freely from the cannula, confirming correct placement.

Attach the fluid ingress line to the cannula and insert the arthroscope. Inspect the medial compartment for evidence of inflammation and then the cranial compartment. Thoroughly inspect the region of the biceps tendon for inflammation or free cartilage pieces (Fig. 33-16).

Direct the arthroscope caudally, and position the light post to inspect the caudal articular surface and joint capsule. Once the OCD lesion has been identified, a guide needle should be passed to position the instrument portal (Fig. 33-17). Use an 18-gauge, 1½-inch needle or in larger dogs a spinal needle or catheter stylet. Insert the needle into the joint from a point approximately 2 cm caudal to the arthroscope portal. The needle should be inserted so it can be visualized at the site of the lesion.

The needle should be directed to the site of the OCD lesion. The most common error is overangling the needle and crossing the needle over the arthroscope.

Once the position for the instrument portal has been established, decide if you are going to work through an open instrument portal, an instrument cannula, or a combination of the two. If you choose to work through an open portal site, use a No. 11 Bard-Parker scalpel blade to make a 0.5- to 1-cm soft tissue tunnel adjacent to the guide needle. If the cartilage flap is still attached (generally cranial and/or medial), insert

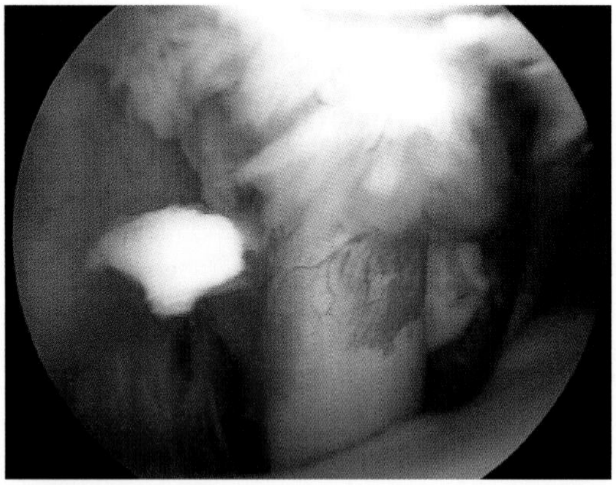

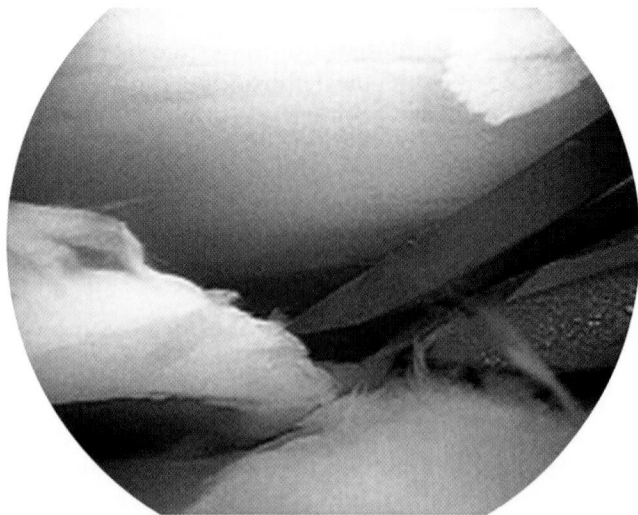

FIG. 33-16
View of the biceps tendon; note the free cartilage fragments adjacent to the tendon.

FIG. 33-17
Arthroscopic triangulation within the shoulder joint for removal of an OCD fragment.

a probe or elevator to free the edge of the flap. Do not free the cartilage flap completely; leave it attached at one or more sites. Insert grasping forceps and hold the cartilage flap with the forceps and remove it (Fig. 33-18). To facilitate removal of the flap, twist the forceps to fold the flap longitudinally, and ease passage through the joint capsule. Remove the cartilage flap as a single large fragment or, as is often the case, in two or three smaller pieces.

If working through an instrument cannula, insert the small instrument cannula with a sharp trocar into the joint adjacent to the guide needle. Place larger cannulas with the use of switching sticks, but use the smallest instrument cannula through which the lesion can be treated. Pass a hand curette, hand burr, or motorized shaver through the cannula, and use it to break the cartilage flap into small pieces.

The pieces generally are small enough to flow out the instrument cannula.

If a cartilage piece is too large to pass freely through the cannula, insert small grasping forceps and capture the fragment. Pull the fragment next to the instrument cannula, and remove the cannula and forceps at the same time. Reestablish the instrument port by placing a switching stick into the joint followed by the cannula. Continue to break the cartilage flap into small pieces until the cartilage lining the periphery of the lesion bed is firmly attached to the underlying subchondral bone. Next, treat the lesion bed by surface abrasion or microfracture (most surgeons use surface abrasion) (Fig. 33-19).

Whether using an open portal or instrument cannula to facilitate removal of the cartilage flap, treatment of the lesion bed is best accomplished through an instrument cannula.

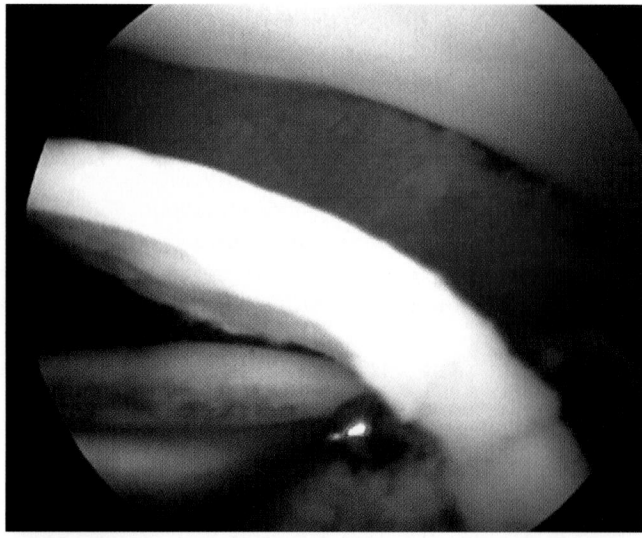

FIG. 33-18
OCD cartilage fragment raised from the underlying bone surface.

If an open portal was used to remove the cartilage flap, insert an instrument cannula over a switching stick. Treat the surface of the lesion with aggressive abrasion using a hand-held curette, hand-held burr, or motorized shaver. Continue to abrade the surface until the underlying bone bleeds freely. Stop ingress fluid as needed to observe the extent of bleeding bone. Upon completion of surface abrasion or microfracture, flush small bone or cartilage fragments from the joint by increasing the ingress flow and allowing egress through a large instrument cannula. Inspect the joint for

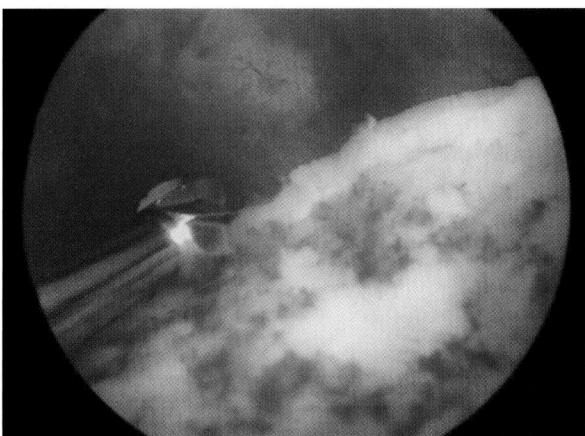

FIG. 33-19
Abrasion arthroplasty of the surface of an OCD lesion on the humeral head using a hand burr.

remaining bone or cartilage fragments, and then remove the arthroscope and instrument cannula. Suture the portals with nonreactive, nonabsorbable suture.

POSTOPERATIVE CARE AND ASSESSMENT

The animal usually can be released to the owner the day of surgery or the following day. The client should be instructed to limit the animal's activity for 1 month to allow soft tissue to heal and to provide time for formation of fibrocartilage in the OCD lesion. The dog can then be returned gradually to full activity. The portal sites should be observed for drainage, which usually resolves without therapy.

Open Surgical Techniques for Osteochondritis Dissecans

Surgical treatment involves exploratory arthrotomy and removal of the cartilage flap. The goals of surgery are to remove the cartilage flap from the humeral head and curette the edges of the bony defect to ensure removal of all affected cartilage. Subchondral bone that appears pale and sclerotic should also be curetted. The joint should be carefully explored and flushed extensively to identify and remove any pieces of dislodged cartilage.

One of several different approaches may be used to expose the scapulohumeral joint surgically, depending on the location of the defect and any detached cartilage flaps. Infraspinatus tenotomy affords excellent exposure of the humeral head and access to both the cranial and caudal joint compartments. However, because the infraspinatus tendon is cut and the joint is subluxated during the procedure, this approach is more traumatic than approaches that do not involve tenotomy. Longer postoperative recovery periods should be expected than with other techniques. A caudal approach to the joint affords good exposure of the humeral head (with adequate retraction) and excellent access to the caudal ventral joint

compartment without tenotomy; however, it does not allow the cranial aspect of the joint to be explored.

> NOTE: In animals with unilateral lameness that have bilateral radiographic lesions, surgery should be performed on the lame leg. The other leg may require surgery if lameness subsequently develops in that limb.

Surgical Anatomy

Important anatomic landmarks for identifying the location of the scapulohumeral joint are the acromion process of the scapular spine, the greater tubercle, and the acromial head of the deltoid muscle. The omobrachial vein is located superficially over the acromial head of the deltoid muscle. The caudal circumflex humeral artery and vein and axillary nerve are encountered and must be protected during the caudal approach to the shoulder.

Positioning

The dog is positioned in lateral recumbency with the affected limb up. The limb should be prepared from the dorsal midline to below the elbow.

SURGICAL TECHNIQUE
Infraspinatus Tenotomy for Exposure of the Scapulohumeral Joint

Make an incision in the skin and subcutaneous tissue from just proximal to the acromion process to the proximal humerus (Fig. 33-20, A). Curve the incision over the joint along the palpable cranial margin of the deltoid muscle's acromial head. Incise the deep fascia along the cranial margin of the acromial portion of the deltoid muscle, and retract the muscle caudally (Fig. 33-20, B). Isolate the infraspinatus tendon, and place a stay suture in its proximal portion. Incise the tendon 5 mm from its insertion on the humerus and retract it caudally (Fig. 33-20, C). Incise the joint capsule midway between the glenoid rim and the humeral head (Fig. 33-20, D). Internally rotate the humerus until the head subluxates, exposing the caudal surface of the humeral head (Fig. 33-20, E). Remove the cartilage flap from the humeral head and curette the edges of the bony defect to ensure removal of all affected cartilage (Fig. 33-20, F). Flush all parts of the joint thoroughly to remove any cartilage debris or joint mice. Close the joint capsule with 3-0 absorbable suture in a simple interrupted pattern. Reappose the infraspinatus tendon with an absorbable suture in a Bunnell or locking-loop pattern (see p. 1320). Close the muscular fascia, subcutaneous tissue, and skin separately.

Caudal Approach to the Scapulohumeral Joint

Make an incision in the skin, subcutaneous tissue, and deep fascia that extends from the midscapular spine to the midhumeral diaphysis (Fig. 33-21, A). Incise the intermuscular

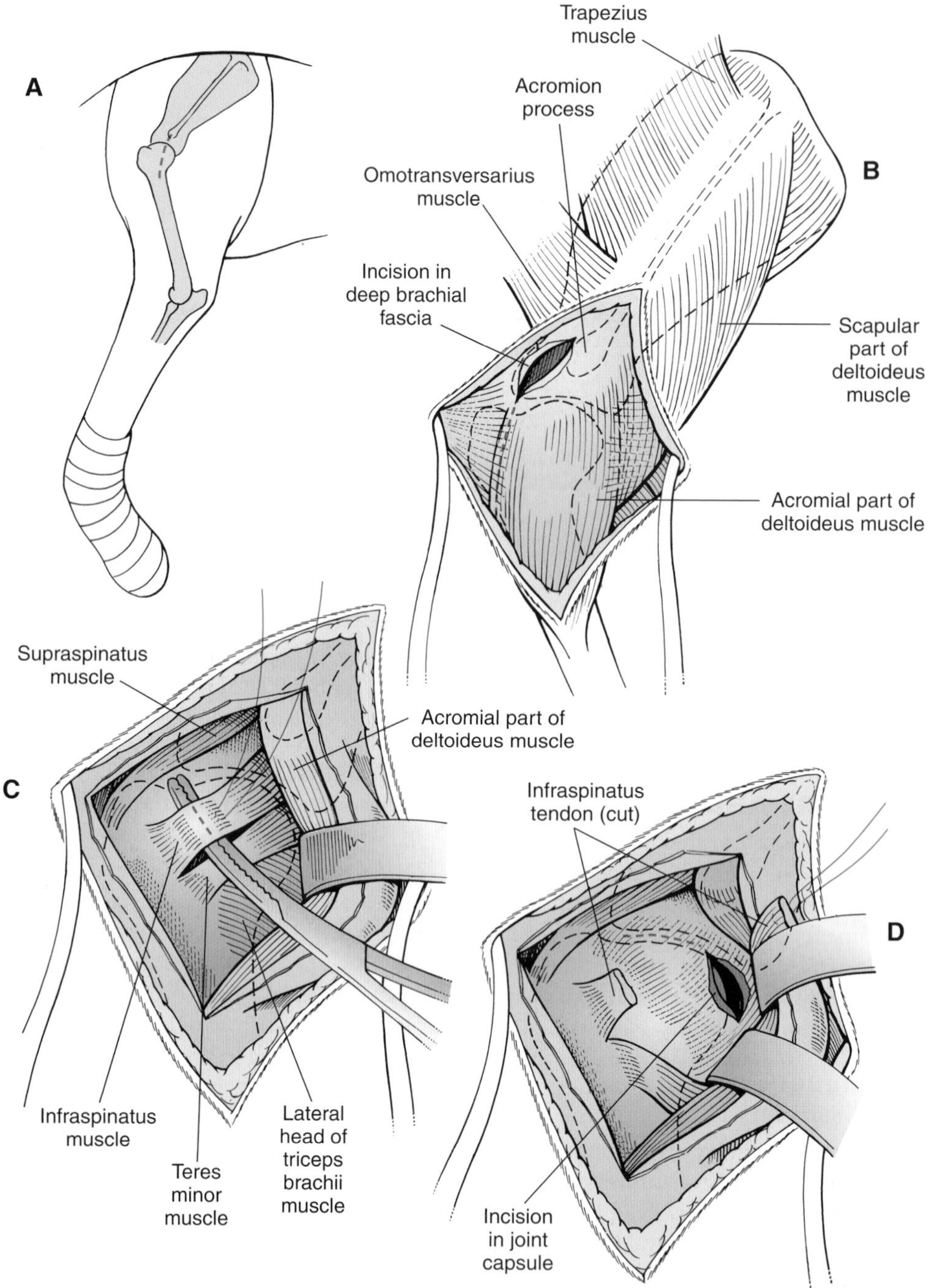

FIG. 33-20
Craniolateral approach to the shoulder. **A,** Make an incision in the skin and subcutaneous tissue from just proximal to the acromion process to the proximal humerus. **B,** Incise the deep fascia along the cranial margin of the acromial portion of the deltoideus muscle and retract the muscle caudally. **C,** Isolate the infraspinatus tendon, place a stay suture in its proximal portion, and incise the tendon. **D,** Incise the joint capsule midway between the glenoid rim and the humeral head.

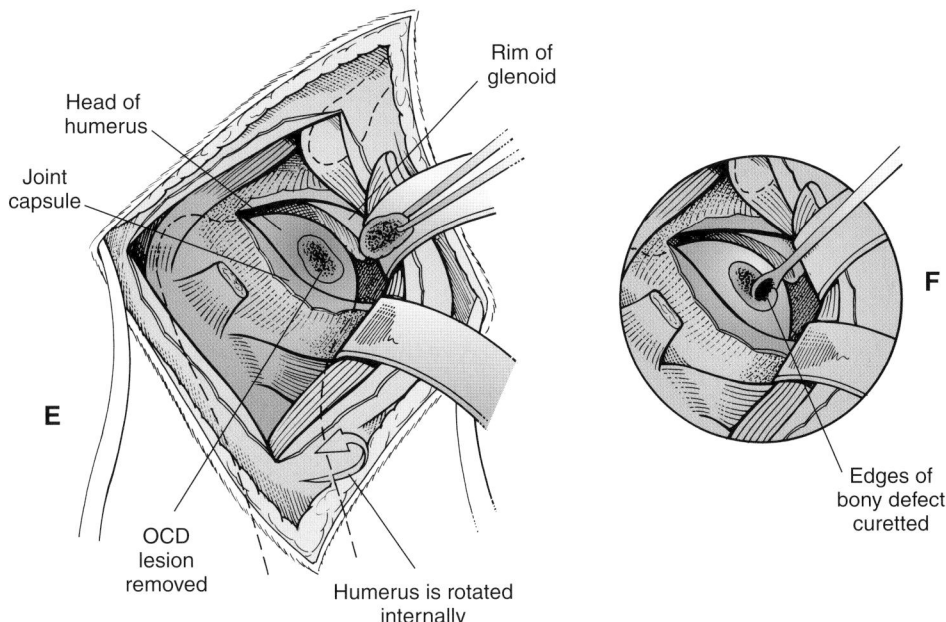

FIG. 33-20, cont'd
Craniolateral approach to the shoulder. **E,** Internally rotate the humerus until the head subluxates and remove the cartilage flap. **F,** Curette the edges of the bony defect to ensure removal of all affected cartilage.

septum between the caudal border of the scapular portion of the deltoid muscle and the long head of the triceps muscle and separate the muscles (Fig. 33-21, B). Use blunt dissection to free the deltoid muscle and expose the caudal circumflex artery and vein, the muscular branch of the axillary nerve, and the teres minor muscle (Fig. 33-21, C). Elevate and retract the teres minor muscle cranially, exposing the axillary nerve and joint capsule. Place a Penrose drain around the nerve, and gently retract it caudally (Fig. 33-21, D). Incise the joint capsule 5 mm from and parallel to the glenoid rim to expose the humeral head (Fig. 33-21, E). To expose OCD lesions of the humeral head, internally rotate the humerus and flex the shoulder. Explore the joint and remove the cartilage as described above. Close the joint capsule in an interrupted pattern with 3-0 absorbable suture. Then suture the intermuscular septum, deep fascia, subcutaneous tissue, and skin as separate layers.

POSTOPERATIVE CARE AND ASSESSMENT

The animal usually can be released to the owner within 1 or 2 days after surgery. The client should be instructed to limit the animal's activity for 1 month to allow soft tissue to heal. The dog then can be returned gradually to full activity. The incision site should be observed for seroma formation, which usually resolves without therapy. Healing of shoulder OCD lesions following flap removal benefits from rehabilitation therapy. The most commonly applied treatments are passive and active range of motion and controlled therapeutic exercises. See Table 33-7 (p. 1185) for an example of a detailed, appropriate exercise regimen.

SUTURE MATERIALS AND SPECIAL INSTRUMENTS

Army-Navy retractors or Gelpi retractors are used to retract soft tissue and improve visualization of the humeral head. A bone curette is used to remove damaged articular cartilage from the humeral head.

PROGNOSIS

Prognosis for normal limb function with OCD of the shoulder is good. After surgery, most dogs become sound within 4 to 8 weeks. Approximately 75% of dogs have excellent function after fragment removal on long-term evaluation. Despite the absence of lameness in these dogs, DJD may develop; owners should be forewarned of this.

Suggested Reading

Beale BS, Hulse DA, Schulz KS et al: *Small animal arthroscopy,* Philadelphia, 2003, Saunders.
This comprehensive textbook on arthroscopy has detailed information regarding instrumentation and techniques of small animal arthroscopy. It also contains a thorough discussion of the indications and disease processes treated.

SCAPULOHUMERAL JOINT LUXATION

DEFINITION

Scapulohumeral joint luxation occurs when loss or damage of supporting structures of the joint is sufficient to cause separation of the humerus from the scapula. Synonyms include a *dislocated shoulder* or a *shoulder luxation*.

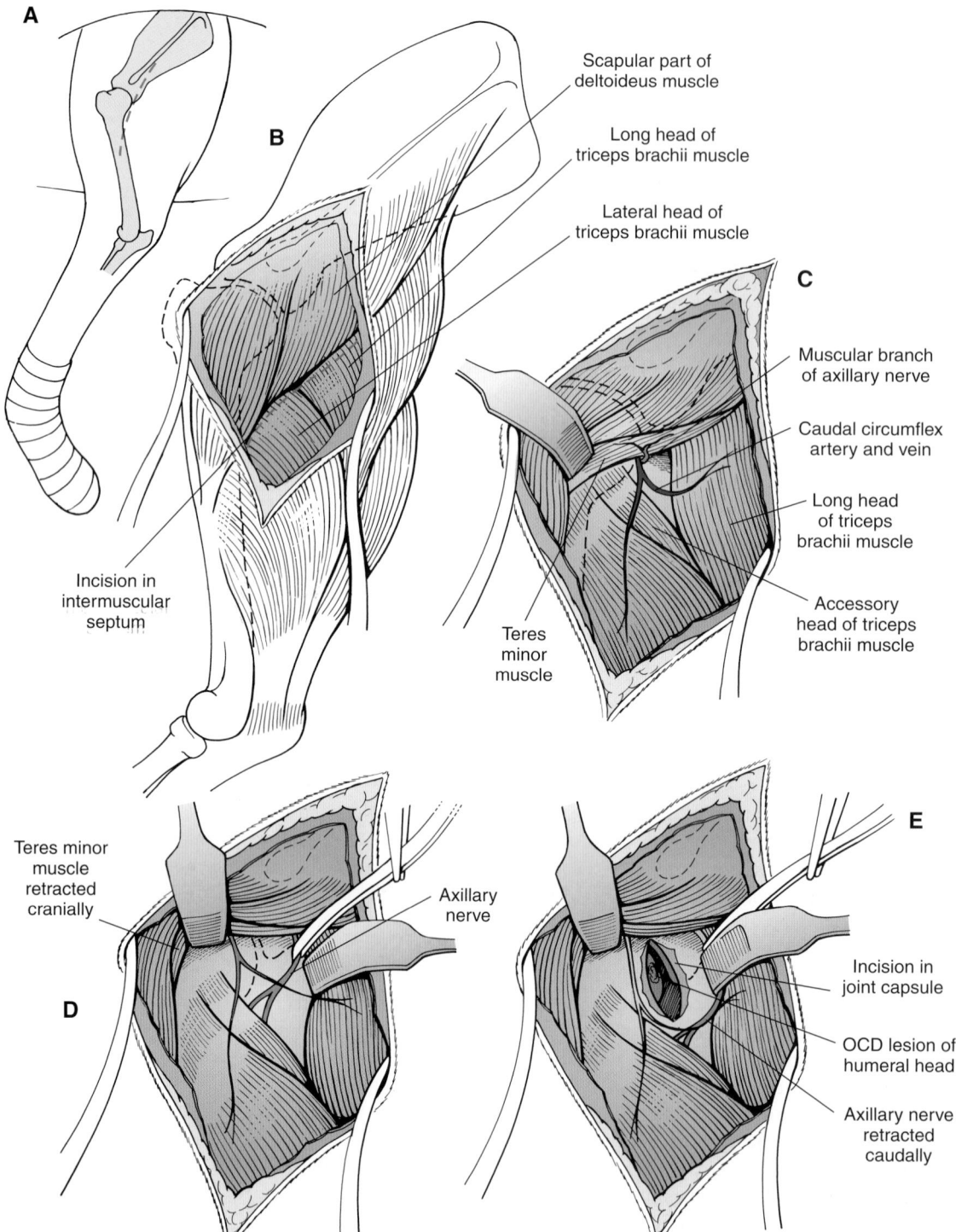

FIG. 33-21

Caudal approach to the shoulder. **A,** Make an incision in the skin, subcutaneous tissue, and deep fascia that extends from the midscapular spine to the midhumeral diaphysis. **B,** Incise the intermuscular septum between the caudal border of the scapular portion of the deltoideus muscle and the long head of the triceps muscle. **C,** Elevate and retract the teres minor muscle cranially, exposing the axillary nerve and joint capsule. **D,** Place a Penrose drain around the nerve and gently retract it caudally. **E,** Incise the joint capsule 5 mm from and parallel to the glenoid rim to expose the humeral head.

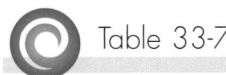 Table 33-7

Physical Rehabilitation Protocol for OCD of the Elbow or Shoulder

ALL TREATMENTS BID	DAY 1 TO DAY 14	DAY 15 TO DAY 24	DAY 25 UNTIL HEALED	HEALED TO RETURN TO FUNCTION
Heat therapy		10 min	10 min	
Passive range of motion/ stretching (repetitions)	20*	20*	10–15*	Stop—when ROM N
Therapeutic exercise- total time	10 min	15 min	20 min	25–45 min
Walk/land treadmill	10 min	5 min	10 min	>10 min
Balancing	+	+	+	
Obstacles	+	+	+	+
Weaving				+
Circles				+
Hills				+
Stairs				+
Jog				+
Underwater treadmill		10 min	10 min	>15 min
Swimming		5 min	5 min	5–10 min
Cryotherapy	15 min	15 min	15 min	PRN

BID, Twice a day; *ROM N,* range of motion normal; +, perform modality; *PRN,* as needed.
*Passive range of motion to all joints of the affected limb.

GENERAL CONSIDERATIONS AND CLINICALLY RELEVANT PATHOPHYSIOLOGY

Scapulohumeral luxations may be caused by trauma or may be congenital in origin. The scapulohumeral joint is supported by the joint capsule, glenohumeral ligaments, and surrounding tendons (supraspinatus, infraspinatus, teres minor, and subscapularis). Significant structures include the biceps tendon and medial glenohumeral ligament (Sidaway et al, 2004). When these structures are torn or deficient, humeral head luxation may occur. Scapulohumeral luxations are named for the direction in which the humeral head deviates. Medial or lateral deviations are most common; cranial and caudal luxations are rare.

Traumatic luxations usually are the result of shoulder injury. Traumatic lateral humeral luxations occur after lateral glenohumeral ligament and infraspinatus tendon rupture, whereas traumatic medial humeral luxations are associated with tearing of the medial glenohumeral ligament and subscapularis tendon. Concurrent thoracic trauma is common (i.e., pneumothorax, hemothorax, pulmonary contusions, or fractured ribs). Congenital or developmental laxity of the capsule and ligaments may result in medial instability and medial luxation of the humeral head. The glenoid cavity may be sufficiently deformed or hypoplastic to prevent reduction of the humeral head. This condition often occurs bilaterally in affected animals. Subluxation or shoulder instability associated with incomplete tearing of the medial

glenohumeral ligament, biceps tendon, or glenoid labrum; distention of the joint capsule; synovitis; and varying degrees of DJD may cause chronic shoulder pain and lameness in dogs.

NOTE: Be sure to differentiate traumatic from congenital luxations because the treatment and prognosis are different.

DIAGNOSIS
Clinical Presentation

Signalment. Traumatic luxation may occur in any age or breed of dog; it is rare in cats. Congenital, medial luxation usually occurs in small and miniature dog breeds, such as toy poodles and Shetland sheepdogs; lameness usually appears when the animal is young.

History. Dogs with traumatic luxation usually have a history or evidence of trauma. Chronic forelimb lameness that first becomes evident at a young age and without a history of trauma suggests congenital luxation.

Physical Examination

With traumatic luxation, affected animals may be non-weight bearing, and the limb often is carried in a flexed position. With lateral luxation, the foot is rotated internally, and the greater tubercle is palpable lateral to its normal position. With medial luxation, the foot is rotated externally and the greater tubercle is palpated medial to its normal location. Pain and crepitation are evident with shoulder manipulation.

Dogs with chronic, congenital medial luxation often are lame. The joint is easily luxated and reduced, but manipulation does not usually cause pain. If the glenoid cavity is deformed, reduction of the humeral head may be impossible. Some small dogs with chronic medial luxation show only mild intermittent lameness and minimal DJD.

Diagnostic Imaging

Lateral and craniocaudal radiographs of the shoulder are evaluated to confirm the diagnosis (Fig. 33-22). With traumatic luxation, special attention should be given to identifying concurrent scapular fractures or thoracic injuries.

Laboratory Findings

Specific laboratory abnormalities are not seen with traumatic or congenital luxation. Traumatized animals undergoing surgery should have sufficient measurement of blood values to determine the optimum anesthetic regimen. Analysis of synovial fluid from affected animals may reflect associated inflammation and the development of DJD.

DIFFERENTIAL DIAGNOSIS

DJD, humeral osteosarcoma, and contracture of the infraspinatus or supraspinatus tendons must be differentiated from luxation on the basis of physical findings and the results of radiography.

MEDICAL MANAGEMENT

Dogs with chronic medial luxation, only mild intermittent lameness, and minimal DJD may be managed with exercise restriction and administration of aspirin during acute exacerbations. Closed reduction can be attempted for a traumatic luxation presented for treatment soon after injury provided the condition is not associated with humeral or scapular fractures. General anesthesia is required for closed reduction. A lateral luxation is reduced with the leg held in extension. Medial pressure is applied to the humeral head, and lateral pressure is applied to the medial surface of the scapula (Fig. 33-23). The humeral head should remain in place when it is gently moved through a normal range of motion. If the luxation appears stable, a lateral spica splint should be applied for 10 to 14 days (see p. 949). A medial luxation caused by trauma is reduced in the opposite manner and immobilized by placing the limb in a Velpeau sling (see p. 949).

SURGICAL TREATMENT

If a traumatic luxation is unstable enough after closed reduction that reluxation occurs or if the luxation is chronic, open reduction and stabilization with capsulorrhaphy or tendon transposition are required. Surgery is warranted in animals with congenital luxations that cause severe or persistent lameness. In cases of severe joint dysplasia or DJD,

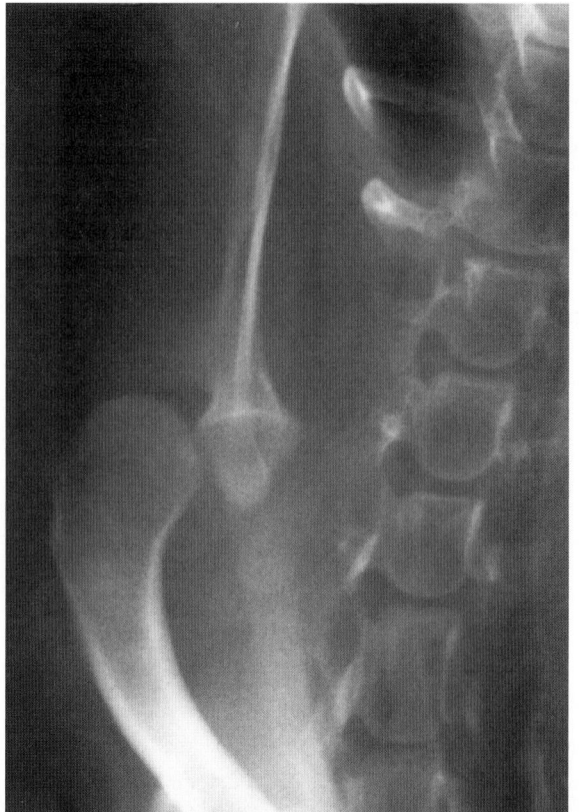

A

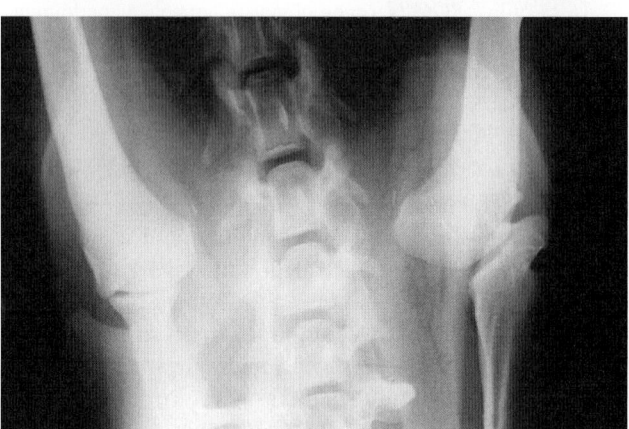

B

FIG. 33-22
Ventrodorsal radiographs illustrating lateral **(A)** and medial **(B)** luxation of the humeral head. (A from Olmstead ML: *Small animal orthopedics,* St Louis, 1995, Mosby.)

open reduction and stabilization are unsuccessful, and salvage procedures (glenoid excision or arthrodesis) must be performed.

Surgical arthrodesis of the shoulder is reserved for animals with chronic intractable luxation, comminuted fractures of the humeral head or glenoid, or severe DJD that precludes primary fixation. This is considered a salvage procedure and should be done only as a last resort and only when other joints are normal. Because scapular mobility compensates for

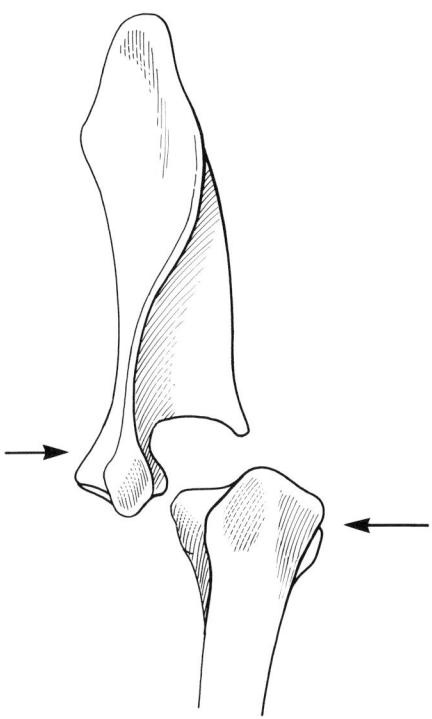

FIG. 33-23
For closed reduction of a lateral luxation, apply medial pressure to the humeral head and lateral pressure to the medial surface of the scapula.

loss of motion in the scapulohumeral joint, most animals have good limb function after shoulder arthrodesis.

Excision arthroplasty is a salvage procedure that causes a pseudoarthrosis to form between the scapula and the humerus, allowing limited scapulohumeral joint motion. This procedure does not require implantation of orthopedic hardware (plates, screws), and most dogs are pain free and bear weight on the limb at a walk or run. However, gait abnormalities and mild or moderate atrophy of shoulder muscles usually are noted after surgery.

Preoperative Management

The animal's overall health should be determined before surgery. Thoracic radiography and electrocardiographic analysis are warranted in animals with traumatic luxation.

Anesthesia

General anesthesia is required for closed or open reduction. A variety of anesthetic regimens can be used in young, healthy animals (see p. 944). Special care should be exercised in anesthetizing older animals or those with concurrent injuries.

Surgical Anatomy

Important landmarks used to identify the location of the scapulohumeral joint are the acromion process of the scapular spine, the greater tubercle, and the acromial head of the

deltoid muscle. Anatomic landmarks for positioning the skin incision include the acromion of the scapula, the greater tubercle of the humerus, and the pectoral muscles. The suprascapular nerve courses over the craniolateral surface of the scapula, and the caudal circumflex humeral artery and axillary nerve pass on the caudolateral aspect of the shoulder and should be avoided.

Positioning

For either medial or lateral luxation, the animal is positioned in dorsal recumbency with the affected leg draped. The prepared area should extend from the dorsal and ventral midlines to below the elbow.

SURGICAL TECHNIQUE
Surgical Stabilization of a Medial Luxation

A craniomedial approach to the shoulder joint is used to expose the luxated joint. It may be helpful to reduce the joint before the approach is made to reestablish normal anatomic relationships.

Beginning at the medial aspect of the acromion, incise the skin and subcutaneous tissue over the greater tubercle, and continue the incision medially to the midhumeral diaphysis (Fig. 33-24, A). Incise the fascia along the lateral border of the brachiocephalicus muscle, and retract the muscle medially (Fig. 33-24, B). Incise the insertions of the superficial and deep pectoral muscles from the humerus, and retract them medially. Carefully incise the fascial attachment between the deep pectoral muscle and supraspinatus muscle to prevent damaging the suprascapular nerve (Fig. 33-24, C). Retract the supraspinatus muscle laterally. Transect the tendon of the coracobrachialis muscle to expose the subscapularis muscle tendon (Fig. 33-24, D). If the joint capsule is not torn, incise it to inspect the joint and assess the condition of the humeral head and medial labrum of the glenoid (Fig. 33-24, E).

If the labrum is worn, the prognosis for successful stabilization of the shoulder is poor. The tendon of the coracobrachialis muscle may be torn and retracted with traumatic luxation.

Reduce the joint, and imbricate the capsule and subscapularis tendon with nonabsorbable mattress sutures. If this does not sufficiently stabilize the joint, incise the transverse humeral ligament over the biceps tendon. Make a small incision in the joint capsule under the biceps tendon to free it, and move the tendon medially. Secure it to the humerus with a bone screw and spiked washer (Fig. 33-24, F). To prevent external rotation of the humeral head during healing, place a rotational suture of heavy, nonabsorbable material from the medial labrum of the glenoid through a bone tunnel in the greater tubercle. For closure, suture the joint capsule, and then suture the pectoral muscles to the deltoid fascia. Suture the subcutaneous tissue and skin separately.

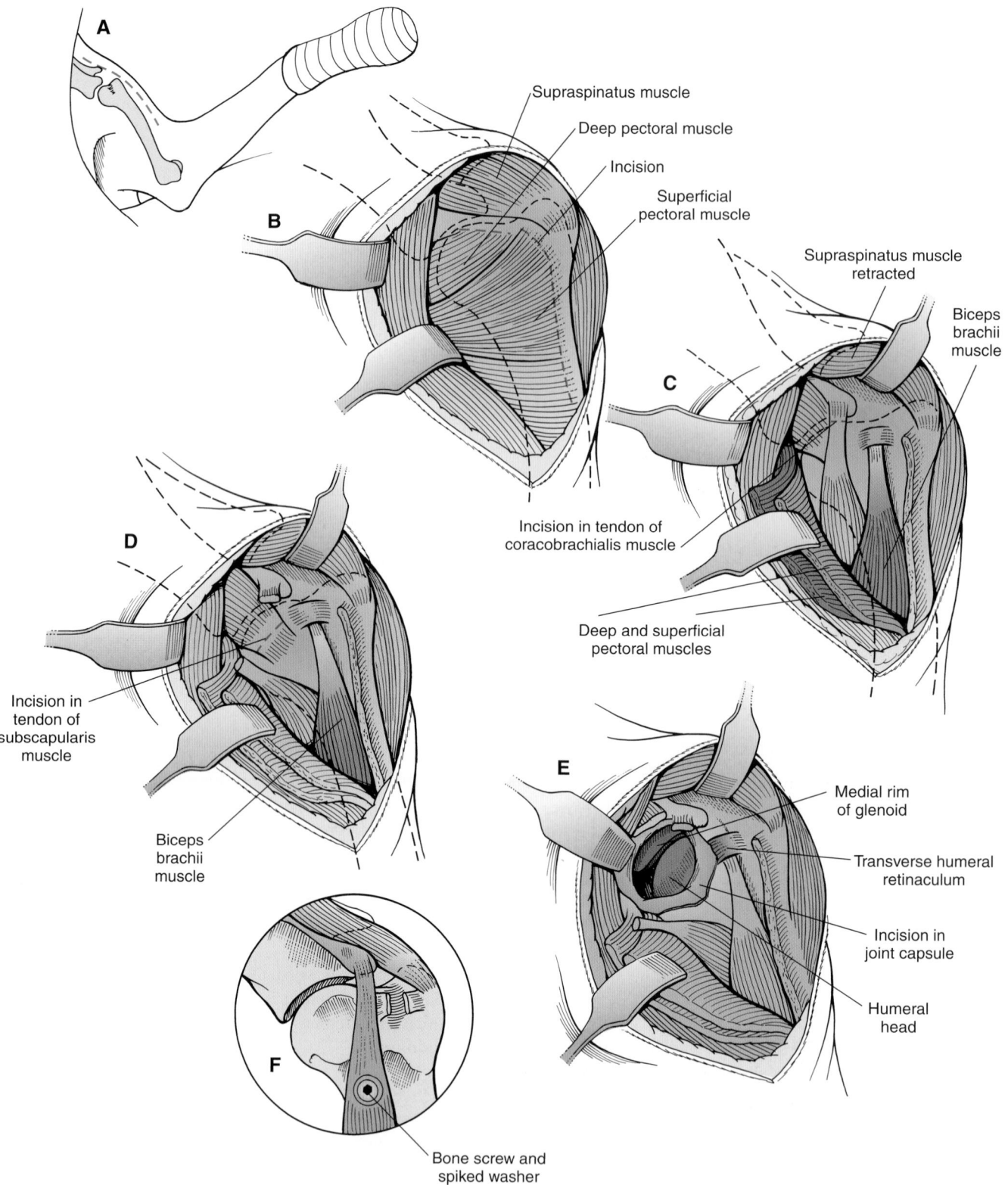

FIG. 33-24

Surgical stabilization of a medial shoulder luxation. **A,** Perform a craniomedial approach with biceps tendon transposition. Incise the skin and subcutaneous tissue over the greater tubercle and continue the incision medially to the midhumeral diaphysis. **B,** Incise the fascia along the lateral border of the brachiocephalicus muscle. **C,** Incise the insertions of the superficial and deep pectoral muscles from the humerus and retract them medially. Retract the supraspinatus muscle laterally. **D,** Transect the tendon of the coracobrachialis muscle to expose the subscapularis muscle tendon. Incise the tendon of the suprascapularis muscle. **E,** Incise the joint capsule to inspect the joint. **F,** To transpose the biceps tendon, incise the transverse humeral ligament. Make a small incision in the joint capsule under the biceps tendon to free it and move the tendon medially. Secure it to the humerus with a bone screw and spiked washer.

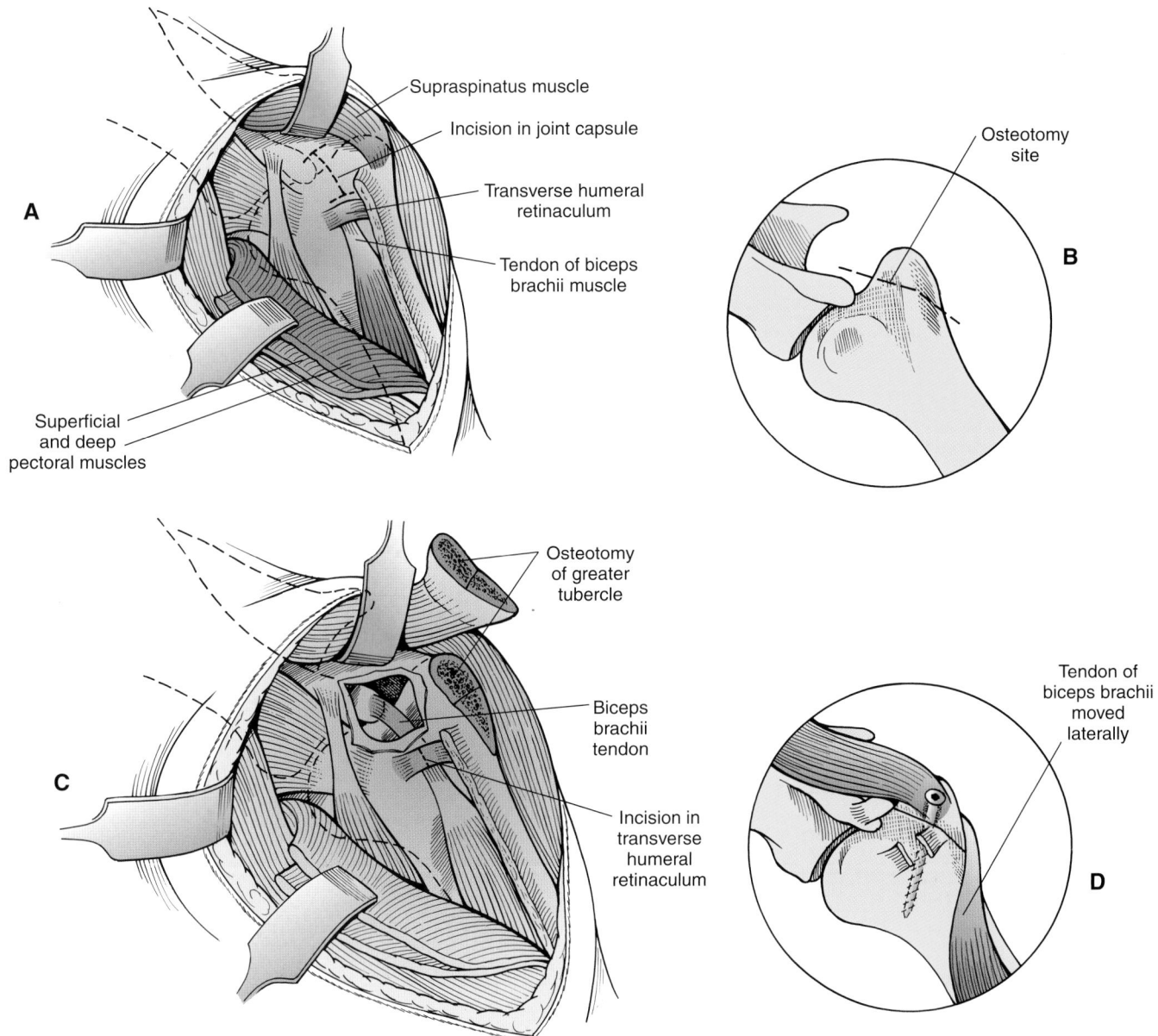

FIG. 33-25
To surgically stabilize a lateral shoulder luxation, perform a cranial approach with biceps tendon transposition. **A,** Expose the joint. **B,** Perform an osteotomy of the greater tubercle, including the supraspinatus muscle insertion. **C,** Incise the joint capsule and the transverse humeral ligament over the biceps tendon. **D,** Free the biceps tendon, and move it laterally across the osteotomy site. Hold the tendon in place, and reduce and stabilize the osteotomy with Kirschner wires and a tension band wire or lag screw.

Cranial Approach to the Shoulder Joint

The biceps brachii tendon is transposed to stabilize a lateral luxation. An approach to the cranial region of the shoulder joint is used to expose the luxated joint (it also is used to approach a cranial luxation of the shoulder). It may be helpful to reduce the joint before the approach is made to reestablish normal anatomic relationships.

Incise the skin and subcutaneous tissue, and deepen the incision through the pectoral muscles as described above for a medial luxation (Fig. 33-25, A). Perform an osteotomy of the greater tubercle that includes the supraspinatus muscular insertion (Fig. 33-25, B). If the joint capsule is not torn, incise it to inspect the joint, and assess the condition of the humeral head and lateral labrum of the glenoid (Fig. 33-25, C).

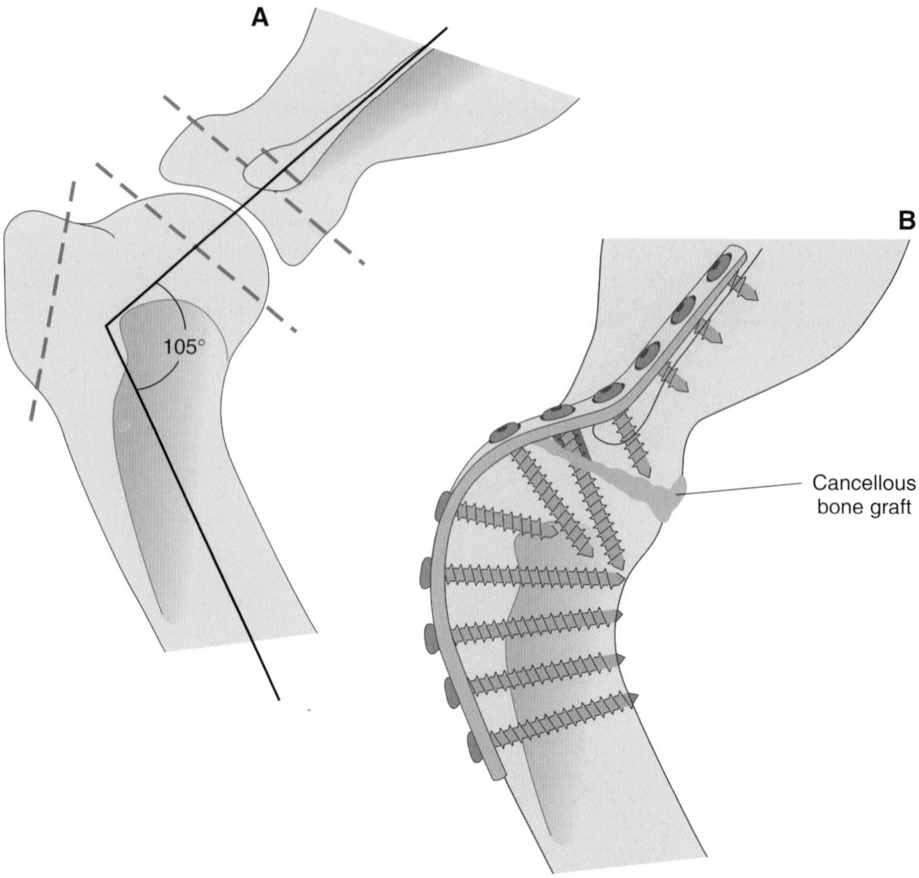

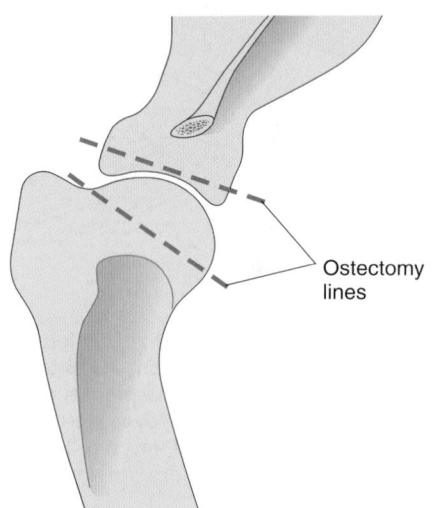

FIG. 33-26
Shoulder arthrodesis. **A,** Osteotomize the greater tubercle and acromion process. Make the ostectomy lines for the glenoid and humeral head parallel to each other when the humerus is held at 105 degrees to the scapula. **B,** Compress the bone surfaces with a contoured compression plate. Place a lag screw across the fracture line. A cancellous bone autograft may be added.

Surgical Stabilization of a Lateral Luxation

If the labrum is worn, the prognosis for successful stabilization of the shoulder is poor.

Reduce the joint and imbricate the capsule with nonabsorbable mattress sutures. If sufficient stabilization is not achieved, incise the transverse humeral ligament over the biceps tendon. Make a small incision in the joint capsule under the biceps tendon to free it, and move the tendon laterally across the osteotomy site. While the tendon is held in place, reduce and stabilize the osteotomy with Kirschner wires and a tension band wire or lag screw (Fig. 33-25, D). Suture the biceps tendon to the deltoid fascia. Close as described above.

Shoulder Arthrodesis

Perform a combined craniolateral and cranial approach to the shoulder with osteotomy of the acromion process (see p. 1034) and greater tubercle (see p. 1189). Detach the biceps tendon from the supraglenoid tubercle. Using an oscillating saw or osteotome, perform ostectomies of the glenoid process and humeral head, which parallel each other when the humerus is held at an angle of approximately 110 degrees to the scapula (the exact angle should be customized to the individual animal). Take care to preserve the suprascapular nerve and caudal circumflex humeral artery. Appose the flat surfaces and temporarily

FIG. 33-27
Ostectomy lines for glenoid excision.

stabilize the bones with a Kirschner wire driven through the cranial aspect of the humerus and into the glenoid. Contour an 8-or 10-hole plate to fit from the dorsocranial junction of the spine and scapula over the cranial aspect of the humerus (Fig. 33-26). Be sure that the plate does not impinge on

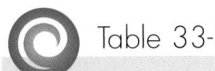

Table 33-8

Physical Rehabilitation Protocol Following Repair of Shoulder Luxation

ALL TREATMENTS BID	DAY 1 TO DAY 14	DAY 15 TO DAY 24	DAY 25 UNTIL HEALED	HEALED TO RETURN TO FUNCTION
Heat therapy		10 min	10 min	
Passive range of motion/ stretching (repetitions)	20*	20*	10–15*	
Therapeutic exercise- total time	10 min	15 min	15 min	25–45 min
Walk/land treadmill	10 min	5 min	10 min	>10 min
Balancing	+	+	+	
Obstacles	+	+	+	+
Weaving		+	+	+
Circles			+	+
Hills			+	+
Stairs				+
Jog/run				+
Underwater treadmill		10 min	10 min	>15 min
Swimming			5 min	5–10 min
Cryotherapy	15 min	15 min	15 min	PRN

BID, Twice a day; +, perform modality; *PRN*, as needed.
*Passive range of motion to all other joints of the affected limb.

the suprascapular nerve. If necessary, contour the cranial humerus with rongeurs to obtain a better fit for the plate. Insert one of the screws across the apposed ostectomy lines as a lag screw. Remove the Kirschner wire and attach the biceps tendon to the surrounding fascia or attach it to the humerus with a bone screw and spiked washer. Secure the greater tubercle to the humerus lateral to the plate with Kirschner wires or bone screws. Suture the soft tissue and close the skin routinely.

Excision Arthroplasty

Perform a craniolateral approach to the shoulder with oste-otomy of the acromion process (see Fig. 32-20 on p. 1033). Detach the biceps tendon from the supraglenoid tubercle, and incise the joint capsule. Using an oscillating saw or osteotome, perform an ostectomy of the glenoid (Fig. 33-27). Take care to preserve the suprascapular nerve and caudal circumflex humeral artery when performing the excision. Bevel the glenoid so that the lateral edge is longer than the medial edge. Part of the humeral head can be ostectomized to create a vascular surface to promote pseudoarthrosis. Pull the teres minor muscle over the glenoid ostectomy site, and suture it to the medial joint capsule and biceps tendon to provide soft tissue interposition between bone surfaces. Pull the acromion process proximally until the deltoid muscle is taut. Wire the process to the scapular spine (see p. 1033), then close the soft tissue.

SUTURE MATERIALS AND SPECIAL INSTRUMENTS

Stabilization techniques for scapulohumeral luxations re-quire retractors, a periosteal elevator, osteotome and mallet, Kirschner wires, orthopedic wire, wire driver, wire twister, bone screw and spiked washer, drill, drill bit, tap, depth gauge, and screwdriver. Plating equipment is required for arthrodesis. Excision arthroplasty requires instruments similar to those for luxations.

POSTOPERATIVE CARE AND ASSESSMENT

Postoperative radiography is performed to document the position of the humeral head and any implants used. After lateral luxation, the limb should be supported in a spica splint (see p. 949) for 10 to 14 days; after medial luxation, it should be supported in a Velpeau sling (see p. 949) for a similar period. Owners should be cautioned to limit activity and protect the bandage. After removal of the bandage, reha-bilitation exercises can begin; however, uncontrolled activity should be limited for an additional 6 to 12 weeks. An ex-ample of a physical rehabilitation exercise protocol is pro-vided in Table 33-8.

After shoulder arthrodesis, postoperative radiographs should be made to evaluate the implant's position and to serve as a comparison for subsequent evaluations. A spica splint is applied until radiographic signs of bone union are seen, usually in 6 to 12 weeks. Once bone union is evident, the splint can be removed and the animal gradually returned to full activity.

After excision arthroplasty, postoperative radiographs are assessed to document alignment of the scapula and humeral head. Early postoperative use of the limb should be encouraged. The animal should be walked on a leash and physical therapy (range of motion exercises) should be performed beginning 1 or 2 days after surgery. Once the sutures have been removed (10 to 14 days after surgery), activity should be encouraged to promote rapid formation of a pseudoarthrosis. Lameness often is evident for 4 to 8 weeks after surgery. Physical therapy may be of particular benefit following excision arthroplasty. Programs usually consist of passive range of motion and cryotherapy postoperatively followed by swimming and walking beginning at 3 weeks.

COMPLICATIONS

The major complication associated with surgical repair of scapulohumeral joint luxations is reluxation of the humeral head. With traumatic luxation, most dogs regain normal limb use; however, some DJD may occur and require periodic treatment with analgesics.

PROGNOSIS

After closed reduction, the prognosis is good for maintenance of reduction and return of limb function if the joints are stable during forelimb manipulation. However, the prognosis is guarded if the joints appear unstable; open reduction and joint stabilization should be considered in such cases. The prognosis is guarded for dogs with congenital or developmental medial luxation. When it is not possible to maintain reduction of scapulohumeral joints, a salvage procedure may be indicated (i.e., shoulder arthrodesis, excision arthroplasty, or amputation).

Reference

Sidaway BK, McLaughlin RM, Elder SH et al: Role of the tendons of the biceps brachii and infraspinatus muscles and the medial glenohumeral ligament in the maintenance of passive shoulder joint stability in dogs, *Am J Vet Res* 65:1216, 2004.

Suggested Reading

Talcott KW, Vasseur PB: Luxation of the scapulohumeral joint. In Slatter D, editor: *Textbook of small animal surgery*, Philadelphia, 2003, Saunders.
This chapter provides a comprehensive review of the causes and treatments of shoulder luxation.

SHOULDER INSTABILITY

DEFINITION

Shoulder instability is characterized by a pathologic increase of the range of motion of the shoulder joint, most commonly in the mediolateral plane. Synonyms include *shoulder subluxation* and *glenohumeral instability*.

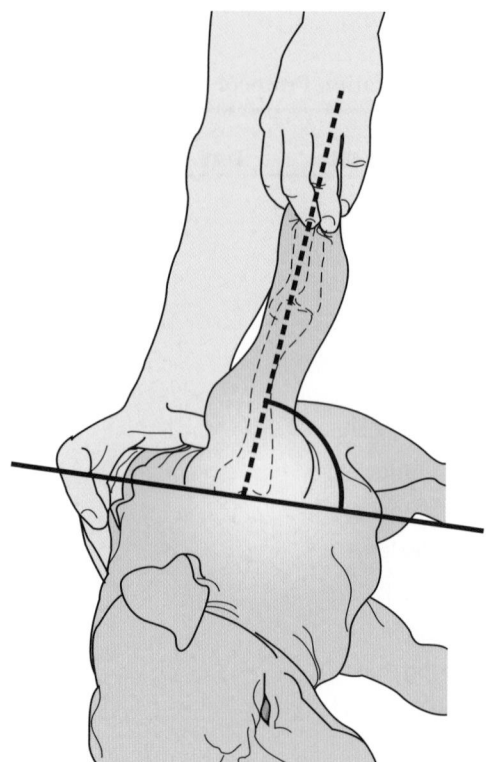

FIG. 33-28
Abduction palpation of the shoulder joint to evaluate for medial instability.

GENERAL CONSIDERATIONS AND CLINICALLY RELEVANT PATHOPHYSIOLOGY

Shoulder instability is due to tearing or stretching of the medial or lateral supportive structures of the shoulder joint. The injury likely is due to low-grade chronic trauma rather than acute blunt trauma, resulting in instability and subluxation of the joint without complete luxation. Damaged structures may include the medial or lateral glenohumeral ligaments and subscapularis tendon. Damage to the biceps tendon may also be apparent. Dogs with shoulder instability may have varying degrees of osteoarthritis.

DIAGNOSIS
Clinical Presentation

Signalment. Shoulder instability is primarily a disease of medium- and large-breed dogs.

History. This disease occurs most commonly in active dogs, but may be diagnosed in older animals after years of exercise and activity. The animal typically has a history of moderate chronic lameness. Less commonly, there may be an acute onset of lameness and a history of mild trauma.

Physical Examination Findings

A moderate weight-bearing lameness is usually observed on gait analysis. Orthopedic examination may reveal moderate muscle atrophy of the affected limb. Palpation of the limb

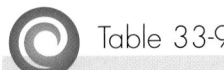 Table 33-9

Physical Rehabilitation Protocol for Shoulder Instability and Elbow Dysplasia

ALL TREATMENTS BID	DAY 1 TO DAY 14	DAY 15 TO DAY 24	DAY 25 UNTIL HEALED	HEALED TO RETURN TO FUNCTION
Heat therapy		10 min	10 min	
Passive range of motion/ stretching (repetitions)	20*	20*	10–15	stop—when ROM N
Electrical stimulation†	10 min	10 min	10 min	10 min
Therapeutic exercise- total time	10 min	20 min	25 min	30–45 min
Walk/land treadmill	10 min	10 min	10 min	>15 min
Balancing	+	+	+	
Obstacles	+	+	+	+
Weaving		+	+	+
Circles			+	+
Hills			+	+
Stairs				+
Jog				+
Underwater treadmill		10 min	10 min	>15 min
Swimming				5–10 min
Cryotherapy	15 min	15 min	15 min	PRN

BID, Twice a day; *ROM N,* range of motion normal; +, perform modality; *PRN,* as needed.
*Perform passive range of motion to all joints of the affected limb.
†Electrical stimulation is most beneficial in these cases to strengthen flexors/extensors if nerve damage is present. See Chaper 12 for further specifications.

may demonstrate increased angles of abduction in cases of medial shoulder instability (Cook et al, 2005) (Fig. 33-28). Most dogs have pain on manipulation of the shoulder joint.

Diagnostic Imaging

Radiographs are usually normal in shoulder instability, although some cases may have changes compatible with osteoarthritis. Dogs with concurrent bicipital tenosynovitis may have osteophytosis and sclerosis of the bicipital groove on skyline views.

Arthroscopy. Definitive diagnosis of shoulder instability is made by arthroscopy. Arthroscopic findings may include tearing or laxity of the medial glenohumeral ligament, lateral glenohumeral ligament, or subscapularis tendon. Tearing or inflammation of the biceps tendon may also be evident.

Laboratory Findings

Specific laboratory abnormalities are not seen. Arthrocentesis of the shoulder joint will show changes compatible with osteoarthritis.

DIFFERENTIAL DIAGNOSES

Shoulder instability must be differentiated from OCD, osteoarthritis, other trauma, and neoplasia.

MEDICAL MANAGEMENT

Medical management consists primarily of rest and physical therapy. Rehabilitation programs are designed to maintain range of motion while strengthening the muscles around the shoulder joint to minimize instability. Physical rehabilitation for shoulder instability should focus on strengthening periarticular structures and improving comfortable active range of motion. Table 33-9 provides an example of a physical rehabilitation protocol.

SURGICAL TREATMENT

Treatment of shoulder instability is an advanced technique that should be performed by an individual with significant experience in the management of joint disease and surgery. Treatment of shoulder instability has been performed with either arthroscopic or open surgery, and neither method has been shown to be superior.

Arthroscopy for Shoulder Instability

Perform standard lateral shoulder arthroscopy, and examine the medial glenohumeral ligament and subscapularis tendon and the biceps tendon and cartilage surfaces. Observe for tearing or significant laxity of the medial supporting structures. If tearing or laxity is not apparent, switch to a craniomedial arthroscope portal for examination of the lateral supporting structures. To perform a craniomedial arthroscope portal, insert a switching stick through a standard instrument portal, advance the tip of the stick to the medial aspect of the biceps tendon, and push the skin out. Incise the skin over the switching stick, and advance the stick out of the joint. Remove the arthroscope from the lateral portal, and pass the arthroscope cannula over the switching stick. Evaluate the lateral collateral ligament for tears and stretching.

If a pathologic condition is identified, use a radiofrequency probe with a shrinkage tip on standard settings. Brush the stretched ligament and adjacent joint capsule, shrinking the tissue using the probe sensor setting.

Open Surgery for Shoulder Instability

Perform a craniomedial approach to the medial aspect of the shoulder joint (see p. 1187). Place two bone anchors in the distal scapula at the sites of origin of the medial glenohumeral ligament (Fig. 33-29) and a single bone anchor in the humerus at the point of insertion. Connect the humeral and scapular bone anchors with heavy gauge nylon. Tighten the sutures to minimize abduction of the joint but not so tightly as to limit joint motion. Close the surgical site routinely (Fitch et al, 2001).

SUTURE MATERIALS AND SPECIAL INSTRUMENTS

Arthroscopic management of shoulder instability requires a radiofrequency system with shrinkage probes. Thorough knowledge of the mechanism and precautions of this equipment is imperative before its use. Radiofrequency can cause severe and permanent damage to cartilage and soft tissue structures around the joint. Open repair of shoulder instability requires bone anchors or bone screws and heavy nylon suture material for stabilization.

POSTOPERATIVE CARE AND ASSESSMENT

Postoperative care requires placement of the affected limb in a Velpeau sling for up to 8 weeks depending upon the technique (see p. 949). The sling may be used for 2 to 4 weeks for the open surgical technique. The arthroscopic technique relies on capsular shrinkage, which results in weakening of the tissue for 4 weeks or more. It is subsequently imperative that the limb be protected from loading for up to 8 weeks in a Velpeau sling. The sling can result in significant complications, particularly contracture of the carpus, so extreme care and observation must be used. The use of physical therapy in the management of this disease may be very beneficial and is highly recommended. Re-

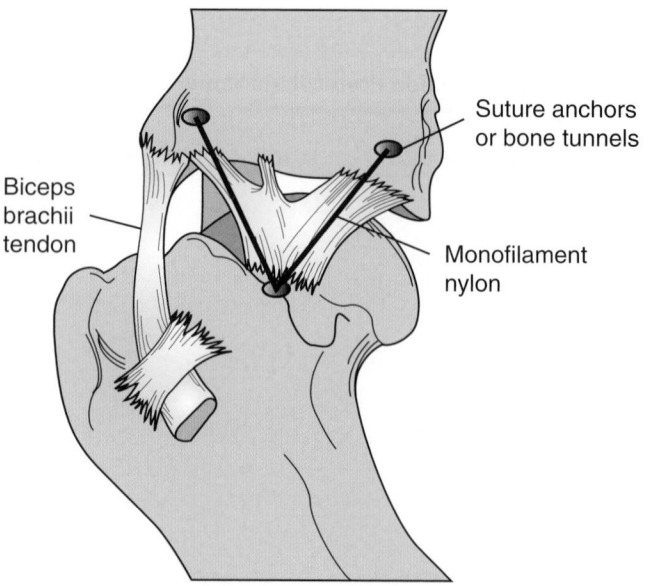

FIG. 33-29
Positioning of bone anchors for stabilization of medial glenohumeral instability.

evaluation includes lameness evaluation and palpation of the joint for stability.

PROGNOSIS

Prognosis for treatment of shoulder instability is variable depending upon the severity of the soft tissue injuries and the osteoarthritis. Reports of both open and arthroscopic techniques have suggested favorable results.

References

Cook JL, Renfro DC, Tomlinson JL et al: Measurement of angles of abduction for diagnosis of shoulder instability in dogs using goniometry and digital image analysis, *Vet Surg* 34:463, 2005.

Cook JL, Tomlinson JL, Fox DB et al: Treatment of dogs diagnosed with medial shoulder instability using radiofrequency-induced thermal capsulorrhaphy, *Vet Surg* 34:469, 2005.

Fitch RB, Breshears L, Staatz A et al: Clinical evaluation of prosthetic medial glenohumeral ligament repair in the dog (10 cases), *Vet Comp Ortho Trauma* 14:222, 2001.

BICEPS TENDON DISEASE

DEFINITIONS

Biceps tendon disease is a general term that incorporates various types of injury, including tearing of the tendon and inflammation of the tendon and surrounding synovial sheath. **Bicipital tenosynovitis** is an inflammation of the biceps brachii tendon and its surrounding synovial sheath. **Bicipital tendon tenodesis** involves surgically moving the origin of the bicipital tendon.

GENERAL CONSIDERATIONS AND CLINICALLY RELEVANT PATHOPHYSIOLOGY

The cause of bicipital tenosynovitis is either direct or indirect trauma to the bicipital tendon. Repetitive injury or overuse may be an inciting factor. Chronic inflammation causing synovial hyperplasia and dystrophic mineralization of the tendon may occur. The tendon may be partly or completely ruptured. Proliferative fibrous connective tissue and adhesions between the tendon and sheath limit motion and cause pain. Osteophytes may form in the intertubercular groove. Mineralization of the supraspinatus tendon may cause a secondary mechanical tenosynovitis and lameness that is refractory to steroid injection, but responsive to curettage of the mineralization. The biceps is a significant stabilizer of the shoulder joint, and biceps tenosynovitis may occur in conjunction with generalized shoulder instability (see p. 1192).

DIAGNOSIS
Clinical Presentation

Signalment. Affected dogs usually are medium- to large-sized and middle-aged or older. There is no predisposition in either gender. Working, active dogs and sedentary dogs may be affected.

History. Intermittent or progressive forelimb lameness that worsens after exercise is common. The owner may relate the lameness to trauma, but usually the onset of clinical signs is slow. Less commonly, biceps tendon disease (particularly tearing of the tendon) may be associated with an acute onset of lameness and a history of blunt trauma.

Physical Examination Findings

Lameness of one forelimb usually is evident. The animal usually stands on the limb, but is lame during gaiting. Pain may be evident during palpation of the bicipital tendon, especially with concurrent flexion of the shoulder and extension of the elbow. Pain may also be evident during palpation of the biceps muscle while the dog is standing. In some cases the condition is bilateral. Atrophy of the supraspinatus and infraspinatus muscles may be palpable.

Diagnostic Imaging

Radiographic views should include standard lateral projections of both shoulders. A craniocaudal projection of the humerus (skyline) with the shoulder flexed can be used to identify the bicipital groove. Calcification of the biceps tendon and osteophytes in the intertubercular groove may be evident. Arthrography (see p. 1177) can be used to outline the tendon and reveal irregularities and filling defects suggestive of synovial hyperplasia, tendon rupture, and joint mice. Caution is indicated in interpretation of arthrography because the biceps tendon sheath is a continuation of the shoulder joint capsule, and any disease that causes inflammation of the shoulder joint may also cause synovial proliferation of the biceps tendon sheath. Radiographic findings of synovial proliferation within the sheath therefore are not diagnostic for biceps tendon disease.

Ultrasound is used extensively in other species (humans, horses) for evaluation of tendon injuries and is superior to radiography in its ability to visualize tendons. Both transverse and longitudinal views should be obtained. The normal biceps tendon has an echogenic linear echotexture in a uniform pattern. Acute trauma results in fiber pattern disruption and fluid accumulation within or around the tendon. Chronic trauma may demonstrate dystrophic mineralization. Fluid accumulation and synovial proliferation of the tendon sheath are easily appreciated, but cannot be differentiated between those caused by bicipital disease and those associated with shoulder joint inflammation of other causes (Kramer et al, 2001).

Arthroscopy. Arthroscopy provides direct visualization of the biceps tendon and sheath and definitive diagnosis of disease in most cases. From a standard lateral arthroscopy portal, the biceps tendon is observed and visualization of the tendons is maximized by flexing the shoulder and elbow to approximately 90 degrees each. The normal biceps tendon has a small cuff of proliferative tissue around the origin of the biceps tendon, which should not be interpreted as disease. Moderate to severe fibrous proliferation at the origin of the tendon or obvious tearing is compatible with disease. The joint should be carefully observed for damage to other supporting structures.

Laboratory Findings

The results of hematologic and serum biochemical analyses reflect the dog's general health. The results of arthrocentesis typically are normal or may suggest mild inflammation and DJD, with higher concentrations of monocytes and macrophages in the joint fluid. Evidence of sepsis is a contraindication to arthrography or intraarticular corticosteroid therapy.

DIFFERENTIAL DIAGNOSIS

Bicipital tenosynovitis must be differentiated from osteoarthritis of the shoulder, shoulder instability, supraspinatus tendonitis, OCD, early osteosarcoma or other bone tumors of the proximal humeral metaphysis, synovial osteochondromatosis, cervical disk disease, or neurofibroma of the brachial plexus. Definitive diagnosis is confirmed with arthroscopic examination of the shoulder joint (see p. 1178).

MEDICAL MANAGEMENT

Medical therapy generally is used initially to treat dogs with bicipital tenosynovitis. Methylprednisolone acetate (10 to 40 mg) can be infiltrated into the bicipital tendon sheath or injected into the scapulohumeral joint. This treatment is followed by confinement for 6 weeks. After the confinement period, exercise should be increased gradually to strengthen the surrounding musculature. Oral administration of corticosteroids does not appear to be effective.

Pulsed mode therapeutic ultrasound may be used in the treatment of biceps disease (see Chapter 12). Response to this therapy is uncertain.

SURGICAL TREATMENT

Bicipital tendon tenotomy or tenodesis is performed to eliminate movement of the biceps tendon in the inflamed tendon sheath. This procedure is indicated in dogs with ruptured bicipital tendons and chronic bicipital tenosynovitis, if the condition has not responded to medical therapy. As an alternative, surgical or arthroscopic exploration and resection of mineralization and inflamed synovium may be effective. Confirmation of the disease and evaluation of the other supporting structures of the shoulder joint should be performed before surgical therapy. Tenotomy or tenodesis should only be performed when either there is confirmation of a partial tear of the biceps tendon or there is evidence of chronic biceps tenosynovitis with documentation of normalcy of the other supporting structures of the shoulder joint, including the medial and lateral glenohumeral ligaments, subscapularis tendon, and supraspinatus tendon. Tenodesis or tenotomy of the biceps tendon in a shoulder with other significant soft tissue injuries may contribute to irreversible instability of the joint.

Preoperative Management

The overall health of the animal should be determined before surgery.

Anesthesia

Anesthetic management of dogs with orthopedic disease is discussed on p. 944. Postoperative analgesics are discussed on p. 944 (see also Table 13-4 on p. 133).

Surgical Anatomy

Surgical anatomy of the shoulder is discussed on p. 1033. The bicipital tendon arises from the supraglenoid tubercle and crosses the cranial portion of the scapulohumeral joint. The tendon courses through the intertubercular groove of the humerus and is held in position by the transverse humeral ligament. The tendon is surrounded by a synovial sheath that communicates with the scapulohumeral joint.

Positioning

For arthroscopic treatment, the dog is positioned in lateral recumbency. For open surgery, the dog is positioned in dorsal recumbency with the affected leg draped. The prepared area should extend from the dorsal and ventral midlines to below the elbow.

SURGICAL TECHNIQUE
Arthroscopic Treatment

Standard lateral arthroscopy is performed on the affected shoulder joint (see p. 1178).

Examine the entire joint, paying particular attention to the medial glenohumeral ligament and subscapularis tendon. If a pathologic condition of the biceps tendon is identified and the remainder of the joint is normal, tenotomy of tendon may be performed. Establish a cranial portal using either an out-to-in or in-to-out method. For an out-to-in method, insert a

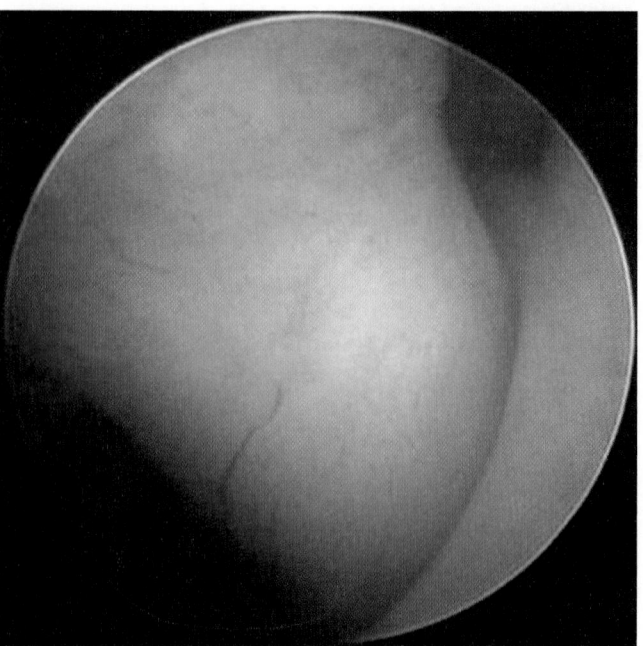

FIG. 33-30
Arthroscopic visualization of the biceps tendon.

needle adjacent to the biceps tendon. Once the needle can be visualized through the arthroscope, incise adjacent to the needle to establish the cranial portal. To perform an in-to-out technique, pass a switching stick from a standard caudolateral instrument portal past the biceps tendon on either the medial or lateral side. Tent the skin, and incise the skin over the switching stick to establish the portal.

Transection of the biceps tendon may be performed with or without cannulas (Fig. 33-30).

Insert an arthroscopic blade through a cannula or an No. 11 blade without a cannula, and transect the tendon below the site of disease. Resect the remaining origin of the tendon with a power shaver or biter.

Open Surgical Treatment

An approach to the cranial region of the shoulder joint is used to expose the bicipital tendon and bicipital groove (see p. 1188). Incise the transverse humeral ligament and joint capsule to expose the tendon and intertubercular groove. Transect the tendon near the supraglenoid tubercle. Reattach the tendon to the humerus distal to the groove with a bone screw and spiked Teflon washer. As an alternative, redirect the tendon through a bone tunnel created in the humerus, and suture it to the supraspinatus muscle.

SUTURE MATERIALS AND SPECIAL INSTRUMENTS

No special arthroscopic equipment is required for arthroscopic treatment. For open surgical treatment, equipment for placing a screw and spiked washer is needed.

POSTOPERATIVE CARE AND ASSESSMENT

Following arthroscopic treatment, the dog should be rested without significant activity for 2 to 3 weeks. Use of a sling is not necessary. After open surgery, the limb should be supported in a Velpeau sling (see p. 949) for 2 to 3 weeks. The animal should be closely confined for 6 weeks, after which gradual resumption of normal activity should be encouraged. Postoperative physical therapy can aid in the rehabilitation after biceps surgery. Therapy involves cryotherapy, passive range of motion, and short leash walks followed by gradual muscle strengthening exercises.

PROGNOSIS

The results of medical treatment range from excellent to poor. The results of arthroscopic and surgical treatment generally are good to excellent. The time required for dogs to regain optimum function ranges from 2 to 9 months.

Reference

Kramer M, Gerwing M, Sheppard C et al: Ultrasonography for the diagnosis of diseases of the tendon and tendon sheath of the biceps brachii muscle, *Vet Surg* 30:64, 2001.

Suggested Reading

Bardet JF: Lesions of the biceps tendon diagnosis and classification: a retrospective study of 25 cases in 23 dogs and one cat, *Vet Comp Orthop Traum* 12:188, 1999.
This study provides a large case series with arthroscopic findings and treatment of biceps tendon disease.

Beale BS, Hulse DA, Schulz KS et al: *Small animal arthroscopy,* Philadelphia, 2003, Saunders.
This book has detailed descriptions on the arthroscopic findings and treatment of biceps disease.

Bruce WJ, Burbidge HM, Bray JP et al: Bicipital tendonitis and tenosynovitis in the dog: a study of 15 cases, *N Z Vet J* 48:44, 2000.
This article describes the clinical radiographic and sonographic findings of 15 dogs with biceps disease and the efficacy of treatment.

Wall CR, Taylor R: Arthroscopic biceps brachii tenotomy as a treatment for canine bicipital tenosynovitis, *J Am Anim Hosp Assoc* 38:169, 2002.
This article provides the first description of the arthroscopic technique of biceps transection.

ELBOW JOINT

CANINE ELBOW DYSPLASIA

Elbow dysplasia likely represents the leading cause of forelimb lameness in the dog. Several diseases have been designated as components of inherited canine elbow dysplasia (Box 33-14). These diseases (e.g., FCP, OCD, UAP, articular cartilage disease, and joint incongruity) differ in terms of pathophysiology, but all are causes of elbow arthrosis. Breed dispositions to the development of these diseases indicate

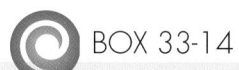

BOX 33-14

Important Considerations for Treatment of Elbow Dysplasia

- Elbow dysplasia is a set of diseases that include osteochondrosis, fragmented coronoid process, and ununited anconeal process.
- There is strong evidence of a hereditary component in the etiology of elbow dysplasia.
- Loss of elbow range of motion is evidence of DJD; in immature large dogs, this finding usually indicates the presence of elbow dysplasia.
- Careful attention to positioning for radiographs is essential for the diagnosis of subtle lesions and for differential diagnosis.
- Both elbows should be radiographed.
- Surgical removal of bone and cartilage pieces usually results in improved limb function.

that they are genetically influenced, and evidence now indicates that canine elbow dysplasia, like hip dysplasia, is a polygenic trait with both hereditary and environmental influences playing a part in its development. Selective breeding in Sweden has reduced the prevalence of elbow arthrosis in rottweilers and Bernese mountain dogs. Several groups have been organized to review elbow radiographs to determine the presence of elbow dysplasia (similarly to hip radiographs for hip dysplasia). In one study of submitted screening radiographs of Labrador retrievers, the bone dysplasia lesion most often detected was elbow dysplasia (17.8%), followed by hip dysplasia (12.6%) (Morgan et al, 1999).

> NOTE: Because all forms of canine elbow dysplasia are hereditary, breeding dogs identified with this condition should be strongly discouraged.

FRAGMENTED CORONOID PROCESS

DEFINITION

Fragmented coronoid process (FCP) usually occurs as a separation of a small portion of the medial coronoid process of the ulna that results in lameness and DJD. Synonyms include *ununited coronoid process, fractured coronoid process, elbow dysplasia, medial compartment disease,* and *jump-down syndrome.*

GENERAL CONSIDERATIONS AND CLINICALLY RELEVANT PATHOPHYSIOLOGY

The etiology of FCP is unknown. However, several theories have been proposed. (1) FCP may result from an osteochondrosis lesion in which disruption of endochondral ossification of the coronoid process leaves it vulnerable to cartilage degeneration, necrosis, and fissure formation. (2) Developmental elbow incongruity may play a role in the pathophysiology of FCP. Asynchronous growth of the radius and ulna (causing the ulna to be longer than the radius at some time during the growth process) may result in an increase in weight-bearing forces on the medial coronoid process, which precipitates fissuring and fragmentation. Also, trochlear notch dysplasia or malformation, resulting in joint incongruity, may contribute to mechanical overloading and fragmentation of the coronoid. (3) Incongruence between the radial head and the radial notch has also been proposed as a cause of fragmentation. (4) FCP may result from vascular abnormality of the medial coronoid that leads to osteonecrosis and fragmentation.

FCP may be characterized by complete fragmentation and separation, partial fissuring of the coronoid, or osteonecrosis. Fissures that develop in the coronoid may or may not progress to fragmentation. When fragmentation occurs, it results in a separated piece of cartilage and trabecular bone that is attached to the annular ligament with fibrous tissue. Separation occurs through calcified trabeculae that are then covered in part with a thin layer of fibrous tissue. The end result is coronoid fragmentation and development of DJD. Cartilage of the opposing medial humeral condyle may be eroded by the loose coronoid fragment. The degree of cartilage damage associated with FCP varies tremendously, and the specific cause of the cartilage wearing is uncertain. Some cartilage damage may be due to abrasion against the loose fragment; however, elbow joint pathology with severe cartilage loss cannot be explained by this mechanism alone. The greatest cartilage damage is almost always concentrated in the medial portion of the joint (medial coronoid and medial portion of the humeral condyle) and is commonly described as *medial compartment disease*. Periarticular osteophytes increase and soft tissue fibrosis develops over time.

DIAGNOSIS
Clinical Presentation

Signalment. Large dogs (Labrador retrievers, rottweilers, Bernese mountain dogs, Newfoundlands, golden retrievers, German shepherds, and chows) usually are affected. The disease process starts when the animal is immature, with clinical signs first becoming apparent at 5 to 7 months of age. However, dogs may be brought in at any age for osteoarthritis secondary to FCP and elbow dysplasia.

　History. Forelimb lameness that worsens after exercise may be acute or chronic. Owners frequently complain that the dog is stiff in the morning or after rest. There may be a coincidental history of trauma.

Physical Examination Findings

Lameness of one forelimb usually is evident. The gait may appear stiff or stilted if bilateral lameness is present because the animal may walk with shortened steps. Palpation of the dog standing may demonstrate symmetrical or asymmetrical muscle atrophy associated with chronic pain and decreased muscle use. Joint effusion and periarticular soft tissue swelling may be palpable and are most easily felt while the dog is standing. Palpation of the elbows should include an evaluation of range of motion. Pain on hyperextension of the elbow

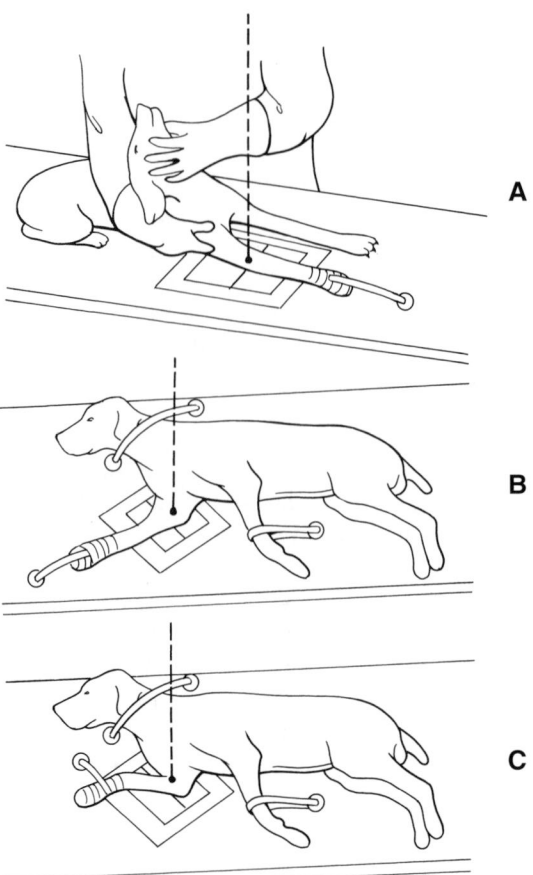

FIG. 33-31
A, For a craniocaudal radiograph of the elbow, position the dog in sternal recumbency with the elbow flexed 30 degrees and slightly medially rotated. For standard lateral **(B)** and flexed lateral **(C)** views, position the dog in lateral recumbency with the elbow against the cassette.

joint may be one of the earliest signs of FCP. Decreased ability to flex the elbow is indicative of more severe osteoarthritis. Crepitation during elbow flexion and extension may be felt if advanced osteoarthritis is present. Manipulation of the joint is often painful. It is important that the shoulder not be inadvertently flexed and extended during elbow manipulation to prevent mistaking shoulder pain for elbow pain.

Diagnostic Imaging

In many cases, diagnosis of FCP is made on the basis of radiographic signs of DJD. Radiographic views should include a standard lateral of the elbow, flexed lateral (joint positioned at 45 degrees' flexion) to expose the anconeal process, a standard craniocaudal view, and an oblique craniocaudal view made with the elbow flexed 30 degrees and slightly rotated medially (15 degrees) to evaluate the lateral profile of the medial coronoid process (Fig. 33-31). Radiographs of both elbows should be made because bilateral disease is common. The earliest radiographic sign is often sclerosis of the distal aspect of the trochlear notch. This is visible as a loss of the fine trabecular pattern and an in-

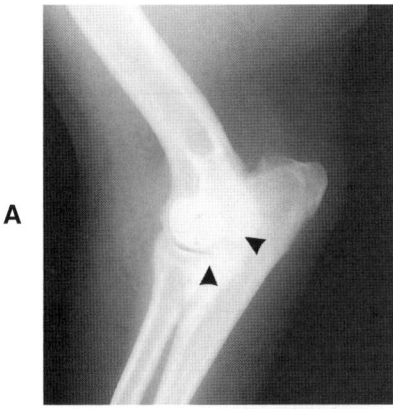

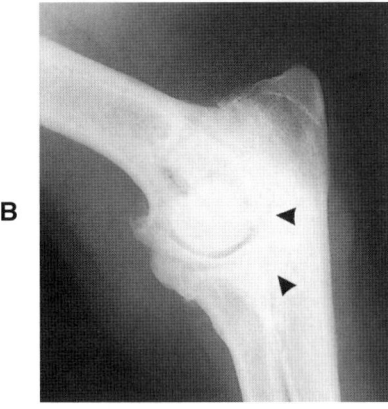

FIG. 33-32
A, Preoperative radiographs of a dog with FCP and DJD. There is subchondral bone sclerosis caudal and distal to the trochlear notch of the ulna *(arrowheads)*. **B,** Radiographs of the same dog 8 years after surgical removal of the FCP. Note the progression of degenerative changes *(arrowheads)*.

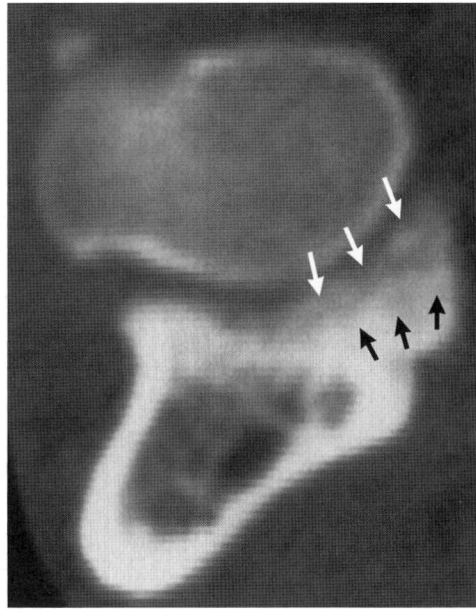

FIG. 33-33
CT scan showing in situ osteomalacia of the medial coronoid process *(arrows)*.

crease in opacity (Fig. 33-32). Blunting of the medial coronoid process is also an early radiographic finding. These radiographic findings may be subtle, and evaluation by a radiologist or orthopedic surgeon may be helpful. Visible fragments are rarely seen. Later, osteophytes associated with the coronoid process and tip of the anconeus may be visible (see Fig. 33-32). The fragmented process cannot always be observed and the diagnosis may be made by inference from the presence of osteoarthritis. Joint incongruence may be evaluated on radiographs, but evidence suggests a high rate of false positives and negatives for incongruence less than 3 mm.

> Note: Radiographs in dogs with elbow dysplasia may have very subtle changes (occult elbow dysplasia) even in the presence of significant elbow arthrosis.

CT is helpful for identifying FCP and can be used to evaluate other aspects of the articular surfaces for defects and incongruity (Fig. 33-33). CT scans are more accurate for identifying FCP than survey radiographs. Although older CT scanners required use of general anesthesia, newer machines (which are significantly faster in acquisition time) often allow images to be obtained under heavy sedation. CT has the advantage over arthroscopy of being able to diagnose incomplete fragmentation of the medial coronoid that does not reach the cartilage surface. The greatest value of CT may be in evaluating the elbow joint for incongruence (Gemmill et al, 2005; Holsworth et al, 2005).

Arthroscopy. Arthroscopy is the most valuable tool for diagnosing FCP and medial compartment disease (Fig. 33-34). Unlike other modalities, arthroscopy enables direct visualization and assessment of the cartilage surface. Fragmentation is clearly visible except with incomplete fragments that do not reach the cartilage surface. Osteonecrosis may be diagnosed by firm palpation of the medial coronoid process.

Laboratory Findings

Results of hematologic and serum biochemical analyses are normal in most affected animals. Results of arthrocentesis may include decreased synovial fluid viscosity, increased fluid volume, and increased numbers of mononuclear phagocytic cells (up to 6000 to 9000 WBC/μl).

DIFFERENTIAL DIAGNOSIS

Other conditions affecting the elbow of immature dogs (OCD, UAP, combined UAP and FCP, and subluxation resulting from premature physeal closure) may produce similar clinical signs and must be differentiated from FCP. Other diseases that affect the forelimb of young growing dogs

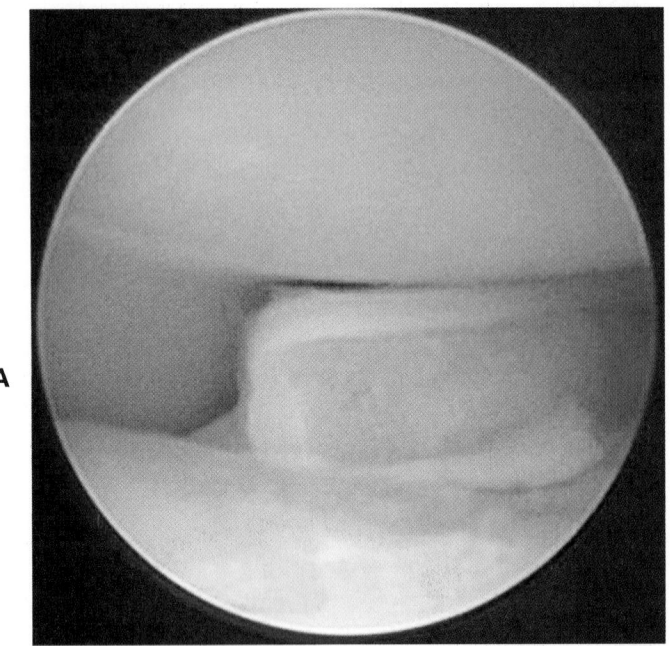 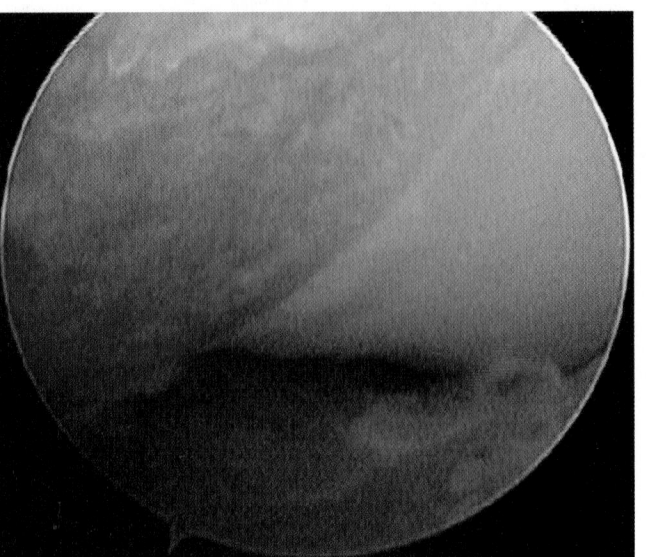

FIG. 33-34
A, Arthroscopic view of the elbow demonstrating an osteochondral fragment of the medial coronoid process. **B,** Arthroscopic view of the elbow demonstrating medial compartment disease with full thickness (Grade IV) cartilage damage.

(OCD of the shoulder, panosteitis) should also be differentiated from FCP. These conditions usually can be differentiated radiographically.

MEDICAL MANAGEMENT

Dogs with FCP may be treated conservatively; however, owners should be cautioned that delay in surgical removal of a loose fragment can allow continued cartilage damage by the fragment. Exploration of the elbow joint with arthroscopy should be encouraged, particularly for young patients with mild to moderate osteoarthritis. Patients that benefit most from surgical treatment are those that have only fragmentation, but no significant cartilage damage. In these patients, fragment removal can result in complete resolution of clinical signs and eliminate the possibility of cartilage damage caused by abrasion from the fragment. If surgery is to be performed, it should be done as early in the disease process as possible to minimize progression of osteoarthritis.

Alternatively, because cartilage damage cannot be attributed to the fragment alone in all cases, surgery may not necessarily affect the progression of osteoarthritis. The value of surgical or arthroscopic treatment of dogs with advanced osteoarthritis is questionable as the pain coming from the osteoarthritis is likely greater than that caused by the presence of the fragment.

When conservative management is elected, it should include focusing on the five principles of medical management of osteoarthritis (see p. 1145), particularly weight management, nutritional supplementation, exercise moderation, and antiinflammatory medication. Many dogs with radio-

graphic signs of osteoarthritis are asymptomatic and remain so for several years. Although owners should be apprised of the problem, they should also be reassured that the dog may function as a pet with minimal treatment (Box 33-15).

SURGICAL TREATMENT

Affected animals are candidates for surgery when they have intermittent or chronic lameness and minimal to moderate degenerative changes. Occasionally, animals with advanced osteoarthritis and persistent lameness not amenable to medical therapy may benefit from joint exploration and removal of a loose fragment. However, surgical treatment does not halt the progression of osteoarthritis, and continued medical therapy may be required in these patients. There does not appear to be any correlation between the severity of lameness before treatment, the severity of radiographic signs, and the type of lesion found at surgery.

The basis of treatment of FCP is fragment removal by either arthroscopy or open arthrotomy. Arthroscopic treatment of FCP has numerous advantages over open surgery. Arthroscopy provides superior visualization and magnification of the joint, is less invasive, has lower postoperative morbidity, and provides greater opportunity for topical treatment of osteoarthritic lesions (Meyer-Lindenberg et al, 2003).

Additional surgical treatments for FCP depend upon the specific lesions diagnosed. Incongruence has been suggested as a likely cause of FCP and associated osteoarthritis, and several surgical treatments for incongruence have been described. These procedures are relatively invasive and their

BOX 33-15

Important Information for Clients With Dogs That Have Elbow Dysplasia

- There is strong evidence for a hereditary component in the etiology of fragmented coronoid process and osteochondrosis.
- Bilateral elbow radiographs should be made because of the frequency of bilateral disease; however, unless the animal shows clinical signs, surgery of the opposite limb is not performed.
- Surgical removal of the bone and cartilage pieces usually results in improved function of the limb if the dog is treated before extensive secondary degenerative changes occur in the joint.
- After surgery, the dog is confined and exercise is limited to short walks on a leash for 2–4 wk.
- Surgical treatment does not appear to alter the progression of DJD (osteoarthritis); if the elbow is incongruent, changes may be moderate or severe, and the dog may require medical therapy after surgery.
- Dogs usually function well as pets with osteoarthritis of the elbow, but they may not be appropriate as working or competitive sporting dogs.

efficacy has not been demonstrated; therefore it is important to definitively diagnose incongruence before application of these techniques. Incongruence of the joint may be investigated with either plain film radiography or CT. Routine radiography using standard medial-lateral positioning has been reported to be an inaccurate means of diagnosis of mild incongruity (Mason et al, 2002); however, incongruence may be more accurately evaluated on flexed lateral views (Blonde et al, 2005). CT is a more accurate means of evaluating incongruence (Gemmill et al, 2005; Holsworth et al, 2005). Surgical procedures that have been described for incongruence include proximal and distal ulnar osteotomies and proximal radial osteotomy.

Arthroscopy of the elbow joint may demonstrate mild to severe cartilage damage to the articular surfaces. FCP or OCD with cartilage damage is termed medial compartment disease. In cases of full thickness cartilage loss, topical treatments—including abrasion arthroplasty or microfracture—may be warranted. These are advanced arthroscopic techniques. Coronoidectomy has also been described for treatment of FCP and medial compartment disease. Indications and outcomes for this procedure have not been completely described.

Preoperative Management

Most affected animals are young and require minimal preoperative workup (see Chapter 5).

Anesthesia

These dogs usually are young and healthy, thus a variety of anesthetic regimens may be used (see p. 944).

Arthroscopic Treatment of FCP and Medial Compartment Disease

Indications. Elbow arthroscopy is most commonly used for diagnosis and treatment of elbow dysplasia. Further indications for arthroscopic surgery of the elbow include treatment of OCD, biopsy of inflamed synovium, and biopsy of abnormal intraarticular tissue.

Instrumentation. A 30-degree foreoblique 1.9- or 2.4-mm arthroscope commonly is used in the elbow joint. Both sizes are easily inserted into the joint space without introducing significant damage to the articular cartilage. The surgeon must be aware of the diameter of the arthroscope sheath (cannula) because it, too, must enter the joint. Each arthroscope cannula can be fitted with a blunt obturator or a sharp obturator (trocar point). Although either can be used to enter the joint, the blunt obturator is preferred because it is safer.

An assortment of hand instruments is necessary for elbow arthroscopy (please see Chapter 14). Instruments to assist in the inspection of intraarticular structures (probes), grasping forceps for removal of free bodies (FCP, OCD), biopsy forceps, and instruments for surface arthroplasty are recommended. Instruments commonly used for surface arthroplasty are hand-held burrs, curettes, or a motorized shaver. Instruments commonly used for microfracture are micropicks and a mallet. Instruments can be inserted into the joint through an open instrument port or instrument cannulas or a combination of the two. If one chooses to work through an instrument cannula, different-size cannulas and switching sticks are necessary.

Portal sites and technique. *Clip and prepare the medial aspect of the elbow joint.*

Beginning arthroscopists should clip and prepare the area as if an open arthrotomy were to be performed so that the arthroscopy procedure can be aborted and an open arthrotomy performed if necessary. Advanced arthroscopic techniques, including use of caudal and cranial portals, also require circumferential preparation of the limb. One of two methods for limb preparation may be used, depending on the limb maneuverability desired.

If you wish to have maximum maneuverability of the limb during surgery, use a hanging limb preparation. As you become more experienced and adept at elbow arthroscopy, less maneuverability is needed, and you may wish to perform a medial limb preparation for each limb. Use two or three portal sites for elbow arthroscopy, depending on the purpose of arthroscopic intervention. If visual exploration of the elbow joint is all that is required, use an egress portal and an arthroscope portal. If tissue biopsy or treatment of a pathologic joint condition is undertaken, use an additional instrument portal. Position the dog in dorsal recumbency because both elbows may need intervention. As one elbow is operated on, lean the body toward that limb. Position the limb such that the elbow joint can be centered over the edge of the table (padded) or over an elbow brace (Fig. 33-35).

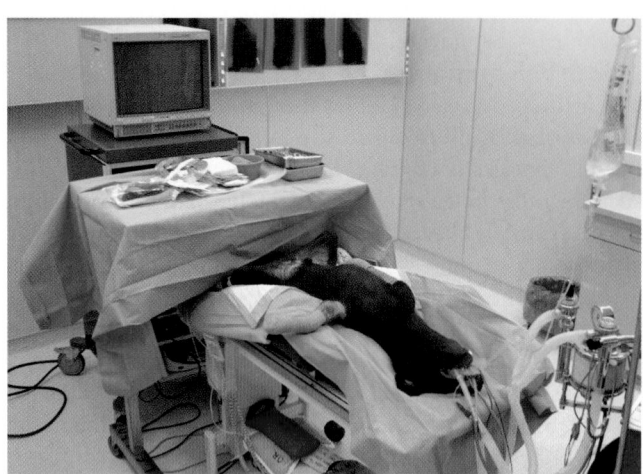

FIG. 33-35
Positioning for elbow arthroscopy.

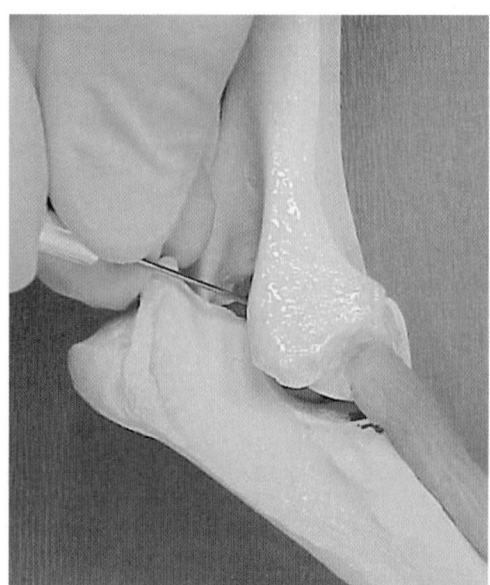

FIG. 33-36
Specimen showing the location of the egress portal into the condylar fossa.

This allows the assistant to externally rotate the paw and apply a valgus stress to the limb. These maneuvers help open the medial joint space, allowing increased mobility of the arthroscope and instruments. The joint may also be positioned with self-retaining retractors. This allows the surgeon to move freely around the limb and prevents problems of movement by the assistant.

As with other joints, accurate placement is essential for the egress, arthroscope, and instrument portals.

Establish the egress portal first (Fig. 33-36), then the arthroscope portal (Fig. 33-37), and finally the instrument portal. Establish the egress portal by inserting an 18- or 20-gauge needle between the medial epicondyloid ridge and the ridge of the anconeal process. Once the needle is in place, aspirate joint fluid to ensure proper positioning of the needle in the joint. Instill lactated Ringer's solution through the needle to distend the joint. With the joint distended, use a second needle to determine the correct position of the arthroscope portal. Insert the needle perpendicular to the joint line approximately 1 cm distal and 0.5 cm caudal to the medial epicondyle.

Once the joint is entered, fluid will flow from the needle, confirming proper placement in the joint.

Use a No. 11 Bard-Parker blade to make a small entry wound through the skin and superficial soft tissue adjacent to the needle.

It is not advisable to enter the joint with the scalpel blade because extravasation of fluid from the joint cavity is more likely if the blade enters the joint.

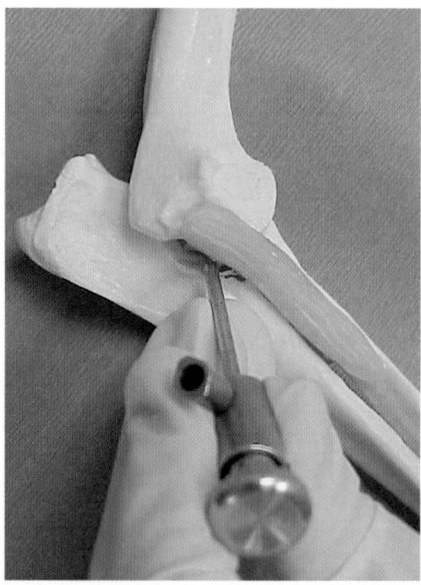

FIG. 33-37
Specimen showing the location of the arthroscope portal site. The position is caudal to the medial epicondyle at the level of the joint line.

Remove the needle, and insert the arthroscope cannula with the attached blunt obturator. Once in the joint, remove the obturator from the cannula.

Fluid will flow freely from the cannula, confirming correct placement.

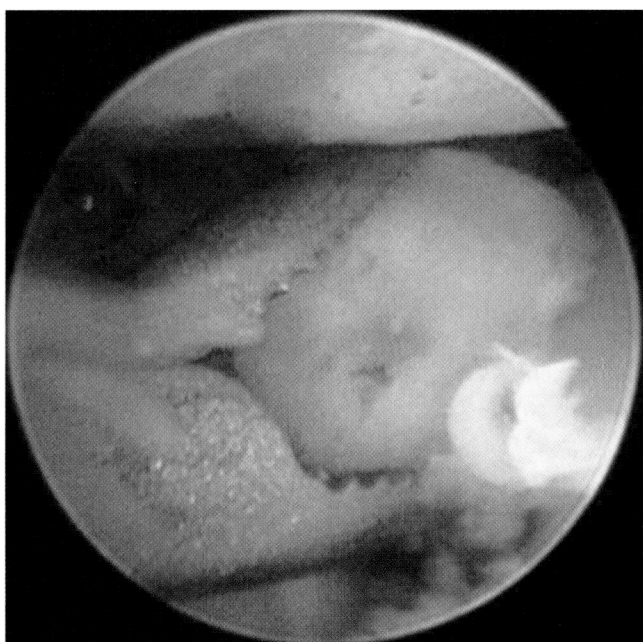

FIG. 33-38
Arthroscopic view showing a fragmented medial coronoid process.

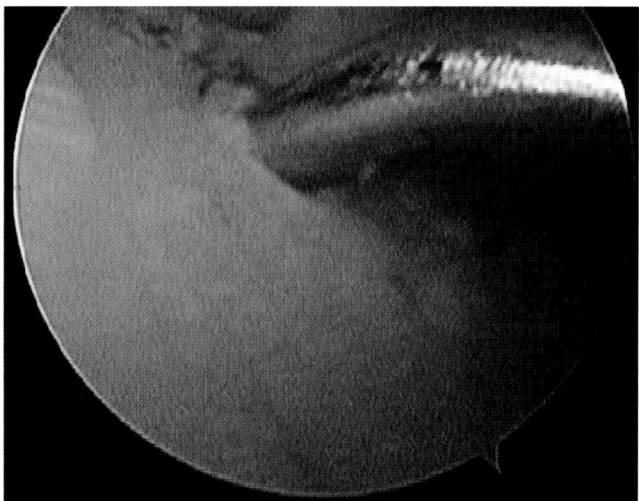

FIG. 33-39
Arthroscopic microfracture of the medial coronoid process of the elbow.

Attach the fluid ingress line to the cannula and insert the arthroscope.

If treatment of a pathologic joint condition (FCP, OCD) or biopsy of intraarticular structures is required, establish an instrument portal approximately 1 to 2 cm cranial to the arthroscope portal.

This distance is only an approximation because it will vary with the size of the dog.

Learn to triangulate the instrument portal relative to the arthroscope portal for best results. To triangulate the position for the instrument portal, position the arthroscope to view the medial coronoid process. Insert a 20-gauge needle at the estimated position for the instrument portal. Insert the needle perpendicular to the skin surface, and maintain this orientation as it passes through the soft tissue. As the needle enters the joint, observe it on the monitor.

The most common reason for not seeing the needle as it enters the joint is crossing the needle over the scope. This is caused either by inserting the needle too close to the arthroscope portal or by inserting the needle such that the point is angled toward the arthroscope.

Once the position of the instrument portal has been confirmed by the triangulation needle, make a 3-mm incision through the skin and superficial soft tissue. If working through an open instrument portal, lengthen the incision (4 to 6 mm) and carry it into the joint. If working through an instrument cannula, do not lengthen the incision and do not carry it into the joint. Instead, insert a cannula with appropriate obturator into the joint. Use switching sticks to place increasing-sized cannulas

and instruments. Remove in situ or free fragments, and perform surface arthroplasty (microfracture or abrasion) through the open or cannulated instrument portal (Fig. 33-38).

To perform abrasion arthroplasty, insert a power burr or hand burr, and evenly abrade any exposed subchondral bone, removing 1 mm of bone at a time. Check for bleeding by shutting off the inflow fluids. If bleeding is inadequate, remove more subchondral bone. If bleeding is adequate, flush the joint and close routinely.

To perform microfracture, insert an angled micropick (Fig. 33-39). Position the tip of the pick on the subchondral bone, and force the tip into the bone. Have an assistant hit the external end of the micropick lightly with a mallet to form the microfractures. Repeat this technique across the surface of the exposed subchondral bone every few millimeters. Check for bleeding by shutting off the inflow fluids. If bleeding is inadequate, perform more microfractures. If bleeding is adequate, flush the joint and close routinely.

POSTOPERATIVE CARE AND ASSESSMENT

Bandaging is not indicated following elbow arthroscopy. Rest and minimal weight bearing are recommended for up to 8 weeks to allow optimal cartilage healing. Physical rehabilitation may be of significant benefit postoperatively. A sample physical rehabilitation exercise regimen can be found in Table 33-9 on p. 1193. It is particularly important in cases of medial compartment disease with significant cartilage damage. Gradual return to full activity is recommended.

SURGICAL TREATMENT

Affected animals are candidates for surgery when they are persistently lame and have mild degenerative changes. Occasionally, animals with advanced DJD and persistent lameness not amenable to medical therapy may benefit from joint exploration and removal of a loose fragment. However, surgical treatment does not halt the progression of DJD, and continued medical therapy may be required in these patients. There does not appear to be any correlation between the severity of lameness before treatment, severity of radiographic signs, and type of lesion found at surgery. Surgical treatment does not appear to reduce the incidence of lameness compared with medical therapy; DJD progresses with either treatment.

Preoperative Management

Most affected animals are young and require minimal preoperative workup.

Anesthesia

These dogs usually are young and generally healthy, and a variety of anesthetic regimens may be used (see p. 944).

Surgical Anatomy

Landmarks for the surgical incision include the medial epicondyle, epicondyloid crest, and proximal radius. The median nerve and brachial artery and vein course cranially to the medial epicondyle. The ulnar nerve courses caudally to the medial epicondyle over the anconeus muscle. The median nerve and brachial artery and vein are visible in the surgical field and must be identified and protected.

Positioning

The limb is prepared from shoulder to carpus. The dog is positioned in dorsal recumbency with the affected limb suspended for draping. The limb is then released to allow access to the medial surface of the elbow.

SURGICAL TECHNIQUE

Exposure of the medial coronoid process can be obtained with one of several techniques. Tenotomy of the pronator teres muscle and incising the medial collateral ligament offer good exposure but at the expense of the supporting structures. A muscle-splitting technique has been proposed that preserves the joint's supporting tendons and ligaments, but limits exposure. Osteotomy of the medial epicondyle provides the best exposure, but requires implantation of a lag screw or wire to replace the epicondyle and is associated with more postoperative complications than other procedures. Concurrent ulnar osteotomy (see p. 1220) has been proposed as a salvage procedure for treating mature dogs with osteoarthritis and as an adjunct to FCP removal in immature dogs. The procedure allows rotation of the proximal ulna, relieving abnormal contact of the humeroulnar joint. However, it remains to be proven if this technique affords a better outcome than fragment removal alone.

Exposure of the Medial Coronoid Process via Transection of the Pronator Teres Muscle

Make an incision on the medial surface of the joint starting at the medial epicondylar crest and extending distally over the medial epicondyle to the proximal radius. Protect the median nerve and brachial artery. Transect the pronator teres tendon. Make an incision to the humeral condyle through the joint capsule and collateral ligament to expose the joint (Fig. 33-40). Identify the coronoid process and any lesions on the medial humeral condyle. Remove the coronoid fragment.

When removing the coronoid fragment, the line of cleavage of the fragment may not be readily visible and may require prying with an elevator to allow identification. In chronic cases, osteophytes may obscure the line of cleavage and must be removed with a rongeur to allow identification of fragments.

Close the wound by suturing the joint capsule with simple interrupted absorbable sutures. Place several nonabsorbable sutures in the collateral ligament. Reattach the pronator teres tendon with a Bunnell's or locking-loop nonabsorbable suture (see p. 1330). Suture the fascia, subcutaneous tissue, and skin in separate layers.

Exposure of the Medial Coronoid Process via Muscle Splitting

Incise the skin and subcutaneous tissue as described previously. Identify the demarcation between the flexor carpi radialis and superficial digital muscles, and separate and retract them. Expose the joint capsule, and incise it parallel to the muscle-splitting incision to expose the coronoid process (Fig. 33-41). Remove the fragmented coronoid as described above. Suture the joint capsule with interrupted absorbable sutures. Suture the fascia, subcutaneous tissue, and skin in separate layers.

Coronoidectomy

Complete resection of the medial coronoid process has been described for treatment of fragmentation of the coronoid process and associated fissures and osteoarthritis (Puccio et al, 2003).

Perform the pronator teres tenotomy approach described above. Using an osteotome, transect the medial coronoid at its base and remove the entire medial coronoid.

Proximal Ulnar Osteotomy

See p. 1220 for the approach for ulnar osteotomy. Make a transverse osteotomy and do not insert a pin; this allows the proximal ulna to rotate caudomedially, theoretically relieving the joint contact at the medial coronoid ridge.

Distal Ulnar Osteotomy

Perform a 3-cm longitudinal incision over the lateral aspect of the distal third of the ulna, ending at the distal ulnar physis. Dissect between the tendon of the lateral digital extensor muscle and the tendon of the ulnaris lateralis muscle to expose the diaphysis of the ulna. Incise and elevate the periosteum, and isolate the ulna with Hohmann retractors. Remove a 5-mm-length section of the ulna with an osteotome, rongeur, or bone saw. Reappose the periosteum with

Medial View

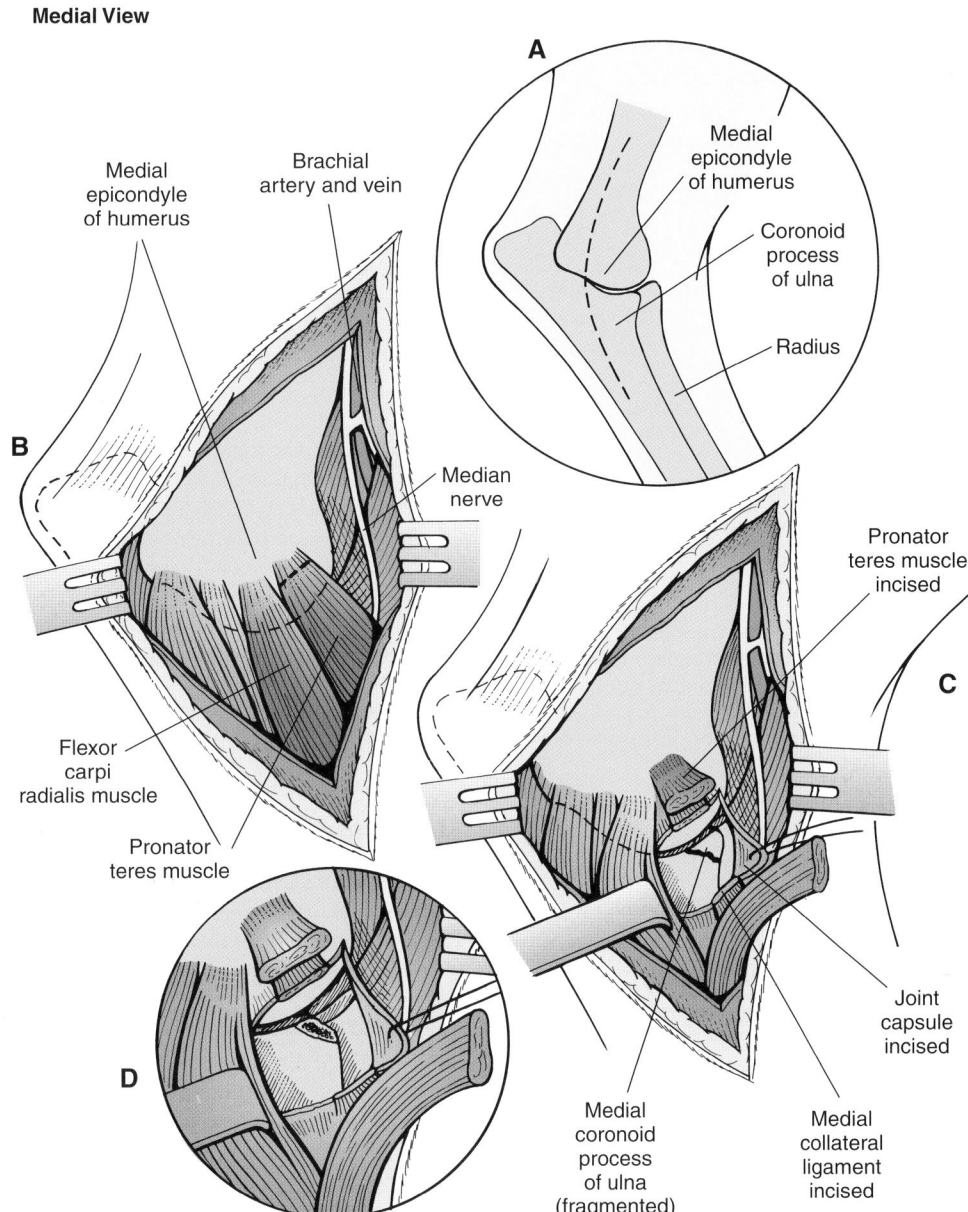

FIG. 33-40
A, To expose the medial aspect of the elbow joint by means of transection of the pronator teres muscle, make a skin incision on the medial surface of the joint, starting at the medial epicondylar crest and extending distally over the medial epicondyle. **B,** Gently retract the median nerve and brachial artery and vein cranially. **C,** Transect the pronator teres tendon and make an incision parallel to the humeral condyle through the joint capsule and collateral ligament to expose the FCP. **D,** Remove the fragment.

3-0 absorbable suture in a simple continuous pattern. Close the deep fascia in a simple continuous pattern with absorbable suture. Apply a caudal spoon splint for 3 to 5 days to aid in patient comfort.

Elevation of the interosseous ligament off of the ulna aids in distal migration of the ulna; however, it may lead to significant hemorrhage.

SUTURE MATERIALS AND SPECIAL INSTRUMENTS

An Oschner forceps is useful for grasping the fragment, and an oscillating bone saw facilitates ulnar ostectomy.

POSTOPERATIVE CARE AND ASSESSMENT

The limb may be bandaged after surgery for up to 1 week to provide soft tissue support, and the animal should be con-

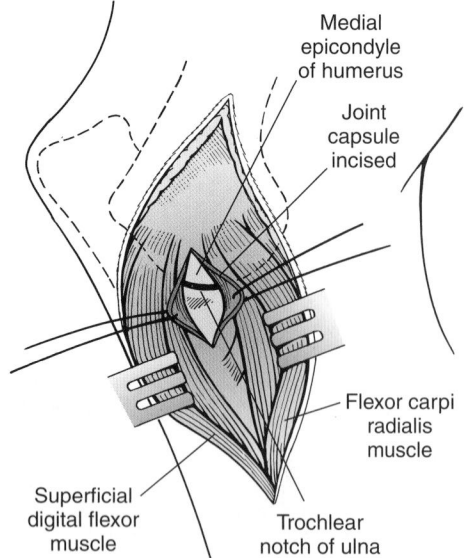

Medial
epicondyle
of humerus

Joint
capsule
incised

Flexor carpi
radialis
muscle

Superficial
digital flexor
muscle

Trochlear
notch of ulna

FIG. 33-41
To expose the medial aspect of the elbow joint using a
muscle-splitting approach, identify the demarcation between
the flexor carpi radialis and the superficial digital muscles
and separate and retract them. Expose the joint capsule and
incise it parallel to the muscle-splitting incision to expose the
coronoid process.

fined for 4 weeks. Physical rehabilitation is beneficial in regaining strength and range of motion, and decreasing overall
lameness. For a sample physical rehabilitation exercise protocol for this condition, refer to Table 33-9.

COMPLICATIONS

Possible surgical complications of fragment removal or coronoidectomy include iatrogenic infection and nerve damage. The risk of infection is likely decreased with arthroscopy. Soft tissue irritation by implants, nonunion, and
infected nonunion are possible complications when an ulnar
osteotomy is performed.

PROGNOSIS

Prognosis for return to full function depends upon the severity of cartilage disease. In cases with fragmentation only
in which the remainder of the joint cartilage appears healthy,
the prognosis after fragment removal is good to excellent.
Minimal osteoarthritis may progress, but in most cases does
not become severe. In cases with significant cartilage damage, the prognosis is guarded because of progressive osteoarthritis, which develops regardless of the treatment method;
however, most dogs function as pets and are only intermittently lame. The use of physical rehabilitation may dramatically improve joint and limb function in cases of elbow
dysplasia (see Box 33-15). Recurrent lameness can be treated
with antiinflammatory drugs and analgesics (see p. 1149).
Benefits of coronoidectomy over fragment removal have not
been determined, although the outcome of coronoidectomy

in one clinical study appears to be favorable (Puccio et al,
2003).

References

Blond L, Dupuis J, Beauregard G et al: Sensitivity and specificity of
radiographic detection of canine elbow incongruence in an in
vitro model, *Vet Radiol Ultrasound*. 46:210, 2005.

Gemmill TJ, Mellor DJ, Clements DN et al: Evaluation of elbow
incongruency using reconstructed CT in dogs suffering fragmented coronoid process, *J Small Anim Pract* 46:327, 2005.

Holsworth IG, Wisner ER, Scherrer WE et al: Accuracy of computerized tomographic evaluation of canine radio-ulnar incongruence in vitro, *Vet Surg* 34:108, 2005.

Mason DR, Schulz KS, Samii VF et al: Sensitivity of radiographic
evaluation of radio-ulnar incongruence in the dog in vitro, *Vet
Surg* 31:125, 2002.

Meyer-Lindenberg A, Langhann A, Fehr M et al: Arthrotomy versus
arthroscopy in the treatment of the fragmented medial coronoid
process of the ulna in 421 dogs, *Vet Comp Orthop Traum* 16:204,
2003.

Morgan JP, Wind A, Davidson AP: Bone dysplasias in the Labrador
retriever: a radiographic study, *J Am Anim Hosp Assoc* 35:332,
1999.

Puccio M, Marino DJ, Stefanacci JD et al: Clinical evaluation and
long-term follow-up of dogs having coronoidectomy for elbow
incongruity, *J Am Anim Hosp Assoc* 39:473, 2003.

Suggested Reading

Beale BS, Hulse DA, Schulz KS et al: *Small animal arthroscopy*,
Philadelphia, 2003, Saunders.
This comprehensive textbook on arthroscopy has detailed information regarding instrumentation and techniques of small animal
arthroscopy. It also contains a thorough discussion of the indications and diseases processes treated.

Morgan JP, Wind A, Davidson AP: *Hereditary bone and joint diseases in the dog*, Hannover, 2000, Schlutersche.
This book provides an excellent overview of hereditary bone diseases, including elbow dysplasia.

Schulz KS, Krotscheck U: Canine elbow dysplasia. In Slatter D, editor:
Textbook of small animal surgery, Philadelphia, 2003, Saunders.
This chapter contains a detailed description of the pathophysiology,
diagnosis, and treatment of elbow dysplasia in addition to a complete literature review.

Theyse LFH, Hazelwinkel HAW, van den Brom WE: Force plate
analyses before and after surgical treatment of unilateral fragmented coronoid process, *Vet Comp Orthop Traum* 13:1-4,
2000.
This study describes objective findings in surgical management of
FCP and suggests that dogs improve significantly after surgical
treatment.

OSTEOCHONDRITIS DISSECANS OF THE DISTAL HUMERUS

DEFINITIONS

Osteochondrosis is a disturbance in endochondral ossification that leads to retention of cartilage; it occurs commonly
in the shoulder, elbow, stifle, and hock of immature large
dogs. OCD occurs when fissure formation in the abnormal

cartilage leads to development of a flap of cartilage. A loose flap of cartilage in the joint is a **joint mouse.**

GENERAL CONSIDERATIONS AND CLINICALLY RELEVANT PATHOPHYSIOLOGY

Osteochondrosis begins with a failure of endochondral ossification in either the physis or the articular epiphyseal complex, which is responsible for formation of metaphyseal bone. Osteochondrosis has been implicated in the pathophysiology of OCD, FCP, and UAP of the elbow. The origin is unknown, but genetic factors, rapid growth, overnutrition, trauma, ischemia, and hormonal factors are possible causes. Failure of endochondral ossification leads to cartilage thickening. Because developing cartilage is nourished initially by synovial fluid and later by vascularization through subchondral bone, increased cartilage thickness may result in malnourished, necrotic chondrocytes. Chondrocyte loss deep in the cartilage layer leads to formation of a cleft at the junction of calcified and noncalcified tissues. Subsequent trauma caused by normal activity can lead to development of vertical fissures in the cartilage; eventually the fissures communicate with the joint, and a cartilage flap is formed. This communication allows cartilage degradation products to reach the synovial fluid, where they may cause joint inflammation. OCD does not cause apparent clinical signs until a loose flap of cartilage develops. This loose body of cartilage does not ossify. DJD (osteoarthritis) of the elbow is the final outcome.

With OCD of the distal humerus, a flap of cartilage covering a defect in the surface of the trochlear ridge of the medial humeral condyle usually is seen. Opposing joint cartilage of the coronoid process may be eroded. Histologic examination of the lesion confirms that the flap consists of cartilage, that subchondral bone trabeculae in the defect are thickened, and that bone marrow fibrosis is present.

DIAGNOSIS
Clinical Presentation

Signalment. Affected dogs usually are large (Labrador retrievers, golden retrievers). The usual age of onset of lameness is 5 to 7 months.

History. Forelimb lameness that worsens after exercise may be acute or chronic. Owners frequently complain that the dog is stiff in the morning or after rest. There may be a coincidental history of trauma.

Physical Examination Findings

Lameness of one forelimb usually is evident. The gait may be stiff or stilted if forelimb steps are shortened because of bilateral lameness. Pain may be elicited on elbow extension and on lateral rotation of the forearm. Palpation of the elbows should include an evaluation of range of motion. A decrease in the animal's ability to flex the elbow is indicative of secondary osteoarthritis. Crepitation during elbow flexion and extension, joint effusion, and periarticular swelling may be noted if osteoarthritis is present. It is important that the shoulder not be inadvertently flexed and extended dur-

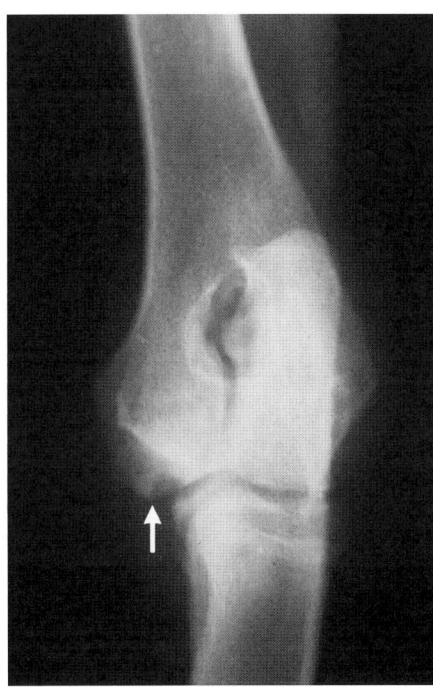

FIG. 33-42
Radiograph of an elbow with OCD of the medial portion of the humeral condyle. There is a radiolucent defect in the humeral condyle *(arrow).*

ing elbow manipulation to avoid confusing shoulder pain and elbow pain.

Diagnostic Imaging

Radiographic views should include a standard lateral view of the elbow, a flexed lateral view to expose the anconeal process, and a craniocaudal view (see Fig. 33-31). Radiographs of both elbows should be made because bilateral disease is common. Oblique views may be necessary to demonstrate the lesion on the humeral condyle. Definitive radiographic diagnosis of OCD is made when a radiolucent concavity is observed on the distal aspect of the medial humeral condyle (Fig. 33-42). This lesion is most often identified on the craniocaudal view. Radiographic signs of secondary osteoarthritis are similar to those seen with the FCP (see p. 1198).

Arthroscopy. Arthroscopy permits confirmation of the diagnosis of elbow OCD and medial compartment disease (Fig. 33-43). Unlike other modalities, arthroscopy enables direct visualization and assessment of the cartilage surface, measurement of the size of the OCD, assessment of the opposing cartilage, and more accurate prognostication.

Laboratory Findings

Results of hematologic and serum biochemical analyses are normal in most affected animals. Results of arthrocentesis may include decreased synovial fluid viscosity, increased

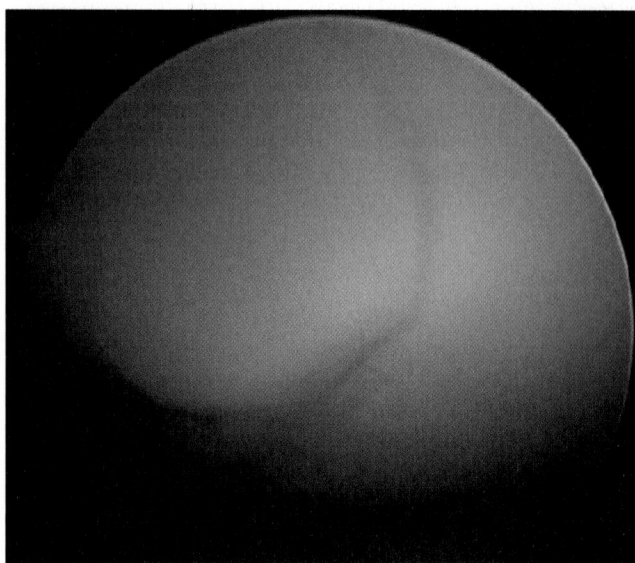

FIG. 33-43
Arthroscopic view of OCD of the elbow.

fluid volume, and increased numbers of mononuclear phagocytic cells (up to 6000 to 9000 WBCs/μl).

DIFFERENTIAL DIAGNOSIS

OCD must be differentiated from FCP, UAP, combined UAP and FCP, and other diseases of young, growing dogs that affect the forelimb (e.g., OCD of the shoulder and panosteitis) and may produce similar clinical signs. These diseases are usually differentiated radiographically. Rarely, OCD and FCP may be identified in the same elbow.

MEDICAL MANAGEMENT

Dogs that have radiographic abnormalities but no symptoms do not require treatment. This is most commonly seen in cases of osteochondrosis that have not progressed to OCD. Dogs with true OCD may be treated conservatively; however, owners should be cautioned that delay in surgical removal of a loose cartilage flap may encourage additional damage to the opposing cartilage. Patients that benefit the most from surgical treatment are those that have only OCD but no significant cartilage damage to the opposing surfaces (kissing lesions). If surgery is going to be performed, it should be done as early in the disease process as possible to minimize the progression of osteoarthritis.

When conservative management is elected, it should include focusing on the five principles of medical management of osteoarthritis, particularly weight management, nutritional supplementation, exercise moderation, and antiinflammatory medication. After lameness has subsided or resolved, exercise should be gradually increased to strengthen the surrounding musculature.

SURGICAL TREATMENT

Surgical removal of the cartilage flap is recommended in young animals when the disease is diagnosed before the onset of osteoarthritis and can also be helpful in treating animals with chronic moderate to severe lameness. Arthroscopic treatment of OCD has numerous advantages over open surgery. Arthroscopy provides superior visualization and magnification of the joint, is less invasive, and provides greater opportunity for topical treatment of osteoarthritic lesions.

Preoperative Management

Most affected animals are young and require minimal preoperative workup (see Chapter 5).

Anesthesia

These animals are usually young and healthy, thus a variety of anesthetic regimens can be used (see p. 944).

Surgical Anatomy

For pertinent anatomy of the elbow joint, see p. 1204.

Positioning for Open Surgery

The limb is prepared from shoulder to elbow. The dog is positioned in dorsal recumbency with the affected limb suspended for draping. The limb is then released to allow access to the medial surface of the elbow.

SURGICAL TECHNIQUE
Arthroscopy

Arthroscopy of the elbow joint is discussed on p. 1201. Moving the arthroscope portal slightly caudally and proximally to the standard positioning permits improved visualization of the OCD lesion.

Insert the needle perpendicular to the joint line approximately 0.75 cm distal and 1 cm caudal to the medial epicondyle. Remove in situ or free cartilage fragments (Fig. 33-44). Using a curette, make the "shoulders" of the lesion right angles to the joint surface. Perform surface arthroplasty through the open or cannulated instrument portal using a hand burr.

Open Surgery

Exposure of the medial portion of the elbow joint can be obtained with several techniques. Tenotomy of the pronator teres muscle and incision of the medial collateral ligament offer good exposure at the expense of the supporting structures (see p. 1204). A muscle-splitting technique preserves the joint's supporting tendons and ligaments, but limits exposure (see p. 1204).

Regardless of the technique used for exposure, examine the medial condyle of the humerus and remove the flap of cartilage. Curette only to remove fragments of cartilage from the edges of the lesion. Repeatedly flush the joint to remove any

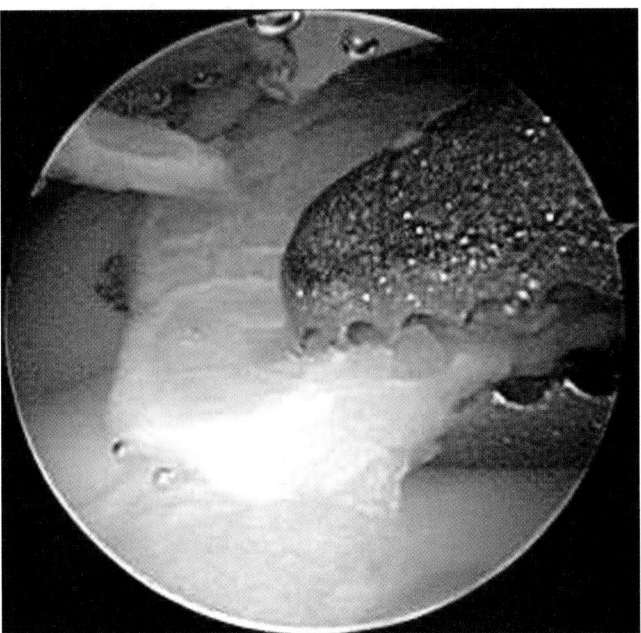

FIG. 33-44
Arthroscopic removal of OCD of the elbow.

*small fragments. Inspect the coronoid process, and remove it
if fragmented (see p. 1204).*

SUTURE MATERIALS AND SPECIAL INSTRUMENTS

An Oschner forceps is useful for grasping the flap, and a
bone curette is needed to curette the defect.

POSTOPERATIVE CARE AND ASSESSMENT

The limb may be bandaged after surgery for up to 1 week to
provide soft tissue support, and the animal should be confined for 4 weeks. Gradual return to normal activity is recommended.

Bandaging is not indicated following elbow arthroscopy.
Rest and minimal weight bearing are recommended for up
to 8 weeks to allow optimum cartilage healing. Physical rehabilitation may be of significant benefit postoperatively.
The primary focus is to retain range of motion and musculature immediately after the surgical intervention (see Table
33-9 on p. 1193; see also Chapter 12). After surgery, cryotherapy, passive range of motion, and controlled leash walks
are the primary methods of physical rehabilitation.

PROGNOSIS

Dogs treated conservatively for OCD of the distal humerus
usually have continued intermittent lameness and progressive osteoarthritis. Dogs treated surgically for OCD of the
distal humerus usually have improved limb function; however, lameness may be evident after exercise. Osteoarthritis
usually is present and requires medical treatment (see previ-

ous discussion), but most dogs are functional pets and are
only intermittently lame. Iatrogenic infection is a possible
surgical complication.

> NOTE: Be sure to warn owners that many affected
> dogs will have progressive osteoarthritis despite
> surgery.

Suggested Reading

Beale BS, Hulse DA, Schulz KS et al: *Small animal arthroscopy,*
Philadelphia, 2003, Saunders.
This comprehensive textbook on arthroscopy has detailed information regarding instrumentation and techniques of small animal
arthroscopy. It also contains a thorough discussion of the indications and disease processes treated.
Schulz KS, Krotscheck U: Canine elbow dysplasia. In Slatter D, editor: *Textbook of small animal surgery,* Philadelphia, 2003,
Saunders.
This chapter contains a detailed description of the pathophysiology, diagnosis, and treatment of elbow dysplasia in addition to a
complete literature review.

UNUNITED ANCONEAL PROCESS

DEFINITION

Ununited anconeal process (UAP) or *elbow dysplasia* is a
disease of large growing dogs in which the anconeal process
does not form a bony union with the proximal ulnar metaphysis.

GENERAL CONSIDERATIONS AND CLINICALLY RELEVANT PATHOPHYSIOLOGY

The anconeal process arises as a secondary center of ossification in the elbow at 11 to 12 weeks of age. It does not fuse to
the ulna until 4 to 5 months of age, therefore the diagnosis
of UAP cannot be made before that age. Several theories
have been proposed for the etiology of UAP. One is that
the UAP may be a manifestation of osteochondrosis in
which failure of timely endochondral ossification of the attachment of the anconeal process to the ulna leads to thickened cartilage, necrosis, and fissures. The stress of weight
bearing on this abnormal cartilage then causes failure of ulnar unification. Other possible etiologic factors include he-
redity, hormonal influences, nutrition, and acute or chronic
trauma.

More recently, developmental joint incongruity has
been theorized to cause increased pressure or trauma to
the anconeal process. Trochlear notch malformation and
disparate radius and ulnar lengths (i.e., a longer radius in
relationship to the ulna) have both been incriminated in
the development of UAP. Pressure of the trochlear notch
against the humeral condyles may cause a shearing stress
on the anconeal process, resulting in a fracture, or simply
may provide enough stress to prevent fusion. The UAP

may be free within the joint, but in most cases it is attached to the ulna with fibrous tissue. Ununited or fractured anconeal processes are unstable and result in secondary DJD. Pathologic changes include joint effusion, chondromalacia, periarticular fibrosis, and osteophyte formation.

DIAGNOSIS
Clinical Presentation

Signalment. Large- to giant-breed male dogs are most commonly affected. German shepherd dogs are overrepresented. The usual age of presentation is 6 to 12 months. Some older animals may be seen for lameness caused by secondary osteoarthritis.

History. The history generally is one of intermittent lameness of one or both forelimbs that worsens after exercise. Owners frequently complain that the dog is stiff in the morning or after rest.

Physical Examination Findings

Lameness of one forelimb usually is evident. The gait may be stiff or stilted because elbow range of motion is decreased. This causes the elbow to circumduct laterally during the swing phase of the gait. The dog may sit and stand with the paw externally rotated. If osteoarthritis is present, there may be crepitation during elbow flexion and extension. Joint effusion and periarticular soft tissue swelling may be palpable. The animal may experience pain during joint manipulation, particularly during palpation over the anconeal process. It is important that the shoulder not be inadvertently flexed and extended during elbow manipulation to avoid mistaking shoulder pain for elbow pain.

Diagnostic Imaging

Radiographic views include a standard lateral view of the elbow, a flexed lateral view to expose the anconeal process, and a craniocaudal view of the elbow made while the elbow is flexed 30 degrees and slightly rotated medially (see Fig. 33-31). Radiographs of both elbows should be made because bilateral disease occurs in 20% to 35% of cases. UAP is visible as a lucent, indistinct line separating the anconeal process from the ulna. It is best visualized on the flexed lateral view (Fig. 33-45). Concurrent FCP can occur. Signs of osteoarthritis may include subchondral bone sclerosis, articular and periarticular osteophyte formation, joint space narrowing, joint effusion, and an increase in periarticular soft tissue.

> NOTE: Be sure the animal is old enough for physeal closure before diagnosing UAP.

Laboratory Findings

The results of hematologic and serum biochemical analyses are normal in most affected animals. The results of arthrocentesis may include decreased synovial fluid viscosity, increased fluid volume, and increased numbers of mononuclear phagocytic cells (up to 6000 to 9000 WBC/μl).

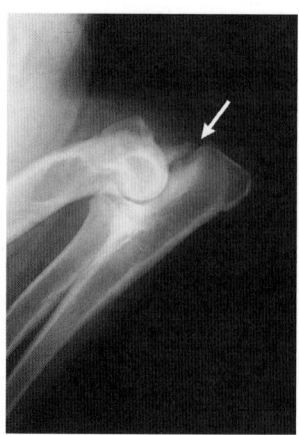

FIG. 33-45
A flexed lateral radiograph of an elbow with an ununited anconeal process. There is a lucent, irregular line between the anconeal process and the olecranon *(arrow)*, with subchondral bone sclerosis of the olecranon.

DIFFERENTIAL DIAGNOSIS

Differential diagnoses include OCD, FCP, combined UAP and FCP, and other diseases of young, growing dogs that affect the forelimb (i.e., OCD of the shoulder and panosteitis). These diseases can usually be differentiated radiographically.

MEDICAL MANAGEMENT

Dogs less than 5 or 6 months old when seen for possible UAP may be treated with confinement and limited exercise. Follow-up radiographs should be made monthly to document either fusion of the anconeal process or UAP. Medical therapy generally is used to treat older dogs with established osteoarthritis. Surgical removal of the anconeal process after extensive development of osteoarthritis does not stop the progression of osteoarthritis.

When conservative management is elected, it should include focusing on four of the five principles of medical management of osteoarthritis: specifically, weight management, nutritional supplementation, exercise moderation, and antiinflammatory medication. After lameness has subsided or resolved, exercise should be gradually increased to strengthen surrounding musculature.

SURGICAL TREATMENT

Surgical removal of the anconeal process has been the standard treatment if UAP is diagnosed before the onset of extensive osteoarthritis, despite concerns regarding loss of normal joint congruity. Surgical reduction and lag screw fixation of the anconeal process have been reported sporadically over the past 30 years, but the outcome is not uniformly successful and implant failure can occur. Ulnar osteotomy has been recommended to relieve pressure on the anconeal process, allowing spontaneous healing of the fragment to the ulna in immature dogs. This procedure initially was proposed for treatment of chondrodystrophic dogs, but more recently has been applied to other dogs with UAP. Ulnar osteotomy may be used concurrently with lag screw fixation of the anconeal process (Meyer-Lindenberg et al, 2001). The success of achieving union with ulnar osteotomy or osteotomy with lag screw fixation is highly dependent upon age. One study reported excellent results with combined lag screw and osteotomy in nearly 85% of cases (Meyer-Lindenberg et al, 2001). These procedures should only be recommended in dogs under 1 year of age with minimal degenerative changes in the joint and at the site of nonunion.

Preoperative Management

Most affected animals are young and require minimal preoperative workup.

Anesthesia

These animals are usually young and a variety of anesthetic regimens can be used (see p. 944).

Surgical Anatomy

Landmarks for the skin incision when performing a lateral approach for removal of a UAP include the lateral humeral epicondyle, epicondylar crest, and proximal radius. The deep branch of the radial nerve runs under the proximal cranial border of the extensor carpi radialis muscle. The superficial branch of the radial nerve lies between the lateral head of the triceps and the brachialis muscle and can be visualized in the proximal portion of the incision. Landmarks for the combined medial approach are the medial epicondyle, epicondylar crest, and proximal radius. The median nerve and brachial artery and vein course cranial to the medial epicondyle and run under the pronator teres muscle. These structures must be identified and protected. The ulnar nerve courses caudal to the medial epicondyle, over the anconeus muscle, and is visualized during the medial approach to the anconeal process. The landmark for ulnar osteotomy is the caudal border of the ulna, which is easily palpated.

Positioning

For a lateral approach to the elbow, the animal is positioned in lateral recumbency, whereas for a medial approach and for ulnar osteotomy, the animal is positioned in dorsal recumbency. The limb should be suspended for draping to facilitate limb manipulation during surgery.

SURGICAL TECHNIQUE
Removal of the Anconeal Process: Lateral Approach

Make an incision in the skin, starting proximal to the lateral humeral epicondyle. Curve the incision to follow the epicondylar crest, and end it over the proximal portion of the radius. Incise the subcutaneous tissue to expose the cranial border of the lateral head of the triceps muscle. Retract the cranial border of the triceps muscle caudally to expose the anconeus muscle. Incise the anconeus muscle and joint capsule along the epicondylar crest, and retract them caudally to expose the

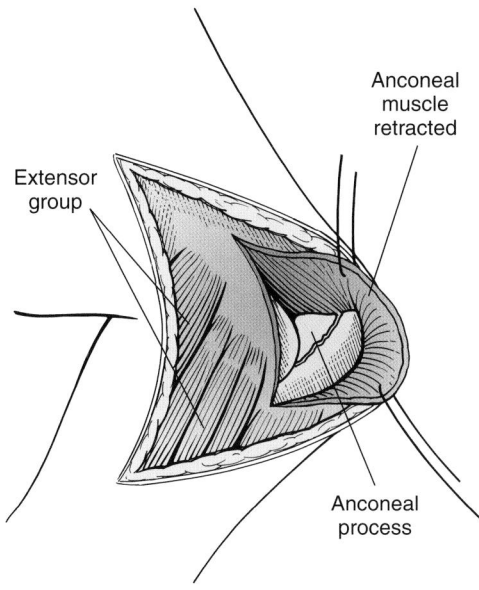

FIG. 33-46
For a lateral approach to the caudal compartment on the elbow, make a skin incision starting proximal to the lateral humeral epicondyle and curving to follow the epicondylar crest. End the incision over the proximal portion of the radius. Incise the anconeus muscle and joint capsule along the epicondylar crest and retract them caudally to expose the anconeal process.

anconeal process (Fig. 33-46). Grasp the process with towel forceps or an Oschner forceps and remove it.

Fibrous tissue attachments to the ulna may have to be incised before the anconeal process can be mobilized.

If necessary, smooth the remaining bone surface with a file. Flush the joint. Suture the joint capsule and anconeus muscle to the extensor carpi radialis muscle. Suture the subcutaneous tissue and skin in separate layers.

Removal of the Anconeal Process and Medial Coronoid Process: Combined Medial Approach

Expose the medial coronoid process using one of the techniques described on p. 1204. After closing the craniomedial compartment of the elbow, approach the caudomedial compartment by retracting the ulnar nerve cranially and exposing the cranial border of the medial head of the triceps muscle. Retract the triceps muscle caudally to expose the caudal border of the medial epicondylar crest and origin of the anconeus muscle. Incise the anconeus muscle and joint capsule parallel to the medial epicondylar crest, leaving 2 to 4 mm of tissue attached to the crest for closure (Fig. 33-47). Remove the anconeal process. Suture the anconeus muscle and joint capsule in one layer to close the joint.

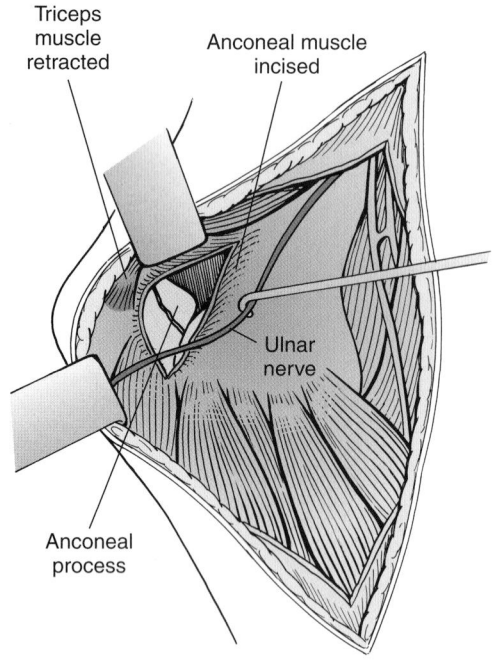

Triceps muscle retracted

Anconeal muscle incised

Ulnar nerve

Anconeal process

FIG. 33-47
For a medial approach to the caudal compartment of the elbow, retract the ulnar nerve cranially and the triceps muscle caudally to expose the caudal border of the medial epicondylar crest and the origin of the anconeus muscle. Incise the anconeus muscle and joint capsule parallel to the medial epicondylar crest to expose the anconeal process.

Ulnar Osteotomy

Make a skin incision along the caudal border of the ulna, beginning medial to the tuber olecranon and ending at the middiaphysis of the ulna. Incise the subcutaneous tissue and fascia along the same line. Incise the attachments of the flexor carpi ulnaris and ulnaris lateralis muscles along the medial and lateral borders of the ulna, and elevate the muscles to expose the joint capsule. Make an osteotomy of the ulna 20 to 30 mm distal to the trochlear notch with an oscillating saw or Gigli wire.

The osteotomy is performed in a caudoproximal to craniodistal direction. A gap should occur at the osteotomy site.

If necessary, elevate the interosseous ligament to free the proximal ulna so that it can move into position. Remove a 2- to 4-mm section of the ulna if there is concern that the osteotomy will heal before the dog has stopped growing. Suture the flexor carpi ulnaris fascia to the ulnaris lateralis fascia over the caudal border of the ulna. Suture the subcutaneous tissue and skin separately.

Lag Screw Fixation of the Ununited Anconeal Process

This technique may be performed open or closed with arthroscopic guidance. Screw placement is critical, as there is only limited bone stock available in the ununited portion and inadvertent placement of the screw in the joint will lead to hemarthrosis and crippling osteoarthritis. Results with this technique are best when combined with a proximal ulnar ostectomy.

To perform the procedure open, begin with a medial or lateral approach to the olecranon (see previous discussion). Roll the skin incision caudally to expose the proximodistal aspect of the ulna. Drive a small Kirschner wire beginning at the caudal aspect of the ulna perpendicular to the nonunion line and into the ununited portion. Drill a 3.5-mm hole parallel to the Kirschner wire, from the caudal aspect of the ulna towards the tip of the anconeus, stopping when the drill reaches the nonunion site. Place a centralizing drill guide in the hole, and drill through to the tip of the anconeus with a 2.5-mm drill bit. Measure the depth of the hole and place a 3.5-mm screw several millimeters shorter in the hole and observe for compression of the nonunion site.

It is important to use a screw several millimeters shorter than the measured length to prevent exposure of the tip of the screw as the nonunion site compresses (Fig. 33-48).

Close the joint routinely and perform a proximal ulnar osteotomy.
To perform lag screw fixation with arthroscopic guidance, begin with standard arthroscopy portals and visualize the nonunion site. Make a small incision on the caudal aspect of the proximal ulna at the level of the anconeus. Place a lag screw as described above.

SUTURE MATERIALS AND SPECIAL INSTRUMENTS

An Oschner forceps is useful for extracting the UAP. Rongeurs and bone files are used to smooth the area. A Gigli wire or oscillating saw is needed for ulnar osteotomy. Bone screws and a power drill are required for lag screw fixation.

POSTOPERATIVE CARE AND ASSESSMENT

Immediate postoperative radiographs should be made if implants are used. The limb may be bandaged after surgery for up to 1 week to provide soft tissue support, and the animal should be confined for 4 weeks. Repeat radiographs are recommended 6 weeks after surgery if an osteotomy or lag screw fixation was performed. Physical rehabilitation may be beneficial in management of osteoarthritis and in improving the range of motion associated with UAP (see Table 33-9). After surgery, cryotherapy, passive range of motion, and controlled leash walks are the primary methods of physical rehabilitation.

COMPLICATIONS

Possible surgical complications include iatrogenic infection, nonunion of the ulnar osteotomy, nonunion of the anconeal process, and implant complications.

PROGNOSIS

Prognosis for dogs with UAP is guarded for normal limb function because secondary osteoarthritis will occur. The prognosis for limb function is good in most dogs less than 1

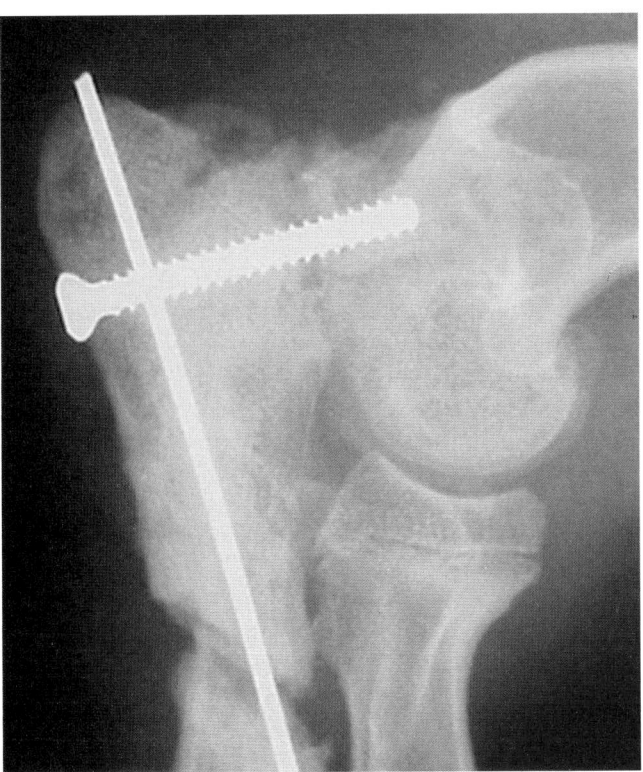

FIG. 33-48
Postoperative radiograph of lag screw fixation of a UAP.

year old when treated surgically by removal of the anconeal process. However, despite treatment, loss of range of motion, crepitation, and progressive osteoarthritis occurs. Ulnar osteotomy may be more successful in young dogs than in older dogs.

NOTE: Counsel owners about the probability of progressive osteoarthritis in these dogs even after surgery.

Reference

Meyer-Lindenberg, Fehr M, Nolte I: Short and long-term results after surgical treatment of an ununited anconeal process in the dog, *Vet Comp Orthop Traum* 14:101, 2001.

Suggested Reading

Krotscheck U, Hulse DA, Bahr A: Ununited anconeal process: lag screw fixation with proximal ulnar osteotomy, *Vet Comp Orthop Traum* 13:212, 2000.
This article provides a detailed description of the technique of lag screw fixation and ulnar osteotomy for the management of UAP and a case series review.
Schulz KS, Krotscheck U: Canine elbow dysplasia. In Slatter D, editor: *Textbook of small animal surgery*, Philadelphia, 2003, Saunders.
This chapter contains a detailed description of the pathophysiology, diagnosis, and treatment of elbow dysplasia in addition to a complete literature review.

 BOX 33-16

Important Considerations in Traumatic Elbow Luxation

- Closed reduction of the elbow should be attempted as soon as possible.
- The stability of the elbow should be carefully evaluated after reduction.
- The elbow's response to trauma is DJD and diminished range of motion.
- The prognosis is good if the elbow is quickly reduced and stabilized.

TRAUMATIC ELBOW LUXATION

DEFINITION

Traumatic elbow luxation (or *dislocated elbow*) usually is associated with blunt trauma of the elbow joint, causing lateral displacement of the radius and ulna with respect to the humerus.

GENERAL CONSIDERATIONS AND CLINICALLY RELEVANT PATHOPHYSIOLOGY

Elbow trauma that results in rupture or avulsion of one or both collateral ligaments allows luxation of the radius and ulna (Box 33-16). The radius and ulna usually luxate laterally because the large medial condyle of the humerus generally prevents medial luxation. The bone to which the collateral ligaments attach may be avulsed, or rupture of the ligaments may occur. In severe injuries, origins of the extensor or flexor muscles may be ruptured or avulsed from the humeral condyle as well. Cartilage damage may occur at the time of injury. Chronic luxation results in chondromalacia, articular cartilage destruction, and secondary DJD.

DIAGNOSIS
Clinical Presentation

Signalment. Any age or breed of dog may be affected, although traumatic elbow luxation is rare in cats. Immature animals tend to have physeal fractures rather than joint luxation.

History. The history usually includes trauma, such as a vehicular or dog fight encounter. The animal usually is acutely lame on the affected limb.

Physical Examination Findings

Affected dogs are unable to bear weight on the affected limb, and the elbow is carried in a flexed position. The forelimb is abducted and externally rotated. Palpation of the elbow reveals a prominent radial head, indistinct lateral humeral condyle, and lateral displacement of the olecranon. Most animals are in pain and resist elbow extension.

Diagnostic Imaging

Lateral displacement of the radius and ulna is apparent on a craniocaudal view of the elbow (Fig. 33-49). The lateral view shows an uneven joint space between the humeral condyle

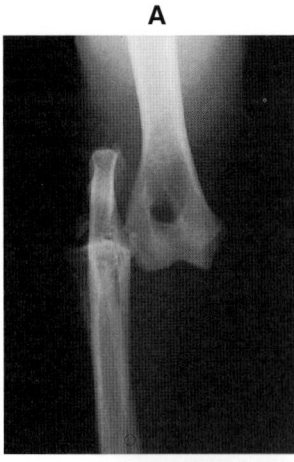
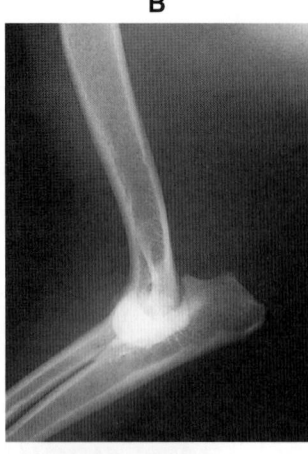
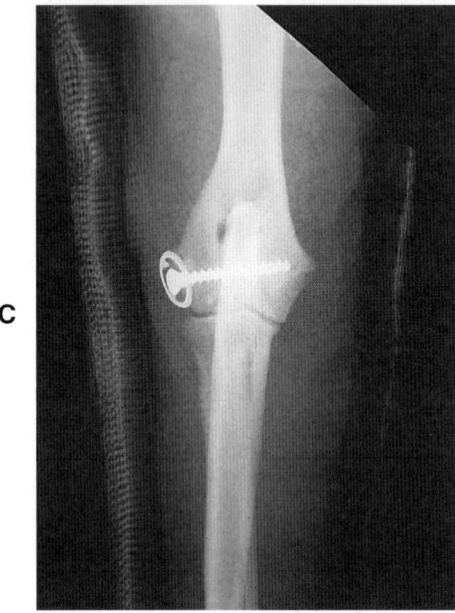

FIG. 33-49
Craniocaudal **(A)** and lateral **(B)** radiographs of a luxated elbow in a dog. The radius and ulna are luxated laterally. On the lateral view, there is loss of the humeroradial joint space. **C,** Open reduction and stabilization of the collateral ligament with a screw and Teflon washer were performed.

and the radius and ulna. Avulsion fractures of the medial or lateral condyle of the humerus may be evident. Because of the traumatic cause, thoracic radiographs before surgery are indicated.

Laboratory Findings

Significant laboratory abnormalities are not associated with elbow luxation, but may be associated with the trauma that caused the injury.

DIFFERENTIAL DIAGNOSIS

Traumatic elbow luxations must be differentiated from articular fractures and Monteggia fractures.

MEDICAL MANAGEMENT

Most luxated elbows can be reduced by closed manipulation if treated within the first few days after injury. However, dogs with avulsion fractures may be candidates for open reduction and stabilization of the fractured bone to provide greater immediate stability. Closed reduction may be facilitated by suspending the limb from an IV drip stand for 5 to 10 minutes and using the dog's body weight to distract the joint and encourage muscle relaxation; the dog is then placed in lateral recumbency with the affected limb up. The objective during manual reduction is to hook the anconeal process between the condyles.

To reduce the elbow, determine the position of the anconeal process in relation to the humeral condyles (Fig. 33-50, A). Flex the elbow to about 100 degrees and inwardly rotate the antebrachium (Fig. 33-50, B). After the anconeal process hooks over the lateral condyle, extend the elbow slightly. Abduct and inwardly rotate the antebrachium while placing medial pressure over the head of the radius to force it under the humeral capitulum and into the reduced position (Fig. 33-50, C). After the elbow has been reduced, evaluate stability provided by the collateral ligaments by flexing the elbow and paw to 90 degrees and rotating the paw medially and laterally.

If the lateral collateral ligament is intact, the paw can be rotated medially to about 70 degrees (140 degrees if it is ruptured). If the medial collateral ligament is intact, the paw can be rotated laterally to 45 degrees; rupture allows the paw to be rotated laterally to about 90 degrees.

After the elbow has been reduced, radiographs should be performed to document the location of the radius and ulna and to evaluate joint stability. Mild subluxation, or widening of the joint space, usually responds to immobilization. Notable subluxation is an indication for open reduction and internal stabilization. If reduction is achieved, the limb should be positioned with the elbow in extension and supported with a soft, padded bandage and spica splint or a cast that prevents elbow flexion for 2 weeks (see p. 948). After removal of the bandage, range of motion exercises should be performed daily. Exercise should be limited for 3 to 4 weeks after bandage removal. Complications of closed reduction may include reluxation and osteoarthritis.

SURGICAL TREATMENT

Open reduction of a luxated elbow is indicated when it is impossible to achieve closed reduction. This is most common when the luxation is chronic. Open reduction should also be considered when the elbow is unstable after closed reduction or when stabilization of an avulsion fracture will improve joint stability. Elbow arthrodesis should be considered with severe damage to the cartilage from the trauma of luxation. It is also performed when fixation of articular fractures of the elbow is unsuccessful and with chronic osteoarthritis that is unresponsive to medical management. Elbow

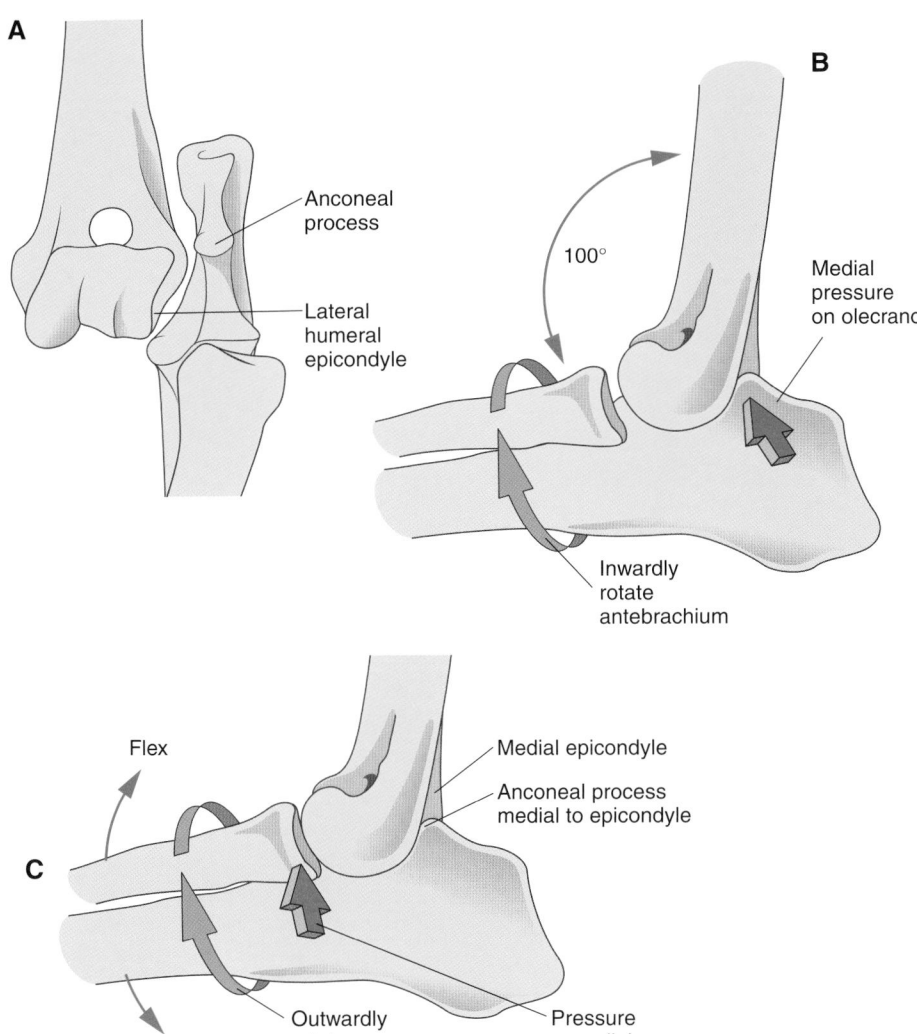

A

Anconeal process

Lateral humeral epicondyle

B

100°

Medial pressure on olecranon

Inwardly rotate antebrachium

C

Flex

Medial epicondyle

Anconeal process medial to epicondyle

Outwardly rotate antebrachium

Pressure on radial head

Extend

FIG. 33-50
A, For closed reduction of a laterally luxated elbow **(B)**, flex the elbow and inwardly rotate the antebrachium to hook the anconeal process into the olecranon fossa. **C,** Then extend the elbow slightly and abduct and outwardly rotate the antebrachium while placing pressure on the radial head.

arthrodesis limits the dog's function because a normal range of motion in this joint is essential for a normal gait. It is a salvage procedure that is done as a last resort and as an alternative to amputation.

> NOTE: Excessive instability of the joint indicates the need for open stabilization of surrounding joint tissue. If the joint is stable despite collateral ligament damage, immobilization will allow periarticular fibrosis and some degree of stability; however, this may not provide sufficient stability for large, active dogs.

Preoperative Management

The extent of the preoperative workup depends on the animal's overall health. Laboratory evaluation, thoracic radiographs, and an electrocardiogram evaluation may be indicated before traumatized animals are anesthetized. Stabili-

zation of the trauma patient's condition is more important than reduction of the elbow. However, as soon as the patient's condition has been stabilized, reduction should be attempted.

Anesthesia

General anesthesia is necessary for closed reduction to achieve the profound muscle relaxation necessary for manipulating the elbow into position. Neuromuscular blockage may be helpful in recent fractures or luxations. Special care should be exercised in anesthetizing older animals or those with concurrent injuries.

Surgical Anatomy

Anatomic landmarks for open reduction of an elbow luxation are the radial head, olecranon and anconeal processes, and lateral humeral condyle. The deep branch of the radial nerve runs under the proximal cranial border of the extensor carpi radialis muscle. The superficial branch of the radial

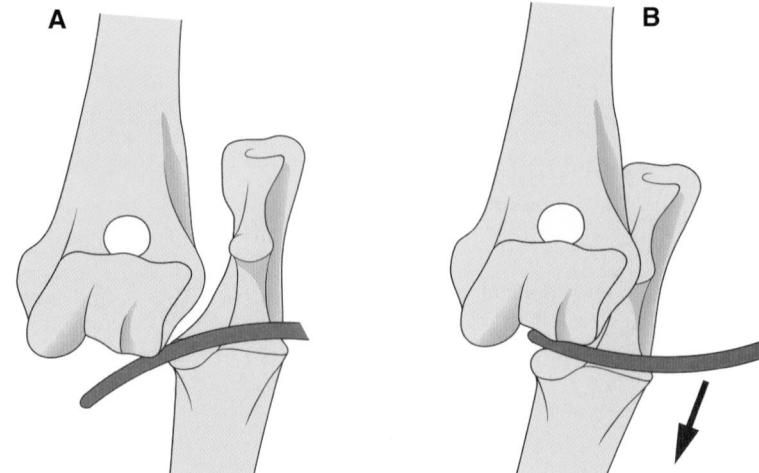

FIG. 33-51
A and **B,** Open reduction of the elbow may be accomplished using a blunt, curved instrument as a lever. **C** and **D,** As an alternative, perform an olecranon osteotomy to eliminate the pull of the triceps muscle during reduction.

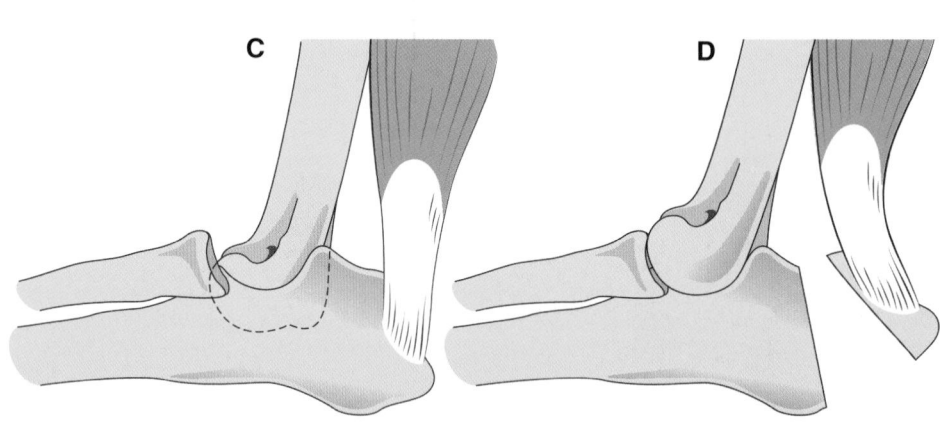

nerve lies between the lateral head of the triceps and the brachialis muscle and may be exposed in the cranial portion of the incision; it must be identified and protected during surgery. The median nerve and brachial artery and vein course cranially to the medial epicondyle, and the ulnar nerve courses caudally to the medial epicondyle, over the anconeus muscle. These structures must be visualized and protected if a medial approach is made to repair the medial collateral ligament.

Positioning

The dog is positioned in lateral recumbency with the affected leg up. The leg should be prepared from shoulder to carpus.

SURGICAL TECHNIQUE
Open Reduction of an Elbow Luxation

Perform a lateral approach to the caudal compartment of the elbow (see p. 1211). Reduce the elbow as described previously for closed reduction. Protect the articular cartilage during reduction. If muscle contraction and subsequent overriding are severe, use a blunt instrument to gently lever the radial head into position (Fig. 33-51, A and B). If reduction is not achieved, perform an olecranon osteotomy to eliminate the pull of the triceps muscle (Fig. 33-51, C and D). After reduction, flush the joint and assess its stability.

Stability may be enhanced by primary repair of the lateral collateral ligament.

Identify the ends of the ligaments, and appose them with nonabsorbable sutures in a locking-loop or Bunnell pattern (see p. 1320). If the ligament has torn from its attachment to the bone, secure it to the bone with a screw and spiked Teflon washer (see Fig. 33-49) or use a suture anchor. If the collateral ligament is beyond repair, replace it with two screws and a figure-eight wire or heavy (No. 1 or No. 2) nonabsorbable suture (Fig. 33-52, A and B). Reduce avulsion fractures of the humeral condyle, and secure them with a lag screw (Fig. 33-52, C and D). Suture torn muscles. Reattach the olecranon (if osteotomized) with a tension band wire (see p. 990). Suture the fascia, subcutaneous tissue, and skin in separate layers. If additional stability is neces-

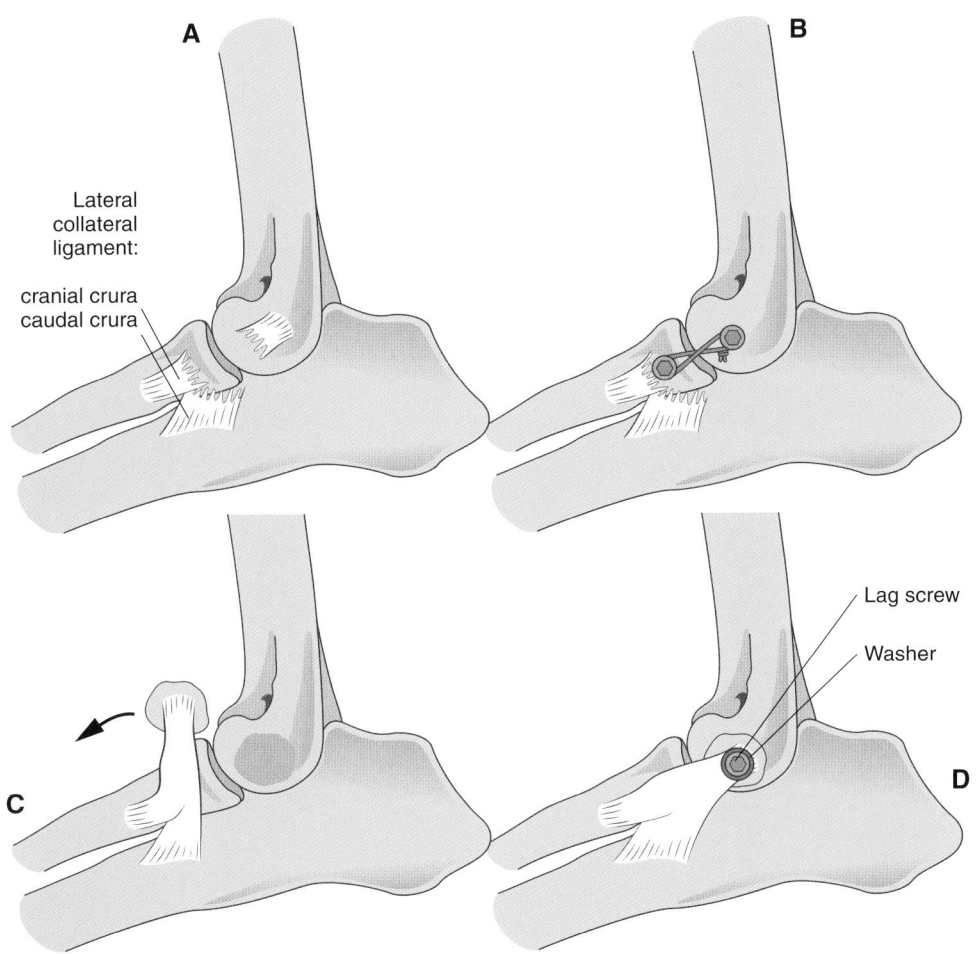

FIG. 33-52
A and **B,** To stabilize the elbow, replace collateral ligaments by using two screws and a figure-eight wire.
C and **D,** To secure an avulsed fragment, use a lag screw with a spiked Teflon washer.

Lateral collateral ligament:
cranial crura
caudal crura

Lag screw
Washer

sary, expose the medial surface of the elbow (see p. 1204) and repair or replace the medial collateral ligament.

Elbow Arthrodesis

Predetermine the angle of arthrodesis by measuring the standing angle of the opposite elbow. Make a caudolateral approach to the joint (see p. 1211), and osteotomize the olecranon (Fig. 33-53, A). Expose the joint by incising the lateral collateral ligament and elevating the origins of the extensor muscles. Remove the cartilage from the distal humerus, radial head, and trochlear notch with a high-speed burr. Follow the contours of the joint. Temporarily stabilize the elbow in the correct position with a pin placed through the humerus and into the ulna. Contour a plate to fit onto the caudal surface of the humerus, over the joint, and onto the caudal surface of the ulna. Place at least three screws in the humerus and three in the ulna. Use additional screws as lag screws to gain compression where they cross the arthrodesis site (Fig. 33-53, B). Check limb alignment, rotation, and angulation before securing fixation. Harvest and place a cancellous bone graft at the arthrodesis site. The most accessible site for cancellous bone harvest is the ipsilateral proximal

humerus (see p. 962). Reattach the olecranon to the ulna on either side of the plate with a lag screw (see p. 944).

> NOTE: Be sure to remove articular cartilage and rigidly stabilize the joint, or arthrodesis will not occur.

SUTURE MATERIALS AND SPECIAL INSTRUMENTS

Instruments needed for open reduction of the elbow include an osteotome and mallet, pin chuck, suture anchors, Kirschner wires, orthopedic wire, and bone screws, and instrumentation for their insertion. For arthrodesis, a high-speed drill, burrs, and plating equipment are necessary.

POSTOPERATIVE CARE AND ASSESSMENT

After open reduction, postoperative radiographs should be made to document the location of the radius and ulna and to evaluate the implant's position. After surgery, the limb should be positioned with the elbow in extension and supported with a soft, padded bandage for several days. If questionable stability was achieved, a spica splint can be applied

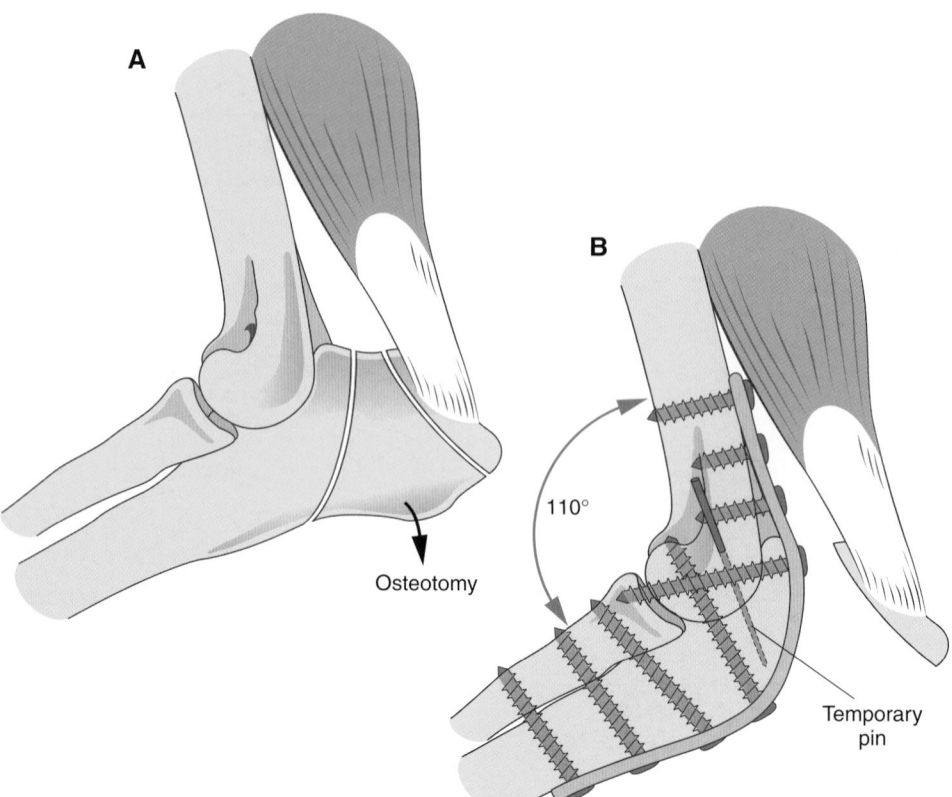

FIG. 33-53
Arthrodesis of the elbow.
A, Make two osteotomies and remove a portion of the proximal ulna. Temporarily stabilize the elbow in the correct position with a pin placed through the ulna and into the humerus.
B, Contour a plate to fit onto the caudal surface of the humerus and the caudal surface of the ulna. Place at least three screws in the humerus and three in the ulna. Use additional screws as lag screws to gain compression across the arthrodesis site.

to the limb for 2 weeks. After removal of the bandage, passive range of motion should be performed daily, but exercise should be limited for 3 to 4 weeks.

After arthrodesis, radiographs of the elbow should be taken to evaluate the implant's position and limb alignment. A soft, padded bandage should be applied for a few days after surgery. If there is concern about stability of the implants, a spica splint can be applied for 6 weeks or until radiographic evidence of bone healing is seen. Activity should be limited until the arthrodesis has healed.

COMPLICATIONS

Complications of arthrodesis include iatrogenic infection, delayed union or nonunion, implant migration, implant irritation of soft tissue, fracture of the bone at either end of the plate, and increased degenerative changes in the limb's distal joints, which are forced to compensate for the loss of elbow range of motion. Possible surgical complications include recurrent luxation, infection, decreased range of motion of the elbow, irritation or migration of implants, and secondary osteoarthritis.

PROGNOSIS

The prognosis is good for normal limb function after a stable closed reduction; however, variable development of osteoarthritis and limited range of motion will occur. The prognosis is fair for normal limb function after an unstable closed reduction. Smaller, less active dogs have a better prognosis because the periarticular fibrosis that occurs is likely to be adequate to maintain the elbow in position, whereas it may

not be adequate in large or active dogs. Osteoarthritis and limited range of motion are also more likely to occur in larger dogs. The prognosis after surgical reduction and stabilization of the elbow depends on chronicity of the luxation and severity of joint damage. Most dogs have good limb function after surgery. Smaller, less active dogs have a better prognosis than larger, more active dogs. Varying degrees of osteoarthritis and limited range of joint motion commonly develop after surgery.

The prognosis following arthrodesis depends upon the size and activity level of the dog. Smaller dogs have fewer complications and less noticeable gait abnormalities. Larger dogs have a higher rate of complications, including delayed union or nonunion and implant failure. The gait abnormalities tend to be more apparent in larger dogs. Active dogs will tend to use the limb at a walk and while standing, but may hold the limb to the side when running. Elbow arthrodesis in very active dogs may be a source of exercise restriction when compared with amputation.

ELBOW LUXATION OR SUBLUXATION CAUSED BY PREMATURE CLOSURE OF THE DISTAL ULNAR OR RADIAL PHYSES

DEFINITIONS

Elbow luxation or **subluxation** may be associated with asynchronous radial or ulnar growth caused by premature closure of one of the distal physes. An **osteotomy** is a cut made through bone. An **ostectomy** is removal of a section of bone.

BOX 33-17

Important Considerations in Elbow Incongruity

- Elbow incongruity is the most likely cause of elbow pain and lameness in dogs with asynchronous radial and ulnar growth.
- Elbow incongruity may contribute to FCP and a UAP.
- Elbow incongruity leads to secondary DJD.

GENERAL CONSIDERATIONS AND CLINICALLY RELEVANT PATHOPHYSIOLOGY

Two syndromes are grouped under elbow subluxation or incongruity. One syndrome is observed as a part of the pathophysiology of premature closure of the distal ulnar or radial physes after trauma in immature dogs (see p. 1073). The other occurs in chondrodystrophic breeds and is caused by asynchronous growth of the radius and ulna with no overt injury to the growth plate (Box 33-17). This asynchronous growth results in incongruity of the elbow joint because either the radius or ulna is inappropriately short. Untreated, elbow incongruity causes instability of the joint and development of secondary DJD.

When the ulna is too short, the trochlear notch is pulled distally and the anconeal process impinges on the humeral trochlea. In some dogs, this may be associated with a UAP (see Fig. 33-45). It is often associated with angular limb deformity (see p. 1076), including radius curvus, valgus, and external rotation. When the radius is too short, the radial head is pulled distally and does not articulate with the humeral capitulum (Fig. 33-54). The trochlea of the humerus then rests directly on the coronoid process of the ulna. This incongruity has been implicated in the etiology of FCP. Shortening of the radius usually is not associated with angular limb deformity.

Clinical Presentation

Signalment. This condition occurs in immature dogs with open physes. Any breed of dog affected with premature closure of the physes after trauma may have subluxation of the elbow. Basset hounds and other chondrodystrophic dogs are more frequently affected with asynchronous growth of the radius and ulna that is not attributable to trauma. The animal may be presented for examination at the onset of the problem or as an older animal with established secondary osteoarthritis.

History. Affected animals often have a history of intermittent lameness.

Physical Examination Findings

Affected dogs show varying degrees of lameness. A gross deformity of the limb may be present, depending on the physeal plate affected and the relationship of the injury to

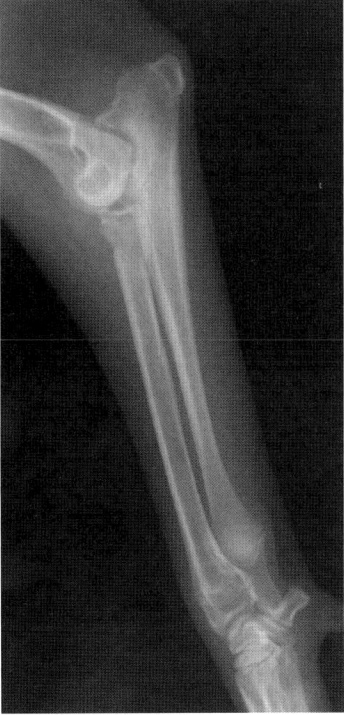
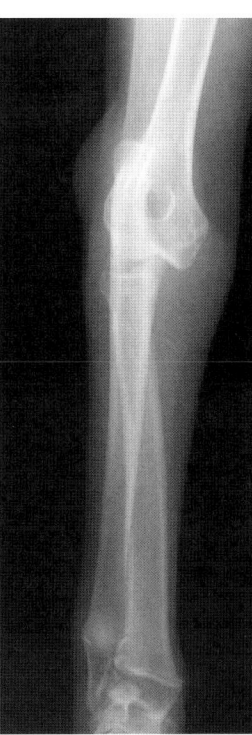

FIG. 33-54
Radiograph of elbow incongruence due to radial shortening.

the animal's growth. Even if there is no limb deformity, the animal usually is lame and sensitive to joint manipulation because of the elbow incongruence. Crepitation and limited range of motion may be present during elbow manipulation.

Diagnostic Imaging

Radiographs of the radius and ulna should include the carpus and elbow to determine the exact configuration and cause of the elbow incongruity. Radiographs of the contralateral forelimb often can be used to compare the affected limb with a normal one; however, bilateral disease may be present.

Laboratory Findings

Specific laboratory abnormalities are not found with this condition.

DIFFERENTIAL DIAGNOSIS

Differential diagnoses in large dogs include FCP, UAP, or OCD. Other conditions that may show similar clinical signs in small dogs include trauma and osteoarthritis.

MEDICAL MANAGEMENT

Medical treatment should address the five principles of medical management of osteoarthritis; however, response to medical therapy is unpredictable, and correction of the subluxation should be attempted to minimize additional joint damage, slow the progression of osteoarthritis, and decrease lameness.

SURGICAL TREATMENT

Surgical treatment is directed at restoring elbow congruity by performing a corrective osteotomy of either the radius or the ulna. Ulnar-lengthening osteotomy is indicated when the cause of elbow incongruity is an ulna that is too short. Ulnar-shortening ostectomy and/or radial lengthening osteotomy are performed when subluxation (widening) of the humeroradial joint is caused by radial shortening.

Preoperative Management

Affected animals are young and require minimal preoperative workup (see p. 943 and Chapter 5).

Anesthesia

These animals usually are young and healthy, thus a variety of anesthetic regimens can be used (see p. 944).

Surgical Anatomy

Landmarks for ulnar osteotomy include the caudal border of the ulna, which is palpable, and the trochlear notch, which can be exposed surgically by muscle elevation and must be avoided when the osteotomy is performed. Landmarks for radial lengthening osteotomy are dependent on the size of the bone plate to be applied.

Positioning

The dog is positioned in dorsal recumbency with the affected leg suspended for draping. The leg is prepared from shoulder to carpus.

SURGICAL TECHNIQUE
Lengthening Osteotomy

Make a skin incision along the caudal border of the ulna, beginning medial to the tuber olecranon and ending at the ulnar middiaphysis. Incise the subcutaneous tissue and fascia along the same line. Incise the attachments of the flexor carpi ulnaris and ulnaris lateralis muscles along the medial and lateral borders of the ulna, and elevate the muscles to expose the joint capsule. Incise the joint capsule on both sides of the ulna to expose the distal trochlear notch area (see p. 1070). Make an oblique osteotomy of the ulna distal to the trochlear notch, running from caudal proximal to cranial distal, with an oscillating saw or Gigli wire (Fig. 33-55).

A gap should form at the osteotomy site. The gap may be increased by prying apart with an osteotome. If necessary, elevate the interosseous ligament to free the proximal ulna so that it can move into position.

Drive a smooth pin or Kirschner wire from the tuber olecranon down the medullary canal, across the fracture gap, and into the medullary canal of the distal ulna. The smooth pin and the oblique direction of the osteotomy allow the forces

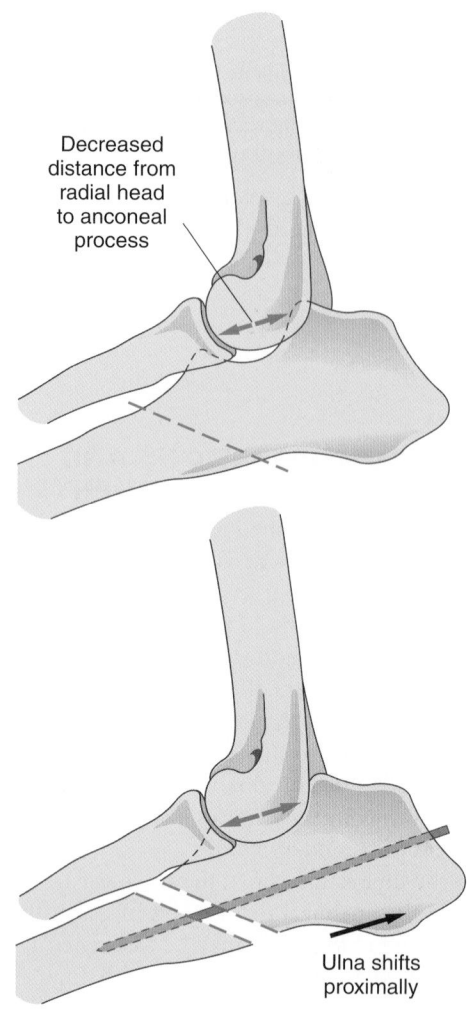

FIG. 33-55
For an ulnar-lengthening osteotomy, make an oblique osteotomy of the ulna distal to the coronoid process. Stabilize the ulna with a small intramedullary pin.

of the surrounding musculature to exert a dynamic effect on the proximal ulna and slide it into position with the humerus without causing angular distraction of the proximal ulna. Suture the joint capsule. Suture the flexor carpi ulnaris fascia to the ulnaris lateralis fascia over the caudal border of the ulna. Suture the subcutaneous tissue and skin separately.

Shortening Ostectomy

Shortening the ulna allows the radial head to come into contact with the humeral capitulum.

Approach the ulna as described earlier for the ulnar-lengthening osteotomy. Using an oscillating saw or Gigli wire, resect a segment of ulna that is longer than the measured distance from the radial head to the humeral capitulum. Drive a small, smooth pin or Kirschner wire from the tuber olecranon down the medullary canal, across the fracture gap, and into the medullary canal of the distal ulna (Fig. 33-56). The smooth pin allows the forces of the sur-

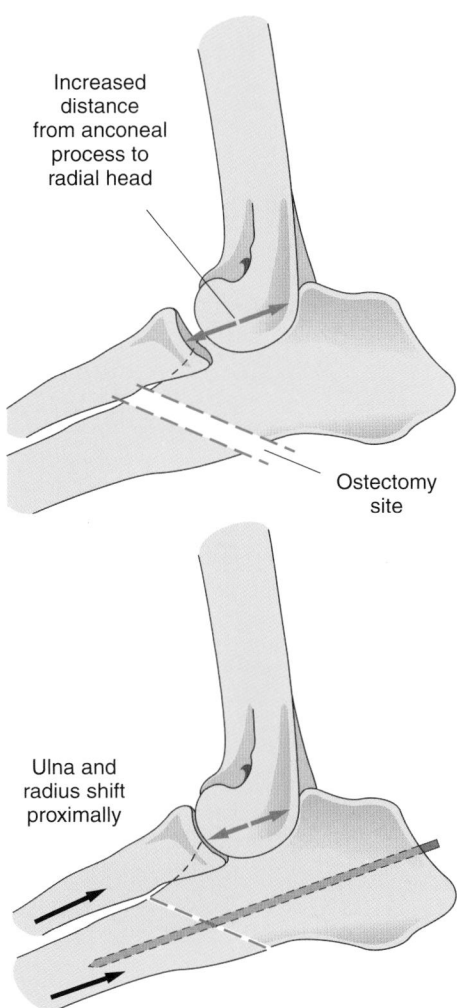

FIG. 33-56
For an ulnar-shortening ostectomy, make two oblique osteotomies of the ulna distal to the coronoid process. Remove a length of bone sufficient to allow reduction of the radial head. Stabilize the ulna with a small intramedullary pin.

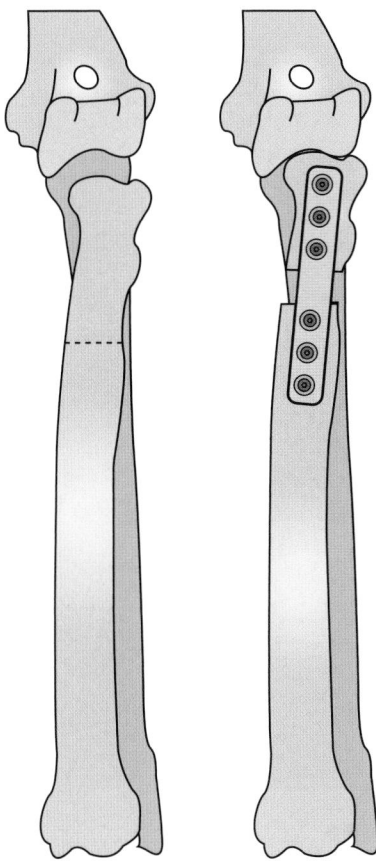

FIG. 33-57
Radial lengthening of the radius using a transverse osteotomy.

rounding musculature to exert a dynamic effect on the proximal ulna, causing it to collapse into the ostectomy site.

Radial Lengthening

Radial lengthening is performed by transposing a segment of ulna into an osteotomy site on the radius to lengthen the radius while permitting the ulna to shorten.

Perform a caudal approach to the central third of the ulna. Dissect down to the bone and around the diaphysis. Using a bone saw, remove a segment of bone equal to or just shorter than the length discrepancy of the radius. Close the ulnar incision routinely. Perform a cranial approach to the radius over the proximal and central thirds of the diaphysis.

Operative planning for the site of the radial osteotomy requires determining the length and location of an appropriate-

sized bone plate. In small dogs, a 2.7-mm bone plate may be used, whereas in large dogs a 3.5-mm bone plate may be used. The osteotomy should be planned so that three holes of the bone plate may be placed proximal to the osteotomy.

Perform a transverse osteotomy of the radius at the location that permits stabilization with a bone plate. Using an osteotome, lever the radial osteotomy apart, and insert the ulnar bone fragment or a portion of it (Fig. 33-57). Secure the osteotomy with a 2.7-mm or 3.5-mm bone plate using standard ASIF technique.

As an alternative, an oblique osteotomy of the radius may be performed using a bone sliding technique.

Perform an oblique osteotomy in the radius, then slide the proximal segment further proximally. Secure temporarily with a Kirschner wire or bone clamp (Fig. 33-58). Secure the

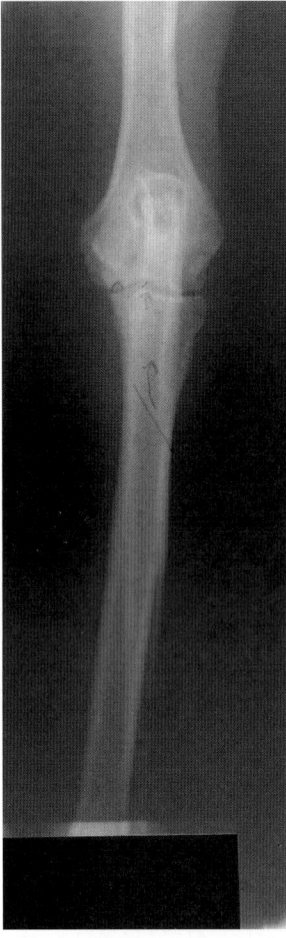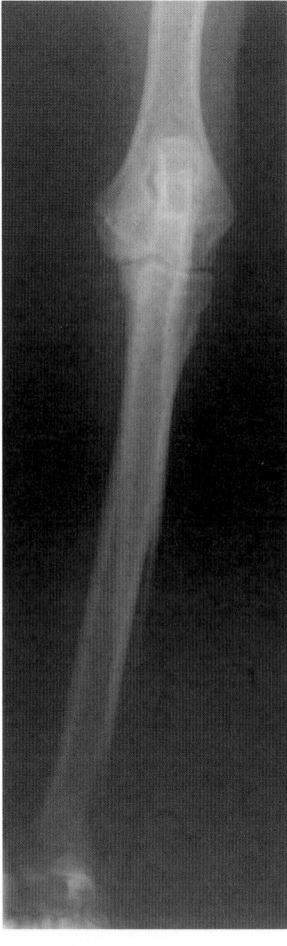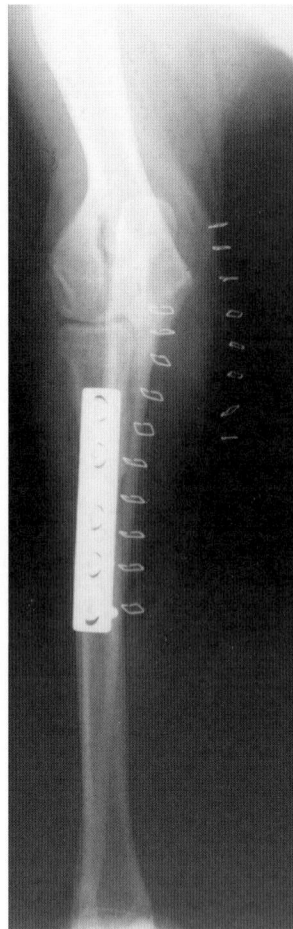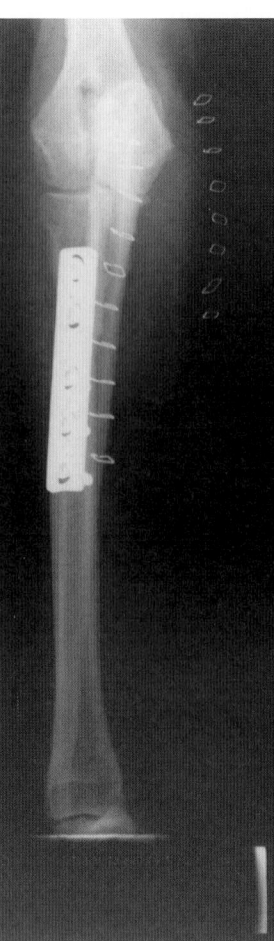

FIG. 33-58
Radial lengthening of the radius using an oblique osteotomy.

osteotomy with a 2.7-mm or 3.5-mm bone plate using the standard ASIF technique.

SUTURE MATERIALS AND SPECIAL INSTRUMENTS

Instruments for ulnar osteotomy include a Gigli wire or oscillating saw, Steinmann pins, and a pin chuck or power drill for pin insertion. Instruments for radial lengthening include a power saw and bone plating equipment.

POSTOPERATIVE CARE AND ASSESSMENT

Postoperative radiographs should be taken to evaluate the position of the ulna and congruence of the joint. Obvious changes in position may not be evident until several days after surgery. A soft, padded bandage should be applied to the limb postoperatively. Early motion of the elbow is important for dynamic reduction of the subluxated elbow, therefore leash activity should be encouraged; however, excessive activity may lead to implant failure and nonunion. Serial radiographs should be made until the area of osteotomy or ostectomy has healed. The implant can be removed after the bone has healed. Following healing, rehabilitation consists of passive range of motion, muscular strengthening,

and aquatic therapy. Physical rehabilitation can be key in maintaining range of motion of the other joints of the limb after this type of procedure, along with decreasing lameness and improving overall function. For a sample physical rehabilitation exercise protocol, please refer to Table 33-9 on p. 1193.

> NOTE: Radiographs taken 48 to 72 hours after surgery can demonstrate the effect of motion on the position of the ulna.

COMPLICATIONS

Possible surgical complications include iatrogenic infection, implant migration, implant failure, delayed union or nonunion of the osteotomy, and implant irritation of soft tissue. If the intramedullary pin irritates the triceps tendon, it should be removed.

PROGNOSIS

Without surgery, abnormal anatomy of the elbow will cause osteoarthritis and lameness. If surgery is performed before osteoarthritis is established, the prognosis is good for relatively normal limb function, although some osteoarthritis usually occurs. The amount of correction after surgery varies and appears to be directly related to the amount of displacement; that is, less displacement results in better correction. Despite the lack of radiographic correction, most dogs appear to be more comfortable after surgery. After osteoarthritis is established, periodic treatment with analgesics and antiinflammatory drugs may be necessary (see Table 33-4 on p. 1149).

CONGENITAL ELBOW LUXATION

DEFINITION

Congenital elbow luxation results in lateral rotation of the proximal ulna and subluxation or luxation of the humeroulnar joint. Synonyms include *congenital elbow luxation* and *congenital elbow malformation*.

GENERAL CONSIDERATIONS AND CLINICALLY RELEVANT PATHOPHYSIOLOGY

The etiology of congenital elbow luxation is unknown. The bone malpositioning occurs at a young age, and because the bones do not articulate normally, congruent joint surfaces do not form. At approximately 3 months of age, secondary remodeling occurs and degenerative changes begin to develop. Pathologic conditions vary with the chronicity of the condition. The olecranon is rotated lateral to the distal humerus, and the trochlear notch does not contact the humeral condyles. The result or results may be (1) hypoplasia and remodeling of the trochlea and trochlear notch; (2) hypoplasia of the medial humeral condyle with stretching of the medial collateral ligament and joint capsule; (3) hyperplasia of the lateral humeral condyle with contracture of the lateral joint capsule and lateral collateral ligament; (4) contracture and displacement of the triceps muscle; and (5) degenerative changes of the articular cartilage.

DIAGNOSIS
Clinical Presentation

Signalment. Small breeds of dogs are affected: pugs, Yorkshire terriers, Boston terriers, miniature poodles, Pomeranians, Chihuahuas, cocker spaniels, and English bulldogs are overrepresented. The condition can be unilateral or bilateral and usually is recognized when the puppy begins to walk at 3 to 6 weeks of age.

History. The history describes inability to extend one or both front legs and difficulty walking because of the crouching position. Smaller dogs tolerate the deformity better and in some cases show minimal or no gait abnormality or pain.

Physical Examination Findings

Puppies with this condition carry the affected forelimb in flexion and internal rotation (external rotation of the elbow). If the condition is bilateral, the puppy supports weight on the caudomedial aspect of the forelimbs. The elbows cannot be extended. The olecranon is located on the lateral aspect of the limb and may be mistaken for the lateral humeral condyle. The condition usually is not painful.

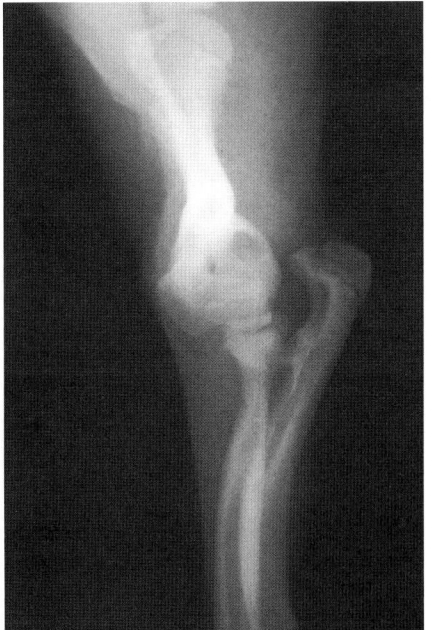

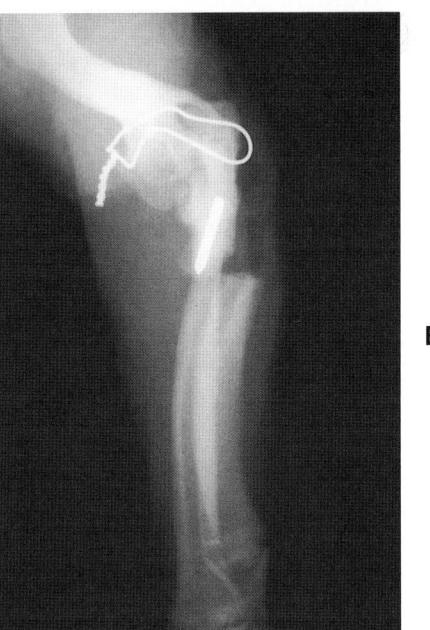

FIG. 33-59
A, Preoperative craniocaudal radiograph of the forelimb of a dog with congenital elbow luxation. **B,** Craniocaudal radiograph of the forelimb after reduction of the elbow and translocation of the olecranon.

Diagnostic Imaging

Lateral and craniocaudal radiographs of the elbow show lateral displacement and rotation of the olecranon with varying degrees of contact between the ulna and the humerus (Fig. 33-59). The radial head usually is in contact with the humerus, although this may change as the animal matures. Secondary DJD is apparent in chronic cases.

Laboratory Findings

Abnormal laboratory findings are uncommon.

DIFFERENTIAL DIAGNOSIS

Differential diagnoses include hemimelia (congenital segmental deficiency of the radius or ulna), ectrodactyly (congenital splitting of the limb), and previous fracture and malunion of the limb.

MEDICAL MANAGEMENT

Conservative therapy (splints and bandages) does not alter the course of the disease. Joint reduction and stabilization should be performed as soon as possible, before secondary degenerative changes and joint remodeling occur (usually before the animal is 4 months of age). The type of reduction technique used depends on the pathologic condition present. Closed reduction can be successful if the joint can be manipulated into position. Closed reduction is indicated in dogs that have only mild changes in bone and soft tissue. The olecranon should be rotated medially into position and secured by placing a transarticular pin from the caudal aspect of the olecranon, through the olecranon, and into the humerus. The pin is left in place for 10 to 14 days (Fig. 33-60).

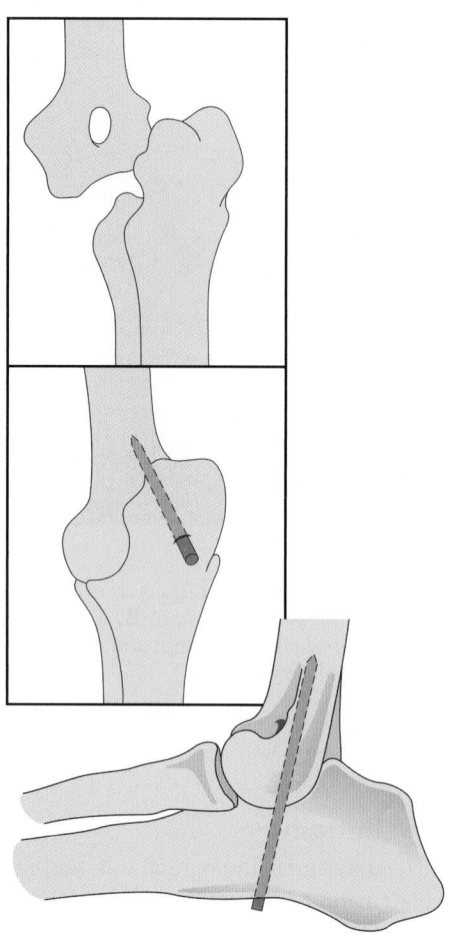

FIG. 33-60
A transarticular pin can be placed to hold the ulna in position after manual reduction of a congenitally luxated elbow.

SURGICAL TREATMENT

Open reduction and corrective osteotomy are used when the joint cannot be manually replaced (Box 33-18). Techniques for open reduction and stabilization vary, depending on the severity of the pathologic condition. Techniques used include lateral release of soft tissue (including the joint capsule and anconeus muscle), medial support of the olecranon using capsular imbrication and stay sutures, olecranon or ulnar osteotomy and transposition to reconstruct the joint, and redirection of the pull of the triceps muscle to allow joint extension. The osteotomy is stabilized with Kirschner wires and, if necessary, a tension band wire (see Fig. 33-59, *B*).

Preoperative Management

Affected animals are young and require minimal preoperative workup.

Anesthesia

General anesthesia is required for both closed and open reduction. Pediatric anesthesia techniques should be used. Anesthetic management of animals with orthopedic disease is discussed on p. 944.

Surgical Anatomy

Anatomic landmarks are the olecranon and the medial and lateral humeral condyles. The ulnar nerve is on the medial aspect of the surgical site and should be identified and protected.

Positioning

The dog is placed in dorsal recumbency with the affected limb prepared from shoulder to carpus.

SURGICAL TECHNIQUE

Make an incision on the lateral surface of the joint, starting on the lateral epicondylar crest and extending distally over the lateral epicondyle to the proximal radius, as described on p. 1211. Incise the subcutaneous tissue, and retract the skin medially to expose both the medial and lateral surfaces of the elbow. Incise the soft tissue on the lateral aspect of the humeroulnar joint (including the anconeus muscle and joint capsule) to expose the joint and reposition the ulna. If repositioning is possible, stabilize the ulna by imbricating the medial joint capsule and placing a large (No. 0 to No. 2) nonabsorbable suture from the proximal ulna to the humeral condyle through tunnels drilled in the bone with the needle

 BOX 33-18

Important Considerations in Congenital Elbow Luxation

- Immediate surgical treatment provides the best outcome.
- Repositioning the ulna results in improved limb function because the pull of the triceps muscle is redirected.
- Limited range of motion and DJD occur even with surgery.

or a small Kirschner wire. Perform an olecranon osteotomy, and transpose the osteotomized bone to a position on the ulna that best redirects the pull of the triceps muscle to extend the joint. Stabilize the osteotomy with Kirschner wires and possibly a tension band wire (see p. 990). Reposition the skin to the lateral aspect of the elbow, and close the subcutaneous tissue and skin with interrupted sutures.

SUTURE MATERIALS AND SPECIAL INSTRUMENTS

Instruments needed for open reduction include a general surgery pack, pin chuck, Kirschner wires, and orthopedic wire.

POSTOPERATIVE CARE AND ASSESSMENT

Postoperative radiographs should be made to evaluate the location of the ulna with respect to the humerus and the position of any implants. The limb should be bandaged to support the fixation for 2 to 3 weeks. Splint the elbow in a functional position. Activity should be restricted to leash walking for 4 to 6 weeks. The Kirschner wires should be removed when the osteotomy has healed. Physical rehabilitation can be key in maintaining muscle mass, range of motion, and comfort. See Table 33-9 on p. 1193 for a recommended physical rehabilitation exercise protocol.

COMPLICATIONS

Possible surgical complications include loss of joint reduction, iatrogenic infection, implant migration, and irritation of soft tissue.

PROGNOSIS

Without surgery, the dog may learn to compensate for loss of normal forelimb function by using the rear limbs for support and locomotion; however, ambulation will always be abnormal. The prognosis is good for return of satisfactory function after surgery, but poor for development of a normal joint.

CARPAL LUXATION OR SUBLUXATION

DEFINITIONS

Carpal luxation or **subluxation** results from loss of palmar ligamentous support of the antebrachial, carpal, middle carpal, and/or carpometacarpal joints. Carpal subluxation may also result from severe end-stage polyarthritis. **Pancarpal arthrodesis** involves fusion of all three carpal joints, whereas **partial arthrodesis** is a selective fusion of one or more of the carpal joints.

GENERAL CONSIDERATIONS AND CLINICALLY RELEVANT PATHOPHYSIOLOGY

Carpal hyperextension injuries are sorted into three categories based on injury location. *Category I injuries* are subluxations or luxations of the antebrachial carpal joint. *Category II injuries* include subluxation of the middle carpal and carpometacarpal joints and are associated with disruption of the accessory carpal ligaments, palmar fibrocartilage, and palmar ligaments of the middle carpal and carpometacarpal joints. Dorsal displacement of the free end of the accessory carpal and ulnar carpal bones occurs. *Category III injuries* are disruptions of the accessory carpal ligaments, carpometacarpal ligaments, and palmar fibrocartilage. However, in these injuries subluxation of the carpometacarpal joint occurs without disruption and displacement of the accessory carpal and ulnar carpal bones.

Polyarthritis often affects smaller joints, such as the carpus or tarsus (see p. 1164). Chronic joint inflammation may lead to severe cartilage and soft tissue damage with progressive collapse of the joint to a palmigrade stance.

DIAGNOSIS
Clinical Presentation

Signalment. Any age or breed and either gender of dog or cat may be affected with traumatic luxation or subluxation. Smaller dogs, particularly Shetland sheepdogs, are overrepresented for idiopathic or immune-mediated collapse of the carpal joints.

History. Acutely affected animals usually have a non–weight-bearing lameness. Because the animal is not using the limb, the extent of hyperextension may not be apparent initially. Most animals return to using the leg within a week, but are lame and have a plantigrade stance. Chronically affected dogs with idiopathic or immune-mediated polyarthritis and carpal joint collapse have a history of progressive degeneration of the carpi.

Physical Examination Findings

Acute injuries show clear indications of swelling, pain, and instability. With category I injuries, the animal usually remains unable to bear weight until definitive treatment is given. With category II or III injuries, the animal may begin to bear weight on the limb after the injury. However, as increased weight is placed on the limb, collapse and hyperextension of the carpus become evident.

Dogs with idiopathic or immune-mediated polyarthritis and carpal subluxation have a plantigrade stance and may have other visible deformity of the carpi. There is mild to moderate pain on manipulation of the joints. The disease is often bilateral.

Diagnostic Imaging

Standard craniocaudal and medial-to-lateral radiographs are needed to detect bone fractures or joint malalignment associated with complete luxation of the joints. However, stress radiographs should be made to assess carpal integrity accurately and identify the joint level of the hyperextension injury (Fig. 33-61). With the patient under heavy sedation or general anesthesia, it should be positioned in lateral recumbency with stress applied to the foot to place the carpus in maximum extension. A medial-to-lateral radiograph is produced with the carpus in maximal extension. If the contralateral limb is normal, similar images may be made for comparison. Isolated instability at the level of the antebrachial carpal joint allows an increase in extension without altering the relationships of the

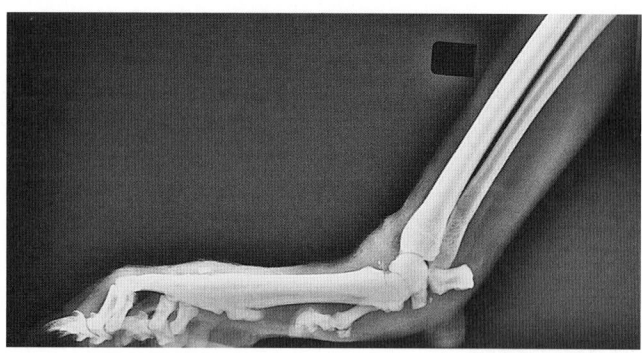

FIG. 33-61
Stress radiograph of a dog with a category II carpal hyper-extension injury. Stress radiographs should be obtained to help classify hyperextension injuries.

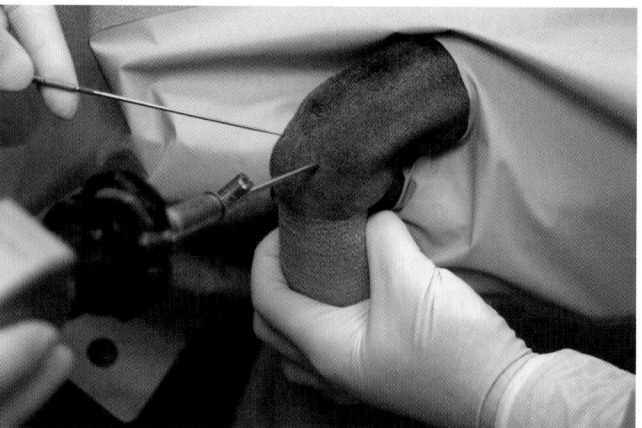

FIG. 33-62
Instrument positioning for arthroscopy of the carpal joint.

carpal and metacarpal bones. Instability at the middle carpal joint, including loss of integrity of the accessory carpal bone, results in widening of the space between the palmar process of the ulnar carpal bone and the base of metacarpal V. The accessory carpal bone deviates dorsally. The proximal carpal bones may appear to override the distal row of carpal bones with instability at the carpometacarpal level. In chronic cases, radiographic evidence of osteoarthritis is evident.

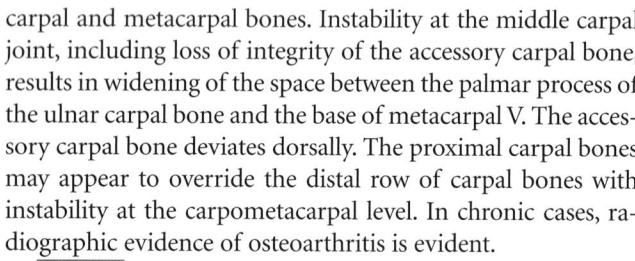**Arthroscopy.** Arthroscopy may be useful in the assessment of cartilage in animals with mild carpal joint disease. It is also used to remove chip fractures in the radiocarpal joint. Arthroscopy of the carpal joint is a relatively simple technique; however, care must be taken to avoid pulling the arthroscope and hand instruments out of the limited space within the joint.

Have an assistant hold the radiocarpal joint in complete flexion. Palpate the distal aspect of the radius and the radio-carpal joint distal to it. Insert a 20-gauge needle into the joint and infuse the joint with saline. Incise the skin on the craniomedial or craniolateral surface, avoiding incision of the joint capsule. Insert the cannula and obturator of a 1.9-mm arthroscope into the joint. Insert a needle opposite the arthroscope (craniolateral or craniomedial) for fluid outflow. Examine the radiocarpal joint. If an instrument portal is needed, remove the outflow needle, and make a stab incision into the joint at the same location. Dilate the instrument portal with a small straight hemostat, then insert the necessary hand instruments (Figs. 33-62 and 33-63).

Laboratory Findings
No consistent laboratory abnormalities are seen.

DIFFERENTIAL DIAGNOSIS
Differential diagnoses of traumatic carpal injuries include acute sprains, collateral ligament tears, distal radial fractures, and fractures of the metacarpal bones. These conditions can

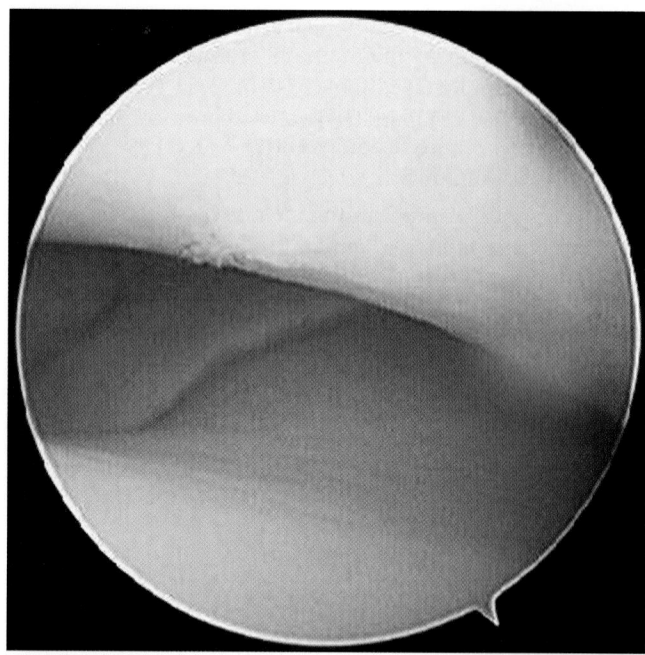

FIG. 33-63
Internal view of arthroscopy of a normal carpal joint.

be differentiated from carpal luxation or subluxation radiographically by use of standard and stress views.

Differential diagnoses for progressive collapse of the carpal joints include any form of polyarthritis or joint collapse due to chronic steroid administration.

MEDICAL MANAGEMENT
Medical or conservative management of carpal hyperextension injuries often is unrewarding. External coaptation may be tried in younger patients, but gradual hyperextension often occurs as weight bearing returns.

For medical management of polyarthritis, see page 1169. Medical management of end-stage carpal collapse due to idiopathic or immune-mediated joint disease is often unrewarding, as the animals usually have severe problems ambulating because of biomechanical failure of the carpal joints.

SURGICAL TREATMENT

Carpal luxations are best treated with pancarpal arthrodesis. Pancarpal arthrodesis is most commonly performed with a dorsally placed bone plate; however, application of a specially designed medial bone plate has also been described (Guerro and Montavon, 2005). Carpal hyperextension injuries are best treated with either pancarpal arthrodesis or partial arthrodesis through a cranial approach to the joint. Antebrachial carpal injuries should be treated with a pancarpal arthrodesis accomplished by removing articular cartilage at all joint levels, placing a cancellous bone autograft at the joint surfaces, and stabilizing with a bone plate. Pancarpal arthrodesis or partial carpal arthrodesis may be used to manage injuries of the middle carpal joint; however, partial arthrodesis that does not reestablish the accessory carpal moment arm may eventually fail because of breakdown of the radiocarpal joint. Partial arthrodesis for treating this injury should include fusion of the middle carpal and carpometacarpal joints with selective fusion of the accessory carpal–ulnar carpal articulation. This procedure may be accomplished with a bone plate, cross pins, or placement of longitudinal metacarpal pins. With isolated carpometacarpal instability, a partial arthrodesis is recommended. Although the accessory carpal ligaments may be compromised, the ligaments between the base of the accessory carpal bone, ulnar carpal bone, and fifth metacarpal bone are intact, preserving integrity of the accessory carpal moment arm. Articular cartilage should be removed, cancellous bone placed in the fusion site, and the site stabilized with a T-plate or intramedullary pins.

End-stage carpal joint collapse due to idiopathic or immune-mediated joint disease is best treated with pancarpal arthrodesis. It is important to verify with arthrocentesis and cytology that the inflammatory stage of the disease is no longer active.

Arthroscopy (see previous discussion) may be useful for evaluation of cartilage damage in mild to moderate cases to determine if medical management or arthrodesis is most appropriate. Arthroscopy may also be used for removal of chip fractures in the radiocarpal joint.

Preoperative Management

An external coaptation splint or bandage should be applied to protect the limb until definitive surgical treatment is undertaken. The animal's activity should be strictly limited to prevent further joint damage.

Anesthesia

Anesthetic management of animals with orthopedic disease is presented on p. 944.

Surgical Anatomy

The carpus consists of seven bones arranged in two rows. The radiocarpal and ulnar carpal bones make up the proximal row, and the first, second, third, and fourth carpal bones make up the distal row. The accessory carpal bone lies caudally and articulates with the ulnar carpal bone. The radiocarpal and ulnar carpal bones articulate with the radius and styloid process of the ulna to form the antebrachial carpal joint. The middle carpal joint, formed by articulation of the proximal and distal rows of carpal bones, has the greatest movement—accounting for 10% to 15% of carpal motion. Very little motion occurs in the carpometacarpal and intercarpal joints. Palmar support is from the flexor retinaculum proximally and palmar fibrocartilage distally. Multiple small ligaments cross the intercarpal articulations between carpal bones to provide additional collateral and palmar support. Two accessory ligaments originate from the free end of the accessory carpal bone and insert onto the palmar surface of the fourth and fifth metacarpal bones. The caudal position of the free end of the accessory carpal bone, in conjunction with the accessory carpal ligaments, acts as a moment arm to balance the vertical force produced when the paw strikes the ground.

Positioning

For arthroscopy, the animal should be positioned in sternal recumbency with the limb that is to be operated pulled forward and off the side of the table. For open surgery, the animal should be positioned in dorsal recumbency. A hanging-leg preparation allows maximum manipulation of the limb during surgery (see p. 36). The leg should be clipped and prepared from the proximal humeral region to the tips of the toes. The proximal humerus serves as the donor site for cancellous bone.

SURGICAL TECHNIQUE

Considerable collagenous and bony tissue proliferation often occurs with carpal luxation or subluxation. Increased vascularity, which accompanies the fibrous proliferation, can make surgical dissection difficult. Use of a tourniquet is helpful. The joint is approached dorsally, where proliferative tissue is pronounced. Sharp dissection through scar tissue and the joint capsule creates the least trauma.

Approach to the Carpal Bones

Make a skin incision over the midline of the dorsal surface of the carpus, extending from 4 cm proximal to the radiocarpal joint line to 4 cm distal to the carpometacarpal joint line (Fig. 33-64, A). Incise the subcutaneous tissue, proliferative fibrous tissue, and joint capsule overlying the radiocarpal, middle carpal, and carpometacarpal joints (Fig. 33-64, B).

The proliferative fibrous tissue will be confluent with the joint capsule proximally and distally.

Using sharp dissection, reflect the synovial joint capsule incision from the cranial face of the carpal bones both medially

A

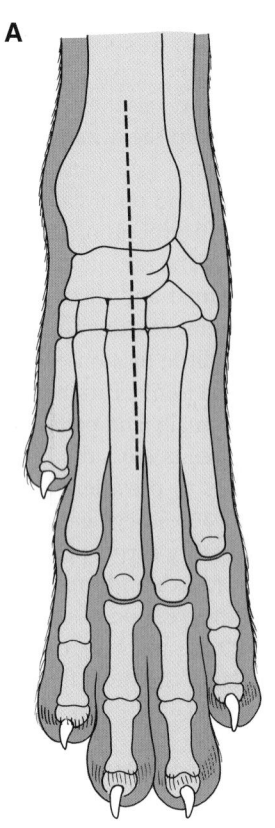

FIG. 33-64
A, To approach the dorsal surface of the carpus, make a skin incision over the midline, extending from 4 cm proximal to the radiocarpal joint line to 4 cm distal to the carpometacarpal joint line. **B,** Incise the subcutaneous tissue, proliferative fibrous tissue, and joint capsule overlying the radiocarpal, middle carpal, and carpometacarpal joints. Remove articular cartilage (indicated as shaded areas).

B

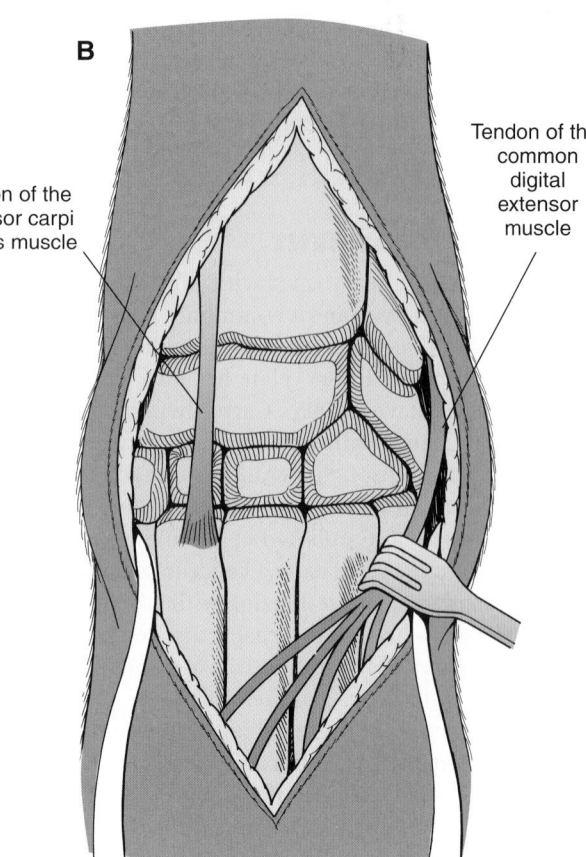

Tendon of the extensor carpi radialis muscle

Tendon of the common digital extensor muscle

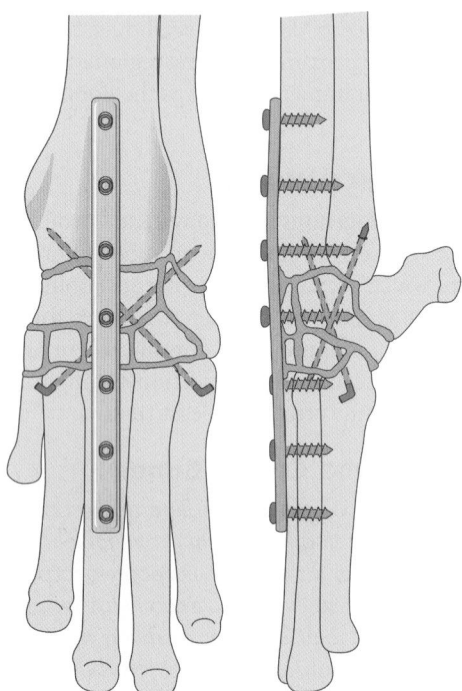

FIG. 33-65
Pancarpal arthrodesis for stabilization of category I carpal hyperextension injuries. Note the cranial application of a bone plate and caudal placement of cross pins. The plate should be contoured 10 degrees in extension.

and laterally. Place Gelpi retractors to maintain exposure of the joint surfaces, and position a small Hohmann retractor between joint surfaces to help visualize the articular cartilage of each joint. Use a low-speed power burr to remove articular cartilage from the surface of the carpal bones in each joint. Attempt to preserve the tendon of the extensor carpi radialis muscle as it crosses the craniolateral aspect of the joint. Harvest a cancellous bone graft from the proximal humerus (see p. 962), and insert the graft within the denuded surfaces of each joint. Stabilize the arthrodesis with an implant as discussed below. Suture the wound in layers; tension may be needed to appose the tissue over a plate. If tension is excessive, perform release incisions on the medial and/or lateral aspects of the limb to permit closure of the primary incision.

Excessive tension during closure of the primary incision can lead to severe limb swelling, wound dehiscence, and in severe cases necrosis and death of the foot. Performing full thickness incisions on the medial or lateral surfaces (release incisions) results in formation of a bipedicle flap that permits closure of the primary wound without tension. The release incisions will heal quickly by secondary intention.

Pancarpal Arthrodesis

Expose the joint surfaces of the radiocarpal, middle carpal, and carpometacarpal articulations, and remove articular cartilage as described above. Use a small Kirschner wire to carpal joint) and the dorsal surface of metacarpal III. Cut the tendon of insertion of the extensor carpi radialis muscle from metacarpal III to facilitate placement of the plate, and suture it to the similar tendon of insertion on metacarpal II (Fig. 33-66).

Partial Carpal Arthrodesis With Intramedullary Pins

Expose the joint surfaces of the middle carpal and carpometacarpal joints, and remove articular cartilage as described above. Harvest and insert a cancellous bone graft. To stabilize the fusion, create a slot in the dorsal cortex of metacarpals III and IV, and drive a pin proximally into the medullary canal of each bone (see Fig. 33-66). Reduce the carpus by flexing it 90 degrees and placing proximal and palmar pressure on the metacarpal bones. Drive the pins proximally into the radiocarpal bone, but do not penetrate the proximal articular surface. Bend the distal ends of the pins into a hook, cut the excess pin, and turn the hook into the bone.

> NOTE: Be sure to remove articular cartilage and rigidly stabilize the joint, or arthrodesis will not occur.

Partial Carpal Arthrodesis With Cross Pins and a Lag Screw

Expose the joint surfaces of the middle carpal and carpometacarpal joints, and remove articular cartilage as described above. Harvest and insert a cancellous bone graft. Stabilize the fusion by placing a pin from medial to lateral, entering the bone near the head of the second metacarpal and penetrating the radiocarpal bone. Place a second pin from lateral to medial, entering the bone near the head of the fifth metacarpal and penetrating the ulnar carpal bone. Fuse the accessory carpal–ulnar carpal articulation by removing articular cartilage between joint surfaces of the accessory carpal bone and ulnar carpal bone, placing a cancellous bone graft, and stabilizing it with a compression screw. Make an incision lateral to the base of the accessory carpal bone. Incise the subcutaneous tissue and deep fascia adjacent to the lateral accessory carpal ligament.

The medial and lateral accessory carpal ligaments will be torn.

Continue the incision lateral to the abductor digiti quinti muscle to the joint capsule. Incise the joint capsule to expose and remove articular cartilage from the ulnar carpal and accessory carpal bones. Insert a cancellous bone graft, and stabilize the fusion with a compression screw and wire. Insert the compression screw from the cranial face of the ulnar carpal bone into the accessory carpal bone. Place a wire from the base of the accessory carpal bone through the head of the fifth metacarpal bone (Fig. 33-67).

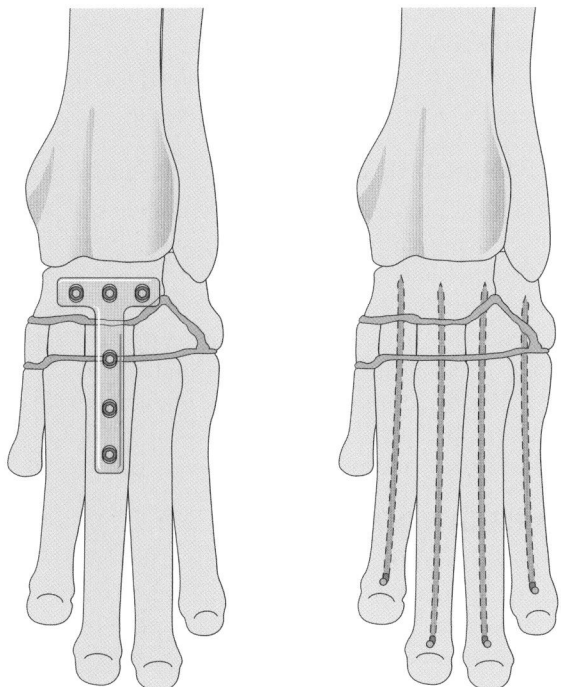

FIG. 33-66
Partial carpal arthrodesis can be stabilized with a T-plate or multiple intramedullary pins or Kirschner wires.

drill multiple holes through the distal radial epiphysis into the marrow cavity to aid vascularization of the fusion. Stabilize the fusion with a bone plate applied as a compression plate to the dorsal surface of the radius.

The plate should be contoured to reflect a 10-degree angle of extension of the carpus.

Apply the plate so that the proximal three plate screws enter the distal radius and the distal three plate screws enter the third metacarpal bone. Place one intermediate plate screw in the radiocarpal bone and the others where bone stock is available. Because the plate is not positioned on the tension surface of the joint, it should be supported with small Steinmann cross pins or external coaptation or both. If pins are selected, place one pin from medial to lateral, entering the bone near the head of the second metacarpal and exiting through the distal ulna. Place a second pin from lateral to medial, entering the bone near the head of the fifth metacarpal and exiting through the distal radius (see Fig. 33-65).

Partial Carpal Arthrodesis With a Plate

Expose the joint surfaces of the middle carpal and carpometacarpal joints, and remove articular cartilage as described above. Harvest and insert a cancellous bone graft. Stabilize the joints with a small T-plate attached to the distal dorsal surface of the radiocarpal bone (as far distally as possible to avoid interference with the antebrachial

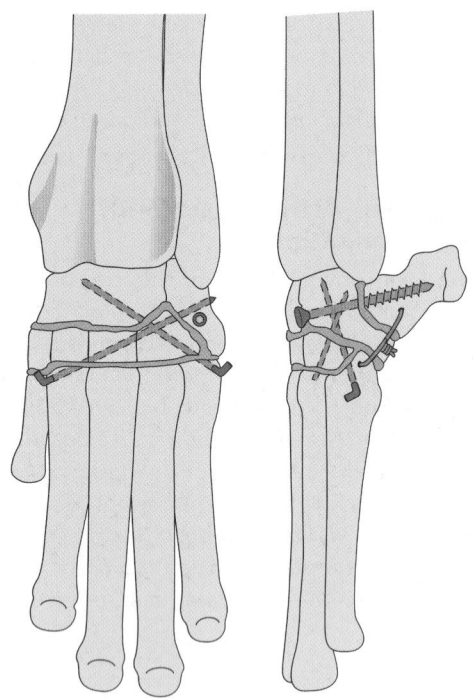

FIG. 33-67
Partial carpal arthrodesis with selective fusion of the accessory ulnar articulation. Note that the pins do not cross the radiocarpal joint.

SUTURE MATERIALS AND SPECIAL INSTRUMENTS

Instruments for arthrodesis include a power drill, burrs, bone curette, Steinmann pins, bone plates, and screws.

POSTOPERATIVE CARE AND ASSESSMENT

A soft, padded bandage with a coaptation splint should be applied postoperatively to reduce swelling and support the internal fixation. Healing of an arthrodesis takes 12 to 16 weeks (Michal et al, 2003) external splint should be worn for 6 to 8 weeks. Once the splint is removed, conservative physical rehabilitation should begin immediately to combat muscle atrophy and loss of range of motion. A sample physical rehabilitation protocol can be found in Table 33-10. Uncontrolled activity should be strictly controlled until union has occurred.

COMPLICATIONS

Occasionally, soft tissue irritation or screw loosening is an indication for removal of the implant. Metacarpal bone fractures may occur in a small percentage of patients with pancarpal arthrodesis, especially if the plate extends only a short distance on the metacarpal bone (Whitelock et al, 1999). Return to function after partial carpal arthrodesis may be compromised if additional instabilities are overlooked or if the plate interferes with the antebrachial carpal joint.

 Table 33-10

Physical Rehabilitation Protocol Following Pancarpal or Pantarsal Arthrodesis, Tarsal OCD, and Carpal or Tarsal Luxation/Subluxation

ALL TREATMENTS BID	DAY 0 TO DAY 14*	DAY 15 TO DAY 24	DAY 25 UNTIL HEALED	HEALED TO RETURN TO FUNCTION
Massage	5 min	5 min	5 min	
Passive range of motion (repetitions)†	15	15		
Therapeutic exercise-total time	10 min	15 min	15 min	25–45 min
Walk/land treadmill	10 min	5 min	5 min	>10 min
Balancing	+	+	+	
Obstacles	+	+	+	+
Weaving		+	+	+
Circles			+	+
Hills				+
Stairs				+
Jog/run				+
Underwater treadmill		10 min	10 min	>15 min
Swimming				5–10 min
Cryotherapy	15 min	15 min	15 min	PRN

OCD, Osteochondritis dissecans; *BID,* twice a day; +, perform modality; *PRN,* as needed.
*Day 0 begins when splint is removed.
†Passive range of motion to all joints of the affected and unaffected limb.

PROGNOSIS

Pancarpal and partial carpal arthrodeses result in excellent limb function in approximately 80% of patients treated for hyperextension injuries. The remaining 20% are substantially improved after surgery, but may have varying degrees of limb dysfunction (lameness) after exercise. A small percentage exhibit continued, slight, weight-bearing lameness, but limb function is vastly improved relative to preoperative function.

References

Guerro TG, Montavon PM: Medial plating for carpal panarthrodesis, *Vet Surg* 34:153, 2005.

Michal U, Fluckiger M, Schmokel H: Healing of dorsal pancarpal arthrodesis in the dog, *J Sm Anim Pract* 44:109, 2003.

Whitelock RG, Dyce J, Houlton JEF: Metacarpal fractures associated with pancarpal arthrodesis in dogs, *Vet Surg* 28:25, 1999.

Suggested Reading

Beale BS, Hulse DA, Schulz KS et al: *Small animal arthroscopy,* Philadelphia, 2003, Saunders.

This comprehensive textbook on arthroscopy has detailed information regarding instrumentation and techniques of carpal joint animal arthroscopy.

CARPAL SUBLUXATION DUE TO COLLATERAL LIGAMENT INJURY

DEFINITIONS

Carpal subluxation may result from loss of collateral ligamentous support of the antebrachial carpal joint. **Pancarpal arthrodesis** involves fusion of all three carpal joints. A **prosthetic ligament** involves replacing the damaged ligament with a synthetic suture.

GENERAL CONSIDERATIONS AND CLINICALLY RELEVANT PATHOPHYSIOLOGY

Carpal collateral ligament injuries are always due to trauma. Either the medial or lateral collateral ligament may be involved. Most injuries involve the radiocarpal joint. Collateral injuries involving other joints of the carpus or other ligaments of the carpus should be treated as described above for carpal luxations.

DIAGNOSIS
Clinical Presentation

Signalment. Any age or breed and either gender of dog or cat may be affected.

History. Acutely affected animals usually have a non–weight-bearing lameness.

Physical Examination Findings

Acute injuries show clear indications of swelling, pain, and instability. Palpation of the carpus demonstrates the ability to "break open" the joint either medially or laterally.

Diagnostic Imaging

Standard craniocaudal and medial-to-lateral radiographs are needed to detect bone fractures or joint malalignment associated with complete luxation of the joints. However, stress radiographs should be made to assess carpal integrity accurately and identify the level of the collateral ligament injury (Fig. 33-68). Integrity of the collateral ligaments is determined by obtaining craniocaudal views of the carpus while a medial and lateral stress is applied to the foot.

Laboratory Findings

No consistent laboratory abnormalities are seen.

DIFFERENTIAL DIAGNOSIS

Differential diagnoses include acute sprains, carpal luxation or subluxation, distal radial fractures, and fractures of the metacarpal bones. These conditions can be differentiated from collateral ligament injuries radiographically by use of standard and stress views.

MEDICAL MANAGEMENT

Medical or conservative management of carpal collateral ligament injuries often is unrewarding. External coaptation may be tried in younger patients, but lameness often persists as weight bearing returns.

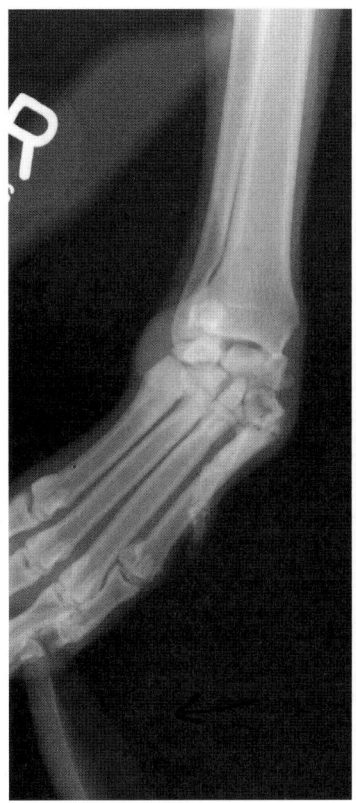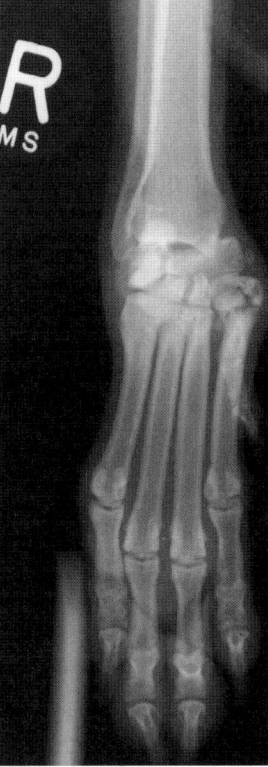

FIG. 33-68
Radiograph of collateral ligament instability of the carpal joint.

SURGICAL TREATMENT

Collateral ligament injuries involving primarily the radio-carpal joint can be treated with prosthetic ligament techniques. A pancarpal arthrodesis may be used to manage these injuries primarily or if the prosthetic ligament fails.

Preoperative Management

An external coaptation splint or bandage should be applied to protect the limb until definitive surgical treatment is undertaken. The animal's activity should be strictly limited to prevent further joint damage.

Anesthesia

Anesthetic management of animals with orthopedic disease is presented on p. 944.

Surgical Anatomy

Collateral ligamentous support arises from the short radial collateral ligament medially and from the short ulnar collateral ligament laterally. Also, sleeves of collagenous tissue that house tendons provide medial and lateral collateral support. Multiple small ligaments cross the intercarpal articulations between carpal bones to provide additional collateral and palmar support.

Positioning

The animal should be positioned in dorsal recumbency. A hanging-leg preparation allows maximum manipulation of the limb during surgery (see p. 36). The leg should be clipped and prepared from the humeral region to the tips of the toes.

SURGICAL TECHNIQUE

Considerable collagenous and bony tissue proliferation often occurs with collateral ligament injury. Increased vascularity, which accompanies the fibrous proliferation, can make surgi-cal dissection difficult. Use of a tourniquet is helpful. The joint is approached medially or laterally depending upon the side of injury. Sharp dissection through scar tissue and the joint capsule creates the least trauma.

Approach To The Carpal Collateral Ligaments

Make a skin incision over the medial or lateral aspect of the radiocarpal joint extending 4 cm proximal and distal to the radiocarpal joint. Incise the subcutaneous tissue, proliferative fibrous tissue, and joint capsule overlying the radiocarpal joint.

The proliferative fibrous tissue will be confluent with the joint capsule proximally and distally.

Using sharp dissection, reflect the synovial joint capsule incision from the medial or lateral face of the distal radius and carpal bone. Place Gelpi retractors to maintain exposure of the joint surfaces. If the remnants of the collateral ligament can be sutured, repair the ligament with interrupted sutures or a locking loop pattern. To place a prosthetic ligament with bone tunnels, drill a small hole from dorsal to ventral through the medial or lateral styloid process and a similar hole through the radiocarpal bone or ulnar carpal bone, being careful to avoid the articular surfaces. For lateral collateral ligament injuries, the suture may be passed between the distal ulna and the distal radius. Thread heavy gauge monofilament nylon through the holes in a figure-eight pattern, and tie to eliminate the collateral instability (Fig. 33-69). Do not tie the suture so tight that range of motion in the joint is sacrificed. To place a prosthetic ligament with bone anchors, insert the bone anchors in the medial or lateral styloid process and the radial or ulnar carpal bone. Pass the suture through the bone anchors in a figure-eight pattern, and tie to eliminate instability.

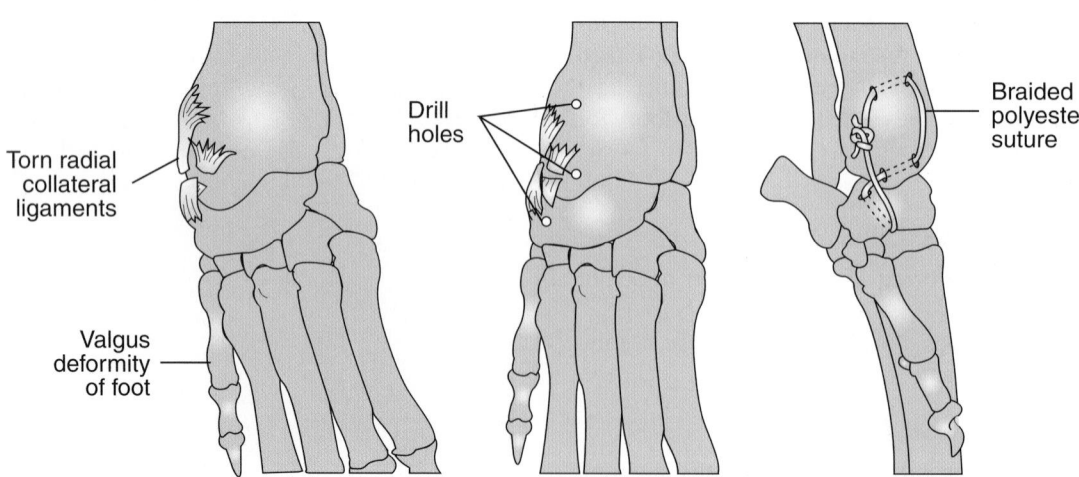

FIG. 33-69
Collateral ligament damage of the carpal joint may be treated by replacement of the ligament with a suture.

Labels in figure: Torn radial collateral ligaments; Valgus deformity of foot; Drill holes; Braided polyester suture

SUTURE MATERIALS AND SPECIAL INSTRUMENTS

Instruments for arthrodesis include a battery- or air-driven power drill, burrs, bone curette, Steinmann pins, bone plates, and screws.

POSTOPERATIVE CARE AND ASSESSMENT

A soft, padded bandage with a coaptation splint should be applied postoperatively to reduce swelling and support the internal fixation. An external splint should be worn for 6 to 8 weeks. Once the splint is removed, conservative physical rehabilitation should begin immediately to combat muscle atrophy and loss of range of motion. For a sample physical rehabilitation protocol, see Table 33-10 on p. 1230. Uncontrolled activity should be strictly controlled until union has occurred.

PROGNOSIS

Prosthetic ligament repair results in excellent limb function in most patients if other injuries to the carpus are not present. Failure of fixation necessitates pancarpal arthrodesis.

COXOFEMORAL JOINT

HIP DYSPLASIA

DEFINITIONS

Hip dysplasia is the abnormal development of the coxo-femoral joint characterized by subluxation, or complete luxation, of the femoral head in younger patients and mild to severe DJD in older patients. **Luxation of the coxofemoral joint** is a complete separation between the femoral head and the acetabulum, whereas **subluxation** is a partial or incomplete separation. The **angle of inclination** is the angle formed between the long axis of the femoral neck and the femoral diaphysis in the frontal plane. The **angle of anteversion** is the angle formed between the long axis of the femoral neck and the transcondylar axis. The **angle of subluxation** is the angle between the femur and the pelvis at which the hip subluxates during limb abduction. The **angle of reduction** is the angle between the femur and the pelvis at which the hip reduces during limb adduction. The **angle of ventroversion** is the angle between the vertical plane and the face of the acetabular cup.

GENERAL CONSIDERATIONS AND CLINICALLY RELEVANT PATHOPHYSIOLOGY

The causes of hip dysplasia are multifactorial; both hereditary and environmental factors play a part in the development of abnormal bone and soft tissue. However, hereditary factors are the primary determining factors. Rapid weight gain and growth through excessive nutritional intake may cause a disparity of development of supporting soft tissue, contributing to hip dysplasia. Factors that cause synovial inflammation (i.e., mild, repeated trauma) may also be important. Synovitis leads to an increased volume of joint fluid, which abolishes joint stability derived from the suctionlike action produced by a thin layer of normal synovial fluid between the articular surfaces. These factors contribute to development of hip joint laxity and subsequent subluxation, which are responsible for early clinical signs and joint changes. Subluxation stretches the fibrous joint capsule, causing pain and lameness. Acetabular cancellous bone is easily deformed by continual dorsal subluxation of the femoral head. The pistonlike action of the femoral head dynamically subluxating from the acetabulum with each step causes tilting of the acetabular articular surface from a normal horizontal plane to a more vertical plane. It also reduces the surface area of articulation, which concentrates the stress of weight bearing over a small area in the hip joint. Fractures of the acetabular trabecular cancellous bone may occur and exacerbate the pain and lameness. Physiologic responses to joint laxity (subluxation) are proliferative fibroplasia of the joint capsule and increased trabecular bone thickness. These changes relieve pain associated with capsular sprain and trabecular fractures. However, the surface area of articulation is still reduced, leading to premature wear of articular cartilage, exposure of subchondral pain fibers, and lameness.

> NOTE: Hip dysplasia is painful in juvenile dogs because wear of articular cartilage exposes pain fibers in subchondral bone and laxity causes stretching of soft tissue. In older dogs, hip dysplasia causes pain through osteoarthritis.

DIAGNOSIS
Clinical Presentation

Signalment. The incidence of hip dysplasia is highest in large-breed dogs. History and clinical signs vary with the patient's age. Two populations of animals are affected: juvenile patients with hip laxity and mature patients with osteoarthritis. Hip dysplasia is rare in cats.

History. Symptoms in young patients include difficulty rising after rest, exercise intolerance, and intermittent or continual lameness. As animals mature, they may develop additional signs attributable to hip joint pain. Progressive DJD in these patients results in difficulty rising, exercise intolerance, lameness after exercise, atrophy of the pelvic musculature, and/or a waddling gait attributed to abnormal movement of the rear limbs. Patients often are seen for evaluation of lameness that has suddenly worsened during or after increased activity or injury.

> NOTE: Exercise intolerance is the most common sign of hip dysplasia.

Physical Examination Findings

Juvenile patients with lameness associated with hip dysplasia are typically first evaluated at 5 to 10 months of age. Physical findings in these patients include pain during extension, external rotation, and abduction of the hip joint,

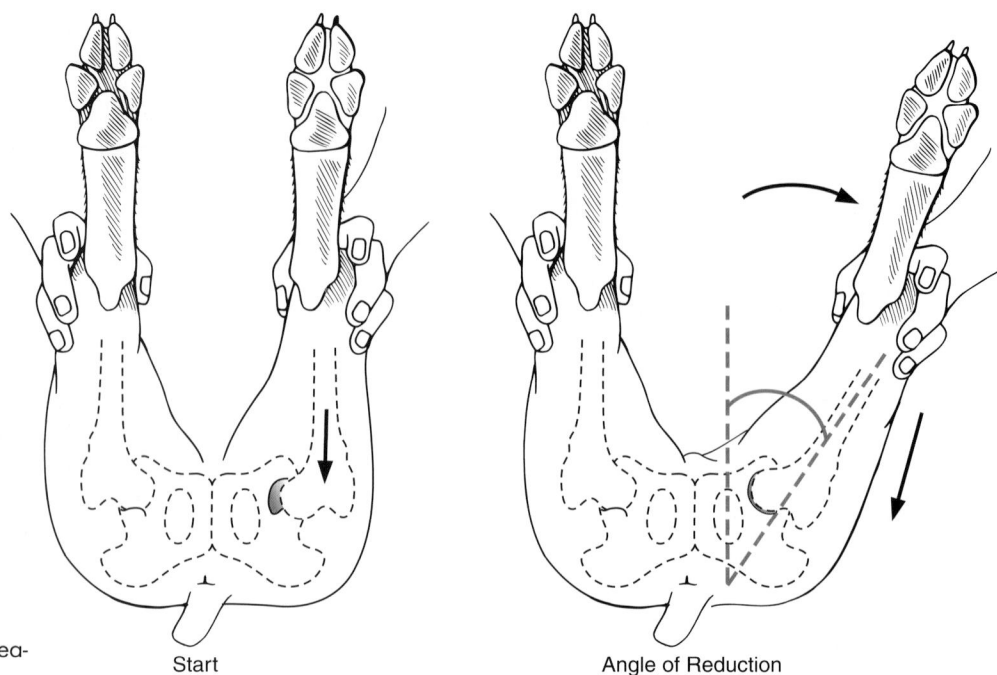

Start

Angle of Reduction

FIG. 33-70
The *angle of reduction* is the measured point where the femoral head slips back into the acetabulum when the limb is abducted. The *angle of subluxation* is the measured point where the femoral head slips out of the acetabulum when the limb is adducted.

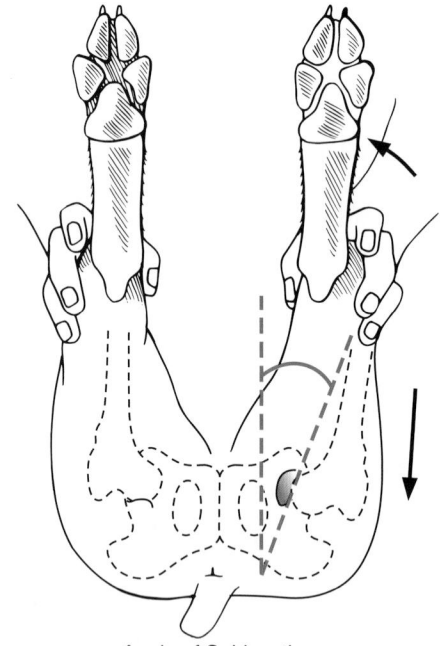

Angle of Subluxation

and poorly developed pelvic musculature. Hip examination (see p. 938) performed under general anesthesia shows increased laxity of the hip joints as evidenced by abnormal angles of reduction and subluxation (Fig. 33-70). Many juvenile dogs spontaneously improve with increasing age after conservative management. This is due to elimination of subluxation by scar tissue formation around the joint.

Physical examination findings in older animals include pain during hip joint extension, reduced range of motion, and atrophy of pelvic musculature. There is generally no detectable joint laxity because of the proliferative fibrous response, but crepitus may be detected on joint manipulation. It is important to note that clinical signs do not always correlate with radiographic findings. A correct diagnosis of hip

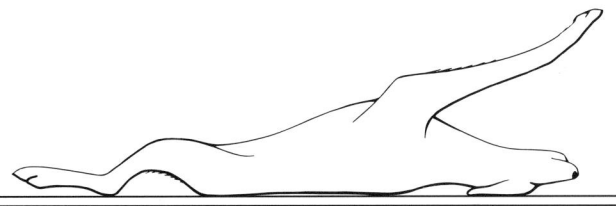

FIG. 33-71
For standard Orthopedic Foundation for Animals–type radiographs to evaluate hip conformation, extend the hips and internally rotate the tibias until the patella lies directly over the trochlear grooves. Be sure the pelvis is straight, with symmetric obturator foramina.

dysplasia as the cause of clinical problems is based on age, breed, history, physical findings, and radiographic changes.

Diagnostic Imaging

The standard radiographic view for diagnosis of hip dysplasia is the ventrodorsal view of the pelvis with rear limbs extended symmetrically and rotated inward to center the patellae over the trochlear grooves (Figs. 33-71 and 33-72, *A*). The dog must be heavily sedated or anesthetized for proper relaxation and positioning. The Orthopedic Foundation for Animals will certify a dog after 2 years of age within seven established grades for categorizing radiographic congruity between the femoral head and acetabulum. Hips determined to be "normal" radiographically may be further classified as excellent, good, fair, or near normal; animals with dysplasia are categorized as mild, moderate, or severe. Stress radiographs can be used to detect breed susceptibility to hip dysplasia as early as 4 months (Penn Hip). Stress radiographs require that the dog be under deep sedation or light anesthesia to eliminate muscle tension. Radiographic views are taken with the hips in both a neutral stance position and distracted (obtained by levering a custom-designed distractor between the legs). A distraction index is calculated from these views and is used to predict the likelihood of development of DJD secondary to hip laxity. Individual logistic regression curves that predict the risk of the development of DJD have been developed for different breeds because it appears that some breeds are more "laxity tolerant" than others. Specialty centers have been certified nationally to determine a patient's distraction index. Older dogs with established DJD do not require perfect positioning or special studies for a diagnosis of hip dysplasia (Fig. 33-72, *B*).

> NOTE: Clinical signs often do not correlate with radiographic findings. Some dogs with moderate or severe dysplasia are asymptomatic.

Arthroscopy. Arthroscopy of the coxofemoral joint is a relatively simple technique in juvenile dogs with significant hip laxity. Arthroscopy of

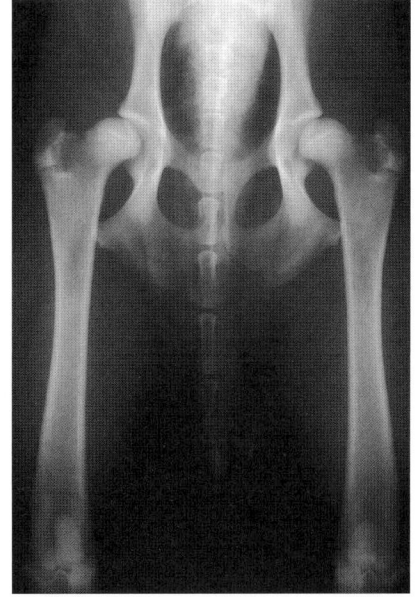

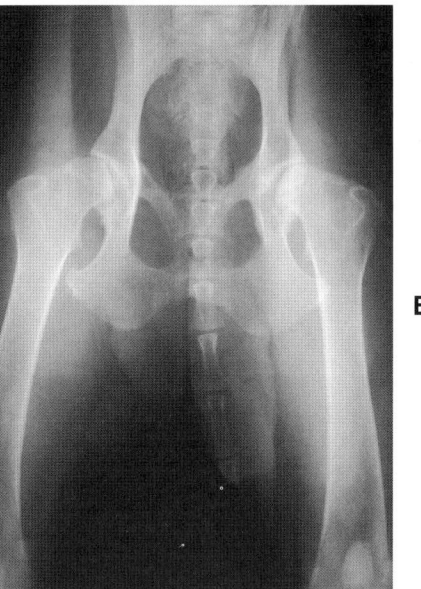

FIG. 33-72
A, Ventrodorsal radiograph of an immature dog with subluxation of the femoral heads and minimal evidence of DJD, typifying a candidate for triple pelvic osteotomy. **B,** Ventrodorsal radiograph of a dog with advanced hip dysplasia and osteophyte formation. This dog may be a candidate for total hip replacement or femoral head ostectomy if clinical signs cannot be managed medically.

juvenile hip dysplasia has been reported in a large case series (Holsworth et al, 2005). Arthroscopy permits direct visualization of cartilage damage, ligament tearing, and damage to the acetabular labrum (Fig. 33-73). Assessment of arthroscopic findings may be of assistance in decision making relative to the appropriateness of triple pelvic osteotomy (TPO) to the treatment of juvenile hip dysplasia; although specific criteria have not been established, arthroscopic evi-

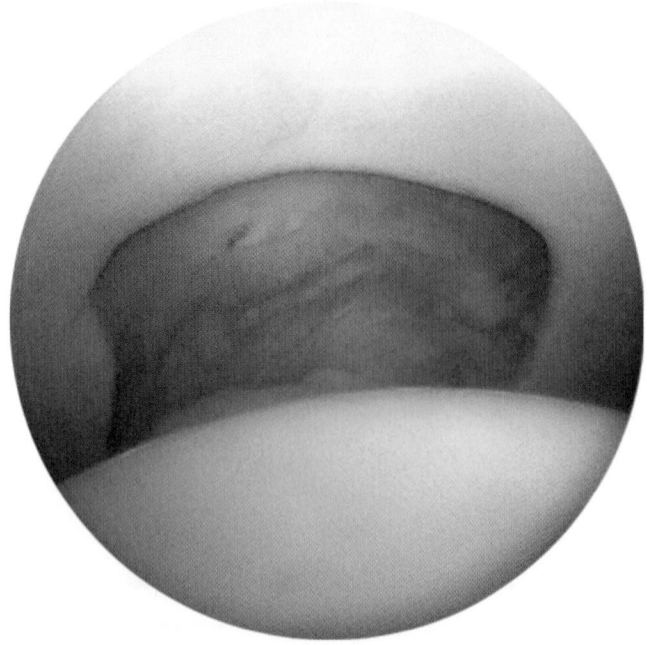

FIG. 33-73
Arthroscopic view of a normal hip joint.

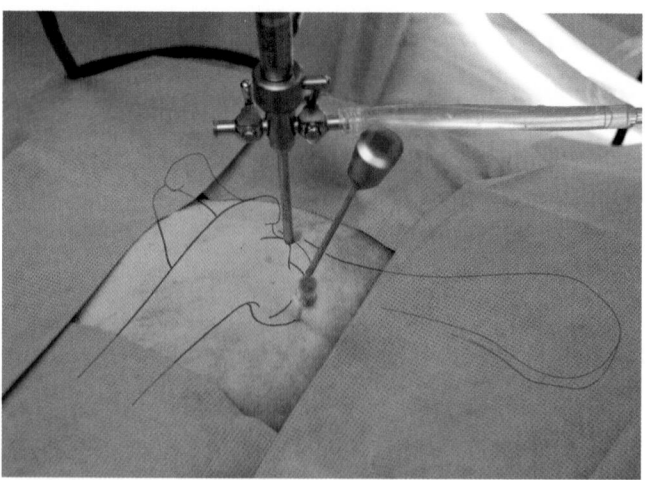

FIG. 33-74
Instrument positioning for arthroscopy of the hip joint.

dence of moderate or severe cartilage damage worsens the prognosis for success of a TPO. Thorough knowledge of hip joint anatomy is important as the joint is deep within the musculature, providing few palpable landmarks for instrumentation of the joint. In most cases, a long 2.7-mm arthroscope is necessary to reach the joint.

Position the patient in lateral recumbency with the affected limb uppermost. Have an assistant hold the limb horizontally, and apply distal distraction of the limb to help open the joint space dorsally. Insert a large 3.5-inch spinal needle or catheter needle just proximal to the greater trochanter and perpendicular to the limb until it enters the joint and contacts the medial wall of the acetabulum. Aspirate joint fluid to confirm that the needle is in the joint, and then infuse saline or lactated Ringer's solution to fill the joint to moderate pressure. Remove the needle and make a 7-mm-long incision at the same location, inserting the blade deeply into the muscles, but do not enter the joint capsule. Insert the arthroscope cannula with a blunt obturator through the incision and into the joint. On a right hip, insert the spinal needle into the joint at the 5 o'clock position (on the left hip insert the needle at the 7 o'clock position) as an outflow cannula (Fig. 33-74). Explore the joint routinely.

Laboratory Findings

Consistent laboratory abnormalities are not seen.

DIFFERENTIAL DIAGNOSIS

A number of neurologic and orthopedic problems cause similar clinical signs. In younger dogs, lameness caused by panosteitis, osteochondrosis, physeal separation, hypertro-

phic osteodystrophy, and partial or complete CCL injury must be differentiated from hip dysplasia. In older patients, neurologic conditions (cauda equina) and orthopedic conditions (rupture of the CCL, polyarthritis, bone neoplasia) must be ruled out before attributing clinical signs to hip dysplasia.

MEDICAL MANAGEMENT

Treatment depends on the patient's age and degree of discomfort, physical and radiographic findings, and client's expectations and finances. Conservative and surgical options are available for juvenile and mature animals with hip pain secondary to hip dysplasia. Although early surgical intervention may increase the prognosis for long-term acceptable clinical function, approximately 75% of young patients treated conservatively return to acceptable clinical function with maturity. The remainder require further medical or surgical management at some point in life. Surgery is indicated in older patients when conservative treatment is not effective or in young patients when athletic performance is desired or the owner wishes to slow the progression of DJD and enhance the probability of good long-term limb function.

Pain relief and clinical improvement associated with conservative treatment are derived from fibrous proliferation of the joint capsule, which strengthens the capsule and prevents further capsular sprain. Concurrently, increased thickness of the cancellous trabeculae in the subchondral bone strengthens the bony trabeculae and prevents fractures. However, these patients are still afflicted with hip dysplasia and have a diminished surface area of hip joint articulation. Clinical signs that develop as the animal matures are attributable to articular cartilage wear and progressive osteoarthritis. Conservative treatment is divided into short- and long-term phases. Initially, these patients should be treated for an acute sprain. Complete rest is mandatory and must be enforced for 10 to 14 days.

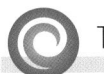 Table 33-11

Rehabilitation Protocol for Osteoarthritis of the Hip Joint

ALL TREATMENTS QID	LAMENESS SCORE 5/5	LAMENESS SCORE 4/5	LAMENESS SCORE 3/5	LAMENESS SCORE 2/5	LAMENESS SCORE 1/5	LAMENESS SCORE 0/5
Heat therapy	10 min	10 min	10 min	10 min	10 min	10 min
Massage	5 min	5 min	5 min	5 min	5 min	5 min
Passive range of motion (repetitions)	15	15	15	15	15	15
Electrical stimulation†	10 min	10 min	10 min	10 min		
Therapeutic exercise-total time	5 min	10 min	15 min	15 min	20 min	20 min
Walk/land treadmill	5 min	10 min	15 min	20 min	20 min	20 min
Balancing	+	+	+	+	+	
Obstacles	+	+	+	+	+	+
Weaving	+	+	+	+	+	+
Circles				+	+	+
Hills					+	+
Stairs						+
Jog/run						+
Underwater treadmill‡	5 min	10 min	15 min	20 min	20 min	20 min
Swimming					5–10 min	5–10 min
Cryotherapy	15 min	15 min	15 min	15 min	15 min	15 min

QID, Four times a day; +, perform modality.
*Passive range of motion to all joints of the affected limb.
†Electrical stimulation to be performed on the semimembranosus/semitendinosus muscle groups in patients with muscle atrophy. See Chapter 12 for specifications.
‡Alternate land treadmill and underwater treadmill during session; do not do both in one session. Do LTM/walk when at home and institute underwater treadmill 2-3 times a week.

Adjunct physical rehabilitation is helpful in maintaining range of motion and providing comfort during this period. Intensive physical rehabilitation should concentrate on strengthening periarticular structures, which can decrease lameness and discomfort. For a sample physical rehabilitation exercise protocol, see Table 33-11. Antiinflammatory drugs are indicated to relieve pain and make administration of physical therapy more tolerable. However, antiinflammatory drugs are likely to make the patient more comfortable, which may make enforcement of rest more difficult. Clients must be advised to continue the rest period even if the patient appears to have returned to normal function.

> NOTE: Be sure to stress to the owners of an animal with an acute injury that they must enforce rest, even if the animal feels like exercising.

A number of NSAIDs are available over-the-counter and through prescriptions. NSAIDs most commonly used in veterinary medicine are presented in Table 33-4 on p. 1149.

Clients should be advised to avoid giving their pets NSAIDs without recommendation of a veterinarian. When administering NSAIDs, begin with the lowest possible therapeutic dosage and administer with small amounts of food.

> NOTE: Administer NSAIDs at the lowest effective dose.

Long-term conservative treatment for pain associated with DJD includes application of the five principles of medical management of osteoarthritis (see p. 1145). Weight management is the single most important aspect of these principles. The animal should be weighed weekly and its caloric intake determined. Feeding bulk diets low in fat and protein may be beneficial. Nutritional supplementation, including omega-3 fatty acids and glucosamine/chondroitin, may be of benefit in many cases. Exercise (e.g., swimming and long walks) is important to maintain an appropriate weight. High-intensity activity should be allowed only for short durations after an adequate warm-up period. Antiinflammatory drugs should be administered only as needed and should not take the place of weight control and a moderate exercise program. Physical rehabilitation may involve sit-to-stand exercises and aquatic therapy, specifically on an underwater treadmill (see Chapter 12).

> NOTE: Stress to owners that weight control is a critical part of managing chronic hip dysplasia. If pain associated with hip dysplasia prevents the animal from exercising normally, the owners should reduce the animal's caloric intake to prevent weight gain.

SURGICAL TREATMENT

In puppies less than 20 weeks of age, **juvenile pubic symphysiodesis** (JPS) may be performed to alter growth of the pelvis and degree of ventroversion of the acetabulum. Most puppies of this age do not show clinical signs of hip dysplasia, so diagnosis depends upon use of a screening technique, such as Penn Hip, to determine which animals may be candidates for the procedure. Although specific criteria for application of JPS have not been developed, puppies under 20 weeks of age that have palpable and radiographic evidence of laxity on a hip distracted view should be considered for the procedure. Risks of complications with the procedure are low and failure of the procedure to reduce hip subluxation does not preclude further surgical treatment in the future.

In immature dogs, a decision must be made early to perform **pelvic osteotomy** for maximum benefits, but this decision must be balanced against the observation that many dogs diagnosed with hip dysplasia at a young age do not have clinical signs at long-term follow-up. Pelvic osteotomy is useful in younger patients to axially rotate and lateralize the acetabulum in an effort to increase dorsal coverage of the femoral head. This procedure is indicated in patients leading athletic lives (i.e., working breeds) or when the client wants to arrest or slow the progress of osteoarthritis. The most favorable prognosis for pubic osteotomy is in patients with (1) radiographic evidence of hip subluxation with minimal degenerative changes in conjunction with (see Fig. 33-72, *A*); (2) an angle of reduction less than 30 degrees and an angle of subluxation less than 10 degrees; (3) a solid feeling of reduction of the femoral head into the acetabulum; and (4) minimal cartilage damage as visualized on hip arthroscopy. The angle of subluxation increases as the acetabular rim is lost to wear. Also, the loss of the acetabular rim can be appreciated as a grating or crepitant feeling as the femoral head slides over the acetabular rim into the acetabulum. The angle of reduction is an indication of the degree of capsular laxity, which increases with increased subluxation of the hip but decreases over time as the capsule becomes thickened with fibrosis. Reduction of the head should produce a solid "clunk." An indistinct reduction indicates filling of the acetabulum. A canine pelvic osteotomy plate is the most effective method of obtaining axial rotation and acetabular lateralization. With this procedure, the amount of axial rotation is set by choosing an angled plate based on previously determined angles of reduction (maximum amount of rotation) and subluxation (minimum degree of rotation). The angle of acetabular rotation commonly used is slightly less than the measured angle of reduction, usually not exceeding 30 degrees. Twenty to 30 degrees of acetabular rotation effectively achieves the maximum increase in articular contact area of the hip. The use of 8 hole TPO plates or double plating may limit implant loosening in larger patients (Fitch et al, 2002).

Total hip replacement (THR) is a highly advanced procedure and should be performed only by experienced surgeons trained in this technique. THR is considered a salvage procedure in that the coxofemoral joint cannot be repaired and so the joint is removed and replaced. Most commonly, THR is performed when medical management of osteoarthritis of the hip can no longer maintain function of the limb and quality of life of the patient. Generally the use of the five principles of medical management should be exhausted before electing THR because of the costs, risks, and complications of the surgery. Traditionally, THR is done as late in life as possible. This philosophy is based on a similar practice in human hip replacement and is based on the concept that a prosthetic joint replacement is in a constant state of degeneration and placement as late in life as possible diminishes the potential need to revise or replace the original hip prosthesis. Some owners and surgeons may elect hip replacement instead of medical management for patients with significant complications from NSAIDs or for clients who are extremely concerned with potential complications from NSAIDS. The advent of cementless THRs has also altered the philosophy of when THR is indicated. Since cementless prostheses are much less inclined to loosen with time, their use in younger patients is more common and acceptable. At a minimum, THR should be delayed until body weight reduction is attempted, particularly in obese patients. Correction of body weight may eliminate or delay the need for THR and will decrease the risks of complications when THR is performed.

Contraindications to THR include septic arthritis and significant or progressive neurologic disease. Sepsis of the coxofemoral joint, although rare, is an absolute contraindication to cemented THR. Cementless THRs have been used for the revision of septic loosening of cemented THRs.

Implant designs. Canine THRs are broadly divided into cemented and cementless designs (Fig. 33-75). Cemented THRs (Fig. 33-76) have been used significantly longer in dogs than cementless designs. The cement serves as a mortar between the implant and the bone. Medical grade bone cement is polymethylmethacrylate (PMMA) and bonds as a cohesive versus an adhesive (i.e., it locks into irregularities in the implant and bone versus forming a chemical bond). Most contemporary cemented implants are modular, meaning that they have interchangeable parts, allowing the surgeon to adjust stem size, neck length, head diameter, and cup size to fit the individual patient. Generally the preparation of the bone (acetabulum and femur) is simpler with a

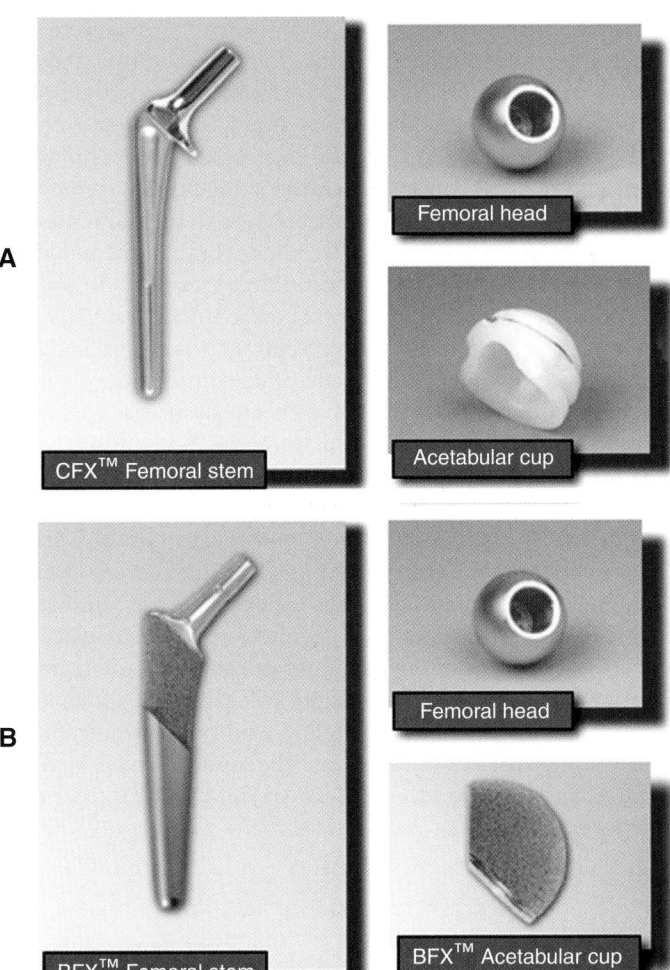

FIG. 33-75
A, Cemented canine THR implants. **B,** Cementless canine THR implants.

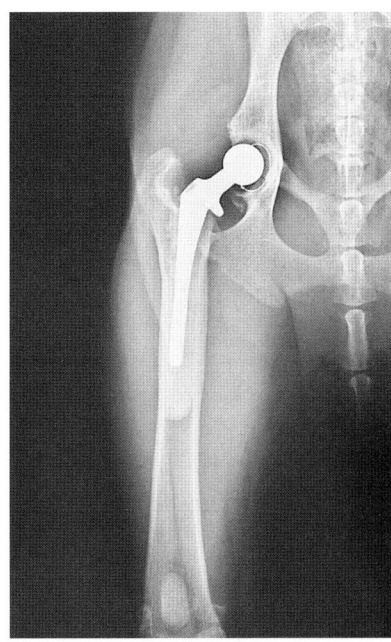

FIG. 33-76
Radiograph of a dog after cemented THR. Note the radiopaque cement mantel surrounding the femoral and acetabular prostheses.

cemented THR than a cementless THR. The use of cement, however, requires strict attention to asepsis, handling characteristics, and implant positioning. Cemented THRs are generally strongest within 2 days of implantation, but then may weaken and loosen over time because the cement cannot adapt to changes in the bone or alteration of loads.

Cementless THRs (see Fig. 33-75) are either press fit–ingrowth or stabilized by monocortical screws. All canine cementless acetabular cups are press fit–ingrowth meaning that initial stabilization is achieved by impacting the cup into an acetabular bed that has been prepared to have a smaller diameter than the cup, resulting in very high friction between the cup and bone after it has been forced (impacted) into the bone bed. Long-term stabilization is achieved by bone growth into the shell of the cup. Most canine THR cups include a metallic shell and a polyethylene liner. The shell is designed to encourage bone ingrowth that locks the implant in place.

The femoral component of cementless THRs is initially stabilized, either by press fit or monocortical screws, into the medial femoral cortex. Reports on the long-term outcome of both these designs is limited and selection between the two designs is based primarily on surgeon preference and experience. In either case, long-term stabilization is achieved by bony ingrowth into the implant or around the screws.

Implant selection is based primarily on surgeon preference and experience. Development of cementless implants was based primarily on concern regarding aseptic loosening in cemented implants. For surgeons using both cemented and cementless varieties, age often plays a major role in the decision-making process. Older patients often receive cemented implants, as their limited life expectancy and lower level of activity suggest that the cemented implant will outlast the patients' lifetime. Older patients may also have slower rates of bone ingrowth and a higher risk of fracture with cementless implants. Younger patients are more appropriate for cementless implants because their higher bone metabolism may result in more rapid and secure bone ingrowth, whereas their longer life expectancy and higher activity levels may lead to aseptic loosening of cemented THRs.

In general, bone preparation for cemented THRs is less exacting than that for press fit cementless THRs. Because the cement serves as a mortar between the implant and the bone, the acetabulum and femoral canal do not need to be prepared as precisely, whereas with a press fit implant, the implant must fit precisely to prevent implant migration during the initial period before bone ingrowth. Cementless femoral components relying on screw fixation also do not require as exacting preparation of the femoral canal as do press fit cementless designs.

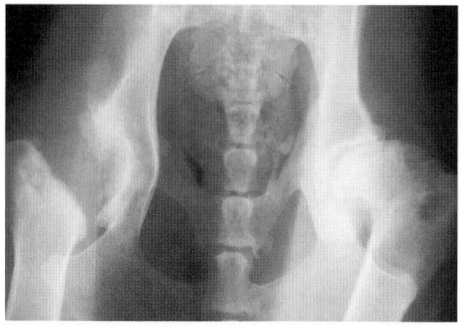

FIG. 33-77
Radiograph of a dog after femoral head and neck ostectomy. Note the complete removal of the femoral neck.

Cement preparation requires thorough understanding of the chemistry and mechanics of bone cement. Issues of temperature, hardening rates, and handling characteristics are critical to successful cemented THRs. The complexities of PMMA and the inability to modify the cement after hardening are other reasons for the increased popularity of cementless implants.

Femoral head and neck excision limits bony contact between the femoral head and acetabulum and allows formation of a fibrous false joint (Fig. 33-77). This procedure can be used when conservative treatment has failed, and when financial, medical, or size constraints preclude alternative methods of surgical intervention. Caution should be used in treating juvenile animals with this procedure because a significant percentage of them improve with maturity. Because fibrous pseudoarthrosis is an unstable joint, clinical function postoperatively is unpredictable. For this reason, most surgeons consider femoral head and neck excision to be a salvage procedure. However, many patients with painful arthritic hips undergoing femoral head and neck excision have improved limb function and quality of life postoperatively. There are no specific weight guidelines for the use of femoral head and neck ostectomy (FHO). Although smaller patients routinely have better results than larger patients, this procedure may yet be indicated in large- and giant-breed dogs in which other treatments have been ineffective or are not feasible.

Preoperative Management

A complete orthopedic and neurologic examination should be performed to correctly attribute the clinical problem to hip dysplasia. Perioperative systemic antibiotics should be administered when pelvic osteotomy or THR is performed.

Anesthesia

Dogs treated with pubic symphysiodesis or pelvic osteotomy are generally young and healthy and can be anesthetized with a variety of protocols. Older dogs treated with THR or femoral head and neck excision should be carefully evaluated and the anesthetic protocol altered if necessary. Epidural administration of analgesics (see Chapter 13) preoperatively is useful for lowering the anesthetic dose requirement and for reducing postoperative discomfort.

Surgical Anatomy

Surgical anatomy of the hip joint is discussed on p. 1099. Special anatomic considerations for pubic symphysiodesis include identification of the pubic symphysis and protection of the urethra and colon. Special anatomic considerations for pelvic osteotomy include identifying the pectineus muscle as a landmark for the ventral approach to the pubis and avoiding the obturator nerve at the caudal limit of the pubic osteotomy. Surgical anatomy encountered during the approach to the iliac body is described on p. 1093. It is important to protect the sciatic nerve ventral to the iliac body during the osteotomy. Special anatomic considerations for FHO are important in patients with hip dysplasia. In patients with atrophied hip musculature, the joint capsule is obvious as soon as the deep gluteal muscle is reflected. If subluxation of the hip joint is moderate or severe, the joint capsule usually appears thickened and bulges outward. In mature patients, thickening of the joint capsule is even more pronounced. To obtain adequate exposure of the femoral head and neck, the vastus lateralis muscle must be released and reflected ventrally. The femoral head and neck often are short and deformed. To perform an FHO in these patients, the juncture of the femoral neck and femoral shaft must be clearly visualized. In young patients, the round ligament may be intact and must be severed; the ligament usually is absent in older patients.

> NOTE: Before performing pelvic osteotomy, review the relationship between the gluteal musculature and iliacus muscle, the position of the sciatic nerve, and the course of the internal pudendal artery and nerve (see p. 1099).

Positioning

The patient is positioned in dorsal recumbency for pubic symphysiodesis. The patient is positioned in lateral recumbency for hip arthroscopy or pelvic osteotomy. Clip and prepare the leg for aseptic surgery from the midline to the tarsal joint on both medial and lateral limb surfaces. For femoral head and neck excision, the patient is positioned in lateral recumbency and the area from the dorsal midline to the stifle is clipped and prepared for aseptic surgery. The patient should be draped in a manner that allows manipulation of the limb during surgery (see p. 36).

SURGICAL TECHNIQUE
Juvenile Pubic Symphysiodesis

In many cases, the patient is spayed or neutered at the same time. The surgical incision should be adjusted as necessary to combine the two procedures. For female dogs, spay them first and then extend the incision over the pubis and perform JPS before closing the abdomen. This enables palpation in the pelvis. In male dogs, perform JPS first as it is a cleaner surgery than the neuter.

With the patient in dorsal recumbency, make a ventral midline incision over the pubic symphysis. In male dogs, make

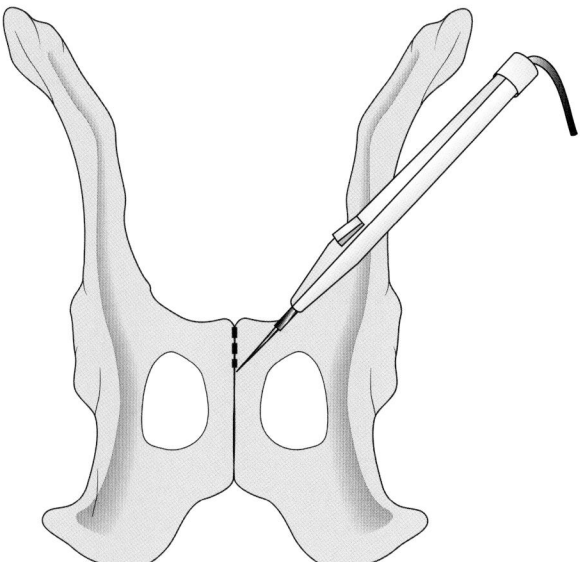

FIG. 33-78
Expose the pubic symphysis with a ventral midline incision over the pubis. Using a spatula electrode set at 40 watts, perform ablation by placing the electrode against the symphysis for approximately 10 seconds, repeating every 2 to 3 mm along the symphysis.

the skin incision parallel to the penis, extending from the scrotum to 3 cm cranial to the pubis. Incise subcutaneous fascia, and ligate any collateral branches of the pudendal artery and vein. Retract the penis past midline. Expose the pubic symphysis by incision of the deep fascia followed by subperiosteal elevation of the adductor and gracilis muscles. Introduce a thin ribbon malleable retractor or finger into the pelvic canal to protect the rectum and urethra from thermal injury (Fig. 33-78). Using a spatula electrode set at 40 watts, perform ablation by placing the electrode against the symphysis for approximately 10 seconds, repeating every 2 to 3 mm along the symphysis. Perform the ablation primarily on the cranial half of the symphysis.

Alternatively, a needle electrode or metal needle may be inserted into the symphysis every 2 to 3 mm using 40 watts for up to 30 seconds.

Perform routine closure in layers starting with reapposition of the adductor and gracilis muscles across the pubic symphysis.

Pelvic Osteotomy

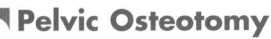

Pelvic osteotomy requires that an incision be made through the pubic brim, ischial floor, and iliac body. The optimum position for pubic osteotomy is adjacent to the medial wall of the acetabulum.

With the patient in lateral recumbency, abduct the leg while keeping the femur perpendicular to the acetabulum. Locate the origin of the pectineus muscle, and center a 6-cm skin incision over this point. Incise the subcutaneous tissue to

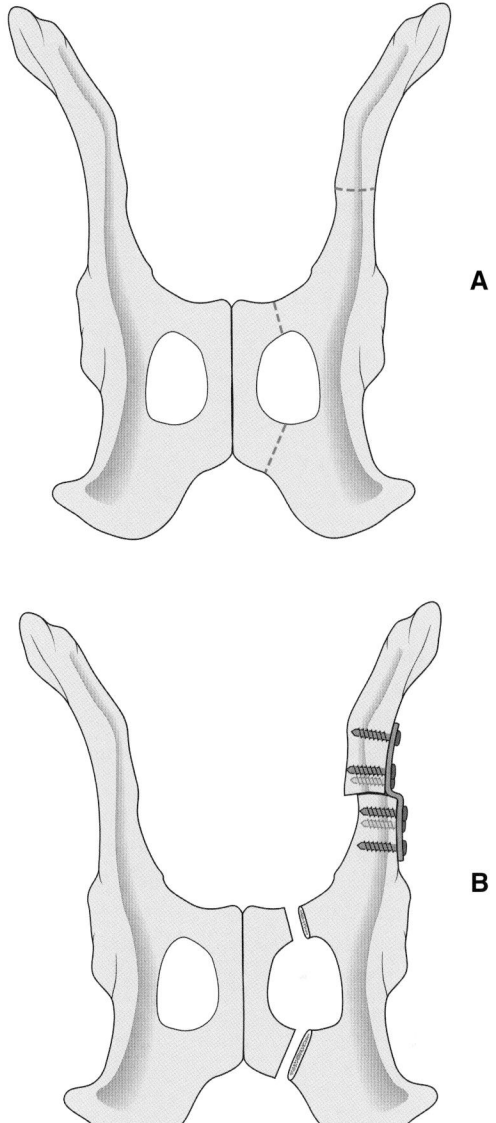

FIG. 33-79
A, Position of osteotomies for completion of a TPO and **(B)** stabilization with a bone plate. Note the axial rotation and lateralization of the hemipelvis.

further isolate the origin of the pectineus muscle at the iliopectineal eminence. Release the origin of the pectineus muscle to expose the cranial brim of the pubis.

The pectineus muscle may be allowed to retract or may be resected.

Reflect the periosteum from the cranial, lateral, and caudal pubic surfaces. To protect soft tissue during the osteotomy, place spoon Hohmann retractors cranial to the pubis and within the obturator foramen caudally. Perform a pubic osteotomy adjacent to the medial wall of the acetabulum (Fig. 33-79). As an alternative, ostectomize a portion of the pubis. Suture soft tissue and skin using standard methods.

Next, perform an osteotomy of the ischial floor. Make a skin incision midway between the medial prominence of the ischium and the lateral tuberosity. Make the incision in the vertical plane, beginning 4 cm proximal to the ischial floor and extending 3 cm distally. Incise the subcutaneous tissue and deep fascia. Make a 3-cm incision through the periosteal insertion of the internal obturator muscle at the dorsal crest of the ischial floor. Elevate the internal obturator muscle cranially to the obturator foramen. Then incise the periosteal origin of the external obturator muscle at the ventral crest of the ischial floor and reflect the muscle from the ventral surface of the ischium cranially to the obturator foramen. Place two spoon Hohmann retractors to protect the soft tissue; insert one into the obturator foramen dorsally and one into the foramen ventrally. Direct an osteotome caudal to cranial in line with the center of the Hohmann retractors; this centers the osteotomy line into the obturator foramen. As an alternative, use a reciprocating saw to perform the osteotomy. Close the incision after the osteotomy of the ilium is completed. At that time, if desired, drill two small holes on either side of the osteotomy adjacent to each other. Place orthopedic wire through the holes and twist them in a figure-eight fashion to stabilize the osteotomy. Suture the fascia of the internal obturator muscle to that of the external obturator muscle, then close the subcutaneous tissue and skin using standard methods.

Perform an osteotomy of the ilium to allow axial rotation of the acetabulum. Make an incision from the cranial extent of the iliac crest caudally 1 to 2 cm beyond the greater trochanter. Center the incision over the ventral third of the iliac wing. Incise the subcutaneous tissues and gluteal fat along the same line to visualize the intermuscular septum between the superficial gluteal muscle and the short part of the tensor fasciae latae muscle. Incise the muscular septum to separate the tensor fasciae latae muscle and middle gluteal muscle cranially and the tensor fasciae latae and superficial gluteal muscles caudally. Cranially, use sharp dissection to separate the middle gluteal muscle and long head of the tensor fasciae latae muscle. Palpate the ventral border of the ilium and make an incision to the bone near the ventral insertion of the middle and deep gluteal muscles. Isolate and ligate the iliolumbar vessels and reflect the deep gluteal muscle from the lateral surface of the ilium. Incise the origin of the iliacus muscle at the ventral border of the ilium and reflect the muscle from the ventral surface. Elevate the periosteum from the medial surface of the ilium with a periosteal elevator. Place two spoon Hohmann retractors to protect soft tissue during the osteotomy; place one medial to the ilium to reflect the iliacus muscle and one over the dorsal crest of the ilium to retract the gluteal muscle mass. Judge the cranial position of the osteotomy by placing the osteotomy plate such that the most caudal plate hole is 1 to 2 cm cranial to the acetabulum. Perform the iliac osteotomy with an oscillating saw titled 20% cranially to a line perpendicular to the long axis of the hemipelvis. Lateralize the caudal segment with bone-holding forceps, and secure an appropriate osteotomy plate to this segment. Next, reduce the osteotomy and apply plate screws in the cranial segment. If the cranial plate screws penetrate the sacrum, they should penetrate well within the sacrum

to prevent premature screw loosening. Remove the sharp spike of ilium dorsal to the plate, fragment it, and use it as bone graft at the osteotomy site. To close the incision, place sutures between the fascia of the middle gluteal muscle and that of the tensor fasciae latae muscle cranially and between the superficial gluteal muscle and the tensor fasciae latae caudally. Approximate the gluteal fascia and tensor fasciae latae, subcutaneous tissue, and skin, using standard methods.

Femoral Head and Neck Ostectomy

Make a craniolateral approach to the hip joint and luxate the hip. If the round ligament is intact, incise it.

Incising the round ligament is facilitated by placing lateral traction on the greater trochanter with bone-holding forceps and subluxating the femoral head. This allows curved scissors to be placed into the joint to cut the ligament.

Perform the ostectomy by externally rotating the limb to where the joint line of the stifle is parallel to the operating table. Identify the line of ostectomy perpendicular to the operating table at the junction of the femoral neck and the femoral metaphysis (Fig. 33-80). To ensure the accuracy of the bony cut, predrill a series of three or more holes along the line of the ostectomy. Use an osteotome and mallet to complete the cut. As an alternative, it may be easier to perform the ostectomy with an oscillating saw.

Ventral reflection of the vastus lateralis muscle facilitates proper placement of an osteotome or saw blade during this procedure.

Once the femoral neck and head have been removed, palpate the cut surface of the femoral neck for irregularities.

The most common finding is a shelf of femoral neck left on the caudal surface of the femur.

Remove any edges with rongeurs. Suture the joint capsule over the acetabulum if possible. To close, suture the vastus lateralis and deep gluteal muscles, tensor fasciae latae, subcutaneous tissue, and skin using standard methods.

SUTURE MATERIALS AND SPECIAL INSTRUMENTS

A 2.7-mm-long arthroscope is necessary for hip arthroscopy. An electrocautery unit is necessary for JPS. An oscillating saw, reciprocating saw, or osteotome and mallet, self-retaining retractors, Hohmann retractors, and instrumentation for insertion of a bone plate and screws are necessary for pelvic osteotomy. FHO requires an osteotome and mallet or oscillating saw.

POSTOPERATIVE CARE AND ASSESSMENT

No restrictions are necessary after diagnostic hip arthroscopy. After prepubic symphysiodesis, the puppy should be restricted until skin sutures are removed. After that time,

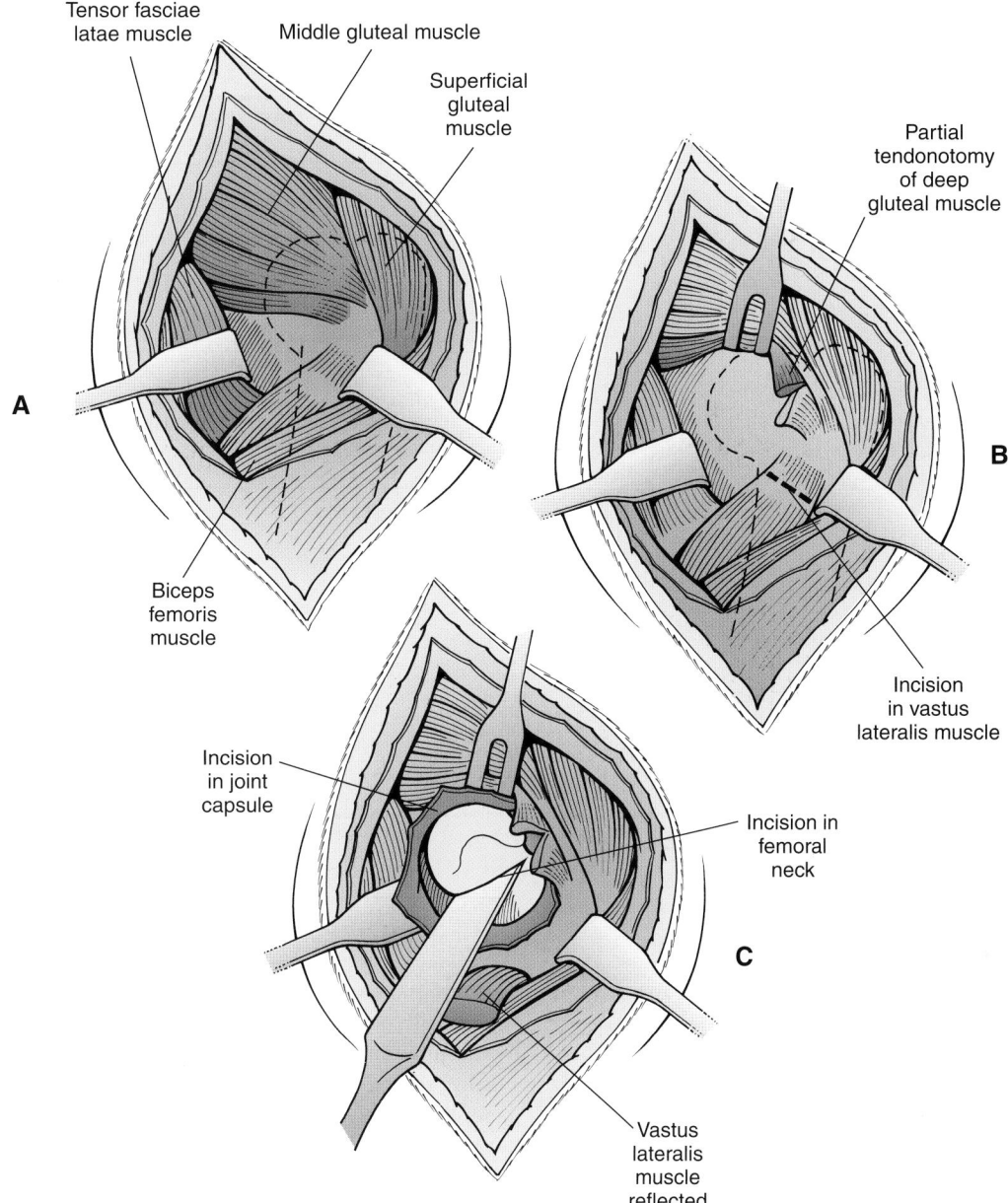

FIG. 33-80
To expose the femoral head for ostectomy, make a craniolateral skin incision centered over the hip joint. **A,** Retract the biceps femoris muscle caudally and the tensor fasciae latae muscle cranially. **B,** Incise the vastus lateralis muscle and reflect it ventrally. **C,** Incise the joint capsule and perform the ostectomy by externally rotating the limb such that the joint line of the stifle is parallel to the operating table. Identify the line of ostectomy perpendicular to the operating table at the junction of the femoral neck and femoral metaphysis.

no special postoperative care is required. Determination of the efficacy of the procedure may be made by follow-up radiographs at skeletal maturity; however, accurate determination of the effectiveness of the procedure in inducing ventroversion requires CT. Complications are rare and include damage to the urethra or colon or failure to achieve symphysiodesis.

After pelvic osteotomy, the patient should be restricted to leash exercise until radiographic evidence of healing of the osteotomies is complete, generally in 6 weeks. The duration of exercise (leash walks) should be increased gradually according to the patient's tolerance. If the contralateral side is to have surgical treatment, the second surgery should be performed when discomfort associated with the first surgery is well tolerated by the dog. Reported complications include implant failure, loss of limb abduction, and pelvic outlet narrowing. However, the incidence of complications is low, and reports of long-term clinical function are good to excel-

Table 33-12

Rehabilitation Protocol Following TPO, THR, Hip Luxation

ALL TREATMENTS BID	DAY 0 TO DAY 14	DAY 15 TO DAY 24	DAY 25 UNTIL HEALED	HEALED TO RETURN TO FUNCTION
Heat therapy		10 min	10 min	
Massage	5 min	5 min	5 min	
Electrical stimulation†	10 min	10 min	10 min	10 min
Therapeutic exercise-total time	5 min	10 min	15 min	25–45 min
Walk/land treadmill	5 min	5 min	5	>10 min
Balancing	+	+	+	+
Obstacles			+	+
Weaving				+
Circles				+
Hills				+
Stairs				+
Jog/run				+
Underwater treadmill		5 min	15 min	>15 min
Swimming				5–10 min
Cryotherapy	15 min	15 min	15 min	PRN

BID, Twice a day; +, perform modality; *PRN,* as needed.
*Electrical stimulation to the semimembranosus/semitendinosus. See Chapter 12 for further specifications.

lent. Recommendations for physical therapy following TPO are provided in Table 33-12.

Early active use of the limb is beneficial after FHO. A recommended physical therapy protocol for FHO patients is provided in Table 33-13. Good return of active limb function depends on the length of time the pathologic hip joint condition was present and on the severity of the degenerative changes. Patients with chronic disease (muscle atrophy and proliferative DJD) are slower to return to function than patients with acute lameness.

COMPLICATIONS

Complications of canine THR vary with the type of implant placed. Complications that are common to all designs include luxation, infection, and aseptic loosening. The incidence of luxation after canine THR is approximately 5%. Luxations may be due to intrinsic laxity of the hip, preexisting luxation, incorrect implant selection or positioning, or trauma. Treatments for luxation include closed reduction and sling application, open reduction with surgical stabilization (see section on hip luxation), implant modification (alteration of cup position, neck lengthening), or implant removal.

Infection is a more significant problem with cemented THRs than cementless THRs; cement appears to be more easily colonized by bacteria than metallic implants. Most surgeons mix antibiotic powder with the bone cement; how-

ever, this does not prevent infection in a small percentage of cases. Treatment of septic loosening in cemented THRs invariably requires removal of the implants and cement to resolve the infection; however, some cases have been treated by replacement of the infected cemented prosthesis with a cementless design. The incidence and specific treatment of infection of cementless THRs have not been reported.

Aseptic loosening of cemented THRs may occur on the acetabular or femoral side or both (Fig. 33-81). The cause for aseptic loosening of cemented implants may be either biomechanical or cytologic. Biomechanical causes occur when bone remodeling leads to loosening of the cement bone interface or when cement cracking initiates loosening between the cement and the bone. Cytologic causes are usually initiated by wear particles of polyethylene, metal, or rarely, cement, which cause macrophage migration and up-regulation of bone resorption. Aseptic loosening of cemented THRs usually occurs years after implantation, but rarely can occur within months of implantation.

Aseptic loosening of cementless implants most commonly occurs during the press fit stage of stabilization. Acetabular implants may rotate or avulse out of the bony bed. Femoral press fit components may rotate or subside and may lead to severe fractures of the femoral diaphysis. Femoral screw fixation components may avulse from the medial wall, or fractures may occur through the screw holes or access

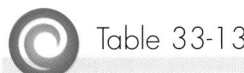

Table 33-13

Physical Rehabilitation Following Femoral Head and Neck Ostectomy

ALL TREATMENTS BID	DAY 1 TO DAY 14	DAY 15 TO DAY 24	DAY 25 UNTIL HEALED	HEALED TO RETURN TO FUNCTION
Heat therapy		10 min	10 min	
Massage	5 min	5 min	5 min	
Passive range of motion (repetitions)	15*	15*	15*	15*
Electrical stimulation†	10 min	10 min	10 min	10 min
Therapeutic exercise-total time	15 min	25 min	30 min	25–45 min
Walk/land treadmill	5 min	10 min	10 min	>10 min
Balancing	+	+	+	+
Obstacles	+	+	+	+
Weaving	+	+	+	+
Circles		+	+	+
Hills		+	+	+
Stairs			+	+
Jog/run			+	+
Underwater treadmill	10 min	15 min	20 min	>25 min
Swimming	5 min	10 min	15 min	20 min
Cryotherapy	15 min	15 min	15 min	PRN

BID, Twice a day; +, perform modality; *PRN*, as needed.
*Perform passive range of motion to all joints of the affected limb.
†Electrical stimulation to be performed on the semimembranosus/semitendinosus muscle groups in patients with muscle atrophy. See Chapter 12 for specifications.

holes. The incidence of delayed loosening of cementless implants has not been reported, but appears to be low.

Results after FHO vary. The prognosis is highly dependent on the patient's size and on postoperative physical therapy. In large patients, approximately 50% of animals have good or excellent function. The remainder have varying degrees of lameness, but function usually is improved compared with the preoperative status. Medium and small patients usually have good or excellent limb function.

PROGNOSIS

Prognosis after JPS is determined by the age of treatment and severity of the dysplasia. Dogs treated after 20 weeks of age have a poor prognosis for increased ventroversion. The degree of ventroversion in dogs treated before 20 weeks is variable and somewhat unpredictable.

Prognosis after pelvic osteotomy is largely determined by case selection. Best results are obtained in patients with acceptable physical findings (see previous discussion) and few or no degenerative changes. Long-term function is good to excellent. Although degenerative changes are radiographically evident after this procedure, they are less than what would be expected without surgery.

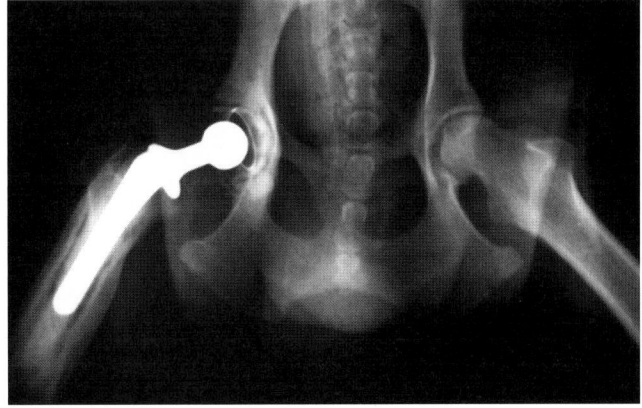

FIG. 33-81
Radiograph of aseptic loosening of a cemented THR.

THR results in excellent return to normal function unless complications occur. Reported rates of successful outcomes of cemented THRs vary from 75 to 95 percent (Braden et al, 2004). Outcomes of cementless THRs have not been adequately reported to date. In the majority of cases, the outcome of THR is either complete resolution of lameness or failure of the technique, resulting in implant explantation. In a small percentage of cases there may be chronic lameness following THR.

References

Braden TD, Olivier NB, Blaiset MA et al: Objective evaluation of total hip replacement in 127 dogs utilizing force plate analysis, *Vet Comp Orthop Traum* 17:78, 2004.

Fitch RB, Kerwin G, Hosgood G et al: Radiographic evaluation and comparison of triple pelvic osteotomy with and without additional ventral plate stabilization in forty dogs-part I, *Vet Comp Orthop Traum* 15:164, 2002.

Holsworth IG, Schulz KS, Kass PH et al: Comparison of arthroscopic and radiographic abnormalities in the hip joints of juvenile dogs with hip dysplasia, *J Am Vet Med Assoc* 227:1087, 2005.

Suggested Reading

Dueland RT, Adams WM, Fialkowski JP et al: Effects of pubic symphysiodesis in dysplastic puppies, *Vet Surg* 30:201, 2001.

This paper describes the mechanics and physiology of JPS in the treatment of juvenile hip dysplasia.

Holsworth IG, Schulz KS, Kass PH et al: Comparison of arthroscopic and radiographic abnormalities in the hip joints of juvenile dogs with hip dysplasia, *J Am Vet Med Assoc* 227:1087, 2005.

This article describes the technique of hip arthroscopy and the clinical findings in a large population of juvenile dogs with hip dysplasia. Arthroscopy was shown to be much more accurate than radiography in the assessment of osteoarthritis.

Patricelli AJ, Dueland RT, Adams WM et al: Juvenile pubic symphysiodesis in dysplastic puppies at 15 and 20 weeks of age, *Vet Surg* 31:435, 2002.

This paper evaluates the effectiveness of JPS at varying ages to determine its effectiveness.

Schulz KS: Application of arthroplasty principles to canine cemented total hip replacement, *Vet Surg* 29:578, 2000.

This review article describes the principles of cemented THR.

Schulz KS, Dejardin LM: Surgical treatment of canine hip dysplasia. In Slatter D, editor: *Textbook of small animal surgery*, ed 3, Philadelphia, 2003, Saunders.

This chapter provides a detailed description of the surgical management of canine hip dysplasia.

Simmons S, Johnson AL, Schaeffer DR: Risk factors for screw migration after triple pelvic osteotomy, *J Am Anim Hosp Assoc* 37:269, 2001.

This paper explores the causes of screw loosening in TPO.

Skurla K, Egger EL, Schwarz PD et al: Owner assessment of the outcome of total hip arthroplasty in dogs, *J Am Vet Med Assoc* 217:1010, 2000.

This paper reports the results of owner surveys on the outcomes of cemented THR in dogs.

Tomlinson JL, Cook JL: Effects of degree of acetabular rotation after triple pelvic osteotomy on the position of the femoral head in relationship to the acetabulum, *Vet Surg* 31:398, 2002.

This paper demonstrates the benefit of the degree of rotation of the acetabulum in TPO, suggesting that 20 degrees of rotation is usually the most appropriate.

COXOFEMORAL LUXATION

DEFINITION

Coxofemoral or **hip luxation** is a traumatic displacement of the femoral head from the acetabulum.

GENERAL CONSIDERATIONS AND CLINICALLY RELEVANT PATHOPHYSIOLOGY

Coxofemoral luxation typically results in craniodorsal displacement of the femoral head relative to the acetabulum. Most affected animals have sustained trauma, such as motor vehicle accidents. Ventrocaudal displacements, in which the femoral head may lodge within the obturator foramen, occur less often. This type of luxation may be associated with fracture of the greater trochanter. Spontaneous luxation has been described and carries a poor prognosis (Trostel et al, 2000). The amount of soft tissue damage surrounding the hip joint depends on the trauma incurred. The round ligament of the femoral head always fails completely; it may be an interstitial rupture or an avulsion of the ligament from the fovea capitis. The fibrous joint capsule must also be completely torn to permit dislocation of the femoral head. The tear in the joint capsule may be a small rent through which the femoral head is dislodged, or complete fraying of the entire capsule may occur.

Hip luxation should be treated as quickly as possible to prevent continued damage of the soft tissue surrounding the hip joint and degeneration of articular cartilage. Articular cartilage derives its nutrients from synovial fluid, which is pumped into the matrix during normal articular movement. Early reduction allows rapid return of the nutrient source of the articular cartilage. Because coxofemoral luxations usually are associated with trauma, as many as half of these patients have a major injury in addition to the hip luxation. A careful physical examination should be performed before induction of anesthesia and treatment of the luxated hip to identify concurrent trauma.

> **NOTE:** Early reduction of luxated hips is essential. Do not delay in treating these animals.

DIAGNOSIS

Clinical Presentation

Signalment. Any age or breed and either gender of dog or cat may be affected.

History. Affected animals usually show a unilateral non–weight-bearing lameness. The traumatic episode may or may not be witnessed by the owner.

Physical Examination Findings

Animals with hip luxation usually are presented for evaluation of a non–weight-bearing lameness associated with trauma. When the femur is displaced craniodorsally, the limb is carried adducted, with the stifle externally rotated (Fig. 33-82). When it is displaced caudoventrally, the limb is carried abducted, with the stifle internally rotated. Manipulation of the limb causes crepitus or pain. A palpable lack of symmetry is noted between the tuber ischii and greater trochanter on the affected side compared with the normal limb. With craniodorsal displacement, the greater trochanter is dorsal to an imaginary line drawn from the crest of the ilium to the tuber ischii, and the distance between the tuber ischii and

greater trochanter is greater than in the normal limb (Fig. 33-83). With a ventrocaudal luxation, the greater trochanter is displaced ventrally, and the space between the tuber ischii and greater trochanter may be narrowed. Hip luxation also causes limb length discrepancy. Craniodorsal luxations cause the affected limb to be shorter than the normal limb, whereas the opposite is true with ventral luxations.

Diagnostic Imaging

Diagnosis of hip luxation should be confirmed with ventrodorsal and lateral radiographs (Fig. 33-84). Before a treatment method is chosen, radiographs should be carefully evaluated for evidence of avulsion of the fovea capitis, associated hip joint fractures, and degenerative changes secondary to hip dysplasia.

Laboratory Findings

Consistent laboratory abnormalities are not seen.

DIFFERENTIAL DIAGNOSIS

Differential diagnoses include acute subluxation or luxation of the hip joint secondary to hip dysplasia, femoral capital physeal fracture, femoral neck fracture, and acetabular fracture.

MEDICAL MANAGEMENT

Coxofemoral luxation may be managed with closed manipulation to replace the femoral head within the acetabulum or with open surgical manipulation. Closed reduction should be attempted before open reduction in most animals, unless there is radiographic evidence of hip dysplasia or a fracture. The animal should be anesthetized for a closed reduction.

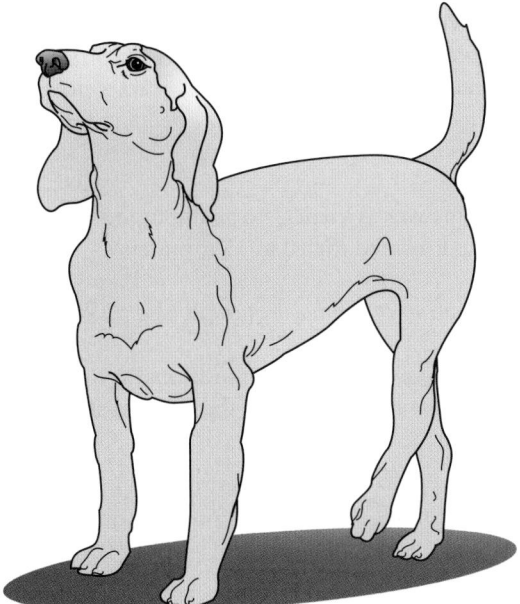

FIG. 33-82
Typical carriage of the limb in a patient with a craniodorsal coxofemoral luxation. Note the position of the paw beneath the body and the external rotation of the stifle.

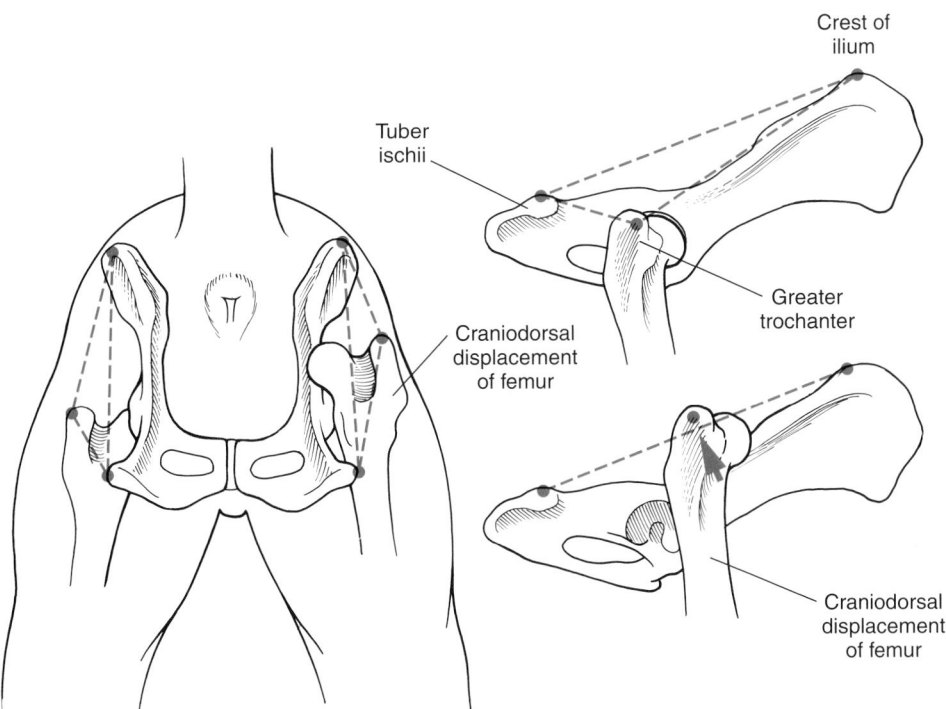

FIG. 33-83
With craniodorsal displacement of the femur, the greater trochanter is dorsal to an imaginary line drawn from the crest of the ilium to the tuber ischii, and the distance between the tuber ischii and the greater trochanter is greater than in the normal limb.

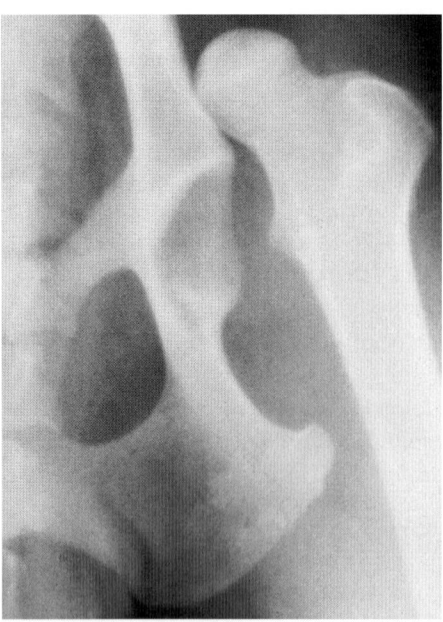

FIG. 33-84
Ventrodorsal radiograph of an animal with a craniodorsal coxofemoral luxation.

Closed Reduction of a Craniodorsal Luxation

Place the patient in lateral recumbency under general anesthesia. Place a rope in the groin of the affected limb, over the back, and secure it to the table to provide resistance. Grasp the affected limb with one hand near the tarsal joint and place the other hand on the greater trochanter to direct the proximal femur (Fig. 33-85, A). Externally rotate the limb, and pull it distally to position the femoral head over the acetabulum (Fig. 33-85, B). When the femoral head lies lateral to the acetabulum, internally rotate the limb to seat the femoral head within the acetabulum (Fig. 33-85, C). Apply medial pressure to the greater trochanter while flexing and extending the joint to help expel debris from the acetabular cup.

This maneuver is critical to maintaining reduction and should be performed for 10 to 15 minutes.

Place the limb in an Ehmer bandage (see p. 949).

If the hip is very stable, or if the animal's conformation or multiple limb trauma prohibits the use of a sling, cage confinement may be adequate.

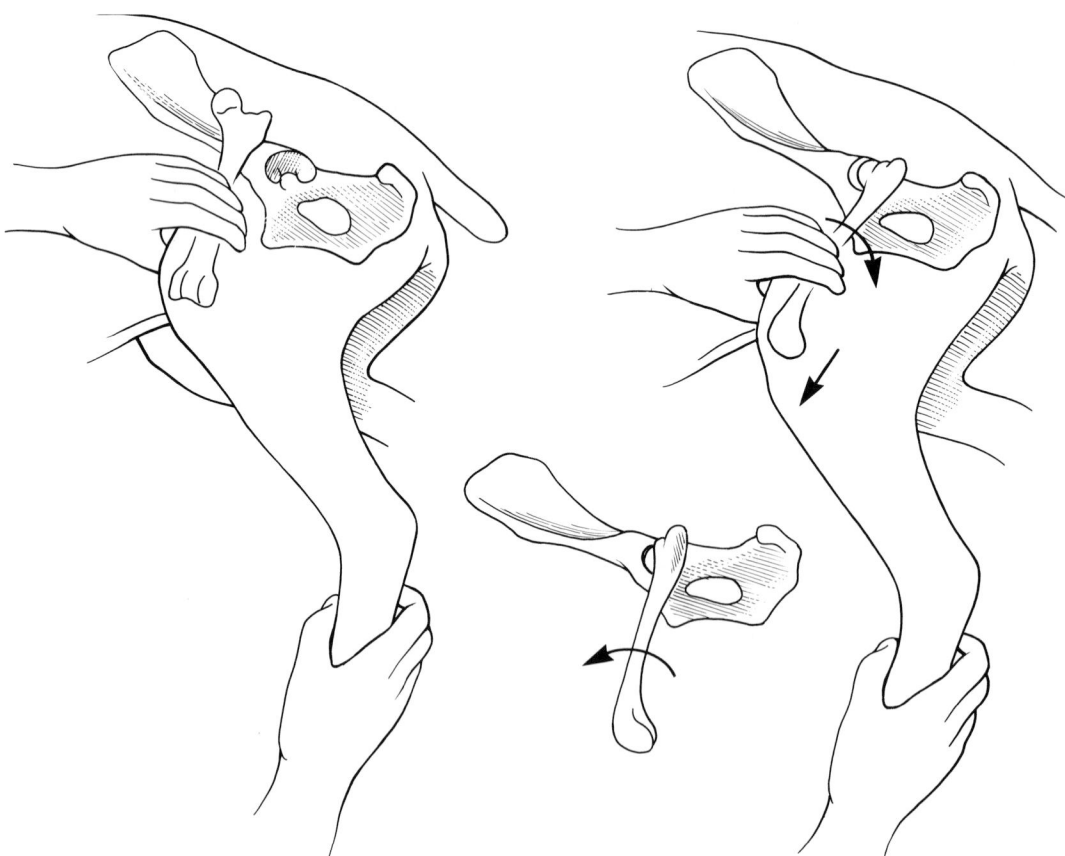

FIG. 33-85
Closed reduction of a craniodorsal hip luxation. **A,** Grasp the affected limb near the tarsus with one hand and place the other hand under the limb against the body wall to provide resistance. **B,** Externally rotate the limb and pull it caudally to position the femoral head over the acetabulum. **C,** When the femoral head lies lateral to the acetabulum, internally rotate the limb to seat the femoral head within the acetabulum.

Limit the animal to cage confinement and controlled activity on a leash until the bandage is removed in 4 to 7 days. After removal of the bandage, limit activity to controlled leash walking for an additional 2 weeks.

Closed Reduction of a Caudoventral Luxation

Place the patient in lateral recumbency with the limb held perpendicular to the spine. Grasp the limb near the tarsal joint with one hand, and place the other hand to stabilize the body (Fig. 33-86, A). Place traction on the limb while simultaneously abducting the leg to pull the femoral head beyond the medial rim of the acetabulum (Fig. 33-86, B). Once the femoral head has cleared the acetabular rim, exert lateral pressure to position the femoral head lateral to the acetabulum. Push proximally and allow the femoral head to fall into the acetabulum (Fig. 33-86, C). After reduction, place the patient in hobbles to prevent abduction

of the limb. Limit activity to controlled walking on a leash until the bandage is removed in 4 to 7 days. Limit activity to leash walking for an additional 2 weeks after the hobbles have been removed.

SURGICAL TREATMENT

Open reduction is indicated with avulsion of the fovea capitis or when closed reduction has failed to reduce the hip or maintain hip reduction. The hip joint should be explored to assess the soft tissue injury and the likelihood of maintaining reduction with a reconstructive procedure. If stability of the hip joint can be achieved through a reconstructive procedure, there are a number of techniques from which to choose. If no reasonable chance exists of maintaining long-term reduction after a stabilization procedure, an alternate procedure must be considered, such as a femoral head and neck ostectomy (see p. 1242) or THR (Pozzi et al, 2004).

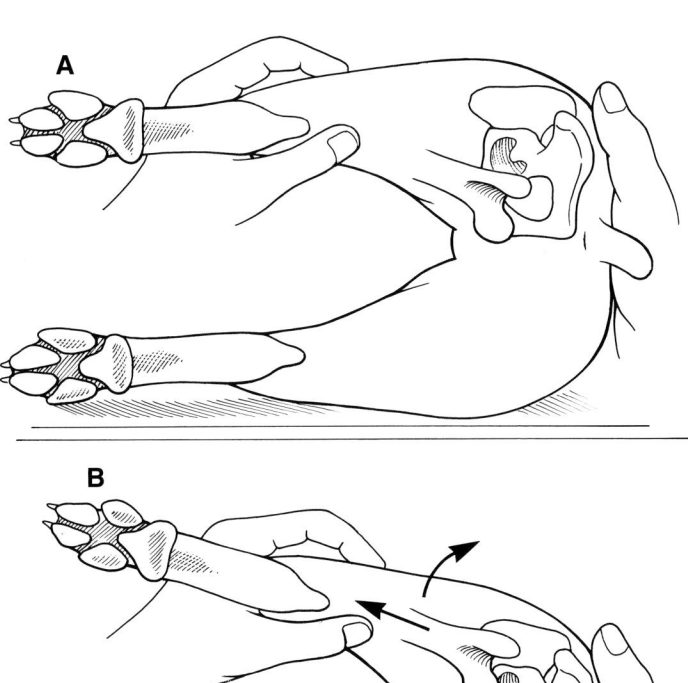

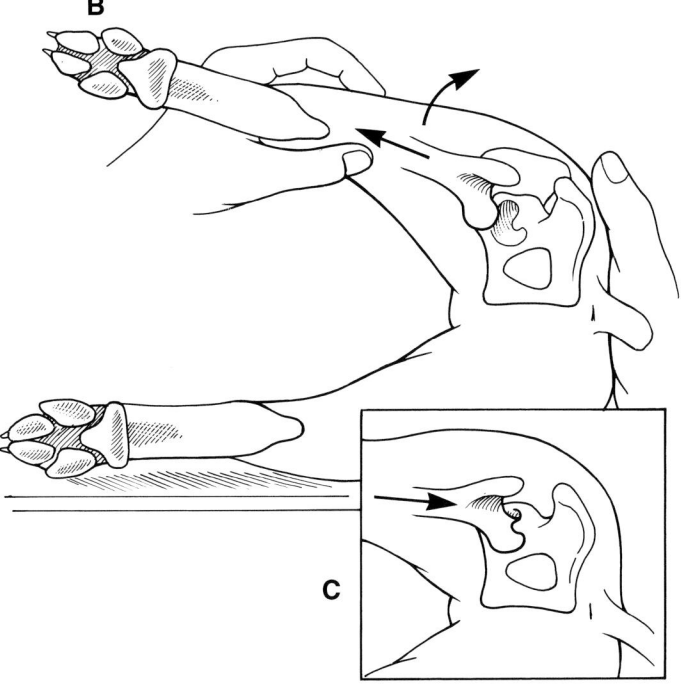

FIG. 33-86
Closed reduction of a caudoventral hip luxation. **A,** Place the patient in lateral recumbency with the limb held perpendicular to the spine. Grasp the limb near the tarsal joint with one hand and use the other hand to stabilize the body. **B,** Place traction on the limb while simultaneously abducting the leg to pull the femoral head beyond the medial rim of the acetabulum. **C,** Once the femoral head has cleared the acetabular rim, exert lateral pressure medial to the hip joint to position the femoral head lateral to the acetabulum. Push proximally and allow the femoral head to fall into the acetabulum.

Preoperative Management

These animals should be thoroughly examined for evidence of concurrent trauma. Surgery may need to be delayed until the animal's condition has been adequately stabilized.

Anesthesia

See p. 944 for anesthetic considerations for patients with orthopedic disease.

Surgical Anatomy

Normal anatomy of the hip is described on p. 1099. With hip luxation, the anatomy may appear abnormal, and tissue may be difficult to identify. Muscles surrounding the joint often are bruised and swollen. It is helpful to reduce the hip before starting the surgical approach to establish normal tissue relationships. The cranial edge of the greater trochanter may be used to help identify the correct plane of surgical dissection. The prominent tendinous insertion of the deep gluteal muscle can also be used for orientation. When the hip is luxated, the femoral head usually lies beneath the deep gluteal muscle. The proximal femur usually is displaced craniodorsally and may obscure visualization of the acetabulum.

Positioning

The patient is positioned in lateral recumbency with the affected limb up. The limb is suspended for surgical preparation to allow limb manipulation during surgery.

SURGICAL TECHNIQUE

Surgical stabilization of hip luxation may be accomplished by capsular reconstruction if the joint capsule is intact. When the capsule cannot be securely closed or if added stability is needed, other reconstructive procedures must be performed to ensure hip stability for 3 to 4 weeks until capsular healing occurs. Reconstructive procedures include synthetic capsular reconstruction with suture and bone screws or suture anchors and toggle pin placement. Additional stability may be gained by translocation of the greater trochanter. If the dog is mildly dysplastic, TPO may be indicated to maintain hip reduction (see p. 1241). TPO may also be useful for nondysplastic dogs when other means are insufficient (Haburjak et al, 2002).

Exploration of the Hip Joint

Perform a craniolateral exposure of the hip joint (see Fig. 32-76, A and B on p. 1099); if additional exposure is necessary, perform a trochanteric osteotomy (see Fig. 32-76, C-E on p. 1100). Reflect the deep gluteal muscle and visualize the femoral head craniodorsal to the hip joint. Visualize and remove remnants of the round ligament and debris from the femoral head and acetabulum; this allows the femoral head to completely seat within the acetabulum. Once the hip has been reduced, assess its stability by viewing the acetabular coverage of the femoral head and placing the hip joint through a complete range of motion. Perform the chosen stabilization technique (see later discussion).

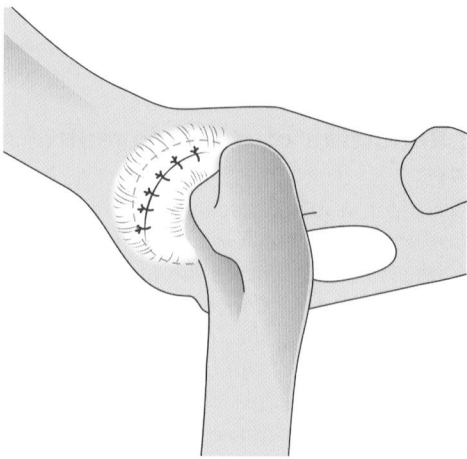

FIG. 33-87
Coxofemoral joint stabilization by means of capsulorrhaphy. Interrupted sutures have been placed to appose the joint capsule.

> NOTE: A Hohmann retractor placed within or just caudal to the acetabulum and used to lever the femur caudally improves visualization of the acetabulum.

Capsule Reconstruction

It is not uncommon for the joint capsule to be intact except for a small rent, through which the femoral head has luxated, or an area where the capsule has torn loose from its insertion site at the femoral neck. In both situations, if after replacing the femoral head the acetabular coverage is adequate and the joint is stable through a range of motion, primary suturing of the capsule can be used as the sole reconstructive procedure.

Suture the joint capsule with nonabsorbable monofilament material using an interrupted pattern (Fig. 33-87). If the capsule has torn from its insertion site, drill small holes in the femoral neck through which the suture can pass or reattach the capsule with suture anchors.

> NOTE: Reconstruction of the joint capsule as the sole means of stabilization requires that the dorsal joint capsule be identifiable and that the conformation of the hip joint be normal.

Joint Reconstruction

The joint capsule may be damaged to a degree that primary suturing is impossible. In such cases, a prosthetic capsule or toggle pin can be used to maintain reduction during healing of the fibrous joint capsule. A prosthetic capsule is made of suture material inserted in the craniodorsal acetabular rim and trochanteric fossa (Fig. 33-88).

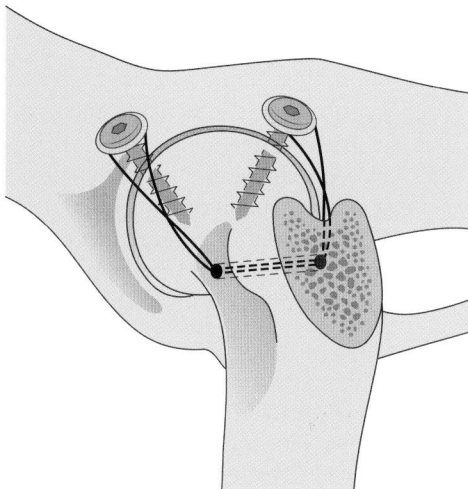

FIG. 33-88
Coxofemoral joint stabilization by placement of a prosthetic capsule. Note the strategic placement of bone screws in the dorsolateral acetabulum. Suture material is passed from the screws through a predrilled tunnel in the dorsal femoral neck and tightened. The presence of suture in this position prevents craniodorsal reluxation. The same procedure may be performed using suture anchors.

Place two screws with flat metal washers or bone anchors in the dorsal rim of the acetabulum. Insert one anchor at the 10 o'clock position and one at the 1 o'clock position (on a left hip). Place a third screw and washer or anchor in the trochanteric fossa (as an alternative, drill a hole through the femoral neck in the trochanteric fossa to accept suture). Pass heavy nonabsorbable suture in a figure-eight pattern between the acetabular anchors and trochanteric fossa. Tie the sutures tight enough to maintain reduction but not so tight that they will tear with normal ambulation.

A toggle pin technique may be beneficial when the capsule is severely damaged or the luxation is chronic, or if multiple limb injuries demand early use of the reconstructed hip. The synthetic round ligament created will not last indefinitely, but if properly placed will provide stability until capsular fibroplasia occurs.

Starting at the level of the third trochanter and centered in the femoral neck, use a C-guide to drill a 2.5-mm hole that exits at the fovea capitis (Fig. 33-89, A). Drill a 3.5-mm hole through the upper end of the acetabular fossa (Fig. 33-89, B). Attach multiple strands of large nonabsorbable suture to a commercial toggle rod or a toggle pin made by bending a Kirschner wire to form a loop and two wings (Fig. 33-89, C). Pass the toggle rod through the acetabular hole, and rotate it by pulling on the suture until the pin is secured against the medial acetabular wall. Pass the suture through the femoral tunnel, reduce the hip, and pull the sutures taut (Fig. 33-89, D). Secure the suture by passing one pair of

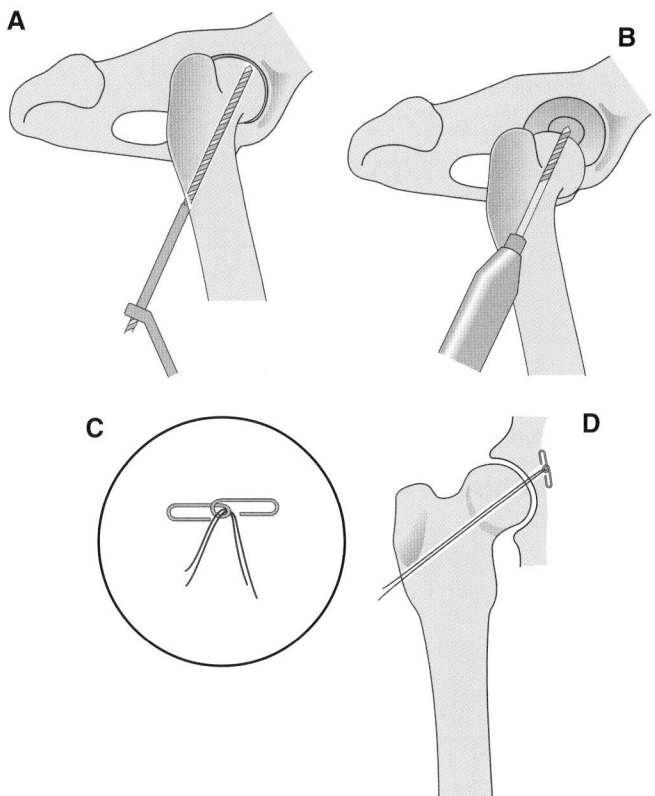

FIG. 33-89
Stabilization of the coxofemoral joint with a toggle pin suture. **A,** Drill a hole centered through the femoral neck and **(B)** through the acetabular fossa. **C,** Attach multiple strands of nonabsorbable suture to a toggle pin formed from a Kirschner wire. Pass the toggle pin through the hole in the acetabular fossa and pull to set the pin. **D,** Pass the sutures through the hole drilled in the femoral neck. Reduce the hip and secure the sutures.

sutures through a drill hole created through the lateral femoral cortex and tying it to the opposite suture pair. As an alternative, pass the suture through a two-hole polypropylene button and tie the suture. Tie the suture tight enough to maintain hip reduction but not so tight that it will rupture with normal ambulation.

Translocation of the Greater Trochanter

If the hip is unstable and if the gluteal musculature is not compromised, a trochanteric osteotomy can be performed to translocate the greater trochanter distally and slightly caudal to add stability to the repair. Relocation of the greater trochanter allows contraction of the gluteal muscles to abduct and internally rotate the femoral head.

Perform a trochanteric osteotomy (see p. 1100), and reflect the gluteal musculature proximally. Once the hip has been cleaned of debris and reduced, place the limb in abduction. Use an osteotome and mallet to create a new surface caudal and distal to the point where the greater trochanter normally seats (Fig. 33-90). Then replace the greater trochanter at its new attachment site, and secure it in position with a pin and tension band technique.

SUTURE MATERIALS AND SPECIAL INSTRUMENTS

Either No. 1 or No. 2 nonabsorbable suture is used for capsule reconstruction. An osteotome, mallet, pins, and wire are needed for translocation of the greater trochanter. Prosthetic capsule reconstruction requires screws and stainless steel washers or suture anchors. Toggle rods are commercially available, or toggle pins may be made of small Kirschner wires; a drill and drill guide are needed to place the toggle pin and suture.

POSTOPERATIVE CARE AND ASSESSMENT

Patients may be placed in an Ehmer bandage to assist hip reduction in the early postoperative period. The bandage is removed 4 to 7 days after reduction. Cage confinement may be adequate for dogs with stable hips. Once the Ehmer sling has been removed, it is beneficial to begin very controlled physical rehabilitation exercises. Refer to Table 33-12 (see p. 1244) for a sample exercise protocol. Reexamination 3 days after removal of the Ehmer bandage and before resumption of unsupervised activity is advised.

PROGNOSIS

The success rate for maintaining reduction and regaining good to excellent limb function with closed reduction is about 50%. The success rate is lower in patients with poor

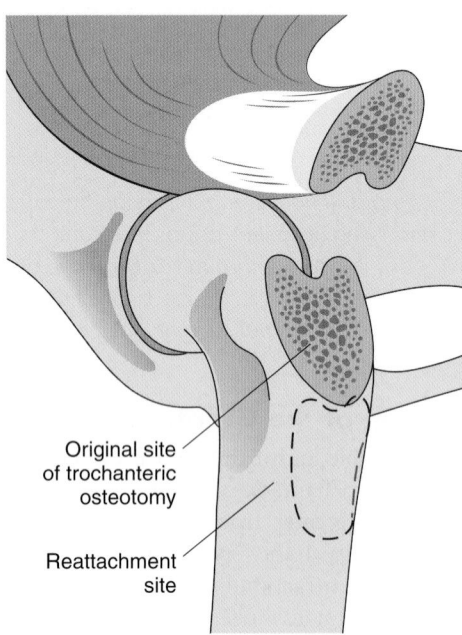

FIG. 33-90
Stabilization of the coxofemoral joint by translocating the greater trochanter. Prepare a new site distal and slightly caudal to the normal anatomic position. Stabilize the greater trochanter in this position with small pins and orthopedic wire (tension band).

Original site of trochanteric osteotomy

Reattachment site

conformation of the hip joint secondary to hip dysplasia or previous trauma. Clinical studies indicate that the success of surgical intervention after failure of closed reduction is not different from the success rate in patients undergoing surgical reduction as a primary treatment. Therefore it is reasonable to attempt closed reduction in patients with a hip luxation. The success rate for maintaining reduction with good to excellent limb function after open reduction is approximately 85% to 90%. The results do not appear to favor any one reconstruction technique.

References

Haburjak JJ, Lenehan TM, Harari J et al: Treatment of traumatic coxofemoral luxation with triple pelvic osteotomy in 19 dogs (1987-1999), *Vet Comp Orthop Traum* 14:69, 2001.

Pozzi A, Kowaleski MR, Dyce J et al: Treatment of traumatic coxofemoral luxation by cemented total hip arthroplasty, *Vet Comp Orthop Traum* 13:198, 2004.

Trostel CT, Peck JN, deHaan JJ: Spontaneous bilateral coxofemoral luxation in four dogs, *J Am Anim Hosp Assoc* 36:268, 2000.

Suggested Reading

Holsworth IG, DeCamp CE: Coxofemoral luxation. In Slatter D, editor: In *Textbook of small animal surgery,* ed 3, Philadelphia, 2003, Saunders.
This chapter provides a detailed description of the pathophysiology, diagnosis, and treatment of canine hip dysplasia.

LEGG-PERTHES DISEASE

DEFINITION

Legg-Perthes disease is a noninflammatory aseptic necrosis of the femoral head that occurs in young patients before closure of the capital femoral physis. Synonyms include *osteochondritis dissecans of the femoral head* and *avascular necrosis of the femoral head.*

GENERAL CONSIDERATIONS AND CLINICALLY RELEVANT PATHOPHYSIOLOGY

Legg-Perthes disease results in collapse of the femoral epiphysis because of an interruption of blood flow. The reason for the loss of blood flow is not known for certain, but several theories have been proposed, including hormonal influence, hereditary factors, anatomic conformation, intracapsular pressure, and infarction of the femoral head. The vascular supply to the femoral head in young animals with open proximal femoral physes is derived solely from epiphyseal vessels; metaphyseal vessels do not cross the physis to contribute to femoral head vascularity. Epiphyseal vessels course extraosseously along the surface of the femoral neck, cross the growth plate, and penetrate bone to supply nourishment to the femoral epiphysis. Synovitis or sustained abnormal limb position may increase intraarticular pressure enough to collapse the fragile veins and inhibit blood flow. An autosomal recessive gene has been proposed as a genetic cause for the development of aseptic necrosis of the femoral head. After cell death occurs, the reparative processes begin. The bone substance is weakened mechanically during the revascularization period, and normal physiologic weight-bearing forces may cause collapse and fragmentation of the femoral epiphysis. When this happens, incongruence of the femoral epiphysis and acetabulum results in DJD. Fragmentation (fractures) of the femoral epiphysis and osteoarthrosis cause pain and resulting lameness.

NOTE: Because this condition has been linked to an autosomal recessive gene, be sure to advise owners to have affected animals neutered.

DIAGNOSIS
Clinical Presentation
Signalment. Legg-Perthes disease is diagnosed in young, small-breed dogs (i.e., under 10 kg). The peak incidence of onset is 6 to 7 months with a range of 3 to 13 months, and males and females are equally affected. This condition occurs bilaterally in 10% to 17% of affected animals.

History. Affected animals usually are presented for evaluation of a slow onset, weight-bearing lameness that worsens over a 6- to 8-week period. Lameness may progress to non–weight-bearing. Some clients report an acute onset of clinical lameness. In these patients, sudden collapse of the epiphysis may cause acute exacerbation of an already present but imperceptible lameness. Other clinical signs can include irritability, reduced appetite, and chewing at the skin over the affected hip.

Physical Examination Findings
Manipulation of the hip joint consistently elicits pain in affected animals. Limited range of motion, muscle atrophy, and crepitus may be present with advanced disease.

Diagnostic Imaging
Radiographs show deformity of the femoral head, shortening and/or lysis of the femoral neck, and foci of decreased bone opacity within the femoral epiphysis (Fig. 33-91).

Laboratory Findings
Consistent laboratory abnormalities are not seen.

DIFFERENTIAL DIAGNOSIS
Differential diagnoses include physeal trauma and luxation of the medial patella. Small dogs may have concurrent bilateral medial patellar luxation (see p. 1289), and the stifle joint must be examined carefully to diagnose this condition.

MEDICAL MANAGEMENT
Because the condition is not painful in most dogs during the early stages of the disease, the diagnosis often is made after collapse and fragmentation have resulted in joint incongruity and DJD. Conservative treatment with antiinflammatory medication and leash-limited or non–weight-bearing exercise, such as swimming, may provide pain relief in a small percentage of dogs, but most dogs require surgical intervention to relieve the lameness. In rare cases the diagnosis is made before collapse of the femoral head, and treatment

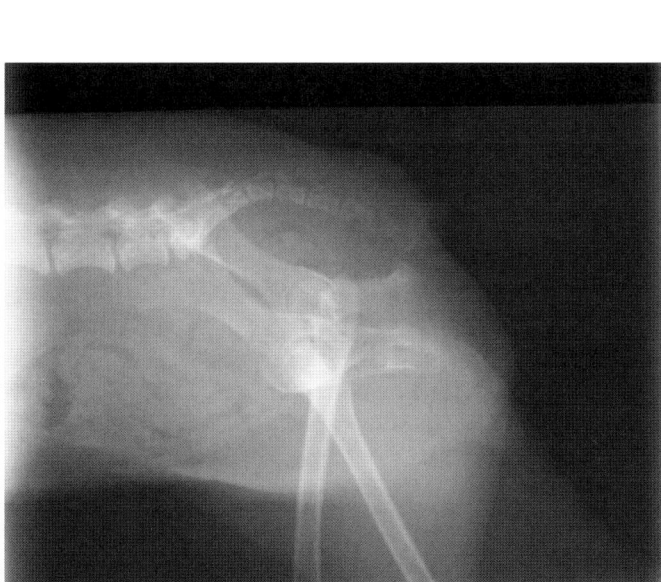
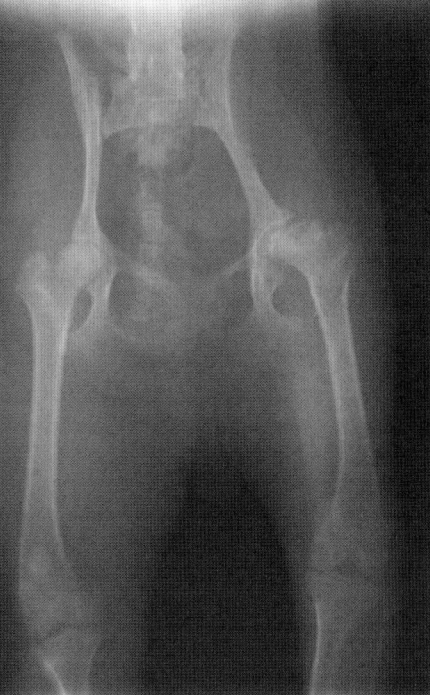

FIG. 33-91
Radiograph of a young dog with Legg-Perthes disease. The femoral head appears moth-eaten and is misshapen.

consists of limiting weight bearing on the limb during the revascularization period to prevent collapse of the femoral head.

SURGICAL TREATMENT
Preoperative Management

Activity is limited until definitive surgical treatment has been performed. Antiinflammatory medications may be administered for pain relief.

Anesthesia

Anesthetic management of animals with orthopedic disease is provided on p. 944.

Surgical Anatomy

Anatomy of the coxofemoral joint is discussed on p. 1240. In animals with Legg-Perthes disease, the joint capsule appears thickened and more vascular than normal. The femoral head and neck often appear misshapen. The bone may be soft and may fragment when the head and neck are excised, requiring that rongeurs be used to remove small fragments.

Positioning

The animal is positioned in lateral recumbency with the affected leg up. A hanging-limb preparation may be used to facilitate manipulation of the limb during surgery. The leg should be prepared from the dorsal midline to midtibia.

SURGICAL TECHNIQUE

Excision of the femoral head and neck is the treatment of choice. See p. 1242 for a description of the technique.

SUTURE MATERIALS AND SPECIAL INSTRUMENTS

Instruments necessary to remove the femoral head and neck in small dogs include an osteotome and mallet, bone cutters, and rongeurs.

POSTOPERATIVE CARE AND ASSESSMENT

The animal should be encouraged to use the limb immediately after surgery. This should include immediate rehabilitation exercises as outlined in Table 33-13 (see p. 1245). NSAIDs should be administered to reduce pain and encourage early function. Passive flexion and extension of the hip joint should be performed twice daily as soon as the animal tolerates it. Physical therapy should be initiated with small movements and the range of motion gradually increased over 5 to 10 minutes.

PROGNOSIS

Prognosis for normal limb use is good after femoral head and neck excision because of the small size of affected dogs; however, owners should be warned that slight, intermittent lameness may still occur in damp weather or after heavy exercise or a period of inactivity. Poor results occur occasionally and have been related to non–weight-bearing before surgery, severe preoperative muscle atrophy, and incorrect surgical technique.

STIFLE

CRANIAL CRUCIATE LIGAMENT RUPTURE

DEFINITIONS

Cranial cruciate ligament injuries are complete or partial tears of the ligament or avulsions of the origin or insertion. **Cranial drawer** is a term used to describe excessive craniocaudal movement of the tibia relative to the femur as a result of cruciate ligament injury. **Cranial tibial thrust** is defined as cranial movement of the tibial tuberosity in the cranial cruciate–deficient stifle when the hock is flexed and the gastrocnemius muscle contracts. **Translation** is defined as movement of a bone parallel to an axis or plane. **Pivot shift** is cranial movement of the tibia combined with internal rotation of the tibia. **Tibial plateau angle** (TPA) is the angle between a line perpendicular to the long axis of the tibia and a line parallel to the tibial plateau. **Medial buttress** is a palpable thickening of the medial aspect of the stifle. **Imbrication** is defined as the tightening of a structure. **Isometry** is defined as maintaining equal distance or tension throughout a range of motion.

GENERAL CONSIDERATIONS AND CLINICALLY RELEVANT PATHOPHYSIOLOGY

The CCL is divided into craniomedial and caudolateral bands, which have different insertion points on the tibial plateau. The CCL functions primarily to limit cranial translation of the tibia relative to the femur (Fig. 33-92). The craniomedial band is taut during all phases of flexion and extension; the caudolateral band is taut in extension, but becomes lax in flexion. The CCL also functions to limit internal rotation of the tibia; as the stifle is flexed, the cranial and caudal cruciate ligaments twist on each other, limiting the degree of internal rotation of the tibia relative to the femur. Interaction of the cranial and caudal cruciate ligaments during flexion also provides a limited degree of varus-valgus support to the flexed stifle joint.

Mechanoreceptors and afferent nerve endings have been identified in the interfiber layers of the CCL. Innervation of the ligament serves as a proprioceptive feedback mechanism to prevent excessive flexion or extension of the stifle joint. This protective action is accomplished through stimulation or relaxation of muscle groups that lend support to the joint.

> NOTE: The craniomedial band of the CCL is the primary check against craniocaudal drawer motion.

CCL failure can result from degenerative and traumatic causes. The categories are interrelated, because ligaments

Normal   Injured

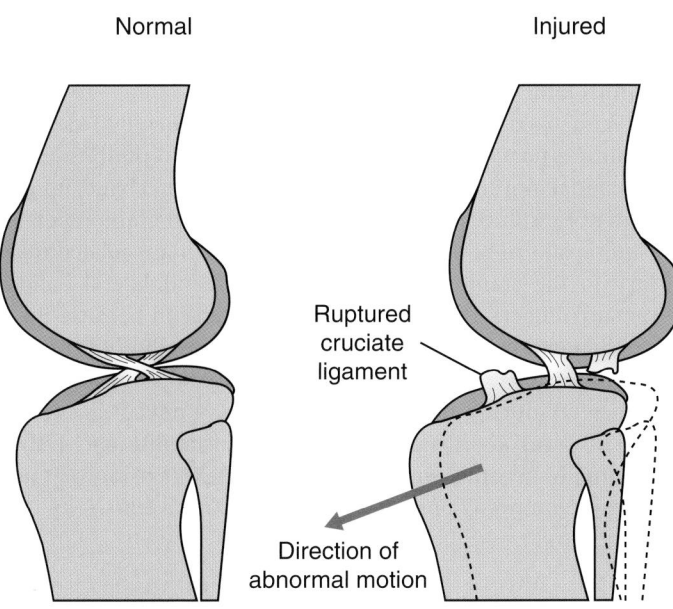

Ruptured
cruciate
ligament

Direction of
abnormal motion

FIG. 33-92
The CCL prevents cranial translation of the tibia.

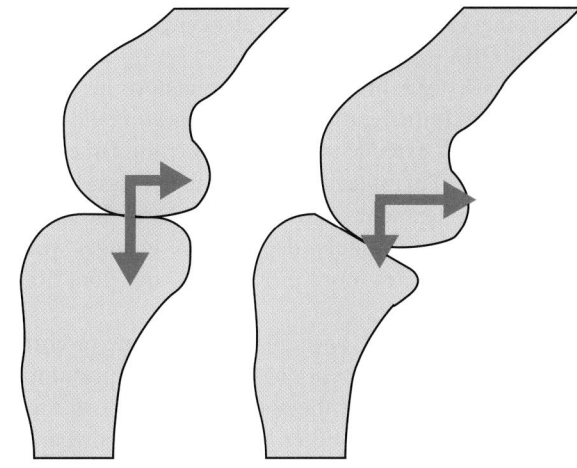

FIG. 33-93
A larger tibial plateau angle results in a greater cranial
force on the tibia during weight bearing.

weakened by degeneration are more susceptible to trauma. The high incidence of CCL failure in dogs suggests that there is an underlying cause of premature degeneration of the cruciate ligament in most cases. Degeneration of the ligament is associated with aging (especially in large-breed dogs), conformational abnormalities (straight rear limbs), and immune-mediated arthropathies. Degeneration of the ligament has also been associated with an increased TPA, although not all studies have identified this correlation (Morris et al, 2001; Reif et al, 2003; Wilke et al, 2002). An increased TPA has been theorized to place chronic excessive loads on the CCL leading to eventual mechanical failure (Fig. 33-93). In cats, excessive body weight may significantly increase the risk of CCL rupture (Harasen et al, 2005).

The mechanism of CCL traumatic injury is primarily a reflection of its function as a constraint to joint motion. Acute injury is most commonly associated with the hyperextension and internal rotation of the leg that occurs when a dog's foot becomes caught in a hole or fence. Jumping can also cause cruciate ligament rupture if the force of the cranial tibial thrust exceeds the breaking strength of the ligament. With ligament degeneration, even repetitive normal activities can cause progressive rupturing of the ligament. In many cases, the underlying pathologic condition is present in both stifles and a high percentage of dogs either have bilateral cruciate ligament rupture, or they rupture the contralateral ligament within 1 to 2 years. Partial rupture of the CCL results in lameness with minimal detectable stifle instability and progressive radiographic signs of osteoarthritis.

Partial rupture generally proceeds to complete ligament rupture with time.

CCL injury with stifle instability is part of a cascade of events that include progressive osteoarthritis and medial meniscus injury. Stifle instability results in synovitis, articular cartilage degeneration, periarticular osteophyte development, and capsular fibrosis. The immobile medial meniscus is subject to injury in the unstable joint (see p. 1285). Progressive osteoarthritis occurs after CCL rupture regardless of the treatment method.

DIAGNOSIS
Clinical Presentation

Signalment. Either gender and any age or breed of dog may be affected; however, most dogs brought in for treatment of CCL injury are young, active, large-breed dogs. CCL injury is uncommon in cats.

History. Acute injury, chronic injury, and partial tears are three clinical presentations associated with CCL injury. Patients with acute tears show a sudden onset of non–weight-bearing or partial–weight-bearing lameness. Lameness usually improves within 3 to 6 weeks after injury without treatment, particularly in patients that weigh less than 10 kg. An exception is dogs with associated meniscal injury. These dogs usually maintain a minimally weight bearing or non–weight-bearing lameness until surgical intervention takes place.

Patients with chronic injury have a prolonged weight-bearing lameness. There may or may not be a history of acute non–weight-bearing lameness followed by gradual improvement to moderate weight bearing. Patients may have a history of difficulty rising and sitting. The owners may report that the dog sits with the affected limb out to the side of the body. Lameness is typically worse after exercise or after sleeping. Chronic lameness is associated with the development of DJD.

Partial CCL tears are difficult to diagnose in the early stages of injury. Initially, affected animals have a mild weight-bearing lameness associated with exercise; the lameness resolves with rest. This stage of the disease may last for many months. As the ligament continues to tear and the stifle becomes increasingly unstable, degenerative changes worsen, and lameness becomes more pronounced and does not resolve with rest.

Dogs of any age may have bilateral subacute or chronic bilateral CCL rupture. These dogs may have a presumptive neurologic disease because the dog may be unable or unwilling to support weight in either hind limb. The owner may also report that the dog is unable to sit normally, but sits on elevated surfaces, such as a stool or step.

Physical Examination Findings

Animals with acute complete tears often are apprehensive during examination of the stifle joint, but pain usually is mild or absent. Instability can be difficult to elicit because of the patient's apprehension and the resulting muscle contraction. Joint effusion may be palpable adjacent to the patellar tendon. A positive tibial compression test may be easier to elicit than a positive drawer test.

Patients with chronic tears may have thigh muscle atrophy (compared with the normal limb), and crepitus may be evident when the stifle is flexed and extended. When the joint is extended from a flexed position, a clicking or popping may be heard and felt; this is commonly associated with a meniscal tear. However, the absence of joint noise does not eliminate the possibility of meniscal injury. An enlargement along the medial joint surface (medial buttress) often can be palpated and is caused by osteophyte formation along the trochlear ridges and fibrous tissue formation along the medial condyle and proximal tibia. Craniocaudal instability can

be difficult to elicit, particularly in large or apprehensive patients with chronic tears, because of proliferation of the fibrous joint capsule.

With partial tears, early instability is difficult to detect because a portion of the ligament is intact and inhibits craniocaudal movement. Tearing of the caudolateral band alone does not produce instability because the intact craniomedial band is taut in both flexion and extension. If an isolated injury to the craniomedial band occurs (caudolateral band remains intact), the joint is stable in extension because the caudolateral band remains taut; however, instability is present in flexion because the caudolateral band normally becomes lax during flexion. Initially, pain, synovial effusion, and crepitus are absent, but signs of instability and DJD eventually become evident. Pain on hyperextension of the joint is commonly present in dogs with partial tears.

> NOTE: Always compare the limb that has the suspected injury with the opposite limb if the instability and stifle swelling are questionable.

Cranial drawer movement is diagnostic of cruciate ligament injury. The **cranial drawer test** is performed with the patient in lateral recumbency. Lack of adequate patient relaxation is a common cause of failure to elicit cranial drawer movement. Therefore if suspicion is high that the lameness is caused by cruciate ligament injury, general anesthesia or heavy sedation may be necessary to negate the influence of muscle tension (see p. 933). Once the dog is in lateral position, the examiner stands to the patient's rear and positions the thumb and forefinger of one hand on the femur (Fig. 33-94). The thumb is placed directly behind the fabella and the forefinger over the patella. The remaining fingers are wrapped around the thigh. The other hand is placed on the tibia with the thumb directly behind the fibular head and the

FIG. 33-94
To examine for cruciate ligament injury, place the thumb of one hand over the lateral fabella and the index finger over the patella. Stabilize the femur with this hand. Place the thumb of the opposite hand caudal to the fibular head with the index finger on the tibial tuberosity. With the stifle flexed and then extended, attempt to move the tibia cranially and distally to the femur.

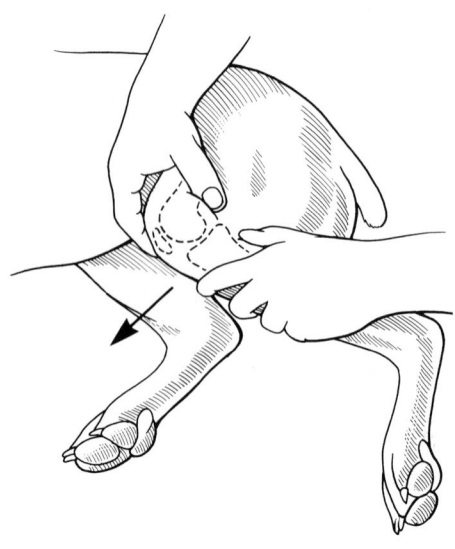
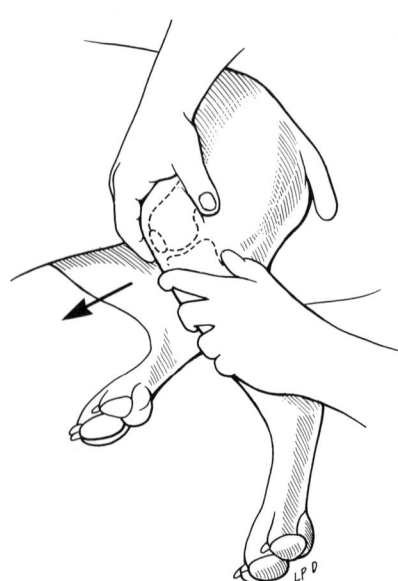

forefinger over the tibial crest. The three remaining fingers are wrapped around the tibial shaft. The femur is stabilized with the one hand while the second hand moves the tibia forward and back in a direction parallel to the transverse plane of the tibial plateau. The pressure to move the tibia forward should be applied through the thumb behind the fibular head.

The tibia must be held in neutral position, as determined by the position of the fingers on the patella and tibial tuberosity, and not be allowed to rotate internally. If this occurs, internal rotation of the joint may appear as cranial drawer movement. The examiner must test for signs of instability with the stifle joint in extension, in the normal standing angle, and in 90 degrees of flexion. If the degree of movement is questionable, comparison with the opposite limb is helpful. A positive test result is craniocaudal movement beyond the 0 to 2 mm found in normal stifle joints. In younger patients, normal craniocaudal translation may be as great as 4 to 5 mm, but ligament rupture is confirmed by the absence of an abrupt stop at the cranial extent of movement. Because most isolated cruciate ligament tears involve the CCL, craniocaudal instability usually is associated with injury of this ligament. If a partial tear is present, the cranial drawer sign may reveal only 2 to 3 mm of instability when the test is done with the stifle flexed and no instability with the stifle in extension. Mild partial tears may have no cranial drawer sign in any position. Upon completion of the cranial drawer test, the stifle should be flexed and extended through a range of normal movement. With the leg in extension, collateral stability should be assessed.

> NOTE: Juvenile dogs have increased joint laxity (4 to 5 mm), but maintain a distinct end point when the tibia is moved cranially.

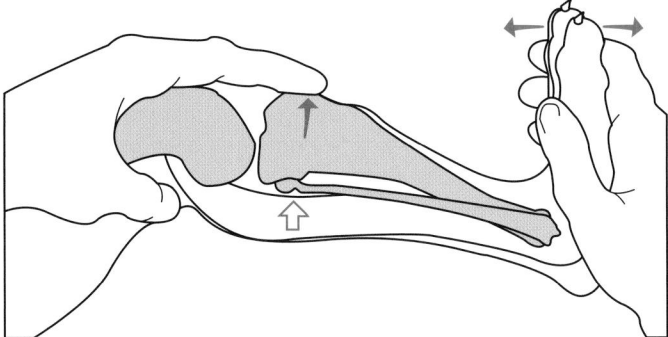

FIG. 33-95
To perform a tibial compression test, grasp the distal quadriceps with one hand from the cranial surface so that the index finger can be extended down over the patella and the tip of the finger is on the tibial crest. Use the second hand to grasp the foot at the metatarsal region from the plantar surface. With the limb in moderate extension, flex the hock with the lower hand and prevent stifle flexion with the upper hand. Feel for cranial movement of the tibia, which is an indication of cruciate ligament damage.

The **tibial compression test** is performed with the patient standing or in lateral recumbency. The examiner stands to the patient's rear and grasps the distal quadriceps with one hand from the cranial surface so that the index finger can be extended down over the patella, and the tip of the finger is on the tibial crest (Fig. 33-95). The second hand grasps the foot at the metatarsal region from the plantar surface. The limb is positioned in moderate extension and as the lower hand flexes the hock, the upper hand prevents stifle flexion. The index finger of the upper hand is used to feel for cranial movement of the tibial crest while the hock is being flexed. In the normal knee, the upper hand will feel pressure from the patella on the index finger. With CCL rupture, the tibial crest will be advanced forward as the hock is flexed. The technique should be repeated in different degrees of stifle flexion to test for a partial CCL rupture.

Diagnostic Imaging

With acute tears, radiographs are helpful in ruling out other causes of stifle joint lameness. Radiographic findings in patients with chronic ligament tears or partial tears include compression of the fat pad in the cranial aspect of the joint and extension of the caudal joint capsule caused by joint effusion and osteophyte formation along the trochlear ridge, the caudal surface of the tibial plateau, and the distal pole of the patella (Fig. 33-96). Thickening of the medial fibrous joint capsule and subchondral sclerosis are also evident. Radiographic changes in patients with CCL rupture are nonspecific and can be seen with other stifle diseases, including infection, soft tissue neoplasia, and osteoarthritis. Avulsion of the CCL attachment may be specific in that a bone fragment may be seen adjacent to this site.

MRI has been investigated for evaluation of the cruciate ligament in dogs; however, the long acquisition times required and lack of availability of MRI have limited the use of this technique in the diagnosis of canine cruciate ligament injury.

AP **Arthroscopy.** A large percentage of the surface of the cruciate ligament can be examined arthroscopically for gross tears, fibrillation, or discoloration associated with cruciate damage. The menisci and cartilage may also be examined. Arthroscopy has been shown to decrease the short-term morbidity for dogs requiring stabilization of CCL injuries (Hoelzler et al, 2004).

Indications. Diagnostic and therapeutic procedures of the stifle joint are performed arthroscopically. Diagnostic arthroscopy is most commonly used to confirm the presence of partial tears of the anterior cruciate ligament and to assess the degree of osteoarthritis; therapeutic arthroscopy is most commonly applied for removal of CCL remnants, assisted reconstruction of the CCL, treatment of meniscal injury, and treatment of stifle OCD and topical treatment of osteoarthritis (abrasion arthroplasty and microfracture). In general the egress portal, arthroscope portal, and instrument portal sites are the same for these procedures.

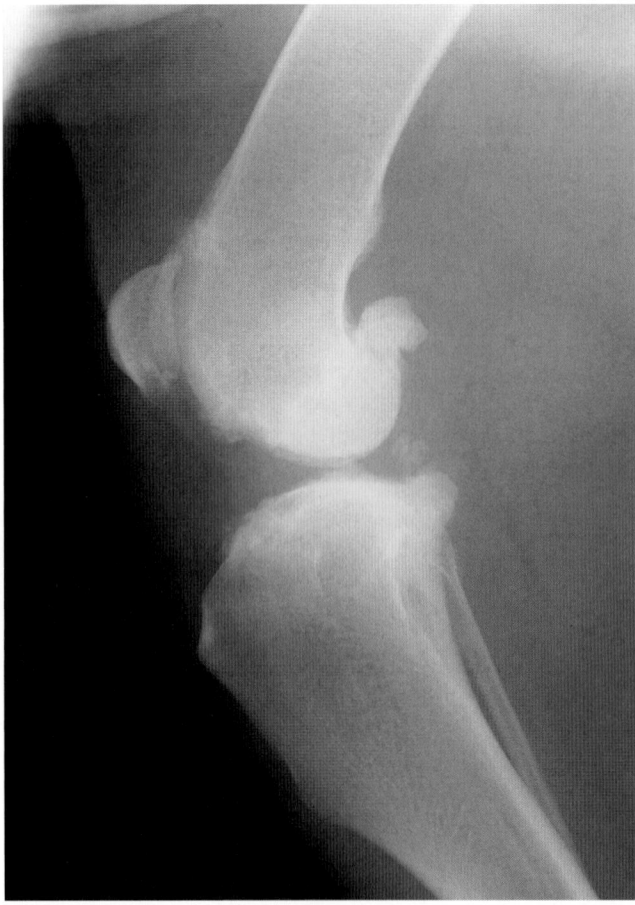

FIG. 33-96
Lateral radiograph of a dog with a chronic cruciate ligament rupture. Note the loss of fat pad definition and distention of the caudal joint capsule. Also note the osteophyte formation along the trochlear ridge and the subchondral bone sclerosis of the tibial plateau.

Instrumentation. A 2.7-mm arthroscope is commonly chosen for use in the stifle joint. A 4-mm arthroscope can be used in larger dogs, but the larger the arthroscope, the more difficult it is to introduce other instruments into the joint. A multifenestrated egress cannula with a flow control valve is preferred over an egress needle because the former is less likely to dislodge from the knee during surgery. A motorized shaver is essential to create a viewing window through removal of an interfering fat pad. The large shaver handpiece with a 3.5-mm or 4-mm full radius shaver blade is preferred. A radiofrequency unit or intraarticular electrocautery is helpful to control hemorrhage and ablate tissue (meniscectomy). Arthroscopic electrocautery handpieces connect to standard electrocautery units. Hand instruments useful for stifle joint arthroscopy include probes, tissue graspers, and tissue biters. Instrumentation designed for canine arthroscopy is readily available; these instruments are preferable to most human small joint instruments because the latter often are too large for use in dogs. Be aware that the smaller the

instrument, the more delicate it is and thus the more easily damaged.

Portal sites and technique. The arthroscope portal and egress portal are established first and simultaneously.

Locate the arthroscope portal lateral to the patellar tendon, approximately midway between the tibial tuberosity and the distal pole of the patella, by incising through the skin and completely into the joint with a No. 15 blade. Pass the obturator of the egress cannula into the arthroscope portal and under the patella so that it tents the skin medial and proximal to the patella. Incise over the obturator and advance it through the skin. Pass the egress cannula over the obturator until the end is approximately under the center of the patella. Remove the obturator, and then move the tip of the egress cannula into the medial joint pouch by extending the stifle joint and levering the cannula over the medial trochlear ridge. Once the egress port has been established, insert the arthroscope in the scope portal. Place the instrument port at the same proximodistal level but medial to the patellar tendon. Systematically examine the suprapatellar compartment and trochlear ridges. As the joint is flexed, position the arthroscope lateral to the intercondylar notch.

Further examination of the joint is limited by the presence of the fat pad, which generally is inflamed and obscures visualization of the cruciate ligaments and menisci.

Make a viewing window through the fat pad so that you can thoroughly examine the ligaments and menisci. Use a motorized shaver to remove the inflamed fat pad (Fig. 33-97). Position the arthroscope to view the intercondylar notch and top of the fat pad. Establish an instrument port as described above, and insert the shaver blade. Visualize the shaver blade and position the shaver window away from the lens of the arthroscope. Remove tissue via the suction and cutting action of the shaver blade. Visualize the cruciate ligaments (often remnants of the CCL) as a viewing window is established through removal of the fat pad (Fig. 33-98). Use a thermal ablation instrument or arthroscopic cautery to remove tissue that obstructs viewing of the internal structures of the joint. Once a viewing window has been established, examine the cruciate ligaments and menisci. Ablate or remove remnants of a torn CCL with the motorized shaver. Examine both the lateral and medial menisci for fraying or classic bucket handle tears.

The medial meniscus is most commonly injured (bucket handle tear, radial tears, or fraying).

To view the posteromedial compartment (medial meniscus), place a Hohmann retractor through the instrument portal (Fig. 33-99). As an alternative, apply a valgus stress to open the medial compartment of the joint. Use small hand instruments, such as a grasper or probe, to hold a torn section of meniscus, then remove the damaged meniscus with

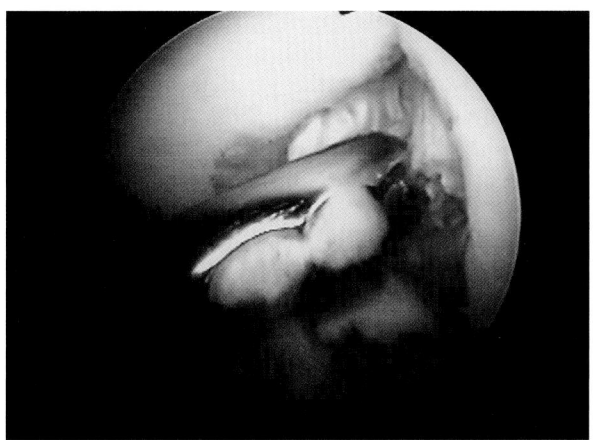

FIG. 33-97
Motorized shaver removing fat pad cranial to the intercondylar notch to create a viewing window.

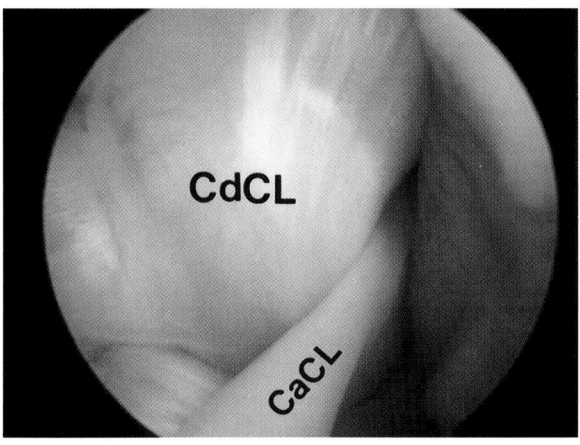

FIG. 33-98
Cranial view of the intercondylar notch. The caudal cruciate ligament (CdCL) is intact. A small cranial medial band is all that remains of the cranial cruciate ligament (CCL).

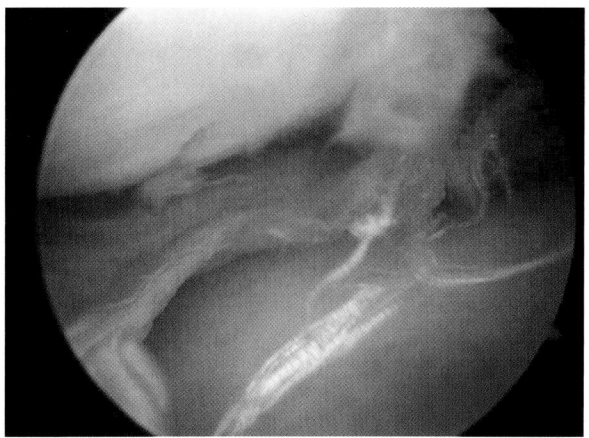

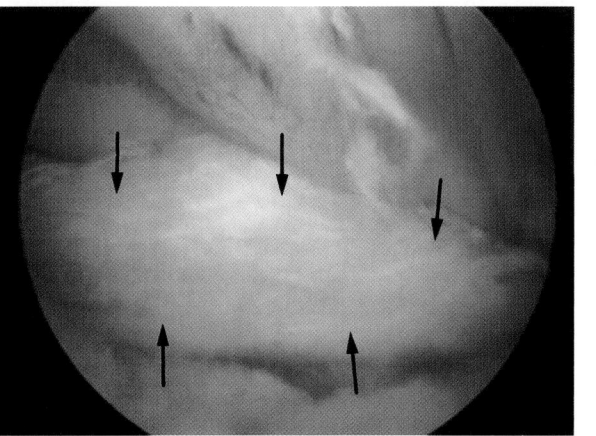

FIG. 33-99
A, Cranial view of a frayed medial meniscus associated with a torn CCL. **B,** Cranial view of a bucket handle tear of the medial meniscus. The torn meniscus is folded cranially *(arrows)*.

the ablation unit or tissue biters. Once the menisci have been inspected and torn sections removed, stabilize the CCL-deficient joint. Use traditional stabilization by extraarticular methods (see p. 1263) or intraarticular methods (see p. 1260) or perform dynamic stabilization with a tibial plateau leveling osteotomy (TPLO) or tibial tuberosity advancement (TTA) (see p. 1260).

Laboratory Findings

If joint palpation and radiographs are inconclusive, joint centesis and synovial fluid examination are helpful. In cases of partial ligament tear, centesis is particularly helpful in identifying stifle joint involvement as the cause of the lameness. Increased amounts of joint fluid and a two- to three-fold increase in cell numbers (6000 to 9000 WBC/µl—

primarily mononuclear cells) are indicative of secondary DJD (see also p. 1145).

DIFFERENTIAL DIAGNOSIS

Differential diagnoses include mild joint sprains or muscle strains, patellar luxation, caudal cruciate ligament injury, primary meniscal injury, long digital extensor tendon avulsion, primary or secondary arthritis, and immune-mediated arthritis.

MEDICAL MANAGEMENT

Conservative treatment is best tolerated in patients weighing less than 10 kg and generally is unsuccessful in larger dogs. Retrospective studies of dogs weighing less than 10 kg indicate that they typically have adequate clinical function with conservative treatment. Conversely, in dogs larger than 10 kg, lameness typically improves, but the animal does not return to preinjury activity without evidence of recurring lameness. Surgical stabilization is recommended in patients of any size to ensure optimum function. Lameness often resolves within 6 weeks in small patients managed conservatively (i.e., rest and antiinflammatory drugs). These patients appear to function normally on the injured leg; however, instability persists and secondary DJD frequently develops. Despite the fact that the animal appears to function adequately after the initial injury, body weight often is merely shifted to the uninjured leg. Abnormal stress, coupled with the increasing mechanical weakness of the cruciate ligament associated with aging, may lead to rupture of the cruciate ligament in the opposite stifle joint within 12 to 18 months. Because these patients are then nonambulatory, they often are incorrectly diagnosed as having an acute neurologic problem. An accurate history and physical examination should alert the clinician to the fact that bilateral cruciate ligament injury, rather than neurologic disease, is the problem. Treatment of patients with bilateral cruciate ligament ruptures is less successful than in animals with only one injured stifle joint.

NOTE: Injury of the contralateral cruciate ligament occurs in 40% of patients. The percentage increases (60%) if radiographic changes are visible in the uninjured joint.

SURGICAL TREATMENT

Surgical therapy is divided into intracapsular and extracapsular reconstruction techniques, corrective osteotomy, or primary repair with augmentation. The surgical method chosen is a matter of the surgeon's preference, patient size and function, and cost of the procedure because most retrospective studies have shown the success rate to be near 90% regardless of the technique used.

Intracapsular and extracapsular surgical procedures have focused on re-creation of the passive constraints of the stifle joint (CCL, joint capsule fibrosis). **Intracapsular reconstruction** consists of passing autogenous tissue through the joint using the "over-the-top" method or passing the tissue through predrilled holes in the femur or tibia or both. The most commonly used material is autogenous fascia lata. Synthetic materials are rarely used because of eventual stretching or rupture and the risk of infection. Allografts with and without bone plugs are available, but are not in widespread use for cruciate ligament reconstruction. An advantage of intracapsular techniques is that they most closely mimic the original position and biology of the original CCL. Disadvantages of these techniques are their invasiveness and the tendency of the graft to stretch or fail.

Extracapsular reconstruction involves placement of sutures outside the joint or redirection of the lateral collateral ligament. Extracapsular reconstruction with sutures is often incorrectly referred to as imbrication sutures. Numerous patterns and combinations of suture origins and insertions have been described. The most commonly used origin for an extracapsular suture is the lateral fabella, and the most com-

mon insertion is the tibial crest. Location of the origin and insertion of an extracapsular suture can have significant effects on the isometry of the joint, thereby affecting the amount of drawer motion throughout the normal range of motion of the stifle joint. Extracapsular sutures may also be secured from bone anchors most commonly placed in the distal femur as the point of origin. This improves the isometry of the suture material. Materials used in extracapsular sutures include monofilament nylon or fishing or leader line manufactured orthopedic wire, or braided orthopedic suture (Sicard et al, 2002).

True **imbrication techniques** have also been described for treatment of CCL rupture, usually in addition to one of the other techniques. Imbrication for cruciate ligament rupture is performed by tightening the fascia lata either through an advancement technique using a vest over pants suture pattern or by partial excision and closure. These techniques are usually performed as part of the routine closure of the fascia lata.

The **fibular head advancement technique** advances the insertion of the lateral collateral ligament to prevent abnormal drawer and internal rotation of the tibia. This procedure may be performed alone or in combination with other stabilizing techniques.

The **tibial plateau leveling osteotomy** (TPLO) changes the mechanics of the stifle to achieve stabilization by active constraint of the joint (Reif et al, 2002; Warzee et al, 2001). The stifle joint normally is stabilized by both passive constraints (ligaments, menisci, joint capsule) and active constraints (muscles and tendons). The CCL functions as a passive constraint to cranial tibial translation and internal rotation of the tibia. Ground reaction forces and muscle forces generate compressive loads on the articular surface of the tibia during weight bearing. As a result of the caudally directed slope of the tibial plateau, when the tibia is loaded, a shear force is generated that induces abnormal tibial translation in CCL-deficient stifle joints. The shear component of the compressive force is referred to as the cranial tibial thrust (CTT) and is passively constrained by the CCL (see Fig. 33-93). The CTT is also proportional to the slope of the tibial plateau. If the slope of the plateau decreases, CTT also decreases. The tibial plateau slope can be reduced such that tibial thrust changes from a cranioproximal direction to a neutral or caudal direction. At the point where the tibial thrust changes direction to a caudal thrust, there is increased reliance on the caudal cruciate ligament as a passive constraint to abnormal caudal translation of the tibia. The intent of TPLO surgery is to attain a tibial plateau slope (approximately 5 to 7 degrees) with which tibial thrust can be effectively controlled by the caudal cruciate ligament and the active constraints of the stifle (e.g., the quadriceps muscle group). Because the CCL also passively constrains excessive internal rotation of the tibia, we must logically question the source of these internally rotatory moments and the role of the TPLO procedure in functionally controlling them. Failure to control the internal rotation resulting in drawer in association with internal rotation is referred to as pivot shift. The significance of this motion to functional outcome following TPLO surgery is uncertain. Slocum introduced the concept of limb malalignment as a leading contributor to internal rotational moments acting about the stifle. That is to say, a dog with a "bowlegged" posture (as a result of tibial or femoral varus) and a pigeon-toed stance (arising from internal tibial or femoral torsion) experiences dramatic internal rotatory moments acting about its stifle compared with a dog with a more aligned pelvic limb. Limb alignment adjustments coupled with the TPLO procedure may help control excessive rotatory moments acting about the stifle in dogs with limb malalignment. TPLO is an effective procedure for dogs with a complete or partial tear of the CCL (Fig. 33-100). Many surgeons prefer TPLO for treating larger, active dogs in which long-term rehabilitation and postoperative control are difficult.

Tibial wedge osteotomy (TWO) is the forebearer of the TPLO and was originally described for the treatment of severely increased TPAs in dogs. The TWO is based on the same principles of biomechanics as the TPLO (Fig. 33-101);

however, the lower location of the osteotomy results in alteration of the relative position of the tibial crest that may be associated with complications of the stifle extensor mechanism. The TWO remains a valuable technique for management of CCLR and increased TPA in young dogs with open proximal tibial physes since the TWO will not affect these physes as the TPLO may.

Tibial tuberosity advancement (TTA) seeks to eliminate tibial thrust by positioning the patellar tendon perpendicular to the shear forces in the stifle. When the paw is loaded on weight bearing, a force is created through the foot to the metatarsus and tarsus that causes the calcanean (Achilles) tendon to react with a second force to maintain the stability of the tarsus at its weight-bearing angle. A vector force (sum of the resulting forces of weight bearing) occurs in the tarsus, creating a simultaneous force through the patellar ligament necessary to stabilize the stifle. A combination of forces in the stifle results in a vector force in a plane almost parallel to the patellar ligament at the standing weight-bearing angle of the stifle (135 degrees) (Fig. 33-102). This is the tibiofemoral force across the stifle joint at normal weight bearing. If the slope of the tibial plateau is not anatomically oriented perpendicular to the patellar ligament on weight bearing, then the vector force does not superimpose the normal compressive tibiofemoral force of weight bearing on the stifle joint. A tibiofemoral shear force (in the direction of cranial

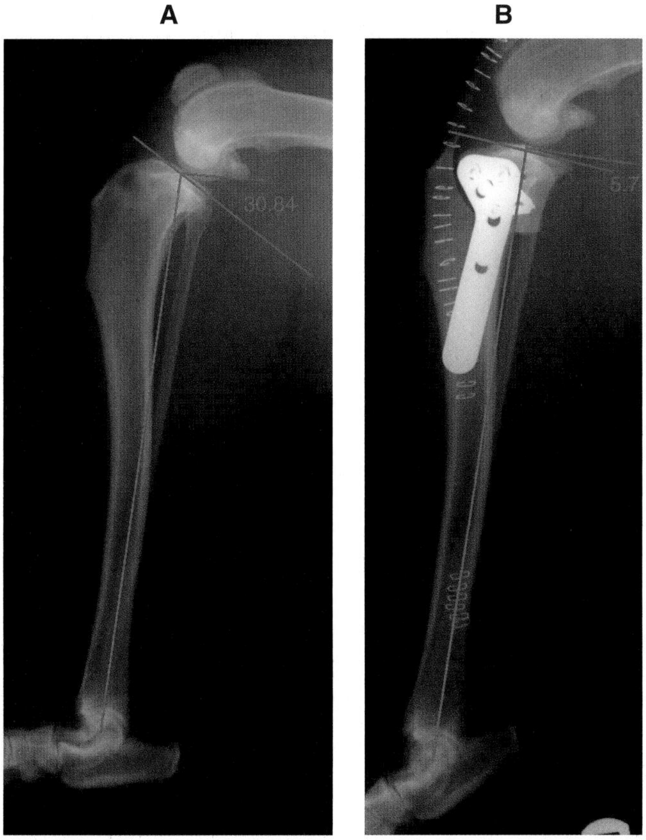

A   **B**

FIG. 33-100
A, Preoperative lateral radiograph of a dog showing measurement of the tibial slope for a TPLO. **B,** Postoperative lateral radiograph showing leveling of the tibial slope (5 degrees) for active stabilization of the cranial cruciate–deficient stifle joint.

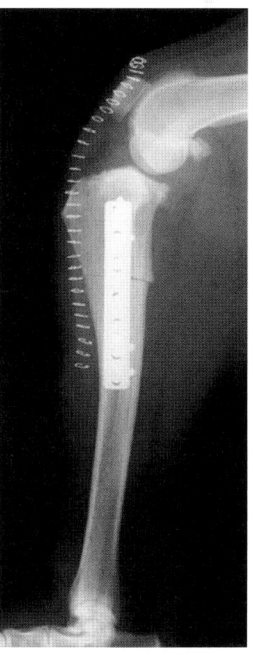

FIG. 33-101
Radiograph of a tibia after a TWO.

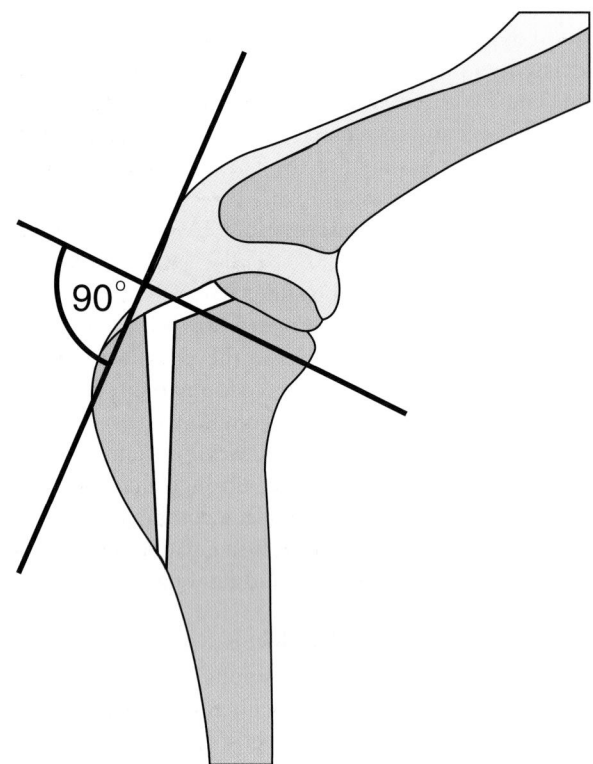

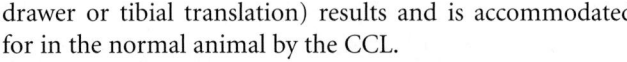

FIG. 33-102
Biomechanics of TTA. TTA positions the patellar ligament perpendicular to the slope of the tibial plateau by advancing its insertion in a cranial direction, eliminating the tibiofemoral shear force with weight bearing and relieving the function of the CCL.

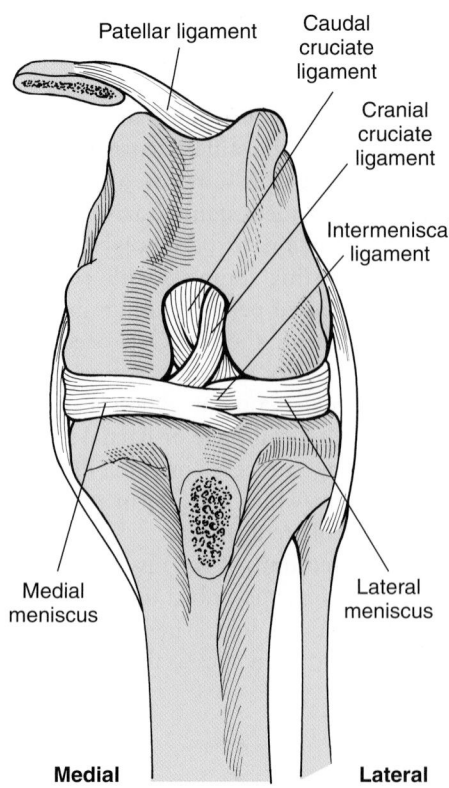

FIG. 33-103
Orientation of the cruciate ligaments and menisci.

drawer or tibial translation) results and is accommodated for in the normal animal by the CCL.

TTA positions the patellar ligament perpendicular to the slope of the tibial plateau by advancing its insertion in a cranial direction, eliminating the tibiofemoral shear force with weight bearing and relieving the function of the CCL. The TPLO procedure accomplishes essentially the same redirection of vector force by rotating the tibial plateau to neutralize the tibiofemoral shear force. However, TPLO may increase the tension on the patellar ligament, whereas TTA theoretically relieves patellar ligament tension. TTA appears to result in less patellar ligament inflammation than the TPLO (Carey et al, 2005). TTA does not affect joint congruency; however, it does increase loading of the caudal cruciate. This may be partially offset by the general reduction of internal joint reactions as a result of a longer patellar ligament lever arm.

Regardless of the technique used to stabilize the stifle, the meniscus should be inspected by open arthrotomy or arthroscopy for tears or other evidence of trauma. Damage to the caudal body of the medial meniscus is seen in 50% to 75% of patients with a torn CCL. Most of these patients have a bucket handle tear (see Fig. 33-99, *B*), which must be excised.

Preoperative Management

Activity of patients with torn CCLs should be limited before surgery to prevent further damage to the articular cartilage or meniscus. Perioperative antibiotics (see p. 945) and preemptive pain management with opiates, NSAIDs, and/or epidural analgesia (see Table 33-4 on p. 1149) are indicated for dogs undergoing stifle reconstructive techniques.

Anesthesia

General anesthesia recommendations for orthopedic patients are discussed on p. 944. Opioid epidural administration reduces postoperative discomfort (see p. 945). Intraarticular administration of 0.5% bupivacaine (0.5 ml/kg) or morphine (0.1 mg/kg diluted with saline to a volume of 0.5 ml/kg) before skin closure also reduces postoperative discomfort.

Surgical Anatomy

Knowledge of the origin and insertion of normal ligamentous structures and menisci of the stifle joint is important when considering arthroscopic exploration or surgery to repair a cruciate ligament rupture. The tendon of the long digital extensor muscle originates from the extensor fossa of the lateral femoral condyle and is located directly below the lateral arthrotomy incision. The CCL originates from the

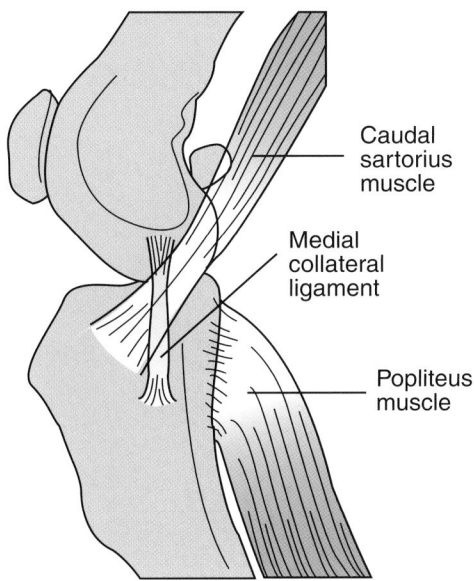

FIG. 33-104
Anatomy of the medial aspect of the stifle for TPLO or TTA surgery.

Labels in figure:
Caudal sartorius muscle
Medial collateral ligament
Popliteus muscle

inside (medial) surface of the lateral femoral condyle (Fig. 33-103), courses distal and medial, spirals 90 degrees, and inserts onto the craniomedial surface of the tibial plateau beneath the intermeniscal ligament. The caudal cruciate ligament is visible as a broad expanse of ligament located in the intercondylar notch. The medial and lateral menisci are fibrocartilaginous disks that have a semilunar shape and are attached to the tibia and surrounding soft tissue (see p. 1285).

If an extracapsular reconstruction is chosen as a method of treatment, care must be taken to prevent injury to the peroneal nerve, which courses lateral and caudal to the stifle. The fabellae are located between the femoral condyles and the distal femoral diaphysis and sit in the origin of the gastrocnemius muscle. Osteoarthritis causes osteophytosis of the fabellae and may complicate passage of a needle and suture around the fabella. The lateral collateral originates on the lateral femoral condyle and inserts on the fibular head. The fibula is connected to the tibia proximally by the ligament of the fibular head.

The medial collateral ligament is used as an approximate landmark for the distal aspect of the TPLO osteotomy. It inserts broadly several centimeters below the tibial plateau at the caudal aspect of the tibia (Fig. 33-104). The popliteal artery and vein are located just caudal to the tibia proximally and must be protected during the osteotomy. The medial saphenous vein lies on the medial aspect of the tibia distally and should be protected during insertion of the distal jig pin.

Positioning

For arthroscopy, the patient is positioned in dorsal recumbency. The limb should be prepared in a suspended position and clipped and prepared for aseptic surgery from the hip

to the tarsus. Prepare the limb as for open surgery in case an arthrotomy is required or for cruciate stabilization following the arthroscopy. The limb may be held by an assistant or placed in an arthroscopy brace to maintain the positioning.

For an intracapsular or extracapsular stabilization, the patient may be positioned in dorsal or lateral recumbency. The limb should be prepared in a suspended position to allow maximum manipulation during surgery. The leg should be clipped and prepared for aseptic surgery from the hip to the tarsus.

For TPLO, TTA, or TWO, the patient may be positioned in dorsal recumbency or dorsolateral oblique tilted towards the side to be operated. Some surgeons prefer to position the patient so that the operated limb can be placed flat on the operating table (or a Mayo stand for giant breed dogs) when the limb is flexed with both the stifle and hock at 90 degrees. The leg should be clipped and prepared for aseptic surgery from the hip to the tarsus.

SURGICAL TECHNIQUE
Lateral Approach to the Stifle Joint

Make a craniolateral skin incision centered at the level of the patella (Fig. 33-105, A). Begin the incision 5 cm proximal to the patella, and continue it distally 5 cm below the tibial crest. Incise the subcutaneous tissue along the same line to visualize the septum between the superficial leaf of the fascia lata and the biceps femoris muscle proximally and the lateral retinaculum distally. Make an incision through the fascia lata proximally, and carry the incision through the fascia lata and lateral retinaculum distally (Figure 33-105, B). Make an incision through the joint capsule, beginning 1 cm distal to the patella. Continue the incision proximally along a line adjacent to the patellar tendon and proximal to the patella. Then incise along the border of the vastus lateralis muscle toward the fabella (Fig. 33-105, C). Displace the patella medially to expose the cranial surface of the joint.

Medial Approach to the Stifle Joint

Make a craniomedial incision centered at the level of the patella (Fig. 33-106). Begin the incision 5 cm proximal to the patella, and continue distally 5 cm below the tibial crest. Incise subcutaneous tissue along the same line to expose the parapatellar medial retinaculum. Make an incision through the medial retinaculum and joint capsule adjacent to the medial ridge of the patellar tendon. Continue the incision proximally to the extent of the suprapatellar joint capsule and distally to the tibial tuberosity.

Intracapsular Repair

For a description of an intracapsular repair, see *Small Animal Surgery,* second edition or the e-dition.

Lateral Retinacular Stabilization

Perform arthroscopy or an arthrotomy as described above, resect the remnants of the CCL, and inspect the meniscus for

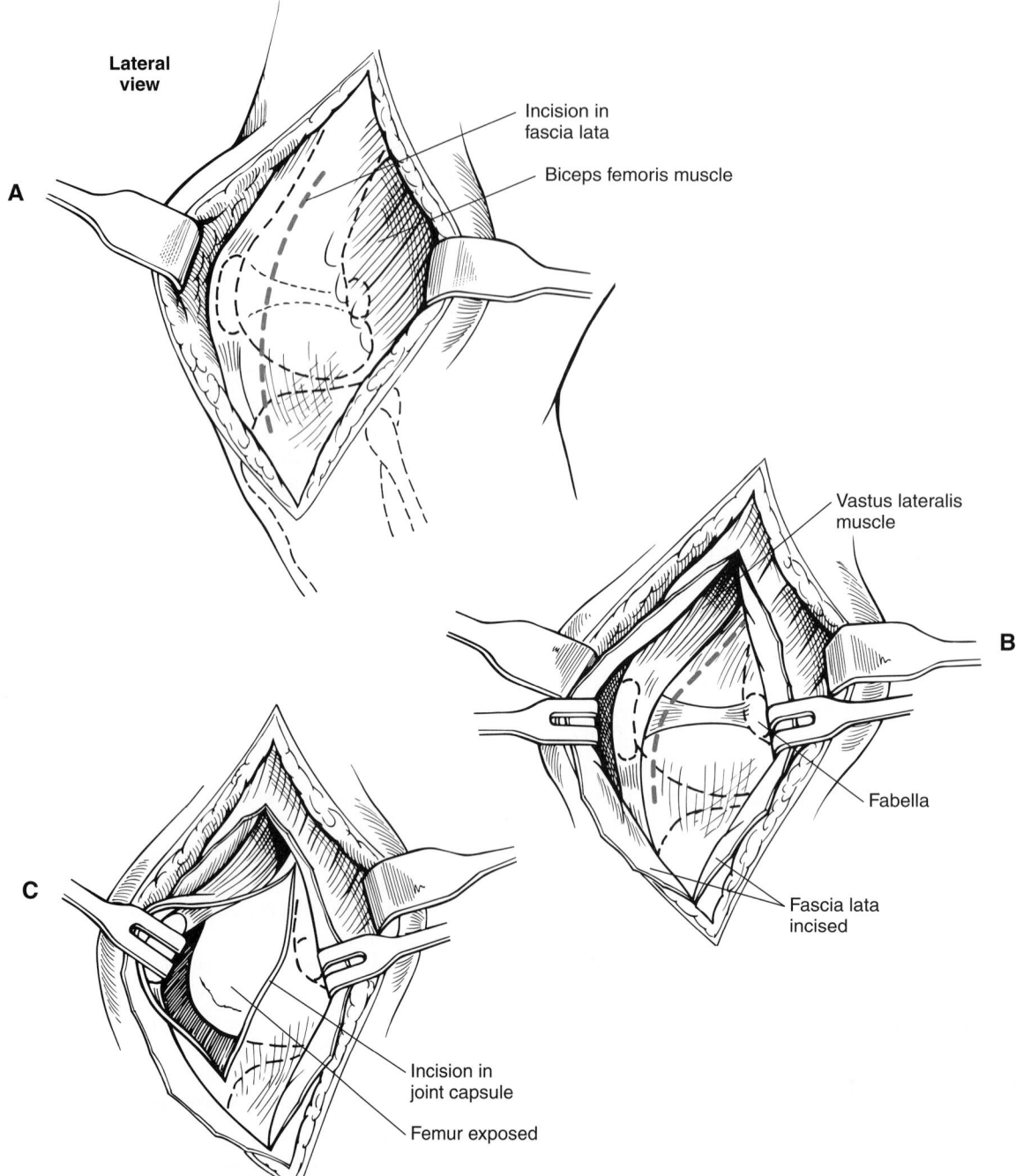

**Lateral
view**

A

Incision in
fascia lata

Biceps femoris muscle

B

Vastus lateralis
muscle

Fabella

Fascia lata
incised

C

Incision in
joint capsule

Femur exposed

FIG. 33-105
Lateral approach to the stifle joint. **A,** Make a craniolateral skin incision centered over the patella. Incise the subcutaneous tissue along the same line to visualize the septum between the superficial leaf of the fascia lata and the biceps femoris muscle proximally and the lateral retinaculum distally. **B,** Make an incision through the fascia lata proximally and carry the incision through the fascia lata and lateral retinaculum distally. **C,** Incise the joint capsule and continue the incision proximally adjacent to the patellar tendon. Then incise along the border of the vastus lateralis toward the fabella. Displace the patella medially to expose the cranial surface of the joint.

Medial View

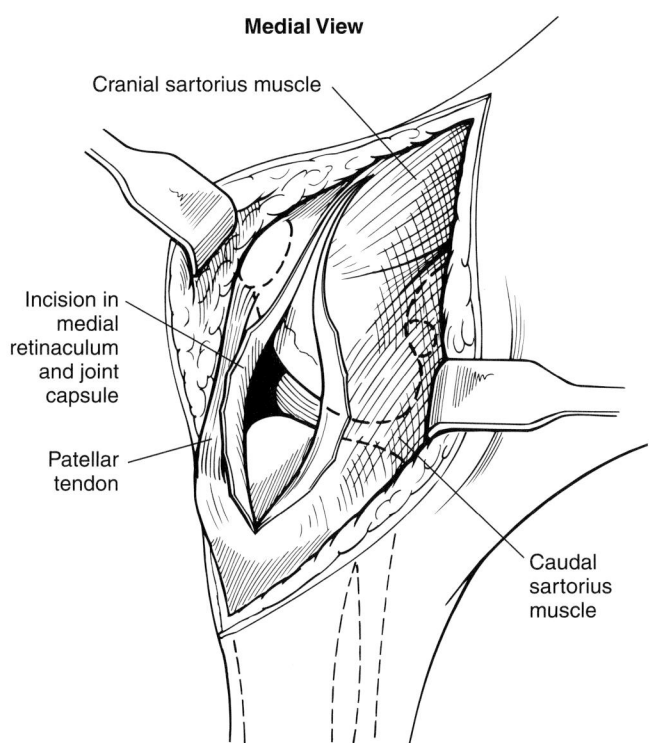

Cranial sartorius muscle

Incision in medial retinaculum and joint capsule

Patellar tendon

Caudal sartorius muscle

FIG. 33-106
Medial approach to the stifle joint. Make a craniomedial incision centered over the patella. Incise the subcutaneous tissue along the same line to expose the parapatellar medial retinaculum. Make an incision through the medial retinaculum and joint capsule adjacent to the medial ridge of the patellar tendon.

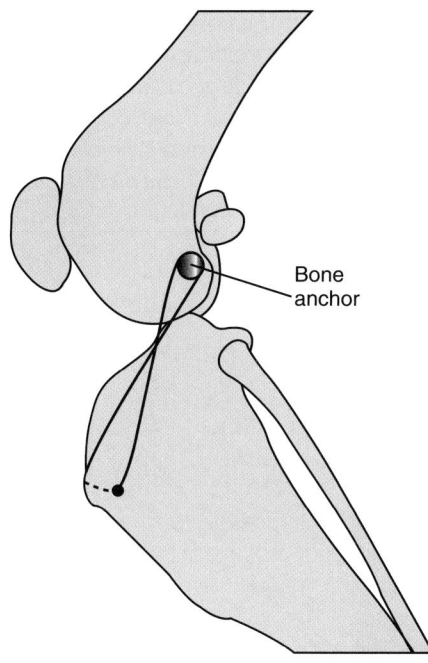

Bone anchor

FIG. 33-107
An extracapsular reconstruction using a heavy, nonabsorbable suture and suture anchors.

tears or damage. Remove the damaged meniscus, if present, and close the arthrotomy or arthroscopy portals.

If not already done, perform the lateral approach to the stifle joint. Retract the skin laterally, and make an incision through the lateral retinaculum and distal fascia lata.

This incision has already been made if the stifle has been approached laterally.

Elevate the biceps femoris muscle from the lateral surface of the joint capsule to expose the gastrocnemius muscle. Pass monofilament nylon sutures or monofilament nylon leader material (No. 2 monofilament nylon suture for dogs up to 10 kg; nylon leader material [27 kg test] for dogs up to 30 kg and 36 kg test for dogs more than 30 kg) through the eye of the appropriately sized "cruciate" needle, and pass the needle around the fabella from proximal to distal. Alternatively, use a swaged-on double line of monofilament nylon designed for cruciate stabilization. The suture may also be anchored using a suture anchor in the lateral femoral condyle (Fig. 33-107). Place the anchor as far caudally as possible at the distal pole of the lateral fabella. Next, pass the suture behind the patellar ligament immediately proximal to the tibial tuberosity. Drill a hole of sufficient size to pass the needle through

the tibial crest from medial to lateral and pass the suture through the hole in the same direction. Cut the suture to remove the needle, obtaining two sutures to tie. Flex the stifle to a normal standing angle, hold the tibia caudally and rotated externally to remove drawer motion, and tie or crimp the sutures (Fig. 33-108).

In addition to the stabilizing suture, advance the lateral retinaculum cranially and distally by placing a series of vertical mattress imbricating sutures (vest over pants). Place each suture through the retinaculum caudal to the arthrotomy line, cross them superficial to the arthrotomy, penetrate in and out of the retinaculum cranial to the arthrotomy and distal to the initial position of the suture on the caudal retinaculum, and return to pass the suture through the caudal retinaculum. Preplace individual sutures and tie when all sutures in the series are in place. Proper placement of sutures draws the caudal retinaculum over the cranial retinaculum. Close as described above.

Fibular Head Advancement

Static advancement of the lateral collateral ligament is a useful technique for eliminating instability in the CCL-deficient stifle joint. This is accomplished by advancing the fibular head, which is the point of insertion of the lateral collateral ligament.

Perform arthroscopy or an arthrotomy as described previously, resect the remnants of the CCL, and inspect the menis-

cus for tears or damage. Remove the damaged meniscus, if present, and close the arthrotomy or arthroscopy portals.

If not already done, perform a lateral approach to the stifle joint and reflect the fascia lata caudally. To facilitate reflection of the fascia lata, make a craniocaudal transverse incision of the fascia lata 2 to 3 cm distal to the joint line.

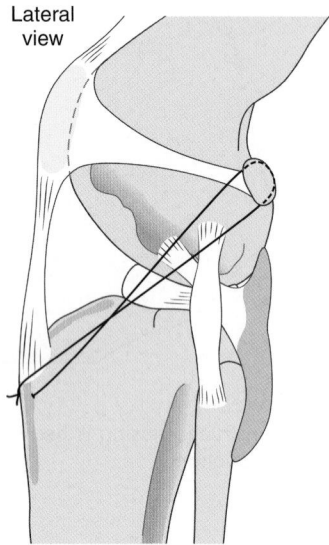

FIG. 33-108
An extracapsular reconstruction using a heavy, nonabsorbable suture (or sutures). The suture passes through deep fascia surrounding the fabella and through a predrilled hole in the tibial crest. Tying the suture eliminates the cranial drawer.

Using sharp dissection and elevation, free the fibular head cranially and caudally from the tibial epiphysis (Fig. 33-109, A). Make an incision along the cranial and caudal edges of the lateral collateral ligament to allow cranial transposition of the ligament-bone complex. Taking care not to injure the popliteal tendon or lateral meniscus, free the deep surface of the ligament from its origin at the femoral epicondyle to its insertion at the fibular head.

This is most easily accomplished with a small periosteal elevator.

Incise the fibularis longus and lateral digital extensor muscles at the joint line and reflect them craniodistally to allow cranial redirection of the fibular head. Externally rotate the tibia, and advance the fibular head and collateral ligament cranially using pointed reduction forceps. Stabilize the fibular head with a small Steinmann pin and tension band wire (Fig. 33-109, B). Suture the extensor muscles and fascia lata with absorbable suture using a simple interrupted pattern. Close the subcutaneous tissue and skin incisions as previously described.

> NOTE: Use extreme care in identifying and protecting the peroneal nerve throughout this procedure.

Primary Repair With Augmentation

Primary repair with augmentation is reserved for a small percentage of patients that have experienced failure of the cruciate ligament at the point of insertion on the tibial pla-

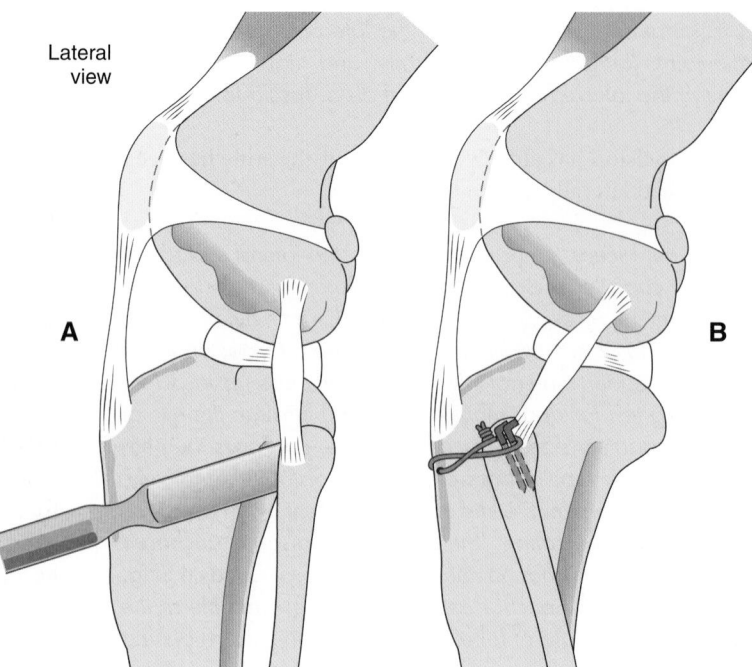

FIG. 33-109
Fibular head advancement. **A,** Free the fibular head cranially and caudally from the tibial epiphysis with sharp dissection and elevation. **B,** Advance the fibular head and stabilize it with a small Steinmann pin and tension band wire.

teau or failure from the origin of the ligament on the femur. This mode of ligament failure may occur after trauma to the stifle joint in patients less than 1 year of age. The most frequent site of failure is the point of insertion of the ligament on the tibial plateau. Surgical exposure is the same as that described for intracapsular or extracapsular reconstruction. A reconstructive procedure is always used in addition to primary repair.

Perform either a medial or lateral approach to the stifle joint as described above. Once the arthrotomy has been made, identify the CCL. A small piece of cancellous bone often remains attached at the site of failure. Pass nonabsorbable suture through the ligament using a locking-loop pattern (see p. 1320). Make two small parallel drill holes from the medial tibial metaphysis to exit within the joint at the insertion point of the CCL. Place wire loops through the holes and pass the free ends of the suture through the wire. Pull the wire through the predrilled holes to exit laterally. Perform a reconstructive procedure to augment the primary repair. When the reconstruction has been completed, tie the sutures from the ligament outside the joint (Fig. 33-110). Close the surgical wound using the technique described above.

Tibial Plateau Leveling Osteotomy

Radiographic assessment. *With the patient under general anesthesia, position the dog in lateral recumbency with the limb to be radiographed dependent. Elevate the opposite limb out of the x-ray beam. Position a radiographic plate to include the distal femoral condyles, the entire tibia, and the tarsal joint (Fig. 33-111). Position the limb so that the femoral condyles overlap and the trochlear ridges of the talus overlap. Complete the radiograph and obtain a craniocaudal radiograph of the limb including the same structures.*

The most accurate measurements of TPA are made when there is less than 2 mm difference between the two femoral condyles and when the beam is centered towards the tibial plateau (Reif et al, 2004).

On the lateral radiograph, mark the center of the trochlea of the talus and the center of the intercondylar eminence of the tibial plateau. Connect these two points with a line (line a) (Fig. 33-112). Draw a second line (line b) to estimate the tibial plateau (Fig. 33-112). Where these two lines intersect, draw a third line (line c) perpendicular to the first line (Fig. 33-112). Measure the angle between lines b and c. This is the tibial plateau angle. Using the conversion chart appropriate to the selected osteotomy blade (Table 33-14), determine the degree of rotation.

The osteotomy should be performed to allow space for the proximal aspect of the bone plate while preserving adequate tibial crest to prevent fracture. The osteotomy should exit the caudal aspect of the tibia perpendicular to the bone without an "uphill" or "downhill" exit.

Surgical technique. Perform arthroscopy or an arthrotomy as described previously, resect the remnants of the CCL, and inspect the meniscus for tears or damage. Remove

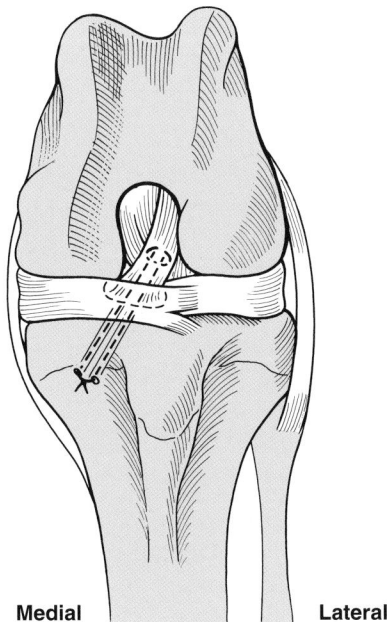

Medial   **Lateral**

FIG. 33-110
For a primary repair of an avulsed CCL, place a suture through the avulsed piece of bone and ligament. Pass the free ends of the suture through parallel tunnels and tie them outside the joint.

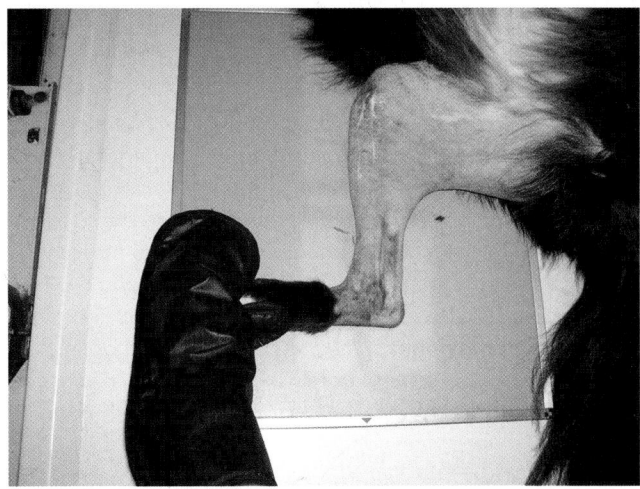

FIG. 33-111
Positioning for radiography before TPLO or TTA surgery.

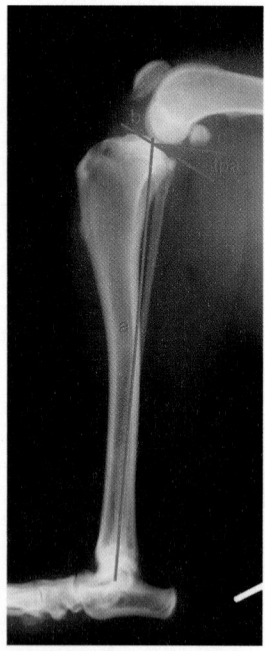

FIG. 33-112
To measure the TPA: On the lateral radiograph, mark the center of the trochlea of the talus and the center of the intercondylar eminence of the tibial plateau. Connect these two points with a line *(line a)*. Draw a second line to estimate the tibial plateau *(line b)*. Where these two lines intersect, draw a third line *(line c)* perpendicular to the first line. Measure the angle between lines b and c. This is the TPA.

 Table 33-14

Rotational Charts for Tibial Plateau Leveling Osteotomy

TPA	ROTATION			
	12 mm	**18 mm**	**24 mm**	**30 mm**
15	2.00	3.00	4.25	5.25
16	2.25	3.25	4.50	5.75
17	2.50	3.75	5.00	6.25
18	2.70	4.00	5.50	6.75
19	2.90	4.25	6.00	7.25
20	3.00	4.50	6.25	7.75
21	3.25	4.75	6.75	8.30
22	3.50	5.00	7.00	8.85
23	3.70	5.50	7.50	9.40
24	3.90	5.75	8.00	10.00
25	4.00	6.00	8.25	10.40
26	4.25	6.25	8.75	11.00
27	4.50	6.75	9.00	11.50
28	4.70	7.00	9.50	12.00
29	4.90	7.25	10.00	12.50
30	5.00	7.50	10.25	13.00
31	5.25	8.00	10.75	13.50
32	5.50	8.25	11.00	14.00
33	5.70	8.50	11.50	14.50
34	5.90	8.75	12.00	15.00
35	6.00	9.00	12.25	15.50
36	6.25	9.50	12.75	16.00
37	6.50	9.75	13.00	16.50
38	6.70	10.00	13.50	17.00
39	6.90	10.25	14.00	17.50
40	7.00	10.50	14.25	18.00

the damaged meniscus, if present, and close the arthrotomy or arthroscopy portals.

Make a medial skin incision centered at the level of the proximal tibia (Fig. 33-113). Begin the incision 3 cm proximal to the tibial plateau, and continue it distally 5 cm below the level of the tibial crest. Incise the subcutaneous tissue along the same line sharply or with electrocautery to visualize the insertion of the cranial head of the sartorius. Incise the insertion of the sartorius, and reflect the muscle caudally to visualize the medial collateral ligament and the caudal aspect of the proximal tibia. Sharply incise the origin of the popliteus muscle from the caudomedial aspect of the tibia. Bluntly dissect the origin of the muscle from the caudal aspect of the tibia to the lateral border. Once elevated, place a moistened sponge in between the muscle and the bone to protect the muscle and popliteal artery and vein during the osteotomy.

Be certain to keep the periosteal elevator against the bone to prevent damage to the popliteal artery and vein.

Insert a jig pin perpendicular to the sagittal and parallel to the transverse planes starting at the proximal-caudal point

that represents the center of rotation for the osteotomy. Advance the jig pin until it engages both cortices of the tibia. Assemble the jig on the proximal jig pin and determine the position for the distal pin. Make a 1-cm skin incision over the center of the tibial diaphysis at the location for the distal jig pin, taking care to protect the medial saphenous vein. Drive the distal jig pin through the jig and through the center of the tibia, engaging both medial and lateral diaphyses. Cut the proximal jig pin short while leaving the distal jig pin long (Fig. 33-114, A and B).

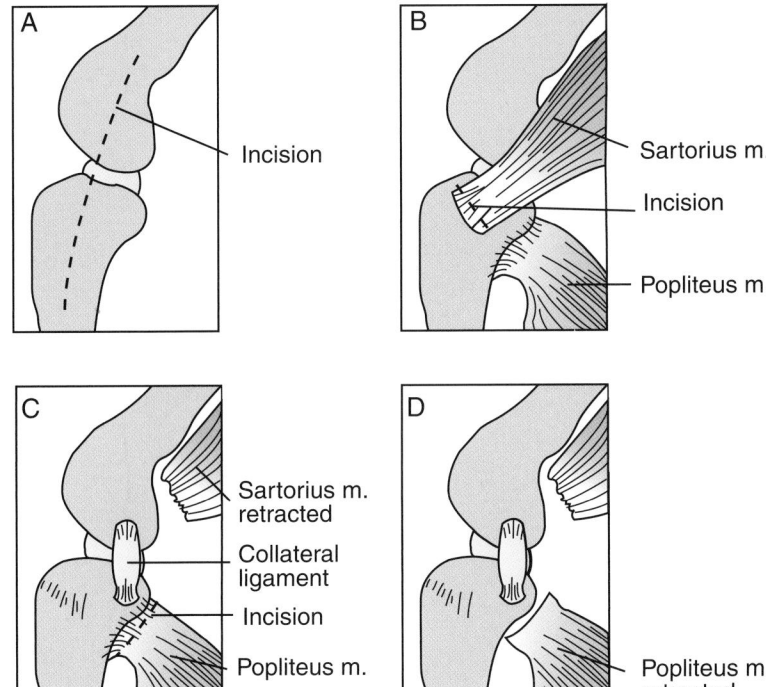

FIG. 33-113
Medial approach to the proximal tibia. **A,** Make a medial skin incision centered at the level of the proximal tibia. Begin the incision 3 cm proximal to the tibial plateau and continue it distally 5 cm below the level of the tibial crest. Incise the subcutaneous tissue along the same line sharply or with electrocautery to visualize the insertion of the cranial head of the sartorius muscle. **B,** Incise the insertion of the sartorius muscle and reflect it caudally to visualize the medial collateral ligament and the caudal aspect of the proximal tibia. **C,** Sharply incise the origin of the popliteus muscle from the caudomedial aspect of the tibia. Bluntly dissect the origin of the muscle from the caudal aspect of the tibia to the medial border. Once elevated, place a moistened sponge in between the muscle and the bone to protect the muscle and popliteal artery and vein during the osteotomy.

Placing the jig pins may be performed with the dog in dorsal recumbency and the limb held up or the dog in oblique recumbency so that the limb may be placed flat on the operating table.

Position the appropriate-sized biradial saw at the location for the osteotomy.

In most cases, the distal aspect of the saw intersects the distal aspect of the insertion of the medial collateral ligament. The patellar tendon may be protected by placing a Hohmann retractor caudal to the ligament and having an assistant retract it cranially. Additional protection may be afforded by elevating the cranial tibial muscle off of the tibia on the lateral side and placing a sponge between the muscle and the bone.

Start the osteotomy by placing the saw at an oblique angle to the bone so only the edges of the bone are initially engaged by the saw. Then bring the saw to a position perpendicular to the bone and parallel to the jig pins. The saw should be roughly centered over the proximal jig pin and parallel to both pins. Make an initial superficial cut with the saw, then stop to evaluate the osteotomy position. Evaluate the thickness of the tibial crest, the area available for the bone plate, and the angle of the osteotomy as it exits the caudal aspect of the tibia.

Cutting the bone may be performed with the dog in dorsal recumbency and the limb held up or the dog in oblique recumbency so that the limb may be placed flat on the operating table. The cut should preserve enough tibial crest to prevent fracture, allow ample room for the bone plate, and exit the bone caudally perpendicular to the bone.

After confirming the correct position of the osteotomy, continue the osteotomy while lavaging the saw blade with cool saline until the tibia is cut approximately 50%. Using an osteotome, make marks on either side of the osteotomy the appropriate distance apart as determined by the TPA, the saw size, and the appropriate rotation chart (Fig. 33-114, C). Complete the osteotomy and remove the protective gauze sponges.

Insert a large pin into the cranial proximal medial aspect of the proximal bone segment, directing the pin distally, caudally, and laterally.

This is the rotation pin.

Rotate the proximal segment distally and caudally so that the marks line up (Fig. 33-114, D).

It may be necessary to pass an elevator between the osteotomy segments and to pry slightly to permit easier rotation.

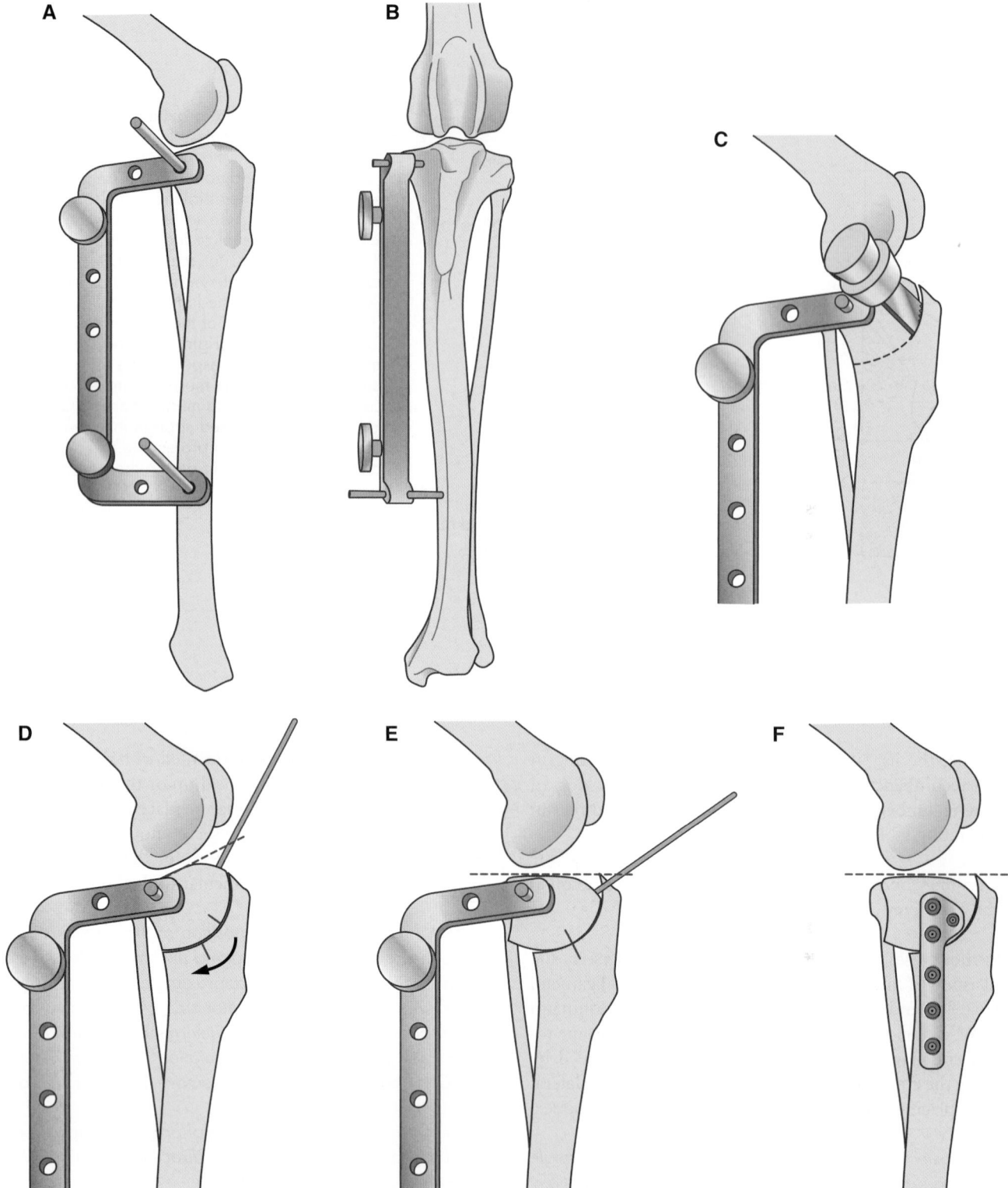

FIG. 33-114

To perform a TPLO: **A** and **B,** Position the jig perpendicular to the long axis of the tibia. **C,** Perform the osteotomy to a depth of one third of the bone, keeping the saw parallel to the jig pins. **D,** Mark the bone for rotation. **E,** Rotate the proximal segment to align the marks. **F,** Secure the osteotomy with the appropriate-sized bone plate.

Do not translate the proximal segment medially to line up the cortices because this may contribute to limb malalignment. Insert a small pin through the proximal tibial crest and into the proximal osteotomy fragment to secure the two bone pieces in the new position. Test for tibial thrust.

It is important to test for tibial thrust before placing the bone plate to ensure that thrust has been eliminated. Adjustments to the degree of rotation may be necessary if thrust still exists at this stage of the procedure. The distance of rotation can be measured at this point by measuring the amount of exposed osteotomy surface at the caudal aspect of the tibia.

Apply the appropriate-sized bone plate beginning with screws in the distal segment followed by screws in the proximal segment (Fig. 33-114, F).

Contouring of the bone plate may be made simpler by removing excessive fibrous tissue on the medial aspect of the stifle joint (medial buttress–butressectomy). When drilling for screw placement in the proximal segment it is useful to have the drill parallel to the jig pin to avoid accidentally entering the stifle joint (Fig. 33-115). The second and third holes of the bone plate may be used in a compressive manner to compress the osteotomy line.

If locking screws are used, apply a nonlocking screw first if contact between the plate and the bone is intended.

Suture the insertion of the cranial head of the sartorius muscle to the deep fascia of the tibia with absorbable suture in a continuous pattern. Suture the remainder of the deep fascia with absorbable suture in a continuous pattern. Suture the superficial fascia and subcutaneous tissues with absorbable suture in continuous patterns. Suture the skin with nonabsorbable suture in a simple interrupted pattern or use skin staples.

Tibial Wedge Osteotomy

Radiographic assessment. *With the patient under general anesthesia position the dog in lateral recumbency with the limb to be radiographed dependent. Elevate the opposite limb out of the x-ray beam. Position a radiographic plate to include the distal femoral condyles, the entire tibia, and the hock joint. Position the limb so that the femoral condyles overlap and the trochlear ridges of the talus overlap. Complete the radiograph and obtain a craniocaudal radiograph of the limb including the same structures.*

The most accurate measurements of TPA are made when there is less than 2 mm difference between the two femoral condyles and when the beam is centered towards the tibial plateau.

On the lateral radiograph mark the center of the trochlea of the talus and the center of the intercondylar eminence of the tibial plateau. Connect these two points with a line (a)

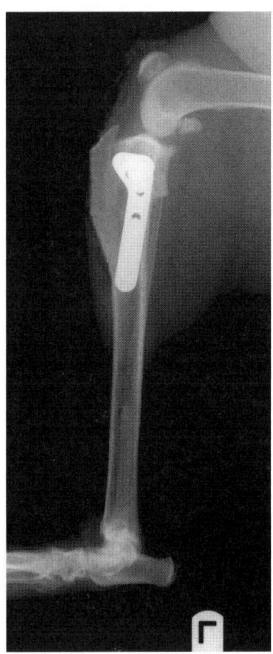

FIG. 33-115
Postoperative radiographs of a TPL.

(Fig. 33-116). Draw a second line (b) to estimate the tibial plateau (Fig. 33-116). Where these two lines intersect draw a third line (c) perpendicular to the first line (Fig. 33-116). Measure the angle between lines b and c. This is the tibial plateau angle. Make a line (d) perpendicular to line a at the base of the flare of the tibial crest (Fig. 33-116). Make another line that intersects line d at the caudal aspect of the tibia and creates an angle equal to the TPA minus six degrees.

The osteotomy should be performed to allow adequate length for the proximal aspect of the bone plate (a minimum of 3 screws) while being as close to the stifle joint as possible. Placing the osteotomy as close to the stifle joint as possible maximizes the biomechanical effect and decreases the risk of fracture.

Surgical technique. Perform arthroscopy or an arthrotomy as described above, resect the remnants of the CCL and inspect the meniscus for tears or damage. Remove the damaged meniscus, if present, and close the arthrotomy or arthroscopy portals.

Make a medial skin incision centered at the level of the proposed osteotomy. Begin the incision 5 cm proximal to the osteotomy site and continue it distally 5 cm below the level of the osteotomy. Incise the subcutaneous tissue along the same line sharply or with electrocautery to expose the tibia. Dissect circumferentially around the tibia and place Hohmann retractors cranially and caudally to protect the lateral structures.

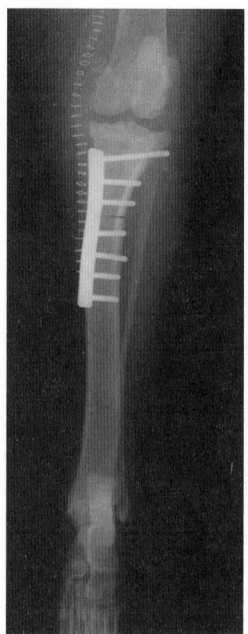

FIG. 33-116
Radiographic measurement for TWO. On the lateral radiograph, mark the center of the trochlea of the talus and the center of the intercondylar eminence of the tibial plateau. Connect these two points with a line (line a). Draw a second line to estimate the tibial plateau (line b). Where these two lines intersect, draw a third line perpendicular to the first line (line c). Measure the angle between lines b and c. This is the tibial plateau angle. Make a line perpendicular to line a at the base of the flare of the tibial crest (line d). Make another line that intersects line d at the caudal aspect of the tibia and creates an angle equal to the tibial plateau angle minus 6 degrees.

Using a straight saw blade, mark both the lines of the osteotomy. Alternating between the two cuts, complete the osteotomy and remove the wedge of bone. Reduce the bone segments and apply an appropriate-sized bone plate (Fig. 33-117).

In larger dogs it may be necessary to apply two parallel bone plates to achieve adequate stability.

Suture the deep fascia with absorbable suture in a continuous pattern. Suture the superficial fascia and subcutaneous tissues with absorbable suture in continuous patterns. Suture the skin with nonabsorbable suture in a simple interrupted pattern or use skin staples.

Tibial Tuberosity Advancement
Radiographic assessment. *With the patient under general anesthesia, position the dog in lateral recumbency with the limb to be radiographed dependent. Elevate the opposite limb out of the x-ray beam. Position a radiographic plate to include the distal femoral condyles, the entire tibia, and the hock joint. Position the limb so that the femoral con-*

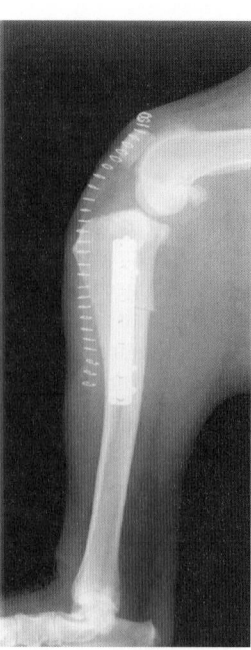

FIG. 33-117
Technique for TWO. Using a straight saw blade, mark both the lines of the osteotomy. Alternating between the two cuts, complete the osteotomy and remove the wedge of bone. Reduce the bone segments and apply an appropriate-sized bone plate.

dyles overlap and the trochlear ridges of the talus overlap. Place the stifle in a weight-bearing angle (135 degrees of extension). Complete the radiograph and obtain a craniocaudal radiograph of the limb including the same structures. Apply the TTA template over the lateral stifle radiograph and determine the amount of advancement necessary (Fig. 33-118).

Surgical technique. *Perform arthroscopy or an arthrotomy as described above, resect the remnants of the CCL and inspect the meniscus for tears or damage. Remove the damaged meniscus, if present, and close the arthrotomy or arthroscopy portals. Make a medial skin incision centered at the level of the proximal tibia. Expose the medial tibial crest by reflecting periosteum.*

NOTE: Be sure to reflect at least half the medial tibial periosteum and related soft tissues cranially to have substantial tissue to close over the implants cranially.

Elevate the fascial insertion of the sartorius muscle and related fascia proximally to the level of the patella. Separate the fascial attachment of the cranial tibial muscle at the level of its attachment to the cranial tibia, just distal to the termination of the tibial crest and insert a moistened gauze sponge. Place the appropriate-sized plate over the tibial crest to assess its proper selection (Fig. 33-119).

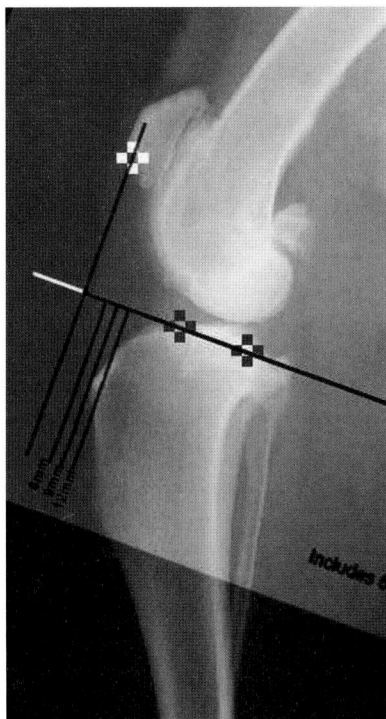

FIG. 33-118
Radiograph of the tibia and overlying TTA template for determining the amount of advancement.

NOTE: Ensure that the distal portion of the plate will not extend beyond the caudal aspect of the tibial shaft after the crest is advanced by the cage.

Determine the exact point for the proximal fork hole in the crest (immediately caudal to the tibial tuberosity), and mark this point with the 2.0 drill bit. Place the fork template over the crest, pass the 2.0 drill bit through the proximal jig hole, and insert the tip of the drill bit into the marked pilot hole. Line the template jig parallel with the tibial crest, and drill the first 2.0 fork hole. Insert the jig pin through the jig and into the first hole. Drill the most distal hole, and place the second jig pin through the jig into this hole. Drill all remaining interposed holes and remove the jig. Identify the proximal and distal crest osteotomy points.

The proximal osteotomy point is the palpable depression at the one third and two thirds junction between the tibial tuberosity and caudomedial tibia. The distal osteotomy point is where the crest terminates by tapering caudally onto the tibial shaft. Make sure the distal point of the proposed osteotomy does not extend distally to the level of the first screw hole in the plate.

Perform a transverse partial crest osteotomy, leaving the lateral cortex intact in the proximal one third of the osteotomy.

The patellar ligament must be carefully protected when carrying the osteotomy proximally, and it is important to make the osteotomy as close to transverse as possible.

Remove the moist sponge from underneath the cranial tibial muscle. Contour and assemble the plate and fork, and seat the plate in the tibial crest holes using the impactor and mallet. Complete the osteotomy. Release soft tissue attachment at the portion of the tubercle of Gerdy remaining on the crest. Measure the width of the proximal tibial crest at the osteotomy site on the tibial shaft to determine the proper cage length. Open the osteotomy gap and insert the cage at the level of the proximal portion of the tibial osteotomy. Drill the hole through the caudal cage ear (2.0 mm, directed slightly caudal and slightly distal), and place the first 2.4-mm screw in the caudal ear of the spacer. Reduce the tibial crest, and hold the distal end of the crest in contact with the tibial shaft using a medium pointed reduction forceps. Check CTT to insure that the TTA is satisfactory before placing screws through the plate. If CTT is present, increase the length of advancement to the next larger cage. Drill, measure, and insert self-tapping plate screws (2.7 mm for 3, 4, 5 hole/fork plate; 3.5 mm for 6, 7, 8 hole/fork plate), placing the most distal screw in the plate first.

NOTE: Add 2 mm to the measurement of each screw because the screw head does not countersink into the plate.

Recheck the position of the patella to ensure it does not luxate and recheck CTT. Insert a 2.4-mm screw in the cranial ear of spacer cage cranially through the tibial crest. Fill the osteotomy gap and cage with a cancellous bone graft obtained from the distal femur. Suture the deep fascia with absorbable suture in a continuous pattern. Suture the superficial fascia and subcutaneous tissue with absorbable suture in continuous patterns. Suture the skin with nonabsorbable suture in a simple interrupted pattern or use skin staples. Obtain postoperative radiographs to confirm correct implant placement (Fig. 33-120).

SUTURE MATERIALS AND SPECIAL INSTRUMENTS

Small Hohmann retractors are useful for inspecting the medial meniscus. Wallace stifle retractors also aid in distracting the stifle joint and visualizing the meniscus. With intracapsular repairs, instruments to drill holes in the tibia, a periosteal elevator, and an osteotome are also needed. For extracapsular repairs, use No. 2 monofilament nylon suture or nylon leader material. Special needles are designed for encircling the fabella. A crimp clamp system may be helpful for securing the large-diameter nylon leader material. Bone anchors may be used to secure the suture proximally. Steinmann pins and wire are used to secure the fibula in a fibular head advancement procedure.

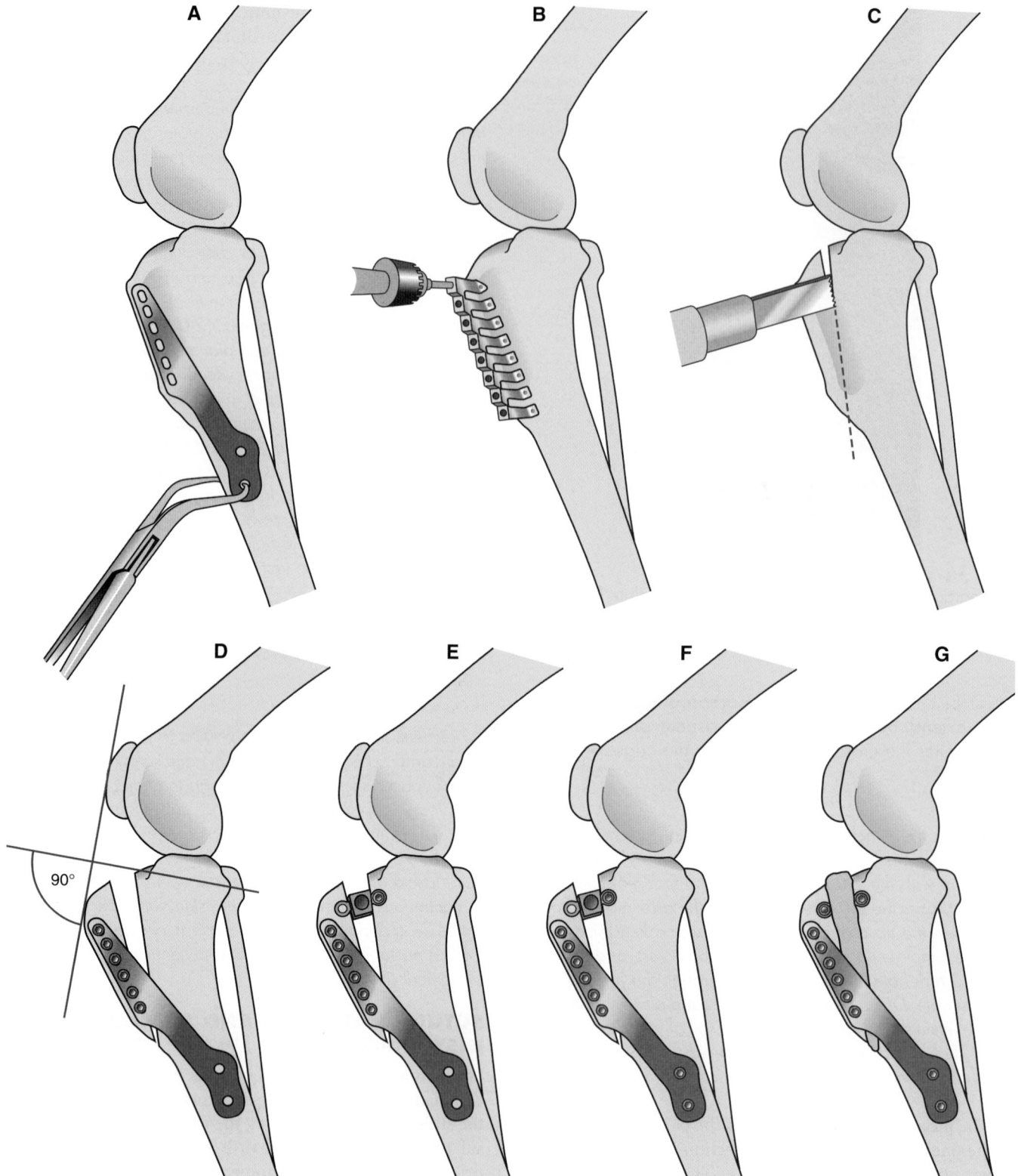

FIG. 33-119
Technique for TTA. **A,** Position the proper-sized plate on the tibial crest to assess its selection. **B,** Place the fork template over the crest and drill the holes beginning with the proximal pilot hole, the most distal hole, and then the remaining holes. **C,** Perform a transverse partial crest osteotomy leaving the lateral cortex intact. **D,** Seat the plate into the tibial crest, then complete the osteotomy. **E,** Open the osteotomy gap and insert the cage at the level of the proximal aspect of the osteotomy and secure with a screw through the caudal cage ear. **F,** Insert the screws through the plate beginning with the most distal screw. **G,** Insert the cranial cage ear screw, fill the gap with bone graft, and close the surgical site.

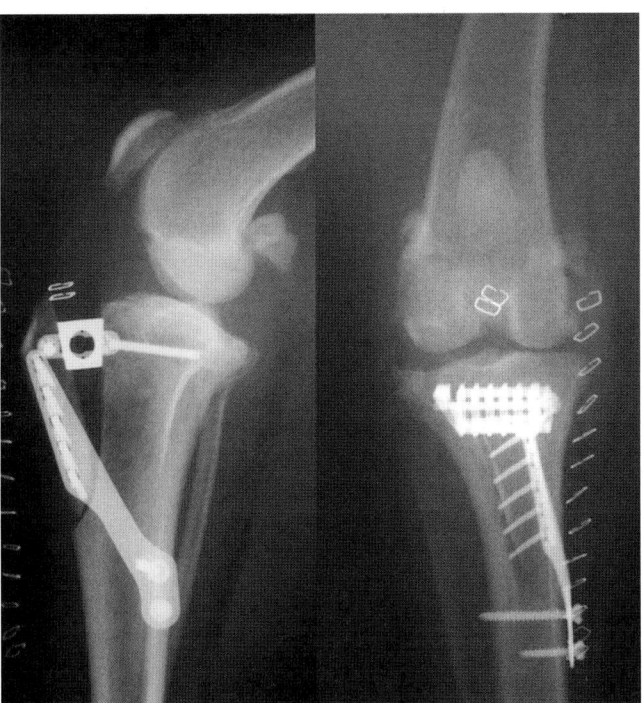

FIG. 33-120
Postoperative radiographs of a TTA. (Photo courtesy Nate Miller, Denver.)

Performance of a TPLO requires a TPLO jig, a biradial saw blade and saw, TPLO bone plates and plating equipment, and a power drill. Performance of a TWO requires a sagittal saw, straight bone plates, plating equipment, and a power drill. TTA requires a sagittal saw, a power drill, and TTA implants.

POSTOPERATIVE CARE AND ASSESSMENT

After intracapsular repairs, a soft bandage with a lateral splint is maintained for 24 to 48 hours. Physical rehabilitation should begin within the first 24 to 48 hours of surgical fixation. These exercises focus on safe weight bearing of the limb and improving usage. A sample physical rehabilitation protocol can be found in Table 33-15. After extracapsular repairs, the limb is placed in a soft, padded bandage for 1 to 2 days after surgery. Physical rehabilitation should begin within the first 24 to 48 hours of surgical fixation. These exercises focus on safe weight bearing of the limb, combating muscle atrophy, and improving range of motion. A sample physical rehabilitation protocol for postoperative extracapsular repairs can be found in Table 33-16.

Following TPLO, TWO, or TTA, strict exercise restriction is required until radiographs demonstrate adequate healing. In young dogs, healing may occur within 4 weeks whereas in older dogs bony union may not occur until 12 weeks postoperatively. Exercise is limited to specific physical rehabilitation exercises and leash walking for several weeks followed by a gradual return to normal activity (see Table 33-15). A rigorous progressive physical rehabilitation program may enhance recovery after stifle surgery (Marsolais et al, 2002).

COMPLICATIONS

Complications of CCL surgery include infection, lack of stabilization, meniscal injury, implant complications, and progressive osteoarthritis (Pacchiana et al, 2003). An additional complication of TPLO is patellar tendon desmitis (Carey et al, 2005). Patients having poor outcome following CCL repair should undergo systematic evaluation for each of these potential complications.

PROGNOSIS

Long-term function for patients that have undergone a reconstructive procedure is good and results are conflicting regarding the influence of the method of reconstruction (Aragon and Budsberg, 2005; Lazar et al, 2005). Most published assessments of outcome state that 85% to 90% of dogs improve after surgery. DJD progresses regardless of treatment. The long-term outcome includes a decline in activity over time, an increasing level of disability, an adverse response to cold weather, and stiffness after inactivity related to progressive DJD (Innes et al, 2000).

References

Aragon CL, Budsberg SC: Applications of evidence-based medicine: cranial cruciate ligament injury repair in the dog, *Vet Surg* 34:93, 2005.

Carey K, Aiken SW, DeResta GR et al: Radiographic and clinical changes of the patellar tendon after tibial plateau leveling osteotomy: 94 cases (2001-2003), *Vet Comp Orthop Traum* 18:235, 2005.

Harasen GLG: Feline cranial cruciate rupture, *Vet Comp Orthop Traum* 18:254, 2005.

Hoelzler MG, Millis DL, Francis DA et al: Results of arthroscopic versus open arthrotomy for surgical management of cranial cruciate ligament deficiency in dogs, *Vet Surg* 33:146, 2004.

Innes JF, Bacon D, Lynch C et al: Long-term outcome of surgery for dogs with cranial cruciate ligament deficiency, *Vet Rec* 147:325, 2000.

Lazar TP, Berry CR, deHaan JJ et al: Long-term radiographic comparison of tibial plateau leveling osteotomy versus extracapsular stabilization for cranial cruciate ligament rupture in the dog, *Vet Surg* 34:133, 2005.

Marsolais GS, Dvorak G, Conzemius MG: Effects of postoperative rehabilitation on limb function after cranial cruciate ligament repair in dogs, *J Am Vet Med Assoc* 220:1325, 2002.

Morris E, Lipowitz AJ: Comparison of tibial plateau angles in dogs with and without cranial cruciate ligament injuries, *J Am Vet Med Assoc* 218:363, 2001.

Pacchiana PD, Morris E, Gillings SL et al: Surgical and postoperative complications associated with tibial plateau leveling osteotomy in dogs with cranial cruciate ligament rupture: 397 cases (1998-2001), *J Am Vet Med Assoc* 222:184, 2003.

Reif U, Dejardin LM, Probst CW et al: Influence of limb positioning and measurement method on the magnitude of the tibial plateau angle, *Vet Surg* 33:368, 2004.

Reif U, Hulse DA, Hauptman JG: Effect of tibial plateau leveling on stability of the canine cranial cruciate-deficient stifle joint: an in vitro study, *Vet Surg* 31:147, 2002.

Reif U, Probst CW: Comparison of tibial plateau angles in normal and cranial cruciate deficient stifles of Labrador retrievers, *Vet Surg* 32:385, 2003.

Table 33-15

Physical Rehabilitation Protocol Following TPLO, TTA, TWO, MPL, LPL, and Other Stifle Ligament Damage

ALL TREATMENTS BID	DAY 1 TO DAY 14	DAY 15 TO DAY 24	DAY 25 UNTIL HEALED	HEALED TO RETURN TO FUNCTION
Heat therapy		10 min	10 min	
Massage	5 min	5 min	5 min	
Passive range of motion/ stretching (repetitions)	20*	20*	10–15*	Stop—when ROM N
Electrical stimulation†	10 min	10 min	10 min	10 min
Therapeutic exercise-total time	10 min	15 min	15 min	25–45 min
Walk/land treadmill	10 min	15 min	15 min	>10 min
Balancing	+	+	+	+
Obstacles	+	+	+	+
Weaving				+
Circles				+
Hills				+
Stairs				+
Jog/run				+
Underwater treadmill				>15 min
Swimming				5–10 min
Cryotherapy	15 min	15 min	15 min	PRN

BID, Twice a day; *ROM N*, range of motion—normal; +, perform modality; *PRN*, as needed.
*Passive range of motion to all joints of the affected limb.
†Electrical stimulation to be performed on semimembranosus/semitendinosus muscle groups for femur fractures in patients with muscle atrophy. See Chapter 12 for specifications.

Sicard GK, Hayashi K, Manley PA: Evaluation of 5 types of fishing material, 2 sterilization methods, and a crimp-clamp system for extra-articular stabilization of the canine stifle joint, *Vet Surg* 31:78, 2002.

Stauffer KD, Tuttle TA, Elkins AD et al: Complications associated with 696 tibial plateau leveling osteotomies (2001-2003), *J Am Anim Hosp Assoc* 42:44, 2006

Warzee CC, Dejardin LM, Arnoczky SP et al: Effect of tibial plateau leveling on cranial and caudal tibial thrusts in canine cranial cruciate–deficient stifles: an in vitro experimental study, *Vet Surg* 30:278, 2001.

Watt P: Tibial plateau leveling, *Aust Vet J* 78:461, 2000.

Wilke VL, Conzemius MG, Besancon MF et al: Comparison of tibial plateau angle between clinically normal greyhounds and Labrador retrievers with and without rupture of the cranial cruciate ligament, *J Am Vet Med Assoc* 221:1426, 2002.

Suggested Reading

Anderson CC, Tomlinson JL, Daly WR et al: Biomechanical evaluation of a crimp clamp system for loop fixation of monofilament nylon leader material used for stabilization of the canine stifle joint, *Vet Surg* 27:533, 1998.

The efficacy of the crimp clamp system of securing a loop of monofilament nylon leader material was compared with knotted loops. The crimp clamp system has the potential for eliminating knot irritation and providing surgeons more consistent initial loop tensions, less loop elongation, and higher load to failure characteristics than knotted monofilament leader material for clinical stabilization of the cruciate-deficient stifle.

CAUDAL CRUCIATE LIGAMENT INJURY

DEFINITION

A **caudal cruciate ligament tear** may be complete or partial, with resultant instability causing progressive DJD.

GENERAL CONSIDERATIONS AND CLINICALLY RELEVANT PATHOPHYSIOLOGY

The caudal cruciate ligament can be functionally separated into two components: the larger cranial portion is taut in flexion and lax in extension, and the smaller caudal section is taut in extension and lax in flexion. The cranial and caudal bands prevent caudal translation (sliding) of the tibia

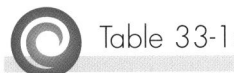 Table 33-16

Physical Rehabilitation Protocol Following Extracapsular Cruciate Repair or Patellar Surgery

ALL TREATMENTS BID	DAY 0 TO DAY 14	DAY 15 TO UNTIL 4/5 LAMENESSS	DAY 15 TO UNTIL 4/5 LAMENESSS	4/5 TO 3/5 LAMENESS	3/5 TO 1/5 LAMENESS
Heat therapy			10 min	10 min	10 min
Massage	5 min	5 min	5 min		
Passive range of motion (repetitions)	15*	15*	15*		
Electrical stimulation†	10 min	10 min	10 min		
Therapeutic exercise-total time	15 min	20 min	25 min		
Walk/land treadmill	10 min	10 min	15 min	20 min	25 min
Balancing	+	+	+	+	+
Obstacles	+	+	+	+	+
Weaving		+	+	+	+
Circles		+	+	+	+
Hills			+	+	+
Stairs				+	+
Jog/run					+
Underwater treadmill		10 min	15 min	20 min	25 min
Swimming					5–10 min
Cryotherapy	15 min	15 min	15 min	15 min	PRN

BID, Twice a day; +, perform modality; *PRN*, as needed.

*Passive range of motion to all joints of the affected limb.

†Electrical stimulation to be performed on the semimembranosus/semitendinosus muscle groups in patients with muscle atrophy. See Chapter 12 for specifications.

during flexion. The caudal cruciate ligament also functions in concert with the CCL to provide rotational stability in flexion and varus-valgus stability in extension.

Isolated caudal cruciate ligament tears are rare in small animals because (1) the caudal cruciate ligament is positioned in the joint such that loads that commonly cause ligament injury are directed toward the CCL; (2) the caudal cruciate ligament is stronger than the CCL; and (3) the types of accidents that might cause caudal cruciate ligament rupture are seldom encountered. Nevertheless, isolated ruptures of the caudal cruciate ligament do occur and generally are caused by a cranial-to-caudal blow directed against the proximal tibia. This type of injury is most commonly associated with an automobile accident or falling on the limb while the stifle joint is flexed. Caudal cruciate ligament injuries are more commonly associated with severe derangement of the stifle joint. In these patients, combinations of primary joint restraints (CCL, caudal cruciate ligament, medial collateral ligament) and secondary joint restraints (joint capsule, muscle tendon units, meniscocapsular ligaments) are ruptured after a severe traumatic episode, such as an automobile accident.

DIAGNOSIS
Clinical Presentation

Signalment. Dogs or cats of either gender and any breed or age may be affected. Isolated tears are more frequently encountered in large-breed dogs. In cats, tears of the caudal cruciate and medial collateral ligaments commonly occur concurrently.

History. Patients with an isolated caudal cruciate ligament rupture initially have a non–weight-bearing lameness. The lameness progressively improves, but the patient seldom regains athletic status. The animal may have a normal gait at a walk, but is lame when undergoing strenuous activity because the caudal cruciate ligament functions to stabilize the joint primarily when it is flexed. During walking, flexion occurs in the swing phase of the gait; during running and turning, the knee is more flexed in the stance (weight-bearing) phase of the gait.

> NOTE: Nonathletic dogs usually function normally with caudal cruciate tears.

Physical Examination Findings

Diagnosis of isolated caudal cruciate ligament tears is based on the presence of craniocaudal instability. Often it is difficult to differentiate craniocaudal movement caused by CCL rupture from that caused by caudal cruciate ligament injury. The following points may help make this differentiation:

- When the joint is held in extension, the degree of palpable instability is less with caudal cruciate ligament tears than with CCL tears.
- With the patient in dorsal recumbency and the limb positioned such that the stifle is flexed and the tibia is parallel to the ground, the tibial tuberosity forms a distinct prominence cranial to the patella. If a caudal cruciate ligament injury is present, the weight of the limb causes a caudal "sag" of the tibia, resulting in loss of the tuberosity prominence.
- When the tibia is moved forward, there is a distinct endpoint to the cranial movement when the caudal cruciate ligament is ruptured.
- With the tibia in an extended position, there is a distinct caudal subluxation of the tibia when the stifle joint is flexed and internally rotated if the caudal cruciate ligament is torn.

Caudal cruciate ligament tears that are part of a multiple ligament injury are diagnosed by the presence of severe instability (see p. 1283).

Diagnostic Imaging

Radiographs may be helpful in the diagnosis of caudal cruciate ligament injuries. Small bone opacities associated with ligament avulsion may be apparent on the lateral projection just caudal and distal to the femoral condyles. With a lateral radiographic projection, the tibial plateau may be seen to be caudally displaced relative to the femoral condyles.

Laboratory Findings

No consistent laboratory abnormalities are seen.

DIFFERENTIAL DIAGNOSIS

Differential diagnoses include CCL injury (see previous discussion) and multiple ligament injury.

MEDICAL MANAGEMENT

Long-term evaluation of dogs having reconstruction of isolated caudal cruciate ligament tears shows the prognosis to be good, regardless of the treatment method. Conservative management of isolated caudal cruciate tears (i.e., activity restricted to leash walking for 8 weeks) is an option for smaller dogs or cats and for dogs leading inactive lives.

SURGICAL TREATMENT

Joints with caudal cruciate ligament injury are treated with resection of the remnants of the ligament and stabilized by one of several extracapsular reconstruction techniques: suture stabilization, redirection of the medial collateral ligament, or popliteal tendon tenodesis. Suture stabilization consists of imbrication of the caudomedial joint capsule and placement of a medial or lateral stabilizing suture. Redirection repair uses existing autogenous tissue, such as the medial collateral ligament.

Preoperative Management

These animals should be evaluated for evidence of other ligamentous or bony trauma.

Perioperative antibiotics (see p. 945) and preemptive pain management with NSAIDs (see Chapter 13), opiates, and/or epidural analgesia are indicated for dogs undergoing stifle reconstructive techniques.

Anesthesia

See p. 943 for the anesthetic management of animals with orthopedic disease and p. 1262 for the anesthetic management of animals with CCL injury. Opioid epidural administration and intraarticular administration of bupivacaine or morphine reduce postoperative discomfort (see p. 945).

Surgical Anatomy

The caudal cruciate ligament originates from the intercondyloid fossa of the craniolateral (inside) surface of the medial condyle (see Fig. 33-103). From the point of origin, the ligament courses distally to insert into the popliteal notch of the tibia.

Positioning

The animal is positioned in lateral recumbency with the affected limb up or in dorsal recumbency.

SURGICAL TECHNIQUE
Exploratory Arthrotomy

Perform arthroscopy or make a standard craniomedial or craniolateral approach to the stifle joint (see p. 1263), and explore internal structures. Resect the remnants of the caudal cruciate ligament.

Suture Stabilization

Drill a hole in the caudomedial corner of the tibial epiphysis. Place a stabilizing suture from the proximal patellar tendon through the predrilled hole (Fig. 33-121). On the lateral side, imbricate the caudal joint capsule, and place a stabilizing suture from the proximal patellar tendon through a predrilled hole in the fibular head.

Use of Autogenous Tissue

Incise through the insertion of the caudal sartorius muscle and medial fascia along the tibial metaphysis. Reflect the muscle and fascia caudally to expose the medial collateral

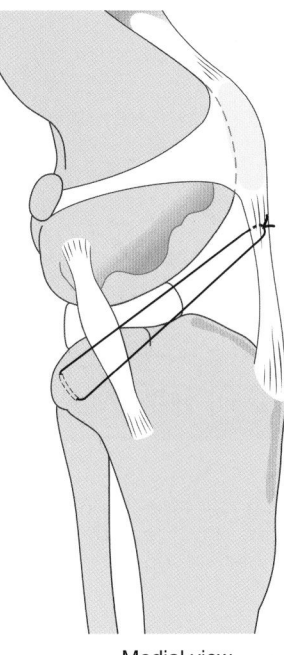
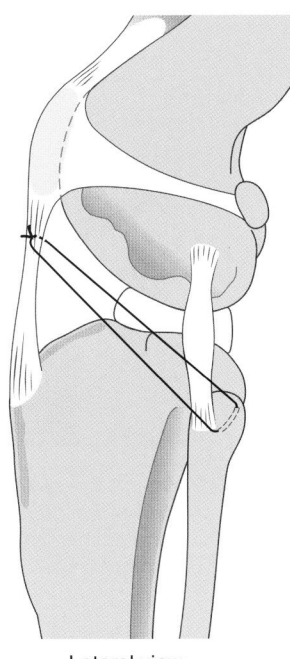

Medial view   Lateral view

FIG. 33-121
For caudal cruciate ligament tears, extracapsular sutures are placed from the patellar tendon just distal to the patella to the caudal tibia (medially) and fibular head (laterally).

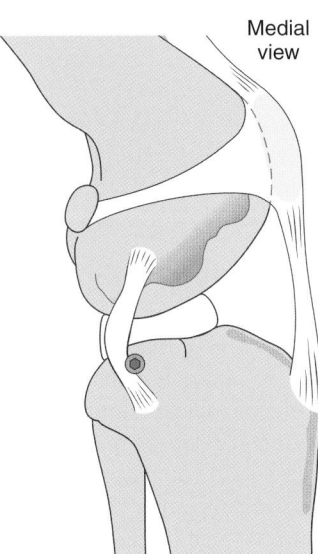

Medial view

FIG. 33-122
The medial collateral ligament may be redirected caudally to stabilize caudal cruciate ligament tears. The ventral surface of the ligament is freed, and the ligament is secured caudally with a bone screw.

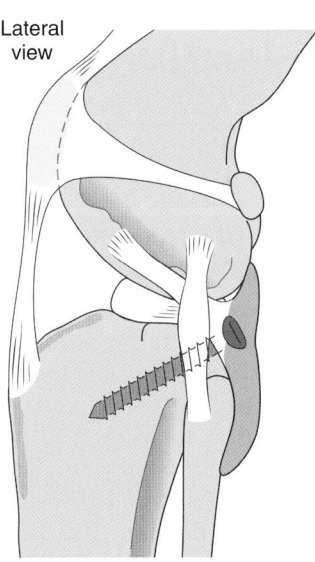

Lateral view

FIG. 33-123
Tenodesis of the popliteal tendon may be performed to stabilize caudal cruciate ligament tears. Entrap the popliteal tendon with a screw as it passes caudal and proximal to the fibular head.

ligament. Free a portion of the body of the ligament with a periosteal elevator and direct the ligament caudally to course in the same sagittal plane as the caudal cruciate ligament. Secure the ligament in this position with a bone screw and spiked washer (Fig. 33-122).

Entrapment (Tenodesis) of the Popliteal Tendon

Make a lateral approach to the stifle joint (see p. 1263), and reflect the fascia lata to isolate the popliteal tendon as it passes beneath the lateral collateral ligament (Fig. 33-123).

Entrap the popliteal tendon with a screw and Teflon or poly-acetyl washer as it passes caudal and proximal to the fibular head.

SUTURE MATERIALS AND SPECIAL INSTRUMENTS

A bone screw and Teflon washer are used to secure the medial collateral ligament or popliteal tendon to bone. Nonabsorbable monofilament suture is preferred for extracapsular stabilization techniques.

POSTOPERATIVE CARE AND ASSESSMENT

Uncontrolled exercise should be restricted to specific physical rehabilitation exercises and leash walking for 6 weeks; the animal should be gradually returned to unsupervised activity over a 6-week period. A sample physical rehabilitation exercise protocol can be found in Table 33-15 on p. 1276.

PROGNOSIS

The prognosis is good to excellent for return to normal limb function in most animals after surgery. Clinically and experimentally, DJD does not appear to progress as rapidly after isolated caudal cruciate ligament injury as it does after CCL injury.

COLLATERAL LIGAMENT INJURY

DEFINITION

A **collateral ligament injury** is a complete or partial tear of the medial or lateral collateral ligament.

GENERAL CONSIDERATIONS AND CLINICALLY RELEVANT PATHOPHYSIOLOGY

As the medial collateral ligament crosses the medial joint surface, it forms a strong attachment to the joint capsule and medial meniscus. This attachment is important in stabilizing the medial meniscus, but it predisposes the caudal body of the meniscus to injury from the medial femoral condyle when CCL rupture is present. The medial and lateral collateral ligaments function in concert to limit varus-valgus motion of the stifle joint. This is most important when the stifle joint is extended and both the medial and lateral collateral ligaments are taut. As the stifle joint flexes, the medial collateral ligament remains tight, but the lateral collateral ligament relaxes to allow internal tibial rotation. This motion permits the foot to turn inward beneath the body during ambulation. As the stifle joint extends, the lateral collateral ligament becomes taut once again to assist in external rotation of the tibia. This motion aligns the foot into proper position for weight bearing.

Isolated medial or lateral collateral ligament tears are rare in small animals. Most injuries that involve the medial or lateral collateral ligaments occur in conjunction with injury to other primary and secondary restraints of the stifle joint. These multiple ligament injuries are often the result of se-

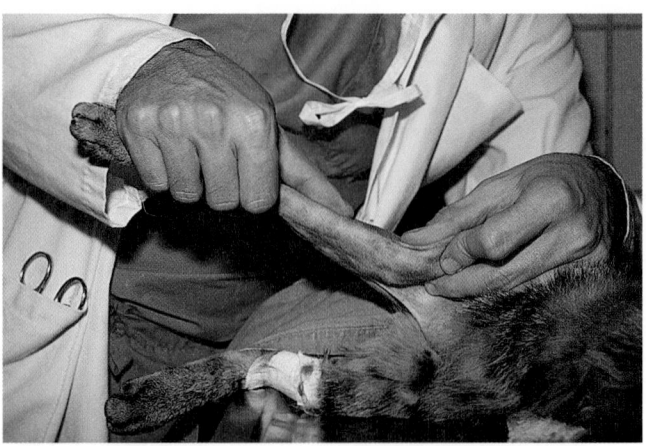

FIG. 33-124
Medial collateral ligament injury in a cat. Note the appearance of the stifle when a valgus stress is applied. The foot displaces upward, and the medial joint line opens.

vere trauma directed to the stifle joint and involve injury to a myriad of stifle joint ligaments.

DIAGNOSIS
Clinical Presentation

Signalment. Any age or breed and either gender of dog or cat may be affected.

History.   This injury may occur while the animal is exercising (without evidence of trauma) or during a traumatic incident (i.e., vehicular accident), in which the animal has sustained major injuries.

Physical Examination Findings

Diagnosis of collateral ligament injury, whether an isolated ligament tear or part of a complex injury, is based on palpation. It is important to remember that the stifle joint must be extended to examine for collateral injury. The *valgus stress test* is used to evaluate integrity of the medial collateral ligament. With the patient in lateral recumbency, one hand is used to stabilize the femur while the other hand grasps the distal tibia and applies an upward force (abduction). If the medial joint restraints (medial collateral ligament, joint capsule, peripheral meniscal ligaments) are torn, opening of the medial joint line is apparent (Fig. 33-124). The *varus stress test* is used to evaluate integrity of the lateral collateral ligament. One hand stabilizes the femur while the other hand grasps the distal tibia and applies an inward force (adduction). If the lateral joint restraints are torn, opening of the lateral joint is apparent. Isolated tears show minimal opening, whereas obvious opening occurs with more extensive injuries (lateral collateral ligament, joint capsule, peripheral meniscal ligaments).

NOTE: Be sure to hold the stifle joint in extension when assessing the medial and lateral restraints.

Diagnostic Imaging

Radiographs should be obtained to determine if bone fragments are associated with ligament damage. Craniocaudal and medial-to-lateral radiographs are indicated to confirm the presence or absence of bony avulsions. Stress radiographs are useful for demonstrating an increase in medial or lateral joint space (Fig. 33-125).

Laboratory Findings

Consistent laboratory findings are not seen. Laboratory evaluation depends on the signalment and physical findings in animals that have sustained trauma.

DIFFERENTIAL DIAGNOSIS

Differential diagnoses include muscle strains or cranial or caudal cruciate ligament tears and nondisplaced physeal fractures in immature animals.

MEDICAL MANAGEMENT

The decision to use conservative or surgical treatment for isolated collateral ligament injury is based on the degree of injury to the ligament and secondary joint restraints (joint capsule, peripheral meniscal ligaments). This assessment is based on palpation and radiographs. Minimal swelling and only slight opening of the joint space when the joint is placed under stress are indications for conservative treatment, which involves a fiberglass cast applied for 2 weeks and then controlled activity for 6 additional weeks.

SURGICAL TREATMENT

Moderate to severe swelling and significant opening of the joint space when the joint is placed under stress indicate significant injury to the collateral restraints. Surgery is recommended for these patients. Treatment includes reconstruction of the collateral and meniscocapsular ligaments and the joint capsule. Primary repair of the collateral ligament is undertaken if the point of failure is the origin or insertion of the ligament or an intrasubstance tear with large segments of the ligament intact. Occasionally a small fragment of bone may be present on the end of the ligament that can be incorporated into the repair.

> NOTE: Be sure to repair all injured ligaments, tendons, and joint capsule.

Preoperative Management

To prevent additional damage to the articular cartilage or menisci, place a modified Robert Jones bandage on the limb (see p. 947) and limit activity to leash walking until definitive surgical treatment can be done. These animals should be evaluated for evidence of other ligamentous or bony trauma. Patients with injuries caused by vehicular accidents should undergo thoracic, cardiovascular, and abdominal evaluation. Perioperative antibiotics (see p. 945) and preemptive pain management with NSAIDs, opiates, and epidural analgesia

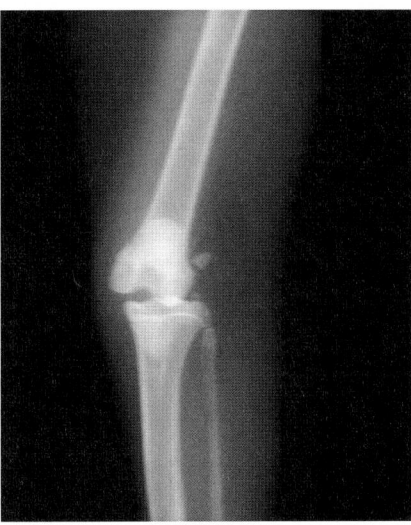

FIG. 33-125
Stress radiograph of a cat with a medial collateral ligament injury. Note the severity of joint opening when a valgus stress is applied to the joint.

are indicated for animals undergoing stifle reconstructive techniques.

Anesthesia

See p. 944 for anesthetic management of animals with orthopedic disease caused by trauma. Opioid epidural administration reduces postoperative discomfort (see Chapter 13).

Surgical Anatomy

Knowledge of the origin and insertion points of the collateral ligaments is important. The medial collateral ligament originates from the medial femoral epicondyle and courses distally to insert onto the proximal tibial metaphysis (Fig. 33-126). As the ligament crosses the medial joint line, it forms a strong attachment to the joint capsule and medial meniscus. The lateral collateral ligament originates from an oval area on the lateral femoral epicondyle; it then courses distally to insert onto the fibular head. The medial collateral ligament lies deep to the caudal sartorius muscle; the lateral collateral ligament lies deep to the fascia lata. The peroneal (fibular) nerve is a branch of the sciatic nerve. It obliquely crosses the distal aspect to the stifle joint, where it lies superficial to the gastrocnemius muscle and sends an articular branch to the lateral collateral ligament. Care should be taken when dissecting near the lateral collateral ligament to preserve this nerve.

Positioning

To repair a lateral collateral ligament injury, position the patient in lateral recumbency with the affected leg up. For medial collateral ligament injuries, position the animal in

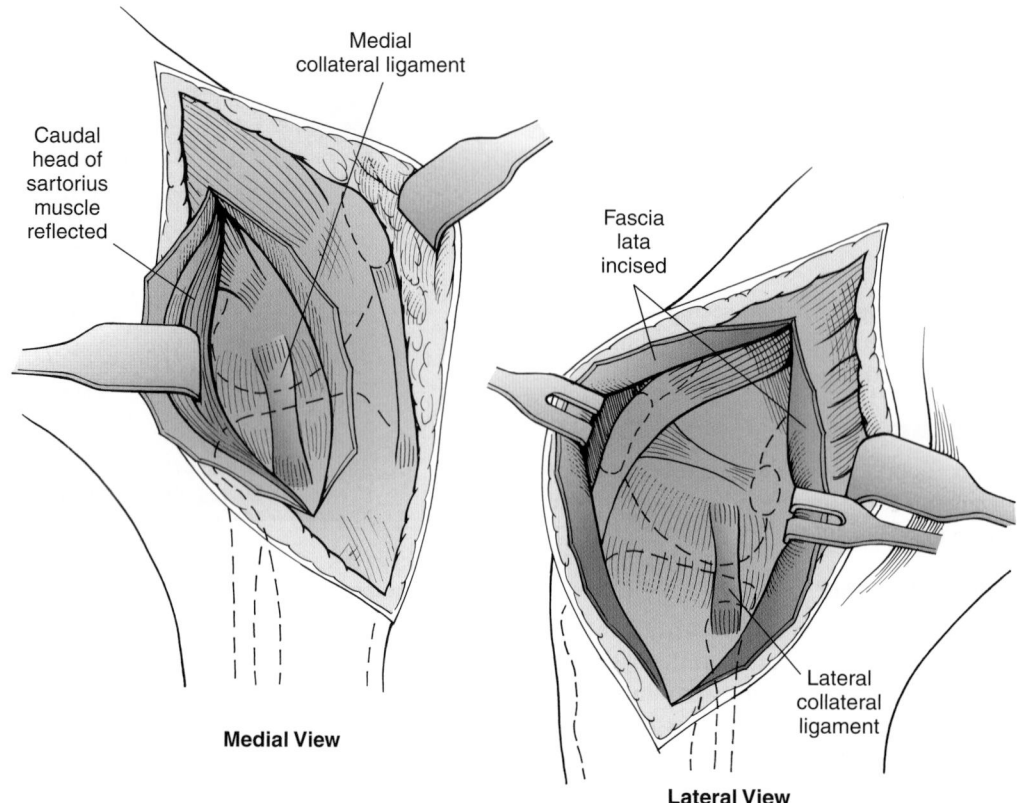

Caudal head of sartorius muscle reflected

Medial collateral ligament

Medial View

Fascia lata incised

Lateral collateral ligament

Lateral View

FIG. 33-126
Medial and lateral views of the stifle showing soft tissue structures surrounding the collateral ligaments.

dorsal recumbency. If multiple ligament tears are present, the animal can also be positioned in dorsal recumbency to facilitate exposure of both sides of the limb. Suspend the limb and prepare it for aseptic surgery (see p. 36).

SURGICAL TECHNIQUE
Medial Collateral Ligament Injury

*Make a medial parapatellar incision. Use a medial approach to expose the medial collateral ligament (see p. 1263). Incise the insertion of the caudal head of the sartorius muscle and deep fascia along the craniomedial border of the proximal tibia (Fig. 33-127, A). Retract the muscle and fascia caudally to expose the collateral ligament and medial joint capsule. Replace the ligament to its anatomic site, and secure it with a screw and polyacetyl spiked washer (Fig. 33-127, B). As an alternative, place a suture anchor at the insertion of the ligament and suture the ligament to the anchor. If the ligament injury is an intrasubstance tear, perform primary repair by suturing the ligament ends; use a locking-loop suture pattern with small, nonabsorbable suture (see p. 1320). Supplement the primary repair with screws or bone anchors and figure-eight support (Fig. 33-127, C). After repair of the collateral ligament, carefully reconstruct the meniscocapsular ligaments and joint capsule using inter-*rupted sutures of small, nonabsorbable suture material (polypropylene or nylon).

Lateral Collateral Ligament Injury

Use a craniolateral approach to expose the lateral collateral ligament (see p. 1263). Make a proximal-to-distal parapatellar incision through the fascia lata. Continue the incision distally 4 cm below the tibial crest, parallel to the joint line. Use caution in isolating the peroneal nerve, and protect it carefully during surgery (see Surgical Anatomy, p. 1264). Reflect the fascia lata caudally to expose the collateral ligament and lateral joint capsule. Repair the ligament as described previously.

SUTURE MATERIALS AND SPECIAL INSTRUMENTS

Bone screws, polyacetyl spiked washers, suture anchors, and heavy, nonabsorbable suture are needed for collateral ligament repair (Robinson, 2000).

POSTOPERATIVE CARE AND ASSESSMENT

The limb is placed in a soft, padded bandage with a lateral splint for 10 to 14 days. Uncontrolled exercise should be restricted to specific physical rehabilitation exercises and leash

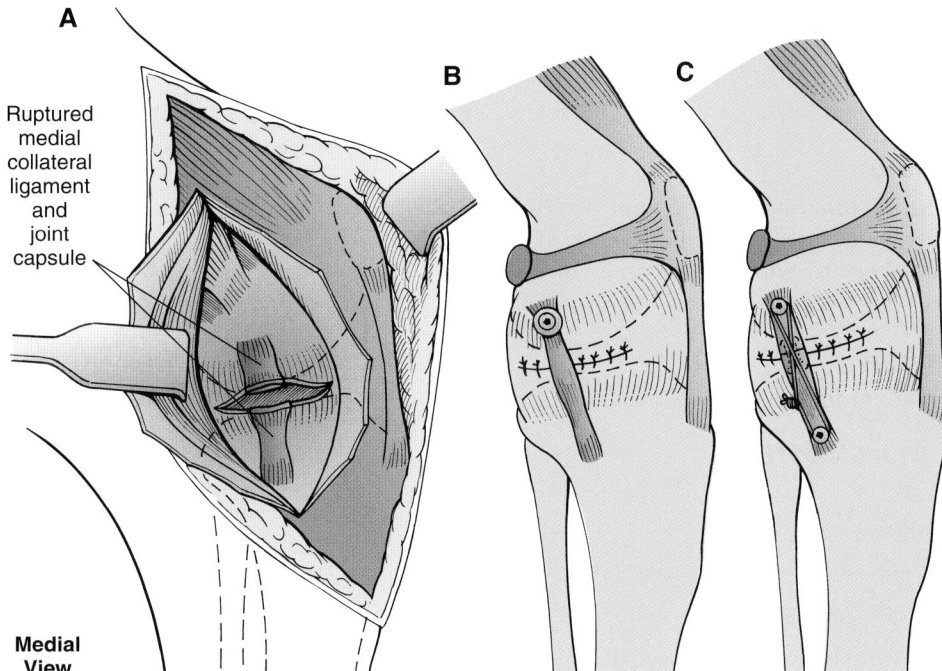

FIG. 33-127
Repair of a medial restraint injury. **A,** Incise the insertion of the caudal head of the sartorius muscle and deep fascia along the craniomedial border of the proximal tibia. **B,** Replace the collateral ligament in its anatomic site and secure with a screw and polyacetyl spiked washer. As an alternative, use suture anchors. **C,** If the ligament injury is an intrasubstance tear, perform primary repair by suturing the ligament ends with a locking-loop suture pattern. Supplement the primary repair with screws and figure-eight support.

walking for 6 weeks; the animal should be gradually returned to unsupervised activity over a 6-week period (see Table 33-15 on p. 1276).

PROGNOSIS

The prognosis for isolated collateral ligament tears is good to excellent. If multiple ligaments are torn, the prognosis is fair.

Reference

Robinson A: Clinical application of prong-type tissue anchors in small animal surgery, *J Small Anim Pract* 41:207, 2000.

MULTIPLE LIGAMENT INJURIES

DEFINITIONS

Multiple ligament injuries are injuries in which the cranial or caudal cruciate ligaments and collateral ligaments are damaged simultaneously. **Varus angulation** is an inward rotation of the leg (toward the midline of the body), and **valgus angulation** is an outward rotation (away from the midline of the body). The **primary stifle restraints** are the cruciate and collateral ligaments; the **secondary stifle restraints** are the joint capsule, meniscus, tendon, and muscle.

GENERAL CONSIDERATIONS AND CLINICALLY RELEVANT PATHOPHYSIOLOGY

Multiple ligament injuries are caused by automobile accidents or other major trauma. A common triad of injuries includes cranial and caudal cruciate ligament tears, failure of the primary and secondary medial restraints, and peripheral medial meniscal tears. Varus angulation of the limb with a medial stress indicates lateral injury, whereas valgus angulation of the limb (with a lateral stress applied to the foot) indicates medial injury.

DIAGNOSIS
Clinical Presentation

Signalment. Either gender and any age or breed of dog or cat may be affected.

History. The animal usually is presented for evaluation of an acute, non–weight-bearing lameness. The trauma may or may not have been observed.

Physical Examination Findings

Combined cranial and caudal cruciate tears are characterized by notable craniocaudal movement of the tibia relative to the femur. Concurrent damage to the collateral ligament and joint capsule complexes usually can be determined by palpation. With the leg in extension, a varus stress applied to the distal tibia causes opening of the lateral joint line if the lateral restraints are injured, whereas a valgus stress causes opening of the medial joint line if the medial restraints are injured.

Diagnostic Imaging

Radiographs reveal subluxation of the stifle joint. Careful assessment of both craniocaudal and mediolateral radiographs may show small bone fragments at the origin or insertion of ligaments.

Laboratory Findings

Consistent laboratory abnormalities are not seen.

DIFFERENTIAL DIAGNOSIS

Distal femoral and proximal tibial metaphyseal fractures may show similar clinical signs and should be differentiated from ligament injuries.

MEDICAL MANAGEMENT

Multiple ligament injuries require surgical intervention. Conservative treatment with external coaptation (splints or casts) is not effective in maintaining alignment of the stifle joint and leads to severe DJD.

SURGICAL TREATMENT

Surgical treatment involves careful reconstruction of the cruciate ligaments, the collateral ligaments, and the menisci. The collateral ligament complex is repaired first, followed by reconstruction of the cruciate ligaments. The specific repair and reconstruction techniques used depend on the surgeon's preference and are described in the discussion of each individual ligament.

Preoperative Management

To prevent damage to the articular surfaces of the joint, a soft, padded bandage with a lateral splint should be applied and activity limited until surgery can be done. Affected animals should be evaluated for evidence of other ligamentous or bony trauma; other fractures are often associated with this injury. Patients with injuries from vehicular accidents should have complete physical examinations, with particular attention to the respiratory and cardiovascular systems. Perioperative antibiotics (see p. 945) and preemptive pain management with NSAIDs (see Table 33-4 on p. 1149), opiates, and/or epidural analgesia are indicated for animals undergoing stifle reconstructive techniques.

Anesthesia

See p. 944 for the anesthetic management of animals with orthopedic disease caused by trauma. Opioid epidural administration (see p. 945) reduces postoperative discomfort.

Surgical Anatomy

The normal anatomy of the stifle joint is described on pp. 1262 and 1281. With multiple ligament injury, moderate to severe swelling and bruising of soft tissue surrounding the

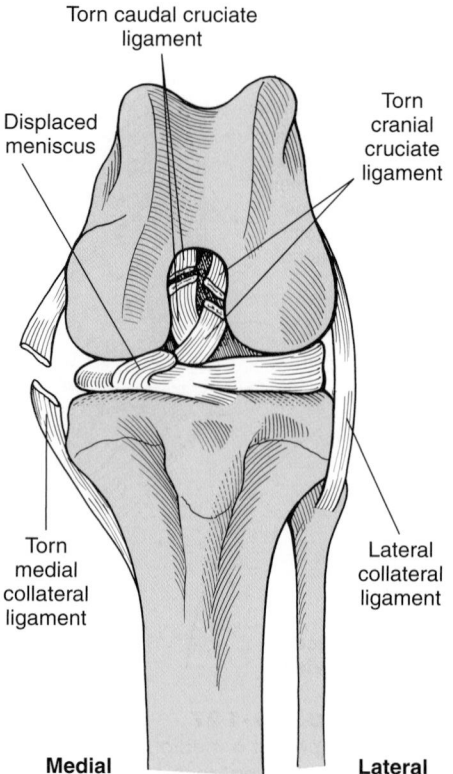

FIG. 33-128
Structures commonly injured with multiple ligament derangement of the stifle joint. Note the loss of the cranial and caudal cruciate ligaments and the disruption of the medial restraints.

joint are seen. A knowledge of the normal origins and insertions of the collateral ligaments, meniscocapsular ligaments, and ligaments in the joint is required. Torn collateral ligaments are difficult to identify because they often are encased in edematous connective tissue. Menisci often are displaced from their normal positions and folded cranially or caudally (Fig. 33-128).

Positioning

The patient is positioned in dorsal recumbency with the affected limb up. The leg is prepared from the dorsal midline to the tarsal joint. A hanging-limb preparation facilitates manipulation of the leg during surgery.

SURGICAL TECHNIQUE

Cruciate ligament repair is discussed on p. 1263, collateral ligament repair on p. 1282, and meniscal injuries on p. 1287.

SUTURE MATERIALS AND SPECIAL INSTRUMENTS

See requirements for cruciate ligament repair discussed on p. 1263, collateral ligament repair on p. 1282, and meniscal injuries on p. 1287.

POSTOPERATIVE CARE AND ASSESSMENT

After surgery, the limb should be placed in a soft, padded bandage with a lateral splint for 3 weeks. The support bandage should be placed before the patient recovers from anesthesia to allow accurate positioning of the bandage with the leg in extension. The bandage provides comfort in the early postoperative period by immobilizing soft tissue and preventing extension and flexion of the stifle joint. It should be changed weekly or more often if necessary. Activity should be limited to leash walks only while the bandage is in place. After removal of the bandage, physical rehabilitation of the stifle is encouraged. Refer to Table 33-15 on p. 1276 for a sample physical rehabilitation exercise protocol.

PROGNOSIS

The prognosis is good for return to nonathletic performance. Animals with subluxated joints have a better prognosis for return to function than animals with luxated joints and failure of secondary stabilizers. Subsequent to extensive ligament injury, loss of flexion beyond 110 degrees and mild to moderate instability are common after surgery. This instability and loss of normal range of motion limit athletic performance. Severe lameness should be expected in animals that are managed without surgery. Physical therapy is helpful for rehabilitation of the stifle (see Table 33-16 on p. 1277). Programs include cryotherapy, passive range of motion, and muscle strengthening exercises.

MENISCAL INJURY

DEFINITIONS

Meniscal injury *(tear)* occurs when excessive crushing or shearing forces associated with stifle injury result in meniscocapsular detachment or separation in the substance of the meniscus. **Radial tears** are those that run in an axial to abaxial direction. **Circumferential tears** are those that follow the curvature of the meniscus. **Bucket handle tears** are circumferential or transverse tears with separation of the meniscus at the site of the tear. **Meniscal release** is a midbody or meniscotibial incision of the medial meniscus intended to prevent future meniscal impingement and damage.

GENERAL CONSIDERATIONS AND CLINICALLY RELEVANT PATHOPHYSIOLOGY

The menisci are important intraarticular structures. They function in load transmission and energy absorption, help provide rotational and varus-valgus stability, lubricate the joint, and render joint surfaces congruent. Isolated meniscal injuries are uncommon in dogs, although isolated meniscal tears involving the midbody of the lateral meniscus occasionally occur during a fall when the leg is twisted. Most meniscal tears causing lameness in dogs occur in conjunction with CCL ruptures. These tears usually involve the caudal body of the medial meniscus because the craniocaudal instability associated with CCL rupture displaces the medial femoral condyle caudally during stifle joint flexion. The caudal body of the medial meniscus becomes wedged between the femur and the tibia and is crushed upon weight bearing and joint extension. The most common type of injury is a bucket handle tear. This is a circumferential or transverse tear in the caudal body of the medial meniscus that extends from medial to lateral. The free portion of the meniscus frequently is folded forward (Fig. 33-129). Peripheral meniscal tears are the second most common type of meniscal injury. These injuries are associated with a severe traumatic episode that results in multiple ligament injuries. Rupture of the medial meniscocapsular ligament commonly occurs, allowing the entire meniscal body to fold forward.

NOTE: Isolated meniscal tears are uncommon; they usually occur in conjunction with cruciate ligament injury. Isolated lateral meniscal tears occur in the caudal horn.

Meniscal release has been advocated as a means of protecting the medial meniscus following surgical stabilization of the stifle for CCL rupture. This procedure was developed in association with TPLO, which provides active stabilization of the stifle during ambulation, but does not prevent cranial drawer in the unweighted limb. The use of meniscal release is controversial based on its effects on the meniscus and its uncertain efficacy. By transecting the meniscus just caudal to the medial collateral ligament, the function of the meniscus is significantly compromised because of the elimination of hoop stresses.

With either midbody release or transection of the meniscotibial ligament, the femoral condyle likely increases contact with the articular cartilage of the tibial plateau, which may contribute to osteoarthritis. Release also impairs the functions of the meniscus in providing stability and congruence. To date, no clinical studies have demonstrated the efficacy of meniscal release in decreasing the incidence of post TPLO meniscal injury; however, the technique remains in widespread use.

DIAGNOSIS
Clinical Presentation

Signalment. Dogs of either gender and any age or breed may be affected. Meniscal tears are rare in cats.

History. Meniscal injury usually is associated with instability of the stifle caused by CCL rupture (see p. 1254). Dogs with meniscal injury and cruciate ligament injury may be substantially more painful than dogs with cruciate ligament injury alone. If a long-standing lameness suddenly worsens in a dog with CCL injury, tearing of the meniscus should be suspected. The client may report hearing a popping sound when the dog walks, or a popping sound may be noted when the stifle is examined. This is caused by movement of the "free" section of the bucket handle tear.

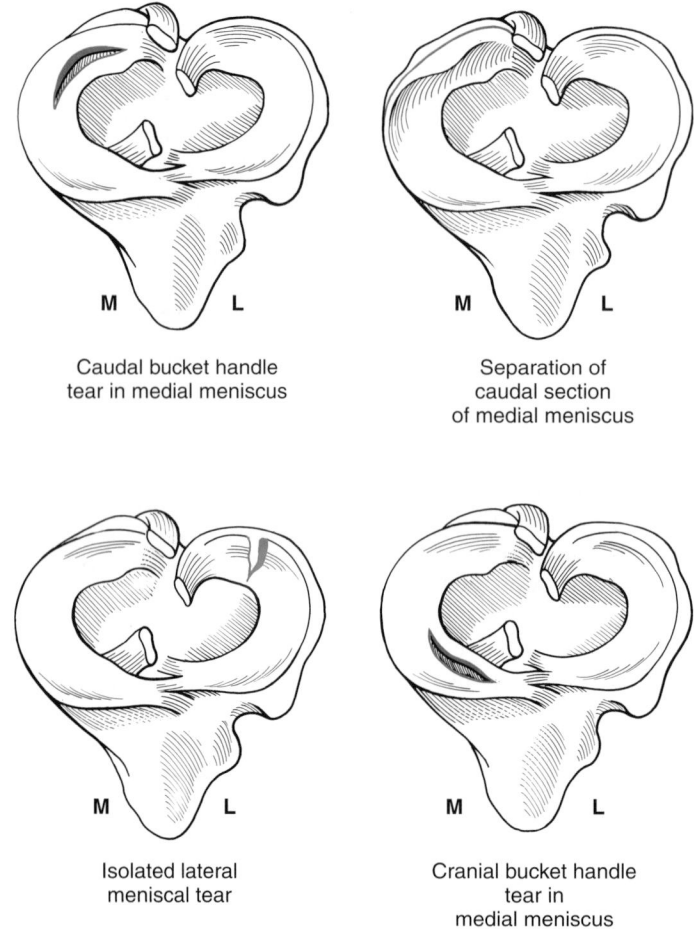

Caudal bucket handle
tear in medial meniscus

Separation of
caudal section
of medial meniscus

Isolated lateral
meniscal tear

Cranial bucket handle
tear in
medial meniscus

FIG. 33-129
Meniscal tears in dogs. Bucket handle tears occur most often.

Physical Examination Findings

Dogs with meniscal injury are frequently in much more pain than dogs with only CCL tears. A meniscal click may be palpable and is most often felt during the later stage of flexion of the joint. Not all patients with meniscal tears have an audible or palpable click. Close inspection of the medial and lateral menisci at surgery provides a definitive diagnosis.

Diagnostic Imaging

Standard craniocaudal and medial-to-lateral radiographs should be taken for diagnostic evaluation of lameness attributed to the stifle joint; however, radiographic findings do not correlate with meniscal injury. Ultrasound of the stifle has been demonstrated in a clinical trial to be effective in the diagnosis of meniscal injury (Mahn et al, 2005). This technique may prove valuable as a minimally invasive technique in cases in which meniscal injury is not otherwise obvious. MRI has been studied for the evaluation of the stifle joint and meniscal injuries. The small size of the meniscus means that strong magnets and/or long acquisition times are necessary for adequate imaging. Artifacts and false negative or positive studies may be a concern. As MRI requires general anesthesia, arthroscopic evaluation may be a more effective means of diagnosis and providing a means of therapy.

Arthroscopy. Arthroscopy provides a minimally invasive means for assessment of the menisci (see p 1257). Arthroscopic examination requires creation of a viewing window by shaving of the fat pad and manipulation of the joint by valgus and varus stress or by positioning of a Hohmann retractor (Ralphs et al, 2002).

Laboratory Findings

No consistent hematologic abnormalities are seen. Joint fluid analysis may be helpful in the diagnosis of partial cruciate tears; patients with meniscal tears may have cell counts that are slightly higher than those in patients with ligament tears alone.

DIFFERENTIAL DIAGNOSIS

Cruciate ligament injury should be suspected in any animal with a meniscal tear. Sprain of the medial restraints should be differentiated from meniscal injury.

MEDICAL MANAGEMENT

Conservative treatment is not an option if meniscal injury is noted on physical examination because continued back-and-forth sliding of the torn meniscus causes severe pain that will not improve with conservative management and accelerates DJD.

SURGICAL TREATMENT

Meniscal trauma. Methods of treatment include partial meniscectomy, primary repair of peripheral meniscal injuries, and total meniscectomy. A partial meniscectomy involves removal of the torn section of the meniscus. Experimentally, partial meniscectomy carries less morbidity than does a total meniscectomy and is the treatment of choice for bucket handle tears of the medial meniscus. Primary repair of a torn meniscal body is advocated by some human orthopedic surgeons. However, because of the low morbidity associated with partial meniscectomy and difficulty in suturing meniscal body tears in dogs, primary repair should be reserved for peripheral tears of the meniscocapsular ligaments. Tearing of the peripheral meniscocapsular ligaments usually occurs after significant trauma and subsequent injury to both primary and secondary restraints of the stifle joint. The medial meniscus is more commonly involved in conjunction with injury of the medial collateral restraints. Meticulous repair with interrupted sutures using an absorbable suture allows meniscocapsular tissue to heal. Total meniscectomy should be considered only when the peripheral rim of the meniscus is so damaged that primary suturing of the meniscocapsular tissue is not possible. For arthroscopy of the stifle joint, see p. 1257.

Meniscal release. Two techniques are available for meniscal release: midbody transection and transection of the meniscotibial ligament. Selection between the two techniques is often based on surgeon preference and surgical approach, although the two approaches do appear to affect the meniscus differently (Kennedy et al, 2005). Midbody release may be performed through an open arthrotomy, arthroscopically, or blind. The latter is performed without opening the joint for examination of the meniscus. This approach is not recommended because of the high incidence of meniscal injury in dogs with cruciate ligament rupture and the possibility of meniscal injury in spite of the absence of meniscal click. The menisci should be thoroughly examined in every case of CCL rupture repair. Transection of the meniscotibial ligament is most readily performed arthroscopically.

Preoperative Management

Perioperative antibiotics (see p. 945) and preemptive pain management with NSAIDs (see Table 33-4 on p. 1149), opiates, or epidural analgesia are indicated for dogs undergoing stifle reconstructive techniques.

Anesthesia

See p. 944 for the anesthetic management of animals with orthopedic disease. Opioid epidural administration reduces postoperative discomfort.

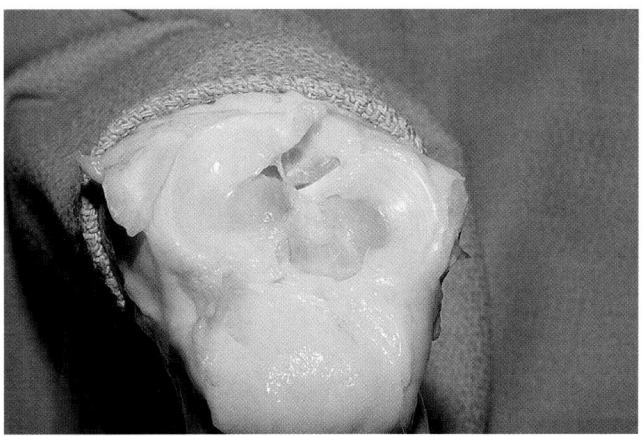

FIG. 33-130
Appearance of menisci and surrounding soft tissue in a cadaver specimen. Note the C-shaped appearance and tibial insertion of the medial meniscus. The lateral meniscus is larger and inserts into the caudal femur.

Surgical Anatomy

The lateral and medial menisci are two semilunar fibrocartilage disks interposed between the femur and the tibia (Fig. 33-130). They are positioned in the joint with the open side of the C facing the midline and are held in place by cranial meniscotibial ligaments, caudal meniscotibial ligaments, and meniscocapsular ligaments. The lateral meniscus has an additional ligament that inserts into the caudal intercondyloid fossa of the femoral condyle. This ligament and loose meniscocapsular ligaments of the lateral meniscus render the lateral meniscus more mobile than the medial meniscus. Clinically the lack of mobility of the medial meniscus predisposes it to injury.

Positioning

For open arthrotomy, the animal is placed in lateral recumbency with the affected limb up, or in dorsal recumbency. For arthroscopy, the animal is placed in dorsal recumbency. The limb is prepared for aseptic surgery from the dorsal midline to the tarsal joint. Preparing the limb in a hanging-leg position facilitates manipulation of the limb during surgery.

SURGICAL TECHNIQUE
Exploratory Arthrotomy

A lateral or medial approach to the stifle may be used (see p. 1263). Visualization of the medial meniscus may be enhanced by a medial arthrotomy.

Partial Meniscectomy

Partial meniscectomy requires that the torn meniscus be adequately exposed. Exposure is facilitated by suction and by levering the tibial plateau down and forward.

Lever the tibia forward by placing the tip of a small Hohmann retractor behind the caudal edge of the tibial plateau and forcing the body of the retractor against the trochlear groove (Fig.

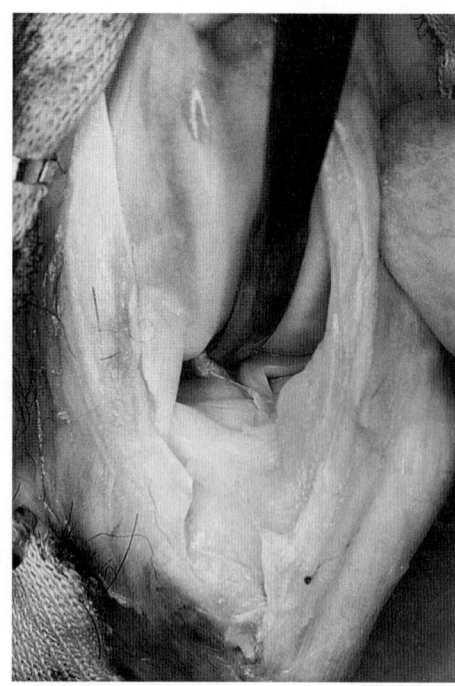

FIG. 33-131
To improve visualization of the caudomedial compartment (where most meniscal tears occur), place a small Hohmann retractor to force the tibia forward and down.

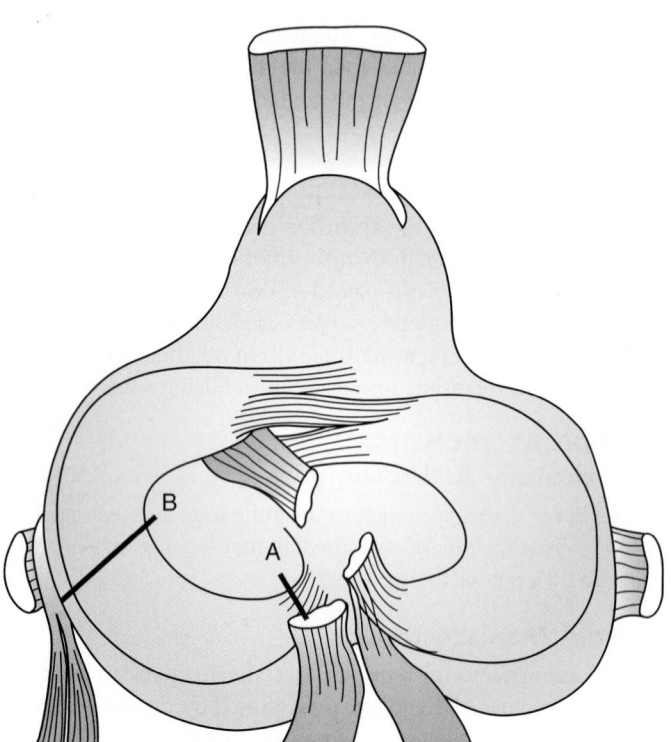

FIG. 33-132
Locations of release of the medial meniscus. Transection of the meniscotibial ligament (line A). Transection of the midbody of the meniscus (line B).

33-131). When the damaged section of meniscus can be seen, remove it with a No. 11 or No. 15 scalpel blade. Incise the most medial attachment of the bucket handle first, then incise the most lateral attachment. After removal of the torn section of meniscus, inspect the remaining meniscus for additional tears.

Meniscal Release

Midbody release. Midbody meniscal release is performed just caudal to the medial meniscus to permit caudal movement of the caudal portion during tibial translation (Fig. 33-132).

Perform an open arthrotomy or arthroscopy. With an open arthrotomy, lever the tibia forward by placing the tip of a small Hohmann retractor behind the caudal edge of the tibial plateau and forcing the body of the retractor against the trochlear groove (see Fig. 33-131). With arthroscopy, place the limb in valgus stress to expose the medial meniscus. On the medial aspect of the limb, estimate the position of the medial collateral ligament. Insert a needle through the skin and joint caudal to the collateral ligament, and visualize it within the joint. The needle should cross the medial meniscus in the midbody region. Chase the needle with a No. 11 blade, and transect the meniscus from dorsal to ventral. Examine the transection to verify that it is complete. Close the joint routinely.

Transection of the meniscotibial ligament. *Perform an open arthrotomy or arthroscopy. With an open arthrotomy, lever the tibia forward by placing the tip of a small Hohmann retractor behind the caudal edge of the tibial plateau and forcing the body of the retractor against the trochlear groove (see Fig. 33-131). With arthroscopy, place the limb in valgus stress to expose the medial meniscus. Identify the meniscotibial ligament of the medial meniscus. Identify and protect the caudal cruciate ligament. Transect the meniscotibial ligament with a No. 11 blade, No. 12 blade, or hook knife. Close the joint routinely.*

SUTURE MATERIALS AND SPECIAL INSTRUMENTS

A small Hohmann retractor is useful for levering the tibia down and forward to allow visualization of the caudal horn of the medial meniscus. A mosquito Oschner forceps is used to grasp the meniscus, and a No. 11 or No. 12 blade is used to resect the damaged tissue or perform a meniscal release. A hook knife is useful for transection of the meniscotibial ligament.

POSTOPERATIVE CARE AND ASSESSMENT

Postoperative management should follow the recommendations given for reconstruction of the CCL (see p. 1275).

PROGNOSIS

The prognosis for recovery in animals with CCL injury is discussed on p. 1275. Total meniscectomy may promote DJD and should be avoided; however, partial meniscectomy or primary repair of the damaged meniscus lessens the degree of DJD and makes the prognosis for return to normal function more favorable. Dogs with meniscal injury associated with CCL rupture have a poorer long-term outcome than dogs with CCL rupture without meniscal injury (Innes et al, 2000).

References

Innes JF, Bacon D, Lynch C et al: Long-term outcome of surgery for dogs with cranial cruciate ligament deficiency, *Vet Rec* 147:325, 2000.

Kennedy SC, Dunning D, Bischoff MG et al: The effect of axial and abaxial release on meniscal displacement in the dog, *Vet Comp Orthop Traum* 18:227, 2005.

Mahn MM, Cook JL, Cook CR et al: Arthroscopic verification of ultrasonographic diagnosis of meniscal pathology in dogs, *Vet Surg* 34:318, 2005.

Ralphs SC, Whitney WO: Arthroscopic evaluation of menisci in dogs with cranial cruciate ligament injuries: 100 cases (1999-2000), *J Am Vet Med Assoc* 221:1601, 2002.

MEDIAL PATELLAR LUXATION

DEFINITION

Medial patellar luxation is a displacement of the patella from the trochlear sulcus.

GENERAL CONSIDERATIONS AND CLINICALLY RELEVANT PATHOPHYSIOLOGY

Medial patellar luxation is a common cause of lameness in small-breed dogs, but also occurs in large-breed dogs. Most patients with patellar luxation have associated musculoskeletal abnormalities, such as medial displacement of the quadriceps muscle group, lateral torsion of the distal femur, a lateral bowing of the distal one third of the femur, femoral epiphyseal dysplasia, rotational instability of the stifle joint, or tibial deformity (Fig. 33-133).

Medial malalignment of the quadriceps muscles in dogs with medial patellar luxation produces sufficient pressure on the distal femoral physis to retard growth. At the same time, there is less pressure on the lateral aspect of the distal femoral physis, which allows accelerated growth. Decreased length of the medial cortex relative to the increased length of the lateral cortex results in the lateral bowing of the distal femur. Abnormal growth continues as long as the quadriceps is displaced medially and the physes are active. Therefore the degree of lateral bowing depends on the severity of patellar luxation and the patient's age at the onset of luxation. With mild luxations, the quadriceps is rarely displaced medially and has minimal abnormal effect on the distal femoral physis. However, with severe luxations, the quadriceps is medially displaced at all times, and maximal effect on the distal femoral physis results in severe lateral bowing of the distal femur in young patients (Fig. 33-134). Tibial deformities seen with patellar luxations are the result of abnormal forces acting on the proximal and distal physes of the tibia. Tibial deformities described with medial patellar luxation include

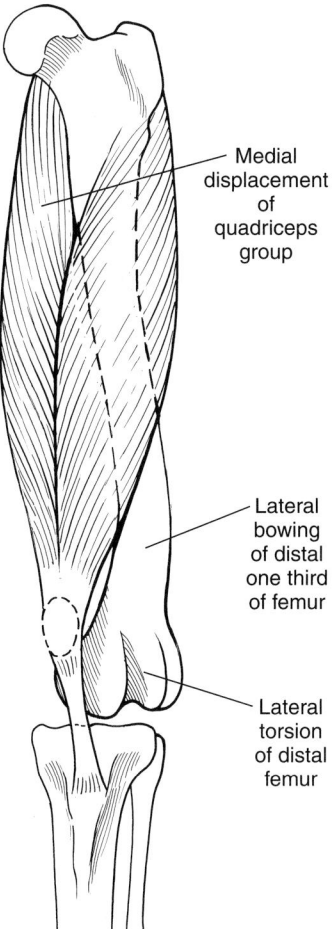

FIG. 33-133
Soft tissue and skeletal abnormalities associated with medial patellar luxation include medial displacement of the quadriceps apparatus, lateral bowing of the distal one third of the femur, and lateral torsion of the distal femur.

medial displacement of the tibial tuberosity, medial bowing (varus deformity) of the proximal tibia, and lateral torsion of the distal tibia.

Articular cartilage is the "physis" for the epiphysis and responds to increased or decreased pressure in the same manner as the metaphyseal physis: increased pressure retards growth and decreased pressure accelerates growth. Dogs with medial patellar luxation have abnormal development of the trochlear groove. The degree of abnormality varies from a near-normal trochlea to an absent trochlear groove. Articulation of the patella within the trochlear groove exerts a physiologic pressure on the articular cartilage that retards cartilage growth. Continued pressure by the patella is responsible for the development of normal depth of the trochlear groove. If the physiologic pressure exerted by the patella is not present on the trochlear articular cartilage, the trochlea fails to gain proper depth. Immature patients with mild luxations show minimal loss of depth to the

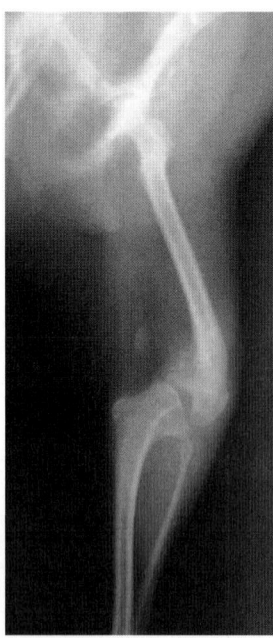

FIG. 33-134
Radiographic appearance of severe skeletal abnormalities associated with medial patellar luxation in a dog.

trochlear groove because the patella is normally positioned during development. However, immature patients with severe luxations have no trochlear groove because the normal pressure responsible for groove development is not present. The degree of the pathologic skeletal condition associated with patellar luxation varies considerably between the mildest and severest forms; therefore a system for classifying canine patellar luxation has been developed (Box 33-19).

Shortening of the limb due to hip luxation or femoral head and neck ostectomy will cause laxity of the quadriceps mechanism, enabling luxation of the patella in some cases. This usually resolves with treatment of the hip luxation and with time after FHO.

DIAGNOSIS
Clinical Presentation

Signalment. Dogs of any age or breed and either gender may have medial patellar luxations, but small- and toy-breed dogs are most frequently affected. Medial patellar luxations are more common than lateral patellar luxations in large-breed dogs; however, large dogs have a higher percentage of lateral luxations than small dogs.

History. Most affected animals have an intermittent weight-bearing lameness. Owners may report that the dog occasionally holds the leg in a flexed position for one or two steps. Dogs with grade IV patellar luxations have severe lameness and gait abnormalities.

Physical Examination Findings

The diagnosis of medial patellar luxation is based on finding or eliciting medial patellar luxation during a physical examination. Physical findings vary and depend on the severity

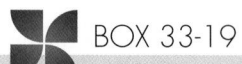 BOX 33-19

Grades of Patellar Luxation

Grade I

The patella can be luxated, but spontaneous luxation of the patella during normal joint motion rarely occurs. Manual luxation of the patella may be accomplished during physical examination, but the patella reduces when pressure is released. Flexion and extension of the joint are normal.

Grade II

Angular and torsional deformities of the femur may be present to a mild degree. The patella may be manually displaced with lateral pressure or may luxate with flexion of the stifle joint. The patella remains luxated until it is reduced by the examiner or is spontaneously reduced when the animal extends and derotates its tibia.

Grade III

The patella remains luxated medially most of the time, but may be manually reduced with the stifle in extension. However, after manual reduction, flexion and extension of the stifle result in reluxation of the patella. There is a medial displacement of the quadriceps muscle group. Abnormalities of the supporting soft tissue of the stifle joint and deformities of the femur and tibia may be present.

Grade IV

There may be an 80- to 90-degree medial rotation of the proximal tibial plateau. The patella is permanently luxated and cannot be manually repositioned. The femoral trochlear groove is shallow or absent, and there is medial displacement of the quadriceps muscle group. Abnormalities of the supporting soft tissue of the stifle joint and deformities of the femur and tibia are notable.

of luxation. Patients with a *grade I luxation* generally show no lameness, and the diagnosis is made as an incidental finding on physical examination. Patients with a *grade II luxation* show occasional "skipping" when walking or running. These patients occasionally stretch the lateral retinacular structures and develop a non–weight-bearing lameness. Lameness in patients with a *grade III luxation* varies from an occasional skip to a weight-bearing lameness. Patients with a *grade IV luxation* walk with the rear quarters in a crouched position because they are unable to extend the stifle joints fully. The patella is hypoplastic and may be found displaced medially alongside the femoral condyle.

Diagnostic Imaging

With a grade III or grade IV luxation, standard craniocaudal and medial-to-lateral radiographs show the patella to be displaced medially, whereas with a grade I or grade II luxation the patella may be within the trochlear sulcus or may be displaced medially (care must be taken to properly position the limb to eliminate artifactual appearing luxations). Full limb radiographs may show varus or valgus deformities and torsion of the tibia and femur. Careful radiographic positioning is critical, as poor positioning results in false positive limb deformity on radiographs. For more severe cases requiring long bone osteotomy and correction, special views (coronal or skyline view of the femur) or CT aid in determining the specific type and degree of deformity.

Laboratory Findings

Consistent laboratory findings are not seen. Arthrocentesis demonstrates changes compatible with osteoarthritis.

DIFFERENTIAL DIAGNOSIS

Differential diagnoses include avascular necrosis of the femoral head, coxofemoral luxation, ligamentous sprain of the stifle, and muscle strain. Careful examination of the hip joint is essential because some patients with patellar luxation also have avascular necrosis of the femoral head (see p. 1252) or hip dysplasia (see p. 1233). Shortening of the limb due to hip luxation (see p. 1246) or FHO (see p. 1240) will cause laxity of the quadriceps mechanism, enabling luxation of the patella in some cases. This usually resolves with treatment of the hip luxation and with time after FHO.

MEDICAL MANAGEMENT

Medial patellar luxation may be treated conservatively or surgically. The choice of treatment depends on the clinical history, physical findings, frequency of luxation, and the patient's age. Surgery is seldom warranted in asymptomatic older patients, whereas young animals or those that are lame usually benefit from surgery. Clients should be advised to observe the animal for the development of clinical signs attributable to medial patellar luxation.

SURGICAL TREATMENT

Surgery is advised in symptomatic immature or young adult patients because intermittent patellar luxation may prematurely wear the articular cartilage of the patella. Surgery is indicated at any age in patients showing lameness and is strongly advised in those with active growth plates because skeletal deformity may worsen rapidly. The surgical techniques used in actively growing animals should not adversely affect skeletal growth. Owners of dogs with bilateral grade IV patellar luxations should be warned of the likely need for multiple surgeries and probable continued lameness even after successful surgery because of the severity of the underlying long bone abnormalities.

Numerous surgical techniques are aimed at restraining the patella within the trochlear groove. Tibial tuberosity transposition, medial restraint release, lateral restraint reinforcement, trochlear groove deepening, femoral osteotomy, tibial osteotomy, antirotational sutures, and transposition of the origin of the rectus femoris have all been advocated for correction of patellar luxation. Generally a combination of techniques is required to achieve intraoperative stability of the patella (Box 33-20). It is important to understand that the primary abnormality is biomechanical, whereby the patella within the straight quadri-

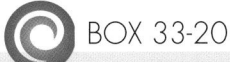

BOX 33-20

Basic Techniques for Repair of Medial Patellar Luxation

Medial fascial release
Trochlear wedge or block recession
Tibial crest transposition
Lateral imbrication

ceps mechanism fails to align with the trochlear groove. Surgeries that involve only deepening of the trochlear groove, capsule and fascial release, and imbrication are more prone to failure, as the patella and trochlear groove have not been permanently realigned.

In most animals, the trochlear groove must be deepened with a trochlear wedge or block recession or a trochlear resection. A trochlear wedge or block recession technically is more demanding, but preserves the articular cartilage (Johnson et al, 2001). Release of the medial retinaculum may be necessary to allow the patella to stabilize in the deepened trochlear groove. Tibial crest transposition must be done to realign the mechanical forces of the extensor mechanism (see p. 1295) unless major corrections of femoral and tibial deformity have been performed. Finally, after the patella is stable, the lateral retinaculum is reinforced with sutures and imbrication of the fibrous joint capsule, placement of a fascia lata graft from the fabella to the parapatellar fibrocartilage, or excision of redundant retinaculum. None of the reinforcement techniques alone is adequate to prevent reluxation permanently. If the mechanical forces pulling the patella out of the trochlear groove have not been neutralized, the reinforced retinaculum eventually stretches.

Osteotomy of the femur is used only in patients with such severe skeletal deformity that maintaining patellar reduction with the previously described techniques is impossible. The deformities usually seen are varus bowing of the distal femur and medial torsional deformity of the proximal tibia. The goal of surgery is to realign the stifle joint in the frontal plane where the transverse axis of the femoral condyles is perpendicular to the longitudinal axis of the femoral diaphysis. This requires accurate preoperative measurement and wedge osteotomy of the femur. Deepening of the trochlear groove, medial restraint release, transposition of the tibial crest, and lateral retinacular reinforcement are also required for success. These techniques require special equipment and training; as such, they should be performed by a trained specialist.

The quadriceps mechanism is a secondary stabilizer of the stifle joint for cranial translation (cranial drawer). Subsequently, chronic luxation of the patella may lead to increased stress on the CCL and eventual rupture. Combination of CCL rupture and patellar luxation is a relatively common finding, particularly in small-breed dogs.

Preoperative Management

Perioperative antibiotics (see p. 945) and preemptive pain management with NSAIDs, opiates, or epidural analgesia (see p. 945) are indicated for dogs undergoing stifle reconstructive techniques.

Anesthesia

See p. 944 for the anesthetic management of animals with orthopedic disease. Opioid epidural administration reduces postoperative discomfort (see p. 945).

Surgical Anatomy

The extensor mechanism of the stifle joint is composed of the quadriceps muscle groups, patella, trochlear groove, straight patellar ligament, and tibial tuberosity (Fig. 33-135). The quadriceps muscle group is formed by the rectus femoris, vastus lateralis, vastus intermedius, and vastus medialis muscles. The vastus medialis and vastus lateralis muscles are fixed to the patella by the medial and lateral parapatellar fibrocartilage. The fibrocartilage rides on the ridges of the femoral trochlea and, along with the medial and lateral retinacula, aids in patellar stability. The medial and lateral retinacula are groups of collagen fibers that course from the fabella to blend with the medial and lateral parapatellar fibrocartilages, respectively. The quadriceps muscle group functions to extend the stifle joint and, along with the entire extensor mechanism, aids in stabilizing the stifle joint. The quadriceps muscle group converges as the patellar tendon on the patella and then continues distally as the straight patellar ligament.

The patella is a sesamoid bone embedded in the tendon of the quadriceps muscle. The inner articular surface is smooth and curved so as to fully articulate with the trochlea. The normal gliding articulation of the patella and trochlea is necessary for maintaining the nutritional requirements of the trochlear and patellar articular surfaces. The patella is also an essential component of the functional mechanism of the extensor apparatus. The patella maintains even tension when the stifle is extended and also acts as a fulcrum in a lever arm, increasing the mechanical advantage of the quadriceps muscle group.

The tibial tuberosity is located cranial and distal to the tibial condyles. Its location and prominence are important for the mechanical advantage of the extensor mechanism. The alignment of the quadriceps, patella, trochlea, patellar ligament, and tibial tuberosity must be normal for proper function. Malalignment of one or more of these structures may lead to patellar luxation.

Special anatomic considerations in patients with medial patellar luxation must be noted. When the patella is positioned medially, the patellar ligament must be identified before making a parapatellar incision to enter the joint. The lateral capsule is stretched and thin, whereas the medial capsule is contracted and thickened. Thickening and contraction of the medial capsule are apparent if medial release is performed. The insertions of the caudal head of the sartorius muscle and the vastus medialis muscle should be identified. The medial ridge of the trochlear sulcus and the ventral surface of the patella may be worn.

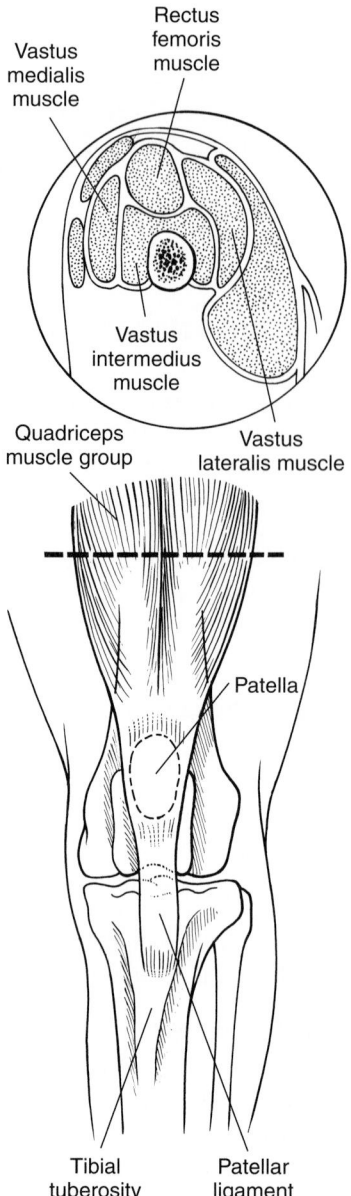

FIG. 33-135
Anatomic diagram of normal soft tissue and skeletal structures associated with the quadriceps extensor mechanism.

Positioning

The animal is positioned in dorsal or lateral recumbency, and the leg is prepared from the dorsal midline to the tarsal joint. Dorsal recumbency allows visualization of unrestrained extensor mechanism deviation and maximum manipulation of the limb to evaluate patellar stability.

SURGICAL TECHNIQUE
Arthrotomy

Make a craniolateral skin incision 4 cm proximal to the patella, and extend the incision 2 cm below the tibial tuberosity. Incise the subcutaneous tissue along the same line.

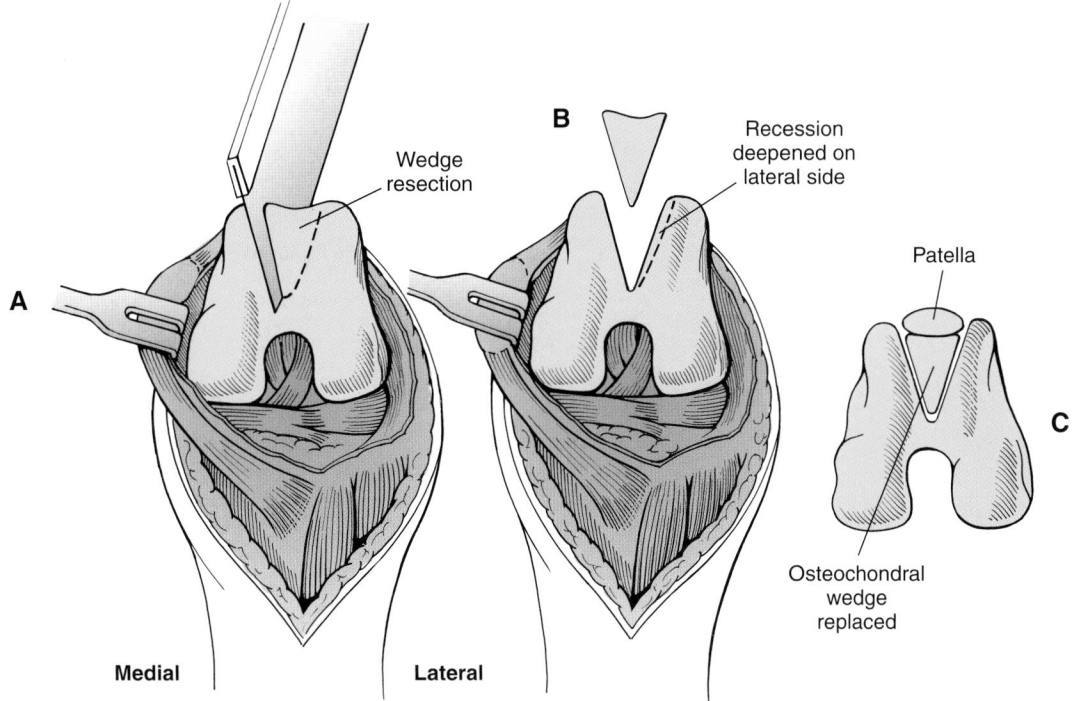

FIG. 33-136
Trochlear wedge recession. **A,** Resect an osteochondral wedge from the patellar groove.
B, Remove bone from the sides of the incised groove to deepen the sulcus. **C,** Replace the
osteochondral wedge.

Incise the lateral retinaculum and joint capsule to expose the joint.

Deepening of the Trochlear Groove

Trochlear wedge recession. Trochlear wedge recession deepens the trochlear groove to restrain the patella and maintain the integrity the patellofemoral articulation. In larger patients, an oscillating saw is often used, but in smaller breeds and toy breeds, a fine-toothed, hand-held saw or the cutting edge of a No. 20 scalpel blade and mallet may be used to make the cuts in the trochlea.

Cut into the articular cartilage of the trochlea, making a diamond-shaped outline. Be sure that the width of the cut is sufficient at its midpoint to accommodate the width of the patella but preserves the trochlear ridges. Using a surgical blade in very small and young patients, a hand saw in small and medium patients, or a power saw in large patients, remove an osteochondral wedge of bone and cartilage by following the outline previously made (Fig. 33-136). Make the osteotomy so that the two oblique planes that form the free wedge intersect distally at the intercondylar notch and proximally at the dorsal edge of the trochlear articular cartilage. Remove the osteochondral wedge and deepen the recession in the trochlea by removing additional bone from one or both sides of the newly created femoral groove.

If necessary, remodel the free osteochondral wedge with rongeurs to allow the wedge to seat deeply into the new femoral groove.

The wedge can also be rotated 180 degrees when it is returned to the femoral groove if doing so aids in heightening the medial ridge.

Replace the free osteochondral wedge when the depth is sufficient to house 50% of the height of the patella.

The osteochondral wedge remains in place because of the net compressive force of the patella and friction between the cancellous surfaces of the two cut edges.

Trochlear block recession. Trochlear block recession deepens the trochlear groove to restrain the patella and maintain the integrity the patellofemoral articulation. In larger patients, an oscillating saw is often used, but in smaller breeds and toy breeds, a fine-toothed, hand-held saw or the cutting edge of a No. 20 scalpel blade and mallet may be used to make the cuts in the trochlea.

Cut into the articular cartilage of the trochlea, making a block-shaped outline. Be sure that the width of the cut is sufficient to accommodate the width of the patella but preserves the trochlear ridges. Using a surgical blade in very small and young patients, a hand saw in small and medium patients,

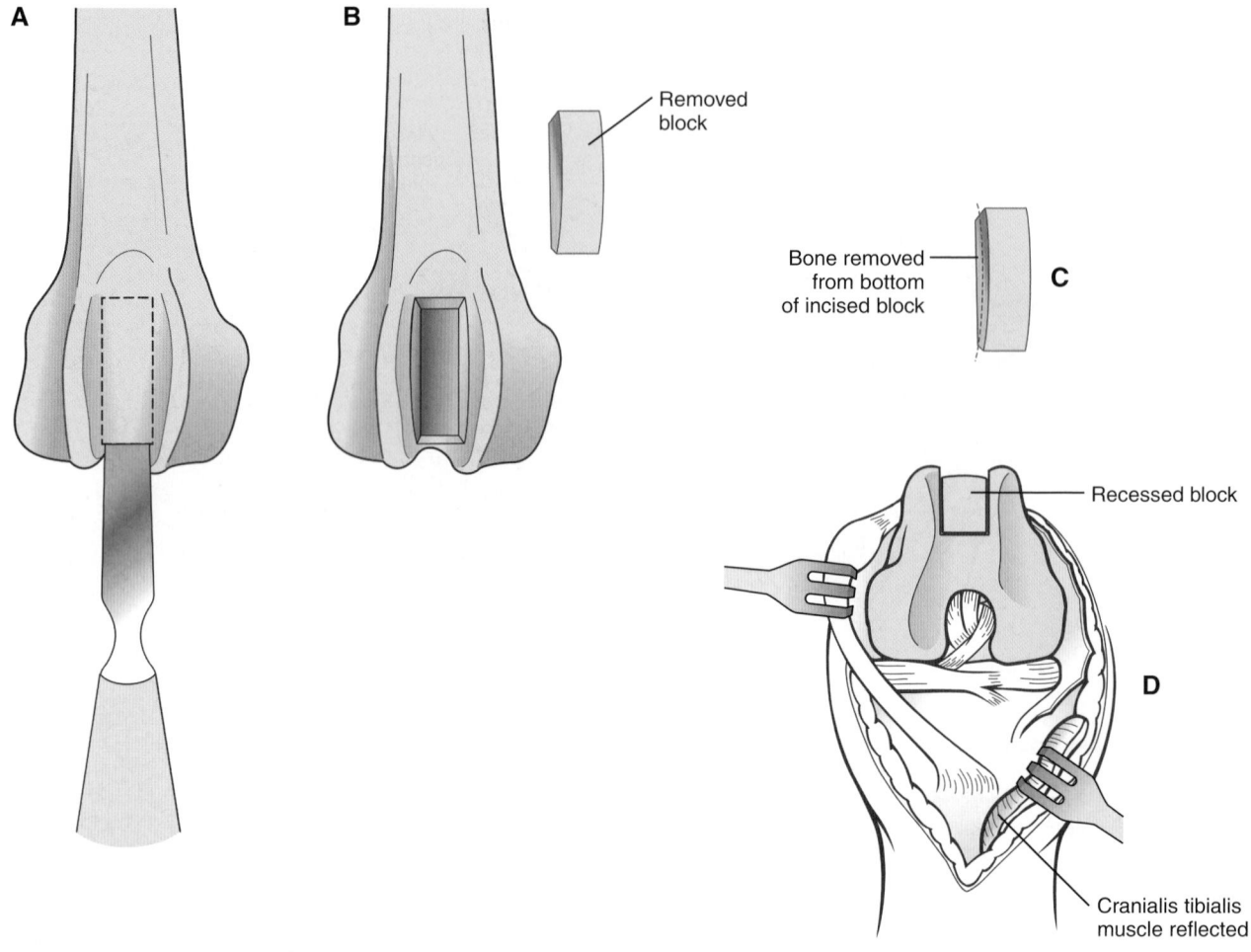

FIG. 33-137
Trochlear block recession. **A,** Use a thin saw blade to make two parallel cuts just axial to both trochlear ridges. **B,** Use an osteotome from proximal and distal to elevate an osteochondral block from the patellar groove. **C,** Remove bone from the bottom of the incised block to deepen the sulcus. **D,** Replace the osteochondral block.

or a power saw in large patients, deepen the proximodistal cuts 2 to 6 mm into the bone (Fig. 33-137). Using an osteotome that is the same width as the osteotomy, elevate the osteochondral segment. Insert the osteotome from both the proximal and distal extents of the osteotomy, meeting in the middle. Take care to remove an appropriate thickness of bone and to avoid cracking or splitting the osteochondral segment. Deepen the recession in the trochlea by removing additional bone from the base of the groove. Replace the free osteochondral fragment when the depth is sufficient to house 50% of the height of the patella.

The osteochondral wedge remains in place because of the net compressive force of the patella and friction between the cancellous surfaces of the two cut edges.

Trochlear resection. Trochlear resection is a method of deepening the trochlear groove through removal of articular cartilage and subchondral cancellous bone. The advantage of this technique is its simplicity. The disadvantage is that it removes the articular cartilage of the trochlea and allows articulation of the patella on the rough cancellous surface, which results in wearing of patellar articular cartilage. This procedure should only be performed when a recession procedure is impossible.

> NOTE: With a medial luxation, it often is best to take more bone from the lateral side of the groove, preserving as much of the medial ridge as possible.

Measure the width of the articular surface of the patella, and use this measurement to determine the proper width of the trochlear resection. Remove articular cartilage and bone with a bone rasp, power burr, or rongeurs (Fig. 33-138). Make the length of the trochlear resection extend to the proximal margin of the articular cartilage and distally to the cartilage margin just above the intercondylar notch. The groove should be deep enough to accommodate 50% of the

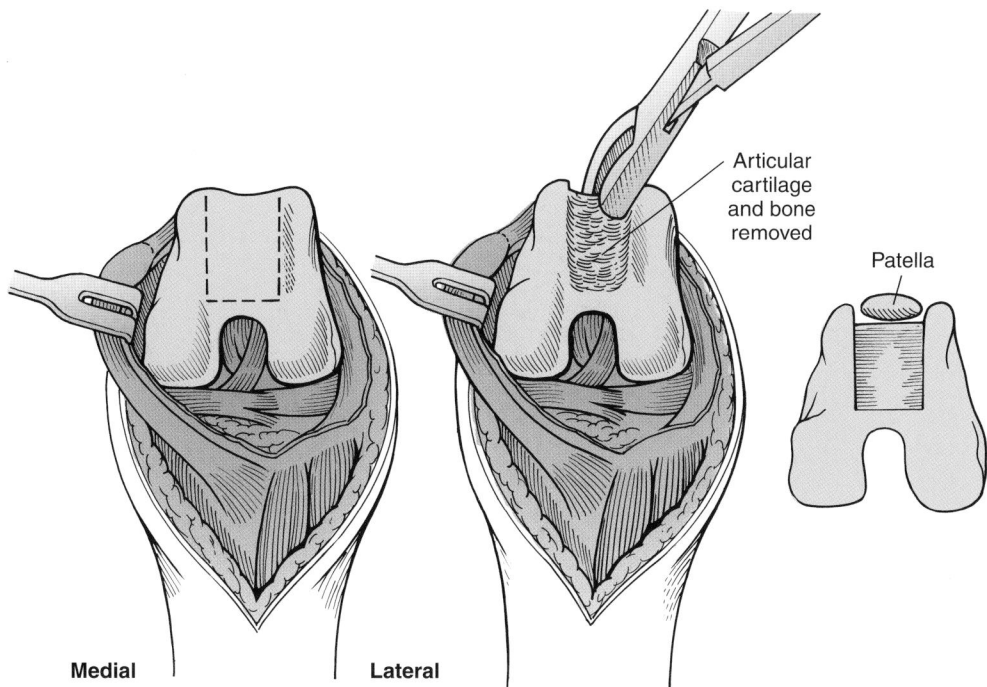

FIG. 33-138
For trochlear resection, remove articular cartilage and bone with a bone rasp, power burr, or rongeurs to a depth at which the patella rides within the new sulcus. Make the medial and lateral trochlear ridges parallel to each other and the base of the groove perpendicular to each trochlear ridge.

height of the patella and allow the parapatellar fibrocartilage to articulate with the newly formed medial and lateral trochlear ridges. Make the medial and lateral trochlear ridges parallel to each other and the base of the groove perpendicular to each trochlear ridge.

Release of the medial joint capsule. The medial joint capsule is thicker than normal and contracted in patients with a grade III or grade IV medial patellar luxation. In these patients, the medial joint capsule and retinaculum must be released to allow lateral placement of the patella.

Using a scalpel, make a medial parapatellar incision through the medial fascia and joint capsule. Begin the incision at the level of the proximal pole of the patella, and extend it distally to the tibial crest. In more severe cases, the release incision needs to be extended proximally on the medial thigh. If dynamic contraction of the cranial sartorius muscle and vastus medialis muscle directs the patella medially, release the insertions of these muscles at the proximal patella. Redirect the insertions and suture them to the vastus intermedius muscle.

Allow the incision to separate and do not suture the cut edges when surgery is complete, but suture medial subcutaneous tissue to the cranial cut edge of the incision. Alternatively, place a cruciate or simple interrupted suture that does not close the tissue gap when the patella is in the

proper position. Placement of a loose suture will prevent iatrogenic lateral luxation.

Tibial tuberosity transposition. *Make a lateral parapatellar incision through the fascia lata, and carry the incision distally onto the tibial tuberosity below the joint line. Reflect the cranialis tibialis muscle from the lateral tibial tuberosity and tibial plateau to the level of the long digital extensor tendon (Fig. 33-139, A). Use sharp dissection to gain access to the deep surface of the patellar tendon for placement of an osteotome, Listen bone cutter, or sagittal saw. Beginning at the level of the patella, make a medial parapatellar incision through the fascia and distally through the periosteum of the tibial tuberosity. Position an osteotome, Listen bone cutter, or sagittal saw beneath the patellar tendon 3 to 5 cm caudal to the cranial point of the tibial tuberosity (Fig. 33-139, B). Complete the osteotomy in a proximal to distal direction. Do not transect the distal periosteal attachment.*

The degree of lateral movement of the tibial tuberosity is subjective, but is based on the longitudinal realignment of the tuberosity relative to the trochlear groove.

Once the site of relocation is chosen, remove a thin layer of cortical bone with a rasp or osteotome. Lever the tibial tuberosity into position, and stabilize it with one or two small Kirschner wires directed caudally and slightly proximally

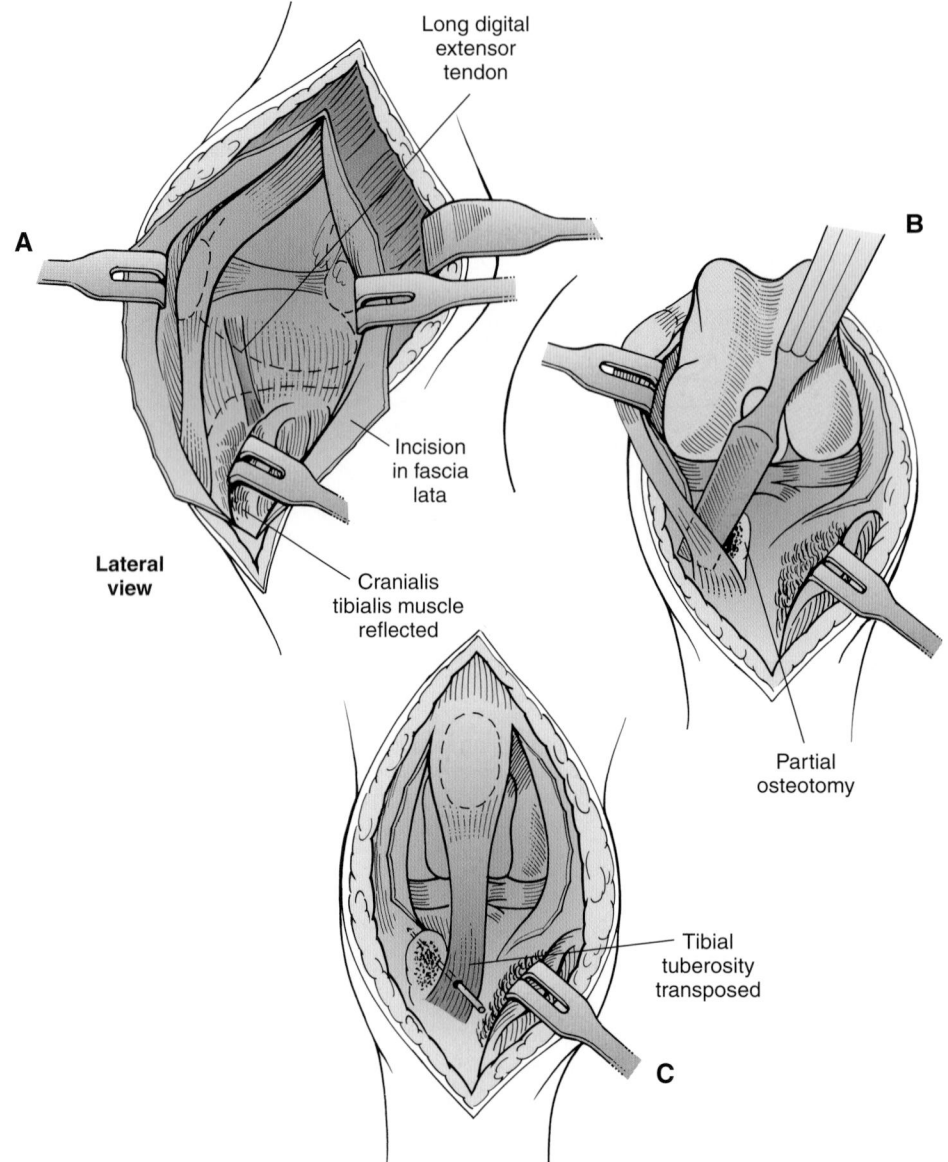

FIG. 33-139
Medial patellar luxations. **A,** Transpose the tibial crest laterally. Make a lateral parapatellar incision through the fascia lata and carry the incision distally onto the tibial tuberosity below the joint line. Reflect the cranialis tibialis muscle from the lateral tibial tuberosity and tibial plateau to the level of the long digital extensor tendon. **B,** Position an osteotome beneath the patellar ligament and partly ostectomize the tibial crest. Do not transect the distal periosteal attachment. **C,** Stabilize the tibial tuberosity in its new location with one or two small Kirschner wires.

(Fig. 33-139, C). Engage the caudal cortex, but do not exit the pin from the tibia caudally; if the pin protrudes too far from the caudal cortex of the tibia, persistent lameness results. Check the stability of the patella as described previously, and relocate the tuberosity if needed.

Security of the tibial transposition is increased by use of a figure-eight wire. The addition of a figure-eight wire is strongly recommended when performing tibial crest trans-

position in large-breed dogs and should be considered in all but the smallest patients. Failure of tibial crest transposition results in proximal displacement of the tibial crest and patella. Restoration of normal anatomy following this complication is difficult, and regardless of treatment, permanent disability often results.

Drill a small hole in the cranial cortex of the tibia several millimeters distal to the distal aspect of the osteotomy. Pass

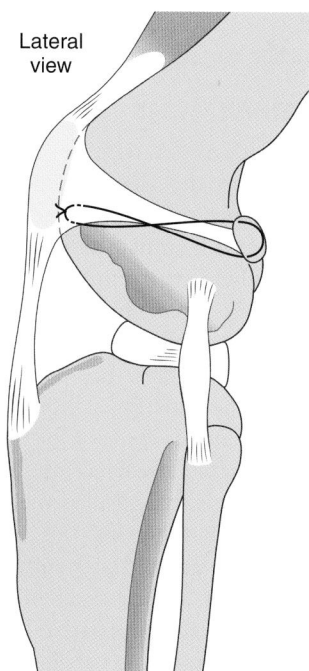

FIG. 33-140
Lateral reinforcement of the retinaculum may be performed by placing a polyester suture through the femoral-fabellar ligament and lateral parapatellar fibrocartilage.

orthopedic wire, or nonabsorbable suture in very small patients, through the hole and over the tips of the pins in a figure-eight pattern. Tighten the wires.

Lateral imbrication. *For suture imbrication, place a polyester suture through the femoral-fabellar ligament and lateral parapatellar fibrocartilage (Fig. 33-140). Next, place a series of imbrication sutures through the fibrous joint capsule and lateral edge of the patella tendon. With the leg in slight flexion, tie the femoral-fabellar suture and imbrication sutures.*

If the patella is out of position most of the time, the retinaculum opposite the side of the luxation will be stretched; with medial luxations, there is redundant lateral retinaculum.

Once the patella has been reduced, excise the excess retinaculum and joint capsule, allowing tight closure of the arthrotomy.

SUTURE MATERIALS AND SPECIAL INSTRUMENTS

A fine-toothed saw (No. 12 X-acto saw, available at most hobby shops) is used for trochlear wedge recession. An osteotome is needed to perform a block recession. An osteotome and mallet, Kirschner wires, orthopedic wire, and a hand chuck or drill are needed to secure the tibial crest when tibial tuberosity transposition is performed.

POSTOPERATIVE CARE AND ASSESSMENT

The limb is placed in a soft, padded bandage for 3 days. Uncontrolled exercise should be restricted to specific physical rehabilitation exercises and leash walking for 6 weeks; then the animal should be gradually returned to unsupervised activity over a 6-week period. A sample physical rehabilitation exercise protocol can be found by referring to Table 33-16 on p. 1277. Radiographs should be obtained at 6 to 8 weeks to evaluate healing of a tibial crest transposition.

PROGNOSIS

Recurrent luxation after surgery has been reported in up to 50% of joints evaluated. However, most are grade I luxations that do not affect clinical function. Most stifle joints function well enough that lameness is not apparent during examination, nor is clinical dysfunction reported by clients. Most patients with recurrent luxation show reluxation only on physical examination when manual force is used to displace the patella. Correlation of reluxation with the method or methods of surgical correction has not been reported. Overall, the prognosis for patients undergoing surgical correction of a grade I to III patellar luxation is excellent for return to normal limb function. DJD progresses despite treatment, but is not as severe as that associated with chronic CCL rupture. Prognosis for patients with grade IV patellar luxation is guarded. Many joints require multiple surgery, and some patellae cannot be reduced without major corrective osteotomies.

Reference

Johnson AL, Probst CW, DeCamp CE et al: Comparison of trochlear block recession and trochlear wedge recession for canine patellar luxation using a cadaver model, *Vet Surg* 30:140, 2001.

LATERAL PATELLAR LUXATION

DEFINITIONS

Lateral patellar luxation is an intermittent or permanent displacement of the patella from the trochlear sulcus. **Anteversion** is excessive external rotation of the proximal femur relative to the distal femur. **Coxa valga** is an abnormal increase in the angle formed by the femoral neck and shaft in the frontal plane.

GENERAL CONSIDERATIONS AND CLINICALLY RELEVANT PATHOPHYSIOLOGY

Lateral patellar luxation is seen most often in large breeds of dogs, but does occur in small and toy breeds of dogs. The cause is unknown, but is thought to be related to anteversion or coxa valga of the coxofemoral joint, which shifts the line of force produced by the pull of the quadriceps lateral to the longitudinal axis of the trochlear groove. This abnormally directed lateral force pulls the patella from the trochlear sulcus. Abnormal force placed on the growth plates of immature patients causes skeletal abnormalities that are mirror images of those seen with medial patellar luxation. For further discussion of the pathophysiology of patellar luxation, see p. 1289.

DIAGNOSIS
Clinical Presentation

Signalment. Dogs of either gender and any age or breed may be affected. Lateral patellar luxations are more frequently seen in large breeds of dogs than in small and toy breeds. Medial patellar luxation, however, is more common than lateral luxation in dogs of all sizes. Lateral patellar luxation has not been described in cats.

History. Affected animals most commonly are seen for evaluation of an intermittent, weight-bearing lameness. Owners may report that the animal occasionally holds the leg in a flexed position for one or two steps.

Physical Examination Findings

Physical examination findings vary and depend on the severity of luxation. The diagnosis is determined by finding or eliciting lateral luxation of the patella and eliminating other causes of rear limb lameness (see later discussion). Patients with a grade I luxation generally show no lameness, and the diagnosis is made as an incidental finding on physical examination. Patients with a grade II luxation show occasional "skipping" when walking or running. These patients occasionally stretch the medial retinacular structures and appear for the first visit showing a non–weight-bearing lameness. Lameness in patients with a grade III luxation varies from an occasional skip to a weight-bearing lameness. Patients with a grade IV luxation walk with the rear quarters in a crouched position because of inability to extend the stifle joints fully.

Diagnostic Imaging

With a grade III or grade IV luxation, standard craniocaudal and medial-to-lateral radiographs consistently show the patella to be displaced laterally. With a grade I or grade II luxation, the patella may be within the trochlear sulcus when the radiographs are made or may be displaced laterally. Varying degrees of osteoarthrosis may be present.

Laboratory Findings

Consistent laboratory findings are not seen.

DIFFERENTIAL DIAGNOSIS

Differential diagnoses include hip dysplasia, osteochondritis of the stifle or tarsal joints, panosteitis, hypertrophic osteodystrophy, capital physeal injury, CCL rupture, and muscle strain. It is important to note that many patients with lateral patellar luxation also have evidence of hip dysplasia. Both conditions may contribute to the lameness and require appropriate treatment for the dog to become sound.

MEDICAL MANAGEMENT

Lateral patellar luxation may be treated conservatively or surgically. The choice of treatment depends on the patient's age, the clinical history, and the physical findings. Older patients that are not lame and that have patellar luxation diagnosed as an incidental finding do not require surgical intervention. Rather the client should be instructed to observe for clinical signs associated with patellar luxation.

SURGICAL TREATMENT

The goals and methods of treatment for lateral patellar luxation are similar to those described for medial patellar luxation on p. 1291. The surgical technique used in animals with lateral patellar luxations is similar to that described for osteotomy of the tibial tuberosity in animals with medial patellar luxations (see p. 1295) except that the tuberosity is repositioned and stabilized medially (Fig. 33-141). Because lateral patellar luxation occurs in large-breed dogs, the use of figure-eight wire with the pins for stabilization of the tibial tuberosity is recommended. Avulsion of the tibial crest following surgery is difficult to correct due to contracture of the quadriceps and proximal displacement of the patella. Limb salvage is difficult following this complication. The medial retinaculum is reinforced with suture reconstruction, fascial lata transposition, and/or excision of the redundant joint capsule. The lateral restraints are released to help neutralize lateral forces acting on the patella. Methods for deepening the trochlear groove are the same as those described for medial patellar luxation. Osteotomies of the femur and tibia may be required to correct severe angular and torsional deformities. Corrective osteotomies are best performed by a specialist with the necessary equipment and training in these complex procedures.

Preoperative Management

Perioperative antibiotics (see p. 945) and preemptive pain management with NSAIDs (see Table 33-4 on p. 1149), opiates, or epidural analgesia are indicated for dogs undergoing stifle reconstructive techniques.

Anesthesia

See p. 944 for a discussion of the anesthetic management of patients with orthopedic disease. Opioid epidural administration reduces postoperative discomfort (see p. 945).

Surgical Anatomy

See p. 1292 for the normal anatomy of the stifle joint. In patients with lateral patellar luxation, abnormal wear of the lateral trochlear ridge may be evident. The patella and patellar ligament lie lateral to the trochlear sulcus in these patients. The patellar ligament must be identified before making a parapatellar incision to enter the joint. The medial retinaculum appears stretched in these patients, whereas the lateral retinaculum appears contracted. Release of the lateral retinaculum (with incision into the joint) reveals a thickened joint capsule.

Positioning

The patient is positioned in dorsal recumbency or in lateral recumbency with the affected leg up. The leg should be prepared from the dorsal midline to the tarsal joint. A hanging-leg preparation and dorsal recumbency facilitate manipulation of the leg during surgery.

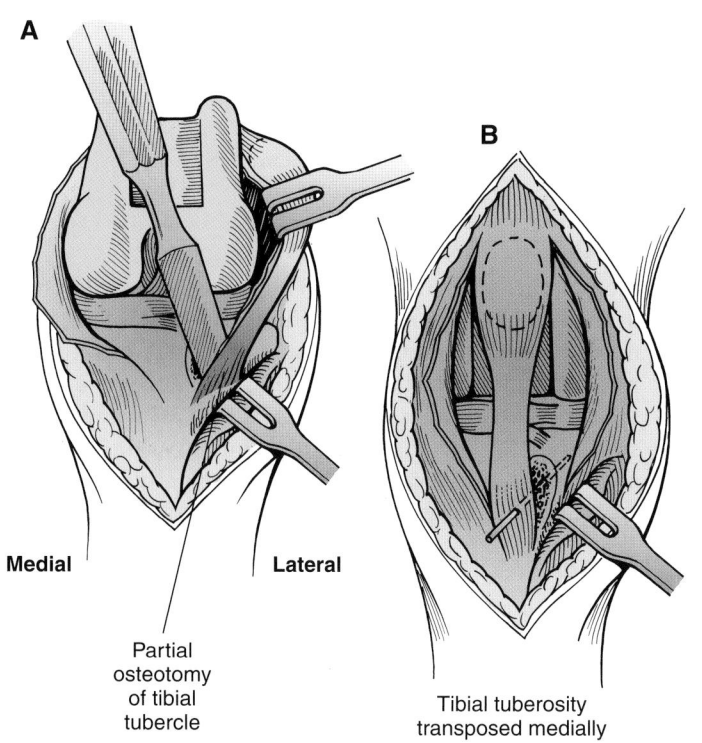

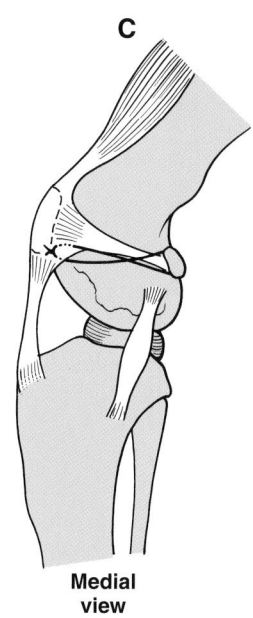

Medial   **Lateral**

Partial
osteotomy
of tibial
tubercle

Tibial tuberosity
transposed medially

**Medial
view**

FIG. 33-141
For lateral patellar luxations,
transpose the tibial crest medially. **A,** Make a parapatellar
incision through the fascia lata
and carry the incision distally
onto the tibial tuberosity below
the joint line. Position an osteotome beneath the patellar ligament and partly ostectomize
the tibial crest. Do not transect
the distal periosteal attachment. **B,** Stabilize the tibial
tuberosity in its new location
with one or two small
Kirschner wires. **C,** Reinforce
the medial retinaculum with
suture placed from the fabella
to the parapatellar fibrocartilage.

SURGICAL TECHNIQUE

A description of the surgical technique for correction of
patellar luxation is given above and on p. 1291.

SUTURE MATERIALS AND SPECIAL INSTRUMENTS

Instruments needed for tibial tuberosity transposition are an
osteotome and mallet, Kirschner wires, and orthopedic wire
to secure the tibial crest transposition, and a hand chuck or
drill. In large-breed dogs, creation of the tibial crest osteotomy is simpler with power sagittal saw. A fine-toothed saw is
needed for trochlear wedge recession. An osteotome is
needed for trochlear block recession.

POSTOPERATIVE CARE AND ASSESSMENT

Exercise should be restricted to specific physical rehabilitation techniques and leash walking for 6 weeks; the animal
should be gradually returned to unsupervised activity over a
6-week period. A sample physical rehabilitation exercise
protocol can be found by referring to Table 33-16 on p.
1277.

PROGNOSIS

The prognosis is less favorable for large dogs with lateral
patellar luxations than for smaller dogs with a medial patellar luxation; however, the prognosis is good for a return to
functional activity with grades I to III. The prognosis with
grade IV patellar luxation in large-breed dogs is guarded due
to the frequent need for multiple surgeries and femoral and/
or tibial correction and the severity of the soft tissue deformity and shortening.

OSTEOCHONDRITIS DISSECANS OF THE STIFLE

DEFINITION

Osteochondritis dissecans (OCD) or *osteochondrosis* is a
disturbance in endochondral ossification that leads to retention of cartilage; it occasionally occurs in the stifle of immature large dogs.

GENERAL CONSIDERATIONS AND CLINICALLY RELEVANT PATHOPHYSIOLOGY

OCD begins with a failure of endochondral ossification in
either the physis or the articular epiphyseal complex, which
is responsible for the formation of metaphyseal bone. This
condition occurs more commonly in the shoulder, elbow,
and hock. The pathogenesis of OCD is discussed on p.
1176. With OCD of the stifle, a piece of cartilage and subchondral bone usually is observed that involves the medial
surface of the lateral femoral condyle (most frequently affected) or the medial femoral condyle. The condition often
is bilateral.

DIAGNOSIS
Clinical Presentation

Signalment. Affected dogs usually are large (e.g., German
shepherds, Great Danes) and young, with the average age at
onset of lameness being 5 to 7 months (range, 3 months to 3
years). Males are affected more often than females.

History. Rear limb lameness, which worsens after exercise, may be acute or chronic and mild or severe. Often the
onset of the lameness is insidious. Owners frequently com-

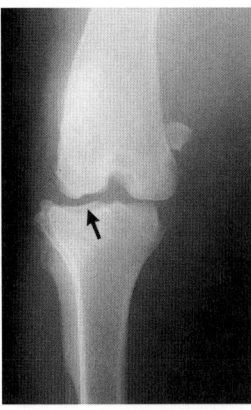

FIG. 33-142
Radiograph of a stifle with OCD of the lateral femoral condyle. There is a radiolucent defect on the distal surface of the lateral femoral condyle *(arrow)*.

plain that the dog is stiff in the morning or after rest, and they generally are concerned that the dog may have hip dysplasia.

Physical Examination Findings

Lameness of one rear limb usually is evident. There may be stifle joint effusion and crepitation, especially if DJD is progressing. In immature dogs, a very slight cranial drawer may be noted, especially with muscle atrophy. However, when the cranial drawer is tested in animals with stifle OCD, drawer motion should stop abruptly, indicating that the CCL is intact (see p. 1255).

Diagnostic Imaging

Radiographic views should include standard craniocaudal and lateral views of the stifle. Oblique views may be needed to observe the extent of the lesion. Radiographs of both stifles should be obtained to identify bilateral disease. Definitive radiographic diagnosis of OCD is made when a radiolucent concavity is observed on the medial or lateral femoral condyle (Fig. 33-142). More subtle radiographic signs include flattening of the articular surface and subchondral sclerosis. Radiographic signs of secondary osteoarthritis usually are seen (see p. 1156).

Arthroscopy. Arthroscopy provides minimally invasive definitive diagnosis of OCD. The site of the lesion is easily visualized following fat pad resection and flap removal; treatment of the underlying subchondral bone is straightforward (see later discussion).

Laboratory Findings

Results of hematologic and serum biochemical analyses are normal in most affected animals. Results of arthrocentesis may include decreased synovial fluid viscosity, increased fluid volume, and an increased number of mononuclear phagocytic cells (up to 6000 to 9000 WBC/μl).

DIFFERENTIAL DIAGNOSIS

OCD must be differentiated from other diseases of young growing dogs that affect the rear limb and may cause similar clinical signs of lameness (hip dysplasia and panosteitis). CCL rupture is ruled out by physical examination and by the presence of radiographic evidence of OCD.

MEDICAL MANAGEMENT

Medical therapy may be used to treat older dogs with established osteoarthritis and dogs with small lesions and minimal lameness. Lame animals should be treated with confinement and administration of NSAIDs (see Table 33-4). After the lameness has subsided, exercise is increased gradually to strengthen the surrounding musculature. Weight control is also important in the management of osteoarthritis. If there is no response, surgery should be considered.

SURGICAL TREATMENT

Surgical removal of the cartilage flap allows the defect to heal by outgrowth of fibrocartilage from underlying subchondral bone. Surgery may be useful in young animals when the disease is diagnosed before the onset of osteoarthritis and in lame animals when the condition is unresponsive to medical therapy. However, surgical management does not usually alter the progression of osteoarthritis.

Many cases of stifle OCD are bilateral, and as the disease occurs most frequently in large- and giant-breed dogs, bilateral arthrotomy may result in significant short-term morbidity. Dogs requiring bilateral surgery are better treated arthroscopically, as the degree of postoperative pain and disability is significantly decreased.

OCD of the stifle may be amenable to treatment with autogenous osteochondral plug transfers to replace the deficient subchondral bone and articular cartilage. This procedure requires advanced equipment and training and should be performed by a surgical expert.

Preoperative Management

Perioperative antibiotics (see p. 945) and preemptive pain management with NSAIDs (see Table 33-4 on p. 1149), opiates, or epidural analgesia are indicated for dogs undergoing stifle exploration (see Chapter 13).

Anesthesia

See p. 944 for a discussion of the anesthetic management of patients with orthopedic disease. Opioid epidural administration reduces postoperative discomfort (see p. 945).

Surgical Anatomy

Surgical anatomy of the stifle is discussed on p. 1292. Either arthroscopy or a standard medial or lateral parapatellar approach can be used to expose the lesion.

Positioning

The dog is positioned in dorsal recumbency with the affected limb suspended for draping. The limb is then released to allow access to the medial or lateral surface of the stifle.

SURGICAL TECHNIQUE
Arthroscopy

Standard arthroscopy portals with fat pad excision provide outstanding visualization and treatment of the lesion with a minimally invasive technique. Dogs requiring bilateral treatment may have less pain and short-term disability when treated arthroscopically than when treated with arthrotomy.

Establish standard craniomedial and craniolateral arthroscopy portals (see p. 1258). Remove the fat pad as needed to visualize the medial and lateral femoral condyles. If working without a cannula, insert a locking grasper through the instrument portal. Grab the flap and twist it, rolling the grasper towards the bone surface until the flap is separated from the bone. Remove the flap. If working through a cannula system, insert a large aggressive power burr, and shave and suction the flap until gone. After flap removal insert a curette and examine the edges of the lesion for loose cartilage. Make the edges of the lesion 90 degrees to the articular surface and subchondral bone to improve healing. Insert a hand burr and perform mild abrasion arthroplasty or perform microfracture on the lesion. Shut off fluid inflow to the joint, and observe for adequate bleeding from the subchondral bone. Flush and close the joint routinely.

Arthrotomy

The surgical approach selected depends on the surgeon's preference (see p. 1263 for the lateral and medial parapatellar approaches).

Regardless of the technique used for exposure, examine the appropriate femoral condyle and remove the flap of cartilage. Perform curettage to remove fragments of cartilage from the edges of the lesion. Repeatedly flush the joint to remove any small fragments before closure.

SUTURE MATERIALS AND SPECIAL INSTRUMENTS

For arthroscopy, a power shaver is required to remove the fat pad. A hand burr or power burr is useful to abrade the subchondral bone. Micropicks and a mallet are necessary for microfracture. For either approach, a bone curette is needed to curette the edges of the lesion.

POSTOPERATIVE CARE AND ASSESSMENT

No bandaging is required following arthroscopic treatment unless there is excessive drainage from the portal sites. Following open arthrotomy, the limb may be bandaged after surgery for 3 to 5 days to provide soft tissue support. Exercise should be restricted to specific physical rehabilitation techniques and leash walking for 6 weeks (see Table 33-16 on p. 1277); the animal should be gradually returned to unsupervised activity over a 6-week period.

PROGNOSIS

The prognosis depends on the size of the lesion and whether DJD is present. Dogs treated conservatively for OCD of the stifle usually have continued intermittent lameness and progressive osteoarthritis. Those treated surgically for OCD of the stifle may have improved limb function, but lameness may be evident after exercise. Osteoarthritis usually is present even after surgery and requires occasional medical treatment (see p. 1300). Most dogs are functional pets and are only intermittently lame. Treatment of the cartilage defects with autogenous osteochondral transfers may improve the outcome.

TARSUS

LIGAMENT INJURY OF THE TARSUS
DEFINITIONS

Ligament injury to the tarsal joint may result from injury within or surrounding the tarsocrural, proximal intertarsal, distal intertarsal, or tarsometatarsal joints. **Luxation** is a complete separation between one of the above joint surfaces, and **subluxation** is a partial or incomplete separation. The term **varus** denotes an inward deviation of the limb, and **valgus** denotes an outward deviation. **Shearing** or **degloving injuries** result from abrasion, which may cause skin, ligament, and bone loss.

GENERAL CONSIDERATIONS AND CLINICALLY RELEVANT PATHOPHYSIOLOGY

Ligament injuries of the tarsus usually result from severe trauma, such as vehicular accidents. Most injuries are open abrasions with moderate to severe loss of soft tissue or bone or both. Shearing injuries usually involve the tarsocrural joint. They typically occur when the limb is caught beneath a tire and are associated with severe abrasion of the soft tissue and malleoli. Shear injuries can involve the lateral or medial surface of the tarsus, but the medial surface is more commonly injured. Subluxation results from injury of the medial or lateral collateral ligament complex or fracture of the medial or lateral malleolus. Luxation generally results from injury of both the medial and the lateral collateral ligament complexes, fracture of both malleoli, or fracture of one malleolus with injury to the contralateral collateral ligament complex. A number of intertarsal injuries have been recognized as resulting from disruption of various ligament complexes between tarsal bones. Proximal intertarsal subluxation, proximal intertarsal luxation, and tarsometatarsal luxation are most common.

DIAGNOSIS
Clinical Presentation

Signalment. Any age or breed and either gender of dog or cat may be affected.

History. Most animals are brought in for evaluation of a non–weight-bearing lameness. Some animals have an associated open wound over the tarsus.

Physical Examination Findings

Complete tarsocrural joint luxation is obvious; the animal is non–weight-bearing, and the paw deviates at an unnatural angle. Pain, swelling, and crepitus are present. Subluxations may be more difficult to diagnose, particularly if only one part of the medial or lateral ligament complex is injured. Animals with very unstable subluxations are unable to bear weight, and the paw deviates to the direction opposite the ligamentous damage (i.e., if the subluxation is medial, the paw deviates laterally). If partial tears of the collateral complex are suspected, varus and valgus forces should be applied to the joint while it is extended and flexed. Laxity in extension denotes injury to the long components of the collateral ligament complex, whereas laxity in flexion only denotes injury to the short component of the collateral ligament complex.

> NOTE: Be sure to place the joint in extension to evaluate medial or lateral restraint injury.

With shearing injuries that cause luxation or subluxation, soft tissue abrasion and bone loss occur. Often the bone surface and articular cartilage are exposed. With intertarsal luxation and tarsometatarsal subluxation, animals usually are in pain and unable to bear weight on the affected limb, and the involved area is swollen. Abnormal rotation and deviation of the foot are seen.

Diagnostic Imaging

Standard craniocaudal and medial-to-lateral radiographs often are sufficient for complete evaluation (Fig. 33-143). If instability is suspected but not confirmed, craniocaudal and varus-valgus stress films performed with the patient anesthetized are useful (Fig. 33-144).

Arthroscopy. For closed injuries, arthroscopy enables visualization of the cartilage of the tibiotarsal joint for assessment of its condition when a decision between reconstruction and fusion is being made.

Laboratory Findings

Consistent laboratory abnormalities are not seen.

DIFFERENTIAL DIAGNOSIS

Differential diagnoses include mild sprain, fractures of one or more tarsal bones, OCD of the talus, and arthritis. These conditions can be differentiated from tarsal luxation or subluxation by radiography.

MEDICAL MANAGEMENT

Medical management is not rewarding with these injuries. Surgery is needed to restore the functional integrity of the joint.

SURGICAL TREATMENT

Each patient needs a thorough neurologic and vascular evaluation to determine the feasibility of treatment. With tarsocrural luxation or subluxation, the objectives of treatment are to reestablish joint stability to achieve pain-free weight bearing. Reconstruction of the short and long collateral ligament components is recommended for optimum results. With severe ligament injuries of the tarsus, partial or complete fusion are alternatives to joint reconstruction. With shearing injuries, the objective of management is to achieve a pain-free, functional patient. If the cartilage and bone damage is limited to the malleolus, reconstruction can be attempted. However, if damage to the cartilage and bone is severe, tarsal arthrodesis should be considered.

Proximal intertarsal subluxation with plantar instability occurs when excessive dorsal flexion causes disruption of the plantar ligament complex between the calcaneus and fourth tarsal bones. Treatment involves selective fusion of the joint surfaces between the calcaneus and fourth tarsal bones.

Proximal intertarsal subluxation can occur with dorsal instability. This injury results from damage to the dorsal ligaments and dorsal joint capsule between the talus and central tarsal bone caused by hyperextension. Treatment in most cases is best accomplished with rigid coaptation. If this is not successful, selective fusion of the talocentral joint can be performed.

Proximal intertarsal luxation occurs when excessive dorsal flexion causes disruption of the plantar ligament complex both between the calcaneus and fourth tarsal bones and between the talus and the central tarsal bone (Fig. 33-145). Complete luxation is differentiated from subluxation by notable dorsal displacement of the distal tarsus at the proximal intertarsal joint. Treatment is by selective fusion of the proximal intertarsal joint.

Tarsometatarsal luxation (Fig. 33-146) occurs when excessive dorsal flexion causes disruption of the plantar ligaments and fibrocartilage. The luxation occurs between the distal row of tarsal bones and metatarsal bones. Treatment is best accomplished with selective fusion of the distal intertarsal joint (tarsometatarsal joint). Occasionally the luxation occurs laterally between the fourth tarsal bone and adjacent metatarsal bones, with the medial separation occurring between the second and third tarsal bones and the central tarsal bone. In these patients, selective fusion of the joint space between the fourth tarsal and adjacent metatarsal bones is accomplished with a bone plate secured to the fourth tarsal bone and fifth metatarsal bone. Medially a small bone plate is secured to the central tarsal bone proximally and the second tarsal and second metatarsal bones distally.

Preoperative Management

Open wounds should be cleaned and a sterile dressing applied before surgery (see Shearing Injuries, p. 1306). Patients with open wounds should be started on therapeutic antibiotics (see p. 945). A bandage with a splint should be applied to support the limb, and the animal should be confined to a small space to prevent further joint damage until definitive surgery can be performed. Preemptive pain management with NSAIDs (see Table 33-4 on p. 1149), opiates, or epidural analgesia is indicated for dogs undergoing tarsal reconstruction.

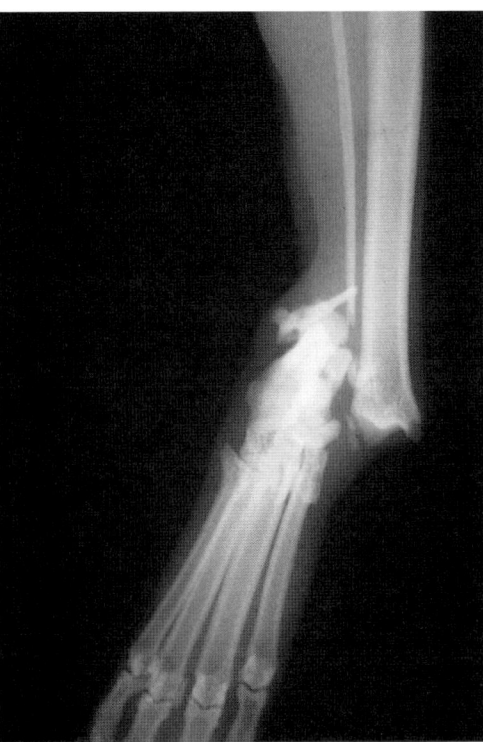

FIG. 33-143
Craniocaudal radiograph of a luxated tarsal joint. Note the fracture of the lateral malleolus and the medial displacement of the tibia.

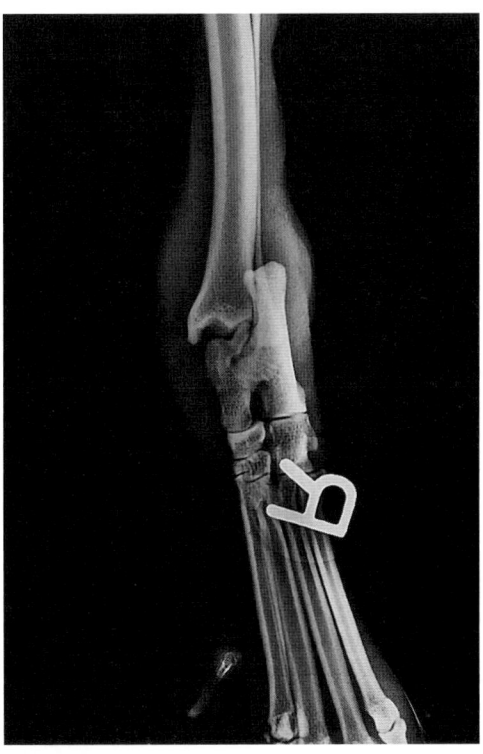

FIG. 33-144
Varus stress radiograph of the tarsus. Widening of the medial joint space indicates damage to the medial collateral ligament and joint capsule.

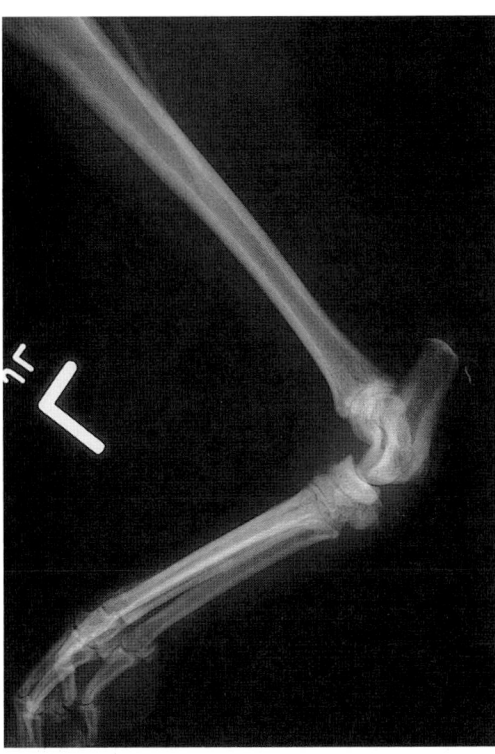

FIG. 33-145
Lateral radiograph of the tarsus of a dog with proximal intertarsal luxation.

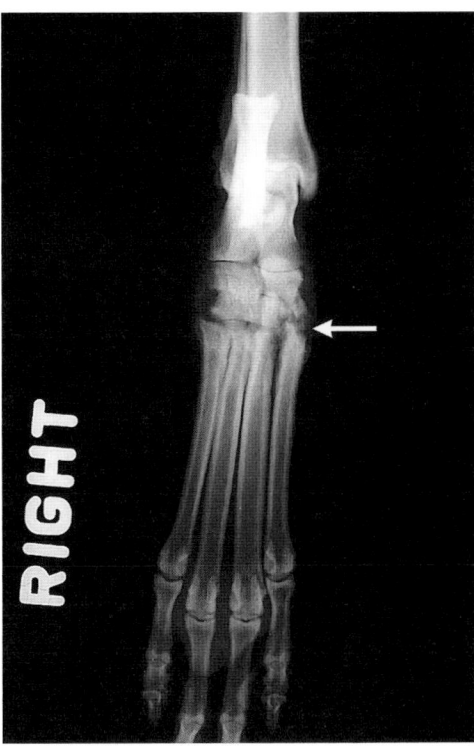

FIG. 33-146
Craniocaudal radiograph of a dog with a tarsometatarsal subluxation. Note the fragmentation of the second tarsal bone *(arrow)*.

Anesthesia

See p. 944 for a discussion of the anesthetic management of patients with orthopedic disease. Opioid epidural administration reduces postoperative discomfort (see p. 945). Traumatized animals should be evaluated for other injuries that may affect the anesthetic protocol.

Surgical Anatomy

The tarsus consists of the tibia, fibula, and proximal tarsal, distal tarsal, and metatarsal bones. These bones form the tarsocrural, intertarsal, and tarsometatarsal joints. The tarsocrural joint is formed by the fibula and cochlea of the tibia proximally and the talus and calcaneus distally. The intertarsal joints are formed by articulations between the tarsal bones, and the tarsometatarsal joints are formed by the articulations between the distal tarsal and metatarsal bones. The tarsal joints are supported by a complex arrangement of ligaments. The major ligaments providing medial support of the tarsocrural joint are the long medial collateral ligament, short medial collateral ligament, and calcaneocentral ligament (Fig. 33-147, *A*). Lateral support is provided by the long lateral collateral ligament and short calcaneofibular ligament (Fig. 33-147, *B*). Knowledge of the anatomic points of origin and insertion of each ligament is

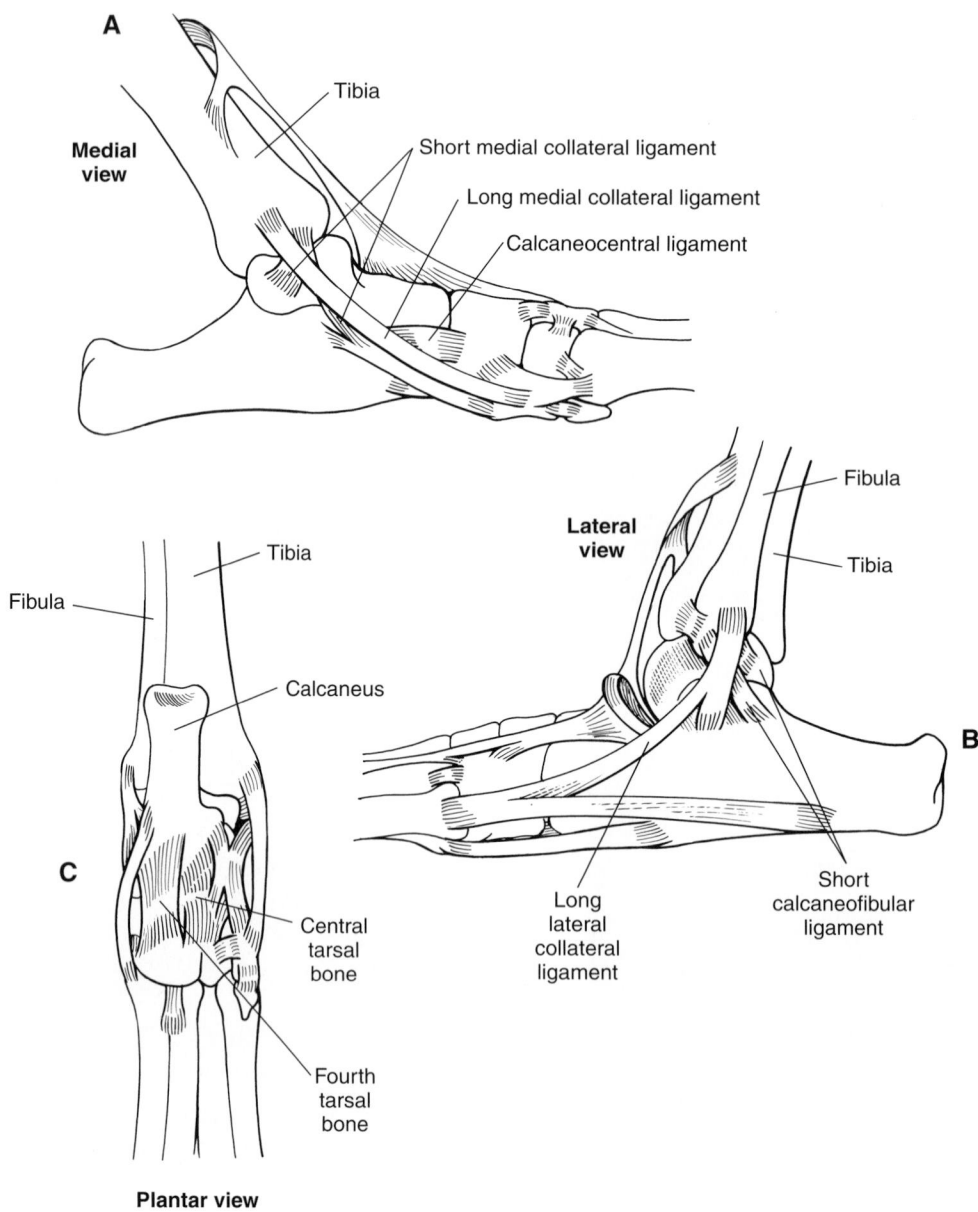

FIG. 33-147
Medial **(A)**, lateral **(B)**, and plantar **(C)** views of ligament structures that provide stability to the tarsal joint.

important for reconstruction of medial and lateral ligament injuries. Most of the stability of the intertarsal and tarsometatarsal joints is provided by a complex network of plantar ligaments, tarsal fibrocartilage, and joint capsule. Plantar ligaments originate from the calcaneus and attach to the central and fourth tarsal bones before inserting on the metatarsal bones (Fig. 33-147, *C*).

Positioning

The limb is clipped from the coxofemoral joint to the digits so that the paw can be included in the sterile field. This allows direct manipulation and visual orientation of the paw during reconstruction. Dorsal recumbency allows exposure of all surfaces of the tarsus. A hanging-leg preparation facilitates manipulation of the limb during surgery (see p. 36). The proximal tibia is available for cancellous bone harvest. As an alternative, prepare the proximal humerus for cancellous bone harvest when arthrodesis is performed. For arthroscopy, the patient is placed in dorsal recumbency for a cranial approach to the tibiotarsal joint and in sternal recumbency for a caudal approach.

SURGICAL TECHNIQUE

AP **Arthroscopy**

The selection between cranial versus caudal portals and medial versus lateral portals depends upon the region of interest. The arthroscope is usually positioned on the same cranial-caudal side as the lesion but on the opposite medial-lateral side as the lesion. If necessary, the arthroscope portals and instrument or egress portals may be switched during the procedure. A 1.9-mm arthroscope is most commonly used.

Insert a 20-gauge needle into the tibiotarsal joint, and infuse the joint with saline or lactated Ringer's solution. Using a No. 15 blade, make a partial thickness incision at the chosen arthroscope site on the same craniocaudal sur-

face, but opposite the mediolateral surface to the lesion. Incise the skin, but do not penetrate the joint capsule. Insert the cannula for a 1.9-mm arthroscope with a blunt obturator into the joint. Be careful not to dislodge the cannula from the joint, as there is limited space between the capsule and the joint surface. Insert a 20-gauge needle mediolaterally opposite the arthroscope for egress (Fig. 33-148). Explore the joint (Fig. 33-149). If bone or cartilage fragments are identified make a full thickness incision adjacent to the needle to create an instrument portal. Enlarge the portal by inserting a straight mosquito hemostat and opening the hemostat to dilate the portal. Insert a grasper and remove any fragments. Close the joint routinely with simple interrupted skin sutures.

Tarsocrural Luxation or Subluxation

Depending on which side is injured, make a curved incision centered over the medial or lateral malleolus. Begin the incision 4 cm above the joint line, and continue distally to a point 4 cm below the tarsometatarsal joint line. Incise the subcutaneous tissue and deep fascia along the same line. Once the deep fascia has been incised, remnants of the collateral ligament complex and joint capsule are exposed, and the articular surface is visible. Reduce and align the joint surfaces. Suture the joint capsule and injured ligaments with small, nonabsorbable suture. Protect the repair with nonabsorbable, heavy (No. 2 to No. 5, depending on the animal's size) figure-eight sutures strategically placed to mimic the short and long components of the collateral ligament complex. Drill bone tunnels in the malleolus where the ligament complex originates. Next, drill tunnels where the short and

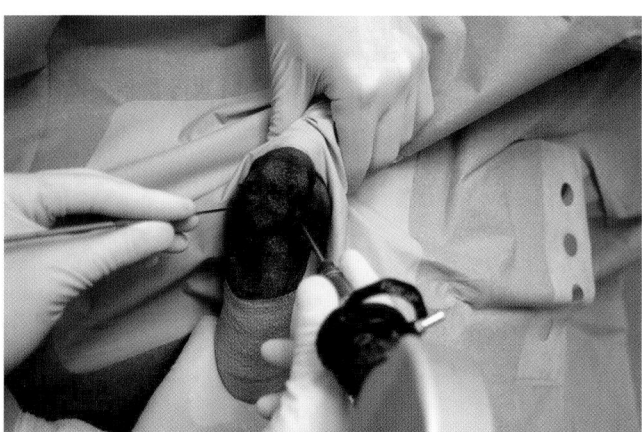

FIG. 33-148
Instrumentation for arthroscopy of the hock.

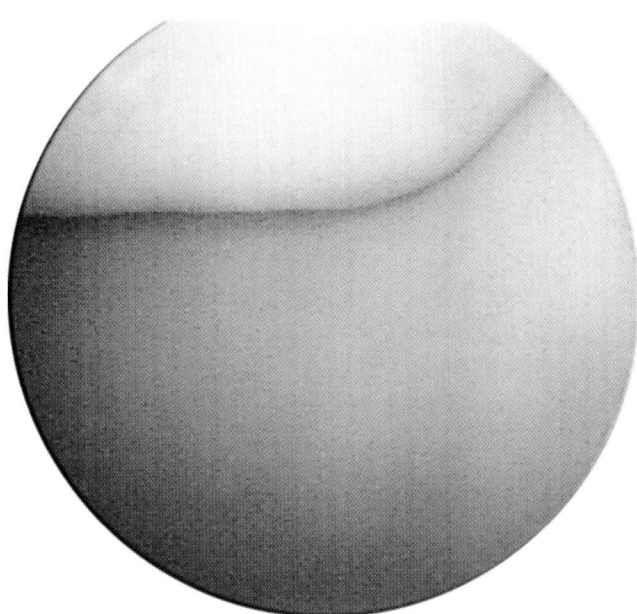

FIG. 33-149
Arthroscopic view of a normal hock joint.

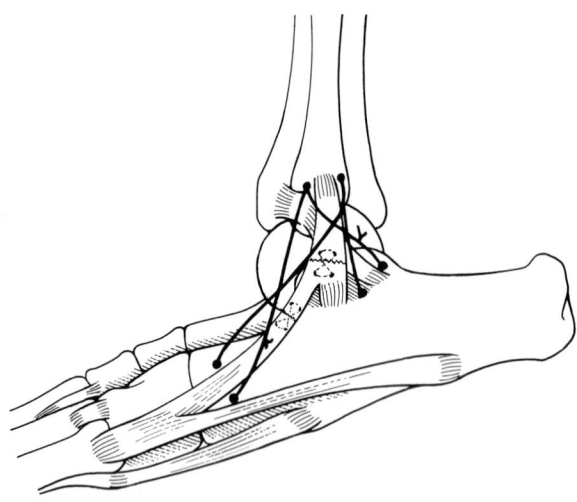

FIG. 33-150
Primary repair of collateral ligaments is supported with heavy suture to simulate the long and short components of the collateral ligament complex.

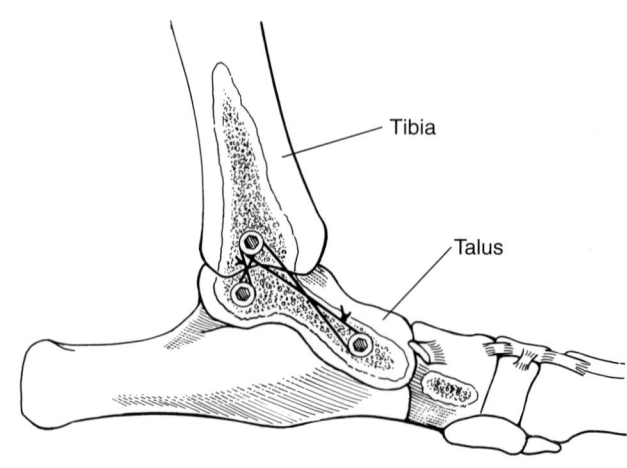

FIG. 33-151
Reconstruction of the medial collateral restraint complex with screws and suture material. Note the proper placement of the proximal and distal talar screws to mimic the insertion points of the short and long components of the restraint complex, respectively.

long components of the collateral ligament complex insert. Place two strands of nonabsorbable polyester suture through the predrilled holes in the malleolus. Pass one end of the suture strand through the tunnel drilled to mimic the insertion of the short component, and pass the end of the other strand through the tunnel drilled to mimic the insertion of the long component of the collateral ligament complex. As an alternative, use bone anchors. Place the sutures in a figure-eight pattern and tie them such that the suture placed as the short component is tied with the joint in 90 degrees of flexion (Fig. 33-150). Tie the suture placed to simulate the long component with the joint in a normal standing angle.

Shearing Injuries

When the animal is first seen, cover the wound with a sterile dressing and temporarily immobilize the limb with an external splint. Once the animal is stable enough to be anesthetized, débride the wound. Liberally flush the wound with 0.05% chlorhexidine. Fill the wound with sterile K-Y Jelly and clip the surrounding area. Transfer the patient to the operating room; débride obvious necrotic tissue and remove foreign material. If the medial surface is abraded, perform ligament reconstruction by inserting bone screws or bone anchors in the malleolus and talus to mimic the origin and insertion of the medial collateral ligament complex (Fig. 33-151). If the lateral surface is abraded, place bone anchors in the malleolus and calcaneus to mimic the origin and insertion of the lateral collateral ligament complex (Fig. 33-152). Place figure-eight, heavy, nonabsorbable suture or wire between the screws. Tie the suture used to mimic the short component of the ligament complex with the joint at 90 degrees and tie the suture used to mimic the long component of the ligament complex with the tarsus in a normal standing

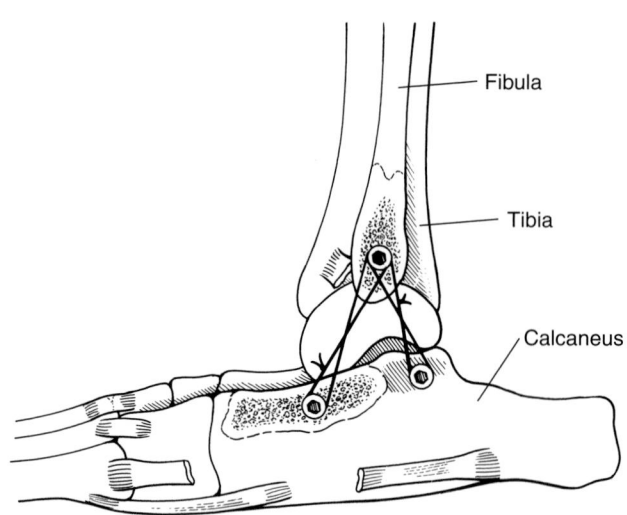

FIG. 33-152
Reconstruction of the lateral collateral restraint complex with screws and suture material. Note the proper placement of the proximal and distal talar screws to mimic the insertion points of the short and long components of the restraint complex, respectively.

angle. If malleolar fracture is present rather than ligament injury, reduce and stabilize the fracture with a tension band technique. Immobilize the reconstruction for 2 to 4 weeks with a transarticular external skeletal fixator. Place one full pin 6 to 7 cm proximal to the malleolus and one full pin through the metatarsal bones just below the tarsometatarsal joint line. Contour medial and lateral external bars to an angle simulating the standing angle of the tarsal joint. Place a half pin 2 to 3 cm above the malleolus and a second half pin through the central and fourth tarsal bones. Tighten the pin clamps. Alternatively, use a bivalve short (mid-tibia) cast (see p. 967).

> NOTE: After placement of the medial and lateral bars, resistance to craniocaudal bending can be improved by adding an additional external bar.

Proximal Intertarsal Subluxation With Plantar Instability

Expose the joint through a caudolateral incision. Remove articular cartilage from the articular surface of the calcaneus and fourth tarsal bones with a curette or pneumatic burr. Use a slightly undersized drill bit (in relationship to the Steinmann pin) to predrill a hole from the proximal calcaneus down the calcaneal shaft. Insert a Steinmann pin to the point where the tip of the pin can be seen exiting where the cartilage was removed. Harvest a cancellous bone graft, and pack it into the space between the calcaneus and fourth tarsal bone. Reduce the joint and drive the pin across it to seat in the body of the fourth tarsal bone. Drill a transverse hole across the distal quadrant of the fourth tarsal bone, and drill a second transverse hole in the proximal quadrant of the calcaneus. Place orthopedic wire through the drill holes in a figure-eight pattern to complete a tension-band wire (Fig. 33-153). Use 20-gauge orthopedic wire for small and medium-sized dogs and cats and 18-gauge for large dogs.

Proximal Intertarsal Luxation

Make a lateral incision beginning at the proximal end of the calcaneus and extending distally 3 to 4 cm below the tarso-metatarsal joint line. Remove articular cartilage from the joint surfaces and insert a cancellous bone graft. Apply a compression plate to the lateral surface of the calcaneus, fourth tarsal bone, and fifth metatarsal bone (Fig. 33-154).

Tarsometatarsal Luxation

Expose the articular surfaces of the joint through a cranial incision. Reflect the extensor tendons laterally to gain adequate exposure. Remove articular cartilage and insert a cancellous bone graft. Reduce the joint and stabilize with cross pins. Place one pin so that it enters the base of the fifth metatarsal bone, crosses the joint, and is seated in the central tarsal bone. Place the second pin so that it enters the base of the second metatarsal bone, crosses the joint, and is seated in the fourth tarsal bone. If the luxation occurs laterally, between the fourth tarsal bone and adjacent metatarsal bones, with the medial separation occurring between the second and third tarsal bones and central tarsal bone, expose the tarsometatarsal joint with two incisions. Make a lateral incision extending 5 cm proximal and distal to the tarsometatarsal joint line. Make a similar incision medially. Remove articular cartilage from all exposed joint surfaces, and insert a cancellous bone graft. Stabilize the fusion with

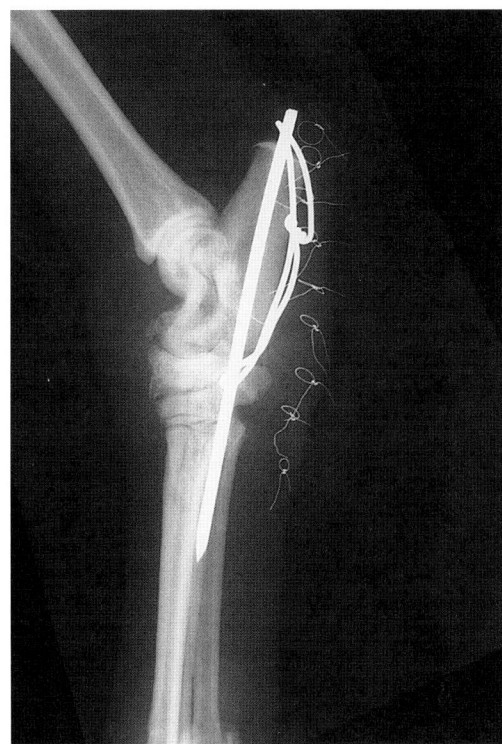

FIG. 33-153
Lateral radiograph showing stabilization of proximal plantar instability with a pin and tension band.

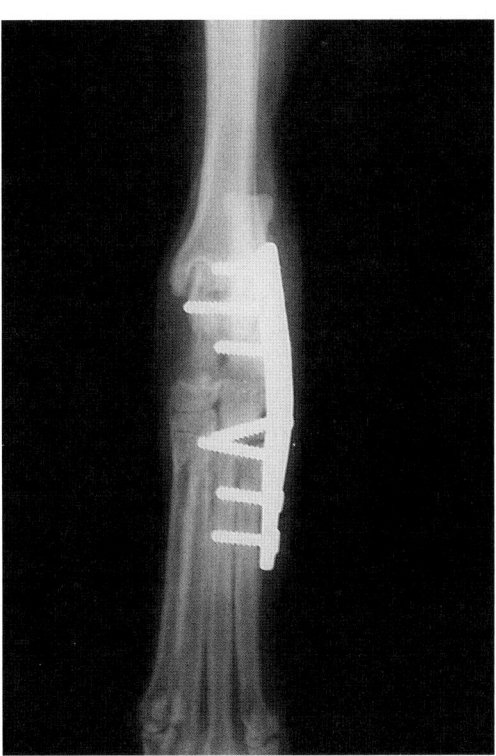

FIG. 33-154
Craniocaudal radiograph showing stabilization of proximal intertarsal instability with a bone plate placed on the lateral surface of the calcaneus and fifth metatarsal bones.

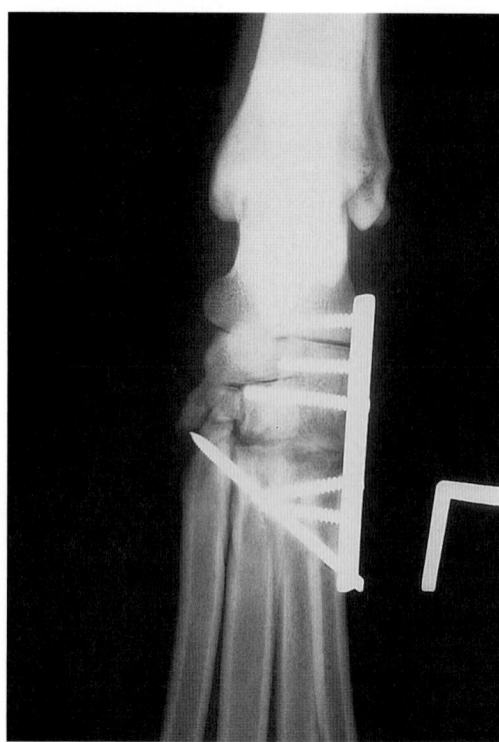

FIG. 33-155
Craniocaudal radiograph showing stabilization of tarsometatarsal instability with a bone plate placed on the lateral surface of the calcaneus and fifth metatarsal bones.

small bone plates. Laterally, secure a plate to the fourth tarsal and fifth metatarsal bones (Fig. 33-155). Medially, secure a small bone plate to the central tarsal bone proximally and to the second tarsal and second metatarsal bones distally.

Tarsocrural Joint Arthrodesis

Tarsocrural joint arthrodesis is indicated for severe injury of the tibial cochlea and condyles of the talus that precludes maintaining a long-term, pain-free articulation. Arthrodesis is also indicated when painful DJD is not responsive to conservative measures. In conjunction with tarsocrural joint fusions, the proximal intertarsal and tarsometatarsal joints are also fused.

Determine the normal standing angle of the opposite limb before surgery, and use it to approximate the fusion angle during arthrodesis of the injured limb. Make an incision over the cranial surface of the joint. Begin the incision over the distal one third of the tibia, and extend it distally midway down the metatarsal bones. Enter the tarsocrural joint to expose the articular surfaces. With a power saw, remove the articular surface of the distal tibia by cutting perpendicular to the long axis of the bone. Cut the trochlea of the talus to achieve the appropriate fusion angle when the cut surfaces rest flush with each other. Alternatively, remove the cartilage of the tarsocrural joint with a pneumatic burr following the joint contours. Use the normal standing angle of the opposite limb to approximate

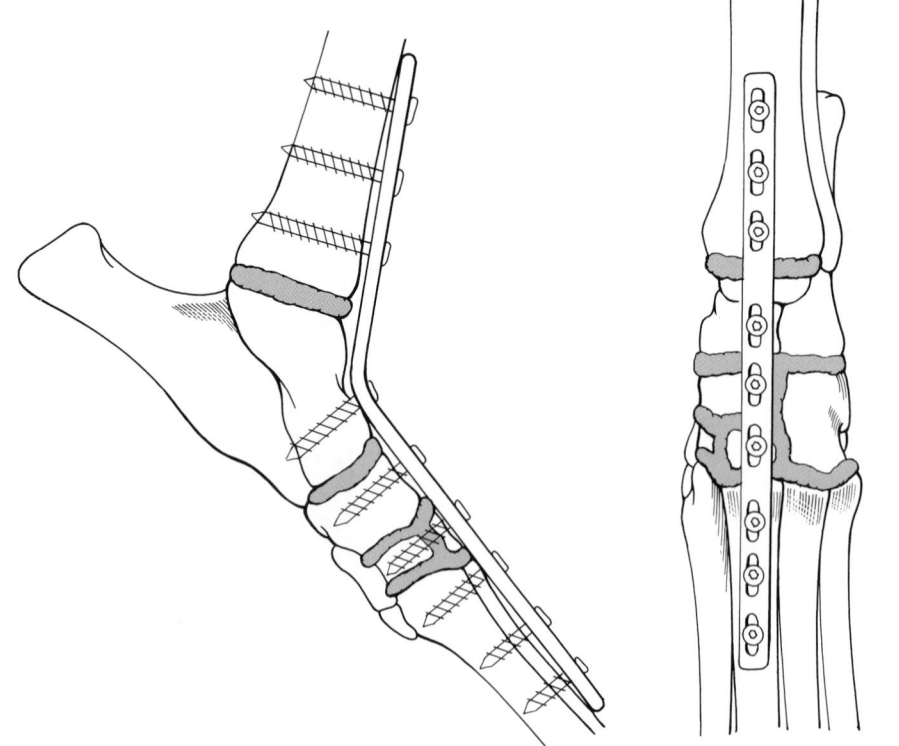

FIG. 33-156
Dorsal placement of a plate for tarsocrural arthrodesis. Because the plate is on the compression surface of the bone, it is subject to failure. If possible, a lengthening plate should be used.

the fusion angle. Maintain reduction of the cut surfaces with small Kirschner pins, and pack a cancellous bone graft around the joint. Open the joint capsule of the proximal intertarsal and tarsometatarsal joints to expose the articular surfaces. Remove the cartilage with a pneumatic burr, and insert a cancellous bone graft. Stabilize the joints with a bone plate applied to the cranial surface. Bend the plate to conform to the established fusion angle, and secure it proximally by placing three screws in the distal tibia, two to four screws in the tarsal bones, and three screws in the third metatarsal bone. As an alternative, if a lengthening plate is used to bridge the tarsus, attach the plate to the distal tibia and metatarsus with three or four screws in each bone (Fig. 33-156).

SUTURE MATERIALS AND SPECIAL INSTRUMENTS

Nonabsorbable suture or wire generally is used throughout the procedures described previously. A power drill, bone plate and screws, and a bone curette and air drill to remove articular cartilage are necessary for arthrodesis and cancellous bone harvest.

POSTOPERATIVE CARE AND ASSESSMENT

After repair of tarsocrural luxation or subluxation, the tarsus should be placed in a normal standing angle and immobilized with rigid external coaptation or a transarticular external skeletal fixator for 3 weeks. During this time, activity should be limited to leash walking, and the coaptation bandage should be checked frequently. Uncontrolled exercise should be restricted to specific physical rehabilitation exercises and leash walking for 6 weeks; then once the splint and bandage are removed and the surgeon deems it safe, the animal should be gradually returned to unsupervised activity over a 6-week period. A sample physical rehabilitation exercise protocol can be found by referring to Table 33-10 on p. 1230.

If a shearing injury is present, treat the wound as an open wound with daily changes of a sterile adherent dressing and liberal flushing with 0.05% chlorhexidine. Once healthy granulation tissue has formed, apply a nonadherent sterile dressing. If an external fixator is used, follow postoperative care guidelines (see p. 974). The external fixator is removed 6 weeks after surgery. After arthrodesis, protect the repair with external coaptation for 6 weeks and restrict activity until radiographic evidence of bone union is seen.

COMPLICATIONS

Complications include infection and loose implants. Implant removal may be indicated. Continued lameness should be expected in animals with subluxation or with luxation that is not adequately stabilized.

PROGNOSIS

Adequate limb function can be expected in most patients with tarsal injuries after appropriate surgical intervention. Dogs with shearing injuries treated with prosthetic ligament or external fixation (or both) have limited range of motion and progressive DJD; however, 75% have good to excellent use of

the limb. After partial tarsal arthrodesis, most dogs resume normal activity. Implant removal may be indicated if lameness persists after bone healing. Long-term outcome after tarsocrural arthrodesis provides good to excellent results in the majority of patients (Benson et al, 2002; McKee et al, 2004).

References

Benson JA, Boudrieau RJ: Severe carpal and tarsal shearing injuries treated with an immediate arthrodesis in seven dogs, *J Am Anim Hosp Assoc* 38:370, 2002.

McKee WM, May C, Macias C et al: Pantarsal arthrodesis with a customized medial or lateral bone plate in 13 dogs, *Vet Rec* 154:165, 2004.

OSTEOCHONDRITIS DISSECANS OF THE TARSUS

DEFINITION

Osteochondritis dissecans (OCD) is a disturbance in endochondral ossification that leads to cartilage retention; it occurs in the hocks of immature large-breed dogs. It is also called *osteochondrosis*.

GENERAL CONSIDERATIONS AND CLINICALLY RELEVANT PATHOPHYSIOLOGY

OCD begins with a failure of endochondral ossification in either the physis or articular epiphyseal complex, which is responsible for the formation of epiphyseal bone. This condition also commonly occurs in the shoulder, elbow, and stifle. The pathogenesis of OCD is discussed on p. 1176. With OCD of the talus, a large piece of cartilage and subchondral bone usually is observed involving the medial (most frequently affected) or lateral trochlear ridge. Histologically the flap consists of cartilage; also, subchondral bone trabeculae in the defect are thickened, and bone marrow fibrosis is noted.

DIAGNOSIS
Clinical Presentation

Signalment. Affected dogs usually are large; rottweilers are most frequently affected. The average age of onset of lameness is 5 to 7 months, and the condition affects both males and females.

> NOTE: There is evidence of a hereditary component in the etiology based on the predilection of rottweilers to develop this condition.

History. Rear limb lameness that worsens after exercise may be acute or chronic. Owners frequently report that the dog is stiff in the morning or after rest.

Physical Examination Findings

Lameness of one rear limb usually is evident. The dog may hyperextend the hocks and have a stiff or stilted gait because of bilateral lameness. Pain may be elicited on hock flexion. Palpation of the hocks should include an evaluation of range

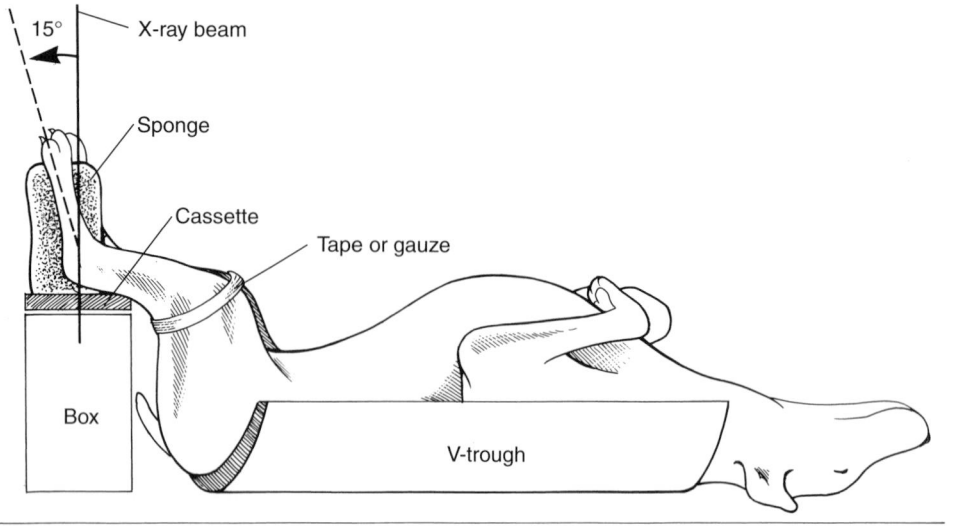

FIG. 33-157
Positioning for a craniocaudal view of the flexed tarsus. This view allows visualization of the lateral trochlear ridge of the talus without superimposition of the calcaneus.

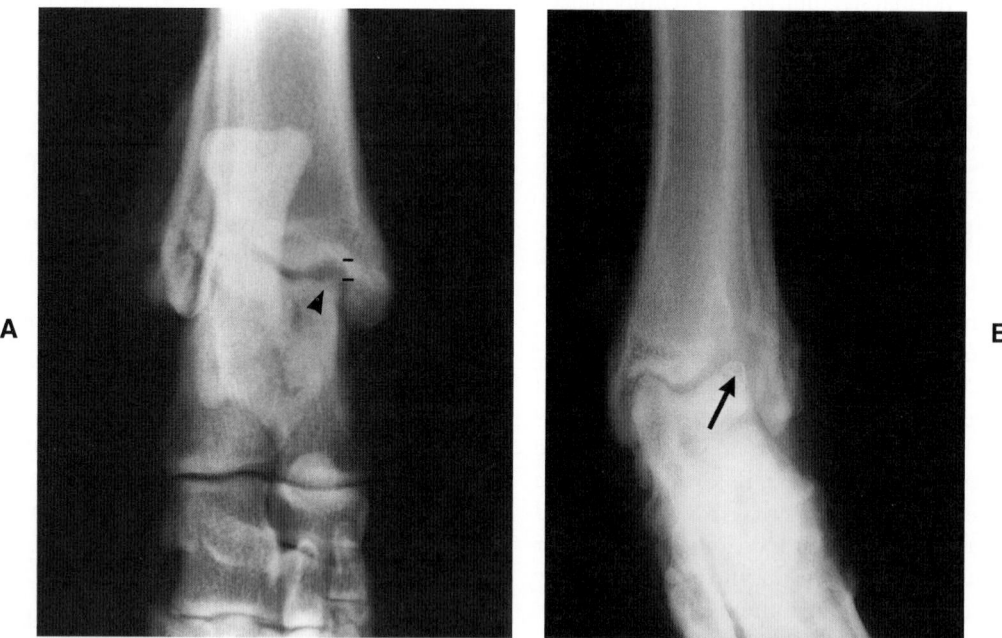

FIG. 33-158
Radiographs of tarsi with OCD. **A,** Standard craniocaudal view with a lesion on the medial trochlear ridge of the talus. There is a flattening of the medial trochlear ridge, and the joint space is widened *(arrowhead)*. **B,** Flexed craniocaudal view with a lesion on the lateral trochlear ridge of the talus. A subchondral fissure is visible at the base of the lateral trochlear ridge *(arrow)*. (From Olmstead ML: *Small animal orthopedics*, St Louis, 1995, Mosby.)

of motion. A decrease in the animal's ability to flex the hock indicates secondary DJD. Crepitation during hock flexion and extension, joint effusion, and periarticular swelling may be noted.

Diagnostic Imaging

Radiographic views of the tarsus should include a standard lateral view of the hock, a flexed lateral view to expose the proximal portion of the talus, a craniocaudal view of the hock (made while the hock is extended to visualize the proximal portion of the trochlear ridges), and a craniocaudal view (made with the hock flexed to visualize the cranial portion of the trochlear ridges and the lateral condylar ridge without superimposition of the calcaneus) (Fig. 33-157). Radiographs of both tarsi should be obtained because bilateral disease is common. Definitive radiographic diagnosis of OCD is made when a radiolucent concavity is observed on the medial or lateral trochlear ridge (Fig. 33-158). Radiographic signs of secondary osteoarthritis usually are seen (see p. 1156). CT can be used to better evaluate the trochlear ridges if OCD is suspected, but cannot be confirmed on survey radiography. CT is valuable because it allows evaluation of the trochlear ridges without superimposition of overlying structures.

> NOTE: Radiograph both tarsi because of the frequency of bilateral disease; however, unless the animal shows clinical signs, surgery of the opposite limb may not be necessary.

Arthroscopy. Arthroscopy provides definitive diagnosis of hock OCD. Arthroscopic approach varies with the location of the lesion (see p. 1305).

Laboratory Findings

Results of hematologic and serum biochemical analyses are normal in most affected animals. Results of arthrocentesis may include decreased synovial fluid viscosity, increased fluid volume, and an increased number of mononuclear phagocytic cells (up to 6000 to 9000 WBC/μl).

DIFFERENTIAL DIAGNOSIS

OCD must be differentiated from other diseases of young growing dogs that affect the rear limbs and may cause similar clinical signs of lameness (i.e., hip dysplasia and panosteitis). Decreased range of motion and swelling in the hock usually identify hock disease as a possible cause of lameness.

MEDICAL MANAGEMENT

Medical therapy is generally used to treat older dogs with established osteoarthritis. Therapy should include each of the 5 principles of management of osteoarthritis. Lame animals are treated with exercise restriction and administration of NSAIDs (see Table 33-4 on p. 1149). After the lameness has subsided, a gradual increase in exercise is indicated to strengthen surrounding musculature. Body weight control is critical to minimization of the clinical signs of osteoarthritis.

SURGICAL TREATMENT

Surgical removal of the cartilage flap allows the defect to heal by outgrowth of fibrocartilage from underlying subchondral bone. Surgery may be useful in young animals when the disease is diagnosed before the onset of osteoarthritis and in lame animals in which the condition is unresponsive to medical therapy. However, surgical management does not usually alter the progression of osteoarthritis.

Preoperative Management

Most affected animals are young and otherwise healthy, therefore only a minimal preoperative workup is necessary (i.e., CBC and serum chemistries). Preemptive pain management with NSAIDs (see Table 33-4 on p. 1149), opiates, or epidural analgesia is indicated for dogs undergoing tarsus reconstruction.

Anesthesia

See p. 944 for a discussion of the anesthetic management of patients with orthopedic disease. Opioid epidural administration reduces postoperative discomfort (see p. 945).

Surgical Anatomy

Surgical anatomy of the hock is discussed on p. 1304. Approaches to the lateral and medial trochlear ridge that do not involve osteotomy of the epicondyle or collateral ligament transection appear to result in less postoperative morbidity and a quicker return to function than do osteotomy approaches.

Positioning

The dog is positioned in dorsal recumbency with the affected limb suspended for draping. The limb is then released to allow access to the medial or lateral surface of the hock.

SURGICAL TECHNIQUE
Arthroscopy

Arthroscopy of the hock is more demanding than arthroscopy of other joints because of the small size and complex anatomy. For a description of arthroscopy of the hock, please see p. 1305.

Arthrotomy

The surgical approach selected depends on the location of the lesion.

Visualize lesions of the medial trochlear ridge using a dorsomedial and/or plantaromedial surgical approach. Lesions of the lateral trochlear ridge are visualized using a dorsolateral and/or plantarolateral surgical approach. Regardless of the technique used for exposure, examine the appropriate trochlear ridge and remove the flap of cartilage. Perform

Dorsomedial approach

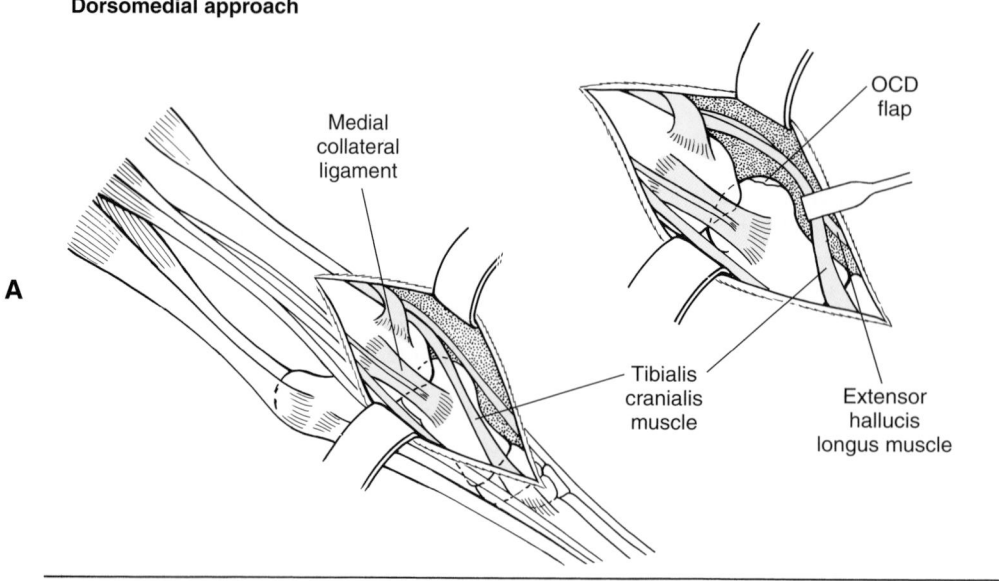

Plantaromedial approach

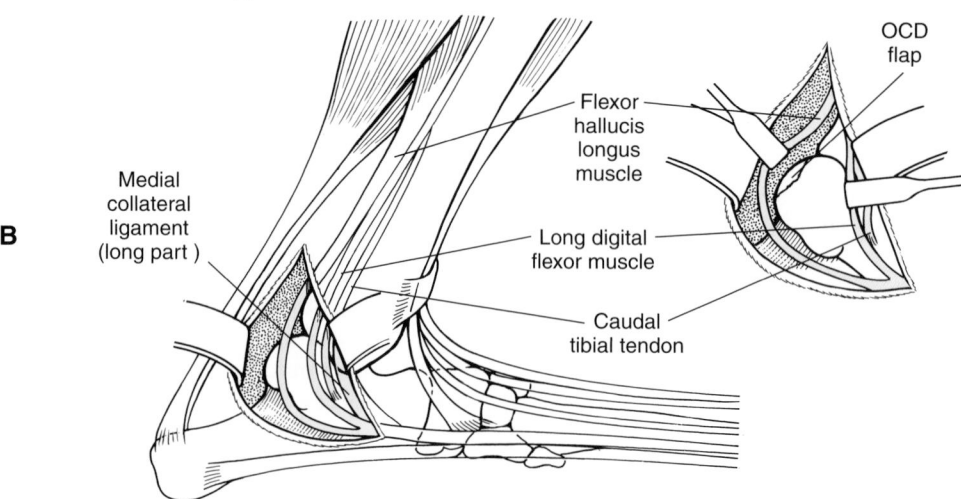

FIG. 33-159

A, For a dorsomedial approach to the hock, make a skin incision starting proximal to the trochlear ridge and extending distally over it. Incise the subcutaneous tissue along the same line. Identify the tendon of the tibialis cranialis muscle, the saphenous nerve, the cranial tibial artery and vein, and the dorsal branches of the saphenous artery and vein and retract them laterally. Incise the deep fascia and joint capsule along the midline of the palpable portion of the medial trochlear ridge. Extend the incision proximally into the periosteum of the distal tibia. **B,** For a plantaromedial approach to the hock, incise the skin and subcutaneous tissue caudal to the medial malleolus over the trochlear ridge. Identify the tendon of the long digital flexor muscle and the distal attachment of the caudal tibial tendon and retract them cranially. Identify the tendon of the flexor hallucis longus muscle, the tibial nerve, the plantar branches of the medial saphenous vein and saphenous artery, and the superficial plantar metatarsal vein and retract them laterally. Incise the deep fascia and joint capsule longitudinally along the midline of the palpable portion of the medial trochlear ridge.

curettage only to remove fragments of cartilage from the edges of the lesion. Repeatedly flush the joint to remove any small fragments before closure.

Dorsomedial Approach to the Tarsus

Extend the hock and palpate the dorsal portion of the medial trochlear ridge. Make a skin incision starting proximal to the trochlear ridge and extending distally over the trochlear ridge. Incise the subcutaneous tissue along the same line. Identify the tendon of the tibialis cranialis muscle, the saphenous nerve, the cranial tibial artery and vein, and the dorsal branches of the saphenous artery and vein and retract them laterally. Incise the deep fascia and joint capsule along the midline of the palpable portion of the medial trochlear ridge. Extend the incision proximally into the periosteum of the distal tibia (Fig. 33-159, A). Visualize the cranial and distal part of the medial trochlear ridge. Extend the hock to increase the amount of visible trochlear ridge. Identify and remove the cartilage flap. Curette the edges of the lesion and flush the joint. Close the wound by suturing the fascia and joint capsule with absorbable suture in a simple interrupted pattern. Suture the subcutaneous tissue and skin in separate layers.

Plantaromedial Approach to the Tarsus

Flex the hock and palpate the proximal or plantar aspect of the medial trochlear ridge. Incise the skin and subcutaneous tissue caudal to the medial malleolus over the trochlear ridge. Identify the tendon of the long digital flexor muscle and the distal attachment of the caudal tibial tendon and retract them cranially. Identify the tendon of the flexor hallucis longus muscle, the tibial nerve, the plantar branches of the medial saphenous vein and saphenous artery, and the superficial plantar metatarsal vein and retract them laterally. Incise the deep fascia and joint capsule longitudinally along the midline of the palpable portion of the medial trochlear ridge (Fig. 33-159, B). Identify and remove the cartilage flap. Flex the hock to increase the amount of medial trochlear ridge visible. Curette the edges of the lesion and flush the joint. Close the wound by suturing the fascia and joint capsule with absorbable suture in a simple interrupted pattern. Suture the subcutaneous tissue and skin in separate layers.

Dorsolateral Approach to the Tarsus

Extend the hock and palpate the cranial portion of the lateral trochlear ridge. Make a skin incision starting proximal to the trochlear ridge and extending distally over the trochlear ridge. Incise the subcutaneous tissue along the same line. Identify the tendons of the long digital extensor muscle, the cranial tibial muscle, the extensor hallucis longus muscle, and the dorsal branch of the lateral saphenous vein and the superficial peroneal nerve, and retract them medially. Identify the tendons of the peroneus longus, lateral digital extensor, and peroneus brevis muscles, and retract them in a plantar direction. Incise the deep fascia and joint capsule longitudinally along the midline of the palpable portion of

the lateral trochlear ridge (Fig. 33-160, A). Visualize the cranial and distal part of the lateral trochlear ridge. Extend the hock to increase the amount of trochlear ridge visible. Identify and remove the cartilage flap. Curette the edges of the lesion and flush the joint. Close the wound by suturing the fascia and joint capsule with absorbable suture in a simple interrupted pattern. Suture the subcutaneous tissue and skin in separate layers.*

Plantarolateral Approach to the Tarsus

Flex the hock and palpate the proximal aspect of the lateral trochlear ridge. Incise the skin and subcutaneous tissue plantar to the lateral malleolus over the trochlear ridge. Retract the tendons of the peroneus brevis muscle, the lateral digital extensor muscle, and the peroneus longus muscle dorsally. It is difficult to retract the tendons of the peroneus brevis, lateral digital extensor, and peroneus longus muscles very far because they are firmly embedded in deep fascia over the lateral malleolus. Retract the plantar branch of the lateral saphenous vein and a branch of the caudal cutaneous sural nerve in a plantar direction, and the tendon of the flexor hallucis longus in a medial direction. Incise the deep fascia and joint capsule longitudinally along the midline of the palpable portion of the lateral trochlear ridge (Fig. 33-160, B). Identify and remove the cartilage flap. Flex the hock to increase the amount of lateral trochlear ridge visible. Curette the edges of the lesion and flush the joint. Close the wound by suturing the fascia and joint capsule with absorbable suture in a simple interrupted pattern. Suture the subcutaneous tissue and skin in separate layers.

SUTURE MATERIALS AND SPECIAL INSTRUMENTS

Oschner forceps are helpful in grasping the cartilage fragment. A bone curette is needed to curette the edges of the lesion.

POSTOPERATIVE CARE AND ASSESSMENT

The limb should be bandaged after surgery for 3 to 5 days to provide soft tissue support. The animal should be confined to leash walks only for 4 to 6 weeks. The use of professional physical therapy can be very helpful in the management of hock OCD. Physical rehabilitation focuses on maintaining range of motion, strengthening the limb, and encouraging healing with healthy fibrocartilage. No or minimal weight-bearing activity is most effective (see Table 33-10 on p. 1230).

PROGNOSIS

Dogs treated conservatively for OCD of the hock usually have continued intermittent lameness and progressive osteoarthritis. Those treated surgically may have improved limb function, but lameness may be evident after exercise. Osteoarthritis usually is present even after surgery and requires medical treatment (see p. 1311); however, most dogs are functional pets and are lame only intermittently. In rare cases, infection of the surgical site may occur after surgery.

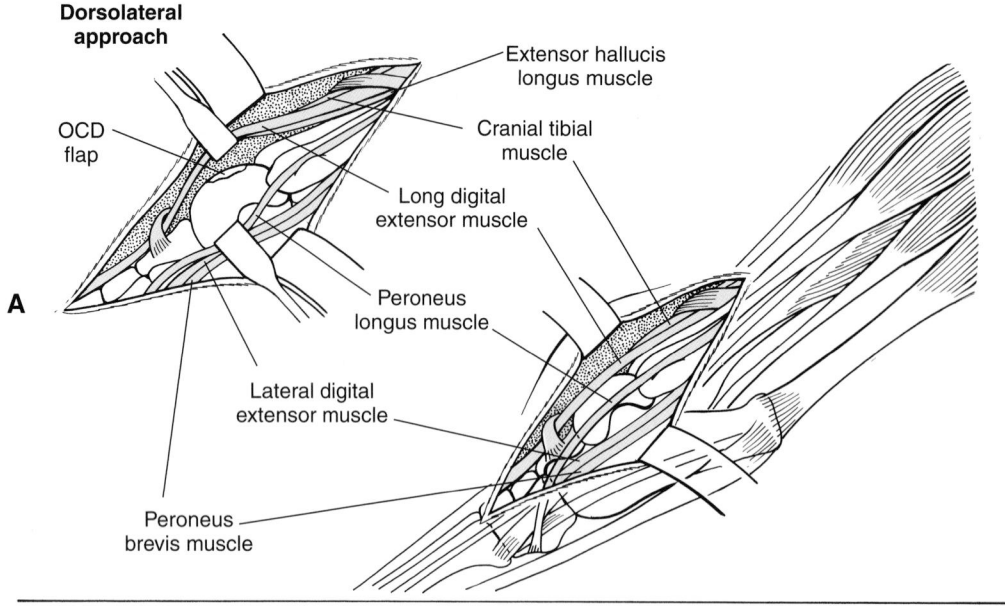

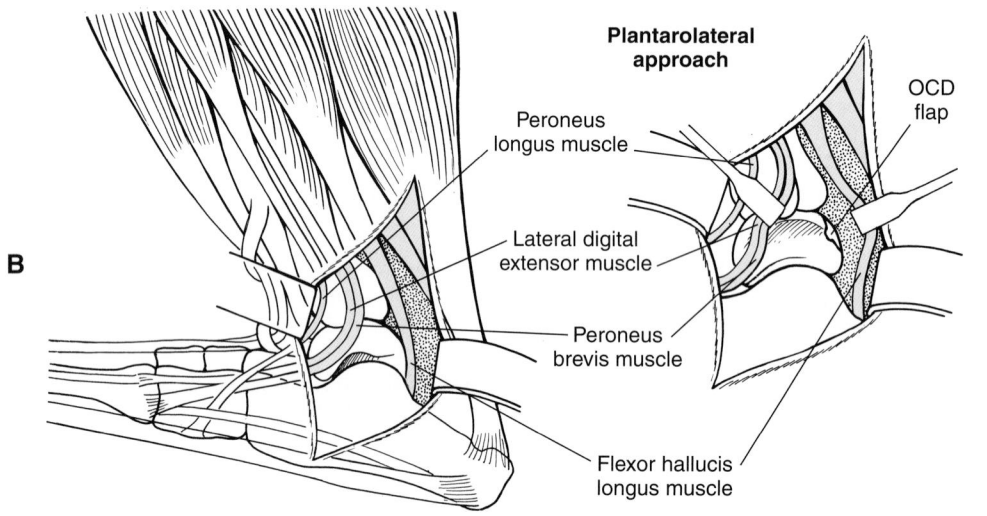

FIG. 33-160

A, For a dorsolateral approach to the tarsus, make a skin incision starting proximal to the trochlear ridge and extending distally over it. Incise the subcutaneous tissue along the same line. Identify the tendons of the long digital extensor, cranial tibial, and extensor hallucis longus muscles; the dorsal branch of the lateral saphenous vein; and the superficial peroneal nerve and retract them medially. Identify the tendons of the peroneus longus, lateral digital extensor, and peroneus brevis muscles and retract them in a plantar direction. Incise the deep fascia and joint capsule longitudinally along the midline of the palpable portion of the lateral trochlear ridge. **B,** For a plantarolateral approach to the tarsus, make a skin incision starting proximal to the trochlear ridge and extending distally over the trochlear ridge. Incise the subcutaneous tissue along the same line. Identify and retract the tendons of the peroneus brevis, lateral digital extensor, and peroneus longus muscles dorsally. Retract the tendon of the flexor hallucis longus in a medial direction. Incise the deep fascia and joint capsule longitudinally along the midline of the palpable portion of the trochlear ridge.

NOTE: Advise owners that surgical treatment does not appear to alter the progression of osteoarthritis, and affected dogs may require medical therapy after surgery.

Suggested Reading

Cook JL et al: Arthroscopic removal and curettage of osteochondrosis lesions on the lateral and medial trochlear ridges of the talus of two dogs, *J Am Anim Hosp Assoc* 37:75, 2001.

Osteochondrosis lesions in the tibiotarsal joint were treated arthroscopically in two dogs. Removal of all osteochondral fragments and curettage of the remaining talar defects were accomplished arthroscopically. Both dogs had excellent short-term outcomes.

Gielen I, van Bree H, Van Ryssen B et al: Radiographic, computed tomographic and arthroscopic findings in 23 dogs with osteochondrosis of the tarsocrural joint, *Vet Rec* 150:442, 2002.

This manuscript provides an excellent review of the diagnostics and treatment of OCD of the hock in dogs.

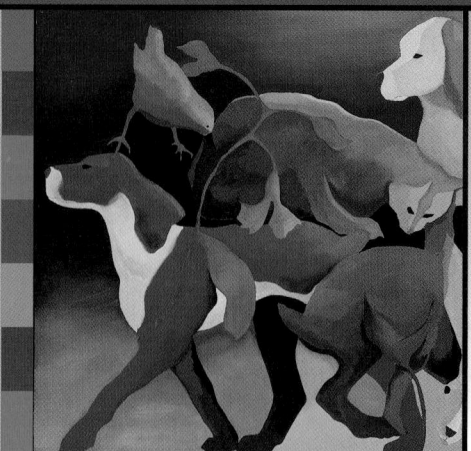

CHAPTER 34

Management of Muscle and Tendon Injury or Disease

MUSCLE CONTUSION AND STRAINS

DEFINITIONS

A **contusion** is a bruise of the muscle with varying degrees of hemorrhage and fiber disruption. A **strain** is a longitudinal stretching or tearing of muscle fibers or groups of fibers. Contusions and strains result in disruption of the normal architecture of the muscle-tendon unit secondary to interstitial edema, hemorrhage, or overstretching.

GENERAL CONSIDERATIONS AND CLINICALLY RELEVANT PATHOPHYSIOLOGY

Muscle contusions are caused by external trauma. An external blow disrupts fibril continuity and the vascular compartment, with subsequent hemorrhage into the interstitial space. Muscle strains are caused by overstretching or overuse. These injuries occur, but are not commonly recognized in animals.

Muscles may span one or more joints and cause a specific joint movement when they contract. For example, the biceps muscle originates from the supraglenoid tuberosity of the scapula and inserts onto the medial tuberosity of the radial head. Contraction causes extension of the shoulder joint and flexion of the elbow. An injured muscle may cause considerable pain during normal body motion. Muscle has intrinsic ability to heal by regeneration of myofibrils if the sarcolemmal cells survive and the endomysial connective tissue sheath is not destroyed. With mild contusions and strains, cells and endomysial sheath are not destroyed, and their preservation allows complete healing. However, if the contusion is severe and causes extensive cell death and hemorrhage precluding muscle regeneration, healing occurs with fibrous interposition between the muscle ends. Excessive scarring may impede muscle fiber regeneration and interfere with muscle contraction.

DIAGNOSIS

Clinical Presentation

Signalment. Any age, breed, or sex of dog or cat may be affected; however, muscle contusion and strain are most commonly diagnosed in athletic dogs (e.g., racing greyhounds and field trial dogs). They are rare in cats.

History. Contusion and strain injuries often occur during strenuous activity. The animal may be brought to a veterinarian because of a noticeable limp or complete inability to bear weight. The trauma is often unobserved by the client. With mild strains, owners may relate that the animal became reluctant to move 12 to 24 hours after strenuous exercise.

Physical Examination Findings

Clinical signs depend on the severity and chronicity of injury. With mild contusions, the animal may exhibit minimal lameness and the source of pain may be difficult to find on examination. With more severe contusions, pain and swelling are present. The majority of severe contusions occur in conjunction with fractures and although the focus is on the fractured bone, injury to the muscle also should be evaluated during surgery. Severe muscle strains are recognized by swelling and pain of the affected muscle unit (Fig. 34-1). Chronic muscle strains occasionally occur in dogs (e.g., bicipital tenosynovitis and iliopsoas muscle injury).

Diagnostic Imaging

Standard craniocaudal and medial-to-lateral radiographs are necessary to rule out bone injury. Ultrasound examination of acute injuries may show no abnormalities or may show disruption of muscle fibers and hematoma formation. Because muscle injuries may be unilateral, comparison with the normal contralateral muscle may help in identification of an abnormality. In chronic stages of a muscle tear, normal muscle fibers may be re-formed or there may be an echogenic scar within the muscle belly.

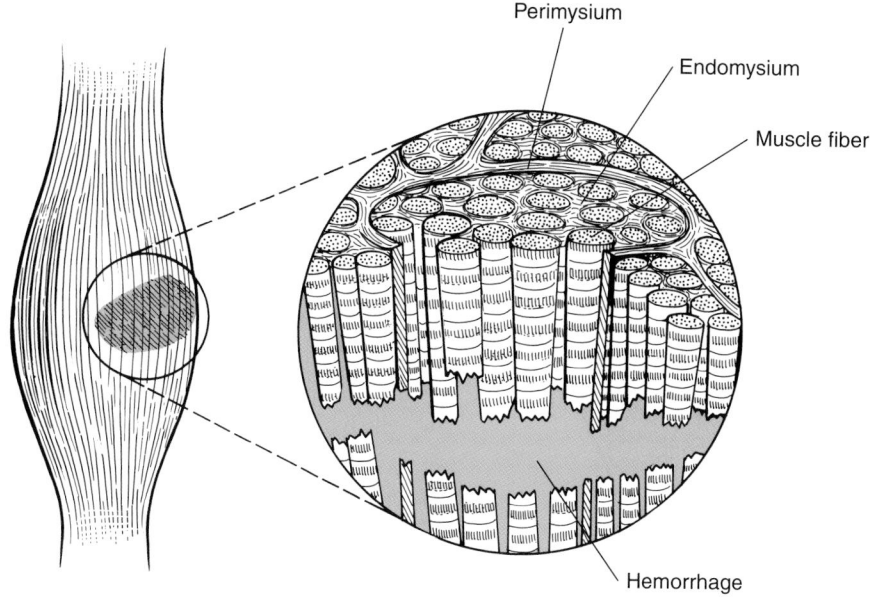

FIG. 34-1
Muscle fibril disruption and interstitial hemorrhage. Blood accumulates between the disrupted fibers.

Laboratory Findings

Consistent laboratory abnormalities are not found.

DIFFERENTIAL DIAGNOSIS

Muscle contusions and strains must be differentiated from joint sprains, fractures, polymyopathies, and polyarthropathies. Physical examination often differentiates muscle injury from joint sprains. Gentle palpation of muscle contusions causes pain and identifies swelling, whereas pain associated with sprains is elicited on manipulation of involved joints. Arthrocentesis (see p. 1145) helps differentiate joint sprain or arthropathy from muscle injury.

MEDICAL MANAGEMENT

The primary treatment for muscle contusions and strains is rest. Enforced rest with controlled activity is necessary for at least 3 weeks. If injury is recurrent or severe, longer periods of enforced rest may be necessary. If the muscle is not allowed to heal adequately, repeated injury is likely. Nonsteroidal antiinflammatory drugs (NSAIDs) (see Table 33-4 on p. 1149) can be administered for the initial 3 to 4 days, but restricted activity must continue even if lameness and pain disappear.

Physical Rehabilitation

With acute injuries (i.e., initial 24 hours), cold compresses can be applied to the affected muscle for 15 minutes, three or four times a day. If the injury is more than 24 hours old, topical heat application is recommended. Use care to prevent burning the patient.

> NOTE: Warn owners that the animal may feel like exercising before it should be allowed, particularly if it has received NSAIDs.

SURGICAL TREATMENT

When a severe contusion is recognized during surgical stabilization of a fracture, decompression of the muscle compartment can be achieved through incision of the epimysium (see p. 1318). Surgical treatment is necessary only if interstitial fluid accumulation causes sufficient pressure to compromise blood flow (i.e., *compartment syndrome*).

Preoperative Management

Surgical intervention should occur as soon as possible. The animal should be confined before surgery to prevent further damage to the muscle.

Anesthesia

Anesthetic considerations for animals with orthopedic disease are given on p. 944.

Surgical Anatomy

Skeletal muscle is made of long, cylindrical fibers encased within connective tissue sheaths (Fig. 34-2). Each individual fiber is enclosed within a sheath called the *endomysium*. Each fiber bundle is also enclosed within a sheath (*perimysium*), as is the entire muscle (*epimysium*). The connective tissue sheaths house blood vessels and nerve fibers that serve to integrate muscle contraction of individual fibers. Muscles

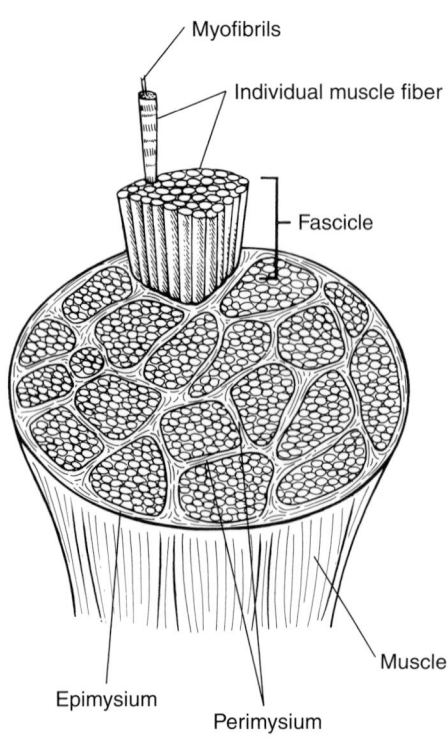

FIG. 34-2
Normal muscle anatomy. Note how the individual muscle fibrils combine to form muscle fibers. Groups of muscle fibers form fascicles, which are surrounded by the perimysium. Groups of fascicles form the muscle, which is covered by a thin fascial layer (epimysium).

[Figure labels: Myofibrils; Individual muscle fiber; Fascicle; Muscle; Epimysium; Perimysium]

are attached to bone by cordlike tendons or flat aponeuroses. The fascial compartment overlying the muscle group appears tight and congested with contusions, and the underlying muscle appears severely bruised and often protrudes from the incision through the fascial compartment.

> NOTE: The cut ends of the tendon (or muscle) often retract and appear frayed. Tendon ends may retract within a tendon sheath and require longitudinal incision to identify the severed ends.

Positioning

The animal should be positioned so that the affected muscle group can be exposed. A generous area should be clipped and prepared for aseptic surgery to allow the incision to be extended beyond the boundaries of the affected muscle if necessary.

SURGICAL TECHNIQUE

Make an incision through the skin and subcutaneous tissue overlying the muscle to be exposed. Once the muscle group is identified, make an incision through the fascia to decompress the muscle compartment. Suture subcutaneous tissue and skin using standard methods.

SUTURE MATERIALS AND SPECIAL INSTRUMENTS

Self-retaining retractors are useful for retracting soft tissue from the area of interest.

POSTOPERATIVE CARE AND ASSESSMENT

The wound should be monitored for swelling and/or drainage for 7 to 10 days after surgery. Suture removal can be performed when the skin incision has healed.

PROGNOSIS

Return to normal function should be expected with most contusions and muscle strains; however, repeat injury is likely if adequate rest is not provided.

Suggested Reading

Millis DL, Levine D, Taylor RA: Canine rehabilitation and physical therapy, Philadelphia, 2004, Saunders.
This book is a comprehensive guide to physical therapy and rehabilitation for dogs. It has detailed descriptions of rehabilitation techniques and how they are applied for specific diseases.
Nielsen C, Pluhar GE: Diagnosis and treatment of hind limb muscle strain injuries in 22 dogs, *Vet Comp Orthop Traum* 18:247, 2005.
This retrospective study evaluated hind limb muscle strains in dogs. The majority of dogs had strains of the hip adductor muscles that were diagnosed by orthopedic examination and ultrasound. Medical management was used in all cases and lameness improved or resolved in almost all dogs.

MUSCLE-TENDON UNIT LACERATION

DEFINITION

Lacerations are tears within the muscle-tendon unit.

GENERAL CONSIDERATIONS AND CLINICALLY RELEVANT PATHOPHYSIOLOGY

Lacerations are usually due to penetration of the muscle-tendon unit by a sharp object. These injuries most commonly involve tendons near the carpometacarpal and tarsometatarsal joints, but may involve muscle units elsewhere.

DIAGNOSIS
Clinical Presentation

Signalment. Any age, breed, or sex of dog or cat may be affected.

History. The animal usually has an open wound and a non–weight-bearing lameness.

Physical Examination Findings

Non–weight-bearing lameness is typical after acute penetration of a muscle-tendon unit by a foreign object. The extent of internal damage can be assessed only through visualizing the wound. The wound should be explored after the patient has been stabilized, and this usually requires general anesthesia. Failure to explore the wound can result in lacerations being undiagnosed until the patient attempts to bear weight. The greater the time span from injury to repair, the more difficult it will be to appose severed tendon ends.

Dogs with chronic tendon lacerations have lameness exacerbated by exercise. Dogs brought in with isolated deep digital flexor tendon lacerations have characteristic hyperextension of one digit.

Diagnostic Imaging

Standard craniocaudal and medial-to-lateral radiographs should be taken to determine whether foreign bodies or concurrent fractures are present. Mild swelling may occur in the area of chronic tendon lacerations. Ultrasonography helps localize the site of tendon injury and may differentiate partial from complete tendon rupture. Tendon injuries have a variable sonographic appearance depending upon severity of the trauma and stage of healing. The normal ultrasound appearance of tendon depends upon the incidence of the ultrasound beam. In a sagittal plane, the tendon or ligament will have a parallel, linear fiber alignment pattern that is hyperechoic. Damaged or torn tendons or ligaments will have disruption of the fiber alignment and edema, which appears as hypoechogenicity between the fibers. In acute injuries, the tendon is often enlarged because of the presence of edema, whereas with chronic injuries thickening of the tendon with focal areas of mineralization may be seen. A complete disruption may be identified by the presence of a hypoechoic band bordered by the retracted hyperechoic tendon ends.

Laboratory Findings

Consistent laboratory abnormalities are not present.

DIFFERENTIAL DIAGNOSIS

Muscle-tendon lacerations must be differentiated from superficial lacerations and muscle strain (see p. 1316).

MEDICAL MANAGEMENT

Lacerations that involve a tendon should be managed with surgery; medical management is not indicated. Minor lacerations of muscle may be treated conservatively.

Physical Rehabilitation

Physical rehabilitation may include cryotherapy and pulsed therapeutic ultrasound. Major lacerations of muscle should be treated with a combination of surgical repair and postoperative physical rehabilitation (see Chapter 12).

SURGICAL TREATMENT

Muscular lacerations require appositional sutures supported with deeper stent sutures. If the laceration goes through the tendon, delicate manipulation and apposition with small-diameter suture are recommended.

Preoperative Management

The wound should be cleaned and a sterile bandage applied until definitive treatment is performed. Exercise should be restricted before surgery.

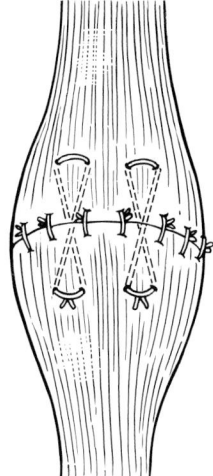

FIG. 34-3
Repair of muscle laceration with appositional sutures supported by tension stent sutures.

Anesthesia

Anesthetic management of animals with orthopedic disease is given on p. 944.

Surgical Anatomy

Tendons are longitudinally oriented bundles of collagen fibers that are surrounded by loose connective tissue sheaths. Blood vessels and nerves also reside within the tendon sheaths. The entire tendon is surrounded by the *epitenon*, which is enveloped by an outer connective tissue sheath called the *paratenon*. Tendons crossing joint surfaces are often encased in a tendon sheath to facilitate movement during joint motion.

Positioning

The animal should be positioned so that the tendon and muscle can be fully exposed. A generous area should be clipped and prepared for aseptic surgery to allow the incision to be extended above and below the injury if necessary.

SURGICAL TECHNIQUE
Muscle Laceration

Thoroughly débride the wound edges to fresh, bleeding muscle (Fig. 34-3). Débride carefully to prevent excess removal of tissue, which makes apposition of the severed ends difficult. Place interrupted sutures in the outer muscle sheath around the circumference of the muscle. Support the appositional sutures with heavy stent sutures placed in a cruciate pattern.

Tendon Laceration

Delicately manipulate and débride the tendon ends. With small, flat tendons, use small-diameter, nonabsorbable material placed in a series as interrupted vertical mattress

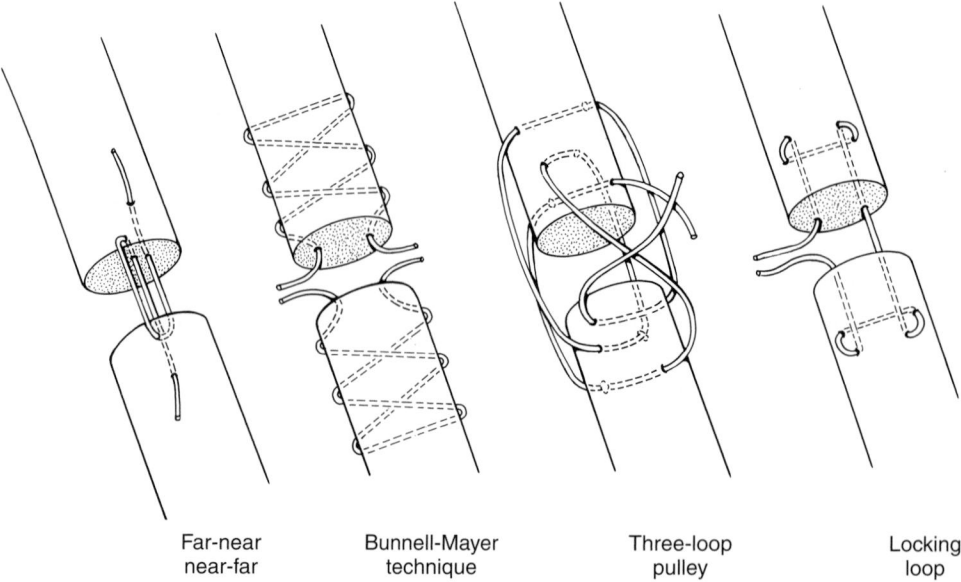

Far-near   Bunnell-Mayer   Three-loop   Locking
near-far   technique   pulley   loop

FIG. 34-4
Suture patterns used to appose tendon ends.

or cruciate sutures. For larger tendons, select the largest suture diameter that will readily pass through the tendon atraumatically.

A locking-loop suture pattern is recommended (Fig. 34-4).

Place each loop of the pattern in a slightly different plane (i.e., a near-far, middle-middle, and far-near pattern). Alternatively, use a three-loop pulley, Bunnell-Mayer, or far-near, near-far suture pattern. Use adjoining fascia to support the tendon appositional sutures.

SUTURE MATERIALS AND SPECIAL INSTRUMENTS

Nonabsorbable or absorbable suture material may be used to repair muscle, provided the material maintains its mechanical strength for 3 to 4 weeks. Nonabsorbable suture material is recommended for tendon repair. Swaged-on needles are helpful in limiting tissue trauma during suturing. Self-retaining retractors are useful for holding surrounding tissue away from the working area.

HEALING OF TENDONS AND MUSCLES

Healing of tendons follows a pattern similar to that of other connective tissue. The inflammatory phase is characterized initially by neutrophils and later by mononuclear cells. Tendon injury is rarely isolated, but exists in a zone with other wounded tissue. Unsuccessful attempts to isolate tendon healing from surrounding tissue have led to the concept of one wound, one scar. This implies that successful healing is dependent on activation of undifferentiated mesenchymal cells, which migrate into the wound. Mesenchymal cells pro-

duce the collagen and matrix that lend strength to the entire wound. The resultant scar unites the tendon ends, which remodel with collagen fibers oriented parallel to lines of stress. Strength is regained through the one-wound, one-scar principle, but function is regained through active and passive postoperative use of the limb.

POSTOPERATIVE CARE

After tendon repair, the limb should be immobilized for 3 weeks by use of rigid external coaptation with the joint positioned to release stress on the repaired tendon (see p. 967). When the splint is removed, the limb should be semirigidly immobilized for an additional 3 weeks with a heavy padded bandage or a half cast (i.e., one side of a split cast applied cranially or caudally to the limb). After muscle repair, the limb should be immobilized for 5 days followed by 4 to 6 weeks of protected activity.

Physical Rehabilitation

During immobilization, pulsed 3-MHz therapeutic ultrasound may aid in collagen repair. After immobilization for muscle or tendon lacerations, physical rehabilitation is vital to reverse the effects of immobilization on the other joints (Table 34-1). The animal should be gradually returned to normal activity; premature weight bearing will result in failure of the tendon to heal.

PROGNOSIS

Return to normal function is expected if postoperative recommendations are followed. Failure generally is associated with the animal being allowed to exercise before the tendon has completely healed.

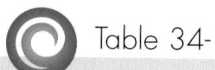 Table 34-1

Sample Physical Rehabilitation Protocol for Patients With Muscle-Tendon Unit Laceration

ALL TREATMENTS BID	WEEKS 6–7	WEEKS 8–9	WEEKS 10–12	HEALED TO RETURN TO FUNCTION
Heat therapy	10 min	10 min	10 min	
Massage	5 min	5 min	5 min	5 min
Passive range of motion (repetitions)	20*	20*	10–15*	Stop-when ROM is normal
Electrical stimulation†	10 min	10 min	10 min	10 min
Therapeutic exercise-total time	20 min	25 min	35 min	25–45 min
Walk/land treadmill	10 min	15 min	15 min	>10 min
Balancing	+	+	+	+
Obstacles	+	+	+	+
Weaving		+	+	+
Circles			+	+
Hills				+
Stairs				+
Jog/run				+
Underwater treadmill	10 min	15 min	15 min	>15 min
Swimming			5 min	5–10 min
Cryotherapy	15 min	15 min	15 min	PRN

BID, Twice a day; *ROM,* range of motion; +, perform modality; *PRN,* as needed; *QID,* four times a day.
Begin no sooner than 6 wk postoperatively, after external coaptation is no longer needed.
*Passive range of motion to all joints of the affected limb.
†Electrical stimulation to be performed on affected muscle groups. See Chapter 12 for specifics.

Suggested Reading

Kramer M, Gerwin M, Michele U et al: Ultrasonographic examination of injuries to the Achilles tendon in cats and dogs, *J Small Anim Pract* 42:531, 2001.
This article reports the ultrasonographic findings of 42 dogs and 7 cats with Achilles tendon injuries. Ultrasonography was shown to be an excellent diagnostic method for these injuries and a means of monitoring healing of the structure.

Lamb CR, Duvernois A: Ultrasonographic anatomy of the normal canine calcaneal tendon, *Vet Radiol Ultrasound* 46:326, 2005.
This article provides a detailed description and pictures of the normal structures of the calcanean tendon as visualized by arthroscopy.

Millis DL, Levine D, Taylor RA: *Canine rehabilitation and physical therapy,* Philadelphia, 2004, Saunders.
This book is a comprehensive guide to physical therapy and rehabilitation for dogs. It has detailed descriptions of rehabilitation techniques and how they are applied for specific diseases.

Moores AP, Comerford EJ, Tarlton JF et al: Biomechanical and clinical evaluation of a modified 3-loop pulley suture pattern for reattachment of canine tendons to bone, *Vet Surg* 33:391, 2004.
This paper describes an alternative method for repair of tendon lacerations or avulsions that may be superior to the locking-loop pattern. It may be more appropriate for use in some clinical cases.

Moores AP, Owen MR, Tarlton JF: The three-loop pulley suture versus two locking-loop sutures for the repair of canine Achilles tendons, *Vet Surg* 33:131, 2004.
This study reports that the three-loop pulley pattern is more resistant to gap formation than two locking-loop sutures. The resistance to gap formation is important in rapid healing of tendon injuries.

Worth AJ, Danielsson F, Bray JP et al: Ability to work and owner satisfaction following surgical repair of common calcanean tendon injuries in working dogs in New Zealand, *N Z Vet J* 52:109, 2004.
This article reported that surgical treatment of calcanean tendon injury combined with rigid immobilization resulted in a satisfactory outcome in 7 of 10 working dogs. A screw and cast method of immobilization was supported by the results of this study.

MUSCLE-TENDON UNIT RUPTURE

DEFINITIONS

Rupture of the muscle-tendon unit is a complete or partial loss of integrity of the muscle-tendon unit caused by extreme overstretching. Synonyms include a *torn muscle* and *dropped hock.*

GENERAL CONSIDERATIONS AND CLINICALLY RELEVANT PATHOPHYSIOLOGY

Muscle ruptures are caused by powerful contraction during forced hyperextension of the muscle-tendon unit. This injury is seen most often in sporting and performance athlete breeds, such as racing greyhounds. The injury most commonly encountered is partial or complete rupture of the Achilles tendon. Injury of the Achilles mechanism may arise from an acute traumatic episode or from chronic progressive stretching of the tendon. Acute injuries are often secondary to a fall or a penetrating wound. Conversely, chronic injuries are often secondary to overuse that causes chronic stretching and deterioration of the tendon. Chronic injuries more commonly occur in sporting breeds (e.g., field trial dogs and bird hunting dogs) and are often bilateral. Bilateral chronic degeneration of the common calcanean tendons is relatively common in Doberman pinschers, although the cause is unknown.

DIAGNOSIS
Clinical Presentation

Signalment. Any age, breed, or sex of dog or cat may be affected. Athletic dogs are most commonly affected. Doberman pinschers may have idiopathic bilateral common calcanean tendon degeneration.

    History. Affected animals usually exhibit weight-bearing lameness after strenuous activity.

Physical Examination Findings

Tarsal hyperflexion is often noted in animals with Achilles tendon rupture. The animal is unable to bear weight if the injury is secondary to acute trauma, and flaccidity of the Achilles tendon is noted on passive dorsal flexion of the tarsus when the stifle is extended. If the injury is secondary to a chronic stretching of the Achilles tendon, the patient will be weight bearing, but will walk plantigrade because of hyperflexion of the tarsus. Patients with chronic Achilles tendon injuries show varying degrees of tarsal hyperflexion, depending on the length of time the injury has been present. If the entire tendon complex is involved, the tarsus and digits hyperflex; if the tendon of the superficial flexor muscle is not involved, the tarsus will hyperflex and the digits will flex. Postural changes associated with a palpable swelling of the Achilles tendon confirm the diagnosis. Occasionally the injury occurs at the myotendinous juncture. Postural changes and careful palpation of the muscle-tendon unit confirm the diagnosis. Doberman pinschers have tarsal hyperextension and swelling of the common calcanean tendon.

Diagnostic Imaging

Ultrasonography can help determine the location of tendon fiber disruption, and may differentiate between partial and complete tears (see p. 1319). Standard craniocaudal and medial-to-lateral radiographs are indicated to determine whether bone avulsion is present or not.

Laboratory Findings

Consistent laboratory abnormalities are not found.

DIFFERENTIAL DIAGNOSIS

Sciatic nerve injury and congenital tarsal hyperflexion must be differentiated from Achilles tendon rupture. Gentle palpation of the muscle-tendon unit reveals loss of continuity and/or an area of swelling with tendon rupture, whereas patients with congenital tarsal hyperflexion lack these findings. When nerve injury is present, neurologic examination will show sciatic reflexes to be absent or decreased.

MEDICAL MANAGEMENT

Surgical repair of completely ruptured tendons is indicated; medical management is not. External coaptation may be tried with partial ruptures, but results are usually unsatisfactory. Doberman pinschers with common calcanean tendon degeneration should be treated conservatively with exercise moderation and bandaging as necessary to protect the tarsus. Splints are rarely beneficial. Physical rehabilitation (see p. 1323) may accelerate tendon healing.

SURGICAL TREATMENT
Preoperative Management

Activity should be limited until definitive treatment is begun. Open wounds (e.g., laceration of the Achilles tendon) should be cleaned and covered with a sterile dressing.

Anesthesia

Anesthetic management of animals with orthopedic disease is discussed on p. 944.

Surgical Anatomy

The Achilles tendon unit is composed of tendons arising from gastrocnemius and superficial digital flexor muscles, and a common tendon from the semitendinosus muscle, gracilis muscle, and biceps femoris muscle. The common tendon of the gastrocnemius muscle is the major component of the Achilles tendon with acute injuries. One can identify each component of the acutely injured Achilles complex, and suture each individually. However, with chronic injuries, the tendon ends retract, leaving a void to be filled with fibrous tissue. Identification of each component is not possible. The complex (fibrous scar and Achilles tendon) is treated as a single structure.

Positioning

Position the patient in lateral recumbency. A hanging-leg preparation facilitates manipulation of the limb during surgery. For Achilles tendon injuries, clip and prepare the limb for surgery from proximal to the stifle joint to the phalanges distally.

SURGICAL TECHNIQUE
Achilles Tendon Rupture

Make an incision over the site of injury on the caudolateral surface of the limb. If the injury is acute, identify the three tendons composing the Achilles complex and suture each tendon separately with an interrupted far-near, near-far pattern (see Fig. 34-4) using nonabsorbable, small-diameter (3-0 to 4-0, depending on the animal's size) monofilament suture. If the injury is chronic, identification of individual tendon units is not possible; continue surgical dissection to expose the circumference of the thickened fibrous band. Then sequentially remove sections of scar tissue from the center of the mass. Remove enough tissue so that tension is present in the Achilles complex when the stifle joint is in a normal standing position and the tarsus is slightly extended. Be careful to not remove too much of the proliferative fibrous tissue.

If excess fibrous tissue is excised, apposition of the cut ends will be difficult.

Suture the cut ends with a three-loop pulley pattern (see Fig. 34-4) or maintain apposition with tendon plating. For tendon plating, appose the cut ends of the tendon with nonabsorbable monofilament suture. Use 3-0 suture for small dogs and cats, 2-0 for medium-sized dogs, and 0 for large dogs. Support the anastomosis by placing a small bone plate adjacent to the tendon (Fig. 34-5). Place interrupted sutures

through the plate holes into the body of the tendon. Use large-diameter, nonabsorbable monofilament suture.

Achilles Tendon Avulsion

Achilles tendon avulsion from the calcaneus is treated by suturing the tendon as described earlier and securing it to the calcaneus by passing the suture through holes drilled through the proximal calcaneus.

Whether the injury is acute or chronic and involves rupture or avulsion of the tendon, support of the tendon anastomosis is critical for a favorable outcome. Support is provided by immobilization of the tarsal joint in slight extension.

Place a raised, threaded transfixation pin through the free end of the calcaneus into the distal tibia. Cut through the pin shaft to leave the pin just below the skin surface. Provide additional support with a fiberglass cast. Alternatively, immobilize the hock in slight extension by placing transfixation pins through the distal tibial diaphysis and the calcaneus, connecting them with bilateral external fixator bars.

SUTURE MATERIALS AND SPECIAL INSTRUMENTS

Nonabsorbable suture material is recommended for tendon repair. Swaged-on needles are helpful in limiting tissue trauma during suturing. Self-retaining retractors are useful for holding surrounding tissue away from the working area. An air-driven or battery-operated drill is useful if a bone screw or transfixation pin is to be inserted.

POSTOPERATIVE CARE

The cast and transfixation pin, or external fixator, are placed for 3 to 6 weeks, after which both may be removed. The limb should then be supported in a padded bandage to prevent full dorsal flexion of the tarsus. Activity should be limited to leash walking for 10 weeks. If tendon plating is performed, the plate should be removed 8 to 10 weeks after surgery. After muscle repair, the limb should be immobilized for a period of 5 days followed by 4 to 6 weeks of protected activity.

Physical Rehabilitation

During immobilization, pulsed 3-MHz therapeutic ultrasound may aid in collagen repair. After immobilization for muscle or tendon ruptures, physical rehabilitation is vital to reverse the effects of immobilization on the joints (Table 34-2). The animal should be gradually returned to normal activity; premature weight bearing will result in failure of the tendon to heal.

PROGNOSIS

Prognosis for return to strenuous athletic activity is unlikely. However, most patients are able to resume normal pet activity.

Doberman pinschers with degeneration of the common calcanean tendon often regain some degree of tendon func-

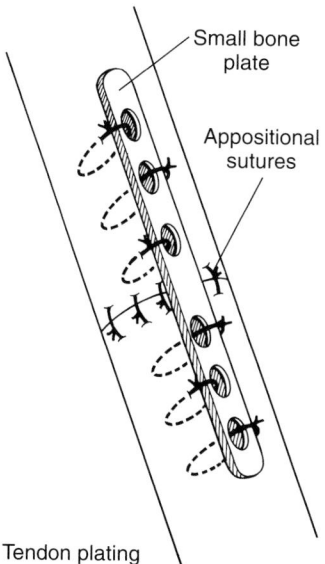

Small bone plate

Appositional sutures

Tendon plating

FIG. 34-5
Tendon anastomosis supported with a small bone plate. The plate serves to neutralize forces acting on the anastomosis.

Table 34-2

Sample Physical Rehabilitation Protocol for Patients With Muscle Tendon Unit Rupture

ALL TREATMENTS BID	WEEKS 10-11	WEEKS 12-13	WEEKS 14-16	RETURN TO FUNCTION
Heat therapy	10 min	10 min	10 min	10 min
Massage	5 min	5 min	5 min	5 min
Passive range of motion (repetitions)	20*	20*	10–15*	Stop-when ROM is normal
Electrical stimulation	10 min	10 min	10 min	10 min
Therapeutic exercise-total time	20 min	25 min	35 min	25–45 min
Walk/land treadmill	10 min	15 min	15 min	>10 min
Balancing	+	+	+	+
Obstacles	+	+	+	+
Weaving		+	+	+
Circles			+	+
Hills				+
Stairs				+
Jog/run				+
Underwater treadmill	10 min	15 min	15 min	>15 min
Swimming			5 min	5–10 min
Cryotherapy	15 min	15 min	15 min	PRN

BID, Twice a day; *ROM*, range of motion; +, perform modality; *PRN*, as needed; *QID*, four times a day.
Begin no sooner than 10 wk postoperatively, after external coaptation is no longer needed.
*Passive range of motion to all joints of the affected limb.
†Electrical stimulation to be performed on affected muscle groups. See Chapter 12 for specifics.

tion spontaneously over time. The tendons often remain swollen, but the degree of hock flexion and disability typically improve over several months of conservative therapy.

Suggested Reading

Kramer M, Gerwin M, Michele U et al: Ultrasonographic examination of injuries to the Achilles tendon in cats and dogs, *J Small Anim Pract* 42:531, 2001.
This article reports the ultrasonographic findings of 42 dogs and 7 cats with Achilles tendon injuries. Ultrasonography was shown to be an excellent diagnostic method for these injuries and a means of monitoring healing of the structure.
Lamb CR, Duvernois A: Ultrasonographic anatomy of the normal canine calcaneal tendon, *Vet Radiol Ultrasound* 46:326, 2005.
This article provides a detailed description and pictures of the normal structures of the calcanean tendon as visualized through arthroscopy.
Millis DL, Levine D, Taylor RA: *Canine rehabilitation and physical therapy,* Philadelphia, 2004, Saunders.
This book is a comprehensive guide to physical therapy and rehabilitation for dogs. It has detailed descriptions of rehabilitation techniques and how they are applied for specific diseases.

Moores AP, Comerford EJ, Tarlton JF et al: Biomechanical and clinical evaluation of a modified 3-loop pulley suture pattern for reattachment of canine tendons to bone, *Vet Surg* 33:391, 2004.
This paper describes an alternative method for repair of tendon lacerations or avulsions that may be superior to the locking-loop pattern. It may be more appropriate for use in some clinical cases.
Moores AP, Owen MR, Tarlton JF: The three-loop pulley suture versus two locking-loop sutures for the repair of canine Achilles tendons, *Vet Surg* 33:131, 2004.
This study reports that the three-loop pulley pattern is more resistant to gap formation than two locking-loop sutures. The resistance to gap formation is important in rapid healing of tendon injuries.
Worth AJ, Danielsson F, Bray JP et al: Ability to work and owner satisfaction following surgical repair of common calcanean tendon injuries in working dogs in New Zealand, *N Z Vet J* 52:109, 2004.
This article reported that surgical treatment of calcanean tendon injury combined with rigid immobilization resulted in a satisfactory outcome in 7 of 10 working dogs. A screw and cast method of immobilization was supported by the results of this study.

MINERALIZATION OF THE SUPRASPINATUS TENDON

DEFINITION

Mineralization is the accumulation of calcified material within the insertional tendon of the supraspinatus. This may also be called *calcification of the supraspinatus tendon.*

GENERAL CONSIDERATIONS AND CLINICALLY RELEVANT PATHOPHYSIOLOGY

The cause of mineralization of the supraspinatus tendon is unknown, but may be associated with excessive exercise. It is commonly seen in active, large-breed dogs. Mineralization may also be associated with tearing of tendon fibers. Severe disease may cause a mass of mineral and fibrous tissue compressing or deviating the biceps tendon in the bicipital groove. Rarely, disease of the biceps and supraspinatus occur together, and in the most severe cases, other diseases of the shoulder (e.g., instability and osteoarthritis) may also be identified. Radiographic mineralization is a common incidental finding and not associated with clinical lameness; therefore, accurate determination of the cause of the lameness is critical.

DIAGNOSIS
Clinical Presentation

Signalment. Athletic large-breed dogs are most commonly affected.

History. Lameness may be mild or severe depending upon the severity of the lesion. Most animals have a chronic history of lameness.

Physical Examination Findings

Mineralization of the supraspinatus tendon must be differentiated from other shoulder diseases. Palpation on the medial aspect of the greater tubercle may cause pain. This response may be magnified by shoulder flexion and internal rotation.

Diagnostic Imaging

Ultrasonography helps evaluate stabilizers of the scapulohumeral joint (i.e., biceps and supraspinatus tendons). In cases of severe injury to the supraspinatus tendon, ultrasound helps determine the degree of tendon fiber disruption. Mineralization of the tendon appears as hyperechoic foci, which cause distal acoustic shadowing. With radiography, mineralization within the supraspinatus tendon may be seen adjacent to the greater tubercle using a skyline view (Fig. 34-6).

Laboratory Findings

Consistent laboratory abnormalities are not found.

DIFFERENTIAL DIAGNOSIS

Differential diagnoses include biceps tenosynovitis, osteochondritis dissecans (OCD), shoulder instability, and shoulder osteoarthritis.

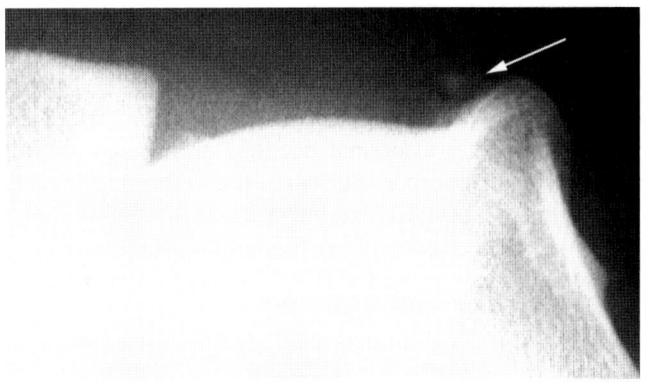

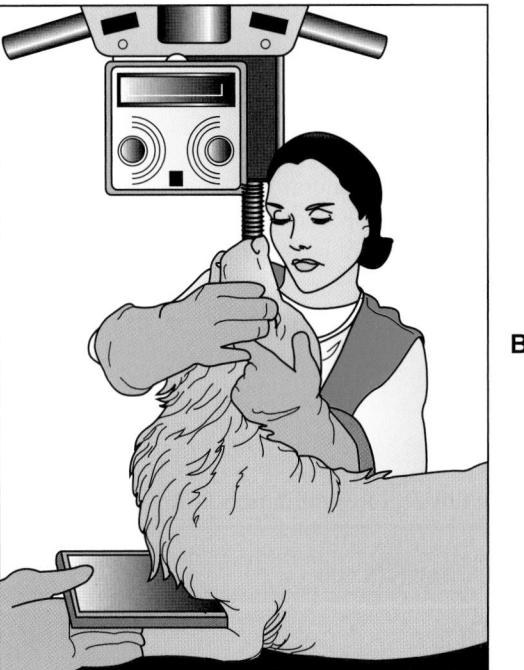

FIG. 34-6
A, Mineralization of the supraspinatus tendon *(arrow).*
B, Radiographic positioning is with the patient in sternal recumbency and the head extended out of the beam. The cassette is placed above the antebrachium with the humerus nearly vertical. The radiographic beam courses down the bicipital groove.

MEDICAL MANAGEMENT

Medical management of supraspinatus mineralization is often attempted first. Corticosteroid injections combined with rest are often attempted and may provide temporary relief. Injection of corticosteroids into the tendon may cause tendon degeneration; therefore multiple injections are not recommended.

Physical Rehabilitation

Physical rehabilitation for mineralization includes cryotherapy and passive range of motion. Therapeutic ultrasound may aid in eliminating mineral deposits in the muscle (see Chapter 12).

SURGICAL TREATMENT

Surgery is recommended for confirmed mineralization of the supraspinatus tendon that is unresponsive to medical management. Complete evaluation of the shoulder joint is needed to rule out other associated diseases. Arthroscopy of the shoulder joint is the most efficient means of thoroughly evaluating the joint. Surgical treatment involves removal of the mineral from the tendon of insertion of the supraspinatus.

Preoperative Management

Activity should be limited until definitive treatment is initiated.

Anesthesia

Anesthetic management of animals with orthopedic disease is discussed on p. 944.

Surgical Anatomy

The supraspinatus tendon has a broad insertion on the medial and lateral aspects of the greater tubercle. The medial portions are adjacent to the biceps tendon.

Positioning

Position the patient in lateral recumbency. A hanging-leg preparation facilitates manipulation of the limb during surgery. Clip and prepare the limb for surgery from dorsal midline to the midantebrachium.

SURGICAL TECHNIQUE

Perform shoulder arthroscopy to evaluate the remainder of the joint. Perform a craniomedial approach to the shoulder joint and biceps tendon (see p. 1187). Identify and remove the mineralized area within the insertional tendon of the supraspinatus. Evaluate the biceps tendon. Close the surgical site routinely (see p. 1187).

SUTURE MATERIALS AND SPECIAL INSTRUMENTS

Gelpi retractors are useful to maintain exposure to the craniomedial portion of the shoulder joint.

POSTOPERATIVE CARE

Activity should be limited to leash walking for 10 weeks.

 Table 34-3

Sample Physical Rehabilitation Protocol for Muscle Contracture and Fibrosis

ALL TREATMENTS QID	DAYS 1 TO 14	DAYS 15 TO 24	DAY 25 UNTIL HEALED	HEALED TO RETURN TO FUNCTION
Heat therapy	10 min	10 min	10 min	
Massage	5 min	5 min	5 min	
Passive range of motion (repetitions)	30*	30*	30*	
Electrical stimulation†	10 min	10 min	10 min	10 min
Therapeutic exercise-total time	10 min	15 min	15 min	25–45 min
Walk/land treadmill	10 min	5 min	5 min	>10 min
Balancing	+	+	+	
Obstacles	+	+	+	+
Weaving	+	+	+	+
Circles				+
Hills				+
Stairs				+
Jog/run				+
Underwater treadmill		10 min	10 min	>15 min
Swimming				5–10 min
Cryotherapy	15 min	15 min	15 min	PRN

QID, Four times a day; +, perform modality; *PRN,* as needed.
*Passive range of motion to all joints of the affected limb.
†Electrical stimulation to be performed on the affected muscle groups. See Chapter 12 for specifics.

Physical Rehabilitation

Physical rehabilitation can be started immediately following surgery and should include cryotherapy for the first 72 hours followed by passive flexion and extension of the limb and heat therapy (see Chapter 12). Specific controlled exercises should be used to regain maximum function (Table 34-3).

PROGNOSIS

The prognosis for return to normal function is fair depending upon the presence of other shoulder diseases. A study of six dogs (four operated; two managed conservatively) showed resolution of lameness in all dogs. However, mineralization recurred in all operated dogs over a mean of 5 years after surgery.

Reference

Laitinen OM, Flo GL: Mineralization of the supraspinatus tendon in dogs: a long-term follow-up, *J Am Anim Hosp Assoc* 36:262, 2000.

Suggested Reading

Millis DL, Levine D, Taylor RA: *Canine rehabilitation and physical therapy,* Philadelphia, 2004, Saunders.
This book is a comprehensive guide to physical therapy and rehabilitation for dogs. It has detailed descriptions of rehabilitation techniques and how they are applied for specific diseases.

FIBROTIC CONTRACTURE OF THE INFRASPINATUS MUSCLE

DEFINITIONS

Muscle contracture or **fibrosis** may occur when there is replacement of normal muscle-tendon unit architecture with fibrous tissue, resulting in functional shortening of the muscle or tendon. This shortening may cause abnormal motion in adjacent joints.

GENERAL CONSIDERATIONS AND CLINICALLY RELEVANT PATHOPHYSIOLOGY

Infraspinatus muscle contracture occurs most often in hunting dogs after irreversible muscle fiber injury. The cause is unknown, but appears to be a primary muscle disorder rather than secondary to neurologic or immune-mediated disorders. Histologic findings (e.g., degeneration, atrophy, and fibroplasia) within damaged areas of the muscle are compatible with severe strain. Disease progression is associated with a breakdown of muscle fibers and replacement by fibrous tissue that causes muscle contracture and external rotation and abduction of the limb.

DIAGNOSIS
Clinical Presentation

Signalment. Contracture of the infraspinatus muscle usually occurs in young, adult, sporting breeds.

History. Acute lameness after strenuous activity in the 3 weeks before evaluation for infraspinatus muscle contracture is typical.

Physical Examination Findings

Animals with infraspinatus muscle contracture initially have a weight-bearing forelimb lameness. Soft tissue swelling around the shoulder joint may be noted. Lameness usually resolves and is absent for 3 to 4 weeks, but then mild lameness and a gait abnormality develop. The characteristic gait abnormality is secondary to progressive fibrosis and contracture of the infraspinatus muscle. As the muscle shortens from contracture, external rotation of the shoulder causes elbow abduction and outward rotation of the paw (Fig. 34-7).

Diagnostic Imaging

The normal infraspinatus tendon should show a typical arrangement of parallel, echogenic striae against a hypoechoic background on ultrasound. Acute injury may demonstrate fiber-pattern disruption with edema and hemorrhage. Chronic muscle contracture varies in appearance depending upon the severity and stage of the disease. Fibrosis of the muscle is visible as increased echogenicity of the tendon.

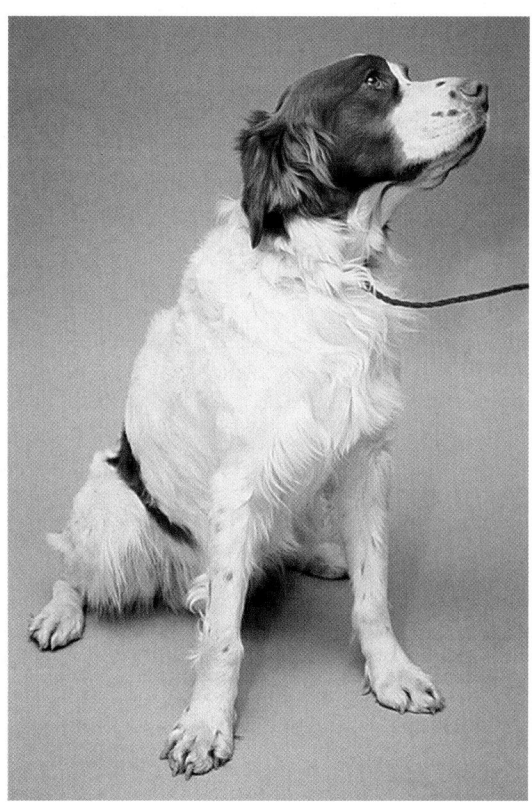

FIG. 34-7
Dog with infraspinatus muscle contracture. Note external rotation of the shoulder and internal displacement of the elbow.

DIFFERENTIAL DIAGNOSIS

Diagnosis of infraspinatus muscle contracture usually is possible from historical and physical examination findings.

MEDICAL MANAGEMENT

Physical rehabilitation may help prevent contracture if the condition is diagnosed and treated early; however, presentation to a veterinarian at this stage is uncommon, and surgical therapy is highly successful. Thus surgical treatment is most commonly performed in affected dogs.

Physical Rehabilitation

Physical rehabilitation entails ultrasound therapy combined with stretching and passive range of motion (see Chapter 12).

SURGICAL TREATMENT

Surgical treatment is directed at releasing the fibrotic myotendinous infraspinatus muscle as it crosses the shoulder joint.

Preoperative Management

These animals otherwise are generally healthy, and minimal preoperative care is necessary.

Anesthesia

See p. 944 for anesthetic management of animals with orthopedic disease.

Surgical Anatomy

The infraspinatus muscle-tendon unit is a cuff muscle of the shoulder joint. The muscle lies next to the scapula, just caudal to the spine. The tendon crosses the joint craniolaterally to insert just distal to the greater tubercle of the proximal humerus. At surgery, the tendon appears thickened and, because of fibrous tissue invasion, has an off-white color rather than the white, glistening appearance typical of normal tendons. The muscle is atrophied and appears pale relative to normal, healthy muscle.

Positioning

Clip the shoulder from the dorsal midline to the elbow and position the patient in lateral recumbency.

SURGICAL TECHNIQUE

Perform a craniolateral approach to the shoulder joint. Isolate the circumference of the infraspinatus muscle with sharp dissection. Transect the fibrotic muscle and any fibrous bands restricting movement of the joint.

Once the fibrous contracture is incised, the limb will assume a normal position, and a normal range of motion of the shoulder will be possible.

SUTURE MATERIALS AND SPECIAL INSTRUMENTS

Self-retaining retractors and a periosteal elevator assist tissue retraction and reflection.

POSTOPERATIVE CARE

Special postoperative care is not required after surgery for infraspinatus muscle contracture. These animals usually begin to use the limb within a few days after surgery. The dog should be allowed to fully bear weight as soon as possible. Physical rehabilitation is important to help the animal regain full usage of the limb (see Table 34-3 on p. 1326).

PROGNOSIS

The prognosis for infraspinatus muscle contracture is excellent, and return to preinjury function is expected after surgery.

Suggested Reading

Millis DL, Levine D, Taylor RA: *Canine rehabilitation and physical therapy,* Philadelphia, 2004, Saunders.
This book is a comprehensive guide to physical therapy and rehabilitation for dogs. It has detailed descriptions of rehabilitation techniques and how they are applied for specific diseases.
Moores AP, Comerford EJ, Tarlton JF et al: Biomechanical and clinical evaluation of a modified three-loop pulley suture pattern for reattachment of canine tendons to bone, *Vet Surg* 33:391, 2004.
This paper describes an alternative method for repair of tendon lacerations or avulsions that may be superior to the locking-loop pattern. It may be more appropriate for use in some clinical cases.

QUADRICEPS CONTRACTURE

DEFINITIONS

Muscle contracture or **fibrosis** *(quadriceps tie down, fracture disease of the rear limb)* may occur when there is replacement of normal muscle-tendon unit architecture with fibrous tissue, resulting in functional shortening of the muscle or tendon. This shortening may cause abnormal motion in adjacent joints. **Myopathy** is another term used to describe muscle disease.

GENERAL CONSIDERATIONS AND CLINICALLY RELEVANT PATHOPHYSIOLOGY

Quadriceps muscle contracture usually occurs after distal femoral fractures in young dogs; however, congenital contracture of the quadriceps muscle has been reported. Inadequate fracture stabilization, excessive tissue trauma during surgery, or prolonged limb immobilization with the stifle in extension may singly, or in combination, contribute to quadriceps contracture. It is often associated with Salter-Harris type I or II fractures in puppies (see p. 951). Quadriceps contracture may occur after splinting in extension for as little as 5 to 7 days. The disease is likely a result of the combination of muscle trauma, rapid bone callus formation, and limb immobilization. Joint stiffness develops because of fibrous adhesions between the quadriceps and fracture callus. With time, adhesions form between the joint capsule and distal femur, limiting limb use and causing the quadriceps muscle to atrophy. In later stages, the disease also causes bone atrophy, atrophy of cartilage in the stifle, intraarticular

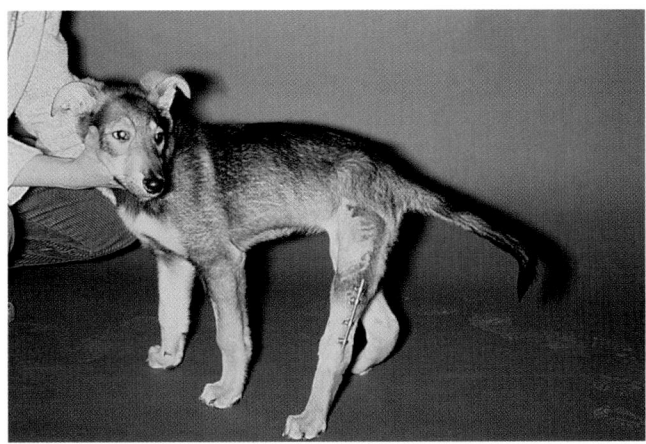

FIG. 34-8
Dog with quadriceps muscle contracture. Note hyperextension of the femur.

fibrosis, and eventual ankylosis of the stifle joint. The cause of congenital quadriceps contracture and why contracture occurs most commonly in young dogs are unknown.

DIAGNOSIS
Clinical Presentation

Signalment. Any age, breed, or sex of dog may develop quadriceps muscle contracture; however, it most commonly occurs in immature patients after distal femoral fracture when inappropriate repair has been done and/or there has been inadequate postoperative physical rehabilitation.

History. Animals with quadriceps muscle contracture usually are evaluated for lameness 3 to 5 weeks after having sustained femoral trauma. Frequently, internal reduction and stabilization of a distal femoral fracture or application of an external splint for stabilization of a femoral fracture has been performed.

Physical Examination Findings

The stifle joint of animals with quadriceps muscle contracture has a limited range of motion (Fig. 34-8). Initially the joint can be fully extended, but can be flexed only 20 to 30 degrees. Gradually the amount of flexion decreases to less than 10 degrees. Contracture may be such that the stifle joint appears hyperextended. Cranial thigh muscles are generally atrophied and palpate as a thickened cord.

Diagnostic Imaging

The normal quadriceps muscle should show a typical echogenic, fibrillar arrangement. Changes in this arrangement vary depending on the type, severity, and stage of trauma (see p. 1316).

Laboratory Findings

Consistent laboratory abnormalities are not present.

DIFFERENTIAL DIAGNOSIS

The diagnosis of quadriceps contracture usually can be made from historical and physical examination findings.

MEDICAL MANAGEMENT

Prevention of quadriceps contracture should begin within 24 hours of surgery for distal femoral fractures in puppies. Therapy should include passive range of motion several times a day, cryotherapy, and massage for edema reduction. Tissue mobilization techniques help prevent fibrosis. Exercises to encourage weight bearing should begin approximately 3 days postoperatively and may include slow leash walking, treadmill walking, and aquatic therapy (see Table 34-3 on p. 1326 and Chapter 12).

Physical Rehabilitation

Physical rehabilitation alone is rarely successful in the management of quadriceps contracture. Forced flexion of the stifle often results in additional fractures to the femur or tibia.

SURGICAL TREATMENT

Treatment of quadriceps contracture is aimed at restoring limb function. Release of fibrous thickening and adhesions between joint capsule and femur and between quadriceps muscle and femur is necessary. If a functional range of motion is not achieved after adhesion release, lengthening of the quadriceps muscle-tendon unit is required. Lengthening may be accomplished by a Z-plasty or by release of the origin of each muscle. Recurrence of contracture with resultant loss of stifle joint motion occurs if preventive rehabilitation measures are not taken after surgery. An effective method to maintain a functional range of stifle motion is to apply a transarticular fixator postoperatively to maintain passive flexion of the stifle joint, but allow active or passive extension. Alternatively, if sufficient flexion is obtained at surgery, a 90/90 bandage can be used (see p. 949).

Preoperative Management

These animals otherwise are generally healthy, and minimal preoperative care is necessary.

Anesthesia

See p. 944 for anesthetic management of animals with orthopedic disease.

Surgical Anatomy

The quadriceps muscle-tendon unit is composed of the *vastus medialis, vastus intermedius, rectus femoris,* and *vastus lateralis* muscles. These muscles all atrophy in patients with quadriceps muscle contracture. Proximally, the *rectus femoris* muscle palpates as a thickened cord. At surgery, all four muscles of the quadriceps appear small and pale in color. In patients with distal femoral fractures, the atrophied muscles lie superficial to, and are intertwined with, proliferative fibrous tissue. Normal range of motion in the stifle joint is from 180 degrees (full extension) to 30 degrees (full flexion).

Positioning

Clip the limb from the dorsal midline to the tarsus, and position the patient in lateral recumbency. A hanging-leg preparation facilitates manipulation of the limb during surgery.

SURGICAL TECHNIQUE

Expose the stifle joint and distal femur through a liberal craniolateral incision (see pp. 1107 and 1115, respectively). Elevate and release adhesions between the quadriceps muscle group and femur with sharp dissection. Release adhesions between the fibrous joint capsule and femoral condyles. Luxate the patella medially, and flex the joint to its full extent. If a functional range of motion (greater than 40 degrees) is not achieved after releasing the adhesions, perform a quadriceps muscle-tendon unit lengthening procedure.

Z-plasty

Make a longitudinal incision through the center of the muscletendon unit beginning 8 to 10 cm proximal to the patella. Extend the incision distally to a point 3 cm proximal to the patella. At the proximal extent of the longitudinal incision, make a transverse incision laterally through the muscle and fibrous tissue. At the distal extent of the longitudinal incision, make a transverse incision medially through the muscle and fibrous tissue. Flex the stifle, and allow the cut edges of the longitudinal incision to slide on each other. When a functional range of flexion is achieved, place interrupted sutures across the longitudinal incision to maintain the desired length of the quadriceps muscle-tendon unit.

Muscle Release

Extend the lateral incision to expose the proximal femur. At the level of the third trochanter, elevate the quadriceps from the medial, lateral, and caudal surfaces of the femur. Incise through the origins of each muscle group to release the quadriceps, and allow distal sliding of the muscle group. Release the vastus intermedius near its point of origin on the ilium. Close the surgical wound using standard methods.

Transarticular Fixator

Insert a half pin just below the third trochanter of the femur using an end-threaded transfixation pin, and insert a full pin through the tibia 4 cm above the tarsus using a centrally threaded transfixation pin. Maximally flex the stifle joint, and maintain this position with a heavy rubber band connecting the proximal and distal transfixation pins. Fashion a bandage around the paw, and connect it to the distal transfixation pin to maintain a functional angle of the tarsus.

SUTURE MATERIALS AND SPECIAL INSTRUMENTS

Self-retaining retractors and a periosteal elevator assist tissue retraction and reflection. Instruments for placement of pins are necessary if a transarticular fixator is placed postoperatively.

POSTOPERATIVE CARE AND ASSESSMENT

After application of a transarticular fixator for quadriceps muscle contracture, pin-to-skin interfaces must be cleaned daily (see p. 974). Passive flexion and extension of the stifle joint and tarsus should begin as soon as the patient allows limb manipulation. Joint movement should be repeated 20 to 30 times and at least three times daily; increased frequency of manipulation improves rehabilitation. The external fixator should be maintained for 3 to 5 weeks. Physical rehabilitation should be continued for an additional 5 weeks after it is removed. If a 90/90 bandage (see p. 949) is applied, it should be maintained for 3 weeks. After bandage removal, passive flexion and extension of the joint should be performed as described previously.

PROGNOSIS

The prognosis after surgery for quadriceps muscle contracture is guarded and depends on the degree of degenerative joint changes present and on whether a functional range of motion is obtained at surgery. The prognosis is fair for functional limb use, but contracture may recur following surgery. A normal range of motion is seldom achieved, and most animals are able to flex the stifle only 45 to 90 degrees.

Suggested Reading

Millis DL, Levine D, Taylor RA: *Canine rehabilitation and physical therapy,* Philadelphia, 2004, Saunders.
This book is a comprehensive guide to physical therapy and rehabilitation for dogs. It has detailed descriptions of rehabilitation techniques and how they are applied for specific diseases.
Moores AP, Comerford EJ, Tarlton JF et al: Biomechanical and clinical evaluation of a modified three-loop pulley suture pattern for reattachment of canine tendons to bone, *Vet Surg* 33:391, 2004.
This paper describes an alternative method for repair of tendon lacerations or avulsions that may be superior to the locking-loop pattern. It may be more appropriate for use in some clinical cases.

FIBROTIC MYOPATHY

DEFINITION

Muscle contracture or **fibrosis** may occur when there is replacement of normal muscle-tendon unit architecture with fibrous tissue, resulting in functional shortening of the muscle or tendon. This shortening may cause abnormal motion in adjacent joints. Synonyms include *hamstring contracture, gracilis or semitendinosis contracture,* and *gracilis or semitendinosis myopathy.* **Myopathy** is a general term used to describe disease of the musculature.

GENERAL CONSIDERATIONS AND CLINICALLY RELEVANT PATHOPHYSIOLOGY

Gracilis or semitendinosis myopathy occurs most often in German shepherd dogs or Belgian shepherds. The cause is unknown, but hypothesized to be either caused by trauma, immune-mediated disease, or is secondary to neuropathy. The musculotendinous junction is consistently thickened and fibrotic. A fibrous band is associated with the caudolateral border of the gracilis muscle. The muscle fibers are replaced with dense fibrous connective tissue, causing a nonpainful lameness. Between 39% and 61% of dogs have bilateral limb involvement.

DIAGNOSIS
Clinical Presentation

Signalment. Gracilis or semitendinosis myopathy occurs in young adult, male German shepherd dogs, and in Belgian shepherds. Traumatic gracilis muscle injuries occur in greyhounds.

History. Usually there is a history of insidious onset of rear limb lameness characterized by an altered gait associated with gracilis or semitendinosis myopathy.

Physical Examination Findings

Dogs with gracilis or semitendinosis myopathy have a shortened stride, a rapid elastic medial rotation of the paw, external rotation of the hock, and internal rotation of the stifle during the mid- to late-swing phase of the stride. The lameness is more pronounced at a trot. Affected muscles are palpable as a distinct taut band and differentiated by the location of origin. Some dogs are painful on muscle palpation. Most dogs exhibit a nonpainful lameness. Abduction of the hip and extension of the stifle and hock may be limited.

Diagnostic Imaging

Radiography is not usually helpful in these cases. Ultrasound examination is typically used to determine the extent and severity of the abnormality.

Laboratory Findings

Consistent laboratory abnormalities are not present.

DIFFERENTIAL DIAGNOSIS

The diagnosis of gracilis or semitendinosis myopathy usually can be made from historical and physical examination findings. Differentials include hip dysplasia, cranial cruciate ligament injury, and neurologic disease.

MEDICAL MANAGEMENT

If muscle trauma is identified early (especially in greyhounds), intermittent rest and ice (15 minutes on, 15 minutes off) may minimize permanent muscle damage. Following acute injury, strengthening and range of motion exercises should be performed while minimizing additional muscle trauma.

Physical Rehabilitation

Physical rehabilitation alone is rarely successful in management of chronic contracture of the hamstring or gracilis muscles; it should be combined with surgery.

SURGICAL TREATMENT

Gait abnormalities observed with gracilis or semitendinosis myopathy can be temporarily reversed by resecting the affected muscles; however, the fibrotic band and subsequent lameness usually recur in 2 to 4 months. When surgery is attempted, it must be combined with aggressive, long-term rehabilitation, particularly during the period of fibrous tissue maturation (approximately 3 to 6 weeks postoperatively).

Preoperative Management

These animals otherwise are generally healthy, and minimal preoperative care is necessary.

Anesthesia

See p. 944 for anesthetic management of animals with orthopedic disease.

Surgical Anatomy

The gracilis muscle originates on the pubic symphysis and inserts along the medial tibial crest, but continues as crural fascia, finally joining with the semitendinosis to contribute to common calcaneal or Achilles tendons, essentially crossing the hip and stifle joints, and inserting on the calcaneus. The semitendinosis muscle originates on the tuber ischium and follows a similar course, inserting on the medial portion of the tibia, continuing as crural fascia and inserting on the tuber calcis. Fibrotic muscle can be palpated before surgery. Affected muscle may be fibrotic throughout its length; more commonly, the distal myotendinous junction of the gracilis muscle is thickened and fibrotic. A thick fibrous band associated with the proximal caudal border of the gracilis may be observed.

Positioning

Clip the rear limb from midline to tarsus and position the animal in dorsal recumbency. Use a hanging-limb technique to facilitate limb manipulation.

SURGICAL TECHNIQUE

Incise the skin directly over the palpated fibrotic band. Expose and isolate the entire muscle and tendon length with sharp dissection. Resect the entire affected muscle to increase joint range of motion.

SUTURE MATERIALS AND SPECIAL INSTRUMENTS

Self-retaining retractors and a periosteal elevator assist tissue retraction and reflection.

POSTOPERATIVE CARE

Postoperative physical rehabilitation is critical if significant fibrosis and contracture are to be prevented. Rehabilitation includes passive range of motion, stretching, and aquatherapy (see Table 34-3 on p. 1326). Use of a temporary cast to maintain limb extension for 8 to 12 hours per day may help in some animals.

PROGNOSIS

Prognosis for gracilis or semitendinosis myopathy is guarded, with recurrence of the fibrosis and restriction of the gait occurring within 4 months in most dogs. Intensive, long-term physical rehabilitation following surgical intervention may improve prognosis.

Suggested Reading

Millis DL, Levine D, Taylor RA: *Canine rehabilitation and physical therapy,* Philadelphia, 2004, Saunders.
This book is a comprehensive guide to physical therapy and rehabilitation for dogs. It has detailed descriptions of rehabilitation techniques and how they are applied for specific diseases.

Moores AP, Comerford EJ, Tarlton JF et al: Biomechanical and clinical evaluation of a modified three-loop pulley suture pattern for reattachment of canine tendons to bone, *Vet Surg* 33:391, 2004.
This paper describes an alternative method for repair of tendon lacerations or avulsions that may be superior to the locking-loop pattern. It may be more appropriate for use in some clinical cases.

CHAPTER 35

Other Diseases of Bones and Joints

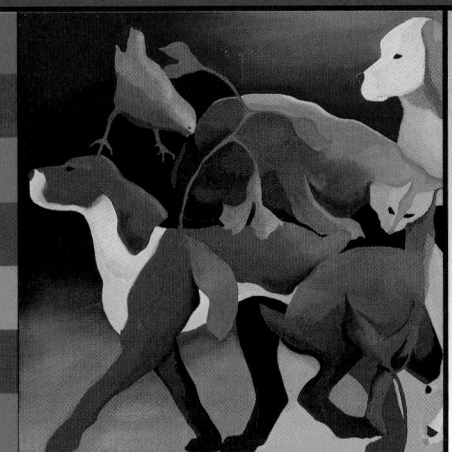

HYPERTROPHIC OSTEOPATHY

DEFINITIONS

Hypertrophic osteopathy is a diffuse periosteal reaction resulting in new bone formation around the metacarpal, metatarsal, and long bones. Synonyms include *pulmonary osteoarthropathy, hypertrophic pulmonary osteoarthropathy,* and *hypertrophic pulmonary osteopathy.*

GENERAL CONSIDERATIONS AND CLINICALLY RELEVANT PATHOPHYSIOLOGY

Hypertrophic osteopathy can affect all four limbs. It can be a paraneoplastic syndrome or can be associated with other diseases (e.g., neoplasia, including primary and metastatic lung tumors, esophageal carcinoma, rhabdomyosarcoma of the bladder, renal transitional cell carcinoma and nephroblastoma; granulomatous lesions; chronic megaesophagus; patent ductus arteriosus; bacterial endocarditis; and heartworm disease) (Anderson et al, 2004; Barrand and Scudamore, 2001; Seaman and Patton, 2003; Watrous and Blumenfeld, 2002). The precise pathophysiology of this disease is unknown. Alterations in pulmonary function have been suggested to increase peripheral blood flow, resulting in connective tissue congestion. The increased peripheral blood flow is thought to be neurally mediated. Periosteum responds by forming new bone on the cortical surfaces of the metacarpal, metatarsal, and long bones. This new bone may appear nodular. Histologically, the affected area is made of bands of new cortical bone that contain small, fibrous marrow spaces.

DIAGNOSIS
Clinical Presentation

Signalment. Any breed or size of dog may be affected; however, because it is most commonly associated with neoplasia, hypertrophic osteopathy is usually seen in older animals. This condition has been reported rarely in cats.

History. Dogs usually are brought in because of lethargy, reluctance to move, and swelling of the distal extremities. Onset of clinical signs may be acute or gradual.

Physical Examination Findings

Affected limbs are warm and swollen. Because this condition is secondary to diseases elsewhere in the body, an effort should be made to determine the underlying etiologic factors. Thorough physical examination is essential when evaluating affected animals.

Diagnostic Imaging

Radiographs of the limbs reveal a uniform periosteal proliferation, which is initially seen on the phalanges, metacarpal, and metatarsal bones (Fig. 35-1). As the disease progresses, periosteal proliferation progresses proximally (i.e., radius/ulna and tibia/fibula). Articular surfaces of long bones usually are spared and appear normal.

Thoracic radiographs are used to identify any underlying pulmonary or mediastinal disease (e.g., primary or metastatic neoplasia, granulomatous lesions, bacterial endocarditis, and heartworm disease). Radiographs and abdominal ultrasonography should also be performed to identify underlying abdominal disease if thoracic disease is not identified.

Laboratory Findings

Results of laboratory analysis usually reflect the underlying disease. Thrombocytosis may occur in some dogs; however, the cause is only poorly understood.

DIFFERENTIAL DIAGNOSIS

This condition should be differentiated from panosteitis and osteochondritis dessicans.

MEDICAL MANAGEMENT

Treatment is aimed at the underlying disease process. Remission of periosteal proliferation may occur after resection of the primary lesion.

PROGNOSIS

Prognosis depends on the possibility for complete resolution of the underlying disease process. If the primary disease can be resolved, the secondary hypertrophic osteopathy often re-

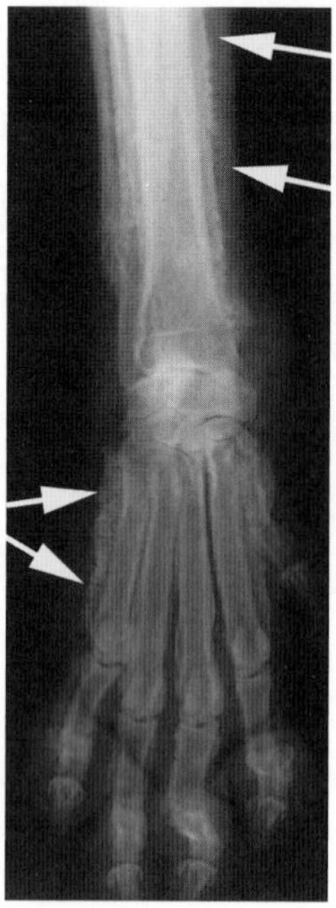

FIG. 35-1
Dorsopalmar view of the forepaw of a dog with hypertrophic osteopathy. Note the periosteal proliferation on the abaxial surfaces of the metacarpal bones and radius and ulna *(arrows)*. Notice that the carpal joints are spared.

solves. Resolution of hypertrophic osteopathy after resection of a renal transitional cell carcinoma that produced granulocyte-macrophage colony-stimulating factor was recently reported in a young bull terrier (Peeters et al, 2001). Although clinical signs often disappear within 1 to 2 weeks after treatment, bone lesions may take months to remodel.

References

Anderson TP, Walker MC, Goring RL: Cardiogenic hypertrophic osteopathy in a dog with right-to-left shunting patent ductus arteriosus, *J Am Vet Med Assoc* 224:1464, 2004.

Barrand KR, Scudamore CL: Canine hypertrophic osteoarthropathy associated with malignant Sertoli cell tumour, *J Small Anim Pract* 42:143, 2001.

Peeters D, Clerxc C, Thiry A et al: Resolution of paraneoplastic leukocytosis and hypertrophic osteopathy after resection of a renal transitional cell carcinoma producing granulocyte-macrophage colony-stimulating factor in a young Bull Terrier, *J Vet Intern Med* 15:407, 2001.

Seaman RL, Patton CS: Treatment of renal nephroblastoma in an adult dog, *J Am Anim Hosp Assoc* 39:76, 2003.

Watrous BJ, Blumenfeld B: Congenital megaesophagus with hypertrophic osteopathy in a 6-year-old dog, *Vet Radiol Ultrasound* 43:545, 2002.

PANOSTEITIS

DEFINITIONS

Panosteitis is a disease of young dogs that causes lameness, bone pain, endosteal bone production, and occasionally subperiosteal bone production. Synonyms include *enostosis, eosinophilic panosteitis, juvenile osteomyelitis,* and *osteomyelitis of young German shepherd dogs.*

GENERAL CONSIDERATIONS AND CLINICALLY RELEVANT PATHOPHYSIOLOGY

Panosteitis is an idiopathic entity that causes endosteal and periosteal new bone formation. Osseous compartment syndrome due to a protein-rich, high-calorie diet has more recently been proposed as a potential cause. Excessive protein may cause intraosseous edema and secondary increased medullary pressure and ischemia (Schawalder et al, 2002). Although some periosteal new bone is often evident, the predominant change is endosteal bone formation as the marrow is invaded by bone trabeculae. The marrow remains highly cellular with varying degrees of fibrosis, and there is no evidence of chronic inflammation, acute infection, or malignancy.

DIAGNOSIS
Clinical Presentation

Signalment. Panosteitis predominantly affects male (80%), large-breed dogs. Young dogs (less than 2 years of age) are most commonly affected; however, older dogs have occasionally been diagnosed with this disease.

History. The hallmark of panosteitis is shifting leg lameness associated with pain on deep bone palpation. Although initial episodes of panosteitis may present as acute lameness in a single limb, typically there is a history of chronic, intermittent, shifting leg lameness.

Physical Examination

Affected dogs are commonly lame in only a single limb. Firm palpation of affected long bones usually elicits pain.

Diagnostic Imaging

Radiographic signs of panosteitis are progressive. Radiographs of affected limbs are often normal during early stages, and clinical signs may precede radiographic abnormalities by up to 10 days. If clinical signs are consistent with panosteitis but radiographs are normal, radiographs should be repeated in 7 to 10 days. Nuclear scintigraphy is a more sensitive diagnostic test of panosteitis than radiographs. In a recent study of bone scintigraphy in 14 dogs with occult lameness, scintigraphy was found to be highly sensitive and relatively specific for localization and characterization or exclusion of skeletal lesions in most dogs (Schwarz et al, 2004). The earliest radiographic signs are a widening of the nutrient foramen and blurring and accentuation of trabecular patterns (which are often difficult to identify except in retrospect), followed by appearance of radiopaque, patchy, or mottled bone within medullary canals (Fig. 35-2). Eventually, remodeling of medullary canals occurs and cortical thickening may remain as the only residual finding.

Laboratory Findings

Consistent laboratory abnormalities are not present.

DIFFERENTIAL DIAGNOSIS

Panosteitis must be differentiated from other orthopedic diseases of large, immature dogs (i.e., osteochondritis dissecans, fragmented coronoid process, and ununited anconeal

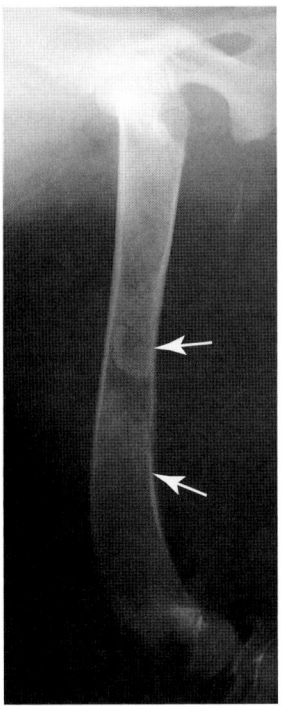

FIG. 35-2
Lateral radiograph of the femur of an immature dog with panosteitis. Note the areas of increased opacity within the medullary canal *(arrows)*.

process in forelimbs; and hip dysplasia and osteochondritis of rear limbs). When radiographic evidence of panosteitis and other orthopedic diseases is present concurrently, panosteitis is usually assumed to be causing the acute clinical signs.

> NOTE: Panosteitis has the best prognosis of all juvenile orthopedic diseases.

MEDICAL TREATMENT

The disease is self-limiting, so treatment consists of controlling pain. Nonsteroidal antiinflammatory drugs (NSAIDs) (see Table 33-4 on p. 1149) are usually administered during acute episodes of lameness. Exercise restriction is recommended when the animal is lame. Owners should be warned of the likelihood of recurrence, but the long-term prognosis is excellent for complete recovery.

SURGICAL TREATMENT

Surgical treatment of panosteitis is not indicated.

PROGNOSIS

The disease is self-limiting and most animals eventually have normal function of affected limbs without evidence of pain. However, the disease may continue to affect different limbs, causing pain and lameness until the dog reaches maturity. Clinical signs rarely persist after maturity.

> NOTE: Advise owners that panosteitis may recur, but it usually resolves by the time the dog is 2 years of age.

References

Schawalder P, Andres HU, Jutzi K et al: Canine panosteitis: an idiopathic bone disease investigated in the light of a new hypothesis concerning the pathogenesis. Part 1: clinical and diagnostic aspects, *Schweiz Arch Tierheilkd* 144:115, 2002.

Schwarz T, Johnson VS, Voute L et al: Bone scintigraphy in the investigation of occult lameness in the dog, *J Small Anim Pract* 45:232, 2004.

CRANIOMANDIBULAR OSTEOPATHY

DEFINITIONS

Craniomandibular osteopathy *(mandibular periostitis, lion's jaw)* is a proliferative bone disease of immature dogs involving the occipital bones, tympanic bullae, and mandibular rami.

GENERAL CONSIDERATIONS AND CLINICALLY RELEVANT PATHOPHYSIOLOGY

The cause of craniomandibular osteopathy is unknown. It is most often recognized in West Highland white terriers, cairn terriers, and Scottish terriers. A genetic predisposition is suspected in many breeds; in West Highland white terriers it is thought to have an autosomal recessive inheritance pattern. A similar syndrome (calvarial hyperostotic syndrome) has been reported in bullmastiffs (McConnell et al, 2006). Craniomandibular osteopathy has been associated with canine leukocyte adhesion deficiency in Irish setters (Trowald-Wigh et al, 2000). A link to canine distemper virus has been postulated but is not supported by epidemiologic studies.

Proliferation of new, coarse, trabecular bone occurs adjacent to the mandibular rami, occipital bones, and tympanic bullae in affected animals. This new bone formation causes irregular enlargement of mandibles and tympanic bullae. Existing lamellar bone is resorbed by osteoclasis and replaced with new bone that expands beyond the periosteal borders. Osteoclastic destruction of the original lamellar bone is accompanied by invasion of inflammatory cells (i.e., neutrophils, lymphocytes, and plasma cells). Normal bone marrow is lost as it is replaced with a vascular fibrous stroma. This proliferative stage of disease occurs when the dog is approximately 5 to 7 months old and is accompanied by intermittent fever, discomfort when eating, and pain when the mouth is forced open. Owners should be warned that multiple relapses may occur; however, bone proliferation decreases as dogs reach maturity and physes close.

DIAGNOSIS
Clinical Presentation

Signalment. Although young West Highland white terriers, cairn terriers, and Scottish terriers are most commonly affected, this disease has been sporadically reported in other breeds (see previous discussion). Clinical signs are usually

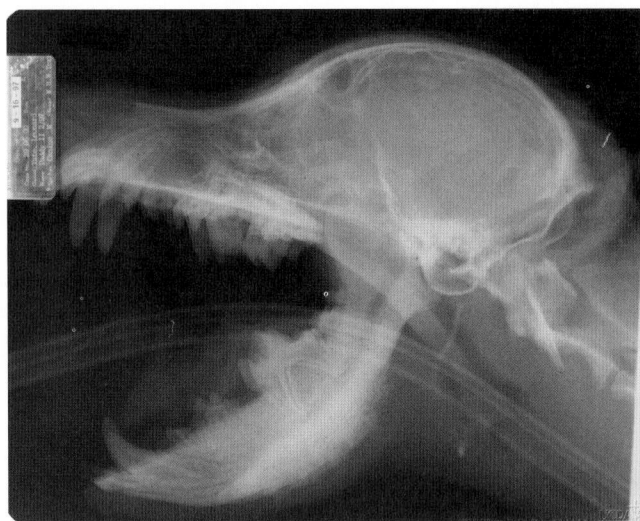

FIG. 35-3
Lateral radiograph of the skull of a dog with craniomandibular osteopathy. Note the areas of periosteal proliferation.

first noted when the dog is 3 to 8 months of age. Males and females are equally affected. There is no seasonal distribution. Calvarial hyperostosis syndrome has typically been considered to be a disease of male bullmastiffs (Pastor et al, 2000); however, a recent report describes this condition in two female bullmastiffs (McConnell et al, 2006).

History. Owners often note that the animal is reluctant to eat, drools, and has trouble chewing food. Pain is often evident when the mouth is opened.

Physical Examination Findings

Affected dogs have bilaterally enlarged mandibles and tympanic bullae. In severe cases, fusion of these structures may occur, preventing the jaws from being fully opened. Pain on opening of the mouth and intermittent fever (body temperature reading of up to 104° F for 3 to 4 days) may be observed.

Diagnostic Imaging

Skull radiographs reveal increased irregular bone density of the caudal mandibles (84% of cases), including tympanic bullae (51% of cases) (Fig. 35-3). Sometimes lesions are confined to the mandibles (33% of cases) and occasionally they are confined to the base of the skull (13% of cases). The calvarium may also be thickened. As dogs reach maturity, edges of the new bone become smooth and affected areas shrink.

Laboratory Findings

Specific laboratory abnormalities are not seen. Blood cultures are negative.

DIFFERENTIAL DIAGNOSIS

Craniomandibular osteopathy must be differentiated from infections (i.e., abscesses or osteomyelitis) that may cause similar signs.

MEDICAL MANAGEMENT

Analgesics (see Table 33-4 on p. 1149) should be given to control pain until the animal reaches maturity. Severely debilitated animals that cannot open their mouths enough to eat solid foods require oral fluid nourishment. Although antibiotics and corticosteroids are often administered during febrile episodes, they will not alter disease progression.

SURGICAL TREATMENT

Surgical therapy is not indicated. Surgical resection of bone bridging the mandible and tympanic bullae in dogs with severely restricted jaw motion has been unsuccessful; however, rostral mandibulectomy may allow the dog to lap gruel. Affected dogs should not be used for breeding purposes.

PROGNOSIS

The prognosis is guarded until the extent of bone production is known (i.e., at maturity). Excessive bone production, leading to fusion of mandibular and tympanic bullae, can restrict mandibular motion sufficiently to prevent dogs from eating. These animals are often euthanized.

NOTE: Warn owners that multiple relapses may occur until maturity.

References

Pastor KF, Boulay JP, Schelling SH et al: Idiopathic hyperostosis of the calvaria in five young bullmastiffs, *J Am Anim Hosp Assoc* 36:439, 2000.

McConnell JF, Hayes A, Platt SR et al: Calvarial hyperostosis syndrome in two bullmastiffs, *Vet Radiol Ultrasound* 47:72, 2006.

Trowald-Wigh G, Ekman S, Hannson K et al: Clinical, radiological, and pathological features of 12 Irish setters with canine leukocyte adhesion deficiency, *J Small Anim Pract* 41:211, 2000.

HYPERTROPHIC OSTEODYSTROPHY

DEFINITIONS

Hypertrophic osteodystrophy is a disease that causes disruption of metaphyseal trabeculae in long bones of young, rapidly growing dogs. Synonyms include *skeletal scurvy, canine scurvy, Moeller-Barlow disease, osteodystrophy Types I and II, metaphyseal osteopathy,* and *metaphyseal dysplasia.*

GENERAL CONSIDERATIONS AND CLINICALLY RELEVANT PATHOPHYSIOLOGY

The cause of hypertrophic osteodystrophy is unknown. Proposed etiologic factors include vitamin C deficiency, oversupplementation of dietary calcium, and infectious organisms. A link to canine distemper virus has been postulated but is not supported by epidemiologic studies. Experimentally, vaccination protocols have been associated with development of hypertrophic osteodystrophy in Weimeraner puppies (Harrus et al, 2002). The pathogenesis is obscure, but an apparent disturbance of metaphyseal blood supply leads to changes in the physis and adjacent metaphyseal bone, causing delayed ossification of the physeal hypertrophic zone. The acute phase lasts about 7 to 10 days. Affected animals show signs ranging from mild lameness to anorexia, pyrexia, lethargy, severe lameness, refusal to rise, and generalized weight loss. Clinical signs may wax and wane.

> NOTE: Affected animals may be very ill and require intense supportive care.

Grossly the metaphyseal regions of long bones are widened with perimetaphyseal soft tissue swelling. A line of separation of metaphyseal trabeculae is present parallel to the growth plate. Histologic microfractures of trabeculae are evident and surrounded by inflammatory cells and necrosis. Failure of bone deposition on the calcified cartilage lattice of metaphyseal bone is evident.

DIAGNOSIS
Clinical Presentation

Signalment. This disease affects young, rapidly growing, large-breed dogs, with males affected more often than females. Clinical signs are usually first noted at 3 to 4 months of age; however, they may occur as early as 2 months. Relapses may occur as late as 8 months of age. The highest incidence is in the fall. Weimeraners may be at an increased risk (LaFond et al, 2002).

History. An acute onset of lameness is often reported, and puppies may be so severely affected that they refuse to walk. Inappetence and lethargy are commonly reported by owners. A history of recent diarrhea may precede the onset of lameness.

Physical Examination Findings

Findings on physical examination range from mild lameness to severe lameness affecting all four limbs. More severely affected animals are often unable to stand or walk. Long bone metaphyses are swollen, warm, and painful on palpation. Swelling is often present in all four limbs; however, forelimb swelling may be more obvious, especially in distal radial metaphyses. Severely affected dogs may be depressed, anorexic, and pyrexic (body temperature of up to 106° F).

Diagnostic Imaging

Radiographs of affected long bones reveal an irregular radiolucent zone in the metaphysis, parallel and proximal to the physis. This gives the appearance of a double physeal line. Metaphyseal flaring with increased bone opacity occurs because of periosteal proliferation in later stages of the disease. This reaction subsides with time, but may leave a permanently widened metaphysis (Fig. 35-4).

Laboratory Findings

Laboratory abnormalities are not usually found. Hypocalcemia has been noted in a few affected dogs, but its significance is unknown. Bacteremia has rarely been reported in association with hypertrophic osteodystrophy.

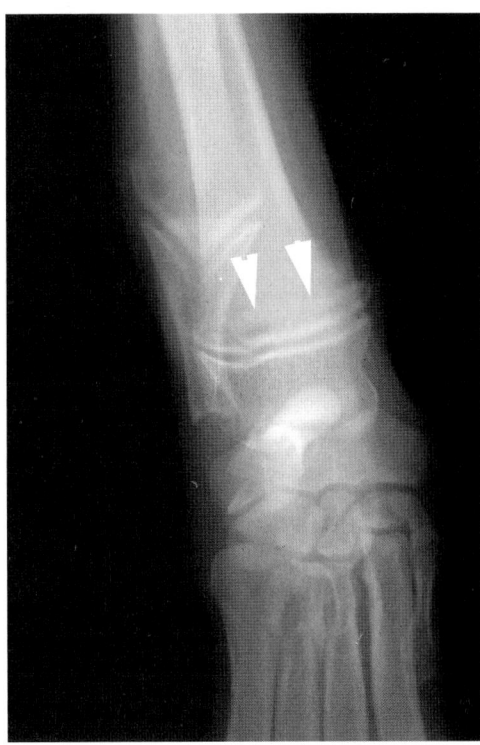

FIG. 35-4
Radiograph of the distal radius and ulna of a dog with hypertrophic osteodystrophy. There is a parallel lucency proximal and adjacent to the physis, which is typical of this disease.

DIFFERENTIAL DIAGNOSIS

This condition should be differentiated from septic arthritis, septic physitis, and panosteitis.

MEDICAL MANAGEMENT

Analgesics should be administered to control pain (see Table 33-4 on p. 1149). Occasionally, severely debilitated animals require fluid support. Corticosteroids, antibiotics, and vitamin C have been administered, but have not proven effective in shortening the disease's course or severity. Bacteremia should be ruled out before corticosteroids are administered.

PROGNOSIS

Most animals recover fully within 7 to 10 days of the onset of clinical signs; however, multiple relapses may occur. Occasionally, severe debilitation or multiple, severe relapses cause owners to request that affected animals be euthanized. Interference with normal physeal development may cause permanent deformity of long bones.

> NOTE: Warn owners that multiple relapses may occur.

References:

Harrus S, Waner T, Aizenberg SN et al: Development of hypertrophic osteodystrophy and antibody response in a litter of vaccinated Weimaraner puppies, *J Small Anim Pract* 43:27, 2002.

LaFond E, Bruer GJ, Austin CC: Breed susceptibility for developmental orthopedic diseases in dogs, *J Am Anim Hosp Assoc* 38:467, 2002.

BONE NEOPLASIA

DEFINITIONS

Primary bone neoplasia arises from cells located within the bone structure. Soft-tissue tumors that spread to bone (metastatic bone tumors) may occur in either the **appendicular skeleton** (i.e., long bones) or **axial skeleton** (skull, vertebrae, ribs, and pelvis).

GENERAL CONSIDERATIONS AND CLINICALLY RELEVANT PATHOPHYSIOLOGY

Primary bone tumors include osteosarcoma, chondrosarcoma, fibrosarcoma, hemangiosarcoma, giant cell tumor, liposarcoma, periosteal osteosarcoma, periosteal fibrosarcoma, parosteal osteosarcoma, osteomas, multilobular osteoma, multilobular chondroma, osteochondroma, and chondroma. Accurate diagnosis of a primary bone tumor requires that an established protocol be followed (i.e., history taking, physical examination, hematologic and serum biochemical evaluation, radiographic examination, and biopsy for histologic evaluation). Primary tumors of the appendicular skeleton most commonly arise in the distal radial metaphysis, proximal humerus, proximal or distal femur, and proximal or distal tibia. Benign bone tumors (e.g., osteoma, ossifying fibroma, multilobular osteomas and chondromas, osteochondromas, enchondromas, and chondromas) are generally slow growing. Depending on tumor accessibility, complete surgical excision of benign bone tumors is usually curative.

> NOTE: Primary bone tumors can be malignant or benign and must be accurately diagnosed for appropriate treatment.

Osteosarcoma is the most common primary bone neoplasm, accounting for approximately 85% of skeletal malignancies; 75% of osteosarcomas originate in the appendicular skeleton (Tables 35-1 and 35-2). Metastasis is common and usually occurs early in the course of disease. Although fewer than 5% of affected dogs have radiographically detectable thoracic metastases at presentation, 90% die or are euthanized within 1 year of diagnosis because of complications associated with pulmonary metastasis. Improved chances for survival are possible with amputation or limb-sparing procedures combined with chemotherapy (e.g., cisplatin).

> NOTE: Osteosarcomas arise most commonly in the metaphyses of the proximal humerus, distal radius, and distal femur.

Osteosarcoma is also the most common tumor of the axial skeleton. Of 116 axial osteosarcomas evaluated, the most common sites of occurrence were mandible (27%), maxilla (22%), spine (15%), cranium (14%), ribs (10%), nasal cavity and paranasal sinuses (9%), and pelvis (6%) (Dernell et al, 2001). Because osteosarcoma is the most commonly diagnosed bone tumor, it is used as the model for evaluation, diagnosis, treatment, and prognosis of bone tumors in this section. Although the workup needed to diagnose neoplasia is similar for all bone tumors, treatment and prognosis vary depending on tumor type (see Tables 35-1 and 35-2).

Extraskeletal osteosarcoma occurs rarely in spleen, mammary glands, gastrointestinal tract, lung, skin, and other sites, without a primary bone lesion. This tumor generally occurs more often in smaller and older dogs. The tumor will metastasize and outcome is generally poor, but may be improved with chemotherapy.

Histologically, osteosarcoma is composed of anaplastic mesenchymal cells that produce osteoid. Histologic subgroups include osteoblastic, fibroblastic, osteoclastic, poorly differentiated, and telangiectatic osteosarcoma. An inflammatory component is often present in fracture-associated sarcoma (i.e., sarcomas that arise in the diaphysis of a long bone at the site of a previous fracture), reflecting altered healing patterns and chronic inflammation associated with these tumors.

The cause of osteosarcoma is unknown. A viral cause is proposed but is currently considered unlikely. Osteosarcoma has been associated with fractures and metallic implants (Boudrieau et al, 2005) and may also occur within radiation fields following radiation treatment of soft-tissue sarcomas. Current studies are investigating potential molecular and genetic causes of osteosarcoma.

DIAGNOSIS
Clinical Presentation

Signalment. Large- and giant-breed dogs have the greatest incidence of appendicular bone neoplasia. The median age of dogs with osteosarcoma is 7 years. Males are more commonly affected than females. Primary bone tumors of the axial skeleton are most common in medium-sized and large-breed dogs. The median age of affected animals is 8.7 years. Osteosarcoma is the most common feline primary bone tumor, primarily affecting older (i.e., 10 years mean age) cats.

History. Dogs with primary bone neoplasia affecting the appendicular skeleton are usually brought in because of lameness and/or localized limb swelling. Pathologic fracture may cause acute lameness. Dogs with primary bone tumors of the axial skeleton usually have pain, reluctance to eat or walk, visible swelling, and/or bleeding from tumor surfaces. Clinical signs may be acute or chronic and progressive.

Physical Examination Findings

Dogs with appendicular tumors are often lame. The limb may be enlarged and firm; cutaneous fistulae are rarely present. Systemic signs of illness (e.g., fever, anorexia, and weight

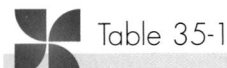 Table 35-1

Malignant Bone Neoplasia in Dogs

TUMOR	INCIDENCE	METASTASIS	TREATMENT	PROGNOSIS
Osteosarcoma of the appendicular skeleton	75% of all bone tumors	High rate of early metastasis to lungs and soft tissue; bone metastasis is a late complication	Amputation and chemotherapy with cisplatin and/or doxorubicin Limb sparing in selected cases Palliative radiation therapy for painful bone lesions	Mean survival time with amputation alone is 12 to 16 wk, median survival time with limb sparing or amputation plus cisplatin and doxorubicin is about 300 to 400 days
Osteosarcoma of the axial skeleton	Less common than appendicular tumors	Highly metastatic, local recurrence except for mandible, which is slower to metastasize	Local resection of tumor (i.e., mandible and rib) Cisplatin, local radiation as adjunct to surgery to reduce local recurrence	Median survival time is 22 wk, 1-yr survival is 26.3%, rate of tumor recurrence is 66.7%
Fibrosarcoma	<5% of bone tumors	Slower to metastasize than osteosarcoma	Amputation (chemotherapy not of proven benefit) Limb sparing in select cases	Poor prognosis (but complete excision of low-grade tumors without metastases may be curative)
Chondrosarcoma	5%–10% of bone tumors	Slow to metastasize	Amputation (chemotherapy not of proven benefit)	May be good after amputation or resection of lesion
Hemangiosarcoma	<5% of bone tumors	May be multicentric, often involves spleen and right atrium, highly metastatic	Amputation (chemotherapy not of proven benefit) Limb sparing in select cases	Poor prognosis because of multiple organ involvement, mean survival time less than 5 mo
Giant cell tumor	Rare	Metastasis to lymph nodes, lung, and bones	Amputation	Poor prognosis
Liposarcoma	Rare	Metastasis to lung, liver, and lymph nodes	Amputation or local resection	Poor prognosis
Fracture-associated sarcoma	Uncommon, associated with fractures in which healing has been complicated; represents 5% of osteosarcomas	Metastasis has occurred in 14% of reported cases	Amputation Limb sparing techniques Chemotherapy	Same as osteosarcoma

loss) are uncommon in acute stages of disease. Tumors of the axial skeleton are often palpable as firm swellings. Tumors affecting the vertebral column may cause acute signs of lameness or paralysis. Respiratory abnormalities associated with pulmonary metastasis may be noted in some animals.

NOTE: Lameness is often the first sign of appendicular bone tumors.

Diagnostic Imaging

Radiographs of affected bones and the thorax should be evaluated. Radiographic signs of osteosarcoma include cortical and trabecular bone lysis, periosteal bone proliferation, and soft-tissue swelling (Fig. 35-5). Thoracic radiographs should include a dorsoventral or ventrodorsal view and both lateral recumbent views (i.e., right bones left lateral views). These radiographs should be carefully evaluated for evidence of tumor metastasis. Alternatively, contrast enhanced

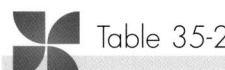

Table 35-2

Malignant Bone Neoplasia in Cats

TUMOR	INCIDENCE	METASTASIS	TREATMENT	PROGNOSIS
Osteosarcoma	Most common primary bone tumor in cats (70%–80%)	Metastasis is uncommon	Amputation, radiation therapy, or excision of skull tumors	Median survival time is 12–50 mo; 12-mo median survival with appendicular osteosarcoma
Fibrosarcoma	Rare, more often due to secondary invasion of bone from soft tissue	Incidence is unknown	Amputation	Long disease-free intervals reported (e.g., 10 to 18 mo)
Chondrosarcoma	4% of bone tumors, reported in the scapula	Incidence is unknown	Amputation	Prognosis guarded
Squamous cell carcinoma	Local bone invasion, occurs in oral cavity, orbit, and digits	See section on oral tumors	Amputation, mandibulectomy, maxillectomy, ± radiation therapy, see section on oral tumors	See section on oral tumors
Multiple cartilaginous exostosis (osteochondromatosis)	Uncommon, usually FeLV positive, benign physeal lesion in dogs	Multiple sites common; scapula, vertebra, mandible in cats, physeal in dogs	Palliative removal of painful lesions	Guarded in cats (favorable in dogs)

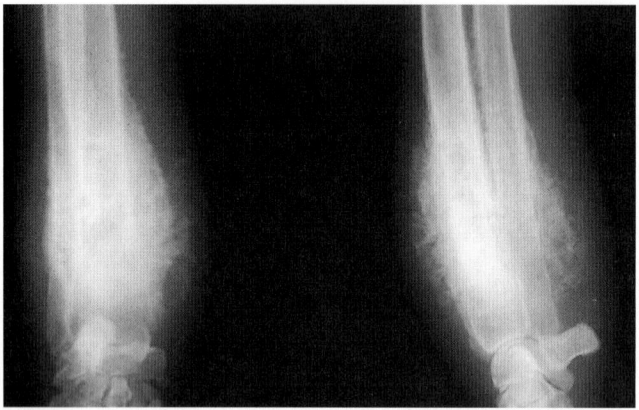

FIG. 35-5
Radiographs of a distal radius of a dog with osteosarcoma. Note the cortical lysis, periosteal proliferation, and soft-tissue swelling.

computed tomography (CT) of the thorax can replace survey radiographs; CT is more sensitive than radiography in detecting small metastatic lesions. Although radiographic signs associated with osteosarcoma cannot be differentiated from those associated with fungal osteomyelitis, coupling radiographic signs with signalment and history can help determine whether neoplasia should be considered likely.

Ultimately, histopathology is necessary for confirmation. If limb-sparing surgery is being considered, magnetic resonance imaging (MRI) should be used to determine the extent of the disease (Wallack et al, 2002).

Bone scintigraphy may help identify multifocal bone lesions in dogs with neoplasia. Osteosarcoma rarely affects multiple bones; however, metastatic lesions have been identified on scintigraphy at initial diagnosis (Janowski et al, 2003). Scintigraphy may also be indicated when other forms of cancer (i.e., multiple myeloma and metastatic bone cancer) are suspected. Nuclear scintigraphy tends to overestimate tumor margins for limb-sparing procedures (Leibman et al, 2001); however, this may be beneficial in that it may ensure more complete tumor excision.

> NOTE: Three view thoracic radiography or contrast enhanced CT is essential to evaluate for pulmonary or thoracic wall metastases.

Laboratory Findings

There are no laboratory abnormalities consistently found with primary or metastatic bone neoplasia. Preoperative findings of elevated total serum alkaline phosphatase and bone isoenzyme of serum alkaline phosphatase are associated with shortened survival and disease-free intervals. A decrease in bone isoenzyme of alkaline phosphatase activity after surgery may be associated with a longer survival times and disease-free intervals.

Fine needle aspiration and cytology may be suggestive of bone neoplasia in a large percentage of cases. Ultrasound guidance may aid in identifying areas of bone lysis, enabling easier aspiration. Cytology of fine needle aspirates may provide adequate evidence of primary bone tumor to initiate treatment; however, definitive diagnosis of bone neoplasia necessitates histologic evaluation of samples obtained by biopsy or excision. Successful identification of a tumor requires that biopsy samples are obtained accurately and that a pathologist accustomed to interpreting bone samples performs the histologic evaluation. Multiple samples should be obtained to increase diagnostic accuracy. Closed trephine biopsy (see p. 1347) from the center of the radiographic lesion is more accurate than biopsy of transitional zones between tumor and normal bone (Dernell et al, 2001). The latter biopsies are more commonly interpreted as reactive bone. Using fluoroscopy or other advanced imaging techniques to choose the biopsy site increases chances of optimal, diagnostic biopsies. Alternatively, radiographs obtained after biopsy can be used to confirm biopsy location.

DIFFERENTIAL DIAGNOSIS

Suspected primary neoplastic lesions must be differentiated from bacterial osteomyelitis, fungal osteomyelitis, metastatic bone tumor (i.e., prostatic carcinoma), direct extension of soft-tissue tumors (i.e., nail bed carcinomas), hypertrophic pulmonary osteopathy, bone infarcts, hypervitaminosis A, periosteal response to trauma, and aneurysmal bone cysts.

MEDICAL MANAGEMENT

Multiple modality treatment (e.g., amputation and chemotherapy) has extended the life span of dogs with osteosarcoma to a median of 300 days with a 40% 1-year survival (Chun et al, 2005; Kent et al, 2004). Adjunctive chemotherapy usually involves administration of cisplatin, carboplatinum, or doxorubicin immediately after amputation. There are numerous protocols for administering one or a combination of these drugs. Adverse side effects of cisplatin therapy (i.e., renal damage, nausea, vomiting, anorexia, and bone marrow suppression) are potentially life-threatening and necessitate that animals be carefully monitored during treatment. Adverse side effects of doxorubicin may involve bone marrow suppression, vomiting, nausea, anorexia, and cardiac toxicity. Extravasation of doxorubicin outside of the vein can cause catastrophic tissue destruction. Complete blood count (CBC), platelet count, blood urea nitrogen (BUN), serum creatinine, and urine specific gravity should be assessed often. In cases in which tumor resection is not possible, palliative radiation treatment may diminish pain (Mueller et al, 2005). Recently, bisphosphonates have also been used to help diminish bone pain associated with osteosarcoma (Fan et al, 2005; Milner et al, 2004). Readers are referred to a medicine text for additional information regarding medical treatment of osteosarcoma.

SURGICAL TREATMENT

Treatment of appendicular bone tumors involves limb amputation (see p. 1342) or tumor resection combined with limb salvage techniques and chemotherapy (see p. 1349). Maxillary and mandibular tumors are treated by mandibulectomy (see p. 343) or maxillectomy (see p. 342), plus appropriate chemotherapy or radiation therapy. Spinal tumors can occasionally be treated with *en bloc* resection, but the procedure is difficult. Tumors of the ribs are treated with *en bloc* resection.

> NOTE: Dogs with severe concurrent orthopedic disease may have difficulty ambulating after amputation; they should be evaluated carefully before amputation.

Preoperative Management

Thorough physical examinations should be performed to identify concurrent problems that might interfere with anesthesia. Limb amputation involves loss of a large amount of tissue, fluid, electrolytes, and red blood cells. Animals should be well hydrated before surgery, and adequate fluids should be administered during surgery. Broad-spectrum antibiotics should be administered perioperatively, particularly during mandibulectomy, maxillectomy, and limb-sparing techniques (see p. 1349).

> NOTE: Perioperative fluid management is essential during limb amputation.

Anesthesia

Bone biopsy, amputation, and limb-sparing techniques are performed under general anesthesia (see p. 944 for suggested protocols). In patients undergoing amputation, analgesia may be provided via a brachial plexus block (see p. 137) or stump injections using bupivacaine and/or with an epidural (see p. 945).

Surgical Anatomy

Surgical anatomy varies with tumor location. Refer to the appropriate bone for an anatomic description.

Positioning

For bone biopsy, scapulectomy, forelimb amputation, rear leg amputation, and limb sparing, the animal is usually positioned in lateral recumbency with the affected leg uppermost. A wide area around the proposed biopsy site is clipped and prepped for aseptic surgery. For the other procedures, the leg is prepped from the dorsal and ventral midline to the foot.

SURGICAL TECHNIQUE
Bone Biopsy

Either a Michele trephine or Jamshidi bone marrow biopsy needle can be used to obtain a bone biopsy. Michele trephines obtain a larger sample of bone; however, there may be

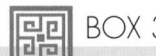

BOX 35-1

Important Considerations for Bone Biopsy

- Obtain samples from the radiographic center of tumors.
- Obtain multiple samples.
- Take radiographs after biopsy to confirm biopsy site.
- Using Jamshidi needles may reduce the risk of pathologic fracture.
- Have pathologists experienced in evaluating bone biopsies perform histology.

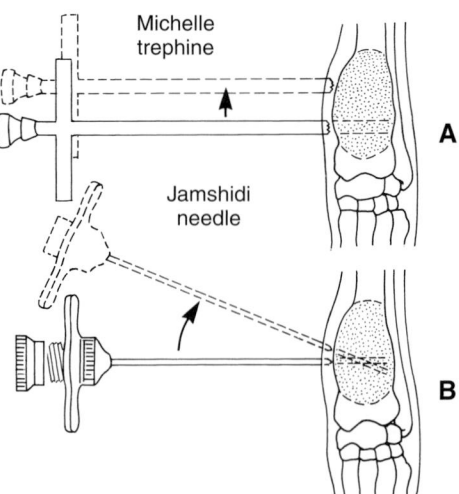

FIG. 35-6
Bone biopsy may be performed with a Michele trephine **(A)** or a Jamshidi needle **(B)**.

an increased risk of fracture through the biopsy site (Box 35-1). Jamshidi needles secure a smaller sample that may decrease the risk of pathologic fracture after biopsy. Accurate diagnoses can be obtained with either technique in greater than 80% of cases.

NOTE: If limb sparing is a goal, take care in locating the biopsy tract in an area that can be easily removed with surgical resection of the tumor. If possible, the same surgeon doing the limb-sparing procedure should also perform the biopsy.

If appropriate, locate the optimal site for biopsy by examining the leg under fluoroscopy while sticking a hypodermic needle into the skin to mark the spot. Once the desired spot for biopsy has been located, make a small skin incision. In large lesions, the incision may be made over the center of the lesion. Locate the skin incision so that biopsy tracts that may be seeded with tumor cells during the biopsy can be removed during the definitive treatment procedure (position the biopsy tract so that it does not interfere with skin flaps developed to cover the amputated bone end, should amputation be necessary). Push the trephine or needle through soft tissue to the bone cortex. Remove the stylet, and advance the trephine or cannula through the bone. Remove the cannula and push the specimen out by inserting the probe into the front opening. Repeat the procedure to obtain multiple specimens (Fig. 35-6).

Amputation

Occasionally, tumors involve only the scapula, so total or partial scapulectomy can be performed. This procedure spares the limb and allows fair to good limb function. Forelimb amputation may be performed by removing the scapula, or alternately, the limb can be removed by disarticulation at the shoulder joint or by resecting the distal humerus. Scapular removal (forequarter amputation) is often preferred because it eliminates the need to cut through bone and is cosmetic because the potential for unsightly muscular atrophy around the scapular spine is eliminated. Midhumeral amputation involves transection of only three tendinous insertions of muscles. The technique can be used for dogs or

cats with neoplasia involving bones of the distal extremities (distal to the elbow).

Rear limb amputation may be performed at the midfemoral diaphysis, or by disarticulating the coxofemoral joint. When tumors affect the femur, the coxofemoral joint should be disarticulated and the entire femur removed. Tumors involving the coxofemoral joint or pelvis require hemipelvectomy. After amputation, the entire tumor should be resubmitted for histologic evaluation to confirm the diagnosis.

Scapulectomy. *Make a skin incision from several centimeters dorsal to the dorsal border of the scapula, over the scapular spine, to the middle third of the humerus (Fig. 35-7, A). Transect superficial muscles (i.e., omotransversarius and trapezius muscles) (Fig. 35-7, B). Maintain a 2- to 3-cm margin between the tumor and site of muscle transection. Expose the medial scapular surface by transecting the rhomboideus muscle (Fig. 35-7, C). Transect the serratus at a point 2 to 3 cm from the tumor margin (Fig. 35-7, D). Protect the brachial plexus and axillary artery and vein during dissection. Transect the suprascapular and subscapular nerves. Transect the teres major and long head of the triceps muscles from their origins on the caudal border of the scapula (Fig. 35-7, E). Transect the coracobrachialis tendon, teres minor, infraspinatus, supraspinatus, and subscapularis muscles close to their humeral origin (Fig. 35-7, F). Incise the joint capsule. Osteotomize the supraglenoid tubercle and remove the scapula (Fig. 35-7, G). To close the wound, suture the tendon origin of the biceps brachii muscle to the joint capsule. Attach the free muscle flaps to adjacent musculature. Suture subcutaneous tissue and skin. Perform partial scapulectomy similarly, but osteotomize the scapula proximal to the scapular notch.*

Forequarter amputation. *Make a skin incision from the dorsal border of the scapula, over the scapular spine,*

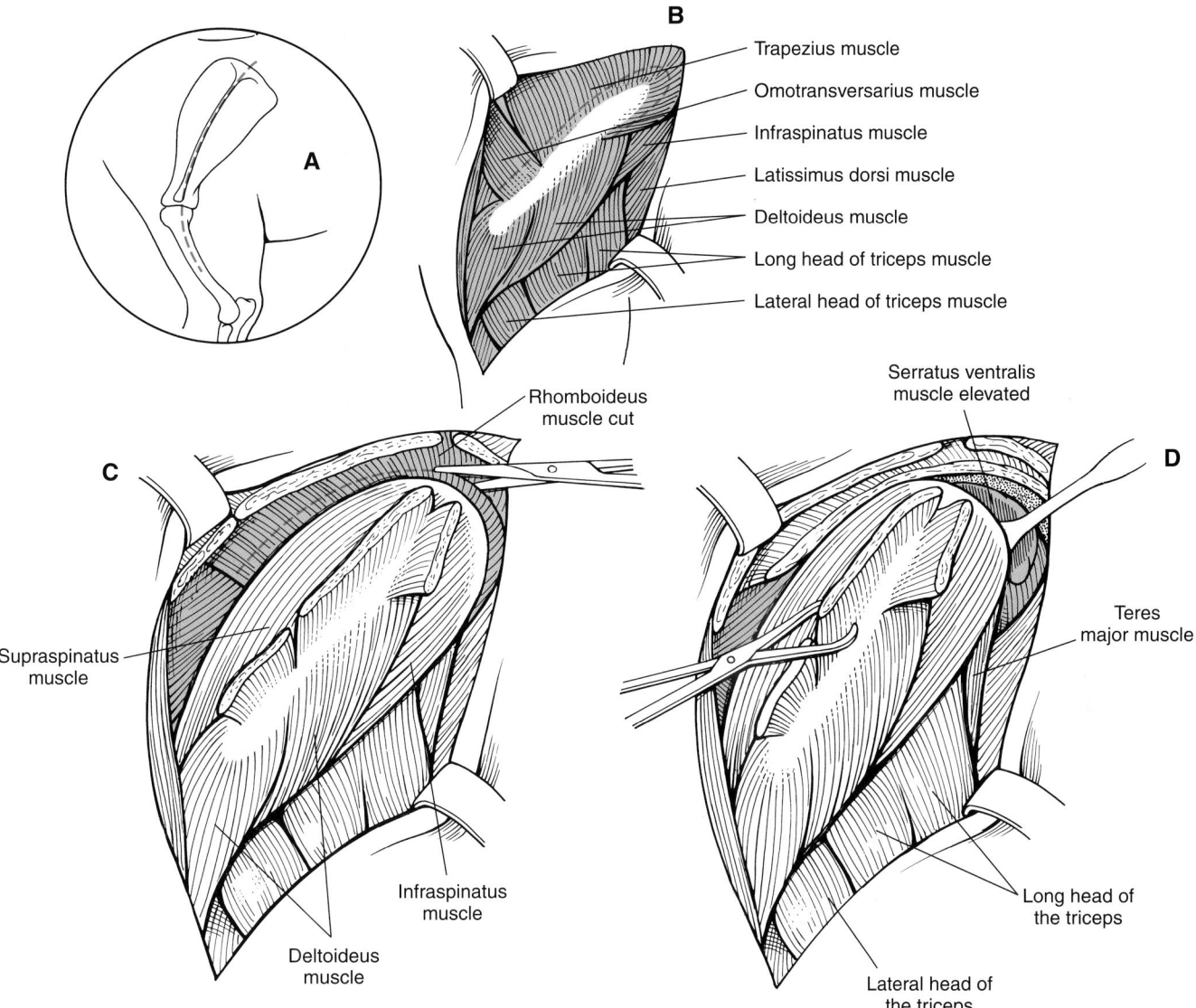

FIG. 35-7
A, For scapulectomy, make a skin incision several centimeters dorsal to the dorsal border of the scapula, over the scapular spine, to the middle third of the humerus. **B,** Transect the omotransversarius, trapezius. **C,** Transect the rhomboideus muscles. **D,** Elevate the serratus ventralis muscle from the scapula.   *Continued*

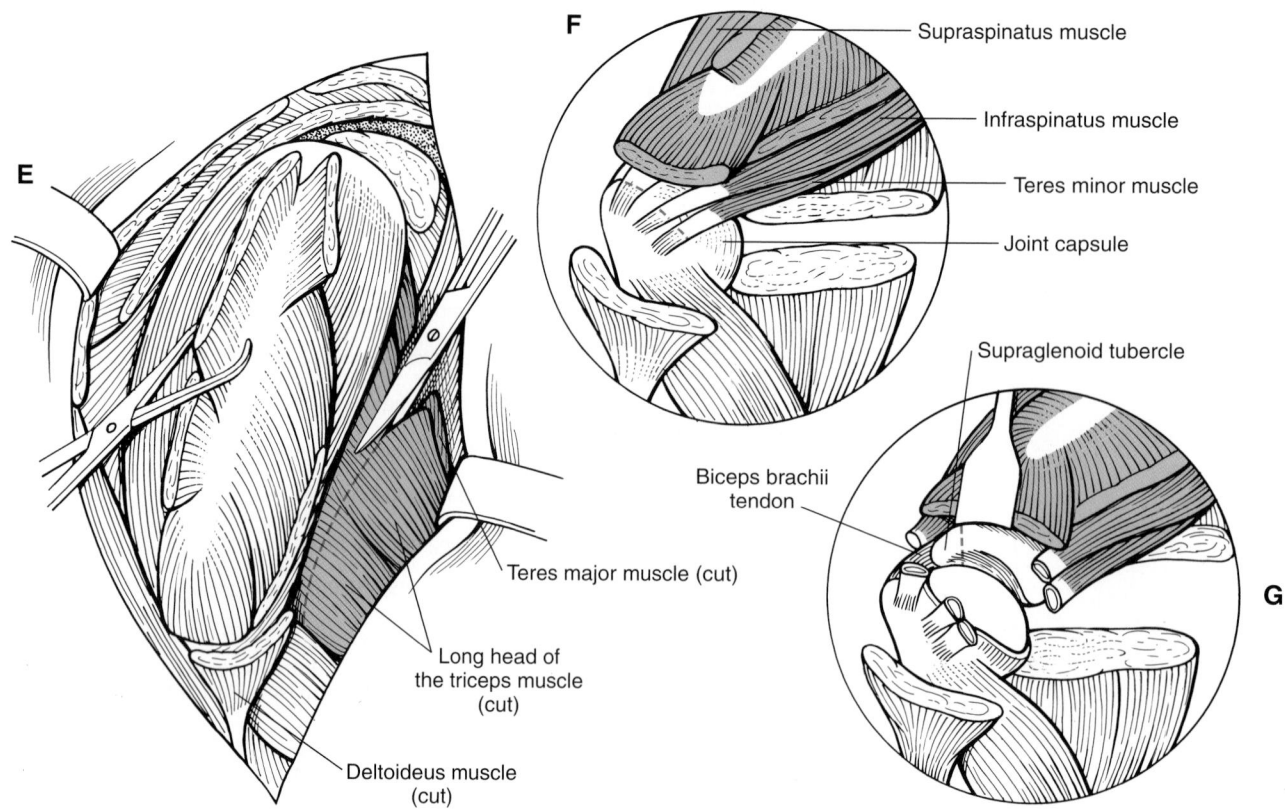

FIG. 35-7, cont'd
E, Transect the acromial and spinous heads of the deltoideus muscle close to the scapula. Transect the teres major and long head of the triceps muscles from the caudal border of the scapula. **F,** Transect the tendons of the teres minor, infraspinatus, supraspinatus, coracobrachialis (not pictured), and subscapularis (not pictured) muscles close to their humeral origins. **G,** Incise the joint capsule, osteotomize the glenoid tubercle, and remove the scapula.

to the proximal third of the humerus. Continue the skin incision around the forelimb at this level (Fig. 35-8, A). Transect the trapezius and omotransversarius muscles at their insertions on the scapular spine. Transect the rhomboideus muscle from its attachment on the dorsal border of the scapula, and retract the scapula laterally to expose its medial surface (Fig. 35-8, B). Next, elevate the serratus ventralis muscle from the medial surface of the scapula (Fig. 35-8, C). Continue to retract the scapula to expose the brachial plexus and axillary artery and vein. Ligate the axillary artery and vein with a three-clamp and transfixation suture technique (Fig. 35-9). Transect the brachial plexus. Transect the brachiocephalicus muscle, deep and superficial pectoral muscles, and latissimus dorsi muscle near their humeral insertions (Fig. 35-8, D and E). Remove the forelimb. To close the wound, approximate the muscle bellies to cover the brachial plexus and vessels, and then suture subcutaneous tissue and skin (Fig. 35-8, F).

Shoulder disarticulation amputation. Make a skin incision around the forelimb at the level of the proximal third of the humerus. The lateral portion of the skin incision should extend further distally than the medial portion of the skin incision. Dissect subcutaneous tissue in the same plane. Transect the brachiocephalicus muscle just below the clavicular tendon. Ligate the cephalic vein in this region. Incise the superficial and deep pectoral muscles close to their insertions on the humerus. Expose the brachial plexus by abduction of the limb and double ligate the brachial artery and vein. Inject the nerves of the plexus with bupivacaine, and then transect them after a delay of several minutes. Transect the acromial head of the deltoideus muscle from its origin on the acromion. Transect the supraspinatus, infraspinatus, and teres minor muscles at their insertions on the humerus. Transect the latissimus dorsi, teres major, and cutaneous trunci muscles near their insertions on the humerus. Open the scapulohumeral joint capsule, and disarticulate the joint by transection of the biceps brachii, coracobrachialis, and subscapularis muscles. Elevate the spinous head of the deltoideus muscle from its insertion on the humerus, and transect the long head of the triceps brachii muscle as distally as possible.

An osteotome may be used to remove the scapular spine and acromion for a better cosmetic effect.

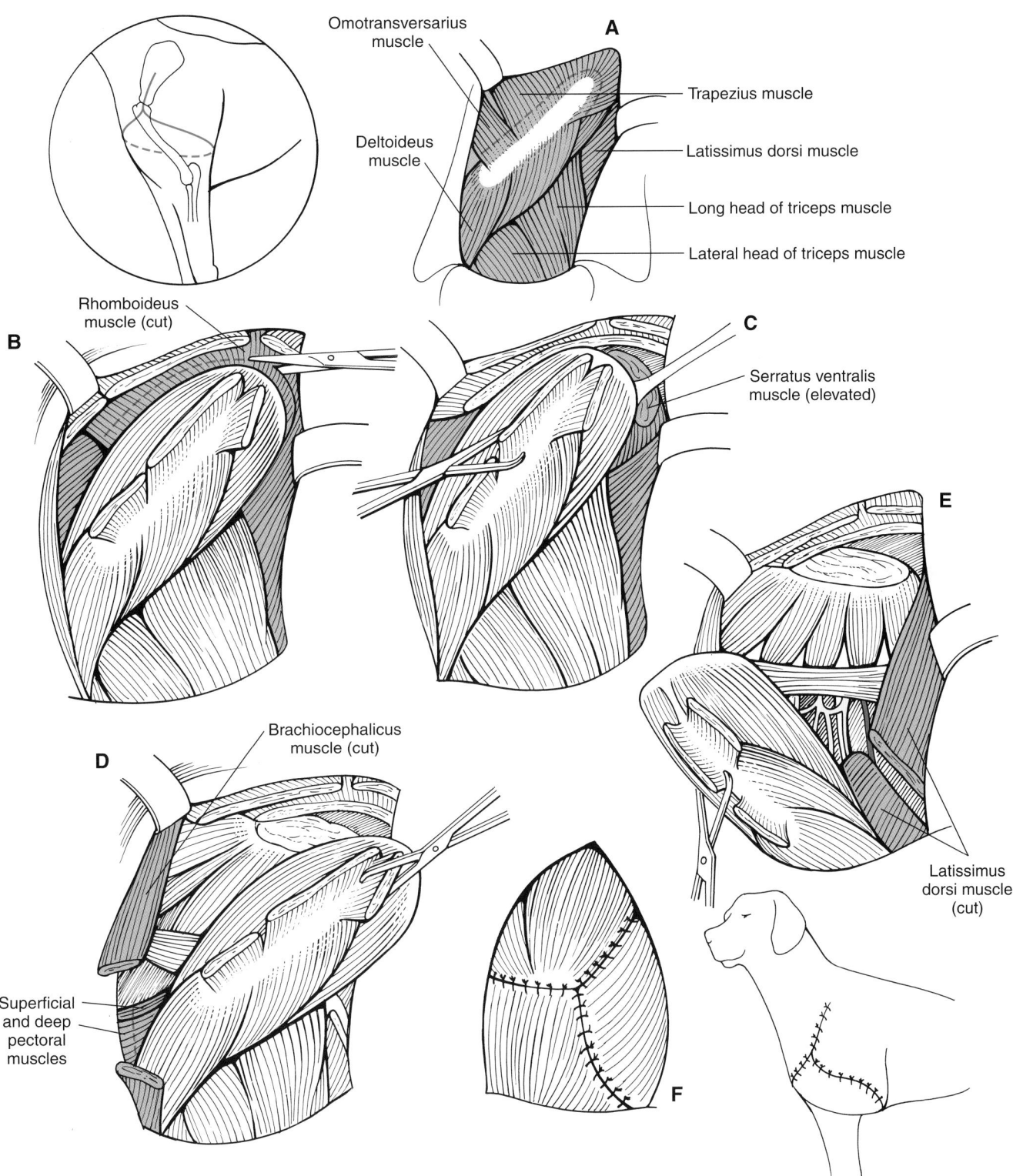

FIG. 35-8

A, For forequarter amputation, make a skin incision from the dorsal border of the scapula, over the scapular spine, to the proximal third of the humerus. Continue the skin incision around the forelimb at this level. Transect the trapezius and omotransversarius muscles at their insertions on the scapular spine. **B,** Transect the rhomboideus muscle from its attachment on the dorsal border of the scapula. **C,** Elevate the serratus ventralis muscle from the medial surface of the scapula. **D,** Retract the scapula laterally to expose the axillary artery and vein for ligation. Transect the brachial plexus. Transect the latissimus dorsi muscle near its humeral insertion. **E,** Transect the brachiocephalicus and deep and superficial pectoral muscles near their humeral insertions and remove the forelimb. **F,** To close the wound, approximate the muscle bellies to cover the brachial plexus and vessels and suture subcutaneous tissue and skin.

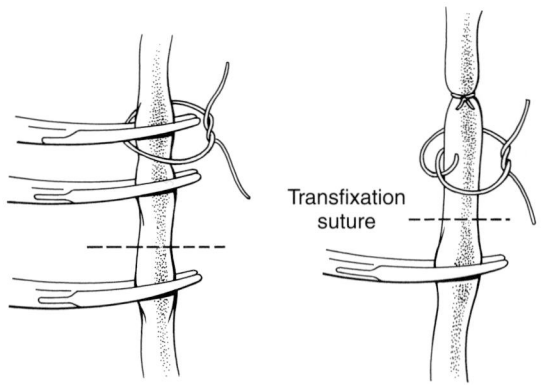

Transfixation
suture

FIG. 35-9
A three-forceps and transfixation suture technique. Place three forceps on the artery and ligate it in the crushed area of the proximal forceps. Place a transfixation ligature distal to the first ligation and cut the vessel between the middle and distal clamps.

Suture the superficial and deep pectoral muscles to the latissimus dorsi, teres major, infraspinatus, and brachiocephalicus muscles. Suture subcutaneous tissue and skin.

Midhumeral amputation. *Make a skin incision around the forelimb at the level of the distal third of the humerus. The lateral portion of the skin incision should extend further distally than the medial portion of the skin incision (Fig. 35-10, A). Dissect subcutaneous tissue in the same plane. Abduct the limb and separate the biceps brachii muscle and medial head of the triceps muscle to expose the brachial artery and vein, and median, ulnar, and musculocutaneous nerves (Fig. 35-10, B). Ligate the artery and vein with a three-clamp and transfixation suture technique (see Fig. 35-9). Transect the nerves; then transect the triceps tendon and reflect the muscles proximally to expose the humerus. Transect the biceps brachii and brachialis muscles at their insertions on the radius and ulna (Fig. 35-10, C). Ligate the cephalic vein, and transect the radial nerve. Elevate the brachiocephalicus muscle from the humerus. Osteotomize the humerus with an oscillating saw, Gigli wire, or osteotome and remove the distal forelimb (see Fig. 35-10, C). Close the wound by suturing the triceps tendon around the humeral stump to the biceps and brachialis muscles. Suture subcutaneous tissue and skin.*

Coxofemoral disarticulation. *Make a skin incision around the rear limb at the level of the middle third of the femur (Fig. 35-11, A). The lateral aspect of the skin incision should extend further distally than the medial aspect. On the medial side, open the femoral triangle by incising between the pectineus muscle and caudal belly of the sartorius muscle to expose and ligate the femoral artery and vein (Fig. 35-11, B) using a three-clamp technique (see Fig. 35-9). Transect sartorius, pectineus, gracilis, and adductor muscles approximately 2 cm from the inguinal crease*

(Fig. 35-11, C). Isolate the medial circumflex femoral vessels over the iliopsoas muscle and ligate them. Transect the iliopsoas muscle at its insertion on the lesser trochanter, and reflect it cranially to expose the joint capsule (Fig. 35-11, D). Incise the joint capsule and cut the ligament of the head of the femur (Fig. 35-11, E). On the lateral side, transect the biceps femoris muscle and tensor fascia lata at midfemoral level, and reflect them proximally to expose the greater trochanter and sciatic nerve (Fig. 35-11, F). Sever the sciatic nerve distal to its muscular branches to the semimembranosus, semitendinosus, and biceps femoris muscles. Transect the gluteal muscle insertions close to the greater trochanter (Fig. 35-11, G). Transect semimembranosus and semitendinosus muscles at the level of the proximal third of the femur. Sever the external rotator muscles and quadratus femoris muscle at their attachments around the trochanteric fossa. Elevate the rectus femoris muscle from its origin on the pelvis. Incise the joint capsule circumferentially and remove the limb. Close the wound by flapping the biceps femoris muscle medially and suturing it to the gracilis and semitendinosus muscles. Flap the tensor fascia lata caudally, and suture it to the sartorius muscle. Suture subcutaneous tissue and skin.

Midfemoral amputation. *Make a skin incision around the rear limb at the level of the distal third of the femur (Fig. 35-12, A). The lateral aspect of the skin incision should extend further distally than the medial aspect. On the medial side, transect the gracilis muscle and the caudal belly of the sartorius at the midfemoral level (Fig. 35-12, B). Isolate and ligate the femoral vessels (see Fig. 35-9). Transect the pectineus muscle through its musculotendinous junction (Fig. 35-12, C). Transect the cranial belly of the sartorius muscle. Transect the quadriceps muscle proximally to the patella (Fig. 35-12, D). Transect the biceps femoris muscle at the same level as the quadriceps muscle. Isolate and cut the sciatic nerve at the level of the third trochanter. Transect the caudal muscles, including the semimembranosus, semitendinosus, and adductor muscles at midfemoral level (Fig. 35-12, E). Elevate the insertion of the adductor muscle from the linea aspera of the femur (Fig. 35-12, F). Cut the femur at the junction of the proximal and middle thirds of the diaphysis and remove the limb. Close the wound by flapping the quadriceps muscle caudally to cover the femoral stump and suturing it to the adductor muscle. Flap the biceps muscle medially, and suture it to the gracilis and semitendinosus muscles. Muscles should be apposed to completely protect the distal end of the femur. Suture subcutaneous tissue and skin.*

Limb-Sparing Techniques

Some dogs with preexisting orthopedic and neurologic disease do not ambulate adequately after amputation. Additionally, some owners will not permit amputation. Limb-sparing techniques that involve *en bloc* resection of the tumor and replacement with a bone allograft can be used in

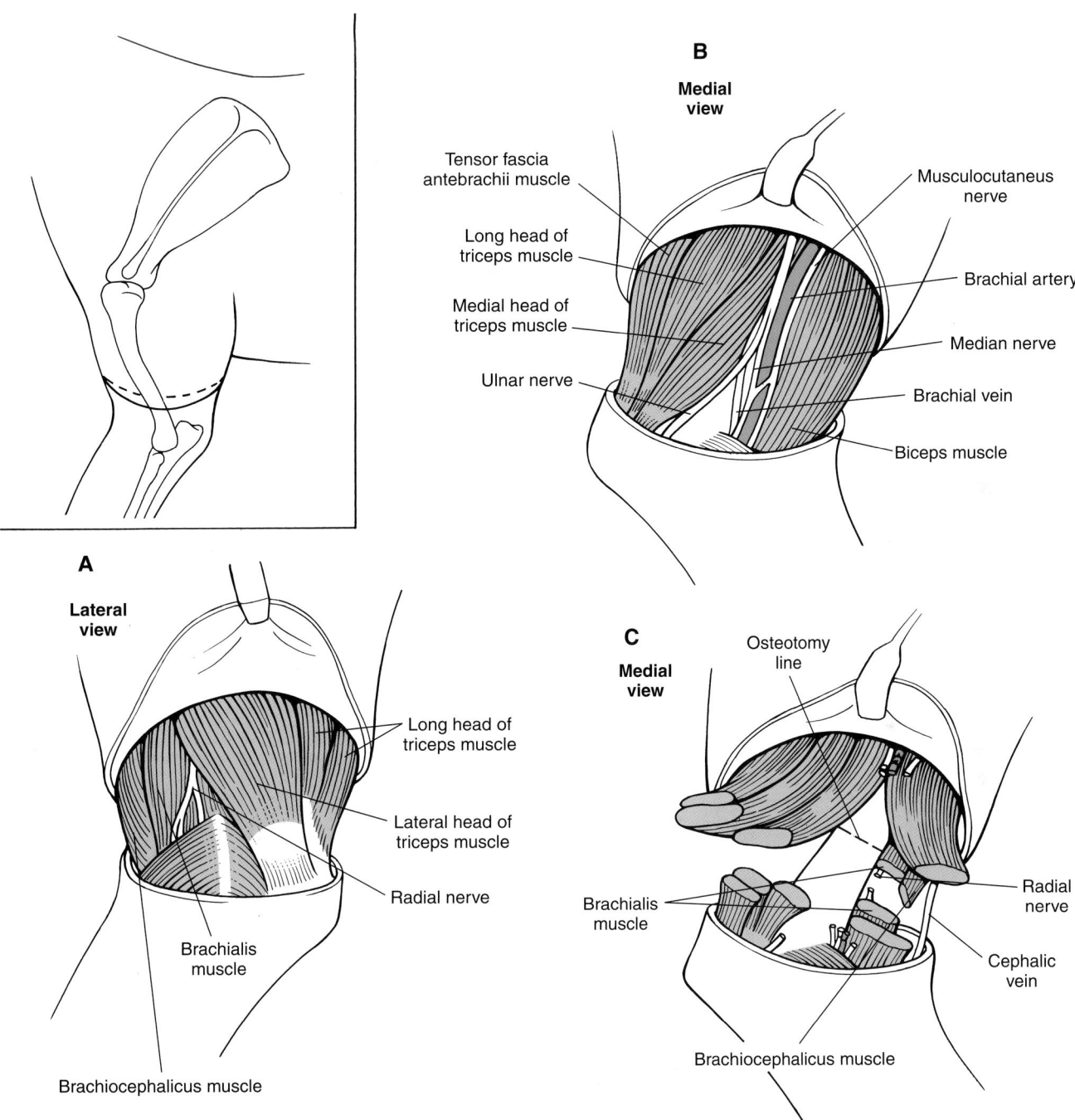

FIG. 35-10
A, For a midhumeral amputation, make a skin incision around the forelimb at the level of the distal third of the humerus. **B,** Abduct the limb and separate the biceps brachii muscle and medial head of the triceps muscle to expose the brachial artery and vein for ligation, and the median, ulnar, and musculocutaneous nerves for transection. **C,** Transect the triceps tendon, cut the biceps brachii and brachialis muscles at their insertions on the radius and ulna, and elevate the brachiocephalicus muscle from the humerus. Ligate the cephalic vein and transect the radial nerve. Osteotomize the humerus and remove the limb.

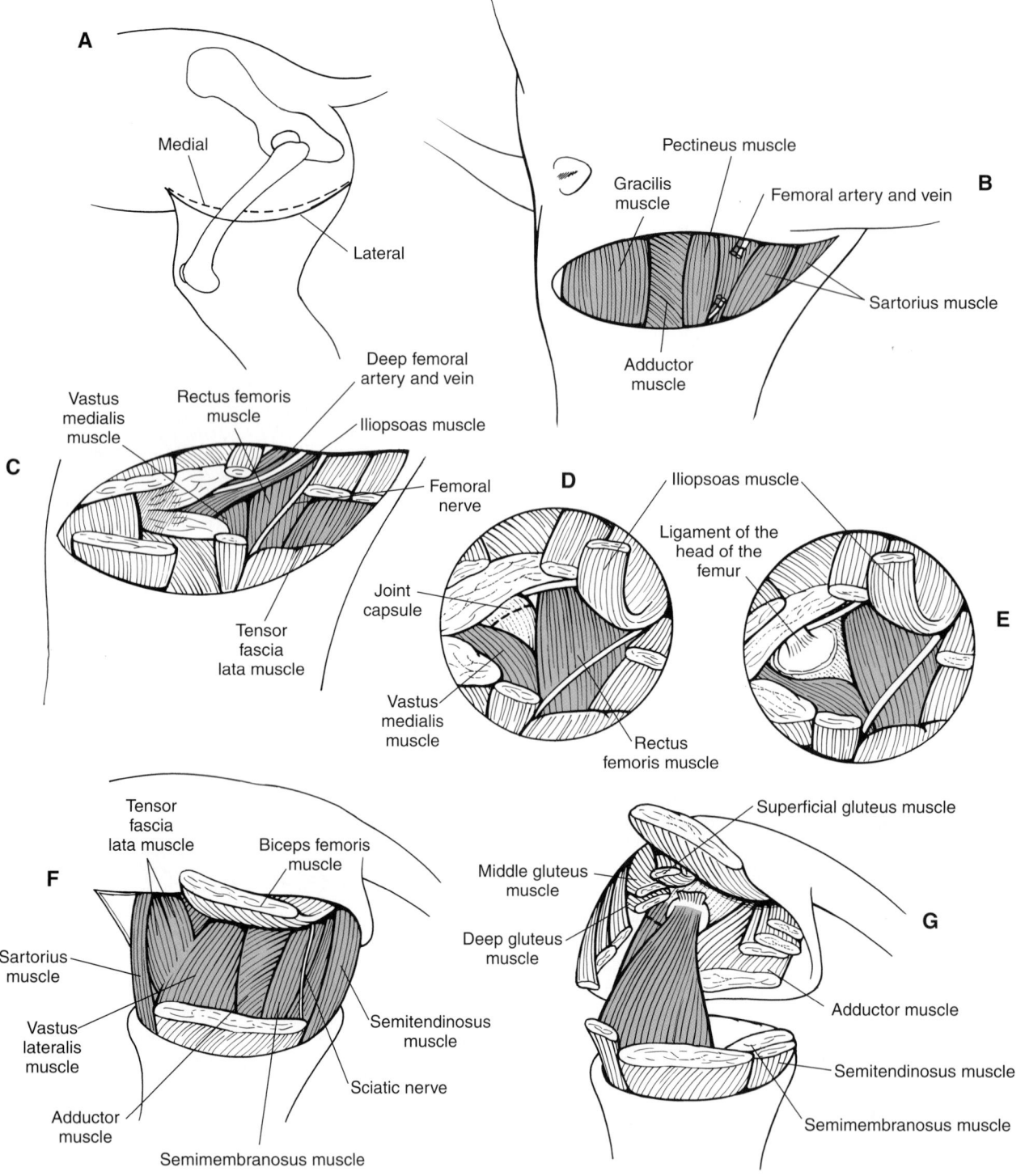

FIG. 35-11

A, For coxofemoral disarticulation, make a skin incision around the rear limb at the level of the middle third of the femur. **B,** On the medial side, open the femoral triangle by incising between the pectineus muscle and the caudal belly of the sartorius muscle to expose and ligate the deep femoral artery and vein. **C,** Transect the sartorius, pectineus, gracilis, and adductor muscles approximately 2 cm from the inguinal crease. **D** and **E,** Transect the iliopsoas muscle at its insertion on the lesser trochanter, and reflect it cranially to expose the joint capsule. Incise the joint capsule and cut the ligament of the head of the femur. **F,** On the lateral side, transect the biceps femoris muscle and tensor fascia lata at the midfemoral level. **G,** Sever the sciatic nerve distal to its muscular branches to the semimembranosus, semitendinosus, and biceps femoris muscles. Transect the gluteal muscle insertions close to the greater trochanter. Transect the semimembranosus and semitendinosus muscles at the level of the proximal third of the femur. Sever the external rotator muscles and quadratus femoris muscle at their attachments around the trochanteric fossa. Elevate the rectus femoris muscle from its origin on the pelvis. Remove the limb.

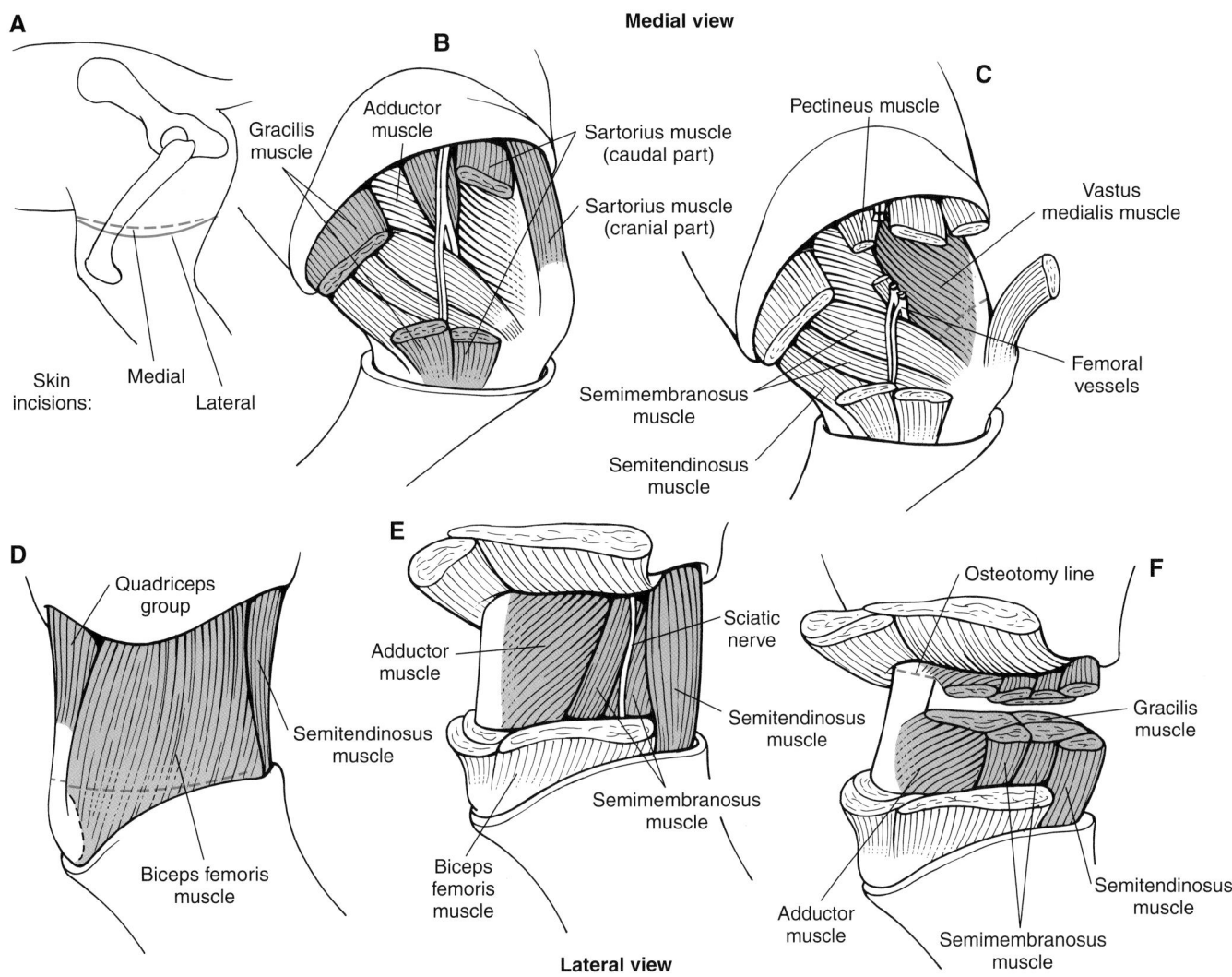

Medial view

A

Skin incisions: Medial Lateral

B

Gracilis muscle
Adductor muscle
Sartorius muscle (caudal part)
Sartorius muscle (cranial part)

C

Pectineus muscle
Vastus medialis muscle
Semimembranosus muscle
Femoral vessels
Semitendinosus muscle

D

Quadriceps group
Semitendinosus muscle
Biceps femoris muscle

E

Adductor muscle
Sciatic nerve
Semitendinosus muscle
Semimembranosus muscle
Biceps femoris muscle

F

Osteotomy line
Gracilis muscle
Adductor muscle
Semimembranosus muscle
Semitendinosus muscle

Lateral view

FIG. 35-12
A, For midfemoral amputation, make a skin incision around the rear limb at the level of the distal third of the femur. **B,** On the medial side, transect the gracilis muscle and the caudal belly of the sartorius at the midfemoral level. **C,** Isolate and ligate the femoral vessels. Transect the pectineus muscle through its musculotendinous junction. Transect the cranial belly of the sartorius muscle. **D,** Transect the quadriceps muscle proximally to the patella. **E,** Transect the biceps femoris muscle at the same level as the quadriceps muscle. Isolate and cut the sciatic nerve at the level of the third trochanter. Transect the semimembranosus, semitendinosus, and adductor muscles at midfemoral level. **F,** Elevate the insertion of the adductor muscle from the linea aspera of the femur. Cut the femur at the junction of the proximal and middle thirds of the diaphysis and remove the limb.

selected cases. The most suitable candidates for limb sparing are dogs with osteosarcoma of the distal radius that affects less than 50% of the bone. Limb sparing for proximal humeral lesions has not been as successful. Numerous limb-sparing techniques have been described (e.g., cortical allograft, cortical allograft with polymethylmethacrylate, cortical ulnar autograft with microvascular transfer, rollover cortical ulnar autograft, intraoperative radiation, bone transport, and stainless steel prosthetic bone substitute). The cortical allograft with arthrodesis of the carpus is the

most common technique. Readers are referred to the Suggested Reading list for specific articles describing other techniques.

AP **Cortical allograft with carpal arthrodesis.**
Position the dog in lateral recumbency. Dissect around the pseudocapsule of the tumor. Osteotomize the bone 3 to 5 cm proximal to the radiographic margin of the tumor. Take a biopsy specimen from the proximal margin of resection to check for tumor. Transect the extensor

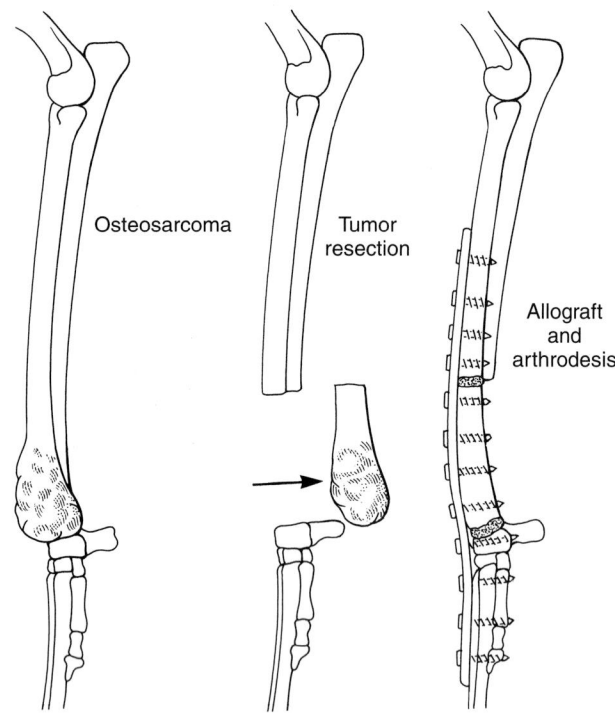

FIG. 35-13
A limb-sparing procedure for distal radial osteosarcoma. Resect the affected bone and soft tissue. Replace the bone with a cortical allograft, and stabilize it with a compression plate. Perform an arthrodesis of the carpus concurrently.

carpi radialis muscle, and remove it with the tumor, along with any other muscles or tendons that are involved.

The distal margin of resection is the joint surface.

Incise the joint capsule and dissect the tumor free. Remove the articular cartilage of the carpal bones in preparation for carpal arthrodesis. Replace the resected bone with a cortical allograft stabilized with a long, dynamic compression plate (see p. 1228).

Filling the graft with polymethylmethacrylate decreases the incidence of implant loosening and allograft fracture, but there are controversial results regarding possible delays in graft incorporation.

Make sure that the plate is of sufficient length that at least four screws can be positioned in the proximal radius and three positioned distal to the graft. Harvest autogenous cancellous bone (or harvest the graft before dissecting the tumor to prevent contamination of the donor site), and place it at the host-graft interface and at the arthrodesis site (Fig. 35-13). If desired, insert a closed suction drain adjacent to the graft before closing the wound. Close subcutaneous tissue and skin routinely.

SUTURE MATERIALS AND SPECIAL INSTRUMENTS

A Michele trephine or Jamshidi needle is needed for a bone biopsy. An osteotome and mallet, oscillating saw, or Gigli wire is used to sever the bone when performing a mid-humeral or midfemoral amputation. Nonabsorbable (polypropylene or nylon) or strong synthetic absorbable (polydioxanone or polyglyconate) suture should be used for vessel ligation during amputation. Plating equipment and an allograft are needed for limb sparing.

POSTOPERATIVE CARE AND ASSESSMENT

Postoperative care after biopsy is minimal, but most dogs are painful after the biopsy, probably because of subperiosteal hemorrhage. Pressure bandages may be needed if there is excessive bleeding. After amputation, the surgical site should be observed for swelling, redness, and/or discharge. If hemorrhage or seroma formation is noted, pressure may be applied to the surgical site by applying a circumferential bandage around the thorax or pelvis. Mobility should be encouraged after surgery so that the animal can learn to walk on three legs; however, some animals require initial support to prevent falling, especially on slick surfaces. Most animals learn to ambulate on three limbs within 4 weeks (many by 1 week after surgery); however, some dogs may require coaxing and encouragement. Pain relief is often evident after amputation of limbs with large neoplastic lesions. Potential complications of amputation include seroma formation, bleeding, infection, and suture line dehiscence.

> NOTE: Many owners are reluctant to accept amputation and must be advised of the animal's ability to adapt to walking on three legs. Keeping a video of a dog with an amputation to show owners considering this procedure may be helpful.

Postoperative care after limb sparing includes care of the closed suction drainage system (if used) and removal of the drain when drainage subsides (usually 1 day after surgery). The leg should be supported in a padded bandage to control postoperative swelling. The incision must be protected from self-mutilation with bandages and/or an Elizabethan collar. Decreased exercise is recommended for 3 to 4 weeks; however, controlled exercise or physical therapy may be necessary to prevent flexure contracture of the digits.

PROGNOSIS

Dogs treated for osteosarcoma with amputation alone have a median survival time of 3 to 4 months (Dernell et al, 2001). Dogs treated with amputation and cisplatin have median survival times of 260 to 400 days and a 38% to 62% 1-year survival rate (Dernell et al, 2001). Carboplatin results in a median survival time of 321 days and 35% survival at 1 year.

In a recent study of 35 dogs with appendicular osteosarcoma treated with cisplatin and doxorubicin combination chemotherapy, median survival time was 300 days; however, 10 dogs that survived to a year lived a median of 510 days (Chun et al, 2005). Although regional lymph node metastasis is rare in dogs with appendicular osteosarcoma, dogs with lymph node metastasis have a poorer prognosis than dogs without (median survival 59 days versus 318 days, respectively) (Hillers et al, 2005). In a recent study, dogs with appendicular osteosarcoma that had strong COX-2 expression had significantly decreased overall survival time. The median survival times for dogs with negative (n = 10), poor (n = 19), moderate (n = 11), and strong (n = 4) expression were 423, 399, 370, and 86 days, respectively (Mullins et al, 2004). Euthanasia is usually requested by owners when pulmonary metastases cause depression, anorexia, and/or respiratory distress. A recent report of canine digital tumors suggested that surgery had a positive impact on survival and early surgical intervention was advised regardless of tumor type or the presence of metastatic disease (Henry et al, 2005).

Limb-sparing procedures in conjunction with cisplatin treatment have resulted in good or adequate limb function in approximately 80% of treated dogs (Morello et al, 2001). There does not appear to be a difference in survival rates between dogs treated with amputation in conjunction with chemotherapy and those treated with limb-sparing procedures in conjunction with chemotherapy. Complications associated with traditional limb sparing vary dramatically according to the study cited and include local tumor recurrence (15% to 28%), implant complications (11% to 60%), and allograft infection (39% to 70%) (Morello et al, 2001). Interestingly, improved survival has been noted in dogs treated with limb salvage when the surgical site became infected (Lascelles et al, 2005). A smaller initial length of radius involved and lower body weight also had a positive influence on survival in the aforementioned study.

References

Boudrieau RJ, McCarthy RJ, Sisson RD: Sarcoma of the proximal portion of the tibia in a dog 5.5 years after tibial plateau leveling osteotomy, *J Am Vet Med Assoc* 227:1613, 2005.

Chun R, Garrett LD, Henry C et al: Toxicity and efficacy of cisplatin and doxorubicin combination chemotherapy for the treatment of canine osteosarcoma, *J Am Anim Hosp Assoc* 41:382, 2005.

Davis GJ, Kapatkin AS, Craig LE et al: Comparison of radiography, computed tomography, and magnetic resonance imaging for evaluation of appendicular osteosarcoma in dogs, *J Am Vet Med Assoc* 220:1171, 2002.

Dernell WS, Straw RC, Withrow SJ: Tumors of the skeletal system. In Withrow SJ, MacEwen EG, editors: *Small animal clinical oncology*, Philadelphia, 2001, Saunders.

Fan TM, de Lorimier L, Charney SC et al: Evaluation of intravenous pamidronate administration in 33 cancer-bearing dogs with primary or secondary bone involvement, *J Vet Intern Med* 19:74, 2005.

Henry CJ, Brewer WG, Whitely EM et al: Canine digital tumors: a veterinary cooperative oncology group retrospective study of 64 dogs, *J Vet Intern Med* 19:720, 2005.

Hillers KR, Dernell WS, Lafferty MH et al: Incidence and prognostic importance of lymph node metastases in dogs with appendicular osteosarcoma: 228 cases (1986-2003), *J Am Vet Med Assoc* 226:1364, 2005.

Kent MS, Strom A, London CA et al: Alternating carboplatin and doxorubicin as adjunctive chemotherapy to amputation or limb-sparing surgery in the treatment of appendicular osteosarcoma in dogs, *J Vet Intern Med* 18:540, 2004.

Lascelles BD, Dernell WS, Correa MT et al: Improved survival associated with postoperative wound infection in dogs treated with limb-salvage surgery for osteosarcoma, *Ann Surg Oncol* 12:1073, 2005.

Leibman NF, Kuntz CA, Stein PF et al: Accuracy of radiography, nuclear scintigraphy, and histopathology for determining the proximal extent of distal radius osteosarcoma in dogs, *Vet Surg* 20:240, 2001.

Milne RJ, Farese J, Henry CJ et al: Bisphosphonates and cancer, *J Vet Intern Med* 18:597, 2004.

Morello E, Buracco P, Martano M et al: Bone allografts and adjuvant cisplatin for the treatment of canine appendicular osteosarcoma in 18 dogs, *J Small Anim Pract* 42:61, 2001.

Mueller F, Poirier V, Melzer K et al: Palliative radiotherapy with electrons of appendicular osteosarcoma in 54 dogs, *In Vivo* 19:713, 2005.

Mullins MN, Lana SE, Dernell WS et al: Cyclooxygenase-2 expression in canine appendicular osteosarcomas, *J Vet Intern Med* 18:859, 2004.

Wallack ST, Wisner ER, Werner JA: Accuracy of magnetic resonance imaging for estimating intramedullary osteosarcoma extent in pre-operative planning of canine limb-salvage procedures, *Vet Radiol Ultrasound* 43:432, 2002.

Suggested Reading

Erhart N: Longitudinal bone transport for treatment of primary bone tumors in dogs: technique description and outcome in 9 dogs, *Vet Surg* 34:24, 2005.

This manuscript describes the use of bone transport for primary treatment of osteosarcoma or after failure of allograft limb sparing. The procedure was successful in almost all dogs and may be an alternative for traditional limb sparing.

Liptak JM, Dernell WS, Lascelles BD: Intraoperative extracorporeal irradiation for limb sparing in 13 dogs, *Vet Surg* 33:446, 2004.

This retrospective study of 13 dogs that underwent extracorporeal intraoperative radiation therapy of tumors other than the distal radius. Complications occurred in 69% of dogs and included deep infection, fracture of the irradiated bone, and implant failure; however, limb function was good or excellent in 10 dogs.

Liptak JM, Dernell WS, Straw RC: Intercalary bone grafts for joint and limb preservation in 17 dogs with high-grade malignant tumors of the diaphysis, *Vet Surg* 33:457, 2004.

In this retrospective study, 17 dogs were identified that underwent limb-sparing surgery with allograft or irradiated autograft for diaphyseal bone tumors. In the vast majority of cases, the procedure resulted in excellent clinical outcome in spite of minor complications.

Liptak JM, Pluhar GE, Dernell WS et al: Limb-sparing surgery in a dog with osteosarcoma of the proximal femur, *Vet Surg* 34:71, 2005.

A proximal femoral allograft and long shaft total hip replacement were used for limb-sparing treatment of a proximal femoral osteosarcoma. The clinical outcome was excellent, although revision of the total hip replacement was necessary due to aseptic loosening.

Seguin B, Walsh PJ, Mason DR et al: Use of an ipsilateral vascularized ulnar transposition autograft for limb-sparing surgery of the distal radius in dogs: an anatomic and clinical study, *Vet Surg* 32:69, 2003.

Viability of a vascularized ulnar autograft for treatment of distal radius osteosarcoma was evaluated in cadavers. The technique was then performed in three clinical cases with good to excellent results.

JOINT NEOPLASIA

DEFINITIONS

Primary joint neoplasms are tumors that arise from synovial linings of diarthrodial joints, tendon sheaths, and/or bursae. The tumors of practical importance are those arising from synovioblastic tissue, called **synovial sarcomas** *(malignant synovioma, synovial cell sarcoma),* **histiocytic sarcomas,** and **synovial myxomas.**

GENERAL CONSIDERATIONS AND CLINICALLY RELEVANT PATHOPHYSIOLOGY

Synovial cell sarcomas are rare tumors arising from synovioblastic mesenchyme in deep connective tissue around joints (Craig et al, 2002). Histiocytic sarcomas likely arise from macrophage/monocyte cell lines. Synovial myxomas arise from fibroblasts in myxomatous tissue. Joints above the carpus and tarsus are more commonly affected than distal joints. Biologic behavior of these tumors ranges from slow growth to aggressive invasion of adjacent tissue. Metastasis occurs to regional lymph nodes, lungs, bone, and other locations.

DIAGNOSIS
Clinical Presentation

Signalment. Synovial sarcomas occur most commonly in large, middle-aged dogs. There is a 3:2 male-to-female ratio. A breed predisposition has not been identified. Rottweilers appear to be affected more commonly with histiocytic sarcomas, whereas Doberman pinschers more commonly have synovial myxomas. The average age at presentation for joint tumors is 9 years (Craig et al, 2002).

History. Affected dogs and cats are usually lame. A mass near a joint may occasionally be noticed by owners. Masses may grow slowly for a period; rapid growth may then occur.

Physical Examination Findings

Masses vary in size, but are usually firm with some fluctuant areas. They are generally nonpainful. The degree of lameness appears to correlate with the amount of bone involvement.

Diagnostic Imaging

Radiographs of involved joints are needed to evaluate extent of bone and soft-tissue involvement. There may be lobulated soft-tissue masses in the joint region. Bone changes (e.g.,

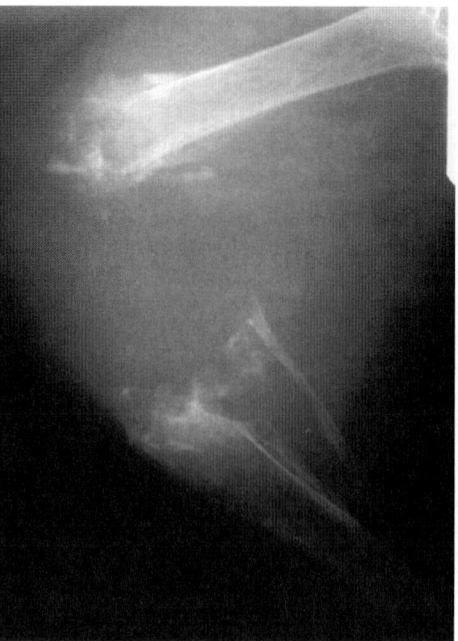

FIG. 35-14
Lateral radiograph of a dog with synovial cell sarcoma of the stifle joint. Notice the extensive lysis of the distal femur and proximal tibia. Because both sides of the joint are affected, a soft-tissue tumor should be suspected.

lysis of subchondral bone and cortex, or new bone production) are often noted on either side of the joint (Fig. 35-14). This contrasts with the appearance of primary bone tumors, which seldom appear to affect the bones on either side of the joint or "cross a joint." Thoracic radiographs or contrast enhanced CT should be performed to evaluate for the presence of pulmonary metastasis.

Laboratory Findings

Consistent laboratory abnormalities are not present.

DIFFERENTIAL DIAGNOSIS

Neoplastic joint lesions must be differentiated from synovial cysts, which are well-circumscribed masses attached to joint capsule, tendon sheath, or bursa (see *Small Animal Surgery,* second edition or e-dition). Synovial cell sarcomas must also be differentiated from fungal and infectious joint diseases (e.g., septic arthritis, erosive arthritis, and villonodular synovitis) and other tumors (e.g., fibrosarcoma, rhabdomyosarcoma, liposarcoma, hemangiopericytoma, malignant fibrous histiocytomas, giant cell tumors of soft tissue, and primary bone tumors). A definitive diagnosis requires a biopsy of the lesion; however, excisional biopsy (limb amputation) rather than incisional biopsy may be warranted if massive bone destruction precludes therapy other than amputation. Fine needle aspiration can reveal malignant cells, but will not allow visualization of tumor architecture necessary for definitive diagnosis of tumor type in many cases.

> NOTE: You should attempt fine needle aspiration or another biopsy technique before amputating the leg because fungal and neoplastic lesions can be radiographically indistinguishable.

SURGICAL TREATMENT

Amputation appears to be the most effective treatment for this tumor (see p. 1342). Local excision is not recommended because of the high recurrence rate. Concurrent chemotherapy may be beneficial.

POSTOPERATIVE CARE AND ASSESSMENT

See p. 1350 for recommendations for the postoperative care of animals following amputation. Periodic examination of affected animals is recommended for early detection of local recurrence or metastasis.

PROGNOSIS

Prognosis is guarded after limb amputation. Although these tumors have historically been considered to be slow-growing tumors that metastasize late in the course of disease, a recent study has suggested that metastasis is common following amputation. In one study, the average survival time for dogs with synovial cell sarcoma was 32 months, 5 months with histiocytic sarcoma, and 30 months with synovial myxoma (Craig et al, 2002). Histiocytic sarcoma has the highest rate of metastasis, whereas synovial myxoma has the lowest. In a recent study of 16 dogs with canine synovial sarcoma, neither clinical stage nor histopathologic grade significantly affected survival (Fox et al, 2002). Dogs receiving surgical tumor excision or amputation had a significantly higher survivability than those receiving no treatment. The authors concluded that aggressiveness of treatment was more useful than clinical staging or tumor grading in predicting survival.

References

Craig LE, Julian ME, Ferracone JD: The diagnosis and prognosis of synovial tumors in dogs: 35 cases, *Vet Pathol* 39:66, 2002.

Fox DB, Cook JL, Kreeger JM et al: Canine synovial sarcoma: a retrospective assessment of described prognostic criteria in 16 cases (1994-1999), *J Am Anim Hosp Assoc* 38:347, 2002.

OSTEOMYELITIS

DEFINITIONS

Osteomyelitis is inflammation of bone marrow, cortex, and possibly periosteum. Acute **osteomyelitis** is characterized by systemic illness, pain, and soft tissue swelling without visible radiographic alterations in bone. **Chronic osteomyelitis** exists when acute and systemic clinical signs have subsided, but infection manifested by draining sinuses, recurrent cellulitis, abscess formation, and progressive destructive and proliferative osseous changes is present. **Sequestra** are fragments of necrosed bone that have become separated from surrounding tissue.

GENERAL CONSIDERATIONS AND CLINICALLY RELEVANT PATHOPHYSIOLOGY

Most bone infections in dogs and cats are bacterial in origin. Many of these are monomicrobial infections, with β-lactamase producing *S. intermedius* or *S. aureus* predominating. Polymicrobial infections are also common and may harbor mixtures of *Streptococcus* spp., *Proteus* spp., *Escherichia coli*, *Klebsiella* spp., and *Pseudomonas* spp. Anaerobic bacteria are an important cause of osteomyelitis, being present in over two thirds of bone infections. Anaerobes may exist alone as the sole causative agent, or more commonly as one organism in polymicrobial infections. Anaerobes isolated from bone infections include *Actinomyces* spp., *Clostridium* spp., *Peptostreptococcus* spp., *Bacteroides* spp., and *Fusobacterium* spp. Characteristics of anaerobic infections include fetid odor, sequestration of bone fragments, and evidence of bacteria with differing morphology on gram-stained smears.

> NOTE: Treatment failures may result from lack of identification and inappropriate treatment of anaerobic bacteria.

Bacterial osteomyelitis is often classified as either hematogenous or posttraumatic; however, the division between the two is often indistinct, since hematogenous seeding of fractures by infectious agents occurs and may induce osteomyelitis. Nevertheless, studies indicate that a common source of bacterial inoculation is surgical site contamination during open fracture reduction. Although the type and quantity of bacteria inoculated are important factors in development of bone infections, bacteria alone do not necessarily cause osteomyelitis. Other important factors in the pathogenesis of posttraumatic osteomyelitis are (1) extent of soft-tissue damage and alteration of blood supply; (2) formation of a biofilm (glycocalyx); (3) and stability of fracture repair. Tissue damage may be caused by the injury or may occur during the surgical procedure. Damaged soft tissue and devitalized bone serve as excellent culture media for bacteria. Bacterial proliferation is also potentiated by foreign materials in the wound (e.g., synthetic suture materials or implants). Glycocalyx is a combination of bacterial slime and host cellular debris that shrouds bacterial colonies and facilitates bacterial adhesion. The biofilm also protects bacteria from phagocytosis, host antibodies, and antibiotic effectiveness. Osteomyelitis is worsened by fracture instability. Continual motion impairs revascularization of spaces between fractured bone ends, which in turn prevents host defense mechanisms from gaining access to the area.

Mycotic bone infections are acquired through hematogenous dissemination of inhaled spores. Offending organisms are endemic in some geographic locations and include *Blastomyces dermatitidis*, *Coccidioides immitis*, and less commonly, *Histoplasma capsulatum*, *Cryptococcus neoformans*, and *Aspergillus* spp. Although viral osteomyelitis is considered uncommon, newer evidence suggests that some canine bone diseases may be viral in origin. Sequences of ribonucleic acid (RNA) homologous with canine distemper viral RNA have been detected in osteoblasts of dogs with metaphyseal osteopathy (hypertrophic osteopathy). It has also been suggested that panosteitis is associated with viral infections. Other causes of osteomyelitis include parasites, foreign bodies, and corrosion of metallic implants. Diagnosis of osteomyelitis is often suspected based on history, clinical signs, and radiographic findings.

DIAGNOSIS
Clinical Presentation

Signalment. Any age, breed, or sex of dog or cat may be affected.

History. Historical findings may include recent open reduction and stabilization of a fracture, bite wounds, open traumatic wounds, or habitation in an endemic fungal region.

Physical Examination Findings

Clinical features of osteomyelitis vary depending on stage of the disease. The initial response of bone to infection is inflammation; soft tissue in the area can become hot, reddened, swollen, and painful (Fig. 35-15). The animal is often pyrexic, depressed, and partially or totally anorexic. Distinguishing between acute osteomyelitis and inflammation associated with surgical intervention is frequently difficult. Persistence of an elevated temperature for longer than 48 hours postoperatively or a neutrophilic left shift increases the likelihood that infection is present rather than only surgically induced trauma. However, lack of either of these findings does not exclude infection. Animals with chronic osteomyelitis usually are brought in for evaluation of draining tracts and/or lameness; pyrexia, anorexia, and other clinical signs associated with systemic disease are frequently lacking.

Diagnostic Imaging

Specific radiographic findings vary depending on the stage of disease, site of infection, and pathogenicity of infective organism. Soft-tissue swelling is the first sign of acute osteomyelitis and may be observed as early as 24 hours postinfection. Radiographic signs may lag behind the clinical presentation. Early radiographic changes include periosteal proliferation with deposition of new bone in a lamellar pattern oriented perpendicular to the long axis of the bone. Lamellated periosteal reactions are typically associated with osteomyelitis, whereas solid periosteal new bone formation is not typically associated with infection (Fig. 35-16). As the infection progresses, lysis of the medullary cavity becomes apparent. Sequestra may develop, and sclerosis and lysis become interspersed throughout cortical and medullary bone at the site of infection as *involucra* (new bone formation around a sequestrum) form. Sequestered bone appears more radiographically opaque than surrounding bone.

Occasionally, fistulography may help confirm that a draining tract leads to a bone lesion when an animal has draining tracts and skeletal lesions that are not confluent. Fistulography is performed by retrograde filling of each draining sinus with a water-soluble iodinated contrast agent. The concentration and volumes of contrast agents used vary; however, they should be diluted (approximately 25% to 60% is recommended) to not obscure identification of associated foreign bodies. Unfortunately, incomplete filling of sinuses and false-negative results are common.

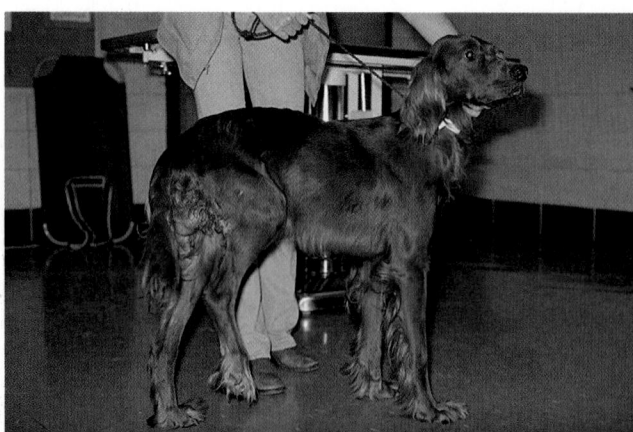

FIG. 35-15
A dog with femoral osteomyelitis. Note the draining tract on the caudolateral aspect of the thigh.

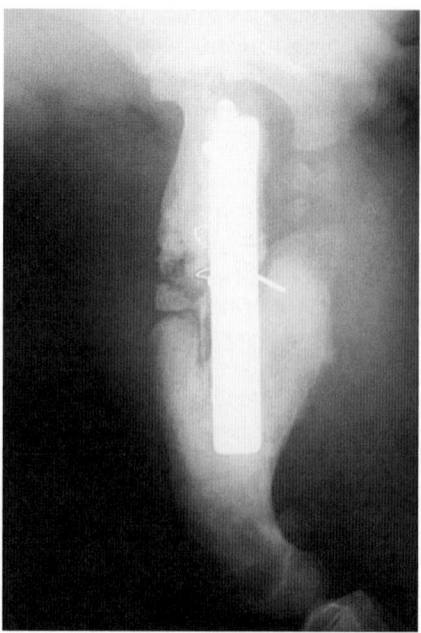

FIG. 35-16
Radiograph of a dog with acute osteomyelitis following open reduction and stabilization of a femoral fracture. Extensive periosteal reaction and sequestrum formation are present.

Laboratory Findings

With acute osteomyelitis, systemic evidence of infection is often present and indicated by an elevated white blood cell count with a neutrophilic left shift. Results of laboratory analysis in dogs with chronic osteomyelitis are usually normal.

DIFFERENTIAL DIAGNOSIS

Microbiologic culturing is definitive for osteomyelitis and is essential in determining the organism's *in vitro* susceptibility to antimicrobial drugs. Sample collection of specimens for culture should not be obtained from draining tracts. Organisms cultured from draining tracts correlate with the pathogen isolated at surgery in fewer than half of patients. Preferably, aerobic and anaerobic cultures should be obtained from bone during surgical intervention. Alternately, collection of culture samples via fine needle aspiration of material directly surrounding the involved bones may be useful. Fungal cultures and cytologic or histologic evaluation of biopsies may be diagnostic of fungal osteomyelitis. Serology may be helpful in diagnosing blastomycosis, coccidioidomycosis, and cryptococcosis. Currently, serology for histoplasmosis or systemic aspergillosis is of dubious sensitivity and specificity.

> NOTE: Collect samples for bacterial culture from deep fine needle aspirates. Do not culture draining tracts.

MEDICAL MANAGEMENT

Medical management consisting of antibiotic therapy and application of warm packs may be effective in patients with hematogenous osteomyelitis or those having postoperative osteomyelitis. Medical therapy may be used when the affected area exhibits signs of inflammation, but sequestra, necrotic tissue, or pockets of exudate should not be present. Additionally, if the patient has postoperative osteomyelitis, implant and bone stability must be present for medical management to be effective. After bone healing, implant removal is usually necessary to resolve the infection. Appropriate antibiotic therapy is determined by culture and sensitivity and is continued for a period of at least 28 days.

SURGICAL TREATMENT

If sequestra or pockets of exudate are present, drainage and débridement of necrotic tissue are necessary. The fracture must be stable, and appropriate antimicrobial therapy should be instituted based on culture and susceptibility testing. Treatment of chronic osteomyelitis entails maintaining or providing fracture stability, removal of loose implants and sequestered bone, cancellous bone grafting of bony deficits, and appropriate antimicrobial therapy.

Preoperative Management

In patients with acute osteomyelitis, antibiotic therapy should be initiated immediately with bactericidal agents having a broad spectrum of activity against aerobic and an-aerobic bacteria (e.g., clindamycin plus enrofloxacin). Definitive antimicrobial therapy is determined through culture and susceptibility testing. Antimicrobial therapy of animals with chronic osteomyelitis is based on culture and sensitivity testing of the offending organisms at surgery. Perioperative antibiotics should not be administered to these patients until intraoperative cultures have been obtained.

Anesthesia

Most animals with osteomyelitis are otherwise healthy and a variety of anesthetic regimens can be used (see p. 944). If preoperative blood work suggests organ dysfunction (i.e., renal or hepatic), refer to Chapter 31 (p. 944) for specific anesthetic recommendations.

Surgical Anatomy

Refer to Chapter 32 for anatomy of the bone involved.

Positioning

Refer to Chapter 32 for exposure of the bone involved.

SURGICAL TECHNIQUE
Acute Osteomyelitis

Open infected wounds and débride necrotic tissue. If a fracture is present, stabilize bone fragments with an appropriate implant system (bone plates and screws or external skeletal fixators are usually preferred).

> NOTE: Stabilization of fractures is the key to successful treatment of osteomyelitis. Bone union will occur in the presence of infection if fragments are stable.

If previous surgery was performed and if the fracture remains stable, leave the original implants in place. If the implants have loosened, choose another fixation system to provide rigid fixation. Establish drainage by treating the surgical site as an open wound. Irrigate the wound with 0.05% chlorhexidine and then pack it with sterile gauze soaked with 0.05% chlorhexidine. Cover wounds with a sterile outer dressing that will absorb drainage products accumulated between bandage changes. Once the infection is eliminated, suture the wound.

Chronic Osteomyelitis

Determine the degree of fracture stability by palpation and radiographic assessment. If fractures and original implants are stable, leave them in place. However, if implants are loose and if fractures have not healed, remove the loose implants and rigidly stabilize the fracture. Identify and remove sequestered bone through radiographic imaging and surgery.

At surgery, sequestered bone is recognized by a yellowish discoloration and has no soft-tissue attachments.

Do not try to stabilize sequestered bone fragments; instead, remove them and place an autogenous cancellous bone graft in areas devoid of bone. Establish drainage as described previously.

Antibiotic-impregnated polymethylmethacrylate beads may be considered for treating chronic infections, especially those associated with cortical allografts used for limb sparing. Bead strings are constructed using a bead mold in which the cement mixture is pressed onto stainless steel or nylon sutures. The strings are secondarily sterilized with ethylene oxide before implanting. The slow elution of the antibiotic can produce wound fluid concentrations up to 200 times that obtained with systemic antibiotics, exceeding the minimum inhibitory concentration for up to 80 days without toxic effects. The beads are usually removed after treatment.

SUTURE MATERIALS AND SPECIAL INSTRUMENTS

Aerobic and anaerobic culturettes should be available. Other instruments needed include those necessary for the insertion of the selected implant, bone curettes, self-retaining retractors, and a selection of absorbable suture material. Nonabsorbable suture material should generally be avoided in infected tissue.

POSTOPERATIVE CARE AND ASSESSMENT

In patients with acute osteomyelitis, antibiotic therapy should be continued for at least 3 to 4 weeks. With chronic osteomyelitis, antibiotics should be administered for at least 4 to 6 weeks. If the wound is managed in an open fashion, the area should be irrigated with 0.05% dilute chlorhexidine twice daily and packed with a chlorhexidine-soaked sponge. Using umbilical tape secured to the skin on either side of the incision that can be tied over the gauze packing facilitates frequent changing of the packing materials. The limb should be bandaged until the wound is closed to decrease likelihood of iatrogenic infection. If a fracture is present, postoperative care is dictated by the fracture configuration and stabilization procedure used. Generally, activity should be restricted to leash walks until the fracture has healed. Affected animals should be observed daily for signs of recurring fever, pain, swelling, and/or draining tracts.

PROGNOSIS

If all bone sequestra are removed and if fractures are adequately stabilized, the prognosis for resolving infection and returning the patient to normal activity is good. Removal of all implants following bone union may be necessary to completely resolve infection. A recent study suggested that crosslinked high amylase starch (CLHAS) matrix used as a biodegradable drug delivery implant was effective for prevention and treatment of osteomyelitis (Huneault et al, 2004). In this study, 32 dogs underwent femoral insertion of a screw inoculated with *Staphylococcus aureus* and were then randomly assigned to four groups: (A) prevention with ciprofloxacin-CLHAS implants, (B) surgical débridement (positive control), (C) surgical débridement and oral ciprofloxacin treatment, and (D) surgical débridement and treatment with ciprofloxacin-CLHAS implants. Osteomyelitis was confirmed at week 4, the infected site débrided, and respective treatments initiated for groups B, C, and D. Radiographs, macroscopic evaluations, bacterial cultures, and histopathologic examinations were used to evaluate the femora at week 10. Femora from preventive group A were almost normal. Dogs of both ciprofloxacin-treatment groups C and D showed better bone healing, less periosteal reaction, and less screw mobility than dogs from group B. Eradication of infection was observed at proximal/distal sites in B: 25%/12%, C: 37%/62%, and D: 62%/75%. Both ciprofloxacin-treated groups improved radiographically from week 4 to week 10. Periosteal and marrow neutrophilic and lymphoplasmocytic infiltrations were less severe in groups C and D versus group B.

Reference

Huneault LM, Lussier B, Dubreuil P et al: Prevention and treatment of experimental osteomyelitis in dogs with ciprofloxacin-loaded crosslinked high amylase starch implants, *J Orthop Res* 22:1351, 2004.

CHAPTER 36

Fundamentals of Neurosurgery

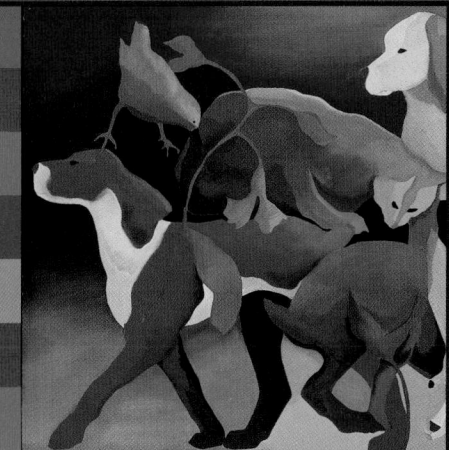

GENERAL PRINCIPLES AND TECHNIQUES

DEFINITIONS

Neurology and neurosurgery have a unique set of terms, the definition of which may vary from one neurologist to another. It is important to establish consistent definitions to ensure accurate communication. **Plegia** and **paralysis** are a complete loss of sensory and motor function to the affected extremity, whereas **paresis** is partial loss of sensation, plus complete or partial loss of motor function to the affected extremity. Terms used to describe anatomic variations of affected extremities include **tetraparesis (tetraplegia),** all four limbs affected; **paraparesis (paraplegia),** both pelvic limbs affected; **hemiparesis (hemiplegia),** front and hind limbs on one side affected; and **monoparesis (monoplegia),** one limb affected.

PROBLEM IDENTIFICATION

A proper systematic examination of animals suspected of having neurologic disorders includes signalment, history, physical examination, and neurologic examination. Signalment (i.e., age, sex, breed, and use of animal), correlated with anatomic localization of the lesion, often helps refine differential diagnoses and indicate appropriate diagnostic procedures.

The history is used to characterize the disorder as acute or chronic, progressive or static, and persistent or intermittent. Previous illnesses, vaccination history, and systems evaluation (i.e., gastrointestinal, cardiovascular, and urogenital) should be considered. Owners should be questioned regarding behavioral changes, seizures, head tilt, circling, or other signs of cranial nerve abnormalities. Careful historical evaluation for the presence or absence of hyperesthesia (pain) and/or paresis can assist in determining differential diagnoses (Box 36-1). If there is spinal hyperesthesia, determine its location (i.e., cervical, thoracolumbar, lumbosacral, and extremity), duration (acute versus chronic), progression (progressive versus static), persistence (persistent versus inter-

mittent), and character (sharp versus dull). It is also important to determine whether affected patients are mono-, para-, hemi-, or tetraparetic and whether the paresis is acute or chronic, progressive or static, and persistent or intermittent. Use of a graph illustrating the patterns of disease may be helpful when obtaining a history. Frequently, historical data suggest the lesion's location within the vertebral canal (i.e., extradural, intradural-extramedullary, and intramedullary). Typically, patients with *extradural* spinal lesions have an acute onset of persistent and sometimes progressive pain and paresis (Box 36-2). Patients with *intradural-extramedullary* spinal lesions generally have histories of chronic, dull pain with slowly progressive paresis. Those with *intramedullary* spinal lesions may have an acute onset of sudden pain and paresis; the pain, if present, is often short-lived and the paresis is persistent, but not progressive. These are general guidelines, but there are some cases that do not fit the classic pattern.

PHYSICAL EXAMINATION

A complete general physical examination should be performed in patients with possible neurologic disease. Some metabolic, cardiovascular, and musculoskeletal disorders mimic the clinical appearance of neurologic disorders (e.g., Addison's disease, toxic pyometra, cardiovascular insufficiency, and bilateral cruciate ruptures). The animal should be observed as it moves around the exam room while obtaining the history from the owner. Visual difficulties may be more apparent when the animal is placed in new surroundings. Proprioceptive loss may also be evident, especially on a slippery floor. Purposeful movements should be noted (e.g., does the animal voluntarily try to move its legs?) Certain components of the neurologic examination are included in a general physical examination, including mental status, gait, posture, evidence of trauma, facial expression, and breathing patterns. Movement of the traumatized patient should be minimized until the presence of a spinal fracture can be eliminated. A thorough physical examination may help establish the presence or absence of neurologic disease.

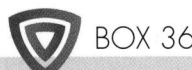

BOX 36-1

Etiology of Spinal Lesions Based on History of Pain and/or Paresis

Acute/Static	Acute/Progressive	Chronic/Progressive
Vascular	**Degenerative**	**Degenerative**
Fibrocartilaginous emboli	IVD—type I	IVD—type I and II
Infarction		Cauda equina
Trauma	**Inflammatory**	Wobbler syndrome
Fracture/luxation	Diskospondylitis	Degenerative myelopathy
	Vertebral osteomyelitis	
Degenerative		**Inflammatory**
IVD—type I	**Trauma**	Diskospondylitis
	Fracture/luxation	Vertebral osteomyelitis
	Anomalous	**Neoplastic**
	Atlantoaxial instability	Meningeal tumors
	Neoplastic	Spinal cord tumors
	Spinal cord tumors	
	Vertebral tumors	

IVD, Intervertebral disk.

BOX 36-2

Etiology of Spinal Lesions Based on Lesion Location

Extradural	Intradural-Extramedullary	Intramedullary
Intervertebral disk extrusion	Meningeal neoplasia	Vascular insult
Vertebral fracture/luxation	Meningioma	Fibrocartilaginous embolus
Extradural neoplasia	Neurofibroma	Parenchymal neoplasia
Wobbler syndrome		
Atlantoaxial instability		
Diskospondylitis		
Vertebral osteomyelitis		

NEUROLOGIC EXAMINATION

The neurologic examination is an extension of the general physical examination and is performed after the signalment and history have been noted and a general physical examination has been completed. The neurologic examination should establish the presence of neurologic disease and help determine its neuroanatomic location. A consistent and methodical approach is necessary to prevent oversight of any abnormalities. A standardized neurologic examination form will keep the examination consistent (Fig. 36-1). Serial neurologic examinations are used to assess patient status (i.e., improving, static, or deteriorating). The neurologic examination should be performed in a quiet area free of distractions that has good footing. Sedatives, narcotics, and/or tranquilizers should not be administered before the examination; however, it is important that the animal be relaxed. Begin the examination by evaluating the patient's mental status, posture, and gait.

Mental status. Allow the animal to move around the examination room. Mental status may be defined as (1) alert (normal); (2) depressed (conscious but inactive; also called *obtunded*); (3) stuporous (sleeps when undisturbed; does not respond to harmless stimuli such as noise, but awakens with a painful stimulus); or (4) comatose (cannot be aroused, even with painful stimulus).

Animals with brain lesions that are unresponsive to their environment usually have diffuse cerebral cortical disease. Those that are stuporous generally have diffuse cerebral disorders or brainstem compression, whereas comatose animals have complete disconnection of the reticular formation and cerebrum.

Posture. Posture is evaluated while the animal is free to move about the examination area and can be further assessed by moving the animal into different positions to observe its ability to regain normal posture. Abnormalities include head tilt, abnormal truncal posture, improper positioning of limbs (proprioceptive deficits), decreased muscle tone in a limb (flaccidity), or increased muscle tone (spasticity). Continuous head tilts are associated with vestibular abnormalities. Abnormal truncal posture may be associated with congenital or acquired spinal cord lesions.

Gait. Evaluation of an animal's gait requires an area with good footing. The animal is observed from the side, moving toward and away from the examiner, in tight circles, and

Signalment

History:

Physical Examination:

Neurologic Examination:

Observation

Mental	Alert		Depressed			Disoriented		Stupor		Coma
Posture	Normal		Head tilt			Tremor		Falling		
Gait	Normal		Ataxia			Hind limbs		All 4		Circling
Paresis	Hind limbs		Tetra			Hemi		Mono		
Other										

Key: 4 = exaggerated clonus: 3 = exaggerated; 2 = normal; 1 = diminished; 0 = none; NE = not evaluated

Postural reactions

	LF	RF	LR	RR
Wheelbarrow				
Hopping				
Ext postural thrust				
Proprioceptive positioning				
Hemistand/walk				
Placing-tactile				
Placing-visual				

Spinal reflexes

	LF	RF	LR	RR
Patellar				
Biceps				
Triceps				
Withdrawal				
Crossed extensor				
Perineal				

Cranial nerves

	L	R			L	R	Comments CN
II, VII - Vision menace				VIII - Nystagmus, resting			
II, III - Pupils resting				VIII - Nystagmus, change			
Stim L				V - Sensation			
Stim R				VII - Facial mm			
II - Fundus				V, VII-Palpebral reflex			
III, IV, VI - Strabismus, resting				IX, X - Gag reflex			
III, IV, VI, VIII - Strabismus, positional				XII - Tongue			

Sensory examination (Locate and describe abnormal)

Hyperpathia	
Superficial pain	
Sensory level	
Deep pain	

Assessment

Anatomic diagnosis

Problem	Rule out location

Neuro-anatomic location of lesion

Etiologic diagnosis

Rule out disease process	Diagnostic plan
Use DAMNIT-V:	Describe plan for each rule out:
Degenerative	D
Anomalous	A
Metabolic	M
Neoplastic	N
Inflammatory/Infectious	I
Trauma	T
Vascular	V

FIG. 36-1
A neurologic examination form is helpful to ensure that your examination is complete.

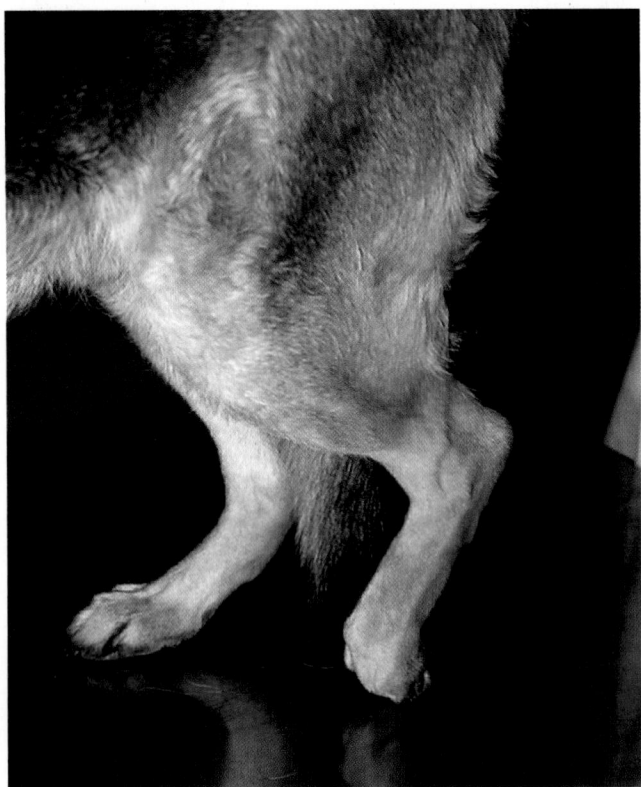

FIG. 36-2
Proprioceptive positioning. The animal should return the paw to a normal position.

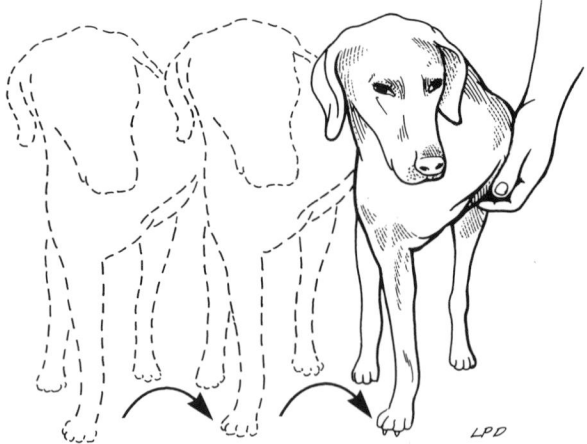

FIG. 36-3
The hopping postural reaction.

backing up. Neurologic organization of gait and posture is complicated, involving brain, spinal cord, and peripheral nerves. *Proprioception* (position sense) is the ability to recognize the location of the limbs in relation to the rest of the body. Deficits cause knuckling, misplacement of the foot, and/or scuffing of the toenails and may be associated with lesions in the brainstem, at any level of the spinal cord, and in the peripheral nerves. *Paresis* is a deficit of voluntary movements; it can be monoparesis, paraparesis, tetraparesis, or hemiparesis (see p. 1357). It is caused by disruption of the voluntary motor pathways, which extend from the brainstem to the spinal cord. Circling in tight circles is usually caused by caudal brainstem lesions; head tilt in association with circling usually indicates involvement of the vestibular system. *Ataxia* is lack of coordination without paretic, spastic, or involuntary movements (although these may be seen in association with ataxia). Ataxia can be caused by lesions at any level, but usually involves cerebellar, vestibular, or spinal cord lesions. *Dysmetria* is characterized by movements that are too long (hypermetria) or too short (hypometria) and are usually caused by cerebellar lesions.

Purposeful movement. Purposeful movement is an animal's conscious attempt to move the legs. It is most applicable to weak ambulatory and nonambulatory animals that drag their legs as they pull themselves along. The legs should be watched for movement, including hip flexion and pushing off with the feet. Assessment of purposeful move-

ments in nonambulatory paraparetic animals can be done by grasping the base of the tail with one hand, lifting the animal, and walking it around. If the legs hang down, purposeful movements are not present, which implies severe, but not necessarily irreversible, spinal cord injury.

Palpation. Careful palpation of the musculoskeletal and integumentary systems while comparing one side with the other is done to check for symmetry. Examiners should look for worn toenails, deep and cutaneous masses, deviation of normal contour, abnormal motion, or crepitation, and should also evaluate muscular size, tone, and strength.

Postural Reactions

Postural reactions are complex responses that maintain an animal's normal upright position. Abnormal postural reactions do not provide precise localizing information, but may indicate neurologic disease.

Proprioceptive positioning. Proprioceptive positioning (knuckling) is performed by flexing the paw so the dorsal surface is on the floor (Fig. 36-2). The animal should immediately return the paw to a normal position. Delayed or absent correction of the knuckled paw indicates neurologic disease. Worn dorsal toenails, skin abrasions, or calluses on the dorsum of the foot may signify long-standing proprioceptive deficits.

Wheelbarrowing. Wheelbarrowing is performed by having the animal bear weight on the thoracic limbs while it is being supported under the abdomen. Normal animals walk forward with coordinated movements of both thoracic limbs. Slow initiation of movement may be due to a cervical spinal cord, brainstem, or cerebral lesion. Exaggerated movements (dysmetria) may indicate cervical spinal cord, lower brainstem, or cerebellar abnormalities.

Hopping. Hopping is tested with the animal positioned as for wheelbarrowing, except one thoracic or pelvic limb is lifted from the ground. The entire weight of the animal is supported on one limb as the patient is moved medially and laterally (Fig. 36-3). Poor initiation of hopping suggests pro-

Table 36-1

Comparison of Common Neurologic Findings in UMN and LMN Disease

SPINAL REFLEXES	LMN	UMN
Patellar	Absent or depressed	Normal or exaggerated
Triceps	Absent or depressed	Normal or exaggerated
Biceps	Absent or depressed	Normal or exaggerated
Pelvic limb withdrawal	Absent or depressed	Normal or exaggerated
Thoracic limb withdrawal	Absent or depressed	Normal or exaggerated
Crossed extensor	Absent or depressed	Normal or exaggerated
Anal sphincter	Absent or depressed	Normal or exaggerated
Tail wagging	Absent or depressed	Normal or exaggerated
Strength	Poor	Variable but stronger than with LMN
Muscle tone	Flaccid	Spastic
Muscle fasciculation	Present	Absent
Muscle atrophy	Early, neurogenic	Late, disuse
Clonus	Absent	Present
Bladder expression	Easy	Difficult
Root signature	Present	Absent

UMN, Upper motor neuron; *LMN,* lower motor neuron.

prioceptive deficits, whereas poor movement suggests motor deficits. Asymmetry may help lateralize a lesion. Generally, testing thoracic limbs yields more reliable information than testing pelvic limbs.

Extensor postural thrust. Extensor postural thrust is performed by supporting the animal under the thorax while lowering it to the floor. When the pelvic limbs touch the floor, they should move caudally in symmetric walking movements to achieve a position of support. Patient assessment is the same as for wheelbarrowing.

Hemistanding/hemiwalking. Hemistanding and hemiwalking are performed by elevating the front and rear limbs of one side so that all of the animal's weight is supported by the opposite limbs. Lateral walking movements are then evaluated. Patient assessment is the same as for wheelbarrowing.

Placing. Placing reactions are evaluated first without vision (tactile placing) and then with vision (visual placing). During tactile placing, the examiner supports the animal under the thorax and covers its eyes with one hand. The distal thoracic limbs (at or below the carpi) are brought in contact with the edge of a table. The normal response is immediate placement of the feet on the table surface in a position that will support weight. Visual placing is tested by allowing the animal to see the table surface. Normal animals reach for the surface before the carpus touches the table. Visual placing requires normal visual pathways to the cerebral cortex, communication from the visual cortex to the motor cortex, and motor pathways to the forelimb periph-

eral nerves. A lesion of any portion of the pathway may cause a deficit in the placing reaction. Normal tactile placing with absent visual placing indicates a lesion in the visual system, whereas normal visual placing with abnormal tactile placing suggests a sensory pathway lesion. Cerebral and diencephalic lesions produce a deficit in the contralateral (opposite) limb. Lesions below the midbrain usually produce an ipsilateral (same side as lesion) deficit.

Spinal Reflexes

Spinal reflexes (myotactic reflexes) test the integrity of sensory and motor components of the reflex arc and the influence of descending motor pathways on the reflex. Three kinds of responses may be seen: (1) absence or depressed reflex, indicating complete or partial loss of either the sensory or motor nerves responsible for the reflex (lower motor neuron [LMN]); (2) normal reflex, indicating that sensory and motor nerves are intact; and (3) exaggerated reflex, indicating an abnormality in the descending pathways from the brain and spinal cord that normally inhibit the reflex (upper motor neuron [UMN]). A list of LMN and UMN signs is given in Table 36-1. In general, the thoracic limb has fewer reliable localizing spinal reflexes than the pelvic limb.

Pelvic Limb

Patellar reflex. The patellar reflex (Box 36-3) is the most reliable pelvic limb reflex. It is performed with the animal in lateral recumbency. The uppermost leg is supported by

BOX 36-3

Spinal Reflexes

Patellar Reflex

- Absent or depressed reflex
  Unilateral—femoral nerve
  Bilateral—lesion at spinal cord segments L4–L6
- Exaggerated reflex
  Bilateral—lesion cranial to spinal cord segment L4

Withdrawal Reflex—Pelvic Limb

- Absent or depressed reflex
  Unilateral—sciatic nerve
  Bilateral—lesion at spinal cord segments L6–S1
- Exaggerated reflex
  Bilateral—lesion cranial to spinal cord segment L6

Triceps Reflex

- Absent or depressed reflex
  Lesion in spinal cord segments C7–T1
  Not always reliable
- Exaggerated reflex
  Bilateral—lesion cranial to spinal cord segment C7

Biceps Reflex

- Absent or depressed reflex
  Lesion in spinal cord segments C6–C8
  Not always reliable
- Exaggerated reflex
  Bilateral—lesion cranial to spinal cord segment C8

Withdrawal Reflex—Thoracic Limb

- Absent or depressed reflex
  Lesion in spinal cord segments C6–T1
- Exaggerated reflex
  Unilateral—peripheral nerves
  Bilateral—lesion cranial to spinal cord segment C6

Anal Sphincter Reflex

- Absent or depressed reflex
  Lesion in spinal cord segments S1–S3
- Normal or exaggerated reflex
  Lesion cranial to spinal cord segment S1

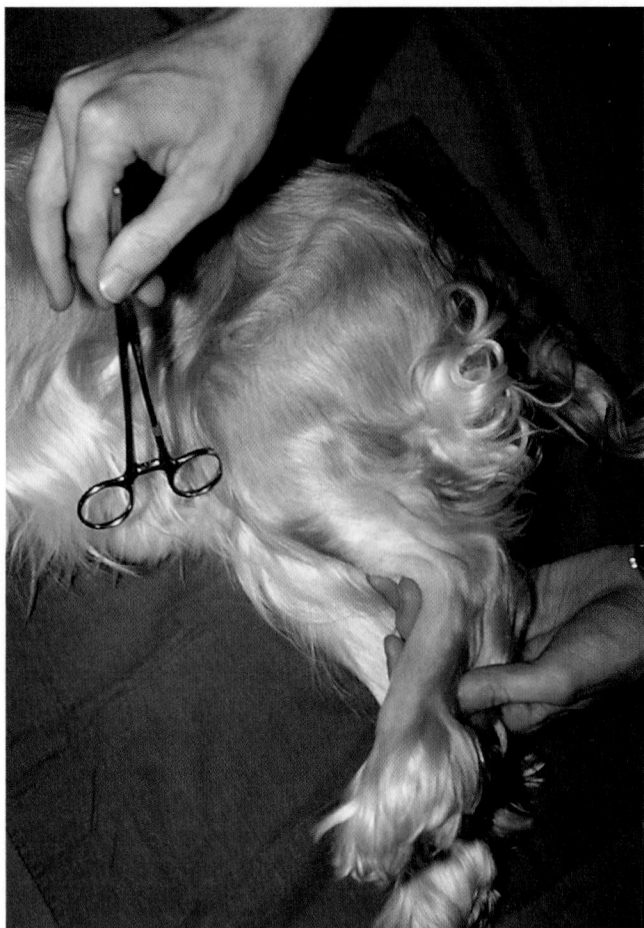

FIG. 36-4
The patellar reflex is initiated by striking the straight patellar ligament with a reflex hammer.

holding the hock with the stifle slightly flexed. When the patellar ligament is struck briskly with a reflex hammer (Fig. 36-4), the response is a single, quick extension of the stifle. Absence or depression of the patellar reflex (hypopatellar reflex) and decreased muscle tone (flaccidity) indicate a lesion of the sensory or motor component of the reflex arc (LMN). Unilateral loss of the reflex suggests a femoral nerve lesion, whereas bilateral loss suggests a segmental spinal cord lesion involving spinal cord segments L4-L6. Occasionally, old dogs lose their patellar reflex yet maintain their ambulatory ability. Exaggerated reflexes (hyperpatellar reflex) and increased muscle tone (spasticity), when associated with other signs of UMN dysfunction, suggest a lesion cranial to the L4 spinal cord segment (UMN).

Withdrawal reflex. Pelvic limb withdrawal reflex (see Box 36-3) is performed with the animal in lateral recum-

bency. The least harmful stimulus possible is applied to the foot; the normal response is flexion of the entire limb (Fig. 36-5). This reflex primarily involves spinal cord segments L6 to S1 and the sciatic nerve. Absence or depression of the reflex indicates a lesion of these spinal cord segments or nerves (LMN). Unilateral absence of the reflex is most likely the result of a sciatic nerve lesion, whereas bilateral absence or depression is more likely the result of a spinal cord lesion. An exaggerated withdrawal reflex indicates a lesion cranial to spinal cord segment L6 (UMN).

Thoracic Limb

Triceps reflex. Triceps reflex (see Box 36-3) is performed with the animal in lateral recumbency. The limb is supported under the elbow; the elbow is fully extended and the entire leg drawn caudally. The triceps tendon is struck with a reflex hammer just proximal to the olecranon (Fig. 36-6). Normal response is slight extension of the elbow. The triceps muscle is innervated by the radial nerve, which originates from spinal cord segments C7-T2. The triceps reflex is difficult to elicit in normal animals; thus absent or depressed

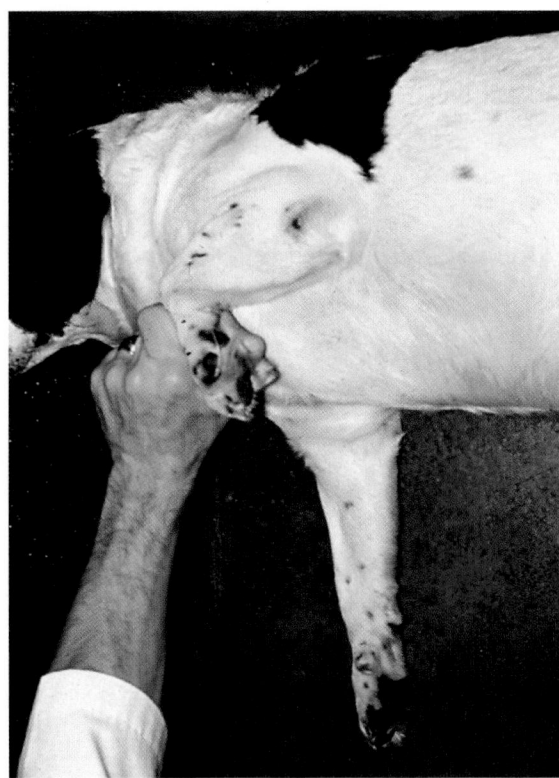
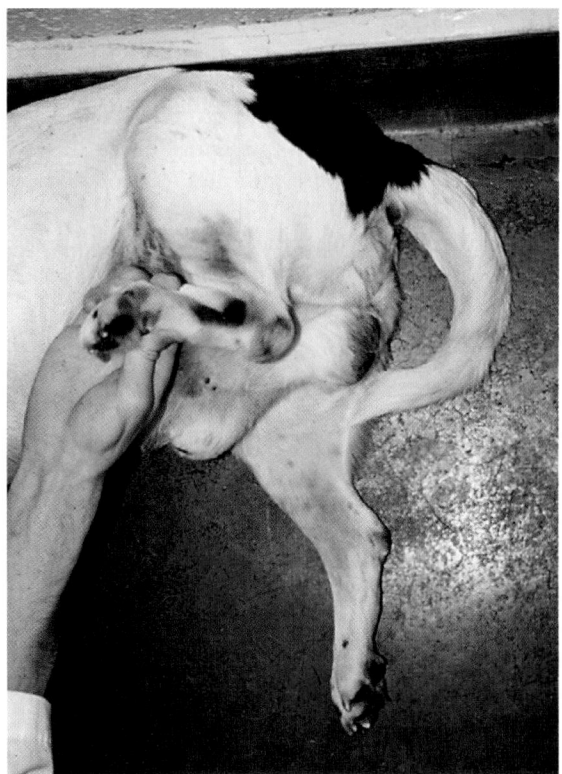

FIG. 36-5
The withdrawal reflex (thoracic and pelvic limbs) occurs when a noxious stimulus is applied to the foot. The entire limb should flex.

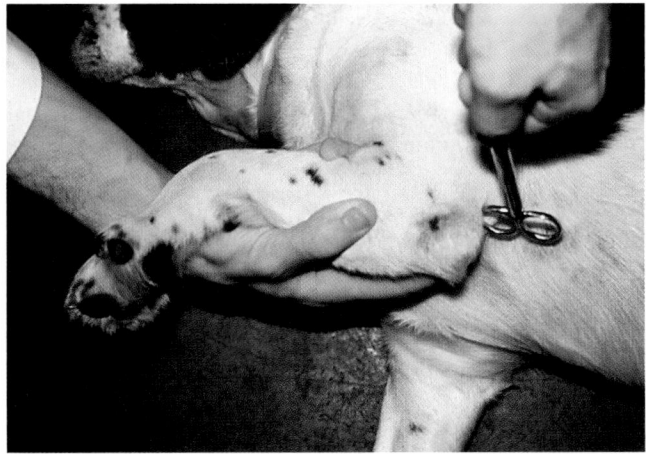

FIG. 36-6
The triceps reflex is initiated by striking the triceps tendon just proximal to the olecranon.

reflexes may not indicate an abnormality. An exaggerated reflex, if elicited, indicates a lesion cranial to C7 (UMN).

Biceps reflex. To perform the biceps reflex (see Box 36-3), the index finger of the examiner's hand that is holding the animal's elbow is placed on the biceps tendon cranial and proximal to the elbow. The elbow is slightly extended and the finger is struck with the reflex hammer. Normal response is slight flexion of the elbow. This reflex is difficult to elicit in the normal animal. Absent or decreased reflexes suggest a lesion involving spinal cord segments C6-T8 (LMN), but may be normal in some animals. An exaggerated reflex, if elicited, indicates a lesion cranial to spinal cord segment C6 (UMN).

Withdrawal reflex. Thoracic limb withdrawal reflex (see Box 36-3) is performed in a similar manner as the pelvic limb withdrawal reflex (see Fig. 36-5). This reflex primarily involves spinal cord segments C6-T2. Absent or depressed reflexes indicate a lesion of these spinal cord segments or of the peripheral nerves (LMN). Exaggerated reflexes, when associated with other signs of UMN dysfunction, indicate a lesion cranial to spinal cord segment C6 (UMN).

Other Reflexes

Anal sphincter reflex. The perineal or anal sphincter reflex (see Box 36-3) is elicited by gentle perineal stimulation with a needle or forceps. A normal response is contraction of the anal sphincter muscle. Sensory and motor innervation occurs through the pudendal nerve (perineal nerve is sensory; caudal rectal nerve is motor) and spinal cord segments S1-S3. The anal sphincter reflex is the best indication of functional integrity of sacral spinal cord segments and sacral nerve roots. Evaluation of this reflex is important in animals with urinary bladder dysfunction. It may be absent, depressed, normal, or exaggerated. Absence or depression of the reflex (failure of the anus to contract) indicates a sacral spinal cord or pudendal nerve lesion (LMN). An exaggerated response indicates a lesion above the S1 spinal cord segment.

Bladder expression. The two general components of urinary bladder innervation are autonomic (hypogastric and pelvic) and somatic (pudendal) nerves. Simplistically, clinical observations of bladder dysfunction can be attributed to spinal cord injury based on the pudendal nerve (S1 and S2). The pudendal nerve innervates urethral striated muscle and helps maintain urinary continence. A lesion above the sacral spinal cord segments causes detrusor spasticity, making the bladder difficult to express (UMN). A lesion involving sacral spinal cord segments causes lack of sphincter tone and an easily expressible bladder (LMN).

Crossed extensor reflex. The crossed extensor reflex may be observed when withdrawal reflexes are elicited. With the animal in lateral recumbency and legs relaxed, the toes of the uppermost limb (thoracic or pelvic) are gently pinched with fingers, eliciting a withdrawal reflex (Fig. 36-7). An abnormal response is flexion of the upper limb and simultaneous extension of the lower limb. The stimulus must be gentle; excessive stimulus causes the animal to attempt to right itself, negating any findings. The crossed extensor reflex results from a lesion that affects descending inhibitory pathways of the spinal cord (UMN). This reflex is commonly associated with chronicity, but does not constitute a poor prognosis.

Tail wag reflex. The significance of tail wagging in patients with spinal cord injuries is often misinterpreted. Animals with a completely transected spinal cord above the sacral and caudal spinal cord segments can wag their tails. This reflex wag is often observed when expressing the bladder or eliciting the anal sphincter reflex. Tail wagging may also be a conscious response to pleasurable stimuli, such as petting the head, calling the animal's name, or seeing the owner. This conscious response implies that some spinal cord pathways are intact. It is important to distinguish between a spontaneous (reflex) and conscious tail wagging.

> NOTE: Do not assume that because the dog can wag its tail, it has an intact spinal cord. It may simply be a reflex.

Panniculus reflex. Panniculus reflex (cutaneous trunci reflex) is elicited by pin-prick stimulus to the skin over the back, beginning at the lumbosacral region and continuing cranially. Normal response is twitching of the cutaneous trunci muscle on both sides of the dorsal midline, at the point of stimulation and cranially. Absence of a response occurs one or two segments caudal to the spinal cord lesion. This reflex must be interpreted with some caution; it may be unreliable with the exception of brachial plexus avulsion

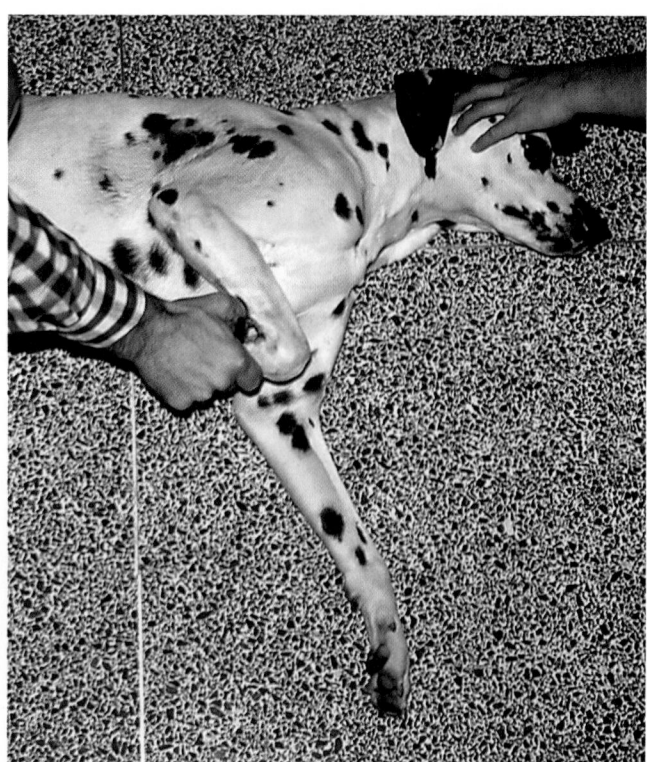

FIG. 36-7
A crossed extensor reflex suggests a lesion afflicting descending inhibitory pathways of the spinal cord (UMN).

injuries, in which it is consistently absent only on the side of the avulsion (ipsilateral).

Clonus. *Clonus* refers to a sustained after-contraction or quivering that may be seen or felt when performing spinal reflexes, especially patellar and crossed extensor reflexes. The hand supporting the extremity being tested may feel this reaction; this reflex is often not visual. Presence of clonus implies a chronic condition.

Sensory Evaluation

Presence or absence of deep pain perception is the most important prognostic test of the neurologic examination and is a reliable indicator of spinal cord integrity. As a general rule, sensory evaluation should be done last. It is performed by applying painful stimuli to each limb and the tail. A significant behavioral response (e.g., animal attempts to vocalize, turns to look or bite, or attempts to get away from the examiner) indicates the presence of sensation. Withdrawal of a limb is not a behavioral response. Progressively stronger painful stimuli (e.g., hemostatic forceps) are used to assess presence or absence of deep pain perception. As a general rule, loss of function after spinal cord injury develops as follows: (1) loss of proprioception, (2) loss of voluntary motor function, (3) loss of superficial pain sensation, and (4) loss of deep pain sensation. Therefore an animal with spinal cord compression that has lost

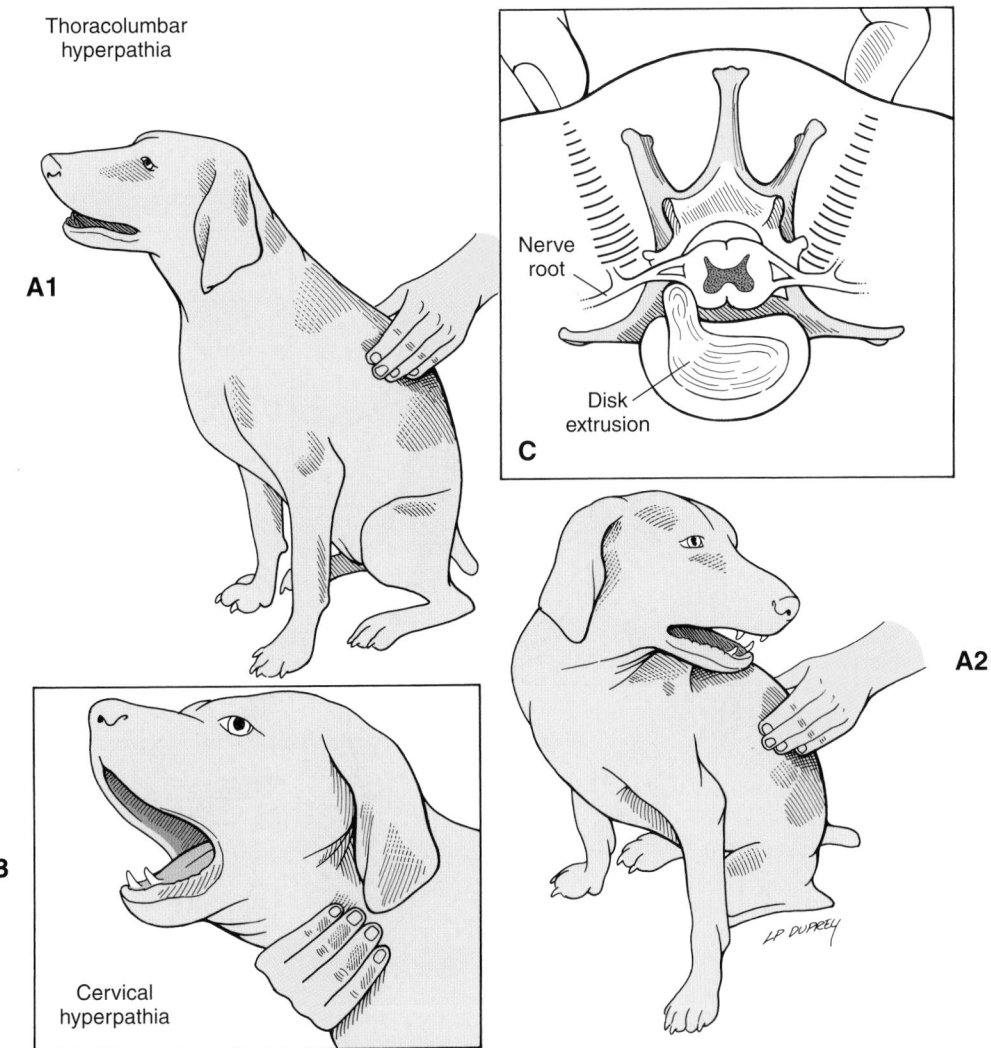

FIG. 36-8
Thoracolumbar and cervical hyperpathia; digital pressure placed over the **(A1)** thoracolumbar paraspinal or **(B)** cervical paraspinal muscles at the site of an extradural lesion results in pain and a behavioral response from the patient **(A2). C,** Pressure placed on epaxial muscles is transferred to the entrapped nerve root *(inset)*, causing nerve root compression and ischemia; the result is pain and a behavioral response.

proprioception and voluntary motor function, but still has superficial and deep pain sensation (paresis), has less severe spinal cord damage than one that has lost all four functions (resulting in plegia and paralysis). Loss of deep pain indicates a severely damaged spinal cord and a poor prognosis. As an animal recovers from spinal cord injury, sensation returns first, then motor function, and lastly proprioception. Because of the prognostic importance of sensory examination, an evaluation of the animal by a second, unbiased examiner or a repeat of the examination in 1 or 2 hours is critical.

Hyperpathia. Hyperpathia is noted when pressure applied to spinous processes and paraspinal muscles of the thoracic and lumbar regions and transverse processes and paraspinal muscles of the cervical region results in pain and

a behavioral response (see previous discussion) (Fig. 36-8). Pain perception occurs at the level of spinal cord involvement, making hyperpathia an accurate localizing feature of the neurologic examination.

Sensory level. Sensory level is determined by pin-prick stimulus applied to the skin over the back, beginning in the region of the L7 vertebrae and continuing cranially. The junction between an area of depressed behavioral response and one of normal behavioral response is the sensory level (Fig. 36-9). Pain perception is noted one or two segments caudal to the level of spinal cord involvement.

Cranial Nerve Examination
Examination of cranial nerves is important, especially when a brain lesion is suspected.

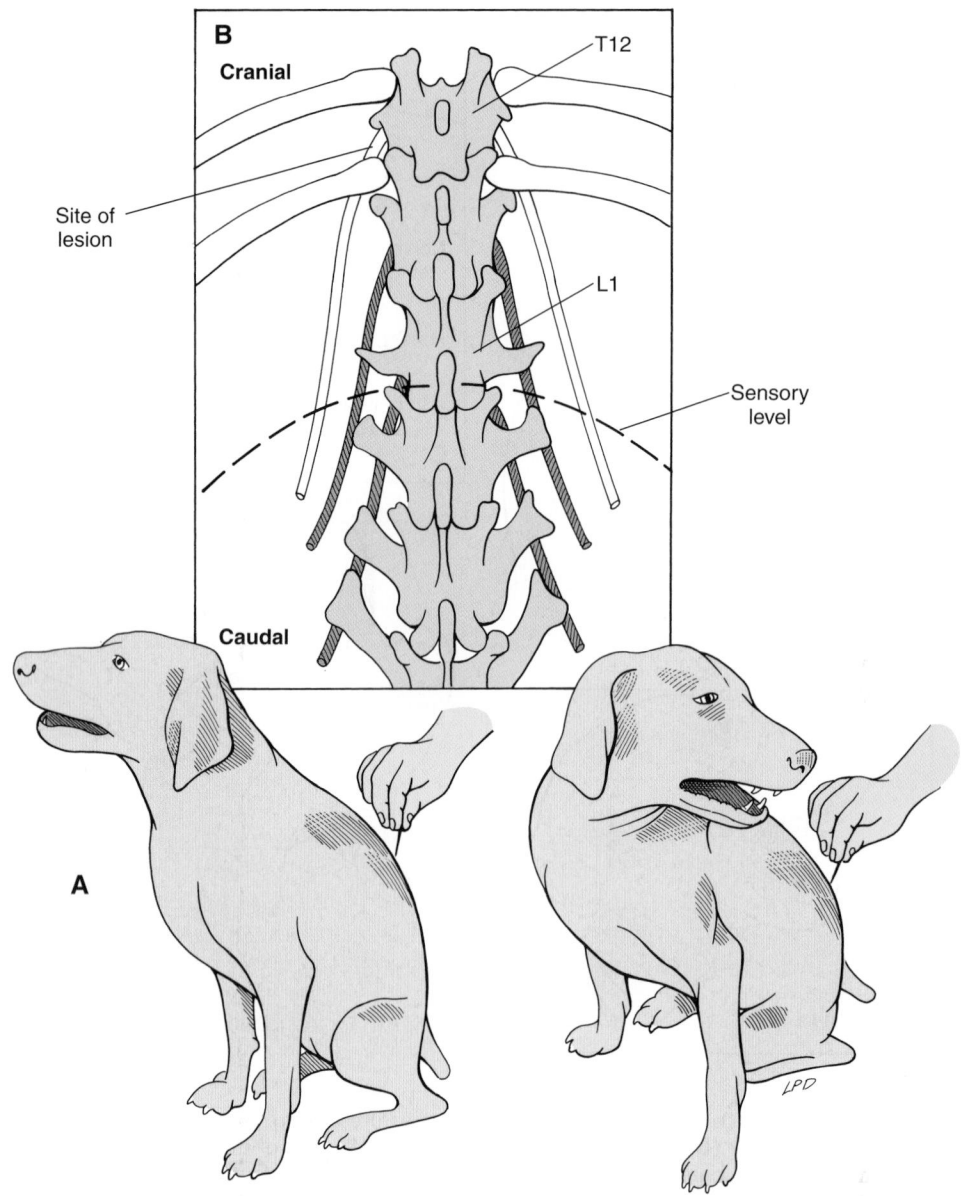

FIG. 36-9
A, Sensory level is the junction between an area of depressed or absent sensation and area of normal sensation. **B,** Because thoracolumbar nerve roots course caudoventrally, the sensory level is one or two vertebral bodies caudal to the spinal cord lesion.

Olfactory nerve. The olfactory nerve is sensory for conscious perception of smell. Rhinitis, tumors of the nasal passages, and diseases of the cribriform plate are the most common causes for loss of olfaction.

Optic nerve. The optic nerve is the sensory pathway for vision and pupillary light reflexes. It is examined by means of three major tests: menace response (elicited by making a threatening gesture with the hand at each eye); visual placing reaction (see p. 1361); and ophthalmoscopic examination. Abnormalities include loss of vision, dilated pupils, and loss of pupillary light response (direct and consensual) when light is shined in the affected eye.

Oculomotor nerve. The oculomotor nerve contains parasympathetic motor fibers for pupillary constriction. It is motor to the extraocular eye muscles and levator muscle of the upper eyelid. After shining a light into each eye, pupils are observed for size and symmetry. Both pupils should constrict symmetrically when a light is shined into either eye (consensual response). Abnormalities include loss of pupillary light response on the affected side (even if light is shined in the opposite eye), fixed lateral deviation (strabismus) of the eye, and dilated pupil.

Trochlear nerve. Lesions of the trochlear nerve cause lateral rotation of the eye.

Abducent nerve. Lesions of the abducent nerve cause medial strabismus, loss of gaze, and inability to retract the globe.

Trigeminal nerve. The trigeminal nerve innervates muscles of mastication and is sensory to the face. Motor function is tested by assessing muscle mass and jaw tone of the masticatory muscles. Sensory function is assessed by checking pain perception of the face, eyelids, cornea, and nasal mucosa. Bilateral motor paralysis produces a "dropped jaw" and muscle atrophy; unilateral paralysis results in unilateral atrophy of the temporalis muscle and decreased jaw tone and strength.

Facial nerve. The facial nerve is motor to the muscles of facial expression and sensory to the inner surface of the pinna, palate, and rostral two thirds of the tongue. Facial paralysis generally causes facial asymmetry (e.g., lips, eyelids, and ears may droop) and loss of ability to blink or retract the lips.

Vestibulocochlear nerve. The vestibulocochlear nerve has two divisions: vestibular (which provides information about the orientation of the head with respect to gravity) and cochlear (which means hearing). Abnormalities associated with nerve dysfunction include ataxia, head tilt, circling, nystagmus, and loss of hearing.

Glossopharyngeal and vagus nerves. Swallowing is controlled by glossopharyngeal and vagus nerves. The swallowing reflex is elicited by gentle external pressure on the hyoid region. The gag reflex is elicited by insertion of the finger into the caudal pharynx. The glossopharyngeal nerve is motor to pharyngeal muscles, and the vagus nerve is motor to pharyngeal and laryngeal muscles. The vagus nerve is sensory to the caudal pharynx and larynx. Abnormalities caused by glossopharyngeal and vagus nerve dysfunction include loss of the gag reflex, dysphagia, and laryngeal paralysis.

Hypoglossal nerve. The hypoglossal nerve is motor to muscles of the tongue. Abnormalities can be observed by wetting the animal's nose and observing its ability to extend the tongue. Strength of tongue retraction, tongue deviation, and presence or absence of atrophy should be evaluated.

LESION LOCALIZATION

Once the neurologic examination has been completed, an attempt is made to determine a single neuroanatomic location that explains all abnormal findings. The lesion is initially categorized as being located above or below the foramen magnum. Lesions suspected of being above the foramen magnum are further localized to one of five locations in the brain: cerebral cortex, diencephalon (thalamus and hypothalamus), brainstem (pons, medulla oblongata), vestibular, or cerebellum. Box 36-4 lists characteristic abnormal neurologic findings that aid in localizing brain lesions.

Lesions suspected of being below the foramen magnum are further localized to one of five locations in the spinal cord: cranial cervical (C1-C5), caudal cervical (C6-T2), thoracolumbar (T3-L3), lumbosacral (L4-S3), and sacral (S1-S3) (Fig. 36-10). The ability to predict the expected UMN and/or LMN signs with lesions at various levels of the spinal cord improves accurate lesion localization. This may be con-

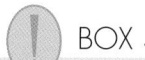 BOX 36-4

Abnormal Neurologic Findings That Help Localize Brain Lesions

Cerebral Cortex

Altered mental status
Ipsilateral circling, pacing, head pressing
Contralateral postural and proprioceptive deficits
Contralateral cortical blindness (normal pupils and pupillary light reflexes)
Contralateral UMN hemiparesis
Seizures

Diencephalon (Thalamus and Hypothalamus)

Altered mental status: aggression, disorientation, hyperexcitability, coma
Contralateral postural and proprioceptive deficits
Bilateral visual deficits
Abnormalities of eating, drinking, sleeping, and temperature (hypothalamus)
Muscle tone, segmental reflexes, and sensation are unaltered

Brainstem (Pontomedullary)

Mental status may be unaltered, to severe depression and coma
Ipsilateral UMN hemiparesis or tetraparesis; may circle if ambulatory
Cranial nerve deficits involving cranial nerves V through XII
  Trigeminal—motor and sensory
  Abducent—medial strabismus
  Facial—facial paralysis
  Vestibulocochlear—central vestibular signs; hearing loss
  Glossopharyngeal/vagus—dysphagia, reduced gag reflex, laryngeal dysfunction
  Hypoglossal—abnormal tongue movement

Vestibular

Disoriented or unaltered mental status
Ipsilateral head tilt, circling, rolling, falling, asymmetric ataxia, and incoordination
Nystagmus (spontaneous or positional) with fast phase away from the side of the lesion
Ipsilateral ventrolateral strabismus
Must differentiate central from peripheral vestibular disease

Cerebellum

Unaltered mental status
Ataxic gait, wide-based stance, dysmetria, head tremor, intention tremor, and truncal ataxia
Visual but may have ipsilateral loss of menace response
Hypermetric postural reactions, goose stepping gait
Muscle tone, segmental reflexes, and sensation are unaltered

UMN, Upper motor neuron.

fusing, however, because a single spinal lesion can be LMN and UMN to various nerve and muscle groups simultaneously. Fig. 36-10 illustrates locations of various spinal cord injuries and the expected UMN and LMN reactions to the front and hind limbs. In the unusual circumstance that an animal has two spinal cord lesions, it is important to predict the expected UMN and LMN signs. Notice also that if an animal has both a UMN and an LMN lesion to a specific site

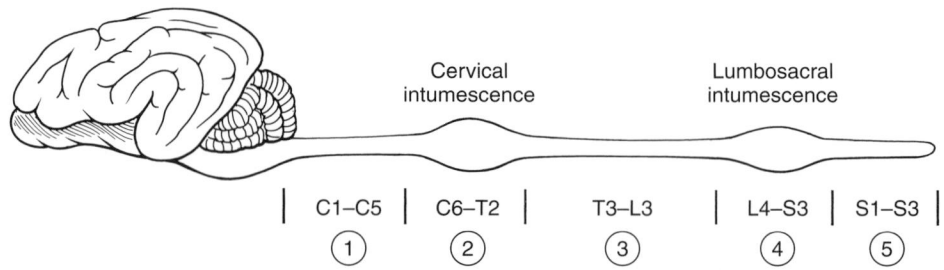

Site number	Spinal cord segments	Expected neurologic response
1 craniocervical	C1-C5	UMN to the front limbs UMN to the rear limbs
2 caudocervical	C6-T2	LMN to the front limbs UMN to the rear limbs
3 thoracolumbar	T3-L3	Normal to the front limbs UMN to the rear limbs
4 lumbosacral	L4-S3	Normal to the front limbs LMN to the rear limbs
5 sacral	S1-S3	Normal to the front limbs Normal to the rear limbs LMN to the tail and anus

FIG. 36-10
Expected UMN and LMN reflex abnormalities caused by lesions located in various segments of the spinal cord.

The expected reflex response to multiple lesions of the spinal cord

Lesion location	Expected neurologic response
Site 1 and 2	LMN front; UMN rear
Site 1 and 3	UMN front; UMN rear
Site 1 and 4	UMN front; LMN rear
Site 1 and 5	UMN front; UMN rear; LMN tail and anus
Site 2 and 3	LMN front; UMN rear
Site 2 and 4	LMN front; LMN rear
Site 2 and 5	LMN front; UMN rear; LMN tail and anus
Site 3 and 4	LMN rear; UMN tail and anus
Site 3 and 5	UMN rear; LMN tail and anus
Site 4 and 5	LMN rear; LMN tail and anus

 Table 36-2

Location of Spinal Cord Segments Within Vertebral Bodies

GENERAL LOCATION	SPINAL CORD SEGMENTS	VERTEBRAL BODIES
Craniocervical	C1–C5	C1–C4
Caudocervical	C6–T2	C5–T1
Thoracolumbar	T3–L3	T2–L3
Lumbosacral	L4–S3	L4–L6
Sacral	S1–S3	L5
	L4	L3–4 interspace
	L5–L6	L4
	L7	L4–5 interspace
Spinal cord ends		L5–6 interspace

(e.g., sites 3 and 4 [see Fig. 36-10]), LMN reflex changes predominate. Lesion localization of spinal cord disorders based on neurologic examination findings should not be limited to spinal cord segments (within the vertebral canal). It is important to be able to localize spinal cord segment abnormalities within a vertebral body (Table 36-2 and Fig. 36-11). Once the neuroanatomic location of the lesion has been identified and signalment, history, and physical examination findings reviewed, differential diagnoses and appropriate diagnostic plans can be formulated.

DIFFERENTIAL DIAGNOSIS OF SPINAL DISORDERS AND DIAGNOSTIC METHODS

Establishing a list of differential diagnoses requires incorporation of historical and physical and neurologic examination findings. The minimum data required for a diagnostic plan include hematology, serum chemistry, and urinalysis. These

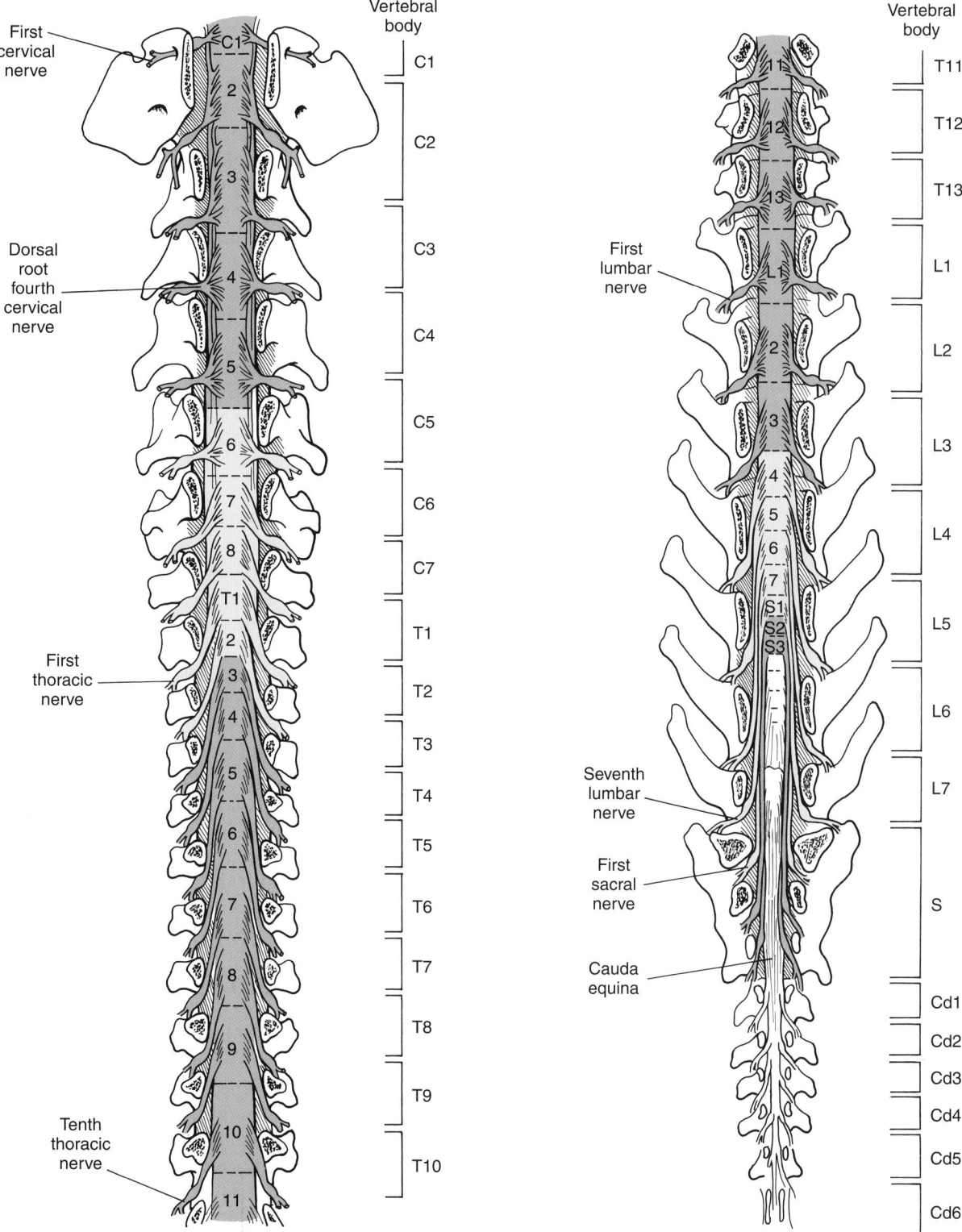

FIG. 36-11

Laminectomized spine showing the relationship of spinal cord segments with vertebral bodies. (Modified from Evans HE, editor: *Miller's anatomy of the dog*, ed 3, Philadelphia, 1993, WB Saunders.)

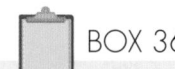

Differential Diagnosis of Spinal Cord Disorders Based on DAMNIT-V Scheme

D—Degenerative

Intervertebral disk disease
Wobbler syndrome
Cauda equina syndrome
Degenerative myelopathy

A—Anomalous

Atlantoaxial instability

M—Metabolic

N—Neoplastic

Spine
Spinal cord
Meninges

I—Inflammatory/Infectious

Diskospondylitis
Vertebral osteomyelitis

T—Traumatic

Vertebral fracture/luxation

V—Vascular

Fibrocartilaginous embolism
Spinal cord infarction

data may vary depending on a differential diagnosis, including an electrocardiogram, echocardiogram, additional laboratory data, and/or chest and abdominal radiographs or ultrasound examination. Patients suspected of having an intracranial lesion may require additional serum chemistry tests, cerebrospinal fluid (CSF) analysis, skull radiographs, computed tomography (CT scan), and/or magnetic resonance imaging (MRI). Those suspected of having a spinal lesion may require a spinal series of survey radiographs, CSF tap, myelography, CT scan, and/or MRI. These diagnostic tests should localize an intracranial (intraaxial, extraaxial) or spinal lesion (extradural, intradural-extramedullary, or intramedullary); help determine the most effective treatment (medical or surgical); and may suggest a cause (see Box 36-2; Box 36-5). The selection of diagnostic tests depends on historical data (i.e., pattern of disease progression: acute/static, acute/progressive, or chronic/progressive), neurologic examination findings (i.e., lesion located above or below the foramen magnum), and initial minimum data.

IMAGING THE SPINE

Initial localization of most spinal disorders can be accomplished with conventional radiographs (spinal radiographs and myelography). The spinal cord, surrounded by CSF, is encased in an osseous spine composed of individual vertebrae connected by complex ligamentous structures (i.e., an-

nulus fibrosus, nucleus pulposus, and diarthrodial facet joints). Each section of the spine (i.e., cervical, thoracic, lumbar, sacral, and caudal vertebra) is anatomically unique. The complexity of the spine demands that careful attention be given to proper radiographic technique, positioning, and interpretation. When spinal radiography is performed, the following guidelines should be followed: (1) general anesthesia should be used; (2) symmetric positioning with care to support the spine during repositioning is required; (3) lateral and ventrodorsal projections of each section of the spine should be obtained; (4) high-quality (detail) radiographic film-screen combinations should be used; (5) each section of the spine should be imaged separately; and (6) high-contrast radiographic technique (less than 70 kVp) with narrow collimation is necessary. Knowledge of normal anatomic variations for each section of the spine is mandatory, and accurate interpretation must be based on minimum data base, historical, physical, and neurologic examination findings.

Survey Radiographs

Survey radiographs allow accurate lesion localization if vertebrae or their ligamentous attachments are directly involved (i.e., congenital anomalies, vertebral fracture/luxation, vertebral body neoplasia, diskospondylitis, vertebral body osteomyelitis, and extruded calcified intervertebral disk). Radiographic signs of spinal disease consist of changes in shape, size, alignment, and opacity (Fig. 36-12). Survey radiographs do not allow one to directly view the spinal cord. Lesion localization in patients with spinal disorders that do not cause visible changes in the vertebrae (i.e., fibrocartilaginous emboli, neoplasia of the spinal cord or meninges, intervertebral disk extrusion, cauda equina syndrome, or wobbler syndrome) requires myelography, CT, or MRI. A recent study showed that the accuracy of determining sites of intervertebral disk protrusion using survey radiography was in the range of 51% to 61% (Lamb et al, 2002).

Stress Radiography

Stress radiography may be used in the definitive diagnosis of spinal disorders. It is performed by placing various sections of the vertebral column in gentle dorsal hyperextension, ventral flexion, and/or linear traction. The end result is to exacerbate or relieve compressive lesions. This information may be important in establishing lesion location and planning therapy. Stress radiography is most commonly used in the diagnosis of atlantoaxial instability (Fig. 36-13), cervical vertebral instability, and lumbosacral instability.

> NOTE: Perform stress radiography carefully so as not to exacerbate the patient's neurologic deficits.

Myelography

Myelography requires subarachnoid injection of contrast media (lumbar or cisternal) to outline the spinal cord. It is indicated when (1) a visible lesion is not identified on survey

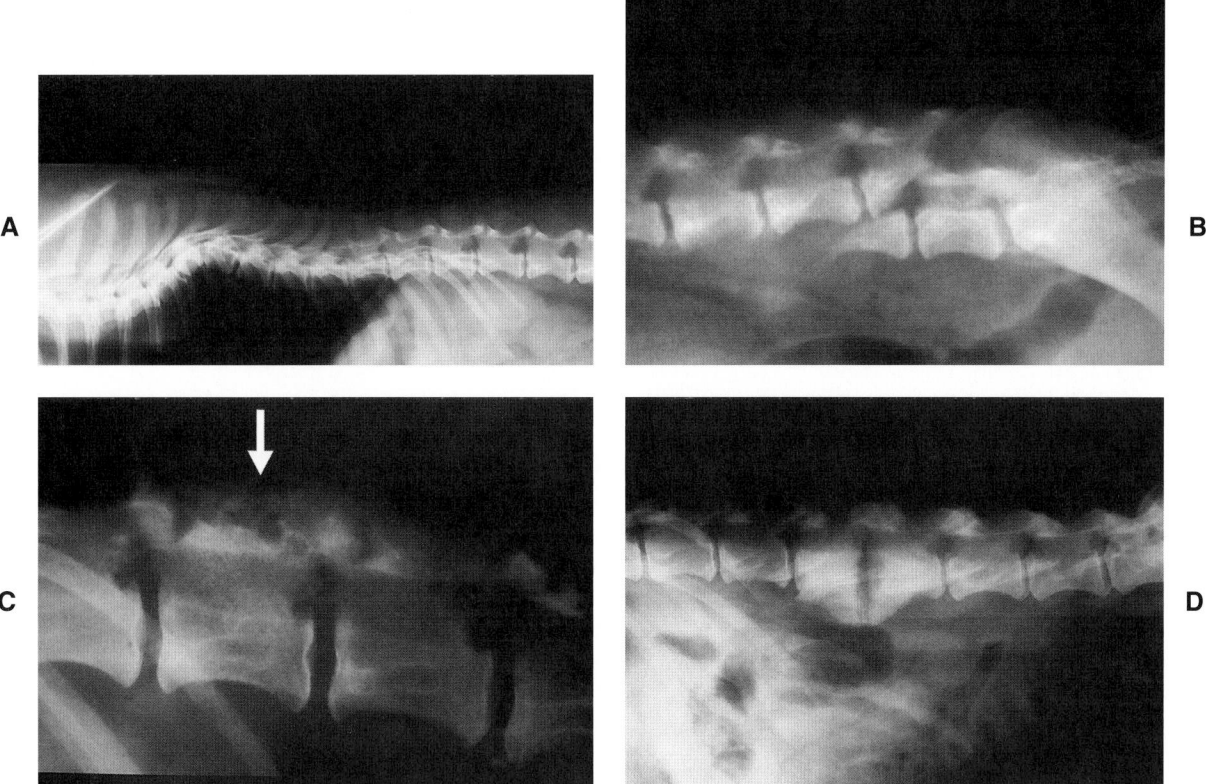

FIG. 36-12
A, Lateral radiography of a dog with a T6–T7 congenital malformation. Notice the elongated dorsal spinous processes, collapse of the intervertebral space, and narrowing of the vertebral canal. **B,** Lateral radiograph of a dog with an L6 spinal fracture. Notice the oblique vertebral body and laminar fracture with cranial displacement and overriding. **C,** Lateral radiograph of a dog with L2 laminar neoplasia. Notice the osteoproduction of the dorsal lamina *(arrow).* **D,** Lateral radiograph of a dog with L3–L4 diskospondylitis. Notice the lysis of the vertebral endplates, spondylosis, and increased bone density of the L3 and L4 vertebral body.

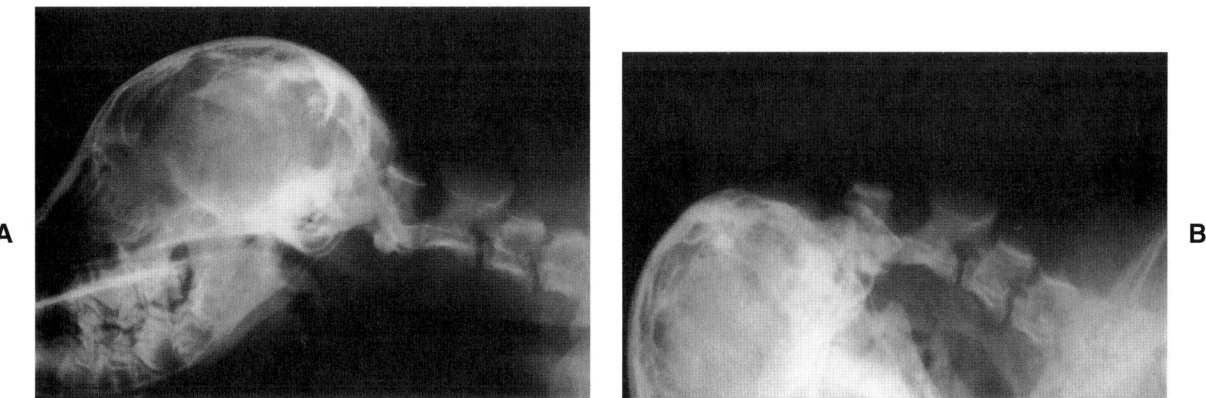

FIG. 36-13
A, Radiograph of a dog with atlantoaxial instability. The head and neck are in normal functional position. **B,** Ventral flexion of the head and neck reveals an increased space between dorsal lamina of C1 and dorsal spinous process of C2, indicating instability.

Table 36-3

Contrast Agents Commonly Used in Myelography

CONTRAST AGENTS	DOSAGE RANGE	CONCENTRATION RANGE	MIDRANGE DOSE	MIDRANGE CONCENTRATION
Iopamidol (Isovue)	0.25–0.45 ml/kg	180–370 mg/ml	0.33 mg/kg	240 mg/ml
Iohexol (Omnipaque)	0.25–0.45 ml/kg	180–350 mg/ml	0.33 mg/kg	240 mg/ml

Table 36-4

Advantages and Disadvantages of Cisternal Versus Lumbar Myelography

CISTERNAL TAP	LUMBAR TAP (L4–L5 OR L5–L6)
Advantages	**Advantages**
Easier to perform	Flows forward under pressure to outline lesions
Excellent view of cervical spine	
Disadvantages	**Disadvantages**
Distribution of contrast depends on gravity and CSF flow	More difficult to perform
Contrast may not pass by compressive lesions	Needle often penetrates spinal cord
Contrast may migrate into the brain	More likely to deposit contrast epidurally

CSF, Cerebrospinal fluid.

radiographs; (2) multiple lesions compatible with the neurologic examination are observed; or (3) a lesion is visualized that is not compatible with the neurologic examination. Contrast agents used in myelographic procedures should be radiopaque, water soluble, miscible with CSF, nontoxic, and rapidly absorbed from the subarachnoid space. The most commonly used myelographic contrast agents are iopamidol (Isovue) and iohexol (Omnipaque). Appropriate doses and concentrations for each contrast agent are given in Table 36-3. Nonionic contrast media up to 350 mg/ml (iohexol) or 370 mg/ml (iopamidol) can safely be used for myelographic examinations and may provide superior image quality compared with concentrations of 300 mg/ml (see Table 36-3). A recent study suggested that myelography with multiple views is 97% accurate with regard to circumferential location of disk material in dogs with thoracolumbar disk herniation (Tanaka et al, 2004).

Myelography is performed with the patient under general anesthesia. Lumbar (L4-L5 or L5-L6) or cisternal puncture can be performed; advantages and disadvantages of each technique are listed in Table 36-4. The skin over the selected injection site is clipped and aseptically prepared.

Complications associated with myelography using iohexol or iopamidol are infrequent (less than 10%) and include exacerbation of neurologic abnormalities, seizures, cardiopulmonary alterations, and death. Anesthetic agent, duration of anesthesia, type of fluid administration, and whether surgery is performed immediately after myelography are not factors associated with complications of myelography; however, patients more than 29 kg (72.5 lb) are more likely to seize.

Cisternal puncture for myelography or CSF analysis. *Position the patient in lateral recumbency. Palpate the wings of the atlas with the thumb and middle finger, and palpate the occiput with the index finger, making a triangle (Fig. 36-14). Gently flex the head, and place a 20- to 22-gauge, 1½- to 2½-inch spinal needle with stylet in the center of the triangle. Place the bevel of the spinal needle in the direction of desired flow of contrast medium.*

As the needle is advanced, a "pop" is felt as it penetrates the dura and enters the subarachnoid space. Return of CSF confirms proper location of the spinal needle.

Slowly withdraw a volume of CSF for analysis, followed by injection of contrast. Elevate the head for 2 to 4 minutes to enhance flow of contrast caudally through all sections of the spine.

Lumbar puncture for myelography or CSF analysis. A successful lumbar puncture requires practice and a lumbar spine skeleton for constant referral to anatomic structures. Fluoroscopy also simplifies accurate needle place-

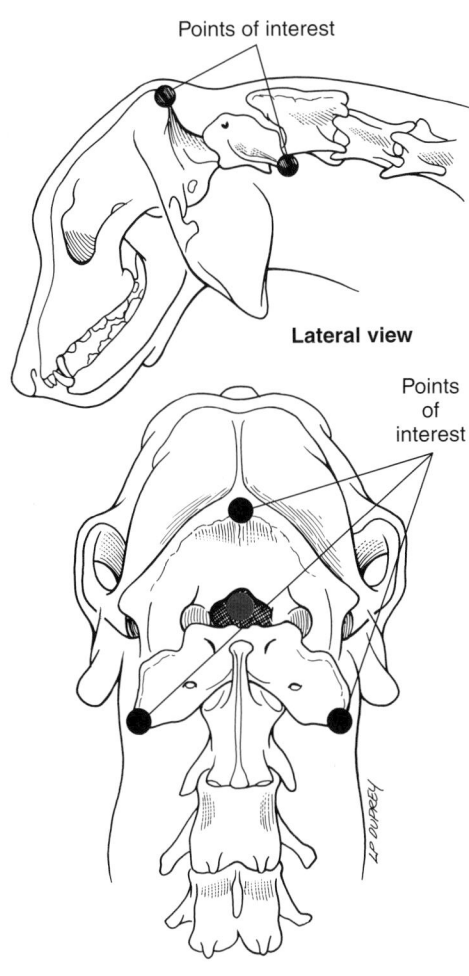

Points of interest

Lateral view

Points of interest

Dorsoventral view

FIG. 36-14
The right and left wings of the atlas and occipital protuberance form a triangle; cisternal puncture is performed by placing a spinal needle in the center of this palpable triangle.

ment. Lumbar myelography typically results in the most diagnostic myelogram.

Position the patient in lateral recumbency. Flex the spine, palpate the caudal dorsal spinous process of L5 or L6 (L5 in an L4-L5 puncture and L6 in an L5-L6 puncture), and place a 20- to 22-gauge, 2½- to 3½-inch spinal needle with stylet at its caudal aspect. Place the needle at a 45-degree angle caudally, and slowly advance cranioventrally and toward the midline in the direction of the L4-L5, or L5-L6 interspace (Fig. 36-15). A characteristic "pop" will be felt as the needle penetrates ligamentum flavum and dura. At this point, withdraw the stylet to examine for flow of CSF. If CSF is visible, remove some for analysis, then slowly inject the calculated dose of contrast. If CSF is not visible, advance the needle through the spinal cord until it contacts the floor of the vertebral canal; occasionally, a tail twitch or leg jerk will result. Withdraw the needle slightly until the flow of CSF is visible.

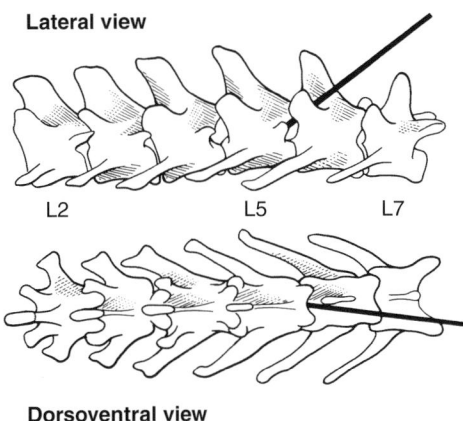

Lateral view

L2   L5   L7

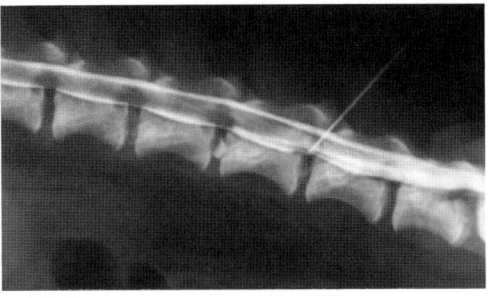

Dorsoventral view

FIG. 36-15
Lumbar spinal puncture is performed at L4–L5, or L5–L6. The needle is placed at a 45-degree angle caudally, advanced to the L4–L5, or L5–L6, midline and passed through the ligamentum flavum and into the dura. The radiograph shows proper needle placement for lumbar myelography.

Place the bevel of the spinal needle in the direction of desired flow of contrast, and slowly inject the calculated dose.

Lesions identified by myelography are classified as extradural, intradural-extramedullary, and intramedullary. Each classification has a list of possible causes (see Box 36-2) and characteristic appearance on myelography. Extradural lesions cause the "contrast column" (subarachnoid space) to be elevated away from the spinal canal on at least one projection (ventrodorsal or lateral) depending upon location of the extradural mass (Fig. 36-16, *A*). On the orthogonal view, the contrast column may appear narrower due to spinal cord swelling (Fig. 36-16, *B* and *C*). Intradural-extramedullary lesions cause the contrast column to become wider on one projection; this widening may resemble a "golf tee" in appearance as the contrast fills around the intradural dural mass, causing a filling defect (Fig. 36-17). From the orthogonal view, the contrast column may appear narrower as a result of spinal cord swelling. Intramedullary lesions cause the contrast column to become narrower on both projections as a result of generalized spinal cord swelling (Fig. 36-18).

Stress myelography. Stress myelography may allow accurate spinal lesion location and help determine treat-

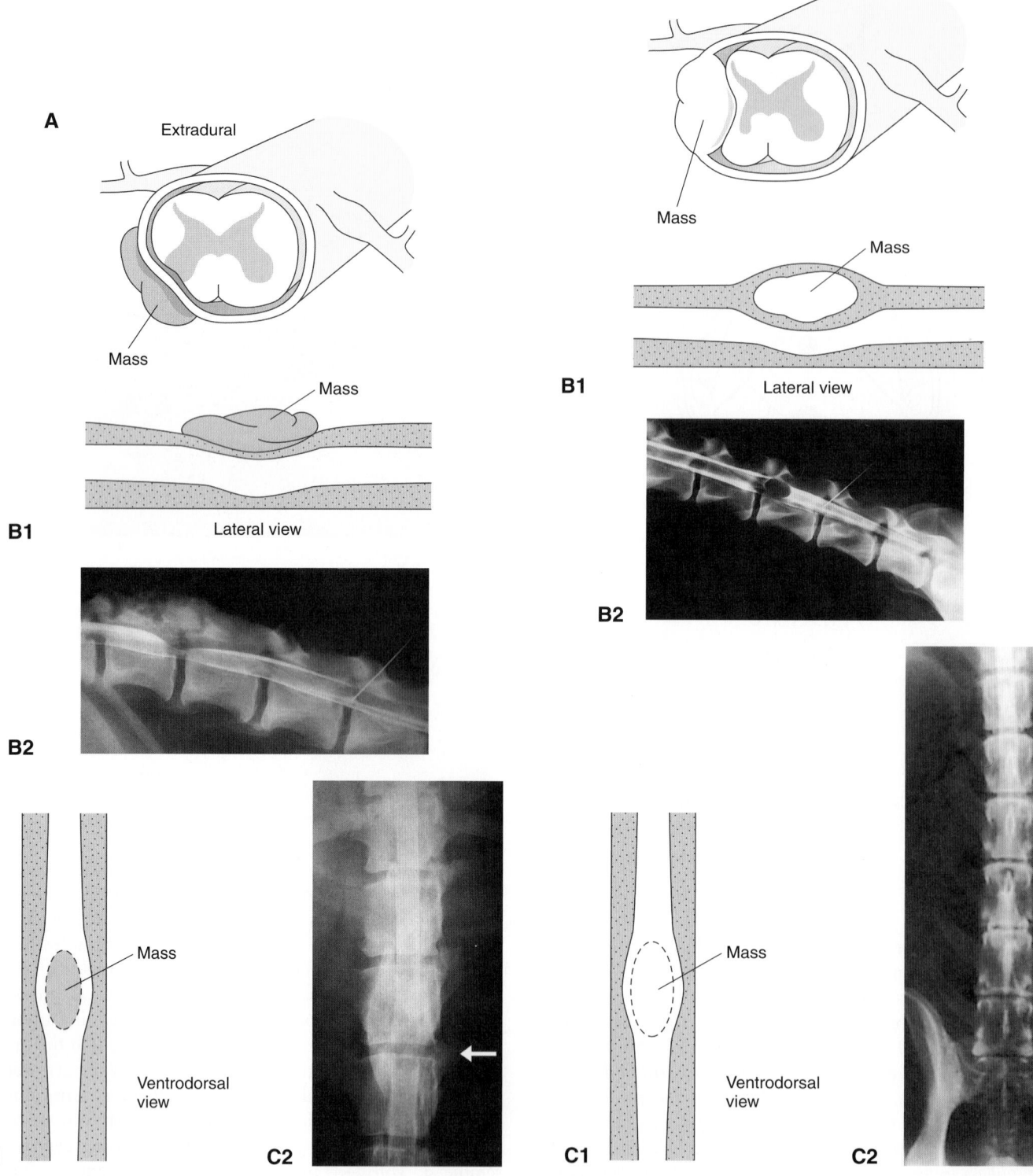

FIG. 36-16
Illustrations and examples of myelographic findings with extradural spinal cord compression. **A,** Schematic showing cross-sectional location of an extradural mass. **B1,** Illustration and **B2,** myelogram showing L2–L3 extradural spinal cord compression *(lateral view).* **C1,** Illustration and **C2,** myelogram showing L2–L3 extradural spinal cord compression *(ventrodorsal view).*

FIG. 36-17
Illustrations and examples of myelographic findings with an intradural-extramedullary lesion. **A,** Schematic showing cross-sectional location of an intradural-extramedullary meningioma. **B1,** Illustration and **B2,** myelogram of a lumbar meningioma causing intradural-extramedullary spinal cord compression *(lateral view).* **C,** Illustration of an intradural-extramedullary compressive lesion on a ventrodorsal view.

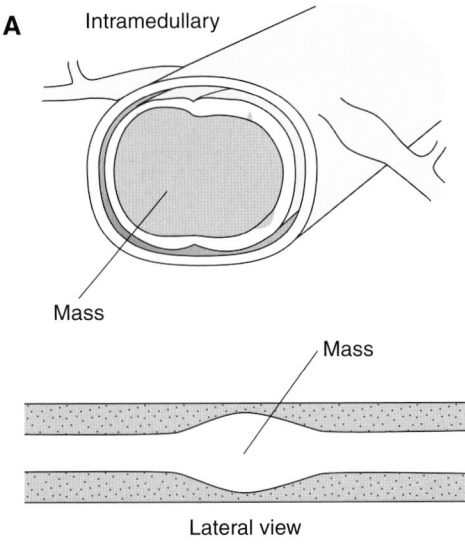

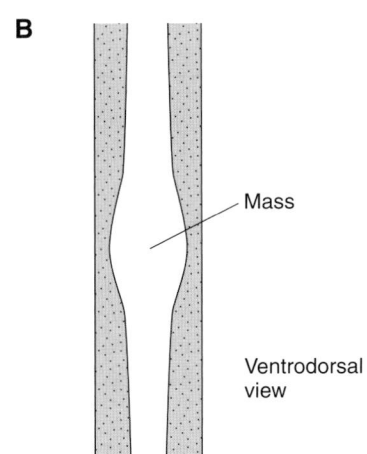

FIG. 36-18
Illustrations of myelographic findings with an intramedullary lesion. **A,** Schematic showing cross-sectional location of an intramedullary lesion. **B,** Illustration of myelographic findings with an intramedullary lesion.

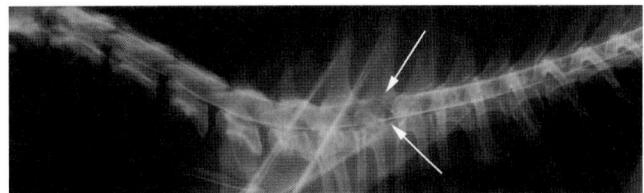

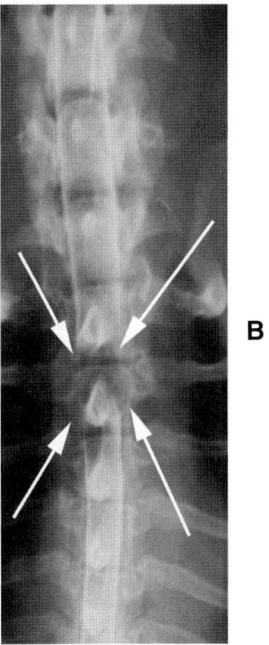

FIG. 36-19
Myelogram of an intramedullary tumor. **A,** Lateral projection shows thinning of the dorsal and ventral aspect of the contrast columns in the cranial thoracic spinal cord *(arrows)*. **B,** Ventrodorsal projection showing widening of the spinal cord and thinning of the left and right aspects of the contrast column *(arrows)*.

ment. It is most commonly used in the diagnosis of wobbler syndrome. Stress myelography is performed by placing segments of the vertebral column in dorsal hyperextension, ventral flexion, and linear traction, thus exacerbating or relieving compressive lesions (Fig. 36-19).

> NOTE: As with stress radiography, perform stress myelography carefully so as not to exacerbate the patient's neurologic deficits.

Other Spinal Imaging Techniques

Epidurography and discography. Epidurography is the injection of a nonionic contrast medium (i.e., iohexol or iopamidol) into the caudal epidural space and recording the image with radiography. Diskography is the injection of non-

ionic contrast into the disk space. These techniques are most commonly used in the diagnosis of cauda equina syndrome.

> NOTE: This procedure is rarely performed since the advent of cross-sectional imaging, although it may be useful in patients that have a dynamic compression of the cauda equina.

For epidurography, insert a 20- to 22-gauge spinal needle between the dorsal lamina of the caudal (coccygeal) vertebra 3-4 or 4-5 and inject 0.15 mg/kg of contrast medium. For diskography, insert a needle into the L7-S1 space and into the disk space. Inject 0.2 to 0.3 ml of contrast medium. Take lateral and ventrodorsal views; for epidurography, inject additional contrast at the rate of 0.1 mg/kg, if necessary. Then obtain neutral, flexed, and extended views of the LS spine.

Significant complications have not been reported with epidurography or diskography. Radiographic abnormalities on an epidurogram include elevation or compression of the

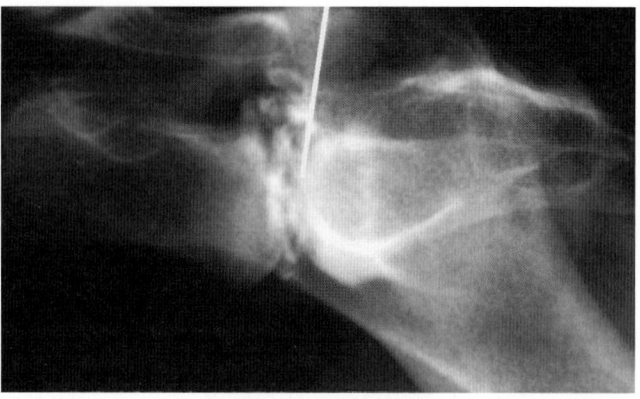

FIG. 36-20
Lateral diskogram of a dog with cauda equina syndrome. Notice the irregular contrast pattern within the L7-S1 nucleus pulposus and extravasation of contrast into the lumbosacral spinal canal.

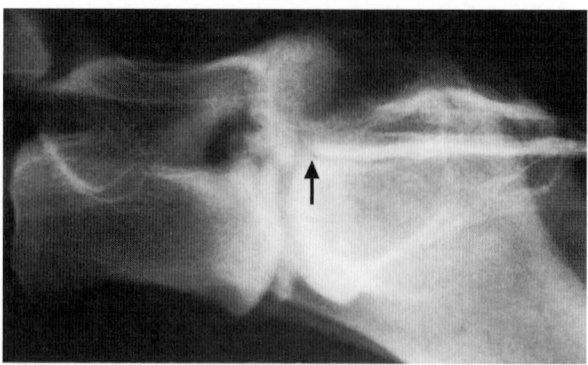

FIG. 36-21
Combination diskogram and epidurogram in a dog with cauda equina syndrome. Notice that the contrast column of the epidurogram is compressed at the lumbosacral junction.

contrast column by the spinal lesion (Figs. 36-20 and 36-21). Radiographic abnormalities for diskography include irregular contrast pattern within L7-S1 nucleus pulposus and extravasation of contrast into the lumbosacral spinal canal (see Fig. 36-20).

Intraoperative ultrasonography. Intraoperative ultrasonography of patients with lesions of the brain or vertebral column can be used to definitively locate the lesion and to evaluate the completeness of removal of these lesions. For patients with brain lesions, ultrasonography is performed following craniotomy.

Perform a craniotomy and fill the resultant space with warm saline. Place an aseptically covered ultrasound transducer adjacent to the dura. Take care to prevent placing pressure on the brain tissue. Assess the ultrasound image for the lesion's location, size, and echogenicity.

Most brain tumors appear hyperechoic compared with the surrounding normal brain tissue.

For patients with vertebral canal lesions, perform ultrasonography after dorsal laminectomy or creation of a ventral slot. Fill the surgical site with sterile saline solution to a depth of 3 to 5 cm, and immerse the head of the transducer in the pool, but do not allow it to come into contact with the tissue. Evaluate the near and far subarachnoid spaces, spinal cord parenchyma, and central canal, and compare their appearance with the appearance of adjacent structures.

Computed tomography and magnetic resonance imaging. Survey radiography has been the mainstay of diagnostic imaging for years. Its advantages include its widespread availability, ease of acquisition, and relative economy.

However, one of its main disadvantages is the superimposition of structures in the image that is generated. Remember that a radiograph is basically a summation of the "shadows" that are created as a result of attenuation of the x-ray beam as it penetrates through the area of interest. With the advent of computers, cross-sectional imaging is now possible. CT and MRI are the current modalities in use to perform cross-sectional imaging. The main advantage of both of these imaging modalities is the lack of superimposition of structures within an image.

CT uses x-rays and their interaction with tissue to create the image; the basic premise is that each type of tissue attenuates the x-ray beam in a unique amount (which is represented by the attenuation coefficient of that tissue). Secondly, the internal structure of an object can be reconstructed from multiple projections of the attenuation of that object. In reality, these projections (which are obtained from a variety of angles) are the amount of transmitted radiation detected passing through the object. All CT scanners are made of some form of x-ray generating device and x-ray detectors. In general, an x-ray beam is passed through the patient. The amount of transmitted radiation is detected on the side opposite the x-ray generator. The x-ray beam is passed through the patient in the same location from a variety of angles. A computer is then used to calculate the attenuation coefficient of the different projections and ultimately can calculate the location of these different tissues. This action produces a single "slice" or cross-sectional image of the patient. Newer CT machines (spiral or helical scanners) scan the patient as a single volume rather than in a single slice and have decreased the scan time to a fraction of the older, single-slice scanners. CT is commonly used to assess the vertebral column because of its high sensitivity to changes in the bony structures. It also is used to assess the brain and spinal cord for abnormalities. Extradural spinal cord lesions are often evaluated via CT after injection of

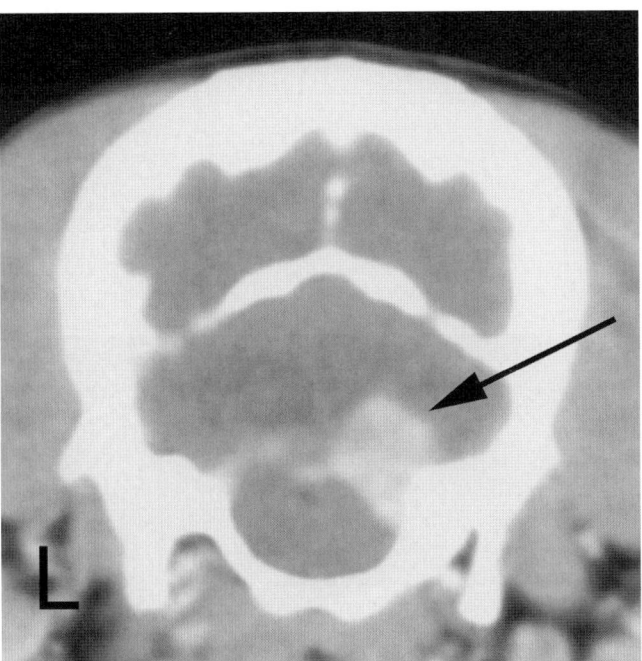

FIG. 36-22
Contrast enhanced CT images of the brain. Extraaxial mass in the right cerebellar-medullary angle *(arrow)*. This mass was a meningioma.

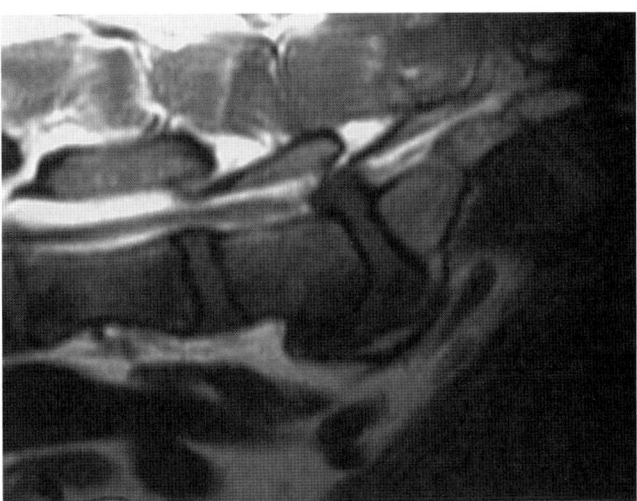

FIG. 36-23
MR image of a patient with extrusion of the dorsal annulus fibrosus of the LS disk.

myelographic contrast. Examples of CT images of patients with spinal disorders are shown in Fig. 36-22.

MRI also provides cross-sectional imaging; however, it does not use ionizing radiation to create the image. Instead, the image is generated by aligning the water molecules of the body within a strong, stable external magnetic field. A second strong radiofrequency (RF) pulse is applied, which causes the water molecules to lose their alignment with the main magnetic field. As the molecules begin to realign themselves after the RF pulse, they emit signals (via Faraday's law of induction), which are then detected by the MRI machine. The types of signals are processed by a computer, which creates the image. In general, portions of the body that do not contain a lot of water (e.g., lung and bone) will not produce a significant signal. MRI is often the diagnostic imaging modality of choice for abnormalities of the brain and intramedullary spinal cord lesions and for any soft tissue (intervertebral disk) that can cause abnormalities of the neurologic system because it can create anatomic images of these soft tissue structures. Examples of MRI of the brain and spinal cord are shown in Figs. 36-23 and 36-24.

IMAGING THE SKULL AND BRAIN

Diagnostic imaging of the skull and brain is indicated when the neurologic examination localizes a lesion above the foramen magnum. Due to the advent of refined diagnostic imaging tools such as CT (without and with contrast) and MRI,

there has been notable improvement in identification and localization of intracranial lesions.

Survey radiographs of the skull may help assess patients with trauma to the calvarium, middle ear infection, neoplasms invading or causing mineralization of the calvarium, or any lesion causing direct involvement of the osseous structures of the skull. When skull radiographs are taken, the following guidelines should be considered: (1) use general anesthesia; (2) position the patient carefully to display bilateral symmetry; (3) take lateral and ventrodorsal projections; and (4) use high quality radiographic film-screen combinations. Knowledge of normal anatomic variation of the skull and results of a minimum database, historical, physical, and neurologic examinations are necessary to allow accurate interpretation. Survey radiographs may be normal in patients with significant neurologic deficits secondary to intracranial disorders (e.g., hematoma, neoplasia, abscess, hydrocephalus, and inflammatory disorders).

CT provides excellent detail of bone and soft tissue, and allows identification and precise localization of many intracranial lesions (see Fig. 36-22). Intravenous contrast medium can be used in conjunction with CT to enhance identification of specific soft tissue structures (e.g., intracranial neoplasia). CT images can be used to determine the extent of a lesion and whether or not the calvarium has been invaded. This procedure is also valuable for planning approaches to the cranial vault.

MRI is noninvasive and does not expose the patient to radiation. Advantages of MRI over CT are improved anatomic detail of soft tissue structures and absence of image degradation because of the thick canine calvarium (see Fig. 36-24). MRI is more sensitive than CT in diagnosing and localizing brain abnormalities in dogs and cats.

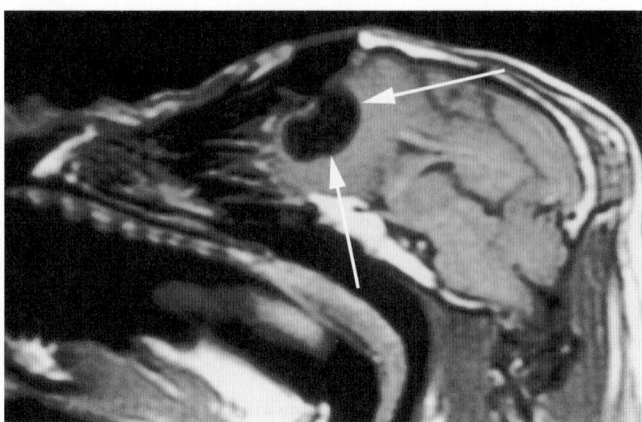

FIG. 36-24
MRI images of a patient with intracranial neoplasia. **A,** Dorsal T2-weighted image of the brain. Notice the high signal mass in the brain *(arrows)*. **B,** Sagittal T1-weighted image of the brain. Notice the low signal mass in the brain *(arrows)*. This was a cystic meningioma.

References

Lamb CR, Nicholls A, Targett M et al: Accuracy of survey radiographic diagnosis of intervertebral disk protrusion in dogs, *Vet Radiol Ultrasound* 43:4, 2002.

Tanaka H, Nakayama M, Takase K: Usefulness of myelography with multiple views in diagnosis of circumferential location of disk material in dogs with thoracolumbar intervertebral disk herniation, *J Vet Med Sci* 66:827, 2004.

Suggested Reading

Bienzle D, McDonnell JJ, Stanton JB: Analysis of cerebrospinal fluid from dogs and cats after 24 and 48 hours of storage, *J Am Vet Med Assoc* 216:1761, 2000.

This prospective study compared CSF samples analyzed immediately with those stored for 24 or 48 hours at 4° C with and without the addition of autologous serum. The authors concluded that CSF samples collected at veterinary clinics remote from a diagnostic laboratory or during nonoperational hours may be preserved through the addition of autologous serum.

CHAPTER 37
Surgery of the Brain

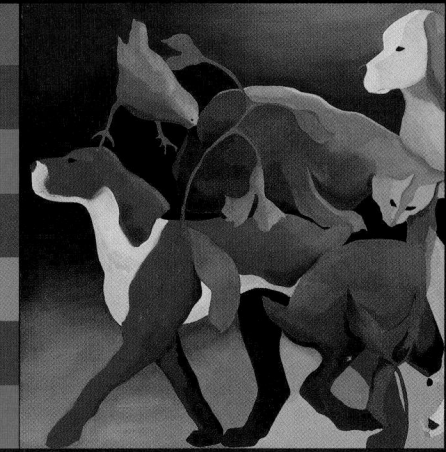

GENERAL PRINCIPLES AND TECHNIQUES

DEFINITIONS

Craniotomy is removal of a portion of the calvarium to expose the cranial vault; the excised bony plate is either replaced during closure or discarded. Right or left **rostrotentorial (lateral) craniotomy** is an approach to the right or left cerebral hemisphere, respectively. **Extended rostrotentorial craniotomy** is a ventral extension of the aforementioned technique with zygomatic arch resection. Right and left cerebral hemispheres may be approached **bilaterally (bilateral rostrotentorial craniotomy). Caudotentorial craniotomy** is an approach to the caudal cerebrum and rostral cerebellum, whereas **transfrontal** and **modified bilateral transfrontal craniotomy** is an approach to the cranial aspect of the cerebrum (olfactory bulb). **Suboccipital craniotomy** is an approach to the caudal aspect of the cerebellum. Various combinations of craniotomy approaches are used when exposure of larger areas of the brain is indicated (e.g., rostrotentorial and transfrontal approaches, caudotentorial and suboccipital approaches, bilateral rostrotentorial approach, and extended rostrotentorial approach).

PREOPERATIVE MANAGEMENT

The most common indications for brain surgery in dogs and cats are trauma and neoplasia. Cerebral edema is a common complication in these patients and may be vasogenic (disruption of tight junctions formed by endothelial cells of brain capillaries), cytotoxic (associated with swelling of cellular elements of the brain), or interstitial (caused by seepage of cerebrospinal fluid [CSF] across the ventricular walls). *Vasogenic edema* may be associated with slow-growing mass lesions (e.g., neoplasia), whereas hypoxia and abnormalities in osmolarity (e.g., acute dilutional hyponatremia, hyperosmolar diabetes mellitus, and salt intoxication) typically cause *cytotoxic edema*. *Interstitial edema* is usually caused by hydrocephalus (obstruction of the ventricular system or reduction in absorption of CSF at the subarachnoid space). Cerebral edema can cause brain herniation. Mannitol is very effective at reducing brain edema by osmotically drawing

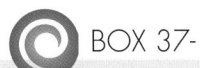 BOX 37-1

High-Dose Methylprednisolone Therapy

1. Initial dose: 30 mg/kg IV*
2. Follow with 15 mg/kg IV*; 2 and 6 hr after initial dose
3. Place on continuous IV infusion at 2.5 mg/kg/hr for 37 hr; then discontinue

IV, Intravenous.
*Give slowly over several minutes.

extravascular fluid into the intravascular space. It has become a popular "first choice" for emergency treatment of increased intracranial pressure caused by moderate to severe head trauma (see p. 1395). Glucocorticoids (e.g., dexamethasone, prednisone, and prednisolone) appear more effective in treating vasogenic and interstitial edema than cytotoxic edema. They also reduce the edema associated with brain tumors. Despite the fact that glucocorticoids have not shown significant benefit in brain trauma patients, they continue to be used in veterinary patients with these injuries. High-dose methylprednisolone therapy (Box 37-1) may reduce nervous tissue destruction and ischemia and improve neurologic outcome in brain trauma; it is recommended in animals that have moderate or severe neurologic dysfunction after trauma or surgery.

Patients with cranial trauma or neoplasia should be stabilized before surgery with intravenous (IV) fluids (Box 37-2); however, overhydration should be avoided, or it could worsen brain edema and further elevate intracranial pressure. Hypertonic saline (see Box 37-2) and hetastarch may benefit patients with brain trauma. Hypertonic saline protects against cerebral edema and increased intracranial pressure, even after subsequent administration of crystalloid solutions. Hyperventilation reduces or prevents brain swelling caused by hypocapnia; hyperventilation reduces cerebral blood volume. Superoxide radical scavengers (e.g., deferoxamine mesylate) may prevent brain tissue damage after injury. Experimentally, deferoxamine mesylate (Box 37-3) is effective if given early to brain trauma patients; however, IV administration is associ-

BOX 37-2

Fluid Administration in Patients With Brain Trauma That Are in Shock

Lactated Ringer's solution (LRS) or 0.9% Saline

40 to 90 ml/kg/hr (use the lower dose in cats); IV shock dose; then decrease to maintenance rate

Hypertonic Saline* (7%)

4–5 ml/kg IV over 3–5 minutes

Hetastarch† (6%)

10–20 ml/kg in lactated Ringer's solution IV (dog); 10–15 ml/kg IV (cat)

IV, Intravenous.
*Do not give to dehydrated patients or those with congestive heart failure, oliguric or anuric renal failure, hypernatremia, or uncontrolled hemorrhage.
†Use with caution in patients with congestive heart failure.

 BOX 37-3

Deferoxamine Mesylate* (Desferal) Administration

25–50 mg/kg IM (single dose)

IM, Intramuscular.
*Do not give concurrently with phenothiazine drugs.

NOTE: Restrict IV fluids to that volume necessary to maintain adequate hydration in patients with cerebral trauma; excessive fluids increase the risk of cerebral edema.

Additional therapy of patients with cranial trauma often includes antibiotics, anticonvulsants, and/or diuretics. Patients with intracranial masses (e.g., neoplasia, abscess, or vascular malformation) are generally treated preoperatively with anticonvulsants, corticosteroids, and diuretics. Mannitol is an osmotic diuretic that draws extravascular fluid into the intravascular space (Box 37-4). It may also reduce CSF production and promote oxygen-free radical scavenging and cerebral arteriolar vasoconstriction. Mannitol's effects last for 2 to 4 hours. To minimize a mild transient rise in intracranial pressure associated with mannitol administration, it should be given slowly over a 10- to 20-minute period with no more than three boluses in a 24-hour period. Mannitol is an excellent choice for emergency treatment of patients with increased intracranial pressure. It is contraindicated in patients that are dehydrated or in hypovolemic shock and should not

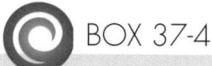 BOX 37-4

Diuretics in Patients With Brain Injury

Mannitol* (20%–25%)

0.25–2 g/kg IV over 10–20 minutes; repeat in 3 to 8 hours if necessary† (limit to three boluses per 24 hours)

Furosemide (Lasix)‡

2.2–4.4 mg/kg IV; repeat in 6 hr if necessary

IV, Intravenous.
*Monitor urine output.
†If the mannitol cannot be excreted because of severe renal disease, it will remain in the bloodstream where it can cause severe hypertension. Use cautiously in animals with congestive heart failure.
‡Can cause hypokalemia if used repeatedly or in high doses, especially in anorexic animals.

be used unless absolutely necessary in patients with congestive heart failure, anuric renal failure, or pulmonary edema because it may cause increased morbidity or even mortality in such patients. Furosemide decreases intracranial pressure by reducing extracellular water and may potentiate the antiedema effects of mannitol (see Box 37-4). It should not be used in dehydrated animals, and overuse may cause electrolyte disturbances (i.e., hypokalemic and hypochloremic metabolic alkalosis). Blood gas analysis should be performed in patients with severe central nervous system (CNS) signs because changes in arterial oxygen and carbon dioxide concentrations may alter cerebral blood flow.

ANESTHESIA

Anesthetic agents alter normal CNS physiology (e.g., cerebral blood flow, CSF production, and intracranial pressure dynamics), which may be deleterious in patients with intracranial disorders. Increased intracranial pressure may worsen cerebral ischemia, prolong cerebral edema, and produce brain herniation. Preoperative medications listed in Box 37-5, coupled with anesthetic protocols that reduce alterations in normal CNS physiology, should be used. For induction of patients with CNS disease, barbiturates are indicated because they significantly reduce cerebral metabolic oxygen requirements, cerebral blood flow, and intracranial pressure. Propofol also decreases cerebral blood flow and decreases cerebral oxygen consumption and may also be used. Although propofol infusion is occasionally associated with seizurelike activity, it is not generally a problem with an induction dose. Anesthesia should be maintained using minimal concentrations of isoflurane or sevoflurane supplemented with opioids or barbiturates, as necessary. Dogs with increased intracranial pressure may have resting bradycardia; blood pressure should be evaluated preoperatively to determine if an anticholinergic is necessary. Preoperative opioids should be avoided in patients with increased intracranial pressure since they cause hypoventilation.

Proper anesthetic management includes arterial catheterization, appropriate induction and maintenance agents, and

ated with profound hypotension, and intramuscular administration is preferred. If given intravenously, it should be administered slowly over a 20-minute period.

BOX 37-5

Selected Anesthetic Protocols for Patients
With Increased Intracranial Pressure

Premedication

Methylprednisolone sodium succinate (30 mg/kg IV) plus
furosemide (1 mg/kg IV) or mannitol (1 mg/kg IV)
   Give 30 minutes before induction

Induction

Diazepam (0.2 mg/kg IV) followed by thiopental (10–12
mg/kg IV) or propofol (4–6 mg/kg IV); moderately hyper-
ventilate the patient with oxygen before exposure to an inhalant

Maintenance

Minimal concentrations of isoflurane or sevoflurane; use
modest hyperventilation to maintain $ETCO_2$ between 28
and 32 mm Hg

IV, Intravenous; *ETCO₂,* end-tidal carbon dioxide.

BOX 37-6

Selected Anesthetic Protocol for Use During MRI
Procedures

Premedication

Butorphanol: 0.2–0.4 mg/kg SC or IM; avoid using opioids in patients with increased intracranial pressure

Induction

Propofol: 4–8 mg/kg IV

Maintenance

Propofol: 0.4 mg/kg/min IV infusion (see Table 37-1)

MRI, Magnetic resonance imaging; *SC,* subcutaneous; *IM,* intramuscular; *IV,* intravenous.

modest hyperventilation (end-tidal carbon dioxide [$ETCO_2$]
approximately 28 to 32 mm of Hg). Arterial catheterization
is used to constantly monitor arterial blood pressure. In patients with increased intracranial pressure, the Cushing reflex may result in hypertension and bradycardia; anesthetized patients may become hypotensive. Arterial blood
pressure should be kept as close to 90 mm Hg as possible.
Periodic arterial sampling for carbon dioxide levels aids anesthetic monitoring (see Box 37-5); additionally, end-tidal
capnography may be used for continuous monitoring. Modest hyperventilation (using a mechanical ventilator) reduces
arterial carbon dioxide, decreases cerebral blood flow (i.e.,
reduces the volatile anesthetic-induced increase in cerebral
blood flow), and lowers intracranial pressure. These patients
should be hyperventilated for 10 minutes before administering inhalant anesthetics. Significant hyperventilation ($PaCO_2$
less than 25 mm Hg or an $ETCO_2$ of approximately 20 mm
Hg) may result in ischemia and should be prevented. Intubation should be done under a deep plane of anesthesia in

patients with increased intracranial pressure to avoid inducing a cough. In patients with CNS dysfunction, ketamine is
a drug that should be avoided because it increases intracranial pressure. Although it has been felt for some time that
acetylpromazine should be avoided because of its effect on
lowering seizure threshold, there is evidence to suggest this
is not the case in clinical patients (Garner et al, 2004). Anesthetic recommendations for animals undergoing magnetic
resonance imaging (MRI) are provided in Box 37-6. Historically, propofol has been used to induce and maintain anesthesia during MRI procedures; however, with the advent of
MRI compatible vaporizers and monitoring equipment,
there are more options. Table 37-1 contains dosages and drip
rates for propofol based on animal weight. With propofol,
the animal is typically intubated and a long Bain system used
to assist ventilation; inhalant anesthetics are not generally
used.

ANTIBIOTICS

Therapeutic antibiotics are indicated in patients with open
cranial trauma (e.g., bite wounds to the cranium and open
skull fractures) or those undergoing craniotomy into a contaminated site (i.e., transfrontal). Use of prophylactic or
therapeutic antibiotics, antibiotic selection, and dose and
duration of therapy are determined by criteria listed in
Chapter 10. Patients undergoing surgical manipulation of
intracranial neoplasia generally do not require prophylactic
or therapeutic antibiotics unless operative times exceed 90 to
120 minutes.

SURGICAL ANATOMY

The brain may be divided into three large regions: cerebrum,
cerebellum, and brainstem. The cerebrum consists of paired
cerebral hemispheres that are separated by a longitudinal fissure. Cerebral hemispheres are composed of cerebral cortex
(gray matter) and underlying white matter. The surface of the
cerebrum contains gyri, separated by grooves known as *sulci.*
Each cerebral hemisphere contains a lateral ventricle that
communicates with the third ventricle through an interventricular foramen. The olfactory nerve originates from the
cerebrum; other cranial nerves arise from the brainstem. The
cerebellum is separated from the cerebrum by a transverse
fissure. It functions to coordinate movement and posture.
The brainstem occupies the middle and caudal fossae of the
floor of the cranial vault and is continuous with the spinal
cord. It contains the third and fourth ventricles. The thalamus, subthalamus, hypothalamus, and epithalamus are components of the brainstem. The hypothalamus controls the
hypophysis and thus the endocrine system. It affects behavior, sleep cycles, temperature regulation, feeding and drinking
behavior, and the autonomic nervous system (i.e., cardiovascular, respiratory, gastrointestinal, and urinary functions).

The major venous sinuses into which the veins of the
brain and its encasing drain are the basilar, paired transverse,
confluens, and dorsal sagittal sinuses (Fig. 37-1, *A* to *C*). The
locations of the sinuses are generally used as borders for the
various surgical approaches to the brain. The middle menin-

Table 37-1

Propofol: Induction and Maintenance

WEIGHT	INDUCTION-DOSE RANGE		INDUCTION-DOSE RANGE		MAINTENANCE PER MINUTE		DRIP CHAMBER		DRIP RATE
KG	4 MG/KG	8 MG/KG	0.4 ML/KG	0.8 ML/KG	0.4 MG/KG/MIN	0.04 ML/KG/MIN	DROPS/MIN	TYPE	DROPS/SEC
1	4	8	0.4	0.8	0.4	0.04	2.4	Microdrip	1/25
2	8	16	0.8	1.6	0.8	0.08	4.8	Microdrip	1/12
4	16	22	1.6	2.2	1.6	0.16	9.6	Microdrip	1/6
6	24	48	2.4	4.8	2.4	0.24	14.4	Microdrip	1/4
8	32	64	3.2	6.4	3.2	0.32	19.2	Microdrip	1/3
10	40	80	4	8	4	0.4	24	Microdrip	1/2.5
12	48	96	4.8	9.6	4.8	0.48	7.2	Standard 15/ml	1/8
14	56	112	5.6	11.2	5.6	0.56	8.4	Standard 15/ml	1/7
16	64	128	6.4	12.8	6.4	0.64	9.6	Standard 15/ml	1/6
18	72	144	7.2	14.4	7.2	0.72	10.8	Standard 15/ml	1/5.5
20	80	160	8	16	8	0.8	12	Standard 15/ml	1/5
22	88	176	8.8	17.6	8.8	0.88	13.2	Standard 15/ml	1/5
24	96	192	9.6	19.2	9.6	0.96	14.4	Standard 15/ml	1/4
26	104	208	10.4	20.8	10.4	1.04	15.6	Standard 15/ml	1/4
28	112	224	11.2	22.4	11.2	1.12	16.8	Standard 15/ml	1/3.5
30	120	240	12	24	12	1.2	18	Standard 15/ml	1/3.5
32	128	256	12.8	25.6	12.8	1.28	19.2	Standard 15/ml	1/3
34	136	272	13.6	27.2	13.6	1.36	20.4	Standard 15/ml	1/3
36	144	288	14.4	28.8	14.4	1.44	21.6	Standard 15/ml	1/3
38	152	304	15.2	30.4	15.2	1.52	22.8	Standard 15/ml	1/2.5
40	160	320	16	32	16	1.6	24	Standard 15/ml	1/2.5
37	168	336	16.8	33.6	16.8	1.68	25.2	Standard 15/ml	1/2.5
44	176	352	17.6	35.2	17.6	1.76	26.4	Standard 15/ml	1/2.5
46	184	368	18.4	36.8	18.4	1.84	27.6	Standard 15/ml	1/2
48	192	384	19.2	38.4	19.2	1.92	28.8	Standard 15/ml	1/2
50	200	400	20	40	20	2	30	Standard 15/ml	1/2

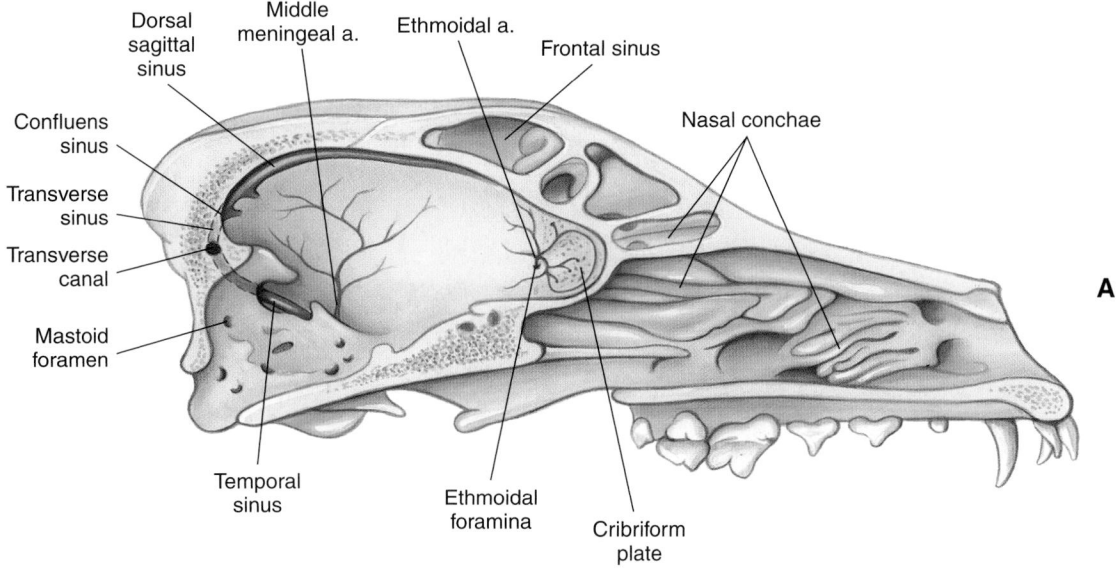

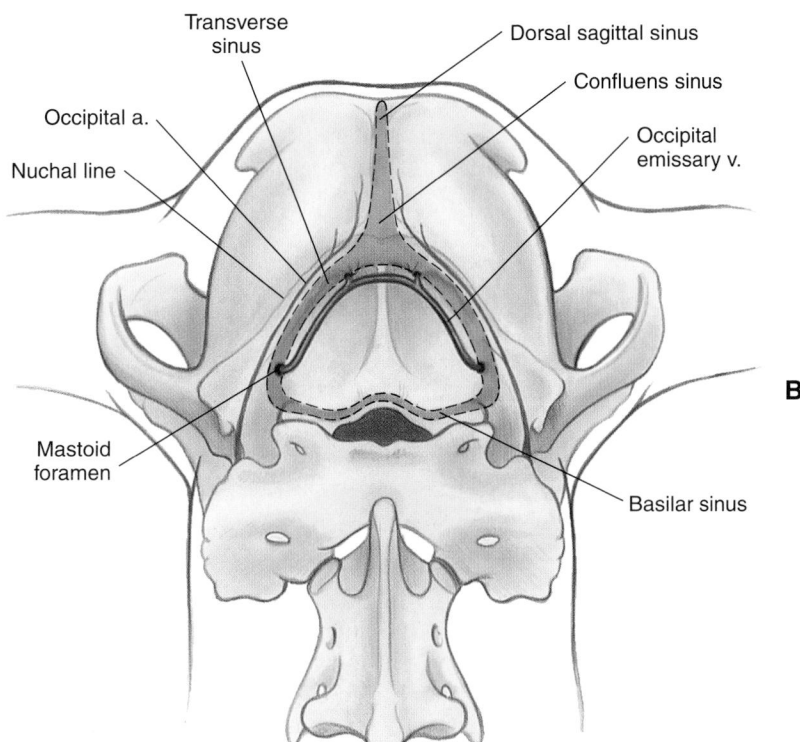

FIG. 37-1
A, Lateral. **B,** Caudal.

Continued

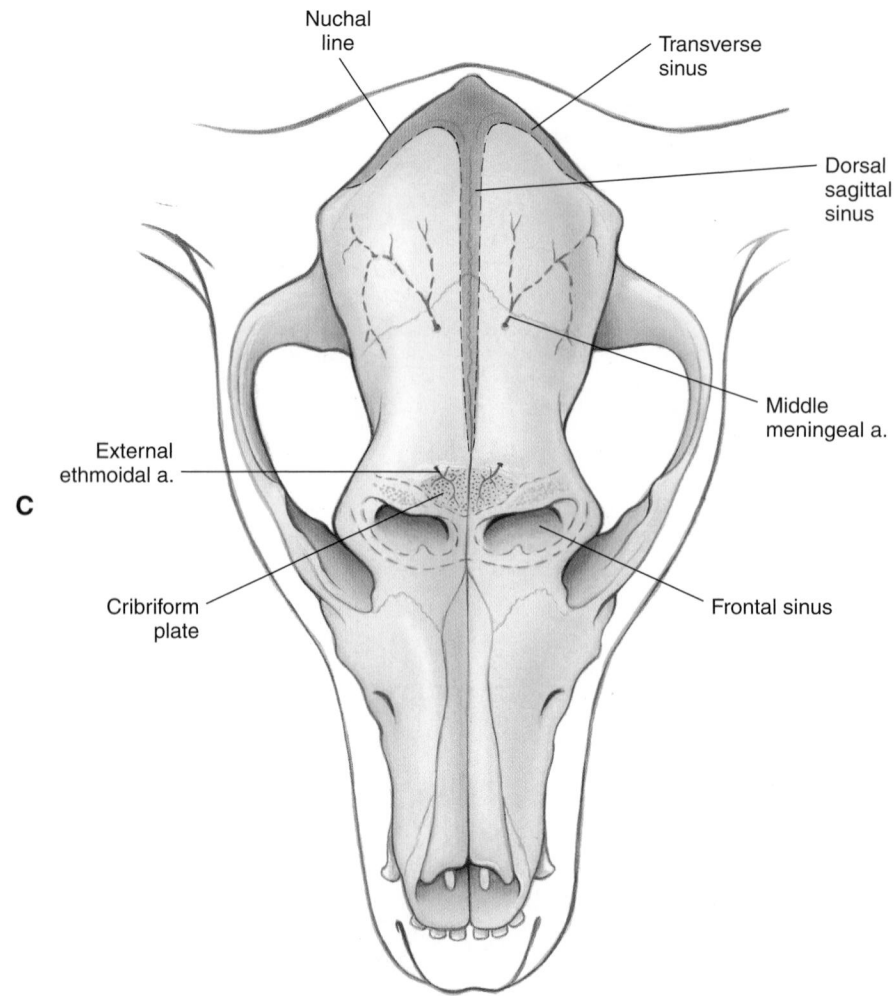

FIG. 37-1. cont'd
C, Frontal aspects of the skull illustrating important surgical landmarks.

geal artery is the largest of the meningeal arteries. Its branches leave at right angles and run both rostrally and caudally, supplying the dura and adjacent portions of the skull (see Fig. 37-1, *A* and *C*). The ethmoidal artery reaches the dura after passing through the ethmoidal foramen and running between the cribriform plate and olfactory bulb (see Fig. 37-1, *A* and *C*).

> NOTE: Be careful to avoid lacerating the dorsal sagittal sinus because this causes considerable hemorrhage; fatal cerebral edema is a common sequela because of poor cerebral venous outflow.

SURGICAL TREATMENT

Surgical approaches to the cranial vault of dogs and cats are generally performed from the frontal (i.e., transfrontal), lateral (i.e., rostrotentorial and caudotentorial), or caudal (i.e., suboccipital) aspect of the skull. Pertinent osseous, ve-

nous, and arterial structures encountered during craniotomy/craniectomy procedures are illustrated in Fig. 37-1, *A* to *C*. The extent of a craniotomy is often determined by location of venous sinuses (i.e., dorsal sagittal sinus and transverse sinus). Location and ligation of the middle meningeal artery is required when approaching the lateral cerebral hemisphere. Removal of the zygomatic arch may facilitate lateral and ventral exposure of the cranial vault.

SURGICAL TECHNIQUE

Most craniotomies are performed with the patient in sternal recumbency. A head stand should be used to stabilize the skull in an elevated position. This minimizes pressure on the jugular veins, thus preventing cerebral venous congestion, impaired venous drainage, and edema, which increase intracranial pressure. This device should allow for adjustments in both height and rotational positioning (Fig. 37-2). Craniotomy approaches can be combined to improve exposure to various aspects of the cerebral hemispheres and cerebellum.

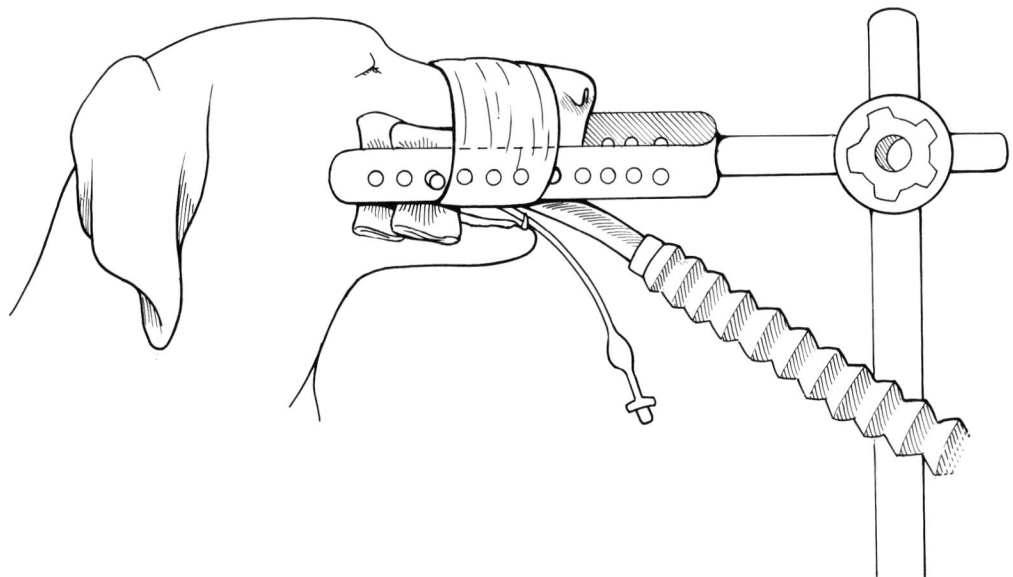

FIG. 37-2
Head stand for intracranial surgery. Notice that the device allows for adjustments in height and rotational positioning.

Table 37-2

Surgical Approach or Combination of Approaches Based on Lesion Location*

LESION LOCATION	CRANIOTOMY APPROACH	COMBINATION APPROACH
Rostral cerebral hemisphere	Rostrotentorial or extended rostrotentorial or transfrontal	Rostrotentorial and transfrontal
Central cerebral hemisphere	Rostrotentorial	
Caudal cerebral hemisphere	Caudotentorial	Caudotentorial and suboccipital
Ventral cerebral hemisphere	Extended rostrotentorial	
Right and left central cerebral hemisphere; corpus callosum; third ventricle	Bilateral rostrotentorial	
Olfactory bulb	Transfrontal	
Rostral and rostrolateral cerebellar		Caudotentorial and suboccipital
Caudal cerebellar	Suboccipital	

*These are general guidelines. Because lesions of the brain may be quite extensive or very discrete, alternate variations of the approaches listed may be required.

Selection of a single approach or combination of approaches depends on the location of the lesion (Table 37-2). Generally, extensive lesions require a combination of approaches, whereas discrete lesions require a single approach. In some instances, however, discrete lesions require combined approaches if they are located at the margin of the exposure provided by a given technique. Careful examination of preoperative MR and/or computed tomography (CT) images should be performed to accurately choose proper surgical approach or a combination of approaches. In addition, in-

traoperative ultrasound can be used to facilitate evaluation of the adequacy of surgical removal of neoplasms.

Rostrotentorial craniotomy exposes the cerebrum. It can be modified to allow increased exposure to the ventral aspect of the cranial vault and cerebral hemisphere by exposing and excising the zygomatic arch. Bilateral rostrotentorial craniotomy allows simultaneous exposure of both cerebral hemispheres. Caudotentorial craniotomy is performed when exposure of the caudal aspect of the cerebral hemisphere or cranial aspect of the cerebellum is indicated. It may be combined with suboccipital craniotomy to examine the cranial (caudotentorial approach) and caudal (suboccipital approach) aspects of the cerebellum. Transfrontal craniotomy is indicated for limited exposure of the cranial aspect of the cerebral hemispheres (e.g., discrete lesions of the olfactory bulb). This approach can be performed unilaterally or bilaterally and may be combined with rostrotentorial craniotomy to facilitate exposure of the cranial aspect of the cerebral hemisphere (i.e., exposure of the rostral compartment of the cranial vault). Suboccipital craniotomy is indicated for exposure of the caudal aspect of the cerebellum. It can be combined with caudotentorial craniotomy to gain access to the rostral and rostrolateral cerebellum.

> NOTE: Unilateral transverse venous sinus occlusion can be safely performed in dogs.

Rostrotentorial Craniotomy

Position the patient in sternal recumbency, and secure the head in a head stand (see Fig. 37-2). Incise the skin in an inverted U shape beginning at a point just caudal to the lateral canthus of the eye. Curve dorsally to the external sagittal crest and then ventrally to a point 1 cm ventral to the external occipital protuberance (Fig. 37-3, A). Incise underlying supporting muscles of the ear and the frontalis muscle to expose the temporalis muscle. Incise the facial attachment of the temporalis muscle along the external sagittal crest, leaving enough dorsal fascia attached to facilitate closure. Subperiosteally, elevate the temporalis muscle, and reflect it ventrally, exposing the lateral aspect of the skull (Fig. 37-3, B). Locate and mark the area of skull to be removed by using a high-speed pneumatic drill with a 2- to 3-mm carbide burr, and drill a hole at each corner of the proposed craniotomy (Fig. 37-3, C). Use a 2- to 3-mm carbide burr, and drill a trough connecting each mark. Drill to a depth that allows penetration to, but does not include, the inner periosteum. Use bone wax to control hemorrhage from the craniotomy trough. Use a periosteal elevator or dental spatula and elevate the craniotomy flap. Either replace the flap in the defect (perform a craniotomy) or discard it (perform a craniectomy). Identify the middle meningeal artery, and ligate it near its base using 5-0 monofilament absorbable suture (Fig. 37-3, D). If the artery is torn during craniotomy flap removal, quickly isolate the vessel with suction and cauterize it with bipolar cautery or ligate it. If the dura is not adherent to the craniotomy flap, tent it with ophthalmic forceps and incise it with a No.11 scalpel blade. Introduce a fine ophthalmic scissors through the incision, and excise the dura to the same opening size as the craniotomy. Make no attempt to preserve dura for closure; discard it after resection. Identify pertinent landmarks (e.g., sulci and gyri) to establish location of the lesion. Control arachnoid, pial, and parenchymal hemorrhage with bipolar cautery or thrombin-soaked sponges. Lavage remaining brain tissue with warmed, sterile physiologic saline solution.

If the bone flap is replaced, drill one or two holes in each edge of the bone flap and craniotomy site. Use 22- to 24-gauge orthopedic wire or 0 to 2-0 nonabsorbable monofilament suture to secure the bone flap to the osteotomy site. Close temporalis muscle dorsally to its remaining dorsal fascial strip with 2-0 or 3-0 monofilament absorbable simple interrupted sutures. Close subcutaneous tissue and skin routinely.

> NOTE: The middle meningeal artery should be located and ligated near its base during this procedure, if possible. Cautery should be available for small bleeders in the arachnoid, pia, and brain parenchyma.

Extended Rostrotentorial Craniotomy

Make an inverted U–shaped skin incision beginning 1 cm distal to the external occipital protuberance. Extend it to the dorsal midline, along the external sagittal crest, over the frontal sinus to the lateral canthus of the eye, and then curve ventrally to the zygomatic arch just caudal to the orbit (Fig. 37-4). Incise the underlying supporting muscles of the ear and frontalis muscle, reflect them ventrally, and expose the temporalis muscle and zygomatic arch. Identify the rostral and caudal aspects of the zygomatic arch, and sever them with a high-speed pneumatic drill and carbide burr. Incise the temporalis muscle from its dorsal, cranial, and ventral attachments. Subperiosteally, elevate the temporalis muscle from its attachment to the skull and reflect it caudoventrally. Reflect the zygomatic arch ventrally with the masseter muscle (Fig. 37-5). Perform a craniotomy as described previously. Discard the craniotomy bone flap or reattach it as described for rostrotentorial craniotomy. Reattach the zygomatic arch with 20-gauge orthopedic wire. Close the temporalis muscle, subcutaneous tissue, and skin as described previously.

> NOTE: This "extended" exposure allows the craniotomy to extend to the anatomic limits illustrated in Fig. 37-5.

Bilateral Rostrotentorial Craniotomy

Incise skin on the dorsal midline of the cranium, beginning 1 cm caudal to the external occipital protuberance and continuing rostrally to a line drawn from the medial canthus of each eye. Incise and reflect the underlying supporting muscles of the ear and frontalis and temporalis muscles (as described previously for rostrotentorial craniotomy) bilaterally. Perform a craniotomy bilaterally as described previously, but leave a 0.5- to 1-cm strip of bone over the dorsal midline to prevent damaging the dorsal sagittal sinus (Fig. 37-6). Use Lempert or Kerrison up-biting rongeurs to carefully remove bone near the dorsal sagittal sinus. Examine the dorsal and lateral aspects of each cerebral hemisphere. Close the craniotomy incisions as described previously.

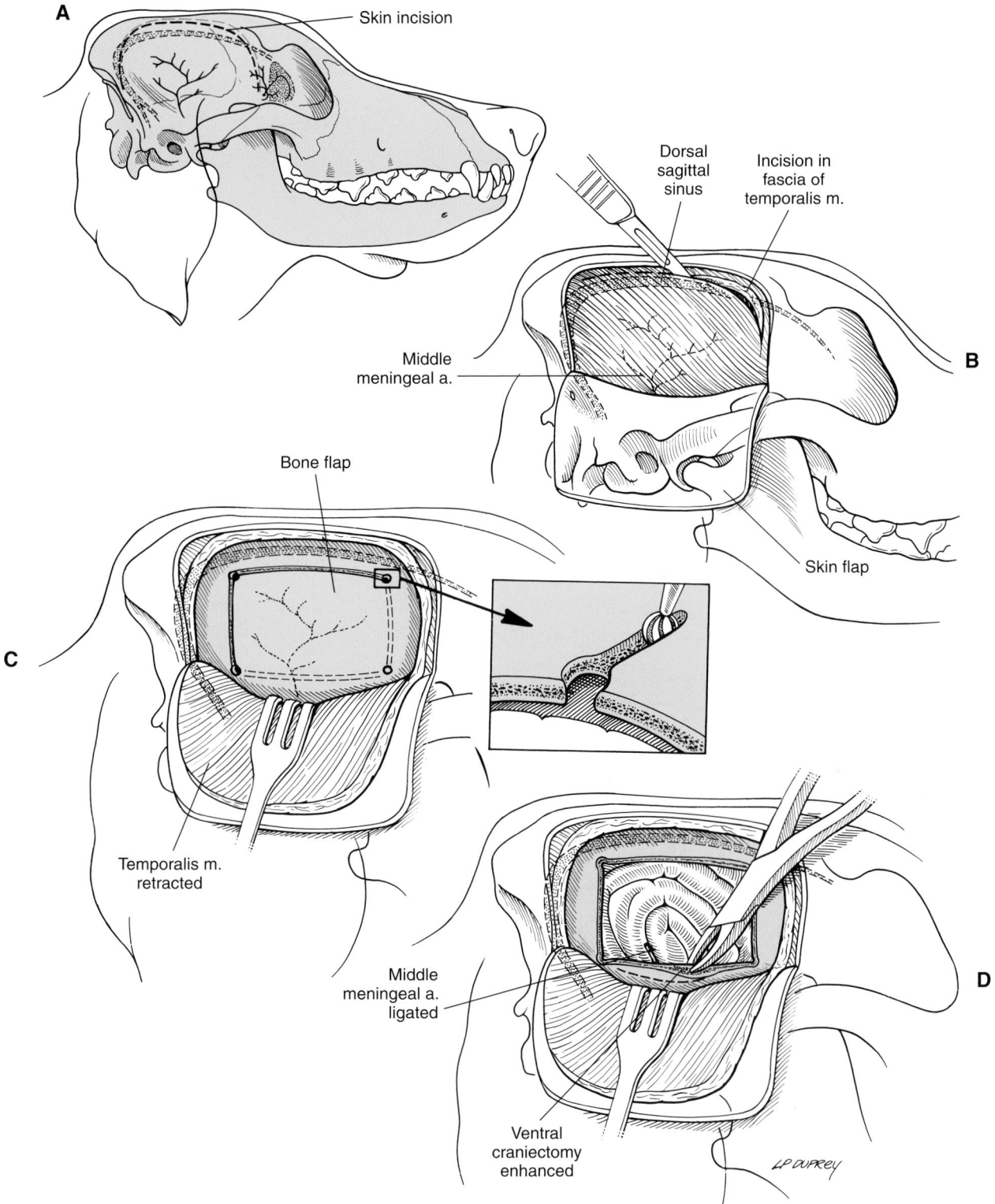

FIG. 37-3

For rostrotentorial craniotomy: **A,** Make a skin incision as illustrated. **B,** Incise the dorsal attachment of the temporalis muscle, subperiosteally elevate it from the lateral aspect of the skull, and retract it ventrally. Using a pneumatic drill, burr a hole at each corner of the proposed craniotomy site and drill a trough connecting each hole. **C,** Notice the location of the middle meningeal artery. **D,** Elevate and remove the bone flap; further exposure can be performed by rongeuring the craniotomy margin.

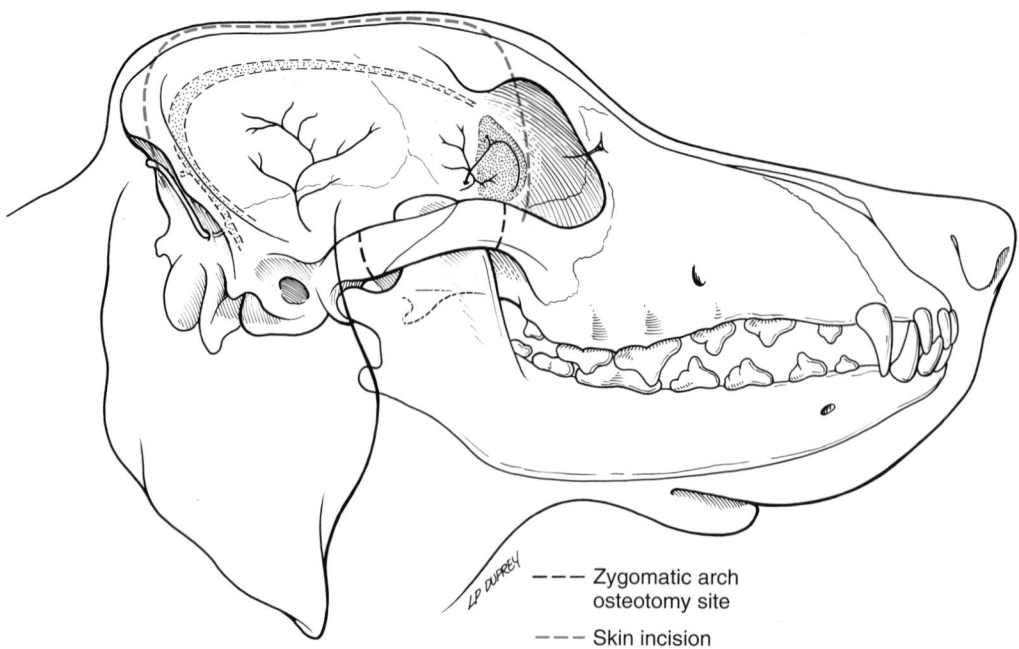

- - - Zygomatic arch
osteotomy site

- - - Skin incision

FIG. 37-4
For rostrotentorial craniotomy, make a U-shaped skin incision. Resect the zygomatic arch for extended exposure (see Fig. 37-5).

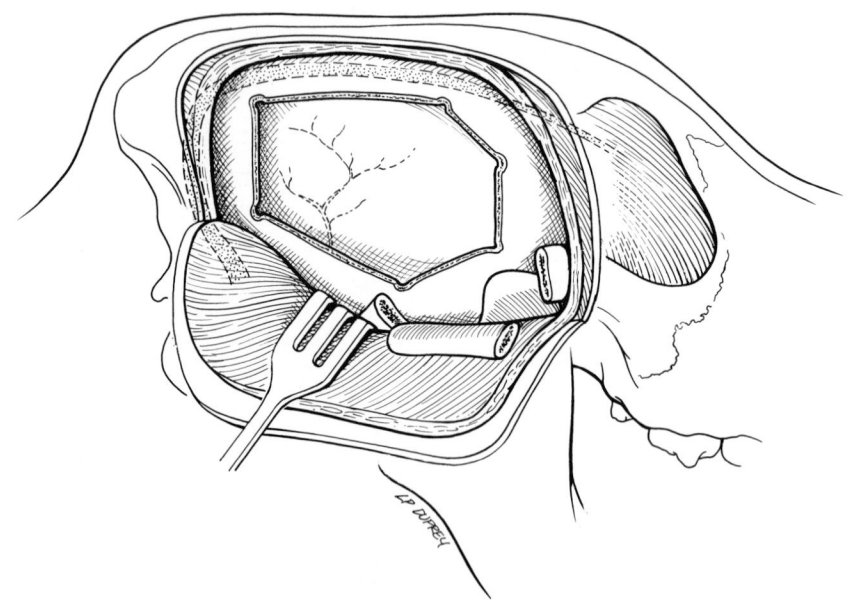

FIG. 37-5
For extended rostrotentorial craniotomy, resect and retract the zygomatic arch ventrally with the masseter muscle.

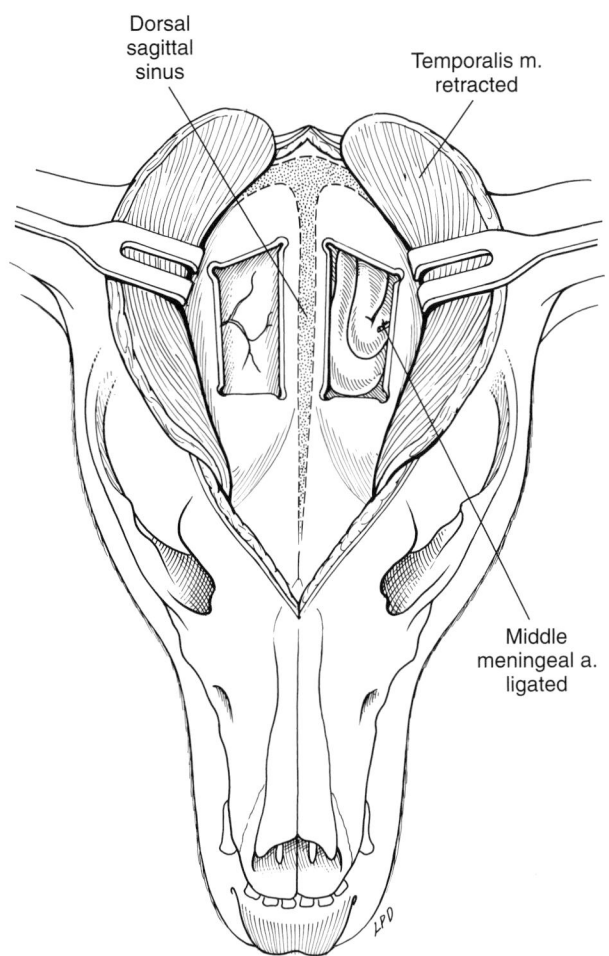

FIG. 37-6
During bilateral rostrotentorial craniotomy, leave a 0.5- to 1-cm strip of bone on the dorsal midline to protect the dorsal sagittal venous sinus.

NOTE: Be sure to leave a strip of bone along the midline to prevent damaging the dorsal sagittal sinus.

Caudotentorial Craniotomy

Perform caudotentorial craniotomy as described for rostrotentorial craniotomy, except center the craniotomy flap further caudally to expose the caudal aspect of the cerebral hemisphere and rostral aspect of the cerebellum. Make the skin incision as described for rostrotentorial craniotomy, but end the caudal aspect of the inverted U, 2 to 3 cm distal to the external occipital protuberance. Expose the cranium similarly to that described previously, except make the nuchal line and transverse sinus the caudal aspect of the craniotomy flap (Fig. 37-7). Close as described for rostrotentorial craniotomy.

Transfrontal Craniotomy

Clip and surgically prepare the entire head from the nasal planum rostrally to an area just behind the ears caudally. Secure the head in a head stand (see Fig. 37-2). Make a semicircular skin incision beginning at the rostral aspect of

the left ear, cross the midline to a point even with the lateral canthus of the right eye, and return to the midline to continue the incision on the dorsal midline to the midpoint of the nasal bones (Fig. 37-8, A). Incise the underlying supporting muscles of the ear, frontalis muscle, and periosteum, and reflect them to the left. Protect this tissue in a saline-moistened laparotomy pad until closure. Use an osteotome and mallet or oscillating saw, and cut a bone flap to expose the frontal sinus. Cut the caudal transverse osteotomy from the left zygomatic process to the right zygomatic process. Then, cut the rostral transverse osteotomy at the level of the caudal one third of the nasal bone, and connect the ends of each osteotomy to complete the trapezoid-shaped bone plate (see Fig. 37-8, A). Remove the bone plate and pack it in a saline-moistened laparotomy pad. Identify the exposed frontal sinuses, internal table of the frontal bone, cribriform plate of the ethmoid bone, and ethmoturbinates (Fig. 37-8, B). Pack off the rostral nasal opening with laparotomy pads, lavage the frontal sinus with sterile physiologic saline solution, and discard any potentially contaminated instruments. Use a Lempert rongeur to remove the ethmoturbinates and cribriform plate to expose the olfactory bulbs (see Fig. 37-8, B). Control hemorrhage with an absorbable hemostatic agent. Lavage the surgical site with sterile physiologic saline solution, and wire the nasal bone plate in place with 24-gauge stainless steel orthopedic wire or 2-0 or 3-0 nonabsorbable monofilament suture. Suture the muscle flap over the nasal bone, and close subcutaneous tissue and skin routinely.*

NOTE: Have an absorbable hemostatic agent available (see later Suture Material and Special Instruments section).

Modified Bilateral Transfrontal Sinus Craniotomy

Modified bilateral transfrontal craniotomy is indicated when both olfactory and frontal lobes require exposure.

Position and aseptically prepare the patient as described for a transfrontal sinus craniotomy. Make a midline skin incision from the caudal edge of the nasal bones at the level of the medial canthus of the eye caudally to the caudal extent of the frontal sinus. Extend the caudal margin of the skin incision to the junction of the median plane of the right and left frontoparietal sutures (i.e., bregma landmark) (Fig. 37-9, A). Reflect the underlying subcutaneous tissue, frontalis muscle, and periosteum laterally on each side of the incision. Elevate periosteum with a Freer periosteal elevator. Remove the diamond-shaped bone flap using an oscillating bone saw starting at the bregma landmark (Fig. 37-9, B). Angle the saw blade 20 to 30 degrees to make a bevel allowing easy and tight closure of the bone plate at the end of the procedure. Extend the bone cut rostrolaterally to the zygomatic process of the frontal bone and rostromedially to the junction of the nasal bones on the midline. Make a similar cut on the opposite

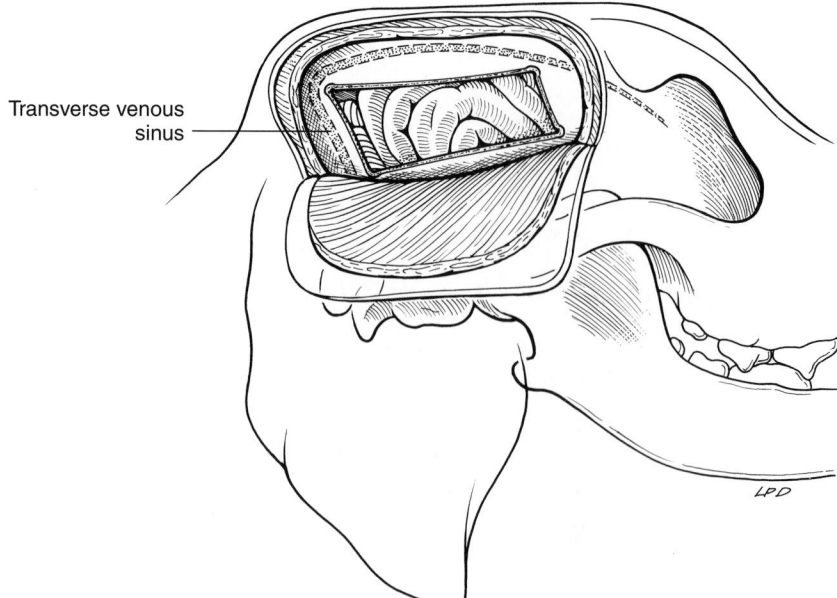

FIG. 37-7
Caudotentorial craniotomy allows exposure of the caudal cerebrum and rostral cerebellum. Notice the location of the caudal osteotomy relative to the transverse venous sinus.

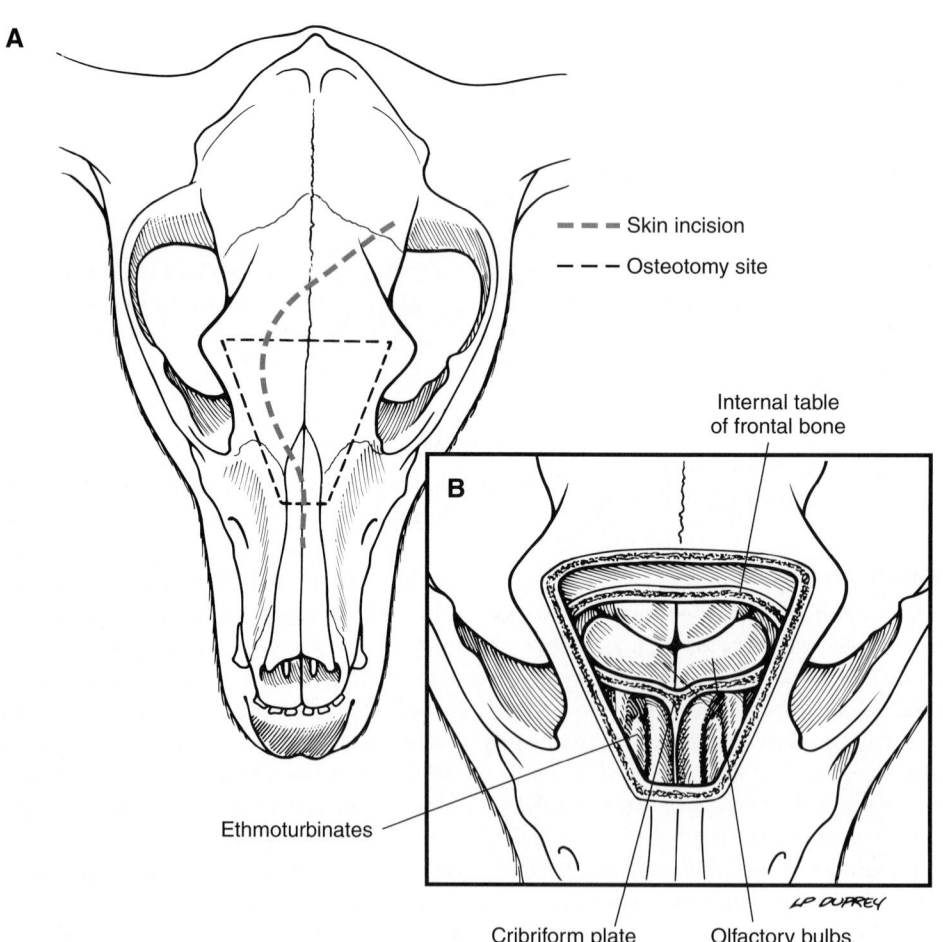

FIG. 37-8
For transfrontal craniotomy: **A,** Make a semicircular skin incision and perform a trapezoid-shaped osteotomy. **B,** The trapezoid-shaped bone flap has been removed. Notice the internal anatomy of the skull, including the cribriform plate, frontal sinuses, ethmoturbinates, internal table of the frontal bone, and craniotomy site.

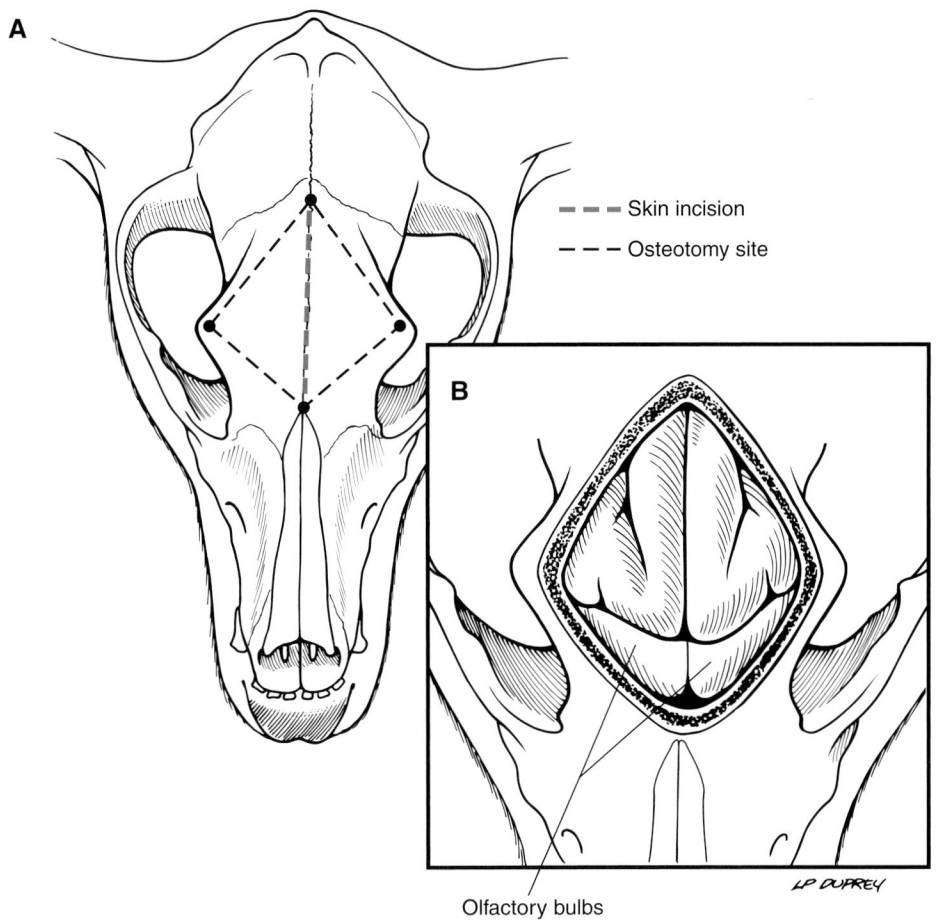

Olfactory bulbs

LP DUPREY

FIG. 37-9
For modified bilateral transfrontal craniotomy: **A,** Make a midline incision from the caudal edge of the nasal bones at the level of the medial canthus of the eye caudally to the caudal extent of the frontal sinus. **B,** Remove a diamond-shaped bone flap using an oscillating bone saw. Then remove the internal table of the frontal bone and a portion of the ethmoturbinates using a rongeur.

side of the skull, uniting the two bone incisions. Remove the bone plate, and wrap it in a saline-moistened sponge. Remove the diamond-shaped bone plate, and identify the frontal sinus, ethmoturbinates, and internal table of the frontal bone. Remove the internal table of the frontal bone and a portion of the ethmoturbinates with a rongeur. Identify the underlying meninges covering the olfactory bulbs and frontal lobes. Close the defect as described for transfrontal sinus craniotomy previously.

Suboccipital Craniotomy

Position the patient in sternal recumbency with the head flexed and secured in a head stand. If the lesion is in a lateral location, rotate the head 30 degrees with the affected side uppermost. Incise skin on the dorsal midline from the external occipital protuberance rostrally to the caudal border of the dorsal spinous process of C2 caudally. Sharply dissect occipital and cervical spinal epaxial muscles to expose the occipital crest and dorsal spine of C2. Elevate muscle from the occipital bone with a periosteal elevator using the nuchal

line as a landmark for lateral dissection. As periosteal dissection approaches the nuchal line, identify the occipital emissary vein and protect or ligate it as it exits the skull. Use self-retaining retractors to facilitate exposure (Fig. 37-10, A). Use a high-speed pneumatic drill and 2- to 3-mm carbide burr to drill a 1-cm diameter opening in the central part of the exposed calvarium. Use rongeurs to remove necessary calvarium for lesion exposure (Fig. 37-10, B). Control hemorrhage with thrombin-soaked gelatin sponge, and lavage the surgical site with warmed, sterile physiologic saline solution. Appose occipital and cervical epaxial muscles with simple interrupted 2-0 or 3-0 monofilament absorbable suture, and close subcutaneous tissue and skin routinely.

> NOTE: The extent of exposure is limited by the following anatomic landmarks: confluens sinus dorsally (external occipital protuberance), transverse sinuses laterally (nuchal line), and ventral occipital sinus ventrally (foramen magnum) (see Fig. 37-10, *B*).

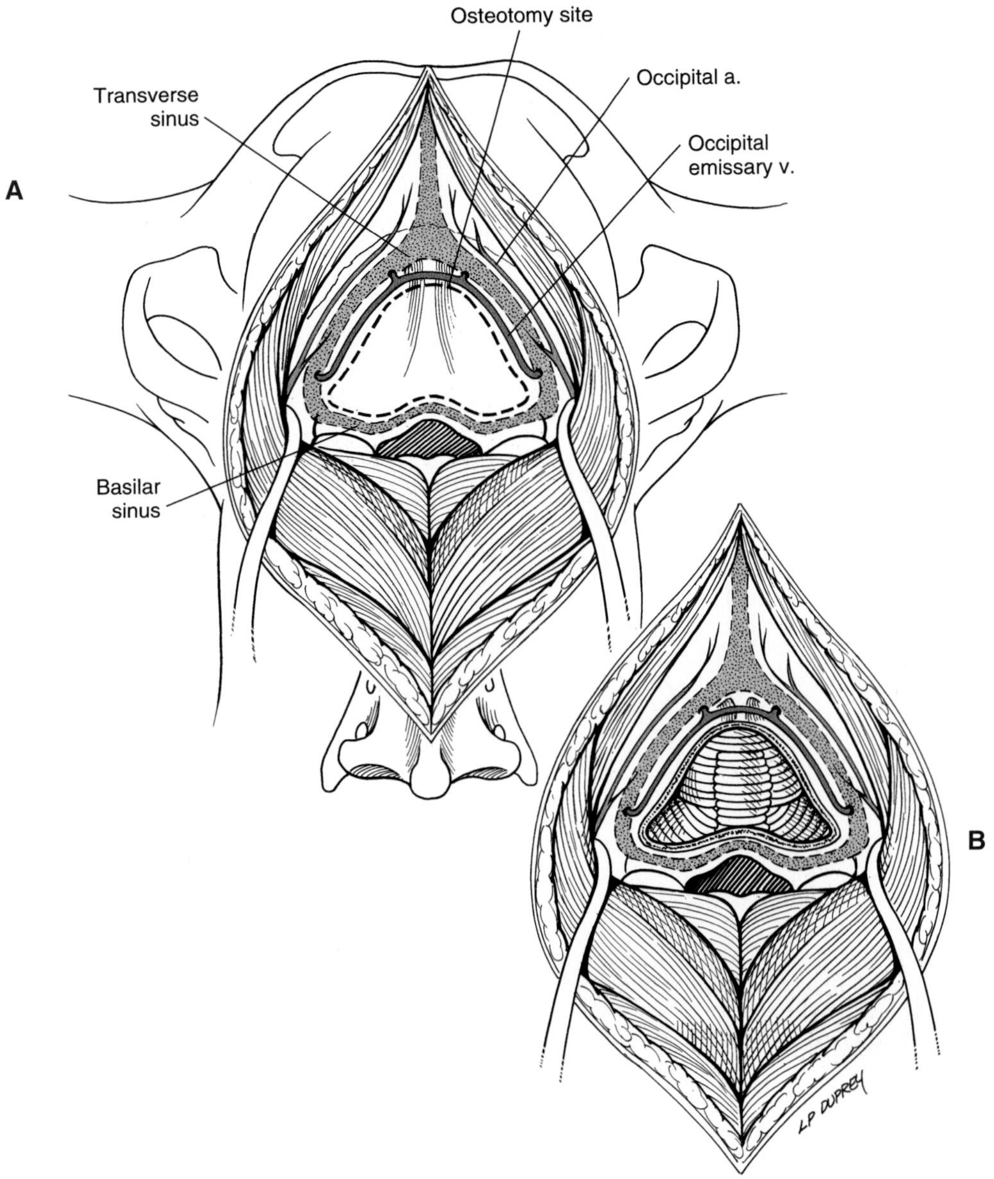

FIG. 37-10
For suboccipital craniotomy: **A,** Elevate the occipital and cervical spinal epaxial muscles, and retract them to expose the caudal aspect of the calvarium. **B,** The extent of exposure provided by suboccipital craniotomy is determined by the confluens sinus dorsally (external occipital protuberance), transverse sinuses laterally (nuchal line), and ventral occipital sinus ventrally (foramen magnum).

HEALING OF THE BRAIN AND SKULL

Within 1 month after craniotomy and bone flap replacement, the flap becomes stable. Occasionally, the flap is slightly depressed (1 to 2 mm). Healing of the osteotomy sites is characterized by fibroplasia and osteoplasia. If dura is replaced during surgery, it becomes thickened and adheres to the bone flap and underlying brain.

Within 6 to 8 weeks after craniotomy, defects are covered with a dense connective tissue membrane that completely separates the cerebral cortex from overlying muscle. At 2 to 3 months postoperatively, the sealing membrane is strong (but without signs of ossification) and offers adequate protection for underlying brain tissue. The temporalis muscle is adhered to the tissue membrane; however, normal brain tissue is separated from the neo-dura mater by a CSF-filled space containing small bridges of fibrous strands.

The meningeal response to resected brain parenchyma is generally characterized by a nonsuppurative meningitis; brain tissue response is a nonsuppurative encephalitis. A reduction in the size of the surgically created defect is initially caused by deviation of remaining brain parenchyma into the surgical site. Later, this area becomes occupied by a web of fibrous connective tissue, blood vessels, and glial scarring.

SUTURE MATERIALS AND SPECIAL INSTRUMENTS

Microsurgical or ophthalmic instruments, including micro-curettes, microneedle holders, microscissors, and microforceps, are invaluable when manipulating dura and brain tissue. Two- or three-power optical loupes or telescopes obviate identification of tissue planes, small vessels, and tumor–normal tissue interfaces. Pediatric brain spatulas (Paton Double Spatula, Storz Instrument Company, St. Louis, Mo.) are used to gently retract brain parenchyma when attempting to expose masses deep to the brain surface. A high-speed pneumatic drill with assorted size burrs is necessary to perform a craniotomy. Various sizes and types of rongeurs (e.g., Lempert, Kerrison, and Ruskin) are used to create and extend craniotomy defects (see p. 52). Small Frazier suction tips (see p. 51) with a controllable degree of suction are used to remove neoplastic tissue and hematomas (e.g., epidural, subdural, and subarachnoid); provide visualization during active hemorrhage; and facilitate hemostasis. Monopolar electrocautery provides hemostasis during the approach to the calvarium. Lint-free cottonoid sponges (Weck-cel, Edward Weck and Co., Durham, N.C.); thrombin-soaked sponges (Johnson & Johnson, Arlington, Tex.); bone wax (Ethicon, Inc., Somerville, N.J.); and bipolar cautery are used to facilitate adequate hemostasis during removal of the bone flap and manipulation of brain parenchyma. Surgical lasers and ultrasonic aspirators facilitate atraumatic removal of abnormal tissue; high cost generally limits their availability. Small vessel ligation and dural retraction require the use of 5-0 and 6-0 monofilament absorbable and nonabsorbable suture.

POSTOPERATIVE CARE AND ASSESSMENT

Patients should be extubated and recovered in a 24-hour intensive care facility for the first 3 to 5 days postoperatively. Blood gas analysis is indicated to evaluate ventilation and oxygenation, and oxygen should be supplemented as necessary. Analgesic medication should be provided (see Table 13-4 on p. 133). Preoperative anticonvulsant therapy should be continued postoperatively or instituted at this time. Corticosteroids may be continued for a variable duration, based on neurologic status (Box 37-7). Antibiotic therapy is dependent on the type of injury, procedure performed, surgery time, and patient status (see previous discussion). Diuretics should be considered in patients that develop deteriorating neurologic signs immediately postoperatively. Serial neurologic examinations should be performed two to three times daily (or more frequently, depending on patient status) for the first 2 to 3 days. Stuporous or comatose patients should be placed in a padded oxygen cage, turned every 2 to 3 hours until alert, monitored for seizure activity, and given IV fluids at two-thirds of the maintenance rate. Alert or obtunded (i.e., depressed) patients should be placed in a padded cage,

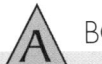

BOX 37-7

Postoperative Corticosteroid Therapy

Dexamethasone (Azium)*

0.25–0.5 mg/kg SC bid; then taper by cutting the dose in half each day over a 2- to 3-day period

SC, Subcutaneous.
*Gastrointestinal bleeding may occur.

monitored for seizure activity, and repeatedly examined for neurologic abnormalities. After discharge from the hospital, patients should be scheduled for routine follow-up examinations at various intervals, depending on patient status and the specific disorder. Reevaluations may include neurologic examination, survey skull radiographs, CT scan, MRI, alteration of anticonvulsant therapy, and/or adjunct therapy (e.g., chemotherapy, immunotherapy, and radiation therapy).

COMPLICATIONS

Reported complications associated with craniotomy, craniectomy, and brain parenchymal resection include uncontrollable brain swelling, deterioration of neurologic signs, increased intracranial pressure, seizures, brain herniation, hemorrhage, and infection. The most commonly reported long-term complication is recurrence of resected neoplastic tissue.

SPECIAL AGE CONSIDERATIONS

Brain tumors (see p. 1397) are most common in older patients that tend to have a greater incidence of dural adhesions to the endosteal surface of the calvarium.

Reference

Garner JL, Kirby R, Rudloff E: The use of acepromazine in dogs with a history of seizures, *J Vet Emerg Crit Care* 14:1, 2004.

SPECIFIC DISEASES

HEAD TRAUMA

DEFINITIONS

Severe **head trauma** generally results in brain ischemia, edema, hemorrhage, and hypoxia. **Ischemia** is caused by disruption and mechanical obstruction of small blood vessels in the traumatized area. **Brain edema** is caused by intracellular accumulation of sodium, chloride, and water and escape of fluid into the extracellular space. **Intracranial hemorrhage** may be epidural, subdural, subarachnoid, or parenchymal. **Epidural hemorrhage** is accumulation of blood between the skull and dura mater, whereas **subdural hemorrhage** is accumulation of blood between the dura mater and arachnoid membrane. **Subarachnoid hemorrhage** is accumulation of blood between the arachnoid membrane and pia mater, and **intraparenchymal hemorrhage** is accumulation of blood within brain parenchyma. Ischemia, edema, and intracranial hemorrhage combine to cause tissue hypoxia and increased intracranial pressure. Other terms for head trauma include *craniocerebral trauma, brain trauma, cranial trauma, head injury,* and *intracranial trauma.*

GENERAL CONSIDERATIONS AND CLINICALLY RELEVANT PATHOPHYSIOLOGY

The most common cause of head trauma in dogs and cats is motor vehicle accidents. Other less common causes include penetrating wounds (e.g., gunshot wounds and bite wounds), falls, and kicks. Because cats and dogs have a relatively thick calvarium and protective musculature covering the brain, severe trauma is generally necessary to cause clinically significant brain injury, although seemingly minor trauma will occasionally be responsible. Greater than 50% of head trauma patients have associated injuries referable to the pulmonary system (e.g., pulmonary edema, contusions, hemorrhage, and pneumothorax). Other major concurrent injuries include spinal cord trauma, pelvic fractures, traumatic myocarditis, and facial fractures (i.e., maxillary and mandibular). Reaction of the brain to trauma can be viewed as a four-stage, self-propagating process. Ischemia and extravasation of blood in the damaged area disrupt cell-membrane integrity by releasing free radicals. Resulting increases in extracellular potassium and bicarbonate cause transport of water into brain cells (brain edema). Cellular swelling increases ischemia and hypoxia, which produce additional brain cell swelling. Edema in the involved region and accumulation of blood increase intracranial pressure, decrease perfusion pressure, and further spread the area of ischemia.

DIAGNOSIS
Clinical Presentation
Signalment. Head trauma may occur in dogs and cats of any age, but is most common in young animals. There is no breed or sex predisposition.

History. The majority of patients are presented with a history of trauma. The animal's state of consciousness is generally altered to some degree (i.e., it is depressed, obtunded, stuporous, or comatose [see p. 1358]), and associated respiratory distress is common.

Physical Examination Findings
Patients with head trauma should have careful and repeated neurologic examinations (see p. 1358) to assess location and degree of intracranial damage. Because the majority of head trauma patients have respiratory system injuries, careful auscultation is necessary. Dogs with significant thoracic trauma should be examined frequently for delayed-onset cardiac arrhythmias caused by myocardial contusion and dyspnea due to delayed pleural and/or pulmonary hemorrhage. Careful physical examination for associated skeletal injuries (e.g., appendicular and spinal) should also be performed.

Diagnostic Imaging
Thoracic radiographs of animals with head trauma should be carefully evaluated for pulmonary edema, hemorrhage, contusion, and/or pneumothorax. Survey skull radiographs may help evaluate patients with suspected skull fractures. Skull fractures may appear as fine radiolucent lines, depressed segments of bone, or radiodense lines if fracture fragments overlap. Although these radiographic findings are indicative of brain trauma, intracranial hemorrhage and brain contusion may occur in the absence of skull fractures. Routine skull radiographs should include lateral, ventrodorsal (or dorsoventral), and lateral oblique projections. Because intracranial space-occupying lesions secondary to trauma (intracranial hematomas) cannot be seen on survey skull radiographs, advanced imaging methods such as CT or MRI should be considered for optimal assessment of patients with head trauma. CT is preferable in patients with head trauma because it is quicker and better at imaging bone and acute hemorrhage. In addition, CT provides an excellent view of the skull, it can be used to diagnose subtle skull fractures, and it is much more sensitive for detecting acute hemorrhage.

> NOTE: Survey radiographs are not helpful in identifying intracranial trauma (e.g., hemorrhage and contusion), and skull fractures may be difficult to identify unless they are displaced.

Laboratory Findings
Laboratory findings in patients with head trauma are nonspecific. Patients with significant pulmonary pathology may show evidence of hypoxia on blood gas analysis or increased hepatic enzymes caused by contusion of the liver.

DIFFERENTIAL DIAGNOSIS
Patients with head trauma must be differentiated from those with intracranial lesions causing ischemia, edema, hemorrhage, hypoxia, and increased intracranial pressure. Differential diagnoses include neoplasia, abscess, congenital malformations (e.g., arteriovenous malformations and hydrocephalus), encephalitis (e.g., viral or granulomatous meningoencephalitis [GME]), and vasculitis (e.g., feline infectious peritonitis [FIP], Rocky Mountain spotted fever, ehrlichiosis, and immune mediated).

MEDICAL MANAGEMENT
Treatment of head trauma patients is based on presenting neurologic signs, serial neurologic examinations, neuroanatomic location of the lesion, and nature of the intracranial injury (e.g., hematoma or parenchymal hemorrhage). Patients with a mildly altered consciousness (i.e., they are depressed or obtunded) are treated medically regardless of le-

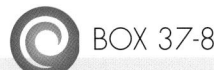 BOX 37-8

Drugs Used to Treat Patients With Intracranial Trauma

Methylprednisolone Sodium Succinate (Solu-Medrol)

30 mg/kg IV once; repeat in 6 hr

Dexamethasone Sodium Phosphate (Azium Sp)*

Initial dose: 1–2 mg/kg IV once or twice
Maintenance dose: 0.25 mg/kg PO tid; tapered over 4–7 days as needed

Prednisone*

1.1–2.2 mg/kg PO bid; tapered over 4–7 days as needed

Furosemide (Lasix)

2.2–4.4 mg/kg IV

Mannitol (20%–25%) (Osmitrol)

0.5–1 g/kg IV over 10–20 min
(limit to three boluses per 24 hours)

Cefazolin (Ancef, Kefzol)

22 mg/kg IV tid

Cephadroxil (Cefa-Tabs)

22–35 mg/kg PO tid

Pentobarbital

5–15 mg/kg IV to effect

IV, Intravenous; *PO,* oral; *tid,* three times a day; *bid,* twice a day.
*Chronic use of prednisolone is less likely to cause gastrointestinal hemorrhage than chronic use of dexamethasone.

 BOX 37-9

Urgent Anticonvulsant Therapy for Patients With Acute Brain Trauma

Diazepam (Valium)*

Dogs: 0.5–1 mg/kg bolus given IV, repeat if necessary or 0.5–2 mg/kg/hr as a CRI
Cats: 0.5 mg/kg bolus given IV, repeat if necessary; give every 5 to 10 minutes if effective (maximum of three doses)†

Pentobarbital

2–15 mg/kg IV to effect until seizure activity stops or 0.5–4 mg/kg/hr as a CRI

Propofol (Dogs Only)*

1–6 mg/kg given as a bolus IV, to effect; then initiate 0.1–0.6 mg/kg/minute as a CRI

Phenobarbital*

2–5 mg/kg given as a bolus IV, to effect, until seizure activity stops or 2–6 mg/dog/hr as a CRI

Potassium Bromide (KBr) (Dogs Only)†

Rectal loading dose 100 mg/kg given every 4 hr for six doses

IV, Intravenous; *CRI,* constant rate infusion.
*Primarily used for cluster seizures/status epilepticus; adjust dose based on serum phenobarbital concentrations.
†Do not use KBr in cats as it may cause serious respiratory problems; with this loading dose steady state and therapeutic levels are reached in 24 hr.

sion location or nature. Those with a moderately to severely altered consciousness (i.e., they are stuporous or comatose) should initially be treated medically and the lesion localized by CT or MRI. If the lesion is located in an area amenable to surgical decompression (i.e., through craniotomy) and is removable (e.g., hematoma and fracture fragment), surgical intervention should be considered. Depressed skull fractures warrant surgical decompression by fracture reduction or fragment removal plus medical therapy. If the lesion is located in an area that is not surgically accessible, such as the brain stem, or not removable, as with parenchymal hemorrhage, medical therapy should be continued; craniotomy should be considered because it may help decrease intracranial pressure.

Medical management is directed at reversing brain edema, hypoxia, ischemia, and increased intracranial pressure and preventing infection. A complete blood count (CBC) and serum chemistry panel are indicated to look for any other problems that could affect therapeutic choices in these critically ill patients. Drugs used to treat patients with head trauma are listed in Box 37-8. Generally, patients admitted with severe head trauma (i.e., they are stuporous or comatose) should be treated initially with appropriate fluid therapy to maintain systolic blood pressure at 90 mm Hg. The

animal should be placed in an oxygen-rich environment (e.g., oxygen cage, nasal oxygen, or ventilator), if necessary (see Chapter 5). If arterial blood gas analysis is available, the partial pressure of oxygen in arterial blood (PaO_2) should be maintained at or above 90 mm Hg for dogs and 100 mm Hg for cats. The most efficient means for oxygen delivery in head trauma patients include face mask, nasal oxygen catheter (see p. 27), or transtracheal oxygen catheter. An oxygen cage may be used, but the constant monitoring required by severe head injury patients necessitates that the cage door be opened frequently. Once the head trauma patient is hemodynamically stable, mannitol should be considered first-line therapy for decreasing intracranial pressure. Administration of furosemide a few minutes before mannitol administration may be synergistic in reducing intracranial pressure. The concern raised about mannitol's effect of exacerbating ongoing brain hemorrhage is unfounded and should be ignored when treating dogs and cats with head trauma. Use of methylprednisolone sodium succinate should be considered as adjunctive treatment in those patients not responding adequately to appropriate resuscitative measures (fluid and oxygen therapy) and appropriate mannitol administration. Induction of a pentobarbital coma (Box 37-9) has been advocated as a "last ditch" effort to decrease metabolic demands of the injured brain; however, there is limited evidence of clinical efficacy. Seizures should be controlled with anticonvulsants (Box 37-9); IV diazepam should be used initially (Box 37-9). If the patient sustained an open head wound or open skull fracture, therapeutic antibiotics (e.g., cefazolin IV at anesthetic induction and 6 hours after surgery [subcutaneously; SC], then cefadroxil for 5 to 7 days [orally; PO] after surgery) should be initiated (see Box 37-8). If the patient is old (greater than 10 years), debilitated, has an associated crush injury, or will have surgery lasting greater than 90 minutes, prophylactic antibiotics (e.g., cefazolin IV at anesthetic induction and every 8 hours for 24 to 36 hours) should be considered.

Initial and serial neurologic examinations establish neuroanatomic localization and patient status, respectively. Patients with severe neurologic deficits or with a deteriorating neurologic status after initial medical therapy should have CT or MRI to establish the presence, location, and size of a possible intracranial mass (i.e., hematoma and skull fragment). If a surgically treatable mass is identified, surgical decompression should be considered. If surgery is not indicated, medical management as described previously should be continued.

SURGICAL TREATMENT

The aim of surgical treatment in patients with head trauma is decompression via mass removal (e.g., hematoma removal, hemostasis, fracture reduction, and skull fragment removal) to reduce intracranial pressure. A prerequisite to performing intracranial surgery is accurate localization of the offending mass with CT or MRI. Indications for surgical intervention include severe neurologic deficits, deteriorating neurologic status, unacceptable response to medical management, and presence of a surgically removable intracranial mass (e.g., hematoma or fracture versus parenchymal hemorrhage). It has been suggested that 100% of patients with severe cranial trauma have some degree of intracranial hemorrhage. Subdural and subarachnoid spaces are relatively common anatomic locations of intracranial hemorrhage in dogs and cats. Although the current mortality rate of patients with severe head trauma is high, accurate localization via CT or MRI and early aggressive surgical decompression via craniotomy may improve patient outcome.

> NOTE: Accurate localization of the brain lesion with CT or MRI is mandatory before surgery.

Preoperative Management

Patients should generally be treated with fluids, oxygen supplementation, mannitol, diuretics, corticosteroids, anticonvulsants (if indicated), and antibiotics (if indicated) on admission and before surgery (see p. 1394). Thoracic radiographs should be taken to detect concurrent pulmonary edema, contusion, hemorrhage, and/or pneumothorax, and an electrocardiogram should be performed to evaluate the patient for traumatic myocarditis.

Anesthesia

Anesthetic management of patients undergoing brain surgery is provided on p. 1380. Recommended protocols for animals undergoing MRI procedures are included in Box 37-6 on p. 1381.

Surgical Anatomy

See p. 1381 for surgical anatomy of the brain.

Positioning

Patients undergoing cranial surgery for head trauma are generally positioned in ventral recumbency with the head stabilized in a specially designed head stand (see p. 1385 and Fig. 37-2). Head rotation is varied depending on desired surgical approach.

SURGICAL TECHNIQUE

A craniotomy approach or combination of approaches that allows adequate visualization of the intracranial hematoma or calvarial fracture should be selected. If bone fragments are present and depressed greater than the thickness of the skull, surgical decompression via fracture reduction or bone fragment removal is recommended. Preoperative CT or MRI is recommended to assess possible intracranial hemorrhage.

Epidural Hematomas

Gently lift off the calvarium and expose the hematoma. Carefully manipulate the hematoma with a brain spatula (see p. 1393), and suction until it separates from the underlying dura. Cauterize dural bleeders with bipolar cautery or use thrombin-soaked sponges and suction. After the hematoma is completely removed and dural hemorrhage controlled, irrigate the surgical field with sterile physiologic saline solution and close as described on p. 1386.

Subdural Hematomas

Gently lift off the calvarium and expose the discolored dura (e.g., deep-red to purple-blue liquid, black "crankcase oil," or black "jellylike" consistency) covering the brain. Incise the dura along the entire length of the hematoma and gently separate it from the underlying hematoma. Use a brain spatula (see p. 1393), and suction to carefully separate the hematoma from the overlying dura and underlying arachnoid membrane. Cauterize small vessels with bipolar cautery or encourage coagulation with thrombin-soaked sponges. Do not attempt to close the dura because it is fragile and generally tears during surgical manipulation. After the hematoma is completely removed and dural, arachnoid, and parenchymal hemorrhage controlled, irrigate the surgical field with warmed, sterile physiologic saline solution and close as described on p. 1386.

Subarachnoid Hematomas

Gently remove the calvarium to expose the dura, arachnoid, and purplish discoloration of the contused brain. Incise dura and arachnoid along the entire length of the hematoma.

Remove any visible clots and pulpified brain tissue with suction. Because the dura and arachnoid are generally fragile and easily torn during surgical manipulation, do not attempt to close them. After the hematoma is completely removed and dural, arachnoidal, and parenchymal hemorrhage controlled, irrigate the surgical field with warmed, sterile physiologic saline solution and close as described on p. 1386.

Skull Fractures

Expose the skull fracture by careful periosteal elevation of overlying muscles as described on p. 1386. Take care to prevent accentuating a depression fracture during exposure. Use a dural hook to carefully elevate the depressed fragment of bone away from the underlying brain. Remove bone fragments and examine underlying dura, arachnoid, and brain parenchyma for hemorrhage. If an epidural, subdural, or subarachnoid hematoma is seen, evacuate the hematoma and control hemorrhage as described previously. Make no attempt to replace fracture fragments.

SUTURE MATERIALS AND SPECIAL INSTRUMENTS

Special instruments recommended for reduction of skull fractures or removal of epidural, subdural, and subarachnoid hematomas are listed and described on p. 1393.

POSTOPERATIVE CARE AND ASSESSMENT

Patients should be recovered in a padded cage in a critical care facility and given analgesics, anticonvulsants, corticosteroids, diuretics, antibiotics, and oxygen supplementation as necessary based on serial neurologic examinations. Discharge from the hospital depends on patient status and owner compliance (see p. 1393). Patients should be scheduled for reevaluation at various intervals after surgery at 1, 3, 6, and 12 months postinjury, depending on their condition and response to therapy. Procedures performed during reevaluations may include neurologic examination, skull radiographs, CT, MRI, and/or alteration of anticonvulsant therapy.

PROGNOSIS

Prognosis for patients with head injury depends on severity of neurologic deficits (i.e., severity of injury), size of the intracranial hematoma, rapidity of hematoma development, ability to accurately localize the compressive mass, and timing of medical and surgical treatment. Patients with mild neurologic deficits admitted within 4 to 8 hours postinjury and managed with appropriate medical therapy have a favorable prognosis, whereas those with severe neurologic deficits have a guarded prognosis, despite appropriate medical therapy and early surgical decompression.

> NOTE: If the prognosis for patients with severe head trauma is to improve, a rapid and aggressive approach using state of the art diagnostic, medical, and surgical techniques must be employed.

Reference

Dewey CW: Head trauma management. In Dewey CW, editor: *A practical guide to canine and feline neurology,* Ames, Iowa, 2003, Iowa State Press.

NEOPLASIA

DEFINITIONS

Brain tumors may be classified as **primary** (originate from neural tissue) or **secondary** (invade the brain via local invasion or hematogenous metastasis). Meningioma, glioma (astrocytoma, oligodendroglioma), choroids plexus tumor, and ependymoma are the most common primary brain tumors. **Gliomas** are primary brain tumors that arise from neuroglial cells; **choroids plexus tumors** arise from vascular elements; and **ependymomas** arise from ependymal cells. **Meningiomas** are mesenchymal tumors that arise from the dura mater, arachnoid, or pia mater, with most meningiomas arising from the arachnoid.

GENERAL CONSIDERATIONS AND CLINICALLY RELEVANT PATHOPHYSIOLOGY

The incidence of intracranial neoplasia in dogs is approximately 14.5 per 100,000. The most common primary tumors in dogs are meningiomas and gliomas (i.e., astrocytomas and oligodendrogliomas) (Box 37-10). Intracranial meningiomas occur more commonly than spinal meningiomas in dogs and cats A recent report states that 80% of meningiomas are intracranial (Axlund et al, 2002). Meningiomas in dogs are generally benign, solitary, slow-growing tumors. They most frequently occur in the frontal lobes, falx cerebri, and cerebellopontine angle. Gliomas are the second most frequently diagnosed primary intracranial tumors in dogs. They usually occur in the cerebrum. Tumor type, biologic behavior, and location of canine and feline primary intracranial tumors are listed in Table 37-3.

> NOTE: Pituitary tumors are discussed in Chapter 22 (see p. 584).

The incidence of intracranial neoplasia in cats is approximately 3.5 per 100,000. The most common primary brain

 BOX 37-10

Most Common Brain Tumors

Primary

Dogs: Meningiomas, gliomas
Cats: Meningiomas

Secondary

Dogs: Nasal adenocarcinoma, mammary adenocarcinoma, prostatic adenocarcinoma, pulmonary adenocarcinoma
Cats: Squamous cell carcinoma, osteosarcoma/osteochondroma, pituitary adenoma, metastatic carcinomas

Table 37-3

Behavior of Canine and Feline Primary Intracranial Neoplasms

NEOPLASM	SPECIES	BIOLOGIC ACTIVITY	COMMENTS
Meningioma	Canine	Locally infiltrates brain parenchyma Has a moderate growth rate 18% to 27% metastasize	Most common intracranial neoplasm Generally solitary Located in cerebrum
Meningioma	Feline	Local growth; rarely metastasizes Well-defined demarcation between tumor and brain parenchyma	Most common intracranial neoplasm Generally solitary Located on cerebral convexity Slow growth rate
Gliomas Astrocytomas Oligodendrogliomas	Canine	Locally infiltrates brain parenchyma Extracranial metastasis is rare	Second most common intracranial neoplasm Located in cerebrum

BOX 37-11

Breeds of Dogs Predisposed to Brain Tumors

Boxers
Golden retrievers
Doberman pinscher
Scottish terriers
Old English sheepdogs

tumor in cats is meningioma. Feline meningiomas are generally solitary; however, multiple tumors are diagnosed more frequently in cats than in dogs. They are most commonly located over the cerebral hemispheres. Slow tumor growth of feline meningiomas accounts for the insidious onset of clinical signs. Primary brain tumors, other than meningiomas, rarely occur in cats. Tumors that have been reported include gliomas, lymphoma, olfactory neuroblastoma, and gangliocytomas. The most common secondary brain tumors in dogs and cats are listed in Box 37-10.

DIAGNOSIS
Clinical Presentation

Signalment. Brain tumors occur in dogs of any age, sex, or breed; however, most affected dogs are greater than 5 years of age. Certain breeds appear to have a higher incidence of specific tumors (e.g., brachycephalic breeds are predisposed to gliomas and dolichocephalic breeds are more likely to develop meningiomas). Breeds most commonly affected are listed in Box 37-11. Sex predilection has not been well established, but it appears that astrocytomas are more common in male dogs and meningiomas in female dogs. The average age of cats with meningioma is 12 years (range 5 to 17 years). A sex predilection has not been definitively identified; however, there are some reports that suggest a higher incidence in male cats. All breeds of cats appear to be affected by meningiomas, although domestic shorthairs may be predisposed.

History. Historical findings in dogs and cats with brain tumors include subtle to overt altered behavior (e.g., hiding, personality changes, lethargy, poor appetite, disorientation, and aggressive behavior); seizures; impaired vision; weakness (e.g., tetra-, mono-, hemi-, or paraparesis); or altered consciousness (e.g., depressed, obtunded, stuporous, or comatose). The severity of clinical signs depends on tumor location, size, invasiveness, and growth rate. Seizures are by far the most common chief complaint in dogs with brain tumors; in cats, behavioral change is most common.

Physical Examination Findings

Abnormal physical examination findings associated with brain neoplasms include weight loss despite normal appetite, hyporexia, decreased thirst, and/or bradycardia. They may occur alone or in conjunction with neurologic abnormalities. Common neurologic abnormalities include seizures, circling, locomotor disturbances, visual deficits, hearing loss, altered states of consciousness, and head pressing. Neurologic signs are generally accurate enough to establish focal neuroanatomic localization of the tumor (see Box 36-5), although some animals with masses have no localizing cranial nerve deficits. Characteristic neurologic signs of focal intracranial lesions affecting the forebrain, cerebellum, brainstem, and vestibular systems (peripheral and central) are provided in Table 37-4. Clinical severity and progression of neurologic signs appear to correlate with survival in dogs with brain tumors; in general, compromised patients with rapidly progressive signs have a shorter survival.

Diagnostic Imaging

Skull radiographs are generally noncontributory to the differentiation or localization of primary intracranial neoplasms. Exceptions include hyperostosis of the calvarium (e.g., with feline meningiomas); invasion of the calvarium by an intracranial neoplasm, causing erosion or complete disruption of the calvarium (e.g., with feline meningiomas); invasion of the calvarium and brain by local extension (e.g., with skull osteo-

Table 37-4

Characteristic Neurologic Findings Associated With Intracranial Lesions in Various Regions of the Brain

REGION OF THE BRAIN	EXPECTED NEUROLOGIC FINDINGS
Forebrain	Seizures
Cerebral cortex	Head pressing
Thalamus	Personality changes Circling to the side of the lesion Visual deficits on the opposite side of the lesion Motor deficits on the opposite side of the lesion Conscious proprioceptive deficits on the opposite side of the lesion Facial palsy on the opposite side of the lesion
Brainstem	Cranial nerve deficits V—loss of facial and ocular sensation VII—loss of blink, sagging of the lip VIII—head tilt, nystagmus, ataxia Altered state of consciousness Depression, stupor, coma
Vestibular-central	Brainstem signs Ataxia Nystagmus Head tilt to the side of the lesion
Vestibular-peripheral	No brainstem signs Ataxia Nystagmus Head tilt to the side of the lesion Horner's syndrome
Cerebellum	Ataxia Dysmetria Intention tremor Wide-based stance

sarcomas, nasal adenocarcinomas, and squamous cell carcinomas of the middle ear); and calcification or mineralization of the intracranial neoplasm (e.g., with feline meningioma). In cats, hyperostotic calvarial lesions are generally adjacent to the meningioma. Because definitive therapy (e.g., surgery, chemotherapy, radiation therapy, and immunotherapy) requires knowledge of precise anatomic location, size, and histologic type of the intracranial neoplasm, preoperative CT or MRI is necessary. These imaging techniques provide information necessary to determine treatment options. Patients with suspected metastatic intracranial neoplasia should have thoracic and abdominal radiographs and abdominal ultrasonography in an attempt to identify the primary tumor.

Laboratory Findings

Results of hematologic and biochemical testing are generally normal. Renal disease (i.e., increased blood urea nitrogen [BUN] and serum creatinine) is surprisingly common in mature to older animals and is always a concern, especially since it is often associated with systemic hypertension. Cats suspected of having intracranial neoplasia are usually feline leukemia (FeLV) negative. CSF analysis should be performed in all patients suspected of having intracranial neoplasia. Approximately 50% to 60% of dogs tested have CSF changes indicative of intracranial neoplasia, including albuminocytologic dissociation (e.g., elevated protein without a concurrent increase in white blood cells [WBCs]), increased protein concentration, normal to increased WBC counts, and/or neoplastic cells. Increased numbers of WBCs in canine CSF may negatively influence survival. CSF analysis in cats with meningioma is generally normal. CSF associated with meningiomas may be unique in that the WBC count may be greater than 50 cells/μl, and the differential often contains greater than 50% neutrophils.

> NOTE: The most common CSF abnormality due to brain tumors is increased protein concentration; however, normal CSF does not preclude neoplasia.

DIFFERENTIAL DIAGNOSIS

It is possible to localize a problem to the brain and, in most instances, determine its neuroanatomic location with signalment, history, and results of physical and neurologic examinations. However, disorders that mimic brain neoplasia (e.g., congenital [arteriovenous malformations, hydrocephalus]; infectious [brain abscess, meningitis, toxoplasmosis]; traumatic; immunologic; metabolic; vascular [stroke]; and idiopathic disorders) must be differentiated. Diagnosis of these diseases requires hematology; serum biochemistry; CSF analysis; survey radiographs (e.g., chest, abdomen, and skull); abdominal ultrasound (e.g., exclude primary malignancy not in the CNS); CT scan; MRI; and/ or biopsy. Definitive diagnosis of intracranial neoplasia requires surgical exposure for incisional or (preferably) excisional biopsy. Although biopsy is desirable in all brain tumor patients, location of the neoplasm (e.g., brainstem) may prohibit surgical exposure due to a high risk of significant postbiopsy neurologic impairment. Refinement of percutaneous CT- or MRI-guided biopsy techniques may reduce these risks.

MEDICAL MANAGEMENT

Treatment of intracranial neoplasia is directed at the primary tumor (biopsy and removal or reduction) and its secondary effects (peritumoral edema, increased intracranial pressure, seizures). Drugs used in patients with intracranial neoplasia include corticosteroids (methylprednisolone sodium succinate or dexamethasone sodium phosphate for initial treatment; dexamethasone or prednisone for maintenance); diuretics (furosemide); hyperosmolar agents (mannitol); and anticonvulsants (phenobarbital) (see p. 1400) (Box 37-12). Corticosteroids decrease peritumoral edema and intracranial pressure and are antineoplastic for lymphoproliferative CNS disorders.

BOX 37-12

Drugs Used to Treat Patients With Intracranial Neoplasia

Methylprednisolone Sodium Succinate (Solu-Medrol)
30 mg/kg IV once; repeat in 6 hr

Dexamethasone Sodium Phosphate (Azium SP)*
Initial dose: 1–2 mg/kg IV once or twice
Maintenance dose: 0.25 mg/kg PO tid; tapered over 4–7 days as needed

Prednisolone*
1.1–2.2 mg/kg PO bid; tapered over 4–7 days as needed

Furosemide (Lasix)
2.2–4.4 mg/kg IV

Mannitol 20%–25% (Osmitrol)
0.5–1 g/kg at 2 ml/minute; IV as a bolus

Phenobarbital
1–2 mg/kg†; PO bid to tid

IV, Intravenous; *PO,* oral; *tid,* three times a day; *bid,* twice a day.
*Adjust dose based on serum phenobarbital concentrations.
†Chronic use of prednisolone is less likely to cause gastrointestinal hemorrhage than chronic use of dexamethasone.

Specific antineoplastic agents are currently being evaluated for treatment of brain tumors. Factors influencing successful treatment of malignant brain tumors with chemotherapeutic agents include the blood-brain barrier (many such drugs cannot cross in therapeutic dosages); variable brain cell sensitivity; and toxicity of normal brain cells to therapeutic dosages. Chemotherapy alone will probably not be curative; however, as part of combination therapy it may prolong remission and improve quality of life. Immunotherapy has been suggested for treating patients with malignant brain tumors. Because most patients with malignant brain tumors have impaired immune function, mechanisms that selectively manipulate the humoral and cellular arms of the immune system against tumor cells may be successful adjuncts to surgical cytoreduction (tumor debulking). Further research in the development of immunotherapeutic techniques and their use in combination with other therapeutic modalities (e.g., surgery, chemotherapy, and radiation therapy) is in progress. Radiation therapy, with or without surgery, appears to enhance survival of dogs and cats with brain tumors. A recent study suggests a significantly longer survival in patients with meningiomas treated with surgical excision and radiation (Axlund et al, 2002). Metastases, pituitary macroadenomas or macrocarcinomas, and meningiomas have been successfully treated with radiation therapy alone or as an adjunct to surgery. Careful treatment planning by a qualified radiation therapist is necessary for successful outcomes. Survival analysis of dogs with intracranial neoplasms showed that patients treated with radiation therapy alone or as adjunctive therapy (combined with surgery or hyperthermia) generally had improved outcomes.

SURGICAL TREATMENT

In addition to providing complete tumor resection or partial removal, surgical intervention affords tissue for histopathology and may substantially decrease the volume of neoplastic tissue, thus facilitating adjunctive therapies. Increased success of surgery in patients with benign or malignant brain tumors is due to (1) improved early diagnosis via neurologic examination and lesion localization; (2) CT and MRI capabilities; (3) improved anesthetic techniques; (4) availability of highly specialized surgical instrumentation (i.e., lasers and ultrasonic aspirators); (5) increased availability of specialty trained surgeons; (6) refinement of surgical approaches to various areas of the brain; and (7) improved postoperative critical care monitoring. Factors have also been identified that help predict ultimate success of surgical excision (e.g., complete versus incomplete tumor resection), including tumor location, type, size, extent, and invasiveness.

Feline cerebral meningiomas are generally completely resectable and result in a favorable prognosis without ancillary treatment. However, if the tumor cannot be completely resected or if it recurs, surgical excision plus radiation therapy is recommended. Other primary or secondary feline brain tumors, particularly those located in the caudal fossa and brainstem, are typically nonresectable and carry a poor prognosis. Canine cerebral meningiomas are invasive, generally being amenable to cytoreduction but not complete resection. With adjunctive therapy (radiation) these patients may have a guarded to favorable prognosis (i.e., median survival time of 16.5 months). Other primary or secondary canine brain tumors are generally nonresectable and have an unfavorable to grave prognosis. Prospective studies are currently being done to establish more successful treatment modalities for feline and canine brain tumors.

Preoperative Management

Patients are generally treated with corticosteroids, anticonvulsants (see Box 37-9), diuretics, oxygen supplementation, and IV fluids before surgery (see p. 1379). Antimicrobial therapy is dependent on age of the patient, predicted duration of surgery, and surgical approach chosen (e.g., transfrontal). See p. 1381 for specific guidelines for prophylactic antibiotic use.

Anesthesia

Anesthetic management of patients requiring brain surgery is given on p. 1380.

Surgical Anatomy

See p. 1381 for surgical anatomy of the brain.

Positioning

Patients undergoing cranial surgery for brain tumors are generally positioned in ventral recumbency with the head stabilized in a specially designed head stand (see p. 1385 and

Fig. 37-2). Slight variations in head rotation are dependent on surgical approach selected.

SURGICAL TECHNIQUE

Select the craniotomy approach or combination of approaches that allows adequate visualization of the intracranial neoplasm (see pp. 1384 to 1393 and Figs. 37-3 to 37-10 on pp. 1387 to 1392). If the neoplasm is located in the cerebrum, perform a durotomy approximately 5 mm to 1 cm beyond the margin of the mass as previously described. Separate tumor tissue from cerebral tissue by gentle blunt dissection using fine thumb forceps and a spatula (see p. 1393). Handle cerebral tissue carefully with small instruments and copiously irrigate with body temperature sterile saline solution. If the mass is located deep in the falx, carefully dissect bluntly with a spatula to separate the cerebral hemispheres from the falx cerebri. Carefully retract the cerebral tissue to allow adequate visualization of the mass. If the mass has invaded cerebral cortex, use a combination of blunt dissection with a spatula and laser or ultrasonic aspirator to facilitate tumor tissue removal. Be careful to remove only neoplastic tissue. If the mass is deep seated, perform cortical extirpation using an electroscalpel to incise leptomeninges, bipolar cautery to control small vessel bleeding, and fine suction to section and remove white and gray matter. Use fine suction to remove exposed neoplastic tissue. If available, use an ultrasonic tissue aspirator or surgical laser to section white and gray matter and remove exposed neoplastic tissue. After complete or partial mass removal, copiously irrigate the surgical site with sterile saline solution, control hemorrhage with bipolar cautery and hemostatic sponges, and close the craniotomy as previously described. If the mass is located in the calvarium (e.g., osteosarcoma, osteoma, chondrosarcoma, and multilobular osteochondrosarcoma), perform a craniotomy to include the affected bone.

SUTURE MATERIALS AND SPECIAL INSTRUMENTS

Special instruments recommended for removal of brain neoplasms are described on p. 1393.

POSTOPERATIVE CARE AND ASSESSMENT

Patients should be recovered in a padded cage in an intensive care facility and given analgesics (see Table 13-4 on p. 133), anticonvulsants (see Box 37-9), corticosteroids (see Box 37-8), diuretics (see p. 1395), and oxygen supplementation as needed based on results of serial neurologic examinations and blood gas analyses. Discharge from the hospital depends on patient status and owner compliance (see p. 1393). Patients should be scheduled for routine follow-up examinations at various intervals depending upon their condition and tumor type. Re-evaluations may include neurologic examination, skull radiographs, CT scan, MRI, alteration of anticonvulsant therapy, adjunct therapy (e.g., chemotherapy, immunotherapy, and radiation therapy), and/or postmortem examination.

PROGNOSIS

Prognosis for dogs and cats with nonmeningioma intracranial neoplasia is generally unfavorable. Prognosis for dogs with meningiomas treated by surgical excision alone is guarded to unfavorable (i.e., median survival time of 7 months); however, postoperative radiation therapy significantly improves survival times (i.e., median survival time of 16.5 months). The main indicators of an unfavorable prognosis include (1) moderate to severe neurologic deficits at initial presentation; (2) rapidly progressive course; (3) increased WBC count in the CSF, particularly in dogs; (4) presence of multiple masses; and (5) inability to provide surgery, with or without radiation therapy. Prognosis for cats with resectable meningiomas (e.g., clean margins on histopathology) is favorable. The cat's age, tumor location, or presence of multiple tumors does not affect final outcome. Median duration of survival is expected to be approximately 26 months with a range of 0.1 months to greater than 54 months (overall survival is approximately 70% at 6 months, 65% at 12 months, and 50% at 24 months). Local regrowth of feline meningiomas after surgical excision occurs in approximately 20% to 30% of cases.

References

Axlund TW, McGlasson ML, Smith AN: Surgery alone or in combination with radiation therapy for treatment of intracranial meningiomas in dogs: 31 cases (1989-2002), *JAVMA* 221:1597, 2002.

Dewey CW: Encephalopathies: disorders of the brain. In Dewey CW, editor: *A practical guide to canine and feline neurology,* Ames, IA, 2003, Iowa State Press.

CHAPTER 38
Surgery of the Cervical Spine

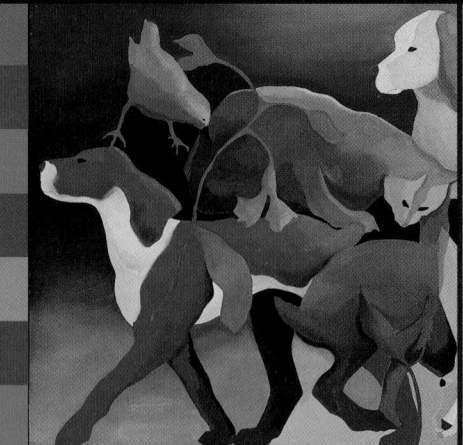

GENERAL PRINCIPLES AND TECHNIQUES

DEFINITIONS

Dorsal laminectomy is removal of dorsal spinous processes, lamina, and portions of the pedicles to expose the dorsal aspect of the spinal cord and nerve roots. **Hemilaminectomy** and **dorsolateral hemilaminectomy** refer to unilateral removal of the lateral and dorsolateral lamina, respectively, in addition to removal of the pedicles and articular facets. **Foraminotomy** refers to the removal of the roof of the intervertebral foramen; **facetectomy** is the complete excision of the cranial and caudal articular facets. Unilateral facetectomy and foraminotomy are commonly performed with dorsolateral hemilaminectomy to expose nerve roots. **Ventral slot** refers to the creation of a bony defect in the ventral aspect of a cervical intervertebral space to gain entrance and visualization of the ventral vertebral canal. The ventral slot provides limited access to the intervertebral foramen. **Fenestration** is the creation of a window or fenestra in the lateral or ventral annulus fibrosus to remove nucleus pulposus from the intervertebral space. **Tetraparesis** is the loss of conscious proprioception and variable motor weakness of all four limbs; **tetraplegia** is the loss of conscious proprioception, motor function, and the ability to perceive superficial and deep pain in all four limbs.

PREOPERATIVE MANAGEMENT

Neurologic function and ambulation should be carefully assessed in patients that require cervical spinal cord surgery. Weakly ambulatory or nonambulatory tetraparetic patients often have subclinical respiratory compromise and require ventilatory support during surgery. Tetraplegic patients usually develop respiratory difficulties as a result of lack of diaphragmatic and intercostal muscle function. Respiratory arrest and subsequent death are more common in patients undergoing dorsal decompressive laminectomy than in those undergoing ventral decompressive procedures (e.g., ventral slot and ventral stabilization). This is probably because dorsal decompressive procedures often require extensive manipulation of the cervical spinal cord.

Preoperative care of patients with unstable cervical fractures, luxations, or subluxations (e.g., palpable crepitus and instability) includes cage rest and serial neurologic examinations. A neck brace should be used to prevent movement of the cervical spine. Weakly ambulatory or nonambulatory tetraparetic patients should be secured to a rigid surface (e.g., board or Plexiglas) until diagnostics have been performed and treatment initiated.

Spinal surgery generally requires that spinal cord and/or nerve roots be carefully retracted to treat the underlying disorder (e.g., removal of disk material or neoplastic lesions, and fracture stabilization). Preoperative administration of corticosteroids may provide some protection to these structures during surgery; however, they should be used cautiously because they may predispose to gastrointestinal ulceration and/or perforation (see p. 1421). Ulceration and/or perforation appears to be associated with the combination of spinal cord trauma, stress of hospitalization or spinal surgery, and steroid administration; the cause remains unknown, however.

During cervical fracture reduction, hemorrhage as a result of laceration of one or both vertebral venous sinuses may be fatal. Blood should be available for transfusion, and techniques to control venous sinus hemorrhage should be employed promptly (Box 38-1). These techniques should be practiced by the surgeon and assistant surgeon before performing a ventral slot procedure.

ANESTHESIA

Animals undergoing cervical spinal surgery should have two cephalic catheters placed to allow rapid fluid administration should venous sinus hemorrhage occur. Blood for transfusion and mechanical ventilatory support should be available; mechanical ventilation or intermittent positive-pressure ventilation is necessary in tetraparetic patients. A balanced electrolyte solution should be administered intravenously (IV) during surgery. Intraoperative measurement of direct arterial blood pressure is recommended. Administration of hypertonic saline (4 to 5 ml/kg IV) and/or positive inotropes (e.g., dobutamine or dopamine) may be necessary if bleeding is severe or if hypotension is profound (Box 38-2). A syndrome characterized by paradoxical bradycardia associ-

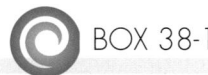 BOX 38-1

Techniques for Controlling Venous Sinus Hemorrhage

Before Procedure Begins:

1. Cut several pieces of Gelfoam into 5 mm × 5 mm pledgets and place them in saline.
2. Cut one or two pieces of cottonoid sponge ~1 cm × 3–4 cm and place them in saline.
3. Have two Brown-Adson thumb forceps readily available.

Once Venous Sinus Hemorrhage Begins:

NOTE: This sequence of events should be practiced by the surgeon and assistant surgeon before performing a ventral slot procedure.

1. Use suction to locate the point of hemorrhage (assistant surgeon).
2. Once the source of hemorrhage is located, quickly remove the suction device and place a Gelfoam pledget at the site (surgeon).
3. Place a cottonoid sponge over the Gelfoam pledget (surgeon).
4. Gently place the suction tip on top of the cottonoid sponge to evacuate blood from the surgical site and draw it through the Gelfoam pledget (assistant surgeon).
5. Continue suctioning; apply gentle pressure with the suction tip to the cottonoid sponge until the hemorrhage subsides.
6. After the hemorrhage is under control, gently remove the cottonoid sponge; leave the Gelfoam pledget to encourage hemostasis.

NOTE: Do not apply suction directly on the Gelfoam pledget as it will disappear into the suction device.

 BOX 38-2

Perioperative Drug Therapy for Hypotension

Dobutamine

2–10 μg/kg/min IV

Dopamine

2–10 μg/kg/min IV

IV, Intravenous.

 BOX 38-3

Selected Anesthetic Protocols for Dogs Undergoing Spinal Surgery

Premedication

Methylprednisolone sodium succinate (30 mg/kg IV) or dexamethasone (1.5 mg/kg IV) plus hydromorphone (0.1–0.2 mg/kg SC or IM), or butorphanol (0.2–0.4 mg/kg SC or IM), or buprenorphine (5–15 μg/kg IM)

Induction

Thiopental (10–12 mg/kg IV) or propofol (4–6 mg/kg IV)

Maintenance

Isoflurane or sevoflurane

IV, Intravenous; *SC*, subcutaneous; *IM*, intramuscular.

 BOX 38-4

Criteria for Use of Antibiotics in Neurosurgery Patients

Prophylactic Antibiotics

- Geriatric patients (i.e., >7 years old)
- Debilitated patients
- Clean, open wounds associated with the surgery site
- Estimated surgical time >90 min
- "Break" in aseptic surgical technique

Therapeutic Antibiotics

- Nonspinal infection that cannot be treated before surgery (e.g., severe dental disease, pyoderma, and open appendicular fracture/luxation)
- Spinal infection requiring surgical intervention (e.g., diskospondylitis and vertebral osteomyelitis)
- Contaminated open wounds associated with the surgical site (e.g., open vertebral fracture/luxation)

ated with hypotension (*acute sympathetic blockade*) can occur intraoperatively in dogs with acute cervical spinal cord trauma (Kube et al, 2003). No effective treatment has yet been described. Animals undergoing surgery of the cervical spinal cord should be premedicated with corticosteroids (methylprednisolone sodium succinate or dexamethasone phosphate) (Box 38-3). Dogs may also be premedicated with an anticholinergic plus oxymorphone, butorphanol, or buprenorphine and induced with a thiobarbiturate or propofol. Isoflurane, halothane, or sevoflurane is preferred for anesthetic maintenance. Acetylpromazine should be avoided because of the risk of hypotension. Acetylpromazine is also contraindicated in animals undergoing myelography because it may promote seizures.

NOTE: Manipulate the neck carefully in these patients during anesthetic induction and positioning for surgery or radiographs, especially if instability is present.

ANTIBIOTICS

Use of therapeutic or prophylactic antibiotics in cervical surgery is based on criteria listed in Box 38-4. Antibiotics selected for prophylaxis should be effective against common causes of postoperative infection (e.g., coagulase-positive *Staphylococcus* and *Escherichia coli*). Cefazolin (22 mg/kg IV at induction, repeat at 2 to 4 hour intervals until completion of surgery) is the antibiotic of choice for antimicrobial prophylaxis in patients undergoing neurologic surgery because of its low toxicity and excellent *in vitro* activity against these bacteria.

Selection of an appropriate antibiotic for therapeutic use (i.e., treatment extending for 7 to 10 days after surgery) should be based on the most probable pathogen. Selection is best determined by culture and susceptibility testing; however, empirical antibiotic selection can be based on published studies of similar cases or on data accumulated from practice records. The most common cause of postoperative wound infection in neurologic surgery is *Staphylococcus* spp.; therefore antibiotics of choice include cefazolin, amoxicillin-clavulanate, cephalothin, or ticarcillin-clavulanate (Box 38-5).

SURGICAL ANATOMY

There are seven cervical vertebrae. Knowledge of anatomic variation of cervical vertebrae enables localization of affected vertebrae. The anatomy of a typical vertebra consists of a body; a vertebral arch, which is composed of right and left pedicles and laminae; and various processes (e.g., transverse,

BOX 38-5

Therapeutic Antibiotics Used in Animals Undergoing Spinal Surgery

Cefazolin (Ancef, Kefzol)

22 mg/kg IV or IM tid

Amoxicillin plus Clavulanate (Clavamox)

Dogs: 12.5–25 mg/kg PO bid
Cats: 62.5 mg PO bid

Ticarcillin Plus Clavulanate (Timentin)

50 mg/kg IV tid to qid

Cephalothin (Keflin)

22–44 mg/kg IV or IM bid to tid

IV, Intravenous; *IM,* intramuscular; *tid,* three times a day; *PO,* oral; *bid,* twice a day; *qid,* four times a day.

spinous, articular, accessory, and mammillary). The first cervical vertebra (atlas) articulates with the skull and axis. The dorsal surface of the body of the atlas contains a depression (fovea of the dens) that articulates with the dens of C2. The dens is a cranioventral, peglike projection from the cranial aspect of the vertebral body. The wings of the atlas are large, lateral projections that are easily palpated. The axis (C2) has a bladelike dorsal spinous process that overhangs the cranial and caudal articular surfaces of the vertebral body.

For dorsal laminectomy, the dorsal spine of C2 is a distinguishing landmark, often overshadowing a short, rudimentary C3 dorsal spinous process. It is the most prominent of the dorsal cervical spinous processes (Fig. 38-1). C3 through C5 differ slightly and are difficult to differentiate. C6 and C7 have fairly prominent dorsal spinous processes that slope cranially. The dorsal spinous process of T1 is prominent, easy to palpate, and allows identification of the adjacent but much shorter cranially facing dorsal spinous process of C7 (see Fig. 38-1).

For ventral procedures, landmarks that can be used to identify the affected intervertebral space are the prominent transverse processes (wings) of C6 and the prominent ventral spinous process of C1. The prominent ventral annulus of the C5-C6 intervertebral space lies on the midline at the most cranial aspect of the transverse process of C6 (Fig. 38-2; see also Fig. 38-1). The prominent ventral spinous process of C1 is palpable just cranial to the C1-C2 intervertebral space (Fig. 38-3).

SURGICAL TECHNIQUE

Patients with surgical disorders of the cervical spine may be treated by ventral decompression via ventral slot, fenestration, dorsal laminectomy, dorsolateral hemilaminectomy, or cervical stabilization via a dorsal or ventral approach. Patients with cervical disk extrusion or cervical vertebral instability should be positioned with the neck in linear trac-

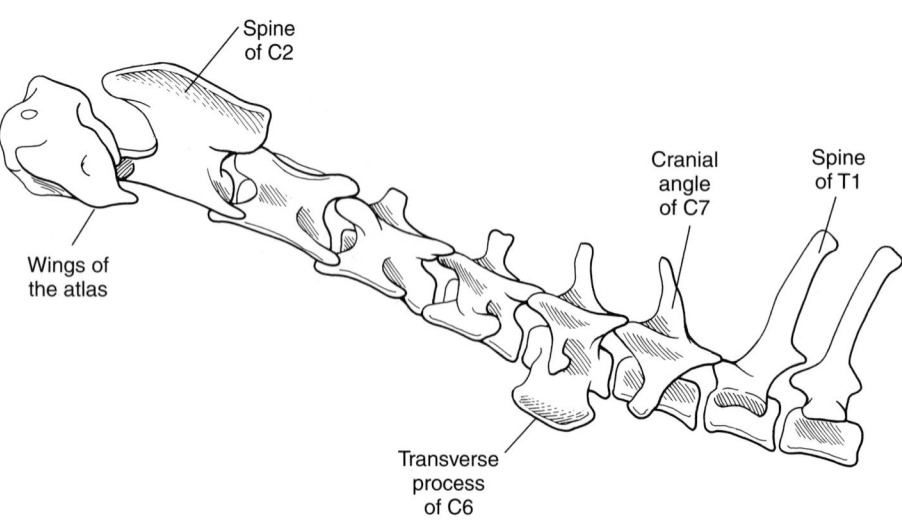

FIG. 38-1
Distinguishing anatomic landmarks of the cervical spine.

tion. This manipulation may enhance visualization of herniated disk material by widening the intervertebral space, or it may decompress the spinal cord during surgery in animals with cervical vertebral instability. Patients with atlantoaxial instability or cervical fracture and/or luxation should be positioned so as to reduce the subluxation or fracture (e.g., linear traction, gentle flexion, or extension) and encourage decompression of spinal cord and nerve roots. Patients requiring dorsal or dorsolateral decompression are positioned with the neck gently flexed to open the articular facets and interarcuate spaces, facilitating laminectomy, foraminotomy, and facetectomy.

> NOTE: Pay special attention to how the patient is positioned for surgery because proper positioning of the cervical spine may encourage spinal cord decompression and enhance surgical exposure.

Ventral Slot

The ventral slot procedure is used to gain entrance and visualization of the ventral cervical vertebral canal for decompression of patients with cervical disk protrusion (Fig. 38-4). This procedure provides adequate visualization of the vertebral canal but only limited access to the interver-

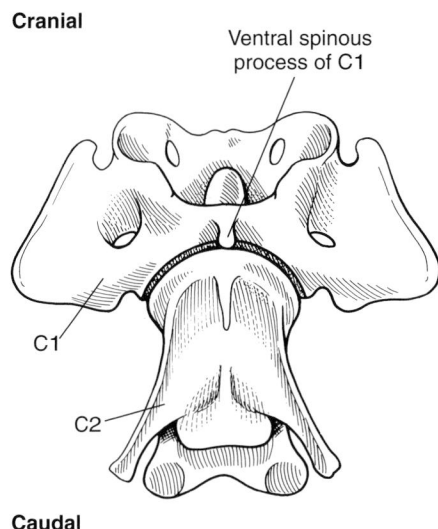

FIG. 38-3
Prominent ventral spinous processes of C1.

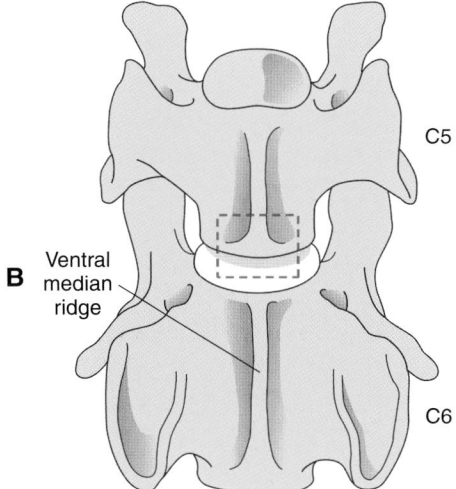

FIG. 38-2
A, Relationship of intervertebral space C5–C6 to the prominent transverse processes of C6. **B,** Notice the prominent ventral median ridge of cervical vertebral bodies.

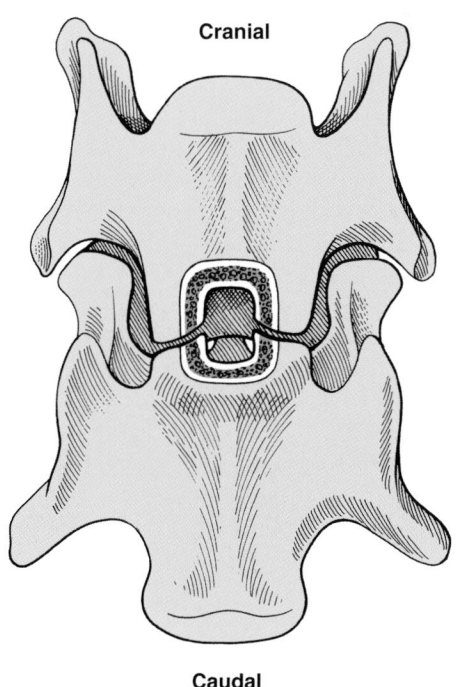

FIG. 38-4
Proper size and location of a completed ventral slot. Notice that the slot is centered just cranial to the intervertebral space.

tebral foramen. The ventral slot procedure may be combined with ventral stabilization procedures in animals with cervical vertebral instability (see p. 1435). Surgical exposure of the ventral aspect of the cervical spine without creating a slot is used for cervical disk fenestration and some cervical stabilization techniques (e.g., atlantoaxial instability and fracture and/or luxation). Ventral slot procedures may be combined with fenestration. Ventral slot procedures require minimal dissection through normal tissue planes and minimal disruption of normal anatomic structures. They provide adequate visualization of the vertebral canal, but only limited access to the intervertebral foramina. Minimal manipulation of the spinal cord is necessary, and recovery is generally rapid, with few complications. Operative time is less than that required for dorsal exposure of the cervical spine.

During the procedure, bipolar cautery, bone wax, Gelfoam pledgets, cottonoid sponges, and suction are used to ensure the meticulous hemostasis necessary to adequately visualize and control venous sinus hemorrhage. Monopolar and bipolar cautery helps control hemorrhage in soft tissue surrounding the bony defect. Bone hemorrhage may be encountered as the cancellous layer of the vertebral body is drilled. If bleeding is excessive, bone wax may be pressed into the bleeding surface to provide adequate hemostasis. Once the vertebral canal is reached, inadvertent damage to the vertebral venous sinuses must be prevented while obtaining appropriate exposure. If a venous sinus is lacerated, suction, Gelfoam pledgets, and cottonoid sponges are used to control hemorrhage (see Box 38-1). Once severe hemorrhage from a lacerated venous sinus has occurred, it is best to avoid further manipulation in the vertebral canal because continued hemorrhage prevents adequate visualization. If hemorrhage can be lateralized and adequately controlled, it may be possible to manipulate within the vertebral canal from the opposite side of the slot.

Clip and prepare the neck from midmandible to caudal to the manubrium sterni for aseptic surgery. Position the animal in dorsal recumbency with the chest in a V-trough. Tape the front legs caudally and tie the head cranially. Apply mild linear neck traction to help stabilize the cervical spine and slightly distract the intervertebral spaces (Fig. 38-5). Make a midline ventral incision from the caudal aspect of the thyroid cartilage to the manubrium sterni (determine the exact length of the incision by the location of the involved intervertebral space or spaces). Separate the paired sternohyoid and sternomastoid muscles on their midline. Identify the esophagus and trachea, and digitally retract them to the left. Locate the carotid sheaths bilaterally and digitally retract them. Determine the location of the affected intervertebral space by palpating the prominent transverse processes (wings) of C6. Locate the prominent ventral annulus of the C5-C6 intervertebral space just midline of the most cranial aspect of the transverse process of C6 (see Fig. 38-2). Alternatively, identify the affected inter-

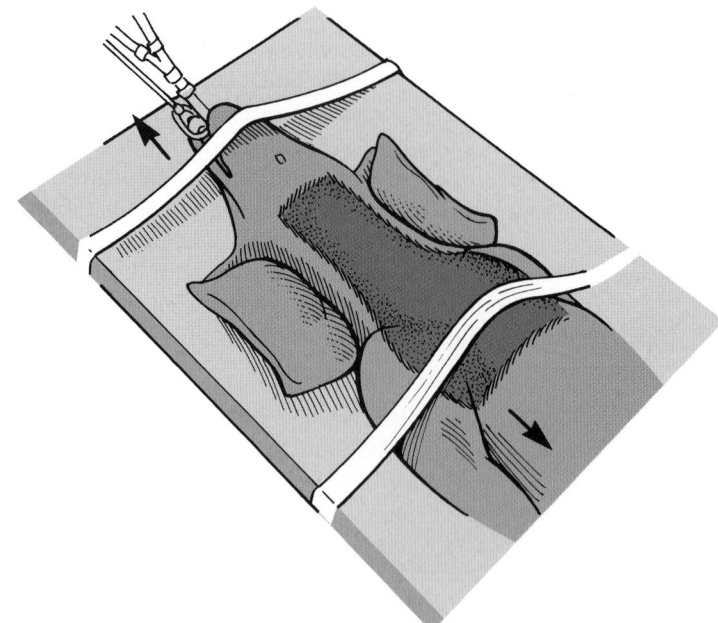

FIG. 38-5
To position the animal for a ventral approach to the cervical vertebrae, place the neck in mild linear traction.

vertebral space by palpating the prominent ventral spinous process of C1 (thus identifying the C1-C2 intervertebral space) and counting caudally (see Fig. 38-3).

Once the involved intervertebral space has been located, bluntly separate the longus colli muscles along their median raphe and cut their tendinous insertions on the ventral spinous processes of affected vertebrae. Subperiosteally elevate longus colli muscle from the ventral surface of affected vertebral bodies or directly adjacent to involved intervertebral space(s). Insert Gelpi retractors to hold the longus colli muscles apart (Fig. 38-6), but take care to protect the carotid sheath and esophagus from inadvertent damage. Meticulously control hemorrhage to prevent pooling of blood in the slot to be created. Remove the ventral spinous process of affected vertebral bodies with rongeurs. Excise the ventral annulus fibrosus with a No. 11 scalpel blade. Remember that intervertebral spaces of cervical vertebrae have a slight caudal-to-cranial angle that must be compensated for when making this cut (Fig. 38-7). Remove the entire ventral annulus fibrosus and any disk material present with a disk rongeur or dental scraper. Use a high-speed pneumatic drill with assorted sizes of carbide- and diamond-head burrs to create a midline rectangular defect in the bodies of the two vertebrae at the level of the affected intervertebral space. Be sure to remain on midline throughout the procedure to avoid lacerating the laterally located vertebral artery and vertebral venous sinuses (Fig. 38-8). Use frequent irrigation with physiologic saline solution to dissipate heat, prevent burning bone, and keep tis-

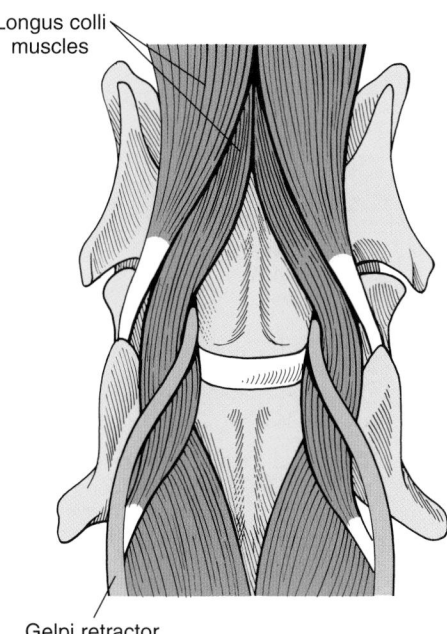

FIG. 38-6
After elevating the longus colli muscle from the ventral surface of affected vertebral bodies, use Gelpi retractors to hold the muscles apart. Take care to prevent damaging the carotid sheath or esophagus.

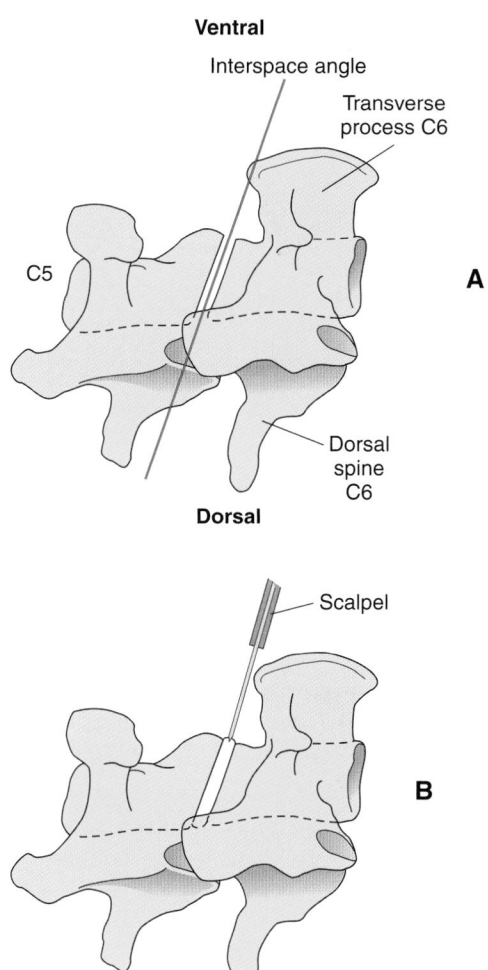

FIG. 38-7
A, Note the slight cranial-to-caudal angle of the cervical vertebral interspaces. **B,** To excise the ventral annulus, the scalpel blade should be inserted at this cranial-to-caudal angle.

sues moist. Do not perform irrigation during drilling because visualization of slot depth is difficult when the drill aerosolizes saline. Extend the slot no further laterally than one half the width of the intervertebral space (Fig. 38-9). Because of the caudal-to-cranial angle of the cervical intervertebral spaces, center the slot slightly toward the cranial vertebral body (Fig. 38-10). This ensures that the slot will be centered directly over the intervertebral space when the vertebral canal is reached. To prevent inadvertent laceration of vertebral venous sinuses, extend the slot no more than one quarter of the length of the vertebra cranially or caudally (see Figs. 38-8 through 38-10).

Gauge the depth of the slot by visualizing three distinct layers of bone while drilling. First, penetrate the hard outer cortical layer of the vertebral body (the white cortical bone exposed when the longus colli muscle is elevated from the vertebral body). Next, visualize the softer, more hemorrhagic marrow layer just below the outer cortical layer. This layer is more easily drilled than the outer cortical layer. Drill the outer cortical and marrow layers with 4- to 5-mm-diameter carbide burrs. Finally, visualize the 1- to 2-mm-thick inner cortical layer of the vertebral body. Once this layer has been reached, drill carefully, using gentle "paint brush" strokes with a 2- to 3-mm-diameter diamond-head burr. Take care not to break into the vertebral canal abruptly. After penetrating the inner cortical layer, use a 3-0 or 4-0 bone curette to enlarge the defect (Fig. 38-11). Carefully curette the dorsal annulus fibrosus and periosteum to expose the dorsal longitudinal ligament. Curette the inner cortical

layer of bone to a diameter sufficient to allow removal of the herniated disk, but avoid excessive lateral curettage lest laceration of a vertebral venous sinus occurs (see Fig. 38-8). Once exposure is adequate, carefully remove the dorsal longitudinal ligament with fine ophthalmic forceps and a No. 11 scalpel blade, allowing access to the vertebral canal (Fig. 38-12). Determine adequate decompression of the spinal cord by visualizing the characteristic bluish hue of dura mater (spinal cord) through the slot (Fig. 38-13). Ensure adequate visualization during manipulation of neural structures. Before closure, irrigate the wound with physiologic saline solution to dislodge any remaining bone fragments from soft tissue. Do not fill the slot with bone graft, fat, or Gelfoam. Appose paired longus colli muscles with simple interrupted sutures. Close subcutaneous tissue and skin routinely.

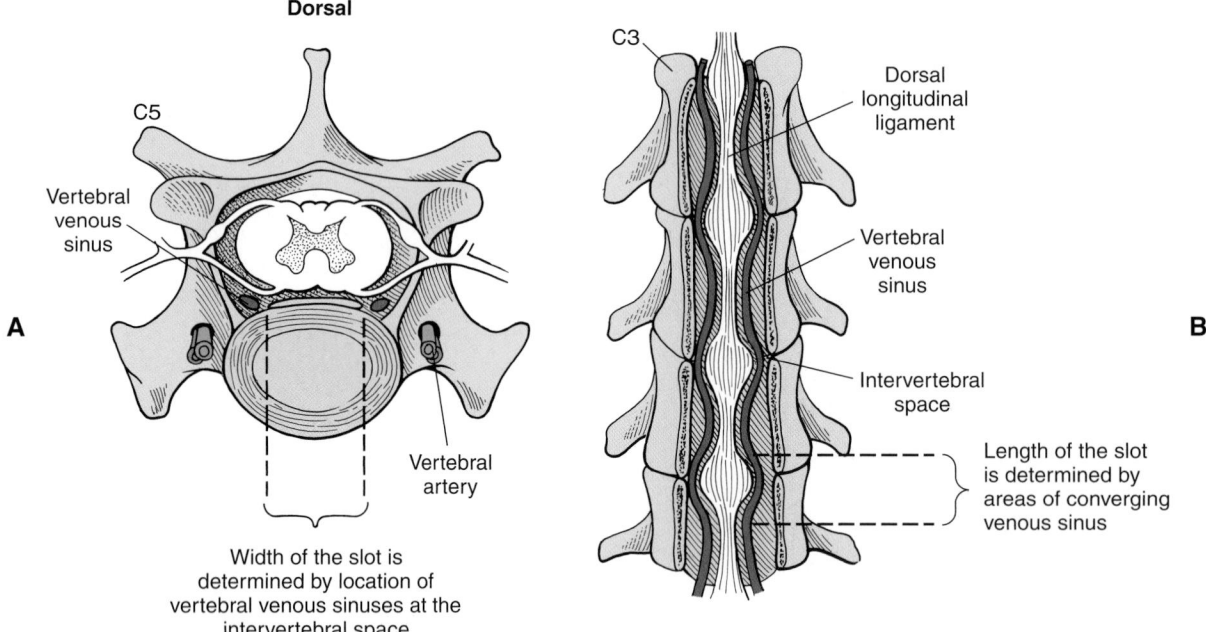

FIG. 38-8
A, Cross section of the cervical spine showing vertebral venous sinus and vertebral artery relative to the intervertebral disk and spinal cord; width of the slot is determined by this relationship. **B,** Laminectomized cervical spine showing the shape of vertebral venous sinus and dorsal longitudinal ligament relative to intervertebral spaces; length of the slot is determined by this relationship.

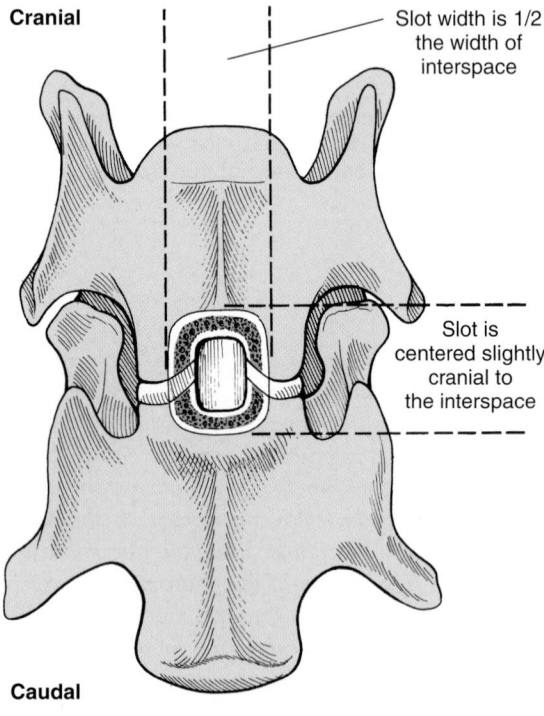

FIG. 38-9
Proper dimensions of a ventral slot, based on length and width of the vertebral body.

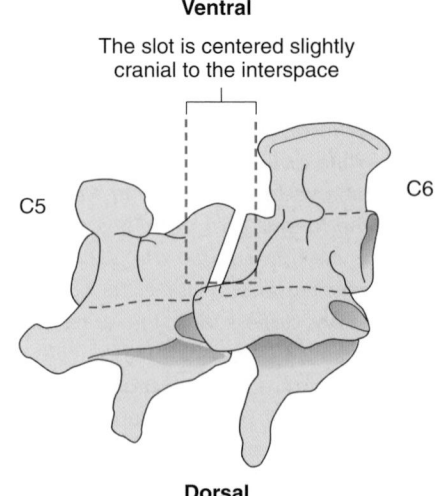

FIG. 38-10
Cranial and caudal extent of the ventral slot defect based on caudal-to-cranial angle of the intervertebral space.

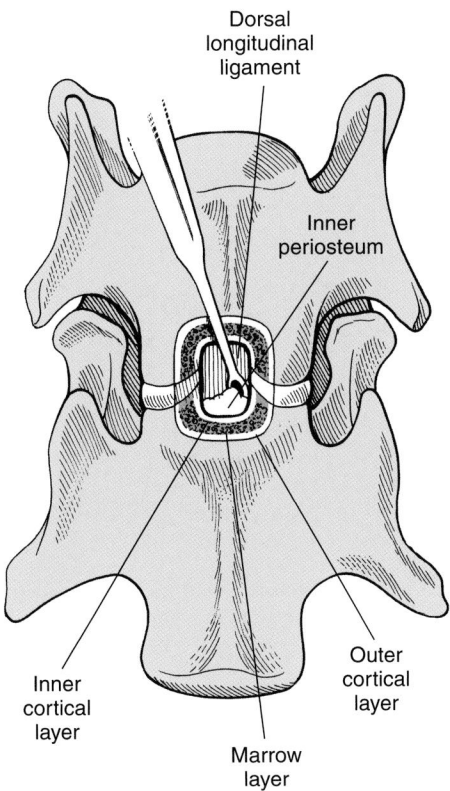

FIG. 38-11
The proper depth of the ventral slot defect is determined by identifying outer cortical, medullary, and inner cortical layers of bone; once the inner cortical layer is reached, use a No. 3-0 or 4-0 curette to expose the dorsal longitudinal ligament.

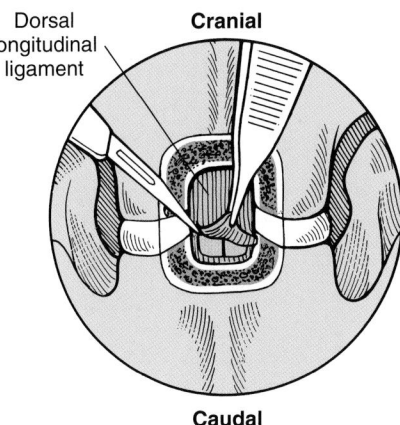

FIG. 38-12
The dorsal longitudinal ligament is grasped with ophthalmic forceps and incised with a No. 11 scalpel blade.

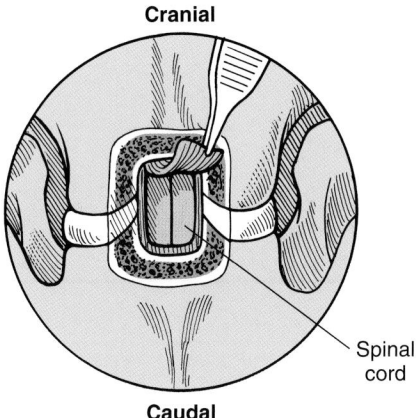

FIG. 38-13
Decompression is complete when the spinal cord is visualized.

Cervical Disk Fenestration

Cervical disk fenestration is performed from intervertebral spaces C2-C3 through C6-C7. It is not indicated for patients with disk material that has herniated into the vertebral canal or intervertebral foramen; however, it may benefit patients with diskogenic pain. There is some suggestion that fenestration of alternate disk spaces after ventral slot procedures may decrease recurrence of disk herniation; however, this is controversial. The author does not recommend disk fenestration after ventral slot procedures.

Position and prepare the patient for surgery as described for a ventral slot procedure. Make an incision from the thyroid cartilage cranially to the manubrium sterni caudally. Expose each intervertebral space in a similar fashion as the ventral slot; however, separate the longus colli muscle only at each intervertebral space. Expose the ventral annulus fibrosus with a periosteal elevator. Use a No. 11 scalpel blade to excise a large, wedge-shaped piece of ventral annulus fibrosus (Fig. 38-14). Hold the scalpel at the proper cranial-to-caudal angle to facilitate excision of ventral annulus and removal of nucleus pulposus (see Fig. 38-7). Remove nuclear

material with an ear loop, tartar scraper, or small bone curette (4-0 or 5-0). Take care to prevent dorsal extrusion of disk fragments into the vertebral canal. Close as described previously for ventral slot procedures.

Dorsal Cervical Laminectomy and Hemilaminectomy

Dorsal cervical laminectomy is the removal of dorsal lamina from cervical vertebrae to expose the spinal cord (Fig. 38-15). Laminectomy is generally indicated when lesions are located in the dorsal or lateral vertebral canal, whereas a ventral procedure slot (described previously) is generally indicated when the compressive lesion is located in the ventral vertebral canal. The specific laminectomy procedure used (i.e., cranial cervical, midcervical, or caudal cervical) depends on location and cause of the compressive

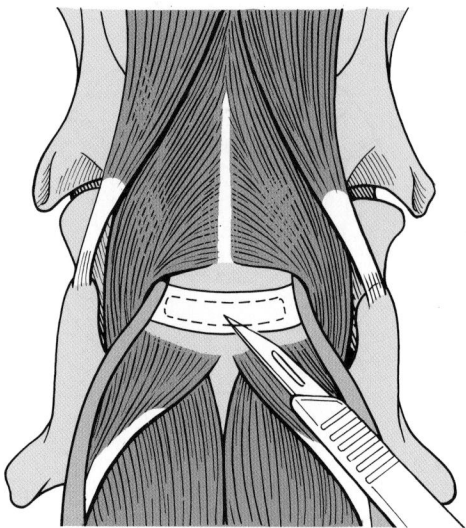

FIG. 38-14
Cut a large rectangular window (fenestration) into the ventral annulus fibrosus to allow exposure and removal of nucleus pulposus.

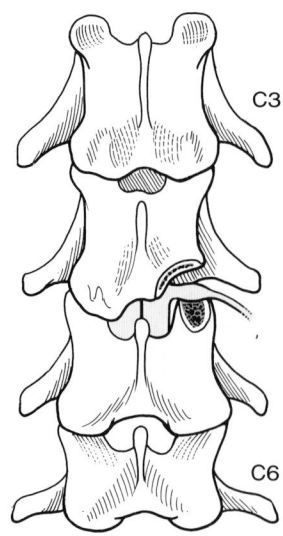

FIG. 38-16
Dorsolateral hemilaminectomy with facetectomy exposing the intervertebral foramen and exiting nerve root.

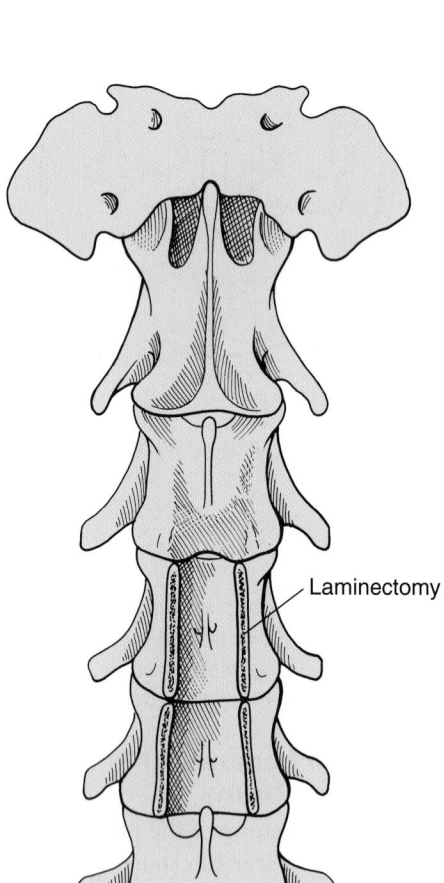

FIG. 38-15
Cervical laminectomy of C4–C5.

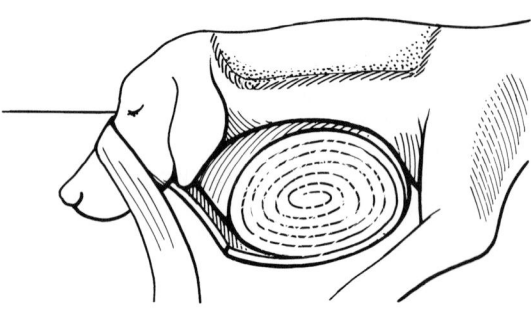

FIG. 38-17
To position an animal for cranial cervical laminectomy, gently flex and support the neck.

lesion. Dorsolateral hemilaminectomy and facetectomy is removal of right or left dorsal lamina, a portion of the right or left pedicle, and portions of the articular facet from affected vertebrae (Fig. 38-16).

Dorsal approach to the cranial cervical spine (C1-C2). *Perform cranial cervical laminectomy with the patient in sternal recumbency, head gently flexed in a neutral position, and head and neck supported by a rolled fleece or rigid vacuum type of apparatus (Fig. 38-17). Make a dorsal midline incision from the occipital protuberance to the dorsal spinous process of C4. Expose the median fibrous raphe between paired splenius muscles and dorsal cutaneous branches of the cervical nerves. Use these structures as a guide to perform midline dissection (Fig. 38-18). Divide the splenius muscles over the spinous process of C2 and retract them laterally. Incise paraspinal epaxial muscles on each side of the*

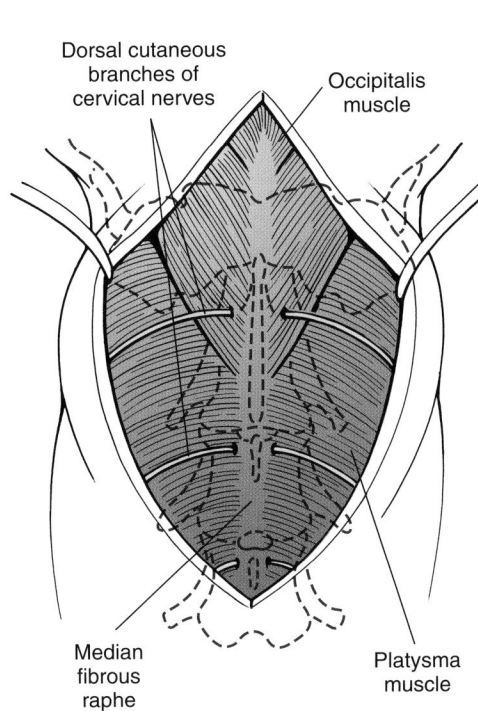

FIG. 38-18
During cervical laminectomy, dissect on the midline of the superficial cervical musculature to expose the median raphe and cutaneous nerves.

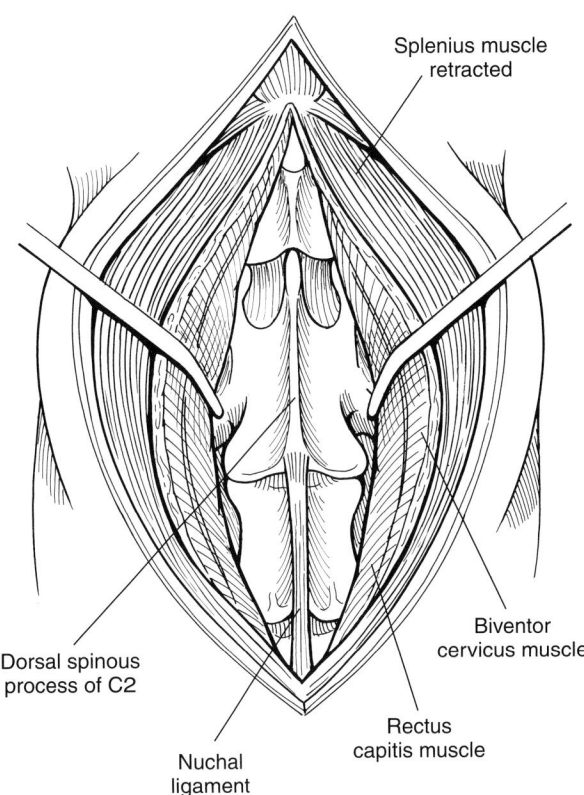

FIG. 38-19
During cranial cervical laminectomy, elevate muscle from the spinous processes and laminae of C1–C2.

spinous process of C2 and reflect them from the spine and dorsal laminae with a periosteal elevator. Elevate muscle to the level of C2-C3 articular facets caudally and the ventral aspect of the C1-C2 intervertebral foramina cranially (Fig. 38-19). If a hemilaminectomy is performed, elevate muscle only on the side to be exposed. Use self-retaining retractors to facilitate exposure. At the cranial end of the dissection, elevate muscles from the dorsal atlantoaxial ligament; wide elevation of muscles from the dorsal arch of C1 may be performed, depending on needed exposure. Caudally, elevate muscle until the multifidus muscle and nuchal ligament are exposed (see Fig. 38-19). From this point, perform a hemilaminectomy, dorsal laminectomy, or axial laminotomy, as needed (Fig. 38-20).

Specific laminectomy techniques are illustrated on p. 1409.

Close the surgical wound by suturing muscles to the tendinous raphe in their respective layers. Close subcutaneous tissue and skin routinely.

Dorsal approach to the midcervical spine (C2-C5).

Position the patient in sternal recumbency. Place rolled padding under the neck at the midcervical region. Flex the neck

over the padding to elevate the cervical vertebrae and open interarcuate spaces (Fig. 38-21). Position the patient carefully to improve palpation of important anatomic landmarks and enhance visualization of interarcuate ligaments. Make a dorsal midline incision from the occiput to the spinous process of the first thoracic vertebra. Identify the median fibrous raphe, and use it as a landmark for midline dissection to the nuchal ligament (Fig. 38-22). Incise along one side of the nuchal ligament and between paired bellies of epaxial muscles. Identify appropriate anatomic landmarks, and use a periosteal elevator to remove epaxial muscles from dorsal spinous processes and lamina of affected vertebrae. Dissect to the level of the articular processes; this depth is sufficient to perform deep dorsal laminectomy and avoid the vertebral arteries.

Specific laminectomy techniques are illustrated on p. 1409.

Close epaxial muscles to the tendinous raphe or nuchal ligament in their respective layers. Close subcutaneous tissue and skin routinely.

Dorsal approach to the caudal cervical spine (C5-T3). Because the scapulae are closely associated with the

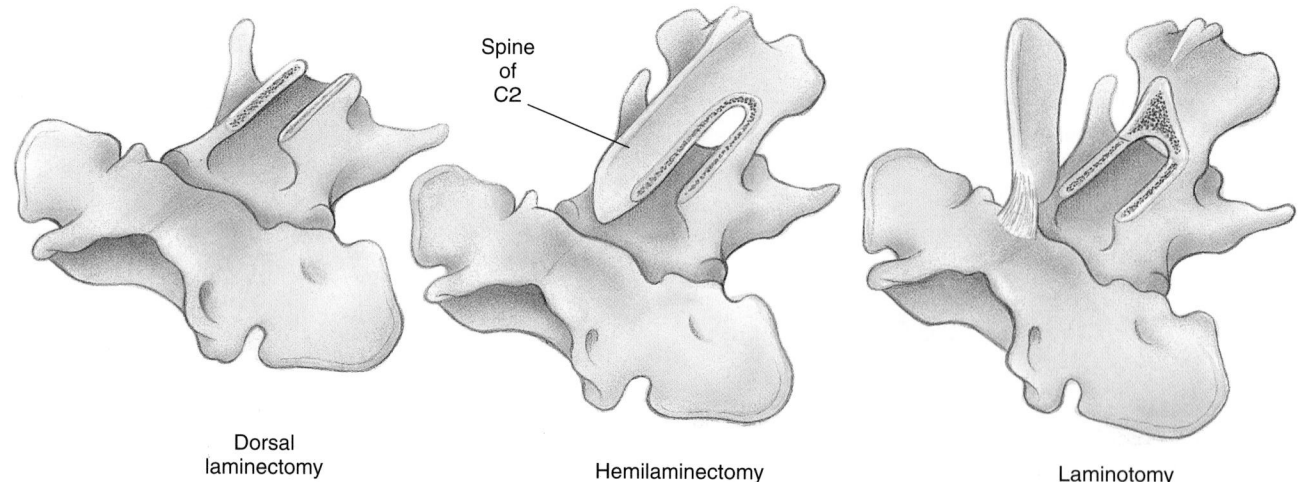

Spine
of
C2

Dorsal
laminectomy

Hemilaminectomy

Laminotomy

FIG. 38-20
Appearance of a completed C2 dorsal laminectomy, hemilaminectomy, and laminotomy.

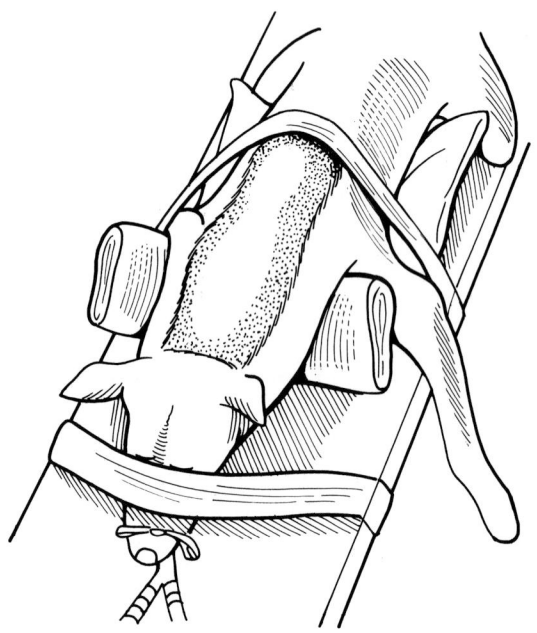

FIG. 38-21
To position an animal for midcervical dorsal laminectomy place the animal in sternal recumbency and flex the neck over padding.

caudal cervical spine and the vertebral laminae are located deep in epaxial muscles, positioning to enhance exposure is recommended.

Position the patient in sternal recumbency. To encourage elevation of the C6-C7 dorsal spinous processes and laminae, cradle the neck by gently flexing and elevating it over rolled fleece, sandbags, or a rigid vacuum type of apparatus (Fig. 38-23). Position the front legs against the body to encourage

abduction of the scapulae from the midline. Do this either by positioning the legs close to the body with sandbags or by tying the front legs across the table (see Fig. 38-23). Make a dorsal midline skin incision from the midcervical region to the dorsal spinous process of T3. Locate the fibrous median raphe and continue midline dissection through epaxial muscles. Retract epaxial muscles with self-retaining retractors to enhance exposure of dorsal spinous processes. Palpate the prominent dorsal spinous process of T1 and cranially slanted smaller dorsal spine of C7 (about half of the height of T1) to determine specific anatomic location (see Fig. 38-1 on p. 1404). Use a periosteal elevator to expose dorsal spinous processes and laminae of affected vertebrae. Remove dorsal spines of T1 through T3 (as needed) for dorsal laminectomy. This will have minimal effect on spinal stability as the nuchal ligament is continuous with the supraspinous ligament. Excise interarcuate ligaments between C6 and T1 (as needed) with a No. 11 scalpel blade to expose the spinal cord.

Specific laminectomy techniques are described on pp. 1414 and 1415.

Close the surgical wound by suturing epaxial muscles to the tendinous raphe or nuchal ligament in their respective layers. Close subcutaneous tissue and skin routinely.

Dorsolateral approach to the cervical spine. Dorsolateral hemilaminectomy is removal of dorsal spinous processes, the dorsolateral portion of lamina, and dorsal articular facets of affected vertebrae. It is indicated in patients with compressive lesions of the lateral aspect of the vertebral canal and intervertebral foramen.

Position the patient in sternal recumbency with the head and neck slightly flexed and elevated. Make a dorsal midline skin incision centered over the affected vertebrae. Identify the

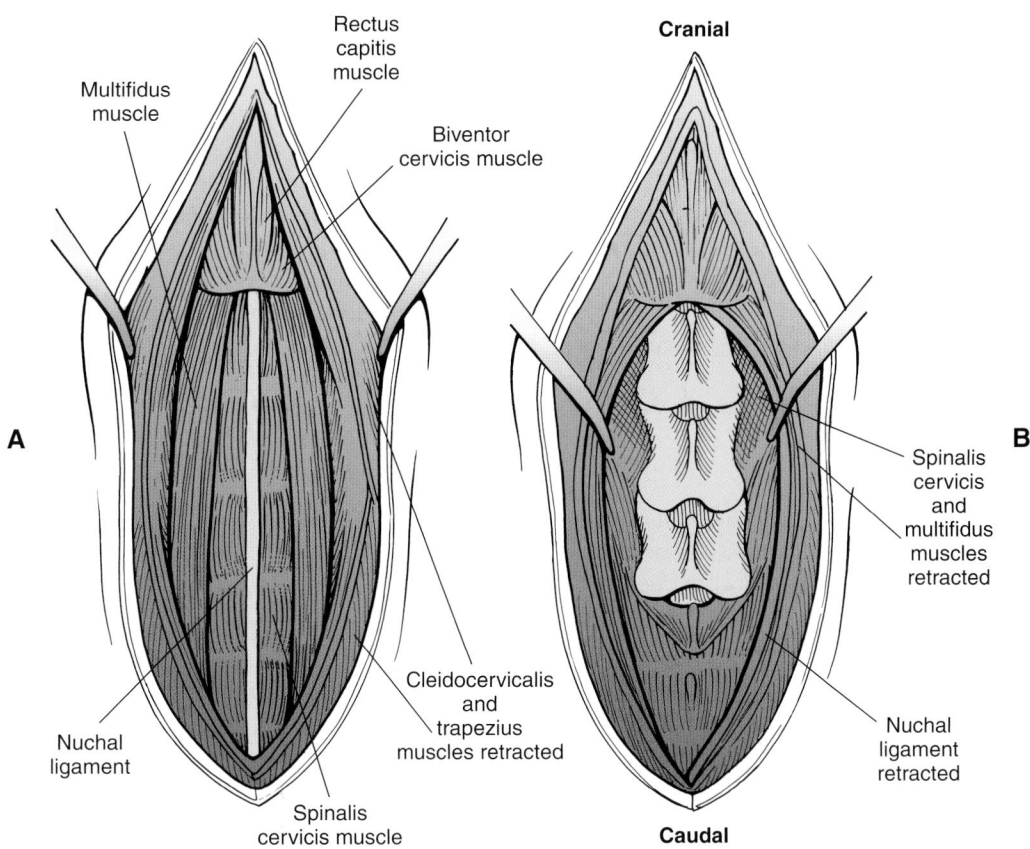

FIG. 38-22
A, Identify the median fibrous raphe and nuchal ligament during dorsal midcervical laminectomy and use them as landmarks. **B,** Elevate the cervical musculature from dorsal spinous processes and laminae of C3, C4, and C5.

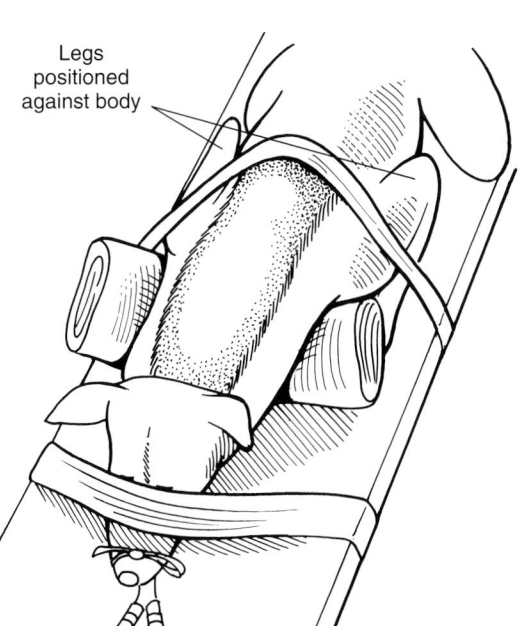

FIG. 38-23
To position an animal for caudal cervical laminectomy, cradle the neck, gently flex it, and elevate it over a rolled fleece, sandbags, or a rigid vacuum type of apparatus. Position the front legs against the body with sandbags or tie them across the table.

median fibrous raphe, and expose the dorsal spinous processes via midline dissection. Elevate epaxial muscles from the dorsal spinous processes, lamina, and dorsal articular facets of affected vertebrae. Continue dissection and periosteal elevation on the lateral aspect of the articular facet and intervertebral foramen to provide full visualization of the lateral aspect of the vertebral body. Carefully dissect and identify the vertebral artery before examination of the intervertebral foramen.

Specific laminectomy techniques are described below.

Close epaxial muscles to the tendinous raphe in their respective layers. Close subcutaneous tissue and skin routinely.

> NOTE: Performing a dorsolateral hemilaminectomy and facetectomy with rongeurs requires careful dissection and visualization of the lateral aspect of the facet joint.

Laminectomy and laminotomy techniques. Laminectomy is performed with a high-speed pneumatic bone drill, rongeurs, or both. Laminar thickness varies with patient size; larger patients generally have thicker lamina. Vertebral and laminar density varies with age; older animals tend to have denser, more compact bone. Disadvantages of dorsal laminectomy and dorsolateral hemilaminectomy include severe disruption of hard and soft tissue, prolonged operating times, poor visualization of ventral and ventrolateral lesions, and excessive spinal cord manipulation to approach the floor of the vertebral canal. It is most efficient to use a high-speed pneumatic drill in conjunction with rongeurs to perform dorsal cervical laminectomy, C2 laminotomy, and dorsolateral hemilaminectomy and facetectomy.

First use a high-speed drill with selected carbide and diamond head burrs to enter the vertebral canal. Then use rongeurs to carefully increase exposure by nibbling away bone from the drilled edge. Remove dorsal spinous processes of affected vertebrae with rongeurs. When using a high-speed drill, identify laminectomy depth by visualizing the white outer cortical layer, the softer red medullary layer, and the white inner cortical layer. Drill the first two layers using 4- to 5-mm carbide burrs (Fig. 38-24, A). Once the inner cortical layer is reached, use a gentle paint brush technique with a 2- to 3-mm diamond-head burr to expose the inner periosteum. Gently elevate periosteum and remaining interarcuate ligament with a dental spatula to expose the vertebral canal and spinal cord (Fig. 38-24, B and C). When performing C2 laminotomy, use

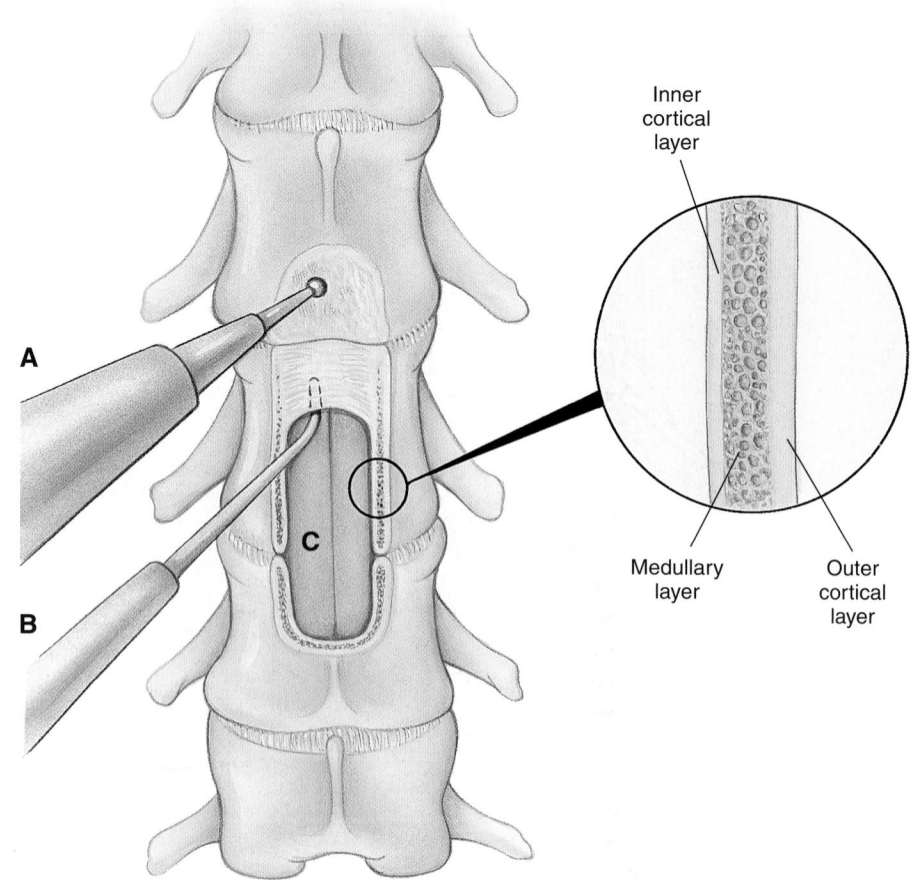

FIG. 38-24
A, Use a pneumatic bone drill to expose outer cortical, medullary, and inner cortical layers of laminar bone. **B,** Elevate periosteum with a dental spatula to gain exposure to the vertebral canal. **C,** Expose the spinal cord and nerve roots.

Inner cortical layer

Medullary layer

Outer cortical layer

a high-speed drill with a 2-mm carbide burr to make fine laminar cuts as necessary to elevate the dorsal spinous process and allow its replacement after exposure of the vertebral canal and spinal cord (Fig. 38-25). When performing dorsolateral hemilaminectomy, use a high-speed drill with 4- to 5-mm carbide and 2- to 3-mm diamond-head burrs to remove lamina and articular facets. Carefully identify outer cortical, marrow, and inner cortical layers of lamina and articular facets while drilling. Once the inner periosteal layer is reached, use a dental spatula and fine ophthalmic forceps to explore the vertebral canal and intervertebral foramen. Identify the vertebral artery located ventral to the intervertebral foramen before manipulating the nerve roots and spinal

cord (see Fig. 38-8 on p.1408). When using rongeurs to perform laminectomy procedures, carefully dissect the interarcuate ligament with a No. 15 blade and ophthalmic forceps to expose the intervertebral space and laminar edge. Accentuate the exposed laminar edge by grasping its dorsal spinous process with towel clamps and gently elevating the lamina (Fig. 38-26). Carefully place rongeurs on this edge, and remove lamina to expose the vertebral canal and spinal cord. Dissect interarcuate ligaments from C6-T1 to expose the vertebral canal and spinal cord.

> **NOTE:** Use of a high-speed drill is recommended.

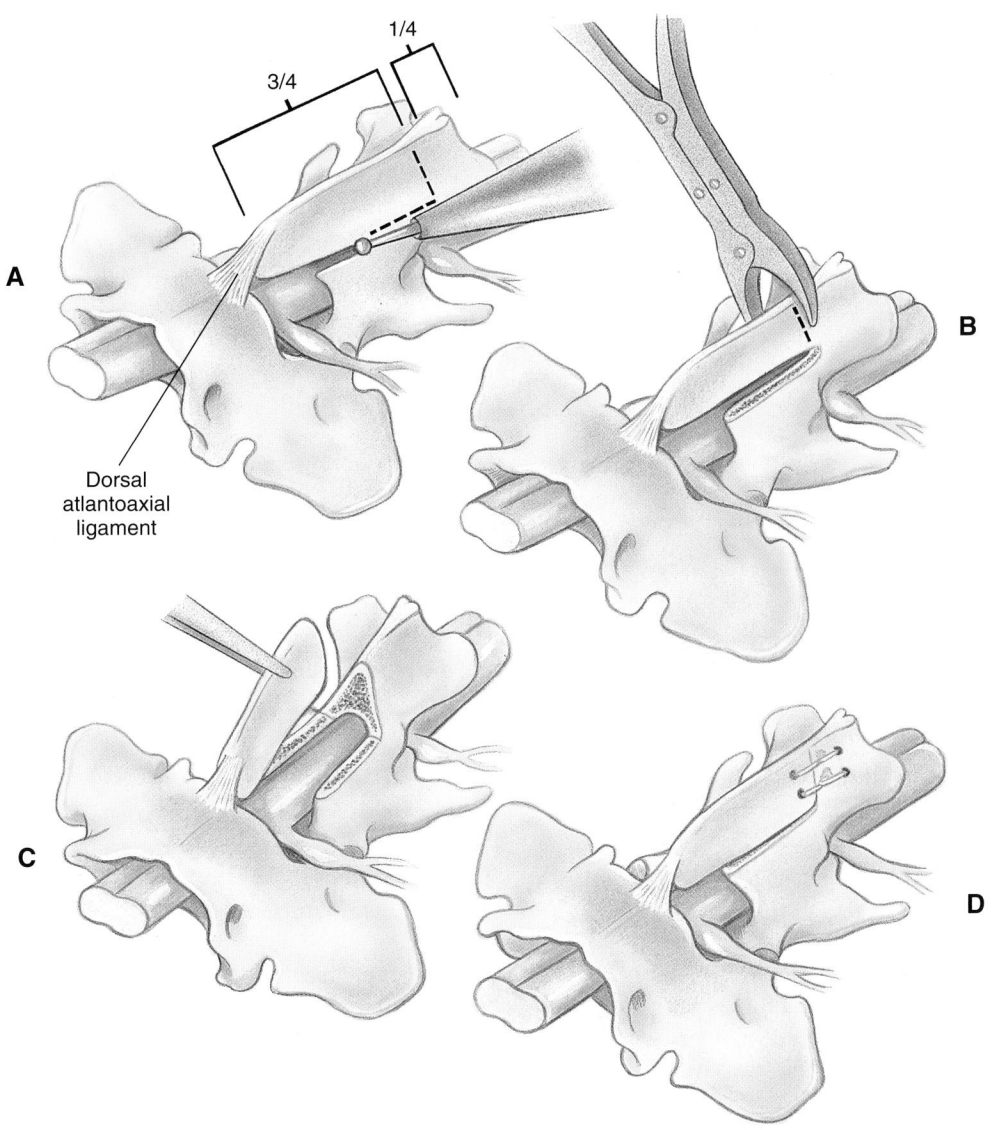

FIG. 38-25
For C2 laminotomy: **A,** Measure the dorsal spinous process of C2 to ensure that three quarters of its length is removed. Use a high-speed pneumatic drill to make the fine laminar cuts needed to elevate the spinous process of C2. **B,** Use bone cutters to transect the spinous process and laminar bone at predetermined sites. **C,** Retract the spine and lamina of C2 cranially, using the atlantoaxial ligament as a hinge. **D,** Wire the dorsal spinous process and lamina in place after examining the spinal cord.

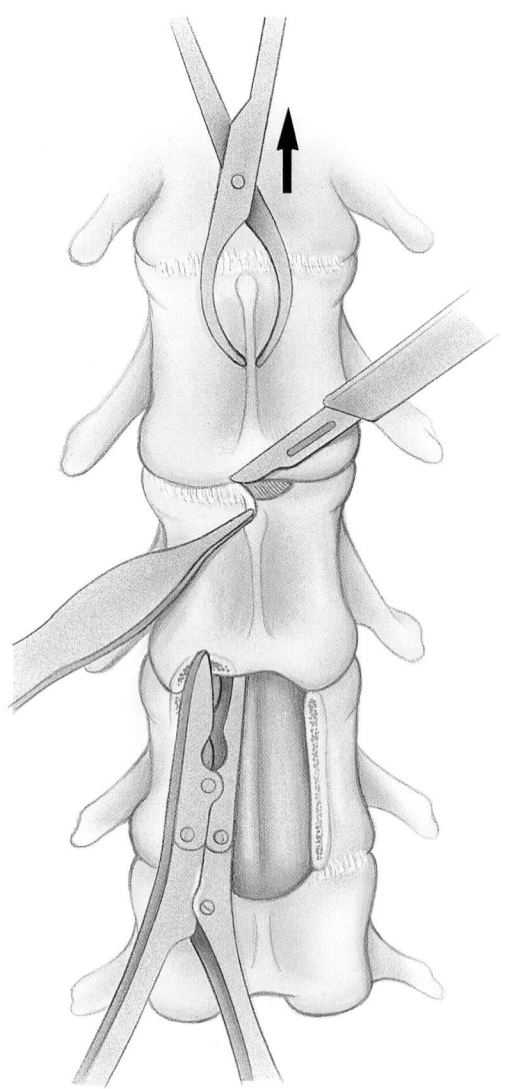

FIG. 38-26
Accentuate the laminar edge by grasping its dorsal spinous process with towel clamps and gently elevating the lamina. Carefully dissect the exposed interarcuate ligament with a No. 15 blade and ophthalmic forceps to reveal the laminar edge. Place rongeurs on this exposed edge and carefully remove the lamina to expose the vertebral canal and spinal cord.

Cervical Spinal Stabilization

Cervical spinal stabilization is a technique used to repair a cervical fracture and/or luxation, malformation, malarticulation, or congenital subluxation resulting in spinal instability. Stabilization can be accomplished by a variety of techniques, including pins and polymethylmethacrylate (PMMA), screws, Lubra plate, cross pins, and orthopedic wire. Surgical exposure is performed by either a dorsal or ventral approach as described previously. The specific stabilization technique used generally depends on location of the instability (see subsequent sections).

HEALING OF THE SPINAL CORD

Three basic categories of change occur after acute injury to the spinal cord: (1) direct morphologic distortion of neuronal tissue and severe axonal injury, (2) vascular changes, and (3) biochemical and metabolic changes. Controversy exists regarding the relative importance of these closely related categories in the production of functional deficits. Direct morphologic damage of spinal cord tissue (e.g., laceration, compression, and stretching) resulting in axonal interruption is felt to be irreversible and untreatable because central axons do not regenerate sufficiently to restore function.

In the case of reversible spinal cord injury, a characteristic series of events occurs during the repair process. Approximately 2 days after injury, a heterogenous population of small cells (most likely of hematogenous origin), including polymorphonuclear, lymphocyte, macrophage, and plasma cells, invades the traumatized tissue. This is essentially an inflammatory response. In a matter of 7 to 20 days, fibroblasts make their appearance and begin laying down scar tissue. A concurrent glial reaction consisting of astrocyte proliferation and expansion of processes occurs. Depending on the extent of spinal cord injury, moderate to extensive fibrosis, nerve fiber degeneration, and multifocal malacia may be seen. Axons that have been severed, compressed, or stretched start to regrow, but will reach the edges of the scar mass and stop. Regeneration of spinal cord axons sufficient to restore function has not been achieved; however, if enough axons remain intact, return to clinically acceptable motor function can be expected.

> NOTE: The pathophysiology of acute spinal cord injury is probably best viewed as being analogous to that of systemic shock; several complicated processes are involved and at some point an irreversible state may be reached.

SUTURE MATERIALS AND SPECIAL INSTRUMENTS

The special instrumentation necessary to perform ventral slot procedures, fenestration, dorsal laminectomy, dorsolateral hemilaminectomy, and spinal stabilization are listed by technique in Table 38-1. It is important to practice each technique, become familiar with regional anatomy, and learn proper use of special instrumentation before performing these surgeries.

POSTOPERATIVE CARE AND ASSESSMENT

Critical care observation for the first 24 hours postoperatively includes monitoring respiration, administration of analgesics, and observation for gastric dilatation-volvulus and seizure activity, particularly if the patient had preoperative myelography. Blood gas analysis is warranted in animals with ventilatory compromise. Postoperative anal-

Table 38-1

Special Instruments Necessary to Perform Cervical Spinal Surgery

PROCEDURE	INSTRUMENTS
Special instruments needed for most procedures	High-speed pneumatic or electric drill burrs: carbide and diamond tip cautery unit (monopolar, bipolar), periosteal elevator/osteotome, suction, hemostatic sponge (Gelfoam), bone wax, dental spatula, dural hook
Ventral slot	Micro suction tip, 3–0 or 4–0 bone curette, vertebral spreaders
Dorsal laminectomy, axial laminotomy, dorsolateral hemilaminectomy, facetectomy	Duck-bill, double-action rongeurs; Lempert rongeurs
Fenestration	Tartar scraper, ear curette, No. 7 Bard-Parker scalpel handle
Spinal stabilization	Steinmann pins, PMMA, small fragment reduction forceps, vertebral spreaders

PMMA, Polymethylmethacrylate.

gesia is provided by low doses of opioids, thus reducing their respiratory depressant effects. Because postoperative pain can result in vocalizing and swallowing air, periodic abdominal girth measurements should be performed to assess presence of gastric dilatation. Fluids should be administered at maintenance rates and the patient turned every 2 hours until sternal. Corticosteroid administration is generally discontinued postoperatively. If neurologic status deteriorates after surgery, corticosteroids may be given until the cause is determined and corrected. Antibiotic therapy (prophylactic or therapeutic) is determined by criteria listed in Box 38-4 on p. 1403.

> NOTE: Respiratory depression or arrest secondary to cervical spinal cord manipulation has been reported; patients must be carefully monitored for this event.

Ambulatory patients may be discharged 24 to 48 hours after surgery and should be confined for 2 to 3 weeks. They should walk on a harness for 4 to 8 weeks. Nonambulatory patients are treated with frequent hydrotherapy, physiotherapy, elevated padded cage rack, frequent turning, and bladder expression three to four times a day. They should be kept clean and dry to prevent decubital ulcers. Avoid indwelling urinary catheters because they are a frequent cause of urinary tract infection. A supporting cart helps nurse patients to an ambulatory status. Advantages of a cart include unhindered eating, drinking, micturition, and defecation. Additionally, animals with motor function are encouraged to ambulate, and an erect position facilitates physiotherapy. Nonambulatory patients may be discharged when owners are able to care for them. Neurologic examinations should be performed at 1, 2, 3, 6, 9, and 12 months postoperatively or until improvement has ceased. Radiographs (of the awake animal) may be performed at 1, 3, 6, 9, and 12 months after surgery or until resolution of the disorder.

COMPLICATIONS

Complications associated with ventral slot procedures include instability and collapse of the intervertebral space as a result of creating a slot that is too wide (Lemarie et al, 2000), laceration of a vertebral venous sinus, and iatrogenic spinal cord trauma. It has been suggested that a slot greater than one half the width of the vertebral body in older small-breed dogs, performed in the caudal spine (C4-C5 to C6-C7), may predispose to vertebral subluxation. Thus performing a distraction and stabilization procedure after ventral slot decompression of small dogs with caudal cervical intervertebral disk disease may be considered. Knowledge of anatomic landmarks and proper neurosurgical instrumentation helps prevent such complications. Complications associated with cervical disk fenestration include inadequate removal of nucleus pulposus; dorsal extrusion of disk fragments into the vertebral canal, causing neck pain and tetraparesis; diskospondylitis; and continued neck pain after fenestration. Complications associated with dorsal laminectomy include excessive hemorrhage from soft tissue dissection, iatrogenic spinal cord trauma, seroma, and surgical wound infection. Complications associated with dorsolateral hemilaminectomy include nerve root damage and laceration of a vertebral artery. Animals with upper motor neuron (UMN) disease are also prone to urinary tract infections, particularly if they are being administered corticosteroids.

SPECIAL AGE CONSIDERATIONS

Softer cortical bone of lamina, pedicles, and vertebral bodies of young animals requires less aggressive drilling and rongeuring than the denser, more compact bone of older dogs.

References

Kube S, Owen T, Hanson S: Severe respiratory compromise secondary to cervical disk herniation in two dogs, *J Am Anim Hosp Assoc* 39:513, 2003.

Lemarie RJ et al: Vertebral subluxation following ventral cervical decompression in the dog, *J Am Anim Hosp Assoc* 36:348, 2000.

CERVICAL DISK DISEASE

DEFINITIONS

Cervical disk disease is associated with disk degeneration and extrusion causing spinal cord compression and/or nerve root entrapment. **Hansen type I disk** degeneration is characterized by chondroid degeneration of the nucleus pulposus, whereas **Hansen type II** disk degeneration is characterized by fibrinoid degeneration of the nucleus pulposus. **Radiculopathy** is pain associated with nerve root compression. **Myelopathy** is a general term denoting functional disturbances and/or pathologic changes in the spinal cord. **Diskogenic pain** is caused by derangement of an intervertebral disk. **Claudication** is a complex of symptoms caused by occlusion of the spinal vasculature. Cervical disk protrusions are also called *slipped disks, herniated intervertebral disks,* and *cervical disk extrusion.*

GENERAL CONSIDERATIONS AND CLINICALLY RELEVANT PATHOPHYSIOLOGY

Intervertebral disk disease is the most common surgical neurologic disorder diagnosed in veterinary patients. Cervical disk disease accounts for approximately 15% of all canine intervertebral disk extrusions. Eighty percent of cervical disk protrusions occur in dachshunds, beagles, and poodles. The most common site of disk extrusion is the C2-C3 intervertebral space; frequency of involvement decreases from C3-C4 through C7-T1.

Disk degeneration is commonly divided into two distinct categories referred to as Hansen type I (Fig. 38-27) and Hansen type II (Fig. 38-28). Both types of disk degeneration occur in the cervical region; however, Type I extrusions are most common. In animals with cervical disk protrusion, the nucleus pulposus undergoes degenerative changes and loses its ability to absorb shock. Continued

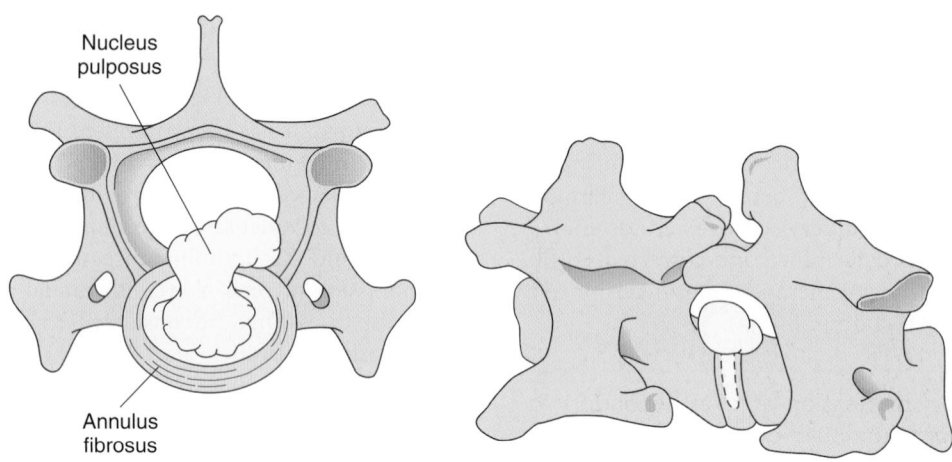

FIG. 38-27
Hansen type I disk degeneration is characterized by an acute massive extrusion of degenerate nuclear material in the vertebral canal.

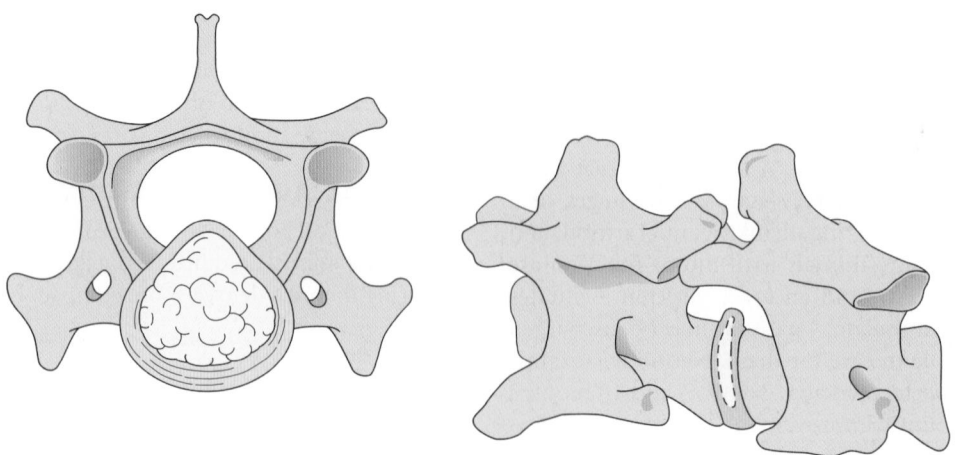

FIG. 38-28
Hansen type II disk degeneration is characterized by a slow chronic protrusion of degenerate dorsal annulus fibrosus in the vertebral canal.

degeneration and subsequent protrusion (Hansen type II) or extrusion (Hansen type I) of disk fragments occur spontaneously or secondary to trauma. Location and force of the extrusion or protrusion dictate the degree of neurologic deficits. Older, nonchondrodystrophic breeds are classically described as having slowly progressive Hansen type II disk disease. However, a recent report suggests that a substantial number of medium- to large-sized nonchondrodystrophic dogs are presented with Hansen type I cervical disk extrusions (Cherrone et al, 2004).

DIAGNOSIS
Clinical Presentation

Signalment. Most animals with cervical disk disease have acute neck pain. Middle-aged (i.e., 4 to 9 years), chondrodystrophic breeds (e.g., dachshunds and beagles) are most commonly affected; however, medium- to large-sized, nonchondrodystrophic dogs may also be affected. There is no sex predilection.

History. A stiff, stilted gait; reluctance to move the head and neck; lowered head stance; and muscle spasm of the neck and shoulder muscles are common. Approximately 10% of affected patients are tetraparetic (ambulatory or nonambulatory).

Physical Examination Findings

The location of extruded disk fragments within the vertebral canal is the most important factor in determining whether affected animals have pain or tetraparesis. If disk material extrudes in a dorsolateral direction (i.e., between the dorsal longitudinal ligament and vertebral venous sinus), nerve root compression and pain occur (Fig. 38-29). This is the most common location of cervical disk extrusion in dogs. If disk material extrudes directly on the midline (i.e., between fibers of the dorsal longitudinal ligament), it causes spinal cord compression and subsequent tetraparesis (Fig. 38-30). These patients may also exhibit neck pain as a result of teth-

ering of nerve roots in the intervertebral foramina. If disk material protrudes against (but not through) the dorsal longitudinal ligament, pain may result from pressure on pain-sensitive fibers of the dorsal annulus fibrosus and dorsal longitudinal ligament (i.e., diskogenic pain) (Fig. 38-31). Diskogenic pain rarely occurs in dogs.

Occasionally, patients have neck pain and front leg lameness (monoparesis) as a result of a dorsolateral disk extrusion in the lower cervical spine (C4-C7) that entraps a nerve root supplying the brachial plexus (see Fig. 38-29). Pressure from disk material on the nerve root causes nerve root ischemia and severe pain and muscle spasm. Pain is often intermittent and generally manifests as foreleg lameness. Presence of a root signature is helpful in localizing the extruded disk (C4-C7). It is important to carefully evaluate patients with forelimb lameness to exclude cervical disk disease. Medium- to large-sized nonchondrodystrophic breeds are more likely to extrude a disk at the C6-C7 intervertebral space.

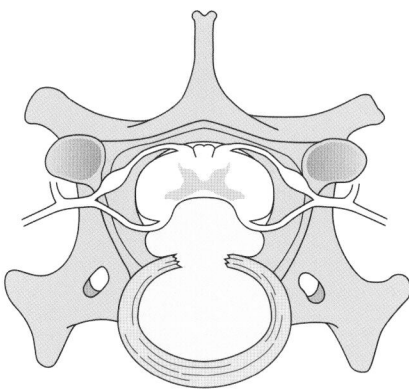

FIG. 38-30
Spinal cord compression by extruded disk fragments, resulting in myelopathy.

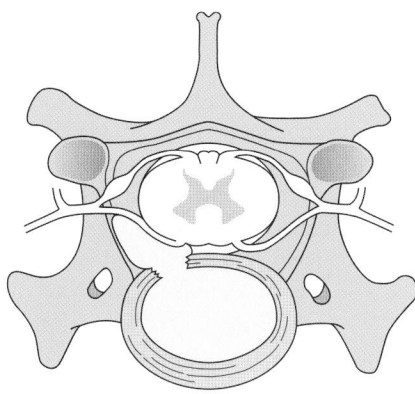

FIG. 38-29
Nerve root entrapment by extruded disk fragments, resulting in radiculopathy.

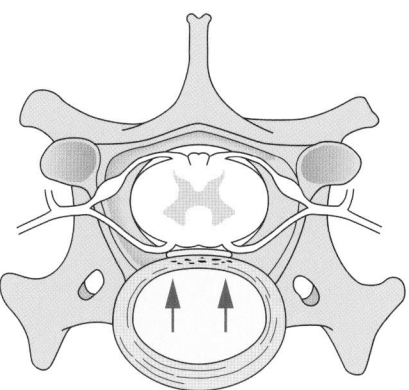

FIG. 38-31
Fibers of the dorsal annulus fibrosus compressed by degenerate nuclear fragments, resulting in diskogenic pain.

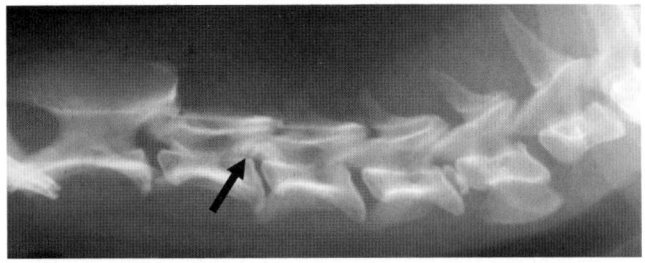

FIG. 38-32
Lateral radiograph of a dog with a C2–C3 herniated intervertebral disk. Notice the increased opacity overlying the plane of the spinal canal *(arrow)*. This is due to herniated, mineralized disk material. Also notice the slightly narrowed intervertebral space.

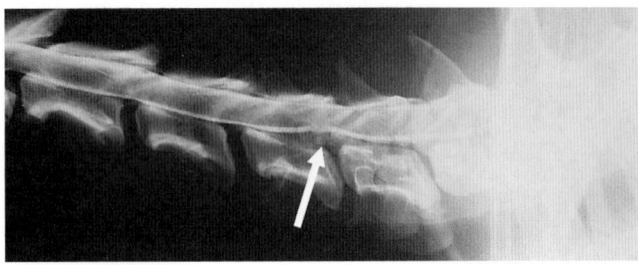

FIG. 38-33
Lateral myelogram of a dog with a C5–C6 herniated intervertebral disk. Notice the elevation of the ventral aspect of the contrast column at C5–C6 *(arrow)*.

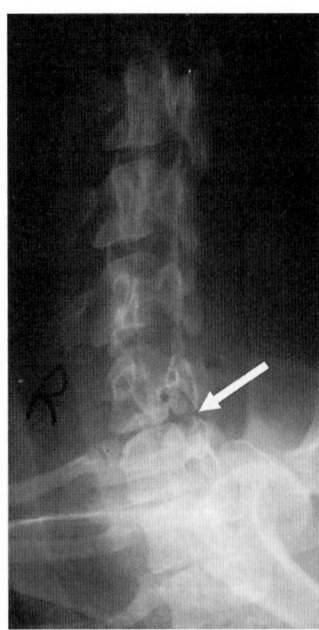

FIG. 38-34
Forty-five- to sixty-degree oblique cervical radiograph showing intraforaminal disk extrusion at C7–T1 *(arrow)*.

> NOTE: General anesthesia is required to obtain diagnostic radiographs in animals with disk protrusion.

> NOTE: Dogs with nerve root signatures (forelimb lameness) are often misdiagnosed as having orthopedic rather than neurologic disease. Performing a complete neurologic examination helps distinguish between the two.

Diagnostic Imaging

Well-positioned lateral and ventrodorsal survey radiographs of the cervical spine may be diagnostic for cervical disk disease. Classic findings on survey radiographs include a narrowed intervertebral space, collapse of the articular facet joints, increased radiopacity of the intervertebral foramen, and/or visualization of calcified disk material within the vertebral canal (Fig. 38-32). Myelography is indicated if abnormalities are noted on survey radiographs or if a lesion is identified that is not compatible with the neurologic examination. A myelogram may help precisely localize the location of the extruded disk material and guide determination of the appropriate surgical approach (e.g., ventral slot versus fenestration; dorsolateral hemilaminectomy versus ventral slot). Myelography is indicated in 90% to 95% of cervical disk patients. Patients with a herniated cervical disk have signs consistent with an extradural compressive lesion on myelography (Fig. 38-33).

An intraforaminal or lateral disk extrusion can cause severe neck pain. However, intraforaminal disk material cannot be seen on survey radiographs unless it is mineralized. It often cannot be observed on contrast ventrodorsal or lateral projections either because the x-ray beam is often not tangential to the extradural mass lesion on the standard lateral and ventrodorsal projections; in these cases, an oblique cervical radiograph may be helpful. To obtain oblique cervical radiographs, the patient is placed in dorsal recumbency, with the entire cervical spine positioned at a 45- to 60-degree angle to the table. Increased radiopacity of the foramen on the survey lateral radiographic projection without concurrent visualization of an opacity in the plane of the vertebral canal on the ventrodorsal projection is suggestive of a lateralized disk extrusion. An extradural compressive lesion may be identified on oblique views (Fig. 38-34).

Cross-sectional imaging (computed tomography [CT], CT after myelography, or magnetic resonance imaging [MRI]) may be used to evaluate cervical disk extrusions. Compression of the spinal cord (which is usually identified by a shape change of the spinal cord and visualization of disk material within the vertebral canal or intervertebral foramen) can be identified on these studies. The advantage of these studies is that there is an unobscured view of the lesion, as superimposition of structures does not occur as it does in radiography. Additionally, MRI provides the added benefit of allowing evaluation of the spinal cord itself (Fig. 38-35, *A* and *B*).

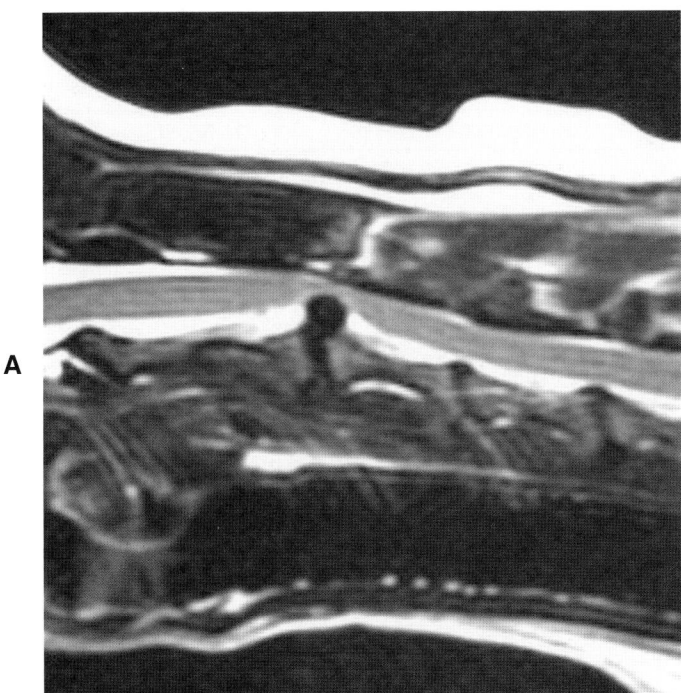
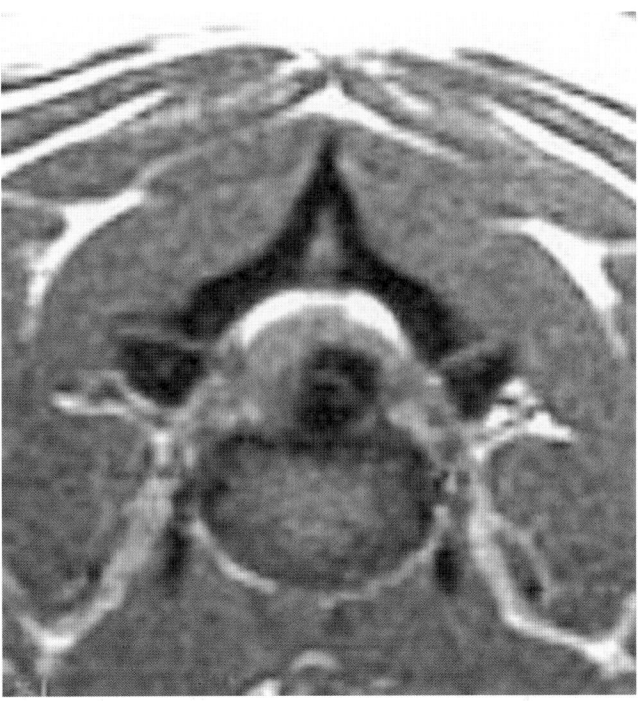

FIG. 38-35
A, Lateral projection of MRI showing herniated disk material at C2–C3 intervertebral space. Notice the disk material in the vertebral canal. **B,** Cross-sectional view. Notice disk material herniated into the vertebral canal, causing spinal cord and nerve root compression.

Laboratory Findings

Patients having cervical disk disease rarely have abnormalities on complete blood count (CBC) or biochemical profile. Because most affected patients have severe neck pain, a stress leukogram may be seen. Patients recently treated with corticosteroids may have elevated hepatic enzymes. If UMN signs have been present, urinalysis should be performed to look for urinary tract infection.

DIFFERENTIAL DIAGNOSIS

Presumptive diagnosis of cervical disk disease is based on signalment, careful historical evaluation, physical examination, and neurologic examination. Potential diseases that mimic cervical disk disease include meningitis, syringomyelia, neoplasia, atlantoaxial instability, diskospondylitis, and spinal fracture and/or luxation. Diagnostic differentials can usually be eliminated by evaluation of physical, hematologic, serum biochemical, cerebrospinal fluid, and radiographic studies. Diagnosis of cervical disk extrusion is confirmed by imaging and/or surgery.

MEDICAL MANAGEMENT

Conservative versus surgical treatment of patients with cervical disk disease is dictated by the patient's history and presenting neurologic signs. A staging system helps determine appropriate therapy (Table 38-2). The most important aspect of conservative management in patients with cervical disk disease is strict cage confinement for 3 to 4 weeks. After this period, 3 to 4 weeks of gradual return to normal activity is recommended. Walks should be restricted to a leash and harness; collars that encircle the neck should be avoided. This duration of forced rest allows resolution of inflammation and facilitates stabilization of the ruptured disk by fibrosis.

Strict confinement and exercise control may or may not be accompanied by administration of antiinflammatories and/or muscle relaxants. It is important to educate the client about potential euphoric effects of antiinflammatory drugs. If strict confinement is not maintained during drug therapy, the patient could potentially worsen because of increased activity leading to further disk extrusion. Antiinflammatory management of patients having pain alone may be instituted multiple times without fear of inducing tetraparesis. Moreover, patients treated conservatively that fail to respond may still benefit from surgery. Therefore most patients with mild to moderate neck pain from cervical disk extrusion should be treated conservatively before surgical intervention. Commonly used antiinflammatories and muscle relaxants and their dosages are provided in Box 38-6. Antiinflammatory drugs and muscle relaxants can be used independently or in combination. The proper drug regimen is dictated by the patient's clinical signs and knowing the outcome of therapeutic trials. Recommended corticosteroid dosages vary dramatically among clinicians. Dosages provided in Box 38-6 should be tapered over a 6-day period and followed with serial neurologic examinations. If there is no response, con-

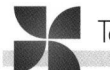 Table 38-2

Staging System to Help Determine Medical Versus Surgical Treatment and Prognosis of Animals With Cervical Disk Disease

STAGE	CLINICAL SIGNS	RADIOGRAPHY	TREATMENT	PROGNOSIS
I	Single or occasional episodes of mild to moderate neck pain	Radiographs not taken Incidental finding of degenerate disks	Conservative Fenestration/ conservative	Favorable Favorable
II	First episode of severe neck pain or second episode of mild to moderate neck pain	Radiographs not taken Extruded disk in canal	Conservative Ventral slot	Favorable/guarded Excellent
III	Uncontrolled neck pain or repeated episodes of neck pain	Extruded disk in canal Intraforaminal disk	Ventral slot Dorsolateral hemilaminectomy	Excellent Excellent/favorable
IV	Ambulatory tetraparesis* with or without neck pain	Radiographs not taken Extruded disk in canal	Conservative Ventral slot	Guarded Excellent/favorable
V	Weakly ambulatory tetraparesis† with or without neck pain	Extruded disk in canal	Ventral slot	Excellent/favorable
VI	Nonambulatory tetraparesis‡ with or without neck pain; absence of forelimb sensory deficits	Extruded disk—C2–C4 Extruded disk—C4–C7	Ventral slot Ventral slot	Excellent Favorable
VII	Nonambulatory tetraparesis‡ with or without neck pain; forelimb sensory deficits present	Extruded disk in canal	Ventral slot	Guarded

*Ambulatory tetraparesis is hind limb weakness with a choppy forelimb gait; the patient can rise without assistance and ambulate with evidence of motor weakness.
†Weakly ambulatory tetraparesis is severe tetraparesis; the patient can rise without assistance and take several steps, but tires easily and assumes a recumbent position.
‡Nonambulatory tetraparesis is severe tetraparesis without the ability to ambulate unassisted; voluntary motor movements may or may not be present.

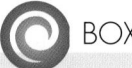 BOX 38-6

Dosages and Regimens of Drugs Used in Patients With Cervical or Thoracolumbar Disk Disease

Corticosteroids

Dexamethasone (Azium)

0.2 mg/kg PO or IM bid for 3 days, then qd for 3 days; reevaluate; may repeat treatment once or twice and consider combining with a muscle relaxant; if no response, consider surgery

Prednisolone

0.5 to 1 mg/kg PO bid for 3 days, then qd for 3 days; re-evaluate; may repeat treatment once or twice; consider combining with a muscle relaxant; if no response, consider surgery

Methylprednisolone (Solu-Medrol)

30 mg/kg IV given once at anesthetic induction; discontinue after one dose

Muscle Relaxants

Methocarbamol (Robaxin-V)

22 mg/kg PO once as a loading dose, then 11 mg/kg PO tid for 10 days; reevaluate; may repeat treatment once or twice and consider combining with steroids; if no response, consider surgery

Diazepam (Valium)

1.1 mg/kg PO bid (not to exceed 20 mg/day) for 10 days; reevaluate; may repeat once or twice; consider combining with steroids; if no response, consider surgery

PO, Oral; *IM,* intramuscular; *bid,* twice a day; *qd,* once a day; *IV,* intravenous; *tid,* three times a day.

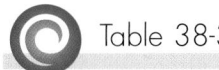 Table 38-3

Recommended Medical/Conservative Therapy Based on Clinical Presentation of Dogs With Cervical Disk Disease*

CLINICAL PRESENTATION	INITIAL TREATMENT†	RESULT	SECOND TREATMENT†	RESULT	THIRD TREATMENT†
Mild neck pain; first episode or multiple episodes	Cage rest only	No improvement	Muscle relaxants for 10 days	No improvement	Steroids plus muscle relaxants for 6 days
Moderate neck pain; first episode or multiple episodes	Muscle relaxants for 10 days	No improvement	Steroids plus muscle relaxants for 6 days	No improvement	Repeat second treatment and consider surgery
Severe neck pain; first episode or multiple episodes	Steroids plus muscle relaxants for 6 days	No improvement	Repeat first treatment	No improvement	Consider surgery
Severe neck pain; first episode or multiple episodes	Steroids plus muscle relaxants for 6 days	Slight improvement to moderate or mild neck pain	Muscle relaxants for 10 days	No improvement	Repeat second treatment and consider surgery
Mild, moderate, or severe neck pain and ambulatory tetraparesis	Recommend surgery, but consider steroid trial for 1 day	No improvement on steroids	Surgery; ventral slot; preoperative steroids		
Mild, moderate, or severe neck pain and nonambulatory tetraparesis	Surgery; ventral slot; preoperative steroids				
Recurrent mild, moderate, or severe pain; unresponsive to medical management	Surgery; ventral slot; preoperative steroids				

*See Box 38-6 for drug dosages and variations on duration of therapy.
†All patients must be placed in strict confinement for 3 to 4 weeks as part of their medical management, regardless of the drug used or duration of drug therapy.

sider repeat corticosteroid therapy, combination therapy, or surgery.

Nonsteroidal antiinflammatory drugs (NSAIDs) may cause severe gastric irritation and ulceration, particularly if the dosage is above recommended levels, given for extended periods, or given in combination with corticosteroids. Newer NSAIDs that preferentially affect COX-2 (e.g., carprofen, meloxicam, and deracoxib) cause fewer problems than the older, nonselective NSAIDs; however, gastrointestinal problems (e.g., ulcers and perforation) may occur when using the COX-2 selective NSAIDS, especially if they are used incorrectly. In particular, it is important to note that if you are going to switch from a nonselective NSAID to a COX-2 selective NSAID, you must allow time for the first NSAID to "wash out" before beginning the new NSAID. Failure to do so can result in severe ulceration and perforation. NSAIDs should not be used in combination with corticosteroids. Muscle relaxants are generally unsuccessful when used alone to treat patients with severe neck or back pain; they should be combined with corticosteroids initially. Muscle relaxants can be

given in combination with prednisolone, dexamethasone, aspirin, phenylbutazone, or flunixin meglumine. A muscle relaxant can be used alone in patients with mild or moderate neck or back pain, or in those with moderate to severe neck or back pain that are improving but require further treatment. Common clinical presentations and suggested therapeutic regimens are listed in Table 38-3. Knowledge of the potential side effects of commonly used antiinflammatory drugs (or combinations of drugs) is important. A list of common side effects of drugs used to treat patients with cervical disk disease is provided in Table 38-4. All patients must be placed in strict confinement for 3 to 4 weeks as part of their medical management, especially if drugs are used.

Patients given antiinflammatory drugs should be monitored carefully for depression, anorexia, abdominal pain, melena, and/or vomiting (especially, but not only, undigested or digested blood [coffee grounds]). If gastrointestinal lesions are suspected, corticosteroids and NSAIDs should be discontinued immediately because gastrointestinal ulceration associated with antiinflammatory medication, spinal

Table 38-4

Side Effects of Commonly Used Antiinflammatory Drugs

DRUG	SIDE EFFECTS
Dexamethasone	When used in combination with NSAIDs, it commonly causes gastric ulceration/perforation and/or colonic ulceration (rare). It should never be used in conjunction with or in close proximity with flunixin. Used at high doses by itself, it can cause gastritis with vomiting and hematemesis, especially in patients with poor visceral perfusion. Bloody stools, ostensibly from colitis, may be seen. Prolonged usage puts the patient at risk for urinary tract infection. Steroids do not cause pancreatitis even though they may increase serum lipase values (but this test is suspect and should not be used to look for pancreatitis).
Prednisolone	Same as dexamethasone, but prednisolone used at routine doses is much less likely to cause such problems as dexamethasone
Aspirin*	Platelet function abnormalities, gastric ulceration/perforation
Phenylbutazone*	Bone marrow suppression, gastric ulceration/perforation
Flunixin meglumine*	Many severe side effects. This drug should not be used in dogs except in very rare circumstances.
Methocarbamol	Slight muscle weakness
Diazepam	Central nervous system depression, potential for client abuse

NSAIDs, Nonsteroidal antiimflammatory drugs.
*These drugs have serious adverse side effects and are not recommended. There are newer and safer NSAIDS and analgesics (see Chapter 13 and Chapter 33).

 Table 38-5

Drugs Used to Treat or Help Prevent Gastrointestinal Complications of Corticosteroids or NSAIDs

DRUG	DOSE	ACTION
Cimetidine (Tagamet)*†	5–10 mg/kg PO, IV, SC tid to qid	Used to treat ulcers; decreases gastric acid formation by the parietal cell, thus preventing further ulceration by HCl
Ranitidine (Zantac)*‡	2 mg/kg PO, IV, IM, SC bid to tid	Same as cimetidine
Famotidine (Pepcid)*, §	0.5 mg/kg PO qd to bid	Same as cimetidine
Omeprazole (Prilosec) *	0.7–1.5 mg/kg PO qd to bid	Used to treat ulcers; blocks proton pump of the parietal cell
Misoprostol (Cytotec)‖	1–5 μg/kg PO tid	A prostaglandin E analog that is used to help prevent NSAID-induced ulcers
Sucralfate (Carafate)*	0.5–1 g PO tid to qid; give 1 hr after other medications	Used to treat ulcers; gastric and duodenal protectant; acts to coat ulcer; acts as a bandage

NSAIDs, Nonsteroidal antiimflammatory drugs; *PO,* oral; *IV,* intravenous; *SC,* subcutaneous; *tid,* three times a day; *qid,* four times a day; *IM,* intramuscular; *bid,* twice a day; *qd,* once a day; *HCl,* hydrochloric acid.
*Although commonly used to protect the stomach of dogs receiving steroids, there are numerous studies showing that these drugs are ineffective for this purpose while there are no studies showing that they are clearly beneficial.
†Cimetidine inhibits hepatic P450 enzymes and decreased hepatic blood flow.
‡Has prokinetic activity in addition to inhibiting gastric acid secretion.
§Is usually the preferred H-2 receptor antagonist; has the longest duration of action and is the most potent.
‖Misoprostol may initially cause diarrhea and abdominal discomfort.

cord injury, and stress of hospitalization may be fatal. Drugs listed in Table 38-5 may be used to treat gastric ulcers; however, there are no medications that will reliably prevent the formation of gastric ulcers in all dogs.

SURGICAL TREATMENT

The objective of surgery in patients with cervical disk disease is to remove extruded disk fragments from attenuated nerve roots and/or spinal cord. This may result in immediate pain relief and eventual restoration of normal motor function. A ventral slot procedure is most commonly performed for removal of disk material in the cervical region; however, midcervical or caudal cervical hemilaminectomy and facetectomy (see p. 1404) are indicated for removal of disk fragments from the intervertebral foramen. Some surgeons prefer to also perform a distraction-stabilization procedure in the slotted intervertebral space in patients with caudal cervical disk extrusions. Dorsal cervical laminectomy may allow suc-

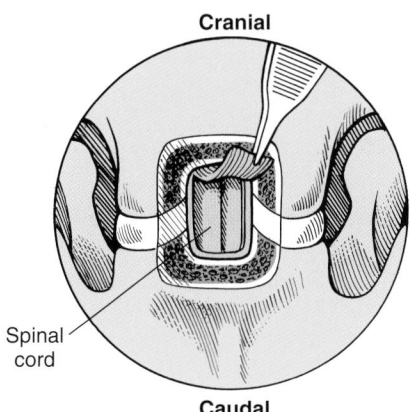

FIG. 38-36
When herniated disk material has been successfully removed, the spinal cord is visible.

cessful decompression in small-breed dogs (see p. 1409). During ventral slot procedures, adequate decompression of the spinal cord is achieved when the characteristic bluish hue of the dural tube is identified through the slot (Fig. 38-36).

Recurrence of cervical disk extrusion at an alternate intervertebral space is rare; routine fenestration of unaffected disks after a ventral slot procedure is unnecessary. Cervical disk fenestration (see p. 1409) may be used to treat patients with neck pain secondary to cervical disk disease. Fenestration relieves pain in some patients, but does not adequately remove compressive disk material from the vertebral canal or intervertebral foramen. Patients that undergo fenestration for cervical disk disease exhibit longer morbidity than those treated with ventral decompression (ventral slot). Tetraparesis may occur from overaggressive fenestration.

Preoperative Management
IV fluids and steroids should be given before surgery. In addition to their therapeutic effect, IV steroids may protect the spinal cord from the effects of surgical manipulation. The steroid of choice is methylprednisolone sodium succinate (30 mg/kg IV).

Anesthesia
Selected anesthetic protocols for animals undergoing cervical spinal cord surgery are provided on p. 1402. The animal's neurologic status and positioning for surgery are important preanesthetic considerations. If the patient is exhibiting motor weakness (e.g., weakly ambulatory or nonambulatory tetraparesis) or will require positioning that may cause respiratory compromise, mechanical ventilatory support should be considered.

Surgical Anatomy
Unique anatomic features of the cervical spine include the following: (1) C1-C2 space does not have an intervertebral disk; (2) C6 has a prominent transverse process; (3) C1 has a prominent ventral spinous process; (4) each vertebral body has a characteristic midline ventral ridge; (5) presence of transverse foramen (for vertebral artery and vein) in each cervical vertebra except C7; (6) characteristic cranial-to-caudal slant of each intervertebral space; and (7) location of the vertebral venous sinuses and dorsal longitudinal ligament on the floor of the vertebral canal.

Positioning
Patients undergoing a ventral slot or fenestration procedure should be placed in dorsal recumbency with their chest in a V-trough. They must be carefully secured with sandbags or a rigid vacuum type of apparatus to prevent lateral motion. The front legs are taped caudally, and a loop of rope is tied around the muzzle, caudal to the maxillary canine teeth. The rope is secured to the table and the front legs are pulled caudally to apply linear traction to the cervical spine (see Fig. 38-5 on p. 1406). Linear traction stabilizes the spine and opens intervertebral spaces and foramina, improving exposure during the ventral slot procedure. An area from cranial to the laryngeal cartilages to caudal to the manubrium sterni should be prepared for surgery (i.e., a ventral midline cervical incision). Patients diagnosed with intraforaminal disk extrusion should be positioned in sternal recumbency with the neck elevated, cradled, and gently flexed (see Fig. 38-17 on p. 1410 and Fig. 38-21 on p. 1412).

SURGICAL TECHNIQUE
Perform a ventral slot procedure as described on p. 1405. Once the vertebral canal has been reached, remove disk material located on the ventral midline first because removal of laterally located disk material increases the risk of lacerating a venous sinus (Fig. 38-37, A). A dull, flat dental spatula is best suited for removal of foraminal disk material. Bend the dental spatula at a 60-degree angle to facilitate removal of laterally extruded disk material and reduce venous sinus laceration. Gently sweep the spatula along the lateral aspect of the vertebral canal (Fig. 38-37, B). Gently tease to loosen disk material from the foramen and encourage fragments to move toward the slot margin where they can either be suctioned using a small suction tip or removed with fine ophthalmic forceps. Take special care when old, calcified disks are encountered because they may be adhered to venous sinus or dura. Carefully tease and manipulate these disks away from the dura with a dental spatula. If severe hemorrhage from a lacerated venous sinus occurs, discontinue manipulation in the vertebral canal and consider closing the incision. The technique for controlling venous sinus hemorrhage is discussed in Box 38-1 on p. 1403. If hemorrhage can be lateralized to one side of the slot, it may be possible to manipulate and remove the disk from the opposite side of the slot, but take care to ensure adequate visualization before manipulation in the vertebral canal.

SUTURE MATERIALS AND SPECIAL INSTRUMENTS
Special instrumentation necessary for ventral slot procedures, disk fenestration, and dorsolateral hemilaminectomy is listed in Table 38-1 on p. 1417.

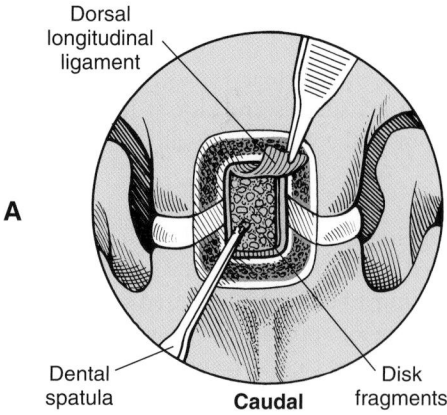

Dorsal
longitudinal
ligament

A

Dental
spatula

Caudal

Disk
fragments

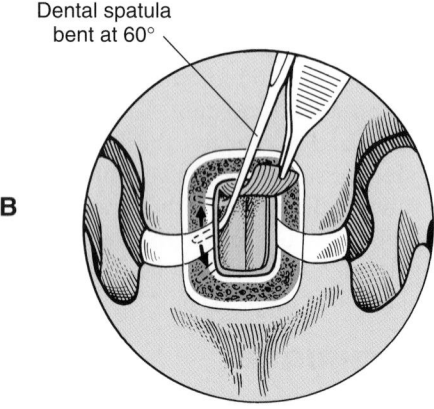

Dental spatula
bent at 60°

B

FIG. 38-37
A, Remove ventrally located disk fragments with ophthalmic forceps and a dental spatula. **B,** Remove laterally located (foraminal) disk fragments with a dental spatula bent at 60 degrees; use a sweeping motion to encourage disk removal.

POSTOPERATIVE CARE AND ASSESSMENT

Respiration should be monitored and animals should be observed for seizures for 24 hours after surgery. Analgesics should be provided as necessary (see Table 13-4 on p. 133) and corticosteroids discontinued immediately postoperatively. Neurologic examination should be performed twice daily. Ambulatory patients are generally discharged by 24 to 48 hours postoperatively. Discharge of nonambulatory patients generally depends on the owner's ability to care for the animal. All patients should be fitted with a harness; neck collars should be avoided. Ambulatory patients should have exercise restricted for 3 to 4 weeks; gradual increase in exercise is allowed over the subsequent 3 to 4 weeks. Stable interbody fusion after a ventral slot procedure requires 6 to 8 weeks, after which return to normal activity is recommended. Care of nonambulatory patients is described on p. 1416. Return of neurologic function is difficult to predict postoperatively; it may take 6 to 8 weeks (or longer) for the animal to regain the ability to ambulate.

COMPLICATIONS

Significant complications in patients treated surgically for cervical disk disease are uncommon. Possible complications include continued neck pain and/or deteriorating motor

status. Treatment of the complication is determined by the cause and surgical treatment used. Successful treatment options are outlined in Table 38-6.

PROGNOSIS

Prognosis for patients treated medically or surgically for cervical disk disease depends on neurologic signs, anatomic location of the disk extrusion, and medical or surgical treatment used, but is generally favorable. Clinical factors and probable patient outcomes are outlined in Table 38-2 on p. 1422. Ambulatory patients with mild, moderate, or severe neck pain should be pain free or significantly improved by 24 to 48 hours postoperatively. Ambulatory, tetraparetic patients (with or without neck pain) should be pain free 24 to 48 hours postoperatively, and motor dysfunction should be resolved by 7 to 10 days. Weakly ambulatory tetraparetic patients (with or without neck pain) should be pain free 24 to 48 hours postoperatively, and motor dysfunction should be resolved by 3 to 4 weeks. Nonambulatory tetraparetic patients (with or without neck pain) should be pain free 24 to 48 hours postoperatively, and motor dysfunction should be resolved by 4 to 6 weeks. Nonambulatory tetraparetic patients have a better prognosis if they do not have foreleg sensory deficits preoperatively, have a C2-C3 or C3-C4 lesion, and regain ambulation within 96 hours postoperatively.

Suggested Reading

Cherrone K, Dewey CW, Coates JR et al: A retrospective comparison of cervical intervertebral disk disease in nonchondrodystrophic large dogs versus small dogs, *J Am Anim Hosp Assoc* 40:316, 2004.

This report suggests that a substantial number of medium- to large-sized, nonchondrodystrophic dogs are presented with Hansen type I cervical disk extrusions.

Fitch RB, Kerwin SC, Hosgood G: Caudal cervical intervertebral disk disease in the small dog: role of distraction and stabilization in ventral slot decompression, *J Am Anim Hosp Assoc* 36:68, 2000.

The authors report a retrospective study of 112 dogs weighing less than 35 lb presented with cervical intervertebral disk disease. Significant improvement in clinical results was seen in caudal disk protrusions when additional surgical distraction and stabilization were provided following ventral slot decompression.

Kube S, Owen T, Hanson S: Severe respiratory compromise secondary to cervical disk herniation in two dogs, *J Am Anim Hosp Assoc* 39:513, 2003.

Respiratory and cardiac complications may occur with cervical spinal injuries. Patients having cervical myelopathies should be screened for respiratory and cardiac dysfunction and treated appropriately.

Lemarie RJ et al: Vertebral subluxation following ventral cervical decompression in the dog, *J Am Anim Hosp Assoc* 36:348, 2000.

Nine dogs with radiographically verified vertebral subluxation following ventral slot procedures were studied. Surgical correction consisting of distraction and stabilization with PMMA and pins resulted in improvement in operated dogs, whereas dogs not undergoing surgical correction did not improve.

Table 38-6

Postoperative Complications in Surgical Patients With Cervical Disk Disease

COMPLICATION	SURGICAL TREATMENT USED	CAUSE (BASED ON RADIOGRAPHY)	COURSE OF ACTION
Continued neck pain	Ventral slot	Slot excessively wide	Neck brace for 2 to 3 wk; pain control; if no improvement, then cervical stabilization
		Disk material remains	Neck brace for 2 to 3 wk; pain control; if no improvement, reoperate
		Normal radiographs	Neck brace and treat medically for diskogenic pain
Continued neck pain	Dorsolateral hemilaminectomy	Disk material remains	Neck brace for 2 to 3 wk; pain control; if no improvement, make oblique radiographs; reoperate if disk present in foramen
Continued neck pain	Fenestration	Disk in canal	Ventral slot, remove disk from canal and foramen
		Disk in foramen	Dorsolateral hemilaminectomy and facetectomy
Deteriorating motor status	Ventral slot	Slot excessively wide	Cervical stabilization
		Disk in canal	Reoperate if disk is in vertebral canal; if second disk, perform ventral slot
Deteriorating motor status	Dorsolateral hemilaminectomy	Disk pushed into canal	Reoperate to remove disk
Deteriorating motor status	Fenestration	Disk in canal	Ventral slot; remove disk from canal

CERVICAL SPONDYLOMYELOPATHY

DEFINITIONS

Cervical spondylomyelopathy, also known as **wobbler syndrome,** is a disorder of the caudal cervical vertebrae and intervertebral disks (i.e., **spondylopathy**) that causes spinal cord compression (i.e., **myelopathy**). Other terms for this condition include *cervical vertebral instability, cervical malformation-malarticulation, cervical spondylolisthesis,* and *cervical spondylopathy.*

GENERAL CONSIDERATIONS AND CLINICALLY RELEVANT PATHOPHYSIOLOGY

Wobbler syndrome is a relatively common disease in Doberman pinschers and other large-breed dogs. The cause is unknown, but may be nutritional, traumatic, hereditary, or acquired. It is a "syndrome" that probably has multiple etiologic factors. Wobbler syndrome has been subdivided into five classifications distinguished by the location of the compressive lesion with respect to the vertebral canal (Table 38-7). Discussion of the proposed pathophysiology of wobbler syndrome is divided into each of the proposed disease classifications (e.g., chronic degenerative disk disease, congenital osseous malformations, vertebral tipping, hypertrophied ligamentum flavum/vertebral arch malformations, and "hourglass" compression).

Chronic degenerative disk disease may originate from either vertebral instability (e.g., stress) or primary degeneration of the intervertebral disk (e.g., Hansen type II disk protrusion). The degenerating annulus fibrosus undergoes hypertrophy and/or hyperplasia. Spinal cord compression

occurs when the disk space collapses and buckles the redundant annulus fibrosus dorsally (Fig. 38-38, *A*). The dorsal longitudinal ligament (located dorsal to the annulus fibrosus on the floor of the vertebral canal) compresses the dura (see Fig. 38-37, *A*). Spinal cord compression in chronic degenerative disk disease is dynamic in that flexion and extension of the neck may vary the degree of spinal cord compression. Generally, dorsal extension of the neck increases spinal cord compression (Fig. 38-38, *B*); ventral flexion (Fig. 38-38, *C*) and linear traction (Fig. 38-38, *D*) decrease compression.

Congenital osseous malformations may occur anywhere along the cervical spine in one or multiple (most common) vertebrae. Malformed vertebrae cause narrowing of the vertebral canal as a result of stenosis of the cranial vertebral canal orifice, articular facet deformities, malformation of vertebral pedicles, and/or deformation of vertebral arches (Fig. 38-39). Diets high in calcium exacerbate the malformations in Great Dane puppies. Congenital osseous malformations may be related to disorders of endochondral ossification.

Vertebral tipping is characterized by displacement (tipping) of the craniodorsal surface of the vertebral body (generally C6 or C7) into the vertebral canal, causing spinal cord compression (Fig. 38-40). Instability secondary to chronic degenerative disk disease (or vice versa) may be the predisposing factor that allows the vertebral body to become malpositioned.

The compressive lesion in hypertrophied ligamentum flavum/vertebral arch malformations occurs on the dorsal aspect of the spinal cord. Patients with isolated ligamentum

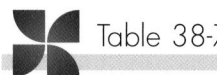

Table 38-7

Classification of Wobbler Syndrome

CLASSIFICATION	AGE/BREED	LESION LOCATION	CAUSE OF COMPRESSION	GENERAL PROGNOSIS
Chronic degenerative disk disease	Adult, male Doberman pinschers	Compresses ventral aspect of spinal cord C5–C7	Disk degeneration and subsequent hypertrophy of ventral annulus fibrosus	Favorable
Congenital osseous malformation	Young Great Danes and Doberman pinschers	Compresses spinal cord laterally or dorsoventrally C3–C7	Congenital malformation of vertebral bodies and articular facets	Unfavorable
Vertebral tipping	Adult, male Doberman pinschers	Compresses ventral aspect of spinal cord C5–C7	Dorsal malposition of the affected vertebral body in the vertebral canal	Favorable
Ligamentum flavum/ vertebral arch malformation	Young Great Danes	Compresses dorsal aspect of spinal cord C4–C7	Hypertrophy and hyperplasia of the ligamentum flavum; vertebral arch malformation	Favorable to guarded
Hourglass compression	Young Great Danes	Compresses spinal cord on all sides C2–C7	Hypertrophy of ligamentum flavum and annulus fibrosus; malformation or degenerative disk disease of articular facets	Guarded

FIG. 38-38
A, Chronic degenerative disk disease produces spinal cord compression because of hypertrophy of the annulus fibrosus. **B,** Mechanism by which dorsal extension of the cervical spine increases spinal cord compression in patients with chronic degenerative disk disease. **C,** Ventral flexion of the cervical spine decreases spinal cord compression in patients with chronic degenerative disk disease. **D,** Linear traction of the cervical spine decreases spinal cord compression in patients with chronic degenerative disk disease.

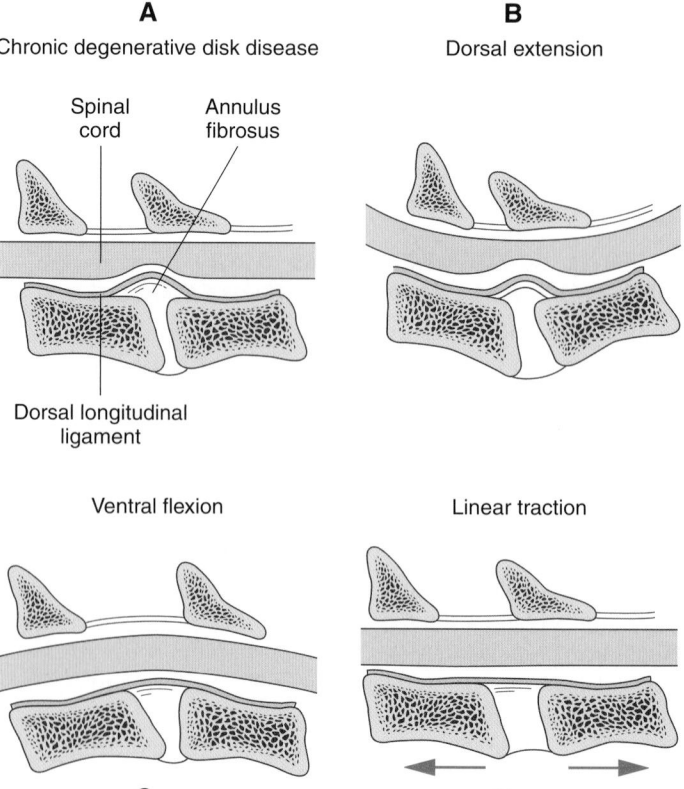

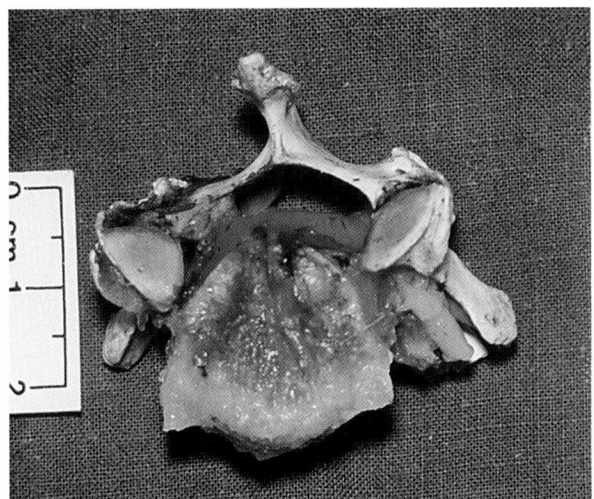

FIG. 38-39
Vertebra with congenital osseous malformation (C7). Notice the malformed facets and deformation of the vertebral canal.

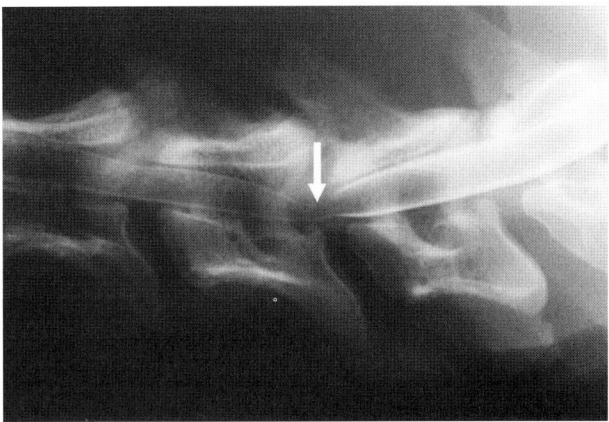

FIG. 38-41
Lateral myelogram of a dog with C5–C6 ligamentum flavum hypertrophy. Notice the ventral deviation of the dorsal aspect of the contrast column *(arrow)*.

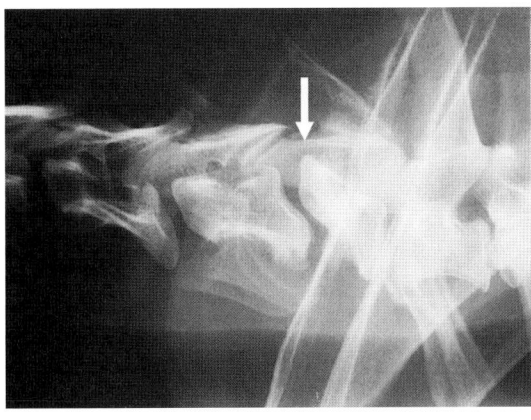

FIG. 38-40
Lateral radiograph of a dog with wobbler syndrome and C6–C7 vertebral tipping. Notice the subluxation of the cranial aspect of C7 into the spinal canal *(arrow)*.

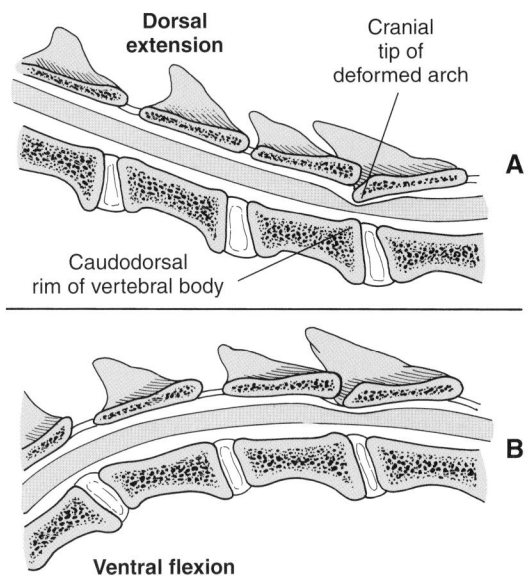

FIG. 38-42
A, Dorsal vertebral arch malformation producing dorsal spinal cord compression. **B,** Ventral flexion causes retraction of the malformed arch, relieving spinal cord compression.

flavum abnormalities will probably develop hypertrophy and/or hyperplasia secondary to instability (Fig. 38-41). Vertebral arch malformations may be genetic and/or nutritional in origin. Whatever the cause, the vertebral arch, articular processes, and facets become plump, deformed, and asymmetric. Spinal cord compression is not the result solely of deformation, but of a combination of static deformation and dynamic compression. In dorsal extension, the cranial tip of the deformed vertebral arch of one vertebra is brought closer to the caudodorsal rim of the body of the adjacent cranial vertebra, increasing spinal cord compression (Fig. 38-42, *A*). When the neck is flexed ventrally, the cranial tip of the elongated vertebral arch is retracted, decreasing spinal cord compression (Fig. 38-42, *B*).

Hourglass compression occurs because the spinal cord compression occurs dorsally, ventrally, and laterally (Fig. 38-43). Annulus fibrosus hypertrophy and/or hyperplasia causes ventral spinal cord compression, whereas hypertrophy and/or hyperplasia of the ligamentum flavum causes dorsal spinal cord compression. Degenerative joint disease or malformation/malarticulation of the articular facets causes lateral spinal cord compression. Dynamic hourglass lesions may occur at any level of the cervical spine.

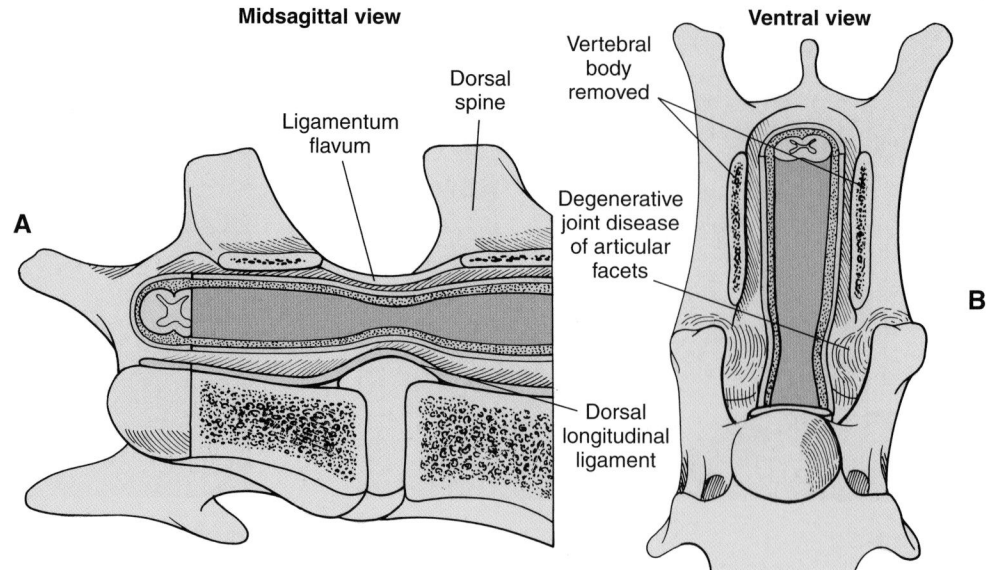

FIG. 38-43
A, Hourglass compression of the ventral spinal cord is caused by redundant dorsal annulus fibrosus; dorsal compression is caused by redundant ligamentum flavum.
B, Lateral compression is caused by degenerative joint disease or malformation and/or malarticulation of articular facets.

DIAGNOSIS
Clinical Presentation

Signalment. Information concerning sex and breed may assist specific classification of wobbler syndrome (see Table 38-7). Doberman pinschers and Great Danes account for 80% of the cases. The incidence of chronic degenerative disk disease is twice as high in males as in females. Variation in age of presentation depends on specific classification (see Table 38-7).

History. Affected animals generally become less coordinated over months to years. All four limbs are affected, but signs are generally initiated and more pronounced in the rear legs. Occasionally an acute exacerbation precipitated by minor trauma may be noted. Approximately 40% of animals have a history of neck pain.

Physical Examination Findings

General physical examination findings are normal in the majority of patients with wobbler syndrome. UMN signs, including a crossed extensor reflex, generally occur in the rear limbs of dogs with chronic disease. A broad-based stance is often noted in the rear legs. Thoracic limb reflex changes are generally mild. A stiff, straight-legged gait and atrophy of the supraspinatus and infraspinatus muscles are common with chronicity. The neck is often carried in ventral flexion because this position produces the least amount of spinal cord compression (see Fig. 38-38, *C*). Dorsal extension of the neck may cause pain and/or accentuate spinal cord compression, with resultant increased motor signs (see Fig. 38-38, *B*). Care should therefore be taken when manipulating the head and neck. Abnormalities noted on neurologic examination vary and may include pain alone, paraparesis, ambulatory tetraparesis, weakly ambulatory

 Table 38-8

Neurologic Classification

NEUROLOGIC FINDING	DEFINITION
Pain	Discomfort on manipulation of the head and neck
Paraparesis	Upper motor neuron deficits and mild-to-moderate motor weakness of the hind limbs; normal thoracic limb function
Ambulatory tetraparesis	Paraparesis with a choppy thoracic limb gait as a result of upper, lower, or upper and lower motor neuron deficits and mild motor weakness
Weakly ambulatory tetraparesis	Severe tetraparesis; patient can still rise without assistance and take several steps, but tires easily and assumes a recumbent position
Nonambulatory tetraparesis	Tetraparesis without the ability to rise or walk

tetraparesis, or nonambulatory tetraparesis. Definitions of each neurologic classification are provided in Table 38-8.

Diagnostic Imaging

Survey radiographs of the cervical spine are not diagnostic for the affected vertebra, intervertebral space, or location of the compressive mass within the vertebral canal (i.e., dorsal, ventral, and/or lateral). Typical changes on survey radio-

Table 38-9

Survey Radiographic and Myelographic Findings With Wobbler Syndrome

CLASSIFICATION	PLAIN FILM CHANGES	MYELOGRAPHIC CHANGES
Chronic degenerative disk disease	Normal; collapse of the intervertebral space; spondylosis deformans; sclerotic endplates; calcified disk; C5–C7 most often affected	Extradural mass compressing the ventral surface of the spinal cord; lesions are generally dynamic
Congenital osseous malformation	Various osseous malformations; C3–C7 most often affected	Extradural mass (bone) compressing the lateral, ventral, and/or dorsal surface of the spinal cord; lesions are generally static
Vertebral tipping	Tipping of the craniodorsal end of a vertebra into the vertebral canal; C6 or C7 most often affected	Normal; extradural mass compressing the ventral aspect of the spinal cord; lesion may be static or dynamic
Ligamentum flavum hypertrophy	Normal; C4–C7 most often affected	Extradural mass compressing the dorsal surface of the spinal cord (soft tissue); lesions are generally static
Vertebral arch malformation	Normal; sclerosis and malformation of affected laminae; C4–C7 most often affected	Extradural mass compressing the dorsal surface of the spinal cord (malformed laminae); lesions often have a static and dynamic component
Hourglass compression	Normal; C2–C7 may be affected	Extradural mass compressing the lateral, ventral, and dorsal surfaces of the spinal cord (soft tissue and osseous); lesions are generally dynamic

graphs for each classification of wobbler syndrome are summarized in Table 38-9.

Although survey radiography may help diagnose wobbler syndrome, myelography, CT imaging, or MRI is essential to determine the following: (1) location and number of affected vertebrae and/or intervertebral spaces, (2) location of lesion(s) within the vertebral canal (i.e., dorsal, ventral, and lateral), (3) degree of spinal cord compression, and (4) occurrence of dynamic compression. Typical myelographic changes expected with each classification of wobbler syndrome are provided in Table 38-9.

Stress myelography is radiographic imaging of the cervical spine in various stressed positions (i.e., ventral flexion, dorsal extension, and linear traction) during myelography. Stress myelography is essential to diagnose dynamic compressive lesions. Classically, spinal cord compression with chronic degenerative disk disease is worsened with the neck in dorsal extension and improved in ventral flexion and linear traction (see Fig. 38-38, *B* to *D*).

> NOTE: Dorsal extension is not recommended in radiographic evaluation of patients with wobbler syndrome because it may exacerbate spinal cord compression.

A complete myelographic examination, including linear traction, allows formulation of a rational therapeutic ap-

proach (see Fig. 38-43). A recent study suggested similar findings using traction during MRI (Penderis et al, 2004). In addition, cross-sectional imaging may be necessary to identify dorsal and lateral compressions, which may not be visualized on myelographic images.

Laboratory Findings

No significant abnormalities are noted in the hemogram or urinalysis of most affected animals. Biochemical analysis may reveal elevated serum cholesterol in Doberman pinschers with subclinical hypothyroidism. Whether hypothyroidism has an influence on wobbler syndrome is unclear.

DIFFERENTIAL DIAGNOSIS

Any disorder causing neck pain, paraparesis, or tetraparesis in large-breed dogs, especially Doberman pinschers and Great Danes, should be considered as differential diagnoses. Diseases that can be mistaken for wobbler syndrome are listed in Table 38-10. Differentiation is usually possible by signalment, neurologic examination, serum chemistry, cerebrospinal fluid (CSF) analysis, and radiography and/or myelography. Diagnosis of wobbler syndrome is confirmed by plain and stress myelography or by standard and stress MRI.

MEDICAL MANAGEMENT

Wobbler syndrome is a chronic, progressive disorder characterized by subtle hind limb weakness that may progress to nonambulatory tetraparesis. Medical therapy may cause

Table 38-10

Differential Diagnoses That Mimic Wobbler Syndrome Using the DAMNIT-V Scheme

CLASSIFICATION	EXAMPLES	DIAGNOSTIC DIFFERENTIALS/TOOLS
Degenerative	Cervical disk disease Bilateral to hip dysplasia Bilateral ruptured cruciate	Static mass on stress myelography Physical exam; neurologic exam; hip radiographs Physical exam; neurologic exam
Anomalous	Atlantoaxial subluxation	Signalment; plain and stress radiography
Metabolic	Any disorder causing generalized weakness (e.g., Addison's disease)	Neurologic exam; laboratory findings
Nutritional	Nutritional secondary hyperparathyroidism	Dietary history; plain radiography
Neoplastic	Tumors of the cervical spine, spinal cord, or nerve roots	Plain and stress myelography
Immunologic	Polyarthritis Polymyositis	Neurologic exam; laboratory data Neurologic exam; laboratory data
Infectious	Cervical diskospondylitis Meningitis	Plain radiographs CSF analysis
Traumatic	Cervical spinal fracture/luxation	History; plain radiographs
Vascular	Fibrocartilaginous embolism	History; CSF analysis; myelography

CSF, Cerebrospinal fluid.

Table 38-11

Conservative Versus Surgical Management for Patients With Wobbler Syndrome

CLASSIFICATION	CLINICAL SIGNS*	NUMBER OF LESIONS	TREATMENT	PROGNOSIS
Chronic degenerative disk disease, vertebral tipping, hourglass compression	Pain alone	Single or multiple lesions	Conservative Surgical	Favorable Excellent
	Paraparesis	Single or multiple lesions	Conservative Surgical	Favorable Excellent
	Ambulatory tetraparesis	Single lesion	Conservative Surgical	Favorable Excellent
		Multiple lesions	Conservative Surgical	Favorable Excellent
	Weakly ambulatory tetraparesis	Single lesion	Conservative Surgical	Favorable Excellent
		Multiple lesions	Conservative Surgical	Favorable Excellent
	Nonambulatory tetraparesis	Single lesion	Conservative Surgical	Favorable Excellent
		Multiple lesions	Conservative Surgical	Favorable Excellent
Ligamentum flavum hypertrophy/vertebral arch malformation	Paraparesis	Single or multiple lesions	Conservative Surgical	Favorable Excellent
	Tetraparesis	Single lesion	Conservative Surgical	Favorable Excellent
		Multiple lesions	Conservative Surgical	Favorable Excellent
Congenital osseous malformation	Paraparesis	Single lesion (rare)	Conservative Surgical	Favorable Excellent
	Tetraparesis	Single lesion (rare)	Conservative Surgical	Favorable Excellent
	Paraparesis	Multiple lesions	Conservative Surgical	Favorable Excellent
	Tetraparesis	Multiple lesions	Conservative Surgical	Favorable Excellent

*The definition of each neurologic classification is given in Table 38-8.

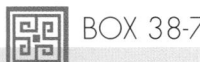 BOX 38-7

Corticosteroids Used in Patients With Wobbler Syndrome

Dexamethasone (Azium)

0.2 mg/kg PO or IM bid for 3 days, then qd for 3 days; reevaluate patient; may repeat treatment once or twice; if no response, consider surgery

Prednisolone

0.5 to 1 mg/kg PO bid for 3 days; then qd for 3 days; reevaluate patient; may repeat treatment once or twice; if no response, consider surgery

Methylprednisolone (Solu-Medrol)

30 mg/kg IV given once at anesthetic induction; discontinue after one dose

PO, Oral; *IM,* intramuscular; *bid,* twice a day; *qd,* once a day; *IV,* intravenous.

temporary improvement; however, progression to an unacceptable neurologic status is common. Whether a patient is treated conservatively depends on classification of the disorder, degree of neurologic dysfunction, and number of affected vertebrae or intervertebral spaces (Table 38-11).

The most important aspect of conservative management is strict confinement for 3 to 4 weeks. During this period, patients should be fitted with a neck brace. Gradual return to normal activity is recommended over the next 3 to 4 weeks. Walks should be restricted to a leash and harness; neck collars should be avoided. Although this duration of forced rest allows resolution of spinal cord inflammation, the long-term beneficial effect on cervical spinal stabilization, malformations, disk degeneration, and tissue hypertrophy and hyperplasia is unknown.

Strict confinement, use of a neck brace, and exercise control may or may not be accompanied by antiinflammatory therapy. Clients must be educated as to the potential euphoric effects of antiinflammatory drugs. If strict confinement is not maintained during drug therapy, the patient may become too active and have increased paresis as a result of acute spinal cord contusion. Commonly used antiinflammatory drugs and their dosages are listed in Box 38-7. Recommended corticosteroid dosages vary among clinicians. NSAIDs may cause severe gastric irritation and ulceration, particularly if given above recommended doses or for excessive durations or when given in combination with corticosteroids. Newer NSAIDs that preferentially affect COX-2 (e.g., carprofen, meloxicam, and deracoxib) cause fewer problems than the older, nonselective NSAIDs; however, gastrointestinal problems (e.g., ulcers and perforation) may occur when using the COX-2 selective NSAIDS, especially if they are used incorrectly. In particular, it is important to note that if you are going to switch from a nonselective NSAID to a COX-2 selective NSAID, you must allow time for the first NSAID to "wash out" before beginning the new NSAID. Failure to do so can result in severe ulceration and perforation. NSAIDs should not be used in combination with corticosteroids. Knowledge of potential side effects of commonly used antiinflammatory drugs (or combinations of drugs) is important (see Table 38-4 on p. 1424).

If conservative treatment is successful, spinal cord edema resolves, remyelination occurs, and the animal recovers function. If no improvement is noted by 3 to 4 weeks or if neurologic deterioration occurs, surgical intervention should be considered.

SURGICAL TREATMENT

The objectives of surgery in patients with wobbler syndrome are relief of spinal cord compression, cervical spinal stabilization (where necessary), and reversal of neurologic deficits. Although numerous surgical techniques have been described for treatment of wobbler syndrome, only a few have long-term prognostic merit. The surgical technique of choice is based on classification, clinical presentation, vertebral body or interspace affected, number of lesions present, location of the lesion within the vertebral canal, and the presence or absence of a dynamic lesion (Table 38-12). Surgical techniques currently used to treat patients with wobbler syndrome include ventral slot procedures, ventral stabilization, ventral traction-stabilization, and dorsal laminectomy.

Techniques that employ decompression and stabilization have improved the outcome of patients with dynamic lesions (Fig. 38-44, *A* and *B*). Based on pathophysiology of the compressive lesion, techniques using linear traction stretch the annulus fibrosus, thus relieving spinal cord compression (see Fig. 38-38, *D*). Once the spine is stabilized in traction, the spinal cord remains decompressed and eventually atrophy of the annulus fibrosus occurs, further improving decompression. Several ventral traction-stabilization techniques have been successfully used to treat patients with wobbler syndrome, particularly those with chronic degenerative disk disease. These include Steinmann pins and PMMA, polyvinylidene spinal plates, Harrington rods, and interbody PMMA plugs. The initial approach for decompression and stabilization is as described for ventral slot procedures (see p. 1405); however, once the affected intervertebral space is located, it and vertebral bodies cranial and caudal to the affected interspace must be exposed. This increased exposure is necessary for placement of the chosen stabilizing device.

> NOTE: The major disadvantages of ventral slot decompression are difficulty in adequately removing the entire compressive lesion and possible instability caused by the slot.

Techniques that employ dorsal decompression without stabilization have also improved the outcome of patients with spinal cord compression secondary to chronic degenerative disk disease, vertebral tipping, ligamentum flavum hypertrophy, and vertebral malformations. Specific procedures employed include dorsal laminectomy of the involved interspaces or continuous deep dorsal laminectomy extending from the dorsal laminae of C3 to the dorsal lamina of C7 (De Risio et al, 2002). Dorsal laminectomy techniques are

Table 38-12

Surgical Techniques for Treatment of Wobbler Syndrome

CLASSIFICATION	CLINICAL PRESENTATION	AFFECTED VERTEBRAL BODY OR INTERSPACE	LOCATION OF LESION WITHIN VERTEBRAL CANAL	DYNAMIC OR STATIC LESION	SURGICAL TECHNIQUE RECOMMENDED	PROGNOSIS
Chronic degenerative disk disease/vertebral tipping	Pain alone	C5-C6 or C6-C7	Ventral	Dynamic	Ventral slot or traction stabilization	Excellent
	Paraparetic	C5-C6 and C6-C7	Ventral	Static	Ventral slot	Excellent
		C5-C6 and C6-C7	Ventral	Dynamic	Ventral slot or traction stabilization	Excellent to favorable
		C5-C6 or C6-C7	Ventral	Static	Ventral slot ± stabilization	Excellent to favorable
	Ambulatory tetraparetic	C5-C6 or C6-C7	Ventral	Dynamic	Ventral traction stabilization	Favorable
			Ventral	Static	Ventral slot and stabilization	Favorable
		C5-C6 and C6-C7	Ventral	Dynamic	Ventral traction stabilization	Favorable
			Ventral	Static	Ventral slot and stabilization	Favorable
		More than two lesions	Ventral	Dynamic/static	Ventral traction stabilization	Guarded to favorable
			Ventral	Dynamic/static	Dorsal laminectomy	Guarded to favorable
	Weakly ambulatory tetraparetic	C5-C6 or C6-C7	Ventral	Dynamic	Ventral traction stabilization	Guarded to favorable
			Ventral	Static	Ventral slot and stabilization	Guarded to favorable
		More than two lesions	Ventral	Dynamic/static	Ventral traction stabilization	Guarded
			Ventral	Dynamic/static	Dorsal laminectomy	Guarded
	Nonambulatory tetraparetic	C5-C6 or C6-C7	Ventral	Dynamic	Ventral traction stabilization	Guarded
			Ventral	Static	Ventral slot and stabilization	Guarded
		More than two lesions	Ventral	Dynamic/static	Ventral traction stabilization	Guarded to unfavorable
			Ventral	Dynamic/static	Dorsal laminectomy	Guarded to unfavorable
Congenital osseous malformation	Paraparesis to tetraparesis	Single lesion (rare)	Lateral, ventral, and/or dorsal	Static	Dorsal laminectomy	Favorable
		Multiple lesions	Lateral, ventral, and/or dorsal	Static	Dorsal laminectomy	Unfavorable
Ligamentum flavum hypertrophy	Paraparesis to tetraparesis	Single lesion	Dorsal	Dynamic	Dorsal laminectomy	Favorable
		Multiple lesions	Dorsal	Static	Ventral traction stabilization	Favorable
			Dorsal	Dynamic/static	Dorsal laminectomy	Guarded
Ventral arch malformation	Paraparesis to tetraparesis	Single lesion	Dorsal	Dynamic	Dorsal laminectomy	Favorable
		Multiple lesions (rare)	Dorsal	Static	Dorsal laminectomy	Favorable
			Dorsal	Dynamic/static	Ventral traction stabilization	Guarded
Hourglass compression	Paraparesis to tetraparesis	Single lesion	Lateral, ventral, and dorsal	Dynamic	Dorsal laminectomy	Favorable
		Two lesions	Lateral, ventral, and dorsal	Static	Dorsal laminectomy	Favorable
		Multiple lesions	Lateral, ventral, and dorsal	Dynamic/static	Ventral traction stabilization	Guarded
			Lateral, ventral, and dorsal	Dynamic/static	Dorsal laminectomy	Guarded

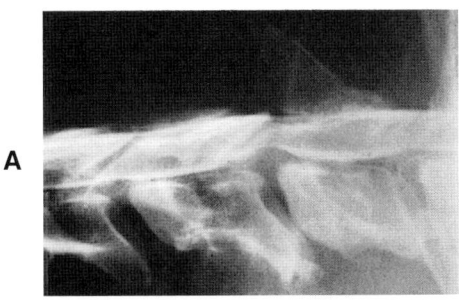

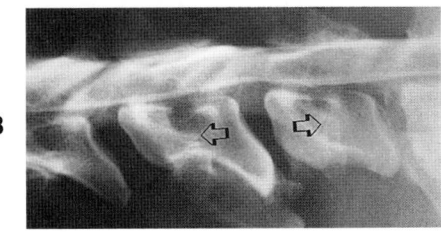

FIG. 38-44
A, Lateral radiograph of a dog with C6–C7 chronic degenerative disk disease and extradural compression of the spinal cord. **B,** Linear traction results in relief of the extradural compression.

effective for patients with dorsal compression or multiple sites of involvement.

Preoperative Management

The dog is premedicated with IV methylprednisolone sodium succinate (30 mg/kg). IV fluids are administered throughout the procedure. Antibiotic therapy is dictated by criteria listed in Box 38-4 on p. 1403.

Anesthesia

Suggested anesthetic protocols for patients with cervical spinal disorders are described on p. 1402. Neurologic status and positioning for surgery are important preanesthetic considerations. If the patient has motor weakness (e.g., weakly ambulatory tetraparetic or nonambulatory tetraparetic) or requires positioning that may cause respiratory compromise (e.g., flexion of the neck or lateral compression of the chest), mechanical ventilatory support should be considered.

Surgical Anatomy

Anatomy of the cervical spine is described and illustrated on p. 1404 (see Fig. 38-1).

Positioning

For a ventral approach, position the animal in dorsal recumbency in a V-trough and carefully secure it to the table to prevent lateral motion. Patients with a dynamic lesion (e.g., chronic degenerative disk disease, hourglass compression, vertebral arch malformation, redundant ligamentum flavum) should be secured to the table with the neck in linear traction. This positioning results in spinal cord decompression. Patients requiring a dorsal approach are

placed in sternal recumbency. The use of dynamic positioning is based on patient classification and results of stress myelography. As a general rule, patients requiring dorsal decompression are positioned with the neck elevated and gently flexed over a rolled fleece or rigid vacuum type of apparatus.

SURGICAL TECHNIQUE
Decompression via a Ventral Slot

Perform a ventral slot procedure as described on p. 1405. Once the vertebral canal is reached, carefully remove redundant dorsal annulus fibrosus (dynamic lesion) or disk material (static lesion). Remove the ventral midline annulus or disk material first so as not to lacerate the vertebral venous sinus. Use ophthalmic forceps and a dental spatula to remove laterally located annular or disk fragments. Continue to remove tissue until the bluish hue of the spinal cord is visible, ensuring adequate decompression of the spinal cord. Lavage the surgical wound and close as described for a ventral slot procedure (see p. 1407).

Stabilization With Pins and Polymethylmethacrylate

This technique can be used to distract and stabilize up to two affected intervertebral spaces. Advantages of this technique include complete spinal cord decompression without entering the vertebral canal and reduced risk of iatrogenic spinal cord trauma. A neck brace is not required postoperatively and a favorable to excellent prognosis can be expected in most ambulatory patients (see Table 38-12).

> NOTE: This is the author's technique of choice for patients requiring dynamic ventral traction-stabilization.

Perform a ventral slot procedure at the affected intervertebral space or spaces to the level of the inner cortical layer (i.e., 75% transdiskal slot) (Fig. 38-45, A). Drill the slot no more than half the width of the vertebral body; slot length is determined by the thickness of the vertebral end plates. Discontinue burring once the cortical end plate of each vertebral body is removed. Place a modified Gelpi retractor (see later under the discussion of special instruments) in defects burred in the vertebral bodies, cranial and caudal to the affected vertebral bodies (Fig. 38-45, B). Create the defects just large enough to accept the blunted tips of the modified Gelpi retractor. Do not fenestrate the intervertebral spaces cranial and caudal to the affected vertebra for placement of the modified Gelpi vertebral spreader; caudal cervical fenestration may result in vertebral instability of the fenestrated space(s). Engage the Gelpi retractor and distract the affected intervertebral space no more than 2 to 3 mm. Harvest autogenous cancellous bone from the heads of the humeri and place just enough graft to fill the distracted slot. Insert two 7/64- or 1/8-inch Steinmann pins into the ventral surface of the vertebral body cranial to the affected intervertebral space. Use nonthreaded or positive profile threaded

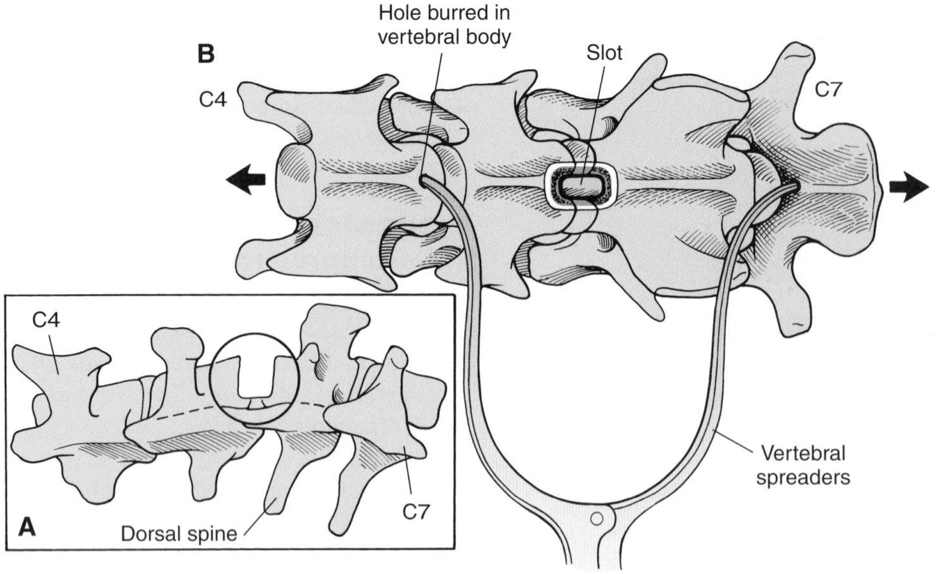

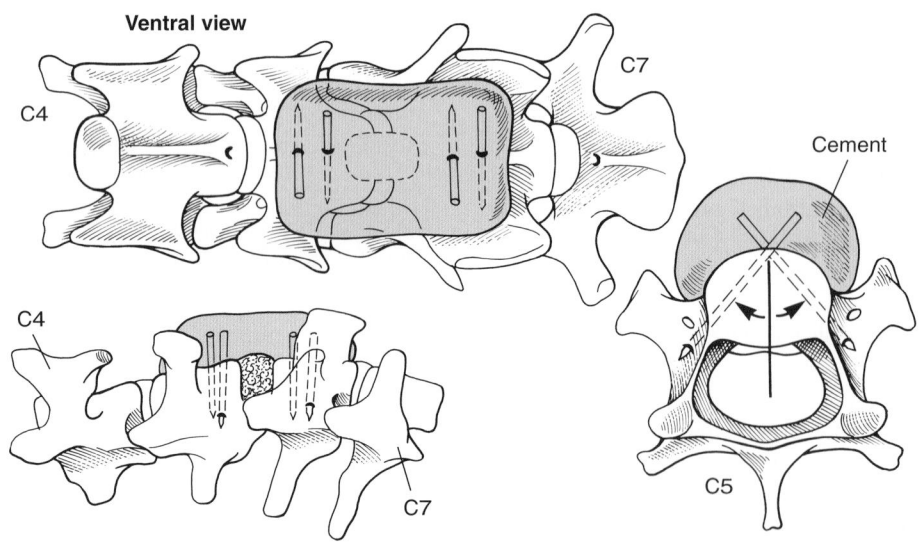

FIG. 38-45
A, To decompress the spinal cord, perform a 75% transdiskal ventral slot at the affected intervertebral space. **B,** Use vertebral spreaders to place the affected intervertebral space in 2- to 3-mm linear traction.

FIG. 38-46
Proper placement of Steinmann pins and PMMA to provide traction and stabilization of the affected intervertebral space.

pins. Insert the pins on the ventral midline of the vertebral body and direct them 30 to 35 degrees dorsolateral to avoid entering the vertebral canal (Fig. 38-46). It is important to engage two cortices with each pin. Cut the pins, leaving approximately 1.5 to 2 cm exposed. If the pins are not positive profile threaded pins, notch the exposed portion of each pin with pin cutters to allow the PMMA to grip the pin and prevent migration. Mix sterile PMMA powder with liquid monomer until it reaches a doughy consistency and can be

handled without sticking to your surgical gloves. Meticulously mold the PMMA around each pin; make sure each pin is completely surrounded and covered with PMMA (see Fig. 38-46). Irrigate the PMMA with sterile saline solution for 5 to 10 minutes to dissipate the heat of polymerization. Remove the vertebral spreaders after the PMMA has hardened. Close the paired longus colli muscles cranial and caudal to the PMMA mass. Close the remainder of the incision routinely.

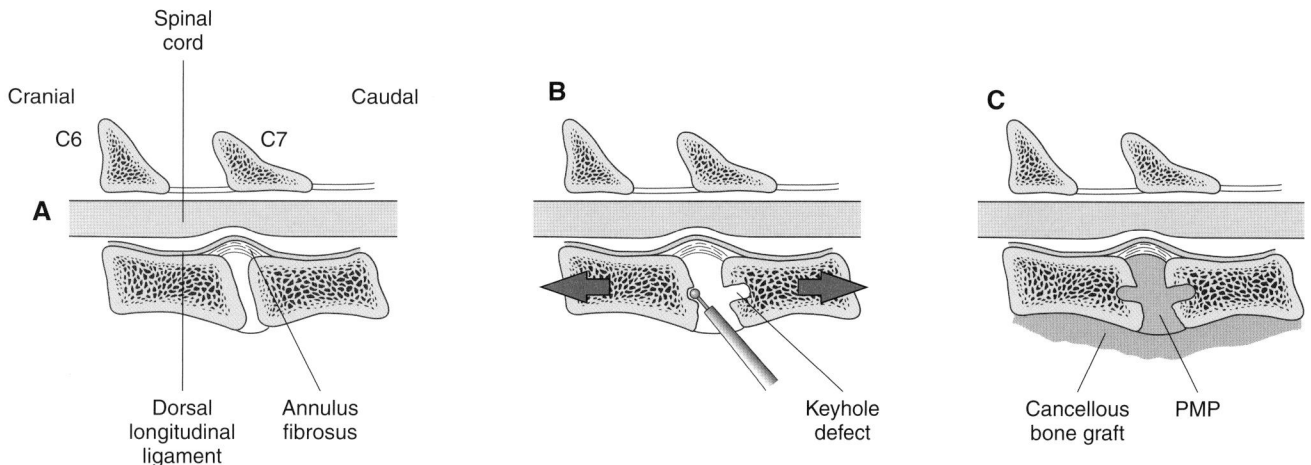

FIG. 38-47
Stabilization with interbody PMMA plug. **A,** Ligamentous hypertrophy resulting in spinal cord compression. **B,** A keyhole defect is made in the cranial and caudal endplates of the affected intervertebral space. **C,** After linear traction is applied to the spine, PMMA is placed in the defect. Once the PMMA has cured, autogenous cancellous bone harvested from the head of the humerus is placed over the exposed cement.

Stabilization With Interbody PMMA Plug

This technique can be used to distract and stabilize up to two affected intervertebral spaces (Fig. 38-47, *A*). Advantages of this technique include complete spinal cord decompression without entering the vertebral canal and reduced risk of iatrogenic spinal cord trauma. A neck brace is not required postoperatively, and a favorable to excellent prognosis can be expected in most ambulatory patients (see Table 38-12).

Identify and expose the affected intervertebral space as described for a ventral slot procedure on p. 1405. Create a fenestration in the affected intervertebral space with a No. 11 scalpel blade, and place the intervertebral space in distraction using a modified Gelpi retractor as described previously. Use a high-speed pneumatic drill to remove annulus fibrosus and end plate cartilage from the vertebral end plates. Leave 3 to 5 mm of the dorsal annulus and bony end plates of each affected disk space intact. With the intervertebral space distracted, use a high-speed pneumatic drill with a 2- to 4-mm burr to create a keyhole defect in the vertebral end plates (Fig. 38-47, B).

Because of the caudoventral to craniodorsal slope of the intervertebral space, the cranial end plate of the caudal vertebra is readily observed, allowing a keyhole of approximately 5 to 10 mm in lateral width × 4 mm in dorsoventral width × 4 mm in depth. Drilling the caudal end plate of the cranial vertebra is accomplished blindly and thus a smaller keyhole often results.

NOTE: This technique is useful in patients with two adjacent lesions (generally C5–C6 and C6–C7).

Inject PMMA in a semiliquid state into the keyhole defect while maintaining the intervertebral space in distraction (Fig. 38-47, C). Apply digital pressure to ensure that the keyhole defect is filled to the level of the ventral aspect of the vertebral bodies. Cool exposed PMMA with room temperature sterile saline lavage until the exothermic reaction is complete and the PMMA is hardened. Harvest an autogenous cancellous bone graft from the heads of the humeri, and place it over exposed ventral surfaces of the vertebral bodies and PMMA. Appose the longus colli muscles over the bone graft to hold it in place. Close the remainder of the incision routinely.

Stabilization With Polyvinylidene Spinal Plates

Advantages of this technique over ventral slot decompression alone include adequate spinal cord decompression without entering the vertebral canal, reduced risk of iatrogenic spinal cord trauma, and improved recovery. Disadvantages include high incidence of implant failure in patients that do not tolerate a neck brace, need for a donor or bone bank, time necessary for allograft incorporation into an interbody fusion, and inability to provide adequate stabilization in patients with multiple lesions.

Identify the affected intervertebral space, and perform a ventral slot procedure as described on p. 1405; however, carry the slot only to the level of the inner cortical layer (i.e., a 75% transdiskal slot) (see Fig. 38-45, A). Place the affected intervertebral space in approximately 2- to 3-mm linear traction using modified Gelpi retractors as described for pins and PMMA stabilization (see Fig. 38-45, B). Create the slot configuration to precisely accommodate a

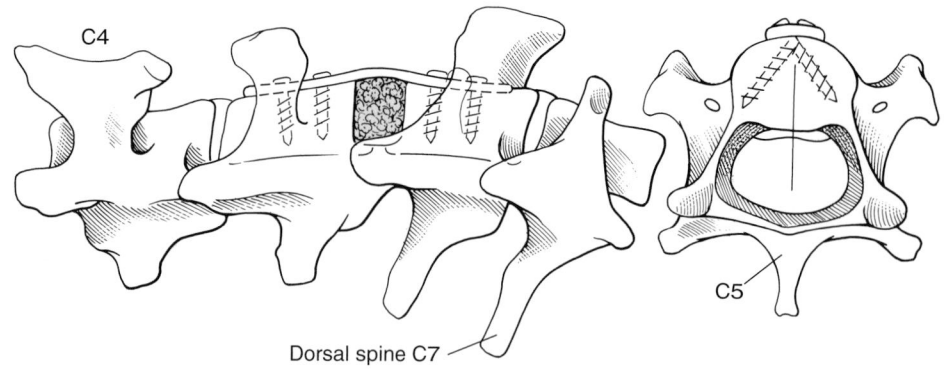

FIG. 38-48
Proper placement of full cortical allograft and polyvinylidene spinal plate to provide traction and stabilization of the affected intervertebral space.

full cortical allograft harvested from the distal third of the tibia of a 15- to 20-lb donor.

The graft maintains the intervertebral space in linear traction, resulting in spinal cord decompression.

Pack the cortical allograft with autogenous cancellous bone harvested from the heads of the humeri before placement in the slot. Once the graft is in place, remove the vertebral spreader. Place the polyvinylidene spinal plate on the ventral surface of the adjacent vertebral bodies to secure the bone graft in the slot. Secure the plate with two screws placed in each vertebral body. Drill and tap holes at a 20- to 25-degree angle from the midline to prevent vertebral canal penetration (Fig. 38-48). Determine screw length by assessing vertebral body width and depth from cervical spinal radiographs. Place autogenous cancellous bone on the ventral surface of the plate. Suture the paired longus colli muscles over the autogenous cancellous bone to hold it in place. Close the remainder of the incision routinely.

Decompression via Dorsal Laminectomy

Identify and expose the dorsal aspect of affected vertebrae as described for dorsal laminectomy on p. 1409. After exposure of the cervical vertebrae, identify affected vertebrae (see the discussion of unique anatomic landmarks of the cervical spine on p. 1404). Remove dorsal spinous processes and laminae with rongeurs and a high-speed surgical burr, respectively.

The laminectomy defect may be from three-quarters the length of each vertebra to a continuous laminectomy extending from C3-C7, depending on the extent of the compressive lesion.

Limit the width of the laminectomy to the medial aspect of the articular facets of the cranial vertebra (Fig. 38-49). First burr the lamina to the level of the periosteum of the inner cortical layer. Use a dental or iris spatula to carefully penetrate the periosteal layer and enter the vertebral canal (see Fig. 38-24 on p. 1414). Use an ophthalmic forceps and No. 11 scalpel

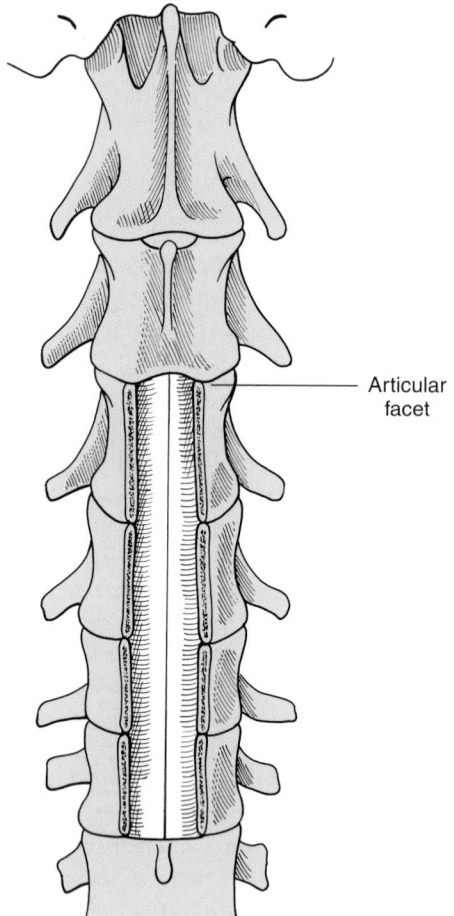

FIG. 38-49
Perform dorsal laminectomy at multiple intervertebral spaces to decompress the spinal cord, if necessary.

blade to gently excise and remove the ligamentum flavum en bloc. If lateral compression exists, use rongeurs to resect the lateral aspects of the vertebral arches to the level of the vertebral artery and vein. Resect hypertrophied joint capsule and ligamentum flavum to achieve lateral decompression of the spinal cord. Place transarticular lag screws for vertebral stabilization if necessary. Drill an appropriate-size hole

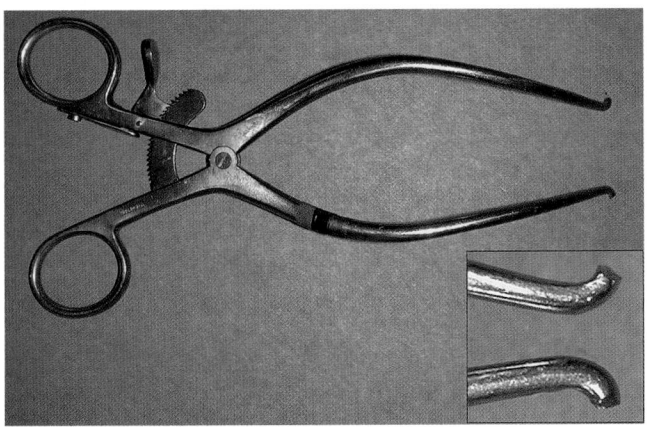

FIG. 38-50
Vertebral spreaders made by cutting the tips off of Gelpi retractors.

through the cranial and caudal articular facets bilaterally. Remove articular cartilage using a high-speed surgical burr, tap the hole, and place a lag screw. Place cancellous bone around the joints to promote arthrodesis. Place an autogenous fat graft over the laminectomy site to help prevent formation of a fibrous laminectomy membrane that could result in spinal cord compression. Approximate paraspinal muscles and fascia; close remaining tissue routinely.

SUTURE MATERIALS AND SPECIAL INSTRUMENTS

See p. 1417 and Table 38-1 for surgical instruments for exposure of the cervical spine. Modified Gelpi retractors with blunted ends are useful for distracting affected vertebrae during stabilization procedures and are made by removing the hooked tips of a Gelpi retractor (Fig. 38-50).

POSTOPERATIVE CARE AND ASSESSMENT

Immediate postoperative care includes administration of IV fluids and analgesics, monitoring cardiovascular and respiratory function, measurement of abdominal girth every 4 hours for 24 hours (i.e., for gastric dilatation-volvulus), and monitoring for seizures (particularly if the patient had immediate preoperative myelography). Steroids should be discontinued immediately after surgery and the neck collar replaced with a body harness.

Postoperative use of a neck brace is generally dictated by the technique chosen and by patient cooperation. Patients that have ventral traction-stabilization using plastic spinal plates or Harrington rods should wear a neck brace for the first 4 to 6 weeks postoperatively. Neck braces should not be used in patients that do not tolerate them because these animals may damage the implant while fighting the presence of the neck brace. These patients should be strictly confined to cages.

Postoperative management of ambulatory patients includes strict confinement with harness walks two to three times daily for the first 2 to 3 weeks, then a gradual increase in exercise over the next 6 to 8 weeks. Slippery surfaces should be avoided. Postoperative management of nonambulatory patients includes physiotherapy (passive range-of-motion exercises), hydrotherapy (swimming), and the use of a supporting cart until the dog has regained the ability to walk.

Patients undergoing dorsal laminectomy procedures are often nonambulatory postoperatively. Return to ambulatory function generally occurs in several days or weeks.

Supporting carts can be constructed from plastic pipe and fabric. Neoprene, nylon, or leather harnesses are useful in weakly ambulatory patients. Special attention to good nursing care of recumbent patients is necessary to prevent decubital ulcers, urinary tract infections, and/or pneumonia. Heavily padded, dry bedding or waterbeds may prevent decubital ulcers.

Patients should be assessed initially by immediate postoperative radiographs to evaluate implants and by neurologic examination 48 hours after surgery. Long-term assessment includes radiographic evaluation at 3, 6, 9, and 12 months postoperatively and neurologic examinations as needed, depending on status (i.e., generally daily until ambulatory, then 1, 2, 3, 6, 9, and 12 months postoperatively).

COMPLICATIONS

Complications may be short term (e.g., immediate postoperative to 1 month) or long term (e.g., greater than 1 month) and vary between procedures. Short-term complications and their most likely causes are listed in Table 38-13. The most common long-term complication in patients treated with ventral slot procedures or ventral traction-stabilization for chronic degenerative disk disease, vertebral tipping, or hourglass compression is development of a second compressive lesion at the interspace adjacent to the previously affected interspace. It is presumed that once an intervertebral space is fused, stress at the adjacent interspaces is increased. It is possible that this increased stress encourages development of spinal instability and subsequent spinal cord compression in some patients or that some patients have a predisposition to disk degeneration in the lower cervical spine that encourages a second lesion. Whatever the cause, this phenomenon is referred to as the *domino effect,* and it may occur in as many as one fourth of patients within 5 to 60 months postoperatively (Fig. 38-51). It is also important to avoid fenestrating the intervertebral spaces cranial and caudal to the affected interspace for placement of vertebral spreaders. Fenestration may cause spinal instability and predispose the patient to a second (domino) lesion.

PROGNOSIS

Prognosis for patients treated conservatively is guarded, but also depends on classification, severity of neurologic signs, and number of lesions (see Table 38-11). The prognosis for surgically treated patients is dependent on disease classification, severity of neurologic deficit, number of lesions, method of therapy available, and quality of aftercare (see Table 38-13).

FIG. 38-51

Interbody fusion from a previous traction stabilization procedure may cause increased stress on the intervertebral spaces cranial and caudal to the fused space. This may result in instability and formation of a second lesion at these stressed spaces.

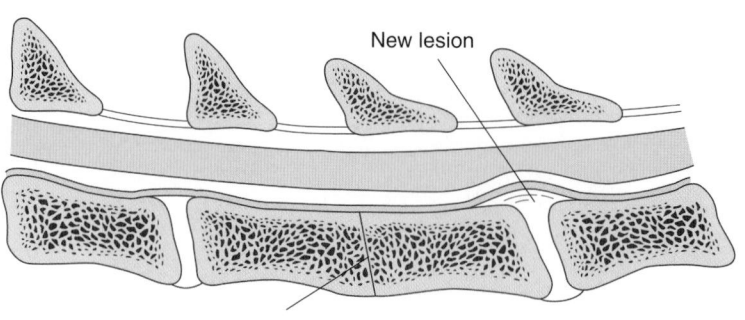

New lesion

Fusion of old lesion

 Table 38-13

Short-Term Postoperative Complications in Wobbler Patients

CLASSIFICATION	SURGICAL TECHNIQUE	SHORT-TERM COMPLICATION	CAUSE OF COMPLICATION
Chronic degenerative disk disease, vertebral tipping, hourglass compression	Steinmann pins and PMMA	Deteriorating neurologic status	Pin in vertebral canal; implant failure
		Pin fracture	Insufficient confinement; pin too small
		Pin migration	Unnotched pin; did not cover pin with PMMA
		PMMA fracture	Never reported
		Implant pulls off vertebrae	Improper angle of pin placement; did not engage two cortices with pins
	Polyvinylidene spinal plates	Deteriorating neurologic status	Screw in vertebral canal; implant failure
		Screw loosening	Insufficient confinement; neck brace not worn
	Harrington rod	Deteriorating neurologic status	Hook in vertebral canal; implant failure
		Rod loosens or slips off	Insufficient confinement; neck brace not worn
	Ventral slot	Deteriorating neurologic status	Slot excessively wide; slot caused spinal instability; entire compressive mass not removed; insufficient confinement
	Dorsal laminectomy	Deteriorating neurologic status	Laminectomy caused increased instability; excessive spinal cord manipulation; insufficient confinement
Ligamentum flavum hypertrophy/vertebral arch Malformation	Dorsal laminectomy	Deteriorating neurologic status	Laminectomy caused increased instability; excessive spinal cord manipulation; inappropriate articular facet stabilization

PMMA, Polymethylmethacrylate.

References

De Risio L, Munana K, Morray M et al: Dorsal laminectomy for caudal cervical spondylomyelopathy: post operative recovery and long-term follow-up in 20 dogs, *Vet Surg* 31:418-427, 2002.

Penderis J, Dennis R: Use of traction during magnetic resonance imaging of caudal cervical spondylomyelopathy ("wobbler syndrome") in the dog, *Vet Rad Ultrasound* 45:3, 216, 2004.

Suggested Reading

Jeffery ND, McKee WM: Surgery for disk-associated wobbler syndrome in the dog—an examination of the controversy, *J Small Anim Pract* 41:574-581, 2001.

This report suggests that wobbler syndrome should be considered a multifactorial disorder. Statistical analysis revealed no significant differences in success rates between the various reported decompressive surgical techniques.

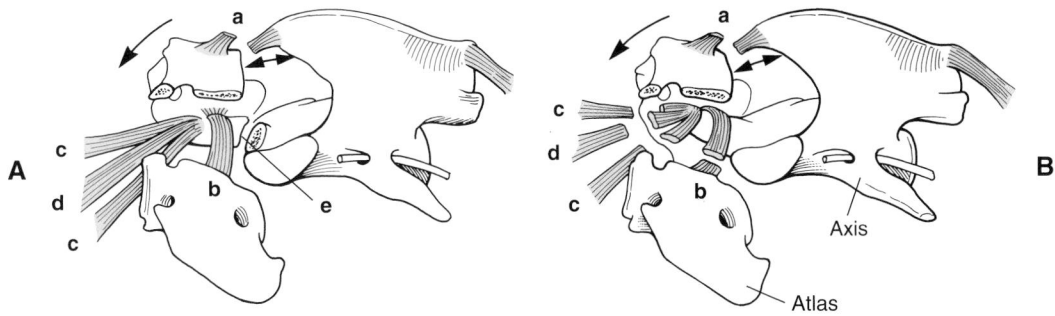

FIG. 38-52
Ligamentous structures associated with the atlantoaxial joint. **A,** Fracture of the dens and rupture of the atlantoaxial ligament result in instability. *(a)* Dorsal atlantoaxial ligament, *(b)* transverse ligament, *(c)* alar ligaments (paired), *(d)* apical ligament, *(e)* fracture and/or malformation of the dens. **B,** Rupture of ligamentous supporting structures of the atlantoaxial joint causes atlantoaxial instability. *(a)* Dorsal atlantoaxial ligament, *(b)* transverse ligament, *(c)* paired alar ligaments, and *(d)* apical ligament.

ATLANTOAXIAL INSTABILITY

DEFINITIONS

Atlantoaxial instability is an alteration of the dens and/or ligaments that span the multifaceted, diarthrodial atlantoaxial articulation and cause instability, vertebral subluxation, and subsequent spinal cord and nerve root compression. Atlantoaxial instability is also known as *atlantoaxial subluxation* and *atlantoaxial luxation.*

GENERAL CONSIDERATIONS AND CLINICALLY RELEVANT PATHOPHYSIOLOGY

Atlantoaxial instability is probably a congenital and/or developmental problem resulting in an unstable articulation between the first two cervical vertebrae. Laxity may result from fracture, absence, hypoplasia, or malformation of the dens, resulting in a nonfunctional attachment of alar, apical, and/or transverse ligaments (Fig. 38-52, *A*), or improper formation, laxity, or rupture of the alar, apical, transverse, or dorsal atlantoaxial ligaments, resulting in lack of ligamentous support between the atlas and axis (Fig. 38-52, *B*). Trauma may elicit clinical signs in animals with laxity as a result of these causes. Instability predisposes the patient to spinal cord and nerve root compression, often resulting in neck pain and ambulatory to nonambulatory tetraparesis.

DIAGNOSIS
Clinical Presentation

Signalment. Atlantoaxial instability primarily occurs in toy-breed dogs. It has occasionally been reported in large-breed dogs and rarely in cats. A majority of the dogs are younger than 1 year of age. Dogs that have clinical signs at an older age generally have had instability since birth, but recent trauma has caused significant spinal cord and nerve root compression.

History. Progressive tetraparesis and incoordination, often associated with neck pain, are expected. Acute presentations can occur after seemingly minor trauma. Owners may report that the dog dislikes having its head touched.

Physical Examination Findings

General physical examination findings are usually normal. Neurologic examination reveals a dog with motor weakness and UMN signs to the front and hind legs. Patients have varying degrees of neck pain. Ventral flexion of the head will often exacerbate neck pain and may worsen the neurologic condition. Care must be exercised during cervical flexion because the dens (if present) can cause spinal cord compression. Forceful flexion must be prevented at all times.

> NOTE: *Do not* forcefully flex the neck of these patients. Flexing the neck may exacerbate neurologic deficits.

Diagnostic Imaging

A preliminary lateral radiograph without anesthesia allows diagnosis of atlantoaxial instability with significant subluxation (Fig. 38-53). A flexed lateral view of the anesthetized animal may be necessary to reveal increased laxity and subluxation of C1-C2. The primary radiographic finding is an increased distance between the dorsal arch of C1 and the dorsal spinous process of C2. A gap of more than 4 to 5 mm between the lamina of C1 and dorsal spine of C2 is usually diagnostic in a small-breed dog (see Fig. 38-53). Ventrodorsal and open-mouth views may show absence or fractionation of the dens. Because the open-mouth view requires flexion of the neck, it is not recommended. Cross-sectional imaging (CT or MRI) can be used to further define the anatomy of the dens, but is usually not necessary for the diagnosis.

Laboratory Findings

Laboratory findings in patients with atlantoaxial instability are generally normal. Young patients or those previously treated with corticosteroids may have slight elevations in serum alkaline phosphatase activity.

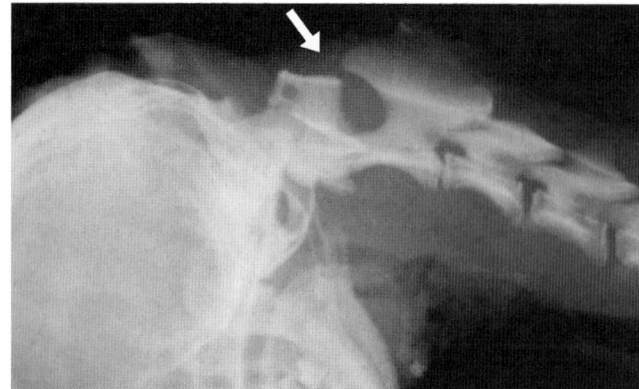

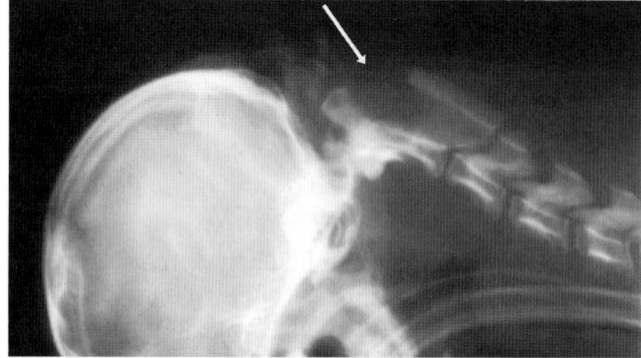

FIG. 38-53

A, Lateral survey radiograph of a normal dog with the neck in ventral flexion. Notice the distance between the dorsal lamina of C1 and dorsal spine of C2 *(arrow)*. **B,** Lateral survey radiograph of a dog with atlantoaxial instability; the neck is in ventral flexion. Notice the distance between the dorsal lamina of C1 and dorsal spine of C2 *(arrow)*. This gap is diagnostic of atlantoaxial instability.

DIFFERENTIAL DIAGNOSIS

Presumptive diagnosis of atlantoaxial instability is made in young, toy-breed dogs with a history of neck pain and acute or progressive, ambulatory or nonambulatory, UMN tetraparesis. Diagnosis of atlantoaxial instability and exclusion of fracture and/or luxation is confirmed by survey radiography.

MEDICAL MANAGEMENT

Medical treatment consisting of strict confinement for 6 to 8 weeks, a neck brace that maintains the neck and head in extension, and short-term corticosteroids may alleviate symptoms. The neck brace, constructed of padded splint material, such as fiberglass casting material, must be worn during the 6 to 8 weeks of confinement, ensuring maximum scar tissue formation. Corticosteroids (e.g., dexamethasone, 0.2 to 1.1 mg/kg intramuscularly [IM] bid) may be used for 24 to 48 hours. Nonsurgical management of dogs with atlantoaxial instability by use of a cervical splint or bandage is associated with a good long-term outcome in greater than 60% of cases. Dogs with an acute onset of clinical signs that have no prior history of neurologic disease, young dogs with immature bone in which surgical fixation may not provide ade-

quate stability, and dogs for which there are financial constraints should be considered as candidates for nonsurgical management (Havig et al, 2005).

SURGICAL TREATMENT

Surgical correction of atlantoaxial instability is indicated when there is a chronic history of clinical signs (greater than 30 days), when clinical signs have relapsed or nonsurgical treatment has failed, and in patients with mature bone capable of supporting surgical implants. In general, surgical management is more likely to be successful if (1) the animal is less than 2 years of age, (2) duration of clinical signs is greater than 30 days, and (3) the animal is ambulatory preoperatively. Objectives of surgery include reduction of atlantoaxial subluxation, decompression of spinal cord and nerve roots, and atlantoaxial joint stabilization. Surgical techniques for decompression and stabilization fall into two major categories (i.e., dorsal and ventral). A ventral approach with placement of Kirschner wires and bone cement (see p. 1443) is preferred by the author.

Preoperative Management

The animal should be given IV fluids and steroids before surgery. Steroids are given to protect the spinal cord from the possible traumatic effects of surgical manipulation. The steroid of choice is methylprednisolone sodium succinate (30 mg/kg IV). Serum glucose concentrations should be assessed before, during (every 30 to 60 minutes), and after surgery in toy breeds. Supplementation with dextrose-containing fluids may be necessary during surgery.

Anesthesia

See p. 1402 for suggested anesthetic protocols for use in dogs with cervical spinal disorders. The patient's neurologic status and positioning for surgery are important preanesthetic considerations. If the patient has motor weakness (e.g., ambulatory tetraparesis, weakly ambulatory tetraparesis, or nonambulatory tetraparesis) or will require positioning that may cause respiratory compromise, mechanical ventilatory support should be considered. Trauma to the cranial cervical spinal cord during reduction of the atlantoaxial instability may cause transient respiratory arrest. Ventilatory support during surgical manipulation of atlantoaxial subluxation is therefore recommended. Care should be taken to prevent hypothermia, and these animals should be actively rewarmed after surgery.

> NOTE: Use extreme care during intubation to prevent excessive neck manipulation in these patients.

Surgical Anatomy

The cervical spine is unique in its variable anatomic configuration from vertebra to vertebra, particularly C1-C2 (see Figs. 38-1 and 38-3 on p. 1404 and p. 1405). Important anatomic variations during surgical repair of atlantoaxial instability are listed in Table 38-14.

Table 38-14

Anatomic Variation of the Atlas and Axis Important to Surgical Repair of Atlantoaxial Instability

VERTEBRAE	ANATOMY	SURGICAL SIGNIFICANCE
C1–atlas	Thin dorsal arch (laminae); no dorsal spinous process	Poor implant-holding power dorsally
	No vertebral body, just thin ventral fovea	Poor implant-holding power ventrally
	Ventrolateral diarthrodial joints	Good purchase for implants ventrally; used to evaluate anatomic reduction
	Prominent ventral tubercle	Landmark for surgical localization
	Prominent wings	Moderate implant-holding power dorsally and ventrally
C2–axis	Prominent dorsal spinous process	Moderate implant-holding power dorsally, patient age and size dependent; landmark for surgical localization
	Thin central vertebral body	Poor implant-holding power ventrally
	Prominent cranial articular processes	Good purchase for implants ventrally; used to evaluate anatomic reduction
	Prominent caudal vertebral body	Good ventral purchase for implants
	Dens	May fracture or displace into vertebral canal
C1–C2	Bilateral ventrolateral diarthrodial joints	Good purchase for implants ventrally; used to evaluate anatomic reduction
	Dorsal atlantoaxial ligament	Moderate purchase of implants used to replace the ligament

Positioning

Patients undergoing a ventral approach are positioned as described for ventral slot procedure on p. 1405 (see also Fig. 38-5 on p. 1406). The neck is placed in a slightly extended position and is fixed in mild linear traction. This position encourages reduction of the subluxation and helps decompress the spinal cord and nerve roots. An area from the intermandibular space to the caudal cervical region, including the heads of the humeri, is aseptically prepared. Patients undergoing a dorsal approach should be positioned in sternal recumbency with the head and neck slightly flexed (see Fig. 38-17 on p. 1410). An area from the occiput to the caudal cervical region is aseptically prepared.

SURGICAL TECHNIQUE
Dorsal Stabilization

The dorsal approach allows reduction of the subluxation and fixation of the dorsal lamina of C1 to the dorsal spine of C2. Bony decompression is provided by hemilaminectomy or reduction of the subluxation. Hemilaminectomy provides dorsal spinal cord decompression, but does not correct the instability or relieve ventral spinal cord compression; in fact, it reduces stability of the fixation. Thus it is not recommended. Rigid immobilization using dorsal lamina of C1-C2 is often unrewarding. Reduction of the luxation and immobilization of the vertebra, without hemilaminectomy, provide adequate decompression. Dorsal fixation is generally provided by a loop of orthopedic wire, synthetic suture material, or autogenous graft (i.e., nuchal ligament). Regardless of the material chosen, it is passed under the lamina of C1, over the spinal cord, and tied to two holes drilled in the dorsal spine of C2. The fixation relies on fibrous tissue to form a solid union. Frequent postoperative complications

with this technique are possible, including breakdown of the suture or bone and tearing out of the suture with minimal strain because the dorsal arch of the atlas and dorsal spinous process of the axis in young toy-breed dogs have the consistency and strength of wet cardboard. Continued micromotion at the atlantoaxial joint may cause the wire to fatigue and break. Additionally, improper placement of fixation material may result in spinal cord trauma. Inadequate reduction of the subluxation and inappropriate stabilization, especially if used in conjunction with hemilaminectomy, are possible.

Perform a dorsal approach to the cranial cervical spine as described on p. 1410. Periosteally elevate epaxial muscle from the dorsal lamina of the atlas and dorsal spine, lamina, and pedicles of the axis. Carefully incise the atlantoaxial fascia caudal to the arch of the atlas and enter the epidural space. Incise the atlantooccipital fascia cranial to the arch of the atlas and enter the epidural space. Gently thread a loop of 25-gauge orthopedic wire under the arch of the atlas in a cranial-to-caudal direction. Thread the suture material through this loop of orthopedic wire, and gently pull it under the arch of the atlas (Fig. 38-54, A). Drill two holes in the dorsal spinous process of the axis, and pass the ends of the suture material through the holes; one from right to left and the other from left to right. Reduce the atlantoaxial joint and tie the suture ends to maintain reduction (Fig. 38-54, B). Close muscle, subcutaneous tissue, and skin routinely.

Ventral Stabilization

The ventral approach allows accurate anatomic reduction for decompression; use of transarticular pins for stability (placed in the most solid portion of the atlas and axis);

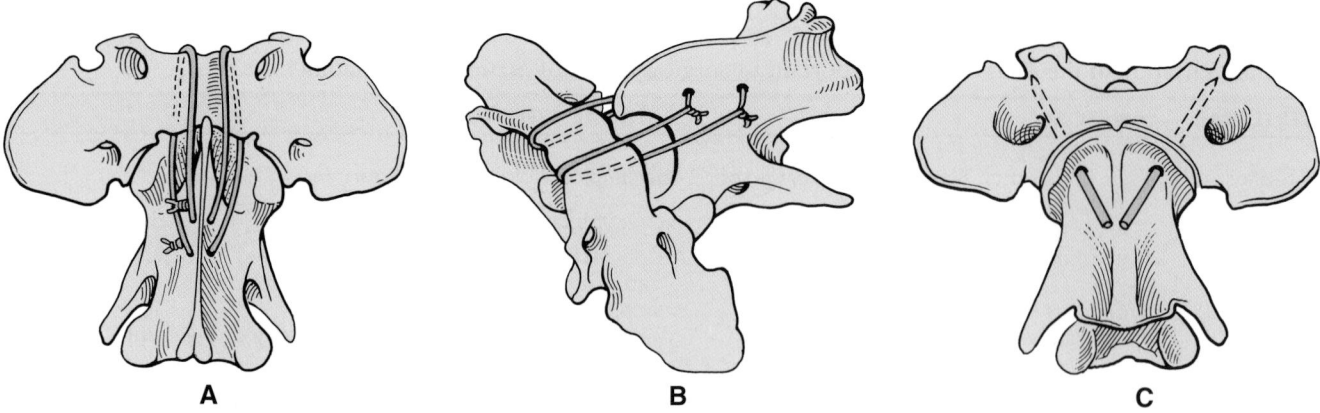

FIG. 38-54
A, For dorsal stabilization of atlantoaxial subluxation, pass wire or suture material under the dorsal arch of C1. **B,** Pass the wire or suture material through holes drilled in the dorsal spine of C2 and secure it. **C,** For ventral stabilization, place Kirschner wires across the atlantoaxial joints.

placement of an autogenous cancellous bone graft to encourage atlantoaxial arthrodesis; and odontoidectomy if indicated (e.g., in the case of a malformed dens). The technique is easy, fast, safe, and effective and involves the placement of Kirschner wires or screws across the C1-C2 articulation (Fig. 38-54, *C*). Placement of Kirschner wires is described later. Screws may be used instead of pins, especially in large-breed dogs with traumatic subluxation. The most common complication has been pin migration. This is effectively prevented by applying PMMA to the exposed portion of the Kirschner pins. Even though this fixation is not on the tension band side, it provides superior fixation to the dorsal approach. Complications associated with the ventral approach include laryngeal paralysis, inappropriate placement of implants causing spinal cord compression or an unstable fixation, implant failure, difficulty swallowing secondary to PMMA mass, and respiratory compromise during the immediate postoperative course.

Approach to the ventral aspect of C1-C2 is as described for ventral slot procedure on p. 1405. Periosteally elevate longus colli muscles from the ventral aspect of the atlas and axis. Be careful not to cause excessive motion of the atlantoaxial joint during exposure. Identify and open the paired atlantoaxial joints. Dissect the joint capsule from the ventral aspect of the vertebral bodies with a No. 15 scalpel blade to visualize articular cartilage. Use an ASIF small fragment forceps or towel clamp to grasp the midbody of C2 (Fig. 38-55). Place caudal traction on C2 to open the atlantoaxial joint, enabling safe removal of articular cartilage. Use a bone curette or high-speed pneumatic drill to remove approximately 50% of the articular surface bilaterally. Expose the head of the humerus, drill a one-eighth-inch Steinmann pin through the outer cortex, and introduce a No. 0 curette to harvest cancellous bone. Transfer the bone graft

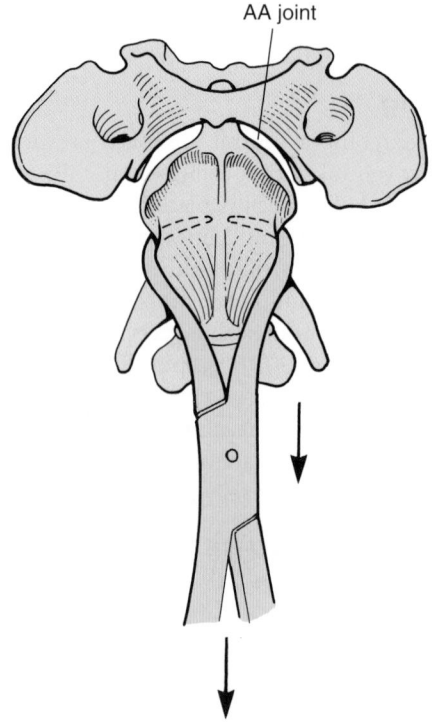

AA joint

FIG. 38-55
Use orthopedic reduction forceps to grasp the body of C2. Use traction and countertraction to reduce the atlantoaxial subluxation.

to the scarified atlantoaxial joints, and reduce the subluxation using the reduction forceps or towel clamps. Select two appropriate-sized, nonthreaded Kirschner wires (0.625 inch or 0.45 inch) or acrylic fixation pins. Start the first pin close to the midline on the caudoventral body of the axis. Direct the pin medial toward the alar notch on the cranial edge of

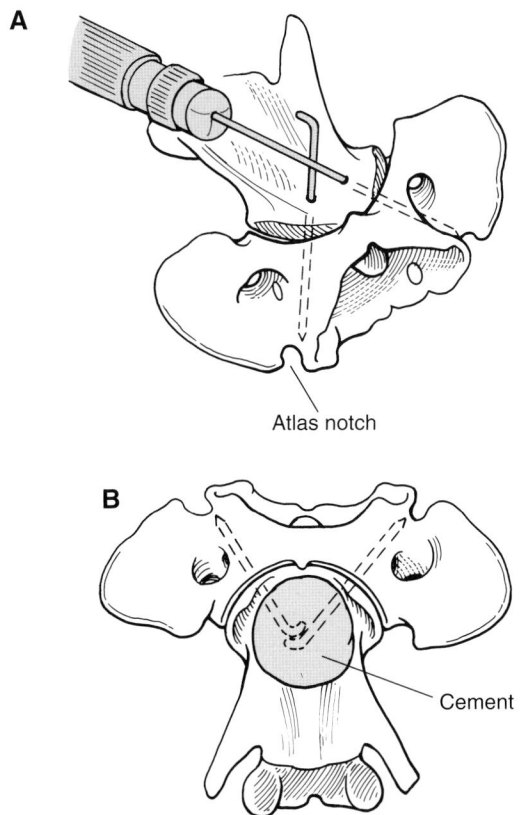

FIG. 38-56
A, Place Kirschner wires in cross-pin fashion; wires are directed toward the alar notch to ensure proper placement. **B,** Notch or bend the exposed ends of the Kirschner wires. Mold PMMA around both pin ends.

the atlas, with the point of the pin angled ventrally (Fig. 38-56, A). An air-driven or electric drill facilitates accurate and easy pin placement. Place the second pin through the opposite joint using similar landmarks. Cut the pins, leaving approximately 5 to 7 mm protruding from the body of C2, and notch or slightly bend the exposed pin. Carefully mold PMMA to incorporate both pins (Fig. 38-56, B). Lavage the PMMA with cool saline to dissipate the heat of polymerization. Close muscle, subcutaneous tissue, and skin routinely.

Several alternative atlantoaxial stabilization techniques using ventral screws, pins, orthopedic wire, and PMMA have been developed (Platt et al, 2004; Sanders et al, 2004). These techniques are similar to the cross pin technique described previously; however, implant placement is designed to distribute forces over a greater implant-bone surface area with a longer moment arm to reduce the risk of joint fixation failure.

Approach to the ventral aspect of C1-C2 is as described for a ventral slot procedure on p. 1405.

Periosteally elevate the longus colli muscles from the ventral aspect of the atlas and axis. Be careful not to cause excessive motion of the atlantoaxial joint during exposure. Identify and open the paired atlantoaxial joints. Dissect the joint capsule

from the ventral aspect of the vertebral bodies with a No. 15 scalpel blade to visualize articular cartilage. Place a 1.5 or 2.0 mm cortical bone screw in the caudal aspect of the body of C2. Estimate screw length from the lateral radiograph to allow the head and a short segment of the threaded portion to remain exposed with the tip of the screw in the dorsal cortex (Fig. 38-57, A). Place a second screw in the cranial aspect of C2. Twist orthopedic wire around the heads of both screws to facilitate traction and reduction of the C1-C2 joint (Fig. 38-57, B). Maintain traction and reduction while passing two transarticular Kirschner wires across the atlantoaxial joints as described previously (Fig. 38-57, C). Remove the orthopedic wire. Next, place three additional 1.5 to 2.0 mm cortical screws in the ventral arch of C1. Leave the heads and a short segment of the threaded portion of the screws exposed. Place a cancellous bone graft from the head of the humeri in the joint space. Mold PMMA over the exposed ends of the implants, and lavage with room-temperature sterile saline to dissipate the heat of polymerization. Close the longus colli muscle over the implant if possible. Close muscle, subcutaneous tissue, and skin routinely.

An alternate technique is to place multiple screws in a slightly different pattern as described previously and attach a Kirschner wire to the protruding heads (Fig. 38-58). Screws, Kirschner wires, and orthopedic wire are incorporated in PMMA, thus providing rigid fixation of the atlantoaxial joint.

SUTURE MATERIALS AND SPECIAL INSTRUMENTS

When using the dorsal approach, braided polyester suture, nonabsorbable monofilament suture, or orthopedic wire is a recommended fixation material. For the ventral approach, PMMA is needed to prevent pin migration, and small fragment forceps or towel clamps aid in reduction and stabilization during pin placement.

POSTOPERATIVE CARE AND ASSESSMENT

Patients with atlantoaxial instability should be evaluated postoperatively in a similar fashion as patients with other cervical spinal disorders. Because of the anatomic configuration of C1-C2 in young toy breeds, any form of fixation should be considered marginal. Regardless of whether a dorsal or ventral approach is used, all forms of internal fixation should be supported with a neck brace, and strict cage confinement should be enforced until radiographic evidence of union.

PROGNOSIS

The prognosis for young patients with a first episode and an acute onset of clinical signs (regardless of severity of neurologic deficits at admission) that are treated medically is favorable. The prognosis for patients treated surgically using a dorsal or ventral approach is related to implant success or failure. If implants fail, the prognosis is unfavorable; if implants succeed, the prognosis is favorable.

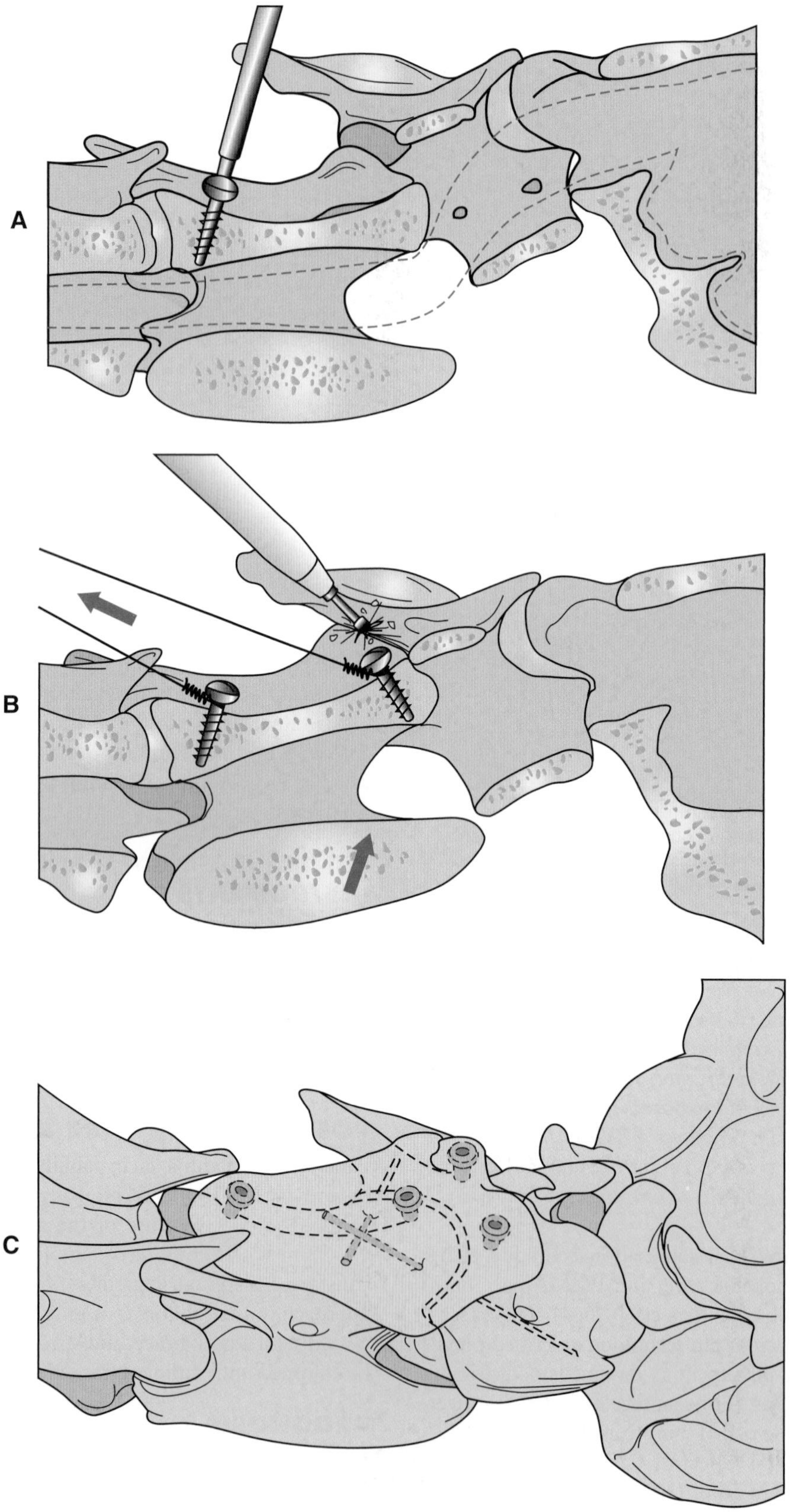

FIG. 38-57
A, Place a cortical bone screw in the caudal aspect of the body of C2. **B,** Place a second screw in the cranial aspect of C2. Twist orthopedic wire around the heads of the screws to facilitate traction and reduction of the C1–C2 joint. **C,** Pass two transarticular Kirschner wires across the atlantoaxial joints. Place three additional cortical screws in the ventral arch of C1. Mold PMMA over the exposed ends of all implants.

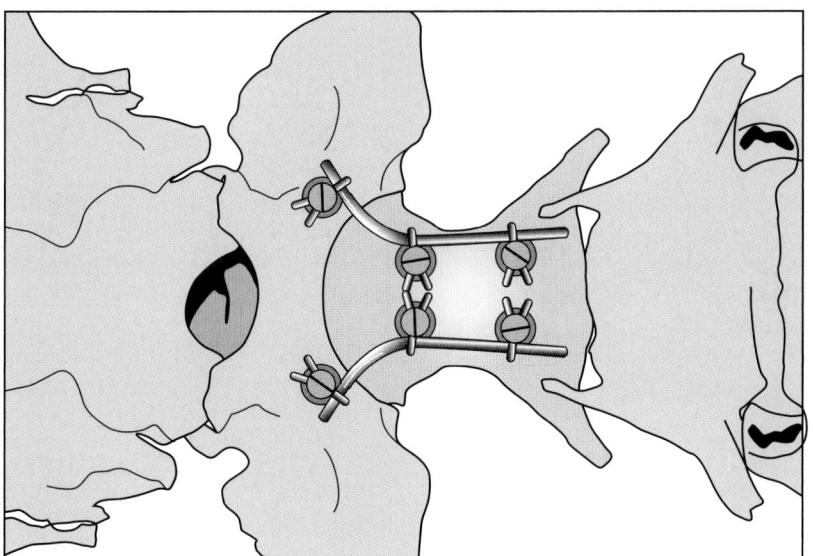

FIG. 38-58
Multiple cortical screws with Kirschner pins wired to the base of the screw heads can be used for atlantoaxial stabilization. Screws wires and pins are incorporated with PMMA.

References

Platt SR, Chambers JN, Cross A: A modified ventral fixation for surgical management of atlantoaxial subluxation on 19 dogs, *Vet Surg* 33:349, 2004.

Sanders SF, Bagley RS, Silver GM et al: Outcomes and complications associated with ventral screws, pins, and polymethyl methylmethacrylate for atlantoaxial instability in 12 dogs, *J Am Anim Hosp Assoc* 40:204, 2004.

Suggested Reading

Beaver DP et al: Risk factors affecting the outcome of surgery for atlantoaxial subluxation in dogs: 46 cases (1978-1998), *J Am Vet Med Assoc* 216:1104, 2000.

Risk factors, such as age of onset and duration of clinical signs, and degree of neurologic impairment tend to influence outcomes of surgery for patients with atlantoaxial instability.

FRACTURES AND LUXATIONS OF THE CERVICAL SPINE

DEFINITIONS

Traumatic or pathologic disruption of osseous and supporting soft tissue structures of the cervical spine may result in **vertebral fracture** or **luxation** and subsequent spinal cord and nerve root compression. Fractures of the cervical vertebrae are also known as *cervical fractures, cervical dislocations,* or a *broken neck.*

GENERAL CONSIDERATIONS AND CLINICALLY RELEVANT PATHOPHYSIOLOGY

Cervical vertebral fractures and luxations occur less often than fractures and luxations of the thoracolumbar spine. The most common cause of cervical fracture and/or luxation is automobile trauma. Other less frequent causes include dog fights, gunshot injuries, running head first into a solid object, hanging by a leash or collar, and underlying metabolic or neoplastic disorders resulting in bone demineralization (e.g., nutritional secondary hyperparathyroidism and osteosarcoma).

Traumatic spinal fractures and/or luxations are induced by forces resulting in severe hyperextension, hyperflexion, compression, and/or rotation. They generally occur at or near the junction of a movable (kinetic) and immovable (static) vertebral segment. In the cervical spine, the skull, atlas, and dens and body of the axis form a unit called the *cervicocranium* (Fig. 38-59). The dorsal spinous process of the axis is secured to the lower cervical spine by caudal articular facets, spinalis and semispinalis muscles, and nuchal ligament. This produces a static-kinetic relationship between the cervicocranium and lower cervical spine; the axis (C2) is the point of stress concentration. Traumatic forces applied to the cervical spine therefore culminate at the axis (Fig. 38-60). Failure of supporting structures of the spine to resist such stress results in mechanical discontinuity (i.e., fracture or luxation) with resultant spinal cord and nerve root compression. Proposed areas of the spine with a static-kinetic relationship include craniocervical, cervicothoracic, thoracolumbar, and lumbosacral junctions.

> NOTE: The most common anatomic location of cervical fracture and/or luxation is the cranial cervical region, with approximately 80% occurring at C1–C2.

Pathologic fractures generally occur when the integrity of bone is compromised because of an underlying disease process. Chronic calcium/phosphorus imbalances, primary and secondary neoplasia (e.g., multiple myeloma, osteosarcoma, and metastatic neoplasia), and osteoporosis are examples of systemic disorders that can result in pathologic fracture. The cause of the underlying disorder must be determined and therapy instituted before spinal fracture and/or luxation repair.

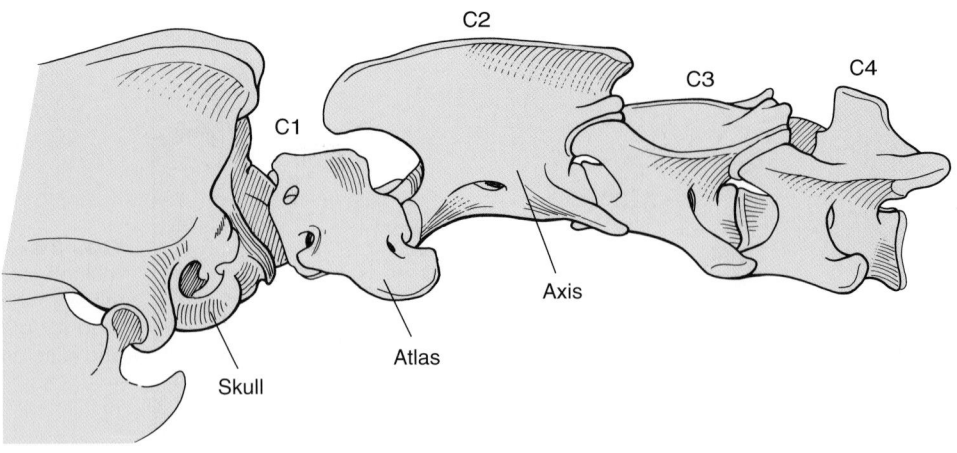

FIG. 38-59
Relationship of the structures (skull, atlas, and dens and body of the axis) that form the cervicocranium.

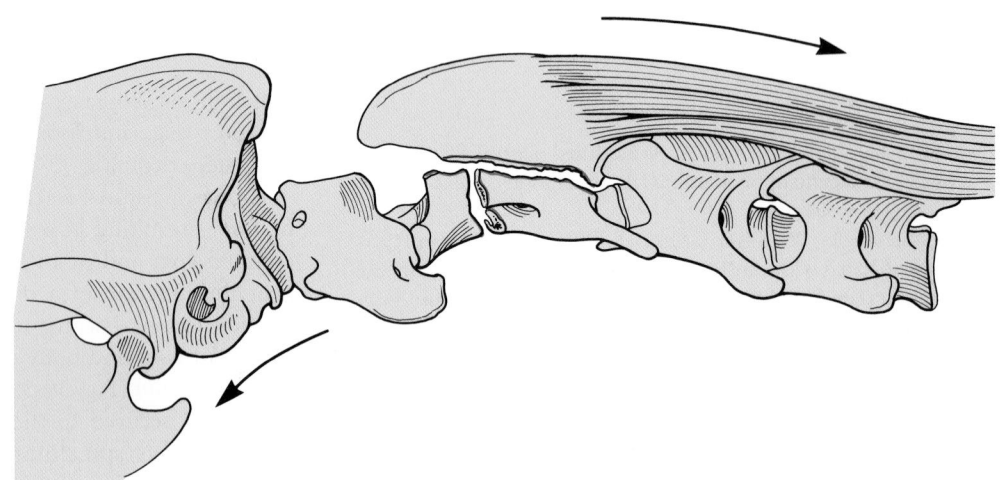

FIG. 38-60
A static-kinetic relationship is produced between the cervicocranium and lower cervical spine; the axis is the point of stress concentration, resulting in fracture and/or luxation.

DIAGNOSIS
Clinical Presentation

Signalment. There is no breed or sex predilection. Cervical spinal fractures may occur in any age dog and cat; however, they are most common in patients younger than 5 years of age.

History. Patients with fracture or luxation of the cervical spine typically have a history of trauma. The majority have been hit by an automobile. They may appear to be in pain; hold their neck in a stiff, protected position; and/or have varying degrees of tetraparesis, depending on the amount of spinal cord contusion and/or compression. Occasionally, patients may have no significant neurologic deficits on initial presentation; however, deficits may occur several days after injury. Careful physical and neurologic examinations are necessary to detect subtle deficits.

Physical Examination Findings

Animals suspected of having cervical fracture and/or luxation should be handled with extreme caution. Because trauma is the most common cause, careful examination of all systems and treatment for shock are important. Patients with no obvious neurologic deficits should undergo a careful cervical spinal examination. Gentle palpation for an area of hyperpathia (i.e., increased sensitivity to pain) can be performed by grasping the ventral aspect of the neck with thumb and fingers and gently squeezing each vertebral body. Discomfort on palpation suggests a lesion and warrants further diagnostics. Careful palpation of the spine may also reveal information as to the type of injury sustained. Crepitus, excessive movement, or anatomic discontinuity of the spine suggests an unstable fracture and/or luxation. These physical findings may be an important factor in assessing inherent stability (or instability) of the traumatized spine.

Patients with neurologic deficits should undergo a careful neurologic examination to localize the fracture or luxation and to determine severity of spinal cord and nerve root compression. Characteristic findings of the neurologic examination (UMN or lower motor neuron [LMN] signs to the front limbs, UMN signs to the hind limbs) allow accurate localization of the fracture and/or luxation. Because the most common location of cervical spinal fracture and/or luxation is

C1-C2, the most likely sign is varying degrees of acute neck pain, with or without UMN tetraparesis.

Diagnostic Imaging

Survey and contrast radiography may be required to accurately diagnose spinal fractures and luxations. Survey radiographs may be taken of conscious or anesthetized animals. Survey radiographs of conscious patients should be taken during the initial workup so that spinal injury may be assessed. Conscious patients may protect the fracture and/or luxation during positioning; however, an uncooperative patient may cause unpredictable radiographic detail. If surgery is necessary or more specific, radiographic evaluation is needed, and the patient should be anesthetized. Advantages of anesthetizing the patient for radiographs include excellent positioning and quality radiographs. The disadvantages are loss of inherent support and increased instability of the spine during transport and positioning.

> NOTE: Anesthetized patients with possible neurologic abnormalities should always be handled carefully.

Typical radiographic findings in patients with cervical spinal fracture and/or luxation include discontinuity of bony structures (i.e., spinous process, lamina, pedicle, and vertebral body), malalignment of the intervertebral space and/or articular facets, fracture lines in the body and/or spinous processes of involved vertebrae, loss of continuity or malalignment of the vertebral canal, or any combination of these (Fig. 38-61). Radiographs of the cervical spine may be difficult to interpret; oblique views are often necessary in addition to standard lateral and ventrodorsal views. Patients with a fracture of C3, C4, or C5 have an 85% chance of a second fractured vertebra. CT is superior to survey radiography in determining the extent and number of fractures involved.

> NOTE: A complete spinal series of radiographs (i.e., cervical, thoracic, lumbar, and sacral) is needed; 20% of patients with traumatic spinal injury have a spinal fracture and/or luxation at a second location.

Fractures may be classified as stable or unstable according to radiographic appearance and the force that caused the injury. Forces resulting in laminar and/or pedicle fracture, dorsal spinous process fracture, articular facet fracture, and supraspinous and/or interspinous ligament rupture (dorsal compartment) are generally considered unstable. Forces resulting in disk rupture, ventral longitudinal ligament rupture, and avulsion fracture of the ventral vertebral body (ventral compartment) are generally considered stable. Forces resulting in a combination of dorsal and ventral compartment injury are generally considered unstable. These are only guidelines; initial neurologic examination, physical examination, and serial neurologic examinations should be

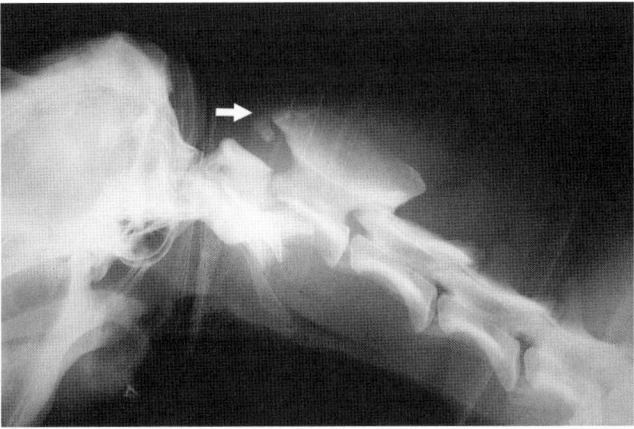

FIG. 38-61
Lateral radiograph of a dog with a C2 fracture. Notice the fracture fragment dorsal to C1 lamina *(arrow)*, malalignment of C1–C2 vertebral bodies, and craniodorsal displacement of C2.

undertaken in combination with radiographic appearance to determine ultimate patient management.

> NOTE: Radiographs only reveal the status of spinal displacement at the time they are taken. It is possible that spinal displacement during the traumatic episode was greater than that seen on radiographs. Evaluating the severity of spinal fracture or luxation radiographically must be done in conjunction with neurologic examination findings.

Myelography or cross-sectional imaging may be necessary if there is suspicion of herniated intervertebral disk material (i.e., annulus fibrosus or nucleus pulposus), bone fragments in the vertebral canal, no evidence of spinal discontinuity, or when radiographic findings do not correlate with neurologic examination. Myelography is infrequently necessary for definitive diagnosis or for surgical planning of patients with cervical fracture and/or luxation.

Laboratory Findings

Patients with cervical fracture and/or luxation rarely have abnormalities on CBC and biochemical profile unless the fracture is secondary to a metabolic disorder (e.g., nutritional secondary hyperparathyroidism). Because most patients have severe neck pain, a stress leukogram may be seen. Patients with a history of trauma or those that have undergone recent treatment with corticosteroids may have elevated concentrations of hepatic enzymes.

DIFFERENTIAL DIAGNOSIS

Presumptive diagnosis of cervical fracture and/or luxation is based on a young dog having a history of trauma and on physical and neurologic examination findings consistent with neck pain and tetraparesis. Other differentials can usually be eliminated by physical, hematologic, serum biochemical, CSF, and/or radiographic evaluations. Diagnosis of cervical fracture and/or luxation is confirmed by radiography.

MEDICAL MANAGEMENT

Patient stabilization is the initial objective. Those patients with severe trauma should be treated for shock. Whenever blunt trauma to the cervical region is suspected, careful examination of the soft tissue structures of the neck is encouraged, including hyoid apparatus, larynx, trachea, and esophagus. The neck should be stabilized with a padded neck brace. Analgesics should be given to control neck pain (see Table 13-4 on p. 133). Cage confinement should be encouraged. After patient stabilization, physical and neurologic examination should localize the fracture and/or luxation. Radiographs of the cervical spine are taken while the patient is conscious for initial assessment. The decision for conservative or surgical management is based on initial neurologic status, radiographic assessment of spinal stability, and serial neurologic examinations.

Stable fractures in patients with strong voluntary motor movements are often managed successfully by conservative means, including strict cage confinement, neck brace, and antiinflammatory agents. Recommended drug treatment regimens are listed in Box 38-8. Serial neurologic examinations should be performed twice daily to determine response to therapy. If the patient does not remain quiet and causes further displacement of the fracture and/or luxation, remains unacceptably static, or deteriorates neurologically, surgical therapy should be considered. Surgery may also be indicated if the fracture and/or luxation appears unstable, if the patient is weakly ambulatory or nonambulatory tetraparetic, or if conservative therapy is unsuccessful.

SURGICAL TREATMENT

Objectives of surgery in a patient with traumatic or pathologic cervical spinal fracture and/or luxation are spinal cord and nerve root decompression and vertebral stabilization. Patients with pathologic fracture must have the cause of the underlying disorder determined and medical therapy instituted before surgical fracture and/or luxation repair. Once the underlying disorder has been controlled, treatment can be performed as described for traumatic fracture and/or luxation.

Factors that should be considered when selecting a stabilization technique are location of the fracture and/or luxation, special anatomic considerations, presence of a compressive lesion within the vertebral canal (e.g., osseous fragment and disk material), patient size, patient age, equipment available, and surgeon's experience. The influence that special anatomic considerations and fracture location have on technique selection is outlined in Tables 38-15 and 38-16, respectively. If a compressive lesion is identified within the vertebral canal, decompression is dictated by lesion location. Ventral lesions are usually removed via a ventral slot technique (see p. 1405)

 BOX 38-8

Antiinflammatory Drugs Used With Cervical or Thoracolumbar Fracture/Luxation

Conservative Management

Dexamethasone (Azium)

0.2–0.5 mg/kg IV at presentation, then 0.2 mg/kg PO bid for 2 days, then qd for 2 days*

Surgical Management

Methylprednisolone (Solu-Medrol)

30 mg/kg IV given once at anesthetic induction; discontinue after one dose

Dexamethasone (Azium)

0.2 mg/kg PO, IM, or IV bid for 1 day, then qd for 1 day*† (if steroids are continued after surgery)

IV, Intravenous; *PO,* oral; *bid,* twice a day; *qd,* once a day; *IM,* intramuscular.

*If the patient is improving, discontinue steroids and enforce strict confinement for 3 additional wk.
†If signs of gastrointestinal upset or hemorrhage develop, discontinue corticosteroids.

and dorsal or dorsolateral lesions via dorsal laminectomy or dorsolateral hemilaminectomy, respectively (see p. 1409). Patient size affects the size and type of implant used to stabilize the fracture and/or luxation: the larger the patient, the larger the implant. Patient age may influence the surgical technique chosen. Younger animals usually have softer, more cancellous bone, whereas older animals have harder, more compact bone. Implant selection will be based on specific holding power in various regions of the cervical spine. Several equally successful techniques for fracture and/or luxation stabilization may be chosen based on availability of specialized equipment or on surgeon experience.

NOTE: Reduction of the fracture and/or luxation may be facilitated and maintained by two techniques: (1) by drilling holes in the ventral bodies of the vertebrae cranial and caudal to the fracture and/or luxation and placing ASIF small fragment reduction forceps in the holes (Fig. 38-62), and (2) by fenestrating adjacent intervertebral disks or drilling holes into adjacent vertebral bodies to accommodate a vertebral distractor to gently distract affected vertebral bodies.

C1-C7 body fractures and/or luxations, traumatic cervical disk extrusions, and atlantoaxial subluxation are generally approached ventrally. The ventral approach to the affected vertebra is performed as described for ventral slot procedures (see p. 1405). An ASIF small fragment reduction forceps may be used to maintain reduction of a cervical fracture and/or luxation (see Fig. 38-62). Steinmann pins and PMMA can be used successfully for selected cervical spinal

Table 38-15

Anatomic Variation of Cervical Vertebrae Important for Surgical Repair of Cervical Spinal Fractures/Luxations

VERTEBRAE	ANATOMY	SURGICAL SIGNIFICANCE
C1–Atlas	Thin dorsal arch (laminae); no dorsal spinous process	Poor implant-holding power dorsally
	No vertebral body, just thin ventral fovea	Poor implant-holding power ventrally
	Ventrolateral diarthrodial joints	Good purchase for implants ventrally; used to evaluate anatomic reduction
	Prominent ventral tubercle	Landmark for surgical localization
	Prominent wings	Moderate implant-holding power dorsally and ventrally
C2–Axis	Prominent dorsal spinous process	Moderate implant-holding power dorsally; landmark for surgical localization
	Thin central vertebral body	Poor implant-holding power ventrally
	Prominent cranial articular processes	Good purchase for implants ventrally; used to evaluate anatomic reduction
	Prominent caudal vertebral body	Good purchase for implants ventrally
	Dens	May fracture or displace into vertebral canal
C1–C2	Bilateral ventrolateral diarthrodial joints	Good purchase for implants ventrally; used to evaluate anatomic reduction
	Dorsal atlantoaxial ligament	Moderate purchase of implants used to replace the ligament
C3–C7	Small dorsal spinous processes	Poor purchase for implants dorsally
	Prominent articular facets	Good purchase for implants dorsally
	Prominent vertebral bodies	Good purchase for implants ventrally
	Prominent transverse processes of C6	Landmark for surgical localization

 Table 38-16

Summary of Surgical Stabilization Techniques for Cervical Spinal Fractures/Luxations, Depending Upon Fracture Location

FRACTURE LOCATION	SPECIAL ANATOMIC AND SURGICAL CONSIDERATIONS	MOST RELIABLE BONY PURCHASE	APPROACH AND FIXATION TECHNIQUE
C1	Respiratory arrest, lack of a vertebral body, thin dorsal arch (laminae)	Dorsal—dorsal arch (laminae) and wings	Dorsal—wire laminae; screw wings and wire between screws
		Ventral—diarthrodial joint and wings	Ventral—pin through joint or wings, with or without PMMA
C1–C2	Respiratory arrest; lack of an intervertebral disk; two lateral diarthrodial joints	Dorsal—dorsal arch of C1; dorsal spinous process of C2	Dorsal—wire or suture spine of C2 to arch of C1
		Ventral—diarthrodial joints	Ventral—pins through joint, with or without PMMA; screws through joint
C2	Respiratory arrest; venous sinus hemorrhage; narrow body (dorsal-ventral); thin spinous process	Dorsal—dorsal spinous process	Dorsal—wire dorsal spinous process with or without PMMA
		Ventral—lateral and caudal aspect of vertebral body	Ventral—pins in body or diarthrodial joint and PMMA; ventral body plate
C3–C7	Venous sinus hemorrhage; small dorsal spinous processes	Dorsal—articular facets	Dorsal—screws (large breed) or wires (small breed) through articular facets
		Ventral—vertebral bodies	Ventral—pins in body and PMMA (to span interspace or stabilize body fracture); ventral body plate (plastic or metal); interbody screw

PMMA, Polymethylmethacrylate.

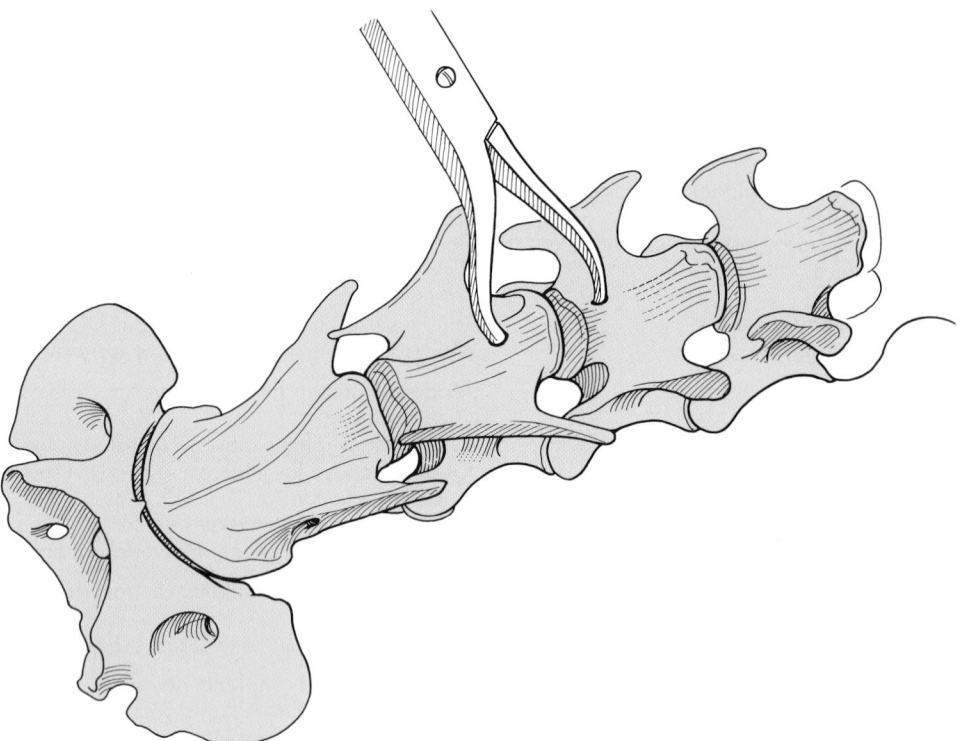

FIG. 38-62
ASIF small fragment reduction forceps may be used to maintain reduction of a cervical fracture and/or luxation.

fractures or luxations. Generally, vertebral body subluxation or body fractures occurring from C1-C7 can be adequately stabilized with this technique (see Tables 38-15 and 38-16). Appropriate exposure for pin and PMMA placement generally requires one or two vertebral bodies cranial and caudal to the fracture and/or luxation to be visible.

> NOTE: The author strongly recommends using a ventral stabilization technique for C3–C7 fracture and/or luxations.

In patients with vertebral luxations, it is advisable to prepare a ventral slot and pack it with autogenous cancellous bone to encourage interbody fusion. Ventral interbody screw fixation should not be used to stabilize vertebral body fracture or luxation because of an unacceptably high incidence of implant failure and vertebral body fracture.

Fractures of the lamina of C1 and dorsal spine and lamina and pedicles of C2 can be approached dorsally as described on p. 1410 and stabilized with orthopedic wire, monofilament or nonabsorbable suture material, or PMMA to reestablish continuity of displaced fragments (see Fig. 38-54, *A* and *B* on p. 1444). Placement of these various implants is described on p. 1443. Decompressive hemilaminectomy is performed only if bone fragments in the vertebral canal cause spinal cord compression. Because laminectomy and hemilaminectomy decrease the stability of an already unstable spine, these procedures should not be routinely performed.

Preoperative Management

Patients should be given IV fluids and steroids before surgery; the latter are given to protect the spinal cord from effects of surgical manipulation. The steroid of choice is methylprednisolone sodium succinate (30 mg/kg IV). Preoperative prophylactic or therapeutic antimicrobial therapy is dependent on criteria listed in Box 38-4 (see p. 1403). Patients with open fractures (e.g., gunshot wounds and bite wounds) require antibiotics. Fracture and/or luxation of the cervical spine often causes laceration of vertebral venous sinuses. Surgical manipulation encourages further hemorrhage. Because venous sinus hemorrhage can be severe and life threatening, blood should be readily available for transfusion.

> NOTE: Thoracic films should be evaluated in trauma patients for evidence of pneumothorax/pneumomediastinum and/or diaphragmatic herniation.

Anesthesia

Suggested anesthetic protocols for use in animals with cervical spinal disorders are provided on p. 1402. The patient's neurologic status and positioning for surgery are important preanesthetic considerations. Those with motor weakness

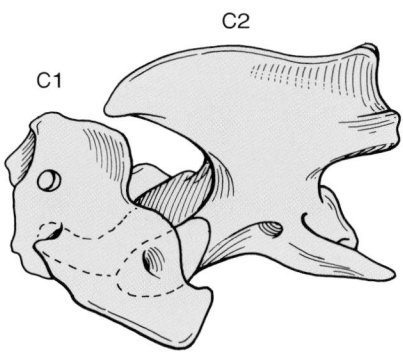

FIG. 38-63
Anatomic configuration of C1–C2.

(i.e., weakly ambulatory or nonambulatory tetraparesis) or those that require special positioning may be predisposed to respiratory or cardiovascular compromise. Reduction of cranial cervical fracture and/or luxations (C1-C3) may also traumatize the cranial cervical spinal cord, causing transient respiratory arrest. Ventilatory support during surgery is therefore recommended.

Surgical Anatomy

The cervical spine has a unique configuration from vertebra to vertebra, particularly C1 and C2 (Fig. 38-63; see Figs. 38-1 and 38-3 on p. 1404 and p. 1405). Anatomic variations and their surgical significance when considering fracture and/or luxation repair are listed in Table 38-15 (see p. 1451).

Positioning

Patients undergoing a ventral approach are placed in dorsal recumbency with their chest in a V-trough and carefully secured with sandbags or a rigid vacuum type of apparatus to prevent lateral motion. Front legs are taped caudally and a loop of rope is tied around the muzzle caudal to the maxillary canine teeth. The rope and tape are used to apply traction or countertraction (based on radiographic evaluation), resulting in complete or partial fracture and/or luxation reduction and stabilization. An area from the laryngeal cartilages to caudal to the manubrium sterni is prepared for midline cervical incision.

Patients undergoing a dorsal approach should be positioned in sternal recumbency with the head and cervical spine positioned to encourage fracture and/or luxation reduction and stabilization (see Fig. 38-17 on p. 1410). Cranial cervical, midcervical, and caudal cervical exposures require slight variation in patient position (see Figs. 38-21 and 38-23 on p. 1412 and p. 1413).

SURGICAL TECHNIQUE
Stabilization With Pins, Screws, and PMMA

The limiting factor of this procedure is the amount of pin or screw purchase in the relatively narrow vertebral bodies of the cranial cervical vertebrae. In patients with a C2 body fracture, pin purchase cranially is established by placing cross

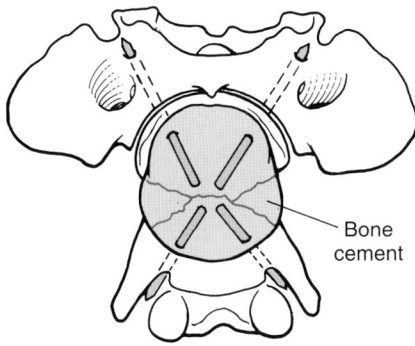

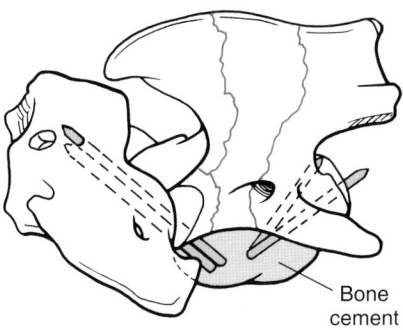

FIG. 38-64
Ventral stabilization of C1–C2 fracture and/or luxation using Steinmann pins and PMMA in the ventral vertebral bodies. Notice that the pins are placed through the C1–C2 articulation and caudal aspect of the C2 vertebral body.

pins bilaterally through the atlantoaxial joints (Fig. 38-64) and caudally by placing pins or screws in the caudal aspect of the C2 vertebral body. This fixation is generally adequate for mid-C2 body fractures. However, if the caudal aspect of the C2 body is fractured, caudal pins or screws are placed in the body of C3.

After fracture and/or luxation reduction, place two appropriate-sized Steinmann or positive profile threaded pins at a 20- to 25-degree angle to the midline on the ventral surface of the vertebral bodies cranial and caudal to the fracture and/or luxation. Drive each pin into the vertebral body to engage two cortices (Fig. 38-65). Cut the pins to protrude 3 to 4 cm from the vertebral body. Notch each pin with a pin cutter, and place PMMA on the protruding pins, taking care to ensure that each pin is completely surrounded and covered with PMMA. Use cool saline lavage to dissipate the heat of polymerization. Close longus colli muscles cranial and caudal to the PMMA mass. Close the sternohyosthyroideus muscle, subcutaneous tissue, and skin routinely.

Pin placement can be substituted with cortical screws.

Place cortical screws as described for pin placement. Allow screw heads and several threads to remain protruding from the ventral surface of the vertebral body. Reduce the fracture

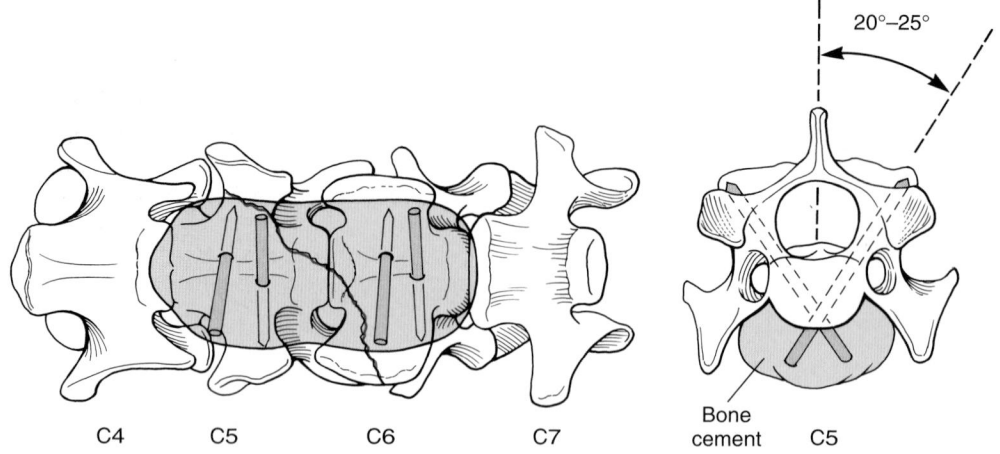

FIG. 38-65
Ventral stabilization of C3–C7 fracture and/or luxation using Steinmann pins and PMMA in the ventral bodies. Notice that the pins are angled away from the vertebral canal.

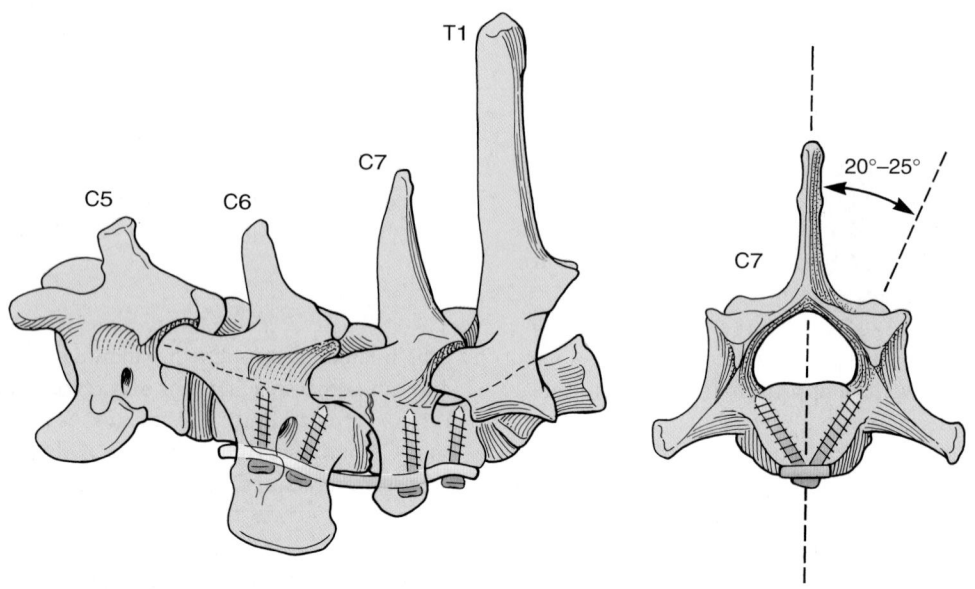

FIG. 38-66
Ventral stabilization of C3–C7 fracture and/or luxation using plastic spinal plates on the ventral vertebral bodies. Notice that the screws are angled away from the vertebral canal.

and incorporate all exposed screw heads and threads with PMMA. Close the wound as described previously.

Stabilization With Ventral Cross Pins

Ventral cross-pin or screw stabilization is performed in patients with C1-C2 luxations or subluxations. The technique is described and illustrated on pp. 1443 to 1445.

Stabilization With Ventral Spinal Plates

Fracture and/or luxations of C2-C7 may be stabilized by the use of ventral spinal plates. The fracture and/or luxation is exposed as described for a ventral slot procedure; however,

the vertebral body cranial and caudal to the fracture and/or luxation is also exposed.

Reduce the fracture and/or luxation as described on p. 1450 and illustrated in Fig. 38-62. Fashion an appropriate size plastic or metal plate to the ventral aspect of the vertebral bodies, allowing for two screws cranial and caudal to the fracture and/or luxation. Determine screw length by evaluating vertebral body size from preoperative radiographs. Drill screw holes 20 to 25 degrees from midline to engage two cortices. Tap the holes and apply the plate across the fracture and/or luxation (Fig. 38-66).

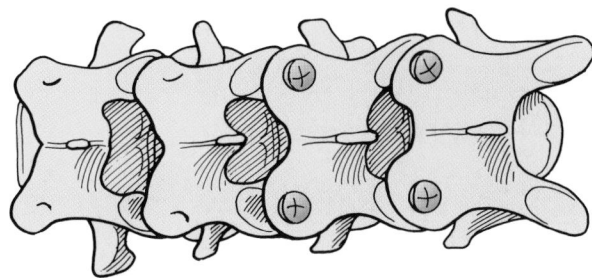

FIG. 38-67
Dorsal stabilization of C3–C7 fracture and/or luxation using articular facet screws.

It is impossible to safely engage two cortices unless screws are placed at an angle.

Harvest autogenous cancellous bone from the heads of the humeri and place it in the fracture defect. Close longus colli muscles over the plate and graft. Close subcutaneous tissue and skin routinely.

Stabilization Using Articular Facet Screws

Fractures and luxations rarely occur from C3-C7. As small dorsal spinous processes in this region preclude the use of dorsal spinous process plates, the only dorsal technique for C3-C7 stabilization is articular facet screwing. The spine is approached as described on p. 1409.

Identify the appropriate articular facets of the fractured or luxated vertebrae. Remove the articular surface of each facet with a curette or high-speed pneumatic drill. Reduce the fracture and/or luxation by grasping the dorsal spinous process cranial and caudal to the fracture and/or luxation with towel forceps. Bring the articular facets into apposition. Drill and tap appropriate-sized holes in each facet. Place one screw in each facet joint in lag screw fashion (Fig. 38-67). Harvest autogenous corticocancellous bone from the dorsal spinous processes of exposed vertebrae. Place the bone graft in and around the stabilized articular facets. Close epaxial muscles, subcutaneous tissue, and skin routinely.

SUTURE MATERIALS AND SPECIAL INSTRUMENTS

Careful reduction and stabilization of cervical fractures are facilitated by the use of ASIF small reduction forceps and modified Gelpi retractors.

POSTOPERATIVE CARE AND ASSESSMENT

Patients with cervical spinal fracture and/or luxation should be evaluated postoperatively in a similar fashion as patients with other cervical spinal disorders. Because of the anatomic configuration of cervical vertebrae, particularly C1 and C2, any form of fixation is marginal at best. It is recommended that all forms of internal fixation be supported with a neck brace and strict cage confinement until radiographic evidence of union.

PROGNOSIS

Prognosis depends on appropriate case management, including assessment of presenting neurologic examination, radiographic classification of the fracture and/or luxation, early stabilization (conservative or surgical), and proper preoperative and postoperative care. Dogs that undergo nonsurgical treatment of cervical fractures have a high likelihood of functional recovery. If adequate and early stabilization is performed (conservative or surgical), a favorable prognosis is possible.

NEOPLASIA OF THE CERVICAL VERTEBRAE, SPINAL CORD, AND NERVE ROOTS

DEFINITIONS

Malignant nerve sheath tumors include neurofibromas, neurofibrosarcoma, and Schwannomas. **Neurofibromas** and **neurofibrosarcomas** arise from nerve connective tissue (medullary layer of a nerve fiber). These are generally very aggressive neoplasms that often recur shortly after surgical resection. **Schwannomas** are benign tumors of the neurilemma (Schwann cells). Schwan cell tumors are rare in dogs. **Meningiomas** are slow-growing tumors that arise from arachnoidal tissue. **Astrocytomas** and **oligodendrogliomas** arise from parenchymal cells, and **ependymomas** arise from ependymal cells lining the ventricular system. Other names for these tumors include *spinal tumors, tumors of the spine, vertebral tumors,* and *nerve root tumors.*

GENERAL CONSIDERATIONS AND CLINICALLY RELEVANT PATHOPHYSIOLOGY

Tumors may arise from numerous sites in and around the spinal cord. They may be classified as primary bone, primary spinal cord, primary peripheral nerve root, primary paraspinal soft tissue, or metastatic tumors. It is important to try to classify the tissue of origin because it affects prognosis. Spinal tumors are also classified according to their location relative to the dura (i.e., extradural, intradural-extramedullary, and intramedullary) (Box 38-9). These locations are usually determined myelographically. The majority of canine cervical vertebral and spinal cord tumors occur extradurally and generally arise from bone (e.g., multiple cartilaginous exostoses, osteosarcoma, fibrosarcoma, multiple myeloma, and chondrosarcoma). Tumors may also metastasize to the vertebra, causing spinal cord compression (i.e., hemangiosarcoma, undifferentiated sarcoma, and lymphosarcoma). Lymphosarcoma is the most common canine soft tissue extradural spinal tumor. The majority of canine intradural-extramedullary tumors are nerve sheath tumors (i.e., neurofibroma, neurofibrosarcoma, and schwannoma) and meningiomas. Nerve sheath tumors arise from nerve roots, but often cause spinal cord compression because of their close proximity. Nerve sheath tumors have a predilection for the cervical spine. Meningiomas can arise from any location along the spinal cord, but are generally near the nerve roots. Intramedullary tumors are rare and include astrocytomas and ependymomas. Lym-

BOX 38-9

Characteristics of Vertebral, Spinal Cord, and Nerve Root Neoplasia

Extradural
- 40% of tumors
- Arise from bone and paraspinal tissue
- Prognosis is unfavorable (less than 50–50 chance of improvement)

Intradural-Extramedullary
- 50% of tumors
- Arise from nerve roots and meninges
- Prognosis is guarded (50–50 chance of getting better)

Intramedullary
- 10% of tumors
- Arise from glial cells
- Prognosis is grave (patient will not get better)

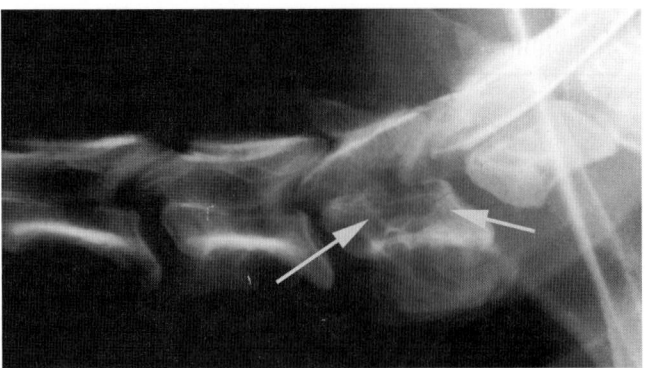

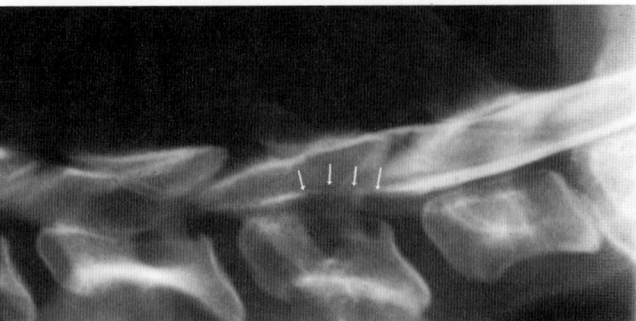

FIG. 38-68
A, Lateral radiograph of a dog with a tumor of C6. Notice the lytic change in the body and transverse processes of C6 *(arrows)*. **B,** Lateral myelogram of the dog in **A.** Notice the extradural compression of the spinal cord at the level of C6 *(arrows)*.

phosarcoma is the most common spinal tumor in cats and generally occurs extradurally. Intradural-extramedullary and intramedullary tumors are rare in cats.

DIAGNOSIS
Clinical Presentation

Signalment. There does not appear to be a sex or breed predilection for cervical vertebral, spinal cord, or nerve root tumors. The majority of patients with cervical spinal tumors are older than 5 years of age; however, benign solitary or multiple cartilaginous exostoses most often occur in patients younger than 1 year of age.

NOTE: When considering differentials in patients with neurologic disorders, remember that "tumors know no age."

History. The classic history of patients with cervical spinal neoplasia is slowly progressing tetraparesis. However, some patients have an acute onset of neurologic abnormalities preceded by insidious, slowly progressing signs. Careful historical evaluation often reveals that subtle neurologic abnormalities occurred before the acute episode. Historical features may also vary, depending on location of the neoplasm with respect to the dura (i.e., extradural, intradural-extramedullary, or intramedullary).

Physical Examination Findings

Physical and neurologic examination findings associated with vertebral, spinal cord, and nerve root tumors depend on tumor location, degree of spinal cord compression, rate of tumor growth, and associated secondary effects of the tumor. Neck pain is often associated with cervical spinal tumors, especially if they involve a nerve root (i.e., intradural-extramedullary), cause bone destruction or destruction of

adjoining soft tissue, or are extradural. Tumors involving nerve roots of the brachial plexus (spinal cord segments C6-T1) often produce forelimb lameness (i.e., monoparesis), progressing to hemiparesis or tetraparesis. Neurologic examination may reveal UMN signs to the hind limbs and LMN signs to the forelimbs with or without neck pain. Patients with an intramedullary tumor have acute paresis but no pain because there are no pain-sensitive fibers within spinal cord parenchyma. The presence of Horner's syndrome (i.e., miosis, ptosis, enophthalmos, and third eyelid protrusion) may help further localize the tumor to spinal cord segments C7-T2.

NOTE: Diagnosis and lesion localization depend on performance and interpretation of the neurologic examination.

Diagnostic Imaging

Survey radiography can be useful in evaluating spinal neoplasia. Osteoproduction and osteolysis from vertebral tumors may be seen on survey radiographs (Figs. 38-68 and 38-69). Some peripheral nerve tumors cause lysis of the intervertebral foramen (Fig. 38-70). Diagnosis of vertebral, spinal cord, and nerve root neoplasms often requires my-

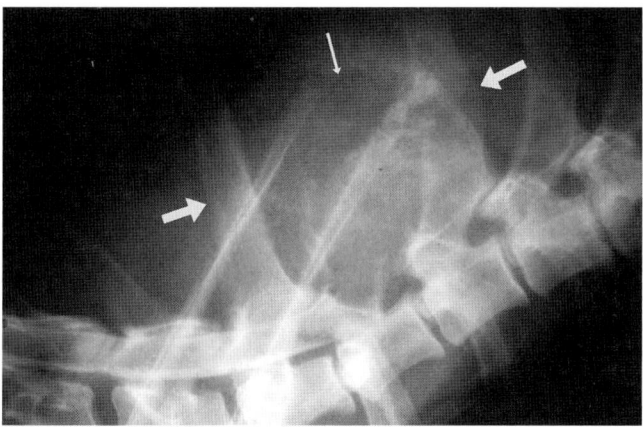

FIG. 38-69
Lateral myelogram of the cervical spine of a dog with a tumor of the T1 spinous process and dorsal lamina. Notice the spinous processes of C7 and T2 *(large white arrows)* and the absence of the spinous process of T1 *(small white arrow)*. Profound spinal cord compression is illustrated by the inability of contrast to move distal to the level of T1.

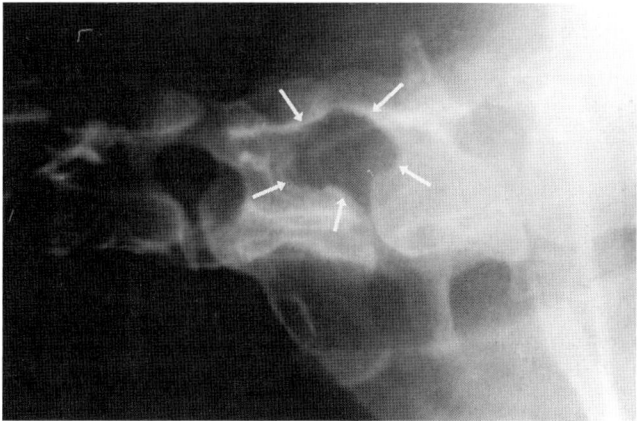

FIG. 38-70
Obliqued (45 to 60 degrees) cervical radiograph of a dog with spinal neoplasia. Notice the enlarged C6–C7 intervertebral foramen *(arrows)*.

elography or cross-sectional imaging. Specific myelographic techniques are described on p. 1370. Myelography identifies the lesion as extradural, intradural-extramedullary, or intramedullary; examples of myelographic abnormalities associated with each classification are described and illustrated on p. 1373 to 1375. CT or MRI may be necessary to accurately determine the extent of a vertebral or spinal cord lesion.

Laboratory Findings

Laboratory findings in patients with vertebral and spinal cord neoplasia are generally normal, but may reflect abnormalities caused by a paraneoplastic syndrome. Changes in CSF are usually noncontributory; however, cell type or evidence of an inflammatory process may suggest neoplasia.

DIFFERENTIAL DIAGNOSIS

A list of differential diagnoses that mimic cervical vertebral and spinal cord neoplasia is provided in Table 38-17. Differential diagnosis of vertebral and spinal cord tumor type is based on location of tumor (i.e., bone, spinal cord, nerve root, or metastasis) and myelographic classification (i.e., extradural, intradural-extramedullary, or intramedullary).

MEDICAL MANAGEMENT

Medical management of cervical spinal tumors is directed at both the primary lesion and secondary effects of the tumor. Corticosteroids are commonly used to decrease peritumoral edema. The steroid of choice is methylprednisolone sodium succinate (30 mg/kg IV, repeated bid if needed, not to exceed two doses). Definitive medical treatment, without surgery, is rarely recommended unless the tumor is inaccessible or the tumor type can be more effectively treated with chemotherapy or irradiation alone. Surgical exposure and inci-

sional or excisional biopsy is usually necessary to determine tumor type and plan adjunct therapy.

SURGICAL TREATMENT
Preoperative Management

The animal should be given IV fluids and steroids before surgery. Steroids are given to protect the spinal cord from the effects of surgical manipulation. The steroid of choice is methylprednisolone sodium succinate (30 mg/kg IV).

Anesthesia

See p. 1402 for suggested anesthetic protocols to use in animals with cervical spinal disorders. The patient's neurologic status and positioning for surgery are important preanesthetic considerations. If motor weakness (e.g., ambulatory tetraparesis, weakly ambulatory tetraparesis, or nonambulatory tetraparesis) is present or if positioning may cause respiratory compromise (e.g., sternal recumbency, flexed neck, or lateral chest wall compression), mechanical ventilatory support should be considered.

Surgical Anatomy

The cervical spine has unique and variable anatomic configuration from vertebra to vertebra, particularly C1 and C2 (see p. 1404 and Figs. 38-1 and 38-3 on p. 1404 and p. 1405). Important anatomic variations are described on p. 1404 and in Table 38-15 on p. 1451.

Positioning

Generally, patients with cervical vertebral, spinal cord, or nerve root tumors require a dorsal approach because ventral approaches do not provide sufficient exposure for tumor resection. Patients are positioned in sternal recumbency with the head and cervical spine gently flexed. Choice of

Table 38-17

Differential Diagnoses That Mimic Cervical Vertebral and Spinal Cord Neoplasia Using the DAMNIT-V Scheme

CLASSIFICATION	EXAMPLES	DIAGNOSTIC DIFFERENTIALS
Degenerative	Cervical disk disease	Plain and contrast radiography; CT; MRI
	Wobbler syndrome	History; plain and stress myelography; stress MRI
Anomalous	Atlantoaxial instability	Plain and stress radiography; CT; MRI
	Congenital malformation	Plain and stress radiography; CT; MRI
Metabolic	Any disorder causing generalized weakness (e.g., Addison's disease)	History; neurologic exam; laboratory findings
Nutritional	Nutritional secondary hyperparathyroidism (may cause pathologic fractures)	Dietary history; plain radiography
Neoplastic	–	–
Immunologic	Polyarthritis	Neurologic exam; laboratory data
	Polymyositis	Neurologic exam; laboratory data
Infectious	Cervical diskospondylitis	History; plain and contrast radiographs; CT; MRI
	Vertebral osteomyelitis	History; plain and contrast radiographs; CT; MRI
	Paraspinal abscess	History; plain and contrast radiographs; CT; MRI
	Meningitis	History; CSF analysis
Traumatic	Cervical spinal fracture/luxation	History; plain radiographs
Vascular	Fibrocartilaginous embolism	History; CSF analysis; myelography; MRI

CT, Computed tomography; *MRI,* magnetic resonance imaging; *CSF,* cerebrospinal fluid.

cranial cervical, midcervical, or caudal cervical laminectomy is based on tumor location and may require slight variation in patient positioning (see Figs. 38-17, 38-21, and 38-23 on pp. 1410, 1412, and 1413, respectively).

SURGICAL TECHNIQUE

Surgical objectives include exposure of the vertebral, spinal cord, or nerve root tumor; wide resection of neoplastic tissue; spinal cord and nerve root decompression; and vertebral stabilization. If wide resection is not possible, biopsy and decompression should be attempted. Definitive diagnosis of tumor type may suggest appropriate adjunct therapy. Patients with tumors of the cranial cervical, midcervical, or caudal cervical vertebrae, spinal cord, or nerve roots are approached via cranial cervical, midcervical, or caudal cervical laminectomy, respectively, as described on pp. 1409 to 1415.

Wide laminectomy, laminotomy, facetectomy, and/or foraminotomy are required for adequate exposure of most extradural and intradural-extramedullary tumors. Dorsal laminectomy and durotomy are necessary for exposure and removal of intramedullary tumors. If stabilization is necessary, articular facet screws are placed as described on p. 1455.

SUTURE MATERIALS AND SPECIAL INSTRUMENTS

Ultrasonic aspirators use high-frequency ultrasonic vibration to fragment (phacoemulsify) tissue; they reduce dense masses to a nearly liquid state that can be atraumatically aspirated. Ultrasonic aspirators are an invaluable addition to neurosurgical instrumentation, especially in removing neoplastic tissue; however, cost may be prohibitive ($90,000 to $100,000).

POSTOPERATIVE CARE AND ASSESSMENT

Patients with cervical spinal neoplasia should be evaluated postoperatively in a similar fashion as patients with other cervical spinal disorders. Adjunct chemotherapy, irradiation, immunotherapy, or combination therapy is based on results of histopathology and surgical margins.

PROGNOSIS

Prognosis for patients with cervical vertebral, spinal cord, and nerve root tumors depends on preoperative and postoperative neurologic status, tumor type, degree of surgical resection, and sensitivity to adjunct chemotherapy, radiation, immunotherapy, or a combination of any of these factors. Malignant extradural neoplasms usually have an unfavorable prognosis, benign extradural neoplasms have a favorable prognosis, malignant and benign intramedullary neoplasms have an unfavorable-to-grave prognosis, and extradural-intramedullary neoplasms have a guarded prognosis. Generally, patients with a better preoperative and postoperative neurologic status have a more favorable prognosis.

Suggested Reading

Dernell WS et al: Outcome following treatment of vertebral tumors in 20 dogs (1986-1995), *J Am Anim Hosp Assoc* 36:245, 2000.

This study evaluated the outcome after treatment of dogs with various vertebral tumors. The authors concluded that a guarded prognosis is warranted in dogs with vertebral neoplasia and that better combinations of surgery, chemotherapy, and radiation therapy need to be defined for these tumors.

Table 38-18

Sample Physical Rehabilitation Protocol for Patients After Surgery for Cervical Disk Disease*

| | DISABILITY INDEX | | | |
TREATMENT	0–2 STEP 1	3–8 STEP 2	9–11 STEP 3	12–14 STEP 4
Heat therapy		10 min	10 min	
Massage	5 min	5 min	5 min	5 min
Passive range of motion (repetitions)	15†	15†	15†	15†
Electrical stimulation‡	10 min	10 min	10 min	
Therapeutic exercise-total time	10 min	20 min	20 min	25–45 min
Assisted standing	+	+	+	
Sit to stands	+	+	+	+
Balancing	+	+	+	+
Obstacles			+	+
Weaving			+	+
Circles			+	+
Underwater treadmill with gait patterning or wading pool/water walking	10 min (after 36–48 hr)	15 min	20 min	>25 min
Swimming§	2–5 min	5–10 min	5–10 min	5–10 min
Cryotherapy	15 min			

Modified from Development of a functional scoring system for dogs with acute spinal cord injuries, *Am J Vet Res* 62:10, 2001.

Disability index (DI):

0-2, *0,* no limb movement and absent deep pain; *1,* no limb movement and present deep pain; *2,* no limb movement, but voluntary tail movement.

3-8, *3,* minimal non–weight-bearing activity of one limb (one joint); *4,* non–weight-bearing activity in more than one joint <50% of the time; *5,* non–weight-bearing activity in more than one joint >50% of the time; *6,* weight-bearing activity of the limb <10% of the time; *7,* weight-bearing activity of the limb 10% to 50% of the time; *8,* weight-bearing activity of the limb >50% of the time.

9-11, *9,* weight-bearing activity 100% of the time, but with reduced strength, and mistakes made >90% of the time, including crossing of the limbs, knuckling of the paws, standing on the dorsum of the paws and falling; *10,* weight-bearing activity 100% of the time, but with reduced strength and above mistakes made 50% to 90% of the time; *11,* weight-bearing activity 100% of the time, but with reduced strength, and mistakes made <50% of the time.

12-14, *12,* ataxic gait with normal strength, but mistakes made >50% of the time, including lack of coordination, crossing of hind limbs, skipping steps, bunny-hopping, and knuckling of the paws; *13,* ataxic gait with normal strength, but mistakes made <50% of the time; *14,* normal gait.

*All treatments should be done three times a day.
†Passive range of motion to all joints of all limbs.
‡E-Stimulation: Electrical stimulation to be performed on the semimembranosus/semitendinosus muscle groups in patients with muscle atrophy. See Chapter 12 for specifications.
§Swimming is most beneficial if patient is moving all four limbs and is controlled. If not getting functional response, return to underwater treadmill or water walking instead. It is safer and more controlled.

PHYSICAL REHABILITATION FOR PATIENTS WITH CERVICAL DISK DISEASE, CERVICAL VERTEBRAL INSTABILITY, ATLANTOAXIAL INSTABILITY, OR FRACTURE/LUXATIONS

Used in conjunction with standard medical and surgical treatment plus proper pain management (see Chapter 13), rehabilitation can facilitate early and more complete recovery of neurologic patients after surgery. For a general description of techniques for optimizing physical rehabilitation in animals after neurologic surgery, see Chapter 12 (p. 127). Table 38-18 provides a sample physical rehabilitation protocol for patients after surgery for cervical disk disease (begin within 12 to 24 hours after surgery), after cervical vertebral instability surgery (if a brace is needed, begin the therapy after the brace has been removed), after surgery for stable atlantoaxial instability (if a brace is used, begin the therapy after it has been removed), and after repair of cervical fractures. After repair of fractures or luxations, only steps one and two should be performed until a bony union has formed and fixation is considered stable, regardless of the disability index.

CHAPTER 39

Surgery of the Thoracolumbar Spine

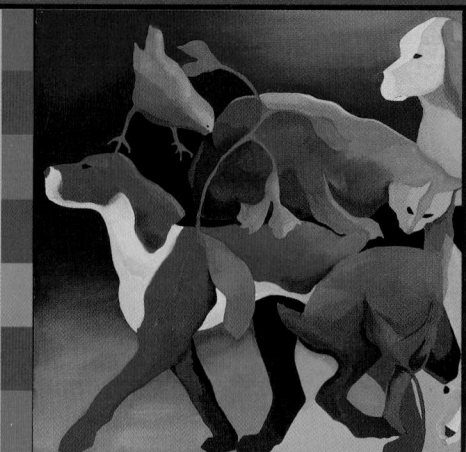

DEFINITIONS

Dorsal laminectomy is the removal of the dorsal spinous processes and portions of the lamina, articular facets, and pedicles of affected vertebrae. **Funkquist A dorsal laminectomy** refers to removal of the vertebral lamina, articular facets, and pedicle to a level corresponding to the middle of the dorsoventral diameter of the spinal cord, whereas a **Funkquist B dorsal laminectomy** is removal of the lamina above the dorsal aspect of the spinal cord (articular facets and pedicles are not removed). A **modified dorsal laminectomy** is similar to a Funkquist B procedure; however, the entire caudal articular processes are removed and the laminectomy edges undercut, causing additional exposure of the vertebral canal. **Deep dorsal laminectomy** involves removal of dorsal lamina, articular facets, and pedicles to the ventral aspect of the vertebral canal. **Hemilaminectomy** is unilateral removal of lamina, articular facets, and portions of the pedicle of affected vertebrae. **Minihemilaminectomy** or **pediculectomy** is removal of portions of the pedicle at the level of the intervertebral foramen.

PREOPERATIVE MANAGEMENT

Serial neurologic examinations should be done to determine surgical urgency. Patients with severe neurologic deficits, deterioration, or unacceptably static neurologic examinations may require immediate surgery. Patients with possible unstable spinal fractures or luxations should be immobilized on a rigid platform or placed in a back brace until definitively diagnosed. Spinal surgery generally requires spinal cord and/or nerve root manipulation to treat the underlying disorder (e.g., removal of disk material or neoplasm, fracture stabilization). Preoperative corticosteroid administration may partially protect these structures during surgery; however, steroids may predispose to gastrointestinal ulceration and/or perforation (see Table 38-4 on p. 1424).

ANESTHESIA

Anesthetic management for thoracolumbar spinal cord surgery is similar to that described for animals with cervical lesions. A selected anesthetic protocol is given in Box 38-3 on p. 1403. Mechanical or intermittent positive-pressure ventilation may help patients with respiratory compromise (e.g., pulmonary hemorrhage).

ANTIBIOTICS

Use of prophylactic or therapeutic antibiotics should be based on criteria provided in Box 38-4 on p. 1403. Cefazolin (22 mg/kg intravenous at induction, repeat at 2- to 4-hour intervals)) is the antibiotic of choice for neurologic surgery patients because of its low toxicity and excellent in vivo activity against common pathogens.

SURGICAL ANATOMY

The vertebral body, lamina, pedicle, dorsal spinous process, transverse processes, accessory processes, and articular facets of each vertebra are unique in anatomic configuration. Figs. 39-1 and 39-2 illustrate the unique anatomy of T11 and L5, respectively. Vertebral venous sinuses run longitudinally on the ventrolateral floor of the vertebral canal. The dorsal longitudinal ligament lies directly on the ventral floor of the vertebral canal with venous sinuses running on each side (see Fig. 38-8). This is also the location of the intervertebral foramen, its exiting nerve root, and the radicular artery. Neurosurgeons should have an appropriate anatomic specimen (in addition to a thorough knowledge of regional anatomy) available for reference.

SURGICAL TECHNIQUE

Patients with surgical disorders of the thoracolumbar spine may be treated by dorsal laminectomy, hemilaminectomy, fenestration, or thoracolumbar spinal stabilization via a dorsal approach. Proper positioning is often critical. Patients with spinal fracture/luxation should be positioned to encourage reduction of the fracture/luxation and spinal cord decompression. Towels or sandbags placed under the abdo-

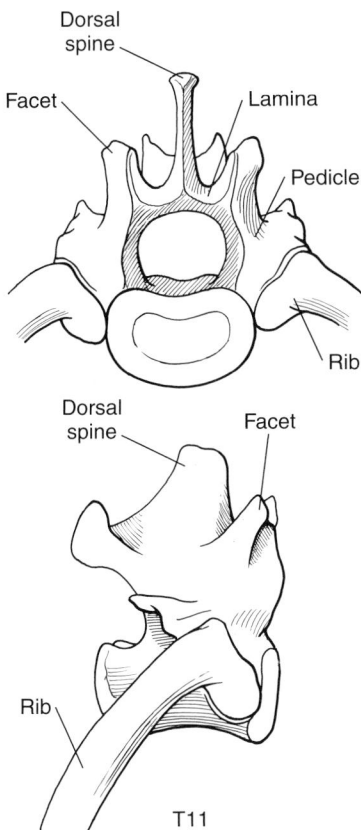

FIG. 39-1
T11 vertebra showing vertebral body, lamina, pedicle, dorsal spinous process, rib, and articular facets.

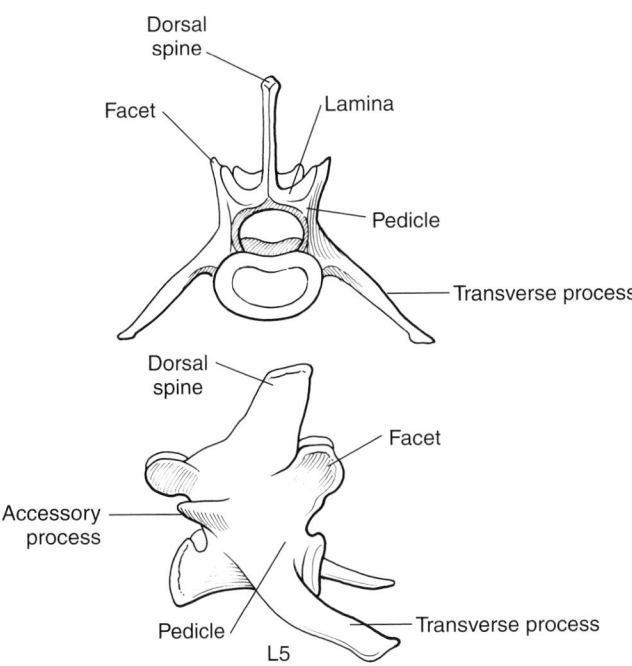

FIG. 39-2
L5 vertebra showing vertebral body, lamina, pedicle, dorsal spinous process, accessory process, transverse process, and articular facet.

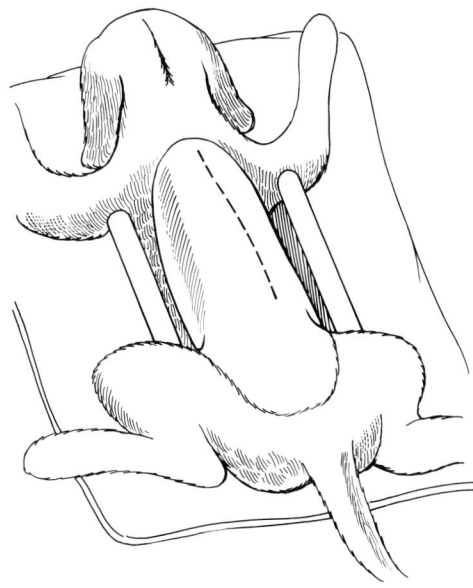

FIG. 39-3
When positioning a dog for dorsal thoracolumbar laminectomy, avoid hyperextending the spine.

men may divert venous return through vertebral venous sinuses and should be avoided. Prevent hyperextending the spine during positioning (Fig. 39-3). Dorsal laminectomy patients should have their backs gently flexed to open articular facets and interarcuate spaces. For hemilaminectomy, the affected side should be gently rotated dorsally (about 15 degrees) to facilitate lateral exposure of vertebral lamina and articular facets (Fig. 39-4).

Dorsal laminectomy allows entrance to all areas of the thoracolumbar vertebral canal and spinal cord (i.e., dorsal, lateral, and ventral). Dorsal decompressive approaches (in order of most commonly to least commonly performed) include modified dorsal, Funkquist A, deep dorsal, and Funkquist B laminectomies. These techniques are indicated for removal of herniated disk fragments; resection of vertebral, spinal cord, and nerve root tumors; and exposure of fracture/luxation.

Modified Dorsal Laminectomy

Modified dorsal laminectomy is indicated for exposure of compressive masses in the ventrolateral and dorsal aspect of the vertebral canal (e.g., disk fragments, fracture fragments, vertebral and spinal cord neoplasms). Laminectomy of no more than two consecutive vertebrae should be performed using this technique.

Make an incision over the dorsal midline to include two spinous processes cranial and caudal to the lesion. Use a periosteal elevator or small osteotome to subperiosteally elevate epaxial muscles from dorsal spinous processes, laminae, articular facets, and pedicles of affected vertebrae (Fig. 39-5). Use Gelpi retractors to facilitate gentle retraction

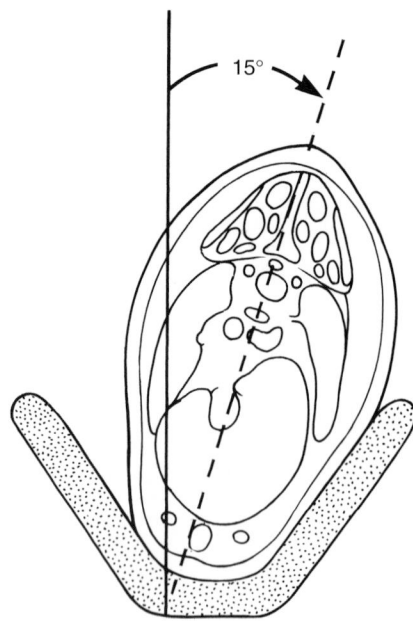

FIG. 39-4
For hemilaminectomy, position the patient with a 15-degree rotation to facilitate lateral exposure of vertebral lamina, pedicle, and articular facets.

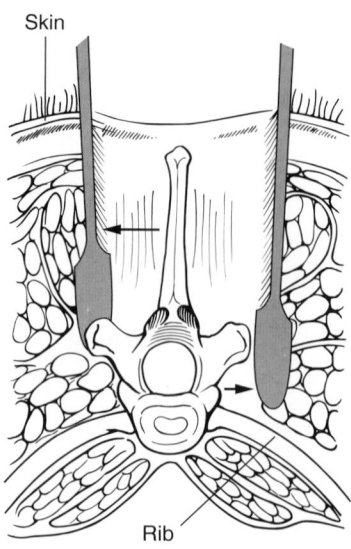

FIG. 39-5
Use a periosteal elevator or small osteotome to subperiosteally elevate epaxial muscles from affected vertebrae.

of epaxial musculature during dissection. Control soft tissue hemorrhage with bipolar cautery. Remove the exposed dorsal spinous processes to the level of the dorsal lamina with large, single-action duckbill rongeurs (see Fig. 8-18 on p. 52). Use a pneumatic air drill to begin burring the outer cortical (white) layer of bone from the lamina of both vertebrae. Remove articular processes of the cranial vertebrae with the drill, working carefully so as much of the cranial articular processes is left intact as possible (Fig. 39-6). Continue drilling the dorsal lamina until the medullary layer of bone is encountered (it is red in appearance, soft, and easily drilled). Carefully burr this layer until the white inner cortical layer is visualized (Fig. 39-7). The inner cortical layer is easily recognized in the midlaminar portion of each vertebral body; however, it becomes more difficult to recognize at the intervertebral space, where bone appears white throughout drilling (see Fig. 39-7). Before drilling over the intervertebral space, remove the interarcuate ligament (i.e., ligamentum flavum and yellow ligament) using sharp dissection with a No. 11 Bard-Parker scalpel blade. Do not use a pneumatic bone drill because it tends to grab soft tissue and force the drill downward toward the vertebral canal. Estimate drilling depth at the intervertebral space first by reaching the inner cortical layer at the midlaminar portion of the vertebral body cranial and caudal to the interspace. Drill remaining bone at the intervertebral space to the same level. Once the inner cortical layers of both laminae have been reached, use careful paint brush–like burring until soft periosteum can be palpated with a dental spatula. Continue to burr until periosteum is palpable over both vertebrae and the interverte-

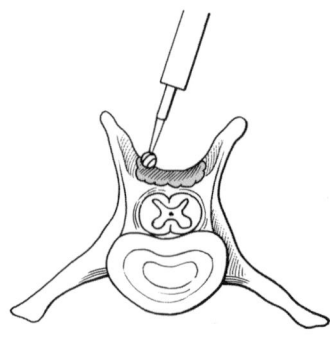

FIG. 39-6
Then performing dorsal laminectomy, use a high-speed pneumatic drill to remove the white outer cortical layer of lamina.

bral space. Use a dental tool and Lempert rongeurs to gently penetrate periosteum, and carefully pry the remaining inner cortical layer away (see Fig. 39-7). If necessary, undercut the dorsal laminae to gain additional exposure. Use a 2- to 3-mm-diameter carbide or diamond burr to carefully drill away the inner layer of laminar bone (Fig. 39-8).

This is the recommended modification because it provides greater exposure, ensuring atraumatic removal of compressive lesions.

If hemorrhage from soft tissue occurs, use suction and bipolar cautery for control. If hemorrhage from bone occurs,

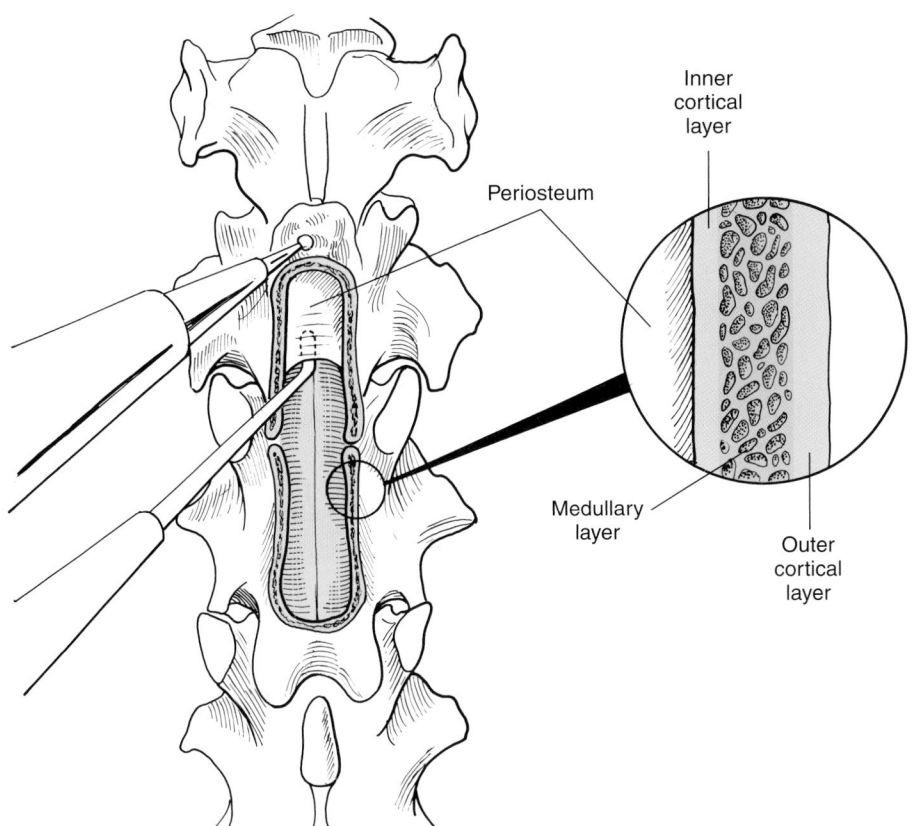

FIG. 39-7
For dorsal laminectomy, carefully drill through outer cortical and medullary layers of bone until the inner cortical layer is reached, then use a paint brush stroke until periosteum is reached. Three layers of bone are drilled: a thick white outer cortical layer, a soft red medullary layer, and a thin white inner cortical layer. Use a dental spatula to penetrate the inner periosteum to expose the vertebral canal.

apply bone wax to the tip of a periosteal elevator and gently press it on the bleeding surface.

Lesions near the vertebral venous sinus should be manipulated with great care. Occasionally, venous sinus hemorrhage is incurred. Proper use of hemostatic agents (e.g., Gelfoam, Surgicel, and Avistat) with cottonoid sponges and suction helps control hemorrhage (see Box 38-1 on p. 1403 for technique to control venous sinus hemorrhage).

Before closure, irrigate the wound with room-temperature physiologic saline solution to dislodge any remaining bone fragments from soft tissue. Span the dorsal spinous processes cranial and caudal to the laminectomy site with 20-gauge, stainless steel orthopedic wire (wire is used for cosmetic purposes only). Harvest a piece of subcutaneous fat, and place it over the laminectomy site to help prevent dural adhesions. Débride any devitalized muscle, and close fascia and epaxial muscles with a simple interrupted pattern over the spanning wire. Close subcutaneous tissue and skin routinely.

Funkquist A Dorsal Laminectomy

Funkquist A dorsal laminectomy provides improved exposure of the lateral aspect of the vertebral canal and spinal cord compared with a modified dorsal or Funkquist B laminectomy. This procedure is indicated when compressive masses are located in the dorsal, lateral, or ventrolateral aspect of the vertebral canal (e.g., lateral disk extrusions; lateral vertebral, spinal cord, nerve root neoplasms; and lateral fracture fragments). Exposure of the vertebral canal is limited to two consecutive vertebrae (one intervertebral space). The approach is as described previously for modified dorsal laminectomy to the level of laminar and facet exposure.

Remove exposed dorsal lamina and cranial and caudal articular facets with rongeurs or a pneumatic drill. Identify outer cortical, medullary, and inner cortical layers of exposed lamina. Enter the vertebral canal by carefully penetrating periosteum with a dental spatula or Lempert rongeur. Use double-action duckbill and Lempert rongeurs to remove remnants of the lamina, articular facets, and pedicles to a level corresponding to that of a dorsal plane through the middle of the dorsoventral diameter of the spinal cord (Fig. 39-9, A). Carefully explore the dorsal, lateral, and ventrolateral aspect of the vertebral canal, spinal cord, and nerve roots. Close as described previously for modified dorsal laminectomy.

Funkquist B Dorsal Laminectomy

Funkquist B dorsal laminectomy (Fig. 39-9, *B*) exposes the dorsal aspect of the vertebral canal and spinal cord. It is indicated when compressive masses are located in the dorsal aspect of the vertebral canal (e.g., dorsal disk extrusion, dorsal extradural neoplasia, and dorsal laminar neoplasia). Laminectomy of up to three consecutive vertebrae can be

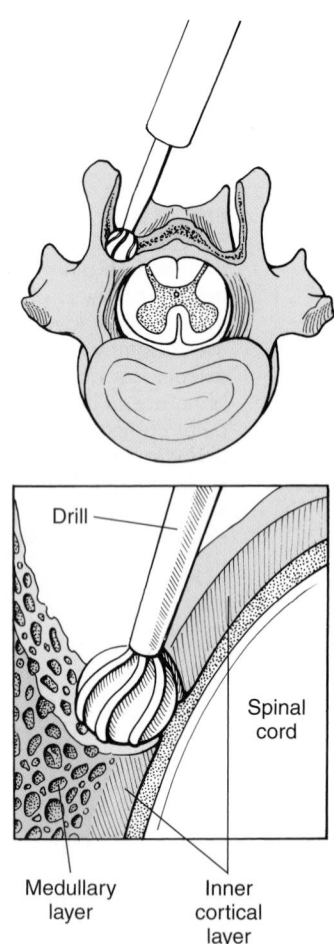

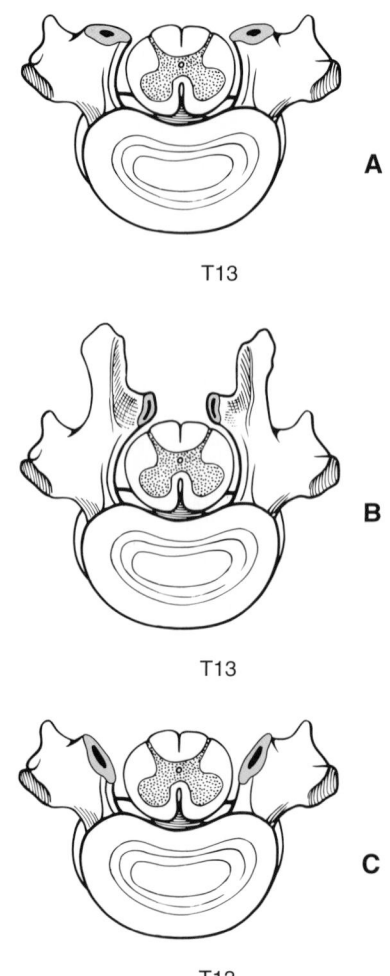

A

T13

B

T13

C

T13

FIG. 39-8
When performing modified dorsal laminectomy, gain additional lateral exposure by carefully undercutting dorsal lamina and cranial articular facet.

FIG. 39-9
A, During Funquist type A dorsal laminectomy, remove articular facets and pedicles to expose the dorsal one half of the spinal cord. **B,** When performing deep dorsal laminectomy, remove the dorsal lamina, cranial and caudal articular facets, and pedicles to the level of the ventral aspect of the vertebral canal. **C,** During Funquist type B dorsal laminectomy, remove the dorsal lamina, taking care to preserve cranial and caudal articular facets.

performed using this technique. The approach is as described previously for modified dorsal laminectomy to the level of laminar exposure.

Remove laminar bone with a pneumatic bone drill, taking care to preserve the cranial and caudal articular facets. Identify the outer cortical, medullary, and inner cortical layers as you drill. Remove periosteum from the dorsal lamina with a dental spatula or Lempert rongeurs. Carefully explore the dorsal aspect of the vertebral canal and spinal cord. Close as described previously for modified dorsal laminectomy.

Deep Dorsal Laminectomy

Deep dorsal laminectomy provides excellent exposure of the dorsal, lateral, and ventral aspects of the vertebral canal, spinal cord, and nerve roots. It is indicated when maximal decompression within the limits of one vertebral length is required (e.g., vertebral, spinal cord, or nerve root tumors, and severe disk herniation). This procedure is performed as

described for Funkquist A laminectomy to the level of articular facet and pedicle removal.

Carefully rongeur the remaining pedicles to the level of the ventral aspect of the vertebral canal (see Fig. 39-9, B). Identify vertebral venous sinuses bilaterally and avoid them if possible. Control venous sinus hemorrhage as described in Box 38-1 on p. 1403). Gently manipulate beneath the spinal cord to remove ventrally located masses. Close as described previously for modified dorsal laminectomy.

Hemilaminectomy

Hemilaminectomy is indicated when the spinal cord is compressed by mass lesions in the lateral, dorsolateral, or ventrolateral vertebral canal (e.g., disk extrusion, extradural mass,

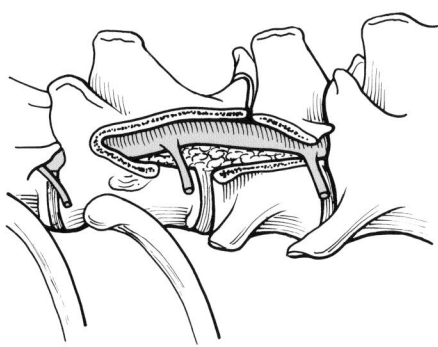

FIG. 39-10
Remove right or left articular facets and pedicles to the level of the ventral floor of the vertebral canal during hemilaminectomy.

intradural-extramedullary mass, nerve root tumor, and fracture fragment) (Fig. 39-10). Hemilaminectomy is preferable to dorsal laminectomy because it best preserves the structural and mechanical integrity of the spine, is less traumatic, is more cosmetic, and reduces the chance of scars causing spinal cord compression. However, the lesion must lateralize myelographically to ensure complete mass removal. Bilateral hemilaminectomy may be performed when the compressive lesion is on both sides of the spinal cord. A recent biomechanical evaluation of multiple site hemilaminectomy suggests that unilateral hemilaminectomy can be performed along three consecutive vertebrae without producing clinically significant spinal instability, whereas bilateral hemilaminectomy can be performed along two consecutive vertebrae (Corse et al, 2003). Hemilaminectomy may be performed with a high-speed pneumatic drill, high-speed electric drill, or rongeurs.

Make a dorsal midline incision to include two dorsal spinous processes cranial and caudal to the affected intervertebral space or vertebral body. Use a periosteal elevator or small osteotome to elevate epaxial muscles from their attachments on the lateral aspect of the dorsal spinous processes, lamina, articular facet, and pedicle to the level of the accessory process. Use a Gelpi retractor to maintain muscle retraction. Use a drill or rongeur to enter the vertebral canal. Regardless of technique used to enter the vertebral canal, be careful when manipulating lesions involving the ventral and ventrolateral aspects of the vertebral canal because the vertebral venous sinuses are in close proximity. If venous sinus hemorrhage occurs, control hemorrhage as described in Box 38-1 on p. 1403. Control soft tissue hemorrhage with bipolar cautery, and hemorrhage from bone with bone wax. Lavage the surgical site with room-temperature physiologic saline solution to dislodge any loose bone fragments. Harvest a fat graft from the subcutaneous area, and place it over the laminectomy site. Close epaxial muscles to the dorsal midline. Close subcutaneous tissue and skin routinely.

If a drill is used, remove articular processes of the involved intervertebral space with a high-speed drill. Visualize a rectangular area from the base of the dorsal spinous processes dorsally, accessory process ventrally, articular facet of the cranial vertebra, and articular facet of the caudal vertebra (Fig. 39-11, A). Drill the outer cortical bone of this rectangle, beginning cranially and working caudally. Continue to drill through the soft, red, medullary layer to the inner cortical layer. Once the inner cortical layer is reached, use a "paint brush" action to expose the soft inner periosteum. Use a dental spatula or Lempert rongeur to carefully enter the vertebral canal (Fig. 39-11, B).

If rongeurs are used, remove articular processes of the involved intervertebral space with rongeurs (Fig. 39-12, A). Have an assistant grasp and elevate the dorsal spinous process of the vertebra cranial to the involved intervertebral space with towel forceps (Fig. 39-12, B).

This maneuver will open the intervertebral space and facilitate exposure of the foramen.

Place one blade of a Lempert rongeur into the opening, and remove a small amount of bone (Fig. 39-12, C). Continue to enlarge the opening cranially and caudally with rongeurs until the laminectomy defect is an appropriate size to allow adequate decompression.

Pediculectomy

Pediculectomy (modified lateral hemilaminectomy) is indicated for lesions confined to the lateral and ventral aspects of the vertebral canal (e.g., ventrolateral intervertebral disk extrusion). The initial surgical approach is as described for hemilaminectomy.

Continue epaxial muscle dissection to the level of the caudomedial one fourth of the transverse process at the affected intervertebral space.

This allows complete exposure of the intervertebral foramen and associated structures.

Using the accessory process as a landmark, drill the slot defect just dorsal and ventral to the accessory process, and extend it half the vertebral lengths cranial and caudal. If the radicular artery is encountered, control hemorrhage with bipolar cautery. Determine depth of drilling by identifying outer cortical, medullary, and inner cortical layers. Use caution when drilling the inner cortical layer and removing inner periosteum.

Identify the spinal nerve from its origin within the vertebral canal and its exit from the intervertebral foramen. Retract the nerve with a small blunt hook, and remove the remaining portion of the pedicle to extend the defect to the floor of the vertebral canal (Fig. 39-13). After removal of disk fragments, harvest a fat graft from the subcutaneous area and place it over the pediculectomy site. Close epaxial muscle, subcutaneous tissue, and skin as described for hemilaminectomy.

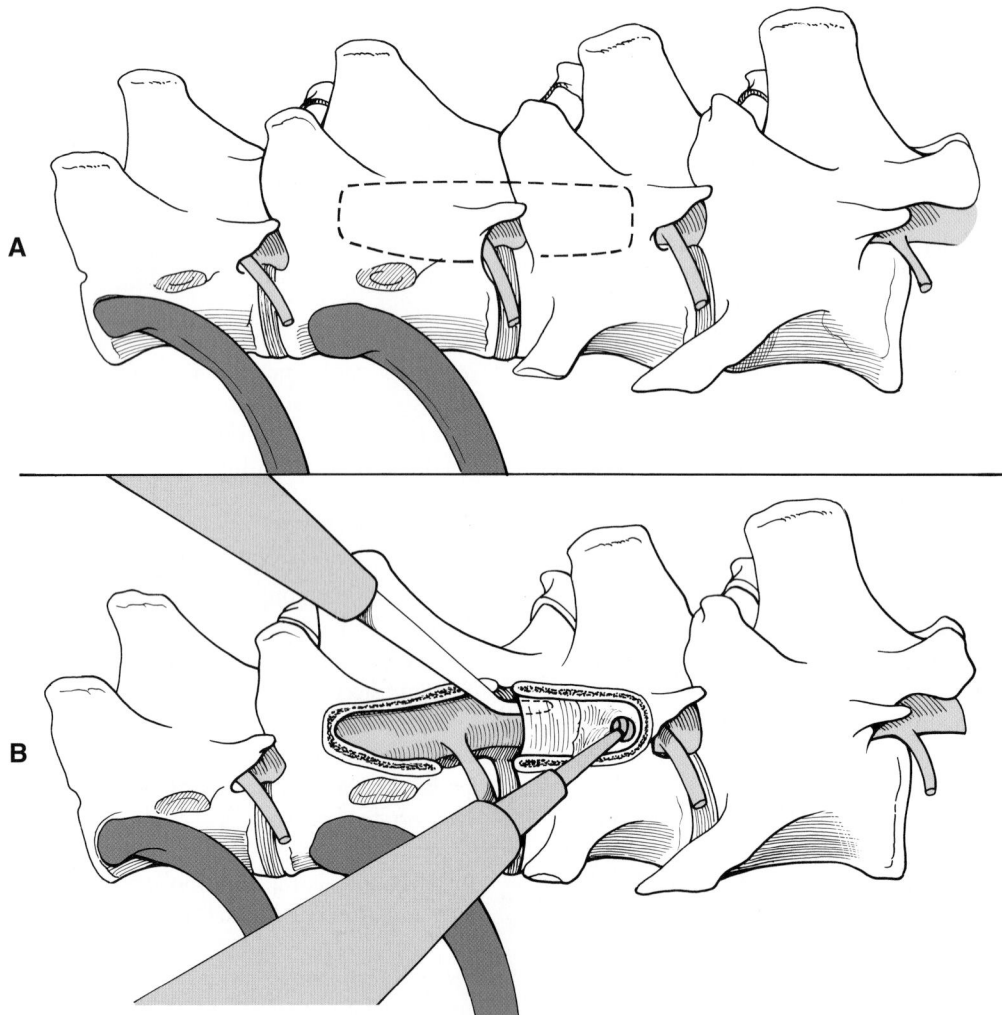

FIG. 39-11
A, During hemilaminectomy, visualize the area of the proposed hemilaminectomy. **B,** Drill outer cortical, medullary, and inner cortical layers of lamina and pedicle to the level of the inner periosteum. Use a dental spatula to remove periosteum and enter the vertebral canal.

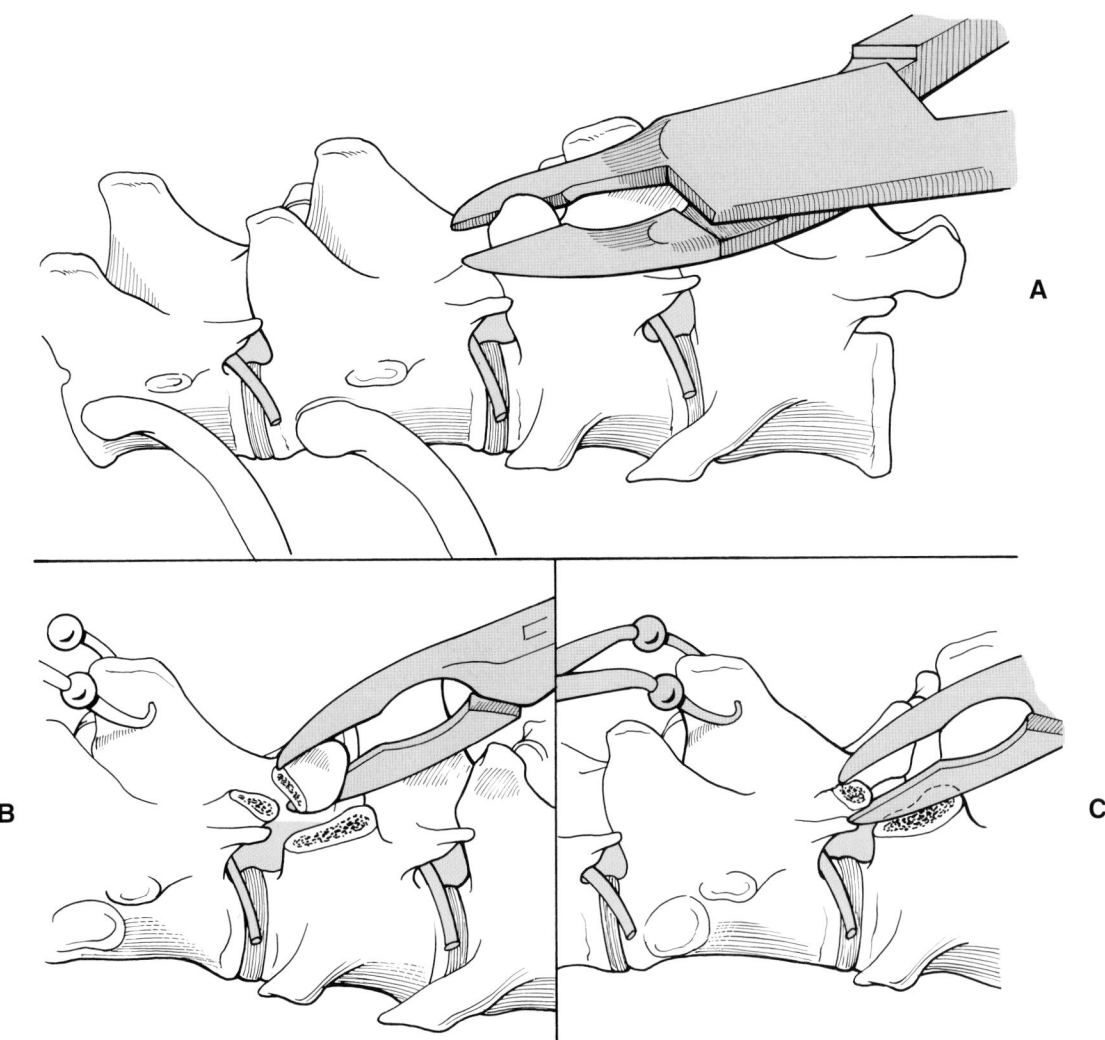

FIG. 39-12
A, During hemilaminectomy, remove cranial and caudal articular facets with rongeurs.
B, Grasp the dorsal spinous process of the vertebra cranial to the affected intervertebral space with towel forceps and retract it in a dorsocranial direction. **C,** This will accentuate the articular space and intervertebral foramen, allowing placement of a rongeur into the opening and facilitating removal of the lamina and pedicle.

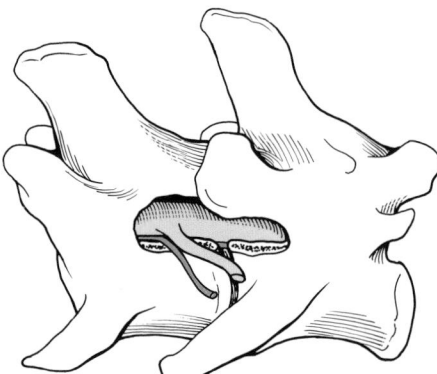

FIG. 39-13
Remove pedicular bone cranial and caudal to the intervertebral foramen during pediculectomy. Cranial and caudal articular facets are preserved.

HEALING OF THE SPINAL CORD

Healing of the thoracolumbar spinal cord is similar to that described for the cervical spinal cord on p. 1416. The surface plexus of arteries is not as dense in the thoracic spinal cord as in the cervical and lumbar regions. The effect this may have on healing of traumatic lesions is unclear.

SUTURE MATERIALS AND SPECIAL INSTRUMENTS

Special instrumentation necessary to perform dorsal laminectomy, fenestration, and spinal stabilization is shown by technique in Box 39-1. It is important to practice each technique, become familiar with regional anatomy, and learn proper use of special instrumentation before performing these surgeries.

POSTOPERATIVE CARE AND ASSESSMENT

Immediate postoperative care is determined based on underlying diseases or conditions in Table 39-1. Neurologic status should be determined when the animal has fully recovered from anesthesia, and complete neurologic examinations should be performed daily until discharge. Postoperative care of ambulatory and nonambulatory patients is described in Box 39-2. Ambulatory patients may be discharged 24 to 48 hours postoperatively. Nonambulatory patients require frequent hydrotherapy, physiotherapy, elevated padded cage racks, and bladder expression three to four times a day. Indwelling urinary catheters should be avoided to help reduce urinary tract infections. If necessary, intermittent urinary catheterization can be performed 3 to 4 times a day. Keep patients clean and dry to prevent decubital ulcers. A supporting cart helps patients return to an ambulatory status. Advantages of a cart include unhindered eating, drinking, micturition, and defecation. Animals with motor function can be encouraged to ambulate, and an erect position facilitates physiotherapy. Nonambulatory patients

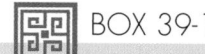 BOX 39-1

Special Instruments Necessary to Perform Thoracolumbar and Lumbosacral Spinal Surgery

Special instruments needed for most procedures	High-speed pneumatic or electric drill
	Drill burrs: carbide and diamond tip
	Cautery unit (monopolar and bipolar)
	Periosteal elevator/osteotome
	Suction
	Hemostatic sponge (Gelfoam)
	Cottonoid felt sponge
	Bone wax
	Dental spatula
	Dural hook
Dorsal laminectomy, hemilaminectomy, facetectomy, foraminotomy	Duck bill, double-action rongeurs
	Lempert rongeurs
	Microsuction tip
	Dental spatula
	Iris spatula
Fenestration	Tartar scraper
	Ophthalmic forceps
	Ear curette
	No. 7 Bard-Parker scalpel handle
	14- to 20-gauge hypodermic needle
Spinal stabilization	Steinmann pins
	PMMA
	Plating equipment
	Dorsal spinous process plates
	External skeletal fixator

PMMA, Polymethylmethacrylate.

should remain in the hospital until recovery of bladder function or until clients can provide appropriate aftercare.

Follow-up neurologic examinations should be performed at 1, 2, 3, 6, 9, and 12 months postoperatively or until the patient makes a full recovery. In patients requiring a spinal stabilization procedure, spinal radiographs (taken without anesthesia) are recommended at 1, 3, 6, 9, and 12 months postoperatively or until there is radiographic evidence of healing.

COMPLICATIONS

Potential complications associated with thoracolumbar surgery depend on the type of surgery performed, number of sites operated on, knowledge of regional anatomy, availability of appropriate neurosurgical instruments, and surgical expertise. Complications associated with dorsal laminectomy, hemilaminectomy, and pediculectomy include iatrogenic spinal cord trauma, seroma, infection, and/or dehiscence. Potential complications associated with fenestration include iatrogenic spinal cord trauma (either from pushing disk into the vertebral canal or trauma from inappropriate instrumentation), pneumothorax, scoliosis, ventral abdomi-

Table 39-1

Postoperative Care and Assessment of Patients With Thoracolumbar and Lumbosacral Spinal Disorders

IMMEDIATE CARE (FIRST 24 HOURS)	DISK	FX/LUX	NEOPLASIA
Intravenous fluids	Yes	Yes	Yes
Analgesics (see Chapter 13 and Table 13-4 on p. 133)	PRN	PRN	PRN
Corticosteroids	No	No	Based on tumor type
Antibiotics	No	See Box 38-5	See Box 38-5
Observe for seizures (particularly if myelogram was performed)	Yes	Yes	Yes
Back brace (thoracolumbar only)	No	Based on postoperative stability	Based on postoperative stability
Neurologic exam	q 24 hrs	q 24 hrs	q 24 hrs

PRN, As needed.

 BOX 39-2

Postoperative Care and Assessment After Thoracolumbar and Lumbosacral Spinal Cord Surgery

Ambulatory Patients
- Strict confinement for 2 to 3 weeks postoperatively
- Physiotherapy for 2 to 3 weeks postoperatively
- Leash walks only for 4 to 8 weeks postoperatively

Nonambulatory Patients (Perform Until Ambulatory)
- Physiotherapy
- Hydrotherapy
- Supporting cart
- Padded bedding
- Elevated cage rack
- Bladder expression—tid-qid (avoid urinary catheters)
- Neurologic exams daily

tid, Three times a day; *qid*, four times a day.

nal muscle paralysis, diskospondylitis, and recurrence of disk herniation. Urinary tract infections may occur secondary to neurologic deficits causing urine stasis. Spinal instability, muscle fibrosis, and/or contracture over the spinal cord may occur if excessive amounts of lamina, articular facets, and pedicles are removed. Guidelines for maximum exposure for each technique were discussed previously. Occasionally, inadvertent trauma or resection of a lumbar or thoracic spinal nerve root causes bulging of the abdominal muscle innervated by that nerve. The resulting abnormality may resemble an abdominal hernia in appearance.

SPECIAL AGE CONSIDERATIONS

Care should be taken when performing laminectomy procedures on young dogs because their cortical and cancellous bone is much softer. Less pressure on the drill or rongeur is needed to safely enter the canal.

THORACOLUMBAR DISK DISEASE

DEFINITIONS

Thoracolumbar disk disease is associated with chondroid degeneration of the nucleus pulposus of intervertebral disks producing extrusion, spinal cord compression, and nerve root entrapment. **Fenestration** is creation of a window or "fenestra" in the lateral or ventral annulus fibrosus to gain access to the nucleus pulposus. **Durotomy** is an incision through dura mater to expose spinal cord parenchyma. Synonyms for thoracolumbar disk disease include a *slipped disk* or *herniated disk*.

GENERAL CONSIDERATIONS AND CLINICALLY RELEVANT PATHOPHYSIOLOGY

Thoracolumbar disk disease is the most common cause of small animal neurologic dysfunction. Significant advances have been made in establishing history, signalment, clinical presentation, and radiographic, myelographic, computed tomography (CT), and magnetic resonance imaging (MRI) findings. However, management methodology remains controversial and is generally determined by clinical experience, rather than critically analyzed data. Many clinicians recommend early surgical spinal cord decompression and mass removal in most cases. Causes of disk degeneration are unknown, and the pathogenesis of spinal cord changes following compressive injury is unclear. Consequently, therapeutic approaches to spinal cord injury remain unsettled. Pathophysiology and pathogenesis of thoracolumbar disk disease are identical to cervical disk disease discussed on p. 1418 (see Figs. 38-27 and 38-28 on p. 1418).

NOTE: The most commonly involved sites of thoracolumbar disk extrusion are intervertebral disk spaces between T11 and L2; these sites make up approximately 65% to 75% of all disk extrusions.

DIAGNOSIS
Clinical Presentation

Signalment. Thoracolumbar disk disease primarily occurs in chondrodystrophic breeds, such as dachshunds, Pekingese, beagles, miniature and toy poodles, cocker spaniels, Shih Tzus, Lhasa apsos, and Welsh corgis. Dachshunds have 10 times the risk of all other breeds combined. Both sexes are equally affected. About 80% of disk problems occur in animals between 3 and 7 years of age. Although disk protrusion occurs in cats, it is uncommon.

Diagnosis of thoracolumbar disk disease in large-breed, nonchondrodystrophic dogs is becoming more common (Macias et al, 2002). The clinical, radiographic, and myelographic features are very similar to those described for small chondrodystrophic dogs. Decision making concerning conservative and surgical treatment is similar to that made for chondrodystrophic dogs.

History. Dogs with thoracolumbar disk disease have various clinical signs. The classic presentation is acute to subacute back pain only or back pain in addition to varying degrees of paraparesis. Although thoracolumbar disk extrusions are variable, many are acute and disruptive. Variables affecting the ultimate severity of spinal cord pathology and subsequent clinical signs are listed in Box 39-3. Acute, rapid extrusions tend to be more deleterious than slow extrusions (i.e., days to weeks). A recent study suggests that the rate of onset (i.e., the speed with which clinical signs develop) significantly and negatively influences clinical outcome in thoracolumbar disk disease patients (Ferreira et al, 2002). Disk material in the vertebral canal may cause inflammation, further exacerbating neural deficits. Onset of clinical signs may occur in minutes or weeks after disk extrusion. Signs may be rapidly progressive, slowly progressive or remain static, or disappear and then later recur. Recurrences are usually caused by further extrusion of the previously affected disk. Patients with a laterally extruded disk in the lumbar intumescence (i.e., intraforaminal) may have hind limb lameness, with or without back pain.

Physical Examination Findings

Physical examination findings are usually normal in thoracolumbar disk disease patients. Neurologic examination findings vary depending on the anatomic location of the extrusion, duration of compression, and force of compression at the time of disk extrusion. Varying degrees of back pain and upper motor neuron (UMN) ambulatory or nonambulatory paraparesis are the most common neurologic abnormalities. Patients with an intraforaminal disk extrusion may have a unilateral hind limb lameness only. The origins of pain (e.g., radiculopathy) and paresis (e.g., myelopathy) caused by disk extrusion are discussed on p. 1418. Accurate localization of the affected intervertebral space requires careful neurologic examination (see Chapter 36). It is not uncommon to confuse thoracolumbar pain with abdominal pain when the patient does not have obvious neurologic deficits. Severity of spinal cord trauma is assessed by neurologic examination; profound neurologic deficits suggest severe spinal cord insult. Finally, determining the pres-

BOX 39-3

Variables That Affect Neurologic Signs

- Location of extrusion (UMN versus LMN)
- Acuteness of disk extrusion
- Velocity of disk extrusion
- Mass of material extruded
- Vertebral canal diameter to spinal cord diameter ratio

UMN, Upper motor neuron; *LMN,* lower motor neuron.

ence or absence of deep pain perception is an important prognostic tool; patients with preservation of deep pain perception generally have a favorable prognosis, whereas those without deep pain perception generally have a guarded to unfavorable prognosis.

> **NOTE:** It is extremely important that deep pain be properly assessed. A withdrawal reflex does not verify the presence of deep pain. If the animal has deep pain, it should vocalize or otherwise indicate (e.g., through dilation of pupils, turning of head, and increased heart rate) that the pain was felt.

Diagnostic Imaging

Location of an extruded thoracolumbar disk is confirmed by radiographic/myelographic, CT, and/or MR imaging. When performing radiographic/myelographic studies, highly collimated lateral, ventrodorsal, and oblique projections of the entire thoracolumbar spine obtained under general anesthesia are often required. Survey radiographic findings indicative of disk extrusion include narrow or wedged intervertebral space, narrow intervertebral foramen, increased opacity of the intervertebral foramen (because of radiopaque herniated disk material), collapse of the articular facets, and calcified material in the spinal canal (Fig. 39-14). Although survey radiographs may suggest the affected intervertebral space, they are rarely definitively diagnostic.

Myelography, CT, or MRI is indicated if there are no visible narrowed interspaces, disk material is not visible in the spinal canal or intervertebral foramen, a lesion is found that is incompatible with the neurologic examination, or when precise localization of the disk is necessary (e.g., left versus right side hemilaminectomy or hemilaminectomy versus dorsal laminectomy). Patients with a herniated thoracolumbar disk exhibit myelographic signs consistent with an extradural compressive lesion (Fig. 39-15, *A-C*). Myelography is described in Chapter 36. Patients with an intraforaminal disk extrusion may have normal survey radiographs and a normal myelogram. CT or MRI may be necessary to establish a definitive diagnosis (Fig. 39-16).

> **NOTE:** The author performs myelography in greater than 90% of patients with thoracolumbar disk extrusions.

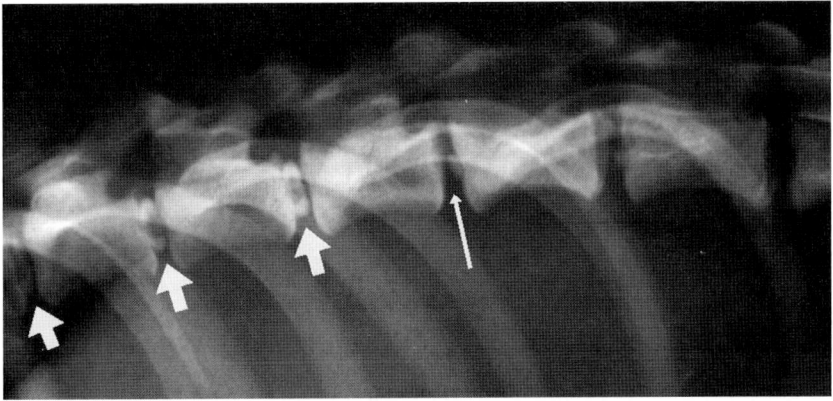

FIG. 39-14
Lateral radiograph of a dog with a T12–T13 herniated intervertebral disk *(small arrow).* Notice the collapsed and slightly wedged intervertebral space, fragmented calcified disk, narrowing of the intervertebral foramen, and collapse of the articular facets. Note also the calcified intervertebral disks in situ *(large arrows).*

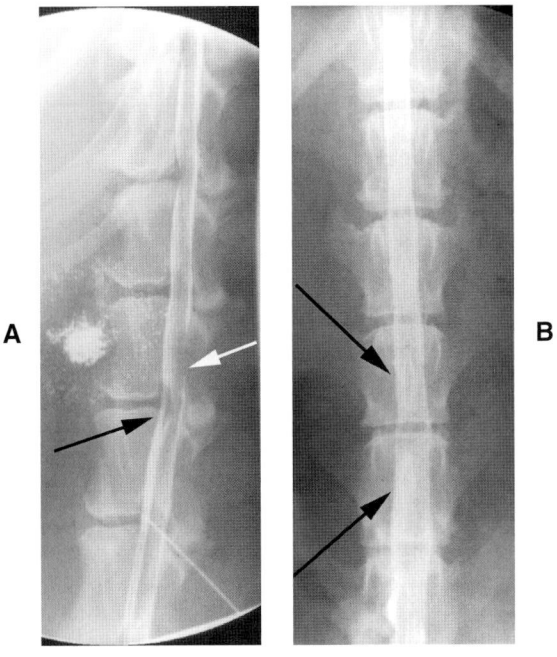

FIG. 39-15
A, Lateral projection of a myelogram showing splitting of the ventral aspect of the contrast column at L3–L4 *(black arrow).* There is attenuation of the dorsal aspect of the contrast column in the body of L3 *(white arrow).* **B,** Ventrodorsal projection of the same myelogram in B; There is shifting of the spinal cord towards the left *(arrows).*

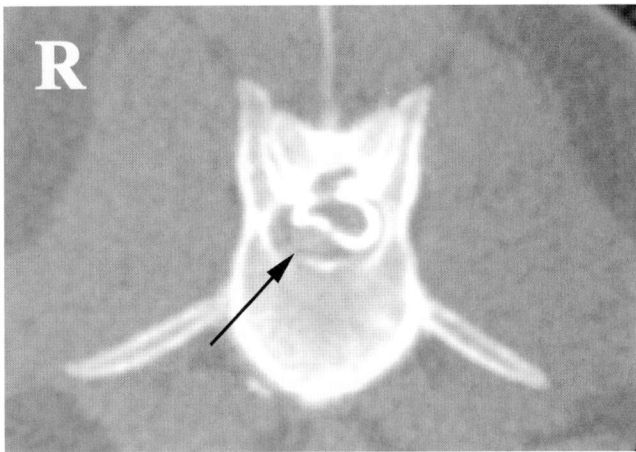

FIG. 39-16
Axial CT myelogram image taken at the level of L3 of the same animal in Figure 39-15. There is a soft tissue attenuating mass within the spinal canal along the right ventral aspect. This is extruded disk material that is causing severe deformation of the spinal cord because of the extradural compression. The CT image shows the severity of the compression to a much greater extent than does the myelogram.

Laboratory Findings

Complete blood count and serum biochemical profile abnormalities are rare. Recent corticosteroid therapy may elevate the level of hepatic enzymes in the serum.

DIFFERENTIAL DIAGNOSIS

Presumptive diagnosis of thoracolumbar disk disease is based on signalment, history, physical examination, and neurologic examination. Possible causes of spinal disorders are based on history, the DAMNIT-V scheme, and myelographic classification given in Chapter 36 on p. 1370. The most likely differential diagnoses for extradural compressive lesions are intervertebral disk extrusion, fracture/luxation, diskospondylitis, congenital malformation, neoplasia, and

Table 39-2

Staging System to Help Determine Medical Versus Surgical Treatment and Prognosis in Animals With Thoracolumbar Disk Disease

STAGE	CLINICAL SIGNS	RADIOGRAPHY/ LESION LOCATION	TREATMENT	PROGNOSIS
I	Single or occasional episodes of mild, moderate, or severe back pain, ± slight CP deficits, no motor weakness	Radiographs not taken Incidental finding of degenerate disks	Conservative Conservative ± fenestration	Favorable Favorable
II	Second episode or persistent and severe back pain, ± CP deficits, ± ambulatory paraparesis*	Radiographs not taken	Conservative ± fenestration Decompression	Favorable/guarded Excellent
III	Uncontrolled severe back pain, ± CP deficits, ± ambulatory paraparesis	Extruded disk in canal	Decompression	Excellent
	Weakly ambulatory† or nonambulatory‡ paraparesis, ± back pain	Extruded disk in canal	Decompression	Excellent/favorable
IV	Paraplegia, § ± back pain			
	Duration <48 hr	Extruded disk in canal	Decompression	Guarded/unfavorable
	Duration >48 hr	Extruded disk in canal	Conservative or decompression	Guarded/Unfavorable

CP, Conscious proprioception.
*Ambulatory paraparesis: patients with hind limb motor weakness that can rise and ambulate without assistance.
†Weakly ambulatory paraparesis: patients that can rise without assistance, take several steps, tire easily, and assume a sitting or recumbent position.
‡Nonambulatory paraparesis: patients that have lost the ability for unassisted hind limb ambulation (voluntary motor movements may or may not be present).
§Paraplegia: patients that have complete loss of both motor and sensory function.

vertebral body osteomyelitis. Diagnostic differentials can usually be narrowed by appropriate use of physical examination, hematology, serum chemistry panel, cerebrospinal fluid (CSF) analysis, and radiography or cross-sectional imaging. Thoracolumbar disk extrusion is confirmed by radiography/myelography and surgery.

Evaluation of history and serial neurologic examinations are needed to formulate appropriate management plans. Establishing onset, course, duration, and severity of motor and sensory impairment helps define prognosis and direct therapy. A staging system may help determine the most appropriate therapy (nonsurgical or surgical) (Table 39-2).

MEDICAL MANAGEMENT

The most important aspect of medical management in ambulatory patients is strict cage confinement for 3 to 4 weeks. Next, 3 to 4 weeks of gradual return to normal activity is recommended. Home confinement means discouraging the animal from jumping up and down on furniture, avoiding stairs, confinement to one room when the owner is absent, and restricted leash walks. This forced rest aids resolution of spinal cord and intradiskal inflammation and facilitates stabilization of the ruptured disk by fibrosis. Nonambulatory patients should have easy access to water and food; a soft, dry area to lie down; bladder expression or intermittent catheterizations

three to four times daily; bowel management; and physiotherapy to maintain muscle mass and joint range of motion. A paraparetic cart may speed recovery by allowing freedom of movement and by improving the patient's attitude.

> NOTE: The most common mistake made in managing animals with disk extrusions is administration of analgesics or antiinflammatories without appropriate concurrent confinement. Strict cage confinement is mandatory in these patients.

Strict confinement and exercise control are sometimes accompanied by drug therapy. It is important to educate the client regarding the analgesic and possible euphoric effects of various medications. If strict confinement is not maintained, excessive activity could cause further disk extrusion with catastrophic neural deficits. Medical management is successful approximately 80% to 90% of the time in patients with just back pain. Commonly used antiinflammatory and muscle relaxant drugs and their dosages are listed in Box 38-6 on p. 1422. These medications can be used independently or in combination. The choice of drugs is dictated by the patient's clinical signs at presentation and by therapeutic trials. Common clinical presentations and suggested thera-

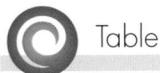 Table 39-3

Recommended Therapy* for Patients With Thoracolumbar Disk Disease Based on Neurologic Signs

CLINICAL PRESENTATION	INITIAL TREATMENT	RESULT	SECOND TREATMENT†	RESULT	THIRD TREATMENT†
Mild to moderate back pain only; first episode or multiple episodes	No drug therapy; cage rest only	No improvement in 5 to 7 days	Muscle relaxant; follow daily	No improvement in 2 to 3 days	Steroids and muscle relaxant; follow daily
Severe back pain only; first episode or multiple episodes	Muscle relaxant; follow daily	No improvement in 2 to 3 days	Steroids and muscle relaxant; follow daily	No improvement in 2 to 3 days	Repeat second treatment or consider surgery
± Back pain and ambulatory paraparesis	Steroids for 1 day	Improvement	Continue steroids for 6 days	Improvement	Observe
		Static	Steroids for 1 day	Improvement	Observe, consider surgery
		Deterioration	Consider surgery	Deterioration	Consider surgery
± Back pain and weakly ambulatory or nonambulatory paraparesis	Recommend early surgery; administer steroids preoperatively				
Recurrent mild, moderate, or severe back pain; unresponsive to medical management	Recommend surgery; administer steroids preoperatively				

*See Box 38-6 on p. 1422 for drug dosages and variations on duration of therapy.
†All patients are placed in strict confinement for 3 to 4 weeks as part of their medical management regardless of the drug used or duration of drug therapy.

peutic regimens are listed in Table 39-3. Knowledge of potential side effects of commonly used antiinflammatory drugs is important; they are listed in Table 38-4 on p. 1424.

Patients treated with antiinflammatory drugs should be monitored for depression, anorexia, abdominal pain, melena, and vomiting of undigested or digested blood (coffee grounds). Many times, anorexia is the only sign in patients with severe gastrointestinal ulceration. If gastrointestinal lesions are suspected, antiinflammatory drugs (see Table 38-4) should be discontinued immediately because ulceration associated with antiinflammatory medication, spinal cord injury, and stress can be catastrophic.

NOTE: Concurrent administration of H_2 receptor antagonists, proton pump inhibitors, Carafate, and/or misoprostol does not negate the adverse gastrointestinal effects of nonsteroidal antiinflammatory drugs (NSAIDs) and steroids. Although these gastroprotective drugs are beneficial in patients that are no longer receiving the NSAIDs or steroids, ulceration/erosion is seldom cured or prevented when the patients continue to receive the NSAIDs or steroids.

SURGICAL TREATMENT

Surgical treatment objectives for patients with thoracolumbar disk disease include gaining access to the vertebral canal and removal of disk fragments causing spinal cord and nerve root compression. Surgical treatment is determined by the patient's neurologic status, results of serial neurologic examinations after admission, and response to medical therapy (see Tables 39-2 and 39-3). If presenting signs warrant surgical intervention or if the patient fails to respond to appropriate medical management, surgery should be considered.

Fenestration has been proposed to eliminate back pain as well as prevent further disk extrusion. Because pain is usually due to a combination of nerve root compression and ischemia from extruded disk fragments, fenestration alone is not the procedure of choice (see Fig. 39-19); removal of extruded disk fragments via laminectomy/pediculectomy is preferred. In rare patients with diskogenic pain (i.e., pressure on the pain-sensitive dorsal longitudinal ligament and dorsal annulus fibrosus), fenestration may alleviate back pain. Evidence of effectiveness of fenestration in prevention of IVDD recurrence is variable. Part of the problem may be that the effectiveness of fenestra-

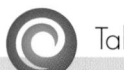

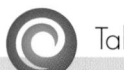Table 39-4

Course of Action if Disk Material Is Not Found at Surgery

SURGICAL PROCEDURE PERFORMED	SURGICAL FINDING	COURSE OF ACTION	RESULT	SECOND COURSE OF ACTION
Hemilaminectomy, pediculectomy, dorsal laminectomy	Epidural fat	At correct space? (recount)	Yes	Close; reevaluate: neurologic exam, myelogram
			No	Operate correct space
Hemilaminectomy	Swollen cord, no disk	Look for ventral extrusion	Ventral disk identified	Remove disk
			No disk	Perform hemilaminectomy on opposite side
Dorsal laminectomy	Swollen cord, no disk	Look on lateral aspect of canal	Disk identified	Extend dorsal to include pediculectomy
			No disk	Extend laminectomy on one side to floor of vertebral canal

tion appears to be dependent on surgical technique. Prophylactic fenestration does not guarantee avoidance of recurrence. In addition, because the prognosis is favorable for the small percentage of dogs that suffer a second episode of IVDD (5% to 20%), performing a second decompressive surgery on this small subgroup may be preferable to performing unnecessary fenestrations in the larger group of dogs (80% to 95%) that were never destined to have recurrence (Mayhew et al, 2004). Moreover, recurrence of clinical signs in dogs undergoing fenestration is reported to be between 5% and 16%. One report suggested that prophylactic percutaneous laser disk ablation results in a 3.4% recurrence of clinical signs (Bartels et al, 2003).

> NOTE: The role of prophylactic fenestration remains unclear. Because the possibility of multiple disks causing recurrent episodes of back pain is unlikely, laminectomy and mass removal of the single offending disk, rather than prophylactic fenestrations of all disks, are warranted (see Tables 39-3 and 39-4).

Decompression in addition to prophylactic fenestration to prevent recurrent disk extrusion at a second site is also controversial. Recurrence of disk extrusion at an adjacent intervertebral space after decompression of the active disk is rare (less than 5%); thus prophylactic fenestration is probably not warranted.

It is generally accepted that patients with even mild paraparesis (i.e., motor weakness) should be treated by early decompression and mass removal via dorsal laminectomy, hemilaminectomy, or pediculectomy. Paresis is a strict function of the forces, mechanical deformation, and pressure exerted on the spinal cord. Fenestration does not remove disk material from its extruded location in the vertebral canal. The decision to pursue surgical intervention is based on the pa-

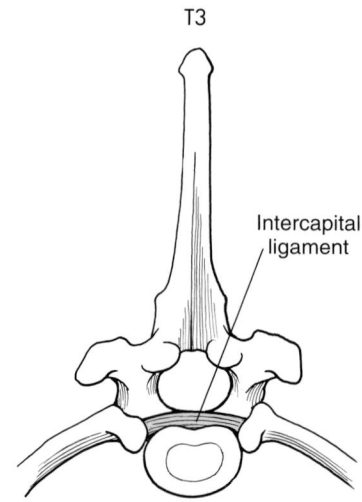

FIG. 39-17
Attachment of the intercapital ligament to each rib head. It spans the dorsal annulus fibrosus.

tient's clinical signs. Generally the earlier spinal cord decompression is undertaken, the better the chance for complete neural recovery. Patients requiring surgery should be operated on within 24 to 48 hours of disk extrusion. Surgery is still a viable option in patients with severe neurologic deficits (i.e., weakly ambulatory or nonambulatory paraparesis) that have been treated medically for 72 to 96 hours before referral; however, they may not recover to a normal neural status (but are often acceptable pets; ambulatory with urinary and fecal continence). Patients with several weeks to months of weakly ambulatory or nonambulatory paraparesis may benefit from surgical intervention if there is myelographic evidence of a compressive mass that can be surgically removed. Although the prognosis is guarded to unfavorable for complete recovery, the animal may become weakly ambulatory paraparetic with voluntary control of bowel and bladder.

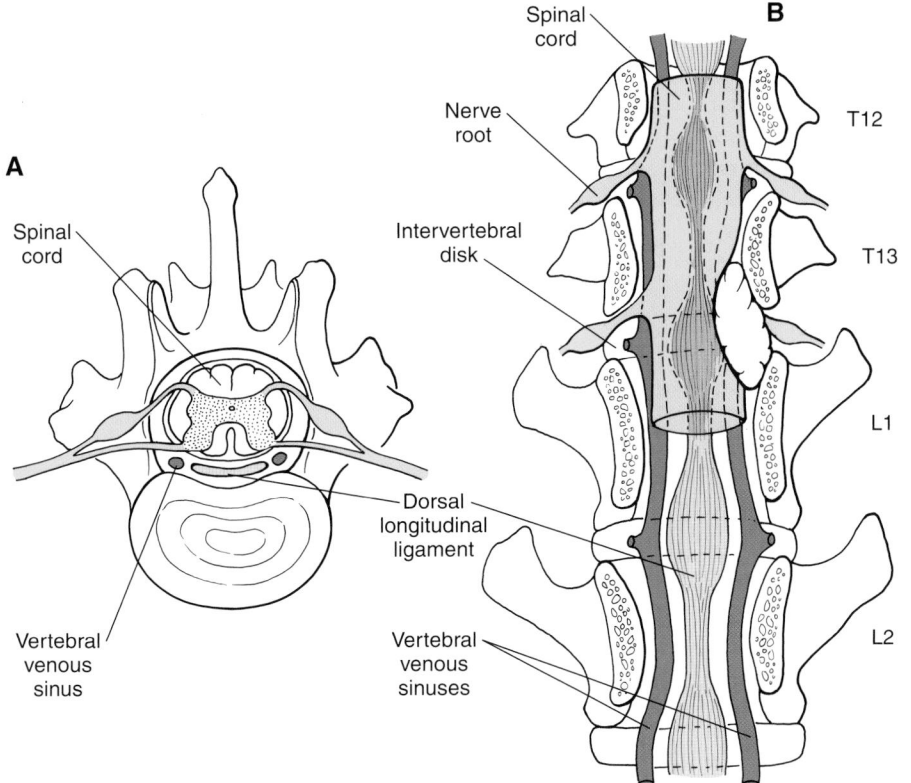

A

Spinal cord

Vertebral venous sinus

B

Spinal cord

Nerve root

Intervertebral disk

Dorsal longitudinal ligament

Vertebral venous sinuses

T12

T13

L1

L2

FIG. 39-18
A, Anatomy of thoracolumbar spinal cord and associated ligaments and vessels. Notice the relationship of the vertebral venous sinus and dorsal longitudinal ligament at the level of the intervertebral space and midvertebral body. **B,** Notice the location of extruded disk relative to the nerve root, vertebral venous sinus, and dorsal longitudinal ligament.

NOTE: It is not sufficient to remove lamina, articular facets, and pedicles; laminectomy, hemilaminectomy, or pediculectomy alone without mass removal can be compared with making a hole in the roof of a house to let water out of the basement. The offending compressive mass lesion (i.e., disk material) must be removed.

Preoperative Management

The animal should be given IV fluids and steroids before surgery. IV steroids should be given to protect the spinal cord from the effects of surgical manipulation. The steroid of choice is methylprednisolone sodium succinate (30 mg/kg IV).

Anesthesia

Suggested anesthetic regimens for dogs with spinal cord injury are given on p. 1402. If the patient requires positioning that may cause respiratory compromise, mechanical ventilatory support should be considered.

Surgical Anatomy

The most common sites for thoracolumbar disk extrusion are between T11 and L2. The tough intercapital ligament from T1-T2 to T9-T10 attaches to each rib head and extends over the dorsal annulus fibrosus (Fig. 39-17), acting as a natural dorsal buttress that helps prevent disk extrusion. The

intercapital ligament at T10-T11 is smaller than the others; disk herniation may occur at this intervertebral space.

Disk extrusions generally occur at the junction of the vertebral venous sinus and dorsal longitudinal ligament (i.e., area of least resistance), resulting in a ventrolateral location of extruded disk fragments (Fig. 39-18). Disk extrusions may therefore cause varying degrees of nerve root compression and ischemia, spinal cord injury, and venous sinus hemorrhage. Extreme care must be used when manipulating and evacuating disk fragments from the floor of the vertebral canal. Occasionally, disk material may extrude laterally into the intervertebral foramen. Removal of the disk requires facetectomy and foraminotomy to expose disk fragments entrapping the nerve root.

Positioning

Patient positioning is dependent upon the surgical procedure selected and is described on p. 1460. Generally, patients undergoing dorsal laminectomy, hemilaminectomy, pediculectomy, or dorsolateral fenestration are positioned in sternal recumbency, whereas those undergoing lateral or ventral fenestration are positioned in lateral recumbency.

SURGICAL TECHNIQUE
Spinal Cord Decompression

The most common procedures used to decompress spinal cord and nerve roots (in order of the author's preference) are hemilaminectomy, pediculectomy, modified dorsal laminectomy, Funkquist B laminectomy, Funkquist A laminectomy, and deep dorsal laminectomy. These procedures are described on pp. 1460 to 1467.

Occasionally, no evidence of extruded disk is seen after entering the canal. Several possibilities exist when this occurs and are listed in Table 39-4, along with a proper course of action for each. Myelotomy, local hypothermia with cool saline, dimethyl sulfoxide (DMSO), naloxone, and thyrotropin releasing hormone are not routinely used in patients with thoracolumbar disk extrusions.

The location of spinal cord compression (right or left lateral) cannot be reliably determined based on lateralization of neurologic signs. A study showed that presenting neurologic signs in 35% of acute and lateral disk extrusions did not correlate with location of disk material in the vertebral canal.

Regardless of the decompression procedure chosen, enter the vertebral canal by carefully lifting off periosteum with a dental spatula, iris spatula, or Lempert rongeur.

At this point, disk material, black venous blood ("crankcase oil"), swollen spinal cord, or epidural fat will be visible.

Acute disk protrusions. Acutely extruded disk material may take on various forms. It may be white flecks of disk incorporated in an organized clot that when incised looks like crankcase oil. This type of disk is often easily suctioned and removal results in full decompression. Extruded material may include portions of the dorsal annulus fibrosus. These fragments are white, firm, and cartilaginous in nature, easy to grasp with ophthalmic forceps, and often can be completely removed as a long continuous strand, resulting in full decompression. Occasionally, hard, white, chalky disk material is found. Removal is accomplished by continually chipping away at the mass with a dental or iris spatula. Take care to protect the spinal cord, nerve root, and venous sinus during dissection because the majority of disks extrude ventrally and laterally (see Fig. 39-18, *B*). Mild-to-moderate shifts of the dural tube back to its normal position following laminectomy and disk removal indicate appropriate decompression.

> NOTE: If approached within hours or days, acute disk extrusions are generally easily removed with carefully applied suction and manipulation using ophthalmic forceps and dental spatulas.

Chronic disk protrusions. Patients with a chronic history (months or more) of medically treated pain and ambulatory paraparesis that finally develop severe motor weakness and require surgery, often have a firm, encapsulated, protruded mass that may be adherent to venous sinus and dura mater (Hansen type II). Disk removal is difficult because of its hard, encapsulated nature; ventrolateral location; and adhesions to dura and venous sinus. If venous

sinus hemorrhage occurs, control it with hemostatic sponges using the techniques described in Box 38-1 on p. 1403.

Lateral intervertebral disk extrusions. Patients with a history of hind limb lameness, with or without back pain, may have a disk that has extruded completely into the intervertebral foramen. There is no evidence of disk in the vertebral canal. Disk removal should be performed via hemilaminectomy, facetectomy, and foraminotomy to expose and remove disk fragments (see p. 1464).

If the disk can be lateralized, perform a hemilaminectomy, including complete removal of the pedicle. If the disk cannot be lateralized, perform a deep dorsal laminectomy (see p. 1464) and visualize the protruded disk. Remove the entire pedicle to the level of the floor of the vertebral canal. Expose the vertebral venous sinus at the level of the affected intervertebral space and transect the sinus, if necessary, to expose the encapsulated disk. Once the disk is adequately exposed, use a No. 11 scalpel blade to incise the disk capsule. Use a dental spatula, iris spatula, and tartar scraper to evacuate the firm disk material.

It is rarely necessary to place dural sutures to manipulate the spinal cord and allow adequate visualization and removal of the disk.

If the protruded disk is located on the ventral midline and cannot be adequately removed as described previously, transect the nerve root at the site of extrusion (permissible only at T3-L3 spinal cord segments). Gently expose the nerve root and radicular vessels and cauterize them with bipolar cautery. As the spinal cord releases, gently roll it off the offending disk for better visualization and less traumatic disk removal. Remove disk material as described previously. Do not attempt to reattach the severed nerve root.

Durotomy

Durotomy is rarely indicated. It is not recommended as a therapeutic modality, but may be useful in determining prognosis. Patients that have paraplegia (i.e., complete loss of motor function and sensory perception) generally have a poor prognosis. Durotomy to evaluate presence or absence of myelomalacia may be useful in deciding patient outcome.

Carefully tent the dura with fine ophthalmic forceps. Use a gentle longitudinal stroke along the dura with a No. 11 or No. 12 scalpel blade.

Penetration of the dura is obviated by the flow of CSF. A 1.5- to 2-cm-long incision allows adequate visualization of spinal cord parenchyma.

Observe the spinal cord for evidence of central hemorrhagic necrosis, loss of anatomic integrity, and toothpastelike consistency.

BOX 39-4

Advantages and Disadvantages of Ventral Fenestration

Advantages
- Avoids the spinal nerve roots
- Minimal hemorrhage

Disadvantages
- Need for a thoracotomy
- Dissection is near major vessels
- Cannot be combined with a decompressive procedure
- Increased risk of pushing disk material into the vertebral canal
- Does not provide spinal cord decompression

 BOX 39-5

Advantages and Disadvantages of Lateral Fenestration

Advantages
- Limited muscle dissection
- Minimal hemorrhage
- Does not require abdominal or thoracic surgery
- Can be combined with a hemilaminectomy

Disadvantages
- An assistant is required
- Exposure is difficult in obese animals
- Thoracic disks are difficult to visualize
- Requires dissection near spinal nerves and vessels
- Does not provide spinal cord decompression

These findings are compatible with complete loss of spinal cord function.

Leave the dural incision open. Harvest a subcutaneous fat graft and place it over the laminectomy site.

Disk Fenestration

Three approaches are commonly used to perform disk fenestration: ventral, lateral, and dorsolateral. Advantages and disadvantages of these techniques are listed in Boxes 39-4 through 39-6.

Ventral approach. *Place the patient in right lateral recumbency and make a paracostal incision. Enter the abdominal cavity, identify the left kidney, and retract it ventrally. Pack off abdominal viscera caudally with moistened laparotomy pads. Elevate the iliopsoas muscle, and locate the short transverse process of L1 for orientation. Digitally depress the aorta and sympathetic trunk to expose the ventral annulus fibrosus of intervertebral disks L1-L2 through L5-L6 (Fig. 39-19, A).*

Using a No. 11 scalpel blade or high-speed pneumatic or electric drill, create a window in the ventral annulus. Use a hypodermic needle (14- to 20-gauge), tartar scraper, or curved spatula to remove as much nucleus pulposus as possible. Place the patient through positional changes (i.e., lateral flexion and extension) to encourage evacuation of nuclear material. After all disks have been fenestrated, close abdominal musculature with absorbable suture material. Move the skin incision to the tenth intercostal space and make a thoracotomy incision. Place self-retaining retractors to hold the ribs apart, pack the lungs cranially with moistened laparotomy pads, and dissect parietal pleura from intervertebral disks T9-T10 through T13-L1. Avoid aorta, sympathetic trunk, and intercostal vessels (Fig. 39-19, B). Perform disk fenestration as described previously. Close the thoracotomy incision routinely.

Lateral approach.
This approach is satisfactory for exposing disks T13-L1 through L5-L6. Fenestration of disks T10-T11 through T12-T13 is more difficult.

 BOX 39-6

Advantages and Disadvantages of Dorsolateral Fenestration

Advantages
- Can be easily combined with a hemilaminectomy procedure

Disadvantages
- Excessive muscle dissection
- Requires dissection near spinal nerves and vessels
- Does not provide spinal cord decompression

Clip and aseptically prepare an area from T6 cranially to the greater trochanter caudally, dorsal spinous processes dorsally to midabdomen ventrally. Place the patient in right lateral recumbency if you are right handed, and left lateral recumbency if you are left handed. Place a 4-inch-diameter sandbag or rolled towel under the L2-L6 vertebrae to create an arch effect that helps open the intervertebral spaces. Make a skin incision from the dorsal spine of T9 to the ventral aspect of the iliac wing. Continue the incision through subcutaneous fat, lumbar fascia, a second layer of fat, and to the longissimus dorsi and iliocostalis lumborum muscles. Palpate the short transverse process of L1 for orientation, and with a pair of Kelly forceps, dissect overlying muscle fibers to expose its dorsocranial surface. Identify the lateral annulus fibrosus, located just cranial and slightly ventral to the junction of the transverse process and vertebral body (Fig. 39-20). Use a blunt retractor to expose the lateral surface of the annulus fibrosus; retract muscle fibers dorsally and muscle fibers, spinal nerve, and spinal vessels ventrally. Use a No. 11 scalpel blade to make a window in the lateral aspect of the annulus fibrosus. Be careful not to incise dorsal to the junction of the transverse process and vertebral body

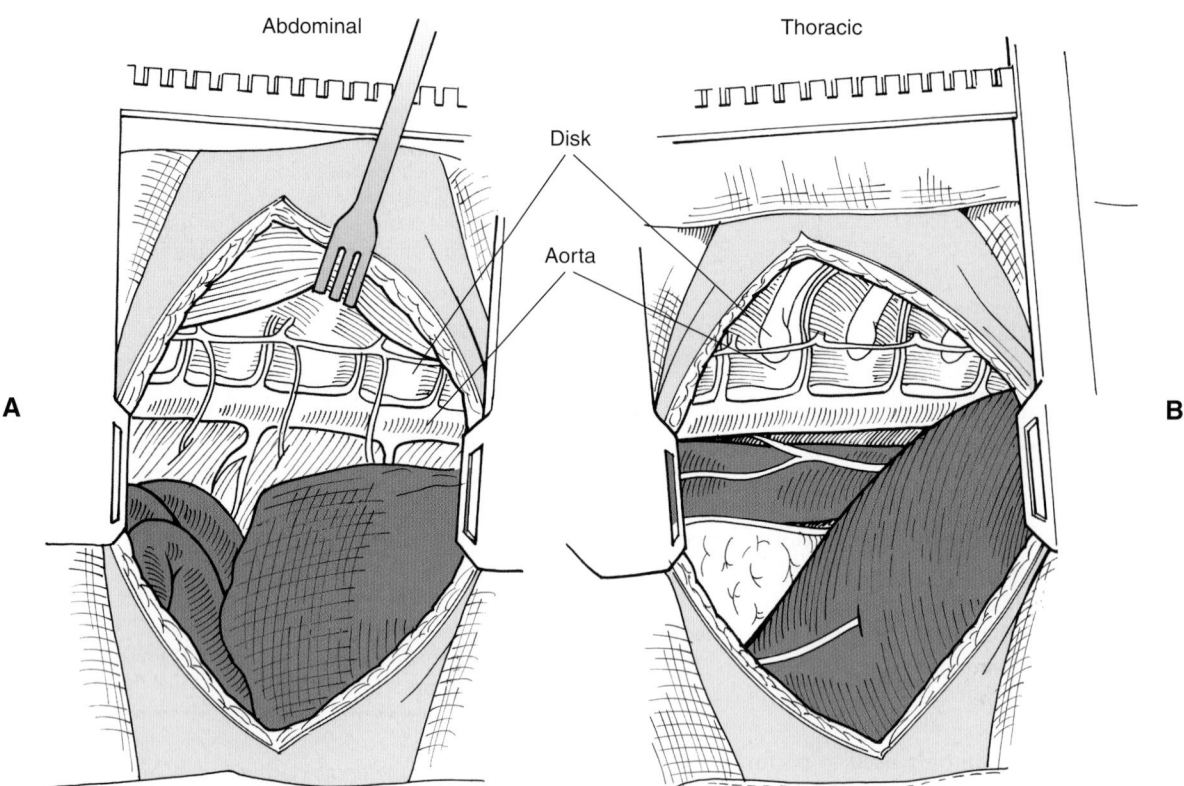

FIG. 39-19
For ventral disk fenestration, perform an **A,** abdominal or **B,** thoracic approach.

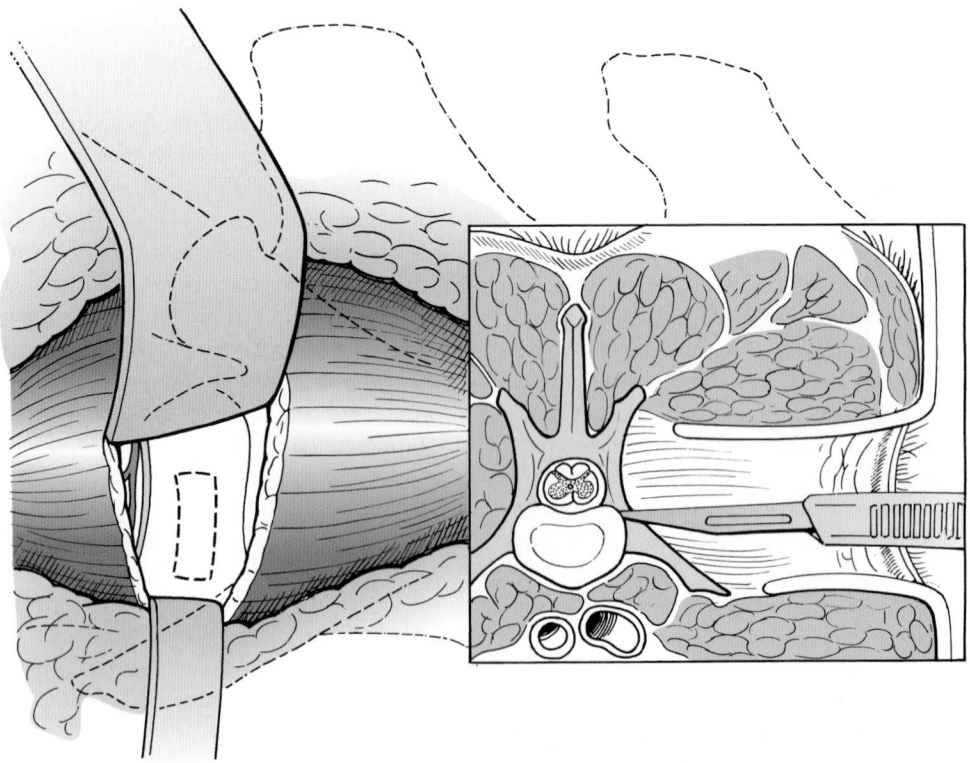

FIG. 39-20
For lateral disk fenestration, perform a lateral epaxial muscle-splitting approach.

because this may result in spinal cord damage. Perform disk fenestration as described for ventral fenestration. To fenestrate disks T10-T11 through T12-T13, elevate the iliocostalis lumborum muscle off the craniodorsal aspect of the rib to the level of the vertebral body and retract it craniodorsally. Retract the remaining musculature on the cranial aspect of the rib ventrally, exposing the lateral annulus.

The thoracic pleura is just ventral to this dissection.

Visualization is limited; be careful to stay below the arch of the rib when incising the annulus fibrosus. After all disks have been fenestrated, use positional changes to encourage further evacuation of nuclear material. Close muscle, subcutaneous tissue, and skin routinely.

Dorsolateral approach. *Place the patient in ventral recumbency with the spine gently arched dorsally. Make a dorsal midline skin incision from the dorsal spinous process of T9 to the dorsal spinous process of L6. Continue dissection to the level of the thoracolumbar fascia. Incise the thoracolumbar fascia along the dorsal spinous processes on the side toward the surgeon. Using a periosteal elevator or small osteotome, elevate epaxial muscles from the lateral aspect of the dorsal spinous processes, working in a caudal to cranial direction. Elevate a second level of epaxial muscle from articular facets. Begin by elevating musculature from the caudal aspect of the articular process and progress to the cranial aspect. Use curved scissors to sever muscular attachments close to their tendon of origin to minimize hemorrhage. Place Gelpi retractors to hold muscles apart and improve exposure. Elevate remaining musculature from the dorsal aspect of the transverse processes of lumbar vertebrae and cranial surface of the ribs of thoracic vertebrae. Identify muscular attachments to the accessory process, spinal nerve, and vessels (Fig. 39-21). Retract these structures cranially to expose the lateral surface of the annulus fibrosus. Perform fenestration as described for ventral fenestration. Close muscle, subcutaneous tissue, and skin routinely.*

SUTURE MATERIALS AND SPECIAL INSTRUMENTS

Special instruments necessary to perform laminectomy and fenestration procedures are listed in Box 39-1 on p. 1468.

POSTOPERATIVE CARE AND ASSESSMENT

Patients with thoracolumbar disk disease should be evaluated postoperatively in a similar fashion as patients with other thoracolumbar spinal disorders (see p. 1469 and Box 39-2). As no inherent or acquired spinal instability is created, physiotherapy is encouraged as soon as the patient has recovered from postoperative discomfort—generally 24 to 48 hours. As the majority of thoracolumbar disk patients are small-breed dogs, clients should be instructed in home management and these patients can often be sent home within 72 hours of surgery, even if they are weakly ambulatory or nonambulatory paraparetic.

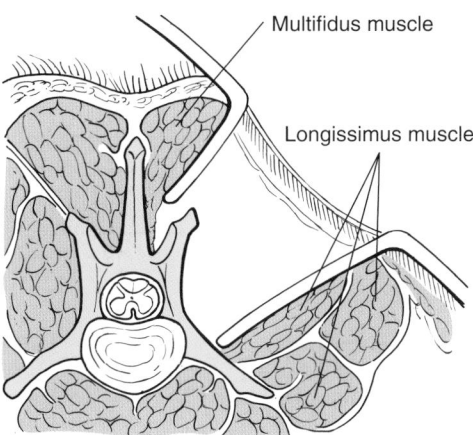

FIG. 39-21
For dorsolateral disk fenestration, perform a dorsolateral epaxial muscle-splitting approach.

NOTE: If these animals are unable to urinate on their own, express their bladder three to four times daily until voluntary urinations occur. Otherwise the bladder may become atonic.

PROGNOSIS

Prognosis for patients treated medically or surgically for thoracolumbar disk disease is generally favorable and is dependent on neurologic signs and the medical or surgical management selected. Clinical factors and probable patient outcome are outlined in Box 39-3 and Table 39-2. The prognosis for surgically treated patients is generally related to the presenting neurologic signs: the better the presenting neurologic status, the quicker the time to complete recovery. A recent study looking at prognostic indicators for time to ambulation after surgical decompression in nonambulatory dogs suggests that recovery is more rapid in patients with postoperative voluntary motor movements (Davis et al, 2002). Patients with voluntary motor movements postoperatively regained ambulatory status within 8 days compared to 14 days in patients without voluntary motor movements. The prognosis for thoracolumbar disk disease patients with no deep pain perception on clinical presentation is variable. Various studies suggest an acceptable recovery rate from 20% to 70%.

References

Bartels KE, Russel GH, Bahr RJ et al: Outcome of and complications associated with prophylactic percutaneous laser disk ablation in dogs with thoracolumbar disk disease: 277 cases (1992-2001), *J Am Vet Med Assoc* 222:1733, 2003.

Corse MR, Walter CR, Friis EA: In vitro evaluation of biomechanical effects of multiple hemilaminectomies on the canine lumbar vertebral column, *Am J Vet Res* 64:1139, 2003.

Davis GJ, Brown DC: Prognostic indicators of time to ambulation after surgical decompression in nonambulatory dogs with acute thoracolumbar disk extrusions: 112 cases, *Vet Surg* 31:513, 2002.

Ferreira AJA, Correia JHD, Jaggy A: Thoracolumbar disk disease in 71 paraplegic dogs: influence of rate of onset and duration of clinical signs on treatment results, *J Sm Anim Pract* 43:158, 2002.

Macias C, McKee WM, May C et al: Thoracolumbar disk disease in large dogs: a study of 99 cases, *J Sm Anim Prac* 43:439, 2002.

Mayhew PD, McLear RC, Ziemer LS et al: Risk factors for recurrence of clinical signs associated with thoracolumbar intervertebral disk herniation in dogs: 229 cases (1994-2000), *J Am Vet Med Assoc* 225:1231, 2004.

Suggested Reading

Amsellem PM, Troombs JP, Laverty PH et al: Loss of deep pain sensation following thoracolumbar intervertebral disk herniation in dogs: treatment and prognosis, *Compend Cont Ed Pract Vet* 25:266, 2003.

In the absence of ascending-descending diffuse myelomalacia, and with surgical decompression and appropriate medical and supportive treatment, more than 50% of these dogs may recover acceptable ambulation and urinary continence as evaluated by owners.

Brisson BA, Moffatt SL, Swayne SL et al: Recurrence of thoracolumbar intervertebral disk extrusion in chondrodystrophic dogs after surgical decompression with or without prophylactic fenestration: 265 cases (1995-1999), *J Am Vet Med Assoc* 224:1808, 2004.

Prophylactic fenestration is generally successful in preventing future disk extrusions at fenestrated disk spaces. Prospective evaluation is still required to determine whether fenestration decreases the overall rate of disk extrusion at adjacent, nonfenestrated disk spaces.

Olby N, Levine J, Harris T et al: Long-term functional outcome of dogs with severe injuries of the thoracolumbar spinal cord: 87 cases (1996-2001), *J Am Vet Med Assoc* 222:762, 2003.

Results suggest that prognosis of paraplegic dogs without deep pain perception because of trauma was guarded, whereas dogs with disk herniation had a better chance of recovering motor function.

FRACTURES AND LUXATIONS OF THE THORACOLUMBAR SPINE

DEFINITIONS

Fractures or **luxations** of the **thoracic or lumbar spine** are caused by traumatic or pathologic disruption of osseous and supporting soft tissue structures, producing spinal cord and nerve root compression. Synonyms for fractures of the thoracolumbar spine include a *broken back, spinal fracture, vertebral fracture, vertebral column fracture,* or *dislocated spine.*

GENERAL CONSIDERATIONS AND CLINICALLY RELEVANT PATHOPHYSIOLOGY

The thoracolumbar spine is the most common site for spinal fractures and luxations. Fractures and luxations occur between T11 and L6 in approximately 50% to 60% of patients with blunt spinal trauma. It appears that the higher incidence of fracture/luxation at certain sites along the vertebral column may not correlate with a difference in muscular or ligamentous attachments, but rather with mobile areas of the vertebral column adjacent to more stable areas of the axial skeleton (e.g., caudal thoracic and caudal lumbar spine). Fractures of the thoracic spine involving T1 through T9 are relatively uncommon, and when they do occur are generally stable and nondisplaced because of the inherent stability gained by massive epaxial muscle mass, rib attachments, ligamentous support, and intercostal muscle attachments. The most common cause of vertebral fractures is automobile trauma (i.e., approximately 90%) (Selcer et al, 1991). Other causes include bite wounds, gunshot injuries, and underlying metabolic or neoplastic disorders resulting in bone demineralization (e.g., nutritional secondary hyperparathyroidism and osteosarcoma).

> NOTE: A complete physical examination should be done. Approximately 39% to 50% of patients with vertebral fractures have associated problems (e.g., pneumothorax, lung contusions, diaphragmatic hernia, urogenital injuries, and other orthopedic injuries).

Fractures and luxations of the thoracolumbar spine are classified as pathologic or traumatic. Pathologic fractures/luxations generally occur when hereditary or congenital ligamentous instability decreases spinal support (e.g., atlantoaxial instability) or when bone integrity is compromised because of an underlying disease process (e.g., metabolic bone disease and neoplasia). Traumatic fractures/luxations are induced by forces resulting in severe hyperextension, hyperflexion, axial compression, and rotation, often occurring at or near the junction of a mobile and more rigid vertebral segment. Failure of supporting structures of the spine to resist such forces causes mechanical discontinuity with resultant spinal cord and nerve root compression.

> NOTE: Approximately 20% of patients have a second spinal fracture/luxation.

DIAGNOSIS
Clinical Presentation

Signalment. There is no breed or sex predisposition; however, dogs more commonly sustain vertebral fracture/luxation than cats. Vertebral fractures may occur at any age, but are more common in younger animals (e.g., 1 to 2 years of age).

History. Patients with thoracolumbar vertebral fractures typically are brought in because of trauma associated with automobiles. They suffer varying degrees of back pain and paraparesis, depending on severity of spinal cord and nerve root compression. Occasionally, patients have subtle neurologic deficits, and careful physical and neurologic examinations are necessary to detect abnormalities.

Physical Examination Findings

Vertebral fracture patients often have concurrent injuries (e.g., pneumothorax, pulmonary contusion, diaphragmatic hernia, and fracture/luxation of the pelvis, ribs, appendicular skeleton, and second vertebral fracture). Thorough physical examination is necessary to recognize these injuries before an appropriate course of action can be planned. Extreme care must be taken during physical examination to prevent exacerbating the spinal injury by excessive movement. Patients with profound neurologic deficits should be secured to a rigid platform during examination and preoperative management. Careful palpation of the spine may reveal a depression over its dorsal aspect, a displaced dorsal spinous process caused by rupture of the supraspinous and interspinous ligaments, or fracture of the dorsal spinous processes. If the patient is ambulatory, the back should be palpated for crepitus or excessive movement as the patient moves. These findings also help assess inherent stability or instability of the traumatized spine. A thorough neurologic examination should be performed to locate the fracture, determine the best therapy, and provide prognostic information (i.e., presence or absence of deep pain perception). Specific neurologic examination techniques are discussed in Chapter 36 on p. 1357.

Diagnostic Imaging

Radiographs are of limited use for evaluating thoracic and lumbar spinal trauma. Survey radiographs may reveal the location of the fracture/luxation and severity of vertebral displacement at the time the radiograph is taken. However, radiographs may not show the maximum displacement at the time of injury; spontaneous reduction of subluxations, luxations, and fractures often occurs before radiography. The amount of spinal cord damage may therefore differ in patients with radiographically similar lesions. Radiographs may help determine prognosis when vertebral displacement is severe enough to reduce vertebral canal diameter more than 80% in the lateral and ventrodorsal projections; these patients generally have irreversible spinal cord and nerve root compression (Fig. 39-22).

> NOTE: Neurologic examination findings are more useful than radiographic findings in discerning extent of spinal cord injury and prognosis. Notably displaced fractures may be found in ambulatory animals and no discernible radiographic lesion may be evident in animals without deep pain.

Survey radiographs may be taken on the awake or anesthetized patient. Advantages and disadvantages of each are discussed on p. 1370. Awake lateral and cross-table ventrodorsal projections are recommended. This evaluation, coupled with neurologic examination findings, aids in determining therapy. If surgery is considered, preoperative anesthetized radiographs or a CT scan should be obtained for critical evaluation of the vertebral injury (see p. 1370). Because up to 20% have a second spinal fracture/luxation, all patients with traumatic spinal injury should have a complete spinal series of radiographs. Typical radiographic findings in patients with thoracic and lumbar spinal fracture/luxation are listed in Box 39-7 (Fig. 39-23, *A* and *B*). A rough idea of spinal stability can be judged by whether the dorsal compartment, ventral compartment, or a combination of dorsal and ventral compartment injury exists. Myelography or cross-sectional imaging may be required if there is a suspicion of herniated intervertebral disk material, bone fragments in the vertebral canal, no evidence of vertebral discontinuity, or when radiographic findings do not correlate with neurologic examination (see p. 1370). Typical myelographic findings in patients with thoracic and lumbar spinal fracture/luxation are consistent with an extradural mass and are described and illustrated in Fig. 36-16 on p. 1374.

Laboratory Findings

Patients having just thoracolumbar fracture/luxation generally have stress leukograms and elevated hepatic enzyme levels. However, if concurrent injuries are present, labora-

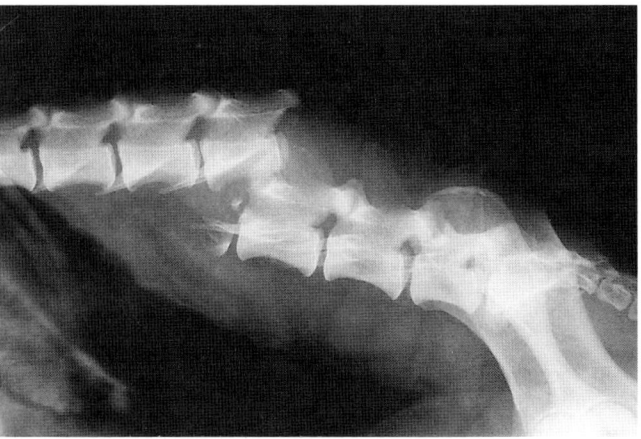

FIG. 39-22
Lateral radiograph of a dog with an L4 fracture. Notice the severe vertebral displacement.

 BOX 39-7

Typical Radiographic Findings With Thoracic and Lumbar Spinal Fracture/Luxation

- Discontinuity of bony structures (i.e., dorsal spinous process, lamina, pedicle, and vertebral body)
- Malalignment of intervertebral spaces and/or articular facets
- Fracture lines in the body, lamina, and/or spinous processes of involved vertebrae
- Loss of continuity or malalignment of the vertebral canal
- Combination of the above

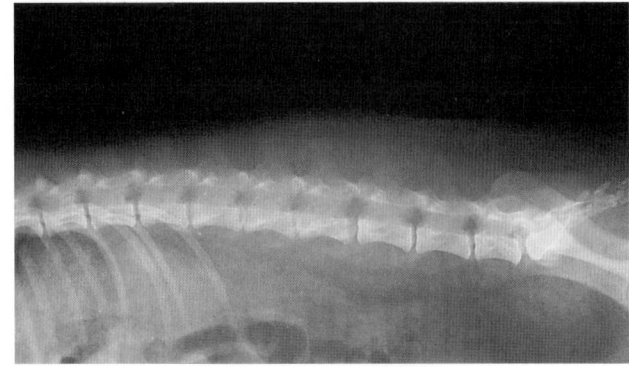

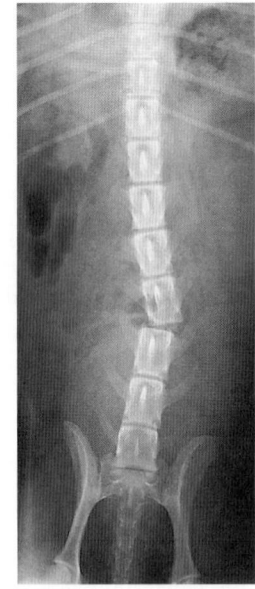

FIG. 39-23

A, Lateral and **B,** ventrodorsal radiographs of a dog with L4–L5 luxation. Notice the accentuated intervertebral space at L4–L5 on the lateral view and lateral vertebral body displacement on the ventrodorsal view.

tory abnormalities (e.g., elevated blood urea nitrogen [BUN] and electrolyte abnormalities with uroabdomen, and blood gas abnormalities with pneumothorax or pulmonary contusions) may occur.

DIFFERENTIAL DIAGNOSIS

Possible etiology of spinal disorders based on history, the DAMNIT-V scheme, and myelographic classification is given in Chapter 36. The most likely differential diagnoses for an extradural mass are intervertebral disk extrusion, fracture/luxation, diskospondylitis, congenital malformation, neoplasia, and vertebral body osteomyelitis. Diagnostic differentials can usually be eliminated by appropriate use of physical, hematologic, serum chemistry, CSF, and radiographic evaluations. Diagnosis of thoracolumbar fracture/luxation is confirmed by radiography.

Because concurrent injuries are common in patients with thoracolumbar vertebral fracture/luxation, physical examina-

tion and patient stabilization, with management of life threatening injuries, is the initial objective. Patients with severe trauma should be treated for shock and the thoracolumbar spine stabilized by securing the patient to a rigid platform. After initial stabilization, neurologic examination is performed to localize the fracture/luxation and help determine therapy. Radiographs of the thoracic and lumbar spine should be taken while the patient is conscious for initial assessment. Conservative or surgical management is based on initial neurologic status, serial neurologic examinations, radiographic assessment of spinal stability (i.e., is the fracture stable or unstable?) (see Box 39-7), and presence of concurrent injuries.

MEDICAL MANAGEMENT

Medical management includes strict confinement, a back brace, antiinflammatory medication, appropriate use of analgesics, and serial neurologic examinations (Table 39-5). Ambulatory patients should be restricted to a cage or a small room or kennel for 2 to 3 weeks. A comfortable, well-padded back brace or body splint constructed from basswood or lightweight, moldable fiberglass supports the spine. Although the efficacy of a back brace may be questioned, it appears useful to counteract excessive ventral and lateral flexion of the torso while the patient is confined. Generally, patients are treated with antiinflammatory drugs. Commonly used antiinflammatory and muscle relaxant drugs and their dosages are listed in Boxes 38-6 and 38-8 on pp. 1422 and 1450. These medications can be used independently or in combination. Knowledge of potential side effects of commonly used antiinflammatory drugs is important (see Tables 38-4 and 38-5 on p. 1424). Choosing the proper drug regimen is dictated by the patient's clinical signs and therapeutic trials. Common clinical presentations and suggested medical therapies are listed in Table 39-6.

Neurologic examinations should be performed twice daily for the first week, then daily until the patient is released from the hospital. Nonambulatory patients are treated with strict cage confinement, a back brace, antiinflammatory medications, and serial neurologic examinations. In addition, nonambulatory patients should have easy access to water and food; a soft, dry area to lie down; bladder expression or intermittent catheterization three to four times a day; bowel management; and physiotherapy to maintain muscle mass and joint range of motion. A paraparetic cart is not recommended because of the pressure placed on the thoracolumbar spine by the cart's supporting bars.

SURGICAL TREATMENT

Patients that fail to respond to an appropriate course of medical management or that have profound neurologic deficits (see Tables 39-5 and 39-6) are surgical candidates. Objectives of surgical treatment include spinal cord and nerve root decompression and vertebral fracture/luxation stabilization. Decompression is generally provided by fracture/luxation reduction. Laminectomy and mass removal (e.g., disk material and bone fragments) are rarely needed. Stabilization can be provided by multiple procedures; however, only techniques and various configurations of techniques that have been clinically or biomechanically proven to provide adequate vertebral stabilization are discussed here. These include Steinmann pins and polymethylmethacrylate (PMMA), vertebral body plates, dorsal spinous process plates, modified segmental spinal fixation, or a combination of the previous techniques. Choice of technique is dictated by location of the fracture; size, age, and disposition of the patient; equipment available; and experience of the surgeon.

> NOTE: It is important to remember that patients retaining even minimal neurologic function deserve the benefits of conservative treatment if surgery is unacceptable to the owner.

Preoperative Management

The animal should be given IV fluids and steroids before surgery. IV steroids may be administered to protect the spinal cord from surgical manipulation. The steroid of choice is methylprednisolone sodium succinate (30 mg/kg IV).

Anesthesia

Suggested anesthetic regimens for animals undergoing spinal surgery are on p. 1403. If the patient requires positioning that may cause respiratory compromise, mechanical ventilatory support should be considered.

Surgical Anatomy

Anatomy of the thoracolumbar spine is described on p. 1460.

Positioning

Techniques used for surgical stabilization for thoracic and lumbar fracture/luxation require a dorsal approach. Patient positioning is generally sternal recumbency and is described and illustrated in Figs. 39-3 and 39-4 on pp. 1461 to 1462.

SURGICAL TECHNIQUE
Steinmann Pins and Polymethylmethacrylate

This technique provides an effective means of spinal stabilization. It can be performed on any area of the spine (e.g., thoracic, thoracolumbar, lumbar, and lumbosacral) and in any age or size animal of any disposition; is performed easily; and requires a minimum of special equipment. It does necessitate a thorough knowledge of vertebral anatomy and constant reference to an appropriate anatomic specimen. Dogs weighing less than 15 kg with luxations or fractures close to the end plate can be stabilized with one 20-g package of PMMA. Dogs weighing more than 15 kg require two 20-g packages. Generally, two or three 20-g packages of PMMA are required when spanning a vertebral body fracture or when a laminectomy has been performed. Because pin placement is critical and anatomic landmarks vary from

vertebra to vertebra, a skeleton should be available for reference during this procedure.

Approach the spine as described for modified dorsal laminectomy (p. 1461). Place towel forceps in the dorsal spinous processes of the vertebrae cranial and caudal to the fracture/luxation; apply traction and countertraction during epaxial muscle elevation from lamina and pedicles.

This helps avoid fracture/luxation displacement during dissection.

Continue dissection ventrally to the level of the costal fovea of the transverse processes if a thoracic vertebra is involved, or the base of the transverse processes if a lumbar vertebra is involved. If a dorsal laminectomy or hemilaminectomy is indicated, perform one as described on pp. 1461 and 1464, respectively. Reduce the vertebral fracture/luxation using bone-holding forceps or towel clamps applied to the dorsal spinous processes. Facilitate reduction by having two nonsterile assistants apply gentle traction on the head and tail. Maintain reduction of the fracture/luxation with traction on towel clamps, or if a dorsal laminectomy is not performed, place a 0.45-inch Kirschner wire across each articular facet. Use an electric or air-driven drill to place Steinmann pins into the vertebral bodies on each side of the fracture/luxation. In the thoracic vertebrae, place pins into the pedicle and drive them into the vertebral body, using the tubercle of the ribs and base of the accessory processes as anatomic landmarks. In the lumbar vertebrae, place pins into the vertebral bodies, using the accessory processes and transverse processes as landmarks. Direct the Steinmann pins cranioventrally and from lateral to medial in the vertebral body cranial to the fracture/luxation, and caudoventrally and from lateral to medial in the vertebral body caudal to the fracture/luxation (Fig. 39-24). Drive each Steinmann pin to exit 2 to 3 mm from the ventral aspect of the vertebral body. Cut the pins 3 to 4 mm below the level of the dorsal spinous processes. Notch each pin at its dorsal aspect with a pin cutter. If a laminectomy was performed, cover the defect with an autogenous fat graft. Thoroughly mix the liquid monomer with polymer powder. Once the PMMA can be handled without sticking to the surgeon's gloves, pack it around the Steinmann pins, making sure it contacts all surfaces of each pin and covers the dorsal aspects. If a dorsal laminectomy or hemilaminectomy has been performed, mold the PMMA into the shape of a doughnut as it is packed around the Steinmann pins (Fig. 39-25). Take care not to allow PMMA to contact spinal cord or nerve roots. If a laminectomy was not performed, apply a circular mass of PMMA, incorporating Steinmann pins, articular facets, lamina, pedicles, and adjacent dorsal spinous process (Fig. 39-26, A). If a fractured vertebral body must be spanned, place pins in the body cranial and caudal to the fractured body (Fig. 39-26, B). Use the same technique as described previously. Lavage the PMMA with cool saline for 5 minutes to dissipate the heat of polymerization. If necessary, excise portions of epaxial muscles

Table 39-5

Conservative Versus Surgical Management of Patients With Thoracolumbar Spinal Fracture/Luxation

INITIAL NEUROLOGIC EXAM*	SERIAL NEUROLOGIC EXAM	RADIOGRAPHIC ASSESSMENT	TREATMENT	PROGNOSIS
Back pain; normal ambulation	Static or improving	Minimal displacement; stable	Conservative	Favorable
	± Back pain; ambulatory paraparesis	Moderate or severe displacement; unstable	Improve conservative management Surgical stabilization†	Favorable to guarded Favorable
	± Back pain; weakly ambulatory or nonambulatory paraparesis	Minimal, moderate, or severe displacement; unstable	Surgical stabilization†	Favorable to guarded
Back pain; conscious proprioceptive deficits	Static or improving	Minimal, moderate, or severe displacement; unstable	Conservative	Favorable
	± Back pain; ambulatory paraparesis	Moderate or severe displacement; unstable	Improve conservative management Surgical stabilization†	Favorable to guarded Favorable
	± Back pain; weakly ambulatory or nonambulatory paraparesis	Moderate or severe displacement; unstable	Surgical stabilization†	Favorable to guarded
Back pain; ambulatory paraparesis	Static or improving	Minimal displacement; stable	Conservative	Favorable
	± Back pain; weakly ambulatory or nonambulatory paraparesis	Minimal, moderate, or severe displacement; unstable	Surgical stabilization	Favorable to guarded
Back pain; weakly or nonambulatory paraparesis	Improving	No displacement; stable	Conservative	Favorable to guarded
	Static or deteriorating	No displacement; myelogram shows no compressive lesion	Conservative	Favorable to guarded
		Myelogram shows compressive lesion	Surgical decompression-stabilization†	Favorable to guarded
		Minimal, moderate, or severe displacement; unstable	Surgical stabilization†	Favorable to guarded
Back pain; paraplegia	Static	Mild displacement; stable	Paraplegic cart or euthanasia	Guarded to unfavorable
	Static	Severe displacement; unstable	Spinal stabilization and paraplegic cart; or euthanasia	Guarded to unfavorable

*Definition of neurologic status (ambulatory, weakly ambulatory, and nonambulatory paraparesis) is given in Table 38-8 on p. 1430.
†Patients retaining even minimal neurologic function deserve the benefits of conservative treatment if surgery is unacceptable to the owner.

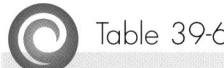 Table 39-6

Recommended Therapy* for Patients With Thoracolumbar Vertebral Fracture/Luxation Based on Neurologic Signs

CLINICAL PRESENTATION	INITIAL TREATMENT†	RESULT	SECOND TREATMENT†	RESULT	THIRD TREATMENT†
Back pain; no paraparesis	No drugs	No improvement	Steroids	Improvement Deterioration; paraparesis	Continue steroids Consider surgical§ stabilization
Back pain; CP deficits	Steroids for 1 day	Improvement	Continue steroids	Improvement	Follow—taper steroids
		Static Deteriorating	Continue steroids Consider surgical stabilization	No improvement	Consider surgical stabilization
Ambulatory paraparesis	Steroids for 1 day	Improvement	Continue steroids	Improvement	Follow—taper steroids
		Static	Steroids for 1 more day	Improvement	Follow—taper steroids
		Deteriorating	Consider surgical stabilization	Static or deteriorating	Consider surgical stabilization
Weakly ambulatory paraparesis	Recommend early surgery; administer preoperative steroids	Follow radiographically			
Nonambulatory paraparesis	Recommend early surgery; administer preoperative steroids	Follow radiographically			
Paraplegia	See Table 39-5				

CP, Conscious proprioception.
*See Box 38-6 on p. 1422 and Box 38-8 on p. 1450 for drugs, dosages, and variations on duration of therapy.
†All patients are placed in strict confinement for 3 to 4 weeks, fitted with a back brace, and given a neurologic examination daily as part of their medical management regardless of drug used or duration of drug therapy.

 BOX 39-8

Advantages and Disadvantages of Dorsolateral Vertebral Body Plating

Advantages
- Can be performed on any age, size, or disposition of patient
- Provides a rigid means of spinal stabilization

Disadvantages
- Need for nerve root resection at the spanned intervertebral space precludes its use below the fourth lumbar vertebra
- Approach to thoracic vertebrae is difficult
- Difficult to ensure the proper drill angle for screw placement
- Requires plating equipment

adjacent to PMMA to facilitate closure. Close lumbodorsal fascia to the dorsal midline with nonabsorbable monofilament suture material in a simple interrupted pattern.

Rarely, relief incisions in the lumbodorsal fascia lateral to the PMMA are necessary to facilitate closure.

Close subcutaneous tissue and skin routinely.

Dorsolateral Vertebral Body Plating

This technique provides effective spinal stabilization. It is recommended that an anatomic specimen be available for reference during placement of plates and screws. Advantages and disadvantages of this technique are listed in Box 39-8. Dorsolateral vertebral body plating requires dorsolateral exposure of lamina, pedicles, facet, and transverse process of lumbar vertebrae or lamina, pedicle, facet and rib head of thoracic vertebrae; the approach is as described for hemilaminectomy on p. 1464. Exposure of articular processes of the vertebra to be plated and articular processes of vertebrae cranial and caudal to these is recommended. If the luxation, subluxation, or fracture is close to the intervertebral space, stabilization of the two adjacent vertebrae is adequate. If a midbody fracture exists, three vertebral bodies are spanned by the plate.

Identify and protect spinal nerve roots encountered cranial and caudal to the fracture/luxation. Using bipolar cautery, carefully cauterize the vessels and nerve root emerging from the intervertebral foramen between the vertebrae to be plated. Carefully sever the vessels and nerve root. If a hemi-

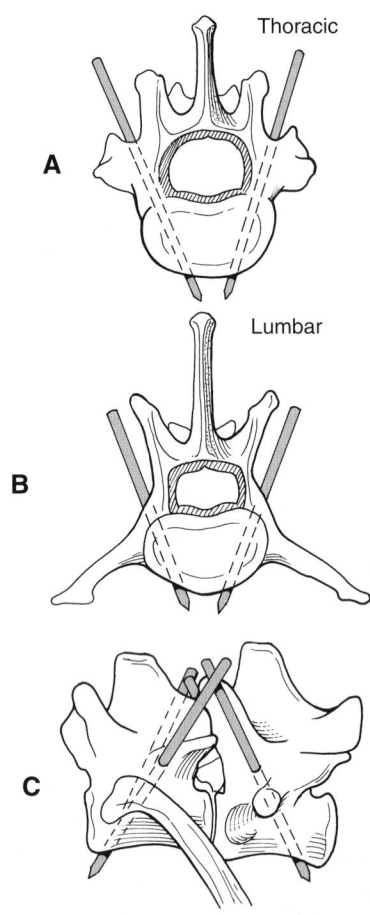

FIG. 39-24
Proper location and direction of Steinmann pins in the
A, thoracic and **B,** lumbar vertebral bodies. **C,** Lateral view
showing proper direction and angle of Steinmann pin placement in two adjacent vertebrae.

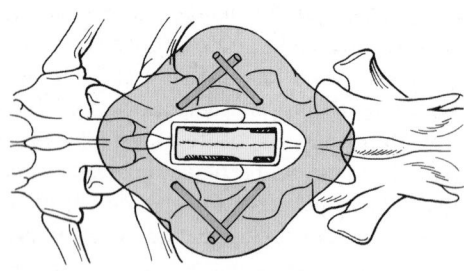

FIG. 39-25
When performing a laminectomy in conjunction with
Steinmann pin and PMMA stabilization, mold bone cement
in the shape of a doughnut to prevent contact of cement and
spinal cord.

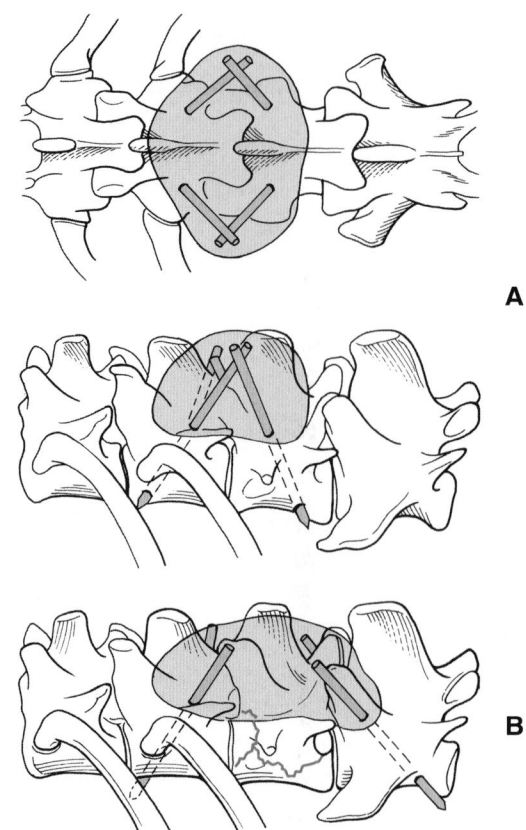

FIG. 39-26
A, If a laminectomy is not performed in conjunction with
Steinmann pin and PMMA stabilization, mold PMMA around
pins, dorsal spinous processes, articular facets, lamina, and
pedicles of affected vertebra. **B,** If a vertebral body fracture
must be spanned using Steinmann pin and PMMA, place
pins in the vertebral bodies cranial and caudal to the fractured vertebra.

*laminectomy is indicated, perform it now (see p. 1464).
Select a bone plate that will allow placement of two screws
in each vertebral body cranial and caudal to the affected
intervertebral space (luxation, subluxation) or affected vertebral body (fracture). Reduce and stabilize the fracture/
luxation by placing towel clamps in the dorsal spinous processes of the vertebrae cranial and caudal to the fracture/
luxation to provide a means of traction and countertraction.
If a laminectomy is not performed, place a 0.45-inch
Kirschner wire through the reduced articular facet to maintain reduction. Lay the plate on the dorsolateral surface of
the reduced vertebral body, ventral to the articular facet or
laminectomy defect. Drill and tap screw holes to ensure that
four cortices are engaged cranial and caudal to the involved
fracture/luxation. Judge the proper angle for each hole by
referring to an anatomic specimen (Fig. 39-27, A). If a
laminectomy is performed, use the anatomic location of the*

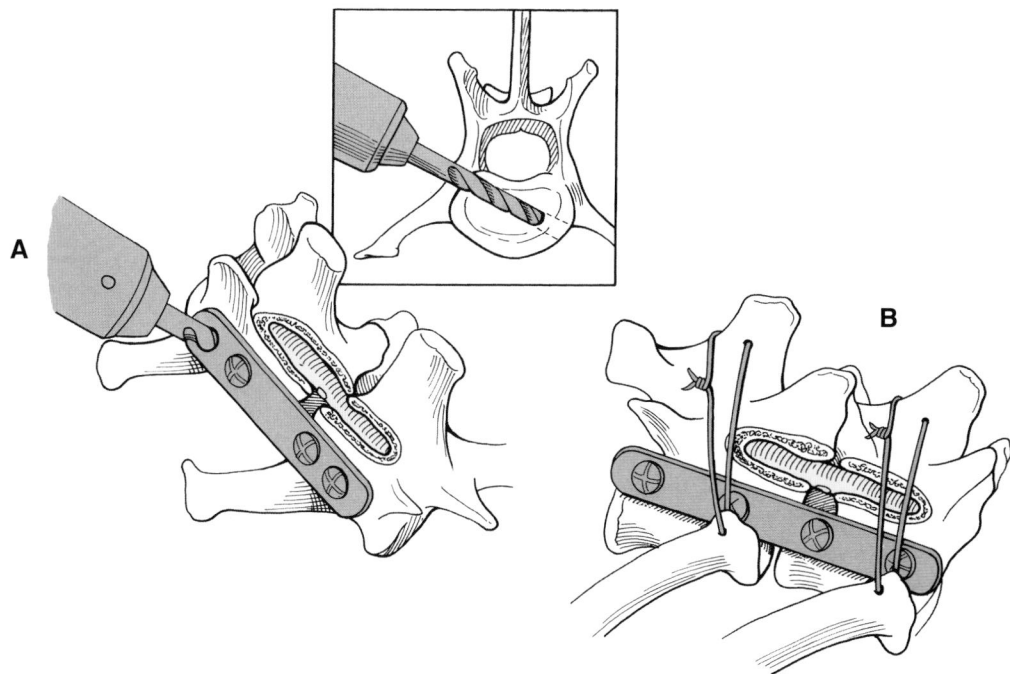

FIG. 39-27
A, Proper placement of a spinal plate on lumbar vertebrae. Notice that nerve root resection (rhizotomy) is required. **B,** For spinal plating of thoracic vertebrae, resect involved ribs to allow placement of the plate against the vertebral bodies. Wire ribs to the dorsal spinous processes after placement of the spinal plate.

spinal cord and vertebral canal as reference points to determine proper drill angle. After the hole is drilled, measure the depth with a depth gauge, tap the hole, select an appropriate length screw, and secure the plate to the vertebral body.

For thoracic vertebrae, expose the rib heads of the vertebral bodies to be plated. Use a bone cutting forceps to cut the rib head from its attachment to the vertebral body. Contour the transverse process with rongeurs until the plate lies flat against the vertebral body. Secure the plate as described previously. Reattach the severed ribs to the dorsal spinous processes with orthopedic wire (see Fig. 39-27, B). Lavage the surgical site with sterile saline solution, harvest an autogenous fat graft and place it over the laminectomy site, appose epaxial muscles with nonabsorbable monofilament suture, and close subcutaneous tissue and skin routinely.

Dorsal Spinous Process Plating

Dorsal spinous process plating using plastic plates provides effective spinal stabilization. Advantages and disadvantages are listed in Box 39-9. Plastic plates are designed to conform to the normal curvature of the spine and come in various sizes. Plate application requires exposure of the dorsal spinous processes and articular facets as described for modified dorsal laminectomy on p. 1461. The technique for reducing and maintaining reduction of the fracture/luxation is as described previously.

Make an incision on each side of the dorsal spinous processes, being careful to preserve supraspinous and interspi-

BOX 39-9

Advantages and Disadvantages of Dorsal Spinous Process Plating

Advantages
- Provides a secure means of spinal stabilization
- Limited exposure helps retain inherent spinal stability
- Easily performed
- Is compatible with hemilaminectomy

Disadvantages
- Cannot be used in soft bone of younger animals
- Requires a series of three prominent dorsal spinous processes on each side of the fracture/luxation strong enough to support the stresses encountered by an unstable spine
- Not rigid enough to use in hyperactive large-breed dogs
- Cannot be used in patients with small dorsal spinous processes
- Requires specialized equipment

nous ligaments. Elevate epaxial muscles from the dorsal spines and articular facets of at least three vertebrae cranial and caudal to the fracture/luxation. Do not sever muscle attachments from the lateral aspect of the articular processes. Select two appropriately sized plates and lay them along the space between the dorsal spine and articular facet on each side of the vertebrae (Fig. 39-28, A). Be sure the plates are long enough to grip spinous processes of three vertebrae on each side of the fracture/luxation. Place them such that the

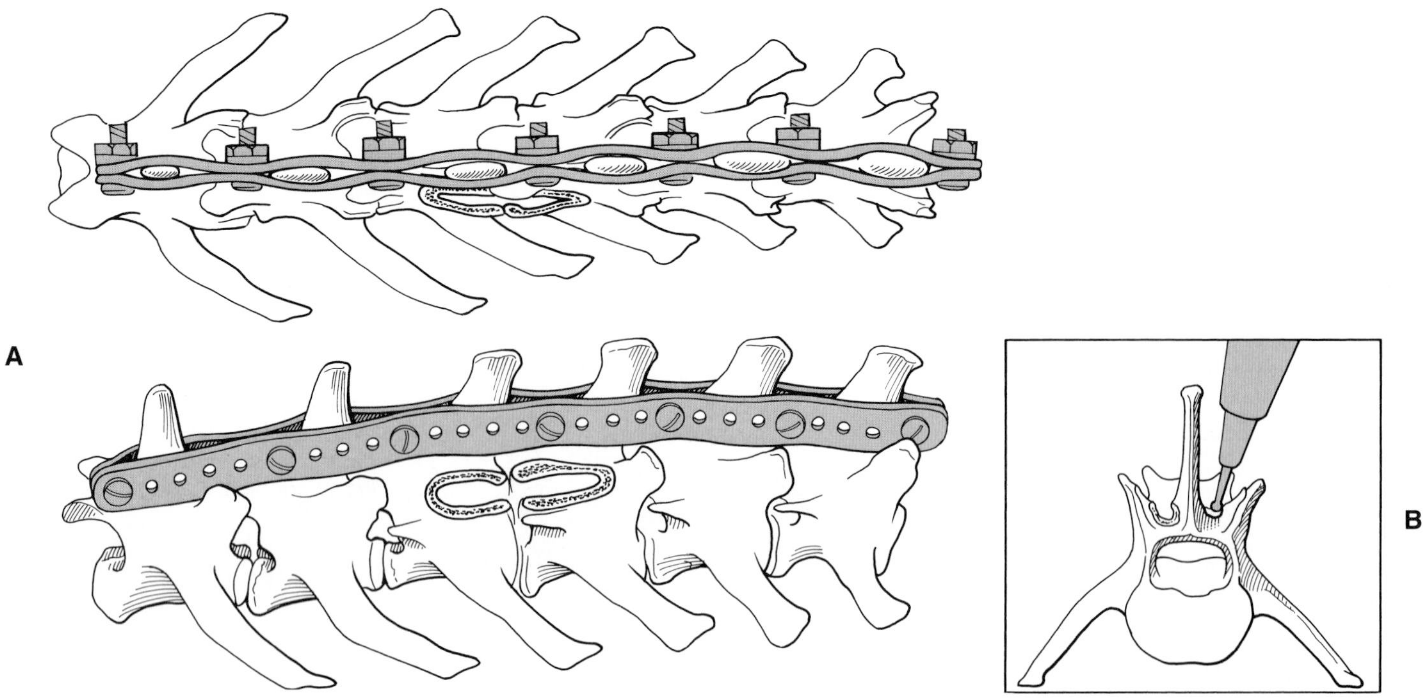

FIG. 39-28
A, Place plastic dorsal spinous process plates on each side of the dorsal spinous processes. Place nuts and bolts through the plates and between spinous processes. **B,** To facilitate uniform plate contact of all dorsal spinous processes spanned by the plate, remove any high points of laminar or articular facet contact by the plates with a high-speed pneumatic drill.

roughened surface lies against the dorsal spinous processes. Identify areas of contact that will keep the plates from lying uniformly on the lamina. Remove the plates and use a high-speed air drill to deepen these areas (see Fig. 39-28, B). Replace the plates, pass stainless steel bolts through predrilled holes in each plate and between spinous processes, and place washers and nuts on each bolt (see Fig. 39-28, A). Hold the fracture/luxation reduced, and tighten the nuts until plates are in contact between the spinous processes. Lavage the surgical site with sterile saline, débride any devitalized muscle, close epaxial muscles with a nonabsorbable monofilament suture, and close subcutaneous tissue and skin routinely.

Modified Segmental Spinal Fixation

Modified segmental spinal instrumentation provides a simple, versatile, and strong repair of vertebral fracture/luxation. Advantages and disadvantages are listed in Box 39-10. Pin and wire application requires exposure of dorsal spinous processes and articular facets as described for dorsal laminectomy procedures on p. 1461. Number and size of longitudinal and central pins (see later) used are dependent on size and activity of the patient and relative stability of the fracture/luxation. Generally, large patients with an unstable fracture/luxation are stabilized with relatively large central pins and a greater number of longitudinal pins (i.e., three to six pins). Moreover, central and longitu-

---

BOX 39-10

Advantages and Disadvantages of Modified Segmental Spinal Fixation

Advantages

- Can be performed in any area of the spine (i.e., thoracic, thoracolumbar, lumbar, and lumbosacral)
- Can be performed in any age, size, or disposition of animal
- Relatively easy to perform
- Requires no special equipment
- Less muscle dissection is required than with Steinmann pins and PMMA or body plating
- Is compatible with dorsal laminectomy procedures
- Provides a strong repair

Disadvantages

- Pin migration and fatigue fracture of orthopedic wire or pins may occur

---

dinal pin size may be varied and the length of longitudinal pins may be sequentially decreased to achieve a leaf spring effect (Fig. 39-29). If further stiffness is desired, muscular and tendinous attachments lateral to the articular facets are dissected free and a second set of pins is placed in a similar fashion lateral to the facets.

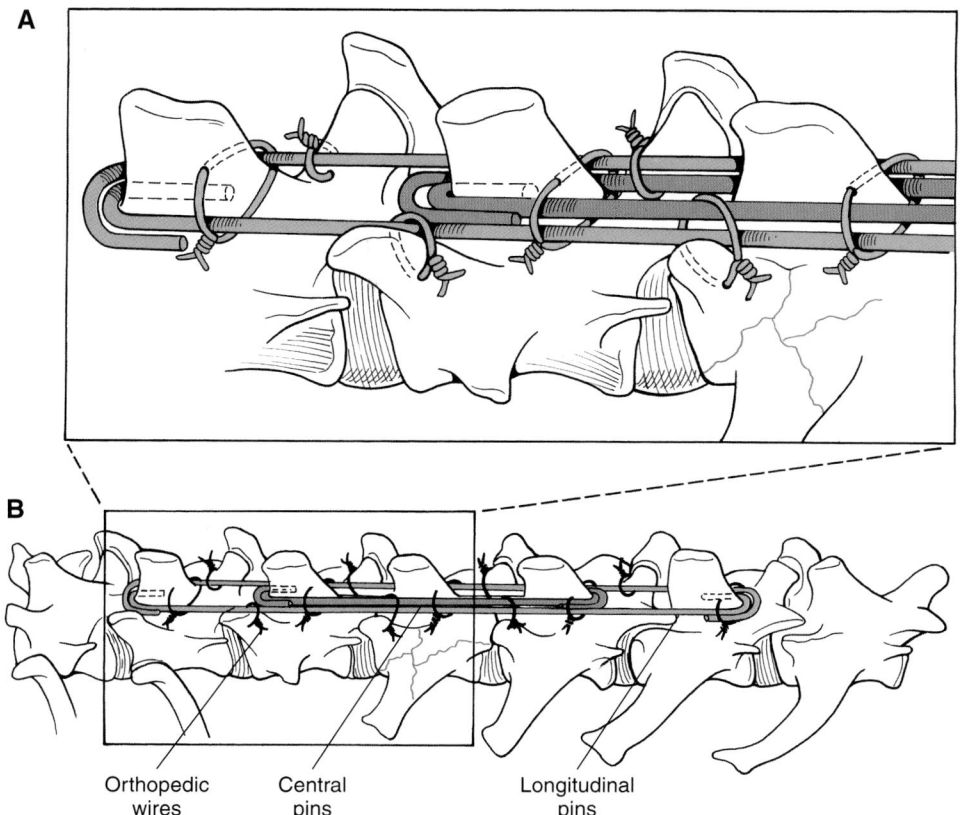

FIG. 39-29
A, Perform modified segmental spinal fixation by wiring central and longitudinal pins to the base of dorsal spinous processes and articular facets. **B,** Place the orthopedic wire through the dorsal spinous process and articular facets.

Orthopedic wires   Central pins   Longitudinal pins

Expose two to three spinous processes and articular facets cranial and caudal to the fracture/luxation, depending on patient size and activity, and inherent stability of the fracture/luxation. Perform a dorsal laminectomy if indicated, as described on p. 1461. Reduce the fracture/luxation and maintain reduction as described previously. Drill holes through the bases of articular facets (do not cross the articulation), bases of dorsal spinous processes, and tangentially through the dorsal lamina. Make the holes large enough to accommodate 18- or 20-gauge orthopedic wire. Preplace orthopedic wire through each hole, leaving the ends long enough to wrap around several Steinmann pins. Select two Steinmann pins long enough to include at least two vertebrae cranial and caudal to the affected vertebra (fracture) or intervertebral space (luxation, subluxation), called longitudinal pins. Bend the ends of the longitudinal pins at right angles to extend either into the interspinous space or through holes drilled transversely through the base of the dorsal spinous process. Place longitudinal pins in the space between dorsal spinous processes and articular facets (see Fig. 39-29, A). Place one central pin on each side of the dorsal spinous processes nearest the fracture/luxation. Bend the ends of the central pins to hook around the base of the dorsal spinous processes. Wire the central and longitudinal pins to the base of the articular facets, dorsal lamina, and dorsal spinous processes with the preplaced stands of orthopedic wire (see Fig. 39-29, B).

Lavage the surgical site with sterile saline, débride any devitalized muscle, close epaxial muscles with a nonabsorbable monofilament suture, and close subcutaneous tissue and skin routinely.

SUTURE MATERIAL AND SPECIAL INSTRUMENTS

Special instruments needed are dictated by the stabilization technique chosen. When using PMMA, an assortment of Steinmann pins of various sizes should be available. Vertebral body plating requires special orthopedic plating equipment; dorsal spinous process plating requires specially constructed plastic spinal plates; and modified segmental spinal fixation requires assorted Steinmann pins and orthopedic wire.

POSTOPERATIVE CARE AND ASSESSMENT

Patients with thoracic and lumbar fracture/luxation should be evaluated postoperatively in a similar fashion as patients with other thoracolumbar spinal disorders (see Box 39-2). See Chapter 13 for suggested analgesics and dosages (see Table 13-4 on p. 133 for opioid doses).

COMPLICATIONS

Complications associated with use of Steinmann pins and PMMA include iatrogenic injury to the spinal cord or pin migration. Complications associated with vertebral body plating include iatrogenic spinal cord injury, inappropriate screw placement, iatrogenic pneumothorax, or screw and plate migration. Complications associated with dorsal spinal plating include plate slippage and fracture of the dorsal spinous process. Complications associated with modified segmental spinal plating include fatigue fracture of pins or wires or pin migration.

PROGNOSIS

Prognosis for patients treated medically or surgically for thoracic and lumbar fracture/luxation is generally favorable and is dependent on assessment of apparent neurologic signs and subsequent medical or surgical management chosen. Clinical factors and probable patient outcome are outlined in Tables 39-5 and 39-6.

NEOPLASIA OF THORACOLUMBAR VERTEBRAE, SPINAL CORD, AND NERVE ROOTS

DEFINITIONS

Neoplasms involving the thoracolumbar vertebrae, spinal cord, and nerve roots are similar to those of the cervical region (see p. 1455). These neoplasms are also referred to as *spinal tumors, spinal cord tumors, tumors of the spine, vertebral tumors,* and *nerve root tumors.*

GENERAL CONSIDERATIONS AND CLINICALLY RELEVANT PATHOPHYSIOLOGY

Tumors of the thoracolumbar vertebrae, spinal cord, and nerve roots are classified by location in and around the spinal cord (e.g., primary bone, primary spinal cord, primary peripheral nerve root, primary paraspinal soft tissue, or metastatic) and by location relative to the dura (e.g., extradural, intradural-extramedullary, or intramedullary). Most canine thoracolumbar vertebral, spinal cord, and nerve root tumors are extradural, generally arising from bone. Tumor types for each location in dogs (e.g., extradural, intradural-extramedullary, and intramedullary) are similar to tumor types for cervical vertebrae, spinal cord, and nerve roots (see p. 1455). Lymphosarcoma is the most common spinal tumor in cats and generally occurs extradurally. Intradural-extramedullary and intramedullary tumors in cats are rare. Spinal neoplasia, regardless of location or classification, becomes clinically significant when the enlarging mass compromises neural tissue (i.e., the spinal cord or nerve roots) or when its invasive growth undermines the vertebra and its supporting structures, leading to pathologic fracture.

DIAGNOSIS
Clinical Presentation

Signalment. There does not appear to be a general sex or breed predilection for patients with thoracolumbar vertebral, spinal cord, or nerve root neoplasia. Most patients are older than 5 years of age. An exception is solitary or multiple cartilaginous exostoses, which usually occur in patients younger than 1 year of age.

> NOTE: When considering differentials in patients with neurologic disorders, remember that "tumors know no age."

History. Historical findings depend on location of the neoplasm relative to the dura. Animals with extradural neoplasia generally are brought in because of acute pain and varying degrees of UMN or LMN paraparesis, whereas those with intradural-extramedullary neoplasia have a chronic history (months to years) of dull back pain or hind limb lameness plus varying degrees of monoparesis or paraparesis. Patients with intramedullary neoplasia have acute paraparesis (often after a long, insidious onset), with or without back pain. Careful historic evaluation often reveals subtle neurologic abnormalities before the acute presenting episode.

Physical Examination Findings

Physical and neurologic examination findings associated with thoracolumbar spinal tumors vary depending on tumor location (see Fig. 36-10 on p. 1368), degree of spinal cord and nerve root compression, rate of tumor growth, and secondary effects of the tumor (i.e., paraneoplastic syndrome). Some generalizations concerning presenting signs can be made for various classifications of vertebral tumors and are discussed on p. 1456. Patients with tumors involving spinal cord segments T3-L3 have varying degrees of back pain and UMN paraparesis, whereas those with tumors involving spinal cord segments L4-S3 have varying degrees of low back pain and LMN paraparesis (see Chapter 36 on p. 1457).

Diagnostic Imaging

Abnormal survey radiographs suggesting vertebral, spinal cord, or nerve root neoplasia include osteoproduction, osteolysis, or lysis of the intervertebral foramen (see Figs. 38-68 to 38-70 on p. 1456). Diagnosis of most spinal cord and paraspinal vertebral neoplasms requires myelography or cross-sectional imaging. Specific myelographic techniques are described in Chapter 36 (see Figs. 36-14 and 36-15 on p. 1373). Myelography classifies neoplasms as extradural, intradural-extramedullary, or intramedullary. Myelographic abnormalities associated with each classification are illustrated in Figs. 36-16 to 36-18 on pp. 1374 to 1375. CT and MRI is often more sensitive in accurately determining the extent of vertebral, spinal cord, or nerve root involvement (Fig. 39-30).

Laboratory Findings

Laboratory findings are generally normal or reflect paraneoplastic syndromes. CSF analysis rarely contributes to a specific diagnosis; however, cell type or evidence of an inflammatory process may support a diagnosis of neoplasia.

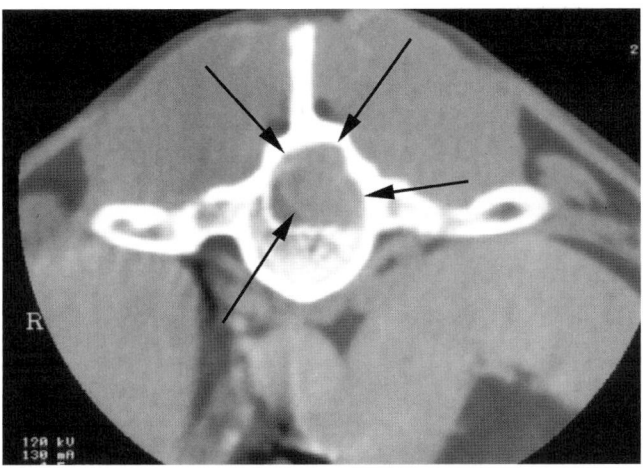

FIG. 39-30
Axial noncontrast CT image of T12. There is a large soft tissue attenuating mass within the spinal canal *(arrows)* causing severe compression of the spinal cord. Notice the enlargement of the spinal canal and corresponding thinning of the laminae in the region of the mass.

DIFFERENTIAL DIAGNOSIS

Differential diagnosis of tumor type is based on location of tumor (e.g., bone, spinal cord, nerve root, or metastasis) and myelographic classification (e.g., extradural, intradural-extramedullary, or intramedullary).

MEDICAL MANAGEMENT

Medical management is directed at the primary lesion and secondary tumor effects. Generally, definitive medical treatment requires surgical exposure and incisional or excisional biopsy to determine tumor type and plan adjunct chemotherapy, irradiation, or combination therapy.

SURGICAL TREATMENT
Preoperative Management

Patients are given IV fluids and steroids before surgery. Steroids help protect the spinal cord during surgical manipulation. The steroid of choice is methylprednisolone sodium succinate (30 mg/kg IV).

Anesthesia

See p. 1403 for suggested anesthetic protocols to use in animals with thoracolumbar spinal disorders.

Surgical Anatomy

Surgical procedures to approach and resect thoracic or lumbar vertebral, spinal cord, and nerve root tumors include dorsal laminectomy and hemilaminectomy, with or without facetectomy and foraminotomy. Each procedure removes various portions of dorsal spinous processes, laminae, pedicles, and articular facets (see p. 1460). Commonly encoun-

tered anatomic landmarks of thoracic and lumbar vertebrae are illustrated in Figs. 39-1 and 39-2 on p. 1461.

Positioning

Generally, patients with thoracolumbar vertebral, spinal cord, or nerve root tumors require a dorsal or dorsolateral approach. Patients requiring dorsal laminectomy are positioned with the back gently flexed to open articular facets and interarcuate spaces, facilitating exposure (see Fig. 39-3 on p. 1461). Patients requiring hemilaminectomy should have the affected side gently rotated (about 15 degrees) to facilitate dorsolateral exposure of affected vertebrae (see Fig. 39-4 on p. 1462).

SURGICAL TECHNIQUE

Surgical objectives include exposure of the tumor, wide resection or biopsy of the tumor, spinal cord and nerve root decompression, and occasionally vertebral stabilization. Thoracolumbar vertebral, spinal cord, or nerve root tumors are generally approached via dorsal laminectomy or hemilaminectomy as described on pp. 1461 to 1467. Wide laminectomy, facetectomy, and foraminotomy are required for adequate exposure of extradural and intradural-extramedullary tumors. Dorsal laminectomy or hemilaminectomy and durotomy are necessary for exposure and removal of intramedullary tumors. If spinal stabilization is indicated, techniques described for stabilization of thoracic and lumbar spinal fracture/luxation are used (see pp. 1483 to 1489).

SUTURE MATERIALS AND SPECIAL INSTRUMENTS

Ultrasonic aspirators are invaluable, especially when removing neoplastic tissue closely associated with, or invading, neural tissue. Other special instruments necessary to perform thoracolumbar dorsal laminectomy and hemilaminectomy are listed in Box 39-1.

POSTOPERATIVE CARE AND ASSESSMENT

Patients with thoracic and lumbar vertebral, spinal cord, and nerve root neoplasia are evaluated postoperatively just like patients with other thoracolumbar spinal disorders. Adjunct chemotherapy, irradiation, immunotherapy, or combination therapy is based on tumor type and surgical margins. See Chapter 13 for suggested analgesics and dosages (see Table 13-4 on p. 133 for opioid doses).

PROGNOSIS

Prognosis depends on tumor location (e.g., spine, spinal cord, or nerve root), myelographic classification (e.g., extradural, intradural-extramedullary, or intramedullary); tumor type (e.g., biologic activity); degree of surgical resection; and tumor sensitivity to adjunct therapy. Generally, malignant extradural neoplasms have an unfavorable prognosis, benign extradural neoplasms have a favorable prognosis, malignant and benign intramedullary neoplasms have an unfavorable to grave prognosis, and extradural-intramedullary neoplasms have a guarded to unfavorable prognosis (see Box 38-9 on p. 1456).

Table 39-7

Sample Physical Rehabilitation Protocol for Patients After Surgery for Thoracolumbar Disk Disease or Fracture/Luxation*

TREATMENT	DISABILITY INDEX			
	0–2 STEP 1	3–8 STEP 2	9–11 STEP 3	12–14 STEP 4
Heat therapy		10 min	10 min	
Massage	5 min	5 min	5 min	5 min
Passive range of motion (repetitions)	15†	15†	15†	15†
Electrical stimulation‡	10 min	10 min	10 min	
Therapeutic exercise: total time	10 min	20 min	20 min	25–45 min
Assisted standing	+	+	+	
Sit to stands	+	+	+	+
Balancing	+	+	+	+
Obstacles			+	+
Weaving			+	+
Circles			+	+
Underwater treadmill with gait patterning or wading pool/water walking	10 min (after 36–48 hr)	15 min	20 min	>25 min
Swimming§	2–5 min	5–10 min	5–10 min	5–10 min
Cryotherapy	15 min			

Modified from Development of a functional scoring system for dogs with acute spinal cord injuries, *Am J Vet Res* 62:10, 2001.
Disability index (DI):
 0–2, *0*, no limb movement and absent deep pain; *1*, no limb movement and present deep pain; *2*, no limb movement, but voluntary tail movement.
 3–8, *3*, minimal non–weight-bearing activity of one limb (one joint); *4*, non–weight-bearing activity in more than one joint <50% of the time; *5*, non–weight-bearing activity in more than one joint >50% of the time; *6*, weight-bearing activity of the limb <10% of the time; *7*, weight-bearing activity of the limb 10% to 50% of the time; *8*, weight-bearing activity of the limb >50% of the time.
 9–11, *9*, weight-bearing activity 100% of the time, but with reduced strength, and mistakes made >90% of the time, including crossing of the limbs, knuckling of the paws, standing on the dorsum of the paws and falling; *10*, weight-bearing activity 100% of the time, but with reduced strength and above mistakes made 50% to 90% of the time; *11*, weight-bearing activity 100% of the time, but with reduced strength, and mistakes made <50% of the time.
 12–14, *12*, ataxic gait with normal strength, but mistakes made >50% of the time, including lack of coordination, crossing of hind limbs, skipping steps, bunny-hopping, and knuckling of the paws; *13*, ataxic gait with normal strength, but mistakes made <50% of the time; *14*, normal gait.
*All treatments should be done three times a day.
†Passive range of motion to all joints of all limbs.
‡*E-Stimulation:* Electrical stimulation to be performed on the semimembranosus/semitendinosus muscle groups in patients with muscle atrophy. See Chapter 12 for specifications.
§Swimming is most beneficial if patient is moving all four limbs and is controlled. If not getting functional response, return to underwater treadmill or water walking instead. It is safer and more controlled.

PHYSICAL REHABILITATION FOR PATIENTS WITH THORACOLUMBAR DISK DISEASE AND FRACTURE/LUXATION

Rehabilitation can facilitate early and more complete recovery of neurologic patients after surgery (see Chapter 12; p. 127). It should be used in conjunction with standard medical and surgical treatment plus proper pain management (see Chapter 13). Table 39-7 provides a sample physical rehabilitation protocol for patients after surgery for thoracolumbar disk disease (begin immediately postoperatively), or spinal fractures or luxations. After repair of fractures or luxations, only steps one and two should be performed until a bony union has formed and fixation is considered stable, regardless of the disability index.

CHAPTER 40
Surgery of the Lumbosacral Spine

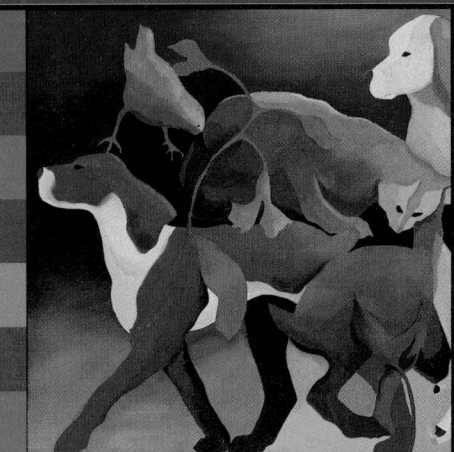

DEFINITIONS

Dorsal laminectomy of the lumbosacral spine is removal of dorsal spinous processes, lamina, pedicles, and articular facets of L7 and S1, S2, and/or S3. **Hemilaminectomy** is removal of lamina and pedicles on the right or left side. **Facetectomy** is removal of articular facets, either unilaterally (hemilaminectomy) or bilaterally (dorsal laminectomy), to increase exposure to the vertebral canal, and **foraminotomy** is removal of the bone forming the intervertebral foramen, allowing unobstructed passage of the exiting nerve root. **Cauda equina** refers to the nerve roots that course through the lumbosacral vertebral canal (e.g., L7, S1-S3, and Cd1-Cd5). **Dysesthesia** is the sensation of burning or tingling in areas supplied by entrapped nerve roots.

PREOPERATIVE MANAGEMENT

Traumatized patients (e.g., victims of automobile accidents) should receive intravenous fluids and be secured to a rigid platform until fractures/luxations are stabilized. Careful physical examination should rule out concurrent trauma to other organ systems (e.g., urinary, cardiopulmonary, and associated vertebral or appendicular skeletal fractures/luxations). Surgical urgency is determined by initial and serial neurologic examinations. Generally, patients with acute signs and severe neurologic deficits (e.g., fracture/luxation, acute intervertebral disk extrusion, and neoplasia) should have surgery as quickly as possible, whereas those with chronic signs (e.g., congenital lumbosacral stenosis, diskospondylitis, vertebral osteomyelitis, and chronic degenerative disk disease) should be carefully evaluated and staged before medical or surgical treatment. Steroids are generally not administered because their efficacy in nerve root injury is uncertain.

ANESTHESIA

Suggested anesthetic protocols used in patients with spinal disorders are given on p. 1403.

ANTIBIOTICS

Criteria for use of prophylactic or therapeutic antibiotics are given in Box 38-4 on p. 1403. Selection of an appropriate antibiotic and dose is determined by criteria given in Chapter 10.

SURGICAL ANATOMY

The lumbosacral spine is unique in its anatomic configuration from vertebra to vertebra, particularly L7 and S1. The anatomic variations and surgical significance of each are listed in Table 40-1.

SURGICAL TECHNIQUE

Positioning is critical in patients with lumbosacral disorders. Animals with lumbosacral stenosis (cauda equina syndrome) should be positioned with the hind legs tucked under the abdomen, thus stretching the interarcuate ligament (also called the *ligamentum flavum* or *yellow ligament*) and accentuating the dorsal lumbosacral space (Fig. 40-1). This facilitates exposure for dorsal laminectomy and hemilaminectomy and may decompress the cauda equina. Patients with lumbosacral fracture/luxation should be positioned to encourage fracture/luxation reduction. Generally, this is accomplished by positioning the patient as illustrated in Fig. 40-1.

Patients with surgical lumbosacral disorders are treated by dorsal laminectomy, hemilaminectomy, facetectomy, or dorsal lumbosacral spinal stabilization. Dorsal laminectomy is most commonly used for decompressing lumbosacral stenosis (cauda equina syndrome) and exposing and removing herniated disk material, fracture fragments, neoplasms, or paraspinal abscesses at L6-L7 or L7-S1. Unilateral or bilateral facetectomy and foraminotomy is performed with laminectomy if the compressive lesion is located laterally. Hemilaminectomy is most commonly used to expose unilateral extradural or intradural-extramedullary lesions involving L6-L7.

Dorsal Laminectomy

Position the patient in sternal recumbency (see Fig. 40-1). Make a dorsal midline incision from the dorsal spinous process of L6 to the first caudal vertebra. Incise the superficial

Table 40-1

Anatomic Variation of L7 and S1 and Its Surgical Significance

VERTEBRAE	ANATOMY	SURGICAL SIGNIFICANCE
L7	Thick dorsal lamina compared with S1	Has distinct outer cortical, medullary, and inner cortical layers
S1	Thin dorsal lamina compared with L7	Outer cortical, medullary, and inner cortical layers are not distinct
L7–S1 articulation	Most mobile joint in the thoracolumbar spine	Positioning in slight ventral flexion results in significant widening of the interarcuate space during surgery
	Large interarcuate space	Allows limited exposure of the cauda equina before laminectomy
	Spinal cord terminates at L5–L6	Only nerve roots course through the L7–S1 vertebral canal
	Close association with wings of the ilium	Makes foraminotomy and facetectomy difficult to perform
S1,2,3	Sacral vertebrae are fused	No intervertebral disk spaces; nerve roots exit through separate dorsal and ventral foramina

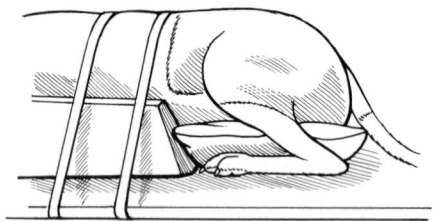

FIG. 40-1
Positioning patients with the hind legs tucked under the abdomen helps accentuate the L7–S1 interarcuate space.

and deep sacral fascia parallel to the skin incision. Using a periosteal elevator or small osteotome, elevate epaxial muscles from their attachments on dorsal spinous processes, lamina, articular facets, pedicles, and accessory processes of L7-S3. Remove the dorsal spinous process of L7 and S1 with rongeurs. Identify the wide interarcuate space of L7-S1; carefully incise and remove associated soft tissue structures (i.e., remaining muscle attachments and interarcuate ligament) with a No. 11 scalpel blade. Use a high-speed pneumatic or electric drill to remove the outer cortical and softer medullary layer, and identify the inner cortical layer from the midbody of L7 to the midbody of S2-S3 (Fig. 40-2).

The dorsal laminar thickness of L7 and S1 varies greatly; L7 is two to three times thicker than S1.

Carefully drill through the inner cortical layer until it becomes soft. Detailed illustrations of each drilled layer are given on p. 1461 and in Fig. 39-7 on p. 1463. Penetrate and remove the inner periosteum with a dental or iris spatula until the

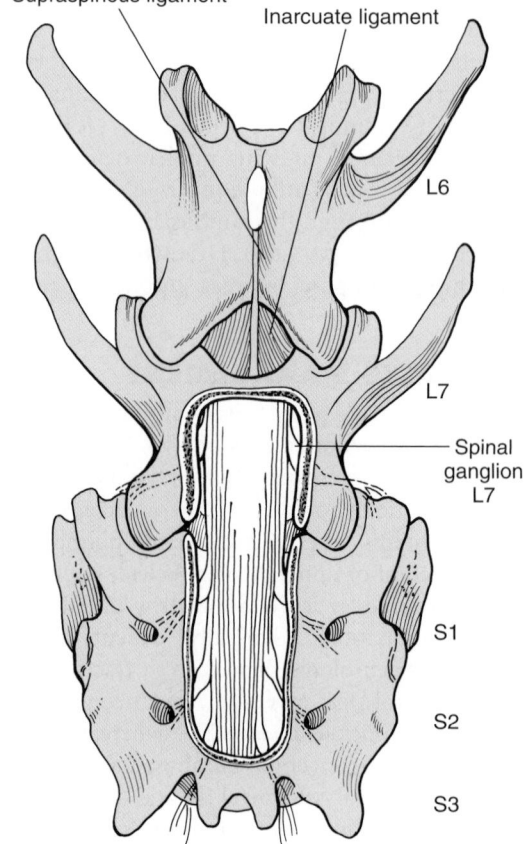

FIG. 40-2
L7, S1, S2 dorsal laminectomy provides exposure of the filum terminale and cauda equina.

entire laminectomy site is exposed. Structures present include nerve roots of L7, S1, S2, S3, and caudal nerve roots, vertebral venous sinus, dorsal longitudinal ligament, and dorsal annulus fibrosus. If the L7 or S1 nerve roots appear to be compressed within the foramen or by enlarged facets, perform a facetectomy and/or foraminotomy, respectively, to establish complete nerve root decompression. Using a high-speed drill, remove the cranial articular process of S1 and caudal articular process of L7. Use the drill to approach the intervertebral foramen and Lempert rongeurs to enter the foramen by removing any remaining articular facet.

This exposure allows visualization of the intervertebral foramen and exiting L7 nerve root. A recent study suggested the use of an endoscope to assist in the relatively difficult technique for L7-S1 foraminotomy (Brett et al, 2004).

Lavage the surgical site with warm saline. Harvest a free subcutaneous fat graft and position it over the laminectomy site. Close epaxial muscles with interrupted, monofilament, nonabsorbable suture. Close subcutaneous tissue and skin routinely.

Hemilaminectomy

Hemilaminectomy and facetectomy are indicated for exposure of the lateral aspects of the lumbosacral vertebral canal. It is used to remove compressive lesions, such as neoplasms, fracture fragments, herniated intervertebral disk material, bulbous articular facets, or paraspinal abscesses.

NOTE: Proper technique for controlling venous sinus hemorrhage is discussed in Box 38-1 on p. 1403.

Position the patient as for dorsal laminectomy (see Fig. 40-1). Make a dorsal midline skin incision from the dorsal spinous process of L6 to the first caudal vertebra, and continue it through the dorsal sacral fascia. Elevate epaxial muscles from the right or left lateral aspect of the dorsal spinous process, lamina, articular facet, pedicle, and accessory process of the L7-S1 intervertebral space. Visualize the dorsal aspect of the transverse process of L7. Use a high-speed drill to remove lamina, articular facet, and pedicle to the level of the accessory process. Identify outer cortical, medullary, and inner cortical layers while drilling (see p. 1461 and Fig. 39-7 on p. 1463). Carefully break through the inner periosteal layer with rongeurs and a dental or iris spatula to enter the vertebral canal. Identify the vertebral venous sinus located on the floor of the vertebral canal. Be careful not to lacerate the sinus while manipulating lesions within the vertebral canal. After complete decompression and mass removal, lavage the surgical site with warm saline. Harvest a free subcutaneous fat graft and position it over the laminectomy site. Close epaxial muscles to the dorsal sacral fascia with interrupted, monofilament, nonabsorbable suture. Close subcutaneous tissue and skin routinely.

Spinal Stabilization

Lumbosacral spinal stabilization is a technique that stabilizes a lumbosacral fracture or luxation, or a congenital or acquired stenosis causing spinal instability (see p. 1505). Spinal stabilization can be successfully accomplished by various techniques, including transiliac pins, transiliac pins and plastic dorsal spinous process plates, Steinmann pins and polymethylmethacrylate (PMMA) bone cement, a combination of external skeletal fixation and dorsal spinous process plates, and modified segmental spinal fixation.

HEALING OF THE CAUDA EQUINA

Nerve roots of the cauda equina respond to injury in a similar fashion as peripheral nerves. Healing of peripheral nerves depends on the extent of injury (e.g., neurotmesis, axonotmesis, or neurapraxia). *Neurotmesis* occurs if the entire peripheral nerve with all its bundles of fibers is severed or ruptured with a gap between severed nerve ends. *Axonotmesis* occurs if some axons in the nerve are ruptured, but anatomic continuity is maintained. *Neurapraxia* is an acute transient physiologic dysfunction of a peripheral nerve after trauma; nerve conduction is blocked, but degeneration does not occur. Full return of function is expected.

Regrowth of axons is spontaneous, but the time until return of function depends on the extent of injury and the distance from denervated end-organs. Peripheral nerves sustaining mild injury that causes neurapraxia develop transient physiologic dysfunction without anatomic disruption of axons. The nerve regains normal function within 3 months or less (peripheral nerve regeneration occurs at 3 cm per month or approximately 1 mm per day). Peripheral nerves sustaining injury sufficient to cause axonotmesis or neurotmesis undergo immediate degeneration at the site of injury. Degeneration toward the cell body over a distance of two to three nodes of Ranvier generally occurs, and regeneration begins from that site. Nerve processes distal to the injury degenerate completely (Wallerian degeneration), and after 1 week a connective tissue framework called the *neurilemmal sheath* is left. Within 2 days, "sprouting" of the proximal end of the severed axon occurs. Axonal regeneration and return of function depend on several factors. If continuity of the nerve is maintained (axonotmesis), the distance from injury site to end-organ becomes the most important variable. Little function will be achieved if the distance is more than 25 to 30 cm; the best chance for functional regeneration is a distance of less than 10 to 15 cm. If anatomic nerve continuity is not maintained (neurotmesis), recovery depends on the distance from the injury to the end-organ, wounding mechanism, time between injury and surgical repair, patient's age and condition, and surgical technique.

Clean, sharp lacerations generally heal better than avulsion, crush, open, or chronic injuries. The earlier a nerve is repaired (see Surgery of Peripheral Nerves in e-dition), the better the chance for healing, reinnervation, and normal function of the end-organ. Young, well-nourished, healthy patients usually have faster nerve regeneration. Anatomic alignment of nerve ends and attention to surgical detail ensure that regenerating axons will find their way along the neurilemmal tube to the end-organ, producing functional recovery (see Surgery of Peripheral Nerves in e-dition).

SUTURE MATERIALS AND SPECIAL INSTRUMENTS

Special instrumentation necessary to perform dorsal laminectomy, hemilaminectomy, facetectomy, foraminotomy, and spinal stabilization is listed by technique in Box 39-1 on p. 1468. It is important to practice each technique, become familiar with regional anatomy, and learn proper use of special instrumentation before performing these surgeries.

POSTOPERATIVE CARE AND ASSESSMENT

Critical postoperative care for the first 24 hours typically includes IV fluids, analgesics, antibiotics, seizure alert (if work-up required a myelogram), and neurologic examinations. Specific care requirements are similar to those for patients with thoracolumbar spinal disorders. Immediate and long-term postoperative care and assessment for ambulatory and nonambulatory patients are given in Table 39-1 and Box 39-2 on p. 1469.

COMPLICATIONS

Complications associated with lumbosacral spinal surgery are uncommon. Seroma of the surgical site may occur, but it is generally resolved with intermittent or continuous drainage. Bladder function is often impaired, and urinary tract infection (UTI) occurs if an upper motor neuron (UMN) or lower motor neuron (LMN) dysfunction occurs. The bladder needs to be manually emptied four times daily until normal function returns; however, it must not be inappropriately traumatized by rough technique. If dorsal laminectomy is performed, excessive removal of lamina, articular facets, and pedicles bilaterally could predispose the patient to muscle fibrosis and contracture over the spinal cord and nerve roots, causing compression; however, this rarely occurs. Spinal instability has not been observed, even when multilevel exposure is indicated (e.g., L6-S3). If a spinal stabilization technique is used, complications are generally associated with the specific technique. Patients undergoing hemilaminectomy rarely have significant complications. Iatrogenic nerve root trauma may occur, but nerve roots can tolerate careful surgical manipulation without developing clinically significant neural deficits.

SPECIAL AGE CONSIDERATIONS

Care should be taken when performing laminectomy procedures on young patients because their cortical and cancellous bone is much softer than in older patients. Less pressure is required when drilling or rongeuring lamina and pedicles in younger patients, and a greater flexibility of the lumbosacral junction allows increased accentuation of the dorsal lumbosacral space during positioning.

Suggested Reading

Brett CW, Lanz OI, Jones JC et al: Endoscopic-assisted lumbosacral foraminotomy in the dog, *Vet Surg* 33:221-231, 2004.
Endoscopic-assisted foraminotomy could be used to improve intraoperative visualization in dogs with foraminal stenosis as a component of degenerative lumbosacral stenosis.

SPECIFIC DISEASES

CAUDA EQUINA SYNDROME

DEFINITIONS

Cauda equina syndrome is a complex of neurologic signs caused by compression of the nerve roots (i.e., cauda equina) coursing through the lumbosacral vertebral canal. **Transitional vertebrae** are vertebrae that possess properties of lumbar and sacral vertebrae. Synonyms for cauda equina syndrome include *lumbosacral stenosis, cauda equina compression, lumbosacral spondylosis, lumbosacral malformation-malarticulation,* and *lumbosacral instability.*

GENERAL CONSIDERATIONS AND CLINICALLY RELEVANT PATHOPHYSIOLOGY

Cauda equina syndrome is relatively common and can be categorized as acquired (degenerative) or congenital (developmental). Potential causes are listed in Box 40-1. The respective nerve roots involved are L7, S1-S3, and Cd1-Cd5 (Fig. 40-3).

The cauda equina consists of nerve roots originating from L7 to Cd5 as they travel through the vertebral canal to exit through their respective intervertebral foramina. The caudalmost part of the *conus medullaris* (caudal end of the spinal cord) in dogs is generally located at L6; however, this depends on the animal's size (the conus medullaris in all cats and in dogs under 7 kg may be L7-S1). Vertebral bodies that contain the cauda equina are L5-Cd5. Bony and ligamentous boundaries of the cauda equina are: dorsally (lamina, interarcuate ligament, and articular facets); laterally (pedicles); and ventrally (dorsal longitudinal ligament, vertebral venous sinus, dorsal annulus fibrosus, and vertebral body). Congenital or acquired defects causing abnormalities in the skeletal or soft tissue boundaries may produce cauda equina compression and cauda equina syndrome.

DIAGNOSIS
Clinical Presentation

Signalment. Although there is no breed predilection for congenital cauda equina stenosis, acquired cauda equina syndrome is most commonly diagnosed in large-breed dogs (mean body weight 35 kg), with German shepherd dogs being overrepresented. Males are more often affected than females (2:1). Most dogs are middle-aged when clinical signs of acquired or congenital cauda equina become apparent; even congenital stenosis often causes clinical signs later in life. A

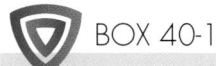

BOX 40-1

Causes of Cauda Equina Syndrome

Acquired

Vertebral fracture or luxation
Diskospondylitis
Vertebral osteomyelitis
Chronic intervertebral disk disease
Acute intervertebral disk extrusion
Fibrocartilaginous emboli
Neoplasia of the L7–S1 vertebra, surrounding soft tissue, or
 nerve roots

Congenital

Transitional vertebra
Congenital vertebral canal stenosis
Breed-influenced vertebral canal stenosis
Developmental sacral osteochondrosis

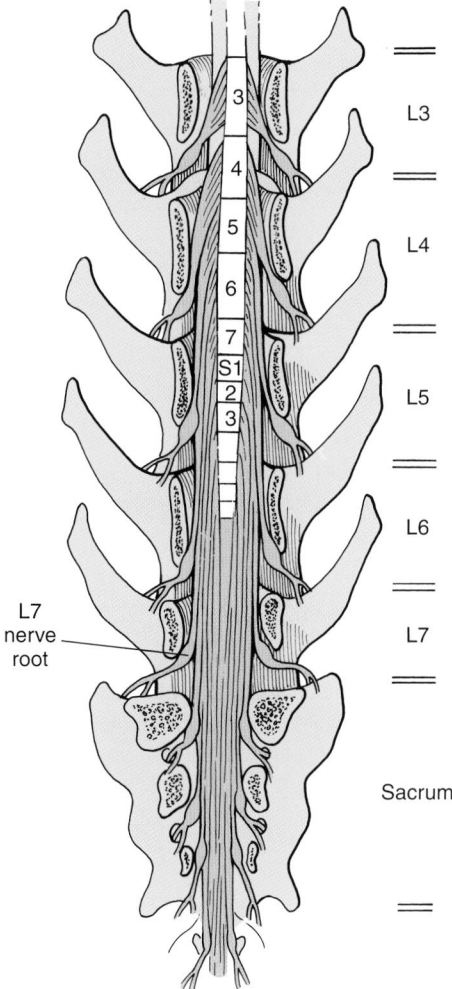

FIG. 40-3
Anatomic relationship of vertebral bodies to spinal cord termination and cauda equina.

recent article reported cauda equina compression in a cat secondary to degenerative disk disease (Jaeger et al, 2004).

History. Dogs with cauda equina syndrome typically have a chronic history of back pain and hind limb lameness, with or without hind limb weakness. Sometimes patients show urinary incontinence. Back pain is due to attenuation of nerve roots, and lameness is due to either pain originating from nerve root entrapment/compression, neurologic deficits secondary to cauda equina compression, or both. However, clinical signs do not generally correlate with the severity of compression as seen on magnetic resonance imaging (MRI) (Mayhew et al, 2002). Other historical findings may include scuffing hind limb toenails, difficulty climbing stairs, a reluctance to jump or sit up on hind legs, urinary or fecal incontinence, abnormal tail carriage, hind limb muscle atrophy, and excessive chewing on the tail and/or lateral aspect of the hind feet. Greater than 50% of affected dogs are considered to be very active, partaking in obedience competition, hunting, or military, police, or security work.

Physical Examination Findings

General physical examination findings vary depending on the cause of cauda equina compression. Patients with fracture/luxation may have associated life-threatening injuries (e.g., cardiopulmonary and urinary) and signs associated with shock (weak peripheral pulses, tachycardia, prolonged capillary refill time, pale mucous membranes), and/or dyspnea. Patients with infectious causes may have fever and depression; sepsis is unusual. Those with neoplasia may have systemic signs associated with secondary effects of the tumor (e.g., paraneoplastic syndrome). Animals with congenital stenosis, chronic degenerative disk disease, or acute disk herniation may have signs that mimic other nonneurologic disorders, including musculoskeletal disorders (hip dysplasia, chronic stifle instability, polyarthritis), vascular disorders

(iliac thrombosis), peripheral neuropathy or myopathy, metabolic disorders causing generalized weakness, primary urogenital tract disease (incontinence, UTI), primary rectal or anal disorders (anal sacculitis, anorectal neoplasia), or distemper radiculopathy.

Neurologic examination findings are related to ischemia and/or compression of nerve roots coursing through the lumbosacral junction (i.e., L7, S1-S2, and Cd1-Cd5). Pain is generally due to nerve root ischemia; paresis is from progressive nerve root ischemia and attenuation. Neurologic signs vary depending on cause and severity of compression, and may be acute or chronic, intermittent or persistent, static or progressive (Table 40-2). The most common neurologic abnormality is lumbosacral hyperpathia (i.e., pain on deep palpation of the lumbosacral junction). Back pain may be accentuated by hyperextension of hind limbs or tail during lumbosacral manipulation. Unilateral or bilateral pelvic limb

Table 40-2

Neurologic Deficits Possible With Cauda Equina Compression

NERVE INVOLVED	NERVE ROOTS INVOLVED	NEUROLOGIC EXAM FINDINGS POSSIBLE
Cauda equina*	L6, L7, S1–3, Cd1–5	Back pain with or without any of the findings below
Sciatic nerve	L6, L7, S1, ± S2	Sensory: loss of sensation on lateral digit; licking and chewing of lateral digit; knuckling Motor: decreased withdrawal reflex, especially hock flexion; hind limb atrophy; motor weakness
Perineal nerve	S1, S2, S3	Sensory: decreased sensation to perineum and caudal thigh; licking perineum
Caudal rectal nerve	S2, S3	Motor: decreased to absent anal sphincter tone on rectal exam
Pelvic nerve	S1, S2, S3	Parasympathetic: loss of bladder control
Pudendal nerve	S1, S2, S3	Motor: varying degrees of urinary incontinence
Caudal nerves	Cd1–5	Sensory: decreased sensation to the tail; pain upon tail manipulation; excessive tail linking Motor: change in tail carriage and tail wag
Femoral nerve†	L4, L5, L6	Sensory: no change expected Motor: patellar reflex appears brisk as a result of the absence of sciatic innervated antagonist muscles

*All neurologic abnormalities involving cauda equina ischemia and/or compression are LMN signs.
†Although the femoral nerve is not supplied by nerve roots of the cauda equina, when the patellar reflex is performed, it appears brisk (UMN); this is caused by loss of antagonist muscles innervated by sciatic nerve and is not a UMN sign.

lameness due to referred pain from attenuation of the L7 and/or S1 nerve root is common. This finding often progresses to loss of conscious proprioception, development of motor weakness, and hind limb atrophy as nerve root ischemia and compression increase. Patellar reflexes may be normal or exaggerated due to loss of antagonism from sciatic innervation (i.e., attenuation of L7, S1-2 nerve roots). This should not be misinterpreted as a UMN sign. Urinary and anal sphincter disturbances may accompany back pain and paraparesis when the S1, S2, and S3 nerve roots become compressed. Patients rarely have sphincter disturbances alone; sometimes the urinary bladder is inappropriately easy to express. Initial presenting signs of urinary sphincter disturbance may resemble chronic UTI (e.g., increased urgency and frequent urination). As nerve root compression progresses, urinary incontinence (i.e., dribbling) becomes evident. Generally, clinically apparent anal sphincter dysfunction occurs after urinary sphincter dysfunction, and is manifested by fecal incontinence and anal sphincter hypotonia or atonia on rectal examination. The degree of sphincteric incontinence may be a prognostic indicator; as incontinence increases, the prognosis becomes more unfavorable. Tail carriage or function may be affected as the caudal nerve roots are affected. Abnormalities may include the following: (1) breeds with an erect tail will carry it in a lower position; (2) ability to wag the tail is decreased or absent; (3) tail manipulation results in pain (e.g., hyperextension); and (4)

there is loss of tail sensation. Paresthesia and dysesthesia (burning or tingling sensations in areas supplied by entrapped nerve roots) may occur in the tail, lateral digits, perineum, or genitals and are manifested by the patient's constant licking and chewing of the affected area. Paresthesia and dysesthesia usually occur in the tail and lateral digits.

> NOTE: Exaggerated patellar reflexes may be a result of a loss of antagonism from sciatic innervation (i.e., attenuation of L7, S1–S2 nerve roots), not a UMN lesion.

Diagnostic Imaging

Specific imaging techniques used to diagnose cauda equina syndrome vary depending on the cause of cauda equina compression. Patients with fracture/luxation may have survey radiographic findings listed in Box 40-2. Those with neoplasia of the lumbosacral spine, surrounding soft tissue, or nerve roots have survey radiographic and myelographic signs dependent on tumor location (e.g., extradural, intradural-extramedullary, and intramedullary) (see Fig. 40-11 on p. 1510). Patients with infectious cauda equina compression (e.g., diskospondylitis and vertebral osteomyelitis) may have osteolysis and/or osteoproduction of the vertebral body, intervertebral space, or both (see Fig. 41-1 on p. 1515).

BOX 40-2

Potential Radiographic Findings in Dogs With Cauda Equina Syndrome Associated With Fracture/Luxation

Discontinuity of bony structures (i.e., spinous process, lamina, pedicle, and vertebral body)
Malalignment of intervertebral space and/or articular facets
Fracture lines in the vertebral body and/or spinous processes of L7, S1–S3
Loss of continuity or malalignment of the vertebral canal
Combination of above

BOX 40-3

Factors Influencing Ability to Accurately Image the L7–S1 Junction

Superimposed density of the wings of the ilium obscuring L7-S1 intervertebral foramen, intervertebral space, and vertebral bodies
Inconsistent termination of the dural sac (i.e., filum terminale)
Exclusively soft tissue changes not evident on many imaging procedures
Technical difficulty of performing specific imaging procedures (e.g., intraosseous venography and diskography)
Cost of special imaging techniques (e.g., CT scan and MRI)
Inconsistent findings (i.e., false-negative results)
Difficulty in interpretation of findings

CT, Computed tomography; *MRI,* magnetic resonance imaging.

The process of imaging the lumbosacral spine to diagnose cauda equina compression secondary to chronic degenerative disk disease, intervertebral disk extrusion, or congenital lumbosacral stenosis is often a challenge. Factors influencing the ability to accurately image the L7-S1 junction are listed in Box 40-3. Imaging techniques must be evaluated in light of historical and neurologic examination findings. Commonly performed imaging procedures include survey radiography, stress radiography, myelography, epidurography, and now more frequently, computed tomography (CT) and MRI. Results depend on the cause of compression (i.e., chronic degenerative disk disease, intervertebral disk extrusion, congenital lumbosacral stenosis, or lumbosacral instability) and are listed in Table 40-3. Techniques for performing these procedures are discussed and illustrated in Figs. 36-12 to 36-24 on pp. 1371 to 1378.

Cross-sectional imaging techniques, such as CT and MRI, are the techniques of choice to definitively diagnose cauda equina syndrome caused by chronic degenerative disk disease, intervertebral disk extrusion, congenital lum-

bosacral stenosis, or lumbosacral instability (see Fig. 36-21 on p. 1376). It is imperative that cross-sectional imaging be performed with the hind limbs in an extended position as this will exacerbate any instability that is present. The lumbosacral region may appear normal in neutral or a flexed position in these animals. Results of imaging techniques consistent with cauda equina compression are listed in Table 40-3.

Electromyography, particularly of the tail base, pelvic diaphragm, and muscles of sciatic distribution, can reveal spontaneous electrical activity indicative of LMN disease. Electrodiagnostic findings, coupled with typical historical, neurologic, and imaging results, may support a diagnosis of cauda equina compression.

Laboratory Findings

Laboratory findings are generally nonspecific. Patients with cauda equina compression secondary to an infection may have leukocytosis, with or without left shift. Patients previously treated with corticosteroids may have a stress leukogram and elevated hepatic enzymes.

DIFFERENTIAL DIAGNOSIS

Differential diagnoses for cauda equina compression include fracture/luxation; diskospondylitis; vertebral osteomyelitis; fibrocartilaginous emboli; neoplasia of the spine, surrounding soft tissue, or nerve roots; chronic degenerative disk disease; herniated intervertebral disk extrusion; or congenital lumbosacral stenosis. Disorders not associated with the lumbosacral junction that mimic cauda equina syndrome include hip dysplasia, metabolic disorders causing weakness, and degenerative myelopathy. Diagnostic tools include careful historical, physical, and neurologic examinations; laboratory data; multiple imaging procedures; and electrodiagnostics. Surgical exploration may be necessary for a definitive diagnosis.

MEDICAL MANAGEMENT

Medical management of patients with cauda equina compression depends on causal factors. The treatment for patients with fracture/luxation is described on p. 1503; for diskospondylitis or vertebral osteomyelitis on p. 1514; and for neoplasia of the spine, surrounding soft tissue, or nerve roots on p. 1509.

Medical management of patients with cauda equina compression secondary to chronic degenerative disk disease, intervertebral disk extrusion, and congenital lumbosacral stenosis is based on severity and duration of neurologic signs, and serial neurologic examinations (Table 40-4). Medical management consists of strict confinement for 4 to 6 weeks. In addition, a change in the patient's life style may improve outcome. Instruct owners to retrain their dogs to limit activities that result in hyperextension of the lumbosacral junction (i.e., jumping up to elevated structures or jumping down from elevated platforms). Steroids are of little benefit to patients with nerve root injury.

Table 40-3

Results of Various Imaging Techniques Based on Etiologic Factors of Cauda Equina Compression

ETIOLOGY	IMAGING TECHNIQUE	POSSIBLE FINDINGS
Chronic degenerative disk disease (DDD)*	Survey radiographs	Transitional vertebrae†; varying degrees of spondylosis‡; may be normal
	Stress radiographs	Perform flexion and extension; combine with epidurography *Extension:* vertebral canal diameter reduces, contrast is obliterated *Flexion:* vertebral canal opens, contrast fills previous compression May be normal
	Myelography	Usually normal; extradural compression may be seen if lesion is large and filum terminale reaches far enough caudally; rules out lesion cranial to L6
	Diskography	Irregular contrast pattern within the nucleus pulposus; can inject greater than 0.1 ml volume of contrast medium; may be normal (i.e., cannot inject greater than 0.1 ml, smooth contrast pattern)
	Epidurography	Contrast flow is stopped or elevated at L7–L1 interspace; combine with stress positioning; may be normal (i.e., contrast flows unobstructed along floor of canal at L7–S1)
	Computed tomography	Bone spurs; spondylosis‡; loss of epidural fat; disk bulging; thecal sac displacement; vertebral canal stenosis
	Magnetic resonance imaging	Attenuation of epidural fat; disk bulging; loss of signal intensity at disk space (indicative of severe disk degeneration); spinal stenosis; location of compressive tissue; vertebral subluxation
Acute intervertebral disk extrusion*	Survey radiographs	Normal; may see fogged L7–S1 intervertebral foramen; early spondylosis‡
	Stress radiographs	Normal
	Myelography	Normal; if disk fragments are large, extradural compression; rules out lesion cranial to L6
	Diskography	Extravasation of contrast medium; can inject greater than 0.1 volume of contrast medium
	Epidurography	Contrast flow is stopped or elevated at L7–L1 interspace
	Computed tomography	Loss of epidural fat; disk bulging; thecal sac displacement; vertebral canal stenosis
	Magnetic resonance imaging	Attenuation of epidural fat; disk bulging; loss of signal intensity at disk space (indicative of severe disk degeneration); spinal stenosis; location of compressive tissue; vertebral subluxation
Congenital stenosis*	Survey radiographs	Narrow canal diameter; transitional vertebra†; enlarged articular facets; rarely see signs consistent with DDD
	Stress radiographs	Normal early; may see signs consistent with DDD later; combine with epidurography
	Myelography	Normal; may see signs consistent with DDD later; rules out lesion cranial to L6
	Diskography	Normal early; may see signs consistent with DDD later
	Epidurography	Normal early; contrast flow is stopped or elevated at L7–L1 interspace; combine with stress positioning
	Computed tomography	Vertebral canal stenosis; vertebral subluxation
	Magnetic resonance imaging	Attenuation of epidural fat; spinal stenosis; location of compressive tissue; vertebral subluxation

*Neurologic examination is the interpretation of results of imaging procedures that must be performed in light of historic, physical, and neurologic examination findings.

†Transitional vertebrae are vertebrae that possess properties of two major divisions of the vertebral column. Lumbosacral anomalies include the following: (1) sacralization of L7 (L7 becomes fused, unilaterally or bilaterally, to the sacrum); (2) lumbarization of S1 (S1 becomes a lumbar vertebra and S2 is fused to the sacrum) and Cd1 may become fused to S3.

‡Spondylosis is characterized by any combination of the following survey radiographic signs: collapse of the intervertebral space, sclerosis of vertebral end plates, ventral and lateral proliferation of bony spurs from the vertebral body in an attempt to bridge the intervertebral space (ankylosis), degeneration and collapse of the articular facets.

 Table 40-4

Recommended Medical Therapy* for Patients With Cauda Equina Compression (i.e., chronic degenerative disk disease, intervertebral disk herniation, congenital lumbosacral stenosis, or lumbosacral fracture/luxation) based on Clinical Presentation

CLINICAL PRESENTATION	INITIAL TREATMENT†	RESULT	SECOND TREATMENT†	RESULT	THIRD TREATMENT†
Back pain only, with or without paresthesia or dysesthesia	Cage rest only	Improvement	Continue cage rest	Cage rest/follow	
		Static	NSAID	Static/deteriorating	Consider surgery
		Deteriorating	Consider surgery‡		
Back pain; mild paraparesis; no urinary incontinence	NSAID	Improvement	Cage rest/NSAID	Improvement	Cage rest/ follow
		Static	Continue NSAID	Static/deteriorating	Consider surgery
		Deteriorating	Consider surgery		
Back pain; mild paraparesis; early urinary incontinence	NSAID	Improvement	Cage rest/NSAID	Improvement	Cage rest/ follow
		Static	Consider surgery		
		Deteriorating	Consider surgery		
Back pain; moderate paraparesis; no urinary incontinence	NSAID	Improvement	Cage rest/NSAID	Improvement	Cage rest/ follow
		Static	Consider surgery		
		Deteriorating	Consider surgery		
Back pain; severe paraparesis; no urinary incontinence	Consider surgery				
Back pain; moderate or severe paraparesis; urinary incontinence	Consider surgery				

NSAID, Nonsteroidal antiinflammatory drug.
*All patients are strictly confined (4-6 weeks) as part of their medical management regardless of the drug used or duration of drug therapy.
†Initial treatment may be the first 24-48 hours or 3-5 days depending upon results of serial neurologic examinations. Second and third treatments are also dependant on neurologic status.
‡Regardless of clinical presentation, if a client cannot afford surgery, a course of cage rest and NSAID therapy should be attempted.

SURGICAL TREATMENT

Surgical objectives include nerve root decompression and vertebral stabilization. Specific surgical procedures for patients with cauda equina compression depend on the cause. Treatment for patients with fracture/luxation is described on p. 1503; diskospondylitis or vertebral osteomyelitis on p. 1514; and neoplasia of the spine, surrounding soft tissue, or nerve roots on p. 1509. The surgical treatment of patients with cauda equina compression secondary to chronic degenerative disk disease, intervertebral disk extrusion, and congenital lumbosacral stenosis is based on severity and duration of neurologic signs (see Table 40-4), outcome of medical management (see Table 40-4), results of imaging (see Table 40-3), EMG findings, and serial neurologic examinations

(see Table 40-4). It is important to consider the patient's clinical signs when evaluating MRI because of the lack of correlation in the degree of compression determined by MRI and the severity of signs demonstrated by the patient (Mayhew et al, 2002). In addition, mild bulging of the L7-S1 intervertebral disk on CT imaging can be associated neuropathy in normal, medium-sized dogs (Axlund et al, 2003).

Preoperative Management

Preoperative management of patients with cauda equina compression is similar to that described for patients with other lumbosacral compressive lesions (see p. 1493). Preoperative steroids are not recommended because they likely do not have a protective effect on nerve roots.

Anesthesia

Suggested anesthetic protocols for use in patients with lumbosacral spinal disorders are discussed on p. 1403.

Surgical Anatomy

Knowledge of topographic anatomy of the cauda equina and its relationship to lumbar, sacral, and caudal vertebrae will facilitate an understanding of possible neurologic findings in patients with cauda equina compression, and the surgical manipulation necessary for decompression (see Fig. 40-3). Dorsal lamina, articular facets and joint capsule, vertebral canal diameter, dorsal annulus fibrosus, interarcuate ligament, and dorsal longitudinal ligament are all points of anatomy that may play a role in cauda equina compression.

Positioning

Because patients are generally treated via laminectomy, they should be positioned in sternal recumbency with the hind legs tucked under the abdomen to encourage flexion and facilitate exposure of the dorsal lumbosacral intervertebral space (see Fig. 40-1).

SURGICAL TECHNIQUE

Surgical techniques for dorsal laminectomy, hemilaminectomy, facetectomy, and foraminotomy are described on pp. 1493 to 1495.

Chronic Degenerative Disk Disease

Patients diagnosed with chronic degenerative disk disease require enough exposure of the vertebral canal to decompress all attenuated nerve roots. Depending on neurologic examination findings and results of imaging, adequate decompression involves dorsal laminectomy, with or without foraminotomy and facetectomy.

Perform a dorsal laminectomy on patients with dorsal compression from lamina and interarcuate ligament. Use a No. 11 scalpel blade and ophthalmic forceps to carefully resect the ligament. In patients with lateral compression, perform a facetectomy to decompress the L7 and S1 nerve roots from the bulbous articular facets. In patients requiring further lateral decompression of the L7 nerve root, perform a foraminotomy to establish complete decompression. Perform unilateral or bilateral facetectomy/foraminotomy based on neurologic examination findings, results of imaging, and surgical findings. Approach nerve root compression from the ventral floor of the vertebral canal (i.e., protrusion of dorsal annulus fibrosus) through careful retraction of nerve roots, sharp annular incision, and mass removal (Fig. 40-4).

Patients may require all or a variety of the above decompressive techniques. Spinal stabilization is not indicated unless spinal instability is documented (Linn et al, 2003) (see p. 1505).

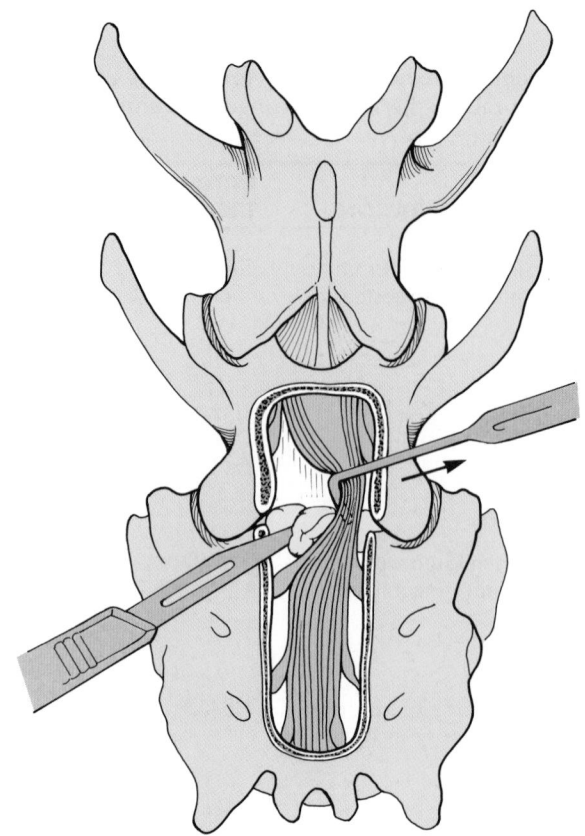

FIG. 40-4
Retract nerve roots laterally with care to facilitate excision of hypertrophied dorsal annulus fibrosus.

Acute Intervertebral Disk Herniation

In patients with herniated intervertebral disk material, perform a dorsal laminectomy if disk fragments are located on the midline or bilaterally, or a hemilaminectomy if neurologic signs and imaging results lateralize disk fragments to one side. Adequately expose the vertebral canal to achieve complete mass removal.

Spinal stabilization is generally not indicated unless spinal instability is documented (see p. 1505).

Congenital Lumbosacral Stenosis

In patients with congenital lumbosacral stenosis, perform a dorsal laminectomy with unilateral or bilateral facetectomy based on neurologic signs, imaging results, and surgical findings. If stenosis is radiographically or surgically demonstrated extending from L6-S1, perform a multilevel dorsal laminectomy and bilateral facetectomy from L6-S1. Remove interarcuate ligaments dorsally and facets laterally to provide complete decompression. Place a free fat graft over the entire laminectomy defect.

Spinal stabilization is generally indicated, as spinal instability is likely (see p. 1505).

SUTURE MATERIALS AND SPECIAL INSTRUMENTS

Special instruments necessary for laminectomy of the lumbosacral junction are similar to those listed in Box 39-1 on p. 1468. It is important to practice each technique, become familiar with regional anatomy, and learn proper use of special instrumentation before performing these surgeries.

POSTOPERATIVE CARE AND ASSESSMENT

Critical care observation for the first 24 postoperative hours includes IV fluids; analgesics; antibiotics; seizure alert (if the work-up required a myelogram); and neurologic examination. A guide to immediate and long-term postoperative care and assessment for ambulatory and nonambulatory patients is given in Table 39-1 and Box 39-2 on p. 1469.

PROGNOSIS

Prognosis for cauda equina compression depends on the causal factors, neurologic deficits on presentation, and treatment regimen chosen (i.e., medical or surgical). The prognosis for medically managed patients with mild to moderate back pain, mild lameness, absent or mild paraparesis, and/or no urinary incontinence is favorable to excellent, particularly if life style changes can successfully be incorporated into the treatment regimen. Prognosis for medically managed patients with severe back pain, moderate to severe lameness, moderate to severe paraparesis, and/or urinary incontinence is guarded to unfavorable. If patients with mild neurologic deficits show static or deteriorating signs or loss of urinary continence during medical management, early surgical decompression should be considered.

Generally, prognosis for surgically treated patients 6 to 8 years of age with acute back pain, mild to moderate lameness, mild to moderate paraparesis, and no urinary incontinence is favorable to excellent. Prognosis for patients greater than 8 years of age with chronic back pain, severe lameness, severe paraparesis, and urinary incontinence is guarded to unfavorable (Linn et al, 2003). Regardless of other presenting signs, urinary incontinence implies an unfavorable prognosis if decompression is delayed.

References

Axlund TW, Hudson JA: Computed tomography of the normal lumbosacral intervertebral disk in 22 dogs, *Vet Radiol Ultrasound* 44:630, 2003.

Jaeger GH, Early PJ, Munana KR et al: Lumbosacral disk disease in a cat, *Vet Comp Orthop Traumatol* 17:104, 2004.

Jones JC, Banfield CM, Ward DL: Association between postoperative outcome and results of magnetic resonance imaging and computed tomography in working dogs with degenerative lumbosacral stenosis, *J Am Vet Med Assoc* 216:1769, 2000.

Linn LL, Bartels KE, Rochat MC et al: Lumbosacral stenosis in 29 military working dogs: epidemiologic findings and outcome after surgical intervention (1990-1999), *Vet Surg* 32:21-29, 2003.

Mayhew PD, Kapatkin AS, Wortman JA et al: Association of cauda equina compression on magnetic resonance images and clinical signs in dogs with degenerative lumbosacral stenosis, *J Am Anim Hosp Assoc* 38:555-562, 2002.

Schwarz T, Owen MR, Long S et al: Vacuum disk and facet phenomenon in a dog with cauda equina syndrome, *J Am Vet Med Assoc* 217:862, 2000.

Suggested Reading

Chen AV, Bagley RS, West CL et al: Fecal incontinence and spinal cord abnormalities in seven dogs, *J Am Vet Med Assoc* 227:1945, 2005.

The authors found that spinal cord problems causing fecal incontinence were often cystic, and that surgery could benefit the incontinence.

FRACTURES AND LUXATIONS OF THE LUMBOSACRAL SPINE

DEFINITIONS

Traumatic or pathologic disruption of osseous and supporting soft tissue structures of the caudal lumbar, sacral, and first caudal vertebrae (e.g., L6-Cd1-5) may result in vertebral fracture or luxation and subsequent nerve root compression (i.e., cauda equina). Fractures of the lumbosacral spine are also called a *broken back, caudal lumbar fractures,* and *vertebral fractures.*

GENERAL CONSIDERATIONS AND CLINICALLY RELEVANT PATHOPHYSIOLOGY

Fractures and luxations of the caudal lumbar vertebra, lumbosacral articulation, sacrum, and caudal vertebrae generally result from direct flexional trauma to the hind quarters. Fractures are usually oblique or short oblique involving the vertebral body of L6 or L7 and may be accompanied by luxation of articular facets. Cranioventral displacement of the caudal segment typically occurs because of muscular forces acting on the sacrum and pelvis, along with the weight of the pelvic mass (Fig. 40-5). Lumbosacral fractures are fairly common as a result of the static-kinetic relationship of the relatively fixed sacrum to the mobile caudal lumbar and caudal vertebral bodies. The most common cause of fracture/luxation is vehicular trauma. The spinal cord terminates in the body of L6; therefore neurologic signs are usually associated with trauma to nerve roots of the cauda equina (e.g., L6-L7, S1-S3, and Cd1-Cd5) instead of the spinal cord. Due to the ability of nerve roots to resist traumatic injury, substantial displacement of the fracture or luxation may still leave the patient neurologically intact. Conversely, fractures or luxations may occur in which severe displacement of the fracture/luxation segments causes tethering or avulsion of nerve roots and will occasionally produce trauma to the caudal spinal cord; neurologic deficits in these patients are often profound.

DIAGNOSIS
Clinical Presentation

Signalment. There is no specific age, sex, or breed predilection for canine or feline lumbosacral fracture/luxation. However, dogs are more likely to sustain this injury than cats, and there is a trend with dogs less than 3 years of age being affected more often.

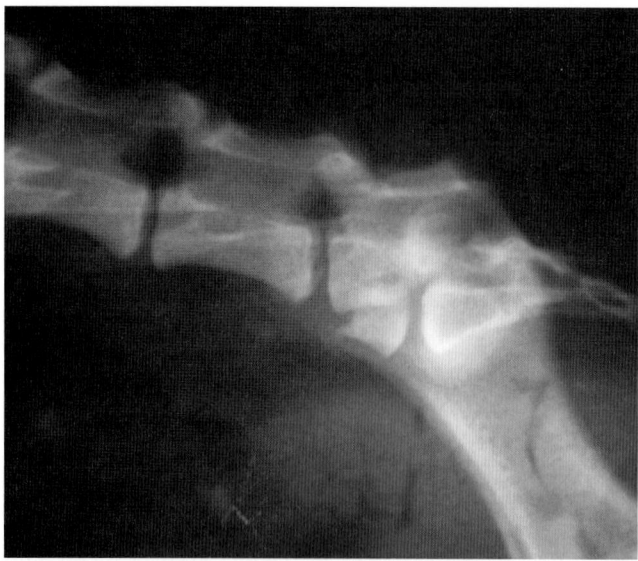

FIG. 40-5
Lateral radiograph of a dog with an L7 fracture. Notice the cranioventral displacement of the sacrum, pelvis, and L7 fracture fragment, which is typical with these fractures.

History. Nearly 80% to 90% of dogs and cats with lumbosacral fracture/luxation have a history of recent vehicular trauma. Patients generally have varying degrees of lumbar pain, ambulatory or nonambulatory paraparesis, and decreased anal and tail tone.

Physical Examination Findings

Severe traumatic injury often produces additional injuries (e.g., cardiopulmonary, urinary, diaphragmatic hernia, appendicular skeleton, and second vertebral fracture/luxation). A thorough physical examination of each system to identify concurrent injury is necessary. Patients that struggle during physical examination or that have profound neurologic deficits should be secured to a rigid platform to prevent further nerve root trauma until a definitive course of action can be taken.

Lumbosacral fracture/luxation may cause trauma and sustained compression to the cauda equina. The most commonly involved nerve roots are L6-L7, S1-S3, and Cd1-Cd5. Major nerves associated with these nerve roots include the sciatic nerve (L6, L7, S1, and/or S2); perineal nerve (S1, S2, S3); caudal rectal nerve (S2, S3); pelvic nerve (S1, S2, S3); pudendal nerve (S1, S2, S3); and caudal nerves of the tail (Cd1-Cd5). Because of the regional anatomy innervated by the cauda equina, ischemia and/or compression may produce a wide variety of neurologic signs (see Table 40-2 on p. 1498). Although a variety of neurologic deficits may occur, the most common presentations are lumbosacral hyperpathia (pain on deep palpation of the lumbosacral junction), LMN ambulatory or nonambulatory paraparesis, varying degrees of anal sphincter atonia, and abnormalities in tail carriage and sensation.

Diagnostic Imaging

Neurologic examination localizes the lesion to the caudal lumbar and sacral region. Survey radiographs are usually diagnostic and generally reveal an oblique or short oblique fracture through the vertebral body of L6 or L7, or a luxation or subluxation between L6 and L7 or L7 and S1 (see Fig. 40-5). The caudal vertebral body is characteristically displaced cranioventral to the cranial vertebral body (see Fig. 40-5). Because of the relatively mild neurologic signs that may be seen with marked fracture/luxation displacement on survey radiographs, prognosis is based on neurologic examination findings, not radiologic findings. Moreover, as LMN signs predominate in patients with multiple spinal fractures, neurologic examination may not identify a second thoracolumbar fracture/luxation. A complete series of spinal radiographs is always recommended in patients with spinal fracture.

> NOTE: Up to 20% of patients with spinal fracture/luxation have a second spinal fracture/luxation.

Laboratory Findings

Patients having lumbosacral fracture/luxation secondary to severe trauma often have a stress leukogram and elevated hepatic enzymes. If patients sustain concurrent injuries resulting in uroabdomen, ruptured spleen, or pulmonary contusion, associated laboratory abnormalities may occur. Laboratory findings are usually nonspecific.

DIFFERENTIAL DIAGNOSIS

Fracture/luxation of the lumbosacral spine must be differentiated from other disorders causing cauda equina compression, including congenital lumbosacral stenosis; diskospondylitis; chronic degenerative disk disease; intervertebral disk extrusion; fibrocartilaginous embolism; and neoplasia of the spine, surrounding soft tissue, and nerve roots. Definitive diagnosis is made by analyzing history, neurologic localization, and radiographic results.

MEDICAL MANAGEMENT

Objectives of medical management include immobilization of the spine and patient confinement until fracture/luxation stabilization and union occur. The following conditions are recommended: strict confinement for 4 to 6 weeks in a dry, elevated padded cage; analgesics/nonsteroidal antiinflammatory drugs (NSAIDs) as needed to control back pain (do not use steroids and NSAIDs concurrently or in close proximity to each other); urinary bladder expression or intermittent catheterization four times daily; passive physical therapy of the hind legs two to three times daily; and serial neurologic examinations twice daily to assess patient response to therapy.

SURGICAL TREATMENT

Objectives of surgical management are decompression of the cauda equina (fracture/luxation reduction), followed by adequate spinal stabilization. Infrequently, patients may require dorsal laminectomy for complete decompression (when bone fragments are present in the vertebral canal) or for its prognostic value in evaluating the severity of cauda equina damage. Surgical reduction and stabilization provides immediate relief of back pain, allows freedom of movement, decreases patient morbidity, and protects spinal roots from further trauma. Surgical versus medical treatment is based on the patient's neurologic status at presentation, response to medical management, and serial neurologic examinations (see Table 40-4 on p. 1501). Adequate stabilization of the lumbosacral junction can be provided by (1) transiliac pins with Kirschner clamps, bent pins, or bone cement; (2) transiliac pins and plastic dorsal spinous process plates; (3) transiliac pin, dorsal spinous process plates, and external skeletal fixation; (4) modified segmental spinal fixation; and (5) Steinmann pins (or screws) embedded in PMMA bone cement. Choice of technique is generally dictated by the surgeon's experience and equipment available.

Preoperative Management

Preoperative management of patients with cauda equina compression is similar to that described for any lumbosacral compressive lesion (see p. 1493). If concurrent spinal cord injury is not present, preoperative steroids are not recommended because they do not protect nerve roots. Lumbosacral instability predisposes the patient to further trauma, and care should be taken to support the patient's pelvis during preoperative manipulations.

Anesthesia

Suggested anesthetic regimens for use in patients with lumbosacral spinal disorders are discussed on p. 1403.

Surgical Anatomy

Refer to the description and illustration of topographic anatomy of the cauda equina in Figs. 40-2 and 40-3 on pp. 1494 and 1497, respectively.

Positioning

The surgical approach for each stabilization technique requires dorsal exposure. Positioning the patient in sternal recumbency with the hind legs tucked under the abdomen encourages flexion of the dorsal lumbosacral region and facilitates fracture reduction and cauda equina decompression (see Fig. 40-1 on p. 1494).

SURGICAL TECHNIQUE
L7 Fracture and L7–S1 Luxation

Transiliac pins. *Expose dorsal spinous processes and lamina of L6, L7, and the entire median sacral crest as described for dorsal laminectomy on p. 1493. Because of the cranioventral displacement of the sacrum, visualization of the cranial aspect of the sacral crest is obscured by the lamina of L7. L7 laminectomy is not compatible with this technique. Use a periosteal elevator or small osteotome to elevate epaxial muscles and expose the articular processes of L7. Use the tip of a Kelly or Carmalt forceps or a Senn retractor, and*

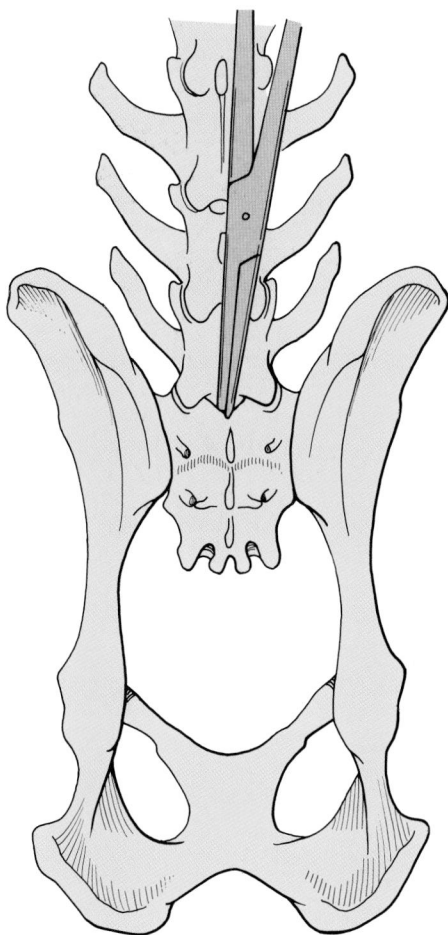

FIG. 40-6
Use of Kelly or Carmalt forceps to aid reduction of an L7 fracture. Hook the tip of the forceps under the cranial lamina of the sacrum and lower the jaws against the caudal lamina of L7.

carefully place it in the lumbosacral junction. Visually monitor the depth of placement of the forceps or retractor to prevent injuring nerve roots. Hook the tip of the forceps or retractor under the cranial lamina of the sacrum to act as a lever against the caudal lamina of L7 (Fig. 40-6). Adequate exposure of the lumbosacral junction is facilitated by reducing the fracture/luxation. Before attempting reduction, place a bone forceps or towel clamp in the wing of each ilium. Have an unsterile assistant available to provide cranial traction on the patient's head or front legs. Reduce the fracture/luxation by making the simultaneous moves listed in Box 40-4.

These manipulations force the sacrum caudodorsally to reduce the fracture/luxation.

Visualize the lumbosacral articular facets; when the articular processes of L7 and S1 are reapposed, reduction is anatomic. Place an 0.062-inch Kirschner wire through each L7-S1 articular facet to maintain fracture/luxation reduction. Next, incise gluteal fascia on the dorsolateral crest of the

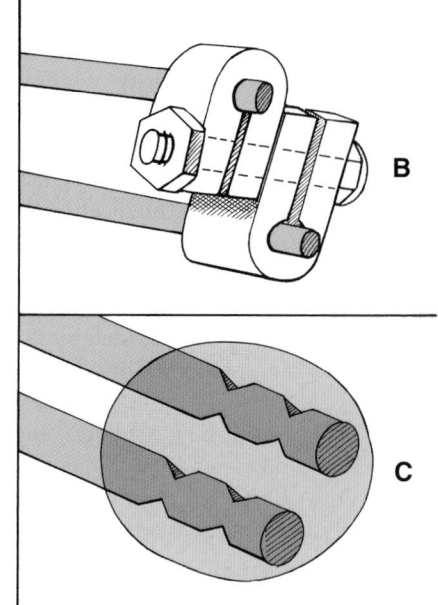

FIG. 40-7
Prevent migration of transiliac pins by **A,** bending the ends of each pin at a 90-degree angle; **B,** connecting the pins on each side with a double Kirschner clamp; or **C,** notching the ends of the pins with a pin cutter and incorporating them with bone cement.

 BOX 40-4

Manipulation of L7-S1 Fracture/Luxation During Reduction

Grasp the towel clamps or bone forceps on the wings of the ilium and pull caudal and slightly dorsal
Have the assistant place counter traction on the head or front legs
Lever the sacrum against the lamina of L7 while pressing ventrally on L6–L7

Table 40-5

Selection of Steinmann Pin Size for Transiliac Pins

ANIMAL WEIGHT (Kg)	PIN SIZE (INCHES)
2.5	7/64
5–10	3/32
10–20	1/8
>20	3/16

wings of each ilium, elevate the middle gluteal musculature, and expose the dorsolateral aspect of each iliac crest. Place an appropriate size Steinmann pin (Table 40-5) through the lateral aspect of the iliac wing, across the dorsal lamina of L7, and through the opposite iliac wing. Place a second pin in a similar fashion starting from the opposite side (Fig. 40-7, A). Be sure both pins cross over the dorsal lamina of L7. Prevent pin migration by employing one of the following techniques: (1) bend the ends of each pin at a 90-degree angle (see Fig. 40-7, A); (2) connect the pins on each side with double Kirschner clamps of the appropriate size (Fig. 40-7, B); or (3) notch the pins' ends with a pin cutter and incorporate them with PMMA bone cement (Fig. 40-7, C). If indicated, remove the interarcuate ligament and perform sacral laminectomy to visualize nerve roots. Lavage the surgical wound with sterile physiologic saline solution, cover the ends of the pins by closing gluteal fascia, and close epaxial muscles by apposing dorsal midline fascia. Close subcutaneous tissue and skin routinely.

Fractures of the Body of L6 and L7 and Luxation of L7–S1

Transiliac pins with dorsal spinous process plates. This technique provides stable fixation by incorporating the caudal lumbar spine to help counteract flexion (plastic plate) and by using multiple points of fixation to prevent rotational instability (transiliac pins). It is compatible with dorsal laminectomy.

Prepare the dorsum of the back, from the midthoracic region to the base of the tail, for aseptic surgery. Make a dorsal midline skin incision such that three dorsal spinous processes

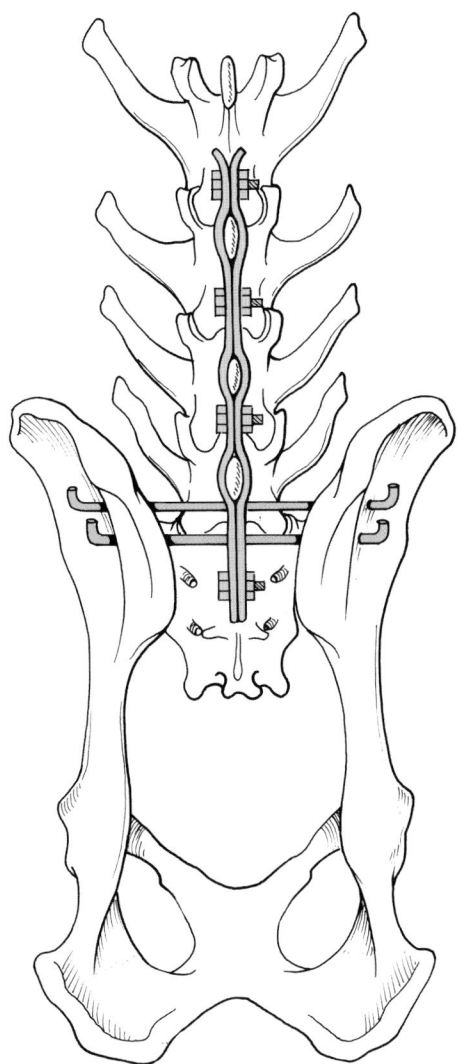

FIG. 40-8
Diagram showing use of transiliac pins and plastic dorsal spinous process plates to repair L7–S1 fracture/luxation.

cranial to the fracture/luxation can be exposed, and extend it caudally to a point midway between the tuber ischii. Preserve the interspinous and supraspinous ligaments cranial to the lumbosacral junction by making two parallel lumbosacral fascial incisions on either side of the dorsal spinous processes. Elevate epaxial muscles to the level of the articular facets bilaterally. Carefully expose dorsal spinous processes; lamina; and articular facets of L6, L7, and/or sacrum, depending on location of the fracture. Reduce the fracture/luxation and maintain reduction with transarticular pins as described previously. Perform a dorsal laminectomy at this time, if indicated (see p. 1493). Select the appropriate size and length of plastic plates, and secure them along each side of the dorsal spinous processes as described on p. 1487. Include a minimum of three dorsal spinous processes cranial to the fracture/luxation. Place two transiliac Steinmann pins as described on p. 1505 (Fig. 40-8). Be sure to place each pin through predrilled holes in each plastic

plate. Prevent pin migration by placing Kirschner clamps on the pin ends, bending the pin ends to 90-degree angles, or notching and covering the pin ends with bone cement as described (see Fig. 40-7). Place a final bolt, washer, and nut through the plates caudal to the transiliac pins (see Fig. 40-8). Lavage the surgical wound, and close dorsal lumbar fascia, gluteal fascia, subcutaneous tissue, and skin routinely.

Modified segmental spinal fixation. Modified segmental spinal fixation can be used in patients of all sizes. It does not require deep exposure, and it is compatible with dorsal laminectomy; simple to perform; versatile (it can be used in combination with other techniques); and results in a stable repair.

Approach the dorsal aspect of the lumbar and lumbosacral spine as described for transiliac pins and dorsal spinous process plates on p. 1505. Expose three dorsal spinous processes cranial to the fracture/luxation. Expose, carefully reduce, and maintain fracture/luxation reduction as described for transiliac pinning on p. 1505. Perform a dorsal laminectomy at this time, if indicated (see p. 1493). Drill holes in the caudal articular processes and bases of dorsal spinous processes of at least two to three vertebrae cranial to the fracture/luxation. Drill holes in the cranial sacral articular facets to ensure a minimum of two points of fixation per pin in the sacroiliac segment. Preplace 3- to 4-inch lengths of 18- to 20-gauge stainless steel wire through each hole. Drill two holes transversely through each iliac wing at the level of the dorsal lamina of the sacrum. Bend four appropriate size and length Steinmann pins at a 90-degree angle, remove the points, and pass the pins through the holes drilled in the wings of the ilia. Place the pins alongside the lamina, and attach them to the articular facets and dorsal spinous processes using the preplaced stainless steel wires (Fig. 40-9).

Fracture of L6 or L7 Vertebral Bodies and Luxation of L6–L7 or L7–S1

Steinmann pins and PMMA. Steinmann pins and PMMA bone cement can be used in patients of all sizes. This technique requires exposure of the dorsal surface of the transverse processes of L6 and L7 and is compatible with dorsal laminectomy; versatile (it can be used in combination with other techniques); requires constant reference to an anatomic specimen (e.g., spine); and produces a stable repair.

Adequately expose the vertebrae cranial and caudal to the fracture or luxation. Incise muscle attachments to articular facets, and periosteally elevate epaxial muscles until the dorsal aspect of the transverse processes of L6 and L7 and dorsal lamina of the sacrum are identified. Reduce the fracture/luxation, and maintain reduction as described for transiliac pinning on p. 1505. If the fracture involves the body of L6, place two pins in the body of L5 and two pins in the body

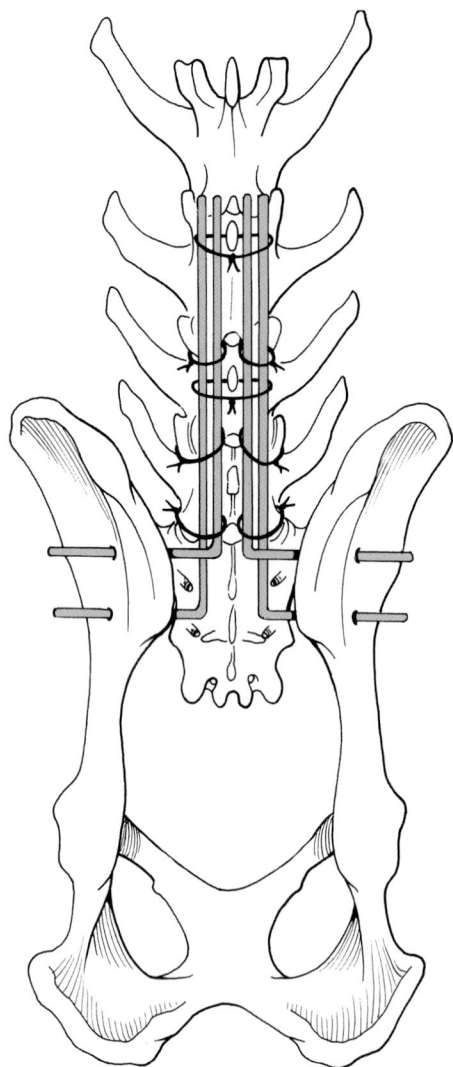

FIG. 40-9
Diagram showing proper pin placement for modified segmental spinal fixation of L6, L7, S1 fracture/luxation.

of L7. If an L6-L7 luxation is being repaired, place two pins in the body of L6 and two pins in the body of L7. Place pins and apply bone cement using the technique described on p. 1483. If the fracture involves the vertebral body of L7 or is an L7-S1 luxation, place two pins in the body of L6, two pins in the body of L7, and two pins in the cranial articular process of S1 with penetration through the ilium. If the fracture involves the vertebral body of L7, pin placement in L7 is dictated by the type of fracture present (e.g., avulsion fracture of the end plate: place two pins in L7; transverse fracture: place one or two smaller pins depending on the size of the fracture fragments; comminuted fracture: no pins should be placed in L7). Insert pins directly into the vertebral bodies of L6 or L7 using the accessory process and transverse process as landmarks. Insert pins into the center

of the cranial articular processes of S1. Drive the pin until it penetrates the gluteal surface of the wing of the ilium. Direct the L6 and L7 pins cranioventral and from lateral to medial, and the S1 pins caudoventral and from lateral to medial. Drive pins to exit 2 to 3 mm from the ventral aspect of the vertebral bodies and wings of the ilia. Cut pins to leave 2 cm protruding and notch the exposed pin heads with a pin cutter. Thoroughly lavage and dry the surgical field (Fig. 40-10). Apply PMMA bone cement as described on p. 1483 (see Figs. 39-24 through 39-26 on p. 1486). If necessary, excise portions of epaxial muscles adjacent to the PMMA to facilitate closure. Rarely, relief incisions in the lumbodorsal fascia lateral to the PMMA are necessary to allow closure of the primary incision. Close subcutaneous tissue and skin routinely.

Transiliac pins with dorsal spinous process plates and external skeletal fixation. Transiliac pins can be used in patients of all sizes. This technique is compatible with dorsal laminectomy, offers dorsal and ventral compartment fixation, requires minimal special equipment, and results in a stable repair.

Performing a dorsal approach, expose three dorsal spinous processes cranial to the fracture/luxation. Expose dorsal lamina and articular facets of affected vertebrae, reduce the fracture/luxation, maintain reduction, and place a dorsal spinous process plate as described on p. 1483. Pull skin and muscle to the center of the incision and percutaneously place a Steinmann pin through skin, muscle, wing of the ilium, holes in the dorsal spinous process plates, opposite iliac wing, and muscle and skin of the opposite side. Place a second Steinmann pin through the vertebral body cranial to the fracture/luxation. Start the pin just caudal to the junction of the transverse process and vertebral body. Pull skin and muscle to the center of the incision, and percutaneously insert the pin through skin, epaxial and body wall muscle mass, vertebral body (i.e., just caudal to the junction of the transverse process and vertebral body), and through muscles and skin on the opposite side. Place single clamps on both ends of each Steinmann pin, and attach connecting bars to each side. Close dorsal lumbar and sacral fascia, subcutaneous tissue, and skin routinely.

SUTURE MATERIALS AND SPECIAL INSTRUMENTS

Depending on the technique chosen, the following special instruments will be needed: plastic dorsal spinous process plates, bone cement, Steinmann pins, skeleton, and Kirschner-Ehmer clamps and connecting bars.

POSTOPERATIVE CARE AND ASSESSMENT

Patients with lumbosacral fracture/luxation should be monitored postoperatively, as are patients with other lumbosacral disorders (i.e., strict confinement, analgesics as needed, short walks using an abdominal sling, frequent urinary bladder

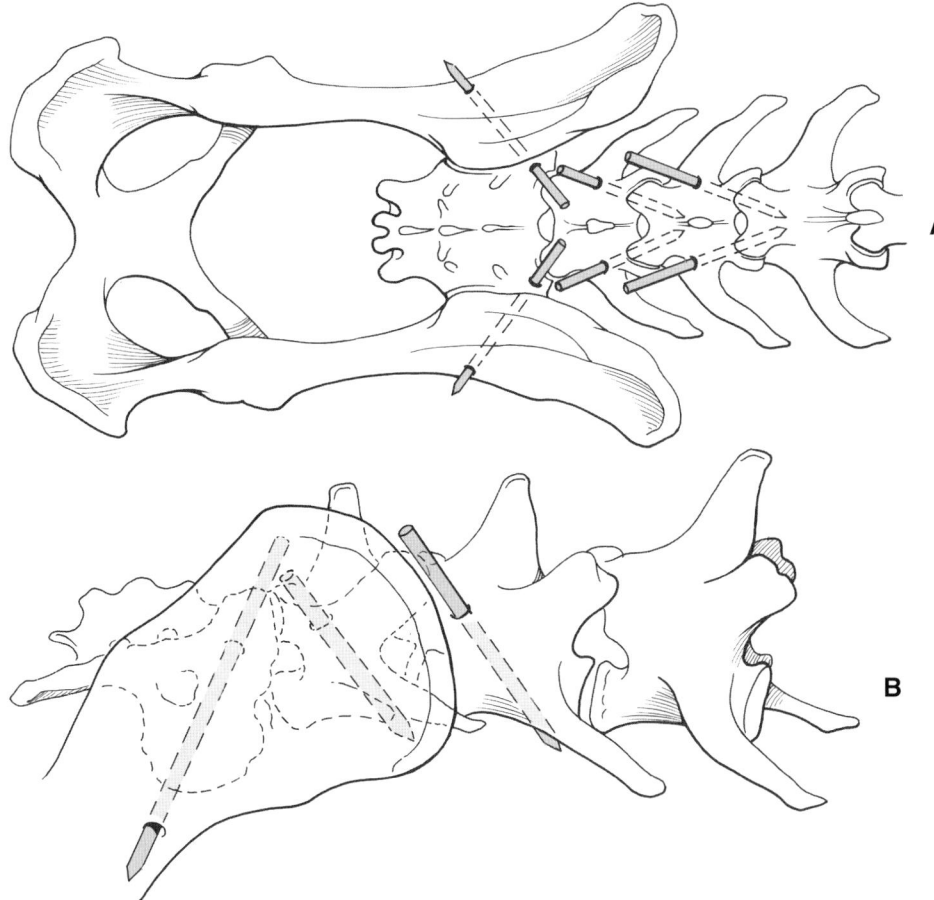

FIG. 40-10
A, Dorsal and **B,** lateral views showing proper pin placement in the iliac wings, articular facets of S1, and vertebral bodies of L6 and L7 when using Steinmann pins and PMMA to repair L6, L7, S1 fracture/luxation.

evacuation, and daily neurologic examinations). Long-term assessment consists of neurologic examinations and unanesthetized spinal radiographs at 1, 2, 3, 6, 9, and 12 months after surgery or when the fracture/luxation resolves.

PROGNOSIS

Prognosis depends on severity of cauda equina compression (i.e., on neurologic examination at presentation) and the treatment regimen chosen. Cauda equina nerve roots withstand considerably more trauma than the spinal cord. Patients with 100% lumbosacral vertebral canal compromise may retain neurologic function of the hind limbs, anus, urinary bladder, perineum, and tail; their prognosis is favorable. However, patients with profound neurologic deficits (e.g., complete loss of motor function and deep pain perception) should be given a guarded prognosis, regardless of the percentage of vertebral canal compromise. As the severity of presenting neurologic deficits increases, early decompression and stabilization allow a more favorable prognosis. If neurologic deterioration during medical management is

determined early, immediate surgical intervention produces a more favorable outcome.

> NOTE: The amount of vertebral canal compromise observed on lateral radiographs should not be used as a prognostic indicator.

NEOPLASIA OF THE LUMBOSACRAL SPINE AND NERVE ROOTS

DEFINITIONS

Neoplasms involving the lumbosacral vertebra and nerve roots are similar to those of the cervical and thoracolumbar regions (see p. 1455). Because the spinal cord terminates in the body of L6, primary spinal cord neoplasms are not encountered in the lumbosacral region. Synonyms include *spinal tumors or spinal cord tumors, vertebral tumors,* and *malignant nerve sheath tumors.*

GENERAL CONSIDERATIONS AND CLINICALLY RELEVANT PATHOPHYSIOLOGY

Tumors of the lumbosacral vertebrae and nerve roots rarely occur. Tumor type, location (e.g., spine, surrounding soft tissue, or nerve root), and classification (e.g., extradural, intradural-extramedullary, or intramedullary) are similar to neoplasms of the cervical, thoracic, and lumbar spine (see p. 1455). Regardless of tumor type or location, once the encroaching mass becomes large enough to cause cauda equina compression and ischemia, any of the neurologic signs associated with cauda equina syndrome or fracture/luxation may occur (see Table 40-2 on p. 1498).

DIAGNOSIS
Clinical Presentation

Signalment. There is no sex or breed predilection for patients with tumors of the lumbosacral spine. Generally, patients with spinal tumors are older than 5 years of age. An exception is solitary or multiple cartilaginous exostoses, which usually occur in patients less than 1 year of age.

History. History depends on the specific location of the neoplasm and the degree of cauda equina compression. Patients may have variable degrees of back pain, with or without LMN ambulatory paraparesis (see Table 40-2 on p. 1498). Anal sphincter atonia and urinary incontinence are inconsistent, but do occur. Patients with nerve root tumors usually have a chronic history of dull hind leg lameness (i.e., monoparesis from root signature). As the tumor enlarges

and compresses more of the cauda equina, paraparesis becomes evident. Patients with vertebral body or surrounding soft tissue (extradural) tumors have an acute history of back pain and ambulatory or nonambulatory paraparesis. Careful historical examination may reveal previous (e.g., weeks to months) subtle back pain or hind limb lameness.

Physical Examination Findings

Physical and neurologic examination findings vary depending on anatomic location of the tumor (e.g., spine, paraspinal soft tissue, and nerve root), degree of nerve root compression/ischemia, specific nerve roots involved, and associated secondary effects (e.g., paraneoplastic syndrome). Generally, patients have any combination of LMN signs associated with cauda equina compression (see Table 40-2 on p. 1498). If a single nerve root is involved (e.g., malignant nerve sheath tumor of L7), neurologic examination findings may allow localization of the tumor to that nerve root.

Diagnostic Imaging

Radiographic findings suggestive of vertebral neoplasia include vertebral body osteolysis and/or osteoproduction. These findings are generally associated with primary bone tumors (e.g., osteosarcoma, chondrosarcoma, and fibrosarcoma). Lysis of an intervertebral foramen suggests a nerve root tumor (e.g., neurofibroma or meningioma) (Fig. 40-11). Diagnosis of lumbosacral neoplasms may require stress radiography, myelography, epidurography, or cross-sectional im-

FIG. 40-11
Lateral radiograph of a dog with L7–S1 intervertebral foramen lysis *(arrow)* suggestive of nerve root tumor.

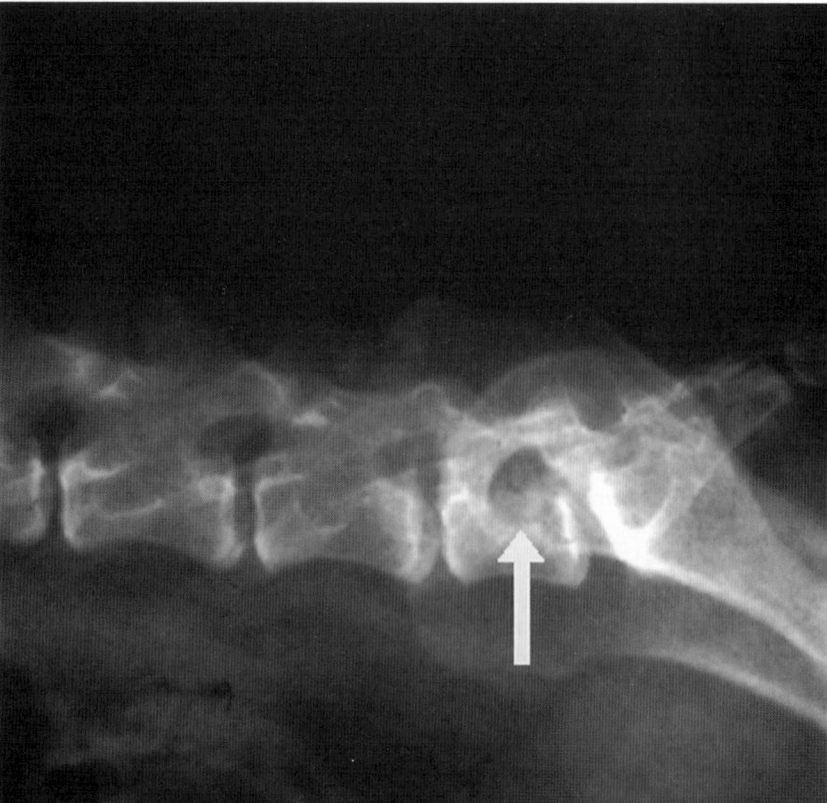

aging. Typically, cross-sectional imaging is more specific and sensitive when compared with radiography in identifying and determining the extent of the tumor. It can be used to determine surgical landmarks and define the margins for surgical resection. Specific techniques for performing these procedures are given in Tables 36-3 and 38-3 (see p. 1372 and 1423, respectively) and Figs. 36-14 through 36-24 (see pp. 1373 to 1378).

Laboratory Findings

Laboratory findings are generally normal or reflect paraneoplastic syndromes (e.g., hypercalcemia or monoclonal gammopathy). Patients with severe back pain and those treated with corticosteroids may have a stress leukogram.

DIFFERENTIAL DIAGNOSIS

Differential diagnoses for cauda equina compression include fracture/luxation; diskospondylitis; vertebral osteomyelitis; fibrocartilaginous emboli; neoplasia of the spine, surrounding soft tissue, or nerve roots; chronic degenerative disk disease; herniated intervertebral disk extrusion; or congenital lumbosacral stenosis. Disorders not associated with the lumbosacral junction that may mimic cauda equina compression include hip dysplasia, metabolic disorders that cause generalized weakness, and degenerative myelopathy. Diagnostic tools include careful historical, physical, and neurologic examinations; laboratory data; multiple imaging procedures; and electrodiagnostics. Surgical exploration may be needed for definitive diagnosis.

MEDICAL MANAGEMENT

Medical management is directed at both the primary lesion and secondary effects of the tumor. Corticosteroid therapy is generally not recommended for primary treatment of nerve root injury. However, steroids may be used for their antitumor effects. With most lumbosacral neoplasms, definitive medical treatment requires surgical exposure and incisional or excisional biopsy to determine tumor type and to plan appropriate adjunct chemotherapy, immunotherapy, irradiation, or combination therapy.

SURGICAL TREATMENT

Surgical treatment objectives include the definitive diagnosis of cauda equina compression (e.g., neoplasia, herniated disk, and abscess), decompression and mass removal, incisional or excisional biopsy (wide surgical excision is preferred if possible), tumor staging, and, if necessary, spinal stabilization. If wide surgical excision creates spinal instability, stabilization is performed as described on p. 1505. Definitive histologic diagnosis is used to plan adjunct chemotherapy, immunotherapy, irradiation, or combination therapy.

Preoperative Management

Patients are given IV fluids before surgery. Preoperative management of patients with lumbosacral neoplasia is similar to that described for patients with any lumbosacral compressive lesion (see p. 1493). Preoperative steroids are not indicated because they do not protect nerve roots. If lumbosacral instability is suspected, care should be taken to support the pelvis during manipulations.

Anesthesia

Suggested anesthetic regimens is for use in patients with lumbosacral spinal disorders are discussed on p. 1403.

Surgical Anatomy

Refer to the description and illustrations of the topographic anatomy of the lumbosacral vertebral canal and cauda equina in Figs. 40-2 and 40-3 on pp. 1494 and 1497, respectively.

Positioning

Exposing neoplasms of the lumbosacral region generally requires a dorsal approach and wide dorsal laminectomy with unilateral or bilateral facetectomy and foraminotomy. If stabilization is needed, a dorsal approach is also recommended. Therefore position the patient in sternal recumbency with the hind legs tucked under the abdomen to gently flex the lumbosacral junction (see Fig. 40-1). This position facilitates exposure of the dorsal intervertebral space.

SURGICAL TECHNIQUE
Nerve Root Tumors

Tumors involving nerve roots of the cauda equina as they course through the lumbosacral vertebral canal are best approached using dorsal laminectomy, facetectomy, and foraminotomy as described on p. 1493 (see Figs. 40-2 on p. 1494 and 40-4 on p. 1502). It is important to identify the specific nerve root or roots to be resected, and have a knowledge of their effect on the patient's neurologic function (see Table 40-2). Neurologic deficits created by single or multiple nerve root resection may incapacitate the patient to an unacceptable degree. In such cases, biopsy for histopathologic diagnosis and adjunct medical management may be indicated.

> NOTE: If possible, excise the tumor so as to include 2 cm of adjacent, normal-appearing tissue.

Enter the vertebral canal by carefully elevating the inner periosteal layer with a dental or iris spatula and ophthalmic forceps. Remove any remaining epidural fat. Identify cauda equina nerve roots on the floor of the vertebral canal. Use a dural hook, dental spatula, or iris spatula to carefully follow the S1 and L7 nerve roots as they course along the floor of the vertebral canal. Identify the L7 nerve root as it lies against the caudal aspect of the L7 pedicle, and follow it as it disappears through the L7-S1 intervertebral foramen. Carefully examine each nerve root for evidence of diffuse enlargement or localized bulging. If the lesion is resectable, identify the nerve root involved, carefully cauterize the root cranial to the lesion using bipolar cautery, transect the root with a No. 11 scalpel blade, and carefully elevate the tran-

Table 40-6

Sample Physical Rehabilitation Protocol for Patients After Surgery for Thoracolumbar Disk Disease or Fracture/Luxation*

TREATMENT	DISABILITY INDEX			
	0–2 STEP 1	3–8 STEP 2	9–11 STEP 3	12–14 STEP 4
Heat therapy		10 min	10 min	
Massage	5 min	5 min	5 min	5 min
Passive range of motion (repetitions)	15†	15†	15†	15†
Electrical stimulation‡	10 min	10 min	10 min	
Therapeutic exercise: total time	10 min	20 min	20 min	25–45 min
Assisted standing	+	+	+	
Sit to stands	+	+	+	+
Balancing	+	+	+	+
Obstacles			+	+
Weaving			+	+
Circles			+	+
Underwater treadmill with gait patterning or wading pool/water walking	10 min (after 36–48 hr)	15 min	20 min	>25 min
Swimming§	2–5 min	5–10 min	5–10 min	5–10 min
Cryotherapy	15 min			

Modified from Development of a functional scoring system for dogs with acute spinal cord injuries, *Am J Vet Res* 62:10, 2001.
Disability index (DI):
   0–2, *0,* no limb movement and absent deep pain; *1,* no limb movement and present deep pain; *2,* no limb movement, but voluntary tail movement.
   3–8, *3,* minimal non–weight-bearing activity of one limb (one joint); *4,* non–weight-bearing activity in more than one joint <50% of the time; *5,* non–weight-bearing activity in more than one joint >50% of the time; *6,* weight-bearing activity of the limb <10% of the time; *7,* weight-bearing activity of the limb 10% to 50% of the time; *8,* weight-bearing activity of the limb >50% of the time.
   9–11, *9,* weight-bearing activity 100% of the time, but with reduced strength, and mistakes made >90% of the time, including crossing of the limbs, knuckling of the paws, standing on the dorsum of the paws and falling; *10,* weight-bearing activity 100% of the time, but with reduced strength and above mistakes made 50% to 90% of the time; *11,* weight-bearing activity 100% of the time, but with reduced strength, and mistakes made <50% of the time.
   12–14, *12,* ataxic gait with normal strength, but mistakes made >50% of the time, including lack of coordination, crossing of hind limbs, skipping steps, bunny-hopping, and knuckling of the paws; *13,* ataxic gait with normal strength, but mistakes made <50% of the time; *14,* normal gait.
*All treatments should be done three times a day.
†Passive range of motion to all joints of all limbs.
‡E-Stimulation: Electrical stimulation to be performed on the semimembranosus/semitendinosus muscle groups in patients with muscle atrophy. See Chapter 12 for specifications.
§Swimming is most beneficial if patient is moving all four limbs and is controlled. If not getting functional response, return to underwater treadmill or water walking instead. It is safer and more controlled.

sected portion of the root. Follow the affected nerve root caudal to the lesion, and complete the resection as described previously. Reexamine the cauda equina to rule out multiple nerve root tumors. Lavage the surgical wound and close the tissue routinely.

Tumors Involving the Vertebral Body or Surrounding Soft Tissue

Tumors involving the vertebral body or surrounding soft tissue are best approached via dorsal laminectomy as described in Figs. 40-2 to 40-4.

Perform a dorsal laminectomy to remove affected bone and provide cauda equina decompression. If bony involvement is extensive and nonresectable, use a trephine to take a biopsy of affected bone and perform a dorsal laminectomy to provide cauda equina decompression. If surrounding soft tissue structures are involved, take a biopsy of representative areas. If neoplastic tissue is cavitated or abscessed, obtain samples for anaerobic and aerobic culture and susceptibility testing. If spinal instability is diagnosed or occurs as a result of decompression, perform spinal stabilization as described on p. 1505.

SUTURE MATERIALS AND SPECIAL INSTRUMENTS

Special instruments necessary for laminectomy and spinal stabilization are listed in Tables 38-1 (see p. 1417) and 39-1 on p. 1468.

POSTOPERATIVE CARE AND ASSESSMENT

Patients with neoplasia of the lumbosacral spine should be monitored postoperatively in a similar fashion as patients with other lumbosacral spinal disorders (see Table 39-1 and Box 39-2). In general, strict confinement, analgesics as needed, short walks using an abdominal sling, frequent urinary bladder evacuation, and daily neurologic examinations are indicated. Long-term monitoring and adjunct medical therapy are dependent on tumor type and surgical margins.

PROGNOSIS

Prognosis depends on tumor type (biologic activity), surgical margins (percent of tumor resection), and sensitivity to adjunct therapy (chemotherapy, immunotherapy, radiation therapy, or combination therapy). Malignant extradural neoplasms tend to have an unfavorable prognosis, benign extradural neoplasms have a favorable prognosis, and extradural-intramedullary neoplasms (nerve root tumors) have a guarded to unfavorable prognosis.

PHYSICAL REHABILITATION FOR PATIENTS WITH LUMBOSACRAL DISK DISEASE AND FRACTURE/LUXATION

Rehabilitation can facilitate early and more complete recovery of neurologic patients after surgery (see Chapter 12; p. 127). It should be used in conjunction with standard medical and surgical treatment plus proper pain management (see Chapter 13) . Table 40-6 provides a sample physical rehabilitation protocol for patients after surgery for lumbosacral disk disease (begin immediately postoperatively), or spinal fractures or luxations. For fractures and luxations, only steps one and two should be performed until a bony union has formed and fixation is considered stable, regardless of the disability index.

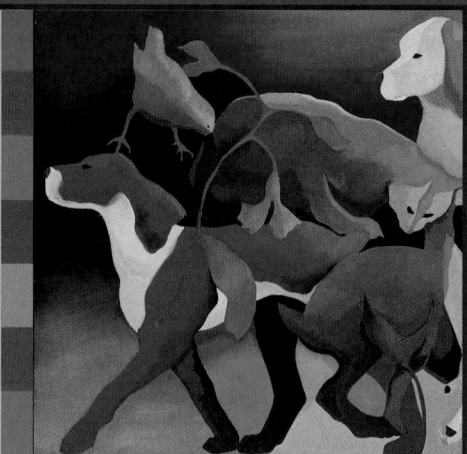

CHAPTER 41

Nonsurgical Diseases of the Spine

DISKOSPONDYLITIS

DEFINITIONS

Diskospondylitis is an infection of the intervertebral disk with concurrent osteomyelitis of adjacent vertebral end plates and vertebral bodies. Infection confined to the vertebral body is referred to as **vertebral osteomyelitis**. Synonyms for diskospondylitis include *intradiskal osteomyelitis, diskitis, intervertebral disk infection,* and *vertebral spondylitis.*

GENERAL CONSIDERATIONS AND CLINICALLY RELEVANT PATHOPHYSIOLOGY

Organisms most commonly associated with diskospondylitis are *Staphylococcus aureus* and *S. intermedius.* They have been cultured from blood, urine, or both in a significant number of patients with diskospondylitis. Other bacteria and fungi isolated from affected animals are listed in Box 41-1. A recent study identified three pathogens that had not been previously reported as causing diskospondylitis; *Pseudomonas aeruginosa, Enterococcus faecalis,* and *Staphylococcus epidermidis* (Adamo et al, 2001). Infection generally originates in a nonvertebral location (i.e., urinary tract infection [UTI], pyogenic dermatitis, valvular endocarditis, and dental disease) and spreads hematogenously. Vertebral infection usually begins in the end plate, where sludging blood in sinusoidal veins predisposes to bacterial colonization. Bacteria diffuse through the cartilaginous end plate of the vertebral body to contact the disk, causing lysis of the adjacent end plate, disk necrosis, and collapse of the intervertebral space. Rarely, bacteria migrate dorsally and cause epidural abscess formation. Vertebral physitis, characterized by bone lysis initially confined to the caudal physeal zone of the affected vertebra and sparing the vertebral end plates, has been reported in some dogs. Immunosuppressed patients may be predisposed to developing diskospondylitis. Areas of the spine most commonly affected include the lumbosacral junction, cervicothoracic junction, thoracolumbar junction, and midthoracic disks. With the exception of the

midthoracic spine, each predisposed area is at a static-kinetic junction of the spine (i.e., an area of spinal stability adjacent to an area of relative spinal mobility), encouraging stress concentration. Infrequently, diskospondylitis is caused by foreign body migration or by postoperative sequelae to disk fenestration.

Because of the public health hazard, animals with diskospondylitis should be tested for *Brucella canis* infection. People are relatively resistant to infection with *B. canis,* however, and the disease is relatively mild compared with infections caused by other *Brucella.* Symptomatic human patients may experience fever, chills, fatigue, malaise, lymphadenopathy, and/or weight loss.

> NOTE: Be sure to inform clients of the potential health hazard of keeping *B. canis*–infected pets.

 BOX 41-1

Organisms Commonly Cultured From Animals With Diskospondylitis

Bacteria

- *Staphylococcus aureus*
- *Staphylococcus intermedius*
- *Brucella canis*
- *Streptococcus* spp.
- *Escherichia coli*
- *Pasteurella multocida*
- *Actinomyces viscosus*
- *Nocardia* spp.
- *Mycobacterium avium*
- *Pseudomonas aeruginosa*
- *Enterococcus faecalis*
- *Staphylococcus epidermidis*

Fungi

- *Aspergillus terreus*
- *Paecilomyces varioti*
- *Mucor* spp.
- *Fusarium* spp.

DIAGNOSIS
Clinical Presentation

Signalment. Diskospondylitis usually occurs in large pure-bred dogs (i.e., 30 to 35 kg or greater), with affected males outnumbering females approximately two to one. Large male purebred dogs may have a higher degree of activity and thus place more stress on the spine, presumably predisposing these areas to infection. Some reports suggest that Great Danes and German shepherds are overrepresented. Dogs are generally older than 1 year, and the risk of diskospondylitis increases with age (i.e., 5 to 9 years) (Burkert et al, 2005).

History. The onset of symptoms is generally insidious, but careful historical evaluation may reveal subtle lameness, difficulty jumping, anorexia, depression, and/or weight loss for weeks to months previously. Varying degrees of chronic paraparesis or tetraparesis may occur later; acute signs may be due to pathologic fracture, epidural abscess, or the protrusion of infected dorsal annulus fibrosus into the vertebral canal.

NOTE: The hallmark of patients with discospondylitis is spinal hyperpathia (i.e., neck or back pain on deep palpation) associated with systemic disease.

Physical Examination Findings

Physical and neurologic examination findings vary, depending on location, severity, and secondary effects of the infection. Patients brought in early in the course of the disease may have systemic signs (i.e., depression, weight loss, and fever); evidence of spinal involvement includes hyperpathia without paresis. Patients brought in later generally have more subtle signs of systemic involvement coupled with more profound neurologic signs (i.e., severe, single or multilevel hyperpathia, with varying degrees of paresis caudal to the lesion). Less frequently, patients may have an acute onset of back pain and ambulatory or nonambulatory paraparesis or tetraparesis, with or without systemic signs. Diskospondylitis should be considered in any patient with signs of spinal disorder and systemic illness. Specific neurologic signs depend on location of the lesion and are discussed on p. 1368.

Diagnostic Imaging

Diagnosis of diskospondylitis is confirmed by survey radiographs or cross-sectional imaging. The earliest radiographic signs may take 2 to 4 weeks to be visible after initial infection and include lysis of one or both vertebral end plates followed by collapse of the intervertebral disk space. As the infection progresses, radiographic signs of continued vertebral end plate lysis, proliferative bony changes adjacent to the disk space, sclerotic margins, and ventral osseous proliferation with varying degrees of bridging spondylosis deformans result (Fig. 41-1). Vertebral body lysis followed by vertebral body shortening and spinal instability occurs infrequently, depending upon the bacterias' virulence. The hallmark of

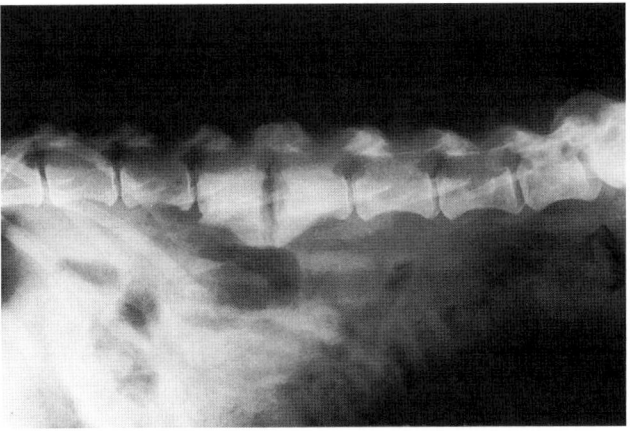

FIG. 41-1
Lateral radiograph of a dog with L3–L4 diskospondylitis. Notice the intradiskal lysis, vertebral end plate lysis, ventral spondylosis, and sclerosis surrounding lytic margins.

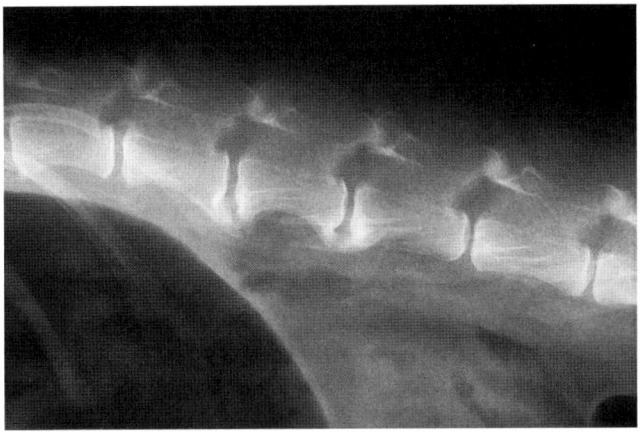

FIG. 41-2
Lateral radiograph of a dog with L2–L3 and L3–L4 spondylosis deformans. Notice the ankylosing spondylitic bridge of mature bone and normal intervertebral space and end plates.

diskospondylitis is end plate lysis. Patients with spondylosis deformans (an asymptomatic and generally incidental radiographic finding) do not have end plate lysis (Fig. 41-2). Bone scintigraphy is helpful in diagnosing early cases of diskospondylitis (i.e., as early as 3 days). Although scintigraphy is extremely sensitive in diagnosing early lesions, false-negative results may occur. Myelography and/or cross-sectional imaging (computed tomography [CT] or magnetic resonance imaging [MRI]) is mandatory in patients requiring surgical intervention. It allows documentation of an extradural mass, dictates the necessary decompressive technique (i.e., dorsal laminectomy versus hemilaminectomy), and may suggest the presence or absence of spinal instability (i.e., stress myelography). However, the degree of spinal cord or cauda equina compression does not predict outcome, nor is there a significant correlation between the degree of spinal cord compression and neurologic status. There is some suggestion that MRI and CT imaging may be more sensitive in early diagnosis of diskospondylitis (Gonzalo-Orden et al, 2000). CT identifies subtle end plate erosion and paravertebral soft tissue swelling and abscess more readily than radiography. MRI is more helpful than survey radiography and most importantly can identify the extent of the soft tissue infection (Thomas, 2000).

Laboratory Findings

Laboratory abnormalities vary considerably. Generally a normal or stress leukogram is seen; leukocytosis does not occur unless other systemic abnormalities are present (i.e., UTI, endocarditis, pyoderma, or prostatic abscess). The serum biochemical profile is usually normal unless other systemic abnormalities are present. UTI may be found in up to 40% of cases; occasionally the same organism is identified in blood and bone cultures. Blood cultures are positive in approximately 50% of patients. Cerebrospinal fluid (CSF) analysis is generally normal, but will occasionally show mild protein elevation. A bone culture is generally not performed, but may be done by a percutaneous, fluoroscopically guided needle biopsy (e.g., similar to a bone marrow aspiration biopsy) or by surgical intervention. Culture results are generally unrewarding, but may identify the same organism in urine and blood cultures. Positive *Brucella* titers are occasionally found. The rapid slide test for *Brucella* has many false-positive reactions, but few false negatives (1%). Therefore if the rapid slide test result is positive, it should be confirmed with a tube agglutination or agar gel immunodiffusion test. Demonstrating the organism by blood culture is definitive.

> NOTE: Because of the public health risk, perform *Brucella* titers in animals with diskospondylitis.

DIFFERENTIAL DIAGNOSIS

Diskospondylitis must be differentiated from spondylosis deformans and spinal neoplasia. Spondylosis and sclerosis are common in both spondylosis deformans and diskospondylitis; however, vertebral end plate lysis only occurs with infection (see Fig. 41-2). Similarly, end plate lysis of adjacent or multiple vertebrae is uncommon in spinal neoplasia; lysis is generally associated with the vertebral body, lamina, pedicles, and dorsal spinous processes of a single vertebra (see p. 1371).

MEDICAL MANAGEMENT

Therapy depends on presenting neurologic examination, laboratory data (i.e., urine, blood, and/or bone cultures and *Brucella* titer), and serial neurologic examinations. Generally, patients that are brought in with pain alone or pain and

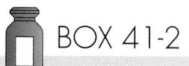 BOX 41-2

Antibiotics for Use in Diskospondylitis*

Amikacin (Amiglyde-V)
20–25 mg/kg IV, IM, SC qd

Clindamycin (Antirobe)
11 mg/kg PO bid to tid

Cloxacillin (Cloxapen, Orbenin, Tegopen)
10–15 mg/kg PO tid

Doxycycline (Vibramycin)
12.5–15 mg/kg PO bid

Enrofloxacin (Baytril)
10–20 mg/kg PO or IV (must be given diluted and slowly over 30 min) qd

Minocycline (Minocin)
12.5 mg/kg PO bid (when used in combination with another antibiotic for treatment of brucellosis)

IV, Intravenous; *IM,* intramuscular; *SC,* subcutaneous; *qd,* once a day; *PO,* oral; *bid,* twice a day; *tid,* three times a day.
*Duration of therapy may be based on one or a combination of the following guidelines:
- Treat for 6 to 8 wk.
- Treat for 2 wk after resolution of clinical signs.
- Treat until radiographic evidence of ankylosing spondylosis appears.
- Treat until *Brucella* titer is negative.

mild paresis are treated with analgesics, antibiotics, and 4 to 6 weeks of strict confinement, regardless of the number of vertebrae affected. Specific antibiotic therapy is based on culture and susceptibility testing of urine, blood, and/or bone and *Brucella* titer. Antibiotics chosen should be bactericidal, achieve minimum inhibitory concentrations in bone, and be effective against the causative organism. If cultures and titers are negative, empirical selection of an antibiotic is based on the most likely causative agent (i.e., *S. intermedius* or *S. aureus*). A β-lactamase–resistant antibiotic (e.g., clindamycin, cloxacillin) should be used in these patients (Box 41-2). A combination of a tetracycline (i.e., doxycycline, minocycline) plus an aminoglycoside (i.e., amikacin) or fluoroquinolone (i.e., enrofloxacin) should be used for diskospondylitis secondary to *B. canis*. Patients should be treated until the *Brucella* titer is negative.

Approximately 80% to 90% of patients respond to appropriate medical management. Patients unresponsive (i.e., continued hyperpathia without paresis) after 7 to 10 days of medical therapy should be treated with a different antibiotic. If pain persists, a third antibiotic may be used, or surgical curettage may be performed to obtain bone samples for culture and susceptibility testing and to débride intradiskal lesions. Analgesics are indicated in animals in pain.

Resolution of radiographic lesions can be used as a guide to therapy, but has some limitations. It may take 2 to 4 weeks after resolution of infection to visualize radiographic improvement (i.e., static end plate lysis). In addition, active areas of lysis may be masked with extensive bone remodeling. In cases with extensive bony proliferation, it may be sensible to extend therapy for 4 to 6 weeks past radiographic resolution of bony lysis. In some cases, the end plate lysis never resolves. In these situations, nuclear imaging, CT, or MRI may be better monitoring methods (Moore, 2000). A recent report suggests that some patients require treatment for 1 year before resolution of clinical signs (Burkert et al, 2005).

SURGICAL TREATMENT

Myelography, CT or MRI, spinal cord decompression, bone samples for culture and susceptibility testing, débridement of intradiskal lesions, placement of an autogenous cancellous bone graft in the intervertebral space, and/or spinal stabilization may be needed in medically treated patients showing neurologic deterioration (i.e., paraparesis or tetraparesis) or patients with an acute onset of spinal hyperpathia and weakly ambulatory or nonambulatory paraparesis or tetraparesis. Myelography, CT, or MRI should be performed to determine the specific location of the compressive lesion (see p. 1370). Spinal cord decompression may be performed via a dorsal laminectomy or hemilaminectomy; hemilaminectomy is preferred because it creates the least spinal instability. Spinal stabilization is performed if decompression and débridement cause spinal instability or if instability is documented radiographically (i.e., stress myelography) before surgery. Techniques for dorsal laminectomy, hemilaminectomy, and spinal stabilization are described and illustrated in Chapters 38 (see p. 1402), 39 (see p. 1460), and 40 (see p. 1493).

Preoperative Management

See preoperative management for each specific location of the spine affected (i.e., cervical, thoracolumbar, and lumbosacral) on pp. 1402, 1460, and 1493, respectively.

Anesthesia

Suggested anesthetic protocols for spinal surgery are provided on p. 1402.

Surgical Anatomy

Anatomic descriptions for each location of the spine affected (i.e., cervical, thoracolumbar, and lumbosacral) are provided on pp. 1404, 1460, and 1493, respectively.

Positioning

Refer to the surgical procedure chosen for recommendations for appropriate surgical positioning.

SURGICAL TECHNIQUE

See surgical technique descriptions for each specific location of the spine affected (i.e., cervical, thoracolumbar, and lumbosacral) on pp. 1404, 1460, and 1493, respectively.

SUTURE MATERIALS AND SPECIAL INSTRUMENTS

Avoid using nonabsorbable multifilament sutures (e.g., silk) in infected surgical sites.

POSTOPERATIVE CARE AND ASSESSMENT

After surgery these patients should be assessed as described on pp. 1416, 1468, and 1496. Antibiotics should be continued for a minimum of 4 to 6 weeks.

PROGNOSIS

Prognosis depends on neurologic examination findings at presentation and the patient's response to initial medical management. Patients with spinal hyperpathia only or spinal hyperpathia plus ambulatory paresis have a favorable to excellent prognosis. Those with spinal hyperpathia and weakly ambulatory paresis have a favorable prognosis if weakness is caused by spinal pain. Patients with either of the previous neurologic findings that do not respond to an initial course of medication have a guarded to favorable prognosis for responding to either a different antibiotic or surgical bone culture and intradiskal débridement.

Patients with acute spinal hyperpathia, weakly ambulatory or nonambulatory paraparesis or tetraparesis, evidence of an extradural lesion, and no evidence of spinal instability have a guarded prognosis when treated surgically. The prognosis is guarded to unfavorable if there is spinal instability.

References

Adamo PF, Cherubini GB: Discospondylitis associated with three unreported bacteria in the dog, *J Small Anim Pract* 42:352, 2001.

Burkert BA, Kerwin SC, Hosgood GL et al: Signalment and clinical features of diskospondylitis in dogs: 513 cases (1980-2001), *J Am Vet Med Assoc* 227:268, 2005.

Gonzalo-Orden JM, Altonaga JR, Costilla S et al: Magnetic resonance, computed tomographic and radiologic findings in a dog with diskospondylitis, *Vet Radiol Ultrasound* 41:142, 2000.

Moore MP: Diskospondylitis, *Vet Clin North Am Small Anim Pract* 30:1027, 2001.

Thomas WB: Diskospondylitis and other vertebral infections, *Vet Clin North Am Small Anim Pract* 30:169, 2001.

Suggested Reading

Auger J, Dupuis J, Quesnel A et al: Surgical treatment of lumbosacral instability caused by diskospondylitis in four dogs, *Vet Surg* 29:70, 2000.

Lumbosacral diskospondylitis may not respond well to conservative treatment because of the mobility of the affected space. Surgical treatment involving distraction and stabilization to obtain intervertebral fusion is very effective in treating lumbosacral instability caused by diskospondylitis.

Davis MJ, Dewey CW, Walker MA et al: Contrast radiographic findings in canine bacterial diskospondylitis: a multicenter, retrospective study of 27 cases, *J Am Anim Hosp Assoc* 36:81, 2000.

Static spinal cord compression is not a significant component of the neurologic dysfunction associated with bacterial diskospondylitis. Identification of vertebral subluxation on some patients may indicate a dynamic lesion that should be evaluated with stress radiography.

Kinzel S, Koch J, Buecker A et al: Treatment of 10 dogs with discospondylitis by fluoroscopy-guided percutaneous discectomy, *Vet Rec* 156:78, 2005.

Bacteria responsible for the infection were cultured from 9 of 10 biopsy specimens, whereas only three urine and four blood cultures grew the pathogens.

GRANULOMATOUS MENINGOENCEPHALOMYELITIS

DEFINITIONS

Granulomatous meningoencephalomyelitis (GME) is an acute, progressive inflammatory disease of the central nervous system (CNS), characterized histologically by large perivascular accumulations of mononuclear cells in the parenchyma and meninges of the brain and spinal cord.

GENERAL CONSIDERATIONS AND CLINICALLY RELEVANT PATHOPHYSIOLOGY

GME may affect any portion of the CNS (i.e., meninges, brain, and spinal cord). The lesion is preponderant in white matter; however, many dogs have meningeal involvement, and occasionally gray matter may be affected. In advanced cases, perivascular lesions extend into the CNS parenchyma and merge with adjacent lesions, forming large coalescent granulomas. The severity of lesions and their regional location (i.e., cerebral, cerebellar, cervical spinal cord, and brainstem) are variable. Three forms of the disorder have been described: disseminated (multifocal), focal, and ocular. History, neurologic examination, laboratory findings, and course of disease may differ depending on the form (Table 41-1). The cause of GME is currently unknown. Suggested hypotheses include a cell-mediated immune response to the sustained presence of an infectious agent, an inflammatory process that may be transformed to a neoplastic one (possibly involving a cell-associated virus), or a genetic predisposition. A recent report suggests that herpesvirus, adenovirus, or canine parvovirus is not present in the brains of dogs with GME (Schatzberg et al, 2005). Currently, there are anecdotal reports of GME being associated with seropositivity to *Bartonella vinsonii*. The incidence of GME ranges from 5% to 25% of all CNS disorders in dogs.

DIAGNOSIS
Clinical Presentation

Signalment. GME occurs in young to middle-aged dogs (i.e., 2 to 6 years); however, occasional reports of dogs as young as 9 months have been described. Females are more often affected than males. This condition occurs most commonly in toy breeds, particularly poodles and terriers; mixed breeds and larger breeds are affected less frequently. GME is rarely diagnosed in cats.

History. Patients generally are brought in with a progressive history of acute, continuous or episodic, multifocal neurologic disease involving brain, meninges, and/or cervical spinal cord. Clinical presentation depends on location of lesions and the form of the disease (i.e., disseminated, focal, or ocular) (see Table 41-1). Occasionally, patients may be brought in for progressive vision loss without other associated neurologic abnormalities (Nuhsbaum et al, 2002).

Physical Examination Findings

Physical and neurologic examination findings are variable and depend on lesion localization and the form of disease present (i.e., disseminated, focal, or ocular) (see Table 41-1). Significant neurologic examination findings include cervical

 Table 41-1

Clinical Signs Associated With Various Forms of GME

FORM*	LESION LOCATION†	CLINICAL SIGNS‡	DURATION OF SIGNS	PROGNOSIS
Disseminated (multifocal)	Lower brainstem Cervical spinal cord Meninges	Acute onset; rapidly progressive; fever may occur early	1 to 8 wk (25% are dead in 1 wk)	Grave; may live 12 to 16 wk
Focal	Brainstem Cerebral cortex Cerebellum Cervical spinal cord	Insidious onset; signs consistent with a space-occupying mass	3 to 6 mo	Unfavorable; may live up to 12 mo
Ocular	Ocular nerve	Sudden blindness; anisocoria	3 to 6 mo§	Unfavorable; may live 12 to 18 mo

*The disseminated and focal forms frequently occur together; the ocular form may occur alone or may be accompanied by the disseminated or focal forms.
†Although lesions can occur anywhere in the CNS, each form of the disease seems to have a predilection for specific locations.
‡Specific clinical signs are associated with lesion location; see p. 1368 for a description of signs expected in each location.
§If the ocular form is present with the disseminated form, duration of signs and prognosis usually follow the disseminated form.

pain evidenced by nuchal rigidity (i.e., suggesting meningeal involvement) or nystagmus, head tilt, blindness, and facial palsy (i.e., suggesting brainstem involvement). Ataxia, paraparesis or tetraparesis, seizures, circling, altered states of consciousness, and behavioral changes are also common. Clinical signs referable to the forebrain are most common with focal involvement, whereas signs referable to the forebrain and brainstem are most commonly seen with the disseminated form. Patients with the disseminated form may be febrile. Animals with the ocular form may have sudden blindness or pupillary abnormalities (i.e., anisocoria, decreased pupillary light reflexes).

Diagnostic Imaging

Survey radiographs of the skull or spine are generally not indicated because they do not provide information about the CNS. Patients that have signs suggesting focal extradural spinal cord lesions (i.e., neck pain and varying degrees of tetraparesis) should have a cerebrospinal fluid (CSF) analysis. MRI is the best imaging technique for use in the diagnosis of focal GME, although contrast enhanced CT may also reveal the lesion. Focal intracranial GME may reveal changes consistent with intracranial neoplasia; multifocal intracranial GME may show signs similar to metastatic neoplasia. Presumptive diagnosis of GME is based on signalment, history, progression of clinical signs, CSF analysis, and results of cross-sectional imaging.

Laboratory Findings

CSF analysis often reveals a mild-to-marked mononuclear pleocytosis consisting of lymphocytes, monocytes, and occasional plasma cells. Neutrophils are seen in up to two thirds of affected animals. They generally make up less than 20% of the total cell count, but occasionally are preponderant. Protein concentrations are usually mildly to moderately elevated, occasionally without an elevated cell count. Previous corticosteroid treatment does not appear to dramatically alter CSF cellularity. Techniques for performing cisternal and lumbar taps are described in Chapter 36 on p. 1372. Patients with disseminated GME may have neutrophilia.

> NOTE: CSF obtained from the cistern is preferable to that obtained from a lumbar tap because the medulla and cervical spinal cord are usually more severely affected than the lumbar spinal cord.

DIFFERENTIAL DIAGNOSIS

GME should be suspected in any mature small-breed dog with acute, progressive, multifocal, or focal disease involving the brain, meninges, or cervical spinal cord. The differential diagnosis of GME must include infectious diseases of the brain (i.e., bacterial, viral, fungal, parasitic, and rickettsial), extradural cervical spinal disorders (i.e., intervertebral disk extrusion, fracture and/or luxation, instability, and malformation), and primary (i.e., meningioma, glioma, and ependymoma) and metastatic neoplasia. Diagnosis is based

on history, signalment, onset and progression of clinical signs, CSF analysis, results of MRI or CT, and postmortem examination of CNS tissue. Definitive diagnosis of GME is based on characteristic histopathologic lesions in affected CNS tissue.

MEDICAL MANAGEMENT

Although an infectious cause has not been completely disproven, recent studies support that GME is an aberrant, autoimmune response caused by the accumulation of preponderantly CD3+ lymphocytes in the perivascular lesions. Corticosteroid therapy makes up the mainstay treatment for GME despite variable clinical response and prognosis. Survival times for dogs with GME treated with corticosteroids range from 7 to greater than 1000 days. The type of steroid, route of administration, dosage schedule, and duration of therapy depend on initial presenting signs. Patients with moderate to severe clinical signs are initially treated with dexamethasone at 2 mg/kg IV; this dosage is decreased to 0.2 mg/kg daily over 3 to 4 days or until neurologic improvement is noted. The patient is discharged on prednisolone (Box 41-3). Variations in the final dosage schedule are dependent upon response to therapy; however, patients should be continued on a maintenance dose indefinitely. If therapy is discontinued, rapid exacerbation of clinical signs often occurs, and it may be difficult to achieve a second remission. Patients with mild clinical signs are treated initially with oral prednisolone (see Box 41-3). Because of the guarded long-term prognosis associated with administration of corticosteroids, alternate therapeutic regimens should be considered. There is current evidence of efficacy for procarbazine, cytosine arabinoside, and cyclosporine. Reports of median survival times are as high as 14 months (Dewey CW, personal communication). Patients with seizures should be treated with anticonvulsant medications.

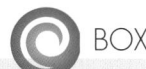 BOX 41-3

Corticosteroid Therapy of Dogs With GME

Moderate to Severe Clinical Signs
Dexamethasone (Azium)*
0.2–2 mg/kg IV (see text)

Prednisolone
1–2 mg/kg PO bid for 2 to 3 wk; taper over a 3- to 4-wk period to 2.5 to 5 mg total dose qod

Mild Clinical Signs
Prednisolone
1–2 mg/kg PO bid for 2 to 3 wk; taper as described above

IV, Intravenous; *PO*, oral; *bid*, twice a day; *qod*, every other day.
*Prolonged use of dexamethasone can be associated with gastrointestinal hemorrhage.

SURGICAL TREATMENT

GME is not generally considered a surgical disorder. There have been isolated case reports describing surgical removal of focal lesions resulting in acceptable long-term survival (Dewey CW, personal communication).

PROGNOSIS

Prognosis for GME is generally unfavorable to grave (see Table 41-1 on p. 1518). Duration of remission with corticosteroid therapy varies with the form of disease: patients with the disseminated (multifocal) form usually do not survive longer than 6 to 8 weeks; those with the focal form may survive for up to 12 months (particularly if the lesion is in the forebrain); patients with purely ocular GME may survive 12 to 18 months. There typically is no significant difference in survival between dogs with focal versus disseminated GME. Patients treated with radiation therapy, particularly those with clinical signs suggesting focal involvement, have a significantly increased survival time.

References

Demierre S, Tipold A, Griot-Wenk ME et al: Correlation between the clinical course of granulomatous meningoencephalomyelitis in dogs and the extent of mast cell infiltration, *Vet Rec* 148:467, 2001.

Nuhsbaum MT, Powell CC, Gionfriddo JR et al: Treatment of granulomatous meningoencephalomyelitis in a dog, *Vet Ophthalmol* 5:29, 2002.

Schatzberg SJ, Haley NJ, Barr SC et al: Polymerase chain reaction screening for DNA viruses in paraffin-embedded brains from dogs with necrotizing meningoencephalitis, necrotizing leukoencephalitis, and granulomatous meningoencephalitis, *J Vet Intern Med* 19:553, 2005.

Suzuki M, Uchida K, Morozumi M et al: A comparative pathological study on granulomatous meningoencephalomyelitis and central malignant histiocytosis in dogs, *J Vet Med Sci* 65:1319, 2003.

DEGENERATIVE MYELOPATHY

DEFINITIONS

Degenerative myelopathy is a neurologic disorder of unknown cause producing progressive demyelination of long-tract fibers, which begins in the thoracolumbar spinal cord.

GENERAL CONSIDERATIONS AND CLINICALLY RELEVANT PATHOPHYSIOLOGY

Degenerative myelopathy is a progressive neurologic disorder causing varying degrees of paraparesis. Pathologic findings include loss of myelin in the spinal cord white matter, a process that generally begins in the thoracic region. The cause is currently unknown. Suggested hypotheses include an immune-related disorder in German shepherds, vitamin B deficiency, trauma, vascular disease, and familial neuronal atrophy. At this time, all suggested causes remain unsupported.

DIAGNOSIS
Clinical Presentation

Signalment. Degenerative myelopathy generally occurs in middle-aged to older (i.e., 5 to 7 years) large-breed dogs, particularly German shepherd dogs. However, there have been rare reports in smaller breeds (e.g., miniature poodles) and cats. There is no sex predilection.

History. Patients usually have a history of slowly progressive hind limb weakness without back pain; signs may have been present for months. Owners commonly complain that the dog has difficulty rising up on the hind legs or that they hear scuffing or clicking of the hind toenails during ambulation.

Physical Examination Findings

The general physical examination results are usually normal. A neurologic examination generally reveals upper motor neuron (UMN), ambulatory or weakly ambulatory paraparesis without spinal hyperpathia (i.e., back pain). Patients generally have symmetric or asymmetric loss of conscious proprioception (i.e., knuckling, wearing of toenails, and stumbling), exaggerated patellar reflexes, and crossed extensor reflexes. Occasionally, patients show lower motor neuron (LMN) (i.e., decreased patellar reflex) and UMN signs. Pain perception and urinary and fecal continence are not lost, even late in the disorder. Thoracic limbs are spared, unless the patient is maintained long enough after complete paraplegia.

Diagnostic Imaging

Survey radiographs and myelography are essentially normal in patients with degenerative myelopathy. Myelography is used to eliminate other spinal cord disorders that mimic degenerative myelopathy (e.g., chronic disk protrusion, spinal neoplasia). If a mild disk protrusion is diagnosed on myelography, the degree of spinal cord compression should be correlated with observed neurologic signs before treatment is considered. Patients, especially German shepherd dogs, may have both diseases simultaneously. Surgical treatment of a mild disk protrusion in the face of degenerative myelopathy may not be warranted. CT and MRI may better help demonstrate spinal cord compressive lesions.

Laboratory Findings

Laboratory findings are generally normal. CSF analysis may show mild increases in protein; however, this can be consistent with chronic disk protrusion or spinal neoplasia.

DIFFERENTIAL DIAGNOSIS

The primary differential diagnoses for patients with degenerative myelopathy are chronic disk protrusion (i.e., Hansen type II), spinal neoplasia, and hip dysplasia. Survey radiographs and myelography differentiate chronic disk protrusion and spinal neoplasia. Because hind leg signs associated with chronic hip dysplasia are caused by joint pain, careful orthopedic and neurologic examination can rule out hip dysplasia. Some patients show signs of degenerative myelopathy and hip dysplasia. A strong presumptive diagnosis of degenerative myelopathy is based on compatible signalment, history, and neurologic examination combined with normal survey radiographs, myelography, and/or cross-sectional imaging. Definitive diagnosis is based on characteristic histopathologic changes in spinal cord parenchyma.

MEDICAL MANAGEMENT

Multiple treatment regimens have been suggested for patients with degenerative myelopathy, including corticosteroids, nonsteroidal antiinflammatory agents, vitamins (i.e., E and B complex), immune modifiers (i.e., suppressors and stimulants), interferon, and enzyme inhibitors (e.g., aminocaproic acid). Presently, no therapy has consistently been effective. Management of ambulatory and nonambulatory patients with thoracolumbar spinal disorders is described on p. 1468.

SURGICAL TREATMENT

Degenerative myelopathy is not a surgical disorder.

PROGNOSIS

Patients with degenerative myelopathy have an unfavorable prognosis. There is no known medical or surgical treatment that successfully halts demyelination. Progression of this condition to a nonambulatory paraparesis may take months to years, depending on the patient's presenting neurologic status.

ISCHEMIC MYELOPATHY

DEFINITIONS

Fibrocartilaginous embolization (FCE) is the ischemic necrosis of a segment of spinal cord (ischemic myelopathy) caused by herniation of intervertebral disk material into the spinal cord microvasculature. Synonyms include *necrotizing myelopathy, spinal cord ischemia, embolic myelopathy, vascular episode,* and *fibrocartilaginous infarct.*

GENERAL CONSIDERATIONS AND CLINICALLY RELEVANT PATHOPHYSIOLOGY

The pathogenesis of canine FCE is poorly understood. Most authors agree that emboli, histochemically identical to the nucleus pulposus of the intervertebral disk, travel to the spinal cord through either arteries or veins. To produce the extent of ischemic myelopathy observed clinically, it is necessary to simultaneously compromise many closely associated small blood vessels. Histopathology usually reveals multiple emboli with staining characteristics much like fibrocartilage found in a degenerating nucleus pulposus. The presence of associated intervertebral disk herniation is variable. Embolization into the ventral spinal artery and its branches and vertebral venous sinuses has been demonstrated (Fig. 41-3). Sudden elevation in central venous pressure, as seen during coughing or vomiting, may be required to propel fibrocartilaginous emboli into the spinal cord's venous drainage. Although other material, such as parasites, tissue, metastatic neoplasia, air, fat, foreign bodies, and bacteria, could embo-

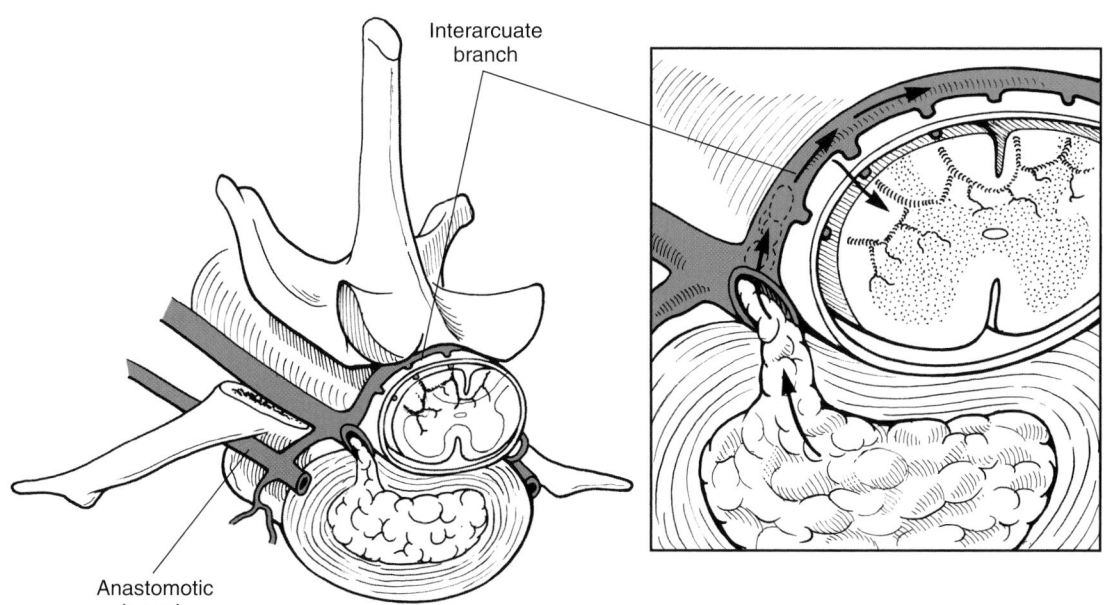

Interarcuate branch

Anastomotic branch

FIG. 41-3
Schematic illustration showing a proposed pathogenesis of a fibrocartilaginous embolism involving extrusion of nuclear material into the vertebral venous sinus or ventral spinal artery and then into small vessels supplying the spinal cord parenchyma.

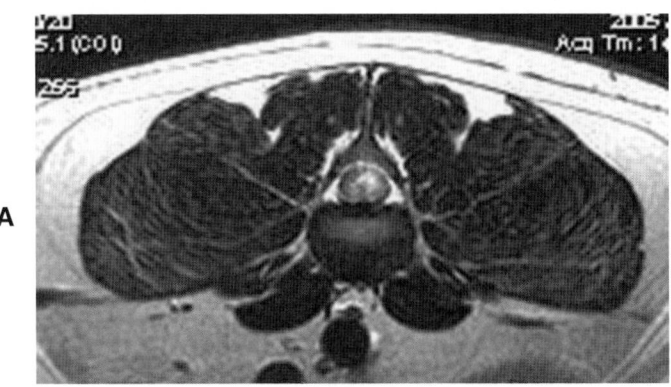
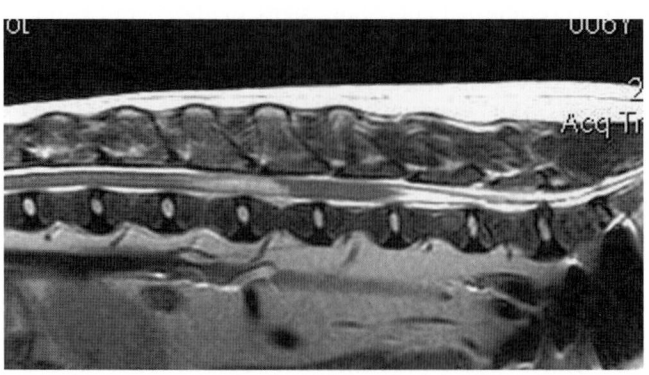

FIG. 41-4

A, Transverse and **B,** sagittal T2-weighted MR image showing a focal, intramedullary, hyperintense lesion suggestive of ischemic myelopathy.

lize the spinal cord, fibrocartilaginous material is most commonly associated with canine embolic myelopathy.

DIAGNOSIS
Clinical Presentation

Signalment. FCE most commonly affects large nonchondrodystrophic breeds (e.g., Great Danes, St. Bernards, Labrador retrievers, and German shepherd dogs). The disease is most common in young adults (3 to 7 years); however, it may be seen at almost any age, including dogs as young as 3 months. FCE has also been reported in cats and horses. There is no sex predisposition.

History. Patients typically have an acute, nonprogressive, ambulatory or nonambulatory tetraparesis, paraparesis, hemiparesis, or monoparesis without spinal hyperpathia (i.e., back or neck pain). In approximately 50% of cases, clinical signs occur after trauma or exercise. Many of these patients have an initial history of pain or discomfort that resolves with time.

Physical Examination Findings

Physical examination findings are generally normal. Neurologic examination findings include an acute onset of nonprogressive UMN or LMN, asymmetric, ambulatory or nonambulatory tetraparesis, paraparesis, hemiparesis, or monoparesis, without spinal hyperpathia. Abnormal neurologic findings are consistent with a focal spinal cord lesion anywhere in the five anatomic divisions of the spinal cord (see Fig. 36-10 on p. 1368). The most common locations for FCE lesions are the cervical (C6-T2) or lumbar (L4-S3) intumescence. Typical neurologic signs for each anatomic division are discussed. A loss of deep pain perception occurs in severe cases of spinal cord ischemia.

Diagnostic Imaging

Survey radiographs are generally normal, although mild collapse of an intervertebral space may occur. Mild spinal cord swelling, suggestive of an intramedullary mass, may be seen if myelography is performed within 12 to 24 hours of the

injury. If myelography is delayed, spinal cord swelling resolves, and a normal study results. CT may document the absence of compressive lesions. MRI is the best antemortem technique for evaluation of this syndrome. The classic finding is an area of high signal intensity within the spinal cord parenchyma on T2-weighted images (Gruenenfelder et al, 2005; Abramson et al, 2005) (Fig. 41-4).

Laboratory Findings

Routine hematologic and serum biochemical analyses are normal. CSF analysis is often normal, but may reveal mild protein elevation with normal or slightly increased numbers of leukocytes. Mild xanthochromia (i.e., a yellowish appearance caused by hemolyzed blood) may be found, particularly if CSF is taken within 24 hours of onset of clinical signs.

DIFFERENTIAL DIAGNOSIS

FCE must be differentiated from disorders causing acute, focal, symmetric or asymmetric (i.e., lateralizing signs), nonprogressive paresis without spinal hyperpathia, including fracture and/or luxation, intervertebral disk extrusion, and spinal neoplasia. Patients with fracture and/or luxation generally have persistent back pain; a diagnosis is based on neurologic examination and survey radiographs. Patients with spinal neoplasia have a variety of clinical and neurologic symptoms; diagnosis is based on myelographic findings compatible with an extradural, intradural-extramedullary, or intramedullary mass (see p. 1374), or on characteristic findings on CT and MRI. A presumptive diagnosis of FCE is based on a compatible history and neurologic examination, combined with normal survey spinal radiographs and characteristic myelographic findings (i.e., normal or mild spinal cord swelling) or high signal intensity within the spinal cord on T2-weighted MRI images. The diagnosis is usually established by eliminating other causes of spinal cord disease; however, definitive diagnosis is based on histopathologic identification of characteristic fibrocartilaginous emboli and resultant spinal cord infarction.

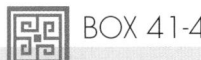 BOX 41-4

Corticosteroid Therapy of Acute FCE

Dexamethasone (Azium)

0.2–0.4 mg/kg PO tid—then bid for 2 days and qd for 2 days

PO, Oral; *bid,* twice a day; *qd,* once a day.

MEDICAL MANAGEMENT

Therapy depends on the time of the patient's examination after the onset of clinical signs. Patients brought in within 72 hours of the onset of clinical signs should be treated with corticosteroids (Box 41-4) and supportive care including physiotherapy; confinement for 2 to 3 weeks in an elevated cage with dry, soft bedding and easy access to food and water; and frequent bladder expressions (i.e., four times a day). Patients brought in after 72 hours are treated with supportive care only. Proper treatment of ambulatory and nonambulatory patients is described on pp. 1393, 1416, and 1468.

SURGICAL TREATMENT

FCE is not a surgical disorder.

PROGNOSIS

Prognosis for recovery depends on the extent and location of spinal cord damage. Generally, patients with less extensive spinal cord damage on presentation (i.e., based on neurologic examination) and those showing improvement within 14 days are more likely to recover. A recent report suggests a positive correlation between a poor prognosis and the involvement of intumescences, symmetrical clinical signs, and decreased deep pain sensation on presentation (Gandini et al, 2003). Of these parameters, absence of deep pain perception was the most important negative prognostic indicator. However, physiotherapy and/or hydrotherapy instituted immediately after the diagnostic work-up seemed to have a major influence on improving the recovery rate.

References

Abramson CJ, Garosi L, Platt SR et al: Magnetic resonance imaging appearance of suspected ischemic myelopathy in dogs, *Vet Radiol Ultrasound* 46:225, 2005.

Gandini G, Xizinauskas S, Lang et al: Fibrocartilaginous embolism in 75 dogs: clinical findings and factors influencing the recovery rate, *J Small Anim Pract* 44:76, 2003.

Gruenenfelder FI, Weishaupt D, Green R et al: Magnetic resonance imaging findings in spinal cord infarction in three small breed dogs, *Vet Radiol Ultrasound* 46:91, 2005.